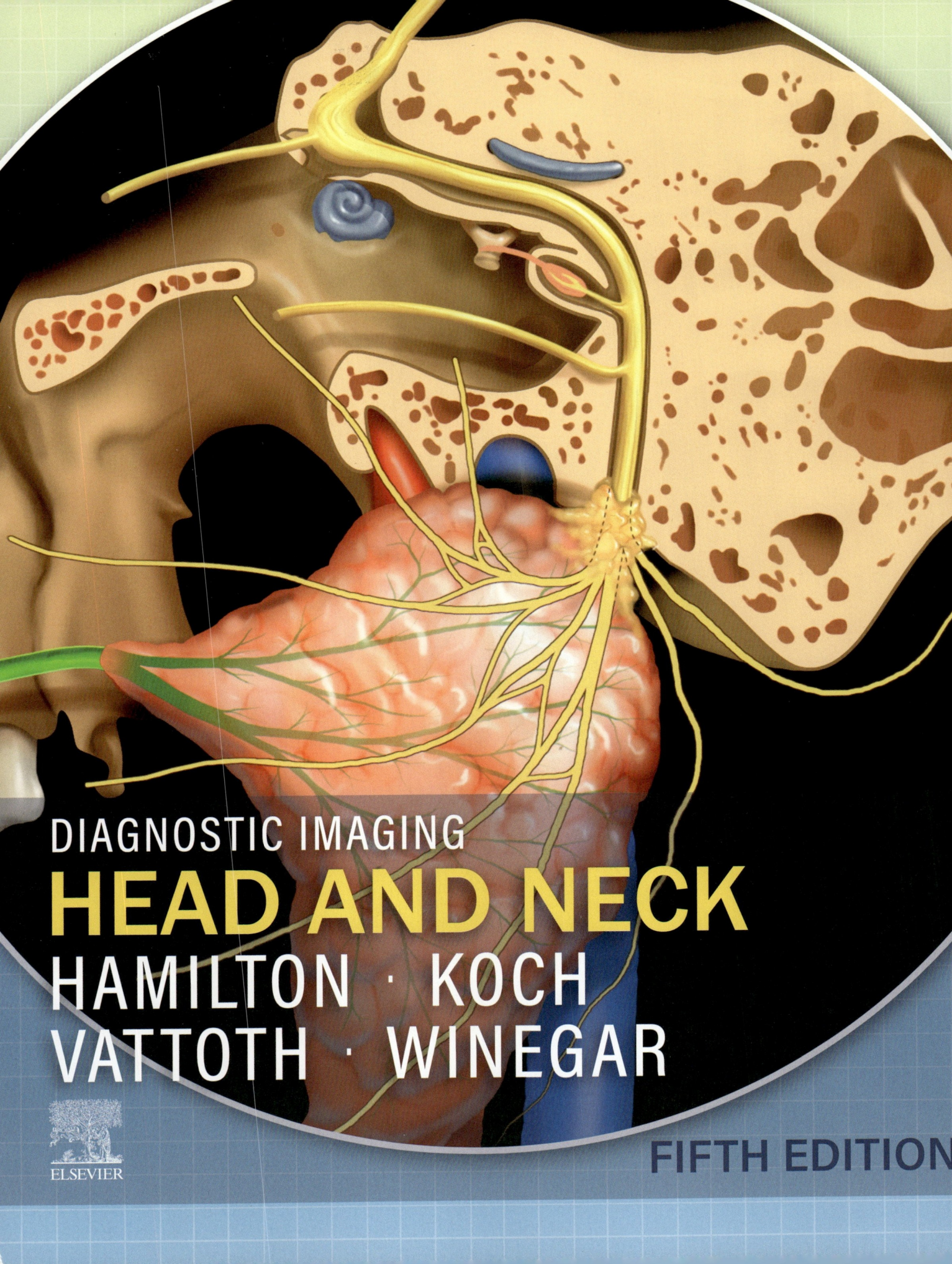

DIAGNOSTIC IMAGING
HEAD AND NECK
HAMILTON · KOCH
VATTOTH · WINEGAR

FIFTH EDITION

ELSEVIER

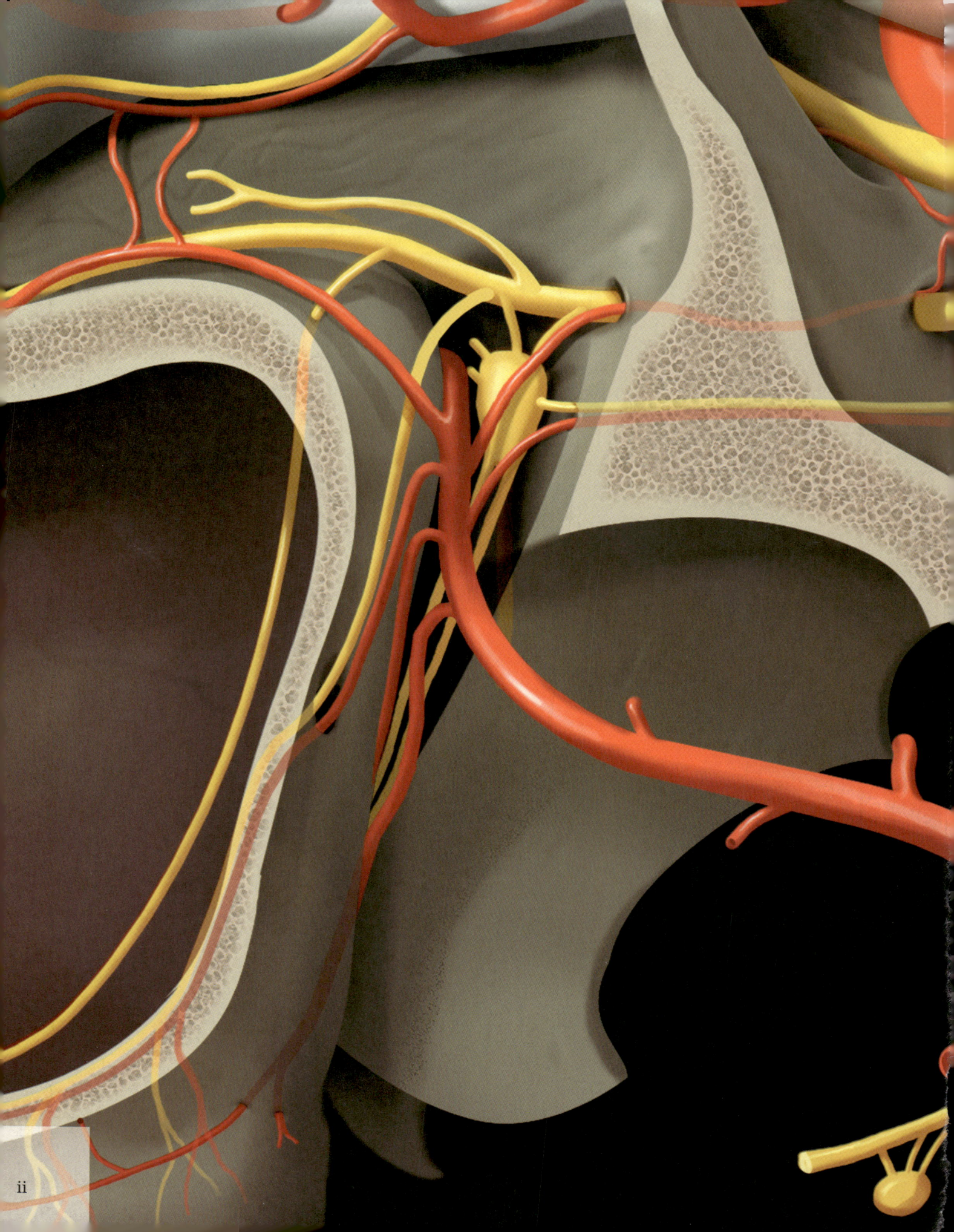

DIAGNOSTIC IMAGING
HEAD AND NECK
FIFTH EDITION

BRONWYN E. HAMILTON, MD
Professor of Radiology
Courtesy Appointment, Otolaryngology - Head & Neck Surgery
Oregon Health & Science University
Portland, Oregon

BERNADETTE L. KOCH, MD
Associate Chief, Radiology
Cincinnati Children's Hospital Medical Center
Professor, Radiology and Pediatrics
University of Cincinnati College of Medicine
Cincinnati, Ohio

SURJITH VATTOTH, MD, FRCR
Professor of Radiology
Director of Pediatric Neuroimaging
Department of Diagnostic Radiology and Nuclear Medicine
Division of Neuroradiology
Rush University Medical Center
Chicago, Illinois

BLAIR A. WINEGAR, MD
Neuroradiology Fellowship Program Director
Associate Professor of Radiology and Medical Imaging
University of Utah School of Medicine
Salt Lake City, Utah

Elsevier
1600 John F. Kennedy Blvd.
Ste 1800
Philadelphia, PA 19103-2899

DIAGNOSTIC IMAGING: HEAD AND NECK, FIFTH EDITION

ISBN: 978-0-443-37890-4

Previous edition copyrighted 2021.

Library of Congress Control Number: 2025944398

Printed in Canada by Friesens, Altona, Manitoba, Canada

Last digit is the print number: 9 8 7 6 5 4 3 2 1

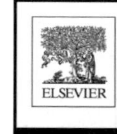

Working together to grow libraries in developing countries

www.elsevier.com • www.bookaid.org

iv

DEDICATIONS

To: Gary, for his enduring love and kindness; Rhiannon, who reminds me to be my authentic self; Kristin, Ryan, and Eric, for their love and acceptance; my parents, for their lifelong love and guidance; and my brother, for always being there and sharing our mutual joy in outdoor adventures.

To many mentors along the way, but in particular "Doc" Jones. I lost the opportunity to share my gratitude for your help in shaping my early path before your untimely passing.

To Ric Harnsberger, for fostering excellence in our head and neck radiology family, and to Bernadette, Surj, Blair, and Nina for their dedication to making our collaborative effort a success.

BEH

Thank you to Bronwyn, Surj, and Blair: It was an honor to work with you on this journey. Thank you to Nina Themann, and the incredible production team for all of your hard work. Thank you to the superb trainees and my colleagues at CCHMC, who inspire me to teach and learn each and every day. And finally, to my family, for their endless love, encouragement, and support.

BLK

Dedicated to Fiju (Dr. Fathima Fijula P. Manzil), my wife and soulmate since childhood; son Lazim, and daughters Lamis & Liya, who happily sacrificed their precious countless hours of evening and weekend family time with me while I was deeply indulged in the work of this book and other projects as a passionate educator. Also indebted to my parents and sisters on the other side of the world who let me fly high and far away from them to fulfill my career dreams and disperse my knowledge in radiology for the betterment of patient care.

SV

First, I would like to thank all of my teachers, mentors, and colleagues who sparked my interest in head and neck imaging and continue to inspire me. I also dedicate my portion of this book to fellows, residents, and students, who provide me with the privilege of teaching head and neck imaging. Your curiosity has kept me humble and focused on a lifelong pursuit of knowledge.

BAW

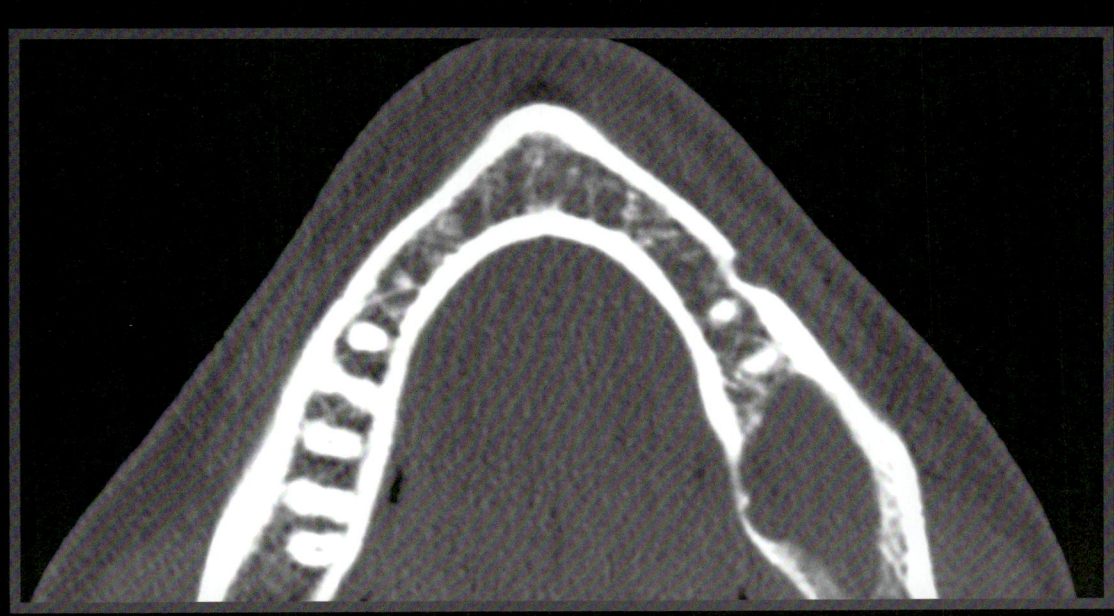

CONTRIBUTING AUTHORS

Shehbaz Ansari, MD
Assistant Professor
Neuroradiology Subdivision
Department of Diagnostic Radiology and
Nuclear Medicine
Rush University Medical Center
Chicago, Illinois

Santhosh Gaddikeri, MD
Associate Professor
Department of Diagnostic Radiology and
Nuclear Medicine
Rush University Medical Center
Chicago, Illinois

Jean Lee, MD
Associate Professor
Medical Imaging Department
St Vincent's Hospital Melbourne
University of Melbourne
Melbourne, Australia

**Melissa Shuhui Lee, MBBS, FRCR,
MMed (Diagnostic Radiology)**
Consultant
Department of Neuroradiology
Singapore General Hospital
Assistant Professor
Duke-NUS Medical School
Singapore

Daniel E. Meltzer, MD
Associate Professor of Radiology
Division of Neuroradiology
Department of Radiology
Icahn School of Medicine at Mount Sinai
New York, New York

William T. O'Brien, Sr., DO, FAOCR
Chief of Pediatric Neuroradiology
Orlando Health
Arnold Palmer Hospital for Children
Orlando, Florida

Michael F. Regner, MD, MS
Assistant Professor of Radiology
Director of Magnetic Resonance Imaging
Director of Fetal Neuroradiology
Oregon Health & Science University
Portland, Oregon

Kalen Riley, MD, MBA
Assistant Professor of Clinical Radiology
and Imaging Sciences
Indiana University School of Medicine
Indianapolis, Indiana

Karen L. Salzman, MD, FACR
Professor of Radiology and Imaging Sciences
Neuroradiology Section Chief
Leslie W. Davis Endowed Chair in
Neuroradiology
University of Utah School of Medicine
Salt Lake City, Utah

Aparna Singhal, MD
Associate Professor
Neuroradiology Section
Department of Radiology
University of Alabama at Birmingham
Birmingham, Alabama

Hilda E. Stambuk, MD
Attending Radiologist
Director of Head and Neck Imaging
Department of Radiology
Memorial Sloan Kettering Cancer Center
Professor
Department of Radiology
Weill Cornell Medical College
New York, New York

Jaclyn E. Thiessen, MD
Associate Professor of Neuroradiology
Neuroradiology Fellowship Program Director
Department of Diagnostic Radiology
Oregon Health & Science University
Portland, Oregon

Ram Vaidhyanath, DMRD, DNB, FRCR
Consultant Radiologist
University Hospitals of Leicester
Leicester, United Kingdom

Melissa B. Warstadt, MD
Assistant Professor of Neuroradiology
Department of Diagnostic Radiology
Oregon Health & Science University
Portland, Oregon

Richard H. Wiggins, III, MD, CIIP, FSIIM, FAHSE, FACR
Director of Head and Neck Imaging
Associate Dean
University of Utah School of Medicine
Professor
Department of Radiology and
Imaging Sciences
University of Utah Health Sciences Center
Salt Lake City, Utah

ADDITIONAL CONTRIBUTORS

Yoshimi Anzai, MD, MPH
Philip R. Chapman, MD
H. Christian Davidson, MD
Kathryn E. Dean, MD
H. Ric Harnsberger, MD
Patricia A. Hudgins, MD, FACR
Troy A. Hutchins, MD
Lisa J. Koenig, BChD, DDS, MS
Nicholas A. Koontz, MD
Joshua E. Lantos, MD
Luke N. Ledbetter, MD
Luke L. Linscott, MD
A. Carlson Merrow, Jr., MD, FAAP
Kevin R. Moore, MD
Kristine M. Mosier, DMD, PhD
Emily S. Orscheln, MD
Anne G. Osborn, MD, FACR
C. Douglas Phillips, MD, FACR
Caroline D. Robson, MBChB
Sara Strauss, MD
Dania Tamimi, BDS, DMSc, FDS, RCPS (Glasg)

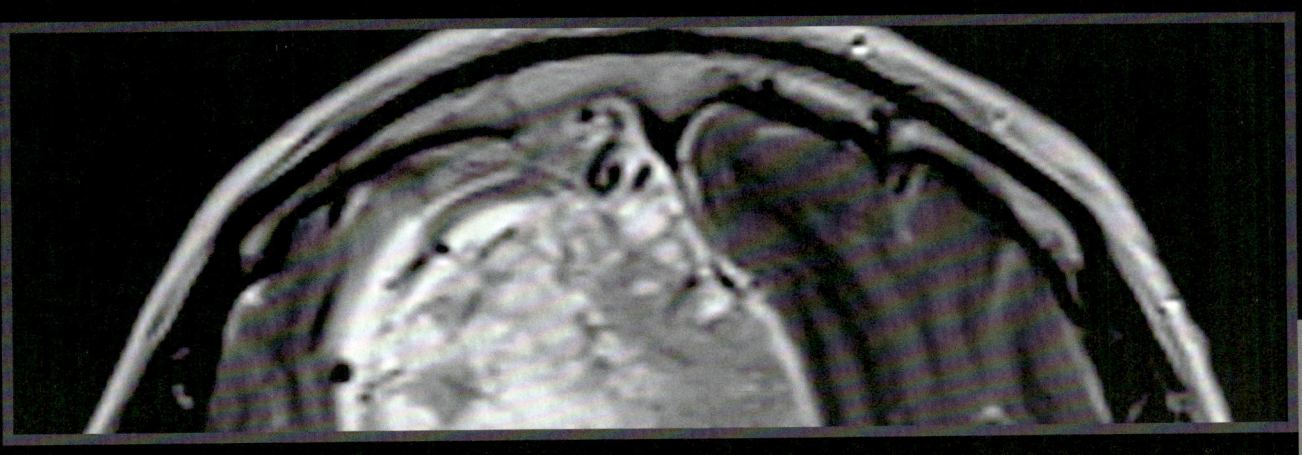

PREFACE

Why *Diagnostic Imaging: Head and Neck*, 5th edition? Medicine continues to evolve at a rapid rate, and this is evident in head and neck imaging, particularly for oncologic imaging. Radiologists need familiarity with changing tumor classifications, nomenclature updates, and newer precision therapies that are in development based on our improved understanding of tumor genomics. The need for multidisciplinary involvement in patient care is greater than ever before. Radiologists and other imaging specialists need to practice with the knowledge that reflects contemporary terminology, diagnosis, and treatment for head and neck disorders. Our current edition comprehensively covers the basics of space-specific imaging diagnosis in the head and neck, and features the most recent changes relevant to head and neck imaging, including:

- Updates from the 5th edition of the World Health Organization (WHO) Classification of Head and Neck Tumours in 2022

  o This includes sinonasal tract tumors that have undergone reclassification with new categories, such as hamartomatous lesions and several newly classified tumors

  o Evolving immunohistochemical techniques and molecular genetics have allowed improved classification of tumors and inflammatory disorders in the head and neck

  o Includes updated nomenclature changes to multiple head and neck tumors and genetic syndromes

  o Improved understanding of genetic disease underpinnings has allowed more precision-targeted therapies that radiologists need to be familiar with, in addition to relevant implications for imaging surveillance and potential complications

  o New diagnoses related to improved higher resolution imaging techniques

- Revised nomenclature from the 2025 International Society for the Study of Vascular Anomalies (ISSVA) for head and neck vascular malformations, important for avoiding misdiagnosis and inappropriate treatment

- Greater use of specific radiotracers in nuclear medicine, such as Ga-68 DOTATATE PET, has applications for neuroendocrine tumors and surveillance

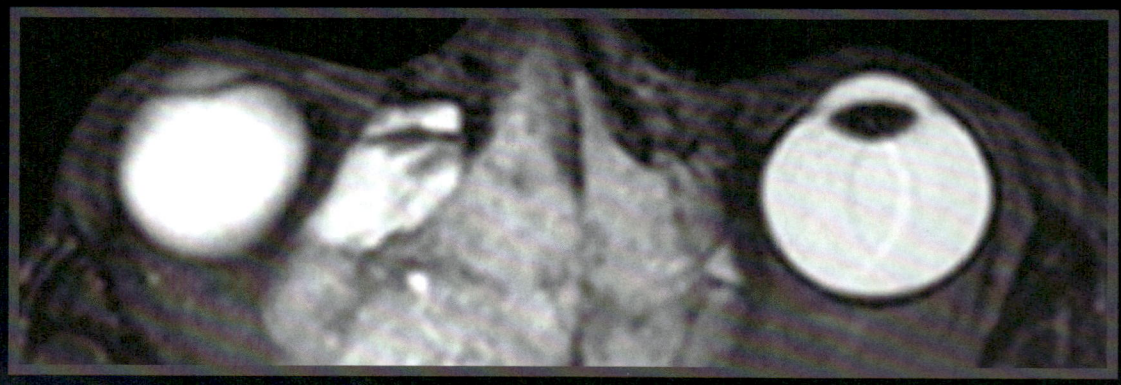

We trust that you will enjoy the same information-dense material in the easily accessible format that appeared in prior editions, augmented by beautiful, enhanced, high-quality illustrations and accompanied by new and updated cases, including 1,000 new images. We are confident that you will enjoy our 5th edition of *Diagnostic Imaging: Head and Neck* as much as we enjoyed writing it for you and know that you will find it to be an invaluable reference in your reading room.

BRONWYN E. HAMILTON, MD
Professor of Radiology
Courtesy Appointment, Otolaryngology - Head & Neck Surgery
Oregon Health & Science University
Portland, Oregon

BERNADETTE L. KOCH, MD
Associate Chief, Radiology
Cincinnati Children's Hospital Medical Center
Professor, Radiology and Pediatrics
University of Cincinnati College of Medicine
Cincinnati, Ohio

SURJITH VATTOTH, MD, FRCR
Professor of Radiology
Director of Pediatric Neuroimaging
Department of Diagnostic Radiology and Nuclear Medicine
Division of Neuroradiology
Rush University Medical Center
Chicago, Illinois

BLAIR A. WINEGAR, MD
Neuroradiology Fellowship Program Director
Associate Professor of Radiology and Medical Imaging
University of Utah School of Medicine
Salt Lake City, Utah

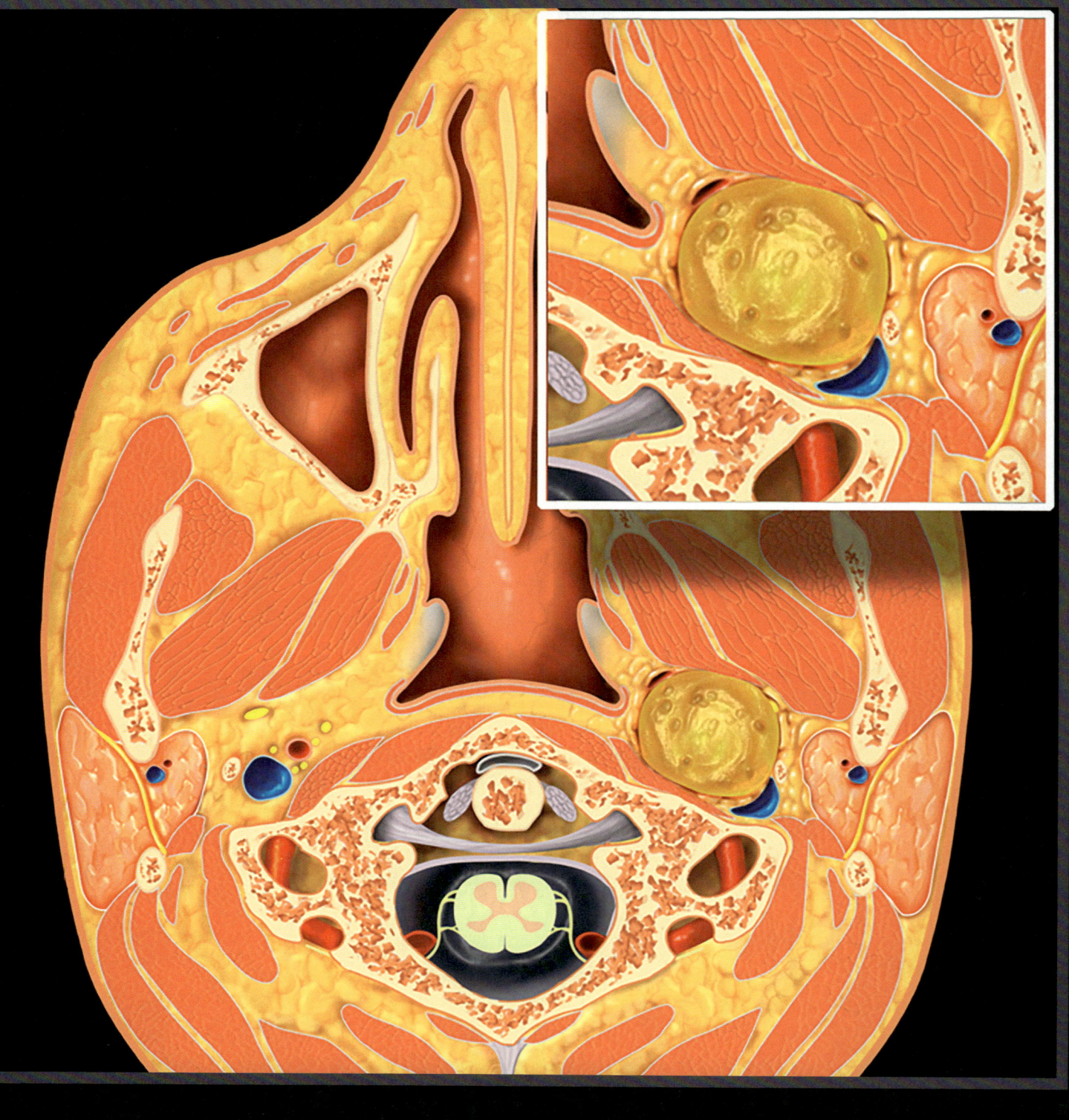

ACKNOWLEDGMENTS

LEAD EDITOR
Nina Themann, BA

LEAD ILLUSTRATOR
Richard Coombs, MS

TEXT EDITORS
Arthur G. Gelsinger, MA
Rebecca L. Bluth, BA
Terry W. Ferrell, MS
Megg Morin, BA
Kathryn Watkins, BA
Shannon Kelly, MA

ILLUSTRATIONS
Lane R. Bennion, MS
Laura C. Wissler, MA

IMAGE EDITORS
Jeffrey J. Marmorstone, BS
Lisa A. M. Steadman, BS

ART DIRECTION AND DESIGN
Sophia Huebel, MS

PRODUCTION EDITORS
Emily C. Fassett, BA
John Pecorelli, BS

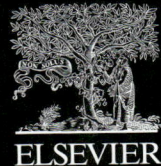

ELSEVIER

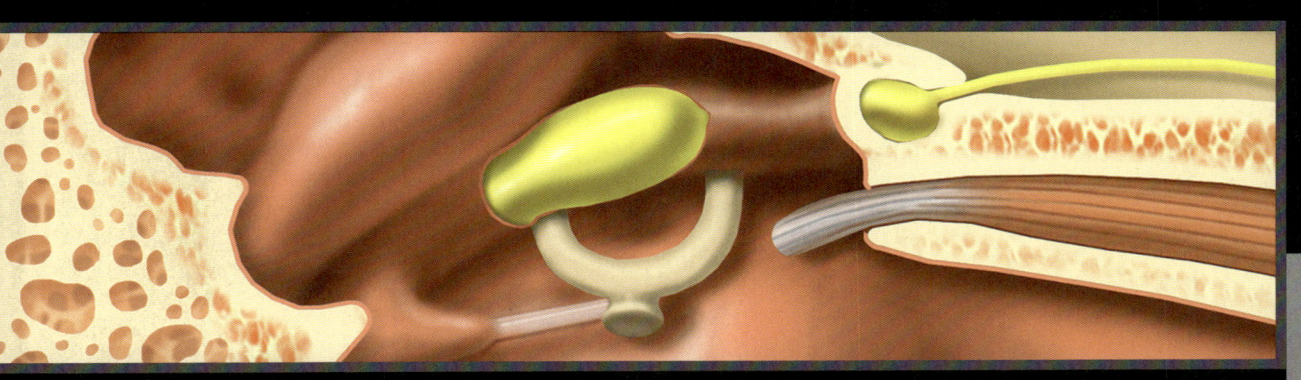

TABLE OF CONTENTS

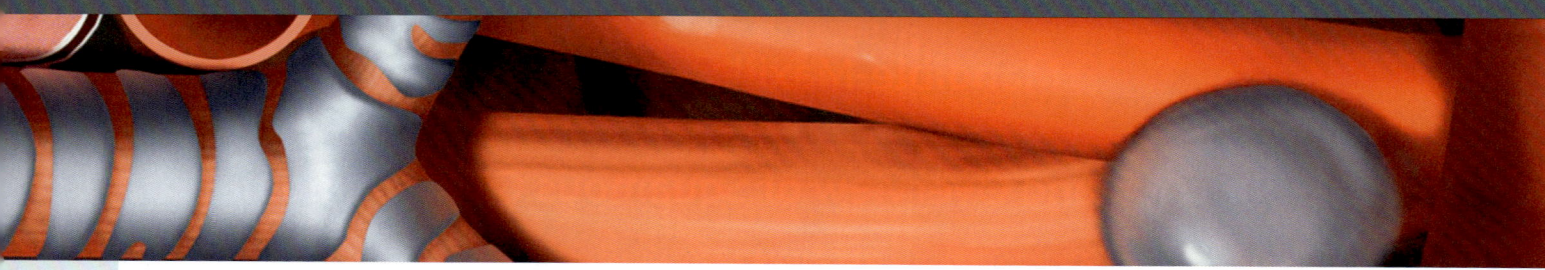

TABLE OF CONTENTS

TABLE OF CONTENTS

TABLE OF CONTENTS

TABLE OF CONTENTS

TABLE OF CONTENTS

TABLE OF CONTENTS

TABLE OF CONTENTS

TABLE OF CONTENTS

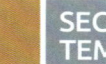

TABLE OF CONTENTS

TABLE OF CONTENTS

TABLE OF CONTENTS

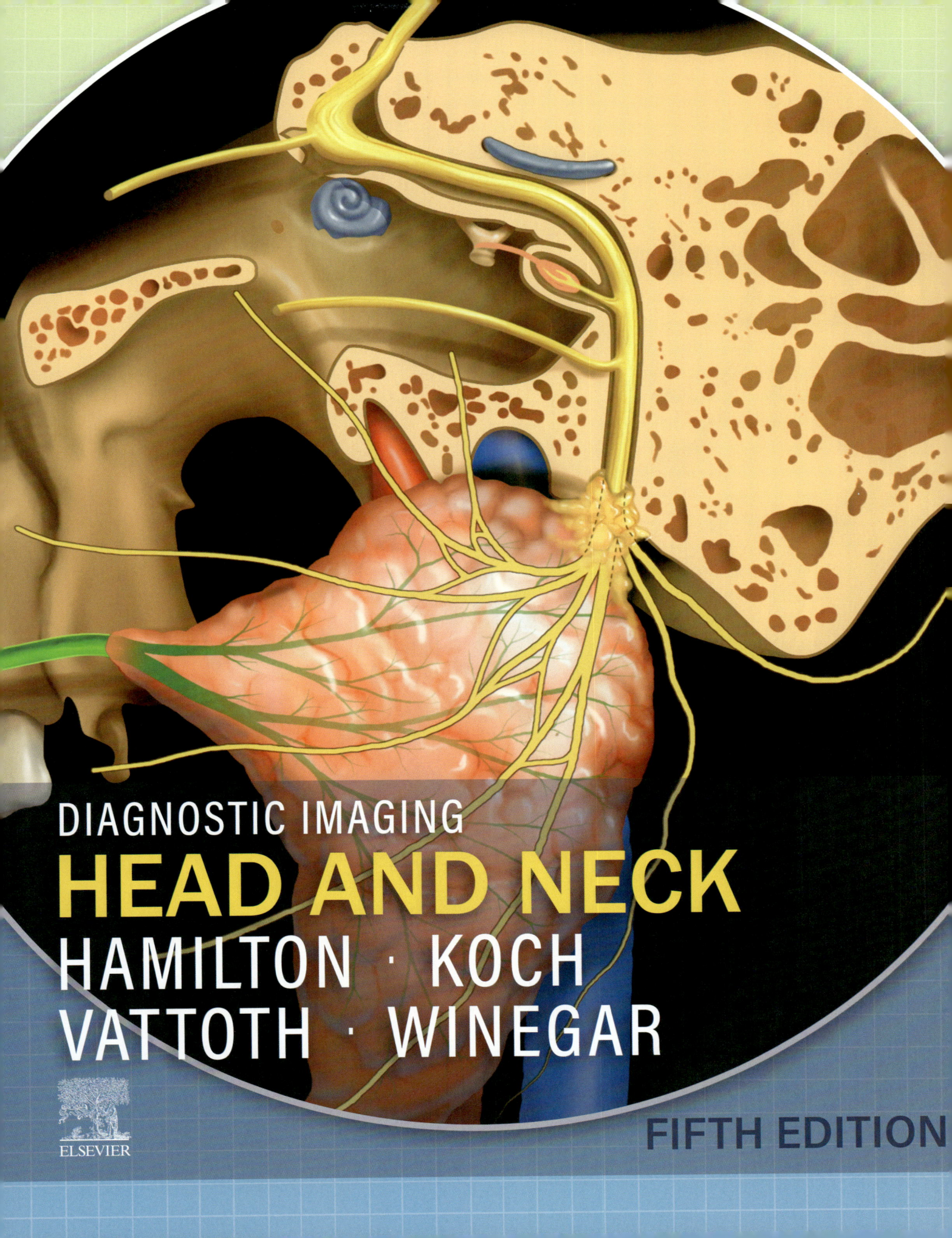

DIAGNOSTIC IMAGING
HEAD AND NECK
HAMILTON · KOCH
VATTOTH · WINEGAR

ELSEVIER

FIFTH EDITION

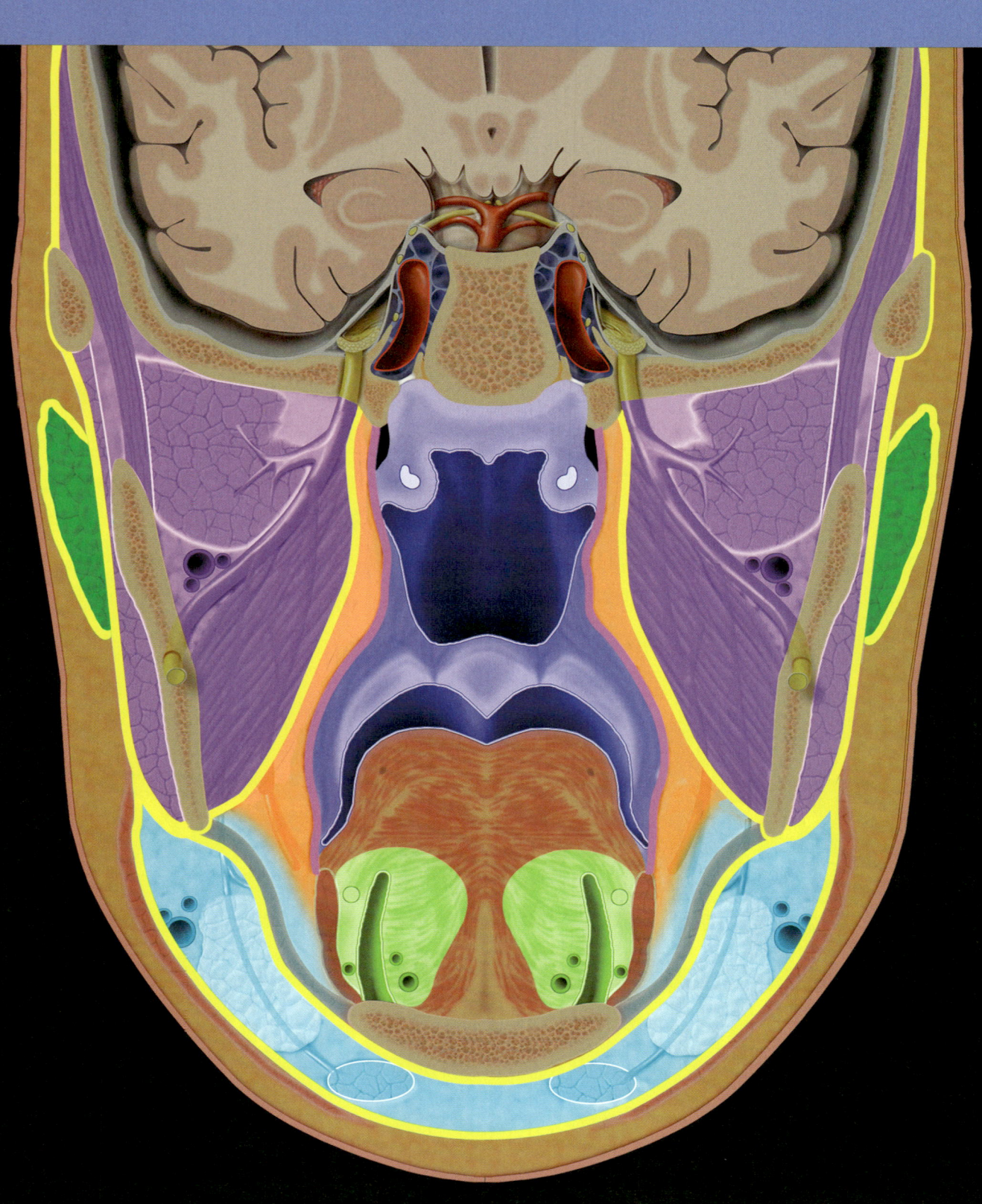

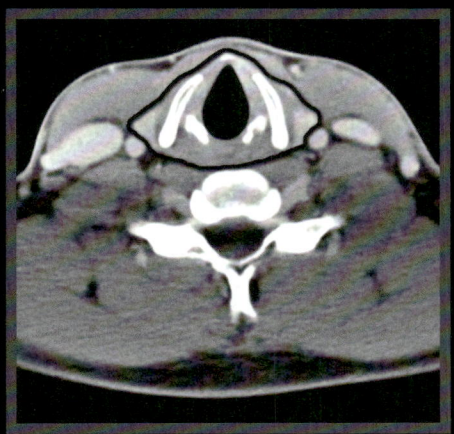

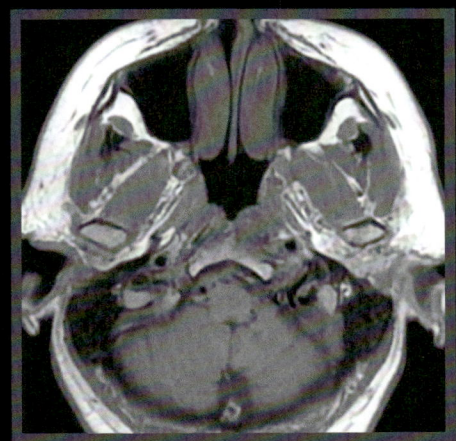

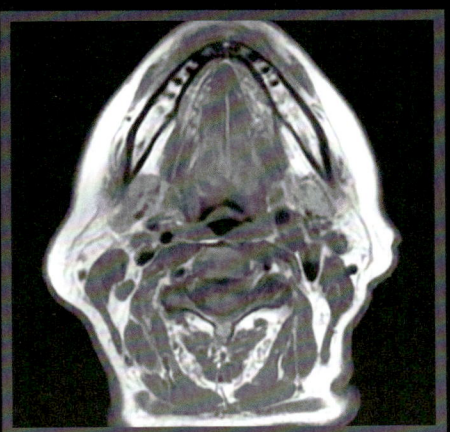

Imaging Approaches and Indications

Many indications exist for imaging the extracranial H&N. Exploratory imaging, tumor staging, and abscess search comprise 3 common reasons imaging is ordered in this area. Global evaluation of the neck from the skull base to the clavicles is most often accomplished using CECT. Axial images can be rapidly obtained after IV iodinated contrast and multiplanar reformations are created. This provides reasonable spatial and contrast resolution.

MR is less readily accessible and used less often but is especially useful in the suprahyoid neck (SHN) because it is less affected by oral cavity dental amalgam artifact. Axial and coronal T1 fat-saturated enhanced MR is superior to CECT in defining the soft tissue extent of a tumor, perineural tumor spread, marrow space invasion, and intracranial spread. When MR is combined with bone CT of the facial bones and skull base, precise preoperative lesion mapping results.

CECT is the modality of choice when infrahyoid neck (IHN) and mediastinum are imaged. Swallowing, coughing, and breathing make this area a "moving target" for the imager. MR quality is often degraded as a result. Multislice CT with multiplanar reformations now permits exquisite images of the IHN unaffected by movement.

High-resolution ultrasound also has a role. Superficial lesions, thyroid disease, and nodal evaluation with biopsy are best done by skilled ultrasonographers.

Squamous cell carcinoma (SCCa) staging is best started with CECT, as both the primary tumor and nodes must be imaged, requiring imaging from the skull base to clavicles. MR imaging times and susceptibility to motion artifact make it a less desirable exam in this setting. Instead, MR is best used when specific delineation of exact tumor extent, perineural tumor, or intracranial invasion is needed. PET/CT is emerging as a useful adjunctive test in complex tumor detection and monitoring.

When the type and cause of H&N infection are sought, CECT is the best exam. CECT can readily differentiate cellulitis, phlegmon, and abscess. CT can also identify salivary gland ductal calculi, teeth infection, mandible osteomyelitis, and intratonsillar abscess as causes of infection.

Imaging Anatomy

In discussing the extracranial H&N soft tissues, a few definitions are needed. The **SHN** is defined as deep facial spaces **above the hyoid bone**, including the parapharyngeal space (PPS), pharyngeal mucosal space (PMS), masticator space (MS), parotid space (PS), carotid space (CS), retropharyngeal space (RPS), danger space (DS), and perivertebral (PVS) space. The **IHN** soft tissue spaces are predominantly **below the hyoid bone** with some continuing inferiorly into the mediastinum or superiorly into the SHN, including the visceral space (VS), posterior cervical space (PCS), CS, RPS, and PVS.

Important **SHN** space **anatomic relationships** include their interactions with the skull base, oral cavity, and IHN. When one thinks about the SHN spaces and their relationships with the skull base, perhaps the most important consideration is to examine each space alone to see what critical structures (cranial nerves, arteries, veins) are at the point of contact between the space and the skull base. Space by space, the

skull base interactions above and IHN extension below are apparent.

- **PPS** has bland triangular skull base abutment without critical foramen involved; it empties inferiorly into submandibular space (SMS)
- **PMS** touches posterior basisphenoid and anterior basiocciput, including **foramen lacerum**; it includes nasopharyngeal, oropharyngeal, and hypopharyngeal mucosal surfaces
- **MS** superior skull base interaction includes zygomatic arch, condylar fossa, skull base, including **foramen ovale (CNV3)**, **and foramen spinosum** (middle meningeal artery); MS ends at inferior surface of body of mandible
- **PS** abuts floor of external auditory canal, mastoid tip, including **stylomastoid foramen (CNVII)**; parotid tail extends inferiorly into posterior SMS
- **CS** meets **jugular foramen (CNIX-XI)** floor, hypoglossal canal (CNXII), and petrous internal carotid artery canal; CS can be followed inferiorly to aortic arch
- **RPS** contacts skull base along lower clivus without involvement of critical structures; it continues inferiorly to empty into DS at T3 level
- **PVS** touches low clivus and encircles occipital condyles and foramen magnum; it continues inferiorly to level into thorax

In addition to skull base interactions, the relationships of the SHN spaces to the fat-filled PPSs are key to analyzing SHN masses. The PPSs are a pair of fat-filled spaces in the lateral SHN surrounded by the PMS, MS, PS, CS, and RPS. When a mass enlarges in one of these spaces, it displaces the PPS fat. Larger masses define their space of origin based on this displacement pattern.

- Medial PMS mass displaces PPS laterally
- More anterior MS mass displaces PPS posteriorly
- Lateral PS mass displaces PPS medially
- Posterolateral CS mass displaces styloid process and PPS anteriorly
- More posteromedial lateral RPS nodal mass displaces PPS anterolaterally

The **IHN** space **anatomic relationships** are defined by their superior and inferior projections. The VS has **no** SHN component, instead projecting only inferiorly into the superior mediastinum. The PCS extends superiorly to the mastoid tip and ends inferiorly at the clavicle. It is predominantly an IHN space, however. The CS begins at the floor of the jugular foramen and carotid canal and extends inferiorly to the aortic arch. The RPS begins at the ventral clivus superiorly and traverses SHN-IHN to the T3 level. The DS is immediately posterior to the RPS but continues beyond the T3 level into the mediastinum. For imaging purposes, RPS and DS can be considered a single entity. The PVS can be defined from the skull base above to the clavicle below. The PVS is divided by fascial slip into prevertebral and paraspinal components.

The **deep cervical fasciae (DCF)** of the neck subdivide and define the spaces we use radiologically to construct space-specific DDx lists and evaluate disease of the neck. It is imperative that a clear understanding of these fasciae be grasped by any imager involved in evaluating this area.

Many nomenclatures have been used to describe the neck fasciae. The following is a practical distillate meant to simplify this challenging subject. There are 3 main DCF in the neck. The same names are used in the SHN and IHN. The superficial layer

Common Tumors in Spaces of Neck

Pharyngeal mucosal space	Warthin tumor	Posterior cervical space
Pharyngeal SCCa	**Carotid space**	Pharyngeal SCCa nodal metastasis
Tonsillar NHL	Vagal paraganglioma	NHL nodal disease
Masticator space	Carotid body paraganglioma	Differentiated thyroid carcinoma nodes
Sarcoma	Schwannoma of CNIX-XII	**Visceral space**
Perineural CNV3 SCCa	**Retropharyngeal space**	Differentiated thyroid carcinoma
Parotid space	SCCa nodal metastasis	Anaplastic thyroid carcinoma
Mucoepidermoid carcinoma	NHL nodal disease	Thyroid NHL
Adenoid cystic carcinoma	**Perivertebral space**	Cervical esophageal carcinoma
Malignant nodal metastases	Vertebral body systemic metastasis	Parathyroid adenoma
Pleomorphic adenoma	Brachial plexus schwannoma	

SCCa = squamous cell carcinoma; NHL = non-Hodgkin lymphoma.

(**SL-DCF**), the middle layer (**ML-DCF**), and the deep layer of DCF (**DL-DCF**) are the 3 important fasciae in the neck.

In the SHN, the **SL-DCF** circumscribes **MS** and **PS** and contributes to the carotid sheath. In the IHN, it "invests" the neck by surrounding the infrahyoid strap, sternocleidomastoid, and trapezius muscles. It also contributes to the carotid sheath of the CS in the IHN.

The **ML-DCF** in the SHN defines the deep margin of the PMS. It contributes to carotid sheath in both the SHN and IHN. In the IHN, it also circumscribes the VS.

In both the SHN and IHN, the **DL-DCF** surrounds **PVS**. A slip of DL-DCF dives medially to the transverse process, dividing the PVS into prevertebral and paraspinal components. Another slip of DL-DCF, the alar fascia, provides the lateral wall to the RPS and DS, as well as the posterior wall to the RPS, separating the RPS from the DS. DL-DCF contributes to the carotid sheath, like the SL-DCF and ML-DCF.

The internal structures of the spaces of the neck are for the most part responsible for the diseases there. Let us begin by defining the **critical contents of the SHN spaces**.

- **PPS** contains fat with rare minor salivary glands
- **PMS** contains mucosa, lymphatic ring, and minor salivary glands; in nasopharyngeal mucosal space, opening of eustachian tube, torus tubarius, adenoids, superior constrictor, and levator palatini muscles can be seen; oropharyngeal mucosal space contains anterior and posterior tonsillar pillars and palatine and lingual tonsils
- **MS** includes posterior mandibular body and ramus, TMJ, CNV3, masseter, medial and lateral pterygoid and temporalis muscles, and pterygoid venous plexus
- **PS** houses parotid, extracranial CNVII, nodes, retromandibular vein, and external carotid artery
- **CS** contains CNIX-XII, internal jugular vein, and internal carotid artery
- **RPS** has fat and medial and lateral RPS nodes inside
- Prevertebral **PVS** contains vertebral body, veins, arteries, and prevertebral muscles (longus colli and capitis); in paraspinal PVS reside posterior elements of vertebra and paraspinal muscles

The **critical contents** of **IHN spaces** are defined next.

- **VS** contains thyroid and parathyroid glands, trachea, esophagus, recurrent laryngeal nerves, and pretracheal and paratracheal nodes
- **PCS** has fat, CNXI, and level V nodes inside
- **CS** houses common carotid artery, internal jugular vein, and CNX
- **IHN RPS** has **no** nodes and contains only fat
- Prevertebral **PVS** has brachial plexus and phrenic nerve, vertebral body, veins, arteries, and prevertebral and scalene muscles within; paraspinal PVS contains only posterior vertebra elements and paraspinal muscles

Approaches to Imaging Issues in SHN and IHN

It is crucial that the imager has a method of analysis when a mass is found in the neck. In the SHN, mass evaluation methodology begins with defining mass **space of origin** (PMS, MS, PS, CS, lateral RPS). When small, this is simple, as the mass is seen within the confines of 1 space. In larger masses, ask, "How does the mass displace the PPS?" Next, utilize a **space-specific DDx** list. Match the imaging findings to the diagnoses within this list to narrow your differential.

With IHN masses, a similar evaluation methodology can be employed. First, determine what space the mass originates in (VS, CS, PCS). Then, review the space-specific DDx list. Match radiologic findings of your case to this DDx list. In all neck masses, knowing the clinical findings can be very helpful.

Lesions of posterior midline spaces (RPS and PVS) of the neck need different image evaluation. When a lesion is defined here, first ask, "How does the mass displace prevertebral muscles (PVM)?" In the case of an **RPS mass**, PVMs are flattened posteriorly or invaded from anterior to posterior. Contrast this imaging appearance to that of the **PVS mass** in which the PVMs are lifted anteriorly or invaded from posterior to anterior. Since most PVS lesions arise from the vertebral body, vertebral body destruction and epidural disease will be linked. The DL-DCF "forces" PVS disease into the epidural space.

Selected References

1. Grani G et al: Thyroid nodules: diagnosis and management. Nat Rev Endocrinol. 20(12):715-28, 2024
2. Rao Y et al: Performance of radiomics in the differential diagnosis of parotid tumors: a systematic review. Front Oncol. 14:1383323, 2024

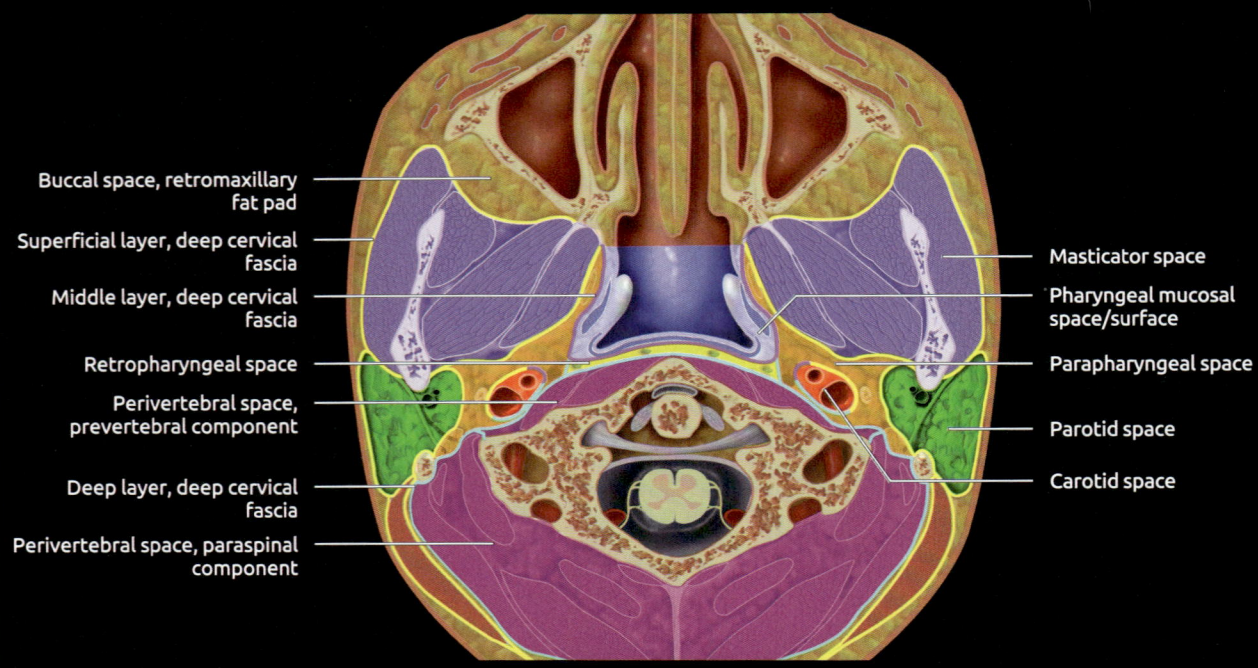

Buccal space, retromaxillary fat pad

Superficial layer, deep cervical fascia

Middle layer, deep cervical fascia

Retropharyngeal space

Perivertebral space, prevertebral component

Deep layer, deep cervical fascia

Perivertebral space, paraspinal component

Masticator space

Pharyngeal mucosal space/surface

Parapharyngeal space

Parotid space

Carotid space

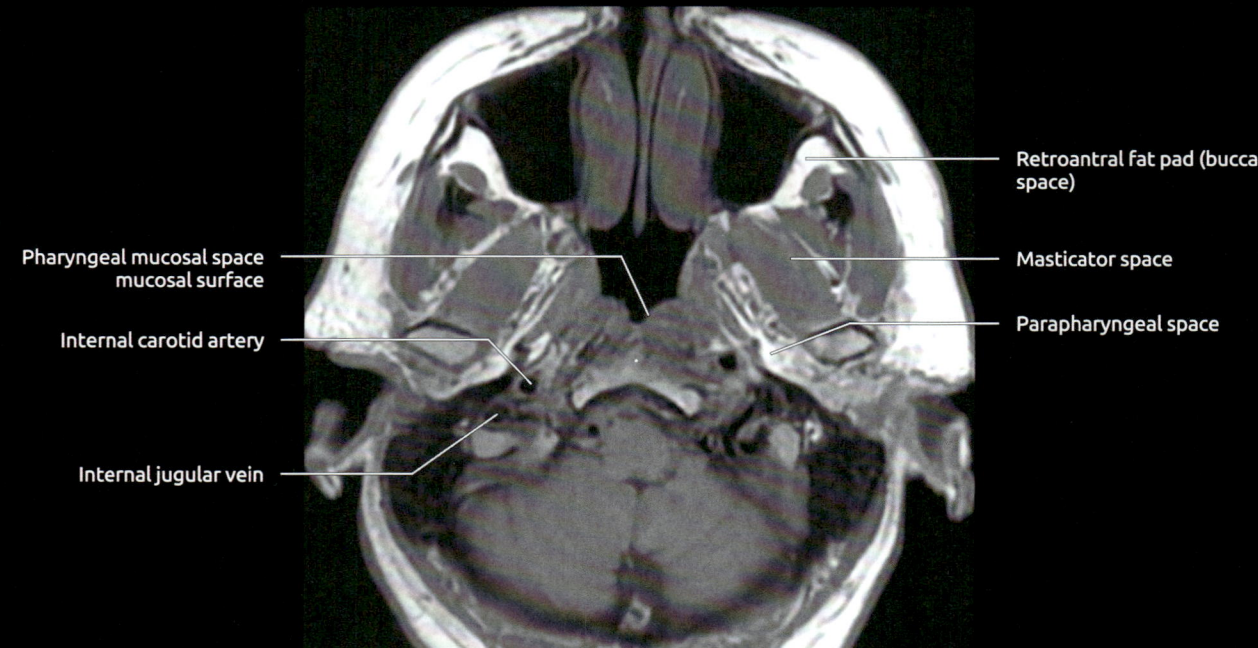

Pharyngeal mucosal space mucosal surface

Internal carotid artery

Internal jugular vein

Retroantral fat pad (buccal space)

Masticator space

Parapharyngeal space

(Top) *Axial graphic depicts the spaces of the suprahyoid neck. Surrounding the paired fat-filled parapharyngeal spaces (PPSs) are the 4 critical paired spaces of this region: The pharyngeal mucosal (PMS), masticator (MS), parotid (PS), and carotid spaces (CS). Retropharyngeal (RPS) and perivertebral spaces (PVS) are the midline nonpaired spaces. A PMS mass pushes the PPS laterally, an MS mass pushes the PPS posteriorly, a PS mass pushes the PPS medially, and a CS mass pushes the PPS anteriorly. A lateral RPS mass pushes the PPS anteriorly without lifting the styloid process. The superficial (yellow line), middle (pink line), and deep (turquoise line) layers of deep cervical fascia outline the spaces. (Bottom) Axial noncontrast T1 MR through the suprahyoid neck at the level of the nasopharynx shows the PMS, MS, PPS, and CS. The retroantral fat pad, which is part of the buccal space, can also be seen.*

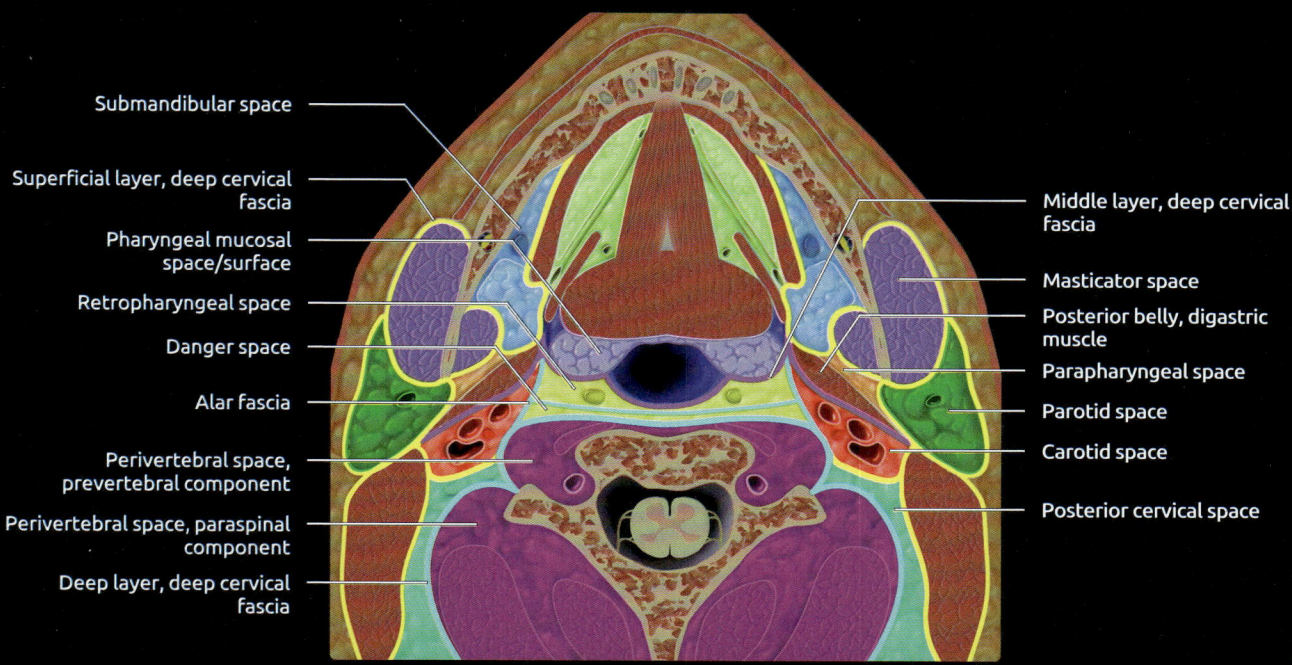

Submandibular space

Superficial layer, deep cervical fascia

Pharyngeal mucosal space/surface

Retropharyngeal space

Danger space

Alar fascia

Perivertebral space, prevertebral component

Perivertebral space, paraspinal component

Deep layer, deep cervical fascia

Middle layer, deep cervical fascia

Masticator space

Posterior belly, digastric muscle

Parapharyngeal space

Parotid space

Carotid space

Posterior cervical space

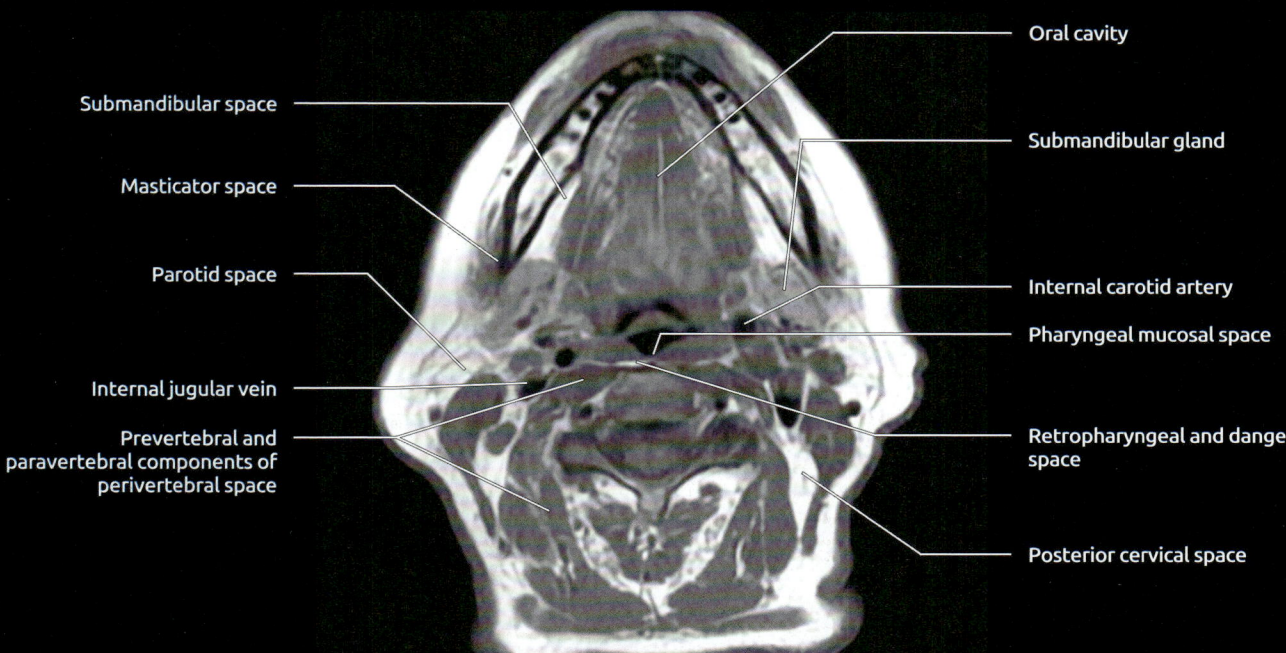

Submandibular space

Masticator space

Parotid space

Internal jugular vein

Prevertebral and paravertebral components of perivertebral space

Oral cavity

Submandibular gland

Internal carotid artery

Pharyngeal mucosal space

Retropharyngeal and danger space

Posterior cervical space

(Top) *Axial graphic shows the suprahyoid neck spaces at the level of the oropharynx. The superficial (yellow line), middle (pink line), and deep (turquoise line) layers of deep cervical fascia outline the suprahyoid neck spaces. Notice that the lateral borders of the RPS and danger spaces are called the alar fascia, which represents a slip of the deep layer of deep cervical fascia. The CS has a tricolored fascial representation for the carotid sheath. This is because all 3 layers of deep cervical fascia contribute to the carotid sheath.* (Bottom) *Axial T1 MR of the suprahyoid neck through the oropharynx shows the oral cavity, submandibular space, parotid space (with fatty infiltration of the parotid tail), PMS, posterior cervical space, perivertebral space, and CS. Note thin fatty signal depicting the retropharyngeal and danger space between the PMS and PVS.*

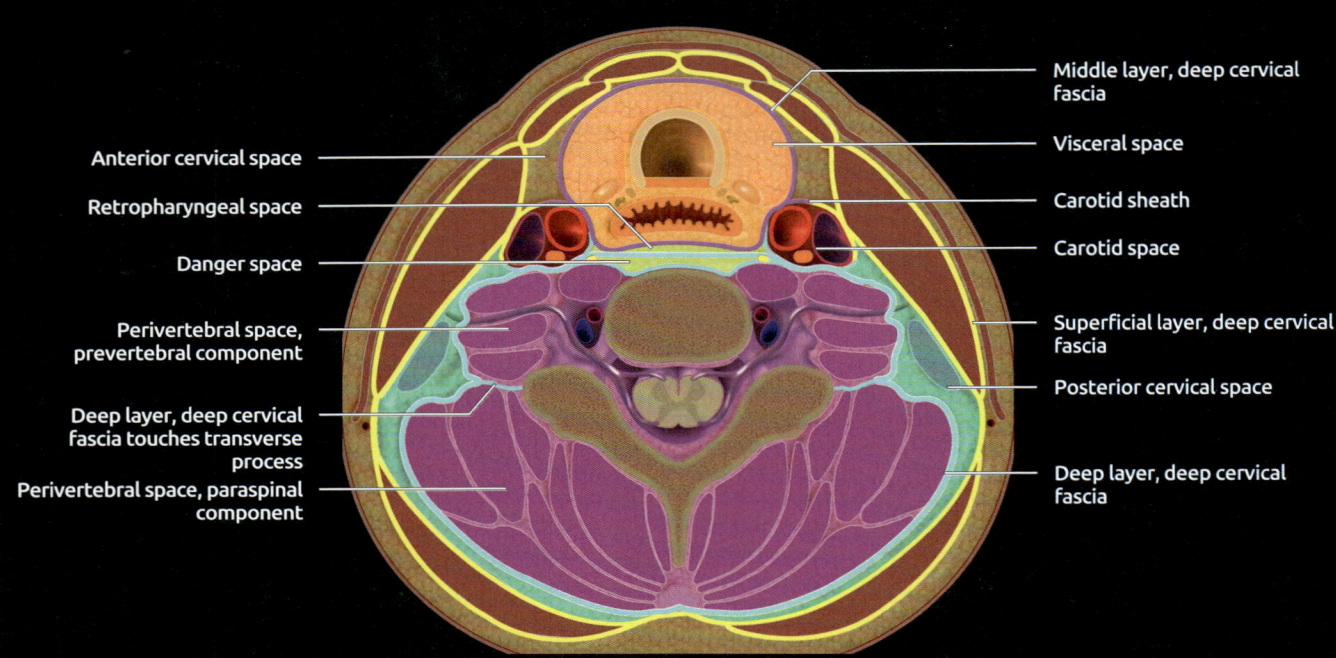

Middle layer, deep cervical fascia

Visceral space

Carotid sheath

Carotid space

Superficial layer, deep cervical fascia

Posterior cervical space

Deep layer, deep cervical fascia

Anterior cervical space

Retropharyngeal space

Danger space

Perivertebral space, prevertebral component

Deep layer, deep cervical fascia touches transverse process

Perivertebral space, paraspinal component

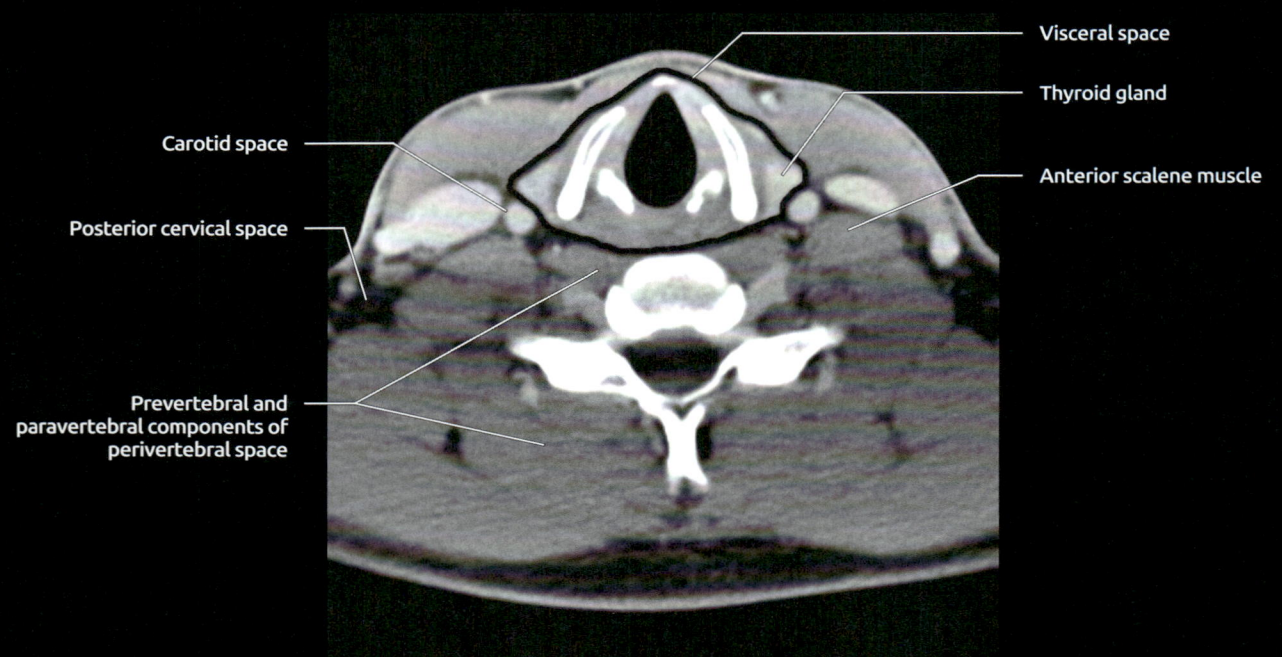

Visceral space

Thyroid gland

Anterior scalene muscle

Carotid space

Posterior cervical space

Prevertebral and paravertebral components of perivertebral space

(Top) *Axial graphic depicts the fascia and spaces of the infrahyoid neck. The 3 layers of deep cervical fascia are present in the suprahyoid and infrahyoid neck. The carotid sheath is made up of all 3 layers of deep cervical fascia (tricolor line around CS). Notice that the deep layer (turquoise line) completely circles the PVS, diving in laterally to divide it into prevertebral and paraspinal components. The middle layer (pink line) circumscribes the visceral space, while the superficial layer (yellow line) "invests" the neck deep tissues.* (Bottom) *Axial CECT through the infrahyoid neck at the level of the larynx shows the visceral space containing the larynx, thyroid gland, CS, posterior cervical space, and prevertebral and paravertebral components of the perivertebral space.*

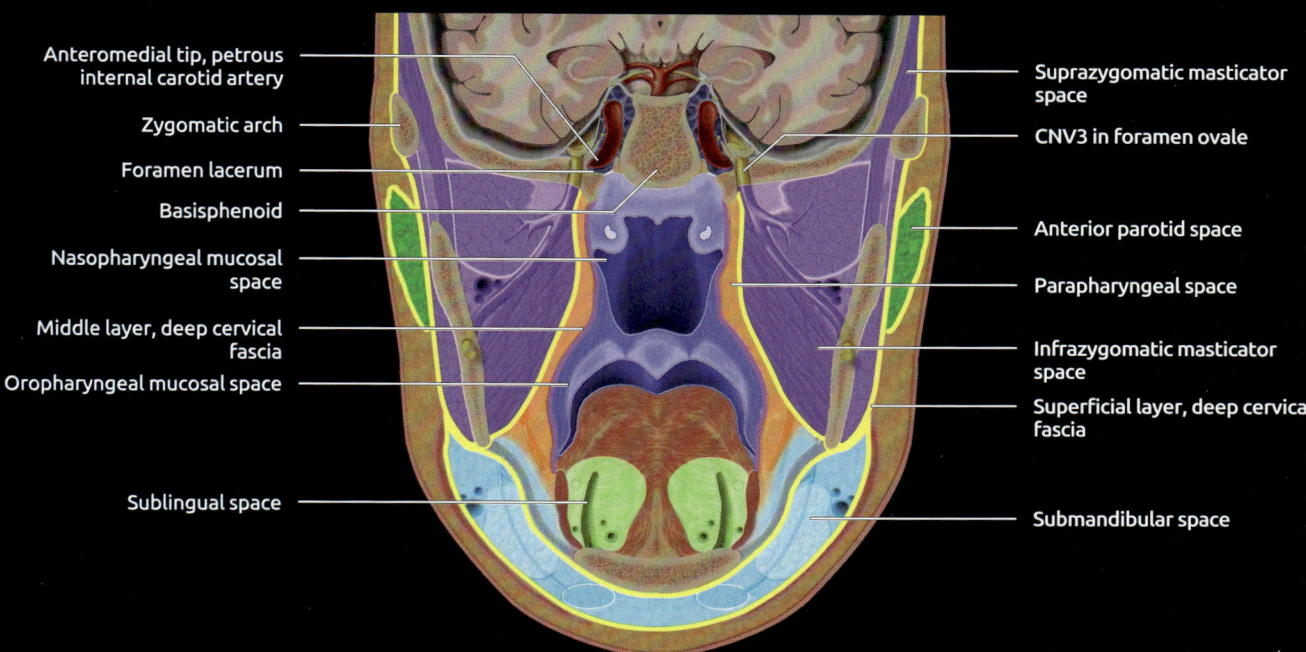

Anteromedial tip, petrous internal carotid artery

Zygomatic arch

Foramen lacerum

Basisphenoid

Nasopharyngeal mucosal space

Middle layer, deep cervical fascia

Oropharyngeal mucosal space

Sublingual space

Suprazygomatic masticator space

CNV3 in foramen ovale

Anterior parotid space

Parapharyngeal space

Infrazygomatic masticator space

Superficial layer, deep cervical fascia

Submandibular space

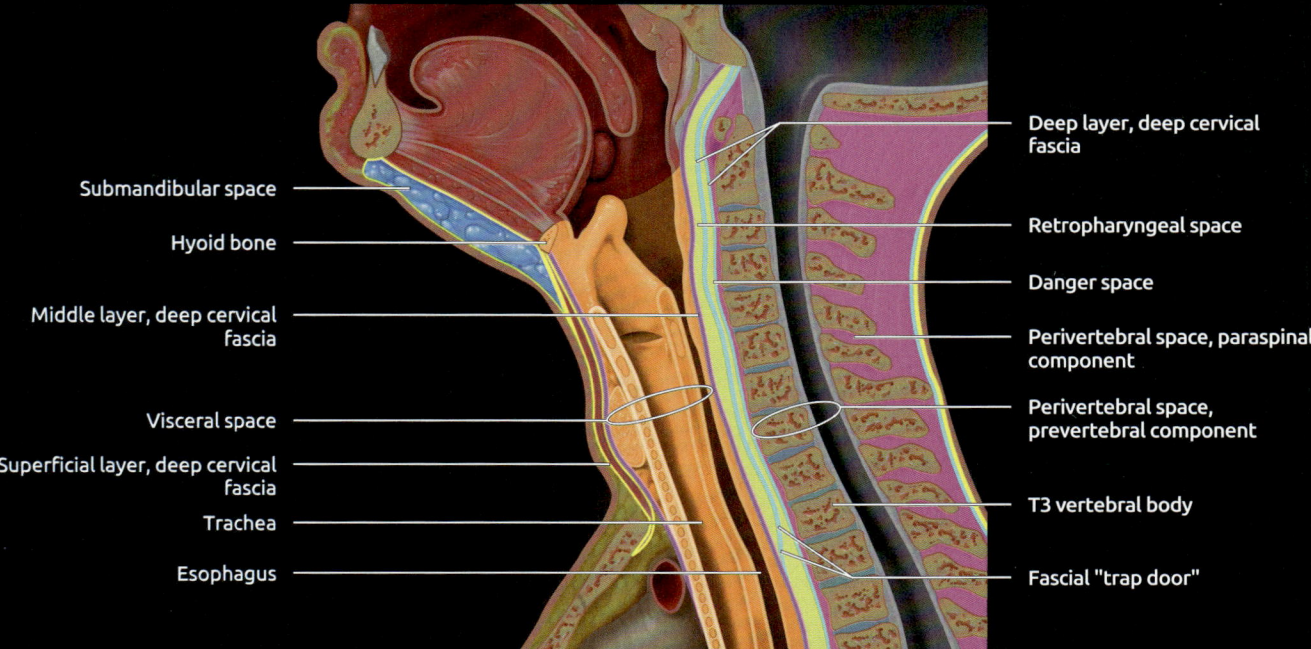

Submandibular space

Hyoid bone

Middle layer, deep cervical fascia

Visceral space

Superficial layer, deep cervical fascia

Trachea

Esophagus

Deep layer, deep cervical fascia

Retropharyngeal space

Danger space

Perivertebral space, paraspinal component

Perivertebral space, prevertebral component

T3 vertebral body

Fascial "trap door"

(Top) *Coronal graphic shows suprahyoid neck spaces as they interact with the skull base. The MS has the largest area of abutment with the skull base, including CNV3. The PMS abuts the basisphenoid and foramen lacerum. The foramen lacerum is the cartilage-covered floor of the anteromedial petrous internal carotid artery (ICA) canal.* **(Bottom)** *Sagittal graphic depicts longitudinal spatial relationships of the infrahyoid neck. Anteriorly, the visceral space is seen surrounded by the middle layer of deep cervical fascia (pink line). Just anterior to the vertebral column, the RPS and danger space run inferiorly toward the mediastinum. Notice the fascial "trap door" found at the approximate level of T3 vertebral body that serves as a conduit from the RPS to the danger space. RPS infection or tumor may access the mediastinum via this route of spread.*

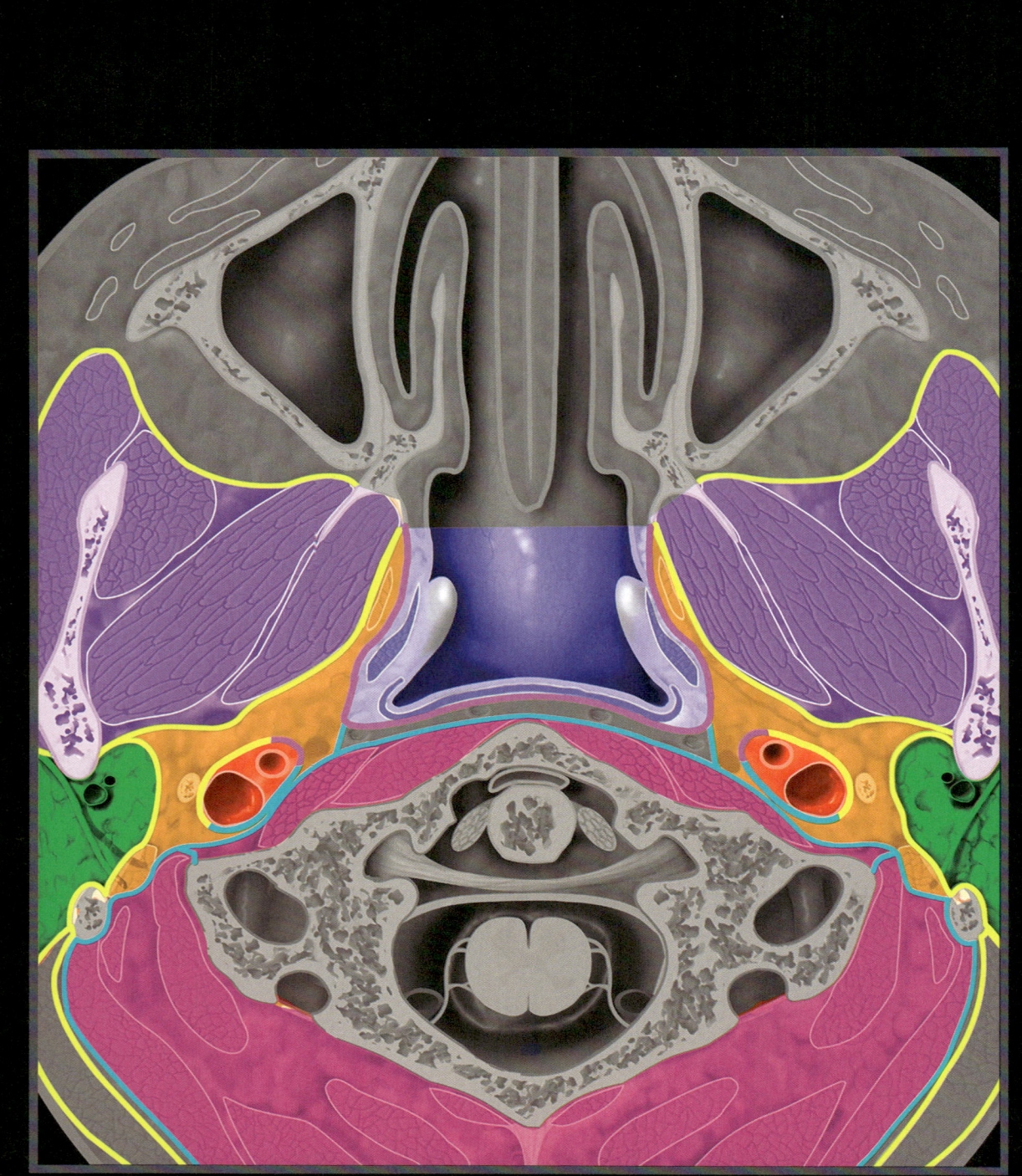

Parapharyngeal Space

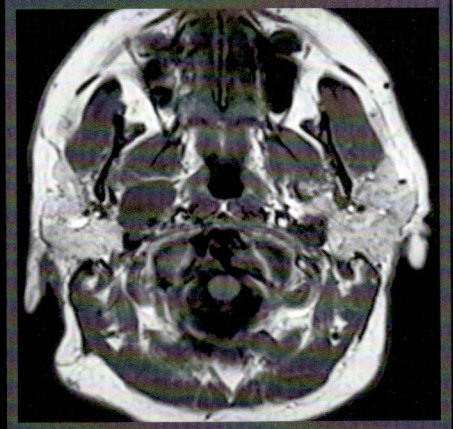
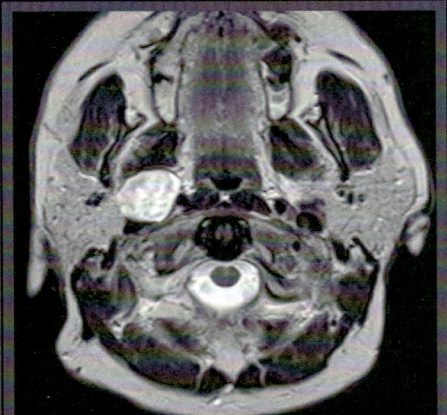
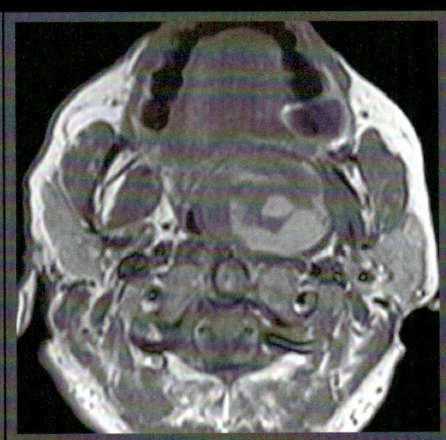

Summary Thoughts: Parapharyngeal Space

The parapharyngeal space (PPS) is an important radiologic landmark in the suprahyoid neck (SHN). It is predominantly fat-filled, which makes it easily identifiable on CT and MR. The PPS is surrounded by 4 key spaces in the SHN, all of which can give rise to pathologic lesions. When a large lesion affects the SHN, it may displace the PPS fat away from the space of origin. Therefore, the displacement of PPS becomes a useful secondary clue to identifying the space of origin of the lesion. Once a space of origin is assigned, the space-specific differential diagnosis can be applied to narrow the diagnostic possibilities.

Imaging Anatomy

The PPSs are paired, central, fat-filled spaces in the lateral SHN around which most of the important spaces are located. These surrounding important spaces are the pharyngeal mucosal space (PMS), masticator space (MS), parotid space (PS), carotid space (CS), and the retropharyngeal space (RPS). The PPS contents are limited; therefore, few lesions actually occur in this space. Diseases (tumor and infection) of the PPS usually arise in the adjacent spaces (PMS, MS, PS, CS) and spread secondarily into PPS.

The importance of the fat-filled PPS is its conspicuity on CT and MR. Even when large lesions are present in the SHN, it is still usually possible to find the PPS. Identifying the direction of displacement of the PPS by a mass lesion from a surrounding space can be a **key finding** in determining its **space of origin**. The PPS displacement direction defines the space of the primary lesion.

- PMS mass lesion pushes PPS laterally
- MS mass lesion pushes PPS posteriorly
- PS mass lesion pushes PPS medially
- CS mass lesion pushes PPS anteriorly
- Lateral RPS mass (nodal) pushes PPS anterolaterally

The PPS is a crescent-shaped, fat-filled space extending in craniocaudal dimension from the skull base superiorly to the superior cornu of hyoid bone inferiorly. As paired, fatty tubes separating other SHN spaces from one another, the PPS serves as a corridor through which infection and tumor from these adjacent spaces can extend to other spaces both vertically and transversely.

The PPS has multiple important **anatomic relationships** with surrounding spaces. As there is no fascia separating the inferior PPS from the submandibular space (SMS), open communication between the PPS and posterior SMS exists. Since the PPS empties inferiorly into the SMS, PPS infection or malignancy spread inferiorly from the upper SHN to present as an angle of the mandible mass. Superiorly, the PPS interacts with the skull base in the bland triangular area on the inferior surface of the petrous apex. No exiting skull base foramina are found in this area of attachment. In the axial plane, the PMS is medial, the MS anterior, the PS lateral, the CS posterior, and the lateral RPS posteromedial to the PPS.

The PPS has limited internal contents aside from conspicuous **fat**. There are no mucosa, muscle, bone, nodes, or major salivary gland tissue within the PPS boundaries. **Minor salivary glands** can be found there but are considered ectopic and relatively rare. While most of the **pterygoid venous plexus** is found in the deep portion of the MS, a part of the plexus can extend to the PPS. The PPS contains no significant lymph nodes, and metastatic disease to PPS is highly unusual.

The **fascia** surrounding the PPS is complex. Different layers of the deep cervical fascia combine to circumscribe the PPS. The medial fascial margin of the PPS is made up of the middle layer of the deep cervical fascia as it curves around the lateral margin of PMS. The lateral fascial margin of the PPS is comprised of the medial slip of the superficial layer of deep cervical fascia along the deep border of the MS and PS. The posterior fascial margin of the PPS is formed by the deep layer of the deep cervical fascia on the anterolateral margin of the RPS and the anterior part of the carotid sheath (made up of components of all 3 layers of deep cervical fascia).

Approaches to Imaging Issues of Parapharyngeal Space

When you discover a lesion in the PPS on CT or MR, answer the following question first: "Is this lesion really primary to the PPS?" This question needs to be answered because there are so few things that actually originate from the PPS. In fact, the vast majority of lesions of the PPS arise in an adjacent space and spread secondarily into the PPS. To conclude that a lesion is primary to the PPS, it must be completely surrounded by PPS fat. In most cases in which a lesion is thought to be primary to the PPS, careful observation will find a connection to one of the surrounding spaces.

Lesions that are primary to the PPS itself include an atypical 2nd branchial cleft cyst and a pleomorphic adenoma and lipoma. All are rare. Far more common lesions can be seen spreading into the PPS, such as an abscess or invasive squamous cell carcinoma of the nasopharynx and oropharyngeal palatine tonsil. When a large primary parotid neoplasm of the deep lobe extends medially into the PPS, it may at first glance appear to be primary to the PPS. Careful inspection will reveal a connection to the deep lobe of the parotid in the vast majority of cases.

Differential Diagnosis

DDx of PPS lesion includes
- Congenital: Atypical 2nd branchial cleft cyst, lymphatic malformation, venous malformation
- Inflammatory: Large diving ranula spreading from SMS into PPS
- Infection: Spreading from PMS, MS, PS, or RPS; most commonly peritonsillar abscess from palatine tonsil (PMS) involves PPS
- Benign tumor: Lipoma, pleomorphic adenoma (from minor salivary gland rest in PPS)
- Malignant tumor: Spreading from PMS, MS, PS, or RPS into PPS; most commonly squamous cell carcinoma spreading from naso- or oropharynx (PMS) into PPS

Selected References

1. Rai P et al: Beyond the throat: imaging of parapharyngeal space lesions. Clin Radiol. 79(12):912-20, 2024
2. Faisal M et al: Neurological complications in benign parapharyngeal space tumors - systematic review and meta-analysis. Int Arch Otorhinolaryngol. 27(1):e158-65, 2023
3. Jiang C et al: Management of parapharyngeal space tumors: clinical experience with a large sample and review of the literature. Curr Oncol. 30(1):1020-31, 2023
4. Rigsby RK et al: Primary pathology of the parapharyngeal space. Clin Neuroradiol. 33(4):897-906, 2023
5. Limardo A et al: The development of a clinical algorithm for the diagnosis of tumours in the parapharyngeal space. A systematic review. Acta Otorrinolaringol Esp (Engl Ed). 73(3):141-50, 2022
6. Zidar N et al: Update from the 5th edition of the World Health Organization Classification of Head and Neck Tumors: Hypopharynx, Larynx, Trachea and Parapharyngeal Space. Head Neck Pathol. 16(1):31-9, 2022

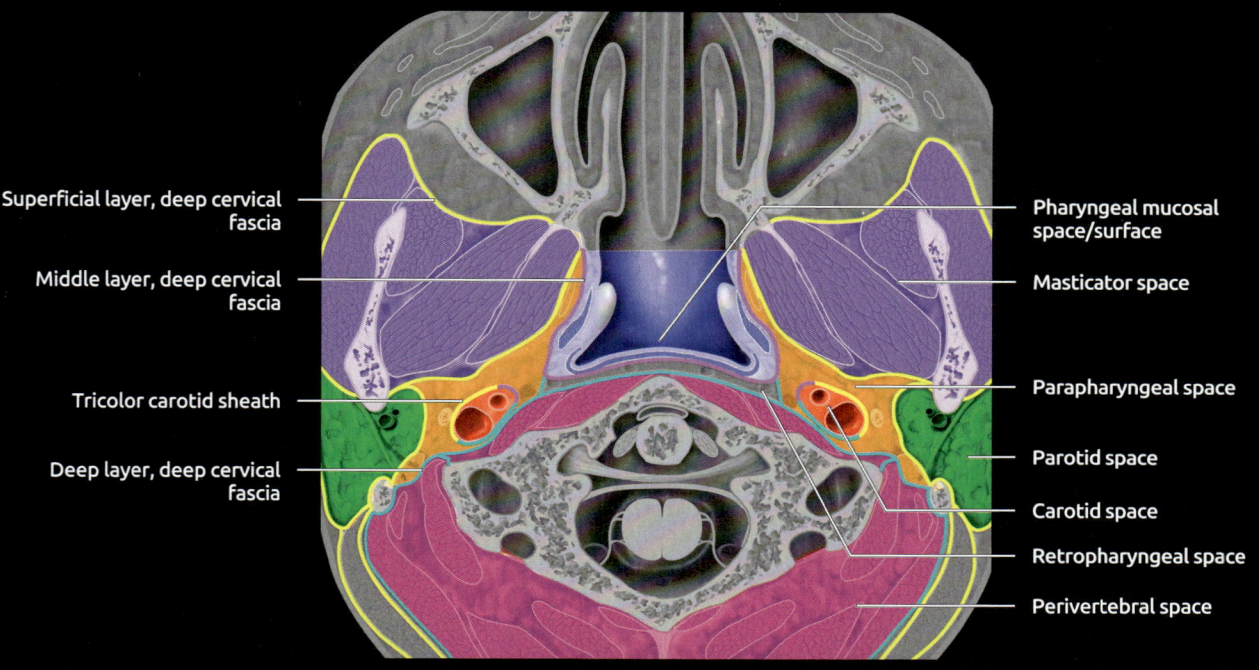

Superficial layer, deep cervical fascia

Middle layer, deep cervical fascia

Tricolor carotid sheath

Deep layer, deep cervical fascia

Pharyngeal mucosal space/surface

Masticator space

Parapharyngeal space

Parotid space

Carotid space

Retropharyngeal space

Perivertebral space

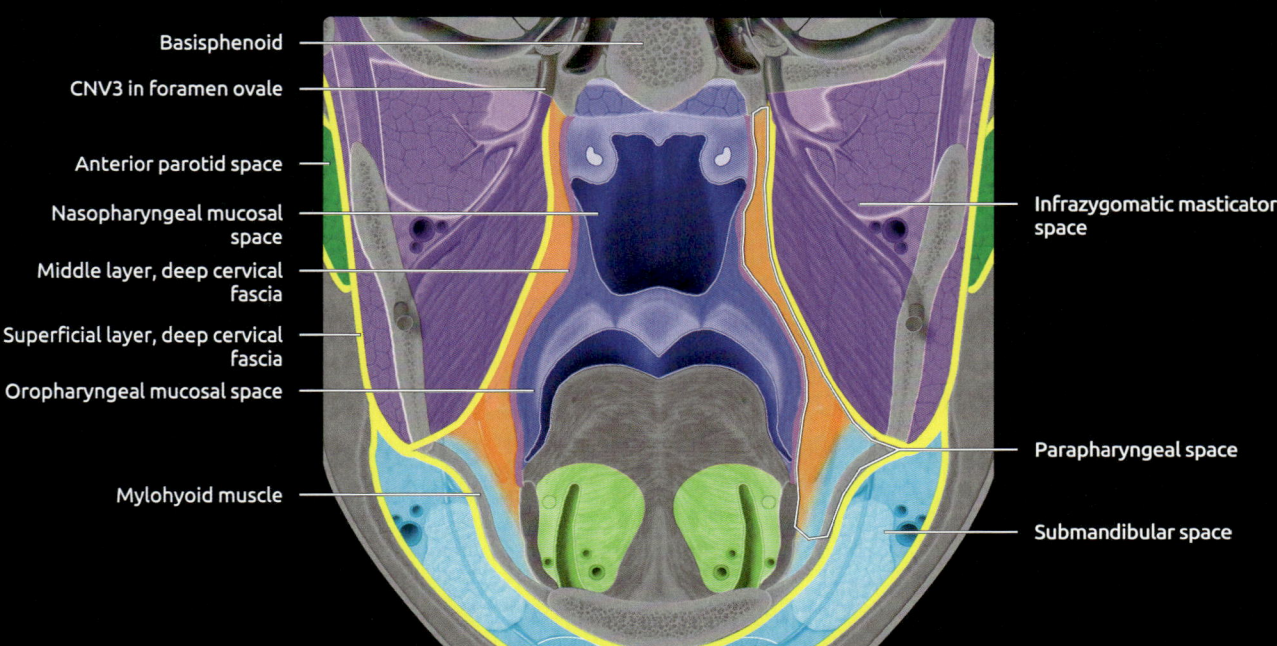

Basisphenoid

CNV3 in foramen ovale

Anterior parotid space

Nasopharyngeal mucosal space

Middle layer, deep cervical fascia

Superficial layer, deep cervical fascia

Oropharyngeal mucosal space

Mylohyoid muscle

Infrazygomatic masticator space

Parapharyngeal space

Submandibular space

(Top) *Axial graphic of the normal parapharyngeal space at the level of the nasopharynx demonstrates the complex fascial margins and the fat-only contents. Mass lesions originating in the surrounding pharyngeal mucosal, masticator, parotid, and carotid spaces can extend into the parapharyngeal space. The resulting displacement pattern of the parapharyngeal space may be helpful in defining the space of origin of a mass in the suprahyoid neck.* (Bottom) *Coronal graphic shows suprahyoid neck spaces as they interact with the skull base superiorly and submandibular space inferiorly. The parapharyngeal space interacts with no critical structures as it abuts the skull base. Inferiorly it empties into the posterior submandibular space along the posterior margin of the mylohyoid muscle. As a consequence of this anatomic arrangement, it is possible for an infection or a malignant tumor that breaks into the parapharyngeal space to present inferiorly as an angle of a mandible mass.*

Pleomorphic Adenoma, Parapharyngeal Space

TERMINOLOGY

- Synonyms: Benign mixed tumor

IMAGING

- Precontrast T1 MR without fat suppression best to identify fat-filled parapharyngeal space (PPS) and identify boundaries
- Rounded, well-defined lesion within PPS fat
  - Distinct from parotid deep lobe
- Rounded, well-defined lesion when small
- More lobulated when larger
- Marked T2 hyperintensity similar to CSF

TOP DIFFERENTIAL DIAGNOSES

- Pleomorphic adenoma, parotid deep lobe
- Neurogenic tumor, PPS
- Pterygoid venous plexus asymmetry
- 2nd branchial cleft cyst

PATHOLOGY

- Benign tumor arising in aberrant salivary gland rests
- Solid but often heterogeneous with hemorrhage, cystic degeneration, or necrosis
- Occasional ossific or calcific degeneration

CLINICAL ISSUES

- Most asymptomatic, or minimally so, because of deep location and slow growth
- Small lesion, usually incidental imaging finding
- Larger lesion may be found at dental/oral exam

DIAGNOSTIC CHECKLIST

- Primary PPS lesions are uncommon
- MR: T2 signal similar to CSF but solidly enhances
- Look for fat plane to distinguish from parotid deep lobe pleomorphic adenoma

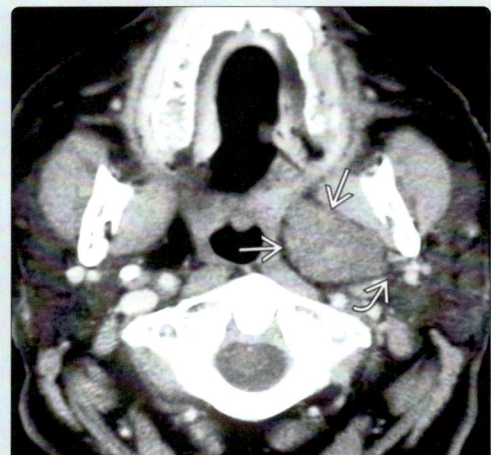
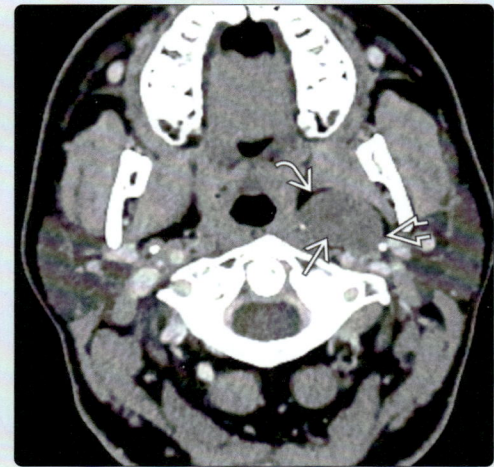

(Left) Axial CECT demonstrates a well-defined, slightly lobulated mass ⇗ within the left parapharyngeal space (PPS). The mass is completely surrounded by fat, separating it from the pharyngeal mucosal space medially, parotid deep lobe laterally ⇗, and carotid space posteriorly. (Right) Axial CECT at PPS level in a 30-year-old woman shows a well-circumscribed lesion ⇗ surrounded by PPS fat ⇗ with separation from the deep parotid lobe ⇒. Biopsy confirmed a pleomorphic adenoma.

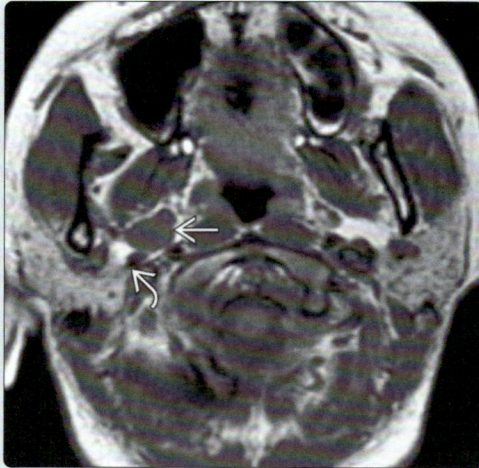
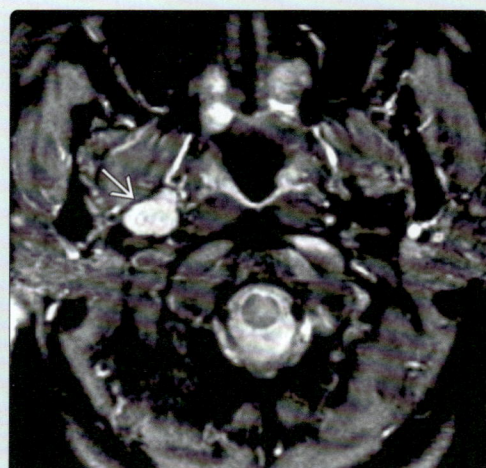

(Left) Axial T1WI MR reveals a well-defined mass within the right deep face ⇒, completely surrounded by parapharyngeal fat. Note the mass is distinct from the medial aspect of the right parotid deep lobe ⇒. (Right) Axial T2WI FS MR shows homogeneous hyperintensity of a slightly lobulated mass ⇒. Hyperintensity similar to CSF is typically seen with pleomorphic adenomas, although postcontrast images confirm it to be a solid mass.

TERMINOLOGY

Abbreviations

- Pleomorphic adenoma (PA), parapharyngeal space (PPS)

Synonyms

- Benign mixed tumor

Definitions

- Benign tumor arising from aberrant minor salivary gland rests in PPS

IMAGING

General Features

- Best diagnostic clue
  - Rounded, well-defined lesion within PPS fat
    - Distinct from parotid deep lobe
- Location
  - Within parapharyngeal fat of deep face
- Size
  - Variable: 1-8 cm
  - If large, often indistinguishable from deep parotid tumor
- Morphology
  - Rounded/ovoid, well-defined lesion when small
  - More lobulated with increasing size

Imaging Recommendations

- Best imaging tool
  - Readily seen on CT or MR; MR allows improved delineation from adjacent structures
    - Parotid deep lobe, internal carotid artery (ICA)
- Protocol advice
  - T1 MR best to delineate fat of PPS and identify boundaries

CT Findings

- CECT
  - Heterogeneous, well-defined lesion within PPS fat
  - Occasional focal ossification or calcification

MR Findings

- T1WI
  - Well-circumscribed, rounded/ovoid lesion within PPS fat
- T2WI FS
  - Marked hyperintensity due to myxoid stroma, can be similar to CSF in signal
- DWI
  - Higher ADC values reflect more myxoid stroma
    - Lesion ADC:normal parotid ADC ratio > 1.3 favors PA; < 1 indicates malignancy (Warthin tumor is exception, however)
- T1WI C+ FS
  - Heterogeneous enhancement, especially when large

DIFFERENTIAL DIAGNOSIS

Pleomorphic Adenoma, Parotid Deep Lobe

- Identical appearance but **within** parotid deep lobe

Pterygoid Venous Plexus Asymmetry

- Tubular enhancing structures in PPS or medial masticator space

Neurogenic Tumor, Parapharyngeal Space

- Well-defined, oval mass, intermediate T2
- Typically within carotid space (displacing ICA anteriorly) vs. PA, PPS ventral to styloid displacing ICA posteriorly

2nd Branchial Cleft Cyst

- Type IV branchial cleft cyst lies within PPS
- Cystic mass abutting lateral pharyngeal wall

PATHOLOGY

General Features

- Etiology
  - Benign tumor arising in aberrant salivary gland rests

Gross Pathologic & Surgical Features

- Solid but often heterogeneous with hemorrhage, cystic degeneration, or necrosis
- Occasional ossific or calcific degeneration

Microscopic Features

- As name implies, morphologically diverse
  - Epithelial and myoepithelial cells, mesenchymal or stromal elements

CLINICAL ISSUES

Presentation

- Most common signs/symptoms
  - Most asymptomatic with deep location and slow growth
    - Small lesion, usually incidental on imaging
    - Large lesion may be seen at dental/oral exam or may have painless oral swelling or dysphagia

Demographics

- Age
  - Adults; peak in 5th decade
- Sex
  - Slight female predominance

Natural History & Prognosis

- Slow growing; may be asymptomatic even when large
- Uncommonly degenerates to malignant mixed tumor (carcinoma ex PA)

Treatment

- Resection for definitive pathology or if symptomatic
- Operative tumor cell spillage may result in recurrence

DIAGNOSTIC CHECKLIST

Image Interpretation Pearls

- Primary PPS lesions are uncommon
  - Should be entirely surrounded by fat
- Look for fat at posterolateral margin to distinguish PA of PPS from parotid deep lobe lesion

SELECTED REFERENCES

1. Douami A et al: Pleomorphic adenoma of the parapharyngeal space. Radiol Case Rep. 20(3):1398-402, 2025
2. Rai P et al: Beyond the throat: imaging of parapharyngeal space lesions. Clin Radiol. 79(12):912-20, 2024
3. Jiang C et al: Management of parapharyngeal space tumors: clinical experience with a large sample and review of the literature. Curr Oncol. 30(1):1020-31, 2023

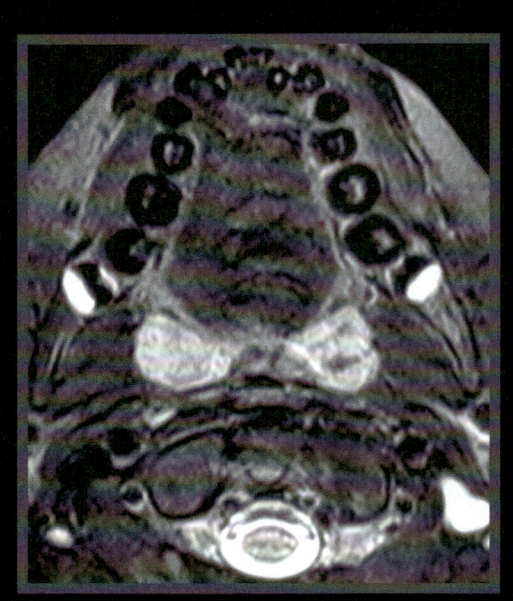

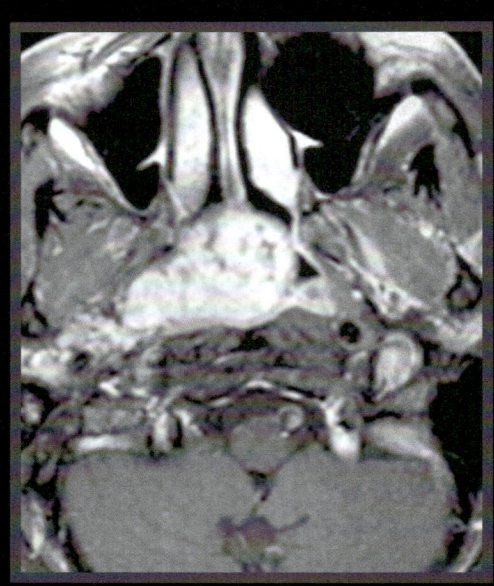

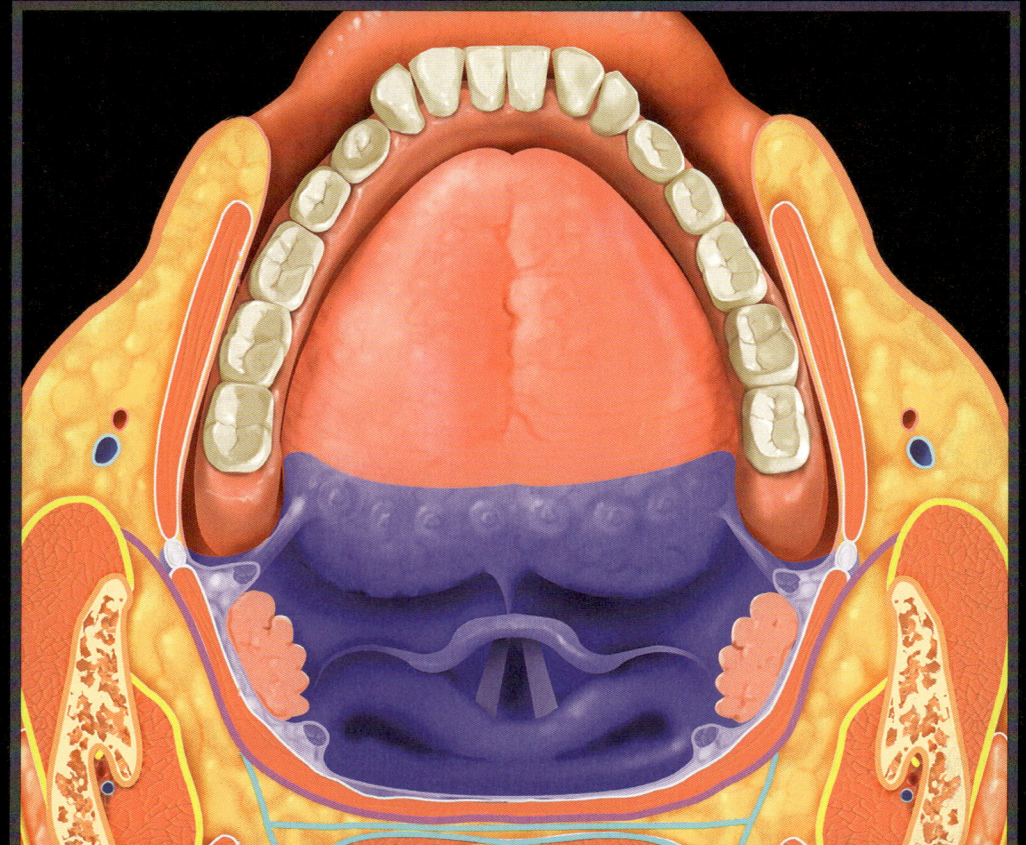

SECTION 3
Pharyngeal Mucosal Space

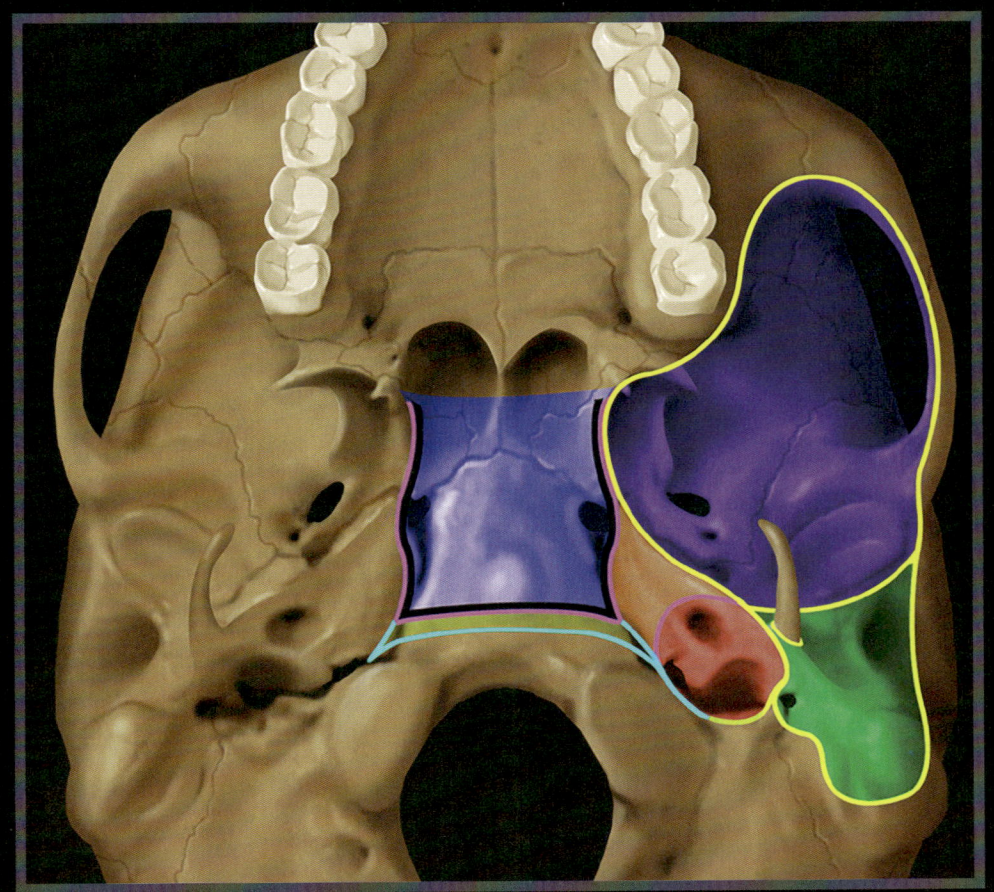

Summary Thoughts: Pharyngeal Mucosal Space

The pharyngeal mucosal space (PMS) is a key conceptual "space" that represents the mucosal surface and superficial elements of nasopharynx, oropharynx, and hypopharynx. Important PMS contents include the mucosa itself, lymphoepithelial tissue of Waldeyer ring, minor salivary glands, and the pharyngeal muscle layer.

An enlarging PMS mass of the palatine tonsil or nasopharyngeal lateral pharyngeal recess displaces the parapharyngeal space (PPS) fat laterally. Disruption of the mucosal and submucosal landmarks also occurs in PMS masses.

Important PMS malignancies include **squamous cell carcinoma (SCCa)** arising from the mucosal surface, **non-Hodgkin lymphoma (NHL)** from the pharyngeal lymphatic ring, and **minor salivary gland carcinoma**. Of these, SCCa is by far the most frequent and the most important. Staging of SCCa primary and nodal disease is one of the most common reasons for imaging studies in the head and neck.

The PMS is not a true space, as it is not enclosed on all sides by fascia. It is an imaging concept to overcome the problems encountered in describing a lesion of the pharynx as nasopharyngeal, oropharyngeal, and hypopharyngeal. These terms, although universally applied to lesions of the PMS surface, do not address the deep tissue component of an invasive PMS mass. Describing a lesion as primary to the PMS with extension into the adjacent suprahyoid neck spaces clearly delineates lesion extent in a radiologic report.

Imaging Techniques & Indications

CECT remains the workhorse for imaging lesions of PMS in a routine radiologic practice. On CECT, neoplasms may present as mucosal thickening or asymmetry, an exophytic mass, an invasive lesion that penetrates the mucosa and muscular layer to enter an adjacent space, or a combination of these findings. Enhanced fat-saturated multiplanar MR can exquisitely demonstrate tumor extent and is useful in some cases when dental amalgam artifact limits CECT or when finer detail is warranted, such as in the search for perineural tumor spread. CE-PET is advocated in some cases in which routine imaging is equivocal.

Imaging Anatomy

The **anatomic relationships** of the PMS and surrounding deep tissue anatomy are extremely important because both PMS malignancy and infection readily spread into these adjacent areas. Directly posterior to the PMS is the retropharyngeal space (RPS). The PPS is lateral to the PMS.

Superiorly, the **PMS** abuts the **skull base** along the roof and posterosuperior portion of the nasopharynx. This broad abutment with the skull base includes the posterior basisphenoid (sphenoid sinus floor) and the anterior basiocciput (anterior clival margin). The **foramen lacerum** [cartilaginous floor of the anteromedial petrous internal carotid artery (ICA) canal] is a key area of abutment of the PMS with the skull base. Nasopharyngeal carcinoma (NPCa) can invade the cartilage of the foramen lacerum and extend intracranially along the ICA and into the cavernous sinus.

The PMS extends from the roof of the nasopharynx above to the hypopharynx below as a continuous superficial sheet that includes the mucosa itself. The PMS mucosal space/surface is subdivided into **nasopharyngeal**, **oropharyngeal**, and **hypopharyngeal** components.

The PMS is a space with fascia on each deep margin but no superficial fascia. With no fascia on the surface of the PMS, it is not a true fascia-enclosed space. In fact, it represents a conceptual construct to complete the spatial map of the suprahyoid and infrahyoid neck. The PMS is often synonymous with the pharyngeal mucosa itself. However, remember that the pharyngeal mucosa is a microscopic layer that cannot be distinguished radiologically. In general, a soft tissue lesion of the mucosa identified on CT or MR is not readily distinguishable from the deeper muscle layer of the PMS. Therefore, in this imaging construct, the **PMS internal structures** include the mucosa, lymphatic ring (of Waldeyer), microscopic minor salivary glands, and the muscular layer.

The **middle layer of deep cervical fascia** (ML-DCF) defines the deep margin of the PMS. Just below the skull base, the ML-DCF encircles the lateral and posterior margins of the pharyngobasilar fascia that connects the superior constrictor muscle to the skull base. More inferiorly, the ML-DCF resides on the deep margin of the superior, middle, and inferior constrictor muscles.

The pharyngeal lymphatic ring is divided into 3 components: The nasopharyngeal **adenoids** and the oropharyngeal **palatine** and **lingual tonsils** (base of tongue). The lymphatic tissue normally declines in volume with age. Microscopic minor salivary glands are found in the submucosa and lamina propria throughout the PMS with the highest concentrations found in the tongue base and palate.

The nasopharyngeal mucosal space also contains the superior constrictor muscle and the **pharyngobasilar fascia**. Along the posterosuperior margin of the pharyngobasilar fascia, there is a notch referred to as the **sinus of Morgagni**. The levator palatini muscle and the distal eustachian tube (torus tubarius) project into the PMS through this notch. NPCa may escape the PMS through this notch.

Approaches to Imaging Issues of Pharyngeal Mucosal Space

The answer to the question, "**What imaging findings define a PMS mass**?" depends on the area of the PMS where the mass originates. The most common PMS mass arises in the lateral pharyngeal recess of the nasopharynx or in the palatine tonsil of the oropharynx. As such, it is medial to the PPS, displacing the PPS fat laterally as it enlarges. A PMS mass of the lingual tonsil projects into the posterior sublingual space of the tongue as it enlarges. The rare posterior nasopharyngeal or oropharyngeal wall mass pushes posteriorly into the RPS as it grows. No matter where in the PMS a mass grows, disruption of the mucosal and submucosal architecture occurs. In addition, the growing airway side of the mass projects out into the adjacent PMS airway.

Traditionally, the pharynx is divided into the nasopharynx, oropharynx, and hypopharynx as a method to describe where on this continuous sheet of mucosa a lesion is found. This **surface of the pharynx** is referred to here as the **PMS**. To unify these 2 terminologies, it is possible to refer to the nasopharyngeal, oropharyngeal, or hypopharyngeal mucosal space. It is not helpful to merely refer to a tumor as either in the oropharynx or found in the oropharyngeal mucosal space. The radiologist must also describe what other deep facial spaces are involved by a PMS tumor. This requires bringing the

Differential Diagnosis of Pharyngeal Mucosal Space

Pseudolesions	Malignant tumor
Asymmetric lateral pharyngeal recess	Nasopharyngeal carcinoma
Fluid in lateral pharyngeal recess	Oropharyngeal squamous cell carcinoma
Asymmetric tonsillar tissue	Palatine tonsil squamous cell carcinoma
Inflammatory lesions	Lingual tonsil squamous cell carcinoma
Mucosal inflammation (pharyngitis, post radiation)	Non-Hodgkin lymphoma
Tonsillar lymphoid hyperplasia	Minor salivary gland carcinoma
Retention cyst	Rhabdomyosarcoma
Postinflammatory dystrophic calcifications	Extraosseous chordoma
Tonsillar inflammation	**Miscellaneous**
Infectious lesions	Tornwaldt cyst
Tonsillar/peritonsillar abscess	Patulous lateral pharyngeal recess + palate atrophy
Benign tumor	In proximal vagal neuropathy
Pleomorphic adenoma, minor salivary gland	

other deep facial spaces affected into the radiologic report, including the PPS, masticator space (MS), parotid space (PS), carotid space (CS), RPS, and perivertebral space (PVS).

When the PMS lesion is identified on CT or MR, there are a limited number of common diseases to consider. If the patient is imaged to evaluate for possible infection, 3 lesions may be identified. **Tonsillar lymphoid hyperplasia** is commonly found in children and young adults, resulting from multiple bouts of tonsillar inflammation. **Tonsillar inflammation** is suggested when enhancing, enlarged tonsils possess "stripes." **Tonsillar abscess** is diagnosed when focal rim-enhancing pus collections are seen. If the abscess has ruptured from the tonsil into the adjacent PPS, RPS, or MS, the term **peritonsillar abscess** may be used.

If the PMS lesion lacks a clinical infectious context but has invasive imaging features, a limited group of **malignant tumors** must be considered. SCCa is by far the most common malignancy of the PMS with NHL next in frequency, followed by minor salivary gland carcinoma. These neoplasms arise from the normal structures found within the PMS.

- Mucosa → **SCCa**
- Pharyngeal lymphatic ring → **NHL**
- Minor salivary glands → **minor salivary gland carcinoma**

The most common **interpretation pitfall** associated with the PMS occurs when the radiologist overcalls large adenoidal tonsillar tissue as a tumor. Recurrent tonsillar inflammation in the young may lead to disturbingly prominent, often asymmetric tonsillar hyperplasia on CT or MR. If the prominent lymphatic tissue in the PMS has no invasive deep margins, demonstrates inflammatory septa, and is found in a patient under 20 years of age, lymphoid hyperplasia is the most likely explanation.

A second common interpretation pitfall occurs when the lateral pharyngeal recess is asymmetric either because of retained secretions, retention cysts, or unevenly distributed adenoidal tissue. Suggesting NPCa in this setting creates great patient and physician consternation. Suggesting normal asymmetry and recommending clinical inspection usually suffice to clear the nasopharynx of significant pathology.

Clinical Implications

Remember that the referring clinician can usually directly visualize a lesion of the PMS. Lesions of the lateral pharyngeal recess of the nasopharynx may be the exception to this rule. In the case of SCCa, the appearance of the mucosal lesion is often diagnostic. Knowing what the physical examination of the pharynx shows at the time of rendering your radiologic report allows for a richly detailed and highly relevant interpretation.

If the requisition requests a staging CT or MR of an **SCCa of the PMS**, the report should comment on both the **primary tumor (T) and nodal (N) stage**. The 9th edition of AJCC/UICC TNM staging manual defining the T and N stages of each of the subsites of the pharynx is an important reference for the radiologist doing this type of work. Familiarity with the routes of spread of SCCa of the PMS by primary site and subsite also permit directed radiologic reports to be rendered.

NPCa, because of its proximity to the skull base, spreads early into the intracranial compartment. The ML-DCF and the pharyngobasilar fascia direct NPCa superiorly, where it will invade directly into the upper clivus, floor of the sphenoid sinuses, and the foramen lacerum. When the tumor invades through the foramen lacerum, it accesses the anteromedial ICA. **Perivascular spread** takes it into the cavernous sinus from there. The proximity of the nasopharyngeal CS to lateral pharyngeal recess NPCa makes early invasion of the ICA and cranial nerves IX-XII likely.

Selected References

1. Nguyen VTN et al: Tonsillitis. Prim Care. 52(1):27-35, 2025
2. Sanders O et al: Hypopharyngeal cancer. StatPearls, 2025
3. Chen Y et al: The role of PTEN in nasopharyngeal carcinoma. Front Biosci (Landmark Ed). 29(5):179, 2024
4. Chowaniec H et al: New hopes for the breast cancer treatment: perspectives on the oncolytic virus therapy. Front Immunol. 15:1375433, 2024
5. Rondi P et al: Magnetic resonance imaging after nasopharyngeal endoscopic resection and skull base reconstruction. J Clin Med. 13(9):2624, 2024
6. Abdel Razek AAK et al: MR imaging of oral cavity and oropharyngeal cancer. Magn Reson Imaging Clin N Am. 30(1):35-51, 2022
7. Akgoz Karaosmanoglu A et al: Anatomy of the pharynx and cervical esophagus. Neuroimaging Clin N Am. 32(4):791-807, 2022

Pharyngeal Mucosal Space Overview

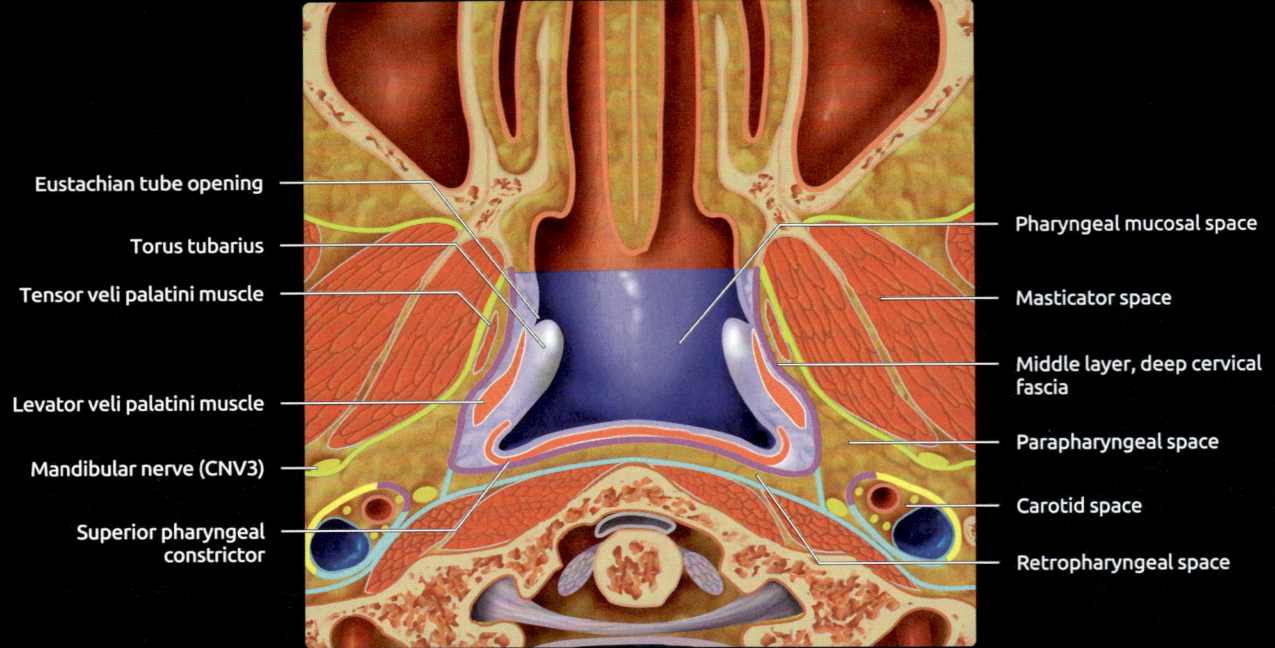

Eustachian tube opening

Torus tubarius

Tensor veli palatini muscle

Levator veli palatini muscle

Mandibular nerve (CNV3)

Superior pharyngeal constrictor

Pharyngeal mucosal space

Masticator space

Middle layer, deep cervical fascia

Parapharyngeal space

Carotid space

Retropharyngeal space

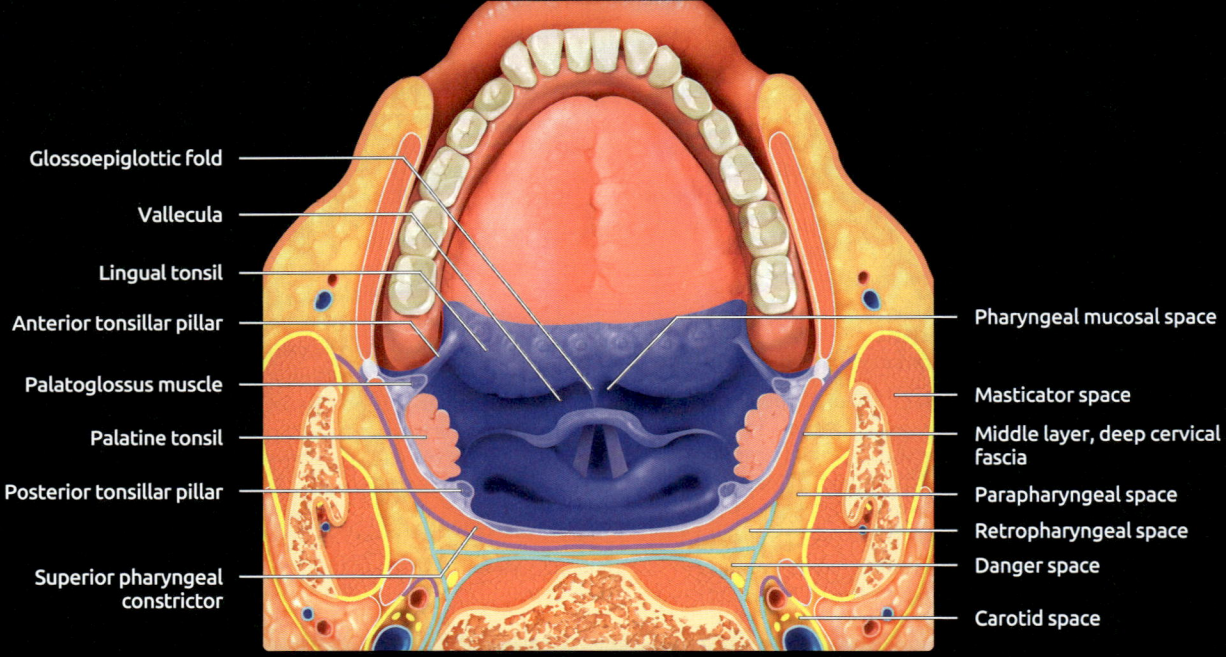

Glossoepiglottic fold

Vallecula

Lingual tonsil

Anterior tonsillar pillar

Palatoglossus muscle

Palatine tonsil

Posterior tonsillar pillar

Superior pharyngeal constrictor

Pharyngeal mucosal space

Masticator space

Middle layer, deep cervical fascia

Parapharyngeal space

Retropharyngeal space

Danger space

Carotid space

(Top) *Axial graphic of the nasopharyngeal mucosal space (in blue) shows that the superior pharyngeal constrictor, levator veli palatini muscles, and the cartilaginous eustachian tube ending (torus tubarius) are within the space. The levator veli palatini and eustachian tube access the pharyngeal mucosal space (PMS) via the sinus of Morgagni in the upper margin of the pharyngobasilar fascia. The middle layer of deep cervical fascia provides a deep margin to the space. The retropharyngeal space is behind and the parapharyngeal space is lateral to the PMS.* **(Bottom)** *Axial graphic of the oropharyngeal mucosal space (in blue) viewed from above reveals that the superior pharyngeal constrictor and the tonsillar pillars along with the palatine and lingual tonsils are all occupants of this space. The middle layer of deep cervical fascia provides a deep margin to the space. The retropharyngeal space is behind, and the parapharyngeal space is lateral to the PMS.*

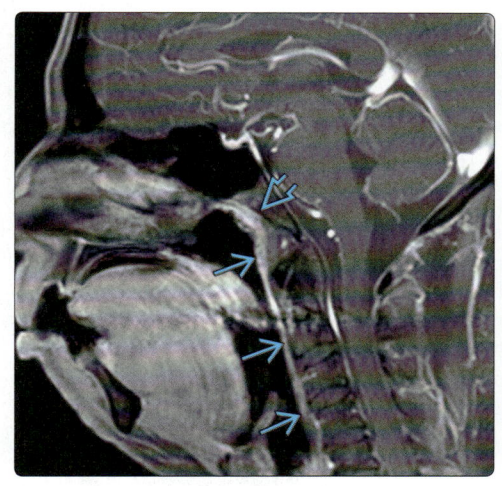

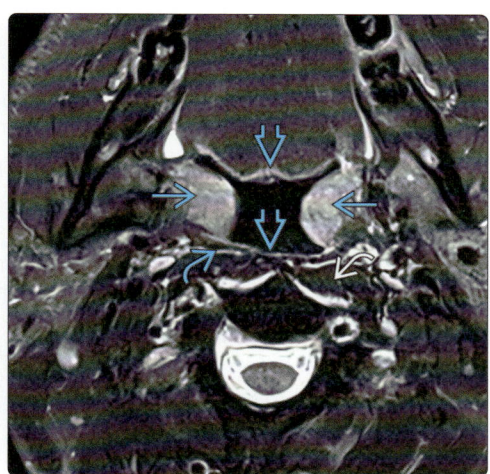

(Left) Sagittal T1 C+ FS MR through the midline of the pharynx shows enhancing mucosa ➡ of the PMS. Note the close relation of the posterosuperior wall of the nasopharynx with the skull base ➡. (Right) Axial T2 FS MR through the oropharynx shows mildly prominent bilateral palatine tonsils ➡ and a thin line of mucosal hyperintensity over the base of the tongue and the posterior wall of the oropharynx ➡. Note immediate posterior relation to the retropharyngeal space ➡ and perivertebral space ➡.

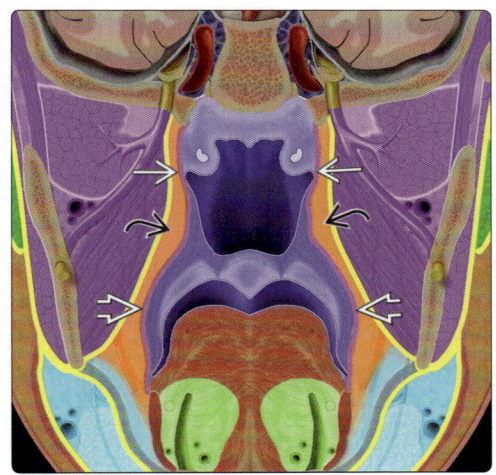

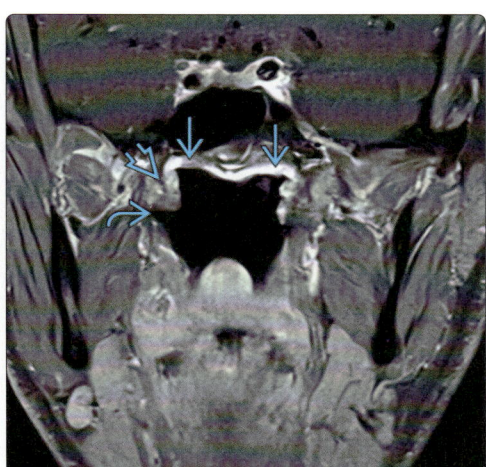

(Left) Coronal graphic shows nasopharyngeal and oropharyngeal mucosal space. Note the middle layer of deep cervical fascia defining the lateral margin of the nasopharyngeal PMS ➡ and the oropharyngeal PMS ➡. The parapharyngeal spaces are paired fatty spaces ➡ lateral to the PMS. (Right) Coronal T1 C+ FS MR through the nasopharynx shows enhancing mucosa lining the nasopharynx ➡. Also note the torus tubarius ➡ and lateral pharyngeal recess ➡.

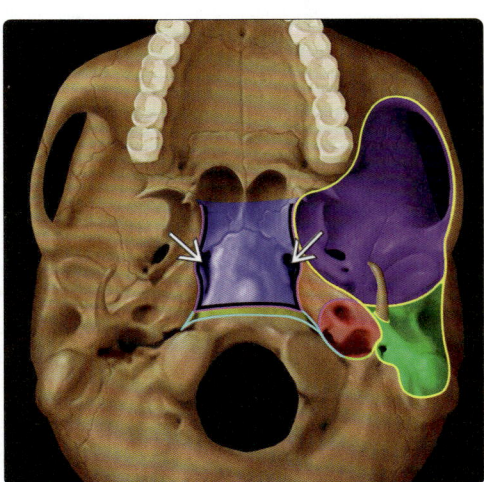

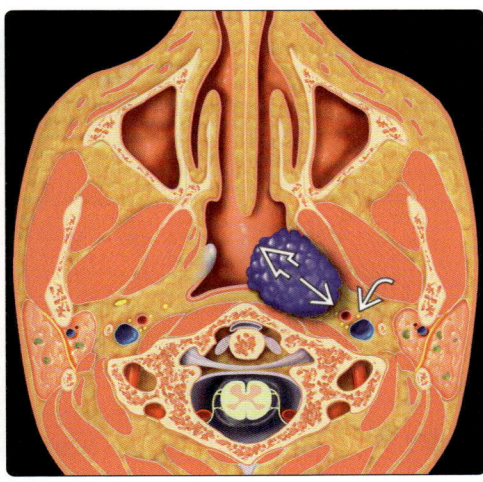

(Left) Skull base graphic viewed from below highlights the area of PMS abutment (blue). Note that the posterior basisphenoid and clival basiocciput both are involved. Foramen lacerum ➡ are both within abutment area. (Right) Axial graphic through the nasopharynx depicts a generic PMS mass. The lesion projects into the nasopharyngeal airway ➡ and pushes from medial to lateral on the adjacent parapharyngeal space ➡. Notice the close proximity of the nasopharyngeal carotid space ➡ with CNIX-XII.

KEY FACTS

TERMINOLOGY

- Tornwaldt cyst (TC): Benign developmental midline nasopharyngeal cyst in pharyngeal mucosal space (PMS) **deep to pharyngobasilar fascia**; covered by mucosa anteriorly & bounded by longus muscles posteriorly

IMAGING

- Ovoid, cystic mass in midline nasopharynx
- MR findings
  - T1: Intermediate to high signal depending on cyst fluid protein concentration
  - T2: Homogeneously high signal with no deep extension into surrounding structures
    - Low signal if contains highly proteinaceous fluid
  - T1 C+: May have minimal enhancement of cyst wall

TOP DIFFERENTIAL DIAGNOSES

- Adenoidal hyperplasia
- PMS retention cyst

- PMS pleomorphic adenoma
- Nasopharyngeal carcinoma

PATHOLOGY

- **Notochordal remnant** where embryologic notochord & endoderm of primitive pharynx come into contact

CLINICAL ISSUES

- Usually asymptomatic & incidental
  - Seen on **5%** of routine brain MR
- Most common symptoms: Postnasal discharge, occipital headache, halitosis
- Most common lesion of nasopharyngeal mucosal space occurring in 4% at autopsy
- Rarely, chronically infected large cyst (> 2 cm) causes periodic halitosis & unpleasant taste in mouth

DIAGNOSTIC CHECKLIST

- If solid components or invasion into prevertebral muscles, think of significant lesions like nasopharyngeal carcinoma

(Left) Sagittal T1WI MR shows an incidental medium-sized Tornwaldt cyst ➡. The cyst is slightly hyperintense due to increased protein content. Subtle internal septation ⇒ is present. (Right) Axial T2WI MR shows a small, ovoid, T2-hyperintense midline nasopharyngeal Tornwaldt cyst ➡. A tiny T2-hypointense left lateral pharyngeal recess (fossa of Rosenmüller) lesion ↗ is also seen, which was hypointense on T1WI MR also (not shown), suggestive of a highly proteinaceous pharyngeal mucosal space retention cyst here.

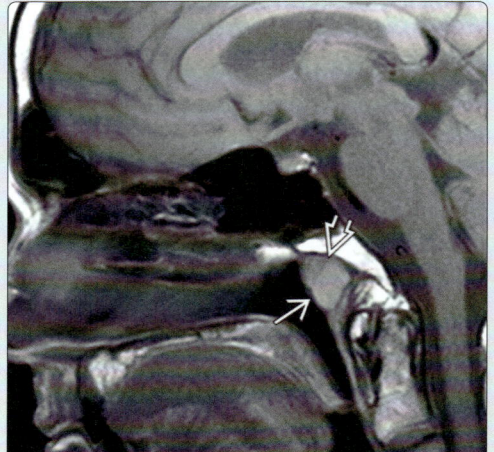
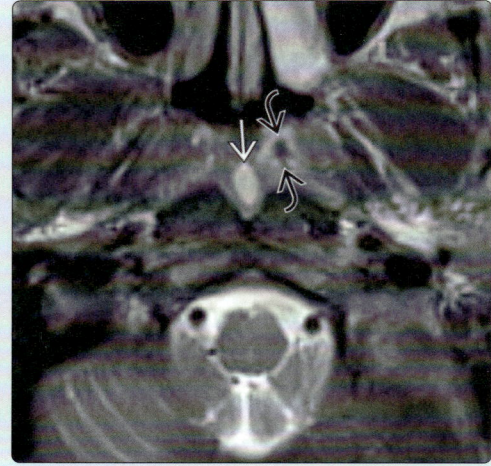

(Left) Axial T2WI MR reveals a Tornwaldt cyst in the midline nasopharyngeal mucosal space that is hypointense on T2WI ➡ and hyperintense on T1WI (not shown) due to proteinaceous contents. When water content is higher, Tornwaldt cysts show high signal on T2WI and low signal on T1WI. These are congenital midline cysts originating deep to pharyngobasilar fascia. (Right) Axial T1WI C+ FS MR demonstrates a classic small nonenhancing Tornwaldt cyst ➡. The mucosal surface enhances ⇒ and is seen as a thin white line.

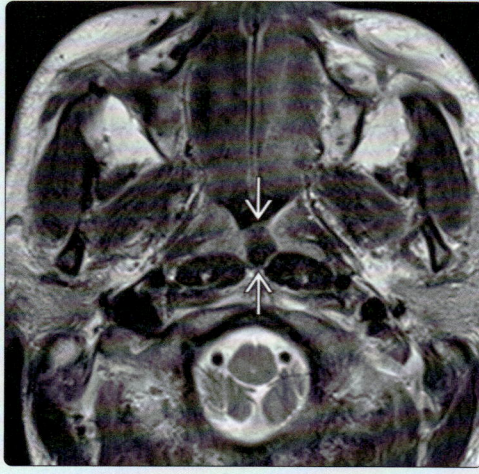
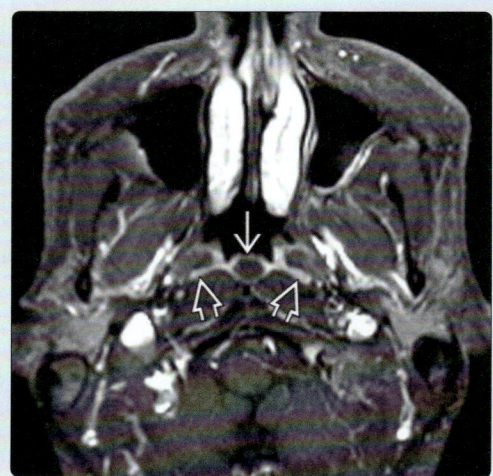

TERMINOLOGY

Abbreviations
- Tornwaldt cyst (TC)

Synonyms
- Nasopharyngeal (NP) bursa, Thornwaldt cyst

Definitions
- Benign developmental NP midline cyst covered by mucosa anteriorly & bounded by longus muscles posteriorly
- TC originates **deep to pharyngobasilar fascia**

IMAGING

General Features
- Best diagnostic clue
  - Midline, well-circumscribed pharyngeal mucosal space (PMS) cyst on posterior NP wall between prevertebral muscles
- Size
  - TC ranges from few millimeters to 2-3 cm in diameter
- Morphology
  - Round or ovoid cyst

CT Findings
- NECT
  - Midline, low-density cyst on posterior NP wall
- CECT
  - Only rim of cyst may enhance; TC remains low density

MR Findings
- T1WI
  - TC intermediate to high signal depending on cyst fluid protein concentration
- T2WI
  - Homogeneously high-intensity NP cyst **without** deep extension into surrounding structures
  - Lower T2 signal possible with high protein content
- T1WI C+
  - May have minimal enhancement of cyst wall

DIFFERENTIAL DIAGNOSIS

Adenoidal Hyperplasia
- ↑ T2, diffuse soft tissue filling NP PMS

Pharyngeal Mucosal Space Retention Cyst
- Often multiple lateral pharyngeal recess (fossa of Rosenmüller) or paramidline NP cysts
- Postinflammatory cyst, originates **superficial to pharyngobasilar fascia**

Pharyngeal Mucosal Space Pleomorphic Adenoma
- Rare, well-circumscribed enhancing submucosal mass

Nasopharyngeal Carcinoma
- Invasive NP mucosal space mass
- T2 intermediate signal
- T1 C+ diffuse enhancement except in necrotic portions

Intraadenoid Cysts
- Cause of midline acquired NP cysts

PATHOLOGY

General Features
- Embryology
  - **Notochordal remnant** where embryologic notochord & endoderm of primitive pharynx come into contact
  - If adhesion occurs at point of contact, small midline diverticulum lined by pharyngeal mucosa is formed as notochord ascends into clivus

Gross Pathologic & Surgical Features
- Smooth, translucent cyst if uninfected
- Thick-walled if prior infection
- Rarely associated with median basal canal

Microscopic Features
- Cyst lining: Respiratory epithelium, little or no lymphoid tissue is seen in cyst wall
- Cyst fluid: Usually with high protein concentration

CLINICAL ISSUES

Presentation
- Most common signs/symptoms
  - Rarely symptomatic, usually no clinical significance
  - Postnasal discharge, occipital headache, halitosis
- Rarely eustachian tube dysfunction with middle ear effusion & hearing loss in large cysts
- Tornwaldt syndrome (rare)
  - Chronically infected large cyst (> 2 cm)
  - Causes periodic halitosis, unpleasant taste
- Extremely rare case of clival osteomyelitis secondary to TC infection in child reported

Demographics
- Epidemiology
  - Most common lesion of NP mucosal space, occurring in 4% at autopsy
  - Seen on ~ **5%** of routine brain MR

Treatment
- Asymptomatic cysts require no treatment
- Chronically infected, painful lesions treated with endoscopic marsupialization

DIAGNOSTIC CHECKLIST

Consider
- TC if **high signal** intensity **midline** NP cyst on T2 MR

Image Interpretation Pearls
- TC on routine brain MR, of **no** clinical significance

Reporting Tips
- If solid components or invasion into prevertebral muscles, think of significant lesions similar to NP carcinoma

SELECTED REFERENCES

1. Konsulov S et al: Symptomatic Tornwaldt cyst: a case report. Cureus. 16(4):e58796, 2024
2. Turan Ş et al: Is transnasal endoscopic marsupialization sufficient in Thornwaldt cysts? J Craniofac Surg. 31(2):e208-10, 2020
3. Benadjaoud Y et al: A case of acute clival osteomyelitis in a 7-year-old boy secondary to infection of a Thornwaldt cyst. Int J Pediatr Otorhinolaryngol. 95:87-90, 2017

Retention Cyst of Pharyngeal Mucosal Space

Pharyngeal Mucosal Space

KEY FACTS

TERMINOLOGY

- Retention cyst (RC) of pharyngeal mucosal space (PMS)
- Postinflammatory cyst: Includes nasopharyngeal RC, tonsillar RC, vallecular cyst
- RC: Benign, asymptomatic PMS cyst

IMAGING

- RC of PMS in nasopharynx or oropharynx
  - Usually < 1 cm
  - Smooth, well circumscribed, round or ovoid
  - **Pear-shaped** when in **lateral pharyngeal recess nasopharynx**
  - Discrete plane between cyst & underlying constrictor muscles; originates superficial to pharyngobasilar fascia
- Simple cyst in PMS on CT or MR
  - T1 MR: Iso to hypointense, may be hyperintense if proteinaceous
  - T2 MR: Homogeneously hyperintense mucosal cyst
    - Low signal if contains highly proteinaceous fluid
  - CT or MR: No significant enhancement in wall

TOP DIFFERENTIAL DIAGNOSES

- Tornwaldt cyst
- Lateral nasopharyngeal branchial cyst
- Thyroglossal duct cyst at foramen cecum
- PMS pleomorphic adenoma

PATHOLOGY

- Epithelial-lined cyst filled with serous fluid

CLINICAL ISSUES

- Incidental PMS lesion usually found on lowest images of routine brain MR
- Common **incidental lesion** found on brain or C-spine MR
- Cyst in lateral pharyngeal recess may rarely obstruct eustachian tube with middle ear-mastoid fluid

DIAGNOSTIC CHECKLIST

- Recognize PMS RC as benign "leave alone" lesion

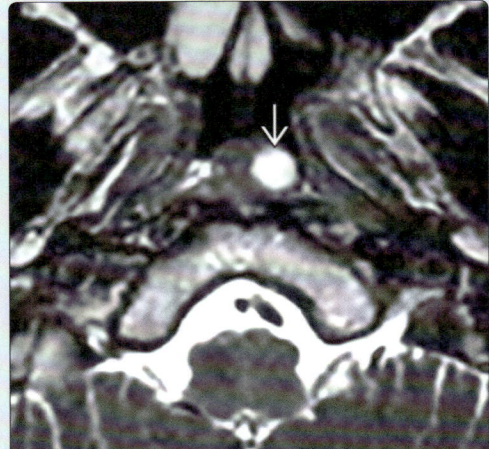 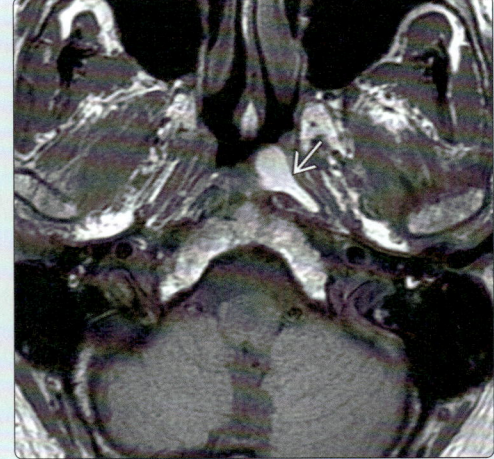

(Left) *Axial 3D T2 CUBE MR shows a left parasagittal nasopharyngeal retention cyst (NRC)* ➡. (Right) *Axial T1 MR shows the characteristic pear-shaped NRC* ➡ *in the left lateral nasopharyngeal recess (fossa of Rosenmüller). Note high T1 signal within the cyst, suggesting proteinaceous contents or, rarely, blood products. NRCs originate superficial to pharyngobasilar fascia, whereas midline Tornwaldt cysts & lateral nasopharyngeal branchial cysts originate deep to the pharyngobasilar fascia.*

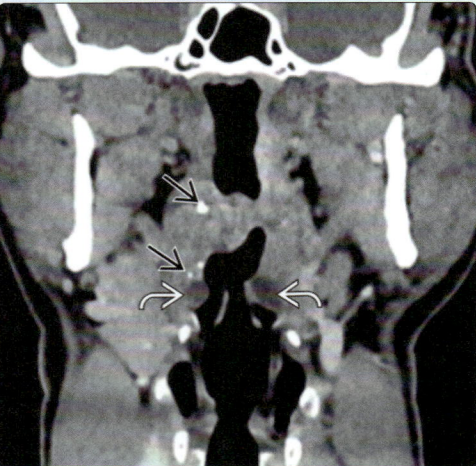 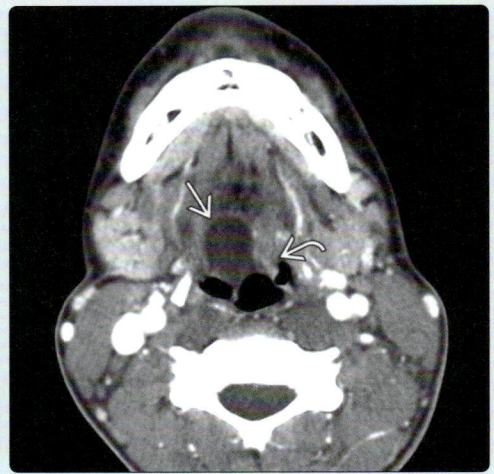

(Left) *Coronal reformatted CECT shows bilateral, bulky palatine tonsils with small RCs at their lower poles* ➡. *Note multiple right tonsilloliths* ➡. (Right) *Axial CECT at the base of tongue in an adult reveals a right vallecular RC* ➡. *The left vallecula is partially filled with enhancing lingual tonsil* ➡. *A foramen cecum thyroglossal duct cyst would be more midline & not fill the vallecula. Obstructed & dilated lingual tonsillar crypt or duct of a mucous gland in adjacent epiglottis or base of tongue gives rise to vallecular cyst.*

24

TERMINOLOGY

Abbreviations
- Retention cyst (RC), pharyngeal mucosal space (PMS)

Definitions
- RC: Benign, asymptomatic PMS postinflammatory cyst
  - Includes nasopharyngeal RC (NRC), tonsillar RC, vallecular RC

IMAGING

General Features
- Best diagnostic clue
  - Simple cyst in PMS on CT or MR
- Location
  - Usually on posterior wall of PMS in nasopharynx or oropharynx
  - Lateral nasopharyngeal recess (fossa of Rosenmüller) common but can occur anywhere on PMS surface, including midline
- Size
  - Usually < 1 cm
  - Occasionally very large; > 1 cm
- Morphology
  - Smooth, well circumscribed, round or ovoid
    - **Pear-shaped** when in **lateral recess of nasopharynx**
  - Usually unilocular but occasionally multiple or septated

CT Findings
- NECT
  - Low-density PMS cyst with no deep extension
- CECT
  - No significant enhancement in cyst wall

MR Findings
- T1WI
  - Difficult to detect when fluid-filled & iso- to hypointense to muscle
  - Hyperintense to muscle if proteinaceous contents
- T2WI
  - Homogeneously hyperintense, superficial mucosal cyst
  - Low signal if contains highly proteinaceous fluid
  - Discrete plane between cyst & underlying constrictor muscles when on posterior wall
- T1WI C+
  - No significant enhancement in wall

Imaging Recommendations
- Best imaging tool
  - T2 MR of PMS best displays RC
- Protocol advice
  - T2 axial & coronal MR images make RC diagnosis straightforward

DIFFERENTIAL DIAGNOSIS

Tornwaldt Cyst
- Benign, embryologic notochordal remnant at midline of posterior nasopharyngeal wall
- Originate deep to pharyngobasilar fascia, whereas NRCs originate superficial to it

Lateral Nasopharyngeal Branchial Cyst
- Originate deep to pharyngobasilar fascia, whereas NRCs originate superficial to it
- Lymphoid aggregation may be seen in subepithelial connective tissue

Thyroglossal Duct Cyst, Foramen Cecum
- Benign embryologic remnant cyst of thyroglossal duct occurring at foramen cecum

Pleomorphic adenoma, Pharyngeal Mucosal Space
- Solid, homogeneously enhancing PMS lesion

Oncocytic Cyst (Warthin Tumor)
- Rare cause of acquired lateral nasopharyngeal cysts

PATHOLOGY

General Features
- Etiology
  - Postinflammatory in origin

Gross Pathologic & Surgical Features
- Soft, discrete, mucous RC lying on mucosal surface of nasopharynx or oropharynx
- Vallecular cysts (epiglottic mucous RCs or base of tongue cysts): Obstructed & dilated lingual tonsillar crypt or mucous gland duct in epiglottis or base of tongue
- Congenital vallecular cyst: Unilocular cyst arising from lingual surface of epiglottis
  - Ductal type of laryngeal cyst due to fluid accumulation secondary to obstructed submucosal glands

Microscopic Features
- Epithelial-lined cyst filled with serous fluid
- May contain proteinaceous fluid or, rarely, old blood

CLINICAL ISSUES

Presentation
- Most common signs/symptoms
  - **Incidental PMS lesion** usually found on lowest images of routine brain MR
  - Cyst in lateral pharyngeal recess may obstruct eustachian tube with middle ear-mastoid fluid
  - Rare large cyst may present with dysphagia
  - Vallecular cysts may present with unanticipated difficulty during intubation in adults or may cause stridor or life-threatening upper airway obstruction in infants
  - Rarely, cysts may get infected

Treatment
- Rarely, large, symptomatic cysts may be surgically excised

DIAGNOSTIC CHECKLIST

Image Interpretation Pearls
- Recognize PMS RC as benign "leave alone" lesion

SELECTED REFERENCES

1. Tomita K et al: Neck point-of-care ultrasound for the identification of tongue-base cysts in infants with stridor: a case series. Pediatr Emerg Care. 40(11):825-7, 2024

Pharyngeal Mucosal Space

TERMINOLOGY

- Synonyms
  - Tonsillitis/tonsillopharyngitis
  - Tonsillar/peritonsillar phlegmon
  - Tonsillar/peritonsillar cellulitis
- Definition: Acute, nonsuppurative tonsillar inflammation

IMAGING

- Bilateral > unilateral tonsillar enlargement with variable attenuation/intensity/enhancement
- CECT to distinguish acute tonsillitis from tonsillar/peritonsillar abscess (TA/PTA)
  - Well-formed capsule and homogeneous internal hypodensity in TA/PTA
- **Striated pattern** of internal enhancement (tiger stripe sign) relatively specific for **nonsuppurative tonsillitis**
- Reactive adenopathy common
- If associated marked enlargement adenoid tonsils and cervical nodes, think infectious mononucleosis

TOP DIFFERENTIAL DIAGNOSES

- Tonsillar/peritonsillar abscess
- Tonsillar hyperplasia (hypertrophy)
- Palatine tonsil squamous cell carcinoma
- Pharyngeal mucosal space non-Hodgkin lymphoma

PATHOLOGY

- Most commonly secondary to respiratory virus
- 30-40% bacterial: Group A β-hemolytic streptococci most common

CLINICAL ISSUES

- Children and young adults
- Large tonsils with 50-100% obstruction of oropharynx can make it difficult to breathe

DIAGNOSTIC CHECKLIST

- Striated pattern of internal enhancement, absence of well-defined capsule help rule out TA/PTA

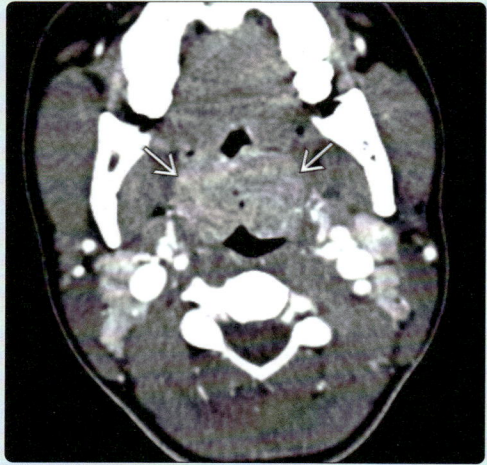
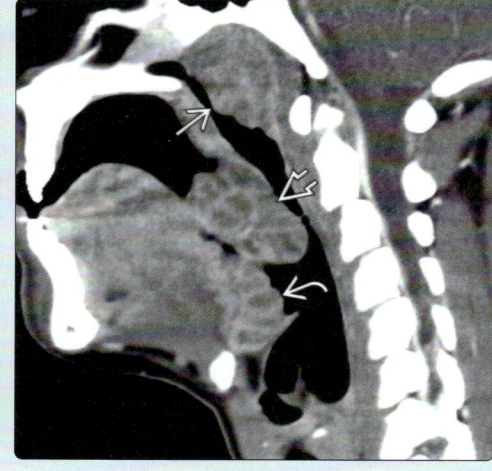

(Left) *Axial CECT in a teenager with sore throat and concern for deep neck infection shows bilateral enlargement of the palatine tonsils, each with striated enhancement ➜ typical of uncomplicated tonsillitis.* (Right) *Sagittal CECT in a teenager shows heterogeneous, striated enhancement in markedly enlarged adenoid tonsils ➜, palatine tonsils ➤, and lingual tonsils ➜. The patient also had marked enlargement of bilateral nonsuppurative cervical lymph nodes, a fairly common constellation of findings in mononucleosis.*

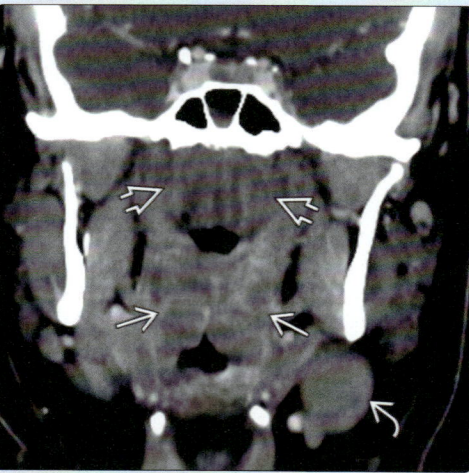
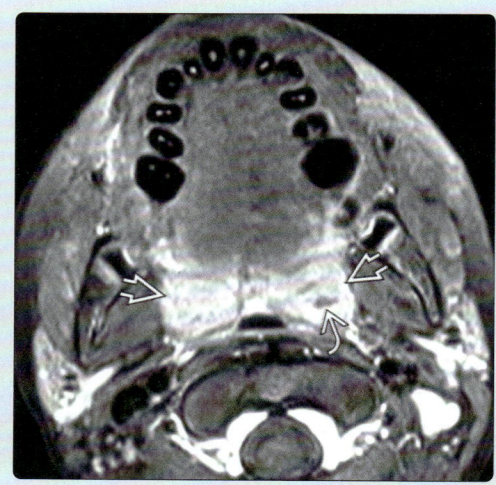

(Left) *Coronal CECT in a teenager with sore throat and fever shows a striated appearance to the palatine ➜ and the adenoid ➤ tonsils, typical of nonsuppurative tonsillitis. Notice also the large left submandibular lymph node ➜ in this patient who tested positive for both Group A streptococcus and EBV.* (Right) *Axial T1WI C+ FS MR shows bilateral tonsillar enlargement and pronounced enhancement ➤. Small internal areas of low signal ➜ are compatible with submucosal edema/exudate.*

Tonsillar/Peritonsillar Abscess

KEY FACTS

TERMINOLOGY

- Definitions
  - Tonsillar abscess (TA): Abscess forming within palatine tonsil (rare)
  - Peritonsillar abscess (PTA): Abscess forming around palatine tonsil between tonsil capsule & superior constrictor muscle ± spread to adjacent parapharyngeal (PPS) ± masticator (MS) ± submandibular (SMS) spaces
  - PTA >> TA

IMAGING

- CECT
  - Clinically suspected PTA: Frequently drained at bedside without imaging
  - TA: Swollen tonsil with peripherally enhancing central low-density
  - PTA: Focal, low-density pus between tonsil & superior constrictor muscle ± spread to PPS ± MS ± SMS
  - Reactive, bulky, bilateral cervical adenopathy common

TOP DIFFERENTIAL DIAGNOSES

- Tonsillar hyperplasia (hypertrophy)
  - Chronic; palatine, ± adenoid, ± lingual tonsil enlargement
  - Tonsils do not significantly enhance or show low-density center (TA)
- Tonsillar inflammation (tonsillitis)
  - Acute; unilateral or bilateral palatine tonsil enlargement with enhancement but without low-density center (TA)
- Tonsillar retention cyst
  - Chronic; incidental CECT finding
  - Focal tonsillar fluid without tonsillar enhancement or enhancing rim
- Retropharyngeal space (RPS) abscess
  - Acute; suppurative RPS node ruptures into RPS
- Palatine tonsil squamous cell carcinoma
  - Chronic; invasive tonsil mass with local invasion

DIAGNOSTIC CHECKLIST

- Carefully differentiate tonsillar edema from TA & PTA

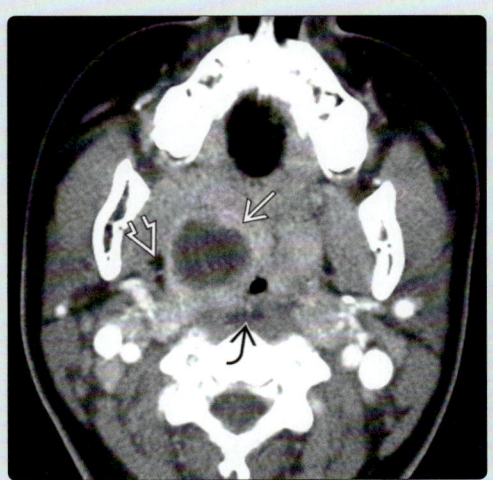
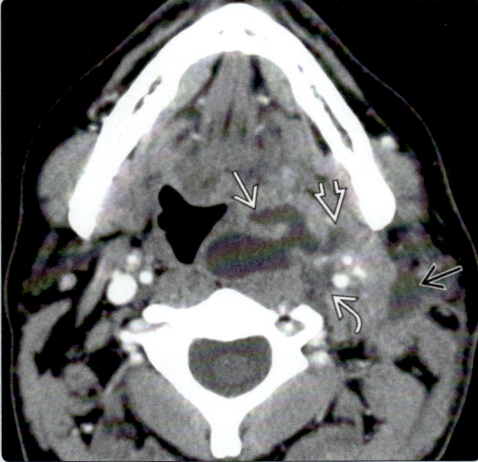

(Left) Axial CECT shows a large, low-density tonsillar abscess ➡. No extension through the capsule into the parapharyngeal space (PPS) ➡ is present. The left tonsil is prominent and enhancing, but no abscess is seen. Note sympathetic effusion in the retropharyngeal space ➡. (Right) Axial CECT reveals a complicated, large, left peritonsillar abscess (PTA) ➡. Infection has ruptured posteriorly into the carotid space ➡, anterolaterally into the upper submandibular space ➡, and laterally into the inferior parotid space ➡.

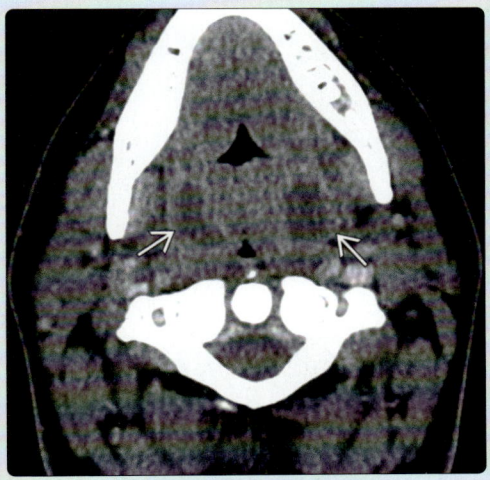
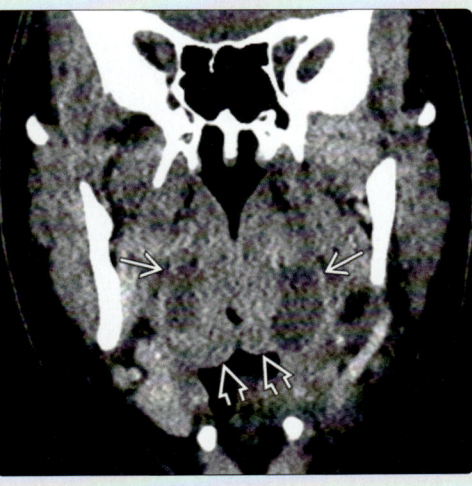

(Left) Axial CECT in a patient with strep throat, not improving on antibiotics, shows bilateral low attenuation collections ➡ in or adjacent to the palatine tonsils, without extension to the PMS or masticator space. (Right) Coronal CECT shows the collections ➡ to be a bit more crescentic in shape along the lateral aspect of the medially displaced palatine tonsils ➡, suggesting a peritonsillar location, which was proven at surgery. This demonstrates the importance of reviewing the coronal images.

Pleomorphic Adenoma of Pharyngeal Mucosal Space

KEY FACTS

TERMINOLOGY

- Pleomorphic adenoma (PA) of pharyngeal mucosal space (PMS); synonym: Benign mixed tumor

IMAGING

- Palate > > oropharyngeal mucosal space (lingual or faucial tonsil) > nasopharyngeal mucosal space
- Size: Variable but usually > 2 cm
- Shape: Oval to round, well-circumscribed mass without invasive margins
- CECT findings
  - Variable enhancing, well-circumscribed **palatal or PMS mass**
- MR findings
  - **T2** signal variable but usually **hyperintense** to muscle
  - **T1 C+ enhancement** pattern variable but most commonly **homogeneous** enhancement
  - Dynamic-contrast MR time-signal intensity curve (TIC) type A: Gradual enhancement with peak time ≥ 150 s

TOP DIFFERENTIAL DIAGNOSES

- PMS retention cyst
- Nasopalatine duct (incisive canal) cyst
- PMS squamous cell carcinoma
- PMS non-Hodgkin lymphoma
- PMS minor salivary gland malignancy
- Thyroglossal duct cyst in foramen cecum

PATHOLOGY

- Interspersed epithelial, myoepithelial, and stromal cellular components must be identified to diagnose PA-PMS

CLINICAL ISSUES

- Submucosal mass of palate or pharyngeal surface

DIAGNOSTIC CHECKLIST

- Submucosal lesion with no deep extension
- T2 MR in multiple planes often best imaging modality for PA visualization

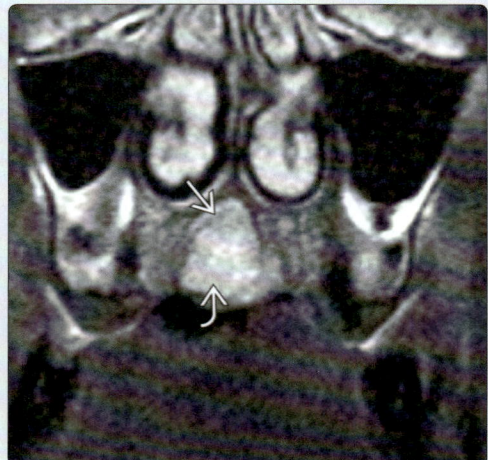
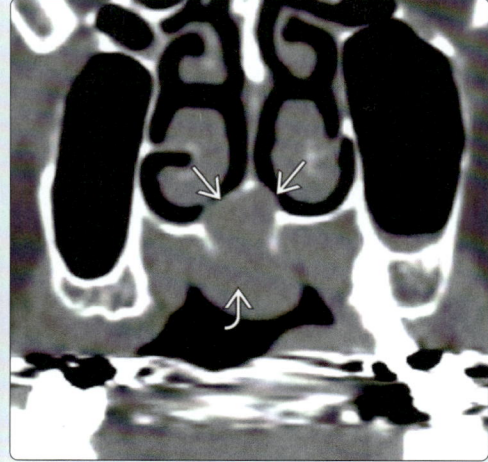

(Left) Coronal T2WI MR shows a well-defined, hyperintense mass ➔, biopsy proven to be a pleomorphic adenoma (PA) of the palate. Note the low signal intensity rim ➔. The mass enhanced with contrast (not shown), excluding palatal or incisive canal cyst. (Right) Coronal NECT in the same patient shows the palatal mass ➔ with smooth scalloping/thinning of the overlying hard palate bone ➔ due to the slow-growing PA. PA of minor salivary glands in the pharyngeal mucosal space occurs in palate > > oropharynx > nasopharynx.

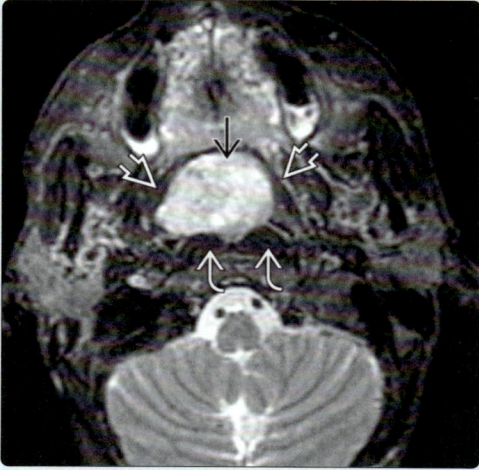
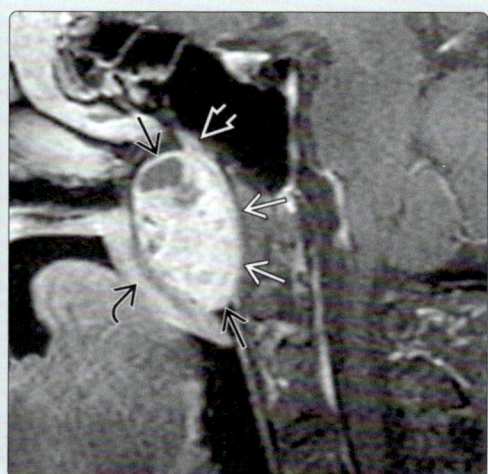

(Left) Axial T2 FS MR shows a hyperintense, well-defined oropharyngeal mucosal space PA nearly filling its airway ➔. There is no invasion of the lateral pharyngeal walls ➔ or prevertebral tissues ➔. (Right) T1 C+ FS MR in a patient with a nasopharyngeal PA shows a heterogeneous enhancing mass ➔ compressing soft palate ➔. No deep invasion into longus capitis muscle ➔ or sphenoid sinus floor ➔ is seen. PA is entirely submucosal without ulceration. Nonenhancing areas in mass are due to cystic changes.

TERMINOLOGY

Abbreviations
- Pleomorphic adenoma (PA)

Synonyms
- Benign mixed tumor (BMT): Older term, as previously considered to be form of teratoma
  - But now known to arise from single layer of germ cells, and purely epithelial

IMAGING

General Features
- Best diagnostic clue
  - Solitary, sharply marginated submucosal mass, often pedunculated when large
- Location
  - Submucosal, anywhere in upper aerodigestive tract
  - Palate > > oropharyngeal mucosal space (lingual or faucial tonsil) > nasopharyngeal mucosal space
  - Buccal mucosa and floor of mouth rare
- Size
  - Variable but usually > 2 cm
- Morphology
  - Oval to round, well-circumscribed, mobile mass

CT Findings
- CECT
  - Variable enhancing, well-circumscribed **palatal** or **pharyngeal mucosal space (PMS)** mass
  - May be heterogeneous with calcifications, hemorrhage, or cystic components
  - If tumor is adjacent to bone (e.g., hard palate), benign-appearing remodeling on bone CT

MR Findings
- T2WI
  - Signal variable but usually **hyperintense** to muscle
    - Dark rim often present
  - Well circumscribed but may be lobulated with **no deep invasion**
- DWI
  - ↑ ADC values compared to malignant salivary tumors
- T1WI C+
  - Variable enhancement, most commonly homogeneous
    - May show nonenhancing, cystic areas
  - Dynamic-contrast MR time-signal intensity curve **(TIC) type A**: Gradual enhancement with peak time ≥ 150 s
  - **Other typical dynamic-contrast TICs in salivary tumors**
    - **Type B**: Early enhancement and high washout with peak time < 150 s and washout ratio (WR) ≥ 30% (Warthin tumor)
    - **Type C**: Early enhancement and low washout with peak time < 150 s and WR < 30% (malignant salivary gland tumors)
    - **Type D**: Flat curve (lymphoepithelial cysts, lymphangiomas)
  - TIC could point to tumor type, but overlaps may happen and have to be correlated with other imaging findings

DIFFERENTIAL DIAGNOSIS

Pharyngeal Mucosal Space Retention Cyst
- Postinflammatory PMS cyst without enhancement

Thyroglossal Duct Cyst at Foramen Cecum
- Midline base of tongue cyst

Nasopalatine Duct (Incisive Canal) Cyst
- Sharply marginated hard palate fissural cyst of incisive canal

Pharyngeal Mucosal Space Squamous Cell Carcinoma
- Mucosal surface has obvious erosive lesion (unless if tumor began in tonsillar crypt)
- Usually only slightly hyperintense on T2 MR

Pharyngeal Mucosal Space Non-Hodgkin Lymphoma
- Diffuse adenoidal prominence or asymmetric faucial or lingual tonsil mass

Pharyngeal Mucosal Space Minor Salivary Gland Malignancy
- Aggressive bone changes when malignancy develops in MSG of hard palate

PATHOLOGY

Gross Pathologic & Surgical Features
- Exophytic, 1-4 cm in size, smooth mass projecting into pharyngeal airway

Microscopic Features
- Interspersed epithelial, myoepithelial, and stromal cellular components must be identified to diagnose PA-PMS
- Malignancy may develop in 2-10% of PA, most commonly carcinoma ex PA

CLINICAL ISSUES

Presentation
- Most common signs/symptoms
  - Painless submucosal mass of palate or pharynx
  - Rare life-threatening bleeding from atypical PA of soft palate reported

Demographics
- Epidemiology
  - 6.5% of H&N PA arise from MSG along oral mucosal space (OMS) and PMS

Treatment
- Complete surgical resection of mass

DIAGNOSTIC CHECKLIST

Consider
- PA-MSG if mucosal space lesion is submucosal with no mucosal ulceration or deep extension

SELECTED REFERENCES

1. Piccinini F et al: Life-threatening bleeding in atypical pleomorphic adenoma of the soft palate. Iran J Otorhinolaryngol. 36(5):627-30, 2024
2. Zar K et al: "The correlation between histopathological pattern and surgical treatment for palatal pleomorphic adenoma. Can we choose a more conservative approach?". J Craniomaxillofac Surg. 52(12):1469-75, 2024

KEY FACTS

TERMINOLOGY

- Minor salivary gland malignancy (MSGM) of pharyngeal mucosal space (PMS)
- Rare, aggressive tumors arising from MSG in PMS
- Most common: Adenoid cystic carcinoma (ACCa) > mucoepidermoid carcinoma (MECa) > adenocarcinoma

IMAGING

- Locations: Oral cavity (**hard palate**) > > oropharynx (**soft palate**, base of tongue) > > nasal cavity/sinus
- Enhancing, infiltrating mass centered in PMS
- Hard palate, skull base, mandible/maxilla invasion common
- MR: Submucosal mass usually **high T2 signal intensity**
- T1 help to detect mandible/maxilla invasion, perineural tumor; T1 C+ FS define perineural spread
- Dynamic contrast MR type C time-signal intensity curve (TIC): Early enhancement (peak < 150 s) & washout ratio < 30%
- FDG PET: High-grade/dedifferentiated tumors high uptake

- Low-grade salivary malignancies (low-grade MECa/ACCa, acinic cell carcinoma, clear cell carcinoma) may not be FDG avid

TOP DIFFERENTIAL DIAGNOSES

- PMS pleomorphic adenoma
- PMS squamous cell carcinoma (SCCa)
- PMS non-Hodgkin lymphoma

CLINICAL ISSUES

- Submucosal pharyngeal surface mass ± ulceration
- ACCa often presents with pain & V2, V3 neuropathy
- Metastatic adenopathy at presentation rare unless high-grade histology
- Preoperative image-guided biopsy usually needed if mass not palpable

DIAGNOSTIC CHECKLIST

- Consider MSGM if T2-hyperintense PMS lesion has bone invasion or perineural spread

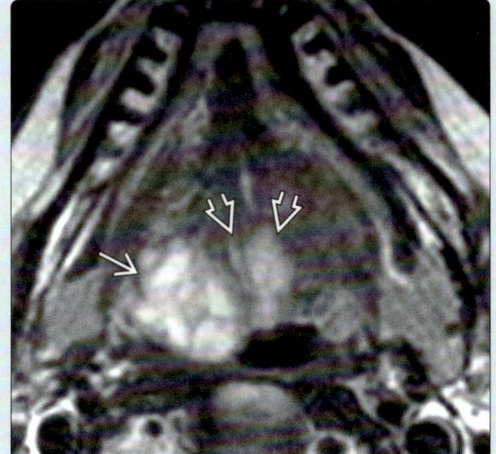
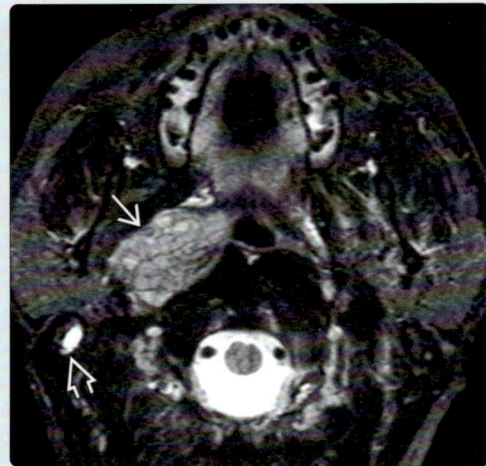

(Left) Axial T2WI MR shows hyperintense, lobulated adenoid cystic carcinoma (ACCa) ➡ involving base of tongue & floor of mouth. Note bilateral genioglossus muscle ➡ invasion. (Right) Axial T2WI FS MR shows hyperintense mucosal-submucosal ACCa in the right nasopharyngeal mucosal space with lateral extension into parapharyngeal space ➡. Note fluid in right mastoid ➡ due to eustachian tube obstruction by the mass. Squamous cell carcinoma is much more common than minor salivary gland malignancy.

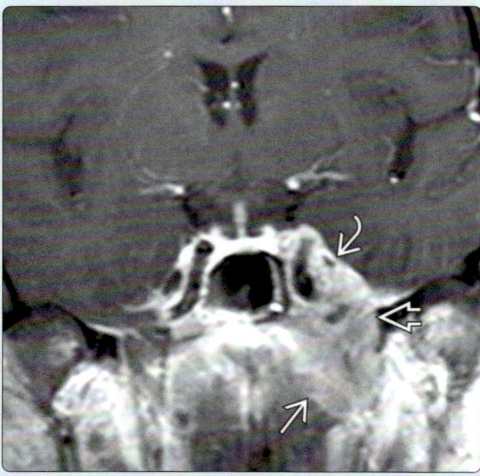
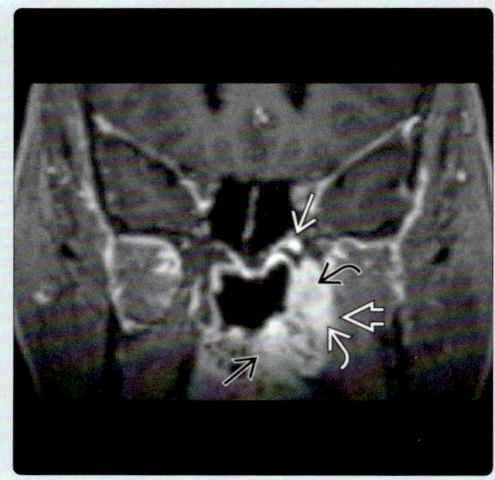

(Left) Coronal T1WI C+ MR shows ACCa of the left nasopharynx ➡ with perineural spread along CNV3 through the widened foramen ovale ➡ into the left cavernous sinus ➡. (Right) Coronal T1 C+ MPRAGE MR shows heterogeneously enhancing ACCa in the soft palate ➡ extending along the left side of nasopharynx ➡ towards the skull base foramen lacerum region. Note enhancing perineural tumor in the left vidian canal ➡. There is invasion into the left parapharyngeal space ➡ & medial pterygoid muscle ➡.

TERMINOLOGY

Abbreviations

- Minor salivary gland malignancy (MSGM), pharyngeal mucosal space (PMS)

Definitions

- Adenoid cystic carcinoma (ACCa) > mucoepidermoid carcinoma (MECa) > adenocarcinoma (ADCa) most common

IMAGING

General Features

- Best diagnostic clue
  - Enhancing, infiltrating PMS mass often with deep extension into adjacent structures
- Location
  - Oral cavity (**hard palate, floor of mouth**) > oropharynx (**soft palate**, base of tongue) > buccal mucosa & nasal cavity/paranasal sinus

CT Findings

- CECT
  - Enhancing, infiltrating mass on pharyngeal surface
  - Hard palate, skull base, mandible invasion common

MR Findings

- T1WI
  - PMS lesion usually isointense to muscle
  - T1 helpful to detect mandible or maxilla invasion, perineural tumor
- T2WI
  - PMS mass hyperintense when low grade
  - ↓ T2 signal mass (more cellular) generally has worse prognosis than high-signal mass (less cellular)
- T1WI C+
  - Enhancing mass with infiltrating margins
  - Fat suppression for **perineural spread**: Hard/soft palate → palatine nerves → pterygopalatine fossa → CNV2
  - Skull base tumor near foramen lacerum can spread into vidian canal → pterygopalatine fossa
  - Dynamic contrast MR time-signal intensity curve (TIC) type C: Early enhancement and low washout with peak time < 150 s and washout ratio (WR) < 30%
  - Other typical dynamic contrast TICs in salivary tumors
  - Type A [pleomorphic adenoma (PA)]: Gradual enhancement with peak time ≥ 150 s
  - Type B (Warthin tumor): Early enhancement and high washout with peak time < 150 s and WR ≥ 30%
  - Type D (lymphoepithelial cyst/lymphangioma): Flat TIC
  - TIC could point to tumor type, but overlaps may happen & have to be correlated with other imaging findings

Nuclear Medicine Findings

- PET
  - High-grade/dedifferentiated salivary tumors can show high F-18 FDG uptake
  - Low-grade salivary malignancies (low-grade MECA/ACCa, acinic cell carcinoma, clear cell carcinoma) may not
  - **Benign tumors can be FDG avid**: Warthin tumor & PA
    - **Warthin tumor** due to epithelial cells with numerous mitochondria, immunoglobulin A, lymphoid stroma

- **PA** due to glucose transporter 1 (GLUT1)

Imaging Recommendations

- Protocol advice
  - T1, T2, & fat-suppressed T1 C+ MR in all planes
  - Perineural spread: Image entire CNV2, CNV3

DIFFERENTIAL DIAGNOSIS

Pharyngeal Mucosal Space Pleomorphic Adenoma

- Well-circumscribed, submucosal, ↑ ↑ T2 mass

Pharyngeal Mucosal Space Squamous Cell Carcinoma

- Nasopharyngeal, palatine tonsil, lingual tonsil carcinoma

Pharyngeal Mucosal Space Non-Hodgkin Lymphoma

- Adenoidal, tonsillar, or lingual lymphoid tissue mass usually ↓ ↓ on T2 MR; large, nonnecrotic nodes in 50%

PATHOLOGY

Staging, Grading, & Classification

- Staged according to anatomic site of origin: Nasopharynx, oral cavity, oropharynx, sinuses

Microscopic Features

- ACCa: Unencapsulated neoplasm of small, darkly staining epithelial cells with cribriform appearance
- MECa: Admixture of epidermoid, mucus-secreting, intermediate & squamous cells
- ADCa: Encapsulated neoplasm composed of cells of glandular origin

CLINICAL ISSUES

Presentation

- Most common signs/symptoms
  - Submucosal, pharyngeal surface mass ± ulceration
  - More invasive lesions, especially ACCa, present with pain & CNV2 & CNV3 neuropathy
- Other signs/symptoms
  - Metastatic adenopathy at presentation most common for higher grade malignancies

Demographics

- Epidemiology
  - Rare, compared to major salivary gland malignancy (1/10 as common)
- Age range: 35-80 yr

Natural History & Prognosis

- Begin as slow-growing tumors that tend to recur late
- 5-yr survival: 80%; 20-yr survival: 20%

Treatment

- Preoperative image-guided biopsy usually needed if mass not palpable
- Wide surgical removal treatment of choice
- Neck dissection controversial but often done for higher grade MSGM

SELECTED REFERENCES

1. Jaber MA et al: Adenoid cystic carcinoma of the minor salivary glands: a systematic review and meta-analysis of clinical characteristics and management strategies. J Clin Med. 13(1): 267, 2024

TERMINOLOGY

- Non-Hodgkin lymphoma (NHL) of pharyngeal mucosal space (PMS)
- Multiple subtypes, usually B- or T-cell categories
- 3 subsites of Waldeyer lymphatic ring
  - Nasopharyngeal adenoids
  - Palatine tonsils
  - Lingual tonsil

IMAGING

- CECT: Minimally enhancing bulky mass filling PMS airway
  - Associated NHL nodal disease present 50% of time
- T2WI MR: Varies in signal intensity depending on cellularity
- DWI MR: Restricted because of high cellularity

TOP DIFFERENTIAL DIAGNOSES

- Tonsillar lymphoid hyperplasia
- PMS pleomorphic adenoma
- Nasopharyngeal carcinoma
- Palatine tonsil squamous cell carcinoma (SCCa)
- Lingual tonsil SCCa
- Inflammatory pseudotumor/IgG4-related disease
- PMS minor salivary gland malignancy

PATHOLOGY

- PMS NHL usually of B-cell origin
- Hodgkin lymphoma of Waldeyer ring and other extranodal sites extremely rare

CLINICAL ISSUES

- Increased incidence in patients with AIDS, Sjögren syndrome, Hashimoto thyroiditis, IgG4-related disease, some autoimmune conditions

DIAGNOSTIC CHECKLIST

- Consider NHL of PMS when imaging shows bulky mass of adenoids, tonsils, or base of tongue
- Note local or deep extension and associated adenopathy for staging and treatment planning

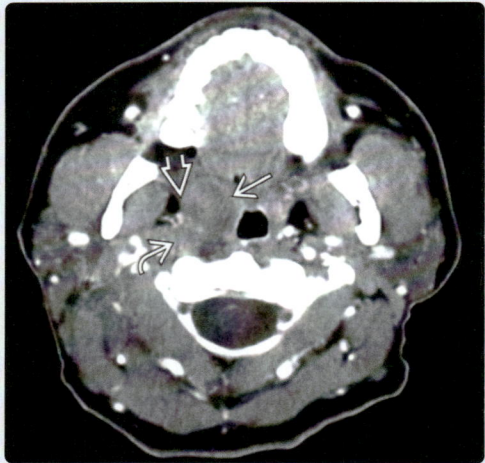
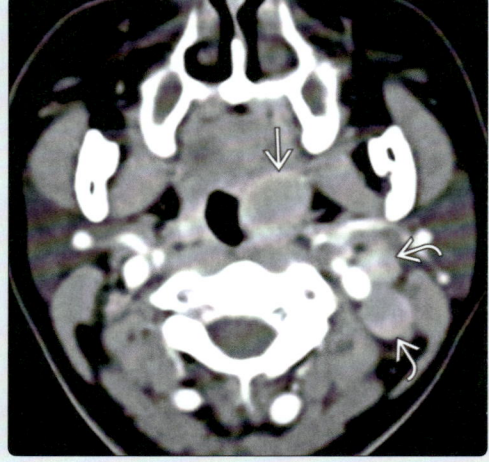

(Left) Axial CECT shows a low-density non-Hodgkin lymphoma (NHL) ➡ in the right tonsil. The smooth interface between parapharyngeal fat ➡ implies no extension through the lateral capsule, but fullness in the right prevertebral muscles ➡ suggests invasion through the posterior tonsillar capsule. (Right) Axial CECT shows a left palatine tonsillar mass ➡ and left level IIA lymphadenopathy ➡, which were later biopsy proven to be diffuse large B-cell lymphoma (DLBCL). Tonsillar infection would have striated enhancement.

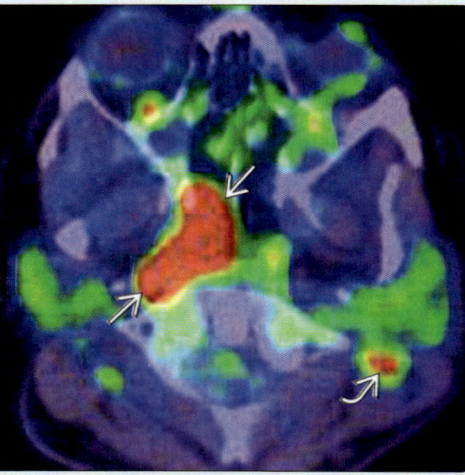
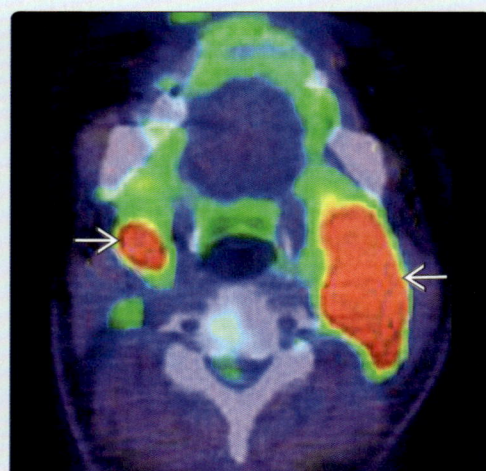

(Left) Axial fused F-18 FDG PET/CT in a patient with DLBCL NHL shows a right nasopharyngeal FDG-avid mass extending into the posterior choana ➡. A small left upper cervical FDG-avid lymph node ➡ is partially visualized. (Right) Axial fused F-18 FDG PET/CT at a slightly lower level through the hyoid bone shows bilateral FDG-avid level II cervical lymphadenopathy ➡, larger on left side. PET/CT is the best for staging and surveillance and differentiates persistent disease from an inactive scar or sterile-treated tumor.

TERMINOLOGY

Abbreviations

- Non-Hodgkin lymphoma (NHL), pharyngeal mucosal space (PMS)

Synonyms

- Multiple subtypes, usually B- or T-cell categories
  - B-cell types: Burkitt, diffuse large B-cell (DLBCL), follicular, immunoblastic large cell, mantle cell, chronic lymphocytic lymphoma (CLL), mucosa-associated lymphoid tissue (MALT)
  - T-cell types: Anaplastic large cell, precursor T-lymphoblastic, mycosis fungoides

Definitions

- 3 subsites of Waldeyer lymphatic ring: Adenoids, palatine tonsils, lingual tonsil

IMAGING

General Features

- Best diagnostic clue
  - Large PMS mass with associated cervical adenopathy > 50% of time
  - Imaging findings **may be identical to squamous cell carcinoma** (SCCa) of PMS
- Location
  - Most common sites of NHL of PMS
    - Palatine tonsil > nasopharyngeal adenoids > lingual tonsil
    - > 1 site often involved
  - Nonnodal, extralymphatic NHL of sinus, orbit, parotid, larynx, or thyroid can rarely occur
- Size
  - Large, usually > 4 cm, at presentation
- Morphology
  - Poorly defined, diffusely infiltrative mass most common (mimics SCCa)
  - Unilateral, asymmetric, smooth mass in tonsil less common (mimics pleomorphic adenoma)

CT Findings

- CECT
  - Minimally enhancing, bulky mass filling PMS airway
  - Associated NHL nodal disease present 50% of time
    - **Nodes** usually **large**, > 2 cm, and nonnecrotic
    - Nodes may be centrally necrotic in high-grade NHL
      - □ Especially AIDS-related NHL

MR Findings

- T1WI
  - Large PMS mass isointense to muscle
- T2WI
  - Varies in signal intensity (SI), depending on cellularity but usually homogeneously intermediate SI
    - Highly cellular lesions generally lower T2 signal
  - Invasion into surrounding structures, including skull base, parapharyngeal space, and prevertebral muscles, may be seen
- DWI
  - Restricted diffusion, especially for FDG-avid lymphoma types
- T1WI C+
  - Enhancing palatine, lingual, or adenoidal tonsillar mass
  - No internal enhancing septa present compared with benign lymphoid hyperplasia or tonsillar infection

Nuclear Medicine Findings

- PET
  - NHL FDG avid
  - MALT-type NHL less FDG avid
  - PET/CT used to stage disease and for surveillance of posttreatment imaging
    - PET/CT limited sensitivity for lower grade NHL

Imaging Recommendations

- Best imaging tool
  - PET/CT best staging and surveillance modality
  - CECT recommended as part of PET/CT imaging
- Protocol advice
  - Imaging (CT or MR) should cover entire extracranial H&N from sellar floor above to clavicles below
    - Coverage should include PMS primary site as well as potential cervical adenopathy

DIFFERENTIAL DIAGNOSIS

Tonsillar Lymphoid Hyperplasia

- Patients < 20 years old (NHL usually > 40 years old)
- Symmetric enlargement of adenoidal and tonsillar tissue
- Internal **enhancing septa** seen on T1 C+ MR

Nasopharyngeal Carcinoma

- Poorly circumscribed nasopharyngeal PMS mass
  - Often mimics NHL on imaging alone
- Associated malignant, often necrotic, adenopathy

Palatine Tonsil Squamous Cell Carcinoma

- Invasive palatine tonsil mass
  - Often mimics NHL on imaging alone

Lingual Tonsil Squamous Cell Carcinoma

- Invasive lingual tonsil mass
  - Often mimics NHL on imaging alone

Pharyngeal Mucosal Space Minor Salivary Gland Malignancy

- May be indistinguishable from H&N SCCa
- Associated nodal metastases are rare

Pharyngeal Mucosal Space Pleomorphic Adenoma

- Well-circumscribed, noninvasive PMS mass

Inflammatory Pseudotumor/IgG4 Disease

- Autoimmune disease, can present as PMS mass
- Spectrum that includes Sjögren syndrome, thyroiditis, autoimmune disease

PATHOLOGY

General Features

- Etiology
  - Primary malignancy of lymphatic system
  - PMS NHL usually of B-cell origin

- Hodgkin lymphoma of Waldeyer ring and other extranodal sites extremely rare
- Genetics
  - Cytogenetics of NHL complicated and related to subtype
  - **Double-hit lymphoma (DHL)**: At least 2 rearrangements involving *MYC*, *BLC2*, &/or *BCL6*
    - HIV-associated DHL of tonsil recently reported
- Associated abnormalities
  - Sjögren syndrome and Hashimoto thyroiditis associated with MALT NHL
  - IgG4-related disease usually associated with MALT lymphoma mostly in Asians
    - MALT and other types, such as DLBCL and follicular lymphoma, reported especially in Western population
  - Posttransplant lymphoproliferative disorders (PTLDs) associated with NHL from iatrogenic immunosuppression used for transplant patients
    - Spectrum of diseases from prominent lymphoid hyperplasia to malignant NHL

Staging, Grading, & Classification

- 2 prognostic groups: Indolent and aggressive
- **Lugano** classification for staging lymphomas (derived from **Ann Arbor** staging system)
  - **Stage I**: Single lymph node or group of adjacent nodes (Waldeyer ring, thymus, and spleen considered nodal structures for staging purposes) (I), or single extranodal organ or tissue (IE) without nodal involvement
  - **Stage II**: 2 or more lymph node regions or nodal structures on same side of diaphragm alone (II), or with involvement of limited, contiguous extralymphatic organ or tissue (IIE)
  - **Stage III**: Lymph node regions or lymphoid structures on both sides of diaphragm (can be nodes on both sides of diaphragm, or nodes above diaphragm with spleen below diaphragm)
  - **Stage IV**: Diffuse or disseminated noncontiguous extralymphatic organ or tissue involvement (more than that can be designated "E"), +/- associated nodal involvement

Gross Pathologic & Surgical Features

- Soft, bulky PMS lesion; may be submucosal or ulcerative

Microscopic Features

- Any NHL patterns and cell types can be seen
- Most common histologic pattern is diffuse with immunoblastic or large cell (B cell) cytologic features, markers
  - Immunochemistry differentiates nasopharyngeal carcinoma (NPCa) from NHL
    - Leukocyte common antigen (LCA) vs. cytokeratin
    - NHL, immunoblastic or large-cell type: LCA (+), cytokeratin (-)
    - NPCa, undifferentiated: LCA (-), cytokeratin (+)

CLINICAL ISSUES

Presentation

- Most common signs/symptoms
  - Presenting signs similar to SCCa
    - Nasopharyngeal adenoidal NHL: Nasal obstruction, serous otitis media

---

    - Palatine or lingual tonsil NHL: Sore throat, otalgia, tonsillar mass
  - Other signs/symptoms
    - B symptoms: Systemic complaints, such as fever, sweats, weight loss
    - Children with large PMS NHL may present with airway compromise
- Clinical profile
  - Most common presentation: Adult with PMS mass, neck mass
  - Increased incidence in patients with AIDS, Sjögren syndrome, Hashimoto thyroiditis, other autoimmune conditions

Demographics

- Age
  - Adult more common than pediatric; > 50 years
- Epidemiology
  - NHL 5x as common as Hodgkin disease in H&N
  - 35% of extranodal NHL in H&N occurs in PMS
  - 50% of PMS NHL have malignant lymph nodes at presentation
  - H&N 2nd most common site of extra nodal lymphoma: Palatine tonsils most common, other sites include nasopharynx and tongue base
  - Recent population-based study in > 60-year-olds: Most common extranodal sites of hematolymphoid neoplasm involvement include salivary glands, mainly parotid gland, followed by tonsil, thyroid, and tongue

Natural History & Prognosis

- Prognosis determined by both stage and aggressive vs. indolent types
  - High histopathologic grade and recurrent disseminated disease have poorest prognosis
  - AIDS-related NHL generally has poorer prognosis
- 2/3 of patients have remission after initial therapy
  - Of these, 2/3 are cured and have no further relapse
- 75% of those relapsing after achieving remission die of NHL

Treatment

- Based on clinical stage and aggressive vs. indolent subtypes at presentation
- Treatment regimens range from "watch and wait" for indolent types (especially in older adults) to combined chemoradiotherapy
- Complete remission and cure rates improved with development of combined chemotherapy options
- **Overall survival rate** for H&N PMS NHL **60%**

DIAGNOSTIC CHECKLIST

Consider

- NHL of PMS when imaging shows bulky mass of adenoidal, tonsillar, or base of tongue (lingual tonsil)

SELECTED REFERENCES

1. S H et al: Unusual presentation of non-Hodgkin lymphoma of two cases: case report. Indian J Otolaryngol Head Neck Surg. 76(4):3717-21, 2024
2. Zheng YH et al: Distribution and survival outcomes of primary head and neck hematolymphoid neoplasms in older people: a population-based study. Clin Exp Med. 23(7):3957-67, 2023

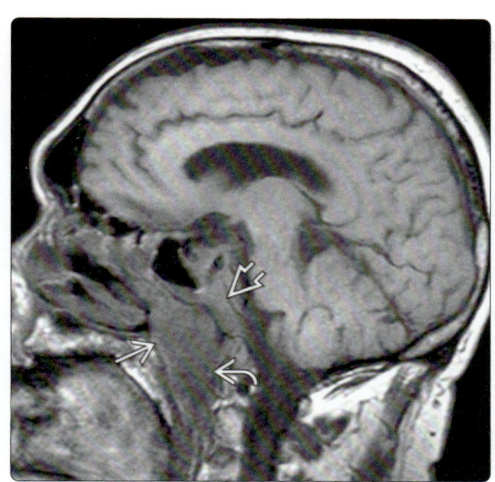

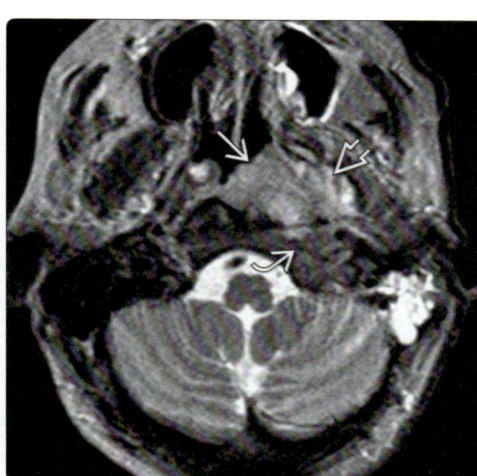

(Left) *Sagittal T1 MR shows a bulky nasopharyngeal mass ➡ extending to oropharyngeal level ➡. Abnormal signal intensity in the clivus ➡ implies central skull base invasion.* (Right) *Axial T2WI FS MR in the same patient reveals the mass ➡ is relatively low signal intensity with invasion of prevertebral muscles ➡ and the parapharyngeal space ➡. Note mastoid opacification from tumor obstruction/invasion of the eustachian tube orifice. Nasopharyngeal carcinoma could exactly mimic this imaging appearance.*

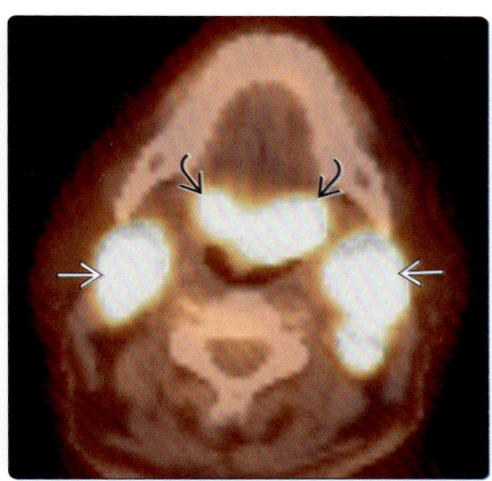

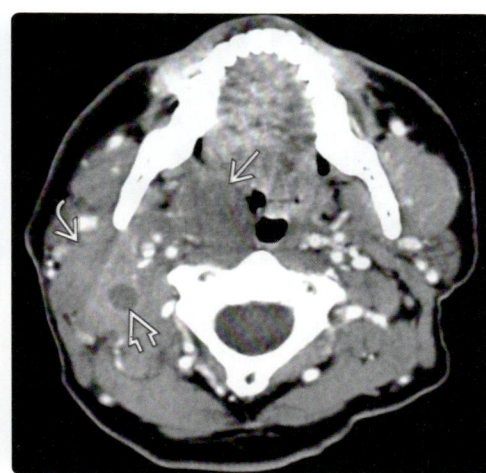

(Left) *Axial fused FDG PET/CT in a patient with NHL shows bilateral, enlarged FDG-avid "kissing" tonsils ➡ touching each other in the midline. Also note the bilateral hypermetabolic level II lymphadenopathy ➡.* (Right) *Axial CECT shows multifocal NHL with involvement in the right tonsil ➡, a level II matted nodal mass ➡ with extranodal extension and partial necrosis ➡. Cervical lymphadenopathy is present > 50% of the time with NHL of pharyngeal mucosal space.*

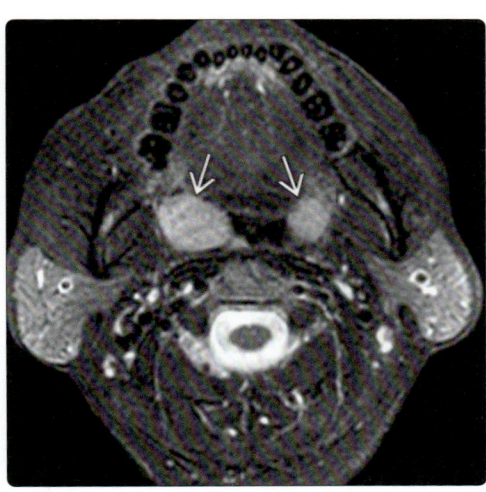

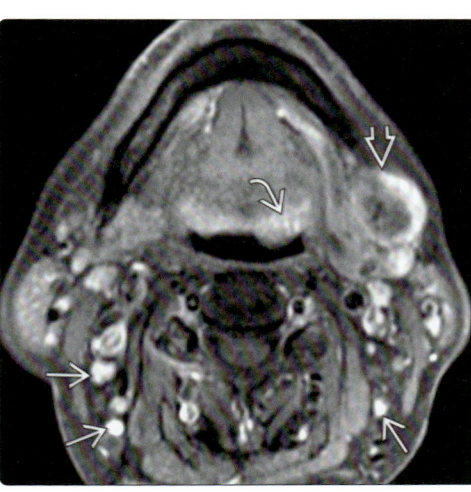

(Left) *Axial T2 FS MR demonstrates multifocal NHL in both palatine tonsils ➡. The well-circumscribed appearance suggests that tumor remains within tonsillar capsules.* (Right) *Axial T1 C+ FS MR in the same patient shows additional sites of NHL in the left base of tongue lymphoid tissue ➡ and a large necrotic left IB node ➡. Multiple small cervical nodes ➡ are seen, which need a metabolic study, like PET/CT, to determine involvement by NHL. Clinically, pharyngeal mucosal space lymphoma may be submucosal or ulcerative.*

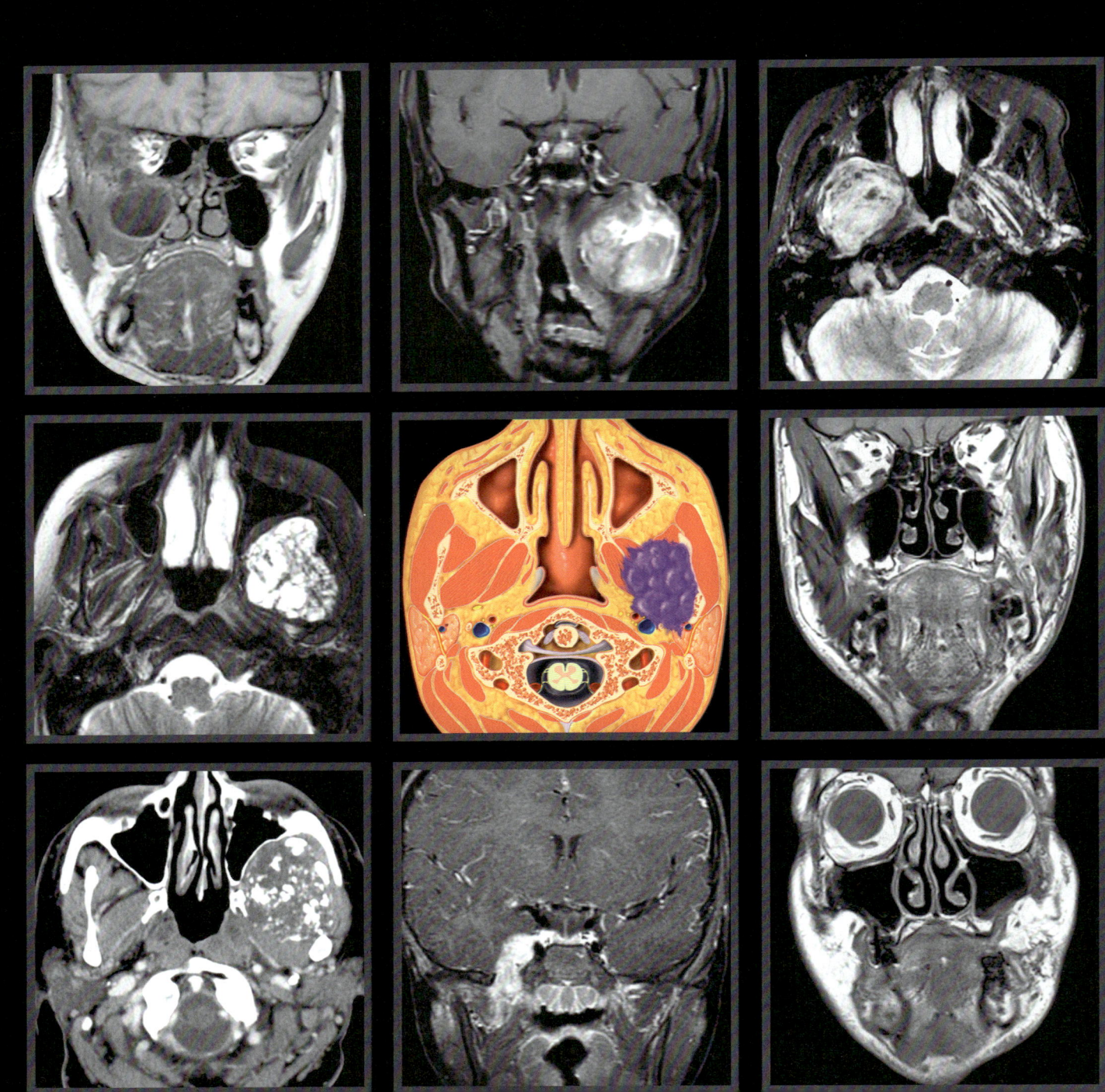

SECTION 4
Masticator Space

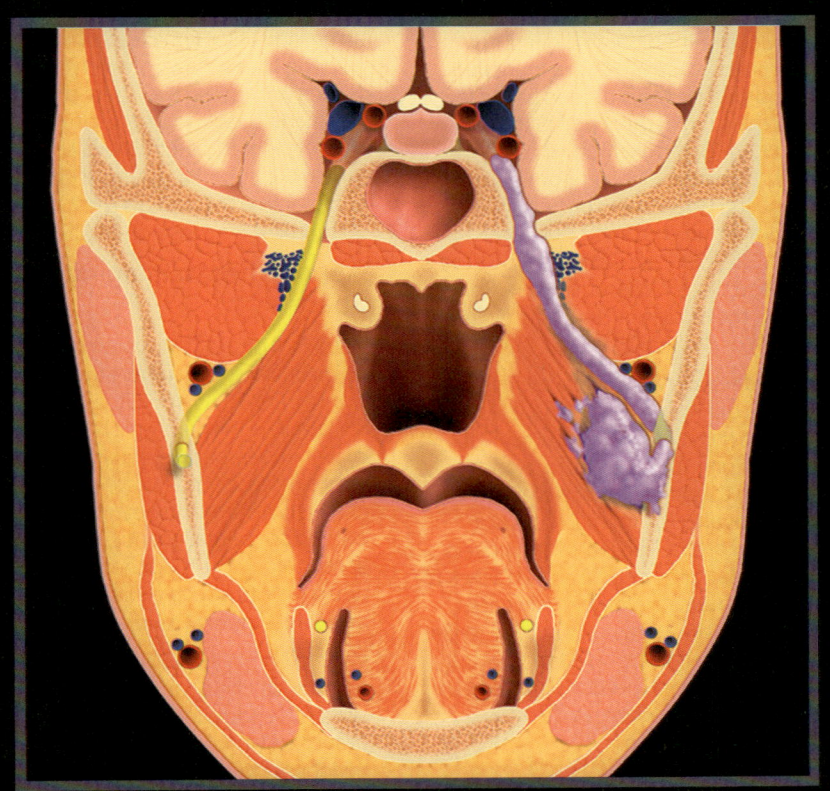

Summary Thoughts: Masticator Space

The 3 most frequently encountered abnormalities in the masticator space (MS) are infection, infection, and infection. Odontogenic infection should always cross the radiologist's mind first when evaluating abnormalities in this space.

When evaluating tumors of the MS, the presence of **perineural CNV3 tumor spread (PNT)** is of critical importance because it is easily overlooked but can have a dramatic effect on treatment and prognosis.

Imaging Techniques and Indications

Odontogenic infection is by far the **most likely pathology** to affect the MS, and over 90% of head and neck infections have a dental origin. CECT is the preferred imaging modality. The responsible tooth is best identified with bone CT. This is important because infection will recur until the offending tooth is treated. To be sure that a worrisome tooth is the true site of origin, look for mandibular cortical erosions that communicate between the apical tooth abscess and the soft tissue MS abscess. Contrast is needed to determine how far the infection has spread into soft tissues. Contrast also helps differentiate cellulitis and phlegmon from a surgically drainable abscess.

When assessing for PNT, any cross-sectional imaging exam should cover the entire length of CNV3 in the MS, from the mandible to the skull base. Ideally, imaging should include the lateral pons, Meckel cave, foramen ovale, mandibular foramen (where the inferior alveolar nerve enters the mandible), the entire inferior alveolar canal, and the mental foramen.

Imaging Anatomy

The MS is the largest suprahyoid neck space. It has greater extension in the craniocaudal dimension than commonly recognized, as it reaches from the bottom of the mandible nearly to the vertex of the skull. The MS is divided at the level of the zygomatic arch into the suprazygomatic MS (**temporal fossa**) and the infrazygomatic MS (**infratemporal fossa**). In the superior direction, its suprazygomatic component extends along the parietal skull almost to the vertex, enclosing the temporalis muscle. There is a broad abutment of the MS to the skull base. Within this area of contact with the skull base is the foramen ovale (CNV3) and the foramen spinosum (middle meningeal artery). Inferiorly, the MS terminates at the inferior margin of the posterior body of the mandible.

The **superficial layer** of the **deep cervical fascia** divides around the inferior margin of the mandible. This split fascia encases the mandible and the muscles of mastication. The medial slip of the fascia runs along the deep surface of the pterygoid muscles to insert on the undersurface of the skull base just **medial** to **foramen ovale**. The medial slip is also known as the medial pterygoid fascia. The lateral slip covers the superficial surface of the masseter muscle and attaches to the zygomatic arch, where the masseter muscle originates. This lateral fascia continues over the temporalis muscle to the top of the suprazygomatic MS. There is no fascia separating the suprazygomatic and infrazygomatic portions of the MS. In fact, there are no horizontal fascia anywhere in the MS, facilitating craniocaudal spread of disease.

MS regional anatomic relationships are important, as both tumor and infection of the MS tend to spread into adjacent spaces. The buccal space is found anteriorly, including the retromaxillary fat pad. The parotid space is posterolateral, while the parapharyngeal space (PPS) is posteromedial to the MS. The relationship between the MS and PPS is important because the PPS fat will be displaced posteromedially by an enlarging MS mass. Medial to the MS is the pharyngeal mucosal space. The subcutaneous fat of the cheek is seen lateral to the MS.

Most of the MS is filled by the **4 muscles of mastication**. The masseter muscle originates at the zygomatic arch and inserts on the inferior mandibular body. The temporalis muscle takes its origin from a semicircular area of bone splayed across parietal skull. Inferiorly, the temporalis inserts on the coronoid process of mandible. The medial pterygoid arises from the medial pterygoid plate and inserts on the lingual surface of mandibular angle and ramus. The lateral pterygoid muscle originates from the lateral pterygoid plate and greater wing of sphenoid and inserts on the pterygoid fovea under the mandibular condyle. The lateral pterygoid is unique among the muscles of mastication because it serves to open the jaw instead of closing it. Additional muscles of MS are tensor tympani and palatini, anterior belly of the digastric, and mylohyoid.

The mandibular division of the trigeminal nerve (**CNV3**) emerges into the MS from the middle cranial fossa via the **foramen ovale**. CNV3 gives off a masticator branch (motor innervation to the muscles of mastication), a mylohyoid branch (motor innervation to the mylohyoid and anterior digastric muscles), and an auriculotemporal branch (sensory innervation to the skin overlying the parotid gland). The nerve continues as the inferior alveolar nerve, entering the mandible via the **mandibular foramen** on the lingual surface of the mandibular ramus.

The remaining contents of the MS are the inferior alveolar artery and veins (which accompany the inferior alveolar nerve into the mandibular foramen), **pterygoid venous plexus** (which lies among the fibers of the pterygoid muscles), and the mandibular ramus and posterior body. The posterior teeth are considered part of the oral cavity, not the MS. The TMJ is within the superior aspect of the infrazygomatic MS; thus, tumefactive TMJ lesions must be considered in the differential diagnosis of an MS mass.

Approaches to Imaging Issues of Masticator Space

The MS is one of the suprahyoid neck spaces that is connected to the intracranial compartment via a major cranial nerve branch, CNV3. As a result, all MS masses should be assessed for possible **PNT** along CNV3 into the middle cranial fossa. MS malignancies, such as squamous cell carcinoma or sarcoma, may demonstrate PNT spread through the foramen ovale into the Meckel cave and beyond. Additionally, when evaluating a parotid space malignancy, consider that tumor may not only spread along the facial nerve (CNVII), but also can spread along CNV (through an interconnection with the **auriculotemporal nerve** branch of CNV3).

When CNV3 is injured, the denervation pattern of the MS muscles can help radiologists identify the potential anatomic site of the pathology. A distal injury affecting the mylohyoid branch will involve the anterior belly of the digastric and the mylohyoid muscles, while sparing the muscles of mastication. In contrast, a more proximal injury, after the nerve emerges from the foramen ovale, would involve all MS muscles. Carefully review these regions to identify potential pathology.

Differential Diagnosis of Masticator Space

Pseudolesions		**Malignant tumor, primary**
Asymmetric pterygoid venous plexus		Chondrosarcoma
Asymmetric accessory parotid lobe		Osteosarcoma
Motor denervation CNV3 (acute or chronic)		Synovial sarcoma
Benign masticator muscle hypertrophy		Rhabdomyosarcoma
Infectious		Malignant schwannoma
Odontogenic abscess		Non-Hodgkin lymphoma (primary head and neck)
Inflammatory		**Malignant tumor, metastatic**
Postradiation scarring		Squamous cell carcinoma from retromolar trigone (direct invasion)
Benign neoplasm		Squamous cell carcinoma from oral cavity (perineural spread along V3)
Schwannoma (CNV3)		Squamous cell carcinoma from nasopharynx (direct spread)
Neurofibroma		Non-Hodgkin lymphoma (systemic)
Infantile hemangioma		Non-Hodgkin lymphoma (direct invasion from jaw primary)
Nodular fasciitis		Systemic hematogenous metastasis
Vascular		**Mandible lesions**
Venous malformations		Odontogenic and nonodontogenic mandible lesions
Lymphatic and mixed lymphovenous malformations		Fibrous dysplasia
Arteriovenous malformations		Osteonecrosis and osteoradionecrosis

There are at least 4 **pseudolesions** that can mimic pathology in the MS. The most challenging of these is the **pterygoid venous plexus** as this structure has a wide range of sizes in normal individuals. Asymmetric pterygoid venous plexus can mimic an infiltrative mass or PNT involving the pterygoid muscles. It lies within and around the pterygoid muscles in the medial MS.

A 2nd pseudolesion of note is **denervation of the muscles of mastication**. In the acute phase of denervation, the affected muscles may be mistaken for tumor infiltration, as they enlarge from swelling and enhance. The sparing of the muscle ligaments is an important clue to the true diagnosis. In late or chronic denervation, the involved muscles lose volume and fatty infiltrate. In these cases, the asymmetric normal muscle bulk on the contralateral side, compared to the denervated muscular atrophy, can be mistaken for a tumor.

A 3rd potential pseudolesion is **benign masticator muscle hypertrophy**. This can mimic a mass lesion clinically due to asymmetric enlargement of the muscles of mastication; however, normal muscle attenuation and signal, lack of enhancement, and preserved internal architecture (with normal striated appearance typical of muscle tissue) helps distinguish this pseudolesion from pathology.

Finally, **prominent or asymmetrical accessory lobe of the parotid gland** can mimic a mass on clinical examination, especially when asymmetrically enlarged on one side. The accessory lobe typically has the same density or signal and enhancement pattern as the remainder of the parotid gland on CT or MR imaging, which helps distinguish this pseudolesion from pathology.

Clinical Implications

A common clinical presentation of a MS mass is **trismus**. Trismus is defined as an inability to open the mouth due to masticator muscle spasm or fibrosis. Patients with trismus are notoriously difficult to examine clinically, so imaging plays an even more important role in assessing these patients.

The most frequent primary neoplasm of the MS is **sarcoma**, either from the mandible or soft tissues. However, extension of **oral cavity squamous cell carcinoma** from the **mandibular alveolar ridge** is far more common than primary MS malignancy; therefore, evidence of a mucosal origin should always be sought.

Tumefactive TMJ lesions must also be considered whenever there is a mass found in the peri-TMJ portion of the MS. While imaging characteristics of **chondrosarcoma** of the TMJ can sometimes appear similar to synovial chondromatosis, pathologic confirmation may be needed. Tenosynovial giant cell tumor and calcium pyrophosphate dihydrate deposition disease are additional TMJ lesions that must be added to the list of tumor-like lesions in the MS.

The presence of PNT is critical to the prognosis and care of cancer patients. PNT may require additional surgery, chemotherapy, &/or radiation therapy. If PNT reaches the intracranial compartment, tumor may be unresectable. Enhanced, fat-saturated MR is far more sensitive for PNT in the soft tissues and extension intracranially, compared to CT. As a result, MR should be recommended in patients who are at risk for PNT. One final caveat regarding PNT: Only a high degree of suspicion during image analysis will allow the radiologist to diagnose subtle PNT.

Selected References

1. Motta G et al: A rare case of extracranial schwannoma in the masticator space removed by endoscopic assisted transoral approach (EATA). Oral Oncol. 161:107164, 2025
2. Young K et al: Infratemporal fossa abscesses: a systematic review of cases. Ear Nose Throat J. 104(6):375-82, 2025
3. Hsieh KJ et al: Perineural spread of tumor in the skull base and head and neck. Oral Maxillofac Surg Clin North Am. 35(3):399-412, 2023
4. Chughtai S et al: Radiographic review of anatomy and pathology of the masticator space: what the emergency radiologist needs to know. Emerg Radiol. 27(3):329-39, 2020

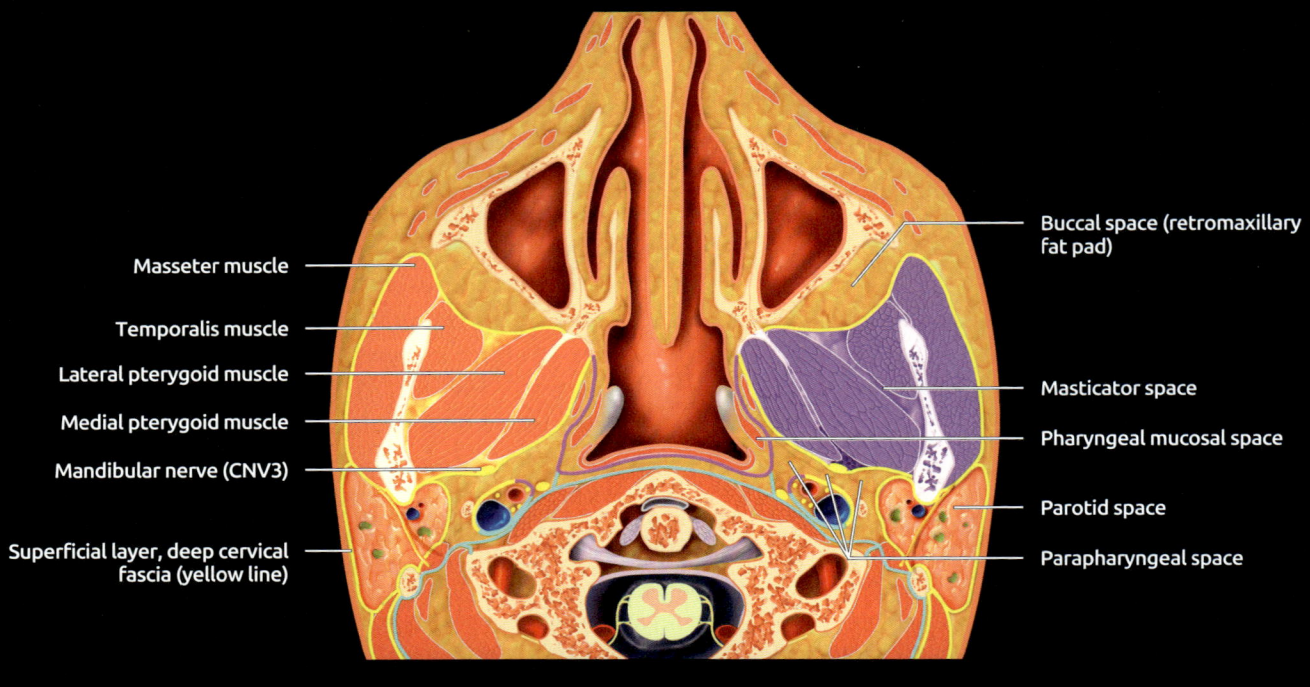

Masseter muscle

Temporalis muscle

Lateral pterygoid muscle

Medial pterygoid muscle

Mandibular nerve (CNV3)

Superficial layer, deep cervical fascia (yellow line)

Buccal space (retromaxillary fat pad)

Masticator space

Pharyngeal mucosal space

Parotid space

Parapharyngeal space

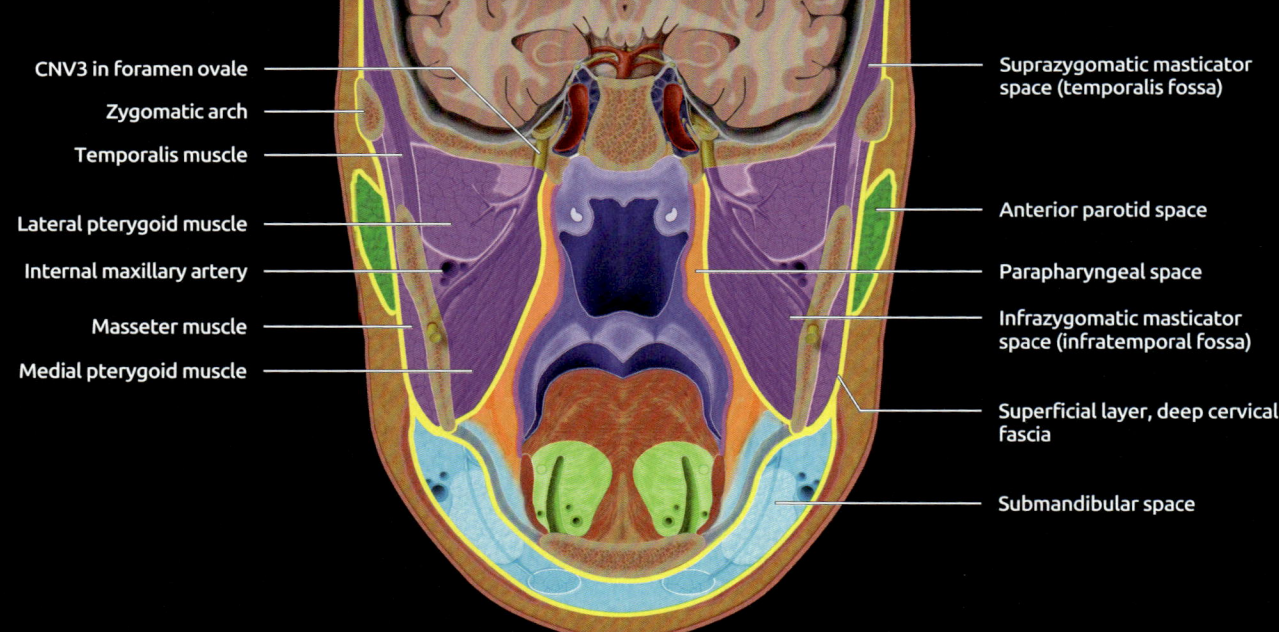

CNV3 in foramen ovale

Zygomatic arch

Temporalis muscle

Lateral pterygoid muscle

Internal maxillary artery

Masseter muscle

Medial pterygoid muscle

Suprazygomatic masticator space (temporalis fossa)

Anterior parotid space

Parapharyngeal space

Infrazygomatic masticator space (infratemporal fossa)

Superficial layer, deep cervical fascia

Submandibular space

(Top) *Axial graphic shows the masticator space (MS) enclosed by the superficial layer (investing layer) of the deep cervical fascia (yellow line). The muscles of mastication from medial to lateral are the medial and lateral pterygoid, temporalis, and masseter muscles. Note the mandibular nerve (CNV3 main trunk) lies just posterior to the medial pterygoid muscle, inside the superficial layer of deep cervical fascia. The buccal space is anterior, while the parapharyngeal and parotid space are posterior to the MS. The pharyngeal mucosal space is medial.* (Bottom) *Coronal graphic of the MS shows the suprazygomatic and infrazygomatic components. Note the medial slip of the superficial layer of the deep cervical fascia attaching to the skull base just medial to the foramen ovale, while the lateral slip continues over the zygomatic arch and up the parietal bone.*

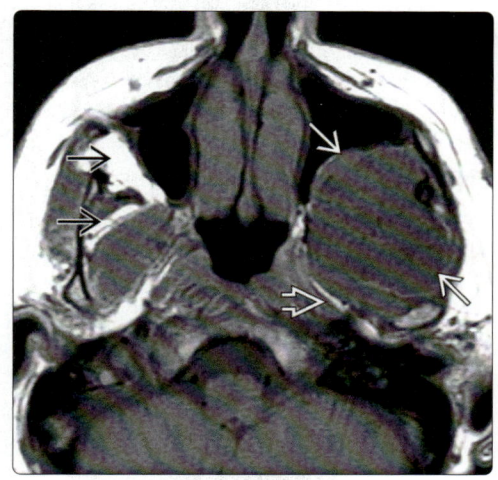

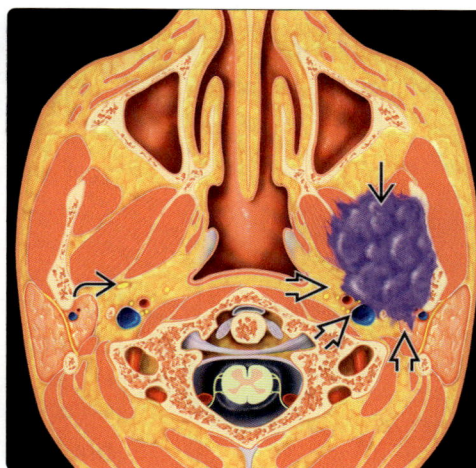

(Left) *Axial T1 MR shows a large MS mass ➡. Parapharyngeal fat ⇨ is displaced posteromedially. The muscles of mastication are invaded, and surrounding fat planes are replaced by tumor. Note the preserved fat planes in the contralateral MS ➡ for comparison.* (Right) *Axial graphic shows a generic MS mass ➡ invading the surrounding parapharyngeal space ⇨ from anterior to posterior. The mandibular nerve is engulfed by the tumor. Note the normal contralateral mandibular nerve ➡ for comparison.*

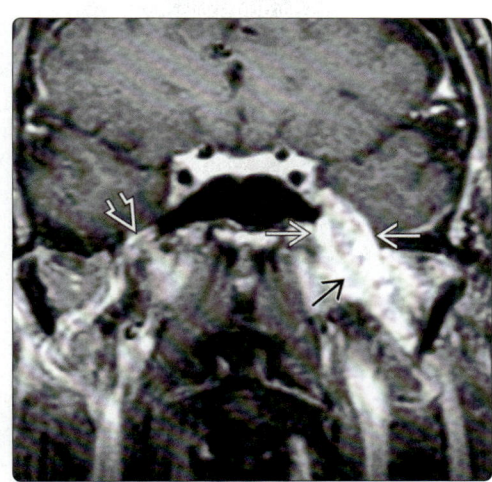

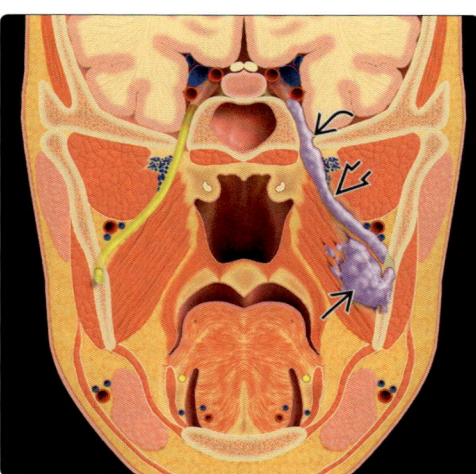

(Left) *Coronal T1 C+ FS MR shows perineural tumor ➡ along CNV3, widening foramen ovale ➡ as it extends intracranially. Compare the perineural tumor to the opposite normal size of the contralateral foramen ⇨, where normal perineural enhancement can be seen.* (Right) *Coronal graphic of the suprahyoid neck demonstrates a generic malignant tumor of the MS ➡ spreading in a perineural fashion along CNV3 ⇨. Notice the tumor traversing the foramen ovale ➡ into the intracranial compartment.*

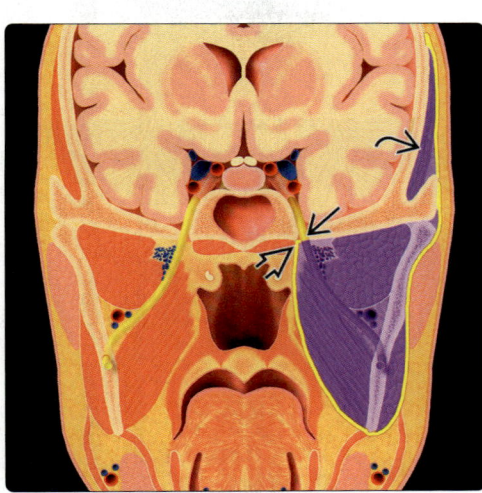

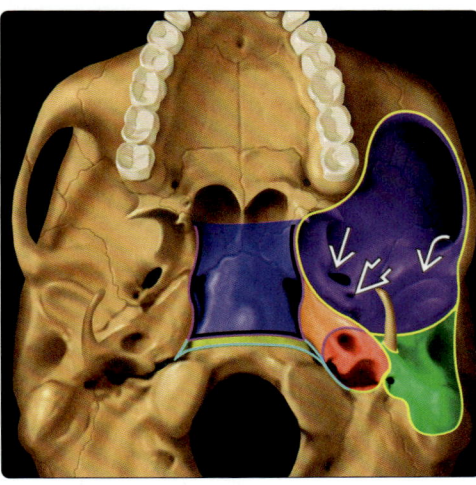

(Left) *Coronal graphic shows craniocaudal extent of MS. CNV3 passes through foramen ovale ➡ near the medial attachment of the superficial layer of the deep cervical fascia ⇨. Note the more superior suprazygomatic MS ➡.* (Right) *Axial skull base graphic depicts the large area of abutment of the MS (purple). The yellow line around the outer MS margin represents the superficial layer of deep cervical fascia. Note the foramen ovale ➡ and spinosum ⇨ and the TMJ ➡ within the MS abutment.*

TERMINOLOGY

- Unilateral prominence of deep facial venous network draining cavernous sinus
- Usually incidental finding at time of brain or neck imaging

IMAGING

- Tubular enhancing structures in medial masticator space (MS) & parapharyngeal space
- Postcontrast imaging shows identical enhancement to other neck veins
- Relevant imaging anatomy
  - Cavernous sinus drains to pterygoid venous plexus (PVP) through foramina ovale, spinosum, & lacerum
  - PVP connects with ophthalmic veins through inferior orbital fissure & anterior facial vein via deep facial branch
  - Receives tributaries correlating to pterygopalatine maxillary artery
  - PVP drainage 1: Maxillary vein → retromandibular vein → internal jugular vein (IJV)
  - PVP drainage 2: Posterior & common facial veins → IJV
- Flow signal is often seen in left > right PVP on 3T MRA images in normal patients
  - This may reflect flow reversal & should not be considered indicative of occult dural arteriovenous fistula
- Protocol advice: Thin-slice CTA/CTV

TOP DIFFERENTIAL DIAGNOSES

- Prominent internal maxillary arterial branches
- Venous vascular malformation
- Perineural V3 tumor, pterygopalatine fossa
- Carotid cavernous fistula (CCF)

CLINICAL ISSUES

- Commonly asymptomatic, incidental/developmental
- Potential intracranial conduit of face/sinus infection

DIAGNOSTIC CHECKLIST

- Consider ipsilateral CCF if there are referable symptoms
- Differentiate PVP asymmetry from CNV3 PNT

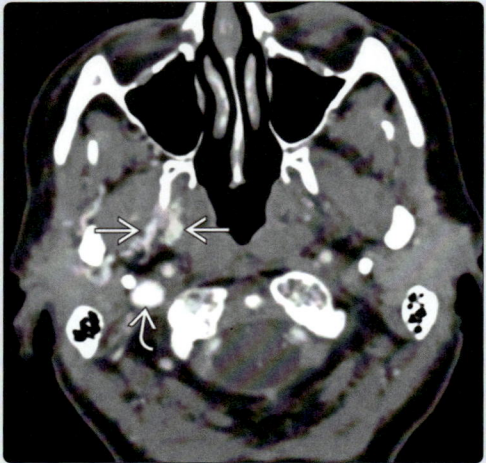
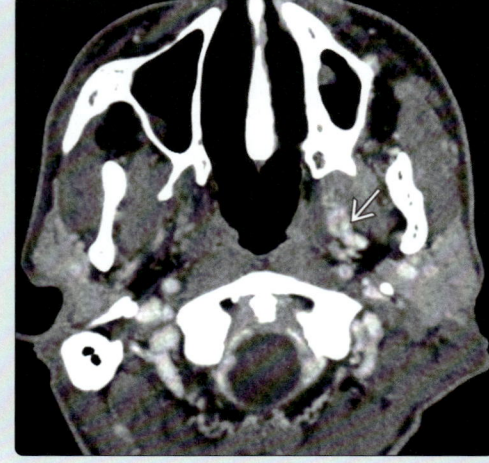

(Left) *Axial venous-phase CTA shows an asymmetric, enlarged right pterygoid venous plexus ➡. Note how enhancement parallels the internal jugular vein ➡.* (Right) *Axial CECT shows curvilinear enhancement in the medial masticator and parapharyngeal spaces ➡ due to an incidental, enlarged, asymmetric left pterygoid venous plexus. Enhancement is similar to other veins.*

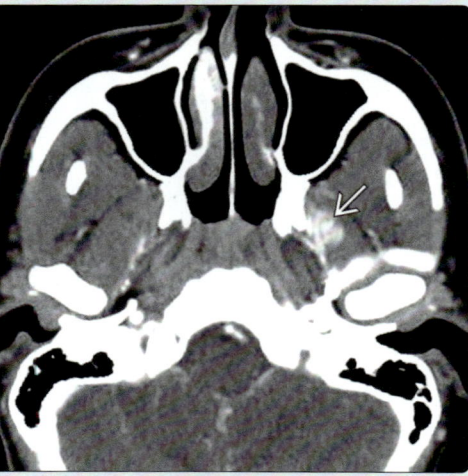
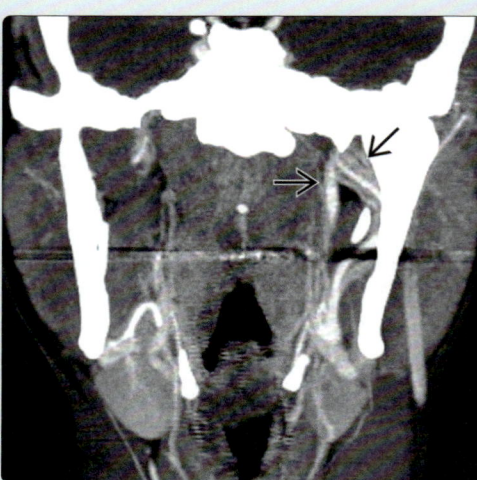

(Left) *Axial CECT shows mass-like enhancement in the medial masticator space ➡, representing incidental, asymmetric enlargement of the left pterygoid venous plexus.* (Right) *Coronal reconstructed CECT in the same patient better demonstrates the linear converging vascular structures ➡, representing incidental, asymmetric enlargement of the left pterygoid venous plexus.*

TERMINOLOGY

Abbreviations

- Pterygoid venous plexus (PVP)

Synonyms

- Pterygoid plexus

Definitions

- Unilateral prominence of deep facial venous network draining cavernous sinus
  - Usually incidental finding on brain or neck imaging
    - Can be misinterpreted as lesion when asymmetric
  - May be secondary to underlying carotid cavernous fistula (CCF) or arteriovenous malformation
    - Angiography indicated in symptomatic patients

IMAGING

General Features

- Best diagnostic clue
  - Tubular enhancing structures in medial masticator space (MS) & parapharyngeal space (PPS)
- Location
  - PVP is medial to pterygoid muscle in MS & in PPSs
- Size
  - Several millimeters in width, runs anteromedially several centimeters
- Morphology
  - Serpiginous structures in deep MS, anterior PPS
- Relevant imaging anatomy
  - PVP drains nasal cavity, paranasal sinuses, & nasopharynx
  - Cavernous sinus drains to PVP through foramen ovale, spinosum, & lacerum
  - PVP connects with ophthalmic veins through inferior orbital fissure & anterior facial vein via deep facial branch
    - Receives tributaries correlating to pterygopalatine maxillary artery
  - PVP drainage
    - Maxillary vein → retromandibular vein → internal jugular vein (IJV)
    - Posterior & common facial veins → IJV

CT Findings

- NECT
  - Poorly seen without contrast
- CECT
  - Asymmetric curvilinear enhancement in MS & PPS near pterygoid muscle
- CTA
  - Thin-slice CTA/CTV may best clarify with venous phase
    - Enhancement identical or similar to other veins

MR Findings

- T1WI
  - Serpiginous flow voids in medial MS & anterior PPS
- T2WI
  - Serpiginous T2 hyperintensity medial MS & anterior PPS
  - May have flow voids; signal depends on flow velocity
- T1WI C+
  - Uniform enhancement of PVP (similar to other veins)
  - Looks like small area of "worms" or curvilinear veins

- MRA
  - Flow signal is often seen in left > right PVP on 3T MRA images in normal patients
    - May reflect flow reversal & should not be considered indicative of occult dural arteriovenous fistula (DAVF)

Angiographic Findings

- AP projection best demonstrates drainage of cavernous sinus through skull base to PVP

Imaging Recommendations

- Best imaging tool
  - Enhanced CT or MR
- Protocol advice
  - Dynamic-phase CTA or CTV if needed to confirm

DIFFERENTIAL DIAGNOSIS

Prominent Internal Maxillary Arterial Branches

- Origin internal maxillary artery of external carotid artery

Venous Vascular Malformation

- Transspatial lobulated or cystic masses with high T2 signal
- Venous component may have phleboliths

Perineural V3 Tumor, Pterygopalatine Fossa

- Search for perineural tumor (PNT) may yield conspicuous PVP asymmetry
  - Must sort out PNT from PVP asymmetry
  - Linear anatomic nerve course in PNT distinguishes from serpiginous veins in PVP

Carotid Cavernous Fistula

- Enlarged, ipsilateral superior ophthalmic vein, cavernous sinus, & inferior petrosal sinus
- Conventional angiography to confirm

CLINICAL ISSUES

Presentation

- Most common signs/symptoms
  - Asymptomatic, incidental CT or MR finding
  - If due to CCF, symptoms reflect high- or low-flow CCF
  - Potential intracranial conduit of face/sinus infection

Demographics

- Epidemiology
  - Reasonably frequent finding on brain or neck imaging

Natural History & Prognosis

- If incidental finding, then of no clinical concern
- If related to CCF, requires interventional treatment

DIAGNOSTIC CHECKLIST

Consider

- Differentiate PVP asymmetry from CNV3 PNT
- Consider ipsilateral CCF if there are referable symptoms

SELECTED REFERENCES

1. Gopal N et al: Ten must know pseudolesions of the head and neck. Emerg Radiol. 28(1):119-26, 2021
2. Tanwar M et al: Mimics of perineural tumor spread in the head and neck. Br J Radiol. 94(1128):20210099, 2021
3. Golub B, Bordoni B. Neuroanatomy, pterygoid plexus. StatPearls, 2020

Benign Masticator Muscle Hypertrophy

IMAGING

- Smooth, diffuse enlargement of masticator muscles
  - Masseter, temporalis, medial, &/or lateral pterygoids
    - Masseter muscle most obviously affected
  - Muscles enhance normally
  - Effacement of adjacent fat
- 50% bilateral, usually asymmetric
- CT: Enlarged, normal-density masticator muscles
  - Cortical thickening affecting mandible and zygomatic arch
- MR: Enlarged, normal-intensity masticator muscles

TOP DIFFERENTIAL DIAGNOSES

- Masticator space (MS) pseudolesion
  - Contralateral MS muscle atrophy
- MS abscess
- MS sarcoma
- MS squamous cell carcinoma (SCCa)
  - MS mass via direct invasion or perineural spread

PATHOLOGY

- **Bruxism** (nocturnal teeth grinding)
- Habitual gum chewing
- TMJ dysfunction
- Anabolic steroids ± unilateral chewing

CLINICAL ISSUES

- Nontender lateral facial mass that enlarges with jaw clenching
  - Masseter muscle most obvious clinical finding
- Benign, slowly progressive muscle enlargement
- Treatment
  - Surgery only for cosmetic reasons
  - Botulinum toxin A injection
  - Treat TMJ dysfunction

DIAGNOSTIC CHECKLIST

- Enlarged muscle(s) of MS are isodense (CT) or isointense (MR) to normal skeletal muscle

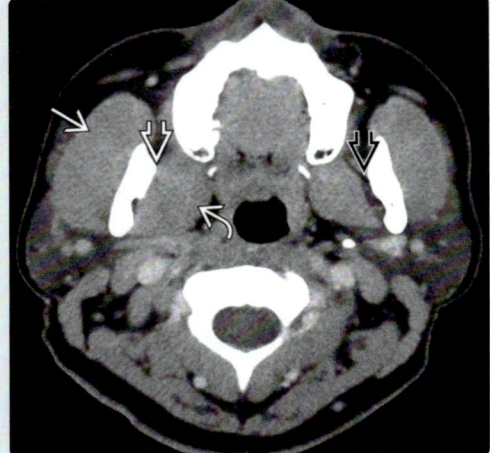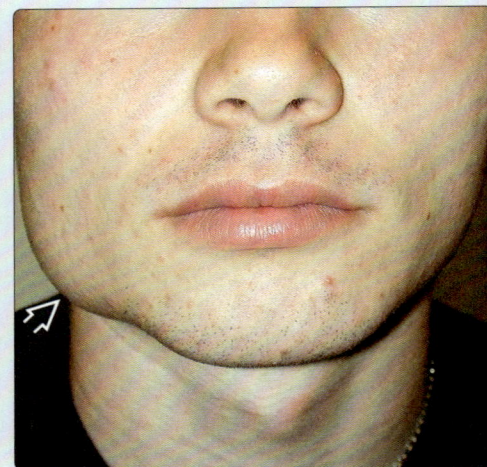

(Left) Axial CECT in a 42-year-old woman with a clinically suspected right parotid mass shows an asymmetric right masseter ⮕ and medial pterygoid muscle enlargement ⬈, consistent with benign hypertrophy. The parotid appears normal. Note effaced fat pads ⮕ compared to the normal side ⬋. (Right) Clinical photograph demonstrates the clinical appearance of a patient with unilateral benign masticator muscle hypertrophy. Note the broad, smooth cheek bulge secondary to the enlarged masseter muscle ⮕.

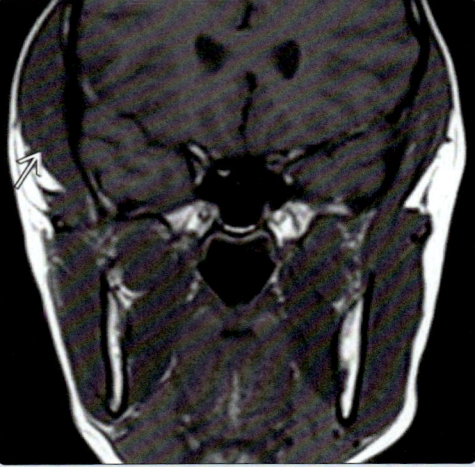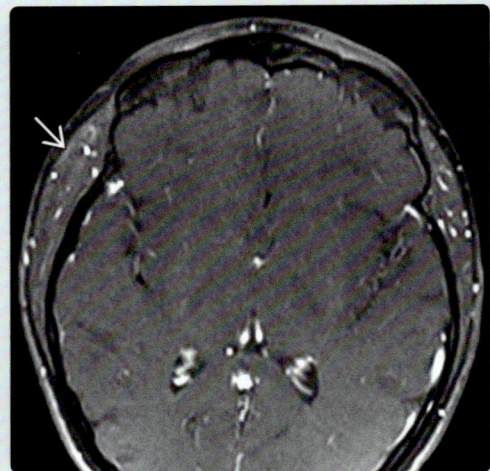

(Left) Coronal T1 MR shows asymmetric enlargement of the right temporalis muscle ⮕ in a young teenager complaining of the cosmetic deformity when wearing her hair pulled back in a ponytail. Although masseter hypertrophy is more common, any muscle can be involved. (Right) Axial T1 C+ FS MR shows normal muscle signal intensity in the enlarged right temporalis without abnormal enhancement ⮕ in the same patient.

TERMINOLOGY

Abbreviations
- Benign masticator muscle hypertrophy (BMMH)

Synonyms
- Benign masseteric hypertrophy

Definitions
- Benign enlargement of muscles of mastication (temporalis, masseter, medial, and lateral pterygoids)

IMAGING

General Features
- Best diagnostic clue
  - Smooth, diffuse enlargement of masticator muscles
- Location
  - Masticator space (MS); masseter muscle most obviously affected
  - 50% bilateral, usually asymmetric

Radiographic Findings
- Radiography
  - May have flaring of mandibular angle with exostosis at masseteric insertion

CT Findings
- NECT
  - Enlarged, normal-density masticator muscles
  - 3D CT may be used to assess response to botulinum toxin type A (Botox) injection
  - Adjacent fat pads effaced due to muscle enlargement
- CECT
  - Enlarged masticator muscles enhance normally
- Bone CT
  - Cortical thickening of mandible and zygomatic arch

MR Findings
- T1WI
  - Enlarged, normal-intensity masticator muscles
  - Less marrow signal in areas of cortical thickening (mandible, zygomatic arch)
- T2WI
  - Enlarged, normal-intensity masticator muscles
- T1WI C+
  - Enlarged masticator muscles enhance normally

Ultrasonographic Findings
- Enlarged masseter muscle with normal echogenicity
- Can be used to guide Botox injection and assess for posttreatment hematoma

Nuclear Medicine Findings
- May have intense FDG uptake on PET

Other Modality Findings
- Sialography: Parotid duct displaced by large masseter

Imaging Recommendations
- Best imaging tool
  - CECT or T1 C+ MR excellent in evaluating MS lesions
- Protocol advice
  - Bone and soft tissue algorithms on CECT data

DIFFERENTIAL DIAGNOSIS

Masticator Space Pseudolesion
- Contralateral small masticator muscles (atrophy) make normal MS appear hypertrophic

Masticator Space Abscess
- Rim-enhancing fluid in MS ± mandibular osteomyelitis

Masticator Space Sarcoma
- Primary malignancy of MS

Masticator Space Squamous Cell Carcinoma, Direct Invasion or Perineural Tumor (V3)
- Enters MS directly (retromolar trigone, faucial tonsil)
- Enters MS via perineural V3 from chin skin squamous cell carcinoma (SCCa) or SCCa (mandibular alveolar ridge)

PATHOLOGY

General Features
- Etiology
  - **Bruxism** (nocturnal teeth grinding), gum chewing, TMJ dysfunction
  - Anabolic steroids ± unilateral chewing

Microscopic Features
- Normal skeletal muscle
- Process may involve hyperplasia (↑ number of fibers) rather than true hypertrophy

CLINICAL ISSUES

Presentation
- Most common signs/symptoms
  - Nontender lateral facial mass
    - Enlarges with jaw clenching
  - Rare cause of parotitis due to kinking of Stensen duct

Demographics
- Age
  - Usually begins in adolescence
- Sex
  - M:F = 2:1

Natural History & Prognosis
- Benign, slowly progressive masticator muscle enlargement

Treatment
- Surgery only for cosmetic reasons
- Botulinum toxin A injection
- Treat TMJ dysfunction

DIAGNOSTIC CHECKLIST

Image Interpretation Pearls
- Enlarged muscle(s) of mastication should be isodense (CT) or isointense (MR) to normal skeletal muscle

SELECTED REFERENCES
1. Ferrillo M et al: The role of botulinum toxin for masseter muscle hypertrophy: a comprehensive review. Toxins (Basel). 17(2):91, 2025
2. Gopal N et al: Ten must know pseudolesions of the head and neck. Emerg Radiol. 28(1):119-26, 2021

TERMINOLOGY

- Abbreviations: Trigeminal nerve (CNV)
- Mandibular nerve: 3rd division of CNV (CNV3)
  - Only division with motor function
  - Involved muscles: Masticator space (muscles of mastication), nasopharynx (tensor veli palatini), and anterior belly digastric and mylohyoid muscles
- CNV3 denervation atrophy: Alteration in appearance of muscle groups from loss of innervation
  - Patterns of muscle involvement determined by location of injury to mandibular nerve ramification
    - Proximal involves all muscles, distal spares masticator

IMAGING

- **Acute**: Slightly enlarged, T2-hyperintense edema of muscles and abnormal contrast enhancement
- **Subacute**: T2 hyperintensity with early fatty replacement and abnormal diminishing contrast enhancement
- **Chronic**: Fatty infiltration of muscles with volume loss

- MR imaging tips
  - FS T2/STIR: T2 hyperintensity more visible
  - FS on T1 C+: Enhancement more visible

TOP DIFFERENTIAL DIAGNOSES

- Masticator muscle hypertrophy
- Masticator space abscess
- Masticator space sarcoma
- Progressive hemifacial atrophy (Parry Romberg) syndrome

PATHOLOGY

- Malignant or benign tumors involving CNV3
- Surgery and trauma frequent causes; pontine causes rare

DIAGNOSTIC CHECKLIST

- 1st confirm that muscles involved reflect CNV3 denervation
- 2nd determine cause of CNV3 denervation
- Review history for obvious episodes of trauma or surgery
- If none, search for malignant CNV3 perineural tumor
  - Evaluate location based on denervation pattern

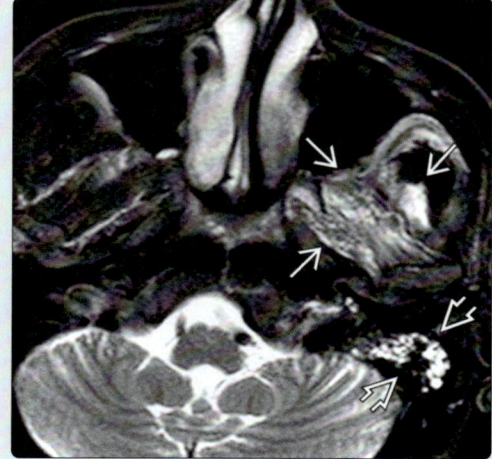
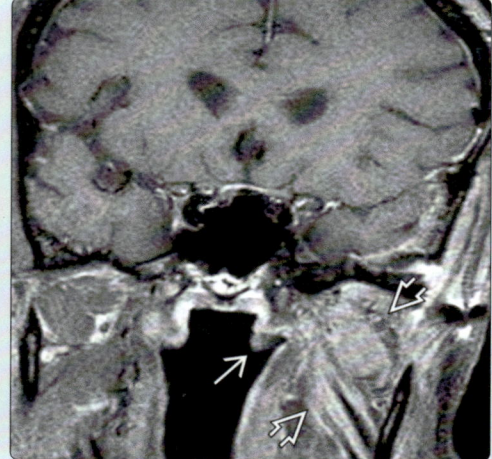

(Left) Axial T2 FS MR demonstrates increased signal in the pterygoid muscles and deep portion of temporalis muscle ➡. Mastoid opacification ⤳ indicates eustachian tube obstruction due to tensor veli palatini dysfunction. This patient had meningioma in Meckel cave (not shown). (Right) Coronal T1 C+ FS MR in the same patient shows mild pterygoid muscle enhancement ➡ as well as small size of left torus tubarius ➡, consistent with subacute denervation atrophy of CNV3.

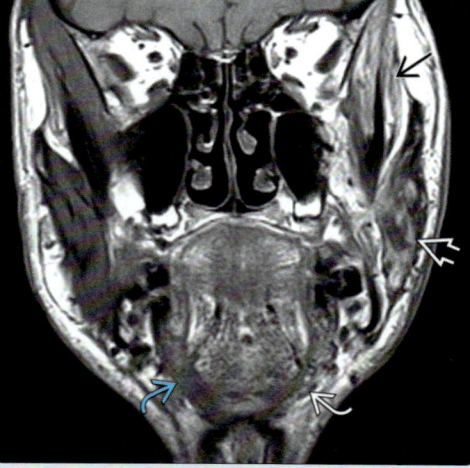
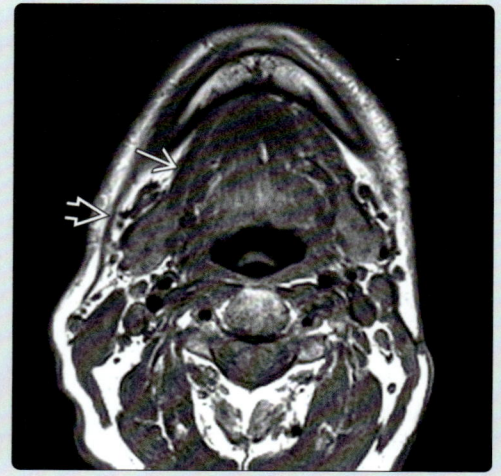

(Left) Coronal T1 MR reveals chronic fatty atrophy of the left temporalis ➡ and masseter ➡ muscle, indicating chronic CNV3 injury. The left mylohyoid muscle ➡ is also small with fatty infiltration compared to the normal right mylohyoid muscle ➡. (Right) Axial T1 MR in the same patient demonstrates the normal right mylohyoid muscle ➡ and platysma muscle ➡. Absence/marked atrophy on the left indicates that both CNV3 (mylohyoid) and CNVII (platysma) are chronically injured.

TERMINOLOGY

Abbreviations

- Trigeminal nerve (CNV)
  o Mandibular nerve: 3rd division (CNV3) of CNV
    – Only division of CNV with motor function

Synonyms

- Denervation atrophy

Definitions

- CNV3 motor denervation: Alteration in appearance of muscle groups from loss of innervation by CNV3
- Denervation pattern identified
  o **Acute** (< 1 month): Muscles slightly enlarged with edema; enhancement seen
  o **Subacute** (≤ 12-20 months): Fatty replacement and atrophy begins
  o **Chronic** (> 12-20 months): Fatty atrophic muscles with significant volume loss

IMAGING

General Features

- Best diagnostic clue
  o Acute: Increased T2 signal intensity with edema of muscles and abnormal contrast enhancement
  o Subacute: T2 prolongation and abnormal contrast enhancement with early fatty replacement
  o Chronic: Fatty infiltration of muscles with volume loss
- Location
  o Most frequently unilateral process
  o CNV3 innervation muscles: **Masticator space** (muscles of mastication), tensor veli palatini in nasopharynx, and anterior belly digastric and mylohyoid muscles
  o Ipsilateral parotid atrophy can accompany chronic CNV3 denervation; proposed theories on etiology
    – Involvement of auriculotemporal nerve
    – Disuse atrophy from decreased ipsilateral mastication and decreased salivary flow
- Size
  o Acute: Muscles slightly enlarged
  o Subacute: Muscles may be normal size
  o Chronic: Muscles atrophic
- Morphology
  o Initially muscle edema; later fatty replacement and atrophy
- **CNV3 motor innervation**
  o Muscles of mastication
    – Medial and lateral pterygoid, masseter, and temporalis muscles
  o Tensor muscles
    – Tensor veli palatini and tensor tympani muscles
  o Mylohyoid and anterior belly digastric muscles

CT Findings

- CECT
  o Acute and subacute CNV3 denervation atrophy
    – Altered density and enhancement may be difficult to identify (MR more sensitive)
  o Chronic CNV3 denervation atrophy
    – Fatty atrophic change readily evident

MR Findings

- T1WI
  o Acute: Reduced muscle signal intensity from edema
  o Subacute: Increased signal intensity starts with fatty replacement
  o Chronic: Increased signal intensity with fatty atrophy
- T2WI
  o Acute: Increased T2 signal intensity of muscles (edema)
  o Subacute: Increased T2 signal intensity (early fat)
  o Chronic: Volume loss and fatty infiltration
- T1WI C+
  o **Acute**: Muscle **enhancement**
  o Subacute: Muscle enhancement more subtle
  o Chronic: No contrast enhancement

Imaging Recommendations

- Best imaging tool
  o MR best characterizes changes of muscles
    – Most sensitive to altered contrast enhancement
  o CT readily identifies chronic fatty atrophic changes
    – Relatively insensitive to earlier changes
- Protocol advice
  o FS
    – STIR/T2 FS: Makes T2 hyperintensity more evident
    – T1 C+ FS: Makes enhancement more evident
  o Contrast distinguishes acute and subacute from chronic

DIFFERENTIAL DIAGNOSIS

Masticator Muscle Hypertrophy

- Clinical: TMJ dysfunction or bruxism (nocturnal teeth grinding)
- CT/MR: Normal side appears "too small" compared to enlarged, hypertrophic muscles
  o Masseter most frequently enlarged of masticator muscles
  o Mylohyoid, anterior belly digastric not affected
  o Normal muscle signal intensity (no T2 hyperintense edema) and no abnormal contrast enhancement

Masticator Space Abscess

- Clinical: Presents with pain, fever, and elevated WBC
- CT/MR: Will not involve all muscle groups
  o Look particularly at temporalis, mylohyoid, and digastric
  o Look for dental source of infection
- Myositis &/or phlegmon most likely to mimic acute denervation since no fluid collection

Masticator Space Sarcoma

- Clinical: History of new or treated deep facial malignancy or enlarging mass unresponsive to antibiotics
- CT/MR: Will not involve all muscle groups

Progressive Hemifacial Atrophy (Parry Romberg) Syndrome

- Diffuse hemifacial atrophy
- Atrophic changes not limited to muscles but also affect fat
- Muscles involved may not follow expected pattern for CNV3 denervation
- Increased seizures, parotid and submandibular gland abnormalities

PATHOLOGY

General Features

- Etiology
  - Masticator space perineural tumor, CNV3
    - Clinical: Usually from squamous cell carcinoma of chin skin, mandible alveolar ridge, deep palatine tonsil
    - CT/MR: Thickened, enhancing CNV3
    - Perineural tumor and CNV3 motor atrophy often coexist if nerve injury present
  - Surgical trauma frequent cause
  - Hemifacial atrophy can rarely occur from unilateral bulbar poliomyelitis infection
  - Hemorrhage/infarcts involving pontine trigeminal nucleus may rarely cause isolated trigeminal motor neuropathy and denervation
- Associated abnormalities
  - Other cranial nerves may also be affected
    - CNVII, X, XI, ± XII (depending on size/location of offending lesion)
- CNV3 denervation patterns due to location relative to branching (just after CNV3 emerges from foramen ovale)
  - Injury **proximal to** mandibular nerve ramification
    - **All muscles** innervated by CNV3 undergo atrophy
      □ Medial and lateral pterygoids, masseter, temporalis
      □ Tensor veli palatini and tensor tympani
      □ Mylohyoid and anterior belly digastric
  - Injury **distal to** mandibular nerve ramification
    - Mylohyoid and anterior belly digastric muscles atrophy
    - Muscles of mastication spared
  - May be helpful in identifying site of injury/lesion
    - If all CNV3 innervated muscles involved, lesion is between root exit zone of lateral pons and foramen ovale
    - If only mylohyoid and anterior belly of digastric muscle involved, lesion is between skull base and mandibular foramen

Gross Pathologic & Surgical Features

- Loss of muscle bulk and tone with fatty change

Microscopic Features

- Denervated muscle shows relatively increased tissue water
- Atrophy of muscle fibers develops in subacute to chronic phases with fatty infiltration
- Denervated, atrophic muscle shows greater concentration of capillaries for muscle volume

CLINICAL ISSUES

Presentation

- Most common signs/symptoms
  - Difficulty chewing
  - Facial asymmetry from masseter muscle volume loss visible in chronic atrophy
  - Denervation difficult to detect clinically
    - Paralysis, loss of tone and reflexes, fasciculations
  - MR STIR signal intensity changes precede electromyography (EMG) changes
- Other signs/symptoms
  - Serous otitis media from eustachian tube dysfunction with tensor veli palatini denervation

Demographics

- Age: Adults are more likely (vs. children) due to increased H&N tumors &/or surgery
- Epidemiology: CNV most frequent of cranial nerves to show motor denervation

Natural History & Prognosis

- With peripheral neuropathies, acute and subacute changes may resolve spontaneously or with nerve grafting
  - Not so with cranial neuropathies
  - Cranial nerve grafting does not significantly reverse CNV3 atrophy
- Acute denervation signal intensity and enhancement pattern to chronic atrophy pattern with time

Treatment

- No effective treatment

DIAGNOSTIC CHECKLIST

Consider

- If CNV3 atrophy is discovered without known cause, search for causal lesion must be completed

Image Interpretation Pearls

- 1st determine that CNV3 denervation is present by analyzing muscles involved
  - Look at all muscles innervated by CNV3
    - Muscles of mastication
    - Mylohyoid, anterior belly digastric muscles
    - Tensor veli palatini dysfunction → small torus tubarius and ipsilateral middle ear/mastoid fluid
    - Tensor tympani dysfunction not apparent by imaging
  - MR best to evaluate muscle signal and size changes for acute, subacute, or chronic denervation
- 2nd determine cause of CNV3 denervation
  - Review history for obvious episodes of trauma or surgery
    - If none, malignant tumor must be excluded
      □ Check for perineural CNV3 malignancy
      □ Follow course of CNV from lateral pons to mandibular foramen
- Finally, look for MR evidence of other CN dysfunction (especially CNVII, X-XII)

SELECTED REFERENCES

1. Gorolay VV et al: Neuroimaging and clinical features of Parry-Romberg syndrome and linear morphea en-coup-de-sabre in a large case series. Acad Radiol. 32(7):4154-63, 2025
2. Saks R et al: Pictorial review of cranial nerve denervation in the head and neck. Radiographics. 44(10):e240023, 2024
3. Kirsch CFE et al: Practical tips for MR imaging of perineural tumor spread. Magn Reson Imaging Clin N Am. 26(1):85-100, 2018
4. Badger D et al: Imaging of perineural spread in head and neck cancer. Radiol Clin North Am. 55(1):139-49, 2017
5. Schellhas KP: MR imaging of muscles of mastication. AJR Am J Roentgenol. 153(4):847-55, 1989
6. Polak JF et al: Magnetic resonance imaging of skeletal muscle. Prolongation of T1 and T2 subsequent to denervation. Invest Radiol. 23(5): 365-9, 1988
7. Harnsberger HR et al: Major motor atrophic patterns in the face and neck: CT evaluation. Radiology. 155(3):665-70, 1985

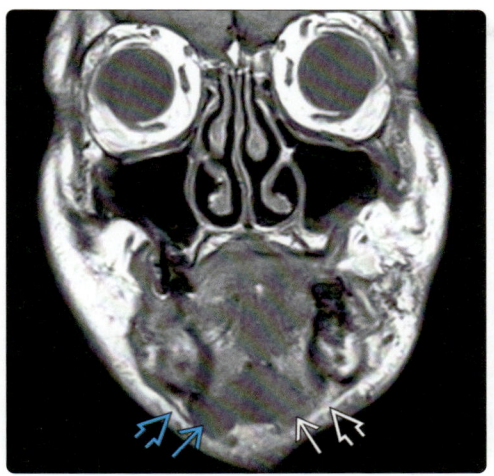

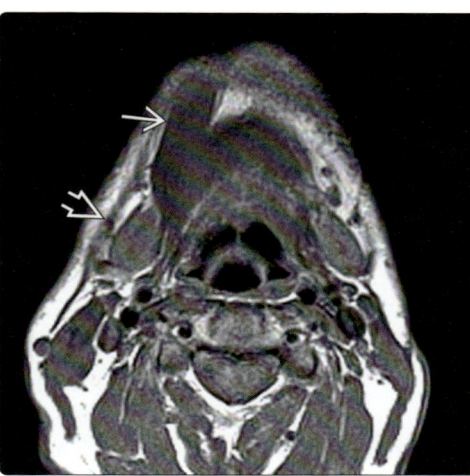

(Left) Coronal T1 MR reveals a normal right anterior belly of the digastric muscle ➡ and platysma muscle ⮕. The left-sided mylohyoid/anterior belly of digastric ➡ and platysma ⮕ are atrophic as a result of chronic CNV3 and CNVII injury, respectively. (Right) Axial T1 MR in the same patient shows a normal right anterior belly of digastric muscle ➡ and normal platysma muscle ➡. Both muscles on the left have undergone fatty atrophy and are not visible. A skull base malignant tumor was found, affecting the foramen ovale and geniculate fossa.

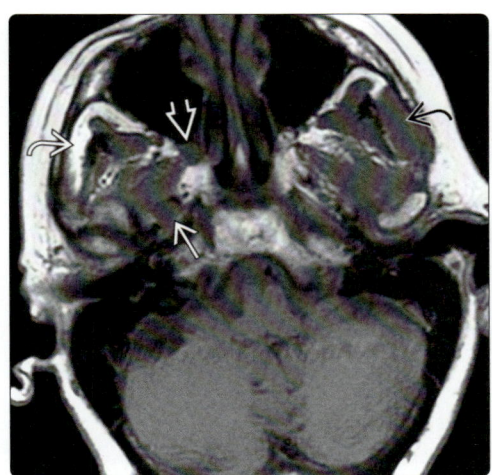

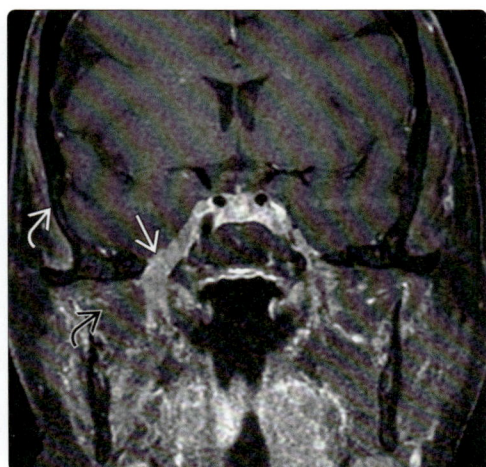

(Left) Axial T1 MR shows enlargement of the right mandibular nerve ➡ from perineural tumor spread. Note denervation atrophy of right masticator space muscles ⮕ compared to normal left side ⮕. Tumor also extends along V2 in the pterygopalatine fossa ➡. (Right) Coronal T1 C+ FS MR in same patient shows an enhancing tumor in the right foramen ovale ➡. Note atrophy of the right temporalis ⮕ and right pterygoids ➡ with little enhancement, supporting late subacute to chronic denervation.

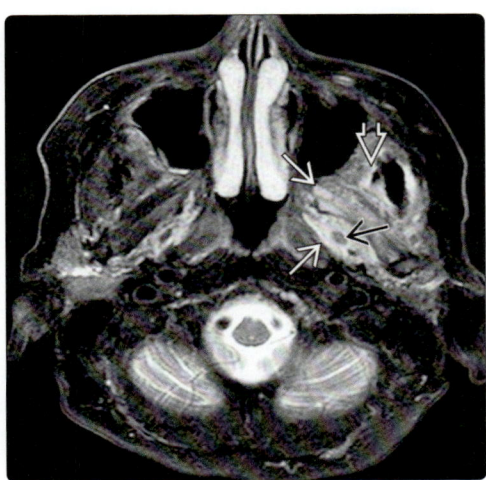

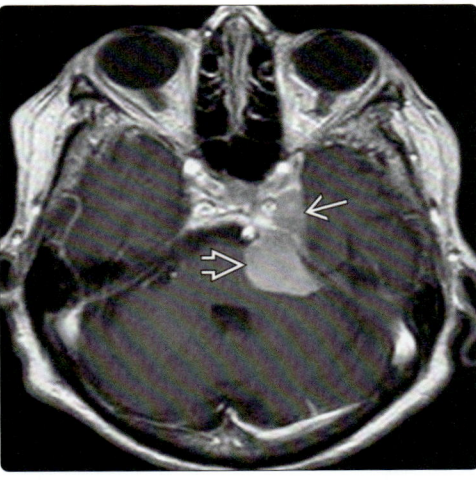

(Left) Axial T2 FS MR demonstrates T2 hyperintensity and swelling in the pterygoid ➡ and temporalis ⮕ muscles, indicating acute to subacute denervation atrophy. The mandibular nerve ➡ is visible here as a lower signal intensity structure within the masticator space. (Right) Axial T1 C+ MR in the same patient shows the cavernous sinus ➡ and prepontine cistern ⮕ meningioma, which is the cause of the denervation changes. Imaging findings of CNV schwannoma could appear similar.

Masticator Space Abscess

TERMINOLOGY

- Abscess in masticator space (MS), commonly from molar tooth infection or following dental procedure

IMAGING

- **CECT** preferred imaging modality in suspected infection
  - Soft tissue and bone algorithm CECT is best imaging approach in acutely infected patients with trismus
- **Focal fluid** with thick, **enhancing rim** within muscles of mastication = MS abscess
  - Adjacent muscles are swollen enhancing without fluid collection = myositis
  - Adjacent fat stranding = cellulitis
- Bone CT findings
  - Tooth: Periapical radiolucency, caries, or extraction socket ± gas
  - Mandibular cortical erosion
  - ± osteomyelitis: Mixed sclerosis and lucency with periosteal elevation, erosion

TOP DIFFERENTIAL DIAGNOSES

- Cellulitis-phlegmon of MS
- Mandibular osteonecrosis
- TMJ degenerative disease
- Masticator muscle hypertrophy
- Sarcoma of MS

CLINICAL ISSUES

- Principal symptom: Trismus, swelling, fever
- Initial presentation may be confused with TMJ disease
- Early MS abscess treated with involved molar extraction + aggressive IV antibiotics
- Late abscess treatment: Surgical drainage + IV antibiotics

DIAGNOSTIC CHECKLIST

- What is potential source (offending tooth)?
- Is mandibular osteomyelitis present?
- Is MS only space with abscess or extension?
- Is suprazygomatic MS involved?

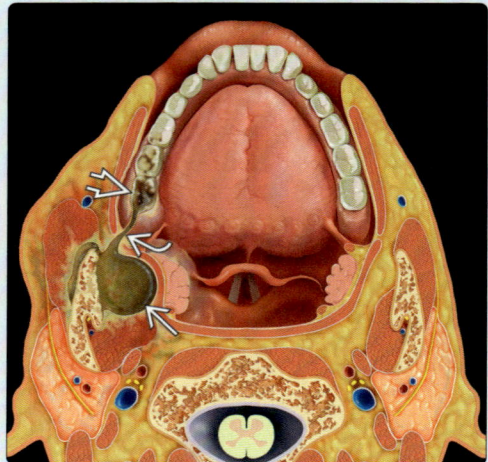 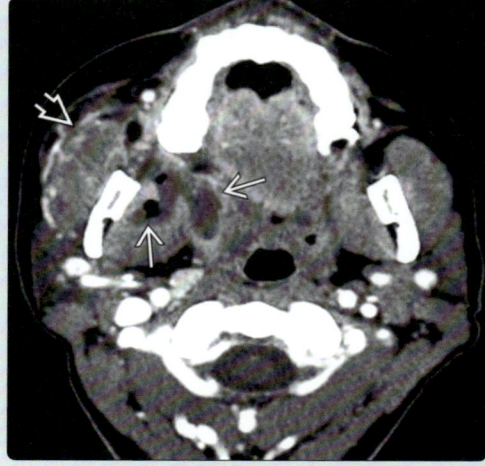

(Left) Axial graphic depicts a masticator space (MS) abscess ➡ arising from an infected posterior mandibular molar tooth ➡. Notice the fistula tract ➡ leading from the tooth to the abscess. (Right) Axial CECT in a 31-year-old with facial swelling, pain, and trismus demonstrates right medial MS abscess containing gas ➡. There is inflammatory change in the lateral MS with edema and enlargement of the masseter muscle ➡.

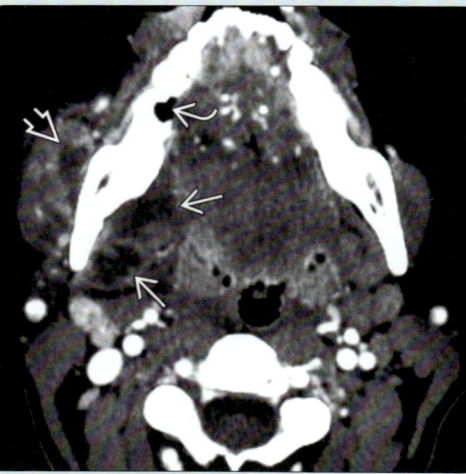 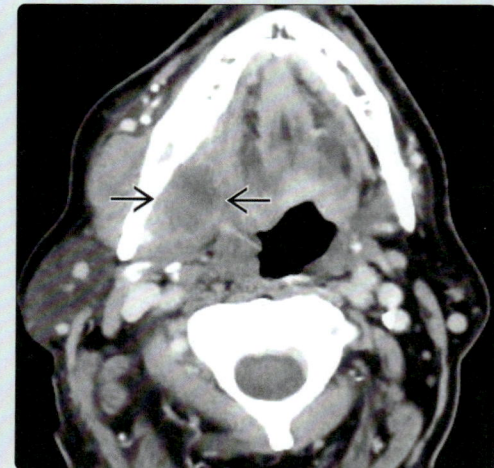

(Left) Axial CECT in the same patient shows further inferior extent of the medial MS abscess ➡ as well as lateral MS abscess ➡. Dental caries involving a posterior molar tooth is the origin of this patient's infection ➡. (Right) Axial CECT shows a well-marginated, peripherally enhancing dental origin abscess in the MS ➡ involving the medial pterygoid muscle, medial to the mandibular ramus.

TERMINOLOGY

Definitions

- Masticator space (MS) abscess: Fluid collection within MS
  - Usually odontogenic source: Arises from molar tooth infection or following dental procedure

IMAGING

General Features

- Best diagnostic clue
  - **Fluid collection with enhancing wall** within MS
- Location
  - Lower MS near posterior body and ramus of mandible
    - If severe, can also spread into nearby spaces
- Size
  - Early abscess: Often small (1-cm) fluid collection adjacent to mandible
  - Late, severe MS abscess: May be many centimeters, filling entire MS and beyond
- Morphology
  - Ovoid to round
  - If breaks into adjacent deep facial spaces, may be lobulated and irregular

CT Findings

- CECT
  - Focal **fluid density** within muscles of mastication with thick, **enhancing rim** = **MS abscess**
    - Adjacent muscles are swollen/edematous, enhancing without associated fluid = **myositis**
    - Adjacent fat stranding ("dirty" fat planes) = **cellulitis**
      □ Linear markings in subcutaneous fat and thickening of skin help differentiate infection from malignancy
  - MS mass lesion with compression of parapharyngeal space from anterolateral to posteromedial
- Bone CT
  - Typically **dental infection**, 2nd or 3rd molar tooth
    - Periapical lucency surrounding molar tooth root
    - Focal cavity/radiolucency ± gas involving tooth itself (caries)
    - Empty socket ± gas (dental extraction)
    - Fistula = radiolucent line leading from tooth area through bone into adjacent soft tissue
  - ± **mandibular osteomyelitis**: Cortical destruction with periosteal elevation
    - Posterior body and ramus mandible usually involved
- CTA
  - If abscess/infection extends to adjacent spaces, proximal internal carotid artery (ICA) may show **spasm**

MR Findings

- T1WI
  - Low-signal fluid adjacent to mandible
- T2WI
  - Focal high-signal fluid collections = MS abscess
- DWI
  - High signal (low ADC) characteristic of abscess
- T1WI C+
  - Focal low-signal area surrounded by **enhancing wall**
  - Sinus tract from mandible may be visible

- MRA
  - If MS abscess/infection has spread to adjacent spaces, proximal ICA spasm may be seen
    - More common in children, usually self-limited

Nuclear Medicine Findings

- Bone scan
  - Can be used to follow mandibular osteomyelitis response to antibiotic therapy

Dental X-Ray or Panorex

- Moth-eaten posterior mandibular body in vicinity of decaying molar tooth
  - Need additional imaging to determine presence and location of abscess

Imaging Recommendations

- Best imaging tool
  - Contrast-enhanced imaging for suspected infection ± abscess
  - **CECT** preferred: Better assessment of dentition, bones, and foci of gas
    - Rapid scan time, important for sick patient
    - MR less specific for dental infection and osteomyelitis
- Protocol advice
  - CECT viewed in soft tissue and bone algorithm is best imaging approach in setting of acutely infected patient with trismus (limited jaw movement)
    - Shows extent of soft tissue abscess cavity
    - Identifies offending tooth and extent of osteomyelitis (if not obscured by dental amalgam artifact)

DIFFERENTIAL DIAGNOSIS

Cellulitis-Phlegmon of Masticator Space

- Clinical: Painful, swollen MS; same as with MS abscess
- Imaging: Swollen MS with cellulitis, myositis ± fasciitis **without** focal rim-enhancing fluid

Mandibular Osteonecrosis

- Clinical: Usually associated with prior H&N radiation therapy or bisphosphonate use
  - **Radionecrosis** in setting of **prior H&N radiation**
    - Imaging: Permeative-destructive change of mandible bone ± soft tissue swelling
    - May have associated abscess
      □ Superimposed infection (osteomyelitis) is common
      □ Needle aspiration to help exclude infection
  - **Bisphosphonate-related osteonecrosis of jaws**
    - Bisphosphonates (IV or oral) are used to treat metabolic bone disorders, primary or metastatic bone tumors, and hypercalcemia of malignancy
    - Imaging: Osseous sclerosis on CT ranging from subtle thickening of lamina dura and alveolar crest to attenuated, osteopetrosis-like sclerosis
      □ May be associated with infection; risk factors include bone trauma, dental extractions or implants, periapical &/or periodontal surgery

TMJ Degenerative Disease

- Clinical: TMJ pain and trismus (no fever)
- Imaging: Degenerative findings in TMJ; no MS abscess

Masticator Muscle Hypertrophy

- Clinical: Asymmetric chewing, TMJ disease, or nocturnal grinding (no fever)
- Imaging: Unilateral enlargement of otherwise normal masticator muscles
  - No focal rim-enhancing fluid, cellulitis, or myositis

Sarcoma of Masticator Space

- Clinical: Hard cheek mass ± trigeminal nerve symptoms
- Imaging: Infiltrating MS mass with significant enhancement and minimal adjacent skin or soft tissue changes
  - Lacks cellulitis, myositis, or fasciitis to suggest infection

PATHOLOGY

General Features

- Etiology
  - Most common source is dental infection (molar) from caries ± periodontal disease or dental manipulation
    - Spreads via cortical dehiscence, rupturing pus into MS ± osteomyelitis of posterior body of mandible
  - May result from spread of infection from adjacent spaces
  - Less common causes include postoperative complications, TMJ arthritis, radiation, bisphosphonates
- Anatomic considerations
  - Superficial layer, deep cervical fascia circumscribes MS tissues
  - MS contains muscles of mastication, posterior body, ramus and condyle of mandible, and CNV3 as it passes into mandibular foramen
  - 2nd and 3rd molars abut anterior surface of MS
  - Temporal fossa = suprazygomatic MS
  - Infratemporal fossa = nasopharyngeal MS + retromaxillary fat pad (high posterior buccal space)

Gross Pathologic & Surgical Features

- Irregular cystic lesion filled with green-white thick fluid (pus) surrounded by thick wall made up of fibrous connective tissue
- Surrounding tissues are edematous

CLINICAL ISSUES

Presentation

- Most common signs/symptoms
  - Principal symptom: **Trismus**
    - Physical exam: Tenderness and limited mouth opening makes examination difficult
      - CECT becomes critical part of physical exam when patient cannot open mouth
  - Fever, high WBC count
  - Tender swollen cheek
  - History of **bad dentition** or recent **dental manipulation** common
- Other signs/symptoms
  - Initial presentation may clinically mimic **TMJ disease** (i.e., TMJ pain and trismus)

Demographics

- Age
  - Increasing incidence with age
    - Dental problems generally increase in older people

- Epidemiology
  - Common cause of MS lesion
  - In countries where antibiotics and dental care are readily available, MS involvement rare
  - When dental care and antibiotics are unavailable, MS abscess from dental decay is common

Natural History & Prognosis

- Commonly originates from infected tooth
- Clinical recrudescence occurs after oral antibiotics (inadequately treated/drained MS infection)
- Adequate drainage of pus leads to rapid cure
- Potential source of deep neck infection or necrotizing fasciitis if untreated

Treatment

- Remove decayed molars first
- Aggressive IV antibiotics for early abscess
- Surgical drainage + IV antibiotics needed in most cases
- Mandibular osteomyelitis may require subperiosteal drain and prolonged IV antibiotics

DIAGNOSTIC CHECKLIST

Consider

- Questions for radiologist to answer in MS abscess
  - What is potential source (offending tooth)?
    - Best to evaluate bone windows on CT
  - Is mandibular osteomyelitis present?
    - If so, requires more extensive surgical intervention and protracted antibiotic therapy
  - Is MS only space with abscess?
    - Surgeon needs 1 drain per space or break through adjacent fascia
  - Is suprazygomatic MS involved?
    - Infection tends to spread upward because superficial layer, deep cervical fascia is firmly attached to inferior margin of mandible below

Image Interpretation Pearls

- Differentiate cellulitis/myositis from abscess in MS
- Dental infections most common cause of MS abscess
- If subtle fluid is seen, consider delayed CECT
  - Multidetector CT may finish data acquisition before contrast reaches abscess wall
  - If so, existing abscess may be missed
- Precise location within MS important to evaluate for potential complications in nearby spaces
  - Infection can potentially spread into nearby spaces: Submandibular, parapharyngeal, retropharyngeal, etc.

SELECTED REFERENCES

1. Pandey AK et al: Medial pterygoid abscess masquerading as a temporomandibular joint disorder: a case report. Indian J Otolaryngol Head Neck Surg. 76(3):2828-32, 2024
2. Patel J et al: Imaging of dental infections. Emerg Radiol. 29(1):197-205, 2022
3. Chughtai S et al: Radiographic review of anatomy and pathology of the masticator space: what the emergency radiologist needs to know. Emerg Radiol. 27(3):329-39, 2020
4. Wabik A et al: Odontogenic inflammatory processes of head and neck in computed tomography examinations. Pol J Radiol. 79:431-8, 2014
5. Faye N et al: The masticator space: from anatomy to pathology. J Neuroradiol. 36(3):121-30, 2009
6. Hardin CW et al: Infection and tumor of the masticator space: CT evaluation. Radiology. 157(2):413-7, 1985

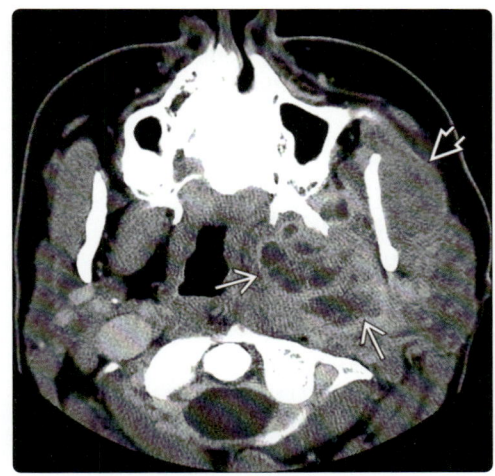
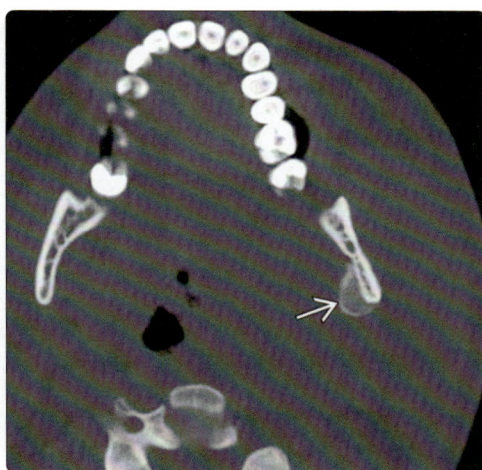

(Left) *Axial CECT demonstrates a large, multiloculated medial MS abscess involving the pterygoid musculature ➡. Note edema and swelling in the masseter muscle in the lateral MS ➡. The patient is a 21-year-old woman who underwent a left molar tooth extraction 9 months previously. Since then, she has complained of trismus and otalgia, misdiagnosed as TMJ syndrome. (Right) Axial bone CT in the same patient reveals periosteal new bone formation indicative of mandibular osteomyelitis ➡.*

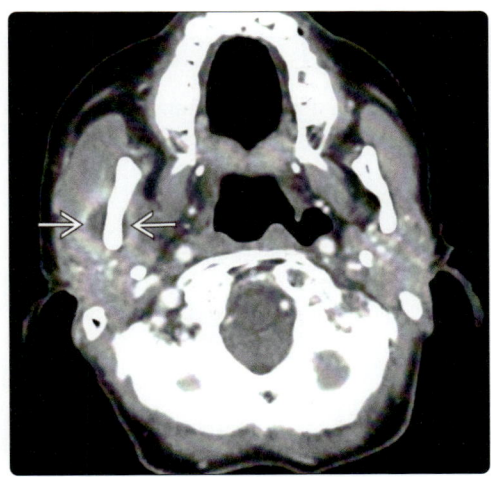
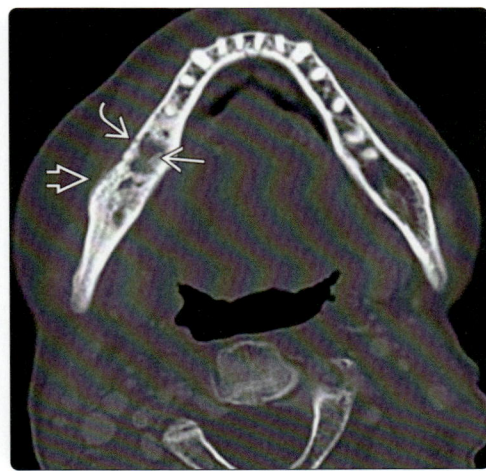

(Left) *Axial CECT shows a small, peripherally enhancing abscess ➡ deep to the masseter and medial pterygoid muscles in a patient with bisphosphonate-related osteonecrosis complicated by infection. (Right) Axial bone CT in the same patient shows mixed osteolytic and osteosclerotic changes in the mandible surrounding tooth #31 (right 2nd mandibular molar) ➡. Note faint cortical lucency ➡ and subtle periosteal reaction ➡.*

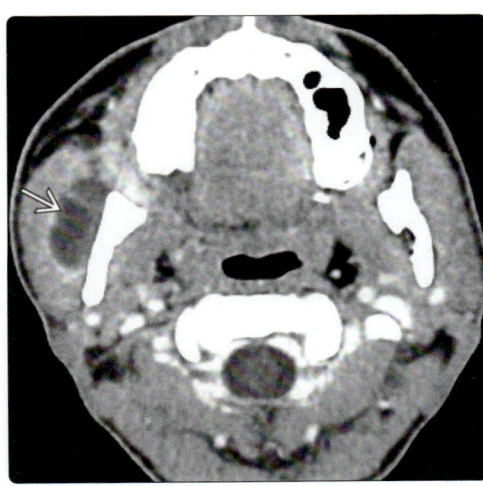
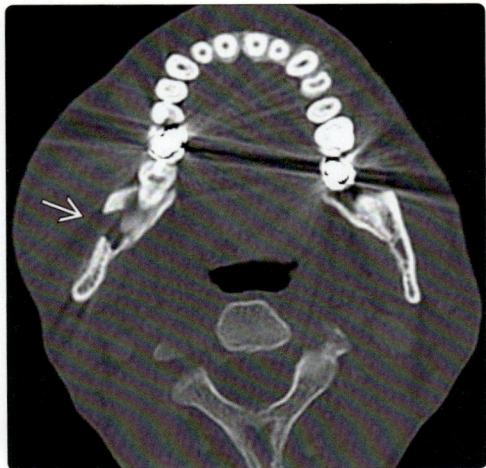

(Left) *Axial CECT shows an abscess ➡ deep to the masseter muscle in this 28-year-old man with an infected right 3rd mandibular molar. (Right) Axial bone CT the same patient demonstrates a well-defined area of lysis with osseous dehiscence ➡ leading to fistula formation and spread of dental infection into the lateral MS from this infected 3rd molar.*

TERMINOLOGY

- CNV3 schwannoma: Encapsulated tumor of Schwann cell origin, which displaces rather than infiltrates fascicles of CNV3 in masticator space (MS)

IMAGING

- Well-circumscribed, smoothly marginated soft tissue mass along course of CNV3
- Bone CT findings
  - **Smooth enlargement/widening of bony foramen**
    - Foramen ovale most commonly enlarged
    - Mandibular foramen, inferior alveolar nerve canal, or mental foramen (in distal CNV3 schwannoma)
- Enhanced MR findings
  - Homogeneous or heterogeneous enhancement
    - Fat saturation may be helpful
  - Rim enhancement with cysts
    - **Intramural cysts** are characteristic of schwannoma
  - Masticator muscle atrophy possible

TOP DIFFERENTIAL DIAGNOSES

- **CNV3 neurofibroma**
- **Perineural tumor** CNV3 in MS
- CNV3 **malignant nerve sheath tumor**
- Odontogenic keratocyst
- Ameloblastoma

CLINICAL ISSUES

- Treatment: Surgery, Gamma Knife, or observation

DIAGNOSTIC CHECKLIST

- **Well-circumscribed, fusiform, or ovoid mass following course of CNV3 suggests schwannoma**
  - Multiple could suggest possible NF2
- Mass in MS without history of H&N squamous cell carcinoma or infection (MS abscess) should suggest sarcoma
  - Sarcoma may mimic schwannoma if centered on CNV3
  - Rapid growth suggests malignancy

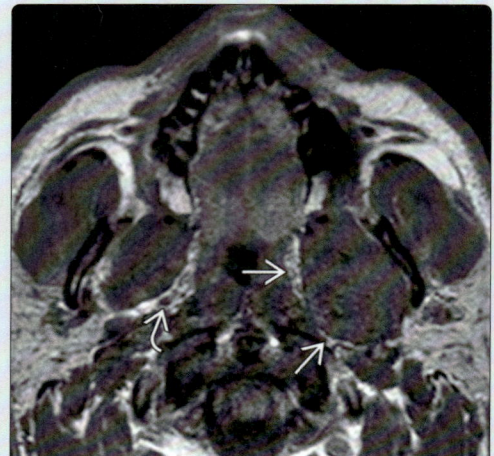
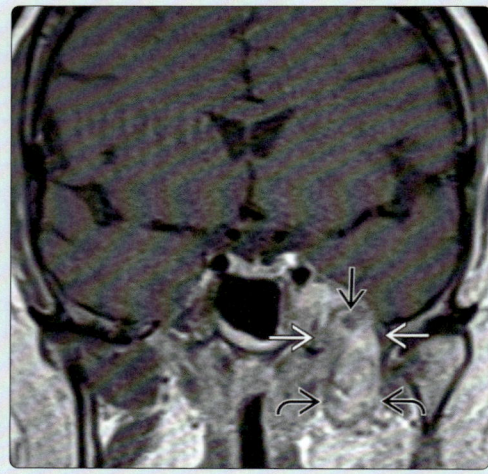

(Left) *Axial T1 MR shows an incidentally found mass in the left masticator space (MS), inseparable from the medial pterygoid and displacing parapharyngeal fat posteromedially* ➡. *Note its location of origin, paralleling the contralateral mandibular nerve* ➡. (Right) *Coronal T1 C+ MR shows a heterogeneously enhancing trigeminal schwannoma expanding the left foramen ovale* ➡ *and extending into the high MS* ➡. *Small intratumoral cystic changes* ➡ *are noted.*

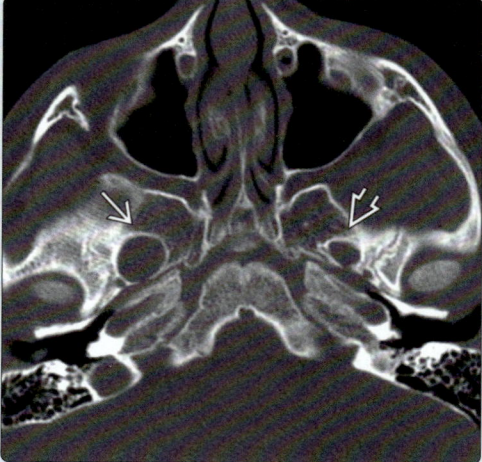
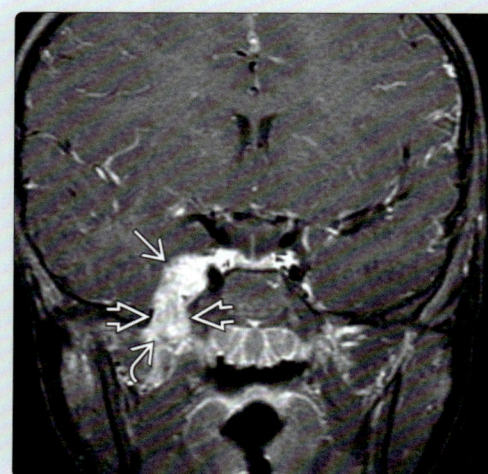

(Left) *Axial bone CT in a patient with known neurofibromatosis type 2 reveals a large right foramen ovale* ➡. *Note the normal left foramen ovale* ➡. *This foraminal enlargement with preservation of its cortical margin is characteristic of benign nerve sheath tumors.* (Right) *Coronal T1 C+ FS MR in the same patient shows a tubular, enhancing CNV3 schwannoma coursing from the parasellar region* ➡ *through the enlarged foramen ovale* ➡ *into the nasopharyngeal MS* ➡.

TERMINOLOGY

Abbreviations
- Masticator space (MS) CNV3 (mandibular branch, trigeminal nerve) schwannoma

Synonyms
- Neuroma, neurilemmoma, neurinoma

IMAGING

General Features
- Best diagnostic clue
  - **Well-circumscribed, smoothly marginated** soft tissue mass along course of CNV3 branch of CNV
  - **Smooth widening**/enlargement of bony foramen ovale
- Location
  - From Meckel cave to MS along CNV3
  - Rarely CNV3 branches: Inferior alveolar or mental nerves
- Morphology
  - Ovoid to fusiform/tubular

Radiographic Findings
- Radiography
  - Enlargement of inferior alveolar nerve canal or mental foramen on plain films, panorex, or bite-wing films

CT Findings
- CECT
  - Lesion enhances mildly to moderately
  - Homogeneous or heterogeneous enhancement
- Bone CT
  - **Smooth enlargement** of bony foramen involved
    - **Foramen ovale** most commonly enlarged

MR Findings
- T1WI
  - Isointense or hypointense to muscles of mastication
  - Variable signal if hemorrhage or cysts present
- T2WI
  - Variable, isointense to hyperintense
    - **Intramural cysts** somewhat characteristic
  - Myxoid or cystic changes: ↑ signal intensity
  - Hypointense foci (blood) common in larger tumors
- T1WI C+
  - Homogeneous or heterogeneous enhancement

Imaging Recommendations
- Best imaging tool
  - T1WI C+ FS MR in axial & coronal plane
- Protocol advice
  - Field of view from lateral pons to mental foramen

DIFFERENTIAL DIAGNOSIS

CNV3 Neurofibroma
- Neurofibromatosis type 1; rarely isolated
- Lesions are usually plexiform type
- More commonly affect CNV1 & V2, not V3

CNV3 Malignant Nerve Sheath Tumor
- Invasive mass centered on CNV3 within MS
- Rapid growth pattern is clinically suggestive

Perineural Tumor CNV3 in Masticator Space
- Typically known squamous cell carcinoma (SCCa) from chin skin, mandibular alveolar ridge, oral tongue, oropharynx
- Imaging shows primary tumor & nearby perineural CNV3 that travels retrograde up nerve

Odontogenic Keratocyst
- Unilocular or multilocular cystic lesion of mandible
- Lesion envelops or incorporates crown & tooth root

Ameloblastoma
- Bubbly, multilocular, cystic-solid tumor, mandible or maxilla

PATHOLOGY

General Features
- Etiology
  - Unknown in sporadic cases
  - Associated with neurofibromatosis type 2 (NF2)
    - Mutation on chromosome 22

Microscopic Features
- Proliferating Schwann cells in collagenous matrix with fibrous capsule that displace rather than infiltrate fascicles
- 2 Antoni tissue types (may coexist in single lesion)
  - Antoni A type: Compact, hypercellular
  - Antoni B type: Looser architecture; cystic changes
- Cystic degeneration (intramural cysts) common

CLINICAL ISSUES

Presentation
- Most common signs/symptoms
  - Most common asymptomatic neoplasm in deep facial soft tissues
  - Other signs/symptoms
    - Atypical facial pain, ↓ chin sensation
    - Masticator muscle weakness ± denervation atrophy

Demographics
- Age: Predominantly 3rd-4th decades
  - Younger in patients with NF2
- Epidemiology
  - Peripheral CNV3 schwannomas account for 5% of all trigeminal schwannomas
  - Most commonly proximal extracranial CNV3

Natural History & Prognosis
- Gradually enlarging MS mass

Treatment
- Some cases may be managed conservatively (observed)
- Surgical resection (open & endoscopic techniques used)
- Gamma Knife

SELECTED REFERENCES

1. Brahmbhatt S et al: Genetic tumor syndromes of the head and neck: update in the genomic era. Neuroradiol J. 38(3):277-90, 2025
2. Li S et al: Intraosseous schwannoma of the mandible: new case series, literature update, and proposal of a classification. Int J Oral Maxillofac Surg. 53(3):205-11, 2024
3. Mak YH et al: Multicompartmental cystic trigeminal schwannoma as an uncommon differential diagnosis of cerebellopontine angle tumors. Radiol Case Rep. 19(6):2552-7, 2024

KEY FACTS

TERMINOLOGY

- Perineural tumor (PNT) of masticator space (MS) is malignant spread along CNV3 (mandibular branch of trigeminal nerve)

IMAGING

- PNT occurs along all or part of V3 from mental foramen to lateral pons root entry zone of CNV
  - Nerve enlarged; may reach 1 cm in diameter
  - CNV3 may be normal size in early PNT
- Bone CT findings
  - **Enlarged neural foramen** mandibular inferior alveolar canal, mandibular foramen, foramen ovale
- MR findings
  - **Abnormal enhancement** of CNV3, commonly enlarged
    - Coronal T1 C+ best shows CNV3 PNT
    - FS ↑ conspicuity of enhancing PNT
  - T1 MR without contrast & **without FS** useful for obliteration of fat pads below foramen ovale

- CECT less sensitive for PNT; MR recommended
- MR very sensitive but not specific for CNV3 PNT

TOP DIFFERENTIAL DIAGNOSES

- Normal pterygoid venous plexus asymmetry
- Normal vasa nervosa, CNV3
- CNV3 schwannoma; CNV3 neurofibroma; skull base meningioma

CLINICAL ISSUES

- **Often asymptomatic (40%)**
- Lower face paresthesias, numbness, MS denervation

DIAGNOSTIC CHECKLIST

- Primary malignancies that may yield CNV3 PNT
  - Skin cancers of chin & jaw [squamous cell carcinoma (SCCa), basal cell carcinoma, melanoma]
  - Oral cavity or pharynx primaries (SCCa, ACCa)
  - MS malignancy (sarcoma, non-Hodgkin lymphoma)
  - Parotid primary (spread via auriculotemporal nerve)

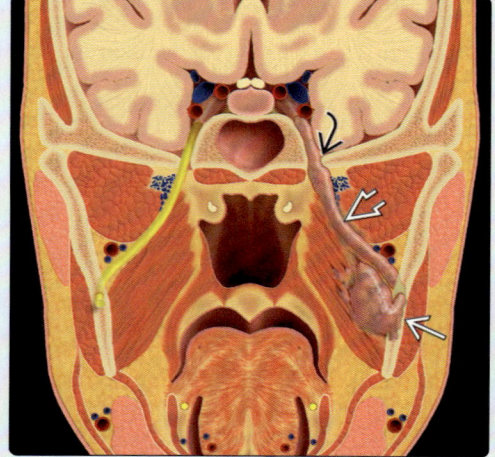
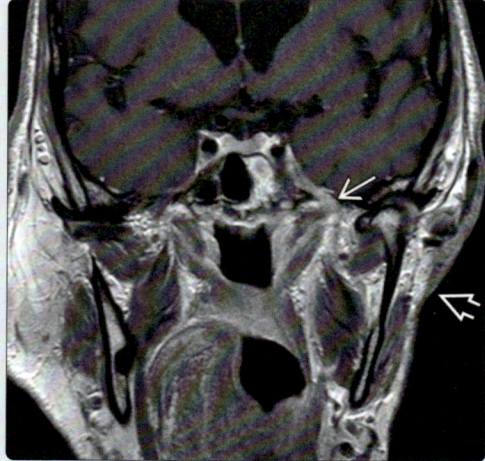

(Left) Coronal graphic depicts a classic example of a malignant masticator space (MS) tumor ➡ with perineural V3 spread ➡ through the foramen ovale ➡ into an intracranial compartment. (Right) Coronal T1 C+ MR shows abnormal asymmetric enhancement and enlargement of V3 as it traverses the foramen ovale ➡ due to perineural tumor spread (PNTS). This patient underwent prior resection for parotid salivary duct carcinoma; note the postsurgical soft tissue defect related to parotidectomy ➡.

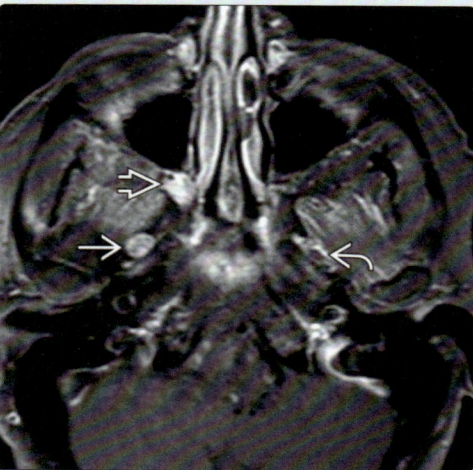
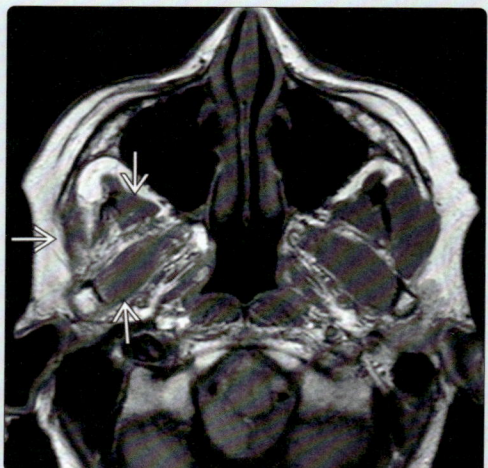

(Left) Axial T1 C+ FS MR shows enlargement and enhancement of V3 on the right ➡ as it enters the foramen ovale in this patient with PNTS from adenoid cystic carcinoma. Note the normal V3 ➡ on the left for comparison. There is also abnormal enhancement along V2 in the right pterygopalatine fossa ➡. (Right) Axial T1 MR in the same patient shows partial atrophy of the right MS muscles ➡ due to chronic denervation.

TERMINOLOGY

Abbreviations

- Perineural tumor (PNT), masticator space (MS)

Synonyms

- PNT spread, PNT invasion

Definitions

- PNT of MS is malignant spread along CNV3 (mandibular branch of trigeminal nerve)
- CNV3: 3rd division of trigeminal nerve (CNV)
- CNV3 PNT: Extension of malignancy along CNV3 allowing spread from MS though foramen ovale into Meckel cave (MC) & potentially intracranially
- MC: Small cistern that contains trigeminal ganglion
  - Trigeminal ganglion = gasserian or semilunar ganglion

IMAGING

General Features

- Best diagnostic clue
  - T1 C+ MR shows **enlarged enhancing CNV3**
- Location
  - PNT can occur along all or segments of CNV3
    - **Inferior alveolar nerve**: In inferior alveolar canal from mental foramen to mandibular foramen
    - **Mandibular branch, CNV3**: Extends from mandibular foramen to foramen ovale in MS
    - **Foramen ovale**: Skull base foramen through which CNV3 passes
    - **MC**: Cistern inferior & lateral to cavernous sinus; contains trigeminal ganglion in anterior aspect
    - **Preganglionic segment CNV**: Spans distance from MC to root entry zone on lateral pons
- Size
  - Nerve usually enlarged; may reach 1 cm in diameter
  - Nerve may be normal in size early
- Morphology
  - Linear, along expected course of CNV3

CT Findings

- CECT
  - CNV3 enhancement & enlargement
  - Enhancement & enlargement of cavernous sinus & MC
  - Fatty atrophy of MS muscles (chronic denervation)
- Bone CT
  - Enlarged/widened inferior alveolar canal in mandible
  - Enlarged/widened mandibular foramen
  - Enlarged/widened foramen ovale

MR Findings

- T1WI
  - Enlargement of CNV3
  - Tissue within mandibular foramen; intermediate to low signal replacing marrow fat of mandibular ramus
  - Infiltration of MS muscle & fat surrounding CNV3
  - Obliteration of trigeminal fat pad
  - MS muscles: Acute edema or chronic fatty atrophy
- T2WI
  - Enlarged MC with loss of normal fluid signal
  - ↑ signal of edematous nerve difficult & unreliable sign

- T1WI C+
  - Enlarged, enhancing extracranial CNV3
    - Inferior alveolar canal of mandible (inferior alveolar nerve)
    - Mandibular foramen to foramen ovale (mandibular nerve)
  - Enhancement of nerve in foramen ovale
    - Normal nerve: Low signal
    - Beware vasa nervosa (veins accompanying nerve)
    - Beware normal pterygoid venous plexus enhancement
  - Enlargement, enhancement of MC
  - Enhancing MS muscles (acute-subacute CNV3 denervation)

Nuclear Medicine Findings

- PET
  - PET/CT useful although uptake along CNV3 often difficult to differentiate from brain & primary tumor
  - PET/MR may be complementary to evaluate PNT

Imaging Recommendations

- Best imaging tool
  - CECT less sensitive for PNT; MR recommended
  - MR very sensitive but not specific for CNV3 PNT
    - Normal nerves asymmetrically enhance in 5% of patients
- Protocol advice
  - Coronal T1 C+ shows CNV3 abnormal enhancing PNT
    - Good quality FS ↑ conspicuity of PNT
    - Beware FS susceptibility artifacts that obscure PNT (e.g., dental amalgam artifact)
  - Coronal T1 MR without contrast & **without FS** useful for obliteration of fat pads below foramen ovale

DIFFERENTIAL DIAGNOSIS

Pterygoid Venous Plexus Asymmetry

- Normal venous plexus in & around pterygoid muscles in MS
- May extend to foramen ovale but does not enter or enlarge
- Asymmetry common

CNV3 Schwannoma in Masticator Space

- Benign neoplasm of CNV3 nerve sheath
- Intermediate T1, heterogeneously bright T2
- Heterogeneous enhancement with intramural cysts possible
- When crossing foramen ovale, dumbbell-shaped on coronal images
- May arise anywhere along course of CNV

CNV3 Neurofibroma

- Uncommon site for neurofibroma
- When crossing foramen ovale, dumbbell-shaped on coronal images
- Uniform enhancement
- May follow branches of CNV3

CNV3 Vasa Nervosa

- Normal small veins accompany CNV3 in foramen ovale
- Vague peripheral enhancement on T1 C+ MR
- Nerve itself remains dark on T1 C+ MR

Normal Skull Base Marrow Around Foramen Ovale

- Marrow fat in skull base around foramen ovale has inherent high T1 signal
- High T1 signal alongside foramen ovale
- Dark cortical bone separates marrow from nerve within foramen
- T1 FS clarifies fat vs. enhancement

Skull Base Meningioma

- Benign neoplasm of brain coverings
- Isointense to brain on T1 & T2 images
- Uniform, brisk enhancement
- May extend into foramen ovale & beyond

CNV3 Normal Fat Pad

- Fat pads normally seen at exit points of cranial nerves
- High inherent T1 signal surrounding nerve
- Does not extend into foramen ovale
- T1 C+ FS MR or compare T1 C+ MR to T1 MR without contrast to clarify fat vs. enhancement

PATHOLOGY

General Features

- Etiology
  - Path of least resistance for tumors predisposed to PNT
  - Tumor expression of nerve growth factor or neural cell adhesion molecules may correlate with propensity to PNT spread
- Tumor may spread outside nerve sheath or involve support tissues (endoneurium, perineurium, epineurium)
- Any malignant tumor may undergo PNT spread

Gross Pathologic & Surgical Features

- Enlargement of nerve complex
- Encasement-replacement of CNV3

Microscopic Features

- Perineural spread = gross pathologic or radiographic diagnosis of tumor along nerve
- Perineural invasion (PNI) = microscopic tumor in nerves
  - Pathologic diagnosis

CLINICAL ISSUES

Presentation

- Most common signs/symptoms
  - **Often asymptomatic (40%)**
  - Paresthesias of lower face
  - Jaw pain or numbness
  - Masticator muscle denervation atrophy

Demographics

- Age
  - 50-80 years (demographics of common primary tumors)
- Sex
  - M > F, because squamous cell carcinoma (SCCa) more common in men
- Epidemiology
  - PNI prevalence 25-80% in head & neck mucosal SCCa
    - PNI in 2.5-5% of cutaneous SCCa
  - Occasionally PNT is presenting finding

- Tumors with greatest propensity for PNT spread
  - **Adenoid cystic carcinoma (ACCa)**; PNI in 50%
  - **SCCa, pharynx or skin**
  - Desmoplastic melanoma, skin; PNI in 36-50%
  - Extranodal lymphoma
  - Mucoepidermoid carcinoma
  - Basal cell carcinoma (BCC)
  - Rhabdomyosarcoma

Natural History & Prognosis

- PNT spread strongly affects patient prognosis
- **PNT** spread is **very poor prognostic sign**
  - ↑ local recurrence
  - ↑ distant metastases
  - ↑ meningeal carcinomatosis
  - ↓ survival
- Cranial nerve defects unlikely to resolve with therapy

Treatment

- Radiotherapy ± surgery & chemotherapy
- Identifying PNT critical to radiation fields & dosing

DIAGNOSTIC CHECKLIST

Consider

- Primary malignancy sites that may yield CNV3 PNT spread
  - **Skin of chin & jaw** (SCCa, melanoma, or BCC)
  - **Alveolar ridge, retromolar trigone** (deep tonsillar & nasopharyngeal SCCa)
  - MS malignancy (sarcoma, non-Hodgkin lymphoma)
  - Parotid malignancy (especially ACCa): May spread CNVII (facial nerve) to **auriculotemporal nerve** of CNV3
- Some CNV3 PNT patients have no known primary
  - Patients with remote skin cancer history may not recall or mention prior diagnosis

Image Interpretation Pearls

- Inspect CNV from mental foramen of mandible to root entry zone of lateral pons
  - Look for asymmetric CNV3 enlargement & enhancement
  - Axial & coronal **T1 C+ FS MR ↑** lesion conspicuity
    - Remove FS if susceptibility artifact obscures PNT
  - Check for trigeminal fat pad effacement
  - Check for denervation changes of MS muscles
- Do not confuse pterygoid venous plexus with PNT
  - Look for CNV3 nerve enhancement to distinguish
- Beware of **skip lesions**: Normal nerve between noncontiguous areas of enhancing PNT
- Beware of PNT spread to other CNs (e.g., auriculotemporal branch of CNV3 spread from parotid malignancy/CNVII)

SELECTED REFERENCES

1. Hassouneh A et al: Intracranial extension of parotid adenoid cystic carcinoma presenting as trigeminal neuralgia: a case report. Radiol Case Rep. 20(5):2346-50, 2025
2. Abdullaeva U et al: Diagnostic accuracy of MRI in detecting the perineural spread of head and neck tumors: a systematic review and meta-analysis. Diagnostics (Basel). 14(1):113, 2024
3. Hsieh KJ et al: Perineural spread of tumor in the skull base and head and neck. Oral Maxillofac Surg Clin North Am. 35(3):399-412, 2023
4. Abdelaziz TT et al: Magnetic resonance imaging of perineural spread of head and neck cancer. Magn Reson Imaging Clin N Am. 30(1):95-108, 2022

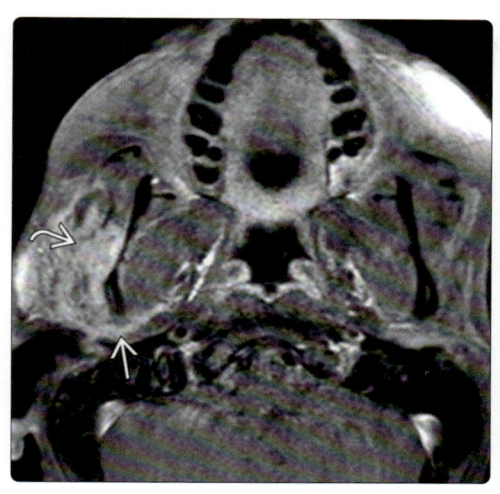

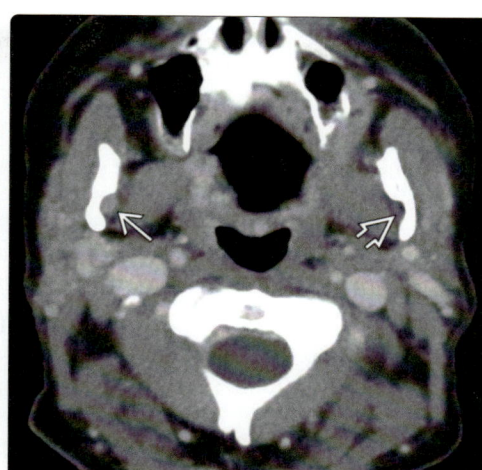

(Left) *Axial T1 C+ FS MR shows thickening and enhancement along the auriculotemporal nerve* ➡ *due to perineural spread from primary parotid adenoid cystic carcinoma. Tumor also invaded directly into adjacent MS musculature* ➚. **(Right)** *Axial CECT shows effacement of the small fat pad in the mandibular foramen due to PNTS along the enlarged inferior alveolar nerve* ➡. *Compare to the normal left mandibular foramen* ➡.

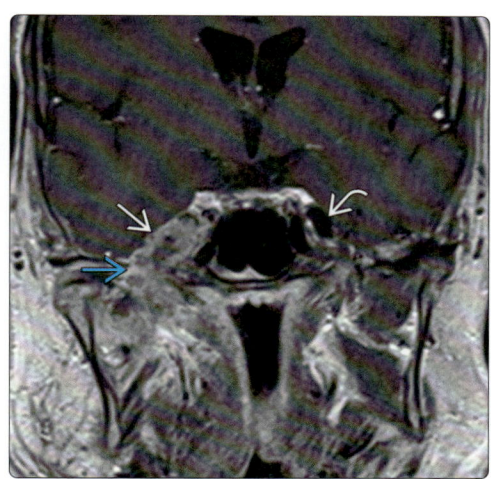

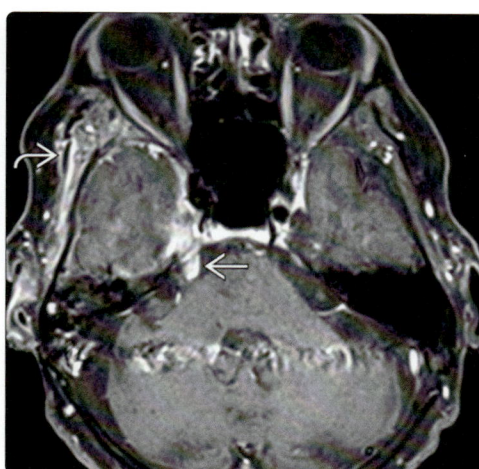

(Left) *Coronal T1 C+ MR in a patient with advanced oral cavity squamous cell carcinoma shows bulky, necrotic-appearing tumor spreading via an enlarged right foramen ovale* ➡ *to Meckel's cave* ➡. *Normal fluid-filled Meckel's cave* ➡ *is noted on the left.* **(Right)** *Axial T1 C+ FS MR in the same patient shows perineural tumor tracking from Meckel's cave along the cisternal CNV* ➡. *Enhancement and asymmetric decreased muscle bulk in the MS are due to late subacute denervation change* ➚.

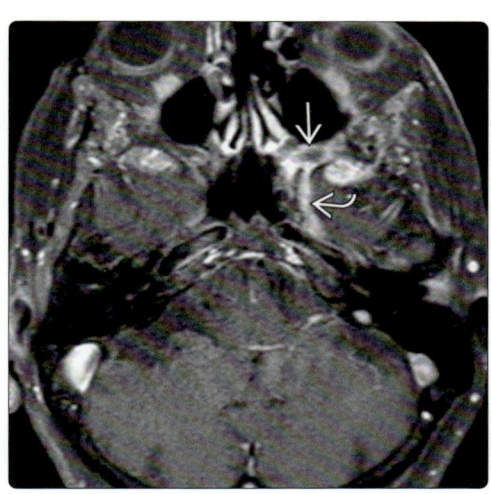

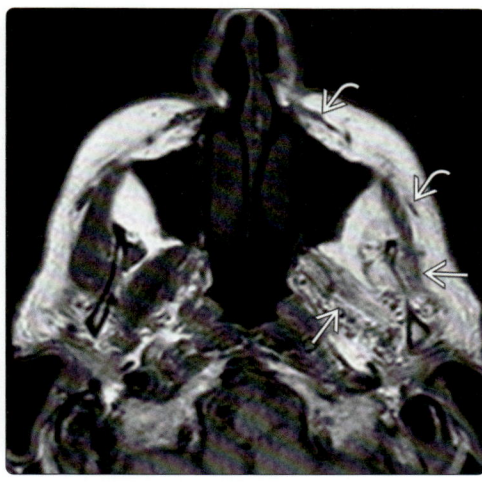

(Left) *Axial T1 C+ FS MR in a patient with PNTS from squamous cell carcinoma shows enhancing tumor along V2 in the pterygopalatine fossa* ➡ *and foramen rotundum* ➚. *PNTS was the presenting symptom in this patient with unknown primary site.* **(Right)** *Axial T1 MR shows chronic denervation atrophy of the muscles of mastication* ➡ *and muscles of facial expression* ➚ *in a patient with PNTS along the trigeminal and facial nerves due to squamous cell carcinoma.*

Masticator Space Chondrosarcoma

TERMINOLOGY

- Chondrosarcoma (CSa), masticator space (MS)

IMAGING

- Enhancing soft tissue mass in MS in or adjacent to mandible with variable Ca^{++} pattern
  - Molar region and ramus most frequent in mandible
  - May extend down from skull base or TMJ
- Bone CT findings
  - **Radiolucent lesion ± areas of Ca^{++}**
    - When using CECT, view bone windows
  - Rings and crescents of calcium: Low-grade tumors
  - Amorphous or no Ca^{++}: High-grade tumors
- MR findings
  - Invasion of bone best delineated on T1 without contrast (without fat sat)
  - T1 C+ heterogeneous, predominantly peripheral enhancement
  - Greater T1 C+ enhancement in high-grade CSa
- High signal typical on T2
  - Extraosseous CSa tends to have intermediate signal
  - Flow voids may be present in extraosseous CSa

TOP DIFFERENTIAL DIAGNOSES

- MS infection
- TMJ synovial chondromatosis
- Odontoma
- Mandibular ossifying fibroma
- Mandibular fibrous dysplasia
- Mandibular osteosarcoma

DIAGNOSTIC CHECKLIST

- CT best to show characteristic Ca^{++}
- MR better delineates extent of tumor
- Infection far more common than sarcoma in MS
  - Consider infection first if no Ca^{++} present
- MS masses should be followed to resolution to ensure that they are not sarcomas

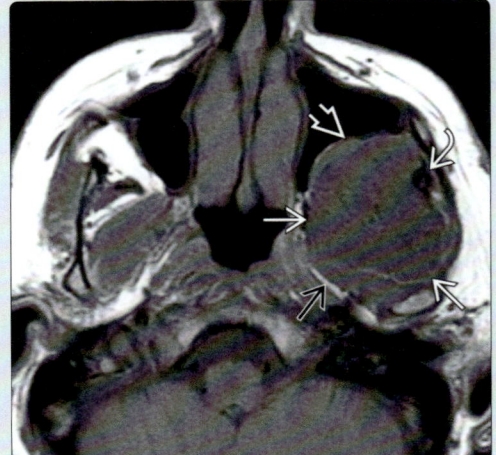
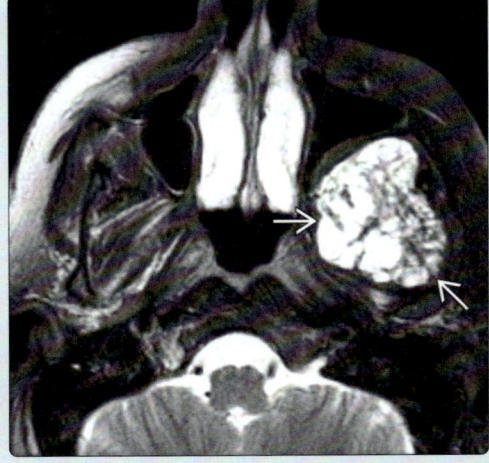

(Left) Axial T1 MR shows an intermediate-signal mass ➡ distending the masticator space and causing anterior bowing of posterior wall of the left maxillary sinus ➡. The parapharyngeal fat pad ➡ is displaced posteromedially. A large focal Ca^{++} ➡ is seen as low signal intensity on all sequences. (Right) Axial T2 MR in the same patient shows the mass ➡ with characteristic pronounced T2 hyperintensity of chondroid tumors.

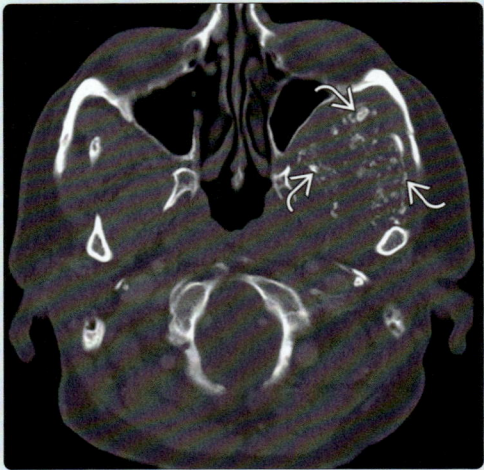
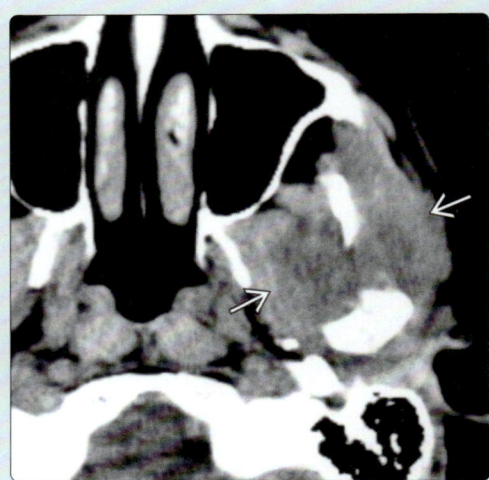

(Left) Axial bone window CECT in the same patient shows a large mass with intrinsic Ca^{++} ➡, which are "fluffy," with rings and arcs. These are typical of chondroid Ca^{++}. Chondrosarcoma with visible well-defined chondroid Ca^{++} usually indicates low-grade tumor. (Right) Axial NECT shows ill-defined, low-density chondrosarcoma ➡ in the masticator space, mimicking an abscess. Although infection is most common in the masticator space, sarcomas should always be considered, and surveillance to ensure resolution is important.

Masticator Space Chondrosarcoma

TERMINOLOGY

Abbreviations

- Chondrosarcoma (CSa)

Definitions

- CSa-masticator space (MS): Malignant tumor of cartilage that originates in MS

IMAGING

General Features

- Best diagnostic clue
  - Enhancing soft tissue mass in MS in or adjacent to mandible with variable Ca^{++} pattern
- Location
  - Adjacent to (inseparable from) bone of origin
  - Mandible, molar region, and ramus most frequent
  - Can also be seen in maxilla
  - May extend down from skull base or TMJ
  - Extraosseous CSa without bony involvement is uncommon (2%)
- Size
  - At presentation, most > 3 cm
- Morphology
  - Round with lobular margin
  - Soft tissue mass may be well circumscribed

Radiographic Findings

- Radiography
  - Symmetrically widened periodontal space on panoral radiographs
  - ± ill-defined radiolucency with mottled Ca^{++}
  - Radiographic imaging not specific for CSa

CT Findings

- CECT
  - Heterogeneous, predominantly peripheral enhancement
- Bone CT
  - Mass with ill-defined osseous borders and wide zone of transition
  - Radiolucent lesion (erosion of bone of origin)
  - ± areas of Ca^{++}
    - **Rings and crescents of Ca^{++}** most characteristic
      - More typical of **low-grade tumors**
    - **Amorphous Ca^{++}** (or no Ca^{++}) are more typical of **high-grade tumors**
    - Presence and degree of Ca^{++} depends on tumor grade
  - Erosion of surrounding bones (e.g., skull base)
  - Widening of temporomandibular joint (when arising from TMJ)
  - Widening of periodontal space
  - Periosteal reaction usually mild, if present

MR Findings

- T1WI
  - Homogeneous, intermediate signal
  - Cartilage matrix or Ca^{++} makes signal heterogeneous
  - Invasion of bone best delineated on unenhanced T1WI (without fat sat)
  - Replacement of normal hyperintense marrow fat with intermediate intensity tumor
- T2WI
  - **High signal** most typical on **T2**
    - Extraosseous CSa tends to have intermediate signal
    - Flow voids may be present in extraosseous CSa
  - Homogeneous or heterogeneous, depending on degree and type of Ca^{++}
  - Marrow, soft tissue edema may be seen
- T1WI C+
  - Enhancement may be focal (often peripheral) or diffuse
  - Extent of enhancement depends on tumor grade
    - Greater T1 C+ MR enhancement in high-grade CSa

Imaging Recommendations

- Best imaging tool
  - CT shows characteristic Ca^{++}
  - MR better delineates extent of tumor
- Protocol advice
  - When using CECT, view bone windows
    - Bone CT most likely to show characteristic Ca^{++}

DIFFERENTIAL DIAGNOSIS

Masticator Space Infection

- Most frequent cause of MS mass
- Usually of dental origin
- Noncalcifying CSa may mimic MS infection on imaging

TMJ Synovial Chondromatosis

- TMJ filled with tiny loose bodies (grain of rice appearance)
- Multiple foci of free cartilage, variably calcified
- Abnormalities usually confined to expanded synovial cavity but can erode skull base
- Pathologic confirmation required; potential for malignant transformation to CSa

Odontoma

- Compound variant: Small teeth identified within mass
- Complex variant: Amorphous Ca^{++} with dense enamel

Mandibular Ossifying Fibroma

- Benign solitary jaw tumor
- Radiodense periphery surrounding fibrous center
- Characteristic stellate Ca^{++} pattern

Mandibular Fibrous Dysplasia

- Expanded bone with characteristic matrix
- Ground-glass and cystic patterns, usually in combination
- Expansile, rather than erosive like CSa-MS
- Confined to bone without soft tissue mass

Mandibular Osteosarcoma

- Most frequent MS sarcoma of bone
- Cumulus cloud pattern of new bone formation
- Sunburst pattern of periosteal reaction
- Osteosarcoma has poorer prognosis than CSa-MS

Mandibular Metastasis

- Ca^{++} seen in lung, prostate, breast, colon metastases
- Amorphous Ca^{++} of mucinous metastases may be confused with chondroid Ca^{++}
- Sites of metastasis include jaw, skull base, soft tissues

PATHOLOGY

General Features

- Etiology
  - CSa-MS mostly sporadic (75%)
  - Predisposing conditions
    – Osteochondroma
    – Enchondroma
    – Ollier disease
    – Maffucci syndrome
    – Paget disease
    – Fibrous dysplasia
    – Synovial chondromatosis
    – Radiation exposure
    – Thorotrast exposure
- CSa-MS may or may not occur at cartilaginous joints (TMJ)
  - TMJ CSa represents tumoral differentiation of pluripotent mesenchymal cells

Staging, Grading, & Classification

- Osseous vs. extraosseous
- Central (medullary) vs. peripheral (juxtacortical)
- Primary vs. secondary (secondary = associated with enchondroma or osteochondroma)
- Histological subtypes
  - Conventional, myxoid, clear cell, mesenchymal, dedifferentiated
- Histologic grade (> 90% of CSa grade 1 or II)
  - Grade I (well differentiated): Ca^{++} and bone formation frequent
  - Grade II (moderately differentiated): Matrix more myxoid than chondroid
  - Grade III (poorly differentiated): No matrix, high mitotic rate (rare)

Gross Pathologic & Surgical Features

- Firm, nodular mass
- Tan-white to opalescent blue-gray
- Gross hemorrhage in high-grade tumors

Microscopic Features

- Matrix of lobular hyaline cartilage
- Multinucleated lacunes with variable nucleoli
- May be difficult to distinguish from chondroblastic osteosarcoma
- Low-grade neoplasms hard to distinguish from enchondroma

CLINICAL ISSUES

Presentation

- Most common signs/symptoms
  - Expanding, painless preauricular mass ±trismus
    – Rate of enlargement depends on tumor grade
    – May be mistaken for parotid mass
  - Other signs/symptoms
    – Headache
    – Loose teeth
    – CNV3 dysfunction
    – CSa arising from TMJ often painful

Demographics

- Age
  - Any age (30-45 years most common)
- Epidemiology
  - 2nd most common malignancy of bone (after osteosarcoma, excluding multiple myeloma)
  - CSa = 15% of malignant bone tumors
  - 5-10% of CSa occur in H&N
    – Larynx, jaws, facial bones, skull base, TMJ affected
    – Orbit more common location in children

Natural History & Prognosis

- Low-grade CSa grows insidiously
- Metastases unusual (7%)
- Overall prognosis depends on tumor grade and size
  - 5-year overall survival: 68% (90% grade I; 50% combined grades II and III)
  - Lower survival if systemic metastases at presentation
- May dedifferentiate into osteosarcoma, malignant fibrous histiocytoma, or fibrosarcoma
- Local recurrence is problematic (50%)
  - Late recurrence (10-20 years) possible

Treatment

- Wide local excision
- Role of radiation, chemotherapy, cryosurgery, and immunotherapy are controversial and evolving

DIAGNOSTIC CHECKLIST

Consider

- Infection far more common than CSa in MS
  - If no Ca^{++}, consider infection first
- If MS mass without clinical suggestion of infection, consider tumor as possibility
  - First consider perineural tumor on V3 from squamous cell carcinoma (SCCa) of chin skin, mandibular alveolar ridge, retromolar trigone
  - If no evidence for SCCa invasion of MS, then consider primary MS sarcoma

Image Interpretation Pearls

- Characteristic Ca^{++} are helpful, but variable appearance of CSa makes precise prospective diagnosis difficult
  - Distinguishing CSa of TMJ from synovial chondromatosis can be difficult
  - If no characteristic Ca^{++} seen within MS tumor, suggestion of CSa is critical
  - Exact pathology can be determined at surgery
- MS masses should be followed to resolution to ensure they are not sarcomas

SELECTED REFERENCES

1. Agosti E et al: Advancing the management of skull base chondrosarcomas: a systematic review of targeted therapies. J Pers Med. 14(3):261, 2024
2. Saucier E et al: Li-Fraumeni-associated osteosarcomas: the French experience. Pediatr Blood Cancer. e31362, 2024
3. Zaleckas L et al: Virtual planning, guided surgery, and digital prosthodontics in the treatment of extended mandible chondrosarcoma. J Prosthodont. 33(5):409-16, 2024
4. Jang BG et al: Differentiation between chondrosarcoma and synovial chondromatosis of the temporomandibular joint using CT and MR imaging. AJNR Am J Neuroradiol. 44(10):1176-83, 2023

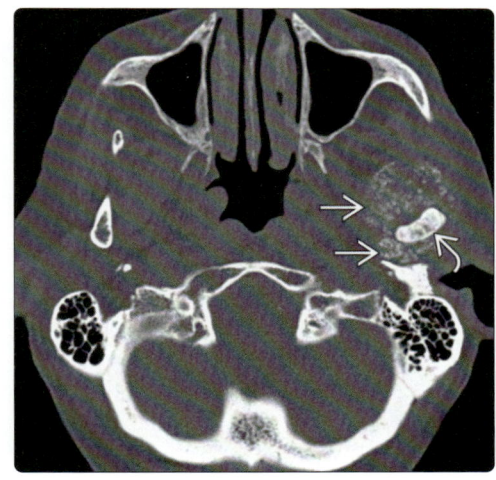

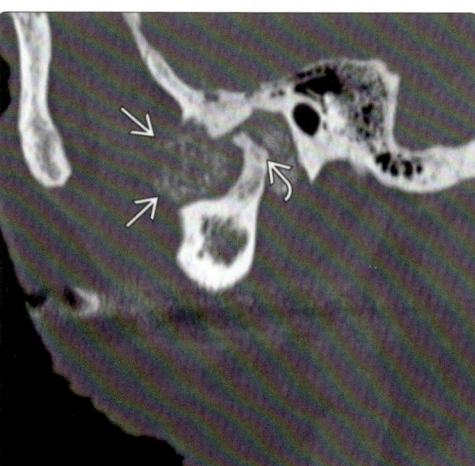

(Left) *Axial bone CT of typical chondrosarcoma through the left TMJ reveals an irregular sclerotic appearance of the mandibular condyle ➔ and multiple small, focal Ca⁺⁺ ➔ around the joint. Although this may be difficult to distinguish from synovial chondromatosis, both are treated surgically, and histology can confirm.* **(Right)** *Sagittal bone CT reformation in the same patient shows condylar deformity ➔ and also suggests that some of the Ca⁺⁺ ➔ reside within a soft tissue component outside of the joint.*

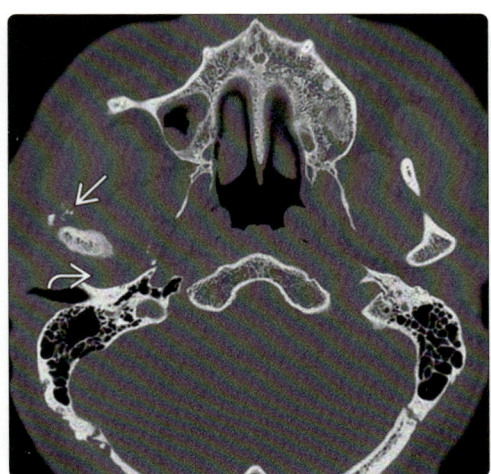

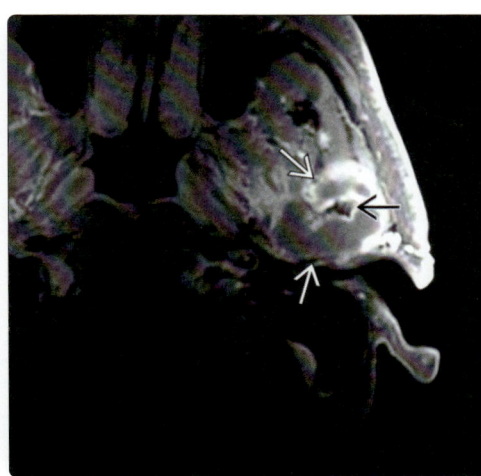

(Left) *Axial bone CT in a case of low-grade TMJ chondrosarcoma shows calcified matrix ➔ within a mass widening the TMJ. Note extensive remodeling and scalloping of the glenoid fossa ➔. ***(Right)*** Axial T1WI C+ MR shows an intermediate signal intensity mass surrounding the eroded condylar head ➔. The tumor shows circumferential peripheral enhancement ➔. Enhancement patterns vary and can be peripheral, diffuse, or focal in chondrosarcoma.*

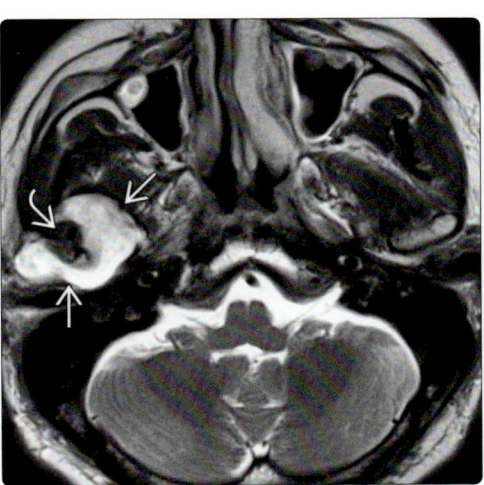

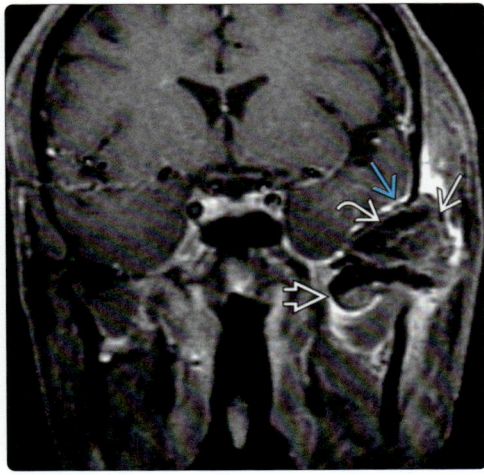

(Left) *Axial T2 MR demonstrates a hyperintense mass ➔ widening the TMJ with well-defined margins. The mass surrounds a deformed-appearing condyle ➔. ***(Right)*** Coronal T1 C+ FS MR shows a heterogeneous enhancing chondrosarcoma arising in the left TMJ with extension into the suprazygomatic ➔ and infrazygomatic ➔ masticator space. Note low-signal foci consistent with areas of mineralized matrix ➔. The mass has remodeled the adjacent calvarium, and dural enhancement ➔ is present.*

Masticator Space Sarcoma

TERMINOLOGY

- Masticator space sarcoma (MS-SA): Malignant tumor of soft tissue origin (fat, muscle, nerve, joint, blood vessel, or deep skin tissues) in MS of suprahyoid neck

IMAGING

- Aggressive, poorly marginated MS mass with bone destruction and invasion of adjacent fascial planes/spaces
- Imaging recommendations: Thin-section bone CT, T1 C+ MR
- Bone CT: Assessment of matrix ± bone changes
  - **Invasive MS mass** with **bone destruction**
  - **Bone production** or **calcification** can be seen in any SA
- MR: Evaluation of soft tissues, possible mandibular invasion
  - Perineural tumor spread along CNV3

TOP DIFFERENTIAL DIAGNOSES

- MS abscess
- Invasive squamous cell carcinoma (SCCa)
  - Palatine tonsil SCCa, retromolar trigone SCCa

- Mandible metastasis
- Mandibular osteomyelitis
- MS venous malformation
- Odontogenic keratocyst
- Perineural tumor of CNV3 in MS

PATHOLOGY

- DNA mutations common in soft tissue SA

CLINICAL ISSUES

- Enlarging soft tissue mass over mandible with ↑ pain
- History of treated facial malignancy with radiation
- SA location and extent, in addition to pathology and TNM stage, is important when planning treatment
- AJCC 8th edition T staging reflects tumor sizes of 2-4 cm

DIAGNOSTIC CHECKLIST

- Absent known malignancy or infectious signs, MS mass should suggest SA

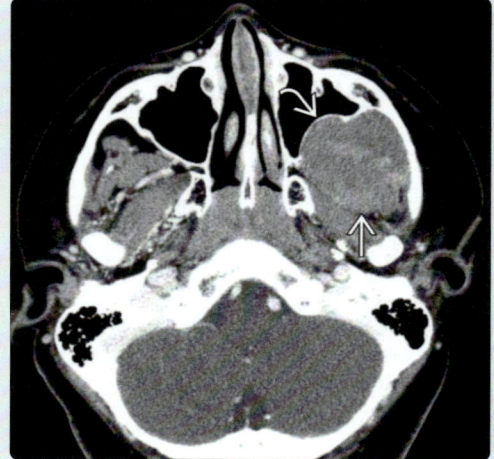
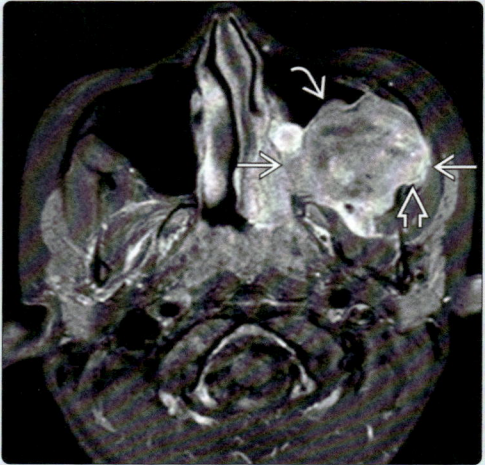

(Left) Axial CECT shows a heterogeneously enhancing rhabdomyosarcoma of the masticator space ➡. There has been pressure erosion and remodeling of the posterior maxillary sinus wall ➡, which belies the aggressive nature of the tumor. (Right) Axial T1WI C+ FS MR shows a heterogeneous rhabdomyosarcoma arising in the left masticator space ➡. Tumor remodels but also locally invades the maxillary sinus ➡ and zygoma ➡.

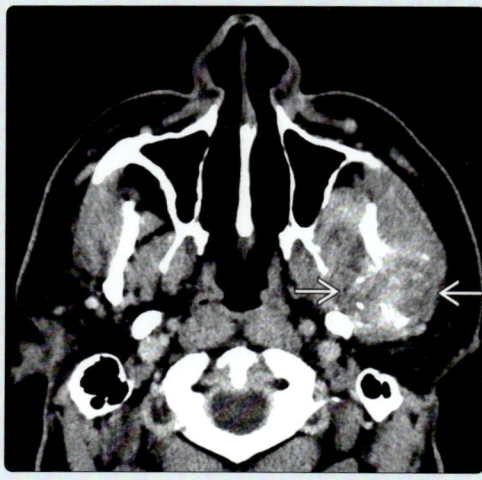
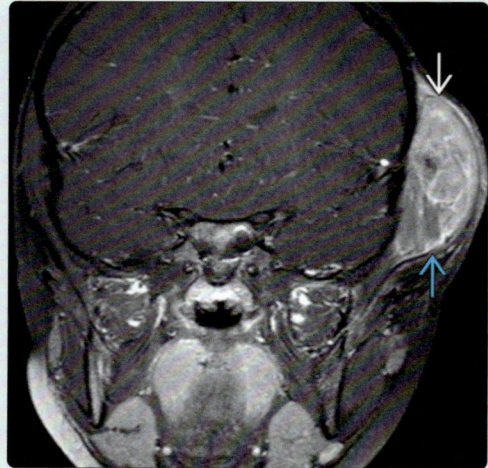

(Left) Axial CECT shows a heterogeneously enhancing masticator space angiosarcoma with highly aggressive invasion of the mandible demonstrating an explosive pattern of bony destruction and fragmentation ➡. (Right) Coronal T1WI C+ FS MR shows a bulky alveolar rhabdomyosarcoma ➡ of the suprazygomatic masticator space ➡ replacing the temporalis muscle. Tumor shows no invasion of the calvarium or intracranial contents.

TERMINOLOGY

Synonyms

- Many types: Rhabdomyosarcoma, leiomyosarcoma, Ewing sarcoma, synovial sarcoma, liposarcoma, fibrosarcoma

Definitions

- Masticator space sarcoma (MS-SA): Malignant tumor of soft tissue origin (fat, muscle, nerve, joint, blood vessel, or deep skin tissues) in MS

IMAGING

General Features

- Best diagnostic clue
  - Aggressive, poorly marginated MS mass with bone destruction and invasion of adjacent fascial planes
- Location
  - MS; frequently within or adjacent to mandible
  - Frequently extends outside of MS
- Size
  - Often **large** (> 4 cm) despite superficial MS location
- Morphology
  - Poorly marginated ± multilobulated

CT Findings

- CECT
  - Variable enhancement pattern; typically heterogeneous
- Bone CT
  - **Invasive MS mass** with mandibular, zygomatic arch, or pterygoid plate **destruction**
    - Jaw osteosarcomas show soft tissue extension in most cases (86%)
  - **Bone production** or **calcification** may occur in any SA
    - Most commonly seen in osteosarcoma (72%), chondrosarcoma, synovial and Ewing SA
    - Periosteal reaction seen in 62% of jaw osteosarcomas
  - Scalloped remodeling of bone in some SAs without aggressive features

MR Findings

- T1WI
  - Iso- to hyperintense to normal muscle, often heterogeneous
  - Mandible involvement shows mass replacing normal hyperintense marrow signal
- T2WI
  - Heterogeneously hyperintense to muscle
  - Flow voids (most visible on T2) may be present
- STIR
  - Heterogeneously hyperintense to muscle
- DWI
  - Quantitative ADC values may help distinguish between infection and SA
  - Suggested ADC value cutoff = $1.20 \times 10\text{-}3 \text{ mm}^2 \text{ s-1}$
    - Higher values suggest infection
    - Lower values suggest malignancy
- T1WI C+
  - Heterogeneous enhancement is typical

Nuclear Medicine Findings

- Bone scan
  - Tc-99m can assist with evaluation
- PET
  - F-18 FDG avid
  - Role in directing biopsy, predicting tumor grade, and assessing treatment response under investigation

Imaging Recommendations

- Best imaging tool
  - Thin-section bone CT combined with T1 C+ MR
    - MR for evaluation of soft tissues, possible mandibular invasion, and evaluation for **perineural tumor spread along CNV3**
    - Bone CT allows assessment of SA matrix ± bone destructive changes

DIFFERENTIAL DIAGNOSIS

Masticator Space Abscess

- Rim-enhancing MS fluid collection ± mandibular osteomyelitis
- Infection history

Invasive Squamous Cell Carcinoma

- Palatine tonsil squamous cell carcinoma (SCCa)
  - Palatine tonsil mass invades subjacent MS
- Retromolar trigone SCCa
  - Retromolar triangle mass invades MS

Mandible Metastasis

- Known primary malignancy ± other metastases
- Aggressive bony destructive changes
- ± periosteal reaction or tumoral calcification

Mandibular Osteomyelitis

- Bony destruction without osteoid formation
- Infection history; may see sequestrum formation

Masticator Space Venous Malformation

- Multiloculated, circumscribed mass ± flow voids and calcified phleboliths

Odontogenic Keratocyst

- Cystic mandible mass with benign expansile changes
  - Smooth, corticated borders without nodular enhancement

Perineural Tumor of CNV3 in Masticator Space

- Chin skin SCCa or SCCa primary of oral cavity or oropharynx
- Malignancy spreads along CNV3 into MS

PATHOLOGY

General Features

- Etiology
  - **Ionizing radiation** (most commonly from XRT to treat other tumors)
    - Account for < 5% of SAs
    - Average time between XRT and SA diagnosis: 10 years
  - Family history
    - Gardner syndrome: Risk of desmoid tumors (low-grade fibrosarcoma) in abdomen
    - Li-Fraumeni syndrome: ↑ risk of developing any soft tissue and bone SAs

- – Retinoblastoma (inherited form): ↑ risk of developing bone or soft tissue SAs
  - o Nodal injury
    - – Lymphangiosarcomas rarely found following surgical nodal dissection or in XRT fields
- Genetics
  - o DNA mutations common in soft tissue SA

Staging, Grading, & Classification

- Histologic grading (G) system: G1, G2, G3
  - o Determined by 3 parameters: Differentiation, mitotic activity, and necrosis
- American Joint Committee on Cancer (AJCC) 8th edition changes
  - o Head and neck SAs have own tumor (T) staging
    - – Reflects typically smaller tumor sizes of head and neck SA (compared to other SA in body) seen in clinical practice
    - – Reflects T4 classification based on invasion of adjacent structures
  - o Based on preliminary data suggesting effectiveness
- T staging in AJCC 8th edition
  - o T1: Tumor < 2 cm
  - o T2: Tumor > 2 cm but < 4 cm
  - o T3: Tumor > 4 cm
  - o T4: Invasion of adjoining structures
    - – T4A: Orbit, skull base, dura, central compartment viscera, pterygoid muscles, or facial skeleton
    - – T4B: Brain, CNS via perineural spread, prevertebral muscle, or carotid encasement
- N staging
  - o N0: No regional lymph node metastases
  - o N1: Regional lymph node metastases
- M staging
  - o M0: No distant metastases
  - o M1: Distant metastases

Gross Pathologic & Surgical Features

- Pathologic findings depend on SA type
- Heterogeneous mass with ossified (yellow-white, firm) and nonossified components (soft, tan foci of hemorrhage ± necrosis)
- Periosteal reaction: New bone lamellae at periphery

Microscopic Features

- Low-grade lesions
  - o Few mitotic figures, little, if any, cellular atypia, and relatively noninfiltrative growth pattern
- High-grade lesions
  - o Marked cellular atypia, hyperchromatism, nuclear pleomorphism, and infiltrative growth pattern

CLINICAL ISSUES

Presentation

- Most common signs/symptoms
  - o Enlarging mass over mandible ↑ pain
  - o Other signs/symptoms
    - – Trigeminal nerve symptoms
    - – Other cranial nerve deficits if skull base involved

Demographics

- Age
  - o Average age depends on histologic subtype
  - o Mean: 35 years old
- Sex
  - o M:F ~ 2:1
- Epidemiology
  - o ~ 8,000 new cases per year in USA
  - o Head and neck is rarer primary site for SA (SA more common in extremities)

Natural History & Prognosis

- Large portion of head and neck SAs are high grade &/or have advanced presentation with perineural tumor spread
- History of treated facial malignancy with radiation
- Propensity for local recurrence

Treatment

- SA location, in addition to pathology and TNM stage, is relevant to treatment planning
  - o Histologic type of SA is important for prognosis and treatment
  - o Optimal treatment strategies undergoing reevaluation following updated T staging in AJCC 8th edition
- Multimodality treatment usually recommended
  - o Typically wide local excision followed by XRT
  - o Chemotherapy added for higher stage tumors, round cell tumors, osteosarcoma
    - – Neoadjuvant or adjuvant depending, or recurrent SA
  - o Several targeted immunotherapies for certain histologies
  - o Possible role for adjuvant chemotherapy in unusual cases
  - o Possible proton and carbon ion radiotherapy

DIAGNOSTIC CHECKLIST

Consider

- Absent known systemic malignancy or signs of infection, MS mass should suggest diagnosis of SA
- Mandibular destruction ± perineural tumor spread along CNV3 toward skull base both suggest SA diagnosis from imaging perspective

Image Interpretation Pearls

- CT or MR invasive MS mass, suspected malignant SA
- Carefully evaluate for perineural tumor spread: Inferior alveolar canal, mandibular foramen, foramen ovale, and remainder of CNV3 course

SELECTED REFERENCES

1. Warren D et al: Head and neck sarcoma tumor board survival guide for neuroradiologists: imaging findings, history, and pathology. Curr Probl Diagn Radiol. 52(4):275-88, 2023
2. Kowa XY et al: Head and neck sarcomas: imaging "pearls" and "mimics". Br J Radiol. 94(1119):20200922, 2021
3. Cates JMM: Staging soft tissue sarcoma of the head and neck: evaluation of the AJCC 8th edition revised T classifications. Head Neck. 41(7):2359-66, 2019
4. Hahn E et al: Ending 40 years of silence: rationale for a new staging system for soft tissue sarcoma of the head and neck. Clin Transl Radiat Oncol. 15:13-9, 2019
5. Scelsi CL et al: Head and neck sarcomas: a review of clinical and imaging findings based on the 2013 World Health Organization classification. AJR Am J Roentgenol. 212(3):644-54, 2019

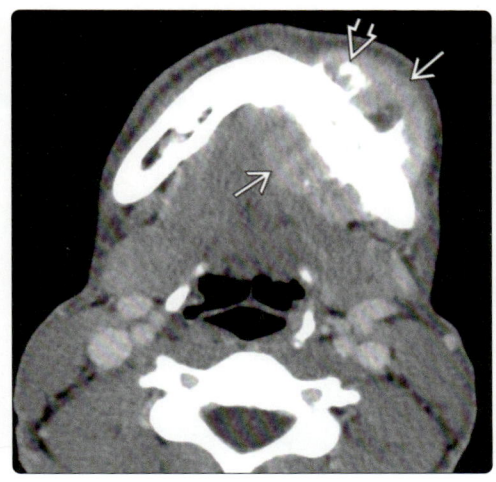

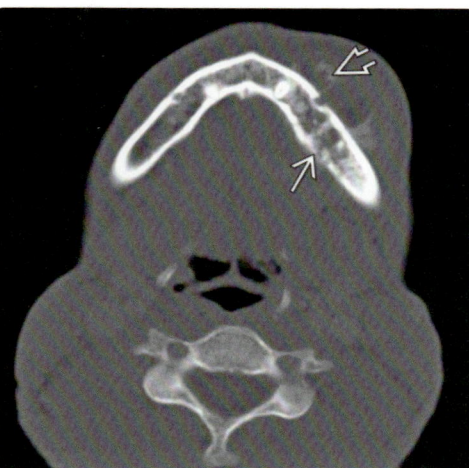

(Left) *Axial CECT shows a destructive, enhancing osteosarcoma arising from the left mandible* ➡️. *Associated periosteal reaction and bone formation are typical* ➡️. (Right) *Axial bone CT in the same patient with osteosarcoma of the jaw shows permeative destructive change in the mandible* ➡️ *with areas of cortical destruction and osteoid matrix* ➡️.

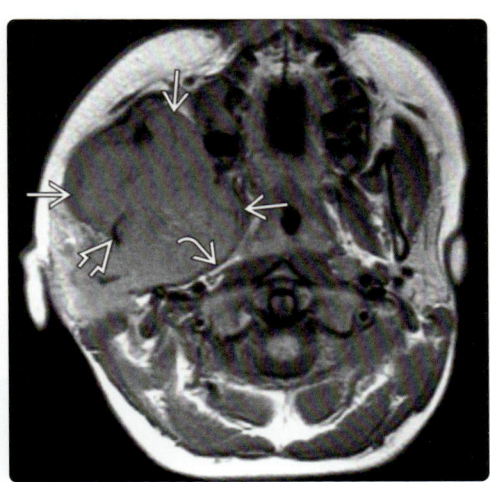

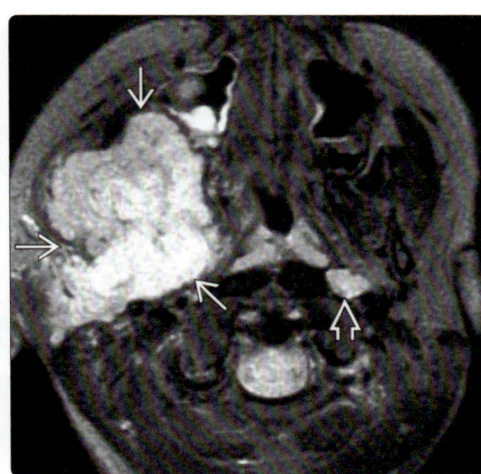

(Left) *Axial T1WI MR shows an Ewing sarcoma arising in the right mandible and spreading to the adjacent masticator space muscles. Notice the very large mass is hyperintense to muscle* ➡️. *Mandible destruction is present with only a small fragment* ➡️ *still visible. The parapharyngeal fat stripe* ➡️ *is displaced medially.* (Right) *Axial T2WI FS MR in the same patient shows the tumor is markedly hyperintense but heterogeneous* ➡️. *A prominent left retropharyngeal node* ➡️ *is incidentally noted.*

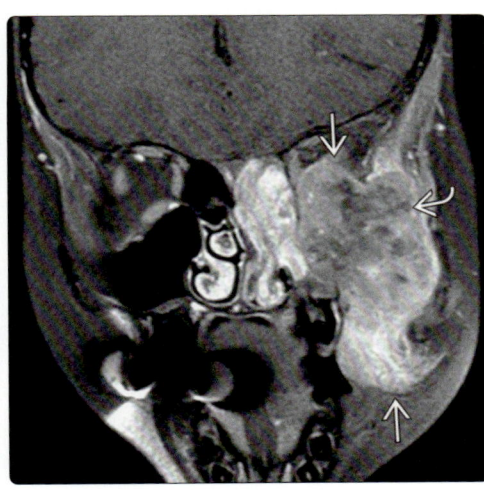

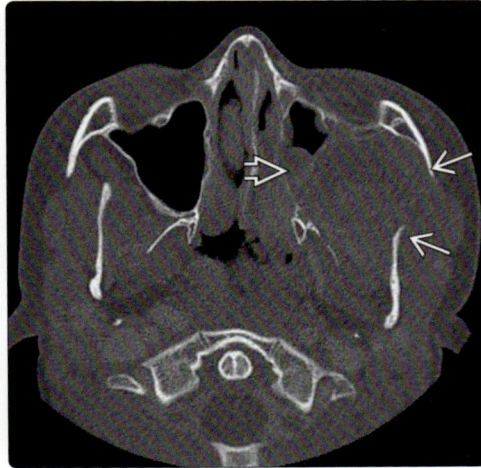

(Left) *Coronal T1WI C+ FS MR shows a masticator space rhabdomyosarcoma invading the inferior left orbit and nasal cavity* ➡️. *The botryoid (grape-like) appearance* ➡️ *of tumor on T1WI C+ MR is a described feature of head and neck rhabdomyosarcomas.* (Right) *Axial bone CT in the same patient shows smooth bony scalloping of adjacent bones* ➡️. *Aggressive tumors, such as this rhabdomyosarcoma, may have relatively benign osseous changes. Note more aggressive local erosion into maxillary sinus with local soft tissue extension* ➡️.

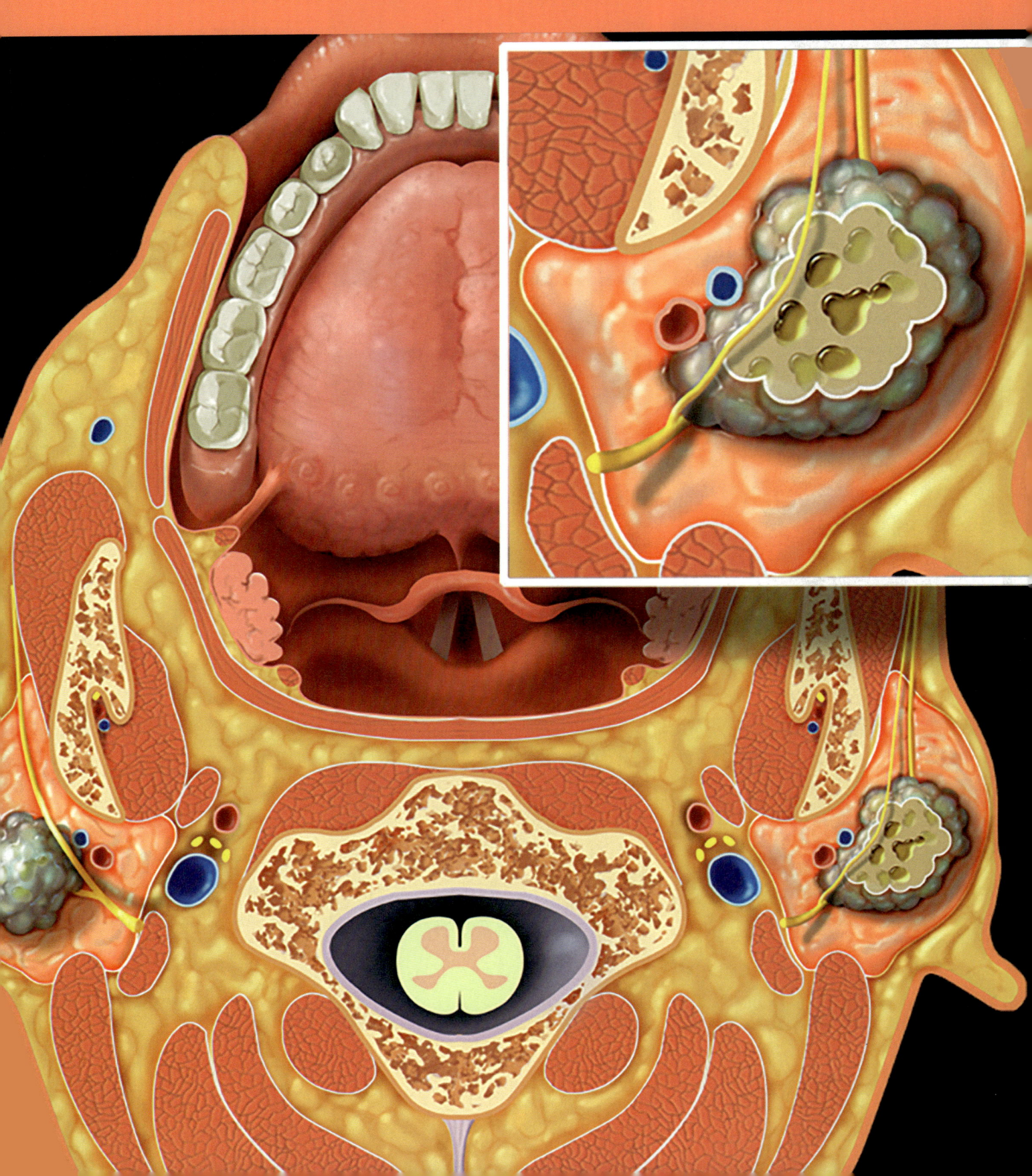

SECTION 5
Parotid Space

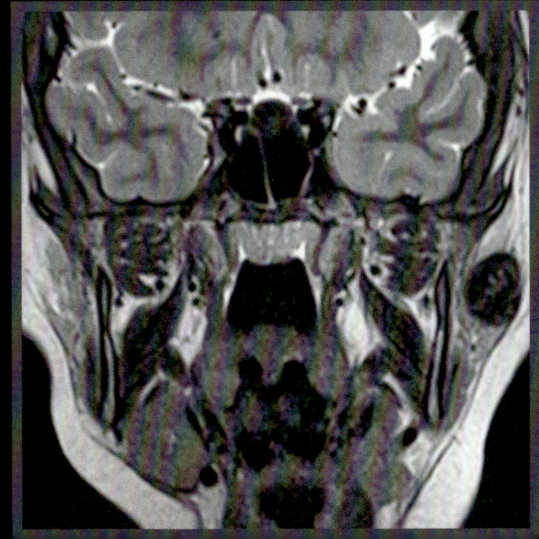
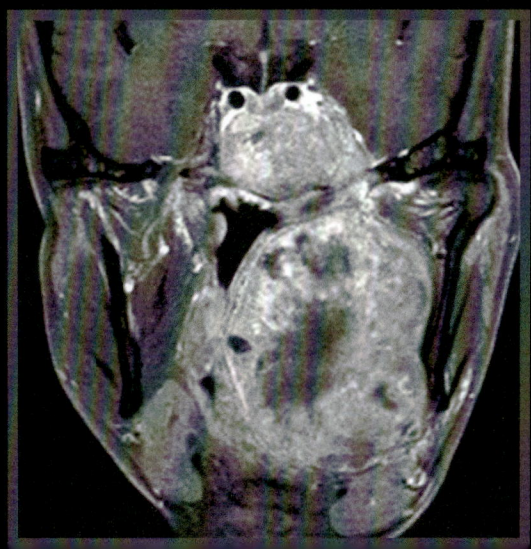

Summary Thoughts: Parotid Space

The parotid space (PS) lies in the lateral suprahyoid neck in the cheek anterior to the external auditory canal (EAC). The main content of the PS is the parotid gland, but many other critical structures, such as the facial nerve (CNVII), external carotid branches, and intraparotid lymph nodes, also lie within the boundaries of this space.

The PS is traditionally divided into **superficial and deep compartments**. The true dividing line between these compartments is the CNVII, but the nerve is not visible radiologically; therefore, an imaginary line between the stylomastoid foramen and the lateral margin of the retromandibular vein serves as a radiologic surrogate.

The deep PS compartment lies anterior to the styloid process and lateral to the parapharyngeal fat. The deep compartment is also called the "**prestyloid parapharyngeal space**" to emphasize these anatomic relationships. Recalling this name may help when determining the site of origin of a parapharyngeal mass; a mass arising anterior to the styloid, displacing parapharyngeal fat medially, is parotid in origin.

In the setting of a PS mass, the key findings are benign vs. aggressive margins, unifocal vs. multifocal, and homogeneity vs. heterogeneity. Potential involvement of CNVII must be carefully sought.

The main goal of imaging a parotid mass is not to provide a precise diagnosis (since this is often difficult). Instead, the **main goal is to guide the next step in the work-up**. For example, would a fine-needle aspiration (FNA) be useful? Does the patient need an oncologic excision with neck dissection?

Key findings in PS inflammation include calculi, ductal dilatation, and the number of glands affected.

Imaging Techniques

Either CECT or MR can be used to evaluate diseases of the PS. The choice is often based on regional preferences. Be aware that, in some patients, a number of parotid tumors can "vanish" or have low conspicuity on either CECT and some MR sequences, including T2 and enhanced T1 MR. Review of the noncontrast T1 MR sequences usually helps avoid this pitfall.

In the setting of suspected inflammatory disease, CT is preferred because it can identify small calculi. Enhanced CT best evaluates for complications, and parotid calcifications are rarely confused for enhancing vessels. The patient's head should be positioned so dental amalgam streak artifact does not interfere with evaluation of the gland or the parotid (Stensen) duct. Since the punctum of the parotid duct lies alongside the second maxillary molar, dental amalgam often interferes with evaluation of the punctum. Open-mouthed images can avoid this pitfall.

MR is preferred in the setting of CNVII paralysis because it can better identify **perineural spread**. MR also allows sialography, in which heavily T2-weighted images emphasize the ductal system in settings like Sjögren syndrome.

Catheter sialography, once a mainstay of parotid radiology, has now become rare because of competition from MR sialography, sialoendoscopy, and ultrasound.

Imaging Anatomy

The PS is a suprahyoid neck space only. PS anatomic relationships include the medial parapharyngeal space (PPS), anterior masticator space (MS), and posteromedial carotid space. The tail of the parotid projects into the posterior submandibular space below. Superiorly, the PS abuts the undersurface of the EAC and the mastoid tip.

The superficial layer of deep cervical fascia circumscribes the PS. This fascia surrounds the **superficial and deep lobes** of the parotid gland. The superficial lobe is ~ 2x as large as the deep lobe. An inconstant 3rd lobe, the **accessory lobe**, is seen in 20% of patients and lies superficial to the masseter muscle.

The parotid duct emerges from the anterior PS and runs along the surface of masseter muscle. It then arches through the buccal space to pierce the buccinator muscle at the level of the maxillary 2nd molar. The normal duct is small and often not appreciable on cross-sectional imaging.

CNVII runs through the center of the PS. Although not usually visible radiographically, its course may be approximated by an imaginary line from the stylomastoid foramen to the lateral aspect of the retromandibular vein. CNVII divides within the parotid, with 5 major branches arrayed in a sagittal plane. Superior to inferior, they are **temporal**, **zygomatic**, **buccal**, **marginal**, **and cervical branches**.

The external carotid artery is the medial and smaller of the 2 vessels behind the mandibular ramus in the PS. The lateral and larger of the 2 vessels is the retromandibular vein.

Because the parotid gland undergoes late encapsulation during development, mature **lymph nodes are present within the parenchyma of the gland**. This differentiates the parotid gland from other salivary glands and results in a longer differential diagnosis for parotid masses [including metastases, lymphoma, benign lymphoepithelial lesion (BLEL)-HIV, and Warthin tumors]. The intraparotid lymph nodes serve as 1st-order drainage for malignancies in the scalp, the EAC, and the deep face. Each gland contains ~ 20 nodes.

The parotid glands undergo progressive fatty degeneration throughout life. In childhood, the glands display density similar to the masseter muscle on CT. With age, gland density progressively decreases due to this process. Occasionally, one gland will undergo premature fatty degeneration.

Clinical Implications

Eighty percent of parotid masses are **benign**. Unfortunately, most parotid masses cannot be diagnosed by imaging alone. As a result, until biopsy or resection is performed, the exact diagnosis remains in question. Some benign lesions [pleomorphic adenoma (PA) in particular] need to be surgically removed because they might degenerate into malignancy, for cosmetic reasons, or to relieve mass effect on surrounding structures.

PA accounts for the majority of parotid masses. Although benign, it can undergo malignant degeneration. Consequently, **all PAs should be surgically removed**. PA also has a high rate of local recurrence, so superficial or total parotidectomy is needed to avoid tumor "spillage."

Parotid masses are a common incidental finding on imaging studies. Parotid malignancies account for 6% of incidentally discovered parotid masses. Because a specific diagnosis is usually not possible radiographically, the goal of imaging is to **determine the next step in the diagnostic process**.

- If discrete PS mass is seen, FNA or biopsy is most frequently employed; goal is not to prevent surgery, but to determine extent of surgery needed; malignancies

Parotid Space Overview

Congenital	Infectious-Inflammatory	Degenerative	Benign Tumor	Malignant Tumor, Primary	Neoplasm, Metastatic
Infantile hemangioma	Acute parotitis	Atrophy	Pleomorphic adenoma	Mucoepidermoid carcinoma	Skin cancer nodal metastasis
Venous, lymphatic and mixed malformations	Reactive adenopathy	Sialosis	Warthin tumor	Adenoid cystic carcinoma	Non-Hodgkin lymphoma nodal metastasis
1st branchial cleft cyst	Chronic parotitis		Oncocytoma	Acinic cell carcinoma	Systemic nodal metastasis
	Sjögren syndrome		Facial nerve schwannoma	Secretory carcinoma	
	Benign lymphoepithelial lesions of HIV		Lipoma	Adenocarcinomas	
	Kimura disease			Primary parotid non-Hodgkin lymphoma	
	Kikuchi disease			Salivary duct carcinoma	
	IgG4-related disease				

often require wider excision ± neck dissection since surgical goal is to perform all procedures in single operative setting; palpable lesions can be needled without imaging guidance; sonographic guidance is most appropriate for superficial lobe lesions; CT guidance is most appropriate for deep lobe lesions

- If aggressive lesion presents that clearly represents malignancy, resection and neck dissection may be performed even without definitive cytologic diagnosis; frozen section guidance is employed in such cases

Advanced imaging techniques, such as dynamic CT/MR, dual-energy CT, or quantitative ADC, may increase diagnostic confidence in the probable diagnosis of a PS mass. However, they cannot provide a definitive diagnosis. Thus, the goal of imaging continues to be guidance of the next clinical step.

Facial nerve palsy in the setting of a PS mass suggests a malignant etiology. Imaging is aimed at determining if the deep PS lobe is affected, if perineural tumor (PNT) is present, and if malignant adenopathy exists. MR is preferred in this setting, as it is particularly sensitive to the presence of PNT. In addition to PNT spread along CNVII, tumors may extend along the **auriculotemporal branch** of the trigeminal nerve. This PNT route runs through the parotid gland, behind the mandibular ramus, joining the main trunk of CNV3 in the MS below the foramen ovale.

Approaches to Imaging Issues of Parotid Space

The answer to the question, "What imaging findings define a PS mass?" is simple for a small parotid mass partly or completely surrounded by parotid tissue. Determining the space of origin for a larger, deep lobe PS mass is more challenging, but typically **PPS fat** is **displaced medially** with MS pterygoid muscles pushed anteriorly. The stylomandibular tunnel is also often widened by a deep lobe mass.

When developing a differential diagnosis for parotid masses, the most important consideration is **multiplicity**.

- **Multiple bilateral lesions** suggest unique differential diagnoses, such as Sjögren syndrome, BLEL-HIV, Warthin tumor, non-Hodgkin lymphoma, or systemic metastases

- For **multifocal unilateral lesions**, primary parotid lymphoma and regional metastases should be more strongly considered; PA is unlikely in this setting
- **Solitary intraparotid lesion** is most often PA; although Warthin tumor may be multifocal, most are solitary

Parotid mass margins can be used to suggest if a lesion is benign or malignant. Ill-defined, aggressive margins suggest a malignant lesion is present. A well-circumscribed lesion is usually benign. However, a **well-defined parotid mass should not be assumed to be benign** since a low-grade malignancy may have an imaging appearance identical to that of PA.

Although there are no truly specific imaging findings to distinguish parotid masses, some diagnoses have characteristic features that may be helpful.

- PA at times will have hyperintense T2 signal (> CSF); when present, this finding strongly suggests PA
- Warthin tumor may appear as well-defined, cystic, rim-enhancing mass; unfortunately, PS carcinoma [especially mucoepidermoid carcinoma (MECa)] may have cystic degeneration mimicking this
- PNT spread is a hallmark of malignancy; while adenoid cystic carcinoma is known for this tendency, lymphoma, MECa, and squamous cell carcinoma can spread this way

Always note the relationship of a PS mass to the CNVII plane. Designate the mass as superficial, deep, or in the same plane as the intraparotid CNVII. Superficial lobe masses are removed by superficial parotidectomy, while deep lobe masses require total parotidectomy. Parotid tail masses must be identified as intraparotid, or their excision may injure CNVII. Remember that the platysma and sternocleidomastoid muscles are the superficial and deep borders of the parotid tail, respectively.

Selected References

1. Singh R et al: Newly discovered parotid lesion: what next? Curr Probl Diagn Radiol. 52(2):134-8, 2023
2. McGeary R et al: Navigating the parotid glands: anatomy, imaging work-up and next steps. Clin Neuroradiol. 32(3):615-23, 2022

Parotid Space Overview

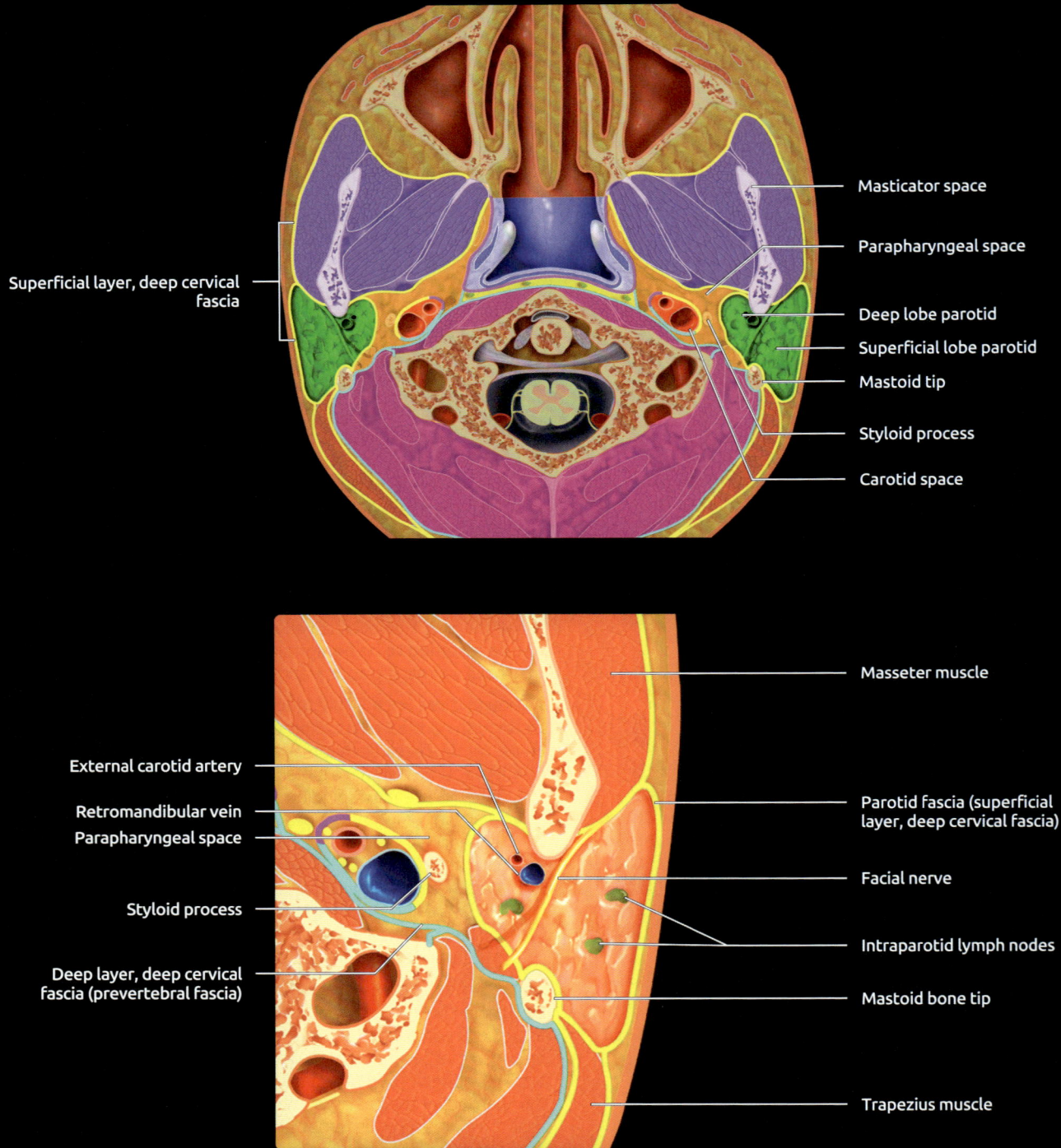

Masticator space

Parapharyngeal space

Superficial layer, deep cervical fascia

Deep lobe parotid

Superficial lobe parotid

Mastoid tip

Styloid process

Carotid space

Masseter muscle

External carotid artery

Retromandibular vein

Parapharyngeal space

Parotid fascia (superficial layer, deep cervical fascia)

Facial nerve

Styloid process

Intraparotid lymph nodes

Deep layer, deep cervical fascia (prevertebral fascia)

Mastoid bone tip

Trapezius muscle

(Top) *Axial graphic of the suprahyoid neck soft tissues shows the relationships between the parotid space (green) and the surrounding spaces on the right. Notice the masticator space is anterior, while the parapharyngeal space is medial, and the carotid space is posteromedial. On the left, the superficial layer of deep cervical fascia (yellow line) is seen to circumscribe both the masticator and parotid spaces.* (Bottom) *Axial graphic at the level of C1 vertebral body shows the contents of the parotid space. The intraparotid course of the facial nerve (not seen with imaging) extends from just medial to the mastoid tip to a position just lateral to the retromandibular vein. Within the superficial lobe (parotid superficial to the facial nerve), only parotid tissue and nodes are present. Within the deep lobe, notice the medial external carotid artery and retromandibular vein. The parapharyngeal space fat lies just medial to the deep lobe of the gland.*

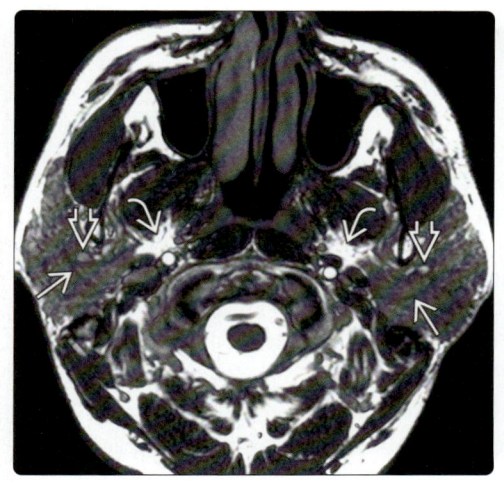
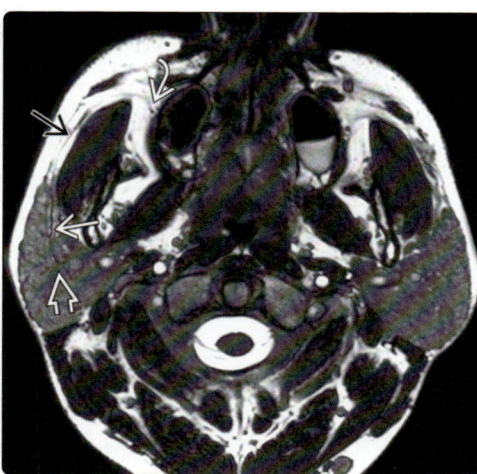

(Left) Axial T2WI high-resolution MR shows the intraparotid facial nerve ⇒ dividing the parotid space into superficial and deep lobes. The retromandibular vein ⇒ is visible just medial to the CNVII projected course. The parapharyngeal space fat ⇒ is immediately medial to the deep lobe. (Right) Axial T2WI high-resolution MR reveals the intraparotid duct ⇒ and radicals ⇒. The duct is seen superficial to the masseter muscle ⇒. It continues anteromedially to pierce the buccinator muscle ⇒.

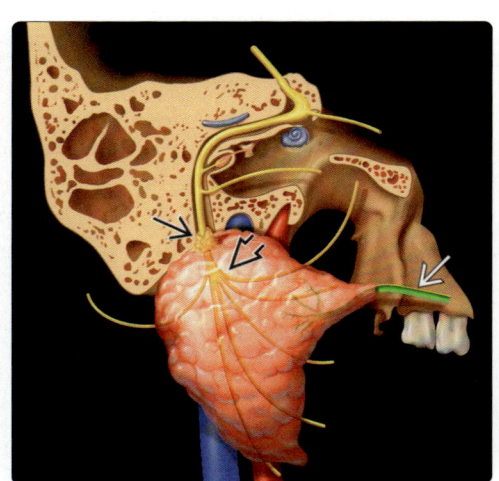
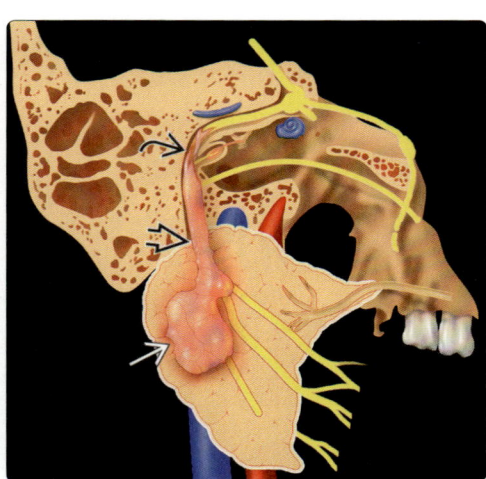

(Left) Sagittal graphic of the parotid shows the facial nerve exiting the temporal bone through the stylomastoid foramen ⇒, then branching ⇒ into its 5 components. The facial nerve plane defines the parotid superficial and deep lobes. Note also the parotid duct ⇒. (Right) Sagittal graphic of a parotid malignancy ⇒ shows perineural tumor spread following the intraparotid facial nerve through the stylomastoid foramen ⇒ along the mastoid segment to the posterior genu area ⇒.

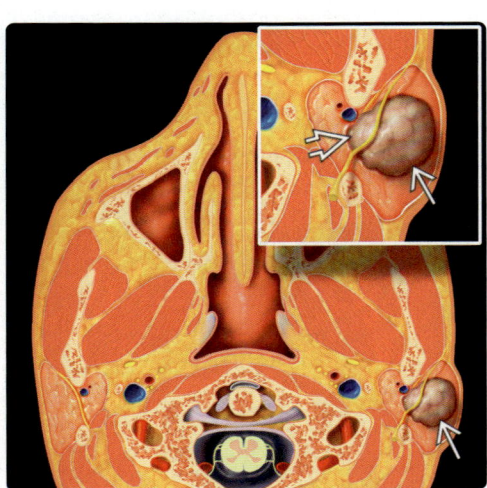
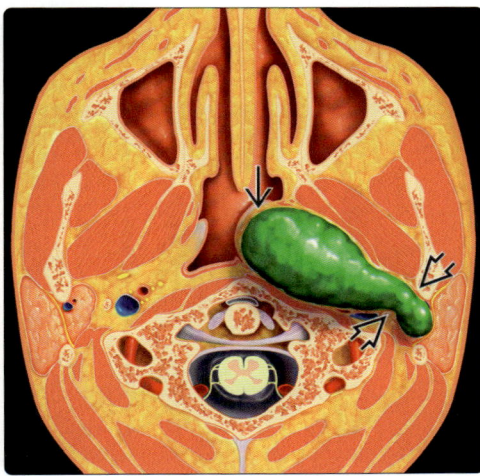

(Left) Axial graphic of intraparotid well-circumscribed tumor ⇒ shows it is primarily in the superficial lobe but has a small component ⇒ crossing the facial nerve plane. If tumor needle biopsy revealed PA diagnosis, it still may be possible to remove it via superficial parotidectomy. (Right) Axial graphic of a deep lobe parotid mass shows medial displacement of the parapharyngeal space fat ⇒. Note widening of the stylomandibular tunnel ⇒. Total parotidectomy is necessary for removal.

KEY FACTS

TERMINOLOGY

- Acute inflammation of parotid gland
  - Bacterial: Localized bacterial infection; ± abscess
  - Viral: Usually from systemic viral infection
  - Calculus induced: Ductal obstruction by sialolith
  - Autoimmune: Acute episode of chronic disease
  - Juvenile recurrent parotitis (JRP): Intermittent, idiopathic; some may have Sjögren syndrome

IMAGING

- Typical appearance: ↑ size and enhancement of parotid ± stranding of surrounding fat; parotid retains normal shape
- Bacterial parotitis: Typically unilateral
  - Periparotid cellulitis/stranding common
  - Intra- or periparotid abscess may occur
- Calculus-induced parotitis: Typically unilateral
  - Large duct with intraluminal stone
- Viral parotitis: Typically bilateral
  - Clinical diagnosis; imaging rarely required

- Autoimmune parotitis: Typically bilateral
  - Diagnose with serum markers
  - Sialography for chronic complications
- JRP: Often unilateral clinically with bilateral imaging abnormalities
  - Normal main duct + dilated intraglandular branches

TOP DIFFERENTIAL DIAGNOSES

- Sjögren syndrome
- Benign lymphoepithelial lesions of HIV
- Parotid sialosis
- Parotid sarcoidosis
- Infected 1st branchial cleft anomaly
- Parotid Infantile hemangioma

DIAGNOSTIC CHECKLIST

- Sialography for recurrent disease to assess complications
- Reimage parotid if residual mass after acute infection resolves to exclude underlying malignancy or abscess

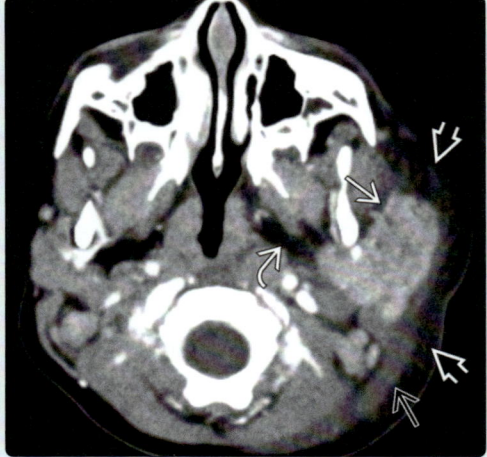
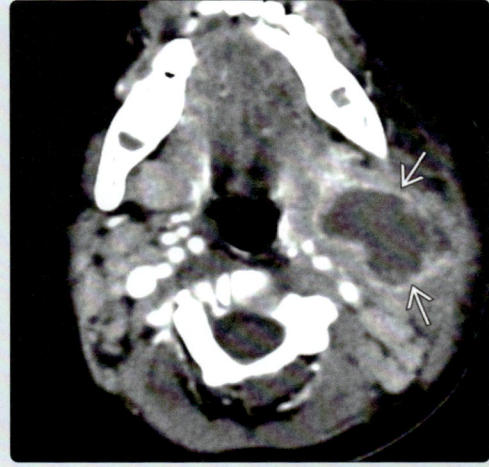

(Left) Axial CECT in a 2-year-old with fever and facial swelling demonstrates diffuse enlargement and asymmetric enhancement of the left parotid gland ➡. There is associated facial cellulitis ⇨, edema in the parapharyngeal fat ➡, and myositis ➡, typical of acute bacterial parotitis. (Right) Axial CECT shows a low-density collection ➡ replacing the left parotid gland. There is substantial surrounding fat stranding, indicating an infectious source. These findings suggest abscess complicating acute bacterial parotitis.

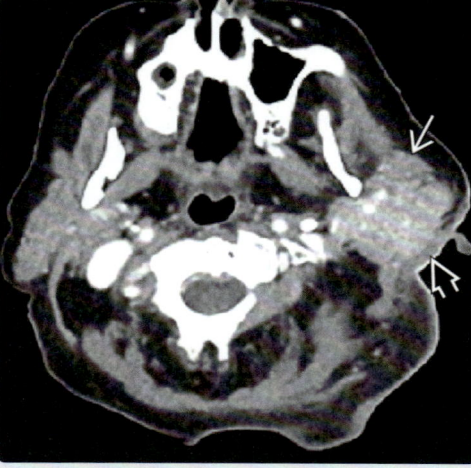
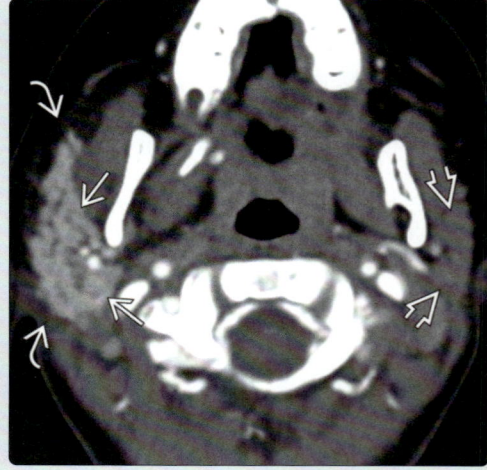

(Left) Axial CECT in an 88-year-old woman with COVID-19 shows typical findings of acute parotitis: Diffuse enlargement and asymmetric enhancement of the left parotid gland ➡ and moderate edema in the adjacent subcutaneous fat ⇨. (Right) Axial CECT in a 4-year-old boy shows diffuse enlargement and hyperenhancement of the right parotid gland ➡ relative to the left ⇨, consistent with unilateral parotitis. There is mild cellulitis involving the adjacent subcutaneous fat ➡.

Acute Parotitis

TERMINOLOGY

Synonyms

- Acute sialadenitis

Definitions

- Acute inflammation of parotid gland
  - Bacterial: Localized infection may become suppurative with central abscess
  - Viral: Usually from systemic viral infection
  - Calculus induced: Ductal obstruction by sialolith
  - Autoimmune: Acute episode of chronic disease
  - Juvenile recurrent parotitis (JRP) or chronic recurrent parotitis of childhood: Intermittent idiopathic episodes of parotid inflammation

IMAGING

General Features

- Best diagnostic clue
  - Enlarged parotid(s) with surrounding fat stranding
- Location
  - Bacterial: Usually unilateral
  - Viral: 75% bilateral; submandibular and sublingual glands may also be involved
  - Calculus induced: Unilateral with radiopaque stone in parotid duct
  - Autoimmune: Usually bilateral
  - Juvenile recurrent: Unilateral or asymmetric clinical presentation with bilateral imaging findings
- Morphology
  - Usually involves entire gland but can be focal
  - Parotid retains normal configuration as it enlarges

CT Findings

- CECT
  - Bacterial: Enlarged, diffusely enhancing parotid
    - Inflammatory stranding of surrounding fat
    - Ring enhancement of low-density abscesses (if present)
  - Viral: Enlarged parotids with mild enhancement
  - Calculus induced: Calcified stone; dilated parotid duct with enhancing walls, otherwise like bacterial
  - Autoimmune: Less stranding of surrounding fat
    - May have ductal dilatation if longstanding disease

MR Findings

- T2WI
  - Diffuse moderately high signal ± focal areas of fluid signal (microabscesses or dilated ducts)
- T1WI C+
  - Enlarged parotid gland with diffuse, moderate enhancement
  - Abscesses: Rim-enhancing fluid collections
- MR sialography (3D SSFP)
  - Exquisite for demonstrating cysts or dilated ducts
  - JRP: Normal main duct with dilated intraglandular branches (sialectasis)

Ultrasonographic Findings

- Enlarged, hypoechoic, heterogeneous, hyperemic gland
- Sensitive for detection of calculi
- Numerous small hypoechoic lesions bilaterally in JRP
- Focal, hypoechoic collection suggests abscess formation
- US can be used to guide aspiration

Other Modality Findings

- Sialography contraindicated in acute suppurative parotitis
  - Useful in evaluating recurrent disease and complications when sialendoscopy not available

Imaging Recommendations

- Best imaging tool
  - Bacterial and calculus-induced inflammation: CECT best for detection of stone or abscess
  - Viral parotitis: Typically clinical diagnosis
    - Imaging rarely required
  - Autoimmune disease: Diagnosed with serum markers
    - Sialography for chronic complications
  - JRP: MR sialography or conventional sialogram

DIFFERENTIAL DIAGNOSIS

Sjögren Syndrome

- Dry eyes and mouth; arthritis
- Cystic and solid intraparotid lesions

Benign Lymphoepithelial Lesions of HIV

- Bilateral heterogeneous glands, ± cystic and solid lesions
- Prominent Waldeyer ring and cervical nodes
- Affects parotid only, not other salivary glands
- May be found prior to HIV seroconversion

Parotid Sialosis

- Bilateral, prolonged, painless, soft parotid (and occasionally submandibular) gland enlargement
- Associated with alcoholism, endocrinopathies (especially diabetes mellitus), malnutrition (anorexia nervosa, bulimia)

Parotid Sarcoidosis

- Rare manifestation of H&N sarcoidosis
- Nodal or parenchymal inflammatory changes

Infected 1st Branchial Cleft Anomaly

- 1st branchial cleft cyst in or adjacent to parotid gland
- Superinfection presents as parotid abscess

Parotid Malignancy

- Firm focal or infiltrative mass without hyperenhancement
  - Benign: Pleomorphic adenoma
  - Malignant: Adenoid cystic carcinoma, mucoepidermoid carcinoma, acinic cell carcinoma

Parotid Infantile Hemangioma

- Diffusely expanded, hypervascular, and homogeneously hyperenhancing parotid; normal surrounding soft tissues
- Presents with swelling in 1st few weeks-months of life

PATHOLOGY

General Features

- Etiology
  - Bacterial: Usually due to ascending infection
    - May result from adjacent cellulitis
    - *Staphylococcus aureus* (50-90%) > *Streptococcus, Haemophilus, Escherichia coli*, anaerobes

- – Neonatal suppurative parotitis may be bilateral, due to bacteremia
  - □ More common in premature infants, males
  - ○ Viral: Mumps paramyxovirus most common cause; so-called epidemic parotitis
    - – Also influenza, parainfluenza, Coxsackie A and B, ECHO, lymphocytic choriomeningitis viruses
    - – CMV, adenovirus reported with HIV infection
    - – COVID-19 recently reported
  - ○ JRP
    - – Recurrent episodes mimic mumps
    - – Usually begin by 5 years of age; resolves by age 10-15
    - – Patient often has unilateral symptoms but bilateral sialographic abnormalities
    - – Sialographically mimics Sjögren syndrome
    - – Etiology unknown; up to 40% of patients may have Sjögren syndrome if alternate pediatric criteria used
  - ○ Other lesions that may have acute parotitis presentation
    - – Sjögren syndrome
    - – Mikulicz syndrome
    - – Sicca syndrome, acute phase
- Bacterial and calculus induced usually unilateral
- Viral and autoimmune more frequently bilateral

CLINICAL ISSUES

Presentation

- Most common signs/symptoms
  - ○ Bacterial: Sudden-onset parotid pain and swelling
  - ○ Viral: Prodromal symptoms of headaches, malaise, myalgia followed by parotid pain, earache, trismus
  - ○ Calculus induced: Recurrent episodes of swollen, painful gland, usually related to eating
  - ○ Autoimmune: Recurrent episodes of tender gland swelling, accompanied by dry mouth
  - ○ JRP: Recurrent episodes ± fever, malaise
- Clinical profile
  - ○ Bacterial: Acutely painful, enlarged parotid in debilitated patient or neonate
  - ○ Predisposing factors
    - – Dehydration, surgery, diuretics, or anticholinergics reducing salivary flow
    - – Duct obstruction by calculus
    - – Immunosuppression, poor oral hygiene, malnutrition
  - ○ Viral: More frequently seen in children who have not received MMR vaccine
  - ○ JRP: Recurrent episodes of painful parotid swelling, often with fever and malaise

Demographics

- Age
  - ○ Bacterial: > 50 years and neonates
  - ○ Viral: Most < 15 years; peak age 5-9 years
  - ○ JRP: Usually begins by 5 years; resolves by age 10-15
- Epidemiology
  - ○ Parotid is most commonly inflamed salivary gland (absence of bacteriostatic mucin in its serous secretions)

Natural History & Prognosis

- Bacterial parotitis mortality may reach 20%
  - ○ Due to occurrence in debilitated older adult patients

- Responds well to early treatment, though number of complications recognized
  - ○ Early complications
    - – Abscess formation → rupture to deep neck spaces, external auditory canal (EAC), or TMJ
    - – Thrombophlebitis of retromandibular or facial veins → internal jugular vein thrombosis
    - – CNVII dysfunction rarely found; usually resolves
  - ○ Long-term complications
    - – Sialectasis (ductal dilation) with recurrent infections, reduced salivation, pain
- Viral parotitis self-limited; swelling lasts ≤ 2 weeks
  - ○ Systemic mumps paramyxovirus has complications
    - – Orchitis, meningoencephalitis, thyroiditis, sensorineural hearing loss, pancreatitis
- Autoimmune: Slowly progressive disease
  - ○ May be complicated by non-Hodgkin lymphoma
- JRP: Usually resolves by age 10-15

Treatment

- Bacterial parotitis
  - ○ Broad spectrum antibiotics, rehydration, good oral hygiene, sialogogues
  - ○ Surgical drainage of abscesses
- Calculus-induced parotitis
  - ○ Extract smaller stones from duct (perorally)
  - ○ Larger proximal stones may require surgical removal ± parotidectomy
- Viral parotitis
  - ○ Supportive treatment with rest, hydration
- Autoimmune parotitis
  - ○ Immunosuppressive medications (steroids)
- JRP
  - ○ Sialography or sialendoscopy ± corticosteroid application

DIAGNOSTIC CHECKLIST

Consider

- Sialography for recurrent disease to assess complications
- Reimage parotid if residual mass after resolution of acute infection to exclude underlying malignancy or abscess

Image Interpretation Pearls

- Carefully inspect entire parotid duct for calculi

SELECTED REFERENCES

1. Boogaard S et al: Interventional treatment for juvenile recurrent parotitis: a 10-year experience in a tertiary centre. Int J Pediatr Otorhinolaryngol. 192:112308, 2025
2. Guhan M et al: Autoimmune etiologies in pediatric recurrent parotitis: a retrospective analysis of patients referred to rheumatology. Int J Pediatr Otorhinolaryngol. 188:112192, 2025
3. Fisher J et al: COVID-19 associated parotitis. Am J Emerg Med. 39:254.e1-3, 2021
4. Lechien JR et al: Parotitis-like symptoms associated with COVID-19, France, March-April 2020. Emerg Infect Dis. 26(9):2270-1, 2020
5. Schiffer BL et al: Sjögren's syndrome in children with recurrent parotitis. Int J Pediatr Otorhinolaryngol. 129:109768, 2020
6. Tucci FM et al: Juvenile recurrent parotitis: diagnostic and therapeutic effectiveness of sialography. Retrospective study on 110 children. Int J Pediatr Otorhinolaryngol. 124:179-84, 2019
7. Guerin JB et al: Pediatric parotid region lesions: an imaging review. Neurographics. 8(6):394-412, 2018
8. Inarejos Clemente EJ et al: Imaging evaluation of pediatric parotid gland abnormalities. Radiographics. 38(5):1552-75, 2018

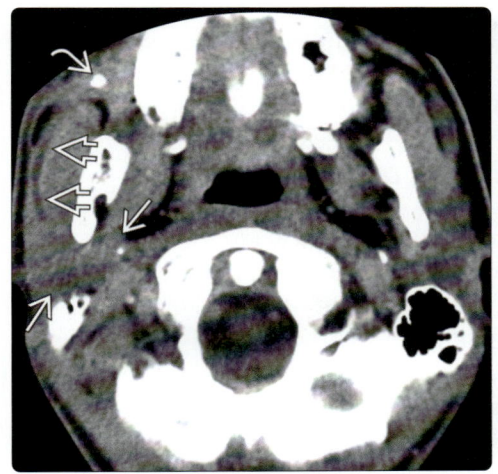

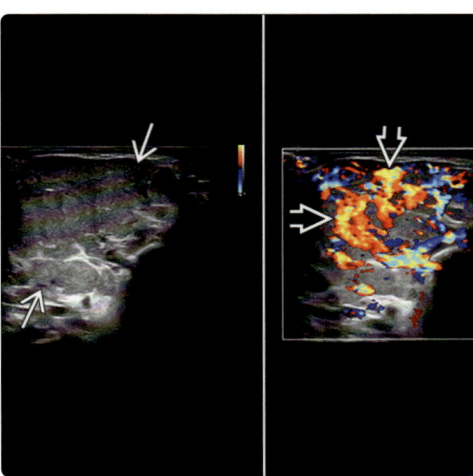

(Left) Axial CECT in a teenage boy with calculus-induced parotitis shows typical enlargement and asymmetric enhancement of the right parotid gland ➡, enlargement of the parotid duct ➡, and distal intraluminal stone ➡. (Right) Transverse grayscale (left) and color Doppler ultrasounds (right) in a 2-month-old infant with facial swelling show diffuse enlargement of a mildly heterogeneous parotid gland ➡ and diffuse hyperemia ➡ without an intraparotid abscess.

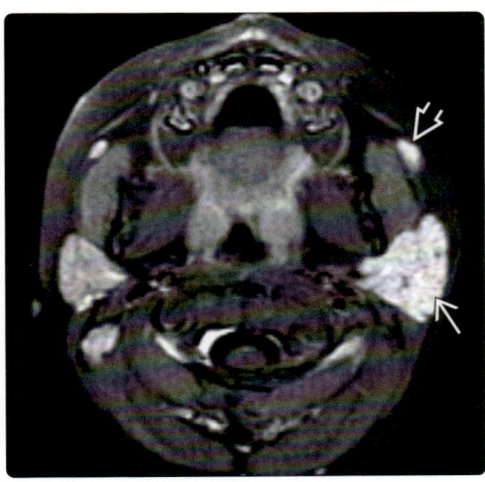

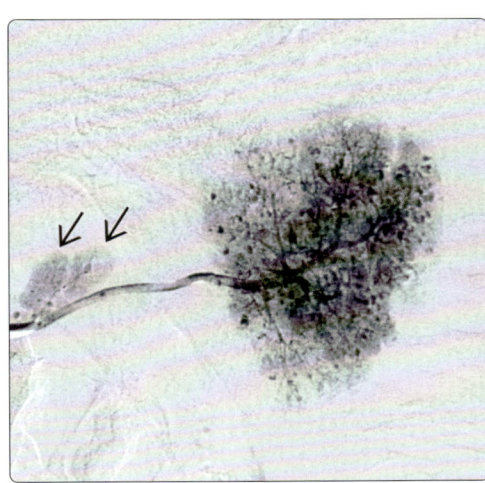

(Left) Axial T1 C+ FS MR in a child with recurrent parotitis shows an enlarged, asymmetrically enhancing left parotid gland ➡ without significant cellulitis. Note moderate enhancement in the ipsilateral accessory glandular tissue ➡ as well. (Right) Lateral sialogram in the same child demonstrates multiple small puddles/collections of contrast throughout the left parotid gland and a few within the accessory parotid tissue ➡. Notice the normal caliber of the ducts.

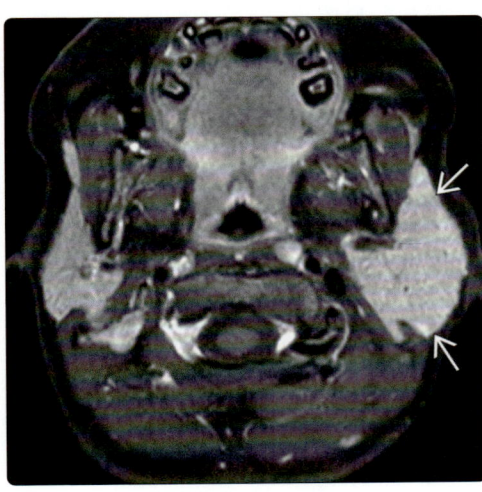

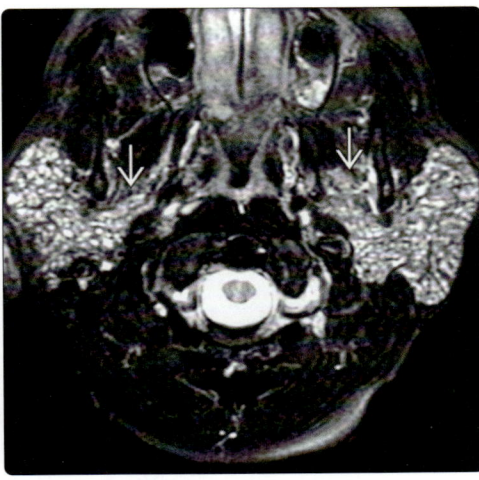

(Left) Axial T1 C+ FS MR in a 2-year-old with facial swelling after viral respiratory infection shows diffuse enlargement of the left parotid gland ➡, which is asymmetrically enhancing relative to the right without cellulitis or abscess. (Right) Axial T2 FS MR shows diffuse enlargement of both parotid glands with numerous foci of increased signal. This patient has an acute exacerbation of autoimmune sialadenitis. Note that the diffuse involvement includes the deep parotid lobes ➡.

Parotid Sjögren Syndrome

TERMINOLOGY

- Sjögren syndrome (SjS): Chronic systemic **autoimmune exocrinopathy** causing salivary & lacrimal gland destruction
  - Primary SjS: Dry eyes & mouth; no autoimmune disorders
  - Secondary SjS: Dry eyes & mouth with autoimmune disorders, most often rheumatoid arthritis

IMAGING

- Imaging appearance depends on stage of disease & presence or absence of lymphocyte aggregates
  - Early-stage SjS: Parotids may appear normal
  - Intermediate-stage SjS: Miliary pattern of **small cysts** diffusely throughout both parotids
  - Late-stage SjS: Larger cysts (parenchymal destruction) & solid masses (lymphocyte aggregates) in both parotids
  - Chronic atrophy with **salt & pepper** micronodularity
- ± punctate diffuse **calcifications** in both parotids
- Conventional or MR sialography
  - Alternating ductal stenosis & dilatation (**string of beads** appearance)
  - Acinar spill into enlarged acini (**apple tree** pattern)
- Ultrasound shows multiple hypoechoic & anechoic foci
  - Small hyperechoic lines & spots
  - ↑ dot-like vascularity on color Doppler

TOP DIFFERENTIAL DIAGNOSES

- Chronic infectious or obstructive parotitis
- Benign lymphoepithelial lesions of HIV
- IgG4-related disease; parotid Warthin tumor; parotid lymphoma; parotid nodal metastases

CLINICAL ISSUES

- Tender, bilateral parotid gland swelling
- Striking **female** predominance (90-95%)
- ↑ risk of malignancy in primary SjS
  - **Relative risk of non-Hodgkin lymphoma = 10-40x**
  - Biopsy if dominant parotid mass ± lymphadenopathy

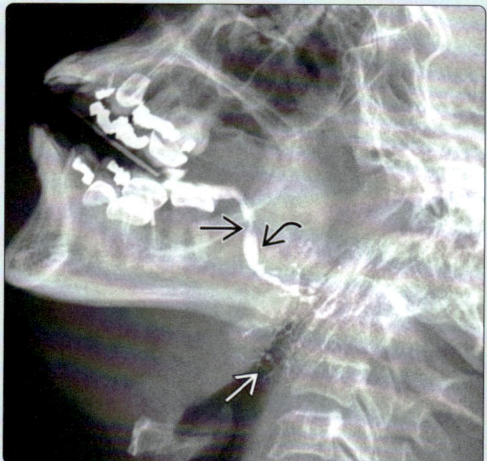
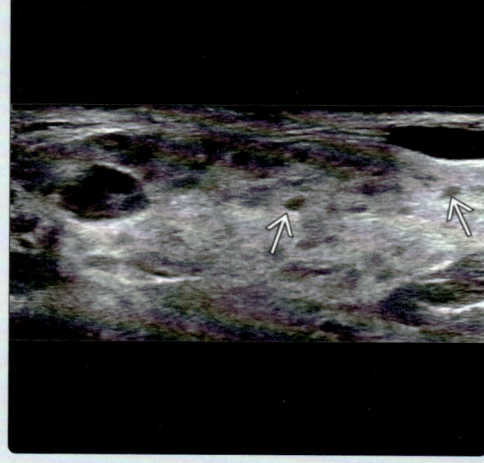

(Left) *Lateral parotid sialogram shows stenosis ➡ and dilation ➡ in the Stensen duct (string of beads appearance). Intraglandular branches are truncated with cystic spaces (apple tree pattern) ➡. Findings can be seen in any chronic sialadenitis but are classic for Sjögren syndrome.* (Right) *Longitudinal ultrasound demonstrates multiple hypoechoic intraparotid nodules ➡, giving a leopard skin appearance. Concurrent CT in this patient appeared normal. Ultrasound is more sensitive to findings of Sjögren syndrome.*

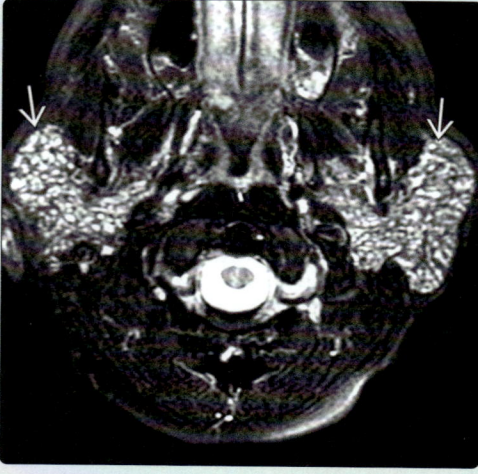
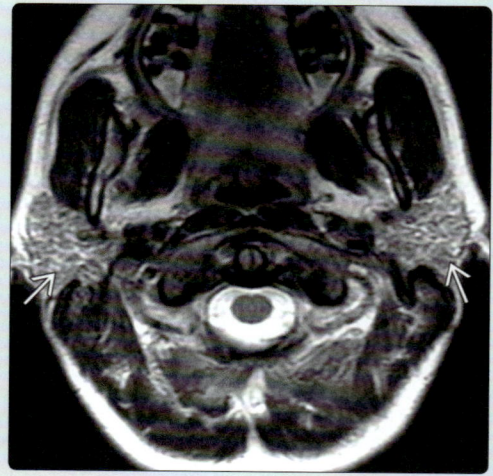

(Left) *Axial T2WI FS MR shows innumerable tiny cysts completely replacing both parotid glands ➡. The glands are markedly enlarged. This represents the acute phase of Sjögren syndrome.* (Right) *Axial T2WI MR in a patient undergoing brain MR for neuromyelitis optica, who also had known Sjögren disease, shows the characteristic salt and pepper appearance of diffuse micronodularity ➡ within the parotids, typical of its chronic form. Primary Sjögren disease is associated with an increased frequency of CNS disorders.*

TERMINOLOGY

Abbreviations

- Sjögren syndrome (SjS)

Synonyms

- Sicca syndrome, sicca complex

Definitions

- SjS: Chronic systemic **autoimmune exocrinopathy** that causes salivary & lacrimal gland tissue destruction
  - Primary SjS: Dry eyes & mouth
    - Usually no other autoimmune diseases
    - ± extraglandular manifestations: Peripheral &/or CNS
  - Secondary SjS: Dry eyes & mouth associated with other autoimmune diseases, most often rheumatoid arthritis (RA)
- Juvenile SjS
  - Predilection for male children until teen years
  - Usually resolves with puberty

IMAGING

General Features

- Best diagnostic clue
  - CT shows **bilateral, enlarged parotids** with multiple **cystic** & **solid** intraparotid lesions ± smooth, round intraglandular calcifications
- Location
  - Bilateral salivary & lacrimal glands
  - Ranula potential early finding in SjS
    - Seen before or at time of diagnosis in 82% of cases
- Size
  - Submillimeters to macrocysts or mixed solid-cystic masses > 2 cm
  - Punctate sialectasis found in early stage/young SjS
  - Adult SjS characterized by atrophy & fatty degeneration
- Morphology
  - Diffuse, bilateral parotid enlargement early, atrophy late
  - Variant: Dominant solid nodule mimics tumor
  - Premature fat deposition progresses over time
- Imaging appearance depends on disease stage & presence or absence of lymphocyte aggregates
  - Early-stage SjS: Parotids may appear normal
  - Intermediate-stage SjS: Miliary pattern of **small cysts** diffusely throughout both parotids
  - Late-stage SjS: Small nodules (lymphocyte aggregates) interspersed with fat ± cysts (parenchymal destruction)
  - Any stage may have solid intraparotid masses that mimic tumor secondary to lymphocytic accumulation
  - Dominant parotid mass ± cervical adenopathy worrisome for **lymphomatous transformation**

CT Findings

- NECT
  - Symmetric parotid enlargement with ↑ CT density & heterogeneity early
  - ± punctate diffuse **calcifications** in both parotids
  - Late fatty atrophy ± micronodularity
    - Fatty atrophy also seen with aging, ↑ BMI, & hyperlipidemia
- CECT
  - Wide range of appearances based on SjS stage
    - Early, diffuse, small fluid-density cysts
    - Cysts mimic HIV lymphoepithelial lesions ± solid nodules, which may mimic neoplasm
    - Chronic SjS shows atrophy & fatty change
  - Heterogeneous enhancement of solid components

MR Findings

- T1WI
  - Discrete collections of low signal intensity, reflecting watery saliva within dilated ducts & acini
- T2WI
  - Diffuse, bilateral, ↑ T2, 1- to 2-mm foci (early stages I & II)
  - Multiple high T2-signal foci > 2 mm (late stages III & IV)
  - Chronic atrophy with ↑ fatty replacement & **"salt & pepper"** micronodularity
- DWI
  - Lower diffusion
- T1WI C+
  - Heterogeneous, mild enhancement of nodular parenchyma & fibrosis with nonenhancing, cystic changes
- MR sialography
  - Approaches 95% sensitivity & specificity for SjS
  - Stages severity of SjS
  - Display punctate, globular, cavitary, or destructive parotid distal ductal changes of SjS as focal high T2 signal
- Changes most evident in parotid > other salivary glands

Ultrasonographic Findings

- Grayscale ultrasound
  - Early-stage miliary (≤ 1-mm punctate cystic changes) may be missed but later stages readily apparent
  - **Leopard skin** or **Tortoise shell** appearance due to multiple hypo- & anechoic foci; may require biopsy to exclude non-Hodgkin lymphoma (NHL)
  - Small hyperechoic lines & spots
    - Hyperechoic bands seen in adults not children
  - Both parotid & submandibular glands involved
- Color Doppler
  - ↑ dot-like vascularity on color Doppler

Nonvascular Interventions

- Conventional sialography
  - Historic reference standard for staging
  - Alternating ductal stenosis & dilatation (**string of beads** appearance)
  - Acinar spill into enlarged acini (**apple tree** pattern)
  - Truncated intraglandular ductal branching pattern
- Sialoendoscopy
  - Accuracy of staging unknown; not widely utilized

Imaging Recommendations

- Best imaging tool
  - MR with sialography
    - Allows cross-sectional analysis & staging

DIFFERENTIAL DIAGNOSIS

Chronic Infectious or Obstructive Parotitis

- Unilateral involvement
- Irregular dilatation & stenosis of ducts

- Lacks solid masses
- Multiple calculi may be present

Benign Lymphoepithelial Lesions of HIV

- Mixed cystic & solid lesions enlarging both parotids
- Tonsillar hyperplasia & cervical reactive adenopathy
- Lack glandular calcifications

IgG4-Related Disease

- Elevated serum &/or tissue IgG4
- May have CNV enlargement & enhancement
- Check for organ involvement outside head & neck

Warthin Tumor

- 20% are multiple; may be unilateral or bilateral
- Tumors characteristically heterogeneous
- Mural nodules present if cystic

Parotid Non-Hodgkin Lymphoma Nodes

- Solid masses in parotid usually without cystic change
- Cervical adenopathy may or may not be present
- Chronic systemic NHL often known

Parotid Metastatic Disease

- Primary malignancy & other metastases often concurrent
- Skin cancers of scalp, face, external ear > systemic disease
- Unilateral or bilateral
- Single or multiple parotid masses with invasive margins

Parotid Sarcoidosis

- Rare manifestation of sarcoidosis
- Cervical & mediastinal lymph nodes
- Mixed cystic & solid masses enlarging both parotids with associated reactive-appearing cervical adenopathy

PATHOLOGY

General Features

- Etiology
  - Poorly understood immune-mediated disease
  - Viral infection, hormonal or epigenetic changes proposed as initiating events
- Periductal lymphocyte aggregates destroy salivary acini
- Autoimmune dysregulation leads to destruction of acinar cells & ductal epithelia of lacrimal & salivary glands
- Activated lymphocytes selectively injure lacrimal & salivary glands, leading to tissue damage

Staging, Grading, & Classification

- Based on conventional or MR sialography
  - Stage I: Punctate contrast/high signal ≤ 1 mm
  - Stage II: Globular contrast/high signal 1-2 mm
  - Stage III: Cavitary contrast/high signal > 2 mm
  - Stage IV: Parotid gland parenchymal destruction
- Modest correlation with disease duration

Gross Pathologic & Surgical Features

- Enlarged parotid glands with multiple small to large cysts & lymphocyte aggregates

Microscopic Features

- Labial biopsy: CD4(+) T-cell lymphocytes
- Periductal lymphocyte & plasma cell infiltration & epimyoepithelial islands
  - Early stages: Lymphocyte-plasma cell infiltration obstructs intercalated ducts with enlarged distal ducts
  - Late stages: Activated lymphocytes destroy salivary tissue, leaving larger cysts & solid lymphocyte aggregates

CLINICAL ISSUES

Presentation

- Most common signs/symptoms
  - Tender, bilateral parotid gland swelling
  - May be incidental finding on imaging
    - Prevalence of SjS in patients with ranulas, parotid cysts, or parotid calcification is 16%, 24%, & 40% respectively
- Other signs/symptoms
  - Dry eyes, mouth, & skin
  - Primary SjS has CNS manifestations in 0.3-48%
    - Overlap with neuromyelitis-optica spectrum disorder
  - Extraglandular manifestations in primary SjS also include pulmonary interstitial lung diseases
  - **Secondary SjS associations**: **RA** > > systemic lupus erythematosus > progressive systemic sclerosis
- Clinical profile
  - Recurrent acute episodes of tender glandular swelling
  - Less common: Chronic glandular enlargement with superimposed acute attacks
  - Less common: Nontender parotid enlargement
- Laboratory
  - **Positive labial biopsy** or **autoantibody against Sjögren-associated A or B antigen**
  - Rheumatoid factor positive in 95%
  - ANA positive in 80%
  - Positive Schirmer test (↓ tear production)

Demographics

- Age
  - 50-70 years old
- Sex: Striking **female** predominance (90-95%)
  - Most common in menopausal women
- Epidemiology
  - Incidence of SjS: ~ 0.5%; prevalence: ~ 0.1-3.0%
  - 2nd most common autoimmune disorder after RA
- Juvenile SjS
  - Males < 20 years old
  - High rate of recurrent parotitis
  - Most resolve spontaneously at puberty

Natural History & Prognosis

- ↑ risk of malignancy in primary SjS
  - **Relative risk of NHL = 10-40x**

DIAGNOSTIC CHECKLIST

Image Interpretation Pearls

- Invasive margins, dominant solid mass, & cervical lymphadenopathy suggest malignant transformation

SELECTED REFERENCES

1. Chandwani A et al: 'Tortoise shell appearance' of parotid gland in advanced Sjogren's syndrome. QJM. 117(10):735-6, 2024
2. Mar D et al: Imaging of the major salivary glands in rheumatic disease. Rheum Dis Clin North Am. 50(4):701-20, 2024

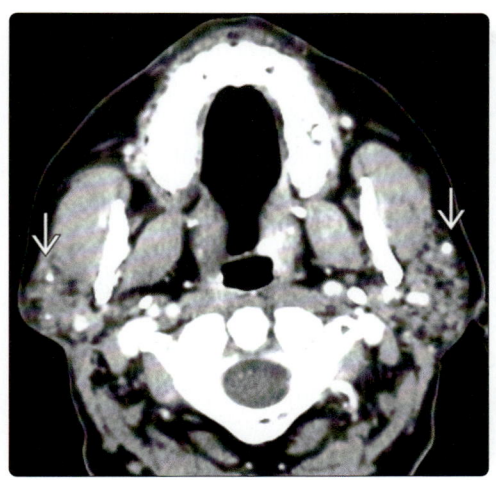

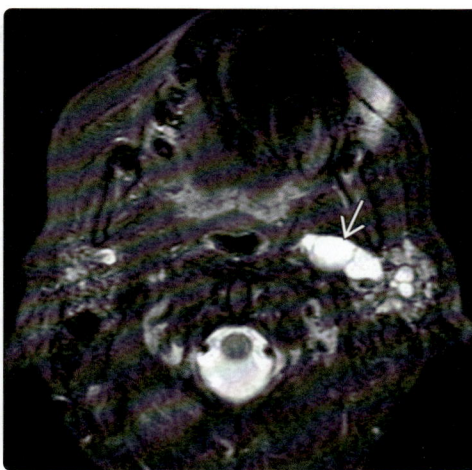

(Left) *Axial CECT shows multiple calcifications ➡ in the bilateral parotid glands with a multilobular configuration and associated fatty involution. Lobules of edematous glandular tissue with intervening fat and scattered calculi are typical of chronic Sjögren syndrome.* **(Right)** *Axial T2WI FS MR shows a septate cystic mass ➡ in the deep lobe of the parotid gland. This is a dilated duct from Sjögren syndrome, but it might be easily mistaken for a neoplasm.*

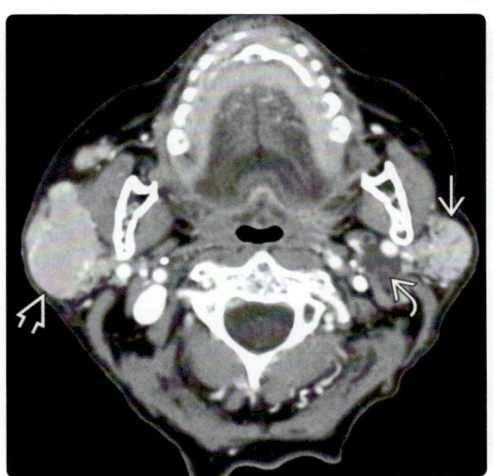

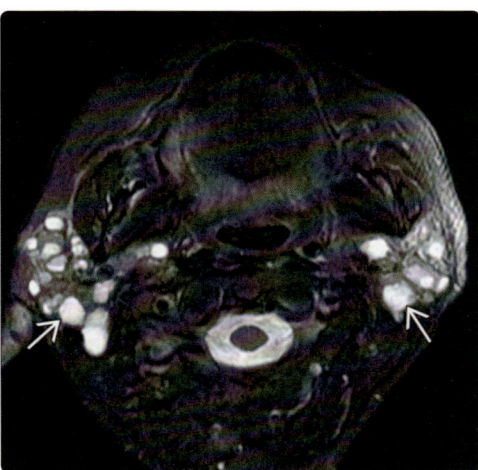

(Left) *Axial CECT shows dense, hyperenhancing parotids ➡ with cystic areas ➡. A solid, uniformly enhancing mass in the right parotid ➡ proved to be lymphoma. Patients with Sjögren syndrome are at high risk for intraparotid lymphoma. Any solid glandular mass should be biopsied.* **(Right)** *Axial T2WI FS MR shows high-signal masses ➡ within both parotids. These represent cystic dilatation of the intraglandular ducts in Sjögren syndrome, but are indistinguishable from lymphoepithelial lesions in HIV.*

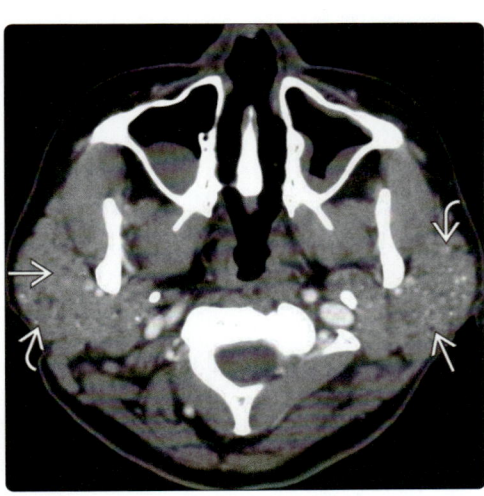

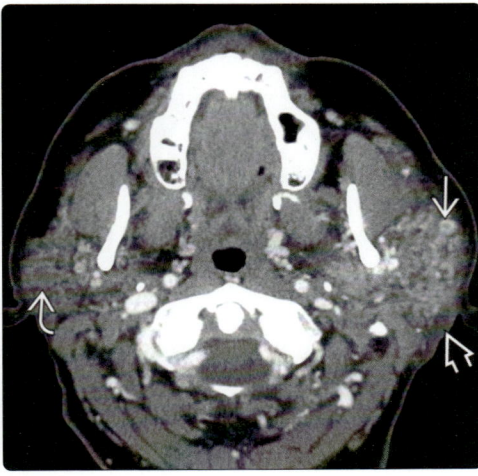

(Left) *Axial CECT shows bilateral parotid gland enlargement and increased attenuation throughout. Note small, hypodense, cystic foci ➡ and punctate glandular calcifications ➡, typical for Sjögren syndrome.* **(Right)** *Axial CECT shows enlargement of the left greater than right parotids due to Sjögren's involvement with a micronodular appearance diffusely ➡. There is active inflammation on the left with stranding of the overlying subcutaneous fat ➡. A focal dominant cyst is noted on the right ➡.*

Benign Lymphoepithelial Cysts of HIV

KEY FACTS

TERMINOLOGY

- **Benign lymphoepithelial cysts associated with HIV (BLEC-HIV)**
  - Generally manifests as painless, bilateral parotid enlargement in HIV(+) patient with clinical, radiologic, or pathologic evidence of cyst formation
- Synonyms: HIV-associated parotid cysts, AIDS-related parotid cysts (ARPC), cystic lymphoid hyperplasia

IMAGING

- Enhanced CT or MR: Multiple bilateral, well-circumscribed cystic and solid masses within enlarged parotid glands
  - BLE cyst wall may be nodular (lymphoid follicles)
- Look for other CECT findings associated with HIV
  - Reactive cervical adenopathy
  - Tonsillar hypertrophy

TOP DIFFERENTIAL DIAGNOSES

- 1st branchial cleft cyst

- Parotid Sjögren syndrome
- Warthin tumor
- Non-Hodgkin lymphoma in parotid nodes
- Metastatic disease to parotid nodes

PATHOLOGY

- Epithelial-lined unicystic or multicystic cavities surrounded by hyperplastic lymphoid tissue, cyst lumen filled with mucoid material

CLINICAL ISSUES

- Historically, **1-10%** of HIV(+) patients develop BLEC-HIV and present with painless, bilateral parotid enlargement

DIAGNOSTIC CHECKLIST

- Painless, bilateral parotid enlargement with cystic or mixed solid-cystic lesions in HIV(+) patient considered diagnostic

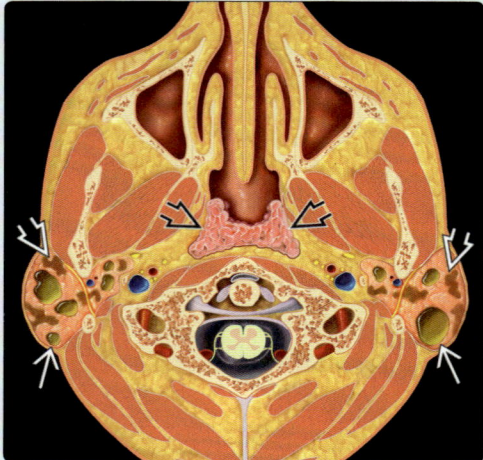
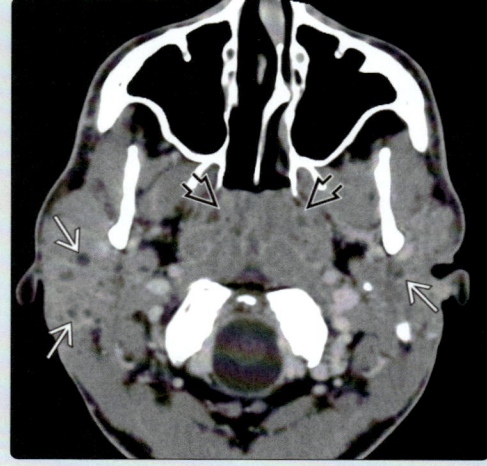

(Left) Graphic shows classic findings of benign lymphoepithelial cysts associated with HIV (BLEC-HIV). Cystic lesions ➡ are mixed with bilateral solid lymphoid aggregates ⊟. Note associated adenoidal hypertrophy ⊟ in the nasopharynx. (Right) Axial CECT shows scattered small cysts ➡ throughout bilateral hyperdense parotid glands in an HIV(+) patient. Note associated adenoidal hypertrophy ⊟.

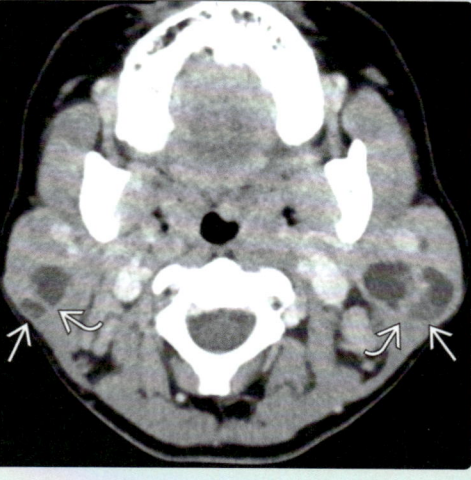
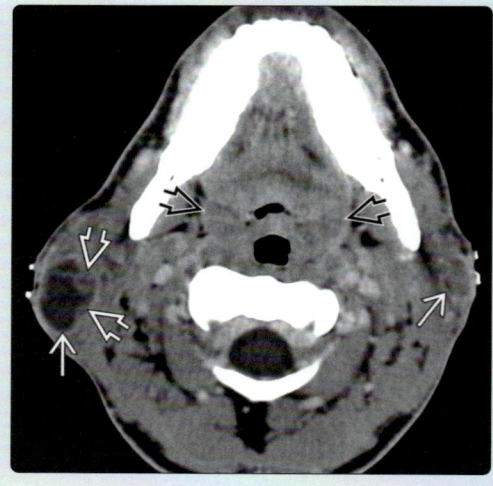

(Left) Axial CECT in an HIV(+) patient demonstrates multifocal, complex, cystic lesions in the bilateral parotid glands ➡ in keeping with benign lymphoepithelial cysts. Septations ⊠ may sometimes be seen within the cysts. (Right) Axial CECT in an HIV(+) patient shows bilateral cystic masses ➡ with mural nodularity ⊟ (lymphoid follicles) in both parotid glands. BLEC-HIV can have both cystic and solid components. Note the associated tonsillar hypertrophy ⊟.

TERMINOLOGY

Abbreviations

- Benign lymphoepithelial cysts associated with HIV (BLEC-HIV)
- Benign lymphoepithelial lesions associated with HIV (BLEL-HIV)

Synonyms

- Cystic lymphoid hyperplasia
- Intraductal epithelial proliferation with cyst formation
- HIV-associated parotid cysts
- AIDS-related parotid cysts (ARPC)
  o Patient need only be HIV(+) to manifest BLEL
    − BLEC-HIV can exist without AIDS
    − Avoid ARPC synonym

Definitions

- **BLEC-HIV**
  o One of most common pathologies of parotid encountered in HIV(+) patients in typical clinical and radiologic practice
  o Generally manifests as painless, bilateral parotid enlargement with clinical, radiologic, or pathologic evidence of **cyst formation**
- **BLEL-HIV**
  o Considered part of spectrum of same entity as BLEC-HIV with similar histopathologic findings of lymphoepithelial proliferation but absence of macroscopic cyst formation
  o Terms BLEL-HIV and BLEC-HIV are used interchangeably by many authors
  o Some authors prefer term BLEL-HIV when lymphoid aggregates predominate, and lesion is predominantly solid

IMAGING

General Features

- Best diagnostic clue
  o Bilateral parotid gland enlargement with underlying cystic (or mixed solid/cystic) lesions in patient with serologic evidence of HIV
- Location
  o Bilateral parotid gland involvement is typical
  o Rarely seen in submandibular or sublingual salivary glands
    − Only parotid has intrinsic lymphoid tissue
- Size
  o Variable: Typically several millimeters, up to 3.5 cm
  o Cyst formation may be microscopic, difficult to identify radiologically but verified at histology
- Morphology
  o Cysts are well circumscribed, rounded
  o Solid lymphoid aggregates may be poorly defined
  o **Bilateral** parotid enlargement
  o Often innumerable small masses

CT Findings

- CECT
  o Multiple bilateral, well-circumscribed cystic and solid masses within enlarged parotid glands
  o Thin rim enhancement of **cystic** lesions with heterogeneous enhancement of **solid** components
  o Bilateral parotid hyperdensity
  o Other CECT findings associated with underlying HIV
    − Reactive cervical adenopathy
    − Adenoidal, palatine, and lingual tonsillar hypertrophy

MR Findings

- T1WI
  o Low-signal cystic lesions
  o Heterogeneous, variable signal in solid lesions
    − Normal parotid fat provides good inherent contrast
- T2WI
  o Hyperintense, bilateral, well-circumscribed round to ovoid intraparotid lesions
  o Hyperintense, bilateral cervical lymphadenopathy
  o Waldeyer lymphatic ring enlargement with high signal
- T1WI C+
  o Thin rim enhancement in cystic lesions with variable, heterogeneous enhancement of solid lesions
    − Cystic lesions solid mural nodules (enlarged lymph follicles)
  o Solid lesions may be less conspicuous on enhanced than unenhanced imaging due to surrounding fat

Ultrasonographic Findings

- Spectrum of sonographic findings ranging from simple cysts to mixed masses with predominantly solid components
  o Cystic lesions not purely anechoic but contain internal network of thin septa supplied by vessel pedicles
    − 40% have mural nodules
  o Solid lesions may resemble parotid neoplasms

Imaging Recommendations

- Best imaging tool
  o Neck CECT shows signature findings of bilateral cystic to solid parotid masses, tonsillar hyperplasia, and cervical adenopathy

DIFFERENTIAL DIAGNOSIS

1st Branchial Cleft Cyst

- Clinical: Recurrent unilateral, inflammatory parotid mass
- Imaging: Unilateral, oval, cystic intraparotid mass

Parotid Sjögren Syndrome

- Clinical: Older female patient with Sicca syndrome (dry eyes, mouth, and skin) and connective tissue disorder (RA); antinuclear antibodies
- Imaging: May be radiologically identical to BLEC-HIV

Parotid Sarcoidosis

- Clinical: Intraparotid sarcoid is very rare
- Imaging: Cervical and mediastinal lymph nodes
  o May be identical to BLEL-HIV

Warthin Tumor

- Clinical: Solitary or multifocal parotid masses
- Imaging
  o Solid or mixed cystic-solid parotid masses with nodular walls
  o 20% are multifocal but never innumerable

○ Lacks associated tonsillar hyperplasia and cervical adenopathy

Non-Hodgkin Lymphoma in Parotid Nodes

- Clinical: Chronic systemic non-Hodgkin lymphoma usually already apparent
- Imaging: Bilateral solid masses in parotid

Metastatic Disease to Parotid Nodes

- Clinical: Primary malignancy and other metastatic deposits already apparent
- Imaging: Unilateral, multifocal, solid parotid masses

PATHOLOGY

General Features

- Etiology
  ○ Term lymphoepithelial is used to denote fact that lesion contains abnormal salivary ductal epithelium as well as abnormal lymphoid proliferation
  ○ Unclear as to whether lesion originates in intraparotid lymph node or in salivary parenchyma as result of lymphoid hyperplasia

Microscopic Features

- Thin, smooth-walled, multicystic cavities measuring few millimeters to 3-4 cm
- Lesion occurs predominantly in intraparotid lymph nodes, but may have secondary parotid parenchymal invasion
- Cyst wall ranges from nondescript thin epithelial lining to nonkeratinizing stratified squamous to pseudostratified respiratory-type epithelium
- Cyst lining surrounded by **proliferative lymphoid tissue** that can contain salivary duct remnants and epimyoepithelial islands
- Cyst aspirate: Mucoid material with various inflammatory cells

Immunohistochemistry

- Lymphoid component includes reactivity for B-cell lineage and T-cell lineage markers
- Epithelial markers (e.g., cytokeratins, EMA, others) delineate squamous epithelial-lined cysts
- **HIV p24** core antigen immunoreactivity found in most cases
  ○ Multinucleated giant cells also S100 protein and p55 positive

CLINICAL ISSUES

Presentation

- Clinical profile
  ○ Bilateral parotid cystic masses in HIV(+) patient
    – Initially seen in HIV(+) patients prior to AIDS onset
      □ BLEC-HIV may actually precede HIV seroconversion
      □ BLEC-HIV not considered precursor to AIDS
  ○ BLEC-HIV may be 1st symptom associated with HIV
  ○ **HIV testing** should be done on any patient with newly diagnosed cystic parotid enlargement to evaluate for **BLEC-HIV**

Demographics

- Age

○ Any age can be infected with HIV, including pediatric age group
○ Most commonly seen in men
- Epidemiology
  ○ Historically, **1-10%** of HIV(+) patients develop BLEC-HIV
  ○ Overall decrease in BLEC-HIV since widespread use of highly active antiretroviral therapy (HAART)

Natural History & Prognosis

- If left untreated, grows into chronic, mumps-like state with significant bilateral parotid enlargement
- Malignant transformation extremely rare

Treatment

- HAART for HIV should be initial management; will completely or partially treat BLEC-HIV
- High-dose radiotherapy (> 22.5 Gy) recommended if HAART fails to control
- Intralesional sclerotherapy for patients in areas with limited access to radiation and medical therapy or poor compliance with HAART

DIAGNOSTIC CHECKLIST

Consider

- Use CECT as 1st imaging modality if suspect BLEC-HIV

Image Interpretation Pearls

- Bilateral cystic and solid masses within enlarged parotids in HIV(+) patient should be considered BLEC-HIV until proven otherwise
- Nonnecrotic cervical adenopathy with tonsillar hypertrophy can be important clue to BLEC-HIV diagnosis

Reporting Tips

- BLEC-HIV may be 1st sign of HIV infection
  ○ Call clinician with HIV testing recommendation in characteristic cases

SELECTED REFERENCES

1. Nkuna T et al: Benign lymphoepithelial cyst of parotid glands in HIV Infected patients on anti-retroviral therapy: a narrative review. Indian J Otolaryngol Head Neck Surg. 75(2):547-56, 2023
2. Iro S et al: Parotid lymphoepithelial cysts revealing HIV infection in a 12-year-old girl: a case report. Ann Med Surg (Lond). 67:102338, 2021
3. Meer S: Human immunodeficiency virus and salivary gland pathology: an update. Oral Surg Oral Med Oral Pathol Oral Radiol. 128(1):52-9, 2019
4. Meer S et al: Human immunodeficiency virus-associated cystic lymphoid hyperplasia: an immunohistochemical description. Indian J Pathol Microbiol. 60(3):336-40, 2017
5. Sekikawa Y et al: HIV-associated benign lymphoepithelial cysts of the parotid glands confirmed by HIV-1 p24 antigen immunostaining. BMJ Case Rep. 2017:bcr2017221869, 2017
6. Mourad WF et al: Management algorithm for HIV-associated parotid lymphoepithelial cysts. Eur Arch Otorhinolaryngol. 273(10):3355-62, 2016
7. Mourad WF et al: 25-year follow-up of HIV-positive patients with benign lymphoepithelial cysts of the parotid glands: a retrospective review. Anticancer Res. 33(11):4927-32, 2013
8. Sujatha D et al: Parotid lymphoepithelial cysts in human immunodeficiency virus: a review. J Laryngol Otol. 127(11):1046-9, 2013
9. Dave SP et al: The benign lymphoepithelial cyst and a classification system for lymphocytic parotid gland enlargement in the pediatric HIV population. Laryngoscope. 117(1):106-13, 2007
10. Kirshenbaum KJ et al: Benign lymphoepithelial parotid tumors in AIDS patients: CT and MR findings in nine cases. AJNR Am J Neuroradiol. 12(2):271-4, 1991
11. Holliday RA et al: Benign lymphoepithelial parotid cysts and hyperplastic cervical adenopathy in AIDS-risk patients: a new CT appearance. Radiology. 168(2):439-41, 1988

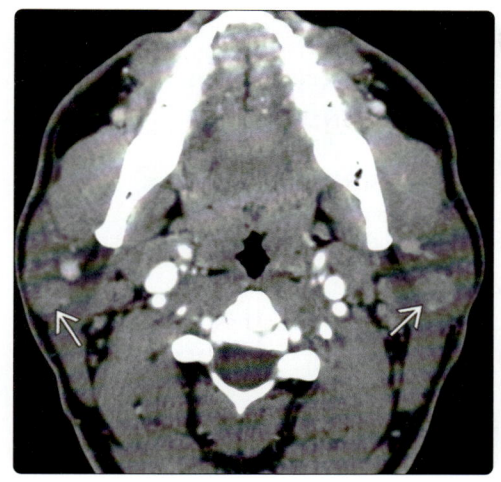

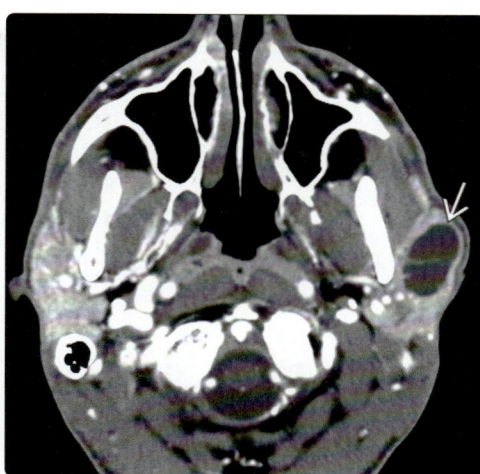

(Left) *Axial CECT shows bilateral, well-defined, enhancing solid masses ➡. The findings are nonspecific; however, in a patient with known HIV, persistent parotid gland lymphadenopathy or BLEL-HIV would be considered.* (Right) *Axial CECT shows a solitary cystic, septated mass ➡ in the left parotid gland. BLEC-HIV are generally multiple but can present as a solitary mass. A 1st branchial cleft cyst may be misdiagnosed in this setting.*

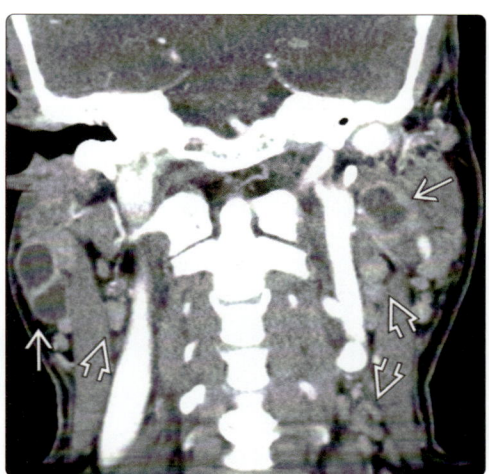

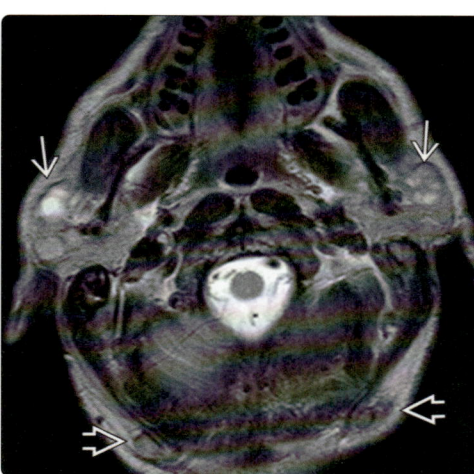

(Left) *Coronal CECT demonstrates bilateral parotid cystic lesions ➡ and partially imaged bilateral multilevel reactive cervical lymph nodes ➡ in this case of BLEC-HIV.* (Right) *Axial T2 MR in an HIV(+) patient shows multifocal cystic lesions ➡ in the bilateral parotid glands compatible with BLEC-HIV. In addition, note bilateral occipital reactive lymph nodes ➡.*

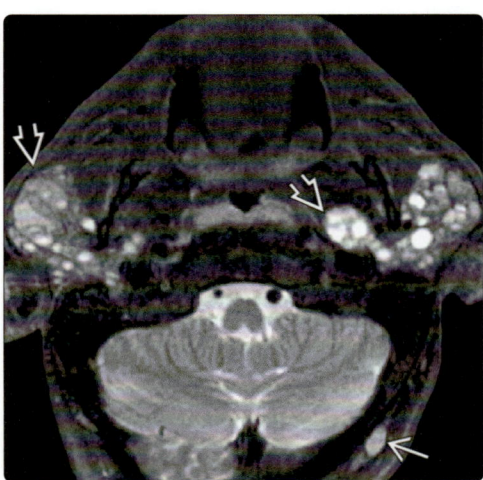

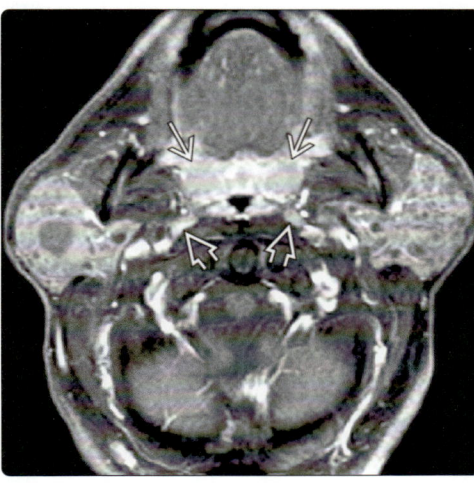

(Left) *Axial STIR MR shows bilateral, intraparotid, hyperintense, cystic lymphoepithelial lesions of HIV ➡. Notice both superficial and deep lobes are involved. Note the associated reactive occipital node ➡.* (Right) *Axial T1 C+ FS MR reveals bilateral cystic and solid intraparotid lesions in a patient with HIV. Findings are typical of BLEC-HIV. Palatine tonsils ➡ are hyperplastic and associated with reactive lateral retropharyngeal nodes ➡.*

Parotid Pleomorphic Adenoma

TERMINOLOGY

- Synonym: Benign mixed tumor (BMT)

IMAGING

- Choice of imaging tool: CECT, MR, or US
  - CT or MR adequate to answer most imaging questions
    - MR best if specific signs (↑ T2 signal, ↑ ADC) present
  - Alternate approach leading with combination of US & FNA cytology (FNAC)
    - If US shows superficial lobe benign lesion & FNAC shows pleomorphic adenoma (PA) cells, no further imaging needed
- CT findings
  - Smooth, variably enhancing, ovoid mass
  - **Pear-shaped** when in deep lobe
- MR findings
  - ↑ T1 signal in hemorrhagic lesions
  - **Very high T2** signal **specific for PA**
  - **ADC values higher** than other parotid tumors

- US findings
  - Well-demarcated, homogeneous, hypoechoic mass with posterior enhancement
  - Larger PA shows heterogeneous hypoechogenicity

TOP DIFFERENTIAL DIAGNOSES

- Warthin tumor
- Parotid nodal metastatic disease
- Primary parotid carcinoma
- Parotid non-Hodgkin lymphoma

CLINICAL ISSUES

- Painless, slow-growing cheek mass most common
- Multifocal primary PA rare (< 1%)
- Rapid enlargement concerning for malignant degeneration

DIAGNOSTIC CHECKLIST

- Infiltrative margins, multicentricity, or hypointense T2 signal suggest malignancy
- Relationship of PA to CNVII critical for surgical planning

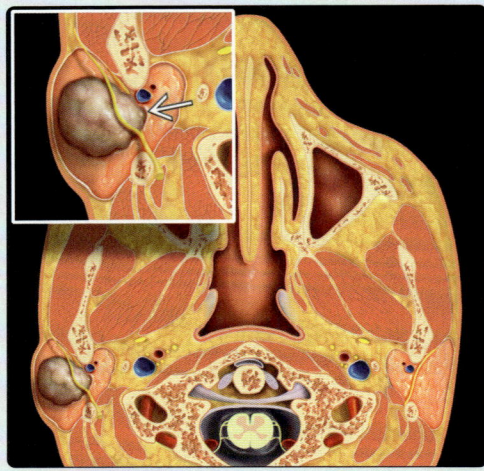 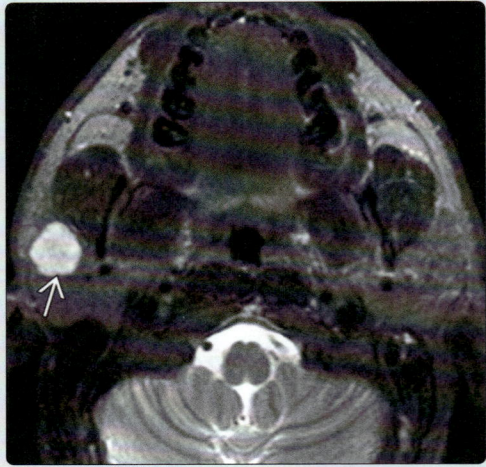

(Left) Axial graphic depicts a small, predominantly superficial lobe pleomorphic adenoma (PA). Notice on the inset, the tongue of the tumor has insinuated itself between 2 facial nerve branches to involve the deep lobe ➡. (Right) Axial T2 FS MR reveals a sharply circumscribed, high-signal PA ➡ in the superficial lobe of the parotid gland. This tumor at the very least abuts, if not crosses, the plane of the intraparotid facial nerve.

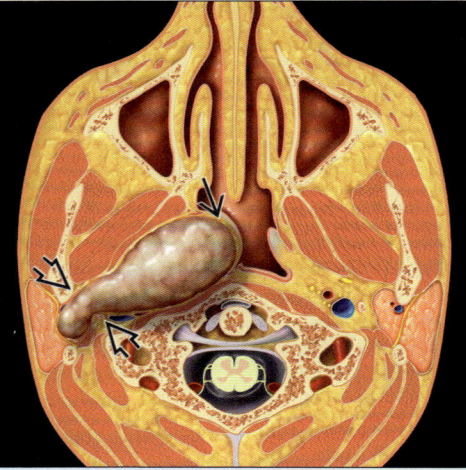 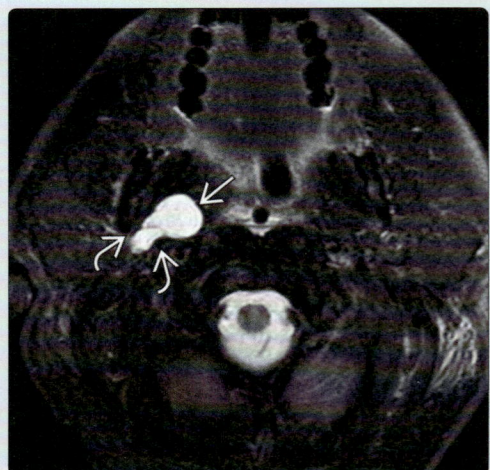

(Left) Axial graphic reveals a pear-shaped PA of the deep lobe of the parotid gland. Despite the size of this tumor, the parapharyngeal fat ➡ can still be seen as it is pushed superomedially. Note the widened stylomandibular notch/tunnel ➡. (Right) Axial T2 FS MR shows a pear-shaped mass ➡ in the parapharyngeal space. The neck of the pear is the portion of the tumor extending through the stylomandibular notch/tunnel ➡. Note the extremely high T2 signal (higher than CSF), which further suggests PA.

Parotid Pleomorphic Adenoma

TERMINOLOGY

Abbreviations
- Pleomorphic adenoma (PA)

Synonyms
- Benign mixed tumor (BMT)

Definitions
- Benign, histologically **heterogeneous** tumor of parotid
- Epithelial, myoepithelial, & stromal components

IMAGING

General Features
- Best diagnostic clue
  - Small PA (< 2 cm): Sharply marginated, intraparotid ovoid mass with uniform enhancement
  - Large PA (> 2 cm): Lobulated mass with heterogeneous enhancement
- Location
  - Parotid space; usually superficial lobe
  - Deep lobe masses present late with oropharyngeal bulging since nonpalpable
- Size
  - Variable; may be > 10 cm if in deep lobe or neglected
- Morphology
  - Round or oval
  - Pear-shaped when arising in deep lobe & extending into stylomandibular tunnel
  - "Bosselated" or lobulated border characteristic

CT Findings
- CECT
  - **Small PA**
    - Smooth, homogeneously enhancing, ovoid mass
  - **Large PA**
    - Inhomogeneously enhancing, lobulated mass with areas of lower attenuation representing foci of degenerative necrosis & old hemorrhage
    - Dystrophic calcification may be present
      - □ Calcifications unusual in other parotid tumors
  - **Deep lobe PA**
    - Variably enhancing, **pear-shaped mass** displacing parapharyngeal space (PPS) fat medially
    - Widening of stylomandibular notch

MR Findings
- T1WI
  - Small PA: Sharply marginated intraparotid mass with uniform hypointensity
  - Large PA: Lobulated intraparotid mass with heterogeneous signal
    - Hyperintense signal can be seen if hemorrhagic
- T2WI
  - Small PA: Well-circumscribed intraparotid mass with **uniform high signal**
  - Large PA: **Lobulated** intraparotid mass with heterogeneous high signal
  - If **very high T2** signal present, **specific for PA**
  - Black ring sign = thick, T2-hypointense rim reflects intact fibrous capsule (usually reflects benign)
  - Corona sign or peritumoral halo is larger on FS T2, & when present, raises concern for invasive carcinoma ex-PA
- STIR
  - Lesions more conspicuous than on standard T2
- DWI
  - On average, PA has **higher ADC value** than other benign lesions & cancers
    - DWI not yet accurate enough to avoid FNA cytology (FNAC)
- T1WI C+
  - Variable, mild to moderate enhancement
  - Dynamic contrast curve shows **quick uptake, then plateau** (contrast retention)
    - Not yet accurate enough to avoid FNAC
  - Presence of corona sign (peritumoral halo) larger on T1 FS or T1 C+ FS MR raises concern for invasive carcinoma ex-PA
- SWI
  - Lower degree of intratumoral susceptibility signal intensity in PA compared to Warthin tumor

Ultrasonographic Findings
- Grayscale ultrasound
  - Well-demarcated, homogeneous, **hypoechoic** mass with **posterior enhancement**
    - Larger PA shows heterogeneous hypoechogenicity
      - □ Secondary to hemorrhage & necrosis
  - Only visible when located in parotid superficial lobe
- Color Doppler
  - ↑ peripheral vessels, mainly venous: Often sparse

Nuclear Medicine Findings
- May be hypermetabolic on FDG PET; mimics malignancy
- Uptake on DOTATATE PET/CT

Imaging Recommendations
- Best imaging tool
  - Either CECT or MR adequate to answer most imaging questions
  - MR best when specific signs (high T2 signal, high ADC) are present
    - May be able to avoid neck dissection without performing FNAC & rely on surgical excisional biopsy as primary treatment
    - Advanced MR sequences (quantitative ADC, dynamic contrast) may become standard of care in future
  - Alternate approach with combination of US & FNAC
    - If US shows **superficial lobe benign lesion** & **FNAC shows PA cells**, no further imaging needed
- Define facial nerve plane
  - CNVII plane projects from stylomastoid foramen, anteroinferiorly to lateral aspect of retromandibular vein, then anteriorly over surface of masseter muscle
  - CNVII plane represents imaging estimation of line dividing superficial & deep lobes of parotid gland
  - Relationship to facial nerve critical for surgical planning; comment in radiology report appropriate
- Risk of malignant degeneration to **carcinoma ex-PA**
  - Features concerning for malignancy: Rapid enlargement, irregular shape &/or margins, low ADC, tumor calcification

DIFFERENTIAL DIAGNOSIS

Warthin Tumor

- Clinical: Adult male smoker
- Imaging: Inhomogeneous but well-circumscribed intraparotid mass
  - Multicentric (20%)
  - Warthin tumor does not calcify, but PA may have calcification

Parotid Nodal Metastatic Disease

- Systemic nodal metastases: Intraparotid nodes may be site of systemic nodal metastases
- Regional nodal drainage
  - Clinical: Known primary periauricular skin malignancy
  - Imaging: Single or multiple pathologic nodes seen

Primary Parotid Carcinoma

- Parotid adenoid cystic carcinoma (ACCa)
- Mucoepidermoid carcinoma (MECa)
  - Clinical for either carcinoma: Gradual-onset facial nerve paresis
  - Imaging for either carcinoma: Heterogeneous, infiltrating mass with poorly defined margins
    - Low-grade malignancy may be well demarcated
    - Perineural tumor spread common for ACCa
    - Adjacent node common for MECa

Parotid Non-Hodgkin Lymphoma

- Clinical: Chronic systemic non-Hodgkin lymphoma may already be present
- Imaging: Solitary, multiple, or bilateral solid masses of parotid gland

PATHOLOGY

General Features

- Etiology
  - Benign tumor arising from distal portions of parotid ductal system, including intercalated ducts & acini
- Genetics
  - Somatic mutation or autosomal dominant transmission
    - PA gene 1 (*PLAG1*)

Gross Pathologic & Surgical Features

- Lobulated, heterogeneous mass with **fibrous capsule**
- Soft tan lobules representing epithelial component interspersed among lobulated firm, white, gritty chondromyxoid component

Microscopic Features

- Interspersed **epithelial, myoepithelial, & stromal cellular components** needed to diagnose PA
- Sites of necrosis, hemorrhage, hyalinization, & calcification may be present

CLINICAL ISSUES

Presentation

- Most common signs/symptoms
  - Painless cheek mass
  - Location-dependent symptoms & signs
    - Superficial lobe or accessory parotid: Cheek mass
    - Parotid tail: Angle of mandible mass
    - Deep lobe: Enlarging mass pushes palatine tonsil into pharyngeal airway
  - Facial nerve paralysis is rare & suggests malignancy
  - May be incidentally discovered on imaging

Demographics

- Epidemiology
  - **Most common parotid space tumor (80%)**
  - 80% of PAs arise in parotid glands
    - 8% in submandibular glands; 6.5% arise from minor salivary glands in pharynx &/or oral cavity
  - 80-90% of parotid PAs involve superficial lobe
  - Multifocal PAs rare (< 1%)
    - Multiple lesions not suggestive of primary PA
    - May be seen in **recurrent PA**
- Age: 30-60 years; most common > 40 years
- Sex: M:F = 1:2
- Ethnicity: Most common in White population, rare in Black population

Natural History & Prognosis

- Slowly growing, painless, benign tumor
- Recurrent tumor typically from incomplete resection or cellular spillage at surgery
  - Recurrent PA **multifocal** (cluster of grapes appearance)
  - Recurrences associated with benign PA metastasis
- Malignant transformation in up to 15% if untreated: **Carcinoma ex-PA**
  - Various histologies

Treatment

- Complete surgical resection of encapsulated mass within adequate margin of surrounding parotid gland tissue to avoid cellular spillage & seeding
- Recurrent tumor difficult to treat
  - Radiation treatment of uncertain effectiveness

DIAGNOSTIC CHECKLIST

Consider

- **Large, asymptomatic** masses arising from **deep lobe of parotid** almost always **PA**

Image Interpretation Pearls

- Define facial nerve plane & identify deep parotid lobe component, as this may be missed clinically
- Infiltrative margins, multicentricity, or hypointense T2 signal suggests malignancy
- Must distinguish deep lobe parotid PA from true parapharyngeal PA
  - Look for fat plane between parotid tissue & PA

SELECTED REFERENCES

1. Johnson F et al: Novel detection of pleomorphic adenomas via analysis of (68)Ga-DOTATOC PET/CT imaging. Cancers (Basel). 16(15):2624, 2024
2. Rao Y et al: Performance of radiomics in the differential diagnosis of parotid tumors: a systematic review. Front Oncol. 14:1383323, 2024
3. Kalwaniya DS et al: A review of the current literature on pleomorphic adenoma. Cureus. 15(7):e42311, 2023
4. Akutsu A et al: MR imaging findings of carcinoma ex pleomorphic adenoma related to extracapsular invasion and prognosis. AJNR Am J Neuroradiol. 43(11):1639-45, 2022

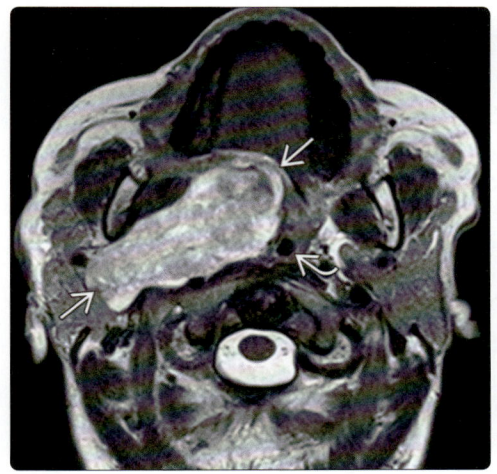

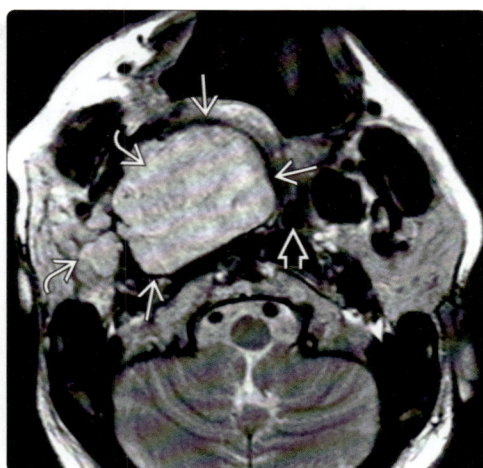

(Left) *Axial T2 MR shows a well-circumscribed deep lobe PA ➡ narrowing the upper nasopharyngeal airway ➡. The tumor is heterogeneous with areas of high and intermediate signal.* (Right) *Axial T2 MR shows a large, well-circumscribed, hyperintense deep lobe parotid PA ➡. This longstanding tumor has an intact, well-developed, hypointense fibrous tumor capsule (black ring sign) ➡. Note mass effect on oropharyngeal airway ➡.*

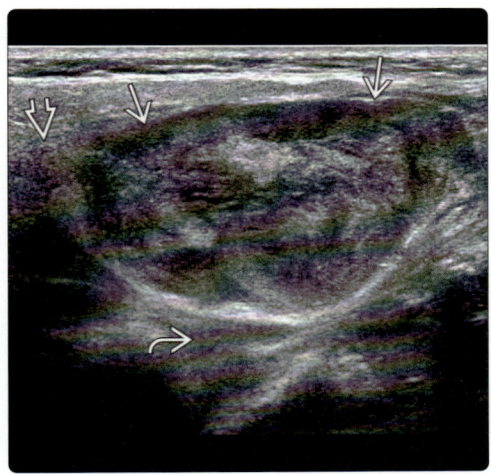

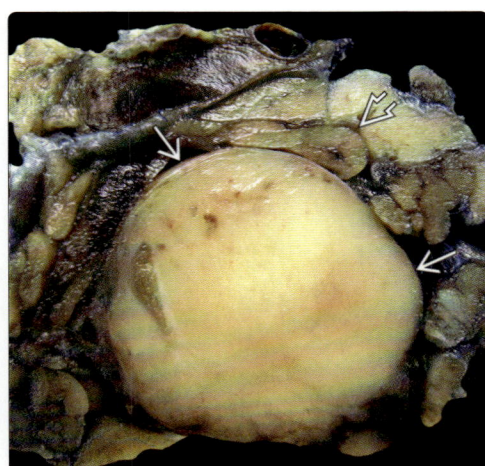

(Left) *Longitudinal grayscale US shows a large parotid PA ➡ in the superficial lobe ➡. Larger PAs often display heterogeneous echo pattern, as on this image, with muted posterior enhancement ➡.* (Right) *Gross photograph shows a formalin-fixed PA with a well-defined fibrous capsule ➡ surrounded by a normal parotid gland ➡. This specimen illustrates why a PA in the parotid gland is so well circumscribed when imaged. Violation of the capsule during surgery may result in multifocal recurrences.*

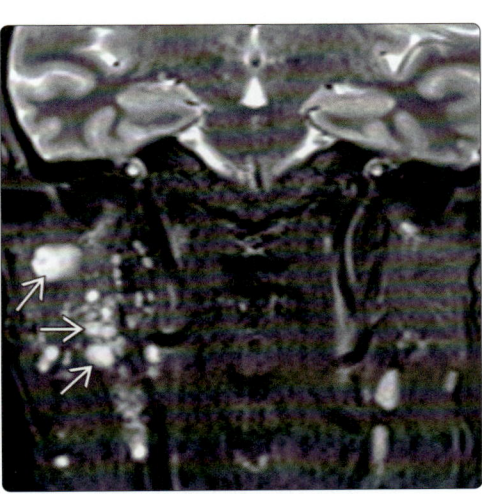

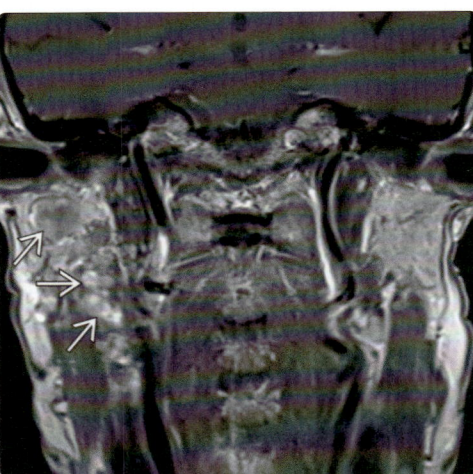

(Left) *Coronal STIR MR shows multiple cystic-appearing nodules ➡ within the left parotid extending into the left parapharyngeal space. This is a typical appearance (cluster of grapes) for a recurrent PA, which occurred due to tumor capsule disruption and seeding of the operative bed during surgery.* (Right) *Coronal T1 C+ MR in the same patient confirms heterogeneous enhancement within the multiple cystic-appearing nodules ➡, consistent with a PA recurrence. Bland parotid cysts would not be expected to enhance.*

TERMINOLOGY

- Benign tumor arising from salivary-lymphoid tissue in intraparotid & periparotid nodes
- Most common mass to arise in parotid tail superficial to angle of mandible

IMAGING

- Enhanced CT or MR provides adequate presurgical information
- **20% multifocal**
  - May be multiple lesions in 1 gland or bilateral lesions
  - May be synchronous or metachronous
- Sharply marginated **parotid tail** mass
- **Parenchymal heterogeneity** is characteristic
- Cystic component in 30% with thin, uniform walls & CT density of 10-20 HU
  - Difficult to differentiate from 1st branchial cleft cyst, infected lymph node, or other cystic mass
- Increased uptake of FDG

- May be incidental PET/CT finding
- Ultrasound can be highly suggestive
  - Well-defined, hypoechoic, noncalcified mass parotid tail
  - Small tumor may mimic intraparotid lymph node

TOP DIFFERENTIAL DIAGNOSES

- Benign lymphoepithelial lesions-HIV
- Parotid pleomorphic adenoma (PA)
- Parotid adenoid cystic carcinoma
- Parotid mucoepidermoid carcinoma
- Parotid metastatic nodal disease
- Parotid non-Hodgkin lymphoma

CLINICAL ISSUES

- Angle of mandible (tail of parotid) mass in **smoker**
- **2nd** most frequent benign parotid tumor
  - PA most common parotid tumor

DIAGNOSTIC CHECKLIST

- Be sure to carefully examine for multiplicity & bilaterality

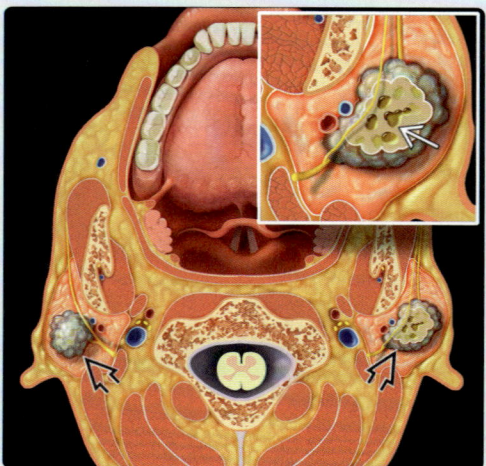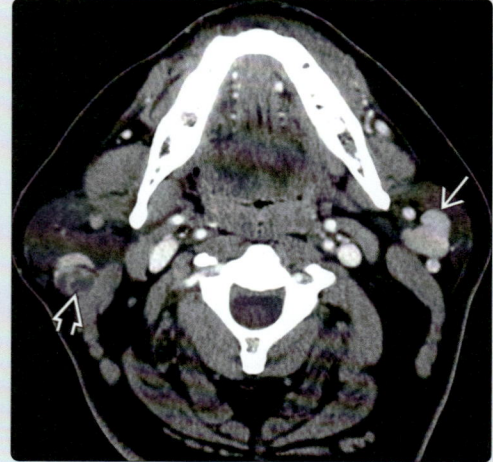

(Left) Axial graphic depicts bilateral, mixed solid/cystic parotid tail Warthin tumors ➡. A larger left intraparotid tumor is cut in the inset to show characteristic parenchymal cystic changes ➡. (Right) Axial CECT shows bilateral parotid masses. The left-sided lesion ➡ is homogeneously enhancing. The right-sided lesion is heterogeneous with small internal cystic changes ➡. Twenty percent of Warthin tumors are multifocal and may be bilateral.

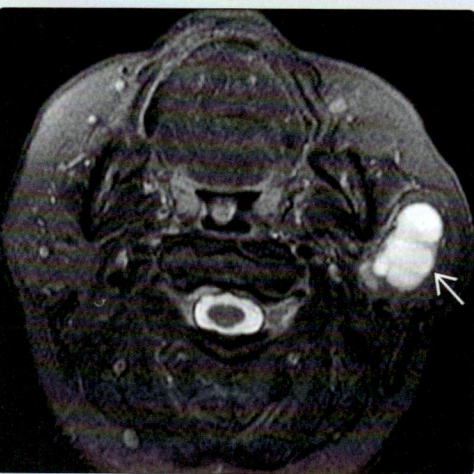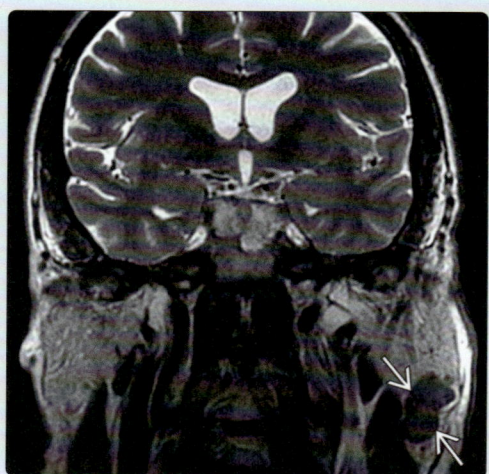

(Left) Axial T2WI FS MR shows a high-intensity mass ➡ with thin septations in the superficial lobe of the parotid gland. Thirty percent of Warthin tumors appear cystic on imaging. (Right) Coronal T2 MR shows (in contrast to prior example) a solid-appearing, hypointense parotid tail Warthin tumor with signal characteristics that could mimic a malignant neoplasm ➡. This tumor was incidentally seen in a patient undergoing brain MR.

TERMINOLOGY

Synonyms
- Papillary cystadenoma lymphomatosum, adenolymphoma, lymphomatous adenoma

Definitions
- Benign tumor with characteristic histopathologic appearance: Papillary structures, mature lymphocytic infiltrate, & cystic changes

IMAGING

General Features
- Best diagnostic clue
  - Sharply marginated parotid tail mass with heterogeneous parenchyma in older male smoker
- Location
  - Intraparotid > > periparotid > upper cervical nodes
  - Most common mass to arise in parotid tail superficial to angle of mandible
  - **20% multifocal**
    - Multiple lesions in 1 gland or bilateral lesions
    - May be synchronous or metachronous
  - Rarely from submandibular or minor salivary glands
- Size
  - Typically 2- to 4-cm diameter
  - Neglected lesions > 10-cm diameter
- Morphology
  - Round to ovoid, well-circumscribed, encapsulated mass or masses
  - **Parenchymal heterogeneity** is **characteristic**

CT Findings
- CECT
  - Solitary small, ovoid, smoothly marginated masses in posterior aspect of superficial lobe of parotid
  - No calcification
  - Cystic component in 30% with thin, uniform walls & CT density of 10-20 HU
    - Large cystic component, septa, or multiple adjacent cystic lesions
      - May be difficult to differentiate from 1st branchial cleft cyst, infected lymph node, or other cystic mass
    - **Mural nodule** more suggestive of Warthin tumor
  - Minimal enhancement of solid components
  - Dynamic CT behavior
    - Rapid enhancement with rapid washout
  - Dual energy may help further characterize

MR Findings
- T1WI
  - Iso- to hyperintense on T1 relative to muscle
  - Variable signal in cystic components (low if bland, high if complicated by proteinaceous debris ± hemorrhage)
- T2WI
  - Variable from low or intermediate signal in solid components to high T2 signal in cystic portions
- STIR
  - Lesions more conspicuous, especially cystic component
- DWI
  - ADC values in solid components lower than pleomorphic adenoma (PA) but similar to carcinoma & lymphoma
- T1WI C+
  - Minimal contrast enhancement of solid components

Ultrasonographic Findings
- Large, clinically obvious tumor
  - Well-defined, hypoechoic, noncalcified mass at lower pole of superficial parotid
- Small, incidental tumor
  - Elliptical, solid reniform mass in parotid tail
  - Heterogeneous architecture & echogenic hilus
  - Mimics appearance of lymph node
- Color Doppler: Prominent hilar (in small tumors) & septal (may be striking) vessels

Nuclear Medicine Findings
- PET
  - Increased uptake of FDG
    - Benign parotid tumors (Warthin, oncocytoma) often incidentally seen on PET (likely due to increased mitochondria)
- Technetium-99m
  - Increased uptake within mitochondrial-rich oncocytes of Warthin tumors
  - Delayed "washout" following sialogogue administration

Imaging Recommendations
- Best imaging tool
  - CECT or MR provides adequate presurgical information

DIFFERENTIAL DIAGNOSIS

Benign Lymphoepithelial Lesions-HIV
- When unilateral & solitary, may strongly mimic Warthin tumor
- Tonsillar hyperplasia & cervical adenopathy help differentiate

Parotid Pleomorphic Adenoma
- Well-circumscribed, homogeneous, intraparotid mass when small
- Larger lesions may be heterogeneous & mimic Warthin tumor

Malignant Parotid Tumor
- Parotid adenoid cystic carcinoma
  - Low-grade tumor may be well demarcated & mimic Warthin tumor
  - High-grade tumor invasive appearance is distinctive
  - Perineural tumor spread common
- Parotid mucoepidermoid carcinoma
  - Low-grade tumor may be well demarcated & mimic Warthin tumor
  - High-grade tumor invasive appearance is distinctive
  - Adjacent malignant nodes common

Parotid Metastatic Nodal Disease
- Primary malignancy on or around skin of ear
- Single or multiple parotid masses with invasive margins
- Central necrosis may mimic cystic change of Warthin tumor

Parotid Non-Hodgkin Lymphoma

- Multiple solid, uniformly enhancing, intraparotid lesions
- Cervical adenopathy helps differentiate from Warthin

PATHOLOGY

General Features

- Etiology
  - 2nd most common parotid tumor
    - Most common tumor on some registries
  - Accounts for 15-30% of parotid tumors
  - **Smoking-induced** benign tumor arising from salivary-lymphoid tissue **in** intraparotid & periparotid nodes
  - Theorized heterotopic salivary gland parenchyma present in preexisting intra- or periparotid lymph nodes
  - Reported association with **EBV**
    - Patients with multifocal or bilateral lesions
- Associated abnormalities
  - Increased incidence in patients with autoimmune disorders
- Embryology
  - Parotid gland undergoes "**late encapsulation**," incorporating lymphoid tissue nodes within superficial layer of deep cervical fascia
    - Warthin tumor arises within this lymphoid tissue

Gross Pathologic & Surgical Features

- Encapsulated, soft, ovoid mass with smooth, lobulated surface
- Tan tissue with cystic spaces that contain tenacious, mucoid, brown fluid or thin, yellow fluid with cholesterol crystals
  - Papillary projections can be seen within cystic areas

Microscopic Features

- Epithelial & lymphoid components dominate histopathologic picture
- Papillary projections are lined with double epithelial layer
  - Inner-luminal layer: Tall columnar cells with nuclei oriented toward lumen
  - Outer-basal layer: Cuboidal or polygonal cells with vesicular nuclei
- Inner lymphoid component of papillary projection is composed of mature lymphoid aggregates with germinal centers
- Electron microscopy shows oncocytes stuffed with mitochondria

CLINICAL ISSUES

Presentation

- Most common signs/symptoms
  - Angle of mandible (tail of parotid) mass
  - Painless
  - Multiple masses ~ 20%
- Other signs/symptoms
  - Facial nerve weakness very rare
    - Suggests malignancy
  - High rate of nonsalivary malignancies (up to 37%)
    - Most often squamous cell carcinomas related to prevalent smoking histories
- Clinical profile

- **90%** of patients with Warthin tumor **smoke**
- Increased incidence with radiation exposure

Demographics

- Age
  - Mean age at presentation: 60 years
- Sex
  - Earlier reports have M:F = 3:1
  - More recent reports show more equal sex incidence (likely related to smoking patterns)
- Epidemiology
  - **2nd** most frequent benign parotid tumor (after PA)
    - Most common tumor in some registries
  - 10% of all salivary gland epithelial tumors
  - 12% of benign parotid gland tumors
  - 20% multifocal: May be unilateral or bilateral, synchronous or metachronous
  - **5-10%** arise in **extraparotid** locations (periparotid & upper neck lymph nodes)

Natural History & Prognosis

- Slow-growing benign tumor
- Malignant transformation reported in < 1%
- "Recurrent" Warthin tumor may be from inadequate resection or metachronous 2nd lesion

Treatment

- Biopsy (or excision) needed to confirm benign nature
- Resection of mass within collar of normal parotid tissue without injury to intraparotid facial nerve is treatment goal
- Surveillance imaging may be important in patients who do not undergo resection due to ~ 4% risk of cytology false-negatives for malignancy

DIAGNOSTIC CHECKLIST

Consider

- Consider CECT to help identify cystic areas within Warthin tumor to help differentiate from small BMT
- Enhanced T1 MR with fat saturation to determine intra- vs. periparotid tumor location & to define plane of facial nerve

Image Interpretation Pearls

- Be sure to carefully examine for multiplicity & bilaterality
- Well-circumscribed, heterogeneous, multiple or bilateral parotid masses in asymptomatic smoker should be considered Warthin tumor

SELECTED REFERENCES

1. Wang Y et al: Evaluation of quantitative dual-energy computed tomography parameters for differentiation of parotid gland tumors. Acad Radiol. 31(5):2027-38, 2024
2. Gökçe E et al: Diagnostic efficacy of diffusion-weighted imaging and semiquantitative and quantitative dynamic contrast-enhanced magnetic resonance imaging in salivary gland tumors. World J Radiol. 15(1):20-31, 2023
3. Luna LP et al: Parotid Warthin's tumor: novel MR imaging score as diagnostic indicator. Clin Imaging. 81:9-14, 2022
4. Borsetto D et al: The diagnostic value of cytology in parotid Warthin's tumors: international multicenter series. Head Neck. 42(3):522-9, 2020
5. Liu YJ et al: Imaging quality of PROPELLER diffusion-weighted MR imaging and its diagnostic performance in distinguishing pleomorphic adenomas from Warthin tumors of the parotid gland. NMR Biomed. 33(5):e4282, 2020
6. Ginat DT: Imaging of benign neoplastic and nonneoplastic salivary gland tumors. Neuroimaging Clin N Am. 28(2):159-69, 2018

Warthin Tumor

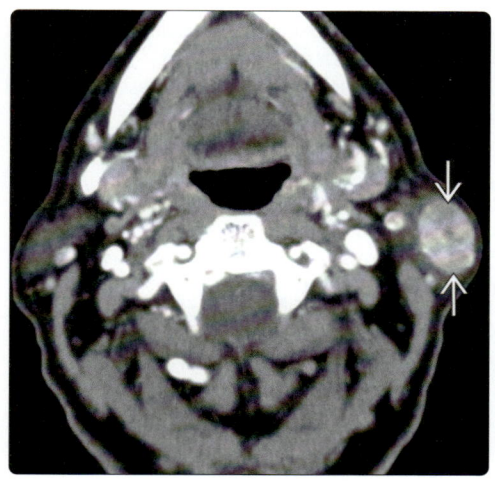

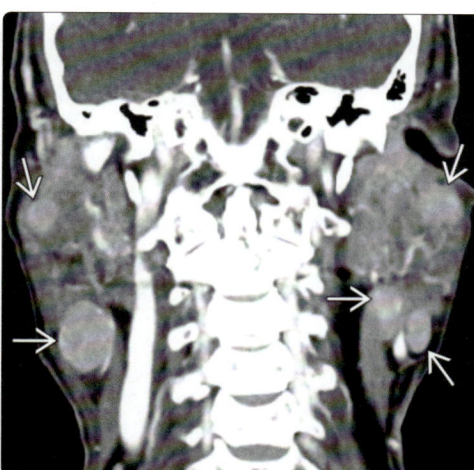

(Left) Axial CECT in a 64-year-old man with a history of tobacco use demonstrates a typical heterogeneously enhancing and well-circumscribed left parotid tail Warthin tumor ➡. A few small low-attenuation areas are noted internally. (Right) Coronal CECT shows multiple bilateral parotid nodules ➡ due to a multicentric Warthin tumor. The parotid tail nodules, bilateral and multifocal in nature, are classic findings in a Warthin tumor although lymphoma could appear similar.

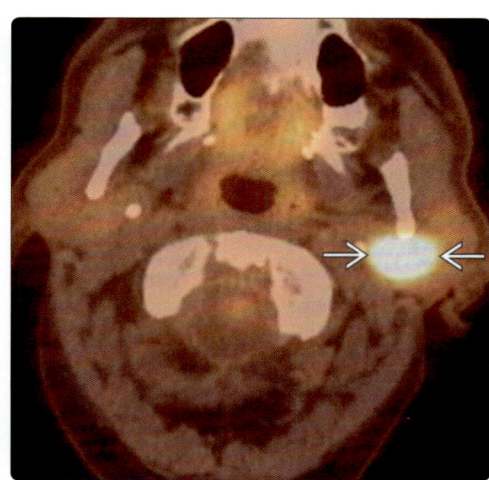

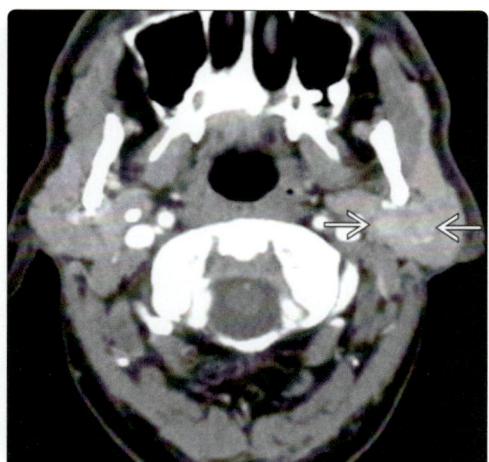

(Left) Axial FDG PET/CT shows an intensely FDG-avid mass in the left parotid gland ➡. Tissue sampling confirmed a Warthin tumor. (Right) Axial CECT in the same patient shows a faintly enhancing mass in the left parotid ➡, a classic "vanishing" tumor that is easily missed on imaging due to its density/enhancement that is nearly isointense to normal gland, along with a lack of heterogeneity or cystic components in this case.

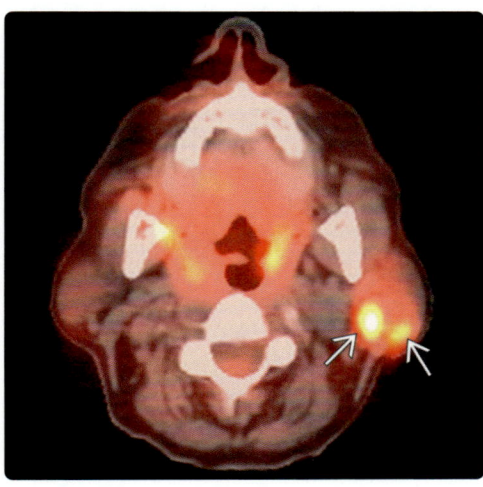

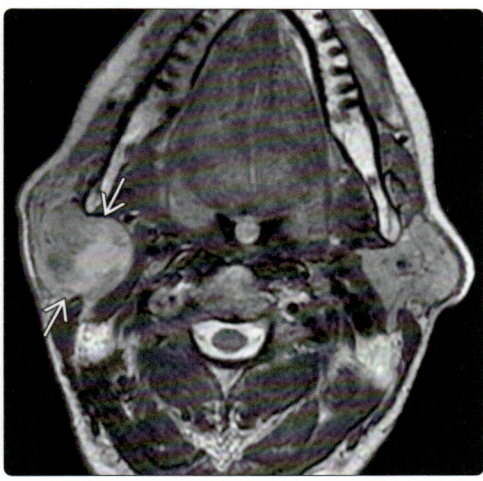

(Left) Axial PET/CT shows marked FDG uptake in 2 adjacent parotid Warthin tumors ➡. Avidity may be related to mitochondria-rich oncocytes in Warthin tumors. Several benign and malignant glandular tumors are FDG avid, but multifocality favors a Warthin tumor. These lesions must be sampled to exclude metastatic disease. (Right) Axial T2 MR shows a well-circumscribed, mixed solid/cystic mass in the right parotid gland at the angle of mandible ➡. Tissue sampling confirmed a Warthin tumor.

Parotid Schwannoma

TERMINOLOGY

- Benign nerve sheath neoplasm from Schwann cells of intraparotid facial nerve (CNVII)

IMAGING

- Heterogeneously enhancing tumor with intramural cystic areas when large
  - Cystic areas may be small, multifocal, or large
- Extension toward or into stylomastoid foramen suggestive, especially if expansile
- Presence of **target sign** suggestive if present
- Similar to schwannomas in other anatomic locations

TOP DIFFERENTIAL DIAGNOSES

- Parotid pleomorphic adenoma
- Warthin tumor
- Parotid metastatic nodal disease
- Parotid mucoepidermoid carcinoma
- Perineural tumor spread, CNVII

PATHOLOGY

- < 10% CNVII schwannoma = extratemporal (intraparotid), remaining = intratemporal or intracranial
- Type A: Exophytic off CNVII branch; no CNVII resection required
- Type B: Intrinsic to facial nerve branch; branch resection required
- Type C: Intrinsic to facial nerve trunk; resection & reconstruction required
- Type D: Encases main trunk & branches; resection & reconstruction required

CLINICAL ISSUES

- Presents like any parotid mass; difficult to differentiate clinically or radiographically
  - Facial nerve palsy uncommon
- Associated with neurofibromatosis type 2
- Treatment goal: Preserve facial nerve function
  - Controversial: Observation vs. surgery vs. radiation

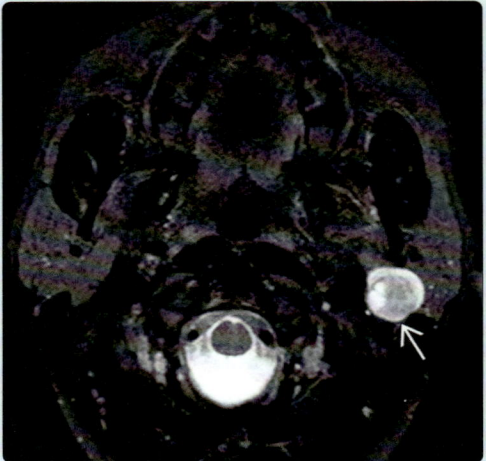
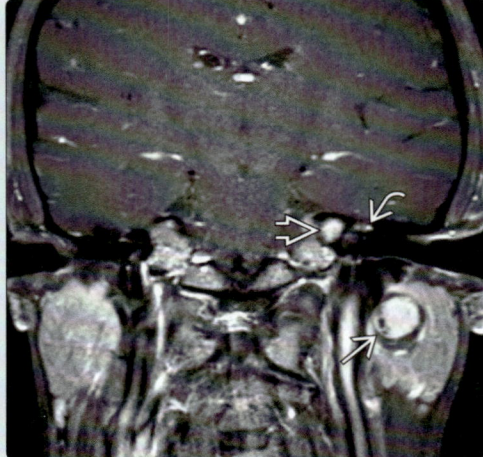

(Left) *Axial T2 FS MR shows a heterogeneous, hyperintense parotid mass wedged into the stylomastoid foramen ➡. The location & characteristic target sign suggest the possibility of facial schwannoma.* (Right) *Coronal T1 C+ FS MR in the same patient shows an enhancing schwannoma along the main trunk of the facial nerve with the target sign & small intratumoral cysts ➡. An additional clue to the Dx is a contiguous enhancing tumor along the intratemporal facial nerve ➡ extending into the internal auditory canal ➡.*

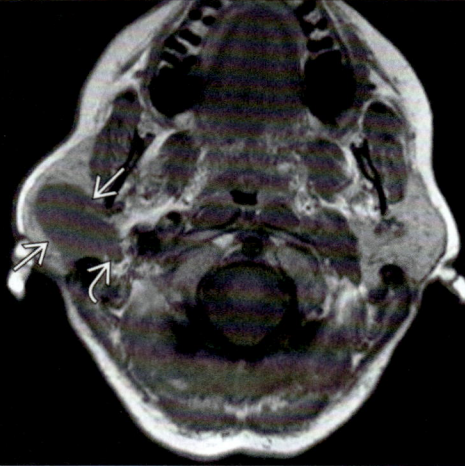
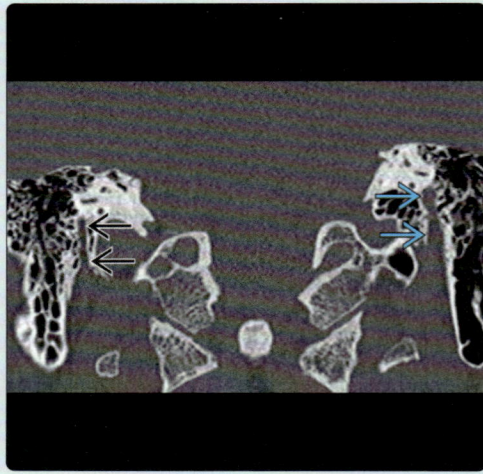

(Left) *Axial T1 MR shows a well-marginated, hypointense mass in the right parotid gland ➡. A small "thumb" of tumor ➡ extending into the stylomastoid foramen is a clue to the tumor origin from the facial nerve, which was confirmed histologically.* (Right) *Coronal bone CT shows asymmetric expansion of the left stylomastoid foramen and lower mastoid segment facial nerve canal ➡ with sharp border delineation and no destructive changes due to local parotid schwannoma extension. Compare to the normal side ➡.*

TERMINOLOGY

Synonyms

- Facial neurilemmoma, intraparotid neurilemmoma

Definitions

- Benign nerve sheath neoplasm from Schwann cells of intraparotid facial nerve (CNVII)

IMAGING

General Features

- Best diagnostic clue
  - Heterogeneously enhancing + **intramural cysts**
- Location
  - Course of intraparotid CNVII ± stylomastoid foramen

Imaging Recommendations

- Best imaging tool
  - T1WI C+ FS MR best demonstrates cystic areas

CT Findings

- CECT
  - Well-defined, round or oval intraparotid mass
  - Intramural cysts within larger (> 2-cm) lesions
  - Enlarged stylomastoid foramen &/or mastoid segment CNVII canal in proximal lesions

MR Findings

- T1WI
  - Tumor isointense to muscle, well defined
- T2WI
  - Slightly hyperintense to brain, muscle
  - Larger lesions with high-intensity cysts
  - **Target sign** (hypointense center with hyperintense rim)
  - High-resolution 3D SSFP may highlight nerve origin
- T1WI C+ FS
  - Enhancing & cystic regions + peripheral enhancement

DIFFERENTIAL DIAGNOSIS

Parotid Pleomorphic Adenoma

- Appears similar to schwannoma on CT & MR

Warthin Tumor

- Cystic areas present as in schwannoma
- Can be multiple, bilateral, & favor parotid tail

Parotid Metastatic Nodal Disease

- Often multiple; have primary lesion (e.g., skin, lymphoma)

Parotid Mucoepidermoid Carcinoma

- Low-grade form of mucoepidermoid carcinoma

Perineural Tumor Spread, CNVII

- Parotid or skin primary lesion

PATHOLOGY

General Features

- Etiology
  - Arises from differentiated neoplastic Schwann cells of CNVII nerve sheath

  - < 10% CNVII schwannoma = extratemporal (intraparotid), remaining = intratemporal or intracranial

Staging, Grading, & Classification

- Type A: Exophytic off CNVII branch; no CNVII resection
- Type B: Intrinsic to CNVII branch; branch resection
- Type C: Intrinsic to CNVII trunk; resection & reconstruction
- Type D: Encases main CNVII trunk & branches; resection & reconstruction indicated

Gross Pathologic & Surgical Features

- Smooth, rubbery, yellow, encapsulated fusiform mass

Microscopic Features

- Same as schwannomas in other anatomic locations

CLINICAL ISSUES

Presentation

- Most common signs/symptoms
  - Painless, slowly enlarging cheek mass
- Other signs/symptoms
  - Presents like any parotid mass; difficult to differentiate clinically or radiographically
    - Rarely diagnosed preoperatively unless biopsied
  - CNVII palsy uncommon: ↑ risk if intratemporal extension
  - Associations: Neurofibromatosis type 2 & schwannomatosis

Demographics

- Can affect any age group

Natural History & Prognosis

- Slow growth; typically 0.5-2.0 mm/year
- May eventually cause mass effect or cosmetic issues

Treatment

- Controversial: Observation vs. surgery vs. radiation
  - Depends on CNVII function & location of tumor
  - Goal: CNVII function preservation & facial cosmesis
  - Can dissect tumor off nerve but may cause CNVII palsy
  - Types C & D lesions at ↑ risk of postoperative CNVII palsy
- Stereotactic radiosurgery may be used if CNVII intact

DIAGNOSTIC CHECKLIST

Consider

- Which branch of facial nerve is involved?
  - Main trunk most common
- Relationship of mass to stylomastoid foramen
  - Involves mastoid segment of bony facial nerve canal

Image Interpretation Pearls

- Difficult to make radiographic diagnosis
  - Tissue sampling required but excisional biopsy risky
  - Image-guided biopsy (CT or US) very useful
    - Core needle biopsy required (FNA inadequate)

SELECTED REFERENCES

1. Huang L et al: Intraparotid facial nerve schwannoma: a comprehensive review of 70 cases at one single institution. Oral Dis. ePub, 2025
2. Wang X et al: Evaluation of multiparametric MRI differentiating pleomorphic adenoma from schwannoma in parapharyngeal space. Eur Arch Otorhinolaryngol. 281(11):5961-9, 2024

Parotid Mucoepidermoid Carcinoma

TERMINOLOGY

- Malignant epithelial salivary gland neoplasm composed of mixture of both epidermoid & mucus-secreting cells arising from ductal epithelium

IMAGING

- Imaging appearance based on histologic grade
  - **Low-grade mucoepidermoid carcinoma (MECa)**: Well-circumscribed, heterogeneous parotid space (PS) mass
  - **High-grade MECa**: Invasive, ill-defined PS mass with associated malignant nodes
- If lesion high grade, infiltrative, or near stylomastoid foramen, be alert for **perineural spread along CNVII**
- High-grade MECa often has **nodal metastases**
- MR findings
  - **Low T2** typical in high grade ± cystic areas common
  - T1 C+ shows heterogeneous tumor enhancement
  - Enhanced images may "hide" lesion
  - Evaluates lesion extent & **perineural tumor spread**

TOP DIFFERENTIAL DIAGNOSES

- Parotid pleomorphic adenoma (PA)
- Warthin tumor
- Parotid adenoid cystic carcinoma
- Parotid non-Hodgkin lymphoma
- Parotid metastatic nodes

PATHOLOGY

- *MECT1::MAML2* **gene fusions** in 50-80% of MECa
- Gene fusions & low histologic grade have better prognosis

CLINICAL ISSUES

- MECa is most common primary parotid malignancy
- Recurrence & survival depends heavily on histologic grade
- Late local recurrence (after 5 years) possible

DIAGNOSTIC CHECKLIST

- Low-grade MECa may exactly mimic PA
- High-grade MECa has invasive appearance

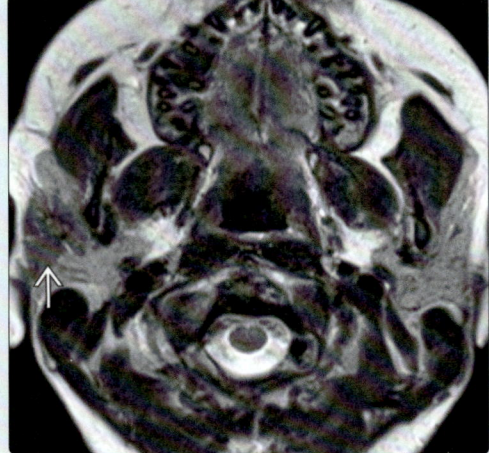
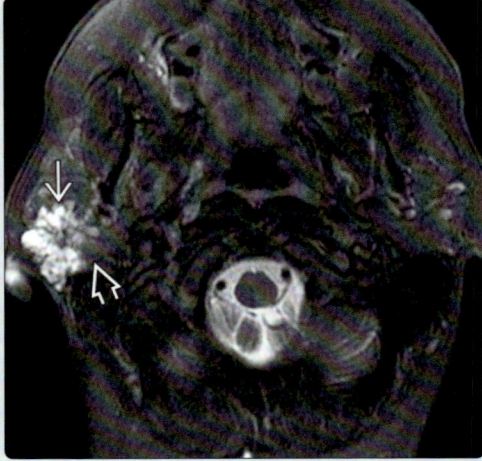

(Left) Axial T2 MR shows an irregular, spiculated-appearing mucoepidermoid carcinoma (MECa) of the superficial right parotid gland ➡. The hypointense signal, infiltrative appearance, and irregular, spiculated borders support malignancy. (Right) Axial T2 FS MR shows an irregular, lobulated mass in the parotid with mixed T2 signal. Laterally, there are high-signal cystic areas ➡, but medially there is a low-signal region ⇒. Low T2 signal within the solid components of the tumor is characteristic of MECa.

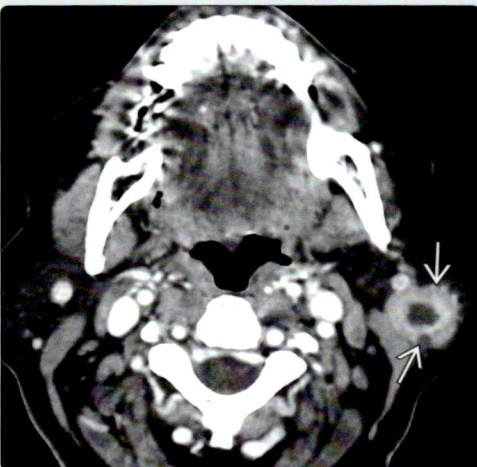
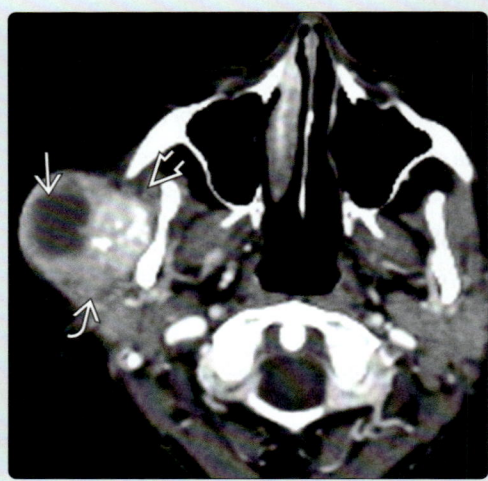

(Left) Axial CECT reveals a well-defined mass ➡ in the superficial lobe of the parotid gland. It has a thick rind of peripheral enhancement and is centrally cystic or necrotic. This is a characteristic imaging appearance for a low-grade MECa. (Right) Axial CECT shows a large, heterogeneous mass with cystic areas ➡, heterogeneous enhancement, and ill-defined borders ➡. The masseter muscle ➡ is invaded. This is a characteristic appearance for a high-grade MECa.

TERMINOLOGY

Abbreviations

- Mucoepidermoid carcinoma (MECa)

Definitions

- Malignant epithelial salivary gland neoplasm composed of variable mixture of both epidermoid & mucus-secreting cells arising from ductal epithelium

IMAGING

General Features

- Best diagnostic clue
  - Imaging appearance based on histologic grade
  - Low-grade MECa: Well-circumscribed, heterogeneous parotid space (PS) mass
  - High-grade MECa: **Invasive**, ill-defined PS mass with associated **malignant nodes**
- Location
  - Superficial lobe > > deep lobe parotid
- Size
  - Usually 1-4 cm at presentation
- Morphology
  - Low grade: Ovoid, well circumscribed
    - Cystic areas may be single & large or small & multifocal
    - Irregular shape
  - High grade: Amorphous, infiltrating mass
- **Malignant adenopathy** often present
  - 1st-order nodes = jugulodigastric nodes (level II)
  - Intraparotid & parotid tail nodes also involved

CT Findings

- CECT
  - Low-grade MECa
    - Enhancing heterogeneous mass with well-defined margins
    - Mucous deposits create cystic areas
    - Calcification or hemorrhage may occur
  - High-grade MECa
    - Enhancing invasive mass with ill-defined margins
    - Intraparotid & cervical metastatic nodes

MR Findings

- T1WI
  - Low-grade: Heterogeneous, well-defined mass with predominantly low signal
  - High-grade: Solid, infiltrative, intermediate-signal mass
- T2WI
  - Low grade: Heterogeneous
    - Cystic areas have high signal
    - Areas of low signal may be present
  - High grade: Intermediate, low signal, infiltrative
- DWI
  - ADC value lower than pleomorphic adenoma (PA) but similar to Warthin tumor
    - Not reliable enough to avoid biopsy
- T1WI C+
  - Heterogeneous enhancement
    - Cystic areas have no enhancement
  - If lesion high grade, infiltrative, or near stylomastoid foramen, perineural spread on CNVII may occur

Nuclear Medicine Findings

- FDG PET useful initially & in restaging
  - High negative predictive value & specificity
  - Metabolic complete response predicts excellent outcome
- DOTATATE PET uptake seen in most salivary malignancies due to somatostatin 2 receptor (SSTR2) expression in tissue & correlates with immunohistochemistry
- While not tumor specific, highest SSTR2 expression in MECa

Imaging Recommendations

- Best imaging tool
  - MR useful for extent of lesion & perineural spread
  - No radiographic modality provides definitive diagnosis
- Protocol advice
  - T1 unenhanced MR best delineates MECa due to inherent lower signal intensity relative to normal hyperintense parotid fat; enhanced images may "hide" lesion even with fat saturation
  - Long-term (at least 10 years) imaging follow-up recommended because of late recurrences

DIFFERENTIAL DIAGNOSIS

Parotid Pleomorphic Adenoma

- Most common parotid mass
- Small: Well demarcated, solid, homogeneous, ovoid
- Large: Heterogeneous, lobulated
- Low-grade MECa may be confused with PA

Warthin Tumor

- Multicentric &/or bilateral (20%)
- CECT: 30% with cystic components
- T1WI C+ MR: Heterogeneous enhancement, well circumscribed
- Cystic areas of low-grade MECa appear similar to cystic areas of Warthin tumor

Parotid Adenoid Cystic Carcinoma

- 2nd most common parotid malignancy
- Homogeneous; well or poorly defined, depends on grade
- Prone to perineural spread

Parotid Non-Hodgkin Lymphoma

- Primary parotid lymphoma: Invasive parenchymal tumor mimics high-grade MECa or adenoid cystic carcinoma
- Primary nodal lymphoma: Multiple well-circumscribed, bilateral intraparotid masses

Parotid Metastatic Nodes

- Primary lesion usually on or around skin of ear [squamous cell carcinoma (SCCa), melanoma]
- Single or multiple parotid masses, often centrally necrotic

Parotid Ductal Carcinoma

- Salivary ductal carcinoma mimics high-grade MECa on CT/MR
- Low T2 signal, infiltrative mass characteristic of both
- Cannot differentiate preoperatively

PATHOLOGY

General Features

- Etiology
  - Exposure risk: Radiation
    - Latency: 7-32 years

Staging, Grading, & Classification

- TNM staging
  - T1: Tumor ≤ 2 cm without extraparenchymal extension
  - T2: Tumor 2-4 cm without extraparenchymal extension
  - T3: Tumor > 4 cm &/or extraparenchymal extension
  - T4: Moderately advanced (T4A) or very advanced (T4B) disease
    - T4A: Tumor invades skin, mandible, ear canal, &/or facial nerve
    - T4B: Tumor invades skull base &/or pterygoid plates &/or encases carotid artery
- Histologic grading (low vs. intermediate vs. high) correlates best with prognosis

Gross Pathologic & Surgical Features

- Gray, tan-yellow, or pink

Microscopic Features

- Mixture of epidermoid & mucus-secreting cells with some cells intermediate between
- Cellular atypia & pleomorphism
- Arises in glandular ductal epithelium

Molecular Features

- *MECT1::MAML2* **gene fusions** in 50-80% of MECa

CLINICAL ISSUES

Presentation

- Most common signs/symptoms
  - Palpable parotid mass, usually rock-hard
  - Other signs/symptoms: Facial pain, otalgia, facial nerve paralysis
    - Other cranial nerve involvement (CNV3)
  - Clinical presentation depends on tumor grade
    - Low grade: Painless, mobile, slowly enlarging
    - High grade: Painful, immobile, rapidly enlarging

Demographics

- Age
  - Patients usually 35-65 years old
  - May be seen in pediatric population
- Epidemiology
  - **MECa is most common** primary parotid malignancy
    - ~ 50% of parotid malignancies
  - MECa: 10% of all salivary gland tumors
  - MECa: 30% of all salivary gland malignancies
  - Majority (60%) occur in parotid
    - Any salivary gland, mucosal surface (especially larynx), bone

Natural History & Prognosis

- Recurrence & survival rates depend on histologic grade
  - Low: 6% local recurrence; 90% 10-year survival rate
  - Intermediate: 20% local recurrence; 80% 10-year survival
  - High: 78% local recurrence; 27% 10-year survival rate
  - Distant metastases common in high grade; uncommon in low/intermediate grade
- Poor prognostic signs
  - Male sex
  - Age > 40 years
  - Fixed tumor, invasion of surrounding structures
  - Higher TNM stage or histologic grade
  - Cellular markers (p53, Ki-67)
- Late local recurrence (after 5 years) possible

Treatment

- Low-grade MECa
  - Wide local excision with preservation of facial nerve
  - Superficial parotidectomy if possible
  - Total parotidectomy often needed if deep lobe involved
  - Postoperative radiotherapy
- High-grade MECa
  - Wide local excision; extended total parotidectomy
  - Facial nerve sacrifice often necessary
  - Neck dissection routine
  - Postoperative radiotherapy with large port

DIAGNOSTIC CHECKLIST

Consider

- Check for **perineural spread along CNVII**
  - Replaced fat in stylomastoid foramen
  - Enhancement of vertical (mastoid) segment of CNVII
  - Extension along CNV3 (foramen ovale) if deep lobe parotid or **auriculotemporal nerve** involved
- Check for invasion of surrounding structures: Mandible, skull base, pterygoid plates, carotid artery

Image Interpretation Pearls

- Low-grade MECa may exactly mimic PA
- High-grade MECa has nonspecific invasive appearance
  - Remember to look for nodal metastases
  - Check stylomastoid foramen & mastoid segment CNVII for perineural tumor spread
- General evaluation of PS masses
  - First decide whether lesion is **intraparotid** (PA, Warthin, MECa, adenoid cystic carcinoma) or **extraparotid** (skin or different suprahyoid space)
  - If intraparotid, distinguish superficial vs. deep lobe
    - Divided by facial nerve plane, just lateral to retromandibular vein
  - Sharp margins helps distinguish benign from malignant
    - Caveat: Benign tumors can incite sialadenitis, & low-grade malignancy may have sharp margins

SELECTED REFERENCES

1. Ban X et al: Morphologic CT and MRI features of primary parotid squamous cell carcinoma and its predictive factors for differential diagnosis with mucoepidermoid carcinoma. Insights Imaging. 13(1):119, 2022
2. Orhan Soylemez UP et al: Differentiation of benign and malignant parotid gland tumors with MRI and diffusion weighted imaging. Medeni Med J. 36(2):138-45, 2021

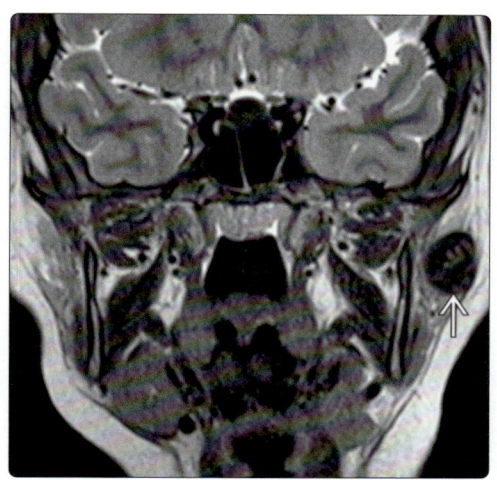

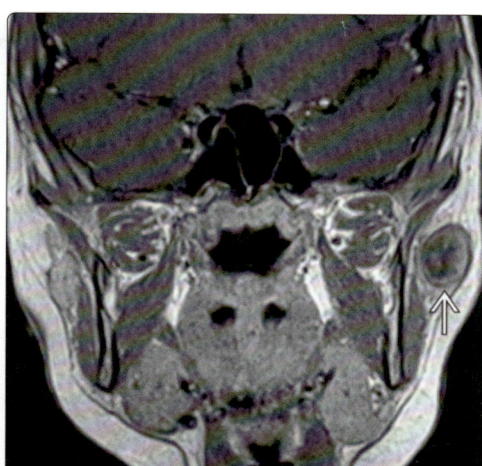

(Left) Coronal T2 MR shows a markedly hypointense, well-circumscribed mass involving the left superficial parotid gland ➔. Initial FNA was benign, but after resection, final pathology disclosed low-grade sclerosing variant MECa. Very low signal in this case may correlate to histologically identified nodular areas of dense keloidal fibrosis with associated lymphocytes and plasma cells. (Right) Coronal T1 C+ MR in the same patient shows heterogeneous postcontrast more peripheral enhancement of the tumor ➔.

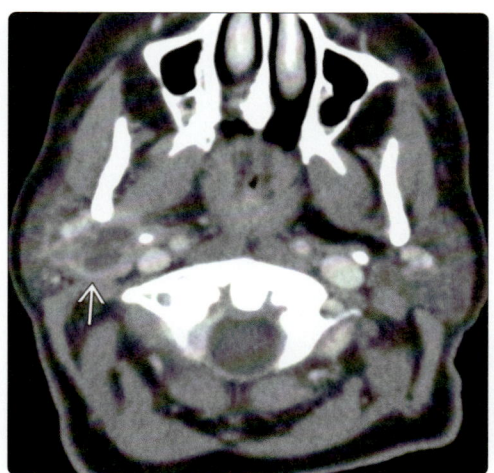

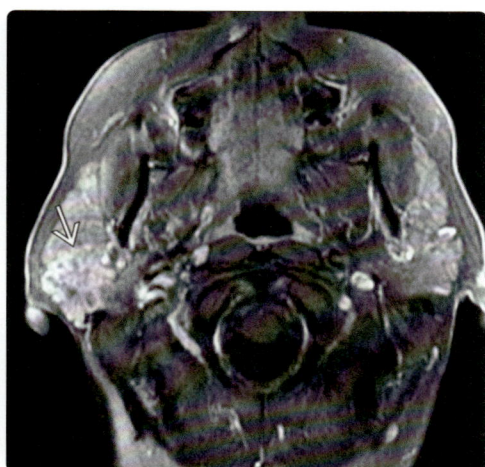

(Left) Axial CECT shows a heterogeneously enhancing MECa of the deep parotid with central cystic &/or necrotic change ➔. Larger size, irregular tumor borders, and findings supporting necrosis favor malignancy. (Right) Axial T1 C+ FS MR shows a lobular, well-defined mass ➔ in the parotid gland with numerous smaller cystic spaces. The cystic areas in MECa can be either 1 large cyst or multiple smaller cysts.

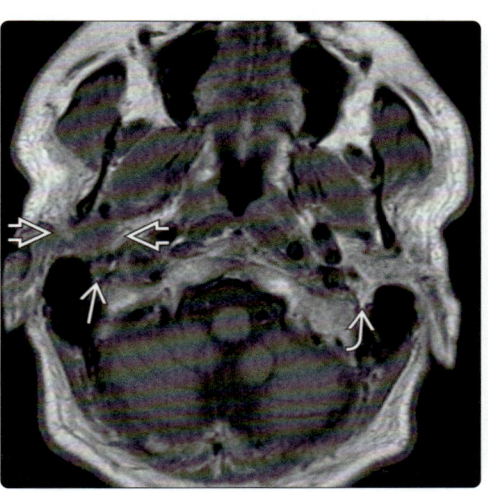

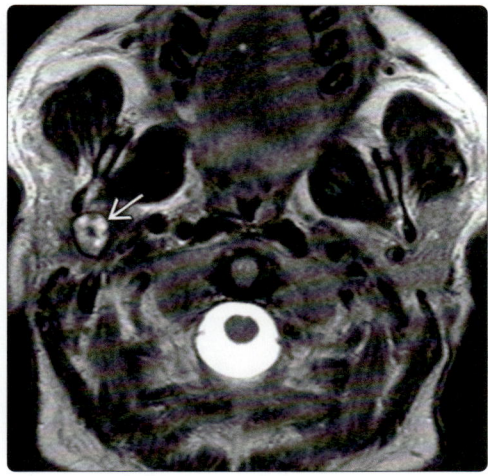

(Left) Axial T1 MR shows an ill-defined mass ➔ invading the stylomastoid foramen ➔, tracking along the main trunk of the facial nerve. Note the normal preserved fat in the left stylomastoid foramen ➔. This proved to be a high-grade MECa with perineural invasion and metastatic adenopathy. (Right) Axial T2 MR in the same patient demonstrates a cystic, well-defined tumor component ➔ in the lower parotid, which was in contrast to the infiltrative tumor appearance seen in the upper gland.

Parotid Adenoid Cystic Carcinoma

KEY FACTS

TERMINOLOGY

- Malignant salivary gland neoplasm arising in peripheral parotid ducts

IMAGING

- **Low-grade adenoid cystic carcinoma (ACCa)**: Well-circumscribed, homogeneously enhancing
- **High-grade ACCa**: Infiltrative, enhancing mass
- MR findings
  - Moderate T2 signal intensity
  - High-grade ACCa: Lower in signal intensity
  - Look for **perineural tumor** CNVII or CNV3
- MR best delineates tumor extent & perineural spread

TOP DIFFERENTIAL DIAGNOSES

- Parotid space pleomorphic adenoma
- Warthin tumor
- Parotid space mucoepidermoid carcinoma
- Intraparotid metastatic nodal disease

PATHOLOGY

- Tumor grading based on dominant histologic pattern
  - Tubular = grade 1
  - Cribriform = grade 2
  - Solid = grade 3
- Most common gene alteration: *MYB::NFIB* fusion (> 50%)

CLINICAL ISSUES

- Greatest propensity of all H&N tumors to spread via perineural pathway
- 33% present with pain & CNVII paralysis
- Treat with complete resection (parotidectomy)
- Postoperative radiotherapy for all but lowest grade
- Favorable short-term but poor long-term prognosis
- Metastases to lungs & bones > lymph nodes
- Nodal metastasis very uncommon
- **Late local recurrence**, up to 20 years after diagnosis, is characteristic

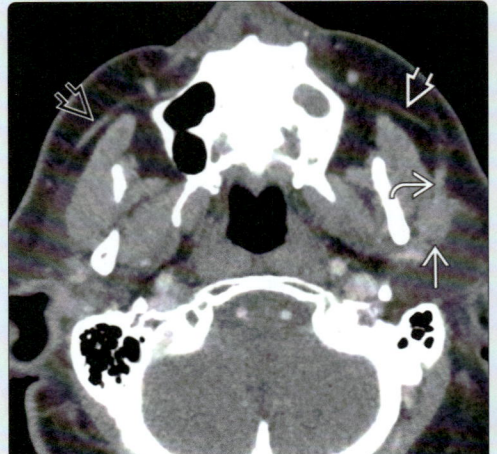 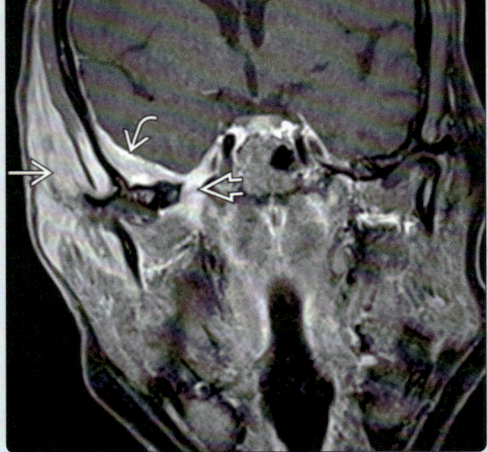

(Left) Axial CECT shows ACCa of the superficial left parotid gland ➡ with linear soft tissue extension along the maxillary division of the facial nerve ➡, confirmed at pathology. Note corresponding denervation atrophy of the ipsilateral zygomaticus major muscle ➡ and compare to normal muscle bulk on right ➡. (Right) Coronal T1 C+ FS MR shows infiltrating parotid ACCa invading masticator space ➡. Gross perineural tumor spread is present along V3 in foramen ovale ➡ and has spread to temporal fossa dura ➡.

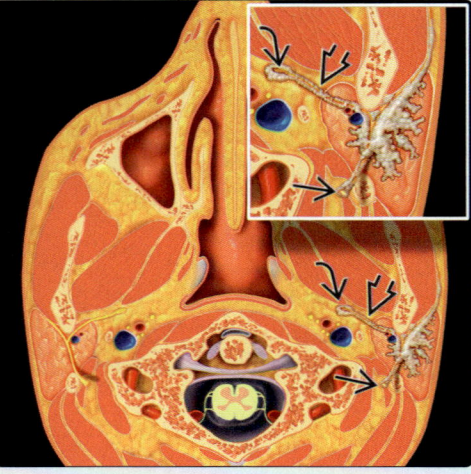 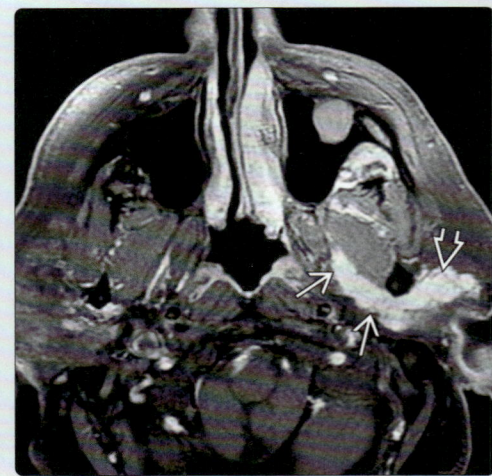

(Left) Axial graphic depicts high-grade parotid ACCa spreading in a perineural fashion along the proximal facial nerve toward the stylomastoid foramen ➡ and via the auriculotemporal nerve ➡ to the mandibular branch (CNV3) of the trigeminal nerve ➡. (Right) Axial T1 C+ FS MR shows marked thickening and enhancement of the auriculotemporal nerve ➡ from perineural spread of ACCa that originated in the superficial lobe of the parotid gland ➡.

Parotid Adenoid Cystic Carcinoma

TERMINOLOGY

Abbreviations

- Adenoid cystic carcinoma (ACCa)

Definitions

- Malignant salivary gland neoplasm arising in peripheral parotid ducts; **2nd most frequent** parotid malignancy (after mucoepidermoid carcinoma)

IMAGING

General Features

- Best diagnostic clue
  - **Low-grade ACCa**: Well-circumscribed, homogeneously enhancing parotid mass
  - **High-grade ACCa**: Infiltrative, homogeneously enhancing parotid mass
- Location
  - May involve superficial or deep lobe

CT Findings

- CECT
  - Homogeneously enhancing parotid space (PS) mass with well- (low-grade) or ill-defined (high-grade) margins

MR Findings

- T1WI
  - Low to intermediate signal intensity PS mass
- T2WI
  - Moderate signal intensity PS mass
  - High-grade tumors usually lower in signal intensity
- T1WI C+
  - Homogeneously enhancing PS mass
  - **Perineural tumor** spread on **mastoid CNVII**

Ultrasonographic Findings

- Irregular borders compared to benign tumors

Imaging Recommendations

- MR best delineates tumor extent & perineural spread

DIFFERENTIAL DIAGNOSIS

Parotid Space Pleomorphic Adenoma

- Well-defined, homogeneous, ovoid, T2-bright PS mass
- May be indistinguishable from low-grade ACCa

Warthin Tumor

- Well-defined PS mass, more heterogeneously enhancing
- Demographic: Older male smokers

Parotid Space Mucoepidermoid Carcinoma

- Well-defined or infiltrative PS mass; depends on grade
- More likely cystic component &/or low T2 signal than ACCa

Intraparotid Metastatic Nodal Disease

- Primary on skin of ear, forehead, or external auditory canal
- Often central necrosis; may be multiple nodes

PATHOLOGY

Staging, Grading, & Classification

- Tumor grading based on dominant histologic pattern
  - Tubular = grade 1, cribriform = grade 2, solid = grade 3

Gross Pathologic & Surgical Features

- Pink-tan with mottled surface; rarely necrotic
- Infiltrative margins; no capsule

Microscopic Features

- 3 distinct histologic patterns
  - Cribriform, tubular, & solid
  - Tumor may have 1, 2, or 3 of these patterns

Genomics

- Most common gene alteration: *MYB::NFIB* fusion in > 50%

CLINICAL ISSUES

Presentation

- Most common signs/symptoms
  - Painful hard parotid mass; present months to years
  - 33% present with pain & CNVII paralysis

Demographics

- Age
  - Peak: 5th-7th decades; rarely < 20 years
- Epidemiology
  - 7-18% of parotid tumors
  - Greatest propensity of all H&N tumors to spread via perineural pathway

Natural History & Prognosis

- **Late local recurrences**
  - ≤ 20 years after diagnosis
- Favorable short-term but poor long-term prognosis
- Metastases to lungs & bones > lymph nodes
- Predictors of distant metastasis: Tumor > 3 cm, solid pattern, local recurrence, node disease
- Tumor seeding along core biopsy tract reported & may be visible on MR

Treatment

- Surgical plan is wide resection with negative margins
- Postoperative radiotherapy for all but lowest grade

DIAGNOSTIC CHECKLIST

Consider

- Look carefully for **perineural tumor** with any parotid neoplasm but particularly ACCa
  - CNVII & CNV
  - **Auriculotemporal nerve** runs behind mandible
    - Alternate course for intracranial spread via CNV3
- Ill-defined margins suggest higher grade lesion

Image Interpretation Pearls

- Imaging findings often nonspecific & similar to other parotid tumors
- Imaging is for extent of mass & perineural tumor

SELECTED REFERENCES

1. Su HZ et al: Polar vessel: a new ultrasound sign for complementary diagnosis of major salivary gland adenoid cystic carcinoma. J Ultrasound Med. 42(3):603-11, 2023
2. Orhan Soylemez UP et al: Differentiation of benign and malignant parotid gland tumors with MRI and diffusion weighted imaging. Medeni Med J. 36(2):138-45, 2021

Parotid Acinic Cell Carcinoma

TERMINOLOGY

- Slow-growing variant of adenocarcinoma arising in parotid glandular tissue
- 3rd most frequent primary parotid malignancy after mucoepidermoid and adenoid cystic carcinoma
- 10-12% of salivary gland malignancies
- Rare in other salivary glands

IMAGING

- Generally indistinguishable from other low-grade parotid neoplasms
- CT: Well defined, usually homogeneously enhancing; may have cystic areas
- MR: Variable signal from cystic areas, necrosis, hemorrhage, but typically hyperintense on T2 and solid component enhances uniformly
- PET: Variable uptake; high-grade acinic cell carcinoma uncommon but has intense FDG uptake

TOP DIFFERENTIAL DIAGNOSES

- Mammary analogue secretory carcinoma
- Parotid pleomorphic adenoma
- Parotid mucoepidermoid carcinoma
- Warthin tumor

PATHOLOGY

- Low-grade tumors; rare high-grade transformation

CLINICAL ISSUES

- Mean age: 44 years (< most parotid malignancies)
- Favorable prognosis: 80% with 10-year survival
- Indolent course; recurrences and metastases may occur many years after treatment
- Histologic grade better predicts survival than TN stage

DIAGNOSTIC CHECKLIST

- Important to describe location, extent, adenopathy
- Always look for CNVII perineural tumor

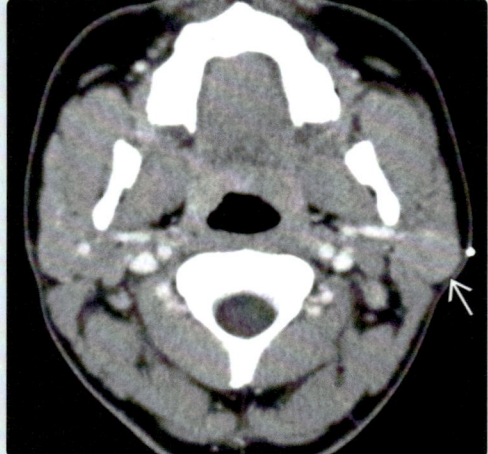 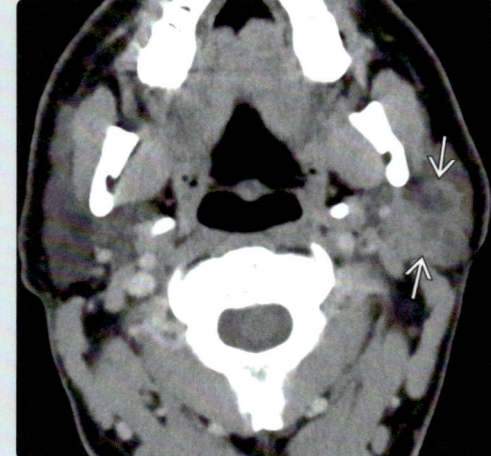

(Left) Axial CECT shows the site of a palpable mass (indicated by the overlying BB). This well-circumscribed mass ➡ mimics a benign neoplasm. This mass could otherwise be easily missed given density close to normal gland. (Right) Axial CECT in a patient with a palpable left cheek mass shows asymmetric enlargement of the left parotid gland due to a heterogeneous partly solid, partly cystic enhancing acinic cell carcinoma ➡. This tumor is more visible due to the lower background gland density and heterogeneity.

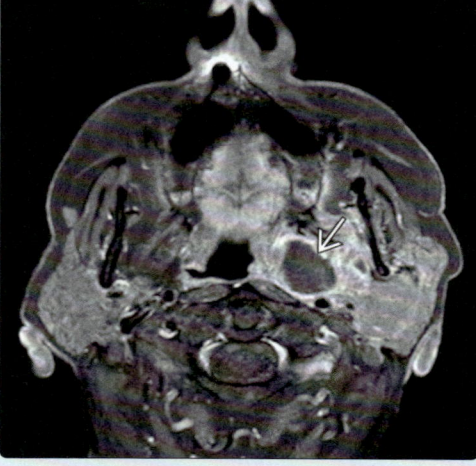 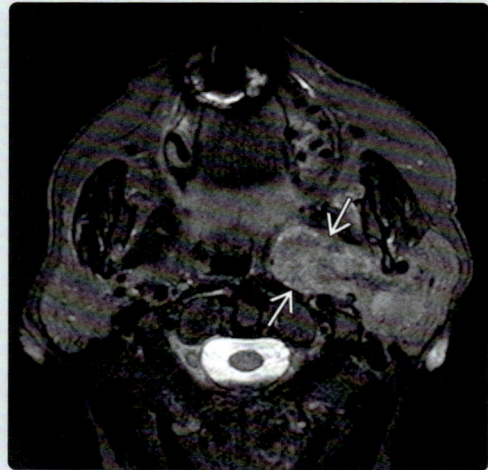

(Left) Axial T1 C+ FS MR shows a heterogeneous tumor with a cystic component in the deep lobe ➡. The patient had longstanding left ear pain and a slowly developing throat bulge on the left. Histology showed low- to intermediate-grade acinic cell carcinoma. (Right) Axial T2 FS MR in the same patient shows a heterogeneous deep lobe parotid mass ➡ that is nearly isointense to normal gland, raising concern for malignancy. The relatively low T2 signal and low ADC (not shown) were concerning for malignancy.

Parotid Acinic Cell Carcinoma

TERMINOLOGY

Abbreviations
- Acinic cell carcinoma (AciCC)

Synonyms
- Acinous cell carcinoma

Definitions
- Slow-growing **variant of adenocarcinoma** arising in parotid
- **3rd most frequent** primary parotid malignancy after mucoepidermoid and adenoid cystic carcinoma

IMAGING

General Features
- Best diagnostic clue
  - Well-circumscribed, lobulated, homogeneously enhancing parotid mass
  - Cystic areas may be present
  - Usually **indistinguishable from other neoplasms**
- Location
  - Most often superficial lobe parotid and parotid tail
  - Rare in other salivary glands
  - Can be multicentric, bilateral
- Size
  - Variable; generally 1-3 cm

CT Findings
- CECT
  - Well-defined, usually homogeneously enhancing ± cysts
  - No calcification
  - Features often benign-appearing

MR Findings
- Tumor conspicuity and characterization better with MR compared to CT
- T1WI: **Varied signal from cystic areas, necrosis, blood**
- T2WI: High signal overall, but varies due to cysts, necrosis, hemorrhage
- DWI: Low ADC values like other malignancies
- T1WI C+: Predominantly uniformly enhancing ± focal, nonenhancing cyst

Nuclear Medicine Findings
- PET
  - Overall, AciCC has variable uptake
  - High grade (uncommon) has intense uptake

DIFFERENTIAL DIAGNOSIS

Mammary Analogue Secretory Carcinoma
- MR may show intratumoral hemorrhage

Parotid Pleomorphic Adenoma
- Well defined, typically markedly T2 hyperintense
- Calcifications may be present

Parotid Mucoepidermoid Carcinoma
- Low-grade variant is well defined, uniform
- Most common parotid malignancy

Warthin Tumor
- Well-defined mass with central low density
- May be multiple, bilateral

PATHOLOGY

General Features
- Etiology
  - Associated with prior radiation, family history
- Epidemiology
  - **10-12% of salivary gland malignancies**

Gross Pathologic & Surgical Features
- Lobular, tan to red, well defined, solid or cystic, 1-3 cm

Microscopic Features
- Polygonal cells in sheets, uniform nuclei, vacuolated cells, locally infiltrative
  - ± microcysts, microhemorrhage, focal necrosis
- **Generally low-grade**, high-grade transformation possible
  - Poorer prognosis if perineural or vascular invasion, many or atypical mitoses, necrosis, or nodal metastasis

Immunohistochemistry
- DOG1, NR4A3 positive, mammoglobulin negative

CLINICAL ISSUES

Presentation
- Most common signs/symptoms
  - Painless parotid mass for several years
- Other signs/symptoms
  - **Facial paresis rare**
  - May be exquisitely painful during FNA

Demographics
- Age
  - Median: 52 years; mean: 44 years
- Sex
  - F:M = 3:2

Natural History & Prognosis
- Favorable prognosis: 80% with 10-year survival
- **Generally indolent course**; recurrences and metastases may occur many years after treatment
  - 35% recur locally
  - Distant metastases occur in lungs, bone
  - May have regional lymph node metastases
- Histologic grade better predicts survival than TN stage

Treatment
- Wide surgical excision ± radiation; chemoresistant

DIAGNOSTIC CHECKLIST

Consider
- Not usually possible to differentiate among malignancies

Image Interpretation Pearls
- Important to describe location, extent, adenopathy
- Look for CNVII perineural tumor

SELECTED REFERENCES

1. Vrinceanu D et al: Parotid gland tumors: molecular diagnostic approaches. Int J Mol Sci. 25(13):7350, 2024

Parotid Secretory Carcinoma

TERMINOLOGY

- Low-grade salivary malignancy
- 90% have specific *ETV6::NTRK3* gene fusion

IMAGING

- Sharp boundaries, regular edges, & uneven density
- CT shows variable cystic areas &/or calcification
- T1: Internal cyst high signal intensity
- T2: Predominantly cystic T2 hyperintensity with solid papillary projection
- C+: Heterogeneous enhancement, often cystic with enhancing mural nodule

TOP DIFFERENTIAL DIAGNOSES

- Pleomorphic adenoma
- Warthin tumor
- Acinic cell carcinoma
- Mucoepidermoid carcinoma
- Parotid facial nerve schwannoma

PATHOLOGY

- Abundant PAS(+) eosinophilic to bubbly secretions
- Historically called acinic cell carcinoma; now reclassified with immunohistochemistry & molecular pathology
  - S-100 & mammaglobin expression
  - Negative DOG-1 staining
  - *ETV6::NTRK3* specific gene fusion

CLINICAL ISSUES

- Slowly enlarging painless nodule in face
- Mean age: 47 years (range 10-86 years)
- M = F
- Surgical resection ± lymph node dissection ± radiation &/or chemotherapy
- Facial nerve palsy uncommon, seen in larger tumors

DIAGNOSTIC CHECKLIST

- Enhanced MR offers best soft tissue characterization
- Cystic parotid mass with ↑ T1 signal & mural nodularity

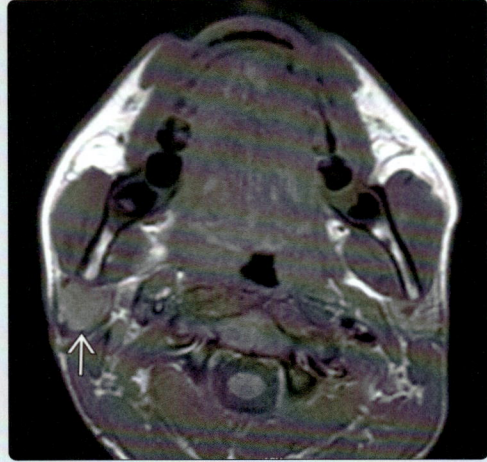
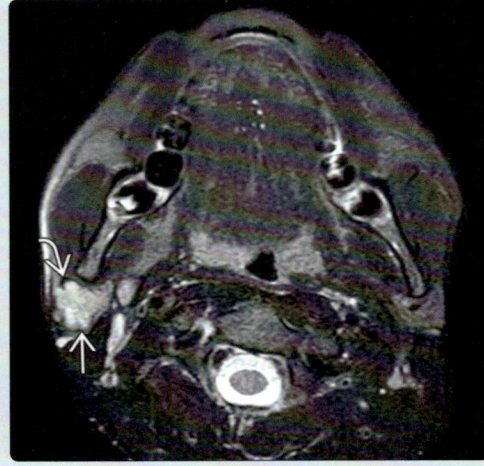

(Left) *Axial T1 MR shows a hyperintense mass enlarging the right parotid gland ➡. Internal T1 hyperintensity is a classic finding that is often due to internal hemorrhage, which is also typically seen at histopathologic analysis. Hemosiderin deposition is often present.* (Right) *Axial T2 FS MR in the same patient shows a cystic, well-demarcated, hyperintense secretory carcinoma in the right parotid gland ➡. Thin, peripheral hypointense signal may be due to hemosiderin deposition ➡ and provides a clue to the diagnosis.*

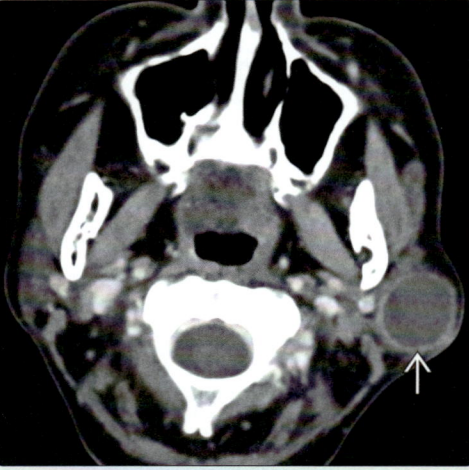
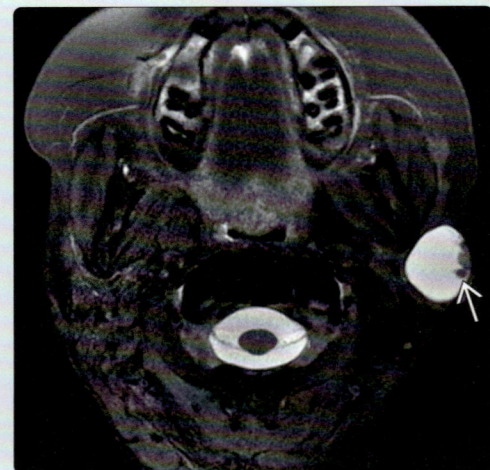

(Left) *Axial CECT demonstrates a cystic left parotid mass with peripheral wall enhancement ➡. This appearance is not specific and could be seen with inflammation or infection as well as cystic benign or malignant neoplasm.* (Right) *Axial T2 FS MR in the same patient offers better soft tissue characterization and demonstrates a characteristic cystic T2- hyperintense secretory carcinoma with peripheral hypointense papillary mural nodularity ➡.*

Parotid Secretory Carcinoma

TERMINOLOGY

Abbreviations
- Secretory carcinoma (SC)

Synonyms
- Mammary analogue secretory carcinoma (MASC)

Definitions
- Low-grade salivary malignancy
- 90% have specific *ETV6::NTRK3* gene fusion

IMAGING

General Features
- Best diagnostic clue
  - Predominantly cystic tumors with solid papillary projection
- Size
  - 2-4 cm
- Morphology
  - Well-circumscribed; may mimic benign tumors
  - Oval or lobulated

CT Findings
- Sharp boundaries, regular edges, & uneven density
- May have cystic areas & calcification
- Up to 25% have cervical adenopathy

MR Findings
- T1: Internal cyst high signal intensity
- T2: Predominantly cystic T2 hyperintensity with solid papillary projection
  - May show focal hypointensities consistent with hemorrhage ± hemosiderin
    - Hemosiderin favors SC over acinic cell carcinoma
  - May have layering blood products
- C+: Heterogeneous enhancement, often cystic with enhancing mural nodule

Ultrasonographic Findings
- Well-demarcated, heterogeneous, & hypoechoic masses with regular morphology
- Cystic to solid, small internal flow may be visible

Imaging Recommendations
- Protocol advice
  - High-resolution parotid ± MR contrast

DIFFERENTIAL DIAGNOSIS

Pleomorphic Adenoma
- Markedly T2 hyperintense, T1 hypointense

Warthin Tumor
- Older male smokers
- Predilection for parotid tail

Acinic Cell Carcinoma
- Predominantly solid tumor; T1 hypointense

Mucoepidermoid Carcinoma
- Low-grade tumors may mimic
- Usually lower signal on T2 & more infiltrative

Parotid Facial Nerve Schwannoma
- Tubular morphology along nerve course
- Target sign morphology

PATHOLOGY

General Features
- Morphologic similarity & gene mutation to breast secretory carcinomas

Staging, Grading, & Classification
- Follows 8th edition AJCC for salivary tumors

Gross Pathologic & Surgical Features
- Solitary, well-circumscribed, & often encapsulated mass, brown to gray with rubbery texture; cystic foci common
- Average size: 2.6 cm

Microscopic Features
- Historically often labeled acinic cell carcinoma
- Abundant PAS(+) eosinophilic to bubbly secretions
- Now reclassified by immunohistochemistry & genetics

Immunohistochemistry
- S-100 & mammaglobin expression
- Negative DOG-1 staining

Molecular Genetics
- *ETV6::NTRK3* gene fusion (seen in 90%) is specific

CLINICAL ISSUES

Presentation
- Most common signs/symptoms
  - Slowly enlarging painless nodule in face
- Other signs/symptoms
  - Facial nerve palsy uncommon, seen in larger tumors

Demographics
- M = F
- Mean age: 47 years (range: 10-86 years)

Natural History & Prognosis
- Prognosis correlated to stage, grade, & surgery
- Ranges from indolent to aggressive
- Mean disease-free survival: 92 months

Treatment
- Surgical resection ± lymph node dissection ± radiation &/or chemotherapy

DIAGNOSTIC CHECKLIST

Consider
- Enhanced parotid/face MR for better soft tissue characterization of parotid neoplasms compared to CT

Image Interpretation Pearls
- Macrocystic T1-hyperintense parotid mass with mural nodularity is suggestive, especially with hemosiderin

SELECTED REFERENCES

1. Kurokawa R et al: Radiological features of head and neck mammary analogue secretory carcinoma: 11 new cases with a systematic review of 29 cases reported in 28 publications. Neuroradiology. 63(11):1901-11, 2021

Parotid Malignant Mixed Tumor

TERMINOLOGY

- Definition: Malignant tumor arising within preexisting pleomorphic adenoma (PA)
- 2 types of malignant mixed tumor (MMT)
  - Carcinoma ex PA (majority); carcinosarcoma (very rare)

IMAGING

- Early: Encapsulated mass, looks like PA
- Late: Extensive aggressive parotid mass with invasion of surrounding structures
  - Encapsulated benign-appearing portion often present
- MR best for lesion extent, invasion, and characterization
  - Unenhanced T1 MR very useful due to inherent contrast from parotid gland fat
  - Native PA has high T2 signal, but most carcinomas have lower T2 signal
  - Native PA has high ADC, but carcinomas have low ADC
- Irregular, lobular mass with uneven margins

- May have well-defined nodule (residual PA) with infiltrative border

TOP DIFFERENTIAL DIAGNOSES

- Parotid PA; Warthin tumor
- Parotid mucoepidermoid carcinoma
- Parotid adenoid cystic carcinoma

CLINICAL ISSUES

- Rapidly enlarging, longstanding parotid mass suggests MMT
- Other signs: Facial nerve weakness and pain
- Early MMT may be found incidentally on PA histology
- Prior radiation may increase risk
- 5-10% of PA degenerate into MMT
  - PA should be removed to prevent this
- Biologic behavior determined by tumor extent and carcinoma subtype
- Larger tumor size, older age at higher risk for malignancy

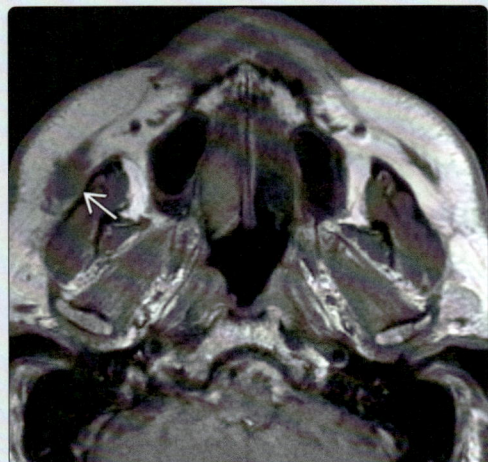 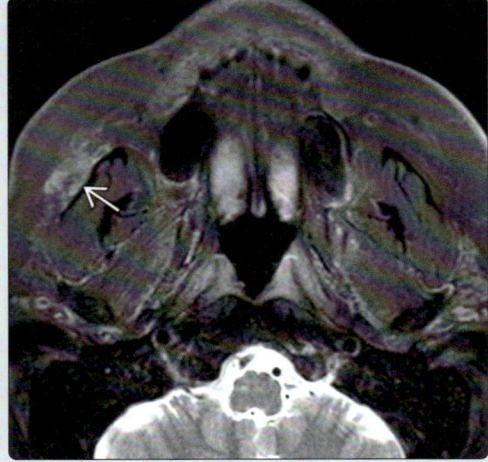

(Left) *Axial T1 MR in an asymptomatic older male referred for imaging after his dentist noted a palpable right cheek mass shows an ill-defined mass* ⮕ *arising along the accessory parotid gland near the distal parotid duct.* (Right) *Axial T2 FS MR in the same patient shows a poorly defined, infiltrative-appearing mass with intermediate signal intensity* ⮕*. The irregular margins on imaging and patient's older age favor malignancy. Pathology disclosed carcinoma ex-pleomorphic adenoma due to myoepithelial carcinoma.*

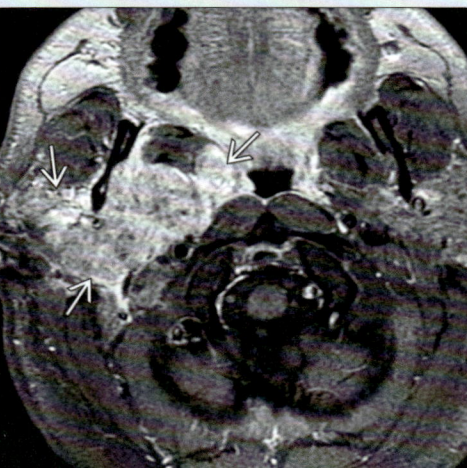 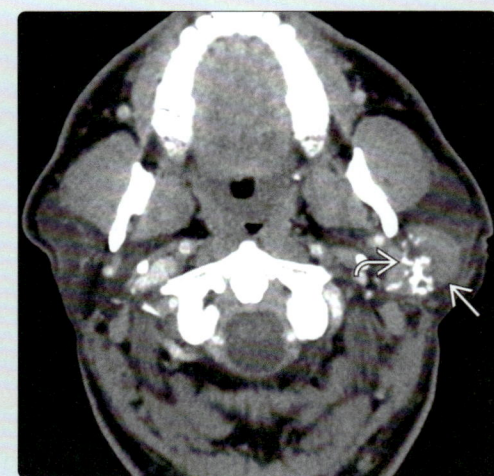

(Left) *Axial T1 C+ FS MR shows an aggressive, heterogeneously enhancing mass* ⮕ *replacing the parotid gland. Histologically, this showed areas of carcinoma and sarcoma as well as residual PA, which confirmed the diagnosis of true malignant mixed tumor (MMT).* (Right) *Axial CECT shows a well-circumscribed parotid carcinosarcoma* ⮕*. Although the sharp margins favor a benign neoplasm, the coarse internal calcifications* ⮕ *are unusual and suggest the potential for malignancy.*

TERMINOLOGY

Abbreviations
- Malignant mixed tumor (MMT)

Synonyms
- Carcinoma ex pleomorphic adenoma (PA)

Definitions
- Malignant tumor arising within parotid PA
- 2 types of MMT
  - **Carcinoma ex PA**
    - Common MMT type
    - Consists of single malignant cell type
  - **Carcinosarcoma** (true MMT)
    - Consists of multiple malignant cell types
    - Very rare (< 70 cases in literature)

IMAGING

General Features
- Best diagnostic clue
  - Early MMT: Not distinguishable from surrounding PA
  - Late MMT: Aggressive parotid mass with extensive invasion of surrounding tissues
    - Tumor has characteristics of malignant cell type
- Morphology
  - Irregular, lobular mass with uneven margins
  - May have a well-defined nodule (residual PA component) with infiltrative border

CT Findings
- Tumor calcifications support malignancy
- Irregular heterogeneously enhancing mass
- Look for metastatic adenopathy

MR Findings
- T2WI
  - Native PA has high T2 signal, often heterogeneous
  - Carcinomas often have low T2 signal
- DWI
  - Native PA has high diffusivity (↓ DWI signal)
  - Carcinomas have low diffusivity (↑ DWI signal)
- T1WI C+
  - Inhomogeneous enhancement

Imaging Recommendations
- Best imaging tool
  - MR best for extent of lesion, invasion, and characterizing different tumor regions
- Protocol advice
  - Unenhanced T1 sequences very useful because of inherent contrast from parotid gland fat

DIFFERENTIAL DIAGNOSIS

Parotid Pleomorphic Adenoma
- Sharp margins; MR: T2 mostly hyperintense

Warthin Tumor
- Demographics: Older male smokers
- May be multiple or bilateral, solid, or cystic

Parotid Mucoepidermoid Carcinoma
- Well-defined or infiltrative parotid space (PS) mass
- Lymphadenopathy common

Parotid Adenoid Cystic Carcinomas
- Well-defined or infiltrative PS mass
- Perineural tumor spread common

PATHOLOGY

General Features
- Biologic behavior determined by tumor extent and carcinoma subtype
- Carcinoma ex PA: Malignant degeneration of 1 cell line in PA
  - Most often salivary ductal carcinoma
  - Need residual PA to diagnose carcinoma ex PA
- Parotid carcinosarcoma: Etiology controversial
  - May arise from pluripotent cell that differentiates in multiple directions while maintaining malignant potential
  - Possibly collision tumor of multiple carcinomas ex PA
  - Carcinoma component of true MMT usually salivary gland carcinoma
    - Sarcoma component usually chondrosarcoma
    - Glandular and spindle cell components common

CLINICAL ISSUES

Presentation
- Most common signs/symptoms
  - Rapid enlargement of longstanding parotid mass
- Other signs/symptoms
  - Facial nerve weakness and pain
  - Early MMT may be incidentally found in PA histology

Demographics
- Prior radiation may increase risk
- 5-10% of PA degrade into MMT
  - PA should be removed before this occurs
- Larger tumor size and older age at higher risk for malignancy

Natural History & Prognosis
- Carcinoma ex PA: Prognosis depends on histologic type, grade, and stage
- Carcinosarcoma: Aggressive tumor with poor prognosis
  - Mean survival: 3.6 years, even with treatment

Treatment
- Trimodal therapy (surgery, chemotherapy, radiation)

DIAGNOSTIC CHECKLIST

Image Interpretation Pearls
- Sudden enlargement of longstanding parotid mass is suggestive; look for CNVII and CNV perineural spread

SELECTED REFERENCES

1. Faur AC et al: Clinical and morphological aspects of aggressive salivary gland mixed tumors: a narrative review. Diagnostics (Basel). 14(17):1942, 2024
2. Levyn H et al: Risk of carcinoma in pleomorphic adenomas of the parotid. JAMA Otolaryngol Head Neck Surg. 149(11):1034-41, 2023

Parotid Non-Hodgkin Lymphoma

TERMINOLOGY

- 3 forms of parotid involvement with non-Hodgkin lymphoma (NHL)
- Nodal NHL
  - **Primary nodal NHL**
  - **Systemic NHL** involving parotid nodes
  - **Primary parenchymal NHL**, often mucosa-associated lymphoid tissue (MALT)

IMAGING

- Nodal NHL: Multiple well-defined, homogeneous parotid masses
- Primary parotid NHL: Infiltrative or focal solid mass, uncommonly cystic
- Often periparotid and upper cervical lymphadenopathy
- Ultrasound shows hypoechoic intraparotid mass(es)
- Color Doppler shows hypervascular mass(es)
- PET/CT typically markedly FDG avid
- Consider NHL with dominant mass if Sjögren

TOP DIFFERENTIAL DIAGNOSES

- Benign lymphoepithelial lesions-HIV
- Parotid Sjögren syndrome
- Warthin tumor
- Parotid nodal metastatic disease
- IgG4-related disease

PATHOLOGY

- Primary Sjögren syndrome has 10-44x ↑ risk of NHL
- Lugano classification uses PET/CT for NHL staging

CLINICAL ISSUES

- Overall 5-year survival: 72%
- Systemic NHL involves parotid in 1-8%
- Primary parotid NHL: ~ 1-5% of parotid malignancies

DIAGNOSTIC CHECKLIST

- Beware: Isodense NHL may be "invisible" on CECT
- Noncontrast T1 (no FS) or T2 FS ↑ conspicuity on MR

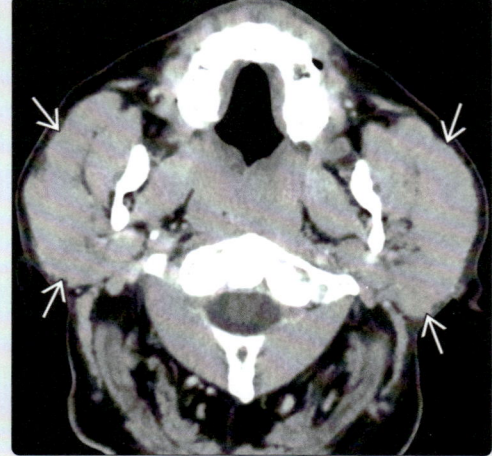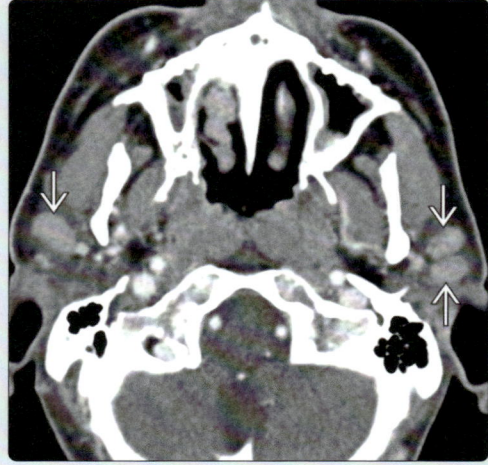

(Left) Axial CECT in a patient with mantle cell lymphoma demonstrates marked homogeneous enlargement of both parotids ⇗ due to involvement by systemic lymphoma. Associated FDG PET hypermetabolism was present (not shown). (Right) Axial CECT shows multiple bilateral, well-defined, homogeneously enhancing masses ⇗. Nodules ≥ 1 cm in parotid gland deserve further evaluation, as they may represent multiple Warthin tumors, metastatic nodes, or lymphoma. The neck should be evaluated for adenopathy.

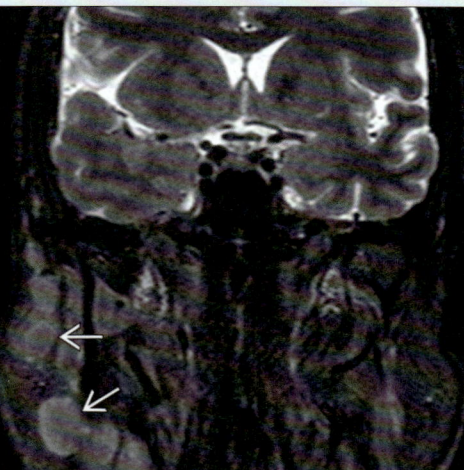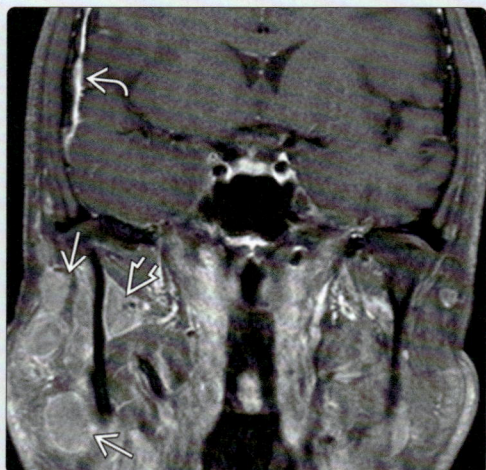

(Left) Coronal STIR MR shows multiple homogeneous low-signal masses within the right parotid gland ⇗ and adjacent tissues in this patient with MALT lymphoma. (Right) Coronal T1 C+ FS MR in the same patient shows multiple homogeneously enhancing enlarged intraparotid lymph nodes ⇗ due to MALT lymphoma. Additional areas of extranodal extralymphatic involvement were noted in the right orbit (not shown) with extension along the right pachymeninges ⇗ and right masticator space ⇗, partly seen here.

Parotid Non-Hodgkin Lymphoma

TERMINOLOGY

Abbreviations
- Non-Hodgkin lymphoma (NHL)

Definitions
- 3 forms of parotid involvement with NHL
  - Nodal NHL
    - **Primary nodal NHL**
    - **Systemic NHL** involving parotid nodes
  - **Primary parenchymal lymphoma**
    - Most often mucosa-associated lymphoid tissue (MALT)-type NHL

IMAGING

General Features
- Best diagnostic clue
  - Nodal NHL: Multiple homogeneous, well-defined parotid masses and upper cervical adenopathy
  - Parenchymal NHL: Infiltrative parotid mass
- Location
  - Parotid gland ± ipsilateral neck nodes
- Size
  - Nodal masses: 1-3 cm
  - Primary lymphoma may involve most or all of gland
- Morphology
  - Most often multiple round or ovoid, well-circumscribed masses
    - Unilateral with primary or systemic NHL
    - Bilateral with systemic NHL
  - Primary parotid lymphoma: Diffusely infiltrating process
    - Occasionally bilateral parotid masses
    - May be solid and cystic mass

CT Findings
- CECT
  - Nodal NHL: Multiple well-defined, solid, intraparotid masses
    - Mild to moderate homogeneous enhancement
    - Necrosis, calcification, and hemorrhage rare
  - Primary parenchymal NHL: Invasive mass or well-defined, solid/cystic mass
  - Periparotid and upper cervical lymphadenopathy often present
  - Background of Sjögren changes in both parotids may be seen; if present with dominant parotid mass, include NHL in differential

MR Findings
- T1WI
  - Homogeneous, intermediate-signal nodules or infiltrative mass; seen in hypointense parotid
- T2WI FS
  - FS or STIR makes parotid lesions more conspicuous
  - Homogeneous, intermediate to low signal intensity nodules or solid/cystic mass
- DWI
  - Lower ADC characteristic but not specific
  - ADC values in Warthin tumor overlap lymphoma due to dense lymphoid tissue
- T1WI C+
  - Mild to moderate, homogeneous enhancement

Ultrasonographic Findings
- Grayscale ultrasound
  - Heterogeneous with multiple **hypoechoic**, intraparotid nodules
  - Allows FNA or core needle biopsy at time if indicated
- Color Doppler
  - **Hypervascular** compared to normal parenchyma

Nuclear Medicine Findings
- PET/CT
  - Negative PET helpful to exclude lymphoma in Sjögren's patients
  - Lugano classification adopted FDG PET/CT as standard imaging modality for staging of FDG-avid lymphomas
  - **Nodal NHL typically markedly FDG avid**
    - Multifocal nodular uptake in parotid ± neck nodes
    - Benign parotid lesions may also be FDG avid
  - **MALT lymphoma variable, often less FDG avid**
- Ga-67 scintigraphy
  - Foci of ↑ activity within normal parotid uptake
  - Improved visualization with SPECT
  - Sialadenitis after chemotherapy or radiation therapy (XRT) may have identical appearance
- Tc-99m pertechnetate
  - Cold lesion(s) within normal uptake of parotid

Imaging Recommendations
- Best imaging tool
  - CECT to identify intraparotid lesions and allow evaluation of cervical lymphadenopathy for staging
    - Beware: Isodense lesions may be "invisible"
  - Intraparotid lesions more conspicuous on T1 or with T2 FS or STIR
- Protocol advice
  - Image skull base to clavicles to aid neck staging
  - PET/CT typically performed for complete staging

DIFFERENTIAL DIAGNOSIS

Parotid Sjögren Syndrome
- Older female patient with connective tissue disease, dry eyes, dry mouth
- Bilateral enlarged parotid glands, small or large cysts ± nodules (lymphoid aggregates)
- Chronic: Atrophied, heterogeneous glands ± calcifications
- Sjögren syndrome has 10-44x ↑ risk of NHL

Warthin Tumor
- Painless parotid mass in older male smoker
- Solid, cystic, or mixed
- 20% multiple, may be bilateral

Parotid Nodal Metastatic Disease
- Multiple unilateral or bilateral masses with invasive margins, often central necrosis
- Often other nodal metastases: Levels II and V
- Periparotid skin and scalp primaries most frequent

Benign Lymphoepithelial Lesions-HIV
- Mixed cystic and solid intraparotid lesions enlarge both parotid glands

- If AIDS patient has NHL, imaging may be complex

IgG4-Related Disease

- Similar to Sjögren with enlarged parotids and nodules
- Dominant nodule in gland mimics NHL
- ↑ risk of lymphoma and pancreatic cancer

PATHOLOGY

General Features

- Etiology
  - Unknown; possibly multifactorial
    - Environmental, genetic, viral, prior radiation
  - ↑ incidence with autoimmune disorders
    - **Primary Sjögren syndrome** has **10-44x** ↑ risk of NHL
    - Rheumatoid arthritis, systemic lupus
  - ↑ incidence with **immunosuppression**

Staging, Grading, & Classification

- **Lugano classification** (based on older Ann Arbor staging) for NHL evaluation, staging, response assessment
  - Stage I: Single node region or lymphoid structure (e.g., spleen) or single extralymphatic site (IE)
  - Stage II: ≥ 2 node regions on same side of diaphragm (II) or contiguous extranodal organ/site + regional nodes ± other nodes on same side of diaphragm (IIE)
  - Stage III: Node regions on both sides of diaphragm (III), spleen (IIIS), extranodal (IIIE), both (IIISE)
  - Stage IV: Disseminated disease: ≥ 1 extranodal organ or tissue, ± nodes or isolated extralymphatic disease with distant nodes
  - Lugano classification incorporated FDG PET/CT into standard staging of FDG-avid NHL
- **WHO** is for NHL histological classification (2016)
  - Based on immunophenotype and morphology
  - B-cell (≤ 85%), T-cell, and putative NK-cell neoplasms

Gross Pathologic & Surgical Features

- Well-circumscribed, encapsulated, soft fleshy masses

Microscopic Features

- Sheets of homogeneous lymphoid cells arranged in diffuse or follicular pattern
  - Subdivided into small-cleaved and large-cell variants
- Primary parotid lymphoma
  - Most often MALT-type NHL
  - Unilateral diffuse invasion of ductal and acinar tissue

CLINICAL ISSUES

Presentation

- Most common signs/symptoms
  - Slowly enlarging, painless parotid mass ± cervical lymphadenopathy
- Other signs/symptoms
  - Systemic "B" symptoms: Fever, weight loss, night sweats
- Clinical profile
  - Middle-aged patient with painless cheek mass

Demographics

- Age
  - Mean at presentation: 59 years
- Ethnicity
  - White > > Black, Hispanic, or Asian
  - Rare T-cell lymphomas more common in young Black males
- Epidemiology
  - Primary parotid NHL uncommon; 1-5% of parotid malignancies
  - Systemic NHL involves parotid in 1-8%

Natural History & Prognosis

- Depends on histology, morphology, and stage
- **Overall 5-year survival: 72%**
  - High-grade disease: Rapidly progressive, aggressive
  - Low-grade lesions: Indolent, minimal treatment, and slow progression over years
    - Best prognosis: MALT, small-cleaved cell and follicular forms
- Generally good prognosis with primary parotid NHL
  - Usually diagnosed early: Stage I or II
  - XRT ± chemotherapy

Treatment

- Parotid tumor debulking may be done for cosmesis
- Chemotherapy and XRT remain mainstays of treatment

DIAGNOSTIC CHECKLIST

Consider

- CECT from skull base to clavicles for intraparotid lesions and to fully evaluate extent of cervical disease
- Beware: Isodense NHL may be "invisible" on CECT
- Noncontrast T1 without FS and T2 MR ↑ conspicuity

Image Interpretation Pearls

- Carefully evaluate for involvement of other salivary glands and lymph nodes
- PET/CT performed as work-up for systemic lymphoma
- If background of Sjögren syndrome changes seen with dominant parotid mass, consider diagnosis of NHL to avoid unnecessary parotidectomy (core biopsy instead)
  - **Sjögren may not be previously diagnosed**

SELECTED REFERENCES

1. Yanagisawa H et al: IgG4-related disease concomitant with diffuse large B-cell lymphoma. Intern Med. 64(6):953-7, 2024
2. Al-Khafaf AE et al: Lymphomas of the salivary glands: a systematic review. Acta Otolaryngol. 143(7):610-6, 2023
3. Jang HB et al: Diagnostic tips for parotid lymphoma. Oral Oncol. 145:106525, 2023
4. van Ginkel MS et al: FDG-PET/CT discriminates between patients with and without lymphomas in primary Sjögren's syndrome. Rheumatology (Oxford). 62(10):3323-31, 2023
5. Gökçe E et al: Advanced magnetic resonance imaging findings in salivary gland tumors. World J Radiol. 14(8):256-71, 2022
6. Kim SY et al: Magnetic resonance imaging of parotid gland tumors: a pictorial essay. BMC Med Imaging. 22(1):191, 2022
7. Yu T et al: The risk of malignancy in patients with IgG4-related disease: a systematic review and meta-analysis. Arthritis Res Ther. 24(1):14, 2022
8. Orhan Soylemez UP et al: Differentiation of benign and malignant parotid gland tumors with MRI and diffusion weighted imaging. Medeni Med J. 36(2):138-45, 2021

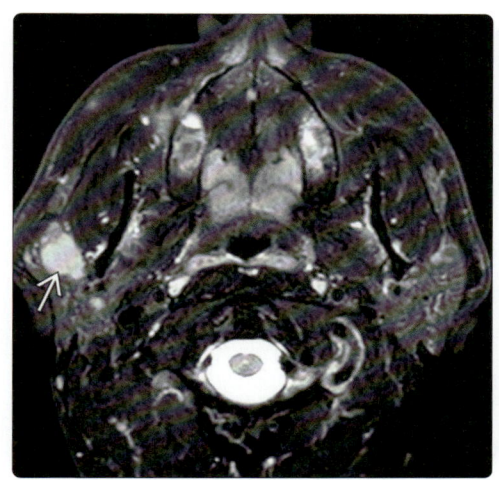

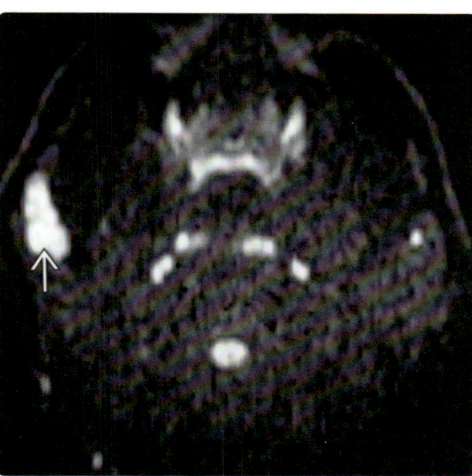

(Left) Axial T2 FS MR in a 39-year-old man initially presenting with nights sweats and weight loss shows a homogeneously hyperintense mass in the superficial right parotid gland ➡. This patient had known stage IV follicular lymphoma with abdominal involvement and additional involvement of both lacrimal glands (not shown). (Right) Axial DWI MR in the same patient shows hyperintensity in the right parotid mass ➡. Although not specific, diffusion restriction is typical of lymphoma.

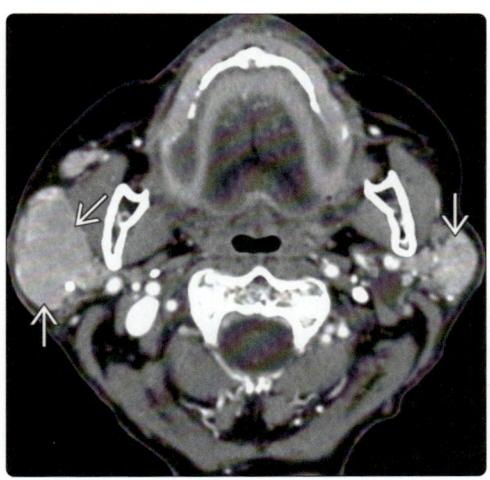

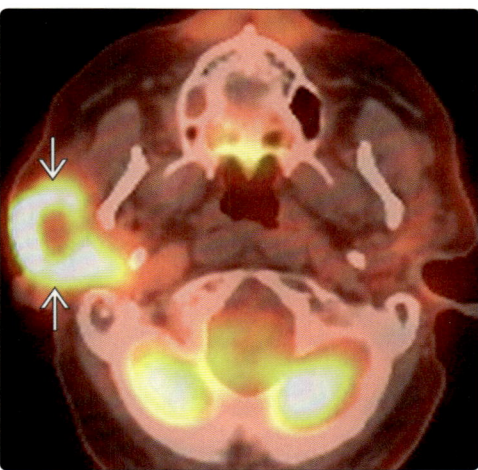

(Left) Axial CECT shows bilateral, homogeneous, enhancing parotid fullness ➡ found to be bilateral primary lymphoma in a patient with longstanding Sjögren syndrome. Primary Sjögren syndrome carries an increased risk of lymphoma. This case is typical of MALT-type parotid lymphoma. (Right) Corresponding axial fused PET/CT shows marked FDG uptake ➡ that is typically found with lymphoma. Interestingly, for such a homogeneous lesion on CT, this lesion has little central uptake, suggesting necrosis.

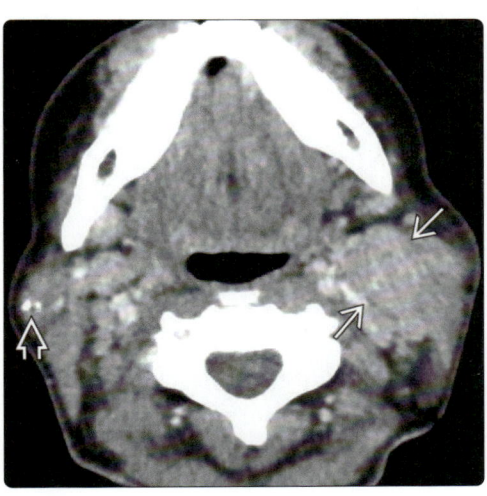

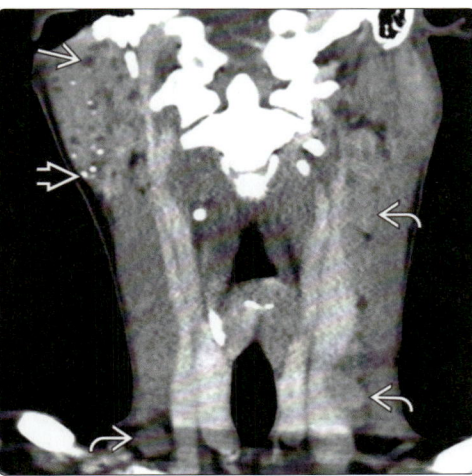

(Left) Axial CECT shows a dominant left parotid tail mass ➡ due to involvement with MALT lymphoma. Punctate calcifications in the right parotid tail are related to underlying Sjögren syndrome ➡. (Right) Coronal CECT in the same patient shows typical small cysts ➡ and calcifications ➡ in the right parotid, consistent with known longstanding Sjögren syndrome. Neck adenopathy was due to additional involvement by MALT lymphoma ➡.

Metastatic Disease of Parotid Nodes

TERMINOLOGY

- Lymphangitic or hematogenous tumor spread to intraglandular parotid lymph nodes
- Parotid and periparotid nodes = **1st-order nodal station for skin** squamous cell carcinoma (SCCa) and melanoma from scalp, auricle, and face ("forgotten nodal station")

IMAGING

- Nodes usually well defined but infiltrative if extranodal spread is present
- Nodes may be homogeneous or heterogeneous with central necrosis
- PET/CT most sensitive for identification of small nodes
- MR most sensitive for extranodal spread and perineural tumor spread on CNVII

TOP DIFFERENTIAL DIAGNOSES

- Benign lymphoepithelial lesions
- Parotid Sjögren disease

- Warthin tumor
- Parotid non-Hodgkin lymphoma

PATHOLOGY

- **Skin cancers** of face, external ear, and scalp account for 75% of primary tumors
- **Metastatic SCCa is 2nd most common parotid malignancy**
- Systemic metastases to parotid nodes rare

CLINICAL ISSUES

- Prognosis depends on presence of extracapsular spread (8% absent vs. 79% local recurrence if present)
- Metastatic SCCa involving parotid gland and neck nodes is aggressive form of SCCa with tendency for infiltrative growth pattern and multiple recurrences

DIAGNOSTIC CHECKLIST

- If asked to image parotid nodal metastases from skin cancer also scan cervical nodes to clavicle

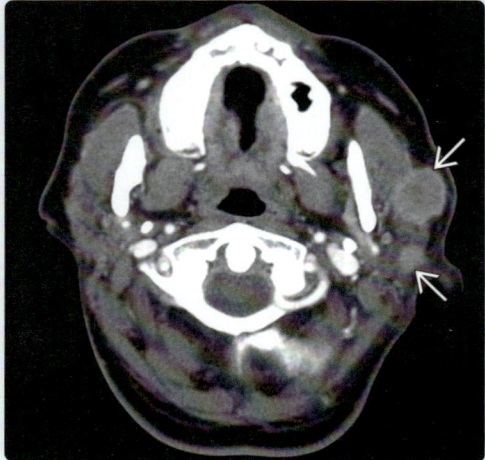
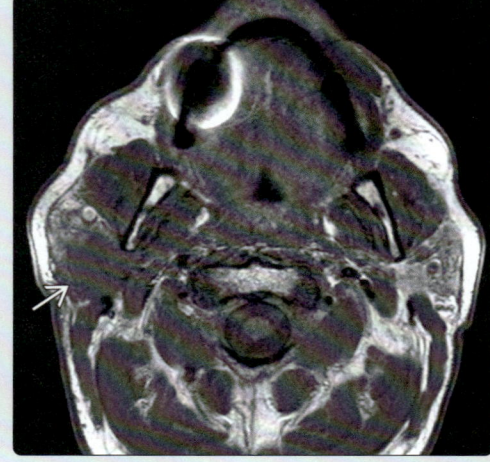

(Left) Axial CECT shows multiple enhancing masses ⇨ of varying size within the left parotid gland. This patient has squamous cell carcinoma (SCCa) of the face, and these nodes represent 1st-order lymphatic drainage. (Right) Axial T1 MR in a patient with p16(+) SCCa of the tonsil shows an invasive hypointense mass due to intraparotid nodal metastasis ⇨. The parotid glands are an uncommon site of oropharyngeal SCCa nodal metastasis.

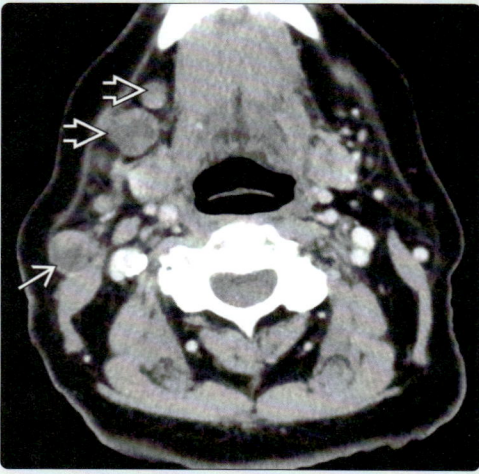
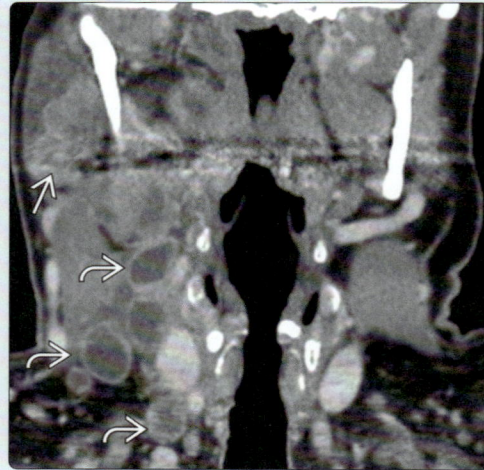

(Left) Axial CECT demonstrates a parotid tail ⇨ and level I ⇨ necrotic adenopathy due to metastatic involvement. Primary skin SCCa arose in the right nasal ala (not shown). (Right) Coronal CECT shows a right parotid nodal mass ⇨ due to melanoma metastasis. Numerous additional nodal metastases were present in the ipsilateral neck ⇨.

Metastatic Disease of Parotid Nodes

TERMINOLOGY

Definitions

- Lymphangitic or hematogenous tumor spread to intraparotid lymph nodes (systemic metastases)
- Parotid and periparotid nodes = **1st-order nodal station** for skin squamous cell carcinoma (SCCa) and melanoma from **scalp, auricle, and face** (regional metastatic disease)

IMAGING

General Features

- Best diagnostic clue
  - Multiple parotid masses in setting of known H&N malignancy
  - 1 or more focal masses in superficial or deep lobe of parotid gland
    - Often with associated preauricular ± cervical nodal masses
- Location
  - Intraparotid ± periparotid
- Size
  - 5 mm to 4 cm, usually 1-3 cm
  - Intraparotid node upper normal size limits
    - 5 to 6 mm short axis
    - 7 to 9 mm long axis
- Morphology
  - Ovoid or round
  - Usually well defined but infiltrative if extranodal spread is present

CT Findings

- CECT
  - 1 or more intraparotid masses with sharp margins (early) or invasive margins (late, extranodal spread)
    - If extranodal, check for perineural tumor on CNVII
    - See if fat in stylomastoid foramen replaced with tumor
  - Nodes may be homogeneous or heterogeneous with central necrosis
  - Preauricular ± cervical nodal metastases may also be present
  - Periauricular or scalp skin thickening (primary skin malignancy)

MR Findings

- T1WI
  - Single or multiple intermediate signal masses
- T2WI
  - Uniform high signal or heterogeneous signal (necrosis)
  - Fat saturation or STIR improves conspicuity
- T1WI C+
  - Enhancing solid or cystic (central nodal necrosis) intraparotid nodal masses
  - If extranodal spread, may appear invasive

Ultrasonographic Findings

- Diagnostic features on US not characteristic enough to avoid biopsy
- US may guide FNA of parotid masses

Nuclear Medicine Findings

- PET
  - If used in staging of primary tumor, may show intraparotid activity

Imaging Recommendations

- Best imaging tool
  - PET/CT most sensitive for identification of small nodes
  - MR most sensitive for extranodal spread and perineural tumor spread on CNVII
- Protocol advice
  - Image primary site, parotid, and remainder of neck nodal chains to clavicles
- MR is best tool to evaluate uncertain parotid masses
  - Deep tissue spread and perineural tumor are better defined by MR
  - T1 non-FS, unenhanced images often best delineate mass (inherent contrast between mass and fatty gland)
- All patients with invasive skin SCCa or melanoma on skin of face, scalp, and auricle should undergo staging PET/CT for intraparotid nodes ± nodes in cervical neck
  - MR obtained if PET/CT is positive

DIFFERENTIAL DIAGNOSIS

Benign Lymphoepithelial Lesions of HIV

- HIV or AIDS patient
- Multiple small, bilateral parotid cystic, and solid lesions

Parotid Sjögren Disease

- Autoimmune disease affecting salivary tissue
- Enlarged salivary glands
- Cystic dilatation of intraglandular ducts + lymphoid aggregates
- Punctate intraglandular calcifications characteristic

Warthin Tumor

- Older male smokers with painless cheek mass
- Often cystic on CT or MR
- 20% multifocal

Parotid Non-Hodgkin Lymphoma

- Patient usually has systemic non-Hodgkin lymphoma (NHL)
- Bilateral multiple intraparotid nodes
- Difficult to distinguish from metastases if no known primary

Recurrent Parotid Pleomorphic Adenoma

- History of pleomorphic adenoma (PA) surgical removal
- Multifocal masses; cluster of grapes appearance

PATHOLOGY

General Features

- Etiology
  - Skin of face, external ear, and scalp accounts for 75% of primary tumors
  - Lymphangitic or hematogenous spread of tumor
    - Systemic metastases to parotid nodes rare
  - Regional spread of upper aerodigestive tract primary SCCa to parotid uncommonly occurs
- Parotid has intraglandular lymph nodes (unlike submandibular and sublingual glands)

- o Normal parotid: ~ 20 intraglandular nodes
- Embryology-anatomy
  - o Parotid undergoes late encapsulation, incorporating nodes within its parenchyma
  - o Parotid is "**forgotten nodal station**"

Gross Pathologic & Surgical Features

- Nodes may remain encapsulated or undergo extracapsular spread
- SCCa node: Tan-yellow nodules within parotid
- Melanoma node: Black, brown, or white rubbery mass

Microscopic Features

- Most common skin carcinomas
  - o **SCCa (60%)**
    - − **Metastatic SCCa is 2nd most common parotid malignancy**
    - − Accounts for ~ 35% of parotid malignancies
  - o Melanoma (15%)
- SCCa: Lymph node is partially or entirely replaced by epithelial-lined structure ± central cystic change
  - o Epithelium lining of cystic spaces is composed of hypercellular and pleomorphic cell population with loss of polarity and ↑ mitotic activity
- Melanoma: Diffuse proliferation of epithelioid ± spindle cells with abundant eosinophilic cytoplasm and prominent nucleoli
  - o Immunochemistry: S100 protein and HMB-45 present
- Systemic metastases: Lung, breast primaries most common
- Parotid nodal metastasis uncommon but may occur in late-stage pharyngeal SCCa
- Parotid nodal metastasis in nasopharyngeal carcinoma is rare (0.4%) but associated with high risk of distant metastasis and regional recurrence

CLINICAL ISSUES

Presentation

- Most common signs/symptoms
  - o External ear, scalp, upper face skin cancer with enlarging parotid mass
  - o CNVII dysfunction
  - o Facial pain
  - o Nonhealing sore (skin SCCa or melanoma) on skin of face, scalp, or auricle-external auditory canal associated with cheek mass

Demographics

- Age
  - o 7th decade most frequent
- Epidemiology
  - o Occurs in 1-3% of patients with H&N SCCa
  - o Metastases = 4% of all parotid neoplasms
  - o Intraparotid nodes more common in geographic regions of ↑ sun exposure

Natural History & Prognosis

- Prognosis depends heavily on presence of **extracapsular spread (8% vs. 79% local recurrence)**
- 5-year parotid control = 78% but overall survival = 54%

- Metastatic SCCa involving parotid gland and neck nodes is aggressive form of SCCa with tendency for infiltrative growth pattern and multiple recurrences
- Some primary subsites (e.g., external ear) have worse prognosis
- Melanoma historically poor prognosis but targeted therapy and immunotherapies are improving survival rates

Treatment

- Parotidectomy, neck dissection + radiation therapy
  - o Elective neck dissection in N0 neck improves disease-specific survival
- SCCa: Parotidectomy and neck dissection dictated by imaging and physical exam
  - o Postoperative radiotherapy
- Melanoma: Parotidectomy and neck dissection dictated by lymphatic mapping and sentinel node identification
  - o Adjuvant radiotherapy ± chemotherapy depends on context
  - o Immunotherapy &/or targeted therapy in melanoma

DIAGNOSTIC CHECKLIST

Consider

- When imaging parotid nodal metastases from skin cancer, also scan cervical nodes to clavicle
- If SCCa or melanoma found in parotid nodes, check external ear and scalp for primary
  - o Patients may not recall prior history of skin cancer
  - o Skin cancer may be hidden above hairline at time of presentation of parotid node

Image Interpretation Pearls

- Multifocal unilateral disease is most suggestive of 1st-order nodal disease from adjacent skin sites
  - o Solitary intraparotid nodal metastasis mimics primary parotid neoplasm
- Presence of bilateral nodes suggests systemic disease or hematogenous metastatic spread

Reporting Tips

- Differential diagnosis for multifocal unilateral parotid masses with cervical adenopathy: Regional metastases, local NHL
- Differential diagnosis for multifocal unilateral parotid masses without cervical adenopathy: Warthin tumor, regional metastases, local NHL, recurrent PA
- Differential diagnosis for multifocal bilateral parotid masses: Systemic metastases, systemic NHL, Warthin tumors, benign lymphoepithelial lesions of HIV, parotid Sjögren disease

SELECTED REFERENCES

1. Furlan KC et al: Utility of UV signature mutations in the diagnostic assessment of metastatic head and neck carcinomas of unknown primary. Head Neck Pathol. 18(1):11, 2024
2. Ai QYH et al: Normal size of benign upper neck nodes on MRI: parotid, submandibular, occipital, facial, retroauricular and level IIb nodal groups. Cancer Imaging. 22(1):66, 2022
3. Kaplanoglu H et al: Normative measurements and apparent diffusion coefficient values of parotid lymph nodes on magnetic resonance imaging. J Coll Physicians Surg Pak. 32(4):435-9, 2022
4. Mayer M et al: Metastases of cutaneous squamous cell carcinoma seem to be the most frequent malignancies in the parotid gland: a hospital-based study from a salivary gland center. Head Neck Pathol. 15(3):843-51, 2021

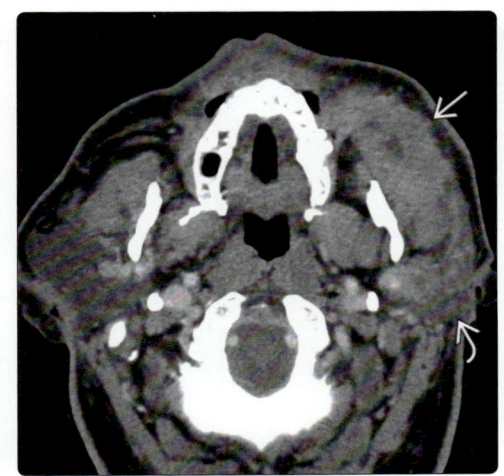

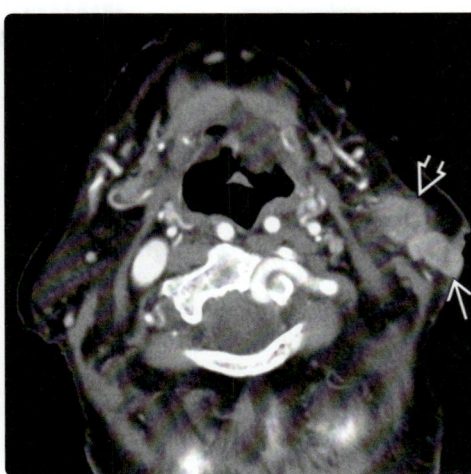

(Left) *Axial CECT shows an infiltrative, heterogeneous enhancing mass involving the left accessory parotid gland* ➡ *due to SCCa, consistent with metastatic disease from primary skin cancer. The main left parotid gland appears atrophic* ➡ *from distal ductal obstruction.* (Right) *Axial CECT demonstrates aggressive primary skin SCCa* ➡ *spreading into deep subcutaneous soft tissues. Note that the 1st-order parotid tail lymph node* ➡ *is affected.*

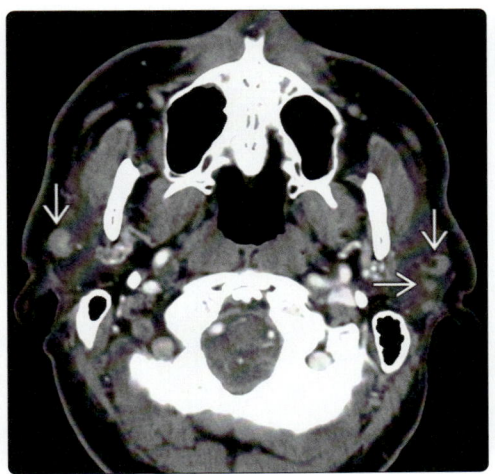

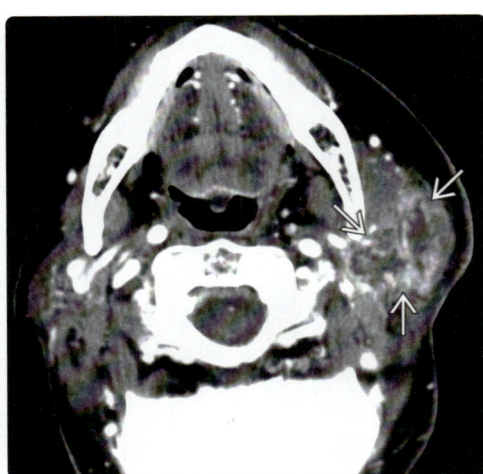

(Left) *Axial CECT reveals bilateral enhancing parotid masses* ➡. *These represent systemic metastatic disease from chronic lymphocytic leukemia. They were accompanied by extensive cervical adenopathy (not shown).* (Right) *Axial CECT shows an ill-defined, heterogeneously enhancing mass* ➡ *in the left parotid gland. The central necrosis and ill-defined margins are indicative of extracapsular spread. These are regional metastases from angiosarcoma of the scalp.*

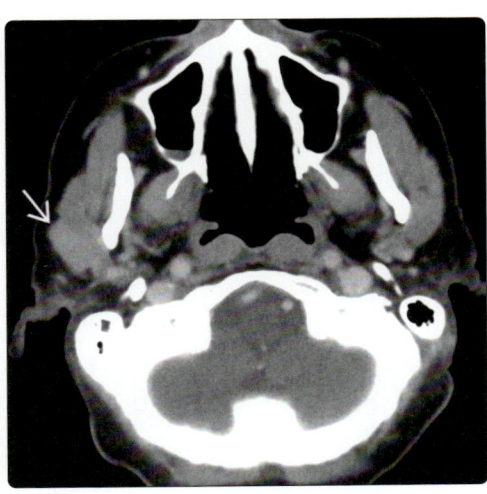

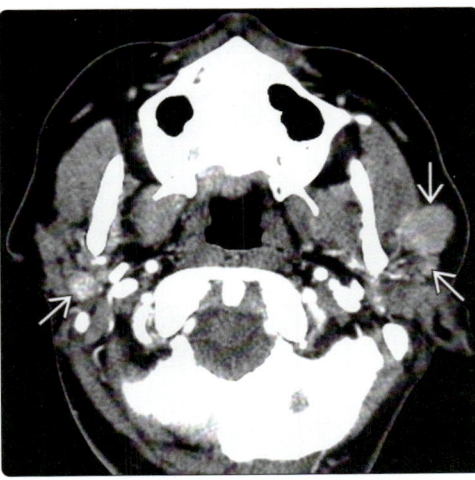

(Left) *Axial CECT shows a difficult to see, homogeneously enhancing nodal metastasis in the superficial right parotid gland* ➡. *Density is close to adjacent masseter muscle, making the mass less apparent. This palpable mass was due to metastatic thymoma.* (Right) *Axial CECT demonstrates numerous bilateral, well-defined, uniformly enhancing parotid masses* ➡ *in a patient with known breast cancer. These masses represent hematogeneous metastases.*

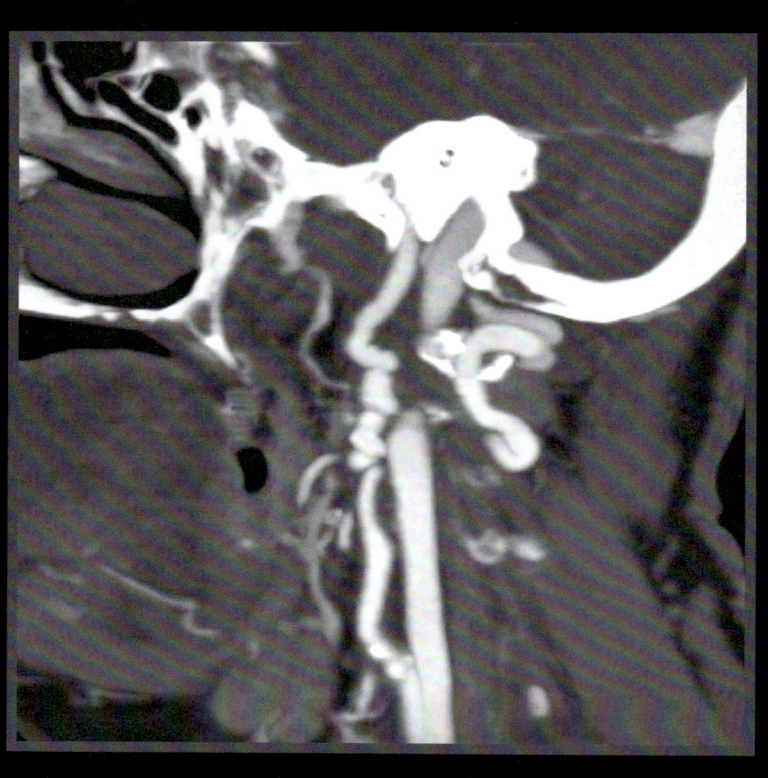
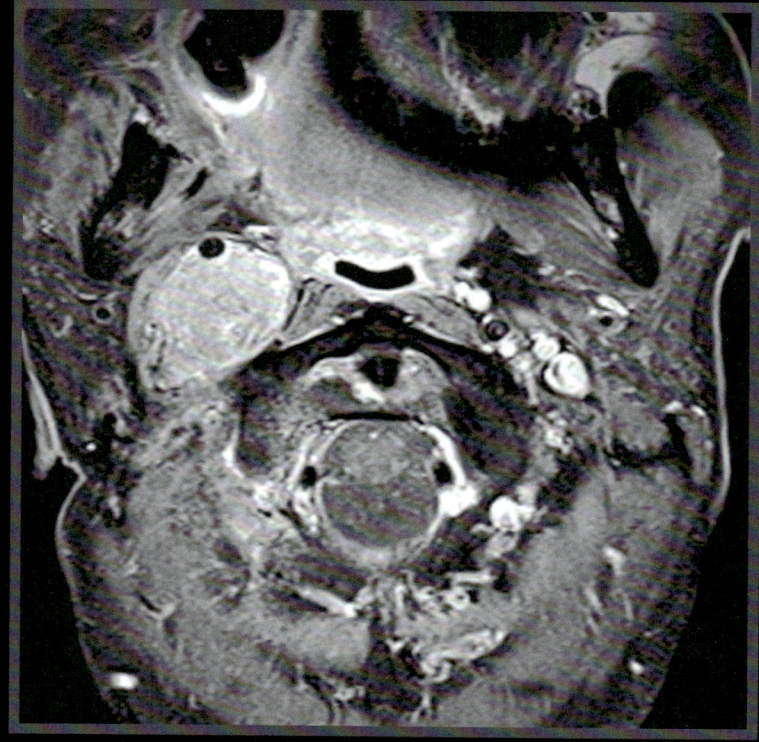

SECTION 6
Carotid Space

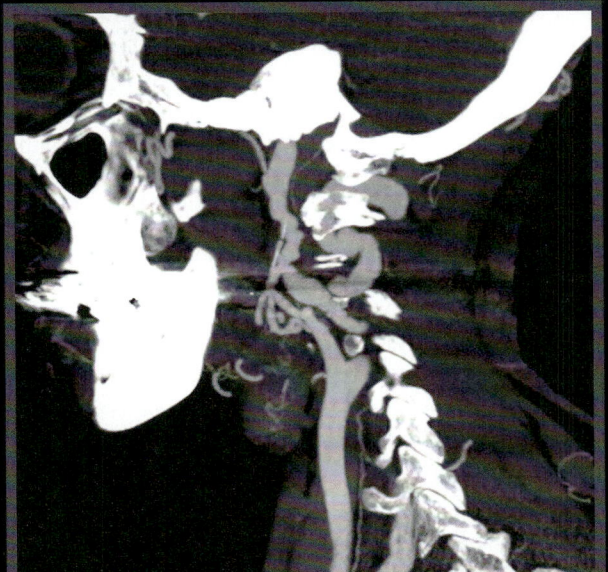
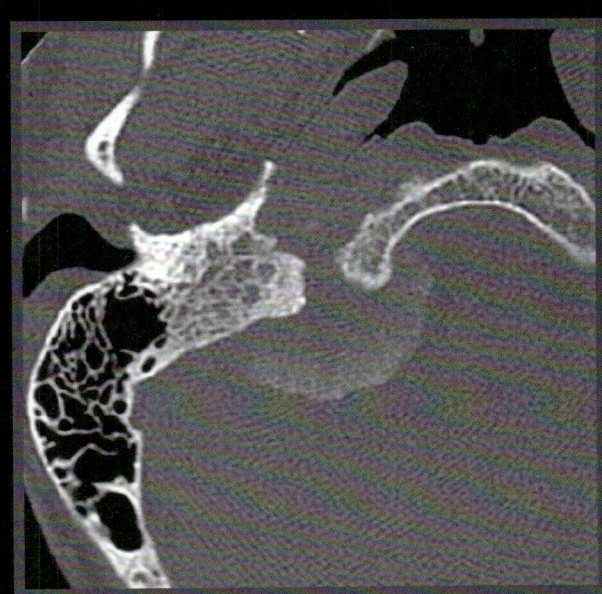

Summary Thoughts: Carotid Space

The carotid spaces (CSs) are paired tubular spaces that traverse the suprahyoid neck (SHN) and infrahyoid neck (IHN) just lateral to the retropharyngeal space (RPS). The CS is enveloped by the **carotid sheath**, which is made up of all **3 layers of deep cervical fascia**. The SHN CS contains the internal carotid artery (ICA), internal jugular vein (IJV), and cranial nerves (CNs) IX-XII. The IHN CS only has the common carotid artery (CCA), IJV, and vagus nerve (CNX) trunk within it.

A **SHN CS mass** displaces the anterior parapharyngeal space (PPS) fat anteriorly as it enlarges. Often, the ICA is also displaced anteriorly by an enlarging SHN CS mass. An **IHN CS mass** engulfs the CCA or splays the carotid bifurcation (carotid body paraganglioma).

Important primary **CS tumors** include paraganglioma, schwannoma, neurofibroma, and sympathetic chain schwannoma. The internal jugular nodal chain is in close proximity to the superficial margin of the CS. As a result, when squamous cell carcinoma (SCCa) metastatic nodes undergo extracapsular spread, they may involve the adjacent carotid artery and vagus nerve.

Imaging Techniques and Indications

CECT (+ CTA ± CTV) or MR (+ MRA ± MRV) easily identify most CS lesions. Certainly, the CS mass lesions are readily seen using either technique. When using CT, CTA gives a multiplanar, arterial-phase view of the intrinsic carotid diseases. Delayed CECT that allows contrast to penetrate into the soft tissues of the neck is better for delineation of CS mass lesions.

When using MR, remember to acquire T1 without contrast to use inherent fat signal for anatomic localization and to look for the high-velocity flow void signature of paraganglioma. MRA and MRV may be helpful in defining a vascular CS lesion (ICA dissection, pseudoaneurysm, or IJV thrombosis).

Imaging Anatomy

The important **anatomic relationships** of the CS can be examined at the SHN and IHN levels. At the SHN level, the CS has the RPS medial, the perivertebral space (PVS) posterior, the deep lobe of the parotid space (PS) lateral, and the PPS anterior. At the IHN level, the CS is bounded by the visceral space (VS) and RPS medially, PVS posteriorly, anterior cervical space anteriorly, and posterior cervical space laterally.

The CS extends from the skull base to the aortic arch. At its superior skull base margin, the **ICA** enters the **carotid canal** just as the **IJV** emerges from the floor of the **jugular foramen** (JF). The sympathetic plexus leaves its position on the medial surface of the nasopharyngeal CS to ascend in the ICA adventitia as the carotid plexus along the ICA course through the temporal bone. At the CS inferior margin, the **CCAs** enter the **aortic arch**, and the **IJVs** merge with the **brachiocephalic veins**. The CS has nasopharyngeal, oropharyngeal, cervical, and mediastinal segments.

The **carotid sheath** surrounds the CS throughout its passage through the soft tissues of the neck. A unique aspect of the carotid sheath is that it is made up of **all 3 layers of deep cervical fascia** (superficial, middle, and deep). In the SHN, the carotid sheath is a considerably less substantial fascia than in the IHN. In the IHN, the sheath is a well-defined, tenacious fascia.

Important **CS internal structures** are best viewed from the perspective of what can be found in the SHN and IHN CSs. The **SHN CS** contains the ICA and IJV along with the glossopharyngeal (CNIX), vagus (CNX), spinal accessory (CNXI), and hypoglossal (CNXII) nerves. Foci of normal neural crest derivative **glomus bodies** are found in the nodose ganglion of the vagus nerve ~ 2 cm below the floor of the JF of the skull base. They are also located in the JF above and the carotid bifurcation below. Along the medial border of the SHN CS is the sympathetic plexus.

All CNs but the vagus nerve have exited the SHN CS by the time it reaches the hyoid bone. **Normal internal structures** of the IHN CS include the vagus nerve, the CCA, and IJV. The **internal jugular nodal chain** is loosely wound into the external fascial layers along the surface of the CS. As such, this nodal chain is considered closely associated, but **not** within, the CS.

Approaches to Imaging Issues of Carotid Space

The answer to the question: "What **imaging findings** define a **CS mass**?" varies depending on the level of the lesion. If the lesion is in the **nasopharyngeal CS**, it displaces the PPS fat anteriorly and lifts the styloid process anterolaterally. At the level of the **oropharyngeal CS**, the PPS is again pushed anteriorly, but an important additional clue is the displacement of the posterior belly of the digastric muscle anterolaterally. At either the nasopharyngeal or oropharyngeal level, lesions in the posterior CS (vagal schwannoma, neurofibroma, paraganglioma) will bow the ICA anteriorly as they enlarge. A mass of the **infrahyoid CS** engulfs the CCA or splays the bifurcation (carotid body paraganglioma).

When a CS lesion is identified on imaging, matching its radiologic findings to common CS lesions is often very rewarding, as many of the lesions have distinctive imaging findings. If the lesion is intrinsic to the carotid artery, ICA tortuosity, dissection, pseudoaneurysm, or thrombosis should all be considered. Intrinsic IJV lesions should suggest IJV asymmetry, thrombophlebitis, and thrombosis. Tumors within the space include paraganglioma (MR high-velocity flow voids), schwannoma (tubular lesions with intramural cysts), and neurofibroma (target appearance on MR; low density on CECT).

Nasopharyngeal CS tumors may "**dumbbell**" inferiorly from the **JF** above. A careful inspection of the JF for imaging signs of simultaneous involvement is in order. If the JF is abnormal, the main differential diagnosis of the CS mass is jugular paraganglioma, JF schwannoma (CNIX-XI), or JF meningioma. **Bone CT** imaging clues that may be helpful include permeative-destructive changes along the margin of the JF (jugular paraganglioma); smooth, expansile JF with sclerotic margins (schwannoma); and permeative-sclerotic or hyperostotic changes (meningioma).

MR clues to consider for a **JF mass** extending into nasopharyngeal CS are plentiful. If the tumor has low-signal, high-velocity flow voids with vector of spread through the floor of the middle ear cavity, jugular paraganglioma is the 1st diagnostic consideration. A fusiform mass with intramural cystic change and a vector of spread that projects upward and medial toward the lateral medulla suggests schwannoma. JF meningioma lacks high-velocity signal voids and spreads centrifugally away from the JF.

Differential Diagnosis of Carotid Space Lesion

Pseudolesions	CCA or ICA aneurysm
Ectatic CCA or ICA	ICA pseudoaneurysm
Carotid bulb ectasia	Fibromuscular dysplasia
Asymmetric IJV	Takayasu arteritis
Congenital	**Benign tumor**
2nd branchial cleft cyst variant	Carotid body paraganglioma
Inflammation or infection	Vagal paraganglioma
CS cellulitis	Jugular paraganglioma, inferior extension
CS abscess	CNIX-XII schwannoma
Acute idiopathic carotidynia	Sympathetic chain schwannoma
Vascular	CNIX-XII neurofibroma
IJV thrombophlebitis	Jugular foramen meningioma, inferior extension
IJV thrombosis	**Malignant tumor**
CCA or ICA atherosclerosis	SCCa primary tumor invasion, perifascial spread
CCA or ICA thrombosis	SCCa extranodal tumor invasion
ICA dissection	Extranodal NHL, internal jugular nodal chain

Above is an exhaustive list of all lesions that can be found in the carotid space. The table is organized by general pathology category. CCA = common carotid artery; ICA = internal carotid artery; IJV = internal jugular vein; CS = carotid space; SCCa = squamous cell carcinoma; NHL = non-Hodgkin lymphoma.

Vascular lesions in the CS arise within the IJV or carotid artery. IJV thrombophlebitis mimics a neck abscess clinically and is easily diagnosed because of the tubular luminal clot and surrounding soft tissue inflammatory changes. The more chronic IJV thrombosis clinically mimics a neck tumor, lacking the soft tissue inflammatory changes on imaging. Important carotid artery lesions include atherosclerosis, dissection with or without pseudoaneurysm, and fibromuscular dysplasia (FMD). This lesion group can be readily diagnosed with CTA with the exception of FMD, which may require angiography to diagnose.

Perhaps the most common image interpretation pitfall associated with CS lesions is the tendency to confuse an SHN CS mass with a lateral retropharyngeal nodal mass. **Lateral RPS mass** lesions displace the ICA-IJV in the CS posterolaterally, whereas SHN CS mass lesions push the ICA anteriorly or anteromedially. As there are no nodes within the CS, if the imaging appearance suggests nodal disease, check to see if the ICA is pushed laterally. If so, you are looking at a lateral RPS lesion.

Clinical Implications

Lesions of the CS often present first with **hoarseness** due to abnormality of the vagus nerve or recurrent laryngeal nerve. Endoscopy or imaging determines which vocal cord is paralyzed. **Left** vocal cord paralysis requires imaging from the posterior fossa to the aortopulmonic window, while **right** vocal cord paralysis only requires the scan to reach the right subclavian artery.

Proximal vagal neuropathy often includes other CN injury (CNIX, XI, or XII). Because the pharyngeal plexus branch of the vagus nerve is injured, the ipsilateral soft palate and superior constrictor muscles fasciculate in the acute phase and become patulous in the chronic phase of injury. In the chronic phase of proximal vagal neuropathy, imaging will show fatty infiltration of the ipsilateral soft palate and a patulous lateral pharynx due to constrictor muscle atrophy. Lesions causing proximal vagal neuropathy can be found involving the brainstem medulla, basal cistern, JF, or suprahyoid CS.

Distal vagal neuropathy is defined as isolated vagal neuropathy without the nasopharyngeal and oropharyngeal findings previously described. In this setting, lesions are sought in the infrahyoid CS. Left-sided lesions may include diseases of the mediastinum, such as lung cancer. Right-sided lesions causing distal vagal neuropathy are usually clinically palpable at the time of imaging.

Postganglionic **Horner syndrome** presents with ptosis (droop of upper eyelid), miosis (decrease in pupil size), and anhidrosis (absence of sweat). The lesion causing Horner syndrome is sought along the segment of oculosympathetic pathway between the superior cervical ganglion and the eye. Much of this pathway is found between the supraclavicular and nasopharyngeal CS. Remember the sympathetic chain passes with the ICA up the skull base carotid canal. The radiologist must interrogate the cervical, oropharyngeal, and nasopharyngeal CSs, the carotid canal in the skull base, cavernous sinus, and orbit. In particular, ICA dissection must be excluded.

Selected References

1. Nimodia D et al: Carotid body tumor imaging: MRI, ultrasound, and elastography with surgical management. Radiol Case Rep. 19(12):6085-92, 2024

2. Roh JL: Postauricular approach for enucleation of cervical vagal schwannomas. Head Neck. 47(5):1433-9, 2024

3. Bond JD et al: The carotid sheath: anatomy and clinical considerations. World Neurosurg X. 18:100158, 2023

4. Sheikh Z et al: The assessment and management of deep neck space infections in adults: a systematic review and qualitative evidence synthesis. Clin Otolaryngol. 48(4):540-62, 2023

5. Zhang CG et al: [Internal carotid artery pseudoaneurysm caused by parapharyngeal abscess: a case report.] Beijing Da Xue Xue Bao Yi Xue Ban. 55(6):1135-8, 2023

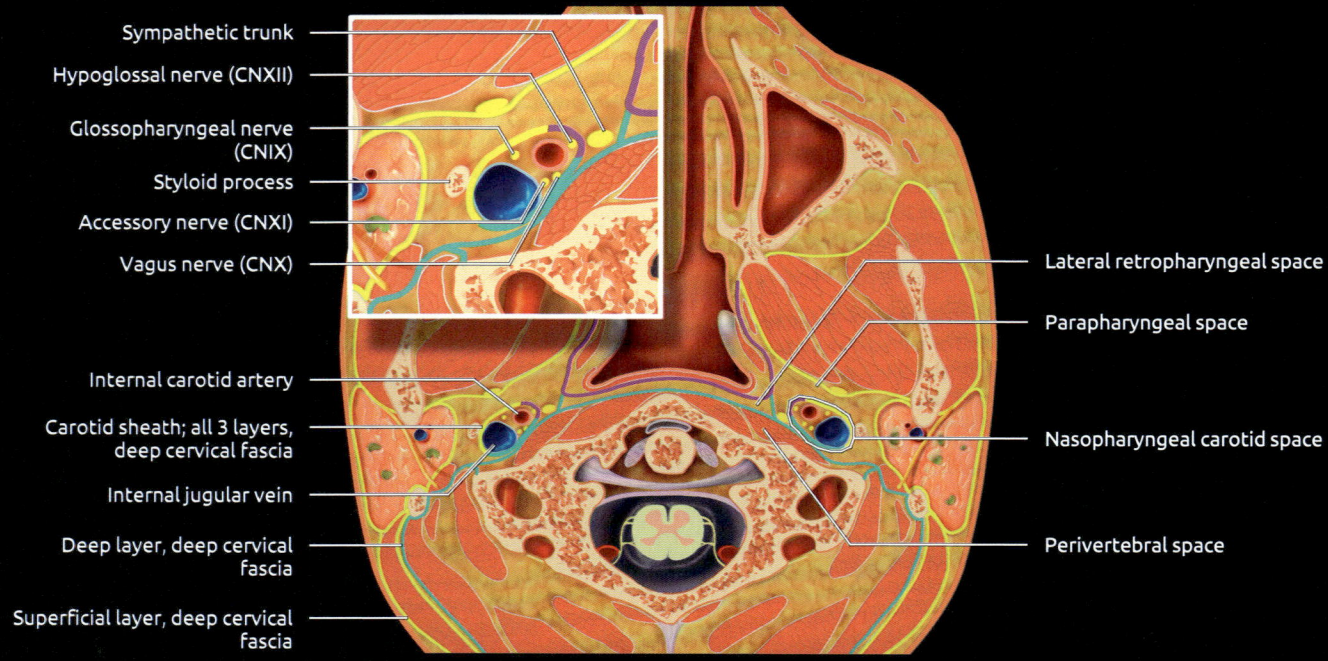

Sympathetic trunk
Hypoglossal nerve (CNXII)
Glossopharyngeal nerve (CNIX)
Styloid process
Accessory nerve (CNXI)
Vagus nerve (CNX)

Internal carotid artery
Carotid sheath; all 3 layers, deep cervical fascia
Internal jugular vein
Deep layer, deep cervical fascia
Superficial layer, deep cervical fascia

Lateral retropharyngeal space
Parapharyngeal space
Nasopharyngeal carotid space
Perivertebral space

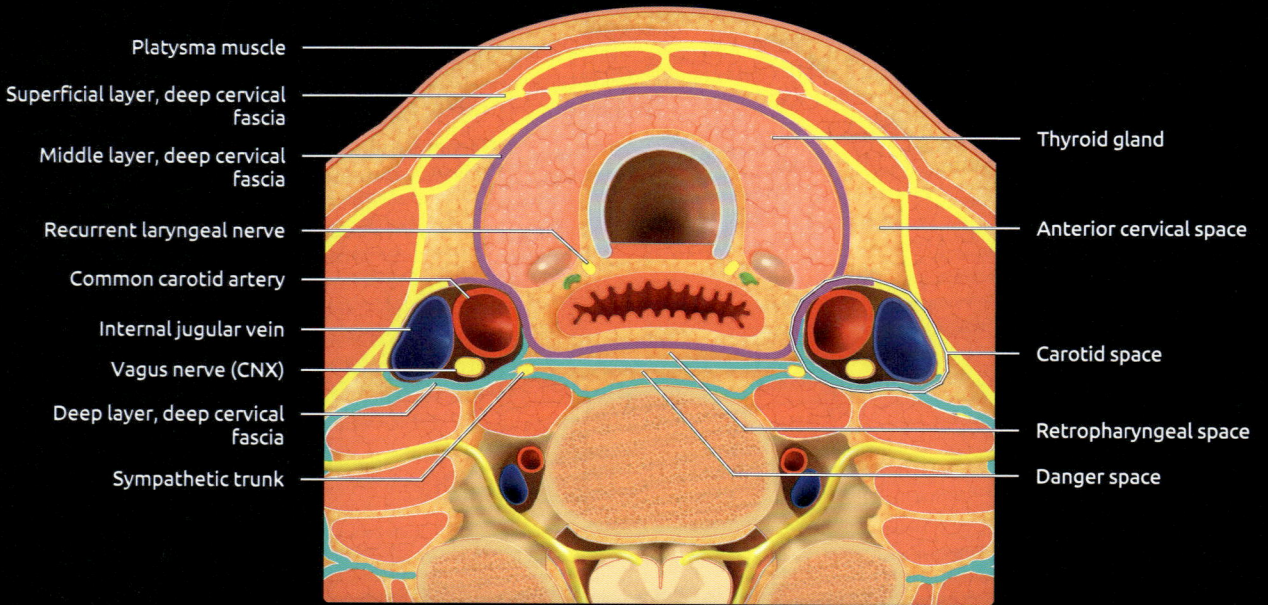

Platysma muscle
Superficial layer, deep cervical fascia
Middle layer, deep cervical fascia
Recurrent laryngeal nerve
Common carotid artery
Internal jugular vein
Vagus nerve (CNX)
Deep layer, deep cervical fascia
Sympathetic trunk

Thyroid gland
Anterior cervical space
Carotid space
Retropharyngeal space
Danger space

(**Top**) *Axial graphic of the suprahyoid neck (SHN) at the level of C1 vertebral body with insert shows a magnified carotid space (CS). The suprahyoid CS contains CNIX-XII, the internal carotid artery (ICA), and the internal jugular vein (IJV). The carotid sheath is made up of components of all 3 layers of deep cervical fascia (tricolor line around CS). In the SHN, the carotid sheath is less substantial than in the infrahyoid neck (IHN). The sympathetic trunk runs just medial to the CS. (**Bottom**) Axial graphic shows the CS in the IHN. Note that the carotid sheath contains all 3 layers of the deep cervical fascia (tricolor line). In the IHN, the carotid sheath is tenacious throughout its length. The infrahyoid CS contains the common carotid artery (CCA), IJV, and only the vagus cranial nerve.*

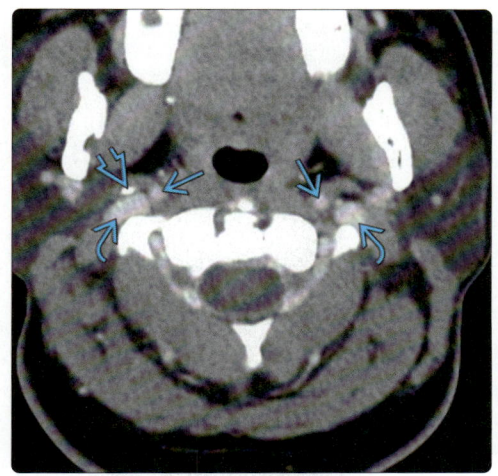

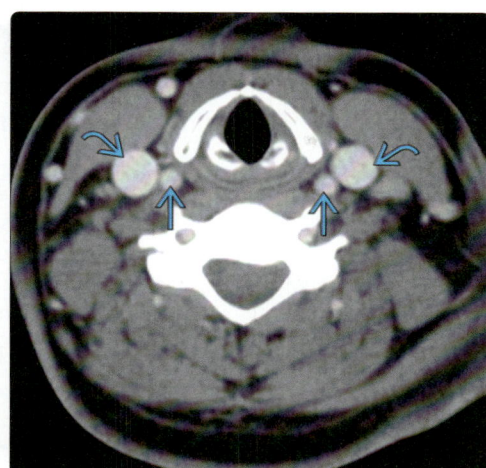

(Left) *Axial CECT at the level of oropharynx shows bilateral CSs containing ICA ➡, IJV ➡, and CNIX-XII (not shown). SHN CS is bound medially by retropharyngeal space (RPS), posteriorly by PVS, laterally by parotid space, and anteriorly by PPS. Styloid process ➡ separates CS from PPS.* (Right) *Axial CECT at the level of larynx shows bilateral IHN CS containing CCA ➡, IJV ➡, and CNX (not shown). CS is related to visceral space and RPS medially, PVS posteriorly, anterior cervical space anteriorly, and posterior cervical space laterally.*

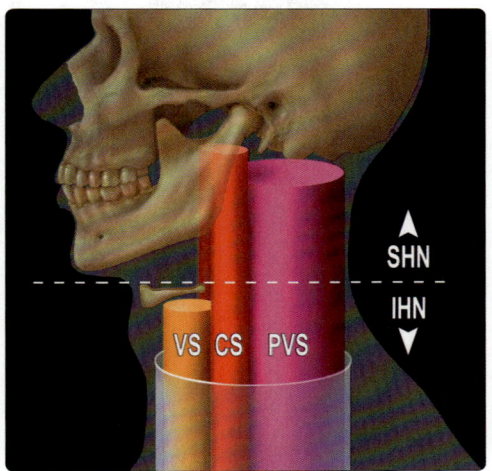

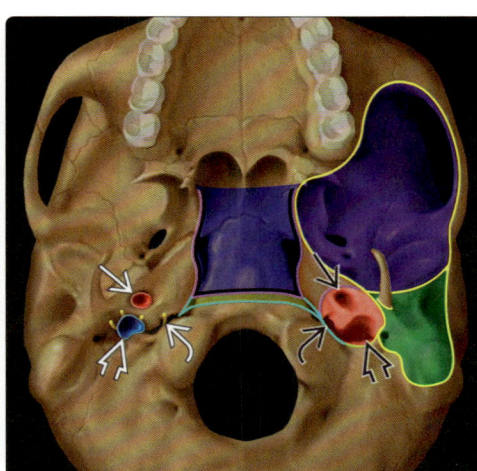

(Left) *Lateral graphic of the cervical neck shows the tubular CS extending from the skull base [carotid canal and jugular foramen (JF)] to the aortic arch.* (Right) *Axial graphic of the skull base viewed from below shows the CS abutting the skull base. The ICA ➡ enters the carotid canal ➡, while the IJV ➡ emerges from the JF ➡. CNIX-XI is exiting the JF. CNXII ➡ is more medial as it enters the CS from the hypoglossal canal ➡.*

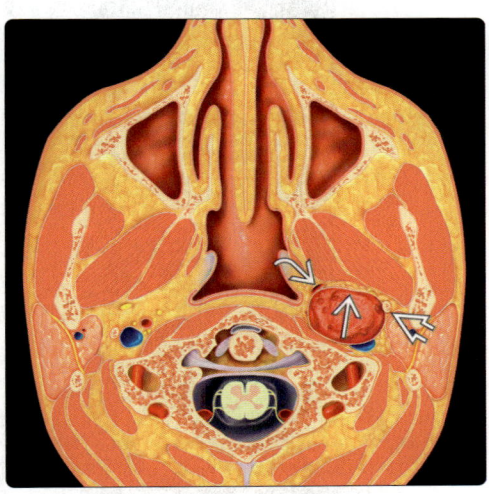

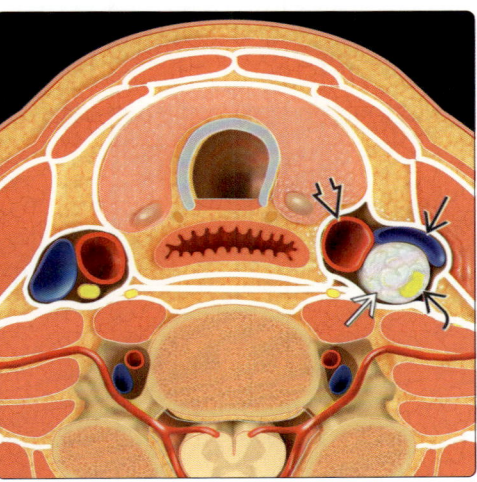

(Left) *Axial graphic reveals a generic nasopharyngeal CS mass. As the CS mass enlarges, it pushes the parapharyngeal space fat anteriorly ➡ as well as lifts the styloid process anterolaterally ➡. Often, the ICA is also lifted anteriorly ➡ by a CS mass.* (Right) *Axial graphic of an infrahyoid CS mass ➡ shows that the CCA ➡ and the IJV ➡ are displaced anteriorly. Note the vagus nerve ➡ is visible in the posterolateral aspect of this vagal schwannoma.*

KEY FACTS

TERMINOLOGY

- Synonyms: Retropharyngeal carotid, carotid transposition, "kissing" carotids, medialized carotid, wandering carotid

IMAGING

- May be unilateral or bilateral
  - **Bilateral = "kissing" carotids**
- **CTA or MRA** easily establishes diagnosis
- CTA/CECT shows enhancing carotid artery (CA) medialized in retropharyngeal space (RPS)
  - Normal round (axial) or tubular (coronal) vessel
  - Contiguous axial images reveal contiguous nature
  - Coronal reconstructions best depict RPS CA
- MR shows normal round CA with flow void

TOP DIFFERENTIAL DIAGNOSES

- CA pseudoaneurysm
- CA dissection
- Carotid body paraganglioma

PATHOLOGY

- CA extends medially from carotid space, bows ± violates **lateral slip of deep cervical fascia** to enter RPS
- Position of carotid can vary scan to scan

CLINICAL ISSUES

- Usually incidental finding on neck CT or MR
- Can cause pulsatile retropharyngeal or retrotonsillar mass
  - Globus sensation
  - May potentiate obstructive sleep apnea
- Common pseudolesion of older population
- Correct imaging diagnosis prevents unnecessary treatment

DIAGNOSTIC CHECKLIST

- Recognize normal **tubular** CA coursing medially in RPS
- Tortuous CA in differential diagnosis of prevertebral soft tissue widening on lateral plain film
- Radiologist must recognize as **nonsurgical** lesion
- **Must report in patients undergoing pharyngeal surgery**

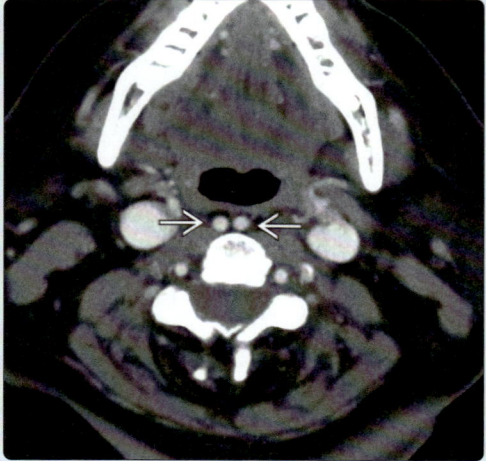
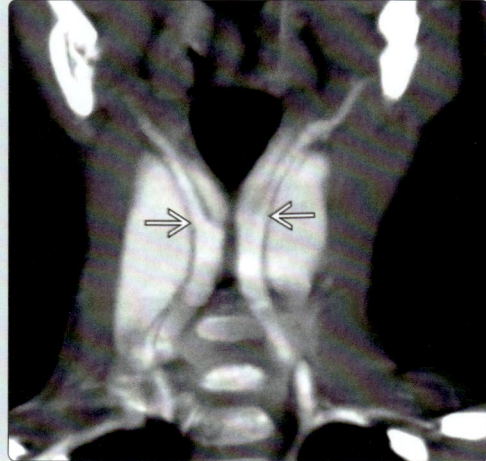

(Left) Axial CECT shows medialization of both cervical internal carotid arteries ➡ displaced medially into the retropharyngeal space. (Right) Coronal arterial-phase CECT MPR shows medialization of the bilateral carotid bifurcations ➡ in a young child imaged for a seat belt sign after trauma. This variant would be important to recognize and document in order to alert the surgeon and avoid iatrogenic injury in the case of planned tonsillectomy.

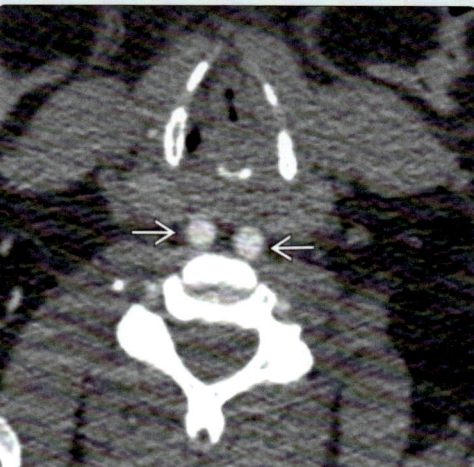
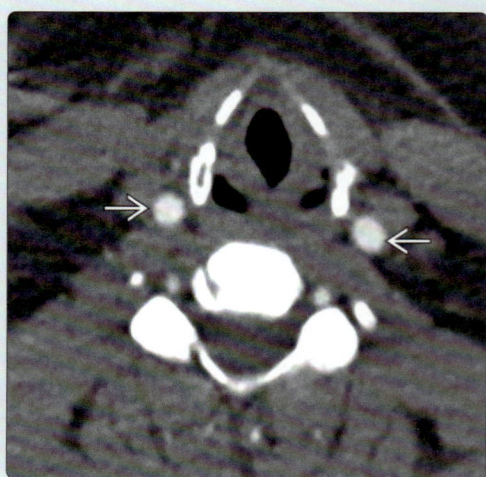

(Left) Axial arterial-phase CECT performed in a 33-year-old woman with neck pain after a car accident shows medialization of both common carotid arteries ("kissing" carotids) ➡. (Right) Axial arterial-phase CECT performed for vertebral artery dissection surveillance 4 days later in the same patient now demonstrates a normal position of the common carotid arteries ➡. This case illustrates the dynamic nature of this variant ("wandering" carotid), which can be transient.

TERMINOLOGY

Synonyms

- Retropharyngeal carotid, carotid transposition, medialized carotid, "kissing" carotids, wandering carotid

Definitions

- One or both carotid arteries (CAs) course medially into retropharyngeal space (RPS)

IMAGING

General Features

- Best diagnostic clue
  - **Normal enhancing CA coursing medially in RPS** on CTA
- Location
  - CA in RPS
- Morphology
  - Tortuous unilateral or bilateral distal common carotid or proximal internal carotid arteries

CT Findings

- CECT
  - Round (axial) or tubular (coronal) enhancing RPS structure
    - Contiguous axial images reveal structure as CA
  - Unilateral or bilateral
    - **Bilateral = "kissing" carotids**
- CTA
  - **Coronal reconstructions** best define tortuous RPS CA
  - Often involves distal common CA + proximal internal CA

MR Findings

- T1WI
  - Round, low-signal retropharyngeal CA
- T2WI
  - Round, low-signal CA due to normal high-velocity flow void
- MRA
  - Coronal MPR best delineates retropharyngeal CA

Imaging Recommendations

- Best imaging tool
  - CTA or MRA easily establishes diagnosis
  - Angiography not necessary to confirm diagnosis
- Protocol advice
  - CTA differentiates ectatic CA from other causes of pulsatile tonsillar or RPS mass

DIFFERENTIAL DIAGNOSIS

Carotid Artery Pseudoaneurysm

- Clinical: History of trauma or CA dissection; pulsatile mass
- Imaging: Complex-appearing CA outpouching

Carotid Artery Dissection

- Clinical: Sympathetic ± vagal neuropathy ± stroke
- Imaging: MR shows abnormal signal in CA wall
- Angiography shows narrowed or occluded vessel

Carotid Body Paraganglioma

- Clinical: Pulsatile angle of mandible mass
- Imaging: Enhancing mass splaying carotid bifurcation

PATHOLOGY

General Features

- Etiology
  - Atherosclerosis causes fusiform enlargement & tortuosity of CA
    - Association with chronic hypertension
    - CA migrates with progressive ectasia
    - Dynamic mobility may occur: Position of carotid can vary from scan to scan
  - May be due to failure of complete descent of dorsal aortic root into chest with persistent embryologic angulation of carotids in children
- Associated abnormalities
  - Can be component of **velocardiofacial syndrome**
- Relevant anatomy
  - As CA pushes medially from normal position within carotid space, bows or violates **lateral slip of deep cervical fascia** (cloison sagittale) to reach RPS

CLINICAL ISSUES

Presentation

- Most common signs/symptoms
  - Usually incidental finding on neck CT or MR
  - May cause pulsatile retropharyngeal or retrotonsillar mass
- Other signs/symptoms
  - May potentiate obstructive sleep apnea
  - Globus sensation, sore throat

Natural History & Prognosis

- CA may protrude further into RPS with advancing age
- Important implications for anesthesiologist when performing transoral block of glossopharyngeal nerve in pharynx or in difficult tracheal intubation
- Risk for CA injury during pharyngeal surgeries: Transoral robotic surgery (TORS), tonsillectomy, adenoidectomy, & velopharyngeal narrowing

DIAGNOSTIC CHECKLIST

Consider

- Tortuous CA in differential diagnosis of prevertebral soft tissue widening on lateral plain film
- Radiologist must recognize **nonsurgical nature** of lesion
  - Big difference between clinical suspicion (suspect vascular tumor) & radiologic impression (tortuous CA)

Image Interpretation Pearls

- Recognize normal tubular, tortuous/medialized CA

Reporting Tips

- Important to report in patients **undergoing pharyngeal surgery** or intubation to avoid iatrogenic carotid injury

SELECTED REFERENCES

1. Steinl GK et al: Variations in the course of the carotid arteries in patients with retropharyngeal parathyroid adenomas. AJNR Am J Neuroradiol. 42(4):749-52, 2021
2. Garrido MB et al: Retropharyngeal internal carotid artery: a review of three cases. Oral Maxillofac Surg. 24(2):255-61, 2020
3. Gerasymchuck M et al: Infrahyoid wandering carotid arteries. Radiol Case Rep. 15(4):400-4, 2020

KEY FACTS

TERMINOLOGY

- Internal carotid artery dissection (ICAD)
- ICAD: Tear in ICA wall allows blood to enter & delaminate wall layers

IMAGING

- Pathognomonic findings of dissection: **Intimal flap** or **double lumen**
- Flame-shaped ICA occlusion (acute phase)
- ICAD most commonly originates in ICA 2-3 cm distal to carotid bulb & terminates before petrous ICA
- Aneurysmal dilatation commonly in distal subcranial ICA
  - Focal pseudoaneurysm unusual
- May show long-segment irregularity of vessel
  - Fibromuscular dysplasia changes in 15% of patients
- T1 FS MR shows hyperintense mural hematomas
- DWI shows mural hyperintensity in 90% of acute ICAD
  - Check cervical ICA on all DWI acute stroke studies

- Although DSA is gold standard, CTA & MRA emerging as best way to image intramural & extraluminal components
  - CTA usually primary modality for diagnosis & surveillance

TOP DIFFERENTIAL DIAGNOSES

- Fibromuscular dysplasia
- Atheromatous plaque
- Traumatic ICA pseudoaneurysm
- Carotid webs
- Carotid artery fenestration
- Vasospasm

CLINICAL ISSUES

- Ipsilateral pain in face, jaw, head, or neck
- Oculosympathetic palsy (partial Horner): Miosis & ptosis
- Bruit (40%), pulsatile tinnitus
- Lower cranial nerve palsies (especially CNX)
- Leading cause of ischemic stroke in patients < 45 years

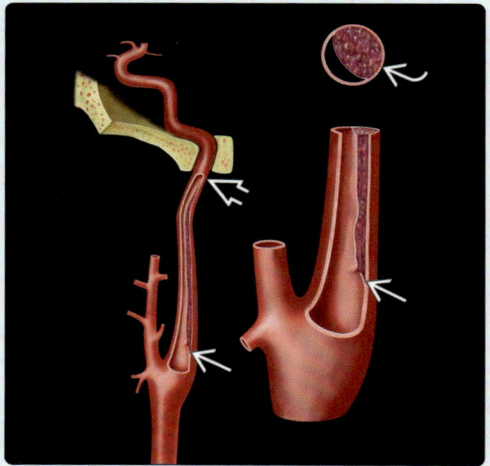
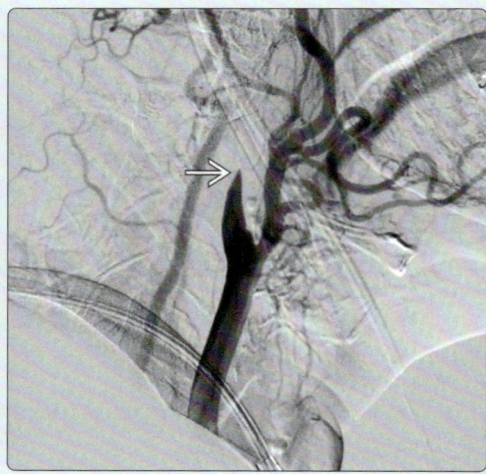

(Left) Lateral graphic depicts typical internal carotid artery dissection (ICAD). Note that the dissection begins above bifurcation ➔ and ends at the skull base ➔. Cross section of a subintimal hematoma ➔ is also shown. (Right) Lateral angiogram shows classic flame-shaped, tapered occlusion of the right ICA ➔ due to acute dissection in this patient after a high-velocity car accident.

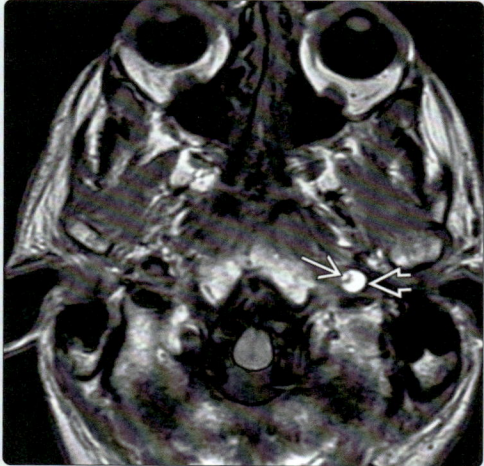
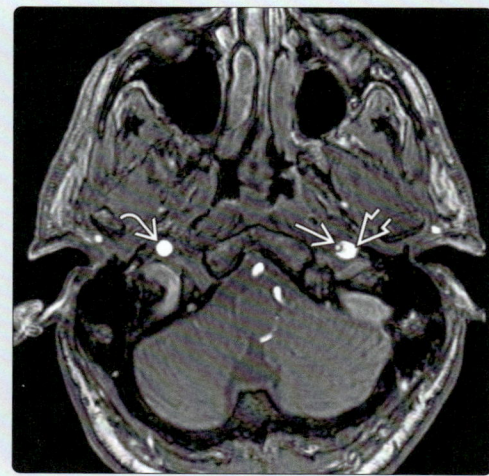

(Left) Axial T1 MR in a 47-year-old man who fell skiing 3 weeks prior to developing left frontotemporal headache shows T1 shortening within a crescentic subacute clot ➔ in the false lumen of the dissected left ICA. Note high-signal thrombus ➔ within the true vessel lumen, which was occluded. (Right) Axial MRA source image in the same patient shows high-signal thrombus in the false lumen ➔ and thrombosed true lumen ➔. Note subtle signal difference in the thrombosed vessel compared to patent flow signal of the right ICA ➔.

Carotid Artery Dissection in Neck

TERMINOLOGY

Abbreviations

- Internal carotid artery dissection (ICAD)

Definitions

- ICAD: Tear in ICA wall allows blood to enter & delaminate wall layers

IMAGING

General Features

- Best diagnostic clue
  - Pathognomonic findings of dissection: **Intimal flap** or **double lumen** (seen in < 10%)
  - **Aneurysmal dilatation** seen in 30%, commonly in distal subcranial segment of ICA
  - **Flame-shaped ICA occlusion** (acute phase)
- Location
  - ICADs most commonly originate in ICA 2-3 cm distal to carotid bulb & variably involve distal ICA
  - Spares carotid bulb & ends prior to entering skull
- Size
  - ICAD extends variable length along distal ICA
  - Stops before petrous ICA
- Morphology
  - ICA luminal narrowing ± focal aneurysmal dilatation
  - Associated pseudoaneurysm develops in 13-49% of ICAD

CT Findings

- CTA
  - Linear hypodense intimal **dissection flap**
    - Double lumen: Contrast in both true & false lumen
    - ± associated contrast filling pseudoaneurysm
  - Intramural thrombus as low-attenuation crescent
  - Narrowed ICA lumen (string sign) ± aneurysmal dilatation
  - Long-segment wall irregularity (alternating caliber)
- Above findings may be seen on CECT as well, although most accurately evaluated on CTA

MR Findings

- T1WI
  - **T1 with fat saturation** (T1 FS): Intramural hematoma as **hyperintense crescent** adjacent to ICA lumen
  - Aneurysmal ICAD: Laminated stages of thrombosis (with intervening layers of methemoglobin & hemosiderin)
- T2WI
  - Aneurysmal ICAD: Laminated stages of thrombosis (with intervening layers of methemoglobin & hemosiderin)
- T2* GRE
  - Hemorrhagic products in vessel wall/aneurysm may cause blooming susceptibility artifact
- DWI
  - Crescentic DWI hyperintensity within mural hematoma
    - Found in ~ 90% of acute ICAD on routine brain MR, in distal cervical/subpetrous segment
    - May avoid need for noncontrast T1 FS MR
- MRA
  - Vessel tapering ± aneurysmal dilatation of dissected ICA
  - Intracranial sequelae of ICAD: Restricted diffusion of acute infarction in ICA distribution ± FLAIR hyperintensity

Ultrasonographic Findings

- Abnormal pattern of flow identified > 90% of cases
- Intimal flap or intramural hematoma seen in < 33% of cases
- Dissection site usually not seen

Angiographic Findings

- Flame-shaped tapered stenosis or occlusion usually acute
- Intimal flap + double lumen (true & false lumens)
  - May have dissecting aneurysm or pseudoaneurysm
- ICA lumen stenosis (string sign) with slow flow
  - ± abrupt reconstitution/dilation (string & pearl sign)
- Fibromuscular dysplasia (FMD) changes in 15% of patients

Imaging Recommendations

- Best imaging tool
  - Angiography (DSA) remains gold standard for ICAD
  - CTA & MRA emerging as superior technologies to image intramural & extraluminal dissection components
    - CTA typically 1st step in imaging evaluation
      - Follow-up angiography generally not performed
    - Surveillance to assess healing (or complications)
- Protocol advice
  - Dedicated arterial imaging preferred (CTA, MRA, DSA)
    - Evaluate for improving or worsening stenosis &/or developing pseudoaneurysm on surveillance
  - T1 FS MR sensitive for hyperintense mural hematoma
  - Brain DWI obtained in acute stroke work-up reveals hyperintense thrombus in 90% of acute ICAD

DIFFERENTIAL DIAGNOSIS

Carotid Fibromuscular Dysplasia

- Clinical: Young female patient with TIA
- Imaging: String of beads sign & long-segment stenoses
  - Look for renal & vertebral artery involvement
  - May have associated ICAD

Atheromatous Plaque

- Clinical: Frequently history of hypertension
- Imaging: ICA narrowing due to eccentric plaque ± vessel wall calcifications, commonly involves carotid bifurcation, MRA/CTA may show prestenotic dilatation

Traumatic Internal Carotid Artery Pseudoaneurysm

- Clinical: History of recent or remote trauma
- Imaging: Dissecting aneurysm can mimic pseudoaneurysm

Carotid Webs

- Clinical: Uncommon cause of ischemic stroke (8x ↑ risk)
- Imaging: Focal, smooth, shelf-like projection into ICA bulb
- Homogeneous & regular without intimal flap or false lumen

Carotid Artery Fenestration

- Clinical: Asymptomatic, normal variant/congenital
- Imaging: Short-segment arterial duplication/division

Vasospasm

- Clinical: ICA vasospasm can occur adjacent to neck infections & with trauma or arterial catheterization
  - Often related to adjacent retropharyngeal neck infections, most commonly in children
  - No treatment needed; typically self-limited
- Imaging: Smooth narrowing without flap or irregularity

PATHOLOGY

General Features

- Etiology
  - Dissections usually arise from intimal tear, blood enters artery wall, **intramural hematoma** forms (false lumen)
    - Intramural hematoma & pseudoaneurysm on heavily T1-weighted MR correlate with stroke risk
    - Enhancing mural hematoma on black-blood T1 MR correlates with stroke risk in spontaneous ICAD
  - 2 types of associated aneurysm
    - **Dissecting aneurysm**: Some normal arterial wall layers present in wall of this aneurysm
    - **Pseudoaneurysm**: Subadventitial dissection causes pseudoaneurysm
      - □ Arterial wall contains no normal layers, just organized clot
  - 3 types of ICAD
    - **Spontaneous dissection**: Most common; etiology unknown
    - **Posttraumatic**: Vertebral artery dissection > ICAD
    - **Predisposed**: Dissection from arteriopathy (FMD, genetic syndromes)
  - Risk factors: Hypertension, migraine, trauma, infection
- Genetics
  - Variation in *PHACTR1* gene may predispose to ICAD
- Associated abnormalities
  - FMD
  - Ehlers-Danlos type IV
  - Marfan syndrome
  - Osteogenesis imperfecta type I
  - Autosomal dominant kidney disease
  - Reversible cerebral vasoconstrictive syndrome
    - Association with ICAD & vertebral artery dissections
    - Clinical: Thunderclap headache presentation
    - Imaging: Intracranial stenoses mimic vasculitis
  - Loeys-Dietz syndrome
    - ↑ risk aneurysms & vessel dissections
    - May have chalice sign (widened carotid bifurcation)
- ICA most common cervical artery to dissect
  - Extracranial ICA more likely to dissect than intracranial
- Pharyngeal portion of extracranial ICA is mobile (carotid bulb to skull base)
  - Vessel tortuosity is associated with ↑ risk of dissection

Staging, Grading, & Classification

- Biffl grading scale for blunt cerebrovascular injury
  - Grade I: Intimal wall irregularity with < 25% narrowing
  - Grade II: Dissection > 25% narrowing
  - Grade III: Arterial pseudoaneurysm
  - Grade IV: Arterial occlusion
  - Grade V: Transection with extravasation
- ↑ risk of stroke with ↑ Biffl grade

CLINICAL ISSUES

Presentation

- Most common signs/symptoms
  - Ipsilateral pain in face, jaw, head, or neck
  - Oculosympathetic palsy (partial Horner syndrome): Miosis & ptosis (specifically associated with ICAD)
  - Ischemic symptoms (cerebral or retinal TIA or stroke)
  - Bruit (40%), pulsatile tinnitus
- Other signs/symptoms
  - Lower cranial nerve palsies (especially CNX)
  - Hyperextension or neck rotation (yoga, vigorous exercise, cough, vomiting, sneezing, resuscitation, neck manipulation)
  - Congenital Horner syndrome with traumatic delivery
- Clinical profile
  - Classic triad seen in ~ 33%: Head & neck pain, partial Horner syndrome, TIA, or stroke

Demographics

- Age
  - 30-55 years; average: 40 years
- Epidemiology
  - Annual incidence 2.5-3 per 100,000
  - Extracranial ICAD > > intracranial ICAD or common CAD
  - 20% of ICADs bilateral or involve vertebral arteries

Natural History & Prognosis

- 90% of stenoses resolve
- 66% of occlusions are recanalized
- 33% of pseudoaneurysms ↓ in size
- Risk of recurrent dissection = 2% (1st month), then 1% per year (usually in another vessel)
- Leading cause of ischemic stroke in patients < 45 years
  - Risk of stroke due to thromboembolic disease ↑; related to severity of initial ischemic insult
- Death from ICAD < 5%

Treatment

- IV heparin + oral warfarin (Coumadin)
  - Unless contraindicated by hemorrhagic stroke
- Antiplatelet therapy in asymptomatic patients & stable imaging findings for 6 months
- Endovascular stenting or occlusion uncommon; used if medical therapy contraindicated or large/enlarging pseudoaneurysm
- Surgical treatment now rare option; used when refractory to maximal medical & endovascular therapy
  - Interposition graft
  - Relatively high morbidity & mortality

DIAGNOSTIC CHECKLIST

Image Interpretation Pearls

- ICAD may present as luminal occlusion, stenosis, or aneurysmal dilatation (pseudoaneurysm)

SELECTED REFERENCES

1. Alalfi MO et al: Assessment of attenuation in pericarotid fat among patients with carotid plaque and spontaneous carotid dissection. AJNR Am J Neuroradiol. 46(2):259-64, 2025
2. Grin EA et al: Atypical carotid webs: an elusive etiology of ischemic stroke. World Neurosurg. 196:123770, 2025
3. Shao S et al: High-resolution magnetic resonance vessel wall imaging in extracranial cervical artery dissection. Front Neurol. 16:1536581, 2025
4. Almohammad M et al: The potential role of diffusion weighted imaging in the diagnosis of early carotid and vertebral artery dissection. Neuroradiology. 64(6):1135-44, 2022
5. Priyadarshni S et al: Carotid webs: an unusual presentation of fibromuscular dysplasia. Cureus. 12(8):e9549, 2020
6. Hakimi R et al: Imaging of carotid dissection. Curr Pain Headache Rep. 23(1):2, 2019

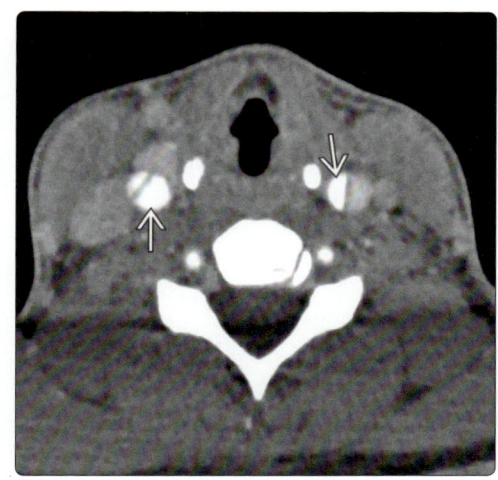
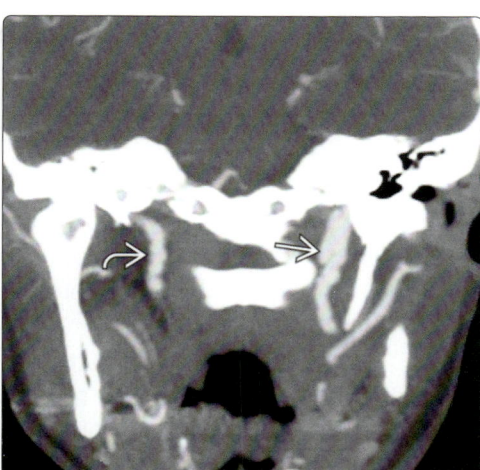

(Left) Axial arterial-phase CECT shows bilateral ICADs in a patient with Loeys-Dietz syndrome and type A aortic dissection. Intimal flaps are present bilaterally with arterial-type enhancement within the true lumen ⮞ of each carotid. (Right) Coronal CTA MPR in a woman with a history of intracranial aneurysm presenting with "worst headache of her life" shows left ICAD associated with a pseudoaneurysm ⮞. Note the standing waves appearance of fibromuscular dysplasia involving the right ICA ⮞.

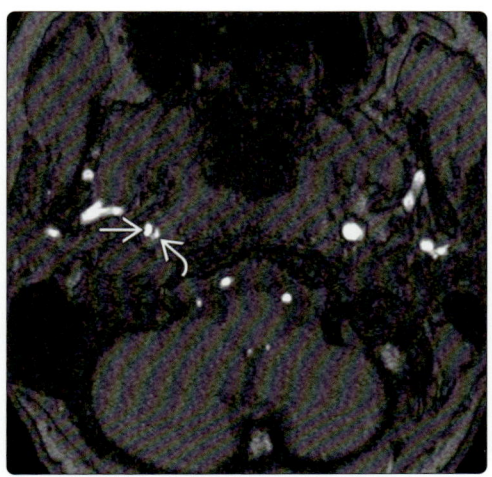
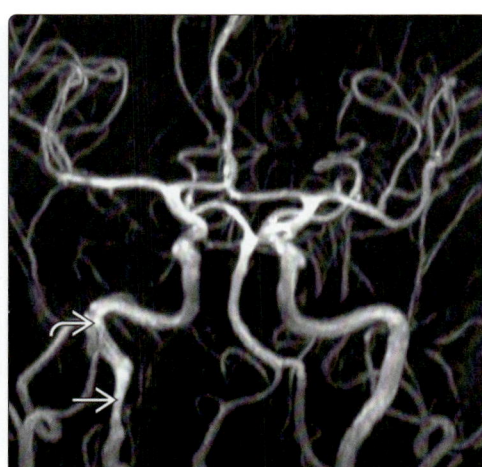

(Left) Axial time-of-flight MRA source image demonstrates a luminal flap with higher signal within the true lumen ⮞ of this right ICAD. Slightly less hyperintense mural hematoma ⮞ is noted medially. (Right) Coronal time-of-flight MRA MIP in the same patient confirms long-segment caliber narrowing ⮞ involving the right ICA distal to the bifurcation. Irregular linear hypointensity is suggested in the distal right carotid ⮞; however, the luminal flap is best seen on the source images.

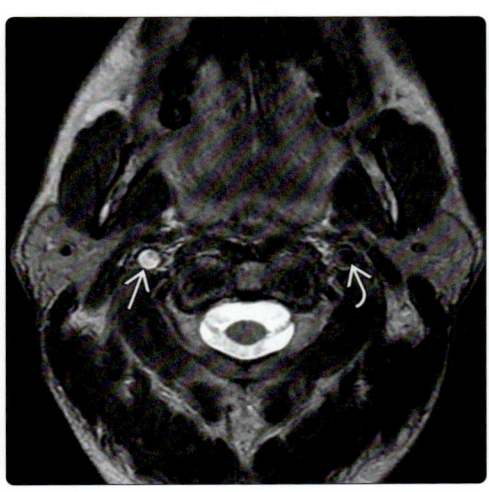
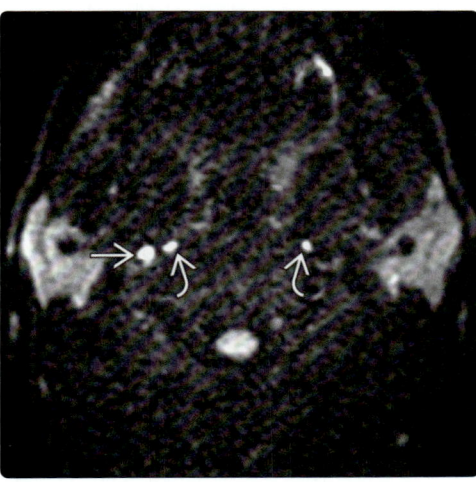

(Left) Axial T2 MR shows loss of flow void ⮞ in right ICAD due to progressive thrombosis. Note normal flow void in the left ICA ⮞. (Right) Axial DWI MR shows hyperintensity ⮞ in the same patient. Routine brain DWI shows hyperintensity in 90% of high cervical ICAD during acute ischemic stroke or CAD work-up, typically in a crescentic or ring-shaped configuration. One must be aware of the normally hyperintense superior cervical ganglia ⮞ and retropharyngeal lymph nodes just medial to the ICA.

Carotid Artery Pseudoaneurysm in Neck

TERMINOLOGY

- Carotid artery pseudoaneurysm (CAPA)
- Synonyms: Carotid artery **false aneurysm**
- CAPA: Outpouching lacking part or all of carotid wall

IMAGING

- Carotid outpouching with extraluminal CAPA
  - Location: Distal cervical internal carotid artery (ICA) just below skull base & common carotid artery
  - CAPA complicates 13-49% of ICA dissections
- **CTA gold standard** to detect CAPA, show size, extent of intraluminal thrombus, & flow ± dissection
  - DSA: Detects CAPA ± dissection but may underestimate CAPA size
  - MR: Detects CAPA ± dissection
    - Partly thrombosed CAPA may require enhanced MRA, as it can have complex wall signal due to stages of thrombosis with methemoglobin & hemosiderin

TOP DIFFERENTIAL DIAGNOSES

- Carotid bulb ectasia
- Tortuous or looping carotid artery in neck
- Carotid artery dissection in neck

PATHOLOGY

- **Posttraumatic (with dissection or direct injury)**
- Sporadic subadventitial ICA dissection
- Atherosclerotic disease (frequently bilateral)
- Iatrogenic: Radiation, carotid endarterectomy
- Infection: Mycotic CAPA
- Congenital arterial wall anomaly

CLINICAL ISSUES

- Pulsatile neck mass
- Smaller CAPA + ICA dissection
  - Anticoagulation + observation ± aspirin
- Large CAPA: Endovascular stent graft, occlusion, or surgery

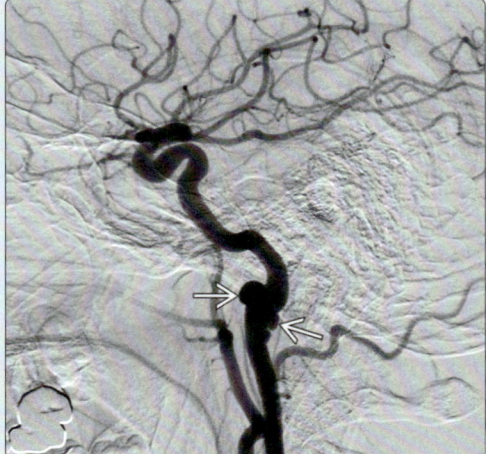
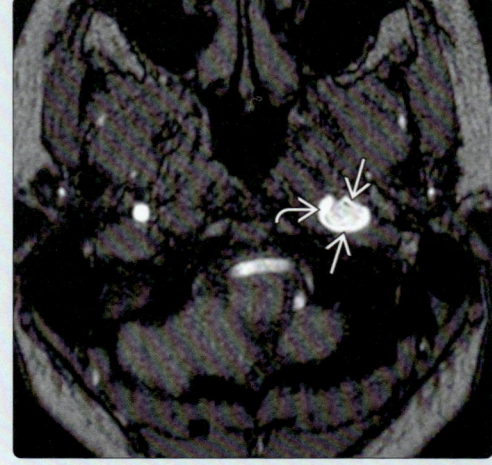

(Left) *Lateral DSA in a 32-year-old man shows a lobulated pseudoaneurysm of distal internal carotid artery (ICA) ➡. Patient had bilateral carotid pseudoaneurysms that were treated conservatively with aspirin.* (Right) *Axial TOF MRA shows a high cervical ICA pseudoaneurysm ➡. Most pseudoaneurysms occur within 1 cm of the skull base. The native lumen is seen as a high-signal area similar to the contralateral ICA ➡, while the pseudoaneurysm has internal heterogeneous lower signal due to more turbulent flow.*

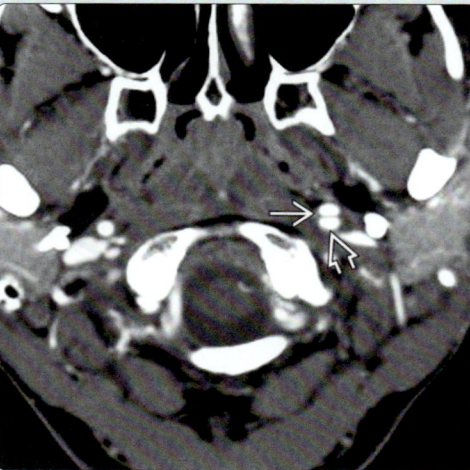
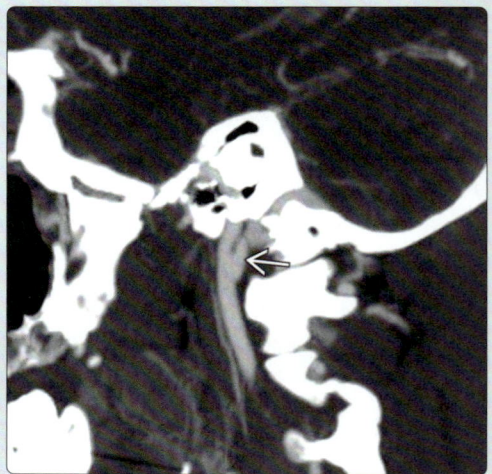

(Left) *Axial CTA in a 29-year-old patient with cervical fractures following a motorcycle crash shows an abnormality involving the high cervical left ICA with evidence of dissection with intimal flap ➡ and focal outpouching along the posterior wall of the vessel ➡.* (Right) *Sagittal reformatted CTA in the same patient clearly demonstrates the pseudoaneurysm related to the ICA dissection ➡. Note that the reformatted image allows clear morphologic characterization, whereas the axial image does not.*

Carotid Artery Pseudoaneurysm in Neck

TERMINOLOGY

Abbreviations
- Carotid artery pseudoaneurysm (CAPA)

Synonyms
- Carotid artery **false aneurysm**; Biffl grade III carotid injury

Definitions
- **Focal carotid artery outpouching** contained by adventitia

IMAGING

General Features
- Best diagnostic clue
  - CTA/CECT: Focal ↑ carotid artery wall/lumen diameter
  - MR: Enlarged carotid with complex wall signal (stages of thrombosis with methemoglobin & hemosiderin)
- Location
  - Carotid space: Distal cervical internal carotid artery (ICA) just below skull base & common carotid artery
- Size
  - 1-3 cm (saccular morphology more likely to enlarge)
- Morphology
  - Saccular or fusiform

CT Findings
- NECT
  - Wall **calcification** if chronic
- CECT
  - Enhancement of central or eccentric lumen of partially thrombosed aneurysm
  - Enhancement irregular with intraluminal thrombus
- CTA
  - CAPA seen as **focal carotid outpouching** with contrast

MR Findings
- T1WI
  - Flow void in patent arterial lumen & residual CAPA lumen
    – Fat saturation may help distinguish thrombus
- T2WI
  - Complex flow in CAPA lumen
- T2* GRE
  - Thrombus may **bloom** (susceptibility effect)
- T1WI C+
  - Luminal enhancement from slow, complex flow
- MRA
  - CAPA seen as carotid outpouching
  - Be aware: Partly thrombosed CAPA may **not** be seen without contrast-enhanced MRA

Ultrasonographic Findings
- Spectral waveform analysis: Characteristic to-&-fro flow

Angiographic Findings
- ICA luminal outpouching with extraluminal CAPA
- Associated ICA dissection often present

Imaging Recommendations
- Best imaging tool
  - DSA detects CAPA but may underestimate its size
  - CTA has largely replaced DSA: CTA shows aneurysm size, extent of intraluminal thrombus, & flow

DIFFERENTIAL DIAGNOSIS

Carotid Bulb Ectasia
- Imaging: Prominent carotid bifurcation without thrombus

Tortuous Carotid Artery in Neck
- Imaging: Tortuous or looping carotid mimics aneurysm

Carotid Artery Dissection in Neck
- Sporadic or posttraumatic narrowed or occluded carotid
  - CAPA frequently develops after ICA dissection

PATHOLOGY

General Features
- Multiple etiologies
  - **Trauma (with dissection or direct injury)**
  - **Sporadic subadventitial ICA dissection**
  - Atherosclerotic disease (frequently bilateral)
  - Iatrogenic: Radiation, carotid endarterectomy
  - Infection: Mycotic CAPA
  - Congenital arterial wall anomaly: **Fibromuscular dysplasia**, cystic medial necrosis, Ehlers-Danlos, Marfan syndrome, Behçet disease

Gross Pathologic & Surgical Features
- CAPA lacks **normal arterial wall layers**
  - CAPA wall contained by adventitial sleeve, surrounding hematoma or soft tissues
  - Adventitia may be disrupted in penetrating trauma or irradiated necks

CLINICAL ISSUES

Presentation
- Most common signs/symptoms
  - Pulsatile neck mass
  - Lower cranial nerve palsy (CNIX-XI)
  - Ischemic symptoms ± stroke
  - Hemorrhage (particularly head & neck cancer patients)

Natural History & Prognosis
- CAPA complicates 13-49% of ICA dissections
- CAPA thrombus may cause transient ischemic attack/cerebrovascular accident
- Risk of rupture of pseudoaneurysm with hemorrhage
  - Acute hemorrhage is often life threatening, requiring emergent embolization
- May be indistinguishable from carotid blowout in postradiotherapy setting for head & neck cancer

Treatment
- Smaller & CAPA + ICA dissection may be treated conservatively with anticoagulation & observation ± aspirin
  - Heparin → warfarin (Coumadin)
- Larger CAPA: Endovascular stent graft treatment of choice
  - Percutaneous thrombin injection is option
  - Surgical repair or vessel sacrifice if other techniques fail

SELECTED REFERENCES

1. Larson AS et al: A review of histopathologic and radiologic features of non-atherosclerotic pathologies of the extracranial carotid arteries. Neuroradiol J. 37(6):678-87, 2024

TERMINOLOGY

- Fibromuscular dysplasia (FMD): Idiopathic, noninflammatory, nonatherosclerotic arteriopathy of medium-sized arteries
  - Most commonly affects renal arteries but can involve cervical internal carotid and vertebral arteries
- Intracranial FMD is rare, typically coexisting with extracranial FMD and presenting with intracranial aneurysms

IMAGING

- Conventional angiography considered gold standard for diagnosis and classification
  - Focal FMD: Focal stenosis
  - Multifocal FMD: Alternating areas of stenosis and dilation produces classic appearance: **String of beads sign**
- CTA/MRA findings
  - Vessel beading/irregularities: **String of beads**
  - **Focal arterial stenosis** without mural Ca++
  - Associations: Dissection, pseudoaneurysm, intracranial aneurysms

TOP DIFFERENTIAL DIAGNOSES

- Atherosclerosis
- Nonatherosclerotic vasculopathies
- Arterial dissection

PATHOLOGY

- Multifocal FMD: Medial fibroplasia, attenuation of elastic fibers, and abnormal collagen synthesis
- Focal FMD: Most commonly associated with intimal fibroplasia

CLINICAL ISSUES

- > 80% of patients are female and have multifocal FMD
- Cervical arterial involvement often asymptomatic
- Symptoms include headache, arterial dissection, cervical bruit, intracranial aneurysm, TIA, stroke

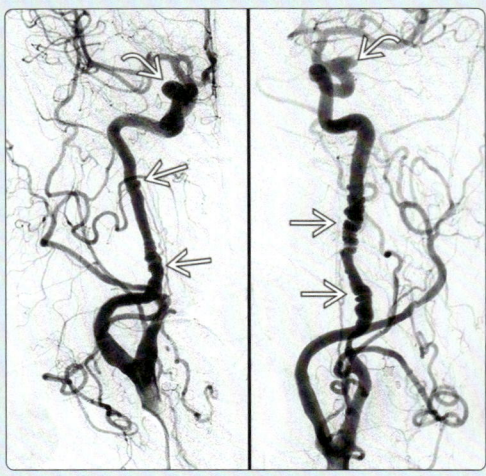
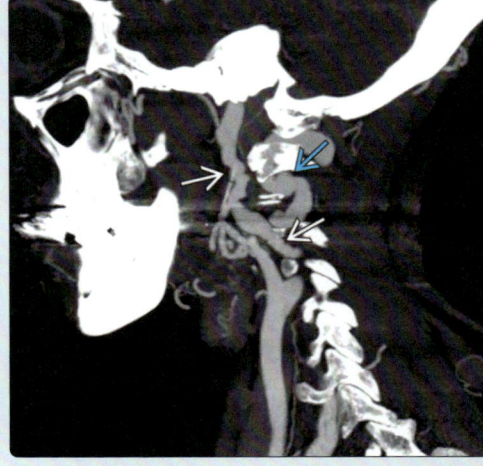

(Left) *Isolated injections of the bilateral carotid vessels in a patient with bilateral internal carotid artery (ICA) multifocal fibromuscular dysplasia (FMD) and bilateral intracranial aneurysms ➡ are shown. The classic angiographic appearance of the string of beads sign ➡ is present bilaterally.* (Right) *Sagittal CTA shows multifocal, diffuse involvement of the right ICA with multiple alternating bands of stenosis and dilation ➡. Note the vertebral artery involvement ➡ as well in this case of multifocal FMD.*

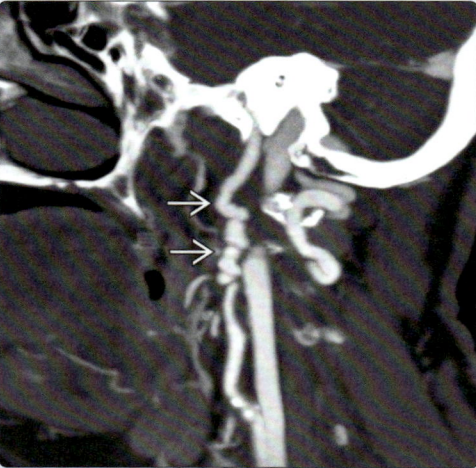
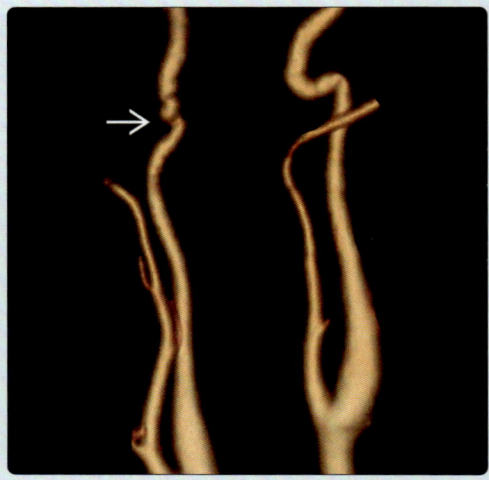

(Left) *Sagittal CTA 2D reformation in a patient with multifocal FMD of the ICA shows multifocal areas of stenosis and dilatation of the mid distal ICA ➡, producing the CTA equivalent of the angiographic string of beads sign. This is a diagnostic appearance of multifocal FMD on CTA.* (Right) *3D CTA in a 54-year-old woman with focal FMD shows focal irregularity and stenosis of the distal ICA on the right ➡. This would fit angiographically into the focal FMD category, which is less common.*

TERMINOLOGY

Abbreviations

- Fibromuscular dysplasia (FMD)

Definitions

- Arterial disease of unknown etiology affecting medium-sized arteries
  - Noninflammatory, nonatherosclerotic arteriopathy with dysplastic arterial wall with overgrowth of smooth muscle and fibrous tissue
  - While FMD most commonly affects renal arteries, term cervicocranial FMD relates to involvement of cervical internal carotid arteries (ICAs) and vertebral arteries and is associated with intracranial aneurysms

IMAGING

General Features

- Best diagnostic clue
  - DSA/MRA/CTA demonstrates segment of tightly spaced alternating regions of stenosis and focal dilation of ICA (or vertebral artery); creates classic string of beads appearance
- Location
  - **Renal arteries** affected 75% (40% bilateral)
  - **Cervicocranial FMD (65-70%)**
    - Mid distal ICA (at level of C1 and C2) is most common location; spares bifurcation
    - > 50% bilateral
    - External carotid arteries (ECAs) and vertebral arteries less common
    - Intracranial involvement manifests as aneurysms

Angiographic Findings

- Remains gold standard for diagnosis of FMD
- Historically attempts have been made to categorize lesions based on angiographic appearance and suspected underlying histopathologic correlate
- More recently consensus statements have simplified approach based on **angiographic appearance** into 2 broad categories
  - Focal: Focal irregularity and stenosis
    - Carotid bulb "web" may represent intimal form of FMD
  - Multifocal
    - Most common type (85%) found in carotid vessels; accounts for string of beads appearance
    - Caused by **medial fibroplasia**, replacement of smooth muscle of media by compact fibrous connective tissue
- Cervicocranial FMD can be associated with arterial dissections and intracranial aneurysms

CT Findings

- CTA
  - Morphologic changes of FMD in carotid and vertebral artery circulations
    - 1st clue is often alternating areas of stenosis and dilation in mid distal ICA viewed on axial source images
    - 2D and 3D reformations more clearly demonstrate classic string of beads morphology

- **Arterial stenosis** without mural Ca^{++} [cf. atherosclerotic vascular disease (ASVD)]
- FMD associations: Dissection, pseudoaneurysm, intracranial aneurysms

MR Findings

- MRA
  - Can demonstrate prominent regions of FMD in cervical vessels but often findings are less conspicuous than CTA or DSA

Imaging Recommendations

- Best imaging tool
  - CTA for noninvasive assessment
  - DSA for definitive diagnosis ± treatment

DIFFERENTIAL DIAGNOSIS

Atherosclerosis, Extracranial

- ASVD affects older vasculopaths
- Typically short-segment stenosis at or above carotid bifurcation with mural Ca^{++}

Carotid Dissection

- Irregular stenosis ± outpouching from associated pseudoaneurysm

PATHOLOGY

General Features

- Histopathology
  - Focal fibrous proliferation and cellular disorganization within arterial wall: May preferentially affect intima, media, or adventia

CLINICAL ISSUES

Presentation

- Most common signs/symptoms
  - For cervicocranial FMD, headache, pulsatile tinnitus, bruit, arterial dissection, TIA, stroke, aneurysm (with mass effect or rupture)
  - Typically affects women 25-50 years of age

DIAGNOSTIC CHECKLIST

Image Interpretation Pearls

- String of pearls sign on DSA/CTA/MRA is classic appearance of multifocal FMD in carotid vessels

SELECTED REFERENCES

1. Porras-Colon J et al: Outcomes of carotid stenting in patients with fibromuscular dysplasia. J Vasc Surg. 77(3):829-35, 2023
2. Abozeed M et al: Screening CT angiography in patients with suspected fibromuscular dysplasia: improved patient care with single-session skull vertex to pelvis coverage. Cardiovasc Diagn Ther. 10(2):201-7, 2020
3. Gornik HL et al: First international consensus on the diagnosis and management of fibromuscular dysplasia. Vasc Med. 24(2):164-89, 2019
4. Harriott A: Idiopathic non-atherosclerotic carotid artery disease. Curr Treat Options Cardiovasc Med. 21(11):64, 2019
5. Kim SJ et al: Carotid webs in cryptogenic ischemic strokes: a matched case-control study. J Stroke Cerebrovasc Dis. 28(12):104402, 2019
6. Soun JE et al: Central nervous system vasculopathies. Radiol Clin North Am. 57(6):1117-31, 2019
7. Choi PM et al: Carotid webs and recurrent ischemic strokes in the era of CT angiography. AJNR Am J Neuroradiol. 36(11):2134-9, 2015

KEY FACTS

TERMINOLOGY

- Synonyms
  - **Translent perivascular inflammation of carotid artery (TIPIC) syndrome**
  - Idiopathic or sclerosing (inflammatory) pseudotumor
  - Idiopathic carotiditis
  - Fay syndrome
- Definition: Self-limited inflammatory disorder of carotid artery causing carotid wall thickening & pain

IMAGING

- **Circumferential thickening of carotid wall**
  - Distal common carotid or carotid bifurcation area
  - Little to no luminal narrowing
- Contrast-enhanced MR: intense wall enhancement
- Contrast-enhanced CT: poor wall enhancement
- Ultrasound
  - Hypoechoic tissue ± intimal plaque
  - Contrast-enhanced ultrasound: Wall enhancement

TOP DIFFERENTIAL DIAGNOSES

- Extracranial atherosclerosis
- Miscellaneous vasculitis
- Carotid artery dissection in neck
- Squamous cell carcinoma extranodal tumor

CLINICAL ISSUES

- Localized tenderness to palpation over carotid
- Pulsatile neck mass, may be indurated
- Typical symptomatic resolution within 2 weeks spontaneously or with antiinflammatory treatment
- If persists after treatment, exclude other pathology

DIAGNOSTIC CHECKLIST

- Contrast-enhanced MR better exam than CECT
- **Diagnosis of exclusion**
  - Confirm absence of other vascular/nonvascular etiology
- If early conservative management fails, histologic confirmation is important

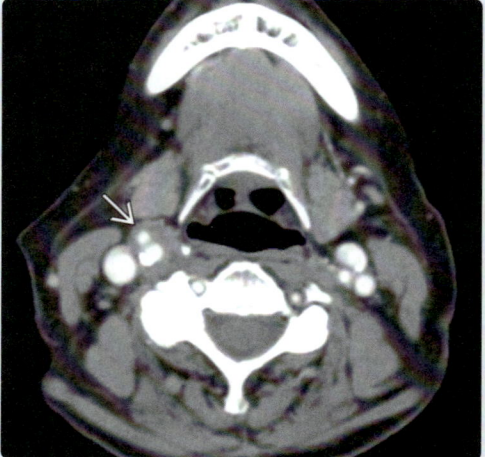
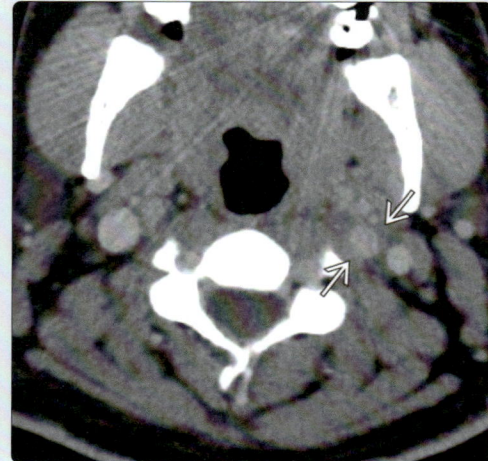

(Left) Axial CECT of the neck reveals circumferential thickening of the common carotid wall ➡ at the carotid bifurcation. This patient was treated with steroids for presumptive diagnosis of carotidynia with symptoms resolving within 36 hours of treatment. (Right) Axial CECT demonstrates ill-defined left internal carotid artery wall thickening ➡, which effaces adjacent fat planes in this patient who presented with severe left-sided neck pain. Symptoms completely resolved after short-term treatment with ibuprofen.

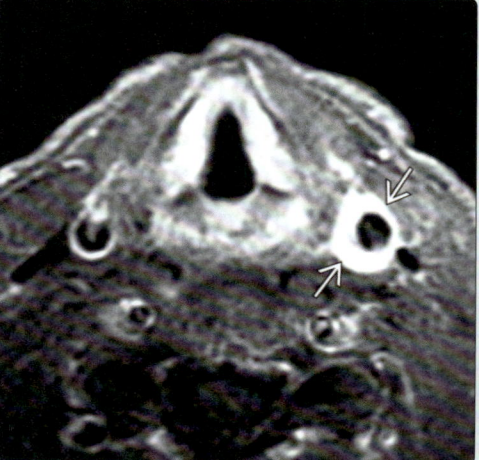
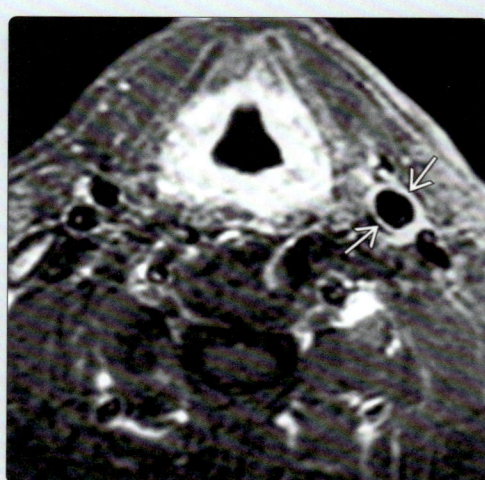

(Left) Axial T1WI C+ FS MR in a patient with painful palpation in the left neck shows a thickened, intensely enhancing common carotid wall ➡, consistent with the diagnosis of carotidynia. Note the lack of luminal narrowing. (Courtesy G. Petermann, MD.) (Right) Axial T1WI C+ FS MR in carotidynia post steroid therapy reveals mild residual wall thickening and enhancement involving the left common carotid wall ➡. (Courtesy G. Petermann, MD.)

TERMINOLOGY

Synonyms
- **Transient perivascular inflammation of carotid artery (TIPIC) syndrome**
- Idiopathic or sclerosing (inflammatory) pseudotumor
- Idiopathic carotiditis
- Fay syndrome

Definitions
- Self-limited inflammatory disorder of carotid artery causing carotid wall thickening & pain
- Proposed TIPIC criteria
  - Acute pain overlying carotid artery ± radiation to head
  - Eccentric perivascular infiltration on imaging
  - Exclude other vascular/nonvascular diagnosis by imaging
- Improvement within 14 days ± NSAIDS

IMAGING

General Features
- Best diagnostic clue
  - Tender mass surrounding carotid near bifurcation
- Location
  - Distal common carotid artery &/or bifurcation
  - Usually unilateral but occasionally bilateral
- Size
  - Craniocaudal extent 1.5 to ~ 3.5 cm
  - ~ 6- to 8-mm thick wall
- Morphology
  - **Circumferential thickening of carotid wall**
  - No or mild lumen narrowing

Imaging Recommendations
- Best imaging tool
  - Contrast-enhanced neck MR &/or ultrasound
    - CECT enhancement is poor
- Protocol advice
  - Contrast-enhanced imaging
  - MR vessel wall imaging technique is optimal
  - Exact site of tenderness can be imaged on ultrasound

Ultrasonographic Findings
- **Hypoechoic** thick soft tissue around carotid wall
- Mild intimal soft plaque seen in > 50%
  - **No significant lumen narrowing** or velocity elevation
- Exact region of tenderness can be imaged
- Contrast-enhanced ultrasound shows wall enhancement

MR Findings
- Enhanced T1 fat-saturated MR
  - **Markedly enhancing tissue involving carotid wall**
    - Intense adventitial enhancement & perivascular infiltration
  - Smoothly marginated, circumferential, without invasion
- T2: Increased intensity of thickened wall
- Vessel wall imaging technique is optimal
- MRA: Absent or mild lumen stenosis; no irregularity

CT Findings
- Poorly or nonenhancing circumferential perivascular infiltration/thickening of carotid wall

DIFFERENTIAL DIAGNOSIS

Extracranial Atherosclerosis
- Eccentric lumen narrowing
- Carotid bulb or internal carotid soft plaque ± calcification

Miscellaneous Vasculitis
- Serum markers; angiography to confirm (± biopsy)
- Multifocal involvement with lumen narrowing

Carotid Artery Dissection in Neck
- Lumen narrowing ± occlusion
- Axial T1 MR: High-signal subintimal hematoma
- Involves internal carotid artery above bifurcation

Squamous Cell Carcinoma Extranodal Tumor
- Suspect if conservative therapy fails; biopsy indicated
- Entire carotid space involved; not just carotid wall

PATHOLOGY

General Features
- Etiology
  - Report of association with COVID-19

Microscopic Features
- Nonspecific chronic inflammation (rarely biopsied)

CLINICAL ISSUES

Presentation
- Most common signs/symptoms
  - Tenderness to palpation over carotid bifurcation
    - May be pulsatile &/or indurated
  - May present with transient neurologic deficits

Natural History & Prognosis
- Self-limited inflammatory condition
- Usually complete resolution within 2 weeks

Treatment
- May respond to NSAIDs ± corticosteroids
- May resolve without treatment

DIAGNOSTIC CHECKLIST

Consider
- Ultrasound & enhanced MR are best exams
- Repeat clinical/imaging assessment after course of antiinflammatories to exclude other pathology
  - Typical symptomatic resolution in days to weeks

Image Interpretation Pearls
- TIPIC/carotidynia is diagnosis of exclusion

SELECTED REFERENCES

1. Ari BC et al: Carotidynia: overview of an uncommon identification for unilateral neck pain. Neuroradiol J. 38(1):124-7, 2025
2. Mumoli N et al: Transient perivascular inflammation of the carotid artery (TIPIC) syndrome in a patient with COVID-19. Int J Infect Dis. 108:126-8, 2021
3. Rafailidis V et al: Role of multi-parametric ultrasound in transient perivascular inflammation of the carotid artery syndrome. Ultrasound. 27(2):77-84, 2019
4. Lecler A et al: TIPIC syndrome: beyond the myth of carotidynia, a new distinct unclassified entity. AJNR Am J Neuroradiol. 38(7):1391-8, 2017

KEY FACTS

TERMINOLOGY

- Jugular vein thrombosis (JVT): Chronic thrombus or clot in internal jugular vein (IJV)
- IJV thrombophlebitis: Acute-subacute thrombosis of IJV with associated adjacent tissue inflammation

IMAGING

- CTV/MRV: **Tubular** filling defect within lumen of IJV
  - Without acute inflammatory changes (thrombosis)
  - Surrounding acute inflammation (thrombophlebitis)
- Acute: Fills vein, enlarged diameter
- Chronic (> 10 days): Variable size ± collaterals
- US shows **noncompressible** thrombus and no flow

TOP DIFFERENTIAL DIAGNOSES

- Slow or turbulent flow in IJV (pseudothrombosis)
- Suppurative adenopathy
- Cervical neck abscess
- Squamous cell carcinoma malignant adenopathy

PATHOLOGY

- JVT pathogenesis: 3 mechanisms for thrombosis (Virchow triad)
  - **Endothelial damage** from indwelling line, IV drugs, infection
  - **Altered blood flow/venous stasis**
  - **Hypercoagulable state**

CLINICAL ISSUES

- Can be asymptomatic or have erythema and tenderness
- Determine/treat etiology of thrombus
- Central venous catheters in neck increase JVT risk
- IJV thrombophlebitis in young, previously healthy patient with sepsis and embolic complications: **Lemierre syndrome**

DIAGNOSTIC CHECKLIST

- Evaluate extent of JVT (i.e., into dural venous sinus)
- Do not mistake JVT with retropharyngeal space (RPS) edema for RPS abscess

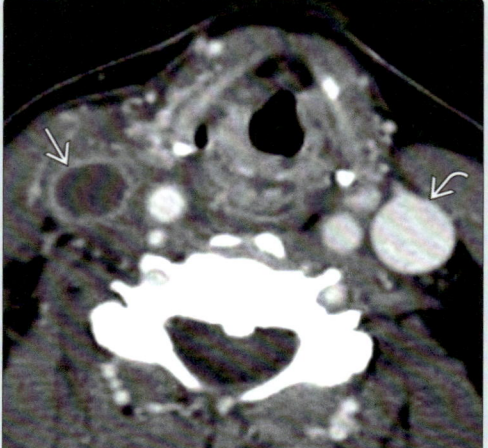
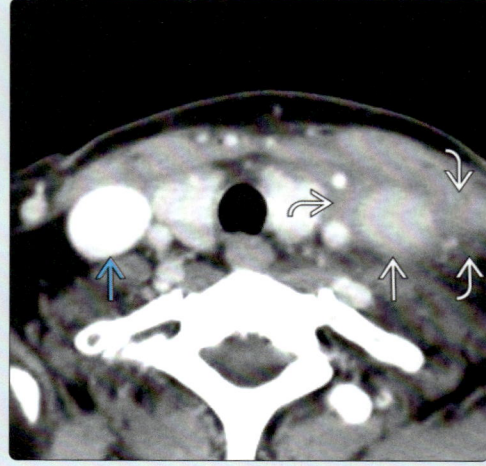

(Left) Axial CECT in a patient with renal failure and a right internal jugular vein (IJV) hemodialysis catheter presents with right neck pain. Note thin wall enhancement of IJV venae vasorum in chronic thrombosis ➡. The patent left IJV ➡ enhances normally. (Right) Axial CECT in a woman with malignancy shows acute hyperdense thrombophlebitis of the left IJV ➡ with surrounding tissue edema ➡. This might mimic patency, but the lower density compared to the normal enhancing right IJV ➡ helps with the diagnosis.

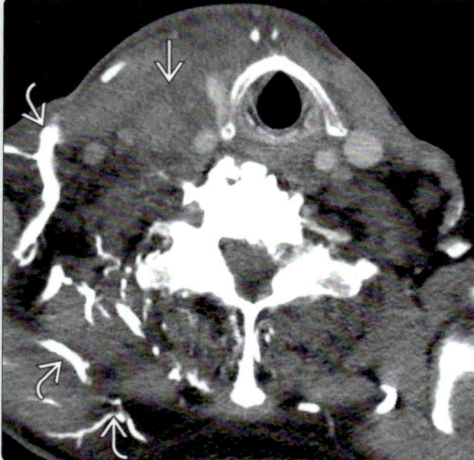
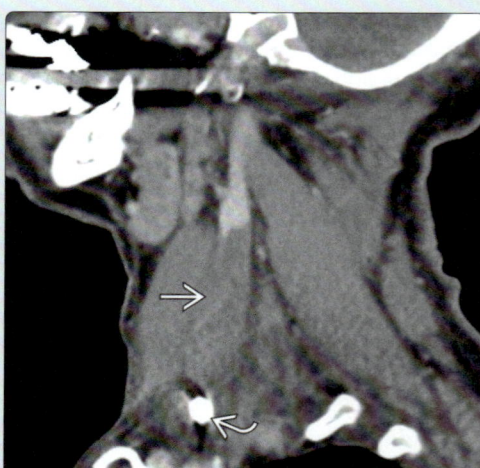

(Left) Axial CECT shows low-density, nonenhancing acute thrombophlebitis of the right IJV ➡. Note surrounding low-density edema effacing adjacent fat planes. Extensive contrast reflux into small collateral veins ➡ is present. (Right) Parasagittal CECT shows long-segment thrombus filling and distending the IJV ➡. An indwelling catheter ➡ in this patient predisposed to thrombosis.

TERMINOLOGY

Abbreviations

- Jugular vein thrombosis (JVT)

Definitions

- JVT: Chronic thrombus or clot in internal jugular vein (IJV), which persists after inflammation is gone (usually > 10 days after acute event)
- Jugular vein thrombophlebitis: Acute to subacute thrombosis of IJV with adjacent soft tissue inflammation

IMAGING

General Features

- Best diagnostic clue
  - **Nonenhancing luminal clot** in IJV
    - With surrounding inflammation of soft tissues (thrombophlebitis) or without associated acute inflammatory changes (thrombosis)
- Location
  - IJV of extracranial head and neck
- Size
  - IJV enlarged in acute-subacute phase
  - IJV may be smaller or normal in chronic phase
- Morphology
  - Ovoid to round, tubular IJV luminal filling defect

CT Findings

- NECT
  - Acute thrombus is hyperdense
    - Hyperdense venous thrombus on noncontrast CT may mimic contrast enhancement but represents thrombus rather than patent lumen
- CECT
  - **Acute-subacute IJV thrombophlebitis** (< 10 days)
    - Nonenhancing central filling defect
      □ Fills vein, usually hypoattenuating
    - Enlarged vein diameter
    - Inflammation of adjacent soft tissues surrounding carotid space (CS) can include
      □ Increased density in fat: Edema/cellulitis
      □ Loss of soft tissue planes: Myositis and fasciitis
    - Peripheral (thickened) enhancement of vessel wall
      □ Wall appears thickened from enhancing venae vasorum
    - Ill-defined fluid may be present in retropharyngeal space (RPS)
      □ Reactive edema, secondary sign of inflammation
  - **Chronic IJV thrombosis** (> 10 days)
    - Well-marginated, eccentric filling defect
      □ Persistent clot without adjacent inflammation
    - Can be normal or smaller size of vein
    - ± tubular/linear enhancement of prominent **collateral veins** bypassing thrombosed IJV
- CT venogram
  - Nonenhancing **filling defect** (thrombus) within IJV
    - Thrombus is low attenuation compared to hyperdense contrast
  - Enhancing venous collaterals may be seen in chronic phase; can be large in size

MR Findings

- T1WI
  - IJV thrombus signal intensity depends on composition or age of clot
    - Acute thrombus is isointense (best seen on fat-suppressed sequences)
    - **Subacute clot** often **high signal** (methemoglobin)
  - Flow voids in collateral veins remain dark
- T2WI
  - Acute thrombus (early hours of acute event) in IJV lumen bright
  - Subacute IJV thrombus low signal
  - High-signal RPS edema may be present
- T2* GRE
  - Luminal thrombus may display susceptibility artifact (blooming) with low signal appearing larger than IJV
- DWI
  - Clot may have diffusion restriction
- T1WI C+
  - **Acute-subacute IJV thrombophlebitis**
    - Hypointense nonenhancing clot fills enlarged IJV
    - IJV wall enhancement with inhomogeneous enhancement of soft tissues surrounding CS
  - **Chronic JVT**
    - Filling defect in normal-sized IJV
    - Partial recanalization may allow contrast to outline clot in IJV
    - Venous collaterals around clotted IJV will be low signal or enhance depending on flow rate
    - No surrounding inflammation or edema
- MRV
  - Acute-subacute IJV thrombophlebitis: Clotted IJV is absent
  - Chronic JVT
    - Eccentric thrombosis in IJV: Absent flow/contrast on that side
    - IJV small and irregular (partially recanalized)
    - Mature venous collaterals, may be prominent

Ultrasonographic Findings

- **Noncompressible** filling defect in IJV
- Intraluminal clot appears as solid mass with midamplitude echoes
- Decreased dynamics: Decrease in venous pulsations and distention on Valsalva maneuvers
- Pulsed Doppler **Absent flow** in affected vessel
- Spectral Doppler: Partial/complete loss of cardiac pulsatility ± respiratory phasicity
- US limitation
  - Nonvisualization of entire vessel: Cephalad to mandible and caudal to clavicle
  - Fresh clot has little inherent echogenicity
- US advantage: Noninvasive means for serial follow-up imaging during treatment of JVT

Imaging Recommendations

- Best imaging tool
  - US is best diagnostic test, complemented by CECT/CTV or MR/MRV where needed
  - CECT/CTV in sick patient permits rapid diagnosis

DIFFERENTIAL DIAGNOSIS

Slow or Turbulent Internal Jugular Vein Flow (Pseudothrombosis)

- MR finding: High signal intensity on T1 may be seen
- Look at all MR sequences; usually 1 will show flow void
  - On CTV, IJV will contrast enhance normally
- Beware nonopacified IJV on CTA: Occurs from technically early imaging post injection, mixing of unopacified blood with IV contrast, or more central venous obstruction

Suppurative Adenopathy

- Multiple focal cystic masses along internal jugular nodal chain (separate from IJV)

Cervical Neck Abscess

- Focal walled-off fluid collection in any neck space

Squamous Cell Carcinoma Metastatic Nodes

- Multiple focal, necrotic, and nonnecrotic masses
- Along internal jugular nodal chain (separate from IJV)

PATHOLOGY

General Features

- Etiology
  - JVT pathogenesis: 3 mechanisms for thrombosis (Virchow triad)
    - **Endothelial damage** from indwelling line (or IV drug use) or infection
    - **Altered blood flow/venous stasis** from compression of IJV in neck (cervical nodes) or mediastinum (superior vena cava syndrome)
    - **Hypercoagulable state**
      - □ Genetic hypercoagulable states, malignancy, oral contraception, pregnancy
      - □ Migratory IJV thrombophlebitis (Trousseau syndrome) associated with malignancy (pancreas, lung, and ovary)
  - Cancer and indwelling catheters most common predisposing factors
  - Complicates necrotizing fasciitis in 21% of cases
  - **Lemierre syndrome**: IJV thrombosis associated with postanginal sepsis/necrobacillosis
    - Young, previously healthy demographic → **sepsis**
    - Septic thrombophlebitis of **ipsilateral** IJV
      - □ Can be isolated to smaller draining veins &/or may be nonocclusive in IJV
    - Develops after oropharyngeal infection (e.g., pharyngitis or tonsillitis), possibly sinuses or mastoids
      - □ Anaerobic infection with *Fusobacterium necrophorum* = most common microorganism
    - Systemic complications due to **septic embolization** with abscesses (pulmonary septic emboli most common, but other organs may be affected)

Microscopic Features

- JVT different from intraparenchymal hematoma
  - JVT: **Lamination** of thrombus occurs
    - No hemosiderin deposition
    - Delay in evolution of blood products (especially methemoglobin)

CLINICAL ISSUES

Presentation

- Most common signs/symptoms
  - Frequently asymptomatic
  - **Acute-subacute thrombophlebitis** phase (< 10 days)
    - Swollen, hot, tender neck mass with fever
    - Radiology request may read "**rule out abscess**"
  - Chronic JVT phase
    - Palpable tender cord in peripheral neck
    - Radiology request may read "**evaluate tumor extent**"
  - Possible patient histories
    - May be spontaneous clinical event
    - Previous neck surgery, central venous catheterization, drug abuse, trauma, recent infection, hypercoagulable state, or malignancy
  - Venous thromboses incidentally found in ICU patients undergoing CT (especially neck and thoracic veins)
    - Frequently missed by radiologists; include vessels in search pattern

Demographics

- Age
  - Typically older, sicker patient population
  - **Lemierre** in **young healthy** population

Natural History & Prognosis

- IJV thrombophlebitis gives way to thrombosis over 7- to 14-day period with decreased soft tissue swelling
- Prognosis related to cause of IJV thrombosis
- IJV thrombosis itself is self-limited
  - Venous collaterals form to circumvent occluded IJV
- Evaluate extent of thrombus into dural venous sinuses
  - Can result in hemorrhagic venous infarctions of brain

Treatment

- Consider anticoagulant therapy in severe or high-risk cases
  - Significant thromboembolism to lungs is rare
- Check for inherited hypercoagulable state
- Aggressive IV antibiotics given to treat any underlying infection

DIAGNOSTIC CHECKLIST

Consider

- Do not mistake JVT with RPS edema for RPS abscess
  - JVT is common cause of reactive **nonabscess RPS fluid**
- Do not mistake IJV thrombophlebitis as tumor
  - Biggest challenge comes with MR; CECT straightforward
- Suspect Lemierre syndrome if persistent neck pain and sepsis after acute pharyngitis in young patient

Image Interpretation Pearls

- Intraluminal nonenhancing **tubular** nature of JVT is key
- Evaluate extent of JVT (i.e., into dural venous sinuses)

SELECTED REFERENCES

1. Shiran SI et al: The clinical value of cranial CT venography for predicting fusobacterium necrophorum as the causative agent in children with complicated acute mastoiditis. AJNR Am J Neuroradiol. 45(6):761-8, 2024
2. Koritala T et al: Internal jugular vein thrombus in Coronavirus disease (COVID-19). AJR Am J Roentgenol. 217(1):257, 2021

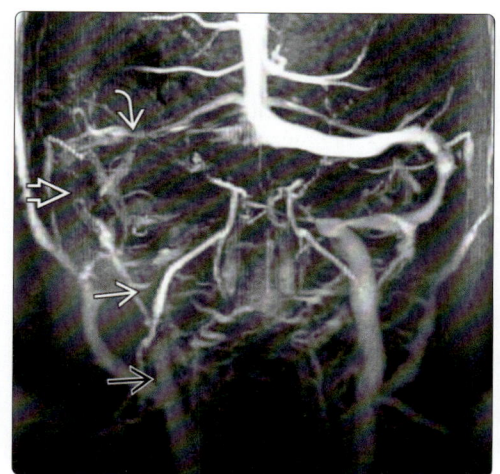
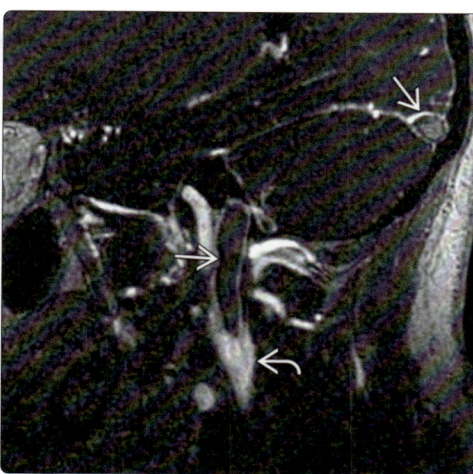

(Left) Coronal MRV shows right transverse ➡ and sigmoid ➡ sinus thrombosis. Note the IJV in the upper neck is also thrombosed ➡. The IJV is patent inferiorly ➡. It is important to confirm thrombosis suspected on MIP images with source images to avoid mistaking hypoplasia for occlusion. (Right) Sagittal enhanced MRV source image in the same patient confirms low-signal acute thrombus extending into the IJV ➡, visible within the patent enhancing portion of the IJV ➡ noted more inferiorly.

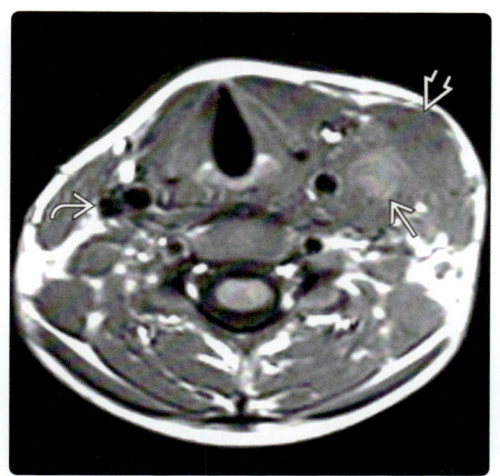
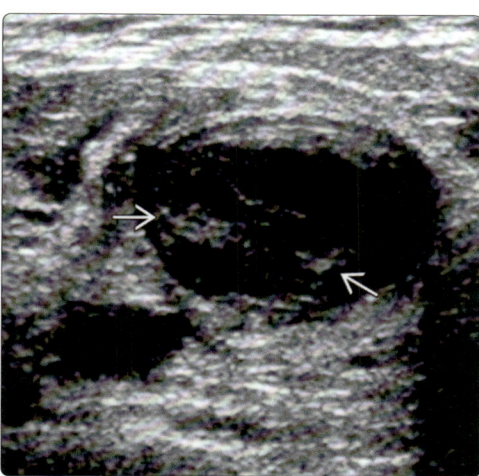

(Left) Axial T1 MR shows a high-signal clot ➡ in the swollen left IJV, indicating acute thrombophlebitis. Adjacent soft tissue planes are obscured by inflammation, including sternocleidomastoid edema ➡. Flow void is visible in the contralateral IJV ➡, although venous signal is variable on MR. (Right) Axial ultrasound shows mixed echogenicity within the IJV, consistent with intraluminal thrombus ➡. The IJV was also incompressible with the ultrasound probe, a key ultrasound clue to diagnosis.

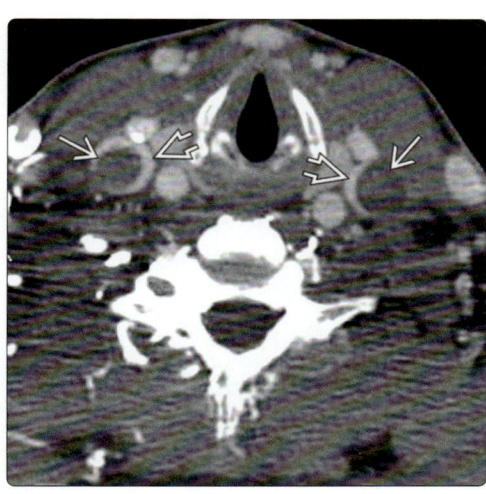
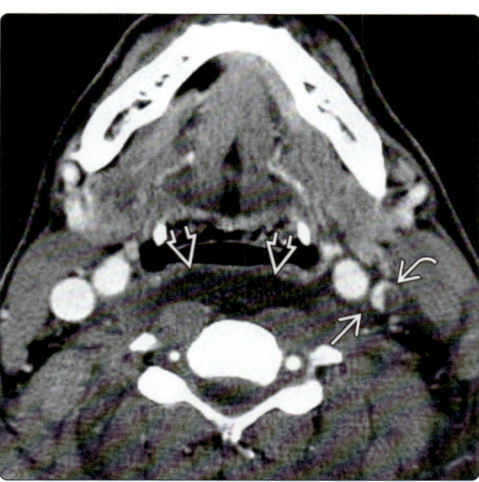

(Left) Axial CECT in a dialysis patient with a history of prior bilateral IJV catheter placement shows an intraluminal low-density clot ➡ in both IJVs. Thin, crescentic enhancement in the patent portion of both IJVs ➡ is visible, indicating partial thrombosis. (Right) Axial CECT of acute left IJV thrombosis shows low-density IJV thrombus ➡. Edema is seen around the left carotid sheath ➡. Extensive retropharyngeal edema is also present without peripheral enhancement ➡. This should not be mistaken for retropharyngeal abscess.

Postpharyngitis Venous Thrombosis (Lemierre)

TERMINOLOGY

- Postanginal sepsis or septicemia, necrobacillosis
- Opportunistic infection causing septic thrombophlebitis & metastatic infection

IMAGING

- CECT: Ipsilateral tonsillar fullness, edema; abscess atypical
  - Internal jugular vein (IJV) ± tributary thrombophlebitis
  - Septic pulmonary emboli
  - Emphysematous osteomyelitis seen in otogenic variant

TOP DIFFERENTIAL DIAGNOSES

- Jugular vein thrombosis; lung metastases

PATHOLOGY

- Usual agent is *Fusobacterium necrophorum*
  - Commensal anaerobic oral cavity bacillus
  - Other agents possible, including *Staphylococcus aureus*
- Historic features
  - Common diagnosis in preantibiotic era
  - Reemergence due to antibiotic resistance
- **Preceding pharyngitis** in **90%** (less frequently, after sinusitis, otitis, dental infection)

CLINICAL ISSUES

- Typical demographic: Teenagers & young adults
  - Usually healthy, immunocompetent patients
- **4-12% mortality** despite aggressive treatment
- **Radiologist often first to suggest diagnosis**
  - May be missed clinically & radiologically

DIAGNOSTIC CHECKLIST

- Classic imaging triad
  - **Pharyngitis + neck vein thrombosis + cavitary pulmonary nodules**
  - Other sites of metastatic infection may occur
- Making this diagnosis is key to accurate antimicrobial therapy & anticoagulation

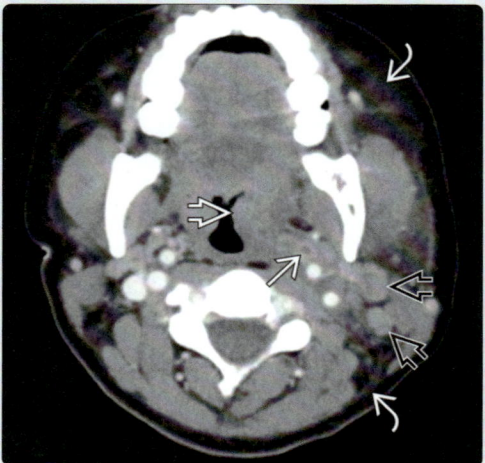
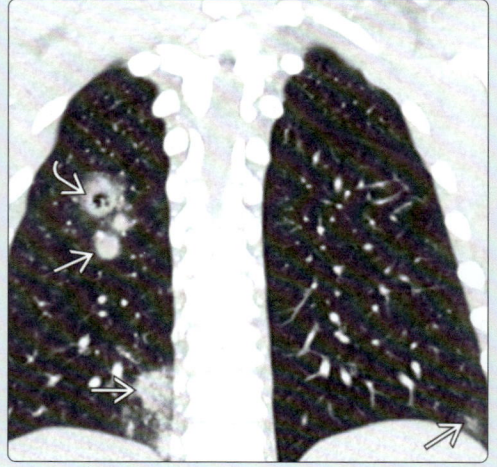

(Left) Axial CECT shows tonsil edema ⮕ and ipsilateral clot in venous tributaries ⮕. Inflammatory changes of fat stranding ⮕ and reactive lymph nodes ⮕ are noted. (Right) Coronal CECT in the same patient shows the characteristic appearance of multiple pulmonary nodules ⮕, some with a cavitary appearance ⮕, in this patient with postpharyngitis venous thrombosis (Lemierre syndrome). Blood cultures grew out of Fusobacterium necrophorum.

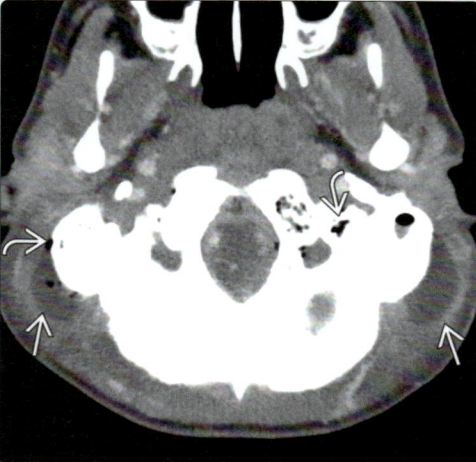
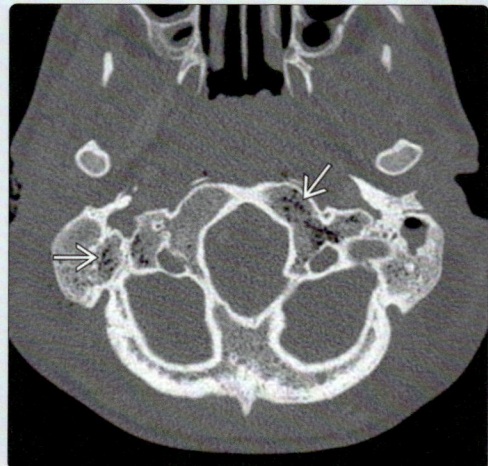

(Left) Axial CECT shows bilateral mastoid tip abscesses ⮕ in a patient with otogenic variant Lemierre syndrome. The presence of gas is a hallmark of this condition and should suggest the presence of Fusobacterium necrophorum. Note areas of gas ⮕ in the abscess and bone (no history of needle intervention). (Right) Axial bone CT in the same patient shows classic findings of emphysematous osteomyelitis with gas in the skull base ⮕, a hallmark of Fusobacterium necrophorum infection in otogenic variant Lemierre syndrome.

Postpharyngitis Venous Thrombosis (Lemierre)

TERMINOLOGY

Synonyms

- Postanginal sepsis, necrobacillosis

Definitions

- Opportunistic infection causing septic thrombophlebitis & metastatic infection
  - Complication of recent pharyngotonsillitis or other upper respiratory infection (sinus, ear)

IMAGING

General Features

- Best diagnostic clue
  - Adolescent or young adult with ipsilateral tonsillar fullness, edema; abscess atypical
  - Internal jugular vein (IJV) ± tributary thrombophlebitis
  - Multiple cavitary pulmonary nodules
- Location
  - **Tonsil** most common **primary source**
  - IJV or venous tributary thrombosis
  - **Metastatic infection** favors **lungs** > joints

CT Findings

- CECT
  - Tonsil fullness, edema, or, less commonly, abscess
  - Ipsilateral vein thrombosis, usually IJV, but other small venous tributaries often involved
  - Neck inflammatory changes
    - Fat stranding, edema, retropharyngeal effusion, reactive adenopathy
  - Metastatic seeding: **Pulmonary** (80%) > joints (15%)
    - Pulmonary septic emboli classically cavitary
  - Otogenic variant *Fusobacterium necrophorum* mastoiditis may occur
    - Bone CT: Look for emphysematous osteomyelitis
    - CTV: Thrombosis beyond sigmoid sinus & jugular
    - CTA: Internal carotid artery narrowing &/or pseudoaneurysm may occur

MR Findings

- CECT best screening exam
- MR best for intracranial & orbital complications
  - Meningitis, abscess, cavernous sinus thrombosis
  - Antegrade or retrograde venous thrombosis possible

Imaging Recommendations

- Best imaging tool
  - CECT: Best for vein thrombosis & pulmonary nodules
  - MR: For suspected intracranial & orbital involvement
  - CT chest for pulmonary septic emboli

DIFFERENTIAL DIAGNOSIS

Jugular Vein Thrombosis

- Secondary to indwelling catheter, tumor compression/invasion, prothrombotic syndromes
- Other causes of septic thrombophlebitis

Lung Metastases

- Primary tumor often known
- Sepsis not part of clinical picture

PATHOLOGY

General Features

- Etiology
  - Usual agent is *F. necrophorum*
    - Pathogenic with altered host defenses
    - Pharyngitis → direct or venolymphatic spread → parapharyngeal & carotid spaces
    - **Preceding pharyngitis** in **90%** (less frequently, after sinusitis, otitis, dental infection)
  - Polymicrobial bacteremia common (33%)
- Reemergence today due to antibiotic resistance

CLINICAL ISSUES

Presentation

- Most common signs/symptoms
  - Antecedent upper respiratory tract infection
    - Pharyngitis > peritonsillar abscess > otitis media
- Other signs/symptoms
  - Sore throat, fever, dyspnea, myalgias
  - Tender swollen neck
  - Sepsis ~ 7 days post resolved pharyngitis
- Clinical profile
  - Most common in 15- to 24-year-old healthy patients

Demographics

- Age
  - Most commonly seen in teenagers & young adults
    - Usually healthy, immunocompetent patients
  - M:F = 2:1

Natural History & Prognosis

- **High mortality**, even with treatment **(4-12%)**
- Radiologist may be first to suggest diagnosis
  - Not recognized in 1/3 of cases, or diagnosed late
- Significant risk of ongoing thromboembolic complications & mortality after initial presentation
  - ↑ risk in patients with intracranial involvement

Treatment

- Antimicrobial therapy
  - Broad-spectrum antibiotics may not cover *Fusobacterium*
- Anticoagulation often used but controversial
- Rare ligation of involved veins & abscess drainage

DIAGNOSTIC CHECKLIST

Image Interpretation Pearls

- Classic imaging triad: **Pharyngitis + ipsilateral neck vein thrombosis + cavitary pulmonary nodules**

Reporting Tips

- Consider this diagnosis with unexplained neck vein thrombosis to allow early treatment

SELECTED REFERENCES

1. Shiran SI et al: The clinical value of cranial CT venography for predicting fusobacterium necrophorum as the causative agent in children with complicated acute mastoiditis. AJNR Am J Neuroradiol. 45(6):761-8, 2024
2. George E et al: Atypical thrombophlebitis patterns in head and neck infections. Neuroradiol J. 36(6):760-5, 2023

Carotid Body Paraganglioma

TERMINOLOGY

- Carotid body tumor

IMAGING

- Vascular mass splaying external & internal carotid arteries
- Rapid dynamic enhancement on CT & MR
- Dynamic contrast-enhanced MR time-signal intensity curve (TIC) immediately follows arterial TIC
  - Rapid peak & early washout
- Serpentine or punctate vascular flow voids ("pepper") on MR, particularly in large lesions
- Hypoechoic, vascular mass on duplex ultrasound
- Arteriovenous shunting on angiography

TOP DIFFERENTIAL DIAGNOSES

- Carotid space schwannoma or neurofibroma
- Carotid artery pseudoaneurysm or ectasia
- Vagal paraganglioma
- Jugulodigastric lymph node

- **Normal carotid body on CTA**: Usually tiny, evaluate for paraganglioma if > 6 mm size

PATHOLOGY

- Multiple gene mutations (familial & sporadic)
  - Paraganglioma syndromes: *SDH* genes
  - Multiple endocrine neoplasia (MEN) syndromes
  - von Hippel-Lindau syndrome, NF1
- Staging: Shamblin grouping (types I, II, III, IIIb)

CLINICAL ISSUES

- Slow-growing, painless, pulsatile mass
- Catecholamine-secreting carotid body paraganglioma rare
- Related to chronic hypoxia in some patients
- Surgical excision treatment of choice
- Preoperative embolization of larger lesions

DIAGNOSTIC CHECKLIST

- CT & MR appearances are diagnostic
- Imaging surveillance with MR for familial disease

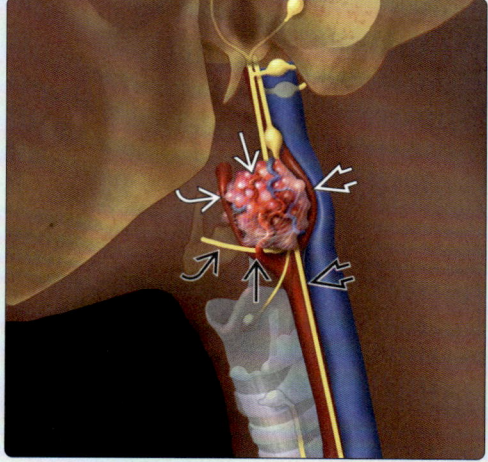
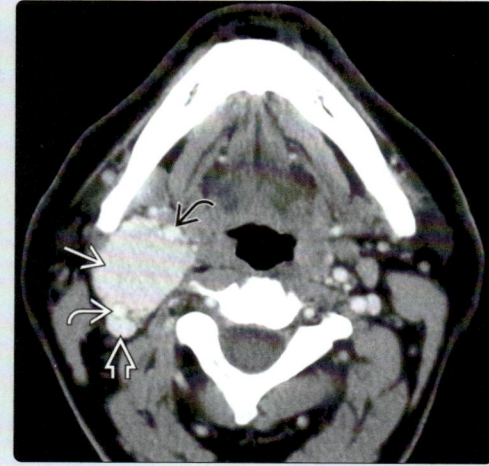

(Left) Lateral graphic depicts a carotid body paraganglioma (CBP) at the carotid bifurcation ➡, splaying the internal carotid artery (ICA) ➡ and external carotid artery (ECA) ➡. The main arterial feeder is the ascending pharyngeal artery ➡. The vagus ➡ and hypoglossal ➡ nerves are in close proximity. (Right) Axial CECT shows a homogeneously enhancing right CBP ➡ between the ECA ➡ displaced anteromedially and the ICA ➡ displaced posterolaterally. Note that the internal jugular vein (IJV) ➡ is displaced posteriorly.

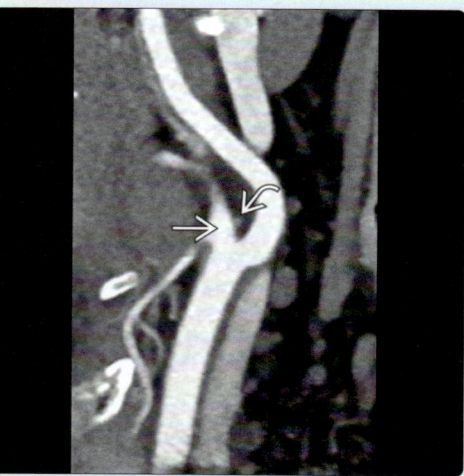
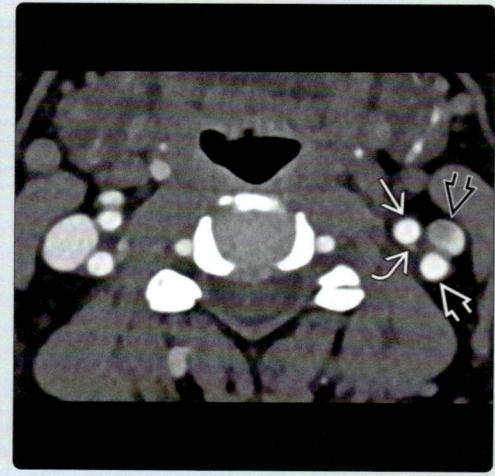

(Left) Sagittal oblique CTA MIP reconstruction shows a tiny normal carotid body ➡ at the left carotid bifurcation towards the ECA ➡ origin. A normal carotid body may be detected on CT angiograms and should not be mistaken for a tiny aneurysm. (Right) Axial CTA source image in the same patient shows the tiny normal carotid body ➡. Note the ECA ➡, ICA ➡, and IJV ➡. The normal carotid body measures 1.1-3.9 mm ± 2 standard deviations (SDs) (~ 2 x 2 mm usually). Lesions > 6 mm (2 SDs) should be evaluated for CBP.

TERMINOLOGY

Abbreviations

- Carotid body paraganglioma (CBP)

Synonyms

- Older terms (better avoided): Carotid body tumor, glomus caroticum, chemodectoma, nonchromaffin paraganglioma

Definitions

- Benign vascular tumor arising in **carotid glomus** body located at carotid bifurcation

IMAGING

General Features

- Best diagnostic clue
  - Vascular mass **splaying external carotid artery (ECA) & internal carotid artery (ICA)**
    - ECA displaced anteriorly (anteromedially or anterolaterally); ICA displaced posterolaterally
    - Internal jugular vein (IJV) compressed & displaced laterally or posteriorly
- Location
  - Mass centered at **carotid bifurcation**
  - Typically unilateral; bilateral in 5-10%
- Size
  - Variable; usually 1-6 cm
  - Do not mistake normal carotid body detectable on CT angiograms for CBP
  - **Normal carotid body**: 1.1 to 3.9 mm ± 2 standard deviations (SDs) (~ 2 x 2 mm usually)
    - Lesions > 6 mm (2 SDs): Evaluate for paraganglioma
  - Do not mistake normal carotid body for tiny aneurysm
- Morphology
  - Ovoid mass with broad, lobular surface contour
  - **Circumferential contact** of tumor to ICA predicts surgical classification
    - Type I: < 180°
    - Type II: > 180° & < 270°
    - Type III: > 270°

CT Findings

- NECT
  - Lobular mass splaying ECA & ICA
  - Density similar to muscles
- CECT
  - **Avidly enhancing** mass at carotid bifurcation
  - Extends cephalad from carotid bifurcation
  - Dynamic enhancement rapid compared to nerve sheath tumors & other masses
- CTA
  - Oblique sagittal reconstruction shows enhancing tumor in "Y" of carotid bifurcation

MR Findings

- T1WI
  - Mass signal similar to muscle
  - **Salt & pepper** appearance in larger lesions
    - "Salt": High-signal areas within tumor parenchyma
      - Secondary to subacute hemorrhage
      - Seen only in larger tumors
      - **Uncommon finding** of limited diagnostic value
    - "Pepper": Hypointense serpentine or punctate vascular channels show **flow void**
      - Expected finding in tumors > 2 cm
      - May be seen on tumor margin or within fibrous matrix of tumor parenchyma
- T2WI
  - Mildly hyperintense compared to muscle with "salt & pepper" heterogeneity
- T1WI C+
  - Intense, **rapid dynamic enhancement**
  - Larger high-velocity flow voids still visible
  - Dynamic contrast-enhanced MR time-signal intensity curve (TIC) immediately follows arterial TIC
    - Rapid peak & early washout due to high vascularity & arteriovenous shunting

Ultrasonographic Findings

- **Hypoechoic** mass at carotid artery bifurcation
- Extensive vascularity on color Doppler images
- **Low-resistance** waveform on duplex scan

Angiographic Findings

- Splaying of ICA & ECA on early arterial images
- Prolonged, intense **tumor blush**
- **Arteriovenous shunting** creates "early vein" phenomenon
- **Ascending pharyngeal** artery is typical arterial feeder
- Lucency between tumor blush & ICA lumen predicts less adherent (type I) lesion
- Angle of bifurcation predicts resectability
  - Splaying > 90° indicates less easily resected

Imaging Recommendations

- Best imaging tool
  - CECT or MR + angiography prior to surgery
- Protocol advice
  - Angiography useful preoperatively
    - Provide vascular **roadmap** for surgeon
    - Embolization for prophylactic hemostasis

DIFFERENTIAL DIAGNOSIS

Carotid Space Neurogenic Tumors

- Sporadic or associated with neurofibromatosis type 1 (NF1) (neurofibroma) or type 2 (schwannoma)
- Fusiform, enhancing mass in carotid space
- **CT low density**, especially neurofibroma
- Does not splay carotid bifurcation, no arteriovenous shunting on DSA
- Dynamic contrast-enhanced MR TIC shows slow, low peak enhancement
  - No rapid peak & rapid washout (which is seen in paragangliomas)

Vagal Paraganglioma

- Older term: Glomus vagale
- Posterolateral high oropharyngeal mass, 1-2 cm below skull base; often asymptomatic but may present with vagal neuropathy

Carotid Artery Pseudoaneurysm

- History of trauma or dissection; pulsatile mass

- Carotid artery mass with complex signal

Ectatic or Tortuous Carotid Artery

- Older patient with atherosclerosis or hypertension

Jugulodigastric Lymph Node

- Asymptomatic "pulsatile" mass
- Enlarged node around carotid space vessels; no ICA/ECA splaying

PATHOLOGY

General Features

- Etiology
  - Arise from carotid glomus bodies (paraganglia)
- Genetics
  - Multiple **gene mutations** in familial & sporadic types
    - *SDH* gene: Paraganglioma syndromes
      - □ Succinate dehydrogenase: Krebs cycle enzyme
      - □ Hypoxia mediators & VEGF lead to hyperplasia, angiogenesis, & neoplasia
      - □ *SDHC* & *SDHD*: Primarily head & neck paragangliomas
      - □ *SDHD* subtype has higher penetrance, especially when inherited from father
      - □ *SDHB* subtype has higher risk of malignant transformation & metastasis
      - □ *SDHB*: Primarily retroperitoneal sympathetic chain paraganglioma & pheochromocytoma
    - *RET* protooncogene: Multiple endocrine neoplasia (MEN) syndromes (MEN2A)
    - *NF1* gene
    - *VHL* gene: von Hippel-Lindau syndrome
      - □ *VHL* & *NF1* associated with pheochromocytomas more commonly
- Associated abnormalities
  - **Paraganglioma syndromes**
    - Multiple head & neck paragangliomas
    - Adrenal pheochromocytoma in some subtypes
  - **MEN type 2 syndromes**
    - Medullary thyroid carcinoma; adrenal pheochromocytoma
  - **von Hippel-Lindau** syndrome
    - Hemangioblastoma, endolymphatic sac tumor
    - Renal & pancreatic tumors & cysts
    - Adrenal pheochromocytoma
  - **NF1**
    - Uncommonly head & neck paragangliomas

Staging, Grading, & Classification

- **Shamblin grouping**
  - Type I: Small tumor, easily dissected within periadvential plane
  - Type II: Larger tumor, adherent to & partially encasing carotid arteries
  - Type III: Large tumor, intimately adherent to & completely encasing carotid arteries
  - Type IIIb: Modification of original description; includes adherent tumors of smaller size

Gross Pathologic & Surgical Features

- Lobulated, reddish-purple mass with fibrous pseudocapsule

Microscopic Features

- **Chief cells** form characteristic nests (**zellballen**)

CLINICAL ISSUES

Presentation

- Most common signs/symptoms
  - Slow-growing, **painless**, **pulsatile** mass
- Other signs/symptoms
  - Vagal ± hypoglossal neuropathy in 20%
  - Catecholamine-secreting CBP rare
    - May include paroxysmal hypertension, palpitations, flushing, & irritability
- Clinical profile
  - **Sporadic**
    - Most common presentation (80-90%)
    - Multicentric paragangliomas in 2-10%
  - **Familial**
    - Variably reported (10-50%)
    - Younger patients (2nd-4th decades)
    - Multiple tumors reported (25-75%)
  - **Hypoxic**/hyperplastic
    - Physiologic response due to chronic hypoxia
    - Cyanotic heart disease, COPD, high altitude

Demographics

- Age
  - Most common in **4th & 5th decades**
- Sex
  - Overall slight male predilection; **hypoxic type 8x** more common in **males**
- Epidemiology
  - CBP most common site for head & neck paragangliomas

Natural History & Prognosis

- Surgical outcome related to Shamblin classification
  - Vagal & other neuropathies in higher group
- Malignant transformation uncommon (5-10%)
  - More common in carotid body than other head & neck paragangliomas
  - Histology unreliable; diagnosed if metastasis seen

Treatment

- Surgical **excision** treatment of choice
- Preoperative **embolization** of larger lesions
- Radiotherapy in poor surgical candidates

DIAGNOSTIC CHECKLIST

Image Interpretation Pearls

- Arterial velocity flow voids ("pepper") suggestive
- When CBP suspected, look for **multiple lesions**
  - Contralateral carotid bifurcation
  - High carotid space (vagal paraganglioma)
  - Jugular foramen (jugular paraganglioma)

SELECTED REFERENCES

1. Verdikhanov NI et al: Long-term results of carotid body tumours surgery and predictive analytics on metastatic disease and recurrence. Vascular. ePub, 2024
2. Nguyen RP et al: Carotid body detection on CT angiography. AJNR Am J Neuroradiol. 32(6):1096-9, 2011

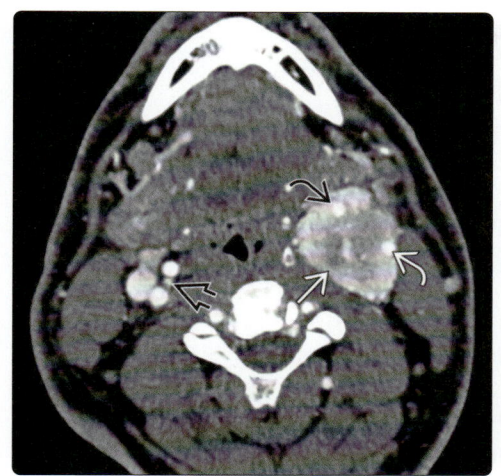

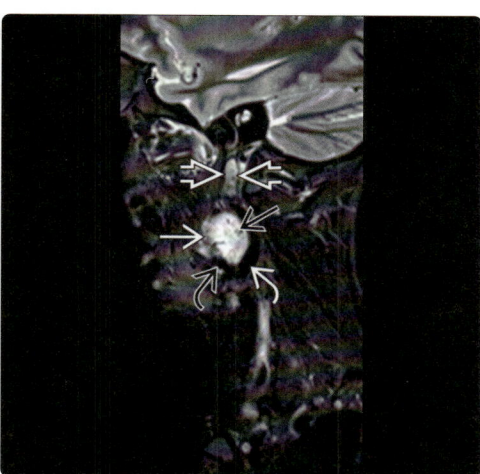

(Left) *Axial CECT with early arterial-phase contrast shows a heterogeneously enhancing left CBP ➡. The mass partially encases the ECA ➡ and ICA ➡, indicating a Shamblin group II or III tumor. A tiny CBP is seen on the right ➡. The patient likely has familial paragangliomas.* **(Right)** *Sagittal T2 STIR MR in another patient shows a hyperintense CBP ➡ with internal flow voids ("pepper") ➡, splaying the ECA anteriorly ➡ and the ICA posteriorly ➡. Also, note a small vagal paraganglioma ➡, located just below the skull base.*

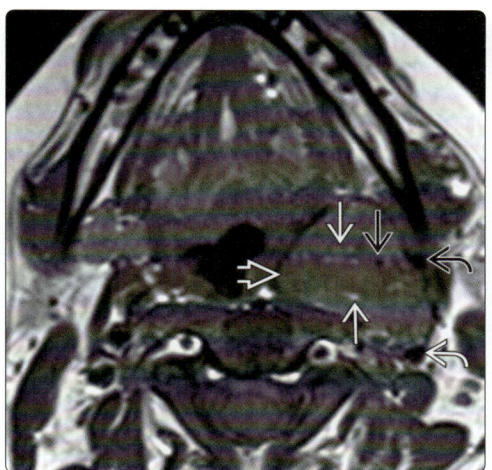

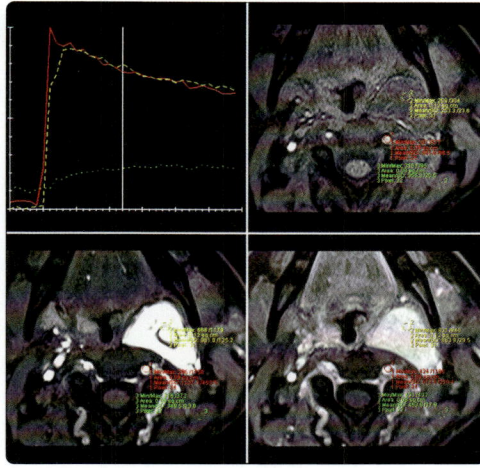

(Left) *Axial T1 MR in the same patient shows the large left CBP ➡ with the "salt" ➡ (subacute blood) and "pepper" ➡ (flow voids) appearance. Note anterolateral ECA ➡ and posterolateral ICA ➡ displacement.* **(Right)** *Axial dynamic T1 C+ MR time-signal intensity curve (TIC) shows that the vascular CBP (yellow ROI and curve) immediately follows arterial TIC (red) with early peak and rapid washout. Early and late arterial- and venous-phase source images show ROIs on CBP (yellow), left vertebral artery (red), and muscle (green).*

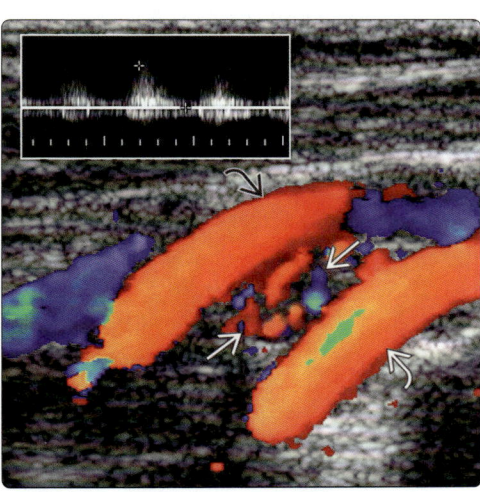

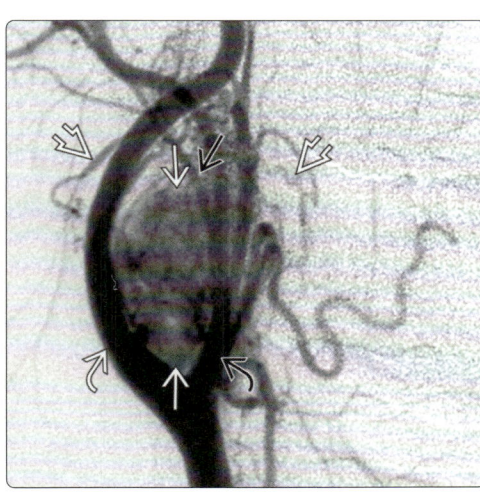

(Left) *Color Doppler US of a carotid bifurcation mass located between the ECA ➡ anteriorly and the ICA ➡ posteriorly shows a highly vascular CBP ➡. Waveform analysis (inset) shows low-resistance characteristics.* **(Right)** *Lateral common carotid angiogram in the late arterial phase demonstrates intense CBP blush ➡ between the ECA ➡ and the ICA ➡. Note enlarged ECA branches ➡ and early enlarged draining veins ➡ due to arteriovenous shunting.*

TERMINOLOGY

- Vagal paraganglioma (PGL): Better term
- Glomus vagale paraganglioma: Older term

IMAGING

- Avidly enhancing mass in nasopharyngeal carotid space centered ~ 2 cm below jugular foramen
  - Displaces internal carotid artery anteromedially
  - Displaces internal jugular vein posterolaterally
  - Displaces parapharyngeal fat anterolaterally
  - Displaces styloid process laterally & slightly anteriorly
- Serpentine or punctate flow voids ("pepper") on MR
- Hyperintense on T2WI & STIR
- Dynamic contrast-enhanced MR time-signal intensity curve (TIC) immediately follows arterial TIC
  - Rapid peak & early washout

TOP DIFFERENTIAL DIAGNOSES

- Carotid space schwannoma/neurofibroma
- Sympathetic schwannoma
- Carotid space meningioma
- Carotid body paraganglioma

PATHOLOGY

- Arises from glomus bodies in nodose ganglion
- Multiple gene mutations (familial & sporadic): PGL, multiple endocrine neoplasia type 2, & von Hippel Lindau syndromes

CLINICAL ISSUES

- Painless, pulsatile lateral cervical mass
- Vagal neuropathy most common
- CNIX, CNXI, & CNXII neuropathies (larger tumors)
- Multicentric PGLs fairly common
- Surgical excision vs. observation
  - Certain loss of vagal function after surgery

DIAGNOSTIC CHECKLIST

- When vagal PGL is suspected, look for multiple lesions
- Imaging surveillance with MR in familial disease

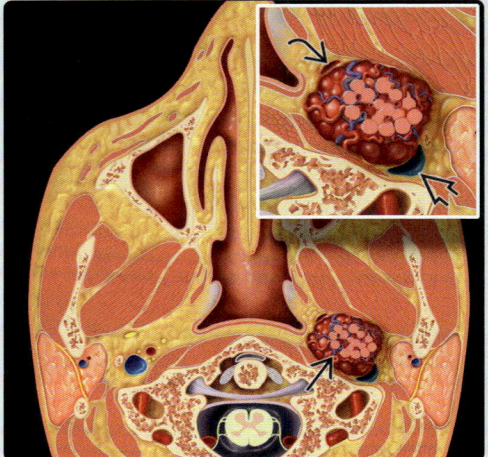
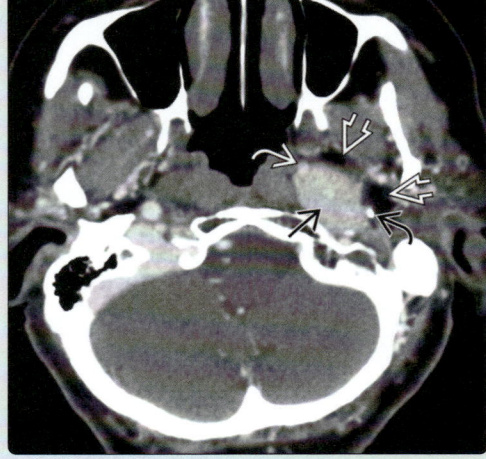

(Left) Axial graphic depicts a vagal paraganglioma (PGL) ⟶ located in the nasopharyngeal carotid space (CS). The mass is interposed between & displacing the internal carotid artery (ICA) ⟶ & internal jugular vein (IJV) ⟶ (inset). (Right) Axial CECT shows a large, ovoid, diffusely enhancing vagal PGL adjacent to the skull base ⟶, centered high in the left CS, medial to the styloid process ⟶, which is displaced laterally & slightly anteriorly. Note displacement of ICA ⟶ anteromedially & parapharyngeal fat ⟶ anterolaterally.

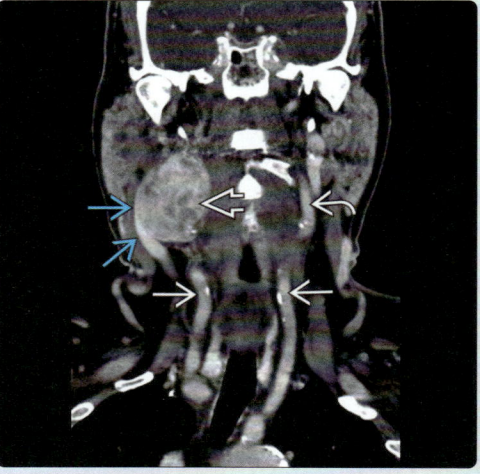
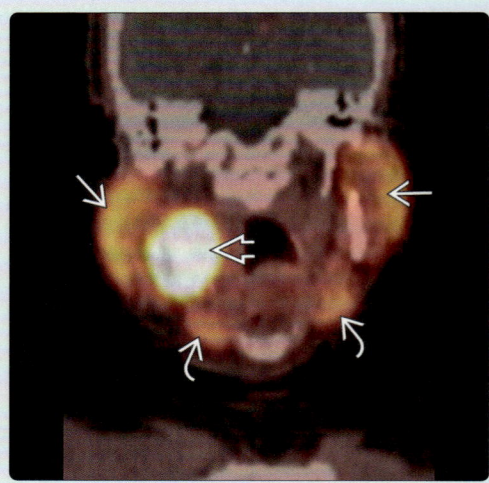

(Left) Coronal CECT shows an enhancing right vagal PGL ⟶ located a few centimeters below the skull base, displacing the right IJV ⟶ laterally. Note that the right ICA is not demonstrated here, as it is displaced anteromedially by the vagal PGL, whereas the left ICA ⟶ & bilateral CCA ⟶ are seen. (Right) Coronal Ga-68 DOTATATE PET shows intense radiotracer uptake ⟶ due to expression of somatostatin receptors in neuroendocrine tumor, PGL. Note physiologic parotid ⟶ & submandibular ⟶ salivary gland uptake.

TERMINOLOGY

Abbreviations
- Vagal paraganglioma (PGL): Better term
  - Better to avoid term glomus vagale PGL, which may be confused with glomus bodies & tumors that arise from them (as in subcutaneous glomus tumors called glomangiomas)

Synonyms
- Glomus vagale PGL: Older term

Definitions
- Benign vascular tumor arising in glomus bodies associated with **nodose ganglion** of vagus nerve

IMAGING

General Features
- Best diagnostic clue
  - Avidly enhancing mass high in **carotid space**
  - Between internal carotid artery (ICA) & internal jugular vein (IJV)
    - Vagus nerve lies within carotid sheath in posterior notch formed by ICA & IJV
- Location
  - Upper (nasopharyngeal) aspect of carotid space
    - Displaces **ICA anteromedially**
    - Displaces **IJV posterolaterally**
    - Displaces **parapharyngeal fat anterolaterally**
    - Displaces **styloid process laterally** &, to lesser extent, anteriorly
  - Arises from glomus bodies (paraganglia)
    - Vagus nerve nodose ganglion
    - 1-2 cm below floor of jugular foramen in nasopharyngeal carotid space
  - Large tumors may extend caudad toward carotid bifurcation or cephalad into jugular foramen
  - **Does not splay** carotid bifurcation
    - Consider multifocal PGL with carotid body tumor if splaying of carotid is seen
  - More common on right side of neck
- Size
  - Variable, usually 2-8 cm
  - Often large at diagnosis
- Morphology
  - Ovoid, lobulated, well marginated
  - Often **elongated** & **fusiform** in craniocaudal direction on coronal or sagittal images

CT Findings
- NECT
  - Soft tissue density similar to muscle
  - Permeative bone change if extension to skull base
- CECT
  - **Avidly enhancing** mass in upper carotid space
  - Bulk of tumor extracranial but may extend into jugular foramen
- CTA
  - Early enhancing mass just below skull base that displaces internal carotid anteromedially

MR Findings
- T1WI
  - Fusiform mass with signal similar to muscle
  - **Salt & pepper** appearance in larger lesions
    - "Salt": High T1 signal foci within vagal PGL
      - Secondary to subacute hemorrhage, seen in larger tumors
      - Uncommon finding, limited diagnostic value
    - "Pepper": Low T1 signal foci with vagal PGL
      - Serpentine or punctate **flow voids**
      - Expected finding in tumors > 2 cm
- T2WI
  - Mildly hyperintense with flow voids
- STIR
  - Moderately hyperintense with flow voids
- T1WI C+
  - Intense, **rapid dynamic enhancement**
  - Larger high-velocity flow voids still visible
  - Dynamic contrast-enhanced MR time-signal intensity curve (TIC) immediately follows arterial TIC
    - Rapid peak & early washout due to high vascularity & arteriovenous shunting
- MRA
  - Displaces ICA anteromedially

Angiographic Findings
- Anteromedial **displacement of ICA** just below skull base (without widening of carotid bifurcation)
- Tortuous, dilated feeding vessels
- Ascending pharyngeal artery is main arterial feeder
- Early, prolonged, intense **tumor blush**
- Arteriovenous shunting creates "early vein" phenomenon
- Angiographic goals
  - Search for multicentric tumors
  - Provide vascular **roadmap** for surgeon
  - Evaluate cervicocerebral circulation in case sacrifice of major vessel necessary
  - **Embolization** for prophylactic hemostasis

Nuclear Medicine Findings
- **Somatostatin receptor** scintigraphy (In-111 octreotide scan, Ga-68 DOTATATE PET)
  - Confirmation of indeterminate lesions
  - Detection of multiple lesions

Imaging Recommendations
- Best imaging tool
  - Contrast-enhanced MR or CT
- Protocol advice
  - Field of view to cover from skull base to carotid bifurcation on MR & CT

DIFFERENTIAL DIAGNOSIS

Carotid Space Neurogenic Tumor
- Sporadic, or associated with neurofibromatosis type 1 (neurofibroma) or type 2/schwannomatosis (schwannoma)
- No arteriovenous shunting on DSA
- **Like vagal PGL, displace** ICA anteromedially & IJV posterolaterally

- Dynamic contrast-enhanced MR TIC shows slow, low peak enhancement
  - No rapid peak & rapid washout (which is seen in PGL)
- Schwannoma: Fusiform mass, uniform enhancement
  - Cystic changes in larger lesions
- Neurofibroma: Fusiform mass, irregular if plexiform
  - CT low-dense, MR T2/STIR hyperintense
  - Variable enhancement, less conspicuous on CT

Sympathetic Schwannoma

- Does not separate ICA & IJV (unlike PGL/schwannoma/neurofibroma)
- Instead, it **displaces** both **ICA & IJV together** anteriorly or anterolaterally
- Sympathetic plexus lies **outside carotid sheath** plastered to prevertebral fascia: Posterior to it or between medial carotid space & lateral retropharyngeal space

Carotid Space Meningioma

- Extension of jugular foramen mass

Carotid Body Paraganglioma

- Located lower than vagal PGL, splaying ICA & ECA

Carotid Artery Pseudoaneurysm

- History of trauma or dissection
- Carotid artery mass with complex signal

Jugular Vein Thrombosis

- Nonenhancing thrombus with edema

PATHOLOGY

General Features

- Etiology
  - Arises from **glomus bodies** (paraganglia)
    - Located in nodose ganglion of vagus nerve
    - Composed of chemoreceptor cells derived from neuroectoderm of primitive **neural crest**
- Genetics
  - Multiple **gene mutations** identified in familial & sporadic types
  - **PGL** syndromes
    - SDH genes; *SDHD* & *SDHB* subtypes
  - Multiple endocrine neoplasia (**MEN**) syndromes
    - *RET* protooncogene (10q11.2)
  - von Hippel-Lindau (**VHL**) syndrome
    - *VHL* gene (3p25-26)
- Associated abnormalities
  - Multiple head & neck PGL
  - Adrenal pheochromocytomas (PGL & MEN2)
  - Medullary thyroid carcinoma (MEN2)
  - Hemangioblastomas, endolymphatic sac tumors, renal & pancreatic tumors & cysts (VHL)

Microscopic Features

- Chief cells form characteristic nests (**zellballen**)
- Electromicroscopy shows neurosecretory granules

CLINICAL ISSUES

Presentation

- Most common signs/symptoms
  - **Painless, pulsatile** lateral upper neck mass (85%)
- Other signs/symptoms
  - **Vagal neuropathy** by far most common
    - Vocal cord paralysis with hoarseness
    - Variable, reported up to 50%
  - CNIX, CNXI, CNXII injury (10-20%)
    - Particularly larger tumors
  - Horner syndrome uncommon (5%)
  - Pulsatile tinnitus; rarely hormonally active

Demographics

- Age
  - Most common in **4th & 5th** decades
  - Younger presentation in familial cases
- Sex
  - **Female** predominance, M:F ~ 1:2
- Epidemiology
  - **Least common** of head & neck PGLs
    - Carotid body > jugular/tympanic > vagal
    - Vagale: **5%** of head & neck PGLs

Natural History & Prognosis

- Progressive vagal dysfunction as tumor grows
- Higher rate of cranial neuropathy in vagal PGL than other head & neck PGLs
- Malignant tumors uncommon (5-10%)

Treatment

- Options, risks, complications
  - **Surgical excision** vs. **observation**
    - Vagal neuropathy generally indicates surgery
    - Larger or growing tumors may indicate surgery
  - Surgical morbidity is unavoidable
    - **100% loss of vagal function**
      - Even if nerve is anatomically intact
    - Adjunctive procedures mitigate vagal dysfunction
      - Teflon injection for vocal fold medialization
      - Cricopharyngeal myotomy
    - Variable risk to CNIX, CNXI, & CNXII
  - Radiation for lesion control in poor surgical candidates
- Bilateral vagal PGL
  - Important to **preserve at least unilateral** vagus function
  - Surgical excision on 1 side only
    - Side with worse vagal deficit operated
  - Radiotherapy or observation on other side

DIAGNOSTIC CHECKLIST

Image Interpretation Pearls

- MR arterial flow voids ("**pepper**") are highly suggestive
- When vagal PGL is suspected, look for **multiple lesions**
  - Contralateral carotid space (vagal PGL)
  - Carotid bifurcations (carotid body PGL)
  - Temporal bones (jugular/tympanic PGL)

Reporting Tips

- Recommend **surveillance** with MR in familial disease

SELECTED REFERENCES

1. Bellamkonda N et al: Management of bilateral head and neck paragangliomas at a single-institution across four decades. Head Neck. 47(1):386-93, 2024

Vagal Paraganglioma

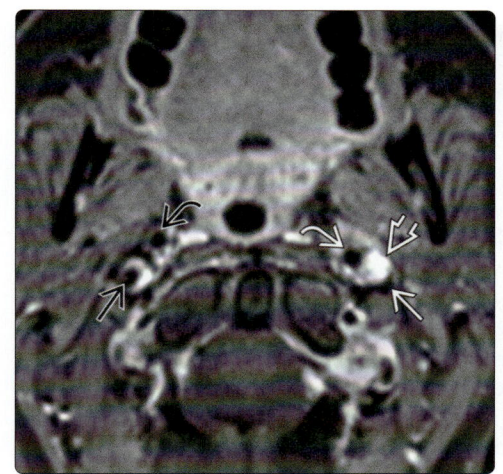

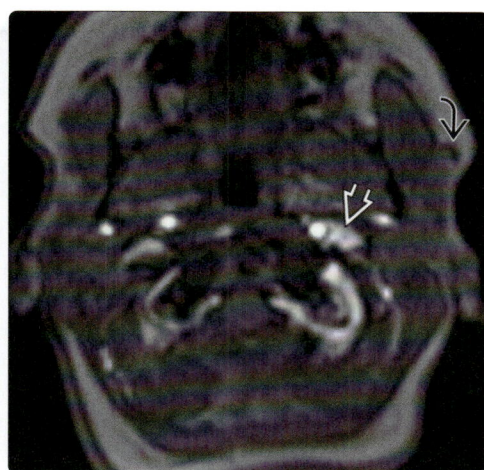

(Left) *Axial T1WI C+ FS MR shows a small, intensely enhancing left CS mass ➡ displacing the left ICA anteromedially ➡ & left IJV posterolaterally ➡. Note the normal right ICA ➡ & right IJV ➡. **(Right)** Axial arterial-phase dynamic contrast-enhanced VIBE MR shows intense enhancement of the left CS mass ➡, suggestive of a hypervascular vagal PGL rather than lymph node or neurogenic tumor. For comparison, note a normal left periparotid lymph node ➡ with no significant arterial-phase enhancement.*

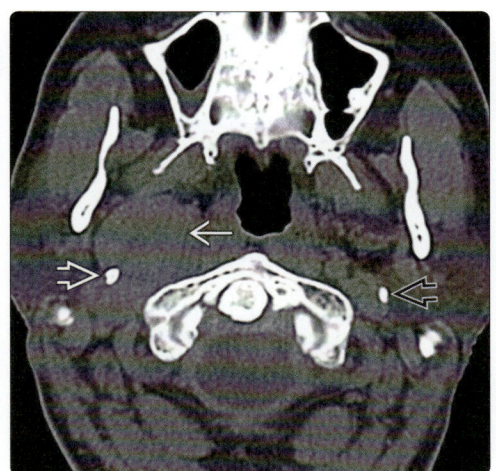

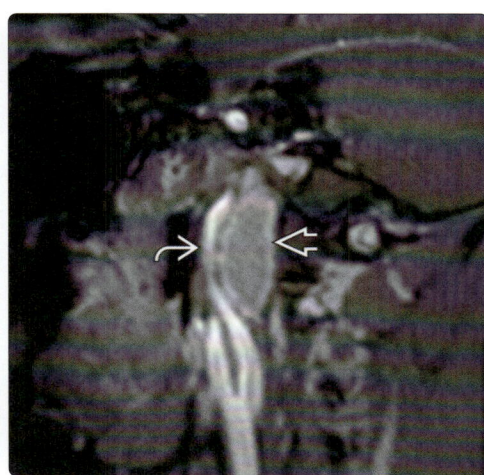

(Left) *Axial NECT shows a vagal PGL centered in the high right CS ➡. The styloid process, even though generally described as located anterior to the CS, is characteristically displaced laterally, & only slightly anteriorly ➡, by vagal PGL. Note the normal location of the left styloid process ➡. **(Right)** Sagittal T1WI C+ MPRAGE MR shows a larger enhancing left vagal PGL ➡, displacing the ICA anteriorly ➡.*

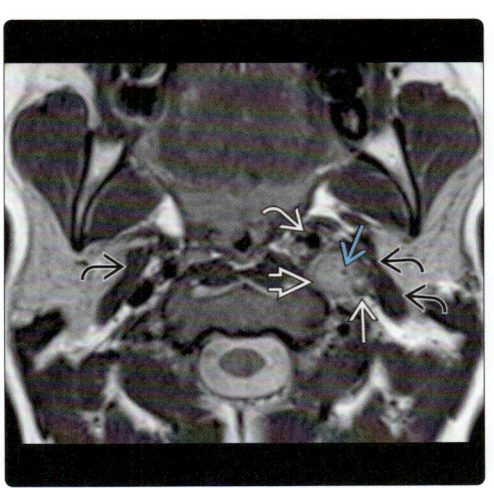

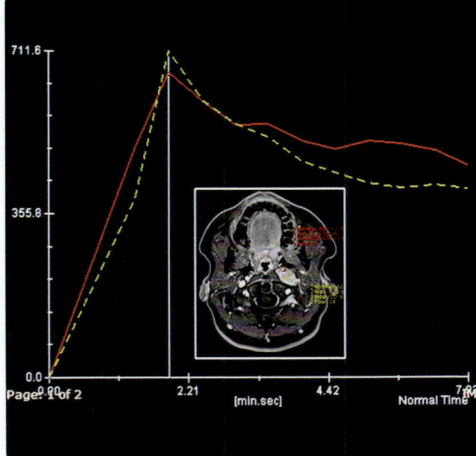

(Left) *Axial T2 MR in the same patient shows hyperintense left CS vagal PGL ➡ with internal tiny vascular flow void ➡, displacing left ICA anteromedially ➡ & IJV posterolaterally ➡. Note the posterior belly of digastric muscle ➡ separating the CS from the deep lobe of the parotid. **(Right)** Axial dynamic T1 C+ MR time-signal intensity curve (TIC) in the same patient shows that vagal PGL (yellow ROI & curve) closely follows ICA arterial TIC (red) with rapid peak & early washout due to high vascularity & arteriovenous shunting.*

Carotid Space Schwannoma

TERMINOLOGY

- **Benign tumor** of **Schwann cells** that wrap around cranial nerve in **carotid space** (CS)
- Nerve of origin: **CNIX-XII**; CNX (vagus nerve) most common

IMAGING

- Fusiform, enhancing CS mass
  - Larger schwannoma: Intramural cystic change
  - **MR: No high-velocity flow voids** characteristic
- Displacement pattern is characteristic
  - Nasopharyngeal CS schwannoma: Displaces parapharyngeal space (PPS) anteriorly and styloid process anterolaterally
  - Oropharyngeal CS schwannoma: Displaces PPS fat anteriorly and posterior belly of digastric laterally
  - Infrahyoid neck CS schwannoma: Displaces to contralateral neck, common carotid artery anteromedially, and posterior cervical space posterolaterally

TOP DIFFERENTIAL DIAGNOSES

- Carotid body paraganglioma; vagal paraganglioma
- CS neurofibroma; CS meningioma
- Vascular lesions (pseudoaneurysm or thrombosis)

PATHOLOGY

- Vagal schwannoma more common than other cranial nerve origins

CLINICAL ISSUES

- Typical presentation
  - Asymptomatic palpable mass
  - May present with dysphagia, internal jugular vein (IJV) occlusion, Horner syndrome, vocal cord paralysis, sleep apnea, sore throat
- Age range: 20-60 years (average: 45)
- **Suprahyoid** CS schwannoma > > infrahyoid
- Preferred treatment: Gross total resection without sacrifice of nerve

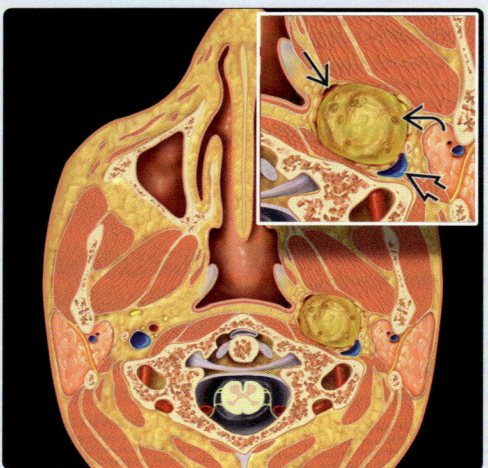
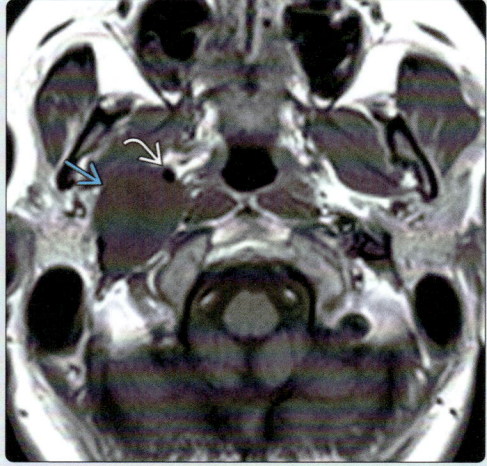

(Left) Axial graphic depicts a typical nasopharyngeal (carotid space) schwannoma. Tumor is seen between anteromedial internal carotid artery (ICA) ➡ and posterolateral internal jugular vein (IJV) ➡. CS schwannomas are typically fusiform, enhancing masses and may contain cystic, nonenhancing areas ➡. (Right) Axial T1 MR shows a right CS mass ➡ isointense to muscle displacing ICA ➡ and PPS fat anteriorly. Lack of flow voids is characteristic of schwannoma and helps differentiate from a paraganglioma.

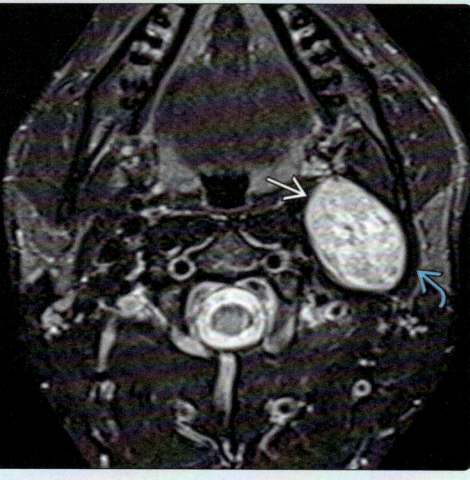
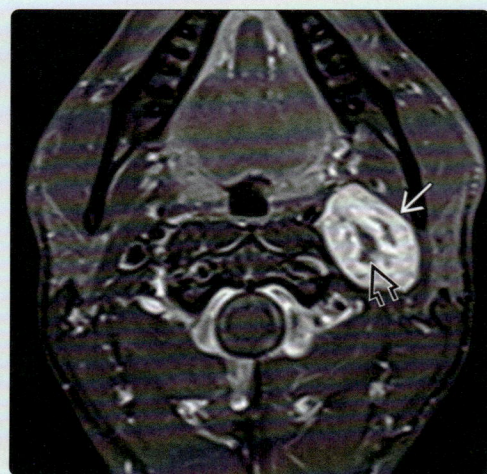

(Left) Axial T2 FS MR shows a circumscribed, hyperintense CS mass ➡ with lateral displacement of the posterior belly of the digastric muscle ➡. The lack of flow voids helps differentiate this schwannoma from a paraganglioma. (Right) Axial T1 C+ FS MR in the same patient shows enhancement of the CS mass ➡ with regions of cystic change ➡, typical of a large schwannoma. CS schwannomas may arise from CNIX-XII or the cervical sympathetic chain but most commonly arise from the vagus nerve (CNX).

TERMINOLOGY

Synonyms

- Neuroma, neurilemmoma

Definitions

- Benign tumor of Schwann cells that wrap around cranial nerve in carotid space (CS)

IMAGING

General Features

- Best diagnostic clue
  - **Fusiform**, enhancing CS mass (CT or MR) **without** flow voids (MR)
- Location
  - CS from nasopharynx above to aortic arch below
- Size
  - Lesions are usually large when clinically detected
  - Range: 2-8 cm
- Morphology
  - Ovoid to fusiform
  - Tumor margins are smooth, sharply circumscribed
- Suprahyoid neck CS schwannoma displacement pattern is characteristic
  - **Nasopharyngeal CS schwannoma**: Displaces **parapharyngeal space (PPS) anteriorly** and styloid process anterolaterally
    - Internal carotid artery (ICA) is usually bowed over anteromedial surface
    - Internal jugular vein (IJV) is often posterolateral and commonly effaced
  - In oropharyngeal CS schwannoma: Displaces PPS fat anteriorly and posterior belly digastric muscle laterally
- Infrahyoid neck CS schwannoma displacement pattern: Thyroid-trachea displaced to contralateral neck, common carotid artery anteromedially, and posterior cervical space posterolaterally
- **Lack of high-velocity flow voids** within tumor allows correct identification of nerve sheath tumor

CT Findings

- NECT
  - Well-circumscribed CS soft tissue density mass
  - Mass density similar to adjacent neck muscles
- CECT
  - Uniform enhancement is rule on CECT
    - Minority are low density even with enhancement
  - Focal areas of absent enhancement seen on CECT if **intramural cystic** change present
- CTA: ICA bowed over anterior surface of schwannoma

MR Findings

- T1WI
  - Variable T1 signal ranging from low to high
    - **No high-velocity flow voids**, even when large
- T2WI
  - Tumor hyperintense compared with muscle
  - **Intramural cysts**, if present, are high-signal foci within tumor
- T1WI C+
  - Dense, homogeneous enhancement is typical

  - Intratumoral nonenhancing cysts often present in larger lesions
- MRA: Anteromedial displacement of ICA without visible arterial supply
  - CS schwannoma itself not visualized on MRA
- MRV: Jugular vein may be flattened or occluded
- DCE may help distinguish schwannoma from paraganglioma

Angiographic Findings

- Angiography is usually unnecessary unless tumor histopathology in doubt
- Scattered contrast "puddles" typical of schwannoma
- No dominant feeding arteries seen
- No arteriovenous shunting or vascular encasement

Imaging Recommendations

- Best imaging tool
  - Enhanced MR best for initial evaluation

DIFFERENTIAL DIAGNOSIS

Carotid Body Paraganglioma

- Mass center: Nestled in common carotid artery bifurcation
- Splays apart external carotid artery and ICA
- MR: High-velocity flow voids in > 2-cm tumor

Vagal Paraganglioma

- Mass center: Nasopharyngeal CS, ~ 2 cm below skull base
- MR: High-velocity flow voids in > 2-cm tumor
- CT: Permeative-erosive bone margins

Carotid Space Neurofibroma

- Mass center: CS
- CECT: Low-density, well-circumscribed CS mass
- MR: Cannot differentiate from vagal schwannoma
- Look for neurofibromatosis type 1 (NF1) association (50%)

Carotid Space Meningioma

- Mass location: Emanates from jugular foramen above into nasopharyngeal CS
- Jugular foramen bony margins on bone CT: Permeative-sclerotic to hyperostotic
- T1WI C+ MR: Centrifugal spread pattern with dural tails

Carotid Artery Pseudoaneurysm in Neck

- Ovoid outpouching of carotid artery
- CECT: Lumen connected to carotid artery lumen
- MR: Complex, ovoid mass in CS

Internal Jugular Vein Thrombosis

- History of IJV instrumentation usually present
- Tubular lesion with central IJV filling defect on enhanced imaging

Sympathetic Chain Schwannoma

- Mass center: Posteromedial to carotid artery and IJV
- Displacement pattern: Pushes both carotid artery and IJV anteriorly/anterolaterally
- MR: No high-velocity flow voids

PATHOLOGY

General Features

- Etiology
  - Arises from Schwann cells wrapping around cranial nerve in CS of extracranial H&N
  - Nerve of origin
    - Nasopharyngeal CS: **CNIX-XII** possible
    - Oropharyngeal CS to aortic arch: **Vagus nerve**
    - **Vagal schwannoma** more common than other cranial nerve origins
- Associated abnormalities
  - Neurofibromatosis type 2

Gross Pathologic & Surgical Features

- White-tan, smooth, encapsulated, sausage-shaped mass

Microscopic Features

- Spindle cells with elongated nuclei
  - Alternating areas of organized, compact cells (Antoni A) and loosely arranged, relatively acellular tissue (Antoni B)
  - Both cell types present in all tumors
- Differentiated neoplastic Schwann cells
  - Malignant transformation is exceedingly rare
  - Melanotic malignant schwannomas have been described as distinct entity
    - May have intrinsic T1 hyperintensity as diagnostic feature
- Immunochemistry
  - Strong, diffuse immunostaining for S100 protein
    - S100 protein: Neural crest marker antigen present in supporting cell of nervous system

CLINICAL ISSUES

Presentation

- Most common signs/symptoms
  - Asymptomatic palpable mass
    - Nasopharyngeal and oropharyngeal CS schwannoma: Posterolateral pharyngeal wall mass
    - Cervical CS schwannoma: Anterolateral neck mass
  - Other signs/symptoms
    - Large suprahyoid schwannoma: May cause dysphagia or IJV occlusion
    - Horner syndrome
    - Vocal cord paralysis (hoarseness)
    - Sleep apnea
    - Sore throat
- Clinical profile
  - Healthy 45-year-old man with asymptomatic suprahyoid, lateral retropharyngeal, or lateral infrahyoid neck mass

Demographics

- Age
  - Range: 20-60 years
  - Average at presentation: 45 years
- Sex
  - Male predominance
- Epidemiology
  - Rare tumor of extracranial H&N

- Suprahyoid CS schwannoma > > infrahyoid CS schwannoma

Natural History & Prognosis

- Delay in diagnosis is frequent due to nonspecific symptoms
- Slow but persistent tumor growth until airway compromise or cosmetic issues supervene
- Vagus nerve preservation is not always possible at surgery
  - If vagus nerve resection required, partial vagal neuropathy is present even if successful reconnection completed

Treatment

- Gross total resection without sacrifice of vagus nerve is treatment of choice
  - Enucleation of tumor with CNX preservation possible in most cases
  - Infrequently, nerve resection occurs at time of tumor removal
    - End-to-end anastomosis of vagus nerve used if short segment removed
    - Nerve graft interposition used if long segment of vagus nerve is removed
  - Severe transient bradycardia may occur during removal
  - Postoperative symptoms in ~ 20% of patients
- Radiation therapy considered for patients who are poor surgical candidates

DIAGNOSTIC CHECKLIST

Consider

- If schwannoma localized to suprahyoid CS, look at jugular foramen for evidence of involvement
  - If jugular foramen involved, imaging findings are characteristic
    - Bone CT: Expanded jugular foramen with sharp, scalloped margins
    - T1WI C+ MR: Enhancing ovoid jugular foramen mass ± intramural cystic change
- Vascular schwannoma may mimic paraganglioma

Image Interpretation Pearls

- Fusiform, sharply circumscribed CS mass **without** high-velocity flow voids = schwannoma/neurofibroma
- Carotid and jugular vessel displacement often predicts likely nerve of origin of CS schwannoma
  - **Vagal nerve** schwannomas typically splay common carotid artery or ICA away from IJV
  - **Sympathetic chain** schwannomas displace vessels together (typically anteriorly/anterolaterally) and do not separate vein and arteries

SELECTED REFERENCES

1. Vasireddi AK et al: The "outline sign": thin hyperenhancing perimeter as an MR imaging feature of meningioma. a useful tool in the temporal bone region for differentiating meningiomas from schwannomas and paragangliomas. AJNR Am J Neuroradiol. 46(2):349-54, 2025
2. Hartmann K et al: 68 Ga-DOTATATE PET to characterize lesions in the neuroaxis. clin Nucl Med. 49(1):9-15, 2024
3. Malla SR et al: Dynamic contrast-enhanced magnetic resonance imaging for differentiating head and neck paraganglioma and schwannoma. Head Neck. 43(9):2611-22, 2021
4. López F et al: Contemporary management of primary parapharyngeal space tumors. Head Neck. 41(2):522-35, 2019

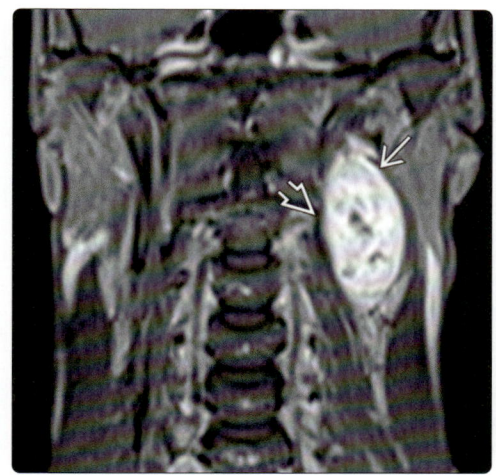

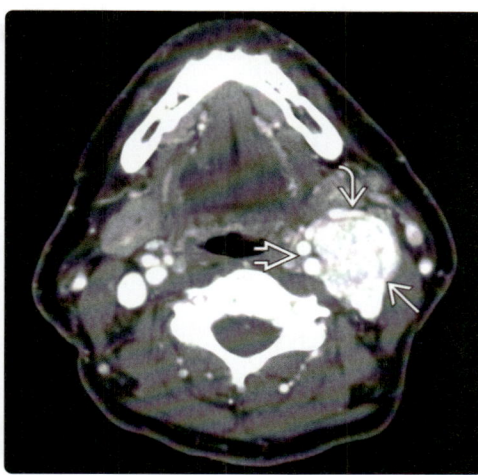

(Left) Coronal T1 C+ FS MR shows a fusiform, enhancing CS ⮕ mass with cystic change, commonly seen in large schwannomas. Note medial location of the ICA ⮕. Vagal schwannomas are more common than other cranial nerve origins in this location. (Right) Axial CECT shows an avidly enhancing, suprahyoid CS mass ⮕. The ICA and external carotid artery ⮕ are displaced medially, typical of schwannoma. Anterior displacement of the IJV ⮕ is unusual. When schwannomas are hypervascular, they may mimic a paraganglioma.

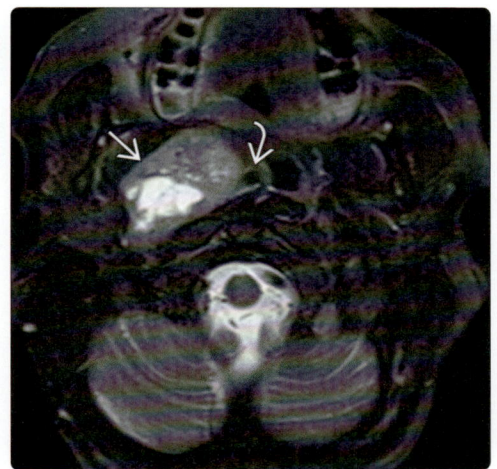

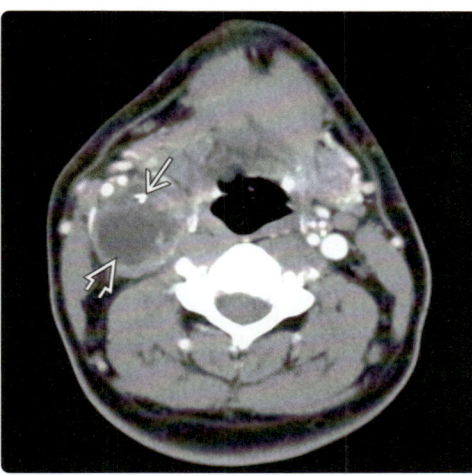

(Left) Axial STIR MR shows a large CS mass ⮕ with cystic change, typical of a CS schwannoma. In this location, the schwannoma may arise from CNIX-XII or the sympathetic chain. Vagal schwannomas are the most common and often splay the common carotid artery or ICA ⮕ away from the IJV. (Right) Axial CECT reveals a mostly cystic schwannoma in the CS just above the hyoid bone. Intramural cystic change ⮕ is a common finding in larger schwannomas. Note the rare calcification ⮕ seen in the anterior tumor wall.

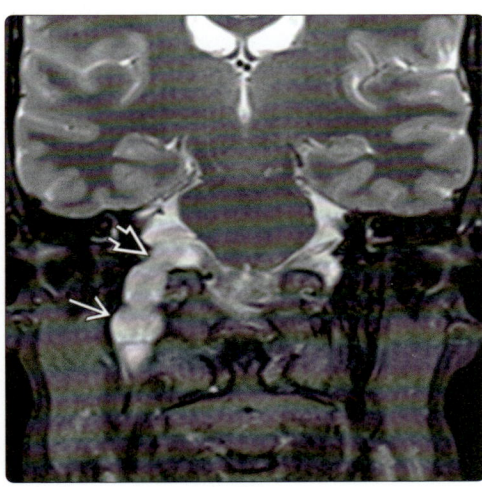

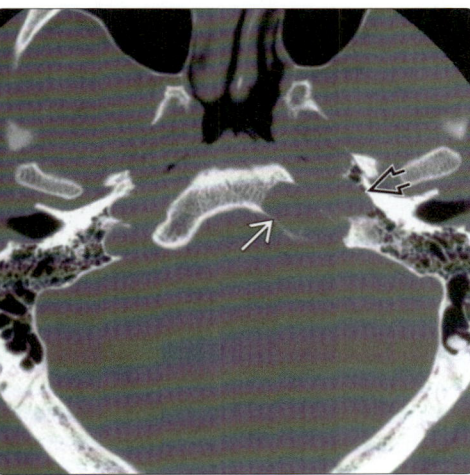

(Left) Coronal T2 FS MR shows a lobular, hyperintense CS mass ⮕ with involvement of the jugular foramen ⮕. The lack of flow voids helps differentiate this schwannoma from the more common paraganglioma in the jugular foramen region. (Right) Axial bone CT in a patient with a CS mass shows a smooth, scalloped appearance of the clivus ⮕, typical of a schwannoma. Nasopharyngeal CS schwannoma remodels the adjacent skull base ⮕. In contrast, a paraganglioma would result in permeative bone changes.

Sympathetic Schwannoma

TERMINOLOGY

- Benign, slow-growing tumor of Schwann cells investing cervical sympathetic chain

IMAGING

- Most common appearance
  - Fusiform enhancing carotid space (CS) mass that displaces both carotid artery and jugular vein anteriorly
- Tumor location
  - Posterior to CS vessels (sympathetic chain lies posterior in CS)
- CECT or enhanced MR findings
  - Ovoid to fusiform enhancing mass in posterior CS
  - Small lesion: Homogeneous enhancement
  - Large lesion: Intratumoral (intramural) nonenhancing cysts may be seen
- CECT often 1st exam for neck mass

TOP DIFFERENTIAL DIAGNOSES

- CS schwannoma/neurofibroma
- Vagal paraganglioma
- Carotid body paraganglioma
- Lateral retropharyngeal lymph node

PATHOLOGY

- Solitary, well-encapsulated tumor arising from peripheral nerve
- Arises from cervical sympathetic chain Schwann cell sheath
- Associated with neurofibromatosis type 2 (multiple schwannomas, meningiomas, and ependymomas)

CLINICAL ISSUES

- Asymptomatic, palpable neck mass
- **Horner syndrome**, headache
- Diagnosing nerve of origin of schwannoma preoperative is crucial in reducing chance of postoperative nerve palsy

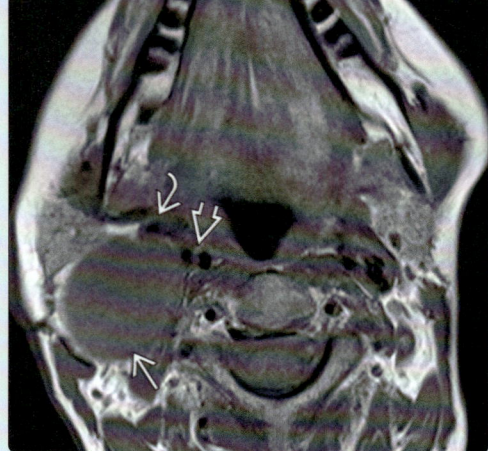
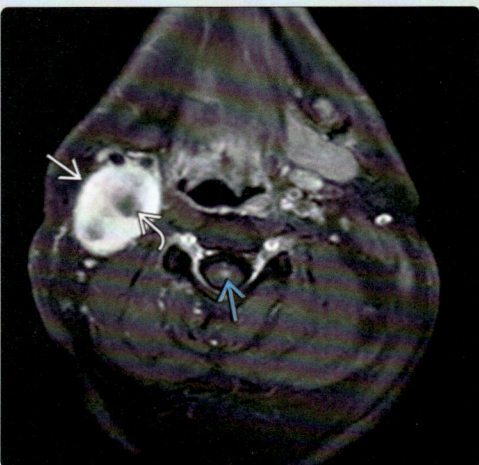

(Left) Axial T1WI MR in a patient with a slow-growing right neck lump shows a well-defined mass ➡ hypo- to isointense to muscle in the right upper neck. The carotid artery ➡ and the internal jugular vein (IJV) ➡ displaced anteromedially suggest sympathetic schwannoma. (Right) Axial T1 C+ FS MR in a patient with a longstanding right neck lump shows more conspicuous enhancement of the lesion in the right neck ➡. There are areas of cystic change ➡ within the lesion. A tiny ependymoma ➡ is seen in the cord.

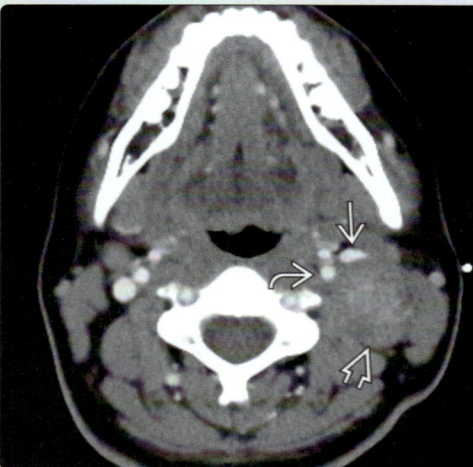
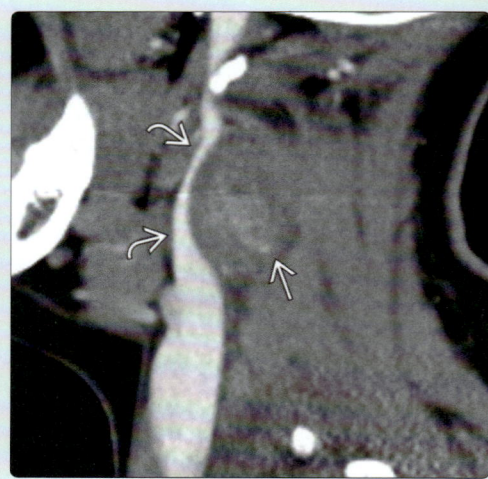

(Left) Axial CECT of a patient with a neck mass demonstrates heterogeneously enhancing, well-defined mass of the suprahyoid neck ➡ underlying the sternocleidomastoid muscle that displaces IJV ➡, internal carotid artery ➡, and external carotid artery branches anteriorly. (Right) Sagittal CECT reformat in the same patient demonstrates a heterogeneously enhancing fusiform mass ➡ that is near isodense to contiguous muscle, displacing the IJV ➡ anteriorly.

Sympathetic Schwannoma

TERMINOLOGY

Synonyms

- Cervical sympathetic chain schwannoma, sympathetic neurilemmoma or neuroma

Definitions

- Benign, slow-growing tumor of **Schwann cells** investing **cervical sympathetic chain**

IMAGING

General Features

- Best diagnostic clue
  - Fusiform enhancing carotid space (CS) mass that displaces both carotid artery and internal jugular vein (IJV) anteriorly
- Location
  - Arises from cervical sympathetic chain in posterior CS
    - Sympathetic chain normally lies posterior to both CS vessels
- Morphology
  - Ovoid, occasionally fusiform lesion

Imaging Recommendations

- Best imaging tool
  - CECT often 1st exam for neck mass

CT Findings

- CECT
  - Ovoid to fusiform mass displacing both carotid artery and IJV anteriorly
  - Smaller lesions may enhance uniformly
  - Intratumor (intramural) **cystic change** in larger lesions with nonenhancing areas

MR Findings

- T2WI
  - Posterior CS mass with intermediate signal intensity, higher than muscle
  - Intratumor cysts, if present, are hyperintense and sharply marginated
- T1WI C+
  - Homogeneous enhancement in small lesions
  - Cystic change in larger lesions demonstrated as nonenhancing areas

DIFFERENTIAL DIAGNOSIS

Carotid Space Schwannoma

- Typical and more common vagal schwannoma will separate carotid artery and jugular vein

Vagal Paraganglioma

- Heterogeneous enhancement with flow voids in larger lesions

Carotid Body Paraganglioma

- Classic location at carotid bifurcation
- Splays internal and external carotid

Nodal Squamous Cell Carcinoma in Retropharyngeal Space

- Lateral retropharyngeal space nodal disease may mimic sympathetic schwannoma

Neurofibroma, Carotid Space

- Low density on CECT

PATHOLOGY

General Features

- Etiology
  - Arise from Schwann cells of CS sympathetic plexus
- Associated abnormalities
  - Neurofibromatosis type 2 (multiple schwannomas, meningiomas, and ependymomas)

Staging, Grading, & Classification

- Benign tumor with rare malignant transformation

Gross Pathologic & Surgical Features

- Solitary, well-encapsulated tumor arising from peripheral nerve

Microscopic Features

- Spindle-shaped cells with elongated nuclei
  - Organized, compact cellular regions (Antoni A) and loose, relatively acellular tissue (Antoni B)
  - Both areas invariably present in tumors

CLINICAL ISSUES

Presentation

- Most common signs/symptoms
  - Asymptomatic, palpable neck mass
- Other signs/symptoms
  - **Horner syndrome**, headache

Demographics

- Epidemiology
  - Very rare tumor of CS; much less common than vagal schwannoma

Treatment

- Surgical excision is curative
  - Postoperative Horner syndrome is common

DIAGNOSTIC CHECKLIST

Image Interpretation Pearls

- Evaluation of position of carotid artery and jugular vein is critical
  - Should both be displaced anteriorly
- Lack of **flow voids** in CS mass on MR suggests schwannoma or neurofibroma
  - If flow voids, paraganglioma most likely diagnosis

SELECTED REFERENCES

1. Das K N et al: Comprehensive analysis of radiological and surgical predictors in cervical sympathetic schwannomas: a novel staging approach and its implications. Eur Arch Otorhinolaryngol. 282(2):1005-15, 2024
2. Li WX et al: Intracapsular enucleation of cervical sympathetic chain schwannoma. Ear Nose Throat J. 103(5):293-7, 2024
3. Dsouza R et al: Cervical sympathetic schwannoma: a forgotten differential for Horner's syndrome. ANZ J Surg. 90(4):638-40, 2020

Carotid Space Neurofibroma

TERMINOLOGY

- Benign nerve sheath tumor in carotid space, arising from vagus nerve, sympathetic chain, or hypoglossal nerve

IMAGING

- Ovoid or fusiform mass centered in carotid space with mild or patchy enhancement
- Interposed between carotid and jugular
  - Displaces carotid anteromedially
  - Displaces jugular posterolaterally
- Infrahyoid lesions typically posterior to vessels
  - Displaces carotid and jugular anterolaterally
- Hypodense and poorly enhancing on CT
- Hyperintense with target sign on STIR or T2WI MR
- Homogeneous or patchy mild enhancement on MR

TOP DIFFERENTIAL DIAGNOSES

- Vagal paraganglioma
- Carotid body paraganglioma

- Carotid space schwannoma
- Carotid artery pseudoaneurysm

PATHOLOGY

- Benign spindle cell neoplasm
- WHO grade 1 tumors

CLINICAL ISSUES

- Asymptomatic solitary or multiple neck masses
- Lower cranial nerve palsies in larger lesions
- Localized neurofibroma (NF): Isolated soft tissue neck mass
- Plexiform NF: Multinodular bag of worms appearance
- 50% associated with neurofibromatosis type 1, 50% solitary
- Surgical removal of symptomatic isolated lesions
- Excision much more difficult for plexiform lesions
  - Recent FDA approval of selumetinib

DIAGNOSTIC CHECKLIST

- Most conspicuous on STIR/FS T2WI
- Often less conspicuous postcontrast enhancement

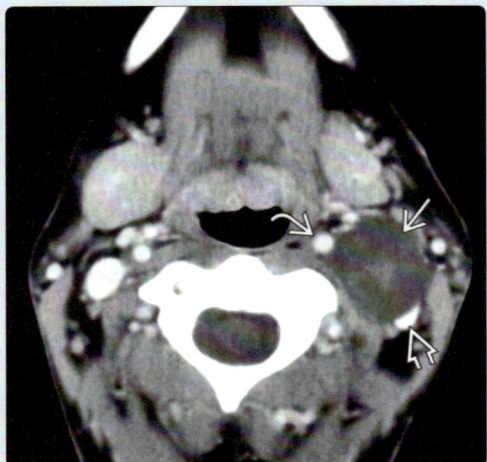 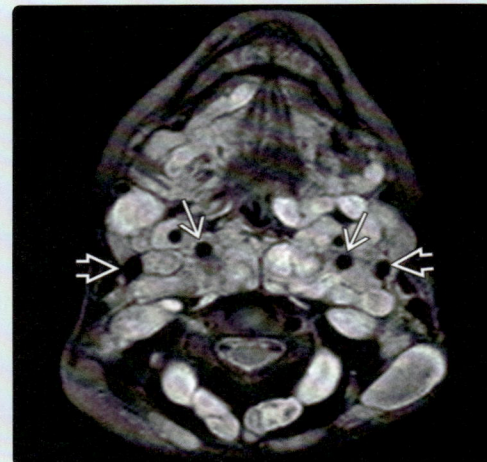

(Left) Axial CECT demonstrates a low-density mass with faint internal enhancement ⮕ located in the left carotid space. The internal carotid artery (ICA) ⮕ is displaced anteromedially, while the internal jugular vein (IJV) ⮕ is displaced posterolaterally. (Right) Axial T2 TSE FS in a 12-year-old girl with neurofibromatosis type 1 (NF1) shows multiple neurofibromas involving all spaces of the H&N. Lesions in carotid sheaths are deviating ICAs ⮕ anteriorly and jugular veins anterolaterally ⮕.

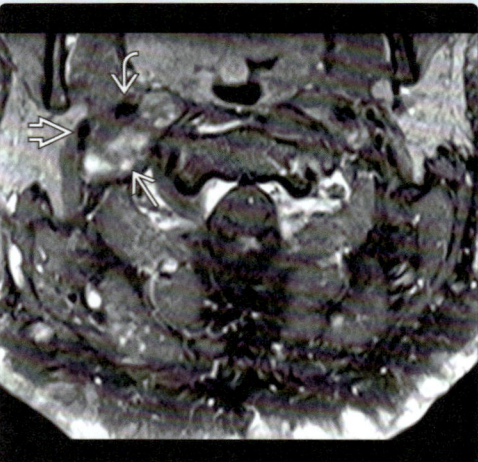 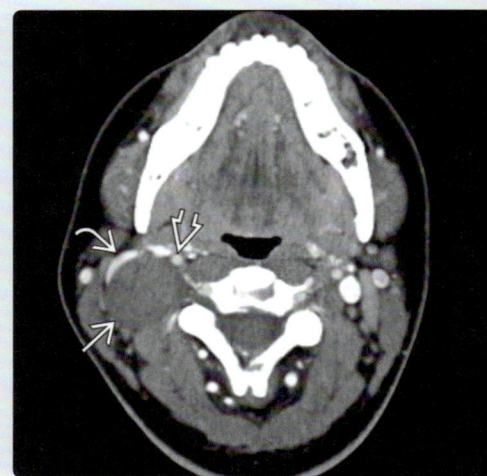

(Left) Axial T1 C+ FS MR in a patient with NF1 demonstrates an ovoid carotid space mass ⮕ with patchy enhancement. The lesion displaces the ICA anteriorly ⮕ and flattens and displaces the IJV anterolaterally ⮕. (Right) Axial CECT shows a right carotid space mass ⮕. Note the ICA pushed anteromedially ⮕ and the IJV anterolaterally ⮕. Clinical symptoms suspicious for malignant peripheral nerve sheath tumor include increased size &/or pain, which this mass histologically proved to be.

TERMINOLOGY

Definitions

- **Benign nerve sheath tumor** in carotid space
- Localized neurofibromas (NFs) arise from **vagus nerve** or **sympathetic** chain; superior lesions may arise from **hypoglossal** nerve
- Plexiform NFs arising from peripheral nerves may also involve carotid sheath

IMAGING

General Features

- Best diagnostic clue
  - **Ovoid** or **fusiform** mass centered in carotid space
- Location
  - Interposed **between carotid artery and jugular vein**
    - Displaces carotid **anteromedially**
    - Displaces jugular **posterolaterally**
  - Infrahyoid lesions typically **posterior** to vessels
    - Displaces carotid and jugular **anterolaterally**
- Morphology
  - Localized NF: **Ovoid or fusiform** shape
  - Plexiform NF: Poorly circumscribed, **multilobulated**

CT Findings

- CECT
  - Hypodense, **poorly enhancing** mass within carotid space
    - May simulate cystic lesion, such as lymphatic malformation

MR Findings

- T1WI
  - Isointense, relatively homogeneous mass
- T2WI
  - Very **hyperintense**, darker centrally (**target sign**)
  - Most conspicuous on T2WI FS
- T1WI C+
  - Homogeneous or patchy **mild enhancement**

Imaging Recommendations

- Best imaging tool
  - Contrast-enhanced FS MR
- Protocol advice
  - Most conspicuous on STIR or FS T2

DIFFERENTIAL DIAGNOSIS

Vagal Paraganglioma

- Clinical: Asymptomatic or vagal neuropathy
- Imaging: Avidly enhancing mass with flow voids
  - Nasopharyngeal aspect of carotid space

Carotid Body Paraganglioma

- Clinical: Asymptomatic or pulsatile neck mass
- Imaging: Splaying of internal and external carotid

Carotid Space Schwannoma

- Clinical: Lateral neck mass
- Imaging: Fusiform, uniform enhancement
  - Intramural cystic changes in larger lesions

Carotid Artery Pseudoaneurysm

- Clinical: History of trauma or dissection
- Imaging: Carotid artery mass with complex signal

PATHOLOGY

General Features

- Etiology
  - Benign **spindle cell** neoplasm
- Genetics
  - Chromosome 17q11.2 in NF1 phenotype

Staging, Grading, & Classification

- WHO **grade 1** tumors

Gross Pathologic & Surgical Features

- Localized NF: Ovoid, **circumscribed** nodule
- Plexiform NF: Infiltrative **bag of worms** texture

CLINICAL ISSUES

Presentation

- Most common signs/symptoms
  - Asymptomatic **solitary** or **multiple** neck masses
  - Enlarging mass, new or increased pain, or neurologic deficit raises question of malignant degeneration
- Other signs/symptoms
  - Lower cranial nerve **palsies** in larger lesions
- Clinical profile
  - Localized NF: Isolated soft tissue neck mass
  - Plexiform NF: Multinodular **bag of worms appearance** with associated NF1 stigmata

Demographics

- Epidemiology
  - 50% associated with NF1, 50% solitary
    - Multiple more likely syndromic

Natural History & Prognosis

- 5-10% **malignant degeneration** in NF1

Treatment

- Surgical removal of symptomatic isolated lesions
- Excision much more difficult for plexiform lesions
  - Recent FDA approval of selumetinib (MAPK 1 and 2 inhibitor): Treatment of plexiform in NF1

DIAGNOSTIC CHECKLIST

Consider

- Assess patient for other **signs of NF1**

Image Interpretation Pearls

- Most conspicuous on **STIR** or FS **T2WI**

Reporting Tips

- Consider dedicated imaging of spine, brain, and orbits

SELECTED REFERENCES

1. Alotaibi HA et al: Selumetinib use as targeted therapy for plexiform neurofibroma: a comprehensive review of the literature. Orbit. ePub, 2025
2. Debs P et al: MRI features of benign peripheral nerve sheath tumors: how do sporadic and syndromic tumors differ? Skeletal Radiol. 53(4):709-23, 2024
3. Mamlouk MD: Solid and vascular neck masses in children. Neuroimaging Clin N Am. 33(4):607-21, 2023

Carotid Space Meningioma

IMAGING

- Enhancing carotid space (CS) mass with **connection to jugular foramen (JF)** above
  - Enhancing, thickened dura around JF
  - Internal carotid artery (ICA) pushed anteriorly by CS mass
- Bone CT: JF margins show **permeative-sclerotic** or **hyperostotic** bone changes
- Protocol: Skull base focused MR with fat-saturated T1 C+
  - Bone CT of skull base to evaluate bones around JF

TOP DIFFERENTIAL DIAGNOSES

- Carotid body or vagal paraganglioma
- Carotid space schwannoma
- ICA pseudoaneurysm

PATHOLOGY

- CS meningioma originates from arachnoid cap cells in JF
- JF meningioma herniates inferiorly into nasopharyngeal CS
- Typically WHO grade 1 (> 90%)

CLINICAL ISSUES

- Patients 40-60 years; M:F = 1:2
- Gradual symptom progression (slow-growing benign tumor)
- Treatment: Surgical resection ± radiation therapy
- Surgical resection limited by degree of ICA & lower cranial nerve involvement
- Radiotherapy for incomplete resection, extensive skull base invasion, or high morbidity patient

DIAGNOSTIC CHECKLIST

- If nasopharyngeal CS mass is associated with JF component, bony margins of JF may predict histology
- CS meningioma: **Permeative-sclerotic** or **hyperostotic**
- CS extension of jugular paraganglioma: **Permeative-destructive** JF margins
- CS schwannoma: **Smooth** JF **enlargement**

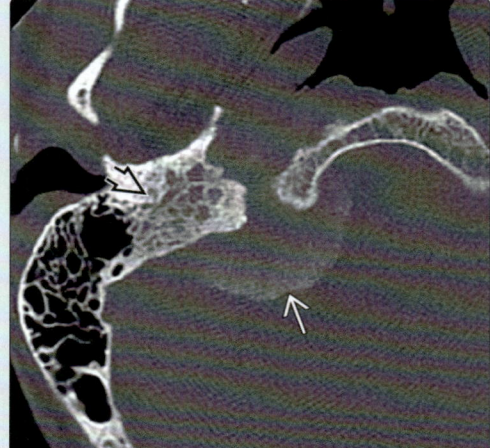
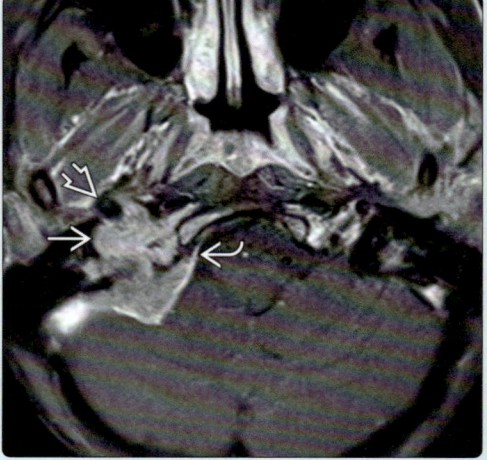

(Left) Axial bone CT shows the typical mixed permeative-sclerotic pattern ⇊ seen in meningiomas of the skull base and jugular foramen. Note the partially calcified ➡ intracranial portion of the tumor. (Right) Axial T1WI C+ FS MR shows a jugular foramen meningioma extending into the carotid space ➡. Note the anterior location of the carotid artery ⇉. These meningiomas originate from arachnoid cap cells within the jugular foramen. Note the intracranial dural tail ➚, characteristic of meningioma.

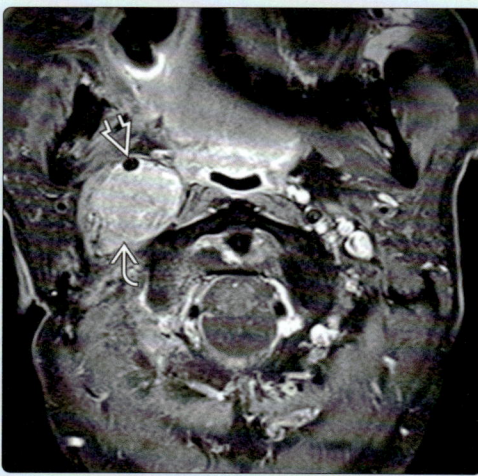
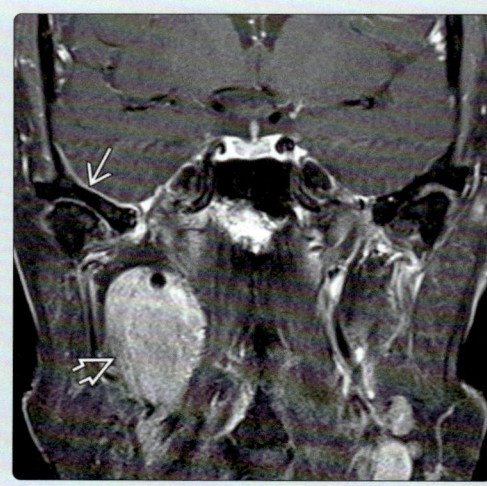

(Left) Axial T1WI C+ FS MR shows a large, enhancing right carotid space mass ➚ displacing the carotid artery anteriorly ➡. Note the lack of flow voids, which can help differentiate this meningioma from the more common paraganglioma. (Right) Coronal T1WI C+ FS MR in the same patient shows the large carotid space meningioma ➚, which originated in the jugular foramen. Note the associated intracranial dural tail ➡, commonly seen in patients who have intracranial extension of a skull base meningioma.

TERMINOLOGY

Abbreviations

- Carotid space meningioma (CSM)

Definitions

- Meningioma of nasopharyngeal carotid space (CS) emanating from jugular foramen (JF) above

IMAGING

General Features

- Best diagnostic clue
  - Connection to JF above with JF margins showing **permeative-sclerotic** or **hyperostotic** bone changes
  - Enhancing CS mass with lack of flow voids
- Location: Nasopharyngeal CS
- Morphology: Dumbbell-shaped (JF ↔ CS)

CT Findings

- NECT
  - Meningioma may be high density from psammomatous calcifications
- CECT
  - Moderately enhancing CS mass
  - Internal carotid artery (ICA) pushed anteriorly by CS mass
- Bone CT
  - JF margins: **Permeative-sclerotic** or **hyperostotic** bone changes

MR Findings

- T1WI
  - Muscle intensity ovoid JF-CS mass
  - Larger lesions may display occasional high-velocity flow voids
- T2WI: Low to intermediate intensity 2° to calcification
- T2* GRE: Susceptibility effect (blooming) possible
- T1WI C+: Mild to moderate enhancement
  - Enhancing, thickened dura around JF
  - May see dural tail
- MRA: ICA draped anteriorly over CSM

Angiographic Findings

- Prolonged capillary tumor blush without arteriovenous shunting or early vein appearance

Imaging Recommendations

- Protocol advice
  - Skull base focused MR with fat-saturated T1 C+ axial & coronal sequences
  - Bone CT of skull base to evaluate bones around JF

DIFFERENTIAL DIAGNOSIS

Carotid Body Paraganglioma

- Mass splays external carotid artery (ECA) & ICA at carotid bifurcation
- T1 MR shows parenchymal high-velocity flow voids

Vagal Paraganglioma

- Enhancing CS mass centered ~ 2 cm below skull base
- T1 MR shows parenchymal high-velocity flow voids

Carotid Space Schwannoma

- Well-circumscribed, enhancing, fusiform CS mass ± intramural cysts

Internal Carotid Artery Pseudoaneurysm

- Narrowed ICA lumen with focal luminal outpouching

Internal Carotid Artery Dissection

- CTA shows linear intraluminal intimal flap or crescent

PATHOLOGY

General Features

- Etiology
  - CSM originates from arachnoid cap cells in JF
  - JF meningioma herniates inferiorly into nasopharyngeal CS

Microscopic Features

- Clustered whorls & lobules of psammomatous calcifications & meningothelial cells

CLINICAL ISSUES

Presentation

- Most common signs/symptoms
  - Lateral posterior pharyngeal mass
  - Other signs/symptoms
    - Complex lower cranial neuropathy (CNIX-XII)

Demographics

- Age: Patients 40-60 years
- Sex: M:F = 1:2
- Epidemiology: Rare manifestation of rare tumor location (JF meningioma)

Natural History & Prognosis

- Gradual symptom progression (slow-growing tumor)
- Surgical treatment often complicated by ↑ cranial neuropathy ± stroke

Treatment

- Surgical resection limited by degree of ICA & lower cranial nerve involvement
- Radiotherapy for incomplete resection, extensive skull base invasion, or high morbidity patient
- Preoperative embolization may ↓ vascularity of tumor

DIAGNOSTIC CHECKLIST

Consider

- If nasopharyngeal CS mass is associated with JF component, bony margins of JF may predict histology
  - CS **meningioma**: **Permeative-sclerotic** or **hyperostotic** JF margins
  - CS extension of jugular **paraganglioma**: **Permeative-destructive** JF margins
  - CS **schwannoma**: **Smooth** JF enlargement

SELECTED REFERENCES

1. Vasireddi AK et al: The "outline sign": thin hyperenhancing perimeter as an MR imaging feature of meningioma. a useful tool in the temporal bone region for differentiating meningiomas from schwannomas and paragangliomas. AJNR Am J Neuroradiol. 46(2):349-54, 2025

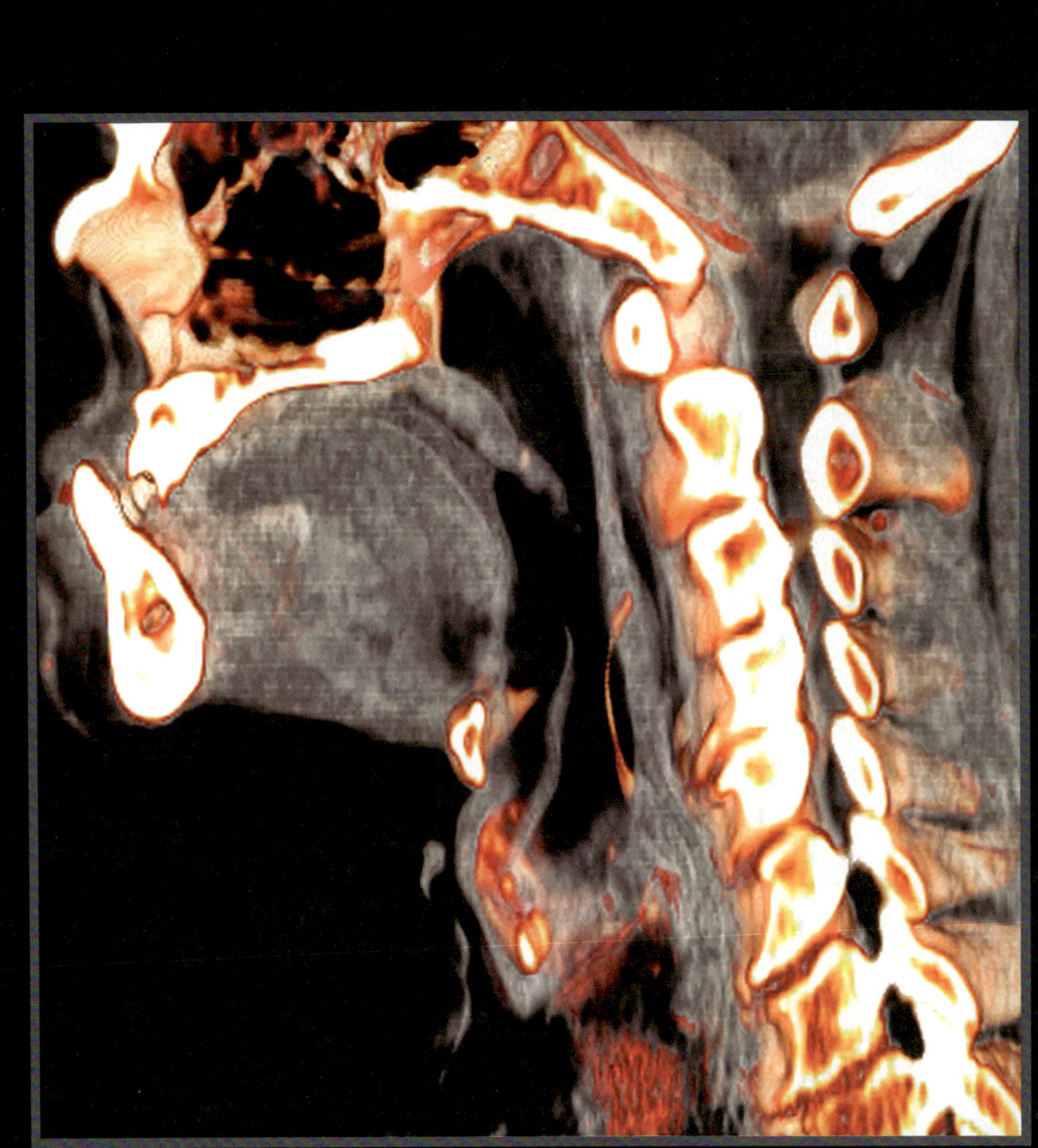

SECTION 7
Retropharyngeal Space

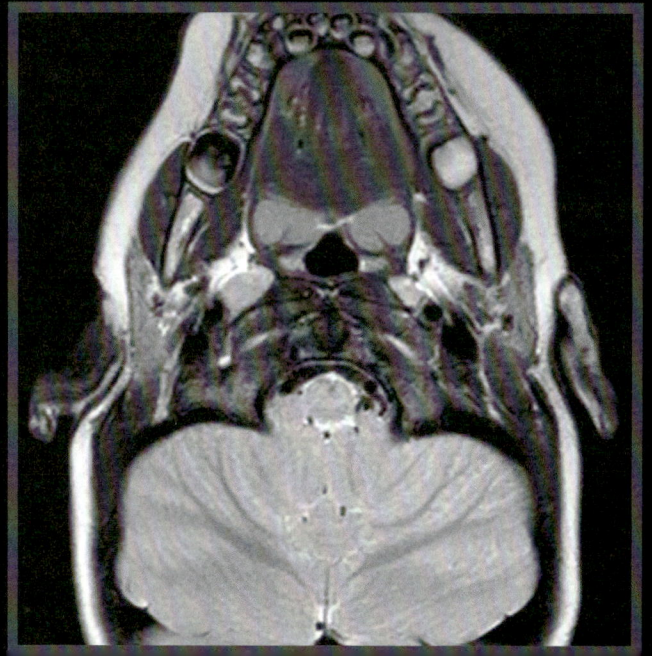
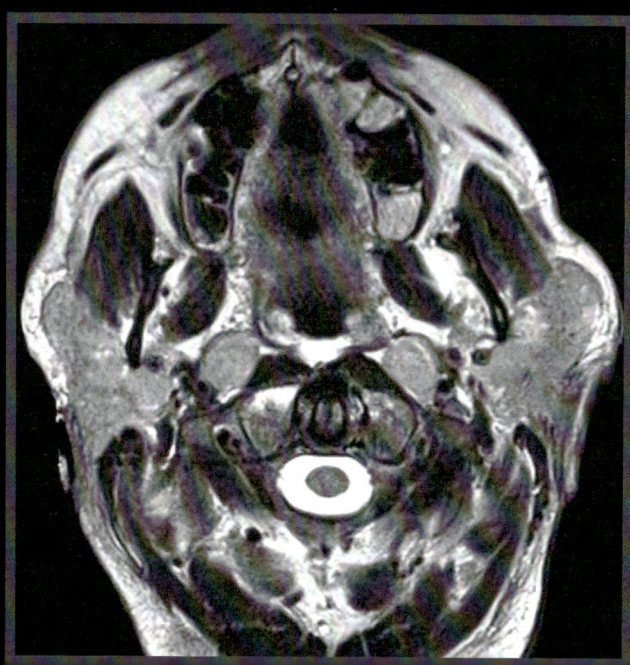

Summary Thoughts: Retropharyngeal Space

The retropharyngeal space (RPS) spans the length of the neck from the skull base to the mediastinum. As its name indicates, it lies posterior to the pharynx. More inferiorly in the neck, it lies posterior to the esophagus. It is located anterior to the cervical and upper thoracic spine and the prevertebral muscles. Anatomically, an additional fascia divides the RPS into 2 components: (1) An anterior true RPS and (2) a posterior danger space (DS). With imaging, it is rare to be able to delineate a lesion as residing in only 1 of these 2 spaces, so for most purposes the 2 are considered 1 RPS.

The RPS contains only **medial** and **lateral** RPS **lymph nodes** and **fat**. This results in a very short differential diagnosis for pathology in this space, primarily a tumor or infection affecting the nodes. While this makes diagnosing easier, the RPS is actually an imaging and clinical "blind spot," with RPS nodes being inaccessible to direct observation or physical examination. Additionally, nonnecrotic nodes often appear isodense to prevertebral muscles on CECT and frequently lie far lateral in the RPS and medial to the internal carotid arteries (ICAs). Therefore, it is critical that the radiologist methodically searches the RPS for adenopathy, particularly in patients with head and neck (H&N) malignancies. This finding can alter radiation treatment planning for H&N malignancies, reducing the risk for local failure.

After nodal disease, the next most common pathology is a frequently seen but poorly understood process known as retropharyngeal edema. While the RPS fluid itself does not require treatment, it is a clue to other pathology in the H&N that may require treatment, and identifying the source is important. Significantly, it may pose a diagnostic challenge, as it mimics the appearance of retropharyngeal abscess, which often requires surgical intervention.

Imaging Approaches and Indications

The presence of fat in the RPS makes this space readily identifiable on CT (due to its low density) and MR (due to its intrinsic T1 and T2 hyperintensity). As CECT is the imaging technique of choice for evaluation of H&N infections, it is often the initial modality for detection of RPS pathology. Imaging of any RPS process must cover from the skull base to the mediastinum because of the potential for craniocaudal and mediastinal spread of disease. IV contrast is important to determine enhancement characteristics of an RPS collection that suggests an abscess and for evaluation of nodal disease and nodal necrosis. It is also important for the evaluation of other neck structures, which may be responsible for RPS infection or edema. Review of the cervical spine for discitis-osteomyelitis as a potential infectious source is important during analysis of the neck CT or MR images.

MR allows excellent delineation of RPS contours but is less often used in evaluation of infection, except for discitis-osteomyelitis. MR is more sensitive than CT for detecting retropharyngeal adenopathy, which is important for the staging of many H&N tumors (particularly nasopharyngeal carcinoma).

Imaging Anatomy

The anterior margin of the RPS is delineated by the posterior pharyngeal wall and inferiorly by the posterior aspect of the esophagus. These structures are enveloped by a middle layer of deep cervical fascia (ML-DCF), also known as the **buccopharyngeal** and **visceral fascia**, respectively. The posterior margin of the RPS is defined by the **prevertebral fascia**, which is a deep layer of deep cervical fascia (DL-DCF).

Superiorly, the ML-DCF and DL-DCF insert on the central skull base, forming the superior boundary of the RPS. Inferiorly, the posterior margin of the RPS is the prevertebral fascia and blends with the anterior longitudinal ligament of the upper thoracic spine.

A 2nd layer of prevertebral fascia (DL-DCF), known as the **alar fascia**, extends in a coronal orientation and divides the RPS into 2 compartments: The more anterior true RPS and the posterior DS. At approximately the T3 level, the alar fascia merges with the visceral fascia on the posterior aspect of the esophagus to form the inferior boundary of the true RPS. The DS extends more inferiorly in the posterior mediastinum and typically reaches the diaphragm. It is usually impossible on imaging to delineate 2 distinct spaces, so for all intents and purposes the RPS and DS are considered 1 RPS. It is important, however, to remember the potential for posterior mediastinal extension of an RPS process to the inferior aspect of the thorax.

The lateral limits of the RPS are defined by sagittally oriented slips of the DL-DCF. This fascia separates the RPS contents from the carotid sheath and generally appears less resistant to the spread of pathology within and from the RPS than the prevertebral and visceral fascia. Consequently, RPS edema frequently extends laterally to the carotid sheaths. Similarly, RPS and DS often appear to communicate freely inferiorly despite the alar fascia.

Pseudolesions of the RPS include medial deviation of the carotid arteries and thyroid gland enlargement due to goiter or malignancy. Both the carotid arteries and thyroid tissue may present in a near midline location in the RPS, which likely occurs from laxity or disruption of this lateral alar fascia. Medial deviation of the carotid arteries is important to report since iatrogenic injury can occur and is particularly at risk during transoral robotic surgery if this anatomic variant is not recognized.

Approaches to Imaging Issues of the Retropharyngeal Space

The answer to the question, "What imaging findings define an **RPS mass**?" varies slightly depending on the level in the neck. Throughout most of the neck, and particularly the infrahyoid neck, an RPS mass is clearly evident as a lesion posterior to the pharynx &/or esophagus and anterior to the prevertebral muscles and spine. The pharynx and the esophagus may be deviated anteriorly, and there may by flattening of prevertebral muscles against the spine. These findings help to clarify an RPS location.

In the suprahyoid neck, and particularly just below the skull base, the RPS contains little fat and frequently appears to be more of a **potential space** with the prevertebral muscles and the pharynx closely opposed. Retropharyngeal nodes are located in the far lateral aspect of the RPS, immediately medial to the ICAs. With a very thin RPS and prominent bellies of the prevertebral muscles, these RPS nodes appear to lie **lateral** to the prevertebral muscles. This is most evident in children, in whom large, nonnecrotic RPS nodes, in association with prominent adenoidal tissue, are normal findings.

Nasopharyngeal or oropharyngeal infection, such as tonsillitis or pharyngitis, will result in reactive enlargement of these already prominent nodes in children. The presence of

Differential Diagnosis of Retropharyngeal Space

Pseudolesion	Congenital	Inflammatory	Infectious	Vascular	Treatment Related	Benign Tumor	Malignant Tumor
Tortuous carotid	Venous malformation	Reactive or inflamed suprahyoid RPS node	Cellulitis or phlegmon from adjacent infection	Jugular vein thrombosis	Radiation edema	Lipoma	SCCa nodal met or direct invasion by SCCa
Thyromegaly (goiter or malignancy)	Lymphatic malformation	Longus colli tendonitis edema	RPS abscess from adjacent infection	Kawasaki disease	Edema from neck or spine surgery	Nerve sheath tumor	Systemic nodal met
			Intranodal abscess	Hematoma		PTH adenoma	NHL node

RPS = retropharyngeal space; SCCa = squamous cell carcinoma; NHL = non-Hodgkin lymphoma; met = metastasis; PTH = parathyroid.

nonenhancing foci within RPS nodes in a child with infectious symptoms indicates **suppuration** (also called intranodal abscess) but does not typically require surgical intervention.

In adults, normal RPS nodes are less frequently found and, when seen, are typically ≤ 5 mm. **Reactive enlargement** of RPS nodes may be found in adults with pharyngeal infection, although reactive nodal enlargement to 1 cm is unusual. RPS reactive adenopathy is distinctly less common in adults, which in part reflects the decreased frequency of pharyngeal infections in adults compared to children.

Enlarged RPS nodes in an adult > 8 mm are concerning for the possibility of **metastatic disease**. This is a 1st-order lymphatic drainage site for nasopharyngeal carcinoma, where unilateral or bilateral RPS metastases are designated as N1 disease. Other H&N tumors also drain to RPS nodes, either primarily or secondarily. Oropharyngeal squamous cell carcinoma (SCCa), sinonasal malignancies, middle ear malignancies, and thyroid carcinoma drain directly to RPS nodes. Other malignancies, such as posterior wall hypopharyngeal SCCa, invade the RPS and then drain through the lymphatic system to the RPS nodes. Non-Hodgkin lymphoma in the H&N frequently involves RPS nodes and may become particularly large without necrosis. Since RPS nodes are not detectable on clinical examination, it is important to pay particular attention to this area. One effective method is carefully searching along the medial aspect of the suprahyoid ICAs.

The differential diagnosis for a **well-defined**, **ovoid mass** in the suprahyoid RPS includes **carotid space (CS)** lesions that mimic RPS nodes by their location medial to the ICA. Schwannoma of the sympathetic chain typically lies medial to the ICA, and vagal paragangliomas may be medial or posterior to the ICA. The lack of other neck adenopathy or the clear demonstration of CS location favors one of these two.

Lymph nodes are not present in the infrahyoid neck; thus, a well-defined, small, oval mass in this location suggests parathyroid adenoma. Arterial-phase imaging showing hypervascularity with intense enhancement is characteristic and can be correlated with clinical findings of hypercalcemia/hyperparathyroidism.

If an RPS abnormality is **diffuse** rather than a focal mass, the diagnostic approach is quite different and can be defined as collections or masses. **Collections** have fluid density (CT) or intensity (MR) and tend to enlarge the entire RPS into either a "bow-tie" or rectangular contour. Whenever a fluid-distended RPS is found, the 1st consideration is to exclude an **RPS**

abscess, which is typically rim-enhancing rectangular distention of the RPS. More frequently evident in neck studies, however, is **RPS edema**, which is nonenhancing and tends to result in less marked RPS enlargement, with a lower volume rectangular contour. Once this diagnosis is suspected, the neck must be searched for an infectious source (typically of pharyngeal origin in children and spinal origin in adults), a vascular source (internal jugular vein thrombosis), inflammation (longus colli tendonitis), or evidence of recent treatment (spine or neck surgery, radiation).

Diffuse masses of the RPS may be lipomatous lesions, such as lipoma or liposarcoma, with fat density/signal on CT or MR imaging, other rare sarcomas, or congenital lesions, such as venous or lymphatic malformations, which share imaging characteristics with such lesions elsewhere in the H&N. These lesions are typically transspatial involving adjacent H&N spaces, as are plexiform neurofibromas, which are characteristic of neurofibromatosis type 1 (NF1).

Clinical Implications

Small lesions of the RPS are typically **not** evident on clinical examination. It is only when lesions become significantly enlarged that bulging of a posterior pharyngeal wall is evident. The radiologist must consider the possibility of RPS metastatic nodal disease in **all H&N cancer patients** and must methodically search along the medial aspect of the cervical ICA for potential adenopathy. Nonnecrotic RPS nodes are more difficult to discern on CECT than MR, so vigilance is key.

Toxic patients with H&N infections, such as pharyngitis or tonsillitis, may be imaged to exclude the development of an RPS abscess. This is a difficult clinical diagnosis because physical examination may not be fruitful. Thus, clinicians must rely largely on a high degree of clinical suspicion. The radiologist must exclude RPS abscess or, if one is found, must delineate the entire craniocaudal extent and specifically exclude mediastinal involvement. Large abscesses may result in airway compromise, though it is rare that a patient presents with airway symptoms secondary to an RPS mass.

Selected References

1. Lääveri M et al: Odontogenic neck abscesses caused by Streptococcus anginosus group bacteria: emergency MRI findings. Oral Surg Oral Med Oral Pathol Oral Radiol. 139(5):594-9, 2025
2. Gomez MA et al: Necrotizing soft-tissue and retropharyngeal space infections and mediastinitis. N Engl J Med. 391(3):e5, 2024
3. Heikkinen J et al: MRI findings in acute tonsillar infections. AJNR Am J Neuroradiol. 43(2):286-91, 2022

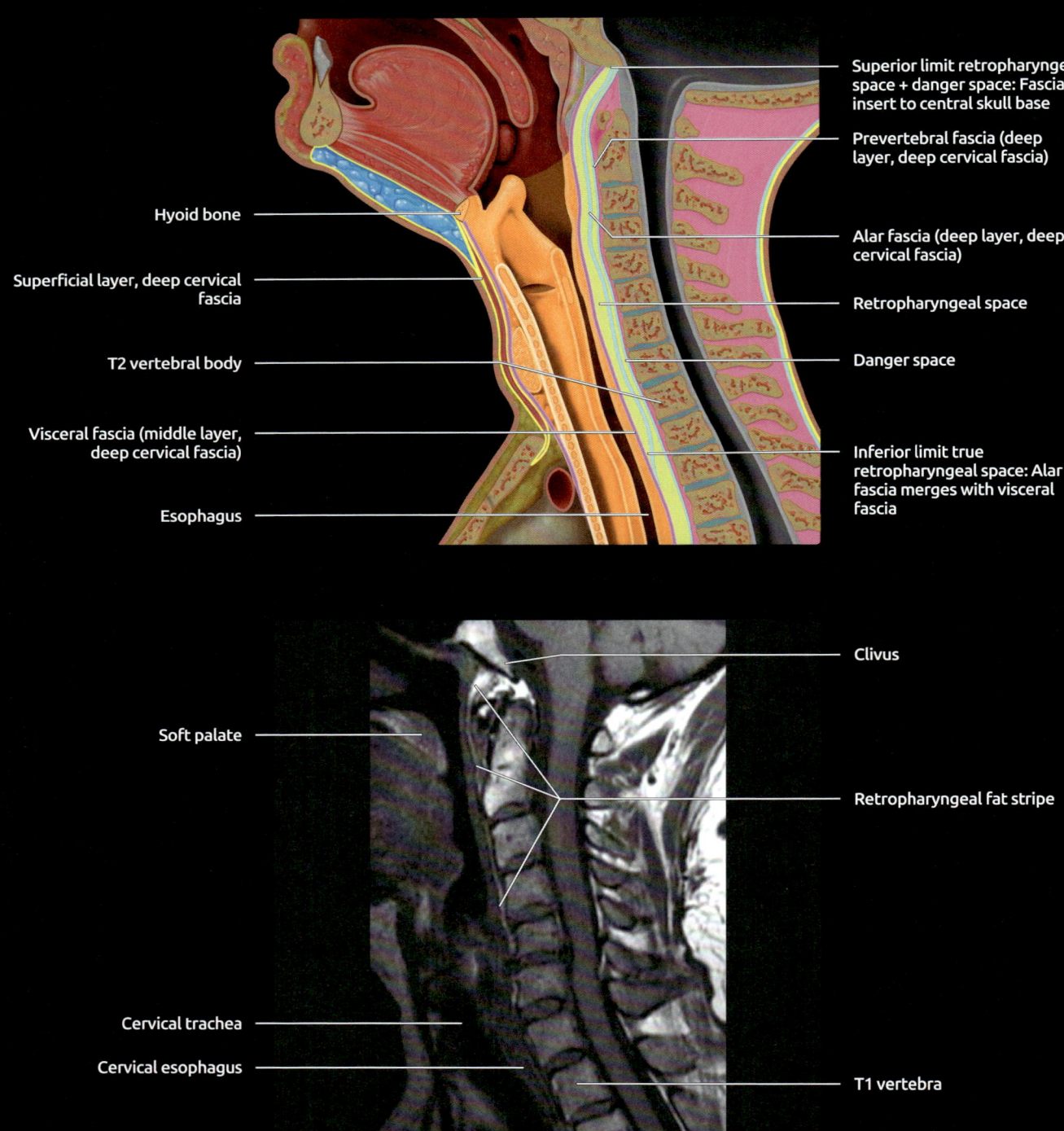

Hyoid bone

Superficial layer, deep cervical fascia

T2 vertebral body

Visceral fascia (middle layer, deep cervical fascia)

Esophagus

Superior limit retropharyngeal space + danger space: Fasciae insert to central skull base

Prevertebral fascia (deep layer, deep cervical fascia)

Alar fascia (deep layer, deep cervical fascia)

Retropharyngeal space

Danger space

Inferior limit true retropharyngeal space: Alar fascia merges with visceral fascia

Soft palate

Cervical trachea

Cervical esophagus

Clivus

Retropharyngeal fat stripe

T1 vertebra

(Top) *Sagittal graphic shows the deep cervical fascia (DCF) layers, which determine and delineate the contours of the retropharyngeal space (RPS). The anterior contour of the RPS is defined by the visceral fascia, the middle layer DCF, which separates the RPS from the pharyngeal mucosal space of the suprahyoid neck (SHN) and visceral space of the infrahyoid neck (IHN). The posterior contour is formed by the prevertebral fascia (deep layer DCF). The alar fascia (also deep layer DCF) anatomically defines an anterior true RPS and more posterior danger space (DS), although this delineation is not typically evident at imaging. Inferiorly, the alar fascia blends with the visceral fascia at ~T3, while superiorly the middle and deep layers of the DCF insert to the central skull base.* (Bottom) *Sagittal T1 MR shows thin, hyperintense signal corresponding to normal fat within the RPS. Contents include this thin fat stripe and the retropharyngeal lymph nodes in the lateral SHN. It can be considered a potential space that is most visible when distended by disease.*

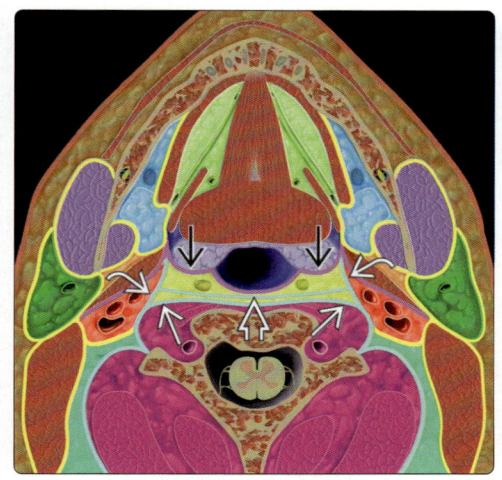

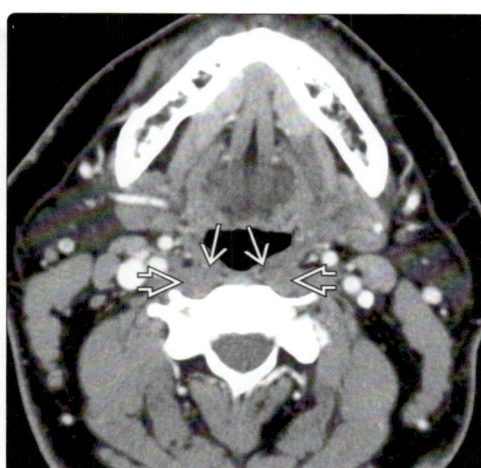

(Left) Axial graphic at the level of the oropharynx illustrates a predominantly fat-filled RPS. The anterior contour is delineated by middle layer DCF ⮕, and the posterior contour by prevertebral fascia (deep layer DCF) ⮕. The alar fascia forms lateral margins ⮕ and the divider ⮕ of RPS into anterior true RPS and posterior DS. **(Right)** Axial CECT shows the typical appearance of RPS in an SHN as a thin, low-density fat stripe ⮕ anterior to prevertebral muscles ⮕.

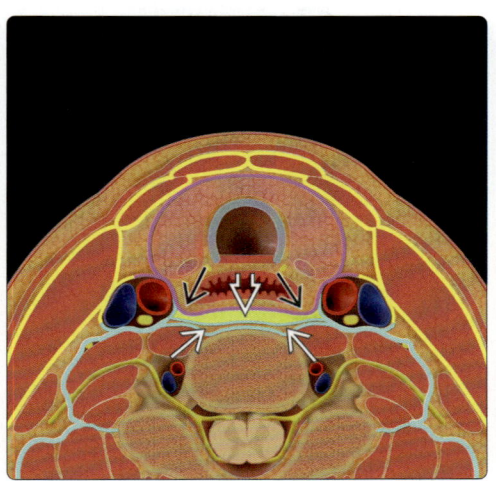

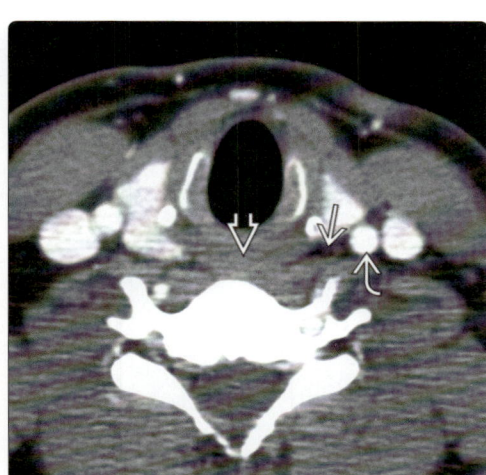

(Left) Axial graphic at the level of the thyroid gland shows infrahyoid continuation of a fat-filled RPS, now posterior to the esophagus and again delineated anteriorly by visceral fascia (middle layer DCF) ⮕. Posterior DS ⮕ separates the true RPS ⮕ from prevertebral muscles and cervical vertebrae. **(Right)** Axial CECT shows RPS as an almost imperceptible fat stripe anterior to the perivertebral space and posterior to the hypopharynx ⮕. Laterally, the RPS has a triangular contour ⮕ immediately medial to the internal carotid artery ⮕.

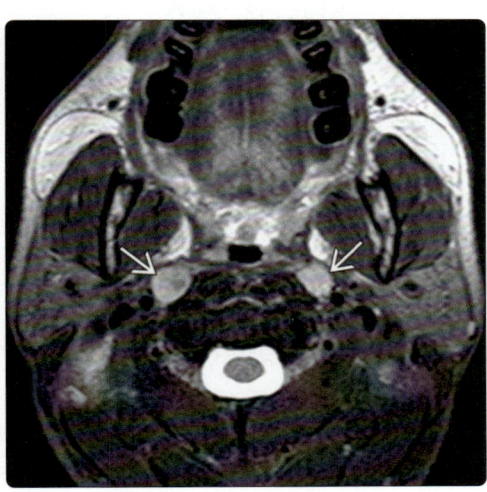

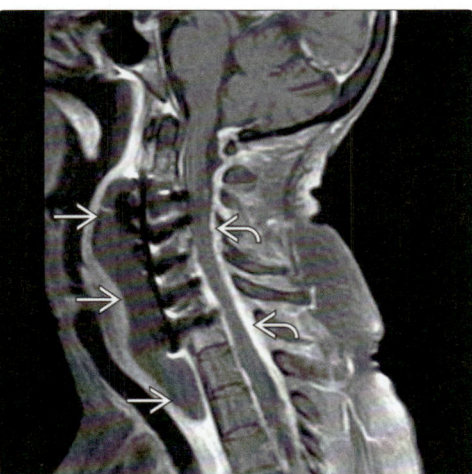

(Left) Axial T2 MR shows solid-appearing retropharyngeal adenopathy ⮕ in a patient with a right-sided nasopharyngeal cancer. Both showed increased uptake on concurrently performed PET/CT (not shown). **(Right)** Sagittal T1 C+ FS MR shows a large, peripherally enhancing fluid collection in the RPS ⮕ due to abscess that developed after anterior cervical spine fusion. Diffuse intraspinal pachymeningeal thickening and enhancement ⮕ are also noted.

Reactive Adenopathy of Retropharyngeal Space

TERMINOLOGY

- Benign enlargement of nodes in response to antigen
- Lateral retropharyngeal space (RPS) nodes known as nodes of Rouvière

IMAGING

- RPS nodes are mildly enlarged
  - Found from skull base to hyoid bone
- Often elongate in craniocaudal direction, so may appear round on axial CT
  - Coronal/sagittal reformats show normal oval shape
- If large or associated with inflammatory change, may deform pharyngeal contour, narrowing airway
- More difficult to detect on CT if no mass effect, as tends to be isodense to prevertebral muscles
  - Contrast (CECT) aids in detection of RPS node & intranodal suppurative change

TOP DIFFERENTIAL DIAGNOSES

- Suppurative RPS node
- Squamous cell carcinoma (SCCa) metastasis to RPS node
- Non-SCCa metastasis to RPS node
- Ectatic internal carotid artery

PATHOLOGY

- Most often in response to infectious agent

CLINICAL ISSUES

- Reactive RPS nodes common in children because of oral exposure to antigens
- Common incidental finding in young patients

DIAGNOSTIC CHECKLIST

- Look for primary infection: Pharyngitis, tonsillitis
- Look for suppurative change/early abscess formation
- Consider metastatic disease in patients > 30 yr if no clinical signs of infection, or persistence/enlargement over time

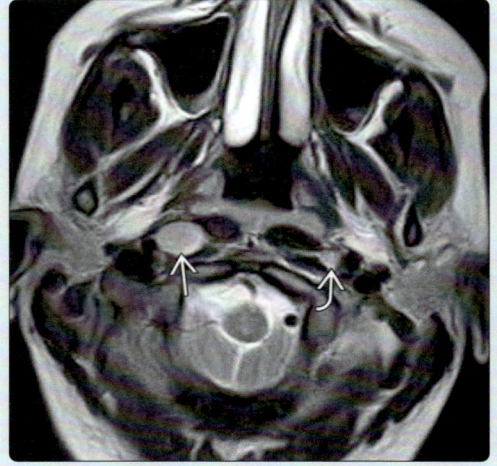
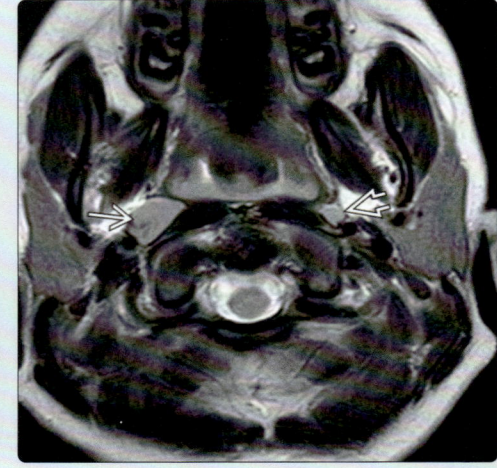

(Left) Axial T2 MR in an 18-year-old woman with headaches is shown. Because the right retropharyngeal lymph node ➡ was asymmetrically enlarged (note small contralateral node ➡) & there was no history of upper respiratory infection, this node was biopsy-confirmed as reactive hyperplasia. (Right) Axial T2 MR shows a slightly heterogeneous & prominent right retropharyngeal lymph node ➡ incidentally noted in an 11-year-old girl imaged for headaches. A smaller node ➡ is seen on the left.

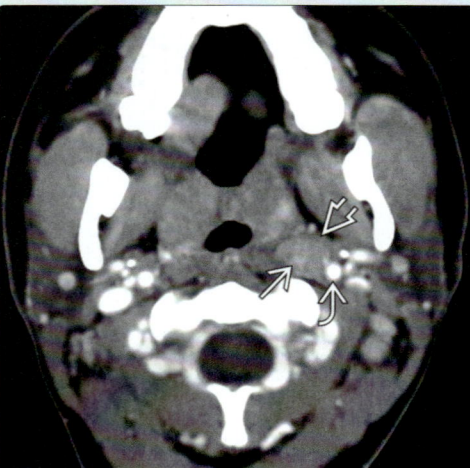
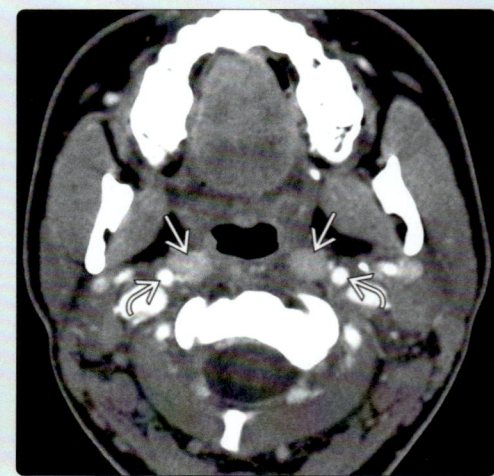

(Left) Axial CECT in a teenage patient with pharyngitis shows a large, reactive left retropharyngeal node ➡ medial to internal carotid artery (ICA) ➡ & lateral to prevertebral muscle. No suppurative change is present, but subtle linear intranodal enhancement ➡ is seen. (Right) Axial CECT shows bilateral, mildly enhancing, reactive retropharyngeal nodes ➡ medial to ICA ➡ in a child with pharyngitis. There is no cystic change to suggest suppuration. Characteristic thin, linear, enhancing septa are noted internally.

Reactive Adenopathy of Retropharyngeal Space

TERMINOLOGY

Abbreviations

- Retropharyngeal space (**RPS**) nodes

Synonyms

- Reactive lymphoid hyperplasia, nodal hyperplasia
- Lateral RPS nodes: Nodes of Rouvière

Definitions

- Benign enlargement of nodes in response to antigen

IMAGING

General Features

- Best diagnostic clue
  - Prominent, mildly enlarged node in RPS
  - Evidence of pharyngeal inflammation as source
- Location
  - RPS nodes found from skull base to hyoid bone
    - Lateral nodes found just medial to high cervical internal carotid arteries (ICA)
    - Medial nodes uncommonly seen
- Size
  - Uncommonly > 1 cm (adults) without suppuration
  - Frequently larger in children normally
- Morphology
  - Well-defined node medial to ICA in RPS

CT Findings

- CECT
  - Variable enhancement, usually mild
  - Tends to be isodense to muscle, so difficult to detect
  - Often long craniocaudally; may appear round on axials
    - Coronal/sagittal reformats show oval shape

MR Findings

- T1WI
  - Homogeneous low to intermediate signal
- T2WI
  - Homogeneous, intermediate signal intensity
- T1WI C+
  - Variable, usually mild enhancement

Nuclear Medicine Findings

- PET
  - Mild FDG uptake may be seen

Imaging Recommendations

- Best imaging tool
  - CECT is study of choice for H&N infection
  - RPS nodes more conspicuous on MR
- Protocol advice
  - Contrast helps to detect node & suppurative change

DIFFERENTIAL DIAGNOSIS

Suppurative Retropharyngeal Space Node

- Low-density RPS node with peripheral enhancement

Squamous Cell Carcinoma Metastasis to Retropharyngeal Space Node

- Nasopharynx, posterior pharynx wall, sinus primary

Nonsquamous Cell Carcinoma Metastasis to Retropharyngeal Space Node

- Thyroid carcinoma, sinus malignancies, & lymphoma

Ectatic Internal Carotid Artery

- Common finding in older adults: ICA bows medially into RPS

PATHOLOGY

General Features

- Etiology
  - Most often in response to infectious agent
    - Often H&N source, such as pharyngitis or tonsillitis
    - Generalized systemic viral infection
- Associated abnormalities
  - If large or associated with inflammatory change, may deform pharyngeal contour, narrowing airway
  - When associated with extensive RPS inflammation, may see narrowed adjacent ICA

Gross Pathologic & Surgical Features

- Retropharyngeal nodes rarely excised

Microscopic Features

- Histologic features of nodal hyperplasia

CLINICAL ISSUES

Presentation

- Most common signs/symptoms
  - Symptoms from primary infection source
  - Common incidental finding in young patients
- Clinical profile
  - Young patient with pharyngeal or systemic viral infection

Demographics

- Age: Usually < 30 yr
- Epidemiology: Common in children from oral exposure to antigens

Natural History & Prognosis

- Node may suppurate (form pus collection)
- Suppurative node can rupture, forming RPS abscess

Treatment

- Primary infectious source should be treated
- Patient monitored clinically for progression of symptoms & reimaged if concern for abscess or malignancy

DIAGNOSTIC CHECKLIST

Consider

- Look for primary infection: Pharyngitis, tonsillitis
- Look for suppurative change/early abscess formation
- Consider metastatic disease in patients > 30 yr
  - If no clinical signs of infection or persistence over time
  - Look for pharynx, thyroid, sinus primary or lymphoma

SELECTED REFERENCES

1. Gozgec E et al: Normal size of retropharyngeal lymph nodes in children on three dimensional magnetic resonance imaging. Pediatr Radiol. 54(12):2006-14, 2024
2. Norris CD et al: Anatomy of neck muscles, spaces, and lymph nodes. Neuroimaging Clin N Am. 32(4):831-49, 2022

KEY FACTS

TERMINOLOGY

- Retropharyngeal adenitis, intranodal abscess
- Formation of pus in retropharyngeal space (RPS) node draining H&N infection

IMAGING

- CECT: 1st-line tool to evaluate extent of deep H&N infection (best demonstrates suppuration)
- RPS node lies medial to internal carotid artery
- Low density within enlarged node
- RPS cellulitis ± internal carotid narrowing
  - Vasospasm more common in children, usually self-limited
- Node may show prominent peripheral enhancement
- Lateral RPS, does not cross midline like abscess
- MR: Restricted diffusion in suppurative node

TOP DIFFERENTIAL DIAGNOSES

- RPS reactive adenopathy; RPS abscess

- RPS nodal squamous cell carcinoma
- RPS schwannoma; RPS edema

PATHOLOGY

- H&N infection seeds RPS nodes
- Node draining infection enlarges = reactive node
- If untreated, progresses to suppurative node
- If still untreated, ruptures = RPS abscess

CLINICAL ISSUES

- More common in children & teens
- Sore throat, odynophagia, fever, neck pain

DIAGNOSTIC CHECKLIST

- Evaluate retropharynx for suppurative change with any H&N infection
- RPS nodes nonpalpable, can rapidly progress to abscess, sepsis, & airway compromise
- Consider metastatic disease if no inflammatory change or clinical infection, or if patient > 40 yr

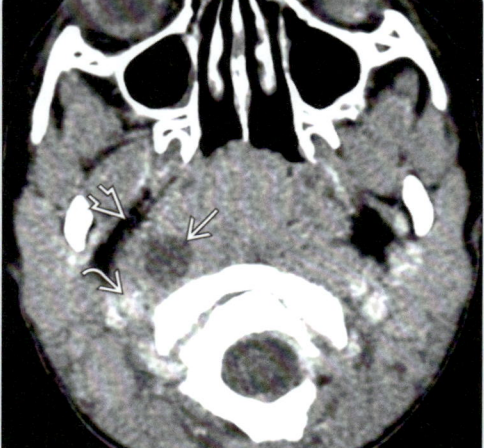
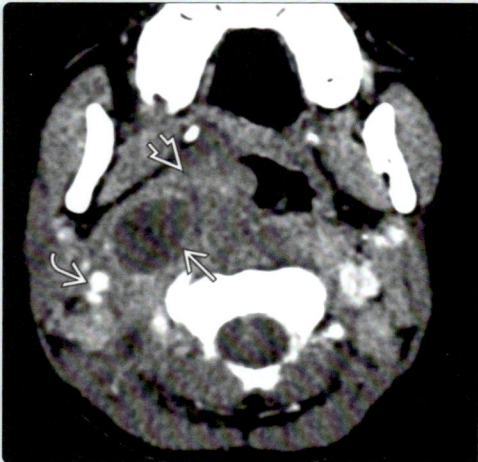

(Left) Axial CECT in a young child demonstrates a well-defined, low-density lesion ➡ anteromedial to the right internal carotid artery (ICA) ➡. This represented pus within the right retropharyngeal lymph node and is associated with effacement of parapharyngeal fat ➡. (Right) Axial CECT in a 6-year-old with sore throat shows a low-density suppurative right lateral retropharyngeal space (RPS) node ➡, surrounding soft tissue swelling ➡, airway asymmetry, and deviation of the carotid sheath vessels ➡.

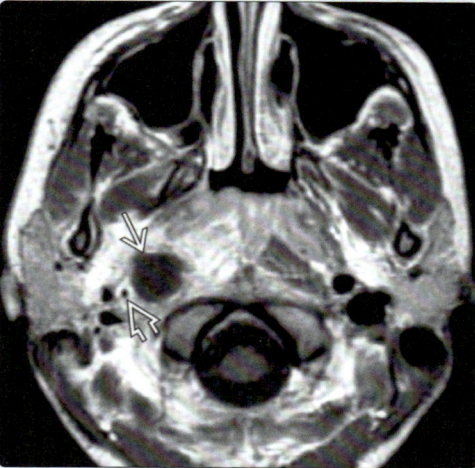
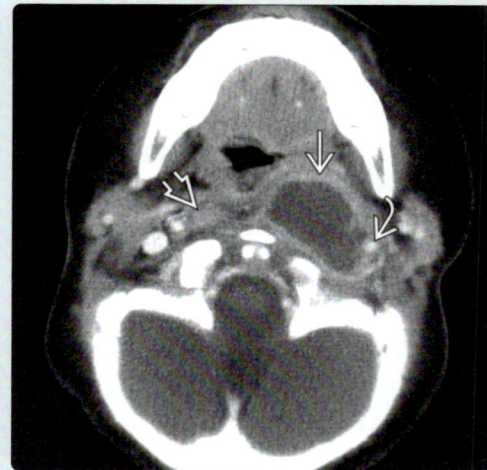

(Left) Axial T1WI C+ MR shows a discrete lateral retropharyngeal suppurative node ➡ with surrounding cellulitis. Note the adjacent internal carotid artery ➡ in spasm due to response to adjacent infection. (Right) Axial CECT shows a hypodense, rim-enhancing collection in the RPS ➡, secondary to extranodal rupture of the suppurative lymph node. There is extension nearly surrounding the left ICA, which is narrowed due to spasm ➡. This is usually self-limited. Note reactive adenopathy in right RPS ➡.

TERMINOLOGY

Abbreviations
- Retropharyngeal space (RPS)

Synonyms
- Retropharyngeal adenitis, intranodal abscess

Definitions
- Formation of pus in RPS lymph node draining H&N infection

IMAGING

General Features
- Best diagnostic clue
  - Central cystic change within enlarged RPS lymph node
  - Surrounding RPS ± pharyngeal inflammatory changes
- Location: RPS between skull base & hyoid bone
  - Medial to internal carotid arteries (ICAs)
  - Lateral RPS suppurative lymph node; does not cross midline (extranodal abscess might)

CT Findings
- CECT: Low density within enlarged lymph node ± peripheral enhancement
  - Well-defined, low-density collection with rim enhancement = drainable pus in only ~ 80% of cases; 20% represent nondrainable phlegmon
  - RPS cellulitis ± ICA vasospasm
    - Vasospasm more common in children, usually self-limited

MR Findings
- T2WI: Diffuse or focal central high intensity in RPS node
  - ↑ signal intensity of surrounding soft tissues
- T1WI C+: Peripheral lymph node & adjacent soft tissue enhancement
- DWI: Restricted diffusion in suppurative lymph node

Imaging Recommendations
- Best imaging tool
  - CECT is 1st-line tool for evaluation of H&N infection
- Protocol advice
  - Image to include upper mediastinum in any patient with suspect deep neck infection

DIFFERENTIAL DIAGNOSIS

Retropharyngeal Space Reactive Adenopathy
- Incidental finding or upper respiratory tract infection
- Homogeneous nodal enlargement, no cystic change

Retropharyngeal Space Abscess
- Toxic patient
- Rim-enhancing fluid collection in RPS

Retropharyngeal Space Nodal SCCa
- Solid or cystic RPS nodal mass without perinodal inflammatory change
- Sinonasal or naso-, oro-, or hypopharyngeal primary

Retropharyngeal Space Schwannoma
- Ovoid mass in RPS, mimics node
- Arises from sympathetic chain

Retropharyngeal Space Edema
- Sterile fluid without rim enhancement, crosses midline RPS
- Between pharynx & prevertebral muscles

PATHOLOGY

General Features
- Etiology
  - H&N infection seeds RPS nodes
    - Spread of infection from site that drains into node, or via direct inoculation secondary to puncture wound
    - Most commonly bacterial pharyngitis
    - Particularly *Staphylococcus aureus* & *Streptococcus*
  - Lymph node draining infection enlarges = reactive node
    - If untreated, progresses to suppuration
    - If still untreated, ruptures = RPS abscess

CLINICAL ISSUES

Presentation
- Most common signs/symptoms
  - Sore throat, odynophagia
- Other signs/symptoms
  - Fever, poor oral intake, neck pain
  - Elevated WBC & ESR
- Clinical profile
  - Young sick patient, upper respiratory infection

Demographics
- Age: More common in children & teens (uncommon > 30 yr)
- Sex: M = F

Natural History & Prognosis
- If RPS cellulitis is extensive, can narrow airway
- Untreated suppurative node can result in RPS abscess

Treatment
- Antibiotics orally; if poor response then intravenously
- Incision & drainage if progression to extranodal abscess

DIAGNOSTIC CHECKLIST

Consider
- Consider malignancy in patient > 40 yr
  - Especially if no inflammatory change or clinical infection

Image Interpretation Pearls
- Evaluate RPS carefully for suppurative change
  - RPS infection can rapidly progress to abscess, sepsis, & airway compromise

SELECTED REFERENCES
1. Loney EL: Non-traumatic head and neck emergencies. Br J Radiol. 97(1154):306-14, 2024
2. Shareef M et al: Critical infections in the head and neck: a pictorial review of acute presentations and complications. Neuroradiol J. 37(4):402-17, 2024
3. Singh S et al: Pediatric head and neck emergencies. Neuroradiology. 66(11):2053-70, 2024
4. Baba A et al: Advanced imaging of head and neck infections. J Neuroimaging. 33(4):477-492, 2023
5. O'Brien WT Sr: Common neck and otomastoid infections in children. Neuroimaging Clin N Am. 33(4):661-71, 2023
6. Stein JM et al: Imaging of head and neck infections. Neuroimaging Clin N Am. 33(1):185-206, 2023

Retropharyngeal Space Abscess

TERMINOLOGY

- Extranodal purulent fluid collection in retropharyngeal space (RPS)

IMAGING

- Lateral radiograph: Wide prevertebral distance with loss of normal contours at hypopharynx-esophagus interface
- CECT best tool for rapid characterization & evaluation of extent/complications
  - RPS distended by defined, ovoid, rim-enhancing, low-density collection with convex anterior margin
  - Complications include airway compromise, jugular vein thrombosis/thrombophlebitis, mediastinal extension/mediastinitis, internal carotid artery (ICA) narrowing common, pseudoaneurysm rare (suggests methicillin-resistant *Staphylococcus aureus*)

TOP DIFFERENTIAL DIAGNOSES

- Pseudothickening of retropharyngeal soft tissues

- RPS edema
- Necrotic/suppurative adenopathy in RPS
- Lymphatic malformation
- Neurofibroma

PATHOLOGY

- Most common etiology: Rupture of suppurative RPS lymph node → abscess

CLINICAL ISSUES

- Dysphagia, sore throat, poor oral intake, dehydration
- Toxic patient: Fever, chills, ↑ WBC & ESR
- Most < 6 years old; ↑ incidence in adults

DIAGNOSTIC CHECKLIST

- Distinction from RPS edema sometimes difficult
  - Oval-shaped collection with convex anterior margin & rim enhancement suggests drainable abscess
    - Rim enhancement may be minimal if early in disease course or if CECT performed with early/arterial timing

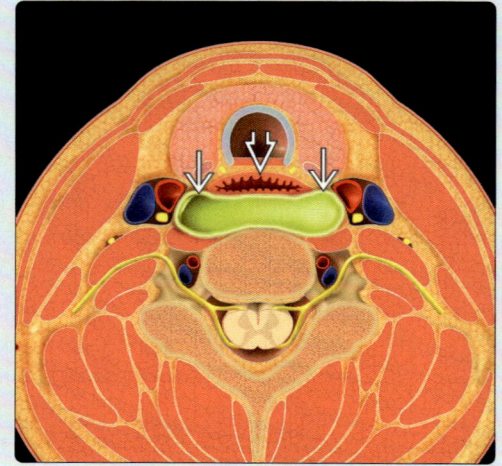
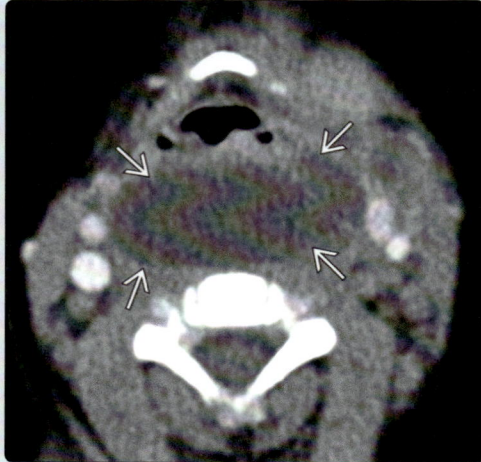

(Left) *Axial graphic illustrates the location & typical contour of a retropharyngeal space (RPS) abscess ➡ displacing the cervical esophagus ➡ anteriorly & flattening the prevertebral muscles.* (Right) *Axial CECT in a 10-month-old infant with a 5-day history of febrile illness reveals a large, low-density, ovoid collection distending the RPS ➡ with anterior displacement of the pharynx & splaying of the carotid sheaths. There is minimal enhancement of the wall of the collection but marked mass effect.*

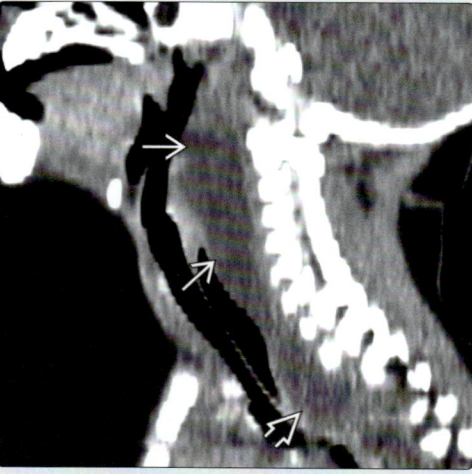
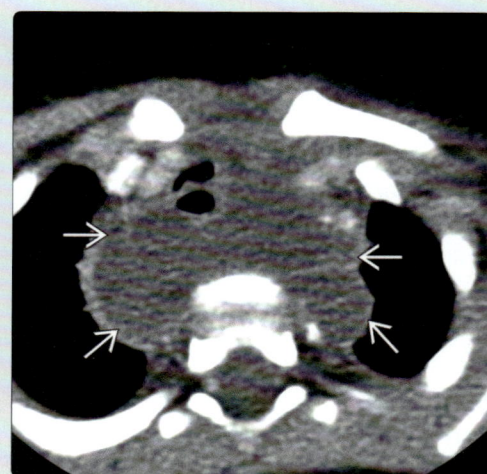

(Left) *Sagittal reformatted CECT in the same infant reveals an abscess ➡ displacing the pharynx & esophagus anteriorly & extending inferiorly to involve the superior mediastinum ➡.* (Right) *Axial CECT reveals the inferior extension of this methicillin-resistant Staphylococcus aureus (MRSA) abscess to the superior mediastinum ➡. This fluid was drained through a cervical approach to the collection. There was no stridor or other sign of airway compromise despite a displaced & narrowed airway.*

Retropharyngeal Space Abscess

TERMINOLOGY

Definitions

- Retropharyngeal space (RPS): Midline space posterior to pharyngeal mucosa & cervical esophagus from skull base to T3 vertebral level in mediastinum
- RPS abscess: Extranodal purulent fluid collection in RPS

IMAGING

General Features

- Best diagnostic clue
  - Midline rim-enhancing RPS fluid collection with mass effect in toxic-appearing patient
- Location
  - Posterior to pharynx & anterior to prevertebral muscles
- Morphology
  - Defined collection, not just infiltrative edema
  - Axial plane: Oval shape with convex anterior margin

Radiographic Findings

- Lateral view critical
  - Normal prevertebral soft tissue thickness
    - C2 (at hypopharynx): ≤ 7 mm at any age
    - C6 (at cervical esophagus): ≤ 14 mm if < 15 years, ≤ 22 mm in adults
  - In children: Must perform lateral radiograph during inspiration **&** with neck extension
    - Neck flexion & expiration → pseudothickening of prevertebral soft tissues in young children
    - Lateral fluoroscopy can distinguish persistent true thickening vs. dynamic pseudothickening
- RPS abscess → thickened prevertebral soft tissues
  - Convex anterior bowing with loss of normal step-off at interface of hypopharynx & esophagus
  - Limited utility for defining extent of collection & differentiating cellulitis/phlegmon from abscess
  - RPS gas rare but diagnostic of abscess (if no trauma)

CT Findings

- CECT
  - RPS markedly distended by rim-enhancing fluid collection
    - In early stages, enhancement may be subtle
    - Thick, enhancing wall suggests mature abscess
    - Prevertebral muscles may also appear edematous
    - Gas rarely present
    - Associated nonsuppurative adenopathy
  - Assess for complications
    - Airway compromise
    - Internal jugular vein (IJV) frequently compressed/effaced, rarely thrombosed
    - Internal carotid artery (ICA) narrowing (spasm) common; pseudoaneurysm rare [suggests methicillin-resistant *Staphylococcus aureus* (MRSA)]

MR Findings

- Rarely utilized emergently
  - Patient may have tenuous airway; patient monitoring more difficult in MR scanner
- Awareness of imaging findings necessary to prevent misdiagnosis as noninflammatory condition

- RPS edema/soft tissue enhancement surrounding fluid-signal intensity, rim-enhancing collection
  - DWI: Diffusion restriction within center of abscess
  - Assess for complications same as with CECT

Ultrasonographic Findings

- Not able to assess full craniocaudal or deep extent of disease
- Limited by operator experience & patient tolerance
- May help evaluate jugular vein patency

Imaging Recommendations

- Best imaging tool
  - CECT
- Protocol advice
  - CT from skull base to carina
  - Contrast loading (split) bolus &/or non-CTA technique improves soft tissue contrast resolution given rapid acquisition times of CT
    - ↑ sensitivity for collections, rim enhancement

DIFFERENTIAL DIAGNOSIS

Pseudothickening of Retropharyngeal Soft Tissues

- Common radiographic mimic of retropharyngeal pathology in young children
- Adequate extension & inspiration or fluoroscopy will confirm as transient finding

Retropharyngeal Space Edema

- Poorly defined, elongated, homogeneous fluid infiltration of prevertebral soft tissues without rim enhancement
- In axial plane: Bow tie shape with concave anterior margin
- RPS vessels may traverse infiltrated tissues
- Drainage not required
- Etiologies include
  - Regional inflammation: Pharyngitis, tonsillitis, longus colli tendinitis
  - Venous or lymphatic obstruction: IJV thrombosis or resection, radiation

Suppurative Adenopathy in Retropharyngeal Space

- Centrally hypodense/necrotic lymph node in lateral RPS with adjacent cellulitis
- May lead to pus formation in reactive node (suppuration): Intranodal abscess
- May progress to extranodal RPS abscess with inadequate medical therapy

Lymphatic Malformation

- Uni- or multilocular, transspatial, cystic neck mass with thin, nonenhancing wall (unless infected)
- Typically involves anterior & lateral neck

Neurofibroma

- Lobular masses of varying size in superficial &/or deep locations (multiple & plexiform in neurofibromatosis type 1)
- May be low attenuation on CT

PATHOLOGY

General Features

- Etiology

- ○ H&N infection (pharyngitis, tonsillitis) seeds RPS lymph node
  - − Reactive node → suppurative intranodal abscess → nodal rupture → RPS abscess
  - − Most common organisms: *S. aureus*, *Haemophilus*, *Streptococcus*
- ○ Pharyngeal penetration by foreign body
  - − Child running with object in mouth
    - □ Lollipop/sucker, toothbrush, stick, toy
- ○ Ventral spread of discitis/osteomyelitis & prevertebral infection
  - − Uncommon in children; pyogenic or tuberculous
- ○ Mediastinal abscess spreading cranially
  - − Esophageal rupture & mediastinitis with danger space (DS) abscess

CLINICAL ISSUES

Presentation

- Most common signs/symptoms
  - ○ Dysphagia, sore throat, poor oral intake, dehydration
  - ○ Septic patient: Fever, chills, elevated WBC & ESR
- Other signs/symptoms
  - ○ Posterior pharyngeal wall edema or bulge
  - ○ Reactive cervical adenopathy
- Clinical profile
  - ○ Toxic-appearing child with marked neck pain & limited movement, especially in extension
  - ○ Uncommonly presents with airway compromise (stridor)

Demographics

- Age: Most often children < 6 years old
  - ○ ↑ frequency in adult population
    - − Immunocompromised states: Diabetes, HIV, alcoholism, malignancy
    - − Discitis/osteomyelitis with perivertebral infection
    - − Trauma with foreign body impaction
    - − Following anterior cervical spine surgery
- Sex: M:F = 2:1
- Epidemiology: ↑ frequency over last decade
  - ○ ↓ incidence of abscess when infection detected & treated in earlier cellulitic stage

Natural History & Prognosis

- Prognosis generally excellent with early diagnosis & aggressive management
- Complications may result from infection spread
  - ○ Narrowing of pharyngeal lumen → airway compromise & stridor
  - ○ Inferior spread via DS to mediastinum → mediastinitis
    - − Up to 50% mortality (much less in infants)
      - □ ↓ mortality rate in recent years with aggressive initial & repeat surgical intervention
    - − MRSA frequent
  - ○ Carotid space involvement
    - − Jugular vein thrombosis or thrombophlebitis
    - − Narrowing of ICA caliber often found; neurologic sequelae infrequent
    - − Rarely ICA pseudoaneurysm &/or rupture; described with MRSA infection
  - ○ Perivertebral space abscess may lead to epidural abscess

- ○ Aspiration pneumonia
- ○ Grisel syndrome rare
  - − Inflammatory, nontraumatic atlantoaxial subluxation
  - − Distention or loosening of atlantoaxial ligaments after H&N inflammation

Treatment

- Early ENT consultation
- IV antibiotics, airway management, fluid resuscitation
- Surgical intervention (I&D) for
  - ○ Significant or complex abscess
  - ○ Lack of improvement/worsening with IV antibiotics

DIAGNOSTIC CHECKLIST

Consider

- Lateral radiograph: Often 1st-line screening tool
- Study of choice: CECT
  - ○ Determine RPS vs. perivertebral space
  - ○ Distinguish RPS abscess from edema
  - ○ Evaluate full craniocaudal extent
  - ○ Evaluate for vascular/airway complications
  - ○ Consider contrast prebolus/split bolus or venous-phase imaging to maximize wall enhancement

Image Interpretation Pearls

- Distinction from RPS edema sometimes difficult
  - ○ Convex anterior margin or oval-shaped collection suggests abscess
  - ○ Rim enhancement suggests abscess
    - − May be minimal early in disease
    - − May not be evident due to early arterial scanning
- Important to evaluate full extent of abscess & presence of complications
- ENT consultation imperative

SELECTED REFERENCES

1. Loney EL: Non-traumatic head and neck emergencies. Br J Radiol. 97(1154):306-14, 2024
2. Shareef M et al: Critical infections in the head and neck: a pictorial review of acute presentations and complications. Neuroradiol J. 37(4):402-17, 2024
3. Singh S et al: Pediatric head and neck emergencies. Neuroradiology. 66(11):2053-70, 2024
4. Baba A et al: Advanced imaging of head and neck infections. J Neuroimaging. 33(4):477-92, 2023
5. O'Brien WT Sr: Common neck and otomastoid infections in children. Neuroimaging Clin N Am. 33(4):661-71, 2023
6. Stein JM et al: Imaging of head and neck infections. Neuroimaging Clin N Am. 33(1):185-206, 2023
7. Carroll W et al: Is vessel narrowing secondary to pediatric deep neck space infections of clinical significance? Int J Pediatr Otorhinolaryngol. 125:56-8, 2019
8. Ho ML et al: The ABCs (airway, blood vessels, and compartments) of pediatric neck infections and masses. AJR Am J Roentgenol. 206(5):963-72, 2016
9. Hoang JK et al: Multiplanar CT and MRI of collections in the retropharyngeal space: is it an abscess? AJR Am J Roentgenol. 196(4):W426-32, 2011
10. Stone ME et al: Correlation between computed tomography and surgical findings in retropharyngeal inflammatory processes in children. Int J Pediatr Otorhinolaryngol. 49(2):121-5, 1999
11. Hudgins PA et al: Internal carotid artery narrowing in children with retropharyngeal lymphadenitis and abscess. AJNR Am J Neuroradiol. 19(10):1841-3, 1998

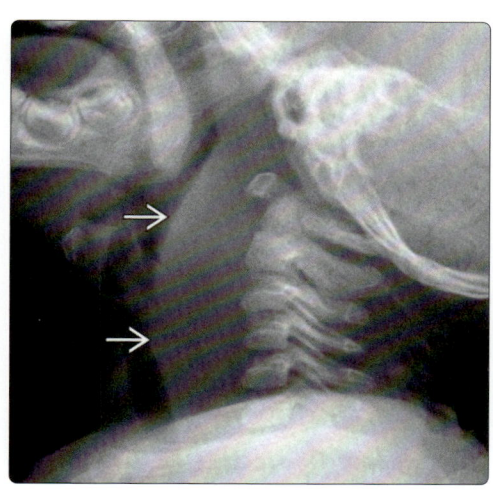

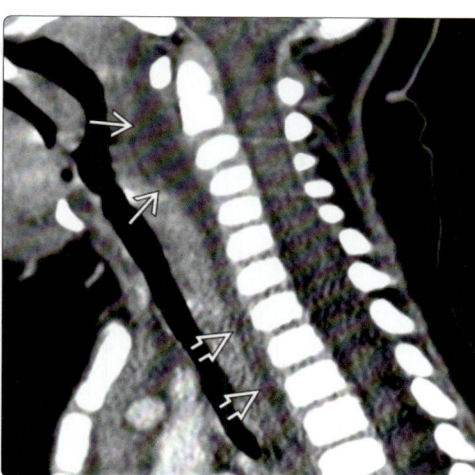

(Left) Lateral radiograph in a 12-month-old boy with sepsis shows significant thickening of the prevertebral soft tissues ➡. The normal step-off at the pharyngeal-esophageal junction is effaced. (Right) Sagittal reformatted CECT in the same child clearly shows the cause of the prominent soft tissues to be a convex anterior RPS abscess ➡ with extension of fluid into the posterior mediastinum ⇉. It is important to image these children from the nasopharynx to the carina in order to evaluate the full craniocaudad extent of the collection.

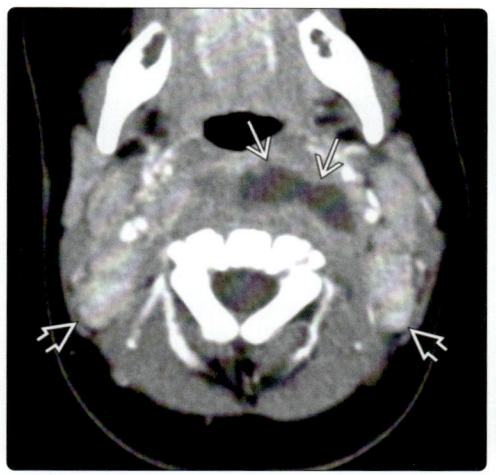

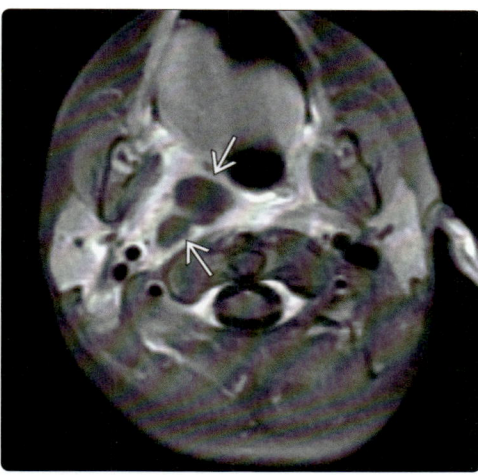

(Left) Axial CECT in a 5-month-old boy shows an irregularly shaped RPS fluid collection ➡ in the midline & left paramidline soft tissues, most likely extranodal spread of a suppurative left lateral RPS lymph node. Notice the bilateral nonsuppurative cervical adenopathy ⇉. (Right) Axial T1 C+ FS MR in a child allergic to iodinated contrast demonstrates a well-defined abscess ➡ in the right lateral RPS with significant surrounding contrast enhancement & mild extension of inflammation medial to the carotid sheath vessels.

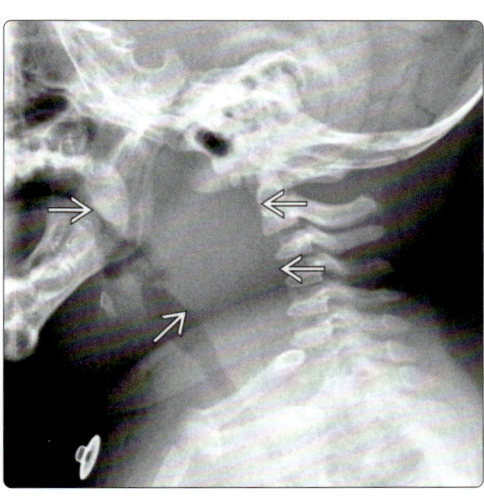

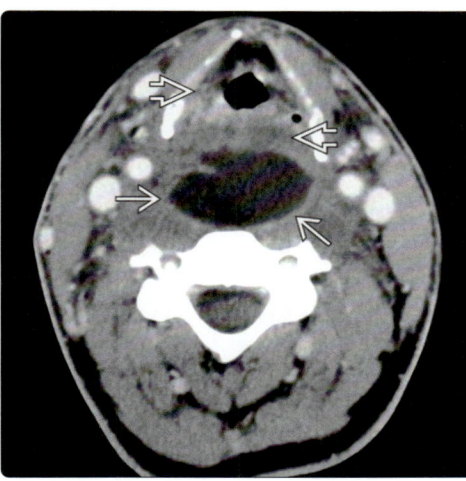

(Left) Lateral radiograph in a 7-month-old child with fever shows marked thickening of the prevertebral soft tissues ➡ with ventral displacement of the pharynx & larynx. There is loss of the normal step-off at the pharyngeal-esophageal junction. (Right) Axial CECT in the same patient shows a faintly enhancing rim ➡ at the periphery of a large RPS abscess, which displaces the hypopharynx & larynx anteriorly ➡. The adjacent carotid sheath vessels are normal in position, enhancement, & caliber.

KEY FACTS

TERMINOLOGY

- Retropharyngeal space (RPS) effusion, benign retropharyngeal fluid
- Accumulation of sterile fluid, effacing RPS fat

IMAGING

- NECT: Smooth expansion of RPS with **water-density fluid**
  - Located between pharynx and prevertebral muscles
- CECT/C+ MR: **No wall enhancement**
- MR: Linear to lenticular ↓ T1 and ↑ T2 (**water signal**) in RPS

TOP DIFFERENTIAL DIAGNOSES

- RPS abscess
- Prominent normal retropharyngeal fat

PATHOLOGY

- Different inciting factors result in RPS fluid
- Infectious/inflammatory, venoocclusive, and noninfectious

CLINICAL ISSUES

- Self-limited or limited by course of causative process
- Does **not** require drainage
- Try to identify primary cause that requires treatment

DIAGNOSTIC CHECKLIST

- Key is to **differentiate from RPS abscess** 1st
  - Rim-enhancing fluid with abscess, not edema
  - Diffusion restriction with abscess, not edema
  - Abscess requires urgent ENT consultation
- CECT pitfall: Beware abscess false-negatives due to early arterial-phase scans (technical lack of rim enhancement)
- Look for underlying cause; may be treatable
  - Current infection: Pharynx, teeth, sinus, spine
  - Venous occlusive disease
  - Recent chemotherapy or radiation therapy
  - Trauma (spine fracture, whiplash injury)
  - Longus colli tendinitis

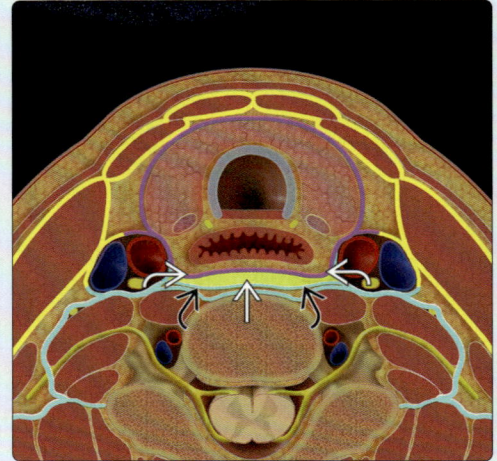
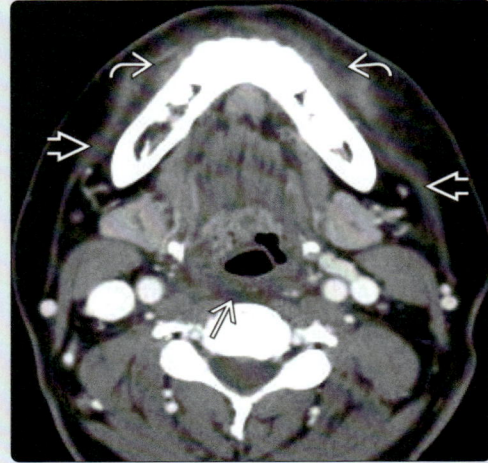

(Left) Axial graphic illustrates retropharyngeal space (RPS) distention with edema ➡. Note fascial delineation of the RPS by a middle layer of deep cervical fascia (DCF) anteriorly ➡ and a deep layer of DCF posteriorly ➡. (Right) Axial CECT shows bland RPS fluid without rim enhancement ➡. Note evidence of source: Cellulitis overlying the mandible ➡ and thickened platysma ➡ from nearby dental infection.

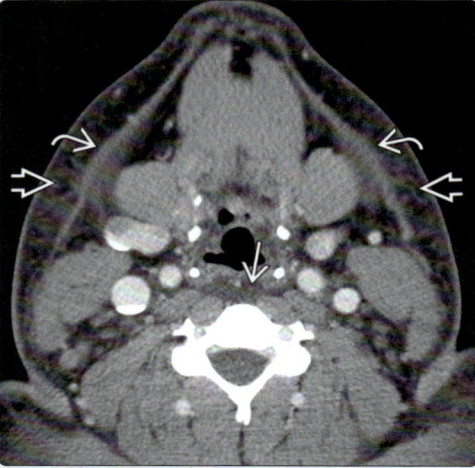
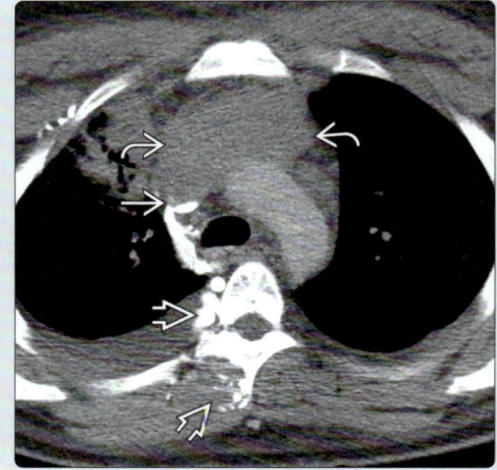

(Left) Axial CECT in a patient with lymphoma shows a small retropharyngeal fluid collection ➡. There are signs of diffuse neck edema with reticulation of subcutaneous fat ➡ and thickening of the platysma muscles ➡ bilaterally. (Right) Axial venous-phase CECT in the same patient demonstrates superior vena cava (SVC) syndrome as the source of RPS edema due to anterior mediastinal lymphoma ➡ invading the SVC ➡. Prominent venous collaterals ➡ drain into the azygous vein, bypassing the SVC.

TERMINOLOGY

Abbreviations
- Retropharyngeal space (RPS)

Synonyms
- Retropharyngeal effusion, benign retropharyngeal fluid

Definitions
- Accumulation of sterile fluid, effacing RPS fat

IMAGING

General Features
- Best diagnostic clue
  - Thin collection of fluid in RPS without enhancing wall
- Location
  - RPS
    - Anterior to prevertebral muscles (prevertebral portion of perivertebral space)
    - Posterior to pharynx (pharyngeal mucosal space)
    - RPS stretches from skull base superiorly to upper mediastinum inferiorly
- Size
  - Several millimeters anteroposterior dimension
  - Variable craniocaudal length of edema (may extend from skull base to upper mediastinum)
- Morphology
  - Smooth expansion of RPS with fluid
  - Sharp demarcation from pharynx and prevertebral muscles
  - Usually lacks bulging contour more typical of abscess

Radiographic Findings
- Radiography
  - Lateral plain film
    - Variably widened prevertebral tissues
    - Cannot distinguish RPS and perivertebral space
    - Cannot distinguish between infected and noninfected RPS collections
  - Look for prevertebral calcification at C1-2 level in longus colli tendinitis

CT Findings
- CECT
  - Uniform low (water-) density fluid collection in RPS without rim enhancement
    - Pitfall: Technical false-negatives occur with early arterial-phase scans where abscess lacks rim-enhancing wall due to inadequate imaging delay
  - Look for possible causative factors
    - **Neck infection** or inflammatory changes
      - Focal rim-enhancing fluid (abscess)
      - Focal area of amorphous enhancing tissue (phlegmon)
    - **Venous thrombosis** or internal jugular vein (IJV) resection
      - IJV distention with luminal clot
    - Superior vena cava **(SVC) syndrome**
    - Acute calcific **longus colli tendinitis**
      - C1-2 level calcifications present acutely

- Calcifications may **not** be present in chronic cases (symptoms > 1 month)
    - **Posttreatment** changes (surgical, radiation)

MR Findings
- T1WI
  - Linear to lenticular low (water) signal intensity bland fluid collection between pharynx and prevertebral muscles
- T2WI
  - High signal intensity similar to CSF
- DWI
  - Helps distinguish between abscess (restricted) vs. edema (facilitated)
- T1WI C+
  - No rim enhancement of fluid collection
  - May see subtle enhancement of edematous tissues or enhancing vessels through fluid

Imaging Recommendations
- Best imaging tool
  - CECT readily evaluates retropharyngeal tissues and assesses contours, contrast enhancement, and potential causes
  - Enhanced MR best for spinal source (early discitis/osteomyelitis)
- Protocol advice
  - Contrast essential; must image from skull base to superior mediastinum
    - Allows detection of enhancement, suggesting abscess
    - Evaluates adjacent soft tissues and vessels for source

DIFFERENTIAL DIAGNOSIS

Retropharyngeal Space Abscess
- Distention of RPS by fluid collection with **convex** margins
- **Rim enhancement** particularly in mature abscess
- Gas + fluid in RPS suggest abscess, or consider necrotizing fasciitis if no history of prior instrumentation
- Prevertebral muscles or pharynx often difficult to delineate from collection
- Diffusion restriction on MR
- Septic patient, neck pain, sore throat

Prominent Normal Retropharyngeal Fat
- Incidental finding
- More often in pediatric or Cushingoid patients
- No distention of RPS
- NECT/CECT: Fat density; negative Hounsfield units
- MR: T1 and T2 hyperintense, signal loss with fat saturation

Retropharyngeal Space Lipoma
- Retropharyngeal lipoma distends RPS
- NECT/CECT: Fat density; negative Hounsfield units
  - Uniform fat density; may be unilateral
- MR: T1 hyperintensity, signal loss with T1 FS

Hypopharyngeal Squamous Cell Carcinoma
- Posterior pharyngeal wall squamous cell carcinoma (SCCa) may infiltrate deeply
- Also possible with posterior oropharyngeal wall SCCa
- **Solid, enhancing**, ill-defined infiltrative mass

PATHOLOGY

General Features

- Etiology
  - Typically due to transudate
  - Inflammatory and infectious processes
    - Pharyngitis, dental infection, sinusitis
    - Acute calcific longus colli tendinitis
      □ Calcium hydroxyapatite deposition in longus colli muscle insertions
      □ Self-limited inflammation responds to NSAIDs ± steroids
    - Kawasaki disease may cause effusion or abscess
    - Multisystem inflammatory syndrome in children (MIS-C) from COVID-19
  - Altered venous flow in neck
    - IJV resection with radical or modified neck dissection
    - IJV thrombosis
    - SVC syndrome
    - Postpharyngitis venous thrombosis (Lemierre syndrome)
    - Neoplasm with venous compression or occlusion
  - Other noninfected fluid collections
    - Current or recent chemotherapy or radiation therapy (**lymphedema**)
    - Trauma (spine fracture, whiplash injury)
    - Pseudomeningocele post anterior cervical discectomy and fusion (ACDF) (CSF leak)
    - Angioedema (anaphylaxis, ACE inhibitors, post-ACDF)
    - Nephrotic syndrome

Microscopic Features

- Should not be aspirated as self-limited or limited by causative factors

CLINICAL ISSUES

Presentation

- Most common signs/symptoms
  - RPS fluid is asymptomatic though patient may have symptoms from primary cause
    - Radiation therapy, SVC syndrome, recent neck surgery, regional infectious/inflammatory process
    - Longus colli tendinitis: Neck stiffness, sore throat, low-grade fever
  - RPS edema is independent risk factor for ICU admission

Demographics

- Age
  - Any; dependent on primary cause
- Sex
  - M = F

Natural History & Prognosis

- Self-limited or limited by course of causative process
  - Venous compromise: IJV thrombosis, resection, or SVC syndrome
    - Effusion improves spontaneously or with resolution of thrombosis
  - Radiation-induced RPS fluid typically appears at 4-6 weeks; resolves spontaneously by 8-12 weeks
  - Adjacent regional infections resolve with antibiotic &/or surgical therapy
    - Some cases can become secondarily infected; imaging may be required for surveillance
  - Calcific longus colli tendinitis resolves with treatment of acute inflammation

Treatment

- Does **not** require drainage
- Try to identify primary cause that requires treatment
  - Treat regional infection with antibiotics ± surgery
  - Treat venous thrombosis with anticoagulants
  - SVC syndrome may require stenting
  - Treat longus colli tendinitis with steroids ± NSAIDs

DIAGNOSTIC CHECKLIST

Consider

- Relatively common lesion seen on CECT in setting of complex neck disease
- Important to **differentiate from RPS abscess**
  - Abscess in RPS
    - **Mass effect** with distention of RPS with convex contours
    - Fluid collection **wall enhances**
    - RPS gas without history of recent instrumentation or pharynx perforation suggests abscess &/or necrotizing fasciitis
    - RPS abscess associated with adjacent cellulitis
    - ENT consultation if RPS abscess suspected
- Confirm that CECT is technically sufficient (i.e., not arterial phase) to expect wall enhancement if present

Image Interpretation Pearls

- Once RPS abscess excluded, look for cause of edema
  - Regional neck inflammatory/infectious process
  - Calcifications at C1-2 level in prevertebral muscles (longus colli tendinitis)
  - Venous compromise: IJV thrombosis, resection, SVC syndrome
  - Recent chemotherapy or radiation therapy

Reporting Tips

- Report should reflect bland fluid without mass effect or rim enhancement
- Do not offer RPS abscess in differential diagnosis as may prompt surgical intervention

SELECTED REFERENCES

1. Vierula JP et al: MRI-based risk factors for intensive care unit admissions in acute neck infections. Eur J Radiol Open. 14:100648, 2025
2. Jenkins E et al: Retropharyngeal edema and neck pain in multisystem inflammatory syndrome in children (MIS-c). J Pediatric Infect Dis Soc. 10(9):922-5, 2021
3. Langner S et al: Differentiation of retropharyngeal calcific tendinitis and retropharyngeal abscess: a case series and review of the literature. Eur Arch Otorhinolaryngol. 277(9):2631-6, 2020
4. Chapman SC et al: Lemierre's syndrome: an atypical presentation. Ann Vasc Surg. 60:479.e1-4, 2019
5. Debkowska MP et al: Acute post-operative airway complications following anterior cervical spine surgery and the role for cricothyrotomy. J Spine Surg. 5(1):142-54, 2019
6. Bhatt AA: Non-traumatic causes of fluid in the retropharyngeal space. Emerg Radiol. 25(5):547-51, 2018

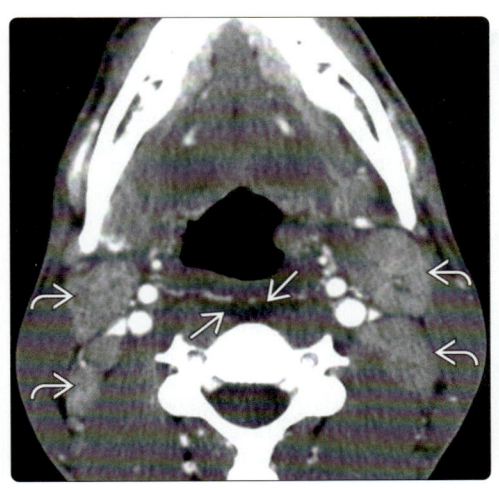

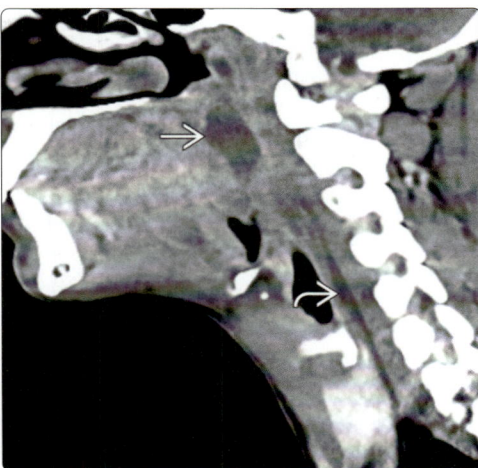

(Left) Axial CECT reveals expansion of the RPS by low-density, nonenhancing fluid ➡. Prevertebral muscles and pharyngeal contours remain sharply defined. Bilateral reactive adenopathy ➡ is also seen in this patient with Streptococcus throat infection. (Right) Sagittal CECT of the neck shows a rim-enhancing peritonsillar abscess ➡ and linear fluid within the RPS without peripheral enhancement ➡. This is a reactive RPS effusion, not an RPS abscess.

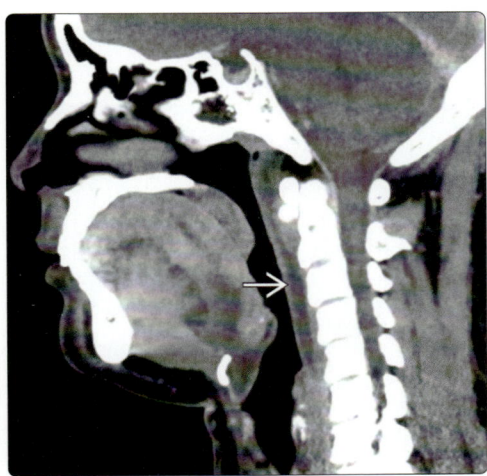

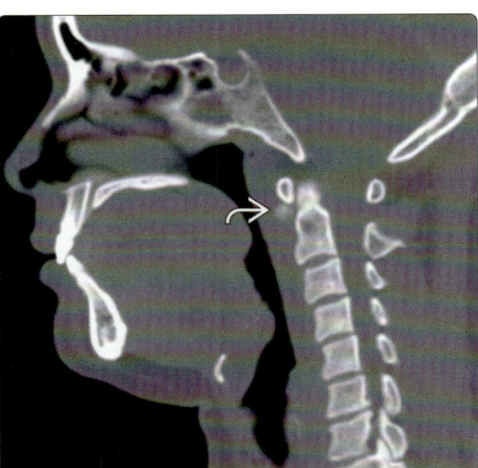

(Left) Sagittal CECT of the neck in a soft tissue window in a patient with 2 days of neck pain shows linear fluid within the RPS without peripheral rim enhancement ➡. Overall mass effect is minimal. (Right) Sagittal CECT of the neck in a bone window in the same patient shows globular mineralization just inferior to the anterior arch of C1 ➡. This is a case of longus colli tendinitis.

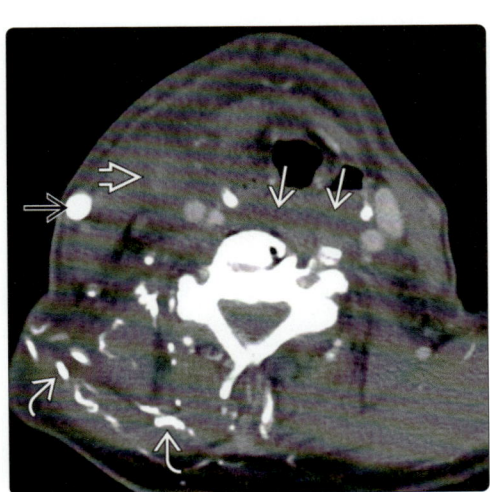

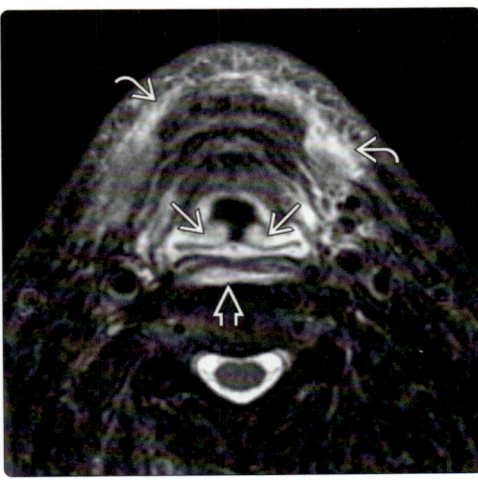

(Left) Axial CECT in a patient with right neck swelling and fevers shows thin RPS fluid ➡ due to right internal jugular vein thrombosis ➡. Note reflux of contrast material into collateral neck veins ➡ and external jugular vein ➡, bypassing the obstruction. (Right) Axial T2 FS MR performed for baseline 8 weeks after chemoradiation for tonsil squamous cell carcinoma shows retropharyngeal edema ➡. Hyperintense edema is seen in subcutaneous fat ➡ and aryepiglottic folds ➡.

KEY FACTS

TERMINOLOGY

- Malignant retropharyngeal space (RPS) nodes: Squamous cell carcinoma (SCCa) RPS nodes from nasopharyngeal carcinoma (NPCa) or posterior wall pharyngeal primary SCCa

IMAGING

- Location: Only present in suprahyoid neck
  - Anterior to prevertebral strap muscles, medial to internal carotid artery
- Oval to round, ± centrally necrotic mass > 0.8 cm in RPS
- Ill-defined margins ± stranding of surrounding fat are features of extracapsular spread
- CECT findings
  - Nodes difficult to identify on CT, especially if small
  - Nodal necrosis: Central low density with variably thick, irregular, enhancing wall
- MR more sensitive to detect RPS nodes than CT
- PET has role in staging & follow-up of H&N SCCa

- Cystic/necrotic nodes may be PET (-)

TOP DIFFERENTIAL DIAGNOSES

- Reactive RPS nodes; suppurative RPS nodes
- Direct RPS invasion by pharyngeal SCCa
- Non-Hodgkin lymphoma RPS nodes
- Thyroid RPS nodal metastasis; systemic RPS nodal metastasis

PATHOLOGY

- RPS nodes = primary drainage for posterior nasal cavity, ethmoid & sphenoid sinus, palate, nasopharynx & posterior wall of oro- & hypopharynx

CLINICAL ISSUES

- RPS malignant adenopathy is often clinically occult
- If large, bulging of posterolateral pharyngeal wall
- 75% of NPCa have RPS adenopathy at presentation
- 8-20% of oro- & hypopharyngeal wall SCCa have RPS nodes
  - Highest risk in posterior wall hypopharynx cancers (24%)

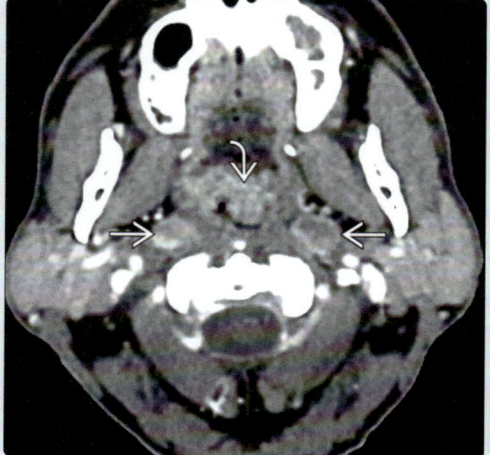
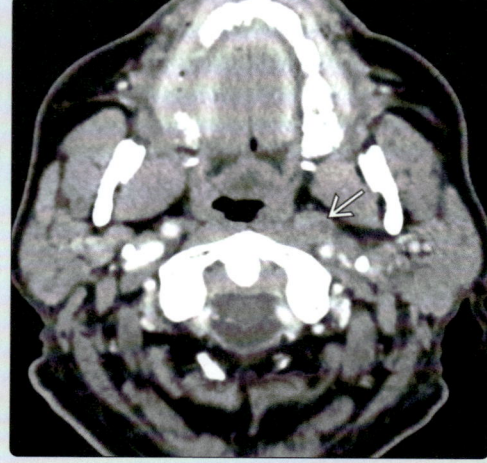

(Left) *Axial CECT shows necrotic retropharyngeal space (RPS) nodes ➡ in a patient with soft palate SCCa ➡. Posterior palate involvement and tumor extension across the midline are predictive of RPS nodal spread. Avid uptake was seen on FDG PET.* (Right) *Axial CECT in a patient with SCCa of the left tongue base reveals a metastatic retropharyngeal lymph node with foci of internal low density due to necrosis ➡. Pharyngeal SCCa is the most likely source of malignant retropharyngeal adenopathy in adults.*

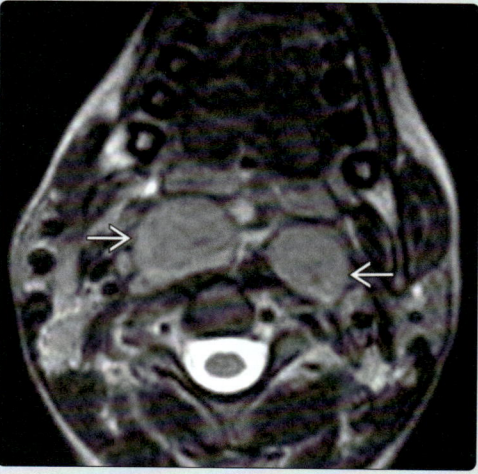
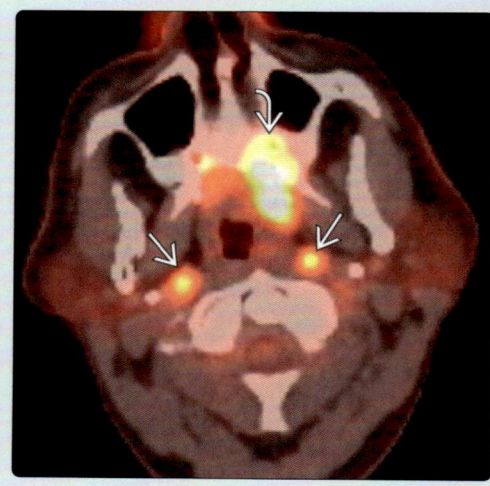

(Left) *Axial T2 MR demonstrates markedly enlarged RPS nodes ➡ due to metastatic involvement in this patient with nasopharyngeal SCCa. RPS nodes > 6 mm on axial imaging are suspicious for metastatic involvement in the context of nasopharyngeal carcinoma.* (Right) *Axial FDG PET/CT shows bilateral RPS nodal metastases ➡ in a patient with a large SCCa of the left tonsil (primary ➡ partly imaged here). RPS lymph nodes are generally clinically occult and critical to proper staging and treatment planning.*

TERMINOLOGY

Definitions

- Malignant retropharyngeal space (RPS) nodes: Squamous cell carcinoma (SCCa) RPS nodes from nasopharyngeal carcinoma (NPCa), posterior wall oropharyngeal, or hypopharyngeal primary SCCa

IMAGING

General Features

- Best diagnostic clue
  - Oval to round, ± centrally necrotic mass **> 0.8 cm** in RPS, medial to internal carotid artery (ICA)
- Location
  - RPS nodes are only present in suprahyoid neck
  - RPS nodes located anterior to prevertebral strap muscles, medial to ICA
- Size
  - Pathologic markers of RPS nodes
    - Size: > 0.8-cm minimum diameter in lateral RPS
    - Any node in medial RPS
    - **Necrosis ± extracapsular spread**, any size

CT Findings

- CECT
  - Often difficult to identify on CT, especially if small
  - Round, mildly enhancing soft tissue density RPS mass
  - Necrosis appears as central low density with variably thick, irregular, enhancing wall
  - Ill-defined margins ± stranding of surrounding fat are features of extracapsular spread

MR Findings

- T1WI
  - Nodes isointense to muscle
- T2WI
  - Nodes hyperintense
- T1WI C+
  - Enhancing lateral or medial RPS node
  - If nodal necrosis, central low intensity with peripheral wall enhancement

Nuclear Medicine Findings

- PET
  - Important role in staging & follow-up of H&N SCCa
    - Cystic/necrotic nodes may be PET (-)
  - Increased metabolic activity may diagnose metastatic SCCa in small, nonnecrotic RPS node

Imaging Recommendations

- Best imaging tool
  - MR best for detection of RPS nodes
    - On CECT, RPS nodes may be missed

DIFFERENTIAL DIAGNOSIS

Retropharyngeal Space Reactive Adenopathy

- Typically in younger patients (< 30 yr old)
- Homogeneous RPS mass < 1 cm
- Multiple other reactive-appearing nodes & adenoidal & palatine tonsillar hyperplasia associated

Retropharyngeal Space Suppurative Adenopathy

- Younger patient (< 30 yr old), pharyngitis, sepsis
- Intranodal abscess: Centrally necrotic, peripherally enhancing node ± RPS edema
- If suppurative node ruptures → RPS abscess

SCCa Direct Retropharyngeal Space Invasion

- Posterior oro- or hypopharynx wall SCCa
- Direct, contiguous invasion into RPS

Non-Hodgkin Lymphoma Retropharyngeal Space Nodes

- Usually large (> 2 cm), homogeneous, solid nodes
- Nodes involving multiple other H&N locations

Nodal Differentiated Thyroid Carcinoma

- CECT: Nodes may be cystic, heterogeneous, calcified
- MR: T1-hyperintense nodes characteristic

Metastatic Node, Non-SCCa, Retropharyngeal Space

- Widespread metastatic disease usually present
- Metastatic nodal melanoma, breast, lung, other

PATHOLOGY

General Features

- Critical RPS nodal anatomy
  - RPS nodes = primary drainage for posterior nasal cavity, ethmoid & sphenoid sinus, palate, nasopharynx & posterior wall of oro- & hypopharynx

CLINICAL ISSUES

Presentation

- Most common signs/symptoms
  - If large, bulging of posterolateral pharyngeal wall
  - RPS malignant nodes are **often clinically occult**

Demographics

- Epidemiology
  - 75% of NPCa have RPS adenopathy at presentation
  - 8-20% of oro- & hypopharyngeal SCCa have RPS nodes
    - Risk highest for posterior wall cancers (24%)
    - Present in 10% of oropharyngeal SCCa

Natural History & Prognosis

- Poor prognosis with RPS metastatic SCCa nodes

Treatment

- For NPCa, nodes included in radiation boost field ± superselective intraarterial chemotherapy
- For oro- & hypopharyngeal SCCa, transoral resection vs. radiation

SELECTED REFERENCES

1. Crompton DJ et al: Beyond the blade: retropharyngeal lymph nodes and an elusive complete resection. Int J Radiat Oncol Biol Phys. 120(1):10-11, 2024
2. Jacomina LE et al: Management of patients with early-stage oropharyngeal cancer with clinically positive retropharyngeal lymph nodes. Int J Radiat Oncol Biol Phys. 120(1):13-14, 2024
3. Roof SA et al: Hiding in plain sight: retropharyngeal lymph node metastasis. Int J Radiat Oncol Biol Phys. 120(1):12-13, 2024

Nodal Non-Hodgkin Lymphoma in Retropharyngeal Space

KEY FACTS

TERMINOLOGY

- NHL is lymphoreticular system malignancy
- Retropharyngeal space (RPS) from skull base to hyoid contains lateral & medial nodal groups
  - Lateral group = nodes of Rouvière
- H&N NHL has multiple forms
  - Nodal, nonnodal lymphatic or extralymphatic

IMAGING

- Oval-round, solid mass > **0.8 cm** (axial) in RPS
  - RPS nodes are medial to internal carotid arteries at or above hyoid
- **Typically associated with other neck adenopathy**
  - May have enlargement of Waldeyer ring
- Necrosis ± extranodal spread suggests high-grade, aggressive NHL
- MR more sensitive than CT for detecting RPS nodes
- CT & MR cannot differentiate normal-sized, nonnecrotic NHL nodes from reactive nodes; PET typically performed

- Most NHL are FDG avid

TOP DIFFERENTIAL DIAGNOSES

- RPS reactive adenopathy
- RPS suppurative adenopathy
- RPS nodal SCCa or systemic metastasis
  - Pharyngeal SCCa > NHL > thyroid carcinoma > melanoma

CLINICAL ISSUES

- Increasing incidence of NHL
- Median age: 50-55 yr
- RPS nodes usually clinically occult
  - If large, may see bulging of posterior pharyngeal wall
- Other manifestations of NHL in H&N
  - Extranodal, lymphatic disease in Waldeyer ring
  - Extranodal, extralymphatic site involvement

DIAGNOSTIC CHECKLIST

- Large, nonnecrotic node more likely NHL than SCCa

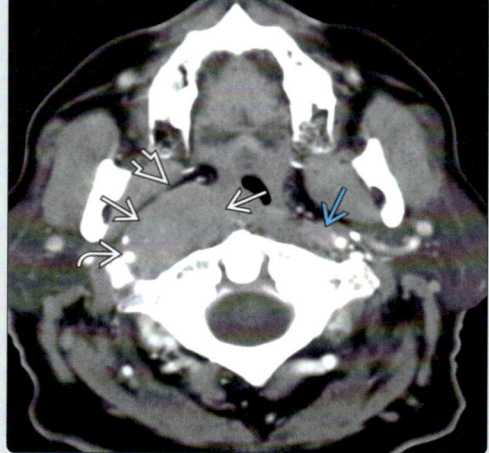
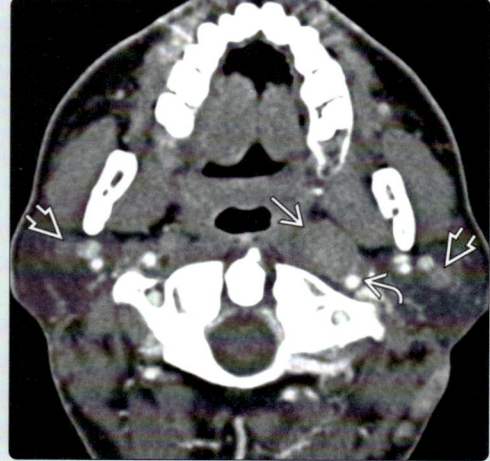

(Left) *Axial CECT in a patient with non-Hodgkin lymphoma (NHL) shows a large, homogeneously enhancing retropharyngeal space nodal mass* ➡ *medial to the internal carotid artery (ICA)* ➡. *This displaces parapharyngeal fat* ➡ *anterolaterally. A small contralateral adenopathy* ➡ *is also present.* (Right) *Axial CECT in a patient with NHL shows a large, oval, homogeneous, nonnecrotic left retropharyngeal node* ➡ *displacing the left ICA* ➡ *posterolaterally. Mildly prominent parotid nodes* ➡ *are also noted.*

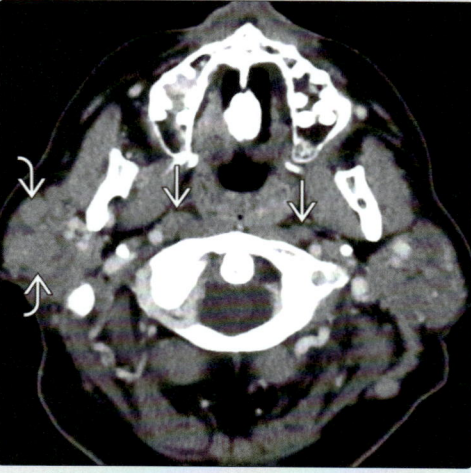
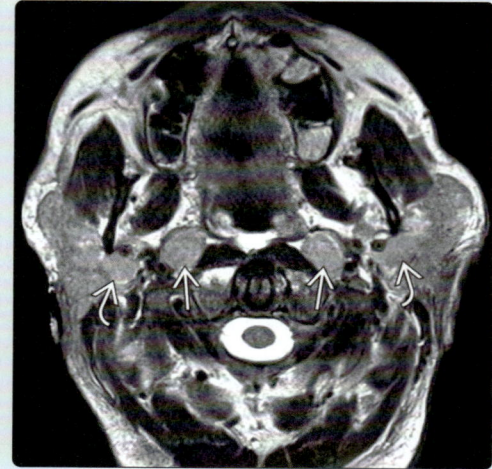

(Left) *Axial CECT shows bilateral retropharyngeal adenopathy due to involvement by lymphoma* ➡. *These might be easily overlooked given their relatively small size. Multiple homogenous-appearing, enlarged parotid lymph nodes* ➡ *are also present.* (Right) *Axial T2 MR demonstrates enlarged bilateral retropharyngeal lymph nodes* ➡ *due to involvement with lymphoma. Bilateral intraparotid adenopathy* ➡ *is also present, which was more conspicuous on T1 MR (not shown).*

TERMINOLOGY

Abbreviations

- Non-Hodgkin lymphoma (NHL) in retropharyngeal space (RPS)

Definitions

- NHL is lymphoreticular system malignancy
  - H&N NHL has multiple forms
    - Nodal, nonnodal lymphatic (tonsils & adenoids), extralymphatic (e.g., thyroid, sinuses)
- RPS skull base to hyoid contains lateral & medial nodes
  - Lateral group = nodes of Rouvière

IMAGING

General Features

- Best diagnostic clue
  - Oval-round, solid mass > **0.8 cm** (axial) in RPS, **typically associated with other neck adenopathy**
- Location
  - RPS nodes only present in suprahyoid RPS
    - **Medial to internal carotid arteries** skull base to hyoid
- Size
  - RPS nodes pathologic if > **0.8 cm (axial)**
- Morphology
  - Typically solid, rounded nodes
  - Necrosis ± extracapsular spread → high-grade NHL

CT Findings

- CECT
  - May be difficult to identify on CT, especially if small
  - Ovoid, mildly enhancing soft tissue mass in RPS
    - Less enhancing than normal nodes (before treatment)

MR Findings

- T1WI
  - Nodes isointense to muscle
- T2WI
  - High-signal nodal masses
- STIR
  - High-signal nodal masses
- T1WI C+
  - Diffuse, mild to moderate enhancement

Nuclear Medicine Findings

- PET
  - Used to stage & follow-up FDG-avid NHL

Imaging Recommendations

- Best imaging tool
  - MR more sensitive for detecting RPS nodes than CT
  - FDG PET: Staging & surveillance of most types of NHL

DIFFERENTIAL DIAGNOSIS

Retropharyngeal Space Reactive Adenopathy

- Homogeneous, ovoid RPS mass ≤ 10 mm
- Multiple other reactive nodes ± tonsillar hyperplasia
- Typically pediatric patients

Retropharyngeal Space Suppurative Adenopathy

- Usually < 30 yr old, septic with pharyngitis

- Central necrosis, peripheral enhancement
- Often associated with RPS edema

Retropharyngeal Space Nodal SCCa

- Most common cause of malignant RPS nodes
- Nodes are round ± central necrosis ± extranodal extension

PATHOLOGY

General Features

- Associated abnormalities
  - Other manifestations of NHL in H&N
    - Extranodal, lymphatic disease in Waldeyer ring
    - Extranodal, extralymphatic site involvement
  - Association of NHL with HIV/infections, posttransplant lymphoproliferative disease, autoimmune disorders

Staging, Grading, & Classification

- **WHO** 5th edition classification (updated 2022)
  - Based on clinicopathologic, molecular, & genetic changes
  - Many types with new subtypes due to genetic features
    - Mature B cell (most common)
    - Mature T & NK cell
    - Hodgkin lymphoma
    - Posttransplant lymphoproliferative disorder
    - Histiocytic & dendritic cell neoplasms

CLINICAL ISSUES

Presentation

- Most common signs/symptoms
  - RPS nodes usually clinically occult
    - May see bulging of posterior pharyngeal wall
  - Other cervical nodes typically present
  - May have enlargement of Waldeyer ring
  - Weight loss, night sweats, fever (more aggressive)

Demographics

- Epidemiology
  - Etiologies include pharyngeal squamous cell carcinoma (SCCa) > NHL > thyroid carcinoma > melanoma
  - Increasing incidence of NHL
- Age: Median 50-55 yr, depends on type
- Sex: M:F = 1.5:1

Treatment

- Treatment depends on stage, cell type, patient age
- Chemo, XRT, or combined modality therapy (CMT)
  - CAR T-cell therapy for relapsed or refractory B cell

DIAGNOSTIC CHECKLIST

Image Interpretation Pearls

- Large, nonnecrotic nodes suggest NHL, not SCCa
- Necrosis &/or extranodal spread or diffuse infiltration suggest high-grade, aggressive NHL

SELECTED REFERENCES

1. Alaggio R et al: The 5th edition of the World Health Organization Classification of Haematolymphoid Tumours: Lymphoid Neoplasms. Leukemia. 36(7):1720-48, 2022
2. Aiken AH et al: Approach to masses in head and neck spaces. In: Diseases of the Brain, Head and Neck, Spine 2020–2023: Diagnostic Imaging. [Internet]. Hodler J et al, editors. Cham: Springer, 2020

TERMINOLOGY

- Definition: Malignant retropharyngeal space (RPS) nodes of nonsquamous cell carcinoma (SCCa) origin

IMAGING

- Best diagnostic clue: Oval to round ± centrally necrotic mass > **0.8 cm** in RPS, **medial to internal carotid artery**
  - Suprahyoid neck RPS **only**
- MR more sensitive for detecting RPS nodes
  - Small nodes may be unseen on CECT
- MR findings
  - Nodes usually isointense to muscle (T1)
  - Differentiated thyroid carcinoma or melanoma may be hyperintense on T1
  - High signal on T2
- CECT findings
  - Oval to round, mildly enhancing soft tissue density mass in RPS ± necrosis
  - Nodal necrosis: Central low density & wall enhancement

- Extracapsular spread: Ill-defined margins ± stranding of surrounding fat
- Thyroid cancer: Cystic or solid, heterogeneous ± calcified
- FDG-avid nodes on PET

TOP DIFFERENTIAL DIAGNOSES

- RPS reactive adenopathy
- RPS suppurative adenopathy
- RPS nodal SCCa

CLINICAL ISSUES

- RPS malignant nodes **often clinically occult**
- If large, bulging of posterolateral wall of pharynx

DIAGNOSTIC CHECKLIST

- RPS non-SCCa nodes prompt search for primary
  - Skull base, posterior sinonasal cavity, nasopharynx, palate cancers (e.g., olfactory neuroblastoma)
  - Neck search for primary thyroid carcinoma in neck
  - Systemic tumor search: Melanoma, lymphoma, other

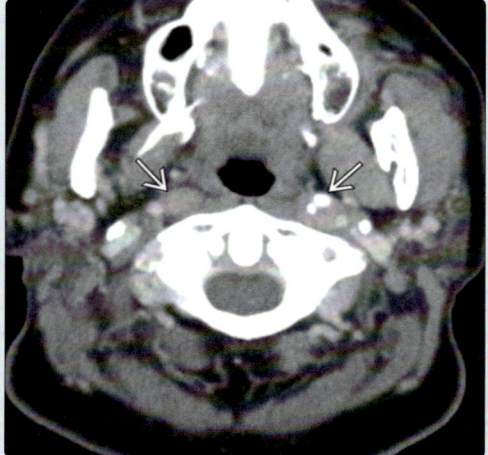
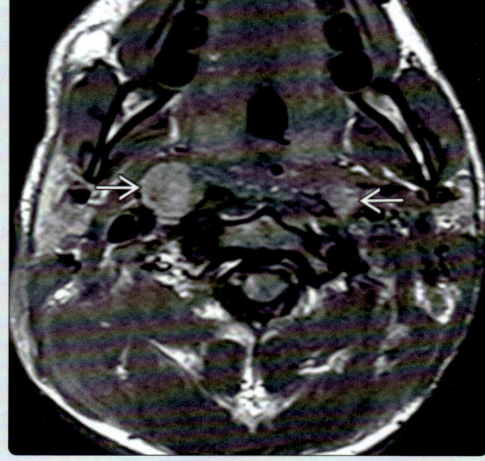

(Left) *Axial CECT shows bilateral retropharyngeal space (RPS) lymphadenopathy ➡. Note calcifications in left RPS node, which raises consideration of differentiated thyroid primary malignancy. Squamous cell carcinoma nodes are rarely calcified.* (Right) *Axial T1 MR shows T1-hyperintense, bilateral RPS lymph nodes in metastatic differentiated thyroid carcinoma ➡. Intrinsic T1 hyperintensity may be due to proteinaceous thyroglobulin or colloid; this can also be seen in melanoma metastasis due to melanin or hemorrhage.*

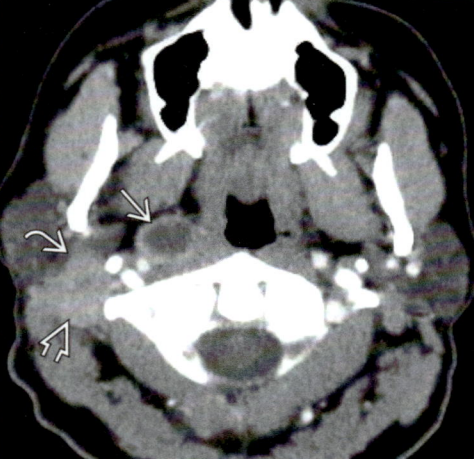
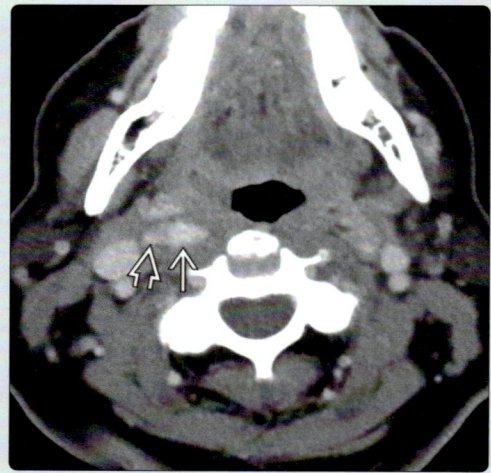

(Left) *Axial CECT shows a necrotic right retropharyngeal lymph node metastasis ➡ due to melanoma. Additional solid metastatic adenopathy in high right posterior cervical space ➡ effaces regional fat planes & has irregular margins concerning for extranodal extension into adjacent parotid gland ➡. (Right) Axial CECT shows a brightly enhancing RPS nodal metastasis ➡ just medial to right internal carotid artery ➡ in a patient with medullary thyroid carcinoma (MTC). Avid hypervascular enhancement is common with MTC.*

TERMINOLOGY

Abbreviations

- Non-squamous cell carcinoma (SCCa) metastatic nodes in retropharyngeal space (RPS)

Definitions

- Malignant RPS nodes of non-SCCa origin
  - Thyroid cancers [differentiated thyroid carcinoma (DTCa), medullary thyroid carcinoma (MTC), & anaplastic], melanoma, olfactory neuroblastoma (ONB), sinonasal undifferentiated carcinoma (SNUC), non-Hodgkin lymphoma (NHL)

IMAGING

General Features

- Best diagnostic clue
  - Oval to round ± centrally necrotic mass > **0.8 cm in RPS**, medial to internal carotid artery (ICA)
- Location
  - Suprahyoid neck RPS **only**
  - Anterior to prevertebral strap muscles, medial to ICA
- Size
  - RPS nodes designated pathologic if > **0.8-cm** minimum diameter in lateral RPS + any node in medial RPS except in children
  - Children may have reactive medial & lateral RPS nodes

Imaging Recommendations

- Best imaging tool
  - MR more sensitive for detecting RPS nodes
    - Small nodes may be unseen on CECT
  - MR & CT unable to differentiate normal-sized, nonnecrotic nodes without extracapsular spread from reactive nodes

CT Findings

- CECT
  - Oval to round, mildly enhancing soft tissue density mass in RPS ± necrosis
  - Nodal necrosis: Central low density with irregular wall enhancement
  - Extracapsular spread: Ill-defined margins ± stranding of surrounding fat
  - DTCa: Cystic or solid, heterogeneous ± calcified nodes
  - MTC: Hypervascular enhancing or calcified nodes

MR Findings

- T1WI
  - Nodes isointense to muscle
  - DTCa may be hyperintense from thyroglobulin or colloid
  - Melanoma may be hyperintense from melanin or hemorrhage
- T2WI
  - Nodes hyperintense
- T1WI C+
  - Nodal necrosis: Central low intensity with wall enhancement

Nuclear Medicine Findings

- PET
  - FDG PET to confirm nodal metastases, especially DTCa
    - Highest sensitivity & specificity in treated patients with rising thyroglobulin & negative radioiodine scan
  - FDG melanoma uptake varies with histology

DIFFERENTIAL DIAGNOSIS

Retropharyngeal Space Reactive Adenopathy

- Homogeneous RPS mass < 1 cm in young patients
- Look for associated reactive-appearing nodes & adenoidal & tonsillar hyperplasia

Retropharyngeal Space Suppurative Adenopathy

- Septic patient with pharyngitis
- Intranodal abscess: Centrally necrotic, peripherally enhancing node ± RPS edema

Retropharyngeal Space Nodal SCCa

- Most common cause of malignant RPS nodes
- Round nodes ± central necrosis

PATHOLOGY

General Features

- Etiology
  - Non-SCCa skull base, sinonasal, palate cancers
    - ONB, SNUC, sarcoma, other
  - Non-SCCa neck malignancy metastases: Thyroid
    - Retrograde lymphatic spread via paratracheal chain, more common after prior neck dissection
  - Systemic cancer with nodal metastases: Melanoma, NHL

CLINICAL ISSUES

Presentation

- Most common signs/symptoms
  - RPS malignant nodes **often clinically occult**
- Other signs/symptoms
  - If large, bulging of posterolateral wall of pharynx

Natural History & Prognosis

- Prognosis on non-SCCa metastasis unknown

Treatment

- Extended radiation field or surgical excision

DIAGNOSTIC CHECKLIST

Consider

- RPS non-SCCa nodes prompt search for primary
  - Posterior sinonasal cavity, nasopharynx & skull base: ONB, SNUC, other
  - Neck search for primary thyroid carcinoma in neck
  - Systemic tumor search for melanoma, NHL, other
- Transoral ultrasound-guided FNA to establish diagnosis

SELECTED REFERENCES

1. Dietz LK et al: Review of retropharyngeal and parapharyngeal nodal metastasis of papillary thyroid carcinoma. Am J Otolaryngol.. 45(5):104438, 2024
2. Panda S et al: In-vivo lymphoscintigraphy of sinonasal tumors identifies retropharyngeal node and level I as predominant sentinel nodes. Rev Esp Med Nucl Imagen Mol (Engl Ed). 42(6):374-9, 2023
3. Mnatsakanian A et al: Anatomy, head and neck, retropharyngeal space. StatPearls, 2020

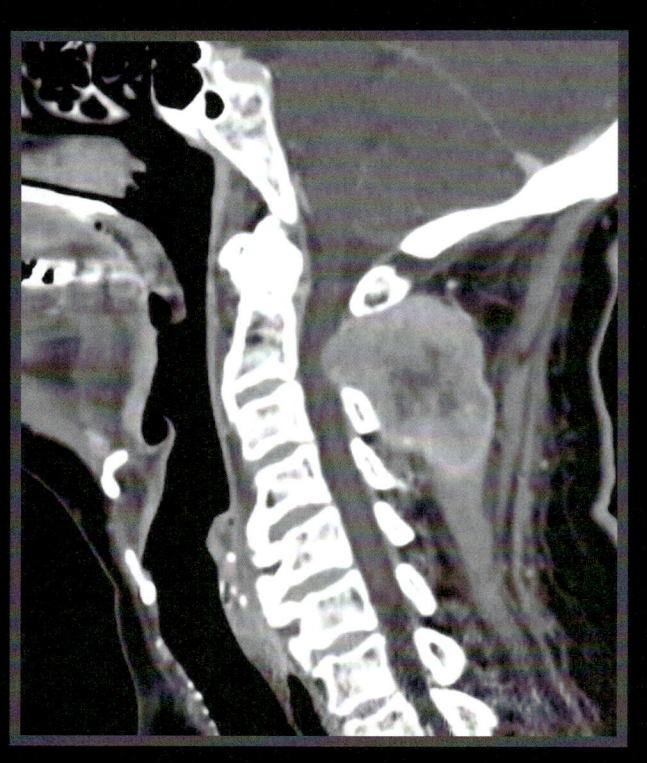
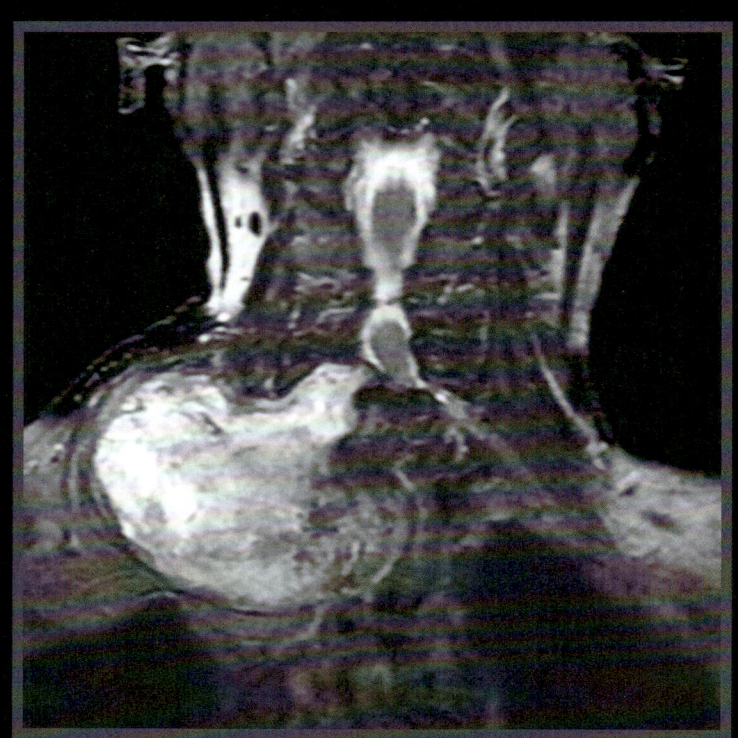
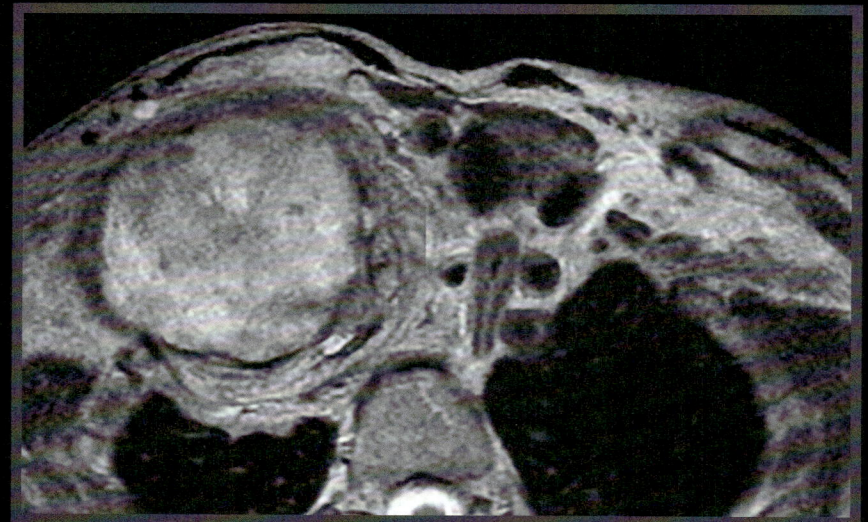
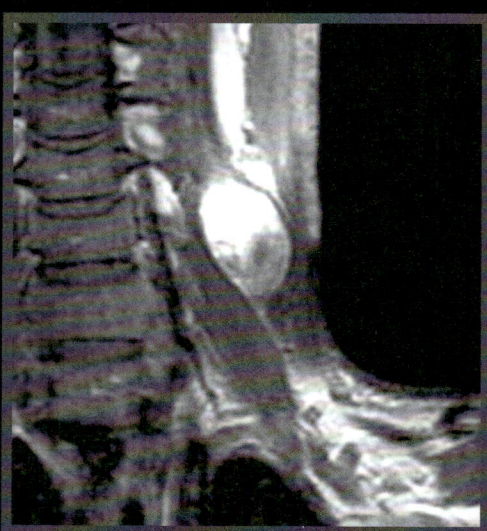

SECTION 8
Perivertebral Space

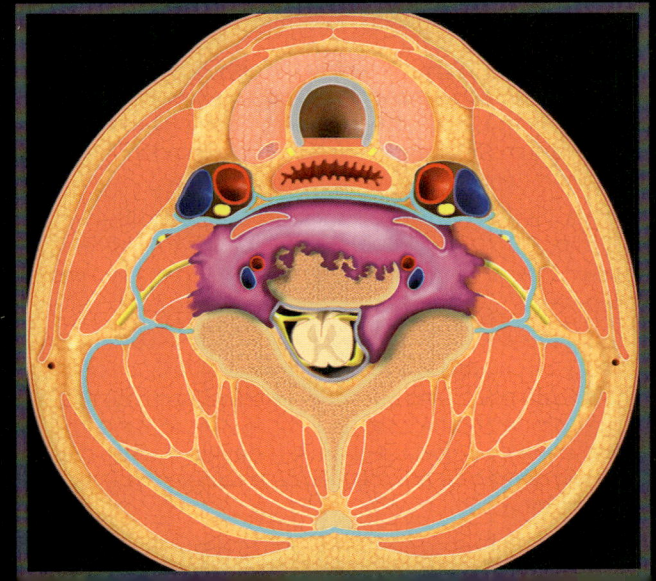
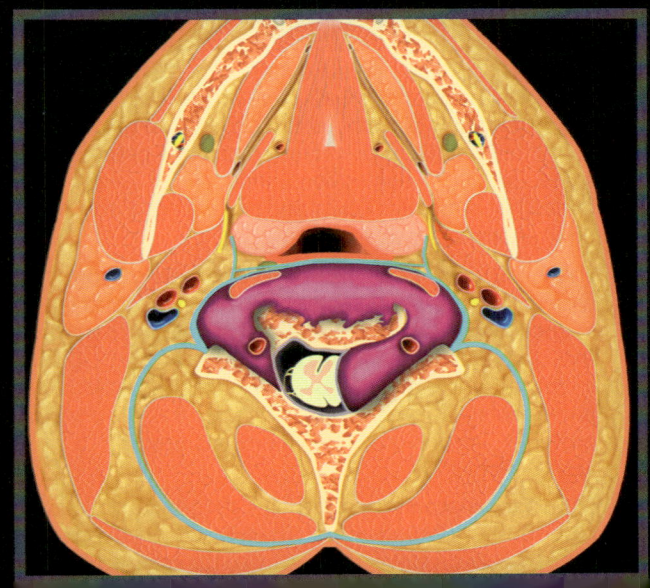

Perivertebral Space Overview

Summary Thoughts: Perivertebral Space

The perivertebral space (PVS) is a cylindrical space surrounding the vertebral column, extending from the skull base to the superior mediastinum. The **deep layer of the deep cervical fascia** (DL-DCF) completely encircles the PVS, which is subdivided into **prevertebral** (prevertebral PVS) and **paraspinal** (paraspinal PVS) portions or spaces.

A **prevertebral PVS mass** will invade, expand, and displace the prevertebral muscles and its ventral fascial margin **anteriorly**, distinguishing it from a retropharyngeal space (RPS) mass, which pushes the muscles and anterior fascial margin posteriorly. A **paraspinal PVS mass** bows the posterior cervical space (PCS) fat away from the posterior elements of the spine.

The DL-DCF serves as a tenacious barrier to the spread of malignancy or infection, and it serves to redirect extension of PVS disease to the **epidural space**.

The vast majority of PVS lesions originate in the **vertebral body or disc space** with **metastatic disease** and **infection** topping the list. Therefore, a PVS lesion is often associated with vertebral disease.

An imaging interpretation pitfall is mistaking a **hypertrophic levator scapulae muscle (LSM)** for a mass. The hypertrophy occurs in response to ipsilateral CNXI denervation and subsequent atrophy of the trapezius and sternocleidomastoid (SCM) muscles.

Imaging Techniques & Indications

A lateral cervical plain film provides a quick check for prevertebral soft tissue swelling and for cervical vertebral body integrity. **CECT** with soft tissue and bone algorithm along with coronal and sagittal reformations is the best exam to evaluate the **cervical soft tissues** and **bones in a single exam**. Contrast-enhanced cervical spine **MR** is the exam of choice to evaluate for **epidural extension** of disease.

Imaging Anatomy

The name PVS nicely describes the anatomy. It is a cylindrical space that quite literally surrounds the vertebral column. This nomenclature has not always been consistent, as the entire region (including portions **lateral** and **posterior to** the vertebrae) was historically referred to as the **pre**vertebral space. Because it seemed counterintuitive to use **pre**vertebral to describe structures lateral and posterior to the vertebrae, a new terminology was applied.

The PVS is bounded by the DL-DCF and extends from the skull base to the superior mediastinum T4 level. It consists of **2 major components**: The **prevertebral PVS** and **paraspinal PVS** portions or spaces. The attachments of the DL-DCF to the vertebral transverse processes mark the division, with the prevertebral PVS lying anterior and the paraspinal PVS lying posterior. The prevertebral PVS extends inferiorly to approximately T4.

Important anatomic relationships can be examined as they relate to these 2 subdivisions. The retropharyngeal and danger spaces are directly anterior to the **prevertebral PVS** in the cervical region. The paired carotid spaces are anterolateral and posterior cervical spaces are lateral to the prevertebral PVS. The **paraspinal PVS** lies deep to the posterior cervical spaces and posterior to the cervical spine transverse processes.

The **DL-DCF** completely encircles the PVS. Its anterior portion (**anterior DL-DCF**) arches in front of the prevertebral muscles from 1 cervical spine transverse process to the opposite transverse process. The posterior portion (**posterior DL-DCF**) arches over the paraspinal muscles to attach to the nuchal ligament of the vertebral body spinous processes.

The **anterior DL-DCF** is often referred to as the "**carpet**" by surgeons because surgical approach reveals a smooth, carpet-like surface on which the pharynx slides up and down. The "carpet" is extremely tenacious and serves as a 2-way barrier to the spread of disease. Therefore, expanding **tumor or infection** of the prevertebral PVS will be redirected by this tough fascia along the path of least resistance to the **epidural space**. Coming from the other direction, pharyngeal malignancy is usually blocked from accessing the PVS. When tumor does invade this fascia and prevertebral PVS, it often leads to fixation and is unresectable.

Only the **brachial plexus** roots pierce the tough DL-DCF. The C1-C5 roots exit the neural foramina, pass between the anterior and middle scalene muscles in the prevertebral PVS, then go out through an opening in the DL-DCF. From there, they traverse the posterior cervical space on their way to the axilla.

A working knowledge of important **PVS internal structures** is key to understanding the pathology and pathology mimics (pseudolesions) found within. The prevertebral PVS contains the prevertebral muscles (longus colli and capitis), scalene muscles (anterior, middle, and posterior), brachial plexus roots, phrenic nerve (C3-C5), vertebral artery and vein, and vertebral body. The paraspinal PVS contains the paraspinal muscles and the posterior elements of the vertebrae.

Approaches to Imaging Issues of Perivertebral Space

When trying to define a lesion in the H&N as in the PVS, one must answer the question, "What **imaging findings** define a mass or lesion as **primary to the PVS**?" A lesion originates from the **prevertebral PVS** if it is centered within the prevertebral muscles or vertebral body. Also, a mass that causes **anterior displacement** of the **prevertebral muscles and anterior fascial margin** is arising from the prevertebral PVS. In most cases, this feature clearly distinguishes a PVS mass from an RPS mass, which pushes the anterior muscle margin posteriorly.

A mass is primary to the **paraspinal PVS** if it is within the substance of the paraspinal musculature or if it bows the posterior cervical space fat away from the vertebral posterior elements.

When prevertebral PVS disease is noted, one should always check for **epidural extension**. Remember that infection or malignancy that breaks out of the vertebral body into the PVS will be blocked by the tough DL-DCF. As a result, the path of least resistance is deep spread into the epidural space through the neural foramen, possibly leading to **spinal cord compression**.

A possible route of disease travel into or out of the PVS is along the **brachial plexus**. Extranodal tumor from the axilla (most frequently breast carcinoma) may access the PVS by retrograde perineural spread along the brachial plexus. Conversely, a PVS invasive malignancy may spread antegrade along this pathway to the axillary apex.

Perivertebral Space Lesion Differential Diagnosis

Pseudolesions	Vertebral body osteomyelitis, pyogenic
Levator scapulae hypertrophy	Vertebral body osteomyelitis, tuberculous
Cervical rib	**Benign tumor**
Large transverse process	Brachial plexus schwannoma
Degenerative	Brachial plexus neurofibroma
Anterior disc herniation	Vertebral body benign bony tumors
Hypertrophic facet joint	**Malignant tumor/metastatic tumor**
Vertebral body osteophyte	Vertebral body metastasis
Vascular	Epidural metastasis
Vertebral artery dissection	Chordoma
Vertebral artery aneurysm	Non-Hodgkin lymphoma
Vertebral artery pseudoaneurysm	Direct invasion, squamous cell carcinoma posterior pharyngeal wall
Inflammatory/infectious	Vertebral body primary malignant tumors
Longus colli tendonitis	

Once a lesion has been identified as originating in the PVS, the differential diagnosis unique to the PVS should be reviewed. Identifying characteristic imaging findings of common PVS lesions often yields a short list of possible diagnoses. By far, the **most common lesions** of the PVS originate in the **vertebral body** with infection and metastatic disease at the top of the list. Therefore, when a PVS lesion is identified, the vertebral bodies should be thoroughly evaluated.

Vertebral body osteomyelitis can be differentiated from other entities on the differential diagnosis list by noting destructive changes of adjacent vertebral endplates with increased T2 signal and enhancement of the intervertebral disc on MR. The disc space will be spared in metastatic disease or non-Hodgkin lymphoma, which are more likely to involve multiple bones than to be solitary. Epidural disease can be seen in either metastatic disease or non-Hodgkin lymphoma.

Longus colli tendinitis occurs as an unusual inflammatory disease in the prevertebral PVS, often producing prevertebral soft tissue swelling and edema with retropharyngeal inflammation or effusion. Focal calcification of the longus colli tendon at C1-2 level and lack of significant infectious signs may be the only clues to separating this from pharyngitis and retropharyngeal abscess.

Diagnosis of chordoma is suggested by a destructive mass centered at the sphenooccipital junction in the clivus or upper cervical vertebral body associated with a large, T2-hyperintense soft tissue mass, commonly with perivertebral and epidural extension. When epidural extension occurs in the neck, cord compression is an early and severe consequence.

Benign neurogenic PVS tumors include brachial plexus schwannoma and neurofibroma. Both appear as circumscribed, fusiform, enhancing masses situated between the anterior and middle scalene muscles.

PVS vascular lesions involve the vertebral arteries, including vertebral artery dissection, aneurysm, or pseudoaneurysm. While all can be usually diagnosed by CTA, axial fat-saturated T1 MR may help in cases of dissection, showing intramural hematoma as a hyperintense crescent.

With most PVS pseudolesions (cervical rib, large transverse process) and degenerative changes (anterior disc herniation, hypertrophic facet joint, and vertebral body osteophyte), there is little diagnostic dilemma on cross-sectional imaging. Probably the biggest potential imaging pitfall when evaluating a PVS lesion is to mistake a hypertrophic LSM for an enhancing mass or recurrent tumor. This "pseudolesion" is secondary to spinal accessory nerve (CNXI) injury, usually from previous neck dissection. The levator scapulae hypertrophies to help lift the arm to compensate for the atrophy of the SCM and trapezius caused by spinal accessory neuropathy. On imaging, the LSM will be enlarged and may enhance. Look for small, fatty infiltrated ipsilateral trapezius and SCM muscles to confirm the diagnosis.

Clinical Implications

Clinical history provides important clues to differentiating PVS lesions. Fever, neck pain, and tenderness herald the onset of **vertebral body osteomyelitis** with possible progression to quadriparesis, if there is epidural abscess. Patients with **metastatic disease** usually have a known primary, and those with **non-Hodgkin lymphoma** have known systemic disease when PVS disease is found. Both can present with neck pain, radiculopathy, or myelopathy.

Brachial plexus **schwannomas** may be seen sporadically or in the setting of neurofibromatosis type 2 (multiple schwannomas). **Neurofibromas** may also be sporadic but are most commonly found in the setting of neurofibromatosis type 1. Typically, both are painless, slow-growing masses.

Vertebral artery injuries can be from minor (chiropractic manipulation) or major trauma and may present with delayed **stroke**, possibly with a lateral medullary (Wallenberg) syndrome if the posterior inferior cerebellar artery is involved.

Longus colli tendonitis is associated with 2-7 days of neck pain and odynophagia. A history of previous surgical neck dissection can usually be elicited in patients with a **hypertrophic LSM**.

Selected References

1. Baran AI et al: A comparative perspective on brucellar, pyogenic, and tuberculous spondylodiscitis. Eur Rev Med Pharmacol Sci. 28(6):2550-7, 2024
2. Mittenzwei R et al: Cytological features of cranial and paraspinal nerve Tumours. Cytopathology. 35(5):572-80, 2024

Perivertebral Space Overview

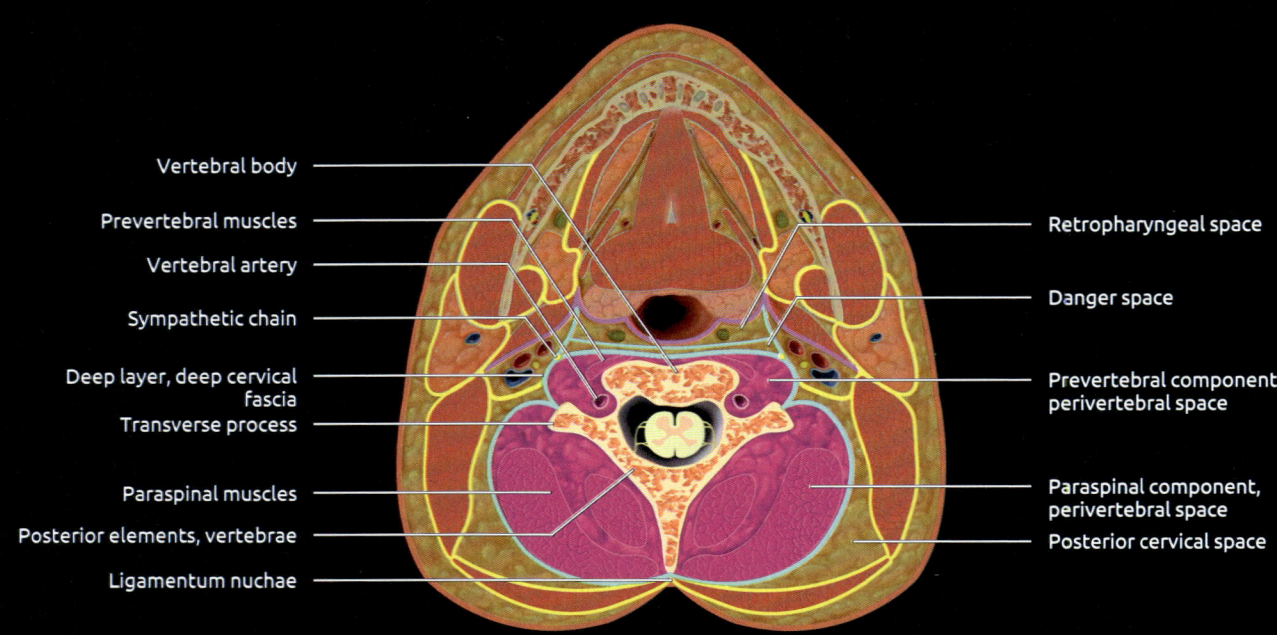

Vertebral body

Prevertebral muscles

Vertebral artery

Sympathetic chain

Deep layer, deep cervical fascia

Transverse process

Paraspinal muscles

Posterior elements, vertebrae

Ligamentum nuchae

Retropharyngeal space

Danger space

Prevertebral component, perivertebral space

Paraspinal component, perivertebral space

Posterior cervical space

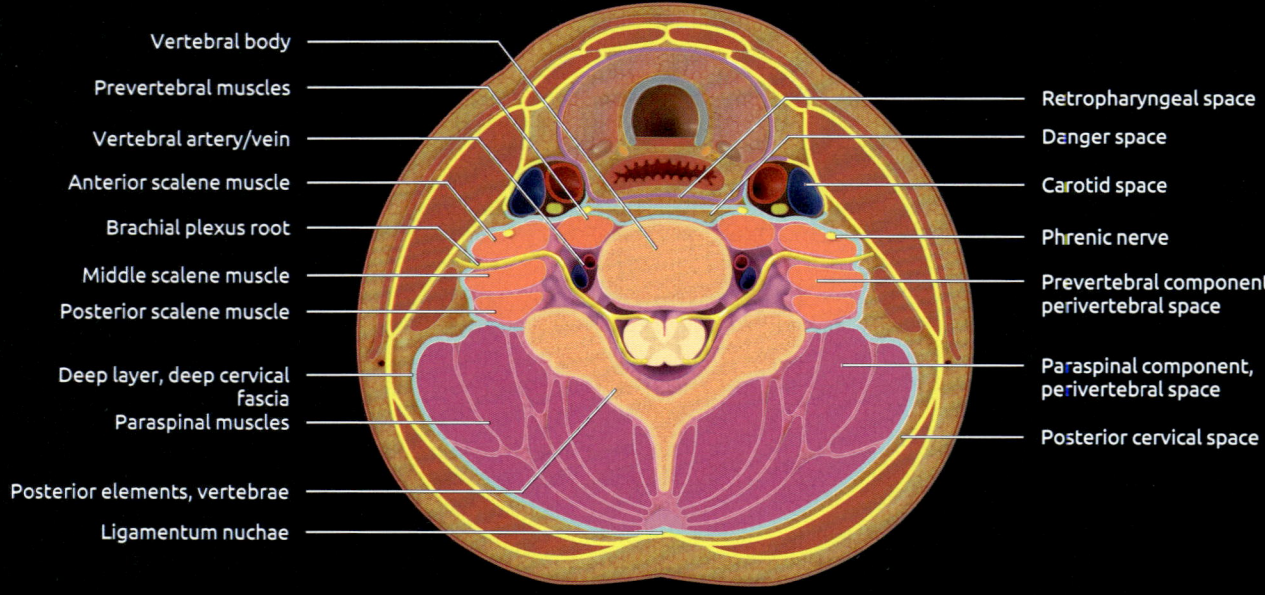

Vertebral body

Prevertebral muscles

Vertebral artery/vein

Anterior scalene muscle

Brachial plexus root

Middle scalene muscle

Posterior scalene muscle

Deep layer, deep cervical fascia

Paraspinal muscles

Posterior elements, vertebrae

Ligamentum nuchae

Retropharyngeal space

Danger space

Carotid space

Phrenic nerve

Prevertebral component, perivertebral space

Paraspinal component, perivertebral space

Posterior cervical space

(Top) *Axial graphic through the level of the oropharynx shows prevertebral and paraspinal components of the perivertebral space (PVS) beneath the deep layer of deep cervical fascia (DL-DCF). Notice this fascia curves medially to touch the transverse processes of the vertebra, dividing the PVS into prevertebral and paraspinal components. The danger and retropharyngeal spaces are anterior to the PVS, whereas the posterior cervical space is lateral and posterior.* (Bottom) *Axial graphic through the thyroid bed shows prevertebral and paraspinal components of the PVS beneath the DL-DCF. The DL-DCF is a tenacious barrier to the spread of infection or malignancy, which will be redirected to the epidural space. The brachial plexus roots pass between the anterior and middle scalene muscles in the prevertebral PVS and serve as a 2-way highway for perineural spread of malignancy between the PVS and axillary apex.*

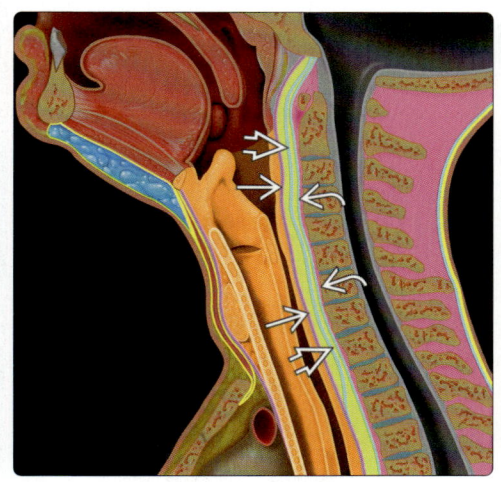

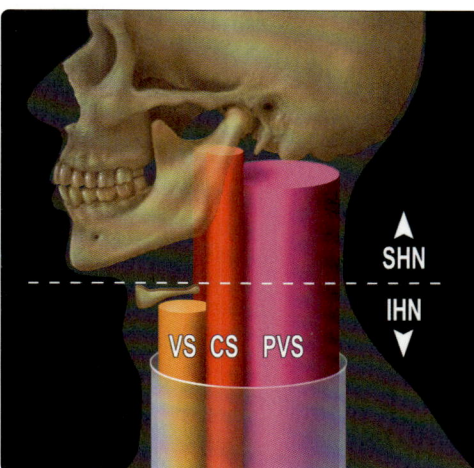

(Left) Sagittal graphic depicts midline spatial relationships of the infrahyoid neck. Just anterior to the PVS (purple) are the danger space ⮊ and retropharyngeal space ➡. The tenacious DL-DCF ⮊ will usually redirect the spread of PVS disease to the epidural space. (Right) Lateral graphic of the extracranial head and neck shows the tubular PVS extending from the skull base to the mediastinum. DL-DCF completely encircles the PVS. SHN = suprahyoid neck; IVN = intrahyoid neck; CS = carotid space; VS = visceral space.

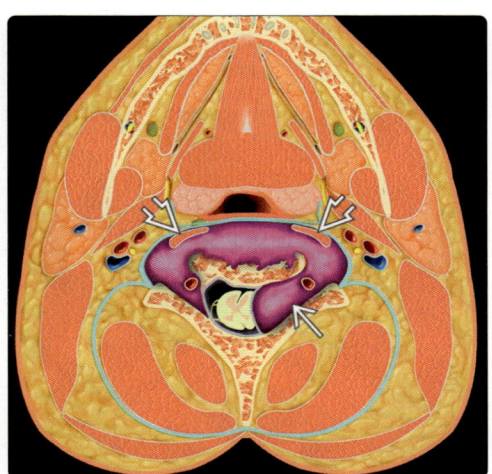

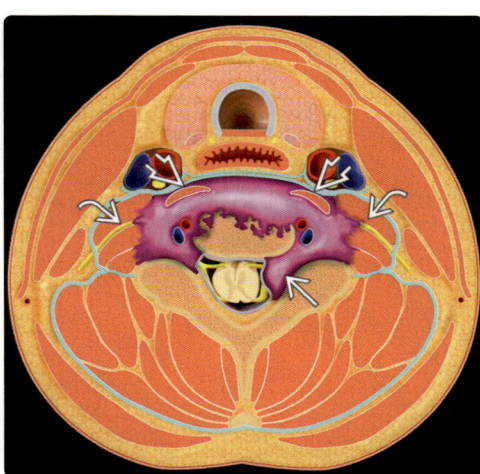

(Left) Axial graphic at the suprahyoid neck oropharyngeal level shows a generic PVS mass that elevates prevertebral muscles ⮊ and destroys the vertebral body. Note the DL-DCF (blue line) confines the mass and "forces" it into the epidural space ➡. (Right) Axial graphic at the thyroid level demonstrates a generic infrahyoid PVS mass arising from the vertebral body and elevating the prevertebral muscles ⮊. Brachial plexus ⮊ & vertebral arteries are engulfed, & epidural disease ➡ is present.

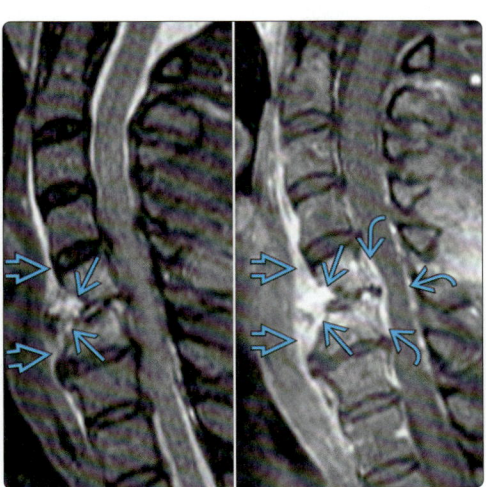

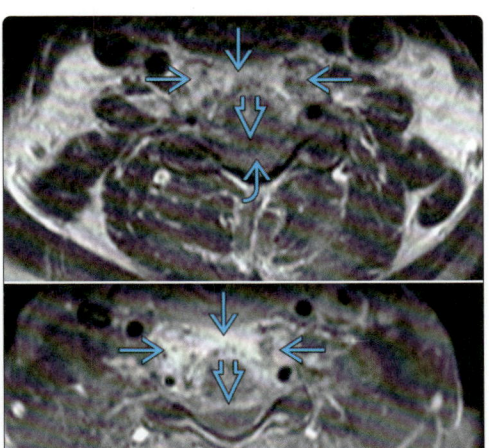

(Left) Sagittal STIR (left) & T1 C+ (right) MR images in a patient with C5-C6 spinal osteomyelitis show anterior adjacent endplate erosions ➡ with prevertebral PVS phlegmon ➡ as well as epidural extension of disease ➡. (Right) Axial T2 (upper) & T1 C+ (lower) MR images in same patient show swelling, edema, and enhancement of longus colli muscles ➡, suggesting prevertebral PVS phlegmon. Also note extension of enhancement to epidural space ➡ through neural foramina resulting is spinal cord compression ➡.

Levator Scapulae Muscle Hypertrophy

TERMINOLOGY

- Levator scapulae muscle hypertrophy (LSMH) in response to trapezius and sternocleidomastoid (SCM) muscle atrophy
- CNXI injury causes denervation atrophy of ipsilateral trapezius and SCM muscles

IMAGING

- CECT: LSMH with normal density of enlarged muscle
- T2WI MR: If acute, LSM may demonstrate ↑ signal
- T1WI C+ MR: If subacute, LSM may enhance slightly more than normal
- If associated with other cranial neuropathies (IX-XII), evaluate for possible skull base mass
- Findings of previous neck dissection (i.e., absence of ipsilateral jugular vein, loss of fat planes contiguous with carotid sheath, and occasional absence of SCM)
- Evidence of trauma to skull base or cervical spine
- Ultrasound can help assess spinal accessory nerve injuries

TOP DIFFERENTIAL DIAGNOSES

- Contralateral LSM atrophy
- LSM mass: Inflammatory or infectious lesion; benign tumor: Lipoma, schwannoma, etc.; malignant tumor: Invasive squamous cell carcinoma (SCCa), sarcoma, etc.

PATHOLOGY

- Damage to spinal accessory nerve leads to denervation atrophy of trapezius muscle with compensatory hypertrophy of LSM

CLINICAL ISSUES

- Palpable "mass" in perivertebral space
- Previous history of radical neck dissection for SCCa
- Pseudolesion recognition avoids potential needle biopsy

DIAGNOSTIC CHECKLIST

- If no previous neck surgery, look for lesion at skull base or brainstem for cause of CNXI neuropathy

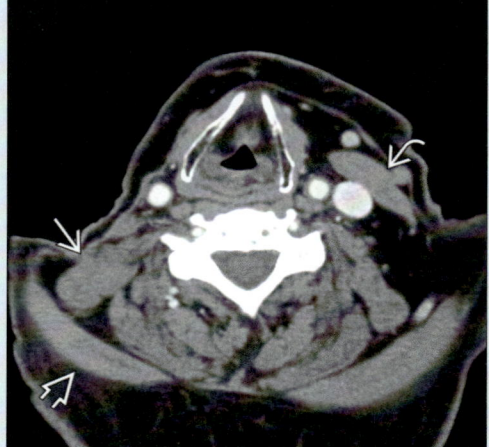 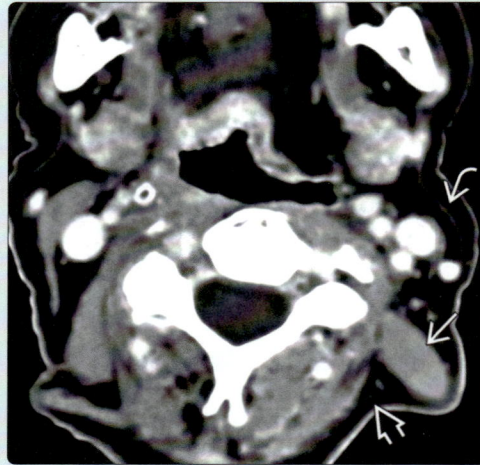

(Left) Axial CECT following right radical neck dissection shows levator scapulae muscle hypertrophy ➡ on the right. The internal jugular vein and sternocleidomastoid muscle ⇨ remain normal on the left. The trapezius ⇥ is also atrophic in comparison to the left. (Right) Axial CECT demonstrates hypertrophy of the levator scapulae ➡ with atrophy of the trapezius ⇥ and sternocleidomastoid ⇥ muscles secondary to jugular foramen paraganglioma (not shown). Ipsilateral tongue atrophy with fatty replacement is also present.

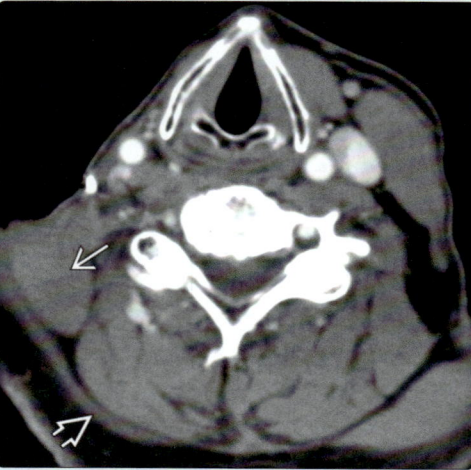 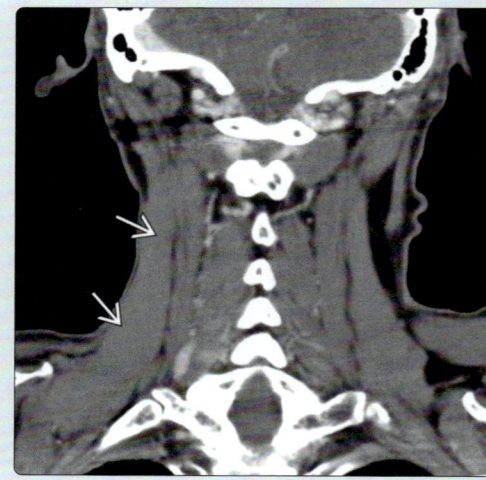

(Left) Axial CECT reveals a right hypertrophic levator scapulae muscle ➡. Note the absence of the right sternocleidomastoid muscle and internal jugular vein from previous right radical neck dissection. The trapezius muscle is atrophic ⇥ as a result of injury to the spinal accessory cranial nerve at the time of surgery. (Right) Coronal CECT reformation in the same patient shows the hypertrophic levator scapulae muscle along its entire length ➡. The muscle otherwise appears normal in density on CT.

Levator Scapulae Muscle Hypertrophy

TERMINOLOGY

Abbreviations
- Levator scapulae muscle hypertrophy (LSMH)

Definitions
- CNXI (spinal accessory nerve) injury causes denervation atrophy of ipsilateral trapezius and sternocleidomastoid (SCM) muscles
  - Most commonly seen following neck dissection
- LSMH: Functional hypertrophy of levator scapulae muscle (LSM) in response to trapezius and SCM muscle atrophy

IMAGING

General Features
- Best diagnostic clue
  - Asymmetric LSM enlargement with denervated trapezius and SCM muscles
    - Findings of previous neck dissection also present (i.e., absence of ipsilateral jugular vein, loss of fat planes contiguous with carotid sheath and occasional absence of SCM)
- Morphology
  - LSM enlarged with convex margins

Radiographic Findings
- Radiography
  - Chest x-ray
    - Demonstrates soft tissue atrophy of trapezius muscle with increased prominence of LSM shadow

CT Findings
- CECT
  - Chronic phase: LSM hypertrophy with normal density
  - Findings of underlying cause
    - Ipsilateral radical neck dissection most common
      - □ Internal jugular vein (IJV), SCM, and spinal accessory nerve sacrificed
      - □ Atrophy of ipsilateral trapezius muscle from denervation
    - Less common causes: Ipsilateral jugular foramen mass (paraganglioma, schwannoma, meningioma, metastasis)
      - □ CNX injury: Ipsilateral vocal cord paralysis
      - □ CNXI injury: Ipsilateral trapezius and SCM muscle atrophy
      - □ CNXII injury: Ipsilateral tongue muscle atrophy with fatty infiltration

MR Findings
- T1WI
  - Enlarged LSM in presence of atrophic trapezius muscle
  - If radical neck dissection, SCM muscle and IJV absent
- T2WI
  - Acute: LSM may demonstrate ↑ signal
  - Chronic: Enlarged LSM with normal signal intensity
- T1WI C+
  - Subacute: LSM may enhance slightly more than normal
  - Chronic: Enlarged LSM with convex margins

Imaging Recommendations
- Best imaging tool

- Post radical neck dissection
  - Follow-up of patients with previously treated squamous cell carcinoma (SCCa) of aerodigestive tract
- Skull base mass
  - If associated with other cranial neuropathies (CNIX-XII), evaluate for possible skull base mass
  - MR with contrast enhancement and fat saturation combined with NECT of skull base is optimal

DIFFERENTIAL DIAGNOSIS

Contralateral Levator Scapulae Muscle Atrophy
- Secondary to denervation
  - C3, C4, ± C5 nerve root compression secondary to cervical spondylosis, disc disease

Levator Scapulae Muscle Mass
- Inflammatory mass
- Benign neoplasm: Lipoma, schwannoma, other
- Malignant tumor: Invasive SCCa, sarcoma, other

PATHOLOGY

General Features
- Etiology
  - Damage to spinal accessory nerve leads to denervation atrophy of trapezius muscle with compensatory hypertrophy of LSM

CLINICAL ISSUES

Presentation
- Most common signs/symptoms
  - Palpable "mass" in perivertebral space
  - Previous history of radical neck dissection for SCCa
- Other signs/symptoms
  - With skull base lesion, may have denervation changes of CNIX-XI

Demographics
- Epidemiology
  - Less commonly seen with more conservative node dissection approaches
  - Should not be seen if CNXI was spared in prior neck dissection

Treatment
- Pseudolesion recognition avoids potential needle biopsy

DIAGNOSTIC CHECKLIST

Consider
- If no previous neck surgery, look for lesion at skull base or brainstem for cause of CNXI neuropathy

Image Interpretation Pearls
- Observing IJV and SCM muscle absence allows radiologist to diagnose radical neck dissection as cause of hypertrophy

SELECTED REFERENCES

1. Hadnadjev Šimonji D et al: ESR Essentials: pseudolesions in head and neck-practice recommendations by the European Society of Head and Neck Radiology. Eur Radiol. ePub, 2025
2. Saks R et al: Pictorial review of cranial nerve denervation in the head and neck. Radiographics. 44(10):e240023, 2024

Acute Calcific Longus Colli Tendonitis

TERMINOLOGY

- Acute calcific prevertebral tendonitis, longus colli tendonitis
- Inflammatory condition due to calcium hydroxyapatite deposition in longus colli tendon

IMAGING

- Process produces 3 distinct findings
  o **Calcifications** in prevertebral muscles at C1-C2
  o Inflammation with swelling of prevertebral muscles
  o Retropharyngeal space (RPS) edema
- Characteristic features best identified with CECT

TOP DIFFERENTIAL DIAGNOSES

- RPS effusion
- RPS abscess
- Perivertebral space infection

PATHOLOGY

- Deposition of **calcium hydroxyapatite crystals** with secondary inflammatory reaction
- Involves superior oblique fibers of longus colli that insert on C1 anterior tubercle

CLINICAL ISSUES

- Subacute neck pain, odynophagia, dysphagia
- Low-grade fever
- Self-limiting condition, although treat pain
- Analgesics and antiinflammatory medications

DIAGNOSTIC CHECKLIST

- Must differentiate from retropharyngeal infection
- 2 key features for diagnosis
  o Calcification at C1-C2 pathognomonic
  o RPS edema is smoothly expansile, nonenhancing

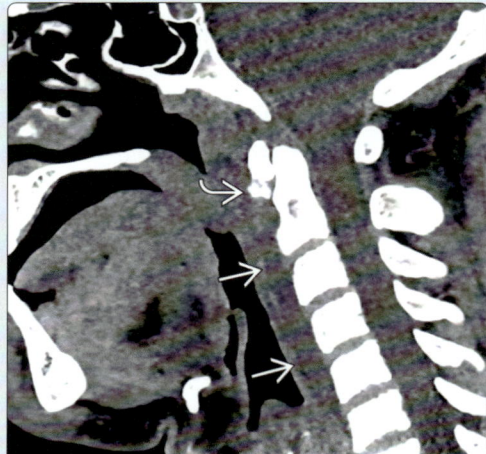
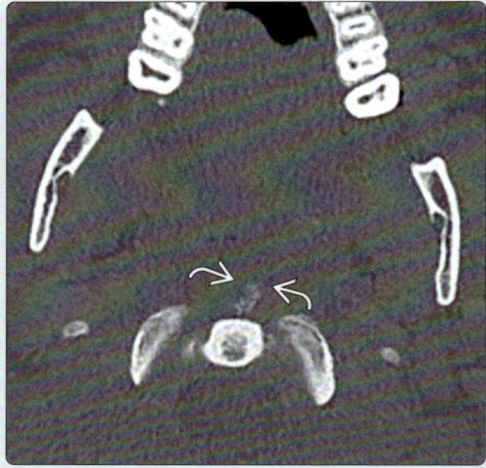

(Left) Sagittal soft tissue window CECT in a 35-year-old man with increasing neck pain shows marked prevertebral soft tissue thickening, edema ➡ and focal amorphous calcification ➡ at C1-C2 junction near longus colli tendon insertion. Note there is no rim enhancement of the prevertebral edema, which helps differentiate this from retropharyngeal abscess. (Right) Axial bone window CECT shows calcification ➡, which is "soft" with irregular margins. This pattern of calcification can be very subtle.

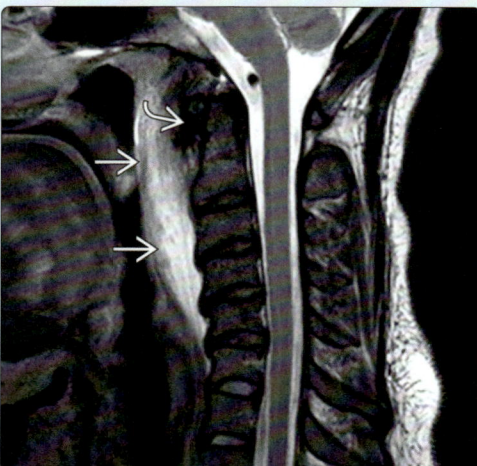
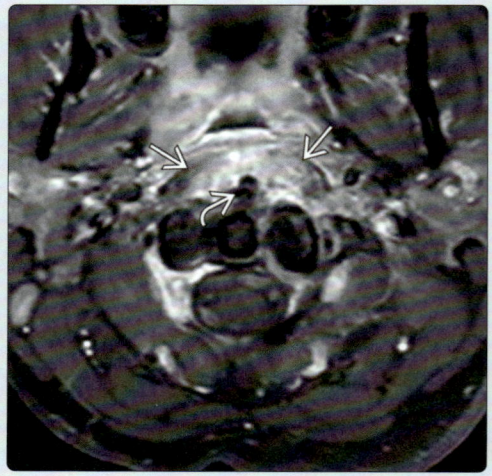

(Left) Sagittal T2 MR in the same patient shows marked T2 hyperintensity in the prevertebral and retropharyngeal spaces with expansion and thickening ➡. The T2 signal can variably represent edema, inflammation, &/or effusion. The calcification is visible as focal hypointensity ➡. (Right) Axial T1 C+ FS MR in same patient at the level of the calcification ➡ shows marked enhancement within the prevertebral soft tissues ➡, indicating marked inflammatory change.

TERMINOLOGY

Synonyms
- Acute calcific prevertebral tendonitis, longus colli tendonitis

Definitions
- Localized inflammation of longus colli tendon insertion associated with calcium hydroxyapatite deposition

IMAGING

General Features
- Best diagnostic clue
  - Focal C1-C2 prevertebral calcification with retropharyngeal edema
- Location
  - Calcifications in prevertebral space at C1-C2
  - Edema in muscles and retropharyngeal space (RPS)

Radiographic Findings
- Radiography
  - Lateral neck: Widening of prevertebral space
  - Frequently see calcification anterior to C1-C2

CT Findings
- CECT
  - Prevertebral **calcification(s)** at C1-C2
  - Variable appearance of calcification(s)
    - Type 1 → well-circumscribed and dense type 2 → ill-defined border and dense type 3 → indistinct border and cloudy
  - Smooth, mild expansion of RPS without peripheral enhancement

MR Findings
- T2WI
  - Inflammation of prevertebral muscles better appreciated than with CT
  - RPS edema also hyperintense
  - ± C1-C2 joint fluid or vertebral body edema
- T2* GRE
  - Hypointense signal of longus colli insertions
- T1WI C+ FS
  - Diffuse prevertebral enhancement
  - No rim enhancement of RPS edema

Imaging Recommendations
- Best imaging tool
  - CT most sensitive to pathognomonic calcification
- Protocol advice
  - CECT with bone and soft tissue algorithm
  - Helps differentiate from retropharyngeal or perivertebral infection

DIFFERENTIAL DIAGNOSIS

Retropharyngeal Space Effusion
- Common feature of longus colli tendonitis
- Also found with pharyngitis, jugular vein thrombosis, neck radiation

Retropharyngeal Space Abscess
- Fluid collection distending RPS
- Peripheral enhancement of collection ± gas
- No prevertebral calcification

Perivertebral Space Infection
- Most commonly due to spondylodiscitis
- Vertebral body endplate erosions
- Often epidural/prevertebral phlegmon or abscess
- No prevertebral calcification

PATHOLOGY

General Features
- Etiology
  - Deposition of **calcium hydroxyapatite crystals** with secondary inflammatory reaction
  - Involves superior oblique fibers of longus colli
    - Tendons insert on C1 anterior tubercle

CLINICAL ISSUES

Presentation
- Most common signs/symptoms
  - Subacute neck pain, odynophagia, dysphagia
  - Low-grade fever
- Other signs/symptoms
  - ± mild elevation of ESR and WBC
  - Limitation of motion

Demographics
- Age
  - Most commonly 30-60 years

Natural History & Prognosis
- Self-limiting condition, although treat pain
- As symptoms resolve, calcifications resolve

Treatment
- Analgesics and antiinflammatory medications

DIAGNOSTIC CHECKLIST

Consider
- C1-C2 calcifications should be sought when RPS edema is present
- RPS edema must be distinguished from RPS infection, which might similarly present with neck pain

Image Interpretation Pearls
- Calcifications at C1-C2 are pathognomonic
- RPS edema is smoothly expanding, nonenhancing

SELECTED REFERENCES

1. Saran S et al: Imaging of calcific tendinopathy: natural history, migration patterns, pitfalls, and management: a review. Br J Radiol. 97(1158):1099-111, 2024
2. Yamamoto N et al: Acute calcific retropharyngeal tendinitis with eggshell-like calcification: case report and literature review on time-course changes in imaging findings. Cureus. 12(4):e7611, 2020
3. Nakagami F et al: Acute non-calcific retropharyngeal tendinitis. Intern Med. 57(23):3499-500, 2018
4. Alamoudi U et al: Acute calcific tendinitis of the longus colli muscle masquerading as a retropharyngeal abscess: a case report and review of the literature. Int J Surg Case Rep. 41:343-6, 2017
5. Silva CF et al: Acute prevertebral calcific tendinitis: a source of non-surgical acute cervical pain. Acta Radiol. 55(1):91-4, 2014

TERMINOLOGY

- Perivertebral space (PVS) infection phlegmon, PVS abscess
- Deep neck infection centered on prevertebral muscles, disc space, vertebral body (VB)
- Most often due to spondylodiscitis
- Uncommonly follows neck or spine surgery
- Increased incidence of TB in immunocompromised patients and IV drug users

IMAGING

- Heterogeneously enhancing prevertebral muscles or rim-enhancing, low-intensity collection
- Anterior displacement of retropharyngeal fat or retropharyngeal fluid
- Large collections more often seen with atypical organisms, especially TB
- Look for epidural phlegmon/abscess
- Bone destruction on CECT and bone CT
- MR C+ for bone and epidural changes

TOP DIFFERENTIAL DIAGNOSES

- Retropharyngeal space abscess
- VB metastasis, PVS
- Lymphoma
- Chordoma

PATHOLOGY

- Spondylodiscitis most often hematogenous infection
- Most common pyogenic organism is *Staphylococcus aureus*
- Worldwide, TB is most common cause

DIAGNOSTIC CHECKLIST

- Differentiate PVS process from retropharyngeal space
- Search for spondylodiscitis as cause
- MR for early identification of disease process even before bone destruction/deformity
- T1 C+ FS MR best evaluates epidural involvement and cord compression
- Whole-spine MR to identify skip/multi focal lesions

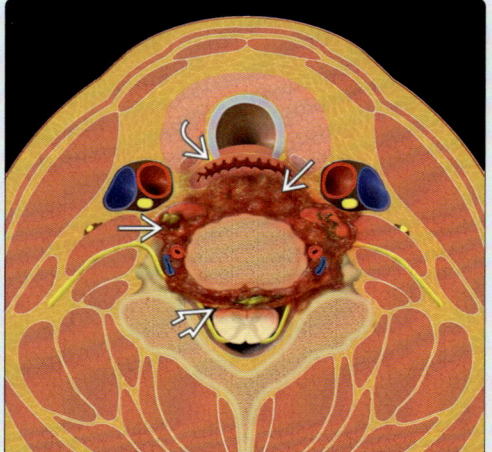

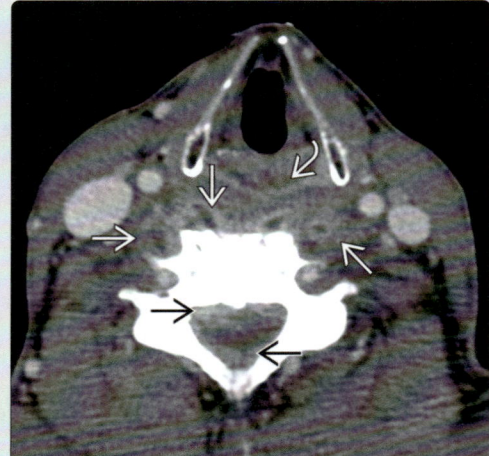

(Left) Axial graphic depicts the typical findings of perivertebral space infection. Phlegmonous soft tissue ➡ surrounds the vertebral body, displacing the esophagus ➡ anteriorly and producing epidural phlegmon/abscess dorsally ➡. (Right) Axial CECT shows heterogeneously enhancing tissue ➡ abutting and surrounding the vertebral body. The hypopharynx ➡ is displaced anteriorly. Careful evaluation of the spinal canal reveals densely enhancing tissue ➡ around the cervical cord, indicating epidural phlegmon.

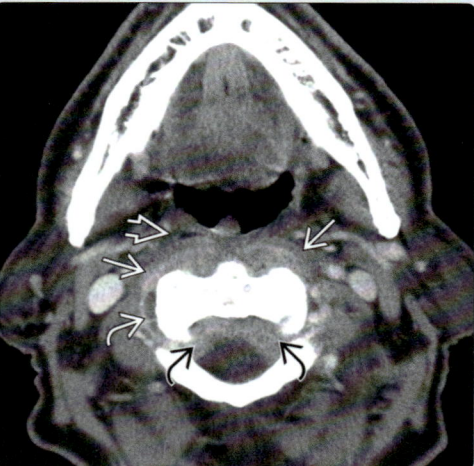

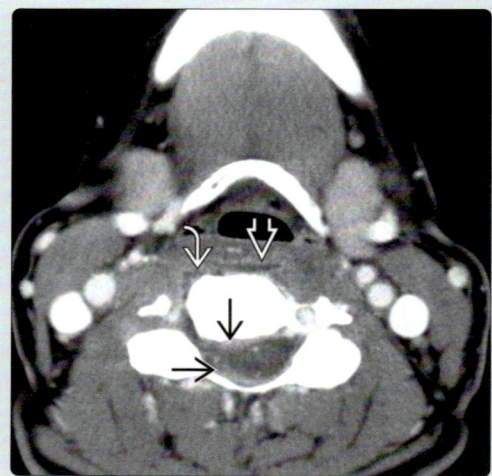

(Left) Axial CECT at the C2 level shows a collar of heterogeneously enhancing tissue ➡ abutting the vertebral body, directly posterior to the thin stripe of retropharyngeal fat ➡. Note the intraspinal epidural component ➡. A small area of early abscess ➡ is present. (Right) Axial CECT reveals heterogeneously enlarged prevertebral tissues with a focal pool of rim-enhancing pus ➡. Inflamed tissues extend from epidural phlegmon ➡. A small retropharyngeal fluid collection ➡ is also noted.

TERMINOLOGY

Abbreviations

- Perivertebral space (PVS) infection

Synonyms

- PVS phlegmon, PVS abscess

Definitions

- Deep neck infection centered at prevertebral muscles, disc space, vertebral body (VB)
  - Most often due to cervical spondylodiscitis
- Phlegmon = inflammation from diffuse tissue infection
- Abscess = marginated collection of pus

IMAGING

General Features

- Best diagnostic clue
  - Prevertebral muscle swelling or collection with destruction or signal change in adjacent VB/disc
- Location
  - Within or posterior to prevertebral muscles, posterior to retropharyngeal space (RPS)
  - Cervical spondylodiscitis most common at C5-C6 level
- Size
  - Variable
    - Phlegmon results in distended PVS muscles
    - Pyogenic infection more commonly phlegmon with small abscesses
    - Atypical organisms, especially TB, may form large (several centimeters) collections
- Morphology
  - PVS infection most often due to **spondylodiscitis**
    - Spread of infection into prevertebral ± paraspinal components
      - Cellulitis with phlegmon → focal then coalescent abscess
    - Infection may simultaneously involve epidural space
      - May result in cord compression ± infarction
      - Common in cervical spondylodiscitis
      - Extensive spinal involvement may be seen
  - **Pyogenic spondylodiscitis**
    - Typically involves disc and adjacent endplates
    - More acute disease presentation and symptoms than TB spondylitis
    - Presents with severe pain, fever ± neurologic deficit
  - **TB spondylitis**
    - Selectively involves VB with relative sparing of endplates and disc
    - May spread under anterior longitudinal ligament to involve multiple VB levels
    - Reactive sclerosis less common
    - Perivertebral soft tissue involvement common, may result in multiple abscesses ± calcification
    - VB collapse with deformity more often than neurologic deficit as presentation
    - Kyphotic deformity may result
  - Atypical infections (e.g., fungus, blastomycosis) usually behave similar to TB

- Spondylodiscitis uncommonly follows neck or cervical spine surgery
- PVS infection usually from osseous or disc infection, rarely from direct muscle seeding

Radiographic Findings

- Radiography
  - Plain films may reveal pyogenic discitis
    - < 7 days: Prevertebral soft tissue swelling
      - Clinical setting to distinguish from RPS mass
    - 7-10 days: Erosion of VB endplate
    - > 2 weeks: Narrow disc space, endplate destruction
    - > 3 weeks: Reactive sclerosis
  - Chronic infection: VB collapse, ± tissue calcifications

CT Findings

- CECT
  - Enhancing heterogeneously enlarged prevertebral muscles
  - Anteriorly displaced RPS and posterior pharyngeal wall
  - May see rim-enhancing abscess
  - Assess for intraspinal epidural phlegmon/abscess
- Bone CT
  - Endplate erosion → frank VB destruction
  - Sagittal or coronal reformats illustrate spine alignment

MR Findings

- T1WI
  - Heterogeneously enlarged prevertebral muscles
  - Loss of normal marrow T1 signal in VB
- T2WI
  - Hyperintensity of prevertebral muscles, disc, and VB
  - Abscess typically markedly hyperintense
  - May also see RPS edema
- DWI
  - Infected disc space often restricts diffusion
- T1WI C+
  - Heterogeneously enhancing prevertebral muscles or rim-enhancing low-intensity collection
  - Diffuse, ill-defined enhancement of prevertebral muscles, disc, VB, and epidural space
  - Look for epidural phlegmon/abscess
  - Enhancement may involve adjacent spaces: Carotid space (CS), RPS

Nuclear Medicine Findings

- Bone scan
  - Sensitive but nonspecific for spondylodiscitis
  - Arterial hyperemia with progressive focal uptake
  - TB infection cold in 35-40%
- PET
  - Usually FDG avid but nonspecific

Imaging Recommendations

- Best imaging tool
  - CECT frequently initial study for neck pain, fever
  - Either CECT or MR good for delineating and distinguishing RPS and PVS processes
  - CT best for bone changes and aspiration guidance
  - MR best for epidural extent ± cord compromise
- Protocol advice

○ If uncertain about epidural involvement on CECT, recommend MR C+
○ Add fat saturation to T1 C+ MR for complete evaluation of epidural extent

DIFFERENTIAL DIAGNOSIS

Retropharyngeal Space Abscess

- Collection between pharynx and prevertebral space
- Flattens anterior aspect of prevertebral muscles
- Most often secondary to pharyngeal infection
- Normal VB and disc spaces

Vertebral Body Metastasis, Perivertebral Space

- VB destruction that typically spares disc space
- Soft tissue extension anteriorly mimics PVS phlegmon but no edema
- Epidural extension ± cord compromise as well
- Other VB lesions may be evident

Lymphoma

- Centered in VB or posterior elements
- May result in associated PVS or epidural mass
- Intermediate to low T2 signal, solid enhancement

Chordoma

- In cervical spine, most often located at C2
- VB mass with lobulated PVS components
- Markedly intense on T2 MR (like CSF signal) but solid enhancement

Ewing Sarcoma

- Rarely arises in VB or sacrum
- Destructive VB soft tissue mass ± PVS and epidural mass
- Disc typically spared

PATHOLOGY

General Features

- Etiology
  ○ PVS infection most often secondary to **cervical spondylodiscitis**
    – Cervical spine is least common site of spondylodiscitis
  ○ Wide variety of causative organisms
    – Most common pyogenic organism is *Staphylococcus aureus*
    – Most common worldwide is TB
      □ Uncommon in cervical spine
  ○ Predisposing conditions
    – Diabetes, IV drug use, transplant or other immunocompromised patients
    – Unwell patients: Older adults; pneumonia; urinary tract infection; skin infection
  ○ Spondylodiscitis uncommonly follows neck or cervical spine surgery
  ○ PVS infection rarely due to direct muscle seeding

CLINICAL ISSUES

Presentation

- Most common signs/symptoms
  ○ Cervical spondylodiscitis
    – Localized severe progressive neck pain and stiffness

    – Fever, malaise, torticollis
    – 20% present with myelopathy from epidural mass
- Other signs/symptoms
  ○ Prevertebral abscess
    – Dysphagia, odynophagia, and shortness of breath

Demographics

- Age
  ○ Any; highest incidence in 6th and 7th decades
- Epidemiology
  ○ Spondylodiscitis represents 2-7% of all osteomyelitis

Natural History & Prognosis

- Epidural spread of PVS infection/spondylodiscitis may result in neurologic compromise
  ○ PVS infection is confined by deep cervical fascia
  ○ Fascia may direct infection into epidural space

Treatment

- Initial treatment
  ○ Aspiration/decompression of abscess collections
  ○ Long-term IV antibiotics
- Other surgical treatment
  ○ Debridement of dead bone
  ○ Supportive bony fusion if VB collapse or kyphosis

DIAGNOSTIC CHECKLIST

Image Interpretation Pearls

- In adult patient with prevertebral muscle inflammation/abscess, carefully assess spine for spondylodiscitis
- Differentiate prevertebral space from RPS process
- Search for spondylodiscitis or VB mass
  ○ Distinguish typical pyogenic spondylodiscitis from atypical or tuberculous spondylitis
- Look for epidural collection, cord compression

Reporting Tips

- Must evaluate for epidural component ± cord compression
  ○ Recommend MR C+ if unsure of epidural extent
  ○ Useful to image entire spine if epidural abscess is present

SELECTED REFERENCES

1. Sareen A et al: Single sequence whole-spine screening magnetic resonance imaging: diagnostic and therapeutic role in multiple-level spinal tuberculosis. Cureus. 16(1):e52757, 2024
2. Shanmuganathan R et al: Active tuberculosis of spine: current updates. N Am Spine Soc J. 16:100267, 2023
3. Hu X et al: Analysis of the diagnostic efficacy of the QuantiFERON-TB Gold In-Tube assay for preoperative differential diagnosis of spinal tuberculosis. Front Cell Infect Microbiol. 12:983579, 2022
4. Almansour H et al: Pyogenic spondylodiscitis: the quest towards a clinical-radiological classification. Orthopade. 49(6):482-93, 2020
5. Chen YC et al: Late deep cervical infection after anterior cervical discectomy and fusion: a case report and literature review. BMC Musculoskelet Disord. 20(1):437, 2019
6. Lawrence R et al: Controversies in the management of deep neck space infection in children: an evidence-based review. Clin Otolaryngol. 42(1):156-63, 2017
7. Mills MK et al: Imaging of the perivertebral space. Radiol Clin North Am. 53(1):163-80, 2015
8. Gonzalez-Beicos A et al: Imaging of acute head and neck infections. Radiol Clin North Am. 50(1):73-83, 2012
9. Rana RS et al: Head and neck infection and inflammation. Radiol Clin North Am. 49(1):165-82, 2011

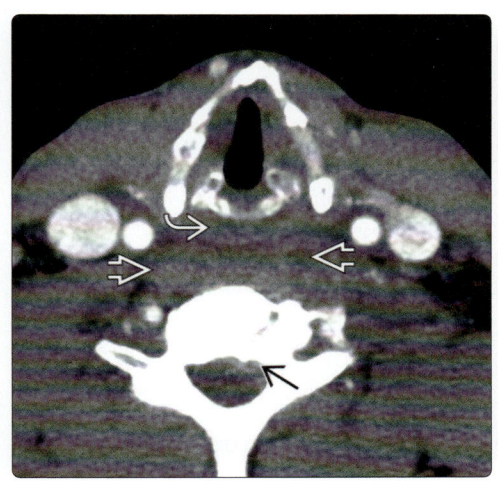

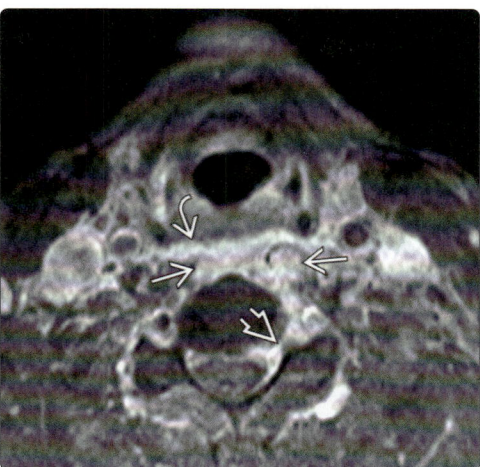

(Left) *Axial CECT in a patient with septicemia, history of drug abuse, and neck pain shows marked prevertebral soft tissue thickening* ➡ *displacing the hypopharynx* ➡ *anteriorly. Note subtle epidural phlegmon* ➡. **(Right)** *Axial T1WI C+ FS MR in the same patient demonstrates extensive soft tissue enhancement in prevertebral space* ➡ *with infiltration of longus colli muscles as well as involvement of retropharyngeal space* ➡. *Subtle left foraminal and epidural enhancement* ➡ *is also evident.*

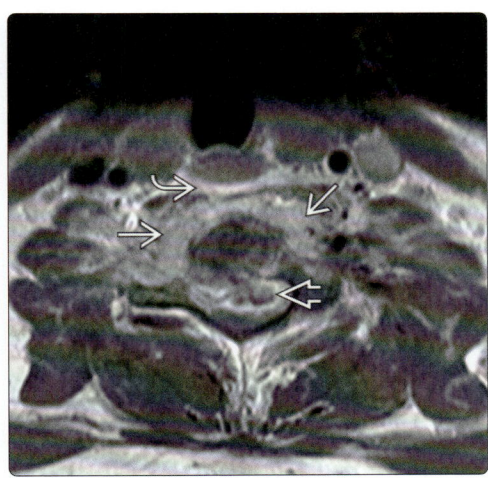

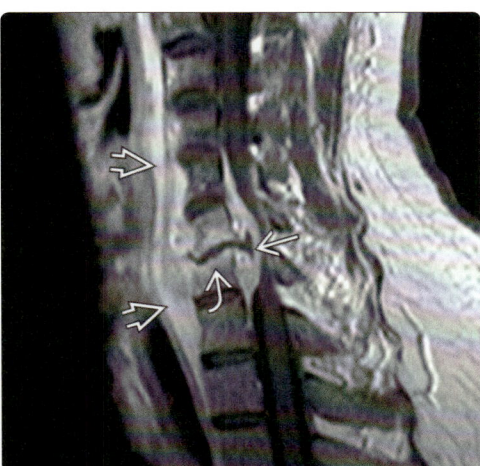

(Left) *Axial T1WI C+ MR demonstrates extensive prevertebral muscle solid enhancement* ➡ *and enlargement, displacing retropharyngeal fat* ➡ *anteriorly. Abnormal epidural enhancement is also noted with rim-enhancing epidural abscess* ➡. **(Right)** *Sagittal T1WI C+ MR demonstrates extensive enhancement of the epidural space with a small, nonenhancing epidural abscess* ➡ *and marked prevertebral soft tissue thickening and enhancement* ➡, *representing phlegmon and abnormal disc space* ➡.

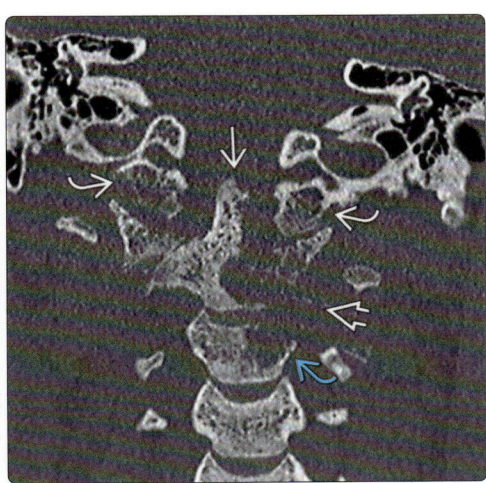

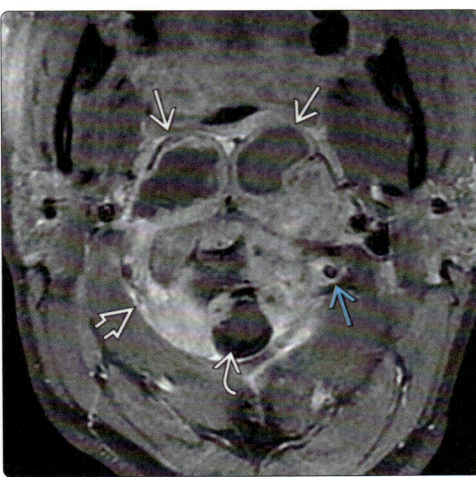

(Left) *Coronal bone CT in a young patient with TB demonstrates extensive bone destruction at C1-C2 vertebral level including the lateral mass of C1* ➡ *odontoid process and body of C2* ➡. *Note involvement of the C2-C3 disk space* ➡ *and the body of C3 vertebra* ➡. **(Right)** *Axial T1WI C+ FS MR in the same patient shows 2 large prevertebral abscess pockets* ➡. *Note enhancing inflammation in perivertebral soft tissue* ➡ *with intraspinal extension, compressing the spinal cord* ➡ *surrounding the left vertebral artery* ➡.

KEY FACTS

TERMINOLOGY

- Vertebral artery (VA) dissection
- Narrowing &/or occlusion of VA secondary to intimal tear and subadventitial hematoma

IMAGING

- 2 typical forms of VA dissection
- **Stenoocclusive dissection**
  - Dissection to subintimal plane with vessel luminal narrowing or occlusion
- **Dissecting aneurysm**
  - Dissection into subadventitial plane with dilatation of outer wall
- Intramural hematoma is pathognomonic
  - Best seen as **bright crescent** on T1 FS MR
- CTA source images show contour changes of lumen
- Conventional angiography is gold standard
- Intimal flap/double lumen are specific

TOP DIFFERENTIAL DIAGNOSES

- Extracranial atherosclerosis
- Fibromuscular dysplasia
- Miscellaneous vasculitis

PATHOLOGY

- **Traumatic** VA dissection
  - Direct or indirect arterial injury
  - Blunt cerebrovascular Injury scale helps guide treatment
- **Spontaneous** VA dissection
  - Many associations and predisposing factors

CLINICAL ISSUES

- Age: Majority < 45 years

DIAGNOSTIC CHECKLIST

- Check other vessels carefully for 2nd dissection
- Evaluate carefully for suboccipital rind sign
- Report degree of luminal narrowing/infarctions in brain

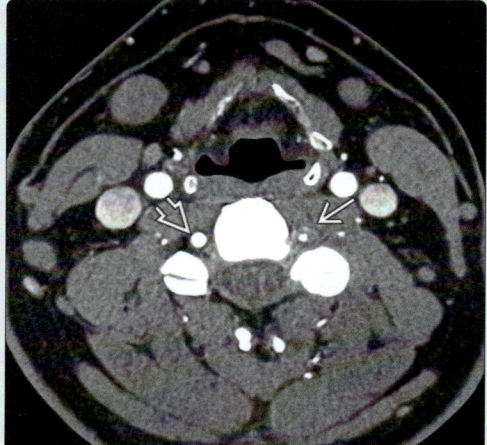
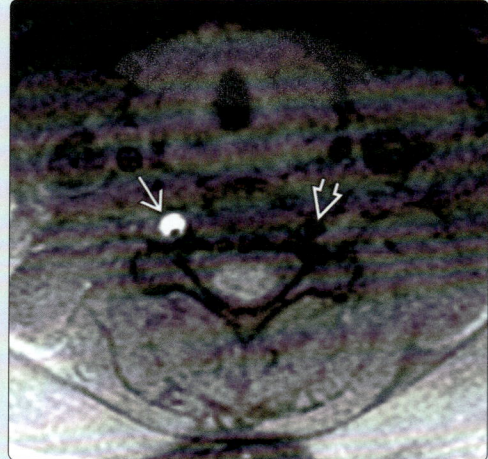

(Left) Axial CTA shows normal symmetric appearance of the common carotid arteries with adjacent jugular veins. The right vertebral artery (VA) ➡ is patent and normal in caliber. The left VA shows markedly diminished lumen caliber ➡ and wall thickening, representing a mural hematoma. (Right) Axial T1WI FS MR in a patient with vertebral dissection reveals a hyperintense crescent within the wall of the right VA ➡, significantly narrowing the VA lumen. This is typical of an intramural hematoma. Note normal left VA flow void ➡.

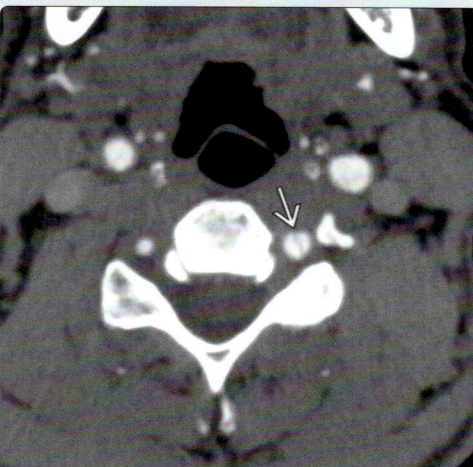
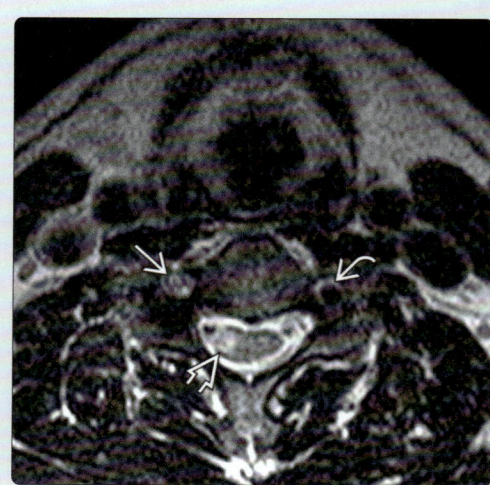

(Left) Axial arterial-phase CECT shows a thin intimal flap within the left VA ➡ due to nonocclusive dissection. A wider soft tissue window setting can be important to best visualize luminal flaps. (Right) Axial T2WI MR in a patient with neck trauma and cervical fractures reveals traumatic VA dissection as loss of a right vertebral flow void ➡ as compared to normal left side ➡. Note right cervical hemicord hyperintensity from infarction ➡.

TERMINOLOGY

Abbreviations
- Vertebral artery (VA) dissection

Definitions
- Narrowing &/or occlusion of VA secondary to intimal tear and subadventitial hematoma

IMAGING

General Features
- Best diagnostic clue
  - Key cross-sectional finding is **crescentic hyperintensity** on T1 FS MR
- Morphology
  - 2 typical forms of VA dissection
  - **Stenoocclusive dissection**
    - Long-segment stenosis → string sign
  - **Dissecting aneurysm**
    - Focal or fusiform aneurysmal dilatation ± stenosis
    - Usually involves intradural VA
    - May present with subarachnoid hemorrhage

CT Findings
- CTA
  - Axial source images show contour changes of lumen
  - **Suboccipital rind sign**
    - Normally opacified VA lumen with mural hematoma

MR Findings
- T1WI
  - Mural hematoma signal varies with time
    - Hyperacute and acute blood
      - Oxy-/deoxyhemoglobin: Iso- to hyperintense
    - Subacute blood (~ 2-3 days)
      - Methemoglobin intrinsically bright on T1 MR
- T1WI FS
  - FS makes mural methemoglobin more conspicuous
  - Inferior presaturation to create black-blood imaging also very useful
- T2WI
  - Loss of normal flow void
- MRA
  - Reveals lumen caliber changes

Angiographic Findings
- Vessel contour changes, including aneurysmal dilatation and stenosis/occlusion
- Intimal flap/double lumen are specific

Imaging Recommendations
- Best imaging tool
  - **Intramural hematoma** is **pathognomonic**
    - Best seen with T1 FS MR with inflow presaturation
  - Conventional angiography is gold standard
    - May miss dissection if subtle change in lumen diameter
- Protocol advice
  - Black-blood MR, MRA, or CTA for VA evaluation
  - Brain imaging to evaluate for infarctions

DIFFERENTIAL DIAGNOSIS

Extracranial Atherosclerosis
- Multiple vessels involved with eccentric, irregular stenoses

Fibromuscular Dysplasia
- Multiple focal, web-like strictures (string of beads appearance) or long-segment stenosis

Miscellaneous Vasculitis
- Stenoses involving multiple variably sized vessels

PATHOLOGY

General Features
- Etiology
  - **Traumatic VA dissection**
    - Direct arterial injury (penetrating trauma)
    - Indirect injury ± cervical fractures
  - **Spontaneous VA dissection**
    - Multiple associations and predisposing factors
      - Hypertension
      - Vascular abnormality: Fibromuscular dysplasia (FMD), Marfan syndrome, collagen vascular disease
      - ↑ dissection risk within 3 months of influenza and influenza-like illness
      - COVID-19 reported association with VA dissection

CLINICAL ISSUES

Presentation
- Most common signs/symptoms
  - Neck pain, headache, or posterior circulation stroke

Demographics
- Age
  - Majority < 45 years
- Epidemiology
  - Dissection → 5-20% of strokes in young patients

Treatment
- Stenoocclusive dissection → anticoagulation
- Dissecting aneurysm → ligation or coil embolization
- Complete resolution of lumen abnormality in ~ 80%
- Stenting may be used in select cases

DIAGNOSTIC CHECKLIST

Image Interpretation Pearls
- Evaluate axial CTA carefully for suboccipital rind sign if normal lumen but high clinical suspicion

SELECTED REFERENCES

1. Bai J et al: Imaging of cerebrovascular complications from blunt skull base trauma. Emerg Radiol. 31(4):529-42, 2024
2. Perez-Roman RJ et al: The role of emboli detection studies in acute inpatient vertebral artery dissection. J Clin Neurosci. 127:110748, 2024
3. Pini R et al: Medical and interventional outcome of dissection of the cervical arteries: systematic review and meta-analysis. J Vasc Surg. 80(3):913-21.e13, 2024
4. Ho AL et al: Predictors of cervical vertebral and carotid artery dissection during blunt trauma: experience from a level 1 trauma center. World Neurosurg. 137:e315-20, 2020
5. Wu Y et al: Predisposing factors and radiological features in patients with internal carotid artery dissection or vertebral artery dissection. BMC Neurol. 20(1):445, 2020

KEY FACTS

TERMINOLOGY

- Benign Schwann cell neoplasm that **arises from brachial plexus** (BP) in perivertebral space (PVS)

IMAGING

- Well-circumscribed, **fusiform mass** along course of BP
- Occurs along course of BP in any segment
- Intra- and extradural and neural foramen
- In PVS between anterior and middle scalene muscles
- 3D STIR to produce MR neurography increasing in utilization to depict BP normal anatomy and schwannomas

TOP DIFFERENTIAL DIAGNOSES

- Nodal metastasis
- Neurofibroma
- Lateral meningocele
- Malignant peripheral nerve sheath tumor

PATHOLOGY

- Cystic degeneration and hemorrhage common
- Firm, encapsulated, fusiform mass attaches to and displaces nerve
- Malignant peripheral nerve sheath tumors (MPNST) comprising 7% of all tumors of BP

CLINICAL ISSUES

- 5% of benign soft tissue neoplasms
- Malignant degeneration rare, more common with multiple schwannoma syndromes
- Development of pain should raise suspicion for malignancy

DIAGNOSTIC CHECKLIST

- Determination that lesion is along course of BP is key
- Roots of BP (C5-T1) emerge into scalene triangle between anterior and middle scalene muscles

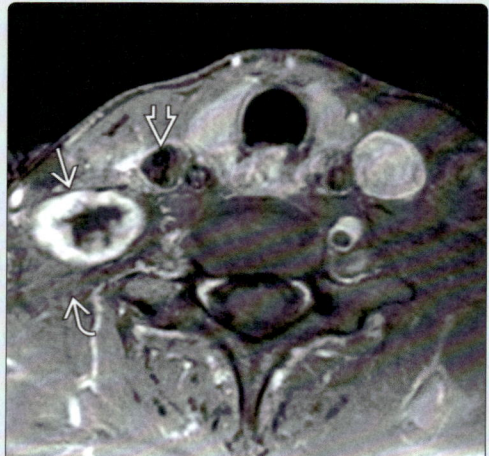
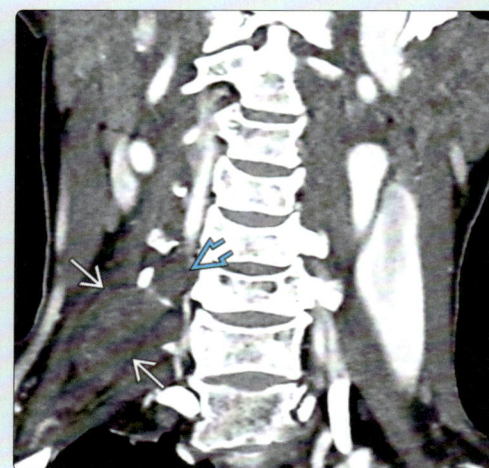

(Left) *Axial T1WI C+ FS MR demonstrates a large schwannoma* ➡ *in the lower right neck overlying the middle scalene muscle* ➡ *with intense, irregular peripheral enhancement. Central nonenhancement represents cystic degeneration. The lesion is more lateral in location than expected for lower cervical nodes, which typically abut the internal jugular vein* ➡. (Right) *Coronal CECT shows a fusiform mass with mild, patchy contrast enhancement* ➡. *Note relation to the C6 root of brachial plexus* ➡.

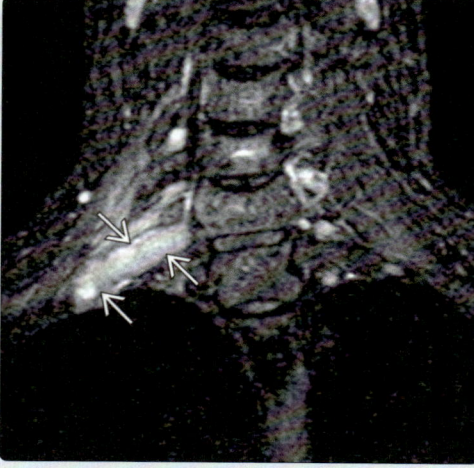
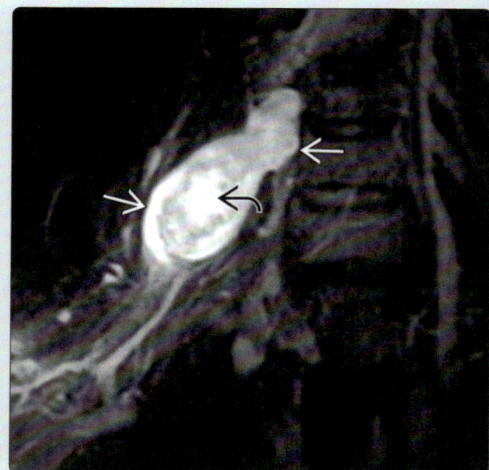

(Left) *Coronal STIR MR (MR neurography technique) demonstrates an asymmetrically enlarged, lobulated right C8 nerve root* ➡ *extending from the C8-T1 neural foramen.* (Right) *Coronal T2 FS MR demonstrates a well-circumscribed, lobulated, fusiform mass* ➡ *oriented along the course of the C6 root of the brachial plexus. The mass is hyperintense on T2WI with areas of heterogeneity, signifying cystic degenerative change* ➡.

TERMINOLOGY

Abbreviations

- Brachial plexus (BP) schwannoma

Definitions

- Benign Schwann cell neoplasm that arises from BP in perivertebral space (PVS)

IMAGING

General Features

- Best diagnostic clue
  - Well-circumscribed, fusiform mass along course of BP
- Location
  - Occurs along course of BP in any segment
    - Intra- and extradural and neural foramen
    - In PVS between anterior and middle scalene muscles
- Morphology
  - Fusiform or dumbbell-shaped mass

CT Findings

- NECT
  - Typically isodense to muscle; calcification uncommon
  - When paraspinal, bony neural foramen shows **smooth enlargement**
- CECT
  - Mild to moderate enhancement

MR Findings

- T1WI
  - **Fusiform mass**, isointense to muscle
- T2WI
  - Heterogeneously hyperintense
  - **Target sign**: Central hypointense, peripheral hyperintense signal
  - **Fascicular sign**: Multiple irregular, central hypointense foci
- STIR
  - 3D STIR to produce MR neurography increasing in utilization to depict BP normal anatomy and schwannomas
- T1WI C+
  - Moderate heterogeneous enhancement
    - **Intramural cysts** common

Imaging Recommendations

- Protocol advice
  - T1WI with FS and STIR improve conspicuity

DIFFERENTIAL DIAGNOSIS

Nodal Metastasis

- Supraclavicular nodes are metastatic site for chest and abdominal disease
- Lower cervical nodes medial to anterior scalene muscle, adjacent to internal jugular vein

Neurofibroma

- May be indistinguishable from schwannoma on MR
- Typically lower density on NECT, approaching water density
- Cystic degeneration and hemorrhage uncommon

Lateral Meningocele

- Fusiform cystic mass follows CSF density/intensity
- Contiguous with spinal canal

Malignant Peripheral Nerve Sheath Tumor

- Progressively enlarging, irregular, heterogeneous mass
- Typically associated with pain

PATHOLOGY

Gross Pathologic & Surgical Features

- Firm, encapsulated, well-circumscribed, gray-tan, fusiform mass attached to and displacing nerve
- Cystic degeneration and hemorrhage common

Microscopic Features

- Tumor arises from Schwann cells of nerve sheath
- Alternating regions of high cellularity (Antoni A) and loose, myxoid component (Antoni B)

CLINICAL ISSUES

Presentation

- Most common signs/symptoms
  - Painless, slow-growing mass in lateral neck ± radiculopathy
  - Pain or dysesthesias on palpation said to be characteristic

Demographics

- Age
  - Peaks at 20-30 years

Natural History & Prognosis

- Slow-growing lesion
- Malignant degeneration rare, more common with multiple schwannoma syndromes
- Development of **pain** should raise suspicion for **malignancy**

DIAGNOSTIC CHECKLIST

Image Interpretation Pearls

- Determination that lesion is along course of BP is key
- Roots of BP (C5-T1) emerge into scalene triangle between anterior and middle scalene muscles

Reporting Tips

- When describing any low neck lesion, always describe relationship of lesion to BP course

SELECTED REFERENCES

1. Madhuranthakam AJ: Advanced techniques on horizon for MR imaging of brachial plexus. Eur Radiol. 34(2):885-6, 2024
2. Davidson EJ et al: Brachial plexus magnetic resonance neurography: technical challenges and solutions. Invest Radiol. 58(1):14-27, 2023
3. Lubelski D et al: Natural history of brachial plexus, peripheral nerve, and spinal schwannomas. Neurosurgery. 91(6):883-91, 2022
4. Gilcrease-Garcia BM et al: Anatomy, imaging, and pathologic conditions of the brachial plexus. Radiographics. 40(6):1686-714, 2020
5. Yonezawa H et al: Structural origin and surgical complications of peripheral schwannomas. Anticancer Res. 40(11):6563-70, 2020
6. Desai KI: The surgical management of symptomatic benign peripheral nerve sheath tumors of the neck and extremities: an experience of 442 cases. Neurosurgery. 81(4):568-80, 2017
7. Jia X et al: Primary brachial plexus tumors: clinical experiences of 143 cases. Clin Neurol Neurosurg. 148:91-5, 2016
8. Lutz AM et al: MR imaging of the brachial plexus. Neuroimaging Clin N Am. 24(1):91-108, 2014

Chordoma in Perivertebral Space

TERMINOLOGY

- Rare, low-grade primary malignant tumor of notochord origin

IMAGING

- Cervical spine: C2-C5 most often
- Lytic vertebral body (VB) lesion without collapse
- CT: Lobulated, low-density soft tissue mass
  - Coarse, amorphous calcifications in 30%
- MR: Marked T2 hyperintensity, similar to CSF
  - Poorly differentiated type: Low T2 signal intensity
  - Typically heterogeneous enhancement
  - DWI: Conventional type: Mean ADC, 1474 ± 117 × 10-6 mm2/sec (higher ADC values in chondrosarcoma)
- FDG PET: Heterogeneous, increased uptake

TOP DIFFERENTIAL DIAGNOSES

- VB metastasis, perivertebral space (PVS)
- PVS infection

- Brachial plexus schwannoma
- Vertebral chondrosarcoma

PATHOLOGY

- Arise from embryonic notochord
- Lobulated, soft, grayish mass with pseudocapsule
- 3-7% all chordomas arise in cervical spine
- Myxoid stroma & characteristic **physaliphorous cells**

CLINICAL ISSUES

- 3rd-6th decades, peaks in 5th decade
- Presents from local pressure effects on cord or prevertebral structures
- May present with nonspecific neck pain
- Treat primarily with surgery, then follow with radiotherapy
- Slow-growing lesion, tendency for local recurrence

DIAGNOSTIC CHECKLIST

- Marked T2 hyperintensity key to diagnosis
- DWI may help distinguish from chondrosarcoma

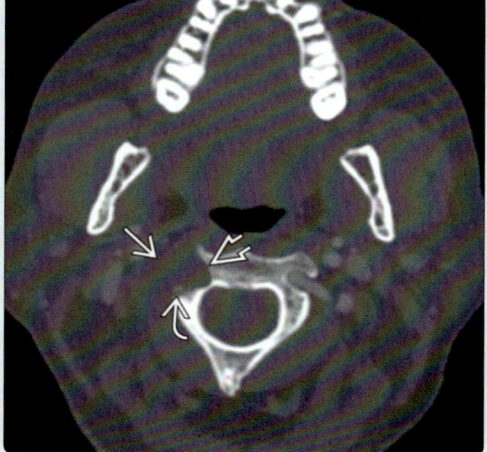 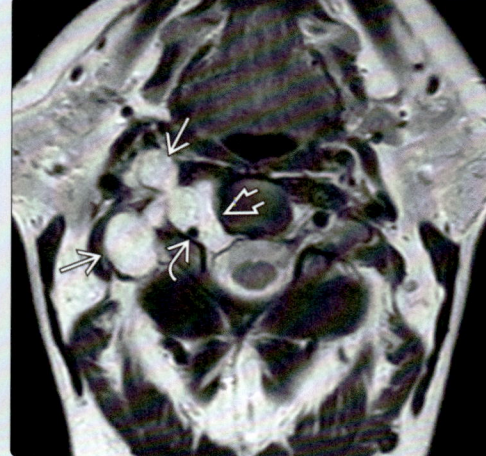

(Left) Axial bone window from a head CT angiogram in a 60-year-old woman demonstrates an incidentally discovered cervical chordoma ➡ involving the lateral mass of C2. The bony margins are relatively smooth ➡. Note the right vertebral artery ➡ is displaced posteriorly. (Right) Axial T2 MR in the same patient shows typical T2 hyperintensity & multilobular nature of cervical chordoma ➡. The medial component extends through & mildly expands the neural foramen ➡. The vertebral artery ➡ was displaced posteriorly.

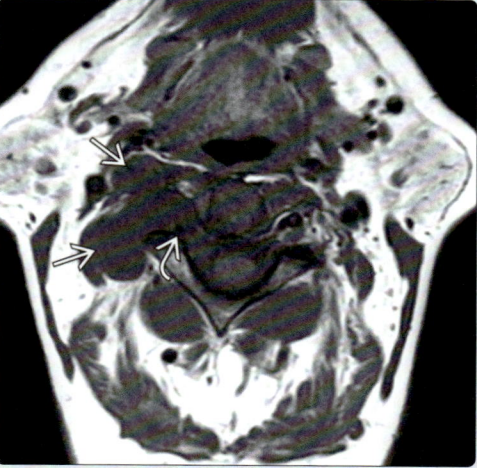 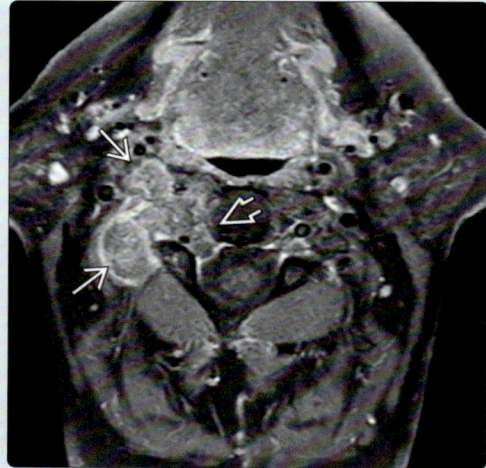

(Left) Axial T1 MR in the same patient shows the soft tissue mass is relatively homogeneous & solid. Flow void from the vertebral artery ➡ is seen displaced posteriorly. The lesion extends anteriorly & laterally into the perivertebral space ➡. (Right) Axial T1 C+ FS MR shows diffuse, moderate enhancement of the lobulated but well-circumscribed chordoma ➡ that arises from the lateral mass of C2 and extends inferior and laterally through the neural foramen ➡.

TERMINOLOGY

Definitions

- Rare, low-grade primary malignant tumor of notochord origin

IMAGING

General Features

- Best diagnostic clue
  - Destructive vertebral body (VB) lesion with well-defined, T2-hyperintense, & enhancing perivertebral mass
- Location
  - Cervical spine: C2-C5 most often
- Morphology
  - VB mass spares posterior elements
  - Associated lobulated soft tissue mass
  - On occasion may involve adjacent vertebra, mimicking spondylodiscitis

Radiographic Findings

- Radiography
  - Lytic, destructive lesion without VB collapse

CT Findings

- NECT
  - Coarse, amorphous calcifications in 30%
- CECT
  - Lobulated soft tissue mass, typically low density

MR Findings

- T1WI
  - Low to intermediate signal intensity
- T2WI
  - **Markedly hyperintense**, similar to CSF
- T1WI C+
  - Typically heterogeneous enhancement

Nuclear Medicine Findings

- PET
  - Heterogeneous, increased FDG uptake

Imaging Recommendations

- Best imaging tool
  - CT & MR are complementary
    - Bone CT best shows VB lysis & occasional calcifications
    - MR for soft tissue extent; T2 hyperintensity of lesion

DIFFERENTIAL DIAGNOSIS

Vertebral Body Metastasis, Perivertebral Space

- Destructive VB soft tissue mass
- Variable signal intensity on T2WI MR

Perivertebral Space Infection

- Disc space narrowing, endplate destruction
- Diffuse marrow, disc, epidural, & perivertebral space enhancement

Brachial Plexus Schwannoma, Perivertebral Space

- Intermediate to high T2 signal follows nerve root
- Smoothly scallops neural foramen

Chondrosarcoma

- Destructive VB ± posterior element lesion
- CT shows chondroid matrix mineralization
- Very high signal intensity on T2WI MR

PATHOLOGY

General Features

- Etiology
  - Arises from embryonic notochord
  - Location parallels distribution of notochordal rests
    - 50% sacrococcygeal region
    - 35% sphenooccipital region
    - 15% spine: Cervical > lumbar > thoracic

Staging, Grading, & Classification

- 4 types: Conventional, chondroid, dedifferentiated and poorly differentiated
- ADC and enhancement pattern seem associated with prognosis

Microscopic Features

- Myxoid stroma & characteristic **physaliphorous cells**
  - Large cells with eosinophilic cytoplasm containing multiple vacuoles & central nuclei

CLINICAL ISSUES

Presentation

- Most common signs/symptoms
  - Typically presents from local mass effect
  - Gradual onset of neck pain, numbness

Demographics

- Sex
  - M:F = 2:1
- Epidemiology
  - 3-7% all chordomas arise in cervical spine

Natural History & Prognosis

- Slow-growing lesion, tendency for local recurrence
- Metastatic disease in 5-43%

Treatment

- Surgery & complete resection is treatment of choice
- Proton beam is favored radiotherapy after surgery

DIAGNOSTIC CHECKLIST

Image Interpretation Pearls

- Marked T2 hyperintensity with heterogeneous enhancement is key to diagnosis
- Carefully evaluate for vascular encasement

SELECTED REFERENCES

1. Park H et al: The clinical outcomes of cervical spine chordoma: a nationwide multicenter retrospective study. Neurospine. 21(3):942-53, 2024
2. Potter GM et al: Skull base chordoma and chondrosarcoma: neuroradiologist's guide to diagnosis, surgical management, and proton beam therapy. Radiographics. 44(10):e240036, 2024
3. Zweckberger K et al: Clivus chordomas: heterogeneous tumor extension requires adapted surgical approaches. Clin Neurol Neurosurg. 199:106305, 2020

Vertebral Body Metastasis in Perivertebral Space

TERMINOLOGY

- Metastatic tumor to cervical vertebral body (VB) ± invasion of perivertebral space (PVS)

IMAGING

- Spinal metastases proportionate to red marrow
- Lumbar > thoracic > cervical spine
- > 50% have multiple level involvement
- Destructive VB mass
- Expanded, infiltrated, or displaced prevertebral muscles

TOP DIFFERENTIAL DIAGNOSES

- PVS infection
- Longus colli tendinitis
- PVS chordoma

PATHOLOGY

- Vertebral metastases may be confined by **prevertebral fascia**, directing tumor to **epidural space**

- Most VB metastases from hematogenous spread
- Adults most often lung, breast, prostate, kidney, GI
- Children most often hematologic malignancies & neuroblastoma
- Rarely, tumor directly penetrates PVS from posterior pharyngeal wall

CLINICAL ISSUES

- Vertebral metastasis is most common malignant spine lesion & vertebra most common site
- Treatment depends on tumor type, symptomatology, & neurologic complications
  - Radiation therapy ± stereotactic radiotherapy, endovascular tumor embolization, vertebroplasty, surgical resection for cord decompression ± spine stabilization; radiofrequency & microwave ablation are emerging options
- Ongoing bone destruction leads to fracture, instability, deformity, & neurologic compromise

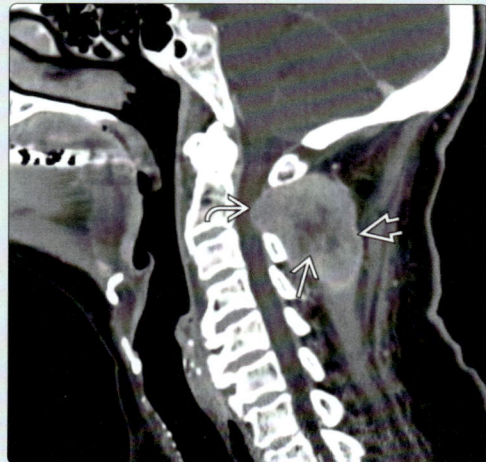
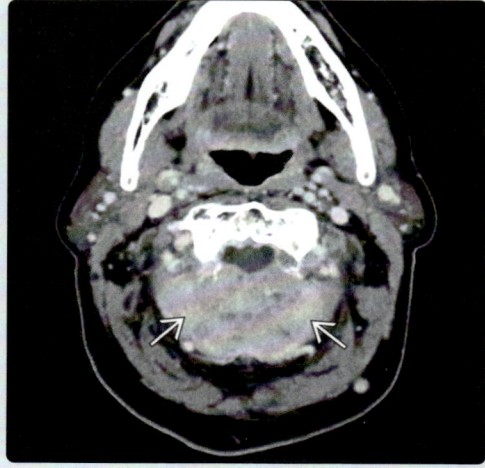

(Left) Sagittal CECT demonstrates a large, expansile lesion ⮕ destroying the posterior elements of C2 in this 60-year-old woman with metastatic melanoma. Tumor encroaches upon the posterior epidural space anteriorly ⮕ and invades the posterior perivertebral space posteriorly ⮕. (Right) Axial CECT in the same patient shows the expansile, enhancing mass that invades the deep musculature of the posterior perivertebral space (PVS) ⮕.

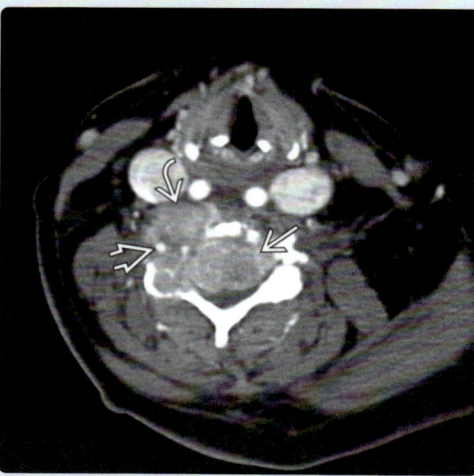
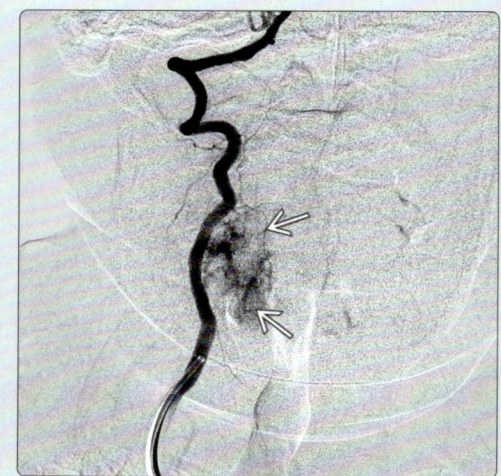

(Left) Axial CECT in a 64-year-old woman with metastatic renal cell carcinoma shows a destructive, heterogeneously enhancing mass involving C5 vertebra ⮕, causing severe spinal stenosis. Extraosseous tumor extends anteriorly into right prevertebral soft tissues ⮕. Laterally, tumor extends beyond the lateral process of C5 to encase the right vertebral artery ⮕. (Right) Anterior DSA of the right vertebral artery in the same patient shows the hypervascular nature of the large metastatic lesion ⮕ at C5.

Vertebral Body Metastasis in Perivertebral Space

TERMINOLOGY

Abbreviations

- Vertebral body (VB) metastasis in perivertebral space (PVS)

Definitions

- Metastatic tumor to cervical VB ± invasion of PVS

IMAGING

General Features

- Best diagnostic clue
  - Destructive mass of VB ± PVS ± epidural or prevertebral extension
  - Often involves multiple VB & multiple spine segments
- Location
  - Cervical VB ± adjacent pre- & perivertebral & epidural tissues
  - Spinal metastases proportionate to red marrow
    - Lumbar > thoracic > cervical spine
  - > 50% have multiple level involvement
- Morphology
  - Destructive VB mass
  - Expanded or displaced prevertebral muscles

Radiographic Findings

- Radiography
  - Increased prevertebral soft tissues
  - Variable destruction of VB ± VB collapse
  - Lytic or sclerotic or mixed destructive changes of VB

CT Findings

- CECT
  - Enhancing, irregular soft tissue involving or displacing prevertebral muscles
  - **Epidural tumor**: Solid intraspinal enhancement posterior to VB
    - May be subtle on CECT
- Bone CT
  - Loss of normal bone trabeculae ± cortex
  - Variable **VB collapse** on sagittal/coronal reformats
  - Irregular sclerosis ± lytic change

MR Findings

- T1WI
  - Focal or diffuse hypointense VB lesion(s)
  - **Disc space** usually **preserved**
    - Appear brighter than marrow when diffuse disease
- T2WI
  - Most metastases iso- to hyperintense; sclerotic metastases hypointense
  - Perivertebral component usually hyperintense
  - Look for flow void of vertebral arteries
- STIR
  - Usually hyperintense with normal fat marrow suppressed
- DWI
  - Low ADC value favors tumor over benign VB edema
- T1WI C+
  - Enhancing VB lesion with soft tissue extension into PVS ± intraspinal epidural space

- Perivertebral involvement has variable appearance but usually solid enhancement
  - Irregular enhancement of tissues mimicking phlegmon
  - Enhancing tissue displacing/invading prevertebral muscles

Nuclear Medicine Findings

- Bone scan
  - Usually seen as focal increased uptake
  - May be negative when metastasis is small & within medullary cavity
- PET
  - FDG uptake in bone & soft tissue metastases

Imaging Recommendations

- Best imaging tool
  - Different modalities have different strengths
  - Bone scintigraphy
    - Cost-effective & readily available whole-body screening test
    - May show other bony metastatic foci
    - Underestimates spine metastases compared to MR
  - Bone CT
    - Helpful for clarifying suspicious MR, bone scan, or PET lesions
    - Useful in guiding needle biopsy
    - Useful in planning spinal stabilization surgery when fusion is contemplated
  - MR
    - Direct evaluation of vertebral, PVS, & epidural involvement
    - Optimal demonstration of cord compromise ± cord signal abnormality
    - Early, noncortical VB metastases may only be seen with MR
- Protocol advice
  - Important to evaluate entire spine, especially when surgery or radiation is considered
    - Ensures treatment of all lesions with potential neurologic compromise
  - MR: Fat-saturation sequences (T2, STIR, & T1 C+) distinguish bone metastases from fatty marrow
    - DWI sequences also helpful in problematic cases

DIFFERENTIAL DIAGNOSIS

Multiple Myeloma

- Lytic lesion, often multiple affecting cervical spine

Perivertebral Space Infection

- Pyogenic discitis: Disc & VB endplate edema & destruction
- Atypical infections (fungal, TB): Centered in VB
- Phlegmon ± abscess in adjacent soft tissues
- Posterior VB elements usually not involved

Perivertebral Space Chordoma

- Markedly hyperintense on T2 MR
- In PVS tends to have lobulated contour
- VB height usually preserved

PATHOLOGY

General Features

- Etiology
  - Most VB metastases from hematogenous spread
  - Adults with PVS metastasis
    - Most often lung, breast, prostate, kidney, GI
    - 15-25% unknown primary
  - Children with PVS metastasis
    - Leukemia, neuroblastoma, Ewing sarcoma
  - Rarely, tumor directly penetrates PVS from posterior pharyngeal wall (squamous cell carcinoma)
  - Vertebral metastases may be confined by **prevertebral fascia**, directing tumor to **epidural space**

Staging, Grading, & Classification

- Tomita surgical classification system for metastases; estimates potential risk for spine instability
  - Type 1: VB
  - Type 2: Pedicle extension
  - Type 3: Body & into lamina
  - Type 4: Epidural extension
  - Type 5: Perivertebral extension
  - Type 6: Extension to adjacent vertebra(e)
  - Type 7: Multiple separate vertebral bodies
- This classification useful for radiologic description of spine metastases
- Tomita grading score for metastases
  - To estimate patient survival with treatment
  - Points given for speed of tumor growth, presence of visceral & bone metastases
  - Final score in range 2-10 (2 = best prognosis)
- Tomita score & classification probably best used together & in conjunction with neurologic symptoms to plan surgery, radiation/chemotherapy

Gross Pathologic & Surgical Features

- Softened, eroded bone ± adjacent soft tissue mass

CLINICAL ISSUES

Presentation

- Most common signs/symptoms
  - 90-95% present with **pain**
    - Local, radicular, or referred
  - Neurologic compromise from cord or nerve root compression
- Other signs/symptoms
  - Fever, sepsis not in clinical picture
- Clinical profile
  - Adult patient with known primary tumor presenting with spine pain & neurologic compromise

Demographics

- Age
  - Most often > 50 years
- Sex
  - M = F
- Epidemiology
  - Vertebral column most common site of bone metastasis

- Vertebral metastasis is most common malignant spine lesion
- 10-40% prevalence with systemic cancer

Natural History & Prognosis

- Ongoing bone destruction leads to fracture, instability, deformity, & neurologic compromise
- If untreated, there is potential for epidural involvement & cord compression
  - Neurologic deficits rarely recover after treatment

Treatment

- Depends on tumor type, symptomatology, & neurologic complications
- Treatment options include
  - Radiation therapy ± stereotactic radiotherapy, endovascular tumor embolization, vertebroplasty, surgical resection for cord decompression ± spine stabilization
  - Minimally invasive techniques, such as CT-guided thermal ablation including radiofrequency & microwave ablation

DIAGNOSTIC CHECKLIST

Consider

- VB metastasis mimics infectious spondylodiscitis
  - Especially atypical infections
    - Fungal & TB tend to also be found in VB center with disc sparing

Image Interpretation Pearls

- Important to obtain & carefully review bone CT images for trabecular loss, cortical destruction
- Carefully evaluate epidural space & spinal cord
- Obtain MR with any neurologic symptoms or when epidural aspect not well evaluated
- Evaluate vertebral arteries for compression or occlusion
- Assess fracture risk

SELECTED REFERENCES

1. Aslan S et al: Evaluating the accuracy and efficiency of imaging modalities in guiding ablation for metastatic spinal column tumors: a systematic review. Cancers (Basel). 16(23), 2024
2. Costa F et al: Incidence, epidemiology, radiology, and classification of metastatic spine tumors: WFNS Spine Committee recommendations. Neurosurg Rev. 47(1):853, 2024
3. Harlianto NI et al: Diagnostic accuracy of imaging modalities for detection of spinal metastases: a systematic review and meta-analysis. Clin Transl Oncol. 27(5):2316-26 , 2024
4. Ong W et al: Application of artificial intelligence methods for imaging of spinal metastasis. Cancers (Basel). 14(16), 2022
5. Pricolo P et al: Whole-body magnetic resonance imaging (WB-MRI) reporting with the METastasis Reporting and Data System for Prostate Cancer (MET-RADS-P): inter-observer agreement between readers of different expertise levels. Cancer Imaging. 20(1):77, 2020
6. Hussain AK et al: The impact of metastatic spinal tumor location on 30-day perioperative mortality and morbidity after surgical decompression. Spine (Phila Pa 1976). 43(11):E648-55, 2018
7. Mesfin A et al: Management of metastatic cervical spine tumors. J Am Acad Orthop Surg. 23(1):38-46, 2015
8. Patel KB et al: Diffusion-weighted MRI "claw sign" improves differentiation of infectious from degenerative modic type 1 signal changes of the spine. AJNR Am J Neuroradiol. 35(8):1647-52, 2014
9. Prince EA et al: Interventional management of vertebral body metastases. Semin Intervent Radiol. 30(3):278-81, 2013
10. Grankvist J et al: MRI and PET/CT of patients with bone metastases from breast carcinoma. Eur J Radiol. 81(1):e13-8, 2012

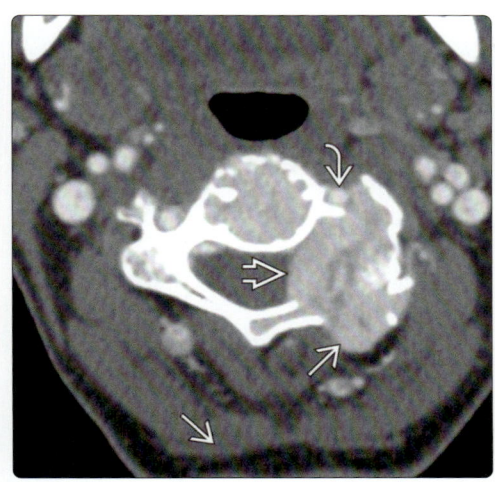
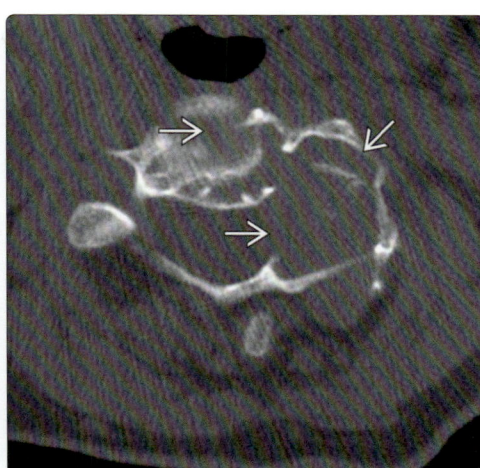

(Left) *Axial CECT demonstrates a large, enhancing mass involving C3 vertebra, left facet, and lamina. Note extension into the paraspinal component of PVS* ➡. *Intraspinal tumor* ⇉ *has a smooth interface with dura. Tumor is around the left vertebral artery* ⬈. **(Right)** *Axial bone CT in the same patient better illustrates the lesion* ⇉ *as predominately lytic and expansile. This destructive lesion was a thyroid carcinoma metastasis and was embolized prior to surgical resection.*

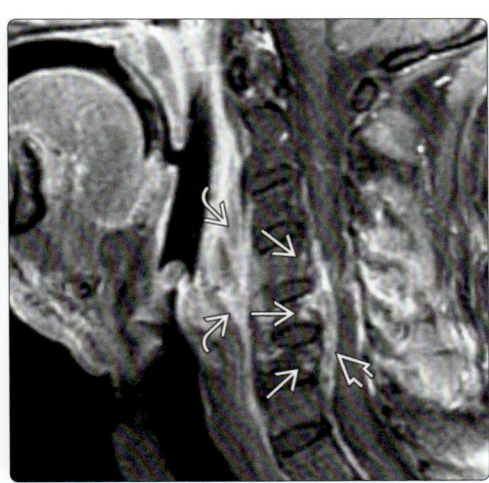
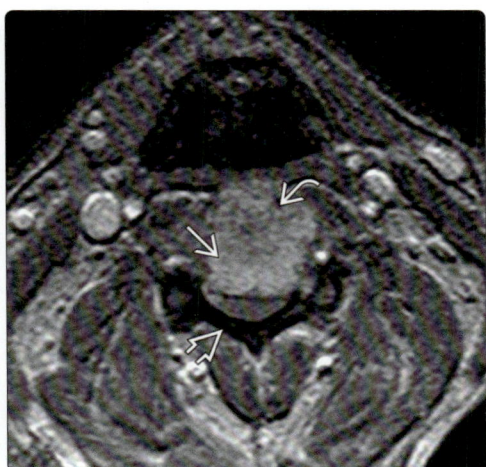

(Left) *Sagittal T1WI C+ FS MR reveals multilevel tumor* ➡ *and extensive epidural* ⇉ *and prevertebral extraosseous tumor* ⬈. *Posterior elements and paraspinous musculature are also diffusely infiltrated. Involvement of multiple adjacent vertebrae is type 6 in the Tomita classification.* **(Right)** *Axial STIR MR shows suppression of normal marrow signal in posterior elements* ⇶ *of the vertebral body (VB) compared to intrinsically bright metastasis involving the VB* ➡ *and extending into prevertebral tissues* ⬈.

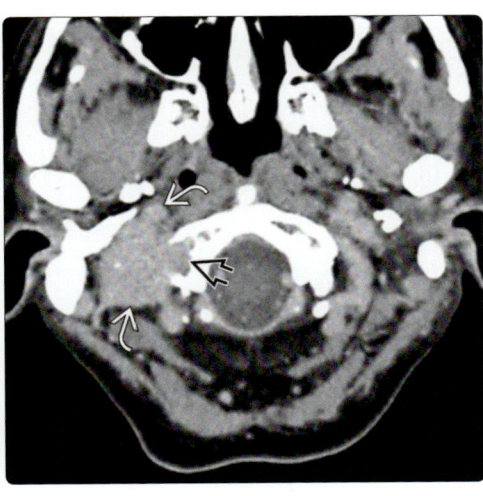
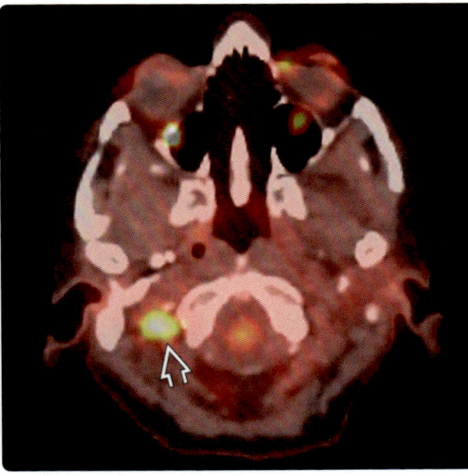

(Left) *Axial CECT in a patient with known metastatic breast carcinoma shows a large, enhancing soft tissue mass* ⬈ *in the skull base confined to right PVS. Note bone destruction at level of foramen magnum/C1 vertebra* ⇶. *The bony component of metastasis can be small. Careful evaluation of skull base in important on routine brain CT.* **(Right)** *Axial FDG PET/CT in the same patient shows avid FDG uptake in the right perivertebral soft tissue mass* ⇉. *Patient also has other multilevel vertebral metastases.*

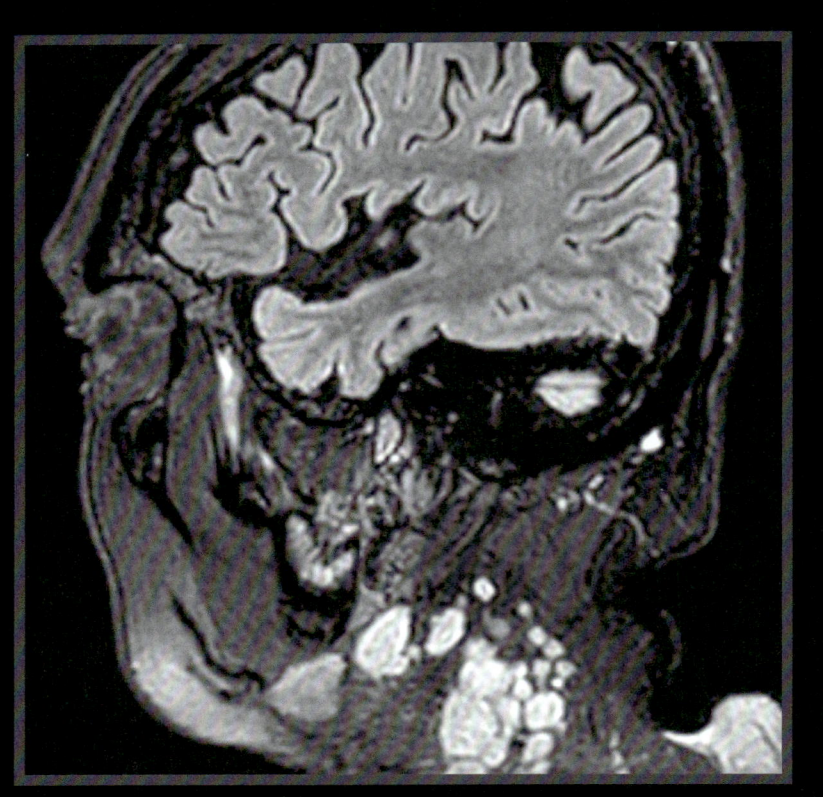
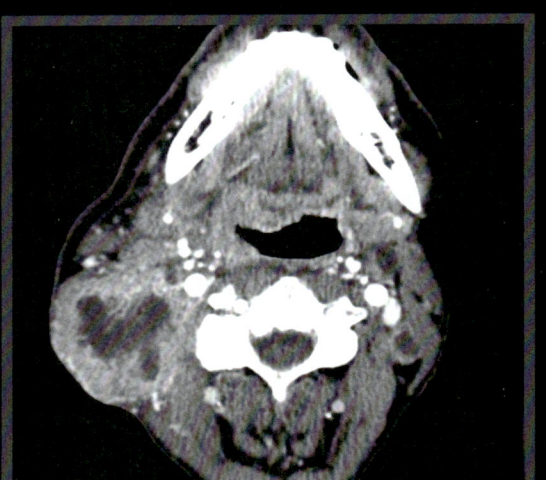
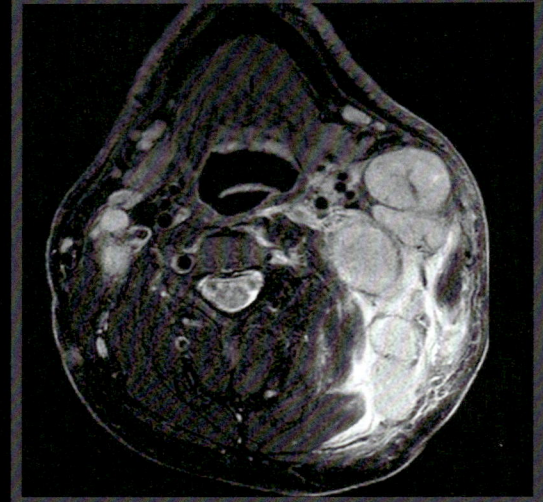
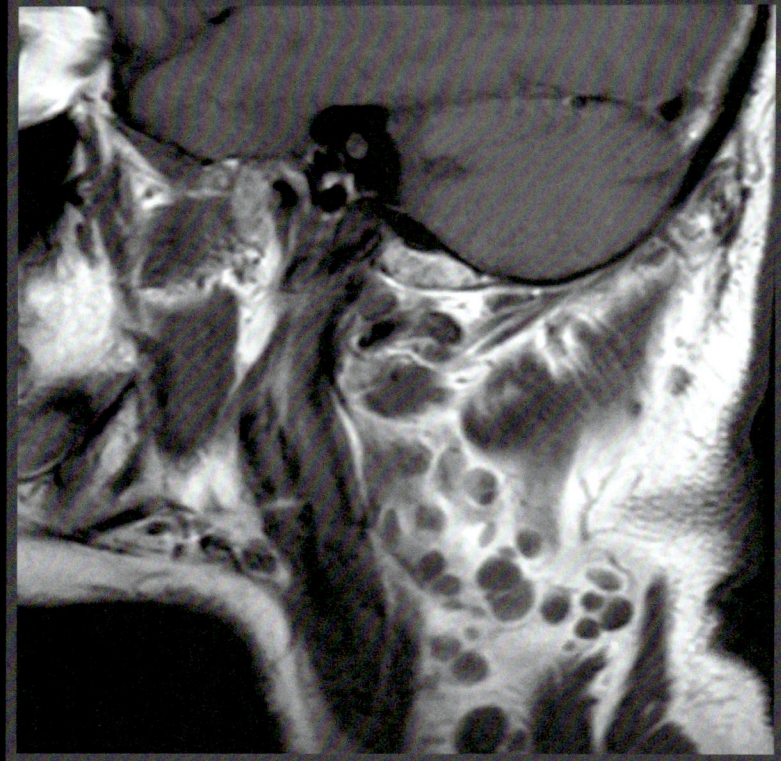
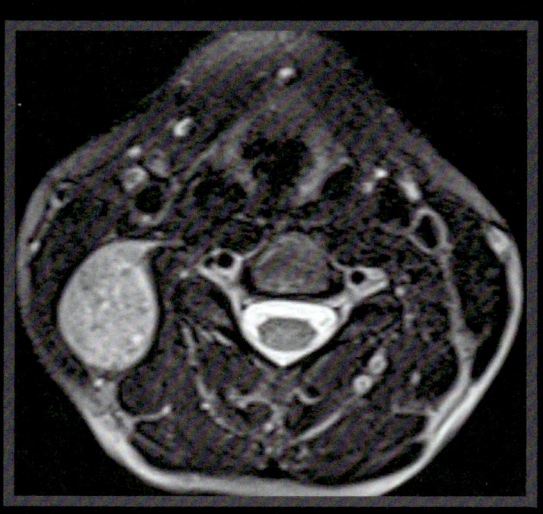

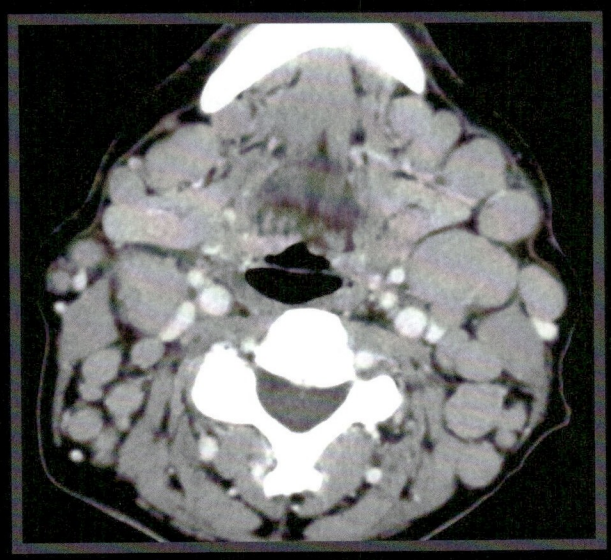

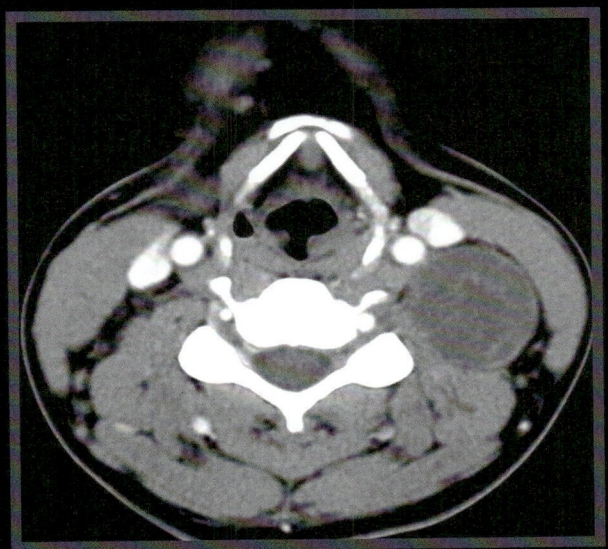

Summary Thoughts: Posterior Cervical Space

The posterior cervical space (PCS) lies in the lateral neck deep to the sternocleidomastoid (SCM) and trapezius muscles and includes the triangle of fat between them. This triangle of fat is superficial to the paraspinal muscles and is known clinically as the **posterior triangle** of the neck. The PCS is small superiorly, encompassing just a region of tissue around the mastoid tip, but it expands inferiorly to encompass most of the lateral neck.

The most frequent pathology to affect the PCS is inflammatory or malignant **lymphadenopathy** in the spinal accessory chain. Identifying the likely source of the primary tumor is of great importance. Other pathology in the PCS is often related to CNXI, which runs obliquely across the PCS, or the brachial plexus, which traverses the lower PCS.

Imaging Approaches and Indications

Masses and inflammation of the PCS may be imaged either with CECT or MR of the neck, depending on regional preferences. Be sure to include the entire PCS, from the mastoid tip through the clavicles.

Imaging Anatomy

Superficial PCS **anatomic boundaries** include the SCM and trapezius muscles and the superficial space (platysma and subcutaneous fat). Deep to the PCS lies the prevertebral (more anteriorly) and paraspinal (more posteriorly) portions of the perivertebral space (PVS). Anteromedial to the PCS, the carotid space (CS) is found.

The PCS has complex **fascial boundaries**. The deep margin of the PCS is separated from the PVS by the deep layer of the deep cervical fascia (DCF); the superficial margin of the PCS is separated from the SCM and trapezius as well as from the superficial space by the superficial (investing) layer of the DCF. The PCS is separated from the CS by all 3 layers of the DCF that make up the carotid sheath.

The main **PCS contents** are fat, lymph nodes, and the spinal accessory nerve (CNXI). The nerve lies along the floor of the space, running obliquely from anterosuperior to posteroinferior. The nodes included are predominantly from the **spinal accessory chain**, along with portions of the transverse cervical chain. This corresponds to **level V** if the nodes are strictly posterior to the posterior border of the SCM, or **levels IIB, III, and IV** if the nodes are deep to the SCM.

Segments of the **brachial plexus** run through the PCS. After the trunks of the brachial plexus emerge from the scalene triangle between the anterior and middle scalene muscles, they ramify into divisions and then cords within the PCS before continuing into the axilla.

The dorsal scapular nerve and segmental cervical nerve roots also traverse the PCS, as does the 3rd portion of the subclavian artery, but the bulk of the PCS is filled with **fat**.

While radiologists divide the neck into fascial-lined spaces, clinicians divide the neck into muscular triangles. The triangle that corresponds to the PCS is the **posterior triangle** of the neck, between the SCM and trapezius muscles. The posterior triangle can be subdivided into the occipital and subclavian triangles using the inferior belly of the omohyoid muscle as the dividing line. The occipital triangle is superior to the omohyoid, whereas the subclavian triangle is inferior.

- Occipital triangle contains fat, CNXI, dorsal scapular nerve, and spinal accessory nodes
- Subclavian triangle contains 3rd portion of subclavian artery and brachial plexus

Approaches to Imaging Issues of Posterior Cervical Space

Multiple imaging findings help answer the question, "What defines a mass as being in the PCS?" First, the lesion should arise within the PCS fat. Larger PCS masses will displace the CS anteromedially, elevate the SCM (aggressive malignancies may invade into SCM, obliterating the intervening fat), and flatten the deeper prevertebral and paraspinal muscles.

The PCS contains nodes from both level V and levels II-IV. This situation yields the question, "How can these nodal stations be distinguished?" Draw an imaginary line from the posterior border of one SCM to the posterior border of the other SCM. If the center of the affected node is posterior to this line, the node is assigned to level V. If it is anterior to this line, it is a level II-IV internal jugular node. The level II-IV nodes are sorted by horizontal landmarks. If the node is above the hyoid bone, it belongs to level II. If it is below the cricoid cartilage, it belongs to level IV, while between these landmarks lies level III.

Clinical Implications

PCS masses can affect function of CNXI, but the most frequent source of CNXI dysfunction is prior surgery. When CNXI is injured or resected, the SCM and trapezius muscles atrophy. Acutely, muscles may enlarge and enhance, but chronically, they shrink and undergo fatty infiltration. The SCM has often been resected in postoperative patients, so trapezius atrophy may be the only clue to CNXI injury.

When the trapezius muscle is dysfunctional, the **levator scapulae muscle** takes over its function in elevating the scapula. The levator scapulae muscle is 1 of the lateral paraspinal muscles. When it hypertrophies, it may be mistaken for a pathologic mass (such as recurrent tumor) both clinically and radiologically.

Differential Diagnosis

PCS Differential Diagnosis by Pathology Category
- Pseudolesion: Cervical rib
- Congenital: Lymphatic malformation, 3rd branchial cleft cyst
- Inflammatory: Reactive or sarcoid adenopathy
- Infectious: TB adenitis, suppurative adenitis, abscess
- Benign tumor: Lipoma, CNXI or brachial plexus schwannoma or neurofibroma
- Malignant primary tumor: Sarcoma, primary non-Hodgkin lymphoma (NHL) of PCS nodes
- Metastatic nodes: H&N squamous cell carcinoma, NHL, differentiated thyroid cancer, melanoma

Selected References

1. Blue M et al: The posterior triangle and posterior muscles of the neck in 3-dimensions: creating a digital anatomic model using peer-reviewed literature, radiographic imaging, and an experienced medical illustrator. S D Med. 77(suppl 8):s17-18, 2024
2. Parker GD et al: Radiologic evaluation of the normal and diseased posterior cervical space. AJR Am J Roentgenol. 157(1):161-5, 1991

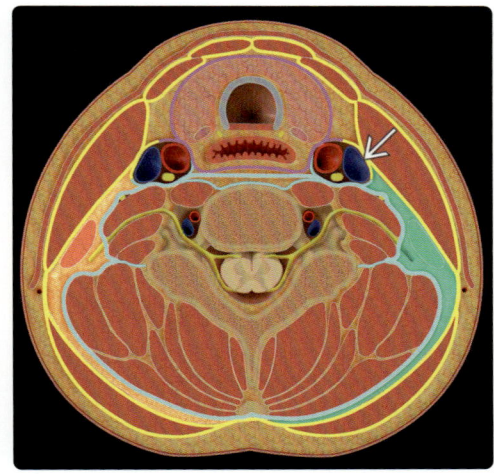

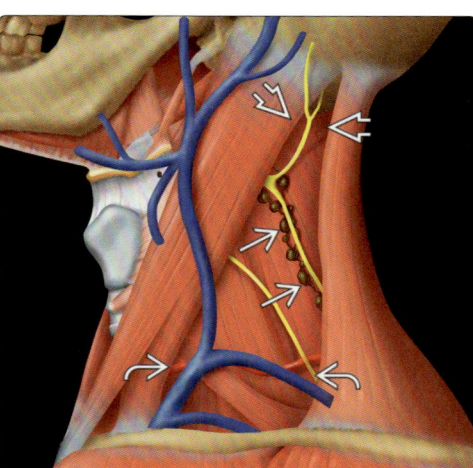

(Left) *Axial graphic depicts the normal posterior cervical space (PCS) (blue-green shading) below the level of the hyoid bone. Complex fascial margins include the superficial layer of the deep cervical fascia (DCF) (yellow line), the deep layer of the DCF (blue line), and the tricolored carotid sheath* ➡️ *(containing all 3 layers of DCF).* (Right) *Lateral graphic shows that the spinal accessory nodal chain* ➡️ *follows the general course of the spinal accessory nerve (CNXI). The PCS is smaller superiorly* ➡️ *than inferiorly* ➡️.

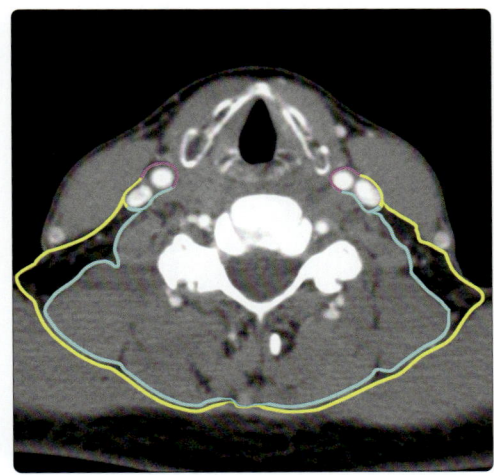

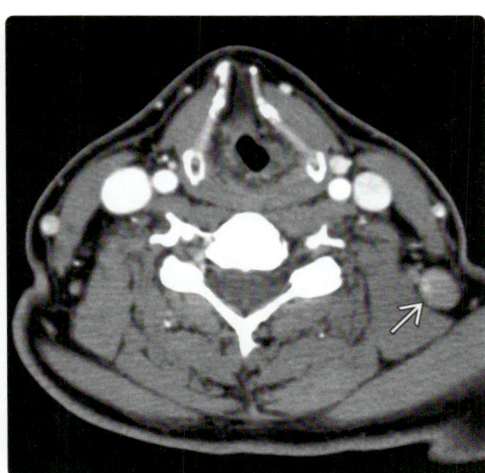

(Left) *Normal axial CECT has the PCS fascial boundaries drawn onto it. The portions of the superficial (yellow) and deep (light blue) layers of the DCF that surround the PCS are depicted.* (Right) *Axial CECT of the infrahyoid neck shows a typical PCS mass. This enlarged lymph node* ➡️ *lies strictly posterior to the posterior margin of the sternocleidomastoid, so it is classified as level V. Clinically, this mass would be within the posterior triangle.*

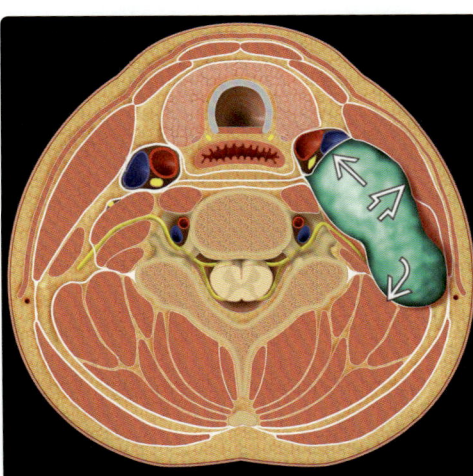

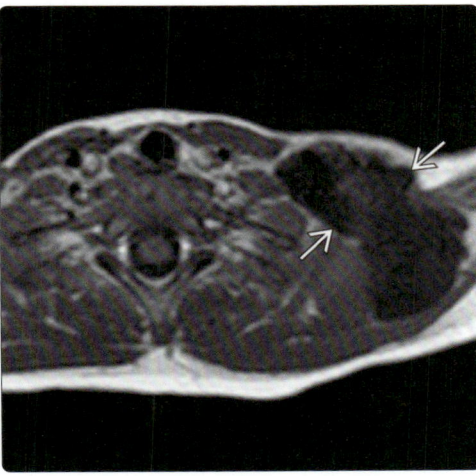

(Left) *Axial graphic of a generic PCS mass reveals compression of the deep paraspinal muscles* ➡️, *elevation of the sternocleidomastoid muscle* ➡️, *and anteromedial displacement of the carotid sheath* ➡️. (Right) *Axial T1 C+ MR shows a lobulated, cystic nonenhancing mass in the infrahyoid PCS* ➡️, *deep to the trapezius muscle. Signal characteristics follow fluid and show no enhancement, consistent with lymphatic malformation.*

TERMINOLOGY

- Synonyms: Neuroma, neurinoma, neurilemmoma, nerve sheath tumor
- Schwannoma in PCS primarily from 3 sites
  - Brachial plexus > cervical sensory nerve > CNXI

IMAGING

- CT: Well-delineated, solitary, fusiform enhancing PCS mass
  - Isodense to hypodense mass
- MR: Modality of choice for presurgical evaluation
  - Contrast-enhanced images critical
  - Large schwannomas often have **cystic** component
  - **Target** sign: ↓ T2 center, ↑ T2 periphery
- US: Hypoechoic mass with posterior acoustic enhancement
  - Marked hypervascularity on color Doppler
- **MR is technique of choice** for presurgical evaluation

TOP DIFFERENTIAL DIAGNOSES

- Spinal accessory reactive node
- Spinal accessory squamous cell carcinoma metastatic node
- Spinal accessory non-Hodgkin lymphoma node
- Differentiated thyroid carcinoma, nodal
- Lymphatic malformation

CLINICAL ISSUES

- Rapid enlargement suggests malignant degeneration
- Core biopsy needed for diagnosis
- Treatment is surgical enucleation
  - Excellent long-term results; goal to preserve function
  - Conservative imaging surveillance another option
- Poor cellularity on FNA common: Core biopsy needed

DIAGNOSTIC CHECKLIST

- **Look for nerve or foramen of origin**
  - Upper neck from jugular foramen (CNXI)
  - Lower neck from brachial plexus (C5-T1)
    - Mass extends between anterior and middle scalenes
- Main differential is solitary PCS nodal mass

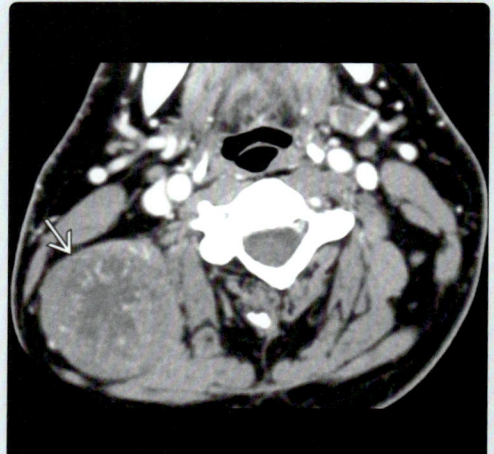
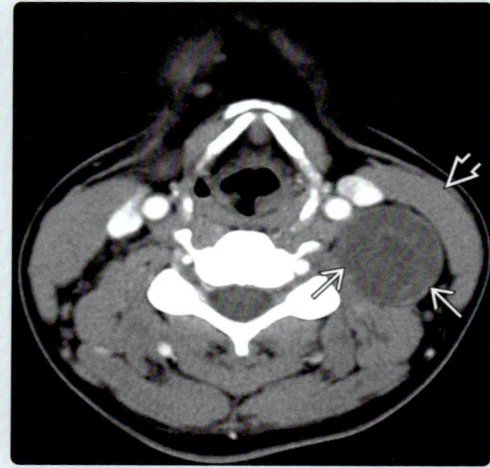

(Left) Axial CECT demonstrates a large, well-defined mass ➡ in the posterior cervical space (PCS) with heterogeneous enhancement. This schwannoma arises from CNXI, which traverses the PCS. (Right) Axial CECT shows a round, well-defined, poorly enhancing mass ➡ in the PCS. Schwannomas in this location will sometimes be entirely cystic. Note lateral displacement of the overlying sternocleidomastoid muscle (SCM) ➡ but sparing of the surrounding fat planes.

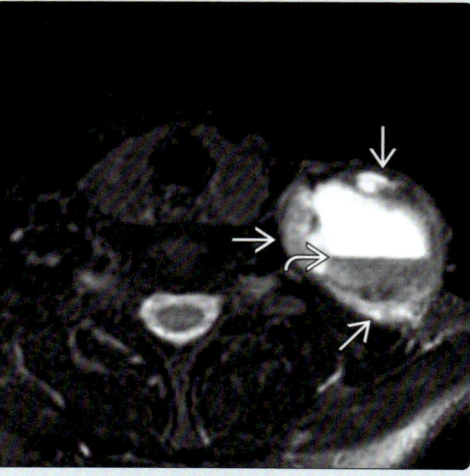
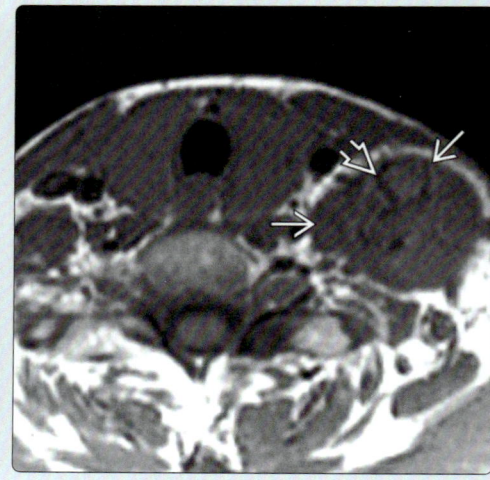

(Left) Axial T2 FS MR shows a large mass ➡ in the PCS with well-defined margins. It is unusual for a schwannoma to have a fluid level ➡, but it does occur occasionally, and this lesion shows internal hemorrhage. (Right) Axial T1 MR shows a large, well-defined mass ➡ with predominantly uniform intermediate signal in the PCS with intact surrounding fat planes. Flow voids ➡ within the mass are suggestive of paraganglioma but may also rarely be seen with schwannoma.

TERMINOLOGY

Abbreviations

- Schwannoma of posterior cervical space (PCS)

Synonyms

- Neuroma, neurinoma, neurilemmoma, nerve sheath tumor

Definitions

- Benign, slow-growing Schwann cell neoplasm arising in PCS from CNXI, brachial plexus, or cervical sensory nerve

IMAGING

General Features

- Best diagnostic clue
  - Solitary, fusiform, enhancing PCS mass
- Location
  - Suprahyoid PCS: Between paraspinous and sternocleidomastoid muscles, posterior to jugular vein
  - Infrahyoid PCS: Between scalene and sternocleidomastoid muscles, lateral to jugular vein
    - May emerge along branchial plexus from between anterior and middle scalene into PCS
  - Schwannoma of CNXI displaces internal jugular vein (IJV) anterior and medial
- Size
  - Variable, may be > 14 cm
- Morphology
  - Well-delineated, solitary, fusiform mass

CT Findings

- NECT
  - Isodense or **hypodense** to muscle
- CECT
  - Homogeneous enhancement of solid component
  - Nonenhancing, **cystic component common** if large
- CTA
  - Helpful to distinguish from paragangliomas
    - Intense arterial-phase enhancement of paragangliomas (light bulb sign)
    - Paragangliomas associated with carotid space

MR Findings

- T1WI
  - Homogeneous signal, isointense to muscle
- T2WI
  - Hyperintense compared to muscle
  - Occasionally fluid-fluid level, hemorrhage present in cystic component
  - **Target sign:** Hypointense center and hyperintense periphery
    - Characteristic of benign nerve sheath tumor
- PWI
  - DCE (4D GRASP) differentiates schwannomas from paragangliomas
    - Schwannomas: Type I inflow with slower wash-in and no washout (continuous enhancement increase)
    - Paragangliomas: Type III showing rapid wash-in, rapid washout, and higher peak enhancement signal intensity
- T1WI C+
  - Homogeneous enhancement of solid component
  - Cystic components best appreciated post contrast as nonenhancing foci

Ultrasonographic Findings

- Grayscale ultrasound
  - Solitary, oval, hypoechoic mass with posterior acoustic enhancement
  - Lacks echogenic hilum of lymph node
- Color Doppler
  - Marked hypervascularity
  - Can be obliterated with transducer pressure

Angiographic Findings

- Angiography not routinely used for diagnosis or management
- Hypovascular ± venous puddling

Nuclear Medicine Findings

- PET
  - Variable FDG avidity

Image-Guided Biopsy

- Schwannomas infamous for poor cellularity on fine-needle aspiration (FNA)
- **Core biopsy** needed for diagnosis
  - Nerve damage very unlikely in lesions > 1 cm

Imaging Recommendations

- Best imaging tool
  - **MR is technique of choice** for presurgical evaluation
    - Extent of lesion
    - Nerve of origin
- Protocol advice
  - Contrast-enhanced images with fat suppression critical

DIFFERENTIAL DIAGNOSIS

Spinal Accessory Reactive Node

- Reniform configuration (central fatty hilum)
- Uniform mild enhancement
- Well-defined margins

Spinal Accessory Squamous Cell Carcinoma Metastatic Node

- Rim-enhancing or solid mass with thick walls, mural nodularity
- Usually multiple, as level V unusual site for solitary metastasis

Spinal Accessory Non-Hodgkin Lymphoma Node

- Uniformly enhancing ovoid mass
- Usually multiple
- Systemic non-Hodgkin lymphoma may not be known

Spinal Accessory Suppurative Node

- Tender posterior triangle masses
- Ovoid, rim-enhancing mass
- Surrounding fat stranding
- If solitary, may mimic schwannoma

Differentiated Thyroid Carcinoma, Nodal

- Cystic or solid nodal mass ± calcifications
- Usually other nodal metastases apparent

Lymphatic Malformation

- **Multilocular cystic spaces** without perceptible wall
- Mixed-signal or enhancing components if venolymphatic
- Multiloculated high T2 signal intensity ± fluid levels

PATHOLOGY

General Features

- Etiology
  - Benign Schwann cell neoplasm **arising from CNXI, brachial plexus, or cervical sensory nerve**
- Genetics
  - Usually sporadic and isolated
  - 1/3 to 1/2 of patients with sporadic schwannomas have deletion at neurofibromatosis type 2 (NF2) locus on chromosome 22
  - May develop in genetically predisposed individuals following nerve injury
  - Increased risk in patients exposed to radiation
- Associated abnormalities
  - **NF2: Multiple schwannomas** with bilateral acoustic schwannomas, meningiomas, and ependymomas
    - Chromosome 22 mutation
  - Schwannomatosis: Multiple schwannomas without acoustic schwannomas or other manifestations of NF2
    - Mutation of NF2 locus found in schwannomas but not in peripheral blood
    - *SMARCB1* and *LZTR1* mutations
- Arises focally from nerve sheath fascicle as eccentric mass displacing nerve
- Schwannoma in PCS primarily from 3 sites
  - Brachial plexus > cervical sensory nerve > CNXI origin

Gross Pathologic & Surgical Features

- Lobulated but smooth, encapsulated, fusiform mass arising eccentrically from nerve
- Gray-tan on cut section; firm, rubbery texture
  - Small intramural cysts may be seen
- Schwannoma variants
  - Plexiform: Morphology mimics plexiform neurofibroma
    - Not associated with neurofibromatosis
  - Melanocytic: Pigmented, poorer prognosis
    - Association with Carney complex
    - Rare genetic disorder with abnormalities of skin, heart, endocrine system, and skin pigmentation

Microscopic Features

- Encapsulated, benign spindle cell tumor
- Differentiated neoplastic Schwann cells within collagenous matrix
- Antoni A areas: Compact cells
  - Verocay bodies: Rows of parallel nuclei and acellular foci
- Antoni B areas: More myxoid, less cellular
- Thick-walled vessels and scattered inflammatory cells
- Nerve axons may be seen at periphery but not within tumor
- Strongly positive for S100 protein stain

CLINICAL ISSUES

Presentation

- Most common signs/symptoms
  - **Slow-growing** posterior neck mass; may be incidental
    - Growth rate unpredictable; surveillance indicated
    - Rapid enlargement suggests malignant degeneration
- Other signs/symptoms
  - May be exacerbated by pressure on lesion
  - Recurring mild neck pain with muscle spasm
  - Denervation atrophy of trapezius and sternocleidomastoid muscles (CNXI)

Demographics

- Age
  - Peak (without phakomatosis): 20-50 years
  - 10% < 21 years
- Epidemiology
  - < 1% of all head and neck neoplasms
  - **Most common solitary neurogenic tumor in neck**
  - 25-45% of schwannomas arise in head and neck

Natural History & Prognosis

- **Malignant degeneration very rare** in isolated lesions
  - Malignant peripheral nerve sheath tumor (MPNST) usually sporadic or associated with neurofibromatosis type 1 (NF1)
  - Rapidly enlarging mass ± pain or nerve dysfunction
- Melanocytic schwannomas very rare but 25% metastasize
- Incompletely excised schwannoma may locally recur

Treatment

- Surgical enucleation
  - Excellent long-term results
  - Aim to preserve nerve function (often impossible)
    - Conservative imaging surveillance another option
  - Complete resolution of symptoms expected
  - Initial neurapraxia is most common complication

DIAGNOSTIC CHECKLIST

Consider

- If multiple schwannomas or child, consider NF2 or schwannomatosis

Image Interpretation Pearls

- Look for nerve or foramen of origin
  - Upper neck: From jugular foramen (CNXI)
  - Lower neck: Brachial plexus (C5-T1)
  - Brachial plexus: Between anterior and middle scalenes
- Evaluate full extent (axillary, intrathoracic, skull base)
- Main differential is reactive, inflammatory, or neoplastic level V (spinal accessory) lymph node

SELECTED REFERENCES

1. Ali MA et al: Outcomes of head and neck neurogenic tumors. Cureus. 16(5):e61156, 2024
2. Ota Y et al: Diagnostic role of diffusion-weighted and dynamic contrast-enhanced perfusion mr imaging in paragangliomas and schwannomas in the head and neck. AJNR Am J Neuroradiol. 42(10):1839-46, 2021
3. El Sayed L et al: Natural history of peripheral nerve schwannomas. Acta Neurochir (Wien). 162(8):1883-9, 2020
4. Helbing DL et al: Pathomechanisms in schwannoma development and progression. Oncogene. 39(32):5421-9, 2020
5. Schraepen C et al: What to know about schwannomatosis: a literature review. British Journal of Neurosurgery. 36(2): 171-4, 2020
6. Boumaza K et al: Peripheral neck nerve tumor: a 73-case study and literature review. Eur Ann Otorhinolaryngol Head Neck Dis. 136(6):455-60, 2019

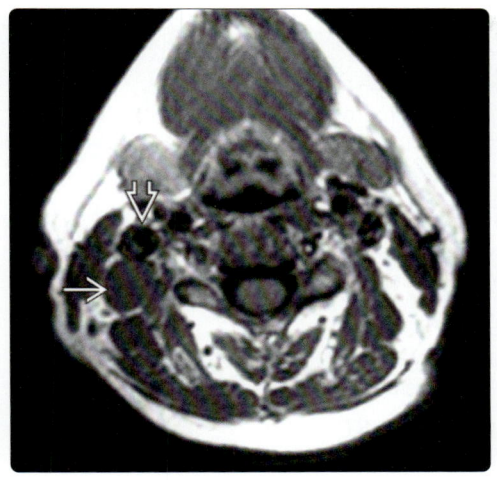

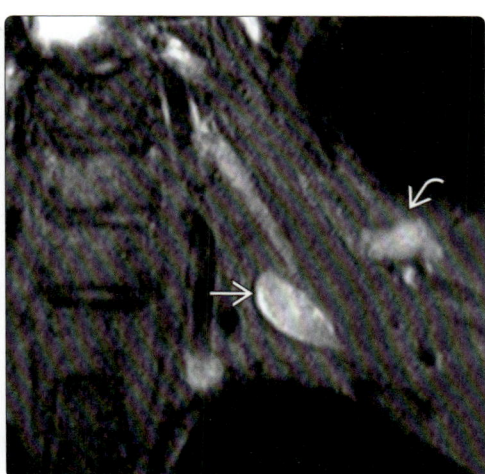

(Left) Axial T1 MR shows a well-defined, intermediate-signal ovoid mass ➡ in the PCS, just posterior to the internal jugular vein ➡. Based on location and imaging characteristics, this schwannoma might be mistaken for an enlarged lymph node. (Right) Coronal STIR MR of the brachial plexus shows hyperintense masses along the left brachial plexus ➡ and peripheral nerves ➡ in a patient with NF2. The larger lesion has a classic targetoid appearance with peripheral T2 hyperintensity and central hypointensity.

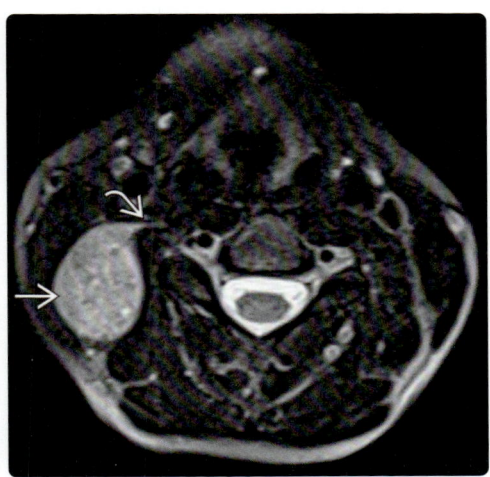

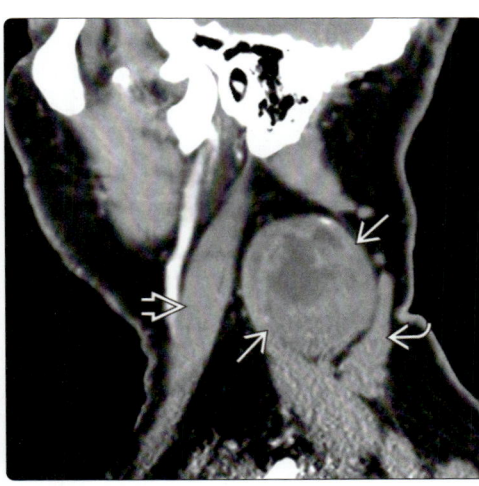

(Left) Axial T2 FS MR shows a well-circumscribed, heterogeneous fusiform mass ➡ deep to the SCM with a tail directed toward the neural foramen ➡. This is a characteristic location for a schwannoma of the sensory cervical roots. (Right) Sagittal CECT reformat shows a heterogeneously enhancing, well-defined, ovoid mass ➡ in the PCS posterior to the SCM ➡ and anterior to the trapezius muscle ➡ with intact surrounding fat planes. This is a characteristic location for a schwannoma of CNXI.

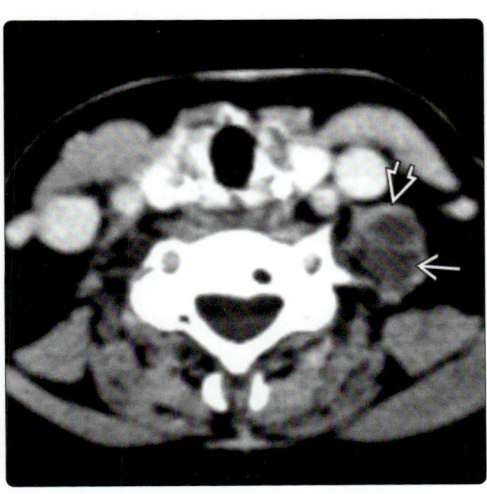

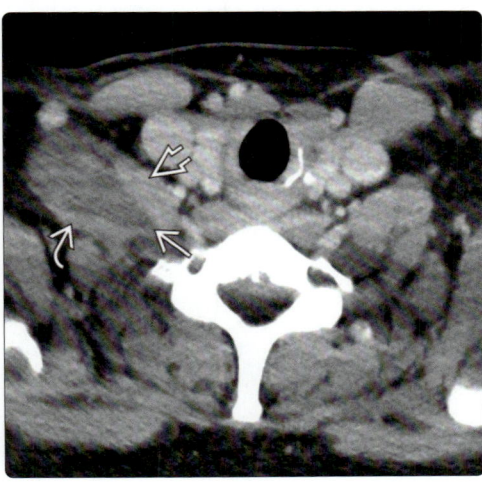

(Left) Axial CECT shows heterogeneous distal brachial plexus schwannoma protruding from between scalene muscles into the medial PCS. Note intramural cystic change ➡ and displacement of the anterior scalene muscle ➡ anteriorly. (Right) Axial CECT shows a teardrop-shaped, smoothly marginated, hypodense posterior cervical space mass ➡ "pointing" between the anterior ➡ and middle ➡ scalene muscles, indicating schwannoma of brachial plexus origin.

Squamous Cell Carcinoma in Spinal Accessory Node

TERMINOLOGY

- Nodal chain accompanying spinal accessory nerve (CNXI)
- Spinal accessory chain divided into level IIB & level V nodes

IMAGING

- **Cervical nodes** concerning for **malignancy** if
  - **Necrosis**
  - **Extranodal extension**: Ill-defined margins ± stranding of surrounding fat (most specific sign)
  - **Round** node with loss of hilar fat
  - Groups of ≥ 3 borderline enlarged nodes
  - > 1 cm in diameter (least specific sign)
- US- or CT-guided biopsy for equivocal nodes
- CECT best 1st tool for indeterminate neck mass
- PET/CT most appropriate for unknown primary or for staging once SCCa diagnosis established
  - Can change nodal stage of disease

TOP DIFFERENTIAL DIAGNOSES

- Reactive adenopathy
- Suppurative adenopathy
- Non-Hodgkin lymphoma nodes
- Thyroid cancer node metastasis
- Skin cancer nodal metastasis from scalp/face
- Posterior cervical space schwannoma

PATHOLOGY

- Nasopharyngeal, oropharyngeal, & hypopharyngeal primaries often present with CNXI nodal metastases

CLINICAL ISSUES

- Single nodal metastasis ↓ survival by 50% in p16(-) SCCa
- Treatment depends on primary site & nodal stage

DIAGNOSTIC CHECKLIST

- **Identification of 1° tumor is important**
- Large (> 2 cm) nonnecrotic nodes suggest NHL, not SCCa

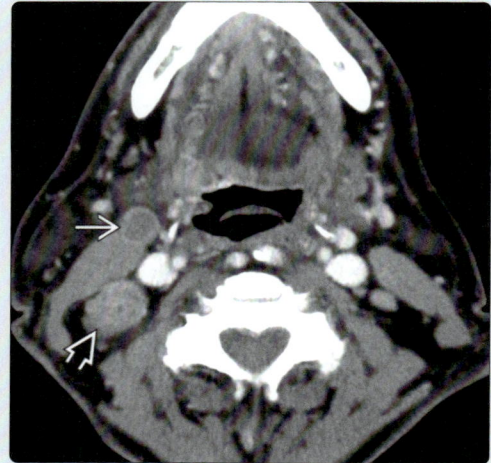 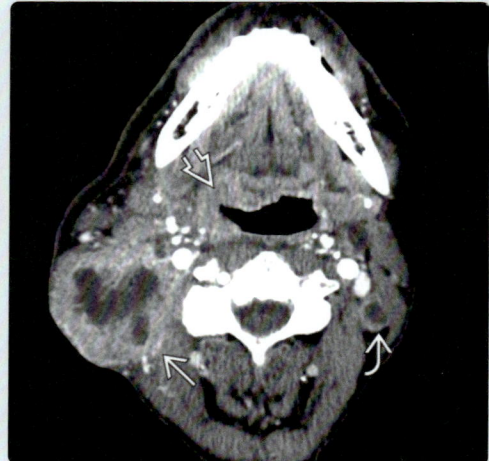

(Left) Axial CECT shows a metastatic necrotic lymph node in level IIA ➡ anterior to the internal jugular vein (IJV) but posterior to the submandibular gland in this patient with tongue base squamous cell carcinoma (SCCa). A level IIB ➡ lymph node has a preserved fat plane posterior to the IJV. (Right) Axial CECT shows metastatic level II adenopathy, likely with extranodal extension given the effaced fat planes ➡. Primary base of tongue SCCa ➡ is partly seen. A necrotic left level II metastatic node ➡ is noted.

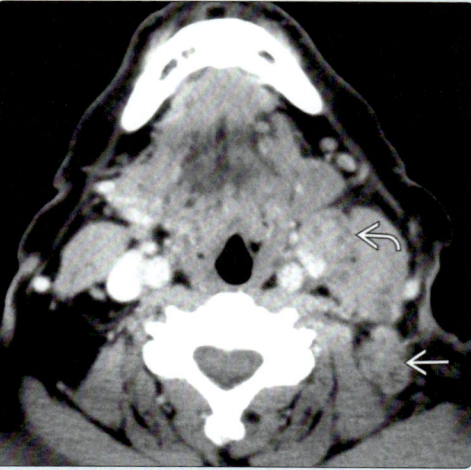 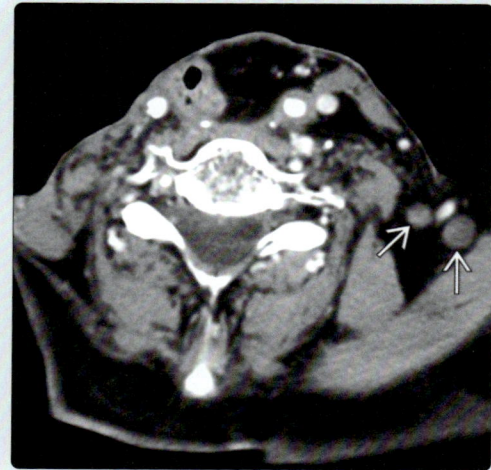

(Left) Axial CECT shows spinal accessory adenopathy ➡ in level V in this patient with base of tongue SCCa. Small foci of necrosis are suggested in this nodal chain as well as in the level II adenopathy ➡. This patient had advanced disease with osseous metastatic disease (not shown). (Right) Axial CECT shows recurrent contralateral spinal accessory nodes ➡ after laryngectomy and right neck dissection. These nodes are low in the neck, such that the spinal accessory nerve is along the posterior aspect of the posterior cervical space.

Squamous Cell Carcinoma in Spinal Accessory Node

TERMINOLOGY

Abbreviations

- Squamous cell carcinoma (SCCa)

Definitions

- Spinal accessory node: Nodal chain accompanying spinal accessory nerve (CNXI)
- Spinal accessory chain divided between 2 surgical levels
  - Level IIB for upper spinal nodes deep to sternocleidomastoid muscle (SCM) but posterior to & not contacting internal jugular vein
  - Level V for posterior cervical space (PCS); strictly posterior to SCM

IMAGING

General Features

- Best diagnostic clue
  - Single or multiple, round/oval, ± **centrally necrotic** soft tissue masses along course of CNXI
  - Cervical nodes concerning for malignancy if
    - **Extranodal extension (ENE)** is most specific
    - Shape: Round node & loss of hilar fat likely pathologic
    - Number: Groups of ≥ 3 borderline enlarged nodes more likely pathologic
    - Size: > 1-cm diameter (least specific sign)

CT Findings

- CECT
  - **Necrosis**: Foci of central low-density with variably thick, irregular peripheral enhancement
  - **ENE**: Irregular nodal margins & lack of perinodal fat plane

MR Findings

- T1WI
  - Nodes isointense to muscle
- T2WI
  - Nodes hyperintense
  - ENE: Ill-defined hyperintensity in perinodal fat
- T1WI C+ FS
  - Necrosis: Central low intensity with peripheral enhancement
  - ENE: Ill-defined perinodal enhancement

Ultrasonographic Findings

- Grayscale ultrasound
  - Typically hypoechoic with loss of hilar definition
  - Poorly defined borders suggests ENE

Nuclear Medicine Findings

- PET/CT
  - Can detect nodal metastases that are negative on CT/MR
  - Useful to stage & evaluate response post treatment

Imaging Recommendations

- Best imaging tool
  - CECT: Initial indeterminate neck mass & node evaluation
  - PET/CT most appropriate for unknown primary or for staging once SCCa diagnosis established

DIFFERENTIAL DIAGNOSIS

Reactive Adenopathy

- **Nonnecrotic** reniform nodes < 2 cm
- Associated adenoidal & tonsillar hypertrophy

Suppurative Adenopathy

- Centrally low density, peripherally enhancing nodes
- Inflammatory stranding of surrounding fat, infection

Non-Hodgkin Lymphoma Lymph Nodes

- Large **homogeneous** lymph nodes
- Bilateral & multispatial typically

Differentiated Thyroid Carcinoma Lymph Nodes

- Avidly enhancing nodes ± Ca++, cystic change

Skin Cancer Nodal Metastasis

- Skin cancers of scalp & face

Posterior Cervical Space Schwannoma

- Well-circumscribed **solitary** mass ± target sign or cysts

PATHOLOGY

General Features

- Nasopharyngeal, oropharyngeal, & hypopharyngeal cancers may present with spinal accessory metastases
- Ultrasound- or CT-guided biopsy for equivocal nodes

CLINICAL ISSUES

Presentation

- Most common signs/symptoms
  - Palpable mass in posterior triangle
  - Extranodal tumor spread results in "fixed" node

Demographics

- Epidemiology: Most common malignant neck nodes (> 80%)

Natural History & Prognosis

- Single nodal metastasis ↓ survival by 50% in p16(-) SCCa
- ENE confers worse prognosis for p16(-) SCCa

Treatment

- Surgery vs. chemoradiation depends on primary site & nodal stage

DIAGNOSTIC CHECKLIST

Consider

- Identification of primary tumor of paramount importance

Image Interpretation Pearls

- Large nonnecrotic nodes favor NHL over SCCa
- Evaluate for imaging findings of ENE

SELECTED REFERENCES

1. Punjabi N et al: A systematic review of occult contralateral neck metastasis in tonsillar squamous cell carcinoma. Laryngoscope. 135(1):27-33, 2025
2. Faraji F et al: Computed tomography performance in predicting extranodal extension in HPV-positive oropharynx cancer. Laryngoscope. 130(6):1479-86, 2020

Non-Hodgkin Lymphoma in Spinal Accessory Node

TERMINOLOGY

- Non-Hodgkin lymphoma (NHL)
- Spinal accessory nodes, a.k.a. posterior triangle or posterior cervical space nodes
    - Level IIB: Posterior to jugular vein
    - Level V: Posterior to sternocleidomastoid muscle

IMAGING

- Nodal NHL may be multiple 1- to 3-cm nodes or dominant, large node may be > 5 cm
- May involve multiple neck nodal groups
- Typically homogeneous, nonnecrotic nodes
- Necrosis/extracapsular spread suggests high-grade, aggressive NHL
- Calcification may be seen post treatment
- Generally FDG avid though some variability
- Standard NHL staging relies on CT/MR & FDG PET

TOP DIFFERENTIAL DIAGNOSES

- Reactive lymph nodes
- Suppurative lymph nodes
- Spinal accessory squamous cell carcinoma (SCCa) node
- Posterior cervical space schwannoma
- Differentiated thyroid carcinoma nodes

CLINICAL ISSUES

- Painless posterior triangle masses ± other nodes
- ↑ risk in immunocompromised patients

DIAGNOSTIC CHECKLIST

- NHL 2nd most common H&N tumor after SCCa
- Some imaging features favor NHL over SCCa
    - Large, solid nodes without necrosis
    - Posterior triangle nodes in isolation
    - Posterior triangle + superior mediastinum nodes

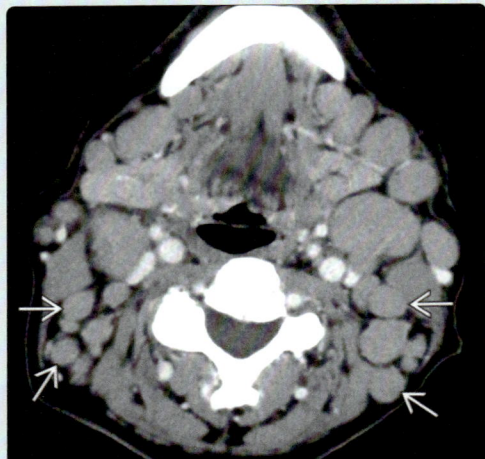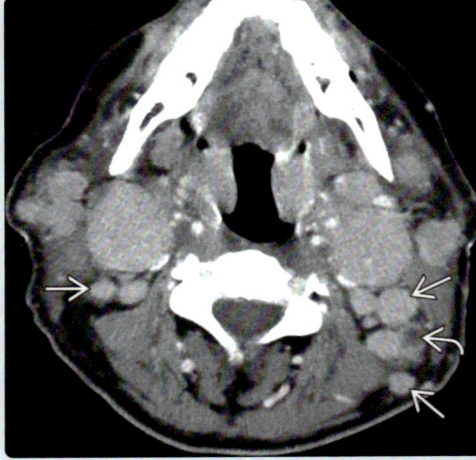

(Left) Axial CECT shows extensive bilateral cervical adenopathy with involvement of both spinal accessory chains ➡ as well as other nodal levels. Note homogeneous density with lack of normal internal nodal architecture. (Right) Axial CECT shows bilateral cervical adenopathy involving the left greater than right spinal accessory lymph nodes ➡. Most are homogeneous in density, but one demonstrates cystic or necrotic change, concerning for higher grade disease ➡.

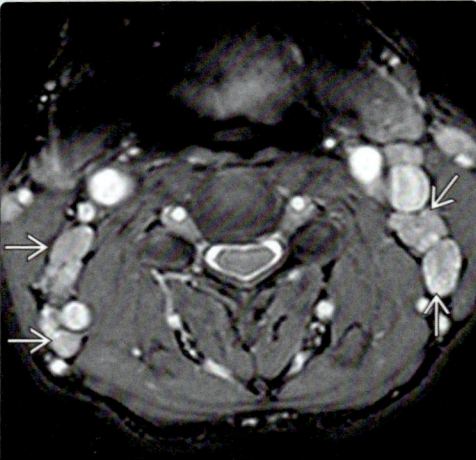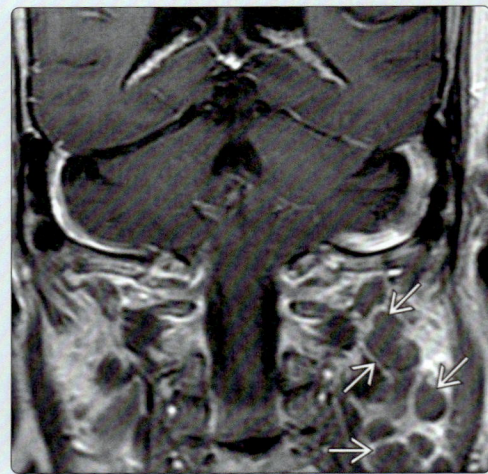

(Left) Axial T2* GRE performed for evaluation of arm pain shows multiple enlarged posterior cervical space lymph nodes ➡ in the neck bilaterally due to lymphoma. Nodes appear homogeneous without necrosis. (Right) Coronal T1 C+ MR shows well-defined, minimally enhancing nodes ➡ in posterior cervical fat. Note that the nodes are only mildly enlarged & show no necrosis but appear round. Asymmetric clustering of nodes also suggests a pathologic nature. This proved to be diffuse large B-cell lymphoma.

TERMINOLOGY

Abbreviations
- Non-Hodgkin lymphoma (NHL)

Definitions
- Spinal accessory nodes, a.k.a. **posterior triangle** or **posterior cervical space** nodes
  - **Level IIB** deep to sternocleidomastoid muscles (SCMs), posterior to jugular vein
  - **Levels VA & VB** posterior to SCM

IMAGING

General Features
- Best diagnostic clue
  - Multiple **homogeneous**, round, enlarged nodes in posterior triangle
  - Level V adenopathy typically is clinically relevant
    - Malignancy most common: Lymphoma > metastases
- Location
  - Uni- or bilateral ± other nodal groups or mediastinal
- Size
  - Multiple 1- to 3-cm nodes, or dominant node up to 5 cm
- Morphology
  - Typically homogeneous, nonnecrotic
  - Necrosis or extracapsular spread (ECS) uncommon
    - More typical of high grade NHL, or seen in immunocompromised patients

CT Findings
- CECT
  - Homogeneous, slightly higher density than muscle
  - Loss of hilar fat & vessels
  - Calcification may be seen post treatment

MR Findings
- T1WI
  - Nodes isointense to muscle
- T2WI
  - Nodes homogeneously hyperintense
- DWI
  - ADC in NHL lower than squamous cell carcinoma (SCCa)
- T1WI C+
  - Uniform mild enhancement

Nuclear Medicine Findings
- PET/CT
  - Generally FDG avid though some variability
  - Useful for both staging & surveillance

Imaging Recommendations
- Best imaging tool
  - CECT best modality for evaluation of neck mass
  - Standard staging for NHL is CT/MR & FDG PET

DIFFERENTIAL DIAGNOSIS

Reactive Lymph Nodes
- Nonnecrotic oval nodes < 2 cm
- Adenoidal & tonsil hypertrophy or active infection

Suppurative Lymph Nodes
- Central low density with peripheral enhancement
- Patient usually septic with tender neck mass

Spinal Accessory Squamous Cell Carcinoma Node
- Central necrosis & ECS findings favor SCCa
- Level V SCCa nodes uncommon without jugular nodes

Posterior Cervical Space Schwannoma
- Ovoid or tubular well-circumscribed, solitary mass

Differentiated Thyroid Carcinoma Nodes
- Cystic, heterogeneous, calcified nodes more typical
- Uncommon in absence of level III/IV nodes

PATHOLOGY

Staging, Grading, & Classification
- WHO classification (2022 update)
  - Based on pathology, genetic, & clinical factors
    - Mature B-cell neoplasms (most common)
    - Mature T- & NK-cell neoplasms
    - Hodgkin lymphoma
    - Posttransplant lymphoproliferative disorder
    - Histiocytic & dendritic cell neoplasms

CLINICAL ISSUES

Presentation
- Most common signs/symptoms
  - Painless posterior triangle masses ± other nodes
  - Systemic: Night sweats, fevers, weight loss

Demographics
- Age
  - Median: 50-55 years
- Epidemiology
  - ↑ risk in immunocompromised patients

Natural History & Prognosis
- May be indolent, progressive but not curable, or aggressive but often curable

Treatment
- Depends on stage, cell type, patient age
- Chemo, XRT, or combined modality therapy

DIAGNOSTIC CHECKLIST

Image Interpretation Pearls
- Some imaging features favor NHL over SCCa
  - Large (> 2-cm), solid nodes
  - Posterior triangle without jugular chain nodes
  - Posterior triangle & superior mediastinum nodes
- Nodal necrosis &/or ECS suggests high-grade NHL

SELECTED REFERENCES

1. Kato H et al: MRI and (18)F-FDG-PET/CT findings of cervical reactive lymphadenitis: a comparison with nodal lymphoma. Pol J Radiol. 90:e9-18, 2025
2. Gamaleldin O et al: Differentiation of benign and malignant neck neoplastic lesions using diffusion-weighted magnetic resonance imaging. J Imaging. 10(10), 2024

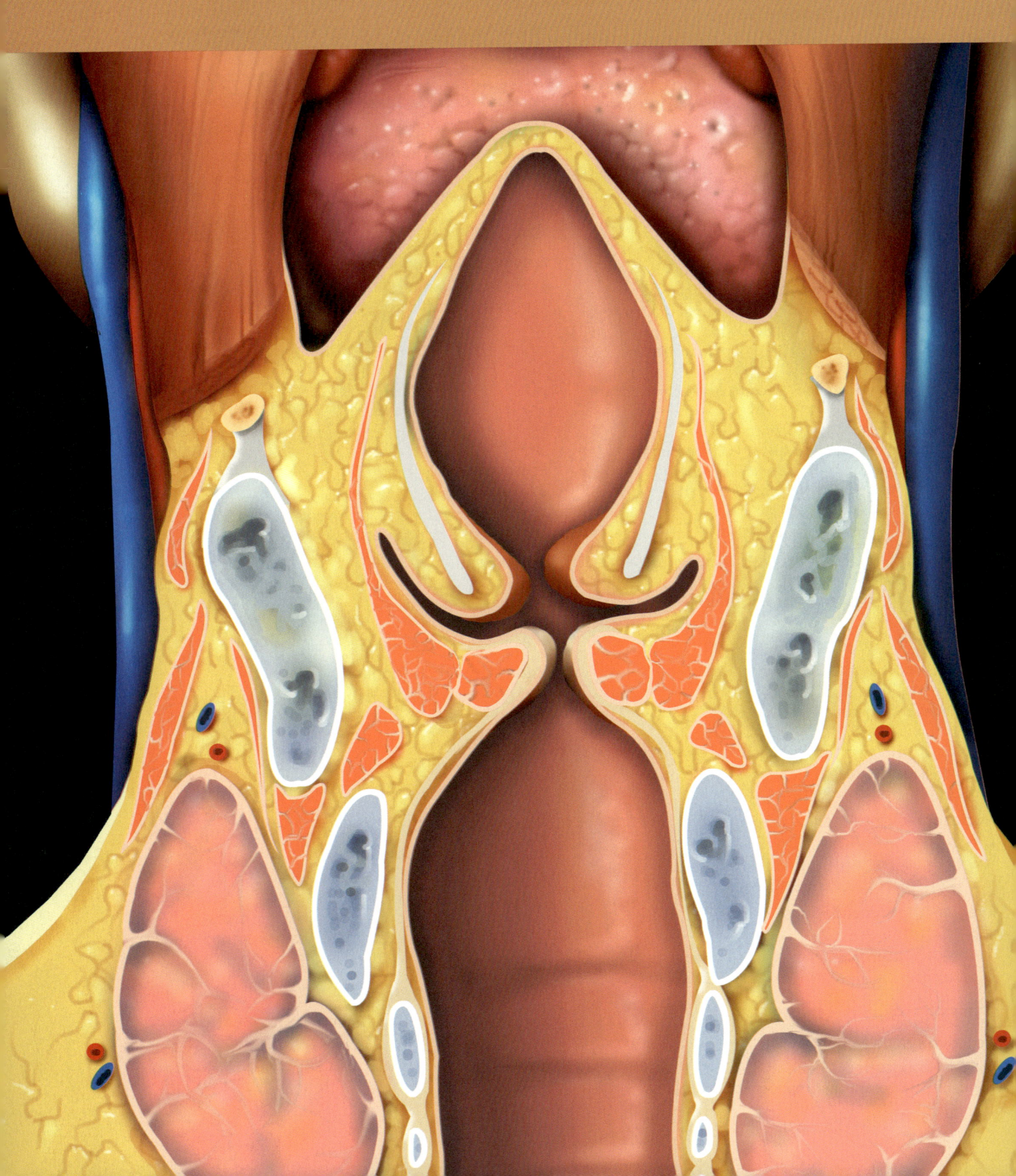

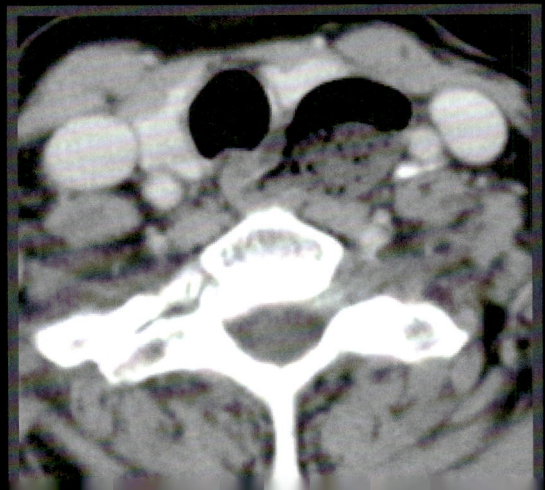
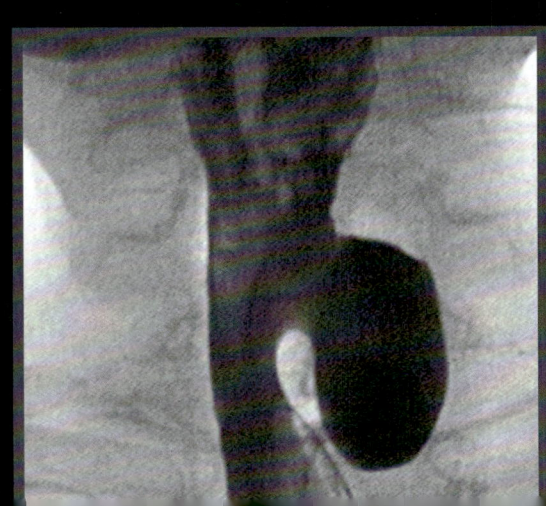

Summary Thoughts: Visceral Space

The visceral space (VS) is a tubular space that occupies the midline anterior aspect of the infrahyoid neck. Extending to the superior mediastinum, the VS lies between the laterally placed carotid spaces (CSs) and is completely encircled by the middle layer of deep cervical fascia (ML-DCF), a.k.a. the **visceral fascia**.

While the largest VS component is the aerodigestive tract (comprised of the hypopharynx, larynx, trachea, and esophagus), the **thyroid gland** most often necessitates imaging of this space. The other key anatomic elements of the VS are less identifiable on routine imaging; the **parathyroid glands** if hyperplastic or neoplastic, and the **recurrent laryngeal nerves** (RLNs) are not seen, although their course through the VS must be carefully evaluated if vocal cord paralysis is present. The aerodigestive tract components are covered elsewhere.

Imaging Techniques & Indications

Both CT and MR are excellent modalities for demonstrating the **thyroid** and its relationship to other VS and neck structures. As there is no inferior fascial limit to the VS, any cross-sectional imaging should continue into the superior mediastinum and preferably to the level of the left pulmonary artery. This encompasses the entire course of the left RLN and superior mediastinal nodes. CT is preferred for evaluation of the left RLN, as it allows better review of any pulmonary pathology.

If there is clinical suspicion of **thyroid neoplasia**, iodinated contrast should not be administered for CT. **Iodinated contrast** is taken up by differentiated thyroid carcinoma (DTCa) and **may delay therapeutic I-131 for 6 weeks**.

US allows excellent high-resolution evaluation of the thyroid, its adjacent nodes, and, when enlarged, the parathyroid glands. **Color Doppler** should always be used when evaluating a thyroid nodule, as increased vascularity is a frequent finding in malignant lesions. It is also important when searching for hypervascular parathyroid adenomas.

Multiphase CECT has supplanted US and Tc-99m sestamibi as a 1st-line imaging modality for localizing **parathyroid adenomas** at many centers. **US &/or Tc-99m sestamibi** are complementary for localization, particularly if equivocal or discordant. Multiphase CT typically includes a noncontrast scan plus arterial and delayed enhancement scans. NECT allows differentiation of a hypodense parathyroid from a normally dense thyroid, although dual-energy CT can aid this distinction for hypodense thyroids. Enhanced phases optimize detection based on the expected pattern of early hypervascular enhancement with delayed-phase washout. CT provides superior anatomic information and is particularly useful for ectopia, multigland disease, and postoperative patients. Craniocaudal coverage from the maxilla to the carina ensures adequate detection of ectopic adenomas. Multiphase enhanced MR may have comparable accuracy but is less often used due to a propensity for greater technical artifacts.

Imaging Anatomy

The VS is the anterior tubular space in the midline of the infrahyoid neck. It is completely encircled by the ML-DCF. The VS shares a common fascial wall with the retropharyngeal space, which is immediately posterior and contains only fat in the infrahyoid neck. The VS is surrounded anteriorly and anterolaterally by the strap muscles, sternocleidomastoid muscles, and the anterior cervical fat. Both muscle groups are enclosed by the superficial layer of DCF (SL-DCF). The CSs are at the lateral margin of the VS with the ML-DCF contributing to the **carotid sheaths**.

The **larynx** and **hypopharynx** are infrahyoid continuations of the oropharynx, and these structures are contiguous with the **trachea** and **esophagus**, respectively, which then traverse the VS to the mediastinum.

The paired thyroid lobes are joined by a midline isthmus. The **thyroid** lobes "cup" the cricoid cartilage and 1st tracheal rings. It is this intimate relation that allows thyroid tumors to invade the trachea.

There are 2 pairs of **parathyroid glands**. The superior glands are consistently found at the posterosuperior aspect of the thyroid, in the lateral aspect of the tracheoesophageal groove (TEG). The inferior glands are in a similar position near the inferior aspect of the thyroid; however, they are less reliably found in this location. They are often found lower in the neck or within the superior mediastinum.

Paratracheal nodes are found in the TEG and are commonly referred to as **level VI** (or central compartment) **nodes**.

Also located in the TEG, the **RLNs** ascend in the neck to the level of the cricothyroid joint, where they enter the larynx to supply the vocal cords. The **right RLN** arises from the vagus nerve in the low neck, then loops around the subclavian artery to enter the inferior VS. The **left RLN** arises more inferiorly, looping beneath the aortic arch before ascending to the VS.

Approaches to Imaging Issues of Visceral Space

Infrahyoid neck lesions differ from suprahyoid masses in that their **space of origin** is typically not an imaging dilemma. The VS has carotid sheaths on either side but is not otherwise surrounded by sources of pathologic processes in the same way that the suprahyoid neck spaces are. The VS does, however, have several common diagnostic dilemmas.

The **incidental thyroid nodule** on CT or MR is the most common imaging dilemma in the VS. Cross-sectional imaging features are not specific. An adult not at elevated risk for thyroid cancer having an incidental thyroid nodule on imaging (without features suspicious for malignancy, such as associated abnormal lymph nodes or signs of local invasion) should undergo further characterization according to the American College of Radiology's Thyroid Imaging Reporting & Data System (**TI-RADS**) recommendations: Perform thyroid US for nodules ≥ 1.0 cm in patients < 35 years old and for nodules ≥ 1.5 cm in patients ≥ 35 years old. Recent data supports that these recommendations should not be applied to the pediatric population where an unacceptably high number of cancers may be missed.

- **Calcifications** are not an uncommon feature in **adenomas**, whereas fine, speckled calcifications are a frequent finding in DTCa, particularly the papillary type. Coarse calcifications may be found in **medullary thyroid carcinoma**. **Hemorrhage** or **cystic degeneration** within a thyroid adenoma results in a very heterogeneous appearance of a mass, which mimics malignant necrotic change. Finally, the size of a thyroid lesion does not indicate any particular pathology. Benign thyroid adenomas can grow to many centimeters in size, whereas malignant thyroid papillary carcinomas may only be several millimeters but already metastatic to nodes.

Differential Diagnosis: Visceral Space

Pseudolesion	Metabolic
Thyroid pyramidal lobe	Multinodular goiter
Patulous cervical esophagus	**Benign tumor**
Inflammatory	Thyroid adenoma
Chronic lymphocytic thyroiditis (Hashimoto)	Parathyroid adenoma
Infectious	Recurrent laryngeal nerve schwannoma
Suppurative thyroiditis	**Malignant tumor**
Congenital	Differentiated thyroid carcinoma
Infrahyoid thyroglossal duct cyst	Paratracheal node from differentiated thyroid carcinoma
Degenerative	Thyroid anaplastic carcinoma
Colloid cyst of thyroid	Thyroid non-Hodgkin lymphoma
Parathyroid cyst	Systemic metastasis to thyroid
Esophagopharyngeal diverticulum (Zenker)	Parathyroid carcinoma
Lateral cervical esophageal diverticulum	Tracheal adenoid cystic carcinoma
Tracheal diverticulum	Cervical esophageal carcinoma

- There is a large overlap of benign and malignant features with **CT** and **MR**. The most concerning characteristics on these modalities are invasive features, such as extrathyroidal extension with infiltration of adjacent tissues or associated neck adenopathy. Such cases should all be referred for **tissue sampling**.
- **US** is able to identify unique imaging features that are most concerning for malignancy and hence is often performed after a lesion is found on CT or MR. Thyroid US will frequently identify characteristics of a **multinodular goiter (MNG)** when only 1 nodule was originally evident on clinical or CECT evaluation. US also allows differentiation between a **cystic**, and therefore benign, thyroid lesion from a **solid lesion** and allows image-guided FNA of the latter.
- On **PET/CT** imaging, diffuse thyroid uptake is relatively common and may be due to **thyroiditis**. Thyroid function tests can determine whether the patient has subclinical hypothyroidism. **Focal** thyroid FDG **uptake** has **~ 20%** chance of **malignancy however**, and FNA should be obtained if incidentally found on PET.

TEG lesions can be a VS diagnostic dilemma. TEG lesions reside in or efface the triangle of fat between the posterior wall of the trachea and anterior margin of the esophagus. Well-defined nodules (< 1 cm and clearly distinct from the thyroid, trachea, and esophagus) may be **level VI lymph nodes**. These are drainage sites for thyroid malignancies, squamous cell carcinomas of the larynx, hypopharynx, and esophagus, and are often involved in lymphomas. Searching for other nodes and a primary source help aid diagnosis. **Parathyroid adenomas** occur here and **hypervascularity** on arterial-phase imaging is distinctive. **Parathyroid carcinomas** are rare but usually hypodense and poorly enhancing with infiltrative borders. **Schwannomas** are rare and may be suggested if a long axis fusiform appearance &/or target sign are seen. The differential for well-defined lesions includes exophytic thyroid or esophageal masses, such as an adenoma or diverticulum, respectively. Multiplanar imaging may clarify these relationships.

- When soft tissue **infiltrates the TEG** and effaces its fat triangle, the differential favors a **malignant process**, such as thyroid, parathyroid, or esophageal carcinoma or thyroid malignancy. These neoplastic processes more often present clinically with disruption of the RLN and **vocal cord paralysis**.

Clinical Implications

Patients may be referred for cross-sectional imaging with either a **midline neck mass** ± **lateral neck mass(es)** from **adenopathy**. When protocoling such a study, it is important to remember that, if DTCa is a possible cause, consideration should be given to US, MR, or even NECT, rather than CECT. Iodinated contrast can delay therapeutic I-131 6 weeks. Clinical indicators of possible thyroid cancer include young women with neck masses, particularly low-neck masses &/or cystic or calcified lymph nodes, and masses associated with vocal cord paralysis.

There are 3 main considerations for a **rapidly growing VS mass**: (1) Hemorrhage or cystic degeneration of thyroid adenoma, (2) anaplastic thyroid carcinoma, and (3) thyroid lymphoma. The latter 2 lesions can appear quite similar on imaging, although lymphoma is more frequently a homogeneous lesion. Calcifications, cystic change, and hemorrhage are much less common in lymphoma than anaplastic carcinoma, which is typically heterogeneous and has a greater tendency to invade the trachea.

When imaging is required for preoperative evaluation of the complete extent of an **MNG**, 2 considerations must be kept in mind: (1) Perform the scan with the patient's arms by their side so as not to exaggerate the substernal extension, and (2) up to 5% of MNGs harbor DTCa. While often these are small foci that have not metastasized, look for adenopathy and invasive thyroid contours that would impact surgery.

Selected References

1. Ponnatapura J et al: The mediastinal visceral space: the central pathway for the spread of mediastinal disease. Indian J Radiol Imaging. 32(3):365-71, 2022
2. Aiken AH et al: Approach to Masses in Head and Neck Spaces. 2020 Feb 15. In: Hodler J et al: Diseases of the Brain, Head and Neck, Spine 2020–2023: Diagnostic Imaging [Internet]. Cham (CH): Springer.16, 2020

Visceral Space Overview

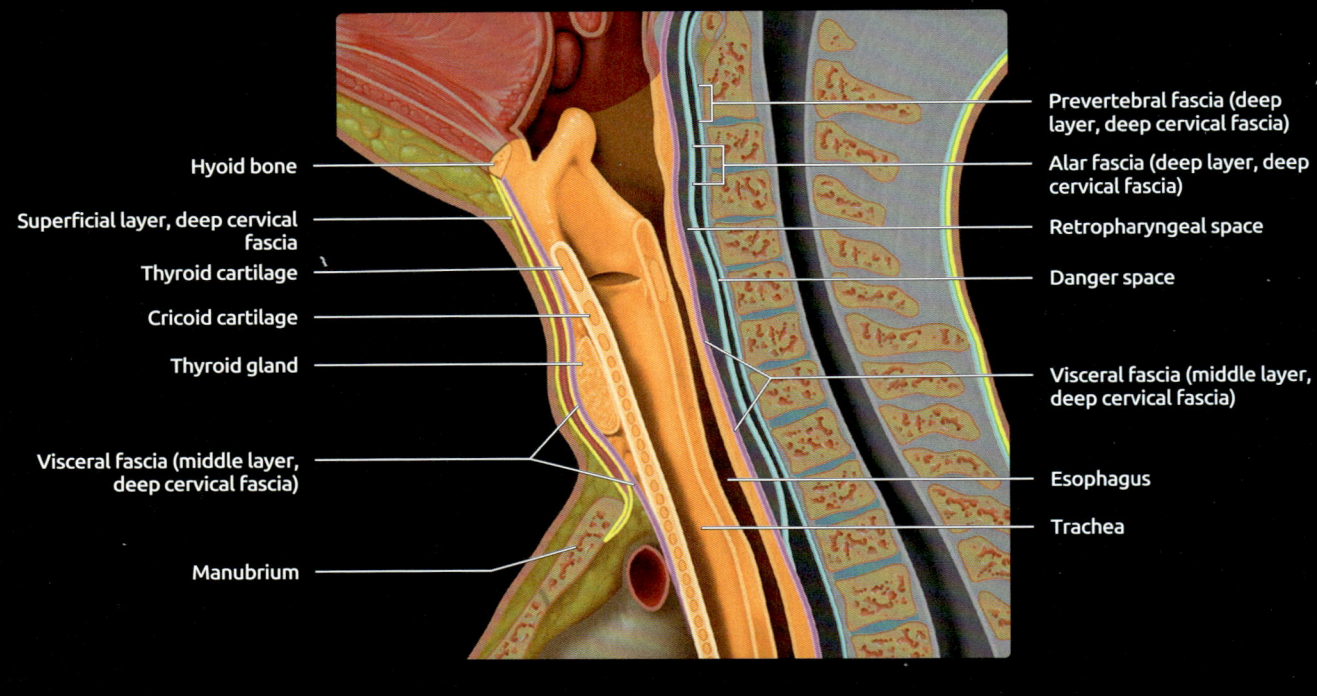

Hyoid bone

Superficial layer, deep cervical fascia

Thyroid cartilage

Cricoid cartilage

Thyroid gland

Visceral fascia (middle layer, deep cervical fascia)

Manubrium

Prevertebral fascia (deep layer, deep cervical fascia)

Alar fascia (deep layer, deep cervical fascia)

Retropharyngeal space

Danger space

Visceral fascia (middle layer, deep cervical fascia)

Esophagus

Trachea

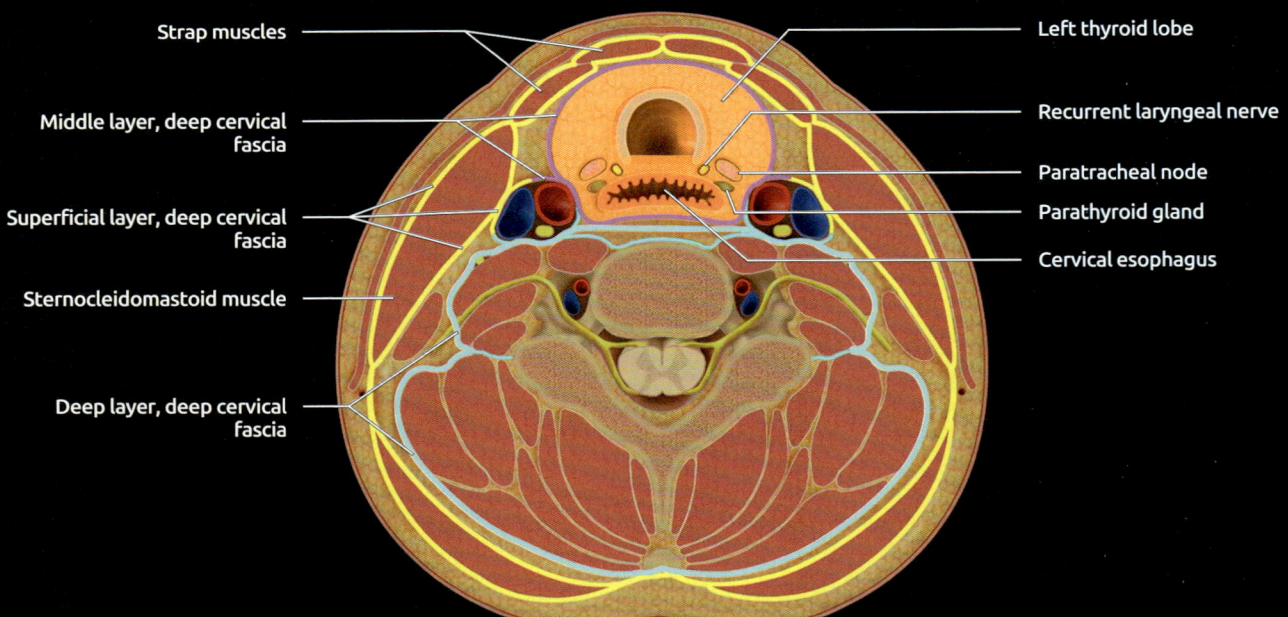

Strap muscles

Middle layer, deep cervical fascia

Superficial layer, deep cervical fascia

Sternocleidomastoid muscle

Deep layer, deep cervical fascia

Left thyroid lobe

Recurrent laryngeal nerve

Paratracheal node

Parathyroid gland

Cervical esophagus

(Top) *Sagittal graphic illustrates the craniocaudal extent of the visceral space (VS) in the anterior aspect of the neck. At the hyoid bone, the superficial and middle layers of deep cervical fascia (DCF) insert. The superficial layer encloses the strap muscles of the anterior neck and sternocleidomastoid muscles of the lateral neck. These muscles surround but are separate from the VS. The middle layer of DCF surrounds the VS. The larynx and cervical trachea and the hypopharynx and cervical esophagus form longitudinal columns within this space from the hyoid to the mediastinum.* **(Bottom)** *Axial graphic depicts the anterior central location of the VS in the infrahyoid neck between the carotid sheaths. Other important VS structures surround the larynx/trachea and the hypopharynx/esophagus, such as the thyroid gland, superior and inferior parathyroid glands, and level VI lymph nodes. The recurrent laryngeal nerves course superiorly to the larynx in the tracheoesophageal grooves.*

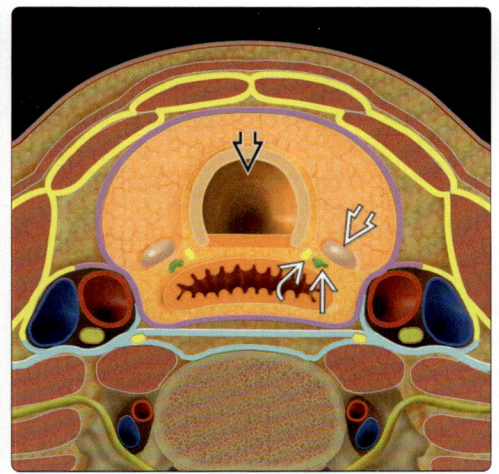

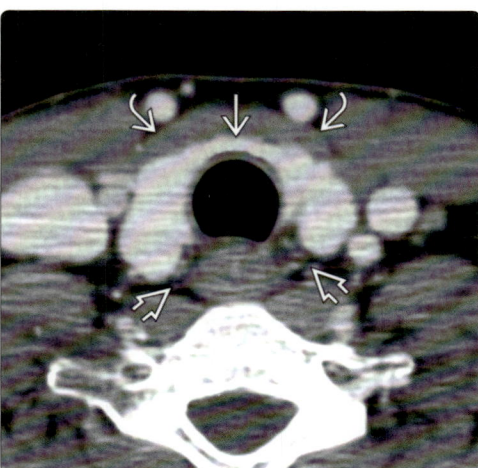

(Left) *Axial graphic depicts the thyroid gland in anterior visceral space (VS) wrapping around the trachea* ➡. *Graphic also illustrates 3 key structures found in tracheoesophageal groove: Recurrent laryngeal nerve (RLN)* ➡, *paratracheal lymph nodes* ➡, *and parathyroid gland* ➡. **(Right)** *Axial CECT at the level of the thyroid gland isthmus* ➡ *(which crosses the anterior surface of the trachea beneath strap muscles* ➡) *shows normal fat, small vessels, and tiny lymph nodes in the tracheoesophageal groove* ➡.

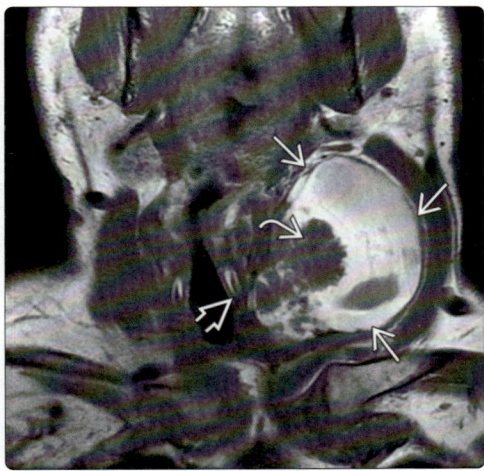

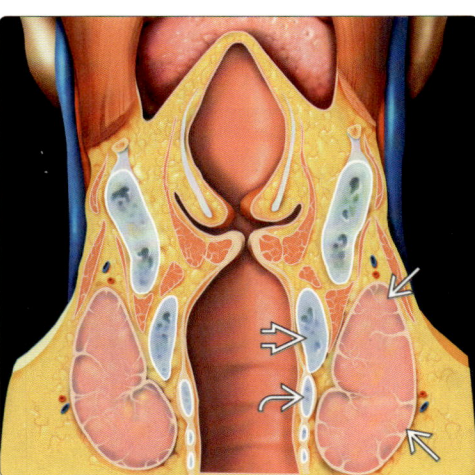

(Left) *Coronal T1 MR shows a heterogeneous solid* ➡ *and cystic* ➡ *infrahyoid neck mass arising from the left thyroid. Note the intrinsic hyperintensity within the cystic component from thyroglobulin. This was found to be papillary thyroid carcinoma, displacing larynx without cricoid* ➡ *invasion.* **(Right)** *Coronal graphic shows the relationship of the thyroid* ➡ *to cricoid cartilage* ➡ *and the 1st tracheal ring* ➡. *It is important to carefully examine the cricoid and proximal trachea for invasion of malignant thyroid tumor.*

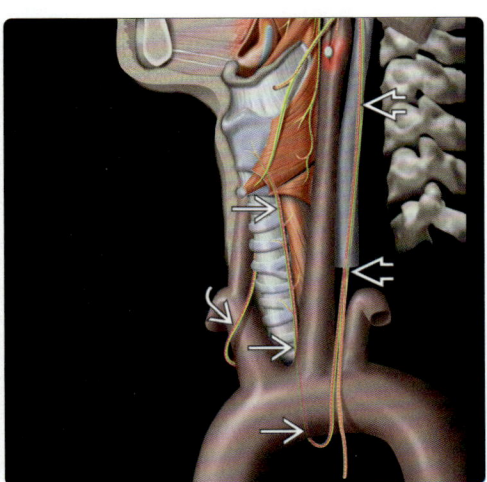

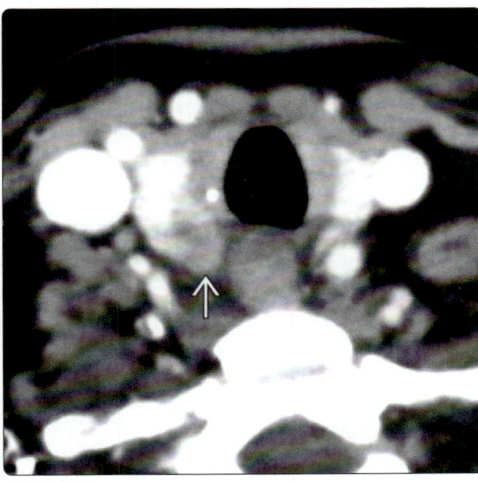

(Left) *Lateral graphic illustrates the ascending course of RLNs in the tracheoesophageal groove of the VS. The left RLN* ➡ *arises from the left vagus* ➡ *in superior mediastinum. The right RLN* ➡ *arises from the vagus at level of subclavian artery.* **(Right)** *Axial CECT in a patient with right vocal cord paralysis shows a small papillary thyroid carcinoma arising in the posterior right thyroid lobe invading the tracheoesophageal groove* ➡. *Tumor was found invading the recurrent laryngeal nerve at pathology.*

Chronic Lymphocytic Thyroiditis (Hashimoto)

TERMINOLOGY

- Chronic lymphocytic thyroiditis (CLT)
- Synonym: Hashimoto thyroiditis

IMAGING

- Best modality is ultrasound for diagnosis & monitoring
  - Early stage shows enlarged, lobulated thyroid with **hypoechoic micronodules** & marked **hypervascularity**
  - Late stage shows small, echogenic fibrosed gland with absent flow signals
- CECT: Diffuse, moderately **enlarged**, **low-density thyroid** without calcifications, cysts, or necrosis

TOP DIFFERENTIAL DIAGNOSES

- Multinodular goiter
- IgG4-related disease (RD) sclerosing thyroiditis
- Thyroid non-Hodgkin lymphoma (NHL)
- Thyroid anaplastic carcinoma

PATHOLOGY

- Antithyroid autoantibodies in serum
- ↑ IgG4 in serum/histology differentiate IgG4 RD from CLT
- Micro: Atrophic follicles, Hürthle cell metaplasia, fibrosis, lymphocyte & plasma cell infiltration
- 13x risk of thyroid **NHL**
  - > 90% of patients with primary thyroid NHL have CLT
- Medullary thyroid carcinoma ↑ risk in CLT (2.7x)
- Papillary thyroid carcinoma ↑ risk in CLT (1.7x)

CLINICAL ISSUES

- Most commonly in women 30-50 years old
- Gradual painless enlargement of thyroid
- Patients most often euthyroid
- Most important complication is thyroid malignancy

DIAGNOSTIC CHECKLIST

- Rapid enlargement of thyroid in patient with history of CLT: NHL until proven otherwise

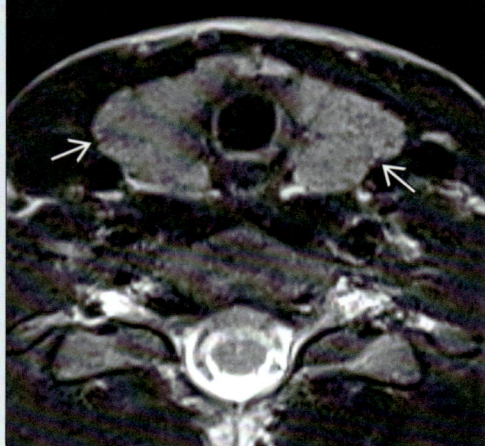 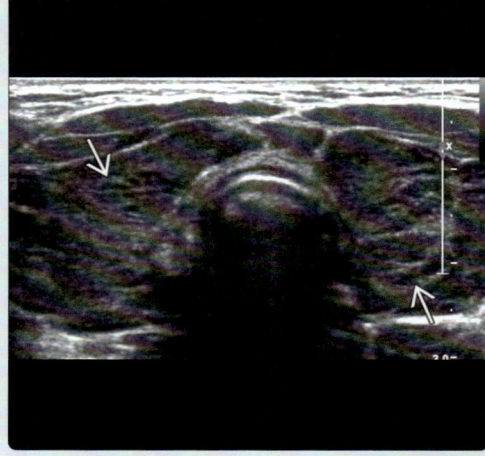

(Left) Axial T2 MR in a 12-year-old boy imaged for dysphagia shows subtle findings of chronic lymphocytic thyroiditis (CLT): Mild thyroid gland enlargement & subtle increased signal intensity with accentuation of lobulated borders due to fibrosis ➡, although the MR findings are not considered specific. (Right) Transverse ultrasound in the same patient illustrates the higher sensitivity for detection of architectural abnormalities in CLT: Heterogeneous thyroid gland parenchyma with numerous hypoechoic nodules ➡ noted diffusely.

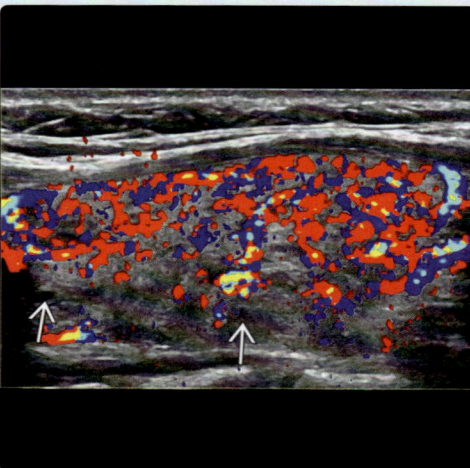 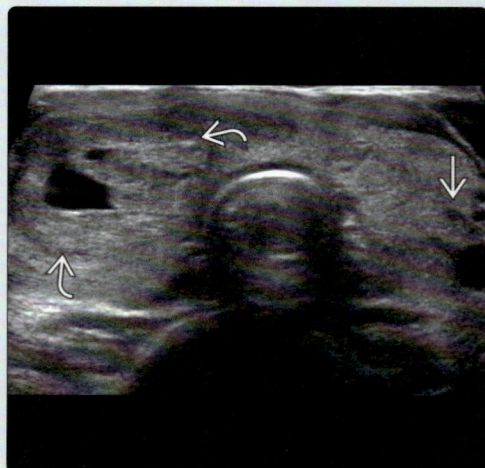

(Left) Longitudinal color Doppler ultrasound shows increased thyroid vascularity (thyroid "inferno") with a background of hypoechoic micronodules ➡ due to CLT. This patient later developed papillary thyroid carcinoma, a less common complication. (Right) Transverse ultrasound shows an enlarged thyroid gland with a few hypoechoic micronodules ➡ typical of CLT. A focal heterogeneous nodule ➡ in the right thyroid lobe had recently enlarged & underwent tissue sampling, which confirmed papillary thyroid carcinoma.

Chronic Lymphocytic Thyroiditis (Hashimoto)

TERMINOLOGY

Abbreviations
- Chronic lymphocytic thyroiditis (CLT)

Synonyms
- Hashimoto thyroiditis (HT), sclerosing lymphocytic thyroiditis

Definitions
- Chronic autoimmune lymphocytic thyroid inflammation

IMAGING

General Features
- Best diagnostic clue
  - Ultrasound: Diffuse, moderately **enlarged thyroid** with **hypoechoic micronodules**
- Size
  - Early phase: Moderate thyroid enlargement
  - Late phase: Diffusely atrophic gland
- Morphology
  - Heterogeneous texture with accentuation of lobular architecture by fibrosis

CT Findings
- CECT
  - Diffusely ↓ density is typical
  - No necrosis, cysts, or calcification

MR Findings
- T2WI FS
  - May see ↑ intensity with lower intensity fibrotic bands

Ultrasonographic Findings
- Grayscale ultrasound
  - Early stages
    - Enlarged, lobulated thyroid with heterogeneous, **diffusely ↓ echogenicity**
    - Diffuse **hypoechoic rounded micronodules**
  - Later stages
    - Small, heterogeneous, & echogenic thyroid
- Color Doppler
  - Early phases: Marked parenchymal hypervascularity
  - Later phases: Blood flow signals are absent

Nuclear Medicine Findings
- PET
  - CLT may show thyroidal uptake
- **Tc-99m pertechnetate & I-123**
  - Early: Diffuse, uniform ↑ activity
  - Later: Coarse, patchy activity

Imaging Recommendations
- Best imaging tool
  - Ultrasound for diagnosis & monitoring

DIFFERENTIAL DIAGNOSIS

Multinodular Goiter
- Diffuse, heterogeneous enlargement of thyroid
- Cystic degeneration, calcification, or hemorrhage

IgG4-Related Sclerosing Thyroiditis
- Invasive fibrous (Riedel) thyroiditis older terminology
- Ultrasound & CT/MR may look similar
- Serum &/or histologic ↑ IgG4 differentiate
- Benign fibrosis with diffuse thyroid enlargement
- Fibrosis extends beyond gland to neck soft tissues
- 1/3 cases involve other organs

Thyroid Non-Hodgkin Lymphoma
- Infiltrative mass diffusely enlarges gland
- Nonnecrotic adenopathy frequently also present

Thyroid Anaplastic Carcinoma
- Heterogeneous, infiltrative thyroid mass
- Necrotic adenopathy frequently present

PATHOLOGY

General Features
- Etiology
  - **Antithyroid autoantibodies**
- Associated abnormalities
  - **Thyroid non-Hodgkin lymphoma (NHL)**
    - 13x risk of developing thyroid NHL
  - Medullary thyroid carcinoma ↑ risk in CLT (2.7x)
  - Papillary thyroid carcinoma ↑ risk in CLT (1.7x)

CLINICAL ISSUES

Presentation
- Most common signs/symptoms
  - Gradual painless enlargement of thyroid
    - Patients most often **euthyroid** with normal T3 & T4 hormones (subclinical thyroiditis)
  - Other signs/symptoms
    - 20% of patients present with hypothyroidism
    - 5% of patients have early hashitoxicosis: Thyrotoxicosis with excess T3/T4 release
- Clinical profile
  - Women > 40 years with gradual thyroid enlargement
- Sex: M:F = 1:9
  - Juvenile form; M:F = 1:2

Demographics
- Age
  - Peak incidence: 4th-5th decades
  - Juvenile form predominantly in adolescents

Natural History & Prognosis
- ↑ incidence of thyroid malignancy
  - Especially lymphoma (MALT or large B cell)

DIAGNOSTIC CHECKLIST

Consider
- **Rapid enlargement** of thyroid in patient with history of CLT: **NHL until proven otherwise**

SELECTED REFERENCES

1. Almahari SA et al: Hashimoto thyroiditis beyond cytology: a correlation between cytological, hormonal, serological, and radiological findings. J Thyroid Res. 2023:5707120, 2023

KEY FACTS

TERMINOLOGY

- Diffuse, multinodular enlargement of thyroid gland in response to chronic TSH stimulation

IMAGING

- Diffuse enlargement of thyroid gland with heterogeneous, nodular appearance
- **40%** have **retrosternal extension**
- CT findings
  - Calcifications, degenerative cysts, & hemorrhage
  - Clear delineation from displaced structures
- MR: Heterogeneous signal & enhancement
- Ultrasound: Multiple iso- to hypoechoic nodules of varying sizes

TOP DIFFERENTIAL DIAGNOSES

- Thyroid colloid cyst
- Thyroid adenoma
- Thyroid differentiated carcinoma

- Thyroid anaplastic carcinoma

PATHOLOGY

- **Sporadic goiter**: Etiology usually unknown, rarely drug induced
- **Endemic goiter**: Associated with iodine deficiency
- 5% have malignant focus at surgery
- Anaplastic thyroid carcinoma may arise from multinodular goiter (MNG)

CLINICAL ISSUES

- Most patients euthyroid, rarely hypothyroid
- Toxic goiter = MNG + hyperthyroidism; uncommon
- Plummer disease = toxic adenoma within MNG

DIAGNOSTIC CHECKLIST

- Well-defined contour of thyroid despite bizarre imaging appearance is key to diagnosis
- Perform presurgical CT with arms by patient's side

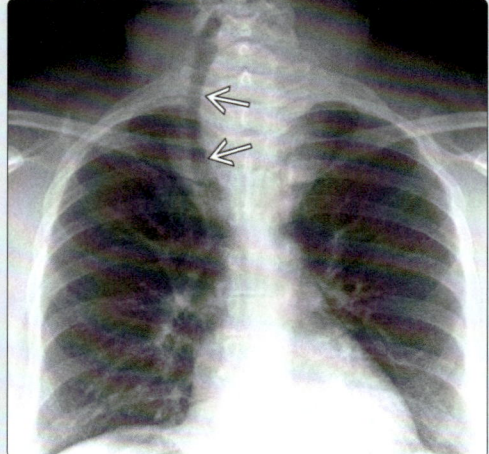
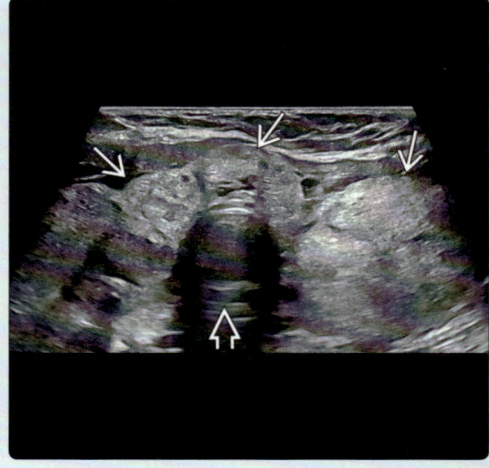

(Left) *PA chest radiograph demonstrates marked displacement of the cervical & thoracic trachea ➡ by a large, left-sided neck & superior mediastinum mass. Even with tracheal compression, patients are often asymptomatic with no clinical evidence of airway compression.* **(Right)** *Transverse grayscale US shows multiple solid, haloed, hyperechoic (compared to adjacent muscle) nodules ➡ in an enlarged thyroid. Note the trachea ➡ is not deviated or compressed. It is difficult to assess retrosternal extension on US.*

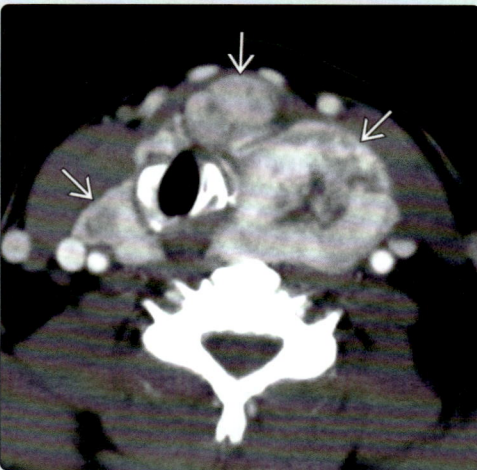
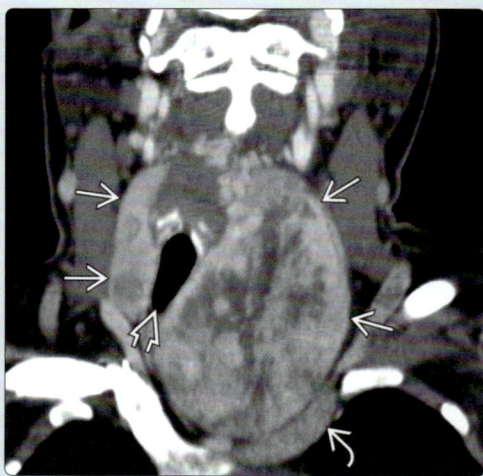

(Left) *Axial CECT shows markedly heterogeneous, lobulated, & enlarged thyroid lobes & isthmus ➡. No calcifications or frank cysts are evident. Gland margins are well defined & adjacent structures merely displaced.* **(Right)** *Coronal CECT shows the craniocaudal extent of a multinodular goiter (MNG) ➡ with heterogeneous thyroid tissue, more marked left lobe enlargement, & marked displacement of the subglottic larynx & trachea ➡. The left brachiocephalic vein ➡ is displaced inferiorly but not compressed by the left lobe.*

TERMINOLOGY

Abbreviations

- Multinodular goiter (MNG)

Synonyms

- Simple nodular goiter, nontoxic goiter

Definitions

- Diffuse, multinodular enlargement of thyroid gland in response to chronic TSH stimulation
- Retrosternal goiter: MNG extends to mediastinum

IMAGING

General Features

- Best diagnostic clue
  - Well-marginated, diffuse enlargement of thyroid gland with heterogeneous, nodular appearance
  - Often **calcifications**, **degenerative cysts**, and **hemorrhage**
- Location
  - Visceral space, thyroid bed
  - **Retrosternal** extension in **40%**
    - Most anterior mediastinum, rarely posterior
    - Retrosternal MNG = most common cause anterior mediastinal mass
- Size
  - May become very large (> 15 cm)
- Morphology
  - Well-marginated, diffuse thyroid enlargement
    - Carotid vessels displaced away from midline
    - Trachea compressed ± displaced

Radiographic Findings

- Radiography
  - Chest x-ray findings
    - If all suprasternal: Normal CXR or tracheal deviation/narrowing
    - If **retrosternal**: Superior mediastinal mass + **tracheal deviation & narrowing**

CT Findings

- NECT
  - **Low-density** areas of **degenerative** & **colloidal cysts**
  - Intermediate-density solid nodules & fibrosis
  - **High-density** foci from **hemorrhage** & **calcification**
    - **90% calcification**: Amorphous, ring-like, curvilinear
- CECT
  - Thyroid parenchyma replaced with multiple variably sized, heterogeneous solid & cystic masses
  - Clear delineation from adjacent displaced structures
  - Diffuse, inhomogeneous enhancement
  - No associated lymphadenopathy
  - Coronal reformats
    - Brachiocephalic vessels "cradle" inferior MNG

MR Findings

- T1WI
  - Generally low intensity, isointense to muscles
  - Focal high signal intensity with fine calcifications or hemorrhage
  - Low signal intensity with cystic degeneration or coarse calcifications
- T2WI
  - Heterogeneous intermediate to high intensity
  - Low signal with fibrosis & coarse calcifications
  - Focal high signal with cystic degeneration & hemorrhage
- DWI
  - Preliminary data: ADC of malignant nodules < ADC of normal tissue < ADC of benign nodules
- T1WI C+
  - Diffuse, heterogeneous enhancement

Ultrasonographic Findings

- Grayscale ultrasound
  - Multiple nodules, bilateral diffuse thyroid involvement
  - Solid nodules usually **isoechoic**, small portions hypoechoic (5%)
  - Nodules unencapsulated but sharply defined, haloed
  - Mass has heterogeneous internal echo pattern with debris, septa, solid/cystic portions
    - Calcification seen as hyperechoic foci with dense shadowing
    - Cystic, hypoechoic regions from hemorrhage, degeneration, or colloid within nodule

Nuclear Medicine Findings

- PET
  - Heterogeneous uptake common
  - Focal uptake within gland requires biopsy
- Tc-99m pertechnetate or I-123
  - No role in initial evaluation of nontoxic goiter
  - Determines mediastinal mass is thyroid in nature
  - Heterogeneously iodine avid with suppression of surrounding parenchyma

Imaging Recommendations

- Best imaging tool
  - CECT is exam of choice for evaluation of MNG
    - Extent & severity of airway compression
    - Presence & extent of retrosternal MNG
    - Unusual extensions of MNG (e.g., retroesophageal, suprahyoid)
  - Ultrasound used to guide needle biopsy of solid nodules
  - If malignancy suspected, MR imaging stages nodal extent without compromising I-131 therapy
- Protocol advice
  - Important to perform neck CT with arms by side
  - Arms elevated, as with chest CT, falsely exaggerates retrosternal extent

DIFFERENTIAL DIAGNOSIS

Thyroid Colloid Cyst

- Variably sized cystic mass within thyroid
- Adjacent normal thyroid tissue

Thyroid Adenoma

- Solitary intrathyroidal mass without local invasion or adenopathy; adjacent normal thyroid tissue seen

Thyroid Differentiated Carcinoma

- Tumor may occupy all or part of thyroid gland

- Thyroid gland margins may be invasive
- 50% have neck or upper mediastinal nodes

Thyroid Anaplastic Carcinoma

- Rapidly enlarging, heterogeneous, invasive tumor originating from thyroid gland

Thyroid Non-Hodgkin Lymphoma

- Large, solid, occasionally invasive tumor originating from thyroid gland
- Typically multiple cervical lymph nodes

PATHOLOGY

General Features

- Etiology
  - **Sporadic goiter**
    - Etiology usually unknown
    - Generally adequate dietary iodine intake
    - Rarely drug induced: Lithium, aminoglutethimide
  - **Endemic goiter**
    - Environmental iodine deficiency → TSH elevation
    - Results in gradual, diffuse thyroid hyperplasia
    - Involution + fibrosis + focal hyperplasia → nodules
- Associated abnormalities
  - 5% have malignant focus at surgery
    - Same incidence as single thyroid nodule
  - Differentiated thyroid carcinoma most common
    - Anaplastic thyroid carcinoma may arise from MNG

Gross Pathologic & Surgical Features

- Aggregate of multiple, partially encapsulated, variably sized colloid & adenomatous nodules

Microscopic Features

- Distended follicles with colloid & hyperplasia
- Follicle degeneration leads to infarction, hemorrhage, fibrosis, cyst formation, & calcification

CLINICAL ISSUES

Presentation

- Most common signs/symptoms
  - Large, multinodular lower neck mass
  - MNG most common cause of asymmetric thyroid enlargement
- Other signs/symptoms
  - Airway compression (55%), hoarseness (15%), dysphagia, & superior vena cava syndrome (10%)
- Clinical profile
  - Most euthyroid
  - Toxic MNG = hyperthyroidism + MNG
    - Either multiple hyperfunctioning areas in MNG or toxic adenoma in MNG (Plummer disease)
    - Iodinated drug (e.g., amiodarone) can induce hyperthyroidism in nontoxic MNG

Demographics

- Age
  - Sporadic goiter has no specific age
  - Endemic goiter occurs during childhood
    - Continues to increase in size with age
- Sex
  - F:M = 2-4:1
- Epidemiology
  - Sporadic
    - 3-5% of population in resource-rich countries
  - Endemic
    - > 13% of world population affected
    - Mild iodine deficiency: Goiter prevalence 5-20%
    - Moderate iodine deficiency: Goiter prevalence 20-30%
    - Severe iodine deficiency: Goiter prevalence > 30%

Natural History & Prognosis

- Growth & nodule production → functional autonomy
- Functional autonomy rarely results in thyrotoxicosis
- Spontaneous regression vs. gradually increasing size with development of multiple nodules, local compression symptoms ± cosmetic complaints

Treatment

- No treatment for asymptomatic, nonpalpable MNG identified on neck imaging done for other reasons
- Patients with prominent growing hard nodule may have aspiration to exclude malignancy
- Large, nontoxic, compressive MNG: Surgical removal
  - Postoperative thyroid hormone replacement
  - Hypoparathyroidism or recurrent laryngeal nerve injury rare complications
- Minimally invasive procedures, such as radiofrequency and microwave ablation, avoid surgery, targeting symptomatic nodules directly

DIAGNOSTIC CHECKLIST

Consider

- **Well-defined thyroid contour** despite **bizarre imaging appearance** is **key** to diagnosis

Image Interpretation Pearls

- Always perform presurgical CT evaluation with arms by patient's side, not above head
- Ensure neck CT covers to inferior limit of MNG

SELECTED REFERENCES

1. Guo R et al: The two-year prognosis of multinodular goiter following radiofrequency ablation: based on all nodule burdens. Eur Thyroid J. 13(1):e230134, 2024
2. Lim H et al: Comparative efficacy and safety of radiofrequency ablation and microwave ablation in benign thyroid nodule treatment: a systematic review and meta-analysis. Eur Radiol. 35(2):612-3, 2024
3. Navin PJ et al: Radiofrequency ablation of benign and malignant thyroid nodules. Radiographics. 42(6):1812-28, 2022
4. Apostolou K et al: Prevalence and risk factors for thyroid cancer in patients with multinodular goitre. BJS Open. 5(2):zraa014, 2021
5. Giovanella L et al: Molecular imaging for thyrotoxicosis and thyroid nodules. J Nucl Med. 62(Suppl 2):20S-5S, 2021
6. Sorensen JR et al: Thyroidectomy improves tracheal anatomy and airflow in patients with nodular goiter: a prospective cohort study. Eur Thyroid J. 6(6):307-14, 2017
7. Bin Saeedan M et al: Thyroid computed tomography imaging: pictorial review of variable pathologies. Insights Imaging. 7(4):601-17, 2016
8. Bombil I et al: Incidental cancer in multinodular goitre post thyroidectomy. S Afr J Surg. 52(1):5-9, 2014
9. Brito JP et al: Prevalence of thyroid cancer in multinodular goiter versus single nodule: a systematic review and meta-analysis. Thyroid. 23(4):449-55, 2013
10. Moalem J et al: Treatment and prevention of recurrence of multinodular goiter: an evidence-based review of the literature. World J Surg. 32(7):1301-12, 2008

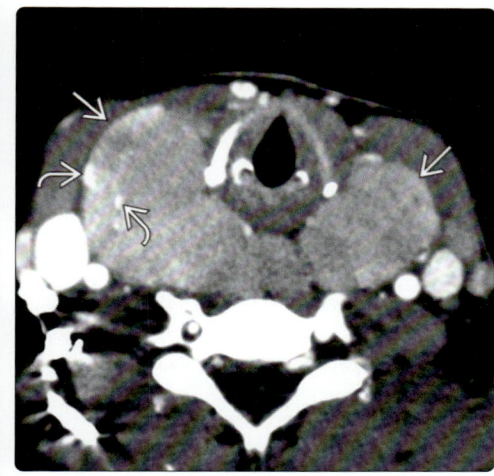
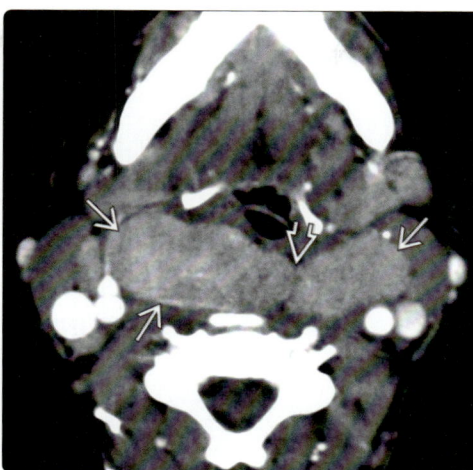

(Left) *Axial CECT through the level of the infraglottic larynx in a patient with MNG shows symmetric enlargement of the thyroid lobes ➡, which appear hyperdense with patchy areas of low density & small focal calcifications ➡. The gland remains sharply demarcated with no evidence of invasion of adjacent soft tissues.* **(Right)** *Axial CECT more superiorly at the level of the hyoid in the same patient shows unusual cranial growth with an MNG extending posteriorly & medially around the pharynx ➡ so that the lobes meet in the midline ➡.*

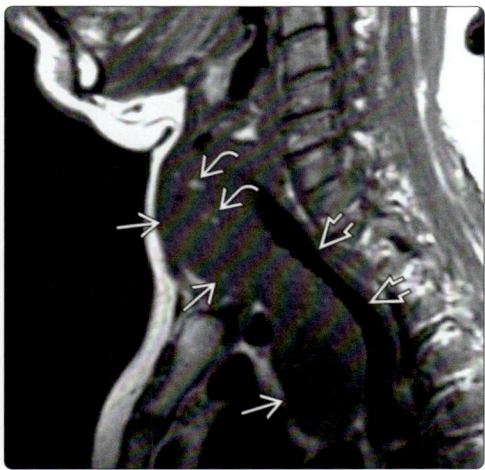
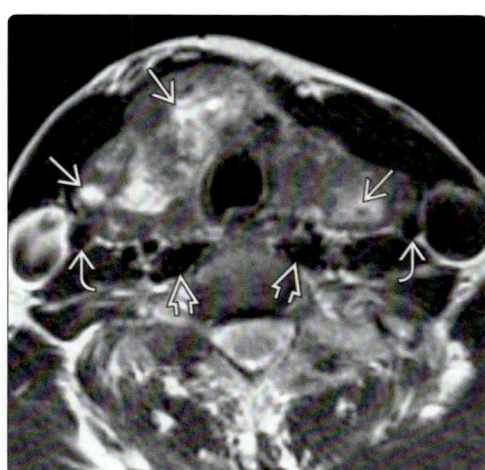

(Left) *Sagittal T1WI MR demonstrates narrowing & displacement of the trachea ➡ posteriorly as a goiter ➡ extends from the lower neck to the superior mediastinum. Focal areas of T1 shortening ➡ within an enlarged thyroid represent calcifications or hemorrhage.* **(Right)** *Axial T2WI MR in the same patient shows a nodular goiter with heterogeneous texture and areas of hyperintense, cystic degeneration ➡. T2 better demonstrates clear delineation of the thyroid from adjacent strap muscles ➡ & carotid arteries ➡.*

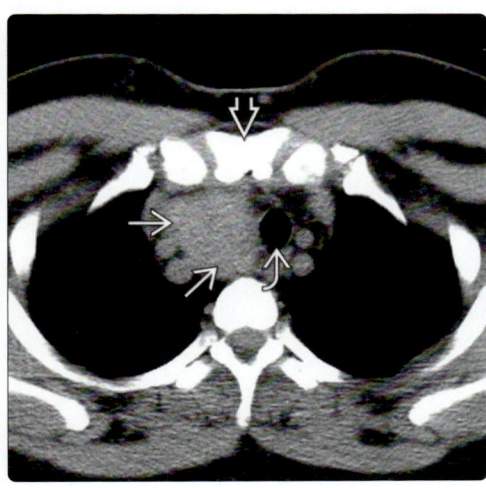
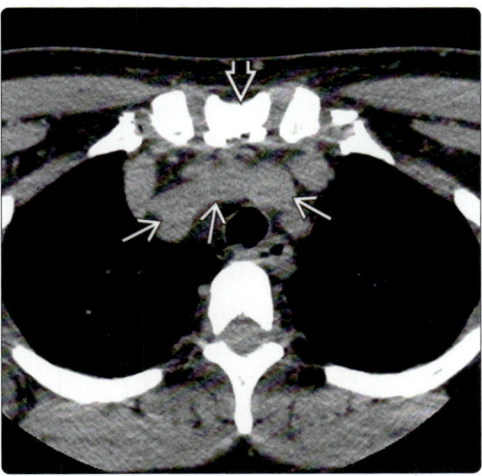

(Left) *Axial NECT for a large MNG shows the inferior aspect of an enlarged right thyroid lobe ➡, posterior to the manubrium ➡ & displacing the trachea ➡ medially. Study was performed as a chest CT with arms above the head.* **(Right)** *Axial NECT in the same patient (on the same day at the same level ➡), performed as a neck study with arms at the patient's side, shows no retrosternal extension of a MNG. Only great vessels ➡ are evident. This illustrates the importance of arms at the side technique for preoperative evaluation.*

KEY FACTS

TERMINOLOGY

- 2 benign categories that present as thyroid nodule
  - True adenoma and adenomatous nodule

IMAGING

- Thyroid adenoma
  - Well-defined nodule compresses adjacent gland
- Adenomatous nodule
  - Less distinct lesion contours; ± multiple lesions
- Calcifications or cystic change may be seen
- Large adenomas often have heterogeneous enhancement with degeneration
- No invasive features or neck adenopathy
- FDG uptake may be seen in adenomas
- Nuclear scintigraphy
  - Hot nodules are usually benign adenomas
  - 20% of cold nodules are malignant

TOP DIFFERENTIAL DIAGNOSES

- Thyroid colloid cyst
- Multinodular goiter
- Parathyroid adenoma
- Thyroid differentiated carcinoma

PATHOLOGY

- Adenomatous nodule > follicular adenoma
- Hürthle cell adenoma least common
- While fine-needle aspiration (FNA) can suggest adenoma, only resection can distinguish from carcinoma

CLINICAL ISSUES

- Typically nonfunctioning, most commonly incidental imaging finding
- Do not evaluate suspected thyroid mass with CECT
  - Iodinated contrast delays iodine treatment of malignant thyroid tumor

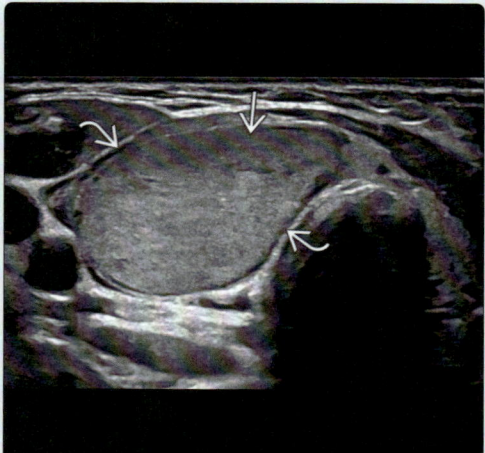
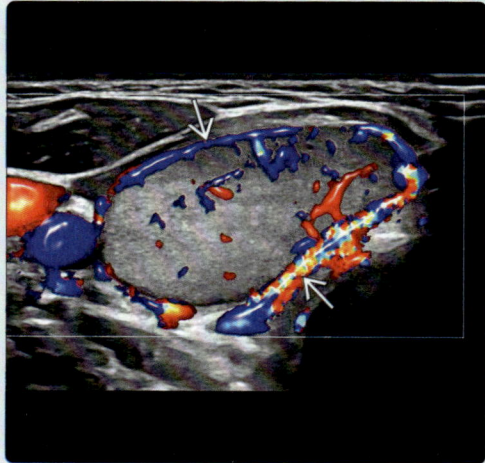

(Left) *Transverse US in a patient with right lower neck swelling shows a well-defined solid lesion ➡ in the right lobe of the thyroid. It is hypoechoic relative to the rest of the thyroid gland. There is no calcification or cystic changes. Note the well-defined halo ➡, which represents the capsule.* (Right) *Transverse color Doppler US in the same patient shows peripheral flow ➡ with patchy central flow. Right hemithyroidectomy was performed later, and pathology confirmed a follicular adenoma.*

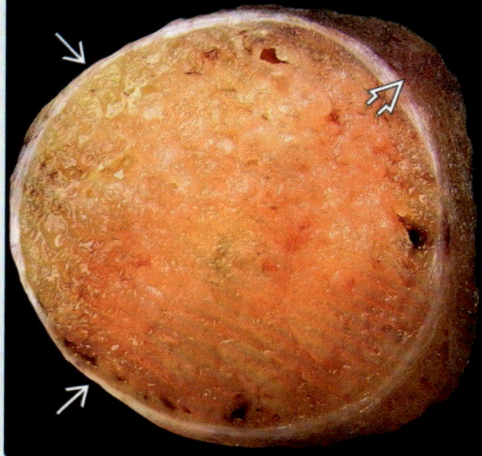
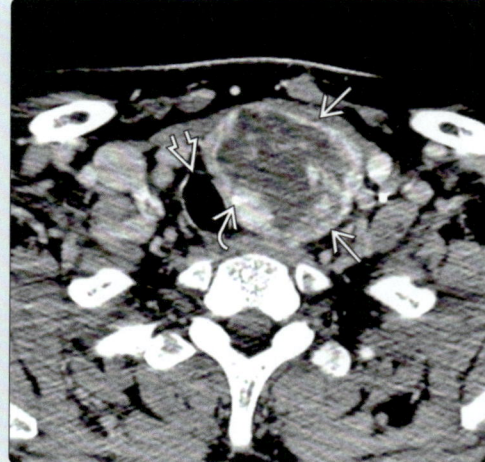

(Left) *Gross pathology shows 1 follicular adenoma. There is a thick, well-formed fibrous connective tissue capsule ➡ separating the adenoma from the surrounding thyroid parenchyma. There is compression of the adjacent thyroid ➡, which is more beefy red.* (Right) *Axial CECT shows a large, heterogeneous mass ➡ with central low density arising within the left thyroid lobe. Focal calcification ➡ is evident. The mass abuts the trachea ➡, but there is no evidence of invasion.*

TERMINOLOGY

Definitions

- **True adenoma**: Benign neoplasm of thyroid glandular epithelium with fibrous encapsulation
  - Follicular adenoma and Hürthle cell adenoma
- **Adenomatous nodule**: Focal adenomatous hyperplasia with incomplete capsule

IMAGING

General Features

- Best diagnostic clue
  - Thyroid adenoma
    - Well-defined nodule compresses adjacent gland
  - Adenomatous nodule
    - Less distinct lesion contours; multiple lesions often present
  - No imaging characteristic highly specific for benign adenoma
- Location
  - Intrathyroidal, though may be exophytic
- Size
  - Usually < 4 cm; palpable if > 1 cm
- Morphology
  - Adenoma: Well-defined, encapsulated, small nodule
  - Adenomatous nodule: Incomplete capsule, less sharp demarcation from adjacent gland

CT Findings

- CECT
  - Findings nonspecific
  - No invasive features or adenopathy
  - Heterogeneous enhancement with degenerative changes
  - Coarse calcifications may be seen

MR Findings

- T1WI
  - Typically iso- or hypointense
  - Foci of increased signal intensity from hemorrhage or calcification
- T2WI
  - Typically hyperintense
- T1WI C+
  - Homogeneous or heterogeneous enhancement

Ultrasonographic Findings

- Grayscale ultrasound
  - Usually **isoechoic**; may be hyper- or hypoechoic
  - Adenoma: Smooth, peripheral, echo-poor halo
  - Adenomatous nodule: Often incomplete halo
  - US features suggesting benign lesion
    - Thin, well-defined halo, regular margin, coarse calcifications
    - Comet-tail artifact within nodule
    - No neck adenopathy
- Color Doppler
  - Thyroid adenoma: Spoke-wheel pattern; peripheral blood vessels extending toward center of lesion
  - Adenomatous nodule has more diffuse vascularity

Nuclear Medicine Findings

- PET
  - FDG uptake can be seen in adenomas
    - Biopsy recommended to exclude malignancy
- Thyroid scintigraphy (Tc-99m pertechnetate or I-123)
  - **Hot nodule**: Focally increased activity
    - Most often hyperfunctioning thyroid adenoma
    - 50% are autonomous adenoma
    - **< 1% are malignant lesions**
  - **Cold nodule**: Absence of activity
    - Most often adenoma/adenomatous nodule or cyst
    - **20% are malignant lesions**

Imaging Recommendations

- Best imaging tool
  - Thyroid nodule common **incidental** CT or MR finding
    - Recommend US if invasive appearance or abnormal lymph nodes
    - If **< 35 years of age**, recommend US for ≥ 1 cm in size
    - If **≥ 35 years of age**, recommend US for ≥ 1.5 cm in size
  - US helpful for differentiating benign and malignant
    - Also allows fine-needle aspiration (FNA) guidance and evaluation of nodes
  - Thyroid scintigraphy can determine if hot nodule; likely benign
- Protocol advice
  - Do not evaluate new thyroid mass with CECT
    - Iodinated contrast delays iodine treatment of malignant thyroid tumor

DIFFERENTIAL DIAGNOSIS

Thyroid Colloid Cyst

- Cystic degeneration of nodule
- Variable MR T1 signal intensity from colloid or hemorrhage

Multinodular Goiter

- Multiple nodules in diffusely enlarged thyroid
- Heterogeneous thyroid texture and coarse calcifications common

Parathyroid Adenoma

- Delineated by fat plane from posterior aspect of thyroid gland
- Rarely ectopic intrathyroidal parathyroid adenoma; diagnosis made by FNA

Thyroid Differentiated Carcinoma

- Focal intrathyroidal mass, may have invasive margins
- Calcifications often seen with papillary type
- Cervical lymphadenopathy frequently found

PATHOLOGY

General Features

- WHO 2022 classification of follicular cell-derived neoplasms: Divided into benign tumors, low-risk neoplasms, and malignant neoplasms
- While FNA can suggest adenoma, lobectomy only can differentiate from carcinoma

Gross Pathologic & Surgical Features

- Thyroid adenoma: Circumscribed, encapsulated lesions of varying color (gray to white to tan)
  - Compress adjacent normal thyroid tissue
  - Hemorrhage, fibrosis, calcification, and cyst formation may be seen
  - FNA can suggest diagnosis but cannot determine malignant capsular or vascular invasion
- Adenomatous nodules: Circumscribed but only partially encapsulated; more often multiple

Microscopic Features

- Several histologic types of adenoma
- Different types may be present in same gland
  - Follicular (simple), macrofollicular (colloid), microfollicular (fetal), trabecular-solid (embryonal)
  - Hürthle cell (oncocytic) adenoma: Granular cells with pink cytoplasm
- Degenerative changes, such as hemorrhage, cyst formation, fibrosis, and calcification may be present
- Significant mitotic activity or necrosis not common in absence of prior FNA or trauma
  - Raises concern for malignancy, though not diagnostic of carcinoma

CLINICAL ISSUES

Presentation

- Most common signs/symptoms
  - Slow-growing, solitary palpable neck nodule
- Clinical profile
  - Usually asymptomatic as nonfunctioning
    - Hyperthyroidism is uncommon presentation ("toxic adenoma")
    - Functional adenomas commonly ≥ 3 cm
  - Clinical factors favoring benign diagnosis
    - Family history of autoimmune disease (Hashimoto), benign nodules or goiter
    - Thyroid hyper- or hypofunction; multinodular goiter without dominant nodule
    - Soft, smooth, mobile nodule; painful or tender
  - Clinical factors favoring malignancy
    - Age < 20 years or > 60 years; male patients
    - History of thyroid carcinoma, prior radiation, family history of multiple endocrine neoplasia
    - Firm, hard, immobile nodule; neck adenopathy

Demographics

- Age
  - May be found in all age groups
- Sex
  - M:F = 1:4
- Epidemiology
  - Thyroid nodules common
    - 25% by US
    - 30-60% at autopsy
  - Adenomatous nodules more common than adenomas

Natural History & Prognosis

- Follicular adenoma: Slow growing; rarely associated with malignancy

- Rapid enlargement may occur with spontaneous hemorrhage
- May degenerate to form thyroid cyst
- Hürthle cell adenoma: Slow growing, may spontaneously infarct
- Adenomatous hyperplasia: More likely to have degenerative changes

Treatment

- Those nodules with "suspicious" or "malignant" features from US criteria should be excised surgically
- Hot nodules followed clinically and with US
- **Cold nodules** have **20%** risk of malignancy
  - Nondiagnostic FNA → repeat aspiration or resection
- Autonomous hyperfunctioning nodules can be treated by several methods
  - I-131 ablation with risk of hypothyroidism
  - Ethanol injection with risk of recurrent laryngeal nerve injury
  - Surgical resection

DIAGNOSTIC CHECKLIST

Consider

- Thyroid nodules common; frequently incidental imaging finding
- 95% benign, clinically not important: Adenomatous nodules, adenomas, thyroid cysts, focal thyroiditis
- Diagnosis of adenoma may be suggested by FNA but not proven without surgical resection

Image Interpretation Pearls

- Imaging cannot differentiate between adenoma and low-grade neoplasm
- Evaluation of suspected thyroid mass with CECT may delay radioactive iodine treatment
- US can determine whether single or multiple, cystic or solid
- Thyroid scintigraphy: < 1% of hot nodules malignant; 20% of cold nodules malignant

SELECTED REFERENCES

1. Cho YY et al: Malignancy risk of follicular neoplasm (Bethesda IV) with variable cutoffs of tumor size: a systemic review and meta-analysis. J Clin Endocrinol Metab. 109(5):1383-92, 2024
2. Ohori NP et al: Follicular neoplasm of thyroid revisited: current differential diagnosis and the impact of molecular testing. Adv Anat Pathol. 30(1):11-23, 2023
3. Jung CK et al: Update from the 2022 World Health Organization Classification of Thyroid Tumors: a standardized diagnostic approach. Endocrinol Metab (Seoul). 37(5):703-18, 2022
4. Alexander LF et al: Thyroid ultrasound: diffuse and nodular disease. Radiol Clin North Am. 58(6):1041-57, 2020
5. Traylor KS: Computed tomography and MR imaging of thyroid disease. Radiol Clin North Am. 58(6):1059-70, 2020
6. Tappouni RR et al: ACR TI-RADS: pitfalls, solutions, and future directions. Radiographics. 39(7):2040-52, 2019
7. Yoon JH et al: Malignancy risk stratification of thyroid nodules: comparison between the thyroid imaging reporting and data system and the 2014 American Thyroid Association Management Guidelines. Radiology. 278(3):917-24, 2016
8. Hoang JK et al: Managing incidental thyroid nodules detected on imaging: white paper of the ACR incidental thyroid findings committee. J Am Coll Radiol. 12(2):143-50, 2015
9. Kamran SC et al: Thyroid nodule size and prediction of cancer. J Clin Endocrinol Metab. 98(2):564-70, 2013
10. Ahn SS et al: Biopsy of thyroid nodules: comparison of three sets of guidelines. AJR Am J Roentgenol. 194(1):31-7, 2010

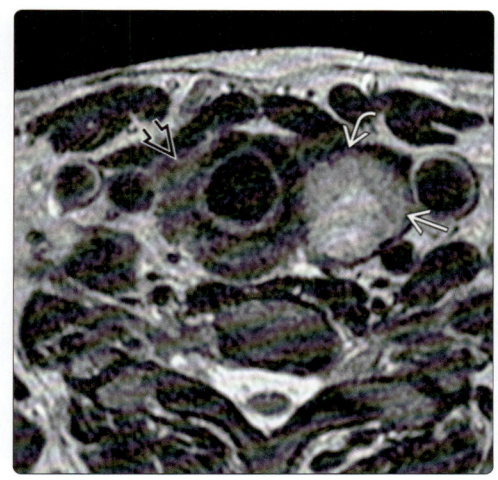 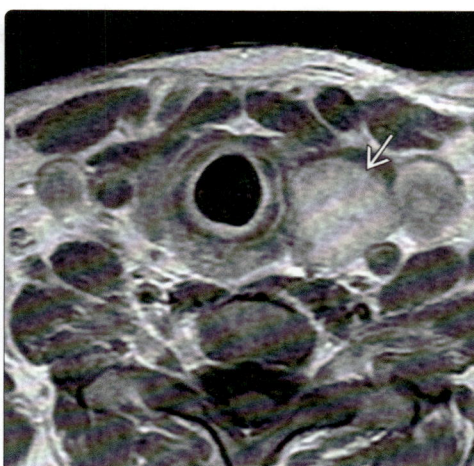

(Left) Axial T2WI MR reveals a mildly hyperintense mass ➡ replacing much of the left thyroid lobe with only a thin rim of normal gland evident at the anterior margin ➡. The mass is well circumscribed and clearly delineated from strap muscles and the adjacent carotid artery and jugular vein. The right thyroid lobe ➡ appears small. (Right) Axial T1WI C+ MR in the same patient reveals diffusely homogeneous enhancement of the mass ➡. There is no neck adenopathy. At resection, the lesion was determined to be follicular adenoma.

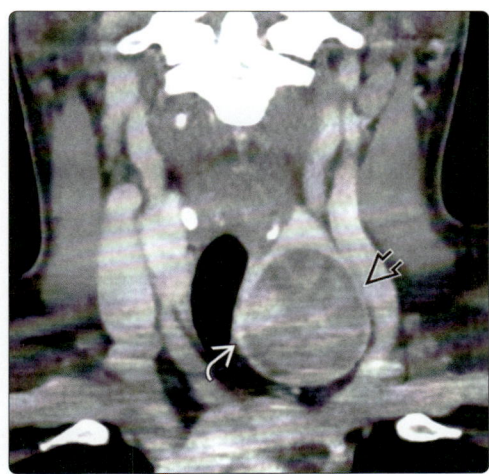 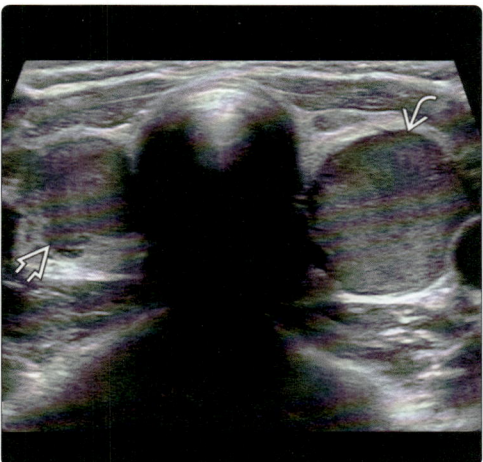

(Left) Coronal CECT reveals a follicular thyroid adenoma. The adenoma is seen as a low-density, heterogeneously enhancing intrathyroidal mass ➡. Note the well-circumscribed margins and mass effect on the trachea ➡ without invasive features. (Right) Midline transverse US shows bilateral thyroid nodules. The left nodule reveals a well-defined capsule ➡ that was a follicular adenoma on excision. The right nodule shows a slightly ill-defined lateral margin ➡ that was a follicular carcinoma on excision.

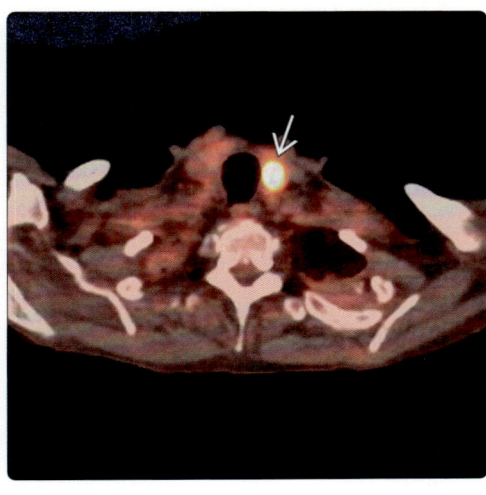 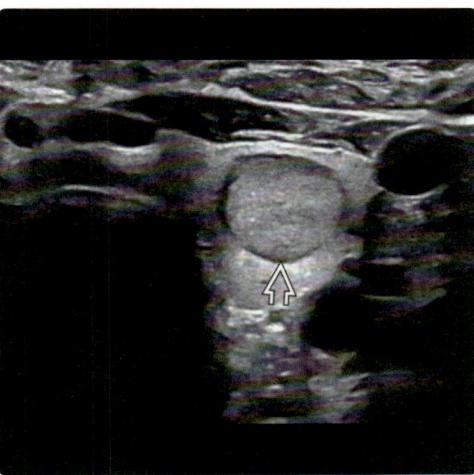

(Left) Staging PET/CT in a patient with malignant melanoma of the left foot shows there is a focus of FDG-avid uptake ➡ in the left thyroid gland. There was no other focus of high FDG uptake in rest of the body and the patient had no previous history of thyroid disease. (Right) Transverse US post PET/CT shows a well-defined nodule ➡ in the left lobe of the thyroid corresponding to the focus of the FDG-avid nodule. FNA suggested a follicular lesion. Following surgery, this was confirmed as a follicular adenoma.

Parathyroid Adenoma in Visceral Space

TERMINOLOGY

- Benign tumor of parathyroid gland producing excess parathyroid hormone, resulting in hypercalcemia

IMAGING

- Parathyroid adenoma (PT Ad) 10-30 mm; normal gland 5 x 3 x 1 mm
- Round or oval, well-circumscribed, solid, hypervascular mass
- **Multiphase CECT** now 1st-line modality at some centers
  - **NECT** differentiates normal thyroid & parathyroid tissue
  - **Arterial-phase** (30 seconds) avid enhancement of PT Ad
  - **Delayed-phase** washout separates PT Ad & nodes
- US &/or nuclear scintigraphy may be 1st-line modalities at some centers
- **US**: Homogeneous, **hypoechoic, hypervascular**
  - Operator-dependent, limited for ectopic/multigland
- **Tc-99m sestamibi: Uptake** on early & **delayed** images
  - SPECT ± CT best to localize; limited for cystic PT Ad
  - Nuclear subtraction scans helpful if thyroid mass

- MR: T2 iso- to hyperintense compared to thyroid
  - Multiphase enhanced MR similar to multiphase CT

TOP DIFFERENTIAL DIAGNOSES

- Reactive lymph nodes
- Thyroid adenoma, multinodular goiter
- Parathyroid cyst, parathyroid carcinoma

CLINICAL ISSUES

- Most patients have asymptomatic hypercalcemia
- Hypercalcemia may have wide range of symptoms
  - "Stones, bones, groans, & psychic moans"

DIAGNOSTIC CHECKLIST

- Compare all modalities available to avoid mistakes
- Base search pattern on knowledge of embryology
- "Classic" multiphase CT enhancement only seen in 20%
- Report all PT Ad candidates by location with relative confidence level, best allows surgeon to plan
- Reporting incidental PT Ad may ↓ long-term morbidity

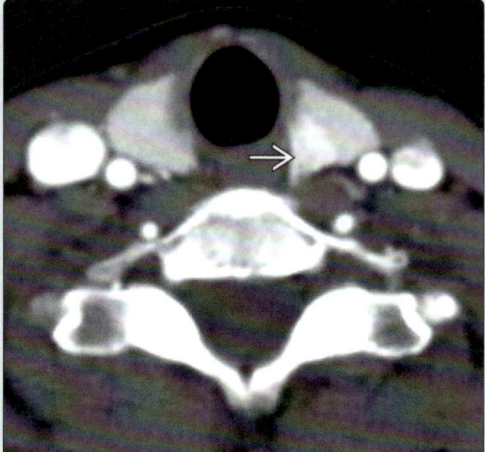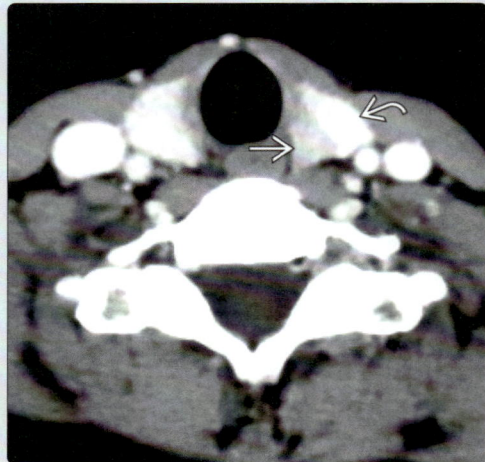

(Left) Axial arterial-phase CECT demonstrates classic intense enhancement in this parathyroid adenoma (PT Ad) ➡, brighter than the normal thyroid gland. (Right) Axial venous-phase CECT demonstrates expected washout of contrast in this typical PT Ad ➡. Compare to the densely enhancing thyroid gland ➡. This classic pattern of intense arterial-phase enhancement with delayed washout is typical of PT Ads but is only seen ~ 20% of the time.

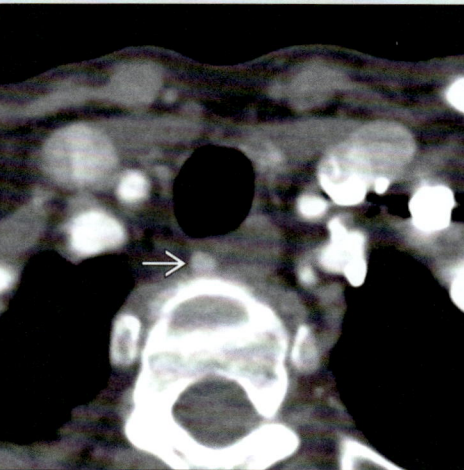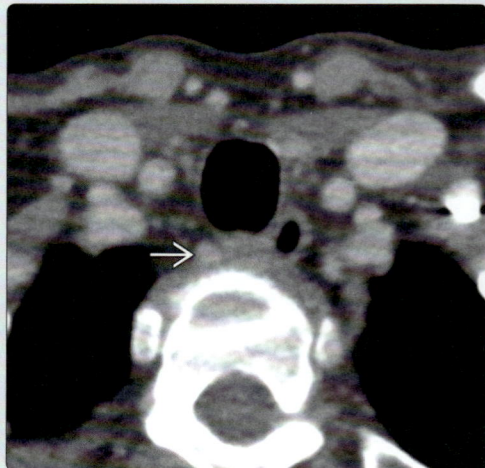

(Left) Axial arterial-phase CECT shows a brightly enhancing solitary PT Ad adjacent to the esophagus ➡. This lesion was not visualized sonographically due to its deep location behind the trachea. Arterial phase improves diagnostic confidence over the venous phase where it is harder to see next to the esophagus. (Right) Axial venous-phase CECT in the same patient shows contrast washout of this PT Ad ➡, which could be easily overlooked without the accompanying arterial phase.

TERMINOLOGY

Abbreviations

- Parathyroid adenoma (PT Ad)

Definitions

- Benign neoplasm of parathyroid gland producing excess parathyroid hormone (PTH), resulting in **hypercalcemia**

IMAGING

General Features

- Best diagnostic clue
  - Intensely enhancing mass on arterial-phase CECT with washout on delayed scan
  - Hypoechoic mass with polar vascularity on US
  - Nuclear scintigraphy shows focal uptake of sestamibi or thallium
- Location
  - Upper parathyroid glands
    - Posterior to upper to midpole of thyroid
    - Rarely posterior to pharynx or esophagus
  - Lower parathyroid glands
    - 65% at inferior thyroid, lateral to lower pole
    - **35%** lower parathyroids **ectopic**, from angle of mandible to lower anterior mediastinum
  - Ectopic locations
    - Hyoid, carotid sheath, mediastinum, intrathyroid
- Size
  - Adenoma typically 1-3 cm in size
    - Normal gland 5 x 3 x 1 mm
    - Gland weight estimated by formula: Length (mm) x width (mm) x height (mm) x π/6
      - □ Correlates well with gland weight at surgery
      - □ Gland weight > 50 g predicts PT Ad
- Morphology
  - Round or oval, well-circumscribed, solid mass
  - Usually homogeneous, but cystic degeneration & hemorrhage may occur
  - Larger cystic PT Ad accounts for 0.5-1.0%, better evaluated by multiphase CT than (99m) Tc-SPECT
- May be incidentally seen on (chest/neck) imaging studies done for other reasons
  - Reporting & indicating correlation for PTH levels may allow earlier identification & potentially ↓ morbidity

CT Findings

- CECT
  - Parathyroid protocol best accomplished using **multiphase CT** having minimum early **arterial-** (CTA) + delayed-phase (venous) CT (2D multiphase)
    - Additional phases include NECT (3D) ± late delayed scan (4D multiphase)
      - □ NECT distinguishes low-density parathyroid tissue from normally radiodense thyroid
      - □ Optional 2nd delayed scan (4D multiphase) helps identify PT Ad having late washout
  - PT Ad mimics lymph node on delayed/venous CECT
  - **Early intense enhancement > > lymph node** (30 seconds post injection)
    - Washout on delayed (90-second) CECT
    - ± central low-density or cystic change
  - Classic enhancement pattern only seen in 20%
  - Dual-energy NECT useful in hypodense thyroids
    - 40 KeV virtual monoenergetic images accentuate contrast of thyroid to parathyroid lesions

MR Findings

- T1WI
  - Iso- to hypointense compared to thyroid
- T2WI
  - Iso- to hyperintense compared to thyroid
- T1WI C+
  - Typically avid enhancement
  - Multiphase (4D) enhanced MR has good localization ability while eliminating radiation dose

Ultrasonographic Findings

- Grayscale ultrasound
  - Operator experience important
  - Common 1st-line localization modality
    - Best for localizing perithyroid PT Ad
  - Homogeneous, well-defined, **hypoechoic** solid mass
  - Look for polar artery &/or trace inferior thyroid artery
  - Typically adjacent to thyroid gland, medial to carotid
  - Limited for ectopic or retrovisceral & mediastinal PT Ad
- Color Doppler
  - Usually **hypervascular**, especially polar

Nuclear Medicine Findings

- **Tc-99m sestamibi alone**
  - Primary localizing modality at some centers
  - Similar sensitivity/specificity compared to US
  - Rapid washout from thyroid, retention in parathyroids
  - Focal ↑ uptake on early & **delayed** images
  - Lower sensitivity for cystic adenomas compared to CT
- **Subtraction techniques**
  - Tl-201/Tc-99m pertechnetate
  - Tc-99m sestamibi/I-123
  - Tc-99m sestamibi/Tc-99m pertechnetate
  - Helpful technique if multinodular goiter, thyroid masses

Imaging Recommendations

- Best imaging tool
  - Multiphase CT (or, less often, MR) evolving as 1st-line modality at some centers vs. 2nd line for discordant localization &/or postoperative neck at others
    - Advantages: Anatomy, ectopia, multigland disease
  - US good for perithyroid PT Ad in experienced hands
  - Tc-99m sestamibi scintigraphy has good sensitivity (> 90%) & specificity (> 90%)
    - Useful for ectopic glands
- Protocol advice
  - **Multiphase CECT** evolving as primary modality
  - **US vs. scintigraphy still 1st exam at some centers**
  - **US** complimentary to scintigraphy or multiphase CT
    - Excellent for **perithyroid location** adenoma
    - Limited in mediastinum & postoperative neck
    - Operator experience is important
- Goal of imaging is **localization**
  - Allows lower risk, minimally invasive procedure
  - Identifying > 1 PT Ad important for surgical planning

DIFFERENTIAL DIAGNOSIS

Reactive Lymph Nodes

- Paratracheal node in tracheoesophageal (TE) groove
- Low density on arterial-phase CECT
- No hypervascular appearance or polar artery

Thyroid Adenoma

- May be exophytic, extend to TE groove
- US, CT, & MR may misinterpret
- Intrathyroid PT Ad misinterpreted as thyroid adenoma

Multinodular Goiter

- Retained sestamibi in hypermetabolic thyroid disease → false-positive
- Exophytic nodules mimic PT Ad

Parathyroid Cyst in Visceral Space

- Cystic lesion in parathyroid location

Parathyroid Carcinoma

- Invasive mass in parathyroid location
- Poorly enhancing, unlike most PT Ad

PATHOLOGY

General Features

- Normal parathyroid distribution
  - 83% of patients have 2 superior & 2 inferior glands
  - 13% of patients have > 4 glands, ~ 3% have only 3 glands
- Relationship of parathyroids to recurrent laryngeal nerve (RLN) approximated by TE groove plane on cross-sectional CT/MR
- Superior parathyroid glands
  - Arise from 4th branchial pouch with thyroid
  - Short descent, close to thyroid, relatively fixed
  - Posterior to plane of RLN
- Inferior parathyroid glands
  - Arise from 3rd branchial pouch with thymus
  - Long descent results in more variable position
  - **35% ectopic**, along thymopharyngeal duct course
    - Locations: Anterior to plane of RLN
    - Perihyoid, carotid sheath, intrathyroid, intrathymic, & mediastinal
- Imaging search pattern based on this embryology

Gross Pathologic & Surgical Features

- Lobulated mass with glistening capsule
- Occasional calcification, cystic or fatty degeneration

Microscopic Features

- Hypercellularity of chief cells with follicular architecture

CLINICAL ISSUES

Presentation

- Most common signs/symptoms
  - Most patients have asymptomatic hypercalcemia
- Other signs/symptoms
  - **Hypercalcemia** may have wide range of symptoms
    - Bone pain related to osseous demineralization
    - Abdominal pain from renal calculi, constipation, peptic ulcer disease, pancreatitis
    - Lethargy, depression, less often, psychosis
      - □ **"Stones, bones, groans, & psychic moans"**

Demographics

- Age
  - Adults; not pediatric neoplasm
- Sex
  - F > M (3:1)
- Epidemiology
  - Primary hyperparathyroidism: 1 in 700 adults
    - 75-85% PT Ad
    - 10-15% parathyroid hyperplasia
    - 2-3% multiple PT Ad
    - < 1% parathyroid carcinoma
  - Secondary hyperparathyroidism
    - More common; from chronic renal failure
  - Associations
    - Multiple endocrine neoplasia (MEN) types 1, 2A, & 4

Natural History & Prognosis

- Surgical excision curative

Treatment

- Surgical excision
  - Bilateral neck exploration before minimally invasive era
  - Minimally invasive era allows unilateral targeted surgery
    - ↓ morbidity, improved success rates
- Minimally invasive parathyroidectomy candidates are those with clearly localizing preoperative imaging
  - Intraoperative serum PTH drop > 50% confirmatory
  - Intraoperative US can also be used to confirm

DIAGNOSTIC CHECKLIST

Consider

- Preferred modality choice controversial
  - Work with your local surgeon; fewer complications, higher success rates using preoperative imaging
  - **Imaging required** if **persistent or recurrent postoperative disease** & with **ectopic PT Ad**
- Reporting incidental PT Ad may ↓ long-term morbidity

Image Interpretation Pearls

- Paratracheal lymph node, protruding esophagus, or exophytic thyroid mass may mimic PT Ad
- Cross correlate available studies: Scintigraphy/US/CT/MR

Reporting Tips

- Report PT Ad location in relation to TE groove & cricoid
- Report PT Ad candidates with relative confidence level
- Note any aberrant subclavian artery (higher risk for non-RLN injury)

SELECTED REFERENCES

1. Bunch PM et al: Opportunistic assessment for parathyroid adenoma on CT: a retrospective cohort study evaluating primary hyperparathyroidism-associated morbidity over 10 years of follow-up. AJR Am J Roentgenol. 1-12, 2025
2. Daoud A et al: Parathyroid cystic adenoma: a systematic review and meta-analysis. Endocr Pract. 29(1):2-10, 2023
3. Gulati S et al: Multi-modality parathyroid imaging: a shifting paradigm. World J Radiol. 15(3):69-82, 2023
4. Kelly HR et al: Parathyroid computed tomography: pearls, pitfalls, and our approach. Neuroimaging Clin N Am. 32(2):413-31, 2022

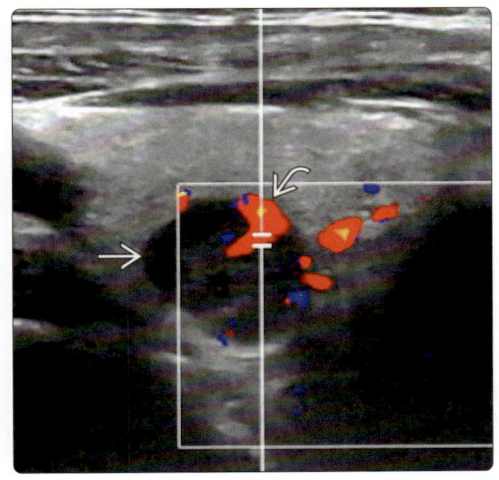

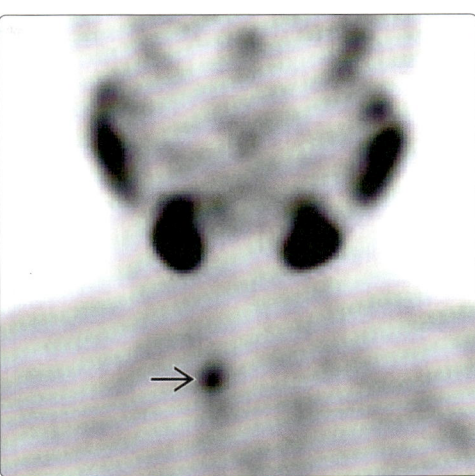

(Left) *Longitudinal color Doppler ultrasound shows a hypoechoic PT Ad* ➡ *posterior to the thyroid gland. Note the associated peripheral increased vascularity* ➡. *A low-resistance waveform was present (not shown). A polar artery sign or tracing the inferior thyroid artery can be helpful to identify a PT Ad.* **(Right)** *Anterior delayed Tc-99m sestamibi scan demonstrates uptake in the inferior right thyroid region* ➡, *compatible with a PT Ad.*

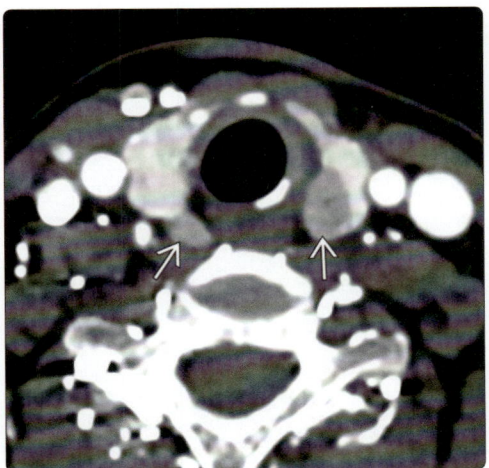

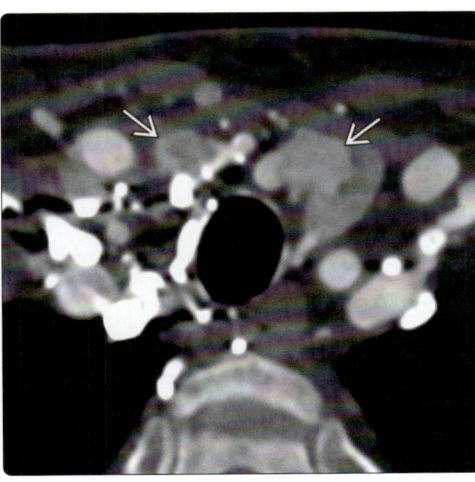

(Left) *Axial arterial-phase CECT shows 2 of this patient's 4 enlarged parathyroid glands* ➡ *due to end-stage renal disease and multigland hyperplasia. This allows the surgeon to develop an appropriate surgical plan with bilateral neck exploration.* **(Right)** *Axial arterial-phase CECT in the same patient shows bilateral, enlarged inferior parathyroid glands* ➡ *anterior to the tracheoesophageal grooves and inferior to the thyroid gland due to multigland hyperplasia.*

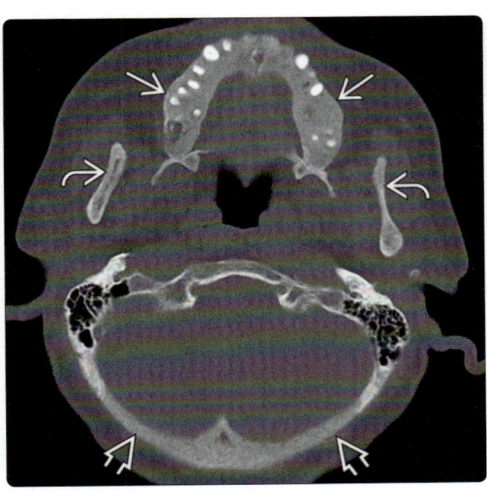

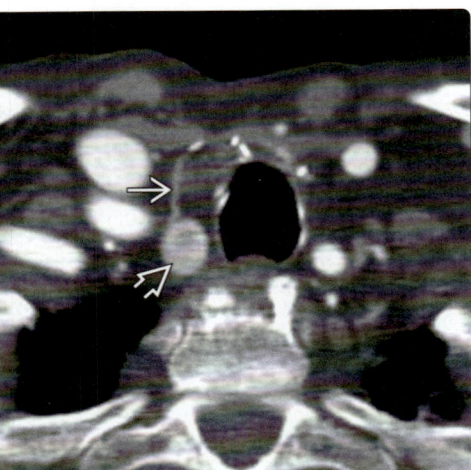

(Left) *Axial bone CT in the same patient shows bony thickening and sclerosis of the maxilla* ➡ *and mandible* ➡. *The skull base* ➡ *demonstrates a classic salt and pepper appearance characteristic of renal osteodystrophy.* **(Right)** *Axial arterial-phase CECT demonstrates a typical "polar artery"* ➡ *supplying a PT Ad* ➡ *inferior to the thyroid gland in the upper mediastinal fat.*

Differentiated Thyroid Carcinoma

TERMINOLOGY

- 2 types of differentiated thyroid carcinoma (DTCa): **Papillary** (more common) and **follicular** carcinoma

IMAGING

- Most often focal thyroid mass ± extracapsular invasion
  - Rarely in ectopic thyroid, thyroglossal duct cyst
  - Microcalcifications suggest papillary carcinoma
- ± metastatic lymph nodes
  - **Cystic** or solid, small or large, ± **calcification**
- US is best modality for initial evaluation and biopsy
  - Concerning US features: Hypoechoic, ill defined, microcalcification, taller than wide, hypervascular
- CT/MR is useful for staging and surveillance
- MR: Intrinsic T1 signal of tumor and lymph nodes due to thyroglobulin &/or hemorrhage
- I-131 diagnostic for recurrence &/or metastasis
  - Can be dosed for treatment of recurrence

TOP DIFFERENTIAL DIAGNOSES

- Thyroid colloid cyst
- Thyroid follicular adenoma
- Multinodular goiter
- Thyroid medullary carcinoma
- Thyroid anaplastic carcinoma
- Thyroid non-Hodgkin lymphoma

PATHOLOGY

- **Papillary** tends to have **nodal** spread
- **Follicular** tends to have **hematogenous** spread

CLINICAL ISSUES

- **Do not give iodinated contrast if suspected DTCa**
  - Delays I-131 therapy by 3-4 months
- 3x more common in women; peaks in 3rd and 4th decades
- 5-year survival: Stages I and II > 90%, stage IV 40%
- **Rising serum thyroglobulin** is indicator of recurrence

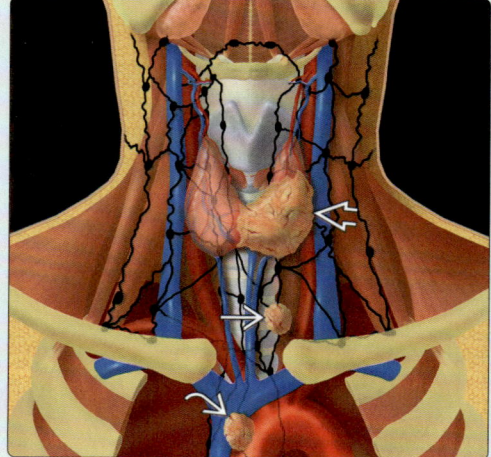
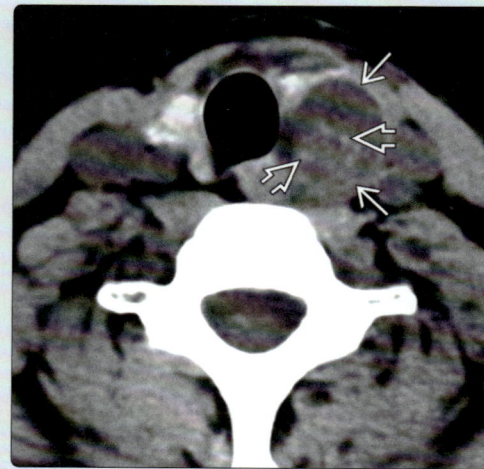

(Left) Coronal graphic illustrates a left thyroid lobe differentiated thyroid carcinoma (DTCa) primary tumor ➡ with metastatic nodal disease in the left paratracheal chain ➡ and superior mediastinum ➡. (Right) Axial NECT shows a well-defined mass ➡ arising from the left thyroid lobe with fine, speckled microcalcifications ➡ centrally. Small calcifications such as these are a suspicious finding for DTCa and especially papillary carcinoma. Intrathyroid tumor is < 4 cm = T2.

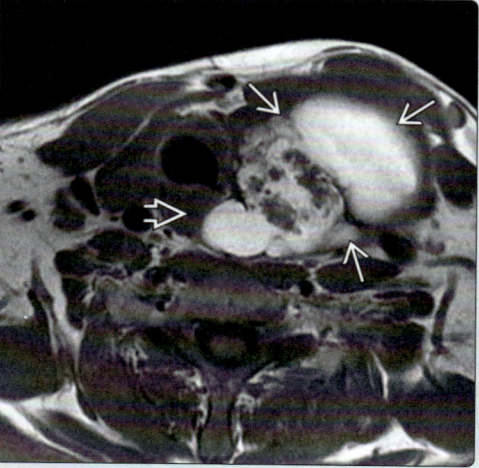
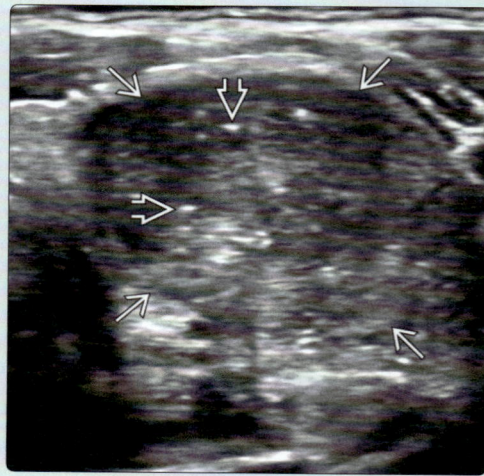

(Left) Axial T1 MR in a 49-year-old man with an enlarging neck mass shows a heterogeneous solid and cystic mass arising in the left thyroid lobe ➡, displacing the esophagus ➡. Note the intrinsic T1 hyperintensity from thyroglobulin. This feature is also present in multiple nodes. Tumor was determined to be papillary thyroid carcinoma. (Right) Longitudinal thyroid US reveals a well-defined mass ➡ with multiple tiny, hyperechoic microcalcifications ➡, found to be a papillary carcinoma.

Differentiated Thyroid Carcinoma

TERMINOLOGY

Abbreviations
- Differentiated thyroid carcinoma (DTCa)

Definitions
- Malignancy arising from epithelial thyroid cells with well-defined histology
- 2 types: **Papillary** or **follicular** with multiple variants

IMAGING

General Features
- Best diagnostic clue
  - Focal intrathyroidal mass ± extracapsular invasion
    - Microcalcifications suggest papillary carcinoma
  - ± metastatic lymph nodes with calcifications
- Location
  - Primary tumor arises within thyroid gland
    - Rarely ectopic thyroid, thyroglossal duct cyst wall
  - Nodal metastases, most often levels VI, IV, and VII
    - Any level possible; check retropharyngeal nodes
- Size
  - Variable: From lesion of several millimeters found at thyroidectomy to tumor replacing whole lobe
- Morphology
  - Variable: Well-defined, solid mass mimicking benign lesion, or heterogeneous, invasive mass

CT Findings
- CECT
  - Role of CECT to evaluate advanced **stage** or **surveillance**
    - If CT for initial/suspected DTCa, do **not** give contrast
  - Primary tumor findings highly variable in thyroid
    - Single or multiple nodules or diffuse infiltration
    - Small to large, well circumscribed to ill defined
    - Heterogeneous, invasive mass: Solid, cystic or mixed
    - ± calcifications; typically tiny, fine, speckled
  - Lymph node findings highly variable, often bilateral
    - Small, solid, reactive-appearing but rounded
    - Large, heterogeneous, high-density cystic nodes
    - Focal calcification may be seen in solid nodes

MR Findings
- Variable
  - T1-hyperintense signal reflects thyroglobulin (Tg) &/or hemorrhage (methemoglobin)
- Primary tumor: Intrathyroidal mass; focal, multinodular, or diffusely infiltrating
  - Typically heterogeneous signal and enhancement
  - Good for extrathyroid extension, especially tracheal
- Nodes: Small, round, solid to large, cystic or mixed
  - Cystic nodes may be **T1 and T2 hyperintense**
  - DWI: Low ADC suggests malignancy/metastases

Ultrasonographic Findings
- Grayscale ultrasound
  - May exactly mimic benign adenoma
  - Findings suggesting malignancy: Hypoechoic, ill-defined margins, microcalcifications, taller-than-wide shape
- Color Doppler
  - **High vascularity** suggests malignancy

Nuclear Medicine Findings
- I-131 scintigraphy
  - Diagnostic scan 4-6 weeks following thyroidectomy
  - If thyroid remnant or metastasis detected, ↑ ablative dose of I-131 administered
- FDG PET/CT
  - Not useful for DTCa, which is I-131 avid
    - Useful in I-131-negative (dedifferentiated) disease
- Tc-99m pertechnetate or I-123 no longer used

Imaging Recommendations
- Best imaging tool
  - US is best for initial lesion characterization (solid vs. cystic), biopsy guidance, and surveillance
  - Cross-sectional imaging used to stage large thyroid tumors (MR preferred over CECT/NECT)
- Protocol advice
  - **Do not give iodinated contrast if initial/suspect DTCa**
    - Contrast delays I-131 therapy for 3-4 months
      - Contrast iodine is taken up by DTCa instead of I-131
  - Cross-sectional imaging must include **superior mediastinal nodes** for complete evaluation
  - If incidental thyroid nodule found on CT/MR, recommended further evaluation with US if
    - ≥ 1-cm diameter (age < 35 years)
    - ≥ 1.5-cm diameter (age ≥ 35 years)
  - If thyroid nodule with clear malignant features (i.e., extracapsular spread) seen on any modality, go directly to image-guided biopsy
  - For detection of recurrent disease
    - I-131 scan ± US
    - FDG PET/CT if ↑ serum Tg but negative I-131 scan

DIFFERENTIAL DIAGNOSIS

Thyroid Colloid Cyst
- Simple cyst; may be hemorrhagic
- US clarifies cystic nature of lesion

Thyroid Follicular Adenoma
- Solitary thyroid mass without local invasion or adenopathy

Multinodular Goiter
- Multiple nodules in enlarged thyroid, no adenopathy

Thyroid Medullary Carcinoma
- May exactly mimic DTCa when imaged

Thyroid Anaplastic Carcinoma
- Rapidly enlarging, invasive, heterogeneous thyroid mass
- Necrotic lymphadenopathy; older patients

Thyroid Non-Hodgkin Lymphoma
- Rapidly enlarging, invasive, homogeneous thyroid mass
- Associated lymphadenopathy; rarely necrotic

PATHOLOGY

General Features
- Etiology
  - Most often sporadic but associated with radiation
  - DTCa arises from endodermally derived follicular cells that are TSH sensitive

Differentiated Thyroid Carcinoma Staging (AJCC 2017)

Patient < 55 Years of Age	Patient > 55 Years of Age
Stage I	**Stage I**
Any T, any N, M0	T1/T2N0M0
Stage II	**Stage II**
Any T, any N, M1	T1/T2N1M0
	T3a/T3b (any N, if M0)
	Stage III
	T4a (any N, if M0)
	Stage IV
	IVA: T4b (any N, if M0)
	IVB: M1 (any T, any N)

Adapted from Amin MB et al: AJCC Cancer Staging Manual. 8th ed. Springer, 2017.

Staging, Grading, & Classification

- **American Joint Committee on Cancer (AJCC) 8th edition (2017)**
  - Primary tumor (T)
    - T1a: Intrathyroidal **≤ 1 cm**; T1b: **> 1 cm and ≤ 2 cm**
    - T2: Intrathyroidal **> 2 cm and ≤ 4 cm**
    - T3a: Tumor **> 4 cm**, limited to thyroid
    - T3b: Tumor any size with gross extrathyroidal extension invading only **strap muscles**
    - T4a: **Marked extrathyroid extension**
      - □ Invades larynx, trachea, esophagus, recurrent laryngeal nerve, subcutaneous tissue
    - T4b: **Very advanced disease**
      - □ Invades prevertebral fascia, surrounds carotid or mediastinal vessels
  - Regional lymph nodes (N)
    - N1a: Level VI (pretracheal, paratracheal, prelaryngeal nodes) and VII (upper mediastinal)
    - N1b: Any other cervical nodes
- **Overall staging (AJCC 2017) reflects patient age**

Microscopic Features

- ± calcification, necrosis, fibrosis, cysts, and hemorrhage
- 50% of papillary carcinoma have calcific psammoma bodies
- Follicular carcinoma has Hürthle cell variant

CLINICAL ISSUES

Presentation

- Most common signs/symptoms
  - Painless, palpable, solitary thyroid nodule
- Other signs/symptoms
  - May present with neck mass from metastatic nodes
  - Rapidly growing thyroid mass, hoarseness
- Clinical profile
  - Female patient with firm thyroid nodule

Demographics

- Age
  - Peak incidence in 3rd and 4th decades
- Sex
  - M:F = 1:3
- Epidemiology

  - Thyroid tumors: Papillary 80%, follicular 10%, medullary 7%, anaplastic 2%, non-Hodgkin lymphoma 1%

Natural History & Prognosis

- Patterns of spread
  - Local invasion of adjacent structures (T3-T4)
  - **Nodes: 50% papillary**, 10% follicular at presentation
    - Paratracheal, deep cervical, spinal accessory, retropharyngeal, superior mediastinal
  - Distant spread: 20% follicular, ≤ 10% papillary
    - Typically hematogenously to lungs, bones, and brain
- Overall good prognosis
  - 5-year survival rate: Stages I and II > 90%, stage IV 40%
  - **Follicular** worse prognosis than papillary
  - **Tall cell variant of papillary** much worse prognosis
- DTCa high likelihood of recurrence, treated with I-131
  - **Rising serum Tg** indicates recurrence

Treatment

- Management of DTCa after diagnosis
  - Total thyroidectomy with central compartment nodal dissection
    - Selective neck dissection for other nodal metastases
    - I-131 scintigraphy to diagnose and treat/ablate recurrent or metastatic disease
    - False-negative diagnostic I-131 possible if tumor dedifferentiates; use PET/CT in this circumstance

DIAGNOSTIC CHECKLIST

Image Interpretation Pearls

- Suspect DTCa when
  - Thyroid mass with calcifications in **young female patient**
  - **Cystic** or mixed cystic/solid neck nodes
  - **Calcified** (CT) or **T1-hyperintense** (MR) nodes

SELECTED REFERENCES

1. Chua WM et al: Differentiated thyroid cancer after thyroidectomy. Radiographics. 44(10):e240021, 2024
2. Fang S et al: Effects of iodinated contrast-enhanced CT on urinary iodine levels in postoperative patients with differentiated thyroid cancer. Curr Med Imaging. 20:e15734056287560, 2024
3. Javid M et al: The evolving role of MRI in the detection of extrathyroidal extension of papillary thyroid carcinoma: a systematic review and meta-analysis. BMC Cancer. 24(1):1531, 2024

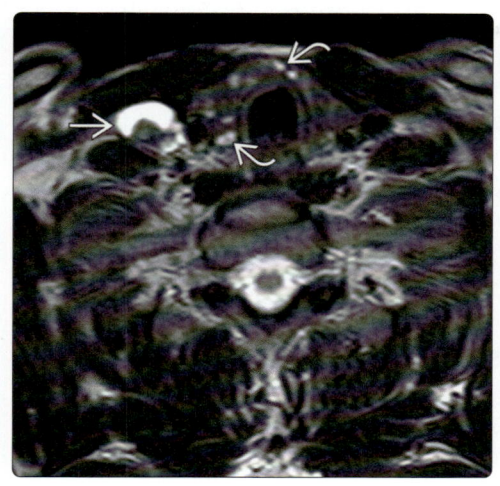
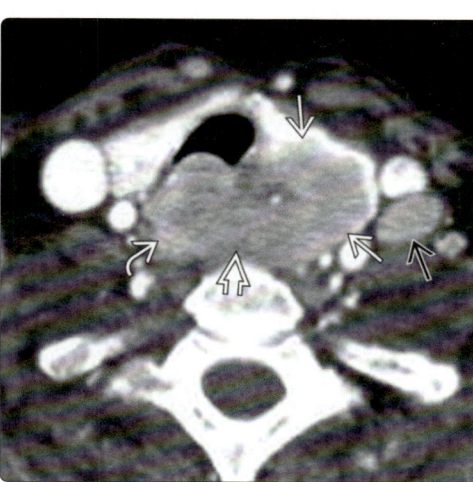

(Left) *Axial T2 MR shows a mixed cystic and solid metastatic lymph node ➡. Multiple small, hyperintense nodules ➡ throughout the thyroid gland are not specific by MR. Surgery confirmed metastatic thyroid cancer with multiple foci of papillary thyroid carcinoma found in both thyroid lobes.* (Right) *Axial CECT in a patient with left vocal cord paralysis due to a papillary thyroid carcinoma ➡ invading the tracheoesophageal groove ➡ is shown. Tumor is inseparable from the esophagus ➡. Note associated adenopathy ➡.*

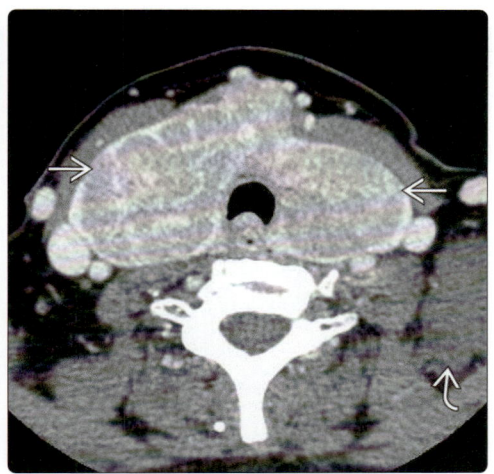
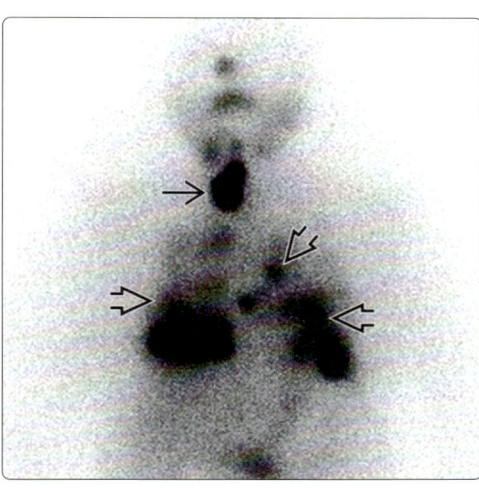

(Left) *Axial CECT shows an enlarged, hypodense thyroid ➡. This patient presented with a spinal metastasis due to this large Hürthle cell carcinoma, a variant of follicular thyroid cancer. A left axillary mass ➡ was an incidental venous malformation.* (Right) *AP projection from a diagnostic I-131 scan in a patient with thyroid follicular carcinoma shows a large area of uptake in the thyroid bed ➡ as well as extensive areas of uptake throughout both lungs ➡.*

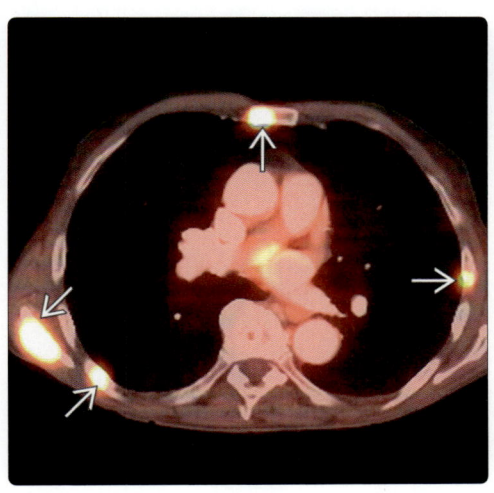
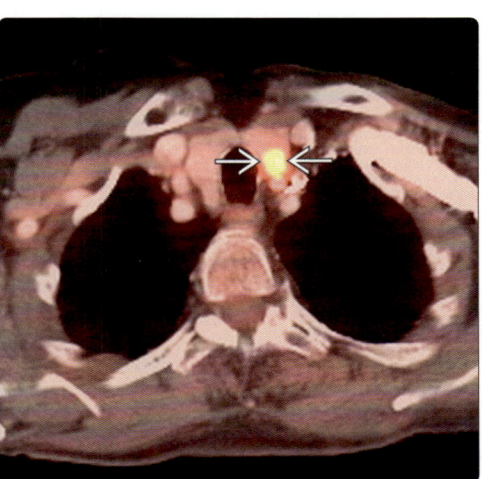

(Left) *Axial FDG PET/CT reveals numerous bone metastases ➡ from follicular thyroid carcinoma. While papillary carcinoma prefers nodal spread, follicular carcinoma is more prone to hematogenous metastases to bone or lung.* (Right) *Axial PET/CT performed for staging of pharyngeal squamous cell carcinoma reveals incidental high uptake in the left thyroid ➡. Diffuse thyroid uptake is usually benign; focal uptake is associated with malignancy in 20% of cases, so incidental masses must be biopsied. This was found to be DTCa.*

TERMINOLOGY

- Medullary thyroid carcinoma (MTC)
- Rare neuroendocrine malignancy arising from thyroid parafollicular C cells that produce calcitonin

IMAGING

- IV iodine is okay to use (not contraindicated for MTC)
- CT/MR: Heterogeneous, well-circumscribed thyroid mass
- Consider familial syndromes if younger patient with multifocal &/or infiltrative tumors
- Most have similar-appearing nodal metastases
  - ± Ca⁺⁺ in tumor &/or nodes
  - Nodal metastasis: Levels VI and VII most common
- Ultrasound best initial test
  - Hypoechoic, irregular mass with hypervascularity
  - Can FNA/biopsy concurrently
- Ga-68 or Cu64-DOTATATE PET for metastatic disease
  - Not reliably FDG avid on FDG PET

TOP DIFFERENTIAL DIAGNOSES

- Multinodular goiter
- Thyroid differentiated carcinoma
- Thyroid non-Hodgkin lymphoma
- Thyroid adenoma

PATHOLOGY

- Type 2 multiple endocrine neoplasia (MEN) syndromes
  - MEN2B: Younger, more aggressive disease
- Familial MTC
  - Later onset, more indolent course than MEN
- Associated with mutations of *RET* protooncogene

CLINICAL ISSUES

- Most MTC sporadic; 15-25% MTC inherited
- Serum calcitonin and CEA usually elevated
- Treatment primarily surgical ± XRT
- Prophylactic thyroidectomy if high-risk *RET* mutation
- Molecularly targeted therapies if progressive

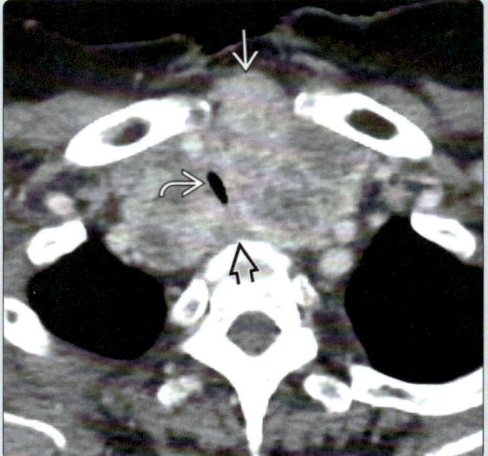
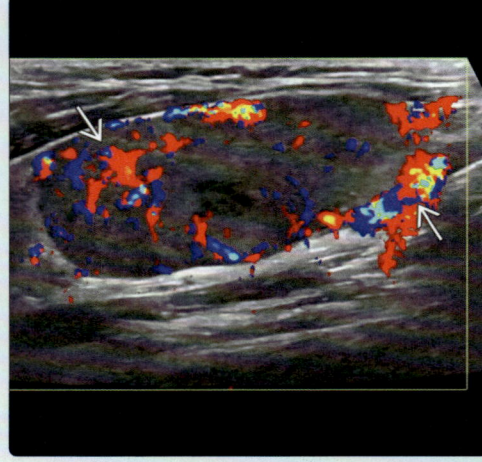

(Left) *Axial CECT shows a heterogeneous, large medullary thyroid carcinoma (MTC) with extrathyroidal extension into the suprasternal notch ➡ narrowing the tracheal airway ➡. Tumor extends into both tracheoesophageal grooves, inseparable from the esophagus ➡.* (Right) *Longitudinal color Doppler ultrasound shows marked increased vascularity within a solid, heterogeneous mass due to metastatic adenopathy ➡ from MTC.*

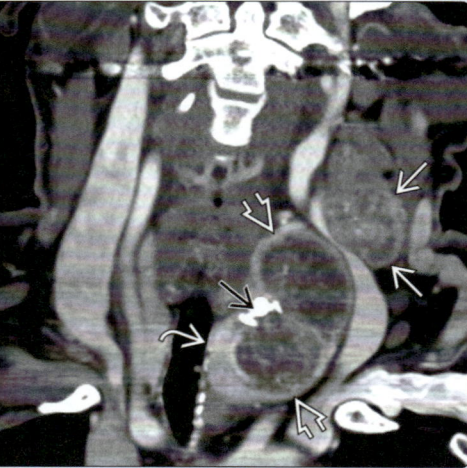
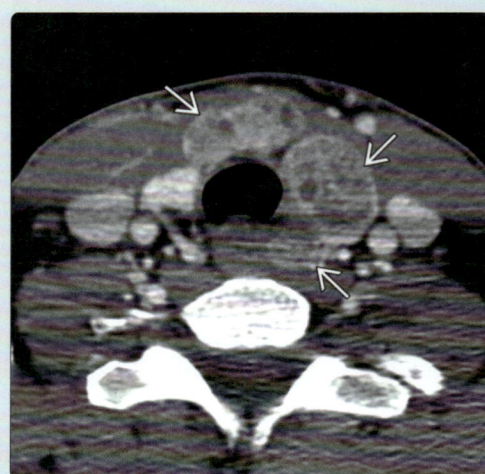

(Left) *Coronal CECT shows a heterogeneous but well-defined thyroid mass ➡ with coarse Ca⁺⁺ ➡ and ipsilateral, similarly heterogeneous, adenopathy ➡. At surgery, tumor was found to have an infiltrated tracheal wall ➡.* (Right) *Axial CECT shows multiple left thyroid and isthmus lesions ➡, found to be multifocal MTC. The lesions are all similarly heterogeneous but well defined and not calcified. Iodinated contrast is not contraindicated with MTC.*

TERMINOLOGY

Abbreviations

- Medullary thyroid carcinoma (MTC)

Synonyms

- Thyroid neuroendocrine carcinoma

Definitions

- Rare neuroendocrine malignancy arising from thyroid parafollicular C cells that produce calcitonin
- Inherited forms of MTC: Multiple endocrine neoplasia (MEN) syndromes, familial MTC (FMTC)

IMAGING

General Features

- Best diagnostic clue
  - Solid lesion in thyroid with ipsilateral nodal metastases
- Location
  - Within thyroid gland
  - Nodal metastasis: Level VI and superior mediastinum
    - Less common: Levels III and IV, and retropharyngeal
- Size
  - 2-25 mm; < 1 cm considered microcarcinoma
  - May be multifocal, particularly inherited forms
- Morphology
  - Solid, usually well-circumscribed mass
  - **Infiltrative variant seen with familial forms**

CT Findings

- CECT
  - Low-density, heterogeneous, circumscribed mass
    - Or multifocal masses (especially with inherited forms)
  - ± fine or coarse Ca++
    - Ca++ in MTC are characteristic of MEN2
    - Fine Ca++ suggests papillary thyroid carcinoma (PTC)
  - Nodal metastases are typically solid ± Ca++

MR Findings

- Usually well-defined mass with ipsilateral nodes
  - May see irregular margins and extraglandular extension
- Nodes solid; less often cystic or T1 hyperintense like PTC

Ultrasonographic Findings

- Grayscale: Hypoechoic, irregular intrathyroidal mass
- Color Doppler: Hypervascularity with irregular arrangement of vessels

Nuclear Medicine Findings

- **Ga-68 DOTATATE PET**
  - Uptake in somatostatin receptor (SSR)-positive disease
    - Neuroendocrine tumors, including MTC, express SSR
  - Highly accurate for detection and metastasis evaluation
  - Similar uptake Cu-64 DOTATATE in MTC, but Cu-64 (newer agent) may have better spatial resolution
- **FDG PET**
  - MTC **not reliably FDG avid**; frequent false-negatives
- **F-18 DOPA PET**
  - Best for MTC recurrence among PET radiotracers
- **I-131 MIBG**
  - Allows whole-body imaging for metastases

Imaging Recommendations

- Best imaging tool
  - US usual initial evaluation of thyroid nodule
    - Fine-needle aspiration (FNA) can be performed at same time
    - Core biopsy preferable due to higher sensitivity
  - CECT required for thorough evaluation of neck and mediastinum for nodes
  - Ga-68 or 64Cu-DOTATATE PET for evaluation of metastasis and recurrence
- Protocol advice
  - CECT extending to carina to evaluate mediastinal nodes
    - Iodinated contrast okay to use for MTC [contraindicated in differentiated thyroid carcinoma (DTCa)]
  - If thyroid nodule with clear malignant features (i.e., extracapsular spread) seen on any modality, go directly to image-guided biopsy

DIFFERENTIAL DIAGNOSIS

Multinodular Goiter

- Enlarged gland with multiple nodules, coarse Ca++
- No neck adenopathy

Thyroid Differentiated Carcinoma

- Most common thyroid tumor
- Solid or cystic nodal metastases

Thyroid Non-Hodgkin Lymphoma

- Diffuse enlargement of gland with infiltrative mass
- Rarely see Ca++ or necrosis

Thyroid Adenoma

- Focal mass without evidence of invasion
- No neck adenopathy

PATHOLOGY

General Features

- Etiology
  - 75-85% of MTCs sporadic
    - No identified exogenous cause
    - Not related to preexisting thyroid conditions
  - 15-25% of MTCs inherited: More often multifocal &/or infiltrative (i.e., MEN and FMTC)
  - **Type 2 MEN syndromes:** inherited autosomal dominant
    - **MEN2A:** Multifocal MTC, pheochromocytoma, parathyroid hyperplasia, hyperparathyroidism
    - **MEN2B:** MEN2A + mucosal neuromas of lips, tongue, gastrointestinal tract, and conjunctiva
      - Younger patients, more aggressive tumors
  - **FMTC:** Inherited autosomal dominant
    - Only neoplasm is MTC
    - Later onset, more indolent course than MEN
- Genetics
  - Associated with mutations of *RET* protooncogene on chromosome 10q11.2
    - 95% of familial and 50% of sporadic cases
    - Screen for *RET* mutations in family of MTC patients

Medullary Thyroid Carcinoma Staging (AJCC 2017)

Tumor Staging (T)	Nodal Staging (N)	Metastases (M)
T1a: Intrathyroidal ≤ 1 cm	**N1a**: Levels VI and VII (pretracheal, paratracheal, prelaryngeal nodes, superior mediastinum)	**M0**: No distant metastasis
T1b: Intrathyroidal > 1 cm and ≤ 2 cm	**N1b**: Any other cervical nodes	**M1**: Distant metastasis
T2: Intrathyroidal > 2 cm and ≤ 4 cm		
T3: Intrathyroidal > 4 cm or minimal extrathyroidal extension		
T4a: Marked extrathyroid extension to larynx, trachea, esophagus, recurrent laryngeal nerve, subcutaneous tissues		
T4b: Invades prevertebral fascia or surrounds carotid or mediastinal vessels		

Adapted from Amin MB et al: AJCC Cancer Staging Manual. 8th ed. Springer, 2017.

Staging, Grading, & Classification

- American Joint Committee on Cancer (AJCC) staging 8th edition (2017)
  - TNM follows that for DTCa
  - **When multifocal tumor, use largest component**

Microscopic Features

- Proliferation of large, atypical round to polygonal cells with granular cytoplasm
- **Stains strongly for calcitoninin in 80%**

CLINICAL ISSUES

Presentation

- Most common signs/symptoms
  - Painless thyroid nodule
  - Less commonly, dysphagia, hoarseness, pain
  - **Elevated serum calcitonin**
    - Used as screening tool for estimation of extent of disease and for posttreatment surveillance
- Other signs/symptoms
  - Diarrhea from elevated calcitonin
  - Paraneoplastic syndromes uncommon: Cushing or carcinoid syndromes
  - Other serum markers may also be elevated
    - CEA, chromogranin A
- Clinical profile
  - Middle-aged patient with low neck mass
  - Family history of MEN with tumor on screening exam

Demographics

- Age
  - Mean: Sporadic = 50 years; inherited = 30 years
  - Pediatric MTC usually inherited, especially MEN2B
- Epidemiology
  - 5-10% of all thyroid gland malignancies
  - 14% of thyroid cancer deaths
  - 10% of pediatric thyroid malignancies (MEN2)

Natural History & Prognosis

- Up to 75% have lymphadenopathy at presentation
- Distant hematogeneous metastasis to lungs, liver, bones
  - Lung metastases frequently miliary, mimics TB
- **Overall 5-year survival = 72%; 10-year = 56%**
- Worse prognosis with certain *RET* genetic mutations
- Indicators of better prognosis
  - Female patients, younger age at surgery
  - FMTC and MEN2A syndromes
  - Tumor < 10 cm, no nodes, early-stage disease
  - Normal preoperative CEA levels, complete resection

Treatment

- Resection of primary tumor and regional nodal disease
  - Total thyroidectomy, level VI ± VII
  - Levels II-V resected if positive lateral neck nodes
- Adjuvant radiation therapy if invasive
- Prophylactic thyroidectomy if familial *RET* mutation (+)
  - FMTC and MEN2A: Thyroidectomy at age 5-6
  - MEN2B: Thyroidectomy during infancy
- Molecularly targeted therapies if progressive

DIAGNOSTIC CHECKLIST

Consider

- Consider familial syndromes if young or multifocal tumor

Image Interpretation Pearls

- Imaging appearance may mimic DTCa, however
  - MTC nodes solid, not often cystic (DTCa more typical cystic with intrinsic T1 hyperintensity)
  - MTC Ca^{++} may be coarser
  - MTC more often multifocal

Reporting Tips

- CT/MR important for detection of nodes/staging
  - Image to carina for superior mediastinum nodes
  - Look for distant metastases

SELECTED REFERENCES

1. Delorme S et al: Medullary thyroid carcinoma: imaging recent results. Cancer Res. 223:129-53, 2025
2. Wang IE et al: Molecular imaging of neuroendocrine tumors: current applications and future trends. Diagn Interv Imaging. ePub, 2025
3. Treglia G et al: Update on management of medullary thyroid carcinoma: focus on nuclear medicine. Semin Nucl Med. 53(4):481-9, 2023
4. Szidonya L et al: Molecular and anatomic imaging of neuroendocrine tumors. Surg Oncol Clin N Am. 31(4):649-71, 2022

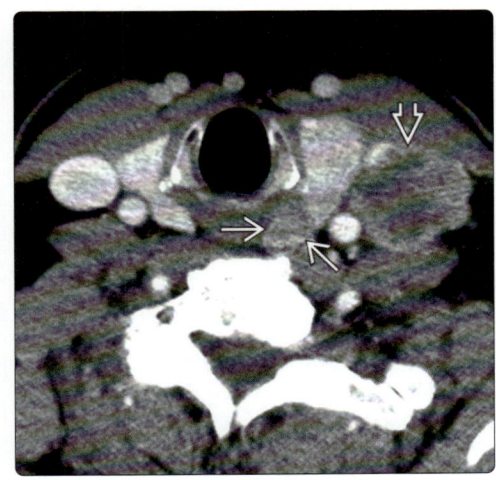
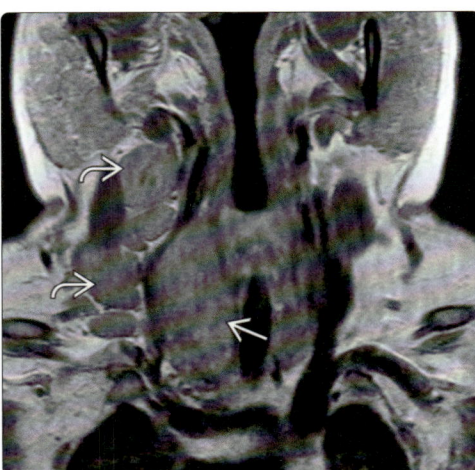

(Left) Axial CECT shows a small left thyroid mass ➡ in the tracheoesophageal groove with heterogeneous ipsilateral adenopathy ➡. This appearance suggests a primary thyroid neoplasm, which is most commonly differentiated carcinoma; however, this was a sporadic form of MTC. (Right) Coronal T1 C+ MR shows an enlarged right thyroid lobe due to MTC ➡. Extensive metastatic right cervical adenopathy ➡ is noted.

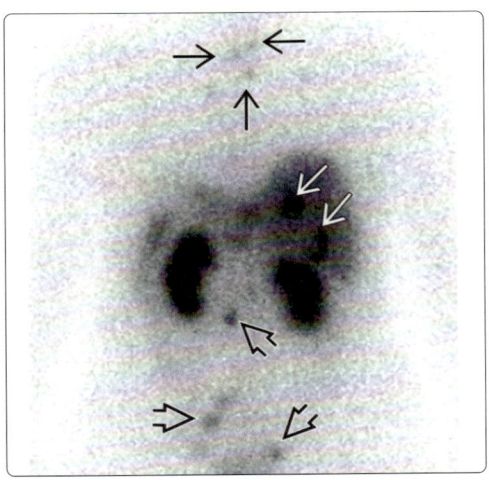
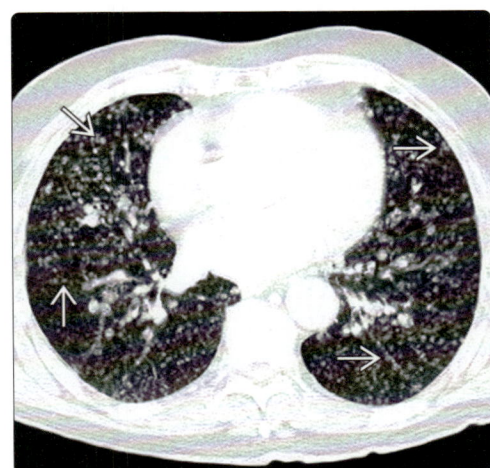

(Left) Posterior view of an octreotide scan shows multifocal medullary uptake within the thyroid bed ➡ from MTC. Multiple foci of uptake within lower spine and sacrum ➡ represent bony metastases, and there are probable liver metastases ➡. (Right) Axial NECT shows innumerable tiny nodules ➡ scattered throughout both lungs. Both MTC and differentiated thyroid carcinoma can produce a miliary pattern of lung metastases that should be distinguished from miliary tuberculosis.

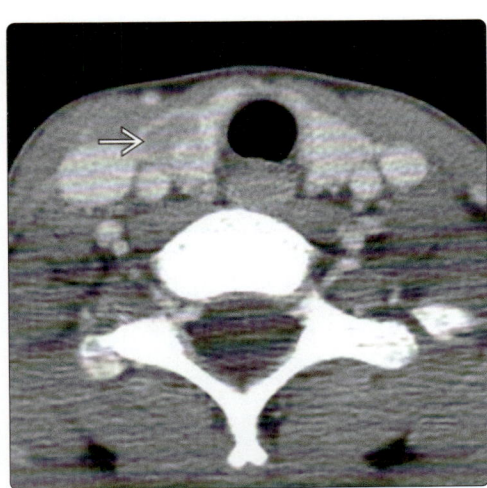
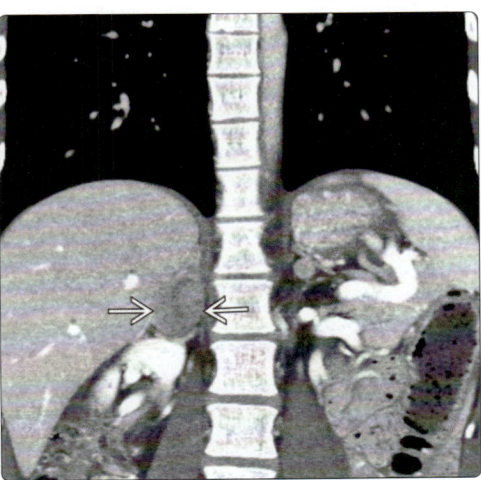

(Left) Axial CECT in a 14-year-old boy with a palpable right thyroid nodule and elevated serum calcitonin of 900 shows a heterogeneously hypodense right thyroid MTC ➡. This patient was found to be positive for the RET protooncogene mutation, and has MEN2B. (Right) Coronal CECT in the same patient shows development of a right adrenal pheochromocytoma ➡, which was surgically resected 18 years after his thyroid cancer.

KEY FACTS

TERMINOLOGY

- Anaplastic thyroid carcinoma (ATCa)
- Synonym: Undifferentiated thyroid tumor
- Often arises from differentiated thyroid carcinoma or multinodular goiter (MNG)

IMAGING

- General findings
  - Large, heterogeneous, infiltrating thyroid mass
  - Necrosis, hemorrhage, calcifications
  - Invades surrounding structures and spaces
  - Common to have nodal metastases at presentation
- CECT for suspected ATCa
  - Iodinated contrast not issue with ATCa
- US: Inadequate for staging purposes
- PET/CT: FDG avid but considered unnecessary tool
- Bone scan: Bone metastases evaluation for staging
- I-123 and I-131 scintigraphy not useful due to lack of iodine concentration

TOP DIFFERENTIAL DIAGNOSES

- Thyroid non-Hodgkin lymphoma
- Thyroid differentiated carcinoma
- Thyroid medullary carcinoma
- MNG
- Thyroid adenoma

PATHOLOGY

- 50% distant metastasis: Lungs, bone, brain
- TNM staging is similar to differentiated thyroid carcinoma
- **ATCa automatically stage IV tumors**

CLINICAL ISSUES

- Rapidly growing, large, painful neck mass
- Tumor of older adults; mean age: 70 years
- Rare thyroid malignancy
- Lethal tumor; mean survival: 6 months
- Aggressive treatment early if possible
- Late presentation typically palliative

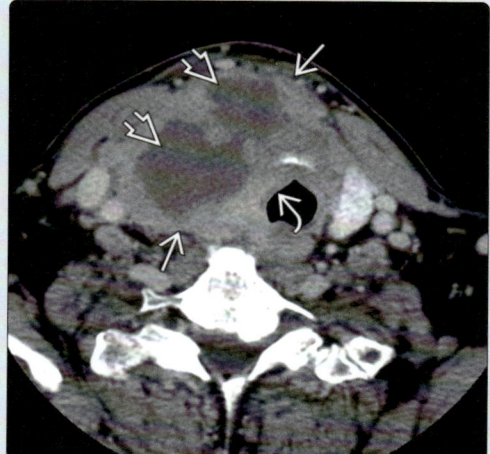
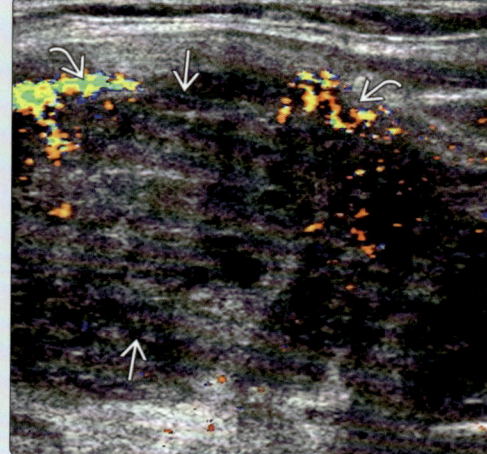

(Left) *Axial CECT demonstrates a large, heterogeneous, predominantly right-sided thyroid mass ➡ with large pools of low-density necrosis ➡. Mass cannot be separated from strap muscles and infiltrates the cricothyroid membrane to tracheal lumen ➡. (Right) Power Doppler US shows the right thyroid lobe appearing completely replaced by a large, heterogeneous, lobulated solid mass ➡ with irregular margins. No internal calcifications are evident; however, color Doppler shows prominent peripheral vascularity ➡.*

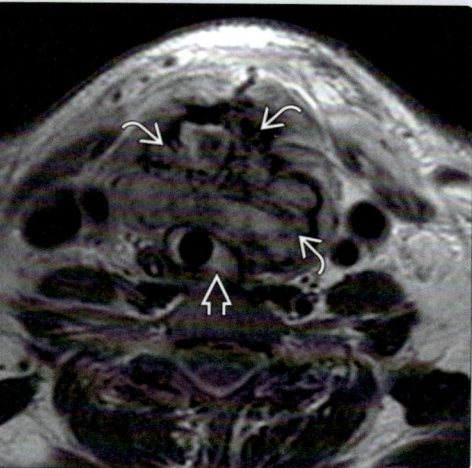
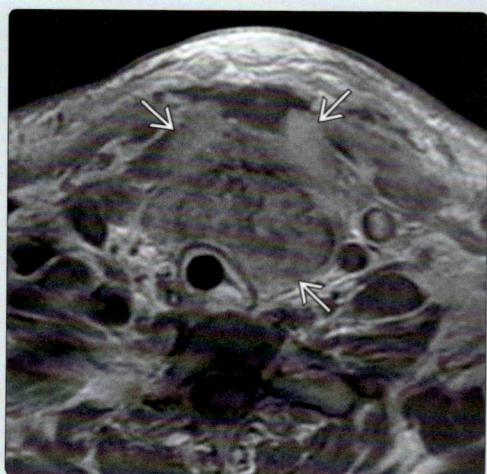

(Left) *Axial T2WI MR in a patient with stridor imaged after tracheostomy shows extensive areas of marked signal loss ➡, suggesting either fibrosis, calcifications (which were not evident on CT), or hemosiderin deposition. T2 signal surrounding tube represents both secretions and infiltrative tumor ➡. (Right) Axial T1WI C+ MR in the same patient illustrates the infiltrative nature of this aggressive, heterogeneously enhancing neoplasm ➡, which involves strap muscles and other extrathyroidal tissues.*

TERMINOLOGY

Abbreviations

- Anaplastic thyroid carcinoma (ATCa)

Synonyms

- Undifferentiated thyroid carcinoma

Definitions

- Aggressive, lethal thyroid malignancy
  - Arises from differentiated thyroid carcinoma (DTCa), multinodular goiter (MNG), or de novo

IMAGING

General Features

- Best diagnostic clue
  - Older adult woman with rapidly growing, heterogeneous, invasive mass arising from thyroid
- Location
  - Begins in thyroid gland but frequently transspatial
- Size
  - Typically > 5 cm at presentation
- Morphology
  - Large, heterogeneous, infiltrating thyroid mass

CT Findings

- CECT
  - Heterogeneous, diffusely infiltrating mass
    - Up to 75% have necrosis and hemorrhage
    - Many demonstrate calcifications; typically dense, amorphous
      - □ Probably from underlying MNG
  - Invades adjacent infrahyoid neck spaces
    - Larynx, trachea, recurrent laryngeal nerve, esophagus
  - Cervical lymphadenopathy very common
    - Up to 50% of metastatic nodes are necrotic

MR Findings

- T1WI
  - Heterogeneous invasive tumor with adenopathy
  - Hemorrhage, necrosis, and calcification may result in heterogeneous mixed signal
- T2WI
  - Variable, typically diffuse iso- to hyperintense
  - May have intratumoral ring-shaped hypointensity
- T1WI C+
  - Heterogeneous enhancement
  - Ill-defined margins with regional invasion
    - Extrathyroidal extension, venous thrombosis, tracheal, esophageal, and vascular invasion, and venous thrombosis all more common than with DTCa

Ultrasonographic Findings

- Grayscale ultrasound
  - Poorly defined, invasive, hypoechoic thyroid mass

Nuclear Medicine Findings

- Bone scan
  - Initial staging for bone metastases
- PET/CT
  - High FDG avidity

- No benefit for staging over CT/MR
- I-123 and I-131 scintigraphy
  - Not used in evaluation or treatment of ATCa
  - Does **not** concentrate iodine because of highly undifferentiated cells

Imaging Recommendations

- Best imaging tool
  - If ATCa diagnosis suspected, then CECT adequate
  - When diagnosis unknown, MR of neck and mediastinum is exam of choice for staging
- Protocol advice
  - Image down to carina for nodal metastases
  - Iodinated contrast is not contraindicated with anaplastic carcinoma

DIFFERENTIAL DIAGNOSIS

Thyroid Non-Hodgkin Lymphoma

- Homogeneous mass, rarely calcified or necrotic
- Associated with Hashimoto thyroiditis

Thyroid Differentiated Carcinoma

- Unilateral thyroid mass ± fine calcifications ± cystic adenopathy

Thyroid Medullary Carcinoma

- May mimic morphology of early ATCa
- Often smaller and more well defined than ATCa

Multinodular Goiter

- Multiple nodules in enlarged thyroid gland
- No invasive features or adenopathy

Thyroid Adenoma

- Noninvasive intrathyroidal mass without adenopathy
- May hemorrhage and rapidly increase in size

PATHOLOGY

General Features

- Etiology
  - Often occurs in iodine-deficient areas and in setting of preexisting thyroid pathology
    - 33% MNG
    - 25% DTCa
    - Possibly arises by prolonged stimulation with TSH
  - Rarely can develop de novo
  - Thought to arise from endodermally derived follicular cells
    - **Does not concentrate iodine or express thyroglobulin**
- Associated abnormalities
  - Distant metastasis present in ≥ 50%
    - Lungs, bones, and brain

Staging, Grading, & Classification

- Adapted from American Joint Committee on Cancer (AJCC) 8th edition
- **For TNM stage, anaplastic thyroid uses same T definition as differentiated thyroid cancer**
- **All anaplastic thyroid considered stage IV**
  - Stage IVA: **Intrathryoid**, N0, M0

- o Stage IVB: **Extrathyroid extension**, any N, M0
- o Stage IVC: Any T, any N, **M1** (distant metastasis)
- N staging
  - o N1a: Levels VI &/or VII
  - o N1b: Lateral compartment (levels I-V) &/or retropharyngeal nodes

Gross Pathologic & Surgical Features
- Invasive mass that extends through thyroid gland capsule

Microscopic Features
- High degree of mitotic activity with substantial infiltration
- Commonly hemorrhagic and necrotic
- Squamoid, spindle cell, and giant cell histologic variants
- 25% have concomitant **DTCa**
- Cytology or histopathology is important to diagnose
  - o Core biopsy preferred due to higher diagnostic accuracy compared to FNA
    - Differentiates ATCa from lymphoma, avoids unnecessary surgical diagnosis if lymphoma
  - o Some pathologists distinguish between anaplastic and undifferentiated carcinoma
    - AJCC considers them to be synonymous

CLINICAL ISSUES

Presentation
- Most common signs/symptoms
  - o **Rapidly growing**, large, painful neck mass
  - o Symptoms from local invasion: Dyspnea, hoarseness, &/or dysphagia
    - Larynx or trachea: Dyspnea
    - Recurrent laryngeal nerve: Hoarseness
    - Esophagus: Dysphagia
- Other signs/symptoms
  - o Predisposing factors: Preexisting MNG, neck radiation
  - o On examination: Firm thyroid mass, typically > 5 cm
    - Nodal disease frequently present at presentation

Demographics
- Age
  - o Older individuals
  - o Mean age: 70 years
- Sex
  - o F:M = 3:1
- Epidemiology
  - o Rare; 1-2% of thyroid malignancies
  - o ~ 20% of thyroid cancer deaths

Natural History & Prognosis
- ATCa is one of most aggressive tumors
  - o **Mean survival: 6 months**
  - o Mortality: 70% at 6 months, 80% at 12 months
  - o Supportive/palliative care can be elected at any point
- Less grave prognosis
  - o Age < 60 years, intrathyroidal tumor, use of combined surgery and radiotherapy
- Death usually from airway obstruction or complications of pulmonary metastases

Treatment
- Aggressive treatment if early diagnosis and tumor not spread outside thyroid
- Multimodality with surgery ± radiotherapy and chemotherapy
- **Late-stage treatment usually palliative** to improve symptoms (i.e., stage IVC)
- Promising molecular-targeted therapies being studied include tyrosine kinase inhibitors

DIAGNOSTIC CHECKLIST

Consider
- If large neck mass, always consider DTCa first; should not use iodinated contrast during CT
  - o Image with NECT, MR, or ultrasound
- Iodinated contrast is not contraindicated with ATCa

Image Interpretation Pearls
- Rapidly enlarging thyroid mass: ATCa, thyroid non-Hodgkin lymphoma (NHL), or hemorrhagic adenoma
  - o ATCa more often is heterogenous with hemorrhage &/or calcifications; found in older patients

Reporting Tips
- Evaluate extent for anaplastic carcinoma staging
  - o Intrathyroidal disease = stage IVA
  - o Gross extrathyroidal extension or cervical lymph node metastasis = stage IVB
  - o Distant metastatic disease = stage IVC

SELECTED REFERENCES
1. Maeda T et al: MRI features of histological subtypes of thyroid cancer in comparison with CT findings: differentiation between anaplastic, poorly differentiated, and papillary thyroid carcinoma. Jpn J Radiol. 43(2):210-8, 2025
2. Boucai L et al: Thyroid cancer: a review. JAMA. 331(5):425-35, 2024
3. Chandekar KR et al: Positron emission tomography/computed tomography in thyroid cancer: an updated review. PET Clin. 19(2):131-45, 2024
4. Bible KC et al: 2021 American Thyroid Association guidelines for management of patients with anaplastic thyroid cancer. Thyroid. 31(3):337-86, 2021
5. Brauckhoff K et al: Multimodal imaging of thyroid cancer. Curr Opin Endocrinol Diabetes Obes. 27(5):335-44, 2020
6. Perrier ND et al: Differentiated and anaplastic thyroid carcinoma: major changes in the American Joint Committee on Cancer eighth edition cancer staging manual. CA Cancer J Clin. 68(1):55-63, 2018
7. Ahmed S et al: Imaging of anaplastic thyroid carcinoma. AJNR Am J Neuroradiol. 39(3):547-51, 2017
8. Molinaro E et al: Anaplastic thyroid carcinoma: from clinicopathology to genetics and advanced therapies. Nat Rev Endocrinol. 13(11):644-60, 2017
9. Ha EJ et al: Core needle biopsy could reduce diagnostic surgery in patients with anaplastic thyroid cancer or thyroid lymphoma. Eur Radiol. 26(4):1031-6, 2016
10. Hahn SY et al: Description and comparison of the sonographic characteristics of poorly differentiated thyroid carcinoma and anaplastic thyroid carcinoma. J Ultrasound Med. 35(9):1873-9, 2016

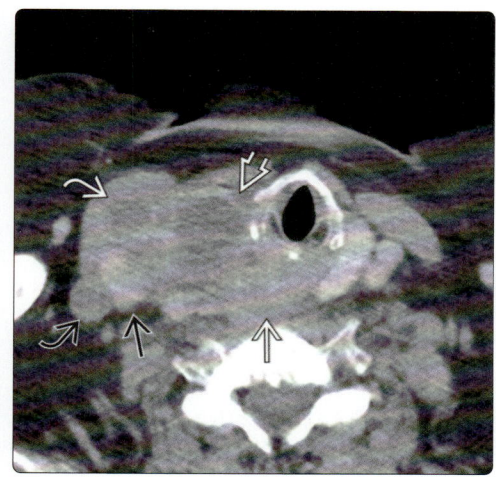

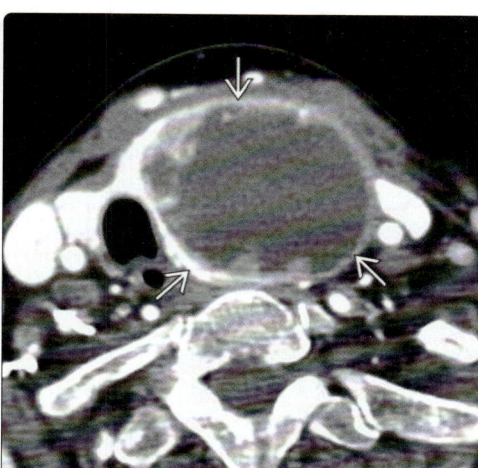

(Left) *Axial CECT shows a lobular, infiltrative, heterogeneously enhancing mass centered in right thyroid lobe* ➡️*, infiltrating into right sternocleidomastoid muscle* ➡️ *and posterior visceral space* ➡️*. Mass displaces right internal jugular vein* ➡️*. Note the pathologic, round, cystic lymph node* ➡️*. (Right) Axial CECT shows a well-defined mass* ➡️ *within the thyroid gland with cystic degeneration and peripheral enhancement, mimicking a colloid cyst. ATCa confined to thyroid gland is unusual and staged as T4a. It has slightly better prognosis.*

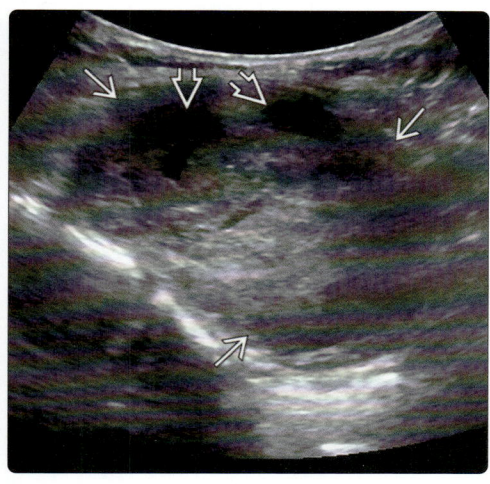

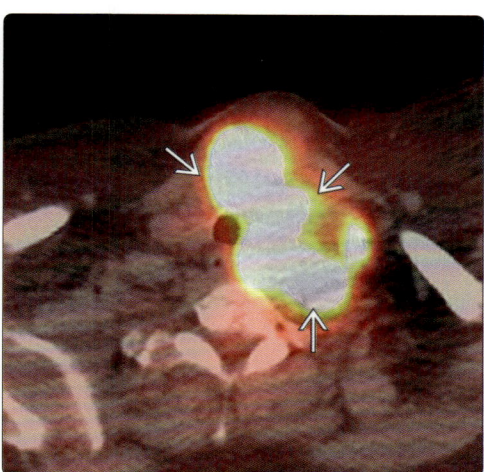

(Left) *Longitudinal oblique US shows a well-defined mass* ➡️ *with heterogeneous echotexture and small focal areas of necrosis* ➡️*. US findings, such as these, are nonspecific but are concerning for tumor and should lead to recommendation for FNA. (Right) Axial fused PET/CT demonstrates a large, markedly FDG-avid mass* ➡️ *extending from the left thyroid into surrounding tissues. PET/CT is not typically used, as all tumors are T4, stage IV disease but can upstage to T4C (stage IVC) if distant metastases are seen.*

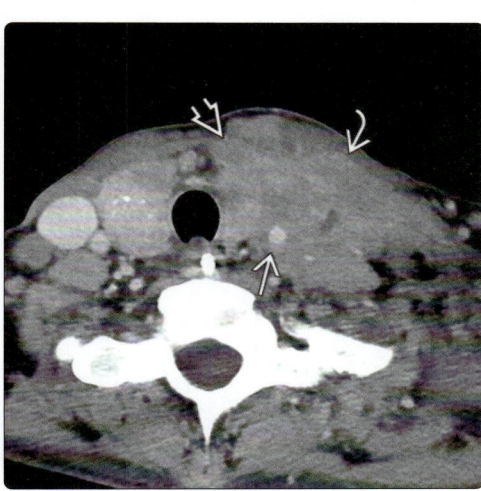

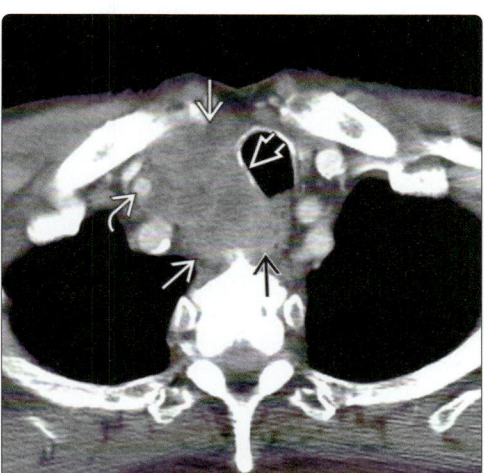

(Left) *Axial CECT demonstrates a large, infiltrating left thyroid and neck mass* ➡️*. There is extrathyroidal extension with involvement of the sternocleidomastoid muscle* ➡️ *and encasement of the left common carotid artery* ➡️*. Carotid involvement upstages this tumor to T4b. (Right) Axial CECT shows a large, heterogeneous, low-density mass* ➡️ *in the right superior mediastinum, displacing the trachea* ➡️*, invading the tracheoesophageal groove* ➡️*, and partly encasing the right common carotid artery* ➡️*.*

Visceral Space

TERMINOLOGY

- Thyroid non-Hodgkin lymphoma (NHL)
  - Primary lymphoma of thyroid gland

IMAGING

- Solid, noncalcified, homogeneous thyroid mass
- 80% solitary; 20% multiple masses or diffuse infiltration
- CECT: Hypodense; necrosis & calcification uncommon
- US: Well-defined, homogeneous, hypoechoic
- PET/CT generally useful except if MALT lymphoma
- Marked hypodensity & linear high-density strand signs favor NHL over chronic lymphocytic thyroiditis (CLT)

TOP DIFFERENTIAL DIAGNOSES

- Anaplastic thyroid carcinoma
- Thyroid differentiated carcinoma
- Chronic lymphocytic thyroiditis (Hashimoto)
- Multinodular goiter

PATHOLOGY

- Most often diffuse large **B-cell lymphoma**
- 40-80% of cases occur in patients with **CLT**
  - CLT has 70x increased risk of thyroid NHL

CLINICAL ISSUES

- Presents as rapidly enlarging neck mass in older female patient with history of CLT
- Rare; 2-5% of all thyroid malignancies
- Frequently associated with neck adenopathy
- Nonsurgical disease unless airway obstruction
- 5-year survival: 75-95%
  - Extrathyroidal spread: Decreases 5-year survival to 35%

DIAGNOSTIC CHECKLIST

- Main differential for rapidly enlarging thyroid mass is **anaplastic thyroid carcinoma**
  - NHL more homogeneous; no necrosis, hemorrhage
  - NHL less likely to invade tissues, such as trachea

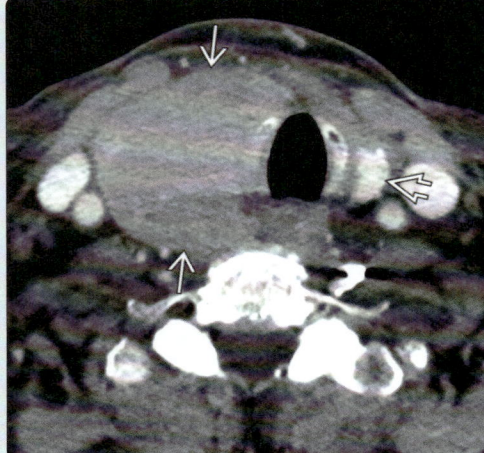
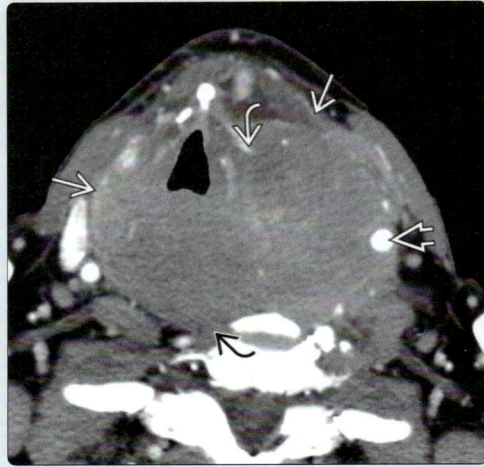

(Left) Axial CECT shows homogeneous enlargement of the right thyroid gland due to diffuse large B-cell lymphoma ⇨. A normal-appearing left thyroid lobe is visible ⇱. The carotid sheath is displaced laterally but not invaded. (Right) Axial CECT shows a large, minimally enhancing mass ⇨ centered in the thyroid gland. Mass invades laryngeal cartilages ⇨ and prevertebral muscles ⇗ and surrounds the carotid artery ⇨. Homogeneous density of the mass suggests lymphoma, but anaplastic thyroid cancer is the main differential.

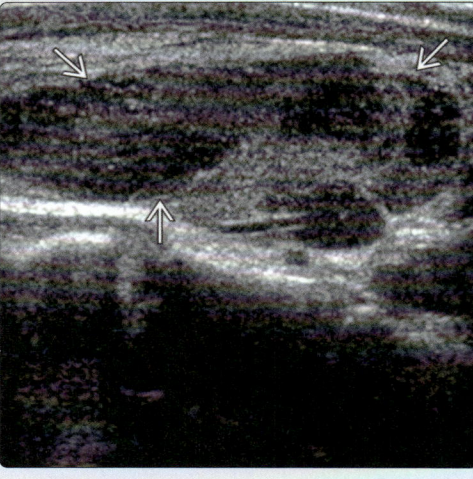
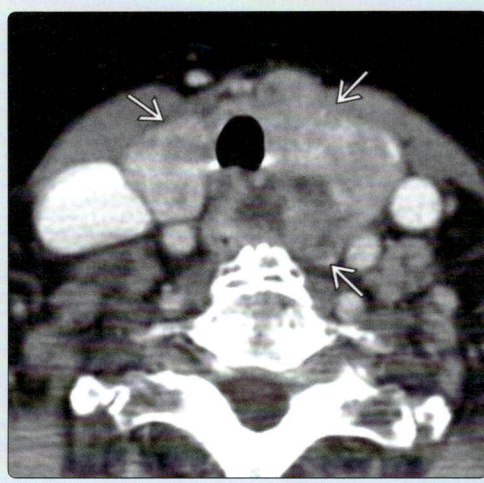

(Left) Longitudinal ultrasound of the thyroid gland shows a low echogenicity lobular mass ⇨. The uniform nature of lymphoma can result in low echogenicity on ultrasound, which may be mistaken for cyst (pseudocyst). (Right) Axial CECT shows multifocal masses ⇨ in thyroid. Although this primary lymphoma might be mistaken for a multinodular goiter, focal loss of definition of thyroid margins, and absence of calcification suggest an alternate diagnosis. Loss of clarity of borders is particularly suspicious for malignancy.

Non-Hodgkin Lymphoma of Thyroid

TERMINOLOGY

Abbreviations
- Non-Hodgkin lymphoma (NHL) of thyroid

Definitions
- Extranodal, extralymphatic primary lymphoma originating from thyroid gland
  - Excludes systemic NHL that secondarily involves thyroid

IMAGING

General Features
- Best diagnostic clue
  - **Rapidly enlarging**, **solid**, **homogeneous, noncalcified** thyroid mass in older female patient with history of chronic lymphocytic (Hashimoto) thyroiditis (CLT)
- Size
  - Often large at presentation; 5-10 cm
- Morphology
  - Diffuse, homogeneous, enlarged thyroid
  - 3 appearances: 80% present as solitary thyroid mass, remainder as multiple masses or diffuse infiltration

CT Findings
- CECT
  - Most often **homogeneous**, solid, hypodense mass
    - Marked hypodensity & linear high-density strand sign favor NHL over CLT
  - Uncommon necrosis, hemorrhage, or calcification

MR Findings
- T1WI
  - Hypointense to normal surrounding thyroid gland
- T2WI
  - Hyperintense to normal surrounding thyroid gland
- T1WI C+
  - Primary tumor lower signal than surrounding thyroid

Ultrasonographic Findings
- Well-defined, homogeneous, markedly hypoechoic mass(es); cystic-appearing but solid mass (pseudocystic)

Nuclear Medicine Findings
- PET/CT
  - Avid (except MALT subtype has low FDG avidity)

Imaging Recommendations
- Best imaging tool
  - Ultrasound with biopsy for initial diagnosis
  - MR or CT neck when thyroid pathology is unknown
  - PET/CT for staging; CECT alone if MALT subtype

DIFFERENTIAL DIAGNOSIS

Anaplastic Thyroid Carcinoma
- Rapidly enlarging, invasive thyroid mass (similar)
- Calcification, necrosis, & hemorrhage common

Thyroid Differentiated Carcinoma
- Poorly marginated thyroid mass ± calcification
- Adenopathy solid or cystic ± calcification

Chronic Lymphocytic (Hashimoto) Thyroiditis
- Chronic, diffuse thyromegaly; no adenopathy

Multinodular Goiter
- Nodules in enlarged thyroid; ± calcification; no adenopathy

PATHOLOGY

General Features
- Etiology
  - In 40-80% of cases, NHL complicates **CLT (Hashimoto)**
    - CLT has 70x increased risk of thyroid NHL

Staging, Grading, & Classification
- Anatomic staging (Ann Arbor staging)
  - Localized to thyroid classified as stage IE
  - Regional lymph nodes changes to stage IIE

Microscopic Features
- 3 main subtypes of NHL involve thyroid gland
  - Diffuse large B-cell lymphoma (most common)
  - Marginal zone B-cell MALT lymphoma
  - Follicular lymphoma
- Rarely, Hodgkin, Burkitt, & T-cell lymphomas
- FNA or core biopsy may be needed
  - Core biopsy usually preferred

CLINICAL ISSUES

Presentation
- Most common signs/symptoms
  - Rapidly enlarging thyroid mass with symptoms from local mass effect or invasion (dysphagia, hoarseness)
  - 30-40% have hypothyroidism clinically or serologically
  - Frequently associated with neck adenopathy

Demographics
- Age range: 50-80 years; peak: Late 60s
- Sex: F:M = 3:1
- Epidemiology: Primary NHL of thyroid is rare
  - 2-5% of all thyroid malignancies
  - 1-2% of all extranodal lymphomas occur in thyroid

Natural History & Prognosis
- MALT has best prognosis: 5-year survival > 95%
- Follicular NHL: 5-year survival = 87%
- Diffuse B-cell has worst prognosis: 5-year survival = 75%
- Extrathyroidal spread reduces 5-year survival to 35%

Treatment
- Rituximab + chemotherapy ± radiation
- Nonsurgical unless airway compromised

SELECTED REFERENCES

1. Harahap AS et al: Variability in primary thyroid lymphoma: a clinicopathological exploration of diffuse large B-cell, marginal zone, and follicular lymphoma. Ann Diagn Pathol. 75:152444, 2025
2. Yang L et al: Contrast-enhanced ultrasound in the differential diagnosis of primary thyroid lymphoma and nodular Hashimoto's thyroiditis in a background of heterogeneous parenchyma. Front Oncol. 10:597975, 2020
3. Luo J et al: Is ultrasound combined with computed tomography useful for distinguishing between primary thyroid lymphoma and Hashimoto's thyroiditis? Endokrynol Pol. 70(6):463-8, 2019

TERMINOLOGY

- Parathyroid carcinoma (PTCa)
- Rare low-grade malignancy of parathyroid (PT) glands

IMAGING

- Multiphase CECT & ultrasonography help localize
- CECT shows poorly enhancing invasive mass
  - Variable tumor calcifications or pathologic adenopathy
- Sonographic features favoring PTCa over adenoma
  - Larger (> 3 cm), irregular shape, poorly marginated, invasive, thick capsule, calcifications
- MR shows heterogeneous signal & enhancement
- Best imaging clue: Invasive, poorly enhancing mass behind thyroid ± adenopathy

TOP DIFFERENTIAL DIAGNOSES

- PT adenoma
- Thyroid adenoma
- Thyroid differentiated carcinoma

PATHOLOGY

- Immunohistochemical loss of parafibromin expression
- Usually due to inactivating mutations of *CDC73* gene

CLINICAL ISSUES

- Patients present with severe hypercalcemia
  - Clinically severe hypercalcemia ± vocal cord paralysis
- PTCa may be younger patients than PT adenoma
- Slow, indolent growth; nodes do not predict outcome
- 5-year survival = 70-85%
- Most are sporadic, but can be familial or syndromic
  - Hyperparathyroidism-jaw tumor or MEN syndrome
- *CDC73* gene has important role in sporadic & familial PTCa
- Mainstay of treatment is surgical resection ± radiation

DIAGNOSTIC CHECKLIST

- PTCa may mimic PT adenoma
  - PTCa usually larger, poorly enhancing, & more invasive
- Consider PTCa if severe hypercalcemia & hoarseness

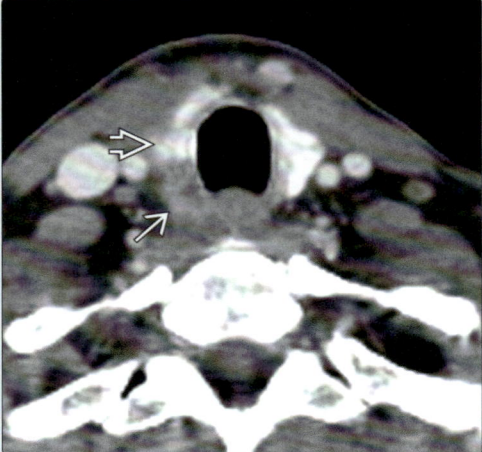
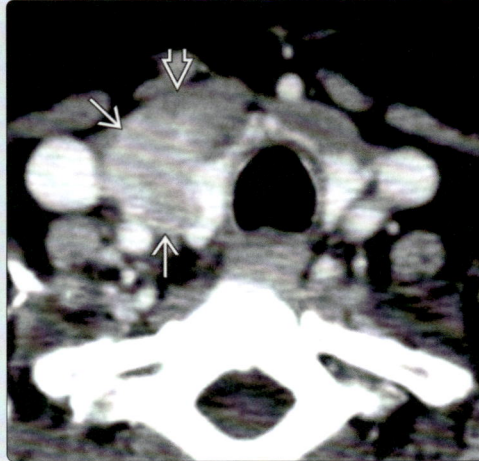

(Left) *Axial CECT shows an ill-defined mass ⟹ in the right tracheoesophageal groove displacing the thyroid gland ⟹ anteriorly, representing parathyroid carcinoma (PTCa). The differential for this lesion is parathyroid adenoma, exophytic thyroid adenoma, or carcinoma.* (Right) *Axial CECT shows a large intrathyroidal mass ⟹ with ill-defined borders invading strap muscles ⟹. Although most PTCas arise posterior to the thyroid, they may also be intrathyroidal and indistinguishable from primary thyroid carcinoma.*

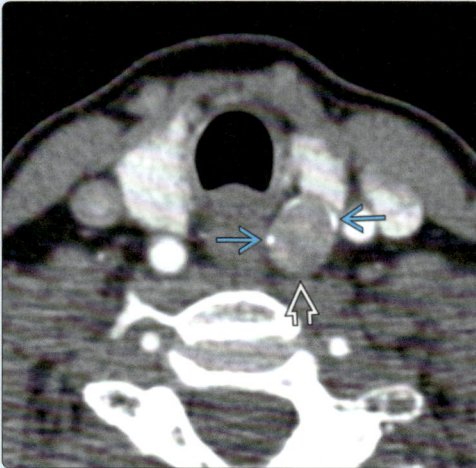
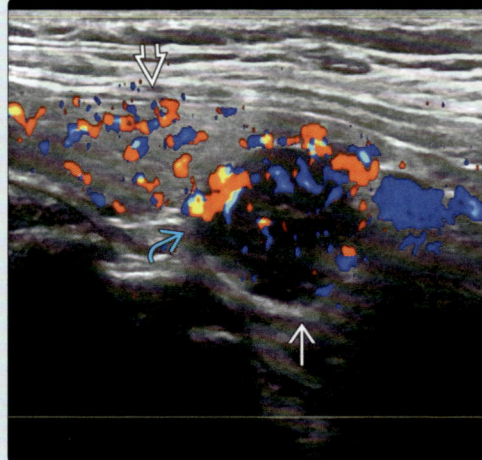

(Left) *Axial neck CECT shows a circumscribed, heterogeneously hypoenhancing lesion ⟹ posterior to the left thyroid with peripheral hyperdense calcifications ⟹. Resection was positive for PTCa.* (Right) *Longitudinal Doppler US shows a prominent, well-circumscribed, heterogeneously hypoechoic mass ⟹ with internal hyperechoic foci of calcium and prominent internal vascularity ⟹, posterior to the inferior left thyroid lobe ⟹. Resection was positive for PTCa.*

TERMINOLOGY

Abbreviations
- Parathyroid carcinoma (PTCa)

Definitions
- Low-grade malignancy arising from parathyroid (PT) gland

IMAGING

General Features
- Best diagnostic clue
  - Uniform mass displacing thyroid gland anteriorly with focal areas of **soft tissue invasion** ± calcifications
- Location
  - Usually **posterior** to thyroid gland; may be within
  - Rarely arises from ectopic PT gland
- Size
  - Typically larger than adenoma at presentation, > 3 cm
- Morphology
  - Usually well defined; ± invasion of surrounding structures

MR Findings
- Heterogeneous signal & enhancement

Nuclear Medicine Findings
- Tc-99m sestamibi
  - Localizes source of hyperparathyroidism by ↑ uptake
    - Similar to PT adenoma
- Uptake on FDG PET & DOTATATE PET

Ultrasonographic Findings
- Grayscale ultrasound
  - Can be similar to adenoma in sonographic appearance
    - Oval hypoechoic mass posterior to thyroid
  - Features favoring PTCa over adenoma
    - **Large size (> 3 cm), thick capsule**
    - Irregular borders, local invasion, heterogeneity, hypoechoic, tumor depth:width ratio ≥ 1
    - ± hyperechoic calcifications
- Color Doppler
  - High vascularity more suggestive of PTCa

CT Findings
- CECT
  - Multiphase CECT (PT adenoma protocol) best
  - Poorly enhancing, usually hypodense compared to thyroid with slow contrast washout
  - Adjacent soft tissue invasion highly suggestive of PTCa
  - High short:long axis ratio, irregular shape, calcification
  - Look for associated pathologic adenopathy

Imaging Recommendations
- Best imaging tool
  - Ultrasonography & multiphase CECT

DIFFERENTIAL DIAGNOSIS

Parathyroid Adenoma
- Smaller arterial-phase hyperenhancement, noninvasive

Thyroid Adenoma
- Well-defined intrathyroidal mass

Thyroid Differentiated Carcinoma
- Poorly defined intrathyroidal mass ± nodes
- Usually appears more aggressive than PTCa

PATHOLOGY

General Features
- Trabecular pattern, mitotic figures, thick, fibrous bands, capsular &/or vascular invasion

Molecular Pathology
- Immunohistochemical loss of parafibromin expression
- Usually due to inactivating mutations of *CDC73* gene

CLINICAL ISSUES

Presentation
- Most common signs/symptoms
  - Primary hyperparathyroidism: Severe hypercalcemia often greater than other causes of hyperparathyroidism
    - Almost unmanageable fatigue, bone & joint pain, headache, depression, digestive symptoms, calculi

Demographics
- Age
  - Usually 4th-5th decades; range: 8-85 years old
    - Younger on average than PT adenoma
- Sex
  - F = M; note that F > > M for adenomas
- Epidemiology
  - Very rare: < 1% of etiologies of hyperparathyroidism
  - Most are sporadic
  - *CDC73* gene has role in sporadic & familial PTCa

Natural History & Prognosis
- Slow, indolent growth; nodes do not predict outcome
- Sporadic, familial, &/or associated with syndromes (hyperparathyroidism-jaw tumor, MEN 1 & 2)
- After resection, can locally recur or metastasize
- 5-year survival = 70-90%
- Death more likely from hypercalcemia than tumor

Treatment
- En bloc resection is mainstay of treatment
  - Level VI dissection usually included

DIAGNOSTIC CHECKLIST

Image Interpretation Pearls
- Poorly enhancing invasive mass on multiphase CECT

Reporting Tips
- Consider PTCa if severe hypercalcemia & hoarseness
- Do not mistake brown tumors for bone metastases

SELECTED REFERENCES

1. Viswanath A et al: Parathyroid carcinoma: new insights. Best Pract Res Clin Endocrinol Metab. 39(2):101966, 2025
2. Liu J et al: Role of ultrasound in the differentiation of parathyroid carcinoma and benign parathyroid lesions. Clin Radiol. 75(3):179-84, 2020
3. Christakis I et al: The diagnostic accuracy of neck ultrasound, 4D-computed tomography and sestamibi imaging in parathyroid carcinoma. Eur J Radiol. 95:82-8, 2017

TERMINOLOGY

- Thyroglossal duct cyst carcinoma (TGDCCa): Cancer of cystic remnant of embryologic thyroglossal duct (TGD)

IMAGING

- Nodularity within cystic mass ± Ca++ adjacent to hyoid
  - Can be midline suprahyoid or midline/paramidline infrahyoid neck
  - Best evaluated with CECT for enhancing nodule and hyperdense Ca++
  - Can also see findings on MR and US

TOP DIFFERENTIAL DIAGNOSES

- TGDC
- Ectopic thyroid
- Delphian or cervical necrotic node
- Thymic carcinoma
- Mixed laryngocele
- Dermoid or epidermoid

PATHOLOGY

- Most commonly papillary thyroid carcinoma as TGDCCa

CLINICAL ISSUES

- Enlarging midline neck mass; usually similar symptoms to benign TGDC
- Most commonly in **adults**; mean = 40 years
- Consider fine-needle aspiration prior to resection as nodularity could be due to inflammation
- Sistrunk procedure: excision of cyst with nodule, tract, and midline hyoid bone (treatment similar to TGDC)

DIAGNOSTIC CHECKLIST

- Nodularity ± Ca++ of cystic mass adjacent to hyoid in midline or paramidline neck suggests carcinoma of TGDC
  - May occur as solid tumor within ectopic thyroid tissue from tongue base to lower neck
- Comment on presence or absence of orthotopic thyroid tissue for preoperative planning

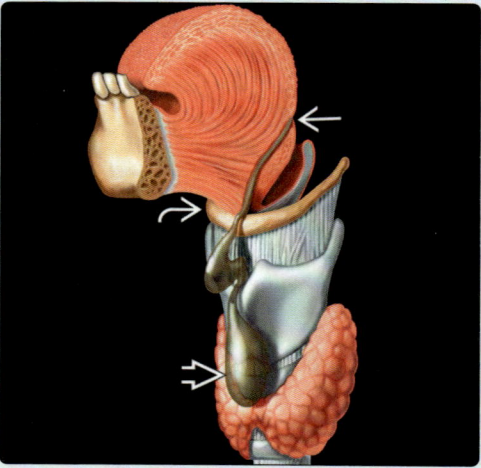
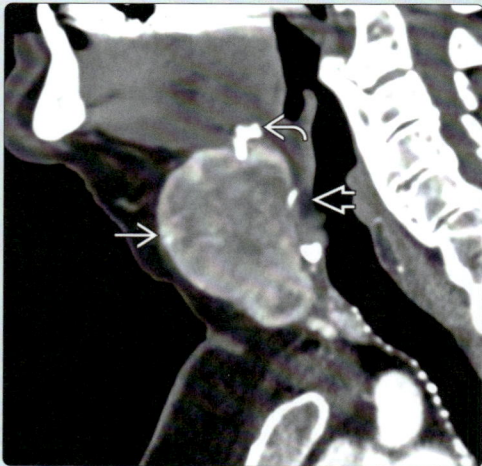

(Left) Sagittal oblique graphic shows the potential sites of a thyroglossal duct cyst (TGDC) from the foramen cecum ➡ to the thyroid bed ➡. Note the close relationship of the midportion of the hyoid bone ➡ to this pathway. A cyst can occur anywhere along this tract and potentially develop TGDC carcinoma (TGDCCa). (Right) Sagittal CECT shows a heterogeneous, enhancing TGDCCa ➡ along the expected course of the TGD near the midline in the upper anterior neck between the hyoid bone ➡ and upper thyroid cartilage ➡.

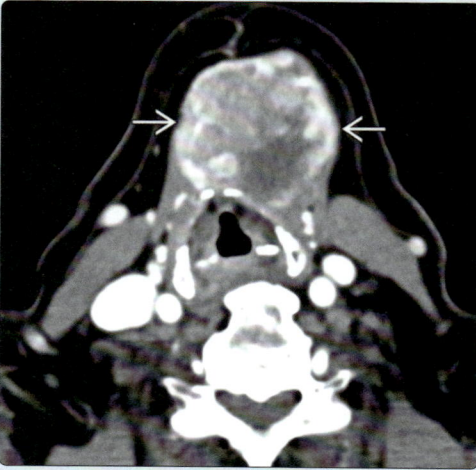
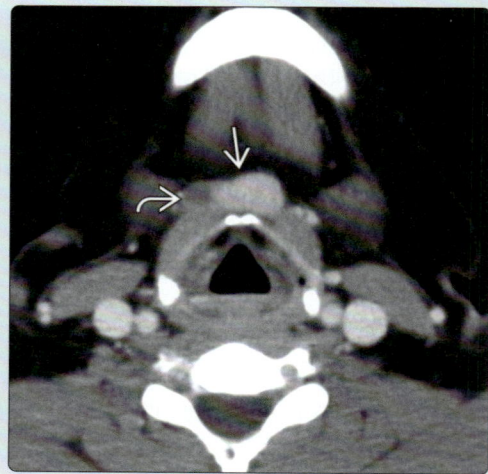

(Left) Axial CECT in the same patient shows a heterogeneous, partly solid, partly cystic enhancing TGDCCa ➡ embedded in the strap muscles anterior to the thyroid cartilage in an expected location along the embryologic thyroglossal duct tract. (Right) Axial CECT shows an enhancing soft tissue mass ➡ located just inferior to the anterior hyoid, an expected location for a thyroglossal duct remnant. A tiny cystic component ➡ is present laterally. Pathology showed papillary carcinoma.

TERMINOLOGY

Abbreviations
- Thyroglossal duct cyst carcinoma (TGDCCa)

Synonyms
- Carcinoma of thyroglossal duct cyst

Definitions
- Malignant tumor arising from remnants of embryologic thyroglossal duct (TGD)
  - Most often occurs within TGD cyst (TGDC)
- TGDC containing thyroid carcinoma
  - Most (94.2%) are papillary carcinoma

IMAGING

General Features
- Best diagnostic clue
  - Solid nodule within cystic mass adjacent to hyoid
- Location
  - TGDCCa with similar location to TGDC
    - Midline suprahyoid neck (base of tongue or within posterior floor of mouth) ~ 25%
    - Around hyoid bone (may project into preepiglottic space) ~ 50%
    - Midline infrahyoid neck or paramidline embedded in strap muscles ~ 25%
- Size
  - Nodule (neoplastic component) is often small (~ 1 cm)
    - Cystic portion (TGDC) variable in size and may be relatively occult
    - Location along TGD with nodular enhancement suggests diagnosis
- Morphology
  - Internal nodularity (carcinoma) within round or ovoid cyst (TGDC), or can be solid mass (carcinoma) ± Ca^{++}

CT Findings
- CECT
  - Enhancing nodularity of cystic neck mass
  - Often with Ca^{++}
  - Can be midline or paramidline infrahyoid mass
    - Midline associated with hyoid bone
    - Paramidline infrahyoid mass embedded in strap muscles may show claw sign

MR Findings
- T1WI
  - Variable within usually hypointense cyst
  - Hyperintense if proteinaceous fluid
- T2WI
  - Variable, within hyperintense cyst
- T1WI C+
  - Enhancing nodularity of cyst, or enhancing solid mass

Ultrasonographic Findings
- Grayscale ultrasound
  - Anechoic or hypoechoic cystic neck mass with heterogeneous nodule
    - Associated with hyperechoic hyoid bone in midline
    - Infrahyoid mass intimately embedded in strap muscle
  - ± echogenic foci of Ca^{++} in mass/nodule

Nuclear Medicine Findings
- PET/CT
  - FDG uptake within nodule (carcinoma) may be found within TGD/TGDC seen on associated low dose CT
  - Not specific for malignancy, can be infectious

Imaging Recommendations
- Best imaging tool
  - CECT shows enhancing nodule within TGDC adjacent to hyoid (also seen on MR)
    - CT better show hyperdense Ca^{++}, if present
- Protocol advice
  - Contrast-enhanced imaging best to evaluate for enhancing nodule or mass
  - Be sure to evaluate for potential lymph node metastases

DIFFERENTIAL DIAGNOSIS

Thyroglossal Duct Cyst
- Midline congenital cystic lesion ± multiloculated
- ± solid components of ectopic thyroid tissue; no Ca^{++}

Ectopic Thyroid
- Solid, round, hyperattenuating mass along TGD
- Homogeneous avid enhancement; no Ca^{++}
- Lingual thyroid only functioning tissue in 75%
  - Associated with absent orthotopic thyroid

Delphian or Cervical Chain Necrotic Node
- Cystic lymph node
- Associated head and neck malignant mass
- No connection to hyoid

Thymic Carcinoma
- Prevascular anterior mediastinal mass
- Necrosis ± Ca^{++}
- Not associated with hyoid

Mixed Laryngocele
- Paramidline fluid-fluid- or air-fluid-containing mass
- Originates from laryngeal ventricle, not hyoid

Oral Cavity Dermoid and Epidermoid
- Cystic or fat-containing mass in floor of mouth or submandibular region
- Not associated with hyoid bone

PATHOLOGY

General Features
- Genetics
  - Carcinoma develops within primary thyroid remnant
- Associated abnormalities
  - Thyroid: Agenesis, ectopia, or pyramidal lobe
    - Or can have normal orthotopic thyroid
- Embryology/anatomy of thyroid
  - TGD originates near foramen cecum at posterior 3rd of tongue and then descends
  - Failure of TGD involution with persistent secretory activity of epithelial cells lining duct → TGDC

○ Presumed microscopic thyroid tissue within TGDC differentiates into carcinoma (TGDCCa)

Gross Pathologic & Surgical Features

- Solid and cystic mass with tract to hyoid ± foramen cecum

Microscopic Features

- Cyst lined by respiratory or squamous epithelium with associated thyroid carcinoma
  ○ Papillary thyroid carcinoma (PTC) is most common
    – PTC often contains psammoma bodies, which can result in Ca^{++} evident on CT
    – Can have other thyroid cancers or squamous cell carcinoma
- TGDC may only have microscopic carcinoma, not identifiable as TGDCCa prospectively with imaging

CLINICAL ISSUES

Presentation

- Most common signs/symptoms
  ○ Midline or paramidline doughy neck mass; can be indistinguishable from TGDC
    – Cystic mass elevates when tongue protrudes if located at hyoid bone
- Other signs/symptoms
  ○ Small lesion may be seen as incidental finding on imaging
  ○ Solid/fixed midline or paramidline neck mass

Demographics

- Age
  ○ Majority of TGDCCa occur in **adults**; mean = 40 years
  ○ Rare pediatric cases of TGDCCa; mean = 13 years
    – Pediatrics usually benign TGDC
- Epidemiology
  ○ TGDC is most common congenital neck mass
    – Rarely associated with carcinoma: TGDCCa < 1%
      □ Most commonly PTC (~ 85%)
      □ Can have other thyroid or squamous call carcinoma

Natural History & Prognosis

- Rapidly enlarging anterior midline mass suggests differentiated thyroid carcinoma of TGDC
  ○ Especially when present with Ca^{++} of nodule
- Consider FNA of solid nodule prior to resection
  ○ Differential can include acute or remote infection of TGDC: Clinical presentation with findings of inflammatory fat stranding, debris, &/or septations helpful
- Many TGDCCa diagnosed on pathologic review of TGDC due to microscopic involvement
- Metastasis from TGDCCa is rare
- Rare local recurrences from incomplete resection

Treatment

- **Sistrunk** procedure: Complete surgical resection of TGD
  ○ Entire TGDCCa, including tract to foramen cecum
  ○ Midline portion of hyoid bone resected
    – Even if imaging shows no obvious connection to hyoid
  ○ Prognosis excellent with complete surgical resection
- Case-dependent additional procedures
  ○ ± lymph node dissection if metastasis; rare

– ↑ risk with adjacent soft tissue extension of carcinoma
○ ± total thyroidectomy if concern for synchronous thyroid carcinoma
  – Allow for potential radioactive iodine therapy
○ ± adjuvant therapy

DIAGNOSTIC CHECKLIST

Consider

- Nodularity ± Ca^{++} of cystic neck mass along TGD suggests associated carcinoma (TGDCCa)
  ○ Can be found in suprahyoid, hyoid, or infrahyoid neck
- Solid mass ± Ca^{++} adjacent to hyoid suggests TGDCCa
- TGDCCa can be found microscopically within TGDC
- Prognosis is excellent with Sistrunk procedure resection

Image Interpretation Pearls

- Any imaging study of TGDC should be carefully evaluated for solid and calcified components
  ○ Nodularity with Ca^{++} suggests malignancy: TGDCCa
  ○ Consider CT or MR to further evaluate complex masses, such as soft tissue invasion and lymphadenopathy
  ○ TGDCCa is rare and usually found in adults
- Nodularity of TGDC may also be due to prior inflammation
  ○ Consider reporting both
  ○ May need FNA of solid component before resection to confirm
- Comment on presence or absence of normal thyroid tissue
  ○ Important for preoperative planning
- Evaluate thyroid for suspicious nodules and possible synchronous carcinoma

SELECTED REFERENCES

1. Podzimek J et al: High-resolution ultrasound of thyroglossal cysts with special emphasis on the detection of cystic portions above the hyoid within the tongue base. Ultrasound. 33(1):20-6, 2025
2. Thimsen V et al: Thyroglossal duct cyst carcinomas - a retrospective study and systematic review of the literature. Virchows Arch. 486(6):1139-51, 2025
3. Chaudhary P et al: Thyroglossal duct cyst carcinoma: our 12-year experience in a tertiary care centre. Indian J Otolaryngol Head Neck Surg. 76(5):4091-5, 2024
4. Colino M et al: Early diagnosis of papillary carcinoma in a thyroglossal duct cyst: a multidisciplinary approach and the crucial role of fine-needle aspiration cytology. Cureus. 16(10):e71254, 2024
5. Lancini D et al: Evidence and controversies in management of thyroglossal duct cyst carcinoma. Curr Opin Otolaryngol Head Neck Surg. 29(2):113-9, 2021
6. Ozturk K et al: Not a pearl necklace: synchronous papillary carcinoma of thyroglossal duct cyst and thyroid gland. Clin Imaging. 73:111-4, 2021
7. Patel S et al: Thyroglossal duct pathology and mimics. Insights Imaging. 10(1):12, 2019
8. Wood CB et al: Papillary-type carcinoma of the thyroglossal duct cyst: the case for conservative management. Ann Otol Rhinol Laryngol. 127(10):710-6, 2018
9. Rayess HM et al: Thyroglossal duct cyst carcinoma: a systematic review of clinical features and outcomes. Otolaryngol Head Neck Surg. 156(5):794-802, 2017
10. Thompson LD et al: Thyroglossal duct cyst carcinomas: a clinicopathologic series of 22 cases with staging recommendations. Head Neck Pathol. 11(2):175-85, 2017
11. Shah S et al: Squamous cell carcinoma in a thyroglossal duct cyst: a case report with review of the literature. Am J Otolaryngol. 36(3):460-2, 2015
12. Wei S et al: Pathology of thyroglossal duct: an institutional experience. Endocr Pathol. 26(1):75-9, 2015
13. Carter Y et al: Thyroglossal duct remnant carcinoma: beyond the Sistrunk procedure. Surg Oncol. 23(3):161-6, 2014
14. Zander DA et al: Imaging of ectopic thyroid tissue and thyroglossal duct cysts. Radiographics. 34(1):37-50, 2014

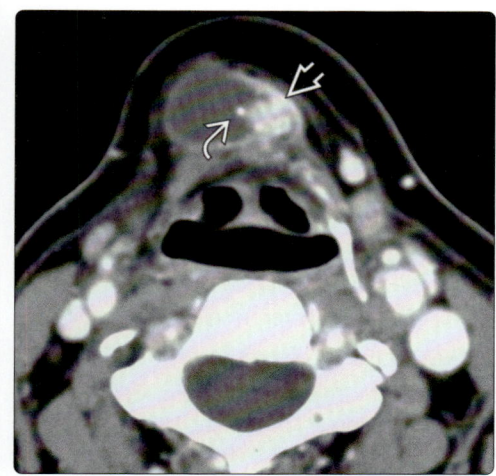

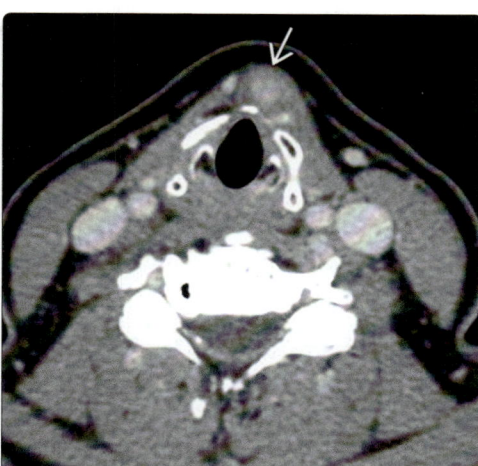

(Left) *Axial CECT shows a TGDCCa with an enhancing nodule* ⇨ *within a cystic mass. Note the associated punctate internal Ca⁺⁺* ⇨ *and invasive component in the adjacent soft tissues.* (Right) *Axial CECT shows a partly cystic, enhancing nodular soft tissue mass anterior to the midline upper thyroid cartilage, embedded in the strap musculature* ⇨*, in a typical location for a TGDC. Enhancing nodularity, present centrally, is worrisome for associated carcinoma, which was confirmed histopathologically.*

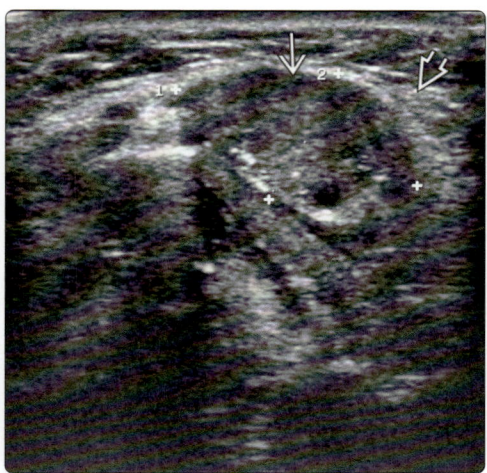

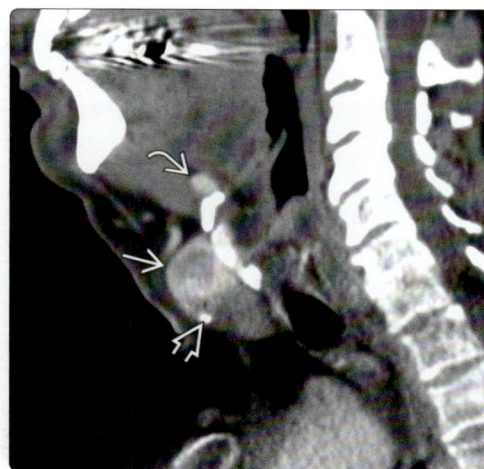

(Left) *Transverse ultrasound shows a heterogeneous hypoechoic nodule* ⇨ *embedded within the left strap muscle* ⇨ *of the infrahyoid neck. This was histologically proven to be papillary carcinoma.* (Right) *Sagittal reformatted CECT of TGDCCa shows a solid, heterogeneous mass* ⇨ *just below the hyoid bone, which contains a focal Ca⁺⁺ at the inferior aspect* ⇨*. An additional small, solid rest of ectopic tissue is present above the hyoid* ⇨*. A normal-appearing thyroid was not present in the lower neck.*

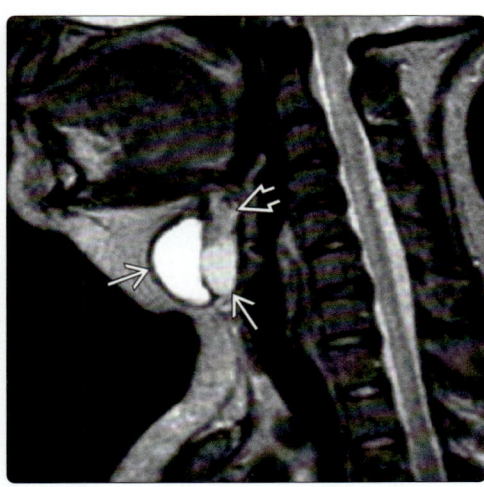

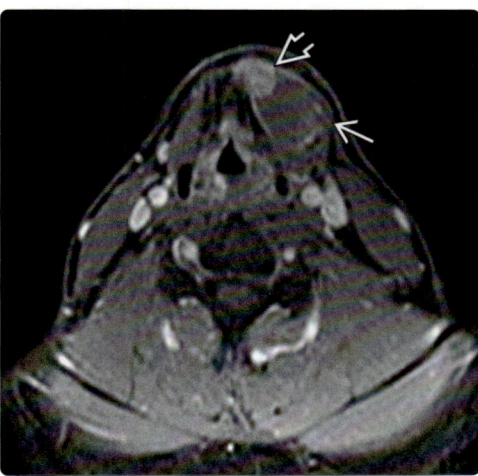

(Left) *Sagittal midline T2WI MR shows an infrahyoid hyperintense, multilobulated cystic mass* ⇨ *with intermediate to low intensity of the superior solid soft tissue nodule* ⇨*. This nodule enhanced with contrast and was proven to be TGDCCa.* (Right) *Axial T1WI C+ FS MR demonstrates an enhancing nodule* ⇨ *within a cystic mass* ⇨ *(TGDC) embedded within the strap muscle of the infrahyoid neck at the level of the thyroid cartilage. Histopathology showed TGDCCa.*

Cervical Esophageal Carcinoma

TERMINOLOGY

- Cervical esophageal carcinoma (CECa)
- > 95% CECa are squamous cell carcinoma (SCCa)

IMAGING

- Cervical esophagus = lower cricoid to thoracic inlet
- **Posterior midline** visceral space focal or invasive mass
- CECT/MR: Both can evaluate invasive extent of tumor
  - Esophageal wall thickened + ill-defined margin
  - Frequent extension to hypopharynx, larynx, thyroid
  - Vocal cord paralysis from recurrent laryngeal nerve involvement
  - Look for level VI & VII (mediastinal) nodes
- PET/CT best tool for staging, monitoring, & surveillance

TOP DIFFERENTIAL DIAGNOSES

- Hypopharyngeal SCCa
- Thyroid anaplastic carcinoma
- Thyroid non-Hodgkin lymphoma

PATHOLOGY

- Strong association with tobacco & alcohol abuse
- AJCC staging as for all esophagus
  - **T1-T3**: Depth of wall invasion
  - **T4**: Invasion of adjacent structures
- Nodal disease present in 70% at diagnosis

CLINICAL ISSUES

- Typically presents with dysphagia, weight loss
- Frequently detected late with poor prognosis
- 5-year survival = 10%
- Definitive chemoradiotherapy preferred if advanced

DIAGNOSTIC CHECKLIST

- Many H&N SCCa patients are smokers, alcoholics
  - Increased risk of 2nd primary malignancy must be considered when imaging these patients
- Also seen with Plummer-Vinson syndrome
  - Iron deficiency anemia, glossitis, esophageal webs

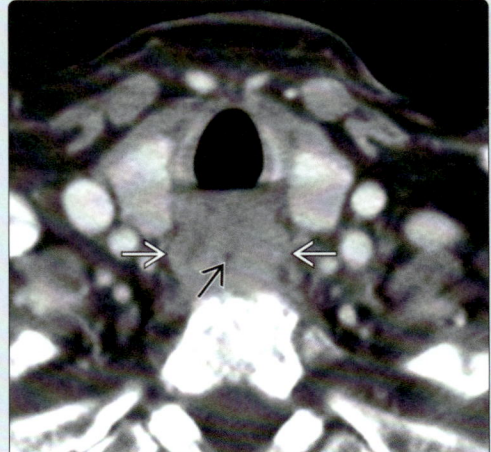
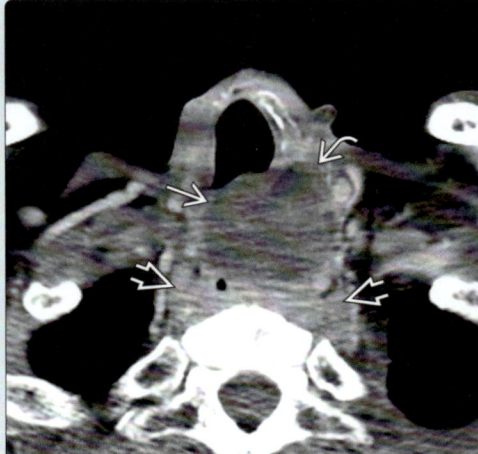

(Left) Axial CECT shows enlargement of the cervical esophagus ➡ due to invasive SCCa with effacement of the soft tissue plane between the esophagus & trachea anteriorly. A tiny central hypodensity suggests the collapsed lumen ➡, emphasizing the nature of the thickened esophageal wall. (Right) Axial CECT at the level of the cervical thoracic junction shows a large posterior midline esophageal SCCa ➡. Anterior invasion on the left ➡ is visible with retropharyngeal-danger space invasion ➡ seen posteriorly.

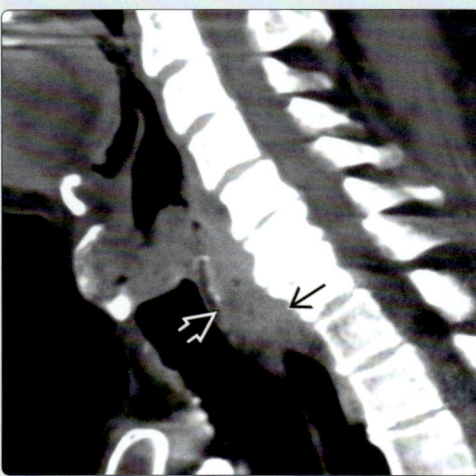
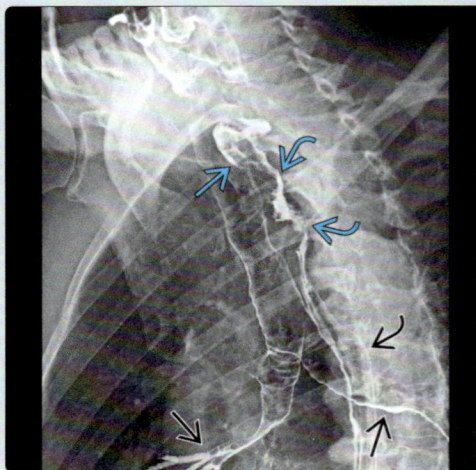

(Left) Sagittal CECT of the neck shows circumferential thickening/mass of the cervical esophagus due to SCCa ➡ with extension into the lower hypopharynx ➡ (tumor extends superiorly above the bottom of the cricoid cartilage). (Right) Oblique spot image from an esophagram with oral contrast outlines irregular narrowing of the cervical esophagus ➡ ("apple-core" lesion with overhanging edges ➡). Note normal mucosa ➡ & aspiration of oral contrast in the bronchi ➡. (CT showed an SCCa mass.)

TERMINOLOGY

Abbreviations
- Cervical esophageal carcinoma (CECa)

Definitions
- Malignancy of epithelium lining of cervical esophagus
  - > 95% are squamous cell carcinoma (SCCa)
  - Adenocarcinomas less commonly

IMAGING

General Features
- Best diagnostic clue
  - **Concentric or eccentric esophageal thickening** with ill-defined outer margins
  - Infiltrative mass in posterior midline visceral space
- Location
  - Cervical esophagus defined from lower border cricoid to thoracic inlet (suprasternal notch)

Fluoroscopic Findings
- Barium swallow
  - Mucosal-based, irregular filling defect
  - Luminal narrowing with larger lesions

CT Findings
- CECT
  - Ill-defined, enhancing, circumferential or eccentric esophageal mass in posteromedial visceral space
  - Often invades hypopharynx, larynx, thoracic esophagus
  - Normal collapsed cervical esophagus dimensions: < 16 mm (anterior-posterior) x 24 mm (lateral)

MR Findings
- T2-hyperintense & enhancing midline posterior visceral space mass of esophagus

Nuclear Medicine Findings
- PET/CT
  - SCCa consistently FDG avid

Imaging Recommendations
- Best imaging tool
  - PET/CT is best for staging, monitoring, & surveillance
    - Local disease extent with CT
    - Regional & distant disease with PET
- Protocol advice
  - Image to **carina** to include mediastinal nodes
  - MR helpful for prevertebral invasion by loss of fat planes

DIFFERENTIAL DIAGNOSIS

Hypopharyngeal Squamous Cell Carcinoma
- Arises in hypopharynx, at or above cricoid level
- May extend into esophagus

Thyroid Anaplastic Carcinoma
- Arises from thyroid; heterogeneous, infiltrative mass
- Older adult patient with rapidly enlarging neck mass

Thyroid Non-Hodgkin Lymphoma
- Arises from thyroid; homogeneous, infiltrative mass
- ± Hashimoto thyroiditis history

PATHOLOGY

General Features
- Etiology
  - Strong association with tobacco & alcohol abuse
  - ↑ incidence in caustic stricture, achalasia, prior radiation
  - Association with **Plummer-Vinson syndrome**
- Associated abnormalities
  - 15% have synchronous or metachronous tumors
    - Especially H&N SCCa, lung carcinoma

Staging, Grading, & Classification
- American Joint Committee on Cancer (AJCC) staging
  - T1-T3 defined by depth of invasion of wall
  - T4a tumor invades resectable structures
  - T4b tumor invades nonresectable structures

CLINICAL ISSUES

Presentation
- Most common signs/symptoms
  - Dysphagia, weight loss (early can be asymptomatic)
- Other signs/symptoms
  - Sensation of fullness, retrosternal pain
  - Hoarseness, if recurrent laryngeal nerve involvement

Demographics
- Age
  - Peak age: 55-65 years
- Sex
  - M:F = 4:1

Natural History & Prognosis
- Tendency to invade local visceral space or hypopharynx
- Frequently detected late with poor prognosis
  - 70% have level VI node involvement at diagnosis
- Overall 5-year survival = 10%

Treatment
- Definitive chemoradiotherapy preferred
  - Possibly augmented with checkpoint inhibitors
- Radical resection of esophagus & hypopharynx with jejunal interposition or gastric pull-up

DIAGNOSTIC CHECKLIST

Consider
- Many patients with H&N SCCa are smokers, alcoholics
- Be aware risk of 2nd primary malignancy on follow-up scan

Image Interpretation Pearls
- Look for paratracheal & superior mediastinum nodes

SELECTED REFERENCES

1. Yang H et al: Oesophageal cancer. Lancet. 404(10466):1991-2005, 2024
2. Morgan E et al: The global landscape of esophageal squamous cell carcinoma and esophageal adenocarcinoma incidence and mortality in 2020 and projections to 2040: new estimates from GLOBOCAN 2020. Gastroenterology. 163(3):649-58.e2, 2022
3. Katsurahara K et al: Clinical significance of the distance between the cricoid cartilage and upper edge of the tumor using PET-CT in cervical esophageal cancer. Oncol Lett. 20(4):40, 2020

Colloid Cyst of Thyroid

TERMINOLOGY

- Synonym: Colloid nodule
- Definition: Fluid lesion of thyroid containing stored form of thyroid hormone (colloid)

IMAGING

- Typically 1-4 cm; when large, usually hemorrhagic
- Sharply defined, fluid-filled lesion
- CECT: Low-density, round to oval lesion
  - Thyroid tissue beaks around cyst
- MR: T2-hyperintense, well-defined lesion
  - T1 frequently hyperintense, may be iso- or hypointense to thyroid
- Ultrasound is key modality for determining nature
  - Shows **thin wall with smooth margins**
  - Typically anechoic, increased through transmission
  - Colloid crystals may be suspended in fluid with **posterior comet-tail artifact (ring-down artifact)**

TOP DIFFERENTIAL DIAGNOSES

- Simple thyroid cyst
- Cystic papillary carcinoma
- Thyroglossal duct cyst

CLINICAL ISSUES

- 15-25% thyroid nodules
- May rapidly enlarge from hemorrhage
- Often incidental imaging finding
  - Smaller cysts commonly seen during thyroid ultrasound
- Benign lesion without malignant potential

DIAGNOSTIC CHECKLIST

- Important to carefully evaluate "cystic" lesion on ultrasound
- Complex thyroid "cyst" may be malignant degenerating lesion
- Difficult to separate microcalcification from comet tail artifacts in solid/cystic lesions

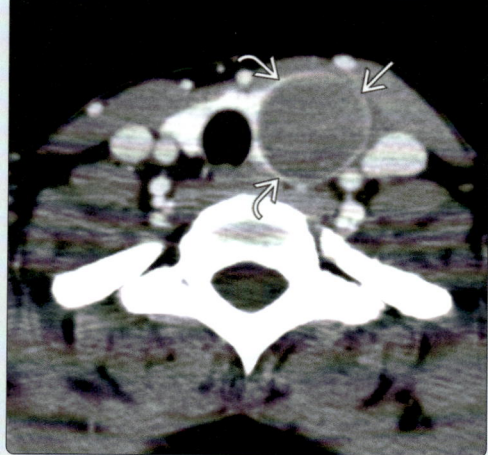
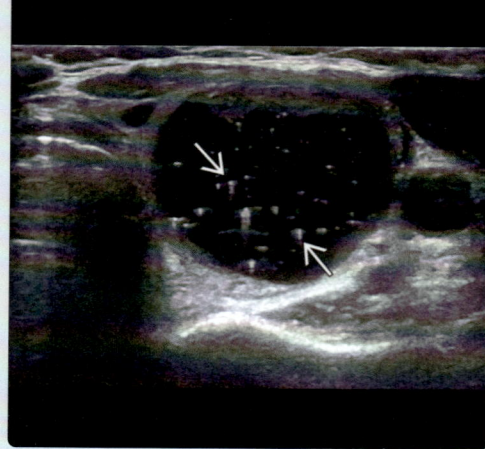

(Left) Axial CECT demonstrates an ovoid, sharply defined, low-density mass ➡ in the left thyroid lobe with thyroid tissue beaking around the anterior and posterior margins of the mass ➡. Needle aspiration revealed a hemorrhagic colloid cyst. (Right) Transverse grayscale US shows a typical colloid nodule with multiple echogenic foci and comet-tail artifacts suspended in the cyst ➡. These represent colloid particles in viscous fluid concentrated with thyroglobulin.

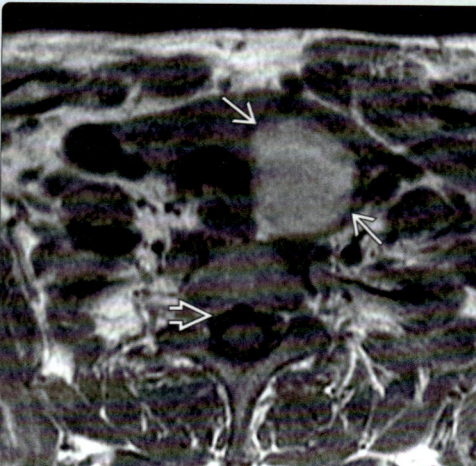
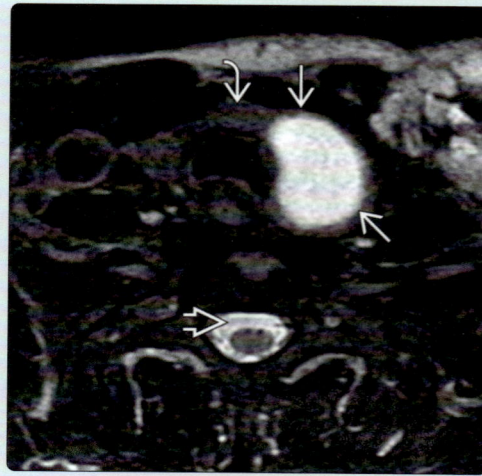

(Left) Axial T1 MR demonstrates a large, well-defined mass ➡ within the left thyroid lobe that is hyperintense to CSF ➡. Mass abuts and displaces left strap muscles anteriorly, but there are no aggressive features to suggest an invasive mass. (Right) Axial T2 FS MR in the same patient shows the mass ➡ to be uniformly, markedly hyperintense, similar to CSF ➡ intensity. Lesion clearly resides within left thyroid lobe and is sharply demarcated from normal adjacent thyroid isthmus ➡. No adenopathy is evident in neck.

TERMINOLOGY

Synonyms

- Colloid nodules

Definitions

- Nonneoplastic lesion of thyroid containing stored form of thyroid hormone (colloid)

IMAGING

General Features

- Best diagnostic clue
  - Ultrasound demonstrates thin rim lesion with anechoic contents ± colloid crystals
- Location
  - Within thyroid gland parenchyma
- Size
  - Typically 1-4 cm; when large, usually hemorrhagic
- Morphology
  - Round or oval cystic lesion

Imaging Recommendations

- Best imaging tool
  - Ultrasound best evaluates thyroid nodules to determine whether truly cystic

CT Findings

- CECT
  - Low-density, round to oval lesion

MR Findings

- T1WI
  - Signal intensity varies with concentration of fluid
  - Frequently hyperintense; may be hypo- or isointense
- T2WI
  - Hyperintense, uniform
- T1WI C+
  - No significant enhancement of lesion

Ultrasonographic Findings

- Grayscale ultrasound
  - Thin wall with smooth margins
  - Anechoic with increased through transmission
  - Colloid crystals may be suspended in fluid with **posterior comet-tail artifact (ring-down artifact)**
    - V-shaped morphology and depth > 1 mm differentiate from microcalcification
  - Thyroid and lesion capsule remain intact
- Color Doppler
  - No significant vascularity of wall
  - May show perilesional blood flow related to perinodular blood vessels

DIFFERENTIAL DIAGNOSIS

Simple Thyroid Cyst

- Uncommon; true cyst with epithelial lining
- Ultrasound: Anechoic with thin, smooth wall

Cystic Papillary Carcinoma

- Rare: Cystic nodule with solid component

- Ultrasound: Solid component: Nonsmooth margin, eccentric configuration, hypoechogenicity, microcalcification

Thyroglossal Duct Cyst

- Congenital, developmental anomaly
- Can occur anywhere from tongue base to thyroid

PATHOLOGY

Microscopic Features

- Rarely, true cyst with epithelial lining
- Usually degenerated macronodule with accumulated serous fluid, colloid substance, or blood

CLINICAL ISSUES

Presentation

- Most common signs/symptoms
  - May be detected as palpable nodule
  - May present with rapid increase in size from intracystic hemorrhage
  - Often incidental imaging finding
- Other signs/symptoms
  - When very large, may displace or distort larynx

Demographics

- Epidemiology
  - 15-25% of thyroid nodules

Natural History & Prognosis

- Benign lesions without malignant potential

DIAGNOSTIC CHECKLIST

Image Interpretation Pearls

- Ultrasound is key modality for determining if lesion is truly cyst and for differentiating from other lesions, including rare cystic papillary carcinoma
- Important to carefully evaluate cystic lesion on ultrasound
  - Solid components may harbor malignancy

SELECTED REFERENCES

1. Clark RDE et al: A clinical practice review of percutaneous ethanol injection for thyroid nodules: state of the art for benign, cystic lesions. Gland Surg. 13(1):108-16, 2024
2. Brigante G et al: De novo lesions frequently develop in adult normal thyroid over almost six years. Front Endocrinol (Lausanne). 11:18, 2020
3. Hoang VT et al: A review of the pathology, diagnosis and management of colloid goitre. Eur Endocrinol. 16(2):131-5, 2020
4. Tessler FN et al: Thyroid imaging reporting and data system (TI-RADS): a user's guide. Radiology. 287(1):29-36, 2018
5. Kim DW: Long-term ultrasound follow-up of thyroid colloid cysts. Int J Endocrinol. 2014:350971, 2014
6. Virmani V et al: Sonographic patterns of benign thyroid nodules: verification at our institution. AJR Am J Roentgenol. 196(4):891-5, 2011
7. Bonavita JA et al: Pattern recognition of benign nodules at ultrasound of the thyroid: which nodules can be left alone? AJR Am J Roentgenol. 193(1):207-13, 2009
8. Cohen JI et al: Thyroid disorders: evaluation and management of thyroid nodules. Oral Maxillofac Surg Clin North Am. 20(3):431-43, 2008
9. Desser TS et al: Ultrasound of thyroid nodules. Neuroimaging Clin N Am. 18(3):463-78, vii, 2008
10. Kabala JE: Computed tomography and magnetic resonance imaging in diseases of the thyroid and parathyroid. Eur J Radiol. 66(3):480-92, 2008
11. Loevner LA et al: Cross-sectional imaging of the thyroid gland. Neuroimaging Clin N Am. 18(3):445-61, vii, 2008

Esophagopharyngeal Diverticulum (Zenker)

TERMINOLOGY

- Mucosa-lined outpouching of posterior hypopharynx
- Posterior pulsion diverticulum **above** cricopharyngeus

IMAGING

- Sac arising from posterior hypopharynx at C5-C6 level
- Extends **posteroinferiorly** and **left** of esophagus
- **Barium esophagram** is best imaging tool
  - Confirms diagnosis and shows diverticular neck
  - Evaluates associated reflux and hiatal hernia
  - Pouch depth correlates with severity and outcome
- On CT/MR usually incidental finding
- CECT: Well-defined mass posterior and to left of esophagus
  - Nonenhancing mass arising from esophagus
  - Containing air, fluid, ± food debris
  - CT esophagram helps rule out postoperative leaks
- MR: Sagittal plane best delineates sac
  - Heterogeneous signal from food debris ± air-fluid level

TOP DIFFERENTIAL DIAGNOSES

- Lateral cervical esophageal diverticulum
- Paratracheal air cyst
- Parathyroid cyst
- Thyroid carcinoma nodal metastasis

PATHOLOGY

- Herniation occurs at Killian dehiscence
- Multiple causes proposed; likely multifactorial
- Almost all have hiatal hernia
- Many have reflux esophagitis

CLINICAL ISSUES

- Dysphagia and aspiration of retained ingested material
- As diverticulum enlarges, symptoms increase
- Complications mostly related to obstruction
- Squamous cell carcinoma is rare complication
- Symptomatic diverticula can be treated by endoscopic or external surgical techniques

(Left) Graphic depicts Zenker diverticulum ⇨ with herniation at Killian dehiscence between the thyropharyngeal ⇨ and cricopharyngeal ⬈ fibers of the inferior constrictor muscle. (Right) Barium esophagram demonstrates a large diverticulum with retained layering contrast ⇨ from the posterior lateral junction of the hypopharynx ⇨ and the cervical esophagus ⬈. The posterior lateral projection confirms this lesion as an esophagopharyngeal (Zenker) diverticulum.

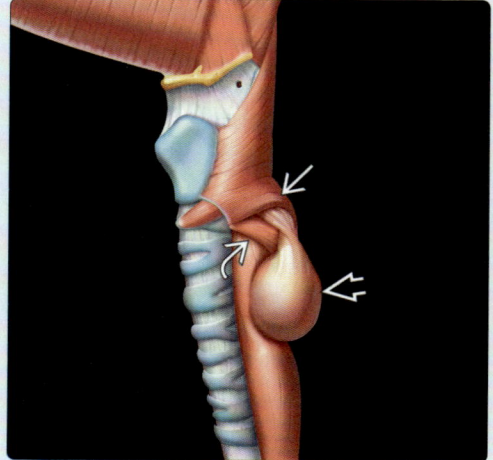
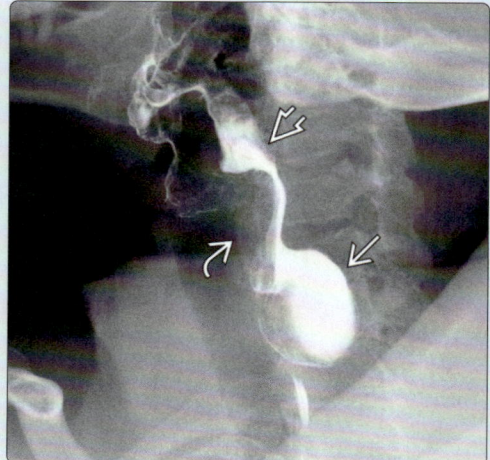

(Left) Parasagittal T2WI MR shows a saccular, well-circumscribed collection of heterogenous signal ⇨ with food debris just below the cricoid cartilage ⇨ at the level of C5-C6. (Right) Axial CT with oral contrast demonstrates a large, well-circumscribed lesion ⇨ posterior and extending predominantly to the left of the esophagus ⬈. This Zenker diverticulum contains layered oral barium contrast ⬈, heterogenous food debris, and air ⬈.

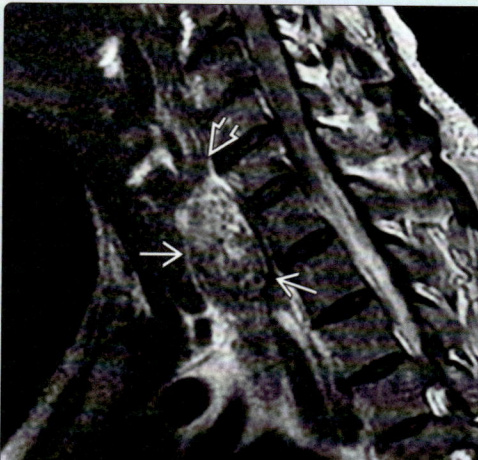
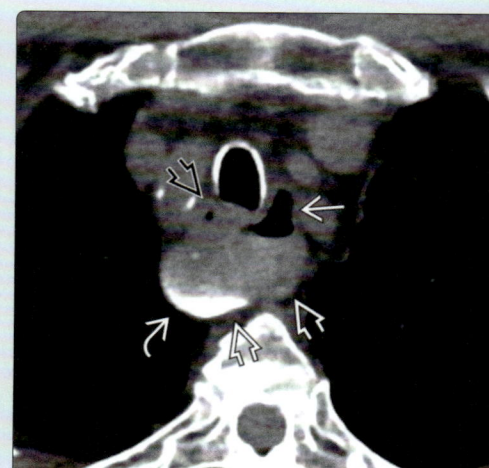

TERMINOLOGY

Synonyms

- Pharyngeal pouch, pharyngoesophageal diverticulum, posterior hypopharyngeal pseudodiverticulum

Definitions

- Mucosa-lined outpouching of posterior hypopharynx
- Posterior pulsion diverticulum **above cricopharyngeus**

IMAGING

General Features

- Best diagnostic clue
  - Well-defined mass **posterior** and to **left** of esophagus
  - Key finding: **Air** within lesion
- Location
  - Arises in posterior hypopharynx, above C5-C6 level
- Size
  - Variable, small to several centimeters
- Morphology
  - Sac-like outpouching descending behind esophagus

Fluoroscopic Findings

- Esophagram
  - Barium-filled sac extends caudally **posterior** and to **left** of cervical esophagus
  - Diverticular neck arise **above** cricopharyngeus
    - Cricopharyngeus may indent posterior esophagus
  - Associated hiatal hernia and reflux esophagitis possible
    - Hiatal hernia predicts worse surgical outcome
  - Irregularity of diverticular mucosal contour suggests inflammation or neoplasia
  - Measurement of pouch depth correlates with clinical severity and surgical outcome

CT Findings

- CECT
  - Nonenhancing thin wall mass with air, fluid, &/or debris
  - CT esophagram protocol helps detect postoperative leaks
    - Look for extraluminal air &/or contrast extravasation

MR Findings

- T2WI
  - Signal depends on contents, often heterogeneous
- T1WI C+
  - May see linear enhancement of mucosa

Imaging Recommendations

- Best imaging tool
  - Barium esophagram best illustrates diverticulum
  - CT esophagram helps rule out postoperative leaks
- Protocol advice
  - Oblique and lateral reveal diverticular neck location

DIFFERENTIAL DIAGNOSIS

Lateral Cervical Esophageal Diverticulum

- Lateral outpouching of proximal cervical esophagus
- Esophagram differentiates this diagnosis from Zenker (esophagopharyngeal) diverticulum

Paratracheal Air Cyst

- Air-filled structure arising from cervical or proximal trachea
- Located posterior and to right of trachea

Parathyroid Cyst

- Degenerative or congenital along parathyroid tract

Thyroid Carcinoma Nodal Metastasis

- Level VI node from differentiated thyroid carcinoma
- Does not contain air or communicate with esophagus

PATHOLOGY

General Features

- Etiology
  - Herniation of mucosa and submucosa of esophagus
    - Occurs at **Killian dehiscence** between thyropharyngeus and cricopharyngeus muscles
  - Multiple causes proposed, likely multifactorial
- Associated abnormalities
  - Hiatal hernia or reflux esophagitis

Staging, Grading, & Classification

- 2 descriptive classifications based on size alone
- Van Overbeek and Groote
  - Small < 1 vertebra in size, large > 3 vertebrae
- Morton and Bartley
  - Small < 2 cm, medium 2-4 cm, large > 4 cm

CLINICAL ISSUES

Presentation

- Most common signs/symptoms
  - Dysphagia as pouch compresses esophagus
  - Regurgitation of contents
  - Respiratory symptoms due to chronic aspiration

Demographics

- Age: Usually > 60 years, rarely < 40 years

Natural History & Prognosis

- As diverticulum enlarges, symptoms increase
- Most complications: aspiration of ingested material
- Squamous cell carcinoma is rare complication (0.3%)

Treatment

- Older adults with few symptoms are often observed
- Symptomatic diverticula can be treated by myotomy via endoscopic or external surgical techniques

DIAGNOSTIC CHECKLIST

Consider

- Barium esophagram is best to confirm diagnosis
- Evaluate for associated hiatal hernia and reflux esophagitis
- Suspect carcinoma if associated irregular mucosa or mass

SELECTED REFERENCES

1. Brown J et al: Surgical nonresponders in Zenker diverticulum and lower esophageal pathology (POUCH Collaborative). Laryngoscope. 134(12):4897-902, 2024

2. Banerjee D et al: Characterizing a CT esophagram protocol after flexible endoscopic diverticulotomy for Zenker's diverticulum: a retrospective series. Transl Gastroenterol Hepatol. 7:34, 2022

Lateral Cervical Esophageal Diverticulum

TERMINOLOGY

- Synonym: Killian-Jamieson diverticulum
- **Lateral outpouching** from **proximal cervical esophagus below cricopharyngeus muscle**

IMAGING

- Small, smoothly marginated lateral sac
- **Usually unilateral, left sided**
- Diameter: 0.2-5.0 cm; average: 1.4 cm
- Barium swallow (frontal & lateral) best imaging tool
  - Lateral sac; overlaps anterior esophageal wall
- Incidental finding on CECT/MR
  - Round or oval mass lateral to esophagus
  - Contents may be air, fluid, food debris, or mixed
- Incidental finding on thyroid US
  - Change in shape & position with swallowing differentiates from thyroid nodule & **avoids unnecessary biopsy**

TOP DIFFERENTIAL DIAGNOSES

- Esophagopharyngeal (Zenker) diverticulum
- Thyroid carcinoma nodal metastasis
- Parathyroid cyst

PATHOLOGY

- Pulsion-type diverticulum through **Killian-Jamieson triangle** in **anterolateral wall** of cervical esophagus
  - Zenker at posterior midline Killian dehiscence

CLINICAL ISSUES

- Less common than Zenker diverticulum
- **Usually asymptomatic**, incidental imaging finding
- Respiratory symptoms uncommon as cricopharyngeus prevents reflux to hypopharynx
- Most not surgically treated due to asymptomatic nature
- Per oral endoscopic myomectomy (POEM) for symptomatic patients

(Left) Axial CECT shows debris within a laterally projecting diverticulum ⇒ interposed between the cervical esophagus, left thyroid lobe ⇒, and common carotid. Note luminal contiguity with the esophagus. (Right) Frontal esophagram shows a prominent diverticular outpouching ⇒ from the left lateral cervical esophageal wall ⇒, compatible with a lateral cervical esophageal diverticulum (Killian-Jamieson). This lesion is below the level of the indentation from the cricopharyngeus muscle ⇒.

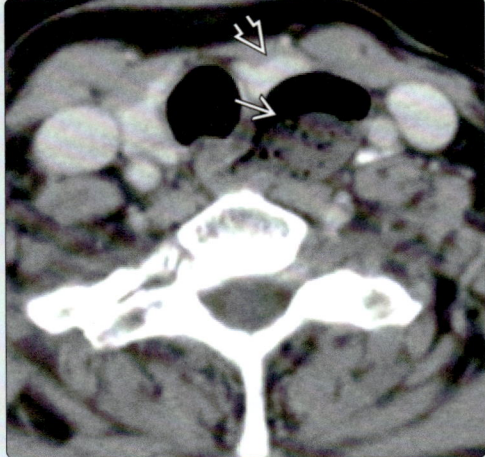
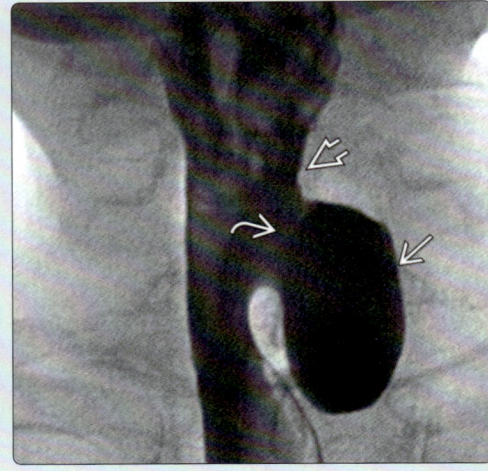

(Left) Transverse US in a patient with a left lower neck mass shows a large, air-filled lesion ⇒ (proven as lateral esophageal diverticulum on CT) posterior to the left lobe of the thyroid ⇒, which is displaced anteriorly, and the trachea ⇒ displaced laterally. (Right) Axial T1 C+ FS MR reveals an esophageal diverticulum as an air-filled, hypointense structure ⇒ in the lower neck posterior to the left thyroid lobe ⇒ and lateral to the cervical esophagus ⇒. Left common carotid artery is also displaced anteriorly, lateral to thyroid.

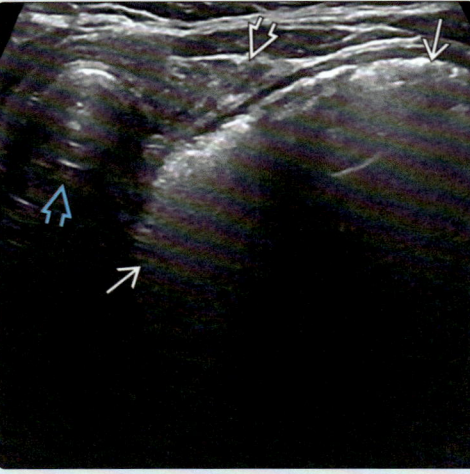
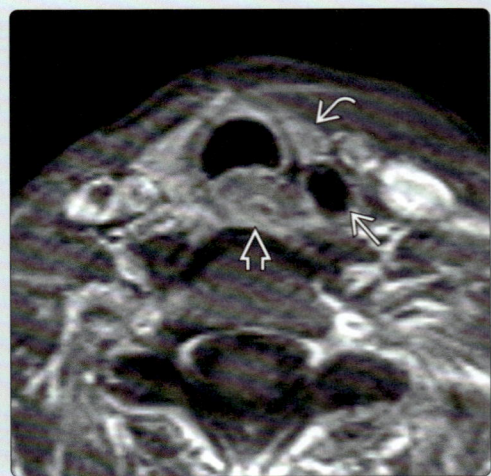

TERMINOLOGY

Synonyms

- Killian-Jamieson diverticulum, proximal lateral cervical esophageal diverticulum
- Lateral pharyngoesophageal diverticulum

Definitions

- Lateral outpouching from proximal cervical esophagus

IMAGING

General Features

- Location
  - **Usually unilateral, left sided**; bilateral up to 25%
- Size
  - Average diameter: 1.4 cm, range: 0.2-5.0 cm
- Morphology
  - Smoothly marginated round-oval sac

Imaging Recommendations

- Best imaging tool
  - Barium swallow best for confirming diagnosis
- Protocol advice
  - True lateral & frontal views should be obtained

Radiographic Findings

- Barium swallow findings
  - Frontal view: Small outpouching from proximal cervical esophagus
  - Lateral view: Arises below cricopharyngeus impression
    - Diverticulum overlaps anterior esophageal wall
- Aspiration rare as cricopharyngeus closes above diverticulum preventing reflux to larynx

CT Findings

- CECT
  - Well-defined, round or oval mass lateral to proximal esophagus
  - Density may be air, fluid, food debris, or mixed; may see air "pointing" toward esophagus
  - Abuts & may displace anteriorly left thyroid lobe & common carotid artery

MR Findings

- T2WI
  - Signal varies depending on luminal contents
  - Well-defined mass lateral to cervical esophagus

DIFFERENTIAL DIAGNOSIS

Esophagopharyngeal (Zenker) Diverticulum

- Arises from **posterior midline above cricopharyngeus**

Thyroid Carcinoma Nodal Metastasis

- Level VI adenopathy from differentiated carcinoma
- Variable density (CT) or intensity (MR)

Parathyroid Cyst

- Degenerative or congenital along parathyroid tract
- Fluid density/intensity

PATHOLOGY

General Features

- Etiology
  - Protrusion through muscular gap (Killian-Jamieson triangle) in anterolateral wall of cervical esophagus
    - Inferior to cricopharyngeus & lateral to longitudinal muscle of esophagus just below insertion on posterior cricoid cartilage
    - Note Zenker diverticulum through Killian dehiscence in posterior portion of cricopharyngeus
  - Pulsion-type diverticulum develops from refluxed pressure against competent cricopharyngeus
- Associated abnormalities
  - May see in association with esophagopharyngeal (Zenker) diverticulum

CLINICAL ISSUES

Presentation

- Most common signs/symptoms
  - Vast majority asymptomatic, incidental imaging finding
  - Dysphagia from pharyngeal dysmotility
- Other signs/symptoms
  - Respiratory symptoms uncommon as diverticulum below cricopharyngeus, preventing reflux to hypopharynx & larynx

Demographics

- Age
  - Usually > 60 years
- Epidemiology
  - Uncommon diverticulum; less common than esophagopharyngeal (Zenker) diverticulum

Treatment

- Typically not treated if asymptomatic
- Diverticulectomy ± esophagomyotomy if symptomatic

DIAGNOSTIC CHECKLIST

Consider

- Arises from lateral cervical esophagus **below cricopharyngeus**
  - Zenker arises just above cricopharyngeus in midline
- Exclude Killian-Jamieson diverticulum before performing fine-needle aspiration for thyroid lesion adjacent to esophagus

Image Interpretation Pearls

- Lateral barium swallow best for distinguishing from Zenker
  - On lateral swallow overlaps anterior esophageal wall

Reporting Tips

- Less common than Zenker & more likely to be asymptomatic

SELECTED REFERENCES

1. Assefa RL et al: Peroral endoscopic myotomy as a treatment for Killian-Jamieson diverticulum (KJ-POEM). Endosc Int Open. 12(10):E1214-19, 2024
2. Constantin A et al: Esophageal diverticula: from diagnosis to therapeutic management-narrative review. J Thorac Dis. 15(2):759-79, 2023

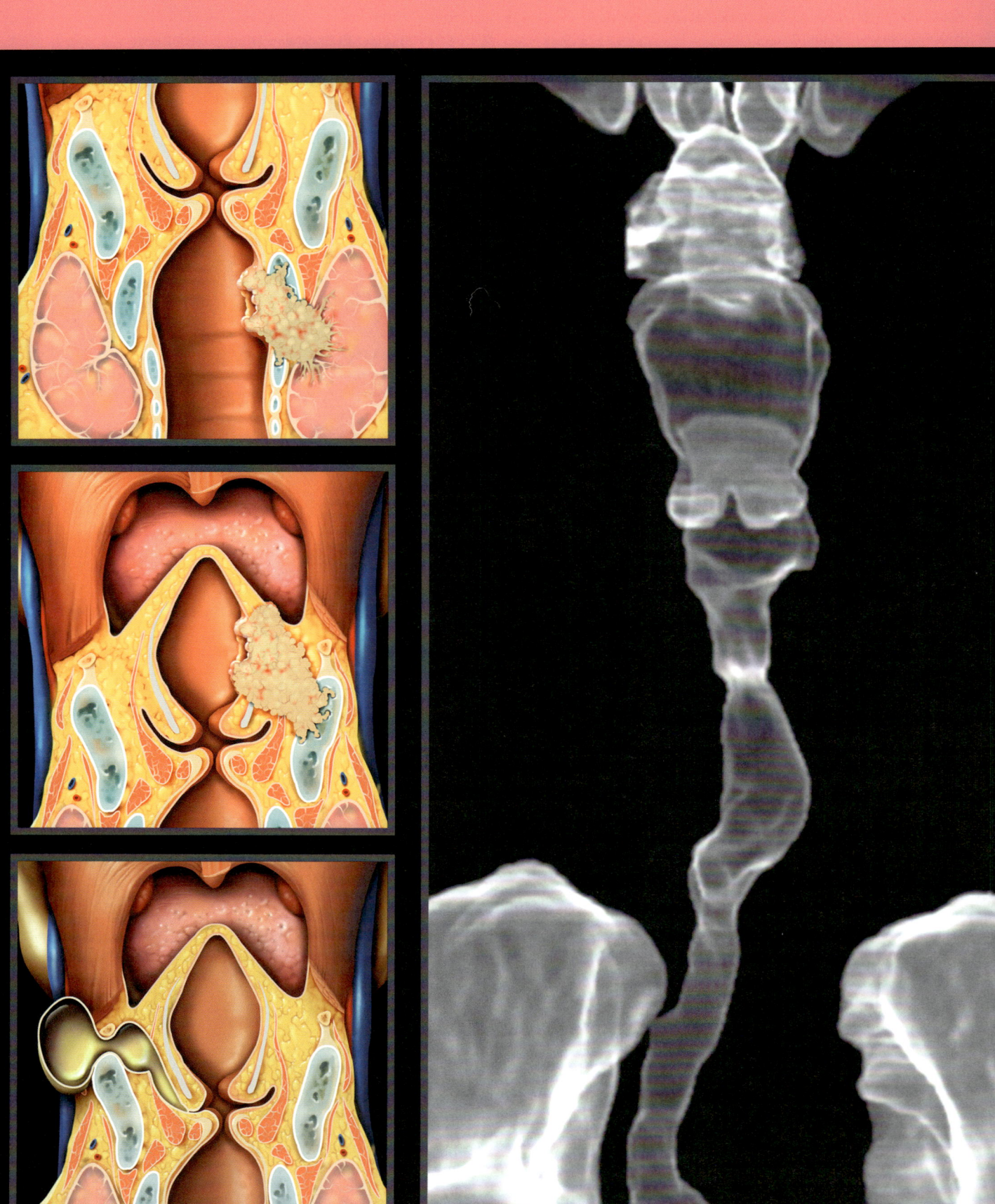

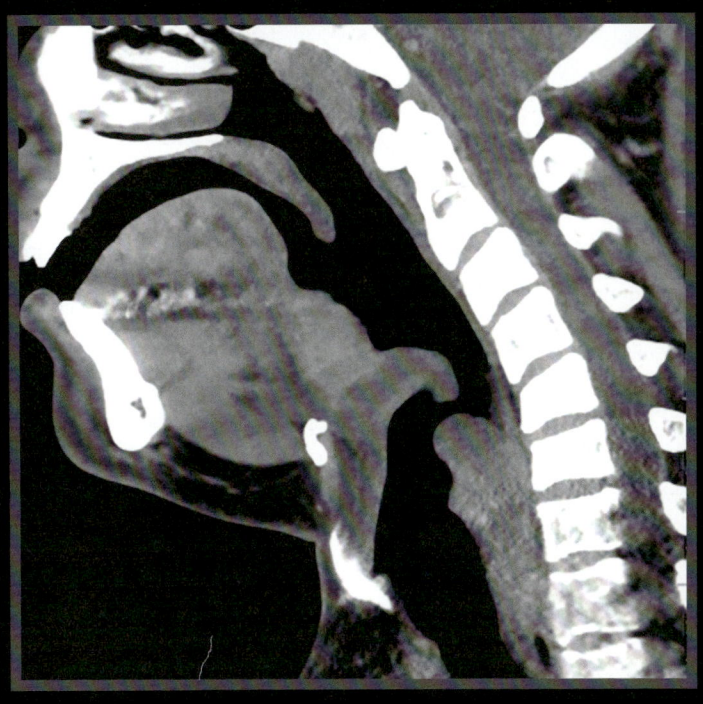

Summary Thoughts: Hypopharynx & Larynx

The hypopharynx and larynx both begin at the lower margin of the oropharynx and end at the lower margin of the cricoid cartilage. The **hypopharynx** is part of the digestive tract, carrying food and liquids to the esophagus. The **larynx** is part of the respiratory tract, connecting to the trachea, creating speech, and preventing aspiration.

Imaging of the **hypopharynx** and **larynx** is commonly performed for evaluation and staging of **squamous cell carcinoma (SCCa)**. Other common pathologies include laryngocele, thyroglossal duct cyst, and trauma. **Important tracheal lesions** include iatrogenic stenosis from intubation or tracheostomy, extrinsic compression or invasion by mass and, less commonly, tracheal inflammatory diseases.

The **larynx** and **hypopharynx** are intimately related anatomically, sharing 2 common walls. This means that pathology in 1 location readily involves the other. One should be able to distinguish the 2 sites and define their anatomic subsites, particularly when **staging SCCa**.

Imaging Techniques & Indications

CECT with sagittal and coronal reformations is the study of choice for the hypopharynx, larynx, and trachea. A standard protocol covers from the alveolar mandible to the clavicles at 1.25 mm or 2.5- to 3.0-mm intervals during quiet respiration, 90 seconds after contrast bolus. Some institutions may employ a biphasic injection technique with a split bolus separated by a variable delay followed by scanning after a slight delay from the 2nd bolus. This technique may provide better lesion and vascular enhancement. For hypopharyngeal or laryngeal SCCa, a **2nd pass** may help assess vocal cord motion. This is performed from the hyoid to cricoid during a breath hold, which opens the pyriform sinuses while the cords adduct.

MR is less commonly used because of breathing artifacts, but it is a useful adjunctive modality for staging of SCCa because it is more sensitive for detection of laryngeal **cartilage invasion**.

FDG PET/CT can help identify 2nd primary malignancies of the lung and upper aerodigestive tract in SCCa patients. It is useful for evaluation of recurrent or residual SCCa but is subject to false-positive results in the 2-3 months after radiation therapy. It increases nodal detection in advanced T tumors but does not consistently identify subcentimeter nodes due to camera resolution limitations.

Embryology

The **laryngeal ventricle** marks the division of 2 embryologically distinct laryngeal components. The **supraglottic larynx** forms from primitive buccopharyngeal anlage, and the **glottic** and the **subglottic larynx** form from tracheobronchial buds. The buccopharyngeal anlage has a much richer lymphatic network compared with the tracheobronchial buds. As a result, **supraglottic SCCa** has a much higher incidence of **nodal metastases** at presentation compared with **glottic** and **subglottic SCCa**.

Imaging Anatomy

The **hypopharynx** is part of the digestive tract, connecting the oropharyngeal mucosal space to the esophagus. At its superior limit, the hyoid bone, glossoepiglottic fold, and pharyngoepiglottic folds demarcate the valleculae, which are part of the oropharynx. The cricopharyngeus muscle defines the inferior limit of the hypopharynx, just below the cricoid cartilage.

The **3 major hypopharyngeal subsites** are the pyriform sinus, posterior wall, and postcricoid region. The **pyriform sinuses** are symmetric pouches hanging behind the larynx. The anteromedial margins of the pyriform sinuses are the posterolateral walls of the supraglottic **aryepiglottic (AE) folds**. The pyriform sinus inferior tip, or pyriform apex, is at the level of the true vocal cords (TVCs).

The **posterior hypopharyngeal wall** is the inferior continuation of the posterior oropharyngeal wall, extending from the hyoid to the inferior cricoid margin. Mucosa covering the posterior surface of the cricoid cartilage is the **postcricoid region**. This is 1 of the "shared walls" of the hypopharynx and larynx but is considered hypopharyngeal.

As part of the respiratory tract and the junction between the upper and lower airways, the **larynx** lies between the oropharynx and the trachea. The thyroid, cricoid, and arytenoid cartilages make up the framework over which the laryngeal soft tissues are draped.

As the largest of the laryngeal cartilages, the **thyroid cartilage** "shields" the larynx. Two laminae meet anteriorly at an acute angle in the midline to form an inverted V appearance on axial images. The posteriorly located **superior cornua** attach to the thyrohyoid membrane, and **inferior cornua** articulate medially with the cricoid cartilage sides, forming the cricothyroid joint. This is a useful imaging landmark for the entry of the recurrent laryngeal nerve to the larynx.

The **cricoid cartilage** provides structural integrity to the larynx as the only complete ring. It has a **signet-ring** shape with a shorter anterior arch and the quadrate lamina forming the signet posteriorly. Paired pyramidal **arytenoid cartilages** perch atop the posterior lamina with true synovial cricoarytenoid articulations. The arytenoid **vocal processes** project anteriorly and are attachments for the posterior margins of the **TVC**. The inferior limit of the cricoid marks the junction between the larynx and the trachea.

There are **3 areas** of the **larynx** with components that become important when staging SCCa. These are the supraglottic, glottic, and subglottic larynx. The **supraglottic larynx** (supraglottis) extends from the tip of the epiglottis above to the laryngeal ventricles below. **Important components** include the vestibule (supraglottic airway), epiglottis, preepiglottic space, arytenoid cartilages, false vocal cords, and paraglottic (paralaryngeal) spaces.

- The **epiglottis** is a leaf-shaped cartilage that serves as a lid to the endolaryngeal "box," which closes to prevent aspiration during swallowing. It has a superior **free margin** that projects above the hyoid bone and is inferiorly fixed to the thyroid cartilage by the thyroepiglottic ligament, just below the midline notch. Anterior to the epiglottis and posterior and inferior to the hyoid bone lies the fat-filled preepiglottic space, a clinical blind spot for submucosal tumor.
- The **false vocal cords** are the mucosal surfaces of the laryngeal vestibule. Deep to the false vocal cords are the paired **paraglottic spaces**. These fat-filled spaces merge superiorly into the preepiglottic space and extend inferiorly deep to the TVC in the glottis.
- The **AE folds** extend from the cephalad tips of the arytenoid cartilages to the inferolateral free margin of the epiglottis. AE folds form the superolateral borders of

Hypopharynx, Larynx, and Trachea Lesion Differential Diagnosis

Congenital	Trauma
Laryngomalacia	Arytenoid cartilage dislocation
Laryngeal web	Cricoid or thyroid cartilage fracture
Thyroglossal duct cyst	Hematoma
Degenerative/Acquired	Laceration
Laryngocele (saccular cyst)	**Benign Neoplasms**
Retention cyst	Hemangioma
Infectious/Inflammatory	Chondroma
Laryngotracheobronchitis (croup)	Lipoma
Epiglottitis/supraglottitis	Squamous papilloma
Tuberculosis	**Malignant Neoplasms**
Sarcoid	Squamous cell carcinoma
Rheumatoid arthritis	Sarcoma (chondrosarcoma)
Amyloid	Minor salivary gland tumor
Wegener granulomatosis	Lymphoma

the supraglottis and also the anteromedial margin of the pyriform sinuses (part of the hypopharynx). They, in effect, form "shared walls." An AE fold SCCa is called a marginal supraglottic laryngeal tumor.

The **glottic larynx** (glottis) consists of the TVCs and their mucosal covering. The **TVCs** are composed of thyroarytenoid muscle with its medial fibers called the vocalis muscle. Medially, there are thick elastic bands known as the vocal ligaments. TVCs meet in the midline anteriorly at the **anterior commissure**, which is only adequately imaged during quiet respiration. The **posterior commissure** is the mucosal surface between the arytenoid cartilages anterior to the cricoid. The mucosa over these areas is normally ≤ 1 mm in thickness.

The **subglottic larynx** (subglottis) includes the undersurface of the TVCs to the lower border of the cricoid cartilage. Its lateral walls are formed by the **conus elasticus**, a fibroelastic membrane extending from the vocal ligaments above to the cricoid below, which is not visible on imaging. Similar to the commissures of the glottis, the mucosa of the subglottis is normally < 1 mm in thickness.

The **trachea** connects the larynx to the lungs, beginning just below the cricoid and ending in the chest at the carina. Each cartilaginous ring surrounds the anterior 2/3 of the trachea with a fibromuscular membrane covering the flat posterior portion. **Important anatomic relationships** include the thyroid lobes laterally, thyroid isthmus anteriorly from the 2nd-4th tracheal rings, and the esophagus posteriorly. Posterolaterally, the tracheoesophageal groove contains the recurrent laryngeal nerves, paratracheal nodes, and parathyroid glands.

Approaches to Imaging Issues of Hypopharynx, Larynx, and Trachea

It is important to distinguish laryngeal and hypopharyngeal anatomic structures when evaluating pathology in this region, especially when **staging SCCa**. Two key "shared walls" are the **postcricoid region**, part of the hypopharynx, and the **AE folds**, part of the supraglottic larynx.

There are **clinical blind spots** in the hypopharynx and larynx, where imaging plays a critical role in tumor detection. In the hypopharynx, the **pyriform sinus apex** is a major site to search in patients presenting with "unknown primary" adenopathy.

In the larynx, the normally fat-filled preepiglottic and paraglottic spaces are clinical blind spots for submucosal spread of SCCa. As no fascia divides these spaces, SCCa can travel freely from one to the other.

Cartilage involvement with SCCa is an important clinical blind spot and also an area of imaging complexity. Irregular cartilage ossification makes determination of cartilage involvement difficult. The diagnosis of invasion should not be made lightly, as it is an indicator for total laryngectomy, as opposed to voice conservation surgery or chemoradiation. Cartilage invasion can only be determined when there is clear medullary invasion, cartilage destruction, or tumor mass on the outer extralaryngeal side of cartilage. Latest advances, such as dual-energy CT and photon-counting CT, have improved the assessment of cartilage invasion.

The clinical endoscopic exam provides useful information that may be essential for imaging evaluation, particularly for early T-stage glottic tumors. Conversely, imaging is very important for staging SCCa and especially for guiding surgeons to biopsy sites when there is an unknown primary tumor.

Clinical Implications

Hoarseness is a common presentation for **laryngeal tumors**. Glottic SCCa usually presents at an early stage with hoarseness. Subglottic SCCa is often discovered at an advanced stage with extralaryngeal spread. Supraglottic SCCa is often diagnosed at an advanced stage because hoarseness does not develop until tumor grows down to vocal cords. Supraglottic and hypopharyngeal SCCa often present with nodal metastases. Other symptoms include sore throat, dysphagia, and referred otalgia.

Tracheal lesions present with **shortness of breath** and **stridor** and may carry Dx of asthma. Primary tracheal tumors are rare; one is more likely to see displacement, compression, or invasion of the trachea by an extrinsic mass.

Hypopharynx, Larynx, and Trachea Overview

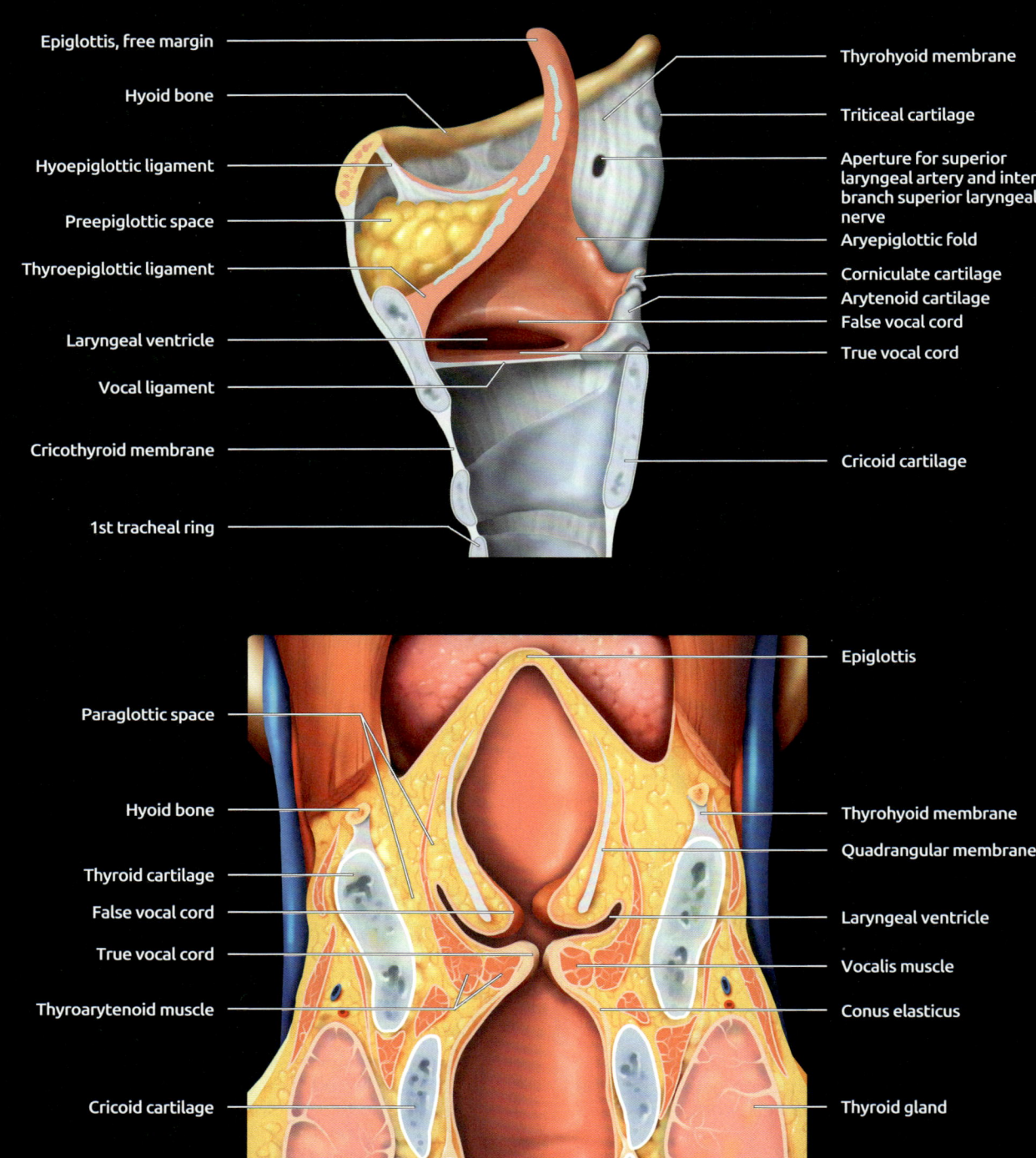

Epiglottis, free margin

Hyoid bone

Hyoepiglottic ligament

Preepiglottic space

Thyroepiglottic ligament

Laryngeal ventricle

Vocal ligament

Cricothyroid membrane

1st tracheal ring

Thyrohyoid membrane

Triticeal cartilage

Aperture for superior laryngeal artery and internal branch superior laryngeal nerve

Aryepiglottic fold

Corniculate cartilage

Arytenoid cartilage

False vocal cord

True vocal cord

Cricoid cartilage

Paraglottic space

Hyoid bone

Thyroid cartilage

False vocal cord

True vocal cord

Thyroarytenoid muscle

Cricoid cartilage

Epiglottis

Thyrohyoid membrane

Quadrangular membrane

Laryngeal ventricle

Vocalis muscle

Conus elasticus

Thyroid gland

(Top) *Sagittal graphic of midline larynx shows the laryngeal ventricle, the airspace that separates the false vocal cords above and true vocal cords below. Aryepiglottic (AE) folds project from the tip of arytenoid cartilage to inferolateral margin of epiglottis and represent a junction between the supraglottic larynx and hypopharynx. The epiglottis attaches to thyroid cartilage by thyroepiglottic ligament and to hyoid bone by hyoepiglottic ligament. Note the aperture in the thyrohyoid membrane for passage of superior laryngeal vessels and the internal branch of the superior laryngeal nerve.* (Bottom) *Coronal graphic, posterior view, of the larynx shows false and true vocal cords separated by laryngeal ventricle. The quadrangular membrane is a fibrous membrane that extends from upper arytenoid and corniculate cartilages to lateral epiglottis. The conus elasticus is a fibroelastic membrane that extends from the vocal ligament of true vocal cord to cricoid. These membranes represent a relative barrier to tumor spread but are not seen on routine imaging.*

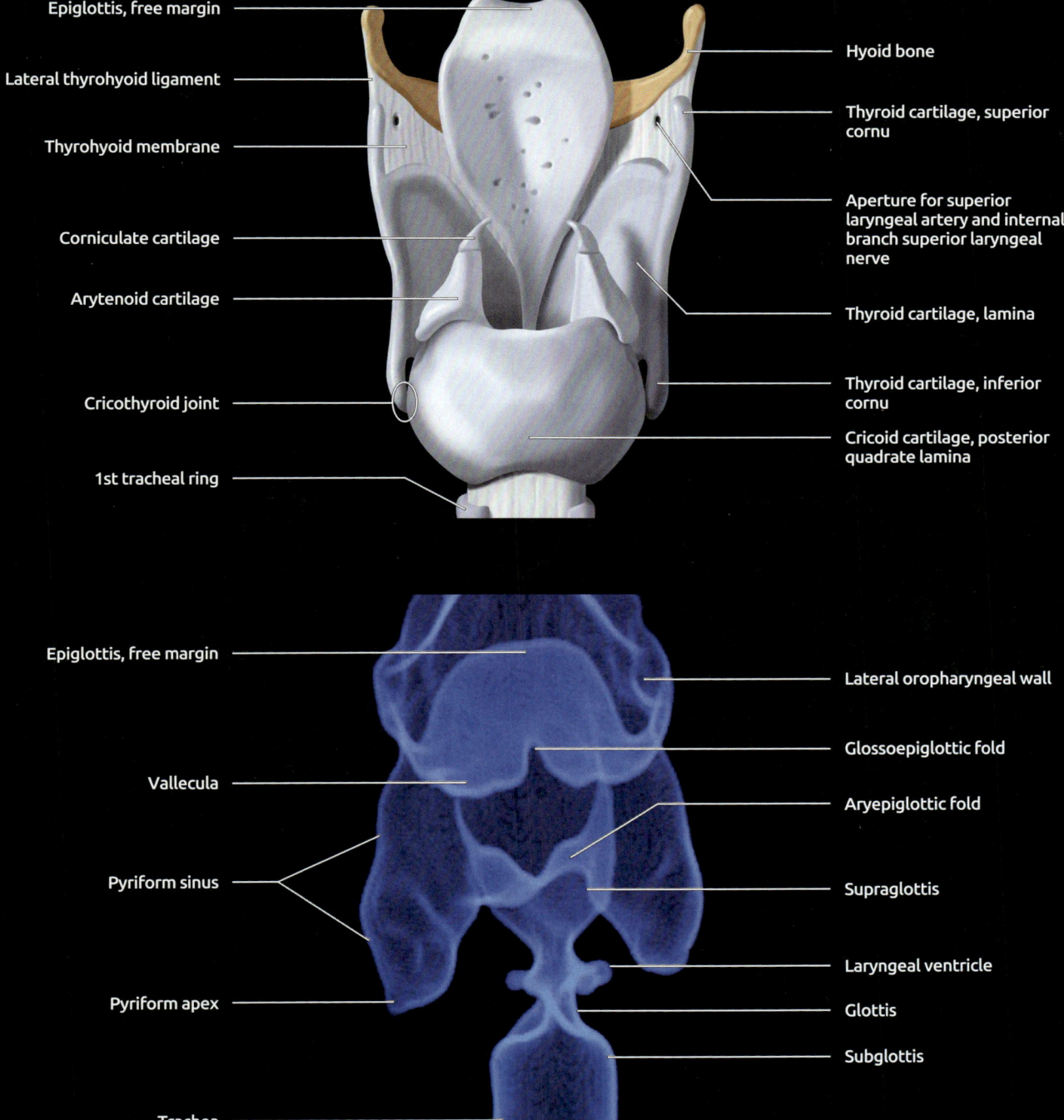

Epiglottis, free margin

Lateral thyrohyoid ligament

Thyrohyoid membrane

Corniculate cartilage

Arytenoid cartilage

Cricothyroid joint

1st tracheal ring

Hyoid bone

Thyroid cartilage, superior cornu

Aperture for superior laryngeal artery and internal branch superior laryngeal nerve

Thyroid cartilage, lamina

Thyroid cartilage, inferior cornu

Cricoid cartilage, posterior quadrate lamina

Epiglottis, free margin

Vallecula

Pyriform sinus

Pyriform apex

Trachea

Lateral oropharyngeal wall

Glossoepiglottic fold

Aryepiglottic fold

Supraglottis

Laryngeal ventricle

Glottis

Subglottis

(Top) *Posterior graphic shows the epiglottis, a leaf-shaped cartilage containing fixed and free margins. The fixed portion has a narrow stem that attaches by thyroepiglottic ligament to internal aspect of thyroid cartilage, just below the superior thyroid notch. Arytenoid cartilages perch on and articulate with the superior aspect of posterior cricoid cartilage. Inferior thyroid cornu articulates with cricoid in synovial-lined cricothyroid joint. Cricoid cartilage is the only complete ring in the endolarynx and provides structural integrity. It is composed of the anterior arch and taller posterior quadrate lamina. The lower border of cricoid represents the junction between larynx and trachea. Thyroid, cricoid, and most of arytenoids are hyaline cartilage and ossify with age. Epiglottis, corniculate, and vocal process of arytenoid are yellow fibrocartilage and do not tend to ossify. **(Bottom)** Frontal 3D surface-rendered CT shows normal mucosal surfaces of oropharynx, hypopharynx, larynx, and trachea when distended during phonation.*

(Left) Axial graphic at the level of the hyoid bone through the roof of hypopharynx shows the anterior preepiglottic space filled with fat ➡️. Midline glossoepiglottic fold ➡️, free margin of epiglottis ➡️, and lateral pharyngoepiglottic folds ➡️ delineate contours of valleculae. **(Right)** Axial CECT at the same level reveals a hypodense, fat-filled preepiglottic space ➡️ and the anterior margin of the glossoepiglottic fold ➡️, which separates valleculae. The free margin of the epiglottis ➡️ is visible.

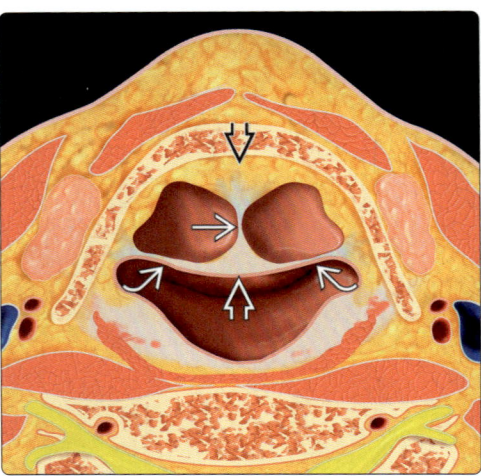
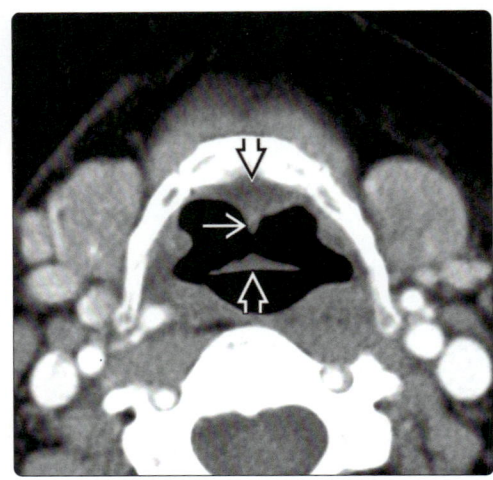

(Left) Axial graphic at the midsupraglottic level shows the hyoepiglottic ligament ➡️ to the fixed portion of the epiglottis ➡️. AE folds ➡️ are part of the supraglottic larynx but also form the anterior wall of the pyriform sinuses ➡️ and therefore form a junction between larynx and hypopharynx. **(Right)** Axial CECT at the same level shows the hyoepiglottic ligament ➡️ and the fixed portion of the epiglottis ➡️ anteriorly. The posterior wall of the AE folds ➡️ forms the anterior wall of the pyriform sinuses ➡️.

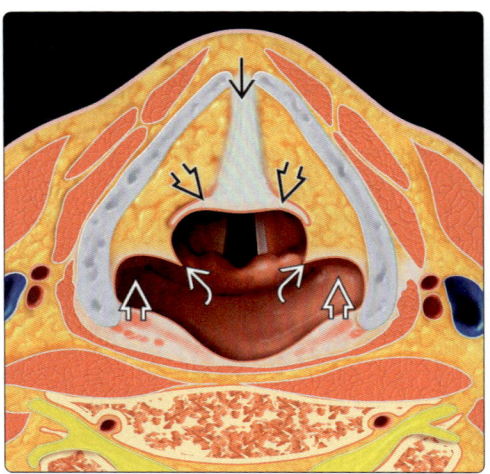
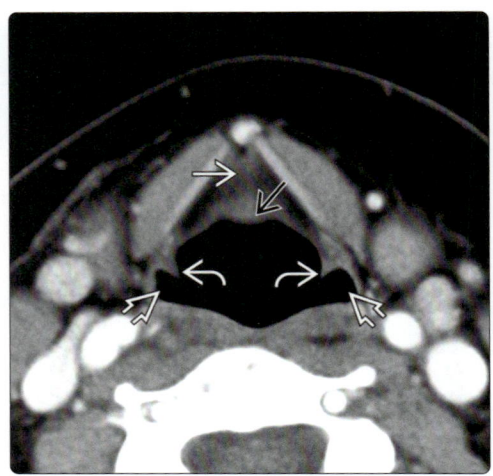

(Left) Axial graphic depicts glottis or true vocal cord level where vocalis ➡️ and thyroarytenoid ➡️ muscles are evident deep to vocal ligaments ➡️. Pyriform sinus apex ➡️ reaches the level of true vocal cord and cricoarytenoid joints ➡️. **(Right)** Axial CECT shows cricoarytenoid joints ➡️, indicating that the scan is at the level of the glottis. True vocal cords ➡️ are abducted, as the study was performed during quiet respiration. Note the thin normal anterior commissure ➡️ during this phase.

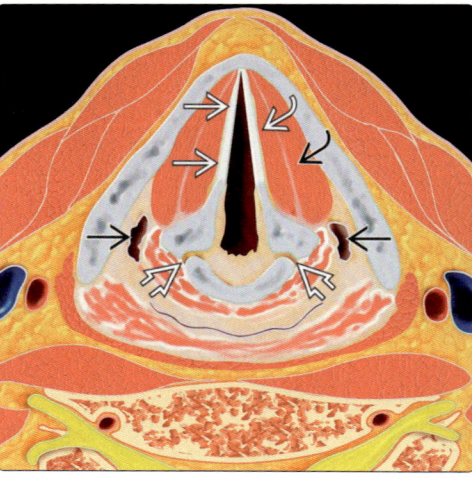
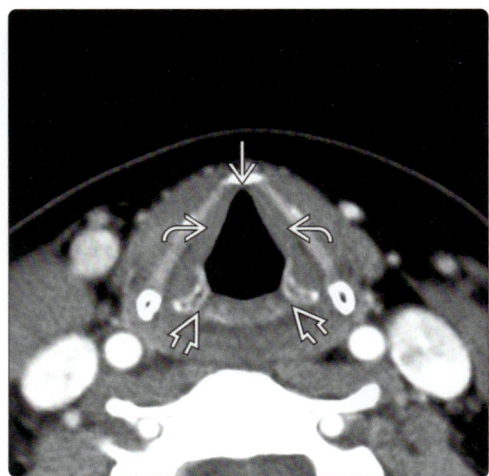

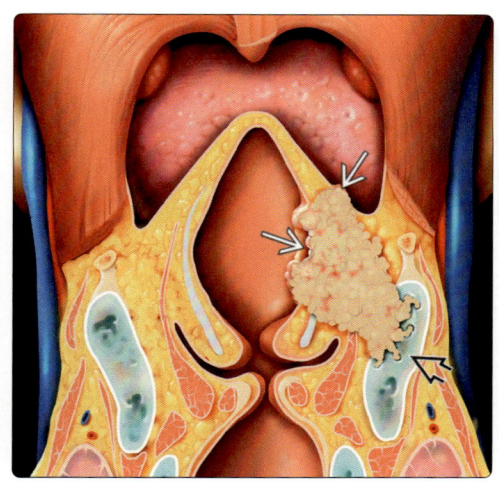 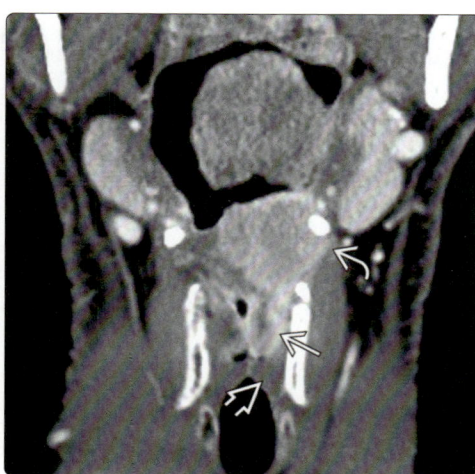

(Left) Coronal graphic depicts a supraglottic squamous cell carcinoma (SCCa) ⮕ centered in the left AE fold and false cord, laterally invading thyroid cartilage ⮕. (Right) Coronal reformatted CECT shows a large, enhancing mass arising in the left supraglottic larynx, extending down paraglottic fat to false cord ⮕. True cord is not involved ⮕. Superiorly, the mass extends to the valleculae, and laterally, protrudes through the thyrohyoid membrane ⮕. Nodal drainage for supraglottic tumors is to levels II, III and IV.

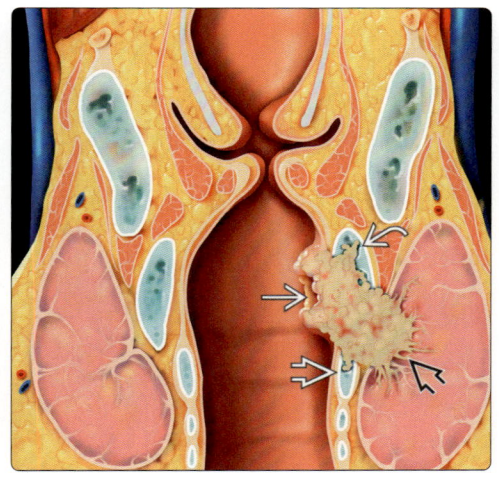 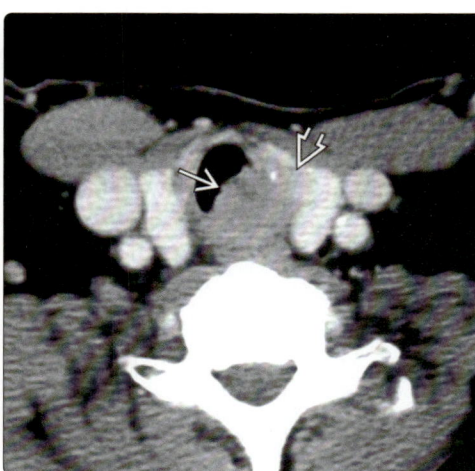

(Left) Coronal graphic depicts a subglottic SCCa ⮕ invading laterally through cricoid cartilage ⮕ into thyroid gland ⮕. First tracheal ring cartilage is also involved ⮕. Nodal drainage for subglottic tumors is to levels IV and VI nodes initially. (Right) Axial CECT through the lower neck reveals the inferior aspect of a subglottic SCCa ⮕ as it invades laterally into the left thyroid gland ⮕. Approximately 50% of subglottic tumors present at this T4 stage.

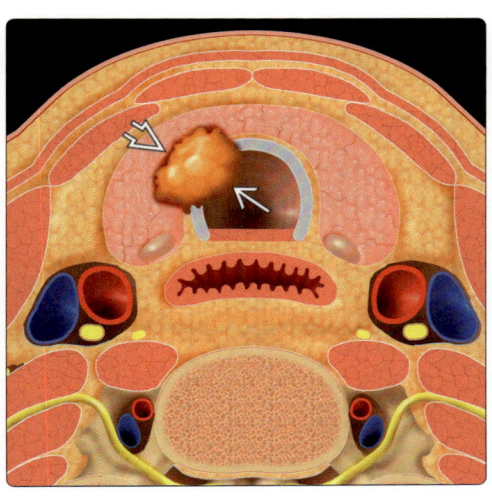 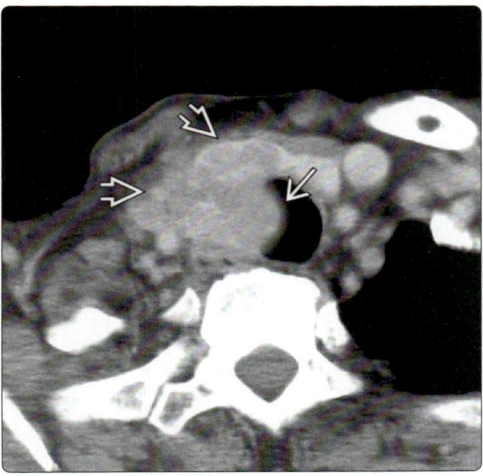

(Left) Axial graphic through the thyroid bed illustrates a tracheal wall mass protruding into tracheal lumen ⮕ and laterally invading the thyroid gland ⮕. Cervical tracheal wall lesions are rare, but diagnosis is often delayed due to nonlocalizing symptoms that may be misinterpreted as asthma. (Right) Axial CECT shows a tracheal wall carcinoma invading laterally and anteriorly into the thyroid gland ⮕. The patient presented with stridor from tumor encroachment on tracheal lumen ⮕.

TERMINOLOGY

- Benign, self-limited viral inflammation of upper airway
- Subglottic edema → stridor & characteristic "barky" cough

IMAGING

- Radiographs to exclude more serious causes of stridor
- Frontal view: Best for typical findings of croup
  - Smooth, symmetric, long-segment subglottic airway narrowing, gradually widens to normal-caliber trachea
    - Steeple or inverted V configuration
    - Loss of normal short segment "shoulders" of subglottic trachea secondary to edema
- Lateral view: Best for excluding other diagnoses
  - Relatively mild narrowing of AP dimension
  - Haziness with loss of subglottic tracheal wall definition
  - ± hypopharyngeal overdistention

TOP DIFFERENTIAL DIAGNOSES

- Foreign body
- Vascular ring
- Bacterial tracheitis
- Infantile hemangioma
- Epiglottitis
- Thermal injury
- Angioedema
- Iatrogenic subglottic stenosis

CLINICAL ISSUES

- Acute clinical syndrome characterized by "barky" or seal-like ("croupy") cough, inspiratory stridor, hoarseness
  - Age range: 6 months to 3 years; uncommon > 6 years
- ± prodrome of low-grade fever, mild cough, rhinorrhea
- Majority are due to parainfluenza virus types 1-3
- Most cases are successfully treated with glucocorticoids ± nebulized epinephrine
- Recurrent episodes or atypical age suggest alternate diagnosis

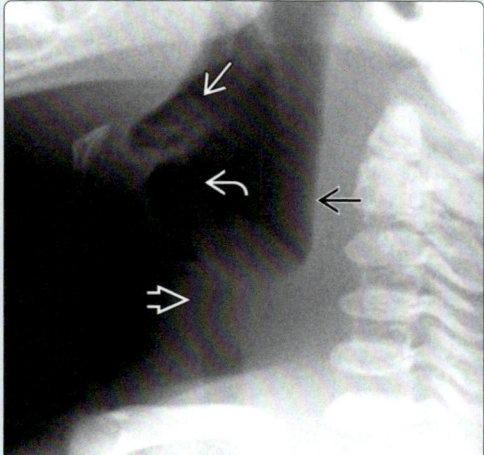
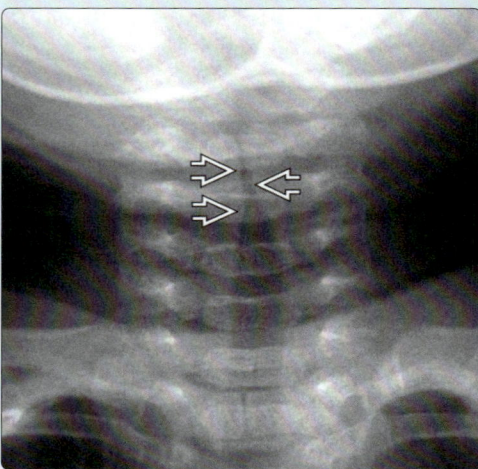

(Left) Lateral radiograph in a 9-month-old infant with stridor shows haziness of the subglottic airway ➡. Overdistention (ballooning) of the hypopharynx ⇨ is noted. The epiglottis ➡ & aryepiglottic folds ➚ are normal. (Right) AP radiograph in the same patient shows symmetric narrowing of the subglottic trachea ➡, typical of croup. The loss of the normal abrupt subglottic/glottic shouldering + gradual tapering of the subglottic airway lumen from inferior to superior is referred to as the steeple sign.

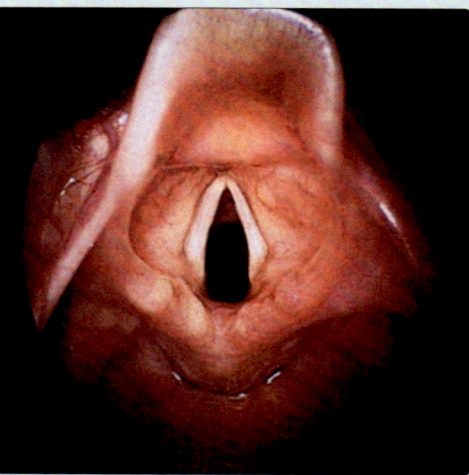
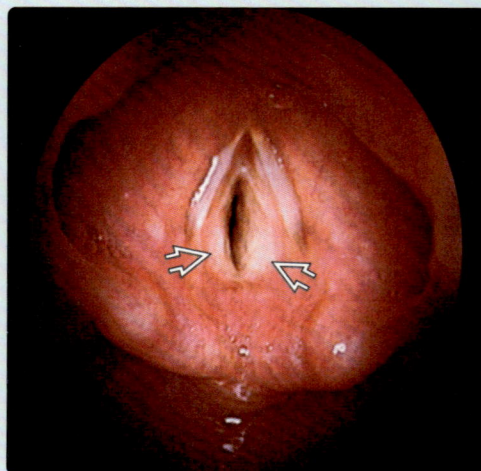

(Left) Endoscopic photograph shows a normal appearance of the subglottic airway. The subglottis is widely patent such that the mucosa is actually hidden beneath the vocal cords. (Right) Endoscopic photograph in a child with viral croup shows edematous subglottic mucosa ➡, which is visualized through the vocal cords. There is marked narrowing of the subglottic airway lumen, predominantly in the transverse dimension.

TERMINOLOGY

Synonyms

- Acute laryngotracheitis

Definitions

- Croup: Self-limited viral inflammation of subglottic airway
- Acute laryngotracheobronchitis: Croup + lower airway involvement
- Spasmodic croup: Recurrent episodes, typically without viral prodrome or fever
- Atypical croup: May refer to recurrent episodes, atypical patient age, prolonged/severe episodes, uncommon pathogen

IMAGING

General Features

- Best diagnostic clue
  - Symmetric subglottic airway tapering/narrowing on frontal radiograph
  - Loss of normal subglottic "shoulders"
- Morphology
  - Normal: Uniform caliber of cervical & thoracic trachea from subglottis to carina
    - Normal subglottic "shoulders": Symmetric, focal, convex, lateral margins at uppermost subglottic airway
      □ ~ 30-45° from horizontal

Radiographic Findings

- Radiography
  - AP/frontal view
    - Steeple or inverted V configuration of subglottic trachea
      □ Smooth, symmetric narrowing of subglottic airway gradually widens to normal-caliber trachea
      □ Loss of normal "shoulders" of subglottic trachea secondary to subglottic edema
      □ Vertical length of narrowing is variable; approximately upper 1/3 of cervical trachea
  - Lateral view
    - Mild narrowing of subglottic trachea in AP dimension
      □ Less than narrowing of transverse dimension on frontal view
    - Haziness & poor definition of subglottic tracheal walls
    - ± hypopharyngeal overdistention
      □ Also seen at end-inspiration in crying child
      □ Hypopharynx may be collapsed with distention of lower cervical trachea on expiratory image
    - Normal epiglottis, aryepiglottic folds, retropharyngeal soft tissues
    - No foreign body

Imaging Recommendations

- Best imaging tool
  - Diagnosis of croup is primarily clinical
    - Radiographs are used to exclude more serious causes of stridor
      □ Atypical or severe course, foreign body concern, recurrent episodes
    - Chest radiographs are sometimes obtained to exclude pneumonia
  - Frontal radiograph is most useful view to confirm croup
  - Lateral radiograph helps exclude other diagnoses
- Protocol advice
  - Ensure that neck is extended with adequate inspiration on lateral view
    - Decreases crowding of airway structures that may simulate disease in young child
  - Avoid image acquisition while child swallows

DIFFERENTIAL DIAGNOSIS

Airway Foreign Body

- Minority of foreign bodies are radiopaque
  - May appear as soft tissue density but with straight, irregular, or pointed margins
- Can lodge anywhere from nasal/oral cavities to bronchi
  - Right main bronchus is most common lower airway site
    - ± asymmetric lung aeration on chest radiographs
- Symptoms & imaging findings depend on location of object
- Esophageal foreign body may cause edema of adjacent trachea, especially if subacute/chronic or button battery ingestion

Vascular Ring

- Intrathoracic tracheal narrowing/deviation
- Double aortic arch, right aortic arch with aberrant left subclavian artery, pulmonary sling

Bacterial Tracheitis

- Synonyms: Exudative tracheitis, membranous croup
- Typically occurs in older child (6-10 years old)
- May be toxic-appearing
- Intraluminal filling defects (pseudomembranes)
- Plaque-like irregularity &/or poor definition of tracheal walls
- Asymmetric subglottic narrowing

Infantile Hemangioma

- Younger child, often < 6 months
  - Develops in 1st few weeks of life → grows rapidly over 6-12 months → slow spontaneous regression
- Asymmetric airway narrowing ± focal tracheal wall contour abnormality
- 50% have another visible hemangioma, most commonly of face/neck in "beard" distribution

Epiglottitis

- Typically occurs in older children
  - Historical mean age (pre-Hib vaccine): 3 years
  - Now teenagers are more common
- Severe, life-threatening condition
- Marked enlargement of epiglottis & aryepiglottic folds
  - Loss of sharp posterior margin of central epiglottis on lateral view
- May cause symmetric subglottic narrowing on frontal view

Thermal Injury

- History of smoke inhalation, burns

Angioedema

- Rapid swelling of facial soft tissues & upper airway
  - ± itching, pain, hives

- May be due to allergic reaction or hereditary angioedema

Iatrogenic Subglottic Stenosis

- History of prolonged or traumatic intubation
- Predisposes to recurrent croup-like episodes

PATHOLOGY

General Features

- Etiology
  - Typical croup is secondary to viral illness
    - Most cases: Parainfluenza virus types 1-3
    - Less frequently: Respiratory syncytial virus, adenovirus, rhinovirus, enterovirus, influenza, herpes simplex, metapneumoviruses, measles, SARS-CoV-2; bacterial forms are uncommon (consider *Corynebacterium diphtheriae* & *Mycoplasma pneumoniae*)
  - Leads to inflammation & edema of subglottic airway
    - Redundant mucosa predisposes to edema & narrowing
      - □ Loose mucosal attachment of conus elasticus
    - Cricoid cartilage is complete ring with inability to expand
    - Swelling of vocal cords → hoarseness
    - Characteristic (but not specific) "barky" cough results from inflammation of larynx & trachea
    - Inspiratory stridor is due to proportionately small subglottic trachea in young children
      - □ Same viral infections & edema do not compromise older child or adult airway
- Associated abnormalities
  - Atypical or spasmodic croup
    - 20-64% incidence of large airway lesions: Subglottic hemangioma, stenosis, laryngeal cleft, laryngeal ulcer, tracheomalacia, laryngomalacia, papillomatosis, laryngeal web, or vocal cord paralysis
    - Additional common disorders in this group: Gastroesophageal reflux, asthma, sleep-disordered breathing, seasonal allergies, chronic cough, prematurity

Staging, Grading, & Classification

- Westley croup severity score (clinical severity score)
  - Mild: Occasional "barky" cough, no stridor at rest, no or mild retractions
  - Moderate: Frequent "barky" cough, stridor at rest, mild to moderate retractions
  - Severe: Moderate criteria + marked retractions, distress, & agitation
  - Impending respiratory failure: Severe criteria + altered mental status, poor air entry, cyanosis or pallor

CLINICAL ISSUES

Presentation

- Most common signs/symptoms
  - Acute clinical syndrome characterized by "barky" or seal-like ("croupy") cough, inspiratory stridor, hoarseness, respiratory distress
- Other signs/symptoms
  - Often prodrome of low-grade fever, mild cough, rhinorrhea

- Typically nontoxic-appearing & able to manage secretions
- More severe cases: Intercostal retractions, tachypnea, pallor, cyanosis, tachycardia, altered mental status
- Symptoms worse at night or with agitation
- May occur with other symptoms of lower respiratory tract infection (wheezing, cough, etc.)

Demographics

- Age
  - Most common range: 6 months to 3 years
    - Uncommon > 6 years
    - Mean age of atypical croup: 2.7-4.8 years
  - If > 3 years, consider other causes of acute stridor
  - If < 6 months, consider predisposing abnormality
- Epidemiology
  - Most common cause of acute upper airway obstruction in young children
    - Affects 5% of children by age 2
    - Affects 3% of children per year
  - Seasonal occurrence with viral disease
    - Most prevalent in fall to winter
    - Historically has shown biennial peaks

Natural History & Prognosis

- Typically benign, self-limited disease
- ~ 85% are classified as mild
- 75% of mild cases resolve within 3 days
- 11% of mild & 49% of moderate cases worsen
- 5% return to emergency department within 72 hours

Treatment

- Mild: Often supportive therapy at home
  - Humidified air, antipyretics if febrile, oral fluids
  - Oral glucocorticoid
- Moderate or severe
  - Oral, IV, or IM glucocorticoid + nebulized epinephrine
  - Supportive measures (antipyretics, humidified air, oxygen, oral or IV fluids)
  - Admission for inadequate response to treatment
    - Downward trend in patients requiring inpatient treatment over last several decades
    - < 5% of patients with croup require hospitalization
  - Intubation is rarely needed, should be performed by skilled provider in controlled setting
  - Death is very rare; < 1% of patients requiring intubation

DIAGNOSTIC CHECKLIST

Consider

- Alternate diagnosis with recurrent episodes or atypical age

SELECTED REFERENCES

1. Akcan Yildiz L et al: Improving croup management at a pediatric emergency department. Postgrad Med. 136(4):438-45, 2024
2. Weinstein R et al: Revisiting dexamethasone use in the pediatric emergency department. Curr Opin Pediatr. 36(3):251-5, 2024
3. Lim CC et al: Croup and COVID-19 in a child: a case report and literature review. BMJ Case Rep. 14(9), 2021
4. Hanna J et al: Epidemiological analysis of croup in the emergency department using two national datasets. Int J Pediatr Otorhinolaryngol. 126:109641, 2019
5. Darras KE et al: Imaging acute airway obstruction in infants and children. Radiographics. 35(7):2064-79, 2015

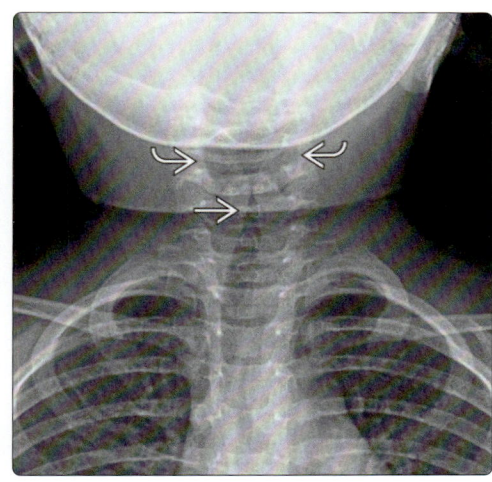

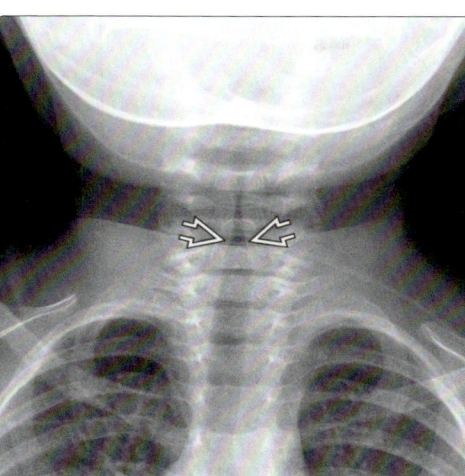

(Left) AP radiograph in a 2-year-old with stridor shows symmetric subglottic narrowing ➡ (steeple sign) & mild overdistention of the hypopharynx ➡. The trachea is otherwise normal in caliber & position. (Right) AP radiograph in a child with viral croup shows symmetric subglottic airway narrowing ➡. The narrowing has the appearance of the steeple sign in which loss of the shouldering normally seen in the subglottic region causes the airway to appear like a steeple.

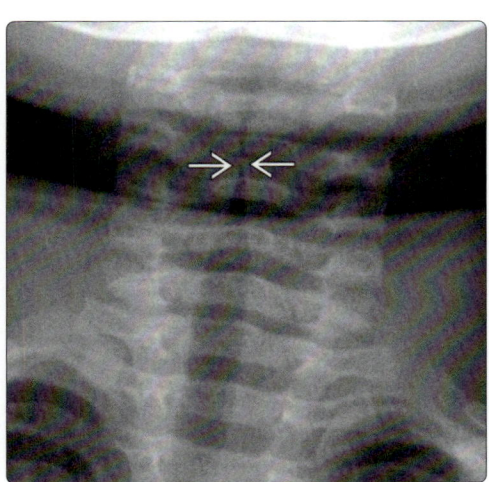

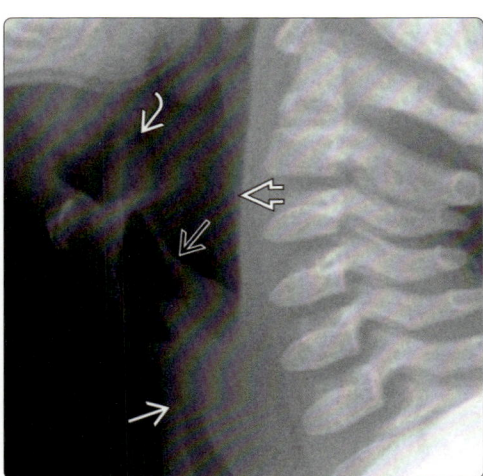

(Left) AP radiograph in a 19-month-old with croup demonstrates the typical steeple appearance of the trachea ➡ & loss of the normal shouldering, secondary to symmetric subglottic tracheal edema. (Right) Lateral radiograph in the same patient shows poor definition/haziness of the subglottic airway ➡, & mild hypopharyngeal distention ➡, findings typical of croup. Notice a normal appearance of the epiglottis ➡ & aryepiglottic folds ➡.

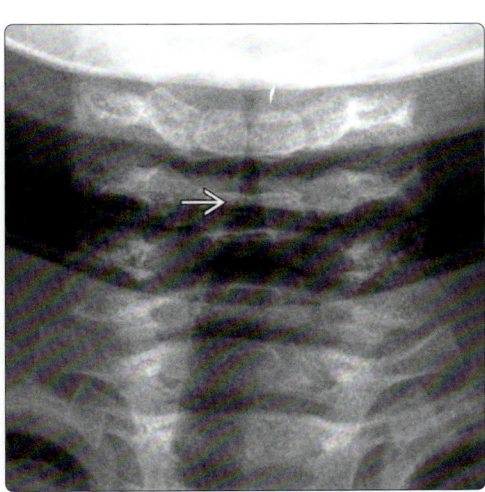

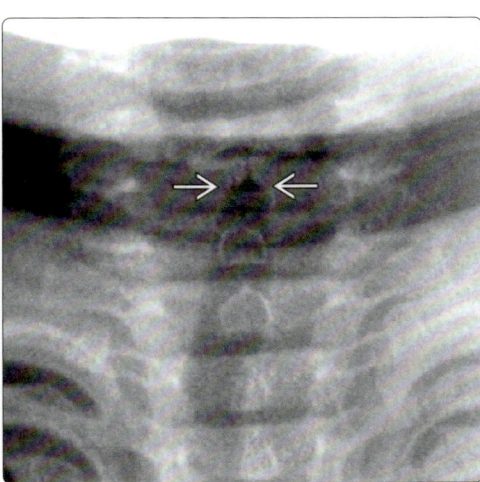

(Left) AP radiograph in a 16-month-old child with stridor shows symmetric subglottic airway narrowing ➡, typical of viral croup. No focal mass or linear/nodular filling defect is identified. (Right) AP radiograph in a normal child shows the typical normal "shoulders" ➡ of the subglottic airway, which are more focal & horizontal than the long, gradual, vertical steepling seen in croup.

Hypopharynx, Larynx, and Cervical Trachea

TERMINOLOGY

- Airway obstruction secondary to inflammation of epiglottis & surrounding tissues
- Synonym: Supraglottitis

IMAGING

- Lateral radiograph: Enlarged epiglottis (**thumb sign**)
  - Aryepiglottic folds thick & convex superiorly
  - Ballooning of hypopharynx
- Frontal radiograph ± symmetric subglottic narrowing
- CECT usually not required: Rarely see phlegmon or abscess

TOP DIFFERENTIAL DIAGNOSES

- Croup
- Exudative tracheitis
- Retropharyngeal abscess

PATHOLOGY

- Most often *Haemophilus influenzae* type b (Hib)

- Decreased incidence after Hib vaccine
- Noninfectious causes: Angioneurotic edema, trauma, foreign body ingestion, Stevens-Johnson syndrome, caustic ingestion, bee stings, vaping/E-cigarettes, thermal injury

CLINICAL ISSUES

- **Acute life-threatening disease**, may require emergent intubation
- **Toxic child** with difficulty breathing & swallowing
- Mean age: 14.6 years after Hib vaccine introduced
- May also occur in adults

DIAGNOSTIC CHECKLIST

- Life-threatening emergency, so may not be imaged
- For radiograph: Child should be upright, comfortable
  - Do not agitate or place in supine position
  - Physician escort + equipment to secure airway if necessary

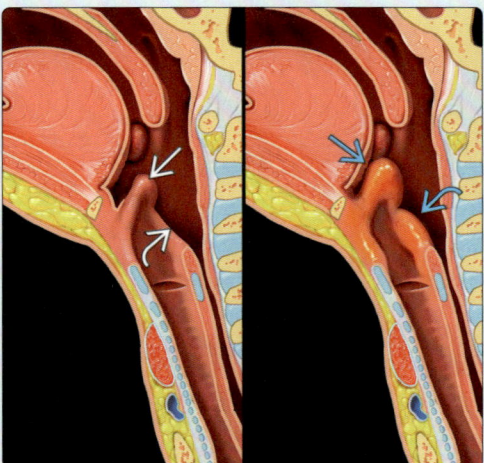
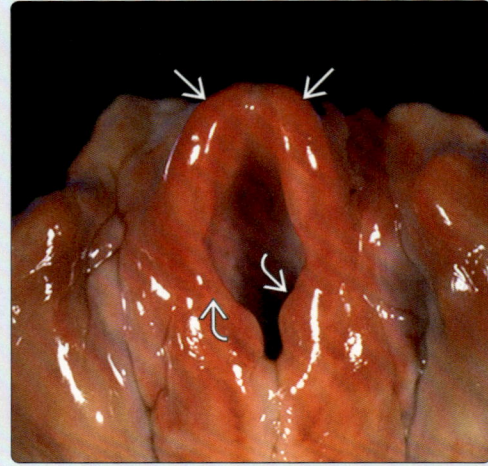

(Left) *Left lateral graphic shows the normal supraglottic larynx on the left with a sharply defined epiglottis ➡ and straight or slightly concave aryepiglottic (AE) folds ➡. Right lateral graphic shows epiglottitis with a thick, swollen epiglottis ➡ and convex, thickened, and inflamed AE folds ➡.* **(Right)** *Gross pathology specimen shows a markedly swollen, reddened epiglottis ➡, and similarly inflamed and thickened AE folds ➡, narrowing the supraglottic lumen.*

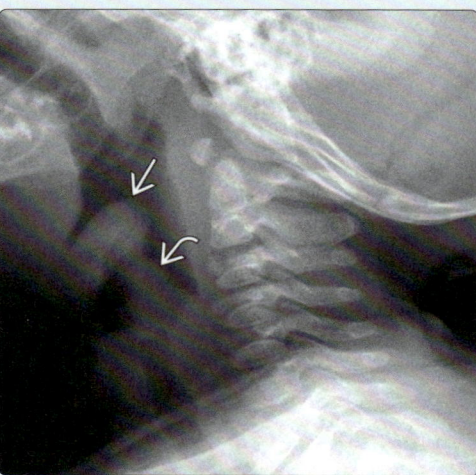
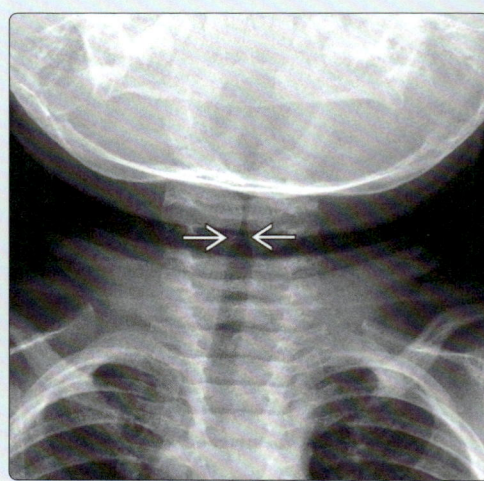

(Left) *Lateral radiograph in a 6-month-old infant with epiglottitis shows diffuse swelling of the epiglottis ➡, resulting in the thumb sign. In addition, the AE folds ➡ are thick with a convex contour, indicating supraglottic inflammation.* **(Right)** *AP radiograph in a child with epiglottitis demonstrates a mildly steepled appearance of the subglottic trachea ➡, which, on AP radiograph alone, is indistinguishable from croup. With epiglottitis, this appearance is due to accompanying subglottic edema.*

Supraglottitis

KEY FACTS

TERMINOLOGY

- Synonym: Adult epiglottitis
- Definition: Relatively uncommon, potentially life-threatening infection/inflammation of supraglottic larynx in adult with sore throat & dysphagia

IMAGING

- CECT: Thickened epiglottis, aryepiglottic folds, obliterated preepiglottic fat
  - + mucosal enhancement
  - Often involves tonsils & base of tongue
- CECT not for diagnosis but to evaluate complications or patients with difficult clinical exam
  - Contraindicated if airway compromise

TOP DIFFERENTIAL DIAGNOSES

- Supraglottic squamous cell carcinoma
- Radiated larynx
- Epiglottitis in child

- Laryngeal trauma
- Caustic or thermal laryngeal injury

PATHOLOGY

- Adult epiglottitis now more common than pediatric
- Etiology: Usually *Streptococcus* or *Staphylococcus* species

CLINICAL ISSUES

- Presentation: Sore throat & dysphagia
- Most resolve with IV antibiotics ± steroids
- Airway management: Observation, intubation, or tracheostomy (15%)
  - Less likely to require airway intervention than children with epiglottitis

DIAGNOSTIC CHECKLIST

- Inflammation affects entire supraglottic larynx ± posterior oropharynx & tongue base, **not** just epiglottis
- Comment if complicated by abscess (ring-enhancing fluid collection) or emphysematous changes (multiple air dots)

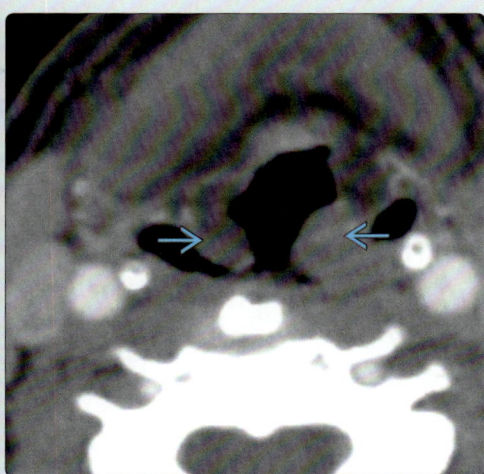

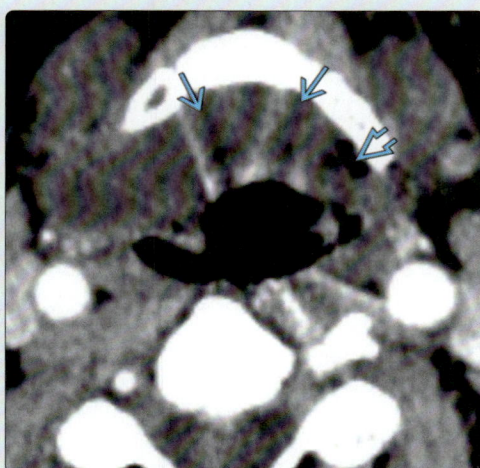

(Left) Axial CECT in a patient with a sore throat and dysphagia due to supraglottitis shows diffuse edematous swelling of bilateral aryepiglottic folds ➡. The most common organisms for adult supraglottic laryngitis include streptococcal and staphylococcal species. (Right) Axial CECT in the same patient shows diffuse preepiglottic low density without rim enhancement, suggesting edema ➡, and tiny air locules ➡. Common complications of untreated cases include abscess formation.

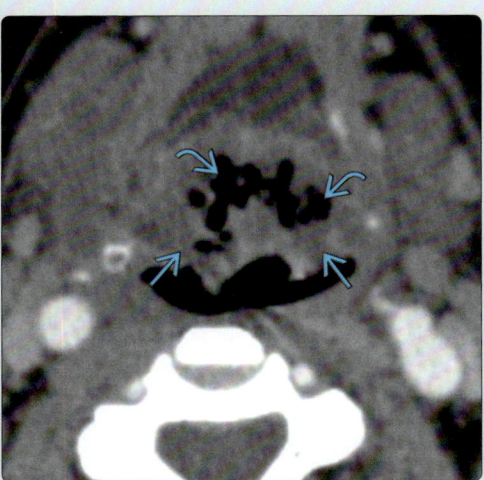

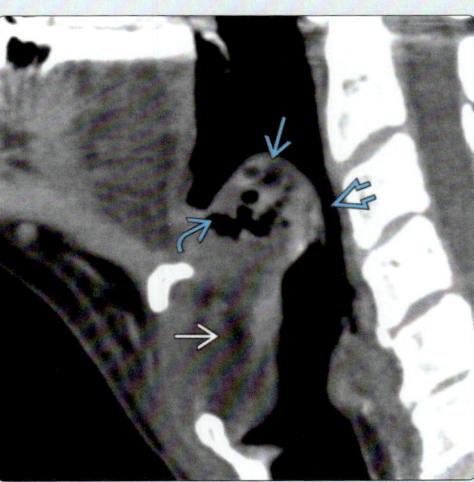

(Left) Axial CECT in the same patient at the level of the epiglottis shows diffuse thickening edematous swelling of the epiglottis ➡ with multiple air locules ➡. (Right) Sagittal reformatted neck CECT in the same patient shows significant swelling and edema of the epiglottis ➡ with air locules ➡, suggesting emphysematous epiglottitis with severe airway narrowing ➡. Note inflammatory changes in preepiglottic fat ➡. Treatment by 2nd-generation cephalosporins and airway management is crucial in these patients.

KEY FACTS

TERMINOLOGY

- Mucosal injury, fracture, or dislocation of larynx
- External blunt trauma or penetrating injury
- Internal iatrogenic injury from intubation or endoscopy

IMAGING

- CT soft tissue windows best evaluate cartilage
- CECT if penetrating injury to evaluate vessels
- May see cartilage abnormalities
- Hematoma can be clue to fracture or dislocation
- Airway may be deformed from fracture or narrowed from hematoma

TOP DIFFERENTIAL DIAGNOSES

- Vocal cord paralysis
- Radiated larynx
- Relapsing polychondritis

PATHOLOGY

- Blunt trauma, especially motor vehicle crashes
- Strangulation or hanging
- Penetrating injury, such as knife or gunshot wound
- Iatrogenic injury secondary to intubation

CLINICAL ISSUES

- Best outcome with early definitive treatment
- Most important initial aim is to stabilize airway

DIAGNOSTIC CHECKLIST

- Thyroid cartilage fractures most frequent
- Arytenoid dislocation can mimic paralyzed cord
- Injury may be subtle; requires high degree of suspicion
- Look for hematoma as clue to fracture/dislocation
- Look for deformity/narrowing of airway
- Always check larynx on trauma C-spine CT
- Soft tissue window best for poorly ossified cartilage
- Soft tissue injuries more common with cricoid fracture

(Left) Axial CECT through the glottic larynx in a patient with dysphonia following a kickboxing bout shows step-off at the superior thyroid notch with internal rotation of fractured cartilage ➡. Note edema of the right vocal cord when compared to the left ➡. (Right) Axial CECT through the supraglottic larynx shows fracture at the superior thyroid notch ➡. Note pockets of air tracking along the right aryepiglottic fold and in the paraglottic space ➡ with mild edema of the right vocal cord ➡.

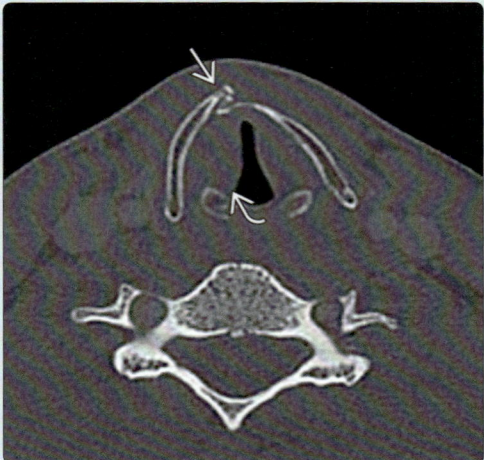 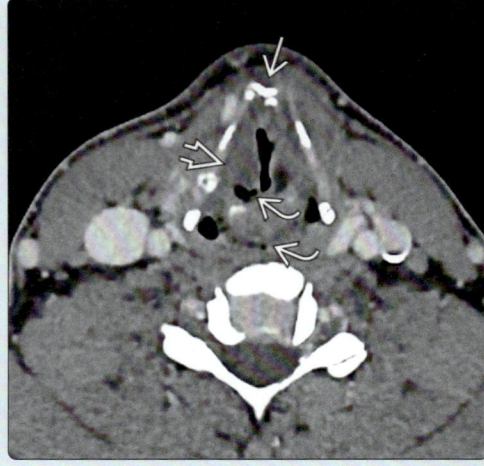

(Left) Axial CTA performed for a pen stabbing through the supraglottic larynx shows a displaced edematous right aryepiglottic fold ➡. The pen tip ➡ terminates adjacent to the left vertebral artery, illustrating the importance of CTA in penetrating injuries. (Right) Axial CTA of a gunshot victim shows diffuse soft tissue emphysema ➡ and shrapnel ➡ adjacent to the cervical vertebra. There are comminuted fractures of cricoid cartilage and the right arytenoid with displaced fragment into the right true vocal cord ➡.

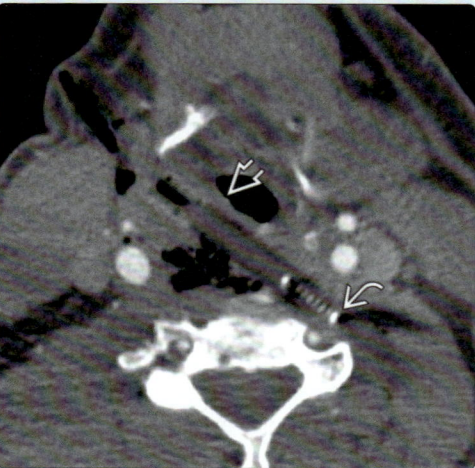 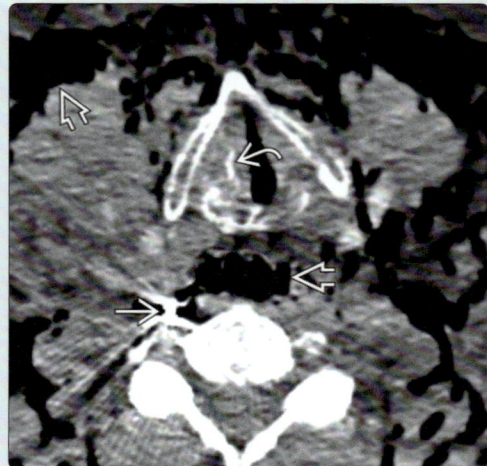

TERMINOLOGY

Definitions

- Mucosal injury, fracture, or dislocation of laryngeal cartilages

IMAGING

General Features

- Best diagnostic clue
  - Edema or hematoma of soft tissues and laryngeal cartilage deformity
- Location
  - Fractures occur to thyroid or cricoid cartilages; hyoid and arytenoid rare
  - Dislocation of cricoarytenoid or cricothyroid joint

Radiographic Findings

- Radiography
  - Deformity of larynx, narrowing of airway
  - Extraluminal gas with mucosal laceration

CT Findings

- NECT
  - Extraluminal gas with mucosal laceration
  - Hematoma can be clue to fracture or dislocation
  - Vocal cord, paraglottic, subglottic swelling
    - Posterior laryngeal and subglottic swelling most likely to cause airway compromise
    - Posterior swelling may expand anteriorly
  - Airway may be deformed from fracture or narrowed from hematoma
  - **Thyroid cartilage fracture: Most common**
    - Vertical: Midline or paramedian alar splaying due to AP compression mechanism
    - Horizontal: Best depicted on coronal images due to strangulation
  - **Cricoid ring fracture**: Usually multiple, disrupt ring, and may lead to airway collapse
  - **Hyoid fracture (rare)**: Separation of hyoid
  - **Cricothyroid joint dislocation**: Widened cricothyroid gap, injury to recurrent laryngeal nerve, secondary to attempted hanging or high-velocity injury
  - **Arytenoid cartilage dislocation**: Typically anterior
  - **Epiglottic injury**: Soft tissue swelling, avulsion at petiole, epiglottic tear
    - Concurrent avulsion of aryepiglottic folds results in complete epiglottis detachment
  - **Laryngotracheal separation**: Horizontal tracheal tear, often acutely fatal
    - Associated with bilateral recurrent laryngeal nerve injury
- CECT
  - Important with penetrating neck injury to evaluate vessels

Imaging Recommendations

- Best imaging tool
  - CT demonstrates soft tissue and cartilage injury best
- Protocol advice
  - Thin axial helical CT slices with multiplanar reformats
  - Soft tissue algorithm/window best for poorly ossified cartilage
  - Penetrating injuries require CECT/CTA to evaluate vessels

DIFFERENTIAL DIAGNOSIS

Vocal Cord Paralysis

- Arytenoid displaced anteromedially
- Enlarged ipsilateral pyriform sinus and ventricle
- Atrophy of ipsilateral cricoarytenoid muscle

Radiated Larynx

- Sclerosis, fragmentation of cartilage
- Evidence of radiation to adjacent tissues

Relapsing Polychondritis

- Autoimmune cartilage destruction associated with collagen vascular diseases (especially SLE)
- Affects ear, nose, articular cartilage, larynx, tracheobronchial tree
- Laryngeal edema, sclerosis, enlargement or demineralization of cartilage

PATHOLOGY

General Features

- Etiology
  - Blunt trauma, especially motor vehicle crashes
    - Larynx compressed against cervical spine, splitting thyroid cartilage and crushing cricoid
    - Soft tissue injuries due to shearing forces
  - Strangulation or hanging
    - Laryngeal fractures without mucosal lacerations
  - Clothesline injury when victim's neck collides with horizontal barrier
    - Laryngeal fractures, laryngotracheal separation
    - High incidence of recurrent laryngeal nerve injury
  - Penetrating injury, such as knife or gunshot wound
  - Iatrogenic injury from intubation or endoscopy
    - Mucosal injury with abrasions or lacerations
    - Arytenoid cartilage dislocation
  - Mortality rate higher for blunt trauma (40%) than penetrating trauma (20%)
    - Delayed presentation for blunt trauma, as patients may be initially asymptomatic
- Associated abnormalities
  - **Often associated with intracranial injuries, cervical spine, or esophageal injuries**
  - Laryngeal injury may not be apparent initially

Staging, Grading, & Classification

- Schaefer system of classifying laryngeal injury
  - Determined by CT and clinical examination
- Directs management and predicts morbidity
  - Group I: Minor hematoma/laceration, no fracture
    - Minor airway symptoms, requires observation
  - Group II: Edema/hematoma, minor mucosal injury, no cartilage exposure, nondisplaced fracture
    - Airway compromise ± tracheostomy
  - Group III: Massive edema, mucosal tear, exposed cartilage, cord immobility

– Above treatment ± exploration
- o Group IV: Group III + > 2 fracture lines, massive mucosal trauma
  – Above treatment ± stent
- o Group V: Laryngotracheal separation
  – Often fatal; requires surgical repair

CLINICAL ISSUES

Presentation

- Most common signs/symptoms
  - o Respiratory distress, stridor, cough, hemoptysis, anterior neck pain
  - o Hoarseness, dysphonia, vocal cord paralysis
  - o Patients with blunt trauma may be initially asymptomatic
- Other signs/symptoms
  - o Subcutaneous emphysema, ecchymosis
  - o Loss of tracheal protuberance (Adam's apple), tracheal deviation
- Clinical profile
  - o Patient with anterior neck trauma, stridor, change in voice, neck ecchymosis, subcutaneous emphysema

Demographics

- Age
  - o Laryngeal cartilage injury less common in children
    – Higher riding larynx sheltered by mandible
- Epidemiology
  - o 1-6 patients per 15,000-42,500 trauma victims
  - o Incidence decreasing in seat belt era
  - o Up to 6% intubated patients

Natural History & Prognosis

- Early definitive surgical treatment associated with better outcome
- Adverse outcomes from laryngeal trauma
  - o Granulation tissue with airway compromise (early), laryngotracheal stenosis (late)
  - o Vocal cord immobility with loss or alteration of voice
    – Vocal cord paralysis or arytenoid dislocation
  - o Disordered swallowing ± aspiration

Treatment

- Most important initial aim is to stabilize airway: Grade II or higher injury usually requires tracheostomy
- Endoscopy &/or surgical exploration to evaluate
  - o Mucosal tears and cartilage exposure
    – Mucosal tears are risk for infection
    – Cartilage exposure predisposes to chondronecrosis, fibrosis, and granulation tissue formation
  - o Cricoid fractures, multiple or displaced fractures, displaced cricoarytenoid joint
  - o Vocal cord immobility or laceration, hemorrhage
- Nonoperative management
  - o Patients with only minor mucosal lacerations sparing free margin of vocal cord and anterior commissure
  - o Hyoid fracture managed conservatively
  - o Single nondisplaced thyroid cartilage fracture; no exposed cartilage
- Endoscopic reduction
  - o Arytenoid cartilage dislocation requires early reduction
- Open reduction and internal fixation

- o Displaced, comminuted laryngeal fractures
- Airway stenting may be required for grade IV injury
  - o From level of false cord to 1st tracheal ring
  - o Helps prevent luminal stenosis, preserve normal shape of endolarynx
- Primary repair or supraglottic hemilaryngectomy for epiglottic injuries

DIAGNOSTIC CHECKLIST

Consider

- Arytenoid dislocation can mimic paralyzed vocal cord clinically and on imaging
- **CECT or CTA** should be performed in penetrating injuries to evaluate vessels

Image Interpretation Pearls

- Evaluate airway, soft tissues, laryngeal skeleton
- Cartilage must be evaluated on bone and soft tissue windows
- Look for hematoma as clue to fracture/dislocation
- Subtle deformity of airway may mean cricoid fracture
- Incomplete cartilage ossification can mimic fracture

Reporting Tips

- Trauma history is key for differential diagnosis
- Injury may be subtle; requires **high degree of suspicion**
  - o Evaluate each cartilage and joint in turn
- Always check larynx on trauma C-spine CT
  - o Look for deformity/narrowing of airway

SELECTED REFERENCES

1. Pincet L et al: External laryngotracheal trauma: a case series and an algorithmic management strategy. Eur Arch Otorhinolaryngol. 281(4):1895-904, 2024
2. DiGrazia GN et al: CT findings in laryngeal trauma and the clinical implications. Clin Neuroradiol. 33(4):1123-31, 2023
3. Nganzeu C et al: Laryngeal trauma. Otolaryngol Clin North Am. 56(6):1039-53, 2023
4. Iarocci AL et al: Laryngeal trauma: a review of current diagnostic and management strategies. Curr Opin Otolaryngol Head Neck Surg. 30(4):276-80, 2022
5. Malvi A et al: Laryngeal trauma, its types, and management. Cureus. 14(10):e29877, 2022
6. Buch K et al: CT-based assessment of laryngeal fracture patterns and associated soft tissue abnormality. Eur Radiol. 31(7):5212-21, 2021
7. Elias N et al: Management of laryngeal trauma. Oral Maxillofac Surg Clin North Am. 33(3):417-27, 2021
8. Adi O et al: Novel role of focused airway ultrasound in early airway assessment of suspected laryngeal trauma. Ultrasound J. 12(1):37, 2020
9. Shi J et al: Multidetector CT of laryngeal injuries: principles of injury recognition. Radiographics. 39(3):879-92, 2019
10. Jain U et al: Management of the traumatized airway. Anesthesiology. 124(1):199-206, 2016
11. Schweiger C et al: Post-intubation acute laryngeal injuries in infants and children: a new classification system. Int J Pediatr Otorhinolaryngol. 86:177-82, 2016
12. Becker M et al: MDCT in the assessment of laryngeal trauma: value of 2D multiplanar and 3D reconstructions. AJR Am J Roentgenol. 201(4):W639-47, 2013
13. Bell RB et al: Management of laryngeal trauma. Oral Maxillofac Surg Clin North Am. 20(3):415-30, 2008
14. Juutilainen M et al: Laryngeal fractures: clinical findings and considerations on suboptimal outcome. Acta Otolaryngol. 128(2):213-8, 2008
15. McCrystal DJ et al: Cricotracheal separation: a review and a case with bilateral recovery of recurrent laryngeal nerve function. J Laryngol Otol. 120(6):497-501, 2006
16. Scaglione M et al: Acute tracheobronchial injuries: impact of imaging on diagnosis and management implications. Eur J Radiol. 59(3):336-43, 2006

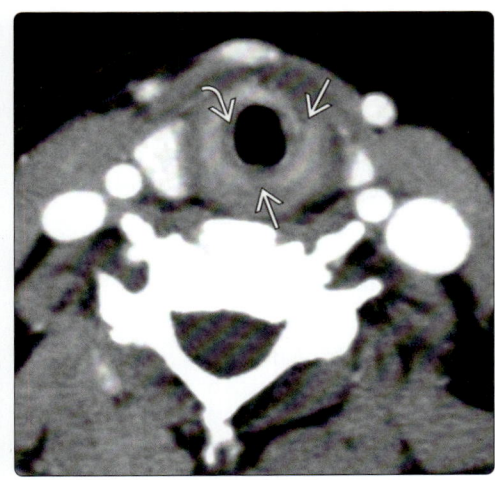

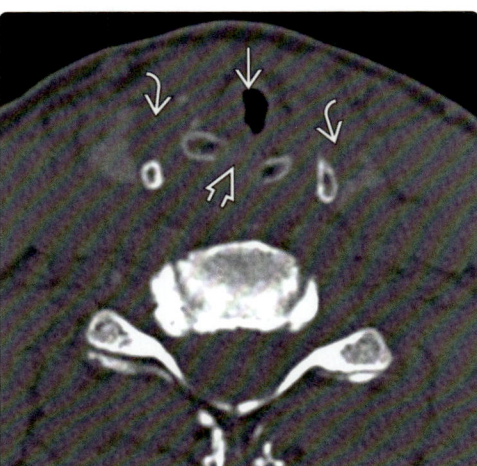

(Left) *Axial CECT depicts 2 fractures of the cricoid ring ➡. Soft tissue windows best evaluate poorly ossified cartilages. Circumferential density internal to the cricoid ring from mucosal hematoma and edema ➡ is a clue to subtle fractures.* (Right) *Axial NECT demonstrates a more obvious displaced posterior midline cricoid fracture ➡ with marked airway deformity and narrowing ➡. Notice subtle but extensive perilaryngeal hematoma and edema displacing thyroid lobes ➡.*

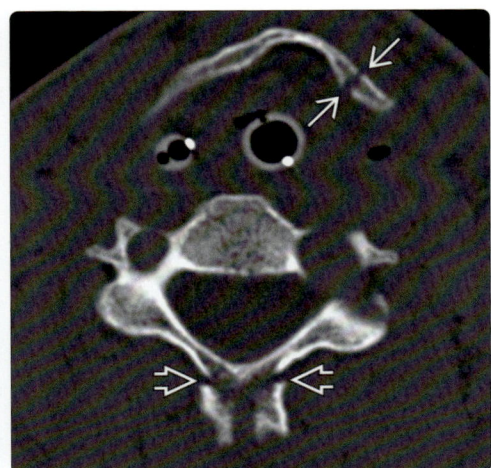

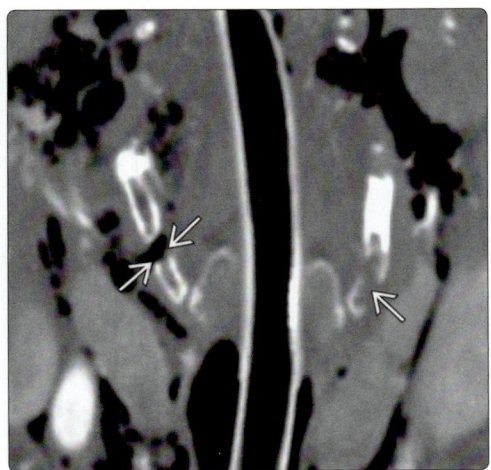

(Left) *Axial NECT shows a rare, minimally displaced hyoid fracture ➡. Note the spinous process fractures ➡ present in this intubated patient who also has extensive edema of neck soft tissues.* (Right) *Coronal CECT reformation reveals bilateral, horizontal thyroid alar fractures ➡. Extensive soft tissue emphysema may be due to pneumomediastinum, but air at the right alar fracture suggests a laryngeal mucosal injury. This requires surgical evaluation.*

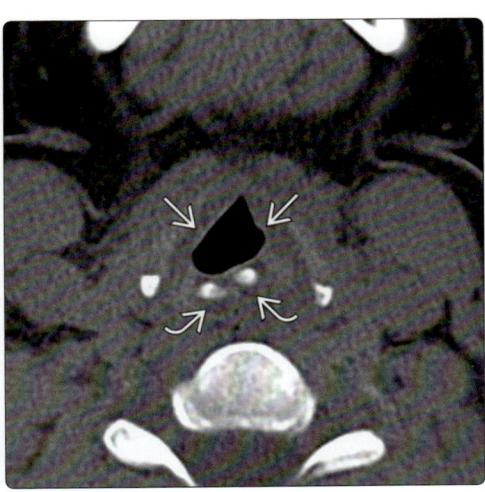

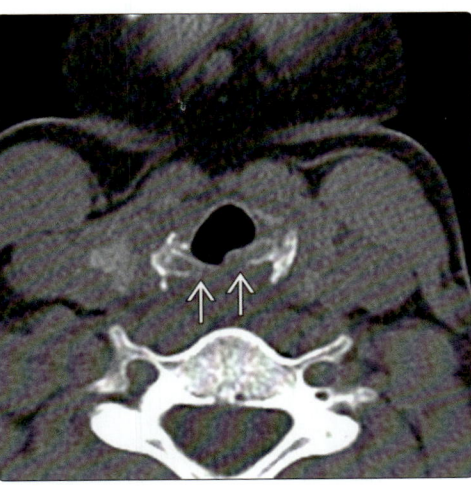

(Left) *Axial NECT in a patient previously in a motor vehicle crash, now presenting with complete aphonia, shows both arytenoid cartilages are dislocated and appear medially rotated ➡. The airway is deformed, and both vocal cords appear atrophic ➡.* (Right) *Axial NECT in the same patient reveals chronic fracture of posterior midline cricoid cartilage ➡ with splaying of fragments and deformity of airway contour. Mucosal irregularity suggests granulation tissue more commonly seen after cartilage exposure.*

KEY FACTS

TERMINOLOGY

- Hemangioma involving subglottic airway

IMAGING

- **Asymmetric** subglottic narrowing in young child
  - Classically subglottic, may be transglottic
- **Enhancing submucosal mass** on CT/MR
  - May be circumferential, bilateral, or unilateral
  - Usually asymmetric or affecting only 1 side, L > R

TOP DIFFERENTIAL DIAGNOSES

- Croup
  - **Symmetric** subglottic tracheal narrowing
- Tracheomalacia
  - Abnormal **dynamic collapse** of intrathoracic trachea
- Congenital subglottic-tracheal stenosis
  - **Symmetric** tracheal narrowing
- Iatrogenic subglottic-tracheal stenosis
  - Prior history of intubation or tracheostomy

- Exudative tracheitis
  - **Intraluminal filling defects**/inflammatory exudates

PATHOLOGY

- Benign **vascular neoplasm**
- **PHACE** syndrome
- 3 phases of growth & regression
  - Proliferative phase begins few weeks after birth
  - Involuting phase shows gradual regression
  - Involuted phase complete by late childhood
- **GLUT1-positive** in all phases

CLINICAL ISSUES

- **Inspiratory stridor** in infants < 6 months
- Usually symptomatic prior to 6 months of age
- Treatment
  - Conservative monitoring, propranolol, corticosteroids, laser therapy, surgical excision rarely required
  - Combination of therapies used in 75% of children

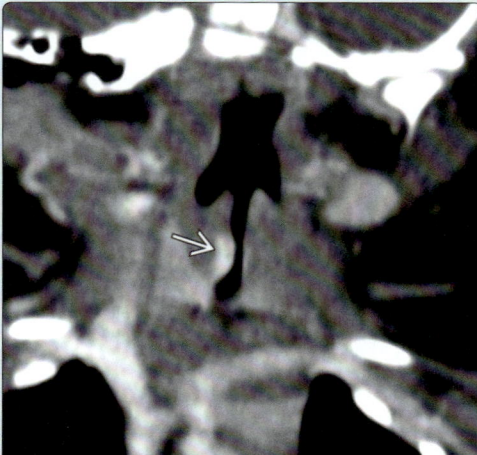
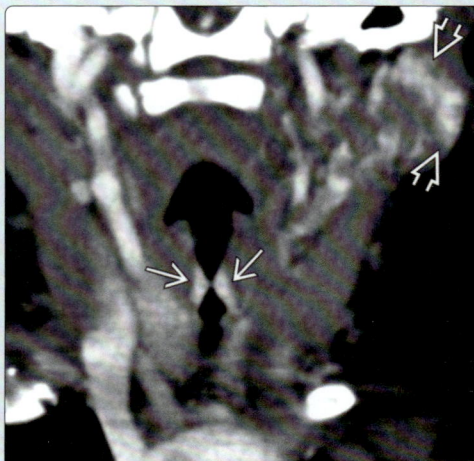

(Left) Coronal CECT in a 4-month-old with stridor and asymmetric right subglottic tracheal narrowing on radiography shows a small, right-sided, enhancing infantile hemangioma ➡ narrowing the airway and causing the stridor. (Right) Coronal CECT in a child with PHACE syndrome shows a circumferential infantile hemangioma ➡ causing symmetric subglottic tracheal narrowing. Notice also the heterogeneously enhancing involuting hemangioma involving the left parotid gland ➡.

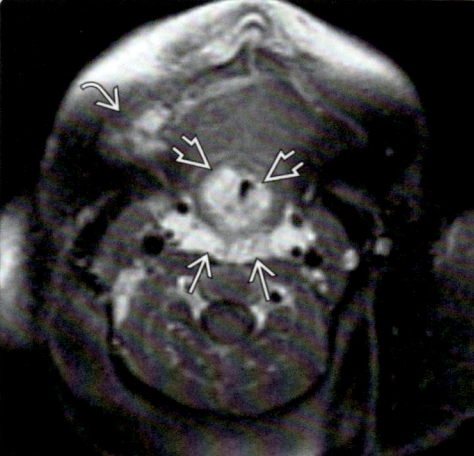
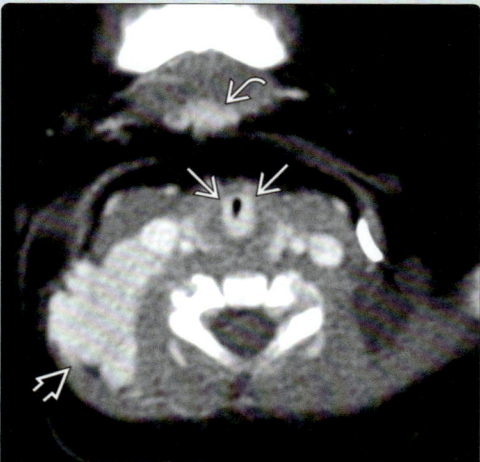

(Left) Axial T1WI C+ FS MR in a child with PHACE syndrome demonstrates multiple enhancing hemangiomas in the retropharyngeal space ➡ surrounding the subglottic trachea ➡ and in the right submental space ➡. (Right) Axial CECT in an 11-week-old girl demonstrates a circumferential, well-defined subglottic hemangioma ➡. Notice also the posterior cervical space ➡ and submental infantile hemangiomas ➡, which should raise the question of PHACE syndrome.

TERMINOLOGY

Definitions

- Infantile hemangioma involving subglottic airway

IMAGING

General Features

- Best diagnostic clue
  - **Asymmetric** subglottic narrowing in young child
    - **Enhancing submucosal mass** on CT/MR
- Location
  - Classically **subglottic**; may be transglottic
  - Usually asymmetric or affecting only 1 side, L > R

Radiographic Findings

- Asymmetric subglottic tracheal narrowing on anteroposterior radiograph

CT Findings

- Usually solitary, enhancing subglottic mass

MR Findings

- Intermediate T1/hyperintense T2, intense enhancement
- Typical high-flow intralesional vessels are uncommon in airway lesions, likely due to small size

Imaging Recommendations

- Best imaging tool
  - 3D CT helps define mass & tracheal compression
    - Quicker than MR & may not need sedation
  - Adjust CT technique for pediatric patient
  - MR more sensitive, but sedation usually needed

DIFFERENTIAL DIAGNOSIS

Croup

- **Symmetric** subglottic tracheal narrowing
- Most common in children 8 months to 3 years

Tracheomalacia

- Abnormal **dynamic collapse** of intrathoracic trachea

Congenital Subglottic-Tracheal Stenosis

- **Symmetric** tracheal narrowing
  - Complete tracheal rings
- ± pulmonary sling or congenital heart disease

Iatrogenic Subglottic-Tracheal Stenosis

- Prior history of intubation or tracheostomy

Exudative Tracheitis

- **Intraluminal filling defects**/inflammatory exudates
- Children usually older than those with viral croup

PATHOLOGY

General Features

- Etiology
  - Benign **vascular neoplasm** of proliferating endothelial cells, **not** vascular malformation
- Associated abnormalities
  - Cutaneous hemangiomas in 50%

  - **PHACE** syndrome: **P**osterior fossa brain malformations, **h**emangiomas of face, **a**rterial anomalies, **c**ardiac anomalies, **e**ye abnormalities, **s**ternal clefts or **s**upraumbilical raphe
    - 7% have subglottic hemangiomas

Staging, Grading, & Classification

- 3 phases of growth & regression
  - **Proliferative phase** begins few weeks after birth & continues for 1-2 years
  - **Involuting phase** shows gradual regression over next several years
  - **Involuted phase** usually complete by late childhood

Microscopic Features

- **GLUT1** immunohistochemical marker: **Positive** in all phases of infantile hemangioma

CLINICAL ISSUES

Presentation

- Most common signs/symptoms
  - **Inspiratory stridor** in infants < 6 months
- Other signs/symptoms
  - **Cutaneous hemangiomas** in **50%**
  - Hoarseness or abnormal cry

Natural History & Prognosis

- Majority of lesions have progressive airway obstruction during proliferative phase
- Symptoms resolve after involution
- Benign condition but can have fatal outcome
- In presence of segmental bearded distribution hemangioma & PHACE syndrome, may have more recalcitrant & complicated natural history
- Diagnosis made at endoscopy

Treatment

- General principles: Combination of therapies used in 75% of children
- Conservative monitoring if < 30% narrowing without respiratory or feeding difficulty
  - Need immediate access to care as lesions may grow quickly & obstruct
- Oral propranolol: Considered 1st-line treatment
- Systemic corticosteroids
  - ± rebound growth when steroids tapered
- Intralesional corticosteroids
- CO_2 laser therapy

SELECTED REFERENCES

1. ISSVA Classification of Vascular Anomalies 2018 International Society for the Study of Vascular Anomalies. Accessed February 15, 2025. http://issva.org/classification
2. Luu J et al: Hemangioma genetics and associated syndromes. Dermatol Clin. 40(4):393-400, 2022
3. Proisy M et al: PHACES syndrome and associated anomalies: risk associated with small and large facial hemangiomas. AJR Am J Roentgenol. 1-8, 2021
4. Schwartz T et al: Efficacy and rebound rates in propranolol-treated subglottic hemangioma: a literature review. Laryngoscope. 127(11):2665-72, 2017
5. Mamlouk MD et al: Arterial spin-labeling perfusion for PHACE syndrome. AJNR Am J Neuroradiol. 42(1):173-7, 2020
6. Merrow AC et al: 2014 Revised classification of vascular lesions from the international society for the study of vascular anomalies: radiologic-pathologic update. Radiographics. 36(5):1494-516, 2016

KEY FACTS

TERMINOLOGY

- Laryngeal chondrosarcoma (CSa): Cartilage-producing chondrocytic neoplasm with cellular atypia, bone destruction, or local invasion

IMAGING

- **Expansile submucosal mass within laryngeal cartilage** with chondroid matrix
- Most arise in cricoid > thyroid cartilage, rare in arytenoid
- CT: **Ring-like or popcorn calcifications** (chondroid matrix) in expansile intracartilage mass
  - Noncalcific component of mass hypodense to muscle
  - Cartilage/bone destruction or local invasion
- MR: **T2-hyperintense** mass, best seen with T2 FS, STIR
  - T1WI C+: Heterogeneous enhancement
- Very high ADC (> 2.0) due to chondroid matrix

TOP DIFFERENTIAL DIAGNOSES

- Chondroma

- Cannot be reliably differentiated from CSa
- Osteosarcoma: Bone-forming or sunburst reaction
  - Other sarcoma: No calcified matrix
- Metastasis to laryngeal cartilage; usually presents in setting of known metastatic disease

PATHOLOGY

- Arise from hyaline cartilage: Cricoid (74%), thyroid (12%), and, very rarely, arytenoid (5%)

CLINICAL ISSUES

- Dysphagia or palpable neck mass (with exophytic growth pattern), dysphonia, stridor
- Symptoms often present for long duration, suggesting indolent process
- Submucosal mass on endoscopy

DIAGNOSTIC CHECKLIST

- If expansile mass arises from laryngeal cartilage, look for arc or ring-like calcifications and T2 high signal

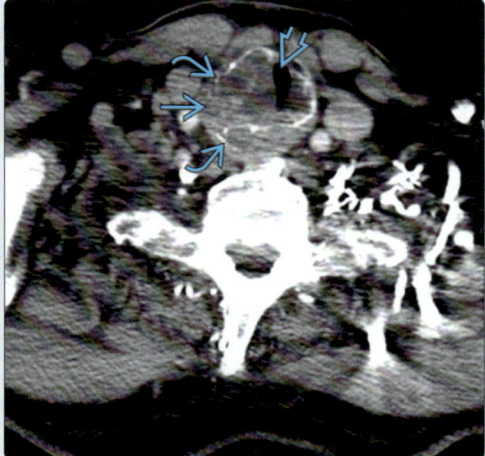
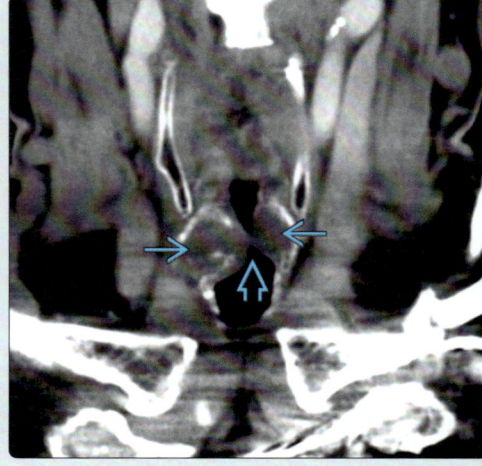

(Left) *Axial CECT in a patient with hoarseness and dysphonia whose endoscopy revealed a large submucosal subglottic mass demonstrates an expansile mass ⊡ centered in the cricoid cartilage with near circumferential involvement asymmetric to the right. Note internal typical calcifications ⊡ and moderate subglottic airway narrowing ⊡.* (Right) *Coronal CECT reformation in the same patient shows a near circumferential mass ⊡ in the cricoid cartilage with subglottic luminal narrowing ⊡.*

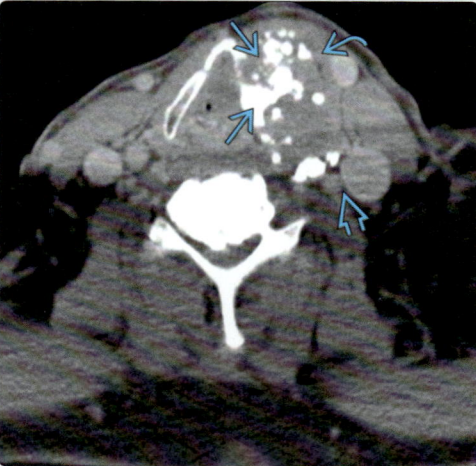
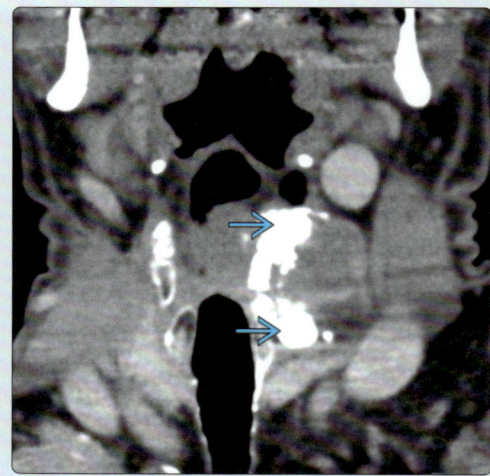

(Left) *Axial CECT in a patient with left anterior midline neck swelling shows a large, heterogeneous, mildly enhancing, partially calcified mass centered in the left lamina of the thyroid cartilage ⊡. There is no intralaryngeal tumor extension. Note lateral displacement of the strap muscles ⊡ and posterolateral displacement of the left carotid space ⊡.* (Right) *Coronal CECT reformation in the same patient better depicts coarse calcification in the mass ⊡. Biopsy of this mass revealed laryngeal chondrosarcoma (CSa) grade I.*

TERMINOLOGY

Abbreviations

- Chondrosarcoma (CSa)

Definitions

- Laryngeal CSa: Cartilage-producing chondrocytic neoplasm with cellular atypia, bone destruction, or local invasion

IMAGING

General Features

- Best diagnostic clue
  - Expansile submucosal mass arising within laryngeal cartilage, popcorn, arc, or ring-like calcifications
- Location
  - In larynx, **most arise in cricoid lamina** (posterior or posterolateral) > thyroid cartilage (inferolateral)
    - Cricoid cartilage: 74%, thyroid cartilage: 12%
  - Rare in arytenoid cartilage (5%) or epiglottis
  - Typically subglottic in location
- Size
  - 1.5-8.5 cm
  - Often large at presentation if airway is spared
    - Tumor growing away from laryngeal lumen
- Morphology
  - Bulky, lobular mass centered in cartilage
  - Chondroid matrix typical

Radiographic Findings

- Radiography
  - Mass of variable density may be exophytic from laryngeal cartilage or grow inward thereby narrowing laryngeal air column
  - Stippled calcification

CT Findings

- NECT
  - 94% of laryngeal CSa show calcifications
  - **Arc and ring-like or popcorn** calcifications (chondroid matrix) in expansile mass arising from cricoid or thyroid cartilage with smooth mucosal covering
  - Not all tumors are calcified
    - Noncalcific (soft tissue) tumor component hypodense to muscle
  - Cartilage/bone destruction or local invasion may be seen in aggressive lesions
  - Presence of soft tissue mass or osteocartilaginous destruction suggests higher grade CSa
  - Often causes airway narrowing
- CECT
  - Minimal, if any, enhancement

MR Findings

- T1WI
  - Intermediate signal intensity; isointense to muscle
- T2WI
  - **Hyperintense** mass; hypocellular tumor, heterogeneity most common with more heavily calcified lesions
- STIR
  - Hyperintense mass
- DWI
  - Extremely high ADC values (due to chondroid matrix)
- T1WI C+
  - Heterogeneous enhancement

Imaging Recommendations

- Best imaging tool
  - CT best shows expansile mass with epicenter in cartilage and demonstrates calcified chondroid matrix of tumor
  - No significant correlation between pathologic grade and imaging findings
- Protocol advice
  - High-resolution axial helical CECT with thin (1.5- to 2.5-mm) collimation
  - Multiplanar reformations help surgical planning

DIFFERENTIAL DIAGNOSIS

Chondroma

- Cannot be reliably differentiated from CSa with imaging
  - Particularly true in noncalcified lesions
- CT: Mass with chondroid matrix
- MR: T2-hyperintense mass and high ADC values > 2.0

Other Sarcomas

- Includes osteo-, fibro-, synovial cell sarcomas, and malignant fibrous histiocytoma
- Osteosarcoma associated with sunburst pattern of periosteal reaction
- Other sarcomas not usually calcified

Relapsing Polychondritis

- Immune-mediated inflammatory destruction of type II collagen in cartilage
  - Typically in many sites: Ear, nose, articular cartilage, larynx, and tracheobronchial tree
  - Look for smooth tracheal and bronchial wall thickening with calcification
- Occurs in patients with vasculitides, collagen vascular diseases (including SLE), other autoimmune diseases
- May cause edema, sclerosis, enlargement or demineralization of cartilage in larynx

Nodular Chondrometaplasia, Larynx

- Posttraumatic condition
- Fibrocartilage (not hyaline cartilage)
- Can be challenging histologically

Metastasis to Laryngeal Cartilage

- Destructive mass centered in laryngeal cartilage, no chondroid matrix

Squamous Cell Carcinoma, Larynx

- Mucosal mass evident endoscopically
- Not arising in, or expanding, cartilage

PATHOLOGY

General Features

- Etiology
  - May arise from pluripotential mesenchymal cells involved in hyaline cartilage ossification
  - Vast majority are low-grade CSa, not distinguishable from benign chondroma

- Arises from hyaline cartilage: Cricoid (74%), thyroid (12%), and, rarely, arytenoid (5%) cartilage
- CSa of elastic cartilage (epiglottis) exceedingly rare

Staging, Grading, & Classification

- Well differentiated (grade I)
  - Most common, account for 67.8% of laryngeal CSa
  - Small, dark nuclei, scant-absent mitoses, calcification common
  - Variable matrix, chondroid and myxoid components resembling hyaline cartilage
- Moderately differentiated (grade II)
  - Accounts for 23.5% of laryngeal CSa
  - Larger nuclei with greater cellularity
  - More prominent myxoid matrix, occasional mitoses (< 2 per 10 HPF)
- Poorly differentiated (grade III)
  - Accounts for 3.8% of laryngeal CSa
  - Still greater cellularity, mitoses common (≥ 2 per 10 HPF)
  - Prominent nucleoli
  - Matrix may contain fusiform spindle cells and necrosis

Gross Pathologic & Surgical Features

- Lobular surface with gritty/crunchy consistency
- White to blue-gray, semitranslucent, with myxoid-mucinous matrix
- Submucosal mass with intact mucosa typical
- Rarely, mucosal erythema ± ulceration in advanced tumors

Microscopic Features

- Overall hypocellular, predominantly small, mononucleated chondrocytes
- Malignant areas may be localized within more benign-appearing lesion (chondroma)
  - May be missed on limited sampling
- Even on complete microscopic review, it may be difficult to differentiate benign from malignant lesion

CLINICAL ISSUES

Presentation

- Most common signs/symptoms
  - Progressive hoarseness and dyspnea
  - Submucosal mass on endoscopy
  - Other symptoms: Dysphagia or palpable neck mass, pain
    - Symptoms often present for long duration, suggesting indolent process

Demographics

- Age
  - Mean: 63 years
- Sex
  - M:F = 3:1
- Epidemiology
  - Laryngeal CSa accounts for ~ 0.2% of laryngeal malignancies
  - Represents < 0.2% of all H&N malignancies

Natural History & Prognosis

- Significantly better prognosis than other laryngeal malignancies with 1-, 5-, and 10-year disease-specific survival rates of 96.5%, 88.6%, and 84.8%, respectively

- No significant difference in outcome based on grade, location, or treatment method
  - Outcome worse in patients with myxoid CSa
- May dedifferentiate, often to malignant fibrous histiocytoma or fibrosarcoma, with poor prognosis
- Metastases are extremely rare

Treatment

- Surgical resection is treatment of choice
  - Voice conservation surgery with complete lesion removal
- Surgical approach is same for benign and low-grade malignant lesions
- Partial resection associated with recurrences in ≤ 20% of cases
  - Patients often do well with salvage laryngectomy
- Total laryngectomy may be required for large lesions or extensive cricoid involvement
- Cricoid resection with thyroid-tracheal anastomosis over stent for large cricoid tumors

DIAGNOSTIC CHECKLIST

Consider

- Determine if mass arises from laryngeal cartilage
- Assess if involved laryngeal cartilage is expanded or eroded/destroyed
- History of prior laryngeal trauma may suggest alternative chondrometaplasia

Image Interpretation Pearls

- If **T2-hyperintense mass** seen on MR arises from laryngeal cartilage
- **Arc- or ring-like calcifications** and chondroid matrix are pathognomonic

Reporting Tips

- Report laryngeal cartilage of origin
- If on benign end of spectrum, report inability to differentiate chondroma from CSa by imaging

SELECTED REFERENCES

1. Piazza C et al: Aggressive subtypes of laryngeal chondrosarcoma and their clinical behavior: a systematic review. Oncol Ther. 13(1):49-67, 2025
2. Vageli DP et al: Laryngeal rare benign non-epithelial tumors and sarcomas emphasizing on chondrosarcomas: a literature review and a case presentation. Pathol Res Pract. 261:155512, 2024
3. MacNeil SD: Non-squamous laryngeal cancer. Otolaryngol Clin North Am. 56(2):345-59, 2023
4. Baba A et al: Imaging features of laryngeal chondrosarcomas: a case series and systematic review. J Neuroimaging. 32(2):213-22, 2022
5. Roch-Zniszczoł A et al: Laryngeal chondrosarcoma treated with conventional radiotherapy - case report and review of the literature. Pol J Pathol. 73(2):176-9, 2022
6. Álvarez-Calderón-Iglesias O et al: Survival outcomes in laryngeal chondrosarcoma: a systematic review. Acta Otorhinolaryngol Ital. 42(6):502-15, 2022
7. Velez Torres JM et al: Primary sarcomas of the larynx: a clinicopathologic study of 27 cases. Head Neck Pathol. 15(3):905-16, 2021
8. Mantilla JG et al: Primary sarcomas of the larynx: a single institutional experience with ten cases. Head Neck Pathol. 14(3):707-14, 2020
9. Chin OY et al: Laryngeal chondrosarcoma: a systematic review of 592 cases. Laryngoscope. 127(2):430-9, 2017
10. Douis H et al: Is there a role for diffusion-weighted MRI (DWI) in the diagnosis of central cartilage tumors? Skeletal Radiol. 44(7):963-9, 2015

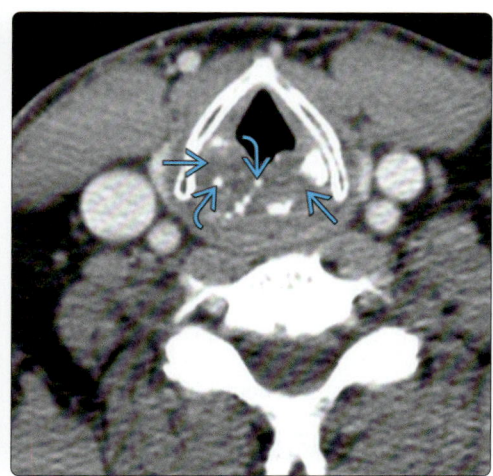
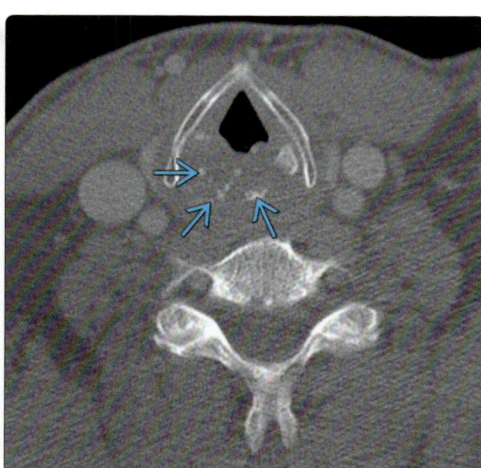

(Left) Axial CECT in a patient with hoarseness whose endoscopy revealed a posterior subglottic submucosal mass shows an expansile mass in the lamina of the cricoid cartilage ➡ with internal multiple calcific densities ➡. (Right) Axial bone window CECT in the same patient demonstrates multiple calcific densities ➡ in the mass centered in the cricoid lamina. Biopsy was consistent with grade I laryngeal CSa. Note that chondroma and low-grade CSa cannot be reliably differentiated on imaging.

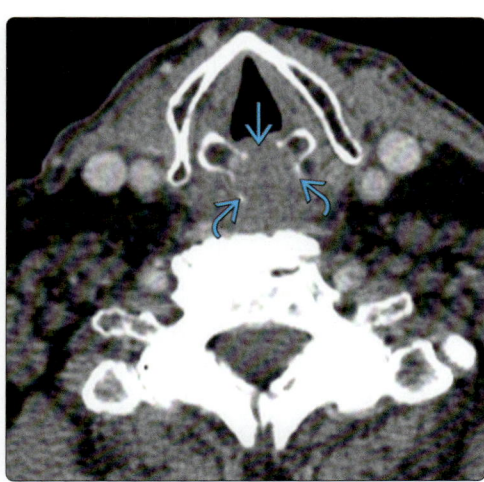
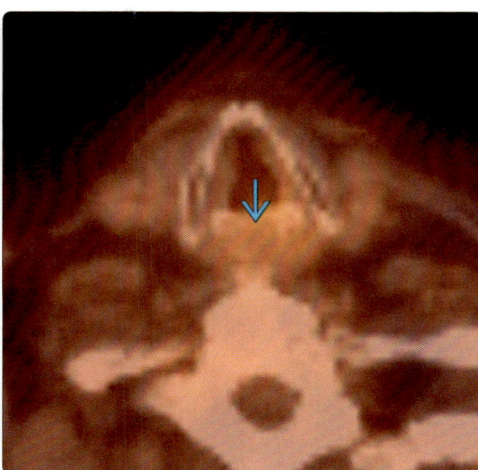

(Left) Axial CECT in a patient with biopsy-proven low-grade CSa involving cricoid cartilage lamina ➡ show a well-circumscribed mass with minimal rim calcifications ➡. Endoscopy revealed a submucosal posterior subglottic mass. (Right) Axial FDG PET/CT in the same patient shows mild low level FDG activity ➡ in this grade I laryngeal CSa. Note that the cricoid cartilage is the most common site for laryngeal CSa followed by thyroid cartilage and arytenoid. Epiglottis CSa is very rare.

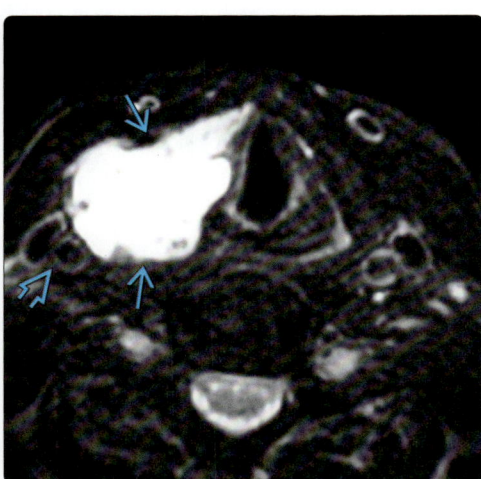
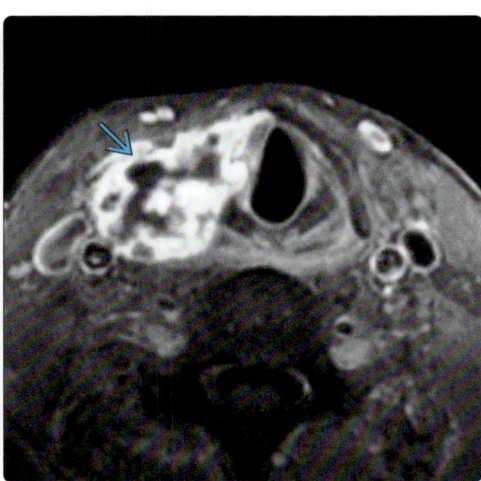

(Left) Axial T2 FS MR shows a hyperintense thyroid cartilage mass ➡ growing away from the laryngeal lumen and displacing the carotid space laterally ➡. T2 hyperintensity would be atypical for carcinoma. Imaging suggests a chondroid lesion, first thought to be a CSa. Chondroma was found at resection. (Right) Axial T1 C+ FS MR reveals heterogeneous enhancement ➡ in this exophytic chondroma. This imaging appearance could represent chordoma or CSa.

KEY FACTS

TERMINOLOGY

- Spectrum of soft tissue and cartilage changes following radiation therapy (XRT) for head and neck tumors
- Changes may be XRT **effects** or **complications**
  - XRT effects seen in all patients
  - Complications seen in minority

IMAGING

- Radiation effects
  - Acute-subacute: Submucosal edema, increased linear mucosal enhancement
  - Chronic: Fibrosis and atrophy
- Radiation complications
  - Persistent edema > 6 months
  - **Chondronecrosis**: Cartilage fragmentation/collapse, sclerosis, adjacent gas
- Treatment failure
  - Persistent mass, solid enhancement, deep ulcerations

TOP DIFFERENTIAL DIAGNOSES

- Transglottic squamous cell carcinoma
- Supraglottitis
- Laryngeal trauma

CLINICAL ISSUES

- Patient symptoms variable, may be minimal
- Higher XRT dose increases severity of XRT effects and increases complication rates
- Baseline CT/MR should be done ~ 8 weeks post XRT

DIAGNOSTIC CHECKLIST

- Submucosal edema and prominent mucosal enhancement are expected findings post XRT
- Chondronecrosis and persistent edema represent XRT complications
- Persistent or enlarged mass on baseline posttreatment scan indicates treatment failure

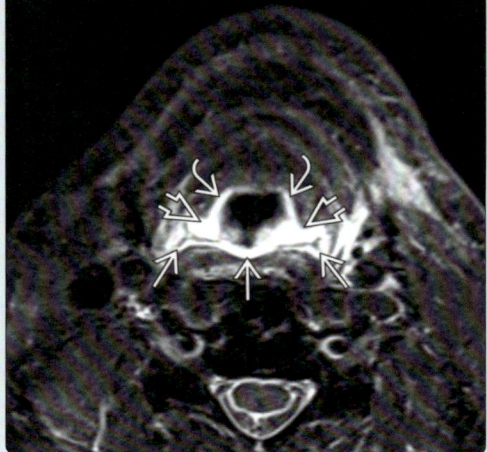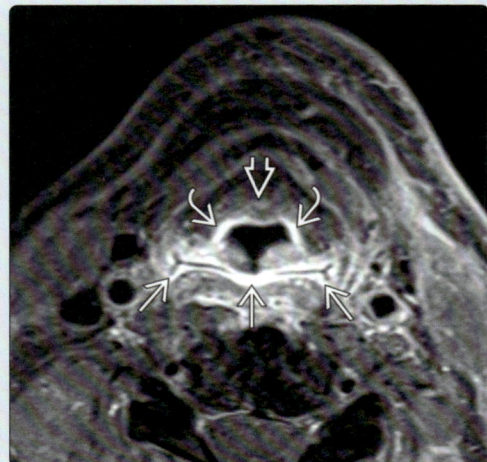

(Left) Axial STIR MR through supraglottic larynx in a patient after XRT for base of tongue cancer shows diffuse edema and skin thickening with thickened aryepiglottic (AE) folds ➡ effacing the piriform sinuses. There is hyperintense signal along mucosal surface of larynx ➡ and hypopharynx ➡, indicating mucositis. (Right) Corresponding axial T1 FS C+ MR (same patient) shows marked enhancement of the mucosal surface of the larynx ➡ and hypopharynx ➡, indicating mucositis. Preepiglottic fat ➡ is infiltrated.

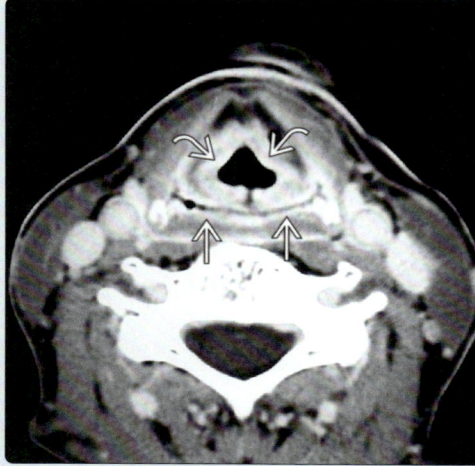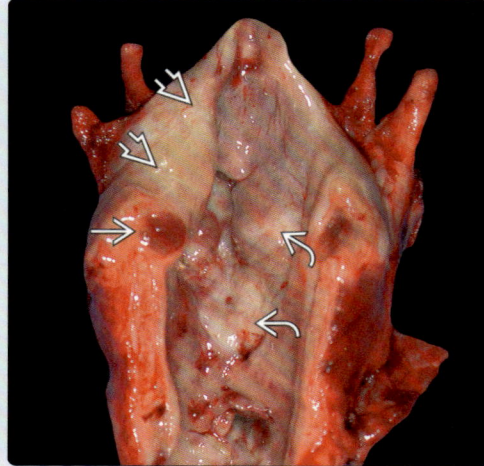

(Left) Axial CECT following XRT for laryngeal SCCa shows there is particularly prominent mucositis manifested as thick but regular enhancement of the mucosal surfaces of the larynx ➡ and hypopharynx ➡. Absence of nodularity or a discrete mass is reassuring. (Right) Gross pathology following laryngectomy with the larynx opened from a midline posterior incision demonstrates diffuse laryngeal swelling ➡, particularly affecting the AE fold ➡. Note focal hemorrhagic necrosis ➡ at the left cricothyroid joint.

TERMINOLOGY

Definitions

- Spectrum of soft tissue and cartilage changes following radiation therapy (XRT) for head and neck tumors
  - **Radiation effects**
    - Acute-subacute: Diffuse edema and inflammation
    - Chronic: Evolves to fibrosis and atrophy
  - **Radiation complications**
    - Persistent laryngeal edema ≥ 6 months
    - Laryngeal chondronecrosis

IMAGING

General Features

- Best diagnostic clue
  - Diffuse laryngeal edema without discrete mass plus radiation changes in neck
- Location
  - **All tissues** in radiation field show XRT changes
    - Supraglottic edema often most prominent
- Morphology
  - Acute-subacute effects: Diffuse edema and mucosal enhancement without discrete mass
  - Chronic effects: Generalized tissue and fat atrophy

CT Findings

- CECT
  - Typical XRT effects: **Acute-subacute**
    - Diffuse laryngeal and pharyngeal **low-density submucosal edema**
      - Thickened epiglottis, aryepiglottic and false folds
      - Effaced pyriform sinuses
      - Anterior and posterior commissure thickening
      - Haziness of paraglottic and preepiglottic fat
    - Mucosa generally shows **increased thin linear enhancement**
    - Mucosal ulceration not uncommon
      - Deep ulcer, solid enhancement suggests tumor
  - Typical XRT effects: **Chronic**
    - Fibrosis + atrophy with decreased volume all neck tissues
    - Decreased low-density edema and enhancement
  - Radiation complications: **Chondronecrosis**
    - Laryngeal cartilage fragmentation/collapse, adjacent gas
    - Cartilage sclerosis concerning for necrosis if not present pre XRT
    - Osteoradionecrosis of hyoid has been reported with similar findings
- CT perfusion
  - Shorter mean transit time in tumor than XRT changes

MR Findings

- MR changes reflect same pathologic stages as CT
- **Acute-subacute** XRT effects
  - Submucosal edema → marked T2 hyperintensity
  - Haziness of fat: Decreased T1 signal, increased T2 signal
  - Prominent diffuse, thin mucosal enhancement
  - DWI: Lower ADC values in tumor compared to XRT change

- **Chronic** XRT effects
  - T2 hyperintensity gradually resolves
  - Fat returns to more normal signal; decreased fat bulk
  - Mucosal enhancement diminishes
- Radiation complications: **Chondronecrosis**
  - Increased T2 signal and enhancement of cartilage
  - Focal gas may be subtle: Low signal on all sequences
  - Fragmentation of cartilage often subtle on MR

Nuclear Medicine Findings

- PET/CT
  - No FDG uptake in normal treated larynx
    - Negative predictive value: 91%
  - Pitfall: False-positive from infection, recent biopsy

Imaging Recommendations

- Best imaging tool
  - Any imaging can be complex in early phase
  - CECT usually significantly easier for patient, as fewer swallowing problems from poorly handled secretions
  - FDG PET may help clarify indeterminate findings
- Protocol advice
  - **Baseline CT or MR** should be obtained ~ **8 weeks post XRT/chemoradiation**
    - Persistent or enlarging mass indicates treatment failure
    - If using CECT, allow delay after contrast injection to maximize enhancement of soft tissue mass

DIFFERENTIAL DIAGNOSIS

Transglottic Squamous Cell Carcinoma

- Solid, enhancing, irregular mass spanning cords
- May see infiltration of paraglottic fat and cartilage
- Frequently see adenopathy as well

Supraglottitis

- Submucosal edema of supraglottic tissues
- In adults, may form small abscesses
- Remaining neck tissues appear normal

Larynx Trauma

- May see cartilage fracture, joint subluxation
- Submucosal altered density from hematoma, edema
- More focal laryngeal changes

PATHOLOGY

General Features

- Etiology
  - Higher dose increases XRT effects and complications
    - Mean dose to larynx should be kept ≤ 43.5 Gy
  - Concurrent chemoradiation improves results but increases severity of acute XRT effects
    - Probably increases frequency of severe late effects
  - Underlying vascular disease, continued smoking, and infection increase complication rates
  - Biopsy may increase incidence of poor outcomes with iatrogenic infection of ischemic tissues

Gross Pathologic & Surgical Features

- Thickening and induration of mucosa and submucosa
- Soft tissue necrosis may also accompany treatment

Microscopic Features

- Acute-subacute: Endothelial damage with increased permeability and interstitial edema, inflammatory infiltrate
- Chronic: Fibrosis, collagen deposition, blood vessel endarteritis, lymphatic fibrosis
  - New blood and lymphatic channels may form with edema resolution
  - Collagen and muscle disorganization, increased collagen and fibronectin
- Decreased perfusion to cartilage may cause ischemic injury, leading to chondritis, possibly soft tissue necrosis or chondronecrosis

CLINICAL ISSUES

Presentation

- Most common signs/symptoms
  - May be minimally symptomatic
  - Hoarseness, mucosal dryness, dysphagia
  - Pain and dyspnea with more severe changes
- Other signs/symptoms
  - Patients with chondronecrosis may have respiratory distress, pain, odynophagia, weight loss
- Clinical profile
  - Patient with history of XRT ± chemotherapy presenting with hoarseness and dysphagia

Natural History & Prognosis

- **Radiation effect**
  - XRT edema and inflammation improve over time
  - Marked symptomatology may necessitate gastrostomy feeding
- **Radiation complications**
  - **~ 10% have persistent late (> 6 months) edema**
    - Increasing incidence with increasing XRT dose
  - **≤ 5% have chondronecrosis**
    - Peaks in 1st year; may occur > 10 years post XRT
    - More common if large tumor, cartilage invasion, or perichondrial disruption
    - Also more common if ongoing smoking, vascular disease, or infection
    - May lead to laryngeal collapse and death
  - Remember that soft tissue necrosis may also complicate XRT
    - Very difficult to distinguish from recurrent disease
    - Nonhealing mucosal lesions and sloughing of soft tissue

Treatment

- Supportive therapy: Humidifier, voice rest, smoking cessation, reflux treatment
- Severe dysphagia/odynophagia may require temporary gastrostomy
- Radiation chondronecrosis may necessitate laryngectomy or tracheostomy
  - Hyperbaric oxygen therapy may be offered for chondronecrosis
  - Total laryngectomy is frequent outcome of severe/progressive radiation chondronecrosis

DIAGNOSTIC CHECKLIST

Consider

- Important to become thoroughly familiar with expected XRT effects
  - Enables detection of tumor or complication
- Any imaging can be complex in early phase

Image Interpretation Pearls

- Radiation treatment → tissue edema and inflammation → fibrosis, scarring, and atrophy
- Check cartilage for fragmentation, gas, or new sclerosis
- All tissues in radiation field show XRT changes
- Chondronecrosis shows cartilage fragmentation and gas
- Persistent or enlarged mass on baseline posttreatment scan indicates treatment failure
- Mucosal ulcers common; deep ulcer with adjacent soft tissue mass or solid enhancement suggests tumor

SELECTED REFERENCES

1. Brahmbhatt S et al: Imaging of the posttreatment head and neck: expected findings and potential complications. Radiol Imaging Cancer. 6(1):e230155, 2024
2. Chakrabarty N et al: Comprehensive review of post-treatment imaging in head and neck cancers: from expected to unexpected and beyond. Br J Radiol. 97(1164):1898-914, 2024
3. Moharrami M et al: Prognosing post-treatment outcomes of head and neck cancer using structured data and machine learning: a systematic review. PLoS One. 19(7):e0307531, 2024
4. Ramsey T et al: Laryngeal preservation strategies. Surg Oncol Clin N Am. 33(4):761-73, 2024
5. Van Hoe S et al: Post-treatment surveillance imaging in head and neck cancer: a systematic review. Insights Imaging. 15(1):32, 2024
6. Zhu Y et al: Systematic review and meta-analysis of the diagnostic effectiveness of positron emission tomography-computed tomography versus magnetic resonance imaging in the post-treatment surveillance of head and neck squamous cell carcinoma. J Laryngol Otol. 137(1):22-30, 2023
7. Alhilali L et al: Osteoradionecrosis after radiation therapy for head and neck cancer: differentiation from recurrent disease with CT and PET/CT imaging. AJNR Am J Neuroradiol. 35(7):1405-11, 2014
8. Saito N et al: Posttreatment CT and MR imaging in head and neck cancer: what the radiologist needs to know. Radiographics. 32(5):1261-82; discussion 1282-4, 2012
9. Berg EE et al: Pathologic effects of external-beam irradiation on human vocal folds. Ann Otol Rhinol Laryngol. 120(11):748-54, 2011
10. Bisdas S et al: Perfusion CT in squamous cell carcinoma of the upper aerodigestive tract: long-term predictive value of baseline perfusion CT measurements. AJNR Am J Neuroradiol. 31(3):576-81, 2010
11. Faggioni L et al: CT perfusion of head and neck tumors: how we do it. AJR Am J Roentgenol. 194(1):62-9, 2010
12. Glastonbury CM et al: The postradiation neck: evaluating response to treatment and recognizing complications. AJR Am J Roentgenol. 195(2):W164-71, 2010
13. Yoo JS et al: Osteoradionecrosis of the hyoid bone: imaging findings. AJNR Am J Neuroradiol. 31(4):761-6, 2010
14. Debnam JM et al: Benign ulceration as a manifestation of soft tissue radiation necrosis: imaging findings. AJNR Am J Neuroradiol. 29(3):558-62, 2008
15. Abdel Razek AA et al: Role of diffusion-weighted echo-planar MR imaging in differentiation of residual or recurrent head and neck tumors and posttreatment changes. AJNR Am J Neuroradiol. 28(6):1146-52, 2007
16. Sanguineti G et al: Dosimetric predictors of laryngeal edema. Int J Radiat Oncol Biol Phys. 68(3):741-9, 2007
17. Mukherji SK et al: Imaging of the post-treatment larynx. Eur J Radiol. 44(2):108-19, 2002
18. Nömayr A et al: MRI appearance of radiation-induced changes of normal cervical tissues. Eur Radiol. 11(9):1807-17, 2001
19. De Vuysere S et al: CT findings in laryngeal chondroradionecrosis. JBR-BTR. 82(1):16-8, 1999
20. Fitzgerald PJ et al: Delayed radionecrosis of the larynx. Am J Otolaryngol. 20(4):245-9, 1999
21. Hermans R et al: CT findings in chondroradionecrosis of the larynx. AJNR Am J Neuroradiol. 19(4):711-8, 1998

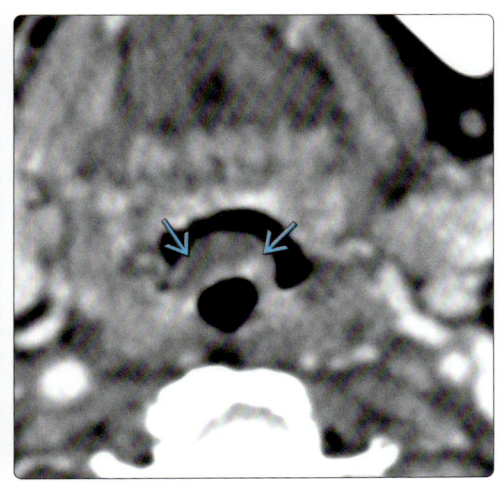
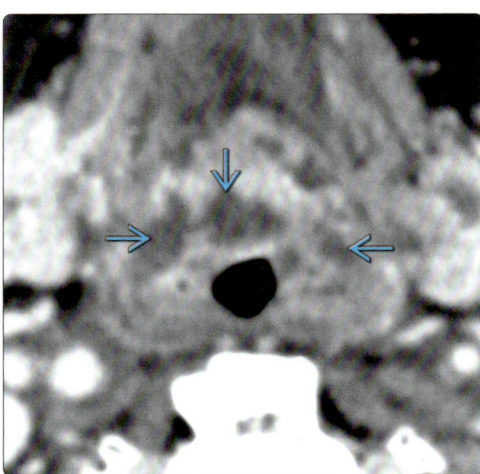

(Left) *Axial CECT in a patient with supraglottic laryngeal cancer after 9 months of definitive chemoradiation treatment shows diffuse edematous thickening of epiglottis ➡. There is no nodular enhancement, a finding consistent with postradiation changes.* **(Right)** *Axial CECT at the level of the inferior part of the epiglottis shows diffuse edema and heterogeneous enhancement of the preepiglottic space ➡. Note that edema and inflammation improve over time.*

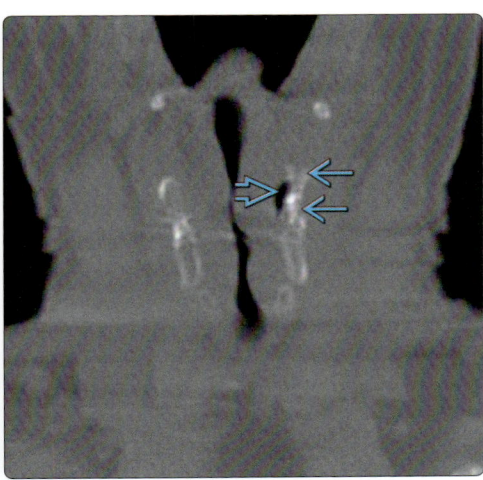
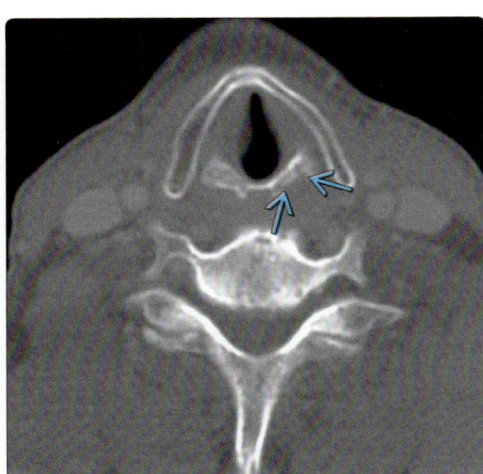

(Left) *Coronal bone window neck MPR CECT in a patient with laryngeal cancer treated with definitive chemoradiation now under surveillance show cortical irregularity of left thyroid lamina ➡ with a locule of air ➡ in and adjacent to it, consistent with chondronecrosis.* **(Right)** *Axial CECT in a patient with laryngeal cancer treated with chemoradiation shows heterogeneous density and cortical erosions in cricoid lamina ➡, consistent with chondronecrosis. Severe cases may warrant laryngectomy.*

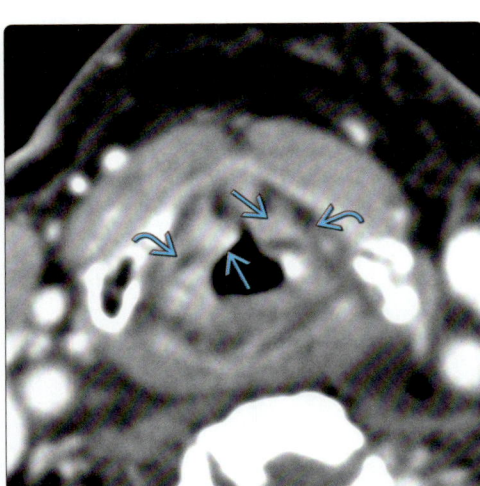
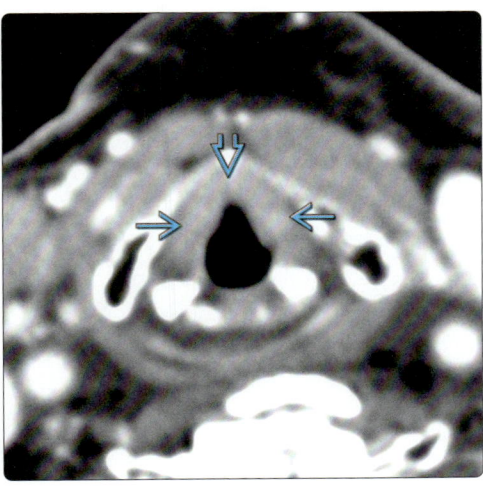

(Left) *Axial CECT at the level of false cords in a patient with glottic cancer post radiation shows diffuse edematous thickening of bilateral false cords ➡ and paralaryngeal fat stranding ➡, consistent with postradiation changes.* **(Right)** *Axial CECT in the same patient at the level of true cords shows diffuse edematous thickening of bilateral true cords ➡ and also an anterior commissure ➡. No nodular enhancement is noted. Edema and mucosal enhancement are typical for acute/subacute postradiation changes.*

KEY FACTS

TERMINOLOGY

- Internal laryngocele: Dilated, air- or fluid-filled laryngeal saccule; located in paraglottic region of supraglottis
- Mixed laryngocele: Extends laterally through thyrohyoid membrane to low submandibular space
- Pyolaryngocele: Pus-containing, superinfected laryngocele
- Secondary laryngocele: Glottic or inferior supraglottic lesion obstructs laryngeal ventricle (15% all laryngoceles)

IMAGING

- Best diagnostic clue
  - Internal laryngocele: Thin-walled, air- or fluid-filled cystic lesion communicating with laryngeal ventricle
  - Mixed laryngocele: Internal + extralaryngeal extension through thyrohyoid membrane
  - Pyolaryngocele: Pus-filled laryngocele with thick, enhancing walls
  - Secondary laryngocele: Glottic or inferior supraglottic lesion causal

TOP DIFFERENTIAL DIAGNOSES

- Thyroglossal duct cyst
- 2nd branchial cleft cyst
- Vallecular cyst
- Lateral hypopharyngeal pouch
- Supraglottitis with abscess
- Laryngeal saccule (normal ventricular appendix)

CLINICAL ISSUES

- Caused by chronic increase in intraglottic pressure
- Seen in glass blowers, wind instrument players, and chronic coughers

DIAGNOSTIC CHECKLIST

- Comment in report if extralaryngeal extension is present
  - If so, mixed laryngocele requires open surgical approach
- Evaluate for infiltrating endolaryngeal mass
  - 5% are secondary laryngoceles
  - SCCa of glottis or low supraglottis is major culprit

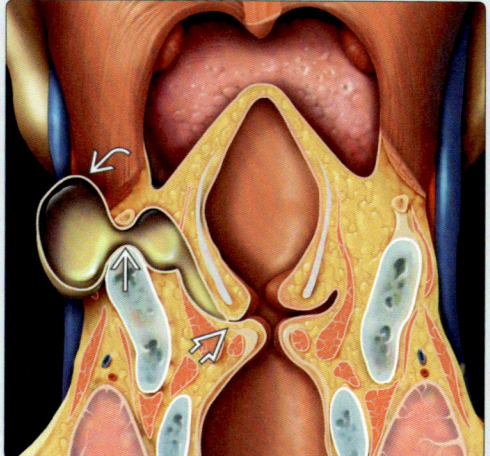
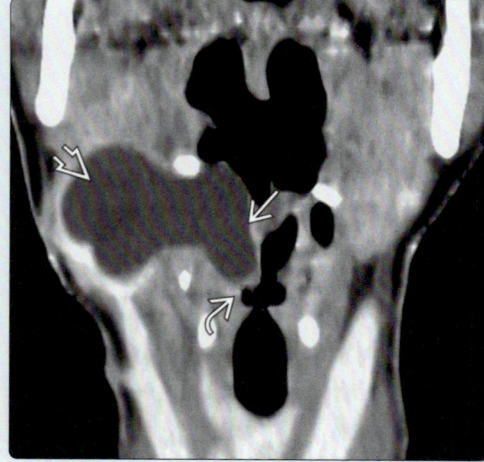

(Left) Coronal graphic shows a laryngocele with extralaryngeal extension. There is an isthmus ➡ where the lesion squeezes through the thyrohyoid membrane to the low submandibular space ➡. Note stenosis at the laryngeal ventricle ➡. (Right) Coronal CECT reformation shows a similar lesion. This is also known as a mixed laryngocele because it contains internal ➡ (intralaryngeal) and external ➡ (extralaryngeal) portions. It can be followed to the laryngeal ventricle ➡.

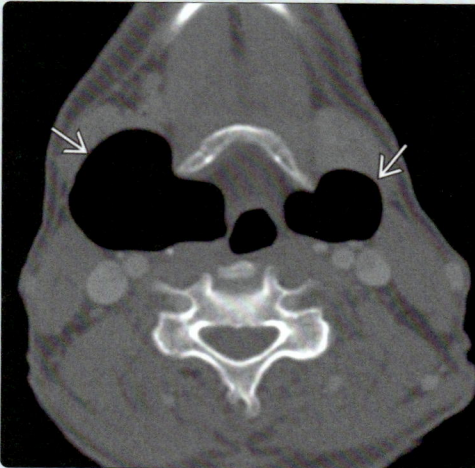
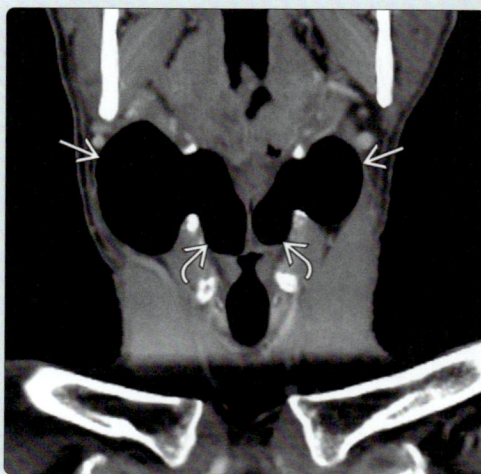

(Left) Axial CECT in a 46-year-old man with complaints of asymmetric fullness in the right neck shows large, bilateral, air-filled laryngoceles ➡. At the level of the hyoid bone, the extralaryngeal components are seen, right greater than left. (Right) Coronal CECT in the same patient again demonstrates large, bilateral mixed laryngoceles, including the intralaryngeal ➡ and extralaryngeal ➡ components. Notice the "waist" created as each laryngocele passes though the thyrohyoid membrane.

TERMINOLOGY

Synonyms

- Internal laryngocele = simple laryngocele
- Mixed (combined, external) laryngocele: Laryngocele with extralaryngeal extension
- Saccular cyst: Currently term best reserved for congenital laryngocele

Definitions

- **Laryngeal saccule**: Appendiceal pouch projecting superiorly from anterior **laryngeal ventricle**
  - Contains numerous mucous glands
  - Functions in lubrication of true cords
- **Internal laryngocele**: Dilated, air- or fluid-filled laryngeal saccule extending above superior margin of thyroid cartilage
  - Located in paraglottic space of supraglottis
  - Synonym: Simple laryngocele
- **Mixed laryngocele**: Extends from paraglottic space through thyrohyoid membrane to low submandibular space (SMS)
  - Synonym: Mixed laryngocele
  - Contains internal (intralaryngeal) and external (extralaryngeal) components
- **Pyolaryngocele**: Superinfected laryngocele containing pus
- **Secondary laryngocele**: Glottic or inferior supraglottic squamous cell carcinoma (SCCa) obstructs laryngeal ventricle
  - 15% of all laryngoceles

IMAGING

General Features

- Best diagnostic clue
  - Thin-walled, fluid- or air-filled lesion communicating with laryngeal ventricle, ± extralaryngeal extension through thyrohyoid membrane
- Location
  - Internal laryngocele: Supraglottic paraglottic space
  - Mixed laryngocele: Paraglottic space → through thyrohyoid membrane → SMS
- Size
  - Variable; may enlarge with Valsalva maneuver
- Morphology
  - Circumscribed, thin walled
  - Mixed lesions have isthmus when passing outside larynx through thyrohyoid membrane
  - If pyolaryngocele, thickened walls with adjacent inflammation
  - If secondary, infiltrating mass seen in low supraglottis or glottis

Radiographic Findings

- Radiography
  - Air pocket seen in upper cervical soft tissues
  - Soft tissue/fluid density projects against air column in supraglottic region

CT Findings

- CECT
  - Internal laryngocele
    - Circumscribed, thin-walled, fluid or air density within **paraglottic space** of supraglottis
    - Absent to minimal peripheral enhancement
    - Paraglottic lesion connects to laryngeal ventricle
      - Coronal plane shows this connection best
    - If does not extend above upper margin of thyroid cartilage, likely prominent saccule and not true laryngocele
  - Mixed laryngocele
    - Paraglottic cyst passes through thyrohyoid membrane into SMS
      - **Isthmus** ("waist") at thyrohyoid membrane
      - Coronal plane shows paraglottic-SMS connection
  - Pyolaryngocele: Thick, enhancing walls with adjacent inflammation
  - Secondary laryngocele: Enhancing, infiltrative glottic or low supraglottic lesion
    - Most commonly from SCCa
    - Amyloid infiltration rare cause

MR Findings

- T1WI
  - Low T1, thin walled, fluid intensity
- T2WI
  - High T2, thin walled, fluid intensity
- T1WI C+
  - Thin walled; absent to minimal linear peripheral enhancement
  - Thick, enhancing walls if pyolaryngocele

Imaging Recommendations

- Best imaging tool
  - CECT of neck soft tissues
- Protocol advice
  - Coronal reformatted images best demonstrate relationship to laryngeal ventricle, thyrohyoid membrane, and SMS

DIFFERENTIAL DIAGNOSIS

Thyroglossal Duct Cyst

- Midline cystic mass adjacent to midportion of hyoid bone
- Extralaryngeal, embedded in infrahyoid strap muscles
- May project into preepiglottic space

2nd Branchial Cleft Cyst

- Cystic mass posterior to submandibular gland at angle of mandible
- Displaces submandibular gland anteromedially, carotid space medially, and sternocleidomastoid muscle posterolaterally
- No connection to larynx

Laryngeal Saccule (Ventricular Appendix)

- Normal structure; pseudolesion when air filled
  - Normal saccule can measure 5- 15 mm in length
- Causes no submucosal deformity
- Located below superior margin of thyroid cartilage

Vallecular Cyst

- Cyst typically displaces epiglottis posteriorly
- Lies anterior to epiglottis, unilateral or bilateral

- Congenital lesion

Supraglottitis With Abscess

- Peripherally enhancing mass with central low density
- No connection to laryngeal ventricle or thyrohyoid membrane

PATHOLOGY

General Features

- Etiology
  - Commonly acquired; rarely congenital
  - Increased intraglottic pressure creates "ball-valve" phenomenon at communication of laryngeal ventricle with saccule
    - Saccule (appendix of laryngeal ventricle) expands
    - Causes: Glass blowing, playing wind instrument, excessive coughing
    - Fills with mucus when obstructed
  - Secondary laryngoceles from proximal saccular obstruction are less common (15%)
    - From **SCCa**, postinflammatory stenosis, trauma, surgery, or amyloid

Gross Pathologic & Surgical Features

- Smooth-surfaced, sac-like specimen

Microscopic Features

- Lined by respiratory epithelium (ciliated, columnar) with fibrous wall

CLINICAL ISSUES

Presentation

- Most common signs/symptoms
  - Principal presenting symptom
    - Internal laryngocele: Larger lesions present with hoarseness or stridor
      - When small, may be incidental and asymptomatic
    - Mixed laryngocele: Anterior neck mass, low SMS just below angle of mandible
      - Expand with modified Valsalva
- Other signs/symptoms
  - Sore throat, dysphagia, stridor, airway obstruction
- Clinical profile
  - Glass blower, wind instrument player, chronic cougher

Demographics

- Age
  - Age at presentation: > 50 years old
- Sex
  - More common in male patients
- Ethnicity
  - More common in White patients
- Epidemiology
  - Bilateral laryngoceles: 30%
  - Internal laryngocele 2x as common as mixed laryngocele

Natural History & Prognosis

- Gradual enlargement over time
- With continued growth, laryngocele penetrates thyrohyoid membrane to enter neck in lower SMS
- Excellent prognosis after removal

Treatment

- 1st, endoscopically exclude underlying lesion of true or false cords obstructing laryngeal ventricle
- Isolated internal laryngocele: Microlaryngoscopic CO_2 laser resection
- Mixed laryngocele: External transthyrohyoid membrane approach, endoscopic or robotic surgery

DIAGNOSTIC CHECKLIST

Consider

- Does lesion change size with Valsalva?
- Is patient glass blower, wind instrument player, or chronic cougher?

Image Interpretation Pearls

- Best diagnostic clue: Fluid- or air-filled, thin-walled lesion communicating with laryngeal ventricle
- Do not forget to look for occult SCCa in low supraglottis or glottic larynx
- Coronal plane best to show relationships to laryngeal ventricle and thyrohyoid membrane
- Differentiate from prominent pyriform sinus or prominent laryngeal ventricle

Reporting Tips

- Extension through thyrohyoid membrane into SMS?
  - Yes: Mixed laryngocele
  - No: Internal laryngocele
- Thickening/prominent enhancement of laryngocele wall?
  - Yes: Pyolaryngocele
- Mass in low supraglottis or glottis?
  - Yes: Secondary laryngocele (accounts for ~ 15%)
  - Remember, endoscopy necessary to fully exclude obstructing mass

SELECTED REFERENCES

1. Verro B et al: CO2 Laser marsupialization for internal and combined laryngocele. Int Arch Otorhinolaryngol. 27(3):e428-34, 2023
2. Hackenberg S et al: Rare diseases of larynx, trachea and thyroid. Laryngorhinootologie. 100(S 01):S1-36, 2021
3. Purnell PR et al: Minimally invasive treatment of laryngoceles: a systematic review and pooled analysis. J Robot Surg. 16(1):1-14, 2021
4. Slonimsky G et al: Terminology, definitions, and classification in the imaging of laryngoceles. Curr Probl Diagn Radiol. 50(3):384-8, 2021
5. Biswas S et al: Blunt trauma to the neck presenting as dysphonia and dysphagia in a healthy young woman; a rare case of traumatic laryngocele. Bull Emerg Trauma. 8(2):129-31, 2020
6. Singh R et al: Systematic review of laryngocele and pyolaryngocele management in the age of robotic surgery. J Int Med Res. 48(10):300060520940441, 2020
7. Madhavan AA et al: Imaging findings related to the valsalva maneuver in head and neck radiology. AJNR Am J Neuroradiol. 40(12):1987-93, 2019
8. Zelenik K et al: Treatment of laryngoceles: what is the progress over the last two decades? Biomed Res Int. 2014:819453, 2014
9. Dursun G et al: Current diagnosis and treatment of laryngocele in adults. Otolaryngol Head Neck Surg. 136(2):211-5, 2007
10. Ling FT et al: Is there a role for conservative management for symptomatic laryngopyocele? Case report and literature review. J Otolaryngol. 33(4):264-8, 2004
11. Ettema SL et al: Laryngocele resection by combined external and endoscopic laser approach. Ann Otol Rhinol Laryngol. 112(4):361-4, 2003
12. Harney M et al: Laryngocele and squamous cell carcinoma of the larynx. J Laryngol Otol. 115(7):590-2, 2001
13. Thabet MH et al: Lateral saccular cysts of the larynx. Aetiology, diagnosis and management. J Laryngol Otol. 115(4):293-7, 2001
14. Nazaroglu H et al: Laryngopyocele: signs on computed tomography. Eur J Radiol. 33(1):63-5, 2000

Laryngocele

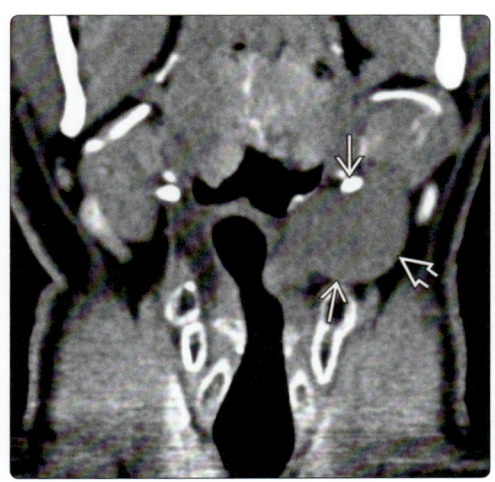 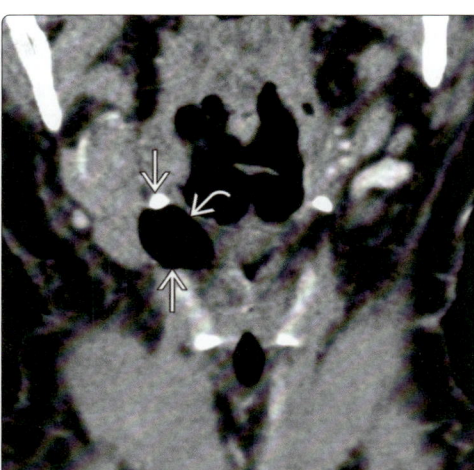

(Left) Coronal CECT reformation in a patient with an anterior neck mass that enlarged with Valsalva reveals a left-sided, fluid-filled laryngocele with extralaryngeal extension (mixed). The lesion passes through the thyrohyoid membrane ➡ to the low submandibular space ➡. (Right) Coronal CECT reformation shows an air-filled sac ➡ traversing the thyrohyoid membrane ➡. An open surgical approach is required to treat this type of mixed laryngocele.

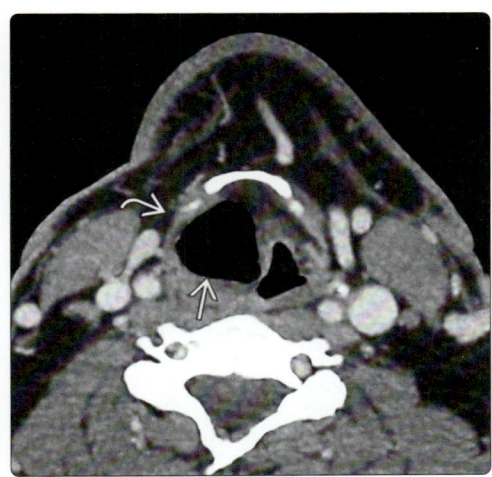 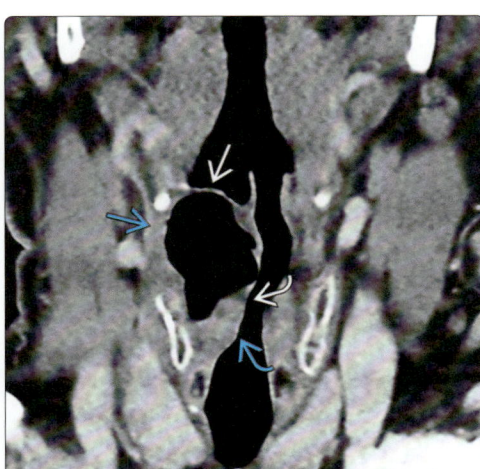

(Left) Axial CECT shows an air-density lesion in the right paraglottic region of the supraglottis ➡. It is contained within the thyrohyoid membrane ➡, suggesting an internal (simple) laryngocele. (Right) Coronal CECT in the same patient shows the relationship of the lesion ➡ to the laryngeal ventricle ➡, glottic larynx ➡, and the thyrohyoid membrane ➡. It is crucial to exclude a small lesion at the laryngeal ventricle/glottis on endoscopy.

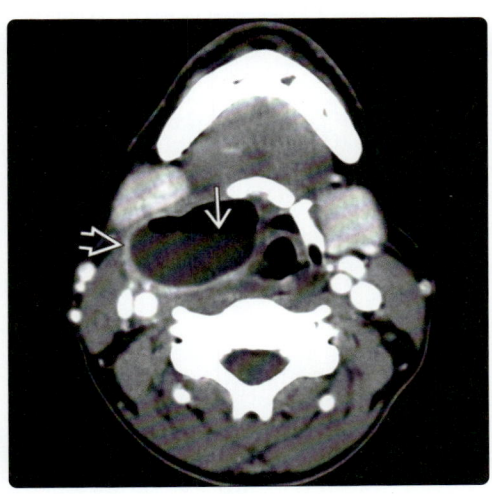 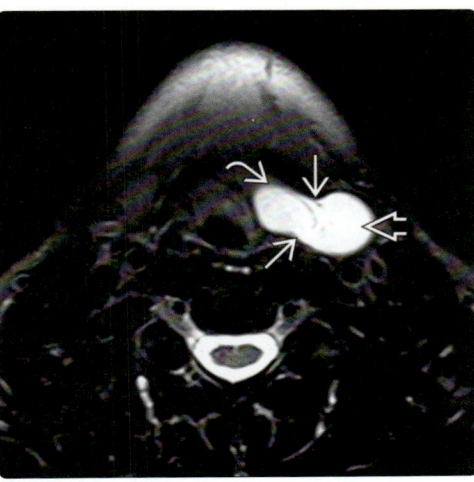

(Left) Axial CECT shows a superinfected laryngocele, also called a pyolaryngocele. Note thickening with prominent enhancement of the laryngocele walls ➡ and the internal air-fluid level ➡. The hypopharyngeal airway is severely compromised. (Right) Axial STIR MR shows typical findings of a laryngocele with extralaryngeal extension (mixed). There is a thin-walled, fluid-intensity lesion extending from the paraglottic region ➡ to the anterior cervical soft tissues ➡. Note isthmus ("waist") at the thyrohyoid membrane ➡.

KEY FACTS

TERMINOLOGY

- Vocal cord paralysis, true vocal cord paralysis, recurrent laryngeal nerve paralysis
- Immobilization of true vocal cord by ipsilateral vagus (CNX) or recurrent laryngeal nerve dysfunction

IMAGING

- Constellation of unilateral laryngeal findings
  - Paramedian position of affected true vocal cord
  - Ballooning of laryngeal ventricle = sail sign
  - Anteromedial rotation of arytenoid cartilage
  - Enlarged pyriform sinus
  - Medially displaced, thickened aryepiglottic fold

TOP DIFFERENTIAL DIAGNOSES

- Laryngeal trauma
- Laryngocele
- Glottic (laryngeal) squamous cell carcinoma

PATHOLOGY

- Injury to or lesion compressing CNX anywhere from medulla to recurrent laryngeal nerve
- Most common etiologies: Neoplasm, trauma, idiopathic, & nonmalignant thoracic pathology
- Can also group by location: Jugular foramen, carotid space, mediastinum, & tracheoesophageal groove

CLINICAL ISSUES

- Hoarseness, dysphonia, "breathy voice"

DIAGNOSTIC CHECKLIST

- Evaluate entire course of CNX & recurrent laryngeal nerve
- **Right** recurrent laryngeal nerve arises from CNX at **subclavian artery**
- **Left** recurrent laryngeal nerve arises from CNX at **aortopulmonary window**

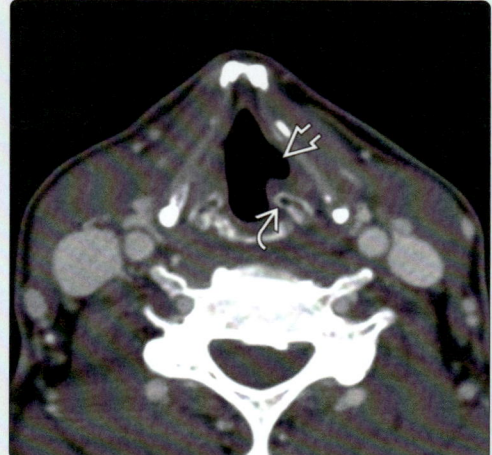
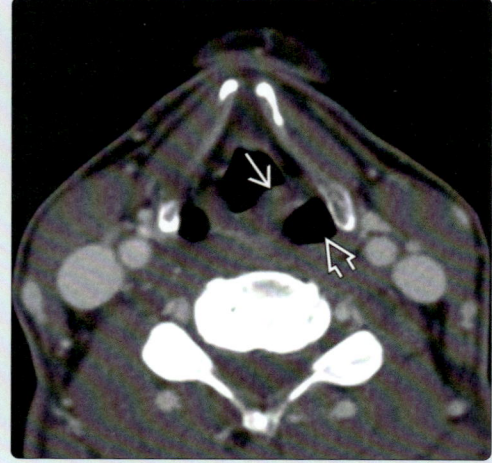

(Left) CECT in a patient with new-onset hoarseness shows slightly medially rotated left arytenoid cartilage ➡ & a more prominent dilated left laryngeal ventricle ➡. This is sometimes referred to as the sail sign, as it mimics the spinnaker of a boat. (Right) Axial CECT in the same patient demonstrates an asymmetrically enlarged left pyriform sinus ➡ & medial position of left aryepiglottic fold ➡, which also appears thickened. Imaging features are consistent with clinical finding of left vocal cord paralysis (VCP).

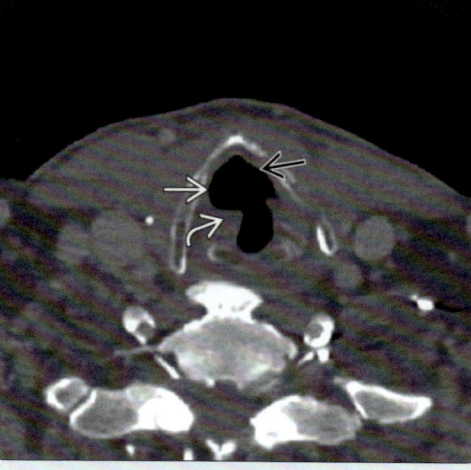
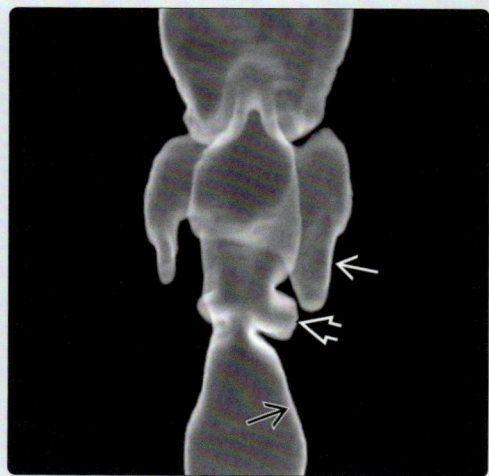

(Left) Axial CT of the neck at vocal cords level shows the mushroom sign, an appearance of the airway due to a combination of ipsilateral laryngeal ventricle dilation ➡ & posterior cord medialization ➡ with anterior contralateral subglottic air ➡. The "head" of the mushroom is tilted towards the side of the VCP. (Right) AP airway 3D volume rendered CT in the left VCP shows an enlarged ipsilateral laryngeal ventricle ➡ & pyriform sinus ➡ with flattening of the subglottic arch ➡ due to a medially positioned vocal cord.

Vocal Cord Paralysis

TERMINOLOGY

Abbreviations
- Vocal cord paralysis (VCP)

Definitions
- Immobilization of true vocal cord by ipsilateral vagus (CNX) or recurrent laryngeal nerve (RLN) dysfunction

IMAGING

General Features
- Best diagnostic clue
  - Paramedian vocal cord & **ipsilateral** findings
    - Ballooning of laryngeal ventricle sail sign
    - Enlarged pyriform sinus
    - Medially displaced aryepiglottic fold
- Location
  - Primary imaging findings are in larynx
  - Causative lesions can be anywhere from medulla (CNX origin) to RLN
    - CNX traverses **jugular foramen**, descends neck in **carotid space**
    - **Right** CNX extends to clavicle, **recurs around right subclavian artery**
    - **Left** CNX extends into mediastinum, **recurs via aortopulmonary window**
    - RLNs ascend to larynx in **tracheoesophageal grooves**
- Morphology
  - Affected cord is flaccid, paramedian in location

Radiographic Findings
- Radiography
  - Chest radiograph less sensitive than CT but often 1st test ordered if left true VCP
    - Pancoast tumor, mediastinal mass/adenopathy, cardiomegaly, enlarged aorta

CT Findings
- CECT
  - **Quiet respiration CT/MR:** Paramedian position of affected true vocal cord with ipsilateral ancillary findings
    - Ballooning of laryngeal ventricle = **sail sign**
      - □ Due to thyroarytenoid muscle atrophy
      - □ **Mushroom sign** on axial: Ipsilateral laryngeal ventricle dilation, medialized posterior cord margin, & contralateral anterior subglottic air
      - □ "Head" of mushroom tilted towards side of vocal cord palsy
    - Anteromedial rotation of arytenoid cartilage
    - Enlarged pyriform sinus (this & aforementioned 2 signs most sensitive)
    - Medially displaced, thick aryepiglottic fold
    - Cricoarytenoid muscle atrophy
  - **Breath-hold CT/MR:** Paralyzed cord does not adduct & contralateral normal cord extends more medially to close glottis with bowed appearance
  - If mass along CNX course from brainstem to jugular foramen
    - CNIX, CNXI dysfunction often also evident
      - □ CNIX injury → loss of ipsilateral pharynx sensation

- □ CNXI injury → ipsilateral trapezius & sternocleidomastoid denervation
  - If mass along CNX in superior carotid space to hyoid
    - CNIX, CNXI + CNXII dysfunction often evident
      - □ CNXII injury → ipsilateral tongue denervation
  - If proximal CNX neuropathy, both pharyngeal plexus motor branches (supplying pharyngeal constrictor muscles & uvula) also affected with RLN
    - Additional ipsilateral oropharynx bowing, pharyngeal constrictor muscles atrophy, & uvular deviation to opposite side
  - Be aware of post thyroplasty vocal cord appearance
    - Procedures add bulk to paralyzed cord, improve voice
    - Vocal cord more midline, no longer patulous
      - □ Low density = fat injected to cord
      - □ High density = Silastic or Gore-Tex implants or Teflon injection
- CTA
  - Helpful to evaluate internal carotid artery for dissection

MR Findings
- MR shows same anatomic findings as CT
  - Medialized cord with patulous enlarged ventricle
  - Ipsilateral medial aryepiglottic fold & large pyriform sinus
- **Pitfall** in MR is acute-subacute denervation
  - T2 hyperintense & enhancing vocal cord muscle
  - May be erroneously interpreted as tumor

Nuclear Medicine Findings
- PET
  - Absent FDG uptake in denervated cord
    - Contralateral normal cord has asymmetric uptake
    - **Pitfall**: If normal side interpreted as abnormal uptake or tumor
  - Teflon injection thyroplasty incites granulomatous reaction in ~ 50% that may take up FDG

Imaging Recommendations
- Best imaging tool
  - CECT is 1st-line imaging tool for evaluation of hoarseness or known VCP
- Protocol advice
  - CECT from skull base to carina
  - Evaluate entire course of both CNX & RLNs

DIFFERENTIAL DIAGNOSIS

Laryngeal Trauma
- Arytenoid dislocation may occur with intubation
- Mimics VCP clinically & on imaging
  - Coronal CT will show difference in height of vocal cords
- Look for other signs of trauma; clinical history is key
- Successful treatment requires early reduction

Laryngocele
- Air-filled internal laryngocele may be misinterpreted as enlarged laryngeal ventricle
- Normal arytenoid & aryepiglottic fold location
- No pyriform sinus dilation

Glottic (Laryngeal) Squamous Cell Carcinoma

- Primary tumor may result in reduced cord mobility (T2 tumor), mimicking VCP
- Direct extension or nodal metastases can cause VCP if injured vagus or RLN

PATHOLOGY

General Features

- Etiology
  - Injury to or lesion compressing CNX from medulla to RLN
  - Most common: Neoplasm, trauma, idiopathic pathology
  - **Neoplastic infiltration** of RLN or CNX
    - Chest: Lung carcinoma, mediastinal adenopathy, aortic pathology
    - Neck: Thyroid carcinoma, neck adenopathy
    - Jugular foramen: Meningioma, jugular paraganglioma, metastases
  - **Traumatic** (including **iatrogenic**) **injury** to nerve
    - Stabbing injury to neck
    - Carotid artery dissection
    - Thyroidectomy, carotid endarterectomy, anterior cervical spine fusion
  - **Idiopathic**
    - Many probably toxic, inflammatory (viral, post viral), or ischemic
    - No causative finding on imaging
    - Toxicity: Vincristine, alcohol
    - Other neuropathies: Radiation-induced, myasthenia gravis, vitamin B12 deficiency, infectious (varicella, Lyme disease), sarcoidosis, SLE
  - **Less common**
    - Neurologic (stroke, demyelination, myasthenia gravis), rarely compression by anterior cervical osteophytes
    - **Nonmalignant thoracic causes**
      - □ a.k.a. cardiovocal (Ortner) syndrome
      - □ Atrial septal defect, Eisenmenger complex, patent ductus arteriosus, primary pulmonary hypertension, aortic aneurysm with stretching of RLN
  - VCP is most commonly unilateral, but, rarely, bilateral VCP also occurs
    - Most common cause of bilateral VCP is surgical trauma (e.g., thyroidectomy, tracheal/esophagus surgery, neck exploration, heart/aorta surgery), less common causes being malignancies, post intubation, neurologic causes, including ALS, Miller-Fisher syndrome, & idiopathic

CLINICAL ISSUES

Presentation

- Most common signs/symptoms
  - Hoarseness, dysphonia, "breathy voice"
- Other signs/symptoms
  - Uncommonly may be asymptomatic with normal voice
  - Aspiration (especially liquids), insufficient cough
  - Foreign body sensation in larynx
  - Shortness of breath sensation, air wasting
- Clinical profile
  - Adult presenting with hoarseness

Demographics

- Sex
  - No known predilection in adults
  - M > F in pediatric age group
- Epidemiology
  - Fewer "idiopathic" cases in CT era

Natural History & Prognosis

- VCP due to recurrent nerve or CNX injury rarely recovers
- Toxic or infectious VCP often self-limited
  - > 80% resolve within 6 months
- Recovery uncommon if no improvement by 9 months

Treatment

- Initially conservative, many "idiopathic" cases will spontaneously improve
- Voice therapy
- **Vocal cord augmentation**: Material injected to paraglottic space
  - Temporary: Resorbable materials (Gelfoam, hyaluronic acid, collagen)
  - Permanent: Fat, calcium hydroxylapatite, Teflon
    - Teflon reserved for terminal patients, as > 50% develop granuloma
- **Laryngeal framework surgery**
  - Medialization thyroplasty with Silastic or Gore-Tex implant
  - Arytenoid adduction
  - Laryngeal reinnervation (hypoglossal nerve, ansa cervicalis)

DIAGNOSTIC CHECKLIST

Consider

- If VCP evident
  - Determine whether vagal neuropathy or RLN paralysis (RLNP)
  - Evaluate for additional cranial neuropathies: CNIX, XI, XII
  - Regardless, evaluate brainstem, jugular foramen, then entire neck ± chest, along entire course of vagus & RLN
- Right RLN arises from CNX at subclavian artery
- Left RLN arises from CNX at aortopulmonary window

Imaging Pitfalls

- MR: Acute-subacute denervation results in T2-hyperintense & enhancing cord
  - May be misinterpreted as vocal cord tumor
- FDG PET: Denervated cord does not take up FDG
  - Contralateral cord may be misinterpreted as tumor
- CECT: Dense medialized cord following thyroplasty
  - Mimics cord tumor with cord paralysis
  - Teflon granuloma will also take up FDG

SELECTED REFERENCES

1. Fadhil M et al: Anterior cervical osteophytes: a rare culprit of unilateral vocal cord palsy. ANZ J Surg. 94(5):967-9, 2024
2. Bashir MH et al: Revisiting CT signs of unilateral vocal fold paralysis: a single, blinded study. AJNR Am J Neuroradiol. 43(4):592-6, 2022
3. Ortega Beltrá N et al: Extralaryngeal causes of unilateral vocal cord paralysis: aetiology and prognosis. Acta Otorrinolaringol Esp (Engl Ed). 73(6):376-83, 2022
4. Din-Lovinescu C et al: Adverse events following injection laryngoplasty: an analysis of the MAUDE database. Am J Otolaryngol. 42(6):103092, 2021

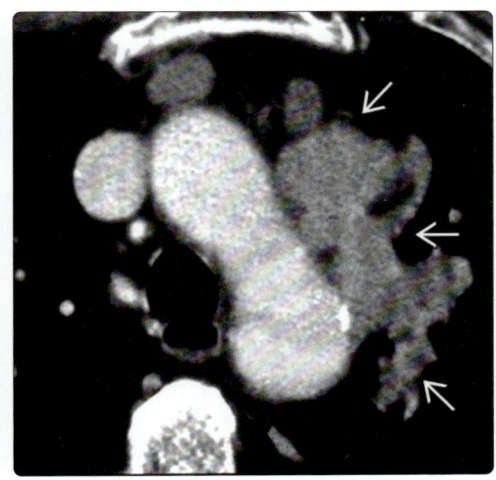
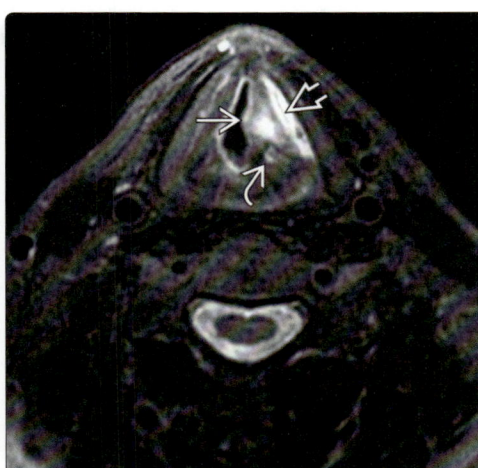

(Left) *Axial CECT stresses the importance of scanning the aortopulmonary window for left VCP. A mediastinal mass (lung carcinoma) ➡ involves left recurrent laryngeal nerve as it courses under aortic arch.* (Right) *T2 MR shows marked T2 hyperintensity of left true cord ➡ in acute/subacute VCP, representing thyroarytenoid denervation change, a potential pitfall in acute/subacute setting, where it can be misinterpreted as neoplasm. Note typical medial cord location ➡ & anteromedial arytenoid rotation ➡.*

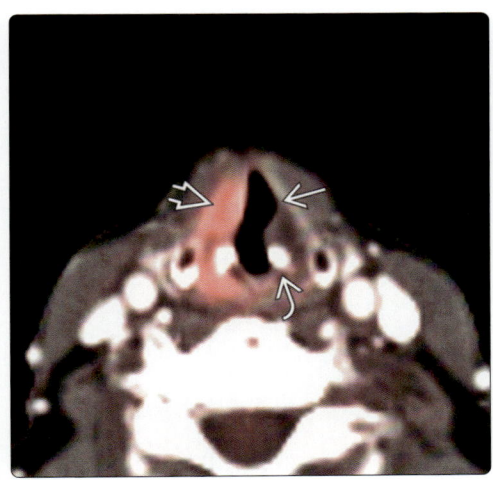
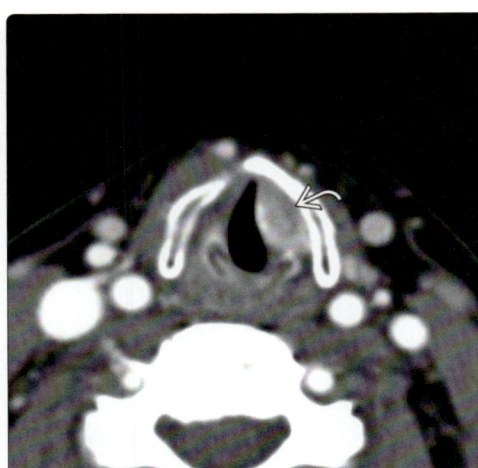

(Left) *Axial PET/CT in a patient with left VCP, as indicated by anteromedial arytenoid rotation ➡ & ballooning of the laryngeal ventricle ➡, is shown. There is asymmetric uptake in the normal right cord ➡, not to be mistaken for tumor.* (Right) *Axial CECT shows the vocal cords with amorphous high density in the left true vocal cord ➡. History revealed prior Teflon injection for left VCP. It is important not to mistake this for malignancy. Note: Teflon can also cause granulomatous reaction, resulting in a false-positive PET scan.*

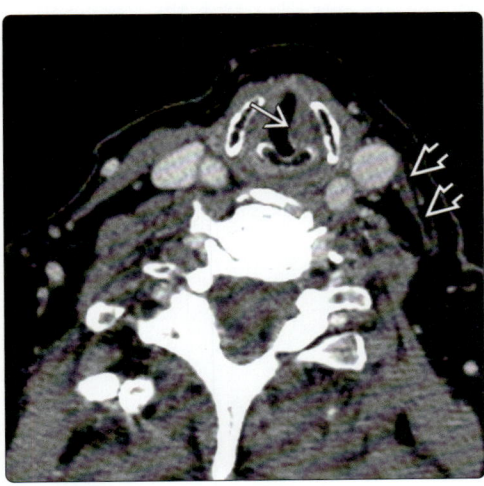
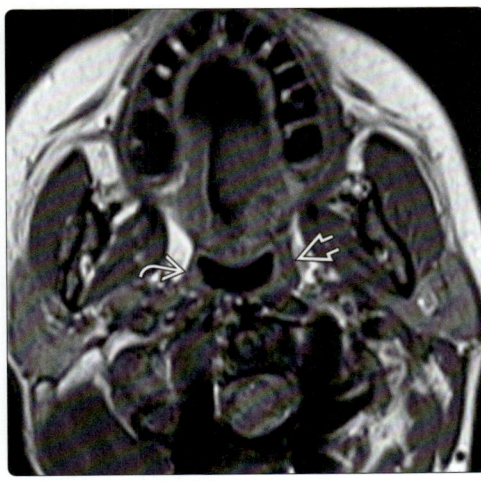

(Left) *Axial CECT demonstrates medialization of the left cord ➡. Note atrophy of the left sternocleidomastoid muscle ➡, indicating concurrent CNXI denervation. VCP, plus CNIX/CNXI involvement, points to a skull base lesion. This patient had a skull base glomus jugulotympanicum.* (Right) *Axial T1 MR shows the soft palate with atrophy of the right superior pharyngeal constrictor muscles ➡ (compare to normal side ➡) due to pharyngeal plexus injury, indicating a vagus nerve lesion above the palate level.*

Hypopharynx, Larynx, and Cervical Trachea

TERMINOLOGY

- Synonyms: Subglottic or laryngotracheal stenosis
- Definition: Nondevelopmental narrowing of cervical airway below vocal cords
  - Due to intrinsic pathology or extrinsic process compressing or invading airway

IMAGING

- **Intrinsic stenosis** usually iatrogenic from intubation or tracheostomy
  - Soft tissue narrows lumen
  - May see irregular, fragmented cartilage
  - Granulomatosis with polyangiitis-related stenoses mostly subglottic and circumferential
- **Extrinsic stenosis** usually due to thyroid mass
  - Multinodular goiter: Enlarged heterogeneous lobes, ± calcifications, hemorrhage, cysts
  - Thyroid carcinoma or non-Hodgkin lymphoma: May compress or invade airway

TOP DIFFERENTIAL DIAGNOSES

- Subglottic infantile hemangioma
- Vascular rings and slings
- Congenital subglottic-tracheal stenosis

CLINICAL ISSUES

- **50%** stenosis before dyspnea on exertion
- **> 75%** airway narrowing before symptoms at rest
- Stenosis misaligned with glottic jet has greater impact on work of breathing

DIAGNOSTIC CHECKLIST

- For intrinsic subglottic/tracheal pathology
  - Evaluate degree and length of stenosis
  - Evaluate for cartilaginous deformity
  - 2D and 3D reconstructed images may help define extent and degree of stenosis
- If tracheal invasion, measure length of airway involvement
  - Determine whether cricoid cartilage involved

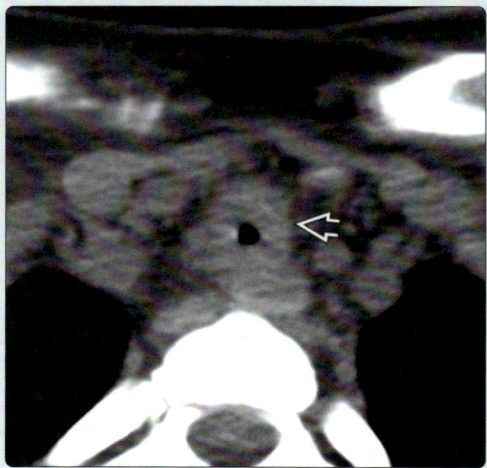
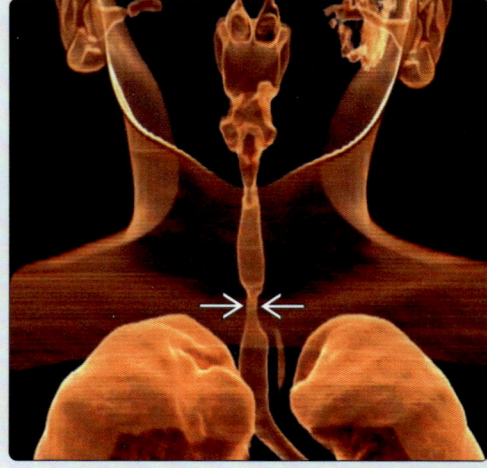

(Left) Axial NECT in a 31-year-old woman with a history of prior intubation and tracheostomy after cardiac arrest demonstrates subglottic airway narrowing with circumferential thickening at the level of the upper trachea with a maximal luminal diameter of 4 mm ➡. (Right) Volume-rendered 3D image from an axial helical NECT demonstrates tracheal stenosis at the thoracic inlet related to a cuffed tube injury. Note the abrupt shelf of stenosis with smooth edges ➡.

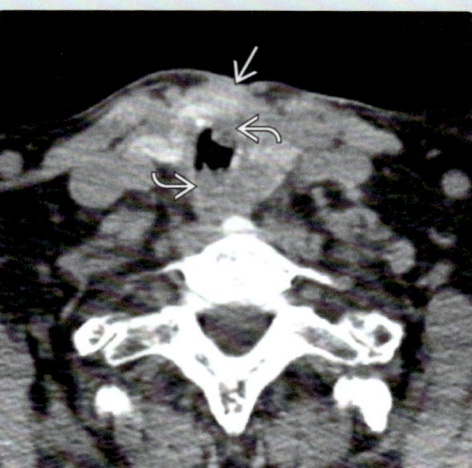
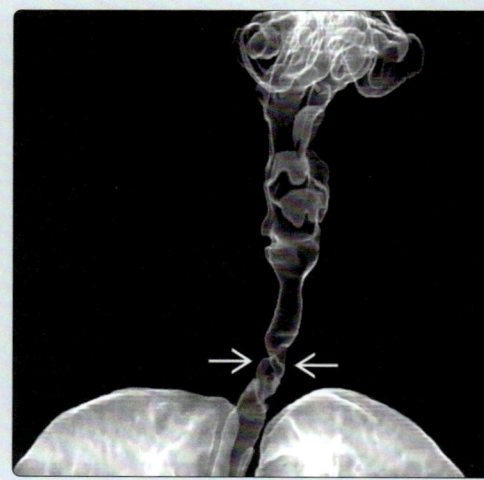

(Left) Axial NECT in a patient with previous tracheostomy reveals subglottic-tracheal narrowing with marked luminal irregularity due to exuberant granulation tissue ➡. Note skin thickening with increased density of subcutaneous fat from scarring along the tracheostomy tract ➡. (Right) Volume-rendered 3D image from an axial helical NECT demonstrates irregular subglottic tracheal stenosis over multiple centimeters due to granulation tissue at a prior tracheostomy site ➡.

Acquired Subglottic-Tracheal Stenosis

TERMINOLOGY

Synonyms

- Subglottic stenosis
- Laryngotracheal stenosis

Definitions

- Nondevelopmental narrowing of cervical airway below vocal cords
  - Due to intrinsic pathology or extrinsic process compressing or invading airway

IMAGING

General Features

- Best diagnostic clue
  - Narrowing of airway below vocal cords
- Location
  - Most commonly subglottic larynx and proximal cervical trachea
- Size
  - Length of stenosis varies with etiology
- Morphology
  - Circumferential or eccentric narrowing, smooth or irregular

Radiographic Findings

- Radiography
  - Narrowing of tracheal air column
  - Trachea may be displaced if asymmetric or unilateral thyroid mass

CT Findings

- Imaging findings depend on cause of stenosis
- **Intrinsic stenosis**: Most often due to **prior intubation** or **tracheostomy**
  - Concentric or eccentric soft tissue internal to cricoid/trachea
  - May be smooth or irregular soft tissue
  - Stenosis from tracheostomy more often irregular and longer segment than stenosis from intubation
- Evaluate carefully for cricoid or tracheal ring deformity or destruction
  - Cartilage necrosis in iatrogenic stenosis
  - Cartilage fracture following trauma
  - Cartilage collapse with relapsing polychondritis (RP), granulomatosis with polyangiitis (GPA)
  - Cartilage invasion with squamous cell carcinoma (SCCa)
- May see calcification of submucosal tissues
  - RP, amyloidosis
- **Extrinsic stenosis**: Most common cause is **thyroid mass**
  - Multinodular goiter: Enlarged heterogeneous lobes, ± calcifications, hemorrhage, cysts
  - Thyroid carcinoma or non-Hodgkin lymphoma (NHL): May compress or invade trachea
    - Evaluate carefully for soft tissue in lumen, cartilage destruction
    - Differentiated carcinoma: ± calcifications
    - Anaplastic: Infiltrative, necrosis common, neck nodes
    - Thyroid NHL: Infiltrative, necrosis uncommon, neck nodes

Imaging Recommendations

- Best imaging tool
  - CT allows best evaluation of airway and cartilage contour and caliber
- Protocol advice
  - Thin-section (1-2 mm) helical imaging allows 2D and 3D reformations
    - Volume rendering and virtual endoscopy views
  - Contrast important for evaluation of tumors and exclusion of vascular rings
  - Inspiratory and expiratory scans helpful if tracheomalacia suspected

DIFFERENTIAL DIAGNOSIS

Subglottic Infantile Hemangioma

- Intensely enhancing submucosal mass internal to cricoid ring
- Circumferential or eccentric
- Symptomatic in infancy with proliferative growth phase

Vascular Rings and Slings

- Vascular rings, pulmonary sling, or innominate artery compression of trachea
- CECT, CTA, or MRA displays vascular anomaly

Congenital Subglottic-Tracheal Stenosis

- Complete tracheal ring(s); no membranous portion
- Trachea develops round contour on axial images
- May be associated with tracheoesophageal fistula

PATHOLOGY

General Features

- Etiology
  - Due to **intrinsic** or **extrinsic** pathology
  - **Intrinsic subglottic or cervical tracheal pathology**
    - Iatrogenic stenosis post tracheostomy or prolonged intubation
      - Most common cause of acquired stenosis **(90%)**
      - Pressure/ischemic necrosis of mucosa and underlying tracheal wall by balloon or tube
    - Laryngeal trauma
      - Acute fracture of cricoid with hematoma
      - Cricoid fracture may heal with distorted contour, fibrosis
    - Laryngeal SCCa
      - Subglottic primary SCCa or transglottic tumor
    - Granulomatous diseases
      - Sarcoidosis, GPA
    - Cartilage or mucosal inflammatory diseases
      - SLE, RP, amyloid
      - Inflammation, fibrosis, ± calcifications
      - Characteristic sparing of posterior membranous tracheal wall in RP
    - Tracheopathia osteochondroplastica
    - Idiopathic
  - **Extrinsic compression or invasion of subglottis/cervical trachea**
    - Thyroid pathology
      - Multinodular goiter compresses or displaces airway

□ Differentiated or anaplastic thyroid carcinoma invades airway

□ Thyroid NHL more commonly compresses airway

– Neck adenopathy

□ Lymphoma or thyroid carcinoma lymph node compresses airway

Gross Pathologic & Surgical Features

- Intubation- or tracheostomy-related stenosis
  - Circumferential scarring with loss of integrity of tracheal cartilage rings and dense fibrosis
  - Mucosal ulceration

Microscopic Features

- Intubation- or tracheostomy-related stenosis
  - Destruction of cartilage rings with loss of type I collagen and aggrecan, dense fibrosis, plasma cell infiltrates
  - Calcification in cartilage rings, ± interruption of elastic fibers, loss of integrity of mucosal basal membrane
  - Hypertrophy of mucosal and submucosal layers, loss of ciliated mucosal epithelium

CLINICAL ISSUES

Presentation

- Most common signs/symptoms
  - Dyspnea, stridor
    - Typically several weeks post intubation
    - May be months to years later
  - 50% airway narrowing required to produce dyspnea on exertion
  - > 75% airway narrowing required before symptoms occur at rest
- Other signs/symptoms
  - Hemoptysis, wheezing, cough
  - Recurrent respiratory infections
- Clinical profile
  - Dyspnea and stridor arising in patient with history of intubation

Demographics

- Epidemiology
  - Post intubation, up to 20% incidence
    - Risk of stenosis declines with softer, more compliant, and low-pressure intubation balloons
  - Post tracheostomy, up to 20% incidence
    - Risk of stenosis declines with good tracheostomy hygiene and frequent tube changes

Natural History & Prognosis

- Depends largely on cause of stenosis
  - Iatrogenic stenosis may slowly progress
  - Multinodular goiter causes slow, gradual stenosis
    - Often minimal airway symptoms
  - Thyroid carcinoma and NHL are rapidly enlarging tumors
    - Secure airway is 1st priority

Treatment

- Endoscopic treatment options (short-segment, soft/mucosal stenosis)
  - For short-segment, mucosal stenosis
  - Balloon dilatation

- Stenting
- Laser resection
- Open surgery options (cartilaginous or framework stenosis, scarring)
  - Resection of stenotic segment with reanastomosis
  - Slide tracheoplasty
  - Cartilage grafts
- Endoscopic treatment has lower morbidity but may require multiple sessions
- Lesions involving subglottic larynx more difficult to treat than pure tracheal lesions
- Longer and multiple stenoses more difficult to treat

DIAGNOSTIC CHECKLIST

Consider

- Most common cause is iatrogenic, prior subglottic/tracheal injury
- Extrinsic masses most commonly thyroid or nodal

Image Interpretation Pearls

- For intrinsic subglottic/tracheal pathology
  - Evaluate degree and length of stenosis
  - Evaluate for cartilaginous deformity
  - 2D and 3D reconstructed images may help define extent and degree of stenosis
- If tracheal invasion, measure length of airway involvement
  - Determine whether cricoid cartilage involved

SELECTED REFERENCES

1. Crane J et al: Tracheal resection for post-intubation/post-tracheostomy tracheal stenosis. Thorac Surg Clin. 35(1):61-72, 2025
2. Perryman MC et al: Laryngotracheal reconstruction for subglottic and tracheal stenosis. Otolaryngol Clin North Am. 56(4):769-78, 2023
3. Catano J et al: Presentation, diagnosis, and management of subglottic and tracheal stenosis during systemic inflammatory diseases. Chest. 161(1):257-65, 2022
4. Gelbard A et al: Comparative treatment outcomes for patients with idiopathic subglottic stenosis. JAMA Otolaryngol Head Neck Surg. 146(1):20-9, 2020
5. Yang MM et al: Subglottic stenosis position affects work of breathing. Laryngoscope. 131(4):E1220-6, 2020
6. D'Andrilli A et al: Subglottic tracheal stenosis. J Thorac Dis. 8(Suppl 2):S140-7, 2016
7. Young E et al: Tracheal stenosis following percutaneous dilatational tracheostomy using the single tapered dilator: an MRI study. Anaesth Intensive Care. 42(6):745-51, 2014
8. Melkane AE et al: Management of postintubation tracheal stenosis: appropriate indications make outcome differences. Respiration. 79(5):395-401, 2010
9. Herrington HC et al: Modern management of laryngotracheal stenosis. Laryngoscope. 116(9):1553-7, 2006
10. Berrocal T et al: Congenital anomalies of the tracheobronchial tree, lung, and mediastinum: embryology, radiology, and pathology. Radiographics. 24(1):e17, 2004
11. Grenier PA et al: Multidetector-row CT of the airways. Semin Roentgenol. 38(2):146-57, 2003
12. Wain JC: Postintubation tracheal stenosis. Chest Surg Clin N Am. 13(2):231-46, 2003
13. Hoppe H et al: Multidetector CT virtual bronchoscopy to grade tracheobronchial stenosis. AJR Am J Roentgenol. 178(5):1195-200, 2002
14. Prince JS et al: Nonneoplastic lesions of the tracheobronchial wall: radiologic findings with bronchoscopic correlation. Radiographics. 22 Spec No:S215-30, 2002
15. Rea F et al: Benign tracheal and laryngotracheal stenosis: surgical treatment and results. Eur J Cardiothorac Surg. 22(3):352-6, 2002
16. Gluecker T et al: 2D and 3D CT imaging correlated to rigid endoscopy in complex laryngo-tracheal stenoses. Eur Radiol. 11(1):50-4, 2001

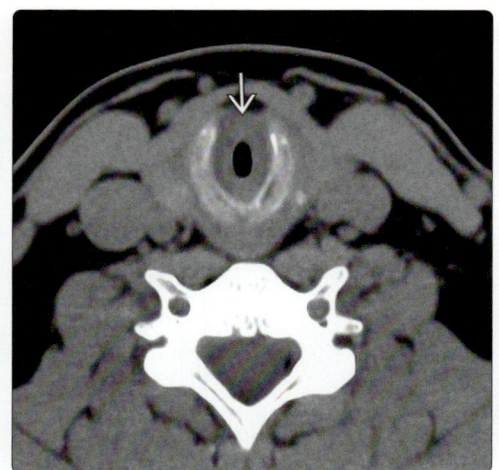
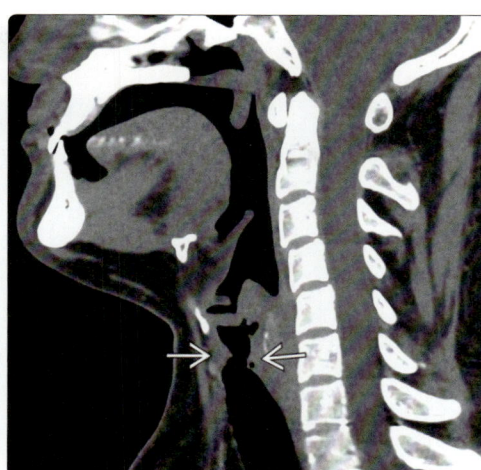

(Left) Axial NECT in a 24-year-old man with increasing shortness of breath with a previous Dx of granulomatosis with polyangiitis (GPA) shows circumferential soft tissue thickening ➡ in the subglottic airway without calcification. (Right) Sagittal NECT shows short-segment narrowing ➡. It is important to measure the length of the narrowed segment on sagittal imaging. GPA-related stenoses are mostly subglottic and circumferential. Relapsing polychondritis-related stenoses are mostly tracheal, anterior, and calcified.

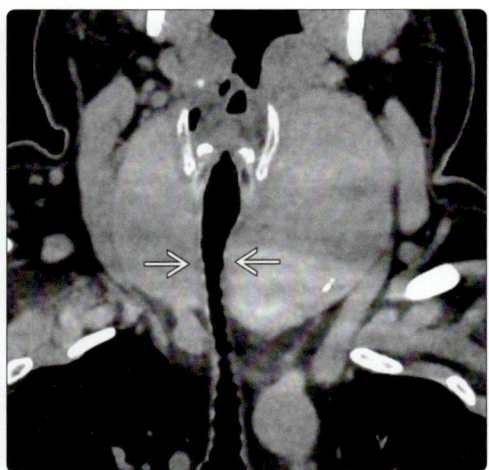
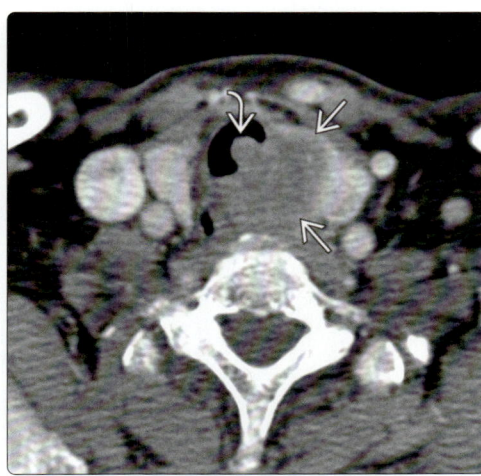

(Left) Coronal 3D rendering of a large thyroid multinodular goiter shows long-segment, smooth, side-to-side subglottic tracheal stenosis ➡ from extrinsic compression. (Right) Axial CECT in a patient presenting with shortness of breath and hoarseness shows homogeneous papillary carcinoma ➡ arising in the left thyroid and invading the cervical trachea. An intraluminal tumor nodule ➡ narrows the airway.

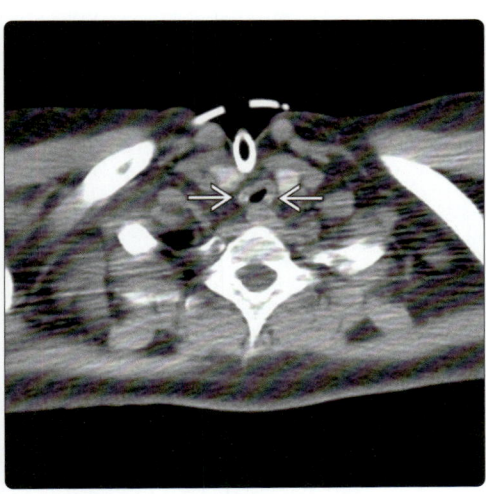
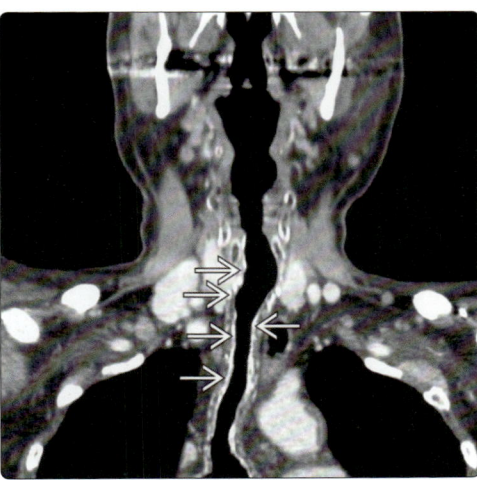

(Left) Axial NECT shows narrowing of the tracheal lumen with thickening and deformity of the tracheal wall ➡ in a patient with relapsing polychondritis. This finding involved most of the trachea. (Right) Coronal CECT curved 2D reconstruction shows irregular narrowing of the trachea with prominent submucosal calcified nodules ➡ due to tracheopathia osteochondroplastica.

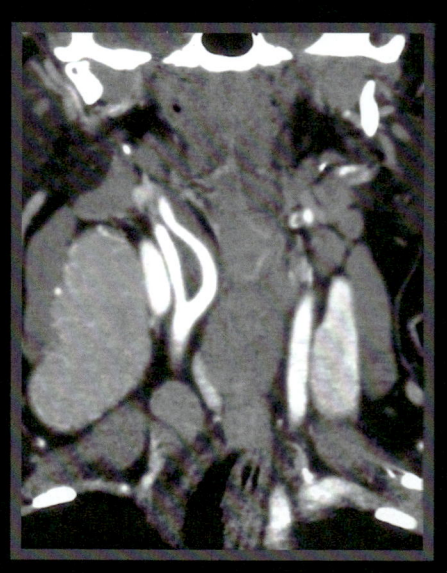
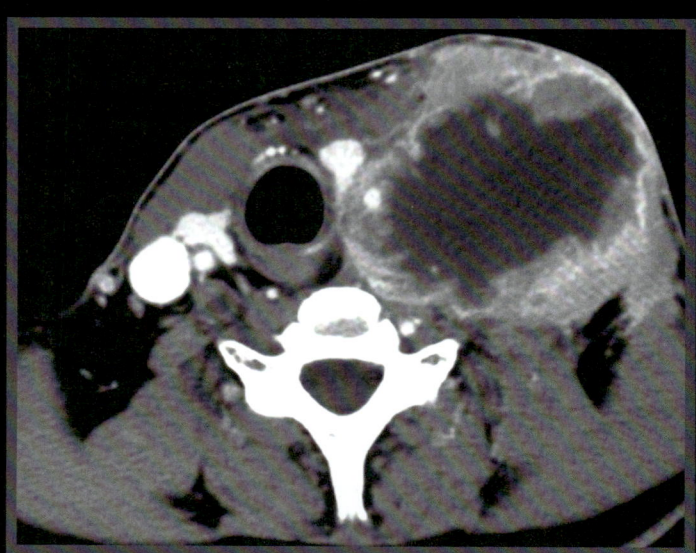
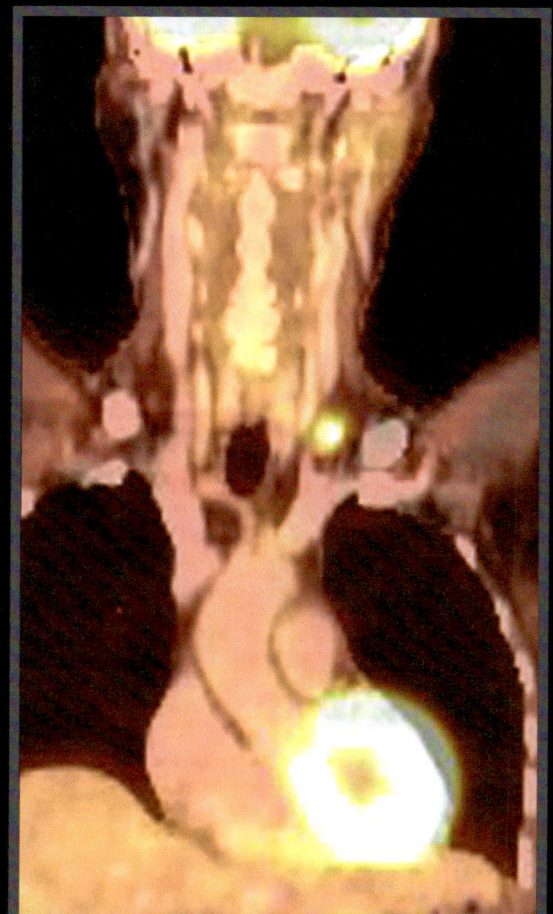
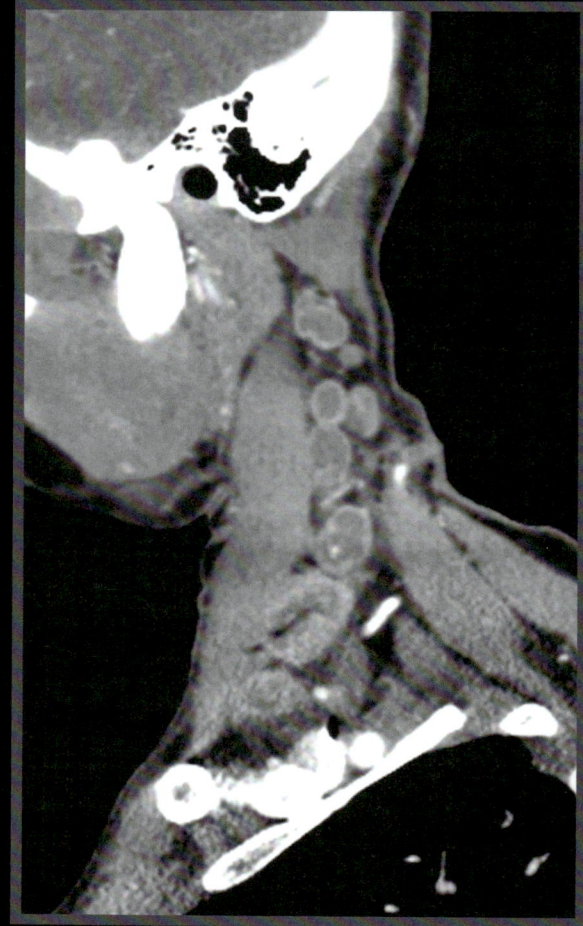

SECTION 12
Lymph Nodes

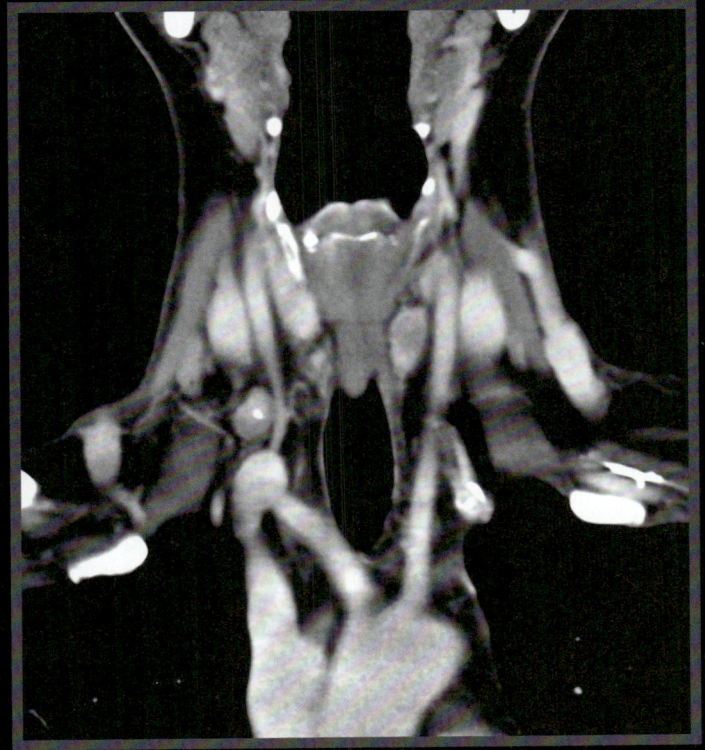

Summary Thoughts: Cervical Nodes

Cervical lymph nodes can be classified based on anatomic distribution or surgical levels used for neck dissection.

The key decision when assessing a lymph node is deciding whether it is **abnormal**. Traditionally, size criteria have been employed, but a multifactorial approach (size, homogeneity, morphology, enhancement, borders, and clustering) is more useful for predicting pathologic adenopathy.

If a lymph node appears abnormal, one must decide whether it harbors inflammation (reactive), pus (suppurative), or tumor [usually squamous cell carcinoma (SCCa)]. This distinction is often quite difficult, especially with uncommon inflammatory diseases.

It is important for radiologists to understand the typical patterns of nodal spread of disease. Particular attention must be paid to subclinical lymph nodes [e.g., retropharyngeal (RP)].

Imaging Anatomy

Anatomically, the cervical lymph nodes are organized into groups (submental, submandibular, parotid, facial, occipital, and RP) and chains (internal jugular, spinal accessory, transverse cervical, paratracheal, and external jugular).

- **Submental** group: Midline, between anterior bellies of digastric muscles
- **Submandibular** group: Anterior to posterior margin of submandibular gland, lateral to anterior belly of digastric
- **Parotid** group: Within parotid gland itself
- **Facial** group: Scattered across face (includes mandibular, buccal, infraorbital, malar, and retrozygomatic)
- **Occipital** group: Posterior and inferior to calvarium
- **RP** group: In RP space
- **Internal jugular** chain (IJC): Surrounding jugular vein from skull base to thoracic inlet
- **Spinal accessory** chain (SAC): Along course of CNXI across posterior cervical space of neck
- **Transverse cervical** chain (TCC): Along transverse cervical artery in supraclavicular fossa; connects inferior aspects of IJC and SAC
- **Paratracheal** (juxtavisceral) chain: Anterior (midline, overlying strap muscles) and lateral to trachea (tracheoesophageal groove)
- **External jugular** chain: Superficial to sternocleidomastoid (SCM)
- Major chains (IJC, SAC, TCC) form triangle of nodes in lateral neck

Surgically, the cervical lymph nodes are organized into **6 levels** (or zones) based on surgical landmarks. Radiologic landmarks are used to approximate the surgical boundaries on imaging.

- Level I: Submental (level Ia) and submandibular (level Ib) groups, located inferior to mandible; receives drainage from lips, floor of mouth, and oral tongue; drains into level II
- Level II: Upper portions of IJC (level IIa) and SAC (level IIb); anterior or deep to SCM, superior to **hyoid bone**; receives drainage from all nodal clusters and from pharynx; drains into level III
- Level III: Mid 1/3 of IJC; anterior or deep to SCM, inferior to hyoid but superior to bottom of **cricoid cartilage**; receives drainage from larynx and level II; drains into level IV

- Level IV: Bottom of IJC and medial 1/2 of TCC; anterior or deep to SCM, inferior to cricoid cartilage; receives drainage from level III, chest, and abdomen
- Level V: Bottom of SAC (level Va) and posterior 1/2 of TCC (level Vb); lies in posterior cervical space, strictly posterior to back edge of SCM; receives drainage from occipital, RP, periauricular, and parotid regions; drains into level IV and mediastinum
- Level VI: Paratracheal chain; superficial to strap muscles, between carotid arteries, and lateral to trachea in tracheoesophageal groove; receives drainage from visceral space (especially thyroid gland), drains into level IV, mediastinum
- In radiation oncology, "supraclavicular nodes" are considered distinct entity, but **in radiology scheme they are part of levels IV and V**

Many nodes found in anatomic classification scheme are not included in the surgical scheme because they are not included in routine neck dissections. These may be overlooked clinically and merit particular attention from radiologists.

- **RP nodes**, in particular, cannot be palpated or clinically visualized; thus, imaging is the primary means of detecting pathology; most commonly seen with nasopharynx, sinonasal tract, and thyroid cancer, RP node metastases can occur with oropharynx and hypopharynx cancer (particularly those involving the posterior wall) as well as esophageal carcinoma
- **Parotid nodes** receive drainage from periauricular region and scalp; most common tumors involved here are skin or external auditory canal (EAC) SCCa and melanoma
- **Facial and occipital** metastases are less frequent but still important when they occur

A few cervical lymph nodes have been singled out and named because of clinical importance or radiologic appearances.

- **Signal (Virchow) node**: Lowest node in IJC; if no primary tumor evident in neck, consider chest or abdomen source with metastasis via thoracic duct; left > right
- **Rouvière node**: Highest node in RP group; lies within 2 cm of skull base; site of spread for nasopharyngeal carcinoma, olfactory neuroblastoma
- **Jugulodigastric (sentinel) node**: Lies within IJC just above hyoid bone; larger than surrounding nodes

Imaging Techniques and Indications

CECT is the 1st-line imaging modality to evaluate an adult with a neck mass of uncertain etiology. In children, US or MR should be considered first to minimize ionizing radiation. If the mass turns out to be metastatic, CECT usually can identify the primary site of origin. In the setting of a known malignancy, CECT or MR can be used to stage the nodes or to search for recurrence. However, whole-body FDG PET/CT or PET/MR are preferred modalities for oncologic imaging, particularly the assessment of metastatic disease of unknown primary.

Advanced imaging techniques, such as quantitative diffusion imaging (DWI), dynamic contrast-enhanced (DCE) MR perfusion, and dual-energy CT/spectral detector CT, show promise for improving the sensitivity and specificity of detecting nodal metastatic disease. While advanced imaging of cervical nodes has increased, reproducible diagnostic thresholds and imaging protocols are not well established. In current practice, these techniques may be complementary to routine imaging protocol but are still investigative.

Lymph Nodes Differential Diagnosis

Inflammatory	Infectious	Regional metastases
Reactive nodes	Viral upper respiratory infection	Squamous cell carcinoma
Castleman disease	Tuberculosis	Non-Hodgkin lymphoma
Kimura disease	Atypical *Mycobacterium* species	Melanoma
Kikuchi disease	Cat-scratch disease	Salivary neoplasms
Rosai-Dorfman disease	HIV adenopathy	Thyroid carcinoma
Inflammatory pseudotumor	**Malignant primary tumor**	Lung cancer
	Hodgkin lymphoma	
	Non-Hodgkin lymphoma	**Systemic metastases**

Approaches to Lymph Node Imaging Issues

Deciding whether a mass arises within a lymph node can be difficult in a few specific locations. In the submandibular space, nodal masses lie anterior to the facial vein, whereas glandular masses lie posterior to the vein. In the lower left neck, the signal node and the distal thoracic duct have a similar location, so a dilated thoracic duct may mimic an enlarged cystic/necrotic node. However, the duct is purely cystic and can be followed proximally into the superior mediastinum. In level II, 2nd branchial cleft anomalies and lymph nodes have a similar location, and metastatic disease from the oral cavity is often purely cystic. In adults, metastatic SCCa should be considered the diagnosis for a cystic mass in this location until proven otherwise. In children, this is typically a 2nd branchial cleft cyst.

Deciding whether a lymph node harbors malignancy is one of the most difficult (and important) issues in head and neck imaging. Traditionally, size criteria have been employed, but, when used in isolation, have poor accuracy. Furthermore, there is limited agreement on which axis of the node to measure and appropriate size thresholds. Instead, a multifactorial approach, including certain imaging findings, should be used to improve the accuracy. In isolation, none of these findings perfectly identify nodal metastases; thus, **all should be taken into consideration**. Also, pretest probability is critical: If a patient has known head and neck cancer, abnormalities of any of these features should be viewed with great suspicion!

- **Homogeneity**: Necrosis in untreated lymph node is highly suspicious for cancer; caveats: (1) Do not mistake normal fatty hilum for necrosis, (2) suppurative nodes can mimic necrotic nodal metastases
- **Morphology**: Normal nodes are reniform (i.e., kidney-shaped) with central hilum containing fat and vessels; malignant nodes are ovoid, round, or show focal cortical expansion
- **Enhancement**: Node that enhances more **or** less than its counterparts is worrisome
- **Borders**: Irregular borders with infiltration of surrounding fat are indicative of cancer and suspicious for **extracapsular spread**

Understanding the usual **patterns of lymphatic spread** from various primary sites is critical for several reasons: (1) Particular attention can be given to areas of likely spread (e.g., RP space nodes in nasopharyngeal carcinoma or lower cervical nodes in lung cancer), (2) equivocal lymph nodes that are outside the usual pattern are less suspicious, (3) likely locations of the primary tumor can be suspected in patients presenting with a nodal mass, and (4) nodal disease outside the usual pattern can prompt a search for a 2nd primary.

The enhancement pattern of a lymph node can help to predict the site of origin. **Necrotic nodes** with a thick, enhancing wall are most likely secondary to tonsillar or tongue base SCCa. **Cystic nodes** with imperceptible walls are associated with papillary thyroid carcinoma. Large, uniformly enhancing nodes are suggestive of lymphoma. Additionally, nodal **microcalcifications** or intrinsic **bright T1 signal** are suspicious for differentiated thyroid carcinoma, often showing a similar appearance to the primary thyroid malignancy.

While lymph node size threshold alone may have limited accuracy in predicting metastatic involvement, it is **not** to say that lymph nodes should **never** be measured. Rather, nodes should be measured judiciously. Measuring nodes is important for: (1) Cancer staging (AJCC instructs measuring nodes in **greatest diameter**, regardless of plane) and (2) assessing for interval change when monitoring treatment response. One must always keep in mind that reactive nodes are frequently enlarged, but not all metastatic lymph nodes are enlarged.

Clinical Implications

Carcinoma of unknown primary occurs when a patient presents with a metastatic SCCa, but a primary site is not identified on physical exam, panendoscopy, or conventional CT or MR imaging. SCCa does not arise within a lymph node; thus, a mucosal primary must be sought. FDG PET/CT and, more recently, PET/MR are helpful in identifying unknown primaries and are the standard of care in these cases. Blind biopsies of likely sites of origin may still be required.

Patients with enlarged upper neck nodes and enlargement of the Waldeyer lymphatic ring usually have an upper respiratory infection. Unfortunately, lymphoma and HIV adenopathy can have an identical appearance, so clinical or radiologic follow-up is needed to exclude these more troubling diseases.

The **signal (Virchow) node** has particular clinical significance. Although sometimes affected by metastatic disease from the neck or upper mediastinum, it may receive metastatic disease from abdominal primaries without intervening nodes in the chest (presumably via the thoracic duct). If a patient presents with a "signal node" metastasis, whole-body imaging is warranted to discover the primary tumor.

Selected References

1. Valizadeh P et al: Diagnostic accuracy of radiomics and artificial intelligence models in diagnosing lymph node metastasis in head and neck cancers: a systematic review and meta-analysis. Neuroradiology. 67(2):449-67, 2025

Lymph Node Overview

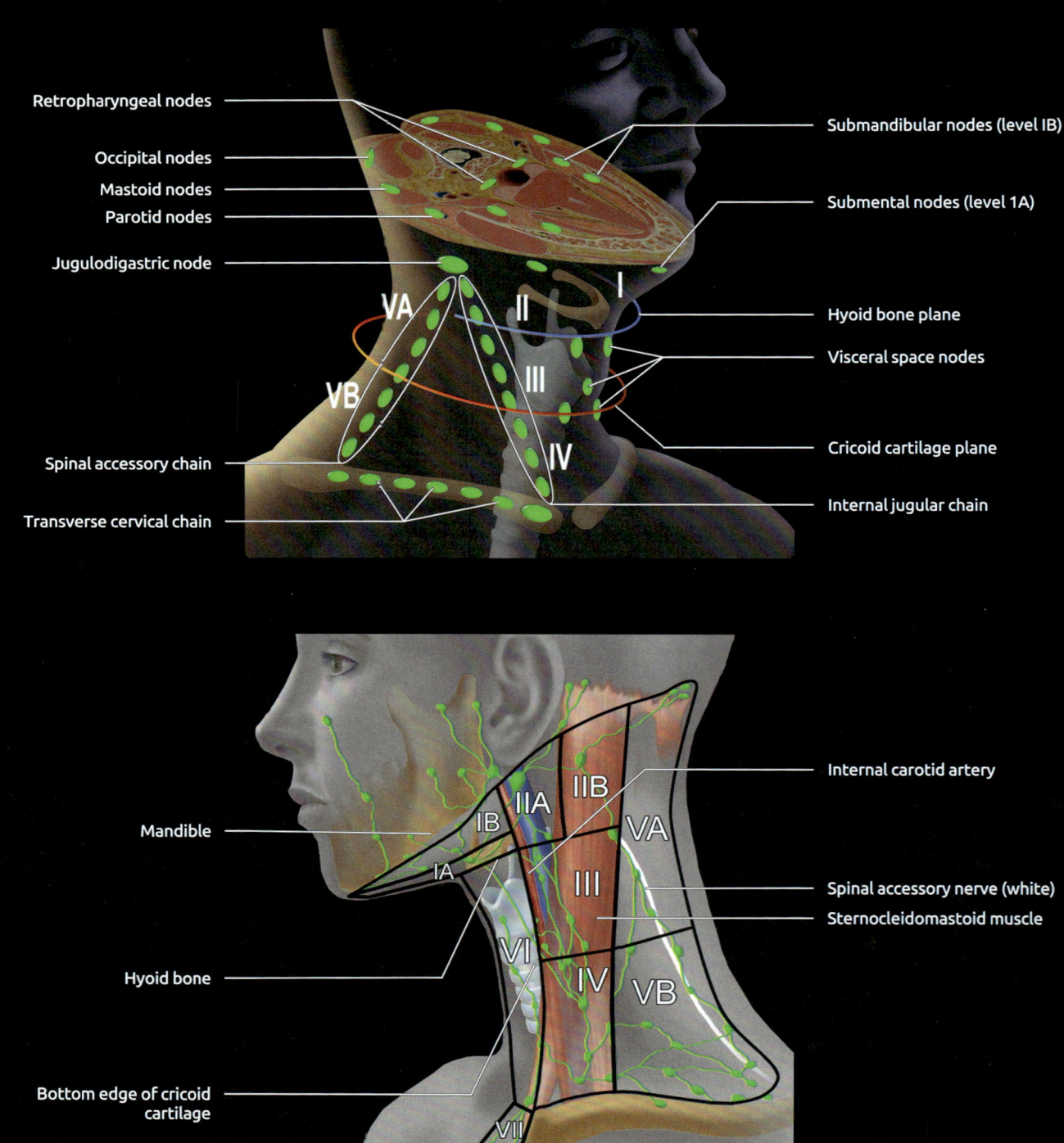

Retropharyngeal nodes

Occipital nodes

Mastoid nodes

Parotid nodes

Jugulodigastric node

Spinal accessory chain

Transverse cervical chain

Submandibular nodes (level IB)

Submental nodes (level 1A)

Hyoid bone plane

Visceral space nodes

Cricoid cartilage plane

Internal jugular chain

VA

VB

II

III

IV

I

Mandible

Hyoid bone

Bottom edge of cricoid
cartilage

Internal carotid artery

Spinal accessory nerve (white)

Sternocleidomastoid muscle

IIA

IIB

IB

VA

IA

III

VI

IV

VB

VII

(Top) *Lateral oblique graphic of the cervical neck depicts an axial slice through the suprahyoid neck. Note that the major node chains [internal jugular chain (IJC), spinal accessory chain (SAC), transverse cervical chain (TCC)] form a triangle in the lateral neck. The planes of the hyoid bone (blue arc) and cricoid cartilage (orange circle) divide the IJC and SAC into surgical levels.* **(Bottom)** *Lateral neck graphic shows the boundaries of the surgical levels. The chains and groups in this image are divided up not by their anatomic groups, as in the previous image, but by surgical landmarks. The hyoid bone separates level LA from level VI and level II from level III. The inferior margin of the cricoid cartilage separates level III from level IV and level VA from level VB. The posterior edge of the sternocleidomastoid muscle (SCM) separates levels II, III, and IV from level V. The carotid artery separates level VI from levels III and IV. The inferior margin of the mandible separates level Ib from the facial lymph nodes.*

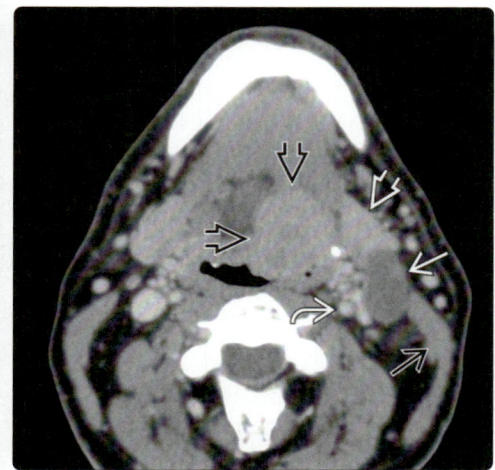
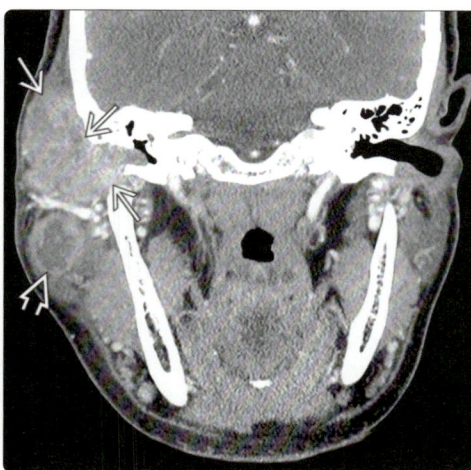

(Left) *Axial CECT in an older adult shows a cystic mass* ⇨ *between the submandibular gland* ⇨*, carotid space* ⇨*, and SCM* ⇨*. While that description fits a 2nd branchial cleft cyst in a younger patient, this is a cystic nodal metastasis from oropharynx squamous cell carcinoma (SCCa)* ⇨ *until proven otherwise in an adult!* (Right) *Coronal CECT shows a necrotic intraparotid lymph node* ⇨*. Intraparotid nodes are the 1st-order nodal drainage of the external ear, which in this case shows a large EAC and external ear SCCa* ⇨*.*

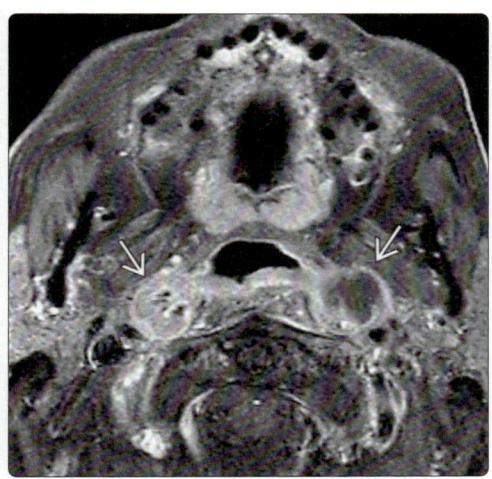
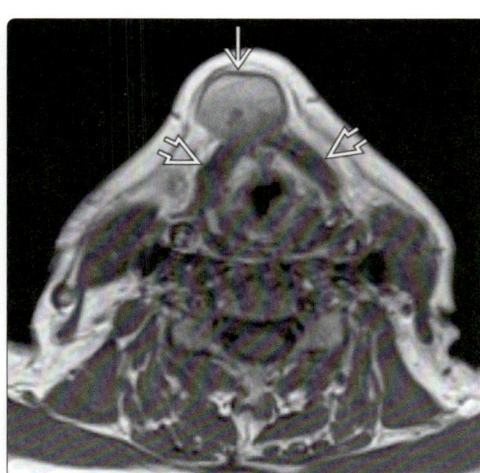

(Left) *Axial T1 C+ FS MR shows bilateral retropharyngeal lymph nodes* ⇨*. The lymph node on the left is cystic. CT-guided FNA revealed metastatic papillary thyroid carcinoma.* (Right) *Axial T1 MR in a patient with papillary thyroid carcinoma shows a large, cystic level VI lymph node* ⇨ *located superficial to the strap muscles* ⇨*. The node is heterogeneously T1 bright, a finding sometimes seen with differentiated thyroid carcinoma and indicating thyroid protein within the node.*

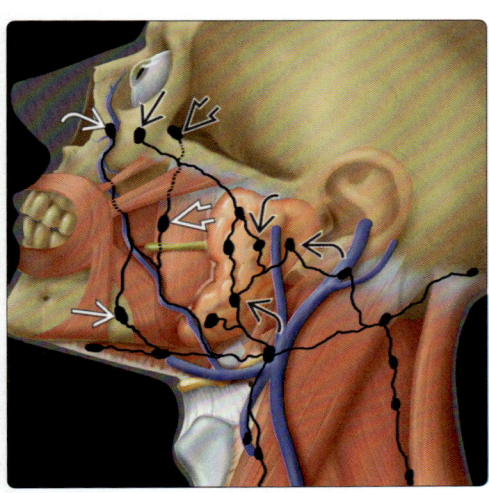
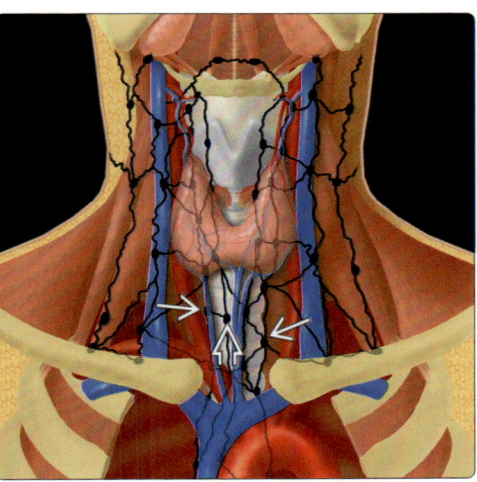

(Left) *Lateral graphic shows facial and parotid nodes. Anteriorly, note mandibular* ⇨ *and infraorbital nodes* ⇨*. The buccinator node* ⇨ *is along the anterior margin of the buccinator muscle. Malar node* ⇨ *and retrozygomatic node* ⇨ *are superior. Note multiple intraparotid nodes* ⇨*, the 1st-order drainage of the ear and portions of the face and scalp.* (Right) *Frontal graphic reveals nodal drainage of the anterior neck. The thyroid gland drains into visceral space nodes (level VI), known as the pretracheal* ⇨ *and paratracheal* ⇨ *nodes.*

TERMINOLOGY

- Reactive nodes: Benign, reversible enlargement of nodes in response to antigen stimulus

IMAGING

- Multiple well-defined, oval-shaped or reniform nodes
- Nodes of normal size or mildly enlarged
  - Size alone is poor predictor of benignity: Must consider **morphology & enhancement pattern**
  - Reactive nodes may be large (≥ 2 cm)
- CECT is 1st-line imaging modality
  - Enhancement minimal to mild, homogeneous
  - Linear enhancement within node is characteristic
- Hilar vascular pattern on US is predictive factor for benign adenopathy

TOP DIFFERENTIAL DIAGNOSES

- Squamous cell carcinoma nodal metastases
- Systemic nodal metastases
- Non-Hodgkin lymphoma nodes
- Tuberculous adenitis
- Sarcoid nodes

PATHOLOGY

- Node reaction seen as specific histologic patterns of hyperplasia: Follicular, sinus, diffuse, or mixed

CLINICAL ISSUES

- Common clinical problem in pediatric age group
- Less common in adults: Consider **malignancy** or **HIV**
- FNA cannot differentiate reactive nodes from lymphoma; consider core biopsy if necessary

DIAGNOSTIC CHECKLIST

- Reactive nodes typically oval-shaped or reniform, clustered
- Adjacent cellulitis suggests bacterial infection
- Focal nonenhancement suggests suppuration or necrosis
- Supraclavicular & posterior cervical location more concerning for malignancy

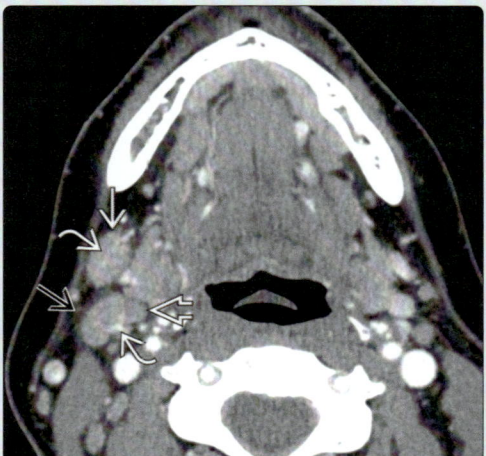
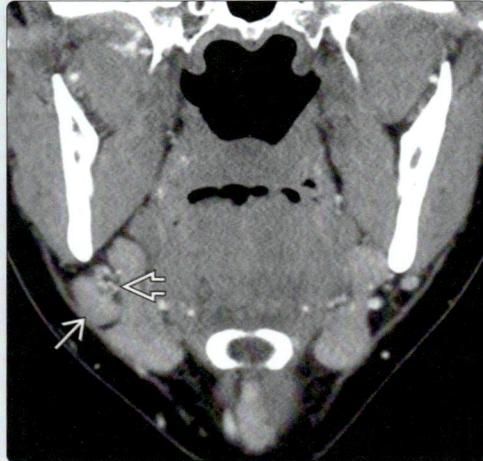

(Left) *Axial CECT in a patient with right preseptal cellulitis shows mildly enlarged, ovoid right level IB ➡ and II ➡ lymph nodes. Note the linear hilar vascular enhancement ➡ and surrounding mild edema ➡, consistent with reactive adenopathy.* (Right) *Coronal CECT in the same patient demonstrates a reniform (kidney-shaped) morphology of the reactive right level IB lymph node ➡. Note the mildly engorged nodal vascularity ➡.*

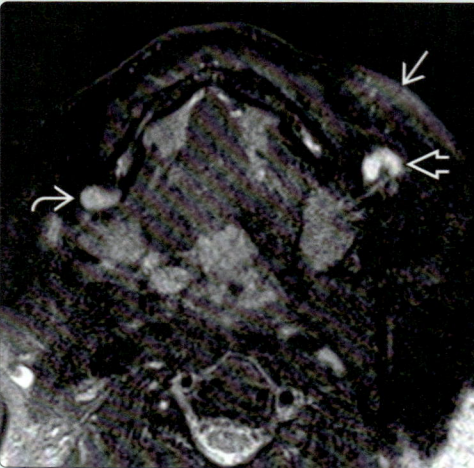
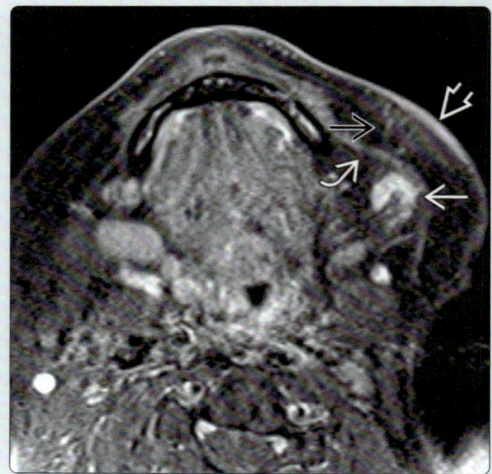

(Left) *Axial T2 FS MR in a patient with left facial cellulitis shows localized subcutaneous edema in the left cheek ➡. A reactive left level IB lymph node ➡ is mildly enlarged and slightly hyperintense compared to a contralateral level IB node ➡ but maintains a reniform morphology without necrosis.* (Right) *Axial T1 C+ FS MR in the same patient shows the reactive left IB node ➡ to be mildly hyperenhancing. Note a thickened platysma ➡ and overlying cellulitis with skin thickening ➡ and subcutaneous edema ➡.*

Reactive Lymph Nodes

TERMINOLOGY

Synonyms

- Reactive adenopathy, reactive lymphoid hyperplasia, nodal hyperplasia

Definitions

- Benign, reversible enlargement of nodes in response to antigen stimulus
  - May be acute or chronic, localized or generalized
- **"Reactive" implies benign etiology**

IMAGING

General Features

- Best diagnostic clue
  - Multiple well-defined, reniform (kidney-shaped) nodes, often with preserved fatty hilum
    - Nodes of normal size or mildly enlarged
- Location
  - Any of nodal groups of H&N
- Size
  - Wide size range
    - Adult: Often up to 1.5 cm
    - Child: Reactive node may be ≥ 2 cm
  - **Size alone is poor predictor of benignity vs. malignancy**
- Morphology
  - Reactive node is typically oval or reniform
    - Rounded morphology, cortical expansion, loss of fatty hilum are concerning for malignancy

CT Findings

- NECT
  - Homogeneous, well-defined nodes, isodense or hypodense to muscle
  - Stranding of adjacent fat frequently associated when acute infectious cause
- CECT
  - Enhancement minimal to mild, homogeneous
  - **Linear enhancement** within node **characteristic**
  - Hyperplasia of pharyngeal lymphoid tissue (Waldeyer ring) often associated, especially in younger patient
    - Caution: Pharyngeal lymphoid tissue may also be enlarged with lymphoid malignancy

MR Findings

- T1WI
  - Homogeneous low to intermediate signal intensity
- T2WI
  - Homogeneous intermediate to high signal intensity
  - Cystic change suggests suppuration vs. tumoral necrosis
- DWI
  - Benign nodes tend to have higher ADC values than neoplastic nodes
    - Optimal ADC thresholds remain undefined; variability between scanners, manufacturers, & field strengths
- T1WI C+
  - Variable enhancement, usually mild & homogeneous
  - **Linear central enhancement favors benign node**
  - Tonsillar enlargement (Waldeyer ring) may be found

Ultrasonographic Findings

- Reniform enlarged nodes (max short-axis diameter > 1cm), hypoechoic, visible hilum, & increased hilar vessels
- US elastography is promising tool for differentiating reactive nodes from metastatic adenopathy
  - Malignant nodes demonstrate higher stiffness than benign lymph nodes

Nuclear Medicine Findings

- PET
  - Mild FDG uptake may be seen
  - Marked uptake more likely with active granulomatous disease or tumor

Imaging Recommendations

- Best imaging tool
  - CECT is 1st-line tool for evaluation of adenopathy
    - Differentiates reactive from suppurative nodes & cellulitis from abscess
    - Allows determination of node extent & evaluation for potential malignant cause
- Protocol advice
  - Contrast enhancement important to detect cystic or suppurative intranodal change
  - Dual-energy CT/spectral detector CT may accentuate differences in nodal enhancement patterns between reactive vs. necrotic/metastatic adenopathy

DIFFERENTIAL DIAGNOSIS

Squamous Cell Carcinoma Nodal Metastases

- Enlarged, **round** node or cluster of nodes
- **Necrosis** suggests nonreactive, malignant node
- Primary pharyngeal lesion should be sought

Systemic Nodal Metastases

- Supraclavicular node suggests infraclavicular primary

Non-Hodgkin Lymphoma Nodes

- Multiple large nodes, usually nonnecrotic
- Enlargement of Waldeyer ring may be seen
- Homogeneous mild contrast enhancement

Tuberculous Adenitis

- Suppurative TB adenopathy in multiple neck nodes
- Rupture with adjacent phlegmon & fistula possible
- Positive chest x-ray common

Sarcoid Nodes

- Homogeneous, well-defined nodes, often > 2 cm
- Intraparotid nodes often involved
- Positive thoracic nodes common

PATHOLOGY

General Features

- Etiology
  - Response to infectious agent, chemical, drug, recent vaccination (including COVID-19), or foreign antigen
    - Includes viruses, bacteria, parasites, & fungi
- Associated abnormalities
  - Hyperplasia of pharyngeal lymphoid tissue (Waldeyer ring) often with viral infections

○ Inflammation of same lymphoid tissue (e.g., tonsillitis) may be cause of adenopathy
○ Associated findings may suggest causative agent
  – **Stranding** of adjacent fat common with bacteria, rare with atypical mycobacteria
  – **Generalized adenopathy** suggests viral infection, collagen vascular disease, or malignancy
  – Parotid lymphoepithelial lesions ± adenoidal hypertrophy suggests **HIV adenopathy**
  – Parotid adenopathy frequently seen with **sarcoid**

Gross Pathologic & Surgical Features
- Firm, rubbery, mobile, enlarged nodes

Microscopic Features
- Node reaction with different histologic patterns of **hyperplasia**
  ○ **Follicular**: Follicles increase in size & number
    – e.g., idiopathic, HIV adenopathy, RA
  ○ **Sinus**: Sinuses enlarge & fill with histiocytes
    – e.g., sinus histiocytosis
  ○ **Diffuse**: Node infiltrated by sheets of cells
    – e.g., viral adenitis
  ○ **Mixed**: Combination of follicular, sinus, & diffuse
    – e.g., TB, cat-scratch disease
- Culture or staining may reveal infectious agent
- Granulomatous pattern shows histiocyte aggregation ± necrotic material
  ○ Response to irritant that histiocytes cannot digest or T-cell-mediated immune response
  ○ Mycobacteria: Acid-fast bacilli with Ziehl Neelsen stain in 25-56%
  ○ Cat-scratch disease: *Bartonella henselae* or *Bartonella quintana*
  ○ Sarcoid: Nonnecrotizing granulomas
  ○ Sarcoid-like: Epithelioid cell granulomas in reaction to tumors
    – Mimic metastases at diagnosis, during treatment, or after treatment completed

CLINICAL ISSUES

Presentation
- Most common signs/symptoms
  ○ Firm, sometimes fluctuant, freely mobile, subcutaneous nodal masses
  ○ Other signs/symptoms
    – Bacterial adenitis & cat-scratch disease usually painful
    – Nontuberculous mycobacteria usually nontender
- Clinical profile
  ○ Child or young adult with nodal enlargement
  ○ Patient with known primary neoplasm may have borderline-sized nodes that are only reactive

Demographics
- Age
  ○ Any age, but most common in pediatric age group
    – Neonatal neck nodes not palpable
- Ethnicity
  ○ High incidence of *Mycobacterium tuberculosis* in developing countries
- Epidemiology

○ Common clinical problem in pediatric age group
  – Pediatric nodes not often imaged
  – Most children have lymphadenopathy at some time
  – Most adenopathy is result of infection, though organism may not be identified
○ Less common in adults
  – Most important differential considerations are malignancy or HIV infection

Natural History & Prognosis
- Bacterial infection, non-TB *Mycobacterium*, & cat-scratch disease frequently progress to necrotic nodes
- Chronic inflammation may result in fatty metaplasia
  ○ Low-density nodal hilus mimics necrosis

Treatment
- Many reactive nodes resolve spontaneously
- Antibiotics if bacterial cause suspected
- Nodal aspiration or biopsy may be necessary
  ○ Failed response to antibiotics
  ○ Rapid increase in nodal size
  ○ Systemic adenopathy or unexplained fever & weight loss
  ○ Features concerning for malignancy
    – Nodes feel hard &/or matted upon examination
    – Supraclavicular or posterior cervical node location
- If needle aspiration shows nonspecific reactive changes, follow clinically for 3-6 months
- Persistent adenopathy requires repeat needle aspiration to rule out lymphoma, metastasis, or TB

DIAGNOSTIC CHECKLIST

Consider
- Adjacent cellulitis suggests bacterial infection
- Always consider metastatic disease, non-Hodgkin lymphoma (NHL), & HIV in adult age group
- Certain locations should raise concern
  ○ Postauricular nodes in child > 2 years likely significant
  ○ Supraclavicular nodes are neoplastic in ~ 60%
  ○ Posterior cervical nodes suggest NHL, skin nodal metastases, or nasopharyngeal carcinoma
- Transient ipsilateral supraclavicular & axillary adenopathy from COVID-19 vaccine has been reported
  ○ Delay routine screening exams at least 6 weeks after final vaccine dose
  ○ Do **not** delay urgent or short-interval treatment monitoring imaging
  ○ Administer vaccine **contralateral** to primary malignancy with both doses to same arm

Image Interpretation Pearls
- Imaging findings often nonspecific with multiple, homogeneous, mildly enlarged or normal-sized nodes
- Oval-shaped nodes more likely benign & reactive
- Central linear vascular enhancement is characteristic
- Focal nonenhancement within node suggests suppuration or necrosis

SELECTED REFERENCES

1. Caliskan E et al: The diagnostic performance of magnetic resonance imaging in the categorization of pediatric neck lymph nodes: radiologic and pathologic correlations. J Pediatr Hematol Oncol. 46(4):188-96, 2024

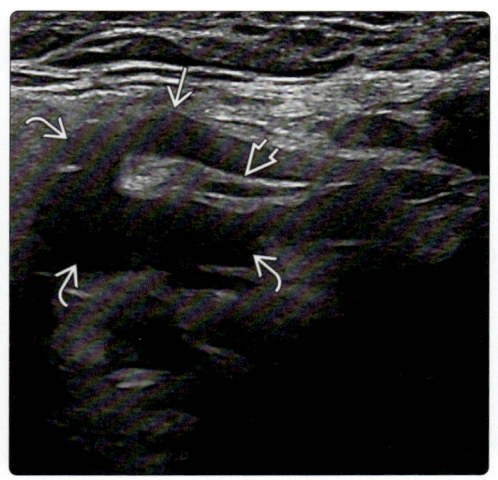

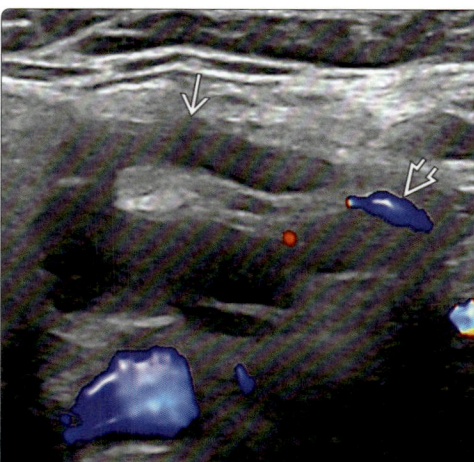

(Left) *Transverse grayscale ultrasound in a young patient with a palpable lump shows the typical appearance of a reactive level II lymph node ➡. Note the overall low internal echogenicity ➡ but preserved echogenic fatty hilum ➡ in this reniform node. Cervical lymph nodes are common in children & can measure more than 1cm along their short axis.* (Right) *Transverse color Doppler ultrasound of the same reactive level II lymph node ➡ shows characteristic vascularity ➡ at the echogenic fatty hilum.*

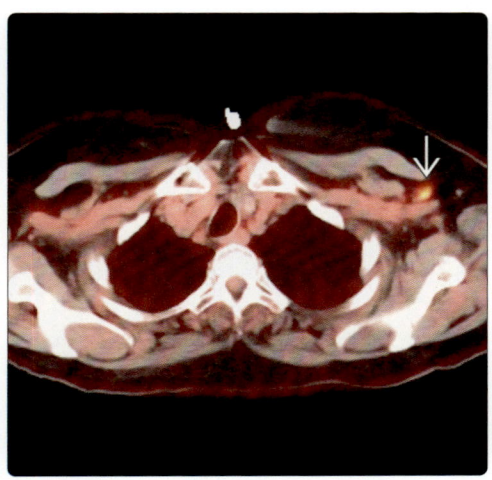

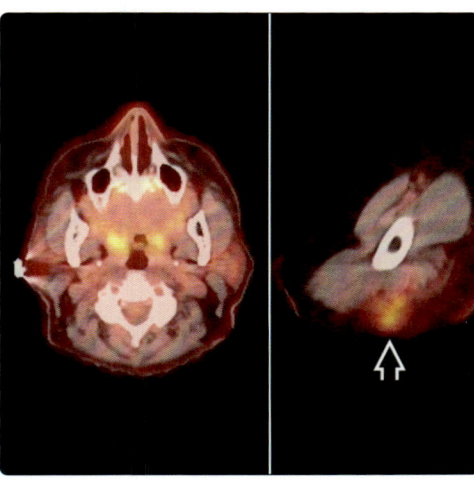

(Left) *Axial F18 FDG PET/CT demonstrates a nonenlarged but moderately FDG-avid left axillary lymph node ➡, which maintains a reniform morphology, suggesting reactive adenopathy.* (Right) *Axial fused F18 FDG PET/CT in the same patient shows an area of localized FDG uptake involving the left deltoid and overlying soft tissues ➡. Review of the medical record identified the culprit etiology: The patient received a COVID-19 vaccine in the preceding week, resulting in reactive adenopathy and local tissue uptake from inflammation.*

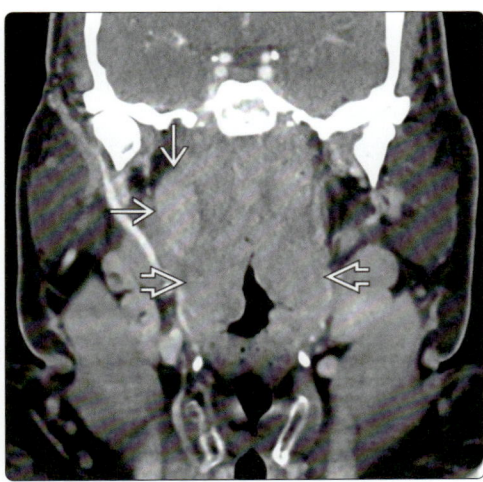

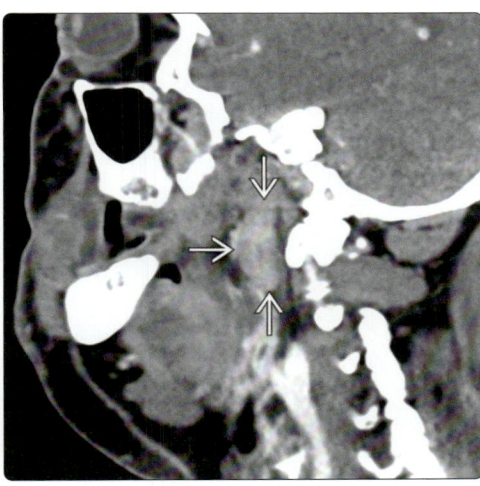

(Left) *Coronal CECT in a patient with nonsuppurative tonsillopharyngitis shows a reactive right retropharyngeal lymph node ➡, which is mildly hyperenhancing. Note hyperemic, enlarged palatine tonsils ➡ without abscess.* (Right) *Sagittal CECT in the same patient shows the 3-cm retropharyngeal lymph node ➡ maintains a reniform morphology without necrosis. While enlarged lymph nodes may indicate metastases, size alone is a poor predictor of malignancy in a lymph node. Morphology and enhancement must also be considered.*

TERMINOLOGY

- Adenitis, acute lymphadenitis, intranodal abscess
- Pus formation within nodes from bacterial infection

IMAGING

- Enlarged node with intranodal fluid and surrounding inflammation (cellulitis)
- Most often jugulodigastric, submandibular, retropharyngeal nodes
- Contrast should be administered to best appreciate extent of suppurative changes
- Consider CT- or US-guided aspiration for diagnosis and minimally invasive therapy

TOP DIFFERENTIAL DIAGNOSES

- Squamous cell carcinoma nodes
- 2nd branchial cleft anomaly
- Nontuberculosis *Mycobacterium* nodes
- Tuberculosis nodes

- Fatty nodal metaplasia

PATHOLOGY

- *Staphylococcus* and *Streptococcus* most frequent causative organisms
- Pediatric infections show clustering of organisms by age range
- Dental infections are typically polymicrobial and predominantly anaerobic

DIAGNOSTIC CHECKLIST

- If no significant cellulitic changes around node
  - In children, consider nontuberculosis mycobacteria
  - In adults, consider squamous cell carcinoma or thyroid carcinoma nodal metastases
- Look for primary infectious source on images
  - Pharyngitis, dental infection, salivary gland calculi
- With any neck infection, must evaluate for airway compromise, thrombophlebitis, and pseudoaneurysm

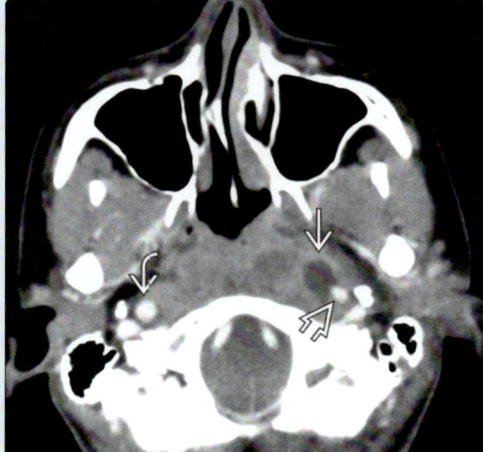
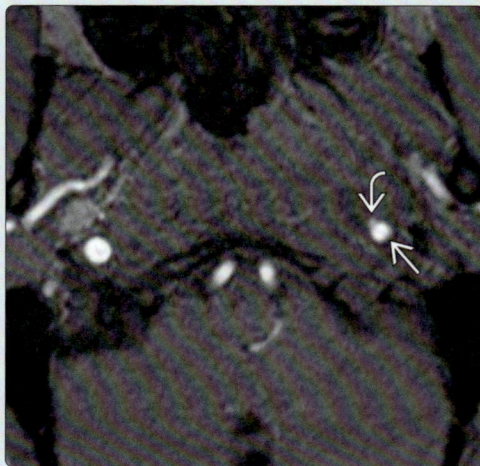

(Left) *Axial CECT in a teenager with neck pain and fever shows a suppurative left retropharyngeal (RP) lymph node* ➡, *which is distended with nonenhancing pus. Note asymmetric caliber and luminal irregularity of the adjacent internal carotid artery (ICA)* ➡ *compared to contralateral ICA* ➡. (Right) *Axial TOF MRA in the same patient shows maintained flow within the left ICA* ➡, *which is narrowed from vasospasm. Anteromedial outpouching of flow-related enhancement* ➡ *represents a small pseudoaneurysm.*

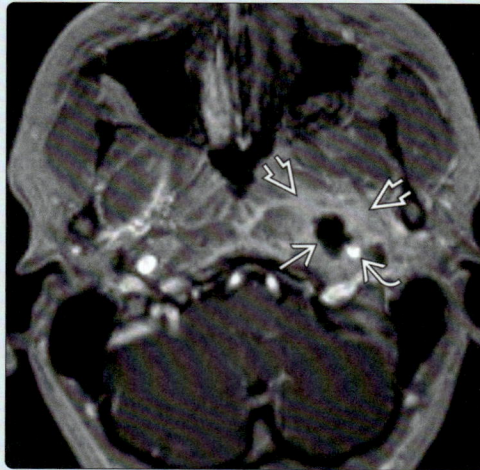
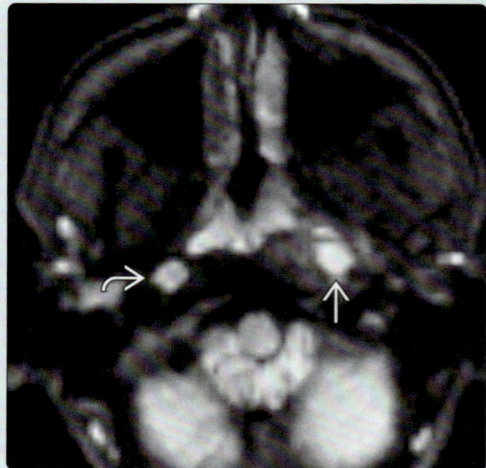

(Left) *Axial T1 C+ SPGR MR in the same patient shows the centrally nonenhancing, suppurative RP node* ➡ *and adjacent phlegmon* ➡. *Left ICA* ➡ *is narrowed and irregular from vasospasm, an important, but usually transient, complication of suppurative RP adenopathy.* (Right) *Axial DWI MR in same patient shows brighter DWI trace signal in suppurative left RP node* ➡ *compared to reactive right RP node* ➡. *ADC map demonstrated matched hypointensity in suppurative node, confirming reduced diffusivity.*

Suppurative Lymph Nodes

TERMINOLOGY

Synonyms
- Adenitis, acute lymphadenitis, intranodal abscess

Definitions
- Pus formation within nodes from bacterial infection

IMAGING

General Features
- Best diagnostic clue
  - Enlarged node with intranodal fluid and surrounding inflammation (cellulitis)
- Location
  - Any of nodal groups of H&N
    - Most often: Jugulodigastric, submandibular, retropharyngeal
  - Unilateral or bilateral
- Size
  - Typically enlarged node or confluence of nodes
  - 1- to 4-cm range
- Morphology
  - Ovoid to round, large node with cystic changes
  - Often poorly defined margins
  - Additional solid or suppurative nodes typically present

CT Findings
- CECT
  - Enhancing nodal wall with central hypodensity/nonenhancement
  - Stranding/edema of adjacent fat and subcutaneous tissues
  - If progresses to abscess: Irregular, ill-defined, peripherally enhancing, low-density collection

MR Findings
- T1WI
  - Node with central low signal intensity
  - Surrounding fat has hazy, decreased signal intensity
- T2WI
  - Node with diffuse or central high signal intensity
  - Fat saturation best demonstrates surrounding hyperintense (edematous or phlegmonous) tissues
- DWI
  - Complementary to routine pulse sequences
  - Suppurative, necrotic nodes have reduced diffusivity (bright DWI trace signal, dark ADC signal)
  - May show higher DWI trace and lower ADC signal relative to metastatic necrotic nodes
    - Optimal ADC thresholds remain undefined
- T1WI C+
  - Marked peripheral enhancement with poorly defined margin
  - Absent central enhancement

Ultrasonographic Findings
- Central decreased echogenicity with increased through transmission
- Color Doppler shows increased peripheral vascularity
  - Very low resistance and pulsatility indices

Nuclear Medicine Findings
- PET
  - Node has increased FDG uptake
    - Larger suppurative nodes may show peripheral increased FDG uptake and central decreased FDG avidity (similar to cystic/necrotic lymph node metastases)

Imaging Recommendations
- Best imaging tool
  - CECT usually 1st-line imaging modality with neck infections
    - To determine site of infection and adenopathy
    - Localizing for aspiration or surgical planning
  - CECT has excellent spatial and contrast resolution
    - Allows determination of focal absence of enhancement, indicating pus
  - Carefully evaluate bone CT images
    - Exclude dental infection and salivary gland calculus disease as cause
- Protocol advice
  - Contrast should be administered to best appreciate extent of suppurative changes
  - Use fat saturation on T2WI and T1WI C+ to best appreciate extent of surrounding inflammation

DIFFERENTIAL DIAGNOSIS

Squamous Cell Carcinoma Nodes
- Usually painless, hard nodes; no hot overlying skin
- On imaging may have nodularity of enhancing wall
- Typically no adjacent inflammation unless extracapsular spread
- Primary tumor mass often evident

2nd Branchial Cleft Anomaly
- 2nd branchial cleft cyst mimics suppurative or metastatic level II node
- Solitary unilateral mass, posterior to submandibular gland
- No inflammation of surrounding tissues unless secondarily infected

Nontuberculosis *Mycobacterium* Lymph Nodes
- Asymmetric, enlarged nodes with adjacent, subcutaneous, necrotic, ring-enhancing masses
- Minimal or absent subcutaneous fat stranding
- Purified protein derivative (PPD) skin test weakly reactive in ~ 55%, interferon-γ release assay usually negative
- Pediatric age group; usually ≤ 5 years of age

Tuberculosis Lymph Nodes
- Painless, low jugular and posterior cervical low-density nodes
- Calcification may be present
- Strongly reactive tuberculosis (PPD) skin test, positive interferon-γ release assay
- Systemically unwell with pulmonary infection

Fatty Nodal Metaplasia
- Chronic inflammation results in fatty change of nodal hilus
- Fat density on CT; fat intensity on MR
- Well-defined node, no inflammatory change

PATHOLOGY

General Features

- Etiology
  - Primary H&N infection
    - Adjacent lymph nodes enlarge in reaction to pathogen: **Reactive nodes**
    - Intranodal exudate forms containing protein-rich fluid with dead neutrophils (pus): **Suppurative nodes**
    - If untreated or incorrectly treated, suppurative nodes rupture, then interstitial pus is walled-off by immune system: **Abscess** in soft tissues
  - Reactive nodes from viral pathogen may have 2° bacterial superinfection, creating suppurative nodes
- Associated abnormalities
  - Primary causes of H&N infection include pharyngitis, salivary gland ductal calculus, dental decay ± mandibular osteomyelitis

Gross Pathologic & Surgical Features

- Fluctuant neck mass with erythematous, warm skin
- Aspiration of pus is diagnostic

Microscopic Features

- Acute inflammatory cell infiltrate in necrotic background
  - Presence of neutrophils and macrophages
  - Negative staining for acid-fast bacilli
- *Staphylococcus* and *Streptococcus* most frequent organisms
  - Increasing incidence of MRSA
- Pediatric infections show clustering of organisms by age
  - Infants < 1 year: *S. aureus*, group B *Streptococcus*
  - Children 1-4 years: *S. aureus,* group A β-hemolytic *Streptococcus*, atypical mycobacteria
  - 5-15 years: Anaerobic bacteria, toxoplasmosis, cat-scratch disease, tuberculosis
- Dental infections: Typically polymicrobial; predominantly anaerobic organisms

CLINICAL ISSUES

Presentation

- Most common signs/symptoms
  - Painful neck mass(es)
    - Often reddened, hot overlying skin
  - Fever, poor oral intake
  - Elevated WBC and ESR
- Other signs/symptoms
  - Other symptoms referable to primary source of infection
    - Pharyngeal/laryngeal infection: May have drooling, respiratory distress
    - Peritonsillar infection: May have trismus
    - Retropharyngeal or paravertebral infection: May have neck stiffness
- Clinical profile
  - Young patient presents with acute/subacute onset of tender neck mass and fever

Demographics

- Age
  - Most commonly seen in pediatric and young adult population
  - Odontogenic neck infections: Adults > > children

Natural History & Prognosis

- Conglomeration of suppurative nodes or rupture of node results in abscess formation
  - Superficial neck abscesses: Anterior or posterior cervical space, submandibular space
  - Deep neck abscesses: Retropharyngeal or parapharyngeal space
- Deep space abscesses can rapidly progress with airway compromise

Treatment

- Antibiotics only for small suppurative nodes and primary infection
- Incision and drainage for large suppurative nodes, abscesses, or poor response to antibiotics
  - Role for CT and US-guided aspiration for minimally invasive management
- Nodes from atypical mycobacteria should be excised to prevent recurrence or fistula/sinus tract

DIAGNOSTIC CHECKLIST

Consider

- Pediatric patient
  - Consider nontuberculous mycobacterial adenitis if no significant inflammatory changes
- Adult patient
  - Consider metastatic squamous cell carcinoma or thyroid carcinoma with necrotic or cystic nodes
    - Especially if inflammatory history or signs are absent
  - Look for tooth infection ± mandibular osteomyelitis if no other cause

Image Interpretation Pearls

- Fatty metaplasia with chronic infection can mimic pus formation
  - Look for fat in node
  - No surrounding cellulitis present
- Look for primary infectious source on images
  - Pharyngitis, dental infection, salivary gland calculi
- Evaluate airway for compromise with any neck infection
  - Bigger problem in deep infections
- Evaluate vascular structures for thrombophlebitis

SELECTED REFERENCES

1. Loney EL: Non-traumatic head and neck emergencies. Br J Radiol. 97(1154):306-14, 2024
2. Shareef M et al: Critical infections in the head and neck: a pictorial review of acute presentations and complications. Neuroradiol J. 37(4):402-17, 2024
3. Singh S et al: Pediatric head and neck emergencies. Neuroradiology. 66(11):2053-70, 2024
4. Baba A et al: Advanced imaging of head and neck infections. J Neuroimaging. 33(4):477-92, 2023
5. O'Brien WT Sr: Common neck and otomastoid infections in children. Neuroimaging Clin N Am. 33(4):661-71, 2023
6. Stein JM et al: Imaging of head and neck infections. Neuroimaging Clin N Am. 33(1):185-206, 2023
7. Park JE et al: Cervical lymphadenopathy in children: a diagnostic tree analysis model based on ultrasonographic and clinical findings. Eur Radiol. 30(8):4475-85, 2020
8. Srivanitchapoom C et al: Suppurative cervical lymphadenitis in adult: an analysis of predictors for surgical drainage. Auris Nasus Larynx. 47(5):887-94, 2020
9. Kimia AA et al: Predictors of a drainable suppurative adenitis among children presenting with cervical adenopathy. Am J Emerg Med. 7(1):109-13, 2018

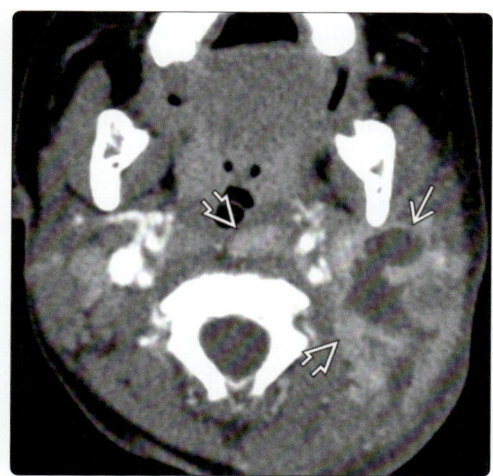

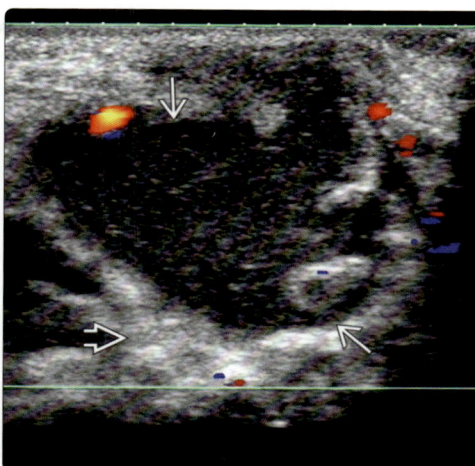

(Left) Axial CECT in a 23-month-old with fever and neck swelling shows an irregularly shaped, rim-enhancing abscess ➡ in the left neck, likely related to the intranodal origin of pus anteriorly, with posterior extranodal extension, cellulitis, and additional adenopathy ➡. (Right) Transverse Doppler US in a 6-year-old with fever and a tender neck mass shows an irregular, hypoechoic abscess ➡ with posterior acoustic enhancement ➡ and no internal vascularity. Swirling of debris upon compression can help confirm drainability.

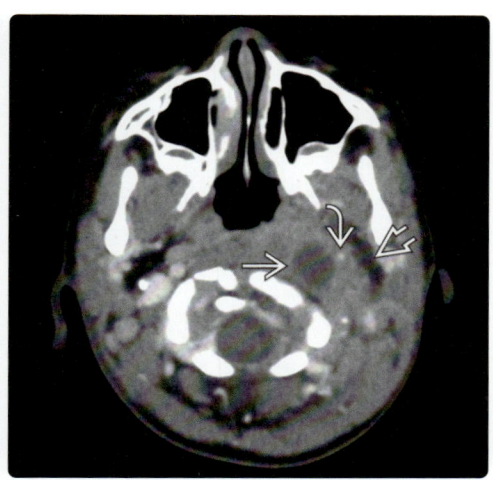

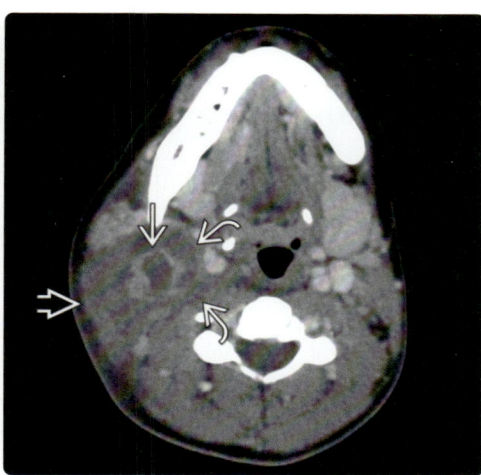

(Left) Axial CECT in a patient with suppurative left RP adenopathy shows an enlarged, centrally nonenhancing left RP node ➡ with edema in the displaced parapharyngeal fat ➡. Critically, do not overlook the small left ICA ➡ from vasospasm! (Right) Axial CECT in a child with suppurative adenopathy shows a peripherally enhancing, centrally necrotic right level II node ➡. Note marked surrounding edema/phlegmon ➡ as well as myositis of the sternocleidomastoid ➡.

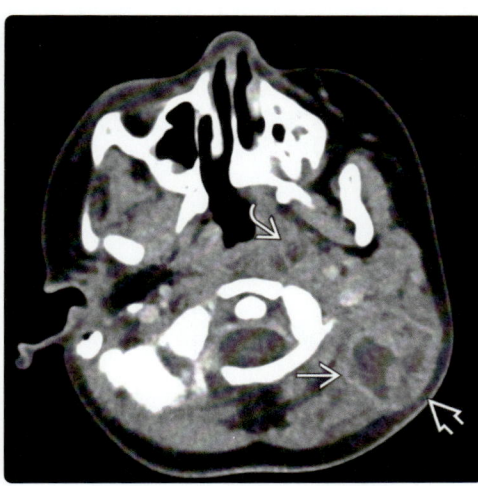

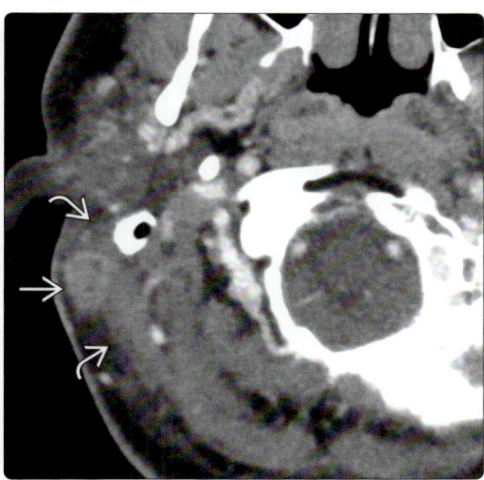

(Left) Axial CECT in a child with neck swelling shows a large suppurative node ➡ with characteristic peripheral enhancement and central nonenhancement. Overlying edema ➡ from cellulitis and a smaller suppurative RP node ➡ are seen. Suppurative nodes are frequently multiple. (Right) Axial CECT shows a suppurative postauricular node ➡. Surrounding edema ➡ is an important secondary sign, as a metastatic node may look similar. Absent extranodal extension of tumor, metastatic nodes rarely show adjacent stranding.

KEY FACTS

TERMINOLOGY

- Cervical adenopathy from *Mycobacterium tuberculosis*

IMAGING

- Conglomerate nodal mass most commonly with **thick**, enhancing rim and central necrosis
- Inflammatory changes often seen
- Obtain chest imaging (CXR vs. CT) if TB suspected
- MRI whole spine for suspected vertebral / spinal canal involvement

TOP DIFFERENTIAL DIAGNOSES

- Non-TB *Mycobacterium* nodes; cat-scratch disease
- Suppurative nodes
- Histiocytic necrotizing lymphadenitis (Kikuchi)

PATHOLOGY

- **Caseating granulomas**, smear for acid-fast bacilli
- Consider core biopsy for TB culture

CLINICAL ISSUES

- Cervical nodes #1 site of extrapulmonary TB adenopathy
- Most common cause of adenopathy worldwide
- Incidence in USA has decreased by 85% since 1990s
  - Vulnerable populations include HIV/AIDS patients, immunosuppressed patients, immigrants from countries with endemic TB, travel to endemic regions
- Systemically unwell patients with pulmonary disease
- 80-100% strongly **reactive skin test (PPD)**, interferon-γ release assay more sensitive
- PPD may be negative with immunodeficiency

DIAGNOSTIC CHECKLIST

- Consider when inflammatory changes associated with necrotic nodal masses
- Rim enhancement most commonly thick and irregular
- Must consider TB if patient is immunosuppressed
- Suspicion for TB warrants **immediate** call to ordering physician and care team

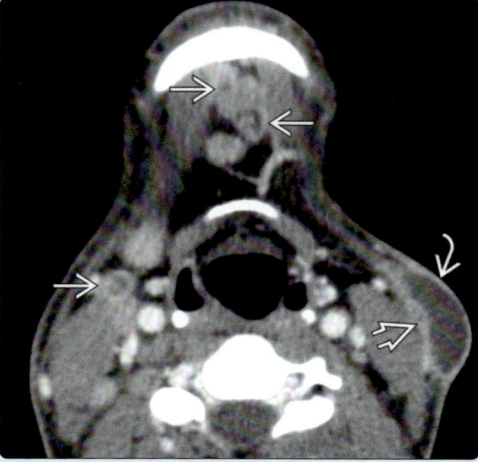
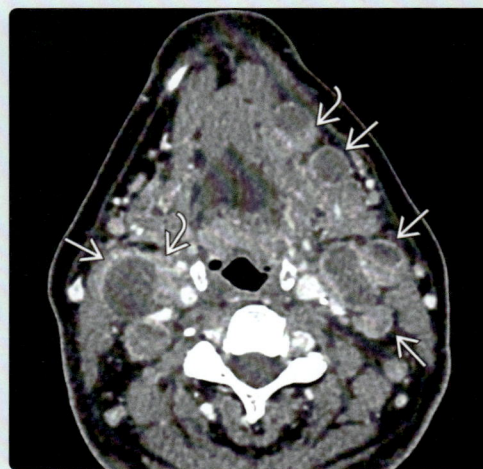

(Left) Axial CECT in a patient with tuberculous (TB) shows multiple abnormal cervical lymph nodes ➡, which are peripherally enhancing with central necrosis. Note the additional left neck subcutaneous mass ➡ with an irregular, enhancing rind ➡ in this patient with scrofuloderma (cutaneous TB). (Right) Axial CECT in a young patient with known pulmonary TB shows multiple bilateral, necrotic, peripherally enhancing lymph nodes ➡. Note extranodular inflammatory changes ➡ typically seen in TB.

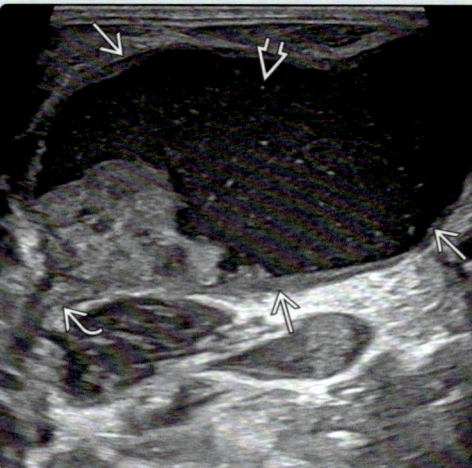
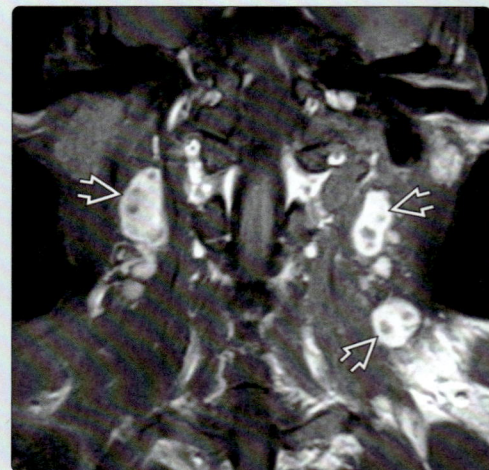

(Left) Transverse US in a patient with TB adenitis shows an enlarged, necrotic cervical lymph node ➡. Note multiple hyperechoic internal debris ➡ with extranodal inflammatory changes ➡ as well as posterior acoustic enhancement. (Right) Coronal T1WI C+ FS MR in a patient with TB adenitis shows markedly enhancing nodes ➡ bilaterally but no surrounding inflammation. Large nodes have focal areas of low signal intensity, representing caseation necrosis. Biopsy revealed granulomas and M. tuberculosis infection.

TERMINOLOGY

Abbreviations
- Tuberculous (TB) lymph nodes

Definitions
- Adenopathy due to *Mycobacterium tuberculosis* infection

IMAGING

General Features
- Best diagnostic clue
  - Most commonly **thick, rim-enhancing nodal mass** with central necrosis and inflammatory changes
- Location
  - Cervical nodes #1 site of extrapulmonary TB adenopathy
  - Cervical nodes ≈ 90% of H&N TB involvement

Imaging Recommendations
- Best imaging tool
  - CECT for nodal necrosis ± calcifications

CT Findings
- CECT
  - Node or nodal cluster with cystic changes
  - Rim enhancement typically **thick** and irregular
  - **Nodal calcification** may be evident
  - Adjacent inflammatory changes typical

MR Findings
- T1WI C+ FS
  - Centrally necrotic nodal mass or multiple nodes
  - Thick, irregularly enhancing nodal periphery

Ultrasonographic Findings
- Grayscale ultrasound
  - Cluster of predominantly hypoechoic nodes with adjacent inflammation

Nuclear Medicine Findings
- PET/CT
  - Increased FDG uptake in active disease; may be valuable for monitoring disease status in HIV patients

DIFFERENTIAL DIAGNOSIS

Nontuberculous *Mycobacterium* Nodes
- Systemically well child, usually < 5 yr
- Persistent preauricular or submandibular node(s)

Cat-Scratch Disease
- Reactive adenopathy in nodes draining skin lesion
- Occurs 1-2 weeks following scratch incident

Suppurative Lymph Nodes
- Typically stranding of fat and adjacent structures
- Systemically unwell with fever, painful mass

Histiocytic Necrotizing Lymphadenitis (Kikuchi)
- Typically Japanese young adults with self-limited fever, lymphadenopathy, rash
- Little or no nodal necrosis, marked perinodal inflammation

PATHOLOGY

General Features
- Etiology
  - Transmission by aerosolized droplets

Gross Pathologic & Surgical Features
- Nodes rubbery or firm and matted with induration of overlying skin
  - ~ 10% have fistula

Microscopic Features
- Caseating granulomas, smear for acid-fast bacilli (AFB)
- Gold standard: AFB culture with sensitivity
- Excisional biopsy more sensitive than fine-needle aspiration

CLINICAL ISSUES

Presentation
- Most common signs/symptoms
  - Painless enlargement of cervical node(s)
  - Systemically unwell with pulmonary disease
    - Fever, night sweats, weight loss, cough
- Other signs/symptoms
  - 80-100% strongly reactive tuberculin skin test with purified protein-derivative (PPD)
  - Interferon-γ release assays more sensitive than PPD

Demographics
- Age
  - Peak: 20-30 yr
- Sex
  - H&N TB has slight female predilection
- Epidemiology
  - Most common cause of adenopathy worldwide
    - 1.7 billion people have been infected with TB (23% of world's population)
  - 85% decreased incidence in USA since 1993
    - Vulnerable populations include: HIV/AIDS patients, immunosuppressed patients, immigrants from countries with endemic TB, those who travel internationally to endemic regions
  - Drug-resistant TB cases stable in USA for 20 years

Treatment
- Medical therapy with 4-drug regimen
- Surgery reserved for residual enlarged nodes, inadequate response to medical therapy

DIAGNOSTIC CHECKLIST

Consider
- Patients typically unwell, ± immunosuppressed, abnormal CXR, abnormal PPD or interferon-γ release assay

Image Interpretation Pearls
- Necrotic nodes most commonly with thick, irregular rim enhancement
- Associated inflammatory changes favor infection

SELECTED REFERENCES

1. Kaur J et al: Otorhinolaryngologic manifestations of tuberculosis: cureus. 16(7):e64586, 2024

TERMINOLOGY

- Nontuberculous *Mycobacterium* (NTM) nodes: Chronic neck infection with NTM
- Many species; commonly *Mycobacterium avium* complex

IMAGING

- Unilateral submandibular or preauricular painless mass in afebrile young child
- CXR: No pulmonary disease
- Ultrasound for neck mass evaluation and FNA
- CECT: Rim-enhancing, cystic-appearing node(s)
  - Minimal surrounding inflammatory changes

TOP DIFFERENTIAL DIAGNOSES

- Suppurative lymph nodes
- Tuberculosis lymph nodes
- Cat-scratch disease
- 2nd branchial cleft anomaly
- Nodal differentiated thyroid carcinoma (DTC)

PATHOLOGY

- Necrotizing granulomatous inflammation with acid-fast bacilli (Z-N stain)
- NTM creates fistula to skin surface if untreated

CLINICAL ISSUES

- Increasing incidence in immunosuppressed patients
- PPD test may be weakly reactive; **interferon-γ release assay usually negative** (may effectively rule out TB)
- Complete excision has > 90% success rate
  - Incision and drainage alone has 16-27% recurrence rate
- Adjuvant antimycobacterial drugs, especially if subtotal excision

DIAGNOSTIC CHECKLIST

- Consider NTM if
  - Cervical nodal mass unresponsive to standard treatment
  - Necrotic node with minimal surrounding inflammation
  - Afebrile child < 5 years with painless nodal mass

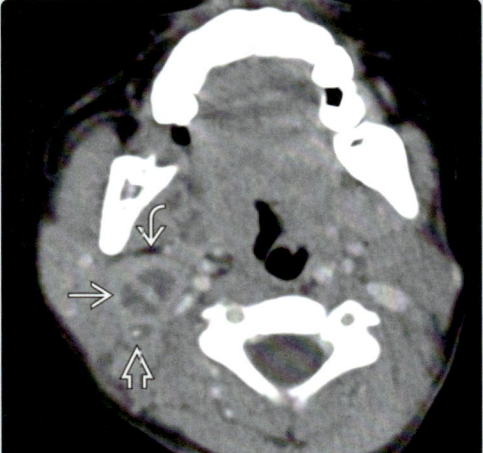
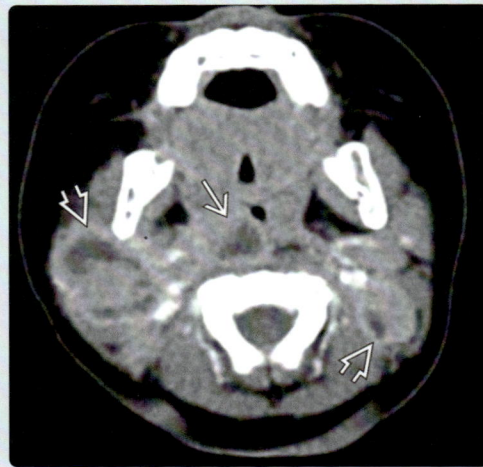

(Left) *Axial CECT in a child with several weeks of painless neck swelling shows a conglomerate of enlarged necrotic right level II lymph nodes ➡, 1 of which contains punctate calcification ⇨. Note a lack of surrounding edema with preserved fat planes ➡. Excision yielded Mycobacterium avium complex.* (Right) *Axial CECT in an afebrile 14-month-old shows right retropharyngeal ➡ and bilateral cervical ➡ necrotic lymph nodes without significant surrounding edema, typical of nontuberculous Mycobacterium (NTM).*

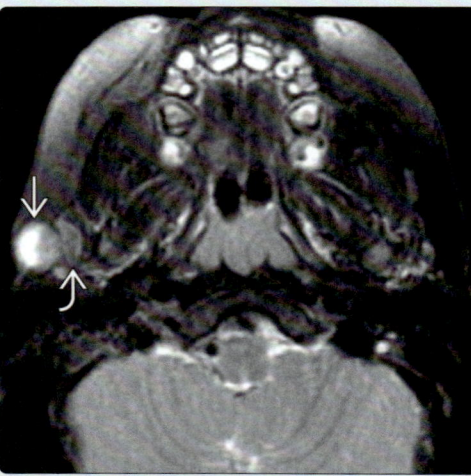
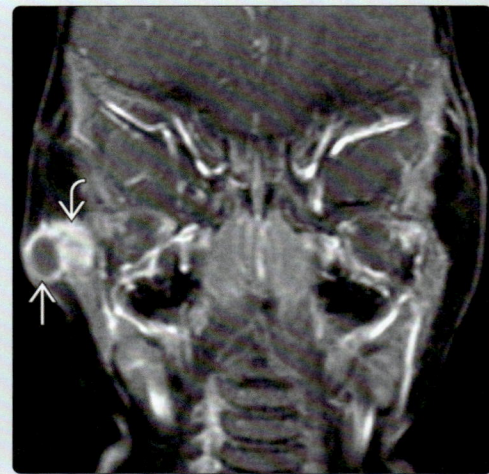

(Left) *Axial T2 FS MR in an 11-month-old with a right preauricular mass demonstrates a well-defined, predominantly hyperintense mass ➡ in the subcutaneous tissues of the right cheek, abutting the superficial lobe of the right parotid gland ➡.* (Right) *Coronal T1 C+ FS MR in the same child reveals the mass ➡ to be cystic/necrotic with peripheral enhancement. Note mild inflammation of the adjacent superficial parotid lobe ➡. FNA revealed M. avium complex.*

Sarcoidosis Lymph Nodes

TERMINOLOGY

- **Noncaseating granulomatous** inflammatory disease of unknown etiology

IMAGING

- Nonnecrotic, homogeneous, enlarged lymph nodes
  Nodal calcification may be present on CT
  Mild nodal enhancement with CT or MR
- PET/CT may be useful for assessing extent of systemic disease or determining site for biopsy
  - Can mimic malignancy due to FDG avidity
  DWI may be of some value in differentiating FDG-avid sarcoidosis nodes from malignancy
  - Typically higher ADC value than malignant nodes; **caution**: Appropriate thresholds not defined

TOP DIFFERENTIAL DIAGNOSES

- Reactive lymph nodes
- Non-Hodgkin lymphoma nodes

- Histiocytic necrotizing lymphadenitis (Kikuchi-Fujimoto)
- Kimura disease

PATHOLOGY

- Unknown cause; probably result of immune response to various environmental triggers

CLINICAL ISSUES

- Usually develops < 50 years, peak at 20-39 years
- F > M
- > 90% of patients have thoracic nodes, pulmonary, skin, ± ocular sarcoid
- Fatigue, night sweats, and weight loss are common

DIAGNOSTIC CHECKLIST

- Diagnosis of exclusion; may require US-guided biopsy
- Include in differential diagnosis when reactive or lymphoma-like nodes seen
- Occurs most frequently in posterior triangle/level V
- Search upper thorax on neck CT for pulmonary disease

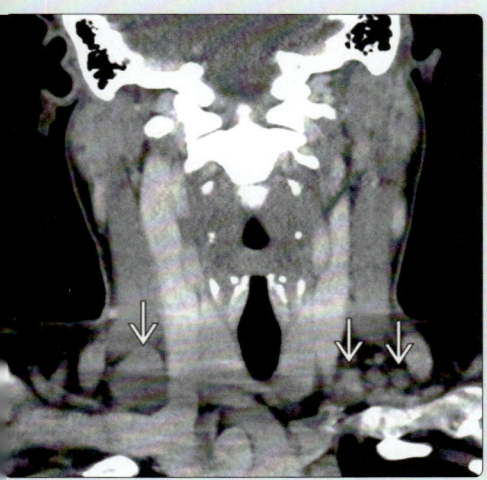
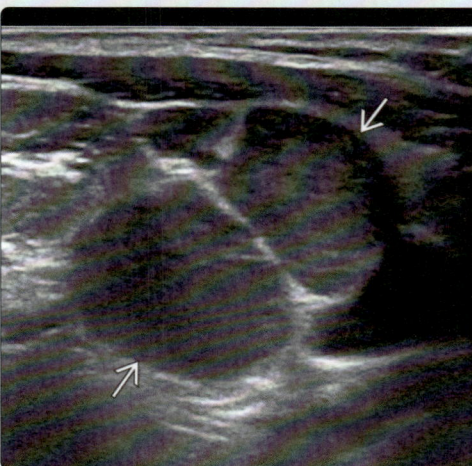

(Left) Coronal CECT in a young adult with palpable adenopathy and dyspnea shows multiple bilateral, ovoid, nonnecrotic supraclavicular lymph nodes ➡ that are asymmetrically enlarged on the right. (Right) Longitudinal grayscale US in the same patient reveals enlarged right supraclavicular lymph nodes ➡ with low internal echogenicity, suspicious for granulomatous disease or lymphoma. Biopsy revealed noncaseating granulomas, confirming the clinically suspected diagnosis of sarcoidosis.

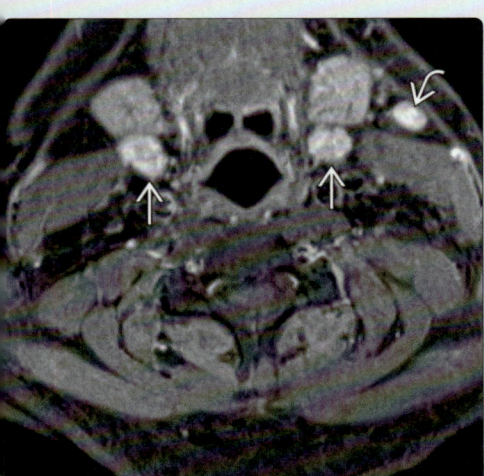
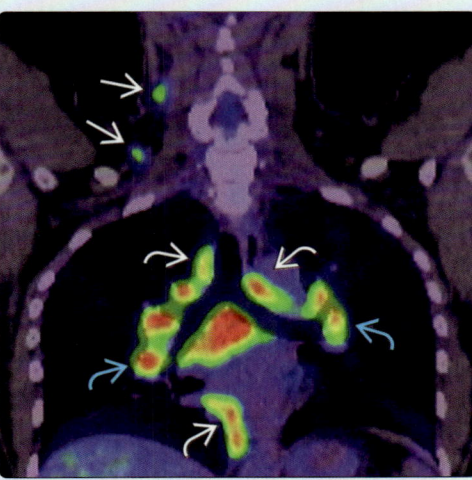

(Left) Axial T1 C+ FS MR shows the typical appearance of sarcoidosis lymph nodes ➡, which are ovoid, mildly enlarged, enhancing, and lack surrounding inflammation. Note hilar vascular enhancement ➡, commonly seen in reactive nodes. (Right) Coronal FDG PET/CT shows ↑ FDG uptake in right level V lymph nodes ➡ as well as FDG-avid bilateral mediastinal ➡ and hilar nodes ➡. US and CT performed prior to PET/CT reported normal-sized lymph nodes in the neck. Core biopsy of neck node confirmed sarcoidosis.

Giant Lymph Node Hyperplasia (Castleman Disease)

TERMINOLOGY

- Castleman disease (CD)
- Multicentric Castleman disease (MCD)
- Uncommon, benign idiopathic hypervascular polyclonal lymphoid hyperplasia
- Morphologic subtypes: **Unifocal** (90%) and **multicentric**
- Histopathogenetic subtypes
  - Hyaline vascular (90%)
  - Plasma cell (< 10%)
  - Human herpesvirus 8 (HHV-8) related
  - MCD not otherwise specified

IMAGING

- Most often mediastinum (70%), then head and neck (15%)
- > 90% of head and neck lesions are unifocal disease
- Moderate to markedly enhancing nodal mass
- CECT: Central **nonenhancing scar**; uncommon
- T2 MR: Hypointense **striations** described; uncommon
- Hypoechoic on US with intense peripheral vascular flow

- PET/CT: Extent and severity

TOP DIFFERENTIAL DIAGNOSES

- Non-Hodgkin lymphoma lymph nodes
- Reactive lymph nodes
- Differentiated thyroid carcinoma
- Carotid body paraganglioma

PATHOLOGY

- Unclear etiology, likely related to interleukin-6
- Most often unifocal, hyaline vascular type, asymptomatic
- Multifocal form rare, plasma cell type, symptomatic
- Diagnosis requires core biopsy or node excision

CLINICAL ISSUES

- Unifocal CD: Surgery curative
- MCD: Variable, aggressive course

DIAGNOSTIC CHECKLIST

- Strongly enhancing lymph nodes on CT and MR

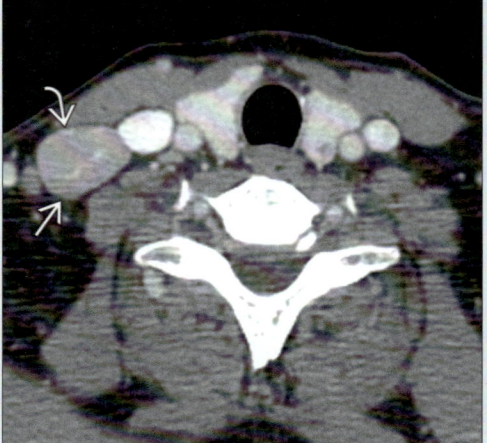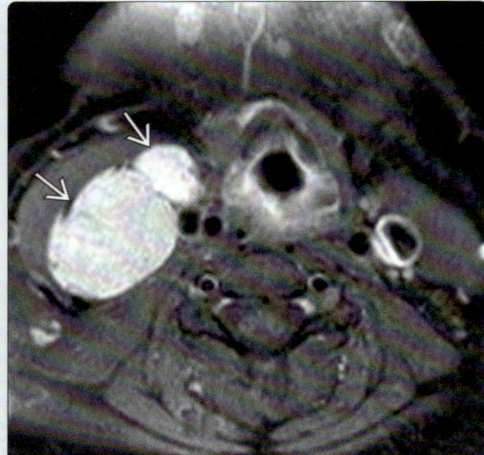

(Left) Axial CECT for a palpable neck mass shows a solitary, mildly enlarged lymph node ➡. There is homogeneous enhancement with associated prominent vessels ➡. This was a unifocal hyaline vascular variant of Castleman disease (CD), cured with surgical resection. (Right) Axial T1 C+ FS MR in a hyaline vascular type of CD reveals right internal jugular chain nodes ➡ with uniform enhancement. The more posterior node is markedly enlarged. There is no evidence of extracapsular spread or inflammation.

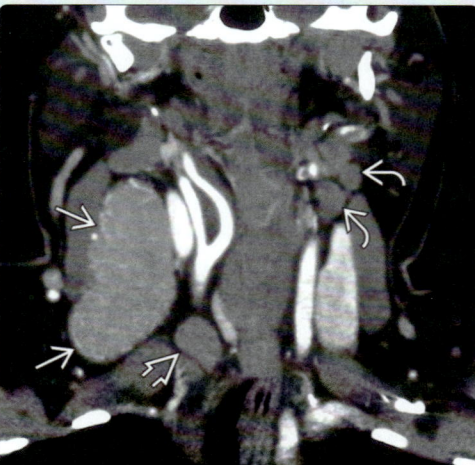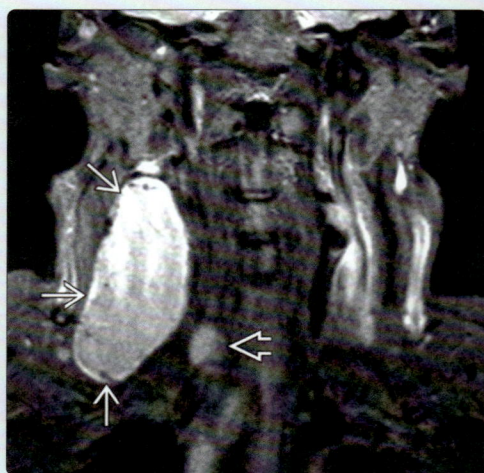

(Left) Coronally reformatted CECT shows a large, homogeneous, moderately enhancing node ➡ along the right internal jugular chain. Also seen are additional smaller, less enhancing nodes in low-level VI ➡ and along contralateral jugular chain ➡. (Right) Coronal T2 FS MR in the same patient shows a large node ➡ to be markedly homogeneously hyperintense with no intranodal necrosis or inflammatory changes surrounding node. A smaller, moderately hyperintense node ➡ is also evident.

TERMINOLOGY

Abbreviations

- Castleman disease (CD)

Synonyms

- Angiofollicular lymphoid hyperplasia, follicular lymphoreticuloma, angiomatous lymphoid hamartoma, lymph nodal hamartoma

Definitions

- Uncommon, benign hypervascular nonclonal lymphoproliferative disorder
  - Clinical subtypes: **Unifocal** and **multicentric** CD (MCD)
  - Histologic classification
    - Hyaline vascular (90%)
    - Plasma cell (< 10%)
    - Human herpesvirus 8 (HHV-8) related
    - MCD not otherwise specified

IMAGING

General Features

- Best diagnostic clue
  - Solitary, **moderate to markedly enhancing** nodal mass
- Location
  - Chest (70%), head and neck (15%), abdomen and pelvis (15%)
  - Single node or adjacent nodes (unifocal) or multiple nodal groups (multicentric)
    - > 90% head and neck lesions are **unifocal** disease
  - Rare extranodal neck locations reported
    - Parotid, submandibular gland, palate, larynx, parapharyngeal space, and floor of mouth
- Size
  - Variable: 5-10 cm
- Morphology
  - Ovoid neck mass

CT Findings

- NECT
  - Well-circumscribed, homogeneous oval mass, isodense to muscle
  - Calcifications uncommon in neck
- CECT
  - Moderate to marked homogeneous contrast enhancement
  - Prominent adjacent vessels are common
  - Central nonenhancing scar described, not often seen

MR Findings

- T1WI
  - Hypointense or isointense to muscle
- T2WI
  - Hyperintense, ovoid nodal mass or masses
  - Branching T2-hypointense **striations** described but not often found
- T1WI C+
  - Moderate to marked homogeneous contrast enhancement

Ultrasonographic Findings

- Grayscale ultrasound
  - Homogeneous hypoechoic mass
  - Posterior acoustic enhancement
- Color Doppler
  - Intense peripheral vascular flow, small scattered foci centrally

Nuclear Medicine Findings

- PET
  - Mild to moderate FDG uptake in unifocal CD
  - Higher FDG uptake in MCD

Imaging Recommendations

- Best imaging tool
  - CT usually initial modality for evaluation of neck mass
  - PET/CT helpful in evaluation of MCD
- Protocol advice
  - Contrast administration essential for CT
  - Evaluate MR carefully for striations on T2WI

DIFFERENTIAL DIAGNOSIS

Non-Hodgkin Lymphoma Nodes

- Usually multiple enlarged nodes, frequently bilateral
- Homogeneous, mild contrast enhancement

Reactive Lymph Nodes

- More often multiple moderate-sized nodes
- Variable enhancement, ± inflammation

Differentiated Thyroid Carcinoma

- May be enhancing nodal mass ± cystic change ± calcifications
- Primary intrathyroidal tumor may be small

Carotid Body Paraganglioma

- Splays internal and external carotid arteries
- CECT: Enhances to same degree as adjacent vessels
- T1WI MR: Flow voids present

PATHOLOGY

General Features

- Etiology
  - Poorly understood; likely exaggerated immune response similar to process with normal antigenic stimuli
  - Related to excessive interleukin-6 (IL-6) production
    - Inappropriate immune response to chronic antigenic stimulation or infectious agent
    - Induces vascular endothelial growth factor production
  - Multicentric form has been associated with HHV-8 and AIDS
    - HHV-8-infected cells secrete viral encoded IL-6
    - HIV infection enhances viral evasion of host immune system

Staging, Grading, & Classification

- Unifocal form most common, most often hyaline vascular histology
- Multifocal form rare, frequently plasma cell histology

Gross Pathologic & Surgical Features

- Smooth to nodular, well-circumscribed mass
- Firm, rubbery texture

Microscopic Features

- Diagnosis requires core biopsy or node excision
- **Hyaline vascular (90%)**
  - Most often unifocal and asymptomatic
  - Irregularly shaped, enlarged nodes with radially arranged capillaries penetrating germinal center
  - Interfollicular stroma with prominent hyalinized vascular network
- **Plasma cell (9%)**
  - Most often multicentric form
  - > 50% systemic symptoms and serologic abnormalities
  - Dense perisinusoidal and interfollicular plasmacytosis
  - Less prominent vascular network and less hyalinization
- Flow cytometry in both types shows polyclonal B-cell lymphocyte expansion

CLINICAL ISSUES

Presentation

- Most common signs/symptoms
  - Most often unifocal form, usually asymptomatic or palpable mass
  - Multicentric form ± plasma cell type frequently symptomatic
    - Fever, diaphoresis, fatigue, weight loss, and hepatosplenomegaly
  - Multicentric form ± plasma cell type often has abnormal serology
    - Anemia, hyperglobulinemia, polyclonal gammopathy, leukocytosis, plasmacytosis, hypoalbuminemia
    - Elevated or reduced platelet count
  - 50% plasma cell types have elevated ESR
- Clinical profile
  - Patients usually present with asymptomatic neck mass

Demographics

- Age
  - Occurs in all age groups, though head and neck disease rare in children
  - Peak incidence: 2nd to 4th decades
  - Older age for MCD: 5th and 6th decades
- Sex
  - M = F
- Epidemiology
  - Rare cause of neck mass
  - Usually unifocal form in neck
    - 98% are hyaline vascular type

Natural History & Prognosis

- Enlargement of masses may result in compression of adjacent structures
- **Unifocal: Benign** course, surgery curative
- **Multicentric**: Variable course, most poor prognosis
  - More rapid progression and poor outcomes in AIDS and HHV-8
  - Not uncommon for multicentric form to have malignant transformation

- Transform into non-Hodgkin lymphoma (10-15%) or Kaposi sarcoma (13%)
  - Thrombocytopenia, anasarca, fever, reticulin fibrosis, and organomegaly (TAFRO) syndrome is considered HHV-8 negative subtype of MCD
    - More aggressive clinical course

Treatment

- Unifocal form
  - Surgical excision treatment of choice
    - 100% cure with complete resection
    - Preoperative embolization can reduce blood loss and facilitate total excision
  - If unresectable, surgical debulking followed by systemic therapy
  - Limited indication for radiation therapy
- Multicentric form
  - Chemotherapy then steroids to prevent relapse
  - Radiotherapy for palliation of obstructive or compressive symptoms
  - Careful observation for recurrence and malignant transformation

DIAGNOSTIC CHECKLIST

Consider

- **Unifocal form** usually hyaline vascular, asymptomatic, and cured with excision
- **Multicentric form** usually plasma cell type, often symptomatic, and aggressive disease course
- Core biopsy or nodal excision required for diagnosis

Image Interpretation Pearls

- Consider with moderate to markedly enhancing mass along jugular nodal chain with prominent adjacent vessels
- Rare findings of focal, **nonenhancing scar** (CECT) or **hypointense striations** (T2 MR) suggest diagnosis
- Also consider when focal, possibly transspatial, large, moderate to markedly enhancing neck mass

SELECTED REFERENCES

1. Wang G et al: (18)F-FDG PET/CT metabolic parameters are correlated with clinical features and valuable in clinical stratification management in patients of Castleman disease. Cancer Imaging. 25(1):12, 2025
2. Hoshiai S et al: Imaging of unicentric hyaline-vascular variant of Castleman disease: emphasis on perilesional fat stranding and fatty proliferation. Glob Health Med. 6(6):375-82, 2024
3. Pelliccia S et al: The application of a multidisciplinary approach in the diagnosis of Castleman disease and Castleman-like lymphadenopathies: a 20-year retrospective analysis of clinical and pathological features. Br J Haematol. 204(2):534-47, 2024
4. Hoffmann C et al: Recent advances in Castleman disease. Oncol Res Treat. 45(11):693-704, 2022
5. Fujimoto S et al: Is TAFRO syndrome a subtype of idiopathic multicentric Castleman disease? Am J Hematol. 94(9):975-83, 2019
6. Zhao S et al: Imaging and clinical features of Castleman disease. Cancer Imaging. 19(1):53, 2019
7. Hill AJ et al: Multimodality imaging and clinical features in Castleman disease: single institute experience in 30 patients. Br J Radiol. 20140670, 2015
8. Jiang XH et al: Castleman disease of the neck: CT and MR imaging findings. Eur J Radiol. 83(11):2041-50, 2014
9. Chen YF et al: Clinical features and outcomes of head and neck castleman disease. J Oral Maxillofac Surg. 70(10):2466-79, 2012
10. Bonekamp D et al: Castleman disease: the great mimic. Radiographics. 31(6):1793-807, 2011

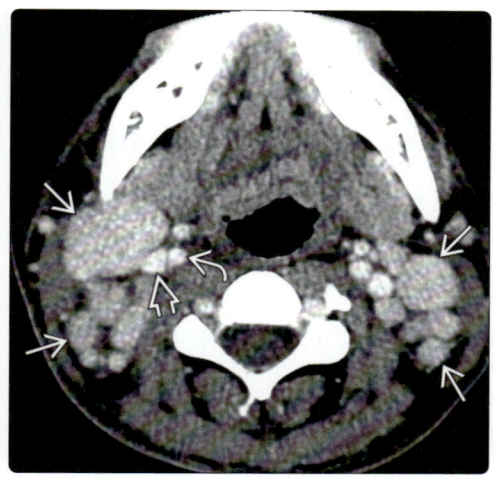

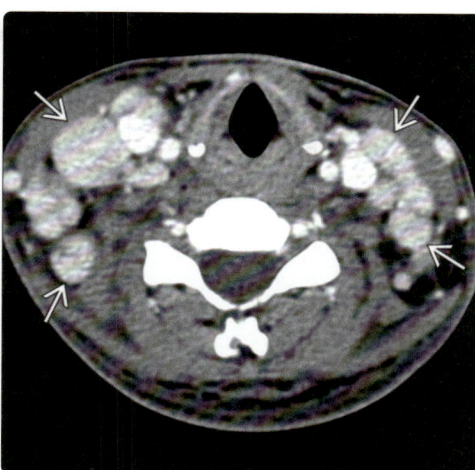

(Left) *Axial CECT in a teenage girl with extensive bilateral cervical adenopathy shows multiple cervical nodes ⮕ of varying size with enhancement nearly as intense as the internal carotid artery ⮕ and jugular vein ⮕.* **(Right)** *Axial CECT in the same patient shows additional adenopathy ⮕ without evidence of necrosis, calcification, or surrounding inflammatory changes. Lymph node biopsy proved CD of mixed hyaline vascular and plasma cell type. This is the rarest form of CD.*

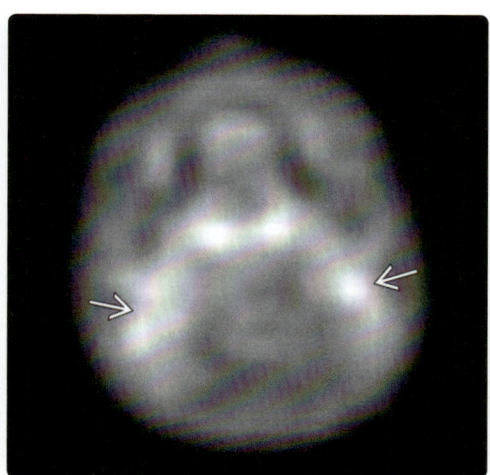

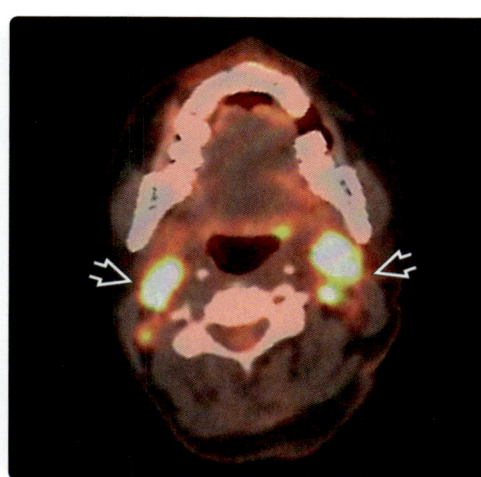

(Left) *Axial FDG PET study performed 2 days after CT in the same patient reveals mild uptake in the neck ⮕.* **(Right)** *Fused axial images for a FDG PET/CT performed in a 26-year-old woman with CD demonstrates FDG-avid bilateral cervical chain lymph nodes ⮕ (e.g., SUV = 9.0). Additional disease above and below the diaphragm is also present in this patient with multicentric CD (not shown).*

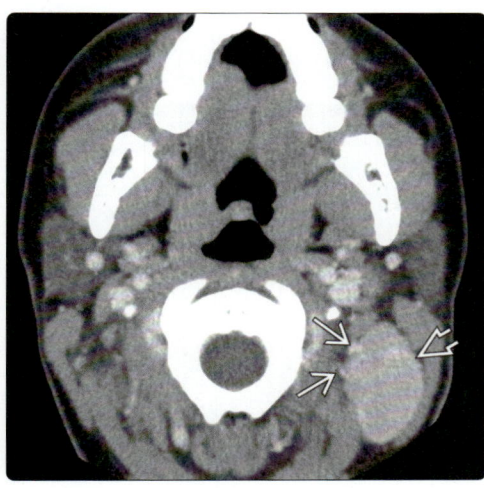

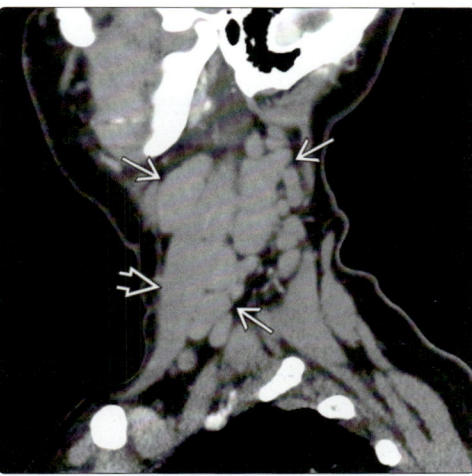

(Left) *Axial CECT in a teenage girl demonstrates an enlarged, avidly enhancing left level IIB lymph node ⮕. Notice the prominent adjacent vessels ⮕. This was the hyaline vascular variant of unicentric CD.* **(Right)** *Parasagittal CECT of the neck shows diffuse enlarged lymph nodes ⮕ surrounding the sternocleidomastoid ⮕. These do not demonstrate the avid enhancement of previous cases. This patient has the plasma cell variant of CD as well as multicentric disease.*

TERMINOLOGY

- Histiocytic necrotizing lymphadenitis
- Synonym: Kikuchi-Fujimoto disease
- Benign, idiopathic, necrotizing cervical adenitis; more common in **young Asian adults**

IMAGING

- **Unilateral**, homogeneous, mildly enlarged nodes with **inflammatory stranding**
- Posterior cervical and jugular chain
- Nodes appear solid or rim enhancing, < 20% necrotic on imaging; indistinct margins of necrotic foci
- Nodes hypermetabolic on PET/CT, mimicking lymphoma

TOP DIFFERENTIAL DIAGNOSES

- Non-Hodgkin lymphoma lymph nodes
- Systemic nodal metastases
- Cat-scratch disease
- Tuberculosis lymph nodes

PATHOLOGY

- Cortical and paracortical coagulative necrosis
- Cellular infiltrate of histiocytes and immunoblasts
- Possibly exuberant T-cell-mediated immune response to variety of nonspecific stimuli
- Associated with increased incidence of systemic lupus erythematosus
- Higher **Japanese** and other **Asian** incidence may be due to *HLA* genes

CLINICAL ISSUES

- Most commonly in Asian women in 3rd decade
- Tender, unilateral posterior neck nodes and high fever
- 30-50% have other systemic symptoms
- Usually resolves without treatment in 1-4 months

DIAGNOSTIC CHECKLIST

- Symptoms, imaging, and histology mimic lymphoma

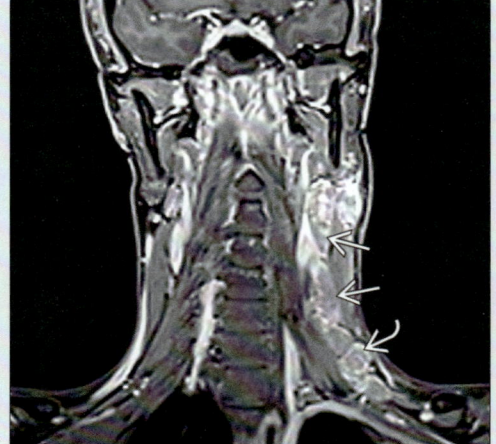
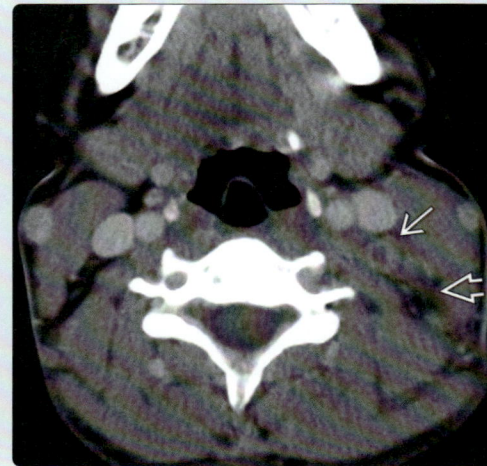

(Left) Coronal T1 C+ FS MR in a young Asian woman with left-sided neck swelling shows predominantly left-sided, well-defined nodes ➡ involving levels 2-5. The nodes appear somewhat matted. Note rim enhancement of the nodes ⤴. (Right) Axial CECT in a middle-aged woman with fever and neck tenderness shows a rim-enhancing left level IIB lymph node ➡ with adjacent fat stranding ➡. This patient has similar nodes throughout levels II, III, and V. Biopsy found histiocytic necrotizing lymphadenitis (HNL).

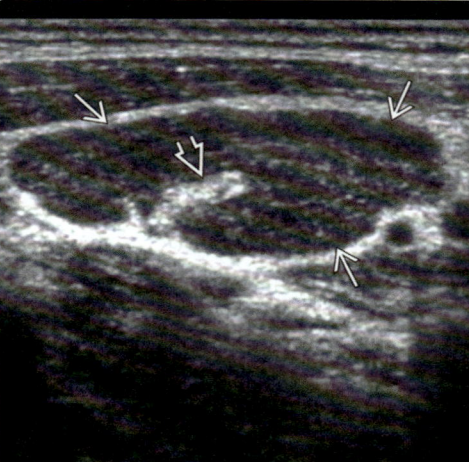
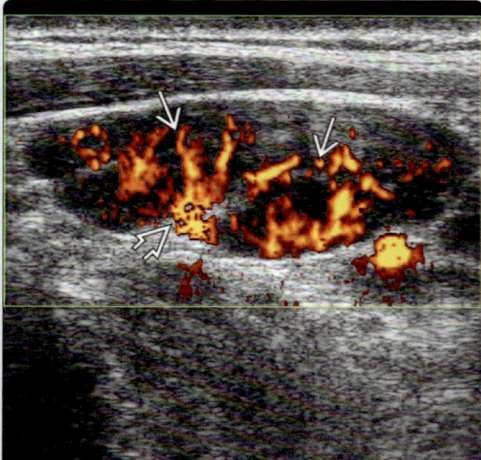

(Left) Longitudinal US obtained in the posterior neck shows a hypoechoic enlarged node ➡ with a hypertrophied cortex but normal hilar architecture ➡ in a patient with HNL (Kikuchi-Fujimoto disease). Note the absence of associated soft tissue edema, intranodal necrosis, or matting of nodes. (Right) Power Doppler US in the same patient reveals prominent vascularity of the perihilar cortex ➡ and hilum ➡. This is a classic appearance of HNL.

TERMINOLOGY

Abbreviations
- Histiocytic necrotizing lymphadenitis (HNL)

Synonyms
- Kikuchi-Fujimoto disease

Definitions
- Benign, idiopathic, necrotizing cervical adenitis more common in **young Asian adults**

IMAGING

General Features
- Best diagnostic clue
  - Unilateral, homogeneous, mildly enlarged nodes, levels 2-5, with inflammatory stranding
- Location
  - Posterior cervical and jugular chain
  - Unilateral > bilateral

CT Findings
- CECT
  - Homogeneously solid (> 80%) or rim-enhancing hypodense
    - 20% internal necrosis
    - Indistinct margins of necrotic foci characteristic
  - Perinodal inflammatory changes

MR Findings
- T2WI
  - Central nonenhancing areas are not hyperintense
- T1WI C+ FS
  - Solidly enhancing or peripherally enhancing nodes

Ultrasonographic Findings
- Grayscale ultrasound
  - Homogeneous, hypoechoic, enlarged nodes with echogenic hilum
- Power Doppler
  - **Hypervascularity** of hilum

Nuclear Medicine Findings
- PET/CT
  - **Increased FDG uptake** in enlarged nodes

DIFFERENTIAL DIAGNOSIS

Non-Hodgkin Lymphoma Nodes
- Non-Hodgkin lymphoma (NHL) nodes are often larger than HNL
- Perinodal inflammation rare in NHL

Systemic Nodal Metastases
- Viral-like illness with HNL, uncommon with mets
- Necrosis in metastatic nodes hyperintense on T2

Cat-Scratch Disease
- Regional adenopathy following scratch incident

Tuberculosis Lymph Nodes
- Typically accompanied by thoracic TB

PATHOLOGY

General Features
- Etiology
  - Unknown but probably viral or autoimmune, may be T-cell and histiocyte response to infectious agent
- Genetics
  - Higher **Japanese** and other **Asian** incidence may be due to *HLA* genes
- Associated abnormalities
  - Associated with autoimmune disorders, increased incidence of systemic lupus erythematosus

Microscopic Features
- Necrosis is microscopic, not often macroscopic

CLINICAL ISSUES

Presentation
- Most common signs/symptoms
  - Tender, unilateral posterior neck nodes and high fever
- Other signs/symptoms
  - 30-50% have extranodal involvement
    - Upper respiratory symptoms, malaise, headache
    - Mouth ulcers, hepatosplenomegaly, arthritis
    - Rare complications, including meningoencephalitis, optic neuritis, panuveitis
  - May have leukopenia, raised ESR and CRP

Demographics
- Age
  - Adults < 30 years
- Sex
  - Female predominance
- Epidemiology
  - Most commonly in Asian, especially Japanese, patients

Natural History & Prognosis
- Usually benign, self-limited over 1-4 months
- Uncommonly complicated course with poor outcome

Treatment
- Symptomatic: NSAIDs or oral steroids

DIAGNOSTIC CHECKLIST

Consider
- Symptoms, imaging, and histology mimic lymphoma

Image Interpretation Pearls
- Some features that should raise possibility of HNL
  - Young Asian woman
  - Unilateral, homogeneous, moderately enlarged nodes, levels 2-5, perinodal inflammation

SELECTED REFERENCES

1. Ahmed HS et al: Neurological manifestations and complications of Kikuchi-Fujimoto disease: a comprehensive systematic review. Clin Neurol Neurosurg. 251:108818, 2025
2. Cheng MH et al: Distinguishing Kikuchi-Fujimoto disease from lymphoma in patients by clinical and PET/CT features. Medicine (Baltimore). 103(16):e37779, 2024
3. Zheng Y et al: Differential diagnosis of pediatric cervical lymph node lesions based on simple clinical features. Eur J Pediatr. 183(11):4929-38, 2024

TERMINOLOGY

- Kimura disease (KD): Angiolymphoid proliferation with **serum eosinophilia** and elevated **IgE**
  - Inflammatory disorder with multiple head and neck masses; rarely involve limbs and groin

IMAGING

- Classic triad
  - Subcutaneous and deep tissue masses of head and neck
  - Salivary gland masses: Parotid > submandibular
  - Solid cervical lymphadenopathy
- CT or MR findings
  - Variable enhancement (CT) and signal (MR)
  - Due to varying vascularity and fibrosis

TOP DIFFERENTIAL DIAGNOSES

- Nodal non-Hodgkin lymphoma
- Plexiform neurofibroma
- Nodal sarcoidosis

- Parotid metastatic nodal disease

PATHOLOGY

- Unknown etiology; allergic and autoimmune theories favored
- ~ 50% have renal dysfunction

CLINICAL ISSUES

- Chronic, slowly progressive course over years
- High recurrence rate after surgical excision

DIAGNOSTIC CHECKLIST

- KD great mimicker, like lymphoma
- Most common in **young Asian male patients**
- Diagnostic triad
  - Painless subcutaneous head and neck masses with regional adenopathy
  - Blood and tissue eosinophilia
  - Markedly elevated serum IgE
- Recommend renal function tests

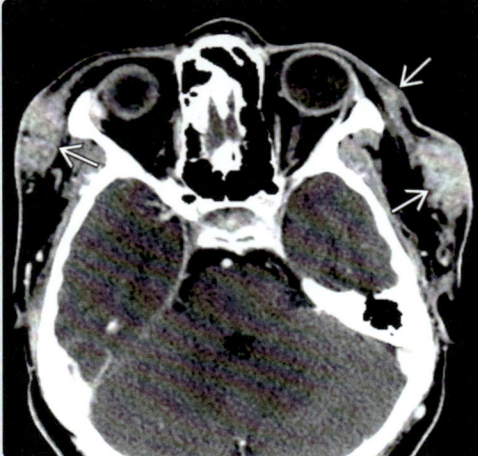
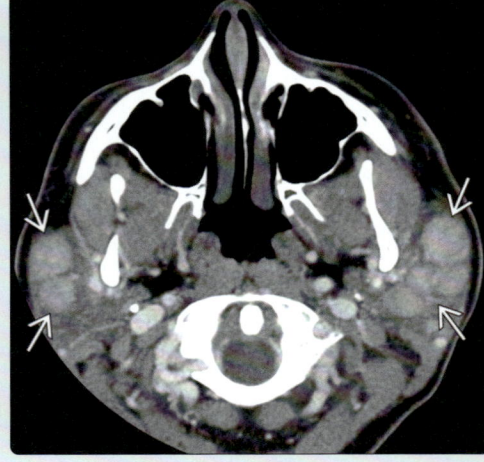

(Left) *Axial CECT in a young Asian woman with a 9-year history of slowly enlarging forehead nodules reveals multiple bilateral, subcutaneous, plaque-like lesions* ➡️ *with significant deformity of the scalp and facial contours.* (Right) *Axial neck CECT in the same patient shows multiple bilateral, enhancing intraparotid nodules* ➡️. *Numerous enlarged cervical nodes were also present bilaterally (not shown). Biopsy of the forehead lesion revealed Kimura disease (KD).*

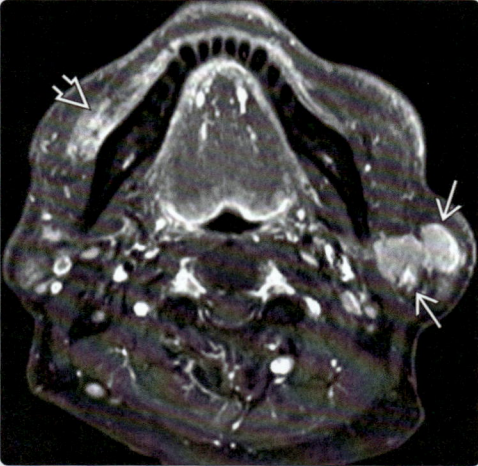
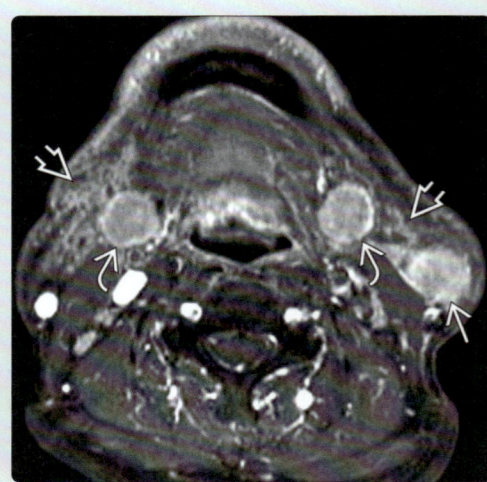

(Left) *Axial T1WI C+ FS MR in a patient with KD demonstrates intensely enhancing left intraparotid masses* ➡️ *within the left parotid gland. Ill-defined, enhancing infiltration of the right cheek deep soft tissues* ➡️ *is evident on the contralateral side as well.* (Right) *More inferior axial T1WI C+ FS MR in the same patient shows bilateral, enhancing submandibular lesions* ➡️ *in addition to a hazy, infiltrated appearance of deep and subcutaneous fat* ➡️ *around them. The tail of parotid enhancing node is evident on the left* ➡️.

TERMINOLOGY

Abbreviations
- Kimura disease (KD)

Synonyms
- Eosinophilic hyperplastic lymphogranuloma, eosinophilic lymphogranuloma, eosinophilic folliculosis

Definitions
- **Angiolymphoid proliferation with peripheral eosinophilia and elevated IgE**
- Benign chronic inflammatory disorder resulting in multiple head and neck masses
  - Primarily in **young Asian male patients**

IMAGING

General Features
- Best diagnostic clue
  - Imaging triad
    - Subcutaneous nodules, salivary gland masses, lymphadenopathy
  - Clinical triad
    - Painless, firm nodes/nodules, blood and tissue eosinophilia, markedly elevated serum IgE
- Location
  - Subcutaneous and deep tissues of head and neck
    - Rare sites: Orbit, lacrimal gland, hard palate, larynx, dura
  - Salivary gland: Parotid > submandibular
    - Less often minor salivary glands
  - Cervical lymphadenopathy very common (60-100%)
    - Occasionally, axillary, inguinal, or antecubital fossa nodes
  - Unilateral > bilateral
- Size
  - Average lesion: 3 cm (range: 2-11 cm)
- Morphology
  - Variable due to variation in vascular elements and fibrosis
  - Subcutaneous masses: Commonly ill-defined borders
  - Salivary gland involvement may be diffuse infiltration, ill-defined mass, or intraparotid nodes
  - Enlarged nodes well-defined, nonnecrotic

CT Findings
- CECT
  - **2 morphological patterns described**: Ill-defined, plaque-like > focal or well defined
    - Plaque-like subcutaneous lesions have moderate or poor enhancement
      - May have overlying tissue atrophy
    - Well-defined lesions typically have intense enhancement
  - Nodes rounded, solid, with moderate-intense enhancement
    - Nodal enhancement tends to mirror lesion enhancement

MR Findings
- T1WI
  - Isointense or hypointense nodal masses compared to parotid glands
- T2WI
  - Usually hyperintense
    - Chronic fibrotic lesions may be hypointense
- T1WI C+
  - Solidly enhancing nodes and masses characteristic
  - Less enhancement with chronic, fibrotic lesions

Ultrasonographic Findings
- Grayscale ultrasound
  - Poorly marginated subcutaneous masses
    - Hypoechoic with hyperechoic bands creates woolly appearance
    - Absent internal cystic spaces
  - Enlarged nodes solid and hypoechoic with homogeneous internal echoes
    - Preserved echogenic hilum
- Power Doppler
  - Prominent intranodal or intralesional vessels with low resistance

Nuclear Medicine Findings
- PET
  - Increased uptake of FDG
- Other nuclear medicine studies
  - Uptake of 111 In-pentetreotide, Tc-99m-labeled autologous granulocytes
  - Uptake of Tl-201 SPECT on early and delayed images

Imaging Recommendations
- Best imaging tool
  - CT or MR demonstrates nodes and masses
- Protocol advice
  - Contrast important for extent of nodal involvement and parotid evaluation

DIFFERENTIAL DIAGNOSIS

Nodal Non-Hodgkin Lymphoma
- Usually bilateral adenopathy
- No subcutaneous masses
- Diffusion restriction, intermediate signal on T2WI

Plexiform Neurofibroma
- Family history
- Characteristic target sign on T2WI
- Lymphadenopathy is uncommon

Nodal Sarcoidosis
- Primary manifestation is multiple enlarged nodes
- Can involve entire parotid gland or intraparotid nodes
- Chest x-ray usually shows mediastinal adenopathy
- No subcutaneous masses

Parotid Metastatic Nodal Disease
- Multiple intraparotid nodes, often with necrosis
- Frequently squamous cell carcinoma or melanoma from local skin primary malignancy
- May develop facial nerve palsy

PATHOLOGY

General Features

- Etiology
  - Unknown, though allergic and autoimmune theories favored because of elevated serum IgE
    - Altered T-cell immunoregulation or IgE-mediated type 1 hypersensitivity
    - Excessive production of eosinophilic cytokines, such as IL-4
  - May be associated with infection: Virus, parasite, *Candida*
- Associated abnormalities
  - 15-60% have renal dysfunction, including nephrotic syndrome
    - Can precede development of subcutaneous lesions
  - Associations with asthma, Loeffler syndrome, and connective tissue diseases reported

Gross Pathologic & Surgical Features

- Tumorous masses of subcutaneous tissues, salivary glands, and adenopathy
- Vascular, rubbery, fibrotic masses
- Nodes may form confluent mass ± adherent to overlying dermis

Microscopic Features

- Abnormal proliferation of lymphoid follicles and vascular endothelium with dense eosinophilic infiltrate
- Lymphoid hyperplasia with germinal centers containing cellular, vascular, and fibrous components
  - **Dense eosinophilic infiltrates** and eosinophilic microabscesses with central necrosis
  - Abundant plasma cells and lymphocytes (proliferation of HLA-DR CD4 cells)
  - Vascular proliferation and variable fibrosis around and within lesion
- Immunofluorescence studies
  - Germinal centers contain heavy **IgE deposits**
  - Variable IgG, IgM, and fibrinogen
- Previously considered 1 entity with angiolymphoid hyperplasia with eosinophilia (ALHE)
  - ALHE differs from KD clinically and histologically
    - Head and neck dermal nodules in middle-aged White women
    - Rarely adenopathy, 20% blood eosinophilia
  - Vascular proliferation and atypia suggest neoplasia more than inflammation

CLINICAL ISSUES

Presentation

- Most common signs/symptoms
  - Insidious onset of solitary or multiple painless swellings of head and neck
    - Predominantly preauricular and submandibular
  - 60-100% cervical adenopathy
  - Laboratory
    - Peripheral eosinophilia and elevated serum IgE
- Other signs/symptoms
  - ~ 50% have renal disease
    - Most often extramembranous glomerulonephritis
    - Proteinuria → nephrotic syndrome
  - Occasional localized or generalized pruritus
  - Melanin pigmentation, skin coarsening
  - Facial nerve palsy not reported with parotid involvement
- Clinical profile
  - 30-year-old Asian man with painless neck masses

Demographics

- Age
  - Onset peaks in 3rd decade
  - Rarer sites of occurrence tend to be in older patients
- Sex
  - M:F = 3-10:1
- Ethnicity
  - Endemic in Asians, particularly Chinese and Japanese
  - Uncommon in Whites, rare in Blacks

Natural History & Prognosis

- Chronic, slowly progressive course over years
- Potentially disfiguring
  - Large (≥ 5 cm) subcutaneous lesions may ulcerate
- Spontaneous resolution reported
- No malignant potential

Treatment

- Resection of mass lesion(s): Up to 30% recurrence
- Intralesional or oral steroids may temporize, though not cure
- Cyclosporine A reported to induce remission
- Consider radiotherapy for persistent/problematic lesions
- Large/recurrent lesions: Surgery with adjuvant monoclonal antibody therapy
- Observation alone if not symptomatic or disfiguring

DIAGNOSTIC CHECKLIST

Consider

- KD is great mimicker, like lymphoma
- KD should be distinguished clinically and histologically from ALHE
- Recommend serology for IgE, eosinophil count, and renal function tests

Image Interpretation Pearls

- KD difficult diagnosis to make by imaging alone
- Chronicity of masses or abnormal serology findings helpful
- Look for **triad of imaging findings**, particularly in Asian male patients
  - Subcutaneous enhancing nodules
  - Salivary gland masses or nodes
  - Cervical adenopathy

SELECTED REFERENCES

1. Zhao F et al: Kimura disease: a detailed analysis of clinical and radiological manifestations in a retrospective case series. J Inflamm Res. 17:3371-81, 2024
2. Bishop C et al: Kimura disease: a rare and difficult to diagnose entity. Head Neck Pathol. 16(1):278-81, 2022
3. Sangwan A et al: Kimura disease: a case series and systematic review of clinico-radiological features. Curr Probl Diagn Radiol. 51(1):130-42, 2020
4. Lin YY et al: Kimura's disease: clinical and imaging parameters for the prediction of disease recurrence. Clin Imaging. 36(4):272-8, 2012
5. Gopinathan A et al: Kimura's disease: imaging patterns on computed tomography. Clin Radiol. 64(10):994-9, 2009

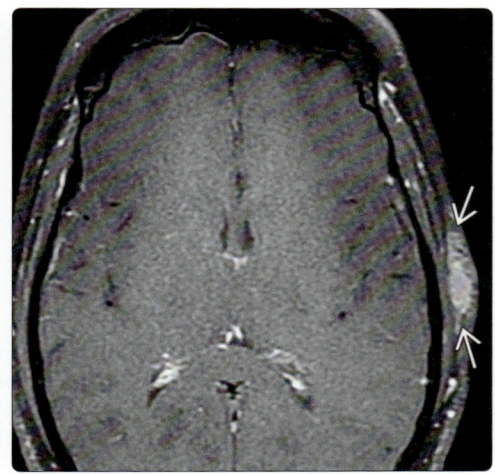

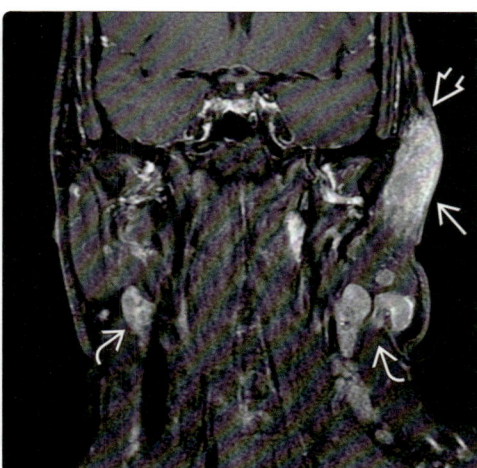

(Left) *Axial T1 C+ FS MR in an Asian patient with known KD demonstrates an infiltrative, moderately enhancing soft tissue subcutaneous lesion ➡ in the left temporal region.* (Right) *Coronal T1 C+ FS MR in the same patient shows a subcutaneous infiltrative lesion ➡ involving the left parotid gland. There was other left intraparotid lymph node involvement as well (not shown). The overlying skin ➡ is intact. Note bilateral enlarged cervical lymph nodes ➡ that are typical of this condition.*

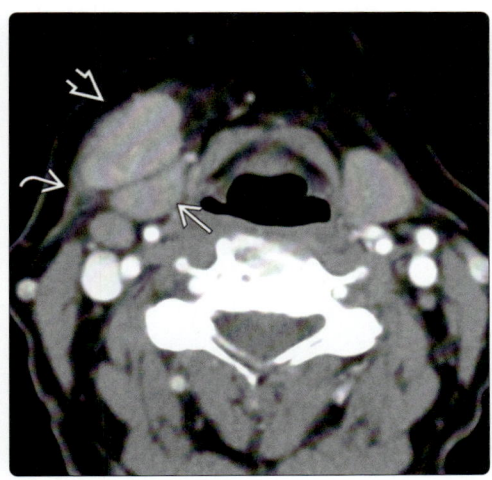

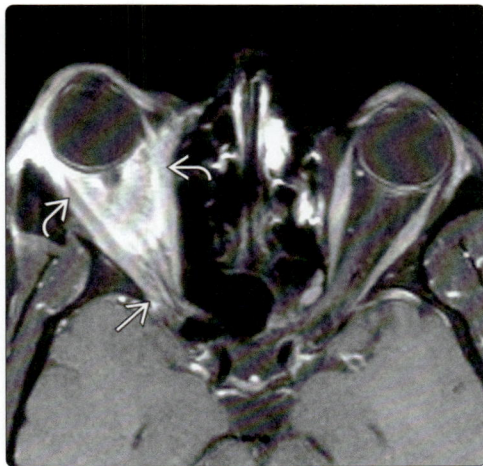

(Left) *Axial CECT shows a heterogeneously enhancing conglomerate nodal mass ➡, resulting in compression and medial displacement of the right submandibular gland ➡ and reticulation of the surrounding fat and thickening of the platysma muscle ➡.* (Right) *Axial T1 C+ FS MR shows an uncommon variant of KD. Infiltrating, intensely enhancing homogeneous tissue ➡ involves the entire right orbit, extending to, but not beyond, the orbital apex ➡, resulting in proptosis.*

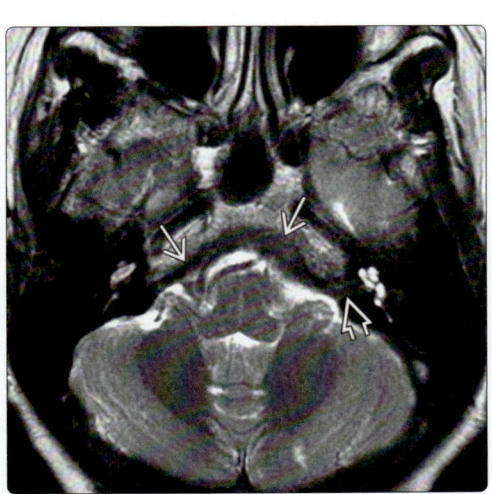

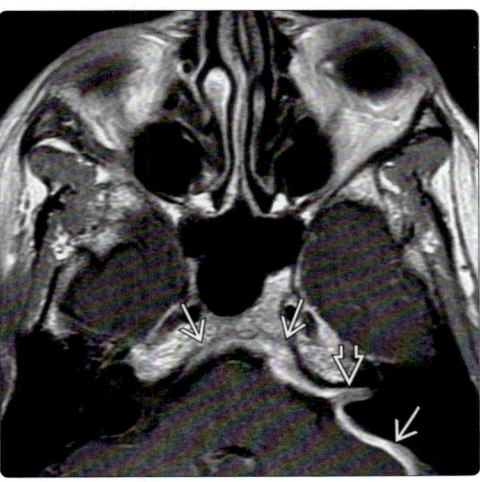

(Left) *Axial T2WI MR shows a rare manifestation of KD in a patient with sensorineural hearing loss who has subtle T2 hypointensity ➡ along the cranial surface of the clivus. Note the filling of the left internal auditory canal (IAC) ➡ with low-signal material.* (Right) *Axial T1 C+ MR in the same patient shows intensely enhancing and thickened dura ➡ overlying the clivus and within the IAC ➡. KD may mimic other entities, such as sarcoid and idiopathic inflammatory pseudotumor.*

Nodal Hodgkin Lymphoma in Neck

TERMINOLOGY

- Hodgkin lymphoma (HL): Classic HL (CHL) with 4 subtypes & nodular lymphocyte-predominant HL (NLPHL)
- NLPHL may be more accurately called nodular lymphocyte predominant B-cell lymphoma (NLPBCL)
- Characterized by presence of **Reed-Sternberg cells**

IMAGING

- Most HL patients present due to **neck adenopathy**
- Uni/bilateral, unilateral in head & neck in 80%
- Single nodal group or contiguous groups; extranodal rare
- Mediastinal nodes frequently involved at presentation
- CECT: Homogeneous, solid nodal masses
  - Necrosis or calcification uncommon
- CECT & FDG PET basic staging modalities
- FDG PET shows **marked activity**
- Persistently positive PET during treatment has high sensitivity for prediction of relapse
- FDG PET differentiates posttreatment inactive scar from residual tumor

TOP DIFFERENTIAL DIAGNOSES

- Reactive lymph nodes
- Nodal differentiated thyroid carcinoma
- Nodal non-HL
- Nodal squamous cell carcinoma

PATHOLOGY

- **WHO** classification (based on pathologic assessment): 95% CHL; 5% NLPHL
- **Lugano** staging (derived from **Ann Arbor** staging)
  - **Waldeyer ring tonsils, thymus,** & **spleen** considered **nodal structures** for staging purposes
- Neoplastic cells: Reed-Sternberg cells
- Tumor bulk nonneoplastic reactive inflammatory cells

CLINICAL ISSUES

- 40% have **B symptoms**: Fever, sweats, weight loss

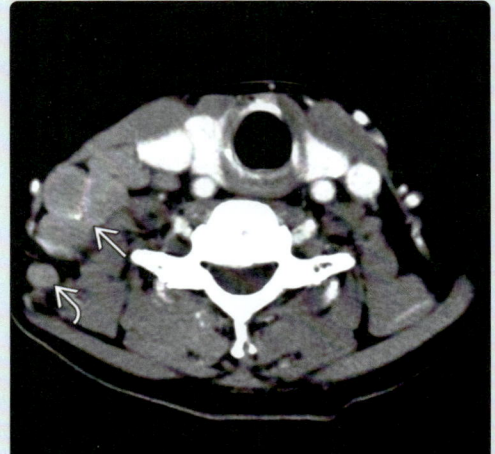
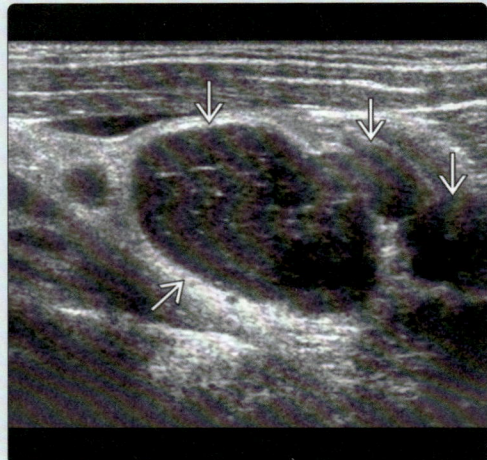

(Left) Axial CECT shows a classic nodular-sclerosis Hodgkin lymphoma (HL) nodal cluster in the right level IV ➡️ & VB ➡️ nodal region. Note the absence of calcification or necrosis. No other regions were involved in the whole body, making this stage I disease. (Right) Longitudinal right lower neck ultrasound shows level IV lymphadenopathy ➡️. Nodes lack normal hilar contour & are variable & heterogeneous, appearing mainly solid & reticular without calcification. The largest lymph node measures 3 cm x 2 cm.

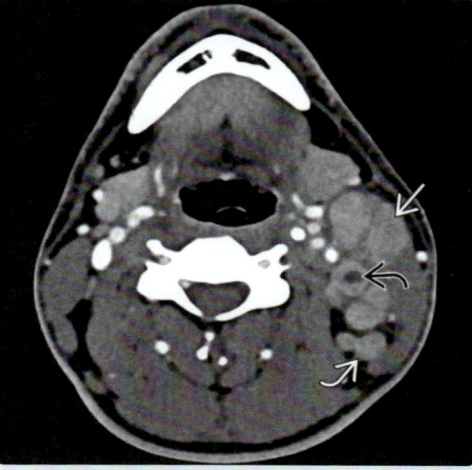
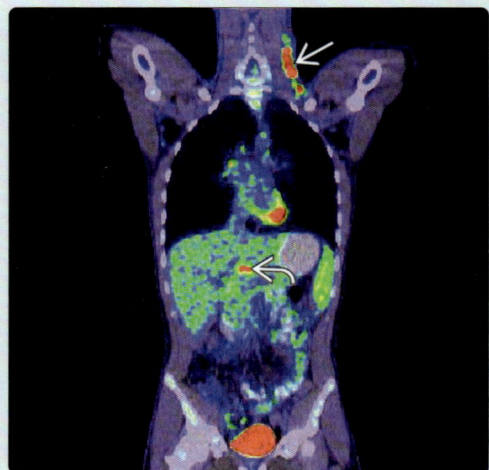

(Left) Axial CECT in a patient with classic mixed cellularity HL shows multiple left level IIA ➡️ & IIB ➡️ enlarged lymph nodes. Most of the nodes show homogeneous mild contrast enhancement, but one has central necrosis ➡️. (Right) Coronal fused whole-body F-18 FDG PET/CT in the same patient shows FDG-avid left cervical lymphadenopathy ➡️. Careful evaluation shows infradiaphragmatic disease in porta hepatis lymph nodes ➡️, upgrading it to stage III (would have been stage I with unilateral cervical lymphadenopathy only).

TERMINOLOGY

Abbreviations

- Hodgkin lymphoma (HL)
  - Classic HL (CHL), nodular lymphocyte-predominant HL (NLPHL)

Synonyms

- Hodgkin disease

Definitions

- Characterized by presence of **Reed-Sternberg (RS) cells**
- **CHL** (95%): More aggressive
  - Nodular sclerosis (60-80%)
  - Mixed cellularity (15-30%)
  - Lymphocyte rich (5%)
  - Lymphocyte depleted (< 1%)
- **NLPHL** (5%): More indolent, tends to respond & relapse
  - Behaves & treated like low-grade non-HL (NHL)
  - 5th edition of WHO classification of hematolymphoid tumors (WHO-HAEM5) maintains terminology for NLPHL
  - NLPHL may be more accurately called nodular lymphocyte predominant B-cell lymphoma (NLPBCL) as its neoplastic cells have functional B-cell program
  - NLPBCL term considered acceptable preparing for future definitive adoption of new nomenclature

IMAGING

General Features

- Best diagnostic clue
  - Young patient with neck & mediastinal adenopathy
- Location
  - HL most commonly **cervical** & **mediastinal** nodes
    - Internal jugular, spinal accessory, & transverse cervical nodal chains
    - **Involves contiguous nodal groups**
    - Uni/bilateral, unilateral in head & neck in 80%
  - Rarely involves Waldeyer ring or other extranodal neck sites (< 1%)
- Size
  - Variable nodal size: 2-10 cm
  - No strict size criteria but nodes usually large & asymmetric
- Morphology
  - Single nodal chain ± spread to contiguous chain
  - 60-80% present with neck/supraclavicular nodes

CT Findings

- NECT
  - Homogeneous, lobulated, round masses
  - Calcification uncommon except after treatment
- CECT
  - Variable enhancement
  - Necrosis may be seen as low-density center

MR Findings

- T1WI
  - Enlarged iso- to hypointense round nodes
- T2WI
  - Nodes hyperintense compared with muscle
- T1WI C+

  - Variable, usually homogeneous nodal enhancement

Ultrasonographic Findings

- Grayscale ultrasound
  - Older transducers: Pseudocystic appearance (hypoechoic with posterior enhancement)
  - High-resolution US: Micronodular/reticular pattern
  - Contrast-enhanced ultrasonography (CEUS) shows homogeneous enhancement in majority
- Color Doppler
  - Mixed central & peripheral high degree of vascularity
  - Variable resistance index (RI)/pulsatility index (PI), can mimic benign or malignant nodes

Nuclear Medicine Findings

- PET
  - FDG PET shows **marked activity**
  - Persistently positive scan during & after treatment has high sensitivity for prediction of relapse

Imaging Recommendations

- Best imaging tool
  - CECT basic staging tool for assessment of disease
  - FDG PET for staging & assessing treatment response

DIFFERENTIAL DIAGNOSIS

Reactive Lymph Nodes

- Multiple nodes; not as large as HL nodes

Nodal Differentiated Thyroid Carcinoma

- Favors level VI neck & superior mediastinum
- Mediastinal nodes not usually bulky
- Variable MR signal: Thyroglobulin, cystic change

Non-Hodgkin Lymphoma in Lymph Nodes

- Imaging cannot distinguish HL & NHL nodes
- NHL more frequently extranodal (30%)

Nodal Squamous Cell Carcinoma

- Central nodal necrosis, extranodal extension common

PATHOLOGY

General Features

- Etiology
  - **Up to 50% EBV(+)**
    - Almost 100% of HIV-associated HL EBV(+)
- Genetics
  - Familial association; 2-9x ↑ risk for siblings
- Associated abnormalities
  - ↑ incidence with **HIV** but not AIDS-defining malignancy: Tend to be more aggressive with poorer prognosis
  - Association with **Castleman disease (CD)**

Staging, Grading, & Classification

- 5th edition of **WHO** classification of hematolymphoid tumors
  - Based on final pathology; CHL (95%) or NLPHL (5%)
- **Lugano classification** for staging, response assessment, & follow-up of lymphomas: Based on **Ann Arbor staging** with **Cotswolds modifications**
  - Based on disease location & clinical symptoms

Lugano Classification for Staging Hodgkin Lymphoma

Based on Ann Arbor Staging With Cotswolds Modifications

Stage I: Single lymph node or group of adjacent nodes (**Waldeyer ring, thymus, & spleen considered nodal structures** for staging purposes) (I); or single extranodal organ or tissue (IE) without nodal involvement

Stage II: 2 or more lymph node regions or nodal structures on same side of diaphragm alone (II); or with involvement of limited, contiguous extralymphatic organ or tissue (IIE) [Number of anatomic regions should be denoted by subscript (e.g., II-2, II-3)]

Stage III: Lymph node regions or lymphoid structures on both sides of diaphragm (can be nodes on both sides of diaphragm; or nodes above diaphragm with spleen below diaphragm)

Stage IV: Diffuse or disseminated noncontiguous extralymphatic organ or tissue involvement (more than that can be designated "E") ± associated nodal involvement

Designation "E": Extranodal contiguous extension in stage I or stage II disease, which can be encompassed within radiation field for nodal disease of same anatomic extent (NB: Further extensive extranocal disease should be designated as stage IV)

Systemic symptoms: Categories A & B
Category A: No systemic symptoms
Category B: Fever, 10% weight loss or night sweats during 6 months period prior to diagnosis

Bulky disease: Single nodal mass of 10 cm, or of longest dimension ≥ 1/3 of transthoracic diameter at any thoracic level on CT scan (NB: Term "X" used in Ann Arbor staging system no longer needed)

Subscript "RS": To designate stage at time of relapse

- **Nodal regions** for lymphoma staging in **head** & **neck** imaging
  - **Waldeyer ring**: Base of tongue, nasopharyngeal & palatine **tonsils**
  - Ipsilateral cervical & supraclavicular nodes
  - Occipital & preauricular nodes
  - Infraclavicular nodes
  - Axillary & pectoral nodes
  - Mediastinal: **Thymus**, prevascular, aortcpulmonary, pre/paratracheal, subcarinal, posterior mediastinal
    - All mediastinal lesions counted as single nodal region
    - Internal mammary nodes considered part of lymphatic system of chest wall; drain diaphragm
    - Paravertebral nodes also drain chest wall & diaphragm; even though in posterior mediastinum
  - Hilar nodes: Right & left hilar nodes considered separate regions; bilateral hilar nodes makes stage II lymphoma

Microscopic Features

- RS cell = multinucleate giant cell; neoplastic B-lymphocyte clonal proliferation: Large lymphocytes with > 1 nucleus
- Tumor bulk nonneoplastic reactive inflammatory cells
- NLPHL: Popcorn lymphocytic & histiocytic cells; few/no RS

CLINICAL ISSUES

Presentation

- Most common signs/symptoms
  - Painless, enlarged, rubbery nodes
  - 25-40% have category **B symptoms**
    - Fever, night sweats, > 10% body weight loss
  - NLPHL rarely extranodal disease or B symptoms
    - Usually presents as early-stage disease (stage I, II)

Natural History & Prognosis

- Poor prognostic features
  - Large mediastinal mass, > 50 years, ↑ ESR, ↑ WBC count, ↓ RBC count, > 4 regions
  - International prognostic factor project on advanced HL: 7 variables: Age ≥ 45 years, stage IV disease, male sex, WBC count ≥ 15,000 cells/µL, lymphocyte count < 600 cells/µL, albumin < 4.0 g/dL, hemoglobin < 10.5 g/dL
  - FDG PET results during or after front line treatment greater prognostic significance than this pretreatment risk stratification
  - For NLPHL, lymphocyte-predominant international prognostic score (LP-IPS): Age ≥ 45 years, stages III-IV, hemoglobin < 10.5 g/dL, splenic involvement

Treatment

- Risk-adapted therapy: Initial therapy based on histology, anatomic stage, & presence of poor prognostic features
  - Early-stage disease: Combined modality strategies, such as abbreviated courses of combination chemotherapy followed by involved-field XRT
  - Advanced stage disease: Longer course chemotherapy, often without XRT
  - Newer agents like brentuximab vedotin & anti-PD-1 antibodies incorporated into front line therapy
- Relapsed/refractory HL: High-dose chemotherapy (HDCT) followed by autologous stem cell transplant (ASCT) standard of care for relapse following initial therapy
  - Failed HDCT with ASCT: Brentuximab vedotin, PD-1 blockade, nonmyeloablative allogeneic transplant or clinical trial participation

DIAGNOSTIC CHECKLIST

Consider

- Posttreatment residual masses: FDG PET differentiates active disease from inactive scar or sterile treated tumor

SELECTED REFERENCES

1. Ansell SM: Hodgkin lymphoma: 2025 update on diagnosis, risk-stratification, and management. Am J Hematol. 99(12):2367-78, 2024
2. Alaggio R et al: The 5th edition of the World Health Organization Classification of Haematolymphoid Tumours: lymphoid neoplasms. Leukemia. 36(7):1720-48, 2022

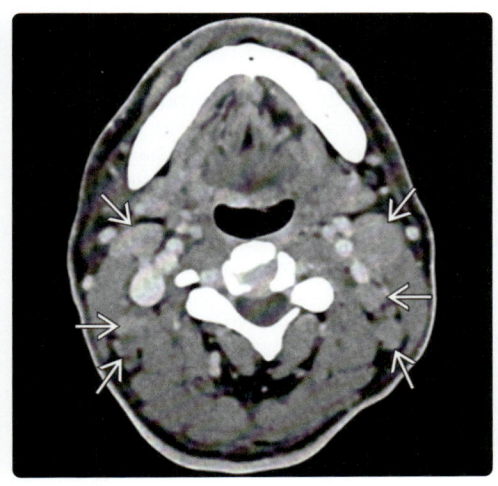

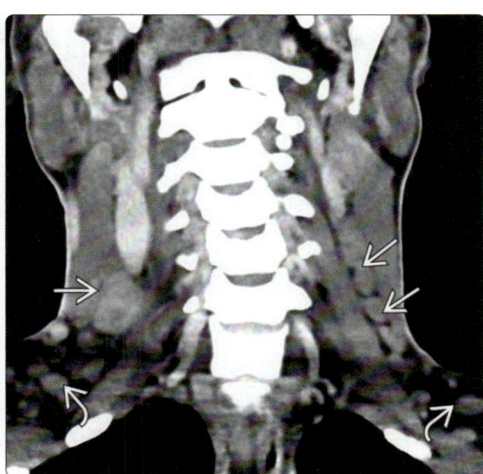

(Left) Axial CECT in a patient with classic nodular sclerosis HL shows bilateral level II cervical lymphadenopathy ➡. (Right) Coronal reformatted CECT in the same patient shows bilateral cervical internal jugular chain ➡ & supraclavicular ➡ lymphadenopathy. No other nodal region or extralymphatic site was involved, making this stage II. Patient had fever, night sweats, & weight loss, hence was designated stage IIB. Cervical & supraclavicular nodes of one side are considered as a single nodal region for staging purposes.

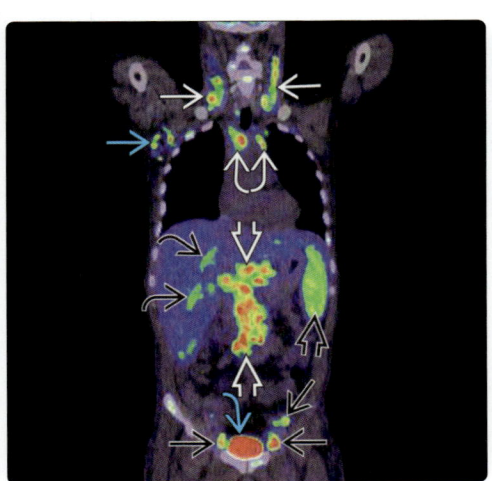

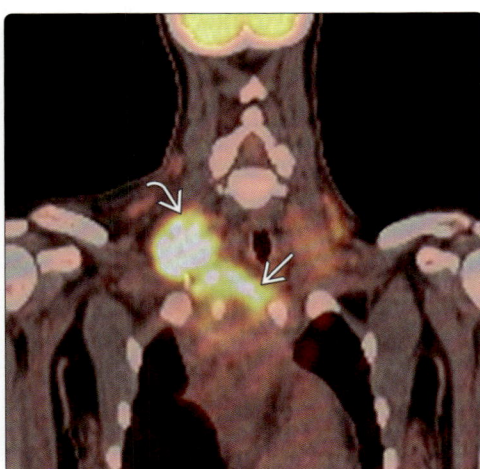

(Left) Coronal fused whole-body F-18 FDG PET/CT shows widespread FDG-avid axillary ➡, mediastinal ➡, abdominal ➡ & iliac ➡ lymphadenopathy, & liver ➡ and spleen ➡ involvement, in addition to bilateral cervical adenopathy ➡, making it stage IV HL. Note normal physiologic FDG excretion into the urinary bladder ➡. (Right) Coronal FDG PET/CT in a 19-year-old woman after front line therapy shows relapsed FDG-avid nodal disease in the supraclavicular region ➡ extending into the mediastinum ➡.

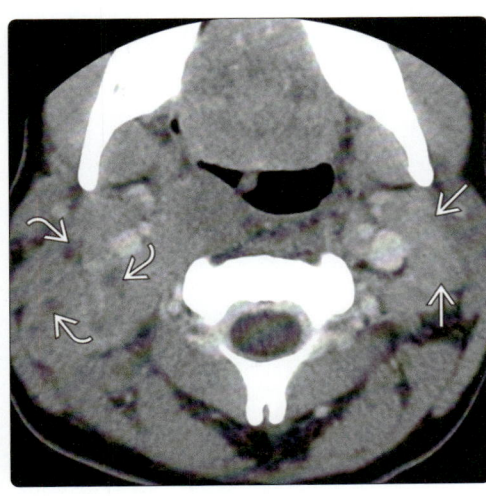

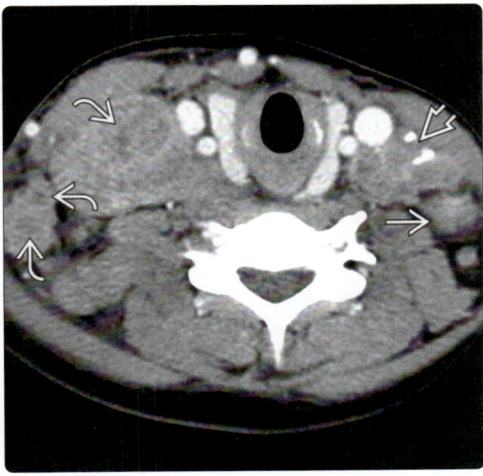

(Left) Axial CECT shows a young adult previously treated with chemoradiotherapy for classic nodular sclerosis HL. Bilateral adenopathy is evident with both homogeneous solid nodes ➡, typical of HL & other more heterogeneous nodes with cystic changes ➡. (Right) Axial CECT more inferiorly reveals additional heterogeneous ➡ & homogeneous solid nodes ➡. Focal calcifications ➡ are unusual in HL & likely reflect previously treated nodes from chemoradiotherapy 18 months earlier.

KEY FACTS

TERMINOLOGY

- Non-Hodgkin lymphoma (NHL)

IMAGING

- Multiple enlarged nodes involving multiple nodal chains
- Uni/bilateral, unilateral in H&N in > 80%
- Typically **large, solid**, round, or oval nodes
- Enhancement may be variable, even in same patient
- **Necrosis/extranodal extension** suggests **aggressive NHL**
- May see different patterns of nodes
  - Multiple mildly enlarged 1- to 3-cm nodes
  - Dominant, markedly enlarged node
- FDG PET shows variable avidity
  - High in aggressive NHL, lower in more indolent NHL

TOP DIFFERENTIAL DIAGNOSES

- Reactive adenopathy
- Tuberculosis lymph nodes
- Sarcoidosis lymph nodes
- Hodgkin lymphoma nodes
- Nodal metastases from systemic primary

PATHOLOGY

- WHO classification of hematolymphoid tumors, 5th edition (WHO-HAEM5)
- **Lugano** classification for staging, response assessment, & follow-up of lymphomas: Based on **Ann Arbor** staging
  - **Waldeyer ring** tonsils, **thymus, & spleen** considered **nodal structures** for staging purposes
- 80-85% B cell: Most common diffuse large B-cell lymphoma
- Often associated with AIDS

CLINICAL ISSUES

- Adult with painless neck masses
- Treat with XRT, chemotherapy, or both
- 5-year survival: Stage I > 82%, stage II 75%, stage III 70%, stage IV > 62%

(Left) Coronal reformatted CECT in a patient with mantle cell lymphoma (MCL) shows bilateral, nonnecrotic cervical lymphadenopathy ➡. MCL non-Hodgkin lymphoma (NHL) usually presents at stage IV with GI & bone marrow involvement, as in this patient. (Right) Coronal whole-body MIP of an F-18 FGD PET in a patient with stage III follicular lymphoma shows bilateral cervical ➡, right axillary ➡, abdominal ➡, iliac ➡ lymphadenopathy, & splenic involvement ➡. Follicular lymphoma is usually indolent NHL but may be high grade.

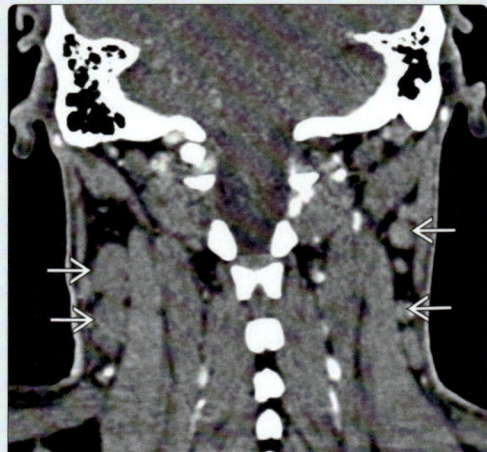
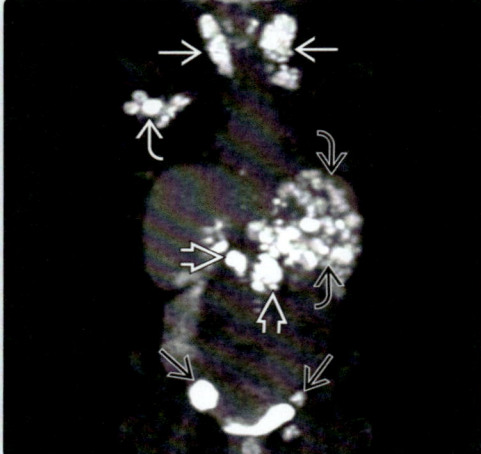

(Left) Axial CECT reveals a large, pedunculated NHL mass involving the left lingual tonsil ➡ & palatine tonsil ➡. Note moderate, diffuse enhancement. Biopsy is necessary to differentiate squamous cell carcinoma (SCCa) from NHL of pharyngeal mucosal space. (Right) Axial T2 FS MR reveals multiple heterogeneous iso- to hyperintense nodal NHL masses ➡. The nodes insinuate around structures with little mass effect & no arterial compression. The largest node wraps around the anterior scalene muscle ➡.

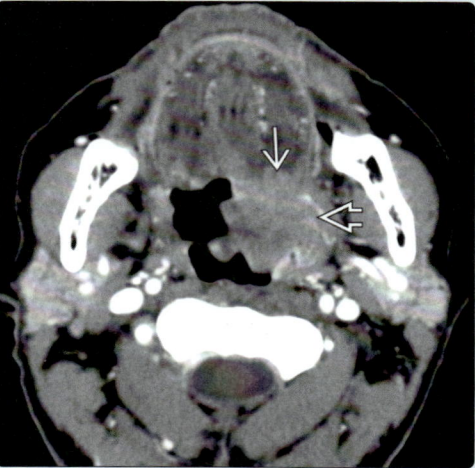
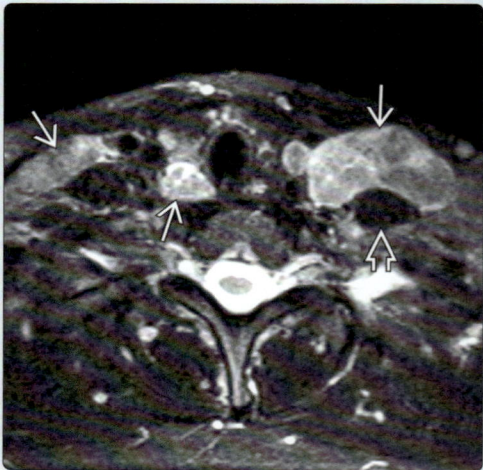

TERMINOLOGY

Abbreviations

- Non-Hodgkin lymphoma (NHL)

Definitions

- Lymphoreticular system malignancy arising from lymphocytes & derivatives
- Multiple different NHL subtypes
  - Most common (20-30%): Diffuse large B-cell lymphoma (DLBCL)
- H&N NHL has multiple forms
  - Nodal, nonnodal lymphatic (tonsils, lingual lymphoid, adenoids), nonnodal extralymphatic (e.g., thyroid)

IMAGING

General Features

- Best diagnostic clue
  - Enlarged nodes involving multiple nodal chains
  - Uni/bilateral, unilateral in H&N in > 80%
- Location
  - All cervical nodal chains may be involved
  - Levels II, III, IV, superficial & parotid nodes often involved
- Size
  - Different patterns of nodes
    - Multiple mildly enlarged 1- to 3-cm nodes
    - Dominant node 3-5 cm in size; may be ≤ 10 cm
- Morphology
  - Round or oval enlarged nodes, typically **solid**
  - **Nodal necrosis ± extranodal tumor** spread suggests **aggressive NHL**
    - AIDS-associated NHL often aggressive: Necrosis & surrounding induration

CT Findings

- NECT
  - Nodal density similar to muscle
  - Calcification rare, usually post therapy
- CECT
  - Bulky, ovoid masses in multiple cervical node chains
  - Enhancement may be variable, even in same patient

MR Findings

- T1WI
  - Nodes isointense to muscle
- T2WI
  - Nodes usually iso- or slightly hyperintense to muscle
- DWI
  - Whole-body DWI useful, but cannot replace PET/CT
- T1WI C+
  - Minimal homogeneous nodal enhancement
  - Necrotic adenopathy enhances peripherally

Ultrasonographic Findings

- High-resolution US: Micronodular/reticular pattern
- Older transducers: Pseudocystic appearance (hypoechoic with posterior enhancement)
- Contrast-enhanced ultrasonography (CEUS) shows homogeneous enhancement in majority
- Color Doppler: Mixed central & peripheral high degree of vascularity
- Doppler: Variable resistance index (RI)/pulsatility index (PI), can mimic benign or malignant nodes

Nuclear Medicine Findings

- PET
  - FDG PET/CT best for staging & treatment assessment
  - **FDG PET** shows **variable avidity**
    - Higher in aggressive NHL, lower in more indolent NHL

DIFFERENTIAL DIAGNOSIS

Reactive Adenopathy

- Patient usually < 20 years of age with viral infection
- Diffuse, nonnecrotic adenopathy, usually < 2 cm

Tuberculosis Lymph Nodes

- Systemically ill patient; strongly positive PPD & abnormal chest x-ray
- Diffuse adenopathy; heterogeneous nodes

Sarcoidosis Lymph Nodes

- Diffuse cervical lymphadenopathy that may exactly mimic NHL
- Calcifications may be seen

Hodgkin Lymphoma Nodes

- Nodal NHL cannot be differentiated from Hodgkin lymphoma (HL) on imaging

Nodal Metastases From Systemic Primary

- Known primary tumor (lung, breast, etc.)
- CEUS of cancerous lymph nodes shows inhomogeneous enhancement in majority

PATHOLOGY

General Features

- Etiology
  - Evidence suggests **viral** cause but yet to be proven
    - Association with EBV or HTLV-1, especially African Burkitt & AIDS-associated lymphomas
- Associated abnormalities
  - Often associated with AIDS in children or adults
    - 2nd most common cancer in AIDS patients
  - Disseminated disease common

Staging, Grading, & Classification

- WHO classification of haematolymphoid tumours, 5th edition (WHO-HAEM5)
  - Genetic-centric approach
  - Hierarchy from benign to malignant with categories such as lineage, family (class), type, & subtype
  - WHO-HAEM5 utilizes triad of attributes: Lineage, dominant clinical attribute, & dominant biologic attribute
    - Dominant biologic attribute encompasses gene fusions, rearrangements, mutations
  - Categories include myeloid neoplasms, lymphoid neoplasms, histiocytic/dendritic neoplasms, & stroma-derived neoplasms of lymphoid tissues
  - Lymphoid neoplasms consist of B-cell lymphoid proliferations & lymphomas & T-cell & NK-cell proliferations & lymphomas
  - **B-cell lymphoid proliferations and lymphomas**

Lugano Classification for Staging Non-Hodgkin Lymphoma

Based on Ann Arbor Staging System

Stage I: Single lymph node or group of adjacent nodes (**Waldeyer ring, thymus, & spleen considered nodal structures** for staging purposes) (I); or single extranodal organ or tissue (IE) without nodal involvement

Stage II: 2 or more lymph node regions or nodal structures on same side of diaphragm alone (II); or with involvement of limited, contiguous extralymphatic organ or tissue (IIE)

Stage III: Lymph node regions or lymphoid structures on both sides of diaphragm (can be nodes on both sides of diaphragm, or nodes above diaphragm with spleen below diaphragm)

Stage IV: Diffuse or disseminated noncontiguous extralymphatic organ or tissue involvement (more than that can be designated "E"), ± associated nodal involvement

Designation "E": Limited extranodal extension (more extensive extranodal disease should be designated as stage IV)

Systemic "B" symptoms (fever, sweats, weight loss) no longer incorporated into non-Hodgkin lymphoma staging; unlike Hodgkin lymphoma staging Systemic "B" symptoms not independent prognostic factor in non-Hodgkin lymphoma

Bulky disease: No cut-off value for largest tumor diameter validated in non-Hodgkin lymphoma; criteria vary by histology (6 cm for follicular lymphoma & 6-10 cm for diffuse large B-cell lymphoma) (term "X" used in Ann Arbor staging system no longer needed)

Disease extent evaluation using PET/CT for avid lymphoma & CT scan for nonavid lymphoma histologies.

Non-Hodgkin lymphoma (NHL) is most frequently spread hematogenously; hence, the NHL staging system is less useful than that for Hodgkin lymphoma (which disseminates mainly by contiguous lymphatic spread). The majority of aggressive NHLs present in advanced stages III/IV, which have similar treatment, & differentiation between these stages offer little therapeutic benefit. NHL staging is mainly to identify the minority of patients with early-stage disease who can be treated with local or combined modality therapy.

- – Tumor-like lesions with B-cell predominance (new in WHO-HAEM5): Includes reactive B-cell-rich lymphoid proliferations that can mimic lymphoma, IgG4-related disease, unicentric Castleman disease, idiopathic multicentric Castleman disease, & Kaposi sarcoma-associated herpesvirus (KSHV)/HHV-8-associated multicentric Castleman disease
  - – Precursor B-cell neoplasms (B-cell lymphoblastic leukemias/lymphomas)
  - – Mature B-cell neoplasms
  - – Hodgkin lymphoma
  - – Plasma cell neoplasms & other diseases with paraproteins
  - ○ **T-cell & NK-cell proliferations & lymphomas**
    - – Tumor-like lesions with B-cell predominance (new in WHO-HAEM5)
    - – Precursor T-cell neoplasms
    - – Mature T-cell & NK-cell neoplasms
- Lugano classification for staging, response assessment, & follow-up of lymphomas: Derived from Ann Arbor staging
- **Nodal regions** for lymphoma staging in **H&N** imaging
  - ○ **Waldeyer ring**: Base of tongue, nasopharyngeal & palatine **tonsils**
  - ○ Ipsilateral cervical & supraclavicular nodes
  - ○ Occipital & preauricular nodes
  - ○ Infraclavicular nodes
  - ○ Axillary & pectoral nodes
  - ○ Mediastinal: **Thymus**, prevascular, aortopulmonary, pre/paratracheal, subcarinal, posterior mediastinal
    - – All mediastinal lesions counted as single nodal region
    - – Internal mammary nodes considered part of lymphatic system of chest wall; drain diaphragm
    - – Paravertebral nodes also drain chest wall & diaphragm, even though in posterior mediastinum
  - ○ Hilar nodes: Right & left hilar nodes considered separate regions; bilateral hilar nodes makes stage II lymphoma

Gross Pathologic & Surgical Features

- Nodes firm & rubbery

Microscopic Features

- Microscopic features depend on cell of origin
  - ○ B- & T-cell lymphomas: Precursor or mature lymphocytes

CLINICAL ISSUES

Presentation

- Most common signs/symptoms
  - ○ Painless large or multiple small, rubbery neck masses
  - ○ Systemic symptoms: Night sweats, recurrent fever, weight loss, fatigue, & pruritic skin rash

Natural History & Prognosis

- Predictors of poorer prognosis: Age > 60 years, > 1 extranodal site, stage III or IV, AIDS related

Treatment

- XRT, chemotherapy, or combined modality therapy
  - ○ Bone marrow transplant may be performed

DIAGNOSTIC CHECKLIST

Consider

- Range of presentations suggestive of NHL
  - ○ Diffuse cervical nodes with variable texture in adult
  - ○ Multiple 1- to 3-cm nodes in multiple nodal chains
  - ○ Large nonnecrotic node without H&N primary; jugular, occipital, retropharyngeal, parotid, submandibular nodes
  - ○ AIDS patient with neck mass
- Imaging cannot distinguish nodal NHL from HL: NHL more common, older patients, extranodal disease suggests NHL

SELECTED REFERENCES

1. Haferlach C et al: Overview on WHO-HAEM5 and the diagnostic relevance of genetic alterations for the classification. Med Genet. 36(1):3-11, 2024

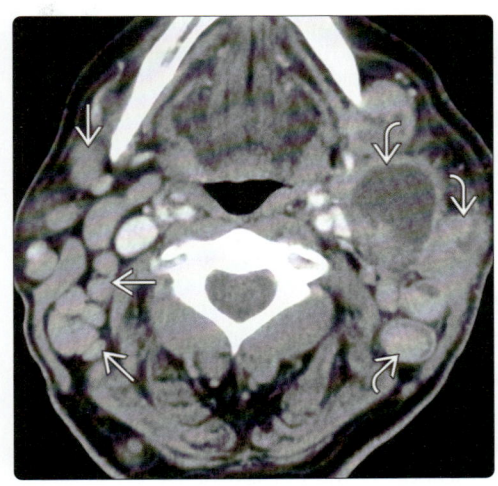

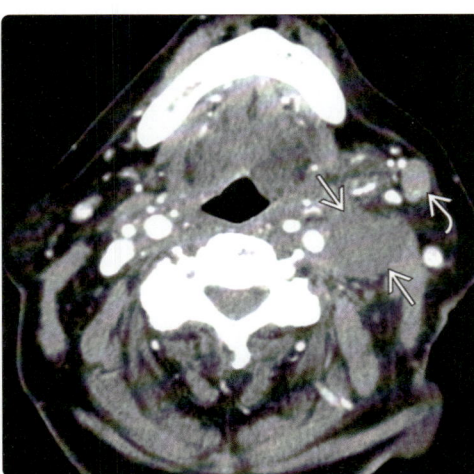

(Left) *Axial CECT in an immunocompromised patient shows multiple small, solid, right-sided NHL nodes* →. *The left-sided large, necrotic nodal masses with surrounding induration & extranodal extension* → *were found to be metastatic SCCa from H&N primary.* (Right) *Axial CECT shows a variable appearance of NHL nodes, which is not uncommon. Note the minimally enhancing lower density left level II node* →, *& a smaller, more enhancing node* → *lateral to the left submandibular salivary gland.*

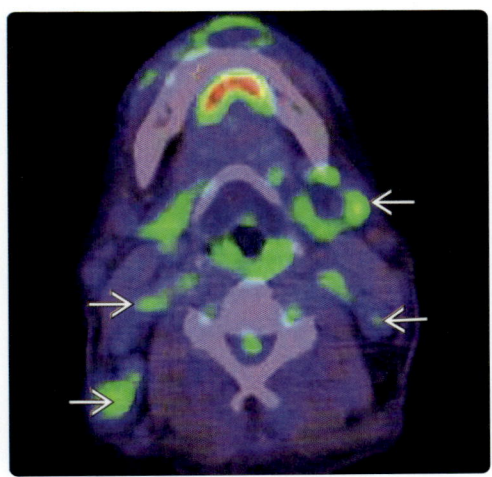

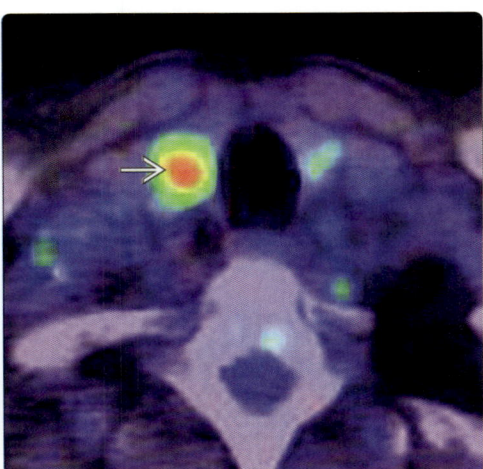

(Left) *Axial fused F-18 FDG PET/CT in a patient with chronic lymphocytic leukemia (CLL) shows bilateral cervical lymphadenopathy, which is only mildly FDG avid* →. *Neck node biopsy showed small lymphocytic lymphoma (SLL) NHL.* (Right) *Axial fused F-18 FDG PET/CT at a lower level in the same patient shows intense FDG uptake in the right lobe of the thyroid gland* →. *FNAC showed a follicular lesion, not NHL. DLBCL & MALT lymphoma are the most common primary thyroid lymphoma. CLL/SLL with a thyroid mass is extremely rare.*

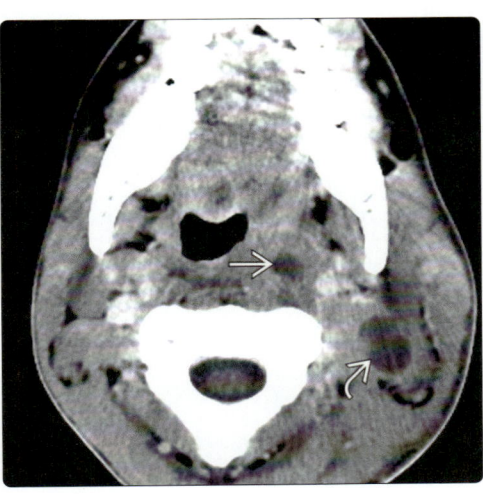

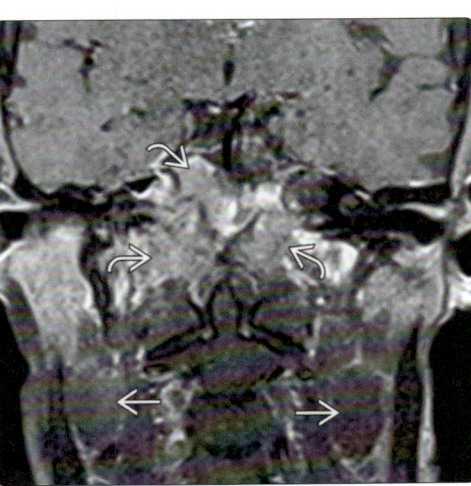

(Left) *Axial CECT in a teenage boy with Burkitt-type NHL shows a necrotic retropharyngeal node* → *deforming pharyngeal lumen. Necrotic left high jugular chain node* → *is evident. Nodal necrosis ± extranodal extension suggests aggressive NHL.* (Right) *Coronal T1 C+ FS MR in a patient with NHL reveals bilateral cervical lymphadenopathy* → *without features to suggest nodal necrosis. The patient also had nonnodal, extralymphatic NHL with an infiltrative, mildly enhancing tumor involving the osseous skull base* →.

Nodal Differentiated Thyroid Carcinoma

TERMINOLOGY

- Differentiated thyroid carcinoma (DTC)
- Metastatic node(s) from papillary thyroid carcinoma (PTC) or follicular thyroid carcinoma (FTC)

IMAGING

- PTC nodal metastases disseminate sequentially, first to **central compartment**, then **lateral neck** nodes
- **Skip metastases** of PTC (~ 7%): Lateral lymph node metastasis without central lymph node metastasis
- **Retropharyngeal** nodal metastases occur, especially when lateral cervical nodes present
- US: Look for cystic change, hyperechoic calcifications, loss of hilar architecture; peripheral vascularity on color Doppler
- CECT may be done, but delays I-131 radioablation
- Solid, cystic, calcified, < 1 cm nodes common
- MR: Nodes heterogeneous in size & signal
- I-123 & I-131 scans: Very sensitive for well-differentiated PTC & FTC

- Sensitivity ↓ as DTC dedifferentiates → FDG PET better
- F-18 FDG PET best when ↑ thyroglobulin with negative radioiodine scan; not sensitive for well-differentiated thyroid carcinoma → radioiodine scans better for these

TOP DIFFERENTIAL DIAGNOSES

- Nodal squamous cell carcinoma, nodal non-Hodgkin lymphoma, nodal tuberculosis, systemic nodal metastases

PATHOLOGY

- Extranodal extension poor prognostic characteristic

CLINICAL ISSUES

- Nodal metastases prognostically significant only if age > 55

DIAGNOSTIC CHECKLIST

- Nodal mass: Features highly suggestive of DTC
  - Heterogeneous **complex cystic** nodes
  - CT/US **calcifications** or MR T1 hyperintensity
- Thyroid primary may not be evident on CT/MR

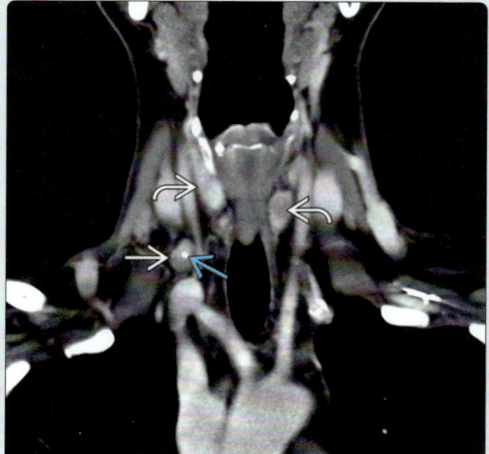
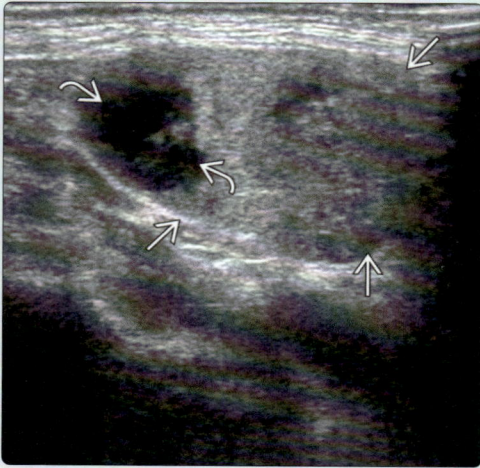

(Left) Coronal CECT shows a mildly enlarged right level IV lymph node ➡ with a speck of internal calcification ➡ in a patient with papillary thyroid carcinoma (PTC) in both lobes of the thyroid gland ➡. PTC nodal metastasis can frequently not be enlarged by size criteria (< 1-cm short-axis dimension) and may show calcifications. (Right) Longitudinal US shows marked internal heterogeneity of an enlarged level III node ➡, which has a cystic area ➡ superiorly. FNA revealed PTC.

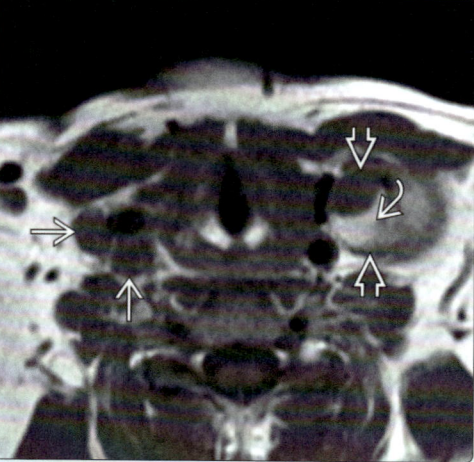
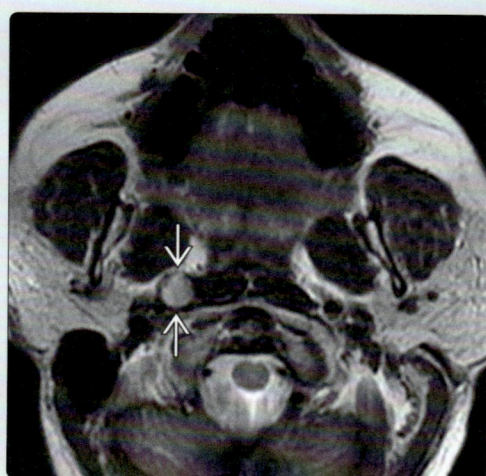

(Left) Axial T1WI MR through the lower neck shows a cluster of round, minimally enlarged homogeneous nodes ➡ on the right at level III and a more complex cystic and solid mass in the lower left neck ➡. T1 hyperintensity within posterior cystic component ➡ makes differentiated PTC most likely primary (bright T1 could be due to thyroglobulin or colloid). (Right) Axial T2WI MR more superiorly in the same patient shows an enlarged, round, right retropharyngeal node ➡. Thyroidectomy revealed PTC in nonenlarged heterogeneous thyroid gland.

TERMINOLOGY

Abbreviations

- Differentiated thyroid carcinoma (DTC)

Definitions

- Metastatic node(s) from DTC [papillary thyroid carcinoma (PTC) or follicular thyroid carcinoma (FTC)]

IMAGING

General Features

- Best diagnostic clue
  - **Heterogeneous, solid & cystic enlarged nodes**
  - Focal **calcifications** (CT/US) or T1 hyperintensity (MR) highly suggestive of DTC
- Location
  - **Central compartment** level VI most common
  - PTC nodal metastases disseminate sequentially, first to central, then **lateral neck** level II-V, supraclavicular
    - Bilateral nodal metastases common
  - **Skip metastases** of PTC (~ 7%): Lateral lymph node metastasis without central lymph node metastasis
  - **Retropharyngeal** nodal metastases occur, especially when lateral cervical nodes present
- Size
  - Variable between patients & in single patient
    - Nodes may be 2-3 cm but **commonly < 1 cm**

Imaging Recommendations

- Best imaging tool
  - US often 1st-line tool for nonpalpable nodes
  - MR useful for retropharyngeal, deep cervical, or mediastinal metastases
  - CECT with iodinated contrast possible but should wait 4-6 weeks before diagnostic I-123 or therapeutic I-131

CT Findings

- CT
  - Overall sensitivity poor, as nodal metastases often small
  - Nodes heterogeneous: Solid, **cystic, calcified,** variable in size & enhancement
  - **Hyperenhancing** nodes may be seen

MR Findings

- T1WI
  - **Frequently bright** from thyroglobulin or colloid
- T2WI
  - Variable; most often hyperintense

Ultrasonographic Findings

- Grayscale ultrasound
  - 3 features concerning for malignancy: Cystic appearance, hyperechoic calcifications, loss of hilar architecture
  - Allows guided FNA
- Color Doppler
  - Peripheral vascularization highly suggest metastasis
  - Metastatic nodes usually show ↑ resistance index (RI) > 0.7 & pulsatility index (PI) > 1.5, but PTC nodes may show lower RI/PI

Nuclear Medicine Findings

- PET/CT

- F-18 FDG PET best when ↑ thyroglobulin with negative radioiodine scan
  - Not sensitive for well-differentiated thyroid carcinoma → radioiodine scans better for these
- I-123 & I-131 scans: Very sensitive for well-differentiated PTC & FTC
  - Sensitivity ↓ as DTC dedifferentiates → FDG PET better

DIFFERENTIAL DIAGNOSIS

Nodal Squamous Cell Carcinoma

- May be heterogeneous, cystic, or solid
- Rarely have calcifications

Nodal Non-Hodgkin Lymphoma

- Usually multiple large, homogeneous nodes
- Calcifications rare except post treatment

Nodal Tuberculosis

- Thick rim of enhancement with central necrosis
- Calcifications may be evident

Systemic Nodal Metastases

- Adenocarcinoma metastases may have calcifications

PATHOLOGY

General Features

- Etiology
  - Thyroid cancers: PTC in 70-80%, FTC in 10-15%, medullary thyroid cancer (MTC) in 5-10%, anaplastic thyroid cancer (ATC) in < 2%

Staging, Grading, & Classification

- **N1a**: Central compartment lymph nodes: Level VI, pre-/paratracheal, prelaryngeal
- **N1b**: Spread beyond central compartment: Uni-/bilateral cervical levels I-V, retropharyngeal, superior mediastinal
- Nodes prognostically significant only if age > **55 yr** in PTC & FTC; any age in MTC
- All ATC classified as stage IV, regardless of tumor size, location, or metastasis
- **< 55 yr**: Nodal disease does not alter staging in **PTC & FTC**
  - As younger patients have ↓ likelihood of dying from DTC
  - Stage I: Any T, **any N**, no metastasis (M0); stage II: Any T, **any N**, with metastasis (M1)
- Age cutoff ↑ from 45 yr to 55 yr in AJCC 8th edition
- **> 55 yr**: PTC/FTC: Stage I: T1 or T2, **N0/NX**, M0; stage II: T1 or T2, **N1**, M0 & T3a or T3b, any N, M0; stage III: T4a, **any N**, M0; stage IVA: T4b, **any N**, M0; stage IVB: Any T, **any N**, M1
- Extranodal extension → poor prognosis

DIAGNOSTIC CHECKLIST

Image Interpretation Pearls

- **Complex cystic** nodes in PTC
- CT/US calcifications or MR T1 hyperintensity suggest DTC
- Thyroid primary carcinoma may not be evident on CT/MR

SELECTED REFERENCES

1. Dietz LK et al: Review of retropharyngeal and parapharyngeal nodal metastasis of papillary thyroid carcinoma. Am J Otolaryngol. 45(5):104438, 2024

Systemic Nodal Metastases in Neck

TERMINOLOGY

- Neck node metastasis from **infraclavicular primary** tumor
- **Virchow node**: Left supraclavicular nodal metastasis

IMAGING

- Nodes generally in **lower** neck, especially on **left**
- Variably sized nodes, often > 1.5 cm
- May be cluster of small nodes
- May form conglomerate mass > 5-6 cm
- Longitudinal length/transaxial width (L:T ratio) < 2
- Ca^{++}: Systemic **adeno**carcinoma or thyroid Ca^{++}
- **Hyperenhancing** metastatic nodes: Renal cell Ca^{++}, neuroendocrine tumors, Kaposi sarcoma, thyroid Ca^{++}
- US: Enlarged, round node, absent echogenic hilus, necrosis
- US: **Early metastasis** with tiny, **subcapsular** nodal deposits → normal echogenic hilus if medullary sinuses uninvolved

TOP DIFFERENTIAL DIAGNOSES

- Reactive lymph nodes

- Sarcoidosis nodes
- Squamous cell carcinoma (SCCa) metastatic nodes
  - Lymph node metastasis & extranodal extension significantly affect prognosis & survival
- Non-Hodgkin lymphoma nodes

PATHOLOGY

- Esophageal, breast, & lung malignancies most common, may be unknown primary
- Neoplastic cells **first** localize **in subcapsular sinus**, then proliferate into body of node
- Focal altered/nonenhancement on CT or MR corresponds to nest of tumor cells or necrosis

CLINICAL ISSUES

- Systemic neck metastases < H&N SCCa nodes

DIAGNOSTIC CHECKLIST

- Neck nodes: Look for H&N primary SCCa first
- If infrahyoid nodal metastasis, suspect systemic primary

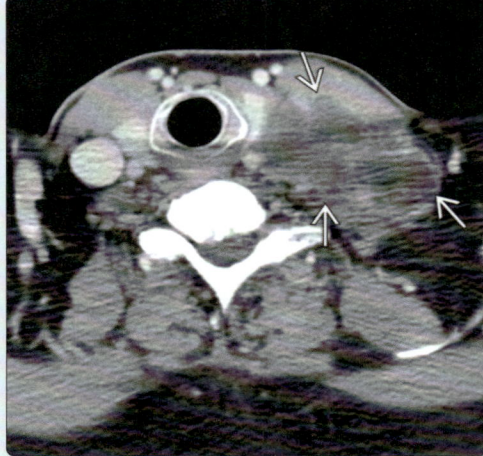
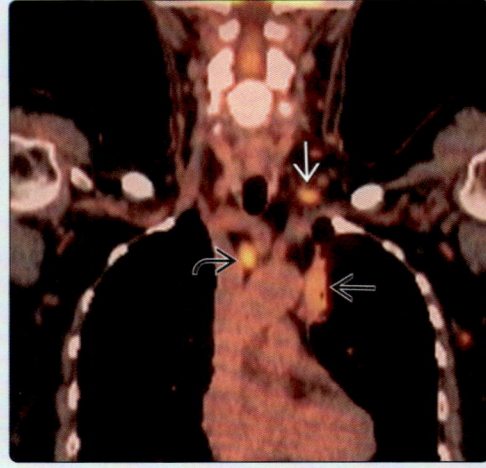

(Left) Axial CECT shows a large, complex conglomerate left supraclavicular nodal mass ➡ with extensive necrosis & infiltration of the scalene & sternocleidomastoid muscles. The patient had neural deficits from invasion of the brachial plexus. FNA revealed metastatic colonic adenocarcinoma. (Right) Coronal fused FDG PET/CT in a 65-year-old woman with a small neck mass shows left lung adenocarcinoma ➡ with mediastinal ➡ & left supraclavicular ➡ lymphadenopathy.

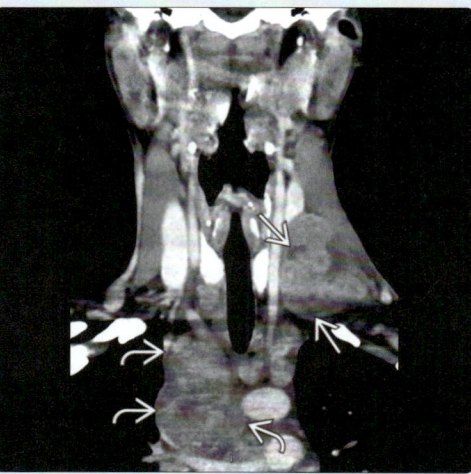
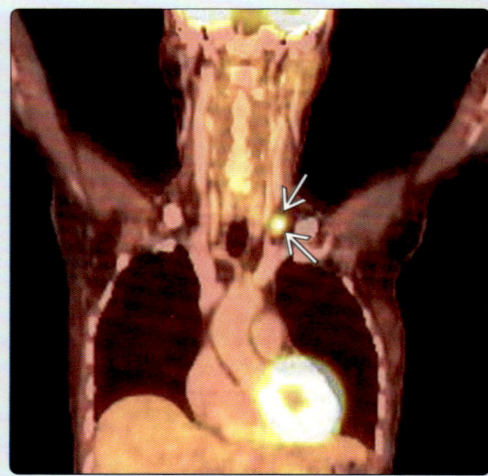

(Left) Coronal MPR CECT in a young man with a metastatic testicular mixed germ cell tumor shows a large left lower neck & supraclavicular confluent lymphadenopathy with some necrotic areas ➡. Also note mediastinal lymphadenopathy ➡. (Right) Coronal PET/CT in a patient with ovarian carcinoma reveals a single, enlarged FDG-avid left supraclavicular node (Virchow node) ➡. Virchow node lies near the junction of the thoracic duct (TD) and left subclavian vein, where lymph from most of the body via TD drains into venous circulation.

TERMINOLOGY

Definitions

- Cervical metastatic adenopathy in systemic malignancy from **infraclavicular primary** tumor
- **Virchow node**: Left supraclavicular nodal metastasis
  - Usually abdominal or pelvic primary malignancy

IMAGING

General Features

- Location
  - Most often lower neck, especially level V
  - Frequently unilateral
- Size
  - Lymph node imaging size criteria for pathology: Maximum **longitudinal** & minimum **axial** diameters
    - Levels I & II nodes: **15 mm** & **11 mm**
    - Retropharyngeal nodes: **8 mm** & **5 mm**
    - All other nodes: **10 mm** & **10 mm**
  - Longitudinal length/transaxial width (**L:T ratio**) < 2 suggest metastasis

CT Findings

- NECT
  - **Ca^{++}**: Systemic **adeno**carcinoma or thyroid Ca^{++}
- CECT
  - Round node > 1.5 cm or cluster of nodes
  - Nodes generally clustered in lower neck, mainly left
  - Homogeneous or heterogeneous enhancement
  - **Hyperenhancing metastatic nodes**: Renal cell Ca^{++}, neuroendocrine tumors, Kaposi sarcoma, thyroid Ca^{++}
  - Coronal reformations help differentiate enhancing node from subclavian vein

MR Findings

- T1WI
  - Cervical nodal mass usually isointense to muscle
- T2WI
  - Nodes slightly hyperintense compared to muscle
- T1WI C+
  - Variable enhancement; peripherally when nodes necrotic

Ultrasonographic Findings

- Grayscale ultrasound
  - Enlarged, round node, absent echogenic hilus, necrosis
  - **Early metastasis** with tiny, **subcapsular** nodal deposits & **normal** echogenic **hilus** if medullary sinuses uninvolved
  - Contrast-enhanced ultrasonography (CEUS): Metastatic lymph nodes show inhomogeneous enhancement in > 80% & centripetal perfusion in > 90%
- Color Doppler
  - Peripheral vascularity with absent or deformed normal hilar vascularity suggests replacement by tumor
  - Aberrant multifocal vessels, capsular vascularity
  - ↑ resistance index (RI) > 0.7 & pulsatility index (PI) > 1.5
  - Papillary thyroid carcinoma nodes may show lower RI/PI

Imaging Recommendations

- Best imaging tool
  - CECT best modality for assessing palpable cervical nodes
  - PET/CECT in known primary malignancy

DIFFERENTIAL DIAGNOSIS

Reactive Lymph Nodes

- Nodes more commonly in suprahyoid neck

Sarcoidosis Lymph Nodes

- Lower neck & mediastinal adenopathy common
- Nodes may be calcified

H&N Squamous Cell Carcinoma Metastatic Nodes

- Most commonly ipsilateral to SCCa in levels II & III nodes
- Worse prognosis in H&N SCCa with ↑ number of nodes & nodal chains, bilateral nodes, & lower level neck nodes
- Lymph node metastasis ↓ survival by 50%, doubles incidence of distant metastasis
- Extranodal extension: Further ↓ survival by 50%, 10-fold ↑ recurrence risk, & 3-fold ↑ risk of distant metastasis

Non-Hodgkin Lymphoma Nodes

- Large, usually nonnecrotic nodes throughout neck

PATHOLOGY

General Features

- Etiology
  - Disseminated malignancy from infraclavicular primary
  - Mainly from lung in males (65%), breast in females (41%)
  - Most prevalent pathology: Adenocarcinoma (65%); males 49% & females 84%
  - Most common site: Level V (85%)
  - Ipsilateral lymph node metastasis (60%), bilateral (27%), & exclusively contralateral (12%)

Gross Pathologic & Surgical Features

- Nodal mass > 3 cm = confluent metastatic nodes
- **Left** > right **lower** neck, probably as thoracic duct on left

Microscopic Features

- Neoplastic cells **first** localize **in subcapsular sinus**, then proliferate into body of node
- Focal altered/nonenhancement on CT or MR corresponds to nest of tumor cells or necrosis

CLINICAL ISSUES

Demographics

- Epidemiology
  - Systemic neck metastases < H&N SCCa nodes

Treatment

- Selective neck dissection may be performed for nodes
- Most patients undergo chemotherapy

DIAGNOSTIC CHECKLIST

Consider

- Screen for lung, breast, urogenital, & gastrointestinal primary malignancy after excluding H&N tumor, especially in levels IV & V lymphadenopathy & with adenocarcinoma

SELECTED REFERENCES

1. Rao JH et al: Cervical lymph nodes metastasis from non-head and neck primary carcinomas: a retrospective analysis of 1448 patients. Head Neck. 47(1):400-9, 2024

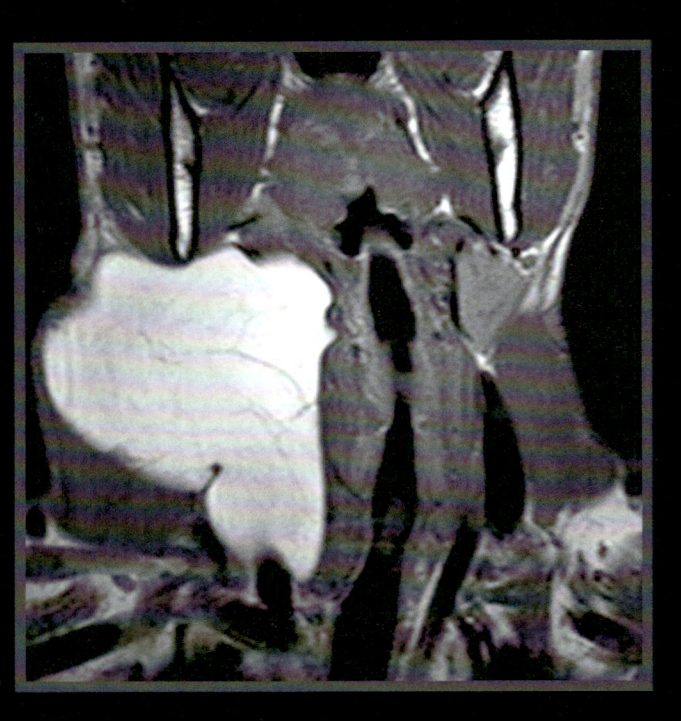

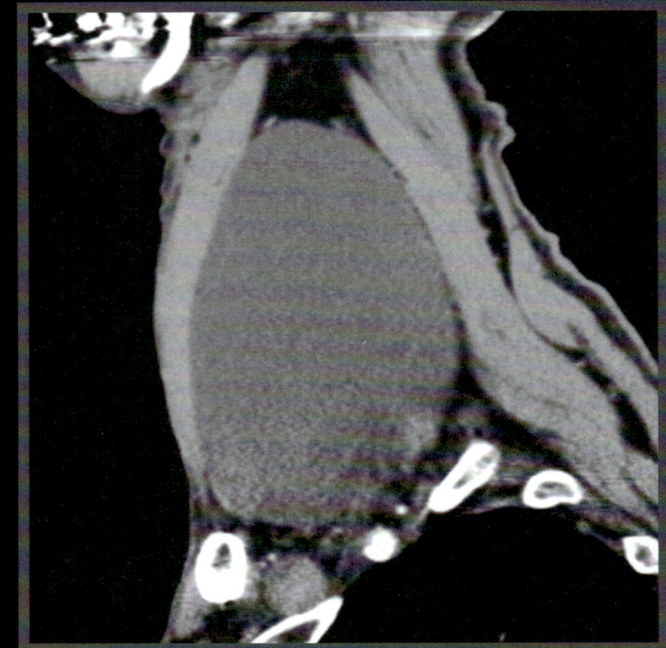

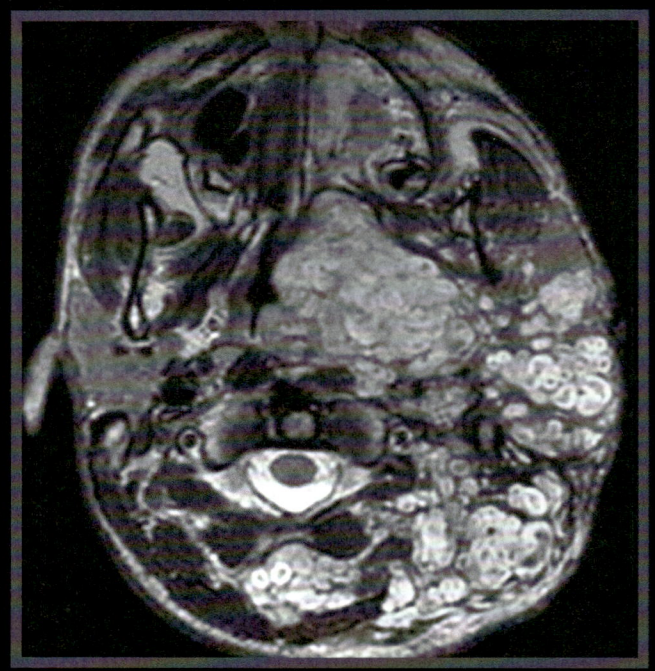

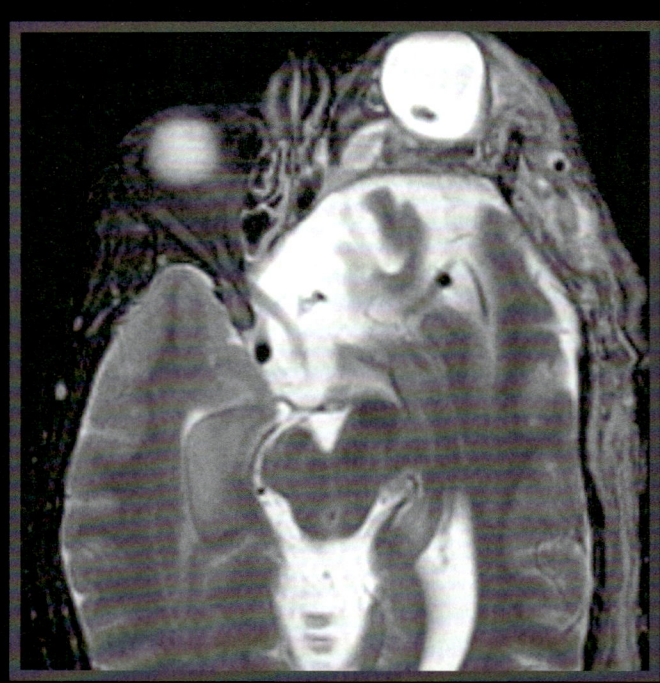

SECTION 13
Transspatial and Multispatial

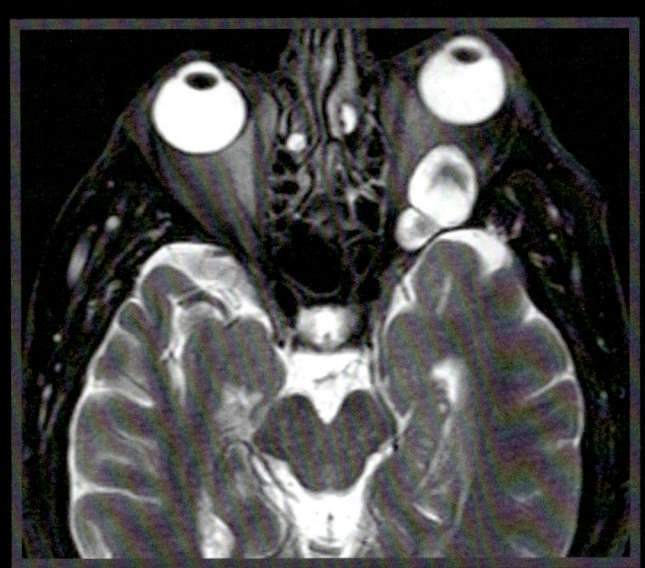

Summary Thoughts: Trans- and Multispatial Lesions

Transspatial and multispatial terms are used to describe specific subsets of lesions found in the head and neck. The **transspatial** descriptor is used to describe a lesion that involves multiple **contiguous** spaces or areas of the extracranial head and neck. **Multispatial** is applied to a lesion that is found in multiple **noncontiguous** spaces or areas.

Approaches to Imaging Issues in Trans- and Multispatial Lesions

Transspatial Lesions

Transspatial lesions are defined as involving multiple **contiguous** spaces or areas in the neck. In the soft tissues of the suprahyoid neck, infrahyoid neck, and oral cavity, where the anatomy can be defined by fascia-circumscribed spaces, this term is directly applicable. However, transspatial can also be used to describe a lesion that is contiguous through the skull base, sinuses, nasal cavity, and orbit where the anatomic areas are distinct but not fascia defined.

Transspatial lesions generally fall into 4 major pathologic categories: Congenital, inflammatory/infectious, benign tumor, and malignant tumor.

- **Congenital lesions** form at the same time or prior to fascia in the extracranial head and neck. As a result, they do not always stay within spatial boundaries and are often transspatial.
- **Inflammatory/infectious lesions** fall within the transspatial group when cellulitis, phlegmon, or abscess involves multiple contiguous spaces. In the case of abscess, defining each space involved for the surgeon ensures that each space is entered with either a probe or a drain.
- **Benign tumors**, such as infantile hemangioma and schwannoma, often involve multiple contiguous spaces. In the case of schwannoma, this is because the nerves that they form from normally run through multiple spaces as they course through the head and neck.
- **Malignant tumors** invade contiguous spaces as they enlarge; in fact, squamous cell carcinoma (SCCa) of the pharynx and oral cavity initially arises from the mucosal space/surface and immediately invades deeply into the surrounding soft tissue spaces. Larger SCCa primary tumors are almost always transspatial at presentation. Along with perineural tumor, the exact spaces invaded by primary SCCa determine tumor resectability and radiation ports.

Multispatial Lesions

Multispatial lesions of the head and neck occupy multiple **noncontiguous** spaces or areas.

Multispatial lesions generally fall into 3 pathologic categories: Congenital, inflammatory/infectious, and malignant tumors.

- **Lesions associated with syndromes**, which may be multispatial, include those found in patients with neurofibromatosis types 1 and 2, PHACE syndrome, and other syndromes that have multiple noncontiguous manifestations.
- **Inflammatory/infectious nodal disease** is commonly multispatial at presentation; reactive nodes may progress to suppurative nodes (intranodal abscesses); tuberculous adenopathy may also be multispatial; any of the many rarer nodal diseases of the head and neck may

also present as multispatial (Castleman disease; IgG4-related disease).
- **Malignant tumors** of the head and neck are often transspatial in their primary site and multispatial in their nodal spread; oral cavity and pharyngeal SCCas and non-Hodgkin lymphoma (NHL) (of Waldeyer lymphatic ring) are both prone to this behavior; Hodgkin lymphoma neck nodes and systemic nodal metastases may also be multispatial in the head and neck.

Transspatial Diseases of Head and Neck

Congenital Lesions
- Venous malformation
- Lymphatic malformation
- Branchial cleft cysts
- Thyroglossal duct cyst
- Thymic cyst
- Neurofibromatosis type 1 (plexiform neurofibroma)

Inflammatory/Infectious Lesions
- Cellulitis
- Phlegmon
- Abscess
- Invasive fungal sinusitis
- Sinonasal granulomatosis with polyangiitis (GPA)
- Fibromatosis

Benign Tumors
- Schwannoma
- Neurofibroma
- Infantile hemangioma
- Solitary fibrous tumor

Malignant Tumors
- Pharyngeal SCCa
- NHL, extranodal
- Rhabdomyosarcoma
- Anaplastic carcinoma of thyroid
- Sinonasal SCCa
- Sinonasal undifferentiated carcinoma (SNUC)
- Olfactory neuroblastoma
- Chondrosarcoma of skull base
- Chordoma of skull base

Multispatial Diseases of Head and Neck

Lesions Associated With Syndromes
- Neurofibromatosis type 1
- Neurofibromatosis type 2
- PHACE association

Inflammatory/Infectious Lesions
- Reactive adenopathy
- Suppurative adenopathy
- Tuberculous adenopathy
- IgG4-related disease

Malignant Tumors
- Pharyngeal SCCa + malignant nodes
- NHL extranodal + nodal
- Systemic metastases
- Metastatic neuroblastoma

Selected References

1. ISSVA Classification of Vascular Anomalies: 2025 International Society for the Study of Vascular Anomalies. Published 2025. Accessed April 25, 2025. https://www.issva.org/classification
2. Charlton A et al: Deep neck space infections: a UK centre, two-year, retrospective review of 53 cases. J Laryngol Otol. 138(12):1161-19, 2024

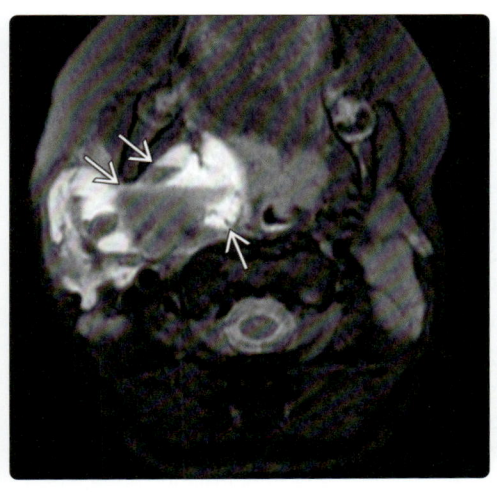

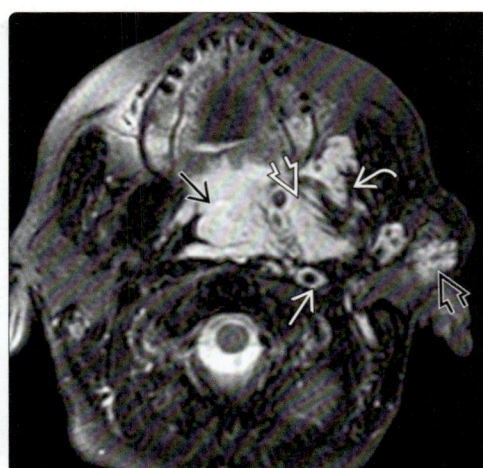

(Left) *Axial T2WI FS MR in a 2-year-old boy shows an extensive, transspatial, macrocystic lymphatic malformation involving the right parapharyngeal, carotid, and parotid spaces, causing moderate mass effect on the oropharynx and containing several fluid-fluid levels ➡ secondary to intralesional hemorrhage.* (Right) *Axial T2WI FS MR in a patient with a large venous malformation shows transspatial involvement of the pharyngeal mucosal ➡, parapharyngeal ➡, masticator ➡, carotid ➡, and parotid ➡ spaces.*

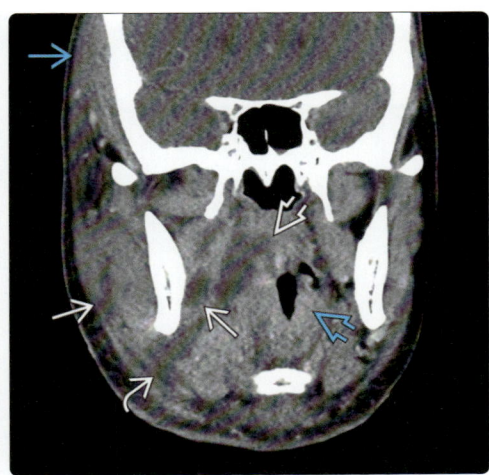

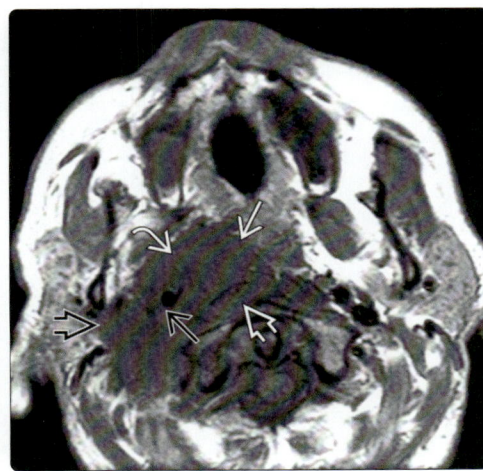

(Left) *Coronal CECT in a septic patient with trismus reveals a transspatial infection in the deep face. There are abscesses in the parapharyngeal ➡, masticator ➡, and submandibular ➡ spaces. Note superior extension of infection ➡ and airway compromise ➡.* (Right) *Axial T1WI MR demonstrates an invasive, transspatial nasopharyngeal carcinoma. This nasopharyngeal mucosal space carcinoma ➡ has directly invaded the parapharyngeal ➡, perivertebral ➡, carotid ➡, and parotid ➡ spaces.*

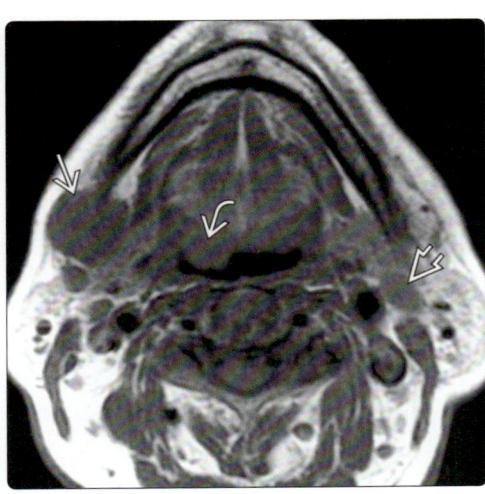

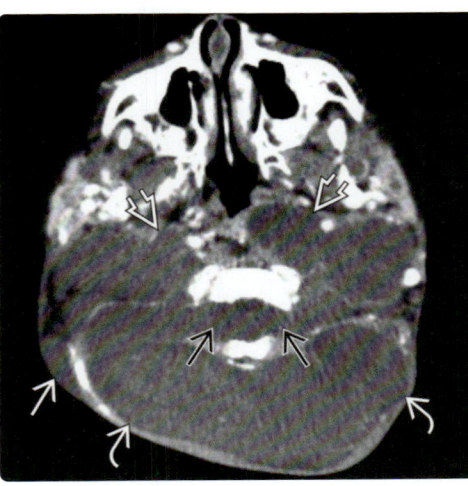

(Left) *Axial T1WI MR in a patient with multiple H&N lesions shows abnormal lymph nodes in the submandibular ➡ and parotid ➡ spaces accompanied by a focal mass in the pharyngeal mucosal space ➡ (lingual tonsil). This example of multispatial disease is caused by non-Hodgkin lymphoma.* (Right) *Axial CECT in a 7-year-old boy with neurofibromatosis type 1 reveals multispatial, low-attenuation neurofibromas in the superficial ➡, carotid ➡, and perivertebral ➡ spaces in addition to the cervical neural foramina ➡.*

TERMINOLOGY

- Synonym: Left lymphatic duct, thoracic duct elements
- Normal anatomic structure draining lymph and chyle from abdomen and left chest to venous circulation

IMAGING

- Tubular structure of fluid density/intensity
- Average diameter: 4-5 mm
- Courses cranially in **left** lower neck posterior to common carotid artery
- Laterally drains into junction of internal jugular vein and subclavian vein

TOP DIFFERENTIAL DIAGNOSES

- Squamous cell carcinoma necrotic (cystic) lymph node
- Necrotic (cystic) nodal metastasis from systemic disease
- Differentiated thyroid carcinoma (cystic) lymph node
- Lymphocele
- 4th branchial anomaly

PATHOLOGY

- Drains lymph and chyle from abdomen and left chest to venous circulation
- Right-sided thoracic duct (very uncommon) drains into right subclavian vein

CLINICAL ISSUES

- Incidental normal finding
- Obstruction results in pleural effusion (chylothorax)
- Probable source of metastasis to left supraclavicular node (Virchow node)

DIAGNOSTIC CHECKLIST

- Key imaging features
  - Tubular structure in left supraclavicular neck
    - Less commonly on right side
  - Isodense/isointense to CSF
- May be mistaken for cystic level IV or VI lymph node
- May be mistaken for 4th branchial anomaly

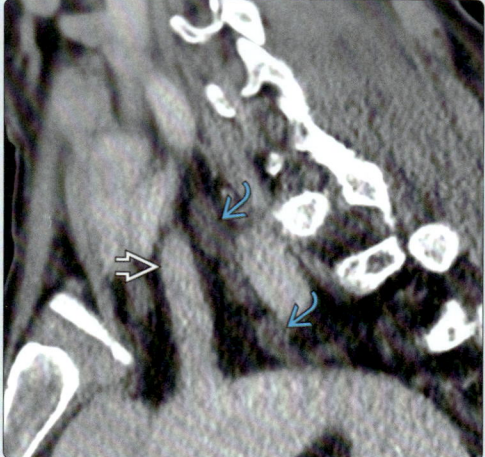 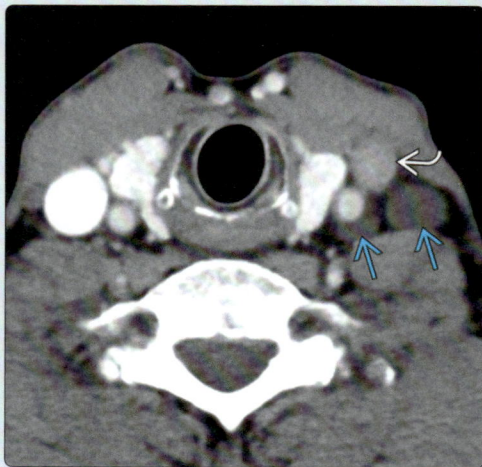

(Left) *Sagittal CECT demonstrates a tubular, varicose, low-density thoracic duct ➦ ascending from the chest posterior to the left carotid artery ➥, which may be mistaken for a thrombosed vessel.* **(Right)** *Axial CECT shows varicose appearances of the thoracic duct in a more lateral location ➦ as it courses toward its terminus at the junction of the internal jugular vein and subclavian vein ➥. The thoracic duct mimics lymph nodes on axial cross-section imaging.*

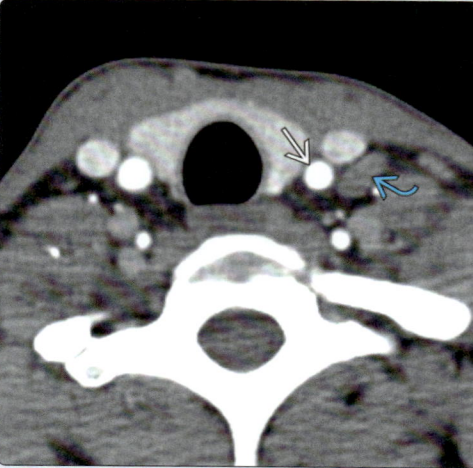 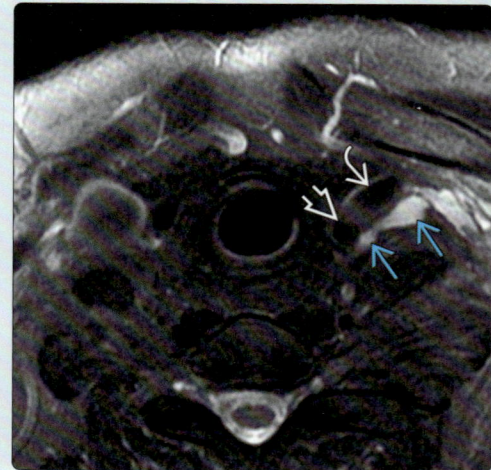

(Left) *Axial CECT shows a typical oval and slightly tubular appearance of the normal thoracic duct ➦ as it curves behind the common carotid artery ➥. The duct could be traced on sequential images (not shown) to its drainage into the left subclavian vein.* **(Right)** *Axial T2FS MR shows the thoracic duct ➦ as a high T2 varicose structure posterior to the left common carotid artery ➥ and internal jugular vein ➥. The thoracic duct appears isointense to CSF on all sequences.*

TERMINOLOGY

Synonyms

- Enlarged cervical lymphatic duct, thoracic duct dilation/distention, thoracic duct elements

Definitions

- Thoracic duct: Normal anatomic structure draining lymph from abdomen and left chest into venous circulation

IMAGING

General Features

- Best diagnostic clue
  - Tubular structure of fluid density/intensity coursing superiorly from chest into neck, posterior to common carotid artery, then laterally into lymphovenous junction (commonly left internal jugular and subclavian vein junction)
- Location
  - Left lower neck posterior to carotid sheath
- Size
  - Average diameter: 4-5 mm
  - Courses 3-4 cm above clavicle in neck
- Morphology
  - Tubular structure
  - Appears varicose, commonly dilating before its termination

Ultrasonographic Findings

- Cystic tubular structure ± flow into lymphovenous junction

Imaging Recommendations

- Best imaging tool
  - Evident on > 80% of CT exams and most US scans
  - Most readily seen on 3D T2 MR with fat saturation

CT Findings

- CECT
  - Nonenhancing, tubular structure
  - On axial images, may be mistaken for node
  - Fluid density without surrounding inflammatory changes

MR Findings

- Always follows fluid signal: ↓ T1, ↑ T2

DIFFERENTIAL DIAGNOSIS

Squamous Cell Carcinoma Nodes

- Squamous cell carcinoma (SCCa) nodes can be necrotic
- Level IV or VI are drainage sites from larynx/hypopharynx or from SCCa nodes more superiorly
- Other nodes usually present

Nodal Metastasis From Systemic Disease

- Left supraclavicular nodal metastasis from chest and abdomen (signal node or Virchow node)

Differentiated Thyroid Carcinoma Nodes

- Thyroid carcinoma nodes may be cystic
- Variable MR signal due to colloid or hemorrhage
  - May be ↑ T1 prior to contrast
- Other nodes usually present

- Differentiated thyroid carcinoma nodes can have variable MR appearances even in same patient

Lymphocele/Thoracic Duct Cyst

- Idiopathic or postsurgical lymph-filled neck cyst
- Supraclavicular fossa, L > R

4th Branchial Anomaly

- More anterior at level of or within left thyroid gland
- Responsible for recurrent suppurative left thyroiditis

PATHOLOGY

General Features

- Etiology
  - Normal anatomic structure
  - Drains lymph from abdomen and left chest into venous circulation

Gross Pathologic & Surgical Features

- Valves at thoracic duct terminus prevent reflux of blood from venous system
- May divide into 2 branches with right lymphatic duct draining into right internal jugular and subclavian vein junction

CLINICAL ISSUES

Presentation

- Most common signs/symptoms
  - Asymptomatic; incidental imaging finding

Demographics

- Age
  - Slightly ↑ in diameter with age
- Sex
  - M = F

Natural History & Prognosis

- Obstruction may result in pleural effusion (chylothorax)
- Probable source of metastases to left supraclavicular nodes

DIAGNOSTIC CHECKLIST

Consider

- Incidental normal finding
- May be mistaken for necrotic (cystic) level IV or VI node
  - Consider history of systemic malignancy or differentiated thyroid carcinoma

Image Interpretation Pearls

- Key imaging features are tubular morphology and fluid intensity/density

SELECTED REFERENCES

1. Kanavaros P et al: The right lymphatic duct: basic anatomy and clinical relevance. Vasa. 53(6):371-7, 2024
2. Negm AS et al: MR lymphangiography in lymphatic disorders: clinical applications, institutional experience, and practice development. Radiographics. 44(2):e230075, 2024
3. Plutecki D et al: The anatomy of the thoracic duct and cisterna chyli: a meta-analysis with surgical implications. J Clin Med. 13(15), 2024
4. Chen L et al: Application of imaging technique in thoracic duct anatomy. Ann Palliat Med. 9(3):1249-56, 2020
5. Johnson OW et al: The thoracic duct: clinical importance, anatomic variation, imaging, and embolization. Eur Radiol. 26(8):2482-93, 2016

KEY FACTS

TERMINOLOGY

- Benign neoplasm composed of mature fat

IMAGING

- 15% of lipomas occur in head & neck
- 5% are multiple, more often in female patients
- May occur in any head & neck space & may be transspatial
- Well-circumscribed, homogeneous mass composed of fat and displacing normal structures
- Homogeneous fat with minimal internal stranding
  - 8% have small, nonfatty soft tissue component
- CT: Homogeneous, well-defined, low-density mass
- MR: Homogeneous signal of subcutaneous fat
- CT or MR: Any enhancement or soft tissue raises concern for liposarcoma
- FDG PET: No uptake in bland benign lipoma
  - Uptake suggests sarcoma or lipoma variant

TOP DIFFERENTIAL DIAGNOSES

- Dermoid
- Teratoma
- Lymphatic malformation
- Liposarcoma
- HIV-associated lipodystrophy

CLINICAL ISSUES

- Asymptomatic lump in neck, more often in male patients
- Clinical differential is lymphatic malformation
- Most often found in 5th-6th decades

DIAGNOSTIC CHECKLIST

- CT: Measure density to determine fat content
- MR: Use chemical-selective fat-saturation techniques, not STIR, to prove fat content
- If lipoma has soft tissue or enhancement, cannot distinguish from well-differentiated liposarcoma

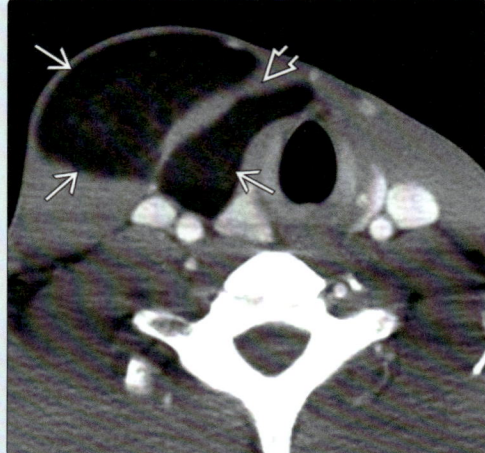
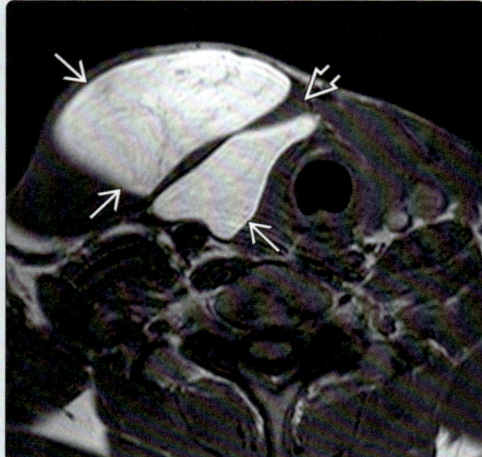

(Left) Axial CECT through the lower neck of a young adult with a prominent neck mass demonstrates a well-defined, low-density right neck mass ➡. Mass herniates around the anterior portion of the omohyoid muscle ➡ and displaces tissues with no evidence of infiltration. (Right) Axial T1WI MR in the same patient 6 weeks later shows an intrinsically hyperintense mass ➡ enveloping the omohyoid ➡ without invasion of adjacent tissues. The mass was thought to have enlarged clinically.

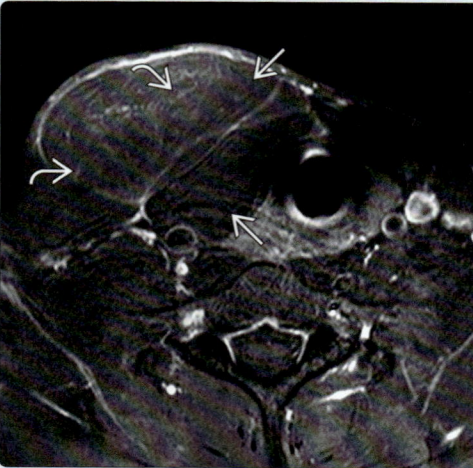
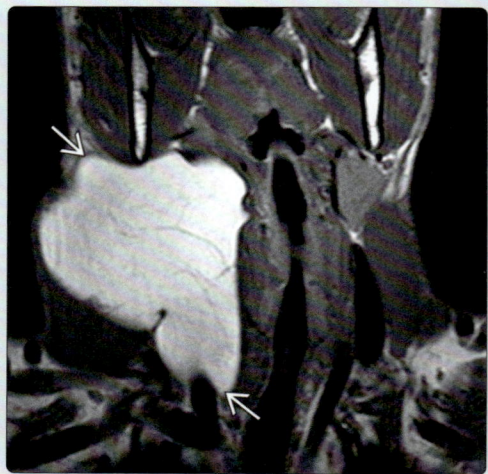

(Left) Axial T1WI C+ FS MR in the same patient reveals suppression of the high-intensity fat within the mass ➡, while also showing mildly complicated, fibrous internal architecture ➡. (Right) Coronal T1WI MR in the same patient illustrates the craniocaudad extent of the mass ➡. Scan also shows mass effect on larynx, which was deviated to a greater extent across midline than on prior CT, raising concern for liposarcoma rather than lipoma. Resection of the mass showed mature adipose tissue of benign lipoma.

TERMINOLOGY

Definitions

- Benign neoplasm composed of mature fat

IMAGING

General Features

- Best diagnostic clue
  - Well-circumscribed, homogeneous mass composed of fat, displacing normal structures
- Location
  - 15% of lipomas occur in head & neck
  - 5% are multiple, more often in female patients
  - May occur in any head & neck space; may be transspatial
  - Most common sites in head & neck
    - Posterior cervical, submandibular spaces
    - Anterior cervical, parotid spaces
- Size
  - Highly variable; may become massive
- Morphology
  - Well-defined mass with thin capsule & smooth contours
  - Majority have homogeneous fat content with **minimal** internal stranding
  - 8% of benign lipomas have small, nonfatty soft tissue component
    - **Cannot be distinguished from well-differentiated liposarcoma** by imaging

CT Findings

- NECT
  - Homogeneous, well-defined, low-attenuation mass
    - Fat density = -65 to -120 HU
- CECT
  - Well-defined, low-density, nonenhancing mass
  - Any significant enhancement raises concern for liposarcoma

MR Findings

- T1WI
  - Homogeneous, hyperintense mass; follows signal of subcutaneous fat
  - Uniform signal loss on FS images
- T2WI
  - Follows signal intensity of subcutaneous fat
- T1WI C+
  - No enhancement on T1WI C+ FS
  - Any significant matrix enhancement raises concern for liposarcoma

Ultrasonographic Findings

- Well-defined, compressible mass
- Multiple echogenic lines oriented parallel to skin
- 75% hyperechoic, 25% iso-/hypoechoic relative to muscle
- No deep acoustic enhancement or attenuation

Imaging Recommendations

- Best imaging tool
  - CT or MR both clearly determine fat content
  - Imaging is diagnostic, defines deep extent & pertinent anatomic relations
- Protocol advice
  - Use **chemical-selective fat-saturation** rather than STIR to prove lipid content

Nuclear Medicine Findings

- PET/CT
  - Typically no uptake in benign lipoma
  - FDG uptake suggests liposarcoma
  - Uptake may be seen in (benign) hibernoma
  - Mild uptake in angiolipoma also described

DIFFERENTIAL DIAGNOSIS

Dermoid

- In head & neck, most often floor of mouth; less commonly, submandibular
- Thin-walled, unilocular cyst with enhancing rim
- Contents usually heterogeneous mixture of fat & fluid
  - Uniform fat, globules of fat, or fat-fluid levels

Teratoma

- Neoplasm arising from all 3 embryonic germ cell layers
- Typically multiloculated, large masses with complex imaging; may contain fat

Lymphatic Malformation

- Key clinical differential diagnosis for lipoma
- Thin-walled, uni- or multilocular cystic mass

Liposarcoma

- Solid mass typically with some fat component; usually enhances
- Well-differentiated liposarcoma may exactly mimic lipoma with stranding
- Plasma D-dimer levels may help differentiate lipoma from liposarcoma

HIV-Associated Lipodystrophy

- Consequence of antiretroviral therapy
- 2 phenotypes: Fat accumulation (lipohypertrophy) or fat loss (lipoatrophy)
- Lipohypertrophy occurs in midline dorsal neck
  - Causes bullfrog neck or buffalo hump appearance

PATHOLOGY

General Features

- Etiology
  - Most common benign mesenchymal tumor
  - Fat in lipoma is unavailable for systemic metabolism
    - Lipoma responds minimally to systemic weight changes
    - Lipoma may become more prominent after systemic weight loss
- Genetics
  - 80% of solitary lipomas have genetic aberration: 12q, 6p, 13q
- Associated abnormalities
  - Several syndromes associated with lipomas/lipomatosis
    - **Benign symmetric lipomatosis (Madelung disease)**
      - Diffuse, symmetric, unencapsulated fatty accumulation
      - Most commonly neck & upper back

□ Posterior superficial, posterior cervical, anterior cervical, & perivertebral spaces

□ Middle-aged men of Mediterranean descent; history of alcohol abuse

– **Familial multiple lipomatosis**

□ Multiple small, well-demarcated, encapsulated lipomas

□ Commonly extremities, sparing neck & shoulders

□ Strong familial component

– **Dercum disease**

□ Rare condition with multiple painful lipomas

□ Typically on extremities of obese postmenopausal women

– **Gardner syndrome**

□ Osteomas, soft tissue tumors, & colonic adenomatous polyps

□ Soft tissue tumors: **Lipoma**, fibroma, leiomyoma, neurofibroma, & desmoid tumors

Gross Pathologic & Surgical Features

- Typically encapsulated, smooth or lobulated, soft yellow masses
- **Benign pathologic variants of lipoma**
  - **Fibrolipoma**
    - Mature fibrous tissue associated with lipoma
  - **Infiltrating lipoma** (intramuscular lipoma)
    - Unencapsulated, mature adipose tissue that infiltrates adjacent tissues
    - High risk of recurrence if intramuscular extensions not meticulously dissected
    - Uncommon in head & neck region
  - **Angiolipoma**
    - Fatty tumor separated by enhancing small vessels
    - Often painful, may be multiple
    - Rare in head & neck region, usually extremities
    - Tend to be found around puberty
  - **Spindle cell lipoma**
    - Variable proportions of mature fat & fibroblast-like spindle cells
    - Typically subcutaneous tissues of posterior neck
    - Indistinguishable from liposarcoma
    - 4th-6th decades, M > > F
  - **Hibernoma**
    - Benign, encapsulated tumor consisting of brown fat, usually mixed with mature adipose tissue
    - Imaging characteristics depends on proportion of mature fat vs. brown fat
    - Brown fat has imaging characteristics similar to muscle ± enhancement
    - FDG uptake reported; may see variable uptake over time
  - **Lipoblastoma**
    - Focal fatty tumor or diffuse lipoblastomatosis
    - Benign pediatric lesion; almost all patients < 5 years age
    - Rarely in head & neck, usually in extremities

Microscopic Features

- Composed of mature adipocytes that are uniform in size & shape
  - No necrosis, atypia, or increased mitotic rate

- Occasional fibrous connective tissue septations

CLINICAL ISSUES

Presentation

- Most common signs/symptoms
  - Asymptomatic lump in neck
    - Clinically may be mistaken for lymphatic malformation
  - Stable size after initial period of discernible growth
- Other signs/symptoms
  - Large masses may present with symptoms attributable to compression of surrounding structures
- Clinical profile
  - Male patient with asymptomatic, compressible neck mass

Demographics

- Age
  - Most often found in 5th-6th decades
- Sex
  - M > F

Natural History & Prognosis

- Benign, slowly enlarging mass
- Recurrence after excision suggests liposarcoma or inadequately resected infiltrating lipoma

Treatment

- Typically not resected unless compressing structures, such as airway, or for cosmetic reasons

DIAGNOSTIC CHECKLIST

Consider

- Carefully evaluate for presence of internal nodularity, enhancement, or stranding
  - These features raise possibility of liposarcoma
  - Be sure to articulate this in report

Image Interpretation Pearls

- Contrast-enhancing components suggest liposarcoma
- CT: Measure HU to prove fat content
- MR: Use **chemical-selective fat-saturation** techniques, not STIR, to confirm fat content

Reporting Tips

- Define full extent of lesion, specifically all spaces involved & tissues displaced

SELECTED REFERENCES

1. Guzman N et al: HIV-associated lipodystrophy. StatPearls, 2025
2. Lee SJ et al: Giant lipoma in the anterior region of the neck: a case report of a rare condition and review of literature. Radiol Case Rep. 20(7):3197-200, 2025
3. Schranz AL et al: Retrospective analysis of radiological investigation of surgically excised head and neck lipomas. Eur Arch Otorhinolaryngol. 281(8):4333-9, 2024
4. Chrysovitsiotis G et al: Retropharyngeal space lipomas. a systematic review of the reported cases in the literature. Indian J Otolaryngol Head Neck Surg. 74(Suppl 3):5630-8, 2022
5. Kale HA et al: Fat: friend or foe? A review of fat-containing masses within the head and neck. Br J Radiol. 89(1067):20150811, 2016
6. Gritzmann N et al: Sonography of soft tissue masses of the neck. J Clin Ultrasound. 30(6):356-73, 2002

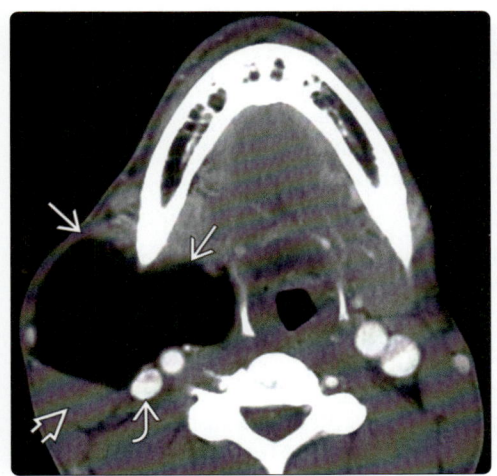
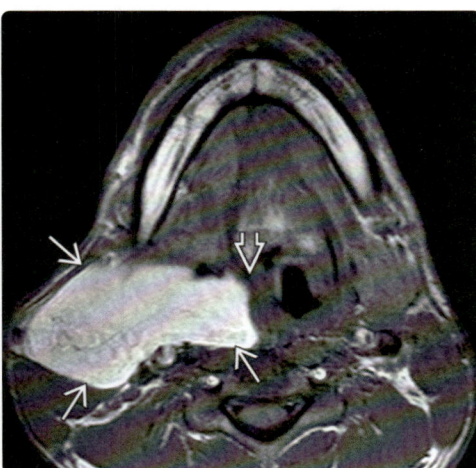

(Left) *Axial CECT shows a very low-density, uniform, well-defined lesion ➡ in the right neck that presented as a "parotid mass." The mass displaces sternocleidomastoid muscle ➡ and carotid and jugular ➡ vessels posteriorly with no aggressive invasive features.* **(Right)** *Axial T1WI MR in the same patient without gadolinium reveals uniform hyperintensity of the mass ➡ abutting pharyngeal wall ➡ and displacing the pharynx to left. Fat-saturated T2 and postcontrast T1 images displayed complete suppression of signal.*

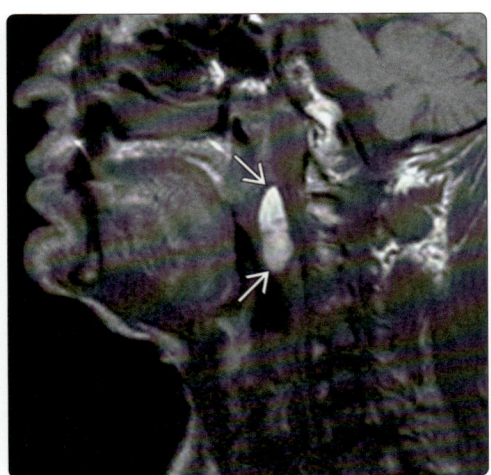
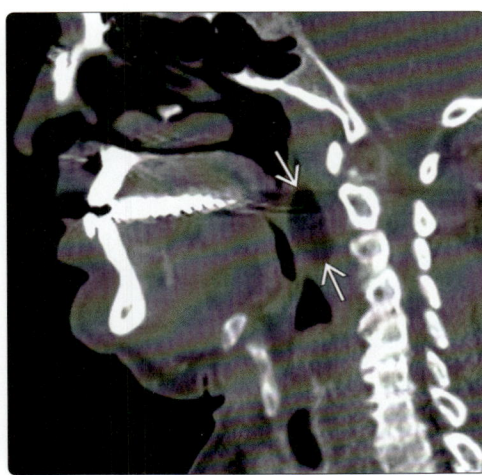

(Left) *Sagittal T1WI MR without gadolinium shows a slightly lobulated, intrinsically hyperintense, well-defined mass ➡ in the retropharyngeal space. The mass was evident on clinical examination as fullness of the right posterior oropharyngeal wall.* **(Right)** *Sagittal CECT reformation in the same patient 5 years later shows no evidence of change in size or contour of mass ➡, which shows homogeneous fat density and no evidence of enhancement within or surrounding it. Stability favors benign lipoma.*

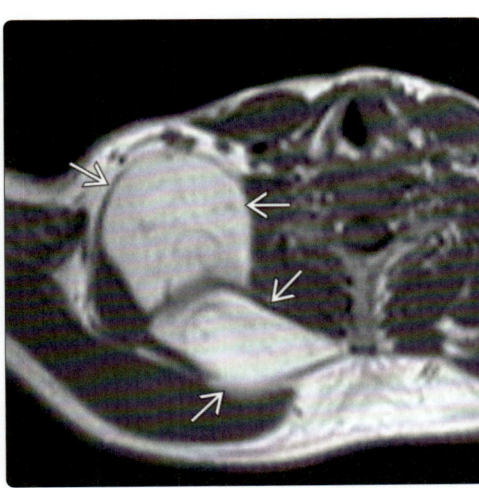
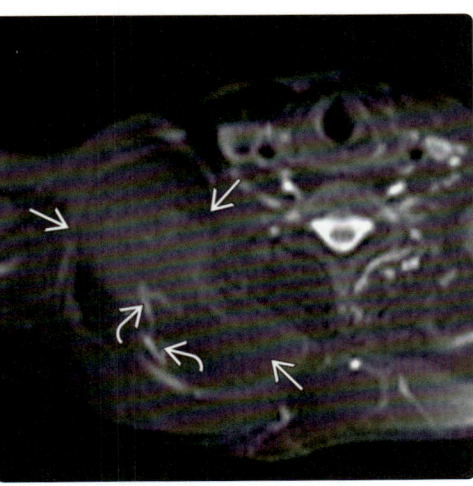

(Left) *Axial T1WI MR in a 53-year-old man with a prior history of coccyx liposarcoma and now a shoulder mass shows a lobulated mass ➡ in the right supraclavicular paraspinal region. The mass is intrinsically hyperintense.* **(Right)** *Axial T2WI FS MR shows almost complete suppression of signal intensity, except for normal vessels ➡ associated with the mass. No abnormal gadolinium enhancement or other features to suggest sarcomatous lesion are evident. The resected mass ➡ proved to be benign lipoma.*

KEY FACTS

TERMINOLOGY

- WHO 2020 solitary fibrous tumor (SFT)
- Uncommon, slow-growing fibroblastic mesenchymal neoplasm with variable degree of malignant potential

IMAGING

- Most SFTs occur in lower extremities, pelvis
- 15% occur in head & neck
  - Intracranial/meningeal: Parasellar & paraclival
  - Orbit, cervical soft tissues, sinonasal cavity
- CT findings
  - Well circumscribed, lobular, avidly enhancing; more invasive behavior if high grade (CECT)
  - May see bone erosion or remodeling (bone CT)
- MR findings
  - Intermediate T1, high T2 signal
  - Vascular **flow voids** common
  - Prominent enhancement, typically uniform

TOP DIFFERENTIAL DIAGNOSES

- Skull base meningioma
- Skull base metastasis
- Skull base trigeminal schwannoma
- Clivus chordoma
- Orbital venous malformation
- Sinonasal angiomatous polyp

PATHOLOGY

- **Non-CNS SFTs graded by histology and tumor behavior**
  - Mitotic activity, necrosis, pleomorphism, aggressive features

CLINICAL ISSUES

- Resection is treatment of choice ± XRT
- Local recurrence in ≤ 50%; 30% metastasize < 10 years
- SFT mimics many more common tumors
- Consider SFT if avidly enhancing, well-circumscribed mass
- Signs and symptoms depend on tumor location

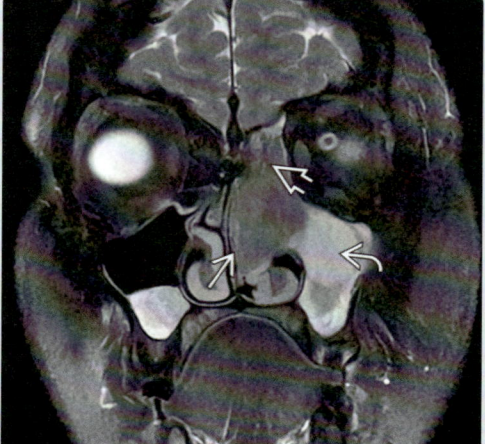
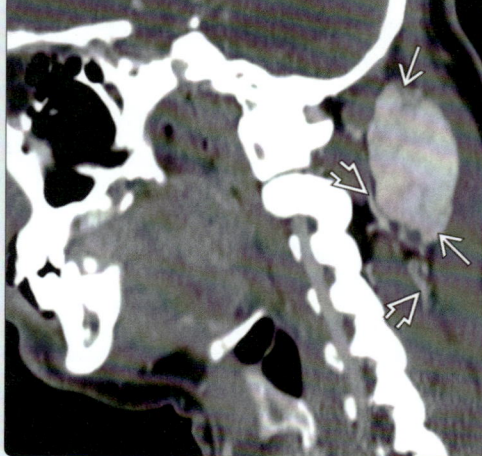

(Left) Coronal T2 MR in a 45-year-old woman with nasal congestion shows a mass in the left nasal cavity ➡ with intermediate signal. Branching curvilinear hypointensity is suspicious for hypervascularity ⮞. Trapped secretions are relatively hyperintense ➡ compared to the mass. (Right) Sagittal reconstructed CECT reveals a densely enhancing mass ➡ in the suboccipital musculature with prominent vasculature adjacent to the lesion ⮞. Paraspinal soft tissues are a characteristic location of cervical solitary fibrous tumor.

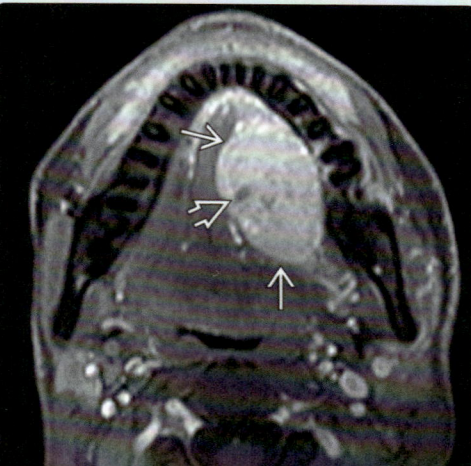
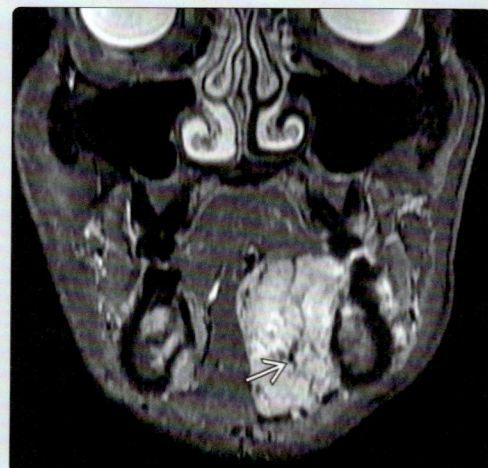

(Left) Axial T1 C+ FS MR in a 36-year-old woman shows a sublingual solitary fibrous tumor ➡. The mass predominantly has marked enhancement, with small areas of relative hypointensity ⮞ representing cystic change. (Right) Coronal T2 FS MR in the same patient shows extensive flow voids ➡ in the left sublingual space mass, consistent with hypervascularity.

Solitary Fibrous Tumor

TERMINOLOGY

Abbreviations
- Solitary fibrous tumor (SFT)

Synonyms
- Hemangiopericytoma (HPC), term no longer recommended

Definitions
- Uncommon, slow-growing fibroblastic mesenchymal neoplasm with intermediate biologic behavior
- WHO 2020 restructured SFT/HPC as SFT

IMAGING

General Features
- Best diagnostic clue
  - Well-circumscribed, avidly enhancing, solid mass
- Location
  - Any location: Most common in lower extremities, retroperitoneum, abdomen/pelvis
  - 15% in head & neck
    - Intracranial/meningeal: Parasellar & paraclival
    - Retrobulbar orbit
    - Cervical paraspinal soft tissues
    - Sinonasal: Nasal cavity, maxillary sinus
- Size
  - SFT of head and neck presents at smaller size than elsewhere in the body, average 4.5 cm

CT Findings
- Lobular, exophytic mass
- May erode or remodel bone
- Prominent enhancement: Homogeneous > heterogeneous

MR Findings
- Intermediate T1 signal
- High T2 signal, frequently with vascular flow voids
- Prominent enhancement: Homogeneous > heterogeneous

Angiographic Findings
- Early florid "blush"
- Enlarged feeding & draining vessels c/w hypervascularity

DIFFERENTIAL DIAGNOSIS

Skull Base Meningioma
- More often sessile + dural tail, calcification, hyperostosis

Skull Base Metastasis
- May be indistinguishable from SFT

Skull Base Trigeminal Schwannoma
- Meckel cave; remodels bone without destruction

Clivus Chordoma
- T2-hyperintense, midline destructive clival lesion

Venous Malformation, Orbit
- Soft, distensible retrobulbar masses
- May enhance but to lesser degree than SFT

Sinonasal Angiomatous Polyp
- Intensely enhancing, noninvasive nasal mass

PATHOLOGY

Staging, Grading, & Classification
- WHO 2020 now uses SFT designation: Non-CNS SFTs classified by histologic features and clinical behavior
  - Benign: Locally invasive, well circumscribed, slow growing, low mitotic activity, no necrosis
  - Not otherwise specified: Not clearly benign or malignant, some aggressive features
  - Malignant: High mitotic activity, pleomorphism, necrosis, higher risk recurrence/metastasis

Microscopic Features
- Arise from pericytes of Zimmerman
- SFT has paracentric inversion at 12q13, fusing *NAB2* & *STAT6* genes, which leads to STAT6 nuclear expression detected by immunohistochemistry

CLINICAL ISSUES

Presentation
- Most common signs/symptoms
  - Presentation depends on site of tumor
    - Skull base: Cranial neuropathy, ophthalmoplegia
    - Orbit: Painless proptosis
    - Cervical soft tissue: Painless mass
    - Sinonasal: Nasal obstruction, epistaxis

Demographics
- Age: Wide range (peaks in 4th decade)
- Epidemiology: Rare tumor

Natural History & Prognosis
- Local recurrence in 50%; 30% metastasize < 10 years
- Metastases, most frequently to lung
- Sinonasal lesions have more indolent course

Treatment
- Wide local excision is main treatment
- Radiation used for high-grade tumor, positive surgical margins, or recurrence
- Monitor for recurrence for > 10 years

DIAGNOSTIC CHECKLIST

Consider
- Include SFT in differential for **avidly enhancing, well-circumscribed masses**
  - **Mimicker** of many more common lesions

SELECTED REFERENCES

1. Laxague F et al: Solitary fibrous tumor of the parapharyngeal space: report of 2 cases and a literature review. Oral Maxillofac Surg. 28(3):1415-21, 2024
2. Ren C et al: Advances in the molecular biology of the solitary fibrous tumor and potential impact on clinical applications. Cancer Metastasis Rev. 43(4):1337-52, 2024
3. Liu H et al: Head and neck hemangiopericytoma: a rare case report and literature review. Ear Nose Throat J. 1455613231191379, 2023
4. Tariq MU et al: Solitary fibrous tumor of head and neck region; a clinicopathological study of 67 cases emphasizing the diversity of histological features and utility of various risk stratification models. Pathol Res Pract. 249:154777, 2023
5. Kallen ME et al: The 2020 WHO Classification: what's new in soft tissue tumor pathology? Am J Surg Pathol. 45(1):e1-23, 2021

TERMINOLOGY

- Plexiform neurofibroma (PNF): Architecturally complex neurofibroma involving multiple nerve fascicles
  - **Pathognomonic for neurofibromatosis type 1 (NF1)**

IMAGING

- **Lobular, serpentine, infiltrative transspatial mass**
- CECT has nonspecific, infiltrative appearance
  - Mild or minimal contrast enhancement
- MR best characterizes and delineates complete extent
  - Lobulated T2 hyperintensity
  - Central T2-hypointense foci: **Target sign**

TOP DIFFERENTIAL DIAGNOSES

- Venous malformation
- Lymphatic malformation
- Sarcoma

PATHOLOGY

- Deletion in *NF1* gene on long arm of **chromosome 17**
- Autosomal dominant inheritance, 50% spontaneous mutation
- ↓ production of neurofibromin (tumor suppressor) protein

CLINICAL ISSUES

- Present at birth or develops with age
- Bag of worms appearance on clinical exam
- PNFs in **~ 30% of patients with NF1**
- 5-10% risk of malignant transformation

DIAGNOSTIC CHECKLIST

- On CECT, appears as infiltrative, solid mass; occasionally appears cystic, may mimic lymphatic malformation
- On MR, may mimic venous malformation; distinguish with target sign and lack of phleboliths
- Look for other manifestations of NF1

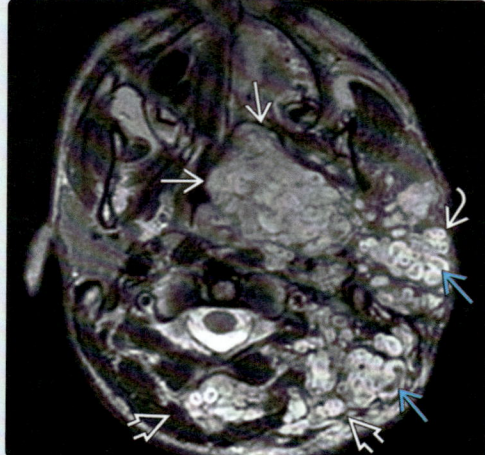
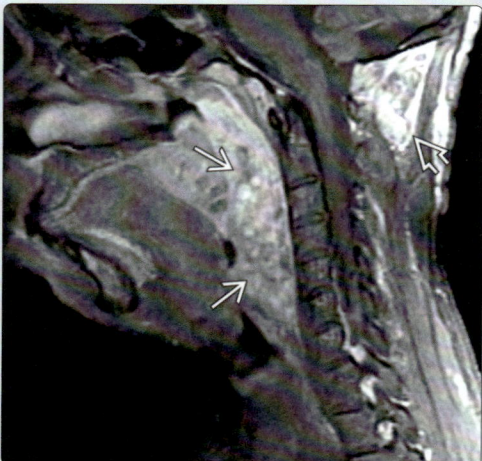

(Left) *Axial T2 MR in a 15-year-old boy with neurofibromatosis type 1 (NF1) shows a plexiform neurofibroma involving the left nasopharynx, ➡, paraspinal tissues ➡, and parotid gland ➡. This multilobulated, transspatial mass is predominantly hyperintense, except for central areas of low T2 signal (target sign) ➡.* **(Right)** *Sagittal T1 C+ FS MR in the same patient shows heterogenous enhancement of the plexiform neurofibroma in both the pharyngeal ➡ and paraspinal ➡ components.*

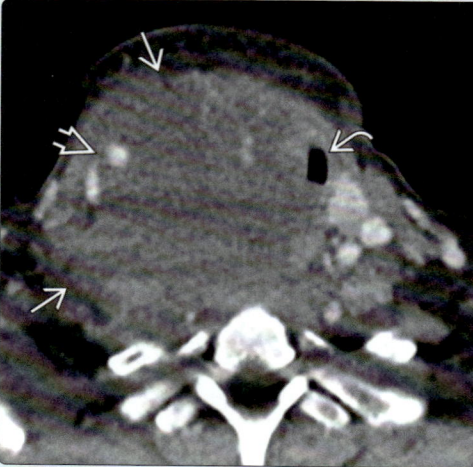
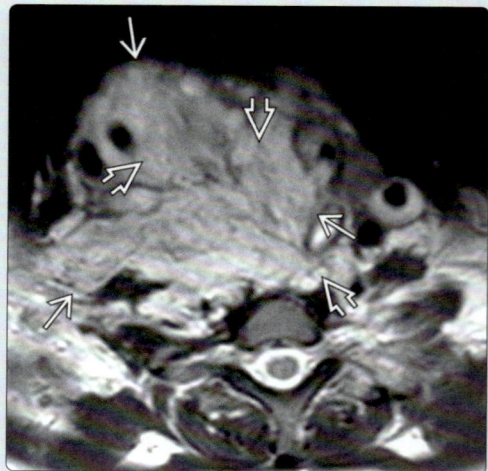

(Left) *Axial CECT in a teenager with NF1 shows an extensive, hypodense, transspatial right neck mass ➡, surrounding the carotid sheath vessels ➡, causing severe leftward tracheal deviation ➡. The hypoattenuation may mimic a cystic, lymphatic malformation.* **(Right)** *Axial T2 MR in the same patient demonstrates a heterogeneous, moderately hyperintense mass ➡ with multiple small intralesional T2 foci of hypointensity, typical of a neurofibroma ➡.*

TERMINOLOGY

Abbreviations

- Plexiform neurofibroma (PNF)

Definitions

- Architecturally complex neurofibroma involving multiple nerve fascicles
  - Often found in areas of branched nerves
  - Pathognomonic for neurofibromatosis type 1 (NF1)

IMAGING

General Features

- Best diagnostic clue
  - T2 FS MR shows lobular, **serpentine contour** of **transspatial mass** with **focal target signs**
- Location
  - Trunk, limbs, or head and neck most common
  - May be superficial cutaneous, subcutaneous, or deep
- Morphology
  - Lobular mass infiltrating along nerve branches

Imaging Recommendations

- Best imaging tool
  - MR best characterizes and delineates complete extent
- Protocol advice
  - Multiplanar imaging best for delineating full extent
    - Fat-saturation sequences helpful for T2 and T1 C+

CT Findings

- CECT
  - Mildly enhancing, infiltrative, solid mass
    - Occasionally no enhancement, simulates cystic mass

MR Findings

- T1WI: Isointense to muscle
- T2WI FS: Hyperintense, lobulated transspatial mass
  - Central low-signal foci are characteristic: **Target sign**
- T1WI C+ FS: Mild to moderate enhancement

DIFFERENTIAL DIAGNOSIS

Venous Malformation

- Close mimic on imaging
- Phleboliths evident in this lesion; best seen on CT

Lymphatic Malformation

- Nonenhancing, cystic transspatial mass

Sarcoma

- Infiltrative, malignant tumor; anywhere in head and neck
- Rapid growth, ± adenopathy

PATHOLOGY

General Features

- Genetics
  - Deletion in *NF1* gene on long arm of chromosome 17
    - Results in ↓ production of **neurofibromin** (tumor suppressor) protein; autosomal dominant inheritance
- Associated abnormalities
  - NF1 has many spine, neck, and brain findings
    - Spinal and dermal neurofibromas
    - Sphenoid wing dysplasia with cephalocele
    - Vascular stenoses and aneurysms
    - Optic nerve glioma
    - Brain and spinal cord astrocytomas
    - Scoliosis

Staging, Grading, & Classification

- WHO grade 1 tumors

Gross Pathologic & Surgical Features

- Diffuse tortuosity, enlargement of nerve and branches

Microscopic Features

- Schwann cells, axons, and endoneural fibroblasts enclosed by perineurium
  - Target sign due to central fibrocollagenous core surrounded by myxomatous tissue

CLINICAL ISSUES

Presentation

- Most common signs/symptoms
  - Superficial lesions palpable, disfiguring
    - Bag of worms appearance on clinical exam
- Other signs/symptoms
  - Specific to tissues infiltrated

Demographics

- Age
  - Variable: Present at birth or develops with age
- Epidemiology
  - NF1 incidence: 1 in 3,000
  - PNFs found in **~ 30% of patients with NF1**

Natural History & Prognosis

- **5-10% risk of malignant transformation** (usually to malignant peripheral nerve sheath tumor)
  - Progressive enlargement/pain suggests degeneration

Treatment

- Impossible to completely resect
- Debulking for cosmetic or functional reasons
- Selumetinib can decrease tumor volume

DIAGNOSTIC CHECKLIST

Image Interpretation Pearls

- CECT: Appears as infiltrative, solid mass
- MR: May mimic venous malformation; look for target sign
- Evaluate for other manifestations of NF1

SELECTED REFERENCES

1. Debs P et al: MRI features of benign peripheral nerve sheath tumors: how do sporadic and syndromic tumors differ? Skeletal Radiol. 53(4):709-23, 2024
2. Gorai S et al: Selumetinib-a comprehensive review of the new FDA-approved drug for neurofibromatosis. Indian Dermatol Online J. 15(4):701-5, 2024
3. Thakur U et al: Multiparametric whole-body MRI of patients with neurofibromatosis type I: spectrum of imaging findings. Skeletal Radiol. 54(3):407-22, 2024
4. Dai M et al: Imaging characteristics of orbital peripheral nerve sheath tumors: analysis of 34 cases. World J Clin Cases. 10(21):7356-64, 2022
5. Gross AM et al: Selumetinib in children with inoperable plexiform neurofibromas. N Engl J Med. 382(15):1430-42, 2020
6. Banks KP: The target sign: extremity. Radiology. 234(3):899-900, 2005

KEY FACTS

TERMINOLOGY

- Posttransplantation lymphoproliferative disorder (PTLD)
- Uncontrolled lymphoid growth in transplant recipient on immunosuppressive therapy
- Disease spectrum ranges from hyperplasia to malignancy

IMAGING

- May also mimic pharyngeal infection & abscesses
- Consider when history of transplant + any nodal or extranodal enlargement or head & neck mass
  - Adenotonsillar &/or nodal enlargement
  - Sinonasal masses or infiltrating tissue to skull base
  - Orbital or oral cavity mass
  - Rarely laryngeal mass, external nasal mass
- ↑ FDG uptake on PET/CT
  - False-negative results may occur, especially in children

TOP DIFFERENTIAL DIAGNOSES

- Tonsillar/peritonsillar inflammation or abscess

- Reactive lymph nodes
- Invasive fungal sinusitis

PATHOLOGY

- Therapeutic T-cell suppression allows proliferation of B cells infected with **EBV**
- WHO Classification of Hematolymphoid Tumors, 5th edition (**WHO-HAEM5**)
  - Under **lymphoid proliferations & lymphomas associated with immune deficiency & dysregulation**

CLINICAL ISSUES

- Solid organ transplant > > bone marrow transplant
- More common in pediatric transplant patients
- Up to 80% 1st year post transplant
- Highest incidence in heart-lung, lung, or small bowel transplant; lowest incidence in renal transplant

DIAGNOSTIC CHECKLIST

- Transplant patient with infection or lymphoma-like lesions

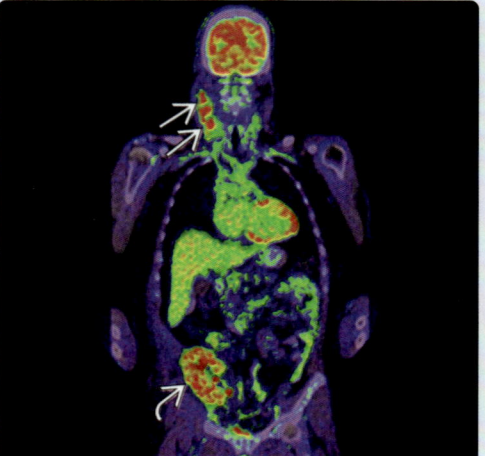
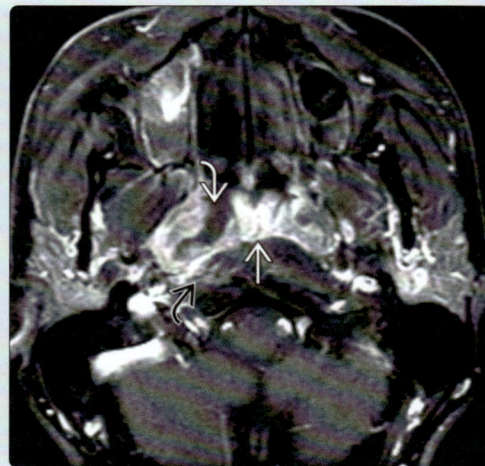

(Left) Coronal FDG PET/CT shows posttransplantation lymphoproliferative disorder (PTLD) in the right internal jugular chain lymph nodes ➡ *(nondestructive plasmacytic hyperplasia subtype). Note the renal transplant ➡. (Right)* Axial T1 C+ FS MR in PTLD *[diffuse large B-cell lymphoma (DLBCL)] shows an asymmetric, enlarged nasopharyngeal tonsil ➡ & a heterogeneous, enhancing mass with internal necrosis ➡. Note deep infiltration into right prevertebral muscles ➡. There was necrotic cervical adenopathy also (not shown).*

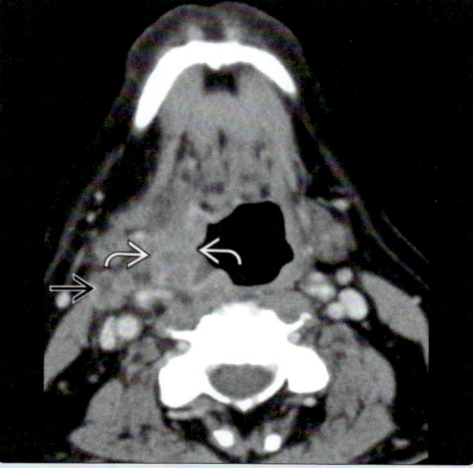
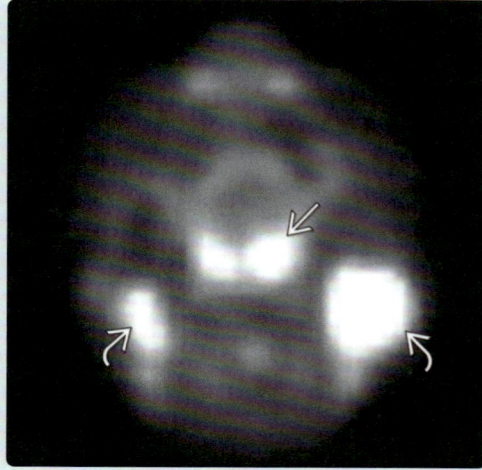

(Left) Axial CECT shows DLBCL PTLD presenting with a necrotic right tonsillar mass ➡ & a level II necrotic node ➡. This patient had chronic lymphocytic leukemia with minimal residual disease & was status post allogeneic stem cell transplant. *(Right)* Axial PET reveals marked FDG avidity in bilateral neck nodes ➡ with asymmetric FDG uptake in the left palatine tonsil ➡. PTLD can mimic tonsillitis with reactive adenopathy, but transplant history is key. Biopsy distinguishes these processes.

TERMINOLOGY

Abbreviations
- Posttransplantation lymphoproliferative disorder (PTLD)

Definitions
- Uncontrolled lymphoid growth in transplant recipient on immunosuppressive therapy
- Spectrum of disease: Hyperplasia to malignancy

IMAGING

General Features
- Location
  - Anywhere in head & neck: Extranodal or nodal
  - Waldeyer ring, sinonasal, orbit, oral cavity, larynx
  - Nodal involvement seen as 2 forms
    - Large nodal masses
    - Clusters of normal-sized nodes

Imaging Recommendations
- Best imaging tool
  - Either CT or MR adequate for delineating H&N mass
  - FDG PET for staging & response to treatment
- Protocol advice
  - Postcontrast imaging best shows necrosis & nodes

CT Findings
- CECT
  - Markedly enhancing, enlarged adenoids or tonsils
    - More often deeply invasive than exophytic
  - H&N mass or infiltrating soft tissue at skull base

MR Findings
- T1WI C+ FS
  - Intensely enhancing, aggressive-appearing masses
  - Necrotic or solid nodes

Nuclear Medicine Findings
- PET/CT
  - ↑ FDG uptake in PTLD
  - Negative FDG PET/CT does not rule out PTLD
  - False-negatives may occur in Waldeyer ring, cervical lymph nodes, or small bowel, especially in children
    - Sensitivity as low as 50% reported in pediatric PTLD

DIFFERENTIAL DIAGNOSIS

Tonsillar Inflammation
- Enlarged, heterogeneously enhancing tonsil

Tonsillar/Peritonsillar Abscess
- Rim-enhancing, low-density focus in or around tonsil

Reactive Lymph Nodes
- Common in children & teens

Invasive Fungal Sinusitis
- Infiltration of perisinus fat, deep facial fat planes

PATHOLOGY

General Features
- Etiology

- Therapeutic T-cell suppression allows proliferation of B cells infected with **Ebstein-Barr Virus (EBV)**
- Greatest risk factors
  - EBV-naïve recipient of EBV-infected donor organ

Staging, Grading, & Classification
- WHO Classification of Hematolymphoid Tumors, 5th edition (**WHO-HAEM5**) classifies PTLD under **lymphoid proliferations & lymphomas associated with immune deficiency and dysregulation**
  - **Hyperplasias arising in immune deficiency/dysregulation**: Encompassing **nondestructive PTLD**, among others
  - **Polymorphic lymphoproliferative disorders arising in immune deficiency/dysregulation**: Encompassing **polymorphic PTLD**, among others
  - **Lymphomas arising in immune deficiency/dysregulation**: Encompassing **monomorphic PTLD** & **classic Hodgkin lymphoma PTLD**, among others

Gross Pathologic & Surgical Features
- Predilection for extranodal sites of disease

Microscopic Features
- **EBV** detectable in tissues: Almost 100% nondestructive PTLDs, & > 90% polymorphic & CHL PTLDs
  - Monomorphic PTLD can be both EBV positive & negative

CLINICAL ISSUES

Presentation
- Most common signs/symptoms
  - H&N: Adenopathy, nasal block, sinusitis, sore throat
  - Generalized: Fever, ↓ weight, night sweats

Demographics
- Age
  - Pediatric patients have 4x incidence of adults
- Epidemiology
  - 2-3% of adult transplant recipients
  - Up to 8% of pediatric transplant patients

Natural History & Prognosis
- Most often after solid organ transplant, less often after bone marrow or stem cell transplant
- Up to 80% in 1st year post transplant
  - Highest incidence: Heart-lung, lung, or small bowel
  - Lowest incidence: Kidney transplant

Treatment
- Reduction of immunosuppression key
- Anti-CD20 monoclonal antibody (rituximab)
- Surgery, radiation, chemotherapy, EBV-specific cytotoxic lymphocytes, anti-EBV peptides

DIAGNOSTIC CHECKLIST

Consider
- PTLD with every transplant patient when imaging suggests infection or lymphoma-like lesions

SELECTED REFERENCES
1. Pollack S et al: Prevention of post-transplant lymphoproliferative disorder in pediatric kidney transplant recipients. Pediatr Nephrol. 40(3):829-34, 2024

KEY FACTS

TERMINOLOGY

- Extraosseous, locally aggressive notochordal tumor
- Very rare; mostly in nasopharynx, occasionally in skull base, foramen magnum, spine, retropharyngeal

IMAGING

- CT findings
  - Nasopharyngeal, heterogeneous, minimally enhancing
  - Dystrophic calcifications common
  - Anterior clival scalloping with well-defined **midline tract** to median (medial) basal canal (MBC)
  - **MBC**: Cephalad exit tract of notochord in lower clivus (basiocciput), extending from intracranial surface into nasopharyngeal soft tissues, rarely seen on imaging
- MR findings
  - Lobular, heterogeneous, nasopharyngeal mass with midline clival tract along course of notochordal remnant
  - Heterogeneous ↑ ↑ T2 signal intensity present
  - ↑ ↑ T2 signal intensity helps differentiate from ↓ T2 signal in other nasopharyngeal malignancies
- Honeycomb pattern heterogeneous enhancement
- More solid enhancement = poorer prognosis

TOP DIFFERENTIAL DIAGNOSES

- Tornwaldt cyst
- Nasopharyngeal carcinoma
- Non-Hodgkin lymphoma
- Benign notochordal cell tumor when retroclival intracranial

PATHOLOGY

- Lobular, bulky mass with fibrous pseudocapsule
- Oval physaliphorous cells predominate

DIAGNOSTIC CHECKLIST

- Consider extraosseous chordoma when ↑ ↑ T2-signal nasopharyngeal mass extends from midline clival cleft
- Preoperative report must note extension along MBC, so complete resection is performed

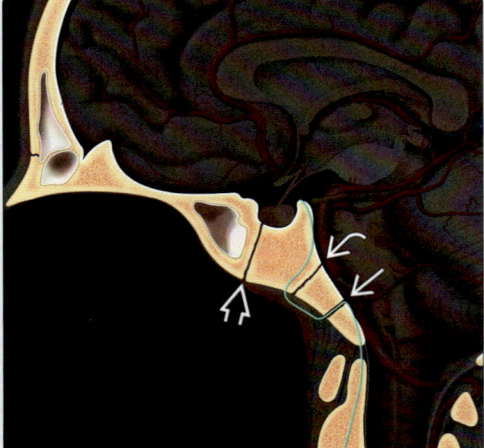 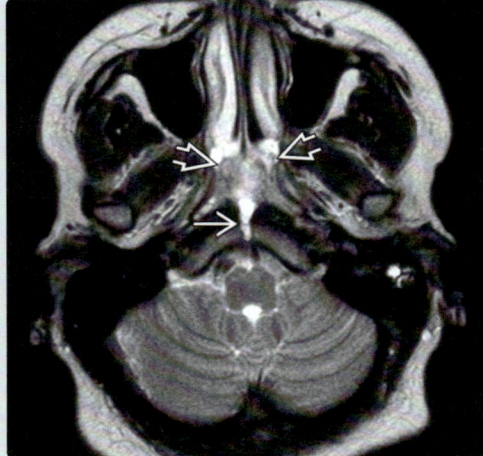

(Left) *Sagittal graphic shows a notochordal remnant pathway (teal line) and its relation to the median basal canal (MBC) ➡ inferiorly in the basiocciput of clivus and sphenooccipital synchondrosis ➡ above MBC. Craniopharyngeal canal ➡ lies more anterosuperiorly. Fossa navicularis magna location is around MBC region in the basiocciput at anterior clival margin.* **(Right)** *Axial T2 MR shows hyperintense nasopharyngeal extraosseous chordoma (EC) obstructing the posterior choanae ➡. Note extension into clival MBC ➡ along notochordal pathway.*

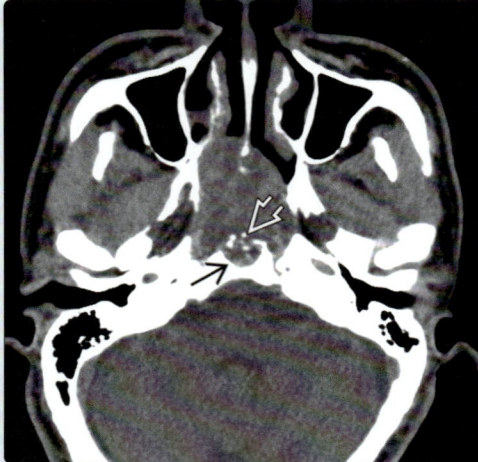 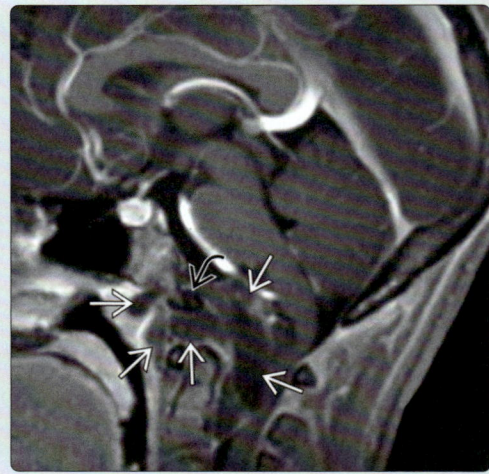

(Left) *Axial CECT shows a large nasopharyngeal EC filling the airway. Note the anterior clival midline scalloping in the area of the MBC ➡. Characteristic bone fragments ➡ are visible in the posterior midline of the tumor.* **(Right)** *Sagittal T1 MPRAGE C+ MR shows a predominant EC ➡ with a minimal heterogeneous honeycomb pattern of enhancement in the nasopharynx, skull base, and craniocervical junction along the notochordal remnant pathway. Only a tiny portion of the clival tip ➡ is involved.*

TERMINOLOGY

Definitions

- Extraosseous, locally aggressive notochordal tumor

IMAGING

General Features

- Best diagnostic clue
  - Very rare; mostly in nasopharynx, occasionally in skull base, foramen magnum, spine, and retropharyngeal locations
  - Submucosal nasopharyngeal mass with **midline clival tract** along course of notochordal remnant
    - Rarely, extension to nasal cavity or maxillary sinus

Imaging Recommendations

- Best imaging tool
  - T2 MR best shows **hyperintense** mass with **sinus tract** extending from mass to midline clival defect

CT Findings

- CECT
  - Lobular, heterogeneous, minimally enhancing nasopharyngeal mass
    - Dystrophic calcifications common
- Bone CT
  - Anterior clival scalloping with well-defined midline tract to **median (medial) basal canal (MBC)**
    - **MBC**: Cephalad exit tract of notochord in lower clivus (basiocciput) below/behind sphenooccipital synchondrosis, from intracranial surface into nasopharyngeal soft tissues, rarely seen on imaging
      - a.k.a. canalis basilaris medianus
  - Fossa navicularis magna [rare, notch-shaped bony depression at anterior margin of lower clivus (basiocciput)] may also be seen around CBM location; may contain lymphoid tissue

MR Findings

- T1WI
  - Hypointense with rare, scattered regions of ↑ signal from intratumoral hemorrhage
- T2WI
  - Heterogeneous ↑ ↑ signal intensity present
    - Helps differentiate from ↓ signal in other nasopharyngeal malignancies
    - **Chondrosarcoma can also be T2 bright** but mostly seen centered at petroclival fissure more laterally and, rarely, only in midline
- DWI
  - Chordomas have lower ADC than chondrosarcomas
    - Solid tumor mean ADC value cut-off point of 1,585 x 10^{-6} mm²/s with 94% sensitivity & 98% specificity
- T1WI C+
  - Honeycomb pattern heterogeneous enhancement
  - More solid enhancement = poorer prognosis

DIFFERENTIAL DIAGNOSIS

Tornwaldt Cyst

- Small, central cyst without discrete clival sinus tract

Nasopharyngeal Carcinoma

- Paramedian mass; much lower T2 signal than chordoma
- Skull base destruction usually off midline; no clival cleft

Pharyngeal Mucosal Space Non-Hodgkin Lymphoma

- Nasopharyngeal mass, lower T2 signal than chordoma
- Associated retropharyngeal, cervical adenopathy common

Benign Notochordal Cell Tumor

- Retroclival intradural nonenhancing, ↑ ↑ T2, ↓ T1 lesion
- Arises from notochordal rests, mostly in prepontine region and rarely within odontoid process

PATHOLOGY

General Features

- Etiology
  - Notochordal remnant with tumor extending from nasopharynx to MBC of clivus
  - Brachyury transcription factor of T-box family expressed in notochord and chordoma
  - mTOR pathway can be activated in chordomas, may render them responsive to mTOR inhibitor therapy
    - Chordomas occasionally seen in tuberous sclerosis

Staging, Grading, & Classification

- Chordomas can be intraosseous/extradural, intraosseous/intradural, extraosseous/extradural, extraosseous/intradural or extraosseous soft tissue (from ectopic rests of notochord)

Gross Pathologic & Surgical Features

- Lobular, bulky mass with fibrous pseudocapsule

Microscopic Features

- Oval **physaliphorous cells** predominate

CLINICAL ISSUES

Presentation

- Most common signs/symptoms
  - Nasopharyngeal fullness or nasal obstruction when nasal cavity extension present
  - Mastoid and middle ear opacification if tumor obstructs eustachian tube

Natural History & Prognosis

- Prognosis generally better for younger patients
- Lower recurrence rate than intraosseous chordoma

Treatment

- Complete surgical extirpation with resection of tumor in MBC to prevent recurrence

DIAGNOSTIC CHECKLIST

Reporting Tips

- Preoperative report must note extension along midline clival tract, so complete resection is performed

SELECTED REFERENCES

1. Tison T et al: A rare case of pediatric extraosseous chordoma of the nasopharynx. Pediatr Blood Cancer. 71(2):e30776, 2024

KEY FACTS

TERMINOLOGY

- **N**on-**H**odgkin **l**ymphoma (NHL)
- Heterogeneous lymphoreticular system malignancy
- Head & neck NHL has multiple forms: **Nodal**, **nonnodal lymphatic** (lingual, nasopharyngeal adenoidal, & palatine tonsils), & **extralymphatic** (e.g., skull base, thyroid, sinuses)

IMAGING

- Intermediate to low T2, diffusion-restricting masses on MR
- **Nodal NHL**
  - Multiple 1- to 3-cm solid nodes, dominant node up to 5 cm; uni-/bilateral, unilateral in head & neck in > 80%; aggressive NHL may have necrosis
- **Nonnodal lymphatic NHL**
  - Enlarged, homogeneously enhancing tonsils &/or adenoids ± enlarged ipsilateral nodes
  - May be heterogeneous & infiltrative
- **Extralymphatic NHL**
  - Focal or infiltrative mass in any tissue in neck

TOP DIFFERENTIAL DIAGNOSES

- Wide differential diagnosis depending on form of NHL: Nodal, nonnodal lymphatic, extralymphatic
- Lymphoma one of great mimickers

PATHOLOGY

- WHO Classification of Hematolymphoid Tumours, 5th edition (WHO-HAEM5)
- **Lugano** classification for staging, response assessment, & follow-up of lymphomas: Based on **Ann Arbor** staging
  - **Waldeyer ring** tonsils, **thymus**, **spleen** considered **nodal structures** for staging purposes

CLINICAL ISSUES

- Disease extent evaluation using PET/CT for avid & CT scan for nonavid lymphoma histologies
- Chemotherapy, radiation, or combined modality therapy
- 5-year survival: Stage I > 82%, stage II 75%, stage III 70%, stage IV > 62%

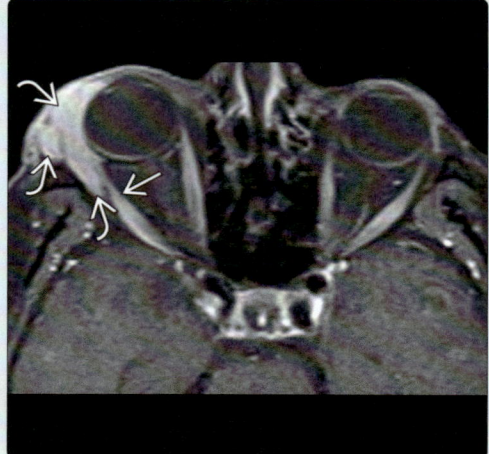
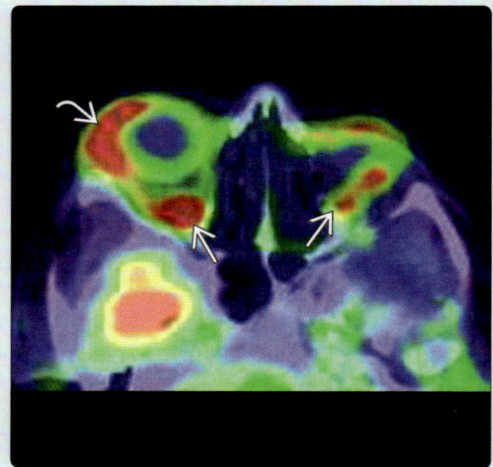

(Left) Axial T1 C+ FS MR shows a right orbital, extraconal, uniformly enhancing mass, including the region of lacrimal gland & eyelid ➡, just lateral to the lateral rectus muscle ➡. (Right) Axial fused F-18 FDG PET/CT shows that the mass is intensely hypermetabolic ➡. High FDG uptake in the retrobulbar orbit is physiologic activity of extraconal muscles ➡. Biopsy of the mass showed mucosa-associated lymphoid tissue (MALT) lymphoma, a subtype extranodal marginal zone lymphoma (MZL) of non-Hodgkin lymphoma (NHL).

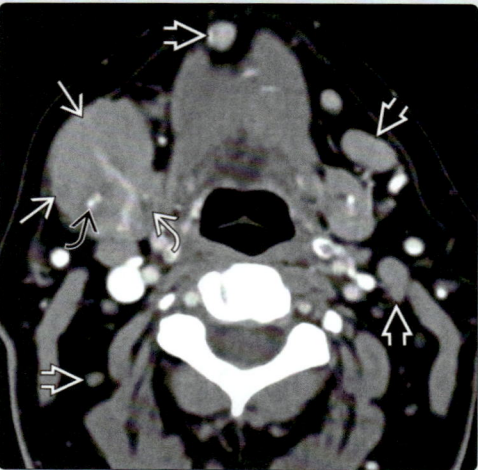
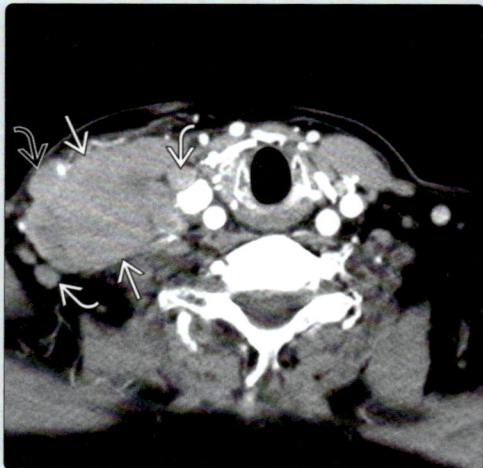

(Left) Axial CECT in low-grade, follicular NHL shows an exophytic, mildly enhancing mass ➡ arising from the right submandibular salivary gland (SMG) ➡ with a vessel contiguous in both the SMG & mass. Calcification ➡ is unusual in untreated lymphoma. Note bilateral, prominent to mildly enlarged lymph nodes ➡. (Right) Axial CECT in a diffuse large B-cell lymphoma (DLBCL) NHL patient shows a homogeneous mass ➡ inseparable from the right sternocleidomastoid muscle ➡ with multiple smaller abnormal nodes ➡.

TERMINOLOGY

Abbreviations

- **N**on-**H**odgkin **l**ymphoma (NHL)

Definitions

- Lymphoma is heterogeneous lymphoreticular system malignancy
  - Many types of lymphoma have been described based on histologic & molecular criteria
- All lymphomas designated Hodgkin lymphoma (HL) or NHL
  - HL: Neoplastic Reed-Sternberg cells with mixed inflammatory cell mass
  - NHL: Multiple subtypes of **B-cell**, **T-cell**, or **NK-cell** lymphomas/leukemias
    - Diffuse large B-cell lymphoma (DLBCL) most common
- **Head & neck NHL has multiple forms**
  - **Nodal**, **nonnodal lymphatic** (tonsils, adenoids, lingual lymphoid), **extralymphatic** (e.g., thyroid, sinuses)

IMAGING

General Features

- Best diagnostic clue
  - Enlarged, nonnecrotic nodes ± tonsillar mass
  - Extralymphatic form appears as infiltrative mass in almost any head & neck area
  - Image-guided core biopsy often required to subtype

CT Findings

- **Nodal NHL**
  - Multiple 1- to 3-cm solid nodes, dominant node up to 5 cm
  - Uni-/bilateral, unilateral in head & neck in > 80% in recent study
  - Aggressive NHL shows necrosis or extranodal extension
- **Nonnodal lymphatic NHL**
  - Enlarged, homogeneously enhancing tonsils ± adenoids
  - May be confined to 1 tonsillar structure, multiple structures, or entire Waldeyer ring
    - Nasopharyngeal **(adenoids)**, **palatine**, **lingual tonsil**
  - ± enlarged ipsilateral nodes
  - Aggressive NHL: Often more heterogeneous enhancement with necrosis
- **Extralymphatic NHL**
  - Appears as focal or infiltrative mass
  - Involves almost any tissue or site in neck
    - Skull base, cranial nerves, lacrimal gland, extraocular muscles, sinonasal, facial bones (especially premaxillary soft tissues), masticator space, parotid or thyroid gland

MR Findings

- T1WI
  - Typically iso- or slightly hyperintense to muscle
- T2WI
  - Intermediate intensity, hyperintense to muscle
  - More aggressive tumors are heterogeneous
- DWI
  - **Low ADC values** (dark) in solid components
  - Necrotic areas show high ADC values
- T1WI C+ FS
  - Intermediate, homogeneous enhancement
  - More aggressive tumors heterogeneous

Nuclear Medicine Findings

- PET/CT
  - Used for initial staging of all NHL
  - FDG PET shows **variable avidity**: Higher in aggressive, lower in more indolent NHL
  - Interim PET/CT, obtained during treatment, assesses response
    - Patients with limited response during treatment will have change in therapy
  - Posttherapy PET/CT used to assess treatment response

Imaging Recommendations

- Best imaging tool
  - Standard staging is FDG PET/CT or PET/CECT

DIFFERENTIAL DIAGNOSIS

Nodal Non-Hodgkin Lymphoma

- Squamous cell carcinoma (SCCa) metastatic nodes
- HL nodes
- Reactive lymph nodes

Nonnodal Lymphatic Non-Hodgkin Lymphoma

- SCCa oropharynx (base of tongue lingual tissue, palatine tonsils)
- Nasopharyngeal carcinoma
- Tonsillar lymphoid hyperplasia
- Minor salivary gland malignancy pharyngeal mucosal space

Extralymphatic Non-Hodgkin Lymphoma

- Orbital idiopathic inflammation (pseudotumor)
- SCCa sinonasal
- Anaplastic thyroid carcinoma
- Fibromatosis

PATHOLOGY

General Features

- Etiology
  - Multiple risk factors: Immunosuppression, infectious agents, genetic mutations, prior ionizing radiation
    - Viral infection: EBV, HIV, human T-cell leukemia lymphoma virus-1, hepatitis C
    - Chronic immune system suppression/stimulation: Sjögren syndrome, celiac sprue, rheumatoid arthritis
- Genetics
  - ↑ incidence in 1st-degree relatives; variable heritability by subtypes

Staging, Grading, & Classification

- WHO Classification of Haematolymphoid Tumours, 5th edition (WHO-HAEM5)
  - Genetic-centric approach
  - Hierarchy from benign to malignant with categories like lineage, family (class), type, & subtype
  - WHO-HAEM5 utilizes triad of attributes: Lineage, dominant clinical attribute, & dominant biologic attribute
    - Dominant biologic attribute encompasses gene fusions, rearrangements, mutations

Lugano Classification for Staging Non-Hodgkin Lymphoma

Based on Ann Arbor Staging System

Stage I: Single lymph node or group of adjacent nodes (**Waldeyer ring, thymus, and spleen considered nodal structures** for staging purposes) (I) or single extranodal organ or tissue (IE) without nodal involvement

Stage II: 2 or more lymph node regions or nodal structures on same side of diaphragm alone (II) or with involvement of limited, contiguous extralymphatic organ or tissue (IIE)

Stage III: Lymph node regions or lymphoid structures on both sides of diaphragm (can be nodes on both sides of diaphragm or nodes above diaphragm with spleen below diaphragm)

Stage IV: Diffuse or disseminated noncontiguous extralymphatic organ or tissue involvement (more than that can be designated "E"), ± associated nodal involvement

Designation "E": Limited extranodal extension (More extensive extranodal disease should be designated as stage IV)

Systemic "B" symptoms (fever, sweats, weight loss) no longer incorporated into non-Hodgkin lymphoma staging; unlike Hodgkin lymphoma staging Systemic "B" symptoms not independent prognostic factor for non-Hodgkin lymphoma

Bulky disease: No cut-off value for largest tumor diameter validated in non-Hodgkin lymphoma; criteria vary by histology (6 cm for follicular lymphoma & 6-10 cm for diffuse large B-cell lymphoma) (term "X" used in Ann Arbor staging system no longer needed)

Disease extent evaluation using PET/CT for avid & CT for nonavid lymphoma histologies.

Non-Hodgkin lymphoma (NHL) is the most frequently spread hematogenously, hence the NHL staging system is less useful than that for Hodgkin lymphoma (which disseminates mainly by contiguous lymphatic spread). The majority of aggressive NHLs present in advanced stages III/IV, which have similar treatment, & differentiation between these stages offers little therapeutic benefit. NHL staging is mainly to identify the minority of patients with early-stage disease who can be treated with local or combined modality therapy.

- Categories include myeloid neoplasms, lymphoid neoplasms, histiocytic/dendritic neoplasms, & stroma-derived neoplasms of lymphoid tissues
- Lymphoid neoplasms consist of B-cell lymphoid proliferations & lymphomas & T-cell & NK-cell proliferations & lymphomas
- **B-cell lymphoid proliferations & lymphomas**
  - Tumor-like lesions with B-cell predominance (new in WHO-HAEM5): Includes reactive B-cell-rich lymphoid proliferations that can mimic lymphoma, IgG4-related disease, unicentric Castleman disease, idiopathic multicentric Castleman disease, & Kaposi sarcoma herpesvirus/HHV-8-associated multicentric Castleman disease
  - Precursor B-cell neoplasms (B-cell lymphoblastic leukemias/lymphomas)
  - Mature B-cell neoplasms
  - Hodgkin lymphoma
  - Plasma cell neoplasms & other diseases with paraproteins
- **T-cell and NK-cell proliferations & lymphomas**
  - Tumor-like lesions with B-cell predominance (new in WHO-HAEM5)
  - Precursor T-cell neoplasms
  - Mature T-cell and NK-cell neoplasms
- **Lugano** classification for staging, response assessment, & follow-up of lymphomas: Derived from **Ann Arbor** staging
- **Nodal regions** for lymphoma staging in **head & neck** imaging
  - **Waldeyer ring**: Base of tongue, nasopharyngeal & palatine **tonsils**
  - Ipsilateral cervical & supraclavicular nodes
  - Occipital & preauricular nodes; infraclavicular nodes; axillary & pectoral nodes
  - Mediastinal: **Thymus**, prevascular, aortopulmonary, pre-/paratracheal, subcarinal, posterior mediastinal

- All mediastinal lesions counted as single nodal region
- Internal mammary nodes considered part of lymphatic system of chest wall; drain diaphragm
- Paravertebral nodes also drain chest wall and diaphragm; even though in posterior mediastinum
- Hilar nodes: Right & left hilar nodes considered separate regions; bilateral hilar nodes makes stage II lymphoma

CLINICAL ISSUES

Presentation

- Most common signs/symptoms
  - **Nodal**: Presentation with neck mass
  - **Nonnodal lymphatic**: Naso- or oropharyngeal mass, but neck adenopathy may be presenting symptom
  - **Extralymphatic**: Mass, pain, cranial neuropathy

Natural History & Prognosis

- Poor outcome predictors: Age > 60, > 1 extranodal site, stage III/IV, ↑ LDH, poor performance status

Treatment

- Treatment depends on cell type, stage, patient age
- Chemo, XRT, or combined modality therapy
- Bone marrow transplant may be performed for recurrent or refractory disease

DIAGNOSTIC CHECKLIST

Image Interpretation Pearls

- Necrosis ± extranodal extension or diffuse infiltration suggests high-grade, aggressive NHL

SELECTED REFERENCES

1. Haferlach C et al: Overview on WHO-HAEM5 and the diagnostic relevance of genetic alterations for the classification. Med Genet. 36(1):3-11, 2024
2. Hough B et al: New and developing first line pharmacotherapies for treating non-Hodgkin lymphoma. Expert Opin Pharmacother. 25(12):1677-89, 2024

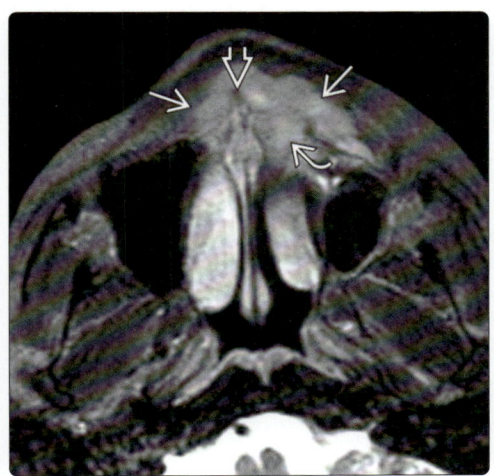

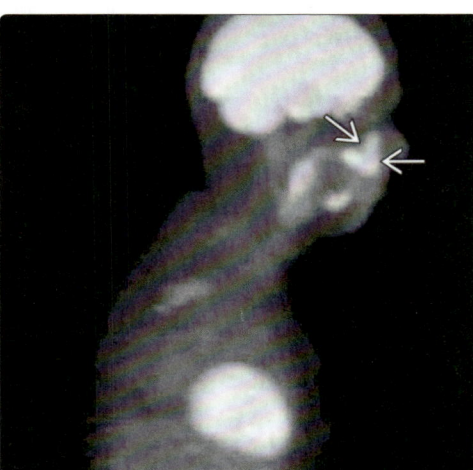

(Left) *Axial T2 FS MR in a young adult with several weeks of maxillary pain that prompted a root canal before biopsy revealed DLBCL NHL. A lobulated, hyperintense mass ➡ involves the anterior aspect of the left maxilla, crossing midline at anterior nasal spine ➡. Premaxillary mass with bone invasion ➡ is classic for extranodal NHL.* (Right) *Lateral projection from FDG PET shows high uptake in the maxillary mass ➡ but no abnormal uptake elsewhere. No B symptoms were present. Patient was treated with combined modality therapy.*

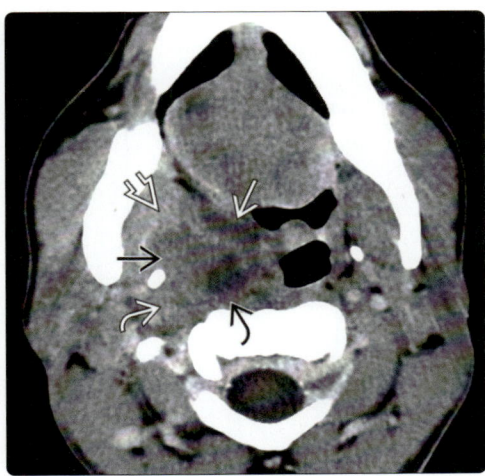

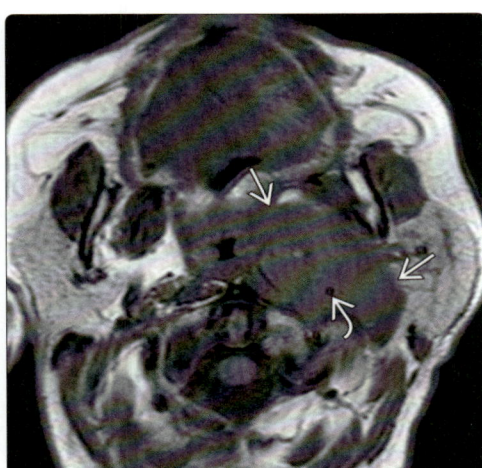

(Left) *Axial CECT in an HIV(+) patient with facial pain shows a large, necrotic, right tonsillar mass ➡ infiltrating the parapharyngeal ➡, masticator ➡, retropharyngeal/prevertebral ➡, & carotid spaces ➡. Biopsy showed atypical Burkitt lymphoma.* (Right) *Axial T1 MR in a patient with DLBCL shows a large, transspatial deep facial & skull base mass ➡. Note that the mass surrounds & narrows the left internal carotid artery ➡ within the carotid space. DLBCL is the most common type of NHL & is usually aggressive.*

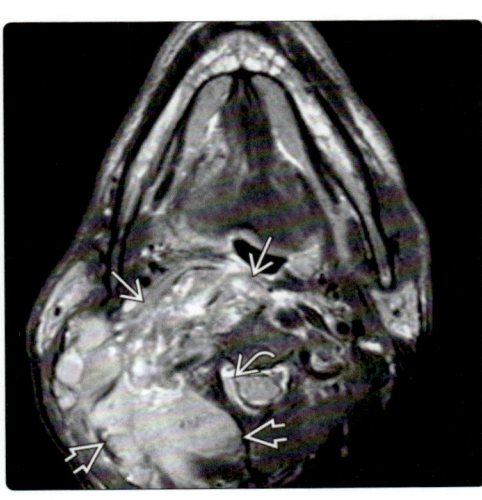

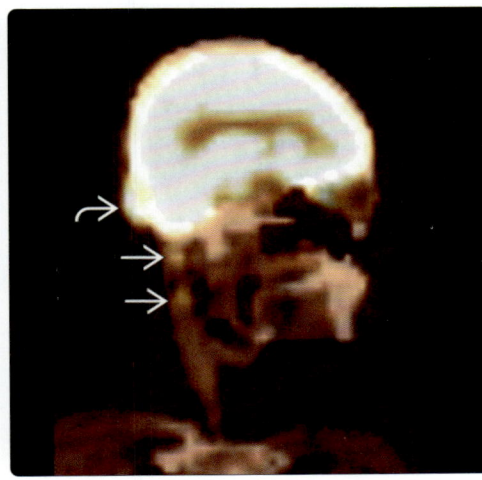

(Left) *Axial T2 MR in an HIV(+) patient with a rapidly enlarging mass shows an extensive, infiltrating mass in the right prevertebral ➡ and paraspinous ➡ muscles. The prevertebral component is heterogeneous & necrotic, whereas the posterior component is solid & homogeneous. There is intraspinal epidural extension ➡.* (Right) *Coronal fused FDG PET/CT in a patient with DLBCL shows FDG-avid right neck lymphadenopathy ➡ & scalp lymphoma deposit ➡. Patient's head was rotated to the left during scanning.*

KEY FACTS

TERMINOLOGY

- Soft tissue malignancy arising from fat tissue
- Tumor with variable pathology, therefore variable imaging
- 4 histological subtypes
  - Atypical lipomatous tumors/well-differentiated liposarcoma (ALT/WDLPS)
  - Myxoid liposarcoma (MLPS)
  - Dedifferentiated liposarcoma (DDLPS)
  - Pleomorphic liposarcoma (PLPS)

IMAGING

- Posterior cervical space most common in H&N
- Well-differentiated liposarcoma
  - Lobulated mass, > 75% fat, septations > 2 mm, enhancing nodules, ± Ca++
  - May mimic complex benign lipoma
- Poorly differentiated liposarcoma
  - Heterogeneous, enhancing, infiltrative mass ± amorphous, fatty foci

- May not see macroscopic fat on CT or MR in poorly differentiated & intermediate grade
- PET: FDG uptake in solid, nonfatty components

TOP DIFFERENTIAL DIAGNOSES

- Lipoma, other sarcomas, teratoma

PATHOLOGY

- Develop de novo, rarely from benign lipoma
- AJCC 8th edition: Anatomic site-specific staging for soft tissue sarcomas: Trunk & extremity/retroperitoneum, H&N, & abdominal & thoracic visceral organs
- H&N: T1-T3 based on tumor size (T1 ≤ 2 cm; T2 > 2 cm to ≤ 4 cm; T3 > 4 cm); T4 invades adjoining structures

CLINICAL ISSUES

- Painless, enlarging, soft, palpable mass in adults
- Local recurrence common
- 5-year survival: Low grade ≤ 90%, high grade 50%
- Wide local resection ± radiation ± chemotherapy

(Left) Axial CECT shows a mixed fat & soft tissue density liposarcoma (LS) mass ➡ in right posterior cervical space. Nodular soft tissue ➡ & thick septa ➡ are seen. Note normal left posterior cervical space fat ➡. (Right) Sagittal reformatted CT shows a well-differentiated LS arising from the posterior hypopharyngeal wall ➡. This mimics a cyst (10-20 HU), but few negative HU fatty areas ➡ are noted. Most LSs in larynx, pharynx, & hypopharynx are of well-differentiated or dedifferentiated types with propensity for recurrence.

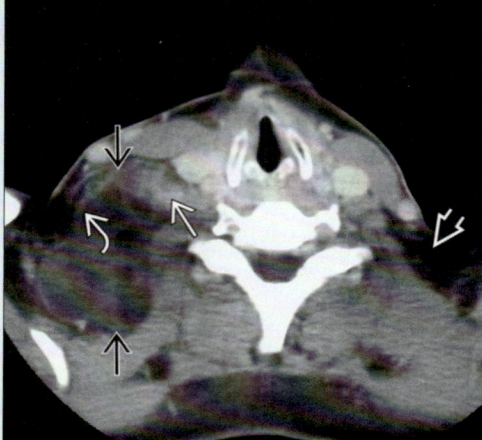
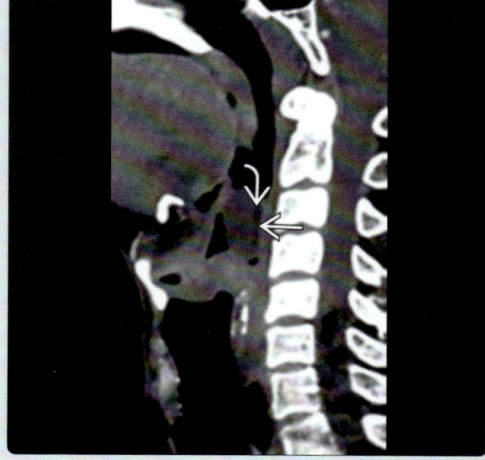

(Left) Axial CECT shows a large, complex LS ➡ distending the retropharyngeal space. The mass is mostly fat density, but fat stranding ➡ is present on the left. Also note enhancement ➡ on the right. (Right) Axial CECT shows bilateral vallecular masses, proven to be well-differentiated LSs. The right-sided mass shows predominant fat densities ➡, whereas the left-sided mass shows predominant soft tissue density ➡ with only a faint focus of hypodensity from fat ➡ within it.

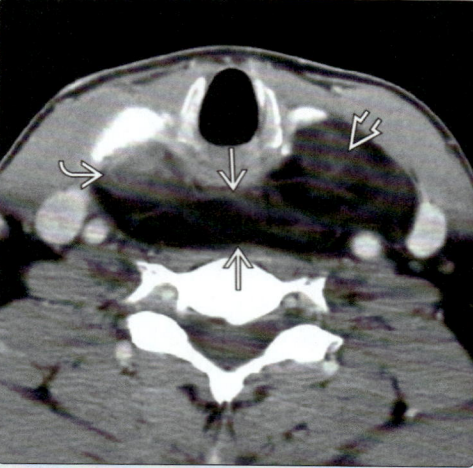
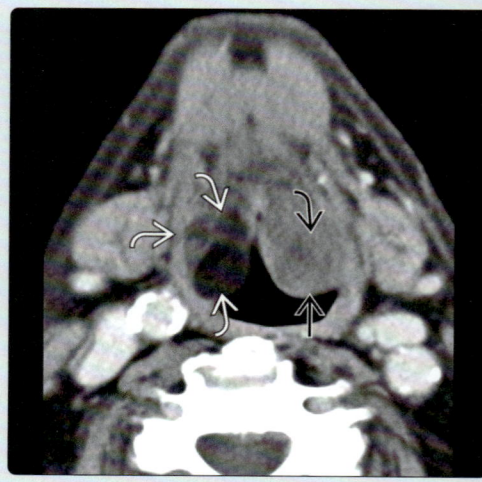

Liposarcoma of Head and Neck

TERMINOLOGY

Definitions
- Soft tissue malignancy arising from fat tissue

IMAGING

General Features
- Best diagnostic clue
  - Soft tissue mass with **variable appearance**
    - From well-defined, predominantly fatty mass with tissue stranding ± nodules
    - To ill-defined, heterogeneous, nonfatty solid mass mimicking any sarcoma
- Location
  - Posterior cervical space most common in H&N
  - Other H&N sites include cheek, larynx, hypopharynx, oral cavity, retropharyngeal space

CT Findings
- CECT
  - Well differentiated: Lobulated mass, > 75% fat, septations > 2 mm, enhancing nodules, ± Ca⁺⁺
  - Poorly differentiated: Heterogeneous, enhancing, infiltrative mass ± amorphous, fatty foci

MR Findings
- MR appearance **variable**, similar to CECT
  - Well differentiated: > 75% intrinsically T1-hyperintense fatty component that suppresses with fat saturation; thick septations, enhancing solid nodules
  - Poorly differentiated: Predominantly solid soft tissue mass, ± fat foci; heterogeneous enhancement, ill-defined contours

Nuclear Medicine Findings
- PET: FDG uptake in solid, nonfatty components

Imaging Recommendations
- Best imaging tool
  - MR best demonstrates soft tissue extent

DIFFERENTIAL DIAGNOSIS

Lipoma
- 8% of benign lipomas have soft tissue component

Sarcoma
- May be indistinguishable from fat-poor liposarcoma

Teratoma
- Multiloculated mass with complex imaging ± fat

PATHOLOGY

Staging, Grading, & Classification
- Most **soft tissue sarcomas** (with some exceptions) **use same latest AJCC 8th edition** system
- **Anatomic site-specific staging** algorithms for soft tissue sarcoma: Trunk & extremity/retroperitoneum, H&N, & abdominal & thoracic visceral organs
- **H&N**: **T**X: Primary tumor cannot be assessed
- T1-T3 by tumor size: T1 ≤ 2 cm; T2 > 2 cm to ≤ 4 cm; T3 > 4 cm

- T4: Tumor with invasion of adjoining structures
  - T4a: Orbital, skull base/dural, central compartment visceral, facial skeleton or pterygoid muscle invasion
  - T4b: Prevertebral muscle invasion, brain parenchymal invasion, CNS perineural spread, carotid encasement
- **N**0: No regional lymph node metastasis or unknown lymph node status; N1: Regional lymph node metastasis
- **M**0: No distant metastasis; M1: Distant metastasis
- Federation Nationale des Centres de Lutte Contre le Cancer/French Federation of Cancer Centers **(FNCLCC) system for histologic tumor grading**
  - Grade determined by sum score of: Differentiation (1-3) + mitotic activity (1-3) + necrosis (0-2)
  - GX: Grade cannot be assessed; grade 1: 2 or 3; grade 2: 4 or 5; grade 3: 6, 7, or 8

Gross Pathologic & Surgical Features
- Varies depending on histology, vascularity, necrosis, proportions of mature fat & fibrous tissue

Microscopic Features
- **Atypical lipomatous tumors/well-differentiated liposarcoma (ALT/WDLPS)**: 30-40% of H&N liposarcomas
- **Myxoid liposarcoma (MLPS)**: **Classic** MLPS & more aggressive **round-cell MLPS** (round-cell component > 5%)
  - Low-grade to moderately aggressive liposarcomas
- **Dedifferentiated liposarcoma (DDLPS)**: ALT/WDLPS with progression, occasionally occur as primary tumor
- **Pleomorphic liposarcoma (PLPS)**: Rarest, most aggressive
  - Highly undifferentiated, 30-50% distant metastasis (mainly lung), 50% tumor-related death

CLINICAL ISSUES

Presentation
- Most common signs/symptoms
  - Painless, enlarging mass; 5% painful

Demographics
- Age
  - Adult tumor: Peak ages 50-65 years

Natural History & Prognosis
- Local recurrence common

Treatment
- Wide local resection ± radiation ± chemotherapy

DIAGNOSTIC CHECKLIST

Image Interpretation Pearls
- **Imaging appearances are variable**
  - Well differentiated with > 75% fat: Complex lipoma
  - **May be solid, invasive mass with no imaging evidence of fat**, mimicking any other sarcoma

SELECTED REFERENCES

1. Kanaris A et al: Transoral excision of a hypopharyngeal liposarcoma. Laryngoscope. 134(11):4688-90, 2024
2. Schranz AL et al: Retrospective analysis of radiological investigation of surgically excised head and neck lipomas. Eur Arch Otorhinolaryngol. 281(8):4333-9, 2024
3. Barisella M et al: From head and neck lipoma to liposarcoma: a wide spectrum of differential diagnoses and their therapeutic implications. Curr Opin Otolaryngol Head Neck Surg. 28(2):136-43, 2020

TERMINOLOGY

- Synovial sarcoma (SSa): Malignant soft tissue tumor with epithelial and mesenchymal components

IMAGING

- Lobular, usually well-circumscribed **nonnodal, nonmucosal** soft tissue mass in head and neck
- CT/MR: Lobular, enhancing mass, ± cysts, Ca^{++}, hemorrhage
- Locations: Hypopharynx > > > masticator space, parapharyngeal space, paranasal sinuses
- Triple sign: Iso-, hypo-, & hyperintense foci (due to solid, cystic, Ca^{++} ± hemorrhagic components)

TOP DIFFERENTIAL DIAGNOSES

- Rhabdomyosarcoma
- Malignant fibrous histiocytoma
- Solitary fibrous tumor
- Nerve sheath tumor, benign and malignant
- Pleomorphic adenoma

PATHOLOGY

- Dual epithelial and mesenchymal differentiation
  - Biphasic: Classic form; mesenchymal and epithelial components
  - Monophasic: Mesenchymal component predominates
  - Poorly differentiated: Epithelioid morphology

CLINICAL ISSUES

- **Young adult** presenting with solitary nonnodal, nonmucosal head and neck mass
- Prognosis for head and neck SSa: More favorable than for extremity
  - ↓ prognosis if poorly differentiated
  - ↓ prognosis in patients > 30 years of age, larger SSa with bony invasion, hemorrhage, or paraspinal location
  - ↓ prognosis for upper aerodigestive tract lesions
  - ↑ prognosis if Ca^{++} present
- Preferred treatment: Complete excision and postoperative radiation

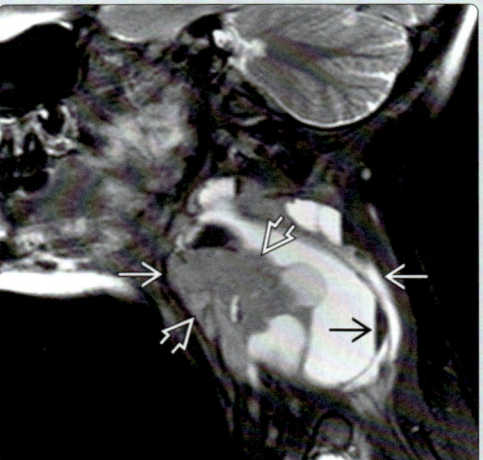 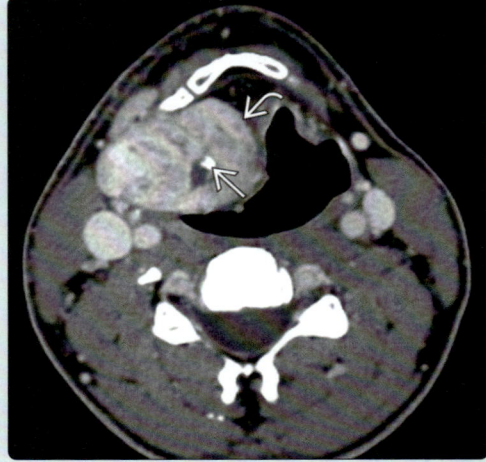

(Left) *Parasagittal T2 FS MR shows a markedly heterogenous but well-circumscribed mass in the posterior cervical space ➡. The mass shows the triple sign with iso-, hypo-, and hyperintense foci: The largely hyperintense cystic component has a focus of hypointense layering hemorrhage ➡, and there is a solid hypointense component ➡ anteriorly. **(Right)** Axial CECT at the hyoid shows a well-defined, heterogeneously enhancing submucosal right paraglottic mass in the supraglottic larynx ➡ with focal Ca^{++} ➡.*

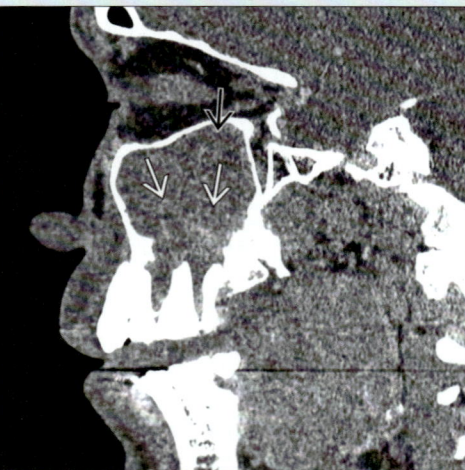 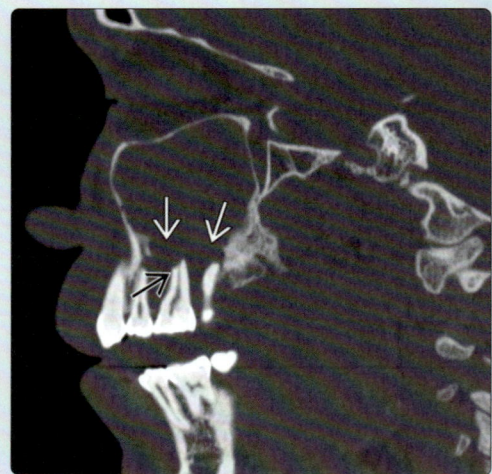

(Left) *Parasagittal CECT shows an aggressive soft tissue mass arising in the maxillary alveolus and extending cephalad into the maxillary sinus ➡. Lower-density post obstructive secretions ➡ are present superiorly. **(Right)** Parasagittal bone CT in the same patient shows an unusual appearance with overt punched-out lytic bone destruction of the involved portions of the maxillary alveolus ➡ with some erosion of the dentition ➡ due to this aggressive synovial sarcoma.*

TERMINOLOGY

Abbreviations
- Synovial sarcoma (SSa)

Definitions
- Malignant soft tissue tumor with epithelial and mesenchymal components

IMAGING

General Features
- Best diagnostic clue
  - Heterogeneous, well-defined, **nonnodal, nonmucosal** soft tissue mass
- Location
  - Hypopharynx > > > masticator space, parapharyngeal space, paranasal sinuses, infratemporal fossa
- Size
  - Variable, 2-8 cm

CT Findings
- CECT
  - Well-defined, lobular mass
  - Mild, heterogeneous enhancement ± cysts, Ca++, hemorrhage
  - Bone invasion extremely rare

MR Findings
- T1WI
  - Iso- to slightly hyperintense to muscle
- T2WI
  - Hyperintense relative to muscle
  - Triple sign: Iso-, hypo-, and hyperintense foci (due to solid, cystic, Ca++ ± hemorrhagic components)
  - Cobblestone sign: Cystic foci with well-defined septa
- T1WI C+
  - Heterogeneous, enhancing mass ± septations

Imaging Recommendations
- Best imaging tool
  - Contrast-enhanced MR

DIFFERENTIAL DIAGNOSIS

Rhabdomyosarcoma
- Middle ear, sinus, nasopharynx, and adjacent spaces
- Aggressive soft tissue mass ± nodes
- Intermediate signal on all MR sequences

Malignant Fibrous Histiocytoma
- Most common sarcoma of head and neck in adults
- Low to intermediate signal on all MR sequences

Solitary Fibrous Tumor
- Sinonasal, dural, perivertebral space
- Locally aggressive mass; prominent vasculature; bone invasion common

Nerve Sheath Tumors
- Benign > > malignant
- Generally well-defined, T2-hyperintense mass

Pleomorphic Adenoma
- Commonly T2-hyperintense, lobulated mass

PATHOLOGY

General Features
- Genetics
  - Translocation t(X;18)(p11.2;q11.2) specific for SSa
  - Misnomer; named for appearance of cells not origin
  - Dual epithelial and mesenchymal cell differentiation
    - Biphasic is classic form with both components

Gross Pathologic & Surgical Features
- Areas of necrosis, hemorrhage, and cysts common

CLINICAL ISSUES

Presentation
- Most common signs/symptoms
  - Palpable mass
  - May have lymph node metastases

Demographics
- Age
  - Adolescents and young adults; typical range: 15-35 years
- Epidemiology
  - 7-10% of all sarcomas (4th most common)
    - Head and neck least common location (3% overall)
    - Far more common in extremities

Natural History & Prognosis
- Prognosis in head and neck more favorable than extremity
  - ↓ prognosis if poorly differentiated
  - ↓ prognosis in patients > 30 years of age, larger SSa with bony invasion, hemorrhage, or paraspinal location
  - ↓ prognosis for upper aerodigestive tract lesions
  - ↑ prognosis if Ca++ present

Treatment
- Complete excision with negative margins
- Postoperative XRT
  - Systemic therapy for disseminated disease

DIAGNOSTIC CHECKLIST

Consider
- SSa unique among sarcomas; well-defined soft tissue mass with heterogeneous signal intensity on T2 MR

Reporting Tips
- Ca++, hemorrhage, septations, solid & cystic
- Lymph node metastases

SELECTED REFERENCES

1. Martín Pérez JA et al: Synovial sarcoma of the larynx, a rare and unusual entity. Case report. Int J Surg Case Rep. 126:110716, 2025
2. Patel RR et al: Oncologic outcomes in patients with localized, primary head and neck synovial sarcoma. Cancers (Basel). 16(23):4119, 2024
3. Lin N et al: Sinonasal synovial sarcoma: evaluation of the role of radiological and clinicopathological features in diagnosis. Clin Radiol. 76(1):78.e1-8, 2021
4. Wang DJ et al: The imaging spectrum of synovial sarcomas: a pictorial review from a single-centre tertiary referral institution. Can Assoc Radiol J. 72(3):470-82, 2021

Transspatial and Multispatial

TERMINOLOGY

- Malignant tumor of Schwann cell or other nerve sheath cell origin

IMAGING

- CECT findings
  - Infiltrating soft tissue mass associated with peripheral nerve
- NECT findings
  - Bone erosion or regressive remodeling/foraminal enlargement
- MR findings
  - Irregular mass with heterogeneous signal
  - Absent target sign on T2; absent split fat sign on T1
  - May see flow voids
- FDG PET
  - In neurofibromatosis type 1 (NF1), ↑ SUV may differentiate known neurofibroma from malignant peripheral nerve sheath tumor (MPNST)

TOP DIFFERENTIAL DIAGNOSES

- Neurofibroma
- Schwannoma
- Solitary fibrous tumor
- Malignant fibrous histiocytoma

PATHOLOGY

- **50%** occur in **NF1** patients
- **10%** of MPNST associated with **radiation exposure**
- ↑ risk of MPNST in SMARCB1-related schwannomatosis
- Nearly 50% arise de novo in normal peripheral nerve

CLINICAL ISSUES

- "Schwannoma recurrence" should suggest MPNST
- Rapidly enlarging mass in NF1 patient raises concern
- Mixed sensory & motor symptom deficits favor MPSNT
- Wide en bloc surgical resection ± radiation therapy
- Distant metastases common: Lung > liver & bone
- Overall poor prognosis

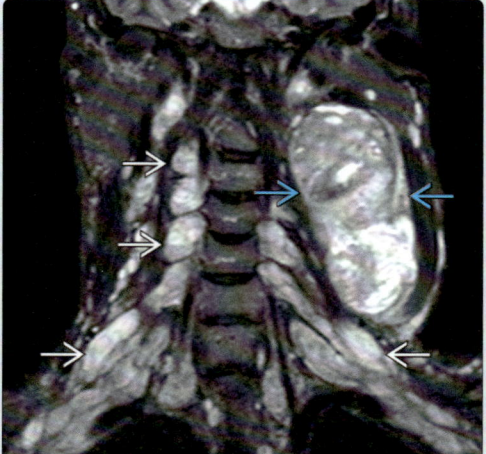
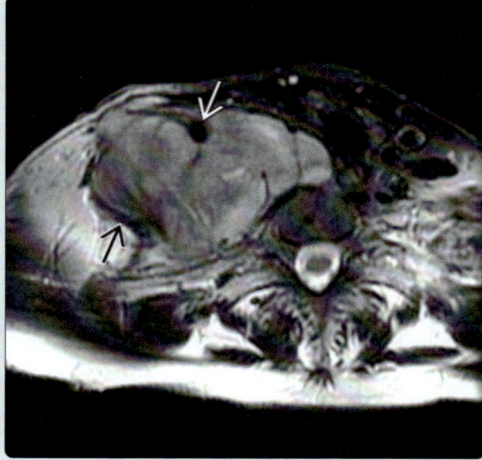

(Left) *Coronal T2 FS MR in a patient with a rapidly enlarging left neck mass shows a heterogeneous left neck malignant peripheral nerve sheath tumor (MPNST) ➡. Extensive plexiform neurofibromas are noted at every cervical nerve root level & the brachial plexus bilaterally ➡. (Right) Axial T2 MR shows heterogeneous, well-defined mass between the right anterior ➡ & middle ➡ scalene muscles along the brachial plexus. No specific imaging findings differentiate this MPNST from a benign nerve sheath tumor.*

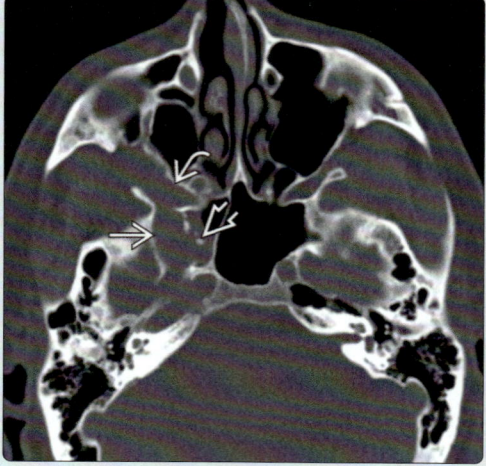
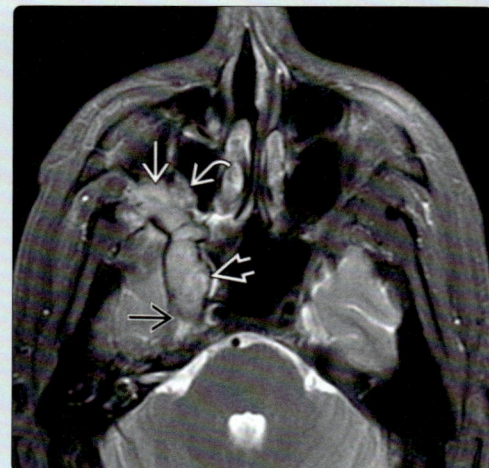

(Left) *Axial bone CT shows an MPNST affecting the 2nd division of the trigeminal nerve (CNV2), causing regressive remodeling & widening of pterygopalatine fossa ➡ & foramen rotundum ➡ & destruction of right lateral sphenoid sinus wall ➡. (Right) Axial T2 FS MR in the same patient reveals a heterogeneously hyperintense CNV2 MPNST invading soft tissues of the pterygopalatine fossa ➡ & right maxillary sinus ➡, indicating aggressive behavior. The mass involves infraorbital nerve, cavernous sinus ➡, & Meckel cave ➡.*

Malignant Peripheral Nerve Sheath Tumor of Head and Neck

TERMINOLOGY

Abbreviations
- Malignant peripheral nerve sheath tumor (MPNST)

Synonyms
- Neurogenic sarcoma, malignant schwannoma, malignant neurolemmoma, neurofibrosarcoma

Definitions
- Malignant tumor of Schwann cell or other nerve sheath cell origin

IMAGING

General Features
- Best diagnostic clue
  - Infiltrating soft tissue mass associated with peripheral nerve
- Location
  - Rare in head & neck region
    - Brachial plexus, sympathetic chain, CNV
    - May arise from preexisting neurofibromas
- Size
  - Larger in neurofibromatosis type 1 (NF1)

CT Findings
- CECT
  - Heterogeneously enhancing mass with no Ca^{++}
- Bone CT
  - Bone erosion, remodeling, foraminal enlargement

MR Findings
- T1WI
  - Tumor is isointense to muscle
  - Absent split fat sign
- T2WI
  - Heterogeneous signal; no target sign
  - Irregular margins & peritumor edema strongly suggest MPNST over benign PNST
- DWI
  - ↑↑ restricted DWI; low ADC (< 1.0-1.1×10^{-3} mm²/s)
- T1WI C+
  - Heterogeneous enhancement

Nuclear Medicine Findings
- PET
  - In NF1, may differentiate neurofibroma from MPNST
    - SUV generally higher in MPNST

Imaging Recommendations
- Best imaging tool
  - Enhanced MR ± bone CT if affecting bone (e.g., skull base)
  - PET + MR = highest specificity differentiating benign PNST from MPNST

DIFFERENTIAL DIAGNOSIS

Neurofibroma
- May have target signal ± central enhancement on T2 MR

Schwannoma
- Heterogeneous; cannot distinguish from MPNST
- May have central enhancement (never in MPNST)

Solitary Fibrous Tumor
- Heterogeneous mass often with flow voids
- Typically lacks bone destruction
- May have Ca^{++}; never present in MPNST

Malignant Fibrous Histiocytoma
- Cannot distinguish from MPNST on imaging

PATHOLOGY

General Features
- Etiology
  - **~ 50%** occur in **NF1** patients
    - Deeper plexiform neurofibromas at higher risk
    - Leading cause of mortality in NF1
  - Nearly 50% arise de novo in normal peripheral nerve
  - **10%** of MPNST associated with **radiation exposure**
  - ↑ risk of MPNST in *SMARCB1*-related schwannomatosis

Staging, Grading, & Classification
- No accepted staging system

Microscopic Features
- Unencapsulated spindle cell tumor
- Histologic diagnosis difficult

CLINICAL ISSUES

Presentation
- Most common signs/symptoms
  - Enlarging soft tissue mass
- Other signs/symptoms
  - Mixed sensory & motor symptoms
    - Neurologic deficit rare in benign tumors

Demographics
- Age
  - 20-50 years (10 years earlier in NF1)

Natural History & Prognosis
- "Schwannoma recurrence" concerning for MPNST
- Nodal metastases rare
- Distant metastases common: Lung (33%) > > liver & bone
- Poor prognosis

Treatment
- Wide en bloc resection ± postoperative radiation therapy

DIAGNOSTIC CHECKLIST

Image Interpretation Pearls
- Infiltrative, fusiform tumor along peripheral nerve
- Never see target sign on T2 MR in NF1 setting

SELECTED REFERENCES

1. Perrino MR et al: Update on cancer and central nervous system tumor surveillance in pediatric NF2-, SMARCB1-, and LZTR1-related schwannomatosis. Clin Cancer Res. 31(8):1400-6, 2025
2. Lucas CG et al: Consensus recommendations for an integrated diagnostic approach to peripheral nerve sheath tumors arising in the setting of neurofibromatosis type 1 (NF1). Neuro Oncol. 27(3):616-24, 2024

Transspatial and Multispatial

TERMINOLOGY

- Benign, lymph-filled cyst due to leaking lymphatic channels
- Lymphatic cyst, lymphocyst, chylocele, chyloma, chylous cyst, (distal) thoracic duct cyst

IMAGING

- Best imaging tools are CECT and US
- Characteristic location is low posterior cervical space in **supraclavicular fossa**
  - Between scalene and sternocleidomastoid muscles
- Unilocular, well-circumscribed cyst with **no visible cyst wall**, enhancement, or septa
  - Cyst wall thickened ± enhancing if complicated by infection/treatment
  - Fluid density (CT HU usually 0-20) or signal (MR)

TOP DIFFERENTIAL DIAGNOSES

- Congenital neck cysts
  - Lymphatic malformation
  - 3rd branchial cleft
  - Thymic cyst
- Postoperative seroma, hematoma, or pseudomeningocele
- Systemic nodal metastases
- Suppurative lymph nodes

PATHOLOGY

- Endothelial-lined cyst with acellular fluid and **fat droplets**

CLINICAL ISSUES

- Growing, painless neck mass without signs of infection
- Treatment options
  - Complete surgical removal is curative
  - Percutaneous sclerotherapy if surgery not possible

DIAGNOSTIC CHECKLIST

- Consider lymphocele in **postoperative** patient with low posterior cervical space supraclavicular cyst pointing toward confluence of internal jugular and subclavian veins
- FNA to confirm ± imaging surveillance if atypical

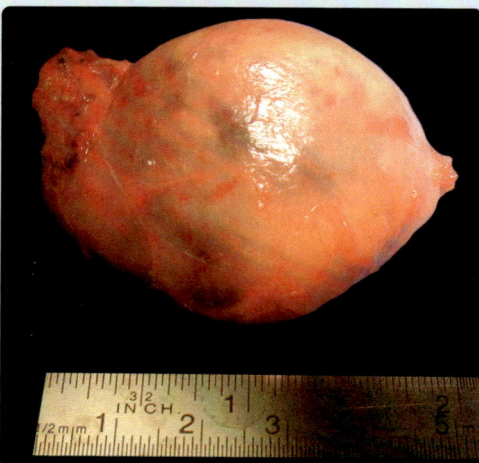
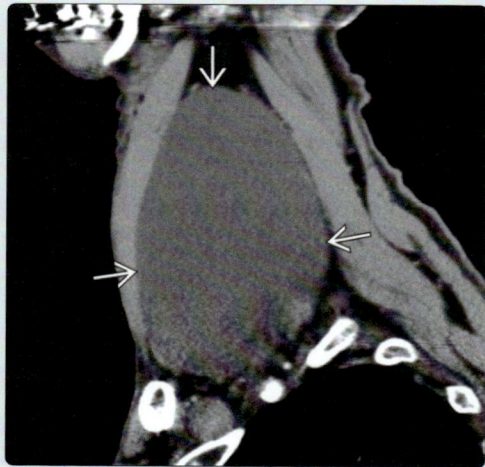

(Left) Gross specimen of a lymphocele shows its typical encapsulated appearance. These masses are usually easy to remove surgically with subsequent cure. (Right) Sagittal CECT MPR demonstrates the typical CT characteristics of a lymphocele: A unilocular, nonseptated, round or ovoid, water-density cyst in the supraclavicular fossa with no perceptible cyst wall ➡ or enhancement.

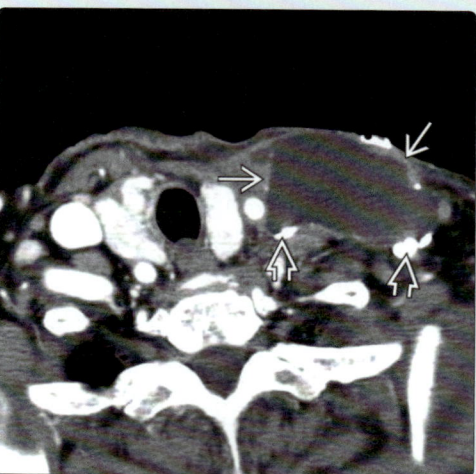
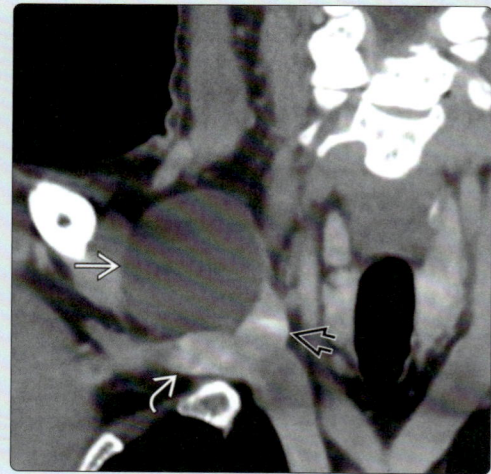

(Left) Axial CECT of a postoperative lymphatic duct lymphocele shows a fluid density cyst in the low posterior cervical space, lateral to the common carotid artery. Cyst wall enhancement ➡ and dependent embolic material ⇨ are related to recent percutaneous sclerotherapy with onyx. (Right) Coronal CECT shows a spontaneously occurring simple unilocular cystic lesion ➡ in the right supraclavicular fossa, centered at the confluence of the internal jugular vein ⇨ and subclavian vein ➡.

TERMINOLOGY

Synonyms

- Lymphatic cyst, lymphocyst, chylocele, chyloma, chylous cyst, (distal) thoracic duct cyst

Definitions

- Benign cyst formed from leaking lymph channels

IMAGING

General Features

- Best diagnostic clue
  - Nonenhancing unilocular fluid-density/signal intensity cyst in supraclavicular fossa
- Location
  - **Posterior cervical space**
  - **Left side** more common
  - **Supraclavicular fossa** most common
    - Distal thoracic duct most common, often at confluence of internal jugular and subclavian veins
    - Rarely high in neck along course of jugular lymphatic trunks
    - Distal thoracic duct cyst may be mediastinal &/or cervical
  - Between scalene and sternocleidomastoid muscles
- Morphology
  - Round, oval, ± lobulations

CT Findings

- NECT
  - Unilocular, fluid density cyst (HU usually 0-20)
  - Well circumscribed
  - No soft tissue nodularity
  - Lack of perceptible cyst wall
    - Lack of septations and surgical history help distinguish from lymphatic malformation
- CECT
  - Nonenhancing cyst wall unless complicated by infection or prior treatment

MR Findings

- T2WI
  - High-signal cyst contents
- T1WI C+
  - No enhancement unless complicated
- Fluid signal intensity on all MR sequences

Ultrasonographic Findings

- Grayscale ultrasound
  - Anechoic or hypoechoic; ↑ through transmission
  - Septa and debris uncommon unless complicated

Imaging Recommendations

- Best imaging tool
  - CECT
- Protocol advice
  - Contrast to exclude infectious or neoplastic causes

DIFFERENTIAL DIAGNOSIS

Congenital Neck Cysts

- Lymphatic malformation
  - Usually transspatial with septa and fluid levels
- 3rd branchial cleft cyst
  - Pediatric age group without surgical history
  - Thin cyst wall; rim enhancing if infected
- Thymic cyst
  - Left cervical-thoracic dumbbell cyst when large

Postoperative Seroma or Hematoma

- Found within surgical bed
- Seroma is CSF signal
- Subacute hematoma is hyperdense on NECT, T1 hyper- and T2 hypointense on MR

Pseudomeningocele (CSF Leak)

- CSF density/signal all sequences
- Enlarging over time with postural headache clinically

Systemic Nodal Metastases

- Cystic nodal metastases usually have perceptible cyst wall with rim enhancement

Suppurative Lymph Nodes

- Enhancing cyst wall with irregular shape or nodularity

PATHOLOGY

Gross Pathologic & Surgical Features

- Bland, acellular fluid with **lipid droplets**
- **Endothelial-lined cyst** ± lymph channel adventitial capsule

CLINICAL ISSUES

Presentation

- Most common signs/symptoms
  - Painless, enlarging supraclavicular neck mass
  - Spontaneous or acquired (surgery or trauma)

Treatment

- Surgical resection curative
- Percutaneous sclerotherapy if patient not surgical candidate or surgery unsuccessful
- Microscopic lymphatic ligation &/or lymphovenous anastomosis for recurrent postoperative lymphocele
- Thoracic duct embolization

DIAGNOSTIC CHECKLIST

Consider

- US, CECT, and MR show bland fluid without cyst wall
- FNA diagnostic with acellular fluid having lipid droplets

Image Interpretation Pearls

- Consider lymphocele in postoperative patient with low posterior cervical space cyst pointing toward confluence of internal jugular and subclavian veins

SELECTED REFERENCES

1. Lee EW et al: Retrograde distal thoracic duct leak embolization via access through lymphocele after thyroidectomy and neck dissection. Korean J Radiol. 25(5):501-3, 2024
2. Uyulmaz S et al: Lymphovenous anastomoses and microscopic lymphatic ligations for the treatment of persistent lymphocele. Plast Reconstr Surg Glob Open. 9(2):e3407, 2021
3. Hamilton BE et al: Characteristic imaging findings in lymphoceles of the head and neck. AJR Am J Roentgenol. 197(6):1431-5, 2011

Sinus Histiocytosis (Rosai-Dorfman) of Head and Neck

KEY FACTS

TERMINOLOGY

- Sinus histiocytosis: Benign pseudolymphomatous clinicopathologic entity of unknown etiology

IMAGING

- **Massive, bilateral cervical lymphadenopathy**
- Head & neck extranodal sites in ~ **50%**
  - Skin, sinonasal, orbits, bone, salivary glands, & dura
- Rare other extranodal sites: Oral cavity, pharynx, trachea, bronchi, & mediastinal lymph nodes
- Imaging findings : CT, MR, PET/CT
  - Homogeneously enhancing, large lymph nodes
  - Enhancing extranodal infiltrates
  - **T2 low signal** of nodal or extranodal lesions common
  - PET/CT: ↑ ↑ FDG uptake

TOP DIFFERENTIAL DIAGNOSES

- Non-Hodgkin lymphoma
- IgG4-related disease

- Skull base meningioma
- Langerhans cell histiocytosis
- Reactive lymph nodes

PATHOLOGY

- Unknown pathophysiology

CLINICAL ISSUES

- Clinical presentation
  - Painless neck masses
- Age at presentation
  - < 20 years old (80%)
- Natural history
  - Long history of benign disease involvement common
  - ↑ morbidity when immunologic dysfunction present (arthritis, circulating autoantibodies)
- Treatment
  - Clinical observation preferred
  - Surgical debulking if vital structure compression

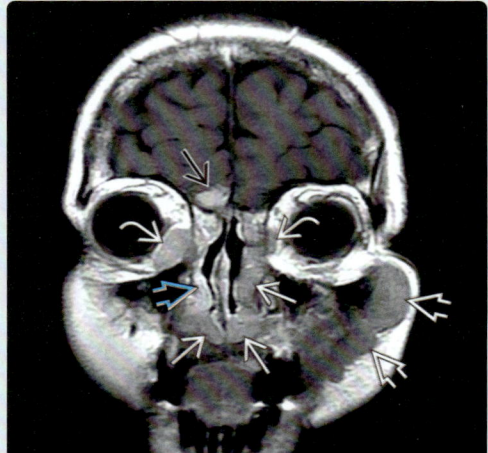
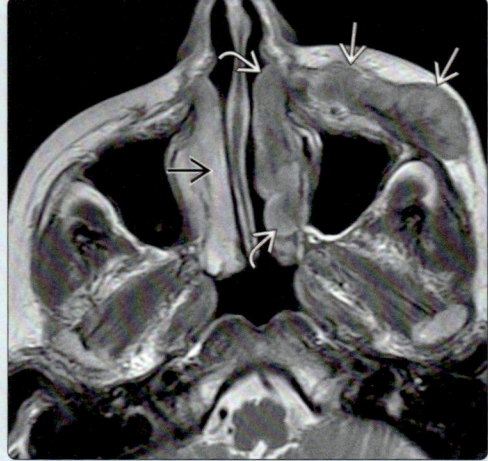

(Left) Coronal T1 C+ MR shows multifocal sinus histiocytosis (SH) lesions extending along the floor of the bilateral nasal cavities & left midnasal cavity ➡, left premaxillary soft tissues ➡, bilateral extraconal orbits ➡, & right frontal dura ➡. Note the lesions are subtly enhancing but much less so than the nasal mucosa ➡. (Right) Axial T2 MR shows lobular SH lesions within left premaxillary soft tissues ➡ also extend into left nasal cavity ➡. Lesions are relatively T2 hypointense to normal sinonasal mucosa ➡.

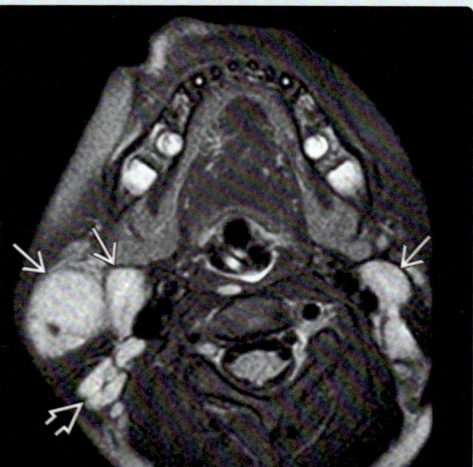
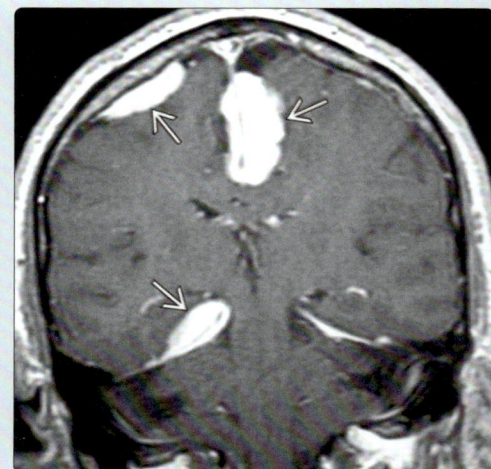

(Left) Axial STIR MR in a child reveals multiple large level 2A ➡ & level 2B ➡ lymph nodes. Notice the right parotid tail large nodal conglomerate mass as well. Nodal biopsy demonstrated SH. (Right) Coronal T1 C+ MR in a patient with documented SH demonstrates multiple smoothly marginated, hemispheric dural-based, avidly enhancing masses ➡, originally thought to be multiple meningiomas. Distinction on imaging alone would be difficult.

TERMINOLOGY

Abbreviations
- Sinus histiocytosis (SH)

Synonyms
- SH with massive lymphadenopathy, Rosai-Dorfman disease

Definitions
- Benign, pseudolymphomatous, clinicopathologic entity of unknown etiology

IMAGING

General Features
- Best diagnostic clue
  - Massive, bilateral cervical lymphadenopathy in patient < 20 years of age
- Location
  - **Bilateral cervical lymphadenopathy**
  - Extranodal sites in ~ 50%: Skin, sinonasal area, orbit, eyelids, bone, salivary glands, & dura

Imaging Recommendations
- Best imaging tool
  - CECT or enhanced MR (suprahyoid lesions)
  - PET/CT: Assessing extent & monitor treatment response

CT Findings
- CECT
  - Homogeneously enhancing, large lymph nodes
    - Bilateral & very large in children
  - Enhancing extranodal infiltrates
    - **Skin, sinuses, nose, orbit, eyelids, bone, salivary glands, & dura**
    - Parotid glands: Low-density foci reported

MR Findings
- T1WI
  - Low signal intensity relative to muscle
- T2WI
  - Relatively **low signal** intensity compared to muscle
    - May help differentiate SH from other causes of lymph node enlargement & extranodal infiltrates
- T1WI C+
  - Homogeneous, enhancing, large neck nodes
  - Enhancing, extranodal, infiltrating masses

Ultrasonographic Findings
- Nonspecific hypoechoic lymph nodes & deposits

Nuclear Medicine Findings
- PET/CT: ↑ ↑ FDG uptake in lymph nodes & deposits

DIFFERENTIAL DIAGNOSIS

Non-Hodgkin Lymphoma
- May exactly mimic

IgG4-Related Disease
- May exactly mimic extranodal SH on imaging

Skull Base Meningioma
- SH of dura may mimic meningioma

Langerhans Cell Histiocytosis
- Nodal disease rare

Reactive Lymph Nodes
- Large, diffuse adenopathy common in children

PATHOLOGY

General Features
- Etiology
  - Unknown pathophysiology
  - Postulated etiologies: Infection, immunodeficiency, autoimmune disease, neoplastic process
- Associated abnormalities
  - ↑ morbidity & mortality when associated immunologic abnormality exists

Microscopic Features
- "Sinusal" lymph node architecture with clustering of lymphocytes simulating germinal centers
- Emperipolesis: Histiocytes phagocytize lymphocytes, plasma cells, erythrocytes, or polymorphonuclear leukocytes
- Immunohistochemical (IHC) analysis
  - SH histiocyte-positive IHC stains: S100, CD68, CD163
  - SH histiocyte-negative IHC stain: CD1a
- Intracytoplasmic eosinophilic globules (Russell bodies) in plasma cells

CLINICAL ISSUES

Presentation
- Most common signs/symptoms
  - Painless neck masses, fevers
  - Elevated erythrocyte sediment rate positive (90%)

Demographics
- Age
  - < 20 years old (80%); < 10 years old (66%)
- Epidemiology
  - More common in African & West Indian heritage

Natural History & Prognosis
- Long history of benign disease involvement common
- ↑ morbidity when immunologic dysfunction present

Treatment
- Most patients do not require treatment
- Surgical debulking in cases of vital structure compression
- Radiation, chemotherapy, & steroids not proven efficacious

SELECTED REFERENCES

1. Solav SV et al: FDG PET scan in cutaneous Rosai-Dorfman-Destombes disease. Indian J Nucl Med. 39(5):396-8, 2024
2. Tran PTC et al: Clinicopathological characteristics of extranodal Rosai-Dorfman disease: a retrospective case series of 25 patients. Ann Diagn Pathol. 73:152377, 2024
3. Li C et al: Clinical features, diagnosis, treatment and prognosis of otolaryngological extranodal sinus histiocytosis with massive lymphadenopathy (Rosai-Dorfman disease, RDD). Eur Arch Otorhinolaryngol. 280(2):861-7, 2023
4. Alwani MM et al: Manifestations of pediatric extranodal Rosai Dorfman disease in the head and neck. Int J Pediatr Otorhinolaryngol. 131:109851, 2020

Fibromatosis of Head and Neck

TERMINOLOGY

- Aggressive fibromatosis, extraabdominal desmoid, infantile fibromatosis
- Rare, infiltrative mass of benign monoclonal fibroblast proliferation

IMAGING

- Well-defined or ill-defined, nonnecrotic, enhancing **transspatial** mass in any head & neck space
- Variable appearance: May be sharply circumscribed or infiltrative; rarely muscle & bone invasion
- CT: No tumor matrix calcification or ossification
- MR: T1 iso- to hypointense compared to muscle
- T2-hyperintense ± hypointense bands
- Generally avid enhancement on MR
- Contrast-enhanced MR is study of choice, as it best shows relationship to critical structures
- If image-guided biopsy performed, always get **core sample** for histology & stains

TOP DIFFERENTIAL DIAGNOSES

- Non-Hodgkin lymphoma, especially nonnodal
- Rhabdomyosarcoma
- Soft tissue fibrosarcoma
- Soft tissue metastases
- Fibromatosis colli (sternocleidomastoid tumor of infancy)

PATHOLOGY

- Infiltrative, unencapsulated growth with uniform spindle cells & collagenous stroma
- In adults, more likely to be associated with Gardner syndrome, familial adenomatous polyposis
- Infantile fibromatosis differs in demographics, genetics, behavior, & treatment

CLINICAL ISSUES

- No nodal or distant metastatic potential but high local recurrence rate
- Complete resection is treatment of choice

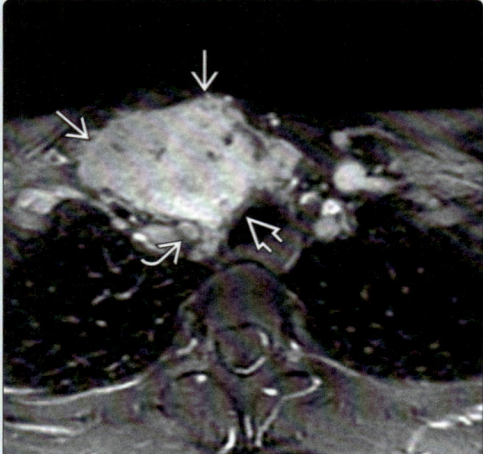
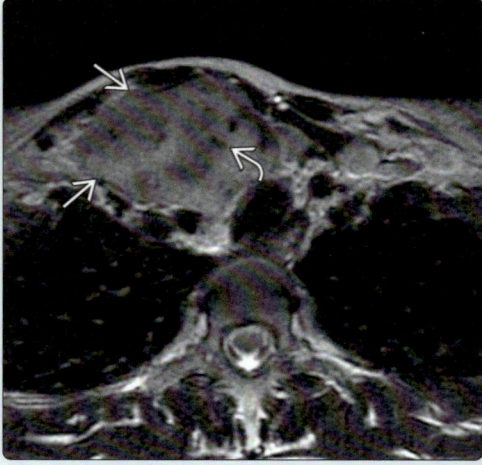

(Left) Axial T1WI C+ FS MR in a young adult with fibromatosis shows a diffuse, enhancing mass ➡ in the lower neck supraclavicular to superior mediastinum region, abutting the trachea ➡ but not infiltrating the tracheal wall. Note the clear plane between the mass & right common carotid artery ➡. (Right) Axial T2WI MR in the same patient delineates the hyperintense mass ➡ from the adjacent sternocleidomastoid & strap muscles & shows focal & linear areas of low signal ➡. The mass is separate from the trachea & vessels.

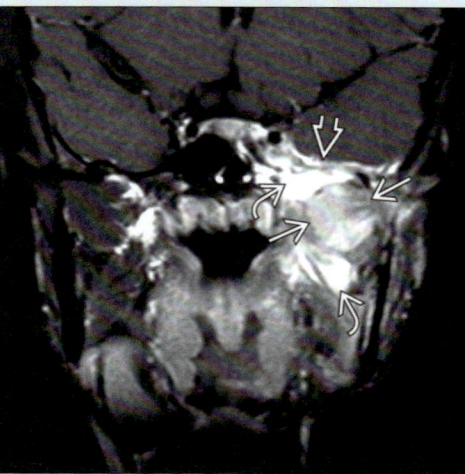
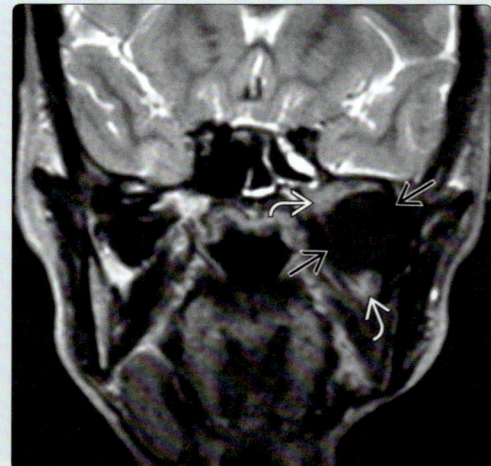

(Left) Coronal T1WI C+ MR shows invasive, aggressive fibromatosis filling the left masticator space with areas of intense ➡ & milder ➡ enhancement. Note skull base involvement of middle cranial fossa dura ➡. (Right) Coronal T2WI MR in the same patient shows diffuse low signal in the milder enhancing portion ➡, compared with remaining T2-hyperintense areas ➡, which showed intense enhancement in the prior image. Lower T2 signal is most commonly seen in older lesions that have stopped growing clinically.

TERMINOLOGY

Synonyms

- Aggressive fibromatosis, extraabdominal desmoid, infantile fibromatosis

Definitions

- Rare, well-defined or infiltrative mass lesion of benign monoclonal fibroblast proliferation
  - In head & neck, deep fibromatoses
  - Superficial fibromatoses most often in extremities

IMAGING

General Features

- Best diagnostic clue
  - Well-defined or ill-defined, infiltrative, nonnecrotic, **transspatial**, enhancing mass
  - Nondesmoid fibromatosis constitutes 60-70%
- Location
  - Any space of extracranial head & neck; often transspatial
  - Most commonly: Salivary glands
  - Supraclavicular area, masticator space, adjacent to mandible, especially if surgical hardware present, deep to sternocleidomastoid muscle
  - Rarely in soft tissue adjacent to cervical spine surgical hardware
  - Infantile desmoid fibromatosis most commonly involves head & neck, especially tongue, mandible, mastoid
    - Rarely larynx & hypopharynx, including postcricoid region, masticator space, face, orbit
- Size
  - Most often 3-10 cm; < 15% of cases are multiple lesions
- Morphology
  - May have well-circumscribed margin
  - More aggressive, & also recurrent, lesions have irregular margins with local muscle & bone invasion
  - May see both well-demarcated & infiltrative margins in same lesion
  - > 1/2 high-grade tumors

CT Findings

- CECT
  - May appear sharply circumscribed or infiltrative
  - Mild to moderate contrast enhancement
  - No tumor matrix calcification or ossification
- Bone CT
  - May erode or invade bone

MR Findings

- T1WI
  - Iso- to hypointense compared to muscle
- T2WI
  - Generally hyperintense; rarely lower T2 signal in older lesions that stopped growing clinically
  - Hypointense bands corresponding to collagen bundles often seen
- T1WI C+
  - Variable but generally avid enhancement
- MRA
  - Larger neck lesions may encircle and compress vessels

- **Recurrent tumor**: After excision, recurrence often has more poorly defined, infiltrative margins
  - Following radiation, tumor ↓ in T1 and T2 signal, becomes more well defined

Imaging Recommendations

- Best imaging tool
  - Contrast-enhanced MR is study of choice
    - Best demonstrates lesion extent & relationship to neural & vascular structures
    - Best study for evaluating response to treatment & recurrence
- Protocol advice
  - Near skull base, both MR & bone CT recommended
    - Contrast-enhanced MR defines soft tissue extent
    - Bone CT identifies bone invasion or erosion
- If image-guided biopsy performed, **core sample** essential so histomorphology & special stains can be performed

Nuclear Medicine Findings

- PET/CT
  - Heterogeneous, mild to moderate FDG uptake
    - FDG may be useful to determine early response to treatment

DIFFERENTIAL DIAGNOSIS

Non-Hodgkin Lymphoma

- May infiltrate multiple spaces when in extranodal, extralymphatic site
- Usually associated with pathologic adenopathy in addition to nonnodal mass

Rhabdomyosarcoma

- Children or young adults, often with cranial neuropathy
- Most often temporal bone, orbit, sinonasal; less often deep face

Soft Tissue Fibrosarcoma

- Very rare malignant tumor of deep face
- If in masticator space, difficult to distinguish from aggressive fibromatosis

Soft Tissue Metastases

- Typically older patient with known primary tumor
- Multiple enhancing, nodular lesions ± nodes

Fibromatosis Colli

- Sternocleidomastoid (SCM) tumor of infancy, associated with muscular torticollis
- Right > left firm, nontender, fusiform mid/lower SCM mass with variable T2 signal and enhancement seen
- Self-limited behavior, microscopic appearance, & treatment distinguish from other forms of infantile fibromatosis
- Mass appears within 2 weeks of delivery, may ↑ in size for days to weeks, & usually regresses by 8 months of age
- Fine-needle aspiration cytology (FNAC) differentiates from other congenital, inflammatory, & neoplastic etiologies

PATHOLOGY

General Features

- Etiology

- ○ Arises from connective tissue, fascia, & musculoaponeurotic structures
  - − Unclear whether **reactive** or **neoplastic growth**
- ○ Unknown cause but various factors proposed: Trauma, surgery, & endocrine
  - − Rare fibromatoses after cervical spine surgery
- Genetics
  - ○ Mutations found in β-catenin protein (*CTNNB1*) or adenomatous polyposis coli (*APC*) gene
    - − Fibromatoses accumulate excess intranuclear β-catenin protein
    - − Mutations not always found in infantile fibromatoses
- Associated abnormalities
  - ○ Most infantile & adult cases are sporadic
  - ○ In adults, more likely to be associated with polyposis syndromes
    - − Familial adenomatous polyposis
    - − Gardner syndrome
      - □ Autosomal dominant: Polyposis coli, osteomas, fibromas, & epidermoid cysts
      - □ Aggressive fibromatosis may be 1st presentation of Gardner syndrome in child

Staging, Grading, & Classification

- No accepted staging system; does not metastasize to nodes or distant sites

Gross Pathologic & Surgical Features

- Whitish, firm, fibrous mass ± adjacent bone & skeletal muscle invasion

Microscopic Features

- Infiltrative, unencapsulated growth with uniform spindle cells & collagenous stroma
- Bland microscopic appearance: No necrosis or abnormal mitoses
- Spindle cell nuclei stain diffusely for **β-catenin**
- Rare reports of thyroid cancer (medullary & papillary) with desmoid-type fibromatosis
- Infantile fibromatosis: 2 microscopic patterns
  - ○ Immature or diffuse pattern, fat often present; called lipofibromatosis if abundant fat
  - ○ Adult pattern identical to adult extraabdominal desmoid fibromatosis, β-catenin positive

CLINICAL ISSUES

Presentation

- Most common signs/symptoms
  - ○ Painless, firm, growing, fixed mass
- Other signs/symptoms
  - ○ Other symptoms depend on tissues involved
    - − Lower neck: Radiculopathy, brachial plexopathy
    - − Deep face: Trismus, dysphagia, airway obstruction
    - − Below skull base: Cranial neuropathies
    - − Orbit: Proptosis
- Clinical profile
  - ○ Adult with firm, painless neck mass
  - ○ Adult with prior history of mandibular or cervical spine surgery

Demographics

- Age
  - ○ Average: 57.4 years
  - ○ Infantile fibromatosis: Usually 1st or 2nd year of life
    - − Upper age limit to differentiate infantile & adult desmoid fibromatosis varies in different series
      - □ 5-10 years of age proposed; most **below 8 years**
- Sex
  - ○ White (≈ 84%) males (≈ 61%)
  - ○ Infantile fibromatosis: M = F
- Epidemiology
  - ○ Rare entity accounting for 0.03% of all neoplasms in human body; head & neck lesions account for 12-15% of all fibromatoses

Natural History & Prognosis

- Unpredictable clinical behavior
  - ○ Teen & adult fibromatosis usually more aggressive than childhood fibromatosis
- Locally aggressive, causing morbidity by invading tissues
- No metastatic potential but high local recurrence rate
  - ○ 10-80% recurrence rate
  - ○ Most recurrences within 2-3 years, up to 6 years
- Cases of spontaneous regression without treatment reported

Treatment

- **Surgery is treatment of choice**
  - ○ Aims to achieve microscopically negative margin
  - ○ Functional considerations in head & neck may limit complete resection
- Radiation for incomplete resection, recurrent tumor, or if lesion not safely resectable
  - ○ Generally not advocated in pediatric patients
- Chemotherapy may be with noncytotoxic or cytotoxic drugs
  - ○ Noncytotoxics: Tamoxifen (antiestrogen) & nonsteroidal antiinflammatory drugs
  - ○ Cytotoxic agents: Vinblastine & methotrexate
    - − Reserved for refractory or severely morbid disease
- For recurrent but stable lesions, clinical observation alone may be considered

DIAGNOSTIC CHECKLIST

Consider

- Fibromatosis of head & neck when large, painless **transspatial** mass
- Infantile fibromatosis behaves somewhat differently
  - ○ Less aggressive, less often associated with gene mutations, polyposis syndromes

Image Interpretation Pearls

- Think of aggressive fibromatosis if malignant-appearing mass in neck of young adult
- Main differential: Sarcoma of deep tissues
- Image-guided biopsy should be **core** so histomorphology & special stains can be performed

SELECTED REFERENCES

1. Raad RA et al: A nationwide analysis of head and neck fibromatoses. Laryngoscope. 134(5):2228-35, 2024

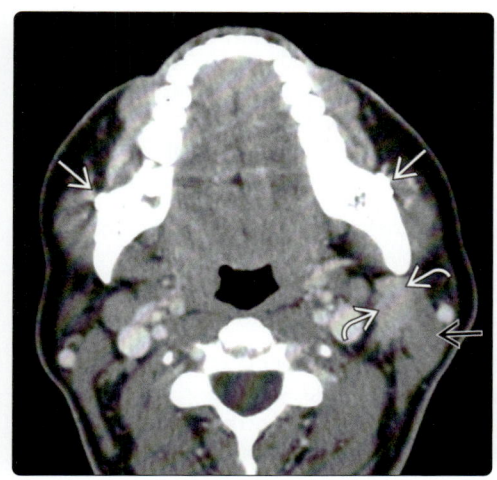

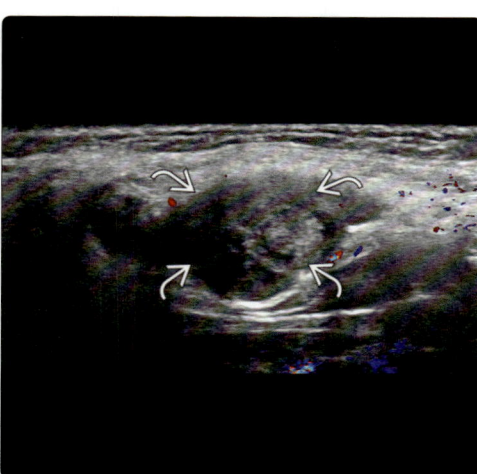

(Left) Axial CECT in a 43-year-old woman who had mandibular reconstruction surgery ➡ 2 years ago and now has a firm to hard mass behind the mandible shows a well-defined, homogeneous, enhancing mass ➡ deep to the left sternomastoid muscle ➡. (Right) Longitudinal color Doppler ultrasound shows a well-circumscribed, heterogeneous, echotexture mass ➡ with no significant internal vascularity. The mass was resected and proven to be desmoid fibromatosis with positive margins at pathology.

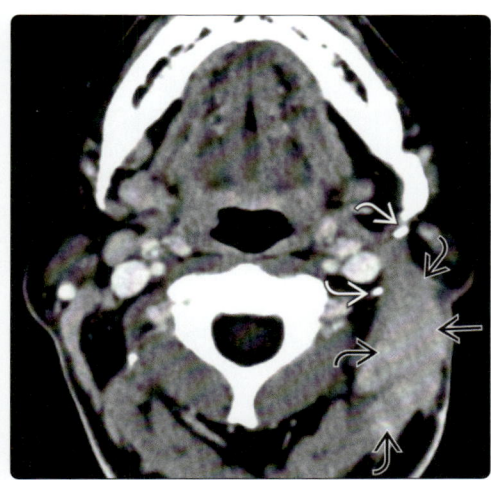

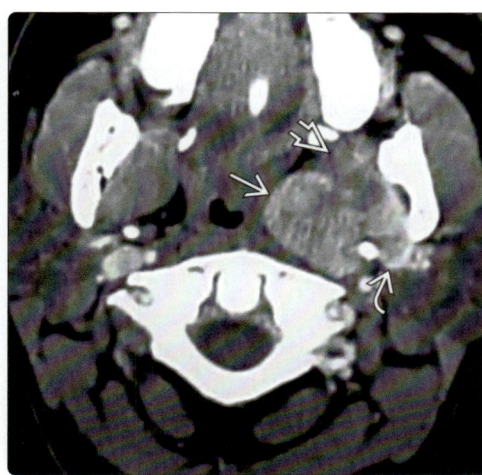

(Left) Axial CECT (same patient, 1 year later) shows recurrent enhancing tumor ➡ in left neck extending more posterior to original tumor, which is more infiltrative, invading the sternomastoid ➡. Note surgical clips ➡ of original desmoid tumor resection. Recurrent fibromatosis is usually more infiltrative. (Right) Axial CECT reveals fibromatosis as a "transspatial" mass invading parapharyngeal ➡, deep masticator ➡, & deep parotid ➡ spaces. Inhomogeneous contrast enhancement is apparent.

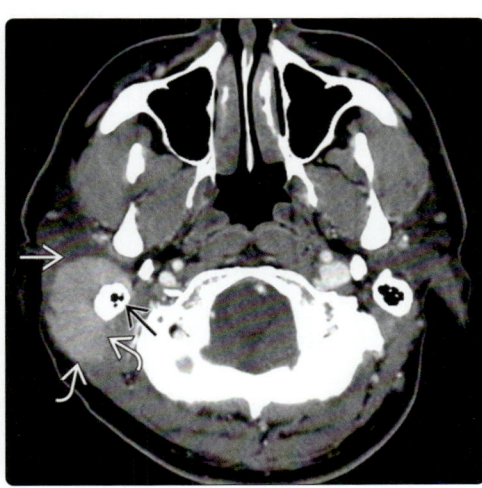

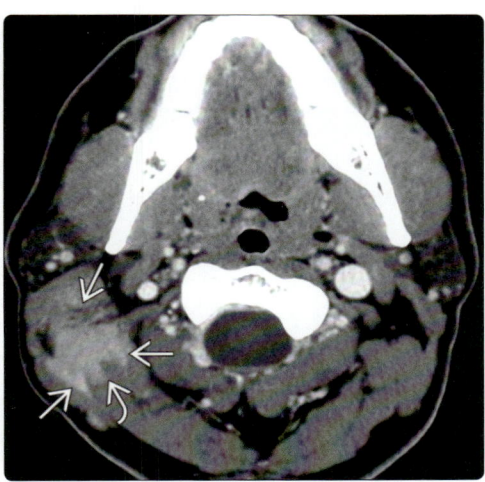

(Left) Axial CECT shows an enhancing mass at right skull base, encircling the mastoid tip ➡. Fibromatosis appears sharply circumscribed from the posterior superficial parotid gland ➡ but has a more ill-defined posterior paraspinous margin ➡. (Right) Axial CECT, more inferior, demonstrates an ill-defined, inferior aspect of enhancing fibromatosis ➡. Note the infiltrative, mass-like appearance with irregular margin at the interface with paraspinal muscles ➡. Both well-demarcated & infiltrative margins may be seen in the same lesion.

KEY FACTS

TERMINOLOGY

- Immune-mediated condition associated with fibroinflammatory lesions at nearly any anatomic site
- Historical terms: Küttner tumor (submandibular), Mikulicz syndrome (parotid & submandibular), Riedel thyroiditis
- Nearly any organ system can be involved: Requires clinical, radiologic, serologic, & histopathologic correlation

IMAGING

- Mass-like or diffuse enlargement of involved organ(s)
  - Enhancing, **enlarged salivary glands**
  - Bilateral, enlarged, enhancing **lacrimal glands**
  - T2 hyperintense acutely, hypointense fibrosis chronically
  - Paranasal sinus inflammation ± **CNV enlargement**
- US for often involved major salivary & thyroid glands
  - Hypoechoic nodules &/or reticular pattern
  - High vascularity in nodal & reticular patterns
- MR > CT for orbit/skull base/intracranial
- F-18 FDG PET useful to assess disease activity

TOP DIFFERENTIAL DIAGNOSES

- Sjögren syndrome, parotid
- Non-Hodgkin lymphoma, parotid
- Idiopathic orbital inflammation (pseudotumor)
- Lymphoproliferative lesions, orbit
- Thyroiditis, chronic lymphocytic (Hashimoto)

PATHOLOGY

- Lymphoplasmacytic infiltrate, storiform fibrosis, obliterative phlebitis, & IgG4(+) plasma cell infiltrate
- Consider in patients with ↑ serum IgG4 level

CLINICAL ISSUES

- Multifocal or systemic involvement in 31-62% of cases
- Age 50-70 years in most cases
- Most commonly affected sites: **Pancreatobiliary system > salivary glands & orbits**; each comprise ~ 25% of all cases
- Treatment: Glucocorticoids &/or rituximab
- Consider if dacryoadenitis/sialadenitis & enlarged CNV

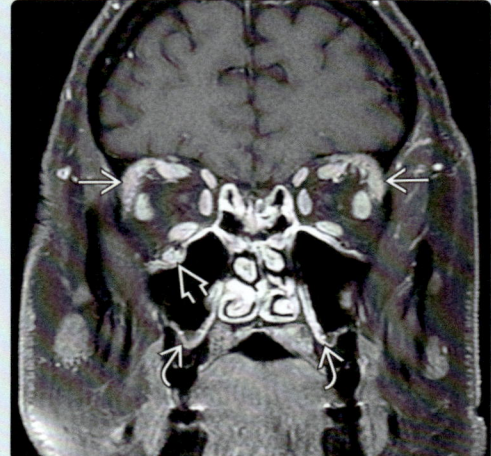
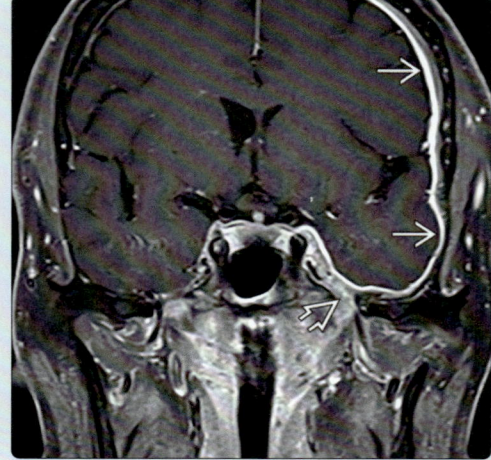

(Left) *Coronal T1 C+ FS MR shows enlarged, enhancing lacrimal glands ➡. Bilateral salivary involvement is most typical, suggesting a systemic etiology. Associated findings of paranasal sinus mucosal thickening ➡ and enlarged, enhancing infraorbital nerve ➡ support IgG4-related disease (IgG4-RD). Patient improved on rituximab.* (Right) *Coronal T1 C+ FS MR shows diffuse pachymeningeal thickening and enhancement ➡ due to IgG4-RD. There is expansion of the foramen ovale with enhancement along V3 ➡, a typical finding.*

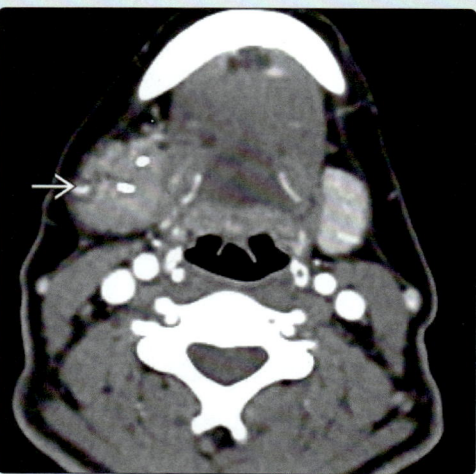
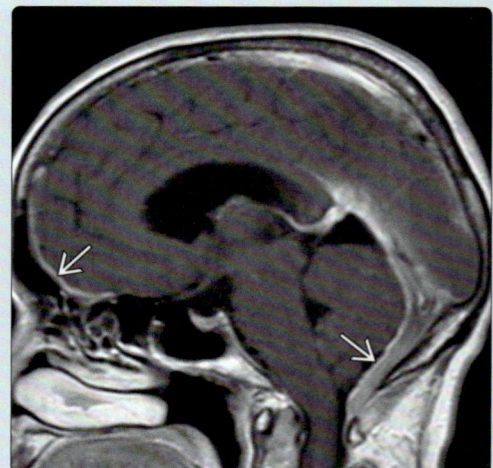

(Left) *Axial CECT shows abnormal enlargement of the right submandibular gland ➡ with calcifications. The historical term for this was Küttner tumor. While the left submandibular gland appears normal in size, it is abnormally dense/enhancing, as expected for a systemic inflammatory process.* (Right) *Midline sagittal T1 C+ MR in a woman with headaches and a history of aortitis shows multifocal pachymeningeal thickening and enhancement ➡. Dural biopsy confirmed dense lymphoplasmacytic infiltrates with increased IgG4.*

IgG4-Related Disease

TERMINOLOGY

Abbreviations
- IgG4-related disease (IgG4-RD)

Synonyms
- Historical terms in various locations include Küttner tumor (submandibular gland), Mikuliçz syndrome (parotid & submandibular), Riedel thyroiditis
- Orbit involvement previously grouped with nonspecific idiopathic orbital inflammation [(IOI), a.k.a. pseudotumor] but now recognized as separate entity
- Skull base "pseudotumor" can be due to IgG4-RD

Definitions
- Systemic immune-mediated disease with fibroinflammatory lesions at nearly any anatomic site (likely autoimmune)
- Requires clinical, radiologic, serologic, & histopathologic correlation; immunohistochemistry has improved characterization of this disease

IMAGING

General Features
- Best diagnostic clue
  - Head & neck manifestations 2nd most common area involved after pancreas
    - Dependent on organ involved
  - Bilateral dacryoadenitis & submandibular sialadenitis
    - Gland involvement usually diffuse with fibroinflammatory change
- Location
  - Endocrine & exocrine glands > other organs
    - Typical head & neck sites include **major salivary glands**, orbits, meninges, pituitary & thyroid gland
    - Sites outside head and neck/CNS: Pancreas, biliary tree, retroperitoneum, aorta, lungs, kidneys
  - Major salivary glands
    - Glands enlarge acutely
    - Findings may mimic Sjögren syndrome
    - Small, T2-hyperintense micronodules
  - Orbit & lacrimal glands
    - Orbital disease usually seen in conjunction with major salivary gland involvement
    - Lacrimal gland enlargement is most common orbital manifestation & is usually bilateral (mimics lymphoma)
    - Trigeminal nerve (CNV) enlargement & enhancement (especially V2)
    - Look for adjacent pan-sinus mucosal thickening
    - Extraocular muscle enlargement or orbital fat involved less frequently (may mimic thyroid-associated orbitopathy)
      - Tendinous insertions tend to be spared
    - Majority of patients with orbital IgG4-RD, especially if bilateral, have extraorbital manifestations
      - Adenopathy > salivary > lung > kidney > hepatobiliary tree > pancreas
      - Thyroid, aorta, meninges/brain, & skin less often
    - Neck, chest, abdominal & pelvic CECT useful to screen
  - Thyroid
    - Enlarged glands with micronodularity
    - US is more sensitive than CT/MR
    - Findings overlap chronic lymphocytic thyroiditis
  - Lymph nodes
    - Adenopathy is typically nonspecific on imaging
  - Pachymeninges
    - Thickened & enhancing
    - ± cranial nerve involvement, especially enlarged CNV
    - Pituitary hypophysitis stalk thickening & enhancement
  - Paranasal sinuses
    - Similar to sinusitis or mass-like with bone destruction
  - Involvement outside CNS + head & neck
    - Most common is pancreatic
- Size
  - Variable; often entire gland/organ involved
- Morphology
  - Linear fibrosis & microcystic changes most often

Radiographic Findings
- IGg4-RD often causes masses that mimic neoplasms, hence historical references to "tumor" or "pseudotumor" in many locations
  - Pseudotumor in orbital inflammation
  - Küttner tumor in submandibular gland
  - Skull base pseudotumor
- Glandular characterization best seen with US > MR/CT

CT Findings
- Orbit and lacrimal glands
  - Lesions with regular borders
  - Multiple lesions, especially bilateral dacryoadenitis
  - Extraocular muscle enlargement (predilection for superior & inferior rectus muscles)
  - Adjacent paranasal sinus mucosal thickening
- PET/CT
  - Areas of active involvement are hypermetabolic
  - F-18 FDG PET useful to assess disease activity

MR Findings
- T1WI
  - Lesions are hypointense
- T2WI
  - Usually iso- to hypointense due to fibrosis
- DWI
  - Typically restricted (unlike idiopathic orbital inflammation), thus difficult to distinguish from lymphoma
- T1WI C+
  - Areas of involvement show enhancement
- Uncommon locations
  - Pituitary infundibulum thickening & enhancement due to hypophysitis
  - Association with other autoimmune diseases

Ultrasonographic Findings
- Grayscale ultrasound
  - Ultrasound is better than CT/MR for major salivary gland & thyroid evaluation
  - Hypoechoic nodules &/or hyperechoic lines & spots with reticular pattern
  - Submandibular > parotid gland involvement
- Color Doppler
  - High vascularity in nodal & reticular patterns

Imaging Recommendations

- Best imaging tool
  - US for major salivary & thyroid glands
    - May guide FNA or biopsy to establish diagnosis
  - MR for orbit/skull base/intracranial
- Protocol advice
  - US > CT for salivary & thyroid gland
  - MR > CT for deep lesions, orbits, brain, cranial nerves

DIFFERENTIAL DIAGNOSIS

Sjögren Syndrome, Parotid

- Small cysts &/or nodules ± punctate calcifications
- Anti-SSA & SSB antibodies

Non-Hodgkin Lymphoma, Parotid

- Parotid soft tissue mass ± adenopathy
- Enlarging mass requires histologic sampling

Idiopathic Orbital Inflammation (Pseudotumor)

- Pain, erythema, proptosis, & restricted ocular motility
- More often unilateral than IgG4-RD

Lymphoproliferative Lesions, Orbit

- Lacrimal gland enlargement mimics IgG4-RD
- CNV involvement ± paranasal sinus inflammation unlikely
- Likely will require biopsy to differentiate

Thyroiditis, Chronic Lymphocytic (Hashimoto)

- Requires biopsy differentiation
- Thyroiditis, invasive fibrous, subtype (Riedel) now recognized as IgG4-RD

PATHOLOGY

General Features

- IgG4:IgG(+):plasma cell ratio of > 40% supports IgG4-RD
- Consider in patients with ↑ serum IgG4 level
- Flow cytometry important to exclude lymphoma

Staging, Grading, & Classification

- American College of Rheumatology/European League Against Rheumatism (EULAR) 3-step criteria for diagnosis
  - ≥ 1 of 11 possible organs involved in manner consistent with IgG4-RD
  - Inclusion criteria from 8 weighted categories of clinical, serologic, radiologic, & pathologic findings
  - Exclusion criteria from 32 clinical, serologic, radiologic, & pathologic items (if any positive, eliminates IgG4-RD)
- Radiologic scoring ≥ 20 points = IgG4-RD
  - Radiologic scoring for lacrimal, parotid, sublingual, & submandibular glands
    - 0 = no involvement
    - 6 = bilateral involvement in 1 of these glands
    - 14 = bilateral involvement ≥ 2 of these glands

Gross Pathologic & Surgical Features

- Tumor-like mass or enlargement of 1 or more organ(s)

Microscopic Features

- Lymphoplasmacytic infiltrate, storiform fibrosis, obliterative phlebitis (least common but most specific), & IgG4+ plasma cell infiltrate

CLINICAL ISSUES

Presentation

- Most common signs/symptoms
  - Multifocal or systemic involvement seen in 31-62%
  - Age 50-70 years in most cases; uncommon in children
  - M:F = 1.6:1 for head & neck manifestations
    - 4:1 for other sites of organ involvement
  - Dependent on location
    - Major salivary glands: Gland enlargement
    - Thyroid gland: Painless thyroid enlargement
    - Orbit: Proptosis, orbital pain
    - Skull base/pachymeninges: Headache & cranial neuropathies
  - Most commonly affected sites: **Pancreatobiliary > salivary glands > orbit**; each comprise ~ 25% of all cases
    - Dacryoadenitis more common in women
    - Pancreatobiliary involvement more common in men
- Other signs/symptoms
  - Elevated serum IgG4 in 55-97%
    - Especially Asian patients
    - Correlates with number of organs involved
  - Other systemic signs & symptoms are infrequent
  - Weakness or weight loss in ~ 25% each

Demographics

- Middle-aged adults

Natural History & Prognosis

- Variable but usually treatment-responsive; however, may cause organ failure & even death if unrecognized
- Limited head & neck or retroperitoneal involvement is more treatment-resistant than pancreatobiliary & systemic

Treatment

- Responds to glucocorticoids &/or rituximab
- Disease-modifying, antirheumatic drugs

Complications

- ↑ risk for malignancy
- ↑ risk for intracerebral aneurysms

DIAGNOSTIC CHECKLIST

Consider

- Tissue sampling to exclude lymphoma if enlarging mass

Image Interpretation Pearls

- Consider IgG4-RD with sialadenitis ± dacryoadenitis &/or enlarged CNV

SELECTED REFERENCES

1. Lai KKH et al: Systemic involvement in immunoglobulin G4-related ophthalmic disease. Ocul Immunol Inflamm. 32(8):1852-8, 2024
2. Gupta L et al: Diffusion-weighted imaging of the orbit: a case series and systematic review. Ophthalmic Plast Reconstr Surg. 39(5):407-18, 2023
3. Naik M et al: Imaging manifestations of IgG4-related disease. Clin Radiol. 78(8):555-64, 2023
4. Behzadi F et al: Imaging of IgG4-related disease in the head and neck: a systematic review, case series, and pathophysiology update. J Neuroradiol. 48(5):369-78, 2021
5. Dragan AD et al: Imaging of IgG4-related disease in the extracranial head and neck. Eur J Radiol. 136:109560, 2021
6. Kurowecki D et al: Cross-sectional pictorial review of IgG4-related disease. Br J Radiol. 92(1103):20190448, 2019

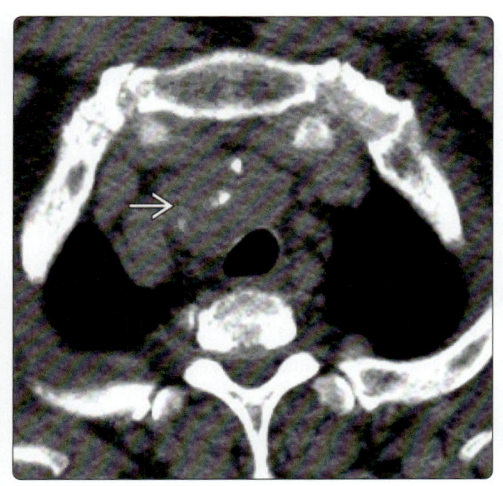

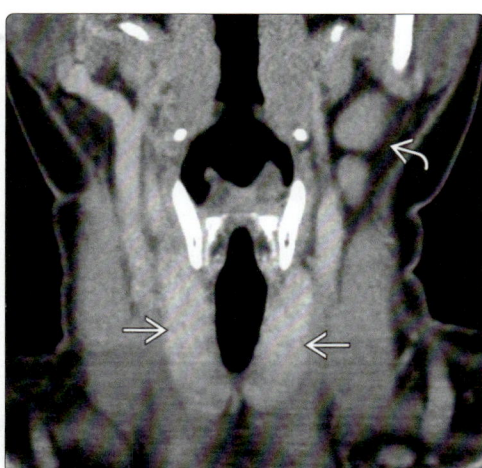

(Left) Axial NECT shows thyroid gland enlargement with coarse calcifications ➡. Although not specific, this patient had IgG4-RD involving the thyroid. Historically, this has been labeled as Riedel thyroiditis. (Right) Coronal CECT MPR demonstrates subtle enlargement of thyroid gland with tiny, granular hypodensities ➡. Findings are more evident on US but overlap with chronic lymphocytic thyroiditis. Associated nonspecific-appearing involved level II lymph nodes ➡ are noted. Biopsy confirmed IgG4-RD.

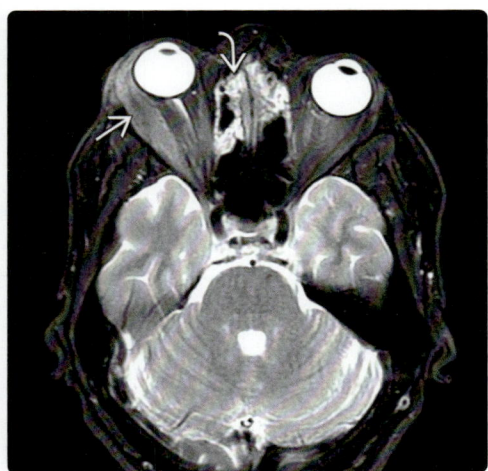

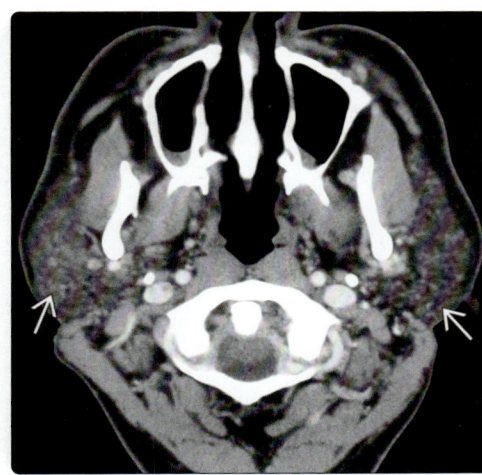

(Left) Axial T2 FS MR shows an enlarged, hyperintense lacrimal gland ➡ due to IgG4-RD. Asymmetric involvement like this is less common and more challenging diagnostically. Associated paranasal sinus mucosal thickening is noted ➡, a common associated finding. (Right) Axial CECT in the same patient demonstrates bilateral parotid enlargement with diffuse micronodularity of the parenchyma ➡. Findings are similar to Sjögren syndrome but lack the cystic changes typical of acute involvement. Findings were due to IgG4-RD.

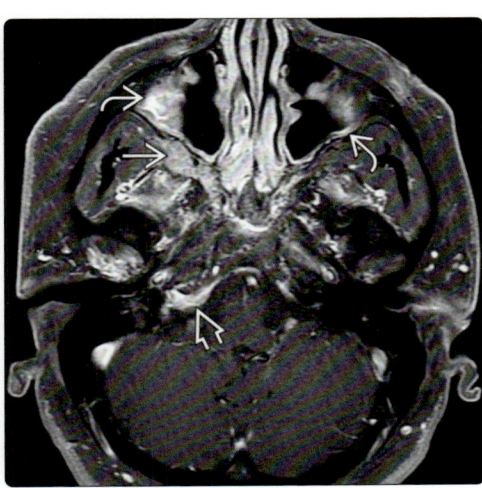

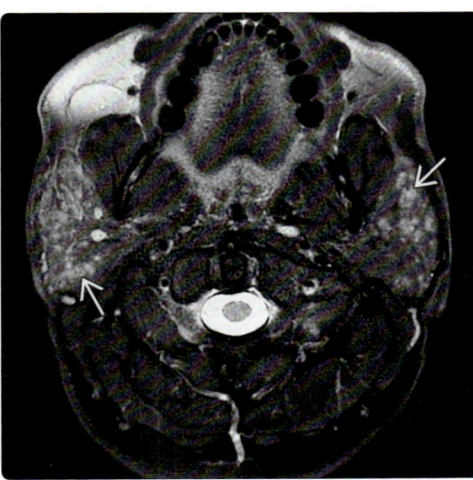

(Left) Axial T1 C+ FS MR show focal soft tissue thickening and enhancement within the pterygopalatine fossa along V2 ➡ due to confirmed IgG4-RD. Paranasal sinus inflammation ➡ is noted. Focal pachymeningeal thickening and enhancement, although not specific, can also be seen with IgG4-RD. Note also dural involvement ➡. (Right) Axial T2 FS MR in the same patient shows bilateral parotid gland enlargement with multiple small, nodular foci of hyperintensity ➡. Findings improved after treatment with rituximab.

KEY FACTS

TERMINOLOGY

- SARS caused by novel SARS-coronavirus 2 (CoV-2) virus, resulting in pandemic COVID-19
- Respiratory infection with viral pneumonia & multiorgan involvement, including head & neck manifestations

IMAGING

- **Head & neck clinical manifestations of COVID-19 often do not have imaging correlate!**
- Anosmia: Signal abnormality &/or enhancement of olfactory bulbs
- Optic neuritis: T2-hyperintense optic nerve(s) ± abnormal contrast enhancement
- Hearing loss: Abnormal enhancement of CNVIII, signal abnormality, &/or enhancement of membranous labyrinth
- Xerostomia & sialadenitis: Edema &/or hyperenhancement of major salivary glands
- Guillain-Barré syndrome: Thickening & abnormal enhancement of affected cranial nerves

- Brachial plexopathy: Edema, thickening, & enhancement of affected brachial plexus
- Postvaccine adenopathy: Transiently enlarged or hypermetabolic regional nodes ipsilateral to vaccine site
- Venous &/or arterial thromboemboli: Tend to be longer segment &/or multifocal
- Cavernous sinus thrombosis: Venous filling defects on enhanced scan
- Invasive fungal sinusitis (↑ risk during/after COVID): Nonenhancing mucosa, effacement of perisinus fat pads

CLINICAL ISSUES

- Cornerstone of management is supportive care
- Preventative measures (e.g., vaccination, mask wearing, & social distancing) remain crucial for disease management

DIAGNOSTIC CHECKLIST

- New ipsilateral axillary or supraclavicular lymph nodes after COVID-19 vaccination may mimic metastasis
- Clinical or imaging follow-up to resolution

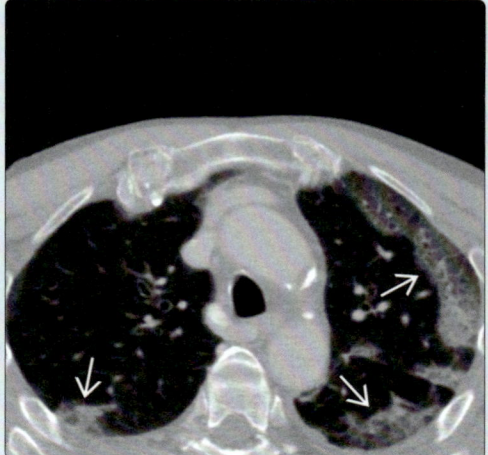
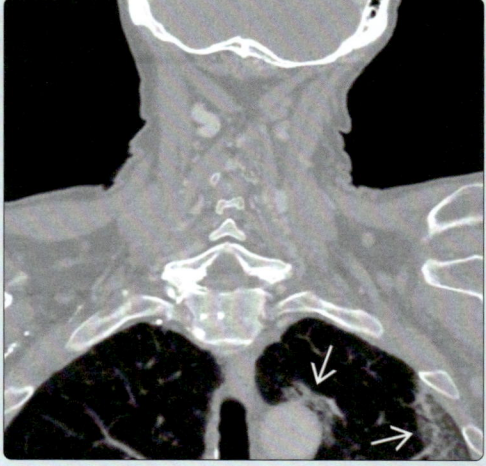

(Left) Axial CECT (lung window) through lung apices included on routine CT of neck in a patient with fever shows multiple bilateral, peripheral (subpleural) ground-glass opacities ➡ with central areas of spared lung. (Right) Coronal CECT (lung window) in the same patient shows the striking subpleural distribution of ground-glass opacities ➡, a pattern highly suggestive of COVID-19. It is critical for interpreting head and neck radiologists to screen the imaged lung apices and rapidly report findings of potential COVID-19 pneumonia.

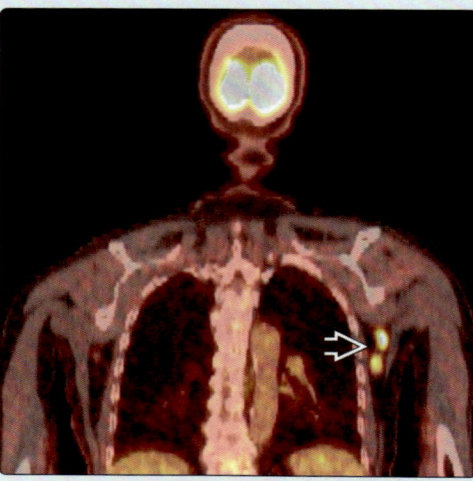
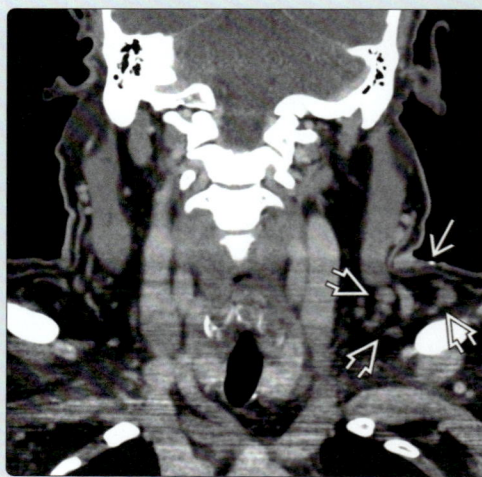

(Left) Coronal F-18 FDG PET/CT in a patient imaged for right parotid squamous cell carcinoma (SCCa) staging shows FDG-avid left axillary adenopathy ➡. Distribution is atypical for contralateral cheek SCCa. Patient received a COVID-19 vaccination (left arm) a few days prior to the PET/CT. (Right) Coronal CECT in a patient with left supraclavicular "swelling" after a COVID-19 vaccination shows a skin marker ➡ that denotes the palpable abnormality. Subjacent is a cluster of reactive lymph nodes ➡.

TERMINOLOGY

Abbreviations

- Coronavirus disease 2019 (COVID-19)

Definitions

- Severe acute viral respiratory syndrome (SARS) caused by novel SARS-coronavirus 2 (CoV-2) virus, resulting in pandemic COVID-19
- Respiratory infection with viral pneumonia & multiorgan involvement, including head & neck manifestations
  - Anosmia
  - Optic neuritis
  - Ageusia & dysgeusia
  - Xerostomia
  - Hearing loss
  - Tinnitus
  - Guillain-Barré syndrome variants
  - Brachial plexopathy
  - Sialadenitis
  - Venous &/or arterial thromboemboli

IMAGING

General Features

- Best diagnostic clue
  - **Head & neck clinical manifestations of COVID-19 often do not have imaging correlate!**
  - Anosmia: Signal abnormality &/or enhancement of olfactory bulbs
  - Optic neuritis: Signal abnormality of optic nerves
  - Hearing loss: Abnormal CNVIII enhancement, signal abnormality, &/or enhancing membranous labyrinth
  - Xerostomia & sialadenitis: Edema &/or hyperenhancement of major salivary glands
  - Guillain-Barré syndrome: Thickening & abnormal enhancement of affected cranial nerves
  - Brachial plexopathy: Adema, thickening, & enhancement of affected brachial plexus
  - Postvaccine adenopathy: Transiently enlarged or hypermetabolic regional lymph nodes ipsilateral to vaccination site
- Location
  - Anosmia: Olfactory bulbs along cribriform plate
  - Optic neuritis: Optic nerves, any segment
  - Xerostomia & sialadenitis: Parotid, submandibular, & sublingual glands
  - Hearing loss & tinnitus: CNVIII cisternal & canalicular segments; cochlea & inner ear structures
  - Guillain-Barré syndrome: Cranial nerves
  - Brachial plexopathy: Brachial plexus
  - Postvaccine adenopathy: Axillary > supraclavicular lymph nodes ipsilateral to deltoid vaccination site

CT Findings

- Xerostomia & sialadenitis
  - Enlarged, edematous major salivary glands
    - May be multifocal & bilateral
  - Hyperenhancing with surrounding edema
- Postvaccine adenopathy

- New reactive axillary or supraclavicular lymph nodes ipsilateral to deltoid vaccination site
  - Typically reniform with linear hilar vascular enhancement
- Venous thrombosis: Filling defects on CECT

MR Findings

- Anosmia
  - Variable imaging findings; commonly negative
  - Intrinsic high T1 signal intensity in olfactory bulbs
    - Thought to represent microhemorrhage
  - Contrast enhancement of olfactory bulbs
- Optic neuritis
  - T2 hyperintensity in any segment of optic nerves ± abnormal contrast enhancement
- Hearing loss & tinnitus
  - Vestibulocochlear neuritis: CNVIII enhancement
  - Labyrinthitis: Intralabyrinthine enhancement
  - Intralabyrinthine hemorrhage: Intrinsic bright T1 signal intensity within membranous labyrinth
- Xerostomia & sialadenitis
  - Edema (↑ T2 signal) & hyperenhancement of major salivary glands: May be multifocal & bilateral
  - Submandibular, sublingual, or periparotid edema
- Guillain-Barré syndrome variants
  - Enhancing ± enlarged affected cranial nerves
- Brachial plexopathy
  - Enlargement, ↑ T2 signal, & hyperenhancement of any portions of brachial plexus
  - Denervation edema of affected shoulder muscles
  - Edema/inflammation surrounding brachial plexus
  - Postvaccination brachial neuritis/Parsonage Turner syndrome
- Cavernous sinus thrombosis: Filling defects on T1 C+
- Invasive fungal sinusitis
  - "Dead" (nonenhancing) turbinate or mucosa
  - Effacement of normal perisinus fat pads with soft tissue
  - Look for spread to orbits/brain

Ultrasonographic Findings

- Postvaccine adenopathy
  - New axillary or supraclavicular lymph nodes ipsilateral to deltoid vaccination site
  - Appear reactive without necrosis; resolves on follow-up

Nuclear Medicine Findings

- Postvaccine adenopathy
  - New hypermetabolic axillary or supraclavicular lymph nodes ipsilateral to deltoid vaccination site
  - Resolves on clinical/imaging follow-up

Imaging Recommendations

- Best imaging tool
  - MR best tool for most head & neck manifestations
  - Ultrasound to confirm resolved vaccine adenopathy
- Protocol advice
  - Clinical question should guide protocol of choice
  - Temporal bone MR with high-resolution T2WI & FS postcontrast imaging for hearing loss or tinnitus
  - High-resolution anterior skull base MR for anosmia; consider including thin coronal T1 precontrast FS to assess for olfactory bulb hemorrhage

DIFFERENTIAL DIAGNOSIS

Hearing Loss and Tinnitus

- Labyrinthitis (non-COVID-19)
- Metastases in cerebellopontine angle-internal auditory canal
- Intralabyrinthine hemorrhage

Optic Neuritis

- Due to MS or other demyelinating disorder

Xerostomia and Sialadenitis

- Sjögren syndrome
- Calculous sialadenitis

Guillain-Barré Syndrome

- Meningitis
- Lymphoma
- Neurosarcoid
- Lyme disease

Brachial Plexopathy

- Metastases
- Neurolymphomatosis

Postvaccine Adenopathy

- Nodal metastasis
- Lymphoma

PATHOLOGY

General Features

- Respiratory infection with human-to-human transmission via respiratory droplets, close contact with affected persons, & potential aerosol & fecal-oral transmission
- Enveloped single-stranded RNA virus belonging to beta subgroup coronavirus family
- Spike S protein of SARS-CoV-2 contains receptor-binding domain that interfaces with human angiotensin-converting enzyme 2 (ACE2), facilitating membrane fusion & uptake into human cells in upper aerodigestive tract
- Within infected cells, nonstructural & structural polyproteins are translated from viral RNA → more viral RNA synthesized → virion precursor formed & transported to cell surface → completed virion released via exocytosis, beginning new replication cycle

Gross Pathologic & Surgical Features

- Consolidated lung with pulmonary edema
- Disseminated intravascular coagulation & endothelial inflammation
  - Systemic complications of prothrombotic state, including cerebral infarction & venous thromboembolism

CLINICAL ISSUES

Presentation

- Most common signs/symptoms
  - Fever or chills; cough; dyspnea, difficulty breathing
  - Headache; new-onset anosmia, dysgeusia, or ageusia
  - Sore throat; congestion, rhinorrhea
- Numerous complications of COVID
  - Venous thrombosis
  - Thromboembolic arterial stroke
  - Invasive fungal sinusitis
  - COVID-associated rhombencephalitis
  - Xerostomia or sialadenitis
  - Optic neuritis
  - Audiovestibular disorders with hearing loss or tinnitus
  - Guillain-Barré syndrome
  - Brachial plexopathy

Demographics

- Indiscriminate infectious disease in any age or sex
  - Worse in older patients & those with medical comorbidities (e.g., hypertension, diabetes mellitus, heart disease)
- ↑ rates of infection- & COVID-19-related deaths in Black, Hispanic, American Indian, Asian American patients
  - Social determinants of health likely influence

Natural History & Prognosis

- Pulmonary involvement with variable severity
  - Viral pneumonia with serous & fibrin exudate
  - Pulmonary edema
  - Interstitial inflammation with lymphocytic infiltrates
  - Diffuse alveolar damage with acute respiratory distress syndrome (ARDS)
- Cytokine storm → ARDS, multiple organ failure, & death
- Life-threatening multisystem inflammatory syndrome in children (MIS-C): Rash, conjunctivitis, hypotension, shock, myocardial dysfunction, pericarditis, coagulopathy, acute gastrointestinal symptoms, & elevated inflammatory markers (ESR, CRP, or procalcitonin)
- Older age & medical comorbidities confer worse prognosis
- COVID-19 symptoms typically last weeks to months with most patients demonstrating full recovery
  - ~ 10% are "long haulers" with persistent symptoms (e.g., cough, dyspnea, fatigue, anosmia, ageusia)

Treatment

- Cornerstone of management is supportive care
  - May necessitate oxygen support via mechanical ventilation or extracorporeal membrane oxygenation
- Steroids antivirals, monoclonal antibodies if severe
- Preventative measures (e.g., vaccination, mask wearing, & social distancing) remain crucial for disease management

DIAGNOSTIC CHECKLIST

Consider

- Head & neck clinical manifestations of COVID-19 frequently do **not** have imaging correlate!
- Postvaccine adenopathy mimics nodal metastases

Image Interpretation Pearls

- New axillary or supraclavicular lymph nodes ipsilateral to recent COVID-19 vaccination are common

SELECTED REFERENCES

1. Kim U et al: COVID-19-associated rhino-orbito-cerebral mucormycosis: a single center prospective study of 264 patients. Orbit. 44(1):24-33, 2025
2. Giordano A et al: Challenging axillary lymph nodes on PET/CT in cancer patients throughout COVID-19 vaccination era. Curr Pharm Des. 30(10):798-806, 2024
3. Farinhas J et al: Imaging of the head and neck during the COVID19 pandemic. Oper Tech Otolayngol Head Neck Surg. 33(2):147-57, 2022

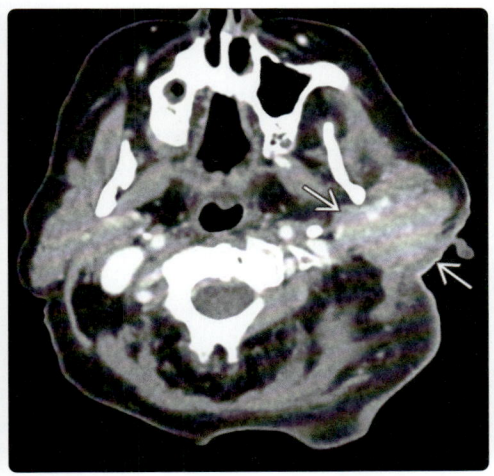

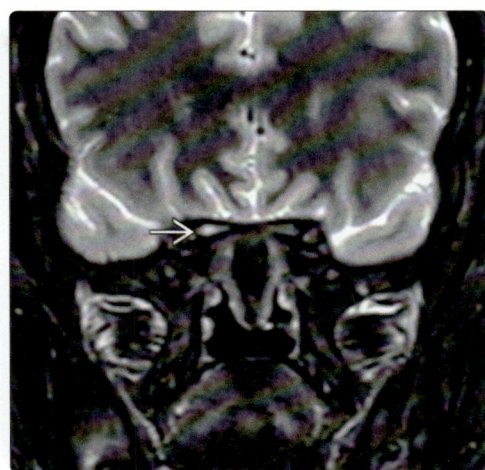

(Left) *Axial CECT demonstrates unilateral parotid enlargement and enhancement due to acute parotitis* ⮕ *in this older adult patient with recent COVID-19 infection. Overlying subcutaneous fat stranding and edema support an inflammatory origin.* (Right) *Coronal STIR MR shows abnormal hyperintensity involving the optic nerve* ⮕ *in a patient with COVID-19 infection. This finding is more often seen in patients with severe COVID-19 infection.*

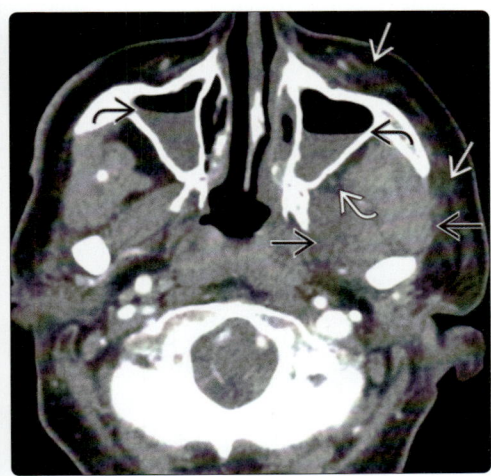

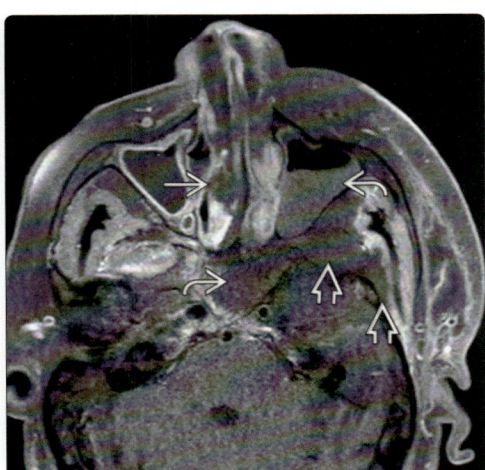

(Left) *Axial CECT in a patient with acute COVID infection and new progressive left facial swelling shows layering fluid* ⮕ *in both maxillary sinuses. Hazy increased density in the retromaxillary fat pad* ⮕ *and swollen masticator space muscles with effaced fat pads* ⮕ *are key findings of invasive fungal sinusitis. There is abnormal infiltration of superficial fat pads* ⮕. (Right) *Axial T1 C+ FS MR in the same patient shows nonenhancing right turbinate* ⮕, *sinus mucosa* ⮕, *and masticator space muscles* ⮕ *due to invasive fungal sinusitis.*

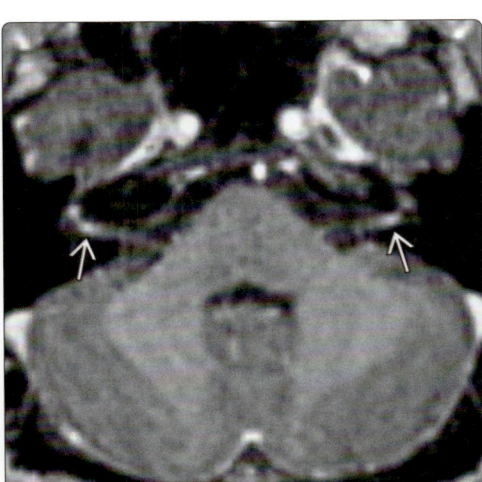

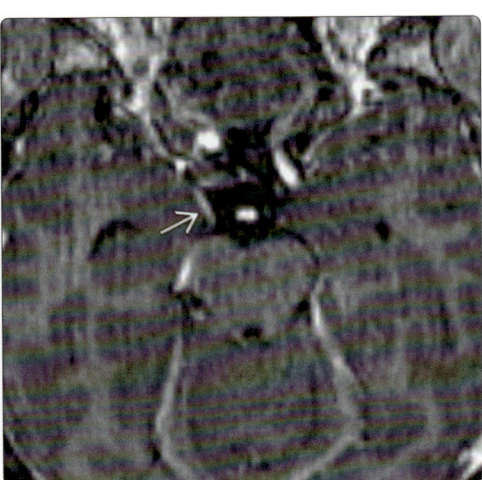

(Left) *Axial SPGR C+ MR in a COVID-19 patient with new bilateral facial weakness shows abnormal enhancement of CNVII bilaterally* ⮕ *extending from the internal auditory canal fundus through geniculate ganglia.* (Right) *Axial SPGR C+ MR in the same patient shows abnormal enhancement of right CNIII cisternal segment* ⮕. *Clinicoradiologic findings, including MR, lab analysis, and electromyography was consistent with COVID-19-mediated bifacial weakness with paresthesia subtype of Guillain-Barré syndrome.*

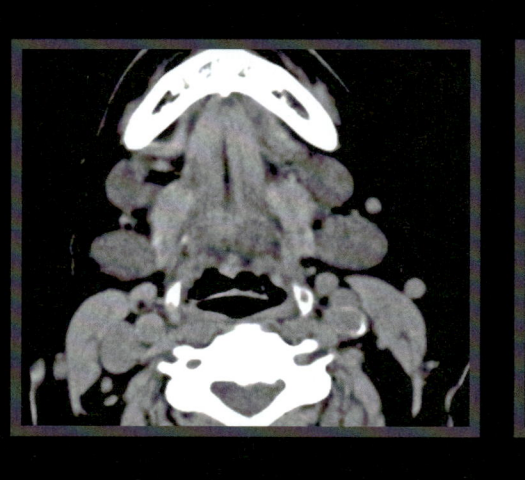
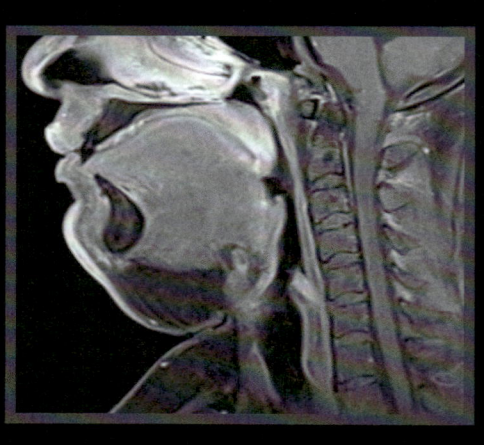
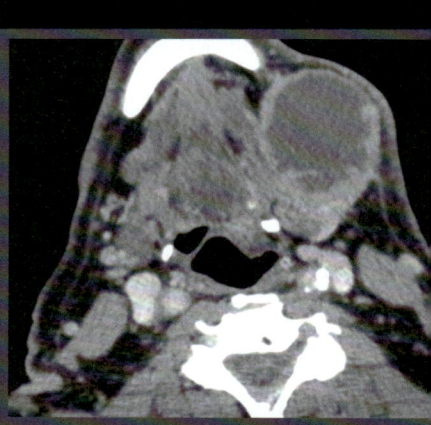

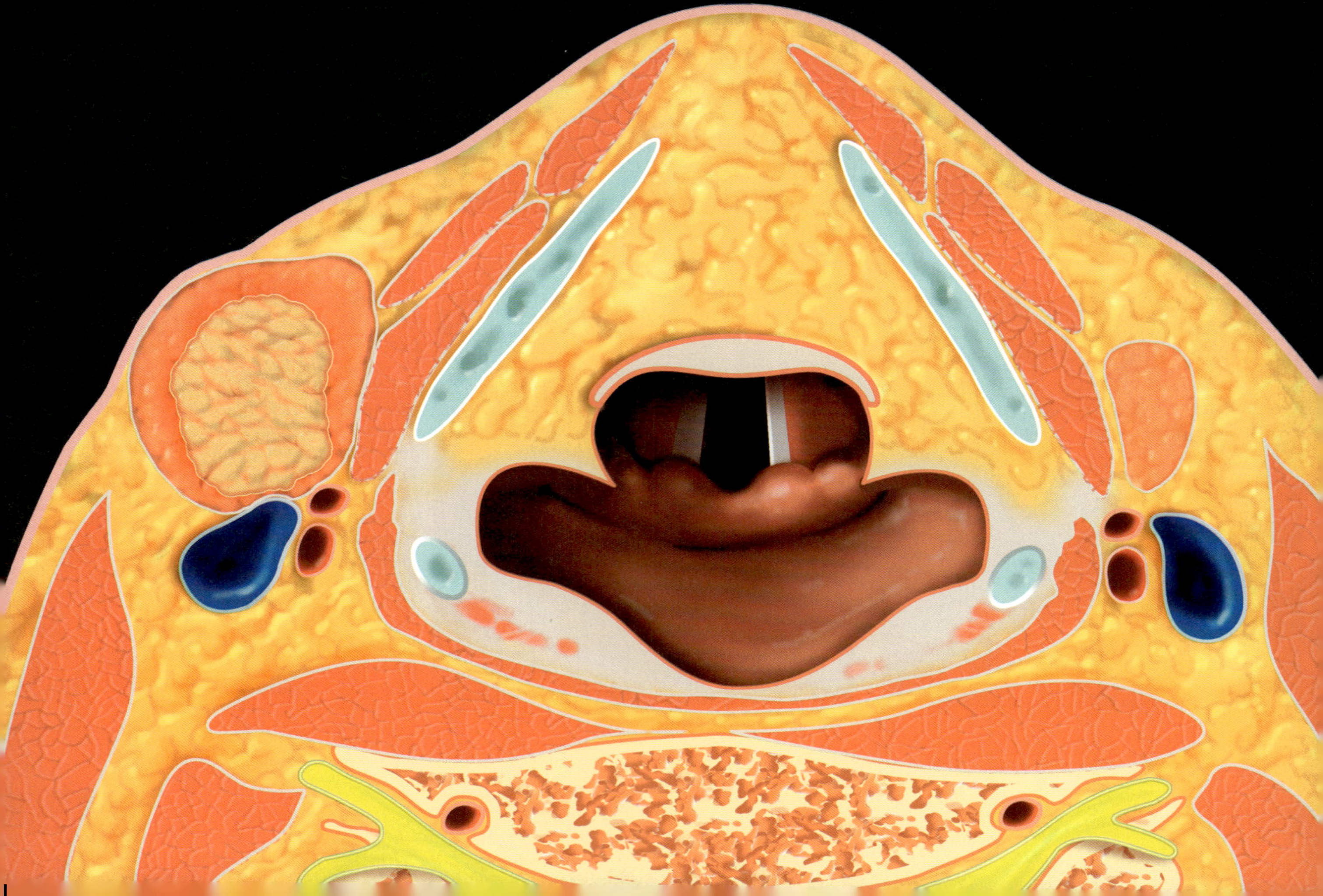

SECTION 14
Oral Cavity

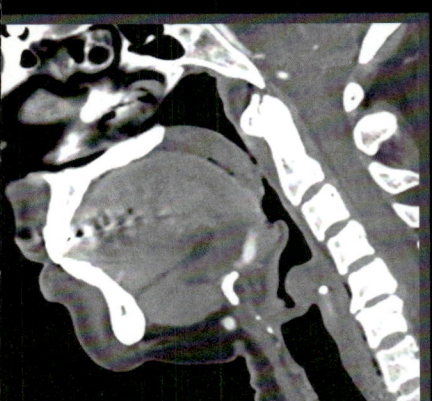
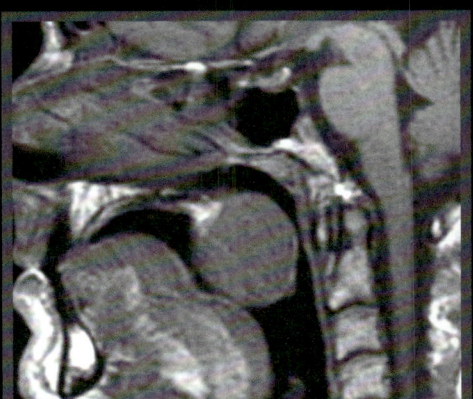
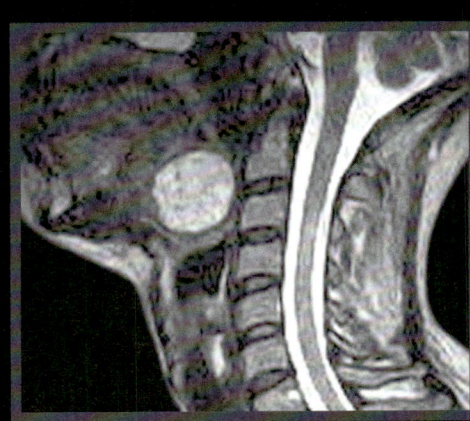

Summary Thoughts: Oral Cavity

The oral cavity (OC) is the area of the suprahyoid neck anterior to the oropharynx and inferior to the sinonasal region. The referring physician can see all mucosal surfaces and palpate most lesions found here. The radiologist's role is to assess the deep tissue extent of OC tumors and provide space-based differential diagnoses when a deep tissue lesion is discovered. Three indications drive the vast majority of CT and MR exams of the OC: (1) Staging OC squamous cell carcinoma (SCCa), (2) evaluation of dental abscess, and (3) differentiating the submandibular nodal lesion and gland mass.

Imaging Techniques and Indications

Tumor Assessment

Both CECT and enhanced MR are used to stage SCCa. Primary tumor and nodal metastases are assessed simultaneously in either case. CT is often compromised by dental amalgam artifact. MR is less affected by dental amalgam and better delineates soft tissue extent of tumor and perineural tumor. As a result, enhanced fat-saturated MR is considered a superior tool for staging OC SCCa.

Infection Assessment

In the clinical setting of suspected OC infection, CECT with mandible and maxilla bone windows is the preferred imaging exam. Abscess of any OC space is easily assessed with CECT. Infectious causes, such as **mandibular teeth decay** with associated apical cyst or mandibular osteomyelitis and submandibular duct **stone**, are more easily seen on bone CTs.

Imaging Anatomy

The OC is the area above the hyoid bone, anterior to the oropharynx and inferior to the sinuses and nose. Its borders are defined superiorly as the hard palate and maxillary alveolar ridge, laterally by the cheek, posteriorly by oropharynx and soft palate, anteriorly by the vermilion border of the lip, and inferiorly by the platysma. The OC contains the oral tongue, mandible body and teeth, maxillary ridge and teeth, and the hard palate.

The OC can be subdivided into 4 distinct imaging areas: (1) **Oral mucosal space/surface** (OMS), (2) **sublingual space** (SLS), (3) **submandibular space** (SMS), and (4) **root of tongue** (ROT). Each area contains unique structures and provides its own space-specific differential diagnosis.

The **OMS** is covered by a continuous mucosal sheet of nonkeratinized stratified squamous epithelium. The mucosal components of the OC are defined according to **SCCa subsites** occurrence, namely, mucosa of the oral tongue, floor of mouth (FOM), retromolar trigone (RMT), upper and lower alveolar ridges with gingiva, buccal (cheek), and mucosa of the lips and hard palate. The OC can also be divided into the oral vestibule, which lies between the cheeks, lips, and teeth with the mucosal surfaces (buccal, lip mucosa, and gingiva, respectively) and into the OC proper. Subepithelial collections of **minor salivary glands** are most commonly located in the inner surface of the lip, buccal mucosa, and palate.

The **SLS** is an area within the deep oral tongue superomedial to mylohyoid muscles and lateral to the genioglossus muscle that is **not** encapsulated by fascia. Anteriorly, the SLS runs into the mandible. The SLS is horseshoe-shaped with the 2 sides communicating anteriorly under the frenulum of the tongue. Posteriorly, the SLS empties into the superior SMS and the inferior parapharyngeal space (PPS). No fascia separates the

posterior SLS from the SMS and inferior PPS. All 3 spaces communicate at the posterior edge of the mylohyoid muscle.

- The SLS contains multiple oral tongue structures. SLS nerves include the **lingual nerve** (sensory branch of CNV3 + chorda tympani branch of CNVII with taste fibers from anterior 2/3 of tongue) and distal **CNIX** and **CNXII**. The tongue's vascular pedicle (lingual artery and vein) passes through the SLS. The sublingual glands and ducts and the deep portion of the submandibular gland and submandibular gland duct are all found in the SLS. Finally, the anterior margin of the hyoglossus muscle projects into the posterior SLS from below.

The **SMS** (surgical synonym is submaxillary space) is located inferolateral to the mylohyoid muscle, superior to the hyoid bone, and deep to the platysma muscle. It is the only fascia-lined OC space. The superficial layer of deep cervical fascia lines its deep and superficial surfaces. The deep slip of fascia is found along the external surface of the mylohyoid muscle, and the superficial slip of fascia lines the deep margin of the platysma muscle. Posteriorly, no fascia separates the SMS from the inferior PPS or posterior SLS spaces.

- The SMS can be conceptualized as a horseshoe-shaped space between the mylohyoid above and the hyoid bone below. There is no fascia blocking the spread of disease from side to side in the SMS.
- The SMS contains the **submandibular gland** and lymph nodes: Submental (level IA) and submandibular (level IB). These structures are responsible for most SMS masses. Other critical structures within the SMS include the facial vein and artery, the caudal loop of CNXII, the anterior belly of the digastric muscle, and fat.

The **ROT** is a term used by surgeons to describe the deep midline oral tongue above the mylohyoid sling and below the extrinsic tongue muscles. The ROT ends anteriorly at the mandibular symphysis. It is made up of the **genioglossus muscle** and the fibrofatty **lingual septum**.

There are 4 additional structures that require specific mention when reviewing the OC anatomy: The **mylohyoid** and **geniohyoid muscles**, the **oral tongue**, and the **RMT**. The **mylohyoid** and **geniohyoid** muscles form the **FOM**. The mylohyoid muscle arises from the mylohyoid line of the medial mandibular body. Anterior and middle fibers insert into median fibrous raphe extending from the symphysis menti to the hyoid bone to its posterior margin. Posterior mylohyoid fibers pass inferomedially to insert into the hyoid bone body. The mylohyoid muscle has been described as the **muscular "sling"** separating the SLS or SMS.

- The OC component of the tongue is referred to as the **oral tongue** and represents the anterior 2/3 of the entire tongue. The posterior 1/3 is called the **base of tongue (lingual tonsil)** and is part of the oropharynx. The **extrinsic tongue muscles** of the oral tongue include the genioglossus, hyoglossus, styloglossus, and palatoglossus. The **genioglossus** is the large, fan-shaped muscle arising anteriorly from the superior mental spine on the inner surface of the symphysis menti of the mandible. It inserts along the entire length of the undersurface of the intrinsic tongue muscles. The **hyoglossus** is a thin, quadrilateral-shaped muscle arising from the body and cornu of the hyoid bone, from there passing vertically upward to insert into the side of the tongue. The **styloglossus** arises from the styloid process and stylomandibular ligament and passes

Differential Diagnosis: Oral Cavity

Pseudolesion	Congenital	Inflammatory-Infectious	Benign Tumor	Malignant Tumor
		Cellulitis (SLS, SMS, ROT)		
CNXII atrophy (SLS, ROT)	Lymphatic malformation (SLS, SMS, ROT)	Phlegmon or abscess (SLS, SMS, ROT)	PA, sublingual gland (SLS)	Oral tongue SCCa
CNV3 atrophy (SMS)	Venous malformation (SLS, SMS, ROT)	Dilated submandibular duct + stone (SLS)	PA, submandibular gland (SMS)	Floor of mouth SCCa
Accessory salivary gland (SMS)	Dermoid/epidermoid (SLS, SMS, ROT)	Sialocele (SLS)	PA, hard palate (OMS)	Retromolar trigone SCCa
	Lingual thyroid (ROT, SMS, PMS-BOT)	Submandibular gland sialadenitis (SMS)	Lipoma (SMS)	Alveolar ridge SCCa
	Thyroglossal duct cyst (ROT, SMS, PMS-BOT)	Sublingual gland sialadenitis (SLS)		Hard palate SCCa
		Submandibular gland mucocele (SMS)		Buccal mucosa SCCa
	2nd branchial cleft cyst (SMS)	Chronic sclerosing sialadenitis (SMS)		Lip SCCa
		Simple (SLS) or diving (SLS-SMS) ranula		Submandibular (SMS) or sublingual gland (SLS) carcinoma
		Reactive or suppurative nodes (SMS)		Nodal SCCa or NHL (SMS)

OMS = oral mucosal space; PMS = pharyngeal mucosal space; SLS = sublingual space; SMS = submandibular space; ROT = root of tongue; BOT = base of tongue (lingual tonsil); PA = pleomorphic adenoma; SCCa = squamous cell carcinoma; NHL = non-Hodgkin lymphoma.

anteroinferiorly between the external and internal carotid arteries to insert into the side of the tongue. Finally, the **palatoglossus** is a thin muscle arising from the anterior surface of the soft palate. From there, it passes anteroinferiorly in front of the palatine tonsil to insert into the side of the tongue. The palatoglossus underlies the anterior tonsillar pillar, which serves as the dividing line between the OC and the oropharynx.

- The **RMT** is a small, triangular-shaped region of OC mucosa behind the last mandibular molar. SCCa of the RMT can spread early into critical proximal locations, such as the masticator space and PPS.
  Pterygomandibular raphe is a fibrous band extending from the hamulus of medial pterygoid plate above to the posterior mylohyoid ridge of mandible below, in close relation to posterior aspect of RMT. The anterior border of pterygomandibular raphe attaches to the buccinator muscle and posterior border to the superior constrictor muscle. RMT SCCa can spread readily in a superior direction along this perifascial route.

Approaches to Imaging Issues in Oral Cavity

There are 3 main OC imaging indications: (1) Staging of primary SCCa and nodes, (2) searching for abscess and its cause, and (3) evaluating an SMS mass to determine whether the mass is nodal or glandular. The clinical context and access to each modality can affect the type of exam (CECT vs. MR) and facilitate the creation of a highly relevant radiology report. Without clinical history, assigning a lesion to a space of origin (OMS, SLS, ROT, SMS) and comparing its radiologic features to those of the **space-specific differential diagnoses** is an alternative approach to analyzing OC images.

OMS SCCa is known at the time of imaging. The mucosal extent of the SCCa is best determined by the clinician. Imaging is critical to evaluate deep soft tissue extent, bone involvement, perineural tumor, and nodal spread. Small tumors may be extremely subtle or even occult to imaging,

and, for this reason, it is very helpful to know the primary subsite when reading OMS SCCa scans. This allows careful evaluation for features that are key to surgical management, such as cortical bone erosion. Each OC primary SCCa subsite has its own set of imaging questions to be considered for staging, which can be found in separate modules on each site.

When a lesion is found in the **SLS**, check to see if it has spread to the contralateral SLS via the connection anteriorly under the tongue frenulum. Also look to see if the lesion has spread posteriorly into the **SMS**.

SMS masses usually arise from either the submandibular gland or the nodal chain (level IA and IB). A smaller submandibular gland tumor, if equivocal on CECT, may benefit from US or MR where the clinician is certain that a lesion is present.

ROT lesions are rare. The differential diagnosis of ROT lesions is short. If a lesion appears to bow the genioglossus muscles laterally away from each other, then it should be considered primary to the ROT.

Differential Diagnosis

Without a history for an OC lesion, assigning a space of origin to review a space-specific differential diagnosis can be a very useful strategy (depicted in the table). This global differential table can be subdivided into 4 distinct lists based on the 4 major OC anatomic areas (OMS, SLS, SMS, and ROT).

Selected References

1. Ansari S et al: Revisiting the "puffed cheek" technique: advantages, fallacies, and potential solutions. Radiol Imaging Cancer. 6(3):e230211, 2024
2. Vutukuri R et al: The pterygomandibular raphe: a comprehensive review. Anat Cell Biol. 57(1):7-12, 2024
3. Choi J et al: Malignant and nonmalignant lesions of the oral cavity. Oral Maxillofac Surg Clin North Am. 35(3):311-25, 2023
4. Famuyide A et al: Oral cavity and salivary glands anatomy. Neuroimaging Clin N Am. 32(4):777-90, 2022
5. Kamrani P et al: Anatomy, head and neck, oral cavity (mouth). StatPearls, 2021

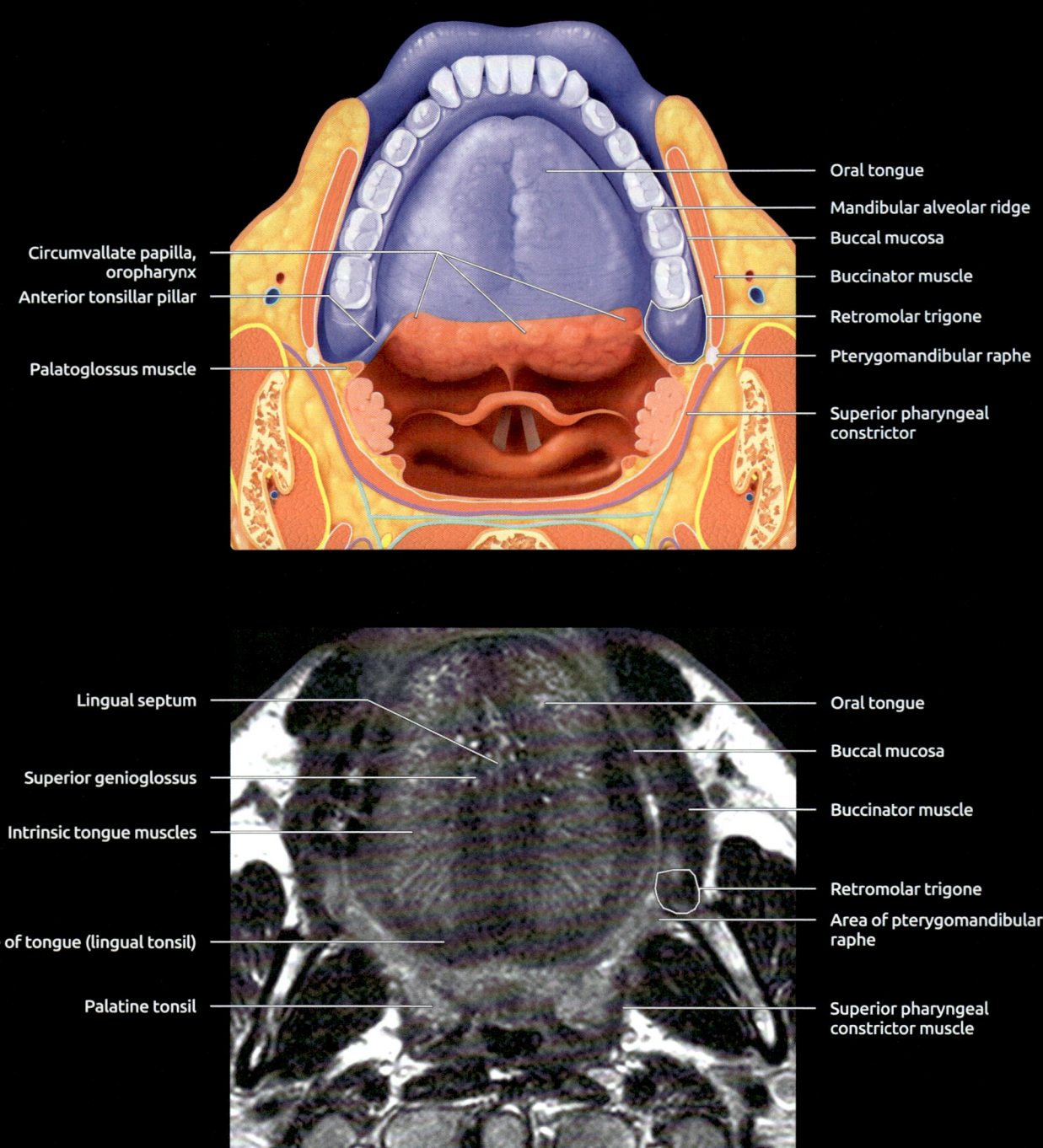

Circumvallate papilla, oropharynx
Anterior tonsillar pillar
Palatoglossus muscle

Oral tongue
Mandibular alveolar ridge
Buccal mucosa
Buccinator muscle
Retromolar trigone
Pterygomandibular raphe
Superior pharyngeal constrictor

Lingual septum
Superior genioglossus
Intrinsic tongue muscles
Base of tongue (lingual tonsil)
Palatine tonsil

Oral tongue
Buccal mucosa
Buccinator muscle
Retromolar trigone
Area of pterygomandibular raphe
Superior pharyngeal constrictor muscle

(Top) *Axial graphic shows oral mucosal space &/or surface (OMS) shaded in blue. Notice that the circumvallate papilla, a superficial line of taste buds, divides anterior oral cavity (OC) from posterior oropharynx. The lingual tonsil is part of oropharynx, not the OC. Four of 7 squamous cell carcinoma (SCCa) subsites are labeled on the right, including the oral tongue, alveolar ridge, buccal mucosa, and retromolar trigone (RMT). The lips, floor of mouth (FOM) and hard palate subsites are not shown. Note that the pterygomandibular raphe (PMR) lies in between and connects to the posterior margin of buccinator muscle and to the anterior margin of the superior pharyngeal constrictor muscle along its anterior-posterior margins. It extends from the hamulus of medial pterygoid plate above to the posterior mylohyoid ridge of mandible below, in close relation to posterior aspect of RMT. The RMT represents a key route of perifascial spread of SCCa of the RMT. **(Bottom)** Axial T2 MR through the superior tongue shows the mucosal subsites on the right along with the buccinator, PMR, and superior constrictor adjacent to the RMT. Note the oropharyngeal palatine and lingual tonsils labeled on the left.*

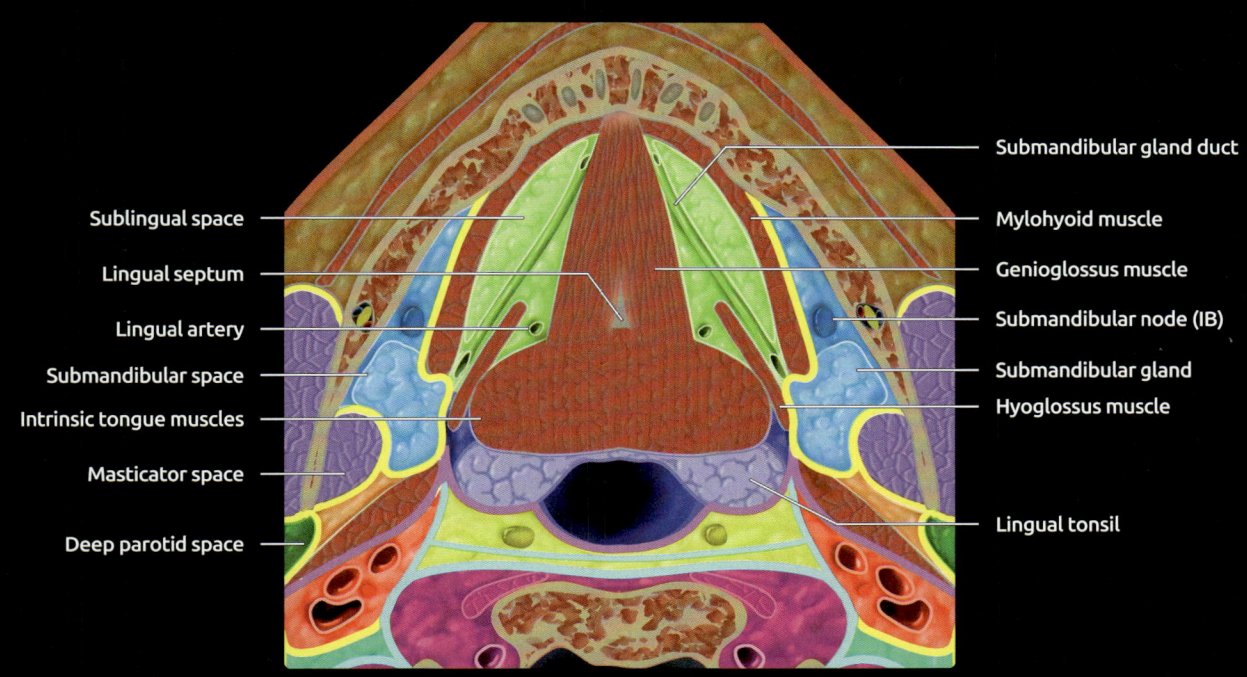

Submandibular gland duct

Sublingual space

Lingual septum

Lingual artery

Submandibular space

Intrinsic tongue muscles

Masticator space

Deep parotid space

Mylohyoid muscle

Genioglossus muscle

Submandibular node (IB)

Submandibular gland

Hyoglossus muscle

Lingual tonsil

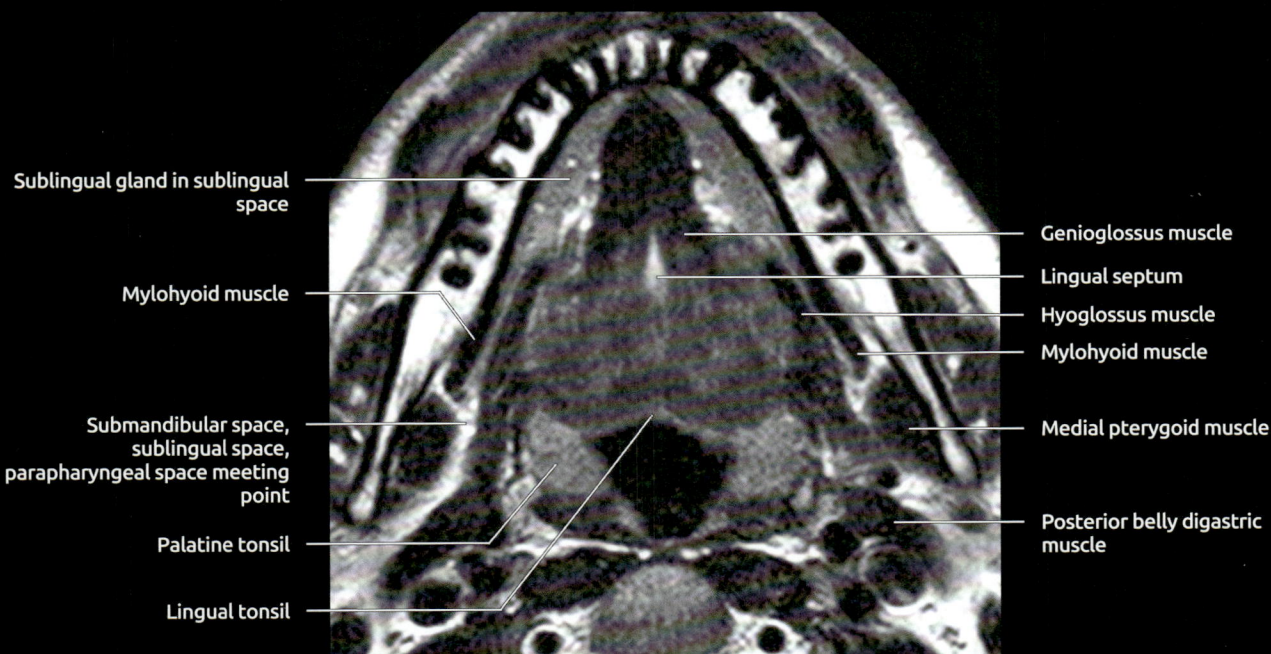

Sublingual gland in sublingual space

Mylohyoid muscle

Submandibular space, sublingual space, parapharyngeal space meeting point

Palatine tonsil

Lingual tonsil

Genioglossus muscle

Lingual septum

Hyoglossus muscle

Mylohyoid muscle

Medial pterygoid muscle

Posterior belly digastric muscle

(Top) *Axial graphic through mid-OC shows superficial layer of deep cervical fascia (yellow line) circumscribing the masticator and parotid spaces posteriorly and defining the deep margin of submandibular space (SMS) (colored in blue). Notice that the principal occupants of SMS are the submandibular gland and level I nodes. The green sublingual space (SLS) has many structures within it, including the sublingual gland, submandibular duct, lingual artery, and the anterior margin of hyoglossus muscle.* **(Bottom)** *Axial T2 MR shows the structures of the FOM and root of tongue (ROT). Notice the symmetric paired genioglossus muscles separated by a fatty lingual septum. The hyoglossus muscles insert into the lateral aspect of the tongue and delineate the location of the submandibular duct, which courses between hyoglossus and mylohyoid and terminates in the anterior aspect of the FOM. The sublingual glands are nestled anteriorly in the FOM also.*

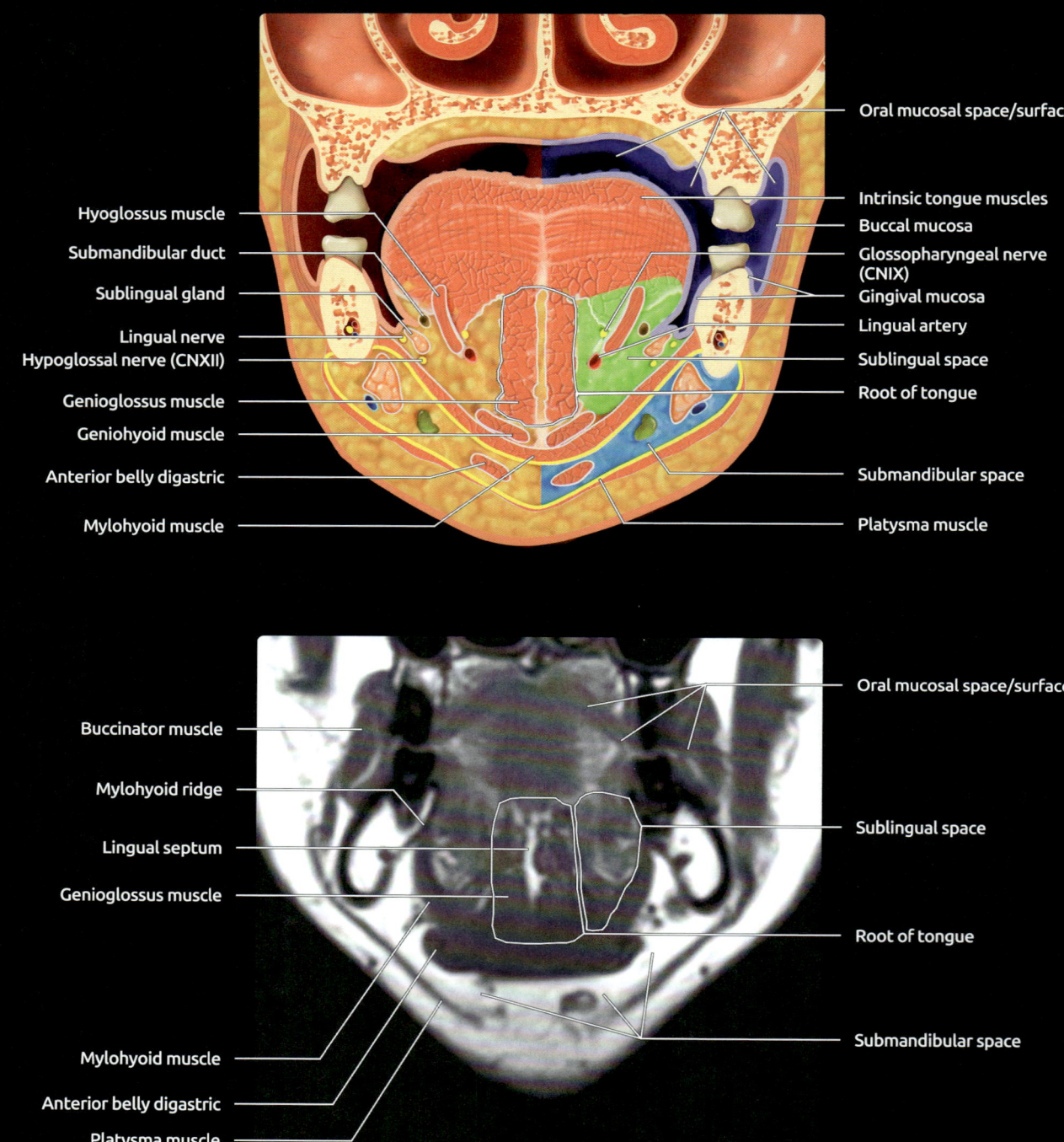

Oral mucosal space/surface

Intrinsic tongue muscles

Buccal mucosa

Glossopharyngeal nerve (CNIX)

Gingival mucosa

Lingual artery

Sublingual space

Root of tongue

Submandibular space

Platysma muscle

Hyoglossus muscle

Submandibular duct

Sublingual gland

Lingual nerve

Hypoglossal nerve (CNXII)

Genioglossus muscle

Geniohyoid muscle

Anterior belly digastric

Mylohyoid muscle

Buccinator muscle

Mylohyoid ridge

Lingual septum

Genioglossus muscle

Mylohyoid muscle

Anterior belly digastric

Platysma muscle

Oral mucosal space/surface

Sublingual space

Root of tongue

Submandibular space

(Top) *Coronal graphic through the OC shows the mylohyoid muscle inserting on each side of the OC along the mylohyoid ridges of the medial mandible. This muscle separates the superomedial SLS (green) from inferolateral SMS (blue). The SLS contains the lingual nerve and artery, submandibular duct, CNIX, CNXII, and sublingual gland. The SMS contains the submandibular gland, facial vein and artery, level I nodes, and anterior belly of the digastric muscle. Genioglossus and the lingual septum form the ROT. The OMS lines the surface of the OC (purple). Buccal and gingival mucosa are separately labeled.* (Bottom) *Coronal T1 MR depicts the mylohyoid muscular sling (FOM) "strung" between the mylohyoid ridges of the mandible. The OMS is difficult to identify on a closed-mouth image, whereas the SLS, SMS, and ROT are all well delineated. On CT, a "puffed cheek" technique can help separate and delineate buccal, gingival, and lip mucosa. Notice that the neurovascular contents of the SLS and SMS cannot be identified.*

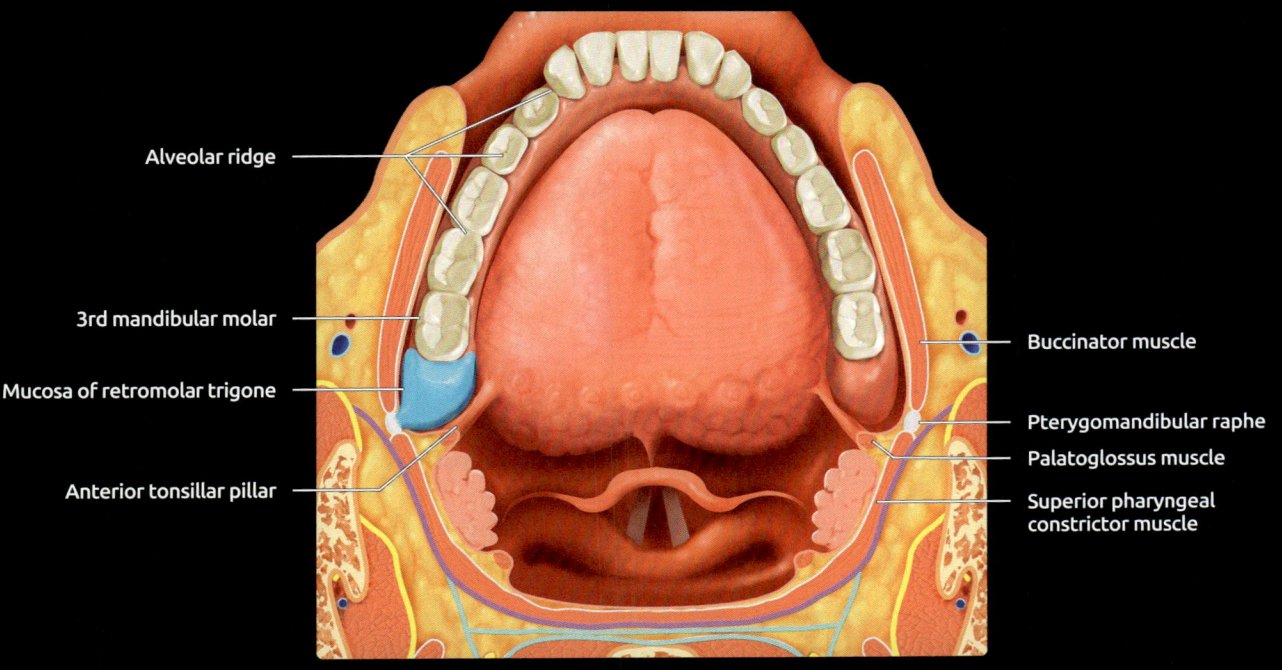

Alveolar ridge

3rd mandibular molar

Mucosa of retromolar trigone

Anterior tonsillar pillar

Buccinator muscle

Pterygomandibular raphe

Palatoglossus muscle

Superior pharyngeal constrictor muscle

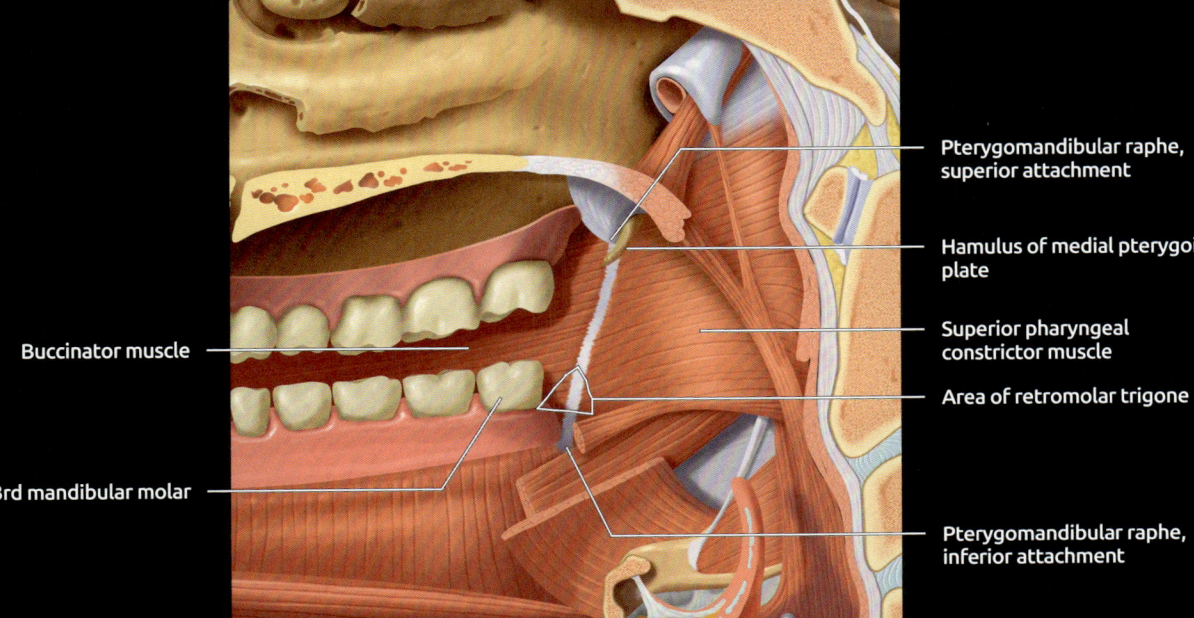

Buccinator muscle

3rd mandibular molar

Pterygomandibular raphe, superior attachment

Hamulus of medial pterygoid plate

Superior pharyngeal constrictor muscle

Area of retromolar trigone

Pterygomandibular raphe, inferior attachment

(Top) *Axial graphic highlights the RMT (shaded in light blue) and the PMR. Notice that the mucosal surface of the RMT is found directly behind the 3rd mandibular molar. The RMT is designated as its own OC subsite for SCCa, but it is really just the most posterior portion of the alveolar ridge. The proximity to the PMR (fascial band connecting buccinator and superior constrictor muscles) is important when SCCa occurs in the RMT because it gives the tumor access to the pterygoid plate above via this perifascial spread route.* (Bottom) *Sagittal graphic viewed from inside the mouth delineates the full extent of the PMR. Note the cephalad PMR attachment to the hamulus of the medial pterygoid plate and its inferior attachment to the posterior aspect of the RMT/posterior mylohyoid ridge on the inner mandibular cortex. Note that inferiorly PMR courses medial to the RMT (between RMT and anterior tonsillar pillar). The PMR "connects" the buccinator muscle to the superior pharyngeal constrictor muscle.*

KEY FACTS

TERMINOLOGY

- Hypoglossal nerve (CNXII)
- Loss of nerve supply to unilateral half of tongue muscles

IMAGING

- Asymmetry of tongue appearance with linear demarcation of abnormality; varies over time
- Acute (typically < 1 month)
  - Hemitongue initially swollen and edematous
  - Enhancement variable
- Subacute (typically 1-20 months)
  - Loss of volume and fatty change of hemitongue
  - ↓ enhancement
- Chronic (typically > 20 months)
  - Fatty atrophy, no enhancement
  - Infrahyoid strap muscle atrophy may be present
    - Innervated by ansa cervicalis, which travels with CNXII in carotid and sublingual space
- Image course of CNXII from skull base to hyoid

TOP DIFFERENTIAL DIAGNOSES

- Oral tongue squamous cell carcinoma
- Oral cavity lymphatic malformation
- Oral cavity venous malformation
- Lingual tonsil squamous cell carcinoma

PATHOLOGY

- Many causes; may be isolated or with CNIX-XI

DIAGNOSTIC CHECKLIST

- Frequent source of mistaken identity
  - Flaccid hemitongue hangs posteriorly into oropharynx, mistaken for (ipsilateral) tongue base tumor
  - Contralateral tongue mistaken as enlarged from tumor
  - Normal uptake in contralateral tongue mistaken for tumor
- Sharp line delineating unilateral changes is key
- Associated infrahyoid strap atrophy indicates carotid or sublingual space lesion

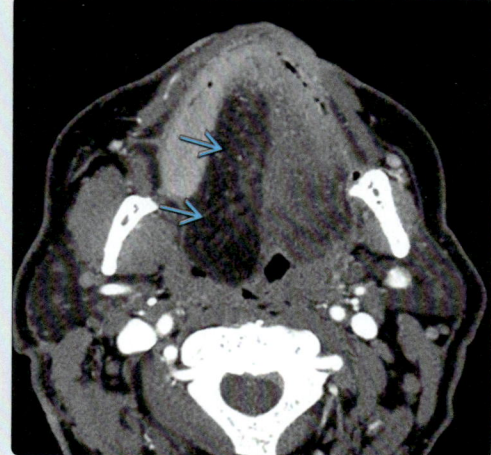
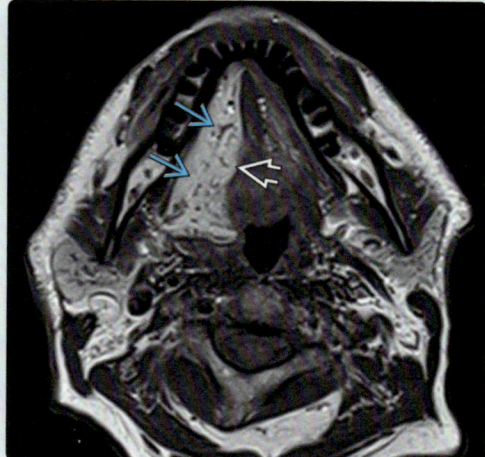

(Left) *Axial CECT shows a classic example of chronic right CNXII palsy. This patient underwent hypoglossal-to-facial cable nerve graft to treat facial palsy and developed hypoglossal denervation, a common sequelae. There is diffuse hypoattenuation in right hemitongue due to muscular atrophy and fatty infiltration ➡.* (Right) *Axial T1 MR shows chronic right hemitongue denervation with hyperintense T1 signal ➡, consistent with fatty replacement. Note linear demarcation of signal change ⇨.*

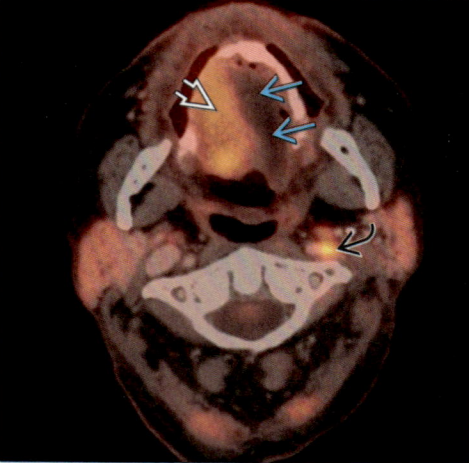
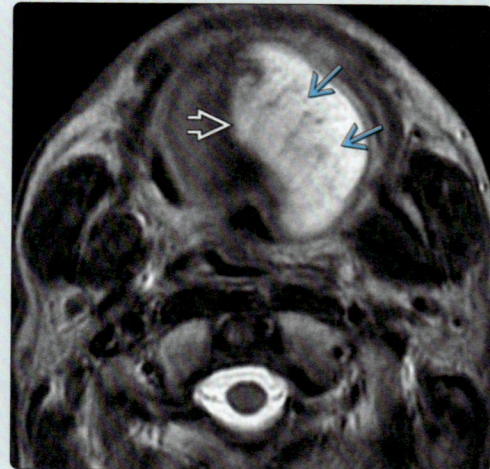

(Left) *Axial fused PET/CT in patient with left carotid space squamous cell carcinoma (SCCa) nodal disease ➡ demonstrates ipsilateral hemitongue denervation fatty atrophy and reduced uptake ➡. Normal contralateral hemitongue uptake ⇨ was misdiagnosed as tumor.* (Right) *Axial T2 MR shows the acute stage of tongue denervation with a swollen left hemitongue and markedly increased signal from edema ➡. Note sharp delineation of abnormality ⇨. Denervation was due to perineural tumor spread along CNXII.*

TERMINOLOGY

Synonyms

- Hypoglossal nerve (CNXII) palsy, hypoglossal nerve paralysis, tongue denervation/paralysis

Definitions

- Loss of nerve supply to tongue muscles
  - Note: Palatoglossus muscle is only extrinsic tongue muscle supplied by CNX

IMAGING

General Features

- Best diagnostic clue
  - Asymmetry of tongue with linear demarcation
- Location: Unilateral tongue musculature
- Morphology: Varies over time
  - Early: Swollen, flaccid, hemitongue; late: ↓ in volume

CT Findings

- CECT
  - Early: Unilateral hemitongue swelling, flaccid
  - Later: Loss of volume and ↓ attenuation, fatty atrophy

MR Findings

- Signal intensity varies over time following denervation
- Acute (typically < 1 month)
  - Unilateral hemitongue swelling, edema, flaccid
  - ↑ T2, subtly ↓ T1 signal, variable enhancement
- Subacute (typically 1-20 months)
  - Swelling resolves, fatty atrophy
  - ↑ T1, ↓ enhancement
- Chronic (typically > 20 months)
  - Hemitongue atrophy
  - Marked ↑ T1, enhancement resolves

Nuclear Medicine Findings

- PET/CT
  - Acute may show ↑ uptake; chronic ↓ uptake
    - May be mistaken for primary tumor

Imaging Recommendations

- Best imaging tool
  - Contrast MR best evaluates CNXII entire course
- Protocol advice
  - Must image entire course of CNXII from skull base to hyoid (orbital roof to just below hyoid)
  - Include heavily T2-weighted 3D, T1-weighted **without** fat suppression and contrast-enhanced T1-weighted with fat suppression

DIFFERENTIAL DIAGNOSIS

Oral Tongue Squamous Cell Carcinoma

- Untreated tumor: Enhancing exophytic, ↑ attenuation mass commonly arising from lateral margin
- Tumor recurrence: ↓ attenuation, peripheral enhancement mimicking abscess

Lingual Tonsil Squamous Cell Carcinoma

- Enhancing tumor at base of tongue with ↑ attenuation

Oral Cavity Venous Malformation

- Enhancing, irregular lesion involving multiple spaces

Oral Cavity Lymphatic Malformation

- Multiloculated, septated, transspatial fluid-filled lesion

PATHOLOGY

General Features

- Etiology
  - Lesion along course of CNXII
  - If isolated CNXII neuropathy, most often 2° skull base lesion or injury
    - Postoperative: Endarterectomy, neck dissection
    - Bone lesion: Metastasis, direct tumor invasion, osteomyelitis
    - Vascular: Carotid dissection, vascular malformation
    - Postradiation: Fibrosis
    - Rarely brainstem or cerebellopontine angle (CPA) lesion
  - With other cranial nerves: CNIX-XI suspect upper carotid sheath lesion, skull base lesion → jugular foramen

CLINICAL ISSUES

Presentation

- Most common signs/symptoms
  - Lower motor neuron signs (infranuclear lesion)
    - Tongue deviation to side of denervation on protrusion
    - Tongue paralysis, fasciculations, loss of tone
  - Dysarthria, difficulty swallowing
- Other signs/symptoms
  - Other cranial nerves may be involved:
    - CNIX: Loss of taste to posterior tongue
    - CNX: Vocal cord paralysis
    - CNXI: Denervation of sternocleidomastoid, trapezius

DIAGNOSTIC CHECKLIST

Consider

- Frequent source of mistaken diagnosis
  - Flaccid hemitongue hangs posteriorly into oropharynx, mimicking (ipsilateral) tongue base tumor
  - Acute swelling and FDG uptake mimics ipsilateral tumor
  - Chronic atrophy and ↓ FDG uptake → contralateral tongue mistaken as tumor

Image Interpretation Pearls

- Key imaging feature = sharp line delineating unilateral tongue changes
- Associated infrahyoid strap muscle atrophy indicates carotid or sublingual space lesion

Reporting Tips

- Carefully review course of CNXII from skull base to hyoid

SELECTED REFERENCES

1. Ragittaran J et al: Imaging of hypoglossal palsy: a pictorial synopsis. Clin Radiol. 81:106754, 2025
2. Pawlukowska W et al: Acute tongue swelling as a still unexpected manifestation of internal carotid artery dissection: a case report. Brain Sci. 13(4):603, 2023
3. Guarnizo A et al: Imaging features of isolated hypoglossal nerve palsy. J Neuroradiol. 47(2):136-50, 2020

Oral Cavity

TERMINOLOGY

- Accessory salivary tissue in mylohyoid boutonnière
- Normal salivary tissue in abnormal position within submandibular space (SMS)

IMAGING

- Benign-appearing SMS mass with CT density and MR signal intensity following normal salivary glands
- SMS; inferior to mylohyoid, most commonly anterior to submandibular gland
- Physiologic uptake may be seen on PSMA PET

TOP DIFFERENTIAL DIAGNOSES

- SMS reactive nodal disease
- SMS lymphatic malformation
- SMS abscess
- Diving ranula
- Submandibular gland mucocele

PATHOLOGY

- Ectopic sublingual or submandibular gland tissue in SMS

CLINICAL ISSUES

- Most commonly **incidental** and discovered on imaging for unrelated indications
- May occasionally present as SMS mass
- Subject to same spectrum of disease as other salivary tissue, including sialadenitis and sialolithiasis, though these occur only rarely

DIAGNOSTIC CHECKLIST

- Include diagnosis of accessory salivary tissue when evaluating submandibular masses
- Accessory SMS salivary tissue focus, when discovered, is "leave alone" lesion
- Look for density/intensity that follows normal submandibular gland

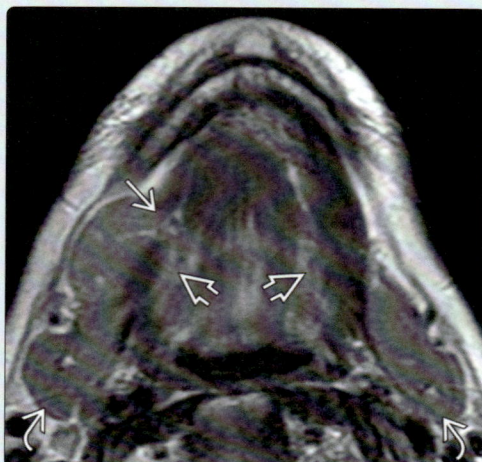 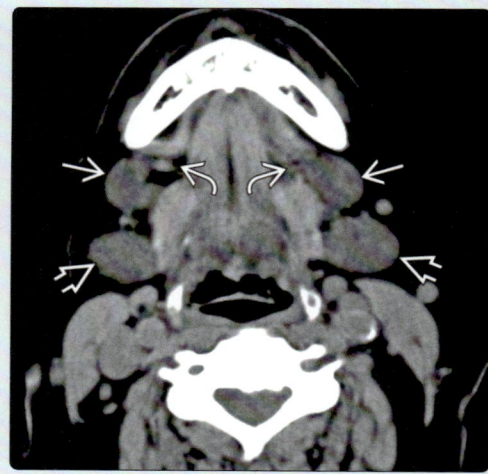

(Left) Axial T2 MR shows an accessory submandibular gland extending through a defect of the mylohyoid muscle ➡. Note that signal intensity is similar to normal sublingual ⬈ and submandibular ⬈ gland tissue. (Right) Axial NECT demonstrates bilateral accessory salivary tissue in the submandibular space ➡. Bilateral mylohyoid dehiscence ⬈ is evident. Note that density of accessory salivary tissue is identical to that of native submandibular glands ⬈.

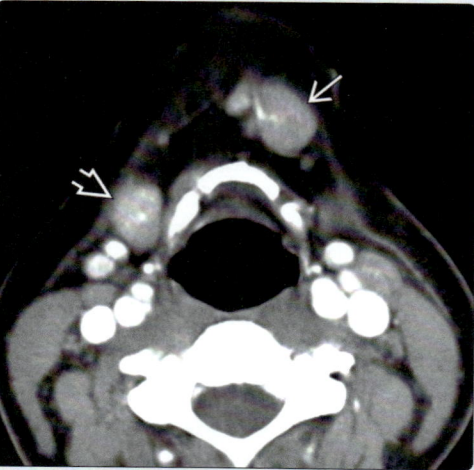 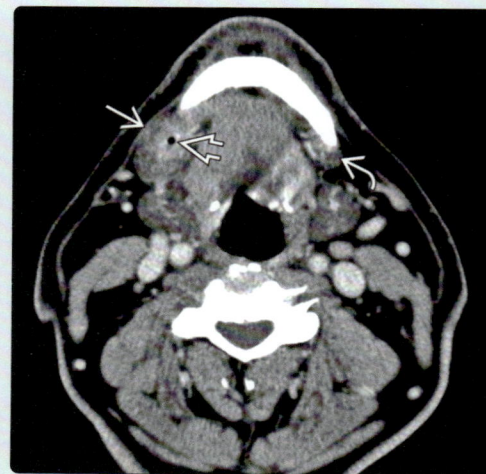

(Left) Axial CECT shows accessory salivary gland tissue ➡ within the anterior midline submandibular space, just to the left of the midline, with density and enhancement similar to the normal submandibular gland ⬈. (Right) Axial CECT shows an enlarged right accessory salivary gland ➡ with increased density and intraductal air ⬈, compatible with the presence of acute sialadenitis. Note the presence of small incidental left accessory salivary tissue ➡.

Submandibular Space Accessory Salivary Tissue

TERMINOLOGY

Synonyms
- Accessory salivary tissue in mylohyoid boutonnière

Definitions
- Normal salivary tissue in abnormal position in submandibular space (SMS)
  - Accessory tissue is separated component of major salivary gland, along external duct (not heterotopia)

IMAGING

General Features
- Best diagnostic clue
  - Benign-appearing SMS mass with density/intensity following normal salivary glands
- Location
  - SMS; inferior to mylohyoid, most commonly anterior to submandibular gland (SMG)
- Size
  - Variable; usually small (< 2 cm)
- Morphology
  - Ovoid to lobulated
  - Pear-shaped when projecting into mylohyoid defect

CT Findings
- NECT
  - SMS mass with density similar to normal SMG
  - Mylohyoid defect may be visible
- CECT
  - Enhances similar to normal SMG
    - Increased density common, indicative of inflammation

MR Findings
- T1WI
  - SMS mass with signal similar to SMG
- T2WI
  - Signal parallels SMG
- T1WI C+
  - Enhancement similar to SMG

Nuclear Medicine Findings
- Physiologic uptake may be seen on PSMA PET

Imaging Recommendations
- Best imaging tool
  - CECT
- Protocol advice
  - Thin images, multiplanar reformations (especially coronal)

DIFFERENTIAL DIAGNOSIS

Submandibular Space Reactive Nodal Disease
- SMS mass distinct from SMG
  - Nodal morphology will vary based on underlying disease

Submandibular Space Abscess
- Rim-enhancing cystic mass with extensive cellulitis

Diving Ranula
- Comet-shaped, unilocular mass with tail in collapsed SLS (tail sign) and head in posterior SMS
- May dive through mylohyoid defect

Submandibular Space Lymphatic Malformation
- Multilocular, transspatial cystic mass

Submandibular Space Mucocele
- Well-circumscribed SMG cystic mass

PATHOLOGY

General Features
- Etiology
  - Ectopic sublingual or SMG tissue in SMS
    - Present in ~ 1/3 of individuals
  - Seen with defect in mylohyoid (boutonnière)
    - Defects occur in ~ 75% of individuals
      - May contain fat, blood vessels, salivary tissue
    - Occasionally, entire sublingual glands may herniate through defect and lie completely below mylohyoid

Gross Pathologic & Surgical Features
- Normal salivary gland parenchyma

Microscopic Features
- Normal salivary gland cellular makeup

CLINICAL ISSUES

Presentation
- Most common signs/symptoms
  - Usually **incidental imaging finding**
  - Other signs/symptoms
    - May occasionally present as SMS mass

Treatment
- Imaging diagnosis allows avoidance of intervention
- When accessory tissue diseased, Tx varies with etiology

DIAGNOSTIC CHECKLIST

Consider
- Include accessory salivary tissue submandibular mass DDx
- Accessory SMS salivary tissue is "leave alone" lesion

Image Interpretation Pearls
- Look for density/intensity that follows normal SMG
- Susceptible to same pathology as orthotopic glands

SELECTED REFERENCES

1. Yazbeck A et al: The clinical anatomy of the accessory submandibular gland: a comprehensive review. Anat Cell Biol. 56(1):9-15, 2023
2. Sabotin RP et al: Conventional and MR-sialography of accessory submandibular glands: a case report. Radiol Case Rep. 17(12):4766-8, 2022
3. Zdilla MJ et al: Clinical implications of the submental and sublingual arteries in relation to the mylohyoid boutonnière. Otolaryngol Head Neck Surg. 164(2):322-7, 2021
4. Zhang W et al: Avid 68Ga-PSMA uptake in accessory submandibular salivary gland. Clin Nucl Med. 44(7):591-3, 2019
5. Desai RS et al: Pleomorphic adenoma of an accessory submandibular salivary gland: a rare entity. Br J Oral Maxillofac Surg. 53(8):e33-5, 2015
6. Kiesler K et al: Incidence and clinical relevance of herniation of the mylohyoid muscle with penetration of the sublingual gland. Eur Arch Otorhinolaryngol. 264(9):1071-4, 2007

Oral Cavity Dermoid and Epidermoid

TERMINOLOGY

- Cystic oral cavity (OC) lesion resulting from congenital epithelial inclusion or rest
- Dermoid: Epithelial elements + dermal adnexa
- Epidermoid: Epithelial elements only

IMAGING

- Dermoid and epidermoid appear as well-demarcated cysts in OC
- Dermoid more often midline
- Dermoid: Complex, cystic mass, often with fat &/or calcification
- MR best reveals foci of fat with chemical shift artifact
  - Fat also bright on T1WI and low signal with fat saturation
- Epidermoid: Fluid contents only
- Both epidermoid and dermoid may have restricted diffusion compared to CSF on DWI

TOP DIFFERENTIAL DIAGNOSES

- Ranula
- Lymphatic malformation of OC
- Submandibular cystic metastatic squamous cell carcinoma node
- Thyroglossal duct cyst
- OC abscess

CLINICAL ISSUES

- Average age at presentation: 30 years
- Painless subcutaneous or submucosal mass (85-90%)
- Often grows rapidly during puberty when sebaceous glands activated
- Surgical resection curative

DIAGNOSTIC CHECKLIST

- OC dermoid, epidermoid, ranula, and lymphatic malformation may appear indistinguishable

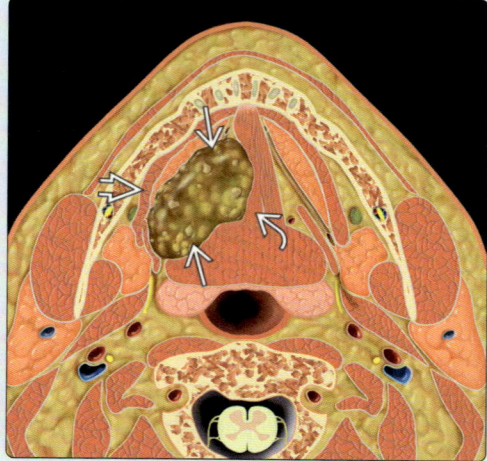
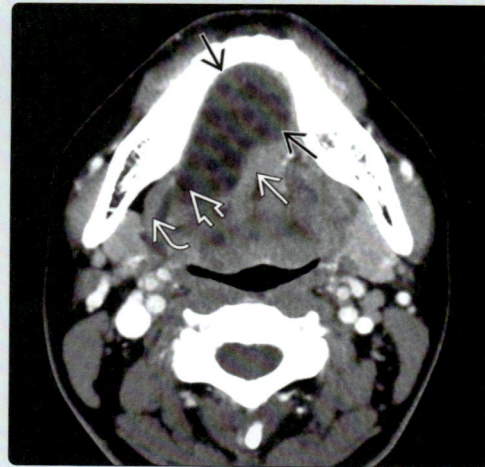

(Left) Axial graphic depicts a dermoid ➡ within the sublingual space that appears well defined and distorts only adjacent anatomy. The mass is complex, containing a mixture of fluid, fat globules, and calcifications. The mylohyoid ➡ and genioglossus ➡ are splayed. (Right) Axial CECT shows a well-circumscribed sublingual mass splaying the mylohyoid ➡ and genioglossus ➡ muscles. This lesion is predominantly fluid density ➡ with multiple lower density intralesional fat globules ➡, consistent with a dermoid.

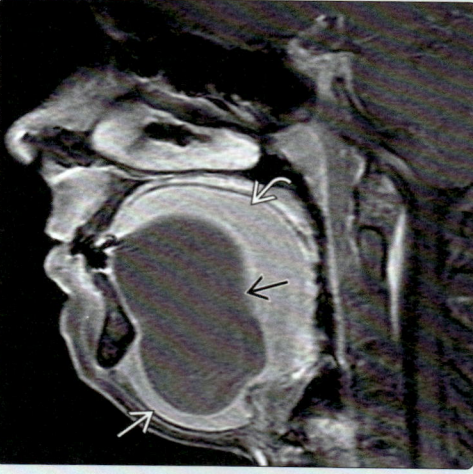
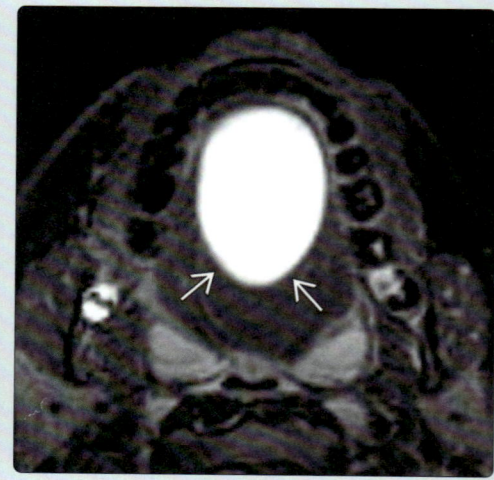

(Left) Sagittal T1 C+ FS MR shows an expansile, homogeneous, hypointense mass ➡ in the floor of the mouth. There is superior and posterior ➡ displacement of the tongue muscles and inferior displacement of the mylohyoid muscles ➡. (Right) Axial T2 FS MR in the same patient shows an expansile, homogeneous, hyperintense mass in the floor of the mouth ➡, pathology proven to be an epidermoid. Both an epidermoid and dermoid could have a similar MR imaging appearance.

Oral Cavity Dermoid and Epidermoid

TERMINOLOGY

Synonyms
- Developmental oral cavity (OC) cyst, ectodermal inclusion cyst, dermoid cyst

Definitions
- Cystic OC lesion resulting from congenital epithelial inclusion or rest
  - **Dermoid**: Epithelial elements + dermal adnexa
  - **Epidermoid**: Epithelial elements only
- Rarer entity is teratoid cyst
  - Epithelial elements + other tissue, such as bone, cartilage, or muscle

IMAGING

General Features
- Best diagnostic clue
  - Dermoid and epidermoid appear as well-demarcated cysts in OC
  - Dermoid: Fatty, fluid, or mixed contents
    - Sack of marbles appearance: Spherical lobules of fat floating in fluid matrix; virtually pathognomonic for dermoid
  - Epidermoid: Fluid only
- Location
  - Submandibular space (SMS), sublingual space (SLS), or root of tongue (ROT)
    - ROT: Potential space in inferior, midline tongue between genioglossus-geniohyoid muscles
  - Dermoid cyst more frequently midline
- Size
  - Typically < 4 cm
- Morphology
  - Ovoid or tubular
    - Most show thin, definable wall (75%)
    - 20% have peripheral nodular soft tissue

CT Findings
- NECT
  - Low-density, unilocular, well-circumscribed mass
    - Dermoid: Fatty internal material, mixed-density fluid, calcification (< 50%)
    - Epidermoid: Fluid density without complex features
- CECT
  - May see subtle enhancement of wall
  - If dermoid has minimal complex elements, can be indistinguishable from epidermoid

MR Findings
- T1WI
  - Well-circumscribed mass in OC
  - Dermoid: Complex fluid signal is characteristic
    - Focal or diffuse high signal suggests fat
      - Fat proven by chemical shift artifact or fat-saturation techniques
  - Epidermoid: Homogeneous fluid signal
    - Diffuse high signal may reflect higher protein content (termed white epidermoid)
- T2WI
  - Dermoid: Heterogeneous high signal
    - Intermediate signal if fat
    - Focal areas of low signal if calcifications
  - Epidermoid: Homogeneous high signal
- DWI
  - Both epidermoid and dermoid may have high diffusion signal
    - Restricted diffusion compared to CSF; ADC map signal typically similar or higher than brain
- T1WI C+
  - Thin rim enhancement often evident

Ultrasonographic Findings
- May be useful for evaluation of superficial lesions
- Dermoid: Mixed internal echoes from fat; echogenic foci with dense shadowing if calcifications
- Epidermoid: Pseudosolid appearance with uniform internal echoes
  - Cellular material in cyst causes pseudosolid appearance
  - Posterior wall echo enhancement is clue to cystic nature

Imaging Recommendations
- Best imaging tool
  - CECT or MR for localization
  - MR best for distinguishing dermoid and epidermoid
    - If complex signal, then lesion most likely dermoid
- Protocol advice
  - CT: Thin section with multiplanar reconstructions aids in specific OC localization
  - MR: Include fat-suppression sequences to prove presence of fat

DIFFERENTIAL DIAGNOSIS

Ranula
- Simple ranula may exactly mimic SLS epidermoid
  - Unilateral, thin-walled SLS cystic mass
- Diving ranula may also mimic SLS-SMS epidermoid
  - Comet-shaped unilocular mass with "tail" in collapsed SLS and "head" in posterior SMS

Oral Cavity Lymphatic Malformation
- Transspatial cystic mass
- May hemorrhage, resulting in fluid levels
- Infected lymphatic malformation may have complex proteinaceous contents

Squamous Cell Carcinoma Nodes
- Cystic metastatic nodal disease
- Submandibular nodes (level IB)
- Most often from OC primary, including lip

Thyroglossal Duct Cyst
- Midline cystic mass between hyoid and foramen cecum
- In posterior tongue root mimics epidermoid

Oral Cavity Abscess
- Clinical setting of septic patient with painful OC mass is distinctive
- Rim-enhancing cystic mass, often with extensive tongue and soft tissue cellulitis-edema

PATHOLOGY

General Features

- Etiology
  - 2 theories: Congenital and acquired
    - Congenital inclusion of dermal elements at site of embryonic 1st and 2nd branchial arches
      □ Sequestration of trapped surface ectoderm during midline fusion in 3rd-4th embryonic weeks
    - Acquired traumatic implantation of epithelial elements within OC mucosa

Staging, Grading, & Classification

- Meyer classification (pathologic)
  - Dermoid: Epithelium-lined cyst containing skin appendages, such as sebaceous and sweat glands, and hair follicles in cyst wall
  - Epidermoid: Lined with simple squamous epithelium and surrounding connective tissue
  - Teratoid: Epithelium-lined cyst containing mesodermal or endodermal elements, such as muscle, bones, teeth, and mucous membranes

Gross Pathologic & Surgical Features

- Oily or cheesy material; tan, yellow, or white
- May contain blood or chronic blood products
- Cyst wall is 2- to 6-mm-thick fibrous capsule

Microscopic Features

- Dermoid
  - Contains dermal structures, including sebaceous glands, hair follicles, blood vessels, **fat** ± collagen
    - Sweat glands in minority (20%)
    - Lined by keratinizing squamous epithelium
  - Dermoid diagnosis can be difficult for pathologist if full cyst lining not available
- Epidermoid
  - Simple squamous cell epithelium with fibrous wall
- Teratoid cyst
  - Contains elements from all 3 germ cell layers
    - Dermoid features + other contents, such as bone, muscle, and cartilage

CLINICAL ISSUES

Presentation

- Most common signs/symptoms
  - Painless subcutaneous or submucosal mass (85-90%)
  - Other signs/symptoms
    - Dysphagia, globus oral sensation
    - Airway encroachment when large
    - Uncommonly acute presentation with cyst rupture and inflammation
- Clinical profile
  - Young man with painless SMS/SLS mass

Demographics

- Age
  - Most often in late teens to 20s
    - Average age at presentation: 30 years
- Sex
  - M:F = 3:1

- Epidemiology
  - Dermoid and epidermoid are least common of congenital neck lesions
  - < 25% of H&N dermoids occur in OC
  - 90% of OC/oropharynx masses are squamous cell carcinoma

Natural History & Prognosis

- Benign lesion with slow growth
- Present during childhood but small and dormant
- May enlarge, become symptomatic when sebaceous glands activated during adolescence
- Sudden growth may also indicate cyst rupture
  - Significant inflammation and increased size

Treatment

- Surgical resection curative
  - Entire cyst must be removed to prevent recurrence
- Extracapsular excision can be performed by intraoral or external approach
- Surgical approach may be decided by lesion position relative to mylohyoid muscle
  - SLS: Superomedial to mylohyoid muscle
    - Intraoral approach with good cosmetic and functional results
  - SMS: Inferolateral to mylohyoid
    - Submandibular approach
- Postoperative complications rare
- Steroids or nonsteroidal drugs calm inflammation in ruptured lesions

DIAGNOSTIC CHECKLIST

Consider

- OC dermoid, epidermoid, ranula, and lymphatic malformation often seem indistinguishable

Image Interpretation Pearls

- Presence of fat ± calcium characterizes dermoid
- When hemorrhagic fluid levels are present, consider lymphatic malformation
- Comet shape with components in SLS and SMS supports diving ranula

SELECTED REFERENCES

1. Bargiel J et al: Giant sublingual, submental, and lingual dermoid cyst restricting tongue movement undiagnosed for several years. Diseases. 12(5):91, 2024
2. Safwan M et al: Unusual giant plunging sublingual epidermoid cyst: a case report and review of literature. Clin Case Rep. 12(6):e9067, 2024
3. Vidit et al: Sublingual dermoid in an adult patient. Cureus. 16(6):e63178, 2024
4. Basla N et al: Imaging features of epidermoid cyst located in the floor of the mouth: case report and narrative review of literature. Acta Otorhinolaryngol Ital. 43(1):3-11, 2023
5. Cunha JLS et al: Clinicopathologic analysis of oral dermoid and epidermoid cysts: a Brazilian multicenter study. Braz Oral Res. 37:e107, 2023
6. Celenk P et al: Imaging features of sublingual dermoid cysts: a report of four cases. Radiol Case Rep. 17(8):2888-93, 2022
7. Sauer A et al: A pediatric lateral submental mass: a rare presentation of dermoid cyst. Ear Nose Throat J. 1455613211019787, 2021
8. Abdel Razek AAK et al: Differentiation of sublingual thyroglossal duct cyst from midline dermoid cyst with diffusion weighted imaging. Int J Pediatr Otorhinolaryngol. 126:109623, 2019
9. Giarraputo L et al: Dermoid cyst of the floor of the mouth: diagnostic imaging findings. Cureus. 10(4):e2403, 2018

Oral Cavity Dermoid and Epidermoid

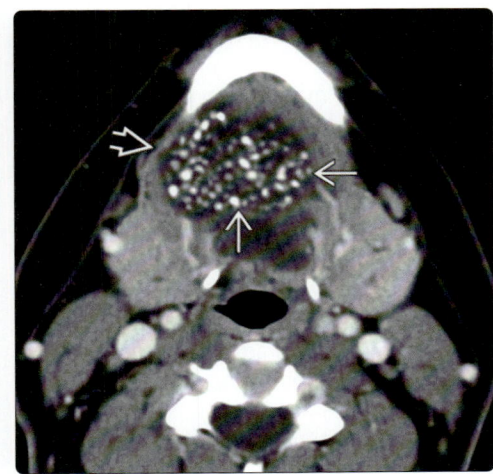

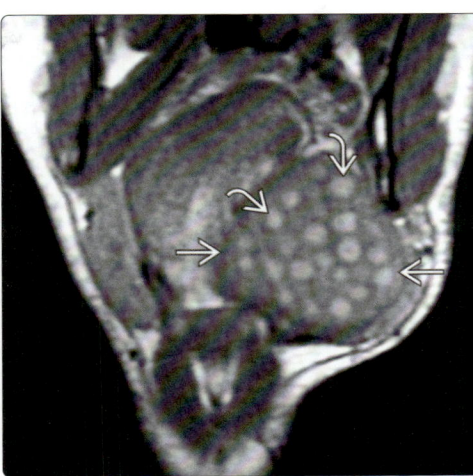

(Left) *Axial CECT reveals a paramedian sublingual space mass ➡, medial to the attenuated right mylohyoid muscle ➡. Multiple stippled calcifications and otherwise heterogeneous low attenuation are evident, consistent with a dermoid cyst.* (Right) *Coronal T1WI MR shows a large sublingual dermoid ➡. Internal round hyperintense foci ➡ are fat lobules. This sack of marbles appearance distinguishes a dermoid from other sublingual cysts, such as an epidermoid, ranula, or lymphatic malformation.*

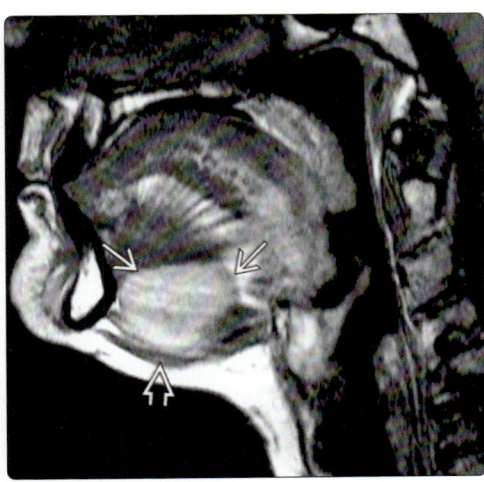

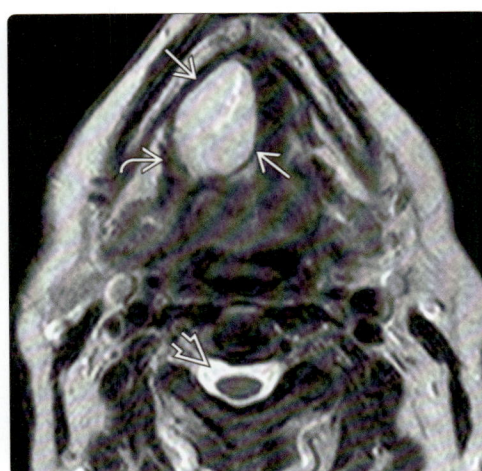

(Left) *Sagittal T1WI MR depicts a hyperintense, well-defined epidermoid ➡ arising in anterior root of the tongue and depressing floor of the mouth muscles ➡. Diffuse high signal suggests increased protein content, termed white epidermoid.* (Right) *Axial T2WI MR reveals mildly heterogeneous high signal within an epidermoid ➡ in the right floor of the mouth. Signal is lower intensity than CSF ➡, reflecting proteinaceous content. Attenuated mylohyoid muscle ➡ is seen along the lateral aspect of the lesion.*

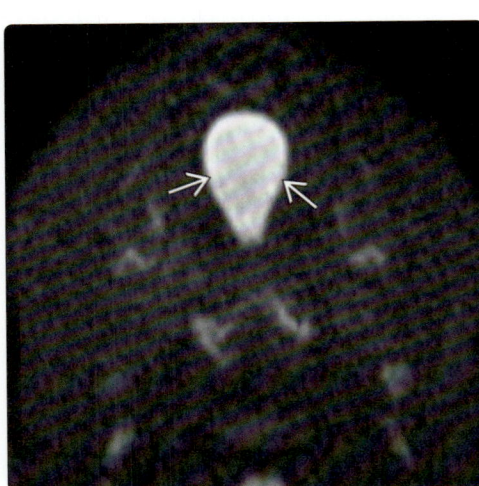

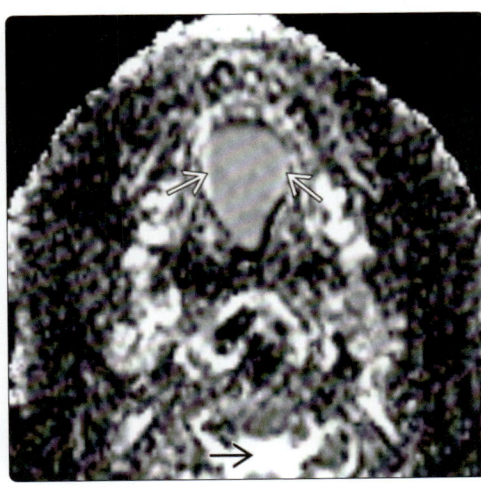

(Left) *Axial DWI MR demonstrates a well-circumscribed, midline floor of the mouth cystic mass with high diffusion signal ➡ in this case of epidermoid.* (Right) *Axial ADC map in the same patient demonstrates corresponding intermediate signal within this midline cystic mass ➡, corresponding to restricted diffusion compared to CSF ➡, typically not present in ranula or lymphatic malformation. Pathology confirmed an epidermoid.*

TERMINOLOGY

- Lymphangioma, cystic hygroma
- Distinguishing lymphatic malformation (LM) from venous or mixed malformations has treatment implications

IMAGING

- Macrocystic (uni- or multilocular) or microcystic
- Microcystic LM more often transspatial
- Submandibular space involvement common
- Typical cystic imaging features on CT/MR
  - Fluid-fluid levels indicate prior hemorrhage
  - Relative paucity of mass effect given size
- Cysts + solid enhancement or phleboliths suggest venous or mixed venolymphatic malformation
- T2 MR best evaluates macro- vs. microcystic nature

TOP DIFFERENTIAL DIAGNOSES

- Ranula
- Oral cavity abscess
- Dermoid & epidermoid, oral cavity
- Thyroglossal duct cyst

PATHOLOGY

- 1 type of slow-flow vascular malformation
- ISSVA classification of vascular anomalies, revised 2025
- Classifies LM into macrocystic, microcystic, or mixed forms

CLINICAL ISSUES

- Percutaneous sclerotherapy appropriate for macrocystic
- Diffuse microcystic malformations often have significant functional/cosmetic impairment
- Potential for airway obstruction
- Internal hemorrhage may cause dramatic enlargement
- Enlargement may occur with upper respiratory infection

DIAGNOSTIC CHECKLIST

- Contrast-enhanced MR to separate venous from LM
- Rim enhancement only in LM (central in venous)
- Fluid-fluid levels in transspatial cystic mass characteristic

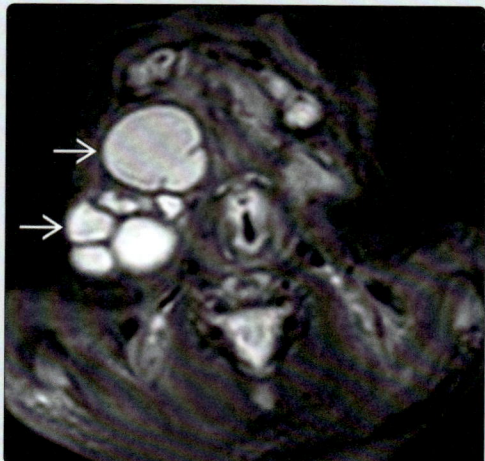
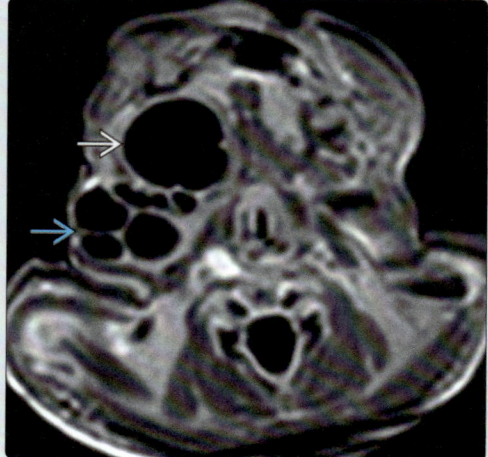

(Left) Axial STIR MR in a 9-month-old with tongue elevation & a right-sided neck mass shows a multilocular macrocystic lymphatic malformation (LM) involving the right sublingual & submandibular spaces ➡. (Right) Axial T1 C+ FS MR in the same patient confirms fluid signal intensity within the large cystic spaces without nodularity ➡. Only thin peripheral enhancement of cyst walls & septations typical of LMs ➡ is seen. The lesion decreased in size after treatment with oral sirolimus.

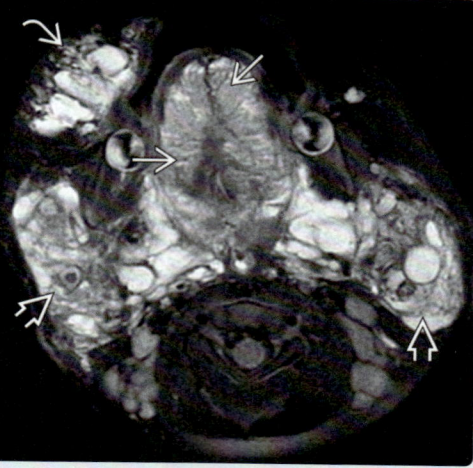
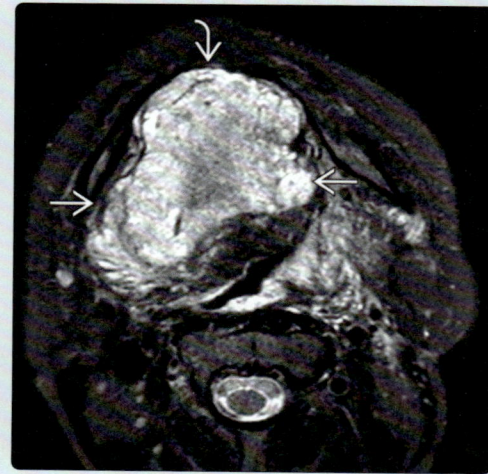

(Left) Axial T2 FS MR shows extensive diffuse microcystic & macrocystic LMs involving many spaces of the neck & oral cavity. Hyperintense components are seen in the tongue ➡, parapharyngeal, carotid, retropharyngeal, parotid ➡, & buccal ➡ spaces. (Right) Axial T2 FS MR shows a microcystic mixed malformation ➡ of the tongue. Faint areas of enhancement were noted (not shown). Patient was tracheostomy tube dependent due to oral & laryngeal airway obstruction. Note bony remodeling of anterior jaw ➡.

TERMINOLOGY

Abbreviations
- Lymphatic malformation (LM)

Synonyms
- Lymphangioma, cystic hygroma

Definitions
- Congenital malformation with lymphatic features
- May be part of venolymphatic (mixed) malformation

IMAGING

General Features
- Location
  - Uni- or transspatial
  - Submandibular space (SMS) involvement common
- Morphology
  - Soft invaginating lesion with little mass effect for size
  - Microcystic (cysts < 1 cm) more often transspatial

CT Findings
- NECT
  - Low-density cystic mass
    - Macrocystic form appears well delineated
    - Microcystic form may appear more infiltrative
    - Fluid-fluid levels indicate prior hemorrhage
  - Phleboliths indicate venous or mixed malformation
- CECT
  - Minimal enhancement of thin peripheral rim

MR Findings
- T1WI
  - Primarily hypointense
  - Fluid-fluid levels & high signal indicate prior hemorrhage
- T2WI
  - Hyperintense septated cystic lesions
  - Circumscribed or infiltrative; often transspatial
  - Microcystic LM only moderate T2 hyperintensity
    - May mimic solid mass
  - No flow voids evident
- T1WI C+
  - Mild enhancement of thin peripheral rim
  - Central enhancement supports venous (or mixed venolymphatic) malformation
  - Microcystic LM may have faint diffuse enhancement

Ultrasonographic Findings
- Primarily hypo- or anechoic transspatial mass

Imaging Recommendations
- Best imaging tool
  - Contrast-enhanced MR for characterization
  - T2WI best to evaluate macrocystic vs. microcystic
- Protocol advice
  - T2 FS MR best delineates lesion extent

DIFFERENTIAL DIAGNOSIS

Ranula
- Unilocular simple (sublingual) or diving (sublingual + SMS)

Abscess, Oral Cavity
- Rim-enhancing, low-density mass with cellulitis

Dermoid & Epidermoid, Oral Cavity
- Unilocular cystic mass with fluid or complex signal

Thyroglossal Duct Cyst
- Unilocular cyst in root or base of tongue

PATHOLOGY

General Features
- Etiology
  - Localized defect of vascular morphogenesis
  - 1 type of slow-flow vascular malformation
- Genetics
  - Somatic mutations often involve dysregulation of PI3K/AKT/mTOR & RAS/MAPK pathways
  - LM common manifestation of *PIK3CA* disorders
  - Most sporadic syndromes: Turner, Noonan, fetal alcohol, Proteus, CLOVES, Klippel-Trenaunay, CLAPO

Staging, Grading, & Classification
- ISSVA classification of vascular anomalies, revised 2025
- Classifies LM as macrocystic, microcystic, or mixed cystic

CLINICAL ISSUES

Presentation
- Most common signs/symptoms
  - Soft, doughy mass
  - May present with airway obstruction
- Other signs/symptoms
  - May enlarge with hemorrhage or URI

Demographics
- Age
  - Present at birth, grow with child

Natural History & Prognosis
- High local recurrence rate with incomplete resection

Treatment
- Oral sirolimus (rapamycin)
- Percutaneous sclerotherapy of macrocystic LM
- Surgical resection most effective if lesion is isolated, unilocular, & not associated with major vessels or nerves
- CO_2 laser useful for tongue lesions
- Microwave ablation for large macrocystic or mixed LM

DIAGNOSTIC CHECKLIST

Image Interpretation Pearls
- Fluid-fluid levels in transspatial mass
- Thin, peripheral rim enhancement only

SELECTED REFERENCES

1. Wang J et al: A real-world study of sirolimus in the treatment of pediatric head and neck lymphatic malformations. J Vasc Surg Venous Lymphat Disord. 13(4):102230, 2025
2. Peiser G et al: Complications of pediatric macrocystic lymphatic malformations of the head and neck: a survival analysis of treated and untreated patients. Emerg Radiol. 31(5):669-75, 2024

TERMINOLOGY

- Thyroid tissue in abnormal location in base of tongue (BOT) or floor of mouth
- Ectopic thyroid tissue

IMAGING

- Well-circumscribed, rounded, solid midline BOT mass
  - Usually at site of foramen cecum, less commonly in sublingual space or tongue root
- Imaging characteristics similar to normal thyroid CT & US, signal & contrast enhancement variable on MR
- High density on NECT due to iodine content, usually avid homogeneous enhancement
- Tc-99m pertechnetate or radioiodine scan confirms diagnosis & determines other sites of thyroid tissue
- US of thyroid bed to look for normal thyroid

TOP DIFFERENTIAL DIAGNOSES

- Venous malformation

- Hemangioma, upper airway
- Tonsillar tissue, prominent/asymmetric
- Non-Hodgkin lymphoma, lingual tonsil

CLINICAL ISSUES

- Most common location of ectopic thyroid (90%)
- In 75% lingual thyroid is only functioning tissue
- Thyroid hormone production may be insufficient, resulting in ectopic thyroid gland enlargement
- Goiter in ectopic gland reported with obstructive symptoms
- Differentiated thyroid carcinoma in lingual thyroid is rare but serious potential complication

DIAGNOSTIC CHECKLIST

- Diagnosis suggested by well-defined, ovoid or round, solid mass in BOT or floor of mouth
- Intrinsic high density on CT characteristic
- Must check for additional cervical thyroid tissue

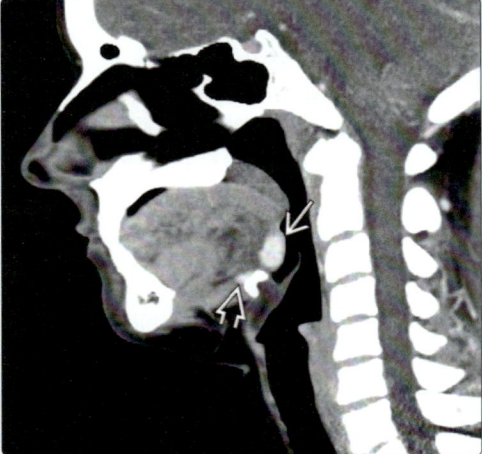
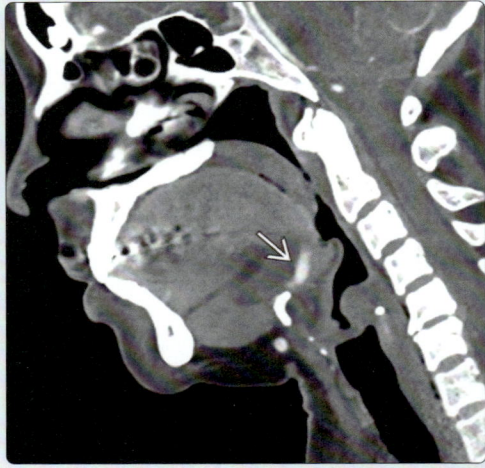

(Left) Sagittal CECT in a 33-year-old woman shows an incidental hyperdense mass in the base of the tongue ➡. There is a similar, smaller mass just anterior to the hyoid body ➡. This patient had no eutopic thyroid tissue. *(Right)* Sagittal CECT in a 54-year-old man shows an incidental hyperdense mass in the root of the tongue ➡. This patient had a normal volume of eutopic thyroid tissue.

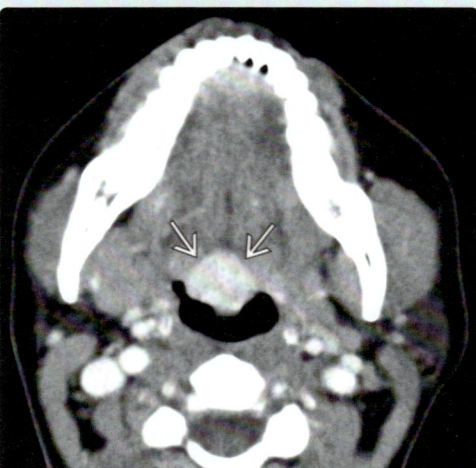
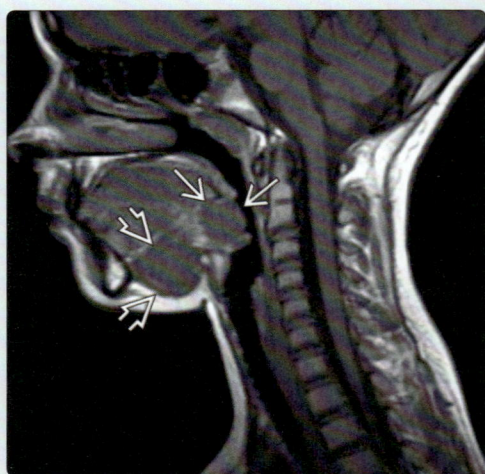

(Left) Axial CECT in a 30-year-old woman shows a hyperdense mass in the midline base of the tongue ➡, consistent with an ectopic lingual thyroid. The majority of patients will not have an orthotopic thyroid in the lower neck. *(Right)* Sagittal T1 MR in an 11-year-old girl demonstrates foci of an ectopic thyroid at the midline base of the tongue ➡ and midline floor of the mouth ➡. Both are well defined and isointense to muscle. Notice also the absence of an orthotopic thyroid in the lower neck.

TERMINOLOGY

Synonyms
- Ectopic thyroid tissue

Definitions
- Thyroid tissue in abnormal location in base of tongue (BOT) or floor of mouth

IMAGING

General Features
- Best diagnostic clue
  - Well-circumscribed, midline BOT mass
  - Imaging characteristics similar to normal thyroid CT & US
    - Signal & contrast enhancement variable on MR
- Location
  - Midline BOT at level of foramen cecum
  - Less commonly in sublingual space or tongue root
- Morphology
  - Well circumscribed, round or ovoid

CT Findings
- NECT: Sharply marginated rounded mass
  - High density secondary to iodine accumulation
- CECT: Avid homogeneous enhancement

MR Findings
- T1WI: Isointense to mildly hyperintense relative to tongue
  - Normal thyroid hyperintense
- T2WI: Isointense to hyperintense relative to tongue
  - Normal thyroid hyperintense
- T1WI C+: Variable; most often homogeneous enhancement

Ultrasonographic Findings
- Well-defined, homogeneous mass with echotexture similar to normal thyroid gland
- Normal bilobed thyroid gland in lower neck usually absent

Nuclear Medicine Findings
- Tc-99m pertechnetate to confirm diagnosis

Imaging Recommendations
- Protocol advice
  - Imaging should include infrahyoid neck to determine if thyroid tissue is present in normal location

DIFFERENTIAL DIAGNOSIS

Venous Malformation
- Vascular malformation, T2 hyperintensity, variable contrast enhancement, ± phleboliths, ± regional fat hypertrophy

Infantile Hemangioma, Upper Airway
- Asymmetric subglottic airway narrowing, intense enhancement

Tonsillar Tissue, Prominent/Asymmetric
- Prominent lingual lymphoid tonsils at entire width of BOT
- Imaging features similar to other lymphoid tissue, such as adenoids & palatine tonsils

Non-Hodgkin Lymphoma, Lingual Tonsil
- Isolated or in association with nodal or tonsillar lymphoma

PATHOLOGY

General Features
- Etiology
  - Arrest of thyroid anlage migration within BOT 3rd-7th weeks of gestation
    - Complete arrest: No thyroid in thyroid bed (variable, reported up to 75%)
    - Partial arrest: High cervical thyroid (25%)
- Associated abnormalities
  - Other thyroid migration anomalies: Thyroglossal duct cyst or 2nd site of ectopic thyroid tissue

CLINICAL ISSUES

Presentation
- Most common signs/symptoms
  - Dysphagia, dysphonia, dyspnea, obstructive sleep apnea
  - Many patients hypothyroid (reports up to 70%), can be euthyroid
- Other signs/symptoms
  - 25% of infants with congenital hypothyroidism will have ectopic gland

Demographics
- Sex
  - Females more often than males (M:F = 1:2-4)
- Epidemiology
  - Lingual location most common ectopic thyroid (90%)
  - Very rare: Estimated incidence (1:10,000 to 1:100,000)

Natural History & Prognosis
- Lingual thyroid may expand rapidly during puberty
  - Goiter in lingual thyroid has been reported
- Carcinoma of lingual thyroid rare
  - Most often follicular thyroid carcinoma, in contradistinction to orthotopic gland (papillary)

Treatment
- Thyroid hormone replacement 1st to shrink gland at BOT
- Surgical resection if obstructive symptoms
- Some advocate radioiodine ablation
- Check for orthotopic thyroid prior to Tx (US)

DIAGNOSTIC CHECKLIST

Consider
- When lingual thyroid identified, must comment on status of infrahyoid thyroid tissue in thyroid bed
  - Only functioning thyroid tissue in up to 75%

Image Interpretation Pearls
- Well-defined midline tongue base mass with intrinsic high density on NECT

SELECTED REFERENCES

1. Al Suqri B et al: Coexistence of eutopic thyroid gland and ectopic thyroid tissue: rare but not uncommon. Cureus. 16(5):e59834, 2024
2. Fakadej T et al: Lingual thyroid: case report and brief review of the literature. Radiol Case Rep. 18(1):312-6, 2023
3. Cruz-Dardíz N et al: Lingual thyroid gland: it's time for awareness. Endocrinol Diabetes Metab Case Rep. ePub, 2020
4. Kumar A et al: Dual thyroid ectopia: a pictorial case series and review of literature. World J Nucl Med. 19(4):336-40, 2020

TERMINOLOGY

- Ranula: Retention cyst of sublingual gland (SLG) or sublingual space (SLS) minor salivary gland
  - Simple ranula (SR): Cyst confined to SLS
  - Diving ranula (DR): SR extends into submandibular space (SMS)

IMAGING

- **SR**: Unilocular SLS cyst
  - Unilateral oval or bilateral horseshoe shape
- **DR**: Comet-shaped unilocular cyst
  - "Body" in SMS & "tail" in SLS
  - **Tail sign** = collapsed SLS component
  - Lateral: Tail in anterior SLS & body anterior to SMG
  - Posterior: Tail medial to mylohyoid, body medial to SMG
- CECT: Unilocular fluid density cyst, thin wall enhancement
- MR: Fluid signal intensity (follows CSF)
- US: Hypoechoic cyst(s) in SLS ± SMS

- SLG herniation through mylohyoid defect or posterior to mylohyoid free edge in DR

TOP DIFFERENTIAL DIAGNOSES

- Oral cavity sialocele
- Oral cavity abscess
- SMG mucocele
- Oral cavity lymphatic malformation

PATHOLOGY

- Retention cyst from gland trauma or inflammation
- SLG or SLS retention cyst herniation through mylohyoid defect may predispose to trauma & DR

CLINICAL ISSUES

- Many imaging & clinical mimics
- SR more common than DR

DIAGNOSTIC CHECKLIST

- **T2 FS MR** best sequence to show subtle tail sign in SLS

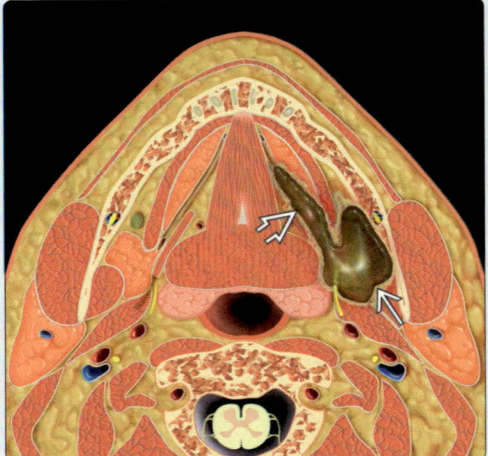
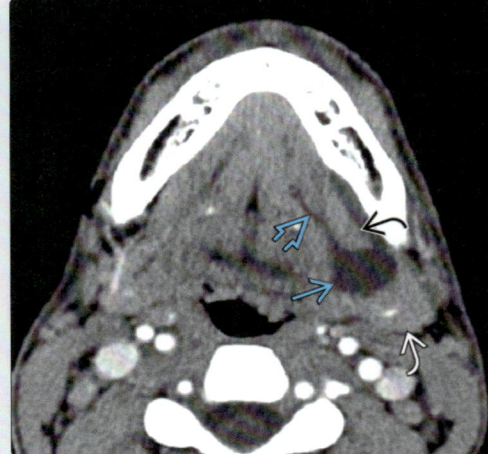

(Left) Axial graphic depicts a diving ranula herniating posteriorly from the sublingual space (SLS) into the submandibular space (SMS) ➡. The tail sign ➡ is the collapsed portion of the cyst in the SLS. (Right) Axial CECT demonstrates a rounded cyst ➡ in the SMS abutting the posterior margin of the mylohyoid muscle ➡ and displacing the submandibular gland (SMG) ➡ posterolaterally. A linear, low-density tail ➡ extends anteriorly within the left SLS, representing the tail sign of collapsed ranula cyst.

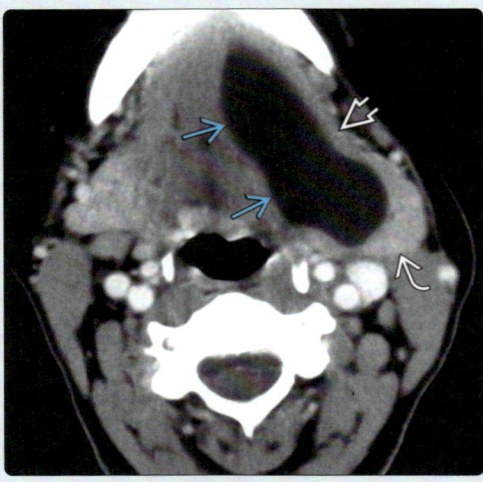
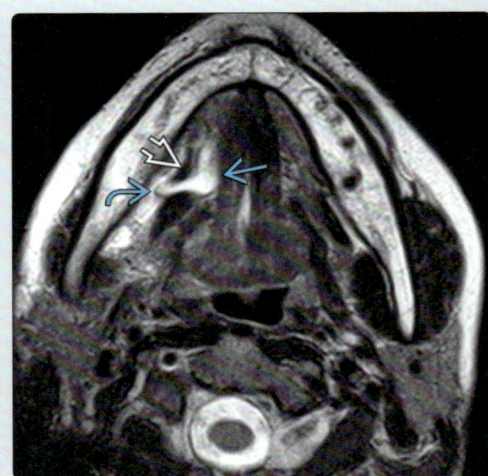

(Left) Axial CECT shows a large simple ranula ➡ distending the right SLS and bowing the mylohyoid muscle ➡ laterally and the SMG ➡ posteriorly. There is no appreciable enhancement or thickening of cyst wall or adjacent inflammatory changes. (Right) Axial T2 FS MR in an adult with sublingual mass shows a small, well-defined, T2 hyperintensity ➡ lateral to the mylohyoid muscle ➡. T2 FS MR best shows the subtle tail sign and the lateral diving ranula through the mylohyoid defect ➡.

TERMINOLOGY

Synonyms
- Simple ranula (SR): Sublingual gland (SLG) mucocele, SLG retention cyst, intraoral ranula
- Diving ranula (DR): Plunging ranula, cervical ranula, retention pseudocyst

Definitions
- SLG or minor salivary gland retention cyst
  - Simple: Cyst confined to sublingual space (SLS)
  - Diving: Extravasated pseudocyst; cyst extending into submandibular space (SMS)
- Term "ranula" derives from Latin "rana," meaning "frog"
  - Sublingual blebs in mouth of frog resemble SR

IMAGING

General Features
- Best diagnostic clue
  - Simple: Well-defined, thin-walled SLS cyst
  - Diving: Thin-walled SMS cyst with **SLS tail**
- Location
  - Simple: SLS (i.e., above mylohyoid muscle)
  - Diving: SMS + SLS
- Size
  - Simple; usually < 3 cm as limited to SLS
  - Diving may be large; usually ≤ 10 cm
- Morphology
  - Simple ranula
    - Unilateral: Oval or lenticular unilocular SLS cyst
    - Bilateral: Horseshoe-shaped unilocular SLS cyst
  - Diving ranula
    - Comet-shaped, unilocular SMS cyst, tail in SLS
    - ± parapharyngeal space (PPS) if large

CT Findings
- CECT
  - Simple ranula
    - Unilocular, low-density SLS cystic mass with subtle or no linear wall enhancement
    - ± extending to contralateral SLS (horseshoe shape)
  - Diving ranula
    - **Tail sign**: Collapsed SLS portion
    - **Laterally** through mylohyoid muscle defect (more common): Tail in anterior SLS & body often anterior to SMG
    - **Posteriorly** over back of mylohyoid: Tail medial to mylohyoid & body often medial to submandibular gland (SMG)
  - Infected ranula (current or recent)
    - Distended cyst with thick, enhancing wall
    - ± septations if recurrent

MR Findings
- T1WI
  - Diffuse low fluid signal (similar to CSF)
- T2WI
  - Markedly high fluid signal (similar to CSF)
- T1WI C+
  - Thin, linear, or nonenhancement of wall if not infected
  - Current or recent infection: Thicker wall; may alter T1 & T2 signal

Ultrasonographic Findings
- Hypoechoic, well-defined cyst in SLS (± SMS if DR) without internal Doppler flow
- SLG herniation through mylohyoid defect or posterior to mylohyoid free edge
- Aspiration of cyst can confirm salivary amylase contents

Imaging Recommendations
- Best imaging tool
  - MR is best study to characterize + define extent of ranula
  - US is good 1st-line test, especially in young patients
- Protocol advice
  - T2 FS MR best sequence to demonstrate SLS cyst & subtle tail in SLS ± SMS
  - Multiplanar reformats help delineate diving component

DIFFERENTIAL DIAGNOSIS

Submandibular Duct Sialocele
- Extravasatved saliva contained within fibrous pseudocapsule
- Possible obstructive stone ± dilated submandibular duct

Oral Cavity Lymphatic Malformation
- Multilocular transspatial cystic mass
- Typically lobulated, septated, & heterogeneous
  - May be transspatial
  - ± Peripheral linear wall enhancement

Oral Cavity Abscess
- Patient usually septic with tender oral cavity
- Single or multiple collections with enhancing wall(s)
- + inflammatory change in fat

Submandibular Gland Mucocele
- Cyst "bubbles" off margin of SMG
- No tail sign to SLS

Oral Cavity Dermoid & Epidermoid
- Unilateral, low density/signal mass in SLS with thin, nonenhancing wall
- In SLS, epidermoid can look identical to SR
  - Fat density/signal diagnostic of dermoid ± bag of marbles appearance
  - Diffusion restriction characteristic of epidermoid

Suppurative Lymph Nodes
- Multiple, cystic-appearing SMS nodes
- Separate suppurative/reactive nodes suggest diagnosis
- Associated inflammation & clinical history are key

PATHOLOGY

General Features
- Etiology
  - Retention cyst/pseudocyst without epithelial lining resulting from trauma or inflammation of SLG or SLS minor salivary gland
  - Congenital ranula from imperforate salivary duct or ostial adhesion, can spontaneously resolve
  - SLS (SR) → SMS (DR)

- Extends laterally through mylohyoid button hole (boutonnière) defect, anterior to SMG (most common)
- Extends posteriorly over posterior margin of mylohyoid to posterior SMS
- Extension to PPS in < 10%

Staging, Grading, & Classification

- SR develops in & confined to SLS
  - May enlarge to fill entire unilateral SLS
  - May extend to contralateral SLS above mandibular insertion of genioglossus muscle
- DR secondary to herniation of SR
  - Herniation of retention cyst into subjacent SMS

Gross Pathologic & Surgical Features

- Simple: Fluctuant sublingual mass, blue tinge or pink
- Diving: Fluctuant mass of extravasated mucus
- Yellow viscous fluid on aspiration

Microscopic Features

- Pseudocyst without epithelial lining, fibrous pseudocapsule + granulation tissue, dense connective tissue, & chronic inflammatory cells
- Contains mucin, salivary amylase

CLINICAL ISSUES

Presentation

- Most common signs/symptoms
  - Painless swelling of floor of mouth (SR)
  - DR typically presents as submandibular mass, which is displaced SMG
    - Displaced SMG may have partially obstructed duct ± inflammatory changes
  - Either can present as waxing & waning masses
- Other signs/symptoms
  - 50% have history of prior neck or oral cavity trauma
  - Can be associated with Sjögren syndrome
- Clinical profile
  - 30-year-old patient with painless floor of mouth mass

Demographics

- Age
  - Any age; median = 30 years
    - SR: 20-30 years; DR: late 30s
    - 20% < 16 years; 90% SR
    - Congenital ranula in infant (rare < 1%)
- Sex
  - M slightly > F
- Ethnicity
  - Increased incidence of DR in Maori of New Zealand & Pacific Island Polynesians (Polynesia, Melanesia, Micronesia)
- Epidemiology
  - SR more common than DR
  - Lateral extension through mylohyoid defect most common type of DR
  - Congenital ranula is rare

Natural History & Prognosis

- Large SR can fill unilateral SLS, may involve contralateral side to be axial plane horseshoe-shape

- Children: May spontaneously resolve in 6 months
- Adults: Tend to extend into SMS as DR
- Recurrence may occur depending on surgical treatment

Treatment

- No consensus, controversial
- Surgical interventions
  - Surgical excision of SLG ± cyst
    - Transoral approach
      - Lowest recurrence rate (< 5%), fewest complications, most recommended
    - Transcervical approach
      - Recurrence & orocutaneous fistula risk if SLG not excised
  - Marsupialization
  - Incision & drainage
    - High recurrence rate (up to 100%)
  - Laser excision & vaporization
- Nonsurgical options
  - Sclerotherapy with intracystic OK-432, ethanol, & bleomycin
  - Cyst aspiration; highest recurrence rate (up to 100%)

DIAGNOSTIC CHECKLIST

Consider

- Many imaging & clinical mimics

Image Interpretation Pearls

- Suspect DR if **tail sign** is present
  - If laterally through mylohyoid defect, SMS cyst anterior to SMG
  - If behind posterior margin of mylohyoid muscle, SMS cyst often medial to SMG
- **T2 FS MR** best sequence to delineate subtle tail sign
- Cyst aspiration for salivary amylase may help in some cases

SELECTED REFERENCES

1. Lazzeroni M et al: Sublingual ranulas, is it time for a new classification? A systematic review and meta-analysis. J Laryngol Otol. 139(2):88-94, 2025
2. Rodrigues Barros C et al: Recurrent plunging ranula due to a sublingual ectopic gland: a rare clinical entity. Cureus. 16(1):e52590, 2024
3. Yun J et al: Diagnostic difficulties of plunging ranula: a review of 18 cases. Laryngoscope. 134(6):2689-96, 2024
4. Song T et al: Amylase as a diagnostic tool for plunging ranula: clinical series and description of the technique. Laryngoscope. 133(3):535-8, 2023
5. Takagi Y et al: Three signs to help detect Sjögren's syndrome: incidental findings on magnetic resonance imaging and computed tomography. J Clin Med. 12(20):6487, 2023
6. Harrison JD: The persistently misunderstood plunging ranula. Am J Otolaryngol. 43(1):103276, 2022
7. Koch M et al: Ultrasound in the diagnosis and differential diagnosis of enoral and plunging ranula: a detailed and comparative analysis. J Ultrasound. 26(2):487-95, 2022
8. Bachesk AB et al: Ranula in children: retrospective study of 25 years and literature review of the plunging variable. Int J Pediatr Otorhinolaryngol. 148:110810, 2021
9. Li J et al: Correct diagnosis for plunging ranula by magnetic resonance imaging. Aust Dent J. 59(2):264-7, 2014
10. Jain P et al: Plunging ranulas: high-resolution ultrasound for diagnosis and surgical management. Eur Radiol. 20(6):1442-9, 2010

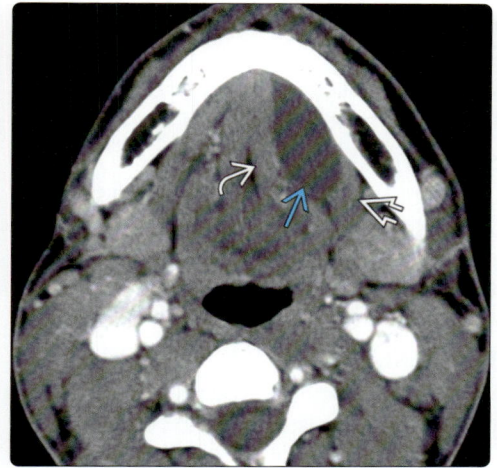

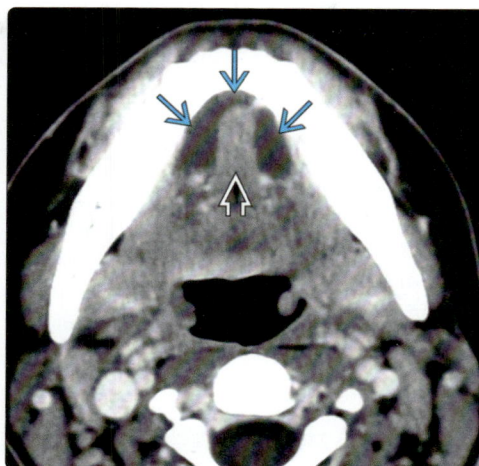

(Left) Axial CECT shows a simple unilateral ranula as an ovoid, low-density lesion in the left anterior SLS ➡. There is no perceptible thickening or enhancement of wall. The mylohyoid is displaced posterolaterally ➡, and the genioglossus ➡ is bowed medially. (Right) Axial CECT demonstrates a cystic, horseshoe-shaped lesion ➡ in the anterior SLS, curving around and above the genioglossus muscle ➡ insertion on the mandible. This is a characteristic simple ranula involving both sides of the SLS.

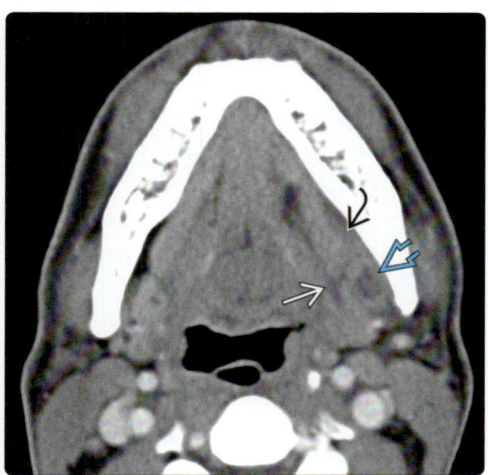

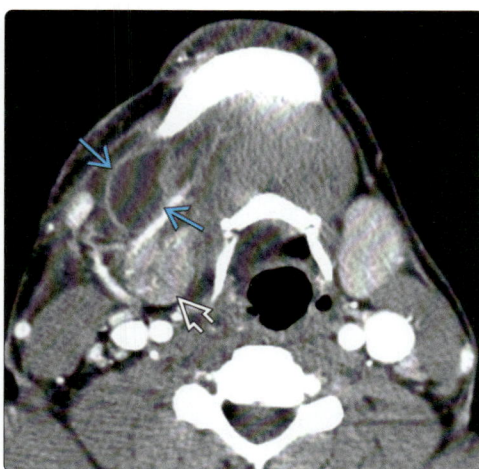

(Left) Axial CECT shows the superior aspect of a ranula ➡ extending toward the posterior margin of mylohyoid muscle ➡, suggesting the diagnosis of a diving ranula, which has become acutely secondarily infected. Note small tail extending to the SLS ➡. (Right) Axial CECT in a young adult patient with marked pain and swelling shows a rim-enhancing, low-density mass ➡ in the right SMS anterolateral to the SMG ➡ with extensive adjacent inflammatory changes.

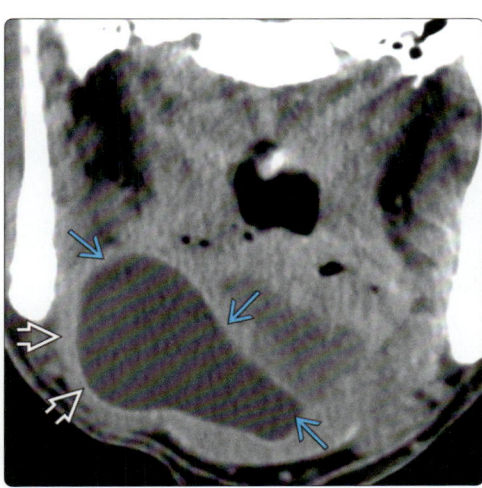

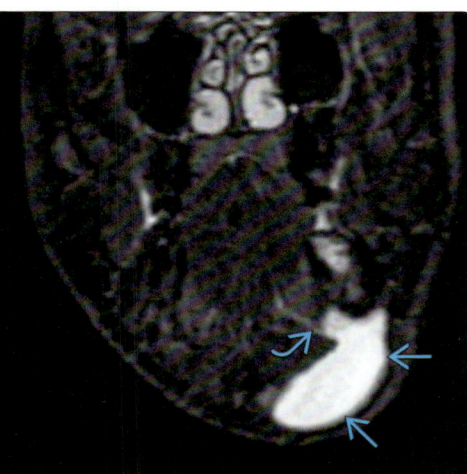

(Left) Coronal delayed CECT shows inferolateral bowing of the mylohyoid muscle ➡ by a large, thin-walled unilocular cyst ➡. A simple ranula appears identical to SLS epidermoid on CT, and definitive diagnosis requires pathology or clear congenital history and restricted diffusion on MR. (Right) Coronal T2 FS MR shows a laterally diving ranula as a large SMS cystic mass ➡ and subtle tail sign ➡ through a boutonnière defect of mylohyoid muscle.

TERMINOLOGY

- Definition: Collection of extravasated saliva
  - Ruptured submandibular duct (SMD) extravasates saliva into sublingual space (SLS)

IMAGING

- CECT findings
  - SLS fluid density focus ± enhancing rim ± adjacent inflammatory change
  - Rarely extends into posterior submandibular space (SMS)
  - ± SMD calculus, SMD dilation + sialadenitis (enhancing, enlarged submandibular gland)
  - Fluid collection is distinct from SMD, but may appear inseparable on imaging
- CECT best delineates sialocele and calculus if present

TOP DIFFERENTIAL DIAGNOSES

- Ranula
- SLS abscess
- SLS epidermoid
- SLS lymphatic malformation

PATHOLOGY

- Etiology: **SMD injury** with leakage of saliva into SLS
  - SMD calculus > trauma or surgery

CLINICAL ISSUES

- Common presentation: Fluctuant, soft, painless SLS mass
  - History of SMD stone, recent oral cavity surgery/trauma
- Sialocele cause: Obstructing SMD calculus > posttraumatic or postoperative
- Sialocele location: Parotid space > > SLS > SMS

DIAGNOSTIC CHECKLIST

- Look closely for possible obstructing calculi
- Consider mimics: Simple ranula, abscess, epidermoid, lymphatic malformation, sialocele without SMD calculus

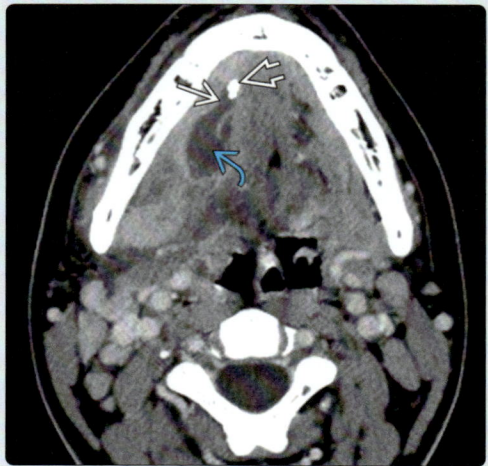
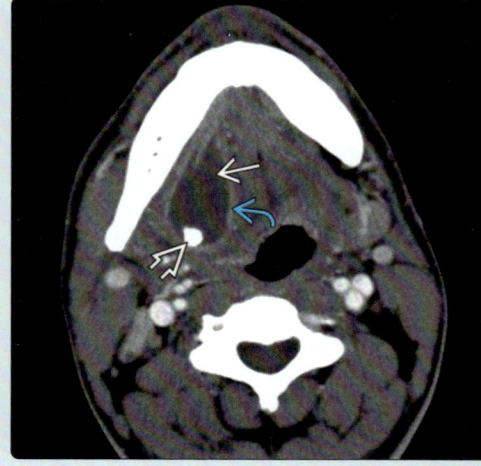

(Left) Axial CECT shows a calculus obstructing the submandibular duct ⇥ at the terminal papilla, causing the submandibular duct to dilate ⇥. Duct rupture has occurred with a sialocele ⇨ visible in the medial sublingual space. (Right) Axial CECT reveals an ovoid cystic sialocele in the right sublingual space ⇨ with a thin enhancing rim (fibrous pseudocapsule) ⇨. Dependent calculus ⇥ is seen posteriorly. This patient likely had a stone obstructing the submandibular duct. When the duct ruptured, the stone fell into the sialocele.

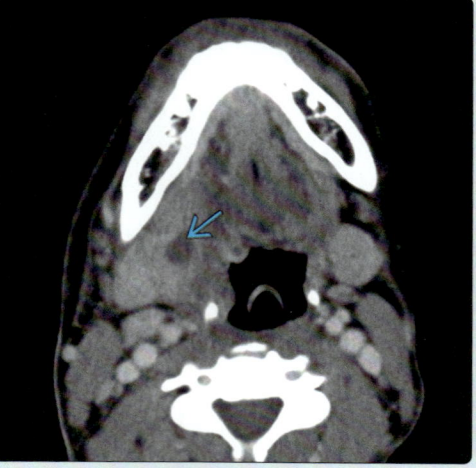
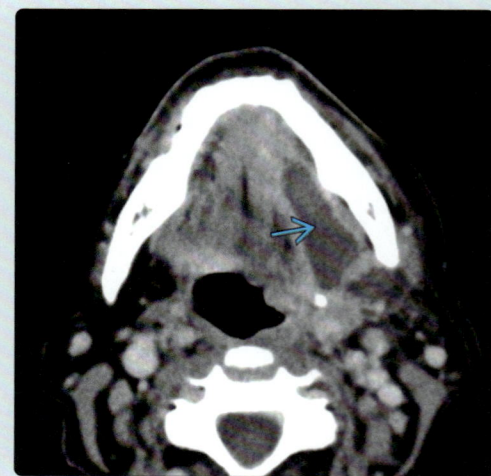

(Left) Axial CECT demonstrates a small cystic mass in the posterior sublingual space ⇨. Ranula, sialocele, and epidermoid were all considered. At surgery, a small pocket of saliva with a fibrous pseudocapsule was found. (Right) Axial CECT in a patient with floor of mouth swelling and history of facial trauma shows a cystic lesion in the left sublingual space ⇨. Both ranula and sialocele were considered; sialocele was found at surgery. History of facial trauma supported a sialocele diagnosis.

Oral Cavity Sialocele

TERMINOLOGY

Synonyms

- Floor of mouth, sublingual, lingual, or submandibular duct (SMD) sialocele, extravasation mucocele

Definitions

- Collection of extravasated saliva from damaged SMD
  - Ruptured SMD extravasates saliva into sublingual space (SLS)

IMAGING

General Features

- Best diagnostic clue
  - Cystic SLS focus along course of SMD
- Location
  - SLS ± submandibular space (SMS)
- Size
  - Variable, usually < 3 cm
- Morphology
  - Ovoid to lenticular

CT Findings

- CECT
  - SLS fluid density focus ± enhancing rim ± adjacent inflammatory change
    - Rarely extends into posterior SMS
  - ± SMD calculus, SMD dilation and sialadenitis (enhancing ± enlarged submandibular gland)
  - Fluid collection is adjacent to but may be inseparable from SMD on imaging ± SMD dilation

MR Findings

- T1WI
  - Low- (fluid) signal in SLS ± dilated SMD
- T2WI
  - High- (fluid) signal in SLS ± dilated SMD
- T1WI C+
  - Rim-enhancing, fluid signal focus
  - ± adjacent inflammatory soft tissue enhancement

Imaging Recommendations

- Best imaging tool
  - CECT best delineates sialocele ± calculus (if present)
- Protocol advice
  - Multislice CT oblique reformations around dental amalgam reduces metallic artifact

DIFFERENTIAL DIAGNOSIS

Ranula

- Smoothly marginated SLS fluid collection, no SMD calculus

Oral Cavity Abscess in Sublingual Space

- Rim-enhancing SLS fluid collection; DWI: Restricted diffusion

Sublingual Space Epidermoid

- Ovoid fluid collection in SLS
- DWI shows restricted diffusion

Sublingual Space Lymphatic Malformation

- SLS-SMS multilocular transspatial cystic lesion
- No perceptible wall unless infected

Submandibular Gland Mucocele

- Retention cyst fluid collection within or on margin of SMG
- SMD may be normal

PATHOLOGY

General Features

- Etiology
  - **SMD injury** with leakage of saliva into SLS
    - SMD calculus > trauma or surgery

Gross Pathologic & Surgical Features

- Saliva outside SMD but within **fibrous pseudocapsule**

Microscopic Features

- Fibrous granulation tissue surrounding saliva ± intact duct

CLINICAL ISSUES

Presentation

- Most common signs/symptoms
  - Fluctuant, soft, painless (if not infected) sublingual mass
- Clinical profile
  - History of SMD stone, recent oral cavity surgery or trauma presents with new SLS mass

Demographics

- Epidemiology
  - Obstructing SMD calculus > > posttraumatic / postoperative
  - Parotid space sialocele > > SLS sialocele > SMS sialocele

Natural History & Prognosis

- Most self resolve; large sialocele may enlarge if untreated

Treatment

- Conservative treatments: Multiple aspirations, pressure dressings, antisialagogues
- Local botulinum toxin type A injection
  - Used for parotid sialoceles
- Surgical treatments: Primary duct repair or stenting, sialocele resection, salivary gland resection
  - Primary treatment or after failed conservative measures

DIAGNOSTIC CHECKLIST

Consider

- Look closely for possible obstructing calculi
- Note history of oral cavity surgery, trauma, or SMD calculus
- Consider mimics: Ranula, abscess, epidermoid, lymphatic malformation, sialocele without SMD calculus

SELECTED REFERENCES

1. Sheykhveisi M et al: The role of botulinum toxin for the management of post parotidectomy sialocele: a randomized controlled trial. Indian J Otolaryngol Head Neck Surg. 77(3):1215-9, 2025
2. Kalaimani G et al: Mucous extravasation phenomenon: a clinicopathologic evaluation of 68 cases. J Oral Maxillofac Pathol. 28(2):182-5, 2024
3. Shupak RP et al: Management of salivary gland injury. Oral Maxillofac Surg Clin North Am. 33(3):343-50, 2021

KEY FACTS

TERMINOLOGY

- Inflammation of submandibular gland (SMG)

IMAGING

- **Acute sialadenitis**
  - Enlarged, enhancing/hypervascular SMG (can be mistaken for node)
  - Adjacent inflammatory change, ± reactive nodes
  - ± duct dilation
  - ± **duct calculus** (most common), stenosis, floor of mouth tumor
  - Complications: Floor of mouth cellulitis, abscess
- **Chronic recurrent sialadenitis** less common
  - Fatty atrophy of SMG
- **US &/or CECT** recommended to assess gland ± calculus
  - NECT unnecessary; calculus and vessel densities differ
  - US for radiolucent calculus, especially young patients
- US and MR more sensitive for gland parenchymal changes

TOP DIFFERENTIAL DIAGNOSES

- Dental infection
- Squamous cell carcinoma nodal metastases
- SMG carcinoma
- SMG pleomorphic adenoma

CLINICAL ISSUES

- SMG calculus more often within duct than gland

DIAGNOSTIC CHECKLIST

- Assess SMG duct for calculus (most common cause); describe location within duct
- Beware: Calculi may be radiolucent or obscured by dental amalgam
- **Look carefully for obstructing floor of mouth tumor**
- If no calculus, consider duct stenosis or gland disease
  - Bilateral: Infection, autoimmune exocrinopathy, sialadenosis, inflammatory
  - Unilateral: Chronic sclerosing sialadenitis, mimics tumor

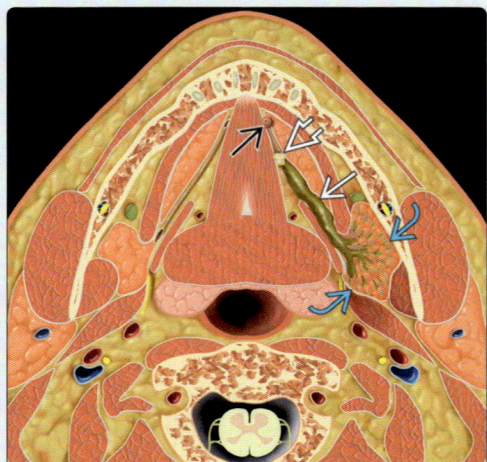
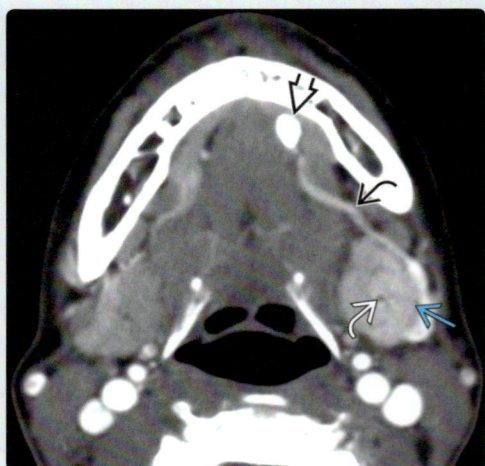

(Left) *Axial graphic shows an inflamed and enlarged submandibular gland (SMG) ➡. Proximal submandibular duct ➡ and intraductal radicles are dilated due to an obstructing calculus ➡ in the distal duct just proximal to the papilla ➡. (Right) Axial CECT shows an asymmetrically enhancing, enlarged left SMG ➡ compared to the right. Hyperdense calculus is evident in distal submandibular duct at the ductal papilla ➡. Only mild prominence of duct at its hilum ➡ is evident. A prominent vessel in floor of mouth ➡ is also noted.*

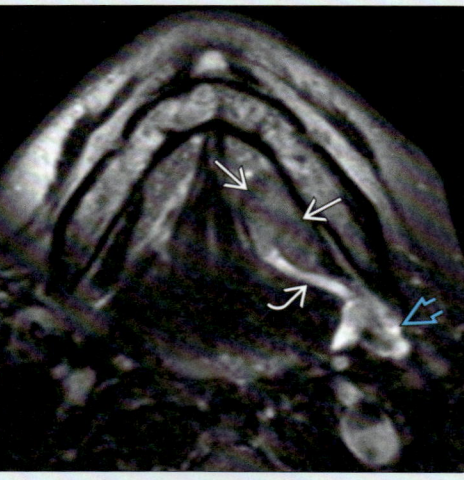
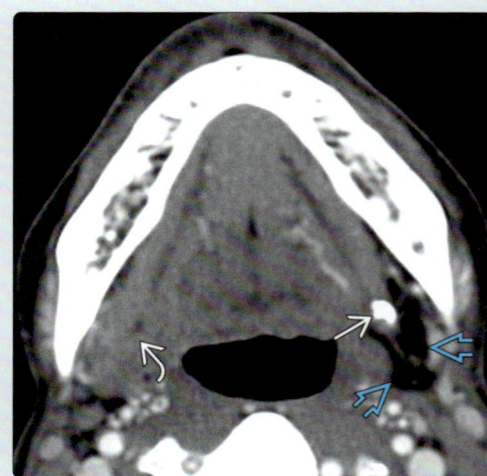

(Left) *Axial T2 FS MR shows a well-circumscribed mass in the left floor of the mouth ➡ in a patient with mucosal squamous cell carcinoma. The mass is obstructing the left submandibular duct ➡, and there is secondary inflammation of the left SMG ➡, which is T2 hyperintense. (Right) Axial CECT through the floor of the mouth in a patient with a right submandibular "mass" shows dense calculus ➡ in the proximal duct at the SMG hilum. Note marked fatty atrophy from left chronic sialadenitis ➡. The right "mass" was a normal SMG ➡.*

TERMINOLOGY

Definitions

- Submandibular gland (SMG) inflammation from any cause
- **Sialolithiasis**: Concretions/calculus within SMG duct(s)
- **Sialadenosis**: Noninflammatory SMG swelling
  - Causes: Diabetes, cirrhosis, hypothyroidism, malnutrition

IMAGING

General Features

- Best diagnostic clue
  - Ductal dilation ± calculus or stenosis
  - Acute: Enlarged SMG + cellulitis
  - Chronic: Fatty atrophy of SMG
- Location
  - SMG calculus can be classified by location
    - Distal: Ductal opening in anterior floor of mouth
    - Proximal: Towards SMG hilum
  - Calculi typically within duct, not SMG parenchyma
- Size
  - Acute-subacute inflammation: SMG enlarged
  - Chronic: SMG small, ± fatty replacement

Radiographic Findings

- Radiography
  - Occlusal views: 90% calculi radiopaque

CT Findings

- CECT
  - **Acute sialadenitis** due to **calculus**
    - Enlarged, enhancing SMG + inflammatory change
    - Duct dilation ± calculus
    - Reactive nodes ± floor of mouth cellulitis
  - **Chronic sialadenitis** ± calculus
    - Fatty atrophy of SMG ± intraductal calculus
  - **Other etiologies**
    - Unilateral: Anterior floor of mouth invasive enhancing mass + duct dilation
    - Bilateral: Systemic cause, e.g., autoimmune (bilateral lymphoepithelial cysts) ± parotid involvement

MR Findings

- MR typically not performed in acute inflammation
- Chronic: Heterogeneous gland, prominent ↑ T2 ducts
  - ± fatty change, ↑ T1 & T2 signal ± ↓ T2 signal calculus

Ultrasonographic Findings

- Enlarged heterogeneous (± hypoechoic) gland, ↑ vascularity
- Duct dilation ± echogenic calculus with acoustic shadowing
  - Can visualize radiolucent calculus (10-20%)
  - Calculus best visualized if > 2 mm, operator-dependent views of distal duct limited by mandible

Imaging Recommendations

- Best imaging tool
  - US &/or CECT to evaluate gland ± calculus
  - US and MR most sensitive to assess gland parenchyma
  - MR sialography useful to visualize ducts

DIFFERENTIAL DIAGNOSIS

Dental Infection

- Bone CT shows periapical lucency
- Spreads from jaw to masticator space/oral cavity

Squamous Cell Carcinoma Nodal Metastases

- Submandibular space (SMS) mass distinct from SMG
- Primary most often oral cavity, lip, nose

Submandibular Gland Carcinoma

- Infiltrating mass arising in SMG

Submandibular Gland Pleomorphic Adenoma

- Well-circumscribed SMG mass ± calcifications

PATHOLOGY

General Features

- Etiology
  - SMG duct obstruction from calculus (most common)
    - Other: Duct stenosis, rarely floor of mouth tumor
  - Infection: Bacterial (e.g., *Staphylococcus aureus*, *Streptococcus viridans*, *Haemophilus influenzae*, E coli, tuberculosis), viral
  - Autoimmune (uncommon)
    - Autoimmune exocrinopathy (Sjögren syndrome)
    - Chronic sclerosing sialadenitis (Küttner tumor): IgG4-related fibrosis and inflammation; SMG > > parotid
  - Inflammatory (post radiation, contrast-induced, radioiodine treatment), drug-induced, granulomatous

CLINICAL ISSUES

Presentation

- Most common signs/symptoms
  - Unilateral, painful SMG swelling associated with eating or psychological gustatory stimulation ("salivary colic")
- Other signs/symptoms
  - 30% of calculi present with painless mass
  - 80% of painful SMS masses due to calculus disease

Demographics

- Age
  - Commonly affects older adults or dehydrated patients
  - SMG calculus: Commonly 30-60 years, M > F

DIAGNOSTIC CHECKLIST

Reporting Tips

- Most common cause: Ductal calculus; describe location
  - Beware: Radiolucent calculus or obscured by dental amalgam
- Look carefully for obstructing floor of mouth tumor
- If no calculi, consider duct stenosis or **gland disease**
  - Bilateral: Autoimmune exocrinopathy, infection, etc.
  - Unilateral chronic sclerosing sialadenitis mimics tumor

SELECTED REFERENCES

1. Hammett JT et al: Sialolithiasis. StatPearls, 2023
2. Kramer JA et al: Utility of point-of-care ultrasound for the rapid evaluation of acute sialadenitis: a case report. Cureus. 14(5):e24881, 2022
3. Abdel Razek AA et al: Imaging of sialadenitis. Neuroradiol J. 30(3):205-15, 2017

TERMINOLOGY

- Oral cavity (OC) abscess
- Synonyms: Submandibular space (SMS), sublingual space (SLS), tongue, lingual, root of tongue (ROT), or OC transspatial abscess
- OC abscess: Focal collection of pus within OC space(s)
- May be in 1 space or multiple contiguous spaces (transspatial)

IMAGING

- CECT best exam for OC abscess
- CECT findings
  - Abscess: Rim-enhancing fluid collection in OC space(s)
  - Found within anatomic spaces (SMS, SLS, &/or ROT)
  - Phlegmon: Enhancing inflammatory tissue without focal fluid/pus
  - Cellulitis: Adjacent soft tissue stranding ± skin thickening
  - Reactive &/or suppurative nodes

TOP DIFFERENTIAL DIAGNOSES

- Oral tongue squamous cell carcinoma (SCCa)
- Simple or diving ranula
- Sialocele
- OC dermoid/epidermoid

CLINICAL ISSUES

- Sublingual or submandibular swelling
- Painful tongue with dysphagia, dysphonia
- Treatment: Eliminate cause, surgical drainage + antibiotics

DIAGNOSTIC CHECKLIST

- Define space(s) with abscess: SMS, SLS, &/or ROT
- Find underlying cause: Tooth abscess ± osteomyelitis, submandibular duct calculus, pharyngitis + suppurative node
- Mimics: OC SCCa, ranula, sialocele, epidermoid/dermoid
- Complications: Floor of mouth cellulitis, necrotizing fasciitis, airway obstruction

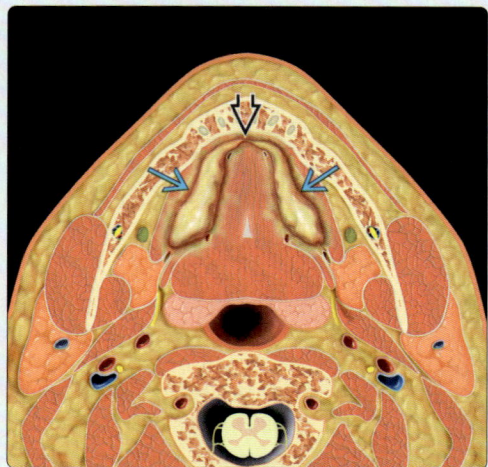
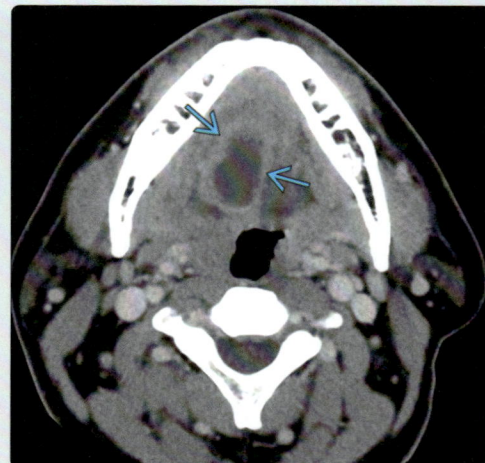

(Left) Axial graphic depicts a bilateral sublingual space abscess ➡. The walled-off, infected fluid collection is seen superomedial to the mylohyoid muscles and has a characteristic midline "isthmus" ➡ anteriorly at the midline. (Right) Axial CECT shows an oral cavity abscess as an oval fluid-density collection ➡ with surrounding enhancement, located within the root of the tongue.

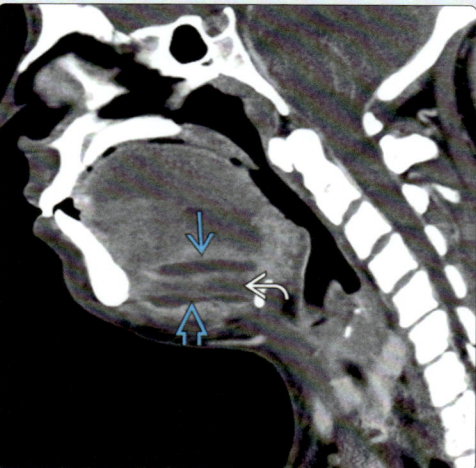
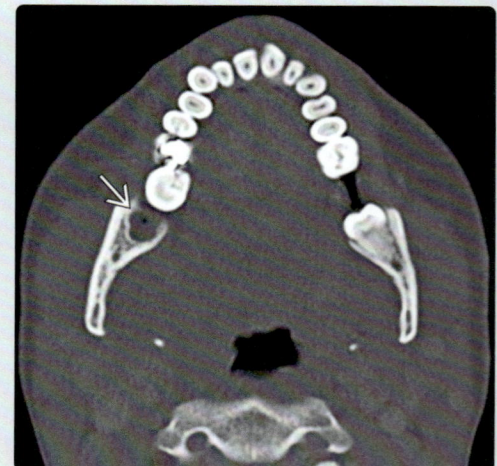

(Left) Sagittal CECT through the midline demonstrates an unusual oral cavity abscess with fluid tracking both above ➡ and below ➡ the geniohyoid and mylohyoid muscles ➡. (Right) Axial bone CT through the mandible in the same patient demonstrates an empty molar tooth socket on the right ➡ at the site of a recently removed tooth, which was the origin of the oral cavity abscess infection in this case.

TERMINOLOGY

Abbreviations

- Oral cavity (OC)

Synonyms

- Submandibular space (SMS) abscess, sublingual abscess, tongue abscess, root of tongue (ROT) abscess, oral abscess, lingual abscess

Definitions

- Focal collection of infected fluid within OC space(s)
  - May involve 1 space or multiple spaces (transspatial)

IMAGING

General Features

- Best diagnostic clue
  - Rim-enhancing, focal fluid collection in OC space(s)
- Location
  - OC space(s): SMS, sublingual space (SLS), ROT (between SLSs); ± parapharyngeal, masticator, buccal spaces
- Size
  - Variable, may become large in deep OC spaces
- Morphology
  - Rim-enhancing fluid collection conforms to surrounding anatomic landscape/spaces (mandible, SMS, SLS, ROT)

Radiographic Findings

- Radiography
  - Dental x-ray or Panorex/OPG
    - Periapical lucency (tooth abscess)
    - May show soft tissue swelling & empty tooth socket
    - Mandibular cortex dehiscence

CT Findings

- CECT
  - Abscess: Rim-enhancing hypodense (fluid) collection
  - **SLS abscess**: Fluid collection superomedial to mylohyoid muscle
    - If bilateral: Axial horseshoe-shaped fluid collection with anterior "isthmus"
  - **SMS abscess**: Fluid collection inferolateral to mylohyoid muscle
    - If bilateral: Coronal horseshoe-shaped fluid collection with inferior "isthmus"
  - **ROT abscess**: Midline fluid collection between SLSs in low lingual septum
  - Associated phlegmon, cellulitis, or myositis
    - Phlegmon: Enhancing inflammatory tissue without focal fluid/pus
    - Cellulitis: Adjacent soft tissue stranding + skin thickening
      □ Ludwig angina: SLS, SMS + submental space
    - Myositis: Enhancing, enlarged muscles
  - If gas is present, consider prior intervention, gas-forming organisms, or necrotizing fasciitis (latter especially if transspatial)
  - Submandibular &/or high internal jugular chain reactive or suppurative adenopathy
- CBCT
  - Often underlying tooth infection

- Dental caries: Erosion of enamel ± dentin of tooth
- Periodontal disease: Periapical lucency
- ± cortical focal dehiscence
  - Osteomyelitis
    - Periosteal reaction ± focal bone erosion of maxilla or mandible

MR Findings

- T1WI
  - Central low signal in fluid collection with adjacent fat stranding
    - Low signal in fatty marrow of mandible at site of infected tooth (if source)
- T2WI
  - Abscess: Central high signal in fluid collection
  - ± adjacent edema
- DWI
  - Diffusion restriction in abscess
- T1WI C+
  - Rim-enhancing fluid collection(s)
  - Nonenhancing central fluid/pus component

Ultrasonographic Findings

- Hypoechoic fluctuant collection within OC musculature is diagnostic in septic clinical setting
- Peripheral hypervascularity, no vascularity in central fluid/pus component
- Needle aspiration for diagnosis could be performed simultaneously

Nuclear Medicine Findings

- Bone scan
  - Increased uptake in regions of maxillary/mandibular osteomyelitis
  - 3-phase bone scan very sensitive for osteomyelitis

Imaging Recommendations

- Best imaging tool
  - CECT
- Protocol advice
  - Routine cervical soft tissue neck CECT study
  - Dental amalgam may obscure OC abscess
  - Soft tissue window: Identify abscess location
    - Coronal plane helps define SLS (superomedial to mylohyoid) from SMS (inferolateral to mylohyoid muscle) abscesses
  - Bone window: Identify tooth abscess, osteomyelitis, or submandibular duct calculus
- Cone beam CT (3D) or CT Panorex (2D) helpful to evaluate dental sources of infection in greater detail

DIFFERENTIAL DIAGNOSIS

Oral Tongue Squamous Cell Carcinoma

- Clinical: Mucosal squamous cell carcinoma (SCCa) lesion usually obvious
- CT-MR findings
  - Enhancing, invasive oral tongue mass
    - Usually untreated SCCa cases show exophytic, high-density oral mucosal surface lesion
  - Cystic-necrotic neoplasm may mimic OC abscess in SCCa recurrence cases following treatment

Simple or Diving Ranula

- Clinical
  - Simple ranula: Sublingual, bluish, translucent mass
  - Diving ranula: Compressible angle of mandible mass
- CT-MR findings
  - Simple ranula: Nonenhancing, low-density, low T1/high T2 signal SLS lesion
    - Mimics SLS epidermoid on imaging
  - Diving ranula: Nonenhancing, low-density, low T1/high T2 signal SMS lesion with SLS "tail"

Sialocele

- Fluid collection adjacent to duct in SLS without enhancing wall
- Possible enlarged proximal submandibular duct ± obstructing calculus

Oral Cavity Dermoid & Epidermoid

- Clinical: Floor of mouth or SMS slow-growing mass
- CT findings
  - Epidermoid: Unilateral low-density, nonenhancing SMS or SLS mass
  - Dermoid: Unilateral fluid ± fat density, nonenhancing SMS or SLS mass
  - No associated cellulitis/edema with either
- MR findings
  - Epidermoid: Low T1/high T2 signal & DWI restriction (DWI can mimic abscess, but clinical presentation is different)
  - Dermoid: If fat macroscopic, high T1 signal within mass
    - **Bag of marbles** appearance classic

PATHOLOGY

General Features

- Etiology
  - Odontogenic infection most common: Molar teeth, especially 1st molar tooth > maxillary central incisor
    - SLS abscess: Tooth root abscess breaks out **above** (superior to) mylohyoid line of medial mandible with pus, then walled off in SLS
    - SMS abscess: Tooth root abscess breaks out **below** (inferior to) mylohyoid line of medial mandible with pus, then walled off in SMS
  - Other causes
    - Submandibular duct calculus: SLS abscess
    - Pharyngitis + suppurative SMS nodes: SMS abscess
    - Penetrating trauma: SLS, SMS, or ROT abscess
    - IV drug abuse: SLS, SMS, or ROT abscess
  - ≥ 20% have no identifiable source

Gross Pathologic & Surgical Features

- Putrid-smelling abscess entered with surgical drain

Microscopic Features

- Oral flora predominate: *Staphylococcus, Streptococcus*
  - Mixed aerobic & anaerobic > aerobic > anaerobic flora

CLINICAL ISSUES

Presentation

- Most common signs/symptoms
  - Sublingual or submandibular swelling
- Other signs/symptoms
  - Painful tongue with dysphagia, dysphonia
  - Elevation & backward displacement of tongue may compromise airway
  - History of recent oral antibiotic treatment & dental procedure common
- Clinical profile
  - Older patients with poor dentition
    - Less commonly, penetrating trauma, especially in immunocompromised patients

Demographics

- Age
  - Older adults
- Epidemiology
  - Primary cause is odontogenic infection

Natural History & Prognosis

- Prognosis for full recovery excellent

Treatment

- Extraction of infected tooth (if present)
- Surgical drainage of abscess cavity
- Antibiotics
  - Amoxicillin is 1st choice; avoided in penicillin allergy
  - 2nd line: Metronidazole, clindamycin, azithromycin

DIAGNOSTIC CHECKLIST

Consider

- Mimics of abscess in OC
  - Ranula, epidermoid/dermoid: No inflammatory changes
  - Sialocele: May be superinfected
  - Cystic-necrotic OC primary SCCa

Image Interpretation Pearls

- 1st define abscess space(s): SLS, SMS, &/or ROT
- Describe unilateral or bilateral, unispatial or transspatial involvement
- Search for underlying cause
  - Review mandible bone window images for **tooth abscess ± osteomyelitis**
  - If teeth normal, check for **submandibular duct stone**
  - In children, look for **pharyngitis + suppurative SMS node**
- Consider complications: Floor of mouth cellulitis (bilateral SLS, SMS, submental), necrotizing fasciitis (gas), airway obstruction

Reporting Tips

- Report abscess location(s) & probable cause

SELECTED REFERENCES

1. Rusinovci S et al: Commensal mouth bacteria are the main cause of dentoalveolar abscesses in the maxillofacial region. J Infect Dev Ctries. 19(1):107-16, 2025
2. Velhonoja J et al: Risk factors and preventive measures for severe orofacial and neck infections: a three-year observational study. BMC Oral Health. 25(1):136, 2025
3. Patel J et al: Infections of the oral cavity and suprahyoid neck. Oral Maxillofac Surg Clin North Am. 35(3):283-96, 2023
4. Mesolella M et al: Clinical and diagnostic aspect of tongue abscess. Ear Nose Throat J. 100(10_suppl):1012S-4S, 2020

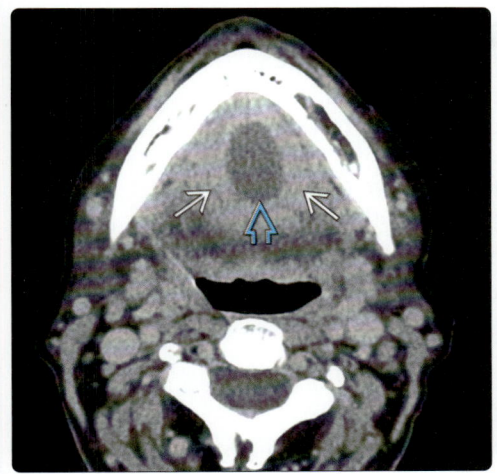

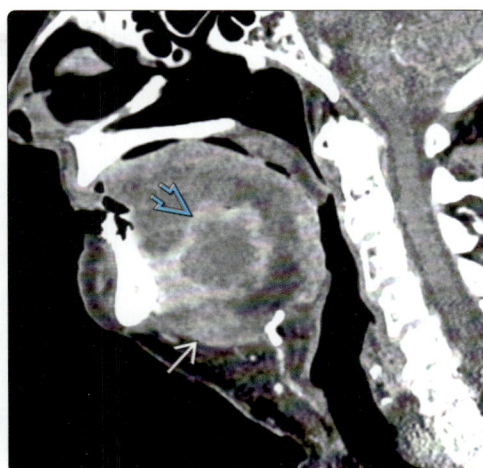

(Left) Axial CECT shows a midline oral cavity abscess as an oval fluid-density collection ⊃ located centrally within the root of the tongue, bowing the genioglossus muscles ➡ laterally. (Right) Sagittal CECT shows a root of tongue abscess ⊃ above the mylohyoid muscle ➡ in the midline deep tongue. This appearance can mimic invasive squamous cell carcinoma but has a different clinical presentation.

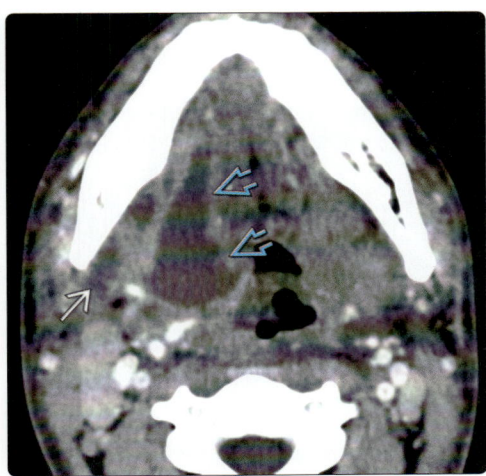

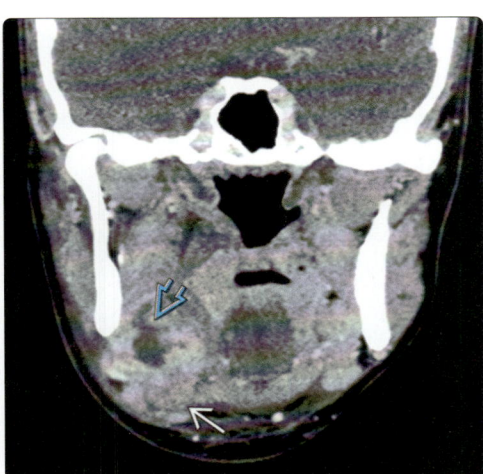

(Left) Axial CECT shows a rim-enhancing fluid collection ⊃ centered within the sublingual space, consistent with a sublingual space abscess, with surrounding inflammatory changes extending posteriorly and lateral to the mylohyoid muscle into the submandibular space ➡. (Right) Coronal CECT shows the posterior submandibular space rim-enhancing abscess ⊃ inferiorly displacing the enlarged, inflamed submandibular gland ➡. Sialoadenitis in this case is due to an adjacent infected socket and abscess (not shown).

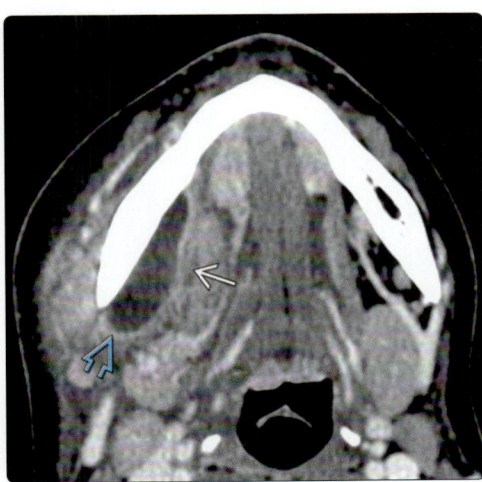

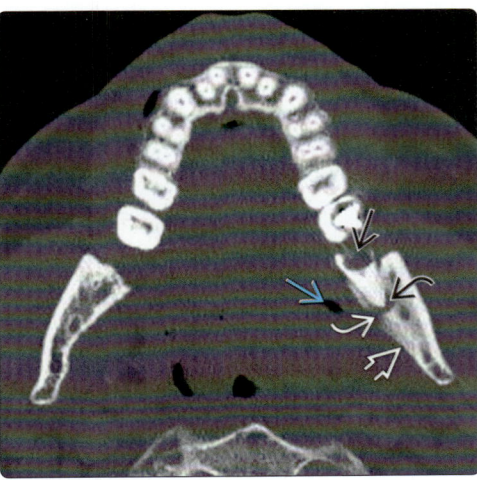

(Left) Axial CECT shows rim-enhancing fluid collection of pus leaking out inferiorly into the submandibular space. The submandibular space abscess ⊃ displaces the mylohyoid muscle ➡ medially as a result. (Right) Axial bone CT of the mandible demonstrates gas ⊃ in an oral cavity abscess caused by tooth decay (enamel and dentin erosion) of the partially erupted left 3rd molar tooth ➡ with periodontal disease (periapical lucency) ➡. Lingual cortical loss ➡ and periosteal thickening indicate osteomyelitis ➡.

TERMINOLOGY

- Synonym: Benign mixed tumor (BMT)

IMAGING

- CECT
  - Enlarged submandibular gland (SMG) with focal or diffuse heterogeneous mass ± calcification
  - Some masses "invisible": Look for contour deformity
  - Dual-phase CECT improves conspicuity
- MR
  - Small: Low T1, high T2, homogeneous enhancement
  - Large: More heterogeneous, ± focal areas of high T2 signal, signal loss with calcification
  - **Marked high T2** intensity characteristic
  - Variable low T2 intensity "capsule"
- US
  - Well-defined, solid, intraglandular lesion
  - Large lesion may show focal cysts, calcification
- Best imaging tool

- **MR > CECT** (some masses poorly seen on CECT)
- **US** affords excellent SMG evaluation

TOP DIFFERENTIAL DIAGNOSES

- SMG sialadenitis
- SMG mucocele
- SMG carcinoma
- Submandibular space lymphadenopathy
- Chronic sclerosing sialadenitis (Küttner tumor)

PATHOLOGY

- Epithelial, myoepithelial, and stromal components

CLINICAL ISSUES

- Most common neoplasm of SMG

DIAGNOSTIC CHECKLIST

- If patient presents with palpable submandibular mass
  - Determine if mass is in SMG or extrinsic (node)
  - If no mass found on CECT, recommend US or MR

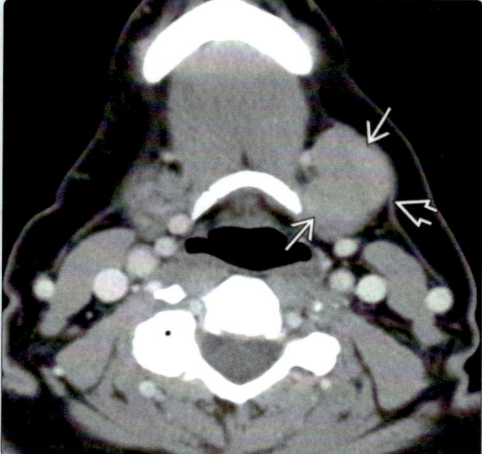
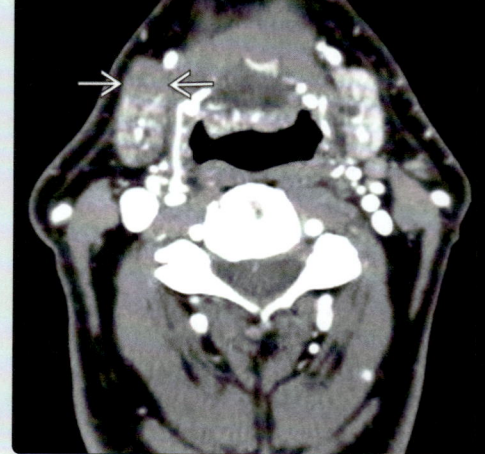

(Left) Axial CECT in a 50-year-old woman with an 8-year history of a slowly enlarging left neck mass (delayed care until obtained insurance) shows an enhancing, solid pleomorphic adenoma (PA) ➡ involving left submandibular gland (SMG), which appears well demarcated and displaces the platysma ➡ laterally. (Right) Axial CECT shows a nearly "invisible" tumor: A small, round, low-density PA with loss of normal internal gland architecture ➡. PET/CT performed for lung cancer staging showed uptake in this incidental nodule.

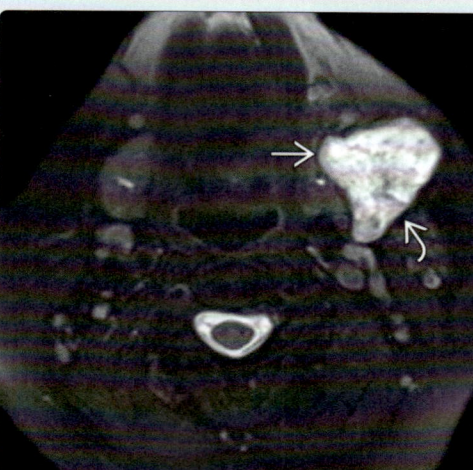
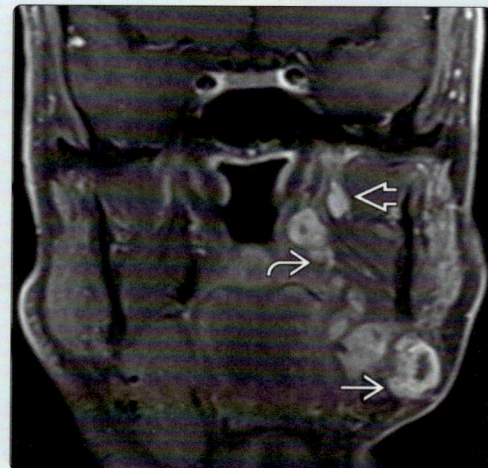

(Left) Axial T2 FS MR shows a circumscribed, T2-hyperintense mass ➡ with lobulated margins and a thin, T2-hypointense capsule ➡. The marked T2 hyperintensity is characteristic of PA. (Right) Coronal T1 C+ FS MR shows multiple heterogeneously enhancing masses within the left submandibular space ➡, masticator space ➡, and parapharyngeal space ➡, representing multifocal recurrence from tumor seeding following intraoperative capsular rupture of a SMG PA.

Submandibular Gland Pleomorphic Adenoma

TERMINOLOGY

Abbreviations
- Submandibular gland (SMG)
- Pleomorphic adenoma (PA)

Synonyms
- Benign mixed tumor (BMT)

Definitions
- Benign, heterogeneous salivary gland primary tumor

IMAGING

General Features
- Best diagnostic clue
  - Enlarged SMG with focal or diffuse heterogeneous mass ± calcification
- Location
  - Submandibular space (SMS)
- Size
  - Variable: Usually 1-4 cm
- Morphology
  - Small: Ovoid, well-demarcated SMG mass
  - Large: Lobulated, heterogeneous mass ± calcification

CT Findings
- CECT
  - Small lesion is usually well defined
  - Large lesion usually heterogeneous density and texture
  - Small or isodense lesions may be inseparable from normal gland or inconspicuous
    - Clues: Symmetric size, deformity of surface contours
    - Dual-phase CECT improves conspicuity
  - Variable calcification, cystic changes in larger PA
  - Mild to moderate enhancement

MR Findings
- Findings largely determined by PA size
  - Small: Low T1, high T2, homogeneous enhancement
  - Large: More heterogeneous, ± focal areas of high T2 signal, signal loss with calcification
  - **Markedly high T2** intensity characteristic
  - Variable, thin low T2 intensity "capsule"

Ultrasonographic Findings
- Grayscale ultrasound
  - Well-defined, solid, intraglandular lesion
  - Large lesion may show focal cysts, calcification

Nuclear Medicine Findings
- Marked FDG avidity on PET/CT mimics malignancy

Imaging Recommendations
- Best imaging tool
  - **MR > CECT** (some SMG masses are poorly seen on CECT)
  - US affords excellent SMG evaluation

DIFFERENTIAL DIAGNOSIS

Submandibular Gland Sialadenitis
- Acute: Enlarged gland that completely enhances
  - Predisposing sialoliths ± sialectasis may be present
- Chronic: Atrophic gland with little enhancement

Submandibular Gland Mucocele
- Fluid collection within SMG

Submandibular Gland Carcinoma
- Enhancing, invasive mass arising from SMG

Reactive Lymph Nodes
- Ovoid mass with fat plane separating it from SMG
- Anterior facial vein separates nodes from SMG

Nodal Squamous Cell Carcinoma in Submandibular Space
- Nodal mass separate from SMG, ± necrosis

Chronic Sclerosing Sialadenitis (Küttner Tumor)
- Inflammatory etiology mimics neoplasm
- Part of IgG4-related disease spectrum

PATHOLOGY

Microscopic Features
- Interspersed epithelial, myoepithelial, and stromal cellular components
  - Calcification, hyalinization, and, rarely, ossification

CLINICAL ISSUES

Presentation
- Most common signs/symptoms
  - Slow-growing, painless SMS mass

Demographics
- Age
  - Most commonly present > 40 years
- Epidemiology
  - PA is most common neoplasm of SMG

Natural History & Prognosis
- Untreated, 5-25% degenerate to malignant tumor
- Usually 15-20 years after initial diagnosis

Treatment
- Complete excision of intact gland and tumor
- Operative rupture of PA capsule seeds surgical bed
  - Results in multifocal recurrence; surgically challenging
  - SMG PA lower recurrence rate than parotid PA

DIAGNOSTIC CHECKLIST

Consider
- Fine-needle aspiration has variable success
  - Sampling and interpretation errors common

Image Interpretation Pearls
- If patient presents with palpable submandibular mass
  - Determine if mass is in SMG or extrinsic (node)
  - If no mass found on CECT, recommend US or MR

SELECTED REFERENCES

1. Sheereen S et al: Pleomorphic adenoma in salivary glands: insights from a 100-patient analysis. J Oral Maxillofac Pathol. 28(1):42-8, 2024
2. Wang C et al: Carcinoma ex pleomorphic adenoma of major salivary glands: CT and MR imaging findings. Dentomaxillofac Radiol. 50(7):20200485, 2021

Palate Pleomorphic Adenoma

TERMINOLOGY

- Palate pleomorphic adenoma (PA): Benign minor salivary gland tumor of palate
- Synonym: Palate benign mixed tumor

IMAGING

- General findings
  - Most commonly found at soft-hard palate juncture
  - Small PA: Well-defined palatal mass with homogeneous, avid enhancement
  - Large PA: Lobulated with heterogeneous enhancement
- Bone CT: Larger PA remodels bony hard palate
- MR findings
  - Intermediate to high T2 signal ovoid palatal mass
  - Very high T2 signal suggests PA
  - Larger PA often with inhomogeneous signal (necrosis, blood products, calcification)
- Best sequences: Sagittal and coronal T2 and T1 C+ FS MR (orthogonal to palate)

TOP DIFFERENTIAL DIAGNOSES

- Palatal minor salivary gland neoplasms
- Palatal squamous cell carcinoma

PATHOLOGY

- Arise in minor salivary glands of palate
- Interspersed epithelial, myoepithelial, and stromal cellular components must be identified to diagnose PA

CLINICAL ISSUES

- Typical presentation is painless palatal mass
- Most common minor salivary gland neoplasm (~ 40%)
- Most common site, minor salivary gland PA (~ 10%)
- Risk factors for malignant transformation (1-6%) include older age, larger PA size, and recurrence
  - Palatal neuropathy suggests malignancy

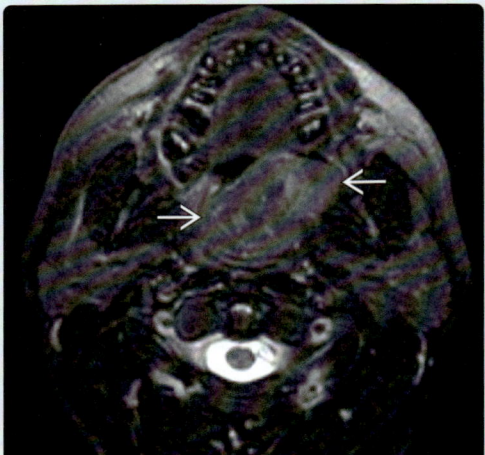
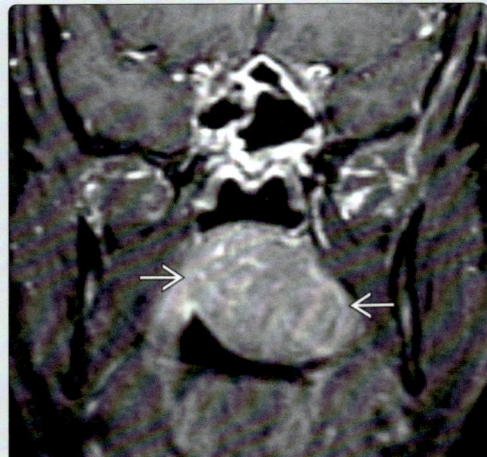

(Left) Axial T2 FS MR shows a heterogeneously hypointense pleomorphic adenoma (PA) ➡ involving the soft palate. While hyperintense signal can be highly suggestive of PA when present, those with low T2 signal, such as in this case, mimic malignancy. (Right) Coronal T1 C+ FS MR in the same patient shows heterogeneous enhancement ➡ in this large, well-marginated soft palate PA. Despite its large size, the tumor does not invade regional soft tissues.

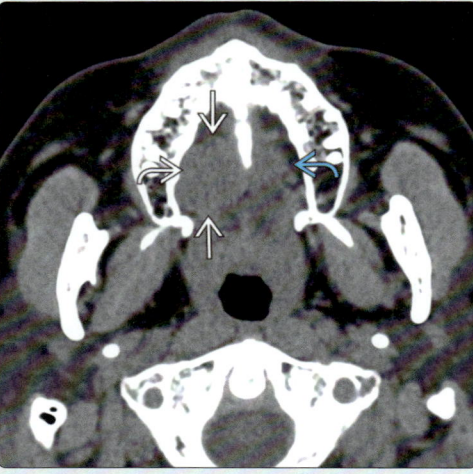
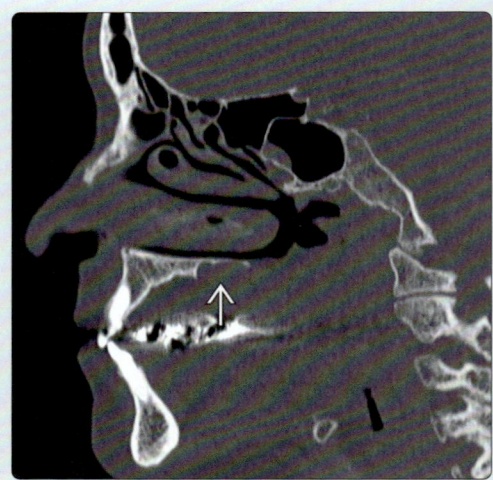

(Left) Axial NECT shows a subtle round mass involving the right soft palate ➡, which could be easily overlooked in the axial plane. Loss of the fat pad laterally is a clue to the presence of a mass ➡. Note the normal fat pad ➡ on the contralateral side. (Right) Sagittal bone CT in the same patient shows smooth osseous scalloping and remodeling ➡ of the posterior hard palate, which serves as an additional clue to the presence of an underlying small soft tissue mass. Orthogonal views can optimize detection of palatal masses.

Palate Pleomorphic Adenoma

TERMINOLOGY

Abbreviations
- Palate pleomorphic adenoma (PA)

Synonyms
- Palate benign mixed tumor

Definitions
- Benign tumor arising from palate minor salivary glands

IMAGING

General Features
- Best diagnostic clue
  - Small palate PA: Well-defined palatal mass with avid enhancement
  - Large PA: Often lobulated mass with heterogeneous enhancement
- Location
  - Soft-hard palate junction
- Size
  - Variable: < 2 cm most commonly

CT Findings
- NECT
  - Hypodense due to myxochondroid stroma
- CECT
  - Small palate PA: Well-defined, homogeneously enhancing, ovoid mass
  - Large palate PA: Lobulated mass with heterogeneous enhancement
    - Calcification or ossification uncommon
    - Low-attenuation areas of degenerative necrosis
    - Old blood products possible
- Bone CT
  - Larger lesions cause remodeling of hard palate
  - CT assesses degree of bone erosion prior to surgery

MR Findings
- T1WI
  - Small PA: Homogeneous, low- to intermediate-signal mass
  - Large PA: Lobulated, heterogeneous mass
    - Hyperintense signal foci if blood products
    - Focal low-signal areas if necrosis present
- T2WI
  - Small PA: Uniform, intermediate- to high-signal mass
  - Large PA: Heterogeneous, high-signal mass
  - **Very high T2 signal** suggests **PA**
    - Reflects chondromyxoid stroma
  - Hypointense rim indicates fibrous capsule
- STIR
  - High signal may be more conspicuous than T2 sequence
- DWI
  - May have ↑ ADC values compared to malignant palatal tumor
    - DWI signal intensity nonspecific
- T1WI C+
  - Variable heterogeneous or avid homogeneous enhancement

Imaging Recommendations
- Best imaging tool
  - Enhanced MR with thin sections through palate
  - Bone CT helps define tumor bony margins
- Protocol advice
  - Best sequences: Sagittal and coronal plane T2 and T1 C+ FS MR (axial suboptimal given parallel to palate)

DIFFERENTIAL DIAGNOSIS

Palatal Minor Salivary Gland Neoplasms
- Malignant minor salivary gland neoplasms
  - Invasive tumor with osseous destruction
  - Perineural tumor CNV2 likely
- Other benign minor salivary neoplasms

Palatal Squamous Cell Carcinoma
- Aggressive tumor + osseous destruction
- May mimic palatal PA when small
- Mucosal lesion usually visible

PATHOLOGY

General Features
- Etiology
  - Benign tumor arising from palate minor salivary glands
  - Risk factors: Genetic predisposition and therapeutic radiation
- Genetics
  - PA gene 1 (*PLAG1*) is specific

Microscopic Features
- Interspersed epithelial, myoepithelial, and mesenchymal components must be seen to diagnose PA
- ± calcification, necrosis, blood products, hyalinization

CLINICAL ISSUES

Presentation
- Most common signs/symptoms
  - Painless palatal mass with normal overlying mucosa
    - Most common minor salivary gland neoplasm (~ 40%)
    - Most common site, minor salivary gland PA (~ 10%)
- Other signs/symptoms
  - Palatal neuropathy suggests malignancy

Demographics
- Age
  - Range: ~ 30-60 years

Natural History & Prognosis
- Slow-growing, painless palatal mass
  - Rapid growth concerning for malignant degeneration
  - Lesion typically submucosal, unlike squamous cell

Treatment
- Complete surgical resection of encapsulated mass
  - Adequate soft tissue margins critical to avoid cellular "spillage" and future seeding of surgical bed

SELECTED REFERENCES

1. Hiyama T et al: Imaging of malignant minor salivary gland tumors of the head and neck. Radiographics. 41(1):175-91, 2021

Sublingual Gland Carcinoma

TERMINOLOGY

- Primary salivary malignancy of sublingual gland (SLG)

IMAGING

- CECT: Well-defined or invasive sublingual space (SLS) mass
  - Mild to moderately enhancing; may be subtle
  - Look for evidence of mandible erosion
- MR: Variable signal & contrast enhancement
  - Well-differentiated tumors may have increased T2 signal
  - Fat saturation & STIR improve conspicuity
- Look for invasion of extrinsic tongue muscles
- PET: Generally low FDG avidity unless high grade

TOP DIFFERENTIAL DIAGNOSES

- Floor of mouth squamous cell carcinoma
- Ranula
- Oral cavity abscess
- Oral cavity lymphatic malformation

PATHOLOGY

- Adenoid cystic carcinoma (ACCa)
  - Strong propensity for perineural spread
  - Tends to hematogenously spread to lungs
  - Slow-growing; may metastasize many years later
- Mucoepidermoid carcinoma (MECa)
  - Tends to spread to lymph nodes
- Malignant degeneration of pleomorphic adenoma

CLINICAL ISSUES

- Painless, hard anterior floor of mouth mass on palpation
- 30-60 years of age, M:F = 1:1
- 70-90% of SLG masses are malignant
- Prognosis depends on stage > histologic grade
- Treatment primarily surgical ± radiation

DIAGNOSTIC CHECKLIST

- Aggressive-appearing lesions within SLS should be considered malignant until proven otherwise

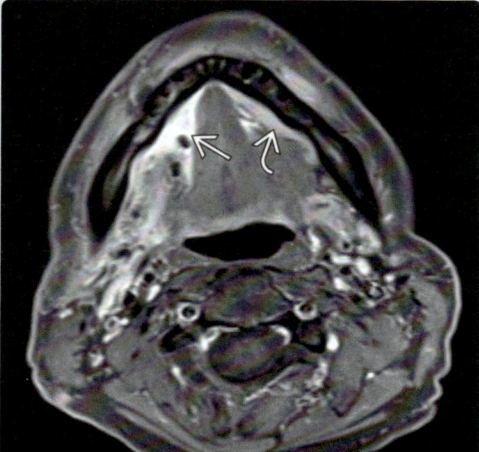
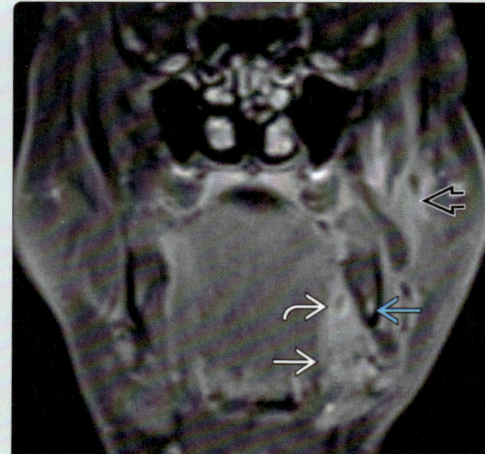

(Left) Axial T1 C+ FS MR shows a heterogeneous, enhancing adenoid cystic carcinoma (ACCa) enlarging the right sublingual gland (SLG) ➡. Compare to the normal size and signal intensity of the left SLG ➡. (Right) Coronal T1 C+ FS MR shows an enhancing left SLG mass, biopsy-proven ACCa ➡. There is enhancing perineural tumor spread to the left lingual ➡ and inferior alveolar nerves ➡ with denervation enhancement in the muscles of mastication ➡. Not shown: Perineural spread to CNVII via lingual nerve/chorda tympani.

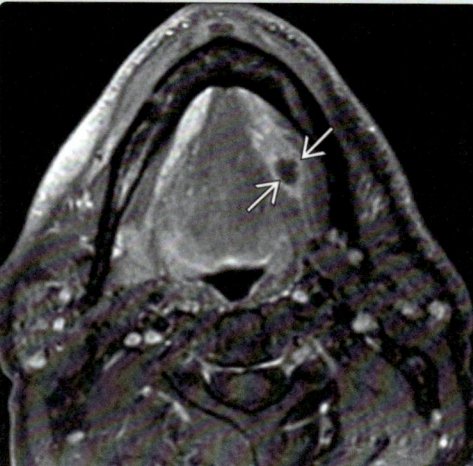
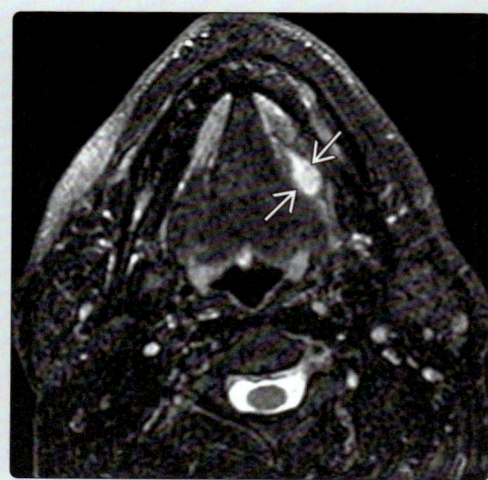

(Left) Axial T1 C+ FS MR demonstrates a small, heterogeneous left SLG mass ➡ with ill-defined borders. The irregular contours suggest this mass may be malignant; however, even well-defined lesions are statistically more likely to be malignant in the SLG. (Right) Axial T2 FS MR in the same patient shows the mass ➡ to be markedly hyperintense. More differentiated salivary malignancies produce fluid/mucin and have high signal. This was found to be mucoepidermoid carcinoma.

TERMINOLOGY

Abbreviations
- Sublingual gland (SLG) carcinoma

Definitions
- Primary salivary malignancy in SLG
  - Adenoid cystic carcinoma (ACCa) > mucoepidermoid carcinoma (MECa) > others

IMAGING

General Features
- Best diagnostic clue
  - Well-defined or invasive sublingual space (SLS) mass
- Location
  - SLS: Potential space superomedial to mylohyoid muscle
- Size
  - Usually < 2 cm

CT Findings
- CECT
  - Mild to moderately enhancing SLS mass
  - May be subtle lesion on imaging
  - Look for invasion of extrinsic tongue muscles, submandibular gland
- Bone CT
  - Look for evidence of mandible erosion

MR Findings
- T1WI
  - Isointense to muscle
- T2WI
  - Variable: Well-differentiated, may be high signal
  - FS or STIR improves mass conspicuity
- T1WI C+
  - Variable contrast enhancement
  - Perineural tumor spread: Especially lingual, inferior alveolar, hypoglossal, facial nerves

Nuclear Medicine Findings
- PET
  - Generally low FDG avidity, unless high grade

Imaging Recommendations
- Best imaging tool
  - CECT is useful 1st-line tool
  - Enhanced MR has fewer dental amalgam artifacts
- Protocol advice
  - Thin-section CECT with bone & soft tissue algorithm

DIFFERENTIAL DIAGNOSIS

Floor of Mouth Squamous Cell Carcinoma
- Not able to distinguish from SLG carcinoma

Ranula
- Unilocular, fluid-filled lesion without enhancement

Oral Cavity Abscess
- Rim-enhancing, cystic mass with cellulitis

Oral Cavity Lymphatic Malformation
- Multilocular nonenhancing cystic mass

PATHOLOGY

General Features
- Etiology
  - ACCa & MECa most common neoplasms
  - MECa associated with radiation exposure

Staging, Grading, & Classification
- Adapted from 8th edition AJCC Staging Manual (2017)
  - **T1**: ≤ 2 cm without extraparenchymal extension
  - **T2**: > 2 & ≤ 4 cm, no extraparenchymal extension
  - **T3**: > 4 cm &/or extraparenchymal extension
  - **T4a**: Invades mandible, ear canal, or skin
  - **T4b**: Invades skull base, pterygoid plates; encases carotid

Microscopic Features
- **ACCa**
  - Unencapsulated; cribriform, tubular, & solid variants
- **MECa**
  - Epidermoid, intermediate, & mucus-secreting cells

CLINICAL ISSUES

Presentation
- Most common signs/symptoms
  - Painless, hard mass in anterior floor of mouth
- Other signs/symptoms
  - Numbness suggests lingual nerve perineural tumor

Demographics
- Age
  - 30-60 years old
- Epidemiology
  - 70-90% of primary SLG masses are malignant

Natural History & Prognosis
- ACCa: Slow-growing tumor
  - Strong propensity for perineural tumor spread
  - Metastasizes to lungs; may be delayed (> 10 years)
- MECa: Less indolent tumor
  - Greater likelihood of node metastases
- Prognosis depends on **stage** > **histologic grade**

Treatment
- En bloc resection of anterior floor of mouth
- Postoperative radiotherapy for high stage, high grade

DIAGNOSTIC CHECKLIST

Image Interpretation Pearls
- Aggressive-appearing lesions within SLS should be considered malignant until proven otherwise

Reporting Tips
- Must search for bone invasion & perineural tumor

SELECTED REFERENCES

1. Miyasaka Y et al: Imaging of salivary gland cancers derived from a sublingual gland herniated into the submandibular space: a report of three cases. Neuroradiology. 66(6):931-5, 2024
2. Otsuka K et al: Low FDG uptake in lung metastasis despite high FDG uptake in a primary adenoid cystic carcinoma of a sublingual gland. Radiol Case Rep. 19(8):3195-9, 2024

Submandibular Gland Carcinoma

TERMINOLOGY

- Primary malignancy arising in submandibular gland (SMG)
- Most commonly adenoid cystic carcinoma (ACCa), mucoepidermoid carcinoma (MECa), adenocarcinoma (AdCa)

IMAGING

- Focal or irregular SMG mass ± adjacent soft tissue invasion
- CECT: Asymmetric &/or heterogeneous SMG
  o Well-defined or ill-defined mass
  o Gland may be focally or diffusely hypodense
  o Mild to moderate contrast enhancement
- MR: Intermediate to high mixed T2 signal
  o Heterogeneous gadolinium enhancement
  o MR: Use fat saturation on T2 & T1 C+
- PET/CT: Low FDG avidity, unless high grade
- US: Ill-defined, hypoechoic lesion

TOP DIFFERENTIAL DIAGNOSES

- SMG sialadenitis, pleomorphic adenoma
- SMG mucocele, reactive lymph nodes
- Nodal squamous cell carcinoma in submandibular space

PATHOLOGY

- Beware FNA sampling & interpretive errors

CLINICAL ISSUES

- Painless submandibular swelling or focal mass
- **45%** SMG neoplasms are **malignant**
- ACCa: Spreads via nerves, also to lungs
- MECa & AdCa: Nodal & hematogenous spread

DIAGNOSTIC CHECKLIST

- 1st determine whether mass is **within SMG or extrinsic**, such as node
- **Beware subtle or occult SMG mass** on CECT
  o If none found on CECT, recommend US or MR

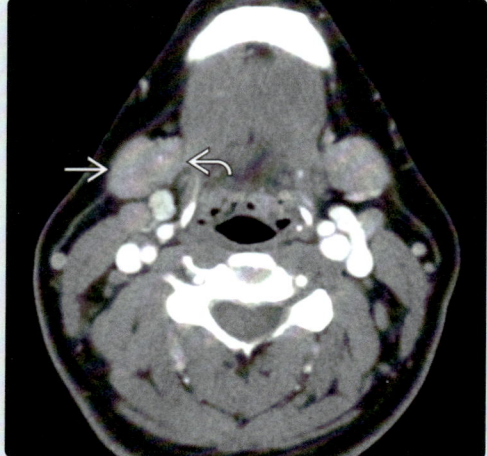
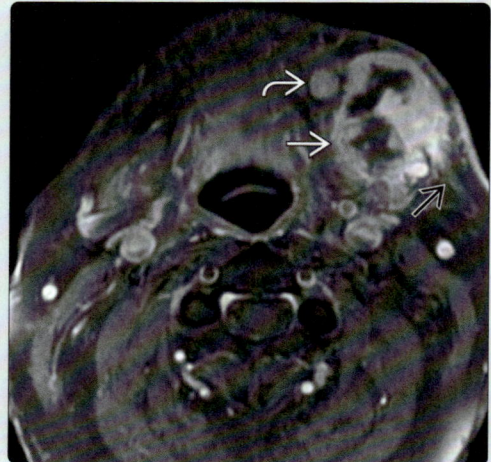

(Left) Axial CECT in a patient with a palpable mass (marked by skin BB) shows a right submandibular gland (SMG) adenoid cystic carcinoma ➡. Tumor enhancement is relatively homogeneous with similar attenuation to normal gland ➡, but the exophytic morphology makes it more visible. (Right) Axial T1 C+ FS MR shows a heterogeneously enhancing, centrally necrotic left SMG mass ➡. There is invasion along the platysma ➡ and adjacent metastatic lymphadenopathy ➡. Pathology showed carcinoma ex pleomorphic adenoma.

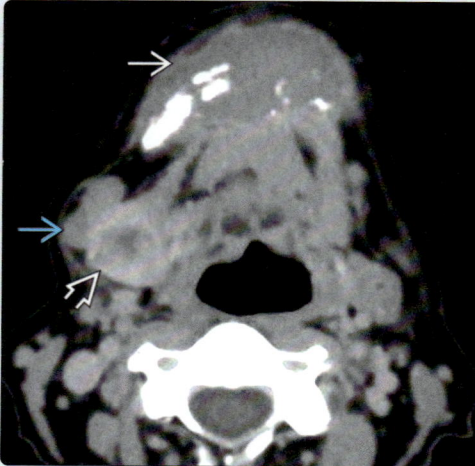
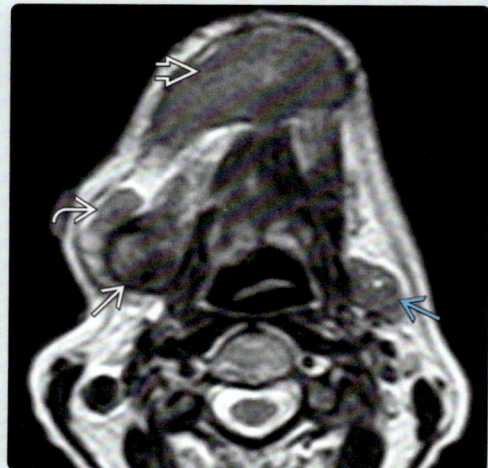

(Left) Axial NECT demonstrates enlargement of the right SMG ➡ with central low attenuation due to adenoid cystic carcinoma. Mandible destruction ➡ was due to extensive perineural tumor spread along the inferior alveolar nerve. Note level I adenopathy ➡. (Right) Axial T2 MR in the same patient shows an asymmetrically large, hypointense right SMG ➡. Note regional adenopathy ➡. Mandible involvement ➡ was due to perineural tumor spread. The left SMG ➡ is normal-appearing.

TERMINOLOGY

Abbreviations
- Submandibular gland (SMG) carcinoma

Definitions
- Primary malignancy arising in SMG
  - Most common: Adenoid cystic carcinoma (ACCa), mucoepidermoid carcinoma (MECa), adenocarcinoma (AdCa)

IMAGING

General Features
- Best diagnostic clue
  - Well-defined or invasive mass arising from SMG
- Location
  - Most often superficial aspect of SMG
- Morphology
  - Well-defined or invasive SMG mass
  - May have homogeneous, enlarged SMG

CT Findings
- CECT
  - Asymmetric &/or heterogeneous SMG
  - Mild to moderately enhancing SMG mass
- Bone CT
  - Bone erosion & calcifications (uncommon)

MR Findings
- T1WI
  - Isointense to muscle, hypointense to gland
- T2WI
  - Intermediate to high mixed signal intensity
  - **High grade** tends to be **intermediate to low signal**
- T1WI C+
  - Variable contrast enhancement
  - Check for perineural tumor spread (PNTS)
    - Lingual, inferior alveolar, hypoglossal, facial nerves

Nuclear Medicine Findings
- PET/CT
  - Generally low FDG avidity, unless high grade

Ultrasonographic Findings
- Grayscale ultrasound
  - Typically ill-defined, hypoechoic lesion

Imaging Recommendations
- Best imaging tool
  - Multiplanar CECT often 1st-line tool
  - US: Excellent for superficial portion of SMG
  - MR offers best delineation of contours
- Protocol advice
  - Thin-section CECT: Bone & soft tissue algorithm
  - MR: Use fat saturation (FS) on T2 & T1 C+

DIFFERENTIAL DIAGNOSIS

Submandibular Gland Sialadenitis
- Enlarged, diffusely enhancing SMG ± stone ± sialectasis
- Chronic disease leads to atrophic SMG
- Chronic sclerosing sialadenitis mimics malignancy

Submandibular Gland Mucocele
- Unilocular, fluid-filled, usually nonenhancing

Submandibular Gland Pleomorphic Adenoma
- Well-demarcated, ovoid SMG mass

Reactive Lymph Nodes
- Ovoid lesion adjacent to normal SMG

Nodal Squamous Cell Carcinoma in Submandibular Space
- Enlarged node adjacent to SMG

PATHOLOGY

Staging, Grading, & Classification
- Adapted from American Joint Committee on Cancer 8th edition staging (2017)
  - **T1**: ≤ 2 cm without extraparenchymal extension
  - **T2**: > 2 & ≤ 4 cm, no extraparenchymal extension
  - **T3**: > 4 cm &/or extraparenchymal extension
  - **T4a**: Invades skin, mandible, ear canal, ± facial nerve
  - **T4b**: Invades skull base ± pterygoid plates ± encases carotid artery

Microscopic Features
- 3 main pathologies: ACCa, MECa, AdCa
- Beware FNA sampling & interpretive errors
  - Biopsy may be necessary to resolve

CLINICAL ISSUES

Presentation
- Most common signs/symptoms
  - Painless submandibular swelling or focal mass
- Other signs/symptoms
  - Chin or lower lip numbness suggests infiltration of inferior alveolar nerve
  - Lower lip weakness suggests facial nerve branch invasion

Demographics
- Age
  - 40-70 years old
- Epidemiology
  - **45%** of SMG tumors are **malignant**
  - **40%** of malignant SMG tumors are **ACCa**

Treatment
- En bloc complete resection of tumor
- Postoperative radiotherapy for high stage, high grade

DIAGNOSTIC CHECKLIST

Image Interpretation Pearls
- **If presentation of mass or fullness**
  - 1st determine if mass is **SMG or extrinsic**, such as node
  - Recommend US or MR if CECT negative

SELECTED REFERENCES

1. Yorita K et al: Macrocystic and non-necrotic salivary duct carcinoma of the submandibular gland: a case report. Radiol Case Rep. 19(8):3049-55, 2024
2. Westergaard-Nielsen M et al: Epidemiology, outcomes, and prognostic factors in submandibular gland carcinomas: a national DAHANCA study. Eur Arch Otorhinolaryngol. 280(7):3405-13, 2023

TERMINOLOGY

- Abbreviation: Minor salivary gland malignancy (MSGM)
- Most common MSGM: Adenoid cystic carcinoma (ACCa) and mucoepidermoid carcinoma (MECa)

IMAGING

- MSGM location: Submucosa of upper aerodigestive tract
  - Hard-soft palate junction > > buccal mucosa
- Well-defined, smooth, submucosal oral cavity mass
- Bone CT findings
  - Bone erosion: Palate, mandible
  - Greater and lesser palatine foramen enlargement
- MR findings
  - T1: Low-signal tumor replaces hard palate marrow fat
    - Noncontrast T1 MR may offer best inherent contrast
  - T1 C+ FS for perineural tumor (PNT) spread
- PET best for staging/restaging
- MSGM uses same TNM staging as squamous cell carcinoma

TOP DIFFERENTIAL DIAGNOSES

- Squamous cell carcinoma
- Pleomorphic adenoma
- Dermoid and epidermoid
- Dentigerous cyst
- Nasopalatine duct cyst

PATHOLOGY

- Prognosis depends on **stage > histologic grade**

CLINICAL ISSUES

- **ACCa**: Tendency for **PNT**, lung metastases
- **MECa**: Tendency for regional malignant **nodes**
- Treatment: Surgical resection ± postoperative radiation

DIAGNOSTIC CHECKLIST

- **May recur late**: Long-term (> 10 year) imaging surveillance
- Check for PNT in MSGM
- Remove FS on T1 C+ MR if susceptibility obscures anatomy

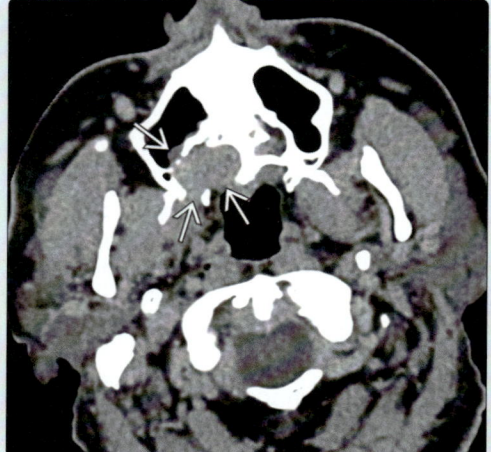
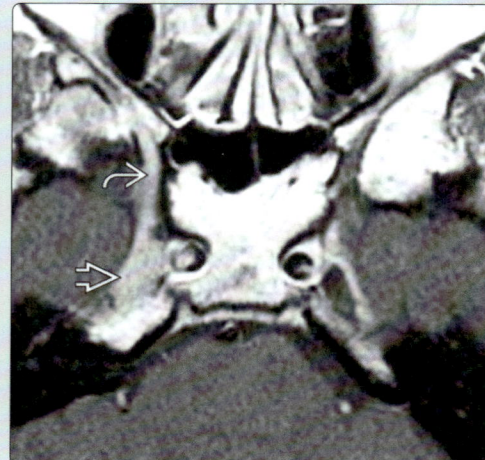

(Left) Axial CECT shows mucoepidermoid carcinoma of right hard palate with multiple areas of osseous erosion ➡. Tumor extends into greater and lesser palatine nerves near their respective foramina at the base of the pterygoid plates. (Right) Axial T1 C+ MR in a patient with hard palate adenoid cystic carcinoma (ACCa) shows perineural tumor along the maxillary division of trigeminal nerve (V2) in foramen rotundum ➡ and cavernous sinus ➡ from contiguous greater palatine nerve and pterygopalatine fossa involvement.

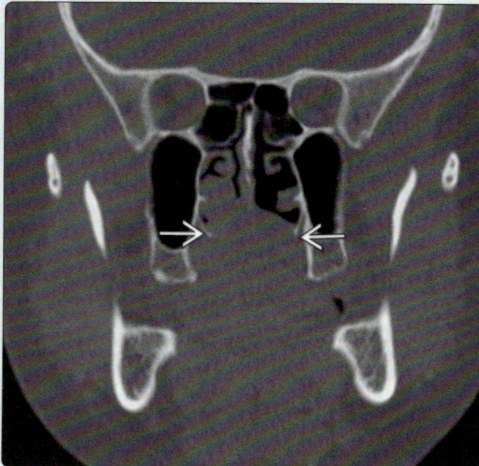
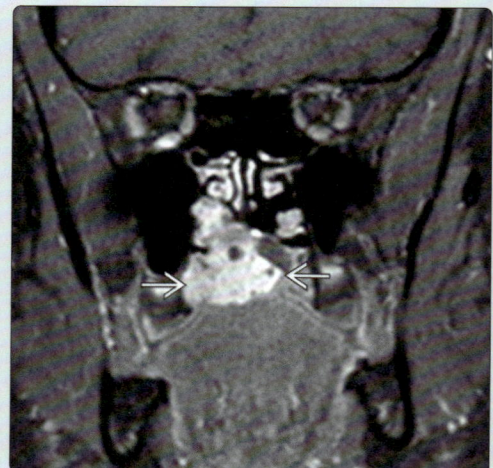

(Left) Coronal bone CT shows a destructive ACCa ➡ from the hard palate that invades the nasal cavity above bilaterally. Bone destruction such as this is the hallmark of a more aggressive process and suggests malignancy. (Right) Coronal T1 C+ FS MR in the same patient better demonstrates the soft tissue component with a heterogeneously enhancing palate mass invading the lower nasal cavity ➡.

Oral Cavity Minor Salivary Gland Malignancy

TERMINOLOGY

Abbreviations
- Oral cavity minor salivary gland malignancy (MSGM)

Definitions
- Primary minor salivary gland malignancy
  - Located in submucosa upper aerodigestive tract

IMAGING

General Features
- Best diagnostic clue
  - Well-defined, smooth, submucosal oral cavity mass
- Location
  - Hard palate > > buccal mucosa > other oral cavity sites
- Size
  - Small (< 2 cm), visible on physical exam

CT Findings
- CECT
  - Homogeneously enhancing mass
- Bone CT
  - Bone erosion (palate, mandible)
  - Greater and lesser palatine foramen enlargement

MR Findings
- T1WI
  - Tumor isointense to muscle
  - Excellent inherent contrast
- T2WI
  - High-signal lesion compared to muscle
- DWI
  - Low ADC compared to benign tumors but lacks specificity
- T1WI C+
  - Homogeneously enhancing tumor
  - Best delineates perineural tumor (PNT) spread

Nuclear Medicine Findings
- PET best for staging/restaging

Imaging Recommendations
- Best imaging tool
  - MR less affected by dental amalgam artifacts than CT
    - T1 C+ FS MR visualizes PNT best

DIFFERENTIAL DIAGNOSIS

Squamous Cell Carcinoma
- May mimic MSGM

Pleomorphic Adenoma of Palate
- Well-circumscribed oral mucosal mass

Dermoid or Epidermoid
- Well-defined oral cavity mass with fatty ± fluid contents
- Nonenhancing oral cavity cystic mass

Dentigerous Cyst
- Maxillary cystic mass ± unerupted tooth

Nasopalatine Duct Cyst
- Anterior, midline hard palate cyst

PATHOLOGY

General Features
- Etiology
  - MECa: Associated with radiation exposure

Staging, Grading, & Classification
- TNM staging now uses pathologic depth of invasion (DOI)
  - T1: ≤ 2 cm, DOI ≤ 5 mm
  - T2
    - ≤ 2 cm with DOI > 5 mm and ≤ 10 mm
    - > 2 cm and ≤ 4 cm with DOI ≤ 10 mm
  - T3
    - > 2 cm and ≤ 4 cm, DOI > 10 mm
    - > 4 cm with DOI ≤ 10 mm
  - T4a: Moderately advanced local disease
    - > 4 cm with DOI > 10 mm
    - Invasion of cortical bone, CNV3, extrinsic tongue muscles, maxillary sinus, &/or skin
  - T4b: Very advanced local disease
    - Invasion of masticator space, pterygoid plates, &/or skull base, ± encases internal carotid artery
- Prognosis depends on stage > histologic grade

Microscopic Features
- Adenoid cystic carcinoma (ACCa): Unencapsulated neoplasm (cribriform, tubular, &/or solid patterns)
- MECa: Epidermoid, intermediate, and mucus-secreting cells

CLINICAL ISSUES

Presentation
- Most common signs/symptoms
  - Painless, slowly enlarging submucosal mass
  - Facial numbness signifies PNT along CNV2

Demographics
- Epidemiology
  - MSGM: 0.5-1.5% of all H&N carcinoma
  - Age: 30-60 years old

Natural History & Prognosis
- **ACCa**: Tendency for **PNT** + lung metastases
- **MECa**: Tendency for regional malignant **nodes**

Treatment
- Tumor resection including perineural extension
- Postoperative radiotherapy for high grade/high stage

DIAGNOSTIC CHECKLIST

Consider
- Long-term (> 10 year) imaging follow-up recommended given **tendency to recur late, especially ACCa**

Image Interpretation Pearls
- Hard palate MSGM: Check for CNV PNT
- Remove FS on T1 C+ MR if susceptibility obscures anatomy
- Noncontrast T1 MR may offer better inherent contrast

SELECTED REFERENCES

1. Hiyama T et al: Imaging of malignant minor salivary gland tumors of the head and neck. Radiographics. 41(1):175-91, 2021

Submandibular Space Nodal Non-Hodgkin Lymphoma

TERMINOLOGY

- Submandibular space (SMS) nodal non-Hodgkin lymphoma (NHL)
- NHL develops in lymphoreticular system

IMAGING

- CECT findings
  - Multiple bilateral, nonnecrotic enlarged level I SMS nodes
  - May see only dominant, single large node
  - Usually large, solid, round nodes
  - Necrosis/extranodal spread indicate aggressive NHL
- PET/CT increasingly used to determine disease extent

TOP DIFFERENTIAL DIAGNOSES

- Reactive lymph nodes
- Nodal squamous cell carcinoma of SMS
- Nodal metastases from systemic primary
- Sarcoidosis lymph nodes

- Tuberculosis lymph nodes

PATHOLOGY

- Unregulated malignant monoclonal lymphocytes in lymphoreticular system
- Multiple different NHL subtypes
  - Most common (> 30%) diffuse large B-cell lymphoma
  - Multiple other subtypes

CLINICAL ISSUES

- Presentation: Multiple painless SMS masses
- 5% all head & neck cancers
- Treatment: Radiotherapy, chemotherapy, or both
- Prognosis
  - 5-year survival: Stages I-II (85%), stages III-IV (50%)

DIAGNOSTIC CHECKLIST

- Consider NHL if imaging reveals multiple 1- to 3-cm cervical nodes in multiple nodal chains, especially if nonnecrotic

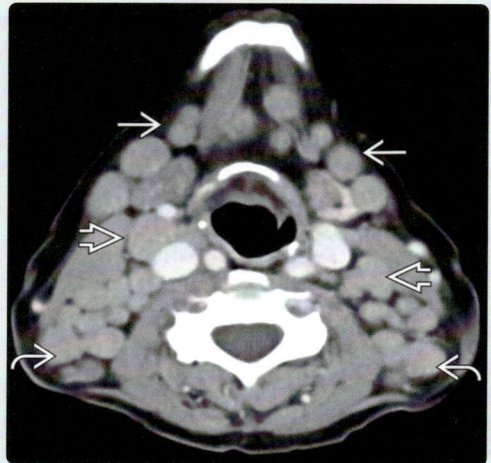
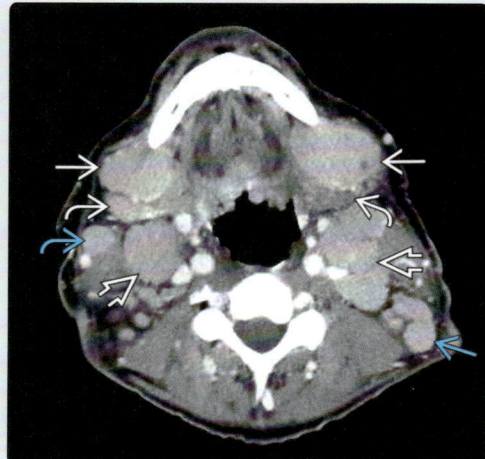

(Left) Axial CECT shows extensive bilateral submandibular space (SMS) level IA & B lymphadenopathy ➡ with a homogeneous, bland appearance. Additional adenopathy is seen in levels II ➡ & V ➡. (Right) Axial CECT shows enlarged, homogeneously enhancing SMS ➡ lymph nodes, characteristic of non-Hodgkin lymphoma (NHL). Submandibular glands ➡ are displaced posteriorly. Additional adenopathy is noted in bilateral level II ➡, left level V ➡, & the right parotid ➡.

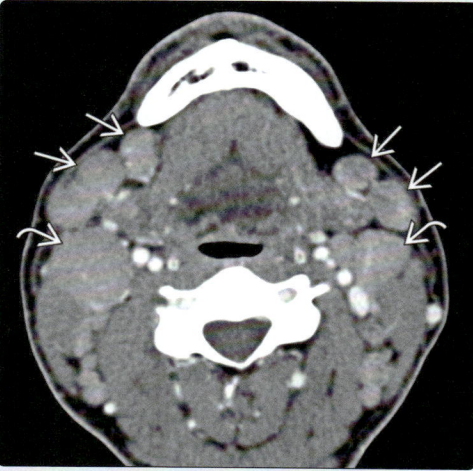
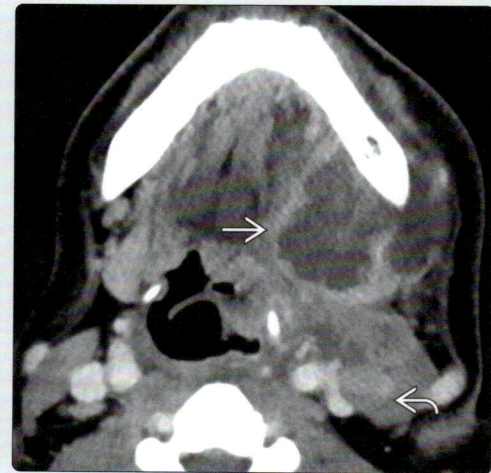

(Left) Axial CECT at inferior mandible level shows large, nonnecrotic NHL nodes in level IB submandibular chain ➡ & bilateral level II jugulodigastric group ➡. (Right) Axial CECT shows a large, peripherally enhancing, centrally necrotic left level IB lymph node ➡ & additional necrotic left level IIA lymph nodes with loss of surrounding fat planes & invasion into the sternocleidomastoid ➡. This was a high-grade diffuse large B-cell lymphoma, which, despite its aggressive imaging & histologic appearance, responded to chemotherapy.

TERMINOLOGY

Abbreviations
- Submandibular space (SMS) nodal non-Hodgkin lymphoma (NHL)

Definitions
- NHL: Lymphoreticular system malignancy, postulated to arise from lymphocytes & derivatives

IMAGING

General Features
- Best diagnostic clue
  - Multiple bilateral, large nodes involving any nodal chain(s)
- Location
  - Any nodal chain may be affected, including level I
- Size
  - Multiple 1- to 3-cm nodes common
  - Dominant node may reach 3-5 cm in size
- Morphology
  - Nodes round or oval, typically solid

CT Findings
- CECT
  - Multiple bilateral round nodes; multiple nodal chains
  - Enhancement pattern variable
    - From isodense to muscle to diffuse enhancement

MR Findings
- T1WI
  - Nodes isointense to muscle
- T2WI
  - Nodes iso- or slightly hyperintense to muscle
- T1WI C+
  - Mild, homogeneous nodal enhancement
  - Necrotic nodes enhance peripherally

Imaging Recommendations
- Best imaging tool
  - CECT usually initial imaging exam
- Protocol advice
  - PET/CT increasingly used to determine disease extent

DIFFERENTIAL DIAGNOSIS

Reactive Lymph Nodes
- Patient < 20-30 years with viral infection
- Diffuse, nonnecrotic nodes; usually < 2 cm

Nodal SCCa of Submandibular Space
- Oral cavity, facial skin squamous cell carcinoma
- Level IA & IB nodes > 1.5 cm ± central nodal necrosis

Nodal Metastases From Systemic Primary
- Known primary tumor (lung, breast, etc.)
- Often unilateral

Sarcoidosis Lymph Nodes
- Diffuse cervical nodes may exactly mimic NHL
- Calcifications may be seen

Tuberculosis Lymph Nodes
- Systemically ill patient, purified protein derivative (+), & abnormal chest x-ray
- Diffuse, heterogeneously enhancing or necrotic nodes

PATHOLOGY

General Features
- Etiology
  - Unregulated malignant monoclonal lymphocytes in lymphoreticular system
  - Evidence suggests viral cause but yet to be proven
- Associated abnormalities
  - Often associated with AIDS in children & adults
    - 2nd most common cancer in AIDS patients
- Multiple different NHL subtypes
  - Most common (>30%) diffuse large B-cell lymphoma (DLBCL)

Microscopic Features
- Microscopic features depend on cell of origin
  - B- & T-cell lymphomas composed of precursor (lymphoblastic) cells or mature lymphocytes

CLINICAL ISSUES

Presentation
- Most common signs/symptoms
  - Multiple painless small, rubbery SMS masses
- Other signs/symptoms
  - Systemic symptoms include night sweats, recurrent fevers, weight loss, fatigue, rash

Demographics
- Epidemiology
  - NHL incidence ↑ with age & immunocompromised state
  - 5% all head & neck cancers
- Age: Median: 50-55 years

Natural History & Prognosis
- May be indolent, progressive but not curable, or aggressive but curable
- Predictors of poorer prognosis
  - Age > 60 years, > 1 extranodal site, stage III or IV, AIDS

Treatment
- Depends on cell type, stage, & patient age
- Usually treated with XRT ± chemotherapy
  - Stage I & II: H&N NHL, XRT alone
  - Stage III & IV: Disseminated NHL, chemotherapy ± XRT

DIAGNOSTIC CHECKLIST

Consider
- NHL: If imaging reveals multiple 1- to 3-cm cervical nodes in multiple nodal chains, especially if nonnecrotic

SELECTED REFERENCES

1. Kwon Y et al: Diagnostic performance and safety of ultrasound-guided core needle biopsy for diagnosing lymphoma: a systematic review and meta-analysis. Cancer Med. 14(1):e70414, 2025
2. Bandargal S et al: Fine needle aspirate flow cytometry's ancillary utility in diagnosing non-hodgkin lymphoma in the head and neck. J Otolaryngol Head Neck Surg. 53:19160216241296127, 2024

Submandibular Space Nodal Squamous Cell Carcinoma

TERMINOLOGY

- Submandibular space (SMS) nodal squamous cell carcinoma (SCCa)

IMAGING

- SMS level IA & IB nodes
  - Level IA: Suprahyoid node(s) between anterior belly of digastric muscles
  - Level IB: Suprahyoid node(s) located lateral & immediately anterior to line tangent to posterior border of submandibular glands
- CECT or MR findings
  - CECT generally preferred over MR for nodal staging
  - CECT improves N staging accuracy over clinical staging
  - SMS nodes **> 1.5 cm** considered malignant in H&N SCCa
  - **Central nodal necrosis** considered sign of malignant involvement in any size node
  - Irregular enhancing margin spread into adjacent tissues implies extranodal extension (ENE)

- PET/CT
  - Superior to CT/MR in clinical N0 neck
- Ultrasonographic findings
  - Round node with loss of hilar echogenicity
  - Main limitation is some nodes are inaccessible

TOP DIFFERENTIAL DIAGNOSES

- Suppurative lymph nodes
- Nodal non-Hodgkin lymphoma

CLINICAL ISSUES

- Treatment: Primary tumor resection vs. chemoradiotherapy ± nodal dissection
- Primary SCCa sites: Oral cavity > pharynx > skin
- **HPV status** impacts **oropharynx** SCCa staging
- HPV(+) SCCa (oropharynx) better overall prognosis
  - Reflected in current AJCC 8th edition staging (2017)
  - Particularly impacts nodal (N) staging
- HPV(-) SCCa has overall worse prognosis

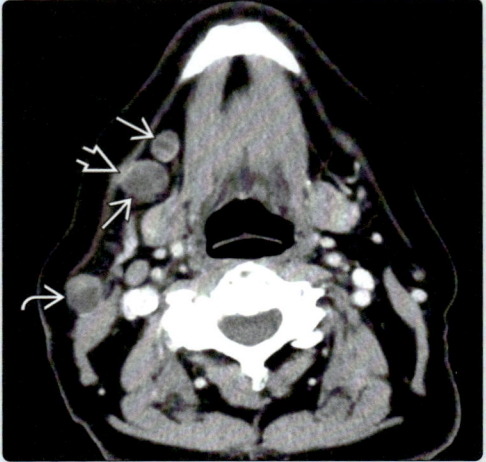
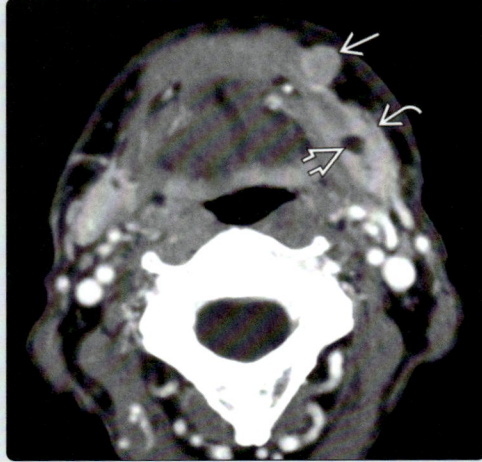

(Left) Axial CECT in a patient with right nasal ala skin cancer shows necrotic right level IB adenopathy ⮕ & a right parotid tail nodal metastasis ⮕. Thickening along the platysma muscle ⮕ is worrisome for extracapsular extension. (Right) Axial CECT through the suprahyoid neck reveals an enlarged, round, enhancing metastatic level IB SCCa node ⮕. The left submandibular gland (SMG) ⮕ is enlarged & enhancing with a dilated hilar duct ⮕. Anterior floor of mouth SCCa (not shown) has obstructed the submandibular duct.

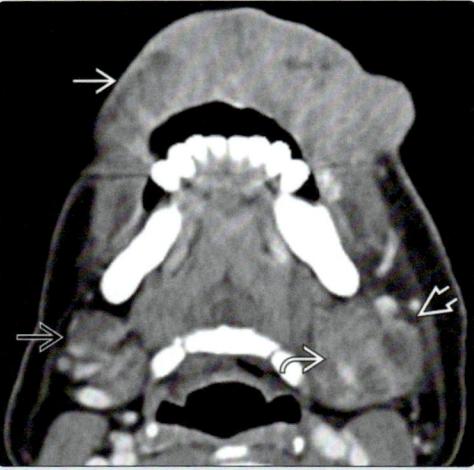
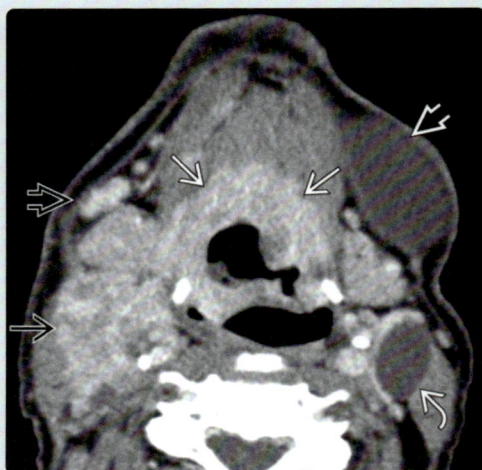

(Left) Axial CECT shows a partially visualized large maxillary mass ⮕ with a heterogeneously enhancing, centrally necrotic left level 1B node ⮕ with extranodal extension into the SMG ⮕. Note a necrotic right level 1B node ⮕. (Right) Axial CECT shows an enhancing base of tongue mass ⮕ & large cystic/necrotic left level 1B ⮕ & 2A ⮕ nodes. There is also a large, heterogeneous right level 2 nodal conglomerate, which is inseparable from sternocleidomastoid muscle ⮕, & a smaller metastatic right level 1B node ⮕.

TERMINOLOGY

Abbreviations
- Submandibular space (SMS) nodal squamous cell carcinoma (SCCa)

Definitions
- Level I nodal metastasis from primary H&N SCCa

IMAGING

General Features
- Best diagnostic clue
  - Enlarged (> 1.5 cm), abnormally rounded, or centrally necrotic SMS node(s)
- Location
  - SMS level IA & IB nodes
    - Level IA nodes: Between anterior digastric muscles
    - Level IB nodes: Lateral to anterior digastric muscles & anterior to posterior border of submandibular glands
- Size
  - SMS nodes > 1.5 cm considered malignant in H&N SCCa
    - Central nodal necrosis abnormal in node of any size
- Morphology
  - Round contour + loss of fatty hilum: Suspicious for malignant involvement
  - Nodal enhancing irregular margins suspicious for extranodal extension (ENE)

CT Findings
- CECT
  - Enhancing level I nodal mass > 1.5 cm ± central necrosis
  - Irregular enhancing margin invades adjacent soft tissues: ENE
  - High prevalence of positive nodes in clinically N0 necks in oral cavity SCCa, especially tongue

MR Findings
- T1WI C+
  - Enhancing level I nodal mass > 1.5 cm ± central low signal
  - Highest specificity for ENE

Ultrasonographic Findings
- Grayscale ultrasound
  - Round node with loss of hilar echogenicity
  - Main limitation is nodes too deep for visualization

Nuclear Medicine Findings
- PET/CT
  - FDG: Focal areas of ↑ uptake matching SMS node indicates malignant nature
    - Superior to CT/MR in clinically N0 neck (↑ sensitivity)

DIFFERENTIAL DIAGNOSIS

Suppurative Lymph Nodes
- Sick or septic patient
- Central fluid density within nodes
- Can mimic SCCa nodes

Nodal Non-Hodgkin Lymphoma of Submandibular Space
- Multiple bilateral, large, usually nonnecrotic nodes

- No primary SCCa on clinical exam

PATHOLOGY

General Features
- Etiology
  - Lymphatic spread of primary SCCa to SMS nodes
  - Common drainage pathways for SCCa SMS nodes
    - All oral cavity sites
    - Anterior facial structures, lips, & skin
    - Oropharynx & hypopharynx SCCa can spread to SMS nodes if ≥ 1 nodes in levels II-IV involved

Microscopic Features
- Metastases 1st lodge in subcapsular sinus → spread through node
- Keratinizing or nonkeratinizing (latter usually HPV related)
- Immunohistochemistry for p16 critical to staging

CLINICAL ISSUES

Presentation
- Most common signs/symptoms
  - Painless, firm SMS mass
    - May be fixed to mandible ± adjacent tissues

Demographics
- Age
  - Most commonly > 40 years

Natural History & Prognosis
- Staging & prognosis depend on primary site
  - Oral cavity SCCa most often metastasizes to SMS nodes
  - Oropharynx & hypopharynx SCCa spread to levels II-IV 1st
  - Cutaneous skin SCCa in advanced cases
- **HPV status** is most important prognostic factor for **oropharyngeal** (OP) SCCa & strongly impacts staging
- HPV(+) SCCa, OP (more common) better overall prognosis
  - Reflected in **current AJCC 8th edition staging (2017)**
- HPV(-) SCCa, OP has overall worse prognosis
  - N stage strongly impact prognosis
  - Single unilateral node ↓ prognosis by 50%
  - Bilateral nodes ↓ prognosis by 75%
  - ENE ↓ prognosis by further 50%
    - Risk of recurrence ↑ 10x

Treatment
- Surgical resection ± chemoradiotherapy ± node dissection

DIAGNOSTIC CHECKLIST

Consider
- Nodal size (> 1.5 cm) or parenchymal inhomogeneity (e.g., necrosis) key to labeling malignant based on imaging

SELECTED REFERENCES
1. Yu YF et al: Frequency of lymph node metastases at different neck levels in patients with oral squamous cell carcinoma: a systematic review and meta-analysis. Int J Surg. 111(1):1285-300, 2025
2. Alsibani A et al: Comparing the efficacy of CT, MRI, PET-CT, and US in the detection of cervical lymph node metastases in head and neck squamous cell carcinoma with clinically negative neck lymph node: a systematic review and meta-analysis. J Clin Med. 13(24):7622, 2024

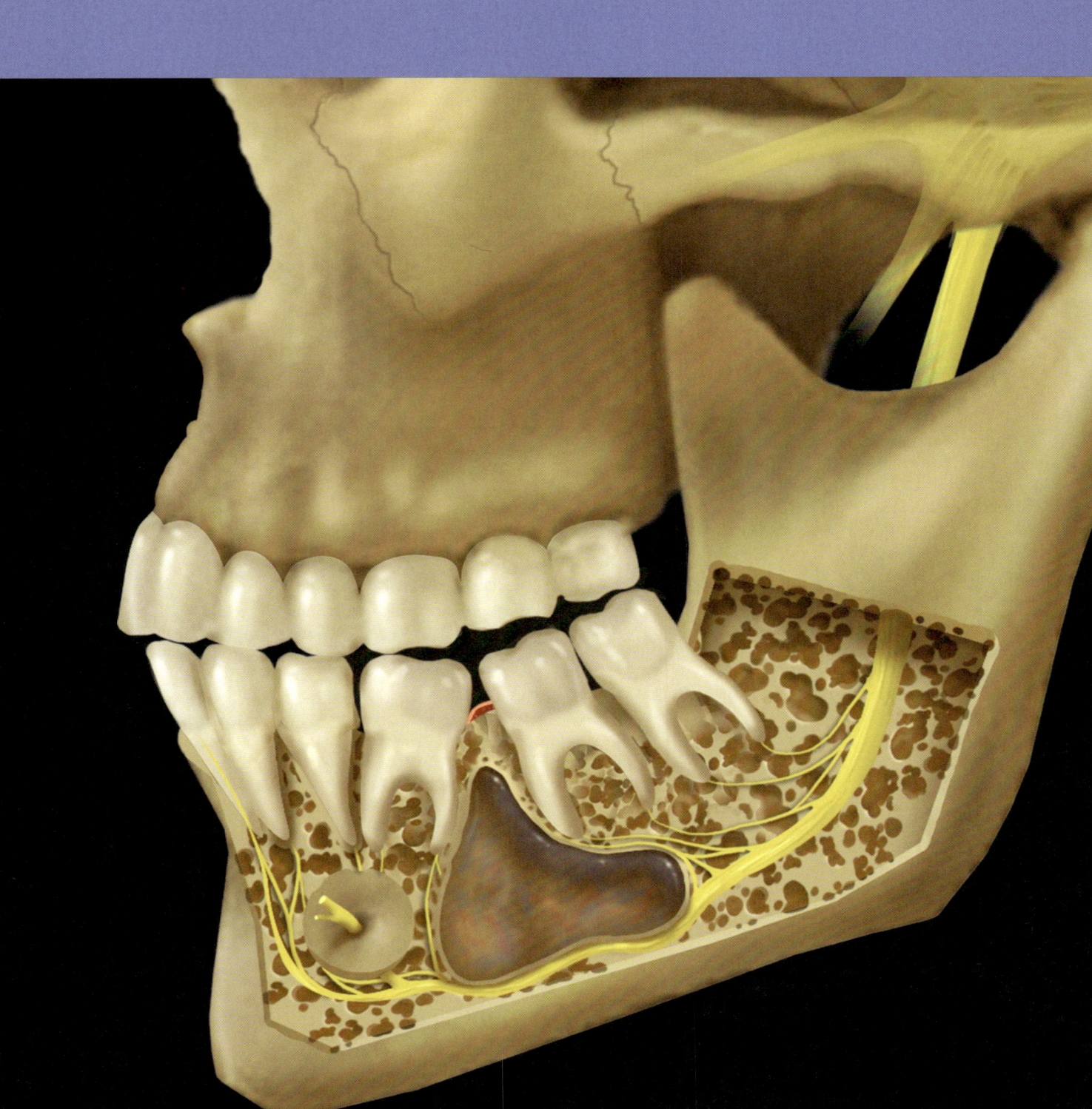

SECTION 15
Mandible-Maxilla and TMJ

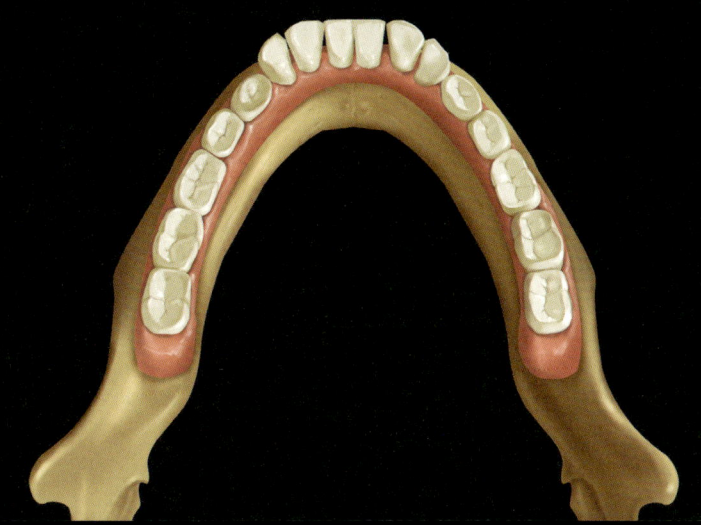

Imaging Techniques & Indications

Mandible and Maxilla

The study of choice for evaluating the mandible and maxilla is **thin-section bone algorithm CT** and **CECT**. **MR** of the maxillofacial complex is used for marrow changes, inferior alveolar nerve, and soft tissues.

- Coverage from orbits to hyoid
- CT: ≤ 1-mm intervals; bone and soft tissue algorithms post processing; can angle maxilla and mandible separately to help avoid artifact from dental restorations; reformats in coronal and sagittal planes, and, if requested, panoramic
- MR: T1-/T2-weighted and contrast-enhanced images, 3 mm, high-resolution/small FOV techniques
- Axial images (CT or MR) should be acquired parallel to inferior border of mandible
- STIR or T2 fat-saturation sequences and contrast enhancement: Sensitive for marrow/nerve changes associated with inflammation or neoplasm

TMJ

MR is the tool of choice for evaluating the TMJ. Small surface, circular (3-in) TMJ coils are ideally used, although multichannel coils (≥ 12 channels) provide adequate signal.

- Sagittal images: Perpendicular to long axis of condyle ("corrected sagittal oblique") at 3-mm intervals; T1-weighted or PD acquired in closed- and open-mouth positions
- Sagittal T2-weighted images: For joint effusions
- Coronal T1-weighted images in closed-mouth position help assess medial or lateral disc displacements
- Contrast-enhanced images: For synovitis or tumors

CT imaging of the TMJ is generally reserved for evaluation of **trauma**, bony abnormalities or **calcified masses**, or **joint reconstruction** with metallic prosthesis.

- Thin-section bone algorithm images are acquired at 1-mm intervals from sella to hyoid and reformatted in coronal and sagittal planes

Imaging Anatomy

Mandible and Maxilla

The **maxilla** consists of a **body** containing the maxillary sinus and 4 processes: **Zygomatic, frontal, alveolar, and palatine**. The maxilla forms the anterior boundary of the infratemporal and pterygopalatine fossae and contributes to formation of the infraorbital and pterygomaxillary fissures. The zygomatic (**malar**) process contributes to the inferior pillar of the zygomatic buttress. The frontal (nasal) process articulates with the nasal bones on the lateral surface with the medial surface forming the lateral wall of the nasal cavity and articulating with the ethmoid bone to enclose the agger nasi cells and anterior ethmoidal cells. The posterior border of the frontal process forms the lacrimal fossa and the anterior lacrimal crest. The **alveolar process** is the thickest and most spongy part of the maxilla and forms the alveolar arches, containing the dentition. The 3D, U-shaped configuration of the maxillary alveolus is such that benign expansile inflammatory or neoplastic processes typically expand it concentrically.

The **maxillary tuberosity** is the rounded, most posterior eminence of the alveolar arch, articulating with the pyramidal process of the palatine bone. The palatine process is a relatively thick, horizontal bone that forms the roof of the mouth and the floor of the nasal cavity. The incisive foramen lies in the anterior midline of the premaxilla and transmits the nasopalatine nerves and descending palatine artery. The premaxillary suture, posterior to the incisive foramen, separates the anterior premaxilla from the more posterior palatine process, which forms the anterior 75% of the hard palate. The horizontal plate of the palatine bone forms the posterior hard palate and contains foramina for the **greater and lesser palatine nerves**.

The **mandible** consists of a horseshoe-shaped body and vertical rami joining in the anterior midline symphysis. On the medial (lingual) surface of the ramus is the **mandibular foramen** for intraosseous passage of the neurovascular supply, namely the inferior alveolar nerve (derived from the mandibular nerve, V3) and artery. The mandibular foramen is bounded by a small bony spine, the lingula. Another branch, the mylohyoid nerve, travels in the mylohyoid groove on the lingual surface of the mandible. On the external surface of the mandible, at roughly the level of the 1st premolar, is the mental foramen for the mental nerve and vessels. Emerging anterosuperiorly from the ramus is the triangular eminence of the coronoid process to which the temporalis and masseter muscles attach. At the posterior-superior termination of the ramus is the condyloid process, consisting of the condyle supported by the more constricted neck. The coronoid process and condyle are separated by a depression, the mandibular (coronoid) notch, through which the masseteric vessels and nerves pass.

Dentition: Dental infection in the form of dental caries or periodontal disease spreads into the alveolus through the root apex or through the **periodontal ligament** (PDL) space. The PDL can be a conduit for the spread of infection following alveolar fracture or intraosseous extension of gingival squamous cell carcinoma.

- **Permanent**: 32 teeth consisting of 2 central and 2 lateral incisors, 2 canines, 4 premolars, and 6 molars in each jaw (numbered 1-16 in maxilla, right to left, and 17-32 in mandible, left to right)
- **Primary:** 20 teeth consisting of 2 central and 2 lateral incisors, 2 canines, and 4 molars in each jaw (lettered A-J in maxilla and K-T in mandible)

TMJ

The **TMJ complex** is a diarthrodial osseous articulation between the mandibular condyle and the glenoid fossa and articular eminence of the temporal bone. The TMJ is the only joint in which articulating surfaces are covered by fibrocartilage. The articular disc is a biconcave, dense, avascular fibrous connective tissue with 3 segments: The anterior band, attached to the capsule and fibers of the superior belly of the lateral pterygoid muscle, the thin intermediate zone, and the posterior band. The bilaminar zone, or retrodiscal tissues, attaches to the posterior band and provides neurovascular innervation.

Approaches to Lesions of Mandible & Maxilla

The 1st step is to try to determine whether the lesion is odontogenic or nonodontogenic in origin. Infectious and inflammatory lesions usually have a dental origin, even if remote. **Odontogenic** cysts and benign and malignant neoplasms are usually centered within tooth-bearing areas of the alveolus. The major exception is gingival squamous cell carcinoma extending through the gingiva or PDL space. **Nonodontogenic lesions** often arise at the tooth root apices or superior (maxilla) or inferior (mandible) to them.

Neurovascular Anatomy

Bone	Nerve Supply	Arterial Supply
Maxillary alveolus and palate	Posterior 2/3 of hard palate and molars: Greater palatine nerve Anterior palate and teeth: Nasopalatine nerve; additional supply to gingiva and teeth from anterior, middle, and posterior superior alveolar nerves	Posterior superior alveolar artery (gingiva, premolar and molar teeth) Anterior &/or middle superior alveolar arteries (incisors and canines) Descending palatine artery (palate)
Mandible	Inferior alveolar nerve: Branches supply teeth as it travels through mandible Mental nerve: Larger branch, supplies skin over mandible and lower lip Incisive nerve: Smaller branch, supplies canines and lateral incisor teeth	Inferior alveolar artery Incisive artery

Mandible-Maxilla Differential Diagnosis

Inflammatory/infectious	Cysts	Malignant neoplasms
Apical rarefying osteitis	**Odontogenic**	**Nonodontogenic**
Radicular cyst	Dentigerous cyst	Gingival squamous cell carcinoma
Osteomyelitis	Odontogenic keratocyst	Osteosarcoma/chondrosarcoma
Osteonecrosis	Glandular odontogenic cyst	Multiple myeloma or metastasis
Osteoradionecrosis	Calcifying epithelial odontogenic cyst	**Odontogenic**
Congenital/developmental	**Benign neoplasms**	Odontogenic carcinoma
Solitary median maxillary central incisor	**Nonodontogenic**	Odontogenic sarcoma
Acquired	Osteoma	**Fibroosseous lesions**
Stafne bone cavity	Ossifying fibroma	Periapical osseous dysplasia
Simple bone cyst	**Odontogenic**	Florid osseous dysplasia
Central giant cell granuloma	Odontoma	Fibrous dysplasia
Cysts	Ameloblastoma	Cherubism
Nonodontogenic	Odontogenic myxoma	**Other**
Nasopalatine duct cyst	Adenomatoid odontogenic tumor	Neurofibroma, schwannoma
Nasolabial cyst	Calcifying epithelial odontogenic tumor	Eosinophilic granuloma

TMJ Differential Diagnosis

Meniscal dislocation	Anterior, medial, lateral, or (rarely) posterior displacement of articular disc
Juvenile idiopathic arthritis	Bilateral flattened, deformed mandibular condyles, joint effusion, synovial enhancement
Synovial chondromatosis	Multiple calcified, small nodules in superior joint space
Tenosynovial giant cell tumor	Locally destructive mass with peripheral hypointense rim on MR
Calcium pyrophosphate dihydrate deposition disease	Chunky, diffuse, calcified mass

Most odontogenic lesions are cystic, cystic-appearing, or relatively hypodense on CT. They are distinguished by their location, loculation, presence of internal calcification, and expansion/erosion of bone. Most dentigerous cysts and odontogenic keratocysts do not become loculated until large; most ameloblastomas demonstrate multiple loculations. The only odontogenic lesions with internal calcification are odontoma, calcifying epithelial cyst/tumor, and adenomatoid odontogenic tumor. Malignant neoplasms generally demonstrate more enhancement than benign lesions.

Assess the following **3 key pieces of information** for any pathology, whether there is involvement of
- Lamina dura (cortical bone forming tooth socket) and PDL space or tooth roots
- Inferior alveolar canal
- Adjacent structures, including maxillary sinus, orbit, pterygopalatine fossa, buccal vestibule and space, masticator space, or sublingual or submandibular space

Selected References

1. Bali A et al: Imaging of radiolucent jaw lesions. Semin Musculoskelet Radiol. 24(5):549-57, 2020
2. Siozopoulou V et al: World Health Organization classification of odontogenic tumors and imaging approach of jaw lesions. Semin Musculoskelet Radiol. 24(5):535-48, 2020
3. Vanhoenacker FM et al: Imaging of mixed and radiopaque jaw lesions. Semin Musculoskelet Radiol. 24(5):558-69, 2020
4. Mosier KM: Lesions of the jaw. Semin Ultrasound CT MR. 36(5):444-50, 2015
5. Mosier KM: Magnetic resonance imaging of the maxilla and mandible: signal characteristics and features in the differential diagnosis of common lesions. Top Magn Reson Imaging. 24(1):23-37, 2015
6. Aiken A et al: MR imaging of the temporomandibular joint. Magn Reson Imaging Clin N Am. 20(3):397-412, 2012

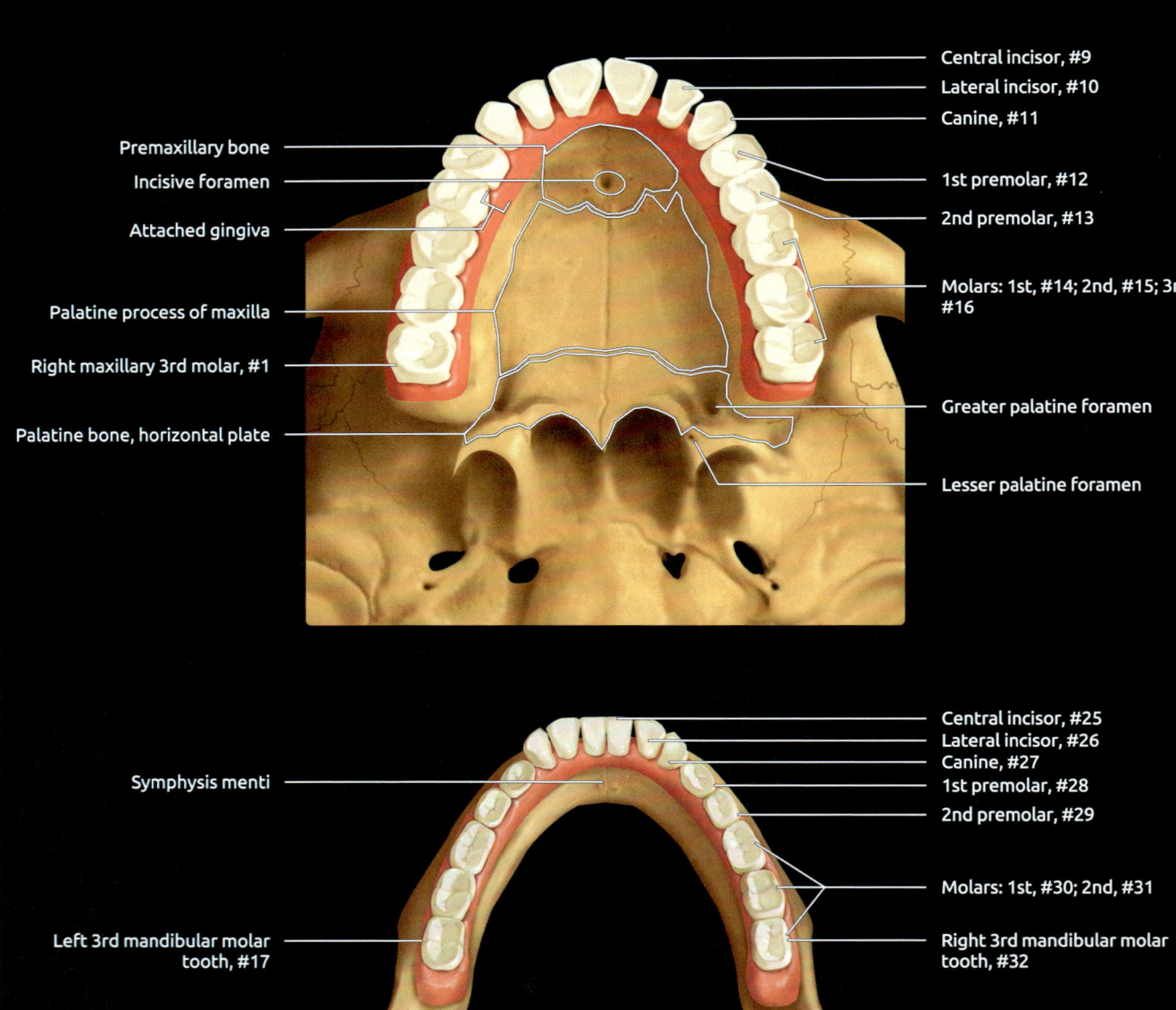

Central incisor, #9

Lateral incisor, #10

Canine, #11

Premaxillary bone

Incisive foramen

1st premolar, #12

2nd premolar, #13

Attached gingiva

Palatine process of maxilla

Right maxillary 3rd molar, #1

Molars: 1st, #14; 2nd, #15; 3rd, #16

Palatine bone, horizontal plate

Greater palatine foramen

Lesser palatine foramen

Central incisor, #25
Lateral incisor, #26
Canine, #27

Symphysis menti

1st premolar, #28
2nd premolar, #29

Molars: 1st, #30; 2nd, #31

Left 3rd mandibular molar tooth, #17

Right 3rd mandibular molar tooth, #32

Lingula

Coronoid process

Mandibular foramen

Condylar neck

Condylar head

(Top) *Axial graphic of the hard palate and maxillary alveolar ridge viewed from below shows the anterior premaxillary bone and the larger palatine process of the maxillary bone. Posteriorly is the horizontal plate of the palatine bone. Note the anterior midline incisive canal and the posterolateral greater and lesser palatine foramina. The alveolus is covered by attached gingiva, which is the oral mucous membrane bound to the tooth and the alveolus. The maxilla has 16 permanent teeth; numbering begins with the right 3rd molar.* **(Bottom)** *Axial graphic of the mandible seen from above demonstrates the cephalad condylar head and neck leading to the more inferior ramus. The mandibular foramen is seen on the inner surface of the mandibular ramus. The cephalad projecting coronoid processes attach to the temporalis muscle tendons. The U-shaped mandibular bodies fuse in the midline at the symphysis menti. There are 16 permanent teeth, numbered beginning at the left 3rd molar from 17 to 32 (right 3rd molar tooth).*

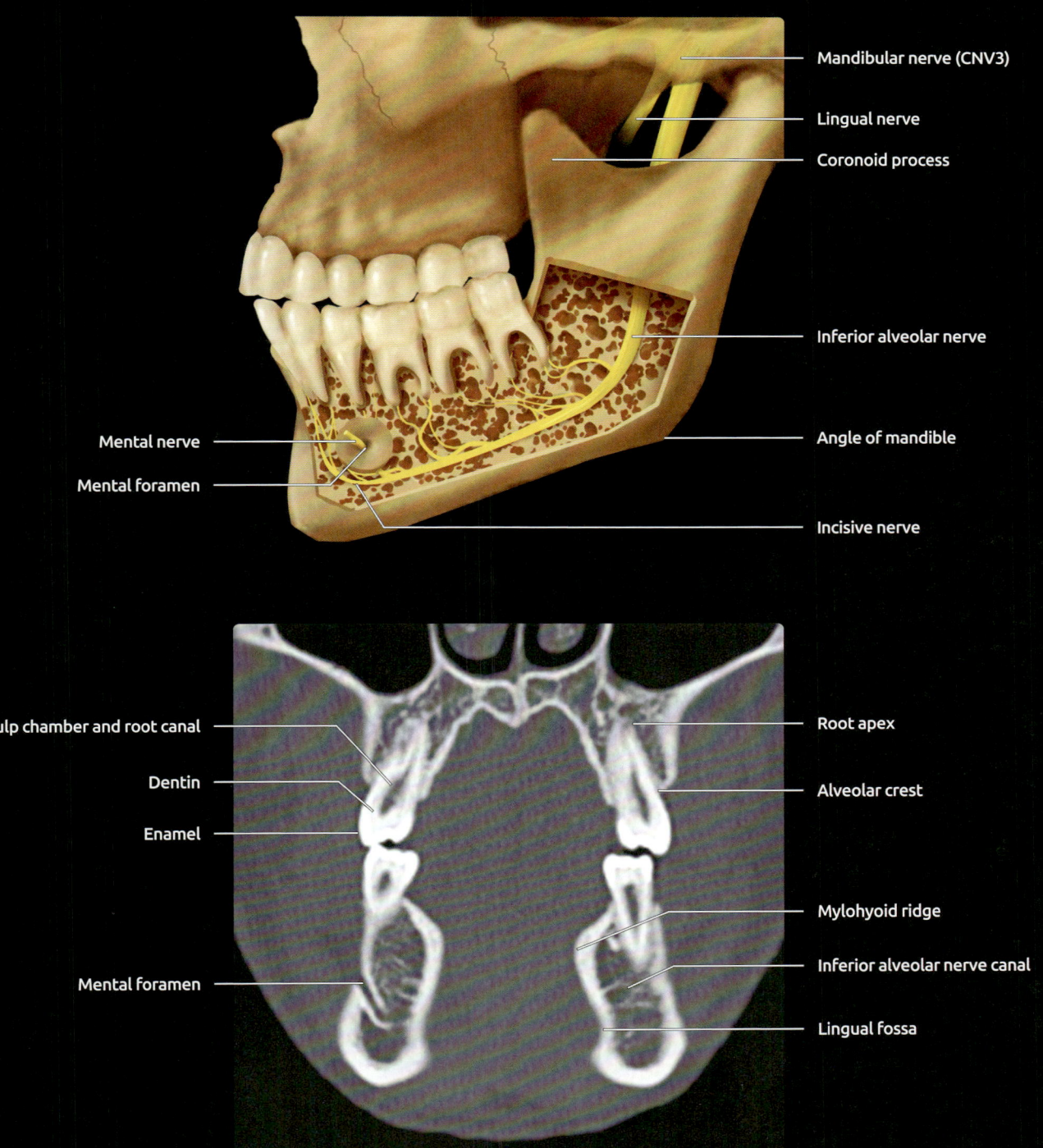

Mandibular nerve (CNV3)

Lingual nerve

Coronoid process

Inferior alveolar nerve

Angle of mandible

Mental nerve

Mental foramen

Incisive nerve

Pulp chamber and root canal

Dentin

Enamel

Mental foramen

Root apex

Alveolar crest

Mylohyoid ridge

Inferior alveolar nerve canal

Lingual fossa

(Top) *Lateral graphic of the mandible with lateral cortex removed shows the mandibular nerve (CNV3) dividing into lingual and inferior alveolar nerves. The inferior alveolar nerve travels anteriorly in the inferior alveolar canal (mandibular canal) and divides distally into a main trunk, mental nerve, which reaches the superficial chin through the mental foramen and smaller, incisive branches.* **(Bottom)** *Coronal bone CT through the anterior mandible is shown. The most common lesion of the maxilla and mandible is dental infection, primarily through carious lesions involving the enamel and dentin with or without extension to the pulp. Lesions at the root apex typically result from infection transgressing the pulp. Apical lesions may also arise from infection of the periodontium with loss of bone at the alveolar crest. The jaws are the only bones with direct exposure to the external environment via the teeth. Infection from teeth may extend through the buccal or lingual cortex to adjacent spaces. The proximity of the lingual fossa to premolar or molar roots predisposes to involvement of the sublingual and submandibular space.*

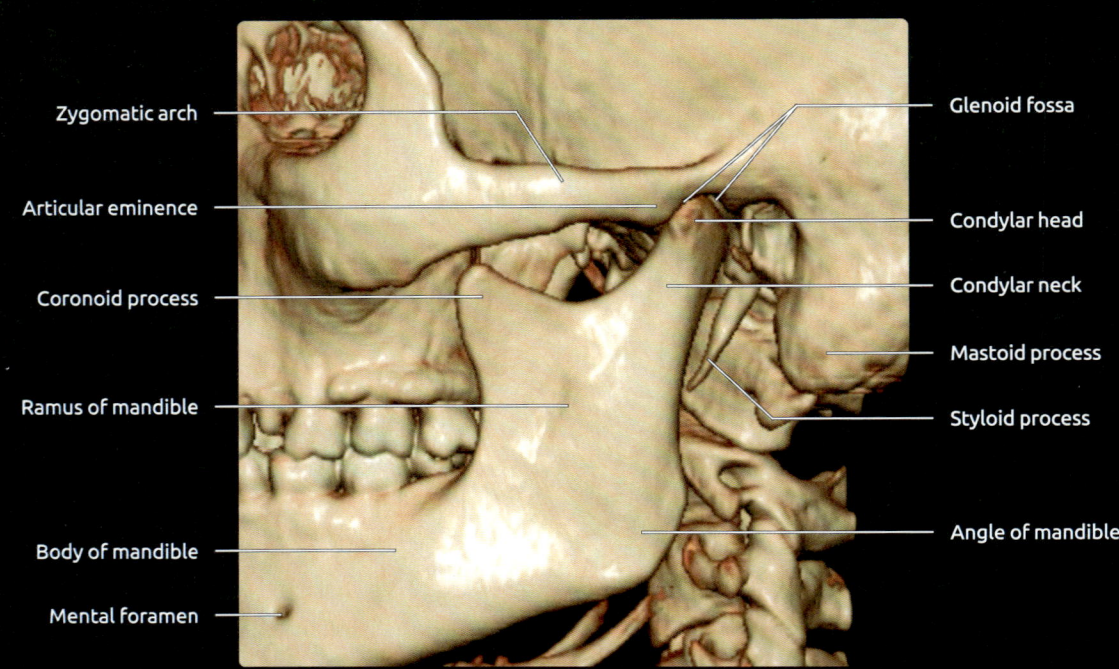

Zygomatic arch

Articular eminence

Coronoid process

Ramus of mandible

Body of mandible

Mental foramen

Glenoid fossa

Condylar head

Condylar neck

Mastoid process

Styloid process

Angle of mandible

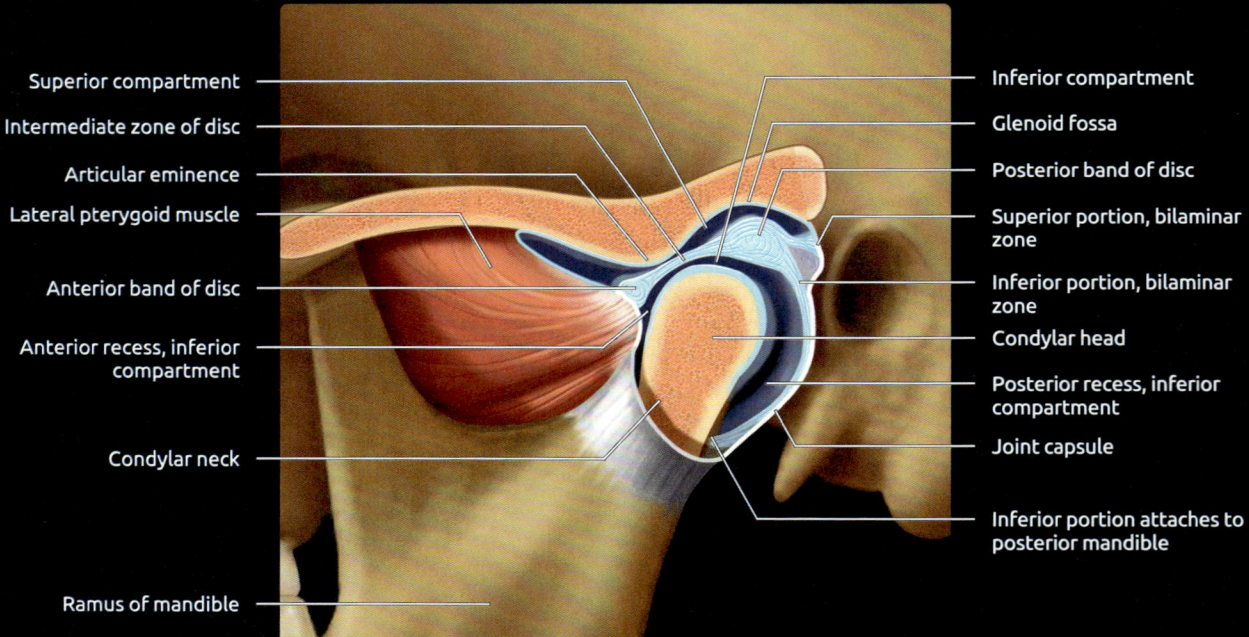

Superior compartment

Intermediate zone of disc

Articular eminence

Lateral pterygoid muscle

Anterior band of disc

Anterior recess, inferior compartment

Condylar neck

Ramus of mandible

Inferior compartment

Glenoid fossa

Posterior band of disc

Superior portion, bilaminar zone

Inferior portion, bilaminar zone

Condylar head

Posterior recess, inferior compartment

Joint capsule

Inferior portion attaches to posterior mandible

(Top) *Sagittal 3D VRT image shows the osseous anatomy of TMJ. The condylar head is situated in the glenoid fossa deep to the posterior zygomatic arch. The zygomatic arch provides some protection laterally for the TMJ in the setting of trauma. The TMJ must be fully evaluated on all mandibular trauma cases to ensure that no dislocation of the mandibular condyle has occurred.* (Bottom) *Magnified lateral graphic of the TMJ shows the articular disc with its anterior and posterior bands. The thinner part of the disc connecting these bands is called the intermediate zone. The disc separates the joint into a superior and an inferior compartment. Note the lateral pterygoid muscle inserting anteriorly on the joint capsule and anterior band. The posterior margin of the posterior band is referred to as the bilaminar zone with the superior strut attaching to the posterior mandibular fossa, while the inferior strut attaches to the posterior margin of the mandibular condyle.*

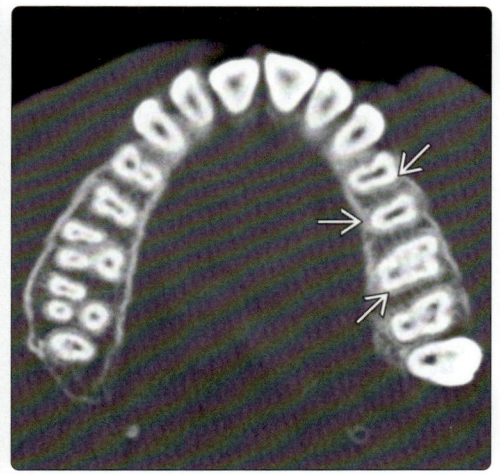

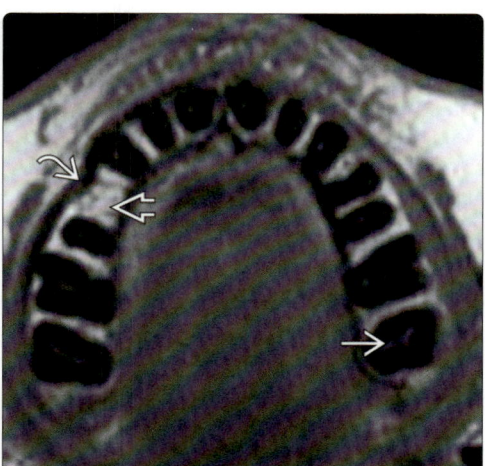

(Left) Axial bone CT shows the normal adult maxilla. Each tooth is surrounded by the periodontal ligament space containing fibers of the periodontal ligament and the lamina dura (cortical bone forming the tooth socket) ➡. (Right) Axial T1 MR shows the normal adult maxilla. Note the slightly hyperintense vascular tissue of the pulp chamber ➡, the normal yellow marrow ➡, and the attached gingiva ➡.

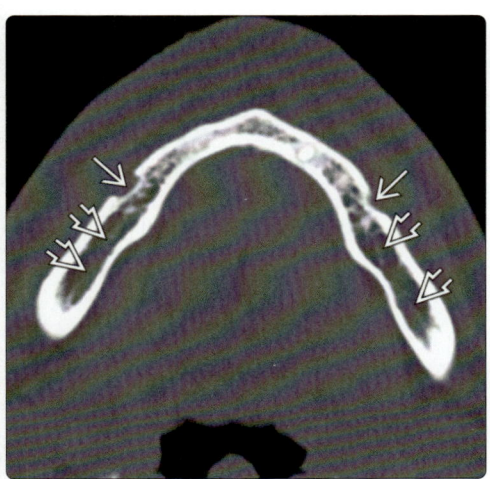

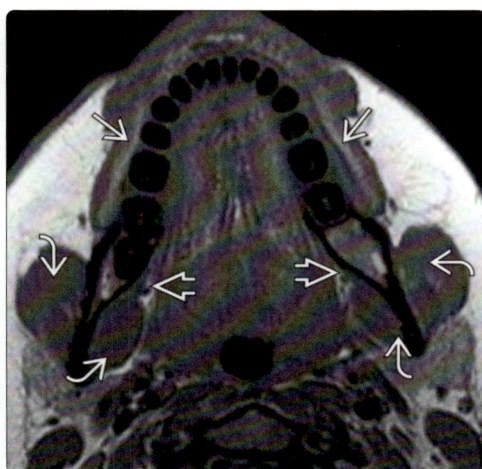

(Left) Axial bone CT of the mandible shows bilateral mental foramina ➡ with inferior alveolar canals ➡ containing inferior alveolar nerves and arteries. The mandible is an end-artery system with ↑ risk relative to the maxilla for development of osteomyelitis, osteonecrosis, or osteoradionecrosis. (Right) Axial T1 MR shows the relationship of the mandible to the buccal vestibule/space ➡, masticator space ➡, and submandibular space ➡, all routes for spread of infection or tumor.

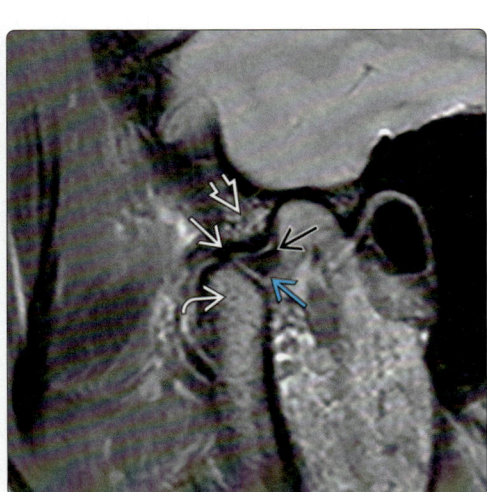

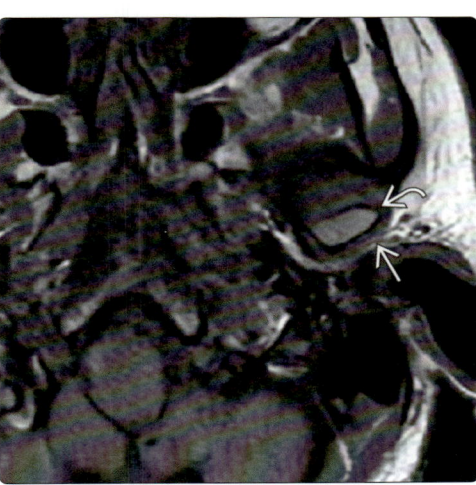

(Left) Sagittal PD MR in open-mouth view shows the thinner intermediate zone of the disk ➡, interposed between the articular eminence ➡ and the condylar head ➡ in a bow tie appearance with the triangular appearance of the anterior and posterior bands, respectively. Note the superior lamina ➡ and inferior lamina ➡ of the bilaminar zone. (Right) Axial T1 MR through the left TMJ demonstrates the joint capsule surrounding the joint ➡. Note the location of the auriculotemporal nerve exiting the joint space posterolaterally ➡.

Solitary Median Maxillary Central Incisor

TERMINOLOGY

- Solitary median maxillary central incisor (SMMCI) syndrome

IMAGING

- Small, **triangle-shaped hard palate**
- **Single maxillary central incisor** in midline
- Congenital nasal pyriform aperture stenosis (CNPAS), midnasal stenosis, or choanal atresia in 90%
- ± **holoprosencephaly (HPE)**

TOP DIFFERENTIAL DIAGNOSES

- Congenital nasal pyriform aperture stenosis
  - Solitary central maxillary incisor in up to 75%
- Choanal atresia
  - Rarely with solitary central maxillary incisor
- Mesiodens
  - Supernumerary midline tooth develops between 2 maxillary central incisors

PATHOLOGY

- Associated with mutations in human sonic hedgehog (*SHH*) gene & deletions on chromosomes 7 & 18
- *SHH* mutations are most frequent etiology of HPE
  - SMMCI can be considered predictor or risk factor for HPE or gene carrier status

CLINICAL ISSUES

- Respiratory distress during feeding
- Hypotelorism, microcephaly, short stature, hypopituitarism
- Treatment initially directed toward relief of associated nasal stenosis, later directed at cosmetic appearance of permanent dentition to include combined orthodontic, prosthodontic, & oral surgical treatment

DIAGNOSTIC CHECKLIST

- Look for SMMCI, CNPAS, &/or choanal atresia when imaging neonates with feeding/breathing difficulties
- If SMMCI diagnosed, be sure to check for findings of HPE

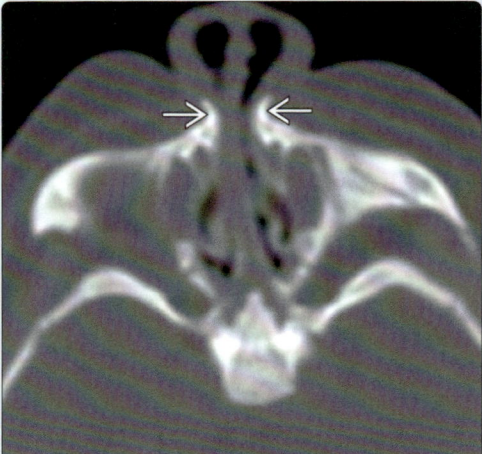
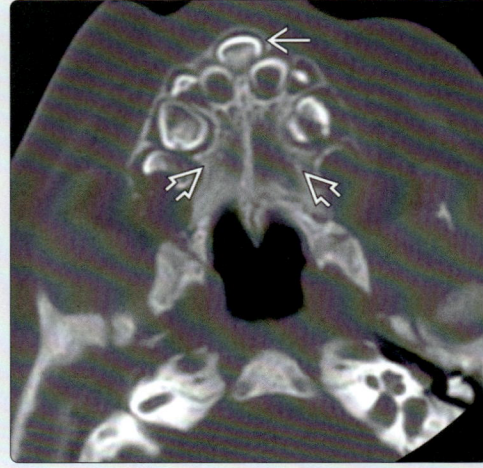

(Left) *Axial bone CT in an infant with respiratory distress (exaggerated during feedings) at the level of the anterior nasal inlet demonstrates narrowing of the nasal inlet, i.e., pyriform aperture stenosis* ➡. **(Right)** *Axial bone CT in the same patient at the level of the hard palate shows a solitary median maxillary central incisor* ➡ *and a small, triangle-shaped hard palate* ➡. *Brain MR in this child, performed to evaluate for potential of intracranial midline anomalies, was normal.*

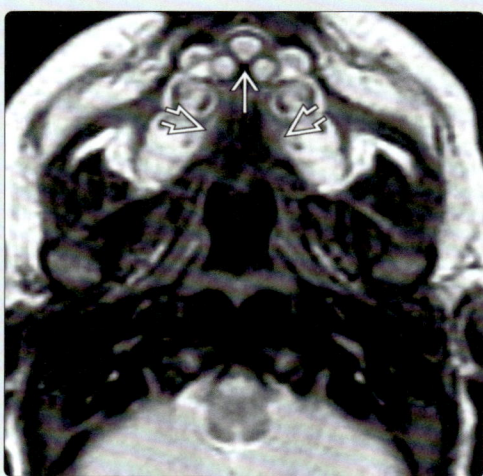
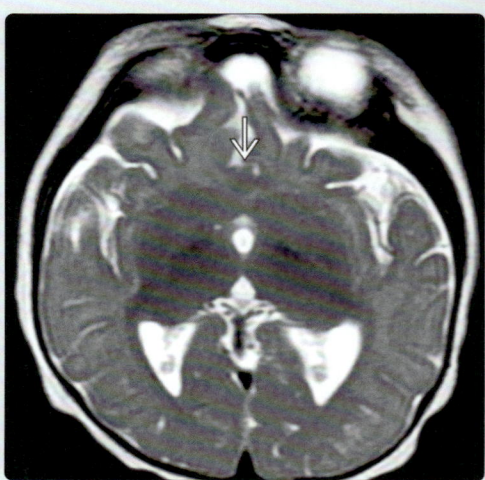

(Left) *Axial T2WI MR through the hard palate in a neonate with pyriform aperture stenosis shows the solitary central incisor* ➡ *and small hard palate* ➡. **(Right)** *Axial T2WI brain MR in an infant with pyriform aperture stenosis and solitary median maxillary central incisor shows very mild lobar holoprosencephaly with incomplete separation of hemispheres at the level of the inferior frontal lobes* ➡. *These patients should also undergo an endocrine evaluation.*

Solitary Median Maxillary Central Incisor

TERMINOLOGY

Abbreviations

- Solitary median maxillary central incisor (SMMCI) syndrome
  - Favored term

Synonyms

- Monosuperoincisivodontic dwarfism: Original term (1976)
- SMMCI, short stature, choanal atresia/midnasal stenosis syndrome
- Shortened to SMMCI syndrome, as other features not necessarily present in all cases
- Single central incisor, single maxillary central incisor syndrome, & single incisor syndrome
  - These terms do not adequately describe peculiarly formed central incisor tooth

IMAGING

General Features

- Best diagnostic clue
  - Triangle-shaped hard palate with solitary central maxillary incisor tooth located in midline

CT Findings

- Narrow anterior palate, **triangular shape**
- **Single maxillary central incisor** in midline
  - May be unerupted
  - Primary and permanent dentition
- **+ congenital nasal obstruction** in **90%**
  - Congenital nasal pyriform aperture stenosis (CNPAS) > midnasal stenosis & choanal atresia
- ± **holoprosencephaly** (HPE)

MR Findings

- Findings often more confusing on MR
  - Tooth buds appear more crowded
- ± HPE, ectopic posterior pituitary, small adenohypophysis

Imaging Recommendations

- Best imaging tool
  - Bone CT
- Protocol advice
  - Look for associated stenosis of pyriform aperture, midnasal cavity, or choanal atresia
  - Consider **MR** to evaluate brain for **midline anomalies**

DIFFERENTIAL DIAGNOSIS

Congenital Nasal Pyriform Aperture Stenosis

- Solitary central maxillary incisor in up to 75%

Choanal Atresia

- Most common congenital abnormality of nasal cavity
  - 1:5,000-8,000 births

Mesiodens

- Supernumerary midline tooth develops between 2 maxillary central incisors

PATHOLOGY

General Features

- Genetics

- Associated with mutations in human sonic hedgehog (*SHH*) gene & deletions on chromosomes 7, 18, & 22
  - *SHH* mutations are most frequent etiology of HPE
  - SMMCI can be considered predictor or risk factor for HPE or gene carrier status
- Associated abnormalities
  - CHARGE (ocular **c**oloboma, **h**eart defects, choanal **a**tresia, developmental **r**estriction, **g**enital/urinary anomalies, **e**ar abnormalities)
  - VACTERL (**v**ertebral defects, **a**nal atresia, **c**ardiovascular defects, **t**racheo**e**sophageal fistula, **r**adial ray or renal anomalies, **l**imb defects)
  - Velocardiofacial, Duane retraction, Goldenhar, & DiGeorge syndromes
  - Clavicle hypoplasia, HPE, pituitary insufficiency, microcephaly, oromandibular-limb hypogenesis syndrome type I, ectodermal dysplasia, congenital cardiac anomalies, spine abnormalities

Gross Pathologic & Surgical Features

- Absent labial frenulum and incisive papilla
- Absent intermaxillary suture
- Prominent midpalatal ridge

CLINICAL ISSUES

Presentation

- Most common signs/symptoms
  - Respiratory distress during feeding
    - When associated with CNPAS, midnasal stenosis, or choanal atresia/stenosis, nasal obstruction hampers breathing when infant feeds
    - Clinical mimic of nasolacrimal duct mucocele → nasal obstruction
- Other signs/symptoms
  - Hypotelorism, microcephaly, short stature, hypopituitarism

Demographics

- ~ 1:50,000 live births

Treatment

- Early treatment directed toward relief of associated nasal stenosis: Sublabial drilling or dilatation
- After permanent dentition, combined orthodontic, prosthodontic, & oral surgical treatment

DIAGNOSTIC CHECKLIST

Image Interpretation Pearls

- Look for SMMCI, CNPAS, &/or choanal atresia when imaging neonates with feeding/breathing difficulties
- Be sure to check for findings of HPE

SELECTED REFERENCES

1. Rosi-Schumacher M et al: Comparison of surgical techniques for the treatment of congenital nasal pyriform aperture stenosis: a systematic review. Ann Otol Rhinol Laryngol. 133(7):639-46, 2024
2. Li J et al: Solitary median maxillary central incisor syndrome: an exploration of the pathogenic mechanism. Front Genet. 13:780930, 2022
3. Garcia Rodriguez R et al: The solitary median maxillary central incisor (SMMCI) syndrome: associations, prenatal diagnosis, and outcomes. Prenat Diagn. 39(6):415-9, 2019
4. Ginat DT et al: CT and MRI of congenital nasal lesions in syndromic conditions. Pediatr Radiol. 45(7):1056-65, 2015

Nasolabial Cyst

TERMINOLOGY

- Rare, benign, developmental cyst in sublabial premaxillary soft tissues, inferior to nasal ala
- Synonyms: Nasoalveolar cyst, Klestadt cyst

IMAGING

- Typically < 2 cm; ≤ 10% bilateral
- Pyriform rim, between upper lip and nasal vestibule
- CT: Nonenhancing hyperdense ± dense fluid levels
  - May cause bone remodeling of maxilla as enlarges
- MR: T2-hyperintense cyst with variable T1 intensity
  - No contrast enhancement of lesion

TOP DIFFERENTIAL DIAGNOSES

- Nasopalatine duct cyst
- Nasolacrimal duct mucocele
- Periapical (radicular) cyst
- Dermoid and epidermoid of oral cavity

PATHOLOGY

- Developmental; 2 theories of pathogenesis
  - Persistence of anlage of nasolacrimal duct or inclusion cyst from formation of facial skeleton
  - Former is favored theory

CLINICAL ISSUES

- Mean age: 40 years; M:F = 1:3
- Presents as facial swelling ± nasal obstruction
- Smooth fluctuant mass, loss of nasolabial fold
- 30% present with infection: Swelling, pain, erythema
- Surgical excision is definitive treatment
- Surgical approaches include intraoral sublabial resection or transnasal endoscopic marsupialization

DIAGNOSTIC CHECKLIST

- Extraosseous origin distinguishes from odontogenic lesions
- Look for bone erosion, extension to turbinate, or nasolacrimal duct obstruction

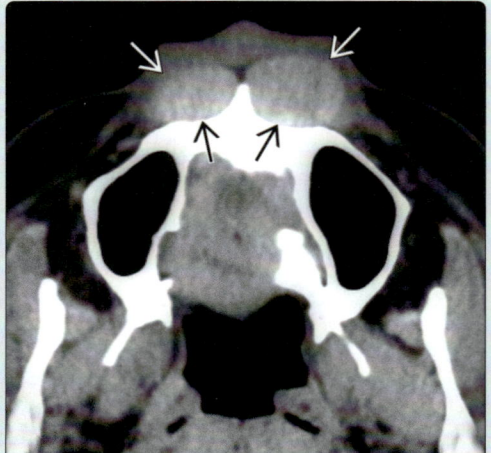
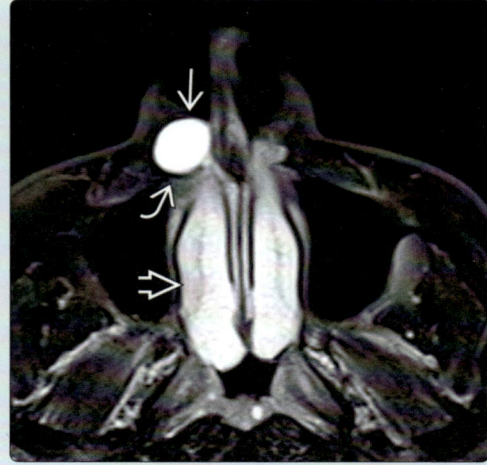

(Left) Axial NECT demonstrates bilateral, well-demarcated, hyperdense, rounded lesions ⮕ anterior to the premaxilla. Lesions result in subtle, left greater than right, remodeling of the maxilla ⮕. Fewer than 10% of nasolabial cyst cases are bilateral. (Right) Axial T2 STIR MR in a patient with right nasolabial swelling shows a well-defined, uniformly T2-hyperintense lesion ⮕ in the right nasolabial region. Note smooth scalloping of the anterior maxillary wall ⮕. The right inferior turbinate ⮕ is not involved in this patient.

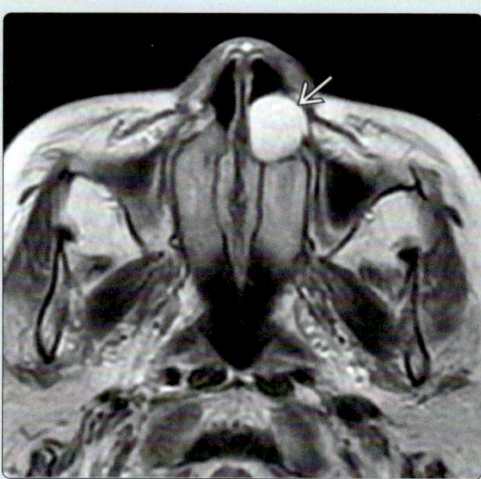
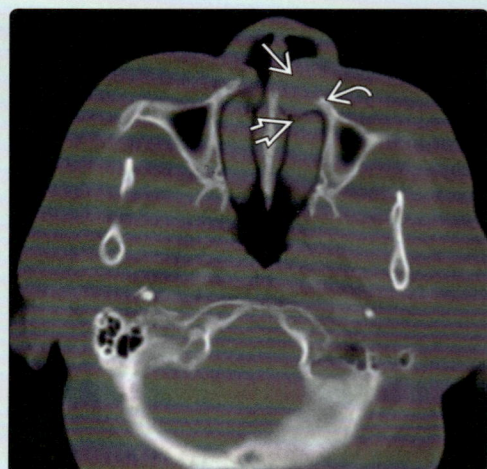

(Left) Axial T1 MR shows an ovoid nasolabial cyst ⮕ along the left piriform rim. T1-hyperintense internal signal likely reflects proteinaceous content. (Right) Axial bony NECT in the same patient demonstrates the ovoid nasolabial cyst ⮕ at the left piriform rim/left nasal vestibule, resulting in mild mass effect on the anterior margin of the left inferior turbinate ⮕. Note the associated smooth remodeling of the frontal process of the left maxilla ⮕.

TERMINOLOGY

Synonyms
- Nasoalveolar cyst, Klestadt cyst

Definitions
- Rare, benign, nonodontogenic, developmental cyst in sublabial premaxillary soft tissues, inferior to nasal ala

IMAGING

General Features
- Best diagnostic clue
  - **Extraosseous** cystic mass in paramedian location at nares
- Location
  - Submucosal, may protrude into anterior nasal floor
  - Pyriform rim, between upper lip and nasal vestibule
- Size
  - Typically < 2 cm; < 10% bilateral

CT Findings
- CECT
  - Iso- to hyperdense nonenhancing soft tissue mass
  - May have dense, dependent fluid levels from calcium oxalate crystals
- Bone CT
  - May cause bone remodeling of maxilla as enlarges

MR Findings
- T1WI
  - Slightly hyperintense from proteinaceous debris
- T2WI
  - Homogeneously hyperintense
- T1WI C+
  - No contrast enhancement of lesion

Imaging Recommendations
- Protocol advice
  - CECT confirms absence of solid component
  - Bone CT images for remodeled bone change

DIFFERENTIAL DIAGNOSIS

Nasopalatine Duct Cyst
- Occurs in nasopalatine duct/incisive foramen → intraosseous midline maxillary alveolus
- Uniform corticated expansion of incisive foramen and nasopalatine canal
- Typically no extraalveolar extension to nasolabial folds unless very large

Nasolacrimal Duct Mucocele
- Failure of canalization of nasolacrimal duct
- Typically appear in infancy
- Usually accompanying dacryocystitis, epiphora, or intranasal mass

Periapical (Radicular) Cyst
- Intraosseous alveolar location ± cortical breakthrough
- Associated with root apex of tooth having caries or periodontal disease

Dermoid and Epidermoid of Oral Cavity
- Usually presents in infancy, childhood
- Very rare in nasolabial area

PATHOLOGY

General Features
- Etiology
  - Developmental; 2 theories of pathogenesis
    - Persistence of anlage of nasolacrimal duct
      - □ Favored theory of formation
    - Inclusion cyst from formation of facial skeleton
      - □ After fusion of medial and lateral nasal processes and maxillary prominence

Gross Pathologic & Surgical Features
- Gray-blue color; thick, fibrous capsule
- Contains mucoid or serous fluid

Microscopic Features
- Pseudostratified, stratified, or mixed respiratory and squamous epithelium with mucous goblet cells

CLINICAL ISSUES

Presentation
- Most common signs/symptoms
  - Swelling of nasolabial fold, upper lip
  - ± nasal obstruction

Demographics
- Age
  - Lesions present in adults; mean age: 40 years
- Sex
  - M:F = 1:3
- Ethnicity
  - More prevalent in Black and Hispanic populations

Natural History & Prognosis
- May grow toward nasolabial fold or vestibule of mouth or nose
- 30% present with infection of cyst

Treatment
- Surgical excision is definitive treatment
  - Sublabial approach; recurrence rare

DIAGNOSTIC CHECKLIST

Image Interpretation Pearls
- **Extraosseous origin** distinguishes from odontogenic lesions

SELECTED REFERENCES

1. Omami G et al: Cysts and benign odontogenic tumors of the jaws. Dent Clin North Am. 68(2):277-95, 2024
2. Liu S et al: Comparative analysis of three common imaging modalities for nasolabial cysts. J Int Med Res. 51(1):3000605221147201, 2023
3. Almutairi A et al: Nasolabial cyst: case report and review of management options. BMC Surg. 20(1):10, 2020
4. Philbert RF et al: Nonodontogenic cysts. Dent Clin North Am. 64(1):63-85, 2020
5. Yeh CH et al: Transcutaneous ultrasonography for diagnosis of nasolabial cyst. J Craniofac Surg. 28(3):e221-2, 2017

Periapical Cyst (Radicular)

TERMINOLOGY

- Synonym = radicular cyst
- **Most common odontogenic cyst**
- Periapical rarefying osteitis = newer term to include periapical cyst, periapical granuloma, and periapical abscess

IMAGING

- **Ovoid cyst (round corticated lucency) at apex of nonvital tooth**
- Millimeters to ≤ 1 cm usually
- May see dental caries: Enamel ± crown erosion
- Nonenhancing lesion at root apex: ↓ T1, ↑ T2

TOP DIFFERENTIAL DIAGNOSES

- Lateral periodontal cyst
- Odontogenic keratocyst
- Dentigerous (follicular) cyst
- Periapical cemental dysplasia

PATHOLOGY

- Develops after inflammation and necrosis of pulp (nonvital tooth)
  - Most often from dental caries, periodontal disease
  - Less often posttraumatic
- Pulp necrosis → growth of epithelial rests of Malassez in periodontal ligament

CLINICAL ISSUES

- Most commonly found on dental radiographs
- Usually asymptomatic unless secondary infection
- Infection → intermittent intense jaw pain
- May progress to periapical abscess ± cellulitis
- Most prevalent in 3rd-5th decades

DIAGNOSTIC CHECKLIST

- Report relationship of lesion to important structures
  - Maxillary teeth: Maxillary sinus
  - Mandible: Inferior alveolar nerve canal

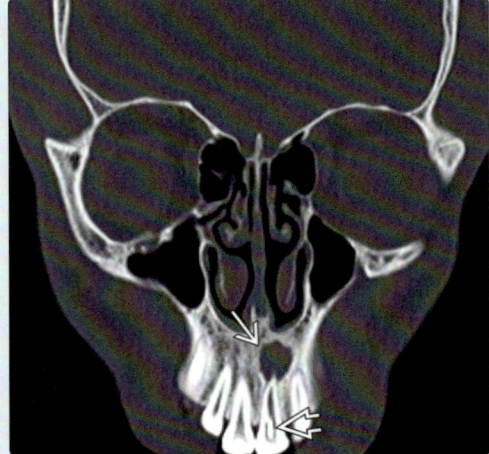
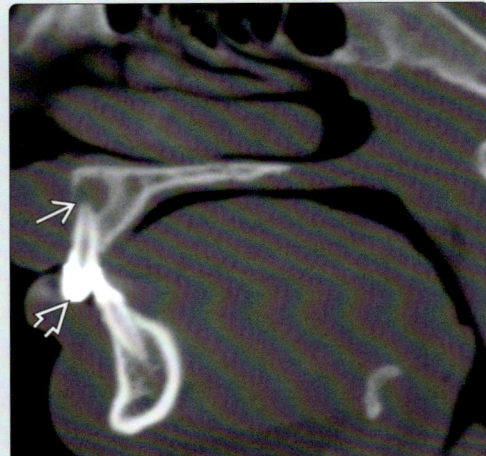

(Left) Coronal bone CT in a 19-year-old who had a head CT after an MVA shows an incidental, well-defined periapical cyst surrounding the apex of the left maxillary central incisor ➡. Note the hyperdense material ➡ in the pulp chamber of the endodontically treated tooth, indicating a nonvital tooth. (Right) Sagittal reformatted bone CT shows a periapical cyst ➡ and dental amalgam ➡ in the same tooth. Periapical cyst occurs secondary to inflammation (or, rarely, trauma) and surrounds the apex of a nonvital tooth.

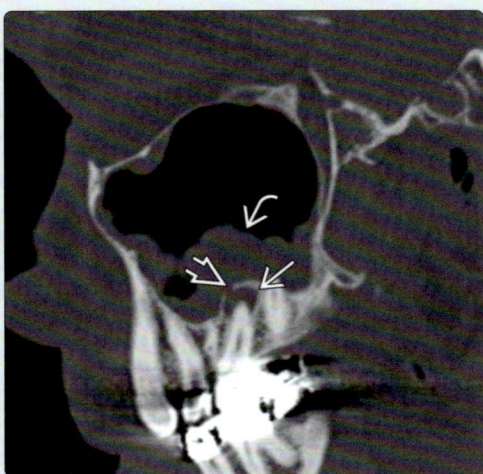
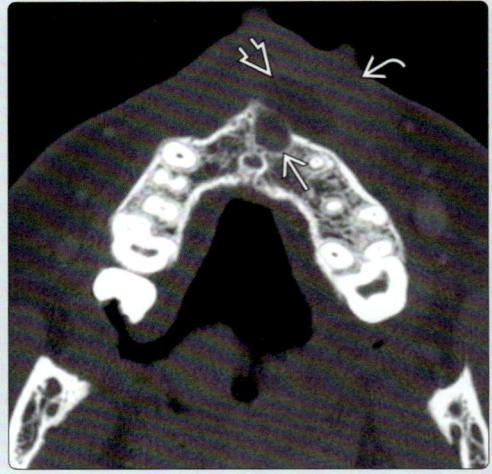

(Left) Sagittal reformatted bone CT shows a moderate-sized maxillary periapical cyst ➡ with a focal dehiscence ➡ in the cyst roof and associated inferior maxillary sinus odontogenic sinusitis ➡. (Right) Axial bone CT in a teenager with facial swelling shows a periapical cyst ➡ surrounding the tip of the left maxillary central incisor root (tip not included in the image). Infection has resulted in buccal surface maxillary cortical disruption, subperiosteal abscess ➡, and surrounding cellulitis ➡.

Periapical Cyst (Radicular)

TERMINOLOGY

Synonyms
- Radicular cyst

Definitions
- Focal cyst at apex (tip of root) of nonvital tooth
- Periapical rarefying osteitis = newer term to include periapical cyst, periapical granuloma, and periapical abscess

IMAGING

General Features
- Best diagnostic clue
  - **Ovoid cyst at apex of tooth with dental caries**
- Size
  - Millimeters to ≤ 1 cm usually; may enlarge to multiple centimeters if neglected
- Morphology
  - Ovoid to round

Imaging Recommendations
- Best imaging tool
  - **Primary imaging modality is dental radiographs**
  - Bone CT best shows lesion for H&N radiologist
- Protocol advice: Thin-section bone CT + 3-plane reformats

CT Findings
- Bone CT: Ovoid to round corticated lucency at **tooth apex**
  - ↑ lucency of pulp
  - May see dental caries: Enamel ± crown erosion
  - Often multiple in cases of extremely poor dentition
  - Maxillary lesions may → maxillary "odontogenic sinusitis"
  - ± cellulitis & abscess

Radiographic Findings
- Corticated cyst at root apex
- Loss of lamina dura
- Widening of periodontal ligament space
- Nonvital tooth + caries, periodontal disease, root resorption

MR Findings
- Nonenhancing lesion at root apex: ↓ T1, ↑ T2

DIFFERENTIAL DIAGNOSIS

Lateral Periodontal Cyst
- Developmental cyst from dental lamina remnants
- Usually associated with lateral root surface of mandibular premolar **vital** teeth
- Asymptomatic tooth; middle-aged men

Odontogenic Keratocyst
- Large, expansile cystic mass, usually within alveolus of posterior mandible
- Small lesions may be **adjacent to root apex**
- WHO 2017 classification reclassified keratocystic odontogenic tumor as odontogenic keratocyst

Dentigerous (Follicular) Cyst
- Developmental lesion around **crown** of unerupted or impacted teeth
- Unilocular cyst, most often mandibular 3rd molar

Periapical Cemental Dysplasia
- Early lesion may be lucent, gradual calcification with maturation
- Tooth is **vital**

PATHOLOGY

General Features
- Etiology
  - **Develops after inflammation and necrosis of pulp (nonvital tooth)**
    - Most often from dental caries, periodontal disease
    - Less often posttraumatic
  - Pulp necrosis → growth of epithelial rests of Malassez in periodontal ligament
  - Central liquefaction necrosis of epithelial rests → cyst formation

CLINICAL ISSUES

Presentation
- Most common signs/symptoms
  - Usually **asymptomatic** unless secondary infection
- Other signs/symptoms
  - Intermittent intense jaw pain or pain with chewing

Demographics
- Age
  - Any age; most prevalent in 3rd-5th decades
- Epidemiology
  - **Most common odontogenic cyst**
  - ~ 15% of all periapical lesions

Natural History & Prognosis
- May progress to periapical abscess ± cellulitis

Treatment
- Treatment depends on degree of inflammation
  - Endodontic therapy (root canal)
  - Tooth extraction with antibiotics if destruction of tooth is severe and tooth is nonrestorable

DIAGNOSTIC CHECKLIST

Consider
- Small odontogenic keratocyst near root apex may mimic radicular cyst

Image Interpretation Pearls
- Ovoid lesion at tooth apex with dental caries

Reporting Tips
- Report relationship of lesion to adjacent structures
  - Maxillary teeth: Maxillary sinus
  - Mandible: Inferior alveolar nerve canal

SELECTED REFERENCES

1. Choi WJ et al: Imaging approach for jaw and maxillofacial bone tumors with updates from the 2022 World Health Organization classification. World J Radiol. 16(8):294-316, 2024
2. Vered M et al: Update from the 5th edition of the World Health Organization Classification of Head and Neck Tumors: Odontogenic and Maxillofacial Bone Tumours. Head Neck Pathol. 16(1):63-75, 2022
3. Mupparapu M et al: Differential diagnosis of periapical radiopacities and radiolucencies. Dent Clin North Am. 64(1):163-89, 2020

KEY FACTS

TERMINOLOGY

- Benign, developmental jaw cyst associated with crown of unerupted tooth
- Synonym = follicular cyst

IMAGING

- Well-circumscribed, expansile cyst **surrounding crown of unerupted or impacted tooth**
- Sclerotic border spares osseous cortex
- Typically displaces teeth, rarely resorbs
- 75% found in mandible
- 3rd molars (mandibular > maxillary) > maxillary canines

TOP DIFFERENTIAL DIAGNOSES

- Odontogenic keratocyst
- Ameloblastoma
- Periapical (radicular) cyst

PATHOLOGY

- Arises after developmental anomaly during formation of enamel (amelogenesis)
- Slow-growing, benign cyst
- 20% of all odontogenic cysts

CLINICAL ISSUES

- Most patients asymptomatic
- Symptomatic if cyst infection or fracture
- Recurrence rare following complete resection
- Ameloblastomas may develop in cyst wall
- Malignant transformation to carcinoma is rare

DIAGNOSTIC CHECKLIST

- When reviewing odontogenic cysts, distinguishing lesions can be difficult
  - Cyst always related to unerupted tooth crown
  - Typically remains unilocular even when large

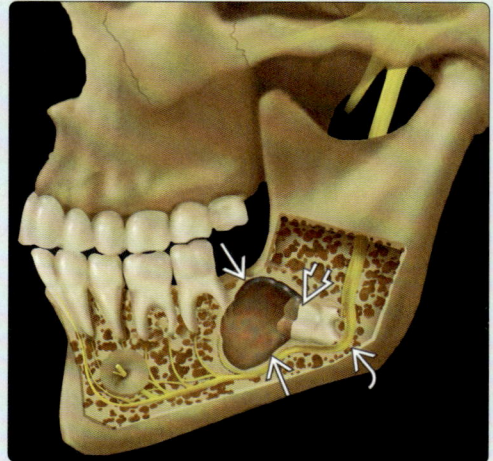
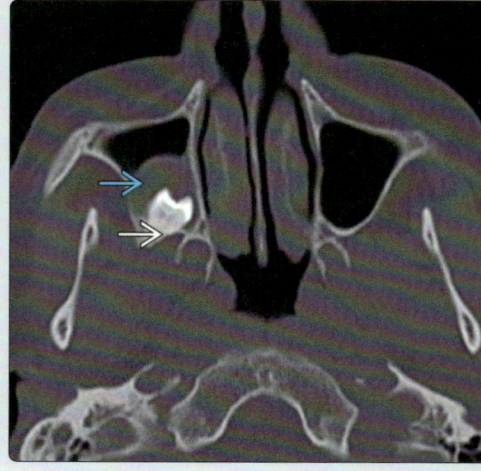

(Left) Lateral graphic of the mandible with the lateral cortical surface removed depicts a classic unilocular dentigerous cyst ⇥ intimately related to the crown ⇥ of the unerupted 3rd mandibular molar tooth. The inferior alveolar canal ⇥ is displaced by the molar. (Right) Axial bone window CT through the maxillary sinuses shows an unerupted maxillary molar tooth ⇥ projecting into the sinus with a dentigerous cyst surrounding the crown ⇥ arising from the cementoenamel junction.

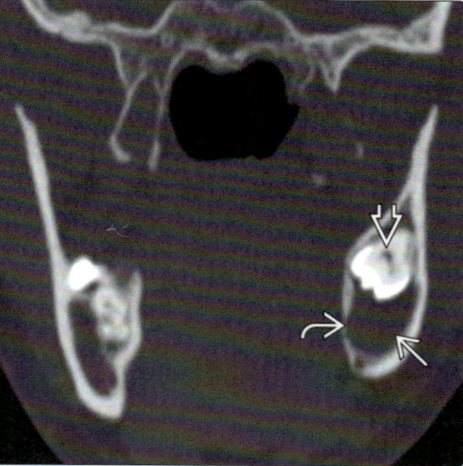
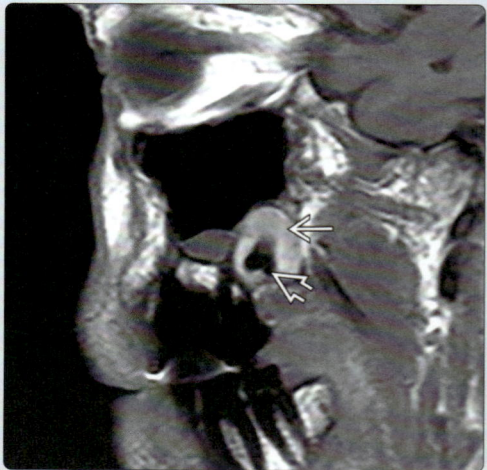

(Left) Coronal bone CT demonstrates an impacted left 3rd mandibular molar ⇥ associated with the smooth-walled cyst ⇥ that expands the mandible and thins the lingual cortex ⇥. The cyst abuts the crown and has no calcifications or periosteal reaction. (Right) Sagittal T1 MR demonstrates hyperintense T1 signal intensity ⇥ within the cystic lesion associated with a right maxillary unerupted molar tooth ⇥. T1 hyperintensity may be due to proteinaceous material or cholesterol crystals within the cyst.

TERMINOLOGY

Synonyms

- Follicular cyst

Definitions

- Benign, developmental jaw cyst associated with crown of unerupted tooth
- Dentigerous means "having teeth;" lesion is intimately associated with tooth

IMAGING

General Features

- Best diagnostic clue
  - Well-circumscribed, expansile cyst around **crown of unerupted or impacted tooth**
- Location
  - **75% found in mandible**
  - 3rd molars (mandibular > maxillary) > maxillary canines
- Size
  - Variable; ≥ 1 cm
- Morphology
  - Unilocular cyst; rarely multilocular

Radiographic Findings

- Radiography
  - Well-demarcated cyst around crown of unerupted tooth
    - Typically displaces teeth
    - Less commonly resorbs apical tooth structures

CT Findings

- Bone CT
  - Thin-walled, well-circumscribed cyst surrounding crown of unerupted tooth with radiolucent area attached to tooth at cementoenamel junction
  - Sclerotic border spares osseous cortex
  - Maxillary lesion may extend into sinus
  - Tendency to displace tooth in opposite direction of cyst

MR Findings

- T1WI
  - Low to intermediate signal intensity cyst
    - May have ↑ T1 signal due to protein or cholesterol
- T2WI
  - Typically hyperintense signal in cyst
  - Thin, corticated rim is hypointense
- T1WI C+ FS
  - No solid enhancement within cyst
  - Cyst wall with thin rim of uniform enhancement

Imaging Recommendations

- Best imaging tool
  - Thin-slice bone CT
- Protocol advice
  - **Bone algorithm** thin-section CT of face with MPR

DIFFERENTIAL DIAGNOSIS

Odontogenic Keratocyst

- Uni- or multilocular cystic mass, not arising from crown
- Envelops entire unerupted tooth
- More likely to have aggressive bone changes

Ameloblastoma

- May be unilocular, exactly mimicking dentigerous cyst
- May be unilocular with enhancing nodule
- May be multilocular expansile mass

Periapical (Radicular) Cyst

- Small cyst at root of tooth (tooth apex)
- Associated with caries or periodontal disease

PATHOLOGY

General Features

- Etiology
  - Developmental anomaly occurring during formation of enamel (amelogenesis)
  - Fluid accumulates between reduced enamel epithelium & surface → cyst surrounding crown

CLINICAL ISSUES

Presentation

- Most common signs/symptoms
  - Most patients **asymptomatic**
- Other signs/symptoms
  - Symptomatic if cyst infection or fracture

Demographics

- Age
  - 2nd-4th decades
- Epidemiology
  - 2nd most common jaw cyst after radicular cysts

Natural History & Prognosis

- Slow-growing, benign cyst
- Recurrence rare following complete resection
- Mural ameloblastomas may occur
- Malignant transformation to carcinoma is rare

Treatment

- Enucleation of cyst & extraction of unerupted tooth
- Marsupialization or fenestration of cyst may preserve permanent tooth in children

DIAGNOSTIC CHECKLIST

Reporting Tips

- Describe bone remodeling secondary to lesion
  - Displacement of inferior alveolar canal
  - Bowing of floor of maxillary sinus, extension to orbit

SELECTED REFERENCES

1. Sueyoshi T et al: Comparison of computed tomographic findings for radiolucent lesions of the mandibular ameloblastoma, odontogenic keratocyst, dentigerous cyst, and simple bone cyst. J Dent Sci. 20(1):605-12, 2025
2. Langä MC et al: Dentigerous cysts in children: clinical, radiological, and healing aspects. Medicina (Kaunas). 60(7), 2024
3. Rajendra Santosh AB: Odontogenic cysts. Dent Clin North Am. 64(1):105-19, 2020
4. Mosier KM: Magnetic resonance imaging of the maxilla and mandible: signal characteristics and features in the differential diagnosis of common lesions. Top Magn Reson Imaging. 24(1):23-37, 2015

Odontogenic Keratocyst

TERMINOLOGY

- Odontogenic keratocyst (OKC)
  - Previously classified as keratocystic odontogenic tumor (KOT)
- Benign cyst of jaw with aggressive behavior and high recurrence rate

IMAGING

- May displace developing teeth or resorb roots of erupted teeth
  - **Not** related to unerupted crown
- Bone CT: Unilocular cystic mass with sclerotic rim
  - Expansile solitary unilocular jaw lesion
  - 75% posterior mandible, often near 3rd molar
  - Extends longitudinally in mandible
- CECT: No solid enhancement
- C+ MR: Cystic with thin, enhancing rim
  - Greater enhancement with recurrent OKC

TOP DIFFERENTIAL DIAGNOSES

- Periapical (radicular) cyst
- Dentigerous (follicular) cyst
- Ameloblastoma

PATHOLOGY

- Thin-walled, friable cyst containing fluid and debris
- Viscosity of contents depends on keratinaceous debris
  - Straw-colored fluid → pus-like → "cheesy" mass

CLINICAL ISSUES

- 50% present with jaw swelling
- Rapid growth and high recurrence rate

DIAGNOSTIC CHECKLIST

- 7% of OKCs are multiple
- If multiple OKCs, consider **basal cell nevus syndrome**
- Look for dural calcifications on same CT scan

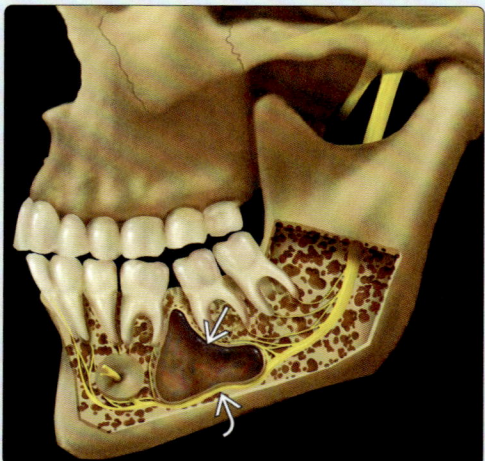
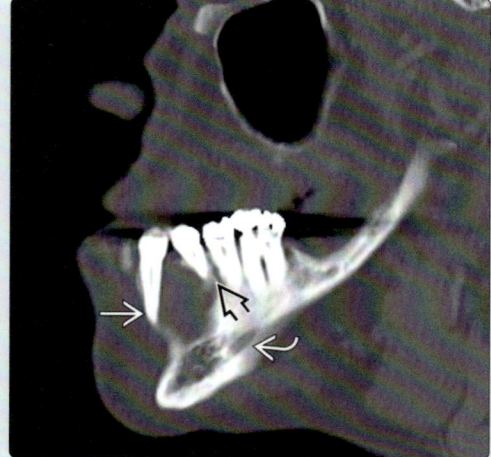

(Left) Lateral graphic of the mandible with the lateral buccal cortex removed illustrates features of a typical odontogenic keratocyst (OKC). A cystic lesion ➡ splays the roots of the 1st and 2nd molar teeth, enlarging the marrow space and displacing the inferior alveolar nerve ➡. (Right) Oblique sagittal NECT shows an expansile cystic mass splaying the roots of the left mandibular canine ➡ and 1st premolar ➡, consistent with OKC. The inferior alveolar nerve canal ➡ is visible posteroinferior to the mass.

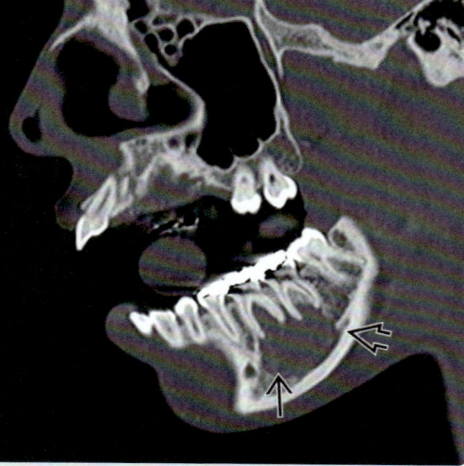
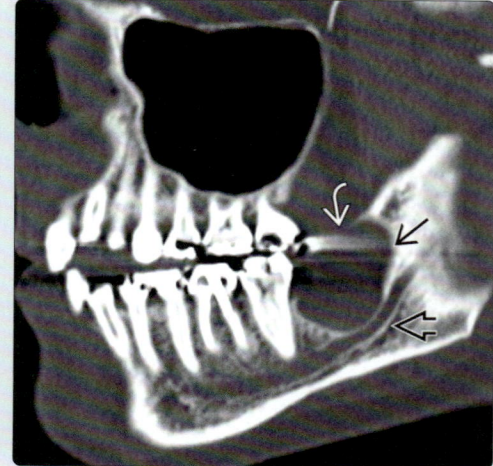

(Left) Oblique sagittal NECT in a 36-year-old woman who felt a "lump under her gum" shows an expansile mass ➡ inferior to the roots of the 1st and 2nd mandibular molars in this case of OKC. The inferior alveolar nerve canal ➡ appears to communicate with the area of bone loss. (Right) Oblique sagittal NECT shows a unilocular cystic lesion ➡ at the former location of the 3rd mandibular molar, found to be an OKC. The inferior alveolar nerve canal ➡ is displaced inferiorly by the lesion. There is cortical dehiscence ➡ superiorly.

TERMINOLOGY

Abbreviations
- Odontogenic keratocyst (OKC)

Synonyms
- Keratocystic odontogenic tumor (KOT), primordial cyst

IMAGING

General Features
- Best diagnostic clue
  - Expansile, solitary, unilocular jaw lesion
- Location
  - **75% posterior mandible**, often near 3rd molar
  - In maxilla, most commonly near canine
- Size
  - 1-9 cm; average: 3 cm

Radiographic Findings
- Radiography
  - Expansile cystic mass; may have "cloudy" lumen
  - 50% unilocular, lucent with sclerotic rim
    - Multilocular jaw cyst favors OKC over dentigerous cyst
  - May displace developing teeth, resorb roots of erupted teeth, cause tooth extrusion

CT Findings
- CECT
  - No detectable enhancement
- Bone CT
  - Corticated **expansile cystic mass**, ± scalloped border
  - Typically extends longitudinally in mandible
    - Typically only mild buccolingual expansion
  - May be near unerupted tooth but **not** crown
  - Density varies with viscosity of contents

MR Findings
- T1WI
  - Intermediate to high signal intensity due to ortho-/parakeratin &/or hemorrhage
- T2WI
  - Heterogeneous, low to high signal intensity
- T1WI C+
  - Thin or no enhancing rim, no solid mass
  - Greater enhancement seen with recurrent OKC

Imaging Recommendations
- Best imaging tool
  - CT allows complete evaluation for diagnosis
    - Bone algorithm best delineates lesion
    - CECT determines no solid enhancement
- Protocol advice
  - Thin-section CT with multiplanar reformats

DIFFERENTIAL DIAGNOSIS

Periapical (Radicular) Cyst
- Unilocular cyst associated with tooth root
- Associated with dental caries and infection

Dentigerous (Follicular) Cyst
- Developmental unilocular cyst

- Arises from unerupted tooth crown

Ameloblastoma
- Expansile, "bubbly" lesion, enhancing wall and nodules

PATHOLOGY

General Features
- Etiology
  - Arises from remnants of **dental lamina**
  - Now reclassified as cyst (WHO 2017)
- Associated abnormalities
  - 7% of OKCs are multiple
    - **50%** have **basal cell nevus syndrome (BCNS)**
  - Associated with Marfan and Noonan syndromes

Gross Pathologic & Surgical Features
- Thin, friable cyst containing fluid and keratin debris
  - Straw-colored fluid → pus-like → "cheesy" mass

Microscopic Features
- Fibrous wall lined by squamous epithelium
- Microcysts or daughter cysts may be seen

CLINICAL ISSUES

Presentation
- Most common signs/symptoms
  - 50% present with jaw swelling
- Other signs/symptoms
  - Pain, paresthesia, trismus

Demographics
- Age
  - Wide range; peaks in 4th decade
- Epidemiology
  - 5-10% of jaw cysts

Natural History & Prognosis
- Rapid growth and high recurrence rate

Treatment
- Enucleation with aggressive curettage

DIAGNOSTIC CHECKLIST

Consider
- If multiple OKCs, consider **BCNS**
  - Look for dural calcifications on CT

Image Interpretation Pearls
- Classic appearance is unilocular mandibular cyst
  - No solid enhancing tissue, often involves 3rd molar

SELECTED REFERENCES
1. Grover S et al: Management regulations for odontogenic keratocyst: a case report and review of the literature. J Med Case Rep. 18(1):152, 2024
2. Castillo-Tobar A et al: Clinical, radiographic, pathological and inherited characteristics of odontogenic keratocyst in nevoid basal cell carcinoma syndrome: a study in three Chilean families. Oral Radiol. 39(3):518-27, 2023
3. Sundaragiri KS et al: Non syndromic synchronous multiple odontogenic keratocysts in a western Indian population: a series of four cases. J Clin Exp Dent. 10(8):e831-6, 2018
4. Mosier KM: Magnetic resonance imaging of the maxilla and mandible: signal characteristics and features in the differential diagnosis of common lesions. Top Magn Reson Imaging. 24(1):23-37, 2015

(Left) *Panoramic plain film in a 12-year-old boy shows an expansile lytic lesion* ⮕ *in the left posterior mandible. The maxillary and mandibular 3rd molars are unerupted, as expected for age.* **(Right)** *Oblique sagittal NECT in the same patient shows an expansile lesion in the posterior mandible, not associated with the crown of the unerupted 3rd molar* ⮕*, consistent with an OKC. This lesion extends into the condylar neck* ⮕ *and the coronoid process* ⮕ *with focal osseous dehiscence* ⮕*.*

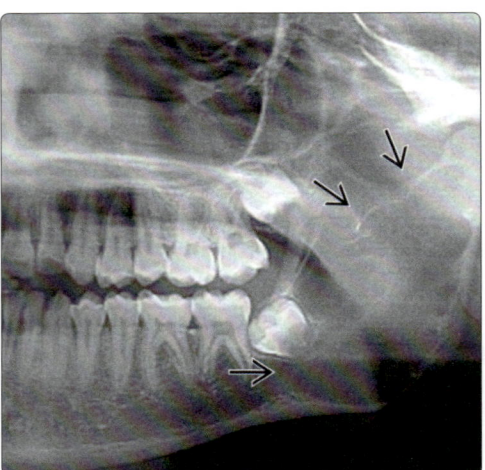
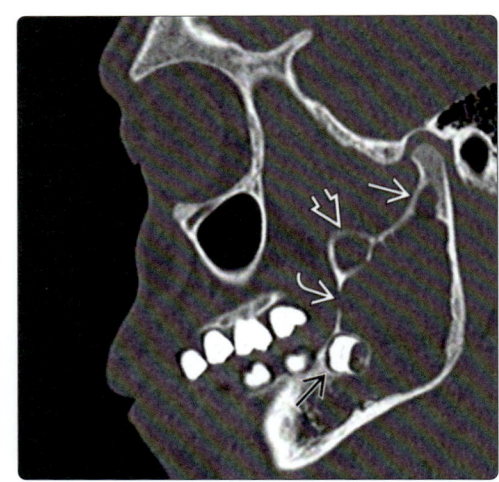

(Left) *Axial CECT in a 41-year-old woman shows an expansile left mandibular mass with an area of marked demineralization of the lingual cortex* ⮕*. Peripherally enhancing fluid density in the masticator space is consistent with superimposed abscess* ⮕*.* **(Right)** *Axial CECT bone window in the same patient shows a 2nd mass more anterior and inferior in the mandible with an irregular, thickened periphery* ⮕*, consistent with chronic inflammation. Both masses were histologically proven to be an OKC.*

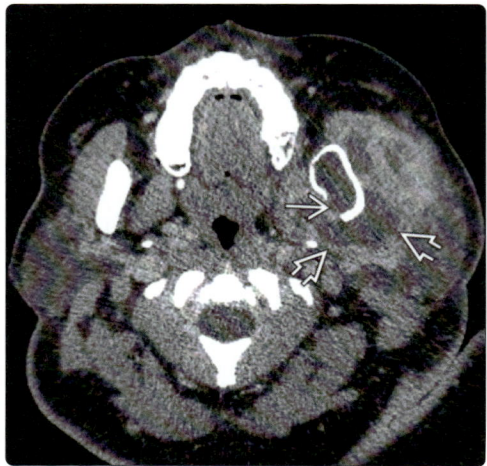
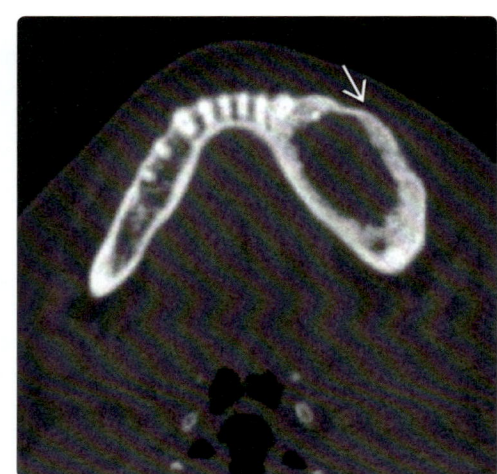

(Left) *Axial bone CT demonstrates an expansile cystic mandibular lesion* ⮕ *associated with an unerupted right 3rd molar* ⮕*, not associated with the tooth crown* ⮕*, and pathology proven to an OKC.* **(Right)** *Sagittal bone CT in a 13-year-old boy with basal cell nevus syndrome (BCNS) shows expansile cystic lesions in the posterior maxilla* ⮕ *and mandible* ⮕*, compatible with OKCs. Tentorial dural calcifications* ⮕ *are also present, an additional imaging feature of BCNS.*

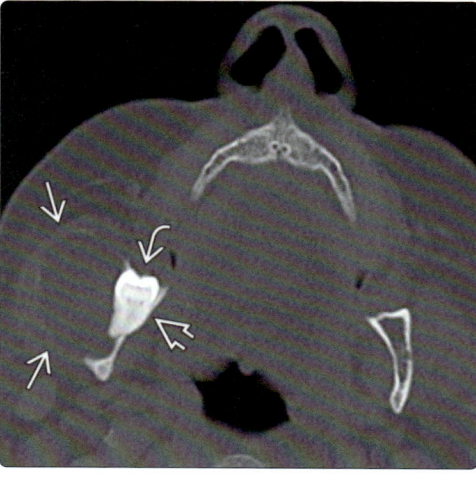
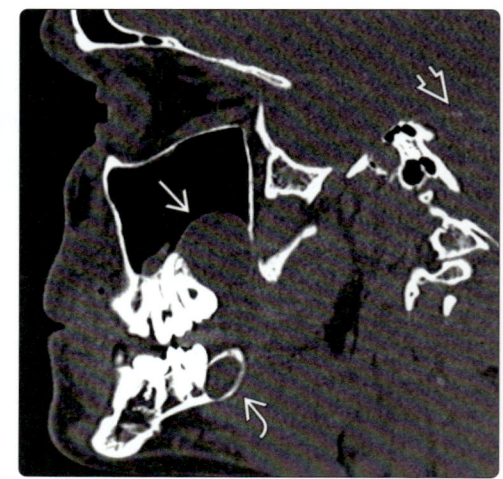

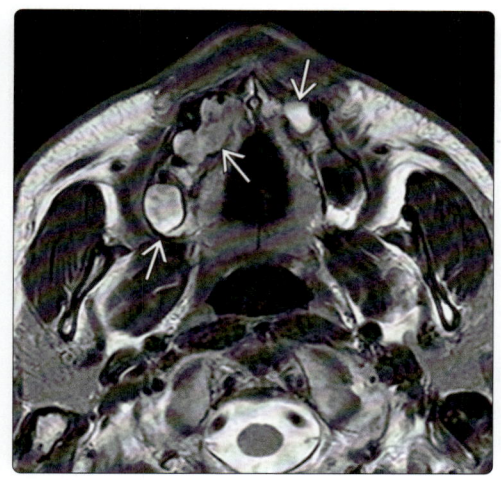

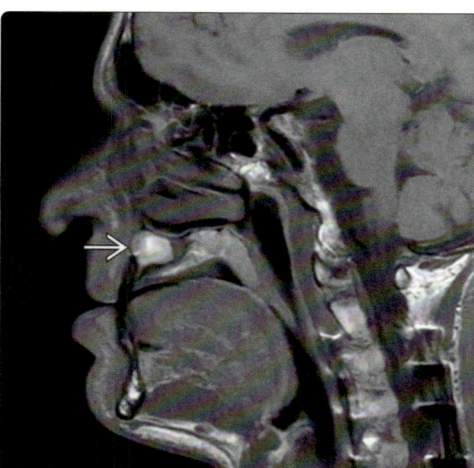

(Left) Axial T2WI MR in a 29-year-old man with BCNS shows multiple expansile hyperintense masses in the bilateral maxilla ➡, consistent with OKCs, more numerous and prominent on the right than on the left. (Right) Sagittal T1WI MR in the same patient shows hyperintensity of one of the maxillary OKCs ➡. The intrinsic T1 signal intensity reflects proteinaceous content of the OKC. Artifact from cervical spine fusion hardware is seen in the lower right-hand corner.

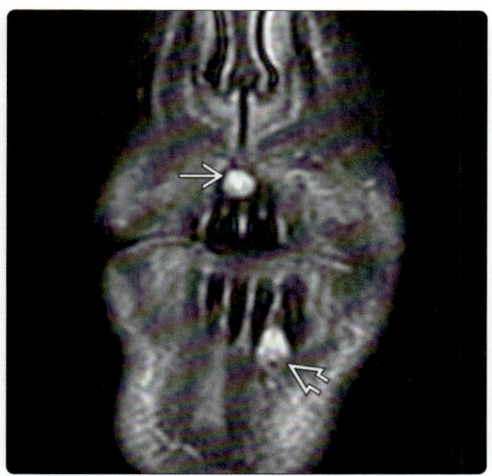

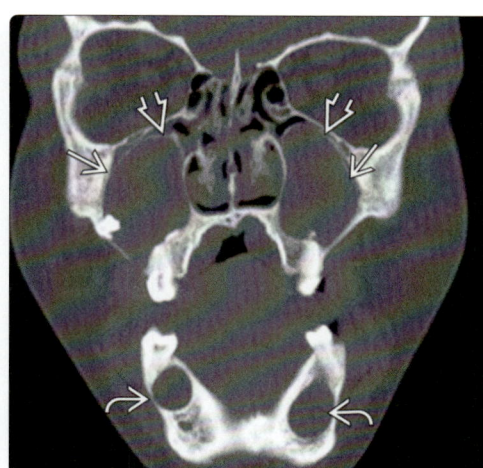

(Left) Coronal T2WI MR in the same patient shows masses consistent with OKCs in the maxilla ➡ and mandible ➡. These OKCs have intermediate T2 signal intensity. (Right) Coronal bone CT in a 15-year-old girl with BCNS shows bilateral expansile OKCs ➡ projecting into the maxillary sinuses. Note osseous margins ➡, inferior to the orbital floors. There are smaller OKCs in the bilateral mandible ➡.

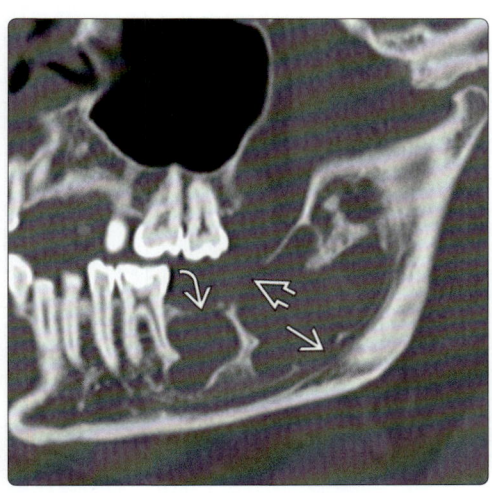

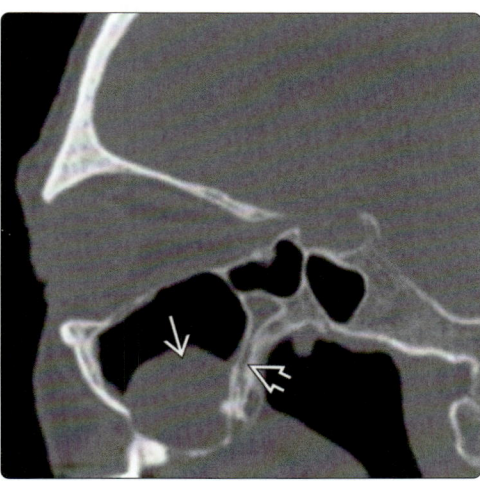

(Left) Oblique sagittal NECT in a 39-year-old man with a remote history of a partially resected OKC is shown. The recurrent OKC is thinning the osseous covering of the inferior alveolar canal ➡. There is also cortical dehiscence ➡ superiorly. There is also a more anterior component of the lesion with similar focal dehiscence ➡. (Right) Oblique sagittal NECT in a 60-year-old man shows an expansile mass in the posterior maxilla ➡, proven to be an OKC. Note the proximity to the greater palatine nerve canal ➡.

Simple Bone Cyst (Traumatic)

KEY FACTS

TERMINOLOGY

- Solitary bony cavity; "cyst" designation is misnomer

IMAGING

- CT: Solitary, unilocular, well-corticated lucent area in body, ramus, or condyle of mandible
  - Homogeneously iso- to hypodense with no internal calcification or matrix
- T2 MR: Hyperintense; no fluid-fluid levels
- T1 C+ MR: Delayed enhancement key

TOP DIFFERENTIAL DIAGNOSES

- Periapical (radicular) cyst
- Giant cell granuloma of mandible-maxilla
- Odontogenic keratocyst
- Aneurysmal bone cyst

PATHOLOGY

- Cystic cavity with connective tissue membrane; no epithelial lining
- "Traumatic" designation misnomer; < 1/2 associated with prior trauma

CLINICAL ISSUES

- Incidental finding on imaging/ less commonly presenting with pain & swelling
- 10-30 years
- Treatment: Surgical curettage ± bone grafting allows both diagnosis & treatment by generation of blood clot in vacant cavity

DIAGNOSTIC CHECKLIST

- Look for association with teeth/teeth roots, cortical thinning & erosion, enhancement pattern to exclude other odontogenic lesions

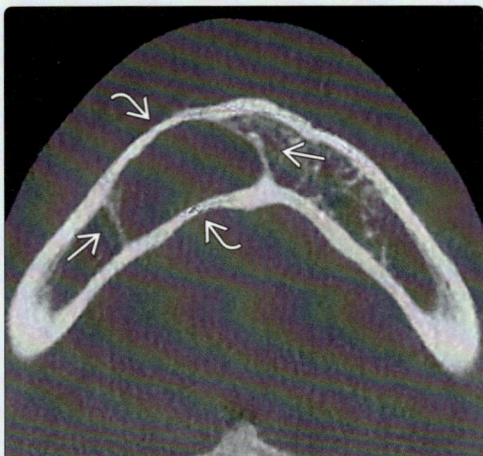
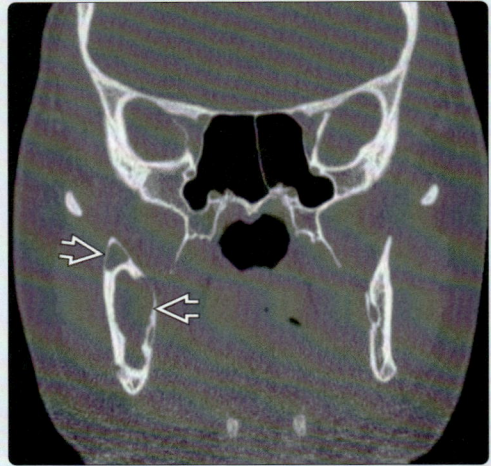

(Left) Axial CBCT shows a unilocular simple bone cyst in the anterior mandible with well-defined, corticated margins ➡. Despite the size, there is no significant bony expansion and the cortex ➡ is intact. (Right) Coronal bone CT demonstrates a lucent ➡ right mandibular lesion involving/expanding the posterior mandibular body, angle, and ramus. The cortex is thinned over the lucent component but intact over the sclerotic component. There is a thin lucent zone surrounding the sclerotic component.

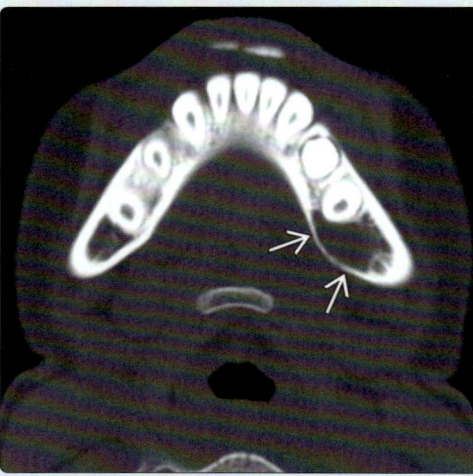
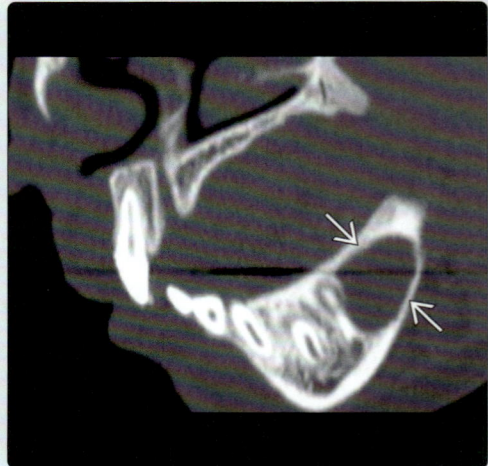

(Left) Axial bone CT in a teenager with an incidental lucency on dental radiographs shows a well-defined, mildly expansile, unilocular cyst in the left mandible ➡. Notice thinning of the lingual cortex without periosteal reaction or associated extraosseous soft tissue mass. (Right) Sagittal bone CT in the same patient again shows a well-defined mandibular cyst ➡ with cortical thinning inferiorly without internal septations or periosteal reaction.

TERMINOLOGY

Abbreviations
- Simple bone cyst (SBC)

Synonyms
- Solitary or traumatic bone cyst

Definitions
- SBC: Solitary bony cavity; "cyst" designation is misnomer, as there is no epithelial lining

IMAGING

General Features
- Best diagnostic clue
  - Single, corticated lucent area in body, ramus, or condyle of mandible
- Size
  - Typically ≥ 1 cm
- Morphology
  - Well-defined, typically nonexpansile; if present, very mild

Radiographic Findings
- Intraoral plain film
  - Well-defined, unilocular radiolucency superimposed over or below root apices
    - May scallop up between teeth
  - Lamina dura & periodontal ligament space intact

CT Findings
- CECT
  - Mildly enhancing at periphery
- Bone CT
  - Solitary, well-corticated lucent area in body, ramus, or condyle of mandible
  - Typically **nonexpansile**; if present, very mild
    - Bone margins uniform, not scalloped
  - Sclerotic margins or osteophytic reaction at cortical surface possible
    - No internal septations
  - No association with teeth

MR Findings
- T2WI
  - Homogeneous hyperintensity without fluid-fluid levels
- T1WI C+
  - Mildly enhancing
  - Dynamic contrast: Enhancement from margin to center on delayed images

DIFFERENTIAL DIAGNOSIS

Periapical (Radicular) Cyst
- Associated with caries & periodontal disease/devitalized teeth
- Lucent or lytic lesion at tooth root apex
- Lamina dura & periodontal ligament space is lost in associated tooth

Giant Cell Granuloma of Mandible-Maxilla
- Large lesions usually have septations
- Tend to be expansile

Odontogenic Keratocyst
- Previously termed keratocystic odontogenic tumor
- Older patients (> 30 years of age)
- Bone margin not as well defined or corticated
- Large unilocular lesions expand longitudinally or concentrically

Unicystic Ameloblastoma
- Older patients (> 30 years of age)
- Bone margin not as well defined or corticated
- Enhancement throughout lesion on CT, MR

Aneurysmal Bone Cyst
- More prevalent in maxilla than SBC
- Multilocular
- Fluid-fluid levels on T2 MR

PATHOLOGY

General Features
- Etiology
  - Unknown; hypothesized etiologies include
    - Medullary infarct following trauma but < 1/2 associated with prior trauma
    - Disturbance in osteoblast differentiation or altered bone metabolism
- Associated abnormalities
  - May be found adjacent to cementoosseous lesions, osteomas, or hypercementosis

Gross Pathologic & Surgical Features
- Empty/partially empty bone cavity with straw-colored fluid or old necrosis

Microscopic Features
- Cystic cavity with connective tissue membrane; **no epithelial lining**

CLINICAL ISSUES

Presentation
- Most common signs/symptoms
  - Incidental finding on imaging
- Other signs/symptoms
  - Pain, swelling if associated with trauma

Demographics
- Age
  - 10-30 years

Natural History & Prognosis
- Recurrence rate variable (~ 2-26%)
- Spontaneous resolution possible

Treatment
- Surgery to exclude other odontogenic lesions

SELECTED REFERENCES

1. Kaygisiz ÖF et al: Evaluation of cyst treatment technique, cyst type, size differences and healing by fractal analysis. BMC Oral Health. 24(1):1271, 2024
2. McLean AC et al: Cystic lesions of the jaws: the top 10 differential diagnoses to ponder. Head Neck Pathol. 17(1):85-98, 2023

TERMINOLOGY

- Definition: Developmental cyst arising from nasopalatine duct

IMAGING

- Bone CT/CBCT findings
  - Well-circumscribed, rounded enlargement of maxillary incisive canal
  - Incisive canal with diameter **> 1 cm** is presumed nasopalatine duct cyst (NPDC)
  - Lamina dura and periodontal ligament space of adjacent teeth intact
  - CBCT better to differentiate NPDC from normal duct
- MR findings
  - Homogeneously iso- to hyperintense T1, hyperintense T2 signal, nonenhancing

TOP DIFFERENTIAL DIAGNOSES

- Periapical (radicular) cyst
- Residual cyst
- Apical periodontitis
- Median palatal cyst
- Odontogenic keratocyst
- Dentigerous (follicular) cyst

CLINICAL ISSUES

- Most common nonodontogenic fissural cyst
- Clinical presentation
  - Incidental finding on CT or MR
  - Less commonly pain, swelling of anterior maxilla
- Treatment: Enucleation via palatine or buccal approach
  - Low recurrence rate: < 2%

DIAGNOSTIC CHECKLIST

- Single, rounded, corticated lucent cyst in midline maxilla
- Look for widening along paired nasopalatine ducts
- Report extension to nasal cavity or displacement of teeth by larger lesions

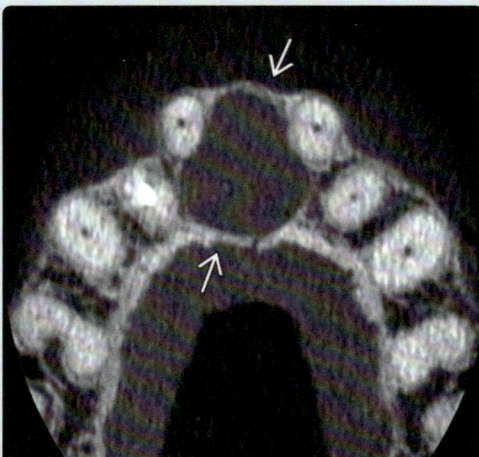
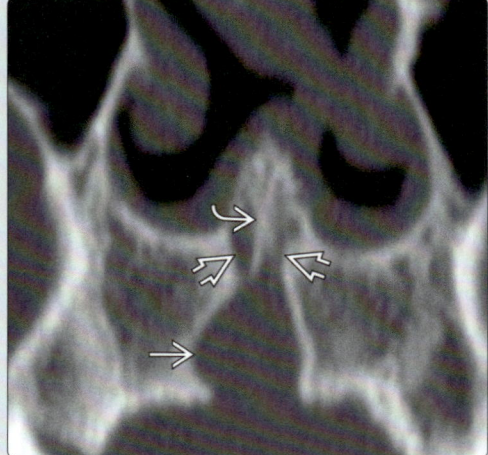

(Left) Axial CBCT shows corticated, concentric expansion of the incisive canal in the midline maxillary alveolus ➡, dorsal to the maxillary central incisor teeth, typical of a nasopalatine duct cyst. (Right) Coronal bone CT shows an expansile nasopalatine duct cyst ➡ extending along the paired nasopalatine ducts ➡, which are seen separated by a thin, bony septation ➡.

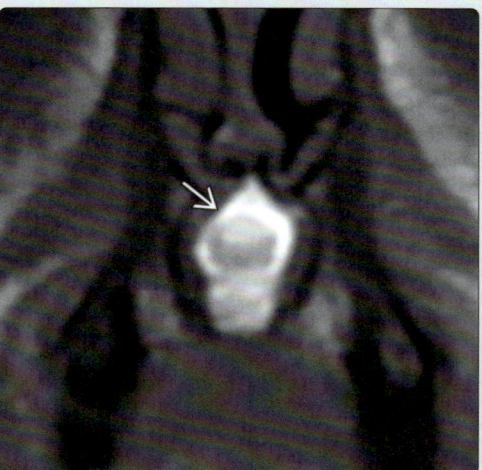
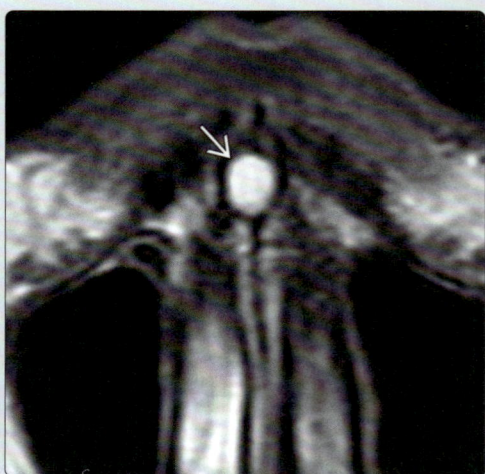

(Left) Coronal T1 MR shows a well-defined, high signal intensity lesion, consistent with a nasopalatine duct cyst in the anterior midline maxilla ➡. (Right) Axial T2 MR shows the classic MR appearance of a nasopalatine duct cyst. Note the uniformly round, homogeneously T2-hyperintense area in the midline maxilla ➡ without cortical disruption or splaying of the teeth.

TERMINOLOGY

Abbreviations

- Nasopalatine duct cyst (NPDC)

Synonyms

- Incisive canal cyst

Definitions

- Developmental cyst arising from nasopalatine duct
- **Most common** nonodontogenic fissural cyst

IMAGING

General Features

- Best diagnostic clue
  - Well-circumscribed, rounded enlargement of incisive canal in maxilla
- Location
  - Incisive canal lingual (posterior) to maxillary central incisor teeth
- Size
  - Incisive canal with diameter **> 1 cm** presumed NPDC

Imaging Recommendations

- Best imaging tool
  - Thin-section bone algorithm CT
- Protocol advice
  - Thin-section facial bone CT with axial, coronal, sagittal reformations

Radiographic Findings

- Dental radiography: Well-circumscribed, corticated radiolucency extending superiorly from between maxillary central incisors

CT Findings

- Bone CT: **Smooth, round > 1-cm incisive canal**
  - ± thinning and dehiscence of lingual cortex maxilla
  - Larger lesions will extend to nasal cavity
  - Lamina dura and periodontal ligament (PDL) space of adjacent teeth intact

MR Findings

- Homogeneously iso- to ↑ T1, ↑ T2 signal
- Typically nonenhancing
  - May enhance with inflammatory component

DIFFERENTIAL DIAGNOSIS

Periapical (Radicular) Cyst

- Cyst arising from infected tooth
- Associated with caries/periodontal disease in teeth
- **Not** centrally located within incisive canal but may involve it secondarily

Residual Cyst

- Persistent radicular cyst remaining after extraction or loss of infected tooth
- Adjacent to, **not** centrally located within, incisive canal

Apical Periodontitis

- Infection at apex of tooth root associated with caries/periodontal disease

- Loss of lamina dura and widened PDL space at/around root apex
- Lytic area millimeters to centimeters in size; noncorticated
- May extend into incisive canal secondarily

Median Palatal Cyst

- Developmental cyst of newborn
- Located at junction of hard and soft palate

Odontogenic Keratocyst

- Expansile, solitary, unilocular jaw lesion
- When large, expands and may erode maxilla
- Typically arises in canine region in maxilla, molars in mandible; rare in midline maxilla

Dentigerous (Follicular) Cyst

- Most common odontogenic cyst
- Arises from around **crown** of unerupted or impacted teeth

PATHOLOGY

General Features

- Etiology
  - Fissural cyst arising from embryologic remnants of incisive canal between oral and nasal cavities

Microscopic Features

- Cyst lined by respiratory ± stratified squamous epithelium

CLINICAL ISSUES

Presentation

- Most common signs/symptoms
  - Incidental finding on CT or MR
- Other signs/symptoms
  - Pain, swelling of anterior maxilla

Demographics

- Age
  - Typically diagnosed at 30-40 years of age

Natural History & Prognosis

- Recurrence rate very low; < 2% when enucleated

Treatment

- Surgical enucleation via palatine or buccal approach

DIAGNOSTIC CHECKLIST

Image Interpretation Pearls

- Single, rounded, corticated lucent cyst in midline maxilla

Reporting Tips

- Extension to nasal cavity important to report if present

SELECTED REFERENCES

1. Lee YP et al: Nasopalatine duct cyst - characteristic histopathological features. J Dent Sci. 19(2):1216-18, 2024
2. Yadav U et al: Assessment of variations in the nasopalatine canal on CBCT: considerations from an anatomical point of view. J Periodontal Implant Sci. 55(1):62-71, 2024
3. Philbert RF et al: Nonodontogenic cysts. Dent Clin North Am. 64(1):63-85, 2020

TMJ Juvenile Idiopathic Arthritis

TERMINOLOGY

- Juvenile idiopathic arthritis (JIA)
- **Autoimmune** musculoskeletal synovial inflammatory disease of childhood

IMAGING

- Bone CT best demonstrates contours of TMJ
  - Flat, deformed mandibular condyles & wide, flat condylar fossae
  - Condyle concavity or bifid
  - Bilateral disease more common than unilateral
  - May have secondary osteoarthritis with osteophytes
- MR may show joint space enhancement & early inflammation before joint destruction
  - TMJ discs thin, perforated, or absent
- In cervical spine, may see atlantoaxial subluxation, vertebral fusion, & ↓ AP vertebral body dimension

TOP DIFFERENTIAL DIAGNOSES

- TMJ condylar hypoplasia
- TMJ degenerative disease
- TMJ synovitis/capsulitis
- Progressive condylar resorption

CLINICAL ISSUES

- JIA affects 1-22 per 1,000 children worldwide
- TMJ involved in 20-90% of children with JIA
  - More likely if systemic disease, young age at diagnosis, & long duration of activity
- TMJ & masticator muscle pain, ↓ range of jaw motion, retrognathia, micrognathia
- **70% asymptomatic** when MR shows acute arthritis
- Treat with local &/or systemic therapy
  - Local: Occlusal devices, arthrocentesis, intraarticular injections
  - Systemic: NSAIDs, methotrexate, sulfasalazine, biologic agents

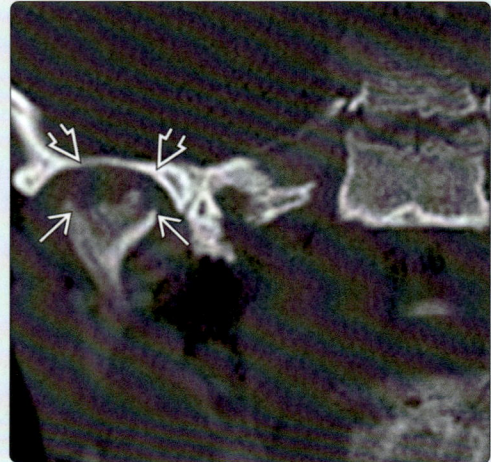
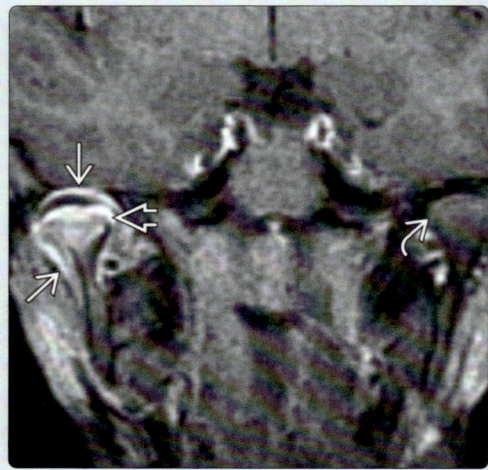

(Left) Coronal bone CT in a 4-year-old girl with juvenile idiopathic arthritis (JIA) demonstrates irregular, chronic erosion of the right mandibular condyle ➡. Note also wide, flattened condylar fossa ➡. (Right) Coronal T1WI C+ FS MR in the same patient with JIA reveals marked inflammatory enhancement involving the joint ➡ & bone marrow of the right mandibular condyle ➡. The left TMJ ➡ shows no inflammatory change, normal condyle, & normal condylar fossa.

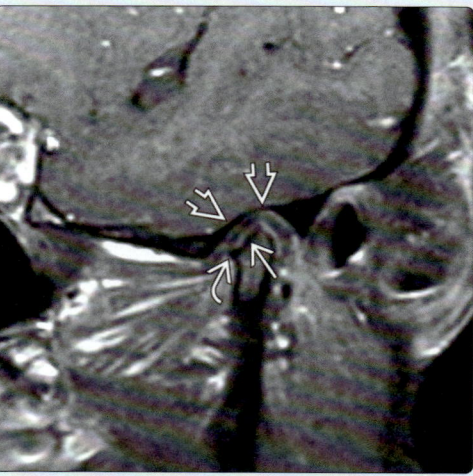
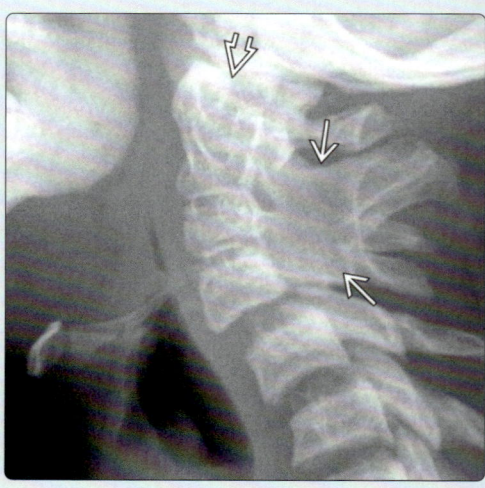

(Left) Sagittal oblique T1WI C+ FS MR in a 21-year-old woman with longstanding JIA reveals a small mandibular condyle with irregular, low-intensity sclerotic margins ➡ & widened, flat condylar fossa ➡. There is no inflammatory enhancement, but note the small anterior osteophyte ➡ from secondary osteoarthritis. (Right) Lateral radiograph in a 19-year-old man shows fusion of the posterior elements & decreased intervertebral disc height C2-C4 ➡, fusion of anterior arch of C1 to the dens ➡, & C4-C5 anterolisthesis.

TERMINOLOGY

Abbreviations
- Juvenile idiopathic arthritis (JIA)

Synonyms
- Juvenile rheumatoid/chronic arthritis

Definitions
- JIA is preferred term of International League of Associations for Rheumatology (ILAR)
- **Autoimmune** musculoskeletal synovial inflammatory disease of childhood
- ≥ 6 weeks of symptoms; begins < 16 years of age

IMAGING

General Features
- Best diagnostic clue: Bilateral, flat, deformed mandibular condyles with wide condylar fossae
- Location: Primarily large joints: Knees, wrists, ankles
  - TMJ, craniovertebral junction, & cervical spine

CT Findings
- Bone CT: Flat & deformed mandibular condyles + wide, flat condylar fossae
  - Condyle concavity or bifid
  - Sclerotic margins when more advanced
  - Bilateral > unilateral
  - May have secondary osteoarthritis with joint space narrowing & osteophyte formation
  - In cervical spine, may see **atlantoaxial subluxation**
    - Fusion & ↓ AP vertebral body dimension

MR Findings
- T1WI: Flat & deformed mandibular condyles + wide, flat condylar fossae
  - Condyle concavity or bifid
- T2WI: Hyperintense joint effusion, bone marrow edema, synovial thickening, &/or subchondral cysts less common
  - TMJ discs thin, perforated, or absent
  - May see early inflammation before joint destruction
  - May be abnormal without symptoms
- T1WI C+: **Joint space enhancement**
- Dynamic imaging: ↓ condyle translation
- Cervical spine & craniovertebral junction
  - Atlantoaxial subluxation
  - Cranial settling, basilar invagination
  - Fusions → ankylosis & ↓ AP vertebral body dimension

DIFFERENTIAL DIAGNOSIS

TMJ Condylar Hypoplasia
- Bilateral: Pierre Robin & Treacher Collins
- Unilateral: Hemifacial microsomia
- Classic condylar hypoplasia

TMJ Degenerative Disease
- Disc displaced anteriorly, joint space narrowing ± osteophyte, subchondral bone cyst, congruent articulation

TMJ Synovitis/Capsulitis
- Enhancing synovium/capsule

Progressive Condylar Resorption
- Postpubertal female patients
- Small condyle, often bilateral

PATHOLOGY

Staging, Grading, & Classification
- ILAR is most widely used classification: 6 subtypes based on clinical features during first 6 months of disease
  - Oligoarticular JIA (50-60%)
  - Polyarticular JIA rheumatoid factor positive & negative (30-35%)
  - Systemic JIA (10-20%)
  - Juvenile psoriatic arthritis (2-15%)
  - Enthesitis-related arthritis (1-7%)
  - Undifferentiated arthritis
- JIA magnetic resonance imaging scoring system for TMJs (JAMRIS-TMJ)
  - Standardized method to measure disease activity
  - ↑ severity grade 0-2; grade each joint separately
  - Inflammatory domain: Bone marrow edema, bone marrow enhancement, joint effusion, synovial thickening, joint enhancement
  - Damage domain: Condylar flattening, erosions, disk abnormalities

CLINICAL ISSUES

Presentation
- Most common signs/symptoms
  - In children with MR findings of acute TMJ arthritis, **70% asymptomatic**
  - TMJ & masticator muscle pain
- Other signs/symptoms
  - **Retrognathia**
  - Mandibular growth disturbance → **micrognathia**
  - Facial asymmetry, unilateral mandibular hypoplasia, malocclusion
  - Chewing difficulties & ↓ mouth opening (↓ maximal incisor opening)

Demographics
- Epidemiology: Most common childhood autoimmune musculoskeletal inflammatory disease
  - F >> M
  - TMJ involved in 20-90% of children & ≤ 70% of adults with longstanding JIA
  - TMJ involvement more likely if systemic disease, young age at diagnosis, & long duration of activity

Treatment
- Systemic therapy: NSAIDs, corticosteroids, methotrexate, sulfasalazine, biologic agents (monoclonal antibodies or soluble receptors), anti-TNF, interleukin-1 & interleukin-6 inhibitors
- Local therapy: Arthrocentesis, intraarticular injections, occlusal devices, & functional appliances

SELECTED REFERENCES

1. Inarejos Clemente EJ et al: MRI of the temporomandibular joint in children with juvenile idiopathic arthritis: protocol and findings. Pediatr Radiol. 53(8):1498-512, 2023

Mandible-Maxilla Osteomyelitis

TERMINOLOGY

- Definition: Polymicrobial bacterial infection, usually odontogenic, of mandible > maxilla

IMAGING

- CECT/bone CT findings
  - Acute osteomyelitis: Bone destruction, tooth/socket abnormality ± associated soft tissue abscess
  - Chronic osteomyelitis: Bone sclerosis with periosteal reaction ± sequestrum
- Enhanced MR findings
  - MR sensitive for acute and chronic osteomyelitis
  - Shows full extent of mandible marrow involvement
  - If dental amalgam obscures CT, MR may show subtle abscess formation not seen by CT
- Serial exams may be necessary to confirm osteomyelitis & document positive clinical response

TOP DIFFERENTIAL DIAGNOSES

- Mandible-maxilla osteoradionecrosis of jaw
- Medication-related osteonecrosis
- Infiltrative neoplasm invading mandible
  - Alveolar ridge or other perimandibular squamous cell carcinoma
  - Mandibular non-Hodgkin lymphoma
  - Mandibular metastasis
- Primary chronic osteomyelitis
- Langerhans histiocytosis, mandible-maxilla

DIAGNOSTIC CHECKLIST

- Identify source of infection
  - Infected tooth ± periapical abscess by far most common source
  - Other sources: Posttraumatic or postsurgical site
- Interrogate soft tissues of masticator & submandibular spaces for abscess & fistulous tract

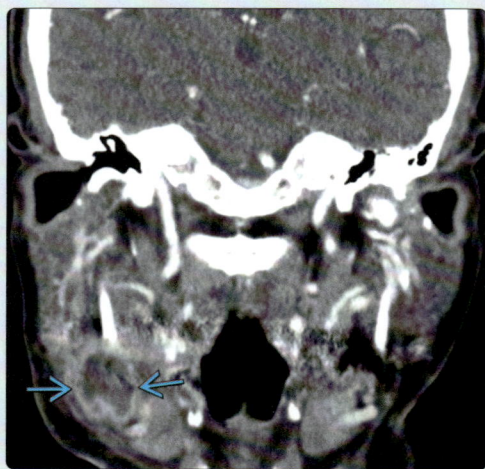
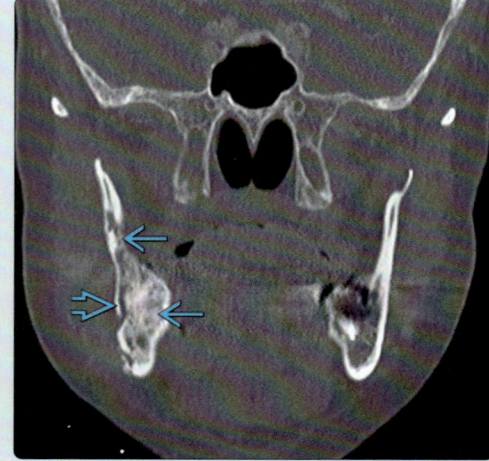

(Left) Coronal CECT MPR in a 27-year-old man with right jaw swelling, fever, & mild leukocytosis shows a rim-enhancing collection ➡ in the right submandibular region with adjacent inflammatory changes suggesting abscess. (Right) Coronal bone window MPR CECT in the same patient shows mixed permeative sclerosis of the right hemimandible ➡ posterior body, angle, & ramus with periosteal reaction ➡, findings consistent with osteomyelitis. Patient was treated with abscess drainage & antibiotics.

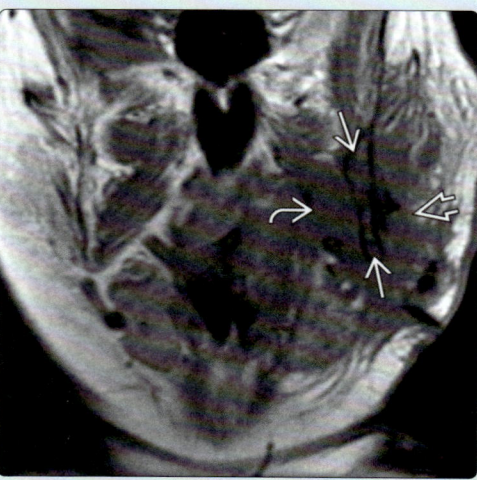
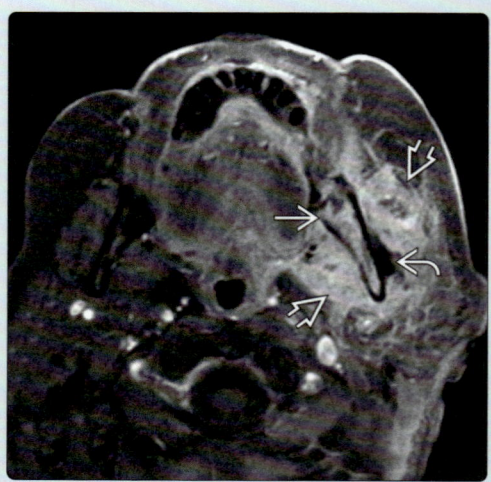

(Left) Coronal T1 MR shows a 79-year-old with recurrent masticator space abscess 12 weeks after initial diagnosis & drainage. Normal high-signal marrow fat has been replaced ➡ in the left hemimandible, consistent with osteomyelitis. Note edema in the medial pterygoid ➡ & masseter ➡ muscles. (Right) Axial T1 C+ FS MR in the same patient reveals diffuse enhancement of the left marrow space ➡ with masticator space enhancement (phlegmon) ➡ & small lateral compartment abscess ➡.

TERMINOLOGY

Synonyms

- Acute or chronic suppurative osteomyelitis

Definitions

- Polymicrobial bacterial infection, usually odontogenic, of mandible > maxilla

IMAGING

General Features

- Best diagnostic clue
  - CECT/bone CT
    - Acute: Lytic, permeative changes in mandible with soft tissue inflammation
    - Chronic: Sclerotic or permeative-sclerotic changes with periosteal reaction & sequestrum

Imaging Recommendations

- Best imaging tool
  - CECT: Use both soft tissue and bone algorithms

Radiographic Findings

- Acute: Ill-defined lucency of bone
- Chronic: Sclerotic or sclerotic-permeative pattern; periosteal reaction

CT Findings

- CECT
  - Phlegmon/frank abscess often present in perimandibular, submandibular, sublingual, & masticator spaces
  - Transspatial induration/enhancement common
- Bone CT
  - Acute: Destruction of cancellous & cortical bone
    - Associated soft tissue edema, phlegmon, or abscess
  - Chronic: Bony sclerosis, laminar periosteal reaction, sequestrum

MR Findings

- T1WI
  - Loss of T1 signal as marrow fat replaced by edema and exudate (acute) or fibrosis/sclerosis (chronic)
- STIR
  - Acute: Marked marrow hyperintensity
  - Chronic: Variable, depending on degree of fibrosis & sclerosis
- T1WI C+ FS
  - Acute: Marked marrow space enhancement
  - Chronic: Variable enhancement

Nuclear Medicine Findings

- 3-phase bone scan with Tc-99m MDP sensitive but not specific
- Indium-111 or Tc99m-HMPAO WBC scan specific

DIFFERENTIAL DIAGNOSIS

Medication-Related Osteonecrosis of Jaw

- Bone loss with intraosseous gas 6-12 months post radiation

Mandible-Maxilla Bisphosphonate Osteonecrosis

- Bone loss occurring with current/previous bisphosphonate therapy

Infiltrative Neoplasm Invading Mandible

- Can produce invasive soft tissue mass & bone destruction
- Alveolar ridge squamous cell carcinoma
- Mandibular non-Hodgkin lymphoma
- Mandibular metastasis
- Sclerotic metastasis can mimic chronic osteomyelitis

Primary Chronic Osteomyelitis

- More insidious course with greater involvement of mandible
- May present as manifestation of systemic disease
  - Chronic recurrent multifocal osteomyelitis
  - Synovitis, acne, pustulosis, hyperostosis, osteitis

PATHOLOGY

General Features

- Etiology
  - Nonodontogenic: Trauma, post surgical, hematogenous (rare)

Staging, Grading, & Classification

- Acute (signs/symptoms < 4 weeks); chronic (> 4 weeks)

Gross Pathologic & Surgical Features

- Acute: Purulent exudate
- Chronic: Devitalized bone, fibrosis, & chronic inflammation

Microscopic Features

- Acute: Marrow exudate with neutrophils, fibrin, necrotic debris, and microorganisms
- Chronic: Marrow fibrosis, periosteal reaction, osteoblastic sclerosis, sequestrum

CLINICAL ISSUES

Presentation

- Most common signs/symptoms
  - Pain, swelling, and tenderness of jaw

Treatment

- Acute: Oral ± IV antibiotics; abscess drainage
- Chronic: Surgical debridement, hyperbaric oxygen

DIAGNOSTIC CHECKLIST

Consider

- Consider malignancy if persistent soft tissue lesion with bone destruction
- Serial physical and CT exams may be necessary to confirm osteomyelitis & document positive clinical response

SELECTED REFERENCES

1. da Silva NC et al: Clinical, radiographic, and histopathological characterization of osteomyelitis of the jaws: a 51-year experience at an oral pathology service. J Stomatol Oral Maxillofac Surg. 102222, 2025
2. Almuzayyen A et al: Osteomyelitis of the jaw: a 10-year retrospective analysis at a tertiary health care centre in Canada. J Can Dent Assoc. 90:06, 2024

KEY FACTS

TERMINOLOGY

- Calcium pyrophosphate deposition disease (**CPPD**)
- **Metabolic disease** resulting in peri- or intraarticular **chondrocalcinosis**
  - **Tophaceous (tumoral)** TMJ form most prevalent
- Synonym: Pseudogout

IMAGING

- Calcified TMJ lesion
  - May involve masticator or parotid space or adjacent skull base
- Bone CT
  - Mild/early CPPD: Subtle calcifications in TMJ
  - Late/severe CPPD →
    - Chunky, **diffusely calcified** mass
    - Calcified mass may have **ground-glass** appearance
    - Associated remodeling, erosion, or mass effect on condyle
  - 50% have involvement of multiple joints

- MR
  - T1: **Low-** to intermediate-signal lesion; capsule and joint space expansion
  - T2: **Hypointense**, somewhat heterogeneous mass
  - T1 C+: Heterogeneously enhancing TMJ lesion

TOP DIFFERENTIAL DIAGNOSES

- Synovial chondromatosis
- Chondrosarcoma
- Chondroblastoma
- Tenosynovial giant cell tumor

PATHOLOGY

- **Calcium pyrophosphate crystals** in synovial fluid are diagnostic
  - In polarized light, crystals are **birefringent**

CLINICAL ISSUES

- Presenting symptoms: Preauricular pain and swelling
- Treatment: Surgical excision + arthrocentesis

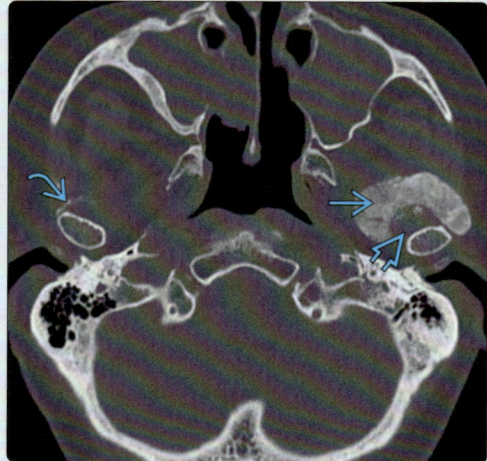
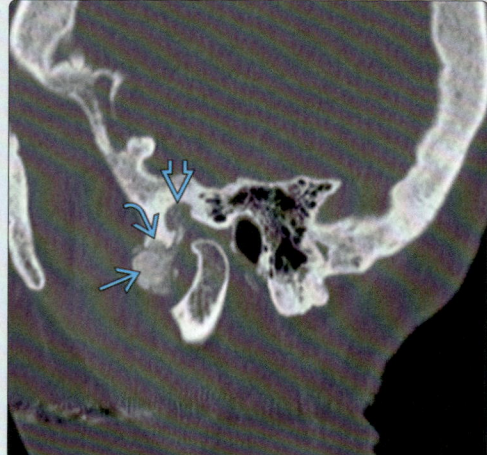

(Left) Axial bone window NECT shows large, calcific density ⮕ in the left TMJ. Note preserved joint space ⮕. Similar subtle calcification is seen in the right TMJ ⮕. (Right) Sagittal bone window MPR NECT shows calcific density in the left TMJ anterior to the condyle ⮕. Note bony remodeling and erosions along the glenoid fossa ⮕ and articular eminence ⮕. Considering the ground-glass appearance of the calcified mass separate from the condyle CPPD is favored.

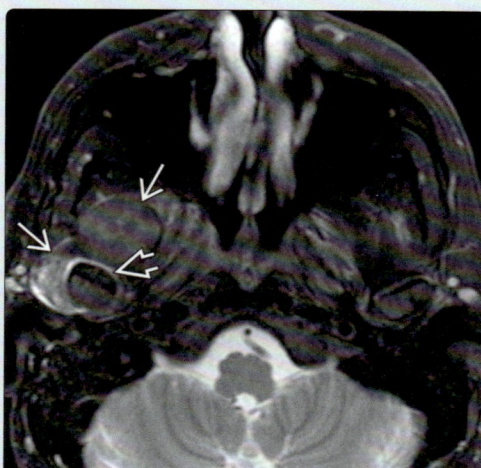
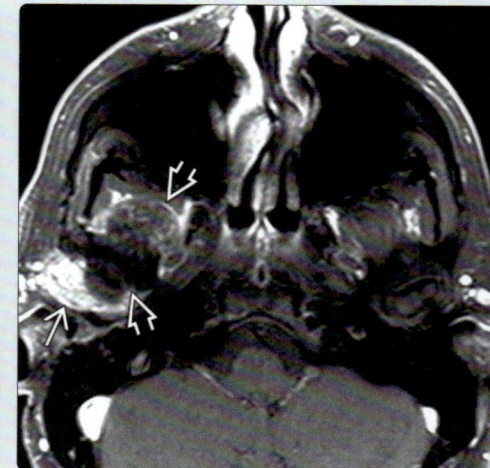

(Left) Axial T2 FS MR in a patient with CPPD in the right TMJ shows a heterogeneous, predominantly low signal intensity lesion ⮕ along the margins of the TMJ. Note joint space fluid around the head of the mandibular condyle ⮕. (Right) Axial T1 C+ FS MR demonstrates enhancement from joint space inflammation of the periphery of the mass ⮕. Notice the bilobed area of low signal ⮕ that represents the area of confluent calcification that is so typical of CPPD.

TMJ Calcium Pyrophosphate Dihydrate Deposition Disease

TERMINOLOGY

Abbreviations
- Calcium pyrophosphate dihydrate deposition disease (CPPD)

Synonyms
- Pseudogout
- Tophaceous pseudogout, pseudotumor, destructive CPPD arthropathy, CPPD deposition disease

Definitions
- **Metabolic disease** resulting in peri- or intraarticular **chondrocalcinosis**
- **Tophaceous (tumoral) CPPD** form most prevalent in TMJ

IMAGING

General Features
- Best diagnostic clue
  - Calcified TMJ mass
- Location
  - Intracapsular > extracapsular
    - May involve masticator space (MS), parotid space (PS), adjacent skull base
- Size: Typically ≥ 1 cm

CT Findings
- Bone CT
  - Mild/early CPPD: Subtle calcifications in TMJ
  - Late/severe CPPD
    - Chunky, **diffusely calcified** mass
    - Calcified mass may have **ground-glass** appearance
    - Associated degenerative changes with remodeling, erosion, or mass effect on condyle
    - May have associated demineralization/erosion of skull base, external auditory canal
      - □ May mimic malignancy
  - **50% involve multiple joints**: Knee, hand, wrist, shoulder, spine

MR Findings
- T1WI
  - **Low-** to intermediate-signal TMJ lesion
  - Expansion of joint capsule and joint space
  - Remodeling or erosion of mandibular condyle
- T2WI
  - **Hypointense**, somewhat heterogeneous mass
- T1WI C+
  - Heterogeneously enhancing lesion

Imaging Recommendations
- Best imaging tool
  - Combination bone CT + TMJ MR
- Protocol advice
  - Thin-section bone CT, enhanced TMJ MR

DIFFERENTIAL DIAGNOSIS

Synovial Chondromatosis
- Multiple small, **calcified loose bodies** in superior joint space
  - Usually do not form contiguous solid mass

- Associated condylar osteoarthritis

Chondrosarcoma
- **Calcified** or partially calcified **TMJ mass**
- Tends to arise from, or be intimately associated with, condyle
- Condylar erosion, resorption
- T2 signal higher than with CPPD; more diffusely enhancing
- Often extends into MS, PS, skull base, temporal bone

Chondroblastoma
- Rare in TMJ
- Lytic condylar expansion ± calcified mass
- May infiltrate through disc and capsule
- 3rd decade; male predilection

Tenosynovial Giant Cell Tumor
- T2-hypointense and noncalcified, locally aggressive benign tumor

PATHOLOGY

General Features
- Etiology
  - Exact pathophysiology unclear
    - Sporadic, familial, and secondary/metabolic forms
  - Unknown noxious event incites cascade that evolves toward hypertrophy and degeneration of chondrocytes
  - Rare in TMJ

Microscopic Features
- Calcium pyrophosphate **crystals** in synovial fluid is diagnostic
  - Crystals **birefringent** in polarized light
    - Gout = nonrefringent crystals of uric acid
- Metaplastic chondroid tissue; pleomorphic hyperchromatic nuclei

CLINICAL ISSUES

Presentation
- Most common signs/symptoms
  - Preauricular pain, swelling, trismus
  - Can cause hearing loss with temporal bone involvement
- Other signs/symptoms
  - Crepitus in TMJ

Treatment
- Surgical excision, arthrocentesis

SELECTED REFERENCES

1. Kachi H et al: Calcium pyrophosphate crystal deposition in the temporomandibular joint associated with temporomandibular joint surgery: Case report. Int J Surg Case Rep. 128:111021, 2025
2. Dang RR et al: Treatment of tophaceous pseudogout in the temporomandibular joint with resection and alloplastic reconstruction: a single-staged approach. Oral Maxillofac Surg. 26(3):505-9, 2022
3. Murahashi M et al: Management of temporomandibular joint diseases: a rare case report of coexisting calcium pyrophosphate crystal deposition and synovial chondromatosis. BMC Oral Health. 22(1):662, 2022
4. Terauchi M et al: Chemical diagnosis of calcium pyrophosphate deposition disease of the temporomandibular joint: a case report. Diagnostics (Basel). 12(3), 2022
5. Marsot-Dupuch K et al: Massive calcium pyrophosphate dihydrate crystal deposition disease: a cause of pain of the temporomandibular joint. AJNR Am J Neuroradiol. 25(5):876-9, 2004

KEY FACTS

TERMINOLOGY

- **Synovial metaplasia** with foci of **hyaline cartilage**

IMAGING

- **Calcified nodules** in superior joint space (SJS)
- Location: Most commonly found in SJS of TMJ
  - Rarely may have extracapsular extension
  - Locations: Masticator space, parotid space, intracranial
- Protocol: TMJ MR + thin-section multiplanar bone CT
- Bone CT findings
  - **Calcified nodules** surround **mandibular condyle**
  - Degenerative changes involving condyle common
- T1/PD MR findings
  - Multiple **hypo-** to **isointense nodules** in SJS
  - Separate from articular disc
- T2 MR: SJS **effusion** ± expansion; fluid surrounds collection of hypointense nodules
- T1 C+ MR: Enhancing synovium

TOP DIFFERENTIAL DIAGNOSES

- Osteochondritis dissecans
- Calcium pyrophosphate dihydrate deposition disease
- Tenosynovial giant cell tumor
- Osteochondroma
- Chondrosarcoma

PATHOLOGY

- **Synovial inflammation** with lymphocytes, macrophages, giant cells
- Milgram staging
  - Phase 1: Synovial metaplasia with no chondroid nodules
  - Phase 2: Active synovial metaplasia & chondroid nodules
  - Phase 3: Chondroid nodules, no active synovial disease
- Fusion between *FN1* & *ACVR2A* genes in > 50%

CLINICAL ISSUES

- Presenting symptoms: Preauricular pain, swelling
- Treatment: Arthroscopy, synovectomy, condylectomy

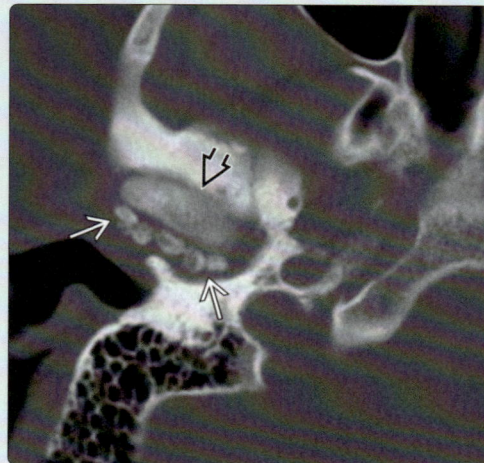
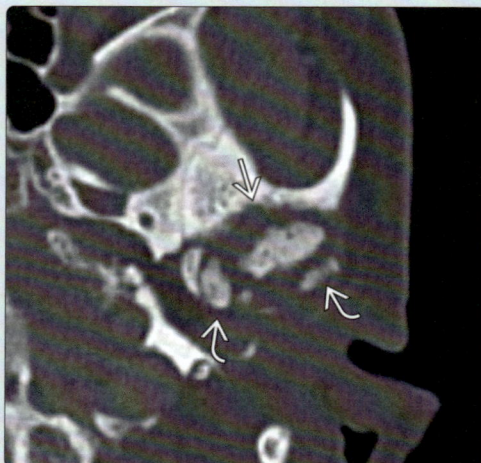

(Left) Axial bone CT demonstrates multiple small, calcified nodules ⇨ within the right TMJ due to synovial chondromatosis. The condyle appears sclerotic and slightly irregular ⇨ with anterior narrowing of the joint space due to chronic degenerative change. (Right) Axial bone CT shows widening of the TMJ with erosive changes on both sides of the joint space ⇨. Multiple ossified joint space loose bodies ⇨ are present.

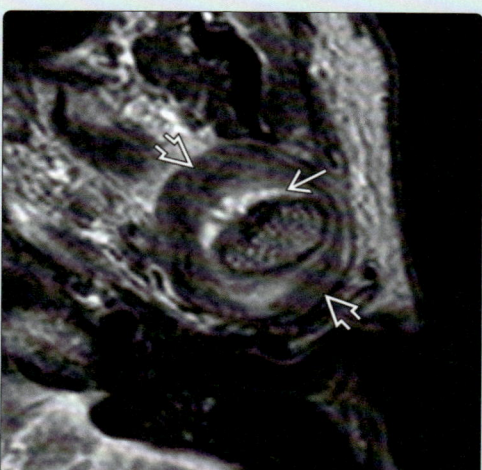
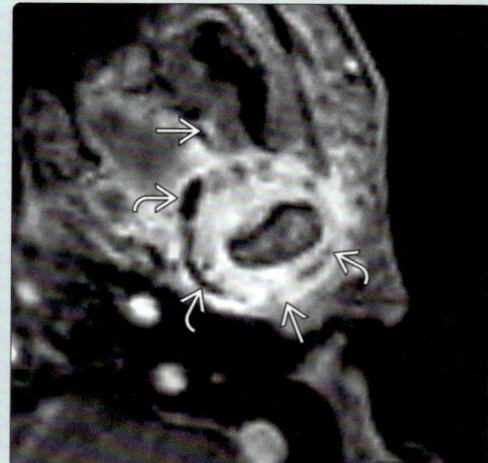

(Left) Axial T2 MR shows widening of the TMJ with fluid ⇨ in this case of synovial chondromatosis. A diffusely thickened synovium with heterogeneous low signal intensity due to patchy, diffuse mineralization is noted widening the joint space ⇨. (Right) Axial T1 C+ FS MR in the same patient shows diffuse thickening and enhancement of the synovium ⇨ with multiple concentric, hypointense joint space calcified nodules ⇨.

TERMINOLOGY

Abbreviations
- Synovial chondromatosis (SC)

Definitions
- **Synovial metaplasia** with foci of **hyaline cartilage**
- Primary SC: Single synovial joint involved, etiology unknown
- Secondary SC: Due to underlying cause (arthritis/trauma)

IMAGING

General Features
- Best diagnostic clue
  - Multiple calcified nodules in superior joint space (SJS)
- Location
  - Most commonly involves SJS (> 90%) of TMJ
  - Most often unilateral; predilection right side
  - Rarely may have extracapsular extension
    - Masticator space, parotid space, middle cranial fossa
- Size
  - Calcifications vary from millimeters to centimeters

Radiographic Findings
- Intraarticular calcified loose bodies

CT Findings
- Bone CT
  - SJS widening & bone sclerosis common
    - Joint space on affected side larger
  - Condylar surface degenerative changes common
    - > 70% show destruction & sclerosis of glenoid fossa
    - Mandibular condyle less often destructive/sclerotic
  - Multiple calcified nodules around mandibular condyle
    - > 80% of patients show calcification
      - □ Ring & arc morphology (26.5%)
      - □ Popcorn-like (38.2%)

MR Findings
- T1WI
  - Multiple **hypointense nodules** in SJS
  - Separate from articular disc
- T2WI
  - Multiple **hypointense nodules** in SJS
  - SJS > inferior joint space (IJS) effusion ± expansion
- T1WI C+
  - Enhancing synovium

Imaging Recommendations
- Best imaging tool
  - MR more sensitive to early-stage disease without calcified loose bodies
- Best imaging tool: TMJ MR ± bone CT

DIFFERENTIAL DIAGNOSIS

Osteochondritis Dissecans
- Condylar erosive defect with adjacent fragment

Calcium Pyrophosphate Dihydrate Deposition Disease
- Tophaceous pseudogout: Rare form, most frequent in TMJ
  - Calcified mass in condyle or joint space

Tenosynovial Giant Cell Tumor
- T1-/T2-hypointense nodules due to hemosiderin are **noncalcified** on CT

Osteochondroma
- Develops from pterygoid muscle tendinous attachments
- Condylar head enlargement often present

Chondrosarcoma
- Associated intra- &/or extracapsular enhancing mass

PATHOLOGY

General Features
- Etiology
  - Primary SC: Unknown
  - Secondary SC: Due to TMJ degeneration or trauma
- Genetics
  - Genetic features in > 1/2: Recurrent fibronectin 1 (*FN1*) & activin receptor 2A (*ACVR2A*) gene rearrangements

Staging, Grading, & Classification
- Milgram staging
  - Phase 1: Synovial metaplasia with no chondroid nodules
  - Phase 2: Active synovial metaplasia & chondroid nodules
  - Phase 3: Chondroid nodules, no active synovial disease

Microscopic Features
- Synovial membrane **inflammation** with lymphocytes, macrophages, giant cells
- Cartilage metaplasia

CLINICAL ISSUES

Presentation
- Most common signs/symptoms
  - Preauricular pain, swelling
- Other signs/symptoms
  - Trismus, limited ability to open mouth, deviated jaw opening or malocclusion, & noise/crepitus of joint

Demographics
- Age
  - Adults (mean: 4th decade)
  - Primary SC younger; secondary SC older
- Sex: F:M = 4:1

Natural History & Prognosis
- Recurrence rate low
- Degeneration to chondrosarcoma very rare but reported

Treatment
- Arthroscopy, synovectomy, condylectomy

SELECTED REFERENCES

1. Vladimír M et al: TMJ synovial chondromatosis - an evaluation of 37 patients. Oral Maxillofac Surg. 28(4):1653-60, 2024
2. Zhang Y et al: Imaging features of temporomandibular joint synovial chondromatosis with associated osseous degenerative changes. Int J Oral Maxillofac Surg. 53(4):311-18, 2024
3. Jang BG et al: Imaging features of synovial chondromatosis of the temporomandibular joint: a report of 34 cases. Clin Radiol. 76(8):627.e1-11, 2021
4. Agaram NP et al: A molecular study of synovial chondromatosis. Genes Chromosomes Cancer. 59(3):144-51, 2020

KEY FACTS

TERMINOLOGY

- Giant cell reparative lesion of mandible > maxilla

IMAGING

- General imaging findings
  - Loculated, expansile mass with wavy septations
  - Anterior mandible ≥ body & ramus > maxilla
- Bone CT findings
  - **Expansile, multiloculated** midline mandibular lesion
  - Septations at **right angle** to cortex
  - Scalloping & cortical dehiscence common in large lesions
- Best imaging tool: CECT
  - Isodense (to muscle); **moderately enhancing** mass

TOP DIFFERENTIAL DIAGNOSES

- Aneurysmal bone cyst (ABC)
  - ~ 15% of central giant cell granulomas contain intralesional ABC
- Cherubism

- Ameloblastoma
- Ossifying fibroma
- Brown tumor of hyperparathyroidism

PATHOLOGY

- Unknown etiology: Likely reactive granuloma
- Histopathology overlaps with giant cell tumor

CLINICAL ISSUES

- Presentation: Pain, swelling of mandible or maxilla
- Age at presentation: Adolescence to 3rd decade
- Treatment of choice: Surgical enucleation with peripheral ostectomy
- Large lesions may be treated with intralesional calcitonin or corticosteroids

DIAGNOSTIC CHECKLIST

- Expansile, septated, moderately enhancing mass in anterior mandible of young adult; septations at right angle to cortex
- Report cortical perforation, root resorption

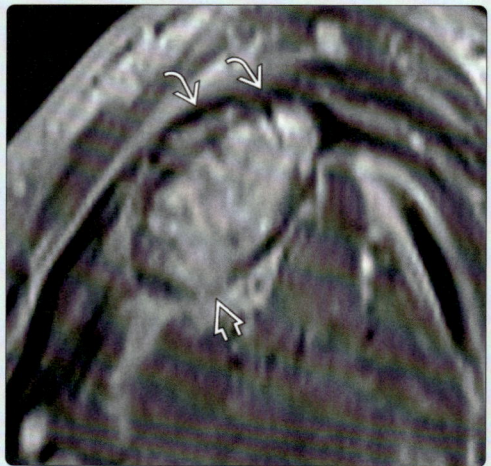
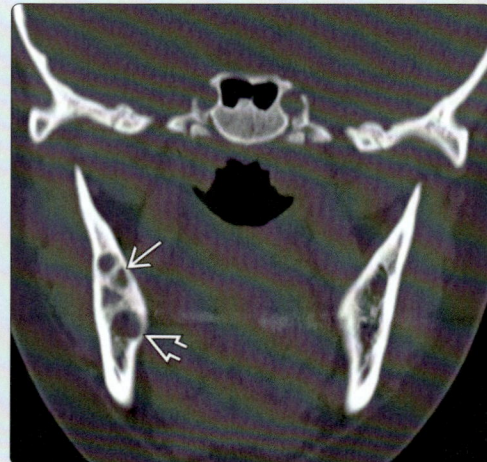

(Left) *Axial T1 C+ FS MR shows a multiloculated, expansile central giant cell granuloma (CGCG) centered in the anterior mandible. Note the multiple thin, wavy septations* ⬈ *at right angle to the cortex characteristic of this lesion, giving the classically described soap bubble appearance. There is perforation of the lingual cortex* ⬈. *(Right) Coronal bone CT shows a loculated, radiolucent CGCG of the mandibular ramus without internal calcifications that thins mandibular cortex* ⬈ *and is distinct from inferior extraction socket* ⬈.

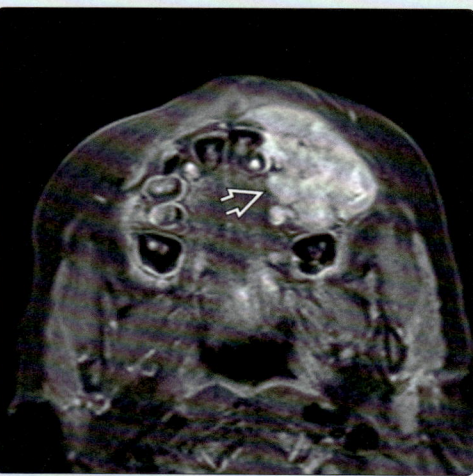
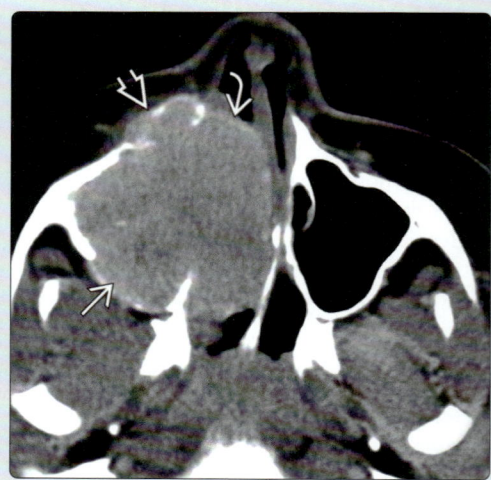

(Left) *Axial T1 C+ FS MR in a 5-year-old girl demonstrates an enhancing, expansile mass arising from the left maxillary alveolus* ⬈. *There is extension to the midline with associated cortical dehiscence and soft tissue extension. This lesion recurred after surgical excision. (Right) Axial CECT demonstrates a large, enhancing, expansile mass filling the right maxillary sinus* ⬈. *This maxillary CGCG dehisces the anterior wall maxillary sinus* ⬈. *Also note obstruction of the right nasal passage* ⬈ *with deviation of the nasal septum.*

TERMINOLOGY

Abbreviations
- Central giant cell granuloma (CGCG)

Synonyms
- Giant cell reparative granuloma

Definitions
- Giant cell reparative lesion of mandible or maxilla

IMAGING

General Features
- Best diagnostic clue
  - **Expansile** mass with **"right angle" septations**
- Location
  - **Anterior midline mandible** ≥ body & ramus > maxilla
    - ~ 50% of lesions anterior to 1st molar in alveolus
    - ~ 35% cross midline
  - Rarely multiple
    - Multiple lesions have been reported in Noonan syndrome & neurofibromatosis type 1
- Size
  - Typically > 1 cm; often large at diagnosis
    - Size > 5 cm suggests aggressive lesion, more likely to recur post surgery

Imaging Recommendations
- Best imaging tool
  - CECT
- Protocol advice
  - Thin-section CECT
  - Bone CT shows septations & relationship to teeth

CT Findings
- CECT
  - Isodense (to muscle), **moderately enhancing** mass
- Bone CT
  - **Loculated, expansile** mass with thin to coarse wavy **septations**
    - Septations often at **right angle** to cortex
    - Smaller lesions: Thicker, coarse septations
    - Large lesions: Thin, wavy septations
  - Center of mass of alveolar lesions typically inferior to root apices
  - May have internal areas of mineralization
  - Scalloping & cortical dehiscence common in large lesions

MR Findings
- T1WI
  - Hypo- to isointense
- T2WI
  - Hypo- to isointense
- T1WI C+
  - Heterogeneously mild to moderate enhancement

DIFFERENTIAL DIAGNOSIS

Aneurysmal Bone Cyst
- ~ 15% of CGCGs contain intralesional aneurysmal bone cyst
- Majority of lesions in molar region of mandibular ramus

- MR: Fluid-fluid levels on T2 sequence

Cherubism
- Mutations in chromosome 4p16.3
- Multifocal giant cell lesions in infants & children
- CT: Multifocal posterior mandible or maxillary expansion

Ameloblastoma
- Predominately 3rd-5th decades
- Most common in tooth-bearing molar regions, mandible > maxilla
- CT: Multiloculated, lucent, expansile mass
  - **Septations** tend to be **coarser than CGCG**

Ossifying Fibroma
- Most common in premolar region of mandible
- Lesions with fibrous component can mimic CGCG
- CT: Calcified/ossified mass with lucent capsule

Brown Tumor of Hyperparathyroidism
- ↑ serum calcification, ↑ PTH, ↑ alkaline phosphatase
- In jaws, CT & MR appearance often identical to CGCG

PATHOLOGY

General Features
- Etiology
  - Unknown: Possibly reparative response to trauma or inflammation

Microscopic Features
- Vascular, fibroblastic, or myxoid stroma
- Heterogeneous **clumps of giant cells** + fibroblastic areas, new bone, hemorrhage
- No necrosis

CLINICAL ISSUES

Presentation
- Most common signs/symptoms
  - Pain, swelling of mandible > maxilla

Demographics
- Age
  - < 30 years
- Sex
  - F:M = 2:1

Natural History & Prognosis
- Recurrence rate: ~ 5-15%
  - Size > 5 cm, rapid growth, root resorption, root displacement, or cortical dehiscence indicates aggressive lesion with ↑ likelihood of recurrence

Treatment
- Surgical excision: Treatment of choice but potential damage to teeth
- Medical treatment includes using drugs like denosumab

SELECTED REFERENCES

1. Alsufyani N et al: Imaging of fibro-osseous lesions and other bone conditions of the jaws. Dent Clin North Am. 68(2):297-317, 2024
2. Puri S et al: Central giant cell granuloma: negotiating the diagnostic and management dilemmas. J Maxillofac Oral Surg. 23(2):316-19, 2024

Mandible-Maxilla and TMJ

KEY FACTS

TERMINOLOGY

- Tenosynovial giant cell tumor (**TGCT**)
- Older term: Pigmented villonodular synovitis (**PVNS**)
- Locally aggressive benign neoplasia of synovium

IMAGING

- CT: **Erosion** of mandibular **condyle** ± glenoid fossa
  - Lobulated, rounded lytic lesions
  - May extend to skull base or intracranially
- T1 MR: **Hypointense** to isointense nodules with peripheral rim of low signal
- T2 MR: **Hypointense** lobulated nodules ± cystic areas of hyperintensity &/or joint effusion
  - Hypointensity due to **hemosiderin** deposition
    - Associated blooming artifact characteristic
- T1 C+ MR: Portions of mass may show mild enhancement
- Best imaging tool: Dedicated C+ MR & thin-section bone CT
- Interpretation pearl: T1/T2 hypointense joint nodules are **noncalcified** on CT

TOP DIFFERENTIAL DIAGNOSES

- Synovial chondromatosis
  - **Calcified nodules** in TMJ joint
- Giant cell tumor
- Chondrosarcoma
- Calcium pyrophosphate dihydrate deposition disease

PATHOLOGY

- Etiology: Unknown
  - Monarticular inflammatory TMJ neoplasia
- Plump histiocytes with **giant cells** + **hemosiderin**
- **Radiologic-pathologic correlation** can be important

CLINICAL ISSUES

- Presenting symptoms: Preauricular pain, swelling, trismus
- Age: 3rd-5th decades
- Sex: F:M = 3:1
- Treatment: Complete surgical resection
  - **Vimseltinib** (CSF1R inhibitor) if poor surgical options

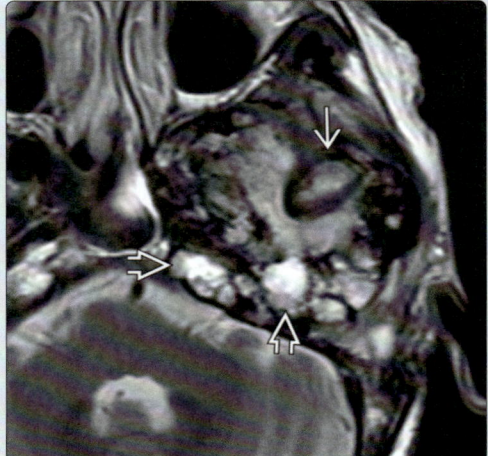
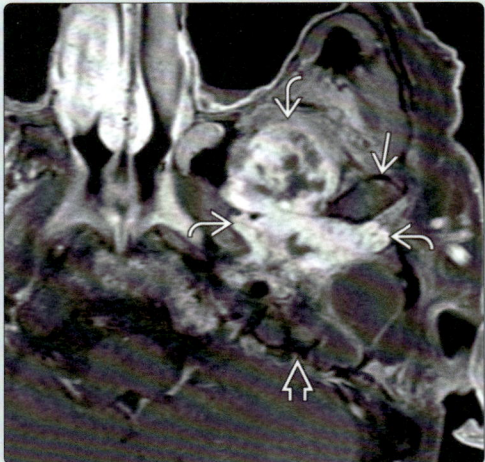

(Left) *Axial T2 MR shows a heterogeneous mass in the joint space surrounding the anteriorly displaced left mandible condylar head ➡. There are foci of cystic T2 signal throughout the involved petrous temporal bone with diffuse peripheral septal hypointensity supporting hemosiderin ➡. (Right) Axial T1 C+ FS MR in the same patient shows heterogeneous cystic and nodular enhancement in the mass ➡ filling the TMJ joint space, surrounding the condylar head ➡, and invading the temporal bone ➡.*

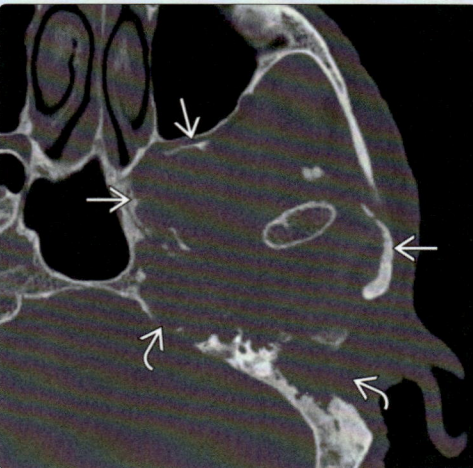
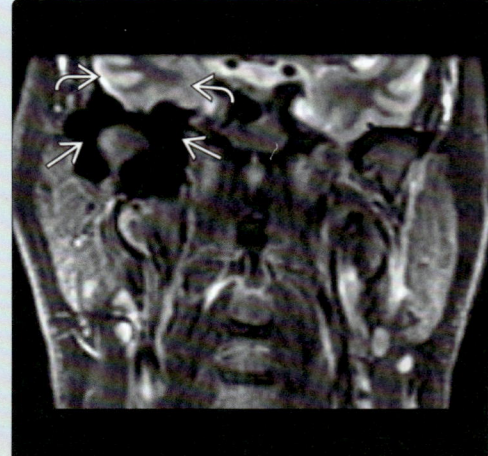

(Left) *Axial bone CT in the same patient shows how the process is centered over the TMJ with remodeling and widening of the joint space ➡. Diffuse erosive changes are noted where locally aggressive tumor invades the temporal bone ➡. (Right) Coronal STIR MR demonstrates nodular foci of markedly hypointense signal ➡ surrounding the right mandible condylar head in this case of tenosynovial giant cell tumor (TGCT). Note the blooming of the adjacent skull base from hemosiderin in these nodules ➡, a nearly pathognomonic finding.*

TERMINOLOGY

Abbreviations

- Tenosynovial giant cell tumor (TGCT)

Synonyms

- Alternative term: Giant cell tumor of tendon sheath
- Older term: Pigmented villonodular synovitis (PVNS)

Definitions

- **Benign**, locally aggressive **neoplasm of synovium**

IMAGING

General Features

- Best diagnostic clue
  - **Monarticular inflammatory benign neoplasia of TMJ**
- Location
  - Rare in TMJ
    - More common in knee, hip, shoulder, ankle, wrist
- Size
  - Typically ≥ 1 cm at diagnosis

Imaging Recommendations

- Best imaging tool
  - T2 & T1 C+ MR
- Protocol advice
  - TMJ & skull base enhanced MR & thin-section bone CT

CT Findings

- Bone CT
  - **Erosion** of mandibular condyle ± glenoid fossa
    - Lobulated, rounded **lytic** lesions
  - May be locally aggressive
  - Large masses erode skull base & intracranially
  - **Joint nodules** are **noncalcified**

MR Findings

- T1WI
  - Hypo- to isointense mass with **peripheral low-signal rim**
- T2WI
  - Hypointense, lobulated mass with peripheral low-signal rim
    - Hypointensity due to **hemosiderin** deposition
  - Synovial fluid will be hyperintense ± joint effusion
- T1WI C+
  - Mild enhancement of portions of mass common

DIFFERENTIAL DIAGNOSIS

Synovial Chondromatosis

- Bone CT: **Calcified nodules** around mandibular condyle
- MR: Multiple hypointense joint space nodules

Giant Cell Tumor

- Most commonly in sphenoid & temporal bones in H&N
- Expansile mass with benign "eggshell" wall on bone CT
  - Multiple lytic lesions may have bubbly appearance

Chondrosarcoma

- Bone destruction ± chondroid calcified matrix
- Hypo- to isointense on T1, hyper- to isointense on T2
- Heterogeneously enhancing on CECT or T1 C+ MR

Calcium Pyrophosphate Dihydrate Deposition Disease

- Diffusely calcified TMJ mass; 50% affect multiple joints

PATHOLOGY

General Features

- Etiology
  - Now considered benign neoplastic process
    - Associated inflammation or reactive synovial infiltrate
- Genetics
  - Recurrent fusions involving colony-stimulating factor 1 (*CSF1*) gene & translocation partners, including collagen type VI alpha 3 chain (*COL6A3I*) or S100 calcium-binding protein A10 (*S100A10*)

Microscopic Features

- **Radiologic-pathologic correlation** can be important
- Plump histiocytes with **giant cells** + **hemosiderin**
- Erosion into surrounding bone; local invasion
- Lymphoplasmacytic infiltrate & chondroid metaplasia

CLINICAL ISSUES

Presentation

- Most common signs/symptoms
  - Preauricular pain, swelling
- Other signs/symptoms
  - Trismus

Demographics

- Age
  - 3rd-5th decades
- Sex
  - F:M = 3:1

Natural History & Prognosis

- Low recurrence rate with complete resection

Treatment

- Complete surgical resection
- FDA approval 2025 of tyrosine kinase inhibitor **vimseltinib** (inhibits CSF1R) for adults with limited surgical options

DIAGNOSTIC CHECKLIST

Consider

- Giant cell tumor & chondrosarcoma usually enhance more

Image Interpretation Pearls

- T1/T2 hypointense joint nodules **noncalcified** on CT

SELECTED REFERENCES

1. Gelderblom H et al: Vimseltinib versus placebo for tenosynovial giant cell tumour (MOTION): a multicentre, randomised, double-blind, placebo-controlled, phase 3 trial. Lancet. 403(10445):2709-19, 2024
2. Ichikawa J et al: Recent advances in immunohistochemical and molecular profiling for differential diagnosis between giant cell-rich lesions and tenosynovial giant cell tumors. Front Oncol. 14:1511127, 2024
3. Aden D et al: FNAC study of giant cell tumor of tendon sheath (localized tenosynovial giant cell tumor): clinico-radiological correlation and cytopathological features. Diagn Cytopathol. 50(12):543-56, 2022
4. Crim J et al: Limited usefulness of classic MR findings in the diagnosis of tenosynovial giant cell tumor. Skeletal Radiol. 50(8):1585-91, 2021

KEY FACTS

TERMINOLOGY

- Benign but locally aggressive neoplasm originating from odontogenic epithelium
- Arises in tooth-bearing areas of mandibular or maxillary alveolus

IMAGING

- CT findings
  - **Expansile, multiloculated**/lobulated, mixed cystic-solid, posterior mandible mass, usually near 3rd molar
  - Maxilla lesions usually arise within premolar-1st molar region
  - Typically associated with **unerupted tooth**
- MR findings
  - T2: ↑ signal intensity of cystic areas
  - Smaller tumors: **Enhancing mural nodule**

TOP DIFFERENTIAL DIAGNOSES

- Periapical (radicular) cyst
- Dentigerous cyst
- Odontogenic keratocyst
- Odontogenic myxoma
- Ossifying fibroma
- Aneurysmal bone cyst

CLINICAL ISSUES

- 3rd-5th decades
- Slow-growing, expansile, painless mass
- Progressive loosening of teeth
  - Nonhealing "tooth abscess"

DIAGNOSTIC CHECKLIST

- Larger dentigerous cyst and odontogenic keratocyst may mimic ameloblastoma
  - Ameloblastomas expand mandible more concentrically than dentigerous cyst or odontogenic keratocyst
- High T2 signal intensity suggests ameloblastoma, rather than more aggressive neoplasm

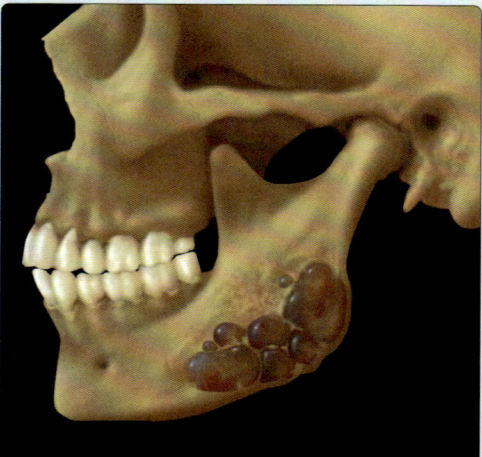
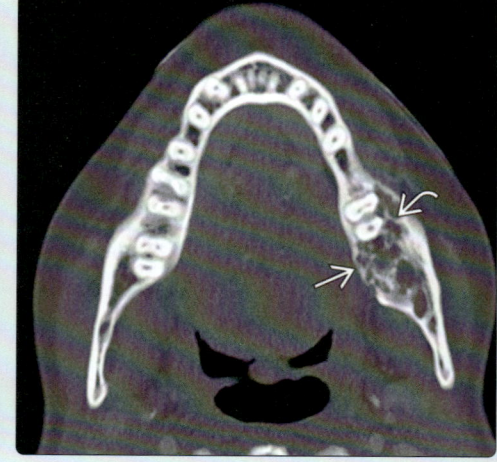

(Left) Lateral graphic shows mandibular ameloblastoma as a "bubbly," multilocular, expansile lesion. The location proximal to the 3rd molar is typical. (Right) Axial bone CT shows the classic appearance of conventional ameloblastoma as a multiloculated, expansile mass in the 2nd-3rd molar region of the mandible ➡. Note the thinned overlying cortex and the characteristic multiple coarse septations ➡.

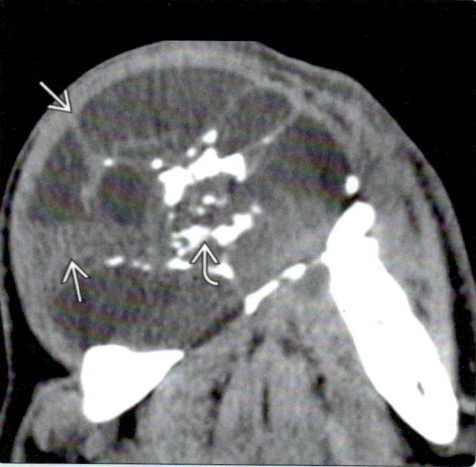
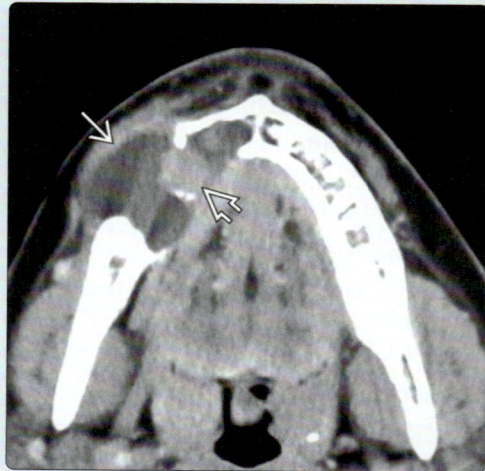

(Left) Axial NECT shows a multicystic mass with soft tissue septations ➡ and cortical fragments ➡ (classified as a conventional ameloblastoma, desmoplastic histologic subtype as per 2022 WHO classification). This type occurs largely in the anterior maxilla and mandible. (Right) Axial CECT of a unicystic ameloblastoma with a mural nodule shows the expansile, hypodense mass ➡ with a central hyperdense and mildly enhancing nodule ➡. Note that the nodule has the potential for involvement of the sublingual space.

Ameloblastoma

TERMINOLOGY

Synonyms

- Adamantoblastoma, adamantinoma (old, nonspecific terms; no longer used)

Definitions

- Locally aggressive, benign neoplasm arising from mandibular or maxillary odontogenic epithelium

IMAGING

General Features

- Best diagnostic clue
  - "Bubbly," multilocular, mixed cystic-solid mass in posterior mandible or maxilla; may be associated with unerupted 3rd molar tooth
- Location
  - Mandible (more common): Usually centered in 3rd molar, mandibular ramus region
  - Maxilla (15%): Usually posterior to premolar/1st molar region
    - Affects maxillary sinus before nasal cavity
- Size
  - > 2 cm at discovery in most cases
- Morphology
  - Mandible: Tumor tends to be confined by thick cortex
  - Maxilla: Tumor more readily extends beyond bone into maxillary sinus and nasal cavity due to thin maxillary cortex

Radiographic Findings

- Radiography
  - Unilocular or multilocular (80%) radiolucent mass with scalloped borders and expanded, thinned cortical margins
  - No calcifications in matrix

CT Findings

- CECT
  - Smaller lesions with marginal enhancement only
  - Larger lesions with extraosseous extension show moderate soft tissue enhancement mixed with cystic (low-density) areas
    - Extraosseous extension is uncommon
- Bone CT
  - Uni- (20%) or **multilocular (80%)** with scalloped borders
  - **Bubbly pattern** is typical; not pathognomonic
  - Unerupted molar tooth association common
  - Resorption of adjacent teeth: More frequent than other cystic lesions
  - Extensive thinning of mandible or maxilla cortex
  - Low-density osteolytic lesion that does not mineralize its matrix

MR Findings

- T1WI
  - Low T1 signal intensity (cystic) typical but high signal occasionally seen
- T2WI
  - Mixed signal intensity

- When large with extraosseous extension, high T2 signal helps differentiate from malignant tumors
- STIR
  - ↑ signal intensity of cystic areas
- DWI
  - Solid areas show ↓ ADC
  - Cystic areas show ↑ ADC > odontogenic keratocyst
- T1WI C+
  - Smaller tumors: **Enhancing mural nodule**
    - May represent tumor growth center, which must be completely resected to achieve surgical cure
  - Enhancement of septations frequently seen
  - Solid regions show rapid enhancement on dynamic MR, reaching maximum contrast by 60 seconds
  - Enhanced imaging may overestimate region of true tumor involvement

Imaging Recommendations

- Best imaging tool
  - Contrast-enhanced thin-section CT with soft tissue and bone algorithm
    - Delineates both focal enhancing mural nodules as well as tumor-bone relationships
- Enhanced MR best defines extraosseous components and association with critical neurovascular structures
  - Especially true in maxilla: Relationships to sinus, nasal cavity, and orbit

DIFFERENTIAL DIAGNOSIS

Periapical (Radicular) Cyst

- Clinically painful with carious lesion or periodontal disease
- Bone CT: Loss of lamina dura and widening of periodontal ligament space
  - Larger lesions are destructive, not expansile

Dentigerous Cyst

- Bone CT: Unilocular cystic lesion surrounding **crown of unerupted tooth**
- No enhancing mural nodule and higher frequency of sclerotic rim from reactive bone

Odontogenic Keratocyst

- Bone CT: Unilocular or multilocular cystic lesion of mandible associated with **unerupted tooth**
  - Lesion envelops around or incorporates crown and tooth root
- Tendency for less buccal-lingual expansion and more sclerotic rim than ameloblastoma
- No enhancing mural nodule

Odontogenic Myxoma (Myxofibroma)

- Uncommon benign tumor arising from dental papilla
- Bone CT: Unilocular or multilocular cystic lesion posterior maxilla or mandible
  - Expansile mass with finer locular septations than typical ameloblastoma
- Myxomatous matrix results in ↑ HU on CT and ↓ T2 on MR relative to ameloblastoma or odontogenic keratocyst

Mandible-Maxilla Ossifying Fibroma

- Bone CT: Fibrotic lytic phase appears as cystic, loculated, or "bubbly" expansile mass

- ○ Tends to scallop around tooth roots
- ○ Wispy septations in expanded cortical bone
- Central ossification, ↑ HU, ↓ T1 and T2

Mandible-Maxilla Aneurysmal Bone Cyst

- More common in children than adults
- Large, round, multilocular mass shows fluid-fluid levels
- No enhancing mural nodule

PATHOLOGY

General Features

- Etiology
  - ○ Benign, epithelial, odontogenic tumor arising from ameloblast (epithelial cell in innermost layer of enamel organ)
  - ○ Previous WHO classification of solid-multicystic, desmoplastic, or unicystic and extraosseous changed to conventional, unicystic, extraosseous/peripheral, adenoid and metastasizing in 2022
  - ○ Recent studies show genetic mutations in mitogen-activated protein kinase (MAPK) pathway (*BRAF*, *KRAS*, and *FGFR2* mutations) and in sonic hedgehog (*SHH*) signaling pathways (*SMO* gene mutations)
- Associated abnormalities
  - ○ 20% may arise from dentigerous cysts
- Mandible:maxilla ratio = 5:1
  - ○ Molar and ramus area > premolar area > symphysis
  - ○ Unerupted 3rd molar tooth often concurrent finding

Gross Pathologic & Surgical Features

- Expansile, multilobular mass in mandible or maxilla
- Mixed lesions, such as ameloblastic odontoma, ameloblastic fibroma, or ameloblastic fibroodontoma, are rare
  - ○ Occur in children

Microscopic Features

- Unencapsulated
- Proliferating sheets or islands of odontogenic epithelium
- Odontogenic tumor of epithelial elements
  - ○ Marginal, palisading, columnar cells with hyperchromatic, small nuclei arranged away from basement membrane
- Histologic types: Plexiform, desmoplastic, follicular (most prevalent), acanthomatous, basal cell, and granular cell
- Malignant variant by histology: Ameloblastic carcinoma
  - ○ Metastasizing ameloblastoma (histologically benign but metastasizes to lungs and lymph nodes)

CLINICAL ISSUES

Presentation

- Most common signs/symptoms
  - ○ Hard, painless mandibular mass
  - ○ Other signs/symptoms
    - – Loose teeth, painless swelling
    - – Bleeding, poorly healing tooth extraction
    - – May be no early clinical symptoms
- Clinical profile
  - ○ Adult with painless, slowly growing mandibular mass

Demographics

- Age
  - ○ Most commonly presents in 30- to 50-year-old patients

- ○ Unilocular lesions often seen in younger age group
- Epidemiology
  - ○ 2nd most common odontogenic tumor (35%)
  - ○ 2nd most common benign mandibular tumor
  - ○ 1% of all lesions of mandible and maxilla

Natural History & Prognosis

- Slow-growing, sometimes indolent, benign neoplasm
- Often takes years to become symptomatic
- Malignant transformation to ameloblastic carcinoma (~ 1%)
- Tumor recurrence is common (33%); more common with multilocularity (85%), sinus destruction or pterygoid erosion in maxillary lesions, root resorption and impacted tooth
  - ○ May require more aggressive 2nd en bloc resection

Treatment

- Complete surgical excision when small or en bloc removal with wide bone margin when large with reconstruction
  - ○ Curettage/enucleation no longer acceptable therapy
- En bloc removal for larger lesions
- Chemotherapy and radiotherapy results have been unpredictable in metastatic settings
- Recent molecular targeted therapies appear to be promising

DIAGNOSTIC CHECKLIST

Consider

- Larger dentigerous cyst and odontogenic keratocyst most difficult to differentiate from ameloblastoma
- Key is relationship to teeth and absence of nodular enhancement in these 2 lesions compared to ameloblastoma

Image Interpretation Pearls

- Ameloblastomas often have resorption of adjacent tooth roots
- **High T2 signal** suggests ameloblastoma, rather than more aggressive neoplasm

Reporting Tips

- Relationship to, or involvement of, inferior alveolar nerve canal in mandible
- Extraalveolar extension to sublingual/submandibular space, buccal space, masticator space, maxillary sinus, pterygopalatine fissure, or orbit

SELECTED REFERENCES

1. Sueyoshi T et al: Comparison of computed tomographic findings for radiolucent lesions of the mandibular ameloblastoma, odontogenic keratocyst, dentigerous cyst, and simple bone cyst. J Dent Sci. 20(1):605-12, 2025
2. Inthong P et al: Factors associated with recurrence of ameloblastoma: a scoping review. Head Neck Pathol. 18(1):82, 2024
3. Rajendra Santosh AB et al: Odontogenic tumors. Dent Clin North Am. 64(1):121-38, 2020
4. Mosier KM: Magnetic resonance imaging of the maxilla and mandible: signal characteristics and features in the differential diagnosis of common lesions. Top Magn Reson Imaging. 24(1):23-37, 2015
5. Sumi M et al: Diffusion-weighted MR imaging of ameloblastomas and keratocystic odontogenic tumors: differentiation by apparent diffusion coefficients of cystic lesions. AJNR Am J Neuroradiol. 29(10):1897-901, 2008

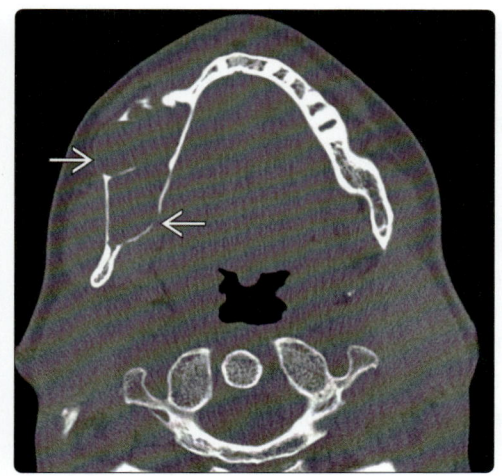

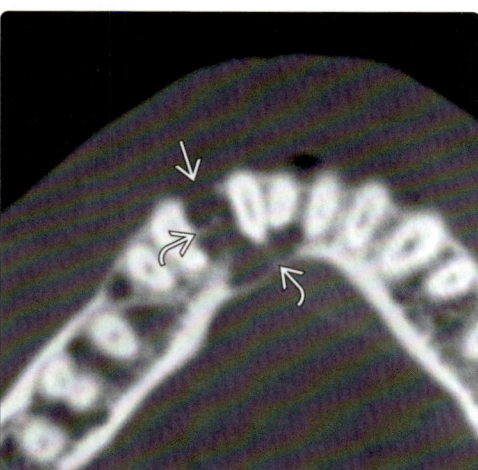

(Left) Axial bone CT shows a large, expansile, multiloculated mass in the body of the mandible on the right. The aggressive character of these lesions is appreciated in the convex expansion of the buccal and lingual cortex, accompanied by marked thinning and focal dehiscence ➡. (Right) Axial bone CT shows a small, multiloculated lesion enlarging between the lateral incisor and the canine teeth. Note the septations ➡ despite its small size and perforation of the buccal cortex ➡.

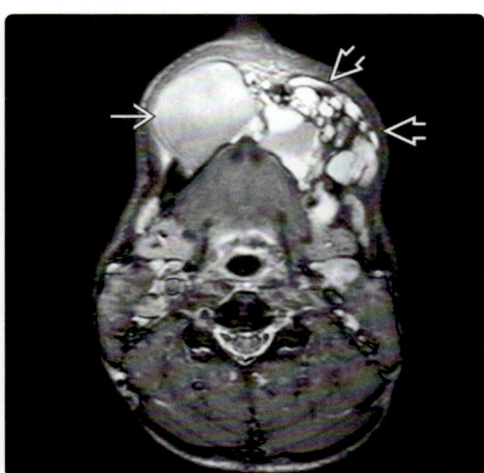

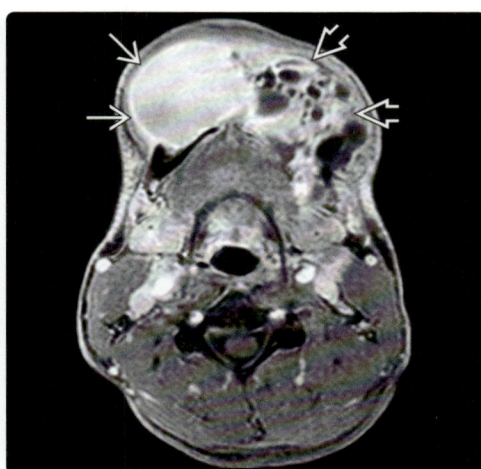

(Left) Axial STIR MR of a large mandibular ameloblastoma suggests a fluid-fluid level in the large, right-sided, cystic component ➡. Note the multilocular, T2-hyperintense component on the left ➡. (Right) Axial T1WI C+ FS MR of the same mandibular ameloblastoma demonstrates prominent enhancement of the walls of both the large, right-sided, unilocular cyst ➡ and of the smaller, multilocular, left-sided, cystic components ➡.

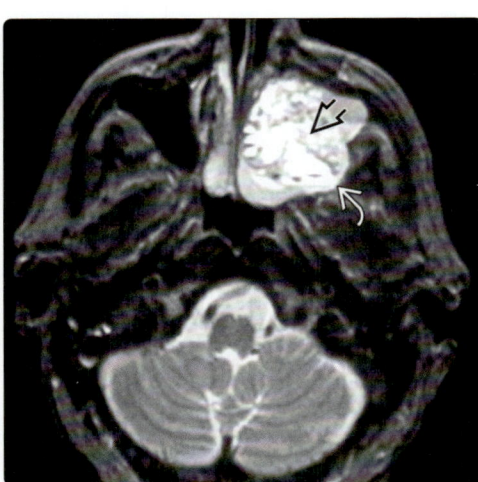

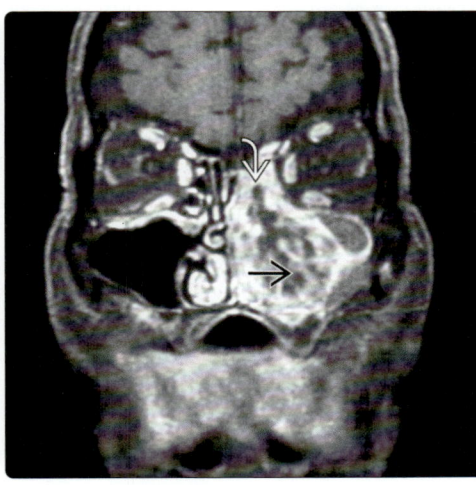

(Left) Axial T2WI FS MR of a maxilla ameloblastoma shows both solid and cystic components in a multiloculated pattern. Note the typical bright T2 signal ➡ of the cystic components and the expansion of the posterior maxillary sinus walls ➡. (Right) Coronal T1WI C+ FS MR of the same ameloblastoma demonstrates the typical enhancement of the septations ➡. The locally aggressive nature of these lesions is likewise evident by the extension into the nasal cavity and ethmoid air cells ➡.

TERMINOLOGY

- Malignant tumor with ability to produce osteoid from neoplastic cells

IMAGING

- Bone CT: Bone destruction with aggressive periosteal reaction and osteoid formation
- MR best evaluates soft tissue component of tumor
  - Intramedullary and extraosseous soft tissues
- US-guided core needle biopsy for diagnosis
- PET/CT: For staging, detection of metastases ± skip lesions
- Bone scan: ↑ tracer uptake

TOP DIFFERENTIAL DIAGNOSES

- Mandible-maxilla osteomyelitis
- Mandible-maxilla osteoradionecrosis
- Mandible-maxilla metastasis
- Ewing sarcoma
- Langerhans cell histiocytosis

PATHOLOGY

- Heterogeneous mass with ossified and nonossified components
- Chondroblastic > osteoblastic > fibroblastic

CLINICAL ISSUES

- Mean age: 35-41 years; M:F = 1.1:1
- Jaw lesions distinct from those occurring in long bones
- Prognosis depends on pathologic type, size, location, and presence of metastases
- 5-year survival: ~ 40-65%
- Complete resection affords best chance of survival
- Local recurrence more common than distant metastasis

DIAGNOSTIC CHECKLIST

- **Aggressive periosteal reaction** suggests osteosarcoma
- If not present, consider infection or metastasis
- Consider XRT-induced sarcoma if patient had radiation years prior

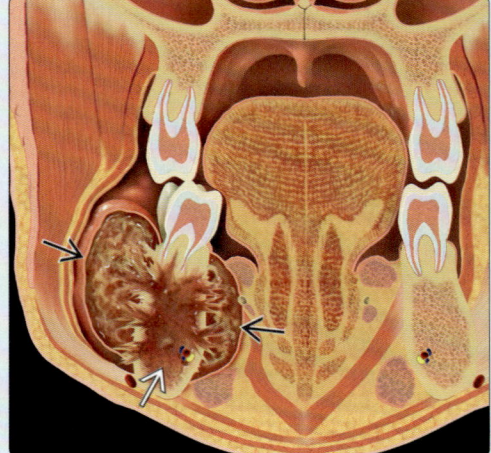
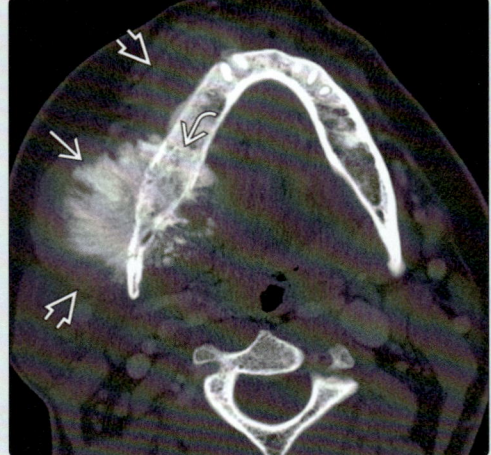

(Left) Coronal graphic shows right mandible osteosarcoma. Note soft tissue mass perforating through cortex ➡ and intramedullary tumor ➡. (Right) Axial bone CT demonstrates a large, dense mass arising from the right mandible ➡. Mass has both osteoid matrix and periosteal reaction. This is classic periosteal reaction associated with osteosarcomas, where periosteum is lifted off perpendicular to bone. Marrow within involved portion of mandible is sclerotic ➡. Note associated soft tissue mass ➡.

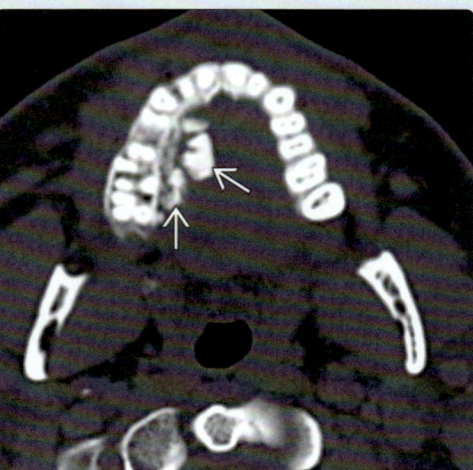
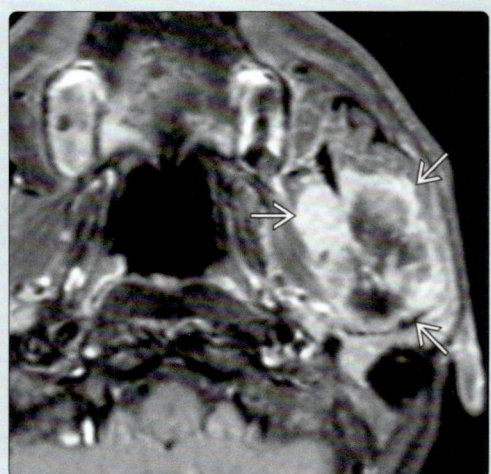

(Left) Axial bone CT through maxilla shows exophytic mass with amorphous, immature new bone ➡ and cortical breakthrough. This is the parosteal form of osteosarcoma. Note absence of significant associated nonossified soft tissue mass. (Right) Axial T1 C+ FS MR shows heterogeneous enhancement of soft tissue component of osteosarcoma arising in mandible. Note tumor has infiltrated the parotid gland, masseter, and pterygoid muscles ➡.

TERMINOLOGY

Synonyms

- Osteogenic sarcoma

Definitions

- Malignant primary bone tumor arising from mandible or maxilla that produces osteoid

IMAGING

General Features

- Best diagnostic clue
  - Bone destruction with aggressive periosteal reaction
- Location
  - Mandible more common than maxilla
    - Angle, ramus, or body of mandible
- Size
  - Variable; usually < 10 cm
- Morphology
  - Destructive lesion with osteoid formation

Radiographic Findings

- Radiography
  - Poorly defined alveolar mass ± tumoral calcification with aggressive periosteal reaction
  - Unilateral symmetric widening of periodontal ligament space of teeth in absence of dental disease

CT Findings

- CECT
  - Moderate enhancement of solid components
- Bone CT
  - Expansile lesion with ↑ density, **aggressive periosteal reaction**
    - Sunburst periosteal reaction most typical

MR Findings

- Heterogeneous signal intensity on T1 & T2
  - Mineralized tumor = low T1, low T2
  - Solid, nonmineralized tumor = intermediate T1, high T2
- Heterogeneous contrast enhancement

Nuclear Medicine Findings

- PET/CT: For staging, detection of metastases ± skip lesions
- Bone scan: ↑ tracer uptake

Imaging Recommendations

- Best imaging tool
  - CT best to show osseous destruction, osteoid matrix
    - Thin-section bone algorithm NECT
  - MR best for soft tissue & intramedullary extent
  - US-guided biopsy for diagnosis
  - PET/CT for staging

DIFFERENTIAL DIAGNOSIS

Mandible-Maxilla Osteomyelitis

- Bony destruction without osteoid formation; ± sequestrum formation
- Garré sclerosing osteomyelitis: Lytic bone destruction with exuberant periosteal reaction
  - Periosteal reaction is typically laminar ("onion skin")

- Chronic recurrent multifocal osteomyelitis (CRMO): Recurrent episodes of multifocal nonbacterial osteomyelitis
  - Chronic recurrent osteomyelitis (CRO) of jaw, almost always in association with CRMO

Mandible-Maxilla Osteoradionecrosis

- Peaks in 2 years following radiation
- Lytic and sclerotic destruction

Mandible-Maxilla Metastasis

- Aggressive bony destructive changes
- No periosteal reaction or tumoral calcification

Ewing Sarcoma

- Irregular, destructive lytic mass
- Does not produce osteoid matrix

Langerhans Cell Histiocytosis

- Punched-out lytic lesion
- ± enhancing soft tissue mass

Fibromatosis

- Irregular, lytic, destructive lesion
- No osteoid matrix or periosteal reaction

PATHOLOGY

General Features

- Etiology
  - Primary etiology unknown in most cases
  - **May occur following radiation to face**
    - Typically > 10 years after XRT

Microscopic Features

- Highly pleomorphic, spindle-shaped tumor cells producing different forms of osteoid
- **Chondroblastic** > osteoblastic > fibroblastic

CLINICAL ISSUES

Presentation

- Most common signs/symptoms
  - Enlarging soft tissue mass over mandible with ↑ pain

Natural History & Prognosis

- Mandibular osteosarcomas less likely to metastasize than long bone tumors
- Prognosis depends on pathologic type, size, location, metastases
- **5-year survival: ~ 40-65%**
  - Greater 5-year survival for mandibular osteosarcomas than maxillary

Treatment

- Complete resection affords best chance of survival
- ± adjuvant chemotherapy, radiation

SELECTED REFERENCES

1. Rodriguez-Molinero J et al: Clinical and pathological features of osteosarcomas of the jaws: a retrospective study. Clin Pract. 14(3):965-79, 2024
2. Sandeep KS et al: Osteosarcoma of head and neck region: tertiary cancer care center experience. Indian J Otolaryngol Head Neck Surg. 76(1):581-6, 2024
3. Brown JM et al: Clinical features and overall survival of osteosarcoma of the mandible. Int J Oral Maxillofac Surg. 52(5):524-30, 2023

Mandible-Maxilla and TMJ

TERMINOLOGY

- **Medication-related osteonecrosis of jaw (MRONJ)**
- Necrosis of mandible or maxilla associated with medications; no history of craniofacial radiotherapy
- **Antiresorptive** medications, such as bisphosphonates & denosumab, & **antiangiogenic** drugs, such as bevacizumab
- **Other names:** Antiresorptive drug-related (**ARONJ**), bisphosphonate-related (**BRONJ**), & denosumab-related osteonecrosis of jaw (**DRONJ**)

IMAGING

- CT: Rare (characteristic, poorly marginated, diffuse low attenuation with bilateral symmetric sclerosis)
- Nonspecific: More common (focal sclerosis, thickened lamina dura, sequestrum, periosteal reaction, gas foci)
  - Early: Nonhealing extraction socket
  - Late: Diffuse destructive changes in alveolar ridge
- Tissue swelling if severe, infected, pathologic fracture
- MR: Variable signal from edema & bone changes

- Enhancement common & does not imply infection
- Typically FDG avid

TOP DIFFERENTIAL DIAGNOSES

- Mandible-maxilla osteomyelitis
- Mandible-maxilla osteoradionecrosis
- Mandible-maxilla metastasis

CLINICAL ISSUES

- Nonhealing exposed bone, after **8 weeks**, no radiation history, **mandible much more common** than maxilla
- Mimics dental infection & follows tooth extraction

DIAGNOSTIC CHECKLIST

- Diagnosis should be considered in patient with nonhealing extraction socket or jaw pain
- Osteonecrosis risk higher with **concurrent steroid** therapy
- Typically mixed lytic-sclerotic mandible-maxilla with edema in surrounding tissues ± reactive adenopathy
- *Actinomyces* infections may be associated

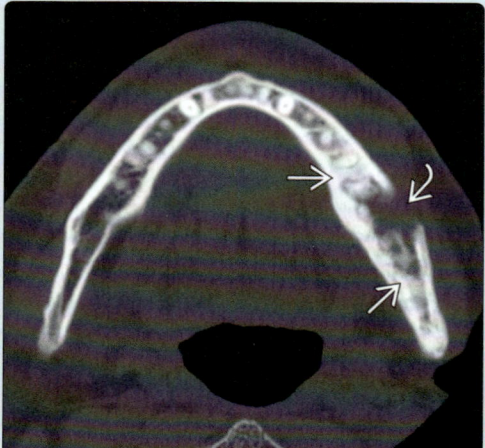
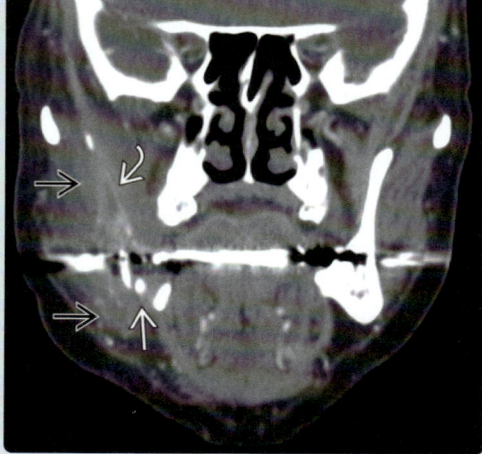

(Left) *Axial bone CT shows medication-related osteonecrosis of jaw (MRONJ) from IV bisphosphonates. Note a mixed sclerotic ➡ & lytic ➡ lesion in left mandible body at site of recent tooth extraction.* (Right) *Coronal CECT shows denosumab-associated MRONJ ➡ in a patient with history of prostate cancer. This advanced MRONJ with extensive lysis of right hemimandible extends into the ramus ➡. Note soft tissue thickening ➡, including masseter muscle, which had inflammatory changes & some pus at surgery.*

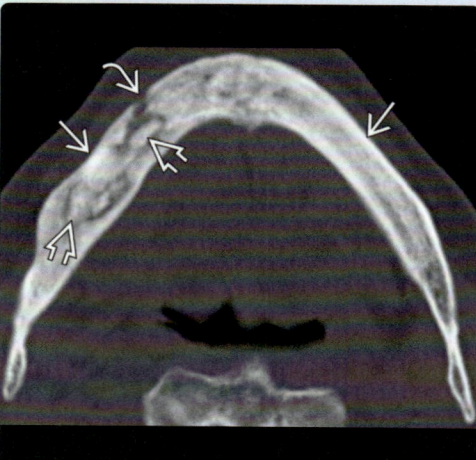
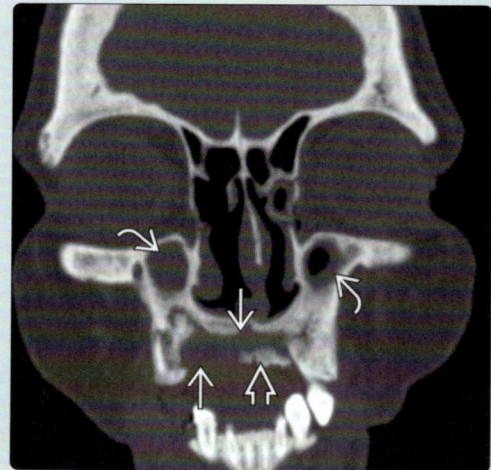

(Left) *Axial bone CT shows marked, diffuse, fairly symmetric sclerosis ➡ in the mandible bilaterally in this patient on bisphosphonates & no history of radiation, consistent with MRONJ. Note the right-sided lucent areas/cortical break ➡ & early sequestrum formation ➡.* (Right) *Coronal bone CT shows severe maxillary medication-related osteonecrosis in a patient with multiple myeloma on IV bisphosphonates. Note bony destruction ➡ & sequestrum ➡. Bilateral maxillary sinus opacification ➡ is seen.*

Medication-Related Osteonecrosis of Jaw (MRONJ)

TERMINOLOGY

Abbreviations

- Medication-related osteonecrosis of jaw (MRONJ)

Synonyms

- **Antiresorptive drug**-related osteonecrosis of jaw (**ARONJ**); terms MRONJ & ARONJ preferred over others
- **Bisphosphonate**-related osteonecrosis of jaw (**BRONJ**)
- **Denosumab**-related osteonecrosis of jaw (**DRONJ**)

Definitions

- Medication-related exposed bone, or bone that can be probed through intraoral or extraoral fistula in maxillofacial region, persisting **> 8 weeks**
  - No history of prior craniofacial radiation therapy
- Induced by **antiresorptive** drugs, such as bisphosphonates (BP) & denosumab, & **antiangiogenics**, such as bevacizumab, sunitinib

IMAGING

General Features

- Best diagnostic clue
  - Spontaneous osteonecrosis usually in mylohyoid ridge, or precipitated by dental surgery/tooth extraction
- Location
  - **Mandible** > > > **maxilla**
  - Often located on alveolar ridge with loss of teeth
  - Advanced disease extends into mandibular ramus
  - Tilted implants with angle ≥ 5.1° relative to occlusal plane of prosthesis show stronger association with periimplant MRONJ

Radiographic Findings

- Radiography
  - Mixed permeative & sclerotic changes with cortical destruction & periosteal reaction
  - Involvement of inferior alveolar canal by lytic process or pathologic fracture in severe cases

CT Findings

- Bone CT
  - Characteristic: Rare (poorly marginated, diffuse, low-attenuation area with bilateral, symmetric sclerosis)
  - Nonspecific: More common (focal sclerosis, thickened lamina dura, sequestrum, periosteal reaction, gas foci)
  - Early: Nonhealing extraction socket
  - Late: Diffuse destructive changes in alveolar ridge
  - Widened periodontal ligament spaces
  - May be associated with **pathologic fracture**
  - Soft tissue swelling if destruction is severe, infected, or associated with pathologic fracture
  - Posttreatment: No new lysis but sclerosis permanent

MR Findings

- T2WI
  - Variable appearance
    - Acute: Bone edema shows high signal intensity
    - Healing phase: Variable or low intensity if sclerotic
  - Surrounding soft tissues, especially muscles of mastication, often hyperintense due to edema
  - Nonnecrotic level I & II **reactive adenopathy** can be seen

- T1WI C+ FS
  - **Enhancement** in healing bone & surrounding soft tissues
    - Does not usually imply infection or tumor

Imaging Recommendations

- Best imaging tool
  - Radiography (panorex) usually 1st imaging utilized
  - Bone CT; CECT/MR if suspected infection

DIFFERENTIAL DIAGNOSIS

Mandible-Maxilla Osteomyelitis

- Periosteal reaction, cortical sinus tract ± adjacent abscess

Mandible-Maxilla Osteoradionecrosis

- Prior radiation for orofacial or oropharynx malignancy
- May mimic nonspecific findings of MRONJ

Mandible-Maxilla Metastasis

- Destructive soft tissue mass in mandible

PATHOLOGY

General Features

- Etiology
  - **Antiresorptive medications: BP & denosumab**
    - To treat metabolic & oncologic bone lesions: Paget disease, multiple myeloma, metastases, osteoporosis
    - BP disrupts osteoclastic function, slowing bone remodeling process & ↑ bone density
    - BP inhibit endothelial proliferation, interrupt intraosseous circulation → BRONJ
  - BP: Non-nitrogen-containing (etidronate, clodronate, tiludronate) or nitrogen-containing BP (pamidronate, alendronate, ibandronate, risedronate, zoledronic acid)
  - Denosumab: Receptor activator of nuclear factor-κ-B ligand (RANKL) antibody
  - **Antiangiogenic drugs**: Used in cancer to prevent metastasis by interfering with new blood vessel formation → ischemia & MRONJ
- Associated abnormalities
  - Osteonecrosis higher with **concurrent steroid** therapy
  - *Actinomyces* infections may be associated

Gross Pathologic & Surgical Features

- Ulcerated lesions in oral cavity, often with exposed nonviable bone; **clinical exam essential** for diagnosis
- **Biopsy may exacerbate** MRONJ

CLINICAL ISSUES

Presentation

- Most common signs/symptoms
  - Jaw pain & ulcers with loose teeth or nonhealing extraction socket

Natural History & Prognosis

- Local debridement & discontinuation of medication/BP should halt progression

SELECTED REFERENCES

1. Jo HG et al: Clinical and Radiographic features of peri-implant medication-related osteonecrosis of the jaw: a retrospective study. Clin Implant Dent Relat Res. 27(1):e13412, 2024

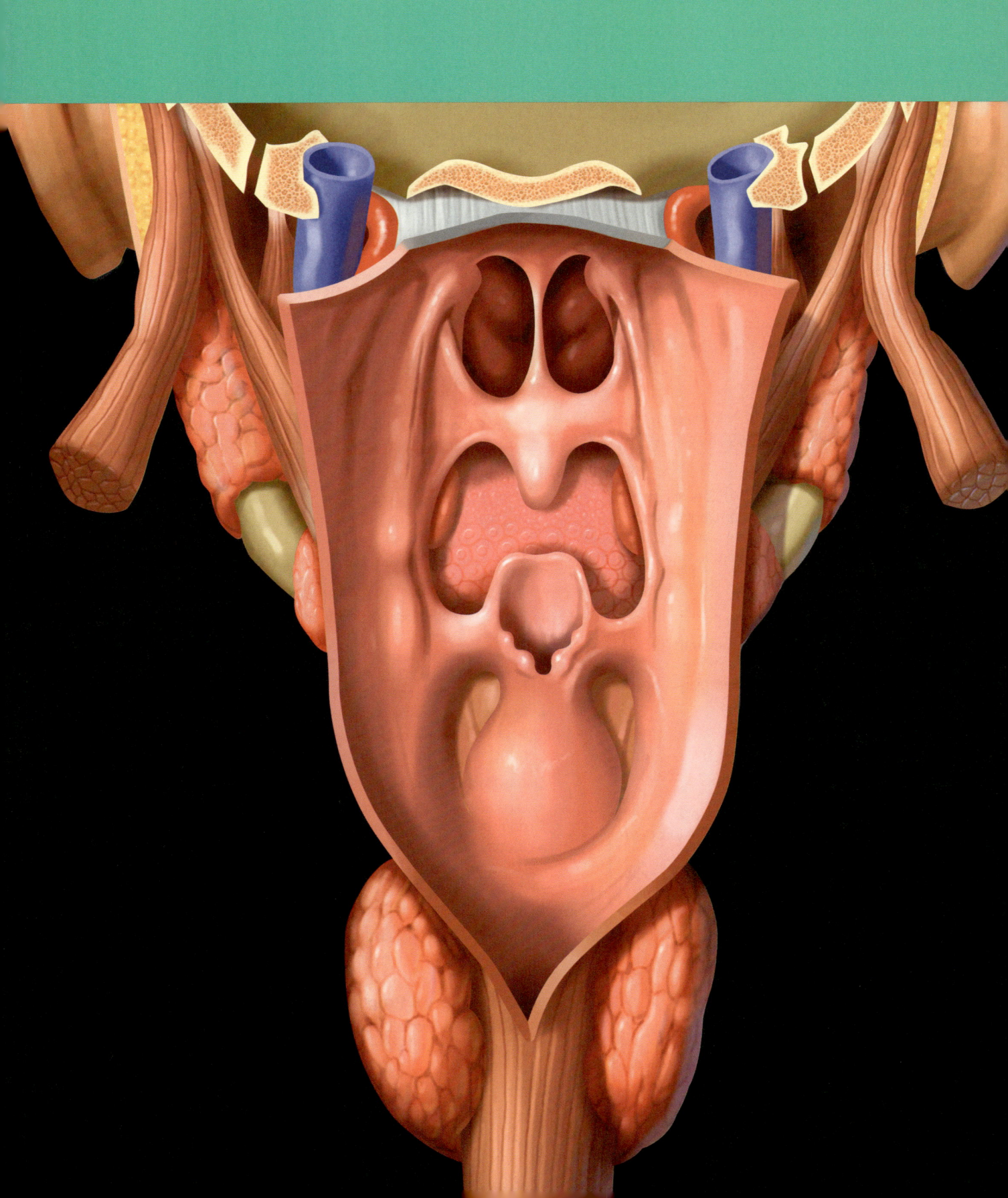

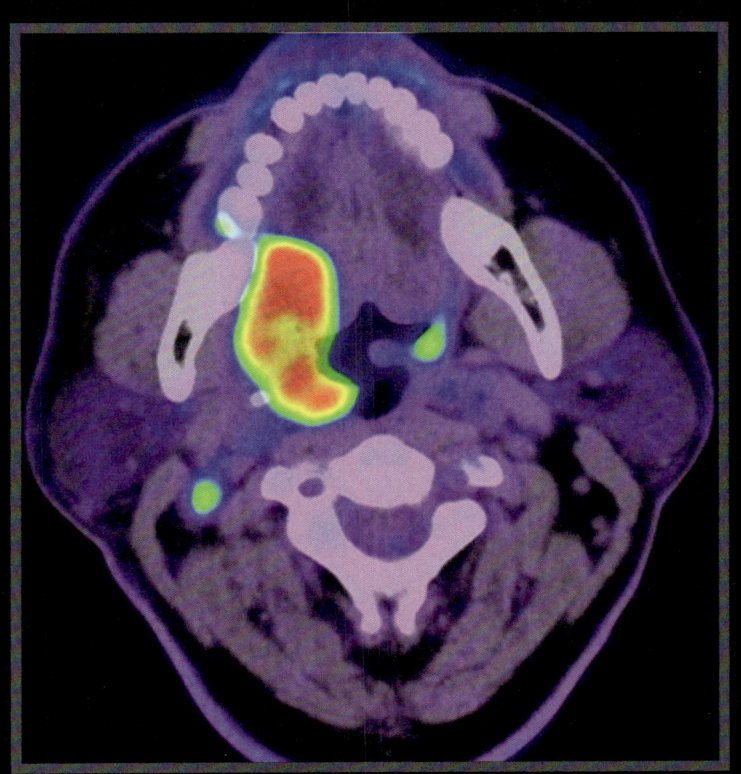

Introduction

Squamous cell carcinoma (SCCa) is the most common malignancy in the head and neck (H&N). Recent developments in the understanding of the molecular nature and causes of SCCa now reveal it to be a heterogeneous malignancy.

In most sites of the H&N, **tobacco** is the most common causative agent of mucosal dysplasia and neoplasia. **Alcohol** is a synergistic cofactor, while poor oral hygiene and genetics are also contributing risk factors. Paralleling the declining trend of smoking over the last few decades, there has been an overall decline in the incidence of H&N SCCa, particularly in the oral cavity, larynx, and hypopharynx.

Conversely, in the oropharynx, there has been a rise in **base of tongue (BOT)/lingual tonsil** and **palatine tonsillar SCCa**, particularly in middle-aged (31-78 years) White (> 90%) males (85%) who may have limited or no history of tobacco and alcohol use. This group of **oropharyngeal SCCa (OPSCCa)** tumors is positive for **human papillomavirus (HPV)**, most commonly HPV-16 subtype, which is also responsible for anogenital neoplasms. The past few decades have seen a 225% increase in HPV(+) OPSCCa and a 50% reduction in HPV(-) OPSCCa. Currently, 80% of OPSCCa in the USA are HPV related with risk directly correlating to number of sexual partners and oral sex practices. HPV(+) OPSCCa is more responsive to chemoradiation than HPV(-) OPSCCa, and patients have an overall better survival rate. Patients who are smokers with HPV(+) tumors carry an intermediate prognosis. A new TNM classification has been added exclusively for HPV(+) OPSCCa in the current (**8th ed.**) American Joint Committee on Cancer (AJCC) staging manual. Previously, AJCC TNM staging was the same for all OPSCCa. Extranodal extension (ENE) of metastatic disease in lymph nodes is a high-risk, poor prognostic factor for most H&N tumors, but ENE is not included in AJCC 8th ed. for HPV(+) OPSCCa staging because pathologic data suggest that perinodal inflammatory changes may simulate ENE. However, advanced radiologic ENE is now used in AJCC 9th ed. (2025) staging for nasopharyngeal carcinoma.

NPCa is a distinctly different neoplasm with the most common histopathologic subtypes associated with **Epstein-Barr virus (EBV)** infection. The least common and most aggressive form (keratinizing NPCa) is related to tobacco and alcohol abuse, although some pathology literature has also suggested an association with HPV infection. **SCCa of the larynx** is strongly associated with tobacco and alcohol abuse, especially in males > 50 years of age. However, recently there is increasing incidence of HPV-related laryngeal cancer cases in younger, < 30-year-old nonsmokers, which is higher in females than males. However, the **College of American Pathologists (CAP) guidelines** suggest not to routinely perform high-risk-HPV testing on oropharyngeal non-SCCas (CAP expert consensus opinion) or on nonoropharyngeal primary tumors of H&N (CAP recommendation). This is due to the fact that HPV positivity does not really affect aggressiveness or prognosis/therapeutic difference in these tumors.

While our current understanding of SCCa is evolving through greater molecular interrogation of these tumors, the radiologist's roles remain largely unchanged. At the time of diagnosis, the radiologist must report details about the primary tumor to assign a **tumor stage**, including **size** and **local extent** of the primary, detecting perineural tumor (**PNT**) spread, and assessing regional **nodes** and **distant** spread of disease. Following treatment, both **baseline** and **surveillance** imaging require careful evaluation to detect **residual** or **recurrent SCCa, treatment complications**, and **2nd primary neoplasms**.

Imaging Approaches & Indications

There is no definitive best imaging modality for all H&N sites when staging SCCa. Some specific tumor sites are better served by either **CECT or MR or PET/CECT**. A patient with copious secretions or pain may not tolerate long MR sequences, and, in that instance, CECT or PET combined with CECT is preferred. Excellent-quality neck imaging is more readily reproducible from patient to patient using CT than MR. Also, large FOV, nonoptimized MR sequences, and lack of familiarity with basic neck anatomy make detection of key findings difficult. A poorly performed, inaccurately reported neck MR is an expensive and unsatisfactory alternative to CT.

MR does offer specific utility in certain areas, e.g., it is the preferred staging tool for **NPCa** because detection of **skull base** infiltration (T3) or **intracranial/cranial nerve** disease (T4) is extremely important for staging and treatment planning. MR offers better soft tissue contrast for detecting small primary tonsillar tumors and evaluating the **deep extent** of a lesion when planning surgical resection or intensity-modulated radiation therapy (IMRT). For this reason, MR may be used in the **oral cavity and oropharynx**. In the **larynx**, MR is so affected by motion artifact that it is largely reserved for determination of **cartilage penetration** (T4a) when CECT is equivocal. **Diffusion restriction** and **dynamic contrast MR** time-signal intensity curves (**TIC**) showing **early enhancement** with a peak time < 150 s and a **low washout ratio** of < 30% may be seen in malignant tumors. After successful treatment, TIC changes from pretreatment rapid rise and washout to posttreatment slow rise and gradual trapping (wash-in) pattern. Lymph node metastasis at any site is almost equally well evaluated with either CECT or MR, but PET is superior to both with the potential to identify FDG-avid metastasis in normal-sized nodes.

Given the complexity of neck anatomy, **FDG PET** in the H&N is best performed as a combined PET/CECT examination. There are variable degrees of normal FDG uptake in muscles, brown fat, salivary and lymphoid tissue, and recent biopsy sites. These all are potential false-positive pitfalls in PET imaging, but routine measurement and reporting of standardized uptake values (SUV) can obviate the pitfalls. A potential false-negative finding is absence of FDG uptake in a cystic/necrotic node, but correlation with neck CECT imaging will allow correct identification of cystic/necrotic nodal metastases.

Ultrasound (US) can be helpful in identifying early subcapsular deposits in normal-sized nodes and ENE of nodal metastasis. US can also serve as imaging guidance for FNA.

Imaging Anatomy

SCCa arises from the mucosal surface of the upper airway and digestive tract, pharynx, and larynx. The pharynx is really a muscular tube encased by the middle layer of deep cervical fascia (DCF) and attached to the skull base by pharyngobasilar fascia. The **pharyngeal mucosal space** is a continuous sheet of tissue on the airway side of the DCF. It is divided into separate sites anatomically. Staging of mucosal SCCa is individualized to each site or subsite.

The **nasopharynx**, posterior to the nasal cavity, extends from the most cranial pharynx at the skull base to the soft palate.

Inferiorly, it is contiguous with the **oropharynx**, which extends caudally to the hyoid bone. Anterior tonsillar pillars and circumvallate papillae of the tongue define the anterior limit of the oropharynx. The anterior 2/3 of the tongue lies in the oral cavity and is known as the oral tongue. The posterior 1/3 is called the tongue base and is part of the oropharynx.

Below the hyoid bone, the pharynx divides to form the larynx, which is continuous with the trachea, and hypopharynx, which joins the cervical esophagus. The **hypopharynx** consists of **3 subsites** starting with the letter "**P**." The **p**osterior wall of the **hypopharynx** (giving rise to 15% of hypopharyngeal SCCa) is a continuation of the posterior wall of the oropharynx. Lateral "pockets" of the hypopharynx form the **p**yriform sinuses and are separated from the larynx by the aryepiglottic (AE) folds. Nearly 65% of hypopharyngeal SCCa arise in the pyriform sinuses. The 3rd subsite of the hypopharynx is the **p**ostcricoid region (20% of hypopharyngeal SCCa). The **larynx** is anterior in the neck and also has **3 subsites**: **Supraglottic** larynx, which includes the epiglottis, AE folds, and false cords; **glottis** with true vocal cords; and **subglottis**, which is contiguous with the cervical trachea. Around 60% of laryngeal SCCa is glottic.

Approaches to Imaging Issues in H&N SCCa

Staging SCCa is performed using the AJCC 8th ed., aside from updated AJCC 9th ed. (2025) for NPCa. Referral to the site-specific tumor (T) and nodal (N) features greatly enhances an imaging report. When the size of a T or N is important for tumor or nodal stage, respectively, the **greatest dimension** is measured. Some superficial oral cavity tumors are best measured on clinical examination. The **puffed-cheek** technique, in which the patient purses the lips and puffs out the cheeks, can be extremely helpful to detect small oral cavity tumors and evaluate the surfaces of larger tumors outlined by more air separating normal structures in the oral cavity. This can be easily done in CT, which is acquired in a few seconds, but may be more difficult in MR, as the patient will have to do the maneuver for a few minutes during the MR sequence acquisition without moving. The key role of cross-sectional imaging is to evaluate features that are not evident on exam, such as deep extent or bone infiltration, which may upstage a tumor or alter treatment options.

Depth of invasion (DOI) was recently introduced into the oral cavity SCCa (OSCCa) clinical T staging (using clinical examination and imaging) in addition to pathologic T staging in AJCC 8th ed., recognizing its prognostic significance and clinical relevance. DOI is measured from the normal mucosal basement membrane adjacent to the tumor to the deepest point of tumor invasion. This is different from tumor thickness (TT), which measures the distance from the tumor surface to the deepest point of invasion. DOI and TT are the same for flat tumors, as the interpreted normal mucosal basement membrane plane is at the same level as the tumor surface. DOI is smaller than TT in exophytic/bulging tumors that extend outward from the interpreted mucosal plane. DOI is larger than TT in endophytic/ulcerated tumors that have a gap between the interpreted mucosal plane and the tumor surface. Practically in tongue SCCa CT/MR imaging (any flat, exophytic/bulging or endophytic/ulcerated tumor) DOI is measured perpendicular to a "plumb line" along the lateral border of the tongue. In axial CT/MR, the "plumb line" connects normal tongue tissue anterior and posterior to the tumor along the tongue lateral border. In coronal CT/MR, the "plumb line" connects the normal lateral border tongue tissue superior and inferior to the tumor. In contrast, TT outer

measurement is along the aforementioned "plumb line" in flat tumor, lateral to the line in exophytic/bulging tumor and medial to the line in endophytic/ulcerated tumor. Pathologic DOI measurement uses adjacent normal mucosal basement membrane as the originating point; however, the basement membrane is invisible on imaging, as the thickness of the oral mucosal epithelium is just 0.5 mm. The difference between the potential originating points of measurement from the mucosal surface on CT/MR and from the normal basement membrane on surgical specimen is negligible. There is a high radiologic and pathologic TT correlation (0.78) in all oral cavity subsite tumors. Pathologic TT (pTT) on a surgical specimen is slightly thinner than radiologic TT (rTT) on CT/MR, apparently due to tumor shrinkage on formalin fixation of the surgical specimen. The shrinkage factor is smaller for the oral tongue (0.91) compared to other oral cavity subsite tumors (0.70), thought to be due to more free margins in the tongue leading to less propensity to shrink than other subsite tumors more deeply embedded in tissues. rTT-pTT correlation is suboptimal when there is > 8 weeks to surgery after imaging, as the tumor would have grown in between. rTT on MR has a slightly higher correlation with pTT in comparison to rTT on CT, but the difference is not statistically significant. As most OSCCa are flat tumors (88%), TT is the same as DOI in most, and both of these are independent predictors of survival, which can stratify death risk in addition to traditional tumor size.

Detection of a **PNT** may significantly alter the surgical resection &/or the radiation treatment field. Both mucosal and skin SCCa exhibit neurotropism, as do some salivary gland tumors and lymphomas. PNT is usually more evident on MR but may be detected on CT with careful evaluation of skull base foramina and known routes of spread.

Metastatic **nodal disease** is the most important prognostic factor in H&N SCCa. Prognosis worsens in H&N SCCa with increasing number of nodes and nodal chains, bilateral nodes, and lower level neck nodes. Lymph node metastasis reduces survival by 50% and doubles the incidence of distant metastasis. **ENE** reduces survival by a further 50% and predisposes to a 10x increased recurrence risk and 3x increased risk of distant metastasis. ENE is considered a high-risk, **poor prognostic** factor for all H&N tumors, **except HPV(+) OPSCCa** and **mucosal melanoma**.

At the time of a staging neck CECT scan, lung apices and the bones should also be evaluated for **metastases**. Finally, many SCCa H&N cancer patients have increased risk of a **2nd primary neoplasm**. Second primary tumors are most frequently found with hypopharyngeal SCCa, and 1/3 are synchronous with the initial SCCa.

After surgery, radiation, &/or chemotherapy, **posttreatment baseline** imaging should be obtained to confirm absence of **residual disease**. This also serves as a roadmap of an anatomically changed neck to aid in detection of **recurrent disease**. The initial posttreatment scan for almost all SCCa is a PET/CECT, which should be delayed ~ 10-12 weeks to minimize false-positive FDG uptake from posttreatment inflammatory changes. A baseline CECT study may be obtained at 8-10 weeks after chemoradiation, while postsurgical studies are often obtained at 10-12 weeks.

The **posttreatment baseline** scan following radiation &/or chemotherapy should show no evidence of residual disease. The presence of enlarged nodes or residual primary mass

Sites and Subsites of Head and Neck Squamous Cell Carcinoma

1. Nasopharynx	3. Oral cavity	4. Hypopharynx
Fossa of Rosenmüller	Oral tongue	Posterior hypopharyngeal wall
	Floor of mouth	Pyriform sinus
2. Oropharynx	Alveolar ridge: Maxilla	Postcricoid region
Palatine tonsil	Buccal mucosa	**5. Larynx**
Posterior oropharyngeal wall	Lip	Supraglottis
Soft palate	Hard palate	Glottis
Lingual tonsil/base of tongue	Retromolar trigone	Subglottis
	Alveolar ridge: Mandible	

following treatment is of concern and is typically surgically resected. Posttreatment neck dissections are ideally performed < 10 weeks to minimize the complexity of surgery that results with neck fibrosis. So-called borderline soft tissue at baseline CT/MR may be carefully watched, may undergo US-guided aspiration, or may be resected.

Radiation therapy has changed enormously in the last 2 decades with increasing use of **IMRT** for H&N cancers. IMRT maximizes dose to tumor, minimizes radiation to normal surrounding tissues, and requires accurate delineation of tumor margins. More input from radiologists to ensure accurate treatment volumes may be needed with MR, PET/CECT, or CECT alone. Radiation ± **chemotherapy** results in significant changes to appearance in neck soft tissues. Radiation results in acute inflammation and edema of all tissues in the radiation field. Over time, this changes to fibrosis, atrophy, and altered appearances on CECT and MR.

Surgical resection of a primary tumor &/or cervical neck nodes also results in changes to normal neck contours. Familiarity with the types of nodal **neck dissections** and common **flap reconstructions** helps evaluate both complications and recurrence. Knowledge of what surgical procedure was performed prior to evaluating posttreatment imaging is critical. Some resections, such as selective neck dissections, can be subtle on imaging, while large resections with flap reconstructions can be quite complex. MR is less affected by hardware artifact and more sensitive for recurrent tumors; however, the muscular component of a flap reconstruction undergoes denervation changes, resulting in variable MR signal intensity and enhancement. On the baseline scan following neck reconstruction, residual or progressive tumors should be described.

Recurrent SCCa most often occurs in the first 2 years after initial treatment. Frequency of **surveillance imaging** during this time is variable and may be performed in 3- to 6-month intervals, depending on initial tumor stage, prognostic features, and clinical course, including physical findings. At the follow-up imaging examination, the possibility of a **2nd primary tumor** must be considered. Remember to look for **residual, recurrent, and new** tumors on each follow-up study.

How to Stage New Tumor With CT or MR
- Determine site of primary; open TNM staging table for specific primary site
- Evaluate size and local extent of tumor; what is deep extent; is there bone marrow infiltration; is there PNT; how far does it go in each direction; primary is best described in dedicated paragraph in report
- Evaluate regional drainage nodes and contralateral node(s); look for any enlarged retropharyngeal nodes
- Evaluate included lungs and bones for metastases
- PET/CT or PET/MR greatly increases staging accuracy

How to Read Posttreatment Scan
- Compare pretreatment scan, history of original tumor stage, treatment and time since treatment; confirm on scans what, if anything, has been resected; be aware that selective neck dissections may be subtle; is there reconstruction flap
- Evaluate effects of radiation and become familiar with posttreatment appearances; look for residual/recurrent tumor at primary site
- Evaluate for adenopathy through entire neck, especially if some levels were dissected previously; drainage patterns may change
- Consider possibility of 2nd primary tumor, especially if history of excessive smoking/alcohol: H&N mucosal SCCa, lungs, cervical esophagus; evaluate lungs and bones for metastases
- Look for **solid, nodular enhancing tumor recurrence** at **anastomotic margins** of grafts and flaps

Clinical Implications

If a primary site is not evident on clinical examination in a patient with a new neck mass that is nodal SCCa (**unknown primary tumor**), 4 key sites should be evaluated for the asymmetric soft tissue of an unknown primary tumor in a neck CECT or MR: (1) Nasopharynx: **Fossa of Rosenmüller**, (2) oropharynx: **Palatine tonsil**, (3) oropharynx: **BOT or lingual tonsil**, and (4) hypopharynx: **Apex of pyriform sinus**. The fossa of Rosenmüller and pyriform sinus apex may be clinical "blind spots," either at the in-office examination or, if very small, even at direct endoscopy. The palatine and lingual tonsils may harbor a tumor in the depths of crypts, so the mucosal tumor may not be evident visually or on palpation.

The rising incidence of HPV(+) OPSCCa makes it imperative that the radiologist is vigilant when evaluating a younger, nonsmoking subset of patients presenting with a new neck mass, which may be a cystic/necrotic or solid metastatic node. Unlike children, a cystic neck mass in an adult, even if in a classic location, of a 2nd branchial cleft cyst should be considered metastatic lymph node unless proven otherwise.

Selected References

1. Ansari S et al: Revisiting the "puffed cheek" technique: advantages, fallacies, and potential solutions. Radiol Imaging Cancer. 6(3):e230211, 2024
2. El Beltagi AH et al: Functional magnetic resonance imaging of head and neck cancer: performance and potential. Neuroradiol J. 32(1):36-52, 2019

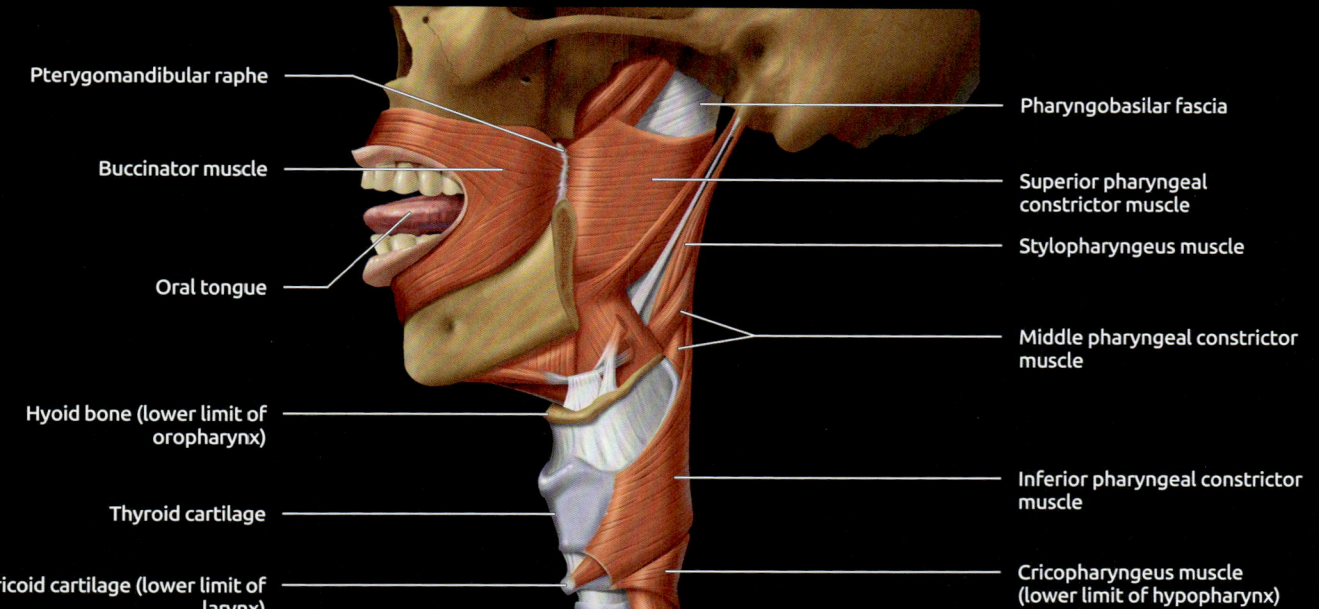

Pterygomandibular raphe

Buccinator muscle

Oral tongue

Hyoid bone (lower limit of oropharynx)

Thyroid cartilage

Cricoid cartilage (lower limit of larynx)

Pharyngobasilar fascia

Superior pharyngeal constrictor muscle

Stylopharyngeus muscle

Middle pharyngeal constrictor muscle

Inferior pharyngeal constrictor muscle

Cricopharyngeus muscle (lower limit of hypopharynx)

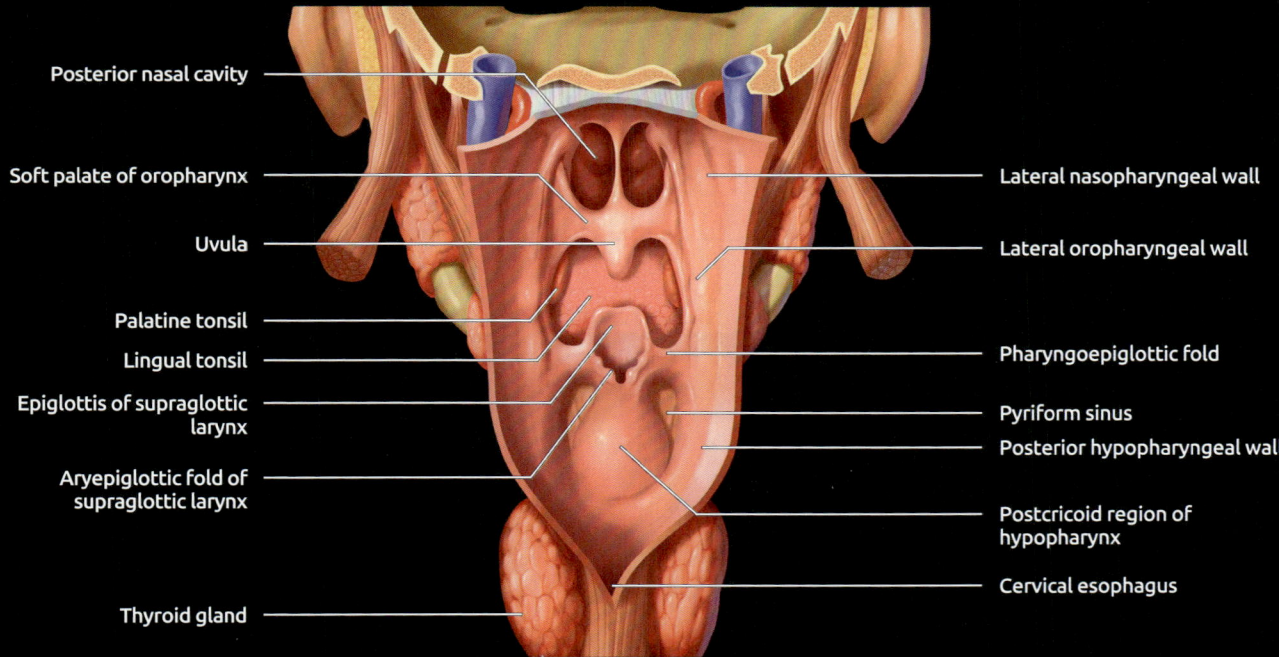

Posterior nasal cavity

Soft palate of oropharynx

Uvula

Palatine tonsil

Lingual tonsil

Epiglottis of supraglottic larynx

Aryepiglottic fold of supraglottic larynx

Thyroid gland

Lateral nasopharyngeal wall

Lateral oropharyngeal wall

Pharyngoepiglottic fold

Pyriform sinus

Posterior hypopharyngeal wall

Postcricoid region of hypopharynx

Cervical esophagus

(Top) *Lateral graphic shows the major muscles of the pharyngeal mucosal space. Notice that the pharynx is essentially a tube attached superiorly to the skull base and formed from the superior, middle, and inferior pharyngeal constrictor muscles. The nasopharynx, oropharynx, and hypopharynx are contiguous segments of this tube with the oral cavity contiguous anteriorly with the oropharynx. The larynx is intimately related to the hypopharynx and originates at the lower aspect of the oropharynx.* **(Bottom)** *Graphic of the pharyngeal mucosal space/surface as if opened from behind shows that this space can be divided into nasopharyngeal, oropharyngeal (OP), and hypopharyngeal areas. The lymphatic ring of the pharyngeal mucosal space (Waldeyer) contains the nasopharyngeal adenoids and the OP palatine and lingual tonsils or base of tongue.*

(Left) Axial graphic of the nasopharyngeal mucosal space (blue) shows superior pharyngeal constrictor ➡ and levator veli palatini muscles ➡ within the space. The middle layer of deep cervical fascia (pink line) provides a deep margin to the space. **(Right)** Axial T1 C+ FS MR in a young Asian woman with trismus shows a large, mildly enhancing nasopharyngeal carcinoma ➡, infiltrating right masticator space & clivus ➡. Note normal left levator veli ➡. MR is better for skull base (T3) & intracranial or cranial nerve (T4) infiltration.

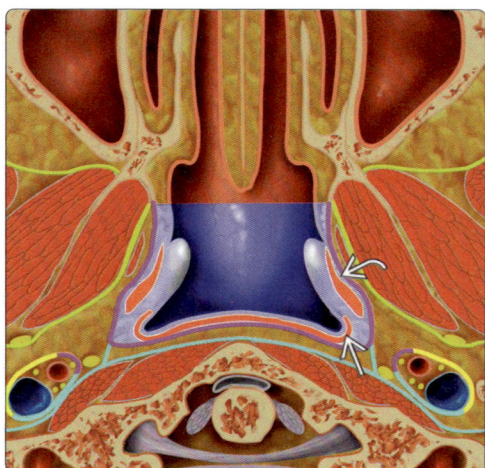
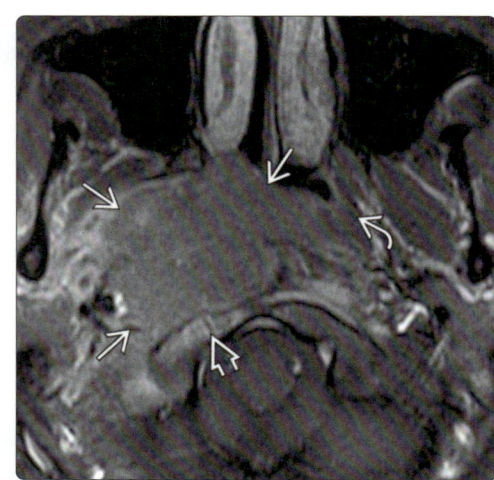

(Left) Axial graphic shows OP mucosal space (blue) and more anterior oral cavity (red). Note anterior tonsillar pillar ➡, palatine tonsil ➡, and lingual tonsil (base of tongue) ➡. The fat-filled (yellow) buccal space ➡ is bounded medially by buccinator muscle ➡, posteriorly by masseter ➡ and parotid, and anterolaterally by facial muscles. **(Right)** Axial fused F-18 FDG PET/CT shows FDG-avid HPV(+) OPSCCa in right palatine ➡ and lingual ➡ tonsils. Note metastatic lymph node ➡. The left tonsil high FDG uptake is physiologic ➡.

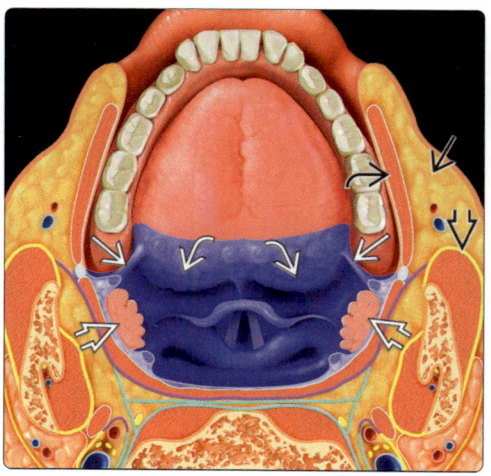
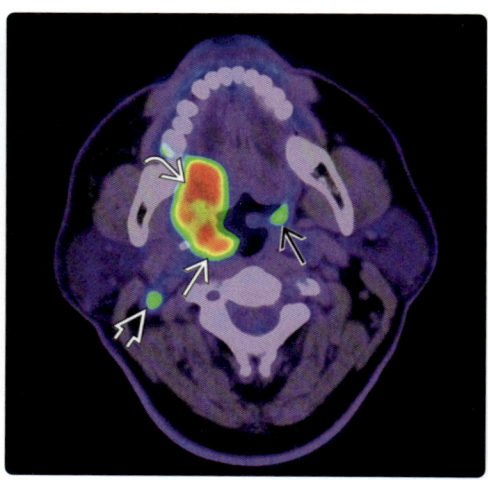

(Left) Axial graphic shows the hypopharyngeal aspect of the pharyngeal mucosal space. At the level of the supraglottis, the hypopharynx is made up of the pyriform sinus (PS) ➡ & posterior hypopharyngeal wall (PHW) ➡. Aryepiglottic (AE) folds ➡ are part of the supraglottis & separate larynx from hypopharynx. **(Right)** Axial CECT shows extensive bilateral adenopathy ➡ with an irregular, superficially spreading mass arising from PHW ➡, involving right PS wall ➡ & the marginal supraglottic AE fold ➡. Note normal left AE fold ➡.

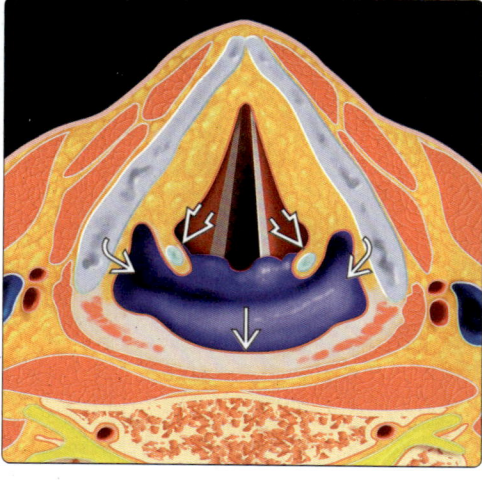
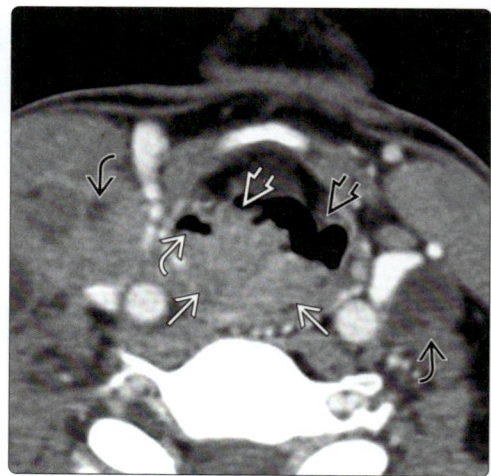

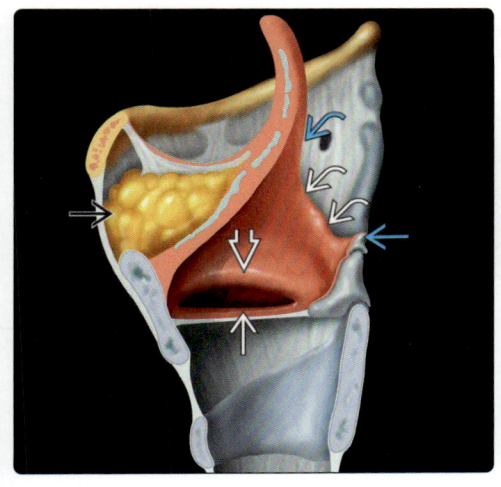

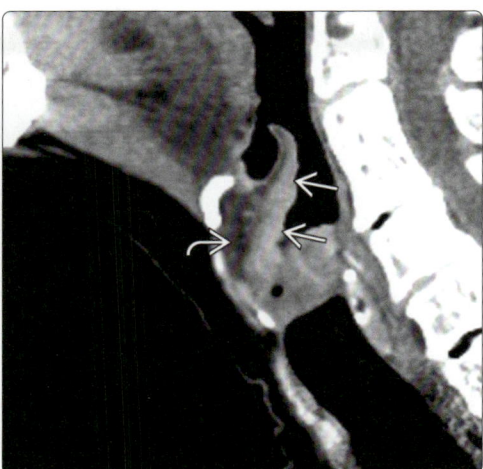

(Left) *Sagittal graphic of larynx shows true vocal cord* ➡️ *of glottic larynx. The false cord* ➡️ *lies above & parallels this, while the AE fold* ➡️ *projects from the arytenoid cartilage tip* ➡️ *to epiglottic inferolateral margin* ➡️. *Note fat in preepiglottic space* ➡️. *Subglottis extends from below true cords to lower cricoid margin.* (Right) *Sagittal CECT shows abnormally thickened laryngeal surface of epiglottis* ➡️ *in SCCa. The supraglottic larynx includes the epiglottis, AE folds, & false cords with fatty anterior preepiglottic* ➡️ *& lateral paraglottic spaces.*

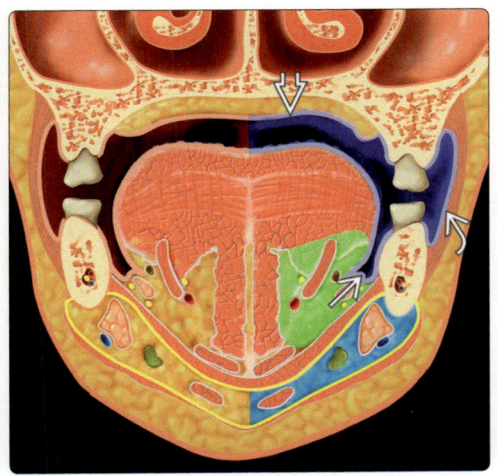

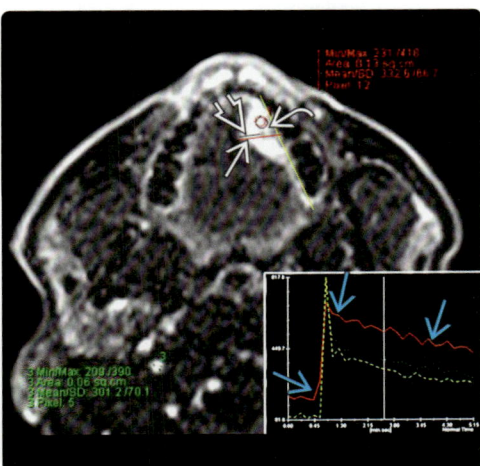

(Left) *Coronal graphic shows oral mucosal surfaces (blue) of hard palate* ➡️, *oral tongue, upper & lower alveolar ridges, buccal space* ➡️, *& floor of mouth* ➡️. (Right) *Axial dynamic VIBE T1 C+ MR shows enhancing left anterolateral tongue SCCa with ulcerated* ➡️ *surface. Tumor thickness (TT, black line)* ➡️ *should be measured from tumor surface (at inner margin of ulcer here), & depth of invasion (DOI, red line)* ➡️ *from tongue mucosal surface, to deepest point of tumor. ROI from tumor shows rapid rise with slow washout time-intensity curve (TIC)* ➡️.

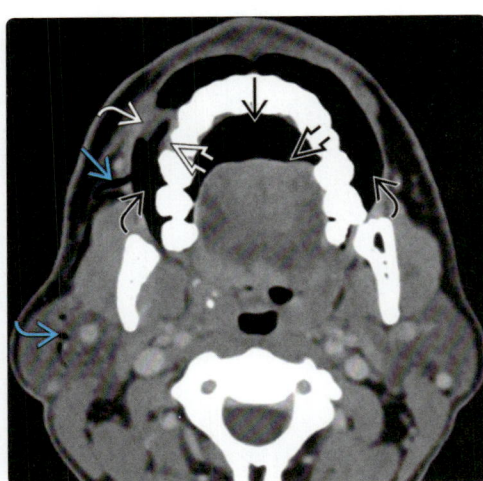

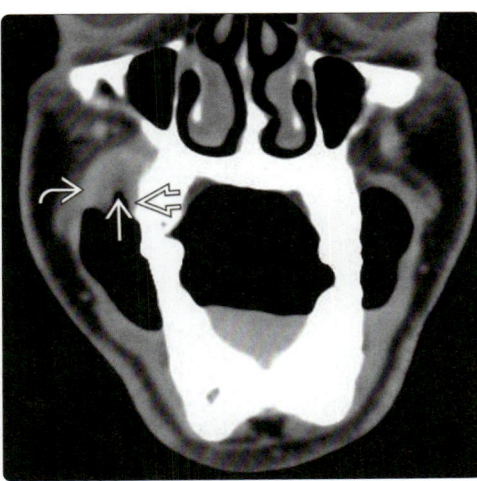

(Left) *Axial puffed-cheek technique CECT shows the small soft tissue of an SCCa along the right maxillary gingival* ➡️ *& buccal* ➡️ *margins. Note air in the central oral cavity proper* ➡️ *outlining the oral tongue* ➡️, *air in lateral oral vestibules* ➡️ *separating buccal & alveolar gingival margins, and air entering the right main parotid duct* ➡️ *& ductules* ➡️. (Right) *Coronal reformatted CECT shows that the tumor spreads from the gingival mucosa* ➡️ *through the superior gingivobuccal sulcus* ➡️ *into the buccal region* ➡️.

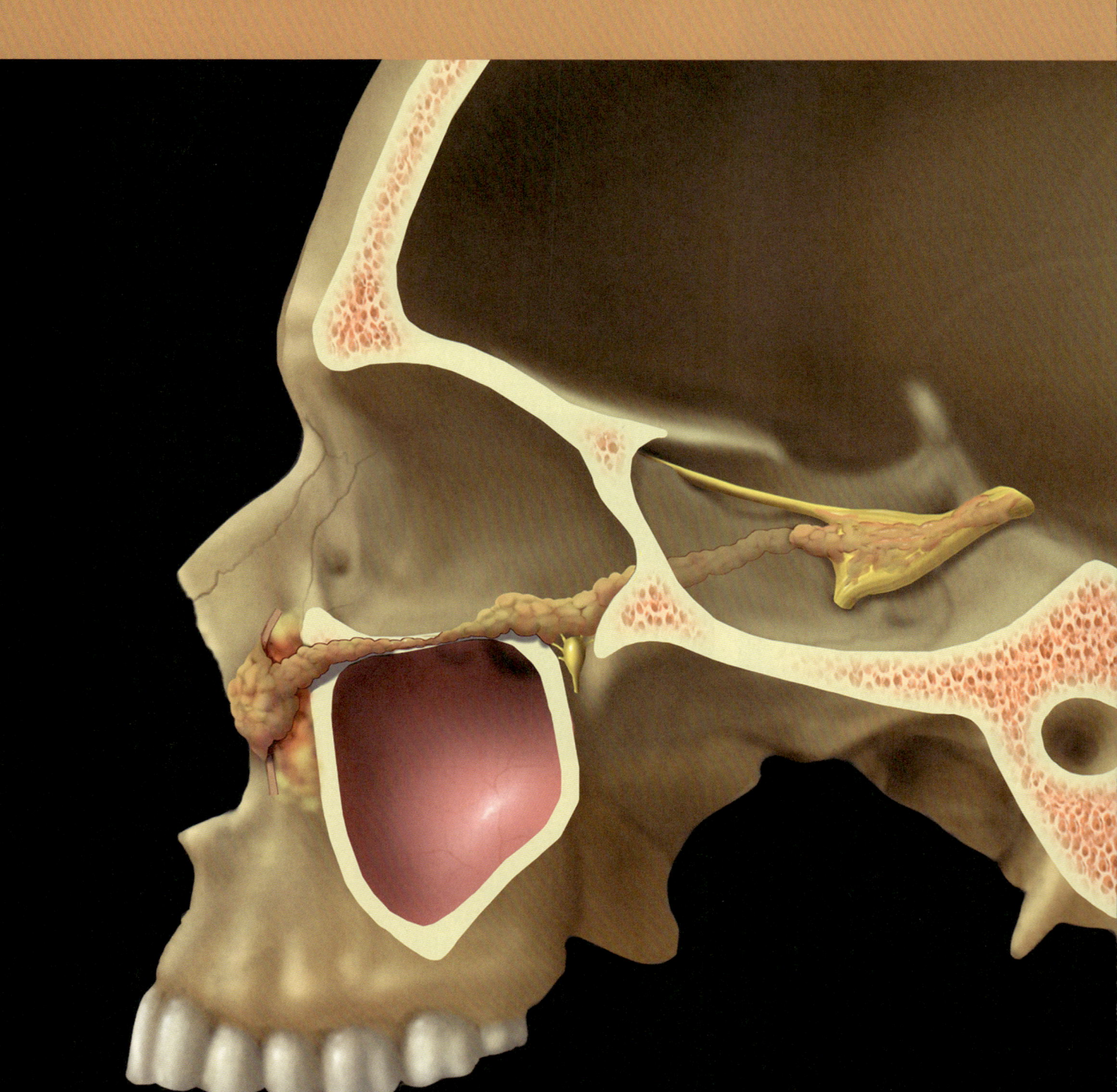

KEY FACTS

TERMINOLOGY

- Nasopharyngeal carcinoma (NPCa): Mucosal tumor of lateral pharyngeal recess (fossa of Rosenmüller), strongly associated with EBV infection

IMAGING

- MR best demonstrates parapharyngeal fat, skull base infiltration, and intracranial tumor
- Nodal disease in 75-90% at presentation: Retropharyngeal, levels II and V most common
- Metastatic nodes often large, ± necrosis
- NPCa is markedly FDG avid

TOP DIFFERENTIAL DIAGNOSES

- Adenoidal benign lymphoid hyperplasia
- Nasopharyngeal non-Hodgkin lymphoma
- Nasopharyngeal minor salivary gland malignancy
- Pituitary macroadenoma
- Skull base metastases

PATHOLOGY

- **25%: Keratinizing NPCa** (previously type I)
- **75%: Nonkeratinizing (NK) NPCa**
  - Strongly associated with EBV
  - **15% differentiated** (previously type II)
  - **60% undifferentiated** (previously type III)
- Rare: Basaloid squamous cell carcinoma

CLINICAL ISSUES

- Peak incidence: 40-60 years
- Pediatric NPCa rare; most often undifferentiated NK
- Clinical presentations
  - Bloody nasal discharge or epistaxis
  - 50-70% present with mass from metastatic nodes
  - Serous otitis from eustachian tube obstruction
- NK NPCa has 5-year survival of ~ 60-70%
- Keratinizing NPCa has 5-year survival of ~ 40%

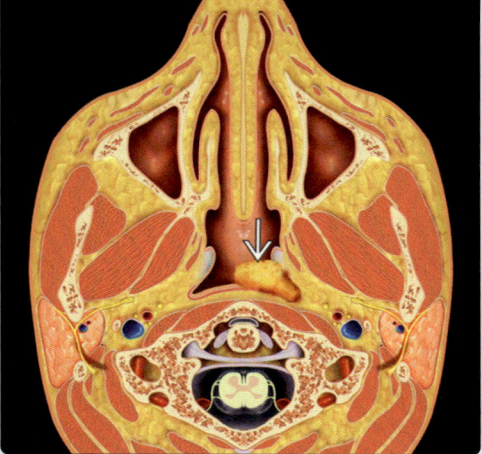
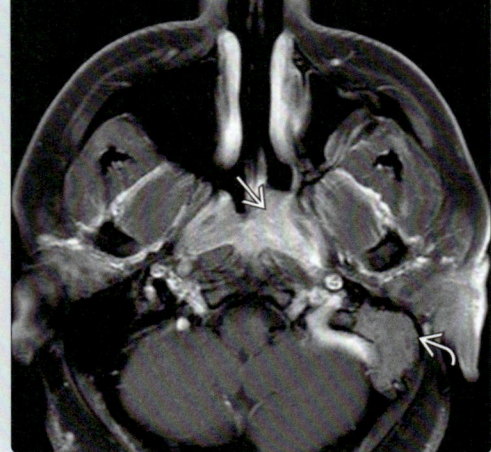

(Left) Graphic shows a typical T1 nasopharyngeal carcinoma (NPCa) with a mucosal-based mass ➡ arising from fossa of Rosenmüller. Tumor does not extend posterolaterally beyond middle layer of deep cervical fascia or pharyngobasilar fascia and does not involve parapharyngeal space. (Right) T1 C+ FS MR in a 43-year-old woman with keratinizing squamous cell carcinoma of nasopharynx shows an enhancing T1 lesion confined to left lateral nasopharynx ➡. Note obstructed fluid in left mastoid air cells ➡.

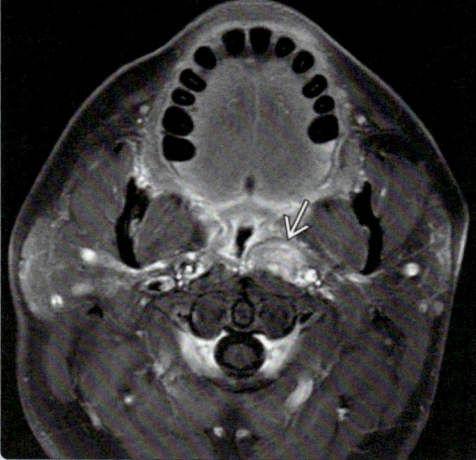
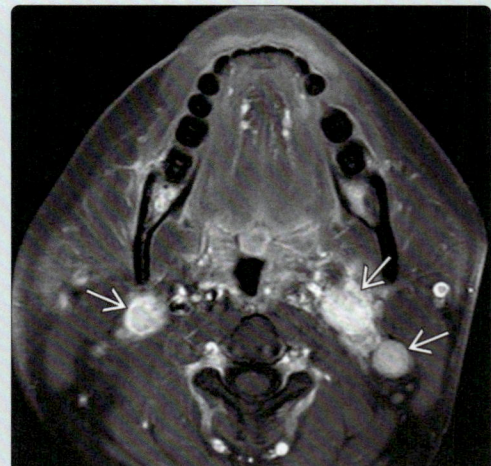

(Left) Axial T1 C+ FS MR shows an enlarged, enhancing left retropharyngeal lymph node, consistent with nodal metastasis ➡. (Right) Axial T1 C+ FS at the level of the oropharynx in the same patient demonstrates enhancing bilateral level II metastatic cervical adenopathy ➡, consistent with N2 disease. There were no nodes below the cricoid. The combination of T1N2M0 disease makes this patient stage II under the latest 9th version of the AJCC/UICC TNM classification.

TERMINOLOGY

Abbreviations

- Nasopharyngeal carcinoma (NPCa)

Definitions

- Primary mucosal malignancy arising in nasopharynx, most strongly associated with EBV infection

IMAGING

General Features

- Best diagnostic clue
  - Lateral pharyngeal recess mass with deep extension and cervical adenopathy
- Location
  - Arises in lateral pharyngeal recess, a.k.a. fossa of Rosenmüller
- Morphology
  - Poorly marginated mucosal mass with deep extension and invasion
  - Nodal disease in 75-90% at presentation

CT Findings

- CECT
  - Mildly enhancing off-midline nasopharyngeal mass
  - Metastatic nodes often large, ± necrosis
  - Retropharyngeal nodes often subtle on imaging, as they appear isodense to muscle
- Bone CT
  - May show destruction of clival cortex or pterygoid plates

MR Findings

- T1WI
  - Asymmetric mass, hypo- to isointense to muscle
  - Sensitive for infiltration of parapharyngeal fat and marrow involvement
- T2WI
  - Moderate hyperintensity of NPCa compared with muscle
- T1WI C+ FS
  - Best illustrates infiltration of deep face and central skull base
    - Coronal images aid in this evaluation
    - Prevertebral space invasion independent prognostic factor; T2 criterion
    - Assess pterygoid muscles (T2), paranasal sinuses and cervical vertebrae (T3) and hypopharynx, intracranial extension, orbit, parotid gland (T4)
  - Mild, homogeneous tumor enhancement

Nuclear Medicine Findings

- PET/CT
  - Markedly FDG-avid tumor, nodes, and metastases
  - Small primary could be missed with thick slices due to brain uptake

Imaging Recommendations

- Best imaging tool
  - MR is recommended by AJCC for staging
    - Most sensitive for skull base and intracranial tumor spread

- More sensitive than clinical exam/US/CT for retropharyngeal nodes
    - CECT is alternative choice
  - PET/CT often obtained if N2/3 disease at staging or recurrent tumor
- Protocol advice
  - T1 MR best shows infiltration of skull base with loss of fat signal
  - Postcontrast axial and coronal images best demonstrate intracranial spread

DIFFERENTIAL DIAGNOSIS

Adenoidal Benign Lymphoid Hyperplasia

- Large adenoids seen in children, teens, and HIV patients
- Symmetric enlargement without infiltration of adjacent tissues

Nasopharyngeal Non-Hodgkin Lymphoma

- Midline symmetric mass, ± deep infiltration to prevertebral muscles
- In clivus, tends to expand rather than infiltrate

Skull Base Osteomyelitis

- Ill defined and infiltrative with osseous and extraosseous abnormalities
- Can be difficult to distinguish if advanced skull invasion

Pituitary Macroadenoma (Invasive)

- Large sella mass extending through sphenoid to nasopharynx
- Expansion of sella is key imaging finding

Skull Base Metastases

- Central skull base metastasis can have extraosseous components that involve sphenoid sinus and nasopharynx

PATHOLOGY

General Features

- Etiology
  - **Nonkeratinizing (NK) undifferentiated subtype** strongly associated with **prior EBV infection**
    - EBV DNA found in tumor and premalignant (dysplastic, in situ) lesions
    - EBV most common but growing prevalence of HPV + NPCa [18% global, 25% in North America]
  - Other proposed factors
    - Carcinogens (nitrosamines) in food eaten in childhood
    - Genetic predisposition
      - Increased risk in 1st-degree relatives
      - Human leukocyte antigen (HLA) genes in major histocompatibility complex (MHC) region on chromosome 6p21 recognized as major risk loci with other non-HLA genes
    - Prior radiation
    - Tobacco and alcohol most associated with basaloid squamous cell carcinoma (BSCCa) and keratinizing NPCa

Staging, Grading, & Classification

- 9th version of AJCC/UICC nasopharyngeal cancer TNM staging classification released in 2025

- No substantial changes to T staging criteria
- Advanced radiologic extranodal extension (with involvement of adjacent muscles, skin, &/or neurovascular bundles) identified as independent adverse factor and added as criterion for N3
- Metastatic disease separated into M1a (≤ 3 metastases) and M1b (> 3)
- **Staging**: Nonmetastatic disease regrouped into stages I-III instead of I-IVA, merging previous I and II, downstaging III to II, IVA to III; and metastatic disease exclusively classified stage IV (A/B)
  - T1-2 N0-1 grouped as stage I (IA/IB), T3/N2 as stage II, and T4/N3 as stage III
- Noteworthy points from prior versions
  - EBV (+) lymph nodes of unknown primary: NPC stage T0
  - N staging very different from other head and neck SCCa

Gross Pathologic & Surgical Features

- Pathologic types classified by WHO
- **Keratinizing NPCa** (previously type I): 20-25%
  - Poorly, moderately, or well differentiated
- **NK NPCa**: 75-80%
  - PCR for EBV (+)
    - Differentiated (previously type II): 10-15%
    - Undifferentiated (previously type III): 60-65%
- **BSCCa**
  - Typically EBV and HPV (-)

CLINICAL ISSUES

Presentation

- Most common signs/symptoms
  - Conductive hearing loss secondary to middle ear obstruction
    - Obstruction or infiltration of eustachian tube
  - Bloody nasal discharge or epistaxis
  - 50-70% present with neck mass from metastatic nodes
- Other signs/symptoms
  - Uncommonly presents with cranial neuropathies

Demographics

- Age
  - Peak incidence: 40-60 years
  - Pediatric NPCa rare; most often undifferentiated NK
- Sex
  - M:F = 2.75:1
- Ethnicity
  - > 70% cases are in East and Southeast Asia
    - Age standardized rate 3 per 100,000 in China to 0.4 per 100,000 in mainly White populations
    - Moderately increased rates in Inuits of Alaska and Canada
  - NK NPCa endemic in southern China (> 95% cases)
  - Decreased risk in 2nd- and 3rd-generation American-born Chinese
  - In children in USA, increased risk in Black population
- Epidemiology
  - Worldwide, most common nasopharyngeal adult malignancy
    - Most common cancer in Asian men

- Declining incidence and improved prognosis over past decades

Natural History & Prognosis

- 5-year survival rates for stage I: ~ 80%, II: ~ 70%, IV: ~ 50%
- Keratinizing NPCa: Poorest prognosis; 5-year survival: ~ 40%
- NK NPCa: Radiosensitive, better prognosis; 5-year survival: ~ 60-70% (undifferentiated better than differentiated)
- BSCCa: Generally poor
- ~ 70% of NPCa present at locally advanced stages
- 75-90% have nodal, 10% have distal metastases at presentation
  - Retropharyngeal nodes followed by levels II and V
- ~ 10-15% recur and most develop distant metastases
  - Bone: Sclerotic or lytic lesions
  - Chest and liver also common sites

Treatment

- Generally radiosensitive, especially NK NPCa
  - Stage I: XRT alone; intensity-modulated radiotherapy (IMRT) most widely used technique (5-year survival: ~ 85-90%), promising role of endoscopic nasopharyngectomy
  - Advanced stages: XRT + chemotherapy
  - M1: Individualized approach, including palliative chemotherapy; ± locoregional radiotherapy and local therapy of metastasis
- Neck dissection for residual/recurrent disease posttreatment, salvage surgery for locally recurrent NPCa

DIAGNOSTIC CHECKLIST

Consider

- Carefully evaluate nasopharynx if middle ear obstruction in adult
- Lymphoma is main differential with nasopharyngeal mass ± adenopathy
  - More often midline and expands clivus

Image Interpretation Pearls

- T1 MR sensitive for parapharyngeal space and bone marrow invasion
- T1 C+ key for intracranial, perineural, and cavernous sinus invasion

Reporting Tips

- Certain key tumor findings should be sought
  - Parapharyngeal fat infiltration (T2)
  - Skull base invasion (T3)
  - Intracranial or cranial nerve involvement (T4)
- Nodal disease is common; nodes often large
  - Retropharyngeal, level II and V nodes most often
  - Extension below caudal border of cricoid cartilage = N3

SELECTED REFERENCES

1. Wu B et al: Advances in nasopharyngeal carcinoma staging: from the 7th to the 9th edition of the TNM system and future outlook. Curr Oncol Rep. 27(3):322-32, 2025
2. Pan JJ et al: Ninth version of the AJCC and UICC nasopharyngeal cancer TNM staging classification. JAMA Oncol. 10(12):1627-35, 2024
3. Zhao BY et al: Human papillomavirus-associated nasopharyngeal carcinoma: a systematic review and meta-analysis. Oral Oncol. 159:107057, 2024
4. Chen YP et al: Nasopharyngeal carcinoma. Lancet. 394(10192):64-80, 2019
5. Perri F et al: Management of recurrent nasopharyngeal carcinoma: current perspectives. Onco Targets Ther. 12:1583-91, 2019

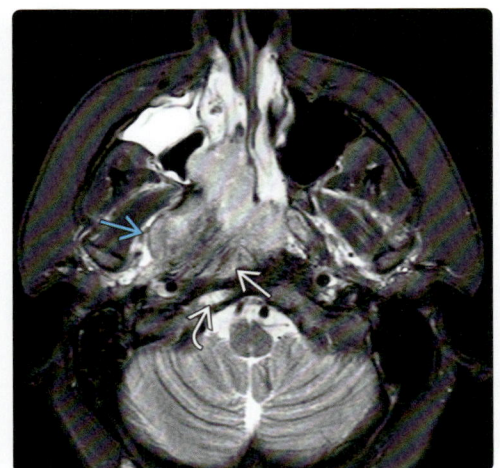

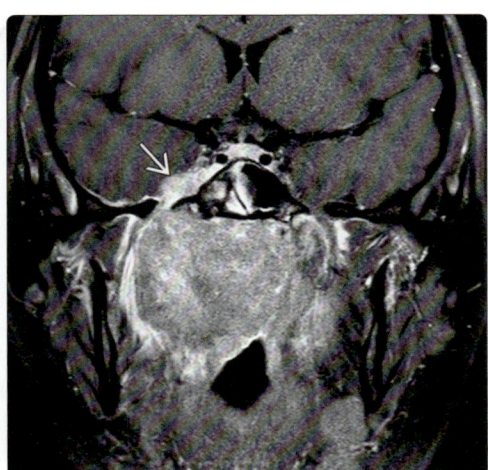

(Left) Axial STIR MR in a 24-year-old woman with EBV (+) NPCa shows a large, enhancing nasopharyngeal mass extending into the posterior choana on the right and invading posteriorly into the longus capitus muscle ➡ and occipital bone ➡. Tumor pushes laterally into the parapharyngeal space, displacing V3 ➡. (Right) Coronal T1 C+ FS in the same patient shows a large, enhancing nasopharyngeal mass invading superiorly through the foramen ovale along V3 ➡. Intracranial disease indicates T4 stage.

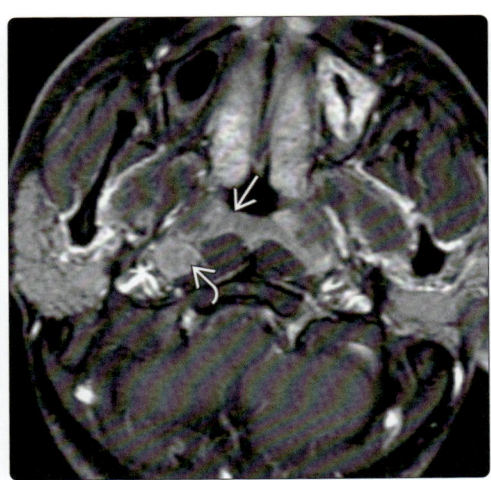

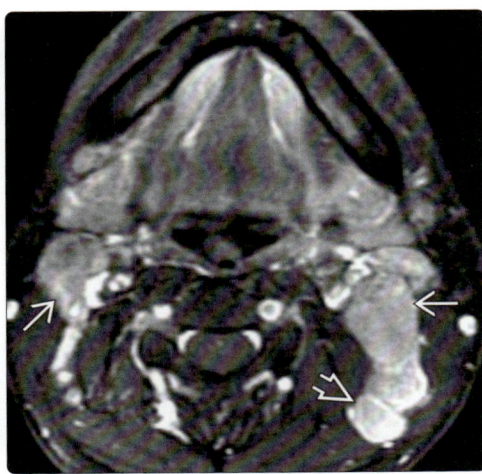

(Left) Axial T1 C+ FS MR in a 26-year-old Asian man with neck masses demonstrates subtly asymmetric soft tissue fullness of nasopharynx mucosa ➡, though without infiltration of the prevertebral muscles. An enlarged right retropharyngeal node ➡ is evident. (Right) Axial T1 C+ FS MR in the same patient demonstrates bilateral enlarged level II ➡ and left level V ➡ nodes [undifferentiated nonkeratinizing carcinoma, EBV (+)]; T1N2, stage II by latest AJCC/UICC TNM classification.

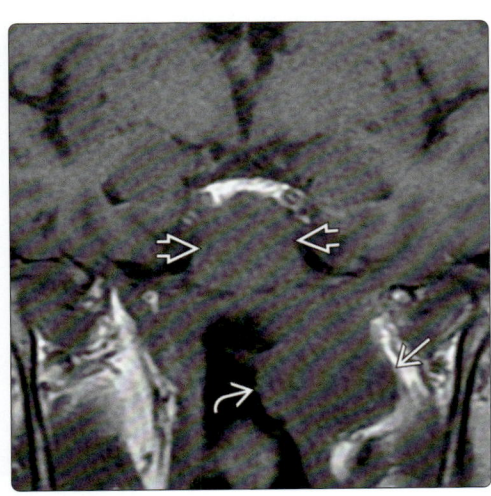

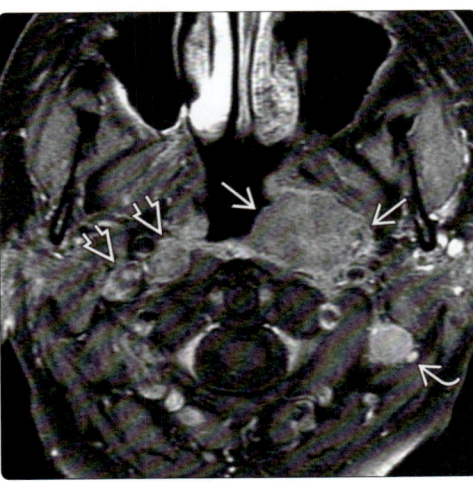

(Left) Coronal T1 MR shows an infiltrative T1-hypointense mass in the superior lateral nasopharynx ➡ extending into the clivus ➡ and the left parapharyngeal space ➡. Endoscopic biopsy showed NPCa. (Right) Axial T1 C+ FS in the same patient shows NPCa in the left lateral nasopharyngeal recess extending in the parapharyngeal space ➡. Contralateral retropharyngeal ➡ and ipsilateral level IIB ➡ nodal metastases are well seen.

KEY FACTS

TERMINOLOGY

- Base of tongue OPSCCa
- Tonsillar tissue at posterior 1/3 of tongue

IMAGING

- Primary tumor may be ulceroinfiltrative or exophytic
- Nodal disease common, even with subtle primary
- CECT most often used but MR more accurate for tumor extent
  - CECT: Scan ≥ 90 seconds after IV contrast to maximize tumor and mucosal enhancement
  - MR: Fat saturation enhances soft tissue contrast: T2 and T1 C+
- PET/CT: Staging, unknown primary search, posttreatment baseline scan
  - Beware of FDG (-) cystic nodal metastasis

TOP DIFFERENTIAL DIAGNOSES

- Lingual tonsil lymphoid hyperplasia

- Lingual tonsil non-Hodgkin lymphoma
- Palatine tonsil SCCa
- Lingual tonsil pleomorphic adenoma
- Lingual tonsil minor salivary gland malignancy

PATHOLOGY

- OPSCCa classically associated with tobacco/alcohol abuse
- Separation of HPV (+) and HPV (-) or p16 (-) OPSCCa in AJCC 8th edition

CLINICAL ISSUES

- Most common presentation is sore throat
- Typically at least 1 node, even when small
- 30% present with bilateral adenopathy
- Increasing incidence of HPV (+) SCCa
  - Patients younger; more commonly nonsmokers
  - HPV is favorable prognostic biomarker
- Overall 5-year survival significantly worse for HPV (-) than HPV (+)

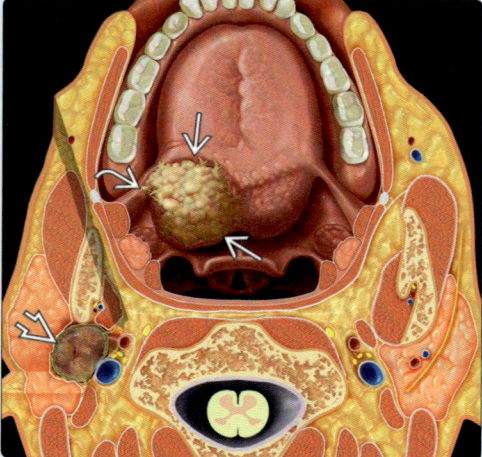
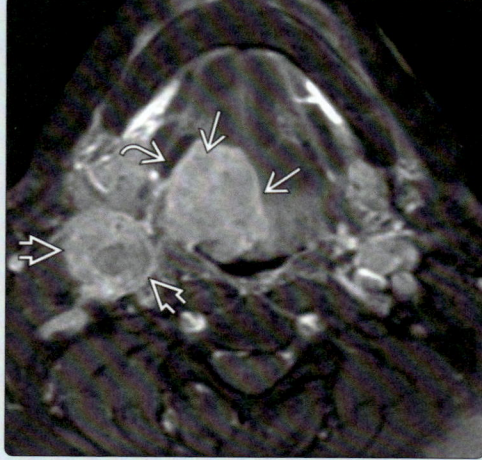

(Left) Axial graphic depicts lingual tonsil SCCa ➡ with ipsilateral adenopathy ➡. Tongue base tumor has predominantly exophytic growth but infiltrates inferior aspect of anterior tonsillar pillar ➡. (Right) Axial T1WI C+ FS MR in a 58-year-old alcoholic presenting with a persistent right neck mass after a dental procedure demonstrates an enlarged, heterogeneous, right level II node ➡. Primary tumor is in ipsilateral lingual tonsil ➡ and infiltrates oral tongue and floor of mouth, medial to hyoglossus muscle ➡.

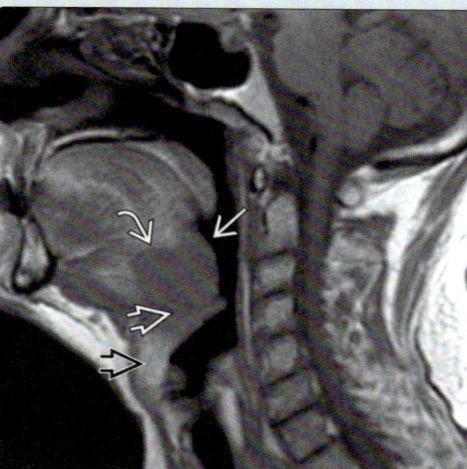
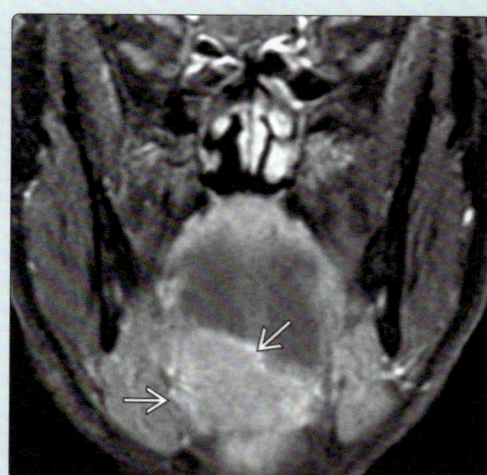

(Left) Sagittal T1WI MR in the same patient shows fullness at the right base of tongue ➡ with a tumor replacing the lingual tonsillar tissue and infiltrating into the floor of mouth ➡. Tumor extends inferiorly to vallecula ➡ but does not extend inferiorly into preepiglottic fat ➡. (Right) Coronal T1WI C+ FS MR shows an asymmetric mass ➡ at the right base of tongue in the same patient infiltrating into the floor of the mouth.

Base of Tongue Squamous Cell Carcinoma

TERMINOLOGY

Abbreviations
- Base of tongue (BOT) squamous cell carcinoma (SCCa)

Synonyms
- Lingual tonsil SCCa

Definitions
- Epithelial tumor in **oropharyngeal (OP)** tonsils at BOT
  - Extends from posterior 1/3 of tongue to valleculae
  - Distinct entity from oral tongue SCCa

IMAGING

General Features
- Best diagnostic clue
  - Asymmetric enlargement of lingual tonsil or invasive BOT mass
  - Early nodal metastasis common (mostly levels II-IV)
- Location
  - Lymphoid tissue, posterior to circumvallate papilla of tongue, extending inferiorly to vallecula
- Size
  - Variable
- Morphology
  - **Ulceroinfiltrative** or **exophytic** mass filling airway
  - Nodal extranodal extension (ENE) designation for staging is determined by clinical examination (not imaging) defined by skin invasion, muscle infiltration, tethering, or nerve invasion with dysfunction
    - Clinical ENE stages p16 (-) OPSCCa to cN3b but is not included in staging of p16 (+) OPSCCa

CT Findings
- CECT
  - Usually moderately enhances, as does lingual tonsil
  - Small lesion: Mucosal asymmetry; often subtle
  - Large lesion: Exophytic or ulceroinfiltrating lesion
  - Nodal disease solid, moderately enhancing, or cystic
    - Spiculation or indistinct nodal margins, irregular capsular enhancement, and fat or muscle infiltration suggest ENE

MR Findings
- T1WI
  - Isointense to tongue musculature
- T2WI
  - Hyperintense to muscle in tongue and floor of mouth
- DWI
  - Variable: ADC values tend to be lower in HPV-mediated OPSCCa (HPV-OPSCCa) than in those not associated with HPV infection [HPV(-) or p16 (-) OPSCCa]
- T1WI C+
  - Moderate to marked enhancement

Nuclear Medicine Findings
- PET
  - FDG avid; generally greater than normal lingual tonsillar tissue
  - Beware of FDG (-) cystic nodal metastasis

Imaging Recommendations
- Best imaging tool
  - CECT most commonly used
    - Cheaper, quicker
  - MR provides more accurate evaluation of tumor extent
    - Superior soft tissue contrast
    - Less affected by dental amalgam artifact
  - PET/CT: 3 main uses in OPSCCa
    - Detection of primary tumor if otherwise occult
    - Staging: For distant metastases
    - Baseline: 3 months post chemo-XRT
- Protocol advice
  - CECT: **Delay imaging ≥ 90 seconds after contrast**
    - Maximizes tumor and mucosal enhancement
  - MR: T2 FS and T1 C+ FS improve tissue contrast

DIFFERENTIAL DIAGNOSIS

Lingual Tonsil Lymphoid Hyperplasia
- Symmetric without deep invasion or discrete mass
- Other lymphoid tissues hyperplastic

Lingual Tonsil Non-Hodgkin Lymphoma
- Exophytic mass or diffusely enlarged tonsil
- Often large, nonnecrotic nodes

Palatine Tonsil Squamous Cell Carcinoma
- Palatine and lingual tonsils meet at glossotonsillar sulcus
- May be difficult to discern site of origin of SCCa

Lingual Tonsil Pleomorphic Adenoma
- Sharply marginated mass in lingual tonsil
- Pedunculates into airway when large

Lingual Tonsil Minor Salivary Gland Malignancy
- Rare; may be indistinguishable from SCCa
- Nodal metastases much less common

PATHOLOGY

General Features
- Etiology
  - **Tobacco and alcohol abuse**
    - Alcohol abuse is independent risk factor and potentiates tobacco effects
    - Results in mucosal metaplasia, dysplasia → neoplasia
    - Ongoing use during treatment reduces survival
  - **HPV infection**
    - Accounts for ~ 70% of all OPSCCa in USA; HPV-16 most prevalent subtype (~ 90%); expected to be preventable by prophylactic HPV vaccination
    - Oncoproteins (E6 and E7) destabilize tumor suppressor proteins (p53 and pRB) → upregulation of cyclin-dependent kinase inhibitor p16
    - 8th edition of American Joint Committee on Cancer (AJCC) Cancer Staging Manual separated OPSCCa into HPV-mediated OPSCCa (HPV-OPSCCa) and those not associated with HPV infection [HPV (-) or p16 (-) OPSCCa]
    - Typically younger patients, often nonsmokers, history of multiple sexual partners; smaller primary

– Overall improved prognosis, despite nodal metastasis at diagnosis
– Majority of HPV-mediated tumors are nonkeratinizing

Staging, Grading, & Classification

- A few important changes made in AJCC 8th edition
- T staging: T criteria for HPV (-) or p16 (-) OPSCCa same as 7th edition; differences from HPV-OPSCCa
  - T4a and T4b tumors combined into T4 category for HPV-OPSCCa (similar prognosis of 2 categories)
  - T0 category present for HPV-OPSCCa but not HPV (-) or p16 (-) OPSCCa
- N staging: Separate tables for clinical and pathologic staging (after nodal resection) different between 2 categories; rationale for change being that HPV-mediated tumors tend to present with multiple nodal metastases, but prognosis improved despite that
- For p16 (-) OPSCCa, clinical N criteria include new criterion of ENE, which is determined by physical examination; after resection, pathologic nodal staging also includes pathologic ENE criterion (not present in HPV-mediated criteria)
- Different prognostic staging tables available for HPV-mediated p16 (+) and p16 (-) OPSCCa
  - For HPV-OPSCCa, no stage IV in absence of metastatic disease
  - Presence of N3 nodal disease or T4 tumor criteria stages disease as stage III; all other stages I or II, again reflecting improved prognosis despite nodal disease
  - Generally, for p16 (-) OPSCCa, staging grades higher for similar T and N criteria as p16 (+) OPSCCa, e.g., bilateral nodes classified as N2c for p16 (-) OPSCCa and staged as IVA or IVB depending on T criteria, compared to p16 (+) OPSCCa, where bilateral nodes also N2 but stage II with T0-3 and stage III with T4

Gross Pathologic & Surgical Features

- Tan or white in color
- Ulceroinfiltrative or exophytic growth pattern

Microscopic Features

- Squamous differentiation with intracellular bridges or keratinization ± keratin pearls
- Further classified into well, moderately, or poorly differentiated
  - **Up to 60% poorly differentiated**

CLINICAL ISSUES

Presentation

- Most common signs/symptoms
  - **Sore throat**; may present with neck nodal mass
- Other signs/symptoms
  - Fullness or throat mass, ipsilateral otalgia (referred pain)
- Clinical profile
  - Classic: 50-year-old patient with heavy tobacco and alcohol use and new neck node mass
  - HPV (+): Middle-aged male nonsmoker with history of multiple sexual partners

Demographics

- Age
  - Adults; typically > 45 years, younger with HPV (+) SCCa
- Sex

  - M > F
- Epidemiology
  - Decreased incidence of tobacco use and related OPSCCa
  - **Rapid increase in incidence of HPV (+) OPSCCa**

Natural History & Prognosis

- Even T1/2 tumors typically present with **at least 1 node**
  - 30% present with bilateral adenopathy
- 10-15% distant metastasis
  - Lungs > bones > liver
- **Overall 5-year survival: ~ 60% for non-HPV-related OPSCCa and ~ 80% for HPV (+) OPSCCa**
- **HPV is favorable prognostic factor biomarker**

Treatment

- Treatments changing with favorable HPV prognosis
- Chemoradiation (CRT) is mainstay, although resection may be performed for exophytic lesion in airway, particularly for HPV (+) OPSCCa
- T1/T2 SCCa usually with surgery or definitive XRT alone
  - Transoral robotic surgery is promising ± nodal dissection
  - XRT: Intensity-modulated radiation therapy
- For locally advanced disease, multimodality options, typically concurrent CRT ± surgery
- Post-CRT surveillance important
  - CECT/MR at 6-8 weeks &/or PET/CT at 3 months
  - Salvage surgery for residual disease

DIAGNOSTIC CHECKLIST

Image Interpretation Pearls

- SCCa may be difficult to delineate on CECT, as both mucosa and tumor enhance
- Do not mistake cystic level II metastatic node as 2nd branchial cleft cyst in adult patient

Reporting Tips

- Measure **greatest diameter** of primary and **define full extent of tumor spread**
- Look for ipsilateral **and** contralateral nodal disease
- Always consider **2nd primary neoplasm** at diagnosis and follow-up
  - Head and neck, esophageal, or lung carcinoma

SELECTED REFERENCES

1. Holsinger FC et al: Transoral robotic surgery in the multidisciplinary care of patients with oropharyngeal squamous cell carcinoma: ASCO guideline. J Clin Oncol. 43(11):1369-92, 2025
2. Hughes RT et al: Predicting extranodal extension with preoperative contrast-enhanced CT in patients with oropharyngeal squamous cell carcinoma. Radiol Imaging Cancer. 7(2):e240127, 2025
3. Suto T et al: Imaging findings of human papillomavirus-positive and human papillomavirus-negative oropharyngeal squamous cell carcinoma associated with recurrence. J Clin Med. 14(3), 2025
4. Chen LL et al: MRI for differentiation between HPV-positive and HPV-negative oropharyngeal squamous cell carcinoma: a systematic review. Cancers (Basel). 16(11), 2024
5. Shenker RF et al: Clinical outcomes of oropharyngeal squamous cell carcinoma stratified by human papillomavirus subtype: a systematic review and meta-analysis. Oral Oncol. 148:106644, 2024
6. Glastonbury CM et al: Head and neck squamous cell cancer: approach to staging and surveillance. In: Hodler J et al: Diseases of the Brain, Head and Neck, Spine 2020-2023: Diagnostic Imaging. Springer, 2020
7. Parvathaneni U et al: Advances in diagnosis and multidisciplinary management of oropharyngeal squamous cell carcinoma: state of the art. Radiographics. 39(7):2055-68, 2019
8. Amin MB et al: AJCC Cancer Staging Manual. 8th ed. Springer, 2017

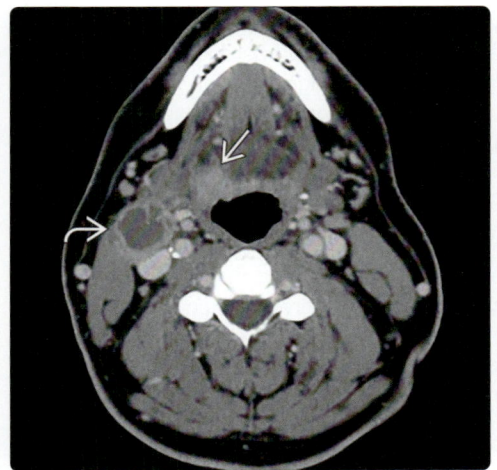
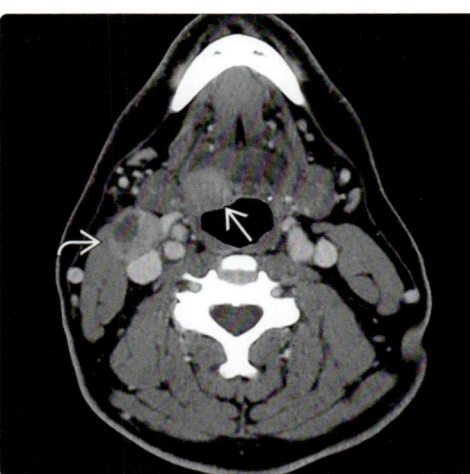

(Left) *Axial CECT through the oropharynx in a 51-year-old man with HPV (-) SCCa of the right tongue base demonstrates a small, enhancing mucosal lesion of the right tongue base ➡ and large right necrotic level II lymph node ➡. The lymph node demonstrated histologic extracapsular extension at the time of surgery.* (Right) *Axial CECT in the same patient, more inferiorly, again shows the enhancing primary tongue base lesion ➡ infiltrating the extrinsic musculature. Necrotic level II node is again seen ➡.*

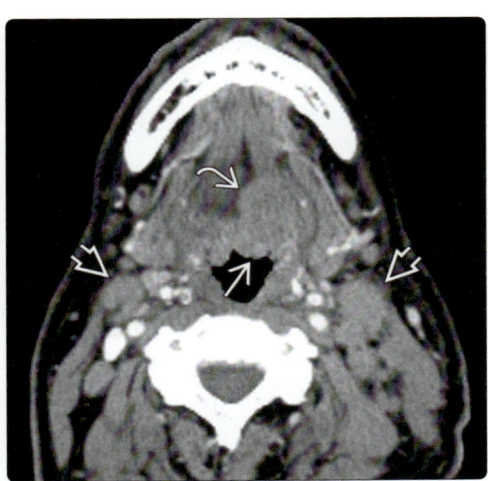
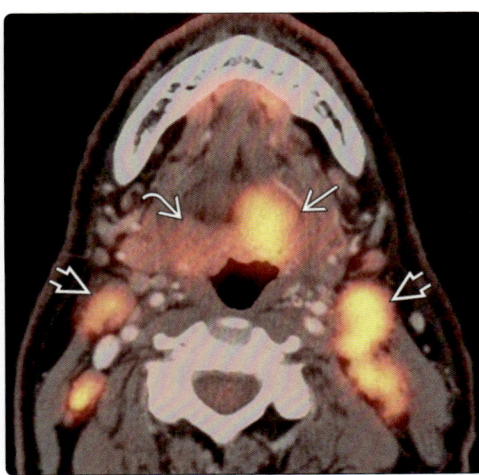

(Left) *CECT in 62-year-old man demonstrates a left base of tongue infiltrative mass ➡ invading the extrinsic muscles ➡. Bilateral lymph nodes with ill-defined capsules are also present ➡, suggestive of extranodal extension. Note, for p16 (-) OPSCCa, clinical criterion of ENE is based on physical examination.* (Right) *Axial FDG PET/CT in the same patient demonstrates elevated FDG uptake within the base of tongue SCCa ➡ compared to normal lingual tonsil ➡. FDG uptake is also present within the bilateral metastatic lymph nodes ➡.*

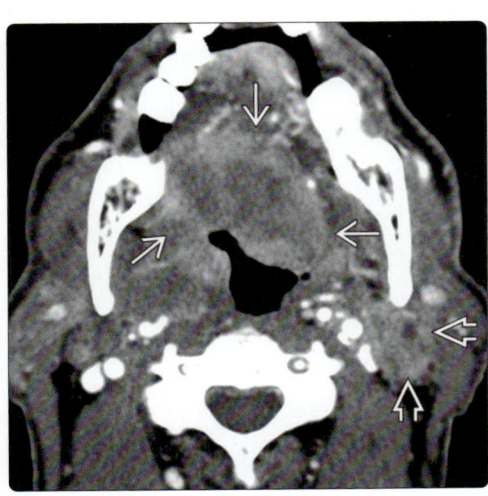
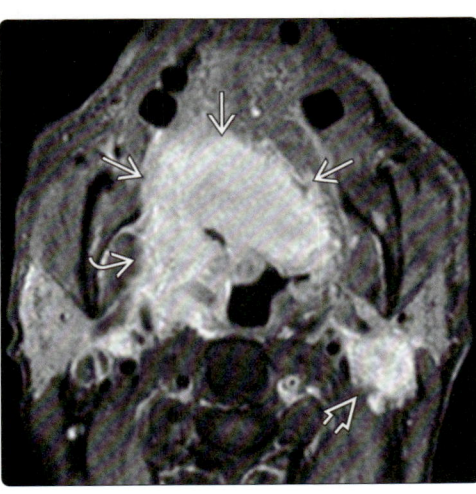

(Left) *Axial CECT obtained in a 65-year-old patient with a history of heavy tobacco and alcohol use and 25-lb weight loss associated with dysphagia and throat pain shows heterogeneous, enlarged left level II node ➡ with large, ulceroinfiltrative mass involving entire tongue base ➡.* (Right) *Axial T1WI C+ FS MR in the same patient better delineates the extent of tumor infiltration into the floor of mouth ➡ and medial pterygoid muscle ➡. Enlarged and irregular left-sided lymph node ➡ is also noted.*

KEY FACTS

TERMINOLOGY

- Palatine tonsil squamous cell carcinoma (SCCa): Most common oropharyngeal SCCa subsite

IMAGING

- Variable appearance & presentation of primary tumor
- Small primary site may be occult on clinical ± imaging
- Larger lesions often exophytic or deeply invasive
- Adenopathy common, most often ipsilateral level II
- MR: Improves detection of small primary & tumor extent
- PET/CT, CECT, or MR to stage primary & nodal extent
- PET/CT: Confirms primary, detects smaller metastatic nodes, distant metastases

TOP DIFFERENTIAL DIAGNOSES

- Tonsillar lymphoid hyperplasia, tonsillar/peritonsillar abscess
- Palatine tonsil non-Hodgkin lymphoma, palatine tonsil pleomorphic adenoma

PATHOLOGY

- **HPV** associated with tonsil SCCa, especially HPV-16
- Tobacco + alcohol abuse also associated with tonsil SCCa
- HPV (+) cancers typically younger patients, smaller primary
- Different staging classification for HPV (+) vs. HPV (-) SCCa
- **Circulating (HPV) tumor DNA** has evolving role in HPV (+) SCCa surveillance with high (> 95%) positive predictive value & negative predictive value

CLINICAL ISSUES

- Presentation: Ipsilateral otalgia, dysphagia, new neck node
- **75-80%** have **adenopathy** at presentation
  - Primary tumor may be clinically & imaging occult
  - 70-80% oropharyngeal tumors arise in tonsil
- Most patients > 45 years; rising incidence < 45 years if HPV (+); HPV (+) SCCa has better prognosis
  - Allows treatment deescalation protocols

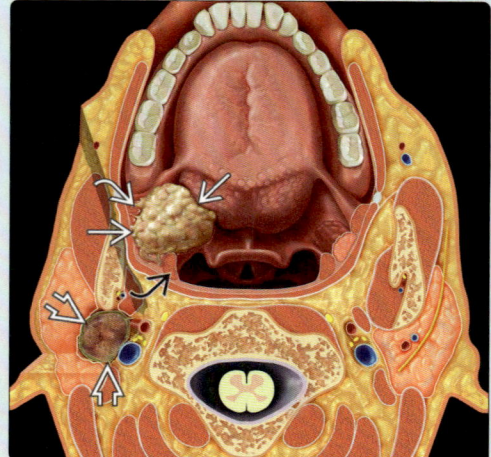
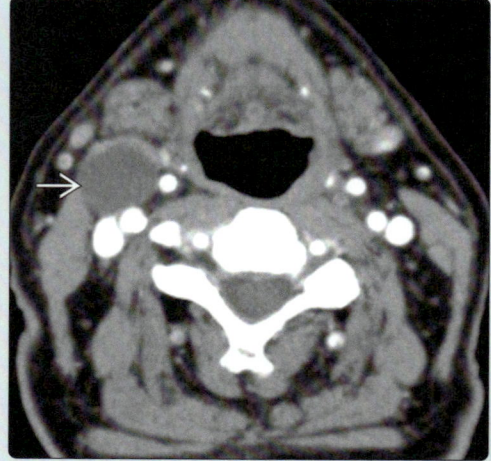

(Left) Axial graphic shows palatine tonsillar primary SCCa ➡ in the lateral wall of oropharynx with involvement of anterior tonsillar pillar ➡. Posterior tonsillar pillar ➡ is not infiltrated. Note ipsilateral level II adenopathy ➡. *(Right)* Axial CECT shows a cystic nodal metastasis ➡. Primary tonsillar SCCa was clinically and radiographically inapparent. A small or occult primary with a cystic level II node is a typical presentation for HPV(+) SCCa that should not be attributed to branchial cleft cyst in an adult without tissue validation.

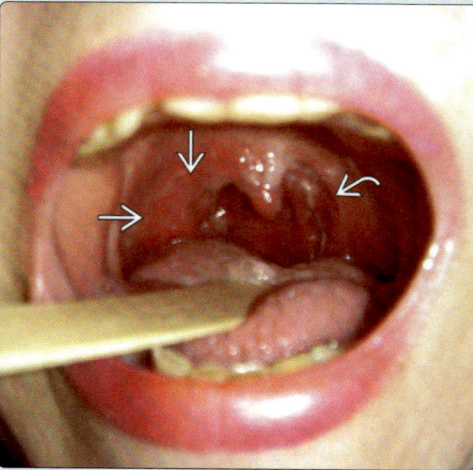
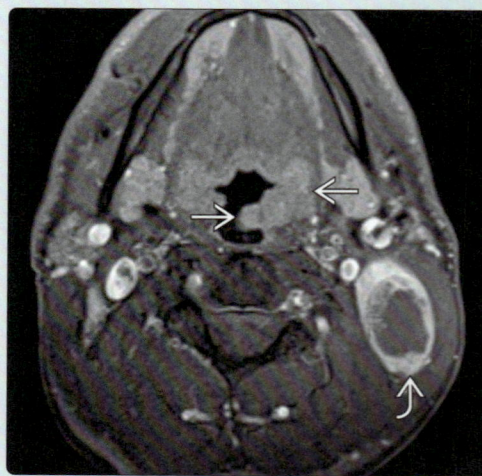

(Left) Clinical photograph in a woman with dysphagia and right throat and ear pain shows an indurated, ulcerated right palatine tonsil ➡. Note effacement of the anterior tonsillar pillar with normal comparison on left ➡. *(Right)* Axial T1 C+ FS MR shows a left tonsil mass ➡ with cystic adenopathy ➡. This p16(+) SCCa was staged as T1N1M0 (stage I), illustrating the lower impact of nodal disease on HPV(+) SCCa staging. Two additional positive neck nodes were present; a p16(-) SCCa would have been stage IVA disease, in contrast.

Palatine Tonsil Squamous Cell Carcinoma

TERMINOLOGY

Abbreviations
- Squamous cell carcinoma (SCCa)

Definitions
- Epithelial malignant neoplasm arising in lateral oropharynx involving tonsillar fossa or pillars

IMAGING

General Features
- Best diagnostic clue
  - Asymmetrically enlarged heterogeneous palatine tonsil, usually with invasive deep margins
- Location
  - Tonsillar fossa > > anterior > posterior tonsillar pillars
- Size
  - Varies from small & occult to large & exophytic
- Morphology
  - Early small tumors may be mucosal only
  - Advanced lesions bulky with local invasion

CT Findings
- CECT
  - Small primary site may be difficult to delineate
    - Human papillomavirus (HPV) (+) tumors often small or occult
  - Larger lesions may be exophytic or deeply invasive
    - Typically moderate or heterogeneous enhancement
  - Adenopathy most common at ipsilateral level II
    - Nodes enlarged, often round, ± central necrosis
    - Cystic level II adenopathy typical of HPV (+) SCCa
    - Interrupted nodal capsule or adjacent soft tissue infiltration suggests extranodal extension (ENE)

MR Findings
- T1WI
  - Tonsil usually enlarged
  - Tumor mildly hypo- to isointense to normal tonsil
- T2WI FS
  - Slightly hyperintense to normal tonsil & muscle
  - Uncommonly small & T2 hypointense
  - Cystic adenopathy more typical if HPV (+)
- T1WI C+ FS
  - Tumor tends to enhance more than normal tonsil

Nuclear Medicine Findings
- PET
  - Locate unknown primary with SCCa node presentation
  - SCCa primary & metastatic nodes FDG avid
  - Tonsil normally has FDG uptake, small lesions occult
  - PET less useful for prognosis in HPV (+) SCCa

Imaging Recommendations
- Best imaging tool
  - PET/CECT: Combination of 2 best stages; primary, metastatic adenopathy, distant metastases
    - Localize unknown primary when occult
  - CECT or MR can stage primary & nodes
    - CECT > MR for nodal metastases
- Protocol advice
  - PET/CECT: Best performed prior to mucosal biopsies, especially when searching for unknown primary tumor

DIFFERENTIAL DIAGNOSIS

Tonsillar Lymphoid Hyperplasia
- Enlarged tonsils without discrete mass or deep invasion

Tonsillar/Peritonsillar Abscess
- Young adult with acute febrile illness
- Intratonsillar or peritonsillar rim-enhancing fluid collection

Palatine Tonsil Pleomorphic Adenoma
- Sharply marginated tonsillar mass
- Usually markedly hyperintense on T2 MR

Palatine Tonsil Non-Hodgkin Lymphoma
- Submucosal mass enlarges tonsil ± deep invasion
- Often associated with large, nonnecrotic neck nodes

PATHOLOGY

General Features
- Etiology
  - Identified causes: HPV infection, tobacco + alcohol
  - **HPV(+)**
    - More common than HPV (-) SCCa
    - Expresses oncoproteins that destabilize tumor suppressor proteins (p53 & pRB)
    - HPV-16 most prevalent subtype (~ 90%)
    - Infection strongly associated with sexual behavior
    - Patients typically younger, often nonsmokers
    - Nodal presentation more common; small primary
    - Overall prognosis better than tumors in smokers
    - Different staging algorithm than HPV (-) SCCa
  - **Tobacco + alcohol abuse** causes metaplasia & dysplasia
- Circulating (HPV) tumor DNA (**ctDNA**) has evolving role in surveillance of HPV (+) SCCa with high (> 95%) positive predictive value & negative predictive value

Staging, Grading, & Classification
- Oropharyngeal cancer staging based on **AJCC 8th edition**
  - Separate classifications depending on **HPV status**

Gross Pathologic & Surgical Features
- Ill-defined, ulcerative, indurated mucosal lesion

Microscopic Features
- Squamous differentiation ± keratin pearls
- Further classified by tumor differentiation

CLINICAL ISSUES

Presentation
- Most common signs/symptoms
  - Ipsilateral otalgia, dysphagia
  - Level II node metastasis may be initial presentation
    - **75-80% have adenopathy at presentation**
- Clinical profile
  - HPV (+): Middle-aged, nonsmoking man ± multiple sexual partners
  - HPV (-): Older man, history of tobacco & alcohol use

American Joint Committee on Cancer (AJCC) Oropharynx Staging, p16(+) (2017)

Tumor (T): Size Measured in Greatest Dimension	Clinical Nodal Metastasis (cN): Size in Greatest Dimension	Pathologic Nodal Metastasis (pN): Size in Greatest Dimension
T1: Tumor ≤ 2 cm	**N1**: Ipsilateral nodes ≤ 6 cm	**pN1**: Metastasis in ≤ 4 lymph nodes
T2: Tumor > 2, ≤ 4 cm	**N2**: Contralateral or bilateral nodes ≤ 6 cm	**pN2**: Metastasis in > 4 lymph nodes
T3: Tumor > 4 cm or extension to lingual surface of epiglottis	**N3**: Node(s) > 6 cm	
T4: Invades larynx, medial pterygoid or extrinsic tongue muscles, hard palate, mandible, or beyond		
Distant metastasis (M): **M0** = no distant metastasis, **M1** = distant metastasis		

Table adapted from American College of Surgeons. Amin, MB et al: AJCC Cancer Staging Manual. 8th ed. Springer, 2017.

American Joint Committee on Cancer (AJCC) Oropharynx Staging, p16(-) (2017)

Tumor (T): Size Measured in Greatest Dimension	Clinical Nodal Metastasis (cN): Size in Greatest Dimension	Pathologic Nodal Metastasis (pN): Size in Greatest Dimension
Tis: Carcinoma in situ	**N1**: Metastasis in single ipsilateral lymph node ≤ 3 cm and ENE(-)	**N1**: Metastasis in single ipsilateral lymph node, ≤ 3 cm and ENE(-)
T1: Tumor ≤ 2 cm	**N2a**: Metastasis in single ipsilateral node > 3 cm but not > 6 cm and ENE(-)	**N2a**: Metastasis in single ipsilateral node ≤ 3 cm and ENE(+); **or** single ipsilateral node > 3 cm but not > 6 cm and ENE(-)
T2: Tumor > 2, ≤ 4 cm	**N2b**: Metastases in multiple ipsilateral lymph nodes, none > 6 cm and ENE(-)	**N2b**: Metastases in multiple ipsilateral nodes, none > 6 cm and ENE(-)
T3: Tumor > 4 cm or extension to lingual surface of epiglottis	**N2c**: Metastases in bilateral or contralateral lymph nodes, none > 6 cm and ENE(-)	**N2c**: Metastases in bilateral or contralateral lymph node(s), none > 6 cm and ENE(-)
T4a (moderately advanced local disease): Tumor invades larynx, extrinsic muscle of tongue, medial pterygoid, hard palate, or mandible	**N3a**: Metastasis in lymph node > 6 cm and ENE(-)	**N3a**: Metastasis in lymph node > 6 cm and ENE(-)
T4b (very advanced local disease): Tumor invades lateral pterygoid muscle, pterygoid plates, lateral nasopharynx, skull base or encases carotid artery	**N3b**: Metastasis in any node(s) and clinically overt ENE(+)	**N3b**: Metastasis in single ipsilateral node > 3 cm and ENE(+); **or** multiple ipsilateral, contralateral, or bilateral nodes, any with ENE(+); or single contralateral node any size and ENE(+)
Distant metastasis (M): **M0** = no distant metastasis, **M1** = distant metastasis		

Table adapted from American College of Surgeons. Amin, MB et al: AJCC Cancer Staging Manual. 8th ed. Springer, 2017.

Demographics

- Epidemiology
  - **70-80% oropharyngeal tumors** are tonsil origin
  - Incidence increasing despite declining tobacco use
  - HPV-related cancers rapidly increasing in USA since 1990
- Sex: M > F
- Age: Adult patients, typically > 45 years
  - Age of presentation decreasing with HPV (+) tumors

Natural History & Prognosis

- **HPV is favorable prognostic biomarker**
  - Overall better treatment response & survival
- Nodal metastasis significantly reduces 5-year survival
  - Worse prognosis with ENE & distal nodal metastasis
- Locoregional recurrence mostly occurs within 24 months
- Distant metastatic disease: Lungs > skeletal > hepatic

Treatment

- Regimens changing given better prognosis in HPV (+) SCCa

- Smaller tumors, T1-T2: 2 options
  - Chemotherapy & radiation to tumor & neck
  - TORS & nodal dissection or radiation to neck
- Larger tumors &/or extensive nodal disease
  - Chemoradiation main treatment regimen

DIAGNOSTIC CHECKLIST

Image Interpretation Pearls

- **Adult with cystic level II mass is unlikely to be 2nd branchial cleft cyst: Assume HPV (+) SCCa first**

SELECTED REFERENCES

1. Suto T et al: Imaging findings of human papillomavirus-positive and human papillomavirus-negative oropharyngeal squamous cell carcinoma associated with recurrence. J Clin Med. 14(3), 2025
2. Agarwal A et al: Preliminary results from retrospective correlation of circulating tumor DNA (ct-DNA) with imaging for HPV-positive oropharyngeal squamous cell carcinoma. AJNR Am J Neuroradiol. 45(8):1135-40, 2024

Palatine Tonsil Squamous Cell Carcinoma

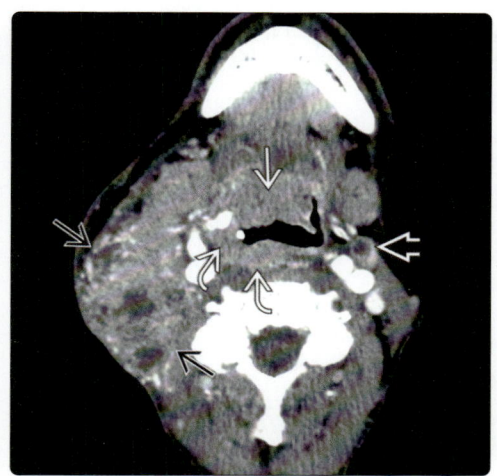

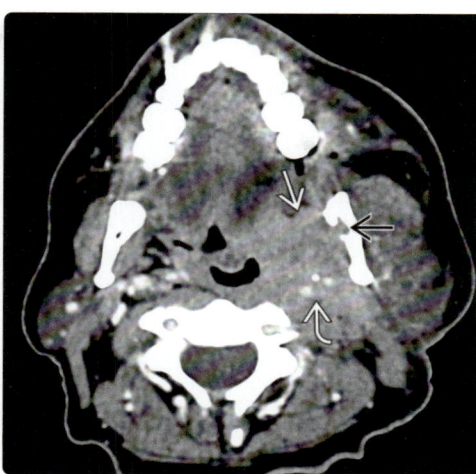

(Left) Axial CECT shows a large p16(-) oropharyngeal primary base of tongue SCCa ⮞ wrapping around posterior oropharyngeal wall ⮡. Note a small cystic nodal metastasis on the left ⮞ and findings concerning for ENE on the right ⮞ with effaced fat planes and irregular soft tissue margins. (Right) Axial CECT shows a bulky left oropharyngeal p16(+) SCCa with invasion into the left masticator space ⮞, making this a T4 lesion. Tumor encases the left carotid sheath ⮞. Note overt tumor spread into the mandibular foramen ⮞.

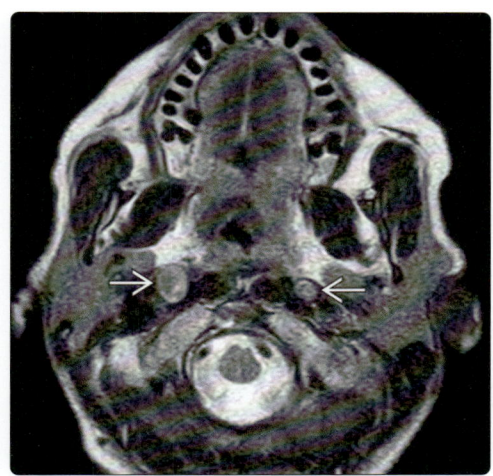

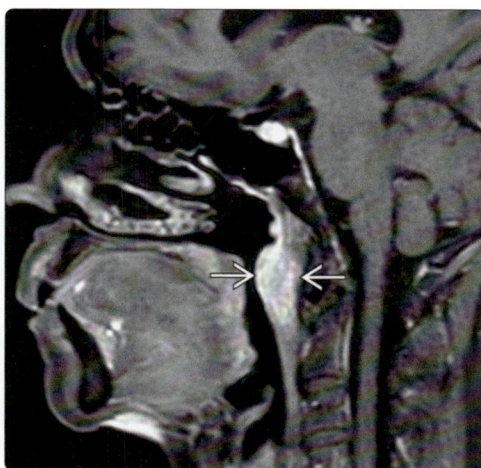

(Left) Axial T2 MR shows a less common pattern of metastatic retropharyngeal adenopathy ⮞ due to posterior oropharyngeal wall SCCa. If not resected transorally, they must be included in radiation treatment field. (Right) Sagittal T1 C+ FS MR in the same patient shows a p16(+) posterior oropharyngeal wall SCCa ⮞ extending across midline. This less common location for oropharyngeal SCCa has a higher propensity for retropharyngeal adenopathy, important to note on imaging as they tend to be clinically occult.

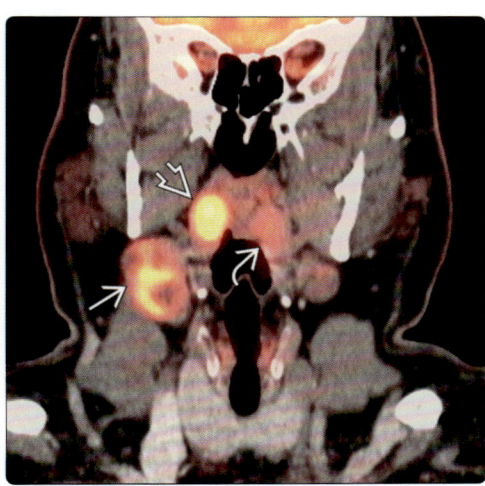

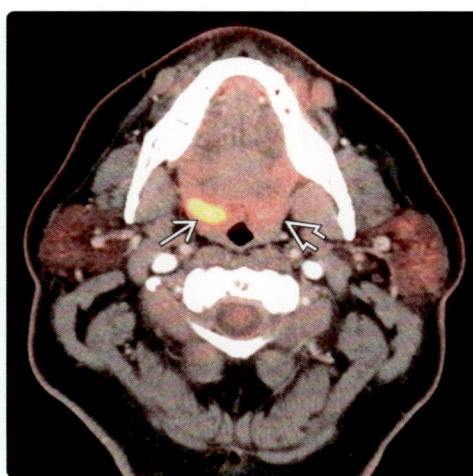

(Left) Coronal PET/CT in a patient with a new right palpable neck mass shows there is increased FDG uptake in a large level II nodal conglomerate ⮞ and asymmetric FDG uptake in right tonsillar SCCa ⮞. Note the normal left tonsil ⮞. (Right) Axial PET/CT in the same patient demonstrates asymmetric increased FDG uptake in the right palatine tonsil ⮞ compared to the left ⮞. CECT did not reveal a lesion in this area. Given an elevated SUV max ratio (> 1.48), the right tonsil was biopsied and revealed SCCa.

Posterior Oropharyngeal Wall Squamous Cell Carcinoma

TERMINOLOGY

- Squamous cell carcinoma (SCCa) arising from posterior oropharyngeal wall
  - **Soft palate** is superior limit; **hyoid** is inferior limit

IMAGING

- Lobulated posterior oropharyngeal wall mass
- CT: Mild to moderately enhancing soft tissue
- MR: Isointense to muscle on T1, moderate T2 signal
  - Moderate contrast enhancement
- Intact retropharyngeal fat plane on MR has high negative predictive value for tumor invasion
- SCCa reliably FDG avid

TOP DIFFERENTIAL DIAGNOSES

- Nasopharyngeal carcinoma
- Posterior hypopharyngeal wall SCCa
- Venous malformation

PATHOLOGY

- 85-90% of oropharyngeal cancers: SCCa
- Most posterior OPSCCa are well differentiated

CLINICAL ISSUES

- Relatively rare; much less common than tonsillar SCCa
- Etiologies: Tobacco & alcohol abuse or HPV-mediated oropharyngeal SCCa
- Typically, relatively asymptomatic until late stage
- May extend posteriorly into retropharyngeal space &/or prevertebral space
- Staging of oropharyngeal SCCa separated into HPV (-) and HPV (+) [p16(+)] SCCa

DIAGNOSTIC CHECKLIST

- Prior to surgery, suggest MR to assess prevertebral invasion
- Nodal metastases should be carefully sought
  - Retropharyngeal, especially if prevertebral invasion
  - Bilateral nodes frequently found

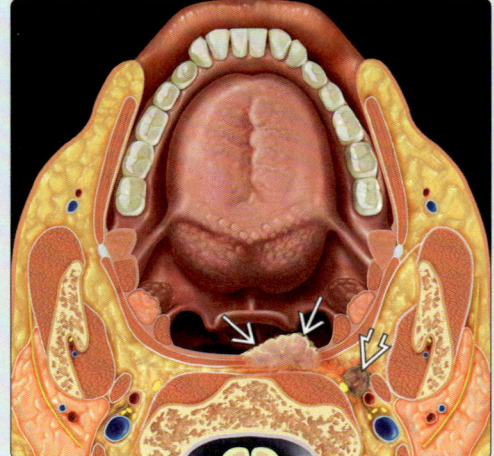
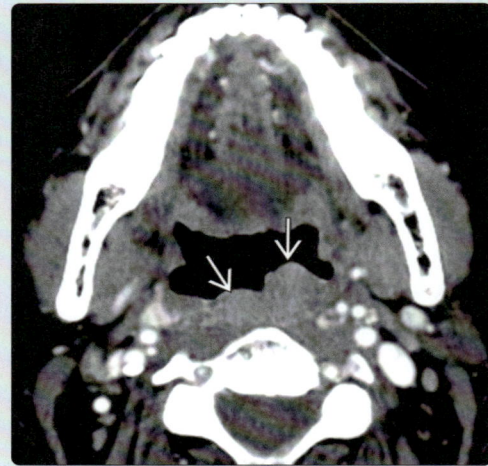

(Left) Transverse graphic depicts irregular SCCa arising from the posterior oropharyngeal wall ➡ & invading the retropharyngeal fat. Invasion of prevertebral muscle indicates a T4 tumor. Note ipsilateral necrotic metastatic retropharyngeal node ➡ medial to the carotid artery. (Right) Axial CECT demonstrates a mildly enhancing soft tissue mass in the left paramedian posterior oropharyngeal wall ➡. Prevertebral muscle invasion & adenopathy are not evident. Patient had extensive tobacco & alcohol history.

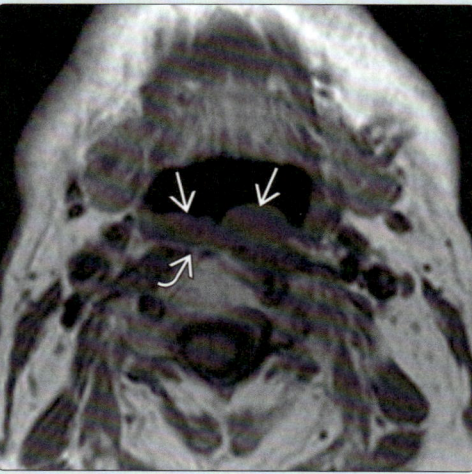
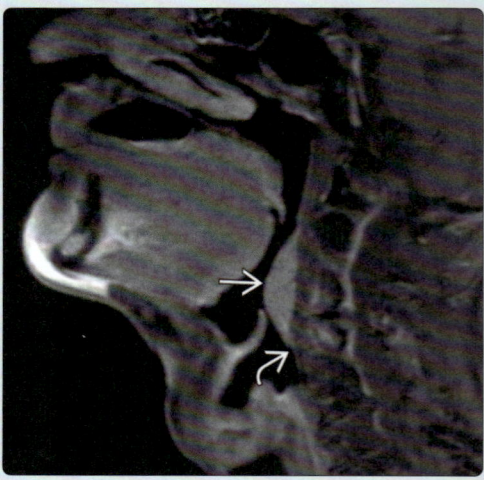

(Left) Axial T1WI MR in a patient with dysphagia shows irregular bilobed thickening of the posterior oropharyngeal wall ➡. Hyperintense retropharyngeal fat is seen on the right side ➡ but is indistinct on the left side. There is no evidence of prevertebral muscle invasion, however. (Right) Sagittal T1WI C+ FS MR shows the left-sided component of a pharyngeal wall tumor that bulges into the posterior oropharynx ➡. Inferiorly, it reaches superior aspect of the hypopharynx ➡ but does not extend superiorly to the nasopharynx.

TERMINOLOGY

Definitions

- Mucosal squamous cell carcinoma (SCCa) of **posterior pharyngeal wall** between soft palate & level of hyoid

IMAGING

General Features

- Location
  - Posterior wall of pharynx from soft palate to hyoid

CT Findings

- Lobulated, posterior oropharyngeal (OP) wall mass
- Mild to moderately enhancing

MR Findings

- T1 isointense to muscle, T2 moderately intense
- Moderate contrast enhancement
- Prevertebral tumor invasion: Intact retropharyngeal fat plane = high negative predictive value, otherwise difficult
  - Surgery often definitive

Nuclear Medicine Findings

- PET/CT
  - SCCa reliably FDG avid

Imaging Recommendations

- Best imaging tool
  - Either CT or MR excellent cross-sectional tools
  - Before surgery, MR done to assess retropharyngeal fat
  - PET/CT for staging or baseline 3 months post treatment

DIFFERENTIAL DIAGNOSIS

Nasopharyngeal Carcinoma

- Typically grows in lateral nasopharyngeal recess
- Can extend inferiorly to oropharynx, still T1 tumor

Posterior Hypopharyngeal Wall Squamous Cell Carcinoma

- Uncommon primary hypopharyngeal SCCa
- Can extend superiorly to oropharynx or vice versa

Venous Malformation

- Heterogeneous mass, moderate/marked enhancement
- Often involves multiple adjacent spaces

PATHOLOGY

General Features

- Etiology
  - Strong association with tobacco & alcohol abuse
  - Human papillomavirus (HPV) infection, especially HPV-16
  - Lower prevalence of HPV (~ 3-30%) for this subsite than for base of tongue (BOT)/tonsils (~ 70%)
    - Typically, HPV-OPSCCa in younger patients with smaller primary = improved prognosis
    - Recent studies suggest poorer survival of p16 (+) nontonsillar/non-BOT SCCa than p16 (+) tonsillar/BOT SCCa but similar to p16 (-) OPSCCa
    - HPV or p16 status may not have prognostic value in nontonsillar/non-BOT subsites of SCCa

Staging, Grading, & Classification

- 8th Edition American Joint Committee on Cancer (AJCC) Staging Manual separated OPSCCa into HPV-mediated and those without HPV [HPV (-) or p16 (-) OPSCCa]

Microscopic Features

- 85-90% OP cancers are SCCa; rarely basaloid type

CLINICAL ISSUES

Presentation

- Most common signs/symptoms
  - Typically relatively asymptomatic until late stage
    - Tend to spread submucosally, 70% present at T3 or T4
  - Dysphagia ± nodal mass
  - Unlike tonsil SCCa, does not present as unknown primary

Demographics

- Age
  - Most patients > 45 years old
- Epidemiology
  - Rare (≤ 5%); much less common than tonsillar SCCa, ~ 2% of OPSCCa

Natural History & Prognosis

- May extend into retropharyngeal &/or prevertebral space
- Because close to midline, often bilateral nodal metastases
  - **Up to 30% have retropharyngeal nodal metastases, generally higher than other subsites**
- Overall 5-yr survival ~ 30%
  - Nontonsillar-related OPSCCa found to have inferior survival outcome compared to tonsillar related

Treatment

- General guidelines; optimal treatment controversial
  - If small, N0: Radiation alone
  - Larger tumors, ≥ N1: Chemoradiation ± neck dissection
- Small tumors may undergo primary resection
  - Increase in transoral robotic surgery (TORS) or laser microsurgery
- Prevertebral invasion indicates unresectable tumor

DIAGNOSTIC CHECKLIST

Image Interpretation Pearls

- Prior to surgery, suggest MR to assess prevertebral invasion

Reporting Tips

- Carefully assess for retropharyngeal nodes, especially if prevertebral invasion & bilateral nodes

SELECTED REFERENCES

1. Kovarik PD et al: Squamous cell carcinoma of the posterior pharyngeal wall: a comparative analysis of oropharyngeal origin versus hypopharyngeal origin. J Laryngol Otol. 1-17, 2024
2. Tirelli G et al: Prevalence and prognostic impact of retropharyngeal lymph nodes metastases in oropharyngeal squamous cell carcinoma: meta-analysis of published literature. Head Neck. 44(10):2265-76, 2022
3. Hammarstedt L et al: The value of p16 and HPV DNA in non-tonsillar, non-base of tongue oropharyngeal cancer. Acta Otolaryngol. 141(1):89-94, 2021
4. De Virgilio A et al: A systematic review of different treatment strategies for the squamous cell carcinoma of the posterior pharyngeal wall. Eur Arch Otorhinolaryngol. 277(10):2663-72, 2020
5. Tham T et al: Anatomical subsite modifies survival in oropharyngeal squamous cell carcinoma: National Cancer Database study. Head Neck. 42(3):434-45, 2020

TERMINOLOGY

- Human papillomavirus (HPV) (+) oropharyngeal squamous cell carcinoma (OPSCCa); most often HPV-16
- TNM classification exclusively for HPV (+) OPSCCa added in 8th edition of AJCC Cancer Staging Manual
- AJCC version 9 for HPV (+) OPSCCA expected in fall 2025 with updates to N staging

IMAGING

- Well-defined, enhancing mass in palatine or lingual tonsil
- ADC lower in HPV (+) compared to HPV (-) OPSCCa
- CECT/MR: Levels II ± III adenopathy; single or multiple, solid or more commonly necrotic/cystic nodes
- PET/CECT to determine small unknown primary

TOP DIFFERENTIAL DIAGNOSES

- 2nd branchial cleft cyst
- Non-Hodgkin lymphoma involving pharyngeal mucosal space or lymph nodes

- Asymmetric lymphoid tissue of pharyngeal mucosal space

PATHOLOGY

- HPV causation determined by staining for HPV DNA, RNA, or p16 kinase inhibitor
- Longitudinal blood sampling to test for association of ctHPVDNA (liquid biopsy): 100% negative predictive value
- Extranodal extension high-risk, poor prognostic factor for all H&N tumors, except for viral-related cancers and mucosal melanoma

CLINICAL ISSUES

- Presentation: Unilateral neck mass, level IIA nodes
- Young/middle-aged, usually nonsmoker White males
- Much better prognosis than HPV (-) OPSCCa seen with tobacco and alcohol abuse

DIAGNOSTIC CHECKLIST

- Consider HPV (+) OPSCCa in adult with new neck mass, even if node looks like 2nd branchial cleft cyst

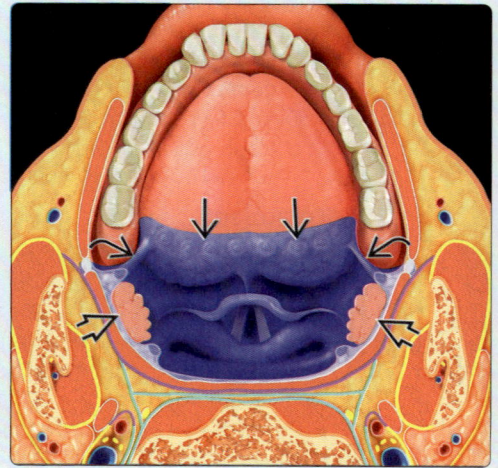
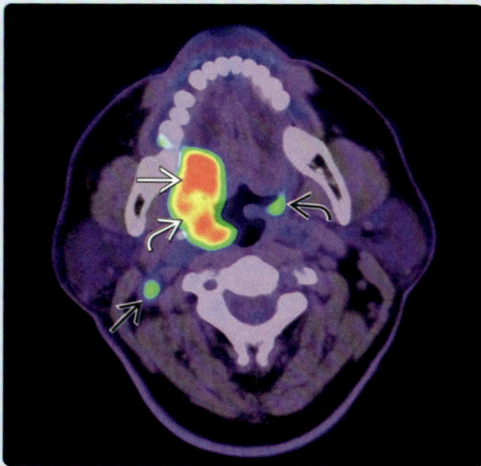

(Left) *Axial graphic of the oropharyngeal mucosal space (blue) is shown. Anterior ➡ and posterior tonsillar pillars, palatine tonsils ➡, and lingual tonsil (base of tongue) ➡ are common oropharyngeal squamous cell carcinoma (OPSCCa) sites.* (Right) *Axial fused F-18 FDG PET/CT in a patient with HPV (+) OPSCCa shows FDG-avid mass in the right palatine tonsil ➡ extending anteriorly into lingual tonsil (base of tongue) ➡, both parts of oropharynx. Note FDG-avid level IIB nodal metastasis ➡. Left tonsil FDG uptake ➡ is physiologic.*

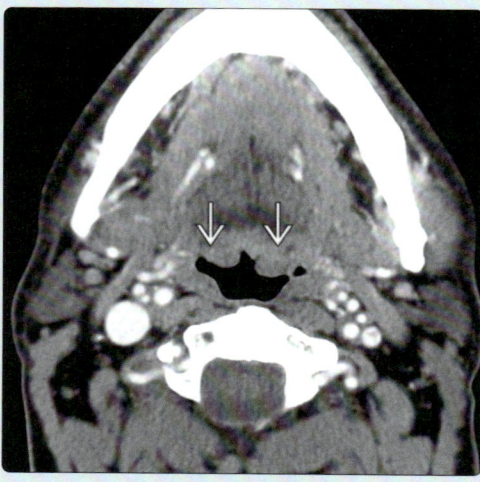
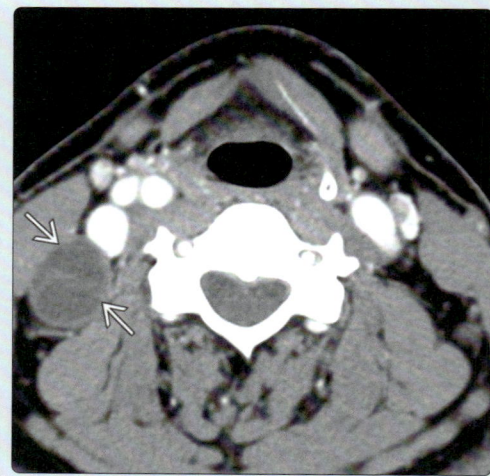

(Left) *Axial CECT shows typical appearance of normal, mildly asymmetric lingual tonsillar tissue ➡ without a discrete mass.* (Right) *Axial CECT (same patient) shows a cystic, septated lymph node in the upper right neck ➡. FNA of node revealed SCCa, and endoscopic biopsy showed primary OPSCCa-HPV in right tongue base. Small tongue base neoplasms may be occult both clinically and on cross-sectional imaging. HPV (+) OPSCCa can have small primary tumors but large and often cystic-appearing nodal metastases.*

TERMINOLOGY

Abbreviations

- Human papillomavirus (HPV)
- Oropharyngeal squamous cell carcinoma (OPSCCa)

Synonyms

- HPV-mediated [p16 (+)] oropharyngeal carcinoma

IMAGING

General Features

- Best diagnostic clue
  - Young/middle-aged, usually nonsmoker White males with level II adenopathy ± mass in palatine/lingual tonsil
  - Imaging appearance may be same as HPV (-) OPSCCa related to tobacco use
  - HPV (+) OPSCCa more likely enhancing and exophytic with well-defined borders and cystic nodal metastases
    - HPV (-) OPSCCa more likely to have poorly defined borders and adjacent muscle invasion
  - On DWI MR, ADC significantly lower in HPV (+) OPSCCa compared with HPV (-) OPSCCa

CT Findings

- CECT
  - **Primary mucosal lesion**
    - Enhancing, variable-sized mass in tonsil/tongue base; other subsites of oropharynx less common
    - Primary lesion may be small and occult
  - **Metastatic adenopathy**
    - Adenopathy variable: Range from single solid or cystic node to bulky, multilevel adenopathy
    - Most commonly, nodes are ipsilateral, involving levels II and III, but can be contralateral, bilateral, and involve lower neck and retropharyngeal sites
    - Contralateral or bilateral lymph nodes more common in tongue base primary tumors
    - Nodes usually levels II and III; may be frankly cystic
    - Morphology of metastatic node ranges from solid → mostly solid → mostly cystic → entirely cystic
    - Although trend toward cystic adenopathy, no particular features can distinguish HPV-related OPSCCa lymph nodes from other metastatic disease
    - Oropharynx rich in lymphatics; 70-80% of oropharynx malignancy presents with clinical or radiologic evidence of nodal metastases
    - Pathologic examination of clinical N0 necks reveals 20-30% rate of occult microscopic metastases
    - Irregular nodal margins with "dirty" fat suggests extranodal extension (ENE), previously known as extracapsular spread (ECS)
    - Pathologic data suggest perinodal inflammatory changes may simulate ENE

MR Findings

- Can be used as primary diagnostic and staging tool; allows for excellent evaluation of primary tumor and nodal drainage pathways
- May be superior to CT if limited by dental amalgam
- T1WI
  - Primary tumor: Homogeneous, isointense mass (to muscle) in tonsil or base of tongue
  - Fat hyperintensity serves as intrinsic contrast to delineate fascial margins
  - Absence of normal fatty tongue muscle striations may delineate infiltration of tongue base tumor
- T2WI
  - Primary tumor: Isointense or minimally hyperintense tonsil or base of tongue mass
  - Metastatic lymph node: Hyperintense to muscle or markedly hyperintense if cystic
- T1WI C+ FS
  - Primary tumor: Enhancing tonsil or tongue base mass
  - Metastatic nodes enhance homogeneously or heterogeneously if nonnecrotic; peripheral enhancement and central low signal if central necrosis
- DWI
  - On DWI MR, ADC significantly lower in HPV (+) OPSCCa compared with HPV (-) OPSCCa
  - Noninvasive prediction of HPV status with good accuracy using ADC and smoking status

Ultrasonographic Findings

- Most commonly see enlarged solid and cystic levels II & III nodes
- Assessment should include lower neck & bilateral nodes

Nuclear Medicine Findings

- PET/CT
  - HPV (+) OPSCCa primary and nodal metastasis FDG avid
  - Highly accurate in detection of primary tumor
  - Small lesions may be difficult to detect
    - Normal tonsillar tissue also FDG avid (normal physiologic uptake)
    - Significant asymmetry of FDG uptake in oropharynx favors primary site
  - False-positive results can occur in oropharynx due to high physiologic activity in lymphoid tissue as well as focal mucosal infection or inflammation
  - Beware: Cystic/necrotic nodal metastases may be falsely negative
  - F-18 FDG PET/CT recommended for initial work-up for H&N cancers of unknown origin; best performed prior to endoscopic biopsies

Imaging Recommendations

- Best imaging tool
  - Most common approach: CECT with ≤ 3-mm slice thickness; delay image acquisition ~ 90 sec to guarantee mucosal enhancement
  - PET combined with diagnostic CECT of neck may be best overall approach, but PET not always readily accessible
    - PET/CT may be only modality to detect occult primary

DIFFERENTIAL DIAGNOSIS

HPV (-) Oropharyngeal SCCa

- Enhancing, mucosal-based mass of tonsil or tongue base will be indistinguishable from OPSCCa-HPV
- More often found in older patient with history of smoking

Non-Hodgkin Lymphoma

- Lymphoma involving palatine or lingual tonsil may present as enhancing, mucosal-based mass
  - OPSCCa usually unilateral, lymphoma often bilateral
  - OPSCCa more common than lymphoma of tonsil
- Cervical lymph nodes with non-Hodgkin lymphoma (NHL) may be indistinguishable from OPSCCa nodal metastases

2nd Branchial Cleft Cyst

- Benign, congenital mass usually in child or young adult
- In adult, 2nd branchial cleft cyst is diagnosis of exclusion—much less likely than HPV (+) OPSCCa nodal metastasis

Asymmetric Lymphoid Tissue of Pharyngeal Mucosal Space

- Palatine tonsils, lingual lymphoid tissue often asymmetric
- Should have no pathologic adenopathy

PATHOLOGY

General Features

- **HPV testing: p16 kinase inhibitor immunohistochemistry (IHC) or HPV-specific tests for HPV DNA or RNA**
- **p16** kinase inhibitor IHC: HPV surrogate marker
- HPV-specific tests for DNA or RNA: Commonly used now as confirmatory tests
- Direct test for **HPV DNA**: In situ hybridization (**ISH**) or polymerase chain reaction (**PCR**)
- Longitudinal blood sampling to test for association of **ctHPVDNA (liquid biopsy)**
  - Primary tumor: Sensitivity 100%, specificity 94.4%, positive predictive value (PPV) 94.4%, negative predictive value (NPP) 100%
    - ctHPVDNA superior to p16 in identification of HPV-OPSCCa at diagnosis
  - Recurrence detection during follow-up: Sensitivity 100%, specificity 98.4%, PPV 90.9%, NPV 100%

Staging, Grading, & Classification

- Staging same as for all OPSCCa in older AJCC systems
- Latest AJCC 8th edition: Clinical TNM (cTNM or TNM) staging prior to treatment, and pathologic TNM (pTNM) if surgery is 1st definitive therapy
- cTNM: Using physical examination/imaging findings
- pTNM: Clinical staging + surgical and pathology findings
- **T staging**: T1-T3 as per greatest dimension of OPSCCa size
  - T0: No primary tumor seen, T1 (≤ 2 cm), T2 (> 2 cm; ≤ 4 cm), T3 (> 4 cm or extension to **epiglottis** lingual surface)
  - T4: Moderately advanced OPSCCa involving
    - Anteriorly to extrinsic tongue muscles or hard palate
    - Laterally to medial pterygoid or mandible
    - Inferiorly to larynx: Extension to epiglottis lingual surface from primary tumors of tongue base and vallecula does not constitute laryngeal invasion
- **N staging (AJCC 8th edition)**
  - **Clinical** (including radiologic) staging based on laterality and size of metastatic nodes, and **pathologic** staging based on actual number of metastatic nodes
  - Levels II and III most commonly involved; retropharyngeal lymph nodes in ~ 10%
  - NX: Regional lymph nodes cannot be assessed

- cN0: No regional lymph node involvement
- cN1: Ipsilateral nodes with no single node > 6 cm
- cN2: Contralateral or bilateral lymph nodes with no single lymph node > 6 cm
- cN3: Lymph nodes > 6 cm
- pN0: No regional lymph node involvement; pN1: 4 or fewer lymph nodes; pN2: > 4 lymph nodes
- **ENE** not **included** in AJCC 8th edition HPV (+) OPSCCa staging
- HPV (+) OPSCCa nodal metastasis more likely to be cystic/necrotic than HPV (-) PSCCa
- **AJCC version 9** for HPV (+) OPSCCa anticipated fall 2025
  - Proposed changes to **N staging** include updated node numbers and **extranodal extension (ENE)**
    - N1a: 1 node, ENE (-)
    - N1b: 2-4 nodes, ENE (-)
    - N2: 1-4 nodes, ENE (+) or > 4 nodes, ENE (-)
    - N3: > 4 nodes, ENE (+)
- **Metastasis staging**
  - cM0: No distant metastasis
  - cM1: Distant metastasis; stage IV reserved for M1
  - pM1: Microscopically confirmed distant metastasis

Gross Pathologic & Surgical Features

- HPV (+) OPSCCa tends to arise from tonsillar crypts, whereas HPV (-) OPSCCa from surface epithelium

CLINICAL ISSUES

Demographics

- Epidemiology
  - ↑ 225% OPSCCa-HPV, whereas ↓ 50% HPV (-) OPSCCa over past few decades
  - 80% of OPSCCa in USA, HPV related
  - Risk directly correlates with number of sexual partners and oral sex practices
- Age: Middle aged (31-78 years), White (> 90%), males (85%)

Natural History & Prognosis

- Overall **better prognosis** than patients with HPV (-), smoking-related OPSCCa
- Survival benefit less pronounced but still present if HPV (+) OPSCCa + significant tobacco history
- ENE high-risk, poor prognostic factor for all H&N tumors, except viral-related cancers and mucosal melanoma

Treatment

- Most often concurrent radiation therapy (XRT) and cisplatin-based chemotherapy
- Transoral robotic surgery (TORS) or transoral laser microsurgery (TLS) ± XRT/chemo-XRT

DIAGNOSTIC CHECKLIST

Consider

- OPSCCa-HPV in adult with new, cystic upper neck mass

SELECTED REFERENCES

1. Ho AS et al: Derivation and validation of the AJCC9V pathological stage classification for HPV-positive oropharyngeal carcinoma: a multicentre registry analysis. Lancet Oncol. 26(8):1113-22, 2025
2. Campo F et al: Circulating tumor HPV DNA in the management of HPV+ oropharyngeal cancer and its correlation with MRI. Head Neck. 46(9):2206-13, 2024

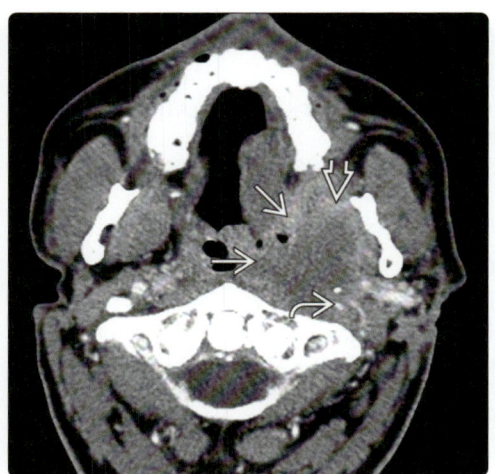

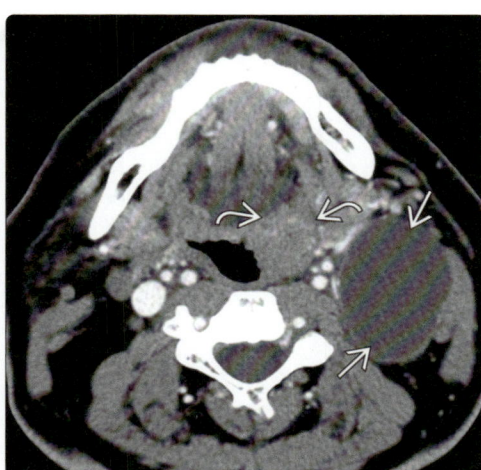

(Left) Axial CECT shows an advanced T4 stage HPV (+) OPSCCa ⇨ extending into the masticator space ⇨ and surrounding and narrowing the left internal carotid artery ⇨. (Right) Axial CECT shows a cystic left neck mass ⇨ mimicking 2nd branchial cleft cyst by location. Note the primary HPV (+) OPSCCa in the left palatine tonsil ⇨, measuring > 2 cm but < 4 cm, making it a T2 tumor. A cystic neck mass in an adult should be considered as nodal metastasis unless proven otherwise.

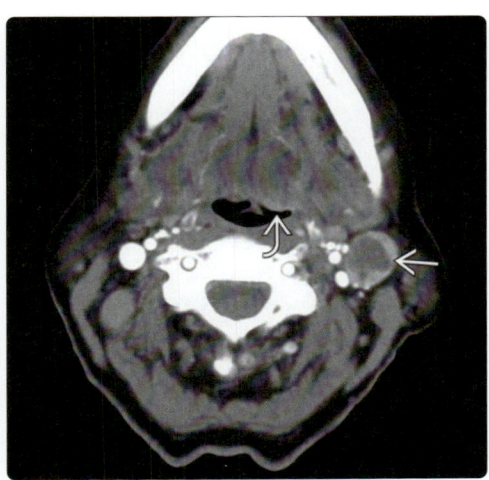

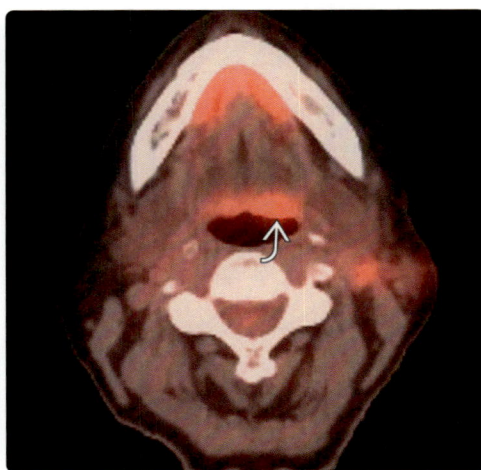

(Left) Axial CECT in a 64-year-old woman shows an enlarged cystic level II node ⇨. Even though this is in the classic location of a 2nd branchial cleft cyst, a metastatic cystic lymph node should be the 1st consideration in an adult (unlike in children), unless proven otherwise. Subtle asymmetry of left tongue base ⇨ is noted, but no lesion was seen endoscopically. (Right) Axial PET/CT after excision of left level II node shows subtle asymmetric increased uptake of the left tongue base ⇨. Excisional biopsy revealed OPSCCa-HPV.

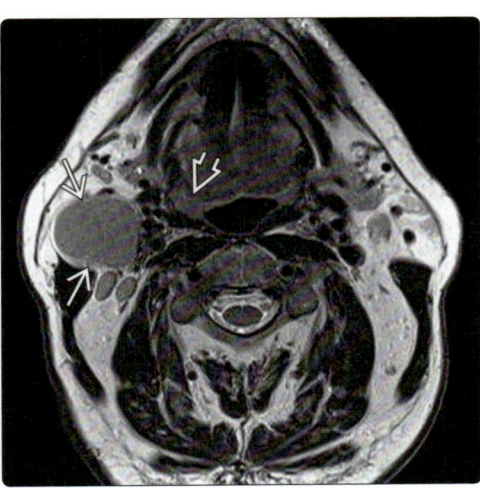

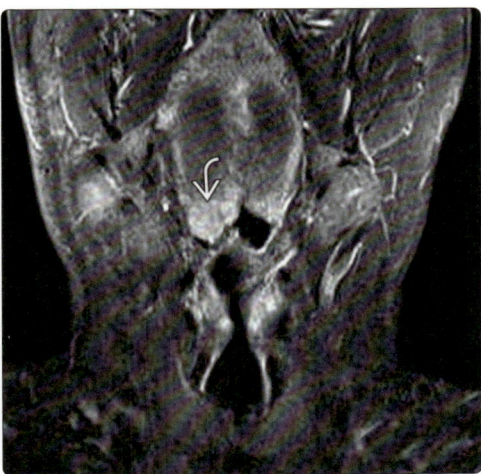

(Left) Axial T2 MR shows an enlarged, solid, pathologic level IIA node ⇨. Subtle asymmetric mucosal thickening of the right tongue base ⇨ is noted. (Right) Coronal T2 FS MR (same patient) confirms asymmetry of right lingual tonsil ⇨. Such asymmetry is nonspecific, but ipsilateral adenopathy increases concern for small mucosal lesion. This proved to be HPV-positive OPSCCa involving lingual tonsil. Primary tumor can be occult on CT and MR, and FDG PET/CT may be only imaging modality to detect the tumor.

TERMINOLOGY

- Mucosal squamous cell carcinoma (SCCa) arising from soft palate (SP) and uvula (tip of SP)
- 5-25% of all oropharyngeal SCCa

IMAGING

- Best evaluated with sagittal and coronal plane rather than axial
- CECT: Mildly enhancing, infiltrative mass; SP may just appear diffusely thickened
- MR: Focal or diffuse, moderately enhancing lesion
- MR allows excellent evaluation of soft tissues, bone involvement, and perineural spread
- FDG PET: SCCa reliably FDG avid

TOP DIFFERENTIAL DIAGNOSES

- Palatine tonsil SCCa
- SP minor salivary gland malignancy
- Expected radiation changes

PATHOLOGY

- AJCC/UICC/TNM staging system (8th edition)

CLINICAL ISSUES

- Patients may present with irritation at back of throat or be asymptomatic
- Strongly associated with tobacco and alcohol abuse
- 5-year overall survival: 51%
- Up to 25% have 2nd primary H&N tumor

DIAGNOSTIC CHECKLIST

- May spread across midline to palatine tonsil
- Look for submucosal spread of tumor and infiltration of parapharyngeal fat
- 60-70% T3/T4 present with nodal metastases
- Strong tendency for bilateral nodal metastases, especially with T4
- Check level 2 and retropharyngeal nodes carefully

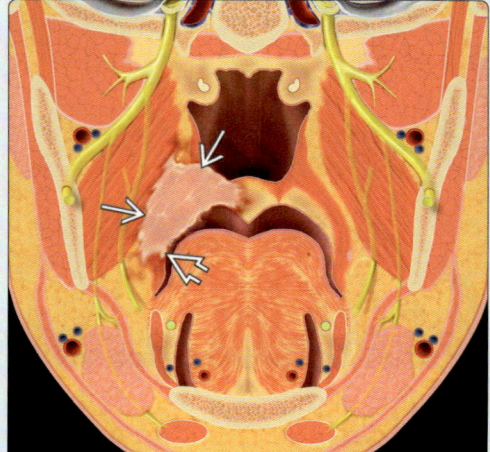 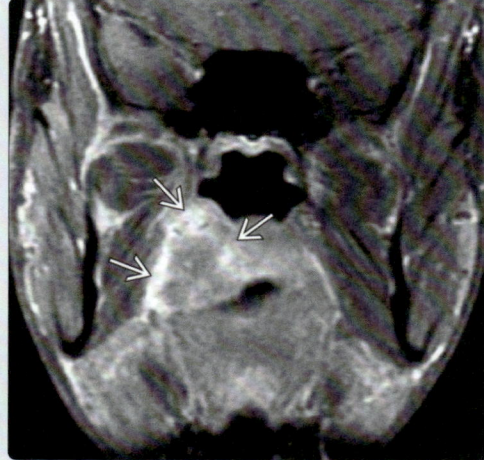

(Left) Coronal graphic illustrates location and growth pattern of soft palate SCCa ➡ that involves the palatal arch and adjacent parapharyngeal fat and extends toward the midline. Laterally, it extends down the pharyngeal wall ➡, where it can involve palatine tonsil. *(Right)* Coronal T1 C+ FS MR in a young patient with heavy tobacco and alcohol use shows a heterogeneously enhancing mass ➡ of the right 1/2 of the soft palate. This proved to be poorly differentiated SCCa with basaloid features (T4a from medial pterygoid invasion).

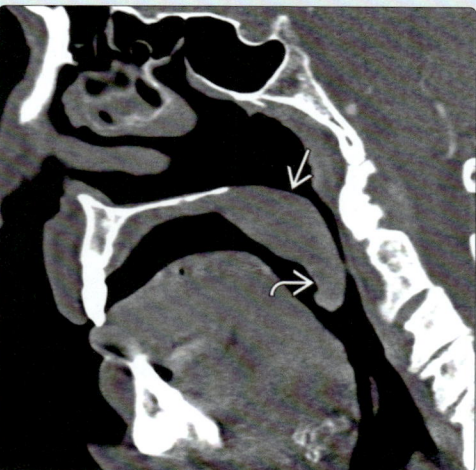 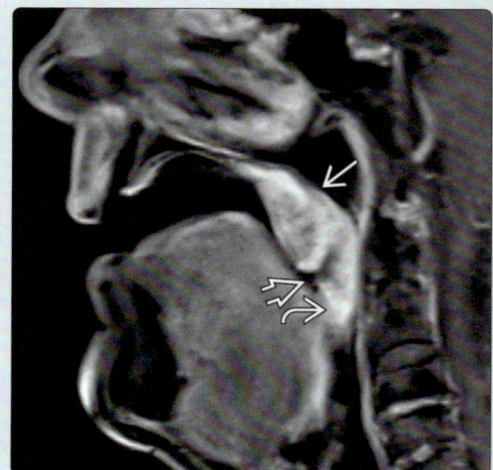

(Left) Sagittal reconstructed CECT in a patient with history of difficulty swallowing shows diffuse thickening and mild enhancement of the soft palate ➡, including uvula ➡. This tumor was staged as T2 N0 M0 on imaging. Pathology confirmed moderate to well-differentiated SCCa of the soft palate. *(Right)* Sagittal T1 C+ FS MR in the same patient demonstrates diffuse thickening and moderate, nonhomogeneous enhancement of the soft palate ➡, including the uvula. ➡ Note an area of necrosis ➡, which is best seen on MR.

Soft Palate Squamous Cell Carcinoma

TERMINOLOGY

Definitions
- Mucosal squamous cell carcinoma (SCCa) arising from soft palate (SP) and uvula (tip of SP)

IMAGING

General Features
- Best diagnostic clue
  - Diffusely or asymmetrically thickened SP
- Location
  - SP; posterior border of hard palate to uvula
  - Tendency to spread across midline &/or to palatine tonsil of lateral oropharynx
- Size
  - Most present T1/T2, therefore ≤ 4 cm
- Morphology
  - Mildly enhancing on CECT, moderately enhancing on MR; ill-defined mass
    - Tendency for submucosal infiltration

CT Findings
- CECT: **Often difficult to fully appreciate in axial plane**
  - Mildly enhancing, infiltrative mass
  - SP may just appear diffusely thickened

MR Findings
- T1WI: Isointense to muscle, slightly hypointense to SP
- T2WI FS: Mildly hyperintense to normal SP
- T1WI C+ FS: Focal or diffuse moderately enhancing lesion

Nuclear Medicine Findings
- PET/CT: SCCa reliably FDG avid

Imaging Recommendations
- Best imaging tool
  - MR allows excellent evaluation of soft tissues, bone involvement, and perineural spread
    - Sagittal and coronal plane more helpful than axial
- Protocol advice
  - CECT: Thin slices with sagittal and coronal reformats
  - MR: Coronal T1, T2 FS, and T1 C+ FS important

DIFFERENTIAL DIAGNOSIS

Palatine Tonsil SCCa
- Tumor arising in tonsil may spread cephalad to SP
- May be difficult to determine primary site on imaging

Soft Palate Minor Salivary Gland Malignancy
- Focal or infiltrating lesion; can be entirely submucosal
- More commonly arises in hard palate

Expected Radiation Changes
- Diffuse SP thickening and enhancement are common findings post XRT + other neck XRT changes

PATHOLOGY

Staging, Grading, & Classification
- Oropharyngeal SCCa American Joint Committee (AJCC) on Cancer TNM staging system (2017), 8th edition

- 2017 update separates HPV-related carcinomas from HPV (-) carcinomas
- Adapted from AJCC
  - Tx = primary tumor cannot be assessed
  - Tis = carcinoma in situ [not stage for HPV (+) SCCa]
  - T1 = tumor ≤ 2 cm in greatest diameter
  - T2 = > 2 cm but ≤ 4 cm in greatest diameter
  - T3 = > 4 cm in diameter
  - T4a = invades medial pterygoid, hard palate, mandible
  - T4b = invades lateral pterygoid, pterygoid plates, lateral nasopharynx, or skull base, or encases internal carotid artery (ICA) [not stage for HPV (+) SCCa]

CLINICAL ISSUES

Presentation
- Most common signs/symptoms
  - Unusual sensation or irritation at back of throat
  - May be asymptomatic

Demographics
- Most commonly arising in 5th-7th decades
- 5-25% of all oropharyngeal SCCa

Natural History & Prognosis
- Strongly associated with tobacco and alcohol abuse
- 75% present with early-stage disease T1/T2
- 5-year overall survival: 51%
- Overall improved survival with HPV-related SCCa

Treatment
- Different schools of thought favor definitive radiation **vs.** surgery ± XRT
- Later-stage tumors probably require chemotherapy in addition to surgery/XRT
- Endoscopic and robotic resection of tumor increasingly used in small tumors

DIAGNOSTIC CHECKLIST

Consider
- Look for submucosal spread of tumor and infiltration of parapharyngeal fat, which may not be clinically evident
- May spread across midline and to ipsilateral/contralateral tonsil
- 60-70% of T3/T4 have nodal metastases at presentation
- Strong tendency for bilateral nodal metastases, especially with T4
  - Check level 2 and retropharyngeal nodes carefully
- Up to 25% have 2nd primary H&N tumor

Image Interpretation Pearls
- Sagittal and coronal images most helpful for evaluating primary site

SELECTED REFERENCES

1. Ding X et al: Endoscopic submucosal dissection for a squamous cell carcinoma of the soft palate and uvula (with video). Gastrointest Endosc. 101(4):905-6, 2024
2. Kim SI et al: A SEER-based analysis of trends in HPV-associated oropharyngeal squamous cell carcinoma. Infect Agent Cancer. 19(1):29, 2024
3. Chebib E et al: Transoral robotic surgery for cancer of the soft palate posterior surface. Ear Nose Throat J. 101(10):660-2, 2022

KEY FACTS

TERMINOLOGY

- Oral tongue squamous cell carcinoma (SCCa) definition: Oral cavity mucosal malignancy that arises from anterior 2/3 of tongue

IMAGING

- Imaging to define deep extent (T4 stage) & nodes
- Lateral margin > undersurface > > tip of tongue
- **Superficial lesion may be occult to imaging**
- CECT/MR: Variably enhancing, invasive lesion
  - Dual-energy CT (DECT)/spectral detector CT (SDCT) may ↑ conspicuity
- MR better evaluates extent of primary than CT
  - MR less affected by dental amalgam artifact
- Growing role of intraoperative transoral US for tumor mapping, predicting depth of invasion

TOP DIFFERENTIAL DIAGNOSES

- Lingual tonsil SCCa

- Tongue schwannoma
- Venous malformation of tongue
- Oral cavity abscess

PATHOLOGY

- Strong association with tobacco & alcohol
- Clinical assessment more accurate than imaging for mucosal size (T1-T3)
- Imaging important for extent of depth & nodes
- 1st-order nodal drainage: Submandibular (IB), then jugulodigastric group (IIA)
- Beware of "skip nodes" where anterior tongue tumors drain directly to levels III or IV

CLINICAL ISSUES

- Painful, nonhealing ulcer of oral tongue
- Median age: 61 years; M:F = 4:1
- Treatment primarily surgical resection ± radiation
- Overall 5-year survival: 60%

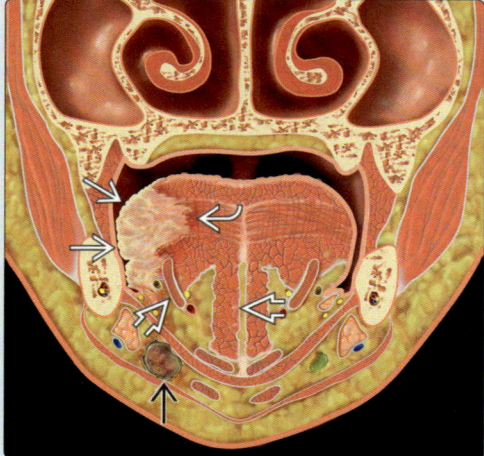
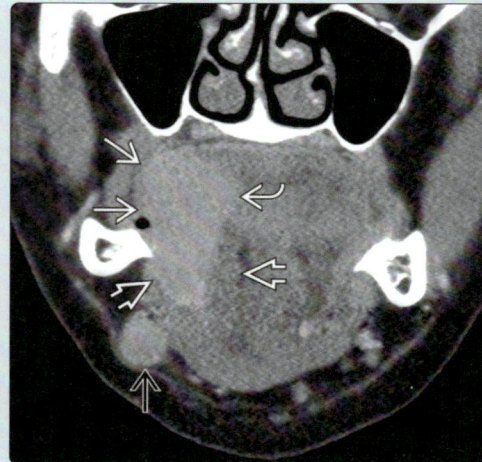

(Left) Coronal graphic illustrates a lateral oral tongue squamous cell carcinoma (SCCa) ➡, which invades the intrinsic tongue muscles ➡. Coronal plane allows scrutiny of extrinsic tongue muscles ➡ and the floor of the mouth. Ipsilateral IB metastatic adenopathy ➡ is shown. (Right) Coronal CECT shows a large, infiltrating right lateral tongue SCCa ➡, which invades the intrinsic ➡ and extrinsic ➡ tongue musculature. An enlarged, round, avidly enhancing IB lymph node ➡ signifies nodal metastatic disease.

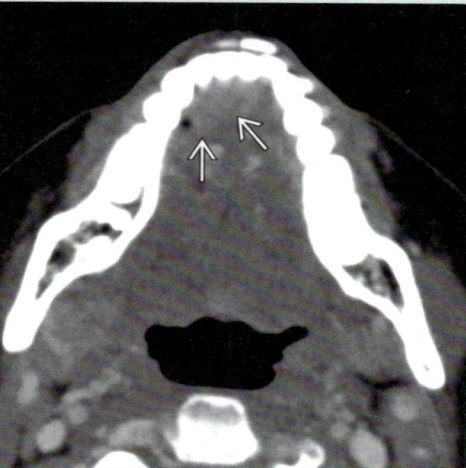
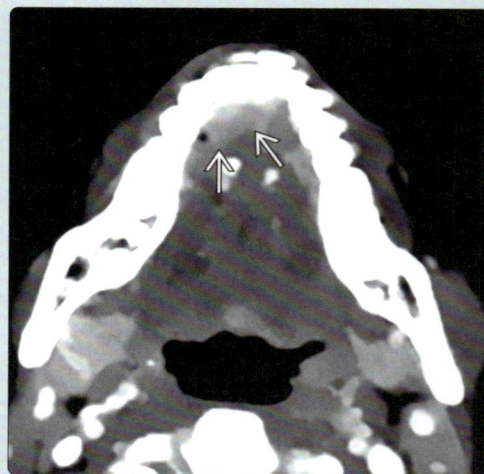

(Left) Axial CECT illustrates a critical challenge of imaging oral tongue SCCa: Clinically overt tumors may be extraordinarily subtle on CT. In this case, a ventral tongue mass ➡ is only faintly visible with exaggerated windowing. (Right) Axial spectral detector CT synthesized monoenergetic (MonoE 40 keV) displayed at identical window level shows the large ventral tongue SCCa ➡ much more conspicuously. By generating an image solely from photons with energies (40 keV) closer to the K-edge of iodine (33.2 keV), contrast enhancement is more robust.

Oral Tongue Squamous Cell Carcinoma

TERMINOLOGY

Abbreviations
- Oral tongue squamous cell carcinoma (SCCa)

Definitions
- Oral cavity (OC) mucosal malignancy arising from anterior 2/3 of tongue
  - Distinct from base of tongue (oropharyngeal SCCa)

IMAGING

General Features
- Best diagnostic clue
  - Asymmetric enhancement ± ulcer of lateral tongue
- Location
  - Oral tongue defined as freely mobile portion
    - Tip, lateral borders, dorsum, & undersurface
  - Most commonly arises from **lateral margin**
    - Next most common is undersurface
- Size
  - Variable, both in superficial & deep extent
    - Mucosal lesion & tumor size are evaluated clinically
- Morphology
  - Irregular ulcer with variable deep invasion

CT Findings
- CECT
  - Variably enhancing oral tongue mucosal lesion
  - **Superficial lesion may be occult to imaging**
  - Dental amalgam streak artifact often problematic
  - Dual-energy CT (DECT) may ↑ conspicuity
- Bone CT
  - May invade mandible (T4 disease)

MR Findings
- T1WI
  - Low signal intensity compared to tongue tissues
- T2WI
  - Typically ↑ signal intensity
  - Most readily observed with fat saturation
- T1WI C+
  - Variable enhancement, mild to moderate
  - Large tumors show ulceration with rim enhancement
  - Imaging role to determine presence of T4 disease

Ultrasonographic Findings
- Growing role of intraoperative transoral US for tumor mapping, predicting depth of invasion
- Hypoechoic tumor with distortion of normal tongue architecture

Nuclear Medicine Findings
- PET/CT
  - SCCa is reliably FDG avid; sensitive for nodal disease
  - Increasing role of PET/MR in staging

Imaging Recommendations
- Best imaging tool
  - MR preferred imaging modality in OC
    - Superior soft tissue contrast
    - Less affected by dental amalgam artifact than CT

- More degraded by motion than CT
- Protocol advice
  - Fat saturation improves T2 & T1 C+ tissue contrast
  - Coronal MPR aid in evaluating deep extent with CECT
  - Consider enhanced DECT to ↑ SCCa conspicuity

DIFFERENTIAL DIAGNOSIS

Lingual Tonsil SCCa
- Invasive tongue base tumor may extend into oral tongue
- More commonly invades floor of mouth, tongue root

Tongue Schwannoma
- Circumscribed mass within oral tongue
- Homogeneous enhancement

Venous Malformation of Tongue
- Congenital vascular lesion
- Calcified phleboliths virtually diagnostic

Oral Cavity Abscess
- Rim-enhancing, cystic mass, often with extensive cellulitis
- Typically associated with dental disease

PATHOLOGY

General Features
- Etiology
  - Strong link with smoking, chewing tobacco, & alcohol
- Genetics
  - SCCa-related oncogene (*DCUN1D1*)
    - May play role in pathogenesis of oral tongue SCCa through amplification of chromosome 3q26
    - May be predictor of regional metastases & marker for aggressiveness & outcome

Staging, Grading, & Classification
- AJCC 8th edition (2017)
- Clinical assessment more accurate than imaging for mucosal size
- Imaging is important for determination of **deep extent: Must look for features that make tumor T4**
  - T4a: Tumor invades through cortical bone, maxillary sinus, skin of face, or extensive bilateral tongue
  - T4b: Tumor invades masticator space, pterygoid plates, skull base, or encases internal carotid artery
  - Contralateral spread important for surgical resection
  - Tumor thickness = radiologic estimate of histologic DOI
    - Measured as tumor depth from line tangent to normal (not ulcerated) plane of surface mucosa
- Anterior tongue SCCa; more often involves floor of mouth
- **Malignant nodes common at presentation**
  - Up to 35% have ≥ N1 disease preoperatively
  - 30% "N0" necks have microscopic nodal metastases
- 1st-order nodal drainage: Submandibular (IB), then jugulodigastric group (IIA)
  - Occasionally, anterior tumors drain directly to midjugular (III) or low jugular (IV): **"Skip nodes"**
  - Midline tumor more likely to have **bilateral** nodes
  - Tongue tip tumors may drain to submental (I)
- Lower nodes more likely to have distant mets
  - Lungs > bones or liver

American Joint Committee on Cancer (AJCC) Oral Cavity Staging (2017)

Tumor (T): Clinical Assessment of Mucosal Extent More Accurate Than Imaging	Clinical Nodal Stage (cN)	Distant Metastasis (M)
TX: Primary tumor cannot be assessed	**NX**: Regional nodes cannot be assessed	**M0**: No distant metastasis
Tis: Carcinoma in situ	**N0**: No regional node metastases	**M1**: Distant metastasis
T1: Tumor ≤ 2 cm, DOI ≤ 5 mm	**N1**: Single ipsilateral node ≤ 3 cm, ENE(-)	
T2: Tumor ≤ 2 cm with DOI > 5 mm and ≤ 10 mm **or** tumor > 2 cm but ≤ 4 cm with DOI ≤ 10 mm	**N2a**: Single ipsilateral node > 3 cm & ≤ 6 cm, ENE(-)	
T3: Tumor > 2 cm and ≤ 4 cm **or** any tumor with DOI > 10 mm or tumor > 4 cm with DOI ≤ 10 mm	**N2b**: Multiple ipsilateral nodes ≤ 6 cm, ENE(-)	
T4a: Tumor invades adjacent structures only (e.g., cortical bone of maxilla or mandible, maxillary sinus, skin of face) **or** bilateral tongue involvement **&/or** tumor > 4 cm with DOI > 10 mm	**N2c**: Bilateral or contralateral ≤ 6 cm, ENE(-)	
T4b: Tumor invades masticator space, pterygoid plates, or skull base, &/or encases internal carotid artery	**N3a**: Nodal mass > 6 cm, ENE(-)	
	N3b: Any nodal metastasis with clinically overt **ENE(+)**	

T = tumor; N = nodal; M = metastasis; DOI = depth of invasion; ENE = extranodal extension. **DOI is not equivalent to tumor thickness**; *lymph nodes are measured in greatest dimension (any plane).*

Adapted from Amin MB et al: AJCC Cancer Staging Manual. 8th Ed. Springer New York, 2017.

Gross Pathologic & Surgical Features

- Red or red & white demarcated areas of roughness/induration
- Ulcerated areas are indurated, firm, painful

Microscopic Features

- Squamous differentiation with intracellular bridges or keratinization, ± keratin pearls
- Further classified by amount of differentiation
  - Well, moderately, poorly, or undifferentiated

CLINICAL ISSUES

Presentation

- Most common signs/symptoms
  - Pain; occurs with smaller size than many OC tumors
  - Nonhealing ulcer of oral tongue mucosa ± bleeding
- Other signs/symptoms
  - Tongue mass + neck masses from regional nodes

Demographics

- Age
  - Median: 61 years
- Sex
  - M:F = 4:1
- Epidemiology
  - > 90% of OC malignancies are SCCa
    - Most common sites: Tongue & floor of mouth
  - Rising incidence of tongue SCCa

Natural History & Prognosis

- Survival significantly impacted by ongoing tobacco & alcohol abuse; adjacent structure invasion ↓ prognosis
- **Overall 5-year survival: 60%** (if no nodal metastases: ~ 77%)

Treatment

- Treatment primarily surgical resection ± radiation
  - Local resection
  - Hemiglossectomy
    - If large tumor not crossing midline
    - Midline determined by fatty lingual septum
  - Total glossectomy: Rarely performed, high morbidity
- To minimize recurrence, 1.5- to 2-cm margin required
  - **Preoperative determination of deep extent crucial!**

DIAGNOSTIC CHECKLIST

Consider

- Mucosal extent better seen clinically than on imaging
  - **Superficial lesion may be occult on MR/CECT**
- Imaging more accurate for **deep extent & nodes**
  - MR typically evaluates extent better than CECT
  - Nodes frequently present, often clinically occult

Reporting Tips

- Determine if tumor crosses to contralateral side (relevant to surgical planning)
- **Look for deeply invasive features (upstage to T4a/b)**
- Evaluate for ipsilateral & contralateral IB & IIA nodes
- Beware "skip nodes" (III or IV without higher levels), especially with anterior tongue tumors

SELECTED REFERENCES

1. See A et al: Radiological sublingual space invasion in tongue squamous cell carcinoma: clinicopathological associations and impact on survival. Otolaryngol Head Neck Surg. 172(3):931-41, 2025
2. Tanaka H et al: Utility of diffusion-weighted MR imaging for evaluating the depth of invasion in oral tongue squamous cell carcinoma. Magn Reson Med Sci. 24(2):210-19, 2025
3. Das R et al: Tumor thickness and depth of invasion in squamous cell carcinoma of tongue as indicators of the loco-regional spread of the disease: a preliminary study. J Oral Biol Craniofac Res. 14(4):423-9, 2024

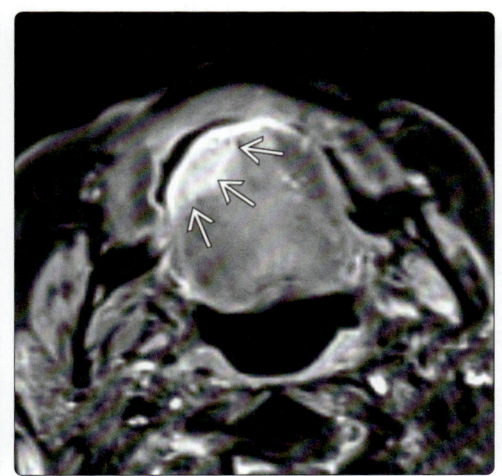
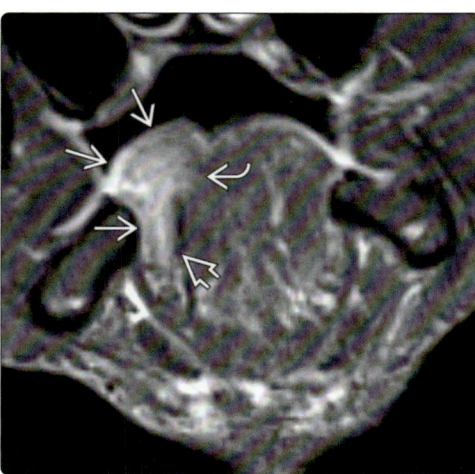

(Left) Axial T1 C+ FS MR in an older patient with tongue pain and bleeding shows an infiltrating right ventrolateral, avidly enhancing mass ➡, which nearly extends to midline. Biopsy revealed moderately differentiated keratinizing SCCa. (Right) Coronal T2 FS MR in the same patient shows the lateral tongue SCCa ➡ to be hyperintense to the tongue musculature. Coronal imaging nicely depicts the extent of invasion into the intrinsic ➡ and extrinsic tongue muscles. In this case, there is early invasion of the hyoglossus ➡.

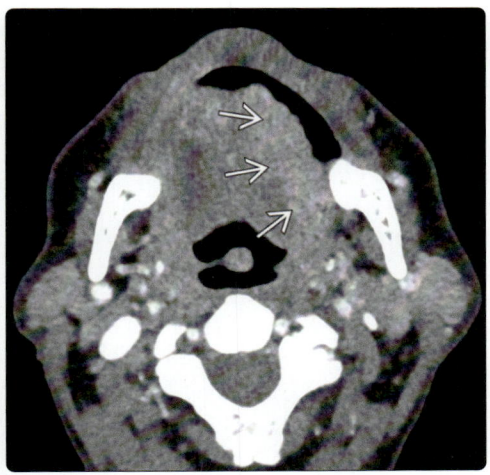
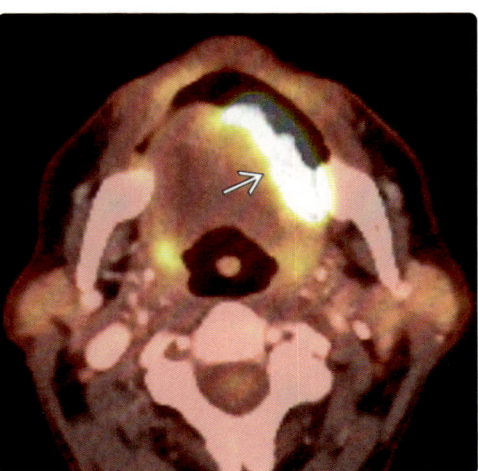

(Left) Axial CECT shows a left lateral tongue SCCa ➡, which despite its size remains quite subtle on CECT imaging. Oral tongue SCCa shows variable enhancement but is typically hyperattenuating compared to the tongue musculature. (Right) Axial fused F-18 FDG PET/CT in the same patient shows the left oral tongue SCCa ➡ to have marked FDG uptake. Oral tongue SCCa is reliably FDG avid, which may be helpful in cases when the primary tumor is not identified on CECT or is obscured by streak artifact from dental amalgam.

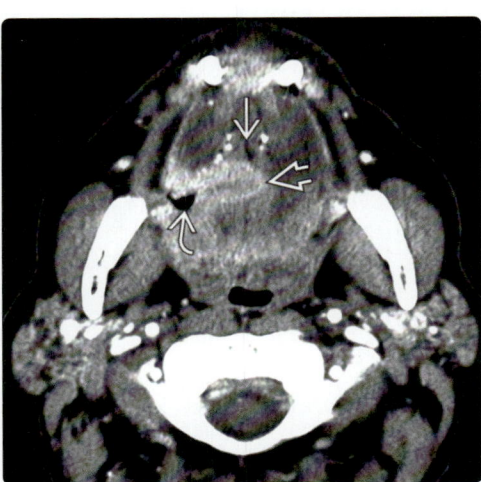
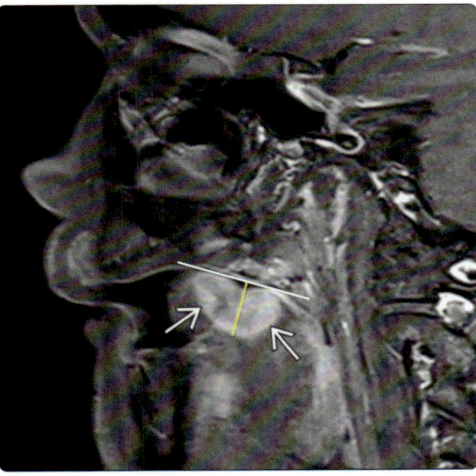

(Left) Axial CECT shows poorly defined lateral tongue SCCa that crosses the lingual septum ➡ into the contralateral tongue ➡. Note a prominent air-filled surface ulceration ➡. (Right) Sagittal T1 C+ FS MR shows an enhancing oral tongue SCCa ➡. Tumor thickness (yellow line) is measured as enhancing tumor depth tangent to the normal mucosal surface (white line). This is a useful staging estimate, although is not equivalent to histopathologic depth of invasion.

KEY FACTS

TERMINOLOGY

- Floor of mouth (FOM) squamous cell carcinoma (SCCa)
  - FOM mucosa overlies mylohyoid and hyoglossus muscles, and body of tongue rests on it

IMAGING

- CECT: Irregular, mild to moderately enhancing mass
- MR: Loss of normal FOM anatomical planes on T1
  - Increased T2 signal intensity and enhancement
- SCCa reliably FDG avid; PET/CT highest sensitivity
- Consider intraoral US assessment for small lesions
- May exactly mimic sublingual gland carcinoma

TOP DIFFERENTIAL DIAGNOSES

- Sublingual gland carcinoma
- Oral tongue SCCa
- Vascular malformation
- Ranula
- Oral cavity abscess

PATHOLOGY

- Strongly associated with tobacco and alcohol abuse
- ≤ 35% have nodes at presentation: Levels I, II
- High incidence of occult nodal metastases

CLINICAL ISSUES

- Most commonly 50-70 years; M:F = 2:1
- Painful, hard ulcer/lesion ± loose teeth
- Overall 5-year survival = 60%

DIAGNOSTIC CHECKLIST

- May present as submandibular gland sialadenitis
- Clinical mucosal size more accurate than imaging
- Imaging is important for identifying deep extent of tumor and nodal metastases
- **Look for and report features that make tumor T4**
  - Erosion through mandibular cortex, marrow infiltration
- Pathologic depth of invasion assessment more accurate than imaging

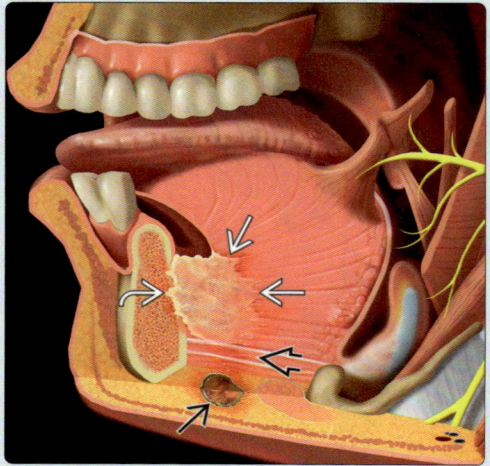
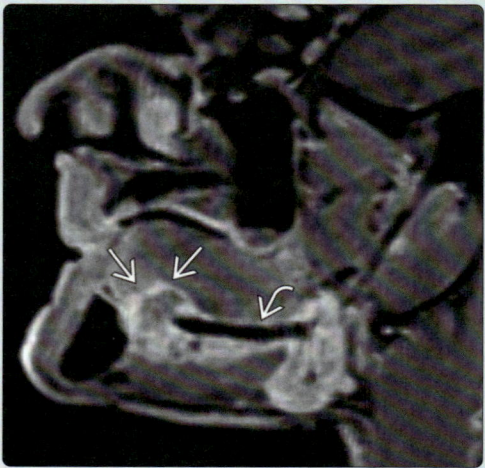

(Left) Graphic shows typical location of a floor of mouth (FOM) SCCa ➡. The primary role of imaging is to determine deep extent of tumor. Note invasion inferiorly to genioglossus & mylohyoid ➡ muscles, posteriorly toward tongue base, & mandibular invasion ➡ anteriorly. The 2nd aim of imaging is to identify nodal metastases ➡. (Right) Sagittal oblique T1 C+ FS MR shows a FOM SCCa ➡. Note dilatation of the submandibular duct ➡ secondary to infiltration of the duct opening by the tumor. Mandible was not involved.

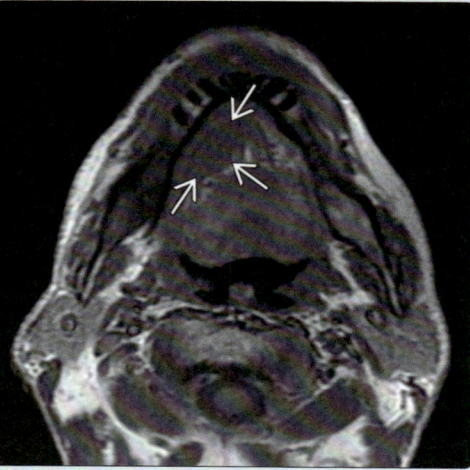
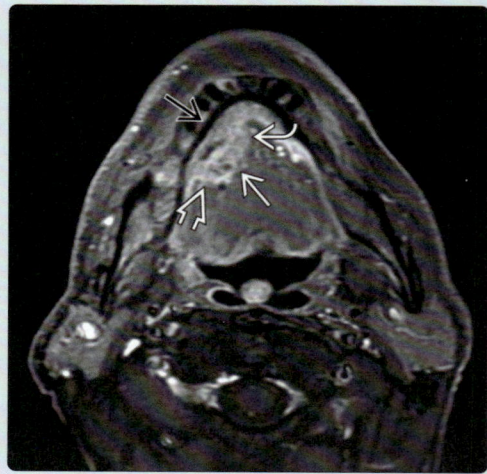

(Left) Axial T1 MR in a patient with FOM SCCa shows a hypointense mass ➡ in the right anterior FOM with loss of the normal fatty signal intensity separating the genioglossus & hyoglossus muscles, which is highly suspicious for invasion of the extrinsic muscles of the tongue. (Right) Axial T1 C+ FS MR shows the mass ➡ to be heterogeneously enhancing with invasion of the genioglossus ➡ & hyoglossus ➡ muscles. Note a maintained dark cortical margin of the parasymphyseal mandible ➡, which is spared.

Floor of Mouth Squamous Cell Carcinoma

TERMINOLOGY

Abbreviations
- Floor of mouth (FOM) squamous cell carcinoma (SCCa)

Definitions
- Oral cavity mucosal malignancy arising from FOM
  - Inner surface of mandibular alveolar ridges to undersurface of tongue

IMAGING

General Features
- Best diagnostic clue
  - Irregular, enhancing mass in anterior FOM
- Location
  - Most within 2 cm of anterior midline FOM
- Size
  - Variable: Several millimeters to several centimeters

CT Findings
- CECT
  - Mild to moderately enhancing, irregular FOM mass
  - May exactly mimic sublingual gland carcinoma
  - May obstruct submandibular duct(s) → sialadenitis
- Bone CT
  - Must evaluate carefully for cortical erosion

MR Findings
- T1WI
  - Low-signal mass in relation to FOM tissues
    - **Subtle loss of normal anatomic contours**
- T2WI
  - Increased signal intensity
    - Fat saturation recommended to improve conspicuity
- T1WI C+
  - Variable enhancement: Mild to moderate
  - Tumor infiltrating marrow typically enhances

Nuclear Medicine Findings
- PET/CT
  - SCCa reliably FDG avid

Imaging Recommendations
- Best imaging tool
  - MR best for determining tumor extent
  - Bone CT important when tumor abuts mandible
  - PET/CT offers highest sensitivity in detection
  - Dual-energy CT (DECT)/spectral detector CT may increase lesion conspicuity
- Protocol advice
  - CECT: Soft tissue and bone algorithm in 2 planes
    - Puffed-cheek CT scan improves mucosal assessment

DIFFERENTIAL DIAGNOSIS

Sublingual Gland Carcinoma
- May be impossible to distinguish by imaging

Oral Tongue Squamous Cell Carcinoma
- Anterior &/or large lesions may invade FOM

Vascular Malformation
- Heterogeneous, moderate to marked enhancement ± phleboliths if venous malformation
- Nonenhancing or thin septal enhancement ± fluid-fluid level if lymphatic malformation

Ranula
- Rim-enhancing fluid mass in FOM

Oral Cavity Abscess
- Rim-enhancing collection(s) + FOM cellulitis

PATHOLOGY

General Features
- Etiology
  - Strongly associated with tobacco (smoking and chewing), alcohol abuse, betel nut, and paan

Staging, Grading, & Classification
- American Joint Committee on Cancer (AJCC) 2017
- Same classification for all oral cavity tumors
  - Tis: Carcinoma in situ
  - T1: Tumor ≤ 2 cm, ≤ 5 mm depth of invasion (DOI)
  - T2: Tumor ≤ 2 cm with DOI > 5 mm and ≤ 10 mm **or** tumor > 2 cm and ≤ 4 cm with DOI ≤ 10 mm
  - T3: Tumor > 4 cm **or** any tumor with DOI > 10 mm but ≤ 20 mm
  - T4a: Tumor invades adjacent structures (e.g., cortical bone of mandible, skin of face, bilateral tongue) &/or DOI > 20 mm
  - T4b: Tumor invades masticator space, pterygoid plates, skull base, or encases internal carotid artery
- Clinical **mucosal extent** more accurate than imaging
- Imaging important for **deep extent: Look for features that make tumor T4**
- Nodal staging: Follows AJCC laryngeal node category
- 1st-order drainage is **level I**, then **level II**
  - **Up to 35%** have nodes found at presentation
- Metastatic disease: Absent = M0, present = M1

CLINICAL ISSUES

Presentation
- Most common signs/symptoms
  - Painful hard ulcer/lesion in FOM
- Other signs/symptoms
  - Invasion of mandible may lead to loose teeth

Demographics
- Age
  - Most commonly 50-70 years

Natural History & Prognosis
- **Overall 5-year survival = 60%**

Treatment
- Primary resection ± reconstruction, ± neck dissection
- ± adjuvant radiation

SELECTED REFERENCES

1. Lin B et al: Imaging and pathology concordance in head and neck cancer: retrospective analysis. Oral Dis. 31(7):2102-18, 2025

KEY FACTS

TERMINOLOGY

- Squamous cell carcinoma (SCCa) arising from gingival mucosa overlying alveolar ridges of mandible or maxilla

IMAGING

- Small lesions may be occult to imaging
- Larger lesions: **Enhancing, infiltrating mass** ± underlying **bone destruction**
- Bone CT: Osseous destruction of mandibular or maxillary alveolar ridge
- MR: Marrow signal and enhancement similar to tumor
  - Less affected by dental amalgam, which may obscure CT
- Coronal plane useful for CT or MR evaluation
- FDG PET/CT to detect nodal and distant metastases

TOP DIFFERENTIAL DIAGNOSES

- Osteomyelitis
- Osteoradionecrosis
- Osteonecrosis
- Metastasis
- Osteosarcoma

CLINICAL ISSUES

- **10%** oral cavity SCCa
- Nonhealing ulcer of jaw, pain, swelling, bleeding, ill-fitting dentures
- Overall 5-year survival ~ 60%
- Surgical resection ± reconstruction ± radiation

DIAGNOSTIC CHECKLIST

- Evaluate local spread, bone infiltration, nodes
- Mandible: Buccal space, masticator space, floor of mouth
- Maxilla: Nasal cavity, maxillary sinus, palate
- Alveolar ridge mucosa attached to bone; allows early marrow infiltration: T4a
- If in bone, evaluate for perineural tumor spread
  - Inferior alveolar (mandible) or palatine (maxilla)
- Metastatic spread favors facial, level I and II nodes

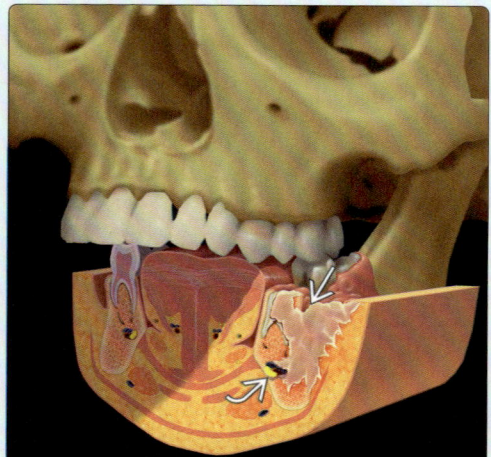
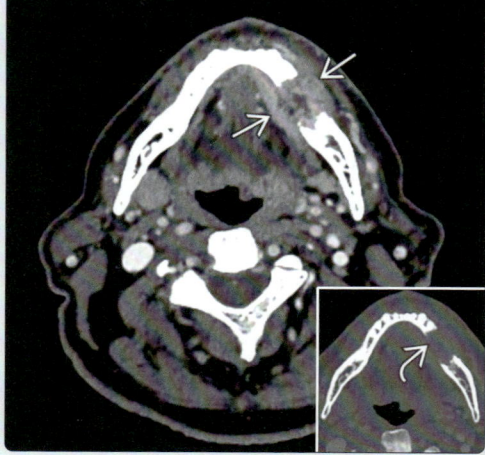

(Left) Graphic illustrates squamous cell carcinoma (SCCa) ➡ arising from the left mandibular alveolar ridge and invading the mandible body, making it T4a. Note involvement of the inferior alveolar nerve ➡, which is important for complete resection. (Right) Axial CECT through the oral cavity demonstrates a left alveolar SCCa as a heterogeneously enhancing mass ➡ invading and destroying mandibular bone. Inset: Corresponding bone window shows lytic destruction of the mandible ➡.

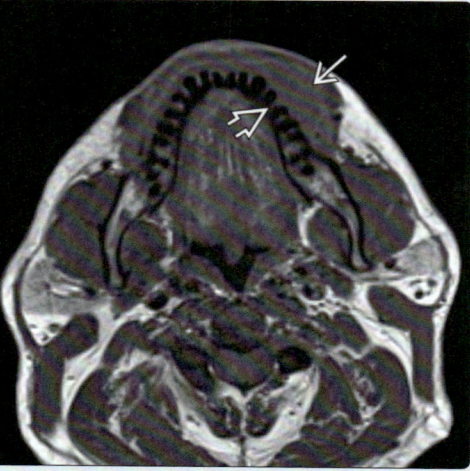
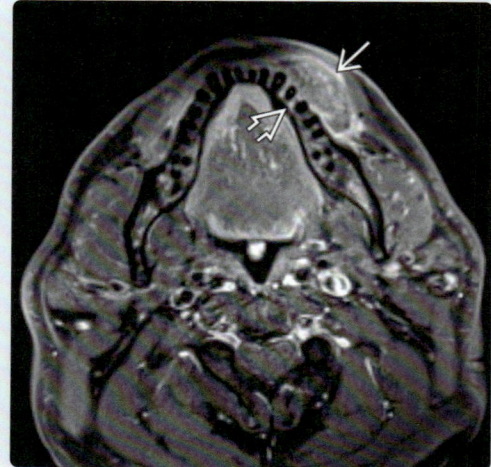

(Left) Axial T1WI MR shows an intermediate signal intensity mass ➡ along the left parasymphyseal mandible, which invades the gingivobuccal sulcus. Loss of dark, cortical signal intensity along the tooth-bearing surface of the mandible ➡ indicates bone invasion. (Right) Axial T1WI C+ FS MR shows a heterogeneously enhancing, exophytic mass ➡ along the left parasymphyseal mandible, which invades the tooth-bearing cortical bone and subjacent marrow space, which has been replaced by enhancement ➡.

TERMINOLOGY

Abbreviations

- Alveolar ridge squamous cell carcinoma (SCCa)

Definitions

- SCCa arising from gingival mucosa overlying alveolar ridges of mandible or maxilla

IMAGING

General Features

- Best diagnostic clue
  - **Enhancing, infiltrating jaw mass; bone destruction**
- Location
  - Mandibular or maxillary alveolar ridge
    - Alveolar ridge = teeth-bearing portion of jaw
- Size
  - Varies from millimeters to several centimeters
- Morphology
  - Poorly marginated mass

CT Findings

- CECT
  - Irregular, mild to moderately enhancing lesion
  - Small lesions may be occult to imaging
- Bone CT
  - Destruction of alveolar bone of mandible/maxilla
  - Enlarged inferior alveolar canal (mandible)/palatine canal (maxilla) suggests perineural tumor

MR Findings

- T1WI
  - Isointense to muscle
  - Loss of normal high marrow signal supports invasion
- T1WI C+
  - Moderately enhancing mass of jaw
  - Marrow enhancement suggests invasion
    - Evaluate entire length of nerve to brainstem

Imaging Recommendations

- Best imaging tool
  - MR preferred for complete tumor extent
    - Bone marrow and perineural tumor spread
    - Less affected by dental amalgam artifact
  - Bone CT to better evaluate for cortical destruction
- Protocol advice
  - MR: Axial and coronal planes, fat saturation on T1 C+
  - CECT: Bone and soft tissue algorithm, axial and coronal

Nuclear Medicine Findings

- PET/CT
  - SCCa reliably FDG avid

DIFFERENTIAL DIAGNOSIS

Mandible-Maxilla Osteomyelitis

- Destructive focus ± adjacent soft tissue abscess

Mandible-Maxilla Osteoradionecrosis

- Destructive mandibular focus, prior XRT

Mandible-Maxilla Osteonecrosis

- Most commonly seen now with bisphosphonate

Mandible-Maxilla Metastasis

- Aggressive mandibular mass, known primary

Mandible-Maxilla Osteosarcoma

- Aggressive mandibular lesion with periosteal reaction

PATHOLOGY

General Features

- Etiology
  - Alcohol and tobacco → epithelial metaplasia → neoplasia

Staging, Grading, & Classification

- American Joint Committee on Cancer (AJCC) 8th Edition (2017)
  - T1: Tumor ≤ 2 cm, ≤ 5 mm depth of invasion (DOI)
  - T2: Tumor ≤ 2 cm with DOI > 5 mm and ≤ 10 mm **or** tumor > 2 cm and ≤ 4 cm with DOI ≤ 10 mm
  - T3: Tumor > 2 cm and ≤ 4 cm with DOI > 10 mm **or** tumor > 4 cm with DOI ≤ 10 mm
  - T4a: Tumor > 4 cm with DOI > 10 mm **or** tumor invades adjacent structures (e.g., cortical bone of mandible or maxilla, maxillary sinus, or skin of face)
  - T4b: Tumor invades masticator space, pterygoid plates, skull base, &/or encases carotid
- **Imaging is critical for determination of T4 status**

CLINICAL ISSUES

Presentation

- Most common signs/symptoms
  - Nonhealing ulcer of jaw

Demographics

- Age
  - Mean: 65 years
- Epidemiology
  - **10%** of oral cavity SCCa

Natural History & Prognosis

- SCCa spreads locally to adjacent spaces
  - Maxilla: Medially to palate, maxillary sinus, nasal cavity
  - Mandible: Medially to floor of mouth, laterally to buccal and masticator spaces
- Lower metastatic rate than other oral cavity sites
- **Overall 5-year survival ~ 60%**

Treatment

- Surgical resection ± reconstruction
  - ± elective neck dissection, adjuvant radiation

SELECTED REFERENCES

1. Asok A et al: Role of diffusion weighted magnetic resonance imaging in oral cancer in predicting response to neoadjuvant chemotherapy. Indian J Otolaryngol Head Neck Surg. 77(6):2352-62, 2025
2. Gopinath Thilak PS et al: Correlation between radiological, macroscopic and microscopic depth of invasion in oral squamous cell carcinoma: a prospective study using contrast-enhanced computed tomography. Oral Oncol. 161:107159, 2025
3. Mukaigawa T et al: Subtraction CT improves detectability of mandibular bone invasion in oral squamous cell carcinoma. Laryngoscope. 135(5):1706-14, 2025

KEY FACTS

TERMINOLOGY

- Retromolar trigone (RMT) squamous cell carcinoma (SCCa)
- RMT has complex shape: Mucosa over mandibular body & ramus posterior to molars, ascends to maxillary tuberosity

IMAGING

- RMT contiguous with anterior tonsillar pillar, buccal mucosa, & alveolar ridge mucosa
  - SCCa primary site may be difficult to determine
- CECT: Variably enhancing mass; may be occult if small
  - Look for asymmetry of fat planes
  - Puffed-cheek technique may improve visualization of mucosal surface tumor in RMT
  - Contrast-enhanced dual-energy CT (DECT)/spectral detector CT (SDCT) may increase conspicuity
  - Dental amalgam artifact may obscure primary tumor or tumor spreading via pterygomandibular raphe
- MR: Allows most accurate delineation of primary tumor, marrow infiltration, perineural & perifascial tumor
  - Look for subtle mandibular invasion by tumor on T1WI
- SCCa reliably FDG avid on PET/CT & PET/MR

TOP DIFFERENTIAL DIAGNOSES

- Masticator space abscess
- Buccal mucosa SCCa
- Oral minor salivary gland malignancy

CLINICAL ISSUES

- Tumor often indolent with late presentation
- Bone/masticator muscle involvement → pain, trismus
  - Both indicate T4 disease; poorest prognosis
  - **Imaging key for determination of T4 disease**

DIAGNOSTIC CHECKLIST

- RMT site results in complex tumor spread patterns
  - Buccal & masticator spaces, oral cavity, & oropharynx
  - Mandible, maxilla, inferior alveolar nerve
  - Via **pterygomandibular raphe** to pterygoid plate
- Must evaluate for all potential spread sites

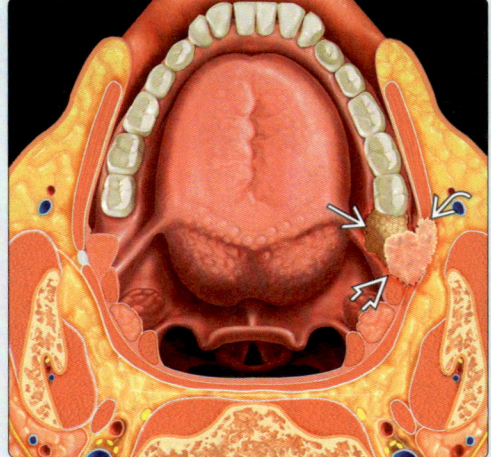
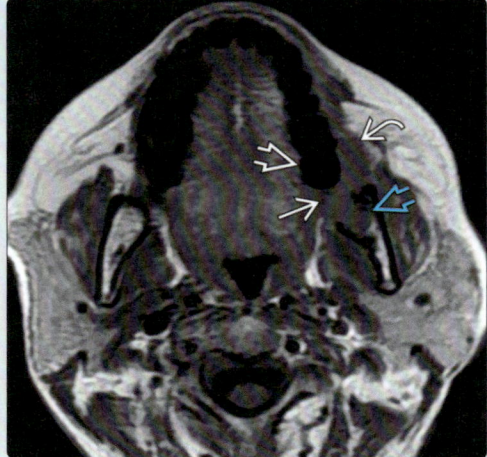

(Left) Graphic illustrates SCCa ➡ arising posterior to the 3rd molar & extending superiorly along the pterygomandibular raphe & laterally onto the buccinator ➡. Tumor encroaches on the anterior tonsillar pillar ➡ of the oropharynx. (Right) Axial T1 MR of the retromolar trigone (RMT) SCCa shows an infiltrating, intermediate-signal mass ➡ centered posterior to the molars ➡. Laterally, the mass invades the buccinator ➡. Note involvement of the mandible ➡ with loss of marrow signal, making this a T4 lesion.

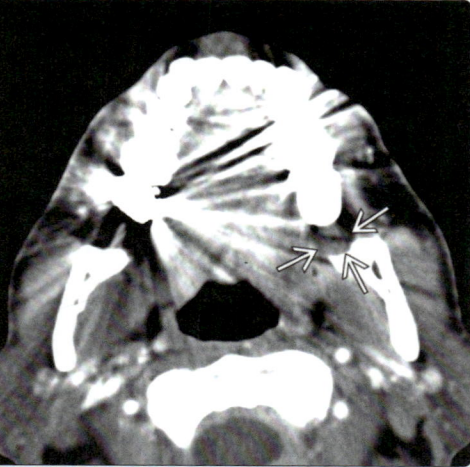
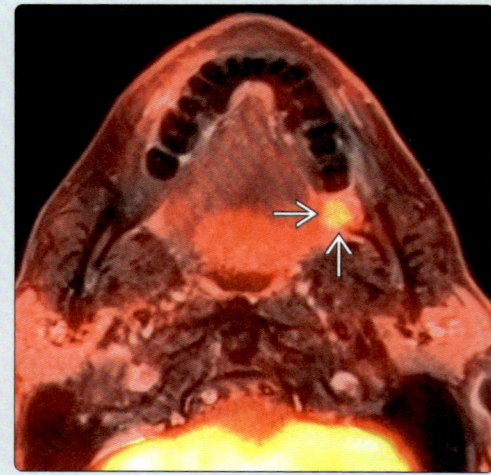

(Left) Axial CECT highlights important pitfalls of imaging RMT SCCa: Lesions are often subtle, & streak artifact from dental amalgam may obscure disease! In this case, the RMT is subtly replaced by soft tissue ➡, which is markedly obscured by streak artifact. (Right) Axial F-18 FDG PET/MR fused to T1 C+ FS MR in the same patient shows the left RMT SCCa ➡ to be FDG avid. The RMT is reliably FDG avid, & MR is much less affected by artifact from dental amalgam, making PET/MR a useful tool for imaging of oral cavity cancer.

Retromolar Trigone Squamous Cell Carcinoma

TERMINOLOGY

Abbreviations
- Retromolar trigone (RMT) squamous cell carcinoma (SCCa)

Definitions
- Oral cavity mucosal malignancy
- RMT: Mucosa overlying ascending ramus of mandible posterior to molars, superior extent to maxillary tuberosity

IMAGING

General Features
- Best diagnostic clue
  - Enhancing mass at RMT ± mandible or maxilla invasion
- Location
  - Mandibular angle, posterior to molars
  - RMT contiguous with anterior tonsillar pillar, buccal mucosa, & alveolar ridge mucosa, so primary site may be difficult to determine
- Size
  - Variable: Tiny lesion to large, infiltrating mass

CT Findings
- CECT
  - Variably enhancing, infiltrative mass
    - May be extremely subtle on CECT; look for asymmetry of fat planes & use MPRs
- Bone CT
  - Important for cortical disruption, marrow infiltration

MR Findings
- T1WI
  - Isointense to muscle; look for loss of marrow intensity
- T2WI
  - Hyperintense as compared to muscle
- T1WI C+ FS
  - Mild to moderately enhancing, infiltrating mass
  - Evaluate for perineural tumor if mandible invaded

Nuclear Medicine Findings
- PET/CT
  - SCCa reliably FDG avid
  - Increasing role of PET/MR; less dental amalgam artifact

Imaging Recommendations
- Best imaging tool
  - MR gives best delineation of tumor extent, marrow infiltration, perineural tumor
    - Small lesion may be occult on CECT
    - MR less affected by dental amalgam artifact
- Protocol advice
  - CECT with coronal reconstructions in bone & soft tissue algorithm
  - Puffed-cheek CT technique may improve visualization of mucosal space tumor in RMT
  - Consider contrast-enhanced dual-energy CT/spectral detector CT (low mono-keV) to increase SCCa conspicuity

DIFFERENTIAL DIAGNOSIS

Masticator Space Abscess
- Heterogeneous enhancement, cellulitis

Buccal Mucosa Squamous Cell Carcinoma
- Lesion arising from inner surface cheeks or lips

Oral Minor Salivary Gland Malignancy
- Often more focal mass but has perineural spread

PATHOLOGY

Staging, Grading, & Classification
- American Joint Committee on Cancer 8th Edition (2017)
  - **T1**: Tumor ≤ 2 cm, ≤ 5 mm depth of invasion (DOI)
  - **T2**: Tumor ≤ 2 cm with DOI > 5 mm & ≤ 10 mm **or** tumor > 2 cm & ≤ 4 cm with DOI ≤ 10 mm
  - **T3**: Tumor > 4 cm **or** any tumor with DOI > 10 mm but ≤ 20 mm
  - **T4a**: Tumor invades adjacent structures (cortical bone of mandible or maxilla, maxillary sinus, or skin of face), bilateral tongue involvement, **&/or** DOI > 20 mm
  - **T4b**: Tumor invades masticator space, pterygoid plates, skull base, **&/or** encases internal carotid artery
- Clinical mucosal extent more accurate than imaging
- **Imaging key for determination of T4 disease**

CLINICAL ISSUES

Presentation
- Most common signs/symptoms
  - Often indolent: Late presentation, high T category
  - Bone/masticator muscle involvement → pain, trismus
  - Trismus can limit clinical assessment & imaging is key

Demographics
- Age: Mean: 67 years
- Epidemiology: 7% of oral cavity tumors

Natural History & Prognosis
- Site of RMT allows for **unique tumor spread patterns**
  - Anterolaterally to buccinator muscle & cheek
  - Posterolaterally to buccal fat & masticator space
  - Posteromedially to tongue
  - Posteriorly to anterior tonsillar pillar & oropharynx
  - Superiorly to maxilla via **pterygomandibular raphe**
  - Inferiorly into mandible ± inferior alveolar nerve
- Poor prognosis if bone or masticator space invasion
- 30% have nodal metastasis at diagnosis
- **Overall 5-year survival ~ 60%**

Treatment
- Typically surgical resection ± adjuvant radiation
  - Surgery + radiation = best 5-year survival

DIAGNOSTIC CHECKLIST

Reporting Tips
- Tumor has **complex potential spread patterns**; scrutinize imaging for tumor spread!

SELECTED REFERENCES

1. Lam V et al: Oral cavity cancer and its pre-treatment radiological evaluation: a pictorial overview. Eur J Radiol. ePub, 2024
2. Yao Q et al: Clinical characteristics and prognosis of patients with primary squamous cell carcinoma of the retromolar trigone: a SEER-based analysis. J Stomatol Oral Maxillofac Surg. 125(2):101675, 2024

KEY FACTS

TERMINOLOGY

- Buccal mucosa squamous cell carcinoma (SCCa)
- Oral cavity mucosal malignancy arising from inner lining of cheek and lips

IMAGING

- Typically difficult to identify with routine imaging
- Mild to moderately enhancing, irregular lesion
- Look for asymmetrically infiltrated buccal fat
- CECT: Puffed-cheek method works well to separate mucosal surfaces and see site of origin
  - Dual-energy CT (DECT)/spectral-detector CT (SDCT) may increase conspicuity
- MR: Hypointense gauze padding works similarly and often better tolerated with long MR sequences
- FDG avid (reserved for advanced nodal disease)
  - Nodes are important prognostic factor

TOP DIFFERENTIAL DIAGNOSES

- Oral cavity infection; oral cavity minor salivary gland malignancy

PATHOLOGY

- Traditionally poorest prognosis of oral cavity SCCa
- Strong association with tobacco, alcohol, betel nut, paan
- **All oral cavity tumors use same TNM classification**
- Imaging important for deep/buccal extent and T4 features
  - T4a: Tumor invades skin of face, through cortical bone, into extrinsic tongue muscles
  - T4b: Tumor invades masticator space, pterygoid plates, skull base, or encases carotid

DIAGNOSTIC CHECKLIST

- Clinical history indicating site of lesion important
- Look for infiltration of buccal space fat
  - If present, evaluate for masticator space infiltration
- 1st-order node drainage: Buccal and level I, II nodes

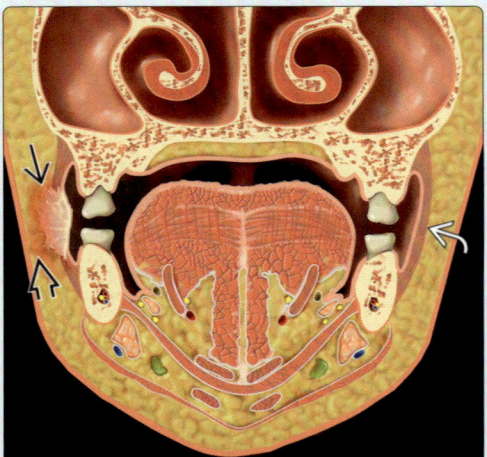
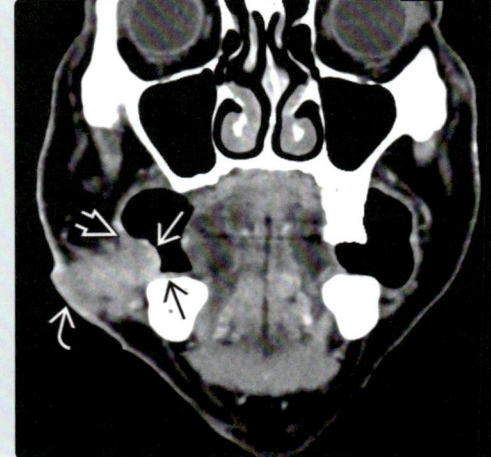

(Left) Coronal graphic depicts a T2 (2- to 4-cm size) buccal mucosal squamous cell carcinoma (SCCa) ➡ that has invaded underlying buccinator muscle and subcutaneous fat ➡. If the lesion had involved the cheek skin, it would be staged as T4. Note normal left buccinator ➡. (Right) Coronal CECT with the puffed-cheek technique shows a mass of the right lower buccal mucosa ➡ involving the mandibular gingiva ➡. There is extension through the buccinator muscle ➡ and subcutaneous fat to the skin ➡, compatible with a T4a lesion.

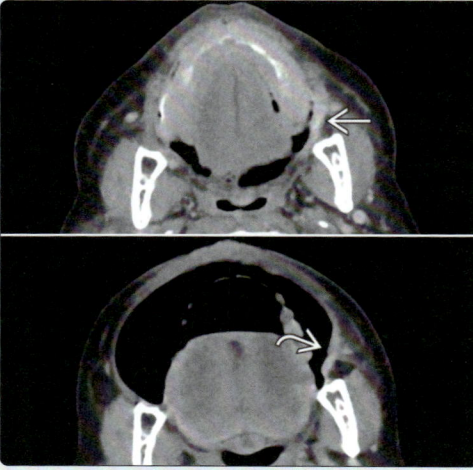
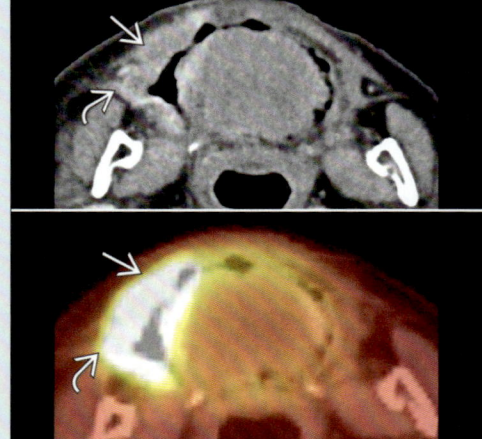

(Left) Axial CECT images without (above) and with (below) the puffed-cheek method show soft tissue thickening of the left posterior buccal mucosa ➡, compatible with buccal mucosa SCCa. The puffed-cheek method increases conspicuity of the lesion ➡. (Right) Axial CECT (above) and PET/CT (below) in a patient with a large right buccal mucosa SCCa shows there is a hypermetabolic mass that invades superficial musculoaponeurotic system ➡ and parotid duct papilla ➡. The mass infiltrates the right buccal space.

TERMINOLOGY

Abbreviations

- Buccal mucosa squamous cell carcinoma (SCCa)

Definitions

- Mucosal malignancy arising from inner lining of cheek, lips

IMAGING

General Features

- Best diagnostic clue
  - May be very subtle, even when infiltrating buccal fat
- Location
  - Most often inner aspect of cheek
- Size
  - Variable: Several millimeters to several centimeters

CT Findings

- CECT
  - Often extremely difficult to see on routine imaging
  - Look for subtle asymmetry of buccal fat
  - Mild to moderately enhancing, irregular lesion
  - Dual-energy CT (DECT)/spectral-detector CT (SDCT) may increase conspicuity

MR Findings

- Hard to see primary lesion without clinical history
  - Isointense on T1, slightly hyperintense T2
  - Look for infiltration of buccal fat
- Variable enhancement: Mild to moderate

Nuclear Medicine Findings

- PET/CT
  - SCCa reliably FDG avid
  - PET/MR may be useful given improved tissue contrast resolution compared to PET/CT

Imaging Recommendations

- Best imaging tool
  - MR generally preferred in oral cavity with better tissue contrast for delineation of tumor extent
- Protocol advice
  - CECT: Soft tissue and bone algorithm in 2 planes
    - **Puffed-cheek method** works well to separate opposed mucosal surfaces
  - MR: Puffed-cheek method not often successful because of sequence time
    - Consider use of **gauze padding** in cheek instead

DIFFERENTIAL DIAGNOSIS

Oral Cavity Infection

- Superinfected traumatic ulcer may result in local inflammation ± cellulitis
- May have reactive buccal adenopathy

Oral Cavity Minor Salivary Gland Malignancy

- Uncommonly arises from buccal mucosa
- Indistinguishable from SCCa on imaging

PATHOLOGY

General Features

- Etiology
  - Strongly associated with tobacco (smoking and chewing) use, alcohol abuse, chewing betel nuts, and paan

Staging, Grading, & Classification

- American Joint Committee on Cancer (AJCC) 8th Edition (2017)
  - T1: Tumor ≤ 2 cm, ≤ 5 mm depth of invasion (DOI)
  - T2: Tumor ≤ 2 cm with DOI > 5 mm and ≤ 10 mm **or** tumor > 2 cm and ≤ 4 cm with DOI ≤ 10 mm
  - T3: Tumor > 4 cm **or** any tumor with DOI > 10 mm but ≤ 20 mm
  - T4a: Tumor invades adjacent structures (e.g., cortical bone of mandible or maxilla, maxillary sinus, or skin of face), bilateral tongue involvement, &/or DOI > 20 mm
  - T4b: Tumor invades masticator space, pterygoid plates, skull base, &/or encases carotid
- **Nodal staging**: Follows AJCC oropharyngeal [p16(-)] node category
- **Metastatic disease**: Absent = M0, present = M1

CLINICAL ISSUES

Presentation

- Most common signs/symptoms
  - Mild discomfort; may "catch" in teeth

Demographics

- Epidemiology
  - In North America, represents 10% of oral malignancies
  - In Taiwan, represents up to 37% (betel nut and paan)
- Age: Mean: 50-70 years
- Sex: M > F

Natural History & Prognosis

- Tendency for submucosal spread, then laterally to skin
- Poor prognosis due to high recurrence rate, invasive spread
  - Overall prognosis: Up to 60% 5-year survival
- Poor prognostic factors: Positive surgical margin, **cervical nodal metastasis (especially if extracapsular spread)**, advanced tumor stage, tumor thickness > 7 mm

Treatment

- Surgical: Resection ± reconstruction ± nodal dissection
- ± adjuvant radiation

DIAGNOSTIC CHECKLIST

Image Interpretation Pearls

- Clinical history indicating site of lesion important
- Look for infiltration of buccal fat
  - If present, evaluate for masticator space infiltration
- Look for buccal and level I, II nodes
  - Level III and IV nodal metastases less common, but not rare

SELECTED REFERENCES

1. De Berardinis R et al: Compartmental surgery for squamous cell carcinoma of the buccal mucosa: description of a new surgical technique. World J Surg Oncol. 23(1):84, 2025

Hard Palate Squamous Cell Carcinoma

TERMINOLOGY

- Hard palate squamous cell carcinoma (SCCa)
- Oral cavity mucosal malignancy of roof of mouth

IMAGING

- Often extremely subtle; may be occult to imaging
- Variable size from several mm to several cm
- **Coronal plane** imaging is **key** for either CT or MR
- CECT: Mild to moderately enhancing soft tissue lesion ± associated bone erosion
- MR: Low T1 tumor signal contrasts against hyperintense palate marrow & mucosa
  - T1 C+ FS & T2 FS aid tumor delineation
  - Look at **greater palatine canal** & **pterygopalatine fossa** for CNV2 perineural tumor (PNT)

TOP DIFFERENTIAL DIAGNOSES

- Hard palate minor salivary gland carcinoma
- Palate pleomorphic adenoma

- Invasive sinonasal SCCa

CLINICAL ISSUES

- Ulcer ± mass on roof of mouth; often painful
- Clinically obvious lesion may be subtle on CT or MR
- Rare tumor; least common oral cavity site
- In this location, SCCa is less common than minor salivary malignancies
- Overall 5-year survival ~ 60%
- Treatment: Surgical resection ± neck dissection ± XRT
  - Elective neck dissection associated with lower recurrence rate, better overall survival

DIAGNOSTIC CHECKLIST

- Must evaluate bone for erosion ± infiltration
- Assess involvement of nasal cavity/maxillary sinus
- MR better evaluates **greater palatine canal** & **pterygopalatine fossa** for CNV2 PNT
- Evaluate carefully for nodal metastases

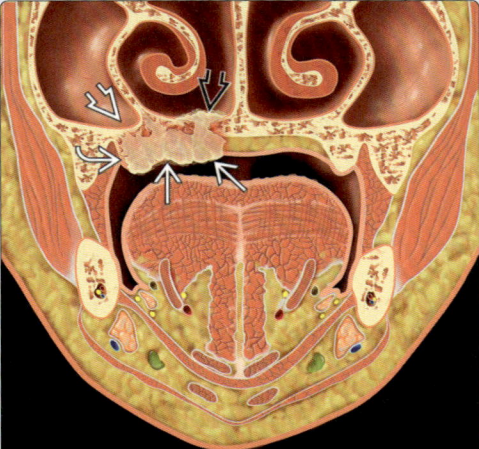
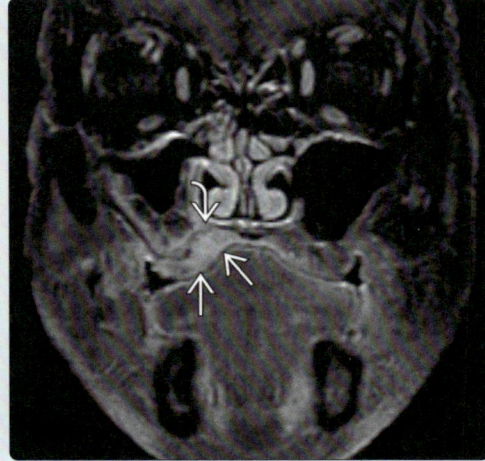

(Left) Coronal graphic shows an oral cavity SCCa ➡ arising from the hard palate mucosa with bone invasion. Tumor may extend through the palatine portion of the maxilla ➡ to the floor of the nasal cavity, through alveolar bone ➡, or into maxillary sinus ➡. Perineural tumor spread may occur along CNV2 branches. (Right) Coronal T1 C+ FS MR of a hard palate SCCa shows an enhancing mass ➡ that extends laterally toward the maxillary alveolus. Thinning of the subjacent cortex ➡ is suspicious for erosion, necessitating CT evaluation.

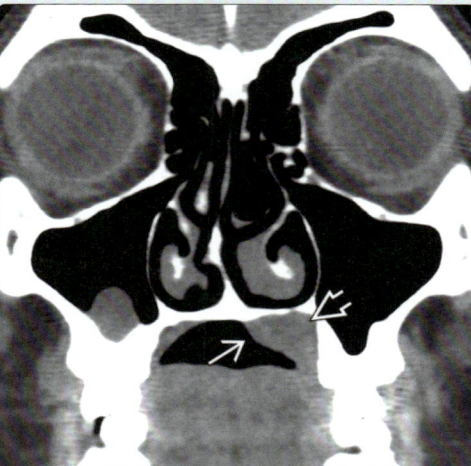
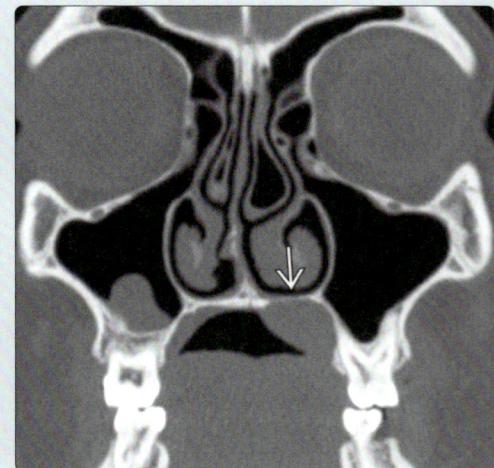

(Left) Coronal NECT (soft tissue window) in a patient with hard palate SCCa shows a mass ➡ centered along left hard palate, which reaches up to midline. Note asymmetric effacement of submucosal fat ➡ on the left, an important clue signifying an invasive mass. (Right) Coronal CECT (bone window) in the same patient shows associated erosion of the hard palate ➡. There is no extension into the left nasal cavity. It is critical to scrutinize the underlying bone for erosions and extension into the maxillary sinus and nasal cavity.

Hard Palate Squamous Cell Carcinoma

TERMINOLOGY

Abbreviations
- Hard palate squamous cell carcinoma (SCCa)

Definitions
- Oral cavity malignancy arising from mucosa overlying hard palate

IMAGING

General Features
- Location
  - Hard palate (a.k.a. roof of mouth)
- Size
  - Variable: Several millimeters to several centimeters

CT Findings
- CECT
  - Often extremely subtle or occult to imaging
  - Mild to moderate enhancement
- Bone CT
  - Erosion of bone often found

MR Findings
- Low T1 signal contrasts against bright palate marrow
- Mild to moderate enhancement

Imaging Recommendations
- Best imaging tool
  - MR allows evaluation of marrow & perineural tumor spread along palatine canals
- Protocol advice
  - Coronal plane essential for either CT or MR
  - CECT: Obtain soft tissue & bone algorithm

DIFFERENTIAL DIAGNOSIS

Hard Palate Minor Salivary Gland Carcinoma
- Mucoepidermoid & adenoid cystic carcinoma most frequent & much more common than SCCa
- Can have smooth bone erosion or aggressive destruction
- Perineural tumor frequently found

Palate Pleomorphic Adenoma
- Circumscribed, T2-intense, round or ovoid mass
- Typically smooth erosion of bone

Sinonasal SCCa
- Maxillary sinus tumor may extend into palate
- Clinically presents as **submucosal** mass

PATHOLOGY

General Features
- Etiology
  - Associated with tobacco & alcohol abuse, but not as strong association as other oral cavity SCCa sites

Staging, Grading, & Classification
- American Joint Committee on Cancer (AJCC) 2017
- All oral cavity malignancies use same TNM staging
- Tis: Carcinoma in situ
- T1: Tumor ≤ 2 cm, ≤ 5 mm depth of invasion (DOI)
- T2: Tumor ≤ 2 cm with DOI > 5 mm & ≤ 10 mm **or** tumor > 2 cm & ≤ 4 cm with DOI ≤ 10 mm
- T3: Tumor > 4 cm **or** tumor with DOI > 10 mm but ≤ 20 mm
- T4a: Tumor invades adjacent structures (e.g., cortical bone of maxilla, maxillary sinus, or skin of face) &/or DOI > 20 mm
- T4b: Tumor invades masticator space, pterygoid plates, skull base, or encases internal carotid artery
- **Size of mucosal component best evaluated clinically**

Gross Pathologic & Surgical Features
- Red & white well-demarcated areas of induration
- Ulcerated areas indurated, tender upon palpation

Microscopic Features
- Squamous differentiation with intracellular bridges or keratinization, ± keratin pearls
- Further classified by degree of differentiation

CLINICAL ISSUES

Presentation
- Most common signs/symptoms
  - Painful ulcer on roof of mouth
- Other signs/symptoms
  - Bleeding, ill-fitting dentures, loose teeth
  - Facial tingling/pain → **V2 perineural tumor**

Demographics
- Age
  - Mean age: 70 years

Natural History & Prognosis
- Survival strongly correlates with T stage
  - Mean survival: T1 = 8 yr, T4 ~ 4 years
- Nodal metastasis significantly impacts survival
  - **Levels I, II** are 1st-order drainage sites
- Overall 5-year survival: ~ 60%

Treatment
- Surgical resection ± neck dissection ± adjuvant radiation

DIAGNOSTIC CHECKLIST

Consider
- Usually clinically apparent but radiologically subtle

Image Interpretation Pearls
- Coronal plane imaging is key for either CT or MR

Reporting Tips
- Must evaluate bone for erosion &/or infiltration
- MR better evaluates palatine canals for greater palatine nerve (CNV2) perineural tumor
- Evaluate carefully for nodal metastases

SELECTED REFERENCES

1. Mohammadzadeh S et al: Comparing diagnostic performance of PET/CT, MRI, and CT in characterization of cN0 head and neck squamous cell carcinoma: a multicenter study. Radiography (Lond). 31(2):102902, 2025
2. Cheval M et al: Oncological outcomes and prognostic factors of squamous cell carcinoma of the upper gingiva and hard palate: a retrospective study. Eur Arch Otorhinolaryngol. 280(10):4569-76, 2023
3. Baba A et al: Relationships between contrast-enhanced computed tomography features of hard palate cancer and pathological depth of invasion. Oral Surg Oral Med Oral Pathol Oral Radiol. 134(5):649-57, 2022

KEY FACTS

TERMINOLOGY

- Mucosal malignancy of hypopharyngeal subsite
  - 2/3 of all hypopharyngeal squamous cell carcinoma (SCCa) arise in pyriform sinus (PS)

IMAGING

- May present as unknown primary with metastatic nodes
- Or large T3-4 tumor, minimal symptoms, metastatic nodes
- Mild to moderately enhancing, irregular mass
- Arises from apex or anterior, posterior, or lateral wall
- May fill PS &/or circumferentially involve walls
- Note that aryepiglottic (AE) fold SCCa considered supraglottic laryngeal SCCa with different staging
- FDG PET/CECT efficient modality to anatomically stage primary PS mass, nodes, and metastatic disease

TOP DIFFERENTIAL DIAGNOSES

- Vocal cord paralysis
- Supraglottitis

- 3rd branchial cleft cyst or 4th branchial pouch anomaly
  - May have sinus or fistula with PS
- Hypopharyngeal minor salivary gland malignancy

PATHOLOGY

- Strong association with tobacco and alcohol abuse
- All 3 subsites of hypopharynx use same latest American Joint Committee on Cancer (AJCC) 8th edition staging
- Extranodal extension (ENE) added as prognostic variable for regional lymph node metastases in AJCC 8th edition
  - Presence of ENE: ENE(+) in pN2a, pN3b, and cN3b

CLINICAL ISSUES

- Often minimal symptoms: Sore throat, dysphagia, otalgia
- Up to 75% have adenopathy at presentation
- Nodes frequently bilateral (N2c)
- 20-40% develop distant metastases
- Overall 5-year survival: ~ 40%
- 16% have 2nd primary malignancies

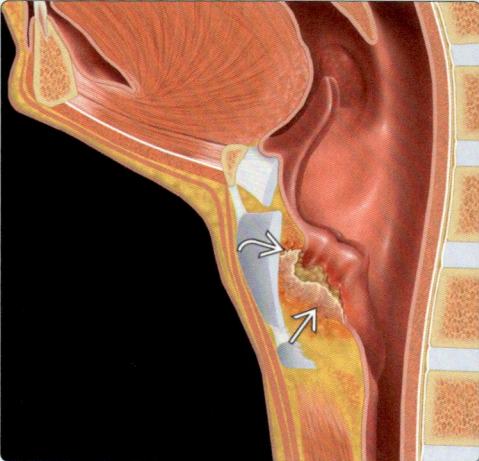
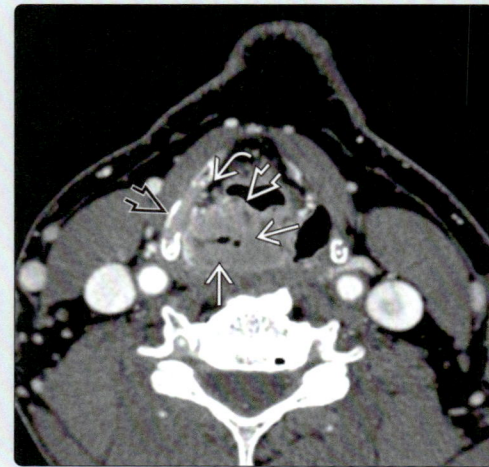

(Left) Lateral graphic illustrates pyriform sinus (PS) squamous cell carcinoma (SCCa) ➡ arising from the anterior wall and extending toward paraglottic fat ➡. Tumor location does not result in airway or swallowing obstruction. (Right) Axial CECT in a 65-year-old man shows a SCCa mass filling the right PS ➡. It involves all walls of PS but does not spread anteriorly to paraglottic fat ➡ or laterally into thyroid cartilage ➡. The right aryepiglottic (AE) fold ➡ is displaced anteriorly, but laryngeal surface is normal.

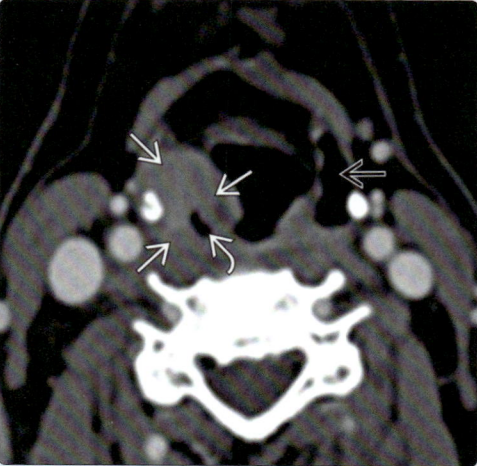
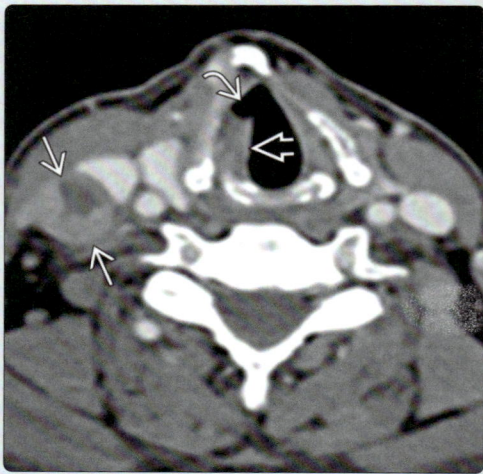

(Left) Axial CECT in a patient with right PS SCCa shows a mildly enhancing mass in the PS walls ➡ with a tiny focus of air in its residual lumen ➡. Note the normal air-filled left PS ➡. (Right) Axial CECT in the same patient shows a right level III necrotic node ➡. Note the medialized right vocal cord ➡ with a dilated right laryngeal ventricle ➡ (sail sign), secondary to right vocal cord paralysis from laryngeal invasion by the right PS SCCa. Inferior tip (apex) of the PS is at the true vocal cord level, and its superior base is at the pharyngoepiglottic fold level.

Pyriform Sinus Squamous Cell Carcinoma

TERMINOLOGY

Abbreviations

- Pyriform sinus (PS) squamous cell carcinoma (SCCa)

Definitions

- Mucosal malignancy of hypopharyngeal subsite

IMAGING

General Features

- Location
  - 1 of 3 subsites of hypopharynx: **P**S, **p**osterior hypopharyngeal wall, **p**ostcricoid region
  - PS: Bilateral anterolateral recesses of hypopharynx
  - Each PS has shape of inverted pyramid with base of pyramid positioned superiorly at level of pharyngoepiglottic fold
    - Inferior tip (PS apex) positioned at level of true cord
  - PS bounded anteromedially by aryepiglottic (AE) fold
    - AE fold separates PS from laryngeal airway
  - PS bounded laterally by lateral pharyngeal wall and inner surface of thyrohyoid membrane (above) and thyroid cartilage (below)
  - PS bounded posteriorly by posterior wall of hypopharynx
- Size
  - Variable: May be small "unknown primary" presenting with adenopathy, or T3-4 tumor with minimal symptoms

CT Findings

- CECT
  - Mild to moderately enhancing, irregular, ulcerative mass
  - May fill PS &/or circumferentially involve walls
  - May arise from apex or anterior, posterior, or lateral wall
    - Apex: Inferior extension can occur to postcricoid region or invade inferiorly to esophageal inlet
      □ If submucosal spread, then occult to clinical exam
    - Anterior: Spread into paraglottic fat of larynx
      □ Can spread into AE fold and laryngeal vestibule
      □ Vocal cord fixation from laryngeal invasion
    - Lateral: Spreads to parapharyngeal tissues (T4a)
      □ May infiltrate through thyrohyoid membrane
      □ Look for thyroid cartilage invasion (T4a)
      □ Look for carotid involvement (T4b), suggested by > 270° encasement
    - Posterior: May invade prevertebral tissues (T4b)
    - Superior extension often occurs to oropharynx
  - Note **AE fold SCCa** considered **supraglottic laryngeal SCCa** with different staging
- Bone CT
  - Look for cartilage erosion, destruction, or sclerosis
    - Sclerosis is sensitive but has poor specificity, as sclerosis alone often represents perichondritis
    - Erosion/destruction more accurate for invasion

MR Findings

- Primary tumor features
  - Low to intermediate T1, intermediate to high T2 signal
  - Heterogeneous gadolinium enhancement
- Cartilage penetration (T4a) on MR
  - Cartilage hyperintensity alone on T2 suggests edema/perichondritis

---

- **Penetration = tumor through cartilage**
  - Cartilage involved if cartilage and tumor signal same in T2 and T1 C+ FS
- Invasion of prevertebral fascia cannot be predicted 100%
  - Intact retropharyngeal fat stripe: Fascia not invaded
  - Loss of fat stripe: Fascia may or may not be invaded
- Adenopathy may be solid or necrotic
  - Look for ill-defined margins suggesting extranodal extension (ENE), a.k.a. extracapsular spread

Nuclear Medicine Findings

- PET/CT
  - Detect unknown PS primary with metastatic nodes

Imaging Recommendations

- Protocol advice
  - CECT: Imaging obtained in quiet respiration; 90-second delay after IV contrast for mucosal enhancement
    - Valsalva or phonation CT as 2nd-pass technique distends PS, which may show exact tumor origin

DIFFERENTIAL DIAGNOSIS

Vocal Cord Paralysis

- Paralyzed side PS dilated, so contralateral PS mimics mass

Supraglottitis

- Inflammatory enlargement of AE folds

3rd Branchial Cleft Cyst/4th Branchial Pouch Anomaly

- PS fistula: From apex of PS to lower neck in younger patient

Hypopharyngeal Minor Salivary Gland Malignancy

- Heterogeneously T2 hyperintense with cystic changes

PATHOLOGY

General Features

- Etiology
  - Strong association with tobacco and alcohol abuse
  - Prior radiation is also risk factor
- Associated abnormalities
  - 2nd primary tumors in 16%
    - 2/3 oral cavity, pharynx, esophagus; 1/3 lung, larynx
    - 2/3 metachronous, 1/3 synchronous

Staging, Grading, & Classification

- All 3 hypopharynx subsites use same latest American Joint Committee on Cancer (AJCC) 8th edition staging
- ENE added as prognostic variable for regional lymph node metastases in AJCC 8th edition
  - Presence of ENE: **ENE(+)** in **pN2a**, **pN3b**, and **cN3b**
  - Absence of ENE: ENE(-) in all other clinical (c) and pathologic (n) nodal stages
- ENE requires unambiguous clinical evidence, such as skin invasion, infiltration of musculature or adjacent tissue leading to fixation or objective dysfunction of cranial nerve, brachial plexus, sympathetic trunk, or phrenic nerve
- Imaging may suggest ENE and support clinical findings but alone is not sufficient to designate ENE

American Joint Committee on Cancer (AJCC) 8th Edition Hypopharynx Cancer Staging

Tumor Stage (T)	Nodal Stage (N)
TX: Primary tumor cannot be assessed	In both clinical (c) and pathologic (P) nodal staging, designation "U" or "L" (above or below lower border of cricoid, respectively) may be used **NX**: Regional lymph nodes cannot be assessed **N0**: No regional lymph node metastasis
Tis: Carcinoma in situ	**cN1/pN1**: Single ipsilateral node ≤ 3 cm in greatest dimension & ENE(-)
T1: 1 subsite &/or ≤ 2 cm in greatest dimension	**cN2a/pN2a**: Single ipsilateral node > 3 cm, ≤ 6 cm, & ENE(-) **pN2a**: Single ipsilateral node ≤ 3 cm & **ENE(+)**
T2: > 1 subsite or adjacent site **or** > 2 & ≤ 4 cm without hemilarynx fixation	**cN2b/pN2b**: Multiple ipsilateral nodes ≤ 6 cm & ENE(-)
T3: > 4 cm **or** fixation of larynx **or** extension to esophagus **mucosa**	**cN2c/pN2c**: Bilateral or contralateral node(s) ≤ 6 cm & ENE(-)
T4a: Moderately advanced local disease: Invades cricoid/thyroid cartilage, hyoid, thyroid gland, central compartment soft tissue, including strap muscles & subcutaneous fat, or esophagus **muscle**	**cN3a/pN3a**: Nodal mass > 6 cm & ENE(-)
T4b: Very advanced local disease: Invades prevertebral fascia, encases carotid, or involves mediastinum	**cN3b**: Any node(s) & clinically overt **ENE(+)** **pN3b**: Single ipsilateral node > 3 cm & **ENE(+)**, or single contralateral node of any size & **ENE(+)**, or multiple ipsilateral, contralateral, or bilateral nodes, any with **ENE(+)**
Distant Metastasis (M): cM0: No metastasis; **cM1**: Distant metastasis **pM1**: Microscopically confirmed distant metastasis	

Midline nodes are considered ipsilateral. Mediastinal nodes are considered regional nodes (level VII). Retropharyngeal nodes should be evaluated, especially if tumor involves posterior wall of hypopharynx. ENE = extranodal extension.

Adapted from Amin MB et al: AJCC Cancer Staging Manual. 8th Ed. Springer, 2017.

- Pathologic classification (pENE) based on microscopic identification of metastatic nodal tumor extending through capsule of lymph node into adjacent tissue

CLINICAL ISSUES

Presentation

- Most common signs/symptoms
  - Sore throat, dysphagia in older adult male smoker/drinker
  - Otalgia as referred pain
    - Internal laryngeal nerve and auricular nerve of CNX to external auditory canal and pinna

Demographics

- Epidemiology
  - 65% of hypopharyngeal SCCa arise in PS
    - 20% postcricoid region, 15% posterior wall

Natural History & Prognosis

- Up to 75% have adenopathy at presentation as rich vascular-lymphatic architecture
  - Most often levels II, III, IV, frequently bilateral (N2c)
- Anterior extension to larynx common
- 20-40% develop distant metastases; lungs > bones and liver
- Overall 5-year survival: ~ 40%
  - Hypopharyngeal has poorest prognosis of head and neck SCCa

Treatment

- Small tumors (T1, some T2): Open or endoscopic partial laryngopharyngectomy or radiation
- Radical radiotherapy can be effective for optimal tumor control in early stage (stage 1 or 2)
- Large tumors: Laryngopharyngectomy ± chemoradiation; however, trend to organ preservation with chemoradiation ± salvage surgery
- T4b tumors typically treated with chemotherapy &/or radiation for palliation

DIAGNOSTIC CHECKLIST

Image Interpretation Pearls

- Small PS apex SCCa may present as unknown primary
- Beware of unilateral collapsed normal PS devoid of air with motion artifacts, secretions, and mucosal enhancement
  - May mimic tumor on imaging, especially MR

Reporting Tips

- Hypopharyngeal SCCa, look for 2nd primary tumor

SELECTED REFERENCES

1. Katano A et al: Early-stage hypopharyngeal squamous cell carcinoma treated with radical radiotherapy at a uniform dose of 70 Gy in 35 fractions: a single-center study. Eur Arch Otorhinolaryngol. 281(8):4401-7, 2024
2. Cho SJ et al: Comparison of diagnostic performance between CT and MRI for detection of cartilage invasion for primary tumor staging in patients with laryngo-hypopharyngeal cancer: a systematic review and meta-analysis. Eur Radiol. 30(7):3803-12, 2020

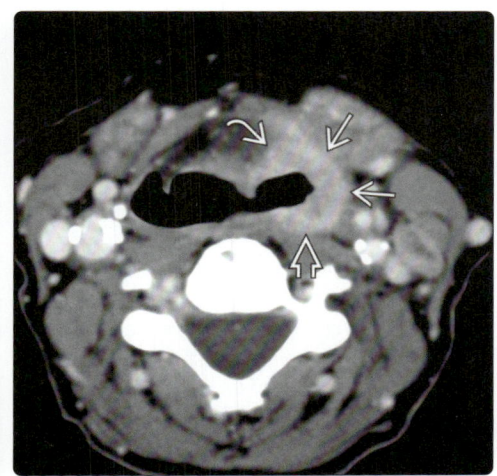

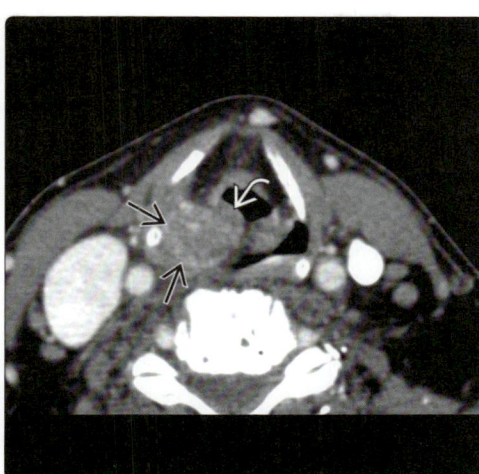

(Left) Axial CECT in a patient with dysphagia and otalgia shows a moderately enhancing SCCa involving all walls of the left PS ➡, extending into the paraglottic & preepiglottic fat ➡. The retropharyngeal fat stripe is lost ➡, which may or may not suggest prevertebral fascia invasion. An intact retropharyngeal fat stripe rules out prevertebral fascia invasion. (Right) Axial CECT shows a right PS SCCa ➡ arising from its lateral and posterior wall, filling the sinus and displacing the AE fold ➡ anteromedially.

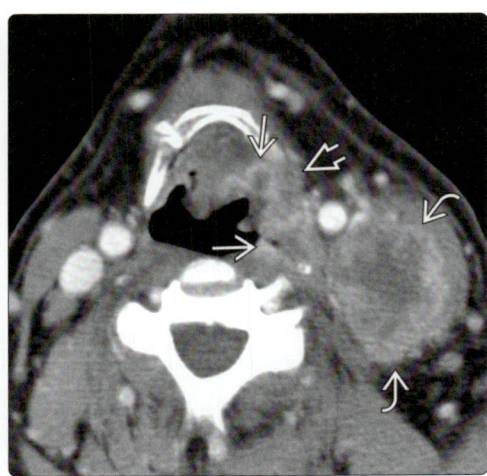

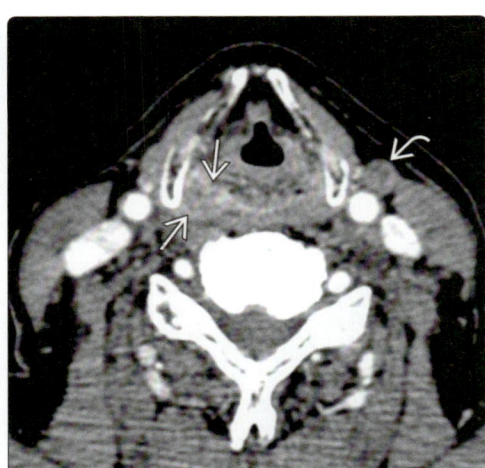

(Left) CECT in a man with irregular, mildly enhancing left PS SCCa ➡ extending up to lateral oropharyngeal wall shows tumor extending through thyrohyoid membrane out to soft tissues ➡. Large ipsilateral metastatic node has extranodal extension (ENE) ➡. ENE was added as prognostic variable in AJCC 8th edition. pN2a, pN3b, and cN3b are ENE(+). (Right) Axial CECT in a man with left level III necrotic lymphadenopathy ➡ reveals a subtle small area of asymmetric enhancement ➡ in right PS apex, proven to be primary SCCa.

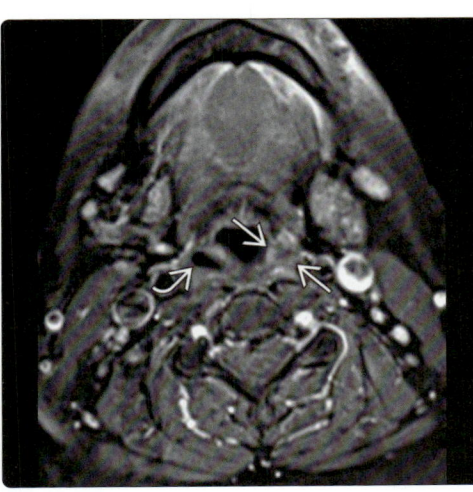

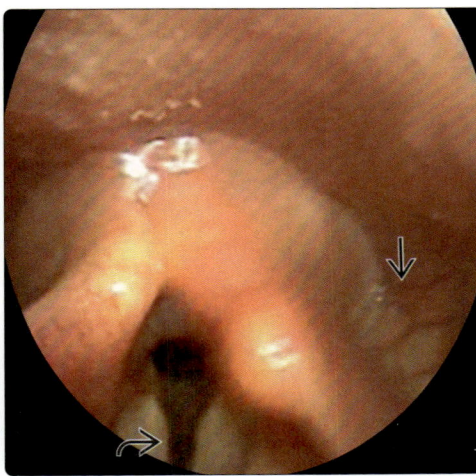

(Left) Axial T1WI C+ FS MR in a 50-year-old woman with throat irritation and blood-stained mucus on coughing shows thickening and enhancement of the left PS ➡, raising the suspicion of PS SCCa. Note the normal right PS with air in its lumen ➡. (Right) Endoscopic view in the same patient shows normal left PS ➡. Note the larynx more anteriorly ➡. MR findings were due to mucosal enhancement of the walls of the unilaterally collapsed left PS, which was devoid of air and had some secretions and motion artifacts.

TERMINOLOGY

- Squamous cell carcinoma (SCCa) arising from hypopharyngeal mucosa located immediately posterior to cricoid cartilage
- Postcricoid region represents 1 of 3 anatomic subsites of hypopharynx that give rise to SCCa: Pyriform sinus (65%), postcricoid (20%), and posterior wall (15%)

IMAGING

- Best clue: CT or MR demonstrates enhancing soft tissue mass in lower hypopharynx posterior to cricoid cartilage
- Axial CECT at cricoid cartilage level shows laminated appearance of multiple tissue layers posterior to cricoid cartilage and anterior to vertebra
  - Normal AP thickness of postcricoid soft tissue < 1 cm
- Metastatic adenopathy common, often bilateral
- Tumor can extend ventrally into larynx, including cartilaginous invasion
- Often spreads submucosally to esophagus

TOP DIFFERENTIAL DIAGNOSES

- Posterior hypopharyngeal wall SCCa

PATHOLOGY

- Strong association with tobacco and alcohol abuse
- Association with Plummer-Vinson syndrome
- Uses same 8th edition American Joint Committee (AJCC) on Cancer TNM staging for all hypopharyngeal carcinoma

CLINICAL ISSUES

- Often presents in advanced stage: T3 or T4
- Postcricoid mucosa normally apposed to posterior wall of hypopharynx mucosa with collapsed lumen in between
  - Makes it very difficult on imaging to distinguish mass arising from these at this location on CT

DIAGNOSTIC CHECKLIST

- Requires critical evaluation of tumor spread into adjacent structures and spaces: Larynx, esophagus, carotid space, and perivertebral space

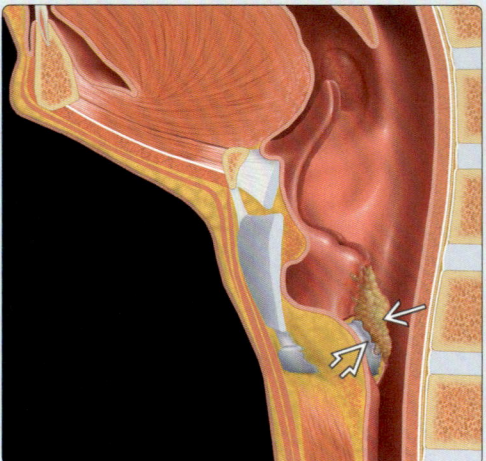
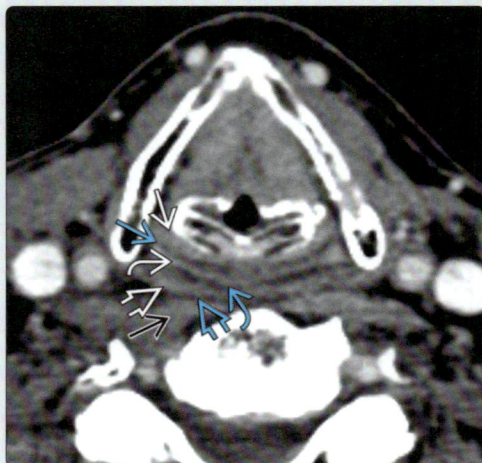

(Left) Lateral graphic of hypopharynx (HP) shows irregular tumor ➡ arising from postcricoid HP (pc-HP) mucosa with cricoid erosion ➡. (Right) Axial CECT shows combined pc-HP (anterior wall) & the posterior wall of HP (pw-HP). Anteroposteriorly lies posterior cricoarytenoid muscles ➡, submucosal fat of pc-HP ➡, combined opposed mucosa of pc-HP & pw-HP ➡ due to collapsed lumen in between, submucosal fat of lower pw-HP ➡, inferior constrictor muscle ➡, retropharyngeal fat stripe ➡, & longus colli muscles ➡.

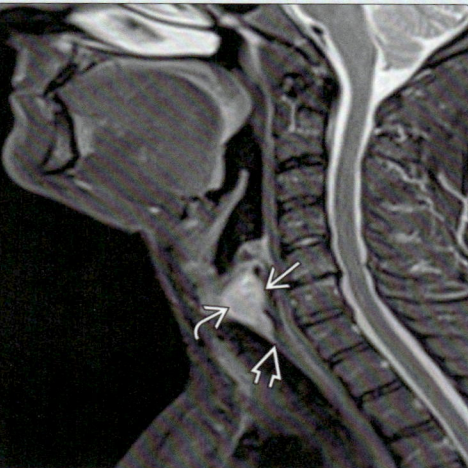
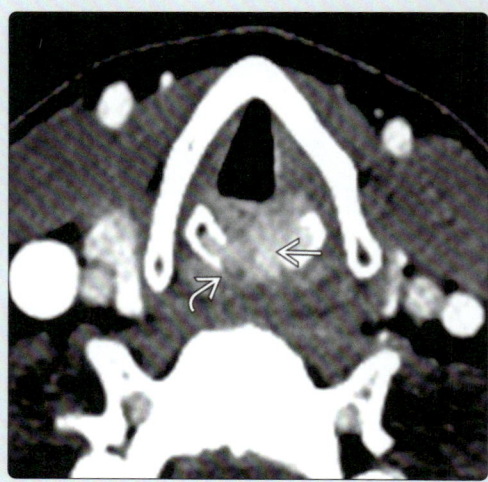

(Left) Sagittal STIR MR in a 55-year-old man shows hyperintense postcricoid SCCa ➡ invading anteriorly into the larynx ➡ & encroaching upon the upper esophagus ➡. (Right) Axial CECT in the same patient shows enhancing tumor straddling the posterior cricoid, protruding into the laryngeal airway & invading the cricoid cartilage ➡. Posteriorly, enhancing tumor can be seen infiltrating the right posterior cricoarytenoid muscle ➡, providing a clue to the postcricoid origin of this SCCa.

TERMINOLOGY

Definitions

- **Postcricoid region of hypopharynx** represents local mucosa and submucosal tissue dorsal to posterior portion of cricoid cartilage; this mucosal surface forms **anterior wall** of lower hypopharynx
  - Mucosa extends superiorly from from level of arytenoid cartilages to inferior margin of cricoid
  - 1 of 3 major subsites of hypopharynx that give rise to squamous cell carcinoma (SCCa): **P**yriform sinus, **p**osterior hypopharyngeal wall, and **p**ostcricoid region

IMAGING

Normal Anatomy of Postcricoid Region and Lower Hypopharynx

- On axial CT and MR at level of cricoid cartilage, normal AP diameter of soft tissue behind cricoid ≤ 1 cm
- ↑ AP thickness: Concern for neoplasm/infiltrative process
- Hypopharynx lumen at level of cricoid typically nondistended and **postcricoid mucosa normally directly apposed to mucosa of posterior wall of hypopharynx**
  - Makes it very difficult on imaging to distinguish mass arising from posterior wall from mass arising from postcricoid mucosa
  - May be necessary to correlate with endoscopic findings

General Features

- Best diagnostic clue
  - Enhancing soft tissue mass in hypopharynx posterior to cricoid cartilage in patient with dysphagia

CT Findings

- CECT
  - Irregular, variably enhancing mass in lower hypopharynx
  - Infiltrates anteriorly to larynx with invasion of cricoid cartilage
  - May spread submucosally toward cervical esophagus
  - Circumferential spread may result in midline soft tissue mass
  - Nodes in 60% at presentation

MR Findings

- T1 isointense to muscle, T2 moderately hyperintense
- Mild to moderate contrast enhancement

Imaging Recommendations

- Best imaging tool
  - CECT often best; patient may not tolerate lengthy MR
  - MR may be helpful for confirming cartilage invasion
- Protocol advice
  - CECT: Imaging obtained in quiet respiration; 90-second delay after IV contrast for mucosal enhancement

Nuclear Medicine Findings

- PET/CT
  - SCCa primary and adenopathy reliably FDG avid

DIFFERENTIAL DIAGNOSIS

Posterior Wall SCCa

- Extension from adjacent hypopharyngeal subsite common

Cervical Esophageal Carcinoma

- Primary upper esophageal neoplasm may spread superiorly to hypopharynx

Pharyngitis/Pharyngeal Edema

- Localized mucosal infection or inflammation
  - Angioedema, radiation-induced mucositis, pharyngitis
- Circumferential, thin, irregular, enhancing mucosa

PATHOLOGY

General Features

- Etiology
  - Strong association with tobacco and alcohol abuse
  - 16% of patients with Plummer-Vinson syndrome develop postcricoid region SCCa

Staging, Grading, & Classification

- Uses same 8th edition American Joint Committee on Cancer TNM staging as for all hypopharyngeal SCCa

CLINICAL ISSUES

Presentation

- Most common signs/symptoms
  - Sore throat, dysphagia
  - Invasion of larynx: Hoarseness, airway obstruction

Demographics

- Typical: Male in 7th decade with history of tobacco or alcohol use

Natural History & Prognosis

- Postcricoid SCCa has tendency for submucosal spread
  - Especially inferiorly to esophagus (T3)
- Often presents late with laryngeal invasion
- 60% nodes at presentation, levels III, IV; often bilateral
- Extranodal extension ↓ disease-free and overall survival
- Hypopharyngeal SCCa has worst prognosis of all H&N SCCa; overall 5-year survival < 40%

Treatment

- Small T1-2: Rare; partial pharyngectomy or radiation
- Larger T2 may be amenable to chemoradiation
- T3, T4a: Laryngopharyngectomy and neck dissection
  - Organ preservation: Chemoradiation is alternative with surgery reserved for salvage laryngopharyngectomy
- T4b: Chemoradiation

DIAGNOSTIC CHECKLIST

Image Interpretation Pearls

- Mass often invades larynx: Look for cricoid invasion
- Imaging useful to evaluate for features that might upstage
  - T3: > 4 cm or esophageal invasion or laryngeal fixation
    - Vocal cord immobility (T3) can be suggested by cord asymmetry on CT/MR, but need endoscopic validation
  - T4a: Cartilage or paralaryngeal invasion
  - T4b: Encase carotid, mediastinal/prevertebral invasion

SELECTED REFERENCES

1. Liao YH et al: The prognostic importance of radiologic extranodal extension in hypopharyngeal carcinoma. Head Neck. 47(2):667-78, 2024

TERMINOLOGY

- Squamous cell carcinoma (SCCa) arising from posterior wall mucosa of hypopharynx (inferior continuation of oropharynx) from hyoid bone to esophageal inlet

IMAGING

- CECT: Irregular, mildly enhancing mass distending lower hypopharynx
- Often, superficial spread superiorly to oropharynx or inferiorly to esophagus
- May invade posteriorly into prevertebral muscles through prevertebral fascia
- SCCa reliably FDG avid
- At level of cricoid cartilage, normal hypopharyngeal soft tissue behind cricoid consists of both postcricoid region (anteriorly) and posterior hypopharyngeal wall (posteriorly)

TOP DIFFERENTIAL DIAGNOSES

- Postcricoid region SCCa (anterior wall)

- Cervical esophageal carcinoma
- Pharyngitis

PATHOLOGY

- Strong association with tobacco and alcohol abuse
- Hypopharyngeal SCCa all use same AJCC TNM staging

CLINICAL ISSUES

- Often asymptomatic until late (stage III-IV)
- ≤ 75% have nodes at diagnosis; often bilateral
- Up to 50% present with neck mass from nodes
- Poor prognosis; overall 5-year survival < 40%

DIAGNOSTIC CHECKLIST

- Commonly spreads superiorly to oropharynx (T2)
- Look for inferior spread to esophagus (T3)
- May infiltrate prevertebral muscles (T4b)
  - Imaging not accurate for predicting invasion
  - Preservation of retropharyngeal fat excludes this
- Carotid encasement or mediastinal invasion (T4b)

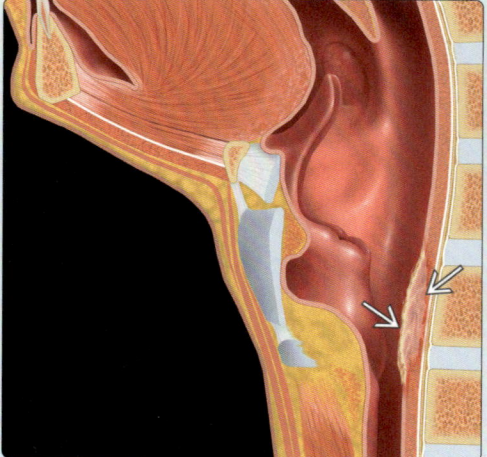
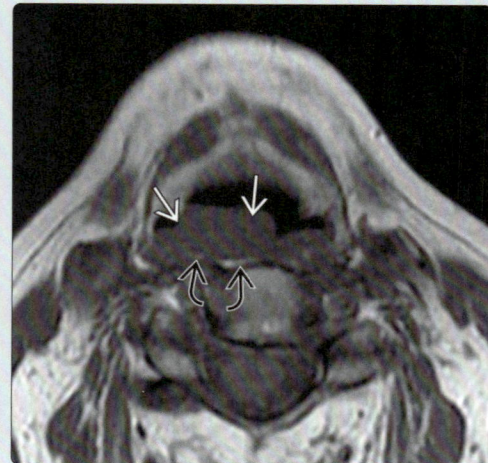

(Left) Lateral graphic illustrates posterior hypopharyngeal wall SCCa ➡. These tumors often spread superiorly to the oropharynx or caudally to the esophagus. Invasion of prevertebral muscles designates T4b. (Right) Axial T1 MR shows posterior hypopharyngeal wall SCCa as a lobulated mass ➡. A retropharyngeal fat stripe ➡ is not clearly defined in its entirety, which may or may not suggest invasion of prevertebral fascia. Intact retropharyngeal fat stripe rules out prevertebral fascia invasion.

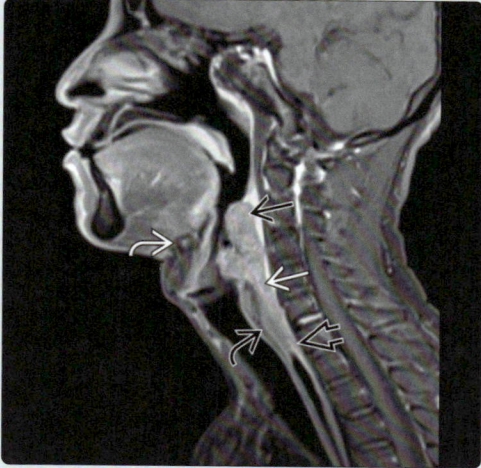
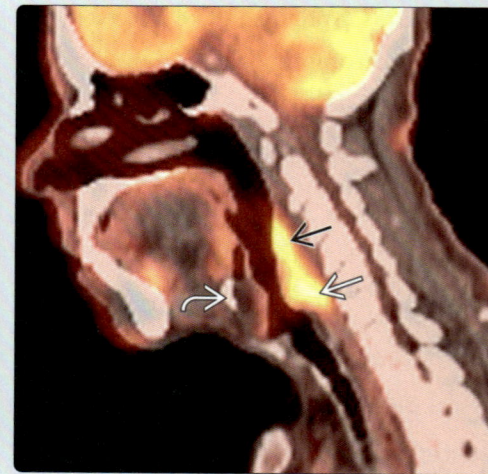

(Left) Sagittal T1 C+ FS MR in a 34-year-old man with enhancing posterior hypopharyngeal wall SCCa ➡ shows extension superiorly into posterior oropharyngeal wall ➡ (above hyoid bone ➡ level) and inferiorly into esophagus ➡. At cricoid cartilage (C6 vertebral) level, the postcricoid region ➡ (anterior wall of hypopharynx) is not invaded by the posterior SCCa. (Right) Sagittal FDG PET/CT shows an FDG-avid SCCa extending from the hypopharyngeal ➡ to the oropharyngeal ➡ (above hyoid ➡) posterior wall.

TERMINOLOGY

Definitions

- Squamous cell carcinoma (SCCa) arising from posterior wall mucosa of hypopharynx (inferior continuation of oropharynx) from hyoid bone to esophageal inlet
  - Subsite of hypopharynx

IMAGING

General Features

- Best diagnostic clue
  - Moderately enhancing posterior hypopharyngeal wall mass, often extending superiorly to oropharynx posterior wall, sometimes inferiorly into esophagus
- Location
  - One of 3 subsites of hypopharynx: **P**yriform sinus, **p**osterior hypopharyngeal wall, **p**ostcricoid region
  - Posterior wall of hypopharynx from level of hyoid/C3 (pharyngoepiglottic fold level) to inferior border of cricoid cartilage/C6 vertebra (cricopharyngeus muscle)
  - Muscular layer of posterior wall of hypopharynx formed by middle and inferior constrictor muscles
  - Note that, at level of cricoid cartilage, hypopharyngeal soft tissue behind cricoid on CT and MR consists of **both p**ostcricoid region (anteriorly) and **p**osterior hypopharyngeal wall (posteriorly)
    - Hypopharynx lumen typically nondistended, and postcricoid mucosa normally directly apposed to mucosa of posterior wall
    - Normal postcricoid soft tissue AP diameter < 1 cm
  - Posterior wall of hypopharynx separated posteriorly from perivertebral space by retropharyngeal space
  - Invasion of prevertebral fascia cannot be predicted 100% on imaging
    - Intact retropharyngeal fat stripe: Fascia not invaded
    - Loss of fat stripe: Fascia may or may not be invaded
    - Paucity of fat in retropharyngeal space in lower neck makes evaluation difficult

CT Findings

- CECT
  - Irregular, mildly enhancing mass distending lower hypopharynx

MR Findings

- T1 isointense to muscle, T2 moderately hyperintense
- Mild to moderate contrast enhancement

Nuclear Medicine Findings

- PET/CT
  - SCCa reliably FDG avid

Imaging Recommendations

- Protocol advice
  - T1 MR best for infiltration of retropharyngeal fat
  - T2 MR helpful for prevertebral muscle invasion

DIFFERENTIAL DIAGNOSIS

Postcricoid Region SCCa

- Arises from **anterior wall** lower hypopharynx

Cervical Esophageal Carcinoma

- Uncommon tumor, may spread superiorly to hypopharynx

Pharyngitis

- Infection/inflammation, often in immunocompromised

PATHOLOGY

General Features

- Etiology
  - Strong association with tobacco and alcohol abuse
  - Association with Plummer-Vinson syndrome

Staging, Grading, & Classification

- Uses same 8th edition American Joint Committee on Cancer TNM staging as for all hypopharyngeal SCCa

CLINICAL ISSUES

Presentation

- Most common signs/symptoms
  - Dysphagia, sore throat
  - Often asymptomatic until late

Demographics

- Age
  - Peak incidence in 7th decade
- Sex
  - M > > F
- Epidemiology
  - Least common hypopharyngeal site (11-15%)
    - Pyriform sinus (65%), postcricoid region (20%)
  - Only 1.6% oropharyngeal SCCa involve posterior wall, 11-15% hypopharyngeal SCCa involve posterior wall

Natural History & Prognosis

- Tendency to present late (stage III-IV)
- ≤ **75%** have **nodal metastases** at diagnosis
- Extranodal extension ↓ disease-free and overall survival
- Nodal drainage often bilateral: Levels III, IV, VI
  - Superior spread to retropharyngeal nodes as well
- Distant metastases develop in 20-40%
- Hypopharyngeal SCCa has poorest prognosis of all H&N SCCa; overall 5-year survival < 40%

Treatment

- Small T1-T2 SCCa: Surgical resection ± radiotherapy (XRT)
- Some T2: ChemoXRT
- T3-T4a: Laryngopharyngectomy ± XRT or organ preservation chemoXRT
- T4b: Palliative chemoXRT

DIAGNOSTIC CHECKLIST

Image Interpretation Pearls

- May infiltrate posteriorly to prevertebral muscles (T4b)
- Look for carotid encasement, mediastinal invasion (T4b)

SELECTED REFERENCES

1. Kovarik PD et al: Squamous cell carcinoma of the posterior pharyngeal wall: a comparative analysis of oropharyngeal origin versus hypopharyngeal origin. J Laryngol Otol. 1-17, 2024
2. Liao YH et al: The prognostic importance of radiologic extranodal extension in hypopharyngeal carcinoma. Head Neck. 47(2):667-78, 2024

KEY FACTS

TERMINOLOGY

- Mucosal squamous cell carcinoma (SCCa) arising in supraglottic (SG) larynx

IMAGING

- CECT: Enhancing mass arising from mucosa of supraglottis subsite: **Epiglottis**, **aryepiglottic fold**, or **false vocal cord**
- Accurate staging requires knowledge of true vocal cord function, clinical & endoscopic finding
- Look for **preepiglottic space** & **paraglottic space** involvement with tumor = T3 disease
- Look for cartilage erosion; describe if inner cortex (T3) or through cartilage (T4)
- Cartilage sclerosis nonspecific, also may be perichondritis from adjacent tumor
- Look carefully for extralaryngeal extension to surrounding soft tissues (T4)
- Supraglottis **rich**, & glottis-subglottis poor **in lymphatics**
  - Nodes frequent; 1st nodal station level II

- Epiglottis SCCa frequently drains bilaterally

TOP DIFFERENTIAL DIAGNOSES

- Laryngocele
- Gastroesophageal reflux
- Rheumatoid larynx
- Laryngeal sarcoidosis
- Laryngeal adenoid cystic carcinoma

CLINICAL ISSUES

- Sore throat, dysphagia, referred ear pain
- May present with metastatic nodes as neck mass
- Typical patient > 50-year-old man with history of tobacco & alcohol abuse
- Overall 5-year survival rate 46%: Localized cancer 61%, regional cancer 47%, distant cancer 30%

DIAGNOSTIC CHECKLIST

- Always search for 2nd primary in patient with tobacco/alcohol history

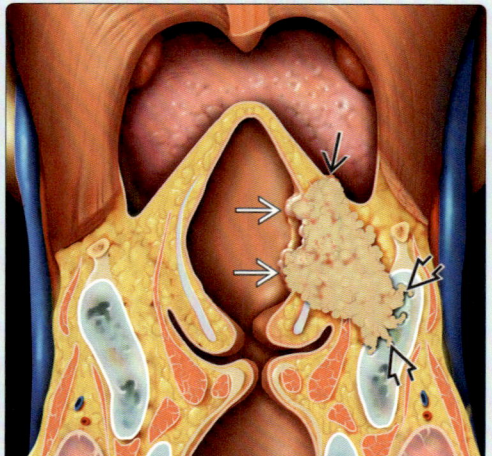
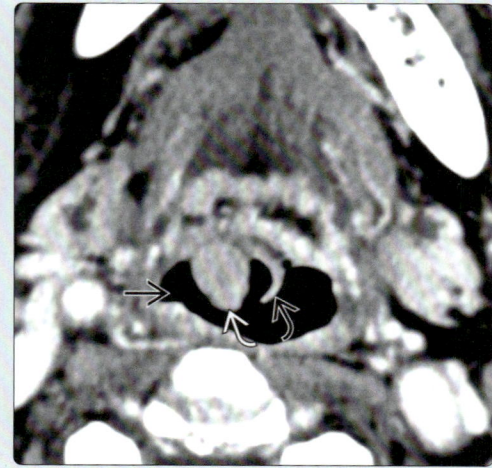

(Left) Coronal graphic shows T3 supraglottic squamous cell carcinoma (SG-SCCa) involving the left false vocal cord (FVC) and aryepiglottic (AE) fold ⟹ with thyroid cartilage invasion ⟹. Only the mucosal portion ⟹ of the tumor is visible on endoscopy. Submucosal extent and cartilage invasion, which are only seen on imaging, are key to staging. (Right) Axial CECT shows an SG-SCCa arising from the right AE fold ⟹. Note the normal left AE fold ⟹. The right pyriform sinus ⟹, which is a subsite of hypopharynx posterolateral to AE fold, is spared.

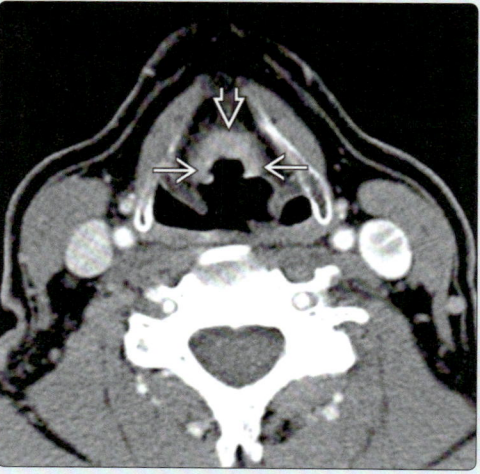
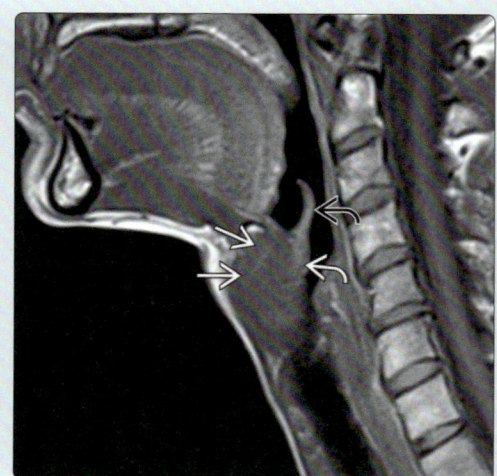

(Left) Axial CECT shows small epiglottic mass ⟹, staged as T3 due to preepiglottic space (PES) invasion ⟹. Mass is symmetric, making it hard to appreciate; however, epiglottis should never be this thick or enhancing. No nodes are evident, but search must be bilateral, especially with epiglottic tumors. (Right) Sagittal T1 MR in a patient with SG-SCCa filling the PES ⟹ shows fixed infrahyoid epiglottis ⟹ is involved, but its suprahyoid free margin ⟹ is spared. Sagittal MR or CECT reformation is best to show PES fat involvement.

TERMINOLOGY

Definitions

- Squamous cell carcinoma (SCCa) from mucosa of any part of supraglottic (SG) larynx
  - SG subsites: **Epiglottis, aryepiglottic (AE) folds, & false vocal cords** (FVCs/vestibular folds)
  - SG deep spaces: **Preepiglottic space** (PES) & **paraglottic space** (PGS)
    - **PES**: Fat-filled space between hyoid bone anteriorly & epiglottis posteriorly
    - **PGS**: Paired fat-containing spaces lateral/deep to FVC (abundant fat) & true vocal cord (TVC) (thin fat layer)
    - Superiorly, PGS merges with PES

IMAGING

General Features

- Best diagnostic clue
  - Moderately enhancing, infiltrating mass of epiglottis, AE fold, or FVC, often with malignant adenopathy
  - Supraglottis rich in lymphatics, regional adenopathy common in SCCa
  - Involvement of PES & PGS associated with higher incidence of regional nodal spread
- Location
  - Any portion of supraglottic larynx: Epiglottis, AE folds, FVCs
  - **Transglottic** carcinoma: SG-SCCa cross laryngeal ventricle from FVC to involve TVC
    - Or involve glottis & extend to subglottis (> 10 mm below free margin of TVC), or both
  - Transglottic spread generally mucosal, but submucosal spread to same anatomic extent through paraglottic pathway can be considered transglottic
  - SG-SCCa can spread anterosuperiorly to involve vallecula & tongue base, & laterally into pharyngeal wall
- Morphology
  - Moderately enhancing mass invades deep tissues of larynx, including PES ± PGS
  - Advanced tumors: Laryngeal cartilage destruction ± malignant nodes
- Size: Variable, larger than glottic or subglottic SCCa usually

CT Findings

- CECT
  - Moderately enhancing mass involving epiglottis, AE fold, FVC, PES, ± PGS
  - **Epiglottic SCCa**: Mass in leaf-shaped cartilage
    - Lid of larynx with **free** margin (suprahyoid), **fixed** portion (infrahyoid)
    - **Petiole**: "Stem" of leaf, which attaches epiglottis to thyroid lamina via **thyroepiglottic ligament**
    - **Hyoepiglottic ligament**: Attaches epiglottis to hyoid
      - □ **Glossoepiglottic fold**: Midline mucous membrane covering superior aspect of hyoepiglottic ligament
    - **Pharyngoepiglottic fold**: Connects free margin of epiglottis to lateral oropharyngeal wall on either side
    - Epiglottic cartilage naturally **perforated**, poorly resistant to tumor penetration into PES
  - **AE fold SCCa**: Spread to FVC (supraglottis itself) or posterolateral spread to pyriform sinus (hypopharynx)

- AE fold represents superolateral margin of supraglottis (hence sometimes called marginal supraglottis), separating it from pyriform sinus
  - **FVC SCCa**: Deep invasion into PGS should be sought, look for replacement of PGS fat density with tumor
  - **PES** spread → extension to **anterior commissure** & **TVC**
  - **PGS** spread → extension to **TVC** or **thyroid cartilage**
  - TVC or **cricoarytenoid joint** invasion → cord fixation
  - **Extralaryngeal extension** to soft tissues outside larynx
    - Most often over or under thyroid cartilage: Anterosuperiorly through **thyrohyoid membrane** or anteroinferiorly through **cricothyroid membrane**
    - Less often: Directly through thyroid cartilage
- Bone CT
  - Cartilage sclerosis, erosion, or destruction
    - Sclerosis alone sensitive but low specificity for tumor invasion; often perichondritis
    - Erosion &/or lysis most specific

MR Findings

- T2WI
  - Intermediate-intensity soft tissue mass
  - Marked T2-hyperintense cartilage suggests cartilage edema/perichondritis
  - Cartilage signal intensity isointense to tumor suggests invasion
- T1WI C+
  - Homogeneous solid tumor enhancement
  - Cartilage enhancement greater than tumor: Suggests cartilage invasion less likely
  - Cartilage enhancement equal to tumor: Suggests cartilage invasion more likely

Nuclear Medicine Findings

- PET/CT
  - Marked FDG uptake in SCCa tumor & nodes
  - Role for PET mainly for nodes & distant mets with advanced T stage or recurrent tumor

Imaging Recommendations

- Best imaging tool
  - PET/CECT preferred imaging tool in staging SG-SCCa
  - Dual-energy CT: Iodinated overlay images compared to weighted average images to assess cartilage infiltration
  - **MR** adjunctive when questionable **cartilage** invasion
- Protocol advice
  - Fast multidetector CT scanners best to prevent motion artifacts caused by breathing, coughing, & swallowing
  - Axial thin slices around 1 mm with coronal & sagittal reconstructions
  - 2-pass method CECT of larynx: Axial images with scan orientation parallel to vocal cords
    - 1st pass: Skull base to mediastinum, quiet respiration
    - 2nd pass: Hyoid to 2nd tracheal ring, during breath hold, to allow imaging of TVC mobility
    - 2nd pass: Alternatively with e-phonation, details laryngeal ventricle, anterior commissure, AE folds
  - MR larynx best with dedicated surface neck coils in phased-array configuration or with parallel imaging
  - Coronal imaging to evaluate laryngeal ventricle involvement & transglottic spread
  - Sagittal plane best delineates PES invasion

DIFFERENTIAL DIAGNOSIS

Laryngocele

- Laryngocele: Dilated air-/fluid-filled ventricular appendix
- Secondary laryngocele: Glottic or SG-SCCa obstructs laryngeal ventricle

Gastroesophageal Reflux

- Reversible edematous changes of posterior larynx, including AE folds & often TVC

Rheumatoid Larynx

- Cricoarytenoid joint swelling in RA

Laryngeal Sarcoidosis

- Glottic & SG thickening, usually without discrete mass

Laryngeal Adenoid Cystic Carcinoma

- Mimics SG-SCCa but is less likely to invade cartilage

PATHOLOGY

General Features

- Etiology
  - Larynx is divided embryologically into 2 parts
    - **Supraglottis**: **Lymphatic rich**, early lymph node mets
    - Glottis-subglottis: Lymphatic poor, late lymph nodes
- Genetics
  - SG-SCCa: Loss in p23 region of chromosome 8 is independent predictor of poor prognosis
  - HER2/neu (*ERBB2*) oncogene expression & positive nodes associated with distant met

Staging, Grading, & Classification

- American Joint Committee on Cancer (AJCC) 8th edition
- Accurate staging requires knowledge of TVC function & clinical & endoscopic finding
- Tis: Carcinoma in situ
- T1: Tumor in 1 SG subsite, normal TVC mobility
- T2: Mucosal-based tumor in > 1 SG subsite, glottis or region outside supraglottis, without laryngeal fixation
  - Extension to mucosa of base of tongue, vallecula, medial wall of pyriform sinus
- T3: Endolaryngeal tumor with fixed TVC ± invasion of any of PES, PGS, postcricoid hypopharynx, or inner cortex of thyroid cartilage
- T4a: Moderately advanced local disease: Tumor invades through thyroid cartilage ± to other extralaryngeal tissues
  - e.g., trachea, cervical soft tissues, strap muscles, deep extrinsic muscles of tongue, thyroid gland, esophagus
- T4b: Very advanced local disease: Tumor invades prevertebral space, encases carotid artery, or invades mediastinal structures
- Clinical N1 (cN1): Metastasis in single ipsilateral node ≤ 3 cm & no extranodal extension [ENE(-)]
- Clinical N2 (cN2): N2a: Metastasis in single ipsilateral node > 3 cm but not > 6 cm in greatest dimension & ENE(-)
  - cN2b: Metastasis in multiple ipsilateral nodes, none > 6 cm in greatest dimension & ENE(-)
  - cN2c: Metastasis in bilateral or contralateral lymph nodes, none > 6 cm in greatest dimension & ENE(-)
- Clinical N3 (cN3): cN3a: Metastasis in lymph node > 6 cm in greatest dimension & ENE(-)
  - cN3b: Metastasis in any node(s) & clinically overt ENE(+)
- Metastatic (M) staging: M0: No met, M1: Distant met

Gross Pathologic & Surgical Features

- Poorly marginated, ulcerative, indurated mucosal lesion

CLINICAL ISSUES

Presentation

- Most common signs/symptoms
  - Sore throat, dysphagia, referred ear pain
  - Presents late with nodes, as SG itself clinically silent
    - 35% have nodal metastasis at presentation
  - Levels II, III, & IV common; **level II** most common
  - Bilateral & contralateral nodal involvement common
  - Epiglottis, midline structure, frequently drains bilaterally
  - Midline nodes considered ipsilateral
  - Anterior & superior mediastinal nodes (level VII) considered regional nodes in larynx carcinoma
  - Other mediastinal & hilar nodes distant metastasis
- Clinical profile: Male > 50 years with history of alcohol & tobacco use

Demographics

- Epidemiology: SG-SCCa: 35% of all laryngeal SCCa

Natural History & Prognosis

- ENE: Important prognostic variable for regional lymph node mets in AJCC 8th edition
- Distant metastasis in laryngeal cancer 3-8%; lung > bone > liver
- Overall 5-year survival rate 46%: Localized cancer 61%, regional cancer 47%, distant cancer 30%
- Prognosis best for inferiorly located tumors
  - Involves TVC, thus presents early with hoarseness
- 22% of clinically node-negative (cN0) SG-SCCa patients have occult lymph node metastasis
  - Elective neck dissection in cN0 SG-SCCa more likely to avoid adjuvant XRT without impacting overall survival

Treatment

- **T1/T2** (smaller tumors): Laser surgery or XRT only
- **T3**: Some may have laser resection or partial laryngectomy
- **T3/T4a** (larger tumors): XRT & chemotherapy
- **T4a**: Extralaryngeal extension or through thyroid cartilage = total laryngectomy
- **T4b**: Palliative nonsurgical treatment

DIAGNOSTIC CHECKLIST

Image Interpretation Pearls

- Cartilage sclerosis nonspecific: Perichondritis or true cartilage invasion
  - T2 & T1 C+ MR best to confirm cartilage penetration
- SG larynx lymphatic rich → frequent metastatic nodes
- Always search for 2nd primary if alcohol/tobacco history

SELECTED REFERENCES

1. Barry E et al: Addressing the neck: an NCDB study of clinically node-negative supraglottic squamous cell carcinoma. Otolaryngol Head Neck Surg. 171(5):1451-61, 2024

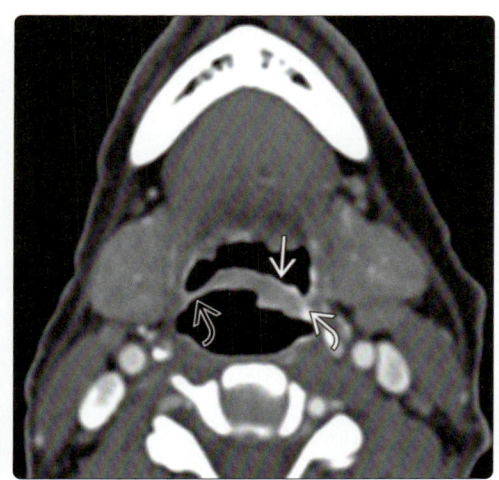

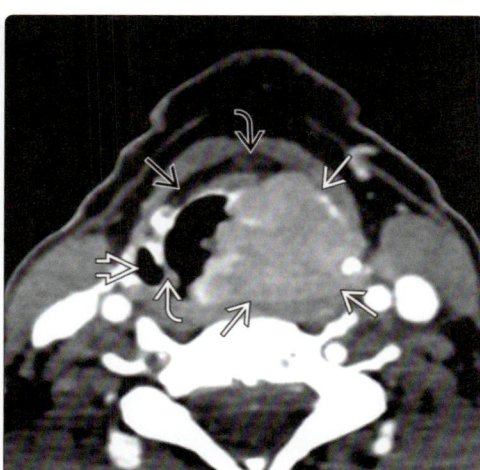

(Left) Axial CECT shows SCCa involving the left side of epiglottis ➡, extending through the thickened pharyngoepiglottic fold into the left lateral pharyngeal wall ➡. Note normal right pharyngoepiglottic fold ➡. (Right) Axial CECT further inferiorly in the same patient shows large SCCa ➡ replacing the region of the left AE fold, filling left side of the laryngeal vestibule and left pyriform sinus. Tumor involves the left paraglottic space (PGS) and left side of PES. Note normal right AE fold ➡, pyriform sinus ➡, PGS ➡, and PES ➡.

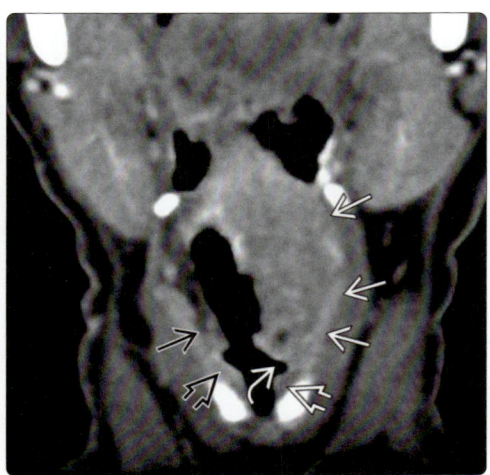

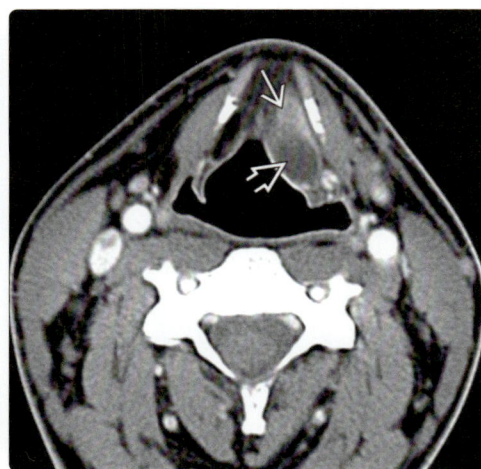

(Left) Coronal CECT reformation in the same patient shows that the enhancing tumor is a transglottic carcinoma, extending from the SG ➡ into the left true vocal cord (TVC) of the glottis ➡, below the laryngeal ventricle ➡. Note normal hypodense right PGS fat ➡ and TVC soft tissue ➡. (Right) Axial CECT shows a mixed-density SG-SCCa distending PGS fat. The nonenhancing mucoid-density portion of the mass ➡ is due to an internal laryngocele from obstruction of laryngeal ventricle by tumor ➡.

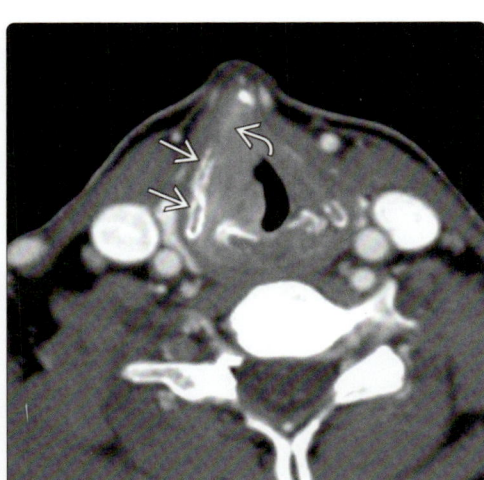

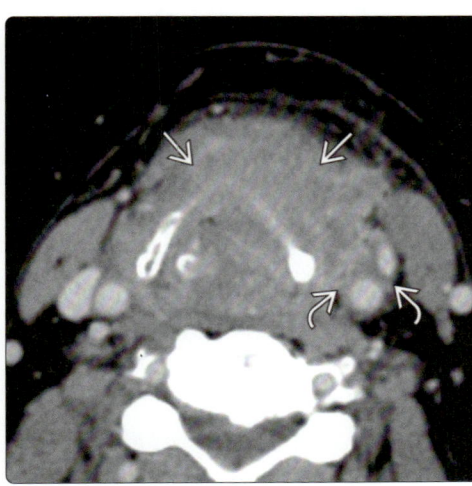

(Left) Axial CECT shows a large right false cord SCCa. Thyroid cartilage is sclerotic ➡, a nonspecific finding that cannot accurately predict cartilage invasion. Tumor penetration ➡ through the inner and outer cortex is present anteriorly. This is a T4a tumor. (Right) Axial CECT shows a large T4a SG-SCCa with complete airway obstruction. The tumor has extended through thyroid cartilage, and bulky extralaryngeal SCCa invades strap muscles ➡. Note the close proximity to the carotid sheath ➡.

KEY FACTS

TERMINOLOGY

- SCCa arising on mucosal surface of glottic larynx
- Vocal cord, anterior & posterior commissures

IMAGING

- Typically, diagnosis known at time of imaging
  - Imaging important to assess supra- or subglottic extension, cartilage invasion, nodes
- CECT/MR findings may be subtle if small tumor
- SCCa typically anterior true vocal cord &/or anterior commissure (> **1-mm** thick **anterior commissure**)
- Supraglottis rich & glottis-subglottis **poor in lymphatics**
  - **Nodal metastasis late** in glottic-subglottic Ca
- CECT: Enhancing infiltrative or exophytic mass
- CECT has fewer motion artifacts than MR; obtain during **quiet respiration** to best assess cords
  - Breath hold will close glottis & cannot assess cords
- MR to assess cartilage invasion if CECT not definitive
- FDG avid on PET; reserved for late-stage tumors

- Transglottic carcinoma: Supraglottic spread across laryngeal ventricle &/or subglottic spread > 1 cm below TVC

TOP DIFFERENTIAL DIAGNOSES

- Gastroesophageal reflux disease
- Laryngeal chondrosarcoma
- Rheumatoid larynx
- Laryngeal adenoid cystic carcinoma

PATHOLOGY

- Keratinizing, well- to moderately differentiated SCCa

CLINICAL ISSUES

- 60% of laryngeal SCCa are glottic tumors
- M >> F; > 50 years; tobacco & alcohol abuse
- Recently ↑ in < 30-year-old nonsmokers: HPV related, F > M
- Often presents early with low T stage because of symptoms of hoarseness or change in voice
- Overall 5-year survival rate: 76%

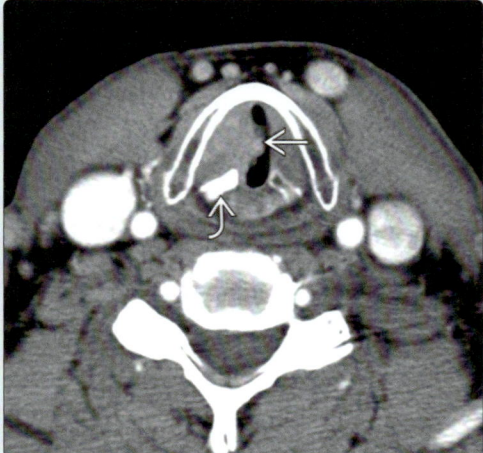
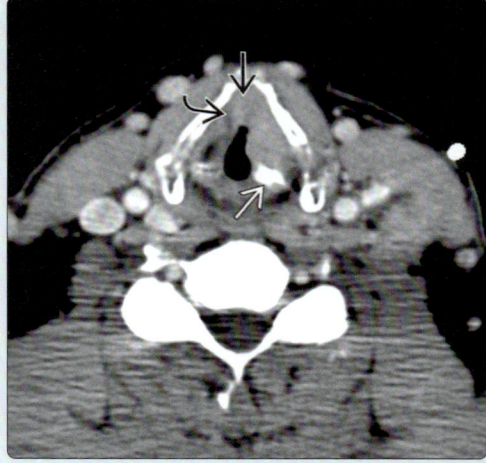

(Left) *Axial CECT shows an enhancing right true vocal cord (TVC) exophytic mass ➡. Anterior & posterior commissures are normal. Right arytenoid cartilage sclerosis ➡ is nonspecific & may be either perichondritis or tumor invasion. Dx was T1a tumor.* (Right) *Axial CECT reveals squamous cell carcinoma (SCCa) involving the entire left TVC, anterior commissure ➡, & anterior 1/3 of the right cord ➡. Left arytenoid ➡ & thyroid cartilages are sclerotic but without destruction or cartilage penetration. This is T1b tumor by imaging.*

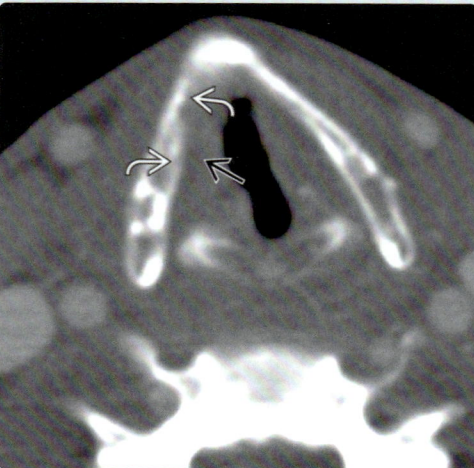
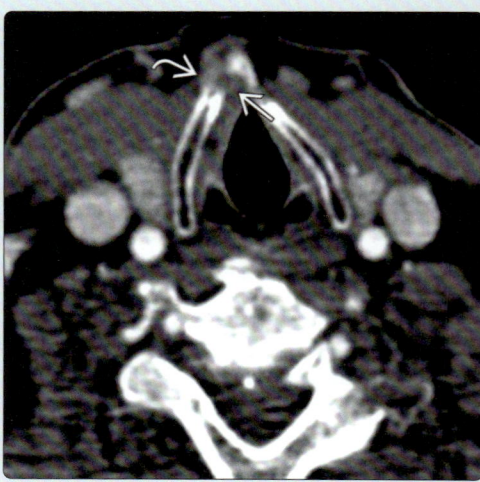

(Left) *Axial CECT shows right vocal cord SCCa ➡ with tumor in the thyroid cartilage eroding through the inner cortex ➡ (but not extending through the outer cortex), upstaging to T3.* (Right) *Axial CECT shows the lower aspect of small glottic-subglottic right vocal cord SCCa ➡ penetrating through the outer cortex of thyroid cartilage ➡ (T4a). Trachea, thyroid gland, esophagus, strap muscles, & deep extrinsic tongue muscle invasion also would be T4a. Mediastinal/prevertebral muscle invasion or carotid encasement would be T4b.*

Glottic Laryngeal Squamous Cell Carcinoma

TERMINOLOGY

Definitions

- SCCa arising on mucosal surface of glottic larynx
  - True vocal cord (TVC), anterior & posterior commissures

IMAGING

General Features

- Location
  - Most often, anterior TVC & anterior commissure
  - Posterior commissure SCCa less common

CT Findings

- CECT
  - Enhancing infiltrative or exophytic TVC mass
  - Imaging findings may be very subtle if small tumor
  - Axial image determined to be at TVC level when
    - Thyroid, arytenoid, cricoid cartilages on same image
    - Thyroarytenoid muscles on image with no fat lateral to muscles (paraglottic fat lies in supraglottic larynx)
    - Apex of pyriform sinus visualized
    - Glottis: 1-cm-thick plane beginning superiorly at level of midpoint of laryngeal ventricles & extending inferiorly through TVCs
  - Metastatic nodes typically late, with large tumor
  - Glottic carcinoma presurgical CT scan depth of invasion (DOI) correlates with perineural invasion, lymphovascular invasion, & nodal metastasis

MR Findings

- T2WI
  - Intermediate-intensity TVC mass
  - Thyroid cartilage invasion likely when T2 signal intensity of cartilage = T2 signal intensity of tumor
- T1WI C+
  - Thyroid cartilage invasion likely when enhancement in cartilage = enhancement in tumor

Nuclear Medicine Findings

- PET
  - Abnormal ↑ FDG uptake by SCCa
  - Note that unilateral TVC uptake may indicate tumor or contralateral TVC paralysis

DIFFERENTIAL DIAGNOSIS

Gastroesophageal Reflux Disease

- Vocal cords edematous with mucosal enhancement

Rheumatoid Larynx

- Cricoarytenoid joint swelling

Laryngeal Chondrosarcoma

- T2-hyperintense submucosal mass of thyroid or cricoid cartilage

Laryngeal Adenoid Cystic Carcinoma

- Typically submucosal & more hyperintense on T2

Laryngeal Sarcoidosis

- Diffusely infiltrative glottic/supraglottic thickening

PATHOLOGY

General Features

- Etiology
  - Tobacco & alcohol abuse in > 50 years
  - Recent ↑ in nonsmokers < 30 years; HPV related, F > M

Staging, Grading, & Classification

- American Joint Committee on Cancer (AJCC) **8th edition**
  - **Tis**: Carcinoma in situ
  - **T1**: Limited to cord(s) or commissures, normal mobility
    - **T1a**: Tumor on 1 cord, **T1b**: Tumor on both cords
  - **T2**: Supra- &/or subglottic spread &/or ↓ cord mobility
  - **T3**: Fixed vocal cord &/or paraglottic space invasion &/or inner thyroid cartilage erosion
  - **T4a**: Moderately advanced: Tumor through outer cortex of thyroid cartilage &/or extralaryngeal extension
    - Involvement of trachea, thyroid gland, esophagus, strap muscles, deep extrinsic tongue muscles
  - **T4b**: Very advanced: Invades prevertebral muscles, encases carotid artery, or invades mediastinal soft tissues

Gross Pathologic & Surgical Features

- **Glottic SCCa spread patterns**
  - Anteromedially to anterior commissure: Worsens prognosis; tendon of anterior commissure may prevent extension to opposite TVC in early stages
  - **Broyle ligament** (BL): Dense connective tissue at insertion of vocal ligaments of TVC to thyroid cartilage
    - Above glottic plane, BL resists glottic Ca invasion
    - Below glottic plane, BL replaced by thin connective tissue layer, & more vulnerable to tumor invasion
    - At BL attachment, thyroid cartilage devoid of perichondrium, & more vulnerable to tumor invasion
  - Posteriorly to arytenoids or cricoid cartilage: Cord fixation with invasion of underlying thyroarytenoid muscle & cricoarytenoid joint
  - Superiorly into supraglottic paraglottic space
  - Inferiorly to subglottis along conus elasticus
    - **Conus elasticus**: Fibroelastic supporting membrane extending from medial margin of TVC (merging with vocal ligament) above to cricoid below
    - Conus elasticus continuous with cricothyroid membrane anteriorly
  - **Transglottic Ca**: Supraglottic spread across laryngeal ventricle &/or subglottic spread > 1 cm below TVC
    - Coronal images best to evaluate transglottic spread
- **Extralaryngeal spread** often anteriorly through cricothyroid ligament
- Supraglottis rich & glottis-subglottis **poor in lymphatics**
  - **Nodal metastasis late** in glottic-subglottic Ca

CLINICAL ISSUES

Presentation

- Most common signs/symptoms
  - Presents early with hoarseness, change in voice

SELECTED REFERENCES

1. Filauro M et al: Depth of invasion assessment in laryngeal glottic carcinoma: a preoperative imaging approach for prognostication. Laryngoscope. 134(7):3230-7, 2024

KEY FACTS

TERMINOLOGY

- Mucosal squamous cell carcinoma (SCCa) originating in subglottic larynx [from inferior aspect of true vocal cord (TVC) to lower border of cricoid cartilage]

IMAGING

- Enhancing mass internal to cricoid ring that fills lumen or invades extralaryngeal tissues
- Local tumor spread patterns
  o May spread superiorly to TVC(s): Transglottic carcinoma
  o Cricoid cartilage invasion common (T4)
- Supraglottis rich & glottis-**subglottis poor in lymphatics**
  o Nodal metastasis late in glottic-subglottic carcinoma
- Nodal spread uncommon (4-21%) except advanced stage
- 50% present as T4 tumor
- Thin-section CECT: Best shows tumor extent
  o Coronal reformats helpful for craniocaudal tumor
- MR: Intermediate T2, enhances with gadolinium
  o If cartilage signal = tumor signal, suggests invasion

- PET/CT: FDG-avid tumor & nodes

TOP DIFFERENTIAL DIAGNOSES

- Larynx trauma
- Larynx adenoid cystic carcinoma
- Larynx chondrosarcoma
- Rheumatoid larynx

CLINICAL ISSUES

- < 5% of laryngeal SCCas are subglottic
- > 50-year-old male smoker &/or drinker
- Stridor, dyspnea, hoarseness if TVC involved
- Subglottic SCCa has long asymptomatic period
- **Subglottic stomal recurrences** common
- Overall 5-year survival rate 52%: Localized cancer 60%, regional cancer 50%, distant cancer 45%

DIAGNOSTIC CHECKLIST

- **Imaging critical**: Clinical & endoscopic staging more difficult than glottic or supraglottic SCCa

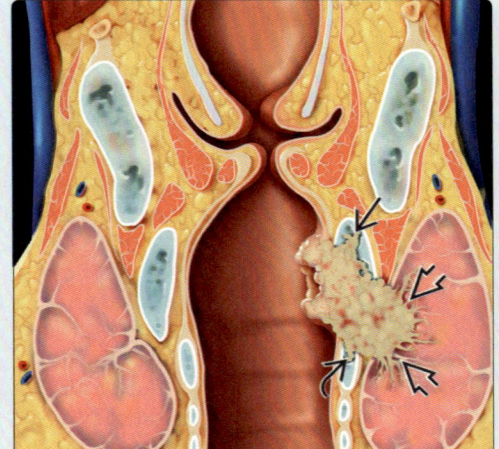
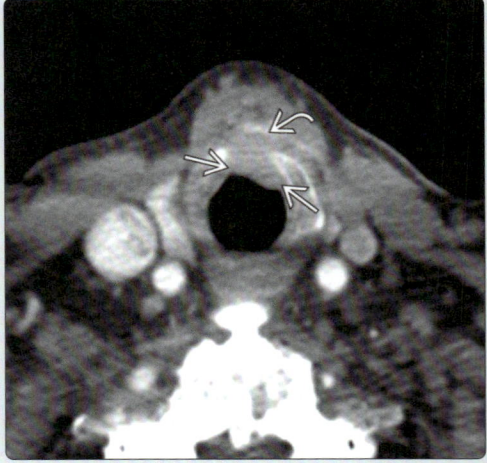

(Left) Coronal graphic depicts left subglottic SCCa tumor invading the cricoid ➡, 1st tracheal ring ➡, and thyroid gland ➡. This is an AJCC stage T4a SCCa tumor. (Right) Axial CECT demonstrates typical subglottic SCCa ➡ in the anterior subglottis. Note midline cricoid cartilage destruction with definite extralaryngeal extension into infrahyoid strap muscles ➡, designating T4a tumor. This is the most common pattern of extension. No soft tissue should be present between the cartilage inner table and airway.

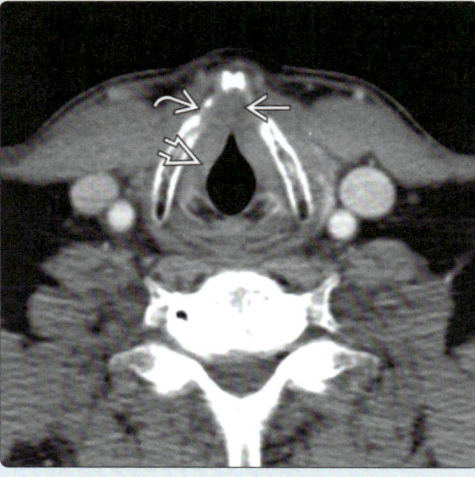
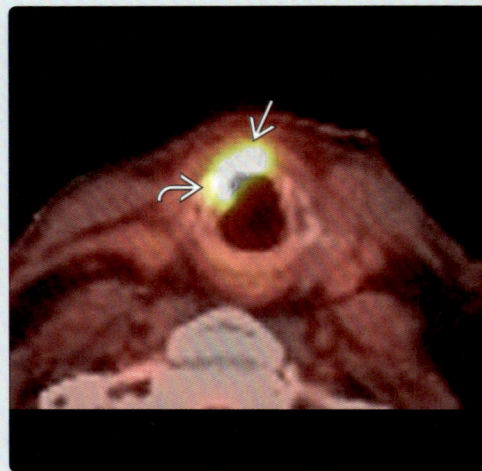

(Left) Axial CECT immediately below the true vocal cord (TVC) ➡ reveals extremely subtle, symmetric, minimally enhancing subglottic SCCa ➡ in the anterior airway. This image is below the TVC, as arytenoid cartilages are not present. There is subtle erosion and sclerosis of right thyroid cartilage ➡. One must know if TVC mobility is normal to stage this tumor. (Right) Axial fused F-18 FDG PET/CT shows a hypermetabolic right anterolateral subglottic SCCa ➡ focally invading the adjacent cricoid cartilage ➡. 50% present as T4 tumor.

Subglottic Laryngeal Squamous Cell Carcinoma

TERMINOLOGY

Definitions

- Subglottic larynx mucosal squamous cell carcinoma (SCCa)
- Subglottic larynx: Inferior aspect of true vocal cord (TVC) to lower border of cricoid cartilage

IMAGING

CT Findings

- CECT
  - Enhancing luminal mass; may spread to TVC
  - **Cricoid cartilage invasion common**
  - Supraglottis rich & glottis-**subglottis poor in lymphatics**
  - Nodal involvement in 4-21%; paratracheal & superior mediastinal nodes most common
    - Can drain to prelaryngeal & delphian nodes
    - Rarely lateral; cervical chain levels III, IV

MR Findings

- T2WI
  - Intermediate signal intensity; if cartilage signal = tumor signal, suggests invasion
- T1WI C+ FS
  - Usually homogeneous enhancement; if cartilage enhancement = tumor enhancement, indicates tumor invasion

Nuclear Medicine Findings

- PET: As with all SCCas, tumor FDG avid

Imaging Recommendations

- Best imaging tool
  - CECT preferred because of motion on MR
  - MR more accurate for detection of cartilage invasion
- Protocol advice
  - Thin-section CECT best shows tumor extent
    - Coronal reformats helpful for craniocaudal tumor

DIFFERENTIAL DIAGNOSIS

Larynx Trauma

- Edema & hemorrhage around fractures

Larynx Adenoid Cystic Carcinoma

- Typically submucosal, T2 hyperintense, less aggressive

Larynx Chondrosarcoma

- Tumor centered in cartilage, chondroid calcifications
- T2-hyperintense submucosal mass on MR

Rheumatoid Larynx

- Cricoarytenoid joint & subglottic swelling

PATHOLOGY

General Features

- Etiology: Tobacco &/or alcohol abuse, > 50-year-old man
- Genetics: p53 overexpression in 50-60%, p16 absence in 90%, loss of Rb protein expression in 20% of glottic & subglottic carcinoma

Staging, Grading, & Classification

- **American Joint Committee on Cancer (AJCC) 8th edition**

- **T stage**
  - Tis: Carcinoma in situ
  - T1: Tumor limited to subglottis
  - T2: Tumor to TVC with normal or impaired mobility
  - T3: Tumor limited to larynx with TVC fixation &/or invasion of paraglottic space &/or inner cortex of thyroid cartilage
  - T4a: Tumor invades cricoid or thyroid cartilage ± invasion of extralaryngeal tissues; e.g., trachea, neck soft tissues, strap muscles, deep extrinsic muscles of tongue, thyroid, esophagus
  - T4b: Tumor invades prevertebral space, encases carotid artery, or invades mediastinum

Gross Pathologic & Surgical Features

- **Subglottic SCCa spread patterns**
  - Circumferential & submucosal internal spread
  - Cartilaginous (cricoid & tracheal) involvement in up to 50%
  - Cephalad to TVC ± supraglottis: Transglottic carcinoma
  - Caudad to tracheal lumen; lateral extension into tracheoesophageal groove, may invade recurrent laryngeal nerve
  - Anteriorly through cricothyroid/cricotracheal membranes; anteroinferiorly to thyroid gland
  - Posteriorly to cricoid, postcricoid hypopharynx, esophagus
- Embryologically, supraglottis rich & glottis-**subglottis poor in lymphatics**; nodal metastasis late in glottic-subglottic carcinoma

CLINICAL ISSUES

Presentation

- Most common signs/symptoms
  - Stridor, dyspnea, hoarseness if TVC involved

Demographics

- Epidemiology: < 5% of laryngeal SCCa subglottic

Natural History & Prognosis

- Subglottic SCCa has long asymptomatic period
  - **50% present as T4 tumor**
- Overall 5-year survival rate 52%: Localized cancer 60%, regional cancer 50%, distant cancer 45%
- **Subglottic stomal recurrences** common
  - Likely from lymphatic spread to paratracheal nodes

Treatment

- Early-stage disease (T1, T2): Either partial laryngectomy or primary radiation with similar overall survival rates
- Advanced-stage disease (T3, T4): Total laryngectomy followed by adjuvant radiation

DIAGNOSTIC CHECKLIST

Image Interpretation Pearls

- Any tissue internal to cricoid ring, view as possible tumor

SELECTED REFERENCES

1. Mann H et al: Management of subglottic cancer. Otolaryngol Clin North Am. 56(2):305-12, 2023

KEY FACTS

TERMINOLOGY

- Secondary laryngocele: Lesion obstructs laryngeal ventricle, causing internal or mixed laryngocele
- Squamous cell carcinoma (SCCa) is most common cause of secondary laryngocele

IMAGING

- CECT with coronal reformats
  - Thin-walled, air- or fluid-filled internal or mixed laryngocele with glottic &/or supraglottic soft tissue mass
  - Obstructing SCCa: Enhancing, infiltrative glottic or low supraglottic mass in area of ventricle
  - Paraglottic laryngocele extends to margin of SCCa
  - Internal laryngocele: Thin-walled, fluid- or air-density paraglottic space cyst
  - Mixed laryngocele: Paraglottic cyst passes through thyrohyoid membrane into submandibular space

TOP DIFFERENTIAL DIAGNOSES

- Primary laryngocele
- 2nd branchial cleft cyst
- Thyroglossal duct cyst

PATHOLOGY

- Lesion obstructs laryngeal ventricle with consequent internal or mixed laryngocele
  - Laryngeal SCCa > > inflammation > trauma: 15% of all laryngoceles

CLINICAL ISSUES

- SCCa: Hoarseness, stridor from fixation of vocal cord
- Small laryngoceles can be removed transorally, but larger laryngoceles require external surgery

DIAGNOSTIC CHECKLIST

- If laryngocele is found in smoker, search for laryngeal SCCa in area of laryngeal ventricle
- Stage primary SCCa as if laryngocele not present

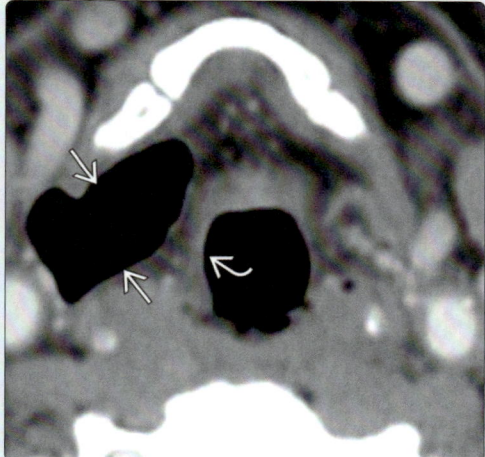
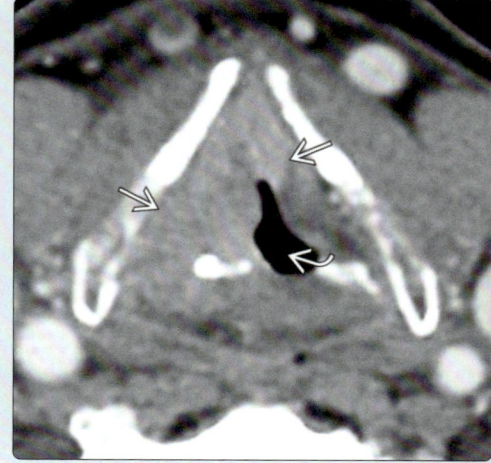

(Left) Axial CECT in a 48-year-old man who is a lifelong smoker with T3 glottic carcinoma shows an air-filled laryngocele ➡ displacing the right aryepiglottic (AE) fold ➡ medially. This is an example of an internal type of laryngocele. *(Right)* Axial CECT at the level of the laryngeal ventricle in the same patient shows large mucosal squamous cell carcinoma (SCCa) ➡ that involved the true cord as well as the false cord. The tumor causes airway narrowing ➡. There was no extra laryngeal extension.

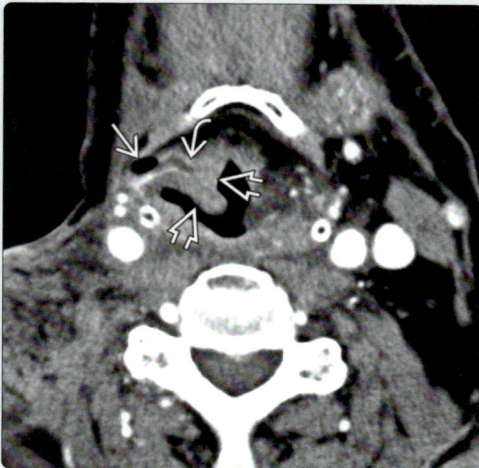
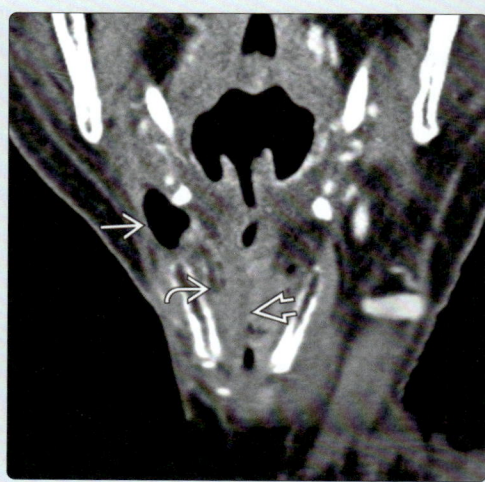

(Left) Axial CECT shows an air-filled mixed secondary laryngocele ➡ with a fluid-filled stalk ➡ obstructed by a supraglottic enhancing SCCa ➡. The SCCa in this image involves the false cord and enlarges the AE fold. *(Right)* Coronal CECT in the same patient reveals the air-filled external secondary laryngocele ➡, the fluid-filled tubular saccule ➡, and supraglottic and glottic SCCa ➡. Remember to search for a laryngeal SCCa in all adults in whom CECT reveals a laryngocele.

TERMINOLOGY

Abbreviations

- Squamous cell carcinoma (SCCa)

Definitions

- **Secondary laryngocele**: Obstruction of laryngeal ventricle causes internal or mixed laryngocele
  - Most common obstructing lesion: Laryngeal SCCa
- **Internal laryngocele**: Dilated air- or fluid-filled laryngeal saccule within paraglottic space
- **Mixed laryngocele**: Paraglottic space internal laryngocele extends through thyrohyoid membrane into low submandibular space (SMS)
- **Pyolaryngocele**: Secondary infection of any laryngocele

IMAGING

General Features

- Best diagnostic clue
  - Thin-walled, air- or fluid-filled internal or mixed laryngocele with ipsilateral glottic &/or supraglottic soft tissue mass (SCCa)
- Location
  - SCCa causing laryngocele: Glottic or low supraglottic lesion involving laryngeal ventricle

Radiographic Findings

- Radiography
  - Air pocket seen in upper cervical soft tissues

CT Findings

- CECT
  - Obstructing SCCa: Enhancing, infiltrative glottic, or low supraglottic mass
    - Involves area of laryngeal ventricle
    - Paraglottic laryngocele extends to margin of SCCa
  - Secondary laryngocele
    - Internal laryngocele: Thin-walled, fluid- or air-density paraglottic space cystic mass
    - Mixed laryngocele: Paraglottic cyst passes through thyrohyoid membrane into SMS

MR Findings

- T2WI
  - Obstructing SCCa: Intermediate signal, infiltrative glottic &/or low supraglottic mass
  - Secondary laryngocele: High-signal paraglottic space lesion ± SMS extension (mixed laryngocele)
- T1WI C+
  - Obstructing SCCa: Enhancing, infiltrative glottic &/or low supraglottic mass involving laryngeal ventricle
  - Secondary laryngocele: Rim enhancing only

Imaging Recommendations

- Best imaging tool
  - CECT often gives least motion-degraded images

DIFFERENTIAL DIAGNOSIS

Primary Laryngocele

- Laryngocele without obstructing lesion found

Thyroglossal Duct Cyst

- Midline cystic lesion embedded in infrahyoid strap muscles
- May project in midline to preepiglottic space

2nd Branchial Cleft Cyst

- Cystic lesion posterior to submandibular gland at angle of mandible
- No connection to larynx

PATHOLOGY

General Features

- Etiology
  - Lesion obstructs saccule or laryngeal ventricle with consequent internal or mixed laryngocele
    - Laryngeal SCCa > > inflammation > trauma
    - 15% of all laryngoceles
    - 5-30% cases of SCCa of larynx

Microscopic Features

- Laryngocele: Lined by respiratory epithelium (ciliated, columnar) with fibrous wall

CLINICAL ISSUES

Presentation

- Most common signs/symptoms
  - SCCa: Hoarseness, stridor from fixation of vocal cord
- Other signs/symptoms
  - Laryngocele: Laryngoscopy shows submucosal supraglottic mass
    - SCCa may be difficult to see
  - Mixed laryngocele: Anterior neck mass at hyoid bone level

Natural History & Prognosis

- Laryngocele will continue to grow slowly until SCCa treated
- Presence of laryngocele does not increase likelihood of transglottic extension

Treatment

- Successful treatment of SCCa may or may not treat secondary laryngocele

DIAGNOSTIC CHECKLIST

Image Interpretation Pearls

- If laryngocele is found in smoker, search for laryngeal SCCa in area of laryngeal ventricle
- Stage obstructing SCCa primary tumor as if laryngocele not present
- Define secondary laryngocele as internal or mixed

SELECTED REFERENCES

1. Litsou E et al: Combined laryngocele and external approach. Maedica (Bucur). 19(1):147-53, 2024
2. Heuveling DA et al: Endoscopic CO(2) laser resection using the inversion technique in 22 combined laryngoceles. Laryngoscope. 133(10):2742-6, 2023
3. Ji YJ et al: [Clinical features and management analysis of 11 cases of laryngocele.] Zhonghua Er Bi Yan Hou Tou Jing Wai Ke Za Zhi. 58(5):470-5, 2023
4. Slonimsky G et al: Terminology, definitions, and classification in the imaging of laryngoceles. Curr Probl Diagn Radiol. 50(3):384-8, 2021

KEY FACTS

TERMINOLOGY

- Perineural tumor (PNT) spread
- Malignant tumor spread along sheath of large, named nerve(s) distant from 1° site

IMAGING

- Most often found along CNV branches & CNVII
- MR more sensitive than CECT for PNT
- CECT: May be extremely subtle
  - Enlarged nerve ± mild enhancement
  - Smoothly widened foramina or canals
  - Muscular denervation atrophy when longstanding (typically muscles of mastication from CNV3 PNT)
- MR: Nerve enlarged & enhancing, loss of normal fat signal along course of nerves
  - T1WI without fat saturation is mainstay of diagnosis with contrast necessary for intracranial PNT
  - Denervated muscles enhance in acute/subacute phase

TOP DIFFERENTIAL DIAGNOSES

- Schwannoma
- Neurofibroma
- Skull base meningioma
- Invasive fungal sinusitis
- Lymphoma

PATHOLOGY

- Neurotropic tumors
  - Adenoid cystic, squamous cell carcinoma, melanoma, lymphoma
  - Skin, parotid, palate, nasopharynx
- Detection is critical for treatment planning (surgery &/or radiation)

DIAGNOSTIC CHECKLIST

- Examine nerve(s) at risk from end organ to nucleus
- PNT may spread anterograde & retrograde, may have "skip lesions," & may cross between nerves

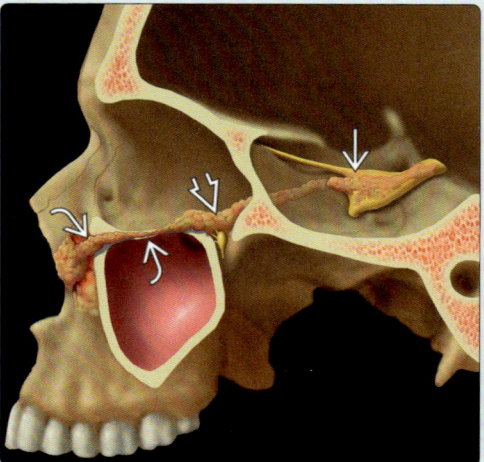
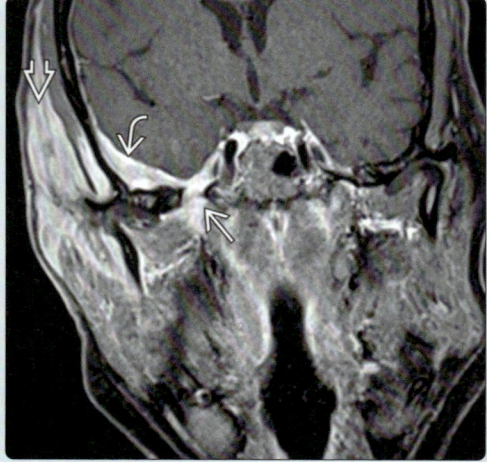

(Left) Sagittal graphic illustrates the classic appearance of perineural tumor (PNT) spread from cheek malignancy. Tumor gains access to the infraorbital nerve ➡ and spreads retrograde to the pterygopalatine fossa (PPF) ➡, foramen rotundum, and into the Meckel cave, involving gasserian ganglion ➡. (Right) Coronal T1 C+ FS MR shows marked enhancement in the right foramen ovale ➡ due to PNT from adenoid cystic carcinoma. Additional tumor spread is noted along the dura ➡ and masticator space ➡.

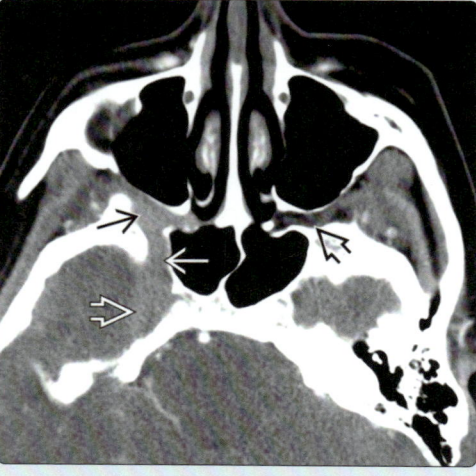
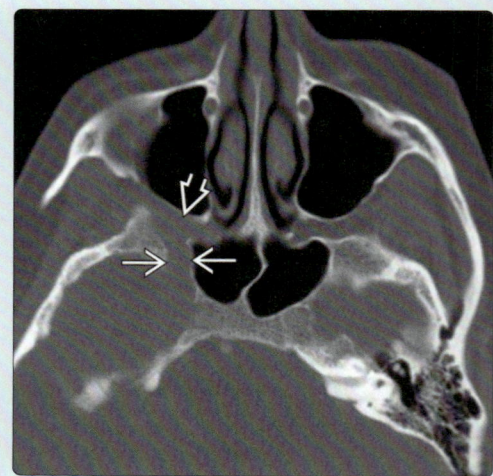

(Left) Axial CECT shows loss of normal fat density in the right PPF ➡, as compared to the normal contralateral PPF containing fat and vessels ➡. Soft tissue density fills the right PPF, and there is widening of the right foramen rotundum ➡ and fullness of the right cavernous sinus and Meckel cave ➡ as tumor spreads retrograde. (Right) Axial bone CT in the same patient demonstrates smooth widening of the right foramen rotundum ➡ and PPF ➡. Findings are typical for extracranial and intracranial PNT along CNV2.

TERMINOLOGY

Abbreviations

- Perineural tumor (PNT) spread

Definitions

- Malignant tumor spread along sheath of large, named nerve(s) distant from 1° site
  - Epineurium & perineurium involved more often than endoneurium

IMAGING

General Features

- Best diagnostic clue
  - Abnormal enlargement & enhancement of nerves
  - Widening of associated neural foramen or canal
  - Muscular denervation atrophy
    - Muscles of mastication (CNV3) > muscles of facial expression (CNVII)
- Location
  - Intracranial & extracranial
  - CNV > > CNVII most frequently involved
    - Maxillary (CNV2) > mandibular (CNV3) > > ophthalmic (CNV1)
- Morphology
  - Tubular enlargement of affected nerve
    - Radiographic "**skip areas**" possible

CT Findings

- CECT
  - CT shows extracranial > > intracranial PNT
    - Enlarged nerve ± mild enhancement
    - Abnormal soft tissue density in foramina, canals
    - Effacement of fat within pterygopalatine fossa (PPF), below skull base, or in premaxillary region
    - Denervation of supplied musculature ranging from acute swelling/enhancement to chronic fatty atrophy
    - Convex, enhancing cavernous sinus
- Bone CT
  - Smoothly widened foramina or canals

MR Findings

- T1WI
  - **Enlarged nerve** replaces high-signal fat
    - Within canals & foramina
    - Along extracranial course of cranial nerve (CN) with obliteration of fat pads
      □ Beneath foramen ovale or medial to mandibular foramen (CNV3)
      □ PPF or premaxillary fat (CNV2)
      □ Superomedial orbit (CNV1)
      □ Beneath stylomastoid foramen (CNVII)
  - High T1WI in chronically denervated muscles, most obvious in masticator space (CNV3)
- T2WI
  - Tumor replaces high-signal CSF in Meckel cave (CNV)
  - High T2WI in acute/subacute muscular denervation
- T1WI C+ FS
  - Abnormal enlargement & enhancement of involved nerve
  - Denervated muscles: Enhance in acute/subacute phase

Nuclear Medicine Findings

- PET/CT
  - Rarely detects PNT
    - Small volume of tumor along nerve not classically FDG avid [e.g., adenoid cystic carcinoma (ACCa)]

Imaging Recommendations

- Best imaging tool
  - MR more sensitive than CECT for PNT
  - If only CECT available, carefully evaluate foramina, fat planes, muscles, & cavernous sinus
- Protocol advice
  - T1WI without fat saturation is mainstay of diagnosis
    - T1WI C+ FS helpful for extracranial tumor
      □ Susceptibility artifact can obscure PNT at skull base foramen: CNV2, CNV3, & vidian nerve
    - T1WI C+ important for intracranial PNT
  - Must image entire nerve from nucleus → end organ

DIFFERENTIAL DIAGNOSIS

Schwannoma

- Tubular, fusiform, lobular mass following nerve
- T2 hyperintense; heterogeneously T1 C+ enhancing
- Larger dimension than perineural tumor

Neurofibroma

- Tubular mass along nerve or plexiform morphology
- T2 shows central target sign
- Homogeneously enhancing

Invasive Fungal Sinusitis

- Infiltrating, diffuse disease in face, not exclusively along nerves
- Immunocompromised patients, including diabetics

Skull Base Meningioma

- Homogeneously enhancing, dural-based mass ± dural tail
- May extend into neural &/or jugular foramen

Lymphoma

- No cutaneous or mucosal 1° lesion as source of PNT

Sarcoidosis

- Dural-based inflammation; may involve CNs
- Typically starts in sinus, mimics PNT

PATHOLOGY

General Features

- Etiology
  - Many head & neck cancers have PNT tendency: Mucosal, skin, salivary origin
  - **Neurotropic tumors**
    - ACCa: Minor or major salivary gland
    - Squamous cell carcinoma (SCCa): Mucosal or skin
    - Desmoplastic melanoma
    - Non-Hodgkin lymphoma
  - 1° sites most at risk for PNT
    - Skin: CNV
    - Parotid: CNVII

- – Hard palate (HP): CNV2
- – Nasopharynx: CNV-XII
- ○ Spread direction: **Retrograde** (toward CNS: Nerve main trunk/brainstem) > > **antegrade** (away from CNS)
- ○ Most common pathways of PNT spread include
  - – **CNV2**: **Maxillary division** → PPF
    - □ **Infraorbital nerve**: Cheek or maxillary sinus tumors
    - □ **Greater & lesser palatine nerves**: HP minor salivary cancer
  - – **CNV3**: **Mandibular division** → foramen ovale → Meckel cave
    - □ **Mental nerve**: Lip or cutaneous SCCa
    - □ **Inferior alveolar nerve**: Mucosal oral cavity SCCa
    - □ **Auriculotemporal nerve (ATN)**: Branch of CNV3: Enters parotid, & its anterior & posterior communicating rami interface with CNVII
    - □ **Mandibular main trunk**: Masticator space 1° or 2° malignancy
  - – **CNV1**: **Ophthalmic division** → cavernous sinus
    - □ Rare; most often forehead SCCa, melanoma
  - – **CNVII**: **Facial nerve**
    - □ **Intraparotid branches** → intratemporal CNVII → internal auditory canal
    - □ **Greater superficial petrosal nerve (GSPN)**: From geniculate ganglion, joins deep petrosal nerve at foramen lacerum to form vidian nerve → PPF
  - – **Direct through sphenopalatine foramen → PPF**
    - □ Nasopharynx cancer, nasal malignancies
  - – **From PPF, tumor may access multiple sites**
    - □ Through inferior orbital fissure to orbital apex
    - □ Along vidian canal to CNVII geniculate ganglion
    - □ Foramen rotundum → cavernous sinus/Meckel cave
- • Associated features
  - ○ GSPN & ATN = central & peripheral connections between CNV & CNVII: Providing important conduits for PNT between nerves
  - ○ CNV3 supplies muscles of mastication + anterior belly of digastric & mylohyoid muscles
  - ○ CNVII supplies muscles of facial expression + posterior belly of digastric muscle

Gross Pathologic & Surgical Features

- • PNT 1st grows along nerve sheath, then invades nerve
- • ACCa: Highest propensity for PNT; SCCa most common source since most common head & neck tumor

Microscopic Features

- • Extension of tumor along nerve via epineurium/perineurium distant from 1° site
- • Perineural invasion (PNI) not = PNT
  - ○ PNI is microscopic finding of nerve invasion at 1° site
- • Immunohistochemical markers associated with PNT
  - ○ Presence of growth factor receptor p75
    - – Abundant in desmoplastic melanoma, maybe ACCa
- • Nerve microenvironment (Schwann cells & macrophages): "Crosstalk" with tumor

CLINICAL ISSUES

Presentation

- • Most common signs/symptoms
  - ○ Commonly asymptomatic but with imaging findings

- ○ CNV: Pain, paresthesia
  - – CNV3: Weakness from denervation atrophy of muscles of mastication
  - – ATN: Preauricular pain & otalgia
- ○ CNVII: Facial weakness or paralysis
- ○ May be confused with trigeminal neuralgia & Bell palsy
  - – High index of suspicion if 1° cancer history

Natural History & Prognosis

- • PNT = poor prognostic sign indicating increased incidence of local recurrence
  - ○ ACCa has tendency for late recurrence, so long-term follow-up recommended

Treatment

- • Surgery combined with postoperative RT ± chemo
- • With PNT, entire course of nerve must be radiated
- • Presence of PNT may preclude 1° surgical therapy; consider immunotherapy for advanced skin cancers
  - ○ 1° RT with proton beam may be indicated for surgically unresectable salivary tumors

DIAGNOSTIC CHECKLIST

Consider

- • Always assess for PNT spread in head & neck cancer
  - ○ Findings are subtle; if it is not looked for, it will not be seen
- • Even if no history of 1° tumor, beware diagnosis of trigeminal neuralgia
  - ○ ACCa: Can present as small HP 1° with extensive PNT

Image Interpretation Pearls

- • Deep face PNT often best seen on precontrast T1 MR without fat saturation
- • Denervated muscles disclose affected nerve
- • If CECT: Check normal fat planes; evaluate for asymmetry

Reporting Tips

- • Examine nerve at risk from end organ to nucleus
  - ○ Knowledge of motor/sensory supply = most effective use of clinical information
- • Remember key facts of tumor spread
  - ○ PNT may spread both anterograde & retrograde
  - ○ Beware possibility of radiographic "skip lesions"
  - ○ Nerves interconnect (e.g., CNV & CNVII)

SELECTED REFERENCES

1. Li KY et al: Pre-treatment and post-treatment nasopharyngeal carcinoma imaging: imaging updates, pearls and pitfalls. Neuroradiology. 67(4):1023-47, 2025
2. Cavanagh K et al: Assessment of perineural spread in advanced cutaneous squamous cell carcinomas treated with immunotherapy. Cancer Imaging. 24(1):37, 2024
3. Doran S et al: Perineural tumour spread in head and neck cancer: a pictorial review. Clin Radiol. 79(10):749-56, 2024
4. Sharma P et al: Diagnostic accuracy of contrast-enhanced MRI for detection of perineural spread in head and neck cancer: a systematic review and meta-analysis. J Neurol Surg B Skull Base. 85(Suppl 3):e97-109, 2024
5. Abdelaziz TT et al: Magnetic resonance imaging of perineural spread of head and neck cancer. Magn Reson Imaging Clin N Am. 30(1):95-108, 2022
6. Kirsch CFE et al: Practical tips for MR imaging of perineural tumor spread. Magn Reson Imaging Clin N Am. 26(1):85-100, 2018
7. Stambuk HE: Perineural tumor spread involving the central skull base region. Semin Ultrasound CT MR. 34(5):445-58, 2013

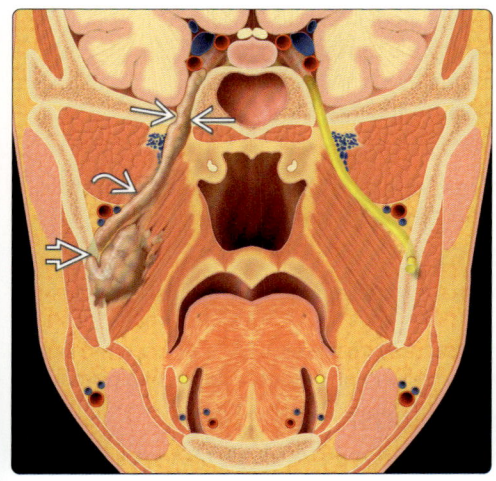

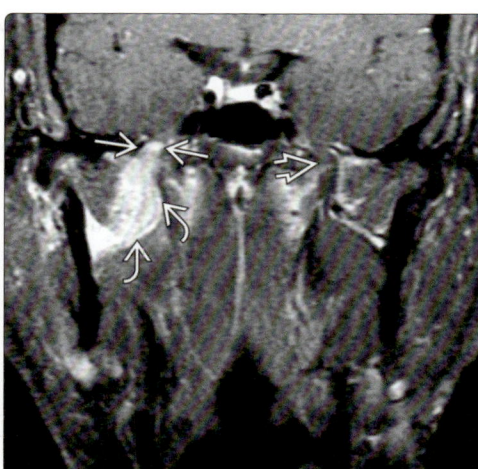

(Left) Coronal graphic depicts PNT extending from the masticator space into the mandible and along the inferior alveolar nerve ➡. Tumor extends along the nerve ➡ through the foramen ovale ➡ to the Meckel cave. (Right) Coronal T1WI C+ FS MR shows markedly enlarged and enhancing mandibular nerve ➡ coursing through the right masticator space to foramen ovale ➡. Note normal appearance of contralateral mandibular nerve ➡ with normal linear enhancement at foramen ovale from veins traversing the foramen.

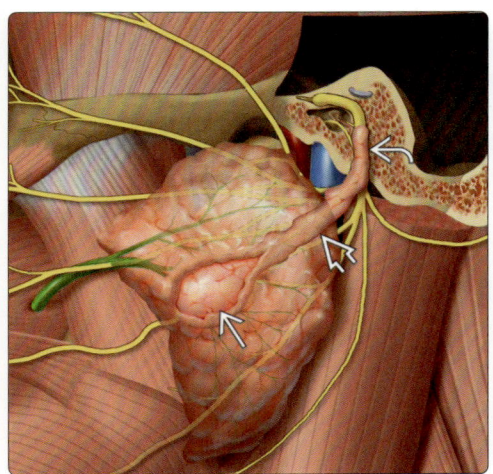

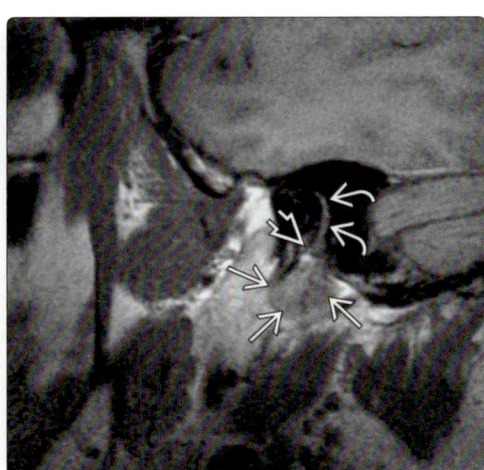

(Left) Sagittal graphic depicts parotid malignancy ➡ engulfing branches of CNVII. PNT extends along the intraparotid CNVII ➡, through the stylomastoid foramen, to the mastoid segment ➡. Any parotid tumor may spread along CNVII, although adenoid cystic carcinoma is the most common. (Right) Sagittal T1WI MR without fat saturation in a patient with facial palsy shows a small parotid mass ➡ immediately beneath the stylomastoid foramen ➡. PNT is evident extending along the mastoid segment of CNVII ➡, which appears enlarged.

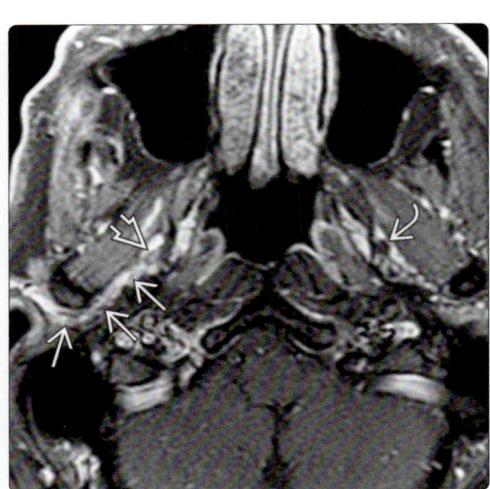

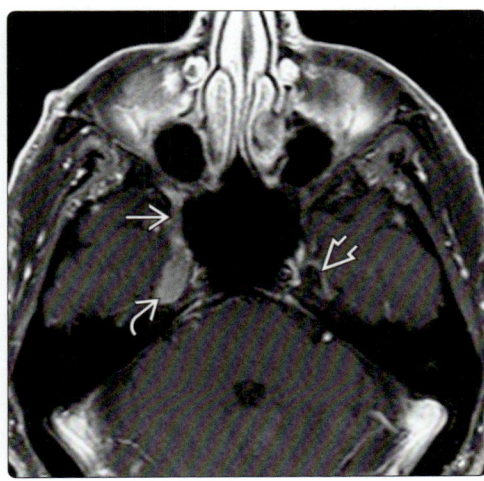

(Left) Axial MR in a patient with multiple prior skin SCCa reveals linear enhancing right auriculotemporal nerve PNT ➡ posterior to the right condyle and medial to lateral pterygoid muscle, joining an enhancing V3 ➡ below the foramen ovale. Note normal left V3 ➡. (Right) Axial MR shows PNT spread along auriculotemporal nerve, filling right Meckel cave ➡, extending antegrade along V2 into cavernous sinus ➡ through foramen rotundum into right PPF. Note normal CSF-filled left Meckel cave ➡. Biopsy proved SCCa.

KEY FACTS

TERMINOLOGY

- Metastatic spread of primary H&N SCCa to nodes

IMAGING

- Change in morphology key to detecting nodal metastasis
- "**Malignant nodal criteria**" best used in combination
  - Nodal enlargement, typically > 10-mm long axis
  - Round node shape rather than oval
  - Clustered nodes: ≥ 3 nodes 8-9 mm
  - Focal nodal defect/necrosis
  - Extranodal extension
- **ENE is determinant of N staging for non-HPV-mediated SCCa**
- **Different N staging for HPV-mediated [p16(+)] oropharynx, nasopharynx, & for non-HPV-mediated [p16(-)] oropharynx & all other sites**

TOP DIFFERENTIAL DIAGNOSES

- Reactive & benign lymph nodes

- 2nd branchial cleft cyst
- Suppurative lymph nodes
- Differentiated thyroid carcinoma nodes
- Non-Hodgkin lymphoma nodes
- Nonhead & neck malignancy nodes

PATHOLOGY

- Lymphatic spread of H&N SCCa follows expected pattern according to primary site of origin

CLINICAL ISSUES

- Nodal metastasis is **most important prognostic factor** for H&N SCCa
- Patient presenting with metastatic SCCa + neck mass with normal clinical & radiographic exam = "**unknown primary**"

DIAGNOSTIC CHECKLIST

- New solid or cystic neck mass in adult is malignant until proven otherwise
- Report should include size, number, laterality, & ENE

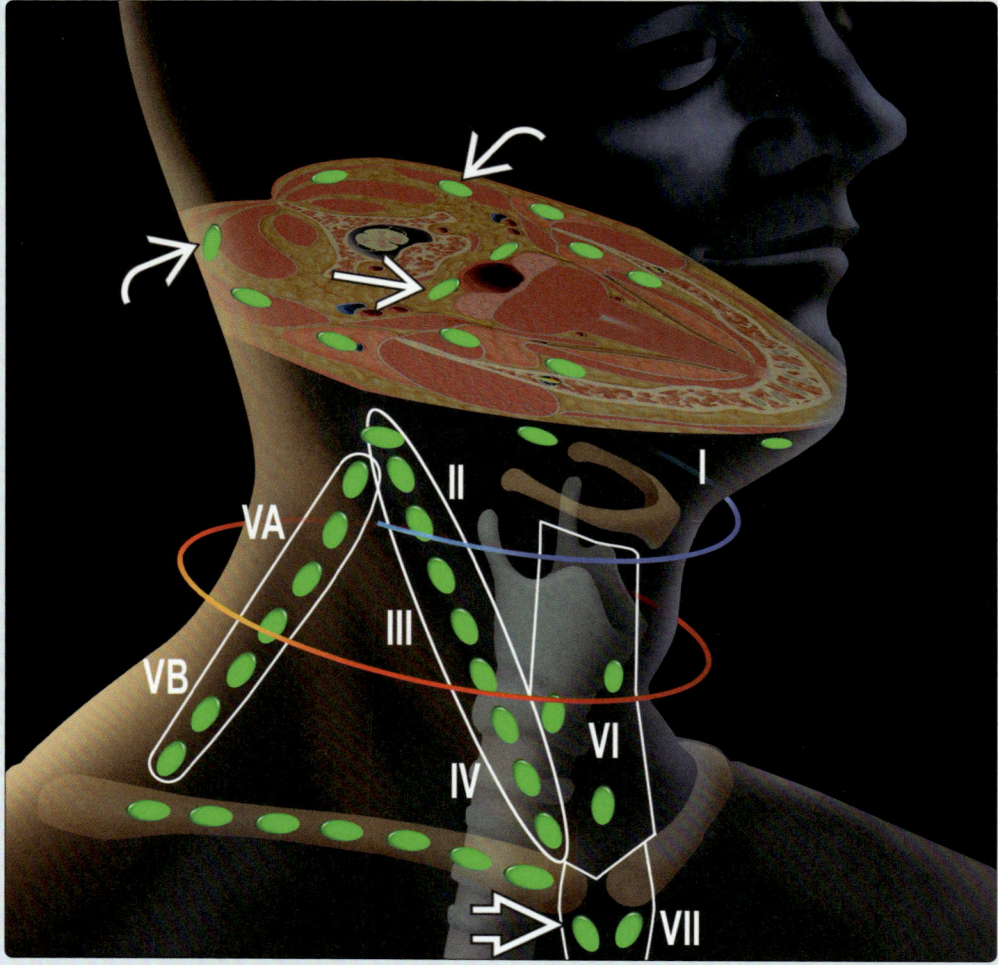

Lateral oblique graphic of the cervical neck depicts the extensive nodal network to which SCCa may metastasize. Superiorly, an axial slice through the suprahyoid neck shows the retropharyngeal nodes ⮕ behind the pharynx and shows multiple superficial nodal groups ⮕. The hyoid bone (blue arc) and cricoid cartilage (orange circle) planes subdivide the internal jugular and spinal accessory nodal group levels. Level II is the most common site of SCCa nodal metastasis, while level VI and level VII are the least common sites. SCCa metastases in level VII ⮕ are considered regional metastases, while nodes more inferiorly in the mediastinum are considered M1 disease.

Nodal Squamous Cell Carcinoma

TERMINOLOGY

Abbreviations

- Nodal squamous cell carcinoma (SCCa)

IMAGING

General Features

- Best diagnostic clue
  - Round, enlarged, &/or heterogeneous node in expected nodal drainage level(s) of head & neck SCCa
  - New neck mass in adult, including cystic mass
- Location
  - Level IIA (jugulodigastric) most often involved
- Size
  - Different nodal size criteria used depending on location
- Morphology
  - Change in morphology is key to detecting nodal metastasis
  - **"Malignant nodal criteria" best used in combination rather than individually**
    - Nodal enlargement; several different limits
      - Levels I & IIA ≥ 15 mm; levels IIB-VI ≥ 10 mm; retropharyngeal ≥ 8 mm
      - Long axis most often used for diameter
    - Round node shape rather than oval
      - Ratio of long axis:short axis < 2
    - Clustered nodes: ≥ 3 nodes 8-9 mm
      - IIA: 9-10 mm
    - Focal nodal defect/necrosis
      - Results in inhomogeneous nodal texture
      - May result in diffuse cystic change
      - Differentiate from fatty hilum
    - **Imaging-derived extranodal extension (iENE) described by Asian and Oceanian Society of Neuroradiology and Head & Neck Radiology (AOSHHNR)/American Society of Head & Neck Radiology (ASHNR)/European Society of Head & Neck Radiology (ESHNR) Joint Task Force**
      - Grade1 = invasion of perinodal fat; grade 2 = coalescent nodes; grade 3 = invasion of surrounding organs
      - Do not call iENE if definitive feature(s) are not detectable on imaging
      - Definitive imaging evidence needed to establish iENE grade
      - If imaging shows criteria for multiple iENE grades, choose highest grade
- Features of surgical unresectability
  - Carotid encasement ≥ 270°
  - Invasion of prevertebral musculature, high skull base extension, &/or dermal lymphatics

CT Findings

- CECT
  - Variable imaging appearance per aforementioned criteria, including iENE

MR Findings

- DWI
  - Do not use DWI to differentiate benign vs. malignant nodes
- MR perfusion: Dynamic contrast enhancement
  - Transfer constant (Ktrans) ↑, treatment responders show early ↓

Ultrasonographic Findings

- Grayscale ultrasound
  - Round node with loss of hilar echogenicity
- Power Doppler
  - Loss of normal hilar flow, ↑ peripheral vascularity

Nuclear Medicine Findings

- PET
  - SCCa is reliably FDG avid
    - Accuracy ~ 75% for detection of positive nodes
    - Accuracy improves as nodes ↑ in size
    - False-negative may occur with cystic nodes
    - False-positive reactive nodes in ulcerative tumor
    - Useful for nodal SCCa & unknown primary site
    - High negative predictive value for posttreatment evaluation
- Lymphoscintigraphy & sentinel node biopsy
  - Has been widely used in Europe for management of oral cavity SCCa with clinically negative neck
  - Ongoing clinical trial (NRG HN006) is investigating sentinel node biopsy vs. elective neck dissection in oral cavity SCCa

Imaging Recommendations

- Best imaging tool
  - CECT or MR
    - CT stages primary tumor & nodes simultaneously
    - CT slightly better than MR for nodal detection, especially for iENE
    - MR better for retropharyngeal node detection
  - US for detailed node exam & FNA

DIFFERENTIAL DIAGNOSIS

Reactive or Benign Lymph Nodes

- Tend to retain nodal ovoid contour; not round
- Typically not high FDG avidity; may be moderate

2nd Branchial Cleft Cyst

- Young patient with recurrent angle of mandible mass
- Thin-walled cystic mass posterior to submandibular gland
- May exactly mimic cystic level II nodal metastasis
- FDG uptake may be present if inflammation present
- Diagnosis of exclusion

Suppurative Lymph Nodes

- Clustered cystic or necrotic-appearing nodes with surrounding inflammatory changes
- Clinically obvious nodes are hot; tender & febrile patient

Differentiated Thyroid Carcinoma Nodes

- May have calcifications, cystic, high CT density
- MR: thyroglobulin may ↑ T1 & ↑ T2 signal
- ↑ FDG uptake as tumor dedifferentiates
- Most often levels VI, III, IV, & superior mediastinum

Non-Hodgkin Lymphoma Nodes

- Multiple well-defined nonnecrotic nodes

- Posterior triangle location alone favors nasopharynx, non-Hodgkin lymphoma (NHL), or scalp SCCa metastases

Nonhead & Neck Malignancy Nodes

- May metastasize to supraclavicular nodes
  - Lung, breast, or abdominal primary tumor

PATHOLOGY

General Features

- Etiology
  - Lymphatic spread of primary SCCa generally follows expected pattern in H&N
  - Skip metastasis: Nodes "miss" level
    - Well described with anterior tongue SCCa

Staging, Grading, & Classification

- Level system useful, as SCCa sites have expected drainage patterns
  - **Nasopharynx**: Retropharyngeal (RPN) > level II, level V
  - **Oropharynx**: Level IIA > IIB, III; RPN common if tonsil or pharyngeal wall
  - **Oral cavity**: Level I & II > III
  - **Hypopharynx**: Level II, III > IV; RPN with pyriform sinus or posterior wall
  - **Larynx**: Level II, III > IV
  - **Scalp skin tumors**: Pre-/post auricular, parotid, suboccipital, level II ± V
- American Joint Committee on Cancer (AJCC) cervical node classification is used when staging most H&N SCCa
  - ENE is now used for N staging of non-HPV-mediated [p16(-)] oropharynx & all other sites
  - Different N staging for HPV-mediated [p16(+)] oropharynx, nasopharynx, & thyroid carcinoma (**see relevant chapters for details**)

Gross Pathologic & Surgical Features

- Enlarged round nodes; frequently multiple
- ENE = tumor infiltration → perinodal fat, adjacent vessels, organs, muscles

Microscopic Features

- Metastases first lodge in subcapsular sinus then spread through whole node

CLINICAL ISSUES

Presentation

- Most common signs/symptoms
  - Cystic level II metastasis often confused with branchial cleft cyst
  - Painless, firm neck mass, may be fixed to adjacent tissues
  - Metastatic node & no obvious primary = "**unknown primary**"
  - Detection of metastatic nodes
    - Clinical exam ~ 75% accuracy, sensitivity 65%
    - Imaging is ~ 80-85% accurate

Demographics

- Epidemiology
  - Presence of nodes varies by primary tumor site
    - Most often: Nasopharyngeal carcinoma (NPCa) (~ 85%)

- Least often: Glottic laryngeal SCCa (< 10%)

Natural History & Prognosis

- **Nodal metastasis is most important prognostic factor for H&N SCCa**
- **ENE is determinant of N staging for non-HPV-mediated SCCa**
  - Carotid artery encasement, prevertebral musculature &/or skull base invasion = surgically unresectable
- Different N staging for HPV-mediated [p16(+)] oropharynx, nasopharynx, & for non-HPV-mediated [p16(-)] oropharynx, & all other sites (refer to appropriate chapters for details)

Treatment

- Resection ± XRT, primary XRT, or chemoXRT

DIAGNOSTIC CHECKLIST

Consider

- New neck mass in adult is malignant until proven otherwise
  - May be solid or cystic node; most often level IIA
  - If calcification, consider thyroid carcinoma
  - If isolated low neck metastasis, consider thyroid or infraclavicular 1°
  - If posterior triangle nodes, consider NPCa, NHL, or scalp SCCa

Reporting Tips

- Look carefully at expected nodal drainage site
- Evaluate contralateral neck nodes & retropharyngeal nodes
- Report iENE & its extent per ASHNR guidance
- Describe extent for surgical resectability

SELECTED REFERENCES

1. American Society of Head and Neck Society: Imaging-Derived Extranodal Extension (iENE) in Head and Neck Cancer. Published 2025. Accessed June 1, 2025. https://ashnr.org/iene/
2. Gupta R et al: International consensus recommendations of diagnostic criteria and terminologies for extranodal extension in head and neck squamous cell carcinoma: an HN CLEAR initiative (update 1). Head Neck Pathol. 19(1):20, 2025
3. Maggialetti N et al: Nodal assessment and extranodal extension in head and neck squamous cell cancer: insights from computed tomography and magnetic resonance imaging. Radiol Med. 130(2):202-13, 2025
4. Mehanna H et al: Accuracy and prognosis of extranodal extension on radiologic imaging in human papillomavirus-mediated oropharyngeal cancer: a Head and Neck Cancer International Group (HNCIG) real-world study. Int J Radiat Oncol Biol Phys. ePub, 2025
5. Alsheikh S et al: The prognostic value of image-identified extranodal extension in laryngeal and hypopharyngeal carcinoma following definitive (chemo-)radiotherapy. Oral Oncol. 158:107007, 2024
6. Caldarella C et al: Role of (18)F-FDG PET/CT in head and neck squamous cell carcinoma: current evidence and innovative applications. Cancers (Basel). 16(10), 2024
7. Duguet-Armand M et al: Radiology-pathology concordance and prognostication of nodal features in pN+ oral cavity cancer. Laryngoscope. 134(12):4947-55, 2024
8. Esce AR et al: Predicting nodal metastases in squamous cell carcinoma of the oral tongue using artificial intelligence. Am J Otolaryngol. 45(1):104102, 2024
9. Henson C et al: Criteria for the diagnosis of extranodal extension detected on radiological imaging in head and neck cancer: Head and Neck Cancer International Group consensus recommendations. Lancet Oncol. 25(7):e297-307, 2024
10. Bhattacharya K et al: Imaging of neck nodes in head and neck cancers - a comprehensive update. Clin Oncol (R Coll Radiol). 35(7):429-45, 2023
11. Jang SS et al: Role of sentinel lymph node biopsy for oral squamous cell carcinoma: current evidence and future challenges. Head Neck. 45(1):251-5, 2023

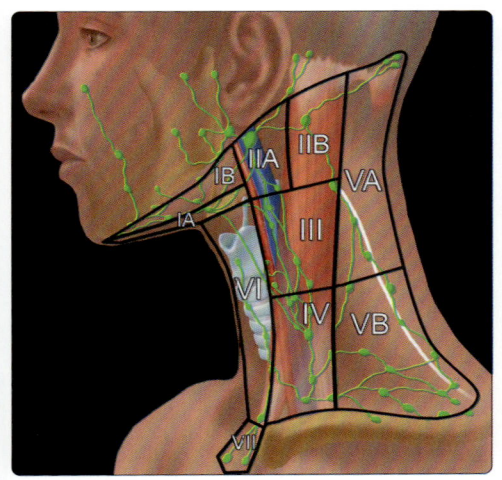

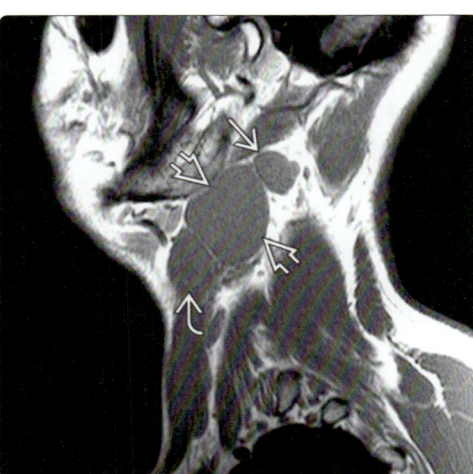

(Left) Graphic of neck node scheme shows submental (IA) and submandibular (IB) nodes below the jaw. The sternocleidomastoid muscle separates jugular chain (II, III, IV) from spinal accessory chain (VA, VB). Midline anterior nodes are included in level VI. (Right) Sagittal T1WI MR shows 3 solid enlarged metastatic nodes from primary tonsillar SCCa. The largest node is level IIA ⮕, beneath the angle of the mandible. Note the smaller adjacent IIB ⮕ and adjacent inferior level III node ⮕.

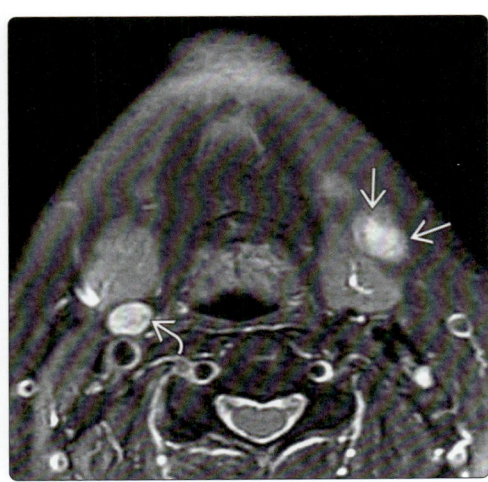

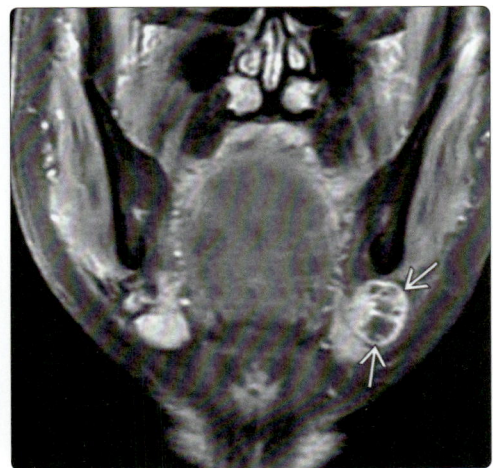

(Left) Axial T2WI FS MR in a 64-year-old woman with large left oral tongue SCCa demonstrates a clearly enlarged heterogeneous, hyperintense left IB node ⮕, which is an expected drainage site for tongue SCCa. Contralateral right IIA node ⮕ is rounded, heterogeneously enhancing & very suspicious for tumor. (Right) Coronal T1WI C+ FS MR in a patient with large left oral cavity SCCa reveals a left IB node ⮕ with cystic necrotic changes & a suspicious right IIA node. Both nodes were positive at resection: T3N2c.

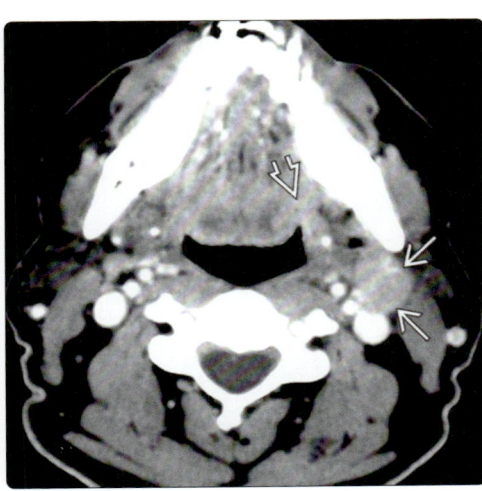

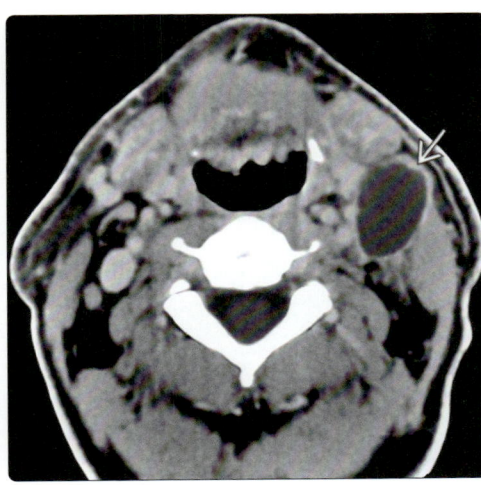

(Left) Axial CECT in a 49-year-old man shows unilateral, enlarged, heterogeneous level IIA node ⮕. FNA revealed SCCa. Panendoscopy was negative, but directed biopsy of left glossotonsillar sulcus mass seen on CT ⮕ showed SCCa. (Right) CECT shows a malignant level II cystic, peripherally enhancing SCCa ⮕ node with a clinically occult lingual tonsil SCCa. Cystic level II mass in an adult is tumor until proven otherwise; do not confuse with a branchial cleft cyst, which is diagnosis of exclusion & rarely presents in adults.

(Left) Axial CECT shows a left base of tongue primary ⇨ exophytic into the left vallecula ⇨. There is a well-defined, cystic, and solid left neck level 2A nodal metastasis ⇨. (Right) Axial fused PET/CT in the same patient shows abnormal FDG activity in the left base of tongue primary ⇨; however, the left neck level 2A cystic and solid node ⇨ shows very little FDG activity and could be missed if CT images were not scrutinized. (Note: Solid component of node merges with the normal FDG uptake of the submandibular gland.)

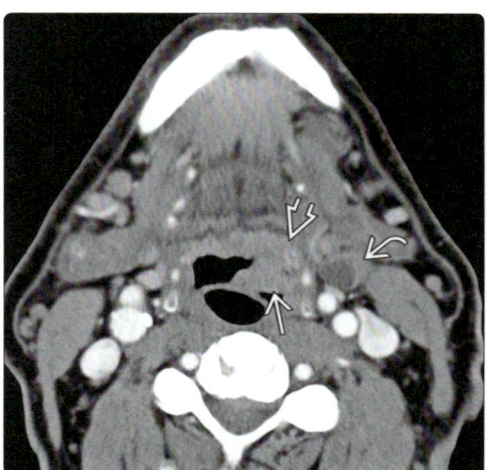
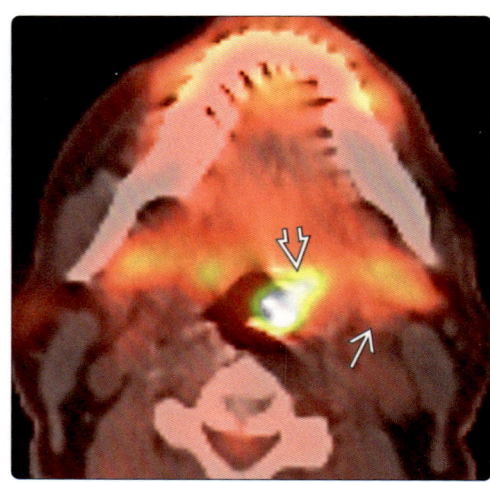

(Left) Axial CECT in 54-year-old man presenting with neck masses shows multiple pathologic left nodes ⇨ secondary to well-defined base of tongue primary SCCa ⇨. Notice ill-defined contours of left IIB node ⇨, indicating extranodal extension (ENE). (Right) Axial T2WI FS MR in 49-year-old patient with lateral tongue SCCa ⇨ shows a large, heterogeneous nodal mass at level II ⇨. Ill-defined margins with infiltration of soft tissues are gross ENE, which involves the carotid sheath ⇨.

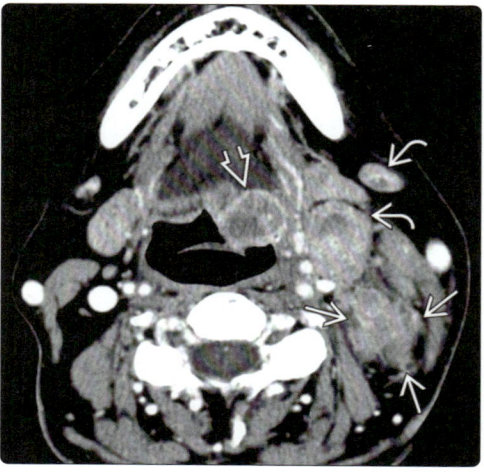
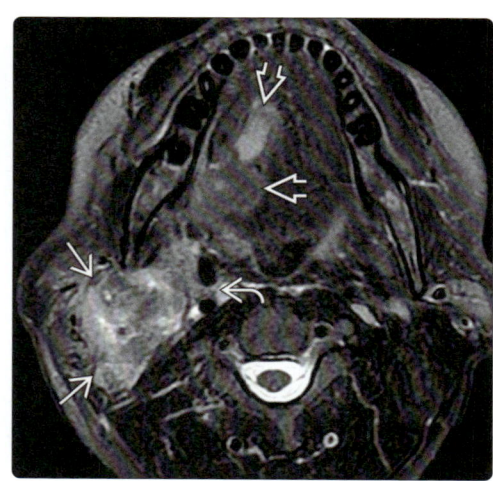

(Left) Axial CECT shows a left common carotid artery ⇨ surrounded by extensive extranodal tumor ⇨ that extends to involve overlying skin ⇨. Air pockets throughout left neck within the necrotic tumor are from skin fistulization. The jugular vein is occluded. (Right) CTA reformation in a patient with extensive extranodal tumor ⇨ reveals multiple outpouchings ⇨ along medial carotid wall, indicating significant carotid wall weakening & imminent arterial rupture. Endovascular carotid occlusion was performed.

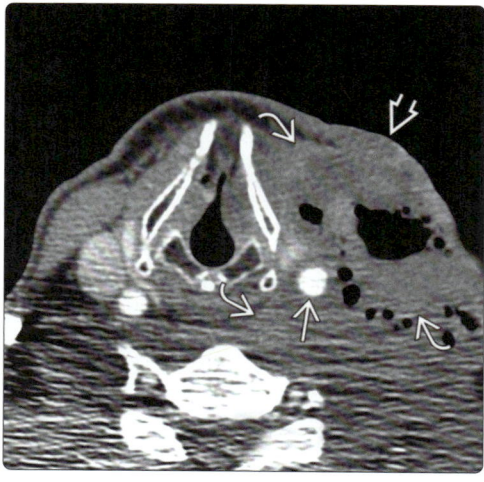
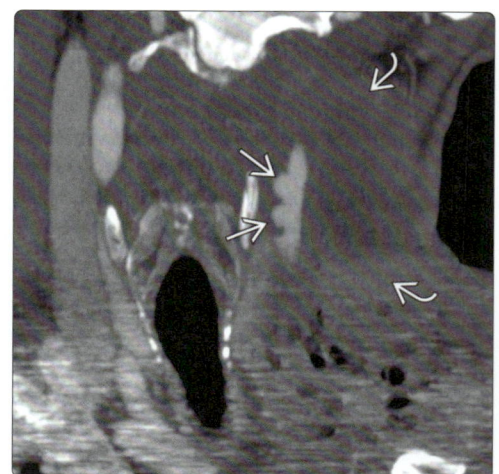

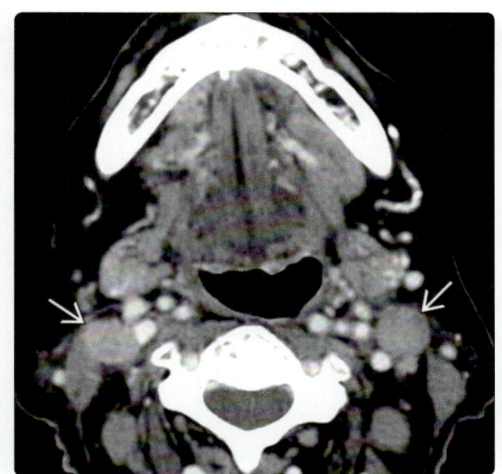

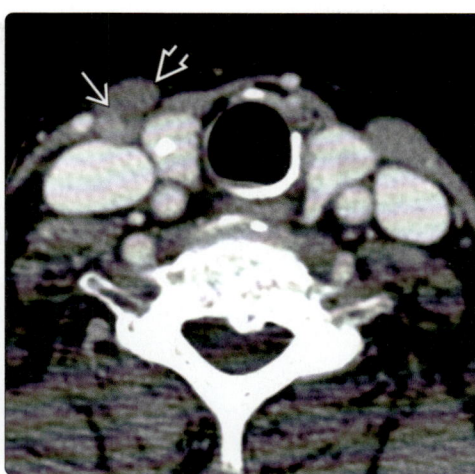

(Left) Axial CECT in an 83-year-old woman with primary SCCa of anterolateral right tongue demonstrates bilateral level 2 adenopathy ➡. While only slightly enlarged, both appear very round in contour and heterogeneous in density. (Right) Axial CECT in a patient with right oral tongue SCCa & IIA nodes shows heterogeneous metastatic level IV node ➡ beneath sternocleidomastoid ➡, confirmed with PET and at excision. No nodes are evident at level III. This is known as skip metastasis.

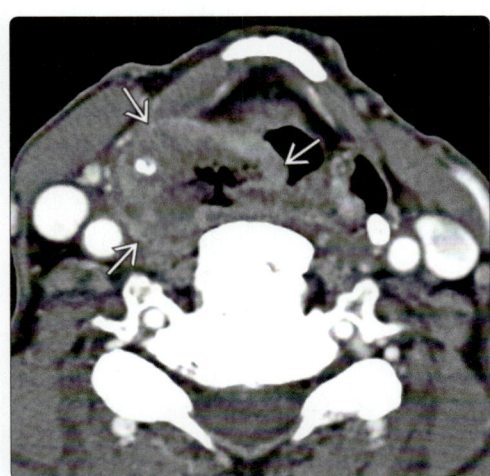

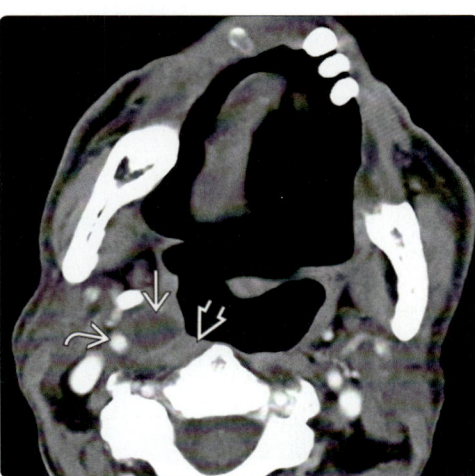

(Left) Axial CECT shows a large, circumferential right piriform sinus primary tumor ➡. Remember to always evaluate for retropharyngeal lymphadenopathy with primary tumors of the hypopharynx, especially in piriform sinus tumors. (Right) Axial CECT in same patient with large, right piriform sinus tumor. Note cystic, nonenhancing right retropharyngeal nodal metastasis ➡ located between the right internal carotid artery ➡ and right prevertebral musculature ➡.

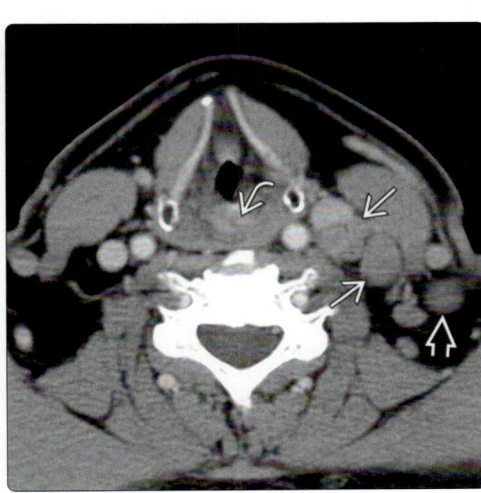

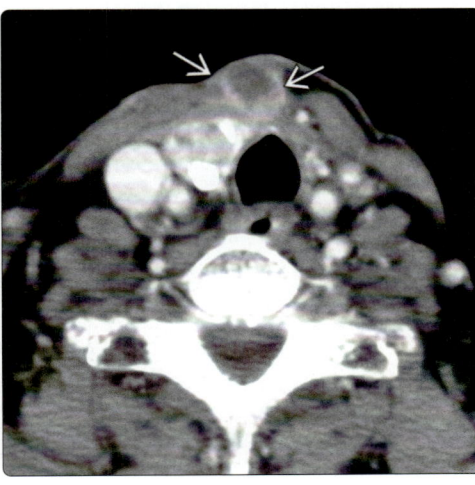

(Left) Axial CECT in a patient shows cluster of nonnecrotic, large rounded nodes in level III ➡. Level VA node ➡ also proved to be metastatic SCCa from subtle postcricoid SCCa ➡, which was apparent on FDG-PET exam. (Right) Axial CECT scan shows a rounded, low-density and rim-enhancing mass in the anterior midline of low neck ➡. This is location of the Delphian, or prelaryngeal node, and, unlike thyroid cancer, SCCa does not often spread here. Ill-defined margins of this node suggest extracapsular spread.

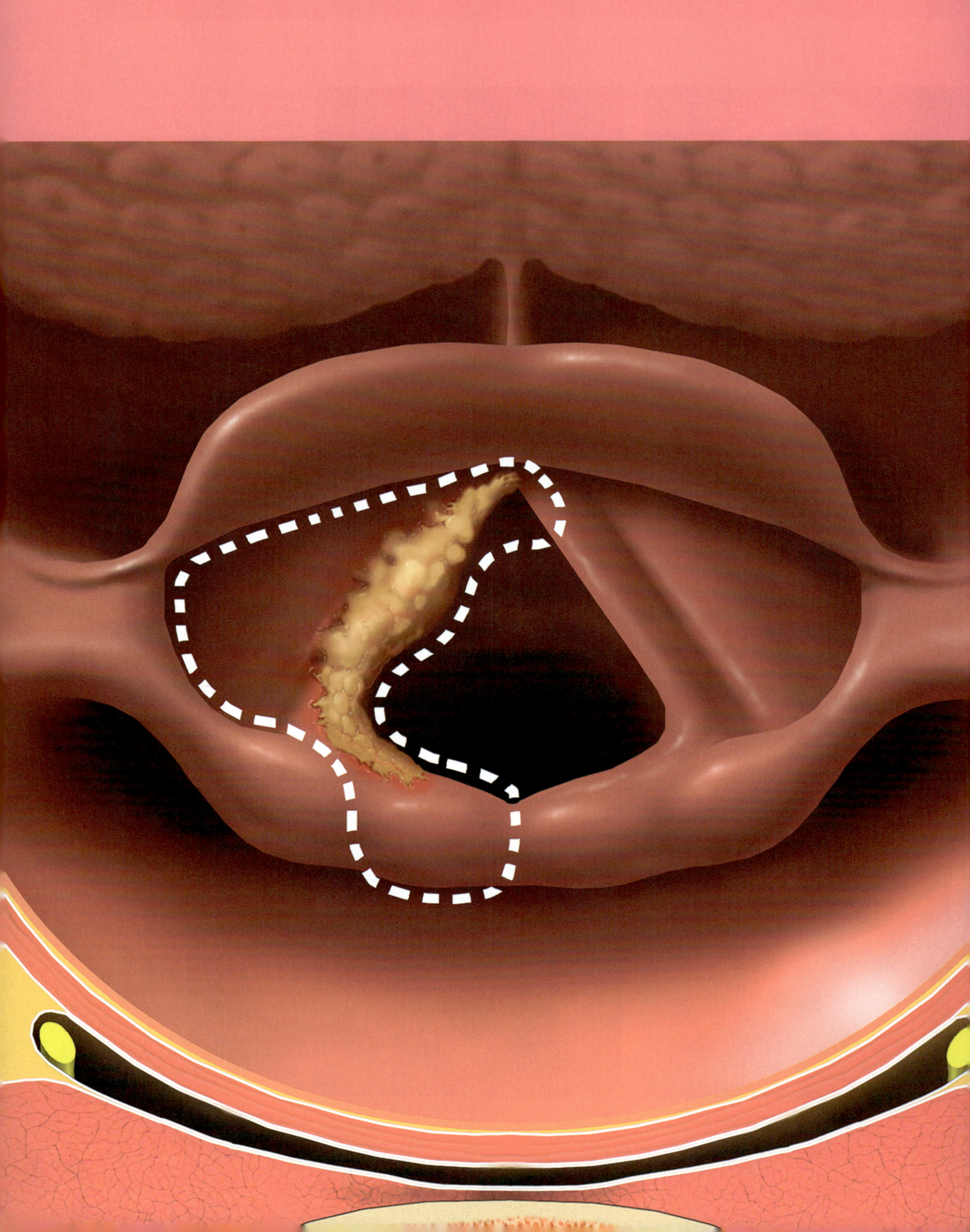

SECTION 18
Posttreatment Neck

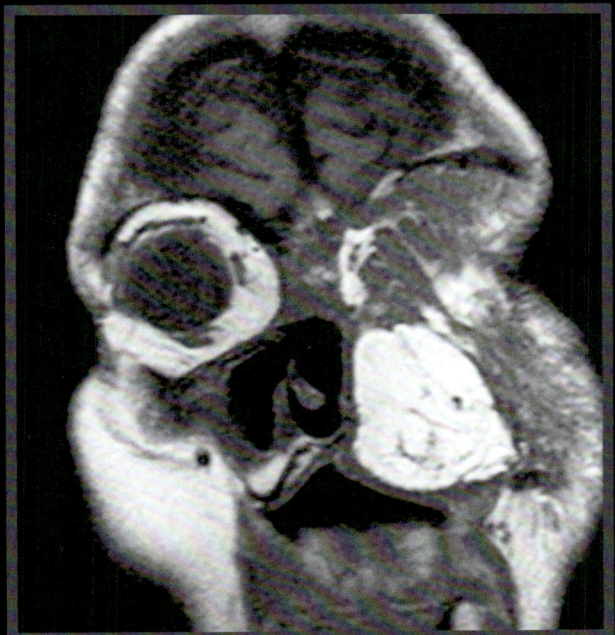
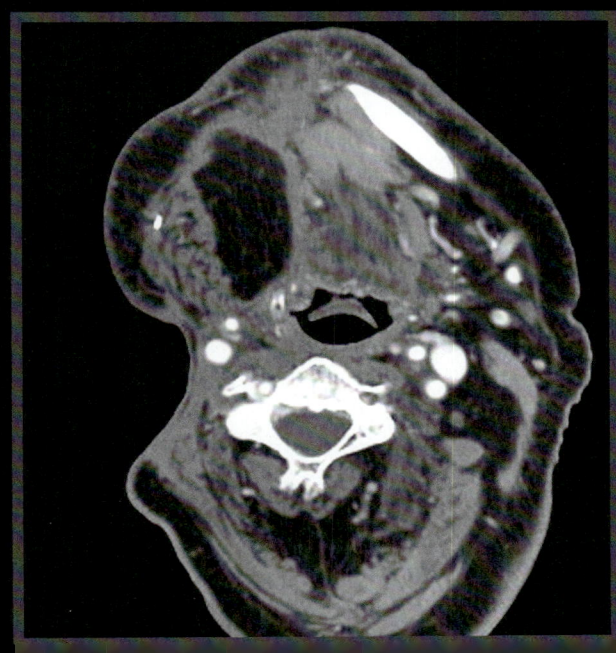

Postreatment Neck

TERMINOLOGY

- Neck dissection (ND) performed to treat or accurately stage head & neck cancer
- **Selective ND (SND)**: Resection of known or potential nodal levels while preserving nonlymphatic structures
  - **SND (I-III)**: Resection of nodes in levels I, II, III
  - **SND (II-IV)**: Resection of nodes in levels II-IV
  - **SND (II-V)**: Resection of nodes in levels II-V
  - **SND (VI)**: Resection of nodes in level VI only
- **Modified (radical) ND (MND)**: Nodal resection levels I-V + preservation ≥ 1 nonlymphatic structure [internal jugular vein (IJV), sternocleidomastoid muscle (SCM), or CNXI]
- **Radical ND (RND)**: Nodal resection levels I-V + IJV, SCM, & CNXI
- **Extended ND**: RND + removal of additional structures, such as internal carotid artery (ICA)

IMAGING

- Fibroadipose tissue resected with all NDs

- Imaging findings reflect different tissues resected
  - SND: Loss of fat around CS & beneath SCM; SCM "draped" over CS; IJV & SCM remain
  - MND: Loss of fat around CS; IJV or SCM resected
  - RND: Fibroadipose tissue removed around CS; IJV & SCM resected
- **Submandibular salivary gland** usually resected **with level IB** nodes in any nodal dissection in neck
- **Atrophy** of ipsilateral & hypertrophy of **contralateral trapezius/SCM** muscle seen in RND; may be present in MND or even SND
- Ipsilateral **levator scapulae** compensatory **hypertrophy**

CLINICAL ISSUES

- ND may be surgical standard of care even if staging CECT, PET/CECT, or MR do not show nodal metastases
- Physical exam for recurrent adenopathy after ND difficult due to scarring
- Imaging often only way to detect nodal recurrence

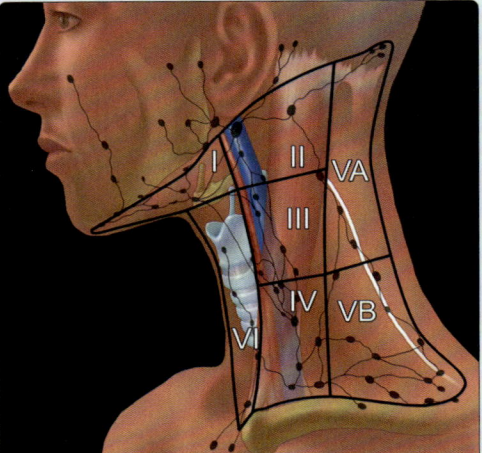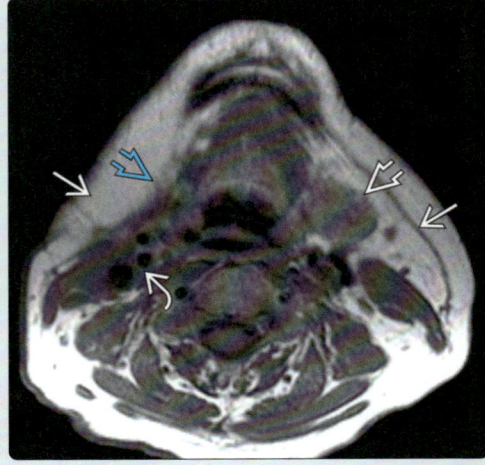

(Left) Graphic illustrates nodal levels that may be removed in different combinations as part of nodal neck dissections (ND), e.g., radical ND (RND) removes all groups & internal jugular vein (IJV), sternomastoid, & CNXI, but selective ND (SND) removes known or potential metastatic nodal groups only. (Right) Axial T1 MR in a patient with right SND shows subtle changes of loss of fat around the carotid space ➡ after nodal groups I-III resection. Note the normal left platysma muscle ➡ & submandibular salivary gland (SMG) ➡, absent on right ➡.

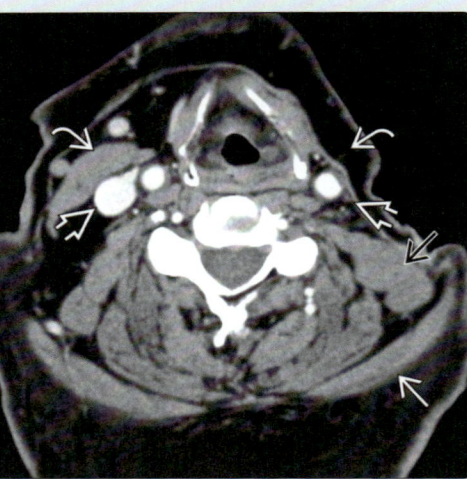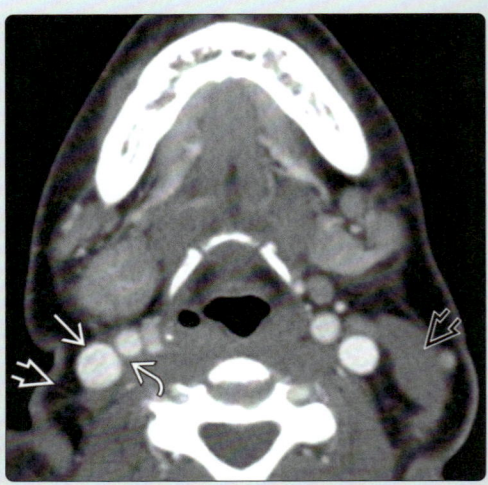

(Left) Axial CECT 8 months after left RND shows absence of the left SCM ➡ & IJV ➡. Note subtle left trapezius atrophy ➡ from CNXI resection with ipsilateral levator scapulae (LS) muscle (supplied by C3, 4, 5 nerves) compensatory hypertrophy ➡. Do not mistake LS as recurrent tumor. (Right) Axial CECT at the level of the hyoid bone reveals modified (radical) ND (MND) on the right level II with surgical resection of SCM ➡ but preservation of the IJV ➡. Subtle loss of fat planes around carotid space is visible ➡. Note normal left SCM ➡.

TERMINOLOGY

Abbreviations

- Neck dissection (ND)
  - Selective ND (SND); modified (radical) ND (MND)
  - Radical ND (RND); extended ND (END)

Synonyms

- Cervical lymph node dissection

Definitions

- **SND**
  - Most common surgical ND performed for head & neck cancer
  - Resection of known or potential nodal levels while preserving functional, nonlymphatic structures
    - **SND (I-III)**: Resection of levels I, II, III nodes (supraomohyoid SND)
      □ Performed in patients with oral cavity squamous cell carcinoma (SCCa)
      □ **Submandibular salivary gland** (SMG) usually **resected with level IB** nodes in any nodal dissection in neck
    - **SND (II-IV)**: Resection of levels II-IV nodes (lateral SND)
      □ Performed in patients with laryngeal & pharyngeal cancer
    - **SND (II-V)**: Resection of levels II-V nodes (posterolateral SND)
    - **SND (VI)**: Resection of level VI nodes only (central ND)
      □ Performed in patients with thyroid carcinoma
- **MND**
  - Resection of levels I-V nodes **&** preservation of ≥ 1 nonlymphatic structure [internal jugular vein (IJV), sternocleidomastoid muscle (SCM), or CNXI]
  - MND type I: Preserves 1 (CNXI)
  - MND type II: Preserves 2 (CNXI & IJV)
  - MND type III: Preserves all 3 (CNXI, IJV, & SCM)
- **RND**
  - Resection of levels I-V nodes **&** IJV, SCM, & CNXI
- **END**
  - RND + removal of additional structures like internal carotid artery (ICA)

IMAGING

General Features

- Best diagnostic clue
  - SND: Loss of fibroadipose tissue of carotid space (CS) & beneath SCM
  - MND: SND + absence of IJV or SCM or CNXI
  - RND: SND + absence of IJV & SCM
- Morphology
  - Contour change of neck from fibroadipose tissue resection
  - Imaging findings may be subtle after SND

CT Findings

- CECT
  - CECT findings depend on type of ND completed
  - **Loss of fat planes around CS & beneath SCM** present in all ND types
    - Fat plane loss secondary to removal of nodes embedded in fibroadipose tissue
  - **SND**: Findings may be **extremely subtle** on imaging
    - Loss of fat around CS & beneath SCM
    - SCM "draped" over CS
    - IJV & SCM remain, but CNXI denervation may be present (atrophy in SCM & trapezius)
    - SMG resected when level IB nodes involved
  - **MND**: IJV **or** SCM removed &/or CNXI
    - CS fibroadipose tissue gone
    - CNXI denervation may be present
  - **RND**: IJV, SCM, & CS fibroadipose tissue all removed
    - Trapezius muscle atrophy secondary to CNXI resection
    - **Compensatory levator scapulae (LS)** muscle **hypertrophy** after 3-6 months; supplied by cervical nerves (C3-C4) & dorsal scapular nerve (C5)

MR Findings

- Like CECT, MR findings reflect type of ND employed
  - Loss of fibroadipose tissue around CS best seen on T1WI
- CNXI denervation **atrophy of trapezius + SCM** & contralateral hypertrophy: RND (CNXI resection), MND (CNXI resection or injury), & **even SND** (CNXI injury)
  - Subacute denervation: Trapezius may enlarge & enhance
  - Chronic denervation: Trapezius fatty atrophy

Ultrasonographic Findings

- Grayscale ultrasound
  - Very high accuracy for detecting recurrent nodal disease when performed by experienced sonographer
  - US not as affected by fatty tissue absence as CECT
    - US better able to detect superficial nodal recurrence
  - Retropharyngeal nodes + level VII not imaged

Nuclear Medicine Findings

- PET/CT
  - Highly FDG-avid tissue suggests post-ND recurrence
  - **Acutely**, could be postsurgical inflammation, or hyperactive denervated ipsilateral trapezius/SCM
  - **Chronically**, asymmetric muscle uptake after ND due to compensatory ↑ normal muscular activity
  - Chronic CNXI denervation: Compensatory **contralateral** trapezius/SCM, & **ipsilateral** LS, rhomboid, & serratus anterior muscle hyperactivity
    - Look for ipsilateral trapezius/SCM atrophy on ND side

Imaging Recommendations

- Best imaging tool
  - CECT or PET/CECT
  - US followed by MR for thyroid carcinoma; CT may be done but can delay I-131 therapy by 6 weeks
- Protocol advice
  - CECT from skull base or through primary tumor to thoracic inlet; 10-cc contrast, 40-s delay
  - Adequate venous opacification essential to assess for IJV patency, if preserved with SND/MND

DIFFERENTIAL DIAGNOSIS

Denervation Atrophy CNXI

- Presence of fibroadipose tissue, IJV, & normal nodes, & no history of prior surgery

- Check jugular foramen for mass causing CNXI injury
  - **Jugular foramen (Vernet) syndrome**: Ipsilateral CNIX-XI symptoms & venous obstruction
    - Loss of gag reflex, ↓ posterior tongue sensations, ↓ parotid secretions (CNIX)
    - Vocal cord palsy initially, soft palate paralysis, & deviation of uvula to normal side later (CNX)
    - Weakness of SCM & trapezius muscles (CNXI)
  - Rarely isolated finding unless posttraumatic

PATHOLOGY

General Features
- Etiology
  - ND performed as treatment or staging for head & neck cancer; usually SCCa or differentiated thyroid carcinoma
  - SND may remove nodes in en bloc manner or piecemeal
  - RND & MND remove nodes in en bloc manner

Gross Pathologic & Surgical Features
- Fibroadipose tissue with nodes embedded within fat

Microscopic Features
- Nodes bisected to determine presence of tumor
- Pathologist determines presence of central nodal necrosis, extranodal tumor extension through nodal capsule, arterial invasion

CLINICAL ISSUES

Presentation
- Most common signs/symptoms
  - Neck scarred with loss of soft tissue volume
  - Physical exam to detect recurrent adenopathy difficult

Demographics
- Epidemiology
  - ND often surgical standard of care even if staging CECT or MR do not show nodal metastases
  - Depth of invasion (DOI), basic T-staging criterion for oral cavity SCCa in AJCC 8th edition, correlates well with nodal metastasis risk & locoregional recurrence
    - Nodal metastasis risk differs with subsite: At DOI 2-4 mm: 11% tongue SCCa, 42% floor of mouth SCCa
  - Oropharynx, supraglottic larynx, hypopharynx SCCa frequently associated with nodal metastases
    - ND or chemotherapy/radiation standard therapy
  - ND performed in more advanced-stage SCCa, either because of malignant nodes on staging CECT/MR or advanced stage
  - Upfront ND before chemoradiation in locally advanced head & neck SCCa: Better 2-year locoregional recurrence-free survival than without upfront ND (93.7% vs. 71%)
    - Typically treated with surgery or chemoradiation therapy & salvage surgery for residual disease
    - Salvage surgery after radiation difficult due to tissue fibrosis

Natural History & Prognosis
- SND by experienced surgeon removes most nodes at risk with less shoulder pain or cosmetic deformity

- Preservation of IJV important in case nodes recur in contralateral neck, & IJV resection is required because of extracapsular disease
- Loss of both IJVs undesirable → leads to venous collateral development, neck & face edema, & swelling

Treatment
- Options, risks, complications
  - **SND**
    - SND 1st-line surgery for uncomplicated nodal disease
    - Removes fewer nodes, but preservation of functional structures reduces morbidity
    - Reported as "SND (levels resected)"
    - **SND (I-III)**: Resection of levels I, II, III + SMG
      - For oral cavity SCCa
      - Previously called "supraomohyoid ND"
    - **SND (II-IV)**: Resection of levels II, III, IV only
      - Performed for all other subsites of neck SCCa that require treatment or accurate staging
      - Previously called "lateral ND"
    - **SND (VI)**: Resection of all level VI nodes
      - Nodes between carotids: Hyoid to sternal notch
      - Performed primarily for thyroid malignancy
      - Previously called "central compartment ND"
  - **MND**
    - When extracapsular extension involves SCM or IJV on CECT or MR
    - Attempt to reduce morbidity of RND by preserving functional structures
  - **RND**
    - When extensive extranodal tumor involves IJV or SCM
    - Marked chronic shoulder pain from CNXI loss is main disadvantage

DIAGNOSTIC CHECKLIST

Consider
- Previous ND if fibroadipose tissue, SCM, or IJV not present in patient with history of H&N cancer, especially SCCa

Image Interpretation Pearls
- Post-ND findings evident on CECT or MR but SND subtle
  - History of type of ND helpful for accurate reporting
- Important to detect recurrent nodes ipsilateral or contralateral to side of ND, **so look carefully**
  - After SND, recurrent nodes have ↓ conspicuity, as they may be isodense to SCM with no surrounding fat
    - Consider using PET/CECT or US in difficult cases
  - Recurrent ipsilateral metastatic adenopathy may occur in level IIB or high submuscular recess

Reporting Tips
- Report should include whether IJV, SCM, SMG, or fibroadipose tissue is present
- After SND, comment on opacification of IJV, as IJV thrombosis is undesired outcome of surgery

SELECTED REFERENCES

1. Okada T et al: Usefulness of upfront neck dissection before chemoradiation therapy for head and neck squamous cell carcinoma. In Vivo. 38(6):2804-11, 2024

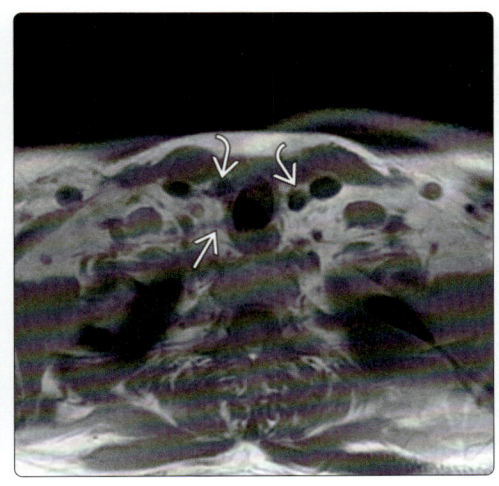

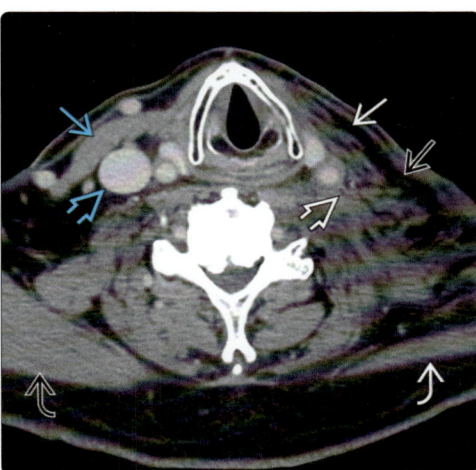

(Left) *Axial T1 MR post thyroidectomy & central compartment neck dissection shows very subtle postoperative changes of medialized common carotid arteries* ➡ *& subtle scarring in the remaining reduced peritracheal fat* ➡. **(Right)** *Axial CECT shows left RND with an absent SCM* ➡ *& IJV* ➡ *(see normal right SCM* ➡ *& IJV* ➡*). The ipsilateral trapezius is atrophic* ➡ *from CNXI resection, & the contralateral trapezius shows compensatory hypertrophy* ➡*. The pectoralis major flap* ➡ *covers the soft tissue defect.*

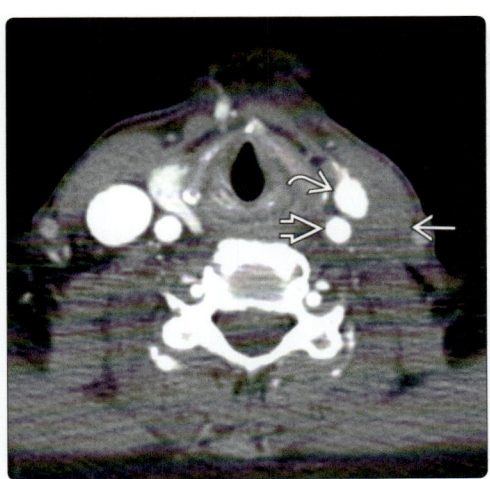

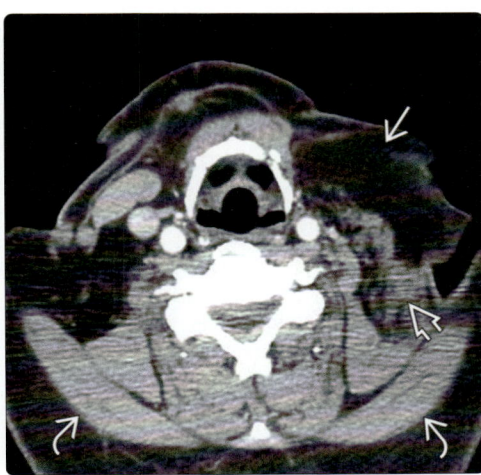

(Left) *Axial CECT shows typical SND findings on the left at level III. The SCM* ➡ *is draped over the common carotid artery* ➡ *& IJV* ➡ *with no fatty tissue beneath SCM. On the right, fat planes around carotid space are preserved. Note contour defect with flattening of the left neck.* **(Right)** *Axial CECT shows left MND with a pectoralis major myocutaneous flap filling the neck defect. The flap has fat* ➡ *& muscular components* ➡*. IJV & SCM were resected, but CNXI was preserved, resulting in symmetric trapezius muscles* ➡*.*

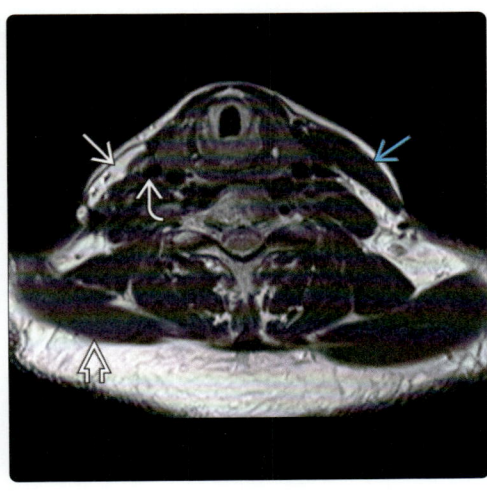

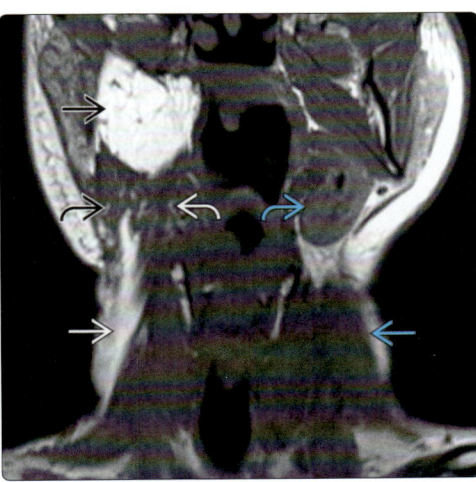

(Left) *Axial T2 MR in a patient with prior right buccal SCCa resection & right MND type II shows an absent right SCM* ➡ *(see normal left SCM* ➡*) but preserved right IJV* ➡*. The right trapezius muscle is atrophic* ➡ *due to CNXI injury during surgery (CNXI & IJV are supposed to be preserved in MND type II).* **(Right)** *Coronal T1 MR in the same patient shows an absent right SCM* ➡ *& SMG* ➡ *(see normal left SCM* ➡ *& SMG* ➡*). Note the right pectoralis major flap with T1 bright fat* ➡ *& isointense muscle* ➡*.*

TERMINOLOGY

- **Flap**: Tissue with intrinsic blood supply transferred from one part of body to another
- Soft tissue or autologous bone used to reconstruct postoperative resection defect in H&N
- **Fasciocutaneous flap**
  - Deep fascia, arterial perforators, & overlying skin
  - Used for smaller surgical reconstructions
  - Donor site radial forearm or anterolateral thigh
- **Myocutaneous flap**
  - Muscle, soft tissue, & skin
  - Used when large surgical defect requires greater tissue volume to fill
  - Donor site usually pectoralis major muscle
- **Osteocutaneous flap**
  - Bone, soft tissue, & overlying skin ± muscle
  - Used when surgical reconstruction requires bone replacement (mandible, maxilla, face)
  - Donor site usually fibula or scapula

IMAGING

- CECT/MR
  - Fasciocutaneous, small myocutaneous flaps: May look like normal soft tissue at surgical defect
  - Myocutaneous flap: Denervated at time of transfer to surgical defect; muscle in flap variable depending on time of imaging
  - Osteocutaneous flap: Bone contoured to approximate shape of excised bone
    - Pedicle ossification in 4-27% fibular free flaps

DIAGNOSTIC CHECKLIST

- Essential that history of flap reconstruction available when interpreting complex follow-up scans
  - Flap may be misinterpreted as recurrent tumor
- Look for new enhancing mass (CECT/MR) or hypermetabolic focus (PET) along deep aspect of flap between surgical defect & flap **at anastomotic site**

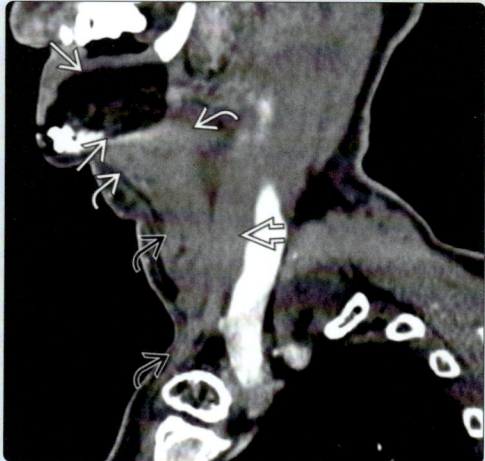
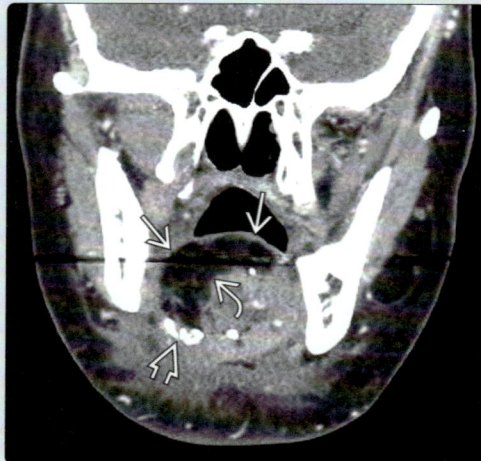

(Left) Sagittal oblique CECT shows a pectoralis major myocutaneous flap with fat superiorly ➡ & muscle inferiorly ➡ filling oral cavity surgical defect. The pectoralis muscle can be traced inferiorly towards its donor chest wall location ➡. Note normal sternocleidomastoid muscle ➡. (Right) Coronal CECT in a patient with fasciocutaneous radial forearm free flap reveals a fatty flap ➡ filling the oral cavity surgical defect, providing soft tissue to reform a smooth contour to the tongue surface ➡. Surgical clips ➡ are visible.

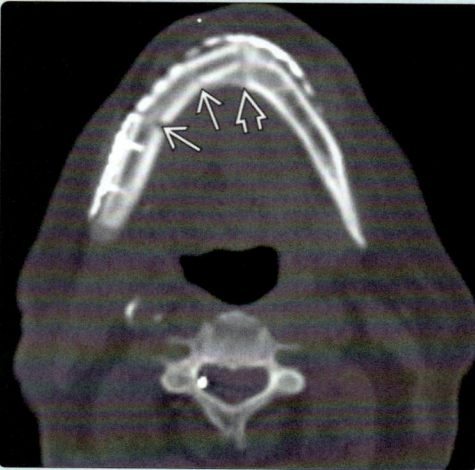
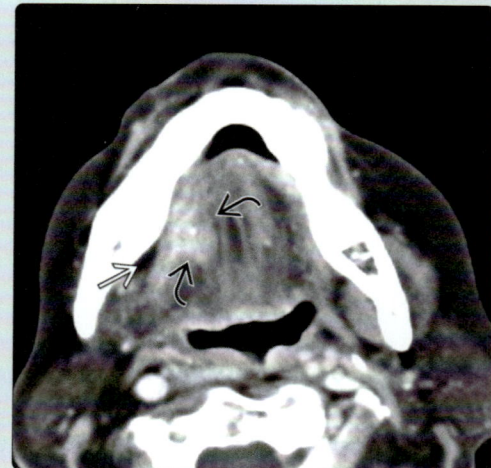

(Left) Axial bone CT shows an osteocutaneous fibular flap used to reconstruct the mandible following partial mandibulectomy. Note osteotomy defects ➡ that allow bone contouring. Donor bone-mandible interface ➡ is present in the midline. Pedicle ossification may be seen in 4-27% of fibular flaps. (Right) Axial CECT in a patient with surgical resection & facial artery myomucosal (FAMM) flap reconstruction ➡ for right lateral oral tongue SCCa shows recurrent tumor deep to the flap in the tongue & sublingual space ➡.

TERMINOLOGY

Definitions

- **Flaps**: Transferred tissue blocks **with own blood supply**
  - **Grafts**: Transferred tissue blocks that need angiogenesis
- Flaps transferred with intact vascular supply or reestablished using microvascular surgery at recipient surgical site
  - Major graft vasculature transected at donor site, & graft placed at recipient site inset without vascular anastomosis
- Flaps: Complex with different types of tissue
  - Grafts: Usually 1 or 2 tissue types
    - Autograft (from patient itself), allograft (from donor, cadaveric or living), alloplastic (man-made)
  - Types: **Skin grafts**, either split thickness (complete thickness epidermis & variable incomplete thickness of dermis) or full thickness (both epidermis & dermis completely), & **bone grafts**
- Flaps heal better & faster with less contracture than grafts
- **Flap**: Tissue with intrinsic blood supply transferred from one part of body to another
- Consists of entire thickness of skin & variable amount of subcutaneous tissue
  - Soft tissue ± muscle ± bone surgical site reconstruction
- Flaps mostly used to reconstruct tumor resection cavity
  - Also to repair posttraumatic defects in H&N
  - Osteocutaneous flap may be used to repair mandibular or maxillary osteonecrosis

Flap Nomenclature

- **According to blood supply**: Random/axial flaps & pedicled/free flaps
- **Random flap**: Supplied by vessels of dermal & subdermal plexus, not supplied by distinct named vessel
  - Contain only skin &/or subcutaneous tissue
- **Axial flap**: Regional areas supplied by specific arteriovenous system (angiosome concept) oriented along axis of flap
  - Can be pedicled, used regionally, or as distant free flap
  - May contain skin, subcutaneous tissue, muscle, &/or bone
- **Pedicled flap**: Blood supply connected anatomically throughout flap; can be distant pedicled flaps also
  - **Submandibular salivary gland flap**: Do not mistake enhancing normal submandibular salivary gland for recurrent/residual tumor at flap site
- **Free tissue transfer (free flap)**: Artery & at least one vein disconnected during transfer
  - Microsurgically reconnected to new artery & vein at recipient site
  - **Perforator flap**: Special type of free flap containing transmuscular &/or transfascial vascular "leash" or pedicle leading to overlying fascia &/or skin only
    - Muscle left behind by dissecting vessels out of muscle, which they perforate
    - ↓ morbidity associated with musculocutaneous flaps
- **According to location: Local, regional, & distant flaps**
- **Local flap**: Use tissue abutting surgical defect: Vasculature preserved

- **Regional flap**: Flap located near defect but not abutting it: Vasculature preserved
  - Pedicled flap with blood supply from same anatomic area of defect
- **Distant flap**: Flap harvested from different part of body: Vasculature transferred & anastomosed
- **According to configuration: Bilobed, rhombic, & Z-plasty**
- **According to tissue content: Cutaneous, fasciocutaneous, myocutaneous, & osteocutaneous**
- **Fasciocutaneous flap**: Constructed of deep **fascia** with its overlying skin
  - Used for smaller surgical reconstructions in H&N
  - Allows harvesting of fasciocutaneous arterial perforators that pass along fascial septa between adjacent muscles
  - Results in larger flap size survival at reconstruction site
  - Sensory cutaneous nerves also harvested when sensory reinnervation desired
  - Donor sites: Radial forearm, lateral arm, temporoparietal, rectus, latissimus dorsi, or anterolateral thigh
- **Myocutaneous flap**: Constructed with **muscle**, soft tissue, & overlying skin
  - Used when larger reconstruction site needs more volume (by muscle) to adequately fill surgical defect
  - Donor sites include pectoralis major, rectus abdominis, or latissimus dorsi muscles
- **Osteocutaneous flap**: Constructed with **bone**, soft tissue, & overlying skin ± muscle
  - a.k.a. **composite** flap
  - Used when reconstruction requires bone replacement
  - Primarily employed in oral cavity squamous cell carcinoma (SCCa) reconstructions
  - Portion of mandible or maxilla removed during tumor treatment surgery
  - Muscle added to osteocutaneous flap if more volume needed for larger surgical defects
  - Donor site usually fibula or scapula

IMAGING

General Features

- Best diagnostic clue
  - Soft tissue or bone present in reconstruction site with **nonanatomic** appearance

CT Findings

- CECT
  - Fasciocutaneous or small myocutaneous flaps
    - May look like normal soft tissue at surgical defect
  - Larger fasciocutaneous, myocutaneous, or osteocutaneous flaps
    - Have **nonanatomic** appearance at surgical defect
    - Muscle portion of myocutaneous flaps denervated at time of transfer to surgical defect
      - □ < 6 weeks: May swell & enhance
      - □ > 6 weeks: Shrinkage & fatty infiltrate
    - Osteocutaneous flaps with bone used for mandible, maxilla, orbital wall reconstruction
      - □ Contoured to approximate normal shape of jaw or orbital wall
    - **Pedicle ossification** in 4-27% of osteocutaneous **fibular** free flap reconstruction

□ Benign finding, does not compromise flap
□ Usually asymptomatic, rarely trismus, or painful neck swelling
○ When looking for **recurrence** in patient with flap
– Carefully inspect interface between surgical defect & flap **at anastomotic site**
□ Most common site of SCCa recurrence
– Focal mass-like enhancement: Likely recurrent tumor
– Check for change in bony component or new erosion
– Carefully assess bilaterally for new cervical nodal mets
• Bone CT
○ Bony portion of flap often contoured to approximate resection site
○ Oral cavity mandible & maxilla most common sites where osteocutaneous flap used
○ Interface between native bone & flap = common site of recurrent tumor

MR Findings

• T1WI
○ Signal intensity of flap depends on type of flap used
– Soft tissue fat (high signal)
– Muscle (intermediate signal)
– Bone (low-signal cortex, high-signal marrow)
• T2WI
○ Muscle portion of flap
– < 6 weeks: Slightly ↑ T2 as denervated at surgery
– > 6 weeks: Intermediate to low signal as muscles scar & fat atrophies
○ Postoperative fibrosis usually low signal
– Fibrosis retracts over time
• T1WI C+
○ Muscle portion of flap
– < 6 weeks: Muscle may swell & enhance
– After 6 weeks: Chronic changes are seen
○ Focal area of mass-like enhancement suspicious for recurrent tumor

Imaging Recommendations

• Best imaging tool
○ PET combined with CECT best imaging study for assessing SCCa flap recurrence
– PET offers physiologic function
□ New nodal recurrence or distant mets have ↑ FDG update
□ Beware: Surgically denervated muscle can have ↑ uptake initially
– CECT best shows new mass or bone destruction at primary site

DIFFERENTIAL DIAGNOSIS

Recurrent SCCa in Reconstruction Flap

• Usually presents with pain or new mass at surgical site months after surgery
○ Neurogenic pain usually implies perineural tumor spread
• Occurs at **anastomotic site** between surgical bed & flap; interface between native bone & flap

Postoperative Infection or Abscess

• Presents after surgery with fever, pain, & surgical site induration days to weeks after surgery

• When rim-enhancing lesion seen immediately after surgery, abscess more likely than tumor recurrence
• Found at surgical site with marked homogeneous (phlegmon) or rim (abscess) enhancement

PATHOLOGY

General Features

• Etiology
○ Surgical defect may be extensive, but only part of cavity may require flap

CLINICAL ISSUES

Presentation

• Most common signs/symptoms
○ Follow-up imaging for recurrence triggered by **pain** or **mass** at surgical site
○ Deep pain without clinical mass suggests recurrence deep to flap or perineural tumor

Demographics

• Age: Most commonly adults with H&N SCCa

Natural History & Prognosis

• Depends on reason for flap transfer
• Expected survival from tumor determines prognosis
• Overall survival rates poor, as flap reconstructions undertaken in late-stage SCCa
○ ~ 50% 2-year, 30% 5-year survival reported in large series

DIAGNOSTIC CHECKLIST

Consider

• Reconstruction flap has nonanatomic appearance (fat, muscle, or bone in defect)
• Initial **baseline PET/CECT** after treatment changes resolve
○ Best acquired 3 months after surgery/end of radiation
• Surveillance CECT in patients post flap

Image Interpretation Pearls

• Essential that flap reconstruction history available when interpreting complex follow-up CECT
○ Anatomic distortion makes scan interpretation challenging
○ Flap may be misinterpreted as recurrent tumor
• Recurrent tumor often occurs at recipient bed **anastomotic site** where flap placed in surgical defect
○ Look for **new enhancing mass** on CECT in fatty portion of flap
– Also look for metastatic cervical adenopathy
○ PET/CT shows recurrent tumor & metastatic cervical adenopathy as high-intensity foci

Reporting Tips

• First describe surgical defect, followed by flap composition: Soft tissue & fat ± muscle &/or bone
• Finally, report surgical site or nodal recurrence if present

SELECTED REFERENCES

1. Farsi S et al: Outcomes of free flap reconstruction for mandibular ORN: systematic review and meta-analysis. Am J Otolaryngol. 46(1):104508, 2025
2. Iwai T et al: Intraoral approach for oral floor reconstruction with the submandibular gland flap. J Dent Sci. 19(1):656-8, 2024

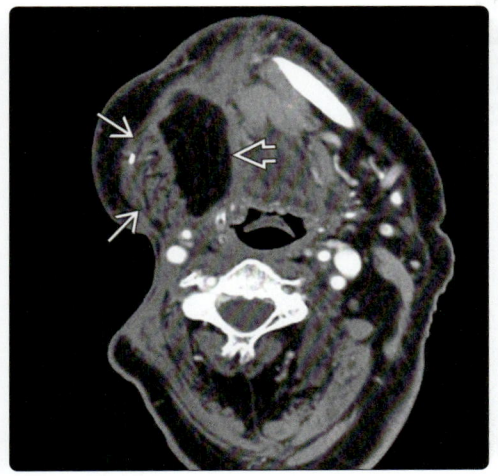
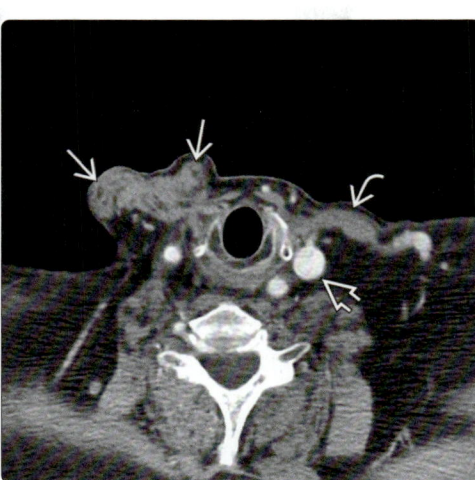

(Left) Axial CECT in a patient with a pectoralis rotational myocutaneous flap following resection of a large retromolar trigone SCCa shows a medial hypodense fat component of the flap ➡ & a lateral striated pectoralis muscle component of the flap ➡. (Right) Axial CECT in the low neck in the same patient shows the flap ➡ coming up from the chest. The normal left internal jugular vein (IJV) ➡ & sternocleidomastoid muscle ➡ are not seen on the right, as the right radical neck dissection was performed as part of the surgical procedure.

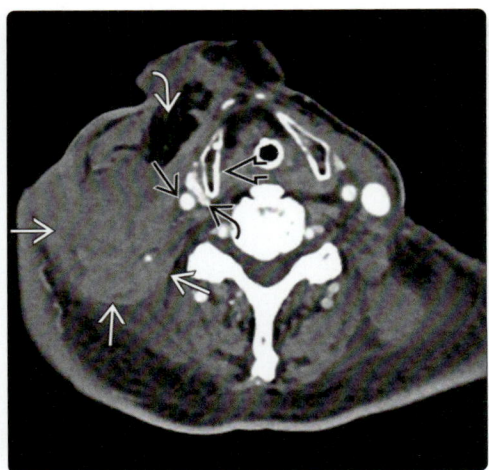
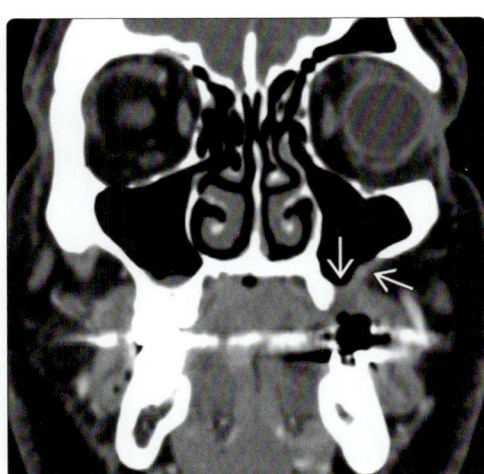

(Left) Axial CECT in a patient with a right pectoralis major myocutaneous flap shows complication by a large flap hematoma ➡. Note part of the fatty component of the flap anteriorly ➡. Right common carotid artery ➡, right lobe of thyroid gland ➡, & thyroid cartilage/larynx ➡ are displaced medially. Right IJV was removed at modified radical neck dissection and is not seen. (Right) Coronal CECT shows surgical repair of an iatrogenic left oroantral fistula (following dental extraction) using full-thickness buccal advancement flap ➡.

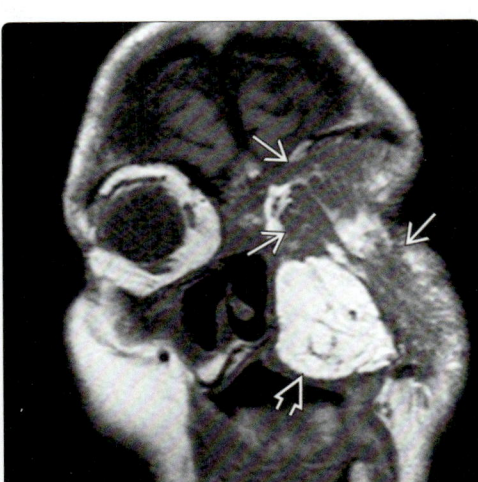
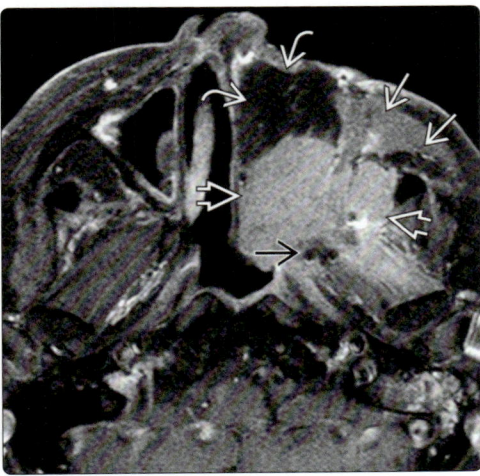

(Left) Coronal T1WI MR shows a typical rectus abdominis myocutaneous flap ➡. Striated, denervated muscular component of free flap fills orbital exenteration defect. Note the fat component ➡, providing further volume to fill the maxillary & left nasal cavity defect. (Right) Axial T1 C+ FS MR (same patient) 18 months later, now with face pain, shows a large, enhancing mass ➡ adjacent to surgical clips ➡. The mass is deep to fatty ➡ & muscular ➡ flap components. This is recurrent SCCa, which typically occurs at anastomotic site.

Expected Changes of Neck Radiation Therapy

IMAGING

- **Early (1-4 months)**: Diffuse edema of all tissues
  - Reticulation of subcutaneous and deep fat planes
  - Thickening and enhancement of mucosa
  - Swollen, ill-defined, enhancing parotid and submandibular glands
  - Subtly swollen muscles, especially pterygoids
- **Late (≥ 12 months)**: Diffuse fibrosis of all tissues
  - Edema and reticulation of fat resolves
  - Mucosal thickening and enhancement may resolve
  - Glandular atrophy but can maintain ↑ enhancement
  - Lymph nodes and lymphoid tissues atrophy
- **MR**: T2 and T1 C+ accentuate changes seen on CECT
  - Marked T2 intensity and enhancement
- **PET/CT**: No high focal uptake unless complication of radiation therapy, infection, or residual/recurrent tumor
- May show asymmetric high FDG uptake on uninvolved area due to ↑ muscular activity with atrophy on side of radiation

TOP DIFFERENTIAL DIAGNOSES

- Retropharyngeal space edema
- Retropharyngeal space abscess
- Acute parotitis
- Submandibular gland sialadenitis
- Superior cervical ganglion vs. retropharyngeal lymph node

PATHOLOGY

- XRT destroys endothelial cells lining small vessels
  - **Early**: Results in ischemia, edema, inflammation
  - **Late**: Results in tissue fibrosis

DIAGNOSTIC CHECKLIST

- 1st post-XRT imaging should be 10-12 weeks after end of treatment
- Careful, systematic imaging evaluation is key
- Severe XRT changes make evaluating scan difficult
  - Residual or recurrent tumor may be easily missed
  - Focal nodular enhancing mass suggests tumor

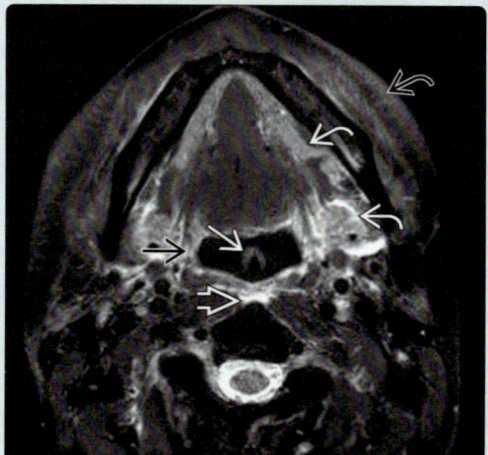
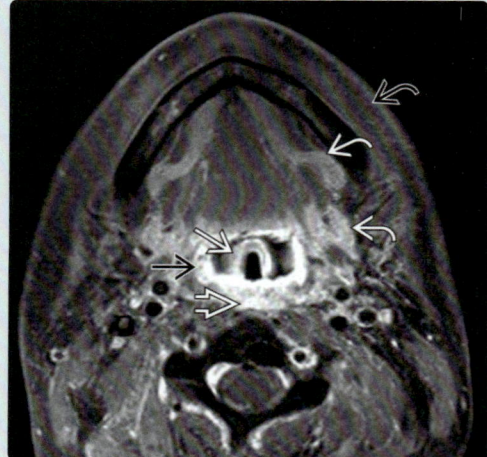

(Left) *Axial T2 FS MR shows expected postradiation baseline appearance at 12 weeks with edema of nearly all of the visible tissues in the neck. There is skin thickening & stranding or "reticulation" of subcutaneous fat ➡. Note edematous, hyperintense pharyngeal mucosa ➡ & epiglottis ➡ with edema fluid in retropharyngeal space (RPS) ➡. Salivary glands ➡ are hyperintense.* (Right) *Axial T1 C+ FS MR in the same patient shows enhancement of fat ➡, pharyngeal mucosa ➡, the epiglottis ➡, RPS ➡, & salivary glands ➡.*

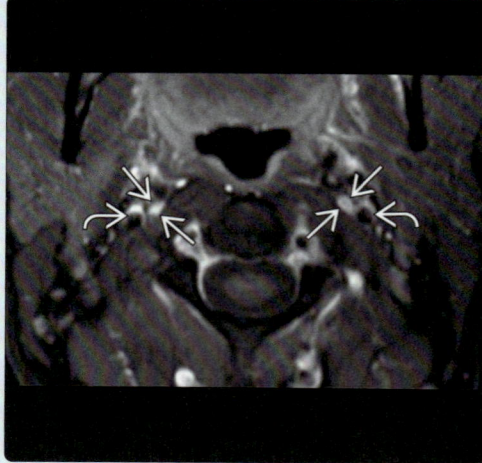
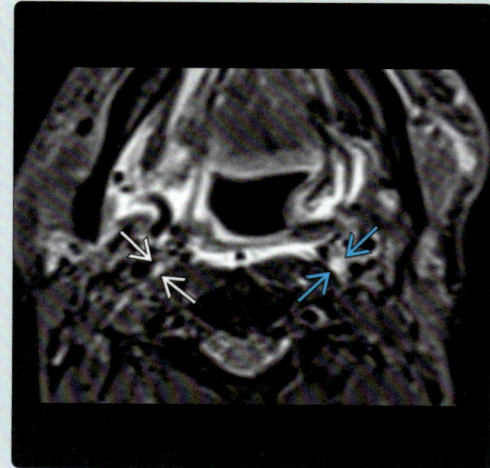

(Left) *Axial T1 C+ MR shows normal superior cervical ganglion (SCG) ➡ at C2-3 level, medial to internal carotid artery ➡, anterior to prevertebral space, & posterolateral to RPS. Note central black dot (cluster of nerve fibers) in SCG. Coronal & sagittal images would show the black dot as vertically oriented along the SCG & the SCG to have tapered upper & lower margins.* (Right) *Axial STIR MR shows a normal T2-hyperintense right ➡ & enlarged brighter left ➡ SCG after chemoradiotherapy for left pharyngeal SCCa.*

Expected Changes of Neck Radiation Therapy

TERMINOLOGY

Abbreviations
- Radiation therapy (XRT)
- Intensity-modulated radiation therapy (IMRT)
  - Reduces radiation dose to uninvolved surrounding tissues & organs

Definitions
- Expected changes in imaging appearances of neck following XRT

IMAGING

General Features
- Best diagnostic clue
  - **Early**: Diffuse edema of all soft tissues of superficial & deep face & neck
    - Tissues appear diffusely "angry"
  - **Late**: Generalized atrophy of all radiated soft tissues & glands

CT Findings
- CECT
  - **Early (1-4 months)**: Diffuse edema of all tissues of neck
    - Thickened skin & platysma
    - Reticulation of subcutaneous & deep fat planes
      - Edema along fascial planes, such as carotid sheath & retropharyngeal space (RPS)
      - Edema of preepiglottic, paraglottic, & parapharyngeal fat
    - Diffuse thickening & enhancement of mucosa, prominent submucosal edema
      - Thickened posterior pharyngeal wall
    - Swollen, ill-defined parotid & submandibular glands (SMGs)
      - Glands usually enhance robustly after XRT
    - Subtly swollen muscles, especially pterygoids
  - **Late (≥ 12 months)**: Diffuse fibrosis of all tissues of neck
    - Edema & reticulation of fat resolves
    - Concave contour of external neck
    - Thinning of subcutaneous & deep fat planes
    - Mucosal thickening & enhancement may resolve
      - Subglottic thickening to 2 mm is common
    - Aryepiglottic (AE) fold & paralaryngeal fat edema remains in ~ 2/3 of patients
    - Retropharyngeal edema resolves by 12 months in 1/3 of patients
    - Glandular tissues (submandibular, parotid, thyroid) atrophy but can maintain increased enhancement
    - Lymph nodes & lymphoid tissues atrophy

MR Findings
- T2 & T1 C+ accentuate changes seen on CECT
  - MR has greater sensitivity to soft tissue inflammation & contrast enhancement
- Early: Extensive T2 hyperintensity & enhancement of most tissues
  - Neck appears "watery" & diffusely inflamed
    - Symmetric T2 hyperintensity & thickening of platysma, reticulation of subcutaneous & deep fat
    - Linear, hyperintense retropharyngeal edema
  - Muscles may show T2 hyperintensity
  - Symmetric, diffuse enhancement of mucosa
  - Increased enhancement of salivary glands
- Late: Most soft tissues return to near-normal signal but appear atrophic
  - Timeline for tissue normalization not defined but likely takes longer than CECT
  - Decrease in enhancement of mucosal & glandular tissues
- T1-hyperintense fatty marrow of cervical vertebrae & skull base
- **Superior cervical ganglion** at C2-3 level (retropharyngeal lymph node mimic): Cross-sectional area (CSA), T2 signal, & ADC of superior cervical ganglion (SCG) ↑ until 1 year → then stable on longer follow-up
- DWI: Benign post-XRT changes mean ADC > 1.3×10^{-3}
  - Always correlate morphologic imaging with physiologic DWI/ADC maps, as overlap exists between benign tissue & recurrent tumor
- Dynamic postcontrast perfusion MR time-intensity curve (TIC): Change from pretreatment rapid rise & slow wash-out → posttreatment slow rise & gradual trapping (wash-in)
  - Posttreatment vascular fenestration functional changes

Nuclear Medicine Findings
- PET/CT
  - No high focal FDG uptake unless complication of radiation therapy, infection, or residual/recurrent tumor
  - Negative predictive value for pathology-proven residual tumor of FGD-PET/CT 3 months after (chemo)radiotherapy for head & neck squamous cell carcinoma ~ 97.5%
    - Spares salvage neck dissection considerably more compared to MR + US-FNA
    - Positive predictive of FDG-PET/CT for detecting pathology-proven residual tumor around 89% compared to only 65% for MR + US-FNA
  - May show high FDG uptake only on uninvolved normal areas due to ↑ muscular activity (as in contralateral hemitongue) with atrophy of radiation site
    - Often compounded by prior surgical resection
    - ↑ uptake especially marked in fasciculating residual muscles after oral cavity/tongue resection
  - Recent research in mice suggests (4S)-4-[3-(18F) fluoropropyl]-L-glutamate [(18F) FSPG] PET as sensitive early marker of response to radiation therapy
    - Tumor retention of (18F) FSPG halved in 7 days after starting treatment, well before radiotherapy-induced tumor shrinkage began

Imaging Recommendations
- Best imaging tool
  - Post-XRT appearance readily identifiable on CT/MR
- Protocol advice
  - CECT: ≥ 90-second imaging after contrast to allow mucosal enhancement & ↑ conspicuity of residual/recurrent mass
  - MR: Fat saturation added to T2 & T1 C+ aids delineation of changes
    - DWI may detect highly cellular tumor recurrence
  - PET/CECT: Complementary to add specificity for differentiating nonneoplastic change from residual/recurrent tumor

– PET/MR improve imaging of skull base/sinus/suprahyoid neck XRT-treated tumor beds

DIFFERENTIAL DIAGNOSIS

Retropharyngeal Space Edema

- RPS edema, including radiation, jugular vein thrombosis, & pharyngeal infection
- No enhancement of fluid or rim

Retropharyngeal Space Abscess

- Defined pus collection in RPS with local mass effect
- Typically lenticular & rim enhancing
- May be associated with narrowing of internal carotid artery (ICA)

Acute Parotitis

- Inflammation of gland often with extensive facial cellulitis
- Typically unilateral; ± calculus

Submandibular Gland Sialadenitis

- Inflammation of submandibular gland (SMG) often associated with calculi
- Typically unilateral with dilated SMG duct

Superior Cervical Ganglion vs. Retropharyngeal Lymph Node

- Superior cervical ganglion (SCG) located at C2-3 level anterior to prevertebral space & posterolateral to RPS
  o Adjacent to ICA, usually (not always) medial to ICA due to ICA tortuosity
  o Anteromedial to ICA (55%), posterolateral to ICA (19%), posteromedial to ICA (10%), & posterior, medial, & anterior to ICA sporadically
- Can be mistaken for retropharyngeal lymphadenopathy
- Fat signal may be seen within SCG in 13% of patients
- SCG seen as oval, enhancing, small (mean CSA: 17.7 mm²) soft tissue with **central black dot** (cluster of nerve fibers) in axial thin postcontrast VIBE & T2 MR
- Coronal & sagittal images show black dot to be actually vertically oriented, wire-like structure passing along central long axis of SCG
- On coronal images, SCG has tapered upper & lower margins
- ADC higher in SCG than in lymph nodes
- **After radiotherapy**: CSA, T2 signal, & ADC of SCG ↑ until 1 year → then stable on longer follow-up MR
  o Apparently due to SCG Schwann cell proliferation &/or perineurial & epineurial thickening

PATHOLOGY

General Features

- Etiology
  o XRT destroys endothelial cells lining small blood vessels
    – **Early**: Results in ischemia, edema, inflammation
    – **Late**: Results in tissue fibrosis
    – Tissues ill-equipped to deal with extreme stressors → XRT complications
    – IMRT goal: Reduce XRT complications in normal tissue surrounding tumor bed
- Associated abnormalities
  o Chemotherapy may be given concurrently to sensitize tissues to XRT

– Increases severity of acute side effects
– Probably increases frequency of late effects
– Improves overall treatment outcome

Microscopic Features

- Histological changes in neck & larynx have been defined
- **Connective tissues (CTs)**
  o Within 2-12 days: Acute inflammatory reaction
  o Within 1-4 months: Inflammatory CT thickening
  o At 8 months: CT fibrosis
- **Muscles**
  o Within 1-4 months: Only minimal abnormalities
  o At 8 months: Waxy degeneration & atrophy
    – Muscle fibers replaced by scar tissue & fat
- **Epithelium**
  o Within 2-12 days: Damage to respiratory epithelium
  o At 8 months: Squamous metaplasia of columnar cells
- **Laryngeal cartilages**
  o Within 2-12 days: Little response as largely hypocellular
  o Within 1-4 months: Mild loss of chondrocytes, giant cells
  o At 8 months: Variable thickening & fibrosis of perichondrium
    – Perichondrium is nutrient source to cartilage
  o Resolution of sclerosis of cartilage abutting tumor correlates with local control
    – Converse is not true; ongoing sclerosis may be evident with no evidence of disease

CLINICAL ISSUES

Presentation

- Most common signs/symptoms
  o Oral pain from mucosal inflammation
    – Reduced saliva flow compounds this
  o Myositis of masticator space → trismus
    – May occur early with myositis or late with fibrosis
  o Glandular atrophy
    – Parotid & SMG atrophy → xerostomia
    – Thyroid atrophy → hypothyroidism; may be subclinical
      □ Seen in 26-48% of H&N squamous cell carcinoma

DIAGNOSTIC CHECKLIST

Image Interpretation Pearls

- 1st post-XRT imaging 10-12 weeks after end of treatment

Reporting Tips

- Image review requires careful, systematic evaluation
  o Look for focal thickening of mucosa or solid neck mass to suggest residual or recurrent tumor/nodes
    – Evaluate specifically along jugular chains, submandibular space, & posterior triangle
  o More focal inflammatory changes suggest secondary infection or other complication

SELECTED REFERENCES

1. Navran A et al: FGD-PET/CT three months after (chemo)radiotherapy for head and neck squamous cell carcinoma spares considerable number of patients from a salvage neck dissection. Radiother Oncol. 198:110407, 2024
2. Sambasivan K et al: [18F]FSPG-PET provides an early marker of radiotherapy response in head and neck squamous cell cancer. Npj Imaging. 2(1):28, 2024
3. El Beltagi AH et al: Functional magnetic resonance imaging of head and neck cancer: performance and potential. Neuroradiol J. 32(1):36-52, 2019

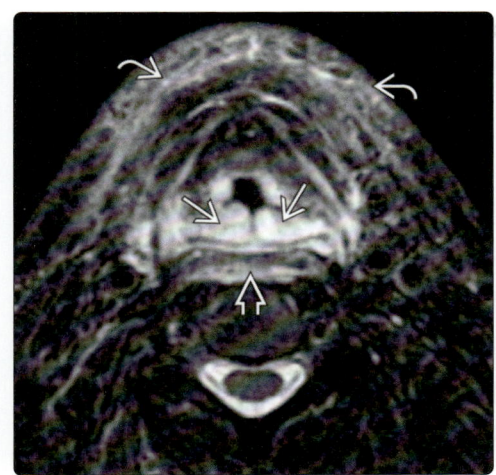

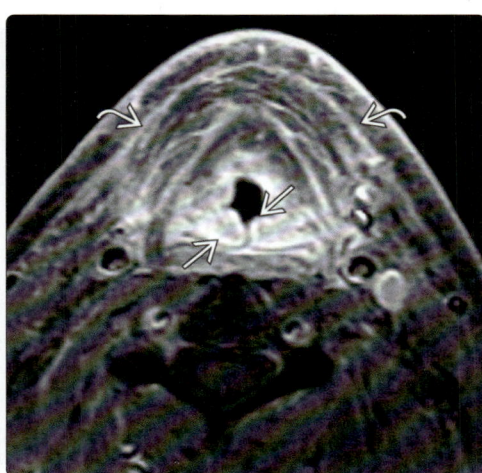

(Left) *Axial T2 FS MR 8 weeks after chemoradiation shows expected changes with hazy, hyperintense edema of subcutaneous ➡ and deep fat. Note the retropharyngeal edema ➡. Both aryepiglottic (AE) folds ➡ are swollen and diffusely hyperintense because of edema.* (Right) *Axial T1 C+ FS MR in the same patient shows extensive enhancement of edematous tissues, particularly thickened skin & platysma muscles ➡, & also smooth linear enhancement of AE fold mucosa ➡. MR shows enhancing submucosa not seen on CECT.*

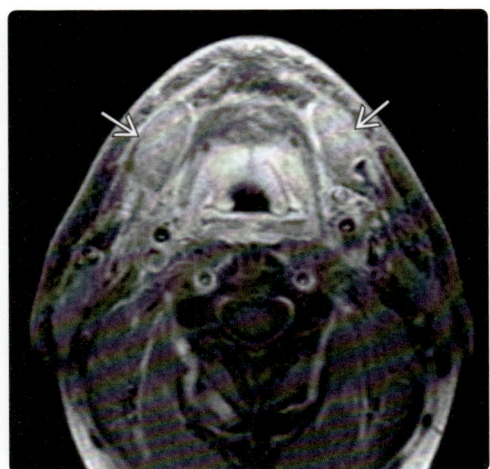

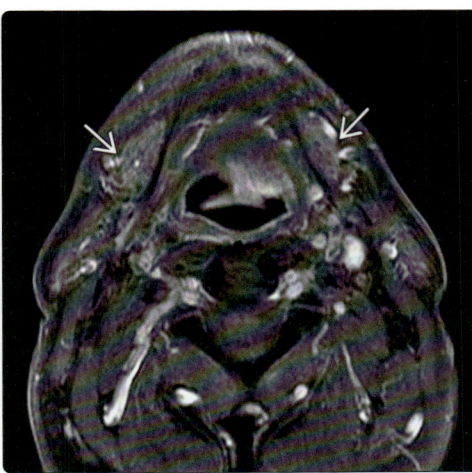

(Left) *Axial T1 C+ FS MR 8 weeks after chemoradiation reveals marked enhancement & thickening of the pharynx & enhancement of deep and subcutaneous fat. Submandibular glands (SMGs) ➡ are swollen and enhancing heterogeneously.* (Right) *Axial T1 C+ FS MR in the same patient 18 months later shows resolution of the diffuse neck XRT changes with a decrease in the enhancement & size of SMGs ➡ due to chronic radiation-induced sialadenitis. Glandular tissues atrophy but can maintain increased enhancement.*

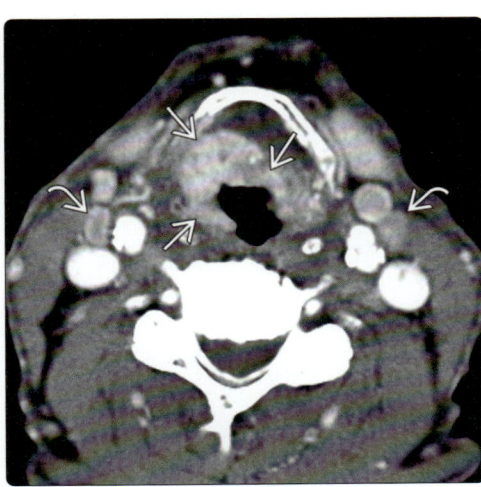

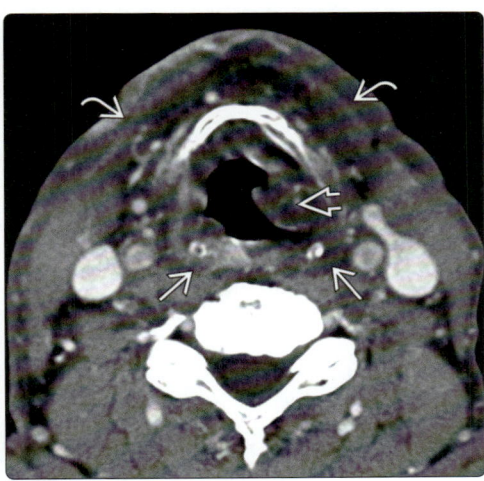

(Left) *Axial CECT shows supraglottic SCCa with an enhancing mass ➡ at the base of the epiglottis, AE fold, & pre- & paraglottic fat. Note bilateral pathologic nodes ➡.* (Right) *Axial CECT in the same patient 3 months following chemoXRT shows no residual enhancing tumor or nodes. All fat planes & submucosal tissues, including left AE fold ➡, are edematous with hazy density. Note retropharyngeal ➡ edema as well as thickened skin and platysma muscles ➡. These are expected posttreatment changes.*

KEY FACTS

TERMINOLOGY

- Uncommon, unintended side effects from radiation therapy (XRT) seen in small proportion of patients

IMAGING

- Potentially involves any radiated neck tissue
  - Excessive inflammation, tissue necrosis, or tumor induction
- CT or MR may be complementary for detection and characterization of abnormality
- CECT typically 1st-order examination; evaluates soft tissues and bones
  - Mucosal ulceration and fistulae, myositis, osteoradionecrosis, chondronecrosis
- MR best for nervous system complications
  - Cerebral radionecrosis, myelopathy, brachial plexitis, cranial neuropathy
- PET may be misleading; intense focal FDG uptake common

TOP DIFFERENTIAL DIAGNOSES

- Recurrent tumor
- Skull base or mandible-maxilla osteomyelitis

PATHOLOGY

- XRT results in obstructive arteriopathy
- Tissues less able to withstand additional stress
- Infection, tumor recurrence, or biopsy may precipitate necrosis

CLINICAL ISSUES

- Uncommon; ~ 1% of patients receiving neck XRT
- Most complications occur ≤ 2 years after XRT
- May occur up to 5-8 years post XRT
- Treatment largely conservative

DIAGNOSTIC CHECKLIST

- Key differential always residual/recurrent tumor
- Look for solid, enhancing mass

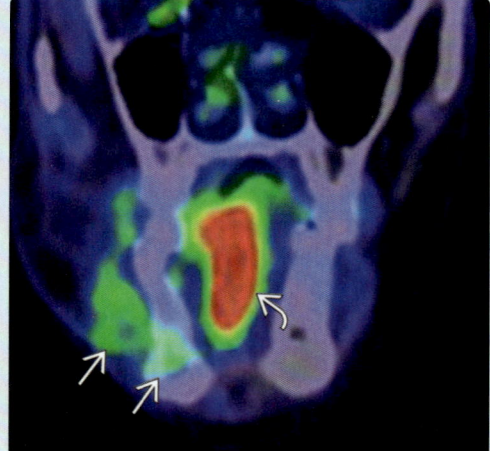
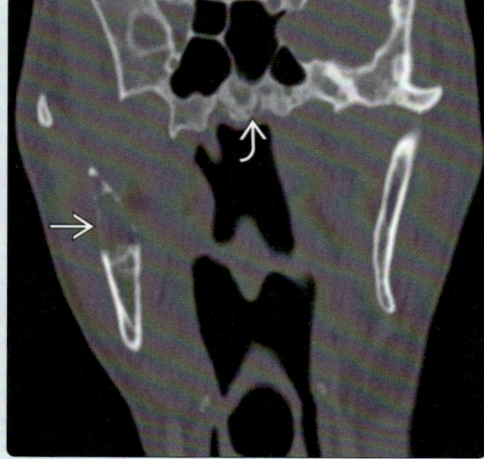

(Left) Coronal fused F-18 FDG PET/CT in a patient with recent chemoradiation for mandibular squamous cell carcinoma (SCCa) ➡ shows radiation-induced right hypoglossal nerve distribution acute denervation changes with intense FDG uptake in right hemitongue ➡. (Right) Bone CT in a patient with history of chemoradiation for right-sided nasopharyngeal carcinoma (NPCa) with skull base invasion shows mixed lytic-sclerotic changes of osteoradionecrosis (ORN) in the right mandible ➡ and skull base ➡.

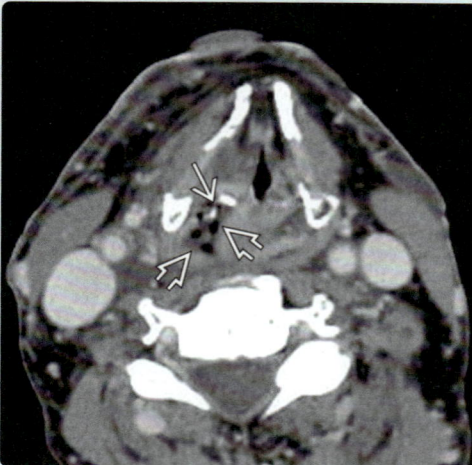
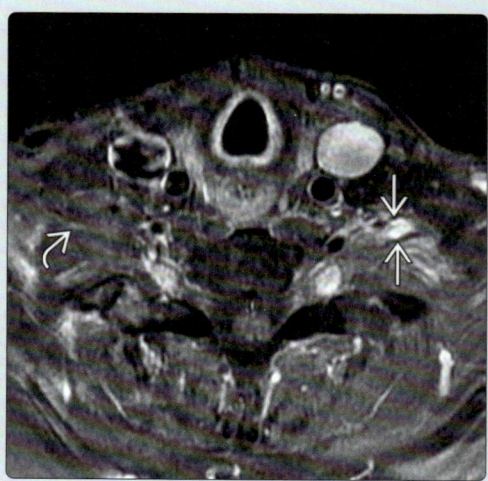

(Left) Axial CECT 4 months after radiotherapy for hypopharynx SCCa shows air and necrotic debris ➡ with soft tissue swelling posterior to right cricoarytenoid joint. Arytenoid cartilage ➡ appears fragmented from chondronecrosis. (Right) Axial T1 C+ FS MR in a patient with left arm weakness 3 years after chemoradiation for left-sided tongue base SCCa shows enlarged, enhancing left brachial plexus nerve roots ➡ compared to the right ➡, consistent with radiation-induced brachial plexopathy.

Complications of Neck Radiation Therapy

TERMINOLOGY

Definitions

- Uncommon, unintended side effects from radiation therapy (XRT) seen in small proportion of patients

IMAGING

General Features

- Best diagnostic clue
  - No single diagnostic feature, as this potentially involves **any radiated tissue** in neck and may have marked inflammation, tissue necrosis, or tumor induction
    - **Tissue necrosis**: Soft tissue, muscle, cartilage, bone, and brain parenchyma
    - **Marked inflammation**: Brachial plexus, cervical cord, and cranial nerves, including optic nerve, muscles
    - **Radiation arteriopathy**: Carotid vessels
    - **Tumor induction**: Radiation-induced neoplasm

CT Findings

- CECT
  - Findings vary with site of complication
  - **Mucosa and submucosa**: Necrosis and ulceration → fibrosis
    - Early: Mucosal ulceration common; if solid enhancement, concern for tumor
      - Rarely, severe edema results in airway narrowing
      - Deep ulceration may lead to fistula
    - Late: May result in fibrotic, stenotic pharynx
      - Smooth, minimally enhancing wall
    - Absence of enhancing mass favors necrosis and ulceration over residual/recurrent tumor
  - **Muscles**: Myositis (acute) to fibrosis (late)
    - Early: Marked swelling and decrease in density
    - Late: Marked volume loss of muscles
  - **Cartilage**: Chondronecrosis
    - Fragmentation of cartilage associated with soft tissue swelling
      - ± gas bubbles adjacent to cartilage
  - **Bones**: Osteoradionecrosis (ORN)
    - Bony cortical disruption, loss of trabeculae
    - Often see sequestrum, fragmentation, fracture, gas
  - **Brain parenchyma**: Cerebral radionecrosis
    - Most often anteromedial temporal lobe(s)
    - Vasogenic edema with mass effect
    - Enhancement may be difficult to detect on CECT
    - Acute brain injury (days to weeks after XRT): No detectable MR changes or diffuse brain swelling
    - Early delayed brain injury (1-6 months after XRT): Nonenhancing white matter T2/FLAIR hyperintensity to new or enlarging enhancing lesions in immediate vicinity of radiated tumor volume
    - Late delayed brain injury (> 6 months after XRT): Leukoencephalopathy, radiation necrosis, arteritis (stenoocclusive and moyamoya-like vasculopathy), aneurysm, cavernoma, stroke-like migraine attacks after radiation therapy (SMART syndrome), mineralizing microangiopathy, chronic expanding encapsulated hematoma, cranial nerve injury, endocrine complications and secondary neoplasm

- **Vessels**: Arteriopathy
  - Calcified, atheromatous plaque
    - Carotid most commonly affected; may be asymmetric and unusual segment

MR Findings

- Also vary with site of complication
- Preferred modality for evaluation of CNS/neural complications
- **Brain parenchyma**: Cerebral radionecrosis
  - Cerebral white matter edema and mass effect with focal, feathery enhancement
  - Anteromedial temporal lobe: Status post nasopharyngeal or sella radiation
  - Inferior frontal lobes: Sinonasal XRT
  - Key differential: Radiation-induced glial tumor
    - Consider if many years (> 10) post XRT
  - MR perfusion shows reduced cerebral blood volume relative to normal white matter
  - MR spectroscopy shows reduced metabolites overall
- **Spinal cord**: Myelitis → myelopathy → necrosis
  - Early: Acute cord injury shows edema ± enhancement
  - Late: Delayed radiation myelopathy has expansion, T2 hyperintensity and enhancement
- **Brachial plexus**: Radiation-induced brachial plexopathy
  - T2 hyperintensity, enhancement, smooth enlargement of nerve roots
- **Cranial nerves**: Radiation-induced neuropathy
  - CNXII most often involved: Tongue atrophy with hemitongue T2 hyperintensity
  - Enlarged and edematous in acute stage, may show contrast enhancement
- **Muscles**: Myositis → fibrosis
  - Acute: ↑ T2 SI and enhancement
  - Chronic: ↓ ↓ T2 SI
- **Bone**: ORN
  - Low T1, high T2, enhancing marrow
  - Diffuse inflammation but no mass
- **Cartilage**: Chondronecrosis
  - Loss of T1 signal; cartilage enhances
  - Focal swelling of surrounding soft tissues

FDG PET Findings

- Acute radiation necrosis in bone and soft tissues, including radiation-induced denervation changes, can be FDG avid
- High FDG uptake on uninvolved side due to ↑ muscular activity (as in contralateral hemitongue) with chronic atrophy on side of radiation
- May mimic tumor or infection: Correlate with CT/MR to exclude tumor and identify acute edema or chronic atrophy changes

DIFFERENTIAL DIAGNOSIS

Recurrent Tumor

- Key differential: Look for solid, enhancing mass

Skull Base or Mandible-Maxilla Osteomyelitis

- Infection often coincident with ORN
- Fragmentation more suggestive of ORN

Timeline for Radiation-Induced Complications

Radiation Complication	Peak Time of Onset
Acute brain injury	Days-weeks
Early delayed cerebral radiation necrosis	1-6 months
Mucosal deep ulceration	1-9 months
Extreme soft tissue swelling	3-6 months
Chondronecrosis	3-12 months
Osteoradionecrosis	6-12 months
TMJ and pterygoid fibrosis	12-15 months
Late delayed cerebral radiation necrosis	12-15 months
Delayed radiation myelopathy	12-24 months
Accelerated atherosclerosis	1-3 years
Cranial neuropathy	≥ 2 years
Radiation plexopathy	2-4 years
Radiation-induced 2nd neoplasm	> 10 years

PATHOLOGY

General Features

- Etiology
  - XRT destroys endothelial cells lining small blood vessels, resulting in obstructive arteriopathy
  - **Tissues less able to withstand additional stress**
    - Infection, tumor recurrence, or biopsy may precipitate necrosis
  - Predisposing factors: Short treatment time, large field, chronic infections, atherosclerosis
    - Many complications seen only with doses **≥ 60 Gy**
    - Ongoing alcohol and tobacco use contribute to mucosal necrosis
  - **Bones**: ORN
    - Most often affects mandible
      - Often precipitated by dental infection or extraction
      - Diseased teeth must be extracted prior to XRT
    - May affect hyoid, sphenoid, temporal, or frontal bone
  - **Cartilage**: Chondronecrosis
    - Perichondrial injury allows infection or tumor to involve cartilage → necrosis
    - Associated with infection &/or recurrent tumor
    - Laryngeal necrosis uncommon, occurs in ~ 1%
      - Peaks in 1st 12 months; may occur years later
  - **Spinal cord**: Radiation myelopathy
    - Extensive demyelination, coagulation necrosis
  - **Radiation-induced neoplasm**
    - Possibly due to imperfect repair of XRT-induced DNA strand breakage in tumor suppressor genes
    - > 5 years after XRT, but most occur > 15 years
    - Long latency makes necrosis or recurrence less likely than new tumor
    - Meningioma
      - Often multiple, more likely higher grade
    - Sarcoma
      - Rhabdomyosarcoma most common
      - Retinoblastoma patients with *RB* gene especially at risk for sarcoma

- Parotid malignancy
  - Mucoepidermoid carcinoma most common
- Glial neoplasm
  - Glioblastoma predominates

CLINICAL ISSUES

Presentation

- Most common signs/symptoms
  - **Pain** common
    - Odynophagia, otalgia
  - Fetor, sputum with cartilage &/or bone fragments
  - Masticator muscle fibrosis → trismus
  - Pharyngeal muscle fibrosis → dysphagia, aspiration
  - Radiation myelitis → paresthesia &/or paralysis

Natural History & Prognosis

- Most complications occur in **1st 2 years** after XRT (peak period for squamous cell carcinoma recurrence as well)
  - May occur up to 5-8 years post XRT

Treatment

- Largely conservative
  - Antibiotics if potentiated or complicated by infection
  - Hyperbaric oxygen therapy if recurrent tumor excluded
  - Soft tissue healing may take ≥ 6 months
- If extensive/fulminant, may require surgical resection

DIAGNOSTIC CHECKLIST

Image Interpretation Pearls

- Key differential always residual/recurrent tumor
  - Recurrent tumor or infection may precipitate necrosis
  - Biopsy may also precipitate necrosis
- Look for solid, enhancing mass to favor tumor over radiation necrosis

SELECTED REFERENCES

1. Lan G et al: [Clinical classification, staging and treatment strategy of radionecrosis of the nasopharynx and skull base.] Lin Chuang Er Bi Yan Hou Tou Jing Wai Ke Za Zhi. 38(6):490-5, 2024

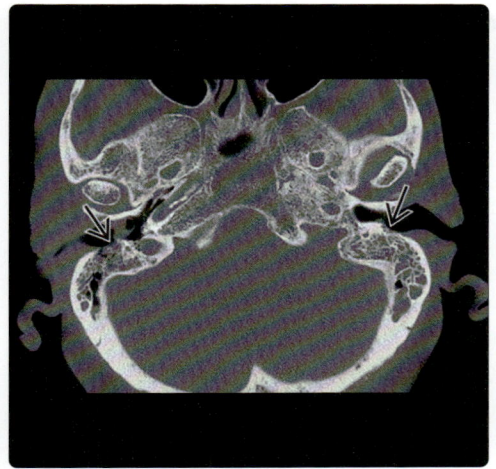
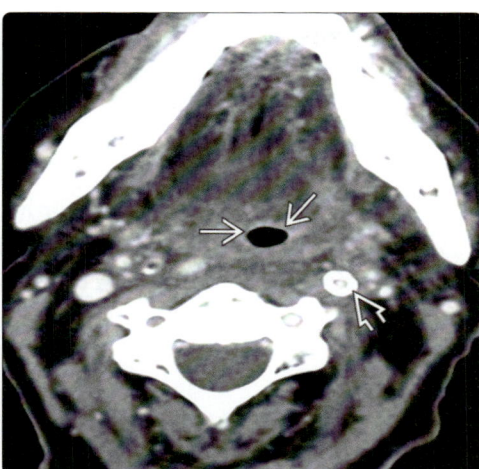

(Left) Axial HRCT temporal bones in an older adult patient with oral cavity cancer and XRT 20 years prior shows features of bilateral external auditory canal (EAC) radiation necrosis. Note erosion ⇨ of posterior EAC wall extending into adjacent mastoid air cells on the right and subtle erosion of EAC posterior wall on the left. (Right) Axial CECT shows radiation-induced fibrosis producing narrowed oropharynx ⇨ and dysphagia. Mucosal contour is smooth, and there is no mass. Carotid calcification ⇨ suggests accelerated atherosclerosis.

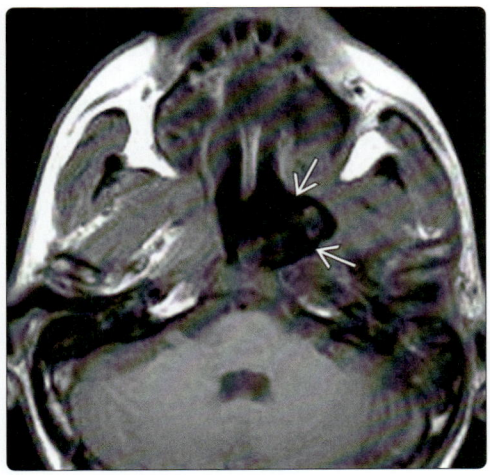
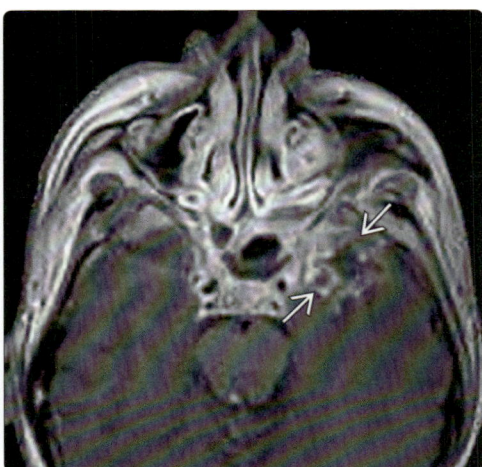

(Left) Axial T1 MR in a patient who received chemoradiation for NPCa a decade ago shows an enlarged nasopharyngeal airway following necrosis of left lateral nasopharyngeal wall tissues ⇨. CT demonstrated ORN of the adjacent skull base sphenoid bone with sequestrum (not shown). (Right) Axial T1 C+ FS MR in the same patient reveals irregular enhancement of the anteromedial left temporal lobe ⇨, indicating brain radiation necrosis. Radiation-induced complications can involve different tissues in radiation field.

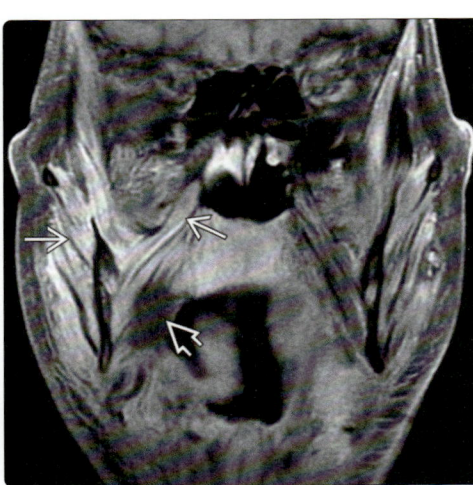
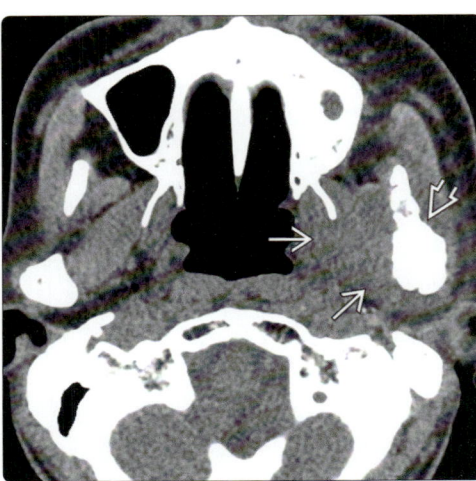

(Left) Coronal T1 C+ FS MR shows marked enhancement of muscles of mastication on the right ⇨ after radiation. Note marked pharyngeal mucosal enhancement and a nonenhancing ulcer at the lateral oropharyngeal wall ⇨. Absence of a mass and enhancement favors ulceration from tissue necrosis. (Right) Axial NECT in a patient treated 14 years prior for NPCa demonstrates swelling of masticator space tissues ⇨ and an irregular, sclerotic, expanded mandible ⇨ due to radiation-induced osteosarcoma.

Osteoradionecrosis

TERMINOLOGY

- Osteoradionecrosis
- Complication of radiation therapy (XRT) with necrosis of bone and failure to heal

IMAGING

- Mandible > > maxilla or skull base
- Associated soft tissue edema and induration common
- Difficult to exclude superinfection
- CT: Mixed lytic/sclerotic bone with sequestra
- MR: Diffuse low T1, high T2 signal from edema
- Diffuse enhancement common

TOP DIFFERENTIAL DIAGNOSES

- Osteomyelitis
- Medication-related osteonecrosis of jaw (MRONJ)
- Alveolar ridge squamous cell carcinoma (SCCa)
- Radiation-induced 2nd primary tumor

PATHOLOGY

- Radiation results in damage to small blood vessels, resulting in hypovascular marrow
- Impairs ability of bone to cope with stressors, such as infection or trauma
- May be precipitated by biopsy or tooth extraction
- Pathologic fracture through bone common

CLINICAL ISSUES

- Most often follows XRT for oral cavity SCCa
- Exposed bone from ulcerated mucosa usually present
- Incidence peaks in first 6-12 months post XRT
- May occur years after XRT

DIAGNOSTIC CHECKLIST

- Jaw pain, nonhealing mucosal ulceration, lytic/sclerotic CT changes
- Must exclude recurrent SCCa as source of changes

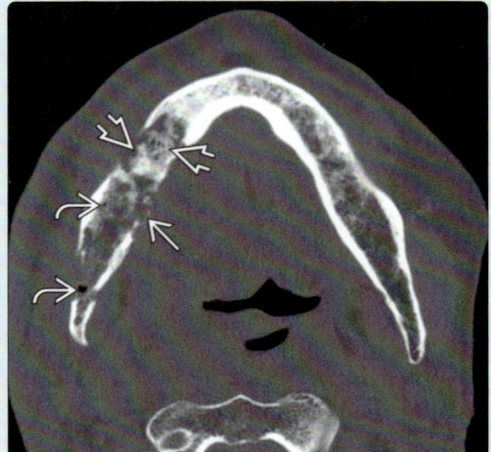
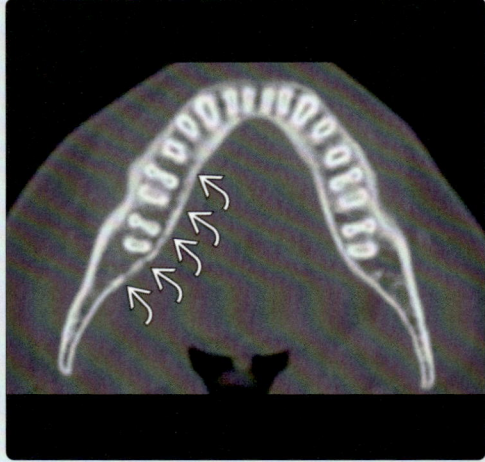

(Left) Axial bone CT demonstrates typical mixed lytic/sclerotic changes & cortical bone interruption ➡ in the right hemimandible following radiation therapy (XRT). Note intraosseous gas bubbles ➡ & evolving bone within bone appearance ➡ due to intraosseous bone sequestra. These findings are consistent with osteoradionecrosis (ORN). (Right) Axial bone window CECT shows subtle findings of ORN with rarefaction/lucencies of the right mandibular buccal alveolar cortex ➡.

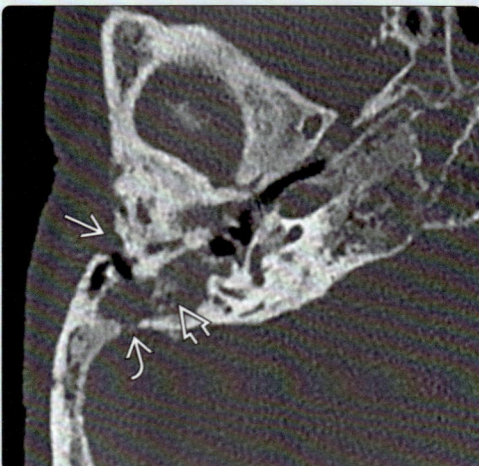
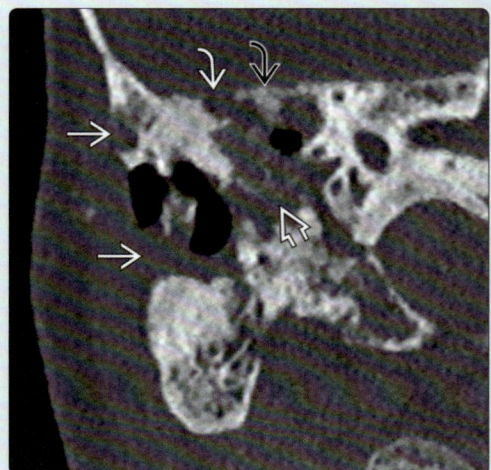

(Left) Axial HRCT of temporal bone in a patient with a prior history of right auriculectomy (ear lobe not visualized) & irradiation for skin cancer shows multifocal lytic lesions due to ORN in the right temporal bone. Note outer cortical defect ➡, sigmoid plate defect ➡, & large opacified lytic mastoid defect ➡ (which was non-diffusion-restricting fluid in MR, excluding cholesteatoma; not shown). (Right) Coronal HRCT in the same patient shows cortical defects ➡, tegmen defect ➡ & sclerosis ➡, & opacified lytic mastoid ➡.

Osteoradionecrosis

TERMINOLOGY

Abbreviations

- Osteoradionecrosis (ORN)

Definitions

- Complication of radiation therapy (XRT) with necrosis of bone and failure to heal

IMAGING

General Features

- Best diagnostic clue
  - Mixed lytic/sclerotic bone in patient previously treated with XRT: Rare if dose < 60 Gy
    - Exposed bone through ulcerated skin or mucosa usually present
    - Often complicated by fracture; may have infection
    - Lack of discrete soft tissue mass helps differentiate from recurrent tumor
- Location
  - In H&N, most often seen in jaw and skull base
    - Mandible > > maxilla or other facial bones
    - Temporal or sphenoid bone of skull base
    - Also described in frontal and hyoid bones
    - Cervical spine ORN rarely, after pharyngeal XRT
    - Buccal cortex > lingual cortex, mandibular body most common
    - Chin and angles of mandible (areas with muscular insertions) relatively spared
- Size
  - May be focal or extensive
  - Bone and soft tissue changes can be more than irradiated area, corresponding to compromised blood supply area of facial vessels in its vicinity

Imaging Recommendations

- Best imaging tool
  - Bone CT best diagnostic modality
  - Soft tissue imaging shows diffuse inflammation, no mass
- Protocol advice
  - Thin bone algorithm CT slices with coronal and sagittal reformations
    - Multiplanar images help plan surgery and potential reconstruction
  - CECT if superimposed infection or recurrent tumor suspected clinically

Radiographic Findings

- Extraoral plain film
  - Mixed lytic/sclerotic bone
  - Extent of involvement and destruction often underestimated by radiography

CT Findings

- CECT
  - Soft tissue edema and induration common, even when no superinfection
  - Focal abnormal enhancement or small abscesses may be evident when infected
  - Fistulization to skin can occur
- Bone CT
  - Cortical bone disruption on background of mixed lysis and sclerosis
    - Loss of trabeculation results in lytic appearance with superimposed sclerosis
  - Sequestered bone spicules and fragmentation often seen
  - Bubbles of air often present within abnormal mandible or in adjacent necrotic tissues
    - ORN, medication-related osteonecrosis of jaw (MRONJ), and mandibular osteomyelitis may contain air/gas
  - Pathologic fractures may be evident; may precipitate patient presentation
- PET/CT
  - Marked FDG uptake typically seen with ORN
    - Probably due to inflammatory component
  - CECT important to interpret with PET study to detect recurrent tumor

MR Findings

- T1WI
  - Diffuse low signal intensity of marrow space
  - Disrupted cortex may be evident
- T2WI
  - Diffuse high signal of marrow space
  - Adjacent tissues may appear edematous also
- T1WI C+ FS
  - Diffuse enhancement of marrow common
  - No adjacent solid mass

DIFFERENTIAL DIAGNOSIS

Osteomyelitis

- Mixed lytic/sclerotic bone in patient with infected tooth or extraction site and no history of XRT
- Osteomyelitis may be found with ORN; frequently difficult to differentiate

Medication-Related Osteonecrosis of Jaw

- a.k.a. bisphosphonate-related osteonecrosis of jaw (BRONJ)
- Induced by bisphosphonates, denosumab, and antiangiogenic drugs, such as bevacizumab
- Mixed lytic/sclerotic bone in patient treated with IV bisphosphonates or other causative medications
- Typically painful; occasionally asymptomatic
- Osteonecrosis of mandible; maxilla unusual due to rich blood supply
- Spontaneous osteonecrosis usually in mylohyoid ridge or precipitated by dental surgery/tooth extraction
- Osteonecrosis risk higher with concurrent steroid therapy
- Actinomyces infections may be associated
- Patient has no radiation history

Alveolar Ridge Squamous Cell Carcinoma

- Primarily destructive bone changes with mucosal ulceration
- Solid soft tissue enhancing lesion
- Recurrent squamous cell carcinoma (SCCa) is main imaging differential when ORN is present

Radiation-Induced 2nd Primary Tumor

- Occurs many years after XRT; typically ≥ 8 years

- Sarcoma most frequent; often with soft tissue mass

PATHOLOGY

General Features

- Etiology
  - Radiation results in damage to small blood vessels
    - Endothelial cells lining blood vessels are destroyed, resulting in obstructive arteriopathy
    - Impairs ability of bone to respond to stressors
  - ORN often precipitated by infection or trauma, including tooth extraction or **tissue biopsy**
- Associated abnormalities
  - Bacterial infection in necrotic bone often present
    - Osteomyelitis not primary event

Staging, Grading, & Classification

- Various staging or clinical grading systems used
- **Store and Boysen staging for jaw**
  - Stage 0: Mucosal defects only
  - Stage I: Radiologic evidence of ORN + intact mucosa
  - Stage II: Radiologic evidence of ORN + denuded bone
  - Stage III: Exposed radionecrotic bone + orocutaneous fistulae

Gross Pathologic & Surgical Features

- Necrotic, fragmented bone with sequestra and spicules
- Fragile, ulcerated mucosa with exposed bone

Microscopic Features

- **Bone necrosis primarily due to hypoxia**
  - XRT results in obliteration of arteries, including inferior alveolar artery
- Bone is hypocellular and periosteum nonviable
- Biopsy specimen may be complicated with osteonecrosis, osteomyelitis, and recurrent/residual tumor

CLINICAL ISSUES

Presentation

- Most common signs/symptoms
  - Ulcerated skin or mucosa with exposed necrotic bone in patient with prior history of H&N XRT
    - Mandible is most common facial bone involved
    - May be exposed through oral ulceration
- Other signs/symptoms
  - Fistulization to skin
  - Oral pain, trismus, dysesthesia, foul breath
  - Masticator space infection with small abscesses

Demographics

- Epidemiology
  - Multiple factors influence incidence of ORN
    - Tumor: Risk increased with stage III/IV primary tumor
    - XRT plan: Risk increased with higher dose, large field size, short treatment time
      - Intensity-modulated XRT (IMRT) with lower bone exposure has lower incidence of ORN
    - Treatment: Risk increased if surgery (mandibulectomy or other osteotomy, tooth extraction) in addition to XRT
    - Patient factors: Risk increased with poor oral hygiene, ongoing alcohol and tobacco exposure

- Age: Typically middle-aged patient with history of XRT
  - Usually oral cavity SCCa

Natural History & Prognosis

- Incidence of ORN ≤ 6%
- Incidence peaks: First 6-12 months post XRT
  - Median time: 10.9 months (range: 1.8-89.7 months) after XRT, 90% within 37.4 months

Treatment

- **Prevention** most important **prior** to XRT
  - Dental extractions and periodontal care prior to XRT
  - Improved nutritional status prior and during XRT
  - Cessation of tobacco and alcohol use
- Conservative treatment includes antibiotics and local irrigation
- Hyperbaric oxygen therapy to promote angiogenesis and aid in treating associated infection
  - Essential to exclude residual/recurrent tumor prior to hyperbaric oxygen treatment
- Sequestrectomy and primary wound closure for early disease
  - Fat grafts and platelet-rich fibrin may be helpful
- Bone resection and reconstruction for severe progressive disease
- Surgery better than medical treatment alone in skull base ORN
  - Vascularized surgical treatment much better than both surgical debridement only &/or medical therapy
  - Surgery should be considered earlier in skull base ORN to prevent severe morbidity & mortality

DIAGNOSTIC CHECKLIST

Consider

- ORN in any patient treated with XRT and new pain, nonhealing mucosal ulceration, lytic/sclerotic CT changes
- Essential to exclude **recurrent SCCa** as source of pain and cortical disruption
  - Tumor favored when solid soft tissue mass present
- While ORN may occur several years after treatment, if ≥ 8 years, consider **XRT-induced sarcoma,** especially if soft tissue mass associated

Image Interpretation Pearls

- Check for local infection or pathologic fracture

Reporting Tips

- Describe extent of disease, cortical bone disruption, exposed bone spicules, and sequestrations

SELECTED REFERENCES

1. Shaari DS et al: Radiation-induced pharyngeal necrosis and cervical spine osteoradionecrosis in patients with oropharyngeal squamous cell carcinoma. Head Neck. 47(1):E11-22, 2024
2. Shah SR et al: Presentation and optimal management of anterior and central skull base osteoradionecrosis: systematic review and meta-analysis. Laryngoscope. 135(3):982-90, 2024
3. Law B et al: Autogenous free fat graft combined with platelet-rich fibrin heals a refractory mandibular osteoradionecrosis. Clin Ter. 171(2):e110-13, 2020
4. El-Rabbany M et al: Interventions for preventing osteoradionecrosis of the jaws in adults receiving head and neck radiotherapy. Cochrane Database Syst Rev. 2019(11):CD011559, 2019
5. Curé JK et al: Radiopaque jaw lesions: an approach to the differential diagnosis. Radiographics. 32(7):1909-25, 2012

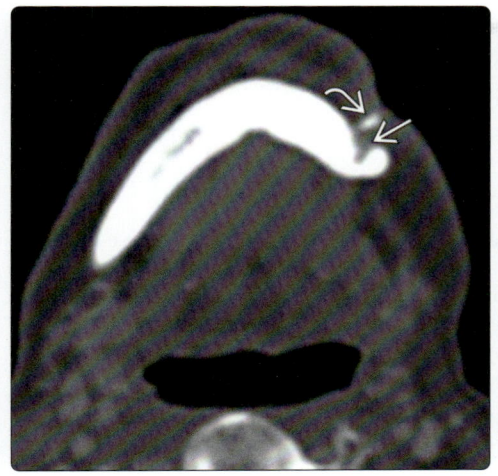

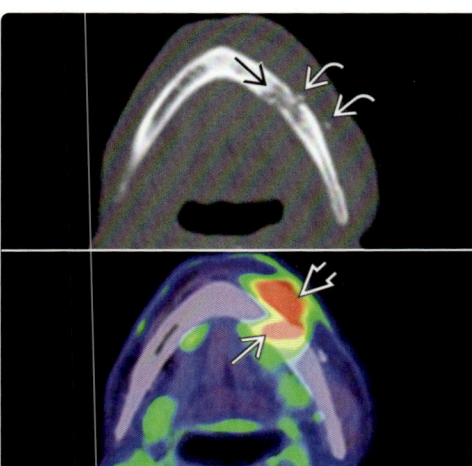

(Left) *Axial CECT in a patient with left maxillary carcinoma post surgery & radiation 6 years prior shows features of mandibular ORN with lytic area ⮕ & a bony sequestrum ⮕ extruding out through a sinus tract toward the skin.* (Right) *Axial bone window NECT (top) shows left mandibular ORN with a mixed lytic/sclerotic lesion ⮕ & bone fragments in soft tissue ⮕. Axial fused FDG PET/CT (bottom) shows intense FDG uptake in the mandible ⮕ & soft tissue ⮕. Biopsy showed ORN without any tumor or infection.*

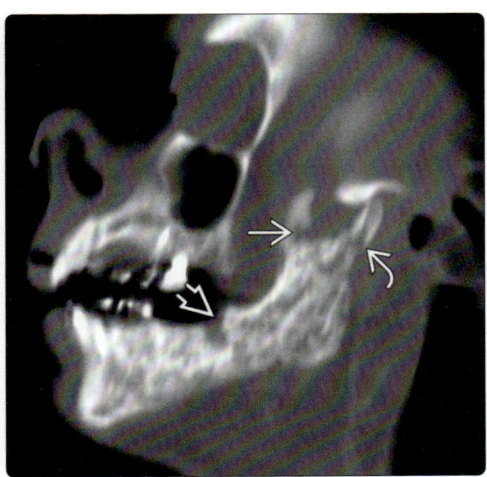

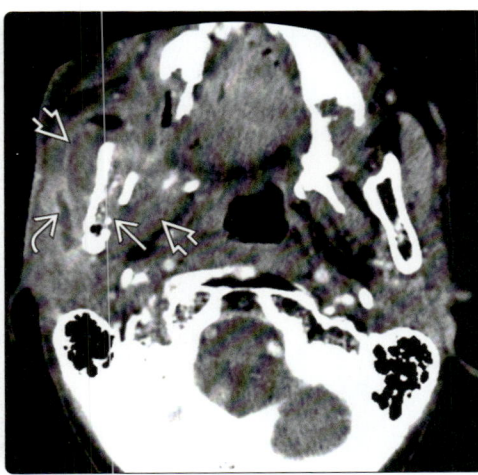

(Left) *Sagittal oblique reconstruction NECT shows heterogeneous multifocal lucency, cortical interruption, & trabecular & cortical thickening & sclerosis due to ORN. Note the deep molar extraction socket ⮕. There is fragmentation of the coronoid process ⮕ & condylar neck ⮕. (Right) Axial CECT shows ORN of the right mandible complicated by infection of the masticator space. There is cortical interruption ⮕, diffuse severe edema of the parotid gland & muscles of mastication ⮕, & a dilated parotid duct ⮕.*

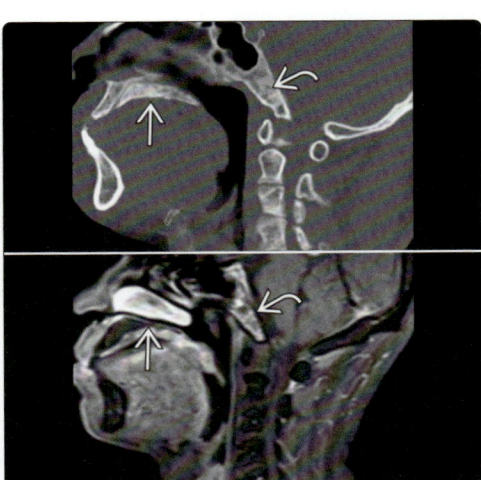

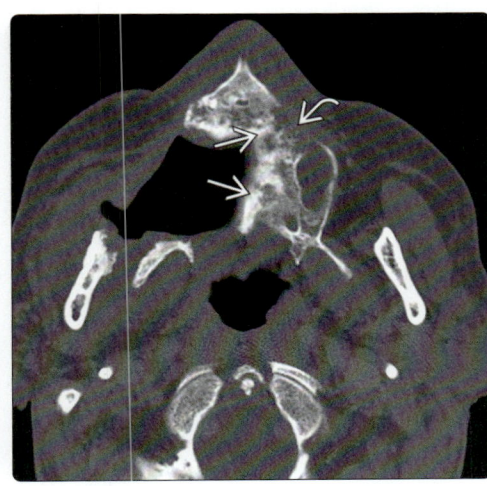

(Left) *Sagittal NECT (top) in a patient who underwent chemoradiotherapy for nasopharyngeal carcinoma shows mixed lytic/sclerotic lesions in the hard palate ⮕ & clivus ⮕. Sagittal T1 C+ FS MR (bottom) shows abnormal contrast enhancement in these bones. Remaining bones are normal. (Right) Axial bone CT shows right surgical palatectomy but mixed sclerotic ⮕ & lytic ⮕ changes in the left maxilla, which was included in XRT field. Maxilla is relatively radioresistant, & ORN is rare.*

Posttreatment Neck

TERMINOLOGY

- Most often performed for neoplasm
- **Total laryngectomy (TL)**: Larynx completely resected & neopharynx created
  - Neopharynx connects oropharynx to esophagus
  - Trachea no longer communicates with pharynx
  - Need tracheostomy to breathe, prosthesis to speak
  - Complications like pharyngocutaneous fistula (PCF)
- **Partial laryngectomy (PL)**: Conservative surgery
  - Aims to preserve voice & breathing, swallowing without aspiration
  - Cordectomy → vertical or horizontal PL → near-TL
  - Imaging varies from near-normal to complex reconstruction & deformity
  - Permanent tracheostomy required only with near-TL

IMAGING

- Abnormal contour of laryngopharyngeal airway, absence of soft tissue ± part or whole of ≥ 1 cartilage(s)

TOP DIFFERENTIAL DIAGNOSES

- Larynx trauma
- Radiated larynx

PATHOLOGY

- Surgeries defined as radical (TL) or conservative (cordectomy or PL)

CLINICAL ISSUES

- **Declining use of both PL & TL** with increasing use of organ preservation chemoradiation
- Laryngectomy also used for cartilaginous laryngeal tumors, invasive thyroid tumors, salvage after failed chemoradiation, chondronecrosis, posttreatment nonfunctioning larynx

DIAGNOSTIC CHECKLIST

- Imaging confusion occurs with complex appearance of PL
- First determine type of procedure
- Look for recurrent mass & lymphadenopathy

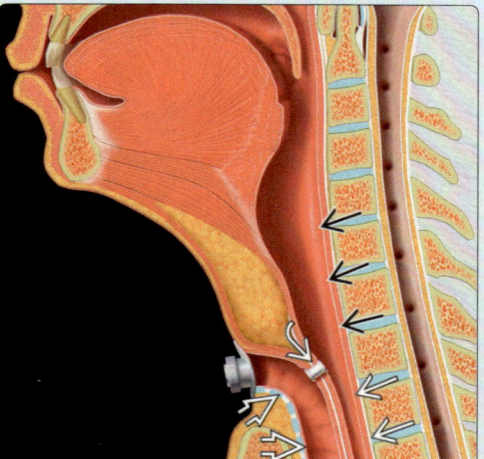
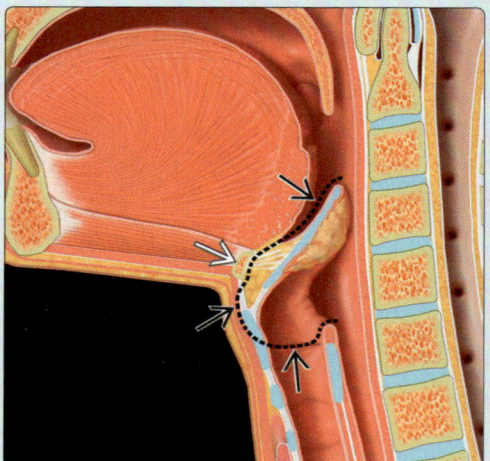

(Left) Sagittal graphic depicts total laryngectomy (TL) with the laryngeal cartilages and hyoid resected. Neopharynx ➡ connects oral cavity to esophagus ➡, while trachea ➡ is brought to skin surface as tracheostomy. Tracheoesophageal voice prosthesis ➡ is a 1-way valve allowing speech when patient manually occludes stoma. (Right) Sagittal graphic shows supraglottic partial laryngectomy (SGL) (a type of horizontal hemilaryngectomy) resection plane ➡. True cord, hyoid ➡, & lower portion of thyroid cartilage are retained.

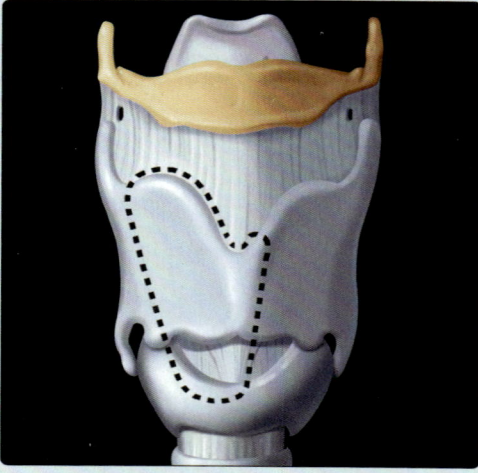
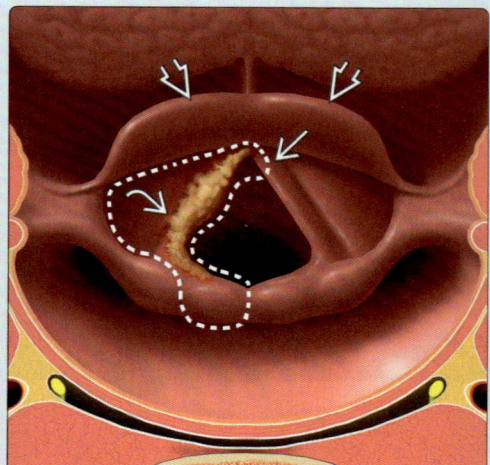

(Left) Coronal graphic shows cartilaginous components resected in right vertical hemilaryngectomy, a type of vertical partial laryngectomy (VPL). Frontolateral laryngectomy (not shown) is another type of VPL with resection of only the midline portion of thyroid cartilage. (Right) Endoscopic graphic of glottic tumor ➡ with dotted white line shows expected resection plan for right vertical hemilaryngectomy. Resection in VPL includes anterior portion of contralateral uninvolved cord ➡ but spares epiglottis ➡.

TERMINOLOGY

Definitions

- Imaging findings following resection of whole or part of larynx, typically for neoplasm
  - Total laryngectomy (TL): Larynx resected, neopharynx created; permanent tracheal stoma
  - Partial laryngectomy (PL): Preserves voice & breathing without permanent tracheostomy
    - Cordectomy, vertical PL (VPL), horizontal supraglottic laryngectomy (SGL), supracricoid laryngectomy (SCL) with cricohyoidopexy (CHP) or cricohyoidoepiglottopexy (CHEP)
      - Term pexy indicates surgical fixation of structure
    - Now more often performed as endoscopic transoral laser surgery (TLS) rather than open surgery

IMAGING

General Features

- Best diagnostic clue
  - Abnormal contour of laryngopharyngeal airway, absence of soft tissue ± part or whole of ≥ 1 cartilage(s)

CT Findings

- CECT
  - Vestibule of neolarynx appears deformed
  - Soft tissue structures &/or cartilages absent
  - Arytenoid soft tissue thickening common with PL
  - **Pseudocord** scar tissue develops between resected true vocal cord (TVC) & anterior portion of contralateral, partially resected cord
    - Usually seen with VPL
  - Not uncommon to see patchy sclerosis or partial resection of cartilages
    - Not often helpful or indicative of recurrence
  - Open resection frequently accompanied by nodal dissection
  - Complications like **pharyngocutaneous fistula (PCF)**, typically after TL

Imaging Recommendations

- Best imaging tool
  - CECT more consistent good-quality larynx imaging
    - MR may have with motion artifacts
  - PET/CECT: Extremely helpful after TL or PL & radiation, as edematous mucosa makes detecting recurrent squamous cell carcinoma difficult
    - Determine systemic disease prior to salvage TL

DIFFERENTIAL DIAGNOSIS

Larynx Trauma

- Deformity of cartilages following open or closed injury
- Cartilage should not be absent
- May have associated hematoma, contusion, vascular injury, & cervical spine fracture

Radiated Larynx

- Mucosal & deep fat space edema
- Cartilages present unless chondronecrosis

PATHOLOGY

Staging, Grading, & Classification

- Surgeries defined as radical (TL) or conservative (cordectomy or PL)
- **Use of chemoradiation & TLS resulted in marked decline of TL & open PL**
- Multiple different forms of PL, but goal always preservation of laryngeal function (breathing, voice, swallowing)
  - Defined by plane of resection & form of reconstruction
- **Cordectomy**
  - Use: Tumor isolated to one TVC without fixation
  - Resected: TVC, vocalis muscle, & tendon
    - Typically performed endoscopically (TLS)
  - Imaging: Very subtle; may appear normal
- **VPL**
  - Use: Early-stage tumor, glottic to anterior commissure (AC) ± arytenoid, **without** cord fixation
  - Frontolateral laryngectomy
    - Use: Tumors to AC without TVC fixation
    - Resected: Vertical midline segment of thyroid cartilage, TVC (± arytenoid) with ventricle & false cord, AC & small part of contralateral anterior cord
    - Reconstruction: Contralateral cord mucosa sutured to perichondrium; ipsilateral side may be left to granulate
    - Imaging: Defect in midline thyroid cartilage, missing aryepiglottic (AE) fold ± ipsilateral arytenoid, dense scar at site of resected cords = **pseudocord**
  - Hemilaryngectomy
    - Use: When more posterior extension of tumor to arytenoid cartilage
    - Resected: As with frontolateral + ipsilateral arytenoid, mucosa of AE fold, & thyroid lamina
    - Reconstruction: Grafts, flap, muscle may be used
- **Horizontal laryngectomy**
  - SGL
    - Use: Supraglottic tumor not involving ventricle; normal cord mobility
    - Resected: Epiglottis, false cords, AE folds, ventricle, upper 1/3 of thyroid cartilage, thyrohyoid membrane
    - Remaining: TVC, arytenoids, lower thyroid cartilage, cricoid
    - Reconstruction: Thyroid sutured to hyoid (thyrohyoidopexy)
    - Imaging: Hyoid & thyroid on same plane, redundant mucosa over arytenoids
  - **Extended SGL**: SGL + 1 arytenoid cartilage, tongue base, or pyriform sinus resected
  - **3/4 laryngectomy**: SGL + ipsilateral TVC & arytenoid cartilage resected
    - Remaining: Hyoid, unilateral glottis, cricoid
  - SCL
    - Use: More extensive tumor, no cord fixation
    - Resected: Thyroid cartilage, paraglottic space, TVC, ventricle, false cords, AC
    - Remaining: Hyoid, 1 or both arytenoids, cricoid
    - Reconstruction: 2 alternative -pexy procedures
      - **CHP** if involvement of preepiglottic or paraglottic space, or thyroid cartilage

□ Imaging: Hyoid sutured to cricoid, no thyroid cartilage, 1 or both cricoarytenoid joints present
□ **CHEP** if epiglottis & preepiglottic fat can be spared
□ Imaging: As previously mentioned but hyoid, cricoid, & epiglottis attached to each other
- **Near-TL**
  ○ Use: Advanced unilateral tumor
  ○ Resected: 1/2 of larynx & anterior part of contralateral TVC **+** hyoid, epiglottis, preepiglottic space, valleculae
  ○ Remaining: 1 arytenoid, part of thyroarytenoid muscle, part of thyroid & cricoid cartilages, recurrent laryngeal nerve
  ○ Reconstruction: Permanent tracheostomy needed for breathing
  ○ Imaging: Only portion of 1 side of thyroid & cricoid cartilages + arytenoid present, tracheostomy
- **TL**
  ○ Use: Advanced extensive laryngeal or hypopharyngeal tumors mainly
  ○ Resected: Entire cartilage framework + endolaryngeal structures, variable thyroid gland
  ○ Reconstruction: Neopharynx created by directly closing pharyngeal surgical defect or with different pedicled/free flaps
  ○ Primary goal of TL: Complete removal of tumor
  ○ Important secondary goals: Preserve swallowing function & restore speech function
  ○ Salvage TL: To manage chronic aspiration, airway compromise, radiation necrosis, & tumor recurrence
  ○ Imaging: No larynx, thyroid remnant, tubular neopharynx, ± tracheoesophageal (TE) valve (voice prosthesis)
  ○ PCF in ~ 14% of primary laryngectomies; 23% in those with radiotherapy & salvage laryngectomies
  ○ Lower rates of PCF & shorter operative time, hospital stay & time to oral feeding with closed stapler-assisted TL compared to traditional manual closure

CLINICAL ISSUES

Presentation
- Most common signs/symptoms
  ○ Typically performed to maximize local control of laryngeal or hypopharyngeal carcinoma
  ○ Chemoradiation often results in better speech preservation than PL
  ○ TL separates trachea from neopharynx & esophagus
    – Speech best with TE valve
    – Breathing occurs through suprasternal stoma
    – Food/liquids swallowed orally then pass through neopharynx to esophagus
  ○ PL aims to preserve **voice & breathing** without permanent tracheostomy
    – Also to allow swallowing without aspiration

Demographics
- Epidemiology
  ○ **Declining use of PL with increasing use of chemoradiation for laryngeal carcinoma**
    – Organ preservation protocols
  ○ **Declining use of open PL in favor of TLS**
    – Less morbidity, better postoperative function

Treatment
- Laryngeal carcinoma most often treated by **radiation, chemoradiation, & endoscopic surgery**, alone or in combination
  ○ Increasing use of radiation ± chemoradiation for T1-T3
  ○ TLS favored over open procedures
- PCF treated conservatively, surgery only in refractory cases
  ○ Surgery like autologous fat injection around hypopharyngeal opening of PCF
- **Glottic carcinoma**
  ○ With early stage, XRT has better voice preservation
  ○ Endoscopic laser resection & cordectomy, VPL, SCL with CHEP
  ○ TL for advanced tumor with poor laryngeal function
- **Supraglottic carcinoma**
  ○ With early stage, XRT has better voice preservation
  ○ Horizontal SGL, SCL with CHP, near-total or 3/4 laryngectomy
  ○ TL for large-volume tumor & transglottic carcinoma if not controlled by/advanced for radiation treatment
  ○ Transglottic carcinoma: Supraglottic carcinoma crosses laryngeal ventricle to involve true & false vocal folds
    – Or involve glottis & extend to subglottis (> 10 mm below free margin of true vocal fold), or both
- **Subglottic**
  ○ TL often; usually advanced presentation
- New directions of surgical management are transoral robotic surgery (TORS) & photodynamic therapy
- Laryngectomies may also be used for **chondronecrosis, invasive thyroid tumors, cartilaginous tumors, caustic destruction of larynx**

DIAGNOSTIC CHECKLIST

Image Interpretation Pearls
- TL typically has straightforward appearance
  ○ Pitfalls: Misinterpretation of residual thyroid as recurrence; failure to identify residual or new nodes
  ○ Recurrence tends to occur at proximal &/or distal anastomosis
- Confusion most often occurs when imaging complex PL
  ○ **Best method to minimize interpretation error is to read surgical notes (if possible)**

Reporting Tips
- **Determine which type of procedure was performed**
  ○ Type of resection: Complete or partial cartilage absence, vertical or horizontal resection plane
  ○ Type of reconstruction: Relationship of remaining cartilages to hyoid
  ○ Additional soft tissue flaps placed
- Look for asymmetric neolaryngeal wall thickening or luminal mass
- Look for **abnormal masses** in remaining tissues, particularly at anastomoses
- Check for neck **adenopathy**, apical lung **metastases**

SELECTED REFERENCES

1. Judd RT et al: Revisiting the closed stapler laryngectomy: technique and review of recent evidence. Am J Otolaryngol. 46(1):104512, 2025
2. da Silva Seidler C et al: Rehabilitation after supracricoid partial laryngectomy: cohort study. Braz J Otorhinolaryngol. 91(2):101532, 2024

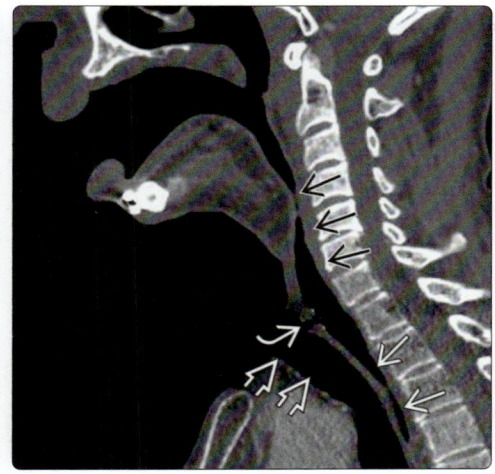
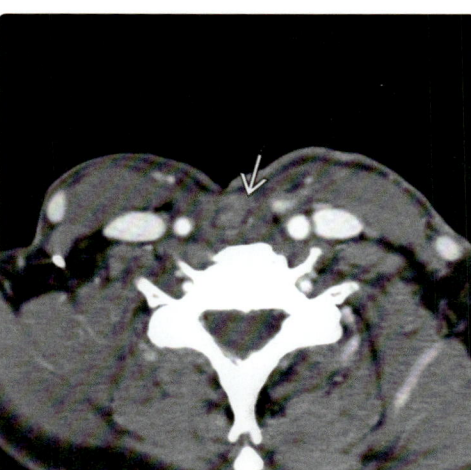

(Left) *Sagittal CECT of TL with total glossectomy in recurrent extensive SCCa shows absence of tongue, hyoid bone, & all laryngeal cartilages. Trachea no longer communicates with pharynx. To eat, the patient's neopharynx* ➡ *connects oral cavity to esophagus* ➡. *To breathe, trachea comes to skin surface with tracheostomy* ➡. *To speak, tracheoesophageal puncture is done for voice prosthesis* ➡. **(Right)** *Axial CECT in another patient with TL, right modified neck dissection, & gastric pull-up shows a multilayered, midline, tubular neopharynx* ➡.

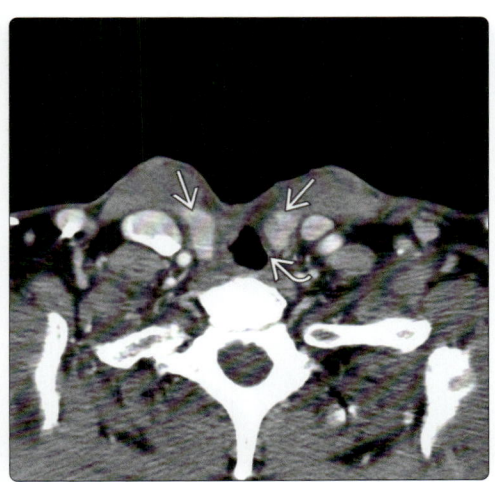
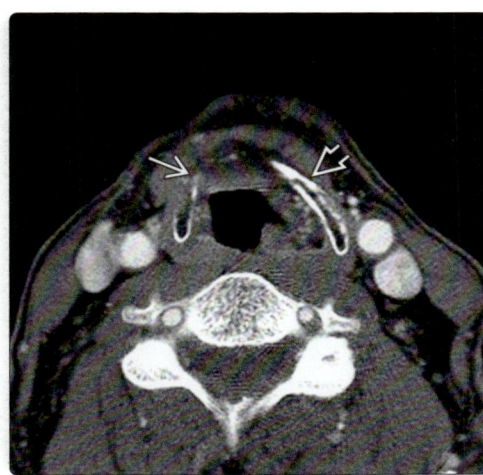

(Left) *Axial CECT in the same patient shows new contour of thyroid lobes* ➡ *after midline splitting of thyroid capsule. If one lobe is resected, other lobe may be mistaken for a recurrent mass, node, or even pseudoaneurysm. Distal anastomosis* ➡ *often has a slightly irregular contour.* **(Right)** *Axial CECT in another patient with open right hemilaryngectomy (VPL) shows resection of anterior right thyroid cartilage* ➡ *& intact superior left thyroid lamina* ➡. *The hyoid bone & epiglottis were present more superiorly (not shown).*

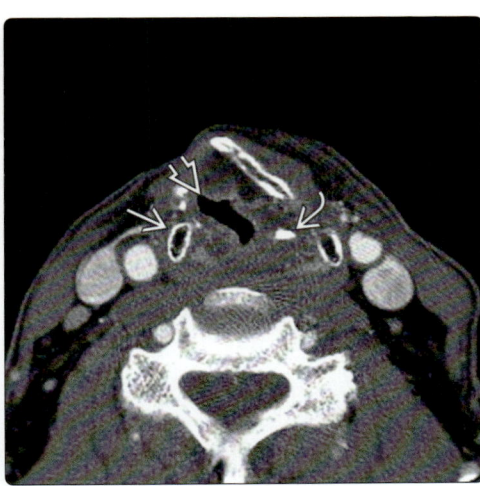
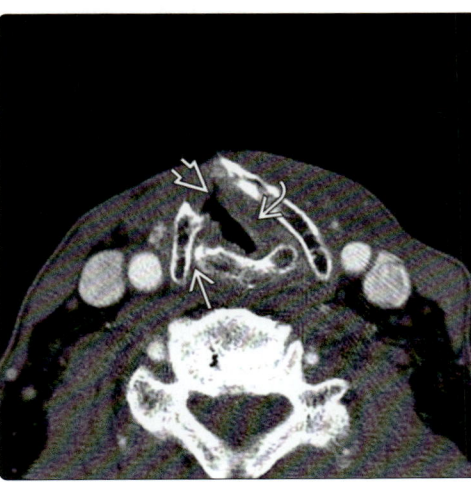

(Left) *Axial CECT in the same patient with right hemilaryngectomy (VPL) shows resection of right true & false cords, ventricle, arytenoid, aryepiglottic fold, anterior commissure, & anterior part of left true vocal cord, along with most of right anterior thyroid lamina* ➡. *Left arytenoid* ➡ *is still present. Note significant airway deformity* ➡. **(Right)** *Axial CECT more inferiorly shows left vocal cord* ➡ *and marked deformity of right glottis from right hemilaryngectomy* ➡. *Right cricothyroid joint is intact* ➡.

(Left) *Axial CECT in a patient with endoscopic resection similar to left frontolateral VPL shows that the left true vocal cord, ventricle, and thyroarytenoid muscle are resected. Anterior commissure and anterior 1/3 of right vocal cord are also removed, but the arytenoid cartilages are present ➡.* **(Right)** *Axial CECT more inferiorly shows nodular soft tissue pseudocord ➡ that was biopsy-proven scar tissue at the site of resected cord. Focal defect of right thyroid lamina was thought to be injury at prior anterior right cord resection ➡.*

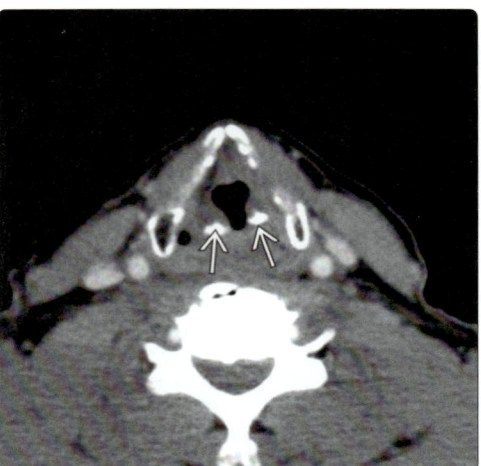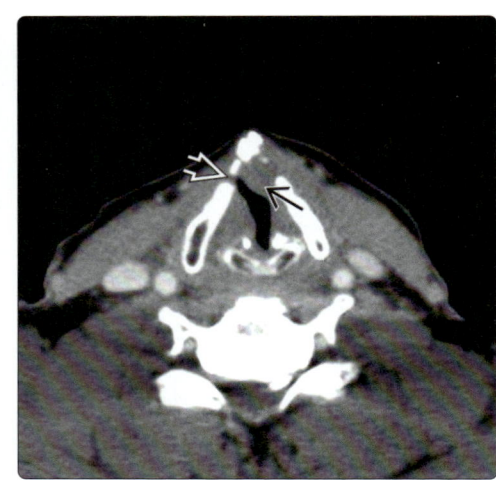

(Left) *Axial T1 MR of the larynx shows subtle changes to the glottis from a right endoscopic cordectomy. Note that the right true vocal cord ➡ is subtly smaller and deformed compared to the normal left cord. Thyroid laminae ➡ and cricoid cartilage ➡ are still present after the cordectomy.* **(Right)** *Axial CECT following open SGL shows resection of anterior midportion of hyoid bone and partial resection of right aryepiglottic (AE) fold ➡. Right modified neck dissection was also done ➡.*

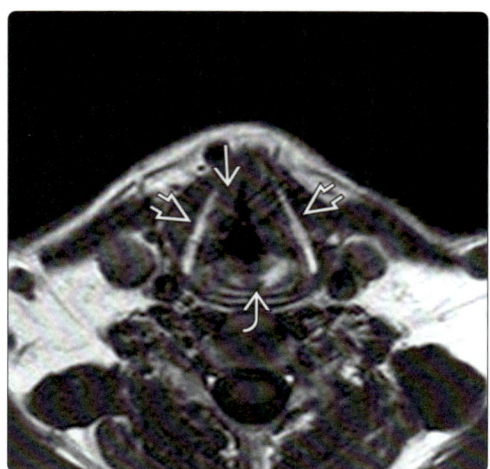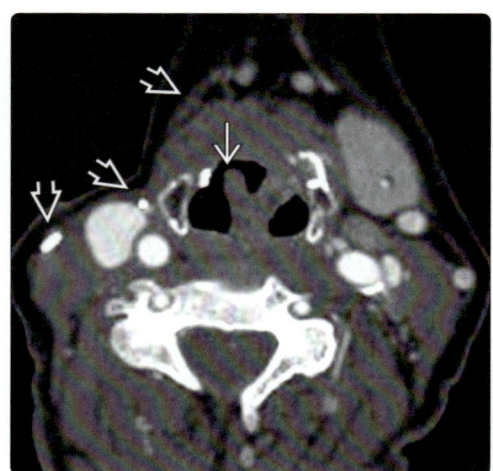

(Left) *Sagittal CECT reformat in the same patient shows absence of epiglottis, which should extend up to oropharyngeal airway ➡. Note elevated location of remaining larynx ➡.* **(Right)** *Sagittal CECT reformat further laterally in the same patient shows new relationship of hyoid ➡ to remaining lower 1/2 of thyroid lamina ➡ following thyrohyoidopexy. This is routine with open SGL with hyoid & thyroid on same plane. Glottis, arytenoid, cricoid, and lower 1/3 of thyroid cartilages are typically preserved in SGL.*

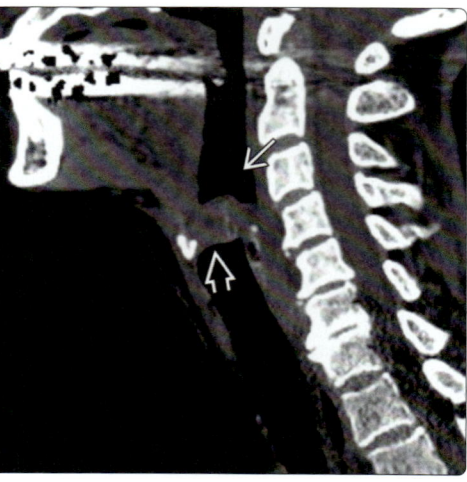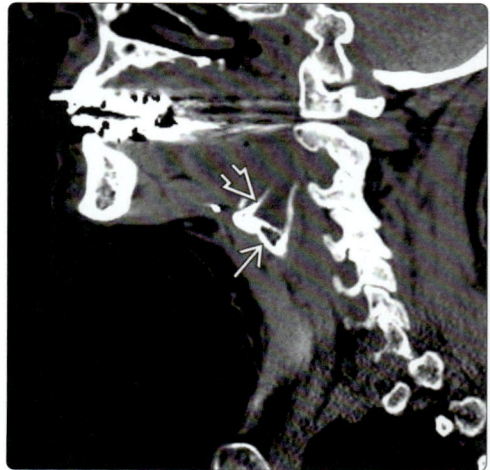

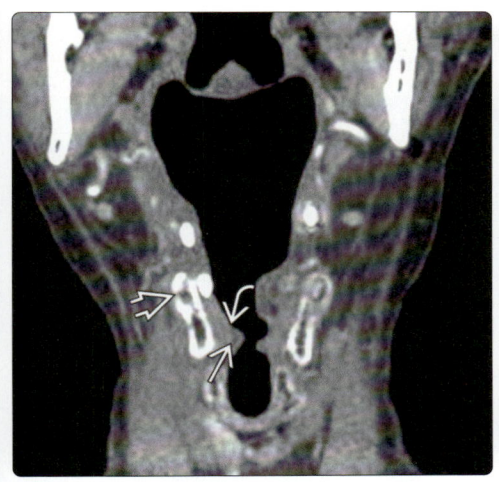
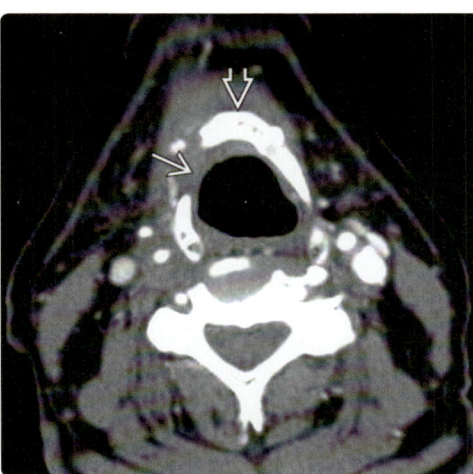

(Left) Coronal CECT reformat following endoscopic right SGL shows resection of the entire epiglottis, right false vocal cord, AE fold, & supraglottic laryngeal mucosa down to the right laryngeal ventricle ➡. There is preservation of the right true vocal cord ➡ and cartilages. Surgical clip lies medial to the thyroid lamina ➡. (Right) Axial CECT in the same patient with endoscopic SGL shows smooth mucosal scar ➡ and demonstrates absence of the superior portion of epiglottis, which should extend above the preserved hyoid bone ➡.

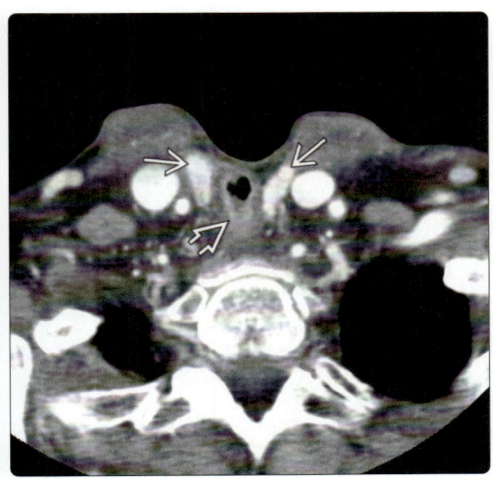
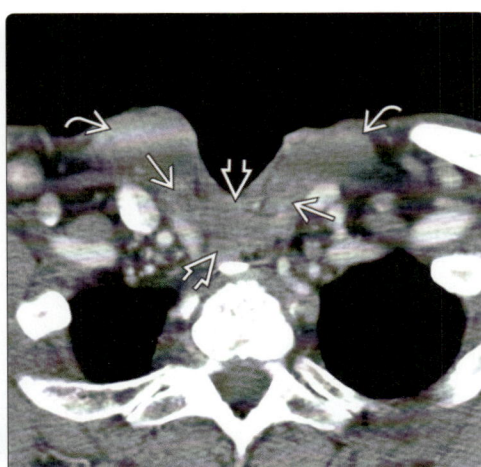

(Left) Baseline axial CECT just above tracheal stoma after TL shows distal anastomosis ➡ of neopharynx to esophagus and both thyroid lobes ➡. Slightly irregular contour of the distal anastomosis is often seen. (Right) Axial CECT in the same patient 9 months later shows new abnormal soft tissue at distal anastomosis ➡. Tumor is infiltrating thyroid lobes ➡, which are now difficult to define from sternocleidomastoid muscles ➡. Recurrent tumor tends to be at proximal or distal anastomosis or is nodal or metastatic.

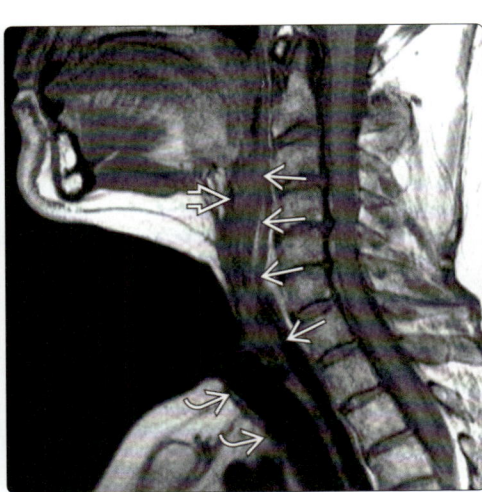
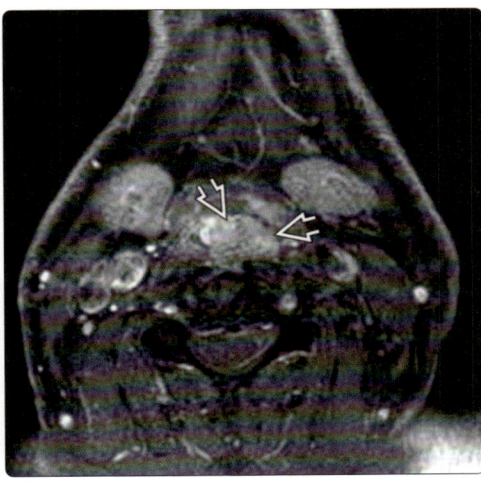

(Left) Sagittal T1 MR in another patient with TL shows resection of all laryngeal cartilages & creation of neopharynx ➡ with cervical trachea ➡ ending at stoma. Neopharynx can be created by directly closing pharyngeal surgical defect or with pedicled/free flaps. Proximal anastomosis appears minimally fuller than expected ➡. (Right) Axial T1 C+ FS MR at the level of "fullness" seen on sagittal T1 MR reveals enhancing, solid, recurrent tumor (biopsy confirmed) at the proximal anastomosis of neopharynx ➡.

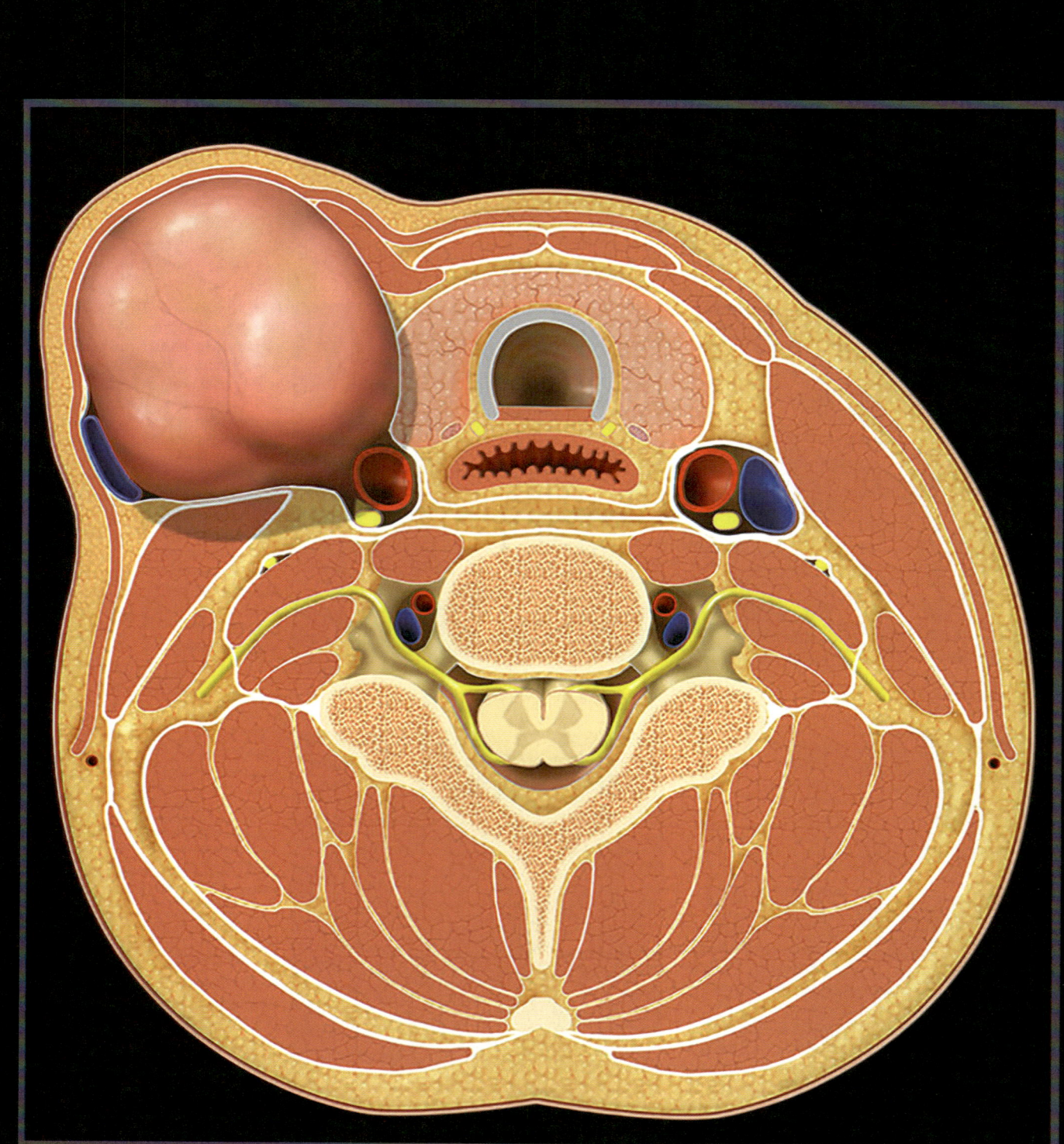

SECTION 19
Pediatric Lesions

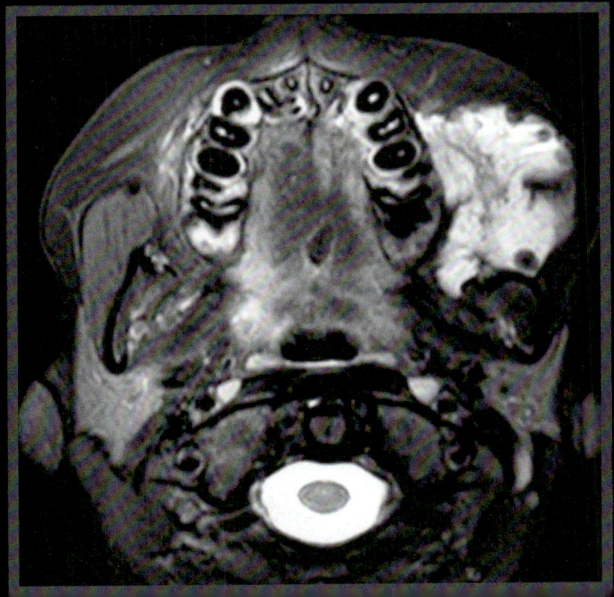
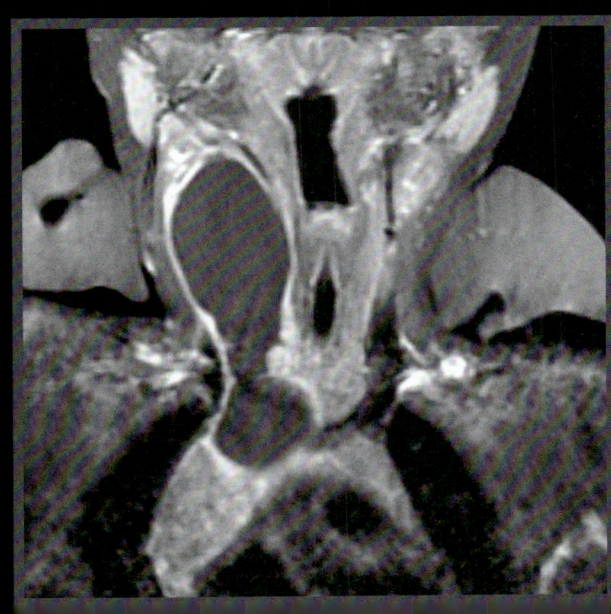

Summary Thoughts: Congenital Cystic Neck Masses

Palpable masses are a common indication for imaging the pediatric head & neck (H&N). Most are congenital or inflammatory in children; only 5% of childhood neoplasms occur in the H&N (excluding the brain). The most common extrathyroid, nonneoplastic **solid** neck masses in children are related to inflammatory disease & do not require imaging at all, unless there is concern for deep neck infection or abscess. The most common **cystic** masses in the pediatric H&N are congenital lesions secondary to abnormal embryogenesis involving the thyroglossal duct (TGD), the branchial apparatus, or the vascular endothelium. TGD cysts (TGDCs) account for 70-90% of all congenital neck abnormalities in children. The most common branchial apparatus lesion is the 2nd branchial cleft or apparatus cyst (BCC/BAC), & lymphatic malformations are the most common vascular malformations in the H&N.

Whenever a cystic neck mass is encountered on a pediatric imaging study, a very reasonable differential diagnosis can be made based on its **location** (midline, paramidline, or lateral as well as location relative to carotid sheath), **imaging appearance** (simple cyst, complicated cyst, enhancement, ± solid component), & **clinical presentation** (present since birth or acute onset ± clinical evidence of infection).

Terminology

A **TGDC** or tract is an anomalous remnant of the TGD that, under normal circumstances, completely involutes. Failure of involution may result in cysts (or solid foci of thyroid tissue) along the tract, anywhere from the midline posterior tongue at the foramen cecum, to the thyroid bed in the lower neck.

Branchial apparatus anomalies can be cysts, sinus tracts, or fistulae. **Cysts** are fluid filled with well-defined walls secondary to the failure of obliteration of a branchial cleft or pouch. **Sinus tracts** are congenital tracts with 1 opening, either externally to the skin surface (or external auditory canal) or internally to the pharynx (2nd branchial cleft), superolateral hypopharynx (3rd branchial cleft), or pyriform sinus (4th or 3rd branchial pouch). **Fistulae** are congenital tracts with 2 openings (1 internal & 1 external) secondary to failure of normal obliteration of the branchial cleft & pouch.

Imaging Techniques & Indications

US, CT, & MR are all reasonable options for imaging of neck masses in children. Modality choice depends on the clinical presentation, the referring clinical service, & the modalities available at the time. For instance, if there is concern that a child with cellulitis & cervical adenitis has a drainable abscess deep to a palpable neck mass, US is ideal for determining the presence of an underlying drainable fluid collection/abscess. Likewise, if a child is thought to have a TGDC, US is the imaging modality of choice to evaluate the suspected TGDC & identify the presence of a normal-appearing thyroid gland in the lower neck. US is also the modality of choice in patients with suspected infantile hemangioma, as color Doppler findings can be quite characteristic. However, CECT is the initial imaging modality of choice to evaluate the total extent of disease in children with suspected deep neck infection & to assess for a possible underlying pyriform sinus tract in children with left-sided neck abscesses that involve the left thyroid lobe.

In children not presenting with signs & symptoms of infection, MR imaging is the preferred modality in many other settings, but frequently requires sedation in children less than 4-6 years of age. MR is also the preferred imaging modality for children with suspected vascular malformations due to its excellent soft tissue contrast resolution, variety of methods of interrogation, lack of limitations regarding depth, & lack of exposure to ionizing radiation.

Embryology

The thyroid gland migrates from the foramen cecum at the midline posterior tongue to the paramidline location in the lower neck via the path of the **TGD**. The TGD normally involutes during the 5th or 6th week of gestation. However, remnant epithelium anywhere along the tract may persist & form a TGDC. As the TGD diverticulum descends caudally, it passes along the anterior surface of the developing hyoid bone; therefore, remnants may be found anterior to the preepiglottic space of the larynx.

Branchial apparatus structures develop between the 4th & 6th week of gestation & consist of 6 pairs of mesodermal arches separated by 5 paired endodermal pouches internally & 5 paired ectodermal clefts externally. During the 6th week of gestation, the 2nd branchial arch overgrows the 3rd & 4th branchial arches, resulting in a combined 2nd, 3rd, & 4th branchial cleft, termed the "cervical sinus of His." Anomalies of the branchial apparatus include cysts, sinus tracts, & fistulae. The most common lesions for which imaging is indicated are BCCs/BACs, & most of these are related to anomalous development of a branchial cleft. However, a few are related to anomalous development of a branchial pouch.

The location of the lesion is the best clue to the origin of a branchial apparatus anomaly. **First BCCs** account for ~ 8% of all branchial anomalies. They are located in or around the external auditory canal, ear lobe, or parotid gland & may extend inferiorly to the angle of the mandible. **Second BCCs** account for up to 95% of all branchial apparatus anomalies & are subclassified by location using the Bailey system: Type I cysts are located deep to the platysma muscle/anterior to the sternocleidomastoid (SCM) muscle; type II cysts are posterior to the submandibular gland/anterior to the SCM (& are the most common); type III cysts protrude between the external & internal carotid arteries; & type IV cysts are directly adjacent to the pharyngeal wall (thought to be a remnant of the 2nd pouch). Fistulas are rare; however, a 2nd branchial apparatus fistula is occasionally identified with an internal opening at the level of the pharynx & an external skin opening anterior to the lower aspect of the SCM.

Third BCCs are rare & located in the posterior compartment of the upper neck or anterior compartment of the lower neck. Third pharyngeal pouch remnants are more common than cleft remnants & are related to descent of the thymic primordium from the lateral margins of the pharynx to the upper anterior mediastinum (via the thymopharyngeal duct) during the 6th-9th weeks of gestation. If the duct does not undergo normal involution, a cervical thymic cyst may form that is in close association with the anterior margin of the carotid sheath. The cyst formation is from interactions between the endodermal primordia & neural crest cells during normal thymic development & migration. Histologically, Hassall corpuscles will be identifiable within the cyst wall. Ectopic foci of solid thymic tissue may also be deposited along the remnant duct.

Types of Congenital Cystic Neck Masses

Thyroglossal Duct Lesions	
Thyroglossal duct cyst: Tongue base to thyroid bed; embedded in strap muscles when infrahyoid	
Ectopic thyroid tissue: Lingual location is most common	
Branchial Apparatus Lesions	
1st branchial cleft cyst (type I): Located anterior, inferior, or posterior to external auditory canal	
1st branchial cleft cyst (type II): Located in or adjacent to parotid gland; may extend inferiorly to angle of mandible	
2nd branchial cleft cyst: Most common location is posterior to submandibular gland, lateral to carotid space, & anteromedial to SCM muscle	
3rd branchial cleft cyst: Posterior cervical space in upper neck or anterior to SCM in lower neck	
3rd branchial pouch remnant → thymopharyngeal duct cyst or ectopic thymus: Along course from pharynx to upper mediastinum	
4th branchial pouch remnant → pyriform sinus tract: Patients present with left-sided abscess involving thyroid gland	
Vascular Malformations	
Venous malformation: Patchy, gradual enhancement; phleboliths are common; ± fluid-fluid levels	
Lymphatic malformation: Multilocular cyst ± fluid-fluid levels; rim/septal enhancement	
Venolymphatic malformation: Mixed enhancing venous & nonenhancing lymphatic components	
SCM = sternocleidomastoid.	

Pyriform sinus tracts, or rarely fistulae, represent a unique congenital anomaly of the **4th (or 3rd) pharyngeal pouch**. This lesion should be suspected in any child presenting with neck infection involving the left thyroid lobe. The inflammation can frequently be traced superiorly to an asymmetric pyriform sinus apex. A post barium swallow CT study is helpful to define the barium-filled tract extending from the pyriform sinus to the anterior lower neck.

Vascular malformations are congenital malformations of endothelial development, divided into simple or combined lesions, combined lesions containing ≥ 2 vessel types. Simple lesions can be divided based on the predominant endothelial characteristics of the lesion into capillary malformations, lymphatic malformations, venous malformations, arteriovenous malformations, & arteriovenous fistulae. The most common vascular malformations in the H&N are lymphatic, venous, & combined venolymphatic lesions.

Imaging Anatomy

Recognizing the defined **location** of a congenital abnormality, particularly congenital cysts, is key to arriving at the correct diagnosis or differential diagnosis. **TGD** remnants may be in the form of cysts or solid ectopic thyroid tissue anywhere from the midline tongue base to the infrahyoid paramidline thyroid bed. **First BCCs** are in or around the external auditory canal or parotid gland. **Second BCCs** are most commonly posteromedial to the submandibular gland & anteromedial to the SCM. Cysts in the posterior upper neck may be 3rd BCCs or lymphatic malformations. Cysts along the lower anterior margin of the SCM may be from the 2nd or 3rd branchial cleft or may be lymphatic malformations. Cysts or solid masses in close association with the carotid sheath along the tract of the thymopharyngeal duct (from the angle of the mandible to the upper mediastinum) should raise the question of cervical thymic cyst or ectopic thymus (**3rd pouch** remnants), & left-sided neck abscesses involving the thyroid gland should raise the question of a pyriform sinus sinus tract as a cause, a **4th (or 3rd) pharyngeal pouch** remnant.

Differential Diagnosis

Thyroglossal Duct Lesions
- TGDC: Tongue base to thyroid bed
- Ectopic thyroid: Lingual thyroid is most common

Branchial Apparatus Lesions
- 1st BCC: **Work type I** lie anterior, inferior, or posterior to external auditory canal; **Work type II** in superficial, parotid, or parapharyngeal space may extend to posterior submandibular space; **IPOG type I** lateral to parotid fascia, **IPOG type II** deep to parotid fascia in gland or between gland & auricular cartilage
- 2nd BCC: Most common posterolateral to submandibular gland, lateral to carotid space, & anteromedial to SCM
- 3rd BCC: Posterior cervical space upper neck, along anterior border of SCM in mid- & lower neck
- 3rd branchial pouch remnant: Thymopharyngeal duct cyst or ectopic thymus
- 4th branchial pouch remnant: Pyriform sinus tract → recurrent thyroiditis or thyroid abscess, usually left sided; some literature suggests this may be 3rd pouch remnant

Vascular Malformations
- Venous malformations: Patchy, gradual enhancement; ± fluid-fluid levels & phleboliths
- Lymphatic malformations: Classically multilocular & transspatial with fluid-fluid levels & minimal rim/septal enhancement
- Venolymphatic malformations: Nonenhancing lymphatic & enhancing venous elements ± phleboliths

Selected References

1. Putra J et al: Advances in vascular anomalies: refining classification in the molecular era. Histopathology. 86(7):1032-43, 2025
2. Heilingoetter AL et al: Comprehensive management and classification of first branchial cleft anomalies: an International Pediatric Otorhinolaryngology Group (IPOG) consensus statement. Int J Pediatr Otorhinolaryngol. 186:112095, 2024
3. Booth TN: Congenital cystic neck masses. Neuroimaging Clin N Am. 33(4):591-605, 2023
4. Mamlouk MD: Solid and vascular neck masses in children. Neuroimaging Clin N Am. 33(4):607-21, 2023

(Left) Anterior graphic of a 6-week embryo shows the 2nd branchial arch ➡ growing inferiorly over the 3rd & 4th arches, resulting in the cervical sinus of His ➡ that combines the 2nd, 3rd, & 4th branchial clefts (BCs). Note that the thymopharyngeal duct is a remnant of the 3rd branchial pouch ➡. **(Right)** Oblique graphic shows the tract of a type I 1st BC anomaly ➡ from the medial bony external auditory canal (EAC) toward the retroauricular area. The tract of a type II 1st BC anomaly ➡ connects the EAC to the angle of the mandible.

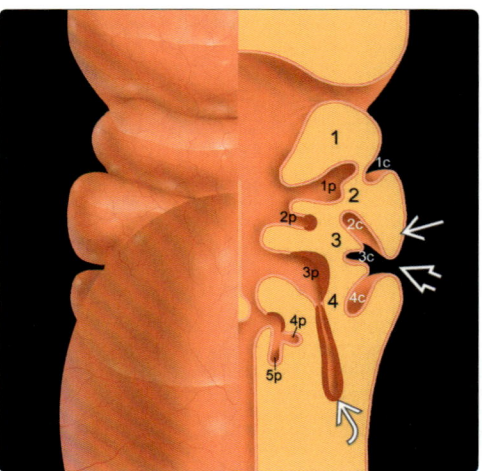

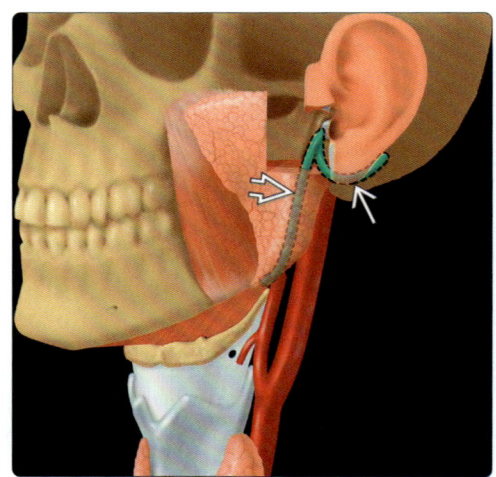

(Left) Oblique graphic of the tract of a 2nd BC fistula ➡ shows a proximal opening ➡ in the faucial tonsil & a distal opening in the anterior supraclavicular neck ➡. Second BC cysts (BCCs) may occur anywhere along this tract & are the most common of the BCCs. **(Right)** Oblique graphic illustrates the tract of a 3rd BC anomaly ➡ extending from the cephalad aspect of the lateral hypopharynx ➡ to the supraclavicular anterior neck skin ➡. Notice cysts would lie in the posterior upper neck or the anterior lower neck.

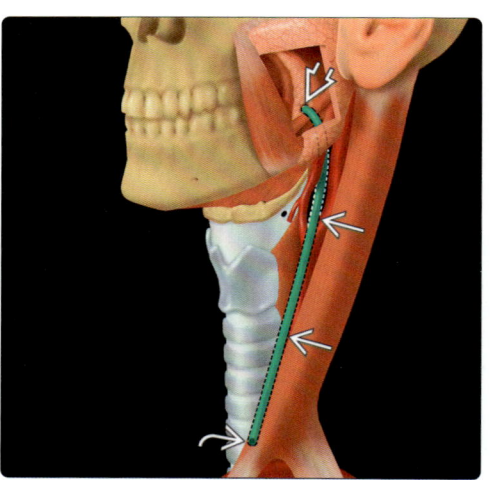

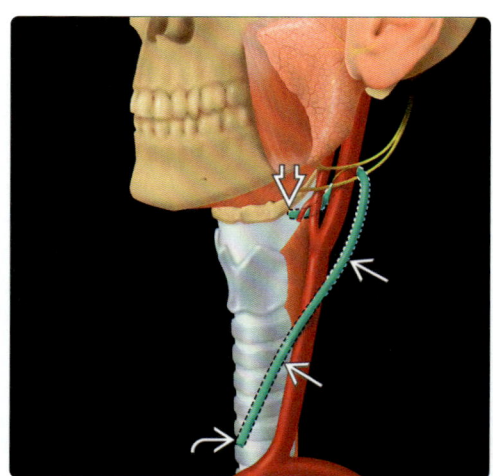

(Left) Anterior graphic shows both thymopharyngeal duct tracts ➡ extending from the lateral hypopharyngeal area ➡ to the location of the normal lobes of the thymus ➡ in the superior mediastinum. Thymic cysts may be cervical, mediastinal, or both. **(Right)** Oblique graphic of the neck shows the tract of a 4th BC anomaly ➡ extending from the hypopharynx ➡ to the location of the left thyroid lobe ➡. This relationship explains why this lesion often presents with thyroiditis or thyroid/perithyroid abscess.

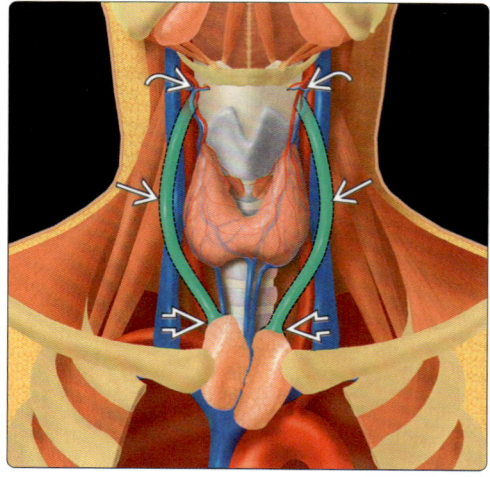

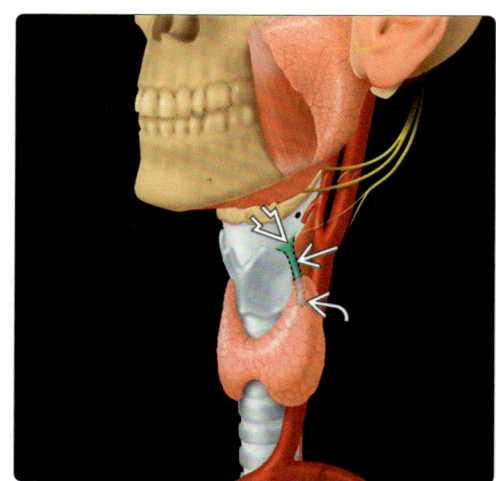

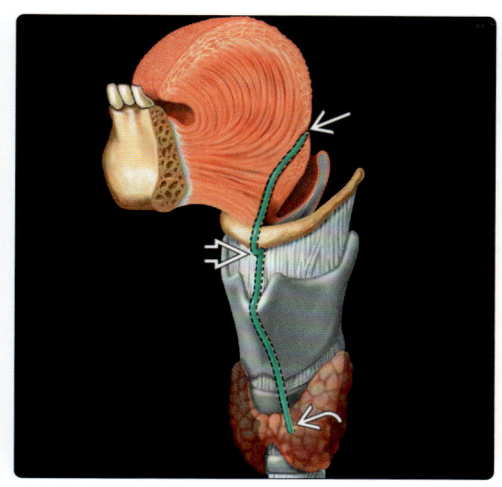

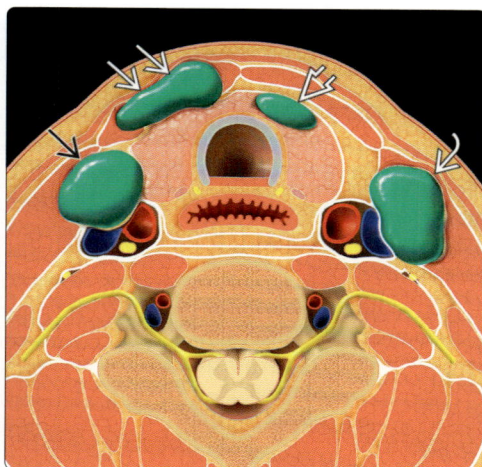

(Left) Oblique graphic illustrates the tract of the thyroglossal duct descending from the foramen cecum ➡ (at the midline tongue base) to the midline hyoid bone ➡ before tracking off-midline to the thyroid lobe ➡. (Right) Axial graphic demonstrates the locations of 4 major congenital cystic lesions of the neck. Shown here are the location of infrahyoid 2nd & 3rd BCCs ➡, infrahyoid thyroglossal duct cysts ➡ (embedded in strap muscle), cervical thymic cysts ➡, & 4th branchial apparatus sinus tracts ➡.

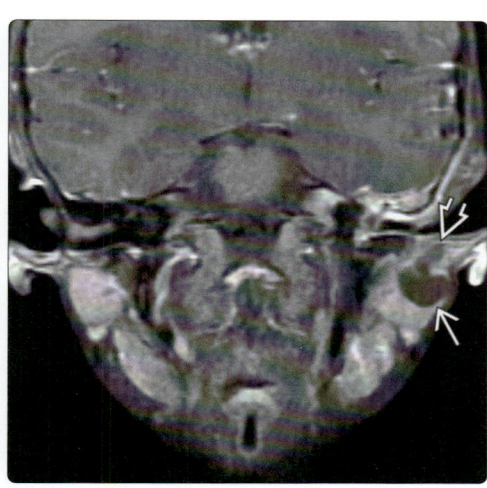

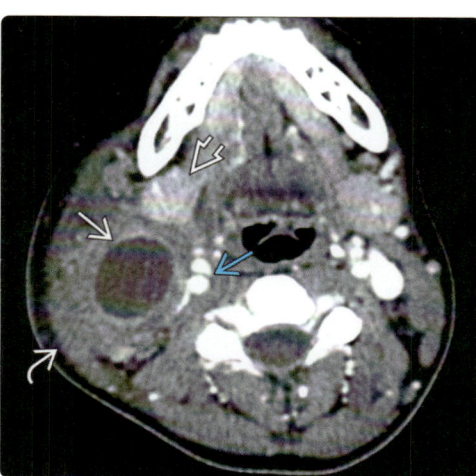

(Left) Coronal T1 C+ FS MR in a 3-year-old patient with a 1st BAC shows a lobulated, nonenhancing periparotid cyst ➡ extending toward the junction of the cartilaginous & bony EAC ➡. (Right) Axial CECT in a teenager with an enlarging mass shows a cystic-appearing lesion ➡ in the typical location of a 2nd BCC: Dorsal to submandibular gland ➡, anterior to sternocleidomastoid (SCM) muscle ➡ & lateral to carotid sheath vessels ➡.

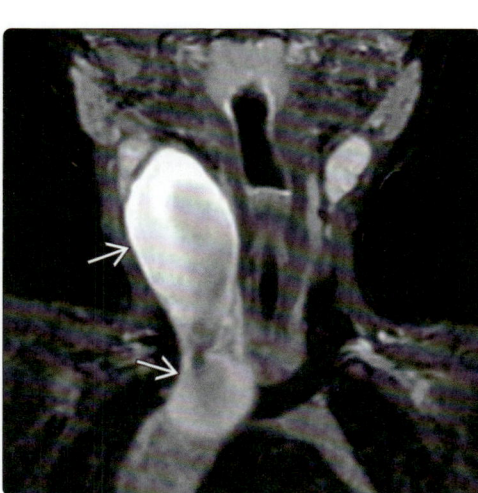

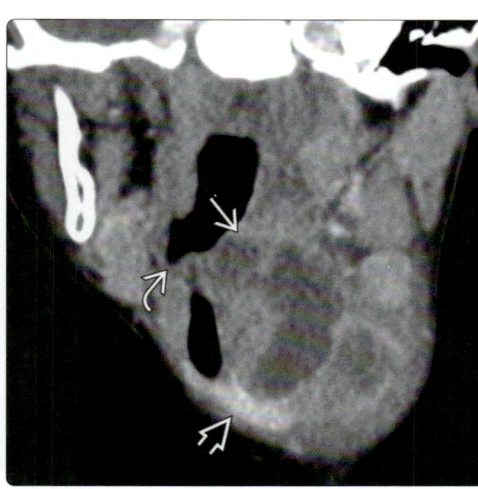

(Left) Coronal FSEIR in a child with a right-sided neck mass shows a bilobed hyperintense cystic mass ➡ extending from the upper neck to the upper mediastinum, the location typical of a thymic cyst. (Right) Coronal CECT in a 2-year-old with a heterogeneously enhancing left neck mass that extends from the region of the effaced left pyriform sinus ➡ to the upper left thyroid lobe ➡, typical of an abscess secondary to congenital 4th (or 3rd) pharyngeal pouch sinus tract, is shown. Notice the air-filled normal right pyriform sinus ➡.

TERMINOLOGY

- Lymphatic malformation (LM): Subtype of slow- or low-flow congenital vascular malformation composed of embryonic lymphatic sacs; not neoplastic
- Composed of macrocysts > 1 cm &/or microcysts < 1 cm

IMAGING

- Macrocystic LM: Multiloculated cystic neck mass with imperceptible wall, thin septations, and fluid-fluid levels
- Microcystic LM: Ill-defined, infiltrative, &/or solid-appearing
- Transspatial, often crosses midline extensively
- Insinuates between vessels and other normal structures
- T2 FS/STIR MR: Hyperintense, frequent fluid-fluid levels
  - Best defines extent, relationship to airway and vessels
- T1 C+ FS MR: No significant or minimal rim enhancement
  - Must compare with precontrast T1, as hemorrhage and protein often show hyperintensity
- US: Cysts can show varying degrees of ↑ echogenicity; Doppler shows no significant internal vascularity

TOP DIFFERENTIAL DIAGNOSES

- 2nd branchial cleft anomaly
- Thyroglossal duct cyst
- Abscess
- Thymic cyst
- Teratoma
- Neurofibroma
- Soft tissue sarcoma

CLINICAL ISSUES

- Nontender, compressible mass
  - Present since birth, grows commensurate with patient
  - May not be clinically apparent until hemorrhage, infection, or hormonal stimulation → rapid ↑ in size
- Depending on size and extent, treatment options primarily include resection, sclerotherapy (for macrocysts), and sirolimus
  - Combination therapy (often staged; may be required)

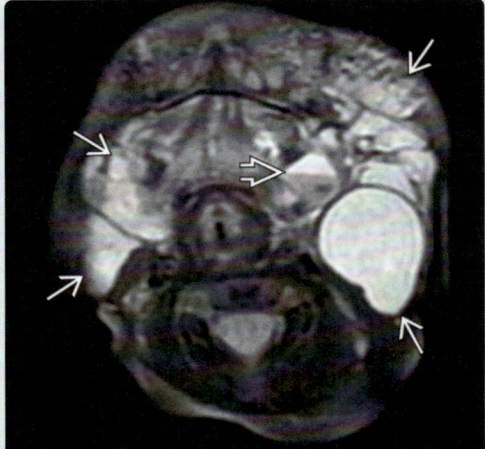
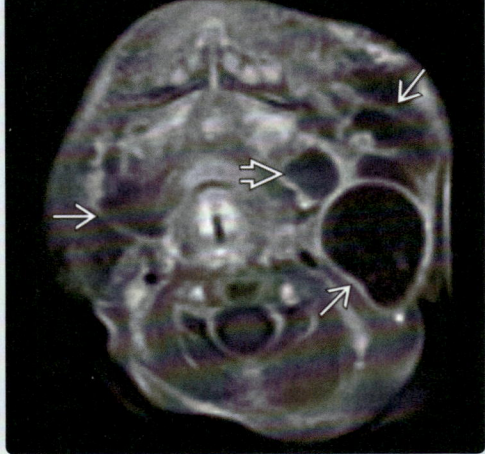

(Left) Axial T2 FS MR in a 1-week-old infant demonstrates a multiloculated, mixed micro- and macrocystic transspatial lymphatic malformation (LM) ⇒ involving the left anterior neck more than the right. A single fluid-fluid level is present in a left-sided submandibular macrocyst ⇒, typical of layering blood products. (Right) Axial T1 C+ FS MR in the same child shows a typical appearance of an extensive LM. The macrocysts show only mild peripheral enhancement ⇒, and the fluid-fluid level ⇒ is much more difficult to discern.

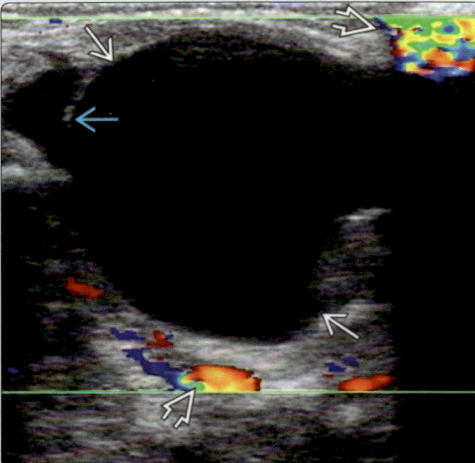
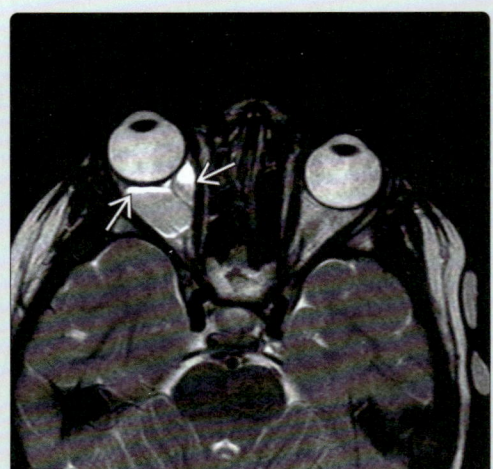

(Left) Transverse color Doppler US in an infant with a macrocystic LM shows the typical anechoic nature of the dominant cyst ⇒ with vessels ⇒ identified adjacent to, but not within, the cyst. Note the thin septation ⇒ peripherally. (Right) Axial T2 MR of the orbit in a 5-year-old with rapid-onset proptosis demonstrates an intraconal, multiloculated lesion with fluid-fluid levels ⇒, consistent with layering blood products, resulting in moderate right-sided proptosis, secondary to the intralesional hemorrhage.

Lymphatic Malformation

TERMINOLOGY

Synonyms
- Vascular malformation, lymphatic type; lymphatic anomaly
- Avoid incorrect terms: Cystic hygroma and lymphangioma

Definitions
- Lymphatic malformation (LM): Subtype of slow- or low-flow congenital vascular malformation composed of embryonic lymphatic sacs; not neoplastic
  - No communication with normal lymphatics
  - Composed of macrocysts > 1 cm &/or microcysts < 1 cm
- Venolymphatic malformation (VLM): Combined elements of venous malformation and LM

IMAGING

General Features
- Best diagnostic clue
  - Macrocystic LM: Multiloculated cystic neck mass with imperceptible wall, thin septations, and fluid-fluid levels
  - Microcystic LM: More ill-defined, infiltrative, &/or solid-appearing
  - Crosses tissue planes, insinuating between vessels and other normal structures
- Location
  - Any face/neck location (not intracranial)
    - Infrahyoid neck
      - Posterior cervical space most common
    - Suprahyoid neck
      - Masticator, submandibular, and parotid spaces most common
    - Orbit, tongue, floor of mouth, buccal space
  - Often in multiple contiguous spaces: Transspatial
    - Soft tissue involvement > > bone; single lesion > > multiple discontinuous lesions
  - Often crosses midline extensively
- Size
  - Individual compartments: Microcystic or macrocystic
  - Overall lesion varies from few cm to massive
  - May suddenly ↑ in size, particularly when intralesional hemorrhage occurs
- Morphology
  - Uni- or multilocular

Radiographic Findings
- LMs may cause mass effect on airway

CT Findings
- NECT
  - Low-attenuation, well-defined, or poorly circumscribed cystic neck mass
  - ± fluid-fluid levels
  - ± phleboliths in venous malformation components of VLM
- CECT
  - Unilocular or multilocular cystic mass with minimal rim &/or septal enhancement
    - In mixed VLM, venous malformation components will show patchy, gradual enhancement ± phleboliths

MR Findings
- T1WI
  - Primarily hypointense fluid; hyperintense if prior hemorrhage or high protein content (± fluid-fluid levels)
- T2WI FS or STIR
  - Best sequence to map lesion extent: Hyperintense throughout
    - Fluid-fluid levels in multiple cysts very common
  - When transspatial, often poorly marginated
- T1WI C+ FS
  - No significant enhancement (± subtle rim enhancement)
  - Patchy enhancement suggests VLM or microcystic LM

Ultrasonographic Findings
- Unilocular vs. septated and multilocular transspatial mass
- Contents predominantly hypo- or anechoic
  - Separate compartments in multicystic mass can show varying degrees of ↑ echogenicity
    - ± swirling debris &/or layering fluid-debris levels
- No true vascular flow in cysts by Doppler
  - ± flow (from encased normal vessels) in septations

Imaging Recommendations
- Best imaging tool
  - US often diagnostic of superficial components
  - MR better for defining deep extent and recognizing characteristic fluid-fluid levels
- Protocol advice
  - Fluid-sensitive sequences (T2 FS or STIR) essential
    - STIR particularly helpful for overcoming poor chemical fat suppression in neck (typical of T2)
  - T1 C+ FS helpful to detect venous malformation component of mixed lesions
    - Subtraction of precontrast T1 FS improves assessment of true enhancement (vs. pseudoenhancement from preexisting T1 shortening of protein/hemorrhage)

DIFFERENTIAL DIAGNOSIS

2nd Branchial Cleft Anomaly
- Ovoid, unilocular cyst at angle of mandible with characteristic displacement pattern

Abscess
- Fluid collection with thick, enhancing, irregular wall
- Adjacent soft tissues show cellulitis > myositis, fasciitis

Teratoma
- Solid and cystic components typical ± internal vascularity
- Frequently contain calcification
- Tend to be more unilateral and focal than LM

Thyroglossal Duct Cyst
- Anterior midline/paramidline unilocular cystic mass
- Tongue base to lower anterior neck
- Embedded in infrahyoid strap muscles

Thymic Cyst
- Unilocular lateral neck cyst
- Closely associated with carotid sheath
- May extend into anterior superior mediastinum

Neurofibroma

- ± lobular, low-attenuation foci on CT without significant enhancement
- T2 MR often confirms characteristic target sign

Soft Tissue Sarcoma

- Well-defined, typically solid; rarely predominantly cystic
  - Cystic mass with discrete solid nodules showing internal vascularity requires biopsy/excision

PATHOLOGY

General Features

- Etiology
  - Congenital error of vessel morphogenesis
  - 2 main theories
    - Failure of embryologic fusion between primordial lymph sac and venous system
    - Abnormal sequestration of embryonic lymphatic sacs
- Genetics
  - Majority sporadic
  - May be part of extensive overgrowth syndrome with capillary VLM
  - Generalized lymphatic anomaly (lymphangiomatosis), kaposiform lymphangiomatosis, and Gorham-Stout disease may have soft tissue LM in association with bone and visceral lesions
  - Confusion regarding anterior neck LM association with Turner syndrome and trisomies
    - Aneuploidy and high mortality in posterior midline cystic neck masses ("cystic hygroma") of early gestation
- Associated abnormalities
  - 70% of patients with periorbital VLM have intracranial vascular and parenchymal anomalies
    - Developmental venous anomaly, cerebral cavernous malformation, dural arteriovenous malformation (AVM), pial AVM, sinus pericranii

Staging, Grading, & Classification

- Microcystic or macrocystic
- Lymphatic alone vs. mixed venolymphatic

Microscopic Features

- Primitive embryonic lymph sacs of varying sizes separated by connective tissue stroma
- Recent recommendation: Use immunohistochemical panel of PROX1, D2-40, VEGFR3, CD31, and CD34 antibodies to differentiate LM from other vascular malformations
  - PROX1 and VEGFR3 most sensitive, specific

CLINICAL ISSUES

Presentation

- Most common signs/symptoms
  - Nontender, soft, compressible mass
  - Present since birth and grows commensurate with patient
    - May not be clinically apparent until hemorrhage, infection, or hormonal stimulation → rapid ↑ in size
  - Larger lesions detected prenatally
- Other signs/symptoms
  - LMs may infiltrate upper airway or cause extrinsic compression

Demographics

- Age: 90% diagnosed < 2 years of age

Natural History & Prognosis

- No clear malignant potential
- Benign disease with potential lifelong morbidity in more extensive cases
- Recurrence may be secondary to redirection of lymphatic fluid into remaining dilated spaces or to growth of truncated lymphatic channels

Treatment

- Surgical resection &/or percutaneous sclerotherapy
  - Sclerotherapy primarily for macrocystic disease
  - Extensive disease often requires combined &/or numerous staged procedures
- Some success with radiofrequency ablation of microcystic LM of oral cavity and laser therapy of tongue lesions
- Medical therapy with mTOR inhibitor sirolimus
  - Future potential with VEGFR3 inhibitors
- Tracheostomy for significant airway involvement

DIAGNOSTIC CHECKLIST

Image Interpretation Pearls

- Transspatial multicystic neck mass with fluid-fluid levels highly suggestive of LM
- Multiplanar T2 FS/STIR MR: Maps extent of transspatial lesion, especially relationship to airway and vessels
- In absence of irritation by infection or hemorrhage, lesion wall should be thin and nearly imperceptible
  - True, solid nodular enhancement in cyst wall must suggest predominantly cystic soft tissue sarcoma over LM → biopsy

SELECTED REFERENCES

1. Azizinik F et al: Vascular lesions of head and neck region: a pictorial review. Eur J Radiol. ePub 2025
2. Zhang C et al: Lymphatic malformation: classification, pathogenesis and therapeutic strategies. Ann Vasc Surg. ePub, 2025
3. Mamlouk MD: Solid and vascular neck masses in children. Neuroimaging Clin N Am. 33(4):607-21, 2023
4. Wiegand S et al: Efficacy of sirolimus in children with lymphatic malformations of the head and neck. Eur Arch Otorhinolaryngol. 279(8):3801-10, 2022
5. Le HDT et al: Generalized lymphangiomatosis-a rare manifestation of lymphatic malformation. Radiol Case Rep. 16(1):66-71, 2021
6. Reis J 3rd et al: Ultrasound evaluation of pediatric slow-flow vascular malformations: practical diagnostic reporting to guide interventional management. AJR. Am J Roentgenol. 216(2):494-506, 2021
7. Crane J et al: Kaposiform lymphangiomatosis treated with multimodal therapy improves coagulopathy and reduces blood angiopoietin-2 levels. Pediatr Blood Cancer. 67(9):e28529, 2020
8. International Society for the Study of Vascular Anomalies: ISSVA Classification for Vascular Anomalies. Reviewed 2024. Accessed May 28, 2025. https://www.issva.org/classification
9. Adams DM et al: Efficacy and safety of sirolimus in the treatment of complicated vascular anomalies. Pediatrics. 137(2):1-10, 2016
10. Merrow AC et al: 2014 revised classification of vascular lesions from the International Society for the Study of Vascular Anomalies: radiologic-pathologic update. Radiographics. 36(5):1494-516, 2016
11. Shiels WE 2nd et al: Percutaneous treatment of lymphatic malformations. Otolaryngol Head Neck Surg. 141(2):219-24, 2009
12. Mulliken JB et al: Hemangiomas and vascular malformations in infants and children: a classification based on endothelial characteristics. Plast Reconstr Surg. 69(3):412-22, 1982

Lymphatic Malformation

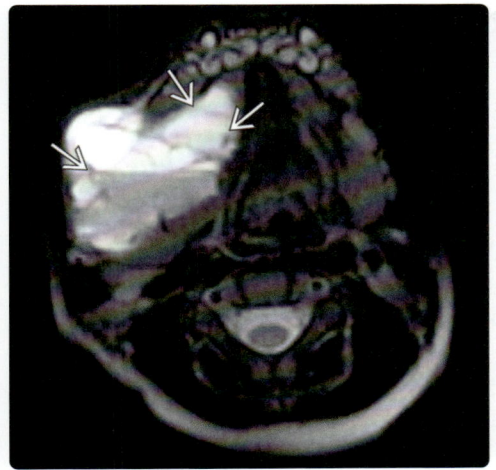

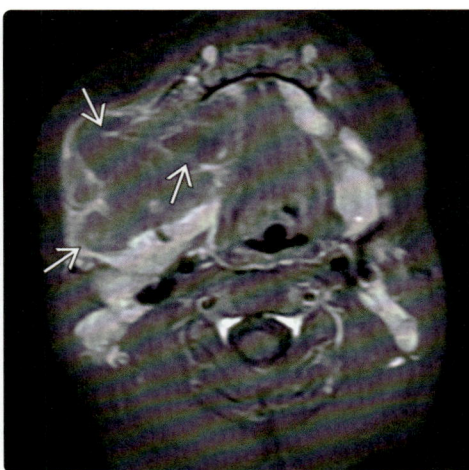

(Left) *Axial TSE FS MR in a 1-year-old child shows a multiloculated, transspatial, macrocystic LM in the right submandibular and sublingual spaces. Notice the multiple fluid-fluid levels ➡ of varying intensities, indicating intralesional blood products.* **(Right)** *Axial T1 C+ FS MR in the same child shows only minimal linear, peripheral, and septal contrast enhancement ➡, typical of macrocystic LM. There is associated mass effect on the submandibular gland and the airway.*

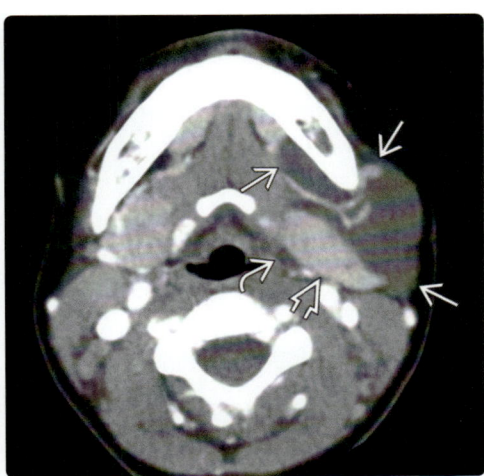

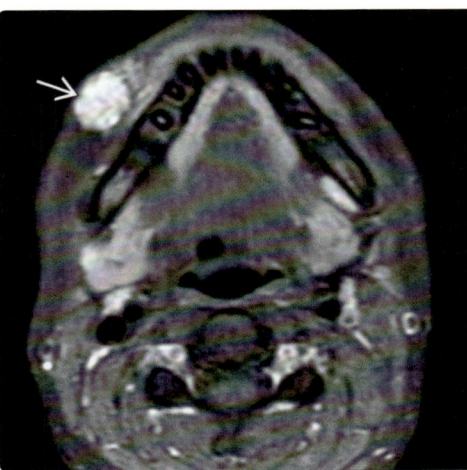

(Left) *Axial CECT in a 3-year-old shows a well-defined, hypodense, macrocystic LM ➡ in sublingual & submandibular spaces, flattening the gland ➡, without phleboliths. There is minimal extension deep to left submandibular gland ➡.* **(Right)** *Axial T1 C+ FS MR in a teenager with a firm, tender lump shows a lobulated, enhancing subcutaneous mass ➡ adjacent to the right mandible, proven to be a microcystic LM. The well-circumscribed morphology and enhancement could also be seen with a sarcoma, thus requiring excision.*

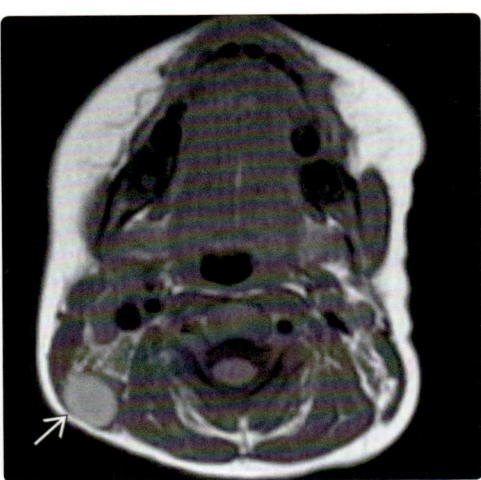

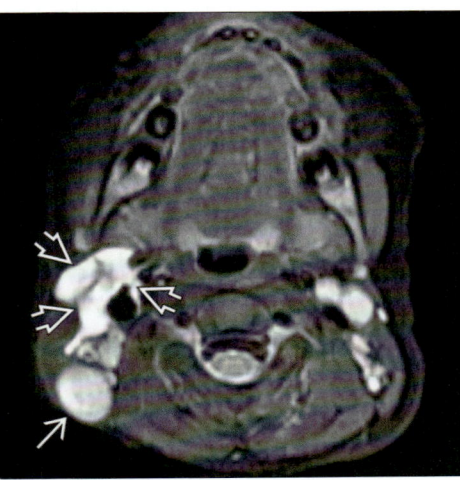

(Left) *Axial T1 MR in a 4-year-old child with an enlarging neck mass shows a multiloculated, macrocystic LM ➡ with a hyperintense locule related to recent intralesional hemorrhage.* **(Right)** *Axial FSEIR MR in the same patient shows the dominant macrocyst contains intermediate signal intensity blood products ➡ and shows to better advantage the more hyperintense, multiloculated, smaller cysts in the anterior neck ➡ with extension into the carotid space.*

589

TERMINOLOGY

- Venous malformation (VM)

IMAGING

- Use MR & US when possible
- General imaging findings
  - Lobulated soft tissue "mass" with phleboliths
  - Solitary or multiple
  - May be circumscribed or transspatial, infiltrating adjacent soft tissue compartments
  - ± combined lymphatic malformation (LM), i.e., mixed venolymphatic malformation (VLM)
- CT findings
  - Rounded calcifications (phleboliths)
  - Osseous remodeling in adjacent bone
  - Fat hypertrophy in adjacent soft tissues
- Enhancement features
  - Variable enhancement pattern reflects sluggish vascular flow to & through lesion

- Patchy & delayed or homogeneous & intense

TOP DIFFERENTIAL DIAGNOSES

- LM
- Infantile hemangioma
- Arteriovenous malformation
- Neurofibroma
- Dermoid & epidermoid
- Soft tissue sarcoma

PATHOLOGY

- Congenital slow- or low-flow vascular malformation
- 70% of patients with periorbital LM or VLM have intracranial vascular & parenchymal anomalies

CLINICAL ISSUES

- Presents as spongy H&N mass that grows proportionately with patient
  - May enlarge suddenly due to hemorrhage, thrombosis, or hormonal changes

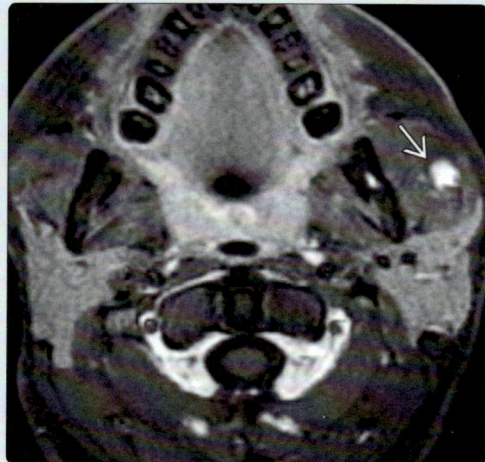
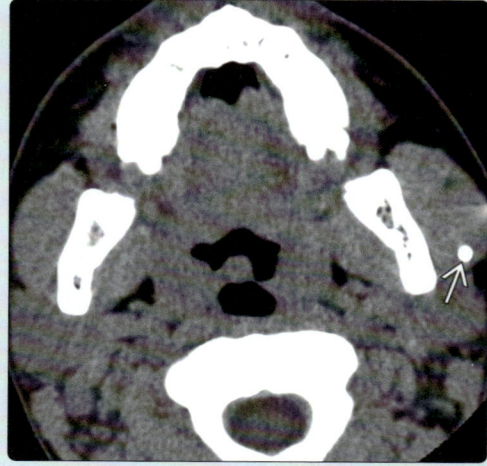

(Left) Axial T1 C+ FS MR in a 14-year-old boy demonstrates a small focal area of enhancement ➡ in an otherwise nonspecific lesion within the left masseter muscle within the masticator space. (Right) Axial NECT in the same patient shows an ill-defined, intramuscular mass with a small phlebolith ➡ representing a calcified intraluminal thrombus, characteristic of a venous malformation (VM). This case seems to be isolated VM without mixed lymphatic malformation.

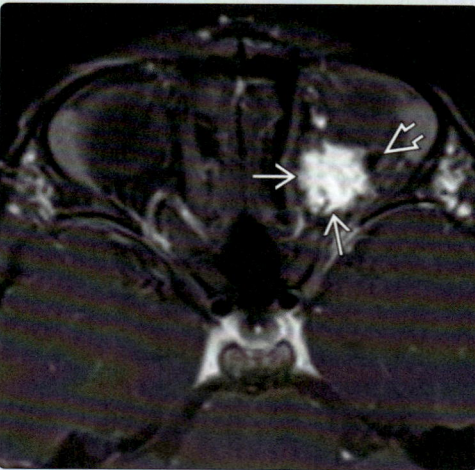
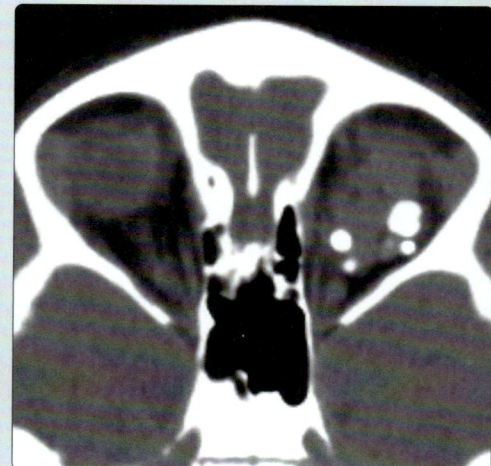

(Left) Axial T1 C+ FS MR in a 5-year-old with proptosis shows an enhancing mass with irregular margins in the left intraconal space ➡. There is a small focus of hypointense signal in the anterolateral aspect of the mass ➡ and a few other punctate foci of nonenhancing, hypointense signal that may represent phleboliths. (Right) Axial NECT in the same patient demonstrates multiple well-defined calcifications within the intraconal space of the left orbit, characteristic of phleboliths in venous VMs.

Venous Malformation

TERMINOLOGY

Abbreviations
- Venous malformation (VM) (preferred term)

Synonyms
- Cavernous malformation, cavernous hemangioma (both terms to be avoided)

Definitions
- VM: Subtype of congenital slow- or low-flow vascular malformation due to error in vein formation; not neoplastic
- Venolymphatic malformation (VLM) combined lesion with venous & lymphatic components

IMAGING

General Features
- Best diagnostic clue
  - Cluster of slow-flow serpiginous vessels + phleboliths
- Location
  - Most commonly subcutaneous &/or intramuscular
  - Focal, multifocal, or diffuse
  - H&N (40%), extremities (40%), trunk (20%)
  - May be in any space(s) in H&N
- Morphology
  - Multilobulated, solitary, or multiple
  - Well circumscribed or transspatial (multiple contiguous spaces), confluent & infiltrative
  - ± combined/mixed VLM
  - ± discrete serpentine venous channels of abnormal number, size, shape, & location (phlebectasia)

Fluoroscopic Findings
- Anatomy & venous drainage best mapped via direct percutaneous injection of venous sinusoids
  - Contrast material pools within clusters of abnormal venous channels/lakes ± connections to normal or abnormal veins
  - Large channels resemble cluster of grapes; smaller channels have more cotton-wool blush appearance

CT Findings
- Lobulated soft tissue mass with fluid attenuation
- Rounded, calcified phleboliths essentially pathognomonic
- Enhancement usually evident but variable: Patchy & delayed or homogeneous & intense
- Lymphatic component of VLM does not enhance
- ± osseous remodeling in adjacent bone
- ± fat hypertrophy in adjacent soft tissues

MR Findings
- T1WI
  - Multilobulated with variable signal intensity
    - Isointense to hypointense relative to muscle typical
    - Hemorrhage, stagnant blood, &/or thrombi → ↑ signal
    - Phleboliths hypointense due to calcification
  - Regional fat hypertrophy, often with fat interspersed within & around lesion
- T2WI FS
  - Vascular channel size influences appearance
    - Large, serpentine vascular channels hyperintense, septated
      - Large varicosities may be hypointense 2° to disturbed flow; may mimic clot
    - Smaller vascular channels appear more solid & intermediate in signal intensity
  - Phleboliths appear as rounded or oval signal voids
  - ± layering fluid-fluid levels 2° to settling of blood products within stagnant cavity
- T1WI C+ FS
  - Enhancement variable: May be delayed, heterogeneous or homogeneous, & mild to intense
  - Variable enhancement pattern reflects sluggish vascular flow to & through lesion
    - No enlarged feeding arteries
    - Lesion often drained by enlarged veins
  - Thrombi &/or intermixed LM components do not enhance
- MRV
  - May show enlarged veins associated with lesion
  - Extracranial VMs may show associated intracranial venous anomalies

Ultrasonographic Findings
- Spongy, compressible mass, heterogeneous echotexture
  - Small vascular channels are more echogenic & less compressible than large, vascular lumina
- ± discrete venous channels of abnormal number, size, shape, & location in surrounding tissues
- Phleboliths = hyperechoic foci with poor acoustic shadowing & twinkle artifact
- Valsalva or compression/release of transducer will ↑ venous flow
- Lack of arterial waveforms or arterialized draining veins; 1-2 normal arteries may be encased by VM

Imaging Recommendations
- Best imaging tool
  - MR best to map full extent & identify combined LM/VLM
  - US to assess response to compression if lesion is superficial
  - CT & radiographs identify phleboliths
- Protocol advice
  - US &/or MR for suspected vascular malformation
  - MR with contrast, fat suppression, & gradient-echo to confirm lack of high-flow vessels

DIFFERENTIAL DIAGNOSIS

Lymphatic Malformation
- Another common slow-or low-flow lesion
- Compressible, fluid-filled, macrocystic soft tissue mass
  - Thin, enhancing internal septations, internal debris, blood-fluid levels
  - Microcystic lesions may enhance & appear solid
- No phleboliths; no enhancement unless mixed VLM or microcystic lesion
- Solitary or multiple; single space or transspatial

Infantile Hemangioma
- Characteristic life cycle: Small at birth, rapid growth during infancy, gradual involution over years

- Benign, vascular neoplasm, GLUT1 (+) marker
- Prominent intralesional vessels
- Rapid, homogeneous, intense enhancement
- Typically intermediate hyperintensity on T2

Arteriovenous Malformation

- Tangle of enlarged, tortuous arteries & veins
- High-flow vessels with shunting by US, MRA/MRV

Neurofibroma

- Elongated, lobular masses along course of nerves
- Multiple adjacent nerves → bag of worms appearance
- Target sign: T2-hypointense center, T2-hyperintense rim
- Variable contrast enhancement

Dermoid & Epidermoid

- Rounded calcifications possible (dermoid)
  - If present, found lying within fat-containing lesion
- Lesion contents very echogenic on ultrasound (dermoid)

Soft Tissue Sarcoma

- Well-defined soft tissue mass with variable enhancement
- ± cystic foci, ± bone destruction

PATHOLOGY

General Features

- Etiology
  - Subtype of congenital slow- or low-flow vascular malformation due to error in vein formation
- Genetics
  - *TEK* mutation in many VM (50% of sporadic VM)
- Associated abnormalities
  - 70% of patients with periorbital LM or VLM have intracranial vascular & parenchymal anomalies
    - Developmental venous anomaly (DVA), cerebral cavernous malformation, dural arteriovenous malformation (AVM), pial AVM, sinus pericranii
- Staging, grading, & classification
  - 2018 revised classification (recent 2025 update) of VM by ISSVA
    - Common VM: Causal genes *TEK*/*PIK3CA*
    - Familial VM cutaneo-mucosal (VMCM): *TEK*
      □ Multifocal lesions of lips, tongue
    - Blue rubber bleb nevus syndrome (BRBNS): *TEK* (TIE2)
      □ Multiple cutaneous, muscular, gastrointestinal VM
    - Glomuvenous malformation (GVM): Chromosome 1p
    - Cerebral cavernous malformation: *CCM1*, *CCM2*, *CCM3*
    - Familial intraosseous vascular malformation (VMOS): *ELMO2*
    - Verrucous VM: *MAP3K3*

Microscopic Features

- Venous channels, variable luminal diameter, wall thickness
- Luminal thrombi, phleboliths
- Immunohistochemical markers: GLUT1 (-), PROX1 (-) [(+) in LM], CD31 (+), CD34 (+) [(-) in LM]

CLINICAL ISSUES

Presentation

- Most common signs/symptoms
  - Spongy soft tissue mass without thrill
    - Bluish skin discoloration when superficial
  - Grows proportionately with patient
  - ↑ ↑ in size with Valsalva, bending over, crying
  - May enlarge rapidly after trauma, thrombosis or under hormonal influences (puberty, pregnancy)
  - May be painful 2° to stasis, intralesional thrombus, or hemorrhage into adjacent tissues

Demographics

- Age
  - VMs are present at birth, but may not clinically manifest until adolescence, or young adulthood
- Epidemiology
  - Most common vascular malformation of H&N

Treatment

- Treatment aimed at decreasing symptoms & improving function, rather than eliminating disease
- Conservative therapy
  - Compression garments, antiinflammatory medications
  - Low-molecular-weight heparin if thrombosis risk ↑
  - Sirolimus may be helpful for lesions with mixed lymphatic components
- Percutaneous procedures
  - Direct injection with sclerosing agent under fluoroscopic/ultrasonic guidance
  - Laser ablation (Nd:YAG laser) of superficial VM
  - Endovascular ablation of varicosities
- Surgical resection of focal lesions
  - Usually in combination with percutaneous sclerotherapy

DIAGNOSTIC CHECKLIST

Consider

- Does lesion enlarge with Valsalva maneuver, crying, or when head is dependent? If yes, suggests VM

Image Interpretation Pearls

- Presence of phleboliths on CT or T2-hyperintense facial mass is most specific imaging finding for VM
  - Rare spindle cell hemangioma may contain phleboliths
- Multiple fluid-fluid levels in pediatric soft tissue mass strongly suggests slow- or low-flow vascular malformation (LM > VM)

SELECTED REFERENCES

1. Azizinik F et al: Vascular lesions of head and neck region: a pictorial review. Eur J Radiol. ePub, 2025
2. International Society for the Study of Vascular Anomalies: ISSVA Classification for Vascular Anomalies. Reviewed 2024. Accessed May 28, 2025. https://www.issva.org/classification
3. Mamlouk MD: Solid and vascular neck masses in children. Neuroimaging Clin N Am. 33(4):607-21, 2023
4. Tasiou A et al: Cavernous malformations of the central nervous system: an international consensus statement. Brain Spine. 3:102707, 2023
5. Cooke-Barber J et al: Venous malformations. Semin Pediatr Surg. 29(5):150976, 2020
6. Van Damme A et al: New and emerging targeted therapies for vascular malformations. Am J Clin Dermatol. 21(5):657-68, 2020
7. Mamlouk MD et al: Vascular anomaly imaging mimics and differential diagnoses. Pediatr Radiol. 49(8):1088-103, 2019

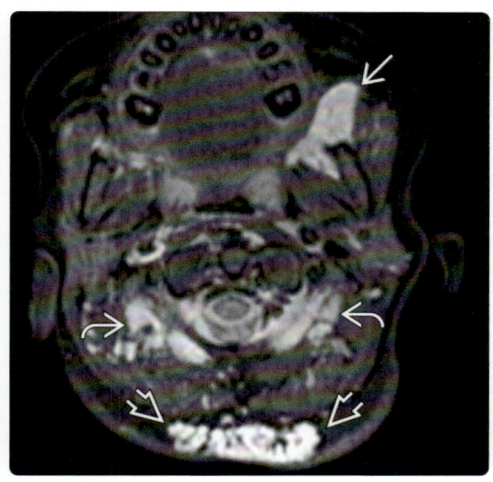

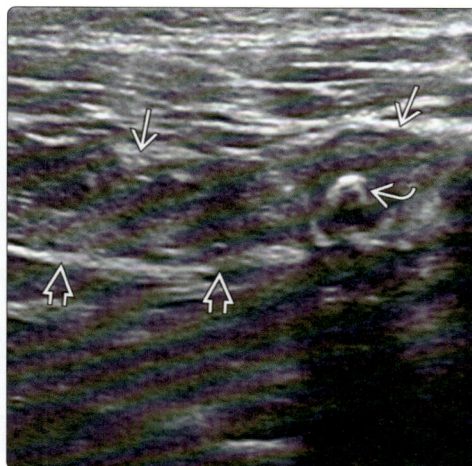

(Left) Axial STIR MR in a 10-year-old girl with multiple VMs demonstrates hyperintense lesions in the left buccal space ➡, the midline posterior subcutaneous neck ➡, and the bilateral paraspinal soft tissues ➡. (Right) Longitudinal ultrasound in a child with known VMs demonstrates a heterogeneous mass ➡ adjacent to the mandible ➡ with a focal echogenic phlebolith ➡ that shows posterior acoustical shadowing.

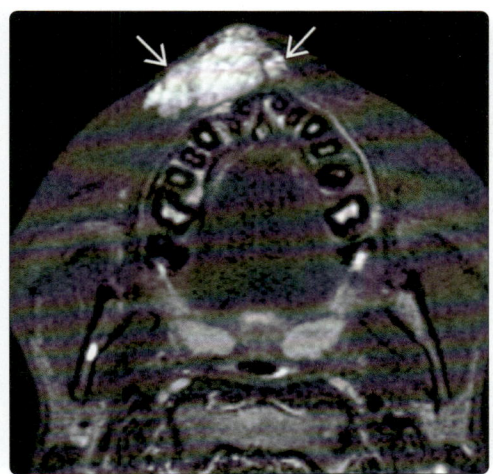

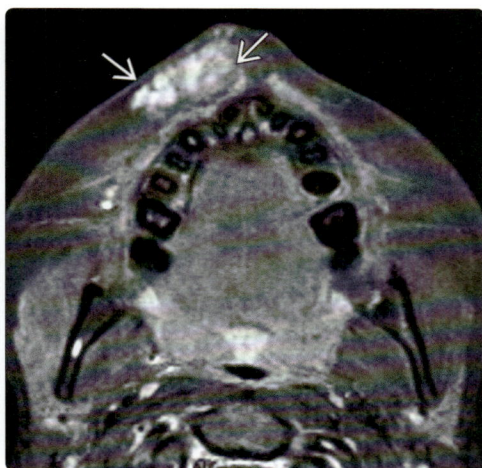

(Left) Axial STIR MR reveals a well-defined, lobulated VM involving the subcutaneous tissues of the upper lip ➡ without an underlying osseous or dental abnormality. (Right) Axial T1 C+ FS MR in the same patient shows moderate, heterogeneous contrast within the abnormal venous lakes ➡, a typical appearance of many VMs.

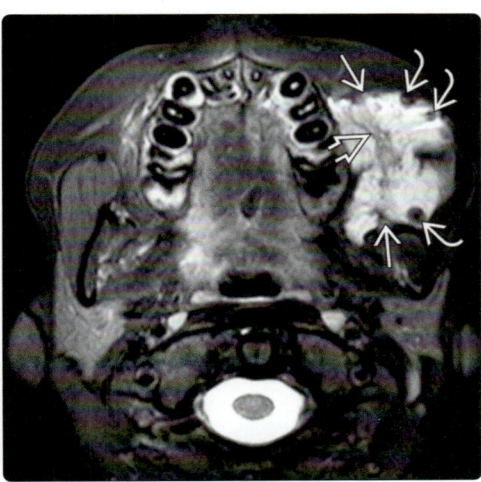

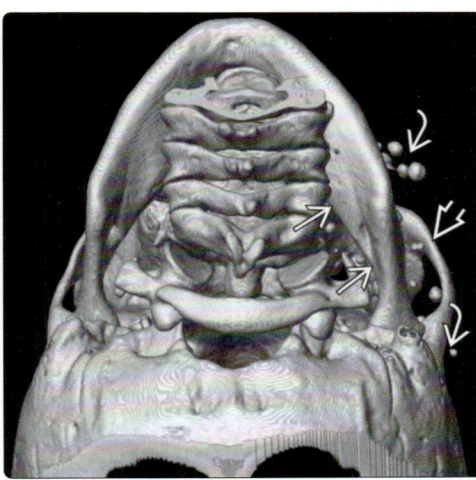

(Left) Axial T2 TSE FS MR in a teenager demonstrates a large, hyperintense left buccal space mass ➡ that contains multiple hypointense septa ➡. Notice also multiple well-defined, round, hypointense foci ➡, typical of phleboliths and nearly pathognomonic of a VM. (Right) 3D surface-rendered MR in the same patient shows mild overgrowth of the left hemimandible ➡, relative to the right, lateral bowing of the thickened left zygomatic arch ➡, and multiple soft tissue phleboliths ➡.

Pediatric Lesions

TERMINOLOGY

- Epiglottic cyst, base of tongue cyst, ductal cyst, saccular cyst
- Congenital cyst arising in vallecula

IMAGING

- Cystic mass in vallecula of child with stridor
- Most diagnosed with direct laryngoscopy

TOP DIFFERENTIAL DIAGNOSES

- **Thyroglossal duct cyst**
  - When midline tongue base cyst (near foramen cecum), may be indistinguishable from congenital vallecular cyst
- **Retention cyst in pharyngeal mucosal space**
  - Benign, postinflammatory retention cyst in nasopharynx or oropharynx
- **Lingual thyroid**
  - Midline solid mass near foramen cecum
  - Increased attenuation on CT
  - Variable signal intensity on MR

- **Lingual hamartoma**
  - Midline posterior tongue mass near foramen cecum
- **Lymphatic malformation**
  - Cystic, usually transspatial congenital lesion
  - Rarely involves vallecula

CLINICAL ISSUES

- Most common signs/symptoms
  - **Inspiratory stridor**
  - Airway obstruction: May lead to life-threatening airway obstruction if left untreated
  - Apnea
- Other signs/symptoms
  - Laryngomalacia
  - Feeding difficulties
  - Failure to thrive
- Treatment
  - Surgical excision, laser-assisted resection, marsupialization, radiofrequency ablation

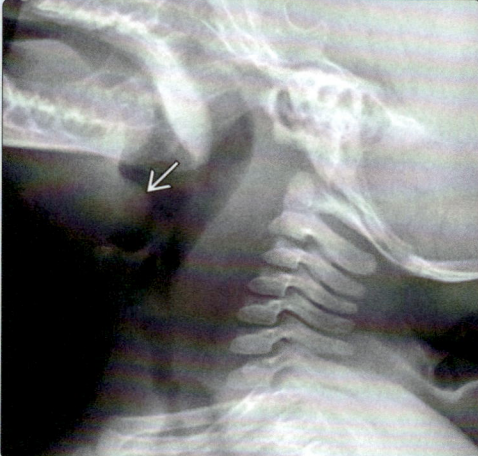
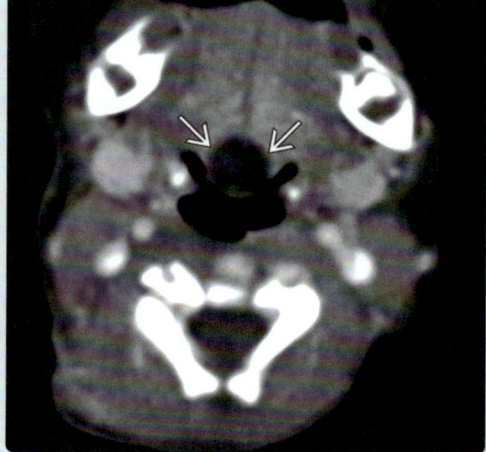

(Left) Lateral radiograph in an infant with stridor shows a well-defined soft tissue mass ➡ at the base of the tongue protruding into the vallecula. (Right) Axial CECT shows a well-defined, low-attenuation, nonenhancing cyst in the midline base of the tongue ➡. Patients present with stridor, airway obstruction, apnea, and feeding difficulties, and may also have laryngomalacia &/or gastroesophageal reflux. Based on CECT findings alone, this lesion is difficult to distinguish from a thyroglossal duct cyst at the foramen cecum.

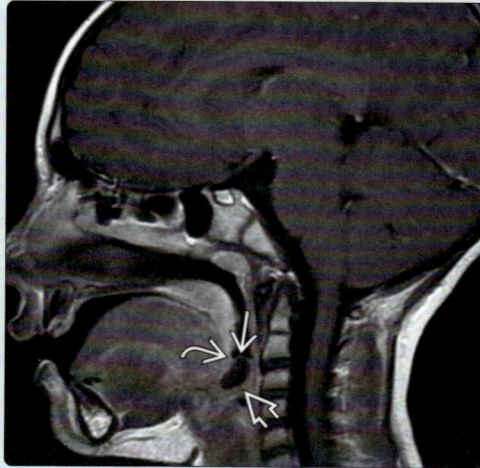
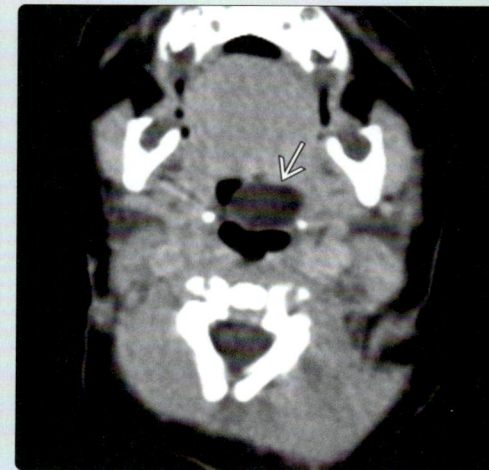

(Left) Sagittal T1 C+ MR in an 8-year-old patient shows an incidental vallecular cyst ➡ between the ventral aspect of the epiglottis ➡ and the dorsal aspect of the base of the tongue ➡. (Right) Axial CECT in a newborn with stridor shows a well-defined hypodense cyst ➡ filling the left vallecula and extending across midline. Stridor is a frequent presenting symptom in infants with vallecular cysts.

TERMINOLOGY

Synonyms
- Epiglottic cyst, base of tongue cyst, ductal cyst, saccular cyst

Definitions
- Vallecula = inferior border oropharynx
  - Anterior to epiglottis, posterior to base of tongue
- Congenital cyst arising in vallecula
  - **Proposed theories of origin**
    - Secondary to obstruction of submucosal glands
    - Secondary to congenital cystic distention of laryngeal saccule

IMAGING

General Features
- Best diagnostic clue
  - **Cystic mass in vallecula of child with stridor**
  - Most diagnosed with direct laryngoscopy
- Location
  - Within vallecula
  - Arises from lingual surface of epiglottis
- Size
  - Variable
- Morphology
  - **Round or lobulated**

CT Findings
- Well-defined, low-attenuation, **nonenhancing** mass in vallecula

MR Findings
- Well-defined, fluid signal intensity mass in vallecula

Ultrasonographic Findings
- Well-defined, anechoic cyst

DIFFERENTIAL DIAGNOSIS

Thyroglossal Duct Cyst
- When midline tongue base cyst (near foramen cecum), may be indistinguishable from congenital vallecular cyst

Pharyngeal Mucosal Space Retention Cyst
- Benign retention cyst in nasopharynx or oropharynx
- More common in older children and adults

Lingual Thyroid
- Midline solid mass near foramen cecum
- Increased attenuation on CT
- Variable signal intensity on MR

Lingual Hamartoma
- Midline posterior tongue mass near foramen cecum

Lymphatic Malformation
- Cystic, congenital, usually transspatial lesion
- Rarely involves vallecula

PATHOLOGY

General Features
- Cyst wall contains respiratory &/or squamous epithelium with mucous glands

CLINICAL ISSUES

Presentation
- Most common signs/symptoms
  - Inspiratory stridor
  - Airway obstruction
- Other signs/symptoms
  - Apnea
  - Coexistent laryngomalacia not uncommon, may complicate clinical picture
  - Feeding difficulties and gastroesophageal reflux
  - Failure to thrive
  - Sleep-disordered breathing

Demographics
- 1.82-3.49/100,000 live births

Natural History & Prognosis
- May lead to life-threatening airway obstruction if left untreated

Treatment
- Surgical excision
- Laser-assisted resection
- Marsupialization
- Radiofrequency ablation

DIAGNOSTIC CHECKLIST

Image Interpretation Pearls
- If well-defined, nonenhancing cystic mass discovered in midline vallecula in infant with stridor, suspect vallecular cyst
- May be difficult to differentiate congenital vallecular cyst from thyroglossal duct cyst in foramen cecum of tongue base

SELECTED REFERENCES

1. Casas T et al: An unusual case of failure to thrive: respiratory failure from a vallecular cyst in a young infant. J Emerg Med. 67(6):e574-7, 2024
2. Cooper DJ et al: Vallecular cyst causing sleep-disordered breathing in an older child. BMJ Case Rep. 17(4):e258824, 2024
3. Singh S et al: Pediatric head and neck emergencies. Neuroradiology. 66(11):2053-70, 2024
4. Wang GX et al: Minimally invasive procedure for diagnosis and treatment of vallecular cysts in children: review of 156 cases. Eur Arch Otorhinolaryngol. 277(12):3407-14, 2020
5. Li Y et al: Vallecular cyst in the pediatric population: evaluation and management. Int J Pediatr Otorhinolaryngol. 113:198-203, 2018
6. Lee DH et al: Clinical characteristics and surgical treatment outcomes of vallecular cysts in adults. Acta Otolaryngol. 1-4, 2015
7. Hsieh LC et al: The outcomes of infantile vallecular cyst post CO_2 laser treatment. Int J Pediatr Otorhinolaryngol. 77(5):655-7, 2013
8. Tsai YT et al: Treatment of vallecular cysts in infants with and without coexisting laryngomalacia using endoscopic laser marsupialization: fifteen-year experience at a single-center. Int J Pediatr Otorhinolaryngol. 77(3):424-8, 2013
9. Suzuki J et al: Congenital vallecular cyst in an infant: case report and review of 52 recent cases. J Laryngol Otol. 125(11):1199-203, 2011
10. Breysem L et al: Vallecular cyst as a cause of congenital stridor: report of five patients. Pediatr Radiol. 39(8):828-31, 2009

1st Branchial Cleft Cyst

TERMINOLOGY

- Most common 1st branchial cleft (BC) anomalies are cysts (BCCs) or sinus tracts

IMAGING

- Best diagnostic clue: Cystic mass near pinna & external auditory canal (EAC) or extending from EAC to angle of mandible
- CECT: Well-circumscribed, nonenhancing or rim-enhancing, low-density mass
  - If infected, may have thickened, enhancing rim

TOP DIFFERENTIAL DIAGNOSES

- Cholesteatoma, EAC
  - Submucosal mass with bone erosion
- Granulomatous infection (nontuberculous *Mycobacterium*)
  - Conglomerate parotid space necrotic nodal mass
  - Necrotic material extrudes into subcutaneous fat
- Parotitis complicated by abscess (rare)
  - Parotitis with thick-walled, ring-enhancing, cystic mass within or adjacent to parotid gland
  - Cellulitis extends to EAC & angle of mandible
- Lymphatic malformation
  - No contrast enhancement, ± fluid-fluid levels
- Venous malformation, EAC
  - Variably enhancing mass, ± phleboliths

PATHOLOGY

- **Remnant of 1st branchial apparatus**
  - Cysts > > sinus or fistula
- Most common location for 1st BCC to terminate is in EAC, between cartilaginous & bony portions

DIAGNOSTIC CHECKLIST

- Think 1st BCC in patient with chronic, unexplained otorrhea or recurrent parotid space abscess
- Look for cyst in or adjacent to EAC, pinna, parotid gland, or, rarely, parapharyngeal space

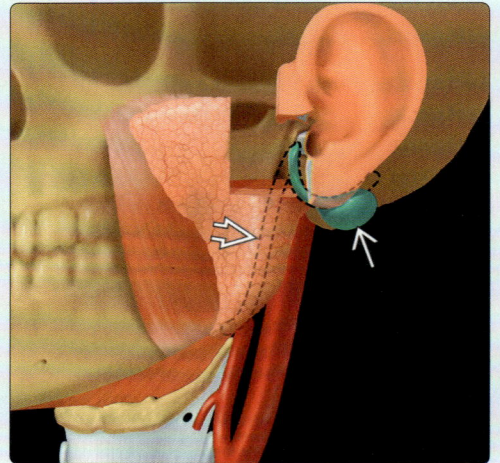
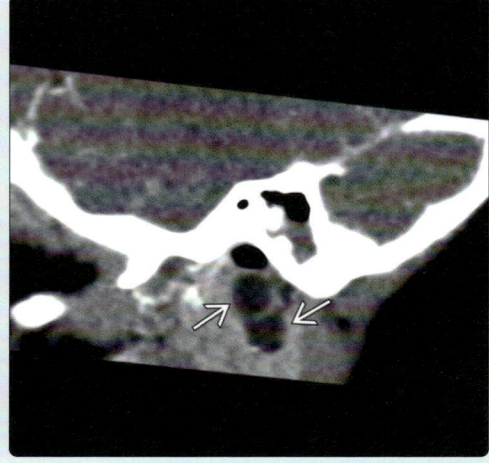

(Left) Oblique graphic of the ear and cheek reveals a Work type I 1st branchial cleft cyst (BCC) ➡ along the tract from the bony-cartilaginous junction of the external auditory canal (EAC) situated just posteroinferior to auricle. The tract of the Work type II BCC ➡ would project inferiorly to the angle of the mandible. (Right) Sagittal CECT in a 2-year-old child shows a well-defined, hypoattenuating 1st BCC ➡ inferior to the left EAC. There is minimal rim enhancement and a single septation.

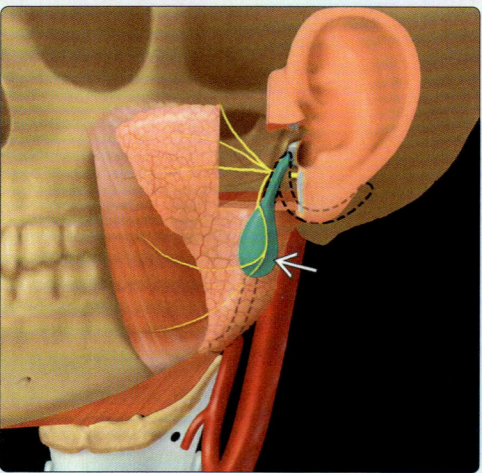
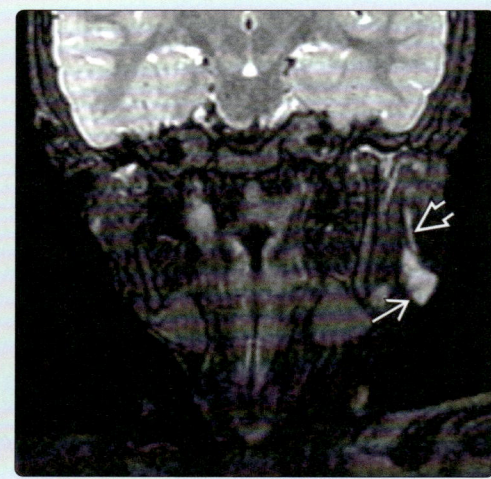

(Left) Oblique graphic of the ear and cheek shows an example of a Work type II 1st BCC ➡ along the course of the tract from the bony-cartilaginous EAC to the angle of the mandible. Note the intimate relationship of the BCC to the facial nerve branches. (Right) Coronal T2WI FS MR demonstrates the cystic inferior component of a type II 1st branchial apparatus cyst ➡ and the sinus tract ➡ extending superiorly toward the EAC. There was a 2nd cyst just inferior to the EAC (not shown), connected to the lower cyst by the sinus tract.

TERMINOLOGY

Abbreviations

- Branchial cleft (BC) cyst (BCC)

Synonyms

- Pharyngeal cleft anomaly = BC anomaly (BCA)
- Pharyngeal apparatus = branchial apparatus (cleft, arch, & pouch)

Definitions

- 1st branchial apparatus anomalies: Most are cysts or sinuses; fistulas from skin to external auditory canal (EAC), eustachian tube, oropharynx, or middle ear are rare
- 1st BCC: Benign, congenital cyst in or adjacent to parotid gland, EAC, or pinna
  - Work classification: Most commonly used classification
    - Work type I: Duplication of membranous EAC; ectodermal (cleft) origin
    - Work type II: Duplication of membranous EAC & cartilaginous pinna
      - Skin (ectodermal cleft) & cartilage (mesodermal arch) origin
      - May also have contribution from 2nd arch
  - Modified Work classification recently proposed by International Pediatric Otolaryngology Group (IPOG)
    - Based on presence or absence of parotid involvement without emphasis on germ layer
    - IPOG type I: Lateral to parotid fascia, do not involve parotid tissue
    - IPOG type II: Deep to parotid fascia with cyst &/or tract within parotid or between parotid & auricular cartilage
- 1st BC sinus tract opens near parotid gland, EAC, parapharyngeal space (PPS), or anterior triangle of neck

IMAGING

General Features

- Best diagnostic clue
  - Cystic mass near pinna & EAC (Work type I) or extending from EAC to angle of mandible (Work type II)
- Location
  - Work type I: Periauricular cyst or sinus tract
    - Anterior, inferior, or posterior to pinna & concha
  - Work type II: Periparotid cyst or sinus tract
    - More intimately associated with parotid gland, medial or lateral to CNVII
    - Superficial, parotid space, or PPS
- Size
  - Variable but usually < 3 cm
- Morphology
  - Well-circumscribed cyst

CT Findings

- CECT
  - Well-circumscribed, nonenhancing or rim-enhancing, low-density mass
  - If infected, may have thickened, enhancing rim &/or intermediate attenuation contents
    - Surrounding fat stranding suggests infection
  - 1st BCC, Work type I
    - Cyst anterior, inferior, or posterior to EAC
    - Cyst may beak → bony-cartilaginous junction of EAC
    - Often runs parallel to EAC
  - 1st BCC, Work type II
    - May be subcutaneous, in parotid space, or in PPS
    - May be as low as posterior submandibular space
    - Deep projection may beak to bony-cartilaginous junction of EAC
  - 1st BC sinus tract: Linear density courses through subcutaneous fat in vicinity of parotid, EAC, or PPS
- If previously infected, can be isodense

MR Findings

- T1WI: Low signal intensity, unilocular cyst
- T2WI: High signal intensity, unilocular cyst
  - May see sinus tract to skin, EAC, or, rarely, PPS
  - Edema in surrounding soft tissues when superinfected
  - Previous or concurrent infection may → thickened, enhancing rim
- T1WI C+ FS: Cyst wall normally does not enhance

Ultrasonographic Findings

- Anechoic mass in periauricular, parotid or periparotid area

Imaging Recommendations

- Best imaging tool
  - CECT or MR for evaluation of cyst
  - MR (T2 FS or STIR) ideal for small lesions & associated sinus tract
- Protocol advice
  - Coronal images best to evaluate relationship to EAC

DIFFERENTIAL DIAGNOSIS

Congenital Cholesteatoma of External Auditory Canal

- Nonenhancing submucosal mass with bone erosion
- Lesion matrix may show bone fragments
- Hole in tympanic plate
- Known association with 1st BCC ± fistula to EAC & stenotic or duplicated EAC

Non-TB *Mycobacterium*, Lymph Nodes

- 4- to 6-week history of minimally tender mass with violaceous skin discoloration
- Conglomerate parotid space necrotic nodal mass
- Necrotic tissue may extrude into subcutaneous fat
- Minimal stranding of subcutaneous fat

Parotitis, Acute

- Presents with marked tenderness & fever
- Enlarged/inflamed, enhancing parotid
- Cellulitis extends to EAC & angle of mandible
- Complicating abscess is rare: Thick-walled, ring-enhancing, cystic mass within/adjacent to parotid gland

Lymphatic Malformation, Periauricular

- Congenital vascular malformation; embryonic lymphatic sacs
- Unilocular or multilocular; microcystic or macrocystic
- Single space or transspatial
- Characteristic fluid-fluid levels are common
- No contrast enhancement or phleboliths unless mixed venolymphatic malformation

Venous Malformation, Periauricular

- Congenital vascular malformation: Endothelial-lined vascular sinusoids
- Single or multiple lobulated mass ± phleboliths
- Variable enhancement pattern reflects sluggish vascular flow to & through lesion
- ± nonenhancing lymphatic component if mixed venolymphatic malformation

PATHOLOGY

General Features

- Associated abnormalities
  - May be seen in association with other 1st branchial apparatus anomalies
  - May occasionally have associated but separate EAC congenital cholesteatoma
    - Small mass in medial EAC with bony remodeling/erosion of EAC & hole in tympanic plate
    - May transgress tympanic membrane (TM) or extend from tympanic plate under TM into middle ear cavity
- Embryology/anatomy
  - Remnant of 1st branchial apparatus
    - Cleft (ectoderm) → EAC
    - Arch (mesoderm) → mandible, muscles of mastication, CNV, incus body, malleus head
    - Pouch (endoderm) → eustachian tube, middle ear cavity, & mastoid air cells
  - Branchial anomaly occurs with incomplete obliteration of 1st branchial apparatus
  - Isolated BCC has **no internal** (pharyngeal) **or external** (cutaneous) communication
  - BC fistula has both **internal & external** connections, from EAC lumen to skin
  - BC sinus tract opens **externally or (rarely) internally**; closed portion ends as blind pouch
  - 2/3 of 1st BC remnants are isolated cysts

Gross Pathologic & Surgical Features

- Cystic neck mass
  - Easily dissected unless repeated infection
- Contents of cyst usually thick mucus
- Cystic remnant may split facial nerve (CNVII) trunk
- CNVII may be medial or lateral to 1st BCC
- Close proximity to CNVII makes surgery more difficult
- Most common location for 1st BCC to terminate is in EAC between cartilaginous & bony portions

Microscopic Features

- Thin outer layer: Fibrous pseudocapsule
- Inner layer: Flat squamoid epithelium
- ± germinal centers & lymphocytes in cyst wall

CLINICAL ISSUES

Presentation

- Most common signs/symptoms
  - Soft, painless, compressible mass: EAC, periauricular, intraparotid, or periparotid suprahyoid neck
- Other signs/symptoms
  - Recurrent EAC, preauricular or periparotid swelling
  - Tender mass ± fever if infected
  - EAC or skin sinus tract rare
  - Chronic purulent ear drainage if EAC sinus tract or fistula

Demographics

- Age
  - Majority present < 10 years old
  - Sinus tracts present earlier
  - When cyst only, may present later, even as adult
- Epidemiology
  - Accounts for 8% of all branchial apparatus remnants
  - Work type II > > Work type I 1st BCC

Natural History & Prognosis

- May enlarge with upper respiratory tract infection
  - Lymph follicles in wall react, wall secretes
- Often incised & drained as "abscess," only to recur
- Prognosis excellent if completely resected
- May recur if residual cyst wall remains
- If multiple BCCs are associated with craniofacial anomalies, think syndromic etiology (e.g., branchiootorenal syndrome)

Treatment

- Complete surgical resection
- Proximity to CNVII puts nerve at risk during surgery
  - Work type I: Proximal CNVII
  - Work type II: More distal CNVII branches

DIAGNOSTIC CHECKLIST

Consider

- Look for cyst in or adjacent to parotid gland, EAC, pinna, or, rarely, PPS
- Think 1st branchial anomaly in patient with chronic, unexplained otorrhea or recurrent parotid gland abscess

SELECTED REFERENCES

1. Heilingoetter AL et al: Comprehensive management and classification of first branchial cleft anomalies: an International Pediatric Otolaryngology Group (IPOG) consensus statement. Int J Pediatr Otorhinolaryngol. 186:112095, 2024
2. Tsur N et al: Management of first branchial anomalies in children: 20 years of experience. Pediatr Surg Int. 40(1):31, 2024
3. Booth TN: Congenital cystic neck masses. Neuroimaging Clin N Am. 33(4):591-605, 2023
4. Koch BL et al: Complete first branchial fistula in a child extending from the external auditory canal to the oropharynx. Neurographics. American Society of Neuroradiology. 11(1):35-7, 2021
5. Liu H et al: Clinical manifestations, diagnosis, and management of first branchial cleft fistula/sinus: a case series and literature review. J Oral Maxillofac Surg. 78(5):749-61, 2020
6. Mehmi N et al: Importance and impact of appropriate radiology in the management of branchial cleft anomalies. Indian J Otolaryngol Head Neck Surg. 71(Suppl 1):953-9, 2019
7. Guerin JB et al: Pediatric parotid region lesions: an imaging review. Neurographics. American Society of Neuroradiology. 8(6):394-412, 2018
8. Johnson JM et al: Syndromes of the first and second branchial arches, part 1: embryology and characteristic defects. AJNR Am J Neuroradiol. 32(1):14-9, 2011
9. Johnson JM et al: Syndromes of the first and second branchial arches, part 2: syndromes. AJNR Am J Neuroradiol. 32(2):230-7, 2011
10. Koch BL: Cystic malformations of the neck in children. Pediatr Radiol. 35(5):463-77, 2005

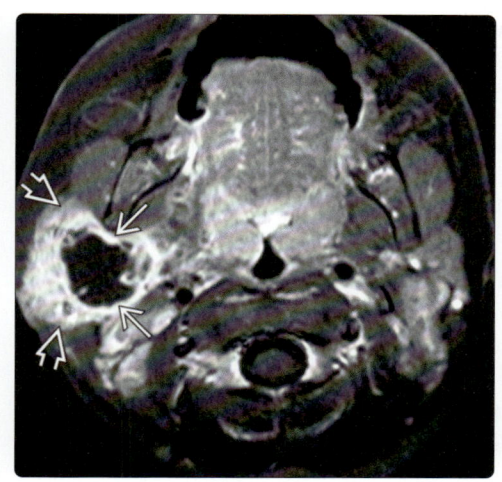
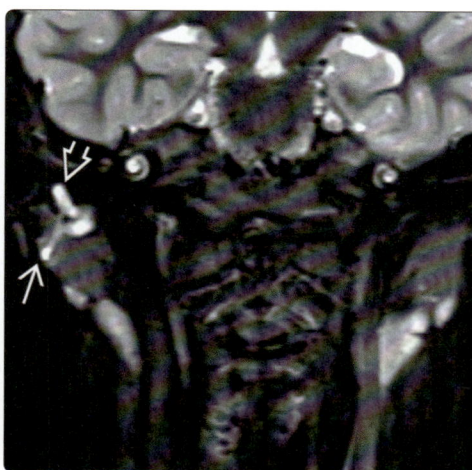

(Left) *Axial T1WI C+ FS MR demonstrates an irregularly shaped, infected 1st BCC ➡ within the right parotid gland with a thick, enhancing wall & diffuse, abnormal enhancement of the surrounding parotid gland ➡.* **(Right)** *Coronal STIR MR in a child with recurrent periauricular abscess and intermittent EAC drainage demonstrates a curvilinear tubular 1st branchial apparatus anomaly in the form of a fluid-filled fistula extending from the skin surface ➡ to the floor of the EAC ➡.*

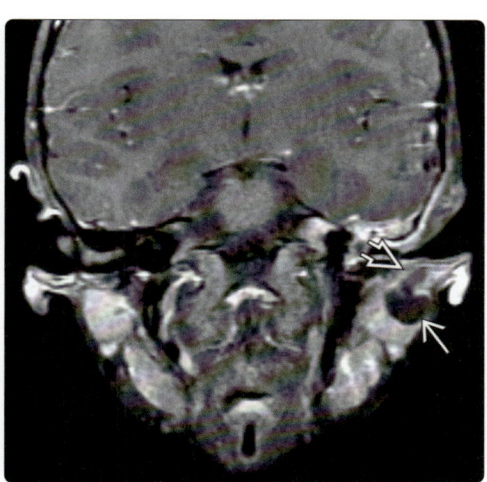
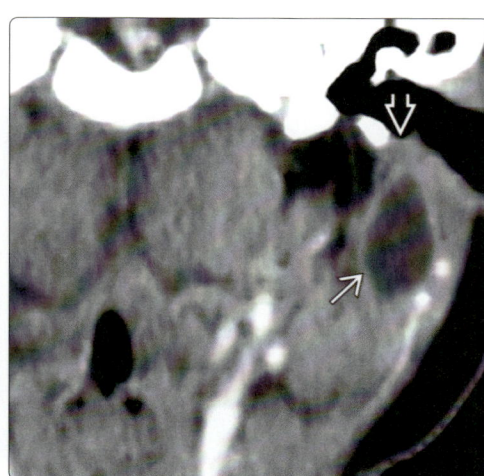

(Left) *Coronal T1WI C+ FS MR in a 3-year-old child with a palpable mass shows a lobulated, hypointense intraparotid mass ➡ with a curvilinear component ➡ extending toward the osseous-cartilaginous junction of the EAC.* **(Right)** *Coronal CECT shows a well-defined intraparotid 1st BCC ➡ with the superior aspect directed toward the bony-cartilaginous junction ➡ of the left EAC.*

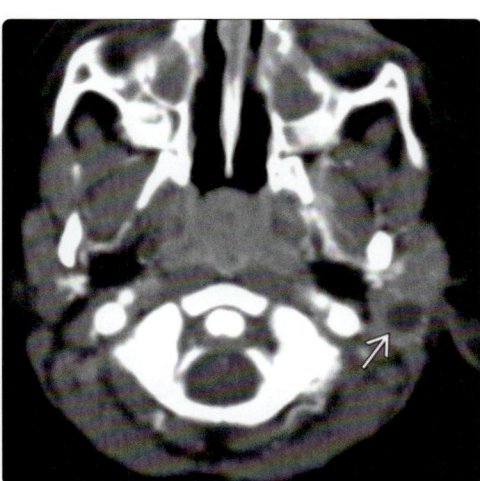
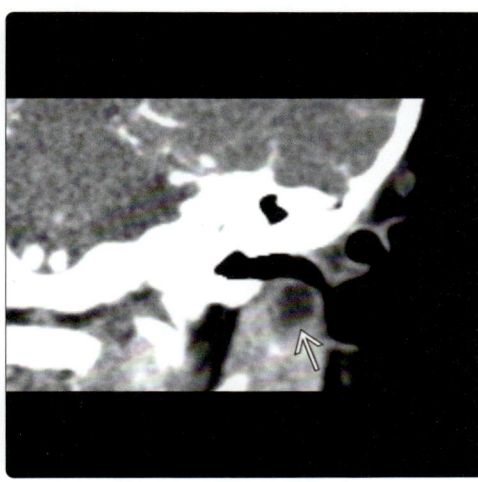

(Left) *Axial CECT in a 1-year-old with a bilobed 1st BCC shows the inferior extent of the cyst to be well defined and intraparotid in location ➡.* **(Right)** *Coronal CECT in the same patient shows the well-defined, nonenhancing upper aspect of the bilobed BCC ➡ along the inferior margin of the left cartilaginous EAC. Any cystic structure in or adjacent to the EAC or parotid gland should be imaged in its entirety and, in a child, should raise the question of a 1st branchial apparatus cyst.*

2nd Branchial Cleft Cyst

TERMINOLOGY

- Cervical sinus of His cystic remnant: 2nd, 3rd, and 4th branchial clefts and 2nd branchial arch derivative
- Synonyms
  - 2nd branchial cleft cyst (BCC) or anomaly
  - 2nd branchial apparatus cyst (BAC) or anomaly

IMAGING

- Best diagnostic clue: Cystic neck mass posterolateral to submandibular gland, lateral to carotid space, anterior (or anteromedial) to sternocleidomastoid muscle
- If infected, wall is thicker and enhances with surrounding soft tissue cellulitis

TOP DIFFERENTIAL DIAGNOSES

- Lymphatic malformation
  - Frequently transspatial
- Cervical thymic cyst
  - Remnant of 3rd pharyngeal pouch

- Lymphadenopathy/abscess
  - Presents with signs and symptoms of infection
- Cystic metastatic nodes
  - Squamous cell carcinoma (SCCa) nodal metastasis
  - Differentiated thyroid carcinoma nodal metastasis
- Carotid space schwannoma
  - Occasional large intramural cysts
  - Thick, enhancing wall
  - Rare in children

PATHOLOGY

- 2nd BAC, sinus, or fistulae
- Epidemiology: 2nd branchial apparatus anomalies (BAAs) account for up to 95% of all BAAs

DIAGNOSTIC CHECKLIST

- Beware of adult with 1st presentation of 2nd BCC
  - May be necrotic metastasis from head and neck SCCa primary tumor

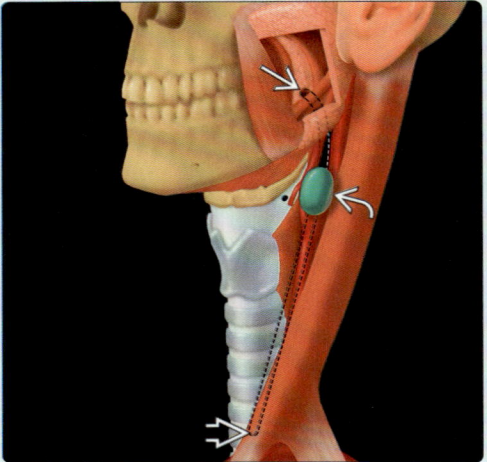
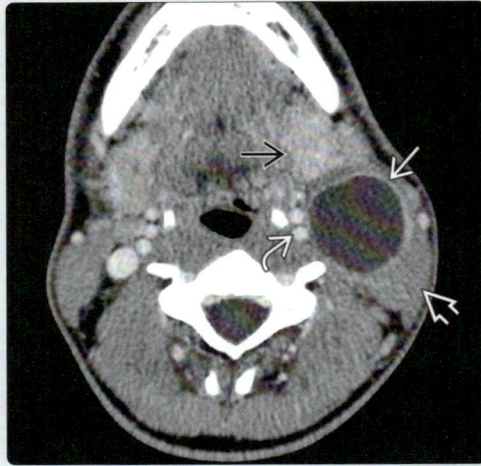

(Left) Sagittal oblique graphic shows a 2nd branchial cleft cyst (BCC) ➡ in its most common location, anterior to the sternocleidomastoid muscle (SCM) and anterolateral to the carotid space. Full tract may extend from the faucial tonsil ➡ to the low anterior neck ➡. (Right) Axial CECT in a 17-year-old boy shows a well-defined, low-attenuation mass ➡ in the typical location of a Bailey type II 2nd BCC: Anterior to the SCM ➡, lateral to the carotid sheath vessels ➡, and posterior to the submandibular gland ➡.

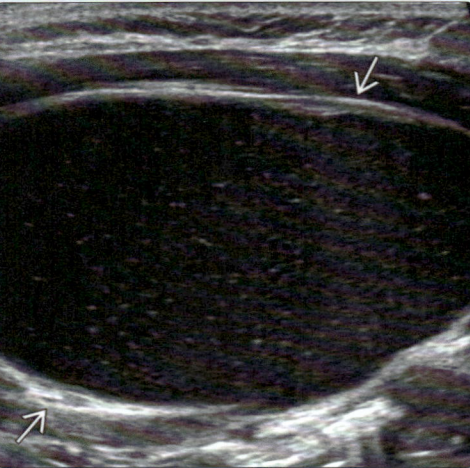
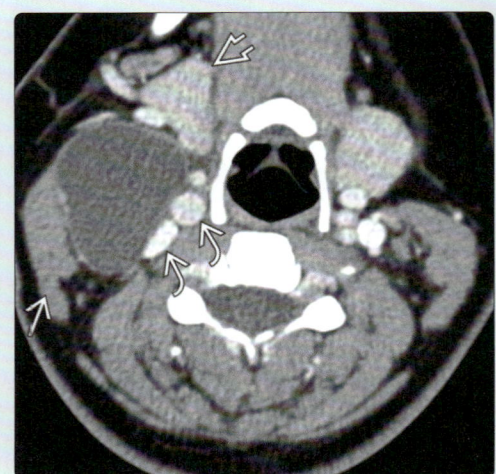

(Left) Longitudinal US in a young adult with VACTERL association and a neck mass with signs or symptoms of infection shows a well-defined, unilocular, hypoechoic anterior right neck mass ➡ with posterior acoustic enhancement and internal echoes. (Right) Axial CECT in the same patient shows to better advantage the typical relationship of a 2nd BCC to the adjacent structures, SCM muscle ➡, submandibular gland ➡, and carotid sheath vessels ➡.

TERMINOLOGY

Abbreviations

- 2nd branchial cleft cyst (BCC)

Synonyms

- 2nd branchial apparatus cyst (BAC)
- 2nd branchial apparatus anomaly (BAA)

Definitions

- 2nd BCC
  - Most common BAC
  - Cystic remnant of cervical sinus of His: Derivative of 2nd, 3rd, and 4th branchial clefts
- Sinus
  - Usually communicates externally along anterior margin of sternocleidomastoid muscle (SCM)
  - Rarely communicates internally to tonsillar fossa
- Fistula
  - Communicates externally and internally
  - Secondary to persistence of both branchial cleft and pharyngeal pouch remnant
- Combinations
  - Cyst + sinus &/or fistula

IMAGING

General Features

- Best diagnostic clue
  - Cystic neck mass posterolateral to submandibular gland, lateral to carotid space, anterior to SCM
  - Most are at or immediately caudal to angle of mandible
- Location
  - Bailey classification of 2nd BACs
    - Type I: Deep to platysma muscle, anterior to SCM
    - Type II: Anterior to SCM, posterior to submandibular gland, lateral to carotid sheath
      □ Most common
    - Type III: Protrudes between internal carotid artery (ICA) and external carotid artery (ECA), may extend to lateral pharyngeal wall or superiorly to skull base
    - Type IV: Adjacent to lateral pharyngeal wall, probably remnant of 2nd pharyngeal pouch
  - 2nd branchial apparatus fistula extends from anterior to SCM, through carotid artery bifurcation, and terminates in tonsillar fossa
- Size
  - Variable; may range from several cm to > 5 cm
- Morphology
  - Ovoid or rounded, well-circumscribed cyst
  - Focal rim of cyst may extend to carotid bifurcation

CT Findings

- CECT
  - Low-density cyst with nonenhancing wall
  - If infected, wall is thicker and enhances with surrounding soft tissue cellulitis

MR Findings

- T1WI
  - Cyst is usually isointense to CSF
  - Infection → increased signal intensity/protein content
- T2WI
  - Hyperintense cyst, no discernible wall
- FLAIR
  - Cyst is iso- or slightly hyperintense to CSF
- T1WI C+
  - No intrinsic contrast enhancement
  - Peripheral wall enhancement if infected

Ultrasonographic Findings

- Anechoic or hypoechoic, thin-walled cyst
  - May give pseudosolid US appearance
    - Real time will demonstrate mobile internal echoes to differentiate from solid lesion
- Thickened cyst wall if infected

Imaging Recommendations

- CT, US, or MR clearly demonstrate location of type I, II, and III cysts
- May be difficult to visualize type IV cysts with US
- CT or MR best demonstrates associated findings of infection and rare type IV cysts

DIFFERENTIAL DIAGNOSIS

Lymphatic Malformation

- Unilocular or multilocular
- Frequently transspatial
- Fluid-fluid levels if intralesional hemorrhage
- Isolation to same location as 2nd BAAs is uncommon

Thymic Cyst

- Remnant of thymopharyngeal duct, derivative of 3rd pharyngeal pouch
- Left side more common than right
- Up to 50% extend into superior mediastinum

Lymphadenopathy/Abscess

- Presents with signs and symptoms of infection
- Irregular, thick, enhancing wall with nonenhancing central cavity
- Surrounding soft tissue induration except with *Mycobacterium*
- Associated ipsilateral nonsuppurative adenopathy

Cystic Metastatic Nodes

- Necrotic mass with thick, enhancing wall
- Rare in children, occasionally in teenagers
- Cystic squamous cell carcinoma (SCCa) nodal metastasis
- Cystic differentiated thyroid carcinoma nodal metastasis

Carotid Space Schwannoma

- Occasional large intramural cysts
- Thick, enhancing wall
- Centered in posterior carotid space

PATHOLOGY

General Features

- Embryology
  - 2nd branchial arch overgrows 2nd, 3rd, and 4th branchial clefts, forming ectodermally lined cervical sinus of His
  - Remnant of 2nd, 3rd, and 4th branchial clefts opens into cervical sinus of His via cervical vesicles

- o Normally developing cervical sinus of His and vesicles involute
- Etiology
  - o Remnants of 2nd branchial apparatus may form cyst, sinus, or fistula
- Associated abnormalities
  - o Usually isolated lesion
  - o May be part of branchiootorenal (BOR) syndrome
    - Autosomal dominant inheritance
    - Bilateral branchial fistulas or cysts and preauricular tag or pit
    - Profound mixed hearing loss
      □ Tapered basal turn of cochlea with offset middle/apical turns → unwound appearance (*EYA1*)
      □ Distinct short protuberant appearance of apical turn of cochlea → "thorny" cochlea (*SIX1*)
      □ Dysmorphic ossicles: Fused, malformed ossicles
      □ Semicircular canal malformations, bulbous vestibular aqueduct, flared internal auditory canal
    - Renal anomalies: Cysts, dysplasia, agenesis
    - Dilated eustachian tubes
  - o Branchiootic syndrome; similar to BOR syndrome without renal involvement

Gross Pathologic & Surgical Features

- Well-defined cyst in locations described by Bailey
- Filled with cheesy material or serous, mucoid, or purulent fluid

Microscopic Features

- Squamous epithelial-lined cyst
- Lymphoid infiltrate in wall, in form of germinal centers
  - o Lymphoid tissue suggests epithelial rests may be entrapped within cervical lymph nodes during embryogenesis

CLINICAL ISSUES

Presentation

- Most common signs/symptoms
  - o Painless, compressible lateral neck mass in child or young adult
  - o May enlarge during upper respiratory tract infection
    - Probably due to response of lymphoid tissue
  - o Fever, tenderness, and erythema if infected

Demographics

- Age
  - o Majority < 5 years; 2nd peak in 2nd or 3rd decade
- Epidemiology
  - o 2nd BAAs account for up to 95% of all BAAs

Natural History & Prognosis

- If untreated, may become repeatedly infected
- Recurrent inflammation makes surgical resection more difficult
- Excellent prognosis if lesion is completely resected

Treatment

- Complete surgical resection is treatment of choice
- Surgeon must dissect around cyst bed to exclude possibility of associated fistula or sinus
  - o If fistula present, usually identified at birth

- Mucoid secretions are emitted from skin opening
  - o If tract proceeds superomedially, it passes through carotid bifurcation into palatine tonsil crypts
  - o If tract courses inferiorly, it passes along anterior carotid space, reaching supraclavicular skin
- Endoscope-assisted resection via retroauricular approach feasible alternative to conventional resection

DIAGNOSTIC CHECKLIST

Consider

- If cyst wall enhances &/or associated cellulitis, consider superimposed infection
- If abscess is recognized posterior to submandibular gland, anterior to SCM, and anteromedial to carotid sheath vessels, think infected 2nd BCC
- Does cyst appear adherent to internal jugular vein or carotid sheath?

Image Interpretation Pearls

- Beware of teenager or adult with 1st presentation of 2nd BCC
  - o Mass may be metastatic node from head and neck SCCa primary tumor
  - o If patient > 30 years of age, 1st consider cystic nodal metastasis

SELECTED REFERENCES

1. Houas J et al: Second branchial cleft anomalies: surgical management and long-term outcomes in a pediatric case series. Int J Surg Case Rep. ePub, 2025
2. Booth TN: Congenital cystic neck masses. Neuroimaging Clin N Am. 33(4):591-605, 2023
3. Gao S et al: Endoscopically assisted transoral resection of a Bailey type IV second branchial cleft cyst: a case report. Medicine (Baltimore). 100(3):e24375, 2021
4. Ginat DT: Imaging findings in syndromes with temporal bone abnormalities. Neuroimaging Cl n N Am. 29(1):117-28, 2019
5. Hsu A et al: The unwound cochlea: a specific imaging marker of branchio-oto-renal syndrome. AJNR Am J Neuroradiol. 39(12):2345-9, 2018
6. Thottam PJ et al: Complete second branchial cleft anomaly presenting as a fistula and a tonsillar cyst: an interesting congenital anomaly. Ear Nose Throat J. 93(10-11):466-8, 2014
7. Chen LS et al: Endoscope-assisted versus conventional second branchial cleft cyst resection. Surg Endosc. 26(5):1397-402, 2012
8. Goff CJ et al: Current management of congenital branchial cleft cysts, sinuses, and fistulae. Curr Opin Otolaryngol Head Neck Surg. 20(6):533-9, 2012
9. Bajaj Y et al: Branchial anomalies in children. Int J Pediatr Otorhinolaryngol. 75(8):1020-3, 2011
10. Buchanan MA et al: Cystic schwannoma of the cervical plexus masquerading as a type II second branchial cleft cyst. Eur Arch Otorhinolaryngol. 266(3):459-62, 2009
11. Hudgins PA et al: Second branchial cleft cyst: not!! AJNR Am J Neuroradiol. 30(9):1628-9, 2009
12. Gupta AK et al: Bilateral first and second branchial cleft fistulas: a case report. Ear Nose Throat J. 87(5):291-3, 2008
13. Koch BL: Cystic malformations of the neck in children. Pediatr Radiol. 35(5):463-77, 2005
14. Lanham PD et al: Second branchial cleft cyst mimic: case report. AJNR Am J Neuroradiol. 26(7):1862-4, 2005
15. Ceruti S et al: Temporal bone anomalies in the branchio-oto-renal syndrome: detailed computed tomographic and magnetic resonance imaging findings. Otol Neurotol. 23(2):200-7, 2002
16. Shin JH et al: Parapharyngeal second branchial cyst manifesting as cranial nerve palsies: MR findings. AJNR Am J Neuroradiol. 22(3):510-2, 2001
17. Benson MT et al: Congenital anomalies of the branchial apparatus: embryology and pathologic anatomy. Radiographics. 12(5):943-60, 1992
18. Harnsberger HR et al: Branchial cleft anomalies and their mimics: computed tomographic evaluation. Radiology. 152(3):739-48, 1984

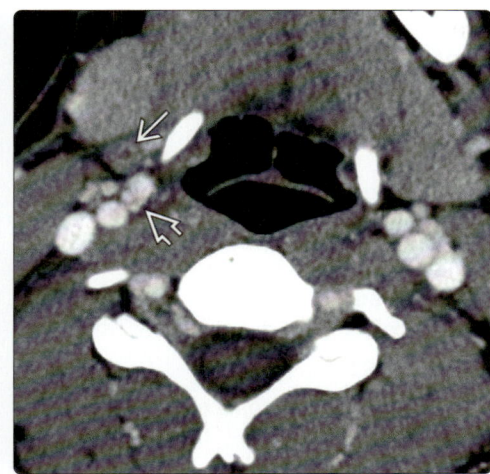

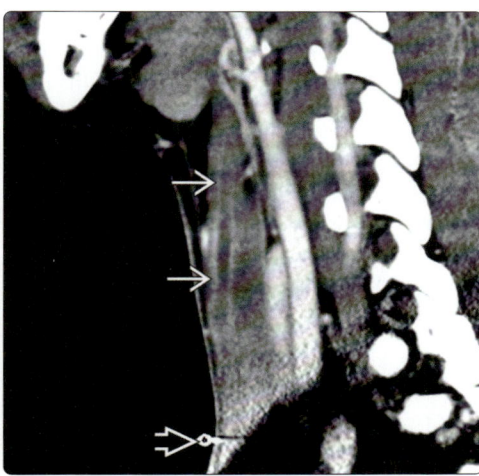

(Left) Axial CECT in a 15-year-old boy with a pit in the lower anterior neck since birth, now draining purulent fluid, demonstrates a well-defined small lesion ⮕ with a thick wall anterior to the carotid vessels ⮕ and posterior to the submandibular gland. (Right) Sagittal CT reconstruction in the same patient demonstrates the course of the infected 2nd branchial cleft sinus tract ⮕, extending from the level of the pit (marked with radiodense marker ⮕) toward the faucial tonsil.

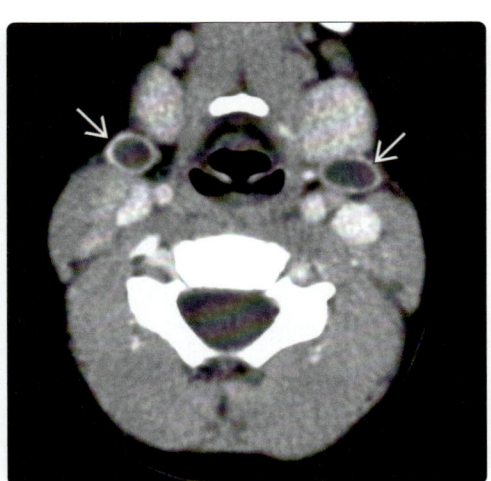

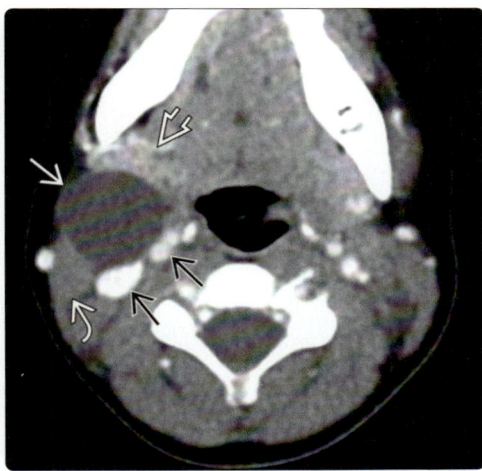

(Left) Axial CECT in a 2-year-old boy with branchiootorenal (BOR) syndrome shows bilateral, well-defined, nonenhancing cysts ⮕ in the typical location of Bailey type II 2nd BCCs. (Right) Axial CECT in a 7-year-old child shows a typical 2nd BCC ⮕: Round, low attenuation with an imperceptible wall without enhancement. Location is also typical: Posterior to the submandibular gland ⮕, anterior to the SCM ⮕, and anterolateral to the carotid sheath vessels ⮕.

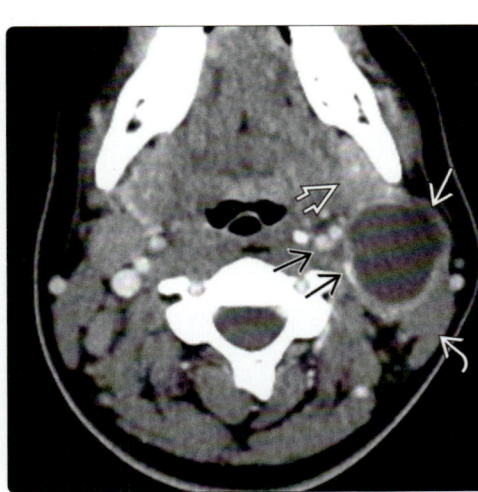

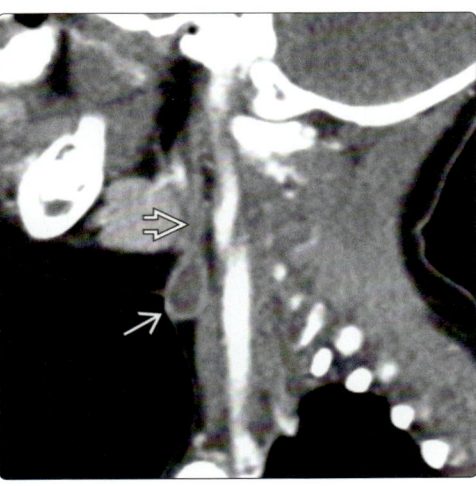

(Left) Axial CECT shows a cyst ⮕ in the typical location of a 2nd BCC: Posterior to submandibular gland ⮕, anterior to SCM ⮕, and lateral to carotid sheath vessels ⮕. Mildly thick wall suggests prior infection. In an adult, differential diagnosis includes a necrotic, metastatic lymph node. (Right) Sagittal CECT in a 2-year-old with BOR syndrome and bilateral anterior neck sinus tracts shows a cyst ⮕ extending from the skin surface, along the left SCM, and a small sinus tract that extends superiorly toward the tonsillar fossa ⮕.

KEY FACTS

TERMINOLOGY

- 3rd branchial cleft cyst (BCC)
  - Epithelial-lined remnant of 3rd branchial cleft

IMAGING

- CT/MR/US
  - Unilocular, thin-walled cyst in upper posterior cervical space or lower anterior neck
  - If infected, cyst wall thickens and enhances
  - ± adjacent cellulitis or myositis
- Barium or water-soluble contrast swallow may outline associated sinus or fistula

TOP DIFFERENTIAL DIAGNOSES

- 2nd BCC: Most common BCC
- Lymphatic malformation: Uni- or multilocular
- Abscess: Signs and symptoms of infection
- Cervical thymic cyst: 3rd pouch remnant

- 4th branchial apparatus anomaly: Pyriform sinus tract and left neck abscess
- Infrahyoid thyroglossal duct cyst: Embedded in strap muscles when infrahyoid
- Cystic-necrotic metastatic lymph node: Usually known primary H&N squamous cell carcinoma or systemic NHL
- External laryngocele: Communicates with laryngeal ventricle through thyrohyoid membrane

CLINICAL ISSUES

- Fluctuant mass in posterolateral upper neck
- Frequently presents in **adulthood**
- Purulent drainage from skin ostium if associated fistula

DIAGNOSTIC CHECKLIST

- Cyst in posterior cervical space of upper neck
  - Think 3rd BCC
- Abscess in posterior cervical space of upper neck
  - Think infected, preexisting, underlying 3rd BCC

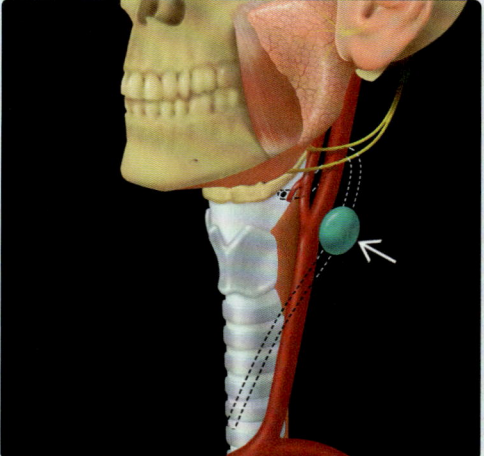
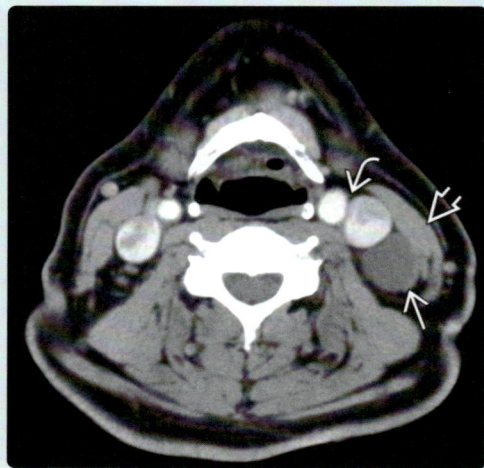

(Left) Lateral graphic illustrates the course of a 3rd branchial anomaly (dashes), along which the 3rd branchial cleft cysts (BCCs) arise, most commonly in the upper posterior neck ➡. (Right) Axial CECT in a man with a posterior left neck mass demonstrates a well-defined, thin-walled unilocular cyst ➡, deep to the sternocleidomastoid muscle (SCM) ➡ and posterolateral to the carotid space ➡. Note that the cyst wall is imperceptible, indicating that the lesion has not been infected.

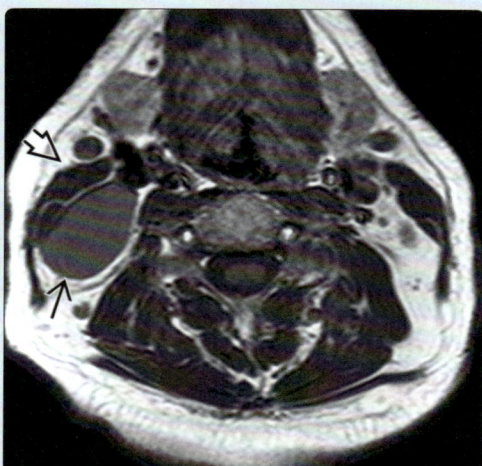
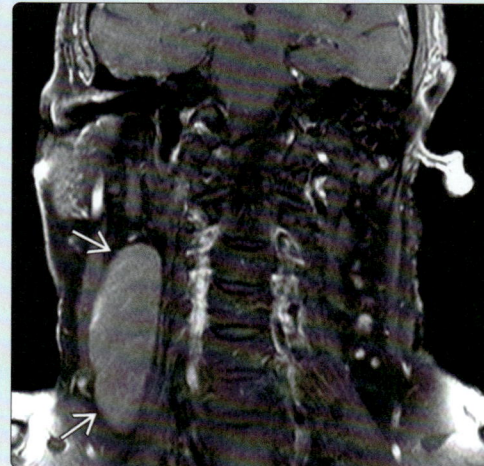

(Left) Axial T1 MR in a 60-year-old man (imaged for other reasons) shows an incidental 3rd BCC in the right posterior cervical space ➡ deep to the SCM ➡. (Right) Coronal T1 C+ FS MR in the same patient shows the cyst ➡ deep to the SCM without significant internal or perilesional enhancement; this is typical of an uncomplicated 3rd BCC.

TERMINOLOGY

Abbreviations
- 3rd branchial cleft cyst (BCC)

Synonyms
- 3rd branchial apparatus cyst (BAC)

Definitions
- Epithelial-lined cystic remnant of 3rd branchial cleft

IMAGING

General Features
- Best diagnostic clue
  - Unilocular, thin-walled cyst in upper posterior cervical space or lower anterior neck
- Location
  - Anywhere along course of 3rd branchial cleft or pouch
    - Upper neck: Posterior cervical space
    - Lower neck: Anterior border of sternocleidomastoid muscle (SCM)
    - Rarely in submandibular space, lateral to cephalad hypopharynx
  - Classically, 3rd branchial fistula would exit base of pyriform sinus and course superior to laryngeal and hypoglossal nerves, inferior to glossopharyngeal nerve
- Size
  - Variable; usually 2-3 cm at presentation
- Morphology
  - Typically ovoid or round cyst

Fluoroscopic Findings
- Barium or water-soluble contrast swallow
  - May outline associated sinus or fistula
  - Point of exit from hypopharynx
    - High lateral margin of pyriform sinus

CT Findings
- CECT
  - Round or ovoid, sharply marginated lesions with central fluid attenuation
  - Cyst wall thin; no calcifications
  - If infected, cyst wall thickens and enhances
    - ± adjacent cellulitis &/or myositis
  - SCM displaced laterally when cyst in high posterior neck
  - SCM displaced posterolaterally when cyst in low anterior neck

MR Findings
- T1WI
  - Homogeneous, hypointense fluid contents
  - Cyst wall thin or imperceptible
- T2WI
  - Homogeneous, hyperintense fluid contents
  - + edema in surrounding tissues if infected
- T1WI C+
  - Thin, uniform, minimally enhancing cyst wall
  - If infected
    - Cyst wall thickened and enhancing
    - Fluid contents hyperintense relative to CSF
    - Strand-like enhancement in soft tissues surrounding 3rd BCC

Ultrasonographic Findings
- Thin-walled, hypoechoic mass upper posterior neck or lower anterior neck
- Lacks internal vascularity

Imaging Recommendations
- Best imaging tool
  - CECT or MR best to evaluate complete extent
- Protocol advice
  - Barium (or water-soluble contrast) swallow may outline associated sinus or fistula
  - Fistula may be outlined by direct injection of cutaneous ostium

DIFFERENTIAL DIAGNOSIS

2nd Branchial Cleft Cyst
- Most common branchial apparatus anomaly
- Most common angle of mandible mass in young adult
- Usually lateral to carotid space, posterior to submandibular gland, and anteromedial to SCM
- Typically nonenhancing fluid signal/attenuation/echogenicity on MR/CT/US
  - If infected, thicker wall with enhancement and surrounding soft tissue cellulitis

Lymphatic Malformation
- Majority diagnosed < 2 years of age
- Unilocular or multilocular
- Focal or infiltrative
- Fluid-fluid levels if intralesional hemorrhage
- Alone or combined with enhancing venous malformation

Abscess
- Presents with signs and symptoms of infection
- Irregular, thick, enhancing wall; low-attenuation center
- Surrounding cellulitis
- If associated with thyroid gland, think 4th branchial pouch anomaly
- If in posterior cervical space of upper neck, think infected underlying 3rd BCC

Cervical Thymic Cyst
- 3rd branchial pouch remnant
- Along course of thymopharyngeal duct
- Left > > right
- Closely associated with carotid sheath
- ± extension to anterior mediastinum

4th Branchial Apparatus Anomaly
- Most often presents with suppurative thyroiditis in children
- Abscess closely associated with anterior left thyroid lobe, thyroiditis
- Sinus tract from pyriform sinus apex to anterior lower left neck
- Prenatal diagnosis suggested if left-sided unilocular neck cyst is identified with tapered medial margin at level of pyriform sinus
- Remnant of 4th (or 3rd) branchial pouch

Infrahyoid Thyroglossal Duct Cyst

- Midline or paramidline anterior neck cyst in child or young adult
- Infrahyoid < suprahyoid, at level of hyoid bone
  - Infrahyoid: Off-midline in strap muscles or anterior to thyroid gland

Metastases, Cystic-Necrotic Lymph Node

- Spinal accessory malignant necrotic adenopathy in posterior cervical space
- Usually known primary head and neck squamous cell carcinoma or systemic non-Hodgkin lymphoma (NHL)
- Almost always in adults; rarely in children

External Laryngocele

- Thin-walled, fluid- or air-filled cystic lesion communicating with laryngeal ventricle + extralaryngeal extension through thyrohyoid membrane
- Most commonly seen in adult glassblowers, trumpet players, or those with chronic coughs
  - Present with enlarging neck mass

PATHOLOGY

General Features

- Etiology
  - Controversial
    - Failure of obliteration of 3rd branchial cleft, portion of cervical sinus of His, or 3rd pharyngeal pouch
- Associated abnormalities
  - 3rd branchial sinus
    - Single opening
      - □ Endopharyngeal in high lateral hypopharynx or cutaneous opening in supraclavicular area anterior to carotid artery
  - 3rd branchial fistula
    - 2 openings
      - □ Endopharyngeal in high lateral hypopharynx and cutaneous opening in supraclavicular area anterior to carotid artery
      - □ Skin opening may be pseudofistula secondary to repeated infection or surgical incision rather than true fistula

Gross Pathologic & Surgical Features

- Smooth, thin-walled cysts
- May contain clear, watery to mucinous material
  - ± desquamated cellular debris

Microscopic Features

- Lined by squamous epithelium (occasionally by columnar epithelium)
- Lymphoid tissue in walls of cyst with reactive lymphoid follicles

CLINICAL ISSUES

Presentation

- Most common signs/symptoms
  - Fluctuant mass in posterolateral neck
  - May enlarge rapidly following upper respiratory tract infection
- Other signs/symptoms

- Recurrent lateral neck or retropharyngeal abscesses
- Draining fistula along anterior margin of SCM

Demographics

- Age
  - Frequently presents in adulthood
  - Presentation of cysts in neonates and infants unusual
  - When sinus or fistula present, early presentation more common
- Epidemiology
  - 3rd branchial cleft anomalies account for only **3%** of all branchial anomalies
  - 2nd BCC > 1st BCC > 3rd BCC

Natural History & Prognosis

- Good prognosis if completely resected
- May become infected and present with neck abscess

Treatment

- Surgical resection
  - If infected, treat with antibiotics prior to surgical resection
  - Surgery includes resection of cyst and any associated sinus or fistula

DIAGNOSTIC CHECKLIST

Consider

- Cyst in posterior cervical space of upper neck, think 3rd BCC
- Abscess in posterior cervical space of upper neck, think infected, preexisting, underlying 3rd BCC

SELECTED REFERENCES

1. Booth TN: Congenital cystic neck masses. Neuroimaging Clin N Am. 33(4):591-605, 2023
2. Castro PT et al: Pre and postnatal diagnosis of a third branchial cleft cyst by sonography and magnetic resonance imaging with three-dimensional virtual reconstruction. J Clin Ultrasound. 49(9):966-8, 2021
3. Li Y et al: Prenatal diagnosis of third and fourth branchial apparatus anomalies: case series and comparison with lymphatic malformation. AJNR Am J Neuroradiol. 42(11):2094-100, 2021
4. Buch K et al: MR imaging evaluation of pediatric neck masses: review and update. Magn Reson Imaging Clin N Am. 27(2):173-99, 2019
5. Mehmi N et al: Importance and impact of appropriate radiology in the management of branchial cleft anomalies. Indian J Otolaryngol Head Neck Surg. 71(Suppl 1):953-9, 2019
6. Goff CJ et al: Current management of congenital branchial cleft cysts, sinuses, and fistulae. Curr Opin Otolaryngol Head Neck Surg. 20(6):533-9, 2012
7. Thomas B et al: Revisiting imaging features and the embryologic basis of third and fourth branchial anomalies. AJNR Am J Neuroradiol. 31(4):755-60, 2010
8. Joshi MJ et al: The rare third branchial cleft cyst. AJNR Am J Neuroradiol. 30(9):1804-6, 2009
9. Koch BL: Cystic malformations of the neck in children. Pediatr Radiol. 35(5):463-77, 2005
10. Liberman M et al: Ten years of experience with third and fourth branchial remnants. J Pediatr Surg. 37(5):685-90, 2002
11. Huang RY et al: Third branchial cleft anomaly presenting as a retropharyngeal abscess. Int J Pediatr Otorhinolaryngol. 54(2-3):167-72, 2000
12. Mandell DL: Head and neck anomalies related to the branchial apparatus. Otolaryngol Clin North Am. 33(6):1309-32, 2000
13. Mukherji SK et al: Imaging of congenital anomalies of the branchial apparatus. Neuroimaging Clin N Am. 10(1):75-93, viii, 2000
14. Koeller KK et al: Congenital cystic masses of the neck: radiologic-pathologic correlation. Radiographics. 19(1):121-46; quiz 152-3, 1999
15. Benson MT et al: Congenital anomalies of the branchial apparatus: embryology and pathologic anatomy. Radiographics. 12(5):943-60, 1992

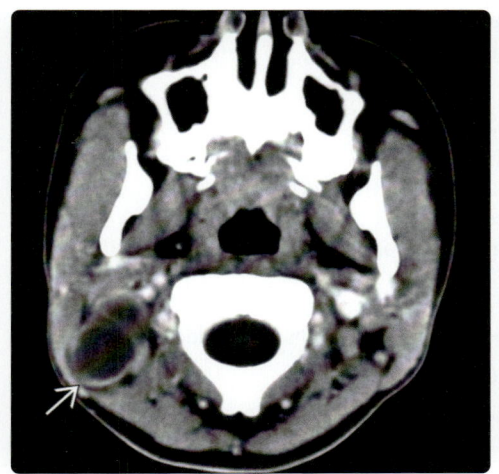
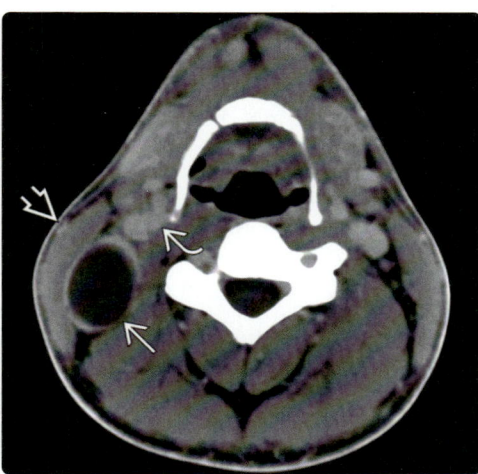

(Left) *Axial CECT demonstrates a 3rd BCC ➡ in the posterior cervical space of the upper neck. Mild enhancement and internal septation are consistent with sequelae of superimposed infection.* (Right) *Axial CECT demonstrates a mildly thick-walled, infected 3rd BCC ➡ deep to the SCM ➡ and posterolateral to the carotid sheath ➡. When occurring in the upper neck, the posterior cervical space is the typical location of 3rd BCCs.*

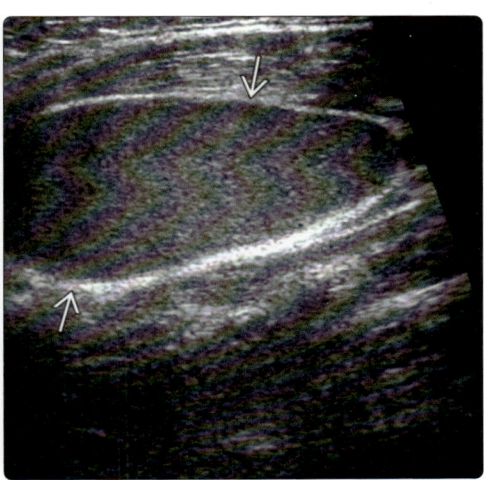
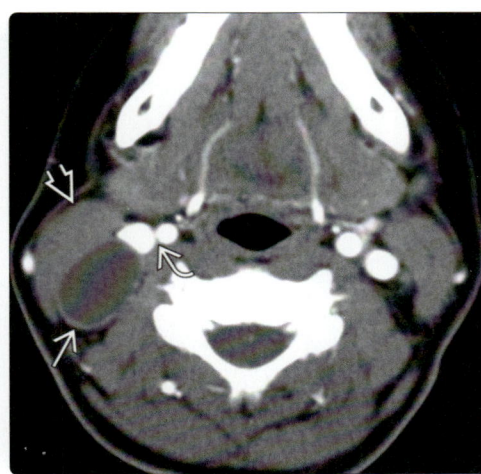

(Left) *Longitudinal US of the neck in a teenager with recent onset of a neck mass demonstrates a well-defined cyst ➡ with internal echoes in the posterior upper neck.* (Right) *Axial CECT in the same child demonstrates the relationship of the well-defined, nonenhancing cyst ➡ to the adjacent structures in the suprahyoid posterior neck, deep to SCM ➡ and posterolateral to carotid sheath vessels ➡. The location and appearance typical of a 3rd BCC DDx would include unilocular lymphatic malformation.*

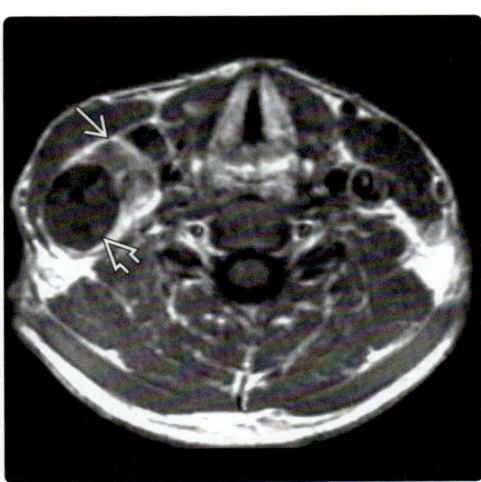
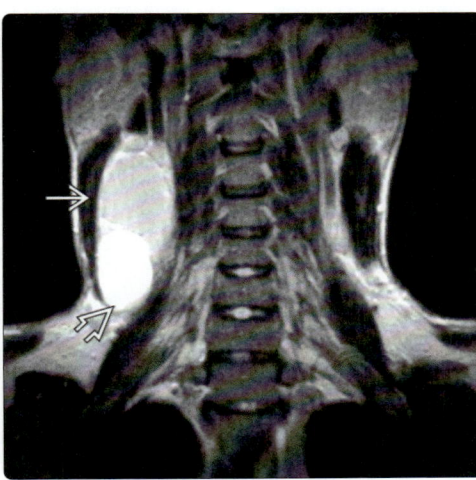

(Left) *Axial T1 C+ MR demonstrates a variant multiloculated 3rd BCC in the right posterior cervical space. The anterior portion ➡ is hyperintense relative to the posterior portion ➡, indicating higher protein content secondary to prior infection or hemorrhage.* (Right) *Coronal T2 MR in the same patient shows the superior portion ➡ to be hypointense relative to the inferior portion ➡. Lymphatic malformation should be included in the preoperative DDx.*

Pediatric Lesions

TERMINOLOGY

- Pyriform sinus "fistula" or 4th branchial apparatus anomaly
  - Most anomalies are actually sinus tracts (not fistulas or cysts) from 4th (or 3rd) pharyngeal pouch remnant
  - Course from apex of pyriform sinus to upper aspect of left thyroid lobe → abscess in anterior lower neck ± thyroid involvement

IMAGING

- Sinus tract extending from apex of pyriform sinus to lower anterior neck after barium swallow
- CECT best demonstrates phlegmon or abscess
  - Abscess in or adjacent to anterior left thyroid lobe
  - CT after barium swallow best identifies sinus tract
- Direct injection of fistula best demonstrates course of fistulous tract

TOP DIFFERENTIAL DIAGNOSES

- Cervical thymic cyst

- Lymphatic malformation
- Thyroglossal duct cyst
- Thyroid colloid cyst
- 3rd branchial cleft cyst

CLINICAL ISSUES

- Recurrent neck abscesses
- Recurrent suppurative thyroiditis
- Treatment options
  - Initial treatment is antibiotics ± incision and drainage of abscess
  - Complete resection of sinus tract or fistula
  - Thyroid lobectomy for lesions in thyroid lobe

DIAGNOSTIC CHECKLIST

- Suspect sinus tract from pyriform sinus in any child with abscess in or anterior to left thyroid lobe

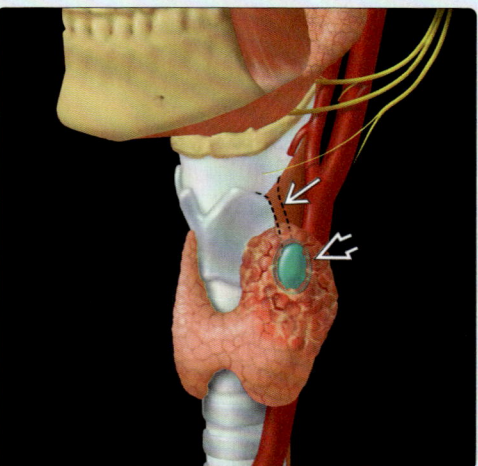
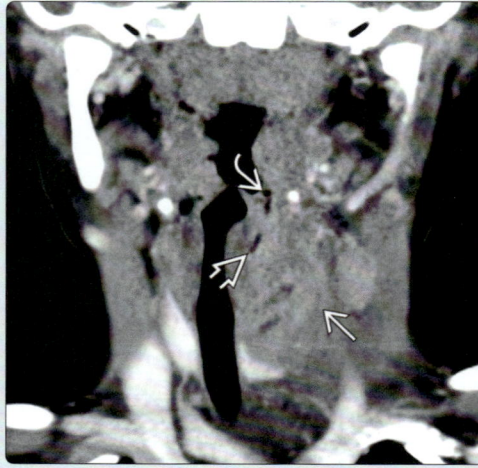

(Left) Sagittal oblique graphic shows a sinus tract ➡ from the pyriform sinus to the left thyroid lobe with associated abscess ➡ and thyroiditis secondary to a 4th pharyngeal pouch remnant. (Right) Coronal CECT shows the classic appearance of an inflammatory mass ➡ deviating the left thyroid lobe inferiorly with inflammation surrounding the sinus tract ➡, extending from the pyriform sinus apex ➡ to the phlegmonous process in the lower neck.

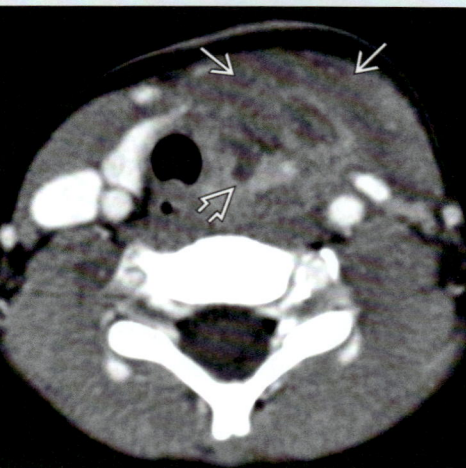
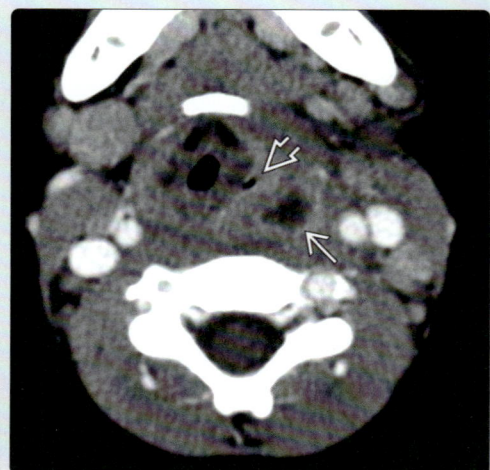

(Left) Axial CECT in a child presenting with acute signs of infection demonstrates a phlegmonous mass ➡ in the anterior left neck, involving the left thyroid lobe ➡ and causing deviation of the airway to the right of midline. (Right) Axial CECT in the same patient shows a rim-enhancing early abscess ➡ deviating an air-filled sinus tract ➡ forward. This constellation of findings should alert the clinician to search for an opening at the apex of the pyriform sinus.

TERMINOLOGY

Synonyms

- Pyriform sinus "fistula"
  - Most 4th branchial anomalies are actually sinus tracts, not fistulas or cysts

Definitions

- 4th branchial apparatus sinus tract
  - Course from apex of pyriform sinus to upper aspect of left thyroid lobe
- Branchial sinus tract: **1 opening** to skin surface, external auditory canal, pharynx **or** hypopharynx
- Branchial fistula: **2 openings** to skin **and** lumen of foregut
  - Arises from epithelial-lined tract left behind when there is persistence of both branchial cleft and its corresponding pharyngeal pouch

IMAGING

General Features

- Best diagnostic clue
  - Sinus tract extending from apex of pyriform sinus to lower anterior neck after barium swallow
  - Abscess in or adjacent to anterior left thyroid lobe
- Location
  - May occur anywhere from pyriform sinus apex to thyroid lobe (> 90% left-sided)
    - Commonly against or within superior aspect of left thyroid lobe or attached to thyroid cartilage
    - Upper end may communicate with or be adherent to pyriform sinus
- Size: Variable
- Morphology: Thick-walled sinus tract ± abscess in or adjacent to left thyroid lobe

Fluoroscopic Findings

- Barium swallow
  - Barium-filled sinus tract extending from apex of pyriform sinus to anterior lower neck
  - If performed during acute infection, may not fill portions of sinus tract
  - Scarring secondary to infection may prohibit filling of sinus tract

CT Findings

- CECT
  - Phlegmonous mass or frank abscess in or adjacent to left thyroid lobe with cellulitis extending around and collapsing ipsilateral pyriform sinus
  - Air within sinus tract or thyroid lobe occasionally present
  - Rarely, fistulous tract identifiable extending to skin at anterior lower neck
- NECT after barium swallow
  - Barium-filled tract extending from apex of pyriform sinus to lower anterior neck
  - If performed during acute infection, may not fill portions of sinus tract
  - Scarring secondary to infection may prohibit filling of sinus tract

MR Findings

- Phlegmon or abscess in left anterior neck with deep neck inflammation extending to pyriform sinus
- Tubular, fluid-filled tract posterior to cricothyroid joint, extending from pyriform sinus apex to left lobe of thyroid in 40%
- Sinus tract may course through thyroid gland or posterior to thyroid gland
- Rarely see unilocular, cystic mass
- Prenatal diagnosis suggested if left-sided unilocular neck cyst is identified with tapered medial margin at level of pyriform sinus

Ultrasonographic Findings

- Heterogeneous, phlegmonous mass or thick-walled abscess with hyperemic wall anterior to or within left thyroid lobe
- Difficult to visualize extent of inflammation surrounding sinus tract communicating with pyriform sinus

Imaging Recommendations

- Best imaging tool
  - CECT best demonstrates phlegmon or abscess as well as inflammation extending craniad to level of asymmetric pyriform sinus
  - CT after barium swallow best identifies sinus tract
  - Fistula course best demonstrated with direct injection
- Protocol advice
  - Thin-section postcontrast helical CT with multiplanar reconstructions very helpful

DIFFERENTIAL DIAGNOSIS

Cervical Thymic Cyst

- Congenital cyst: Remnant of thymopharyngeal duct, derivative of 3rd pharyngeal pouch
- Left side more common than right
- Closely associated with carotid sheath
  - In lower neck: Medial to carotid sheath, posterior to thyroid
  - In upper neck or extending from upper neck to mediastinum: Splay carotid artery and jugular vein
- If confined to visceral space, may mimic 4th branchial apparatus cyst
- Up to 50% extend into superior mediastinum
- May be connected to mediastinal thymus directly or by fibrous cord

Lymphatic Malformation

- Uni- or multilocular
- Microcystic or macrocystic
- Focal or infiltrative
- Isolated or transspatial
- Fluid-fluid levels if intralesional hemorrhage
- ± enhancing venous malformation components if combined venolymphatic malformation

Thyroglossal Duct Cyst

- Anywhere along thyroglossal duct from base of tongue (foramen cecum) to lower anterior neck thyroid bed
  - 20-25% in suprahyoid neck
  - Almost 50% at hyoid bone
  - ~ 25% in infrahyoid neck

– Embedded in strap muscles = claw sign
– Off-midline, anterior to thyroid lobe
– Closely related to thyroid cartilage or strap muscles

Colloid Cyst, Thyroid

- Uncommon in young children, most occur in older children and adults
- Nonneoplastic lesion of thyroid containing stored form of thyroid hormone (colloid)
- May appear bright on T1 MR due to hemorrhage, colloid, or high protein content

3rd Branchial Cleft Cyst

- Unilocular, thin-walled cyst
- Most arise in upper posterior cervical space
- Rarely along lower anterior margin of sternocleidomastoid muscle

Simple Thyroid Cyst

- True thyroid cysts with epithelial lining are rare
  o Most thyroid "cysts" = degenerating adenomas

PATHOLOGY

General Features

- Etiology
  o Controversial
    – Failure of obliteration of 4th branchial pouch or distal cervical sinus of His
    – Literature suggests course of sinus tract does not follow theoretical tract for 3rd or 4th branchial arch remnant
      □ Sinus tract may actually be remnant of thymopharyngeal duct of 3rd branchial pouch
- Associated abnormalities
  o 4th branchial sinus
    – When sinus connection with apex of pyriform sinus is maintained, infection is likely
    – Thyroiditis ± thyroid abscess possible in such circumstances
  o 4th branchial fistula
    – Term fistula denotes 2 openings: 1 in low anterior neck, another into pyriform sinus apex

Gross Pathologic & Surgical Features

- Anterolateral neck cellulitis, phlegmon or abscess
- Direct probing of pyriform apex frequently demonstrates fistula or sinus tract

CLINICAL ISSUES

Presentation

- Most common signs/symptoms
  o Recurrent neck abscesses
  o Recurrent suppurative thyroiditis
  o Fluctuant mass in lower 1/3 of neck anteromedial to sternocleidomastoid muscle
    – Tender if infected
  o Throat pain, dysphagia, stridor, dyspnea

Demographics

- Age

o Most branchial sinuses and fistulae (all types) present in childhood
o Most 4th branchial apparatus anomalies are diagnosed in infants and young children
- Sex
  o More common in female patients
- Epidemiology
  o Rarest of all forms of branchial apparatus anomalies (1-2% of all branchial anomalies)
  o Most cases arise on left

Natural History & Prognosis

- If sinus tract connection to pyriform sinus unrecognized and untreated, recurrent suppurative thyroiditis ensues
- Recurrence likely if tract contains secretory epithelium, is not resected

Treatment

- If infected, initial treatment is antibiotics ± incision and drainage of abscess
- Complete resection of sinus tract or fistula, obliterate opening in pyriform sinus ± hemithyroidectomy
- Endoscopic coblation successful in recent literature

DIAGNOSTIC CHECKLIST

Consider

- Suspect sinus tract from pyriform sinus in child with phlegmon or abscess in or anterior to left thyroid lobe

SELECTED REFERENCES

1. Asimakopoulos AD et al: Acute suppurative thyroiditis extending to retropharyngeal space: report of 2 cases. Ear Nose Throat J. ePub, 2025
2. Booth TN: Congenital cystic neck masses. Neuroimaging Clin N Am. 33(4):591-605, 2023
3. Chen W et al: Endoscopic coblation treatment for congenital pyriform sinus fistula in children. Medicine (Baltimore). 100(19):e25942, 2021
4. Han Z et al: MRI in children with pyriform sinus fistula. J Magn Reson Imaging. 53(1):85-95, 2021
5. Li Y et al: Prenatal diagnosis of third and fourth branchial apparatus anomalies: case series and comparison with lymphatic malformation. AJNR Am J Neuroradiol. 42(11):2094-100, 2021
6. Buch K et al: MR imaging evaluation of pediatric neck masses: review and update. Magn Reson Imaging Clin N Am. 27(2):173-99, 2019
7. Prosser JD et al: Branchial cleft anomalies and thymic cysts. Otolaryngol Clin North Am. 48(1):1-14, 2015
8. Bajaj Y et al: Branchial anomalies in children. Int J Pediatr Otorhinolaryngol. 75(8):1020-3, 2011
9. Ibrahim M et al: Congenital cystic lesions of the head and neck. Neuroimaging Clin N Am. 21(3):621-39, viii, 2011
10. Thomas B et al: Revisiting imaging features and the embryologic basis of third and fourth branchial anomalies. AJNR Am J Neuroradiol. 31(4):755-60, 2010
11. Nicoucar K et al: Management of congenital fourth branchial arch anomalies: a review and analysis of published cases. J Pediatr Surg. 44(7):1432-9, 2009
12. Mantle BA et al: Fourth branchial cleft sinus: relationship to superior and recurrent laryngeal nerves. Am J Otolaryngol. 29(3):198-200, 2008
13. James A et al: Branchial sinus of the piriform fossa: reappraisal of third and fourth branchial anomalies. Laryngoscope. 117(11):1920-4, 2007
14. Koch BL: Cystic malformations of the neck in children. Pediatr Radiol. 35(5):463-77, 2005
15. Wang HK et al: Imaging studies of pyriform sinus fistula. Pediatr Radiol. 33(5):328-33, 2003
16. Park SW et al: Neck infection associated with pyriform sinus fistula: imaging findings. AJNR Am J Neuroradiol. 21(5):817-22, 2000
17. Stone ME et al: A new role for computed tomography in the diagnosis and treatment of pyriform sinus fistula. Am J Otolaryngol. 21(5):323-5, 2000
18. Benson MT et al: Congenital anomalies of the branchial apparatus: embryology and pathologic anatomy. Radiographics. 12(5):943-60, 1992

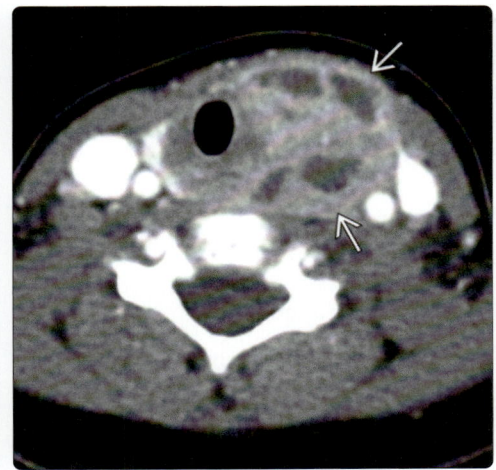

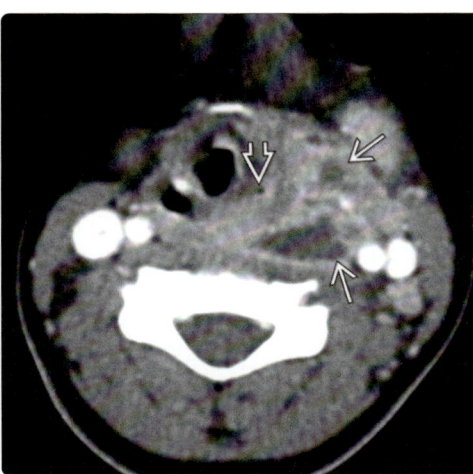

(Left) Axial CECT in a 6-year-old child shows a multiloculated abscess in the left lower neck ➡, causing significant rightward deviation of the trachea. (Right) Axial CECT in the same patient at the level of the pyriform sinus demonstrates the uppermost aspect of the abscess ➡, posterior to the nearly effaced and anteriorly deviated pyriform sinus apex ➡. This appearance should alert the clinician to search for the opening of the sinus tract in the pyriform sinus, which, unless obliterated, may cause recurrent abscess.

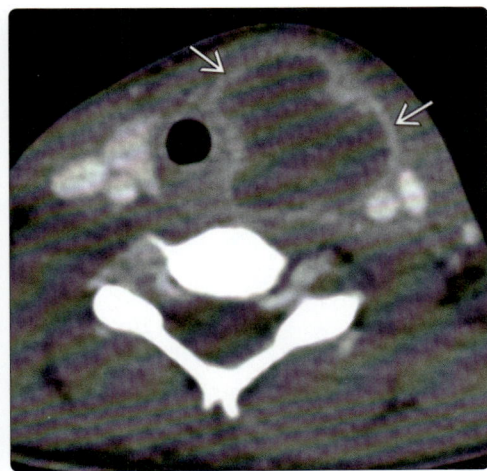

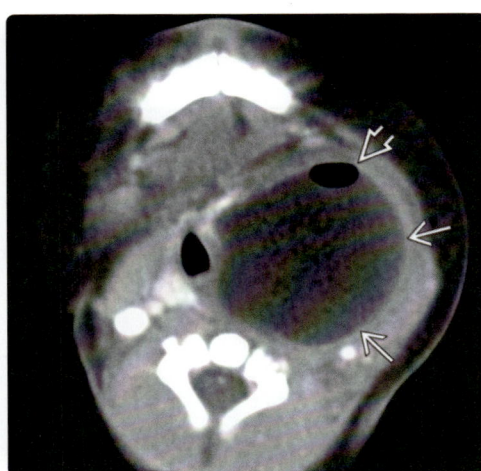

(Left) Axial CECT in a 7-year-old child shows a well-defined, rim-enhancing collection in the left lower neck ➡ with associated myositis and cellulitis. On more inferior images, this involved the left lobe of thyroid and extended superiorly to the level of the pyriform sinus; alerting the clinician to search for the sinus tract is imperative. (Right) Axial CECT shows a large, left-sided cystic mass ➡ at the level of the left thyroid lobe with a small focus of intralesional air ➡, which should suggest connection to the aerodigestive tract.

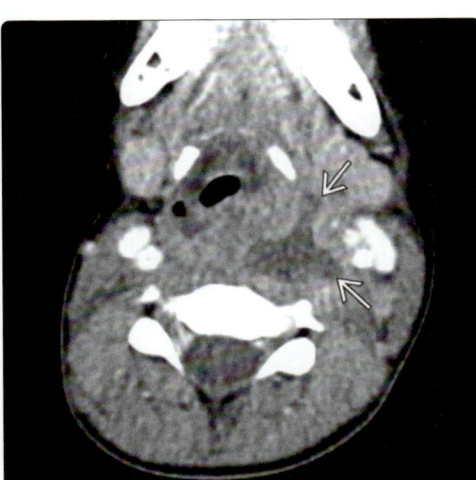

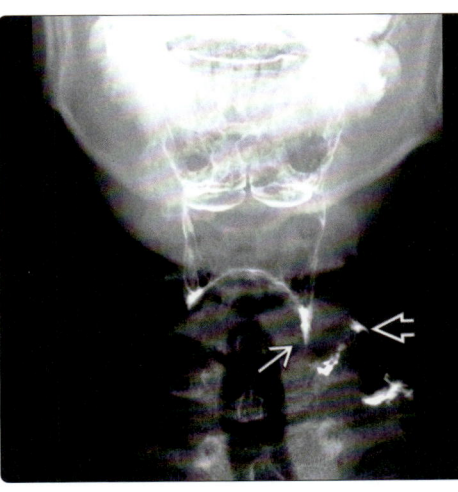

(Left) Axial CECT in a child with fever and a left neck mass shows an irregular-shaped, heterogeneously enhancing abscess ➡ resulting in effacement of the left pyriform sinus and rightward deviation of the airway, the extent of which should raise the question of sinus tract from the pyriform sinus as a cause of the abscess. (Right) AP radiograph in a patient with a perithyroidal abscess confirms a sinus tract ➡ with barium extending from the apex of the left pyriform sinus ➡ to the soft tissues of the lower left neck.

Pediatric Lesions

TERMINOLOGY

- Thyroglossal duct cyst (TGDC): Cystic remnant of embryologic thyroglossal duct (TGD)

IMAGING

- Best diagnostic clue: Round or ovoid midline suprahyoid or midline/paramidline infrahyoid cystic neck mass
- Suprahyoid neck: ~ 20-25%, typically midline
- At hyoid bone: ~ 50%
- Infrahyoid neck: ~ 25%, midline or paramidline
  - Embedded in strap muscles: Claw sign
- ± wall enhancement, soft tissue stranding if infected

TOP DIFFERENTIAL DIAGNOSES

- Dermoid or epidermoid
- Lingual thyroid
- Lymphatic malformation
- Delphian chain necrotic node
- 4th branchial apparatus anomaly

- Cervical thymic cyst

PATHOLOGY

- Failure of involution of TGD + persistent secretion of epithelial cells lining duct → TGDC
- Lies anywhere along TGD route of thyroid anlage descent from foramen cecum at tongue base to thyroid bed in infrahyoid neck

CLINICAL ISSUES

- Most common congenital neck lesion
- Treatment: Sistrunk procedure (excision of cyst, tract, & midline hyoid bone) → ↓ recurrences

DIAGNOSTIC CHECKLIST

- Relationship to hyoid bone important to note: Suprahyoid, hyoid, or infrahyoid in location
- Nodularity or Ca^{++} suggests associated thyroid carcinoma
- Confirm normal thyroid by ultrasound prior to TGDC or lingual thyroid resection

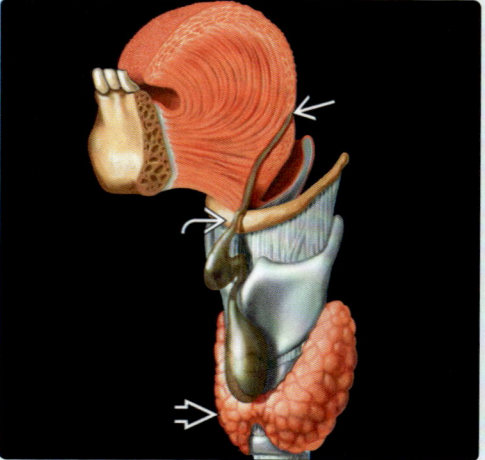
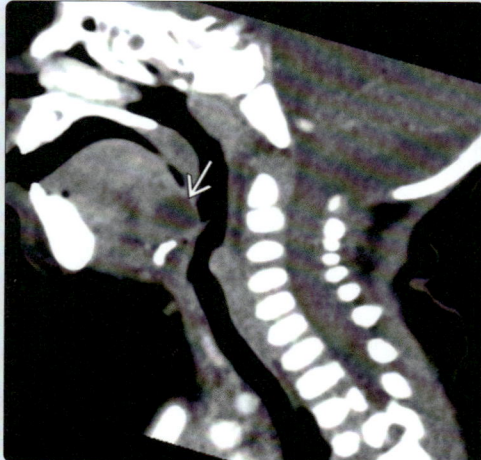

(Left) Sagittal oblique graphic shows the potential sites of a thyroglossal duct cyst (TGDC) from the foramen cecum ➡ to the thyroid bed ➡. Note the close relationship of the midportion of the hyoid bone ➡ to this pathway. A cyst can occur anywhere along this tract. *(Right)* Sagittal CECT shows a well-defined, cystic-appearing mass ➡ at the midline base of the tongue. This mass was incidentally found on a CT performed to evaluate the extent of a deep neck infection (not shown). The mass was subsequently proven to be a TGDC.

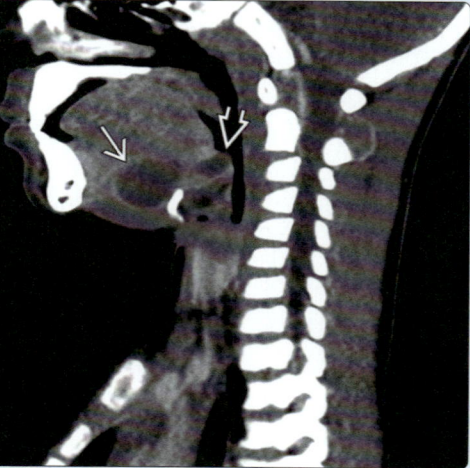
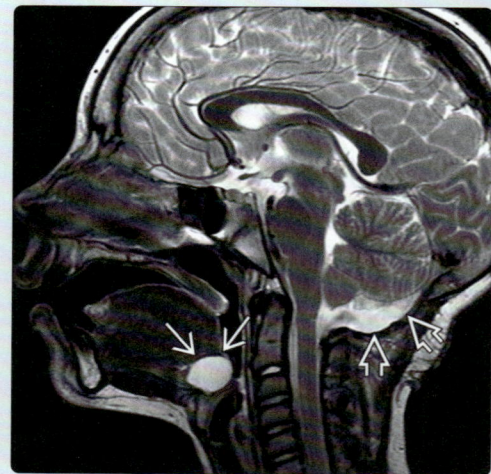

(Left) Sagittal CECT in a child with sore throat & difficulty swallowing shows a lobulated, rim-enhancing, fluid-attenuation mass ➡ in the midline sublingual space with a small posterior extension at the tongue base ➡. Histologically, this proved to be an inflamed TGDC. *(Right)* Sagittal T2 MR incidentally shows a well-defined, hyperintense TGDC ➡ in the midline base of the tongue, at the level of the foramen cecum, in a patient imaged for follow-up after posterior fossa decompression ➡ for treatment of Chiari 1.

Thyroglossal Duct Cyst

TERMINOLOGY

Synonyms
- Thyroglossal duct cyst (TGDC)

Definitions
- Remnant of embryologic thyroglossal duct (TGD) found between foramen cecum at tongue base & thyroid bed in infrahyoid neck

IMAGING

General Features
- Best diagnostic clue
  - Anterior midline suprahyoid or midline/paramidline infrahyoid cystic neck mass
- Location
  - Suprahyoid neck: ~ 20-25%, typically midline
    - Base of tongue or within posterior floor of mouth
  - At hyoid bone: ~ 50%
    - Usually abutting anterior hyoid bone
    - May project into preepiglottic space
  - Infrahyoid neck: ~ 25%, midline or paramidline embedded in strap muscles
    - Further inferior TGDC is more likely to be off midline
- Size
  - Variable, usually 2-4 cm
- Morphology
  - Round or ovoid cyst

Ultrasonographic Findings
- Anechoic or hypoechoic midline neck mass
  - ± internal echoes
    - May or may not be due to hemorrhage or infection
- Must image lower neck to prove presence of normal-appearing bilobed thyroid

CT Findings
- CECT
  - Low-attenuation, cystic midline neck mass with thin rim of peripheral enhancement
    - ± wall enhancement, soft tissue stranding if infected
    - Occasional septations
  - Paramidline infrahyoid TGDC embedded in strap muscles may show claw sign
  - < 1% contain associated thyroid carcinoma (usually papillary carcinoma)
    - Solid mass may have Ca++, and mass is eccentric, within cyst
    - May only be microscopic & not identifiable prospectively with imaging
    - Majority occur in adults but may occur in teenagers
      - Youngest reported: 10 years old

MR Findings
- T1WI: Usually hypointense; hyperintense if proteinaceous fluid
- T2WI: Homogeneously hyperintense
- T1WI C+: Nonenhancing cyst
  - Rim enhancement if infected

Imaging Recommendations
- Children: TGDCs have classic clinical presentation
  - Sonography only to confirm normal thyroid gland
  - CT or MR if infected or diagnosis uncertain
- Adults: CT or MR if cyst suprahyoid or infected
- Nuclear scintigraphy helpful if ectopic thyroid suspected

DIFFERENTIAL DIAGNOSIS

Oral Cavity Dermoid or Epidermoid
- Dermoid: Fat, fluid, or mixed
- Epidermoid: Fluid
- Submandibular space, sublingual space, or root of tongue
- Neither directly involves hyoid bone

Lingual Thyroid
- Most common location of ectopic thyroid
- In 75% of patients, lingual thyroid is only functioning thyroid tissue
- May expand rapidly during puberty
- Solid, round, hyperattenuating mass in base of tongue on NECT, avid enhancement CECT
- Variable T1 & T2 signal, variable contrast enhancement on MR

Lymphatic Malformation
- Unilocular or multilocular
- Microcystic or macrocystic
- Focal or transspatial
- Fluid-fluid levels common secondary to hemorrhage
- Nonenhancing unless infected or part of combined venolymphatic vascular malformation

Delphian Chain Necrotic Node
- Prelaryngeal/precricoid lymph node
  - Located between cricothyroid muscles, anterior to cricothyroid membrane
- Can be difficult to differentiate from infected TGDC
  - Usually in adults, most commonly thyroid & laryngeal cancer nodal metastases

4th Branchial Apparatus Anomaly
- May present with recurrent thyroiditis
- Majority are sinus tracts from apex of left pyriform sinus to lower neck → abscess in or adjacent to left thyroid lobe
- 4th (or 3rd) pharyngeal pouch remnant

Cervical Thymic Cyst
- Congenital cyst, anywhere along thymopharyngeal duct, from pyriform sinus to anterior mediastinum
  - Thymopharyngeal duct is remnant of 3rd pharyngeal pouch
- Left > right
- Close association with carotid sheath
  - May splay carotid artery & jugular vein, particularly near skull base
- May be combined solid thymic tissue & cyst

Mixed Laryngocele
- Off-midline, fluid- or air- & fluid-containing mass
- Traces back to laryngeal origin
- Not embedded within strap muscles

PATHOLOGY

General Features

- Genetics
  - Thyroid developmental anomalies often occur in same family
- Associated abnormalities
  - Thyroid agenesis, ectopia, or pyramidal lobe
  - Occasionally associated with carcinoma
    - Most commonly papillary carcinoma within TGDC
- Embryology/anatomy
  - TGD originates near foramen cecum at posterior 3rd of tongue
  - Thyroid anlage arises at base of tongue → descends around or through hyoid bone → descends along strap muscles → final position in thyroid bed, anterior to thyroid cartilage or cricoid cartilage
  - At 5-6 gestational weeks, TGD usually involutes
    - Foramen cecum & pyramidal thyroid lobe may be left as normal remnants
  - Failure of TGD involution with persistent secretory activity of epithelial cells lining duct → TGDC
  - TGDC or ectopic thyroid tissue may occur anywhere along TGD

Gross Pathologic & Surgical Features

- Smooth, benign-appearing cyst with tract to hyoid bone ± foramen cecum

Microscopic Features

- Cyst lined by respiratory or squamous epithelium
- Small deposits of thyroid tissue with colloid commonly associated
- ± thyroid carcinoma (papillary carcinoma most common)

CLINICAL ISSUES

Presentation

- Most common signs/symptoms
  - Midline or paramidline doughy, compressible, painless neck mass in child or young adult
  - Cyst elevates when tongue protrudes if TGDC located around hyoid bone
- Other signs/symptoms
  - Recurrent midline neck mass with upper respiratory tract infections or trauma
  - ± multiple prior incision & drainage procedures for neck abscess
  - Rarely, lingual TGDC may lead to obstruction in infants
  - Small lesion may be recognized as incidental finding on brain MR, majority lingual location

Demographics

- Age
  - < 10 years at presentation (up to 90%)
- Sex
  - M < F in uncommon familial forms
- Epidemiology
  - Most common congenital neck lesion
    - 90% of nonodontogenic congenital cysts
    - 3x as common as branchial cleft cysts

- At autopsy, > 7% of population will have TGD remnant somewhere along course of tract

Natural History & Prognosis

- Recurrent, intermittent swelling of mass, usually following minor upper respiratory infection
- Rapidly enlarging mass suggests either infection or differentiated thyroid carcinoma within TGDC (< 1%)
  - In recent large systematic review 94% were papillary carcinoma
    - May have co-occurrence of thyroid gland carcinoma
    - Very good prognosis

Treatment

- Complete surgical resection: Sistrunk procedure → ↓ recurrence rate from 50% to < 4%
  - Tract to foramen cecum dissected free
  - Entire cyst & midline portion of hyoid bone resected
    - Even if imaging shows no obvious connection to hyoid bone
    - Exception: Low infrahyoid neck TGDC
- Isolated lingual TGDC may be treated endoscopically
  - Recent reports of success with coblation-assisted transoral endoscopic excision
- Prognosis excellent with complete surgical resection
- Recurrences (from incomplete resection) often complicated & lateral
  - ↑ recurrence in patients with postoperative infection

DIAGNOSTIC CHECKLIST

Consider

- Relationship to hyoid bone important to note
  - Suprahyoid, hyoid, or infrahyoid in location
- Any nodularity or Ca++ suggests associated thyroid carcinoma
- Image thyroid bed with ultrasound to confirm presence of normal thyroid gland prior to TGDC or lingual thyroid excision

SELECTED REFERENCES

1. Negi S et al: Papillary carcinoma of thyroglossal duct cyst-a case series. Indian J Surg Oncol. 16(2):633-8, 2025
2. Niu Y et al: Coblation-assisted transoral endoscopic excision of lingual thyroglossal duct cysts. J Otolaryngol Head Neck Surg. ePub, 2025
3. Thimsen V et al: Thyroglossal duct cyst carcinomas - a retrospective study and systematic review of the literature. Virchows Arch. ePub, 2025
4. Foust AM et al: Congenital and infantile masses of the head and neck. Radiographics. 44(12):e240059, 2024
5. Bertoni DG et al: Diagnosing midline neck masses: comparing clinical exam, the SIST score, and the 4S algorithm. Otolaryngol Head Neck Surg. 169(3):496-503, 2023
6. Booth TN: Congenital cystic neck masses. Neuroimaging Clin N Am. 33(4):591-605, 2023
7. Lancini D et al: Evidence and controversies in management of thyroglossal duct cyst carcinoma. Curr Opin Otolaryngol Head Neck Surg. 29(2):113-9, 2021
8. Lekkerkerker I et al: Pediatric thyroglossal duct cysts: post-operative complications. Int J Pediatr Otorhinolaryngol. 124:14-7, 2019
9. Liaw J et al: Primary papillary thyroid cancer of a thyroglossal duct cyst. Ear Nose Throat J. 98(3):136-8, 2019
10. Hirshoren N et al: The imperative of the Sistrunk operation: review of 160 thyroglossal tract remnant operations. Otolaryngol Head Neck Surg. 140(3):338-42, 2009
11. Glastonbury CM et al: The CT and MR imaging features of carcinoma arising in thyroglossal duct remnants. AJNR Am J Neuroradiol. 21(4):770-4, 2000

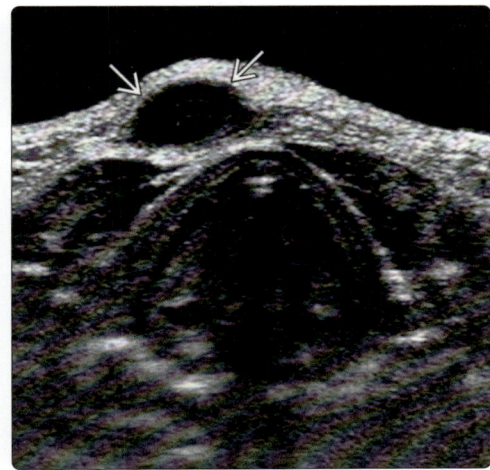

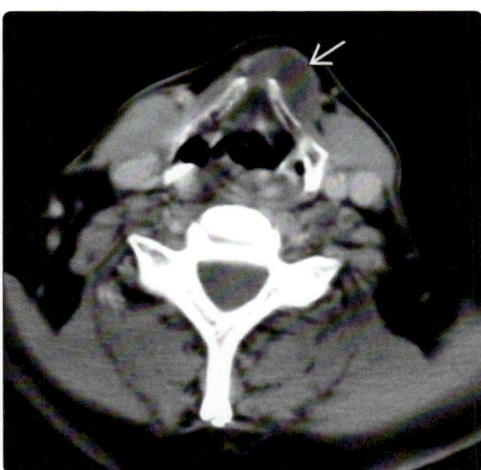

(Left) Transverse US of the anterior neck shows a well-defined, subcutaneous, right paramidline, hypoechoic mass ➡ ventral to the strap muscles. This was surgically removed & confirmed to be a TGDC. (Right) Axial CECT shows a fluid-attenuation TGDC ➡ in the left anterior strap muscles overlying thyroid cartilage. Remember, infrahyoid TGDCs tend to be embedded in the strap muscles.

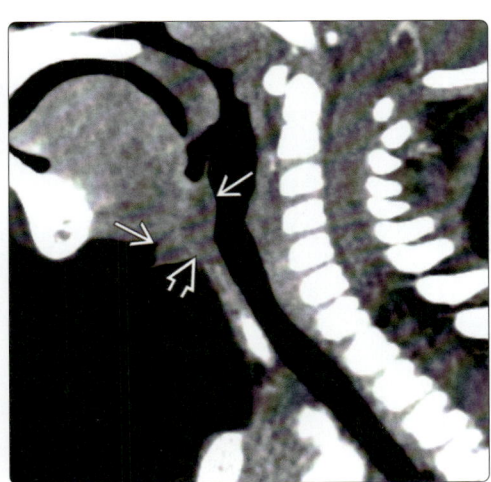

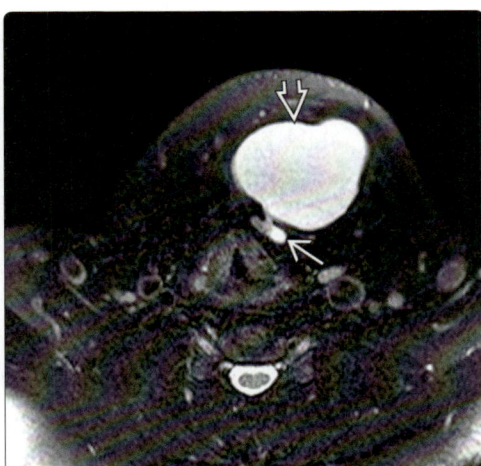

(Left) Sagittal CECT in a child with proven recurrence of a TGDC demonstrates a lobulated, heterogeneous mass ➡ in the midline suprahyoid neck. By imaging, this is indistinguishable from a postsurgical collection. Note the absence of a midline hyoid bone ➡, consistent with a prior Sistrunk procedure. (Right) Axial T2 FS MR of the neck shows a tract ➡ that leads from a large anterior paramidline neck cyst ➡ to the bed of the infrahyoid strap muscles. This is a critical clue to making the correct imaging diagnosis of a TGDC.

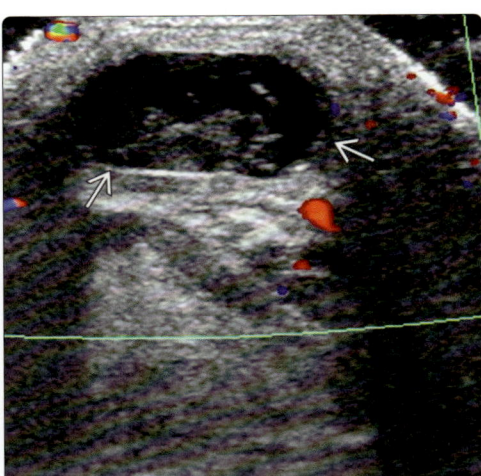

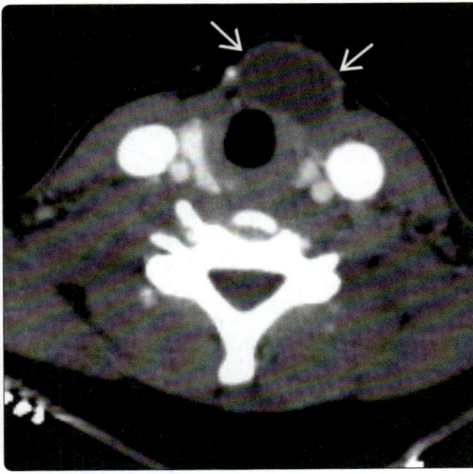

(Left) Transverse color Doppler US in a child with new onset of a paramidline anterior left neck mass shows a heterogeneously hypoechoic lesion ➡ with internal echoes, concerning for dermoid or carcinoma within a TGDC. No internal vascularity is seen. Histologically, the lesion proved to be an uncomplicated TGDC. (Right) Axial CECT of the neck in a teenager with new-onset neck mass demonstrates a low-attenuation infrahyoid mass ➡ embedded within the left strap muscle, typical of a TGDC.

Cervical Thymic Cyst

TERMINOLOGY

- Cervical thymic cyst
- Cystic remnant of thymopharyngeal duct
  - Derivative of 3rd pharyngeal pouch

IMAGING

- Cystic mass closely associated with carotid sheath
- Anywhere along thymopharyngeal duct from pyriform sinus to anterior mediastinum
- Usually lateral infrahyoid neck
- Left > right side of neck
- May splay carotid artery and jugular vein
- Cyst wall may mildly enhance; solid thymic remnants may enhance similar to intrathoracic thymus

TOP DIFFERENTIAL DIAGNOSES

- 2nd branchial cleft cyst; most common: Lateral to carotid sheath, anteromedial to sternocleidomastoid muscle, posterior to submandibular gland

- 4th branchial anomaly
  - Cyst or abscess anterior to left thyroid lobe
- Lymphatic malformation
  - Unilocular or multilocular, focal or infiltrative
  - Fluid-fluid levels common
- Abscess
  - Irregular, enhancing wall with low-attenuation center
  - If associated with thyroid gland, think 4th branchial pouch anomaly

PATHOLOGY

- Hassall corpuscles in cyst wall confirm diagnosis

CLINICAL ISSUES

- Most present between 2-15 years of age
- Only 33% present after 1st decade

DIAGNOSTIC CHECKLIST

- Dumbbell-shaped cervicothoracic cystic mass highly suggestive of thymic cyst (vs. lymphatic malformation)

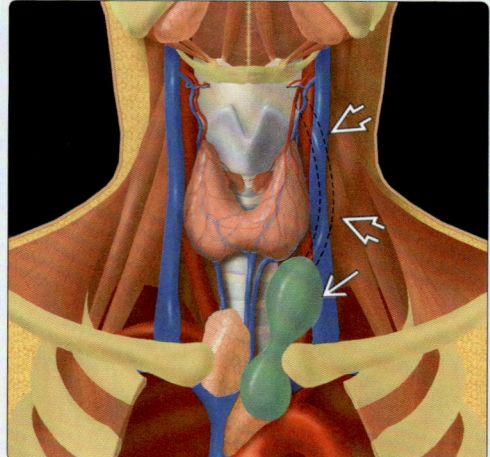
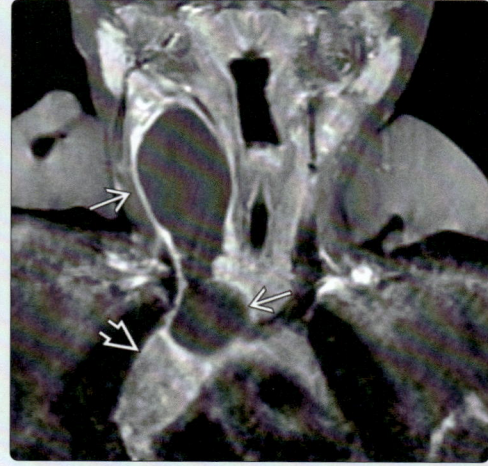

(Left) Coronal graphic shows a typical bilobed cervical thymic cyst ➡ extending from the anterior mediastinum into the lower neck along the course of the thymopharyngeal duct ➡. Notice the close association with the carotid space. (Right) Coronal T1 C+ FS MR in a 16-month-old child shows a cystic-appearing right neck mass ➡ causing mild airway compression. The cyst extends to the otherwise normal-appearing thymus ➡. Mild, diffuse wall enhancement is consistent with chronic inflammation, identified histologically.

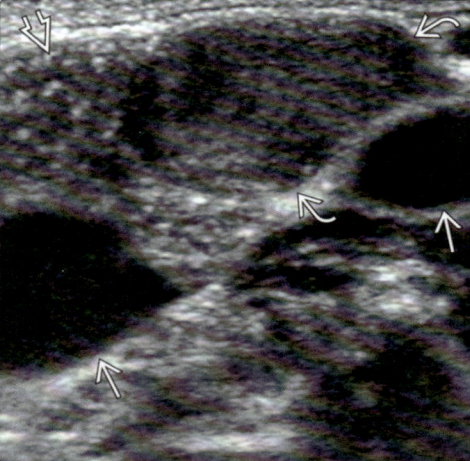
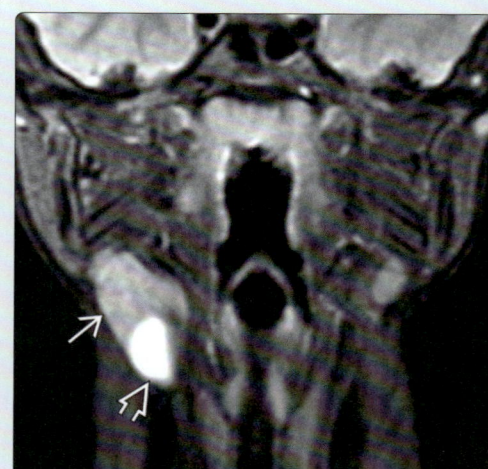

(Left) Transverse ultrasound in a 7-year-old child demonstrates a mixed cystic and solid right thymic remnant splaying the carotid sheath vessels ➡. The lateral component demonstrates echogenicity typical of thymus ➡, and the medial component is cystic with mobile intraluminal echoes ➡ on real-time imaging. (Right) Coronal T2 MR in the same patient shows a mixed solid ➡ and cystic ➡ thymic remnant, the solid portion of which was isointense to intrathoracic thymus on all sequences.

TERMINOLOGY

Abbreviations

- Cervical thymic cyst (CTC)

Synonyms

- Thymopharyngeal duct cyst, congenital thymic cyst

Definitions

- Cystic remnant of thymopharyngeal duct
  - Derivative of 3rd pharyngeal pouch
- Hassall corpuscles in cyst wall confirm diagnosis

IMAGING

General Features

- Best diagnostic clue
  - Cystic mass in left > right lateral neck, in lateral visceral space, or adjacent to carotid space
    - Closely associated with carotid sheath
      - In lower neck: Medial to carotid sheath, posterior to thyroid
      - In upper neck or extending from upper neck to mediastinum: Splay carotid artery and jugular vein
- Location
  - Anywhere along thymopharyngeal duct
    - From pyriform sinus to anterior mediastinum
  - Most common site: Lateral infrahyoid neck, at level of thyroid gland
    - Left > right
  - May parallel sternocleidomastoid muscle (SCM), close to carotid sheath
  - Cervical neck component ± extension to mediastinum
- Size
  - Variable, from several cm to very long, along course of thymopharyngeal duct
- Morphology
  - Usually large, dominant cyst
  - May be multiloculated
  - May splay carotid artery and jugular vein, especially in upper neck
  - Larger CTC may present as dumbbell-shaped cervicothoracic mass, projecting from lower lateral cervical neck into superior mediastinum

CT Findings

- CECT
  - Nonenhancing, low-attenuation, lateral neck cyst
    - Close association with carotid sheath common
    - Solid components rare = aberrant thymic tissue, lymphoid aggregates, or parathyroid tissue
    - May be connected to mediastinal thymus directly or by fibrous cord

MR Findings

- T1WI
  - Homogeneous, hypointense cyst most common
  - May be iso- to hyperintense if filled with blood products, proteinaceous fluid, or cholesterol
  - Thin wall
  - Solid nodules usually isointense to muscle and intrathoracic thymus
- T2WI
  - Homogeneously hyperintense fluid contents
- T1WI C+
  - Cystic component nonenhancing
  - Cyst wall or solid nodules may enhance
    - Solid thymic remnants enhance similar to intrathoracic thymus
  - If infected, cyst wall may be thickened and enhancing; surrounding soft tissue may be inflamed

Ultrasonographic Findings

- Thin-walled anechoic or hypoechoic lateral neck mass
- Rarely has solid nodules in wall

Imaging Recommendations

- Best imaging tool
  - CECT or MR preferable to ultrasound to demonstrate total extent of cyst
  - Ultrasound helpful if solid component has typical thymus echotexture
- Protocol advice
  - **Include upper mediastinum** to demonstrate mediastinal extension

DIFFERENTIAL DIAGNOSIS

2nd Branchial Cleft Cyst

- Most common branchial apparatus cyst
- Most common location
  - Posterolateral to submandibular gland, lateral to carotid space, anterior (or anteromedial) to SCM
- When infrahyoid, anterior to carotid space
- May mimic CTC when found in lower neck
- Rarely protrudes between internal carotid artery and external carotid artery

4th Branchial Anomaly

- Primary location: Sinus tract remnant of 4th (or 3rd) pharyngeal pouch
  - Sinus tract extends from pyriform sinus apex to anterior lower neck → left anterior neck abscess
- Often presents with suppurative thyroiditis
- Inflammation frequently extends to surround apex of pyriform sinus

Lymphatic Malformation

- May affect any space in head and neck
- When in posterior cervical space, abuts posterior carotid space
- Unilocular or multilocular
- Focal or infiltrative and transspatial
- Fluid-fluid levels common, secondary to intralesional hemorrhage

Abscess

- Presents with signs and symptoms of infection
- Irregular, thick, enhancing wall with low-attenuation center
- If associated with thyroid gland, think 4th branchial pouch anomaly

Colloid Cyst, Thyroid

- Primary location: Intrathyroidal, left or right
- Thin wall with smooth margins

- May be large &/or hemorrhagic colloid cyst
- Usually more medial than CTC

PATHOLOGY

General Features

- Etiology
  - Remnants of thymopharyngeal duct → CTC
  - Ectopic thymus may also occur along thymopharyngeal duct
- Embryology
  - Failure of obliteration of thymopharyngeal duct, remnant of 3rd pharyngeal pouch
  - Thymopharyngeal duct arises from pyriform sinus, descends into mediastinum
  - Persistent sequestered remnants may occur from mandible to thoracic inlet
  - Thymus and parathyroid glands arise from 3rd and 4th pharyngeal pouches, respectively
  - Embryologic migration follows caudal course along thymopharyngeal duct during 1st trimester
- No malignant association

Gross Pathologic & Surgical Features

- Smooth, thin-walled cervical cyst, often with caudal fibrous strand extending to mediastinal thymus
- Filled with brownish fluid
- Cyst wall may be nodular
- Associated with lymphoid tissue or parathyroid or thymic remnants
- Rarely may extend through thyrohyoid membrane into pyriform sinus

Microscopic Features

- Hassall corpuscles in cyst wall confirm diagnosis
  - May not always be identifiable if prior hemorrhage or infection
- Cyst wall may contain
  - Lymphoid tissue
  - Parathyroid tissue
  - Thyroid or thymic tissue
  - Cholesterol crystals and granulomas, probably from prior hemorrhage

CLINICAL ISSUES

Presentation

- Most common signs/symptoms
  - Often asymptomatic
  - Gradually enlarging, soft, compressible mid- to lower cervical neck mass
  - When large, may cause dysphagia, respiratory distress, or vocal cord paralysis
- Other presentations
  - Large, infantile, cervicothoracic thymic cyst may present with respiratory compromise
  - Rarely may be associated with disordered calcium metabolism if parathyroid component is functioning

Demographics

- Age
  - Most present between 2-15 years
  - Only 33% present after 1st decade
  - Rare reports of primary presentation in adulthood
- Sex
  - Slightly more common in male patients
- Epidemiology
  - Rare compared with other congenital neck masses
  - Left > right side of neck

Natural History & Prognosis

- Excellent prognosis if completely resected
- Recurrence common if incompletely resected

Treatment

- Complete surgical resection
- Large cervicothoracic thymic cyst may require head and neck and thoracic surgery

DIAGNOSTIC CHECKLIST

Consider

- If cystic mass is intimately associated with anterior carotid sheath, think CTC
- If cystic mass extends from anterior neck to upper mediastinum, think CTC

Image Interpretation Pearls

- Dumbbell-shaped cervicothoracic cystic mass highly suggestive of thymic cyst (vs. lymphatic malformation)
- Unilocular ovoid lesion with discrete margins; may be thymic cyst or unilocular lymphatic malformation

SELECTED REFERENCES

1. Booth TN: Congenital cystic neck masses. Neuroimaging Clin N Am. 33(4):591-605, 2023
2. Chang A et al: Diagnosis and management of ectopic cervical thymus in children: systematic review of the literature. J Pediatr Surg. 56(11):2062-8, 2021
3. Buch K et al: MR imaging evaluation of pediatric neck masses: review and update. Magn Reson Imaging Clin N Am. 27(2):173-99, 2019
4. Mehmi N et al: Importance and impact of appropriate radiology in the management of branchial cleft anomalies. Indian J Otolaryngol Head Neck Surg. 71(Suppl 1):953-9, 2019
5. Prosser JD et al: Branchial cleft anomalies and thymic cysts. Otolaryngol Clin North Am. 48(1) 1-14, 2015
6. Goff CJ et al: Current management of congenital branchial cleft cysts, sinuses, and fistulae. Curr Opin Otolaryngol Head Neck Surg. 20(6):533-9, 2012
7. Thomas B et al: Revisiting imaging features and the embryologic basis of third and fourth branchial anomalies. AJNR Am J Neuroradiol. 31(4):755-60, 2010
8. Sturm-O'Brien AK et al: Cervical thymic anomalies–the Texas Children's Hospital experience. Laryngoscope. 119(10):1988-93, 2009
9. Statham MM et al: Cervical thymic remnants in children. Int J Pediatr Otorhinolaryngol. 72(12):1807-13, 2008
10. Mehrzad H et al: A combined third and fourth branchial arch anomaly: clinical and embryological implications. Eur Arch Otorhinolaryngol. 264(8):913-6, 2007
11. Koch BL: Cystic malformations of the neck in children. Pediatr Radiol. 35(5):463-77, 2005
12. Pereira KD et al: Management of anomalies of the third and fourth branchial pouches. Int J Pediatr Otorhinolaryngol. 68(1):43-50, 2004
13. Liberman M et al: Ten years of experience with third and fourth branchial remnants. J Pediatr Surg. 37(5):685-90, 2002
14. Ozturk H et al: Multilocular cervical thymic cyst: an unusual neck mass in children. Int J Pediatr Otorhinolaryngol. 61(3): 249-52, 2001
15. Koeller KK et al: Congenital cystic masses of the neck: radiologic-pathologic correlation. Radiographics. 19(1): 121-46; quiz 152-3, 1999
16. Benson MT et a : Congenital anomalies of the branchial apparatus: embryology and pathologic anatomy. Radiographics. 12(5):943-60, 1992

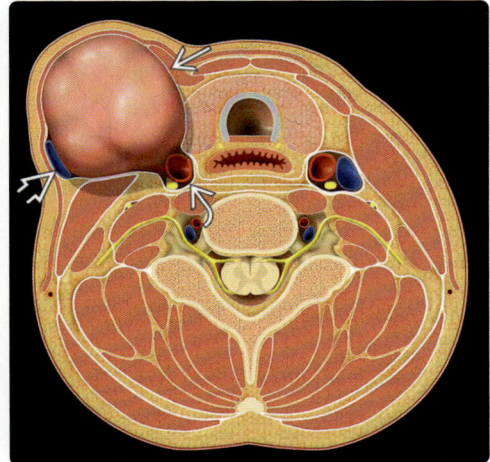
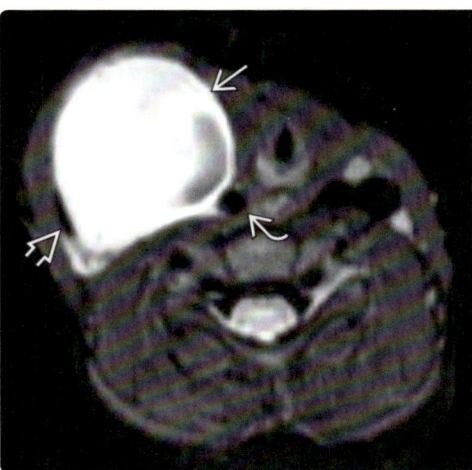

(Left) *Axial graphic of the neck depicts a large right neck cystic mass ➡, representing a cervical thymic cyst. Note that the cyst splays the right jugular vein ➡ and carotid artery ➡, an appearance typical of thymic cysts when they occur in the mid and upper neck.* **(Right)** *Axial FSE-IR MR of the neck demonstrates hyperintense signal within a right neck cystic mass ➡ that characteristically splays the right jugular vein ➡ and carotid artery ➡.*

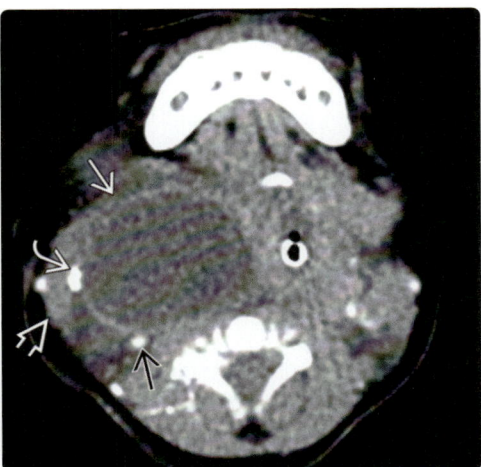
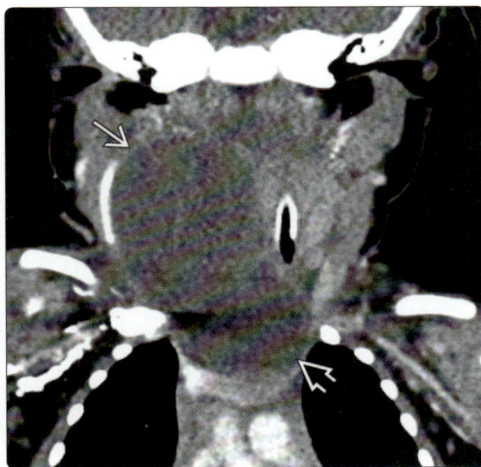

(Left) *Axial CECT in a 4-month-old infant shows a thin-walled cyst ➡ deep to the right sternocleidomastoid muscle ➡ that splays the jugular vein ➡ and carotid artery ➡ and causes significant mass effect on the airway.* **(Right)** *Coronal CECT in the same patient shows the typical bilobed appearance of a thymic cyst with a cervical component ➡ and extension of the cyst to the mediastinum ➡.*

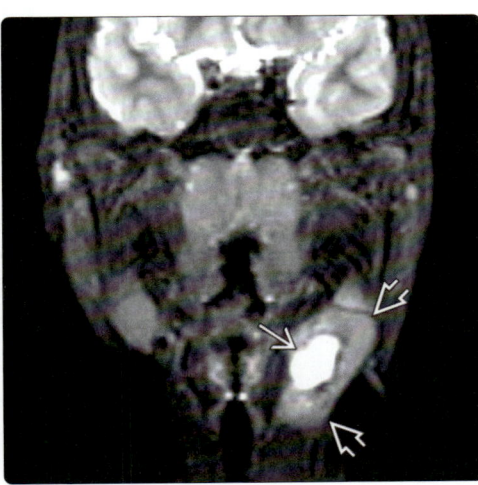
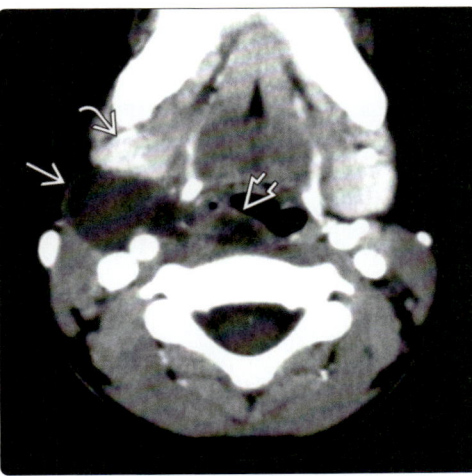

(Left) *Coronal T2 MR shows a rare association of both cystic ➡ and solid ➡ remnants of the thymus in the left neck.* **(Right)** *Axial CECT shows a rare appearance of a thymic cyst extending into the retropharyngeal space ➡. Notice the majority of the cyst is located in the right neck posterior submandibular space ➡, displacing the submandibular gland ➡ anteriorly.*

Dermoid and Epidermoid Cysts

TERMINOLOGY

- Definition: Cystic mass resulting from congenital epithelial inclusion or rest
  - Epidermoid: Epithelial elements only
  - Dermoid: Epithelial elements + dermal substructure, including dermal appendages

IMAGING

- Epidermoid: Cystic, well-demarcated mass with fluid contents only
- Dermoid: Cystic, well-demarcated mass ± fatty, fluid, or mixed contents
- Location
  - Oral cavity: Submandibular space, sublingual space, or root of tongue
  - Anterior neck, usually midline
  - Orbit: Adjacent to frontozygomatic suture > frontolacrimal suture

- Nasal cyst in association with nasal dermal sinus (NDS) ± intracranial extension
- Scalloping or remodeling of bone common
- Subtle rim enhancement of wall sometimes seen
- Restricted diffusion: Epidermoid > dermoid cysts
- Protocol advice
  - Routine CECT of cervical soft tissues
  - MR: T1 precontrast, & use fat-saturation post contrast for orbit, neck, & oral cavity lesions
  - High-resolution anterior skull base MR in NDS; image from tip of nose to posterior to crista galli
  - Sagittal to define tract: Nose → anterior skull base

DIAGNOSTIC CHECKLIST

- If complex lesion with fat, consider dermoid cyst
- Simple lesion (may be proteinaceous fluid) = epidermoid or dermoid cyst

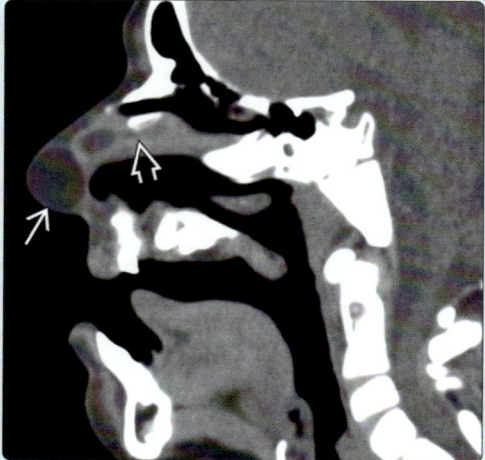
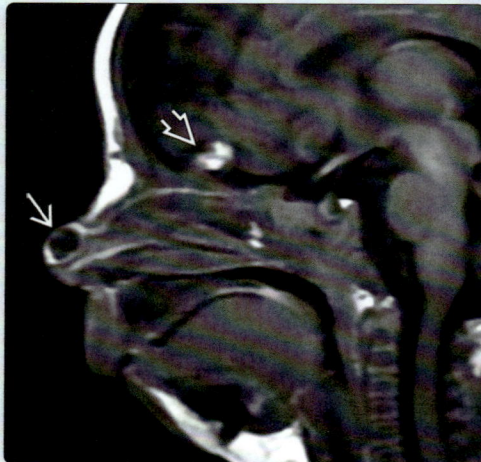

(Left) Sagittal CT reconstruction in a 10-year-old child following cleft palate repair shows a large nasal dermoid ➡ with nasal dermal sinus tract ➡ extending toward the cribriform plate without intracranial extension. (Right) Sagittal T1 MR in a 1-year-old girl with micrognathia shows a fluid signal intensity mass at the tip of the nose ➡ and a fat signal intensity intracranial, extradural mass ➡ superior to the foramen cecum. These were connected via a linear tract, and both histologically proved to be dermoid cysts.

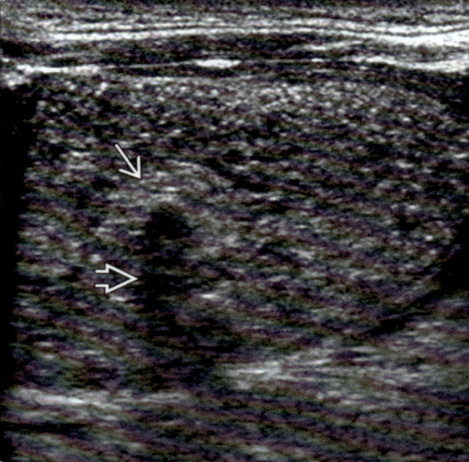
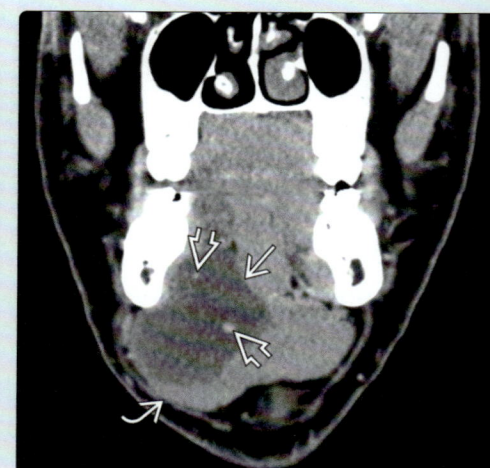

(Left) Longitudinal ultrasound in a 14-year-old boy shows a oral cavity mass with heterogeneous echotexture and minimal increased through-transmission. One hyperechoic focus ➡ has posterior acoustical shadowing ➡, consistent with Ca++, in this dermoid cyst. (Right) Coronal CECT in the same patient shows a low-density oral cavity mass ➡ with a few Ca++ ➡. Inferior displacement of the mylohyoid muscle ➡ indicates this dermoid cyst is in the sublingual space.

TERMINOLOGY

Synonyms

- Developmental cyst, ectodermal inclusion cyst, dermoid cyst

Definitions

- Congenital epithelial inclusion or rest → cystic mass
  - Epidermoid: Epithelial elements only
  - Dermoid: Epithelial elements + dermal substructure, including dermal appendages

IMAGING

General Features

- Best diagnostic clue
  - Epidermoid: Cystic, well-demarcated mass with fluid contents only
  - Dermoid: Cystic, well-demarcated mass ± fatty, fluid, or mixed contents
- Location
  - Epidermoid & dermoid lesions
    - Oral cavity (OC): Submandibular space (SMS), sublingual space (SLS), or root of tongue
    - Anterior neck, usually midline
    - Orbit: Adjacent to frontozygomatic suture > frontolacrimal suture
    - Nasal cyst + nasal dermal sinus (NDS) ± intracranial extension
      - □ Tract or cyst nasal bridge to crista galli
      - □ Large foramen cecum with bifid or deformed crista galli or cribriform plate clue to intracranial extension
      - □ Classification by location: Superficial, intraosseous, intracranial extradural, intracranial intradural
- Morphology
  - Ovoid or tubular

CT Findings

- Low-density, well-circumscribed cystic mass
  - Epidermoid: Fluid-density material inside lesion without complex features
  - Dermoid: Fatty internal material, mixed-density fluid, Ca++ (< 50%) all possible
    - When fluid density without complex features, indistinguishable from epidermoid
  - Scalloping or remodeling of bone common
  - Lesion wall may be imperceptible
  - Subtle rim enhancement of wall sometimes seen

MR Findings

- T1WI
  - Epidermoid: Well-circumscribed mass with homogeneous fluid signal
    - Diffuse ↑ signal if high-protein fluid
  - Dermoid: Well-circumscribed mass with complex fluid signal
    - If fatty elements, focal or diffuse ↑ signal
- T2WI
  - Epidermoid: Homogeneous high signal
  - Dermoid: Heterogeneous high signal
    - Intermediate signal if fat
    - Focal areas of low signal if Ca++
- DWI
  - Restricted diffusion epidermoid > dermoid cysts
- T1WI C+
  - Thin rim enhancement or no enhancement
  - If fat saturation used, fat will be low signal in dermoid

Ultrasonographic Findings

- Epidermoid: Pseudosolid appearance + uniform internal echoes
  - Cellular material in cyst → pseudosolid appearance
  - Posterior wall acoustic enhancement = cystic lesion
- Dermoid: Mixed internal echoes from fat with echogenic foci & dense shadowing if Ca++

Imaging Recommendations

- Best imaging tool
  - CECT is best imaging tool for OC lesions (unless obscured by dental amalgam, then MR best)
  - MR or CECT for neck lesions
  - MR for orbit lesions
  - MR for NDS to better evaluate intracranial extent
    - CT to evaluate skull base & crista galli deformity
- Protocol advice
  - Routine CECT or MR with contrast for cervical soft tissues
  - MR: Include T1 precontrast, & use fat-saturation techniques post contrast for orbit, neck, & OC lesions
  - High-resolution anterior skull base MR in NDS; image from tip of nose to posterior to crista galli
    - Sagittal to define tract: Nose → anterior skull base
    - DWI hyperintensity may diagnose epidermoid

DIFFERENTIAL DIAGNOSIS

Pediatric Sublingual Space, Submandibular Space, or Neck Lesions

- Thyroglossal duct cyst
  - Midline unilocular cystic mass between hyoid bone & foramen cecum
  - No fat or Ca++
- Lymphatic malformation
  - Unilocular or multilocular, transspatial common
  - Fluid-fluid levels common
- Ranula
  - Simple: Unilateral low-density/-signal mass in SLS with thin, nonenhancing wall
  - Diving: Comet-shaped unilocular mass with tail in collapsed SLS (tail sign) & head in posterior SMS
- Abscess
  - Clinical: Fever, erythema, elevated WBC count
  - Imaging: Rim-enhancing cyst often with soft tissue cellulitis, edema, & adenopathy

Pediatric Orbital Lesions

- Orbital Langerhans cell histiocytosis
  - Enhancing soft tissue mass with smoothly marginated lytic bone lesion
- Rhabdomyosarcoma
  - Moderately enhancing mass frequently inseparable from extraocular muscle
  - Frequently without bone erosion when in orbit

- Orbital infantile hemangioma
  - Significant contrast enhancement, no bone erosion, & presents in infancy
- Orbital lymphatic malformation
  - Intraconal, extraconal, or both
  - Nonenhancing; fluid-fluid levels common
- Orbital venous malformation
  - Moderate enhancement
  - Ca^{++}/phleboliths common
  - Positional proptosis may be present
- Orbital venolymphatic malformation
- Orbital idiopathic inflammatory pseudotumor
  - Painful proptosis common
  - Moderately enhancing mass, any area of orbit

Pediatric Nasal Lesions

- Normal fatty marrow in crista galli
  - No mass or pit on nose
- Nonossified foramen cecum
  - Ossifies postnatally in first 5 years of life
  - Normal crista galli
- Frontoethmoidal cephalocele
  - Direct extension of meninges, subarachnoid space, &, sometimes, brain through bone defect in cribriform plate or frontal bone
- Nasal glioma (nasal glial heterotopia is preferred term)
  - Most commonly projects extranasally onto paramedian bridge of nose
  - Less commonly, along anterior nasal septum

PATHOLOGY

General Features

- Etiology
  - Congenital inclusion of dermal elements at site of embryonic fusion
    - Sequestration of trapped surface ectoderm

Gross Pathologic & Surgical Features

- Oily or cheesy material; tan, yellow, or white
- Cyst wall = fibrous capsule; 2-6 mm in thickness

Microscopic Features

- Epidermoid
  - Simple squamous cell epithelium with fibrous wall
- Dermoid
  - Contains dermal structures, including sebaceous glands, hair follicles, blood vessels, fat ± collagen
    - Sweat glands in minority (20%)
    - Lined by keratinizing squamous epithelium
- Teratoid cysts (rare lesion)
  - Contain elements from all 3 germ cell layers

CLINICAL ISSUES

Presentation

- Most common signs/symptoms
  - Painless mass in floor of mouth (FOM), anterior neck, orbit, or nasoglabellar region
- Other signs/symptoms
  - OC lesions: Dysphagia, globus oral sensation, airway encroachment when large

- Orbit lesions: Proptosis, diplopia
- Nasal lesions: Pit on skin of nasal bridge ± protruding hair, recurrent meningitis, intermittent sebaceous material discharged from pit

Demographics

- Age
  - OC lesions: Mean age: Late teens to 20s
    - Most dermoid cysts of FOM present at 5-50 years
    - Average age: 30 years
  - Orbit lesions: Children or early adulthood
  - Nasal lesions: Newborn to 5 years
    - Mean age: 32 months
- Epidemiology
  - Present from birth; spontaneous occurrence
  - Dermoid/epidermoid are least common of all congenital neck lesions
  - Orbit most common dermoid of H&N
  - OC dermoids account for < 25% of all H&N dermoids

Natural History & Prognosis

- Benign lesion, very slow growth
  - Present during childhood but small & dormant
  - Symptomatic during rapid growth phase in young adult
- Sudden growth or change following rupture
  - Significant inflammation & ↑ size (rare complication)

Treatment

- Surgical resection is curative
  - Entire cyst must be removed to prevent recurrence
  - OC lesions: Surgical approach may be decided by lesion position relative to mylohyoid muscle
    - SLS: Intraoral approach
    - SMS: Submandibular approach

DIAGNOSTIC CHECKLIST

Image Interpretation Pearls

- If complex lesion with fat density or signal intensity, consider dermoid cyst
- Simple lesion (may be proteinaceous fluid) = epidermoid or dermoid cyst
- If dermal sinus tract reaches dura anterior cranial fossa, crista galli may be bifid & foramen cecum large
- Foramen cecum normally unossified up to 5 years

SELECTED REFERENCES

1. Ng JJ et al: Surgical management of 2350 pediatric dermoid cysts. Plast Reconstr Surg. 156(1):120-9, 2025
2. Booth TN: Congenital cystic neck masses. Neuroimaging Clin N Am. 33(4):591-605, 2023
3. Naina P et al: Pediatric nasal dermoid- a decade's experience from a South Indian tertiary care centre. Int J Pediatr Otorhinolaryngol. 139:110418, 2020
4. Rodriguez DP et al: Masses of the nose, nasal cavity, and nasopharynx in children. Radiographics. 37(6):1704-30, 2017
5. Hartley BE et al: Nasal dermoids in children: a proposal for a new classification based on 103 cases at Great Ormond Street Hospital. Int J Pediatr Otorhinolaryngol. 79(1):18-22, 2015
6. LaPlante JK et al: Common pediatric head and neck congenital/developmental anomalies. Radiol Clin North Am. 53(1):181-96, 2015
7. Hughes DC et al: Dimensions and ossification of the normal anterior cranial fossa in children. AJNR Am J Neuroradiol. 31(7):1268-72, 2010
8. Hedlund G: Congenital frontonasal masses: developmental anatomy, malformations, and MR imaging. Pediatr Radiol. 36(7):647-62; quiz 726-7, 2006

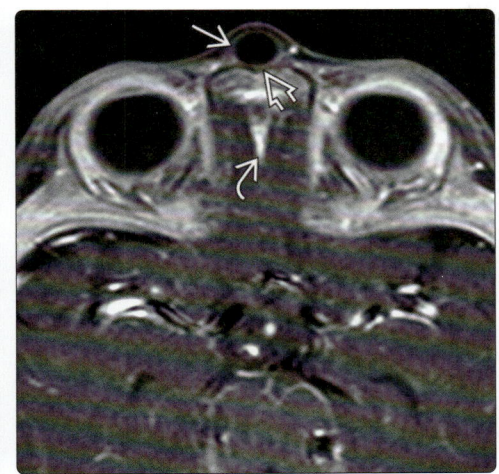

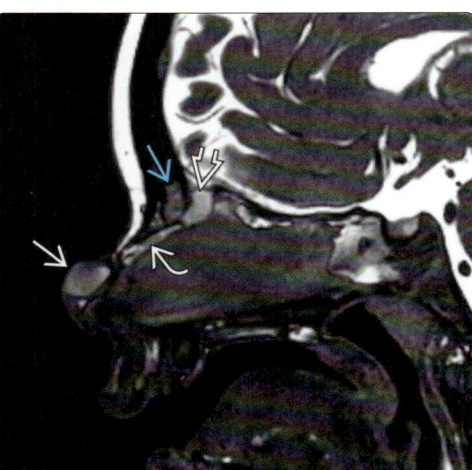

(Left) *Axial T1 C+ FS MR in a 6-month-old infant shows a typical nasal glabella dermoid cyst ➡, well defined and nonenhancing, with adjacent smooth osseous remodeling ➡. Notice the normal appearance of the crista galli ➡.* (Right) *Sagittal FIESTA MR in a 1-year-old girl shows a complex dermoid cyst with a nasal component ➡ and a component extending into the foramen cecum ➡, the 2 connected by a linear tract ➡. In addition, there is another component ➡ that remodels the dorsal aspect of the nasal bone.*

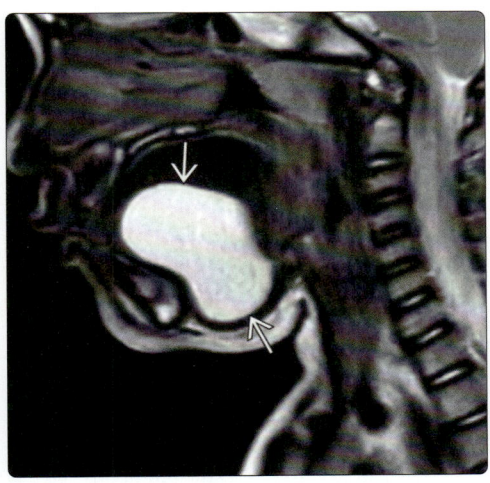

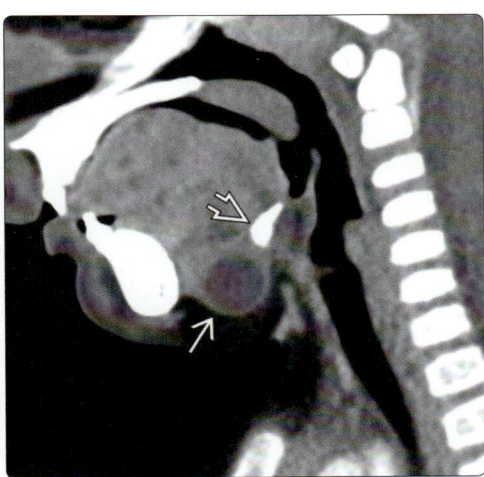

(Left) *Sagittal T2 MR in 5-year-old with recent increase in oral cavity mass shows well-defined, homogeneously hyperintense midline floor of mouth mass ➡, which showed diffusion restriction without contrast enhancement.* (Right) *Sagittal CECT in 20-month-old with midline anterior upper neck mass shows well-defined, round, nonenhancing dermoid cyst ➡ with thin, smooth wall just anterior to the midline hyoid bone ➡. Differential diagnosis at imaging was thyroglossal duct cyst vs. dermoid/epidermoid cyst.*

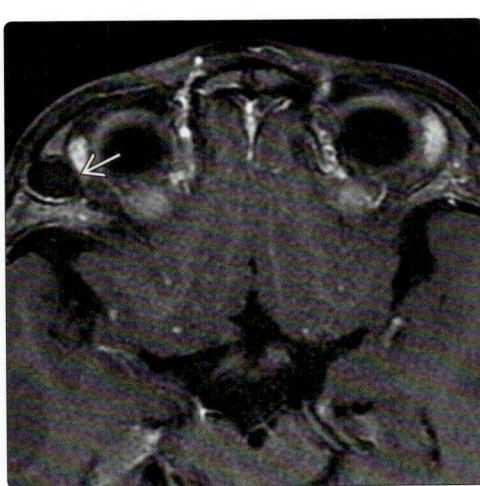

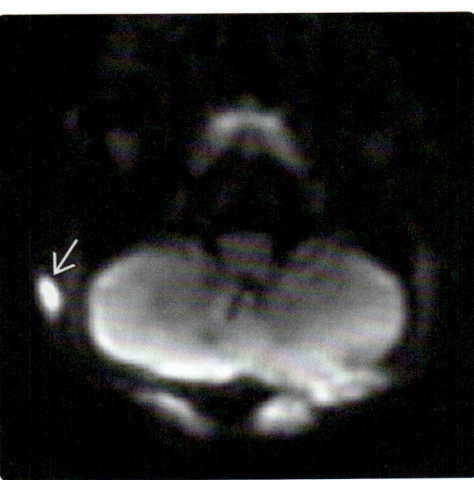

(Left) *Axial T1 C+ FS MR in a 3-year-old shows the typical location and appearance of an orbital dermoid cyst ➡ extending into the zygomaticofrontal suture: Well-defined, cystic-appearing lesion without enhancement and with diffusion restriction (not shown).* (Right) *Axial DWI MR in a young child with a longstanding right retroauricular lesion ➡ demonstrates a well-defined lesion with diffusion restriction. Lesion was fluid signal on other sequences and histologically proven to be epidermoid cyst.*

KEY FACTS

TERMINOLOGY

- Infantile hemangioma (IH): Benign vascular neoplasm of proliferating endothelial cells; **not** vascular malformation

IMAGING

- Doppler US (including spectral): Characteristic flow patterns
  - High vessel density (> 5/cm²) with low-resistance arterial waveforms but no arteriovenous shunting
- Contrast-enhanced CT/MR
  - Well-defined mass with diffuse and intense enhancement during proliferative phase
  - High-flow vessels in/adjacent to mass during proliferation
  - ↓ size with ↑ fatty replacement during involuting phase

TOP DIFFERENTIAL DIAGNOSES

- **Congenital hemangioma**
- **Venous malformation**
- **Soft tissue sarcoma**
- **Plexiform neurofibroma**
- **Arteriovenous malformation**

PATHOLOGY

- **GLUT1** IHC marker (+) in all phases of growth and regression
- In contrast to GLUT1 (-) congenital hemangioma

CLINICAL ISSUES

- Typically inapparent at birth → appears in 1st few weeks of life → grows rapidly for months → spontaneously involutes over years
  - Typically warm, soft, raised reddish or strawberry-like cutaneous lesion
- Majority do not require treatment; propranolol 1st-line therapy in setting of ulceration or vital structure compromise (e.g., airway or orbit)
- If age, clinical/imaging appearance, or growth history are atypical for IH, biopsy recommended

(Left) *Axial T1 C+ FS MR in a 5-month-old shows a large, lobulated, intensely enhancing mass* ➡️ *infiltrating the massively enlarged right parotid gland. Notice the prominent intralesional* ➡️ *and perilesional* ➡️ *flow voids, typical of an infantile hemangioma (IH).* (Right) *Axial 2D SPGR flow-sensitive MR sequence in the same patient shows the typical appearance of multiple high-flow vessels within and adjacent to the primary parotid IH* ➡️.

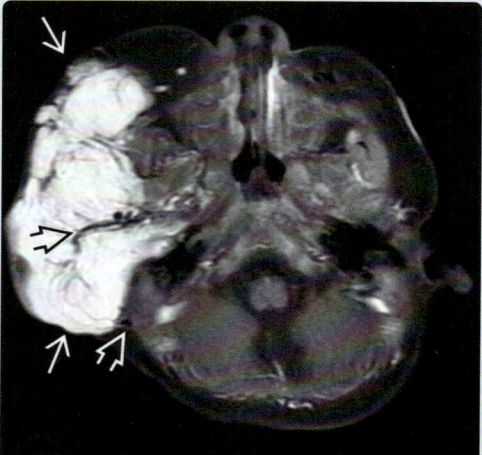
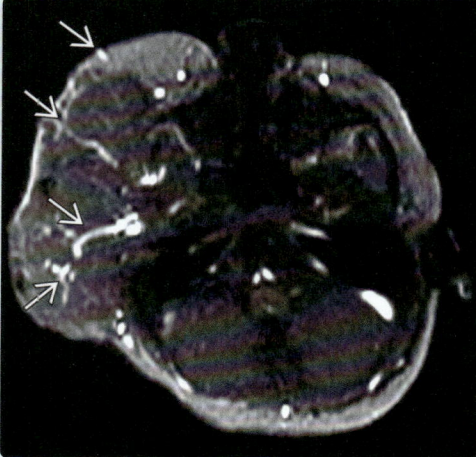

(Left) *Transverse color Doppler US in a 1-month-old child shows a lobular lesion replacing and expanding the parotid gland. Note the high vessel density* ➡️, *typical of a proliferating IH.* (Right) *Transverse color Doppler US spectral tracing through the lesion in the same patient demonstrates low-resistance arterial waveforms, typical of proliferating-phase IH. The waveforms will develop a high-resistance pattern during involution, and there will be a decrease in vessel density.*

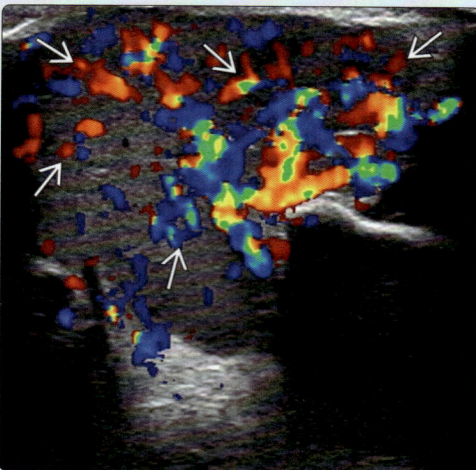
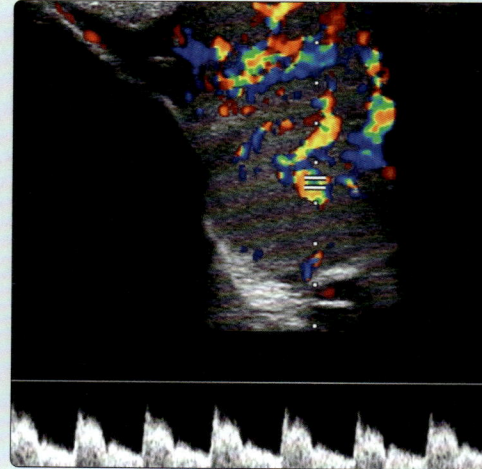

Infantile Hemangioma

TERMINOLOGY

Synonyms
- Capillary hemangioma

Definitions
- Widespread misuse of term hemangioma in literature
- Infantile hemangioma (IH) is different entity from
  - Congenital hemangioma, spindle cell hemangioma, epithelioid hemangioma, lobular capillary hemangioma (pyogenic granuloma)
    - All benign but different vascular neoplasms
  - Hemangioendothelioma: Higher grade vascular neoplasm
  - Cavernous hemangioma, vertebral body hemangioma, and synovial hemangioma = venous malformations
- IH: Benign vascular neoplasm (not malformation) of proliferating endothelial cells
  - Most common soft tissue tumor of infancy
- **Not** vascular malformation
- 2018 revised classification, and more recent update 2025, by International Society for Study of Vascular Anomalies (ISSVA) retains 2 main categories
  - Vascular tumors: True neoplasms with cellular proliferation; grow out of proportion to patient
  - Vascular malformation: Congenital errors of vessel development; grow commensurate with patient

IMAGING

General Features
- Best diagnostic clue
  - During proliferative phase (PP): Lobular, well-defined mass with intense, diffuse enhancement + high-flow vessels in/adjacent to mass
  - During involuting phase (IP): ↓ size, vascularity, and enhancement with progressive fatty replacement
- Location
  - 60% occur in head and neck
    - Any space: Parotid space, orbit, nasal cavity, subglottic airway, face, neck; rarely intracranial
      □ When intracranial &/or multiple, consider PHACE association; typically not intramuscular
- Size
  - Depends on phase of growth and regression; predictable clinical course
    - PP: Rapid growth beginning few weeks after birth and continuing 6-24 months
    - IP: Gradual regression over next several years
    - Involuted phase: Relatively small residual lesion
- Morphology
  - Majority: Isolated, focal, well-circumscribed, lobulated lesions in subcutaneous tissues
    - Tend to displace/efface rather than encase structures
  - Occasionally multiple, transspatial, or deep
    - May be part of PHACE association
      □ **P**osterior fossa malformations (cerebellar hypoplasia most common)
      □ **H**emangioma (infantile) of face and neck, typically segmental or midline, &/or internal auditory canal (IAC)/cerebellopontine angle (CPA)

      □ **A**rterial stenosis, occlusion, aneurysm, hypoplasia, agenesis, aberrant origin
      □ **C**ardiovascular defects (aortic coarctation/aneurysm/dysplasia, aberrant subclavian artery ± vascular ring, ventricular septal defect)
      □ **E**ye abnormalities (persistent hyperplastic primary vitreous, coloboma, morning glory disc anomaly, optic nerve hypoplasia, peripapillary staphyloma, microphthalmia, cataract, sclerocornea)
- CECT
  - Well-circumscribed, lobulated mass with diffuse and intense contrast enhancement in PP
    - Prominent vessels in/adjacent to mass
    - No internal calcification or surrounding edema
  - Progressive fatty infiltration of mass + ↓ size in IP
- MR
  - T1: Isointense to muscle in PP; hyperintense from fatty replacement during IP
  - T2: Mildly hyperintense relative to muscle
  - T2 FS/STIR: At least moderately hyperintense relative to muscle (but not fluid signal intensity) during PP; hypointense to muscle (follows fat) during IP
  - T1 C+ FS: Intense contrast enhancement in PP
  - GRE: High-flow vessels in/adjacent to mass in PP
    - Corresponding serpiginous flow voids in/adjacent to mass on SE/FSE sequences
  - MRA: Stenosis, occlusion, agenesis, aneurysm of craniocervical vessels (PHACE association)
  - Noncontrast arterial spin-labeling (ASL) perfusion MR shows ↑ blood flow on cerebral blood flow (CBF) images
  - DWI: ADC values higher in IHs mm²/sec vs. sarcomas 0.67-0.78 x 10⁻³ mm²/sec
- Ultrasonographic findings
  - Grayscale: Soft tissue mass with variable echogenicity and few macroscopic vessels; ↑ echogenicity during IP
  - Color/spectral Doppler
    - High vessel density (> 5 vessels/cm²), high systolic Doppler shift (> 2 kHz), and low resistive index in arterial vessels without arterialized veins (to suggest shunting) during PP
    - Mean venous peak velocities not elevated (unlike arteriovenous malformation)
  - ↓ vessel density, ↑ resistive index in IP

Imaging Recommendations
- No imaging necessary in majority of patients; characteristic cutaneous appearance and change over time
- Best imaging tool depends on indications
  - US with spectral Doppler
    - Used to establish diagnosis of superficial lesion with atypical history, appearance, or clinical behavior
    - To identify deeper lesions without classic cutaneous manifestations
  - MR
    - To define deep extension of lesion with implications for compromise of vital structures (e.g., orbit and airway)
    - To plan/evaluate therapy pre- and post treatment (if considering medical or surgical/laser therapy)

  - To evaluate for suspected PHACE association (e.g., large segmental facial IH)
  - Search for extracutaneous anomalies: Warranted for children with facial segmental or periorbital IH
- Protocol advice
  o Pulsed/spectral color Doppler US to document characteristic flow throughout lesion
  o MR imaging should include flow-sensitive, fluid-sensitive, and T1 C+ FS sequences

DIFFERENTIAL DIAGNOSIS

Congenital Hemangioma (Rapidly, Non-, or Partially Involuting)

- Present at birth or on prenatal imaging; do not proliferate after birth
  o Rapidly involuting congenital hemangioma (RICH): Involutes by 3-14 months
  o Noninvoluting congenital hemangioma (NICH)
  o Partially involuting congenital hemangioma (PICH)
- Solid, heterogeneous, less well-defined mass ± calcification, hemorrhage, necrosis
- GLUT1 (-) on histology

Venous Malformation

- Congenital vascular malformation composed of large venous lakes
- Fluid signal intensity throughout mass; ± fluid-fluid levels, phleboliths
- Gradual, patchy fill-in with contrast

Soft Tissue Sarcoma

- Rhabdomyosarcoma, extraosseous Ewing sarcoma, undifferentiated sarcoma
- Solid or mixed cystic/solid mass, typically firm
- Mild to moderate enhancement ± osseous erosion
- Internal vascularity present but typically << IH

Plexiform Neurofibroma

- Infiltrative, lobulated masses with target appearance in cross section
- Transspatial involvement ± poorly defined margins
- + additional stigmata of neurofibromatosis type 1

Arteriovenous Malformation

- Congenital high-flow vascular malformation
- Arteriovenous shunting through tangle of feeding arteries and large draining veins; ± other soft tissue components

PATHOLOGY

General Features

- Etiology
  o Proposed theory: Clonal expansion of angioblasts with high expression of basic fibroblast growth factors and other angiogenesis markers
- Genetics: Majority sporadic

Microscopic Features

- Prominent endothelial cells forming small vascular channels (PP), flat endothelial cells + fibrofatty replacement (IP)

Immunohistochemical Features

- GLUT1 (+) during all phases of proliferation and regression

CLINICAL ISSUES

Presentation

- Most common signs/symptoms
  o Growing superficial soft tissue mass in young infant (PP); typically with warm, soft, raised reddish or strawberry-like cutaneous discoloration
  o Occasionally, deeper lesions show bluish skin discoloration secondary to prominent draining veins
- Other signs/symptoms
  o Ulceration of overlying skin
  o Airway obstruction from airway involvement
  o Proptosis from orbital lesion
  o Associated abnormalities in PHACE association

Demographics

- Age
  o Median at presentation: 2 weeks; majority by 1-3 months
    - Typically inapparent at birth
    - Up to 1/3 nascent at birth (i.e., pale or erythematous macule, telangiectasia, pseudoecchymotic patch or red spot)
- Epidemiology
  o Most common head and neck tumor in infants
  o Incidence is 1-2% of neonates; 12% by 1 year of age
  o ↑ in preterm infants and low-birth-weight infants
    - Up to 30% of infants weighing < 1 kg
- Sex: F > M (1.5-4:1)

Natural History & Prognosis

- Majority undergo PP followed by spontaneous regression
  o 90% resolve by 9 years of age
- Large and segmental facial hemangiomas have ↑ incidence of complications if not treated

Treatment

- Majority do not require treatment
- Treatment indications: Compromise vital structures (e.g., optic nerve compression or airway obstruction); significant skin ulceration
- Treatment options: Oral propranolol (β-blocker) primary therapy (instead of oral steroids) due to low side effect profile; less common: Intralesional steroids, laser; rarely, surgical excision
- Recent literature exploring use of everolimus and sunitinib

SELECTED REFERENCES

1. Azizinik F et al: Vascular lesions of head and neck region: a pictorial review. Eur J Radiol. ePub 2025
2. Xie R et al: Everolimus and sunitinib potentially work as therapeutic drugs for infantile hemangiomas. Pediatr Res. ePub, 2025
3. International Society for the Study of Vascular Anomalies: ISSVA Classification of Vascular Anomalies. Reviewed May 2024. Accessed June 2025. https://www.issva.org/classification
4. Mamlouk MD: Solid and vascular neck masses in children. Neuroimaging Clin N Am. 33(4):607-21, 2023
5. Luu J et al: Hemangioma genetics and associated syndromes. Dermatol Clin. 40(4):393-400, 2022
6. Maldonado FR et al: Quantitative characterization of extraocular orbital lesions in children using diffusion-weighted imaging. Pediatr Radiol. 51(1):119-27, 202
7. Proisy M et al: PHACES syndrome and associated anomalies: risk associated with small and large facial hemangiomas. AJR Am J Roentgenol. 1-8, 2021
8. Mamlouk MD et al: Arterial spin-labeling perfusion for PHACE syndrome. AJNR Am J Neuroradiol. 42(1):173-7, 2020

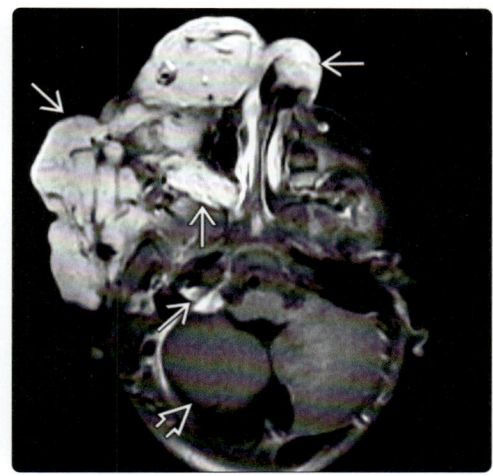
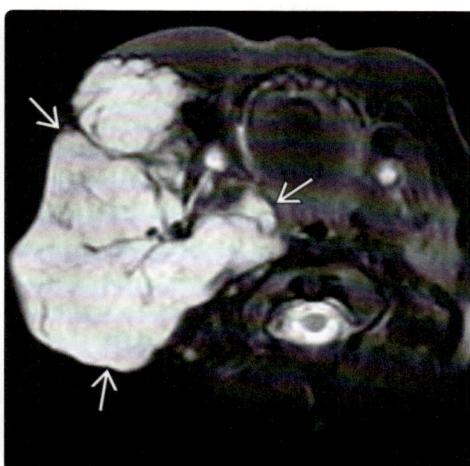

(Left) Axial T1 C+ FS MR in a 4-month-old girl with PHACE association shows multiple enhancing hemangiomas ➡ in the right parotid space, right posterior-inferior orbit, right cheek, nose, and right internal auditory canal (IAC)/cerebellopontine angle (CPA). Also note the ipsilateral right cerebellar hemisphere hypoplasia ➡. (Right) Axial T2 FS MR in a 3-month-old girl shows a holoparotid lesion ➡ with extension to the right cheek with diffuse hyperintense T2 signal and intralesional flow voids, typical of IH.

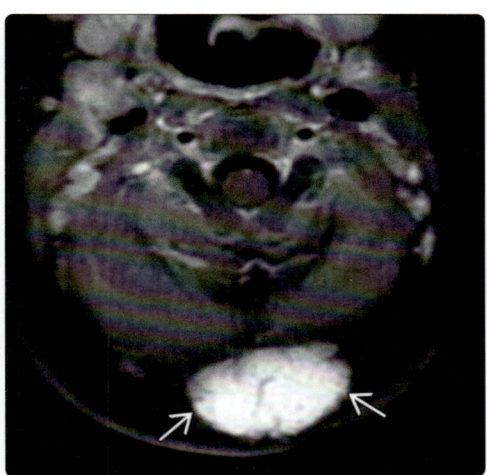
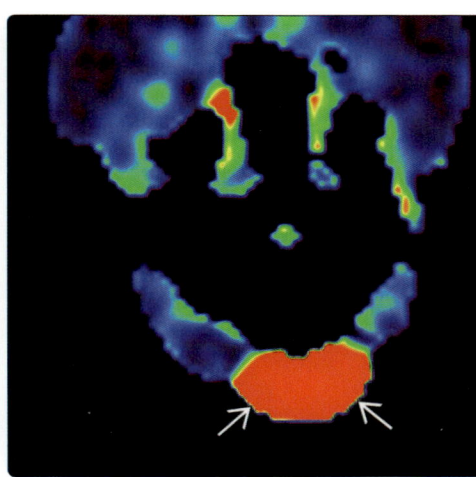

(Left) Axial T1 C+ FS MR in a 5-month-old demonstrates the typical appearance of subcutaneous IH ➡, intensely enhancing but with only a few intralesional foci that may represent high-flow vessels. (Right) Axial noncontrast arterial spin-labeling (ASL) perfusion MR in the same patient shows increased perfusion ➡, typical of an IH.

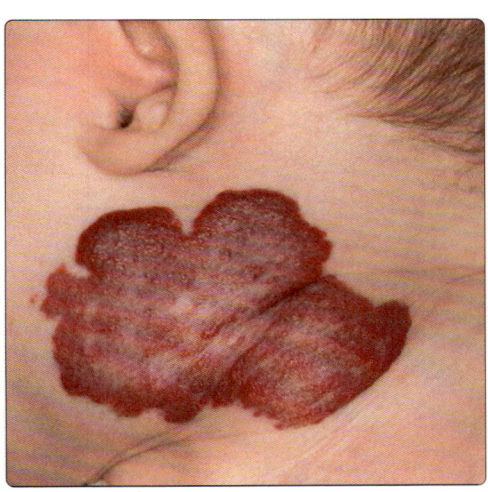
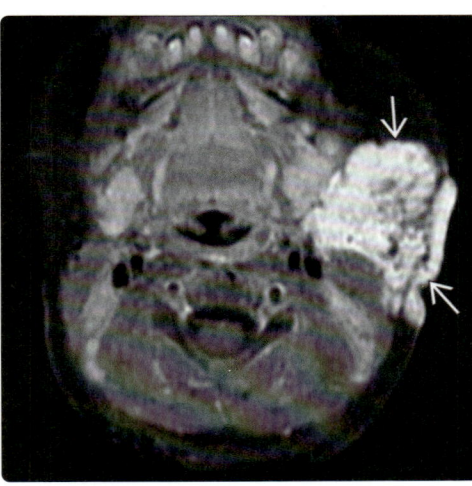

(Left) Clinical photograph in a 6-week-old shows an intensely violaceous lesion with well-defined margins in the left neck, typical of IH. (Right) Axial T1 C+ FS MR in the same child shows the typical intense enhancement of the left face IH ➡. If there is a typical appearance and appropriate clinical scenario of a lesion not present at birth but now growing in size at a few months of age, there is no need for biopsy. If age, history, or imaging are atypical, then biopsy is imperative.

TERMINOLOGY

- **Sternocleidomastoid (SCM) tumor of infancy**
- Nonneoplastic SCM muscle enlargement in early infancy

IMAGING

- **Nontender** SCM muscle **enlargement** in infant
- No adjacent inflammation or significant adenopathy
- Location: Right > left; rarely bilateral
- US: Modality of choice when imaging required
  - Variable echogenicity
- CT: Enlarged muscle has similar attenuation to normal muscle pre- & post contrast
- MR: Variable signal, diffuse or peripheral enhancement

TOP DIFFERENTIAL DIAGNOSES

- Myositis related to neck infection
  - Tenderness, cellulitis evident clinically
  - Adenopathy conspicuous
- Infantile hemangioma
  - Benign, intensely enhancing vascular neoplasm
- Systemic nodal metastases
  - Nodes deep to normal SCM muscle
- Primary cervical neuroblastoma
  - Close association with carotid sheath
- Rhabdomyosarcoma
  - More discrete mass with aggressive margins
- Teratoma
  - Often with fat, calcifications

CLINICAL ISSUES

- **Painless**, **unilateral**, longitudinal cervical neck mass
- Torticollis in up to 30% of cases
- Mass appears within 2 weeks of delivery
- Usually **regresses by 8 months** of age
- ↑ in breech presentation & forceps delivery
- Occasionally, developmental dysplasia of hip
- Treatment: Physical therapy/stretching exercises to ↑ range of motion

(Left) Longitudinal US in a 2-week-old infant shows typical fusiform enlargement of the left sternocleidomastoid (SCM) muscle with mildly increased echogenicity ➡ relative to the uninvolved portion of the muscle ➡. (Right) Longitudinal US in a 24-day-old boy with a right-sided neck mass shows mild increase in echogenicity and fusiform enlargement of the right SCM ➡, consistent with fibromatosis colli. Compare to the normal left SCM ➡.

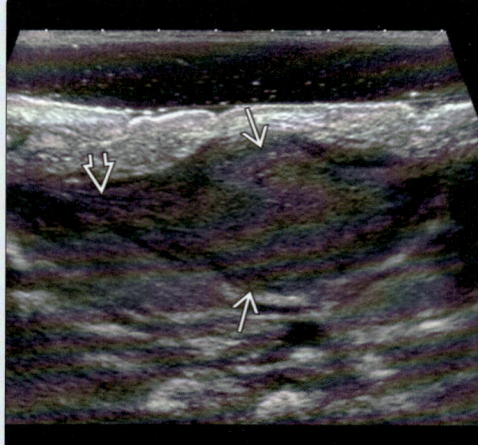 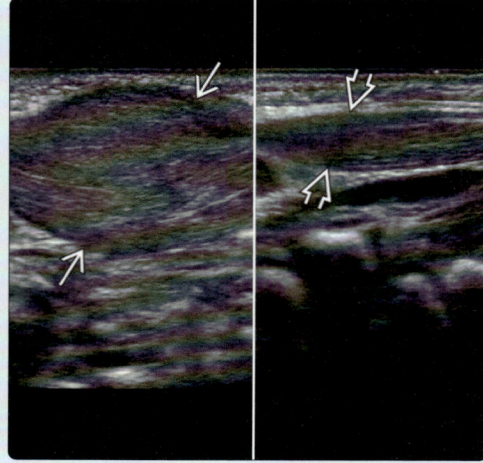

(Left) Axial CECT in a 1-month-old girl with fibromatosis colli demonstrates diffuse enlargement of the right SCM muscle ➡ isodense to the normal contralateral SCM muscle ➡. There is no extramuscular extension, overlying cellulitis, or associated adenopathy. (Right) Coronal T1 C+ FS MR in a 26-day-old boy shows diffuse enlargement and enhancement of the left SCM ➡ compared to the normal right SCM ➡. Also notice mild torticollis with the head tilted to the left.

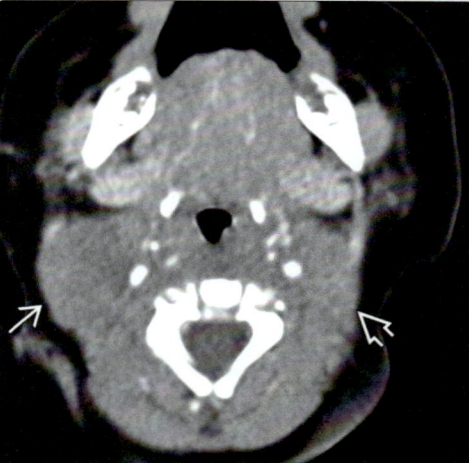 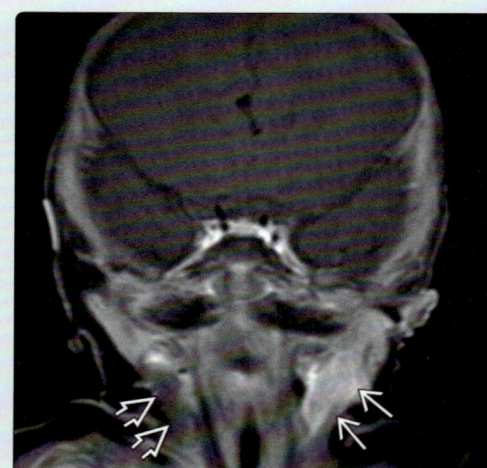

TERMINOLOGY

Synonyms
- **Sternocleidomastoid (SCM) tumor of infancy**
- **Congenital muscular torticollis**
  - Some literature includes 3 clinical subgroups
    - SCM tumor of infancy
    - Muscular torticollis: "Tightness" without mass
    - Postural torticollis: Torticollis without mass or "tightness"

Definitions
- Nonneoplastic SCM muscle enlargement in early infancy
- Postulated to be due to birth trauma, peripartum injury, in utero compartment syndrome, or maldevelopment
- Torticollis ("wry neck"): Twisting of neck such that ear on affected side is positioned lower & more midline than normal & chin turned to contralateral side

IMAGING

General Features
- Best diagnostic clue
  - **Nontender** SCM muscle enlargement in infant
  - Without extramuscular extension, inflammatory changes, or pathologic adenopathy
- Location
  - Mid to lower 1/3 of SCM muscle
    - Rarely, similar process involves trapezius muscle
  - **Right > left; rarely bilateral**
- Size
  - Variable
  - Usually spans much of cervical portion of SCM muscle
- Morphology
  - Fusiform SCM muscle enlargement; lacks surrounding inflammatory change & pathologic adenopathy

Radiographic Findings
- Radiography
  - Cervical spine radiographs may be obtained to exclude congenital or acquired bony abnormalities causing torticollis
  - Lytic changes in clavicular head at muscle attachment are rarely reported x-ray finding

Ultrasonographic Findings
- Grayscale ultrasound
  - Modality of choice when imaging is required
  - **Oval or fusiform SCM muscle enlargement**
  - Variable echogenicity
    - Hyperechoic or mixed echogenicity common
    - Hypoechoic peripheral rim may represent compressed normal muscle
  - **No** discrete extramuscular mass or adenopathy
  - Affected SCM muscle moves with respiration in same fashion as contralateral muscle
  - Affected SCM is shorter & thicker than contralateral side
    - Extended field-of-view imaging useful to show entire length of SCM
    - Comparison to asymptomatic side useful
- Color Doppler
  - Variable hyperemia in acute phase, ↓ blood flow in fibrotic phase

CT Findings
- CECT
  - **Focal or fusiform enlargement of SCM muscle**
  - Similar attenuation to normal contralateral muscle
  - No inflammatory stranding in adjacent fat
  - No adenopathy or calcifications

MR Findings
- T1WI
  - **Focal or diffuse fusiform enlargement of SCM**
  - Variable signal: Iso- to hypointense vs. normal muscle
- T2WI
  - Variable signal intensity
    - Hyper- to isointense vs. other muscles
    - Zones of hypointensity at maximal enlargement, probably due to evolving fibrosis
  - Adjacent soft tissues normal
    - Be aware that incidental reactive nodal enlargement in infants is common
    - Presence of adjacent reactive nodes does not turn this pseudotumor into tumor
- T1WI C+
  - Affected muscle **enhances** heterogeneously
    - May see thick peripheral enhancement

Imaging Recommendations
- Best imaging tool
  - Diagnosis frequently on clinical exam alone without imaging
  - US confirms clinical suspicion
  - MR recommended for atypical cases
- Protocol advice
  - Real-time US + clinical knowledge arrives at correct diagnosis

DIFFERENTIAL DIAGNOSIS

Myositis Related to Neck Infection
- Tenderness, cellulitis evident clinically
- + inflammatory changes & adenopathy

Infantile Hemangioma
- Intensely enhancing, benign vascular neoplasm with characteristic ↑ in size followed by spontaneous resolution
- Characteristic Doppler US appearance: > 5 vessels per cm², shows numerous low-resistance arterial waveforms
- GLUT1 immunohistochemical marker **positive** in all phases of growth & regression
- If multiple, think PHACE association

Systemic Nodal Metastases
- Pathologic appearance &/or number/size of cervical lymph nodes
- Non-Hodgkin lymphoma/leukemia
- Metastatic neuroblastoma

Primary Cervical Neuroblastoma
- Mild to moderately enhancing mass closely associated with carotid sheath
  - Usually posterior → anterior displacement of vessels

- ± calcification &/or adjacent metastatic lymphadenopathy
- Rarely intraspinal extension

Rhabdomyosarcoma

- Rare in newborns
- Up to 40% occur in head & neck
- Invasive soft tissue mass with variable enhancement, not confined to SCM
- ± bone erosion, metastatic adenopathy
- Transspatial mass common

Teratoma

- Complex density (CT) or signal intensity (MR) neck mass
- Solid & cystic components
- Often with fat, calcifications
- Frequently very large
  - May present with airway or feeding difficulties

Congenital Hemangioma (Rapidly, Non-, or Partially Involuting)

- Present at birth or on prenatal imaging; does not proliferate after birth
- Solid, heterogeneous, less well-defined mass
- ± calcification, hemorrhage, necrosis
- GLUT1 immunohistochemical marker **negative**

Pseudomass From Contralateral Sternocleidomastoid Denervation

- CNXI injury → SCM & trapezius muscle atrophy
  - Contralateral normal SCM muscle may appear large
  - Uncommon in infants

PATHOLOGY

General Features

- Etiology
  - Unknown; several trauma theories → degeneration of fibers & fibrosis
    - Trauma → intramuscular hemorrhage &/or edema
    - Traumatic compression of neck during delivery → pressure necrosis or occlusion of venous outflow
    - Possibly precipitated by in utero head position & SCM compartment syndrome
  - ↑ in breech presentation & forceps delivery
- Associated abnormalities
  - Developmental dysplasia of hip, talipes equinovarus (clubfoot)
- When necessary, diagnosis can be confirmed by fine-needle aspiration cytology
  - Cytopathologists must be careful in interpreting cells as benign

Gross Pathologic & Surgical Features

- Seldom resected
- Fine-needle aspirates more common than excisional biopsy; both are uncommon
- Enlargement, fibrosis of affected SCM muscle

Microscopic Features

- Some skeletal muscle fibers atrophy or degenerate & others have fibroblastic-myofibroblastic proliferation
- Cellularity variable: Early on more cellular; later develop ↑ collagen & ↓ cellularity

- Inflammatory changes rare

CLINICAL ISSUES

Presentation

- Most common signs/symptoms
  - Painless, unilateral, longitudinal cervical neck mass
  - Torticollis in up to 30% of cases
- Other signs/symptoms
  - ↓ range of neck motion, facial asymmetry, plagiocephaly
- Clinical profile
  - Infant with nontender neck mass following breech or forceps delivery

Demographics

- Age
  - 70% present by 2 months of age; peak: 24 days
- Sex
  - Male patients slightly > female patients
- Epidemiology
  - Affects 0.4% of infants

Natural History & Prognosis

- Mass appears within 2 weeks of delivery
- Mass may ↑ in size for days to weeks
  - Usually regresses by 8 months of age
- Up to 20% progress to muscular torticollis despite conservative therapy
- Patients with unsuccessfully treated torticollis may develop plagiocephaly

Treatment

- Physical therapy/stretching exercises to ↑ range of motion
- 90% full recovery with conservative treatment, physiotherapy
- Tenotomy for patients with refractory torticollis that fails conservative therapy

DIAGNOSTIC CHECKLIST

Consider

- History of traumatic birth? Mass confined to SCM muscle?
  - If answer to both is yes, DDx = fibromatosis colli
- Mass tender? Other clinical or imaging signs of inflammation?
  - If answer to both is yes, DDx likely neck infection
- Mass extending beyond margins of SCM muscle?
  - Consider rhabdomyosarcoma or other tumor

Image Interpretation Pearls

- Fusiform mass conforming to shape of SCM muscle = fibromatosis colli

SELECTED REFERENCES

1. Saliba T et al: Fibromatosis colli: a thorough description of its MRI characteristics and a review of the literature. J Belg Soc Radiol. 108(1):51, 2024
2. Chauvin NA et al: Musculoskeletal imaging in neonates: use of ultrasound. Pediatr Radiol. 52(4):765-76, 2021
3. Durnford L et al: Bilateral sternocleidomastoid pseudotumors-a case report and literature review. Radiol Case Rep. 16(4):964-7, 2021
4. Rousslang LK et al: Fibromatosis colli leading to positional plagiocephaly with gross anatomical and sonographic correlation. BMJ Case Rep. 14(1), 2021
5. Navarro OM: Pearls and pitfalls in the imaging of soft-tissue masses in children. Semin Ultrasound CT MR. 41(5):498-512, 2020

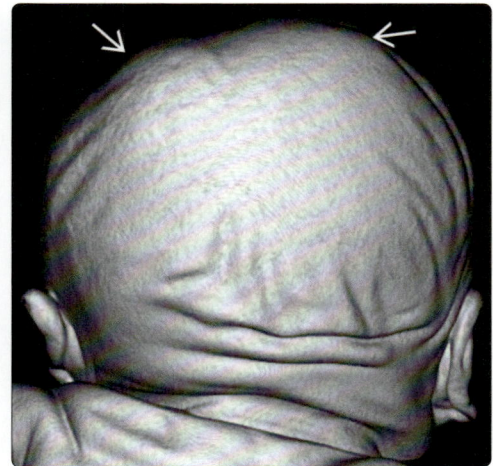
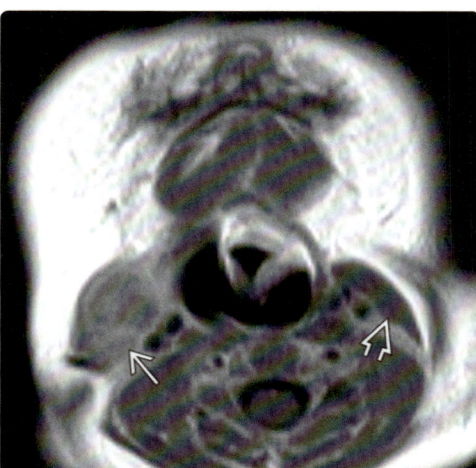

(Left) Posterior 3D surface-rendered soft tissue CT in a child evaluated for bilateral cephalohematomas ➡ demonstrates incidental torticollis secondary to a left SCM tumor of infancy (large left SCM not included). (Right) Axial T1 C+ MR shows prominent mixed heterogeneous enhancement of an enlarged right SCM muscle ➡ in a patient with fibromatosis colli who presented with a right neck mass. Note the normal left SCM muscle ➡.

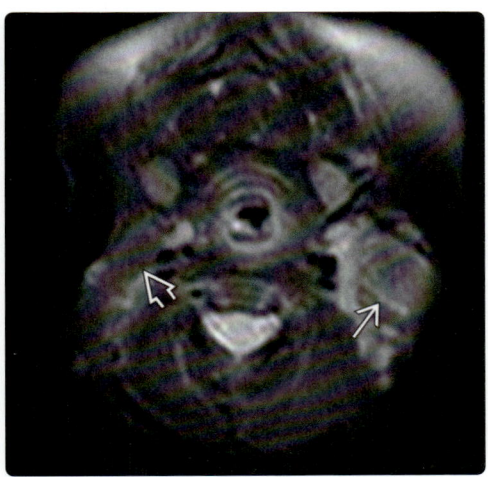
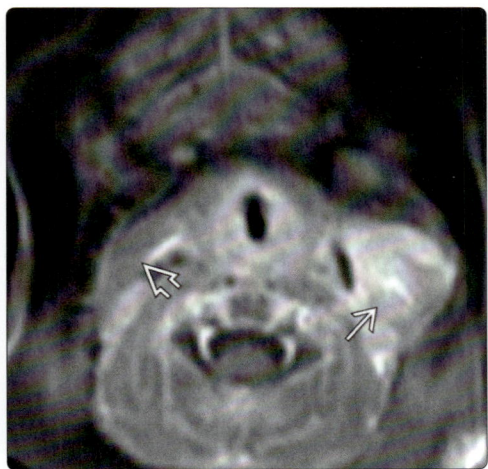

(Left) Axial T2 TSE FS MR in a 1-month-old infant with a hard left neck mass without torticollis shows a heterogeneously hyperintense left SCM ➡ with a few small adjacent reactive lymph nodes. Note the normal size and signal intensity of the right SCM muscle ➡. (Right) Axial T1 C+ FS MR in the same infant shows heterogeneous enhancement of the enlarged left SCM muscle ➡ compared to the normal right SCM muscle ➡.

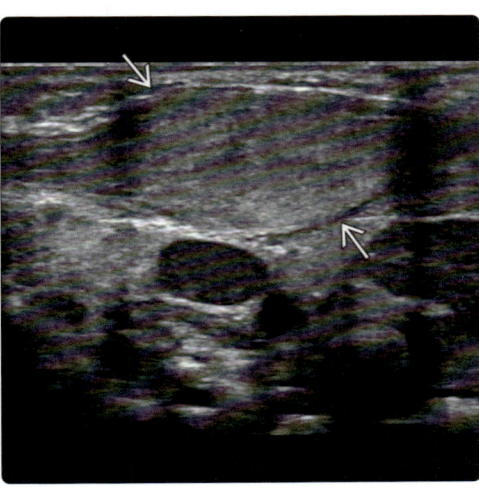
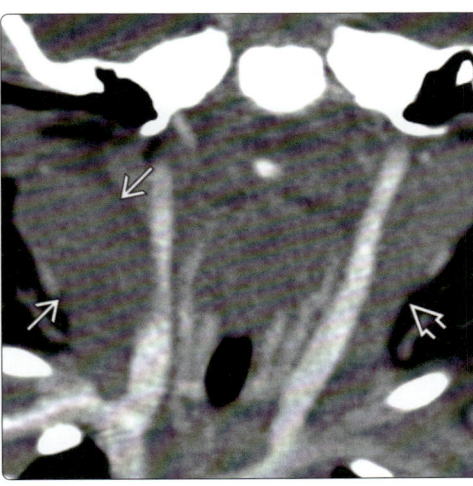

(Left) Longitudinal US in a 21-day-old girl with a nontender neck mass shows fusiform enlargement and heterogeneous mildly hyperechoic echotexture of the SCM muscle ➡, consistent with fibromatosis colli. (Right) Coronal CECT in a 1-month-old infant with facial anomalies shows homogeneous thickening of the right SCM muscle ➡, isodense to the normal contralateral SCM muscle ➡. There is mild associated torticollis with asymmetry at the level of the external auditory canals.

Pediatric Lesions

TERMINOLOGY

- Rhabdomyosarcoma (RMS): Most common childhood soft tissue sarcoma

IMAGING

- Up to 40% occur in H&N
  - Orbital, parameningeal, other sites
- MR is best to
  - Characterize solid soft tissue mass
    - Often intermediate signal on T2 FS or STIR
    - Variable contrast enhancement
    - Typically restrict diffusion
  - Evaluate intracranial spread (requires contrast)
- CT is best to look for bone destruction or remodeling
- Neck imaging for cervical metastatic adenopathy
  - PET/CT may improve staging & treatment evaluation

TOP DIFFERENTIAL DIAGNOSES

- Infantile hemangioma

- Slow-flow vascular malformations
- Fibromatosis colli
- Metastatic neuroblastoma
- Langerhans cell histiocytosis
- Juvenile angiofibroma
- Nasopharyngeal carcinoma
- Non-Hodgkin & Hodgkin lymphoma
- Plexiform neurofibroma
- Leukemia

PATHOLOGY

- 3 histologic subtypes
  - Embryonal RMS: Most common; young children
  - Alveolar RMS: 2nd most common; 15-25 years of age
  - Pleomorphic RMS: Least common; 40-60 years of age

CLINICAL ISSUES

- Presentation: 70% < 12 years of age; 40% < 5 years
- Treatment: Surgery, chemotherapy ± radiation therapy

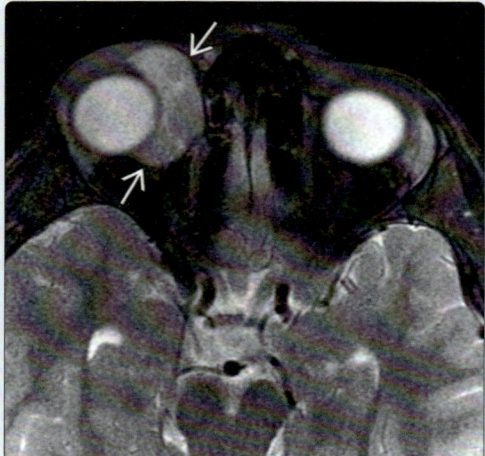
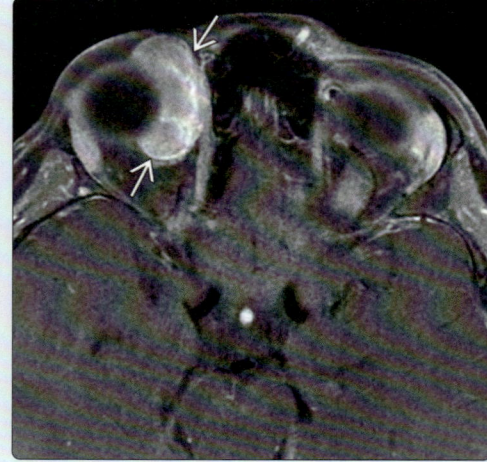

(Left) Axial T2 FS MR in a 10-year-old girl shows an intermediate signal intensity mass ⮕ in the superomedial right orbit, deviating the globe laterally, without bone destruction. (Right) Axial T1 C+ MR in the same patient shows heterogeneous enhancement of the mass ⮕, which demonstrated moderate diffusion restriction (DWI image not shown). Biopsy confirmed embryonal rhabdomyosarcoma (RMS). The absence of bone destruction does not exclude RMS.

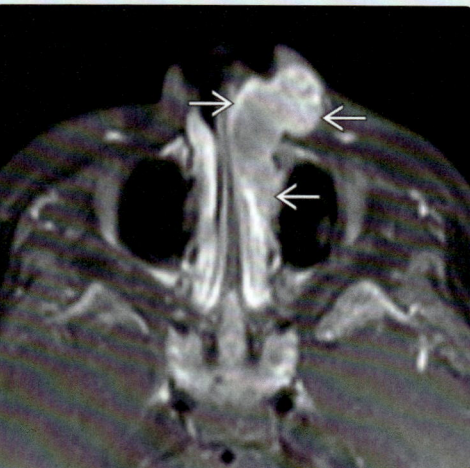
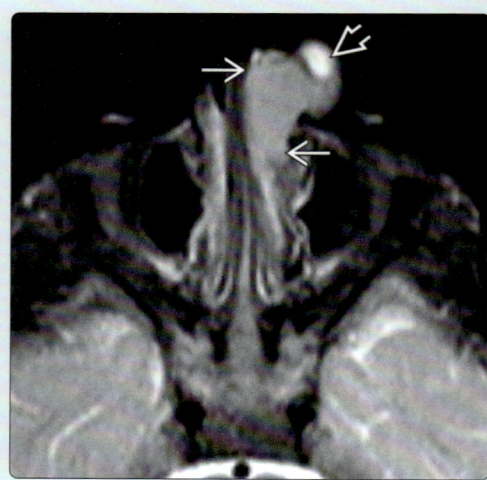

(Left) Axial T1 C+ FS MR in a 15-month-old boy with intermittent epistaxis & swelling of the left nasal ala demonstrates a heterogeneously enhancing left intranasal/nasal alar mass ⮕ obstructing the left nasal cavity. (Right) Axial STIR MR in the same patient demonstrates primarily intermediate signal intensity throughout the mass ⮕ with the exception of a small cystic/necrotic region anteriorly ⮕. Subsequent biopsy revealed an alveolar RMS.

Rhabdomyosarcoma

TERMINOLOGY

Abbreviations
- Rhabdomyosarcoma (RMS)

Definitions
- Malignant neoplasm of mesenchymal origin
  - Most common childhood soft tissue sarcoma

IMAGING

General Features
- Best diagnostic clue
  - Solid soft tissue mass with variable enhancement
- Location
  - Up to 40% occur in H&N, including orbit, parameningeal sites, neck/face soft tissues, nasal cavity
    - Parameningeal sites: Middle ear, paranasal sinus, nasal cavity, nasopharynx, masticator space, pterygopalatine fossa, parapharyngeal space
      - Intracranial extension in up to 55%
      - Temporal bone involvement: Petrous apex & middle ear > mastoid
    - Orbit
    - All other H&N sites: Scalp, cheek, parotid, oral cavity, larynx, oropharynx, hypopharynx, thyroid/parathyroid

CT Findings
- Invasive soft tissue mass with variable enhancement
- Osseous erosion is common but absent in many cases

MR Findings
- Isointense T1, hyperintense T2 signal relative to muscle
  - Not "fluid bright" unless necrotic/cystic components
- Variable contrast enhancement, often mild to moderate
  - Diffuse, intense enhancement is atypical
- Often restricts diffusion
  - ADC values range from ~ 0.5-1.3 x 10^{-3}/mm²
- ASL: Variable, but ↑ perfusion argues against benign low-flow vascular malformations

Nuclear Medicine Findings
- PET/CT
  - Hypermetabolic
    - May improve staging & posttreatment evaluation

Imaging Recommendations
- Best imaging tool
  - CT to evaluate osseous erosion
  - MR is best for soft tissue mass characterization
  - MR to evaluate perineural & intracranial spread of parameningeal RMS
    - Thickening & enhancement of nerves, leptomeninges
  - MR to distinguish between sinonasal tumor & obstructive/inflammatory disease
- Protocol advice
  - T2 FS or STIR MR: ↑ tumor conspicuity
  - Coronal T1 C+ FS MR: Detect intracranial extension
  - DWI MR: ADC values can help separate cellular tumor from benign vascular anomaly
  - Axial & coronal thin-section bone CT: Osseous erosion
  - Image neck: Rule out cervical metastatic adenopathy

DIFFERENTIAL DIAGNOSIS

Infantile Hemangioma
- Benign vascular neoplasm in infants, often with characteristic cutaneous involvement
- Intensely enhancing round or lobulated mass with high-flow vessels during proliferative phase
- ASL MR shows markedly ↑ perfusion
- No bone destruction
- Fatty infiltration during involuting phase

Slow-Flow Vascular Malformation
- May be well defined or extensive/infiltrative
- Fluid signal contents ± layering blood products, retracted clots, or phleboliths (in venous type)
- Venous type shows gradual patchy enhancement; lymphatic macrocystic type shows thin septal enhancement

Fibromatosis Colli
- Benign, self-limited, heterogeneous mass within & expanding midportion of sternocleidomastoid muscle in young infant with torticollis

Metastatic Neuroblastoma
- Most cervical disease is due to metastatic adenopathy rather than primary lesion
- Metastatic disease to skull/skull base is frequently bilateral: Enhancing masses surround aggressive osseous permeation/expansion with radiating spicules of new bone

Langerhans Cell Histiocytosis
- Enhancing soft tissue mass filling sharply marginated, punched-out lytic bone lesion
- Temporal bone: Mastoid > petrous apex & middle ear

Juvenile Angiofibroma
- Highly vascular mass causing nasal obstruction &/or epistaxis in adolescent males
- Intensely enhancing lesion with bone destruction & internal high-flow vessels
- Originates at sphenopalatine foramen on lateral nasal wall
- Often involves nasal cavity, nasopharynx, skull base, masticator space ± orbit, sinus, intracranial extension

Nasopharyngeal Carcinoma
- Nasopharyngeal mass in 2nd decade of life
- Variable contrast enhancement
- Central skull base erosion, widening of petroclival fissure, extension to pterygopalatine fossa + masticator & parapharyngeal spaces
- Unilateral or bilateral cervical & lateral retropharyngeal adenopathy

Non-Hodgkin Lymphoma
- Non-Hodgkin lymphoma (NHL) & Hodgkin lymphoma imaging findings are similar; difficult to differentiate
- Large, nonnecrotic nodes are typical
- Sinonasal, orbital, or nasopharyngeal NHL may cause osseous erosion

Hodgkin Lymphoma
- Extranodal site involvement by Hodgkin lymphoma < < NHL
- Large, nonnecrotic nodes are typical

Plexiform Neurofibroma

- Benign peripheral nerve sheath tumor in NF1
- Lobulated masses with peripherally ↑ T2 signal & centrally ↓ T2 signal (target sign)
- Bone remodeling, typically without destruction

Leukemia

- Soft tissue mass ± aggressive bone destruction, diffuse marrow abnormalities

PATHOLOGY

General Features

- Etiology
  - Originates from primitive mesenchymal cells committed to skeletal muscle differentiation (rhabdomyoblasts)
- Genetics
  - ↑ incidence in children with *TP53* tumor suppressor gene mutation
  - Embryonal MRS: PAX fusion-negative with loss of heterozygosity, most commonly at 11p15 locus
    - Up to 70% of childhood RMS
    - Better prognosis
  - Alveolar RMS: Majority PAX fusion-positive, associated with balanced chromosomal translocations, most commonly t(2;13) have *FOXO1* to *PAX3* (or *PAX7*) gene fusion
- Associated abnormalities
  - ↑ incidence of RMS in Noonan syndrome
    - Hematologic malignancies & neuroblastoma also seen
  - Rarely (~ 5%) associated with underlying cancer predisposition syndromes: Neurofibromatosis type 1, Li-Fraumeni, DICER1, Rubenstein-Taybi, Gorlin basal cell nevus, Beckwith-Wiedemann, or Costello
  - Rarely associated with hereditary retinoblastoma
  - May occur as radiation-induced 2nd primary neoplasm

Staging, Grading, & Classification

- Intergroup RMS Study (IRS) group classification prechemotherapy staging system
  - IRS-I: Tumor completely removed
  - IRS-II: a: Microscopic residual tumor; b: Involved regional nodes; c: Both
  - IRS-III: Gross residual tumor after incomplete resection or biopsy only
  - IRS-IV: Distant metastatic disease
- TNM: Tumor site, size, local invasion, lymph nodes, distant metastases
- Subtypes
  - Embryonal RMS: Most common
    - Up to 70% of all pediatric RMS
    - Occurs in younger children
    - 70-90% occur in H&N or GU tract
  - Alveolar RMS: 2nd most common
    - Usually occurs in patients 15-25 years of age
    - Most common in extremities & trunk
  - Spindle cell/sclerosing RMS
  - Pleomorphic RMS: Least common
    - Usually in adults 40-60 years of age; rarely < 15 years
    - Most arise in extremities; rarely in H&N

CLINICAL ISSUES

Presentation

- Most common signs/symptoms
  - Symptoms in H&N are variable, depend on location
    - Orbit: Mass, proptosis, ↓ vision
    - Sinonasal: Nasal obstruction, epistaxis; may present late with soft tissue facial mass
    - Temporal bone: Postauricular or external auditory canal mass, otitis media, CNVII palsy
    - Neck: Mass, pain, rarely airway compromise

Demographics

- Age
  - 70% < 12 years; 40% < 5 years

Natural History & Prognosis

- Favorable primary tumor sites: H&N, orbital, GU, biliary
- Unfavorable primary tumor sites: Parameningeal, extremities, bladder/prostate, trunk, chest wall, other sites
- Children's Oncology Group risk group assignment: Low, intermediate, & high risk
  - Based on fusion status, stage, & group
    - Fusion negative lower risk

Treatment

- Staging & risk stratification → treatment using risk-adapted approach
- Risk-group assignment based on pretreatment stage, IRS group, tumor biology, & patient age
- Chemotherapy ± surgery &/or radiotherapy
- Research ongoing in proton therapy, immunotherapy, & vaccination
- Sentinel node biopsy may improve treatment stratification

DIAGNOSTIC CHECKLIST

Consider

- Not always associated with bone destruction
  - Beware of enhancing soft tissue mass without bone destruction; may simulate infantile hemangioma (IH)
    - IH is almost always found in 1st year of life; RMS is more common > 12 months
    - IH typically soft/compressible while RMS is more firm
    - IH demonstrates high density of low-resistance arterial vessels on color Doppler
    - IH enhances more intensely & homogeneously
    - IH has higher ADC values on DWI MR

SELECTED REFERENCES

1. Aye JM et al: Nonorbital, nonparameningeal head and neck rhabdomyosarccma: a report from the Children's Oncology Group. Pediatr Blood Cancer. 72(6):e31673, 2025
2. Dehner CA et al: Rhabdomyosarcoma: updates on classification and the necessity of molecular testing beyond immunohistochemistry. Hum Pathol. 147:72-81, 2024
3. Rumboldt Z et al: Retinoblastoma and beyond: pediatric orbital mass lesions. Neuroradiology. 67(2):469-92, 2024
4. Biswas A et al: Extraocular orbital and peri-orbital masses. Neuroimaging Clin N Am. 33(4):643-59, 2023
5. Mamlouk MD: Solid and vascular neck masses in children. Neuroimaging Clin N Am. 33(4):607-21, 2023
6. Maldonado FR et al: Quantitative characterization of extraocular orbital lesions in children using diffusion-weighted imaging. Pediatr Radiol. 51(1):119-27, 2021

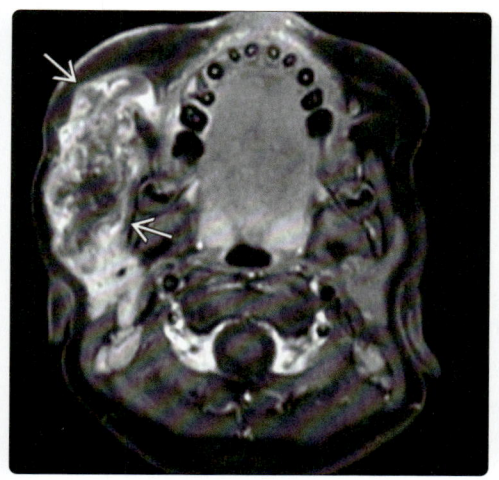

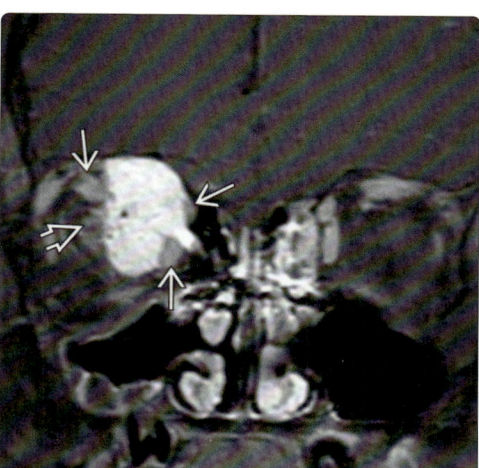

(Left) *Axial T2 C+ FS MR in a 5-year-old with a right-sided facial port-wine stain & recent facial swelling shows a necrotic mass inseparable from the right masseter muscle* ➡. *Lack of overlying cellulitis & unresponsiveness to antibiotics suggest that the lesion is not inflammatory; was biopsy-proven RMS.* (Right) *Coronal T1 C+ FS MR in a 10-year-old boy with intermittent diplopia shows atypical intensely enhancing RMS involving the extraconal space & intraconal space, separate from extraocular muscles* ➡ *& optic nerve* ➡.

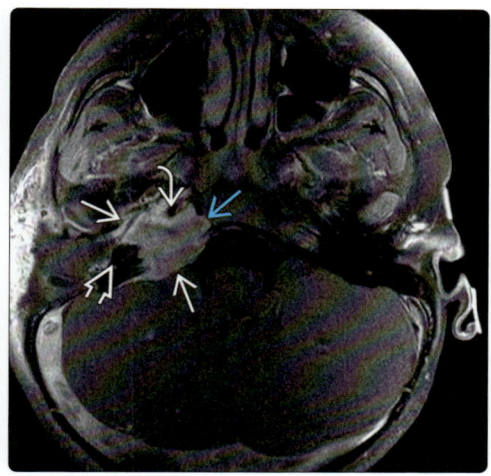

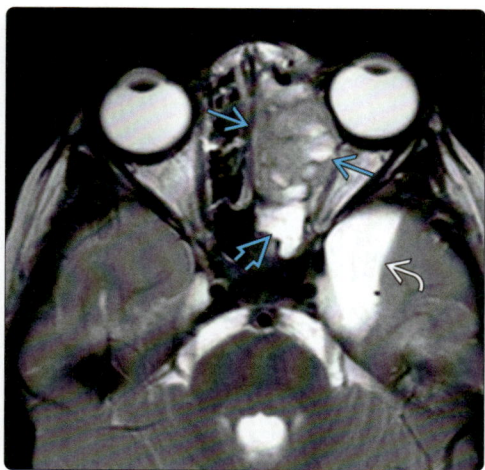

(Left) *Axial T1 C+ FS MR demonstrates a moderately enhancing RMS* ➡ *destroying the right petrous apex & otic capsule bone adjacent to the cochlea* ➡ *& extending along margins of the internal carotid artery* ➡ *into the clivus* ➡. (Right) *Axial T2 MR in a 5-year-old with left proptosis & palpable cervical adenopathy demonstrates a mixed-intensity alveolar RMS* ➡, *as compared to the hyperintense sphenoid sinus inflammatory disease* ➡ *& incidental middle cranial fossa arachnoid cyst* ➡.

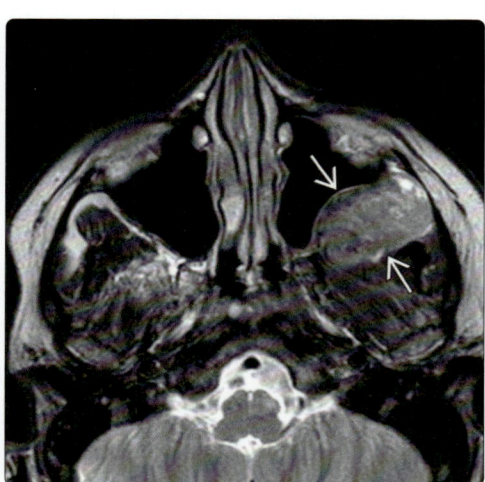

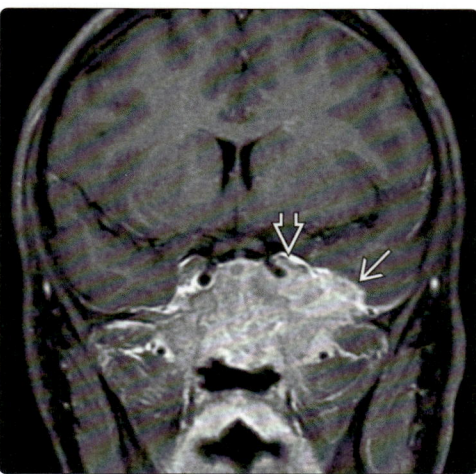

(Left) *Axial T2 MR in a 21-year-old with an embryonal RMS shows anterior bowing of the left maxillary sinus posterior wall by a heterogeneous, mildly hypointense left infratemporal fossa mass* ➡, *consistent with a highly cellular RMS. Although it is relatively hypointense without FS, it is hyperintense relative to skeletal muscle, typical of RMS.* (Right) *Coronal T1 C+ FS MR shows an extensive left skull base RMS with left middle cranial fossa extension (displacing the left temporal lobe* ➡*) & invasion of the left cavernous sinus* ➡.

Primary Cervical Neuroblastoma

TERMINOLOGY

- Neuroblastoma (**NBL**): Malignant tumor of sympathetic chain primitive neural crest cells
- **Primary cervical** in **1-5%** of cases
  - Most cases of NBL arise in adrenal gland (35-48%), extraadrenal retroperitoneum (18-35%), or posterior mediastinum (14-20%)

IMAGING

- CECT or MR: Well-defined, mild to moderately enhancing soft tissue mass in **posterior carotid space**
  - ± adjacent metastatic lymphadenopathy
  - Frequently with calcifications
  - Unlike primary NBL in abdomen, primary cervical NBL often **displaces carotid sheath vessels** rather than engulfing vessels
- I-123 MIBG most specific method of staging & evaluating response to therapy in NBL

TOP DIFFERENTIAL DIAGNOSES

- Reactive lymph nodes
  - Most common neck mass in child
  - ± cellulitis, myositis, abscess
- Neurofibroma
  - Carotid space or brachial plexus common
  - Plexiform "tangle of worms"
- Lymphoma lymph nodes
  - Hodgkin or non-Hodgkin lymphoma
- Metastatic NBL
  - Metastatic H&N disease more common than primary cervical NBL

CLINICAL ISSUES

- **Horner syndrome**
- Palpable mass
- Stridor or feeding difficulties
- Opsoclonus-myoclonus-ataxia syndrome

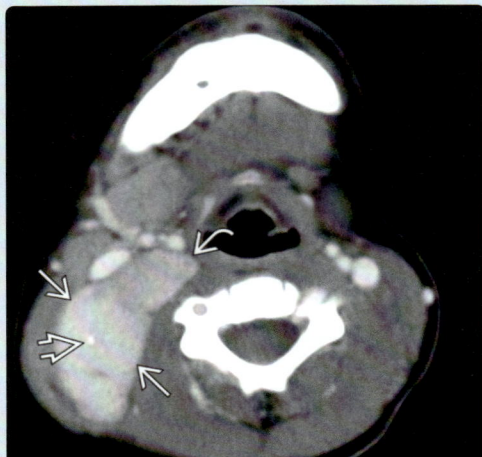
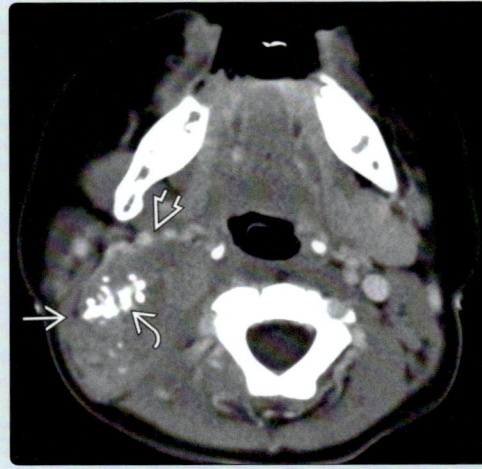

(Left) Axial CECT demonstrates a moderately enhancing right posterior carotid space neck mass ➡ deviating the carotid artery and jugular vein anteriorly. Tiny calcification is present ➡ in a large adherent lymph node ➡, which was positive for neuroblastoma (NBL). (Right) Axial CECT shows a partially calcified right neck mass ➡, deviating the carotid sheath vessels ➡ anteriorly. Coarse calcifications ➡ are present. Final pathology revealed the lesion to be ganglioneuroblastoma.

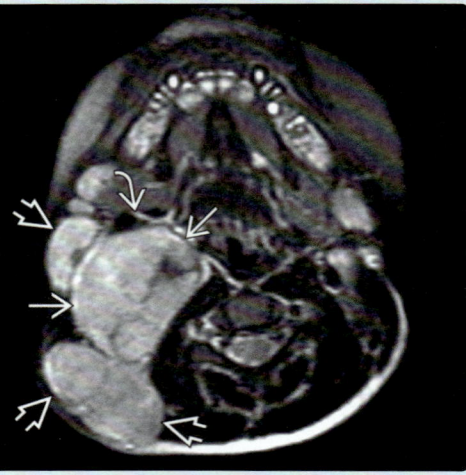
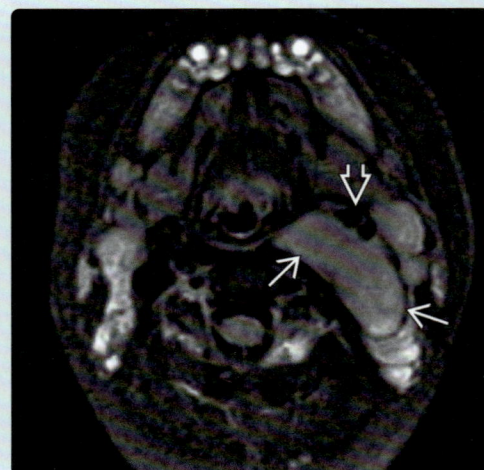

(Left) Axial T2WI FS MR shows a large cervical NBL ➡ situated in the posterior aspect of the carotid sheath. There are multiple large adjacent metastatic lymph nodes ➡. The mass deviates the carotid sheath vessels ➡ anteriorly and deforms the upper airway, both common findings in primary cervical NBL. (Right) Axial STIR MR demonstrates an oblong primary cervical NBL ➡ dorsal to the left carotid sheath vessels ➡ without intraspinal extension.

TERMINOLOGY

Abbreviations

- Neuroblastoma (**NBL**)

Definitions

- Malignant tumor of sympathetic chain primitive neural crest cells
- Increasing degrees of cellular differentiation/benignity along spectrum: Neuroblastoma [(NBL), malignant] → ganglioneuroblastoma (GNBL) → ganglioneuroma [(GN), benign]

IMAGING

General Features

- Best diagnostic clue
  - Well-defined, mild to moderately enhancing soft tissue mass involving sympathetic chain in neck
    - Unlike primary NBL in abdomen, primary cervical NBL often displaces carotid sheath vessels rather than engulfing vessels
    - Unlike thoracic & abdominal NBL, usually lacks dumbbell intraspinal extension
    - Calcifications less common than calcifications in primary NBL in thoracic & abdominal NBL
- Location
  - Primary NBL anywhere from neck to pelvis along sympathetic chain
    - Primary cervical in 1-5% of cases
      - Most cervical disease is nodal metastatic disease from retroperitoneal primary NBL
      - Most cases of NBL arise in adrenal gland (35-48%), extraadrenal retroperitoneum (18-35%), or posterior mediastinum (14-20%), pelvis (2-5%), metastatic disease with no primary identified (1%)
- Size
  - Variable

Imaging Recommendations

- Best imaging tool
  - MR or CECT for diagnosis & presurgical planning
  - **MIBG** for staging & posttreatment surveillance
- Protocol advice
  - Multiplanar enhanced MR for tumor evaluation
  - MR brain & chest if skull or mediastinal extension

Radiographic Findings

- Radiography
  - Rarely identifies calcifications
  - Limited role in evaluation of patients with neck masses

CT Findings

- Mildly enhancing solid mass associated with carotid sheath
- Adjacent vessels displaced
- ± calcification, hemorrhage, or necrosis
- ± extension into mediastinum or skull

MR Findings

- Variably enhancing solid mass closely associated with carotid sheath
- Typically intermediate signal on T1 & moderately hyperintense on T2WI
- May be heterogeneous if intralesional calcification, hemorrhage, or necrosis
- Typically restricts diffusion due to high cellularity
  - ADC helpful to distinguish from GN & GNBL
    - Mean ADC of NBL = 0.81×10^{-3} mm²/s (SD = 0.29×10^{-3} mm²/s, range = $0.39\text{-}1.47 \times 10^{-3}$ mm²/s)
    - Mean ADC of GN/GNBL = 1.6×10^{-3} mm²/s (SD = 0.340×10^{-3} mm²/s, range = $1.13\text{-}1.99\ 10^{-3}$ mm²/s)
    - No GN/GNBL with ADC < 1.1×10^{-3} mm²/s

Ultrasonographic Findings

- Heterogeneous echogenicity with foci of increased echoes (± posterior acoustic shadowing) = calcifications

Nuclear Medicine Findings

- MIBG scintigraphy
  - I-123 MIBG most specific method of staging & evaluating response to therapy in NBL
  - Metaiodobenzylguanidine (MIBG) related to norepinephrine → avid uptake in catecholamine production process
- PET
  - F-18 FDG remains primary PET radiotracer
  - High sensitivity for soft tissue & bony NBL, though generally < MIBG
    - Good for MIBG negative NBL
  - DOTATATE: Somatostatin receptor analog, typically bound with Ga-68
    - May lead to targeted therapies
- Bone scan
  - Tc-99m MDP radiopharmaceutical uptake in cortical > marrow metastases
  - May see uptake in primary mass (up to 74% of cases)
  - Limited role in current era

DIFFERENTIAL DIAGNOSIS

Reactive Lymph Nodes

- Most common neck mass in child
- ± cellulitis, myositis, abscess
- When associated with prominent palatine & adenoid tonsils, think EBV/mononucleosis

Neurofibroma

- Carotid space or brachial plexus common
- Dumbbell neural foramen & intraspinal
- Plexiform "tangle of worms"
- More common in older children

Lymphoma, Lymph Nodes

- Hodgkin or non-Hodgkin lymphoma
- Unilateral or bilateral noncalcified adenopathy

Neuroblastoma, Metastatic

- Metastatic H&N disease more common than primary cervical NBL
- Metastatic disease to orbit, calvarium or skull base → aggressive periosteal reaction
  - More common than lymph node metastases

Rhabdomyosarcoma

- Usually more heterogeneous
- ± bone destruction

Teratoma

- Usually larger, more heterogeneous
- Frequently contains fat & calcification

Thymus, Cervical

- Soft, mildly enhancing mass along path of thymopharyngeal duct, close association with carotid sheath, usually anterior to carotid sheath (NBL usually posterior)
- May extend between carotid artery & jugular vein, especially in upper neck

PATHOLOGY

General Features

- Etiology
  - Malignant tumor derived from embryonic cells that form primitive neural crest
    - Normal development, primitive neural crest cells → adrenal medulla & sympathetic nervous system
- Genetics
  - Some patients inherit genetic predisposition 2° to germline mutation
    - *KIF1B* gene on chromosome 1p36
  - Other patients develop sporadic disease 2° to germline or somatic mutation
  - 1p chromosomal deletion in 70-80% of NB patients
  - Amplification of *MYCN* oncogene correlates with more aggressive behavior
  - Gain on chromosome arm 17q linked with advanced-stage tumors
  - *HER2/neu* oncogene overexpression is unfavorable prognostic indicator
  - Increased CD44 (glycoprotein on surface of NB cells) & expression of TrkA (nerve growth factor) correlate with better prognosis

Staging, Grading, & Classification

- International NBL staging system (INSS)
  - Original 1-4S system based on resection & pathology (1988, 1993)
  - Traditionally used by Children's Oncology Group (COG) for risk stratification as low, intermediate, or high risk
  - Stage 1: Localized tumor completely resected at Dx
  - Stage 2: Localized tumor that cannot be completely resected at Dx
    - May have ipsilateral positive lymph nodes
  - Stage 3: Large tumor spread across midline, cannot be surgically removed at Dx
  - Stage 4: Tumor of any size that has metastasized to distant lymph nodes, bone marrow, bone, or liver
  - Stage 4S: Child < 18 months of age, small localized tumor that has metastasized to liver, skin, &/or bone marrow
- International NBL Risk Group Staging System (INRGSS)
  - More comprehensive, imaging-based system (2009)
  - Utilizes modifying image-defined risk factors
    - L1: Tumor in 1 body compartment, no vital structures involved
    - L2: Tumor in 2 body compartments **or** encasing/invading major structures; rarely resectable at diagnosis
    - M: Distant metastases

- MS: Age < 18 months; metastases confined to skin, liver, bone marrow
    - Bones (including marrow) must be clear by MIBG to qualify for stage 4S/MS (with marrow disease limited to < 10% involvement by biopsy)
  - Used to stratify as very low, low, intermediate, or high risk in conjunction with age, genetics, histology
    - High risk: *MYCN* amplification, metastases if ≥ 18 months of age; additional criteria by some systems
    - "UltraHigh risk": Potential evolving category
- International Neuroblastoma Pathology Classification, a.k.a. Shimada system, distinguishes favorable & unfavorable histology
  - Based on age, grade of neuroblastic differentiation, mitosis-karyorrhexis index, mitotic rate, & presence or absence of calcification

Microscopic Features

- Homer-Wright rosettes
- Spectrum from benign to malignant: GN → GNBL → NBL
  - Determined by degree of cellular maturation
    - GN: Mature neural tissue
    - NBL: Immature neural precursor cells
  - Occasionally with mixed histology

CLINICAL ISSUES

Presentation

- Most common signs/symptoms
  - Horner syndrome
  - Palpable mass
  - Stridor or feeding difficulties
- Other signs/symptoms
  - 95% of patients with NBL have increased urine catecholamines
    - ↑ urine homovanillic acid (HVA) ± vanillylmandelic acid (VMA)
  - ↑ serum neuron-specific enolase (NSE), lactic dehydrogenase (LDH), ferritin
  - Opsoclonus myoclonus ataxia syndrome: Rare in primary cervical NBL
    - Acute-onset chaotic eye movements, myoclonic jerking of limbs/trunk, & ataxia
      - Autoimmune, triggered by viral infection or tumor (paraneoplastic)
    - May lead to devastating neurologic outcome but better overall survival
    - Present in 1-2% of all NBL patients, usually lower stage

Demographics

- Age
  - Most < 5 years
  - Rarely > 10 years
  - Infants more likely to present with thoracic & cervical tumors, older children with abdominal tumors
- Epidemiology
  - Most common extracranial solid malignancy in children
  - Most common childhood cancer diagnosed before 1 year of age
  - 3rd most common malignancy in children
    - After leukemia & primary CNS brain tumors

- 10-15% of all cancer deaths in childhood
- < 5% are primary cervical NBL
  - Most lesions in neck are metastatic from retroperitoneal primary NBL

Natural History & Prognosis

- Risk stratification: Criteria vary by cooperative groups & trials
- In general, prognosis dependent on age, location, & spread of disease
  - < 18 months old: Better prognosis, metastasis to liver & skin
  - > 18 months old: Worse prognosis, metastasis to bone marrow
  - Cervical location favorable prognosis
- INSS: Stage 1 (90%), stage 2 (75%), stage 3 (30%), stage 4 (10%), stage 4S (nearly 100%)
  - Stage 4S: May spontaneously involute without treatment
- *MYCN* oncogene amplification: Worse prognosis
- Increased levels of CD44 (glycoprotein on surface) better prognosis
- Metastatic disease at Dx in up to 70% of patients with NBL
- Segmental chromosome aberrations (loss at 1p, 3p, 11q, 14q): Unfavorable
- *ALK* mutation/amplification: Unfavorable
- DNA index (measure of ploidy)
  - Diploidy or tetraploidy: Unfavorable
  - 1.26-1.76 (near triploid): Favorable

Treatment

- Depends on age at diagnosis, tumor stage, & histology
  - Classified into low-, intermediate-, & high-risk groups
- Primary or secondary resection
- Chemotherapy, radiation
- Myeloablative therapy with stem cell rescue, molecular inhibitors, antibodies, &/or I-131 MIBG therapy especially for refractory/recurrent disease

DIAGNOSTIC CHECKLIST

Consider

- Child with neck mass involving posterior carotid space, think NBL

SELECTED REFERENCES

1. Bacchus MK et al: Neuroblastic tumor recurrence associated with opsoclonus myoclonus ataxia syndrome relapse a decade after initial resection and treatments. J Pediatr Hematol Oncol. 45(3):152-4, 2023
2. Liu Q et al: Clinical and surgical outcome differences on the basis of pathology category in cervical neuroblastic tumors. J Pediatr Surg. 57(12):926-33, 2022
3. Morin CE et al: Imaging for staging of pediatric abdominal tumors: an update, from the AJR Special Series on Cancer Staging. AJR Am J Roentgenol. 217(4):786-99, 2021

KEY FACTS

TERMINOLOGY

- Malignant tumor of sympathetic chain primitive neural crest cells

IMAGING

- Classic imaging appearance of osseous metastases
  - "Hair on end" spiculated periostitis of orbits and skull ± bone destruction
- Cranial metastases
  - Nearly always extradural, calvarial-based mass
- Brain metastases rare
  - ↑ prevalence with improved treatment protocols, stage IV metastatic disease
  - Most parenchymal NB mets supratentorial, hemorrhagic

TOP DIFFERENTIAL DIAGNOSES

- Leukemia
  - Dural- or calvarial-based masses, without aggressive periosteal reaction

- Langerhans cell histiocytosis (LCH)
  - Lytic bone lesions, without periosteal new bone
- Extraaxial hematoma
  - Subdural or epidural hematoma, no periosteal new bone
- Ewing sarcoma
  - Aggressive bone destruction

CLINICAL ISSUES

- Most common extracranial solid malignancy in children
- Most common tumor in neonates/infants < 1 month of age (congenital)
- Metastases in 50-60% at diagnosis, most commonly to bone/marrow, lymph nodes, liver, soft tissues
- Ophthalmic manifestation in 20-55%
  - Proptosis and "raccoon eyes"

DIAGNOSTIC CHECKLIST

- CT can help identify bone spicules, eliminating LCH from differential

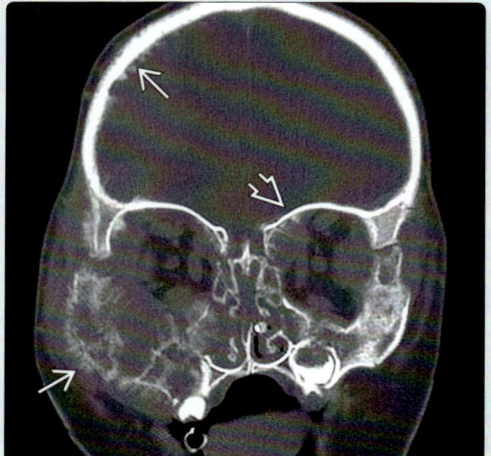
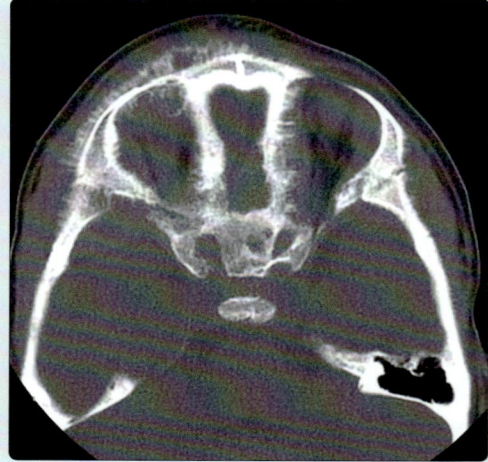

(Left) Coronal NECT of a child with an abdominal mass reveals orbital, facial bone, and calvarial spiculated periostitis, giving rise to a hair on end appearance ➡ with associated large soft tissue masses. Note bilateral disease ➡. Metastatic stage IV neuroblastoma (NB) typically involves the skull and bony orbits. (Right) Axial NECT in the same patient shows the hair on end appearance. Involvement of the orbits often gives rise to proptosis and ecchymosis "raccoon eyes," which may be mistaken for nonaccidental trauma.

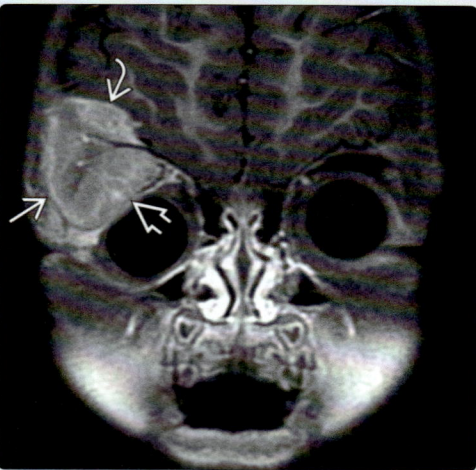
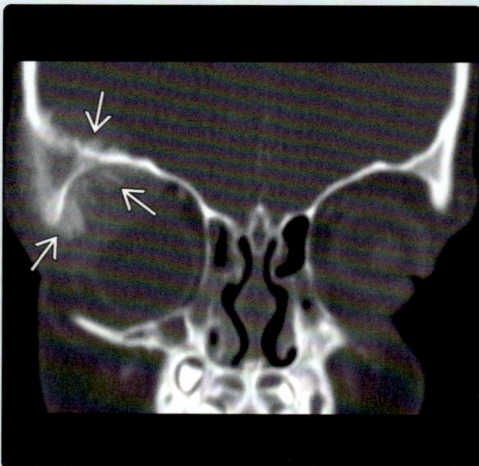

(Left) Coronal T1 C+ FS MR of the orbits in an 18-month-old boy with persistent bruising and swelling a few weeks after trauma shows a heterogeneously enhancing mass ➡ destroying the right superolateral orbital wall with intraorbital extension ➡ compressing the globe and intracranial extension ➡. DDx would include NB and Langerhans cell histiocytosis. (Right) Coronal bone window CECT in the orbits of the same patient clearly shows the aggressive, spiculated periosteal reaction ➡, typical of NB.

TERMINOLOGY

Abbreviations

- Neuroblastoma (NB)

Definitions

- Malignant tumor of sympathetic chain system arising from primitive neural crest cell derivatives

IMAGING

General Features

- Best diagnostic clue
  - Spiculated periorbital bone mass causing proptosis in child with "raccoon eyes"
- Location
  - Cranial metastases nearly always extradural calvarial-based masses
    - Calvarium, orbit, skull base
  - Brain metastases rare, but increased in patients with improved treatment protocols for advanced disease
    - CNS NB is sole site of disease recurrence in 64% of high-risk patients
    - CNS may represent "sanctuary site" for NB
    - Most parenchymal NB metastases supratentorial, hemorrhagic
    - Leptomeningeal, intraventricular lesions also occur

Radiographic Findings

- Classic imaging appearance: "Hair on end" spiculated periostitis of orbits and skull, ± bony destruction

CT Findings

- NECT
  - Best for showing fine spicules of periosteal bone projecting off skull or sphenoid wings
  - Soft tissue mass typically iso- to hyperdense to brain
    - May mimic epidural or subdural hematoma
  - Mass projects into orbit (extraconal) with extension to surrounding spaces, not preseptal space
  - May project through inner and outer tables of skull
- CECT
  - Enhancing dural metastasis if intracranial
  - Rare, ring-enhancing brain parenchymal metastasis

MR Findings

- T1WI: Slightly heterogeneous, hypointense to muscle
- T2WI: Heterogeneous, hypointense to brain, slightly hyperintense to muscle
- FLAIR: Heterogeneous, hyperintense to muscle
- T2* GRE: Hypointense
- T1WI C+: Vigorously enhances, may be heterogeneous
- MRV: May narrow or invade adjacent dural sinuses

Nuclear Medicine Findings

- MIBG
  - I-123 MIBG for diagnosis, staging, follow-up imaging
  - MIBG is related to norepinephrine → avid uptake in catecholamine production process
  - Avid uptake by neural crest tumors
    - NB, ganglioneuroblastoma, ganglioneuroma, carcinoid, medullary thyroid carcinoma

- 99% specific for neuroblastic tumors (NBT)
  - Caveat: Up to 30% of NB not MIBG positive
    - Misses 50% of recurrent tumors
  - Evaluates cortical and bone marrow disease
- PET
  - F-18 FDG remains primary PET radiotracer
    - High sensitivity for soft tissue and bony NB, though generally < MIBG
      - Select populations may benefit from PET, particularly non-MIBG-avid disease
- Bone scan
  - Tc-99m MDP (methylene diphosphonate)
    - ↑ uptake from calcium metabolism of tumor, not specific to neural crest tissue
    - ↑ uptake in bony metastasis (cortical > marrow)
    - Limited role in current era

Imaging Recommendations

- Best imaging tool
  - CT or MR for assessment of primary tumor and adjacent structures to identify Image-defined risk factors (IDRFs)
  - Functional imaging with I-123 MIBG for assessment of disease burden and activity
- Protocol advice
  - MR C+ and FS complementary to CT for assessment of H&N metastases

DIFFERENTIAL DIAGNOSIS

Leukemia

- Dural- or calvarial-based masses, without aggressive periosteal reaction
- More frequent parenchymal masses
- Less heterogeneous on MR

Langerhans Cell Histiocytosis

- Lytic bone lesions + enhancing mass, without periosteal new bone
- Often associated with diabetes insipidus

Extraaxial Hematoma

- Subdural or epidural hematoma, no periosteal new bone
- Bleeding disorder or child abuse to be considered

Ewing Sarcoma

- < 1% of cases involve skull
- Aggressive bone destruction
- Spiculated periosteal reaction

Osteosarcoma

- Rarely primary in calvarium

Rhabdomyosarcoma

- Most common soft tissue malignancy of pediatric orbit
- Less likely bilateral; may invade preseptal space
- In orbit, rarely associated with bone destruction

Beta Thalassemia Major

- Classic "hair on end" calvarial expansion
- Not focal or destructive like NB

PATHOLOGY

General Features

- Etiology
  - Arises from pathologically maturing neural crest progenitor cells
  - Primary tumors arise at sites of sympathetic ganglia
- Genetics
  - ↑ copies of *MYCN* oncogene (*MYCN* or N-myc amplification): Unfavorable prognosis (even stage MS)
  - *ALK* mutation/amplification: Unfavorable
  - Segmental chromosome aberrations (loss at 1p, 3p, 11q, 14q): Unfavorable
  - DNA index (measure of ploidy)
    - Diploidy or tetraploidy: Unfavorable
    - 1.26-1.76 (near triploid): Favorable
  - Only 1-2% of cases are familial, often with multiple primary tumors in infants
- Associated abnormalities
  - Rarely associated with neurofibromatosis type 1, Beckwith-Wiedemann syndrome, Turner syndrome
  - Some association with neurocristopathy syndromes
    - Hirschsprung disease, congenital central hypoventilation, DiGeorge syndrome

Staging, Grading, & Classification

- International Neuroblastoma Staging System (INSS)
  - Original 1-4S system based on resection and pathology (1988, 1993)
- International Neuroblastoma Risk Group Staging System (INRGSS)
  - Presurgical staging based on extent of disease and IDRFs
    - L1: Localized tumor not involving vital structures as defined by list of IDRFs & confined to 1 body compartment
    - L2: Locoregional tumor with presence of ≥ 1 IDRF
    - M: Distant metastatic disease (except stage MS)
    - MS: Metastatic disease in children < 18 months old with metastases confined to skin, liver, &/or bone marrow

CLINICAL ISSUES

Presentation

- Most common signs/symptoms
  - Scalp or periorbital soft tissue swelling related to osseous metastasis may be presenting symptom in child with NB
  - "Raccoon eyes" (periorbital ecchymosis)
    - Secondary to orbital region metastases
  - Palpable calvarial masses
- Other signs/symptoms
  - Palpable abdominal or paraspinal mass
  - Cranial metastatic disease rarely occurs in isolation
- Clinical profile
  - Ophthalmic manifestation in 20-55% at presentation
    - Proptosis and "raccoon eyes," 50% bilateral
    - Horner syndrome
    - Opsoclonus, myoclonus, and ataxia
      - Myoclonic encephalopathy of infancy
      - Paraneoplastic syndrome (not metastatic)
      - Up to 2-4% of NB patients; more favorable prognosis
  - Elevated vasoactive intestinal peptides (VIP)
    - Up to 7% of NBT patients
    - Diarrhea, hypokalemia, achlorhydria
  - Elevated homovanillic acid and vanillylmandelic acid in urine (> 90%)

Demographics

- Age
  - Median age at presentation: 15-19 months
  - 90% < 5 years, 30% within 1st year
  - May be diagnosed prenatally
- Epidemiology
  - Most common extracranial solid malignancy in children
    - Most common malignancy of infancy
  - Metastases in 50-60% at diagnosis, most commonly to bone/marrow, lymph nodes, liver, soft tissues

Natural History & Prognosis

- INRG pretreatment classification scheme: Very low risk, low risk, intermediate risk, or high risk
  - Based on INRG stage, age, histology, differentiation, *MYCN* status, 11q loss of heterozygosity, ploidy
  - At time of strata development, 5-year event-free survival (EFS) for strata were as follows
    - Very low risk: > 85% EFS
    - Low risk: 75% > % to ≤ 85% EFS
    - Intermediate risk: ≥ 50% to ≤ 75% EFS
    - High risk: < 50% EFS
- Non-MIBG-avid tumors more likely extraadrenal and more likely *MYCN* amplified, but have slightly better 5-year EFS
- 15% of cancer-related deaths in children
- MS may spontaneously regress

Treatment

- Ranges from observation to surgery ± chemotherapy, ± radiation, stem cell transplant, I-131 MIBG therapy &/or immunotherapy

DIAGNOSTIC CHECKLIST

Image Interpretation Pearls

- CT without contrast can help identify bone spicules, eliminating Langerhans cell histiocytosis from differential

SELECTED REFERENCES

1. Brown EG et al: Evaluation of image-defined risk factor (IDRF) assessment in patients with intermediate-risk neuroblastoma: a report from the Children's Oncology Group Study ANBL0531. J Pediatr Surg. 60(1):161896, 2025
2. Lai HA et al: Imaging of pediatric neuroblastoma: a COG Diagnostic Imaging Committee/SPR Oncology Committee White Paper. Pediatr Blood Cancer. 70 Suppl 4(Suppl 4):e29974, 2023
3. Liu S et al: Metastasis pattern and prognosis in children with neuroblastoma. World J Surg Oncol. 21(1):130, 2023
4. Yang DD et al: Association of image-defined risk factors with clinical features, tumor biology, and outcomes in neuroblastoma: a single-center retrospective study. Eur J Pediatr. 182(5):2189-96, 2023
5. Irwin MS et al: Revised neuroblastoma risk classification system: a report from the Children's Oncology Group. J Clin Oncol. 39(29):3229-41, 2021
6. Newman EA et al: Update on neuroblastoma. J Pediatr Surg. 54(3):383-9, 2019
7. Chen AM et al: A review of neuroblastoma image-defined risk factors on magnetic resonance imaging. Pediatr Radiol. 48(9):1337-47, 2018

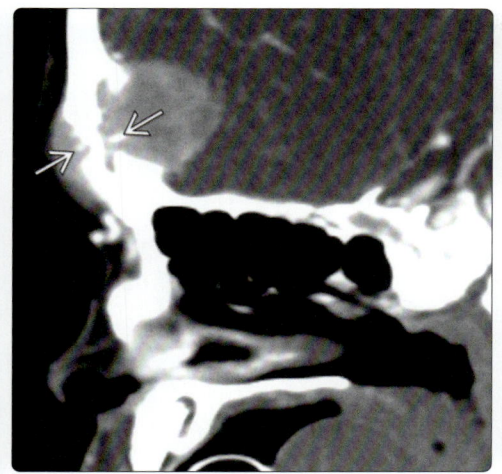

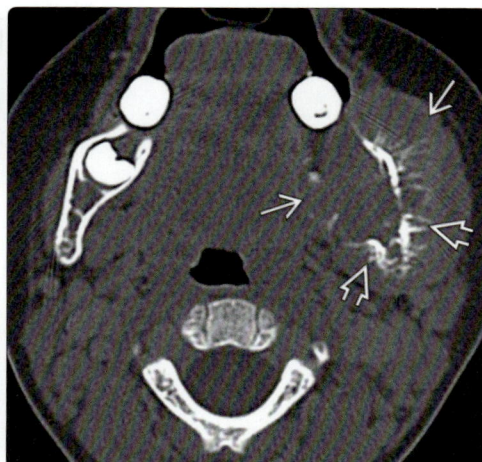

(Left) Sagittal CECT of the orbits in a 1-year-old girl without known NB who presents with forehead swelling shows an aggressive frontal bone lesion with a spiculated reaction ➡ and a heterogeneously enhancing mass with intracranial and extracranial extension. (Right) Axial bone window CECT of the face shows the typical appearance of NB osseous metastasis involving facial bones with a large soft tissue mass ➡, mandible destruction, and aggressive, spiculated periosteal reaction ➡.

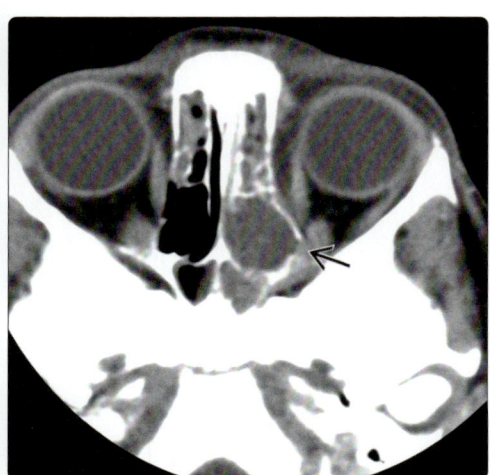

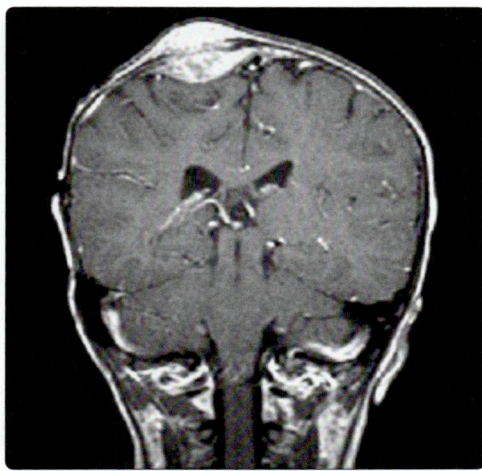

(Left) Axial NECT in a child with NB shows an ethmoid mass. There is a small focus of bony erosion ➡, suggesting the correct diagnosis of NB metastasis. This location is uncommon, as the majority of head and neck osseous metastases involve the orbits, skull base, &/or calvarium. (Right) Coronal T1 C+ MR shows an enhancing convexity mass centered at the diploic space with subperiosteal and epidural components in a child with NB.

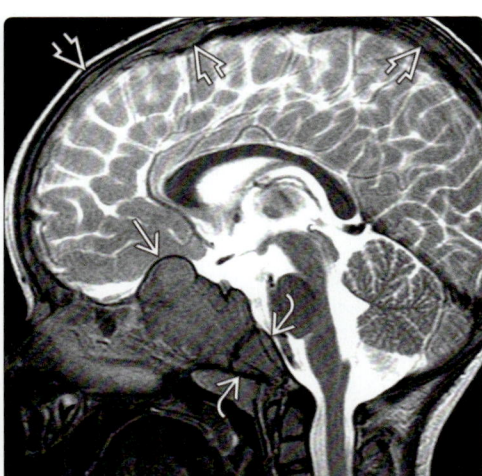

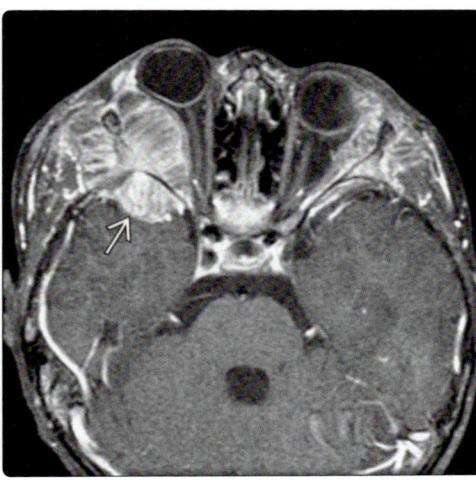

(Left) Sagittal T2 MR shows a large metastasis involving the sphenoid bone ➡. Multiple smaller and less conspicuous calvarial metastases are present ➡. Diffuse spine marrow replacement is present and the large sphenoid mass extends beyond the bony margins ➡. (Right) Axial T1 C+ FS MR shows bilateral, orbital, enhancing soft tissue masses centered on the sphenoid bones. There is marked distortion of the right globe and proptosis. Note the intracranial dural extension ➡.

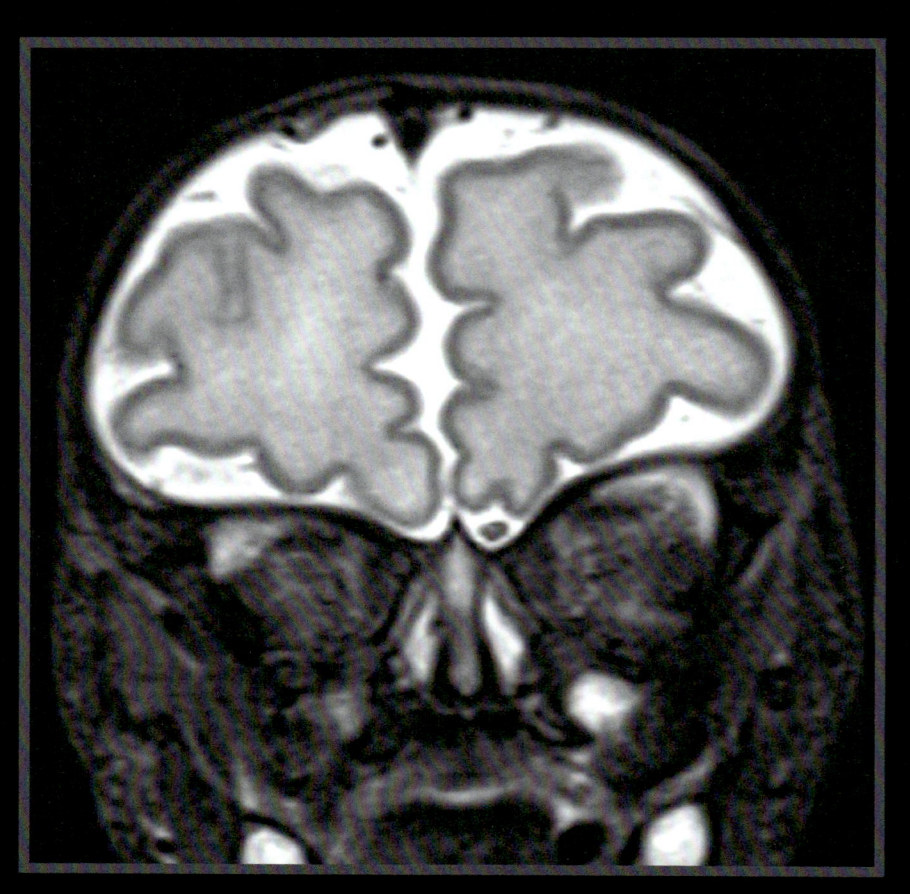
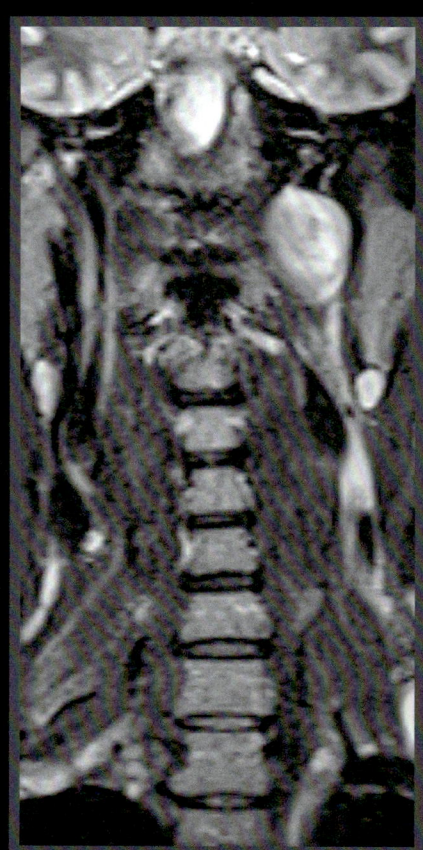
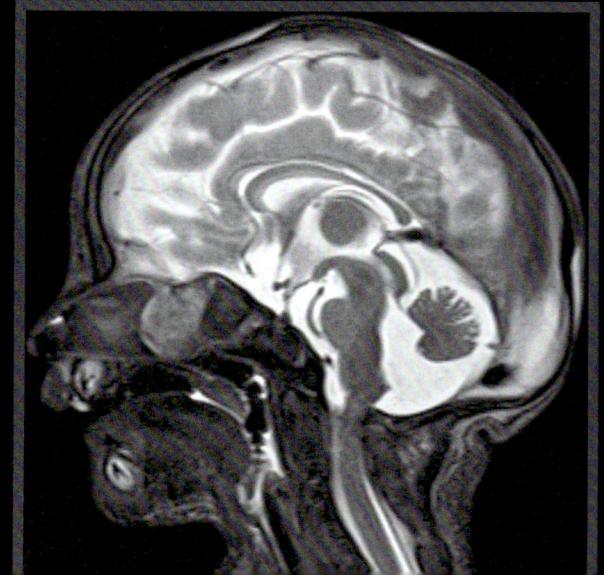
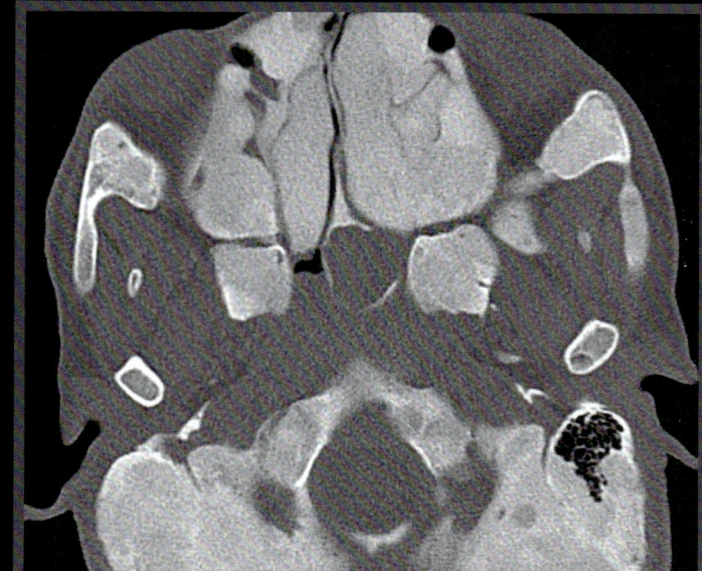

SECTION 20
Syndromic Diseases

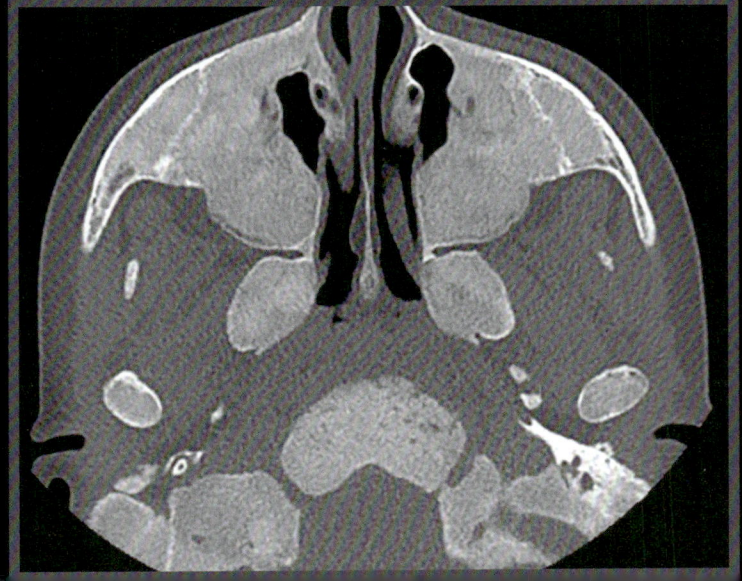

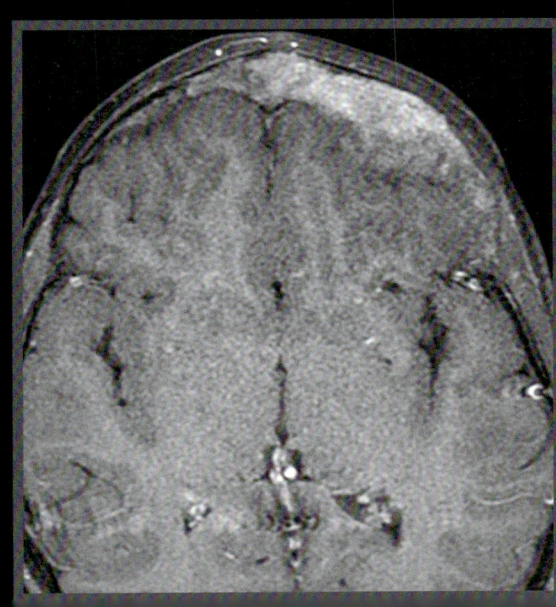

TERMINOLOGY

- Neurofibromatosis type 1 (**NF1**)
- **Neurofibromas**: Multiple localized neurofibromas & plexiform neurofibromas (PNF) in NF1

IMAGING

- Hyperintense T2 signal
  - **Target** = ↓ signal center, ↑ signal periphery PNF
- Postcontrast CT or MR
  - Localized NF: Homogeneous or patchy enhancement, well-circumscribed fusiform mass
  - PNF: Heterogeneously enhancing, lobulated mass along course of peripheral nerve
- Most conspicuous on STIR & FS T2WI
- Other extracranial H&N manifestations of NF1
  - Orbit: **Optic pathway glioma (OPG)**, optic nerve sheath ectasia, Lisch nodules, buphthalmos, large foramina with PNFs

- Skull & skull base: **Sphenoid dysplasia**, smooth enlargement of bony foramina with PNF infiltration, lambdoid suture defect
- Vascular dysplasia: Internal carotid artery stenosis/occlusion & moyamoya; aneurysms & arteriovenous fistula rare

TOP DIFFERENTIAL DIAGNOSES

- Lymphatic malformation
- Venous malformation
- Rhabdomyosarcoma

DIAGNOSTIC CHECKLIST

- Patient with PNF or multiple localized neurofibromas, consider NF1
  - Look for additional findings of brain lesions, OPG, sphenoid wing dysplasia
- Transspatial neurofibroma may be hypodense on CT & mimic lymphatic malformation

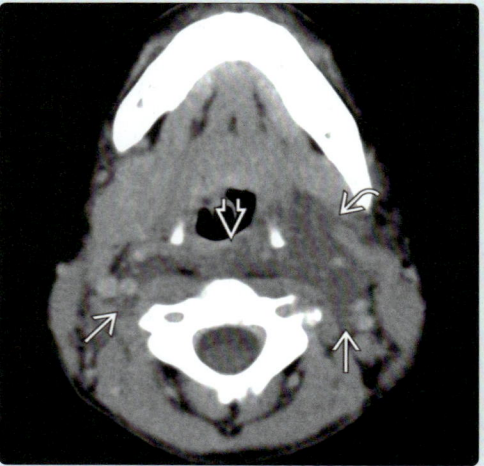
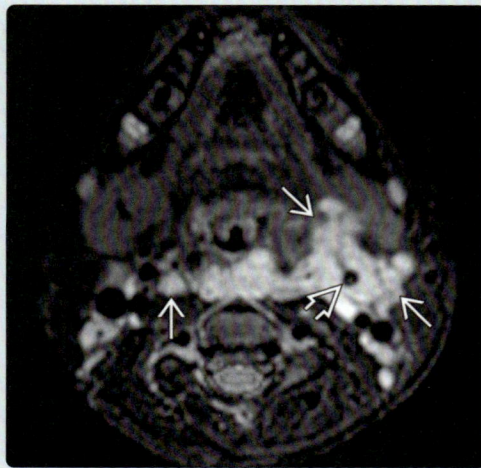

(Left) Axial CECT in a child with neurofibromatosis type 1 (NF1) shows an ill-defined, infiltrative, transspatial plexiform neurofibroma (PNF) involving the bilateral carotid ➡, retropharyngeal ⮢, and left submandibular ➡ spaces. (Right) Axial STIR MR in the same patient better defines the margins of the PNF ➡. Notice the infiltrative pattern with circumferential involvement of the left carotid artery ➡, typical of plexiform lesions.

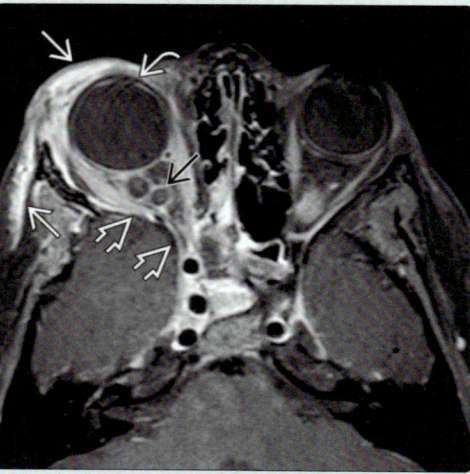
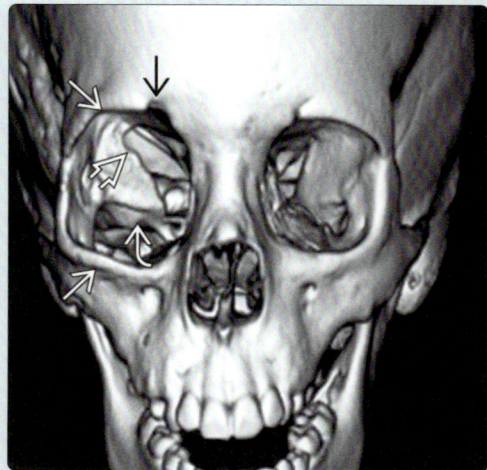

(Left) Axial T1WI C+ FS MR shows a diffusely enhancing neurofibroma ➡ involving the right pre- and postseptal orbit and temporalis scalp. There is also sphenoid wing hypoplasia ➡, buphthalmos ➡, and a tortuous optic nerve ➡. (Right) Frontal 3D reformation in the same patient shows diffuse right orbital expansion ➡. There is also enlargement of the superior ➡ and inferior ➡ orbital fissures and supraorbital foramen ➡ related to sphenoid dysplasia and adjacent PNF.

TERMINOLOGY

Abbreviations
- Neurofibromatosis type 1 (**NF1**)

Synonyms
- von Recklinghausen disease, autosomal dominant neurofibromatosis

Definitions
- Autosomal dominant neurocutaneous disorder (**phakomatosis**)
- Diagnostic NF1 criteria: If ≥ 2 of following present
  - \> 6 café au lait spots measuring ≥ 5 mm in prepubertal & ≥ 15 mm in postpubertal patients
  - ≥ 2 neurofibromas (NFs) or 1 plexiform NF (PNF)
  - Axillary/inguinal freckling
  - Visual pathway glioma
  - ≥ Lisch nodules (optic hamartomas)
  - Distinctive bony lesion
    - Sphenoid wing dysplasia
    - Thinning of long bones
      - ± pseudoarthrosis
  - 1st-degree relative with NF1
- Peripheral nerve sheath tumor (PNST) = schwannoma, NF, & PNF
- **NFs**: Localized, plexiform, & diffuse variants

IMAGING

General Features
- Best diagnostic clue
  - **PNF**
    - Characteristic & diagnostic feature of NF1
  - **Multiple localized NFs**
- Location
  - NFs may involve **any space in H&N**
    - Most common: Carotid, retropharyngeal, & posterior cervical spaces; brachial plexus, oral cavity, cheek
  - PNST
    - Usually major nerve trunks, including brachial plexus
- Morphology
  - **Localized** NF
    - Multiple well-circumscribed, smooth, fusiform, variably enhancing masses along course of nerves
    - Paraspinal NF may be dumbbell-shaped ± smooth enlargement of bony neural foramina
    - Schwannoma may be indistinguishable from NF
  - **Diffuse** NF
    - Plaque-like or infiltrative, poorly defined, reticulated lesion in skin & subcutaneous fat
  - **PNF**
    - Transspatial, lobulated, tortuous, rope-like expansion within major nerve distribution
    - Resembles tangle of worms

CT Findings
- CECT
  - Localized NF & PNF
    - Frequently have low attenuation (5-25 HU) on pre- & postcontrast images; mimic lymphatic malformation
    - Paraspinal NF may be dumbbell-shaped
      - ± enlarged neural foramina

MR Findings
- T2WI
  - Hyperintense
  - Target sign: ↓ signal center, ↑ signal periphery PNF
    - Fascicular sign: Multiple small, irregular hypointense foci (represents fascicular bundles)
- T1WI C+
  - Localized NF: Homogeneous or patchy, heterogeneous enhancement, well-circumscribed fusiform mass
  - PNF: Heterogeneously enhancing, lobulated mass along course of peripheral nerve
  - Malignant PNST
    - Differentiation of benign from malignant PNST difficult on imaging alone
    - If large size (> 5 cm), heterogeneous with central necrosis, infiltrative margins, & rapid growth, consider malignant PNST
  - Diffuse NF: Plaque-like or infiltrative intense enhancement in skin & subcutaneous fat

Imaging Recommendations
- Best imaging tool
  - MR best to characterize & define total extent
    - Most conspicuous on STIR & FS T2WI
  - Bone CT delineates associated bone changes
    - Particularly helpful in patients with sphenoid wing dysplasia & PNF

DIFFERENTIAL DIAGNOSIS

Lymphatic Malformation
- Low attenuation
- Unilocular or multilocular, focal or infiltrative
- No enhancement unless infected or mixed venolymphatic malformation

Venous Malformation
- Phleboliths common

Rhabdomyosarcoma
- Invasive transspatial mass
- Frequently with aggressive bone destruction

PATHOLOGY

General Features
- Etiology
  - *NF1* gene (tumor suppressor gene) normally encodes production of "neurofibromin" that influences cell growth regulation
  - *NF1* gene "turned off" in NF1 → allows cellular proliferation & tumor development
- Genetics
  - **Autosomal dominant; 50% new mutations**
  - Gene locus = **chromosome 17q11.2**
    - Nonsense mutation of this gene leads to NF1
- Associated abnormalities
  - Other extracranial H&N manifestations of NF1

– Orbit: Optic pathway glioma (OPG), optic nerve sheath ectasia, Lisch nodules, **buphthalmos**, **large foramina** with PNFs
– Skull: Lambdoid suture defect
– Skull base findings
  □ Sphenoid dysplasia with PNF, probably sequelae of PNF interaction with developing underlying bone
  □ Smooth, corticated enlargement of skull base bony foramina with PNF infiltration
– Vascular dysplasia: Internal carotid artery stenosis/occlusion & moyamoya; aneurysms & arteriovenous fistula rare
– Neural crest tumors
  □ **Pheochromocytoma** 10x ↑ in NF1 patients
  □ **Parathyroid adenomas** ↑ incidence
○ Other imaging manifestations of NF1
  – CNS findings
    □ Cerebral gliomas, hydrocephalus, cranial nerve schwannomas
    □ Nonenhancing hyperintense T2/FLAIR lesions: White matter, dentate nucleus, globus pallidus, brainstem, thalamus, hippocampus
    □ Spinal cord astrocytomas

Staging, Grading, & Classification

- NFs are WHO grade 1
- Malignant PNSTs are WHO grade 3/4

Gross Pathologic & Surgical Features

- **Localized NF**: Fusiform, firm, gray/white-colored mass intermixed with nerve of origin
- **PNF**: Diffuse, tortuous, rope-like expansion of nerves resembling tangle of worms
  ○ Involves adjacent skin, fascia, & deeper tissues
- **Malignant PNST**: Fusiform, fleshy, tan-white mass with areas of necrosis & hemorrhage
  ○ Nerve proximally & distally thickened due to spread of tumor along epineurium & perineurium

Microscopic Features

- Localized NF
  ○ Schwann cells, fibroblasts, mast cells in matrix of collagen fibers, & mucoid substance
  ○ Axons usually embedded within tumor
- PNF
  ○ Schwann cells & perineural fibroblasts grow along nerve fascicles
- Malignant PNST
  ○ Fibrosarcoma-like growth of spindle cells
  ○ Considered high-grade sarcomas
  ○ PNF: 5% risk of malignant transformation

CLINICAL ISSUES

Presentation

- Most common signs/symptoms
  ○ Majority of NF & PNF asymptomatic
  ○ Cutaneous stigmata of NF1
    – > 95% have skin lesions
  ○ Sudden, painful ↑ in size of stable NF suggests malignant transformation
- Other signs/symptoms

○ ↓ vision with OPG
○ Pulsatile buphthalmos with sphenoid wing dysplasia & PNF

Demographics

- Age
  ○ Any age; most common presentation in late childhood to early adulthood; new lesions may develop at any time
  ○ Malignant PNST: Usually in adults, rare in children
- Epidemiology
  ○ NF1
    – Most common autosomal dominant disorder
      □ 1 in 3,000-5,000
    – **Most common neurocutaneous syndrome**
    – Most common inherited tumor syndrome
  ○ Localized NF
    – **90%** are solitary & not associated with NF1
    – **10%** associated with NF1 → more frequently large, multiple, & involve large deep nerves (e.g., brachial plexus)
  ○ Malignant PNST
    – **50% associated with NF1**
    – **5%** of patients with NF1 develop malignant PNST
  ○ Diffuse NF
    – Majority are in patients **without NF1**

Natural History & Prognosis

- Usually slow-growing NFs unless malignant transformation
  ○ Occasionally, massive enlargement in young kids

Treatment

- Resection of NFs that press on vital structures
- Solitary NF resectable; PNF generally unresectable
- mTOR &/or MEK inhibitors showing promise

DIAGNOSTIC CHECKLIST

Consider

- If patient has PNF or multiple localized NFs, consider NF1
  ○ Look for additional findings of brain lesions, OPG, sphenoid wing dysplasia

Image Interpretation Pearls

- Beware: Transspatial NF may be hypodense on CT & mimic lymphatic malformation

SELECTED REFERENCES

1. Passos J et al: A single-center case study series assessing the effect of selumetinib use in patients with neurofibromatosis-related plexiform neurofibromas. Neurooncol Adv. 6(1):vdae177, 2024
2. Nosé V et al: Update from the 5th edition of the World Health Organization classification of head and neck tumors: familial tumor syndromes. Head Neck Pathol. 16(1):143-57, 2022
3. Galvin R et al: Neurofibromatosis in the era of precision medicine: development of MEK inhibitors and recent successes with selumetinib. Curr Oncol Rep. 23(4):45, 2021
4. Abdel Razek AAK et al: Peripheral nerve sheath tumors of head and neck: imaging-based review of World Health Organization classification. J Comput Assist Tomogr. 44(6):928-40, 2020
5. Ullrich NJ et al: A phase II study of continuous oral mTOR inhibitor everolimus for recurrent, radiographic-progressive neurofibromatosis type 1-associated pediatric low-grade glioma: a Neurofibromatosis Clinical Trials Consortium study. Neuro Oncol. 22(10):1527-35, 2020
6. de Blank PMK et al: Optic pathway gliomas in neurofibromatosis type 1: an update: surveillance, treatment indications, and biomarkers of vision. J Neuroophthalmol. 37 Suppl 1:S23-32, 2017

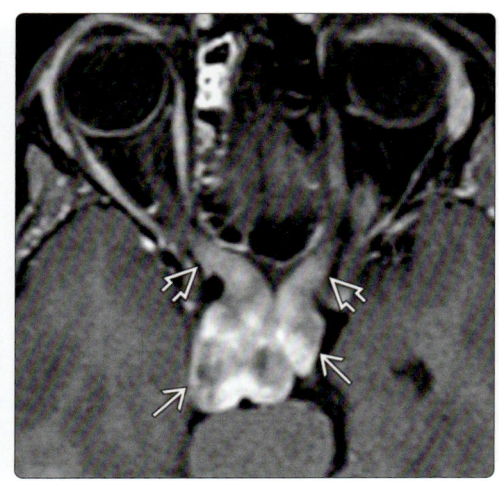
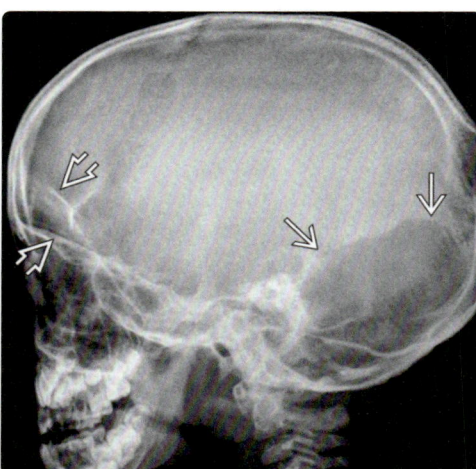

(Left) Axial T1WI C+ MR shows a large optic pathway glioma involving the chiasm ➡ and prechiasmatic optic nerves ➡ in a child with NF1. (Right) Lateral radiograph in a child with a skull base PNF shows a large lambdoid defect ➡, a typical but rare lesion in children with NF1. Notice also the asymmetry in the orbital roofs ➡, secondary to unilateral orbital enlargement, typical of patients with sphenoid wing dysplasia and adjacent PNF.

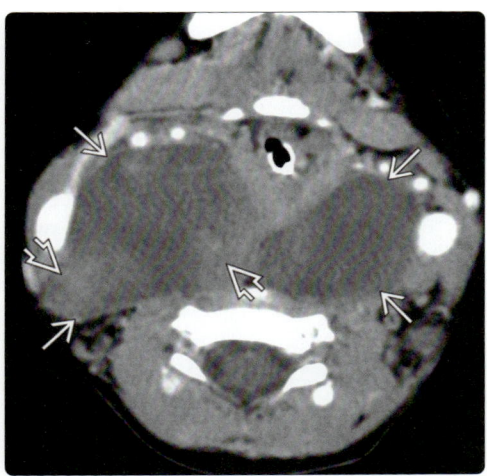
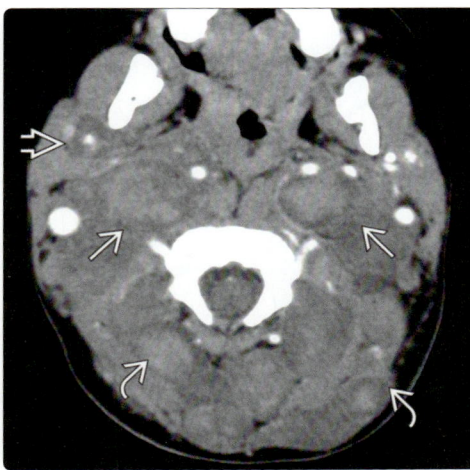

(Left) Axial CECT in a child with NF1 shows the typical appearance of large carotid space neurofibromas ➡: Low in attenuation with only mild patchy contrast enhancement ➡. (Right) Axial CECT in a child with NF1 shows massive tumor burden with numerous neurofibromas involving the bilateral carotid spaces ➡, right parotid space ➡, and posterior cervical spaces ➡. Patchy central enhancement with a peripheral rim of less enhancement is not uncommon.

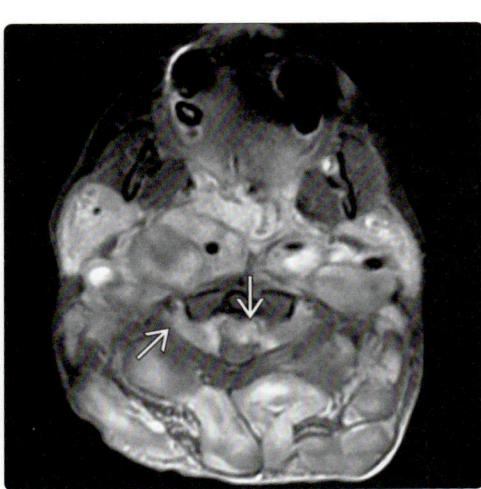
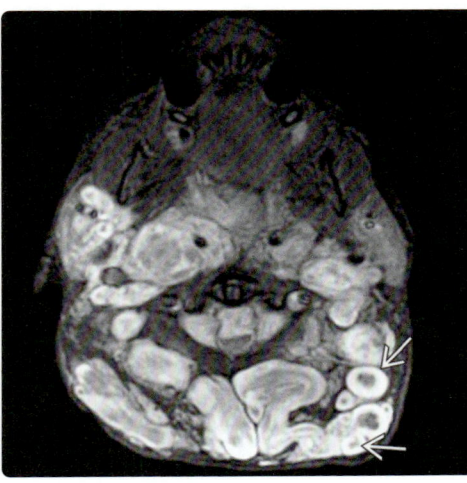

(Left) Axial T1WI C+ FS MR in the same patient shows a similar pattern of contrast enhancement with patchy central enhancement and peripheral decreased enhancement. Notice also neural foraminal extension into the spinal canal ➡, compressing the upper cervical cord. (Right) All lesions are more conspicuous on axial STIR MR. Notice the typical target appearance to several lesions ➡ and a more tram-track appearance to others, imaged along the long axis rather than a cross section through the neurofibroma.

TERMINOLOGY

- Neurofibromatosis type 2 (**NF2**) = inherited syndrome with multiple **schwannomas, meningiomas, & ependymomas**

IMAGING

- Bilateral **enhancing CPA-IAC masses**
  - Ovoid when small; "ice cream on cone" when large enough to fill IAC & CPA
- CNS
  - Calcifications: Choroid plexus, cerebellar hemispheres, & cerebral cortex
  - Other meningiomas & schwannoma (CNIII-XII)
  - Ependymomas > > gliomas
- Spine
  - Meningiomas, schwannomas, & ependymomas

TOP DIFFERENTIAL DIAGNOSES

- CPA-IAC metastases
  - Bilateral IAC enhancing masses in older patient

- Facial nerve schwannoma, CPA-IAC
  - CPA-IAC mass with labyrinthine canal tail of enhancement
- Meningioma, CPA-IAC
  - Dural-based, eccentric CPA mass with dural tail of enhancement projecting into IAC

PATHOLOGY

- Autosomal dominant disorder
  - Mutation of *NF2* gene chromosome 22
  - **50%** result from **new** dominant gene **mutation**

CLINICAL ISSUES

- Unilateral **sensorineural hearing loss**
- Other symptoms: Tinnitus, vertigo, CNVII paralysis
- Mean age at diagnosis: ~ 25 years

DIAGNOSTIC CHECKLIST

- If diagnosis of NF2 made in adult, consider alternative diagnosis of metastases to CPA-IAC

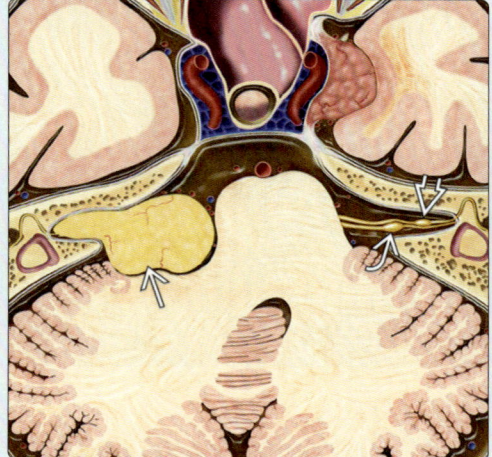

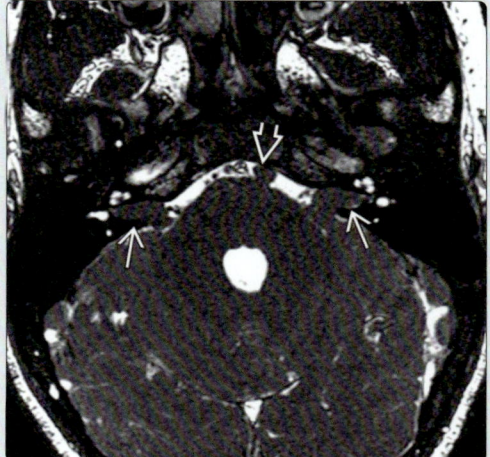

(Left) Axial graphic depicts bilateral cerebellopontine angle-internal auditory canal (CPA-IAC) masses in neurofibromatosis type 2 (NF2). Note a large right vestibular schwannoma ➡. On the left, there is a facial nerve schwannoma ➡ and a vestibular schwannoma ➡. Differentiating a facial from a vestibular schwannoma is important to assess therapy options. (Right) Axial FIESTA in a 12-year-old boy with NF2 shows bilateral hypointense vestibular schwannomas ➡. Note nodular enlargement of left CNVI ➡.

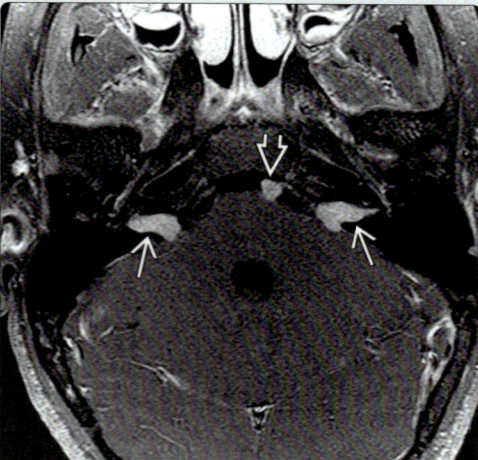

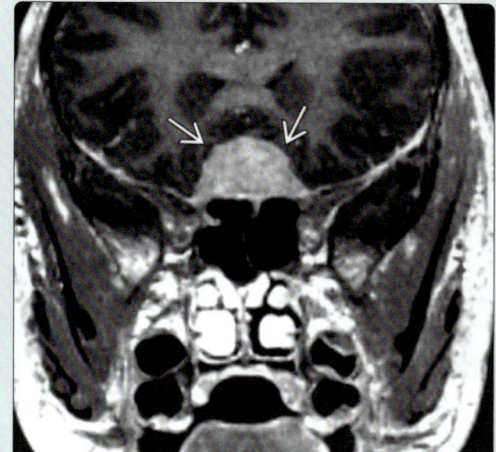

(Left) Axial T1 C+ FS MR in the same patient demonstrates typical diffuse postcontrast enhancement of the bilateral vestibular schwannomas ➡ and the left CNVI schwannoma ➡. (Right) Coronal T1 C+ MR in the same patient demonstrates a broad-based, extraaxial planum sphenoidale mass ➡, proven to represent meningioma. This patient had a very high tumor burden at a young age, including multiple other intracranial and extracranial cranial nerve schwannomas as well as spinal lesions (not shown).

TERMINOLOGY

Abbreviations

- Neurofibromatosis type 2 (**NF2**)

Synonyms

- New nomenclature preferred term is NF2-related schwannomatosis

Definitions

- NF2 = inherited syndrome with multiple **schwannomas, meningiomas, & ependymomas**

IMAGING

General Features

- Best diagnostic clue
  - Bilateral enhancing cerebellopontine angle-internal auditory canal (CPA-IAC) vestibular schwannomas
- Location
  - Schwannomas: CPA-IAC, other cranial or spinal nerves
  - Meningiomas: Dural based
  - Extraaxial tumors: Spinal cord & brainstem
- Size
  - Range from millimeters to centimeters
- Morphology
  - Ovoid when small; "ice cream on cone" when large enough to fill IAC & CPA
- Associated imaging findings
  - CNS: Calcifications: Choroid plexus, cerebellar hemispheres, & cerebral cortex
    - Other meningiomas & schwannoma (CNIII-XII)
    - Ependymomas > > gliomas
  - Spine: Meningiomas, schwannomas, & ependymomas

CT Findings

- CT: May show IAC flaring

MR Findings

- T1WI FS C+: Focal, enhancing mass of CPA-IAC cistern centered on porus acusticus
  - Small: Ovoid-enhancing masses in IAC
  - Large: "Ice cream on cone" shape in CPA & IAC
    - Intramural cysts in 15%
    - Rarely associated with arachnoid cyst/trapped CSF
- High-resolution T2 space, CISS, or FIESTA: Filling defect in hyperintense CSF of CPA-IAC cistern
  - Helps distinguish vestibular from facial schwannoma

Imaging Recommendations

- NF2 screening MR: T1 C+ MR of brain & spine
- High-resolution T2 of CPA used to follow CPA tumors

DIFFERENTIAL DIAGNOSIS

Metastases, CPA-IAC

- Bilateral IAC enhancing masses in older patient

Facial Nerve Schwannoma, CPA-IAC

- CPA-IAC mass with labyrinthine canal tail of enhancement

Meningioma, CPA-IAC

- Dural-based, eccentric CPA enhancing mass with dural tail projecting into IAC

Sarcoidosis, CPA-IAC

- Multiple focal enhancing meningeal masses

PATHOLOGY

General Features

- Etiology
  - Mutation of *NF2* gene (tumor suppressor) creates environment for multiple tumor growth
- Genetics
  - **Autosomal dominant** disorder
  - Mutation of *NF2* gene located on long arm of **chromosome 22**
  - 50% result from new dominant gene mutation
- Associated abnormalities
  - Meningiomas & ependymomas

Staging, Grading, & Classification

- Diagnostic criteria
  - Bilateral vestibular schwannomas, or
  - 1st-degree relative with NF2 & 1 vestibular schwannoma, or
  - 1st-degree NF2 relative & 2 of following: Neurofibroma, meningioma, glioma, schwannoma, juvenile posterior subcapsular lenticular opacity
- Presumptive diagnosis of NF2
  - Early-onset unilateral CNVIII schwannomas (age < 30 years) + 1 of following: Meningioma, glioma, schwannoma, juvenile posterior subcapsular lenticular opacity
  - Multiple meningiomas (> 2) + unilateral vestibular schwannoma or 1 of following: Glioma, schwannoma, juvenile posterior subcapsular lenticular opacity

CLINICAL ISSUES

Presentation

- Most common signs/symptoms
  - Unilateral sensorineural hearing loss (SNHL)
  - Other symptoms: Tinnitus, vertigo, CNVII paralysis

Demographics

- Mean age at diagnosis: ~ 25 years
- 1 per ~ 35,000; much less frequent than NF1

Natural History & Prognosis

- CPA tumor growth results in profound SNHL
- Significant morbidity & ↓ lifespan associated with NF2

Treatment

- Resection with hearing preservation is possible
  - Progressive growth often makes hearing preservation outcome temporary
- Genetic counseling essential

SELECTED REFERENCES

1. Rai P et al: Classification of schwannomas and the new naming convention for "neurofibromatosis-2": genetic updates and international consensus recommendation. Neuroradiol J. ePub, 2025

IMAGING

- Multiple circumscribed masses along course of cranial or peripheral nerves **without** CNVIII involvement
- Rare meningiomas (< 5%)
- C+ MR is mainstay of schwannomatosis imaging

TOP DIFFERENTIAL DIAGNOSES

- Neurofibromatosis type 2 (NF2)
- Sporadic schwannoma
- Neurofibromatosis type 1 (NF1)

PATHOLOGY

- **Schwannomatosis = distinct entity, different from NF2**
- Typically, germline mutation of *SMARCB1* gene
  - *SMARCB1* mutation is **not** found in sporadic (nonsyndromic) schwannomas
  - *SMARCB1* mutation is **not** found in NF2
- Less commonly, germline mutations of *LZTR1* gene

CLINICAL ISSUES

- Incidence thought to be similar to NF2 (~ 1/40,000)
- Typically presents with pain, which may be disabling
  - In contradistinction to NF2, which more frequently presents with neurologic deficits
- Peak incidence between ages 30-60
  - Contrast with NF1 (typically diagnosed in 1st decade)
  - Contrast with NF2 (typically diagnosed in 2nd decade)
- **Normal** life expectancy
  - Contrast with NF2 (↓ life expectancy)

DIAGNOSTIC CHECKLIST

- In patient > 30 years of age with **multiple schwannomas**
  - Consider diagnosis of schwannomatosis
  - Recommend high-resolution temporal bone MR to screen for vestibular schwannomas (and NF2)
- If multiple schwannomas **and** involvement of CNVIII, alternative NF2 diagnosis should be favored

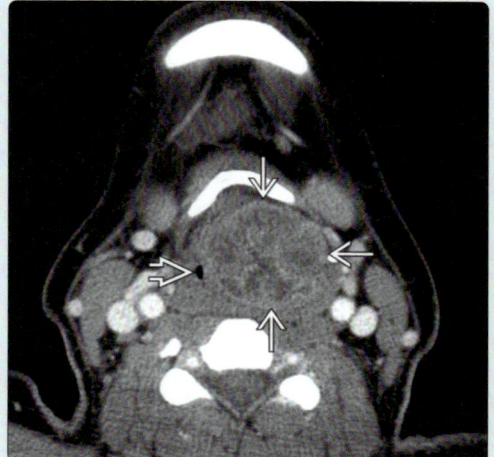
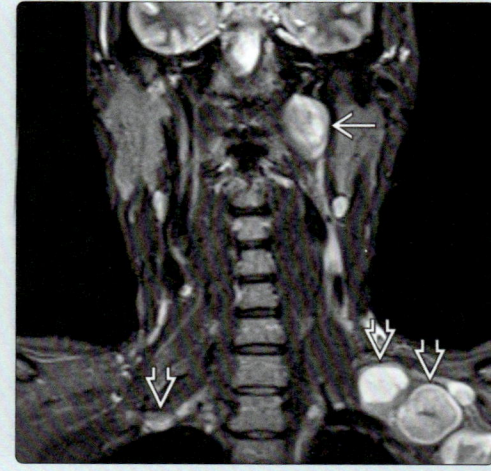

(Left) *Axial CECT of the neck shows a circumscribed, heterogeneously enhancing submucosal mass ⮕ in the supraglottic larynx, which nearly completely effaces the laryngeal airway ⮕. Biopsy demonstrated a schwannoma.* (Right) *Coronal STIR MR in the same patient shows multiple ovoid, heterogeneously hyperintense masses, consistent with additional schwannomas involving the left carotid space ⮕ and brachial plexus ⮕ bilaterally. Genetic work-up confirmed the diagnosis of schwannomatosis.*

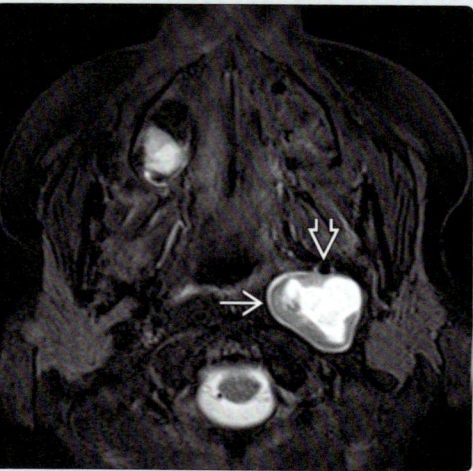
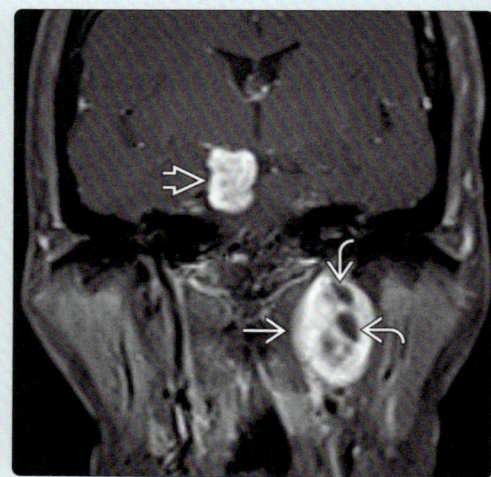

(Left) *Axial T2 FS MR in a patient with schwannomatosis shows a large, circumscribed, heterogeneously T2-bright mass ⮕ centered in the left carotid space at the level of the nasopharynx, which displaces the internal carotid artery ⮕ anteriorly.* (Right) *Coronal T1 C+ FS MR in the same patient shows the left carotid space mass ⮕ to be avidly enhancing with multiple nonenhancing intramural cysts ⮕, commonly seen in large schwannomas. Note an additional avidly enhancing schwannoma of the right oculomotor nerve ⮕.*

TERMINOLOGY

Definitions

- Schwannomatosis: Multiple schwannomas of peripheral nervous system **without** involvement of vestibular nerves

IMAGING

General Features

- Best diagnostic clue
  - Multiple circumscribed masses along course of cranial or peripheral nerves **without** CNVIII involvement
  - Rarely (< 5%) associated with meningiomas

CT Findings

- NECT
  - Iso- to slightly hyperdense compared to brain
  - Benign bone remodeling, smoothly enlarged foramina
- CECT
  - Variable, often heterogeneous enhancement

MR Findings

- Variable signal intensity on all sequences due to varying amounts of Antoni A and Antoni B regions
- Hyperintense on T2WI, PD, FLAIR, and STIR
- Intense, typically heterogeneous enhancement on T1WI C+

Imaging Recommendations

- Best imaging tool
  - C+ MR is mainstay of schwannomatosis imaging
- Protocol advice
  - If multiple schwannomas found during imaging of spine or other body parts, recommend high-resolution temporal bone MR to screen for vestibular schwannomas [and neurofibromatosis type 2 (NF2)]

DIFFERENTIAL DIAGNOSIS

Neurofibromatosis Type 2

- Multiple inherited schwannomas, meningiomas, and ependymomas
  - Bilateral vestibular schwannomas are hallmark

Sporadic Schwannoma

- Identical imaging appearance but typically solitary lesion
- As number of lesions ↑, likelihood of schwannomatosis ↑

Neurofibromatosis Type 1

- Multiple peripheral nerve sheath tumors may have similar imaging appearance
- Typically younger age (1st decade) at time of diagnosis

PATHOLOGY

General Features

- Genetics
  - Complex, incompletely understood genetics involving germline involvement of *SMARCB1* gene, which is **not** found in sporadic, nonsyndromic schwannomas
  - Germline mutations in *LZTR1* gene found in 80% of schwannomatosis patients **without** *SMARCB1* mutation

Staging, Grading, & Classification

- **Baseline criteria** (all must be met)
  - No germline *NF2* gene mutation
  - Must not meet diagnostic criteria for NF2
  - No 1st-degree relative with NF2
  - No evidence of vestibular schwannoma on MR
  - Schwannomas cannot be in prior radiation field
- **Definite** diagnosis
  - ≥ 2 nonintradermal schwannomas (1 histologically proven); **or** 1 pathologically confirmed schwannoma or intracranial meningioma **and** 1st-degree relative meeting diagnostic criteria
- **Possible** diagnosis
  - ≥ 2 nonintradermal tumors without histopathology-proven schwannoma; chronic pain associated with tumor ↑ likelihood of diagnosis

CLINICAL ISSUES

Presentation

- Most common signs/symptoms
  - Pain, typically neuropathic in quality; may be disabling
    - In contradistinction to NF2, which more frequently presents with neurologic deficits
  - Symptom onset typically in 2nd or 3rd decades of life
    - Compared to neurofibromatosis type 1 (1st decade) and NF2 (2nd decade)

Demographics

- Epidemiology
  - Reported incidence from 1/40,000 to 1/1.7 million

Natural History & Prognosis

- **Normal** life expectancy, unlike NF2 patients who have reduced life expectancy

Treatment

- Symptom control with pain management
- Surgical intervention only if spinal cord compression or symptoms clearly due to schwannoma

DIAGNOSTIC CHECKLIST

Consider

- Patient may have schwannomatosis if
  - Age > 30; > 1 schwannoma; no vestibular schwannoma

Image Interpretation Pearls

- **Caution** favoring diagnosis of schwannomatosis in patient < age 30, as vestibular schwannoma may not have formed yet
  - As patient age at time of diagnosis ↑, likelihood of schwannomatosis ↑ and likelihood of NF2 ↓

Reporting Tips

- In patient > 30 years of age, presence of multiple nonvestibular schwannomas should prompt radiologist to
  - Suggest diagnosis of schwannomatosis
  - Recommend high-resolution MR of temporal bones to screen for vestibular schwannomas (and NF2)

SELECTED REFERENCES

1. Plotkin SR et al: Updated diagnostic criteria and nomenclature for neurofibromatosis type 2 and schwannomatosis: an international consensus recommendation. Genet Med. 24(9):1967-77, 2022

TERMINOLOGY

- Basal cell nevus syndrome (**BCNS**)
- Synonyms: Gorlin syndrome, **Gorlin-Goltz syndrome**, nevoid basal cell carcinoma syndrome, nevoid basal cell carcinoma
- **Autosomal dominant** disorder with multiple odontogenic keratocysts, basal cell carcinoma (BCCa), **intracranial dural Ca^{++}**, bifid ribs, palmoplantar pits, ± **medulloblastoma**

IMAGING

- Multiple expansile, lucent lesions of **mandible & maxilla**
- May **displace developing teeth** ± **resorption of roots** of erupted teeth & tooth extrusion
- Variable attenuation/signal intensity depends on protein content &/or hemorrhage

TOP DIFFERENTIAL DIAGNOSES

- Periapical (radicular) cyst
- Dentigerous (follicular) cyst
- Odontogenic keratocyst (nonsyndromic)
- Ameloblastoma

PATHOLOGY

- Etiology: Arise from dental lamina remnants
- Autosomal dominant
  - Up to 40% of cases are new mutations
- Associated abnormalities
  - 3% of patients develop **medulloblastomas**
  - Marked Ca^{++} of falx (80%), dura
  - Multiple skin **BCCas**
  - Bifid ribs & scoliosis

CLINICAL ISSUES

- Syndrome apparent by **5-10 years**
- Patients present by 3rd decade with multiple nevoid BCCas; mean age = 19 years
- Aggressive lesions after puberty; may metastasize

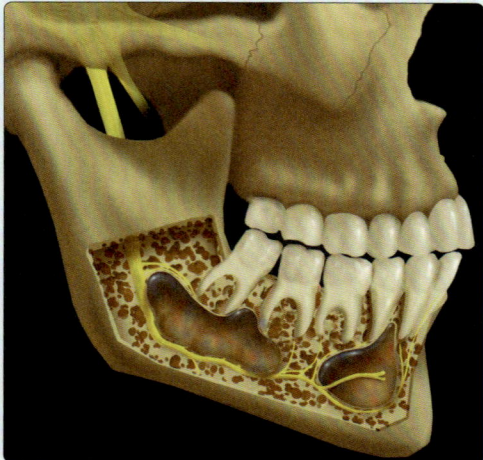
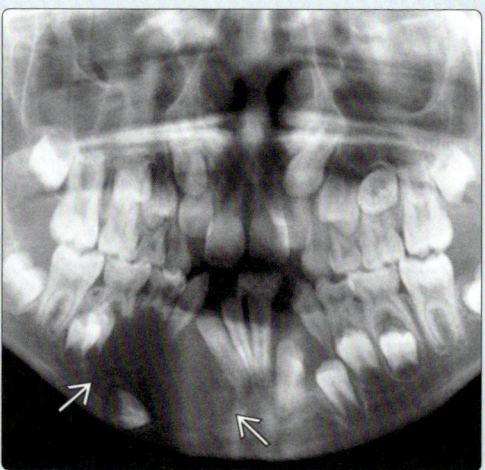

(Left) *Lateral graphic with the mandibular cortex removed shows the classic appearance of multiple odontogenic keratocysts in the basal cell nevus syndrome; lesions tend to splay tooth roots and displace nerves.* (Right) *Anteroposterior panorex radiograph shows a large, expansile radiolucent lesion* ➡ *in the left paramidline mandible with severe crowding and displacement of involved teeth.*

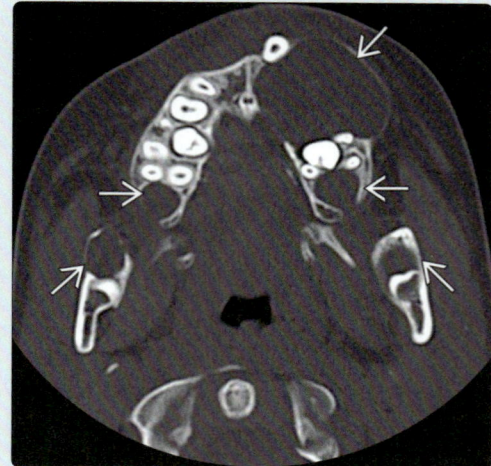
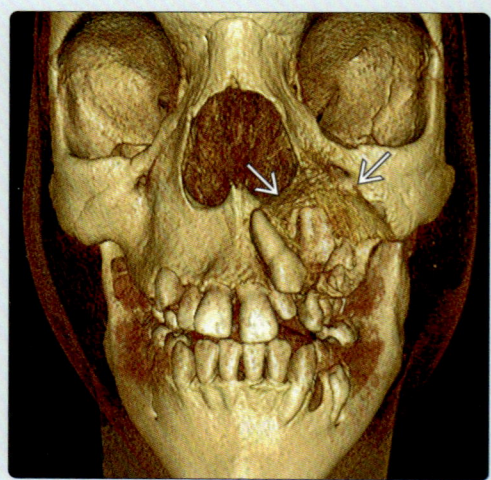

(Left) *Axial bone CT demonstrates multiple bilateral lytic lesions* ➡ *in the maxilla and mandible, typical of odontogenic keratocysts in a 9-year-old boy with basal cell nevus syndrome.* (Right) *Anteroposterior 3D reformation in the same patient shows to better advantage the effect of the largest lesion* ➡ *on the adjacent teeth.*

TERMINOLOGY

Abbreviations
- Basal cell nevus syndrome (**BCNS**)

Synonyms
- Gorlin syndrome, **Gorlin-Goltz syndrome**, nevoid basal cell carcinoma syndrome (NBCCS), nevoid basal cell carcinoma (NBCCa) syndrome

Definitions
- **Autosomal dominant** disorder with multiple odontogenic keratocysts (OKCs), basal cell carcinomas (BCCs), intracranial dural Ca++, bifid ribs ± medulloblastoma

IMAGING

General Features
- Best diagnostic clue
  - Multiple **expansile**, lucent mandible & maxilla lesions
- Location: Mandible >> maxilla
- Size: 1-9 cm, average = 3 cm
- Morphology: unilocular or multilocular

Radiographic Findings
- Radiography
  - Expansile cysts, may have "cloudy" lumen
    - May displace developing teeth ± resorption of roots of erupted teeth & tooth extrusion
  - Rib anomalies, short 4th metacarpals, thick calvarium

CT Findings
- Distinctly corticated expansile cyst, often with scalloped border, extending along mandible length
- High-attenuation precontrast (hemorrhage ± protein)
- Low-attenuation precontrast due to low-protein concentration; no enhancement of wall or matrix

MR Findings
- Variable: Intermediate to high T1, low to high T2 ± thin peripheral contrast enhancement
- GRE/SWI most sensitive for detection of dural Ca++
- ± perineural spread of head & neck BCCs

DIFFERENTIAL DIAGNOSIS

Periapical (Radicular) Cyst
- Unilocular cyst associated with tooth root
- Associated with dental caries & infection

Dentigerous (Follicular) Cyst
- Single unilocular cyst surrounds crown of unerupted tooth

Odontogenic Keratocyst (Nonsyndromic)
- Single multilocular cyst with high attenuation

Ameloblastoma
- Can mimic OKC unless enhancing nodule present

PATHOLOGY

General Features
- Etiology
  - Cysts arise from remnants of dental lamina
- Genetics
  - **Autosomal dominant**
  - Mutations of *PTCH1* gene on chromosome arm 9q
    - 40-80% of patients with BCNS
  - Up to 40% of cases are de novo mutations
- Associated abnormalities
  - 3% of patients develop **medulloblastomas**
  - Marked **Ca++ of falx** (80%), dura
  - Multiple skin **BCCas**
  - **Bifid ribs & scoliosis**
  - May have increased incidence of secondary cancers related to ionizing & ultraviolet radiation
  - Rare ameloblastoma & squamous cell carcinoma, cardiac/abdominal/pelvic mesenchymal tumors

CLINICAL ISSUES

Presentation
- Most common signs/symptoms
  - Multiple enlarging jaw masses; may be asymptomatic or present with pain
    - Multiple OKC seen in 80% of cases of BCNS

Demographics
- Age
  - Syndrome apparent by **5-10 years**
  - Patients present by 3rd decade with multiple nevoid BCCas; mean age = 19 years
    - Aggressive lesions after puberty; may metastasize
- Epidemiology
  - 1 case per 57,000-256,000
    - Prevalence likely higher in patients < 20 years old presenting with BCCas

Natural History & Prognosis
- Morbidity & mortality related to occurrence of neoplasms associated with BCNS
- Aggressive behavior with high recurrence rate of OKC

Treatment
- Surgical methods: Marsupialization, decompression, enucleation, curettage, en bloc resection

DIAGNOSTIC CHECKLIST

Consider
- Long-term follow-up for possible recurrences
- Consider BCNS if precocious dural Ca++ & multiple OKCs

Image Interpretation Pearls
- Can be difficult to differentiate new cyst formation vs. recurrence of treated lesions

SELECTED REFERENCES
1. Choi WJ et al: Imaging approach for jaw and maxillofacial bone tumors with updates from the 2022 World Health Organization classification. World J Radiol. 16(8):294-316, 2024
2. Vered M et al: Update from the 5th edition of the World Health Organization Classification of Head and Neck Tumors: Odontogenic and Maxillofacial Bone Tumours. Head Neck Pathol. 16(1):63-75, 2022
3. Batchala PP et al: Imaging of tumor syndromes. Radiol Clin North Am. 59(3):471-500, 2021
4. Kloth K et al: Defining the spectrum, treatment and outcome of patients with genetically confirmed Gorlin syndrome from the HIT-MED Cohort. Front Oncol. 11:756025, 2021

Branchiootorenal Syndrome

TERMINOLOGY

- Branchiootorenal (BOR) syndrome
- Autosomal dominant syndrome
  - Deafness and ear anomalies
  - Branchial anomalies/preauricular pits
  - Renal abnormalities

IMAGING

- Neck: Branchial cleft cyst/sinus/fistulae
- Temporal bone CT findings
  - Dilated eustachian tubes
  - External ear: Variable stenosis/atresia
  - Middle ear: Dysmorphic; fused, malformed ossicles
  - Cochlea
    - Tapered basal turn, hypoplastic and offset middle/apical turns (*EYA1*)
    - "Thorny" apical turn of cochlea (*SIX1*)
  - Semicircular canal anomaly
  - Dilated, bulbous vestibular aqueduct
  - Flared internal auditory canal; anomalous CNVII canal
- Abdominal CT/US findings: Renal cysts, dysplasia, agenesis
- Variable, asymmetric micrognathia

TOP DIFFERENTIAL DIAGNOSES

- Branchiootic syndrome
  - Normal kidneys; BOR genetic overlap
- Otofaciocervical syndrome: BOR genetic overlap
- Congenital external ear and middle ear malformation

PATHOLOGY

- BOR 1: 8q13.3 locus, *EYA1* gene mutation
- BOR 2: 19q13.3 locus, *SIX1* gene mutation

CLINICAL ISSUES

- Clinical presentation
  - Hearing loss (~ 98%)
  - Preauricular tag, pit (~ 84%)
  - Branchial anomalies (~ 70%)
  - Renal anomalies (~ 40%)

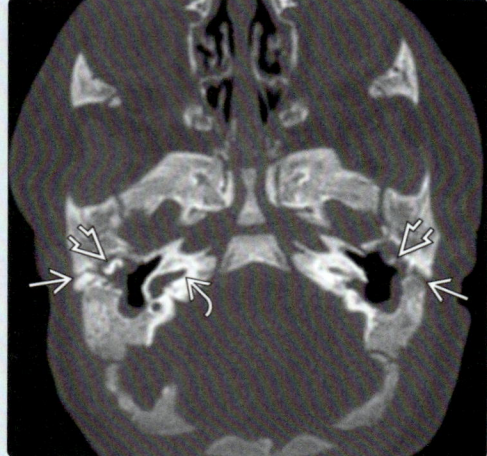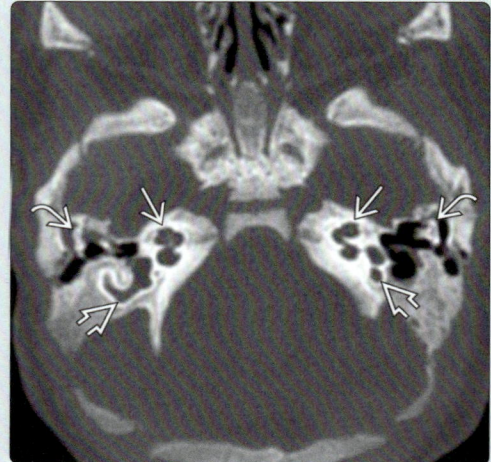

(Left) *Axial bone CT to evaluate microtia in a 10-day-old patient shows bilateral EAC atresia* ➡. *Ossicles* ⇒ *are malformed, fused, and laterally located. Note the tapered basal turn of the right cochlea* ⤴. **(Right)** *Axial bone CT in the same patient shows unwound/offset, hypoplastic middle and apical cochlear turns* ➡ *and deficiency of the right cochlear modiolus. The posterior semicircular canals (SCCs)* ⇒ *and ossicles* ➡ *are malformed. CT findings are characteristic of branchiootorenal (BOR) syndrome.*

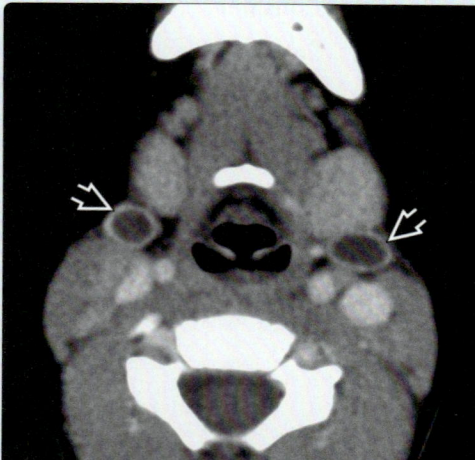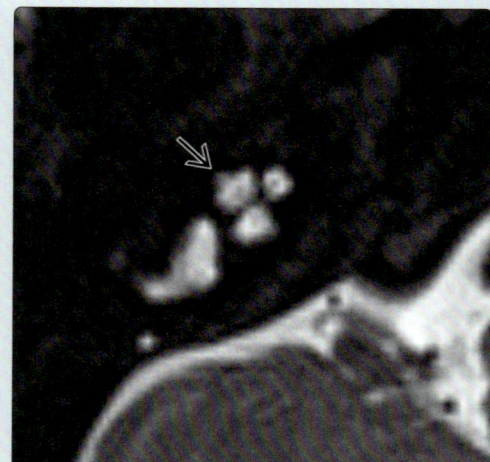

(Left) *Axial CECT in a 2-year-old boy with BOR syndrome shows bilateral, well-defined, nonenhancing cysts* ⇒ *in the typical location of Bailey type II 2nd branchial cleft cysts.* **(Right)** *Axial high-resolution T2 MR in a child with hearing loss shows a recently reported characteristic "thorny" apical turn of the cochlea* ➡ *associated with an SIX1 gene mutation. (Courtesy F. D'Arco, MD.)*

Branchiootorenal Syndrome

TERMINOLOGY

Abbreviations
- Branchiootorenal (BOR) syndrome

Synonyms
- Melnick-Fraser syndrome

Definitions
- Autosomal dominant syndrome
  - Deafness
  - Branchial anomalies/preauricular pits
  - Ear anomalies
  - Renal abnormalities

IMAGING

General Features
- Best diagnostic clue
  - Characteristic cochlear anomalies
    - Tapered basal turn, offset hypoplastic middle and apical turns of cochlea → unwound appearance (*EYA1*)
    - Distinct short protuberant appearance of apical turn of cochlea → "thorny" cochlea (*SIX1*)

CT Findings
- CECT: Preauricular tags, branchial cysts, sinus tracts, and fistulae
- Bone CT
  - Temporal bones findings more common with *EYA1*
  - External auditory canal (EAC): Asymmetric, angulated, and stenotic or atretic
  - Middle ear space: ± underdeveloped and misshapen
  - Ossicles: Dysmorphic, broad incus short process, horizontal orientation long/lenticular process, fusion malleus and incus, ± ossicular fixation
  - Cochlea
    - Tapered basal, offset hypoplastic middle and apical turns of cochlea → unwound appearance (*EYA1*)
    - Distinct short protuberant appearance of apical turn of cochlea → "thorny" cochlea (*SIX1*)
  - Semicircular canals (SCCs): ± globular horizontal SCC, ± absent/hypoplastic posterior SCC
  - Vestibular aqueduct: Dilated, bulbous
  - Internal auditory canal: Flared, widened
  - CNVII canal: Anomalous course labyrinthine segment, obtuse angle anterior genu
  - Skull base
    - Dilated and anomalous eustachian tubes
    - Petrous bone angulation
  - Mandible: Variable asymmetric micrognathia

Ultrasonographic Findings
- Branchial cleft cyst
- Renal abnormalities: Cysts, dysplasia, agenesis

Imaging Recommendations
- Best imaging tool
  - Temporal bone CT
  - US neck and kidneys

DIFFERENTIAL DIAGNOSIS

Branchiootic Syndrome
- Same as BOR except normal kidneys

Otofaciocervical Syndrome
- BOR genetic overlap

Congenital External and Middle Ear Malformation
- CEMEM without syndromic features
- No branchial cleft cyst or renal abnormalities

PATHOLOGY

General Features
- Genetics
  - BOR 1: 8q13.3 locus, *EYA1* gene mutation
  - BOR 2: 19q13.3 locus, *SIX1* gene mutation

CLINICAL ISSUES

Presentation
- Most common signs/symptoms
  - Hearing loss (sensorineural hearing loss, conductive hearing loss, mixed) (~ 98%)
  - Preauricular tag, pit (~ 84%)
  - Branchial anomalies (~ 70%)
  - Renal anomalies (~ 40%)
  - Pinna/EAC anomaly (~ 30%)

Demographics
- Epidemiology
  - 1:40,000; 2% of profoundly deaf children

Natural History & Prognosis
- High penetrance, variable expression: Mild → lethal

Treatment
- Branchial anomalies: Surgical excision
- Ear anomalies: Hearing augmentation, reconstructive surgery as required for microtia, bilateral EAC atresia
- Renal failure: Dialysis, renal transplant

DIAGNOSTIC CHECKLIST

Consider
- Branchiootic syndrome if normal kidneys

Image Interpretation Pearls
- Characteristic **unwound or "thorny" cochlea**
- Look for branchial and renal anomalies

Reporting Tips
- Posterior SCC anomaly often overlooked
- Coronal: Differentiate bulbous VA from jugular vein

SELECTED REFERENCES

1. Lewis M et al: Syndromic hearing loss in children. Neuroimaging Clin N Am. 33(4):563-80, 2023
2. Juliano AF et al: The cochlea in branchio-oto-renal syndrome: an objective method for the diagnosis of offset cochlear turns. AJNR Am J Neuroradiol. 43(11):1646-52, 2022
3. Pao J et al: Re-examining the cochlea in branchio-oto-renal syndrome: genotype-phenotype correlation. AJNR Am J Neuroradiol. 43(2):309-14, 2022

(Left) Axial bone CT in a 4-year-old boy with BOR syndrome shows dilatation of an anomalous eustachian tube ➡ terminating in the sphenoid bone. Some mastoid air cells are opacified ➡. (Right) Coronal bone CT in a 12-year-old boy with BOR syndrome shows angulation of the right EAC ➡ and petrous bones. The right ossicles are malformed and malpositioned in the partially opacified attic ➡. The left EAC is atretic ➡, and the left middle ear cavity is partially opacified.

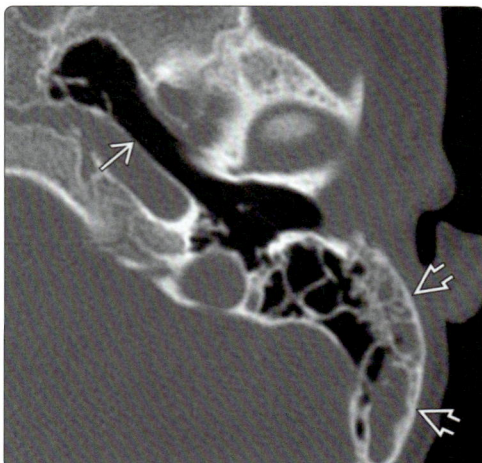
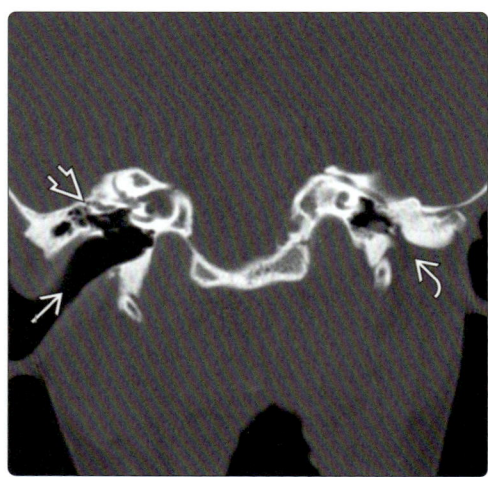

(Left) Axial bone CT in a 5-year-old girl with BOR syndrome shows anterior ligament ossification ➡ fusing the malleus to the attic. Note the hypoplastic middle turn of the cochlea ➡ with an absent modiolus. The vestibular aqueduct is dilated and funnel-shaped ➡. (Right) Coronal bone CT in a 10-year-old boy with preauricular pits and mixed hearing loss shows fusion of malleus to incus and fusion of ossicles to the scutum ➡. Note the horizontal orientation of the cochlear basal turn ➡.

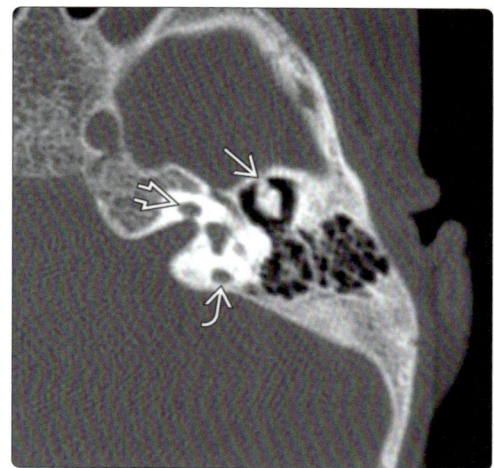
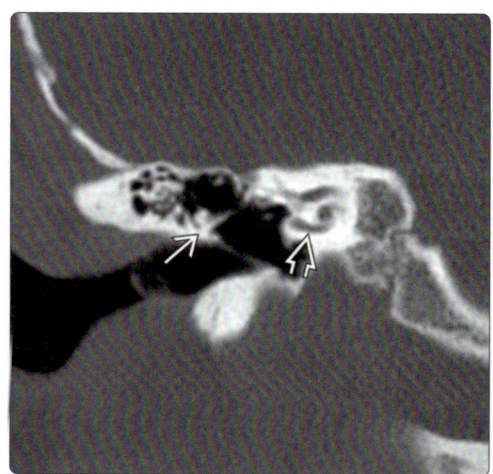

(Left) Axial HRCT in a 4-year-old girl with BOR syndrome shows tapering of the cochlear basal turn ➡ with offset, hypoplastic middle and apical cochlear turns ➡. The ossicles are malformed and partially fused ➡. Mastoid air cells and middle ear cavity are opacified. (Right) Axial HRCT in a 4-year-old boy with BOR syndrome shows similar offset, hypoplastic middle and apical cochlear turns ➡. Malformed ossicles ➡ are partially imaged. Note a small segment of the inferior limb ➡ of the posterior SCC. The superior limb is absent (not shown).

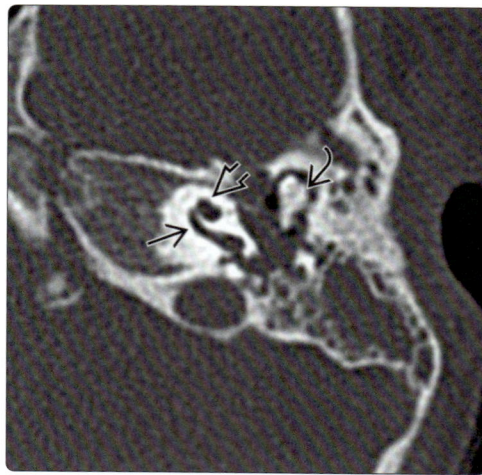
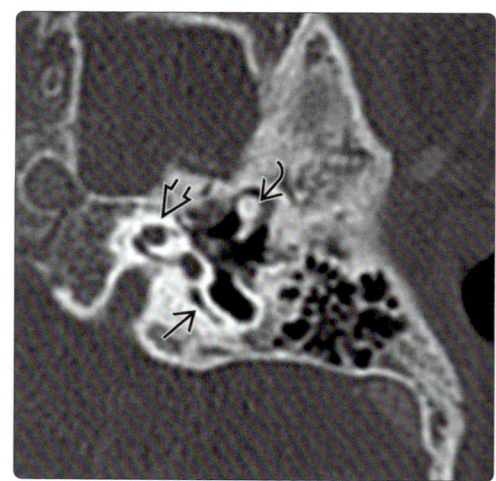

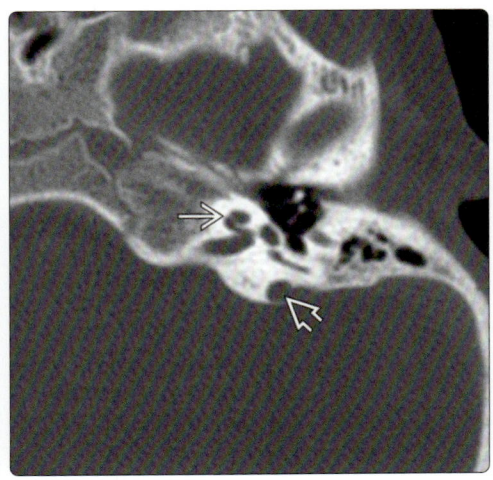

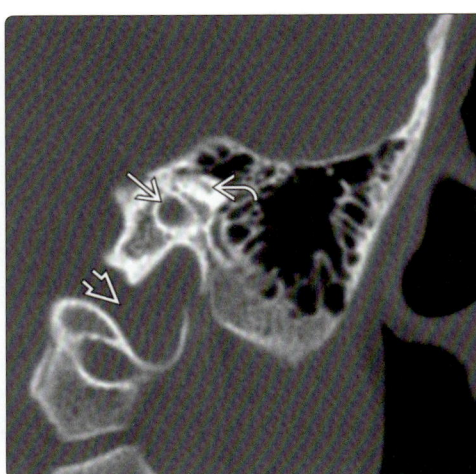

(Left) Axial bone CT in a 5-year-old girl with hearing loss and BOR syndrome shows characteristic hypoplastic middle and apical cochlear turns ➡, which are offset anteriorly. Bulbous enlargement of the vestibular aqueduct ➡ is also seen. (Right) Coronal bone CT in a 5-year-old boy shows the utility of coronal imaging in distinguishing the dilated vestibular aqueduct ➡ above from the jugular fossa below ➡. Note the hypoplastic posterior SCC ➡.

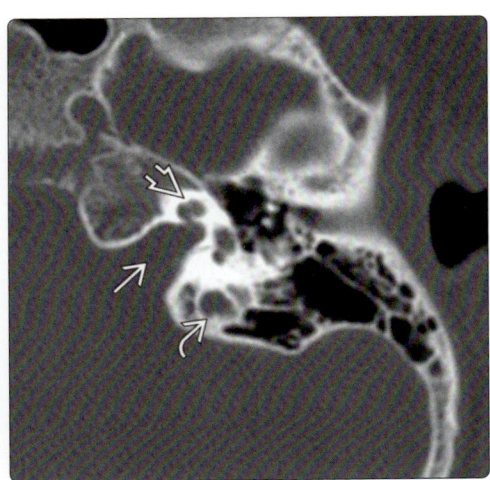

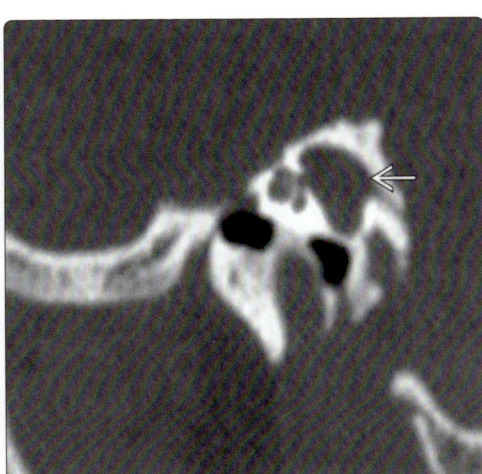

(Left) Axial bone CT in the same patient shows the broad and funnel-shaped internal auditory meatus ➡. Note also the typical hypoplastic middle and apical turns of the cochlea ➡ and rounded enlargement of the vestibular aqueduct ➡. (Right) Sagittal reformatted bone CT in a 14-year-old boy with BOR syndrome shows the bulbous morphology of the internal auditory canal ➡.

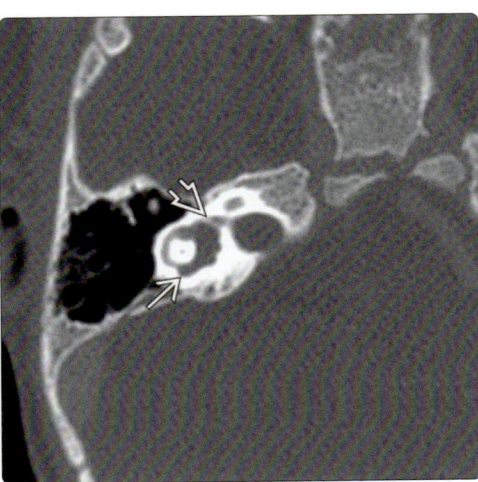

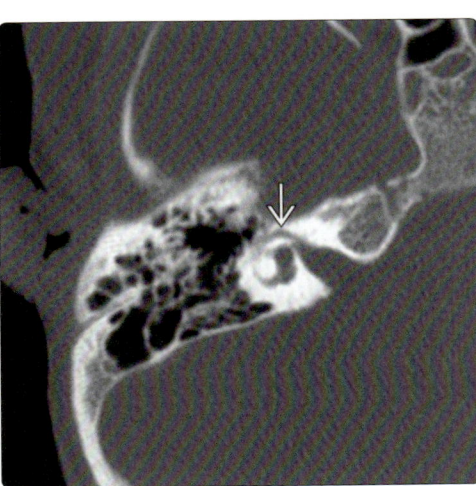

(Left) Axial bone CT in a 19-month-old patient with hearing loss and preauricular pits shows an anomalous posterior SCC ➡. The canal ➡ for the superior vestibular nerve is identified. However, the labyrinthine segment of CNVII is not seen on this image, as it would be in a normal exam. (Right) Axial bone CT in the same patient, more cephalad, shows the anomalous labyrinthine segment of the facial nerve and obtuse angle of the anterior genu ➡.

TERMINOLOGY

- **CHARGE**
  - **C**oloboma
  - **H**eart anomaly
  - **A**tresia choanae
  - **R**estricted growth and development: Mental and somatic development
  - **G**enital hypoplasia
  - **E**ar abnormalities
- Major signs: Coloboma, choanal atresia, semicircular canal (SCC) hypoplasia/aplasia, cranial nerve (CN) involvement
- Minor signs: Hindbrain, external/middle ear, cardiac/esophageal malformations, hypothalamo-hypophyseal dysfunction, intellectual disability

IMAGING

- Choanal atresia, coloboma (variable), cleft lip/palate
- Hypoplastic, misshapen vestibule and markedly hypoplastic or absent SCCs
- Mildly flattened apical ± middle turns + thickened modiolus or single cochlear turn/hypoplasia
- Stenotic/atretic cochlear nerve canal
- Stenotic/atretic oval window ± overlying anomalous tympanic segment of CNVII
- Large emissary veins, hypoplasia basiocciput, clival cleft, basilar invagination, and vertebral anomalies
- Hypoplastic pons, uplifted vermis ± cerebellar malformation; CN hypoplasia/aplasia (mainly CNI, CNVII, and CNVIII)

TOP DIFFERENTIAL DIAGNOSES

- VACTERL association
- Kallmann syndrome: Allelic, less severe
- Branchiootorenal syndrome

PATHOLOGY

- *CHD7* mutation up to 95%
- Highly predictive of CHARGE: Cup-shaped pinna, agenesis/hypoplasia SCC, arrhinencephaly

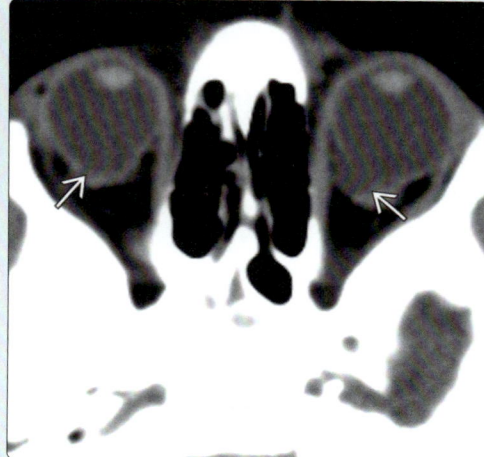
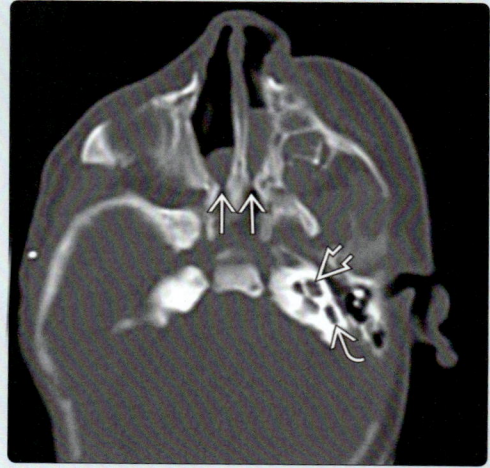

(Left) Axial NECT in an 8-week-old with congenital heart disease and a CHD7 mutation shows bilateral posterior colobomas ➡. (Right) Axial bone CT in a child with CHARGE syndrome shows bilateral bony choanal atresia ➡ and retained fluid in the nasal cavities (right greater than left). Notice also mildly hypoplastic apical/middle turns of the left cochlea ➡ and severe hypoplasia of the left vestibule ➡, all findings typical of patients with CHARGE syndrome.

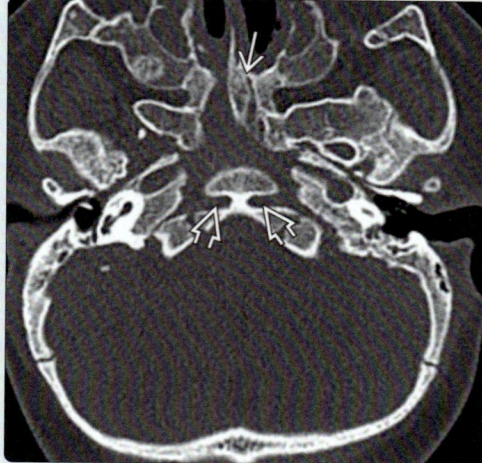
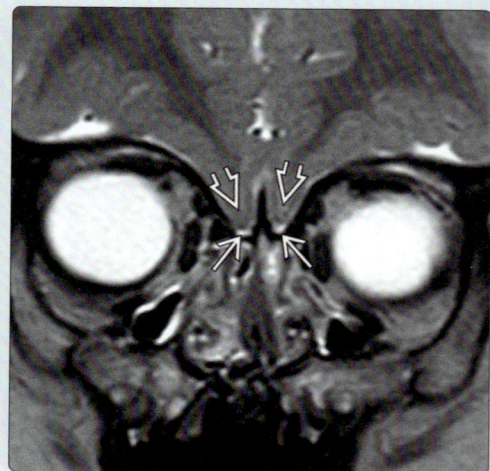

(Left) Axial bone CT in a 1-year-old with CHARGE syndrome, status post repair of bilateral choanal atresia, shows residual bony choanal atresia of the left upper choana ➡ and smooth, bilateral, coronally oriented cleft in the clivus ➡, a common finding in patients with CHARGE syndrome. (Right) Coronal T2 MR in the same patient shows absence of the bilateral olfactory bulbs ➡ and absence of the normally formed olfactory sulci ➡.

TERMINOLOGY

Synonyms

- CHARGE association, Hall-Hittner syndrome

Definitions

- **CHARGE** acronym: **C**oloboma, **H**eart anomaly, **A**tresia choanae, **R**estricted growth and development (mental and somatic development), **G**enital hypoplasia, **E**ar abnormalities

IMAGING

CT Findings

- Bone CT
  - Nose: **Choanal atresia**
  - Eyes: **Coloboma**
  - Face and oral cavity: **Cleft lip/palate**
  - Temporal bones
    - **Vestibule: Hypoplastic and misshapen**
    - **SCC: Markedly hypoplastic or absent**
    - Cochlea: Flattened apical ± middle turns + thickened modiolus or single cochlear turn/hypoplasia
      - Range from normal → hypoplastic upper cochlea → dysmorphic second 1/2 of basal turn + hypoplastic upper cochlear → abnormal first 1/2 of basal turn + severely hypoplastic second 1/2 basal turn and remainder of cochlea
    - Cochlear nerve canal: Stenotic/atretic
    - Vestibular aqueduct: Normal or bulbous endolymphatic duct
    - Oval window: Stenotic/atretic
    - Cranial nerve (CN) VII: Anomalous, hypoplastic, ± dehiscent tympanic segment
    - Ossicles: Dysmorphic, fused
  - Skull base and spine: Jugular foraminal stenosis and large emissary veins; hypoplasia of basiocciput, coronal clival cleft and spinal anomalies

MR Findings

- Hypoplastic pons (common), uplifted vermis ± cerebellar malformation
- Hypoplasia/aplasia of CN: Primarily CNI, CNVII, and CNVIII
- Hypoplasia of basiocciput and vertebral anomalies

Imaging Recommendations

- Best imaging tool
  - CT: Temporal bones, face, nose, clivus, and spine
  - MR: Brain, clivus, orbits, inner ears, CNs, and spine
- Protocol advice
  - Axial bone CT for choanal atresia; MR brain, orbit and 3D T2 (e.g., SPACE, FIESTA) inner ears and CN

DIFFERENTIAL DIAGNOSIS

VACTERL Association

- **V**ertebral/vascular, **a**nal/auricular, **c**ardiac, **t**racheoesophageal fistula, **e**sophageal atresia, **r**enal/radial/rib, **l**imb anomalies

Kallmann Syndrome

- Allelic, less severe

Branchiootorenal Syndrome

- Unwound cochlea distinguishes from CHARGE

PATHOLOGY

General Features

- Genetics
  - Gene map locus 8q12.1, 7q21.11
  - *CHD7* gene mutation in up to 95%
    - > 1000 mutations identified, most de novo
      - Most are frameshift or nonsense mutations → haploinsufficiency

Staging, Grading, & Classification

- Major diagnostic characteristics
  - Coloboma, choanal atresia, CN aplasia/hypoplasia (CNI, CNVII, CNVIII, CNIX-X), temporal bone anomalies (90%)
- Minor diagnostic characteristics
  - Genital hypoplasia, developmental delay, cardiac, growth deficiency, orofacial cleft, tracheoesophageal fistula, abnormal faces
- **Definite CHARGE syndrome**: Child with all 4 major characteristics or 3 major and 3 minor characteristics

CLINICAL ISSUES

Presentation

- Most common signs/symptoms
  - Airway obstruction, feeding difficulty, GE reflux
  - Facial dysmorphism, cleft lip/palate
  - Low-set, cup-shaped ears and deafness
  - Cardiac symptoms (e.g., TOF)
  - Growth retardation
  - Genital hypoplasia (central hypogonadism)
  - Coloboma, microphthalmia, anosmia
  - Developmental delay/autism

DIAGNOSTIC CHECKLIST

Consider

- CHARGE inner ear anomaly highly characteristic

Image Interpretation Pearls

- Oval window atresia ± aberrant/dehiscent CNVII canal: CT
- MR for absent CNs, abnormal pons, and clivus

SELECTED REFERENCES

1. Lewis MA et al: The spectrum of cochlear malformations in CHARGE syndrome and insights into the role of the CHD7 gene during embryogenesis of the inner ear. Neuroradiology. 65(4):819-34, 2023
2. Lewis M et al: Syndromic hearing loss in children. Neuroimaging Clin N Am. 33(4):563-80, 2023
3. Robson CD: Conductive hearing loss in children. Neuroimaging Clin N Am. 33(4):543-62, 2023
4. da Costa Monsanto R et al: Otopathologic abnormalities in CHARGE syndrome. Otolaryngol Head Neck Surg. 166(2):363-72, 2021
5. Ginat DT: Imaging findings in syndromes with temporal bone abnormalities. Neuroimaging Clin N Am. 29(1):117-28, 2019
6. Mahdi ES et al: Clival malformations in CHARGE syndrome. AJNR Am J Neuroradiol. 39(6):1153-6, 2018
7. Hoch MJ et al: Head and neck MRI findings in CHARGE syndrome. AJNR Am J Neuroradiol. 38(12):2357-63, 2017

(Left) Axial bone CT in a 1-year-old boy with CHARGE syndrome shows a prominent modiolus ➔, cochlear nerve canal stenosis ➔, small vestibule ➔, absent semicircular canals (SCCs), abnormal course of vestibular aqueduct ➔, and opacified middle ear cavity and mastoid air cells. (Right) Axial bone CT in a 13-month-old boy with a CHD7 mutation shows a thick modiolus ➔, small vestibule ➔, absent SCCs, narrow malleoincudal joint ➔, middle ear and mastoid air cell opacification, and a large emissary vein ➔.

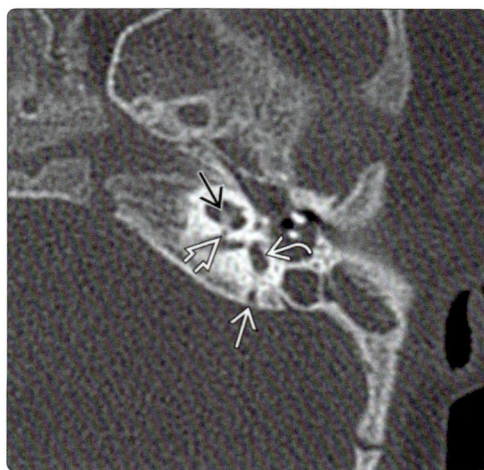
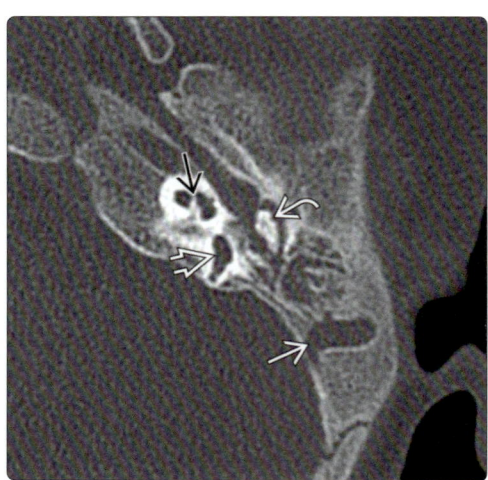

(Left) Axial bone CT in a 16-month-old boy with CHARGE syndrome and a CHD7 mutation shows a single amorphous, unsegmented cochlear turn ➔. The incus and stapes form a single solid bar that is inferiorly angulated ➔. (Right) Axial bone CT in the same patient demonstrates the cephalad aspect of the cochlea ➔, essentially isolated from the internal auditory canal (IAC) ➔. The vestibule is hypoplastic ➔, and the SCCs are absent. The middle ear cavity and mastoid air cells are opacified.

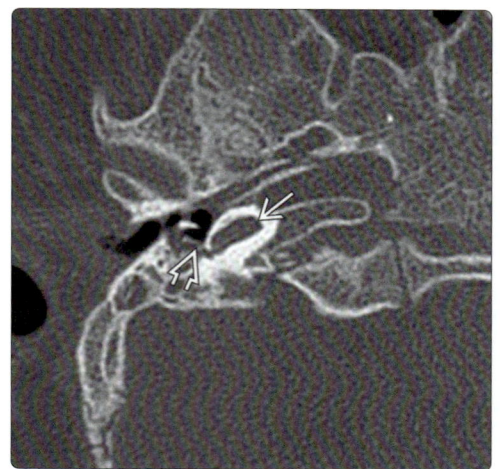
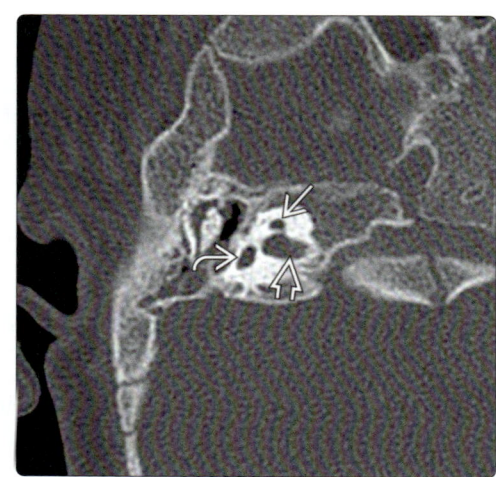

(Left) Coronal bone CT in a 1.5-year-old boy with a CHD7 mutation shows the tympanic segment of CNVII ➔ overlying oval window atresia, hypoplastic vestibule ➔, and absent SCCs. (Right) Coronal bone CT in a 7-year-old girl with CHARGE syndrome shows cervical spine anomaly ➔, petrous angulation, hypoplastic vestibule, and absent SCCs. The facial nerve canal is dehiscent and overlies the atretic oval window ➔. The ossicles contact the facial nerve. A large emissary vein indents the tegmen tympani ➔.

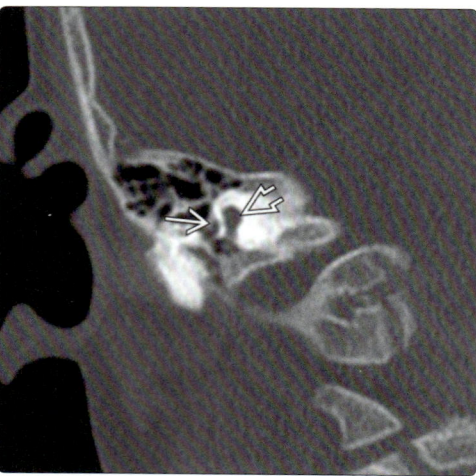
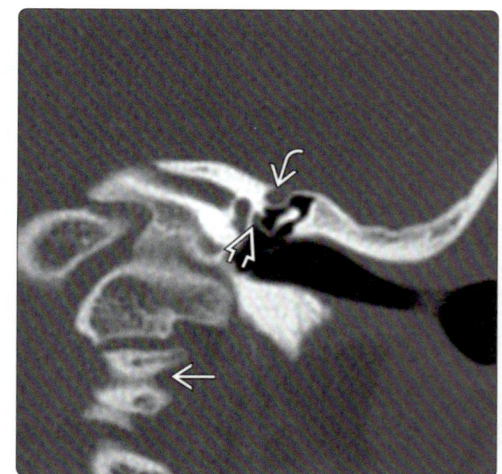

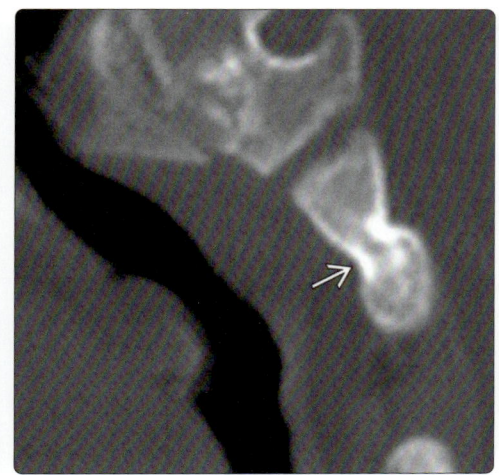

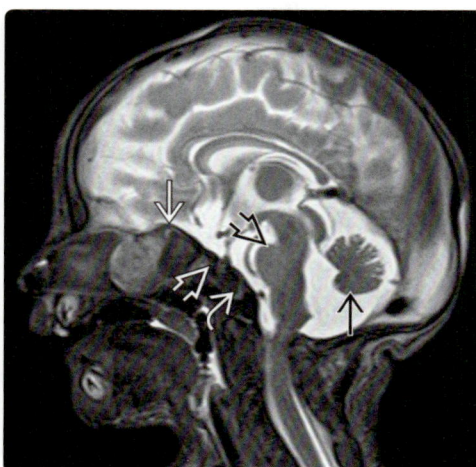

(Left) *Reformatted sagittal bone CT in a 7-month-old boy with CHARGE syndrome shows deformity and constriction of the basiocciput ➡.* (Right) *Sagittal T2 MR in a 4-day-old boy with a CHD7 mutation shows convexity of the planum sphenoidale ➡, inferior placement of the sella ➡, and a hypoplastic basiocciput ➤. There is uplifting of the vermis with mild inferior vermian hypoplasia ➡ and a mildly prominent 4th ventricle. The pons appears shortened ➡ as well, not uncommon in children with CHARGE syndrome.*

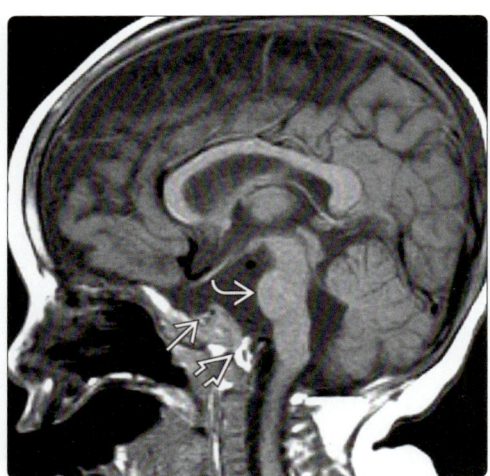

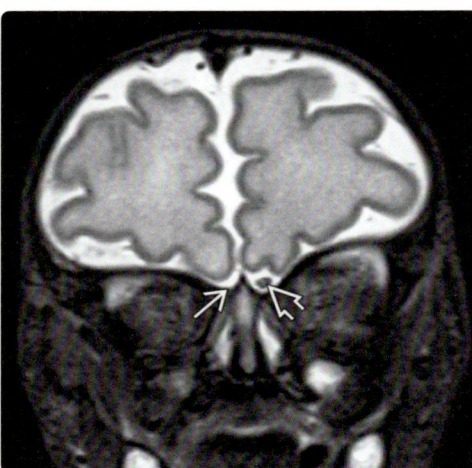

(Left) *Sagittal T1 MR in a 16-month-old boy with a CHD7 mutation demonstrates a partially empty sella ➡, and the infundibulum is not seen. Note the severe hypoplasia of the basiocciput ➡ and basilar invagination. The pons is hypoplastic ➤.* (Right) *Coronal T2 STIR in a 4-day-old boy with a CHD7 mutation reveals absence of the right olfactory bulb ➡. Note the prominent left olfactory bulb ➡.*

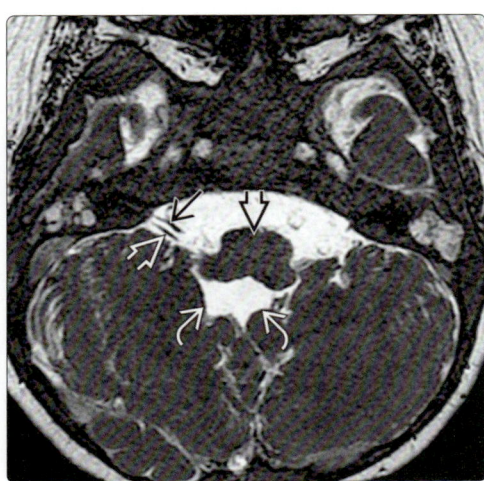

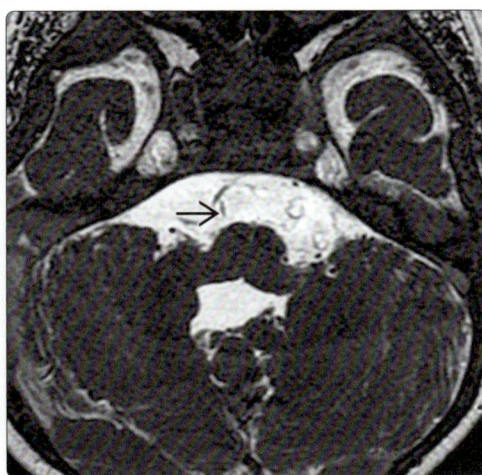

(Left) *Axial 3D FIESTA MR in a 16-month-old patient with CHARGE syndrome shows the right CNVII ➡ and CNVIII ➡. The left CNVII and CNVIII are absent. The pons is hypoplastic and rotated ➡, and the 4th ventricle is asymmetric ➤.* (Right) *Axial 3D FIESTA MR more cephalad in the same patient shows the right CNVI ➡. The left CNVI is absent. CNI, CNVI, CNVII, &/or CNVIII may be hypoplastic/absent in patients with CHARGE syndrome.*

TERMINOLOGY

- Oculoauriculovertebral spectrum, Goldenhar syndrome, facioauriculovertebral sequence
- Defect of 1st & 2nd pharyngeal arch derivatives ± neural crest cells

IMAGING

- Mandibular hypoplasia
  - Unilateral; rarely bilateral & asymmetric
- Zygomatic arch hypoplasia
- Hypoplasia muscles of mastication, facial muscles, & parotid gland
- External auditory canal atresia/stenosis
- Middle ear hypoplasia & ossicular malformation/fusion
- Oval window atresia & CNVII anomaly/hypoplasia
- Cervical spine fusion/segmentation anomalies (Klippel-Feil anomaly)
- CNS (variable): Ventriculomegaly, brainstem cleft, cerebellar hypoplasia, cephalocele

TOP DIFFERENTIAL DIAGNOSES

- Teratogenic embryopathy (e.g., diabetes)
- Townes-Brocks syndrome
- Branchiootorenal syndrome
- Treacher Collins syndrome

CLINICAL ISSUES

- Common disorder, prevalence ~ 1 in 3,500 births
- Microtia/anotia, preauricular skin tags
- Hearing loss (~ 85%; CHL > > SNHL)
- Facial asymmetry; unilateral micrognathia
- Facial nerve weakness (~ 50%)
- Variable facial clefts
- Epibulbar lipodermoid, coloboma
- TEF, cardiac, genitourinary, pulmonary abnormalities

DIAGNOSTIC CHECKLIST

- HFM as cause of facial asymmetry & external ear anomalies
- Facial weakness due to CNVII anomaly/hypoplasia

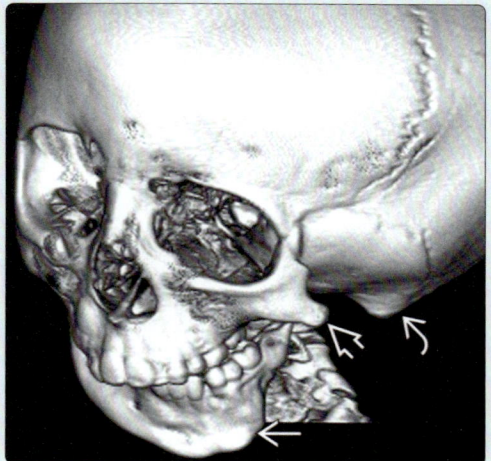
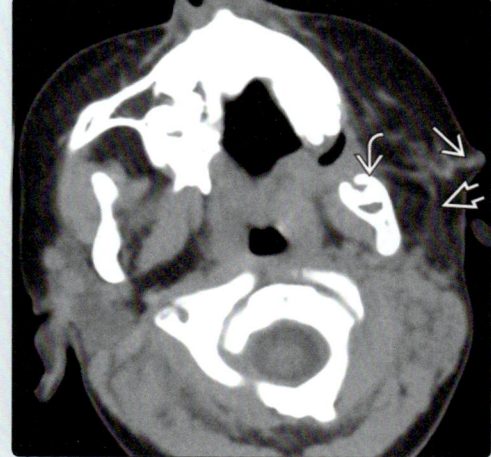

(Left) *3D NECT in a 7-year-old girl with hemifacial microsomia (HFM) reveals a smaller left hemimandible ➡, hypoplasia of the zygomatic arch ➡, underdevelopment of the mastoid process ➡, & external auditory canal (EAC) atresia.* (Right) *Axial NECT in a 4-year-old girl with HFM demonstrates a smaller left mandibular ramus ➡, a preauricular sinus tract, & a skin tag ➡. The left muscles of mastication are underdeveloped, & the masticator muscle and parotid tissue are not seen in their expected location ➡.*

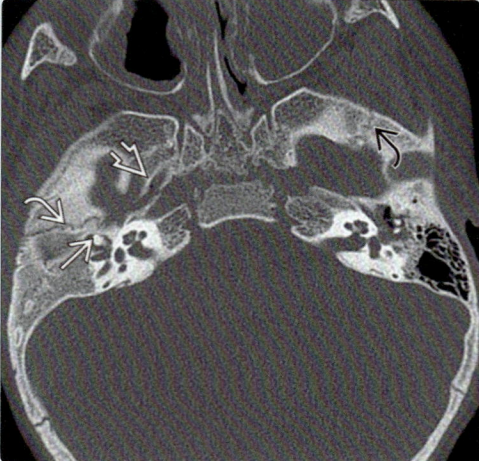
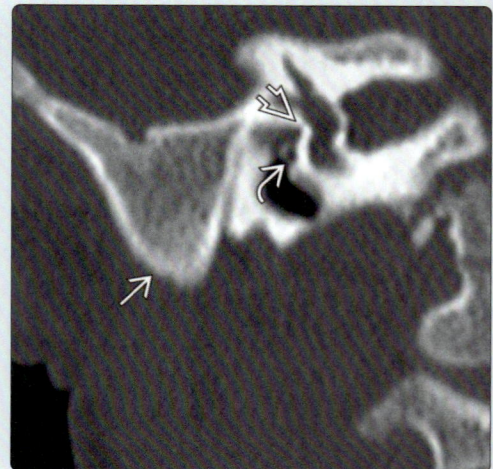

(Left) *Axial bone CT in a 23-month-old boy with HFM shows that the right middle ear cavity is hypoplastic & opacified. The ossicles ➡ are dysmorphic. The right eustachian tube is dilated & anomalous ➡. The right sphenosquamosal suture ➡ is rotated laterally compared with the left ➡.* (Right) *Reformatted coronal bone CT in the same patient shows absent mastoid pneumatization ➡, oval window atresia ➡, and an anomalous inferior course of CNVII tympanic segment ➡ running over the promontory.*

Hemifacial Microsomia

TERMINOLOGY

Abbreviations
- Hemifacial microsomia (HFM)

Synonyms
- Oculoauriculovertebral spectrum, Goldenhar syndrome, facioauriculovertebral sequence

Definitions
- Defect of 1st & 2nd pharyngeal arch derivatives ± neural crest cells
  - **External & middle ear** anomalies
  - Typically unilateral mandibular & TMJ hypoplasia
  - Hypoplastic muscles of mastication & facial muscles

IMAGING

General Features
- Best diagnostic clue
  - **Unilateral** mandibular hypoplasia, deficient zygomatic arch, & external auditory canal (EAC) atresia/stenosis

CT Findings
- Bone CT
  - **Micrognathia**: Typically unilateral; less commonly, bilateral and asymmetric; TMJ hypoplasia or aplasia
  - **Hypoplastic/deficient zygomatic arch**
  - Hypoplasia muscles of mastication & facial muscles
  - Parotid hypoplasia/aplasia ± prominent accessory parotid
  - Temporal bone: **Congenital external & middle ear malformation (CEMEM)**
    - EAC: Stenosis/atresia, small/absent tympanic plate
    - Mastoid: ± variable degrees of ↓ pneumatization
    - Middle ear space: Variable degrees of hypoplasia
    - Ossicles: Malformed, rotated, fused
    - Oval window: ± stenosis or atresia
    - CNVII canal [facial nerve canal (FNC)]: Normal or hypoplastic FNC
      □ Tympanic FNC ± dehiscent/aberrant
      □ Mastoid FNC exits ventrally, sometimes into TMJ
    - Inner ear: Occasional malformation
  - Face: ± facial cleft; ± other structures involved, e.g., orbit
  - Spine: ± fusion/segmentation anomalies

MR Findings
- **Mandibular hypoplasia & small muscles of mastication**
- Spine: ± **vertebral anomalies**
- CNS: ± ventriculomegaly, occasional brainstem cleft, cerebellar hypoplasia, cephalocele
- **CNVII: Normal, hypoplasia, or aplasia,** ± aberrant

DIFFERENTIAL DIAGNOSIS

Teratogenic Embryopathy (e.g., Diabetes)
- Mandibular & temporal bone anomalies depend on etiology

Townes-Brocks Syndrome
- Simulates Goldenhar phenotype; CEMEM; hand, renal, & anal anomalies

Branchiootorenal Syndrome
- Variable asymmetric micrognathia

- CEMEM, large eustachian tubes
- Tapered cochlear basal turn; small, offset middle/apical turns → unwound appearance

Treacher Collins Syndrome
- Bilateral, usually symmetric micrognathia, hypoplastic zygomatic arches, CEMEM

Condylar Hypoplasia
- Abnormally small condyle with normal shape, small mandibular fossa, & ipsilateral hemimandible

PATHOLOGY

General Features
- Etiology
  - Common disorder, prevalence ~ 1 in 3,500 live births
  - 2nd most common craniofacial birth defect after cleft lip & palate
  - Genetic & environmental factors implicated
  - Sporadic, rarely familial

Staging, Grading, & Classification
- **OMENS** clinical classification (for severity score)
  - **O**rbital asymmetry
  - **M**andibular hypoplasia
  - **E**ar deformity
  - **N**erve dysfunction
  - **S**oft tissue deficiency

CLINICAL ISSUES

Presentation
- Most common signs/symptoms
  - Facial asymmetry (~ 100%): Unilateral micrognathia ± maxillary hypoplasia, clefting, ± CNVII weakness
  - Ear (~ 100%): Microtia/anotia, preauricular skin tags, EAC stenosis/atresia, hearing loss [~ 85%; conductive hearing loss (CHL) > sensorineural hearing loss (SNHL)]
  - Eye (72%): Epibulbar lipodermoid, coloboma, microphthalmia, visual impairment (28%)
  - Cervical spine deformity
  - CNS: Hydrocephalus, cephalocele, intellectual disabilities
- Other signs/symptoms
  - Tracheoesophageal fistula (TEF)/esophageal atresia
  - Cardiac, pulmonary, & genitourinary anomalies

Treatment
- Mandibular reconstruction, hearing aids/ear surgery

DIAGNOSTIC CHECKLIST

Consider
- HFM as cause of facial asymmetry & external ear anomalies
- CNVII anomaly/hypoplasia as cause of facial weakness

SELECTED REFERENCES

1. Patino M et al: Fetal head and neck imaging. Magn Reson Imaging Clin N Am. 32(3):413-30, 2024
2. Estandia-Ortega B et al: Proposed clinical approach and imaging studies in families with oculo-auriculo-vertebral spectrum to assess variable expressivity. Am J Med Genet A. 188(5):1515-25, 2022

TERMINOLOGY

- Treacher Collins syndrome (TCS)
- Nager syndrome: TCS + limb anomalies
- Craniofacial malformation: Downslanting palpebral fissures, micrognathia, zygomatic and malar hypoplasia, microtia/anotia, ± limb defects

IMAGING

- Temporal bone findings
  - External auditory canal (EAC): Stenosis/atresia, small/absent tympanic plate
  - Decreased/absent mastoid pneumatization
  - Hypoplastic/atretic middle ear space
  - Malformed or absent ossicles ± fixation
  - Oval window stenosis/atresia
  - Facial nerve canal anomalies/dehiscence
  - Normal or malformed cochlea (flattened turns)
  - Normal or malformed lateral semicircular canal (SCC) ± vestibule

- Relatively symmetric micrognathia, zygomatic/malar hypoplasia
- Coloboma, hypoplastic muscles of mastication, absent or hypoplastic parotid glands

TOP DIFFERENTIAL DIAGNOSES

- Bilateral facial microsomia; nonsyndromic congenital external and middle ear malformation
- Branchiootorenal syndrome

PATHOLOGY

- Autosomal dominant > > recessive, phenotypic variability and genetic heterogeneity, "ribosomopathy"
- TCS: *TCOF1*, *POLR1D*, and *POLR1C* gene mutations
- Nager syndrome: *SF3B4* gene mutation

CLINICAL ISSUES

- Airway obstruction, deafness
- Treatment: Airway support, reconstructive surgery, hearing aids, developmental support

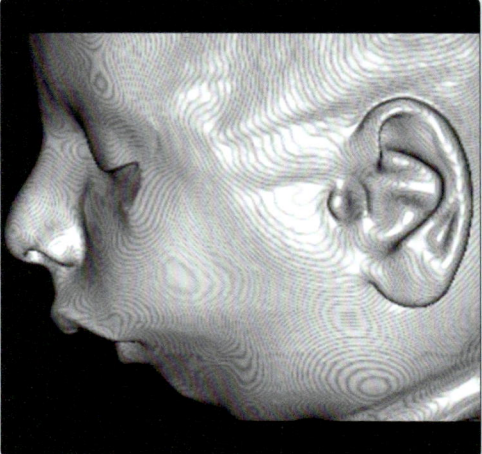
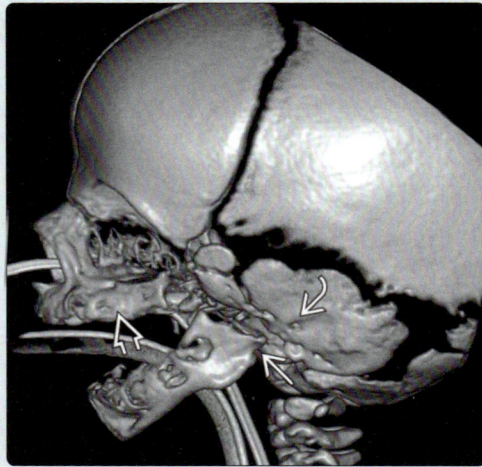

(Left) *3D surface-rendered CT in infant with Nager syndrome [Treacher Collins syndrome (TCS) + limb anomalies] shows micrognathia, malar flattening, mildly low-set ears, & external auditory meatus atresia.* (Right) *3D CT in a 1-month-old shows a broad mandibular angle, hypoplasia of mandibular condyle ➡, flat malar eminence ➡, absent zygomatic arch, & EAC atresia ➡. Abnormalities were bilateral & symmetric; clinically, patient had low-set, malformed pinnae & downslanting palpebral fissures, typical of TCS.*

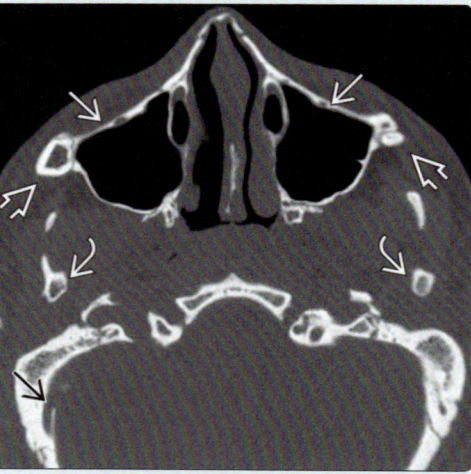
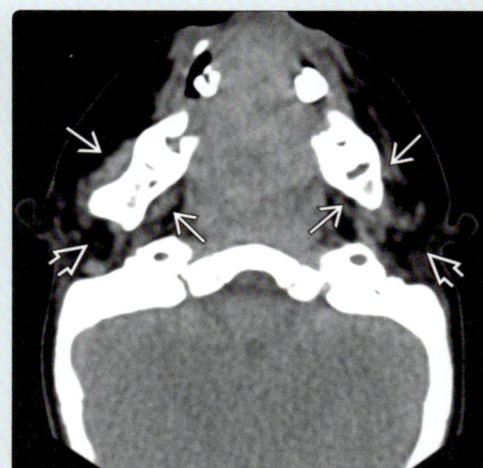

(Left) *Axial bone CT in a 13-year-old girl with TCS shows zygomatic complex hypoplasia with posteriorly slanted maxillae ➡, absent zygomatic arches ➡, & hypoplastic mandibular condyles ➡. Note EAC atresia, absent mastoid pneumatization, & an enlarged mastoid emissary vein ➡.* (Right) *Axial soft tissue CT in a 1-year-old child with TCS shows bilateral mandibular hypoplasia, EAC atresia, microtia with hypoplastic muscles of mastication ➡ & aplasia of the parotid glands ➡.*

Pierre Robin Sequence

TERMINOLOGY

- Pierre Robin sequence (PRS); PRS triad: Micrognathia, glossoptosis, airway obstruction

IMAGING

- Bilateral, usually symmetric **micrognathia**
- **Glossoptosis**: Elevated, posteriorly displaced tongue
- Posterior **U-shaped cleft palate**
- Additional features depend on syndromic etiology
- Temporal bone
  - External auditory canal (EAC): Normal, stenotic (e.g., Stickler syndrome) or atretic [e.g., Treacher Collins syndrome (TCS), Nager syndrome]
  - Middle ear & mastoid: Normal or hypoplastic ± opacification
  - Ossicles: Normal, mildly malformed [e.g., stapes in velocardiofacial syndrome (VCFS)], or severely malformed ± fixation (e.g., TCS)
  - Inner ear: Normal or malformed (e.g., small semicircular canal bone island/anlage anomaly in VCFS & TCS)

TOP DIFFERENTIAL DIAGNOSES

- Stickler & related syndromes (18% of PRS); VCFS (~ 7% of PRS); TCS (~ 5% of PRS)

PATHOLOGY

- Primary micrognathia → glossoptosis → failure of palatal shelf elevation & fusion; 22q11.2 deletion: VCFS
- Collagen (*COL*) gene mutations: Stickler syndromes

CLINICAL ISSUES

- Feeding & breathing difficulties, failure to thrive
- Stickler: Progressive myopia, joint degeneration
- VCFS: Cardiac anomalies, adenoidal hypoplasia, velopharyngeal insufficiency, medial deviation of cervical internal carotid arteries, learning difficulties
- TCS: Malar flattening, downslanting palpebral fissures, coloboma

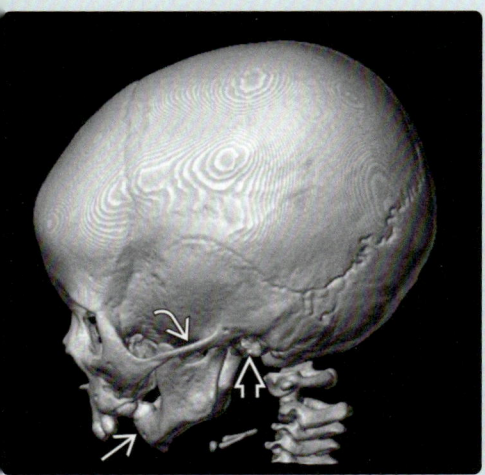
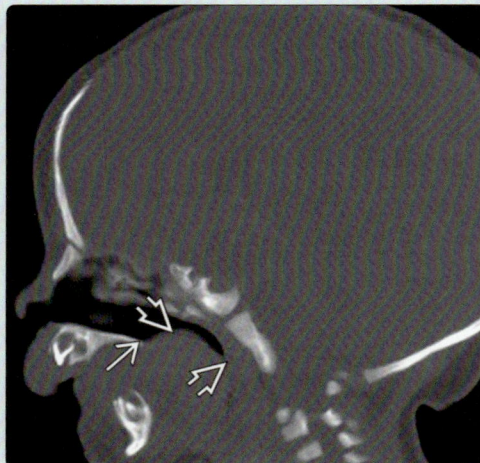

(Left) Lateral 3D surface-rendered image in a 1-year-old with Pierre Robin sequence (PRS) shows significant, symmetric micrognathia ➡ with a normal external auditory canal ➡ & zygomatic arch ➡. (Right) Sagittal CT reconstruction in a 3-week-old with PRS reveals a shortened hard palate ➡ & glossoptosis (abnormal downward or backward displacement of the tongue) ➡. The tongue, which protrudes above & behind the palate, obstructs the oropharynx, resulting in difficulty with breathing & feeding.

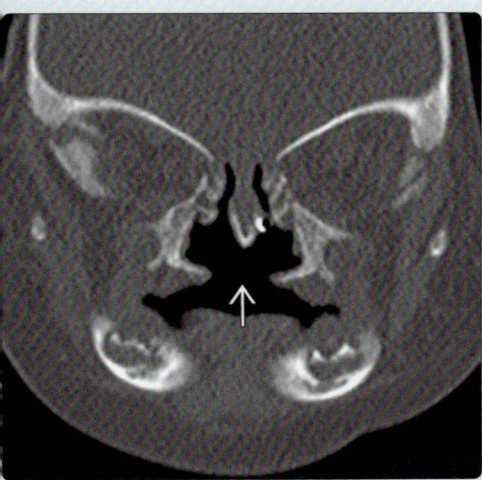
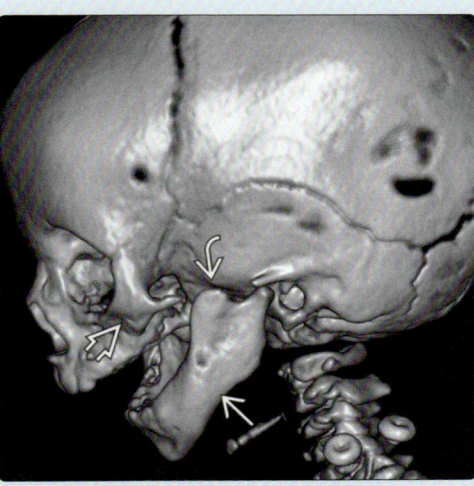

(Left) Coronal bone CT in a 1-week-old infant with bilateral symmetric micrognathia & glossoptosis shows a wide cleft ➡ in the hard palate typical of patients with PRS. (Right) Lateral 3D bone CT in a 6-month-old with glossoptosis shows micrognathia ➡ & airway obstruction typical of PRS. This patient also has associated maxillary hypoplasia ➡, zygomatic arch deficiency ➡, & digit anomalies (not shown). Patient was found to have Nager syndrome.

X-Linked Stapes Gusher (DFNX2)

TERMINOLOGY

- X-linked mixed hearing loss
- Conductive hearing loss (CHL) with stapes fixation (DFN3)
- Cochlear incomplete partition type III (IP-III)
- Profound SNHL ± CHL + bilateral unique inner ear anomaly

IMAGING

- Cochlea: **Interscalar septa present** but **absent modiolus** & cochlear base → **corkscrew cochlea**
- **Cochlea directly at lateral end of IAC**
- IAC: **Bulbous** dilation + deficient lamina cribrosa; vestibule & semicircular canals (SCCs): ± slightly dilated, ± **superior bulge protruding from vestibule** ± SCC ossification
- **Vestibular aqueduct**: More **medial origin** ± large
- CNVII: **Labyrinthine** segment located almost **above cochlea**; superior most structure in temporal bone CT

TOP DIFFERENTIAL DIAGNOSES

- Cochlear incomplete partition type I (IP-I)

- Large vestibular aqueduct + cochlear incomplete partition type II (IP-II)
- Cochlear hypoplasia type II (CH-II)

PATHOLOGY

- X-linked recessive: **Males** affected, female carriers
- Molecular cause: *POU3F4* gene mutation
- Absent lamina cribrosa → communication between CSF & cochlear perilymph → perilymph hydrops
- **Outer** periosteal & enchondral **layers defective** but with thick inner endosteal layer & normal stapes foot plate

CLINICAL ISSUES

- Bilateral profound SNHL (treat by **cochlear implant**) ± CHL
- **Severe gusher** at cochlear implantation surgery & very high chance of **electrode misplacement into IAC**
- IP-III: **Stapes surgery contraindicated** → gusher & ↑ SNHL

DIAGNOSTIC CHECKLIST

- CT/MR: Widened IAC & IP-III (corkscrew cochlea)

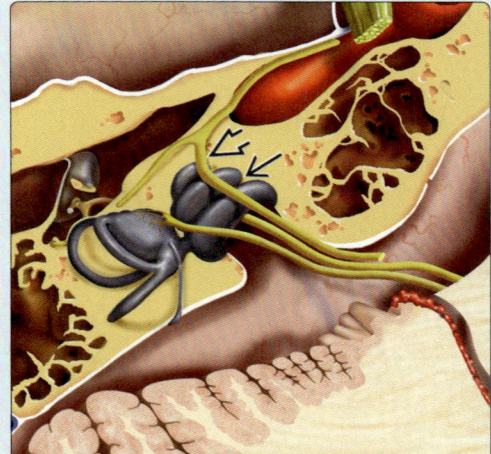 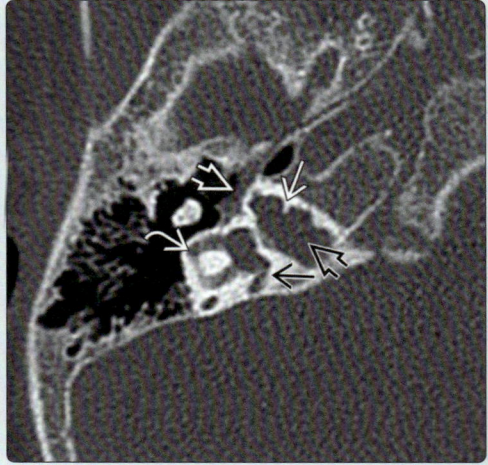

(Left) *Axial graphic of X-linked stapes gusher reveals a corkscrew cochlea (IP-III)* ➡ *with no modiolus. The internal auditory canal (IAC) is small & wide. CNVII labyrinthine segment* ➡ *is superior-most structure in temporal bone located above cochlea.* (Right) *Axial bone CT in a 2-year-old boy with profound SNHL shows a corkscrew cochlea with interscalar septa* ➡ *but absent modiolus. The IAC* ➡ *is wide & merges with cochlea. Note mildly dilated tympanic CNVII canal* ➡*, lateral SCC* ➡*, & vestibular aqueduct (VA)* ➡*. VA has more medial origin.*

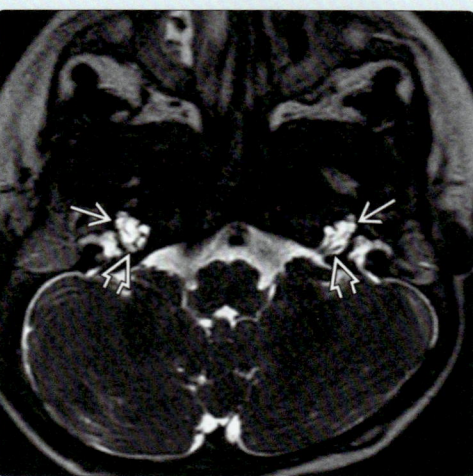 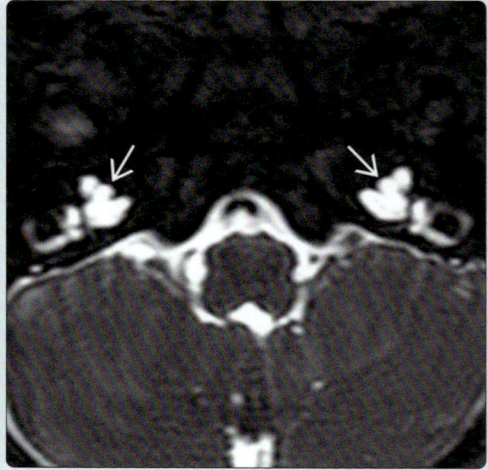

(Left) *Axial FIESTA MR in a 6-month-old with severe SNHL shows corkscrew cochlea with an absent modiolus* ➡*. The IAC is widened* ➡ *& merges with the cochlea.* (Right) *Axial T2 FIESTA MR in a 3-month-old boy with congenital deafness shows a bilateral corkscrew shape to the cochlea* ➡*, typical of X-linked stapes gusher (DFNX2). The IACs were wide & merged with the base of cochlea, & modioli were absent (not shown).*

X-Linked Stapes Gusher (DFNX2)

TERMINOLOGY

Abbreviations
- Deafness X-linked 2 (DFNX2)

Synonyms
- Deafness 3, conductive, with stapes fixation (DFN3)
- X-linked deafness with stapes gusher
- Cochlear **incomplete partition type III (IP-III)**

Definitions
- Profound sensorineural hearing loss (SNHL) ± conductive hearing loss (CHL) + bilateral unique inner ear anomaly
- **IP-III**: Cochlear malformation in X-linked deafness

IMAGING

General Features
- Best diagnostic clue
  - **Bulbous** internal auditory canal (**IAC**) & cochlear **IP-III**

CT Findings
- Bone CT
  - Cochlea: Interscalar septum (ISS) present, absent modiolus & cochlear base → corkscrew appearance (IP-III)
    - Cochlea at lateral end of IAC (vs. usual anterolateral location)
  - Cochlear nerve canal: Widened
  - IAC: Bulbous dilatation laterally, absent lamina cribrosa
  - Vestibule & semicircular canal (SCC): Normal or dilated, ± superior bulge protruding from vestibule ± SCC ossification
  - Vestibular aqueduct (VA): More medial origin than usual with varying degrees of dilatation
  - Facial nerve canal: Labyrinthine segment located almost above cochlea (due to thin otic capsule)
    - Wide labyrinthine & proximal tympanic segments
    - Distal tympanic & mastoid segments normal
  - Oval window/stapes: Normal or atretic

MR Findings
- T2WI
  - Cochlea: **ISS present; modiolus absent**
  - Vestibule & SCC: Usually normal in IP-III ± **superior bulge protruding from vestibule**
    - SCCs may have cystic appearance
  - Endolymphatic sac & duct: **More medial origin** ± large
  - IAC: **Bulbous dilatation laterally**
  - CNVII: Labyrinthine segment above cochlea
  - Hypothalamus may be thickened

DIFFERENTIAL DIAGNOSIS

Cochlear Incomplete Partition Type I (IP-I)
- Absent internal cochlear structure, range from mild (lack of internal cochlear architecture) to severe (figure 8 configuration of cochlea, vestibule SCCs)

Large Vestibular Aqueduct (IP-II)
- Large VA ± absent apical septation & deficient modiolus

Cochlear Hypoplasia Type II (CH-II)
- Defective cochlear modiolus & ISS

PATHOLOGY

General Features
- Genetics
  - Inheritance: **X-linked recessive**
  - Chromosomal locus: **Xq21**; *POU3F4* **gene** mutation

Gross Pathologic & Surgical Features
- Absent lamina cribrosa → subarachnoid space & cochlear perilymph communication → perilymphatic hydrops
- Stapes fixation → perilymph/CSF gusher at stapedectomy
- **IP-III: Defective vascular supply from middle ear**
  - **Outer periosteal & enchondral layers defective** but thick inner endosteal layer & **thickened stapes foot plate**
    - Therefore spontaneous CSF fistula through stapes footplate & recurrent meningitis very rare
- In IP-III, cochlear base defective & modiolus totally absent
  - Cochlear base consists of middle enchondral (main bulk) & inner endosteal layers
  - When enchondral layer absent, inner endosteal layer not enough to form thick base to support modiolus
    - Modiolus cannot form attachment points
  - **Defective cochlear base** & **absent modiolus**, even with normal vascularization of modiolus from IAC

CLINICAL ISSUES

Presentation
- Most common signs/symptoms
  - Males affected; female carriers normal (most) or mild/delayed-onset hearing loss
    - **Bilateral profound SNHL** (may be progressive) ± CHL
- Other signs/symptoms
  - Spontaneous CSF fistula through stapes footplate & recurrent meningitis very rarely in IP-III
    - Due to normal endosteal development, hence normal stapes footplate in IP-III
- **Audiologic evaluation findings**
  - IP-III may have profound SNHL or mixed hearing loss
  - CHL may be due to thin otic capsule, stapes fixation, or perilymphatic pressure on stapes foot plate

Treatment
- Profound SNHL: **Cochlear implantation**
- All IP-III have **severe gusher** at cochlear implant surgery & very high chance of **electrode misplacement into IAC**
- All IP-III (like IP-II) have cochlear nerve, auditory brainstem implant (ABI) not indicated
- IP-III: **Stapes surgery contraindicated** → gusher & ↑ SNHL

SELECTED REFERENCES

1. Lewis M et al: Syndromic hearing loss in children. Neuroimaging Clin N Am. 33(4):563-80, 2023
2. Robson CD et al: Non-syndromic sensorineural hearing loss in children. Neuroimaging Clin N Am. 33(4):531-42, 2023
3. O'Brien WT, Sr et al: Nonsyndromic congenital causes of sensorineural hearing loss in children: an illustrative review. AJR Am J Roentgenol. 1-8, 2021
4. Hong R et al: New imaging findings of incomplete partition type III inner ear malformation and literature review. AJNR Am J Neuroradiol. 41(6):1076-80, 2020

TERMINOLOGY

- McCune-Albright syndrome (MAS); **classic triad**: Polyostotic fibrous dysplasia (FD), hyperfunctioning endocrinopathies, and cutaneous hyperpigmentation
- New recommendations: MAS diagnosis defined as combination of FD and ≥ 1 extraskeletal features **or** presence of ≥ 2 extraskeletal features

IMAGING

- Best diagnostic clues: Expanded ground-glass bone in child with precocious puberty and skin lesions
- Locations in H&N: Skull, skull base, or facial bones
  - Bilateral and asymmetric common
- CT: Imaging appearance depends on degree of fibrous vs. osseous components
  - **Ground glass**: Sclerotic
  - **Mixed** (pagetoid): Radiodensity and radiolucency
  - **Cystic**: Central lucency with thin sclerotic margins
  - Variable enhancement of fibrous component

- MR: Majority ↓ T1, intermediate or ↓ signal T2
  - Rim ↓ signal T2 and central ↑ T2 in cystic lesions
  - Fibrous component may enhance intensely

TOP DIFFERENTIAL DIAGNOSES

- Monostotic FD or polyostotic FD, without MAS
- Paget disease
  - Cotton wool CT appearance
- Jaffe-Campanacci syndrome
  - Nonossifying fibromas, axillary freckling, and café au lait skin lesions, without neurofibromas
- Caffey disease: Usually < 5 months of age
  - Acute-onset fever + hot, tender swelling of bones
- Cherubism
  - Familial, symmetric, bilateral fibroosseous lesions of jaw
- Garré sclerosing osteomyelitis
  - Bony expansion, heterogeneous sclerotic pattern
- Intraosseous meningioma
  - Hyperostosis

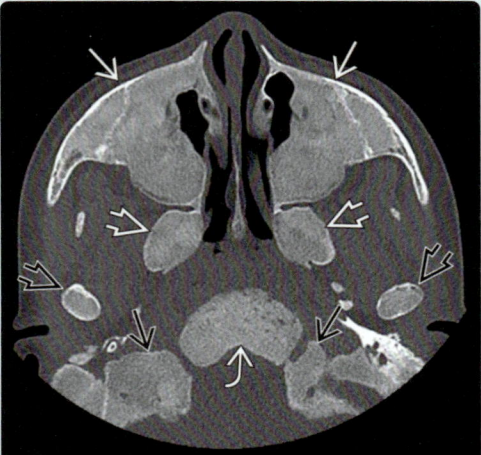
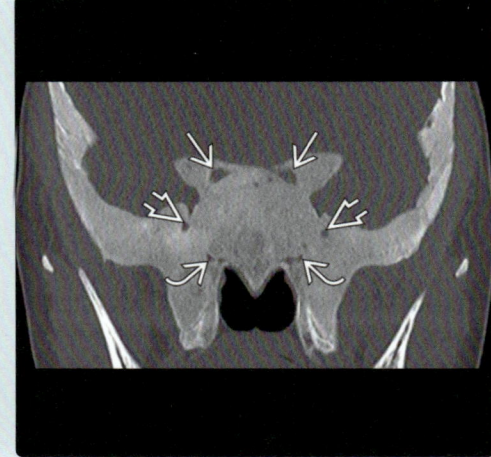

(Left) Axial bone CT in a 14-year-old boy with McCune-Albright syndrome shows multiple areas of fibrous dysplasia with the typical expanded ground-glass appearance. All visualized bony structures are involved, including bilateral maxilla ➡, pterygoid plates ⇥, clivus ➡, occipital condyles ➡, and mandibles ⇥. (Right) Coronal bone CT in the same patient shows extensive involvement of the skull base with narrowing of the bilateral optic canals ➡, foramen rotundum ⇥, and vidian canals ➡.

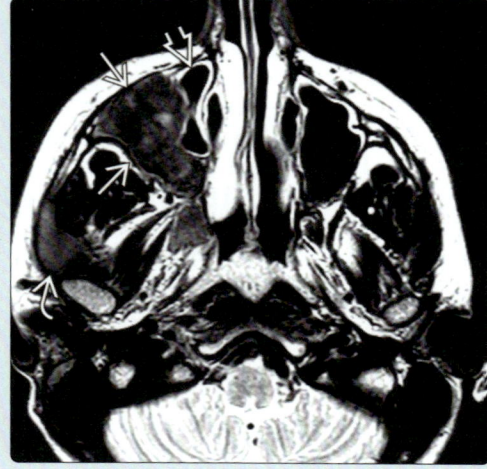
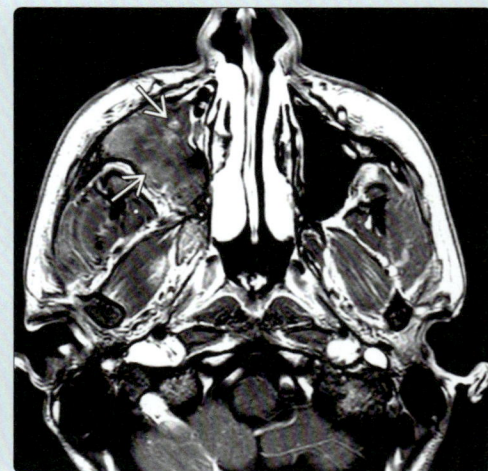

(Left) Axial T2 MR in a teenager with McCune-Albright syndrome shows diffuse thickening and heterogeneous signal in the right maxilla ➡ encroaching upon the lumen of the right maxillary sinus ⇥. There is also involvement of the right posterior zygomatic arch ➡. (Right) Axial T1 C+ MR in the same patient shows heterogeneous contrast; the more focal areas of enhancement ➡ correspond to areas of hyperintense T2 signal, consistent with small areas that are more fibrotic and lucent on CT (not shown).

Cherubism

KEY FACTS

TERMINOLOGY

- Familial, bilateral osteolytic jaw lesions
  - Genetically distinct from fibrous dysplasia (FD)

IMAGING

- **Bilateral** multilocular, **expansile** lucent lesions in **mandible**, displacing teeth
- ± submandibular lymph node enlargement

TOP DIFFERENTIAL DIAGNOSES

- Central giant cell granuloma
  - Expansile lesion with variable septations; single unless related to syndrome or hyperparathyroidism
  - Mandible anterior to molars > maxilla
- FD
  - Ground glass, mixed cystic and sclerotic, or cystic
- McCune-Albright syndrome
  - Subtype of **polyostotic** FD
    - Classic triad of polyostotic FD, precocious puberty, and cutaneous hyperpigmentation
- Brown tumor of hyperparathyroidism
  - May be multiple but not symmetrical

PATHOLOGY

- Autosomal dominant in most

CLINICAL ISSUES

- **Painless**, symmetric, swelling of lower face
- Round face and lower eyelid retraction → eyes raised to heaven or cherub-like appearance
- Begins 14 months to 4 years of age
  - Progresses through puberty, then stabilizes
  - May regress in adulthood
  - Clinical swelling usually abates by 3rd decade
  - Radiographic changes seen until 4th decade
- Treatment: Conservative in most; surgical curettage may improve chances of normal dentition and aesthetics

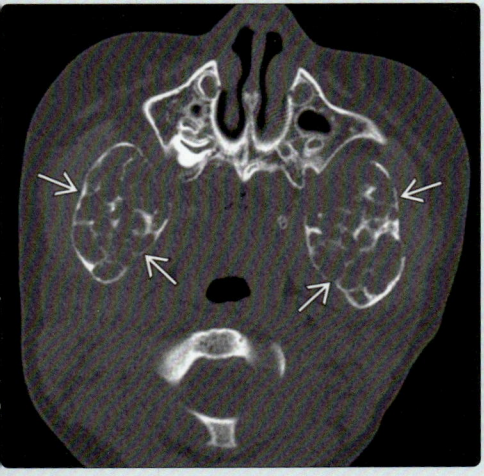
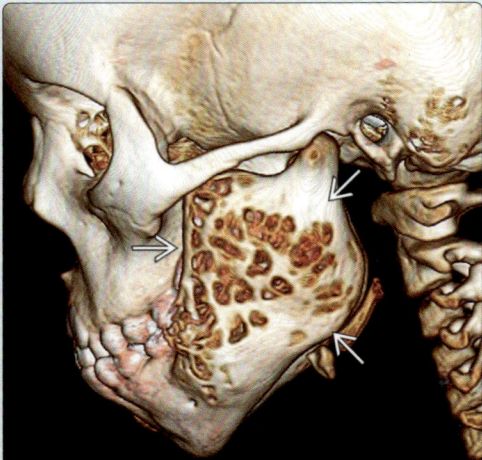

(Left) Axial bone CT in a 17-year-old boy shows bilateral bubbly, expansile lesions ➡ confined to the mandible, a typical appearance of cherubism. Notice there are areas where the cortex appears to disappear without aggressive bone destruction or periosteal reaction. (Right) Lateral 3D reconstruction shows the diffuse expansion of the left mandible ➡ secondary to the multiple bone cysts. (Courtesy J. Cure, MD.)

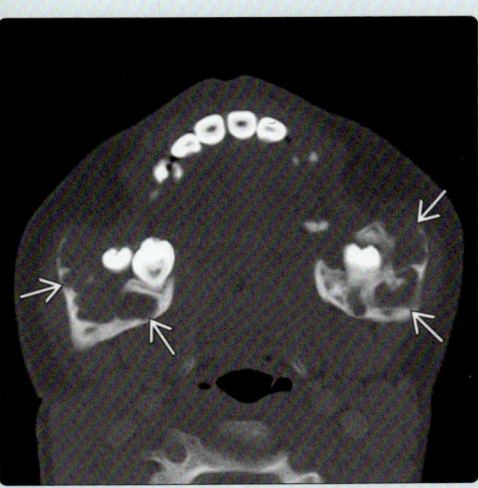
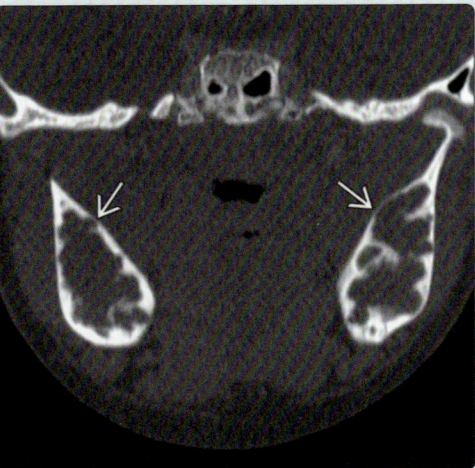

(Left) Axial bone CT in a 4-year-old boy who presented with gradual increase in facial swelling shows bilateral cystic lesions in the mandible ➡ with several areas of diffuse cortical thinning. (Right) Coronal bone CT in the same patient shows bilateral multiloculated cystic lesions ➡ expanding the mandible ➡ without aggressive bone destruction, periosteal reaction, or extraosseous soft tissue masses, typical of cherubism.

Mucopolysaccharidoses

TERMINOLOGY

- Heterogeneous group of hereditary lysosomal storage diseases due to deficiency of enzymes that degrade glycosaminoglycans (GAGs) or mucopolysaccharides
  - Accumulation of partially degraded GAGs → interference with cell, tissue, & organ function

IMAGING

- Skull & face findings
  - Macrocrania
  - Thickened skull base
  - **Large, J-shaped sella**
  - **Macroglossia**
  - **Stylohyoid ligament** with thick Ca++/ossification
  - Underpneumatized mastoid air cells
  - Flat or concave mandibular condyle, TMJ ankylosis
- Craniocervical junction: Dens hypoplasia (95%), atlantoaxial instability, craniovertebral junction stenosis
- Brain findings: Hydrocephalus, large perivascular spaces

TOP DIFFERENTIAL DIAGNOSES

- Down syndrome
  - ± dens hypoplasia without soft tissue dens mass or marrow deposition features
- Achondroplasia
  - Autosomal dominant, abnormal enchondral bone formation
  - Short, broad pedicle & thick laminae → spinal stenosis
- Spondyloepiphyseal dysplasia
  - Flattened vertebral bodies, dens hypoplasia, scoliosis may be present at birth
- GM1 gangliosidosis
  - Shares features of vertebral beaking, upper lumbar gibbus, & dens hypoplasia

CLINICAL ISSUES

- Most common signs/symptoms
  - Course facies at 3-6 months
  - Developmental delay in most

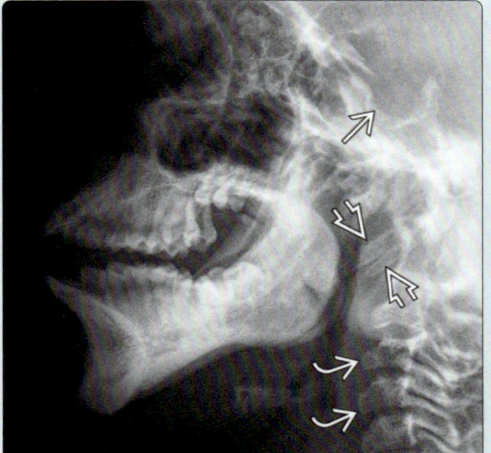
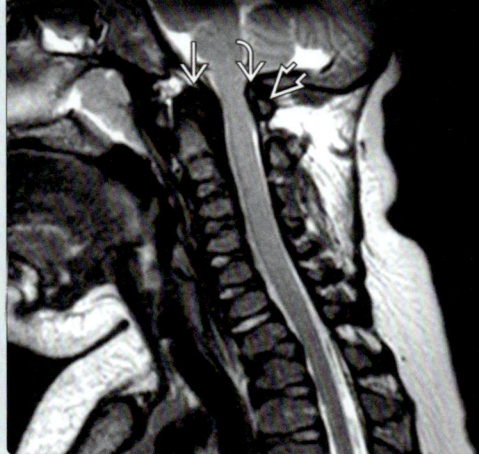

(Left) *Lateral airway radiograph in a 7-year-old boy with Hunter syndrome shows a large, J-shaped sella ➡ & thick/ossified stylohyoid ligaments ➡, typical of patients with MPS & dysostosis multiplex. Note also mild inferior vertebral beaking ➡.* (Right) *Sagittal T2 MR in a 7-year-old girl with Hurler syndrome shows a typical soft tissue "mass" ➡ at the tip of hypoplastic dens, hypoplastic posterior ring C1 ➡, & dural thickening ➡, causing minimal cord compression. Notice also the typical bullet-shaped vertebrae.*

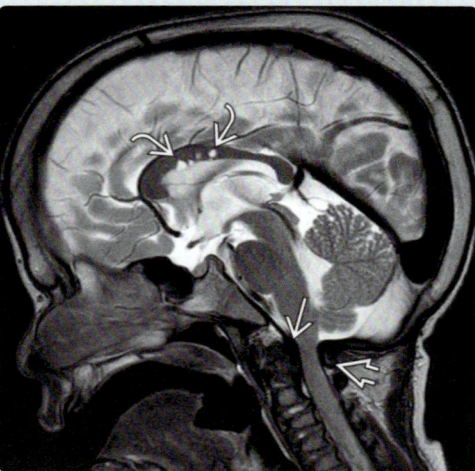
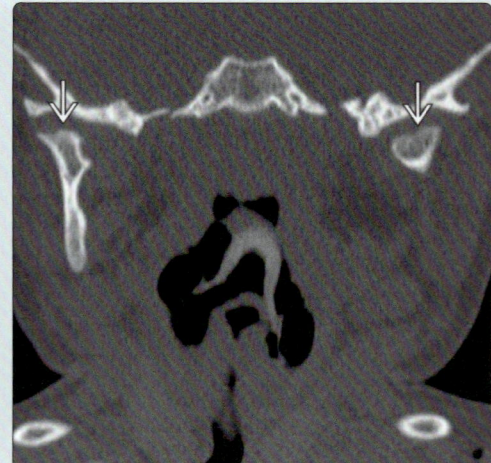

(Left) *Sagittal T2 MR in a child with Hurler syndrome shows CVJ stenosis secondary to a "mass" along the dorsal aspect of the hypoplastic dens ➡ & short posterior ring of C1 ➡. There is also bullet-shaped vertebrae, large craniofacial ratio, & prominent perivascular spaces along the undersurface of the corpus callosum ➡.* (Right) *Coronal bone CT in a 3-year-old boy with Morquio syndrome shows bilateral mandibular condyle flattening & cortical irregularity ➡.*

Mucopolysaccharidoses

TERMINOLOGY

Abbreviations
- Mucopolysaccharidoses (MPS)

Definitions
- Heterogeneous group of hereditary lysosomal storage diseases due to deficiency of enzymes that degrade glycosaminoglycans (GAGs) or mucopolysaccharides
- Dysostosis multiplex (DM): Constellation of bone dysplasia features seen variably in MPS

IMAGING

General Features
- Best diagnostic clue
  - J-shaped sella in child with macrocrania, cervical stenosis, hypoplastic dens, & enlarged perivascular spaces in brain, associated with thoracolumbar gibbus

CT Findings
- Skull & face
  - Macrocrania, large/J-shaped sella, thickened skull base
  - **Macroglossia,** hypertrophy palatine & adenoid tonsils
  - **Stylohyoid ligament calcification**
    - Earlier & thicker than in normal children
  - Underpneumatized mastoid air cells
  - Flat or concave mandibular condyles, TMJ ankylosis
- Craniovertebral junction (CVJ)
  - **Dens hypoplasia** (95%)
  - CVJ stenosis
  - Ligamentous laxity, atlantoaxial instability

MR Findings
- Dens hypoplasia, CVJ stenosis, atlantooccipital instability
- Thickened dural ring at foramen magnum & C2
- Large, J-shaped sella
- CSF signal intensity in large perivascular spaces in cerebral white matter, basal ganglia, & brainstem

Imaging Recommendations
- Skeletal series to assess associated skeletal abnormalities
- MR brain & CVJ

DIFFERENTIAL DIAGNOSIS

Down Syndrome (Trisomy 21)
- ± dens hypoplasia without soft tissue dens mass or marrow deposition features

Achondroplasia
- Short, broad pedicle & thick laminae → spinal stenosis

Spondyloepiphyseal Dysplasia
- Flattened vertebral bodies, dens hypoplasia, scoliosis may be present at birth

PATHOLOGY

General Features
- Coarse facies (formerly referred to as "gargoylism"), ligamentous laxity with reactive change → soft tissue mass around dens
- Etiology: Accumulation of GAGs in most organs/ligaments

- Upper airway obstruction (38%) → difficult intubation
  - Macroglossia, hypertrophy palatine & adenoid tonsils
  - ± thick vocal cords, epiglottis, & aryepiglottic folds
- Dural thickening foramen magnum → cord compression
- Submucosal deposition → small, abnormally shaped trachea & bronchi
- Chronic rhinosinusitis
- Genetics: Majority autosomal recessive (MPS II: Hunter X-linked)
- Associated abnormalities
  - Macrocrania, hydrocephalus
  - Skeletal DM, joint contractures
  - Lumbar gibbus deformity 2° to beaking vertebrae
    - MPS1 H (Hurler): Inferior beaking
    - MPS 4 (Morquio): Middle beaking
  - Dental: Dentigerous cysts, pointed cusps, spade-shaped incisors, thin enamel + pitted buccal surfaces, "rosette" formation of multiple impacted teeth in single follicle

Staging, Grading, & Classification
- MPS subdivisions based on enzyme deficiency
- MPS I-H (Hurler), I-S (Scheie), I-HS (Hurler-Scheie): α-L-iduronidase (4p16.3)
  - Hurler syndrome most severe form of MPS
  - Scheie syndrome mildest form of MPS
- MPS II (Hunter): Iduronate 2-sulfatase (Xq28)
- MPS III (Sanfilippo) A-D: Heparin N-sulfatase (17q25.3)
- MPS IV A-B (Morquio): Galactose 6-sulfatase (16q24.3)
- MPS VI (Maroteaux-Lamy): Arylsulfatase B (5q11-q13)
- MPS VII (Sly): β-glucuronidase
- MPS IX: Hyaluronidase

CLINICAL ISSUES

Presentation
- Most common signs/symptoms
  - Coarse facies at 3-6 months (mild in MPS III, VI, VII)
  - Developmental delay (not in MPS IV & VI)
  - Macrocrania with frontal bossing

Demographics
- Age: Diagnosed in childhood (rare, mild form diagnosed in adult); MPS IH (Hurler) presents in infancy
- Sex: M = F (except MPS II: Hunter X-linked: Male only)

Natural History & Prognosis
- Prognosis varies depending on type & severity
- High spinal cord compression major cause of spinal complications & death

Treatment
- CVJ & spinal surgery for more severe symptoms
- Tracheostomy if severe upper airway obstruction
- Stem cell transplantation
- Enzyme replacement therapy & clinical progress in gene therapies

SELECTED REFERENCES

1. Rossi A et al: Gene therapies for mucopolysaccharidoses. J Inherit Metab Dis. 47(1):135-44, 2023
2. Nicolas-Jilwan M: Imaging features of mucopolysaccharidoses in the head and neck. Int J Pediatr Otorhinolaryngol. 134:110022, 2020

Nose and Sinus

Malignant Tumors

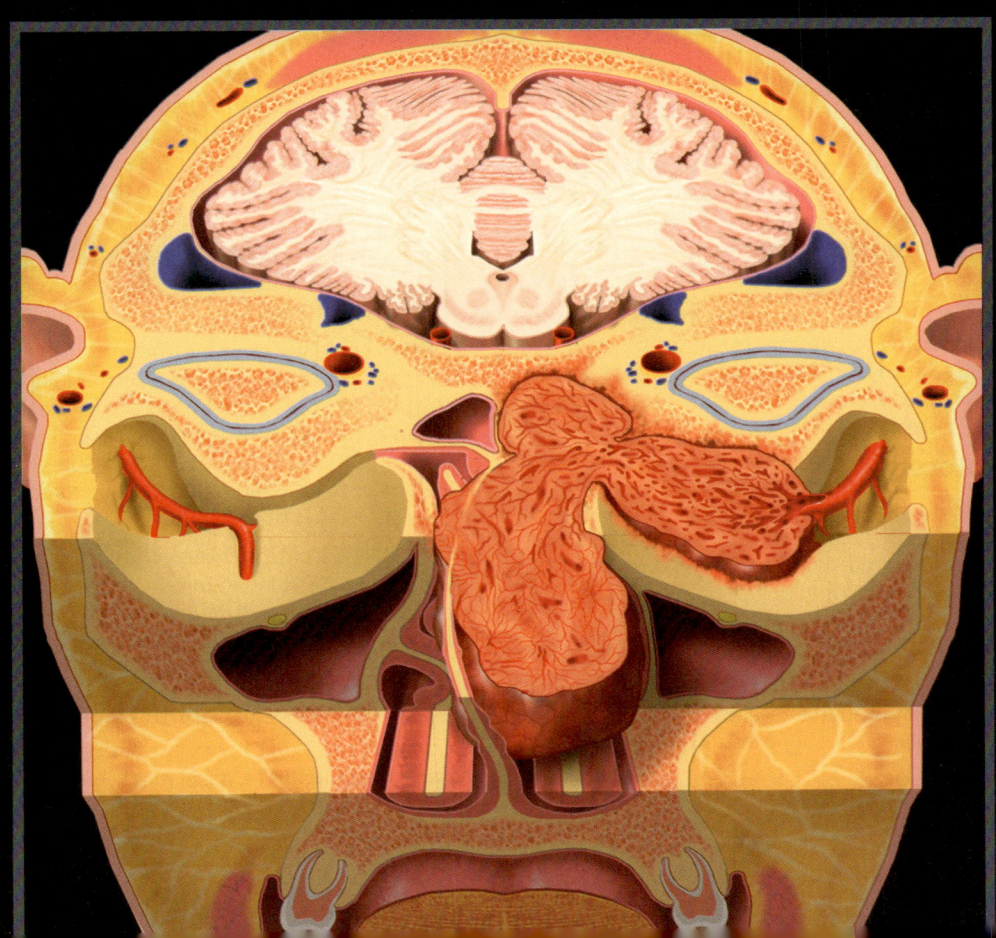

Summary Thoughts: Sinus and Nose

Conditions related to the nose, nasal cavities (NC), and paranasal sinuses (PS) are some of the most common cases encountered by clinicians, with direct costs of chronic rhinosinusitis (RS) estimated at $6.9-9.9 billion annually in the USA. Imaging is required when patients fail 1st-line treatments for inflammatory conditions, when invasive disease or neoplasm is suspected, or when presurgical planning becomes necessary. Given the complex bony architecture and the intervening air-filled spaces, **CT is the most common modality** for evaluating the sinonasal (SN) region. CT determines the extent of disease and is also helpful for surgical planning and intraoperative guidance. MR can be complementary in the evaluation of advanced infectious or inflammatory disease and in the evaluation of neoplasms. Information, such as patient demographics, presenting symptoms, and clinical exam findings, is critical for interpreting imaging studies of this area.

The NC is centrally located and is surrounded by the PS. It is important to understand the drainage pathways of the PS, as one can then predict **patterns of disease** based upon the site of an obstructing lesion. However, this can be challenging due to limitless anatomic variation. Infectious/inflammatory diseases are by far the most common pathologies. Neoplasms, both benign and malignant, are relatively rare. They tend to present at an advanced stage and encroach upon vital structures (orbit, skull base, and cranial nerves). These tumors are difficult to completely resect and are associated with high surgical morbidity. Presurgical tumor mapping in such cases is best accomplished with multiplanar MR.

Imaging Approaches and Indications

CT is the preferred modality to evaluate inflammatory disease, depicting mucosal thickening, opacification, air-fluid levels, and soft tissue masses. CT easily depicts osseous changes, such as remodeling, scalloping, hyperostosis, or erosion, and is sensitive for detecting calcium or bone in lesions, such as osteomas, chronic fungal disease, fibroosseous lesions, chondrosarcoma, or inverted papilloma. **Coronal images** best demonstrate the anatomy of the **ostiomeatal unit** (OMU). CECT is usually reserved for complicated cases in which soft tissue abscess, neoplasm, or vascular complication (cavernous sinus thrombosis) is suspected.

MR is indicated for evaluation of **complex inflammatory disease and neoplasms**. It is optimal for assessing extension or invasion of disease beyond the SN cavities, evaluating perineural tumor spread, and differentiating tumor from postobstructive secretions.

Imaging Protocols

With multidetector CT, a volumetric dataset can be acquired in the supine position, and multiplanar reformatted images can be subsequently generated. Axial images can be used in image guidance systems, obviating additional radiation for "treatment planning" CT prior to surgery. **Sagittal reformatted** images are helpful for delineating **frontal recess** (FR) and the sphenoethmoid region anatomy.

MR protocols generally include axial and coronal T1, STIR, and T1 C+ images, typically with fat suppression.

Imaging Anatomy

The SN region is comprised of the NC and the surrounding PS. There are important anatomic relationships with adjacent structures, including the orbit, oral cavity, pterygopalatine fossa, and both the anterior and central skull bases.

The SN cavities are pneumatized spaces within the maxillary, frontal, sphenoid, and ethmoid bones. Superiorly, the frontal sinuses border the anterior margin of the anterior cranial fossa. The cribriform plate (CP) and fovea ethmoidalis form the roof of the superior NC and ethmoid sinuses, respectively. The hard palate separates the NC from the oral cavity. The NC communicates posteriorly with the nasopharynx via the choanae. The orbits are separated from the ethmoid sinuses by the thin lamina papyracea and are separated from the maxillary sinuses by the orbital floors. Posterior to the maxillary sinuses are the pterygopalatine fossae, which communicate superiorly with the orbital apices, laterally with the masticator space, and posteriorly with central skull base.

The **NC is centrally located** and is divided in the midline by the nasal septum. The posterior septum is bony and formed by the perpendicular plate of the ethmoid superiorly and vomer bone inferiorly. Anteriorly, the septum is cartilaginous. The bony superior, middle, and inferior turbinates project into the NC and divide the NC into inferior, middle, and superior meatuses. The middle turbinate is attached superiorly to the CP via the vertical lamella and posterolaterally to the lamina papyracea via the basal (ground) lamella.

The frontal sinuses are divided in the midline by an intersinus septum. Inferomedially, the frontal sinus narrows toward its ostium, which drains into its FR. The **FR is formed by the walls of surrounding structures**, best visualized on **sagittal reformations**. The drainage of the FR is determined by the insertion of the uncinate process. Most often, the uncinate inserts laterally onto the lamina papyracea, and secretions drain into the middle meatus (MM). Less frequently, the uncinate inserts onto the anterior skull base or middle turbinate.

Paired groups of 13-18 air cells form the ethmoid sinuses. These cells are divided into anterior and posterior groups by the **basal lamella**. The anterior air cells drain into the anterior recess of the hiatus semilunaris and MM via the ethmoid bulla. The posterior air cells drain into the superior meatus and sphenoethmoidal recess (SER).

The maxillary sinuses lie lateral to the NC and inferior to the orbits. Each drains via its maxillary ostium into the infundibulum, then via the hiatus semilunaris into the MM.

The sphenoid sinuses are asymmetric air cells in the body of the sphenoid bone. Important surrounding structures include the maxillary division of CNV in the foramen rotundum laterally, the vidian nerve and artery in the vidian canal inferiorly, the optic nerves and sella superiorly, and the cavernous sinuses laterally. The sphenoid sinuses drain via their ostia into the SER.

The **OMU is a critical intersection** for drainage of the sinuses most affected by inflammatory disease (anterior ethmoid, maxillary, and frontal). Important components of the OMU include the ethmoid infundibulum, uncinate process, hiatus semilunaris, ethmoid bulla, and MM.

Approaches to Imaging Issues of Sinus and Nose

Congenital lesions can be classified as those presenting with a **nasal obstruction vs. nasal mass**. Pyriform aperture stenosis and choanal atresia, for example, cause nasal obstruction without a mass. Frontonasal cephaloceles, dermoids, and

Differential Diagnosis of Sinonasal Lesion

Congenital	Benign tumors and tumor-like lesions	Anatomic variations
Nasolacrimal duct mucocele	Osteoma	Sinus hypo- or hyperpneumatization
Choanal atresia	Fibrous dysplasia	Nasal septal deviation and spurs
Nasal glioma	Ossifying fibroma	Frontal cells
Nasal dermal sinus	Juvenile angiofibroma	**Ethmoid region**
Frontoethmoidal cephalocele	Inverted papilloma	Agger nasi cell
Pyriform aperture stenosis	Hemangioma	Infraorbital (Haller) cell
Infectious and inflammatory	Nerve sheath tumor	Supraorbital ethmoid cell
Acute rhinosinusitis	Pleomorphic adenoma	Large ethmoid bulla
Chronic rhinosinusitis	**Malignant tumors**	Sphenoethmoidal (Onodi) cell
Complications of rhinosinusitis	Squamous cell carcinoma	Asymmetric fovea ethmoidalis
Allergic fungal sinusitis	Olfactory neuroblastoma	Medial or dehiscent lamina papyracea
Mycetoma (fungal ball)	Adenocarcinoma	**Middle turbinate**
Invasive fungal sinusitis	Melanoma	Concha bullosa
Sinonasal polyposis	Non-Hodgkin lymphoma	Paradoxical curvature
Solitary sinonasal polyp	Sinonasal undifferentiated sarcoma	Hypoplasia
Mucocele	Adenoid cystic carcinoma	**Uncinate process**
Silent sinus syndrome	Chondrosarcoma	Pneumatized
Granulomatosis with polyangiitis (Wegener)	Osteosarcoma	Deviated
Sarcoidosis	Rhabdomyosarcoma	Fusion to middle turbinate or skull base
Nasal cocaine necrosis	Metastasis	Atelectatic (approximates orbital floor)

extranasal gliomas present as extranasal masses. Frontoethmoidal cephaloceles, intranasal gliomas, and nasolacrimal duct mucoceles present with an intranasal mass. MR can be very helpful for evaluating any connection to the intracranial space.

RS is the **most common pathology** of the SN region. Acute RS is usually diagnosed clinically and may not require imaging. Because of the anatomy of the PS drainage pathways, predictable patterns of inflammatory disease exist based upon the point of obstruction. For example, obstruction of the MM would lead to disease in the ipsilateral frontal, anterior ethmoid, and maxillary sinuses. SER obstruction might lead to ipsilateral posterior ethmoid and sphenoid disease. Although uncommon, there are several forms of SN fungal disease. Mycetoma and allergic fungal sinusitis occur in immunocompetent patients, and invasive fungal sinusitis (IFS) occurs in the immunocompromised or patients with poorly controlled diabetes. It is important to note that **IFS may appear mass-like** or as **subtle infiltration of fat planes** adjacent to the PS at imaging. Granulomatous disease has a predilection for involving the nasal septum and turbinates.

There are a wide variety of SN neoplasms. Well-marginated tumors that cause bony remodeling suggest benign tumors, while infiltrative masses with osseous destruction suggest malignant lesions. The site of origin may also be predictive of histology. For instance, osteomas most often arise in the frontal and ethmoid sinuses, juvenile angiofibromas (JAF) arise in the posterior NC at the sphenopalatine foramen, inverted papillomas often arise along the lateral nasal wall, and olfactory neuroblastoma (ONB) typically arises near the CP. Squamous cell carcinoma is by far the **most common SN malignancy** and most often arises in the maxillary antrum. The imaging features of adenocarcinomas can be nonspecific, but

they have a predilection for the ethmoid region. Three malignant neoplasms with a **predilection for the NC** include ONB, lymphoma, and melanoma.

Clinical Implications

It is important to note that studies have shown a poor correlation between symptoms of RS and CT findings. The diagnosis of RS is ultimately a clinical one. Lesions located within the NC can be evaluated with endoscopy. Lesions involving the PS are difficult to evaluate with scopes, so imaging is important for full evaluation.

Disease of the SN cavities often presents with nonspecific symptoms, such as nasal obstruction, discharge, and craniofacial pain. Additional symptoms, such as epistaxis, may be indicative of a vascular lesion (JAF or ONB). Pain may also be caused by mucoceles or neoplasms, while paresthesias can be linked to malignancies, such as adenoid cystic carcinoma.

Selected References

1. Agarwal A et al: Update from the 5th Edition of the WHO classification of nasal, paranasal, and skull base tumors: imaging overview with histopathologic and genetic correlation. AJNR Am J Neuroradiol. 44(10):1116-25, 2023
2. Bracigliano A et al: Malignant sinonasal tumors: update on histological and clinical management. Curr Oncol. 28(4):2420-38, 2021
3. McCann MR et al: Emergency radiologic approach to sinus disease. Emerg Radiol. 28(5):1003-10, 2021
4. Agarwal M et al: Sinonasal neoplasms. Semin Roentgenol. 54(3):244-57, 2019
5. O'Brien WT Sr et al: The preoperative sinus CT: avoiding a "CLOSE" call with surgical complications. Radiology. 281(1):10-21, 2016
6. Amine MA et al: Anatomy and complications: safe sinus. Otolaryngol Clin North Am. 48(5):739-48, 2015
7. Charles Burke M et al: A practical approach to the imaging interpretation of sphenoid sinus pathology. Curr Probl Diagn Radiol. 44(4):360-70, 2015

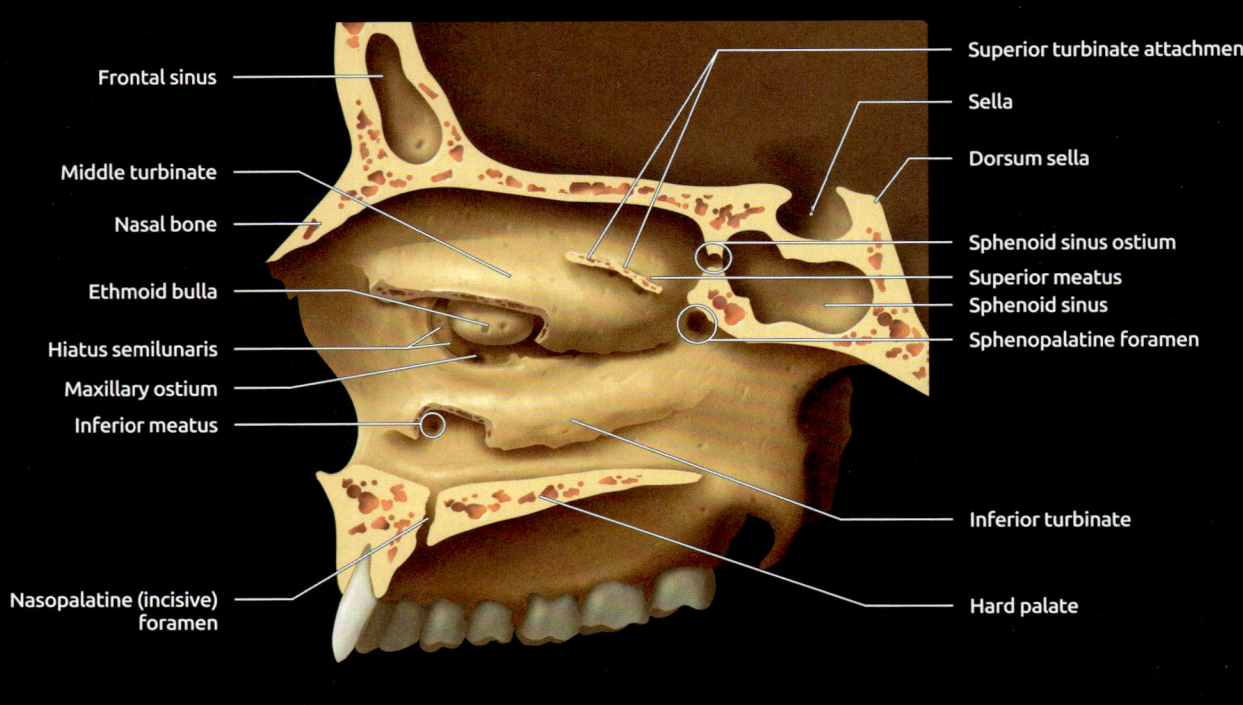

Frontal sinus

Middle turbinate

Nasal bone

Ethmoid bulla

Hiatus semilunaris

Maxillary ostium

Inferior meatus

Nasopalatine (incisive) foramen

Superior turbinate attachment

Sella

Dorsum sella

Sphenoid sinus ostium

Superior meatus

Sphenoid sinus

Sphenopalatine foramen

Inferior turbinate

Hard palate

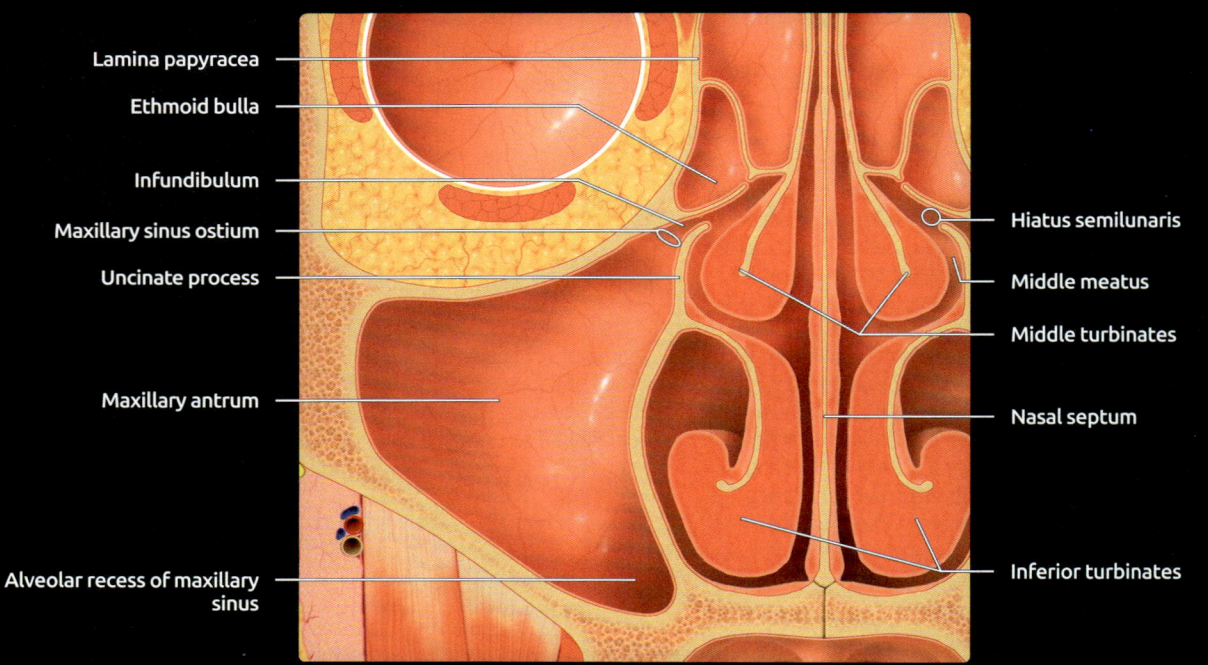

Lamina papyracea

Ethmoid bulla

Infundibulum

Maxillary sinus ostium

Uncinate process

Maxillary antrum

Alveolar recess of maxillary sinus

Hiatus semilunaris

Middle meatus

Middle turbinates

Nasal septum

Inferior turbinates

(Top) *Sagittal graphic demonstrates the osseous anatomy of the lateral nasal wall. The superior turbinate and portions of the middle and inferior turbinates have been resected. The superior, middle, and inferior meatuses drain inferior to their respective turbinates. The ipsilateral frontal, anterior ethmoid, and maxillary sinuses ultimately drain into the middle meatus. The nasolacrimal duct drains into the inferior meatus. The sphenoid ostium is located along the anterior sphenoid sinus wall and drains into the sphenoethmoidal recess. **(Bottom)** Coronal graphic of magnified right sinonasal region shows the important structures around the ostiomeatal unit. The vertically oriented uncinate process is bounded laterally by the ethmoid infundibulum, superiorly by the hiatus semilunaris, and medially by the middle meatus. The ethmoid bulla is the dominant anterior ethmoid cell located superior to the uncinate. The middle meatus drains beneath the middle turbinate.*

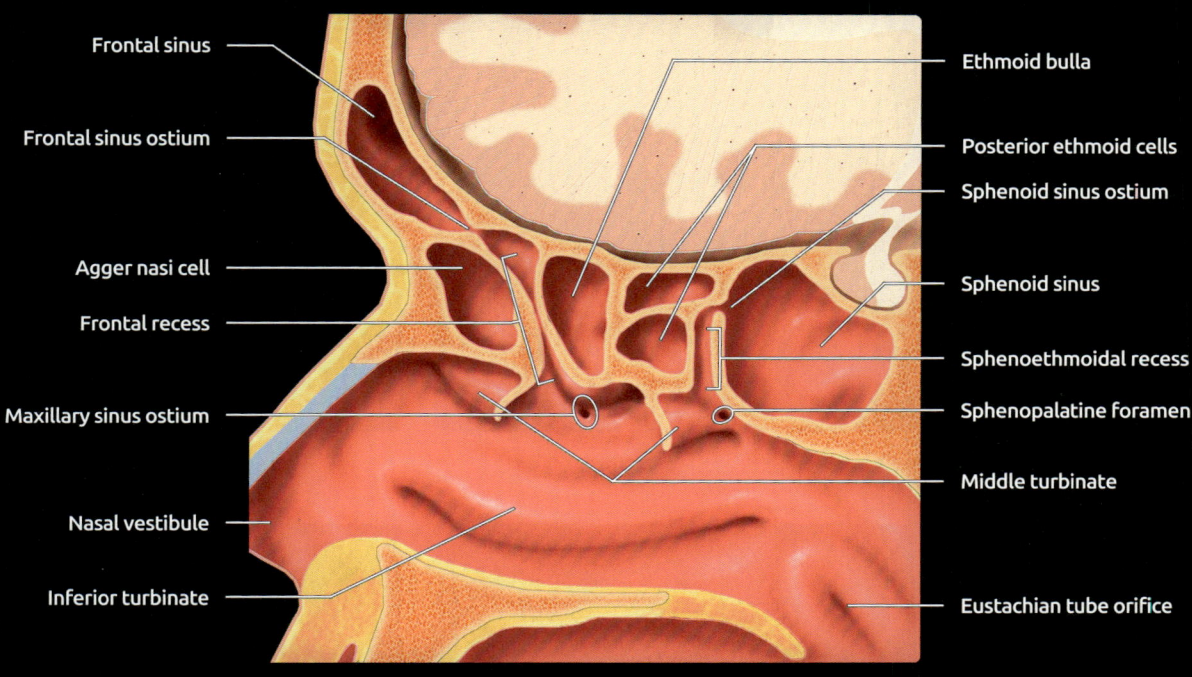

Frontal sinus

Frontal sinus ostium

Agger nasi cell

Frontal recess

Maxillary sinus ostium

Nasal vestibule

Inferior turbinate

Ethmoid bulla

Posterior ethmoid cells

Sphenoid sinus ostium

Sphenoid sinus

Sphenoethmoidal recess

Sphenopalatine foramen

Middle turbinate

Eustachian tube orifice

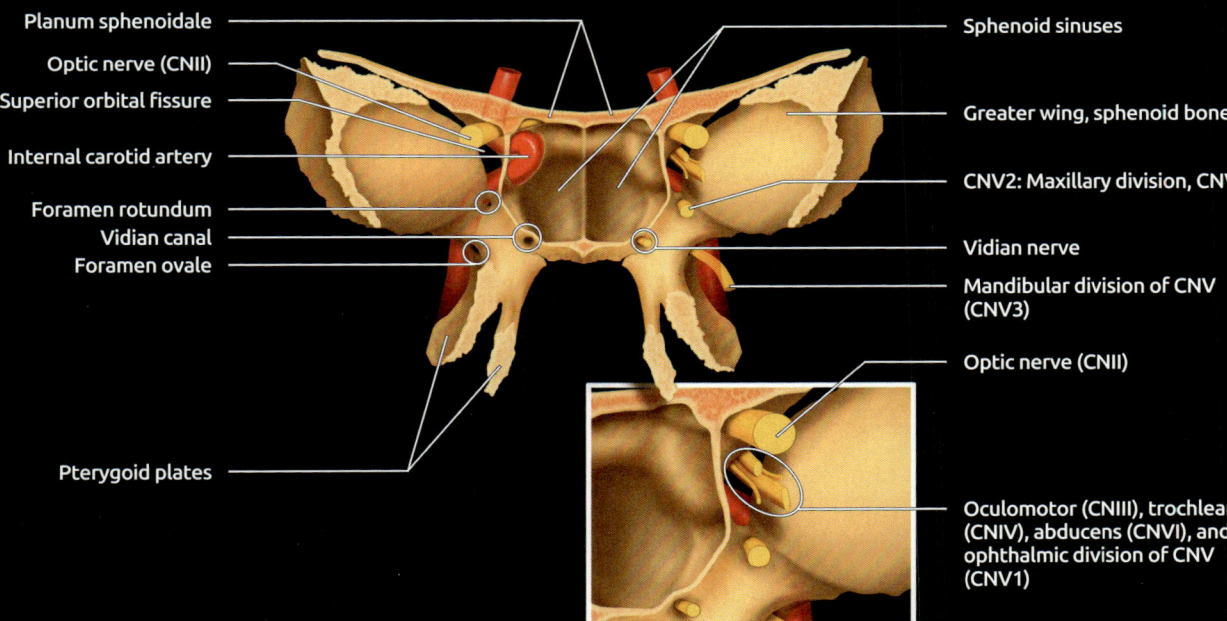

Planum sphenoidale

Optic nerve (CNII)

Superior orbital fissure

Internal carotid artery

Foramen rotundum

Vidian canal

Foramen ovale

Pterygoid plates

Sphenoid sinuses

Greater wing, sphenoid bone

CNV2: Maxillary division, CNV

Vidian nerve

Mandibular division of CNV (CNV3)

Optic nerve (CNII)

Oculomotor (CNIII), trochlear (CNIV), abducens (CNVI), and ophthalmic division of CNV (CNV1)

(Top) *Sagittal graphic shows the frontal sinus drainage pathway. The frontal sinus narrows inferiorly to its ostium. Secretions drain through the ostium into the frontal recess (FR). The FR is not a true duct in that its walls are comprised of adjacent anatomy. In the graphic, the FR is bounded anteriorly by an agger nasi cell and posteriorly by the ethmoid bulla. Note that FR drainage may vary based upon the point of insertion of the uncinate process.* **(Bottom)** *Coronal graphic shows the important anatomy surrounding the sphenoid sinuses. The cavernous portions of the internal carotid arteries lie lateral and posterior to the sinuses. At the orbital apex, the optic nerve can be seen traversing the optic canal. The maxillary division of CNV in the foramen rotundum and the vidian nerve are positioned lateral and inferior to the sinus, respectively. Multiple cranial nerves pass through the superior orbital fissure (see inset) into the orbit, including CNIII, IV, and VI, as well as the ophthalmic division on CNV.*

(Left) *Coronal bone CT shows the paired frontal sinuses ➡ separated by the intersinus septum ➡. The most anterior ethmoid-type cells, the agger nasi ➡, can be seen. Notice the air-filled lacrimal sac ➡ on the left.* **(Right)** *Coronal bone CT shows the medial ➡ and lateral ➡ lamellae of the cribriform plate forming the roof of the nasal cavity. The fovea ethmoidalis ➡ forms the ethmoid sinus roof. Note the patent FRs ➡ leading to the middle meatuses.*

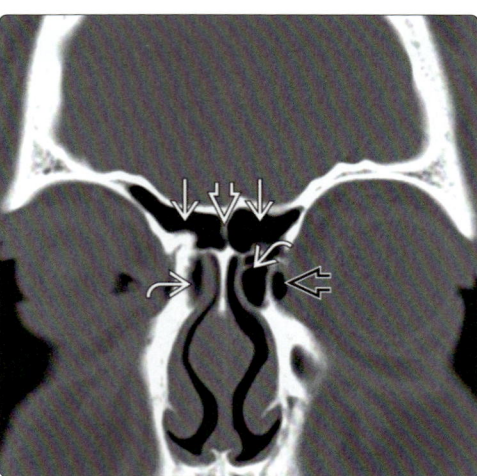
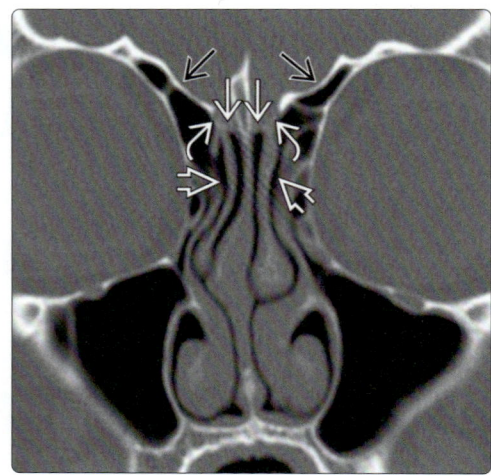

(Left) *Sagittal bone CT shows the frontal sinus drainage pathway. The frontal sinus ➡ drains inferiorly through the frontal ostium ➡ into the FR ➡. The agger nasi cell ➡ is anterior to the recess, and the ethmoid bulla is posterior ➡. The FR drains to the middle meatus adjacent to the middle turbinate ➡.* **(Right)** *Axial T1 MR shows the paired maxillary sinuses ➡ lateral to the nasal cavity. Note the inferior turbinates ➡, midline nasal septum ➡, and air-filled nasolacrimal ducts ➡ above the inferior meatuses.*

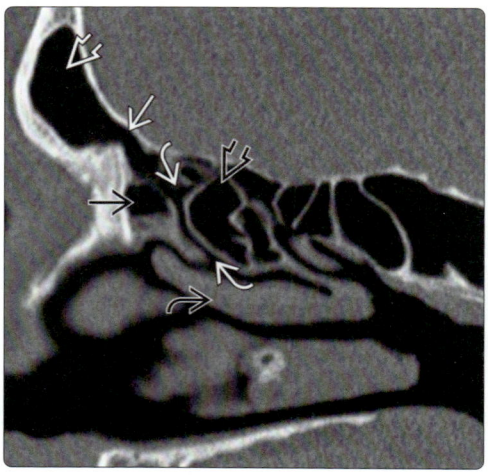
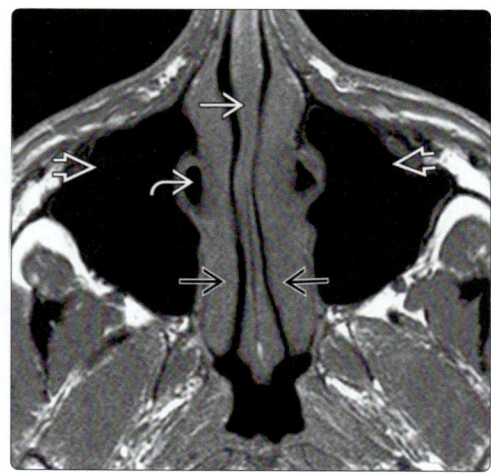

(Left) *Sagittal CT reconstruction shows the nasolacrimal duct ➡ draining into the inferior meatus ➡. Note the pterygopalatine fossa posterior to the maxillary sinus ➡.* **(Right)** *Coronal bone CT at the level of the ostiomeatal units shows the uncinate processes ➡, ethmoid bullae ➡, and middle turbinates ➡. They are pneumatized as is the right inferior turbinate. The middle meatus lies between the uncinate and middle turbinate. A retention cyst blocks the left maxillary ostium.*

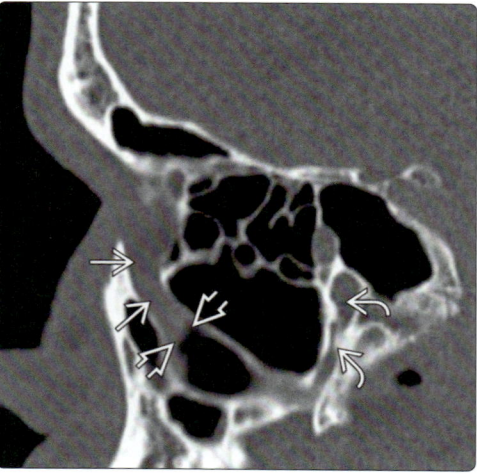
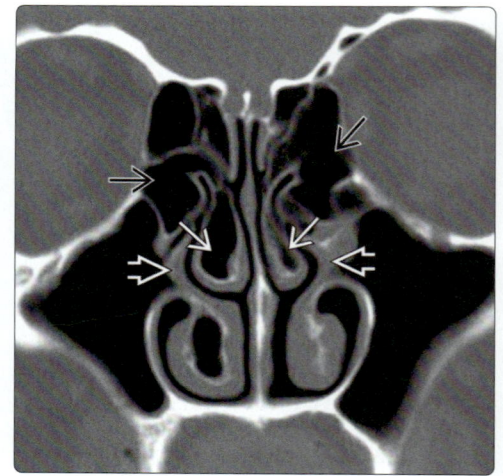

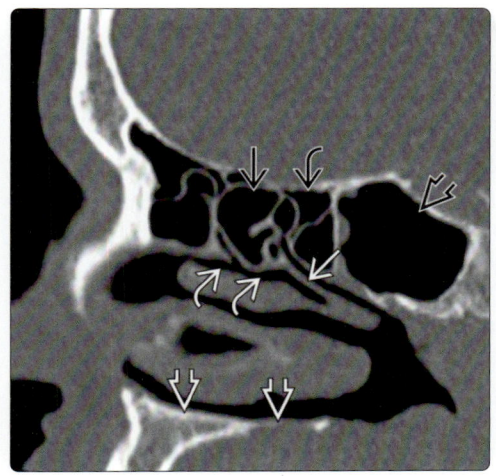

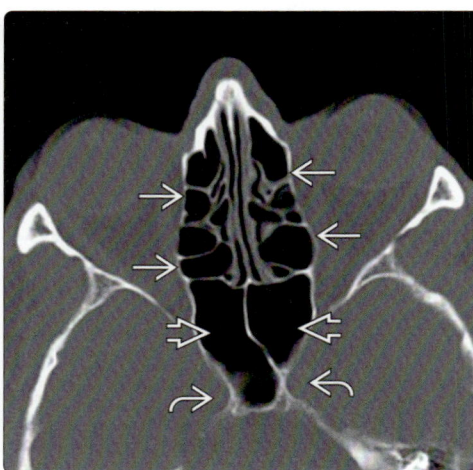

(Left) Sagittal CT reconstruction shows anterior ➡ and posterior ➡ ethmoid cells and the sphenoid sinus ➡. The lateral attachment of the middle turbinate (basal lamella) ➡ is seen. Note the hiatus semilunaris ➡. The palate is noted inferiorly ➡. (Right) Axial bone CT shows the thin lamina papyracea ➡ separating the ethmoid air cells from the orbits. The sphenoid sinuses ➡ are separated by an intersinus septum. The internal carotid arteries ➡ are immediately adjacent to the sphenoid sinuses.

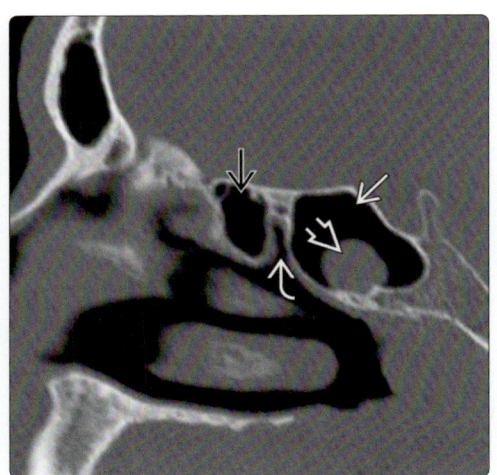

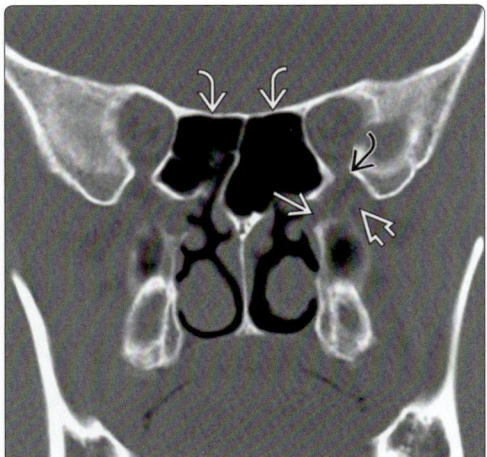

(Left) Sagittal CT reconstruction shows the sphenoethmoidal recess ➡ bounded anteriorly by the most posterior ethmoid air cell ➡ and posteriorly by the sphenoid sinus ➡. A retention cyst is seen in the sphenoid sinus ➡. (Right) Coronal bone CT shows the sphenopalatine foramen ➡ connecting the nasal cavity to the pterygopalatine fossa ➡. The inferior orbital fissure ➡ extends from the pterygopalatine fossa to the orbital apex. Note the planum sphenoidale above the sphenoid sinuses ➡.

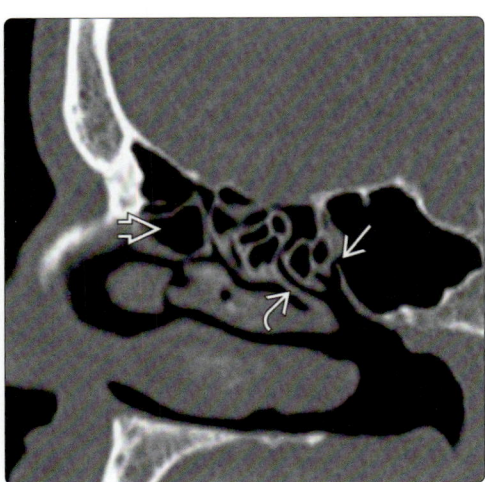

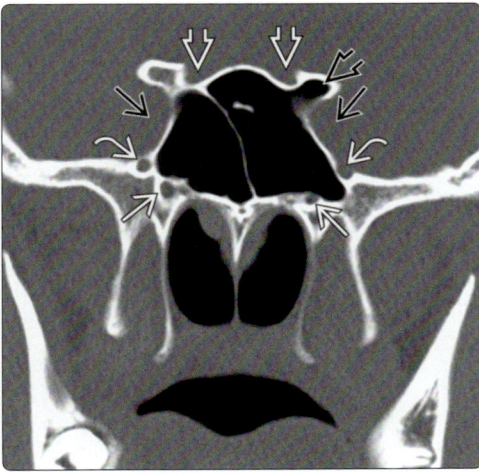

(Left) Sagittal CT reconstruction shows the sphenoid sinus ostium ➡ along the anterior wall of the sphenoid sinus. Agger nasi cell ➡ and the basal lamella ➡ are also seen. (Right) Coronal bone CT shows the important structures around the sphenoid sinuses. The vidian canals ➡ are noted along the sphenoid sinus floors, and the foramen rotundum ➡ is located laterally. The optic nerves lie medial to the anterior clinoids ➡, and the cavernous sinuses lie laterally ➡. Pneumatization of the clinoid ➡ is variant anatomy.

KEY FACTS

TERMINOLOGY

- Synonym: Congenital dacryocystocele if only sac involved

IMAGING

- Well-defined, cystic, medial canthal mass in continuity with enlarged nasolacrimal duct (NLD) in newborn
  - Unilateral or bilateral
- Absent or minimal wall enhancement (unless infected)
- Coronal/sagittal reformatted images show continuity of proximal cyst at lacrimal sac with distal inferior meatus cyst through dilated NLD

TOP DIFFERENTIAL DIAGNOSES

- Orbital dermoid & epidermoid
  - Lateral > medial canthus
- Frontoethmoidal (nasoorbital) cephalocele
  - Swelling at inferomedial orbit connected to brain/meninges on imaging
- Acquired dacryocystocele

  - Typically post traumatic, usually adults

PATHOLOGY

- Tears & mucus accumulate in NLD with imperforate Hasner membrane (i.e., distal duct obstruction)
- Most common abnormality of infant lacrimal apparatus

CLINICAL ISSUES

- Proximal cyst: Small, round, bluish, medial canthal mass identified at birth or shortly thereafter; ± cellulitis
- Distal cyst: Nasal airway obstruction with respiratory distress if bilateral (especially during feeding)

DIAGNOSTIC CHECKLIST

- CT or MR evaluates lacrimal apparatus lesion extent
  - Excludes other sinonasal causes of respiratory distress in newborn
- Comment on full extent of lesion from medial canthus to inferior meatus
- Exclude contralateral lesion

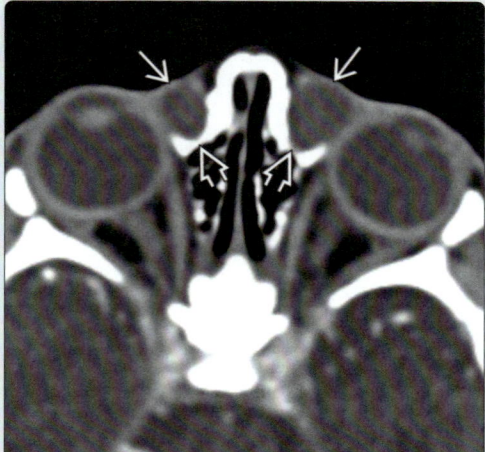
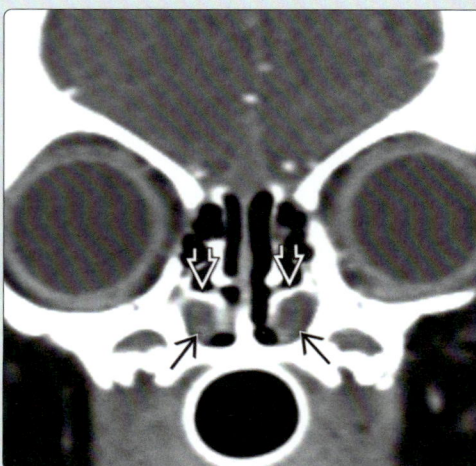

(Left) Axial CECT in a 4-day-old patient with bluish, bilateral medial orbital swelling & left purulent drainage shows bilateral lacrimal sac enlargement ⇨. Note also the bilateral lacrimal sac fossae splaying ⇥. (Right) Coronal CECT in the same patient demonstrates the typical locations of the distal intranasal components of the nasolacrimal duct (NLD) mucoceles in the inferior meatus ⇨, inferior to the inferior turbinates ⇥.

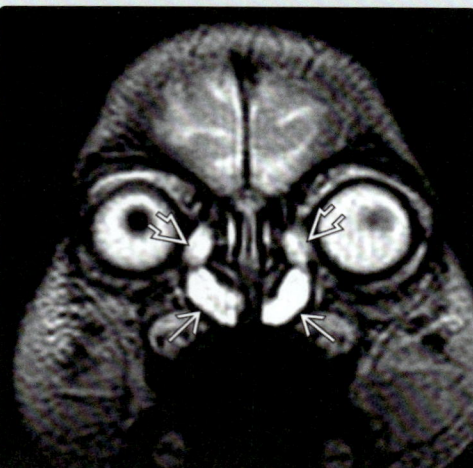
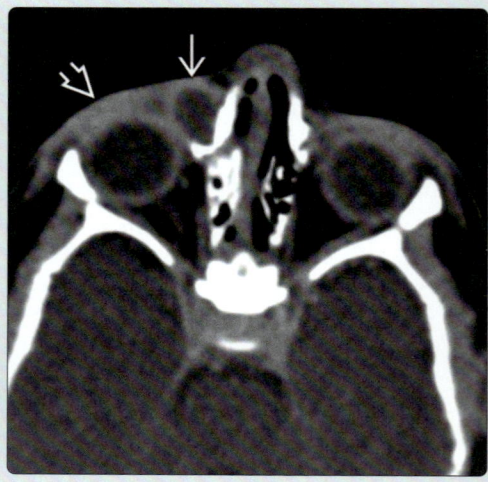

(Left) Coronal T2 MR in an infant shows hyperintense NLD mucoceles extending from the dilated lacrimal sacs ⇨ proximally to protrude inferomedially from the inferior NLDs ⇨. (Right) Axial CECT in a 1-week-old with periorbital cellulitis demonstrates peripheral enhancement of an enlarged right lacrimal sac ⇨ & right preseptal periorbital soft tissue swelling ⇥. More inferior images showed enlargement of the lacrimal canal & an intranasal cystic mass in the inferior meatus, consistent with NLD mucocele.

TERMINOLOGY

Synonyms
- Congenital dacryocystocele if only sac involved

Definitions
- Nasolacrimal duct (NLD) mucocele: Cystic dilation of nasolacrimal apparatus secondary to proximal & distal obstruction of NLD
- Canthus: Corner of eye where eyelids meet

IMAGING

General Features
- Best diagnostic clue
  - Well-defined, cystic, medial canthal mass in continuity with enlarged NLD in newborn
- Location
  - From lacrimal sac at medial canthus to distal aspect of NLD at inferior meatus
  - Unilateral or bilateral

CT Findings
- Hypodense, thin-walled cyst at medial canthus ± bulging cystic component at inferior meatus
  - Cysts communicate through enlarged NLD
- Minimal wall enhancement; if infected, thick rim enhancement ± fluid/debris level

MR Findings
- T1-hypointense/T2-hyperintense, well-circumscribed mass(es)
- Signal intensity varies with protein content &/or infection
- Minimal wall enhancement normally
- If inflamed/infected, then thick rim of enhancement with surrounding poorly defined soft tissue stranding

Imaging Recommendations
- Best imaging tool
  - Thin-section bone CT
  - ± contrast (for better soft tissue characterization)

DIFFERENTIAL DIAGNOSIS

Orbital Dermoid & Epidermoid
- Lateral > medial canthus
- Near suture: Frontozygomatic > frontonasal/nasolacrimal
- 50% show fat density/intensity with thin rim enhancement

Frontoethmoidal (Nasoorbital) Cephalocele
- Swelling at inferomedial orbit connected to brain/meninges

Acquired Dacryocystocele
- Acquired lacrimal sac cyst from trauma, other processes
- Typically in adults with history of prior regional trauma

PATHOLOGY

General Features
- Etiology
  - Tears & mucus accumulate in NLD due to imperforate Hasner membrane at distal duct
  - Distended lacrimal sac may compress lacrimal canaliculi, which bend on themselves → trapdoor obstruction

- Massage cannot decompress lacrimal sac
- Indicates dual obstruction of proximal canalicular-punctal system & distal inferior lacrimal system

CLINICAL ISSUES

Presentation
- Most common signs/symptoms
  - Small, round, bluish, medial canthal mass identified at or shortly after birth = distended lacrimal sac
  - Nasal airway obstruction & respiratory distress (especially during feeding) with bilateral nasal components
    - Obligate nose breathers during infancy
- Other signs/symptoms
  - Tearing & crusting at medial canthus, preseptal cellulitis, dacryocystitis
  - Small NLD mucoceles may be identified incidentally on brain MR in infants

Demographics
- Epidemiology
  - Most common abnormality of infant lacrimal apparatus
  - 3rd most common cause of neonatal nasal obstruction
    - 1st = mucosal edema, 2nd = choanal atresia
- Infancy: Typically 4 days to 10 weeks of age
- M < F (1:3)

Natural History & Prognosis
- 90% of simple distal NLD obstructions (or congenital dacryostenosis) resolve spontaneously by age 1
- Only 50% of patients recognized on prenatal MR ultimately have postnatal symptoms
- Intervene before infection to prevent nasal airway obstruction, dacryocystitis, & permanent sequelae

Treatment
- Daily manual massage ± prophylactic antibiotics
  - Manual massage inappropriate if NLD mucocele infected or causing airway obstruction
- 10% require probing with irrigation ± silastic stent
- If endonasal component & no response to aforementioned treatment, then endoscopic resection with marsupialization
- Excellent prognosis with adequate early treatment
- High success rate for nasal endoscopic surgery: Cure (81.5%), improvement (18.5%), unhealed (0%)
- Theoretical risk of nasolacrimal apparatus scarring, amblyopia, & permanent canthal asymmetry if untreated

DIAGNOSTIC CHECKLIST

Image Interpretation Pearls
- Comment on full extent of lesion from medial canthus to inferior meatus, bilaterality, & signs of infection

SELECTED REFERENCES

1. Pur DR et al: Management of congenital dacryocystocele: a case series and literature review. J Pediatr Ophthalmol Strabismus. 60(3):e31-4, 2023
2. Diab MM et al: Clinico-radiologic characteristics of lacrimal sac area swellings misdiagnosed as dacryocystocele or mucocele. Eur J Ophthalmol. 33(1):152-60, 2022
3. Panda BB et al: Solitary fibrous tumour of lacrimal sac masquerading as lacrimal sac mucocele: a diagnostic and surgical dilemma. BMJ Case Rep. 15(5):e250015, 2022
4. Rodriguez DP et al: Masses of the nose, nasal cavity, and nasopharynx in children. Radiographics. 37(6):1704-30, 2017

TERMINOLOGY

- Congenital obstruction of posterior nasal aperture(s)

IMAGING

- Unilateral or bilateral osseous narrowing of posterior nasal cavity with complete obstruction by associated membrane &/or bony plate
  - Thickening of vomer
  - Medial bowing of posterior maxilla(e)
  - ± air-fluid level in obstructed nasal cavity
- Unilateral in up to 75% (right > left)
- Bilateral in up to 25%
  - 75% of bilateral cases have other anomalies

TOP DIFFERENTIAL DIAGNOSES

- Choanal stenosis
- Congenital nasal pyriform aperture stenosis
- Nasolacrimal duct mucocele

PATHOLOGY

- Choanal atresia is most common congenital abnormality of nasal cavity
- Choanal atresia types
  - Mixed bony & membranous atresia in up to 70%
  - Purely bony atresia in up to 30%

CLINICAL ISSUES

- Typical presentations include
  - Inability to pass nasoenteric tube
  - Bilateral choanal atresia: Significant respiratory distress in newborn
    - Due to their physiologic obligate nasal breather status
  - Unilateral choanal atresia: Chronic, purulent unilateral rhinorrhea with mild airway obstruction in older child

DIAGNOSTIC CHECKLIST

- Respiratory distress & suspected nasal obstruction in newborn should be evaluated with thin-section bone CT

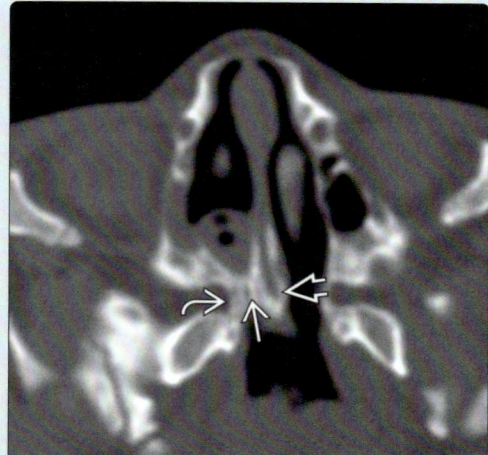
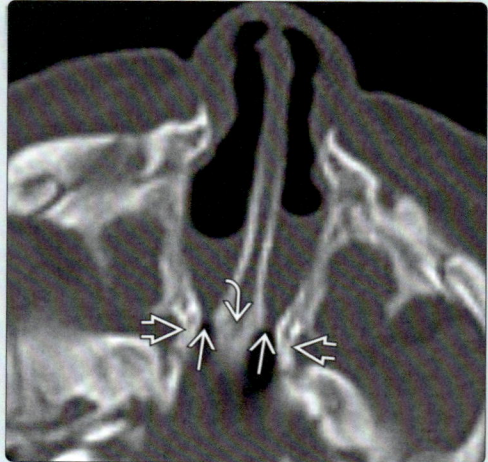

(Left) Axial NECT bone window through the upper choanae shows a complete osseous right choanal obstruction ⇨ secondary to fusion of an enlarged vomer ⇨ to the thickened, medially positioned posterior maxilla ⇨. (Right) Axial bone CT in an infant in whom clinicians were unable to pass a nasoenteric tube shows significant narrowing of the choanae ⇨, medialization of thickened posteromedial maxilla ⇨, a wide vomer ⇨, small membranes traversing the stenotic choana, & bilateral nasal cavity air-fluid levels.

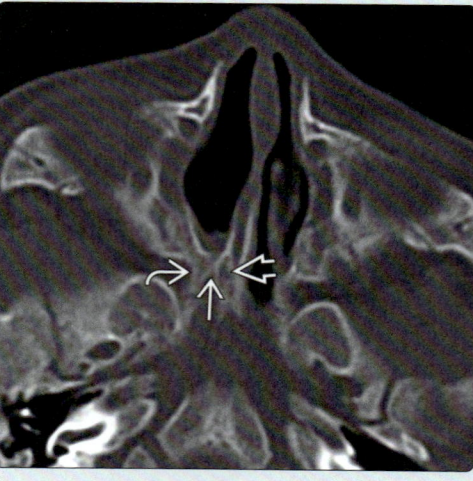
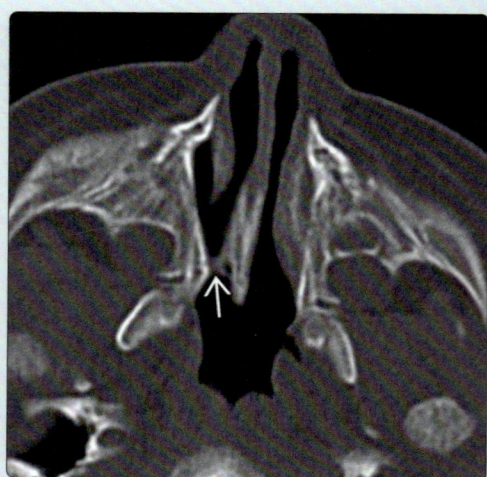

(Left) Axial bone CT obtained at the upper aspect of the choana in a 6-week-old girl with right nasal obstruction demonstrates complete obliteration of the right choana ⇨ by the thickened vomer ⇨ fused to the thickened posteromedial maxilla ⇨. (Right) Axial bone CT 2 mm more inferior in the same patient shows a stenotic choana & crossing membrane ⇨, not an uncommon appearance in patients with mixed atresia, bony (upper) & membranous (low).

TERMINOLOGY

Definitions

- Congenital obstruction of posterior nasal aperture
  - Choana: Junction of posterior nasal cavity & nasopharynx
  - Choanal atresia: Lack of communication between nasal cavity & nasopharynx

IMAGING

General Features

- Best diagnostic clue
  - Bony narrowing of posterior nasal cavity with membranous &/or osseous obstruction of choana
- Location
  - Unilateral in ~ 75% (right > left), bilateral in ~ 25%
- Size
  - Newborn **choanal opening** abnormal if **< 0.34-cm** wide
  - Newborn **vomer** abnormal if **> 0.23-cm** thick
- Morphology
  - Medial bowing of posterior maxilla (lateral nasal wall) & pterygoid plate
  - Large/thickened vomer
  - Bony narrowing ± soft tissue membrane/plug or bony plate obstructing choana
    - Mixed bony & membranous atresia in up to 70%
    - Purely bony atresia in up to 30%

CT Findings

- Bone CT
  - Choanal narrowing by medially bowed posterior maxilla/pterygoid & thickened vomer
  - Narrow gap between maxilla & vomer bridged by continuous bony plate or membrane
    - Membranous atresia may be thin/strand-like or thick/plug-like
  - Air-fluid level frequently present in obstructed nasal passage
    - Nasal cavity may also be filled with soft tissue, hypertrophied inferior turbinates
  - Ipsilateral midnasal cavity may be widened

Imaging Recommendations

- Best imaging tool
  - High-resolution unenhanced bone CT
- Protocol advice
  - Suction secretions from nasal cavity prior to scanning
  - Axial images angled 5° cephalad to palate
    - If angle too great, region of choanae at level of skull base creates false appearance of choanal atresia
  - Edge enhancement bone filters help delineate bone margins in partially ossified skull base
  - Multiplanar reformations as needed
  - 3D reconstructions may be helpful for clinical decision making & surgical planning

DIFFERENTIAL DIAGNOSIS

Choanal Stenosis

- Posterior nasal airway narrowed but not completely occluded
- More common than true choanal atresia

Congenital Nasal Pyriform Aperture Stenosis

- Narrowed pyriform aperture(s) (anterior inferior nasal passage)
- Thickened anteromedial maxilla(e)
- ± anterior nasal septum thinning
- ± solitary median maxillary central incisor
- Must evaluate brain for holoprosencephaly
  - ↑ in patients with pyriform aperture stenosis + solitary median maxillary central incisor

Nasolacrimal Duct Mucocele

- Bilobed cystic mass extending from medial orbital nasolacrimal fossa to inferior meatus
  - Enlargement of lacrimal sac
  - Enlargement of nasolacrimal duct within enlarged nasolacrimal canal
  - Intranasal cystic mass inferior to inferior turbinate

Nasal Foreign Body

- Usually older patient
  - ± unrecognized choanal stenosis or choana atresia

PATHOLOGY

General Features

- Etiology
  - Pathogenesis remains elusive & unproven
    - Misdirected neural crest cell migration
    - Failure of perforation of oronasal membrane (normally perforates by 7th week of gestation)
      □ Bony choanal atresia: Incomplete canalization of choanae
      □ Membranous choanal atresia: Incomplete resorption of epithelial plugs
    - Molecular mechanisms in retinoic acid receptor development recently described in pathogenesis
- Genetics
  - Chromosomal abnormalities, single gene defects, deformations, & teratogens implicated
    - Associated with chromosome 18, 12, 22, XO abnormalities
    - Familial form exists
    - In patients with CHARGE syndrome, 60% have *CHD7* gene mutation
    - De novo mutation of *USP9X* implicated
- Associated abnormalities
  - Unilateral choanal atresia more likely to be isolated
  - Syndromes common in bilateral atresia (up to 75%)
  - CHARGE syndrome: **C**oloboma, **h**eart defect, choanal **a**tresia, **r**estricted growth, **g**enitourinary & **e**ar defects
    - Major diagnostic characteristics: Coloboma, choanal atresia, cranial nerve aplasia/hypoplasias (CNI, VII, VIII, IX-X), & typical outer/middle/inner ear anomalies
    - Minor characteristics: Genital hypoplasia, developmental delay, cardiac anomalies, growth deficiency, orofacial cleft, tracheoesophageal fistula, abnormal face, kidney abnormalities, typical CHARGE faces
  - Other syndromes
    - Acrocephalosyndactyly
    - Amniotic band syndrome

- Apert syndrome
- Craniosynostosis
- Crouzon disease
- Cornelia de Lange syndrome
- Fetal alcohol syndrome
- DiGeorge syndrome
- Treacher-Collins syndrome

Staging, Grading, & Classification

- Types of atresia: Mixed bony & membranous (up to 70%) vs. purely bony atresia (up to 30%)

Gross Pathologic & Surgical Features

- Membranous soft tissue or bony plate occludes choanal opening

CLINICAL ISSUES

Presentation

- Most common signs/symptoms
  - Bilateral choanal atresia: Respiratory distress in newborn
    - Infants breathe through nose (obligate nasal breathers) up to 6 months of age
    - Aggravated by feeding, relieved by crying
  - Unilateral choanal atresia or stenosis: Chronic, purulent, unilateral rhinorrhea in older child
  - **Inability to pass nasogastric tube** through nasal cavity beyond 3-4 cm despite **aerated lungs** on radiograph
- Other signs/symptoms
  - Nasal stuffiness
  - Grunting, snorting, low-pitched stridor
  - May present in older patient with unrecognized atresia/stenosis as nasal foreign body
- Clinical profile
  - Bilateral: Infant with respiratory distress
  - Unilateral: Child/young adult with unilateral purulent rhinorrhea

Demographics

- Age
  - Bilateral choanal atresia presents at birth
  - Unilateral choanal atresia/stenosis may present in infancy or as child/young adult
- Sex
  - F:M = 2:1
- Epidemiology
  - Most common congenital abnormality of nasal cavity
    - 1:5,000 to 8,000 live births

Natural History & Prognosis

- Bilateral choanal atresia
  - Diagnosed & treated in newborn period
  - Prognosis dependent on presence of other associated anomalies
- Unilateral choanal atresia
  - Not life-threatening
  - May present later in childhood
  - Prognosis excellent after surgical therapy
- Some patients prone to restenosis

Treatment

- Establish oral airway immediately to ensure proper breathing
- Membranous atresia may be perforated upon passage of nasogastric tube
- Surgical treatment effective for alleviating respiratory symptoms
  - Transnasal endoscopic/laser-assisted techniques
    - Endoscopic approach frequently used for simple membranous & bony atresias
      □ Minimizes traumatic injury → ↓ scarring, ↓ restenosis
    - ± use of stents
    - In unilateral atresia & **no** respiratory distress, recommend waiting to do surgery after 6 months of age &/or weight > 5 kg when possible
  - ± adjuvant use of stents in selected cases
    - Use of antiproliferative agents debated
    - More commonly used in revision surgery than initial surgery
  - Bilateral bony atresias may require transpalatal resection of vomer with choanal reconstruction
- Postoperative scar & incomplete resection of atresia plate best evaluated with bone CT

DIAGNOSTIC CHECKLIST

Consider

- Once airway established, respiratory distress with suspected nasal obstruction in newborn should be evaluated with thin-section bone CT

Image Interpretation Pearls

- Determine if choanal atresia unilateral or bilateral
- Look for associated anomalies in head & neck

Reporting Tips

- Describe choanal atresia as
  - Unilateral or bilateral
  - Mixed membranous/bony or purely bony
    - Comment on thickness of atretic bone plate

SELECTED REFERENCES

1. Wen JY et al: Navigation-assisted endoscopic U-flap technique and steroid-eluting stent for choanal atresia repair. Int J Pediatr Otorhinolaryngol. 189:112217, 2025
2. Patino M et al: Fetal head and neck imaging. Magn Reson Imaging Clin N Am. 32(3):413-30, 2024
3. Koppen T et al: Diagnostics and therapy of bilateral choanal atresia in association with CHARGE syndrome. J Neonatal Perinatal Med. 14(1):67-74, 2021
4. Qin Z et al: Clinical and genetic analysis of CHD7 expands the genotype and phenotype of CHARGE syndrome. Front Genet. 11:592, 2020
5. Albdah A et al: Choanal atresia repair in pediatric patients: is the use of stents recommended? Cureus. 11(3):e4206, 2019
6. Moreddu E et al: International Pediatric Otolaryngology Group (IPOG) consensus recommendations: diagnosis, pre-operative, operative and post-operative pediatric choanal atresia care. Int J Pediatr Otorhinolaryngol. 123:151-5, 2019
7. Moreddu E et al: Prognostic factors and management of patients with choanal atresia. J Pediatr. 204:234-9.e1, 2019
8. Smith MM et al: Pediatric nasal obstruction. Otolaryngol Clin North Am. 51(5):971-85 2018
9. Zawawi F et al: The pathogenesis of choanal atresia. JAMA Otolaryngol Head Neck Surg. 144(8):758-9, 2018

Choanal Atresia

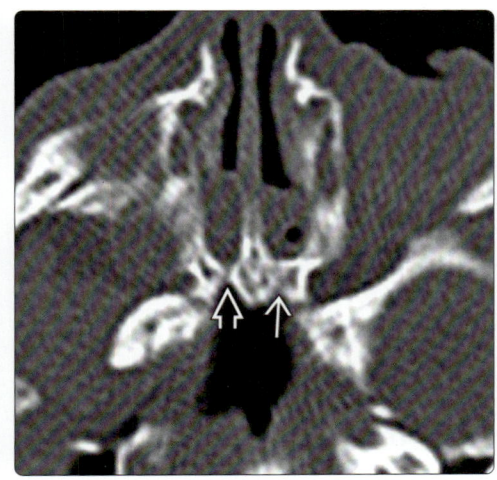

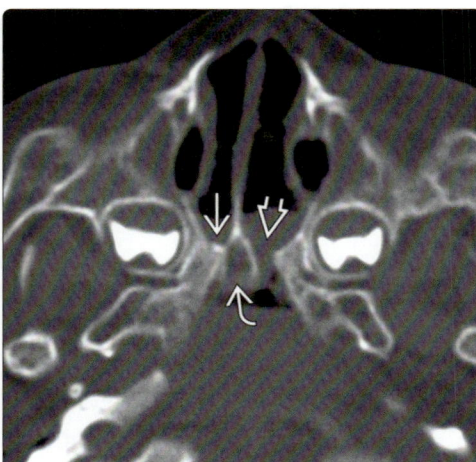

(Left) Axial bone CT in a neonate with severe respiratory distress demonstrates bilateral choanal atresia with thick bony atresia on the left ➡ & near-complete bony bridge on the right ⮞. Notice retained bilateral nasal cavity secretions secondary to noncommunication between the nasal cavity & nasopharynx. (Right) Axial bone CT shows an infant with bony choanal atresia ➡ on the right & membranous choanal atresia ⮞ on the left. The maxillae deviate medially, & the vomer ⮞ is thick.

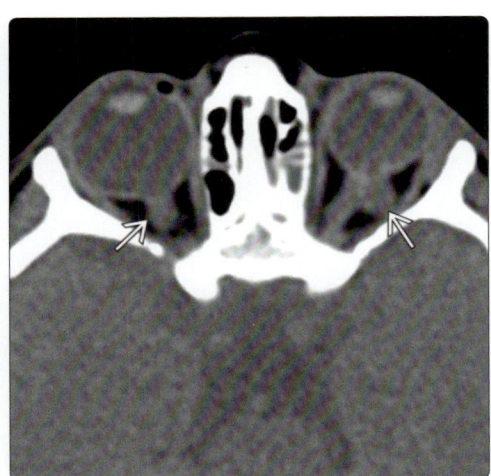

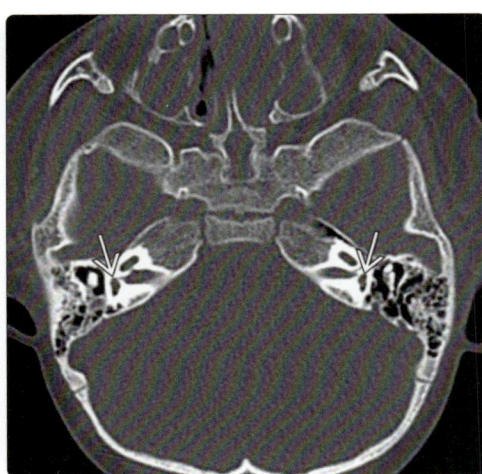

(Left) Axial NECT in a child with unilateral choanal atresia (not shown) & CHARGE syndrome shows bilateral colobomata ➡ & left microphthalmia. (Right) Axial bone CT in the same child shows typical bilateral labyrinthine anomalies with small, diminutive vestibules ➡ & absent semicircular canals. Although semicircular canal hypoplasia/atresia can occur in patients without CHARGE syndrome, absence, or near-complete absence of bilateral semicircular canals should raise the question of CHARGE syndrome.

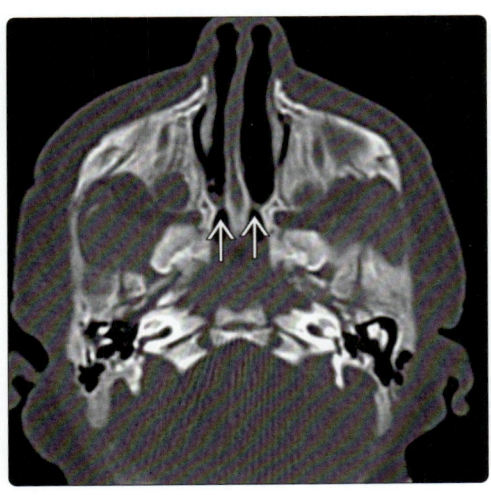

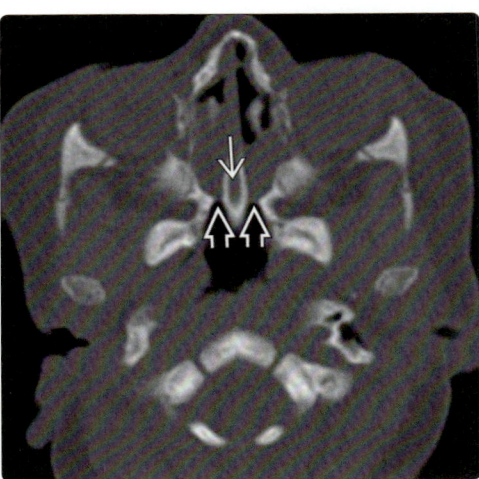

(Left) Axial bone CT in a child with CHARGE syndrome demonstrates bilateral choanal obstructions secondary to linear membranes ➡ extending between the thickened vomer & each medially positioned posterior maxilla, typical of a mixed choanal atresia. (Right) Axial bone CT in another child with known CHARGE syndrome (bilateral colobomas & severe hypoplasia semicircular canals) shows prominent vomer ➡, bilateral bony choanal stenosis, & membranous atresia ⮞.

KEY FACTS

TERMINOLOGY

- Synonym: **Nasal glial heterotopia**; cerebral heterotopia
- Developmental mass of dysplastic neurogenic tissue sequestered & isolated from subarachnoid space
  - **Glioma** is **misnomer**, as this is nonneoplastic tissue
  - Extranasal glioma (ENG), intranasal glioma (ING)

IMAGING

- Well-circumscribed soft tissue mass at superior nasal dorsum (ENG) or within nasal cavity (ING)
  - With no intracranial CSF or brain continuity
- Wide foramen cecum alone not strong indicator of intracranial extension; correlate with MR
- Multiplanar MR
  - May show pedicle of fibrous tissue (not brain parenchyma) between ING & intracranial cavity
  - Better than CT to differentiate from cephalocele or dermoid
  - Gyral structure of gray matter rarely visible
  - Commonly shows hyperintensity related to gliosis

TOP DIFFERENTIAL DIAGNOSES

- Frontoethmoidal cephalocele
- Nasal dermal sinus
- Sinonasal solitary polyp

PATHOLOGY

- Similar spectrum of congenital anomalies as frontoethmoidal cephaloceles
  - Does **not** contain CSF or brain contiguous intracranially
- Rarely associated with other brain or systemic anomalies

CLINICAL ISSUES

- Usually identified at birth
- Treatment of choice is complete surgical resection

DIAGNOSTIC CHECKLIST

- Caution: Anterior skull base **ossification widely variable** in 1st few years of life; do not overcall bony defects

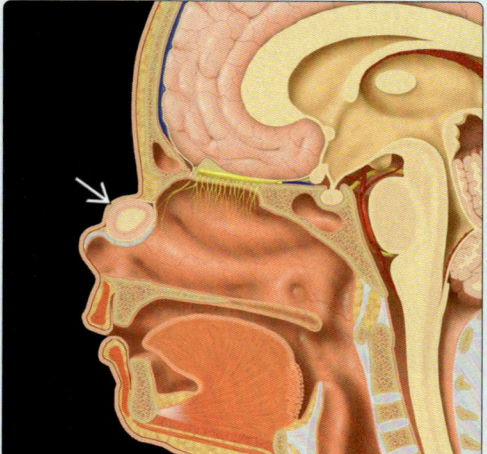
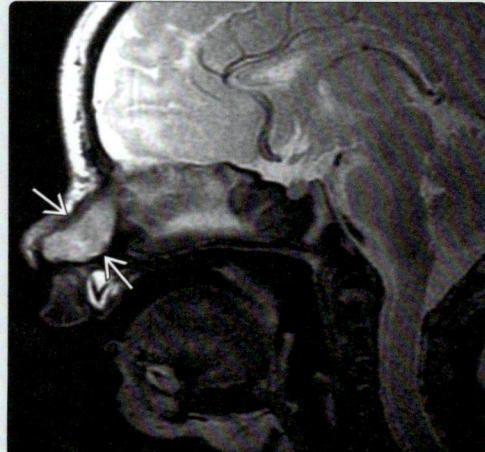

(Left) Sagittal graphic of a nasal glioma shows a mass of dysplastic glial tissue ➡ along the nasal dorsum. Notice the normal foramen cecum, normal crista galli, and absence of a connection to the intracranial contents. (Right) Sagittal T2 MR in a 3-day-old with a nasal mass demonstrates an intermediate signal intensity intranasal glioma ➡ without intracranial extension. Differential diagnosis would include a dermoid cyst. The normal appearance of other midline structures is typical.

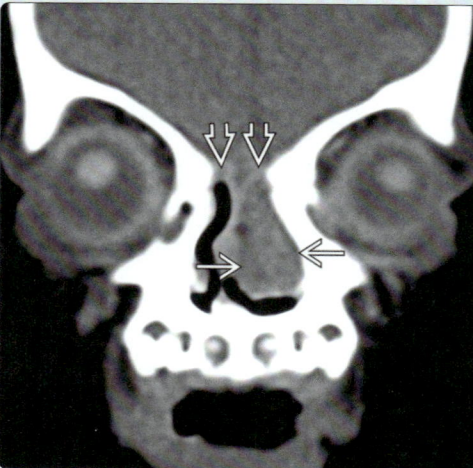
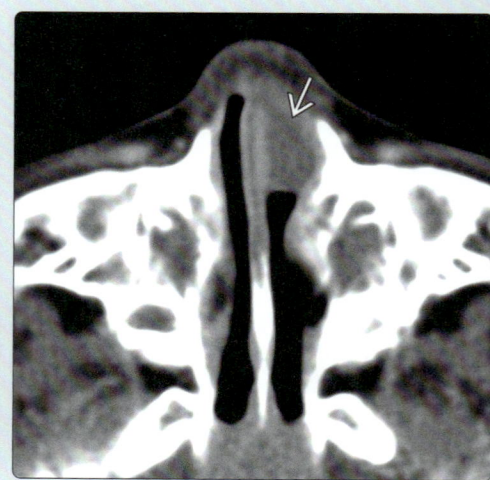

(Left) Coronal NECT shows a well-defined, somewhat polypoid soft tissue mass ➡, consistent with an intranasal glioma, within the left nasal cavity. The nasal septum is slightly deviated toward the right. No definite connection to the frontal lobe parenchyma is appreciated. Anterior skull base defects in an infant should be interpreted with caution; there is wide variation in unossified areas ➡ in the 1st few years of life. (Right) Axial CECT shows a left-sided intranasal glioma ➡ widening the anterior nasal vault.

TERMINOLOGY

Abbreviations

- Nasal glioma (NG)
  - Extranasal glioma (ENG), intranasal glioma (ING)

Synonyms

- **Nasal glial heterotopia**, cerebral heterotopia

Definitions

- Developmental mass of **dysplastic neurogenic tissue** sequestered & isolated from subarachnoid space
  - **Glioma** is **misnomer**, as this is nonneoplastic tissue
  - Best thought of as cephalocele without intracranial connection to brain

IMAGING

General Features

- Best diagnostic clue
  - Well-circumscribed soft tissue mass at superior nasal dorsum (ENG) or within nasal cavity (ING)
    - **No** connection to brain
- Location
  - Most occur at bridge of nose or in & around nasal cavity
  - Usually off midline; right > left side
  - ENG: Mass along nasal dorsum
    - Glabella most frequent location
    - ENG may also be found at medial canthus
  - Other sites of ENG
    - Ethmoid sinus, sphenoid sinus, palate, middle ear, tonsil, nasopharynx, mouth, pterygopalatine fossa (very rare)
  - ING: Nasal cavity mass
    - May be attached to middle turbinate, nasal septum, or lateral nasal wall
- Size: 1-3 cm
- Morphology: Well-circumscribed, round, ovoid, or polypoid mass

CT Findings

- NECT
  - ENG: Well-circumscribed soft tissue attenuation mass at glabella
    - Isodense to brain
    - Superficial to point of fusion of frontal & nasal bones (fonticulus frontalis)
    - Nasal bones may be thinned
  - ING: Soft tissue attenuation mass within nasal cavity
    - Typically high in nasal vault
    - Fibrous pedicle may extend toward skull base but not intracranially
    - Defect in cribriform plate (10-30%)
    - Caution: Anterior skull base **ossification widely variable** in 1st few years of life
      - ☐ Complete ossification by 3 years 10 months (earliest by 14 months)
      - ☐ Foramen cecum (anterior to crista galli) may still persist later
      - ☐ Wide foramen cecum alone not strong indicator of intracranial extension; correlate with MR
  - Calcification rare

- CECT
  - Typically no significant enhancement
  - If intrathecal contrast used
    - Fails to document connection of lesion to subarachnoid space

MR Findings

- T1WI
  - Predominantly mixed to low signal intensity mass
  - Gyral structure of gray matter rarely visible
- T2WI
  - Commonly shows hyperintensity related to gliosis
  - No CSF around lesion connecting to subarachnoid space
- T1WI C+
  - Dysplastic tissue typically does not enhance
    - Perceived enhancement at periphery of intranasal lesions may actually represent adjacent nasal mucosa
    - Internal enhancement may occur rarely

Imaging Recommendations

- Best imaging tool
  - Multiplanar MR
    - May show pedicle of fibrous tissue (not brain parenchyma) between ING & intracranial cavity
    - MR better than CT for differentiating NG from cephalocele or dermoid
    - Avoids radiation to radiosensitive ocular lenses
- Protocol advice
  - Thin-section sagittal T1 & T2 MR important sequences
  - Heavily T2W 3D sequences, such as CISS, FIESTA, or SPACE
    - Better demonstrate lack of brain parenchymal or CSF continuity intracranially
  - Preoperative thin-section axial bone CT with coronal reformatted images may also help in surgical planning
    - Bone only without IV contrast

DIFFERENTIAL DIAGNOSIS

Frontoethmoidal Cephalocele

- Frontonasal (FN) & nasoethmoidal (NE) cephaloceles
- Clinical: Congenital mass on or around bridge of nose (FN) or within nasal cavity (NE)
- Imaging: MR shows connection to intracranial brain parenchyma or CSF
  - Through unobliterated fonticulus frontalis (FN)
  - Through foramen cecum (NE)

Nasal Dermal Sinus

- Clinical: Pit on tip or bridge of nose
- Imaging
  - Associated dermoid or epidermoid along course from tip of nose to foramen cecum, anterior to crista galli
    - Single or multiple
  - Possible intracranial connection via sinus tract in septum from nasal dorsum to skull base

Sinonasal Solitary Polyps

- Clinical: Polyp is less firm, more translucent than ING
  - Unusual < 5 years
- Imaging
  - Typically inferolateral to middle turbinate (ING medial)

o Homogeneous ↑ T2 MR signal with thin enhancement of peripheral mucosa

Orbital Dermoid & Epidermoid

- Clinical: Focal mass in medial orbit near nasolacrimal suture
- Imaging
  - o Dermoid: Fluid or fat density/signal intensity
  - o Epidermoid: Fluid density/signal intensity

PATHOLOGY

General Features

- Etiology
  - o Dysplastic, heterotopic neuroglial, & fibrous tissue separated from brain
    - During development of anterior skull/skull base
  - o Similar spectrum of congenital anomalies as frontoethmoidal cephaloceles but does not contain CSF
    - Not contiguous with subarachnoid spaces
  - o Premature fusion of potential anterior skull base spaces prior to regression of dural diverticulum
  - o ENG: Premature fusion of **fonticulus frontalis** (potential space prior to fusion of frontal & nasal bones)
    - Dysplastic parenchyma sequestered over nasal bones/nasofrontal suture
  - o ING: Premature fusion of **prenasal space** (potential space between nasal bones & cartilaginous nasal capsule)
    - Dysplastic parenchyma sequestered in nasal cavity
- Associated abnormalities
  - o Rarely associated with other brain or systemic anomalies

Gross Pathologic & Surgical Features

- Firm, smooth mass
- Rarely recognized as brain tissue at surgery
- Mixed extra- & intranasal lesions connect through defect in nasal bone
- 10-30% attached to brain by stalk of fibrous tissue through defect in or near cribriform plate
- Cribriform plate ossification begins near vertical attachments of superior & middle turbinates & spreads to reach crista galli by ~ 2 months of age
  - o Only 4% have complete anterior skull base ossification by 2 years
  - o Anterior skull base fully ossified at 3 years 10 months of age (foramen cecum may persist later)

Microscopic Features

- Fibrous or gemistocytic astrocytes & neuroglial fibers
- Fibrous, vascularized connective tissue & sparse neurons
- GFAP & S100 protein positive
- No mitotic features or bizarre nuclear forms

CLINICAL ISSUES

Presentation

- Most common signs/symptoms
  - o ENG
    - Congenital subcutaneous blue or red mass along nasal dorsum (glabella)
    - Usually nonprogressive midfacial swelling
  - o ING
    - Firm, polypoid submucosal nasal cavity mass

- Nasal obstruction & septal deviation may be present
- May be confused clinically with nasal polyp
- Other signs/symptoms
  - o No change in size with crying, Valsalva, or pressure on jugular vein (vs. frontoethmoidal cephalocele)
  - o ENG: Capillary telangiectasia may cover
  - o ING: Respiratory distress; epiphora; may protrude through nostril
- Clinical profile
  - o Firm mass at glabella (ENG) or within nasal cavity (ING) in newborn

Demographics

- Age: Usually identified at birth or within 1st few years
  - o May be detected on antenatal ultrasound & fetal MR
- Epidemiology: Very rare lesion
  - o **ENG: 36%**; **ING: 45%**; mixed: 19%

Natural History & Prognosis

- Grows slowly in proportion to adjacent tissue or brain if attached by pedicle
  - o May deform nasal skeleton, maxilla, or orbit
- May become infected, resulting in meningitis
- Complete resection is curative
  - o 10% recurrence rate with incomplete resection

Treatment

- Treatment of choice is complete surgical resection
  - o ENG without intracranial connection removed via external incision with stalk dissection
  - o ING without intracranial connection may be removed endoscopically
    - Less postoperative deformity than with craniotomy
  - o Stalk removal is imperative to ↓ recurrence rate & minimize CSF leak & subsequent meningitis

DIAGNOSTIC CHECKLIST

Consider

- Most important to **differentiate NG from cephalocele**
- Document lack of connecting brain tissue &/or contiguous CSF space

Image Interpretation Pearls

- Must evaluate images for connection to intracranial cavity through skull base defect (cephalocele)
- Combined use of thin-section MR & bone CT accomplishes this task
  - o Focus imaging to frontoethmoid area

SELECTED REFERENCES

1. Gallego Compte M et al: Nasal glial heterotopia: a systematic review of the literature and case report. Acta Otorhinolaryngol Ital. 42(4):317-24, 2022
2. Yan YY et al: Nasal glial heterotopia in children: two case reports and literature review. Int J Pediatr Otorhinolaryngol. 129:109728, 2020
3. Charles NC et al: Nasal glioma: a rare cause of congenital inner canthal swelling. Ophthalmic Plast Reconstr Surg. 34(3):e93-5, 2018
4. Rodriguez DP et al: Masses of the nose, nasal cavity, and nasopharynx in children. Radiographics. 37(6):1704-30, 2017
5. Hughes DC et al: Dimensions and ossification of the normal anterior cranial fossa in children. AJNR Am J Neuroradiol. 31(7):1268-72, 2010
6. Hedlund G: Congenital frontonasal masses: developmental anatomy, malformations, and MR imaging. Pediatr Radiol. 36(7):647-62; quiz 726-7, 2006

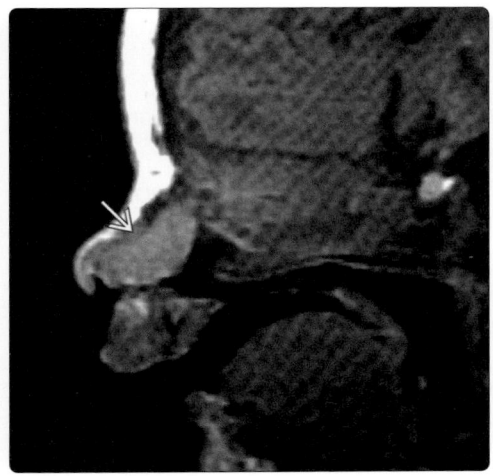

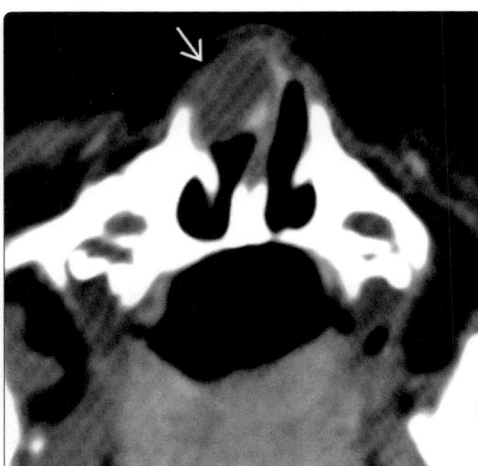

(Left) Sagittal T1 MR in a 3-day-old girl shows a well-defined nasal mass ➡, similar in signal intensity relative to cerebral cortex, without intracranial extension. Differential diagnosis would include cephalocele and epidermoid. Lack of CSF extension into the mass, and lack of diffusion restriction (not shown), would support histologically proven nasal glial heterotopia. (Right) Axial CECT in the same child shows a low-attenuation right nasal mass ➡ without internal enhancement, typical of intranasal glial heterotopia.

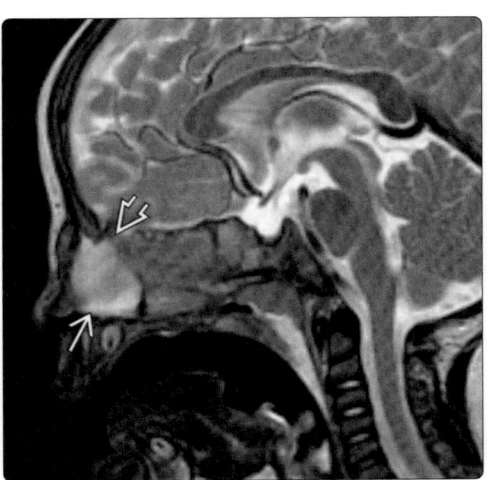

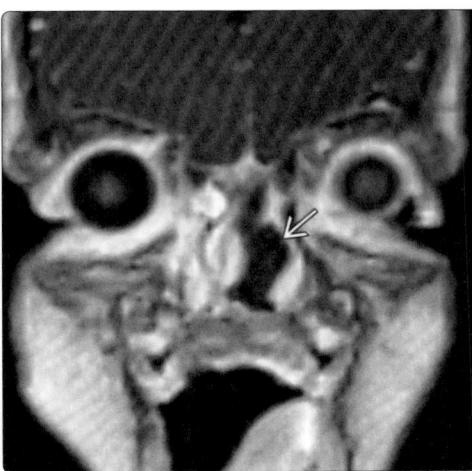

(Left) Sagittal T2 MR in a 10-month-old shows an intranasal mixed, primarily hyperintense nasal mass ➡ extending to the foramen cecum ➡ without intracranial extension. Differential diagnosis would include a dermoid cyst. This lesion was histologically proven to be nasal glial heterotopia. (Right) Coronal T1 C+ MR in the same patient shows a nonenhancing mass without intracranial extension, histologically proven to be nasal glial heterotopia ➡.

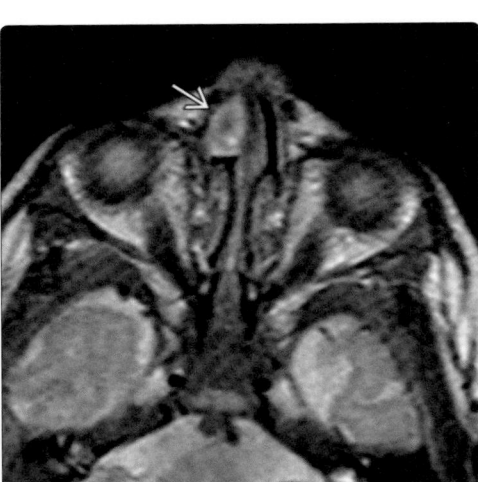

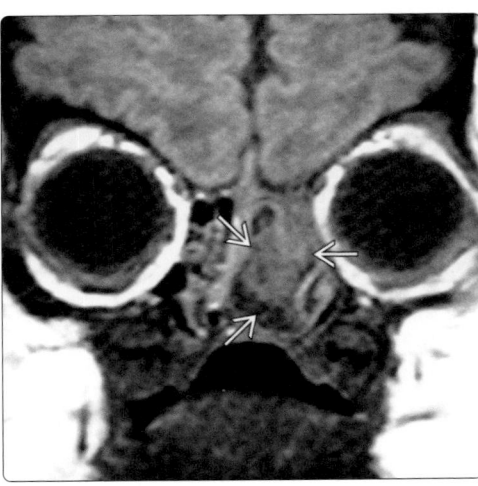

(Left) Axial T2 MR in a 3-month-old with a nasal mass shows obstruction of the right nasal cavity by a small, heterogeneous mass ➡, proven to be glial heterotopia. There was no intracranial extension, which is imperative to report to the surgeon prior to operation. (Right) Coronal FLAIR MR shows mixed signal intensity within an intranasal glioma ➡. There is no connection to the left frontal lobe to suggest that a cephalocele is present.

Nasal Dermal Sinus

TERMINOLOGY

- Defective embryogenesis of anterior neuropore
- Resulting in any mixture of dermoid cyst, epidermoid cyst, &/or sinus tract in frontonasal region

IMAGING

- Midline location anywhere from nasal tip to anterior skull base at foramen cecum
- MR
  - T2: Fluid-signal tract in septum from nasal dorsum to skull base (sinus)
  - T1: Focal low-signal (epidermoid or nonfatty dermoid) or high-signal (dermoid) mass between tip of nose & apex of crista galli
- CT
  - Bifid crista galli with large foramen cecum
  - Fluid-attenuation tract (sinus)/cyst (epidermoid) or fat-containing mass (dermoid)
    - From nasal dorsum to skull base within nasal septum

TOP DIFFERENTIAL DIAGNOSES

- Fatty marrow in crista galli
- Nonossified foramen cecum
- Frontoethmoidal cephalocele
- Nasal glioma (nasal glial heterotopia/cerebral heterotopia)

PATHOLOGY

- Intracranial extension of nasal dermal sinus (NDS) in 20%
  - May rarely lead to meningitis
- Associated craniofacial anomalies in 15%

CLINICAL ISSUES

- Nasoglabellar mass (30%)
- Pit (± protruding hair) on skin of nasal bridge at osteocartilaginous nasal junction

DIAGNOSTIC CHECKLIST

- Nasoglabellar mass or pit on nose sends clinician in search of NDS with intracranial extension

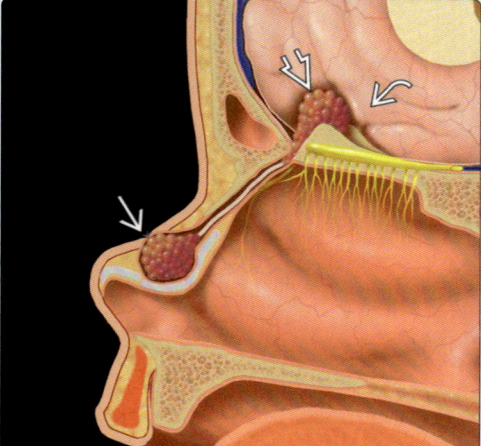
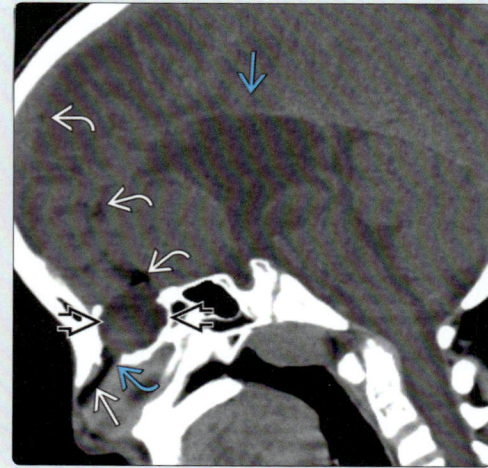

(Left) Lateral graphic depicts a nasal dermal sinus with 2 dermoids. An extracranial dermoid is present just deep to a cutaneous nasal pit ➡. An intracranial dermoid ➡ splits a bifid crista galli ➡. (Right) Sagittal NECT in an 8-year-old child with known midline anomalies shows a fat-lined nasal dermal sinus ➡ deep to the nasal bones. The sinus leads to a large fat and fluid attenuation dermoid ➡. There is a wide foramen cecum ➡ with fatty foci ➡ extending along the falx. Agenesis of the corpus callosum ➡ is also noted.

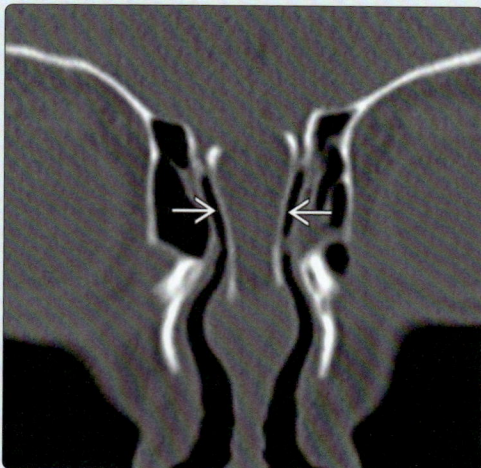
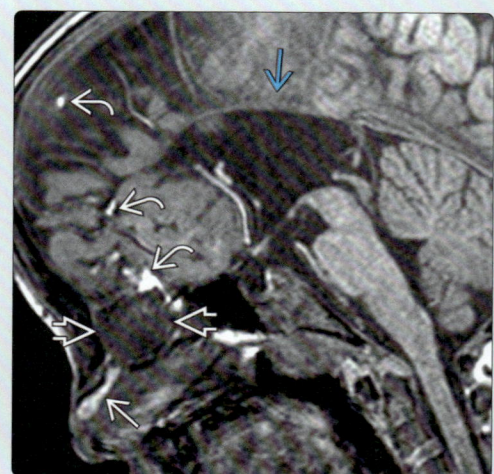

(Left) Coronal bone CT in the same patient shows the bony nasal septum split ➡ by a large fat- and fluid-attenuation dermoid. (Right) Sagittal T1 MR in the same patient shows the fat-lined nasal dermal sinus ➡, large mixed signal intensity dermoid ➡, and falcine foci of fat ➡ (consistent with intracranial extension and rupture). Agenesis of the corpus callosum ➡ is again noted. The dermoid was ultimately resected. Note that the size and extent of findings in this case are greater than typically seen.

TERMINOLOGY

Abbreviations
- Nasal dermal sinus (NDS)

Synonyms
- Nasal dermoid, nasal dermal cyst, anterior neuropore anomaly

Definitions
- Defective embryogenesis of anterior neuropore
- Resulting in any mixture of dermoid cyst, epidermoid cyst, &/or sinus tract in frontonasal region

IMAGING

General Features
- Best diagnostic clue
  - CT
    - Bifid crista galli with large foramen cecum
    - Fluid-attenuation tract (sinus)/cyst (epidermoid) or fat-containing mass (dermoid)
      - From nasal dorsum to skull base within nasal septum
  - MR
    - Fluid-signal tract in septum from nasal dorsum to skull base (sinus)
    - Focal T1 low-signal (epidermoid) or high-signal (dermoid) mass between tip of nose & apex of crista galli
- Location
  - Midline lesion anywhere from nasal tip to anterior skull base at foramen cecum
- Size
  - 5 mm to 2 cm for dermoid/epidermoid
- Morphology
  - Ovoid mass ± tubular sinus tract

CT Findings
- Bone CT
  - Focal tract (sinus) or mass (dermoid or epidermoid) anywhere from nasal bridge to crista galli
    - Fluid-density tract = sinus
    - Fluid-density mass = epidermoid (or dermoid without fat)
    - Fat-density mass = dermoid
  - Signs of intracranial extension
    - Large foramen cecum with bifid or deformed crista galli or sometimes cribriform plate
    - Caution: Anterior skull base ossification widely variable in 1st few years of life
    - Wide foramen cecum alone not strong indicator of intracranial extension; correlate with MR

MR Findings
- T1WI
  - ↓ signal tract = sinus
  - ↑ signal mass = dermoid (fat becomes ↓ on fat-suppressed images)
  - ↓ signal mass = epidermoid or dermoid without fat
- T2WI
  - ↑ signal in sinus, epidermoid, or dermoid

- Coronal plane shows septal lesions to best advantage
- DWI
  - ↑ signal = epidermoid usually; dermoid rarely
  - Susceptibility artifacts at skull base may obscure signal from epidermoid

Imaging Recommendations
- Best imaging tool
  - MR more sensitive for delineating sinus tract, detecting intracranial extension
    - MR characterizes epidermoid/dermoid lesions better
  - Bone CT optimal for identifying skull base defect & crista galli deformity
- Protocol advice
  - Imaging "sweet spot" is small & anterior
    - Focus imaging from tip of nose to back of crista galli
    - Inferior end of axial imaging is hard palate
    - Contrast helps with infectious complications or consideration of other differential diagnoses
      - Not for primary dermoid/epidermoid diagnosis
  - CT
    - Thin-section (1-2 mm) bone & soft tissue axial & coronal images
  - MR
    - Sagittal plane displays course of sinus tract from nasal dorsum to skull base
    - Fat-suppressed T1 images confirm presence of fat in dermoids
    - DWI important additional sequence
    - Heavily T2 3D sequences, such as CISS, FIESTA, or SPACE
      - May demonstrate sinus tract, intracranial continuity, & associated tiny epidermoid/dermoid better

DIFFERENTIAL DIAGNOSIS

Fatty Marrow in Crista Galli
- No nasoglabellar mass or pit on nose
- CT & MR otherwise normal

Nonossified Foramen Cecum
- Small midline pit lying between frontal & ethmoid bones, just anterior to crista galli of ethmoid
- Around 4-mm diameter at birth
- Foramen cecum ossification usually completes by 2 years
  - Sometimes delayed until 5 years
- Crista galli not deformed or bifid

Frontoethmoidal Cephalocele
- Bone dehiscence typically larger, involving broader area of midline cribriform plate or frontal bone
- Direct extension of meninges, subarachnoid space ± brain can be seen projecting into cephalocele on sagittal MR

Nasal Glioma
- Solid mass of dysplastic glial tissue separated from brain by subarachnoid space & meninges
- Preferred terms: Nasal glial heterotopia, nasal cerebral heterotopia
- Most commonly projects extranasally onto paramedian bridge of nose

- Less commonly intranasal & along anterior nasal septum, off midline

PATHOLOGY

General Features

- Etiology
  - Anterior neuropore anomaly: General term for anomalous anterior neuropore regression; 3 main types
    - NDS
    - Nasal glioma (preferred term: Nasal glial/cerebral heterotopia)
    - Frontoethmoidal (sincipital) cephalocele
  - Embryology-anatomy: Development of anterior neuropore in 4th gestational week
    - Dural stalk passes from area of future foramen cecum to area of osteocartilaginous nasal junction
      □ Later regresses completely
    - Failure of involution may leave neuroectodermal remnants along tract of dural stalk
    - Results in dermoid or epidermoid alone, or in association with NDS tract
- Genetics
  - Familial clustering
- Associated abnormalities
  - Intracranial extension of NDS seen in 20%
  - Craniofacial anomalies (15%)

Gross Pathologic & Surgical Features

- Sinus = tube of tissue can be followed through bones
- Epidermoid = well-defined cyst; dermoid = lobular, well-defined mass

Microscopic Features

- Sinus = midline epithelial-lined tract
- Epidermoid cyst contains desquamated epithelium
- Dermoid cyst contains epithelium, keratin debris, skin adnexa

CLINICAL ISSUES

Presentation

- Most common signs/symptoms
  - Nasoglabellar mass (30%)
  - Pit on skin of nasal bridge at osteocartilaginous nasal junction
    - ± protruding hair
- Other signs/symptoms
  - Intermittent sebaceous material discharge from pit
  - < 50% have broadening nasal root & bridge
  - Nasal sinus tract rarely → recurrent meningitis
- Clinical profile
  - Child (mean age: 32 months) with nasal pit ± nasoglabellar mass
  - Rarely presents in adult population
    - Meningitis may be 1st problem leading to diagnosis

Demographics

- Age: Newborn to 5 years old
- Sex: Male patients with dermal sinus more likely to have intracranial extension
- Epidemiology

  - Congenital midline nasal lesions rare (1 in 20,000-40,000 births)
    - Nasal dermoids most common

Natural History & Prognosis

- Isolated problem when surgical correction successful
- Untreated patients have nasal bridge broadening ± recurrent meningitis

Treatment

- 80% require extracranial excision only
  - Local procedure to remove pit
  - Any associated dermoid or epidermoid also simultaneously removed from nasal bridge
    - Open rhinoplasty vs. transnasal endoscopic excision
- 20% undergo combined extracranial & intracranial resection
  - Biorbitofrontal nasal craniotomy approach
    - Dermoid or epidermoid along with involved dura & crista galli removed
    - Primary closure of surgical margins of dura
  - Midline approach via keyhole frontal craniotomy recently described → less blood loss & shorter hospital stay
  - Transnasal approach through midline incision with endoscopic assistance recently reported

DIAGNOSTIC CHECKLIST

Consider

- Nasoglabellar mass or pit on nose sends clinician in search of NDS with intracranial extension
- Focused thin-section MR key to radiologic diagnosis
  - Axial coverage from cephalad margin of crista galli to hard palate
  - Coronal coverage from tip of nose to posterior aspect of crista galli
- Some surgeons prefer to add bone CT if NDS with intracranial extension found on MR

Image Interpretation Pearls

- If dermal sinus tract reaches dura of anterior cranial fossa, then crista galli will be bifid with large foramen cecum
- If foramen cecum large but crista galli not bifid & tract not seen, then foramen cecum normal & not yet closed
  - Foramen cecum may not close before age of 5 years
  - Do not overcall "large foramen cecum," or unnecessary craniotomy may result
  - Repeat imaging in 6-12 months to confirm foramen cecum closure acceptable approach in difficult cases

SELECTED REFERENCES

1. Woodyard De Brito KC et al: Transnasal endoscopic approach for excision of intracranial nasal dermoid sinus cysts. J Craniofac Surg. 36(1):30-6, 2025
2. Shimizu R et al: The necessity of dural resection for nasal dermal sinus cyst with intracranial extension. J Craniofac Surg. 34(6):e589-90, 2023
3. Purnell CA et al: Nasal dermoid cysts with intracranial extension: avoiding coronal incision through midline exposure and nasal bone osteotomy. J Neurosurg Pediatr. 1-7, 2019
4. Rodriguez DP et al: Masses of the nose, nasal cavity, and nasopharynx in children. Radiographics. 37(6):1704-30, 2017
5. Hedlund G: Congenital frontonasal masses: developmental anatomy, malformations, and MR imaging. Pediatr Radiol. 36(7):647-62; quiz 726-7, 2006

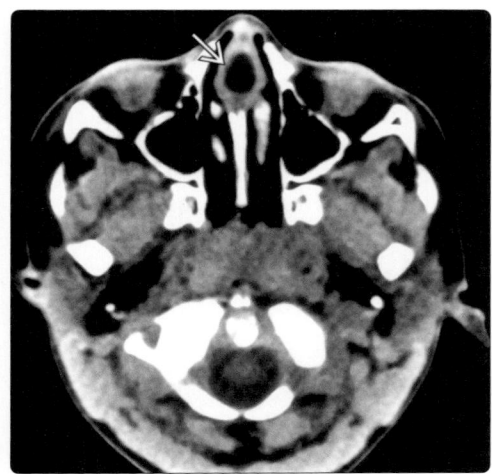

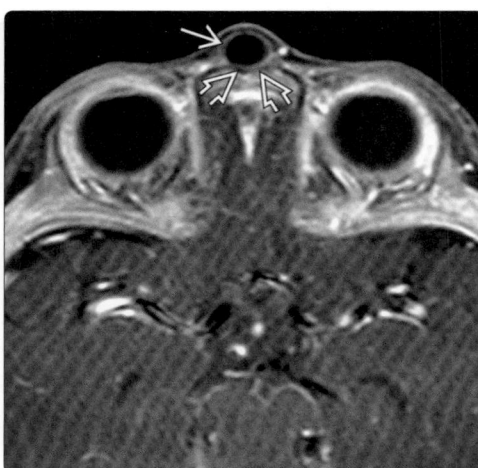

(Left) Axial NECT demonstrates a characteristic low-attenuation dermoid ➔ centered in the cartilaginous portion of the nasal septum. The mass is slightly higher in attenuation than adjacent fat. (Right) Axial T1 C+ FS MR in a 4-month-old infant with a glabellar mass demonstrates a nonenhancing, fluid-signal intensity dermoid cyst ➔ with mild remodeling of the underlying nasal bones ➔. Although dermoid cysts may contain fat, like this lesion, the majority of them do not.

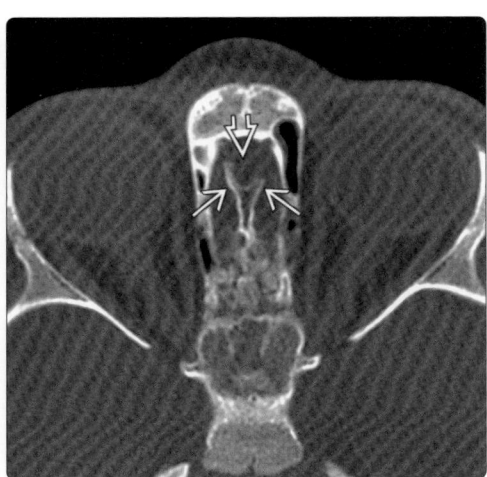

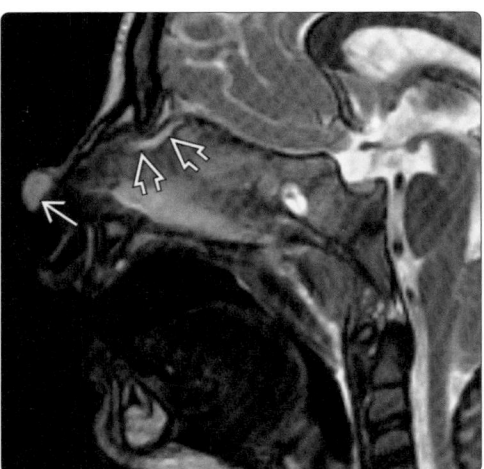

(Left) Axial bone CT demonstrates a bifid crista galli ➔ surrounding an intracranial dermoid ➔ along a persistently large foramen cecum. (Right) Sagittal T2 MR in a 1-year-old child with a mass at the tip of his nose shows an ovoid hyperintense mass ➔ and a tubular lesion ➔ traversing through the nasal septum, extending to the foramen cecum, without intracranial extension. At the level of the foramen cecum, the lesion demonstrated diffusion restriction, typical of dermoid cysts.

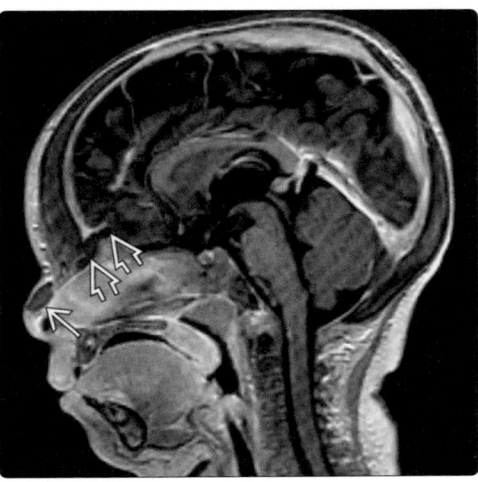

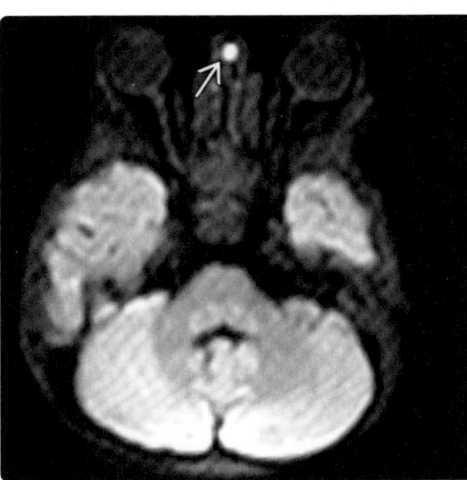

(Left) Sagittal T1 C+ MR in a 1-year-old child with a nasal dorsum mass shows the subcutaneous nonenhancing midline mass ➔ and a midline, fluid-filled lesion extending to the foramen cecum ➔, imaging characteristics consistent with dermoid or epidermoid cysts. (Right) Axial DWI MR in the same patient demonstrates restricted diffusion in the lesion at the level of the foramen cecum ➔, typical of epidermoid cysts, and occasionally present in dermoid cysts.

Cephalocele, Frontoethmoidal

TERMINOLOGY

- Congenital herniation of meninges, CSF ± brain tissue through mesodermal defect in anterior skull/skull base
- Synonym: Sincipital cephalocele

IMAGING

- Heterogeneous, mixed-density mass (variable amounts of CSF and parenchyma) extending through bony defect
  - Midline frontal: **Frontonasal** type (FNCeph)
  - Intranasal: **Nasoethmoidal** type (NECeph)
  - Inferomedial orbital: **Nasoorbital** type (NOCeph)

TOP DIFFERENTIAL DIAGNOSES

- Nasal glioma
- Orbital dermoid and epidermoid
- Nasal dermal sinus
- Nasolacrimal duct mucocele

PATHOLOGY

- **Frontonasal**
  - Protrudes through unobliterated **fonticulus frontalis**
- **Nasoethmoidal**
  - Protrudes through foramen cecum into **prenasal space**
- **Nasoorbital**
  - Protrudes into inferomedial orbit through defect in lacrimal/frontal process of maxillary bones

CLINICAL ISSUES

- Intracranial abnormalities in ~ 80%
- F = 67%, M = 33%
- Most common in Southeast Asian populations

DIAGNOSTIC CHECKLIST

- Sagittal and coronal T1 and T2 MR optimal for showing contiguity of mass with intracranial contents

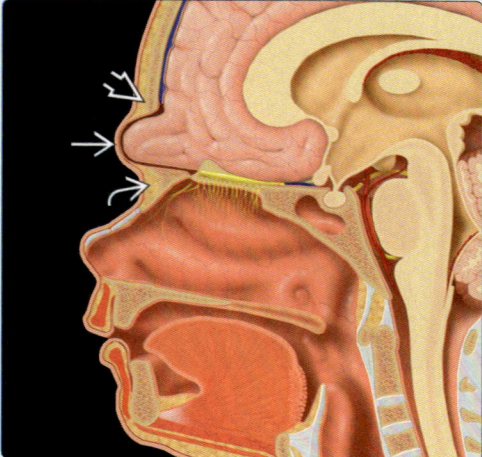
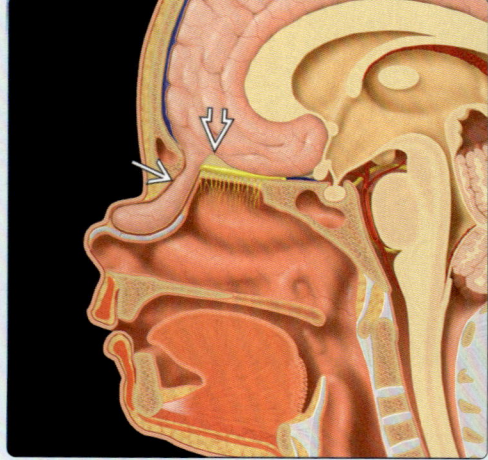

(Left) Sagittal graphic of a frontonasal cephalocele shows herniation of the brain through a patent fonticulus frontalis ➡ between the frontal bones above ➡ and nasal bones below ➡. (Right) Sagittal graphic of a nasoethmoidal cephalocele shows the herniation of brain tissue ➡ into the nasal cavity through a patent foramen cecum. Note that the crista galli is positioned posterior to the skull base defect ➡.

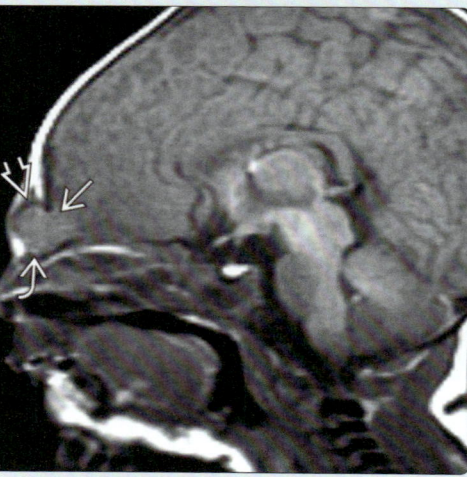
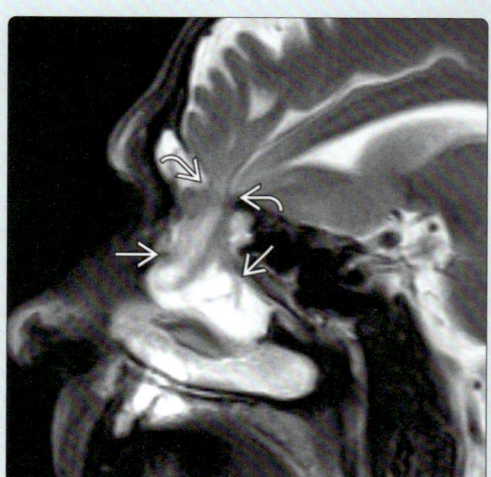

(Left) Sagittal T1 MR in a 1-week-old shows a frontonasal cephalocele ➡ with protrusion of the dysplastic-appearing inferior left frontal lobe through a patent fonticulus frontalis. The frontal bone ➡ is above and the nasal bone ➡ is below the cephalocele. (Right) Sagittal T2 FS MR shows a nasoethmoidal cephalocele with herniation of brain parenchyma and meninges ➡ through a defect in the foramen cecum region of the anterior skull base ➡.

TERMINOLOGY

Abbreviations

- Frontoethmoidal cephalocele (FECeph)
  - Frontonasal cephalocele (FNCeph)
  - Nasoethmoidal cephalocele (NECeph)
  - Nasoorbital cephalocele (NOCeph)

Synonyms

- Sincipital cephalocele

Definitions

- Cephalocele: Outward herniation of CNS contents through defect in cranium
  - Term includes meningocele and meningoencephalocele
- Congenital herniation of meninges and CSF (meningocele) + brain tissue (meningoencephalocele)
- Through mesodermal defect in anterior skull/skull base, presenting as extranasal, intranasal, or medial orbital mass
- **Do not confuse for basal encephaloceles**, which occur through cribriform plate or sphenoid defects
  - Basal cephaloceles: Transsphenoidal, sphenoethmoidal, transethmoidal, sphenoorbital

IMAGING

General Features

- Best diagnostic clue
  - Midline frontal (FNCeph), intranasal (NECeph), or medial orbital (NOCeph) soft tissue mass
  - Contiguous with intracranial brain parenchyma extending through bony defect
- Location
  - FNCeph: Anterior forehead at glabella-dorsum of nose
  - NECeph: Superomedial nasal cavity
    - Intracranially, 90% terminate at single midline defect at foramen cecum
    - 10% terminate at paired openings at anterior cribriform plates separated by midline bony bridge
  - NOCeph: Inferomedial orbit
- Size
  - Variable
  - 1-2 cm to larger than infant head
- Morphology
  - Well circumscribed, round, globular

CT Findings

- NECT
  - Heterogeneous, mixed-density mass (variable amounts of CSF and parenchyma) extending through bony defect
- Bone CT
  - FNCeph: Frontal bones displaced superiorly while nasal bones, frontal processes of maxillae pushed inferiorly
  - NECeph: Nasal bone bowed anteriorly with tract through anterior ethmoid area
    - Crista galli may be bifid or absent
    - Deficient or absent cribriform plate
- CT myelogram
  - Intrathecal contrast: Fills subarachnoid space and surrounds soft tissue extending through bony defect

MR Findings

- T1WI: Soft tissue mass isointense to gray matter contiguous with intracranial parenchyma through bony defect
- T2W: Hyperintense CSF surrounds herniated parenchyma
  - Tissue may show ↑ signal due to gliosis
- T1WI C+: No abnormal enhancement within soft tissue
  - Meninges may enhance if infected/inflamed

Ultrasonographic Findings

- OB US: Frontal (FNCeph), intranasal (NECeph), or medial periorbital (NOCeph) soft tissue mass
  - Widened interorbital distance

Imaging Recommendations

- Best imaging tool
  - MR superior to CT for cephalocele evaluation
    - Differentiates CSF-filled meningocele and parenchymal components
    - Superior for showing other associated brain anomalies
- Protocol advice
  - Thin (3-mm) multiplanar T1 and T2 MR
    - Sagittal and coronal planes optimal for visualizing parenchymal herniation through defects
  - Heavily T2WI 3D sequence (CISS, FIESTA, or SPACE)
    - Better demonstrate intra- and extracranial continuity of CSF and brain
  - Bone CT can provide important information about skull defects for surgical planning
    - CT or MR with intrathecal contrast used only when full MR and bone CT still leave unanswered questions

DIFFERENTIAL DIAGNOSIS

Nasal Glioma (Nasal Cerebral Heterotopia, Glial Heterotopia)

- Clinical: Soft tissue mass along dorsum of nose (extranasal type) or under nasal bones (intranasal type)
- Imaging: MR shows no connection between mass in intracranial contents

Orbital Dermoid and Epidermoid

- Clinical: Focal mass in medial orbit without associated tract
- Imaging: Fat density/intensity if dermoid, fluid density/intensity if epidermoid

Nasal Dermal Sinus

- Clinical: Pit on tip or bridge of nose
- Imaging: Midline sinus from tip of nose to skull base
  - Dermoid or epidermoid may be seen anywhere along tract
  - Possible intracranial connection via sinus tract; does not contain brain parenchyma

Nasolacrimal Duct Mucocele

- Clinical: Small, round, bluish, medial canthal mass seen at birth with submucosal nasal cavity mass at inferior meatus
- Imaging: Nasolacrimal duct dilatation may be present at inferior meatus
  - No connection to skull base or brain parenchyma

PATHOLOGY

General Features

- Etiology
  - Prior to 8th week of gestation, 2 potential spaces
  - **Fonticulus frontalis**: Fontanelle between developing frontal bone superiorly and nasal bones inferiorly
    - Closes when chondrocranium begins to ossify; failure of closure → **FNCeph**
  - **Prenasal space**: Dura-filled space between developing nasal bones anteriorly and nasal capsule posteriorly
  - Chondrocranium of anterior skull base ossifies from posterior to anterior
    - Except small cartilage in front for nasal capsule
  - Nasal bones also ossify further
    - Prenasal space lying in between these becomes encased in bone and obliterates
      - □ Leaves small dural diverticulum, called **foramen cecum**, just anterior to future crista galli
  - Foramen cecum transiently communicates with nasal skin anteroinferiorly
    - Through dura-lined stalk called **anterior neuropore**
  - Anterior neuropore regression failure → **NECeph** via foramen cecum into prenasal space and nasal cavity
  - Defect in lacrimal/frontal process of maxillary bones → **NOCeph** protruding into inferomedial orbit
- Genetics
  - Sporadic occurrence
  - Not linked to neural tube defects, such as occipital cephaloceles
  - Siblings have 6% incidence of congenital CNS abnormalities
- Associated abnormalities
  - **Intracranial abnormalities (~ 80%)**
    - Callosal hypogenesis and interhemispheric lipomas
    - Neuronal migration anomalies
    - Microcephaly
    - Aqueductal stenosis and hydrocephalus
    - Colloid or arachnoid cysts
  - Midline craniofacial dysraphisms and hypertelorism
  - Microphthalmos
  - Morning glory disc anomaly with basal encephaloceles (cribriform plate or sphenoid defects), **not** FECeph

Microscopic Features

- **Meningoencephalocele**: CSF, brain tissue, and meninges
- **Meningocele**: Meninges and CSF only
- **Atretic cephalocele**: Forme fruste of cephalocele with dura, fibrous tissue, and degenerated brain tissue
- **Gliocele**: Glial-lined, CSF-filled cyst

CLINICAL ISSUES

Presentation

- Most common signs/symptoms
  - Externally visible, firm midline forehead (FNCeph), intranasal (NECeph), or medial orbital (NOCeph) mass
- Other signs/symptoms
  - Hypertelorism and orbital dystopia
  - Hyperpigmentation of overlying skin
  - Change in size with crying, Valsalva, jugular compression
  - Seizures and intellectual disability in < 50% of patients

Demographics

- Age
  - Congenital lesion detected on prenatal US or presenting at birth
- Sex
  - F = 67%, M = 33%
- Ethnicity
  - FECeph most common in Southeast Asian populations
- Epidemiology
  - Cephaloceles are uncommon in Western countries
  - 1 in 4,000-5,000 live births in Southeast Asia
  - FECeph account for 15% of all cephaloceles
  - FNCeph (50-61%), NECeph (30-33%), NOCeph (6-10%)

Natural History & Prognosis

- Present at birth, requires surgical repair
- If untreated, may grow with child
- If thin skin covering or no skin, prone to rupture, CSF leak, and infection
- When CSF filled, may ↑ rapidly in size
- Hydrocephalus and presence of intracranial abnormalities are predictors of developmental delay/poor outcome

Treatment

- Biopsy contraindicated: CSF leak, seizures, meningitis
- Complete surgical resection
  - Combined plastic surgery and neurosurgery
  - Herniated brain tissue is dysfunctional (no neurologic deficits result)
- Meningeal and skull base defect repaired or CSF leak, meningitis, or recurrent herniation may result

DIAGNOSTIC CHECKLIST

Consider

- Sagittal and coronal T1 and T2 MR optimal for showing contiguity of mass with intracranial contents
- Bone CT used to evaluate size and location of bony defect prior to surgical repair

Image Interpretation Pearls

- Determine location of lesion relative to nasal bones
  - Above is FNCeph
  - Below is NECeph
- Evaluate brain for associated anomalies

SELECTED REFERENCES

1. Mughal ZUN et al: Letter to the editor: "management of cerebrospinalfluidrelated intracranial abnormalities in frontoethmoidal encephalocele using "shunt algorithm for frontoethmoidal encephalocele" (SAFE), a retrospective cohort study of published cases". Neurosurg Rev. 47(1):119, 2024
2. Nugraha HG et al: Nasofrontal encephalocele: a case report with literature and management review. Radiol Case Rep. 19(5):1907-12, 2024
3. Oley MC et al: Evaluation of long-term results following surgical correction of frontoethmoidal encephalomeningocele. Int J Surg Case Rep. 107:108278, 2023
4. Hedlund G: Congenital frontonasal masses: developmental anatomy, malformations, and MR imaging. Pediatr Radiol. 36(7):647-62; quiz 726-7, 2006
5. Naidich TP et al: Cephaloceles and related malformations. AJNR Am J Neuroradiol. 13(2):655-90, 1992

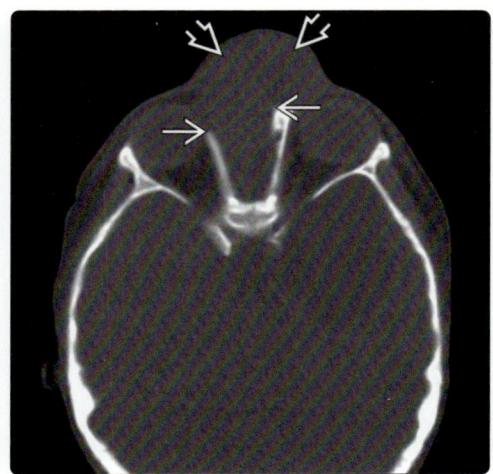

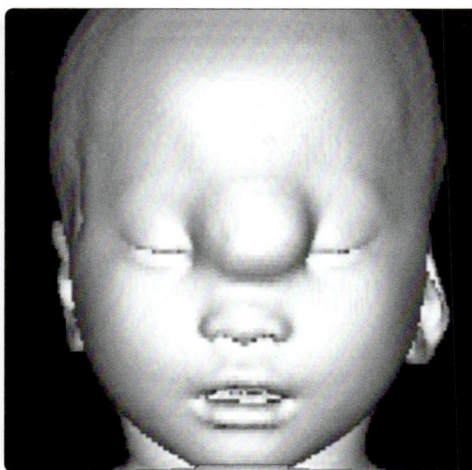

(Left) *Axial bone CT in a newborn with a soft tissue mass in the midline of the forehead shows a large anterior skull defect ➡ through which a large frontonasal cephalocele protrudes ➡.* (Right) *3D surface-rendered CT in the same patient shows the large frontonasal cephalocele protruding through a patent fonticulus frontalis between the eyes.*

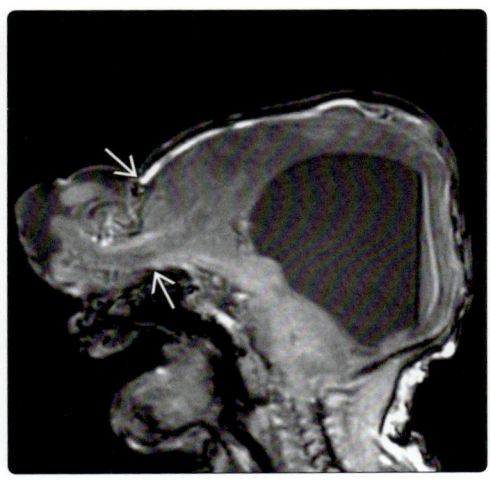

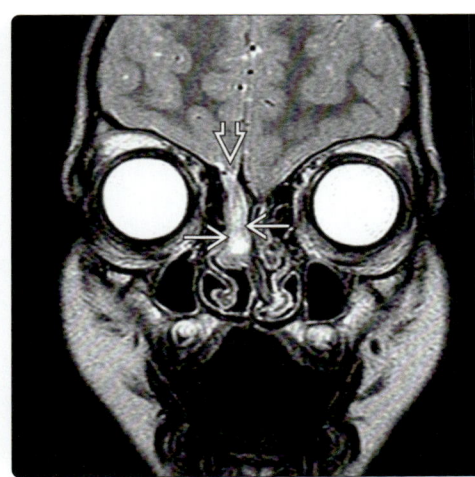

(Left) *Axial T1 MR in a 1-day-old with frontonasal cephalocele shows herniation of the frontal lobes through a frontonasal defect ➡, ventriculomegaly, and crowded/small posterior fossa. The superior sagittal sinus and anterior cerebral arteries extended into the cephalocele (not shown, but important to evaluate).* (Right) *Coronal T2 MR shows a nasoethmoidal cephalocele. Gliotic brain parenchyma ➡ herniating into the nasal cavity is hyperintense. Cephalocele herniates through a skull base defect ➡ to right of midline.*

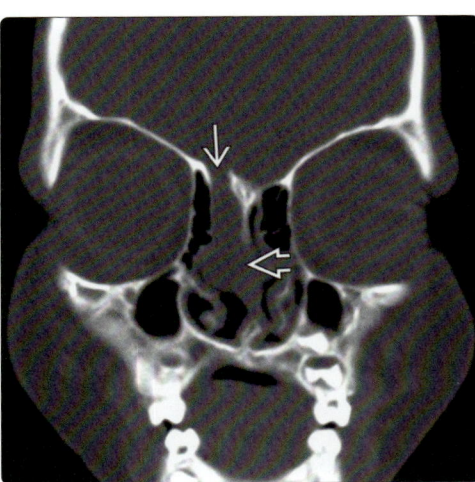

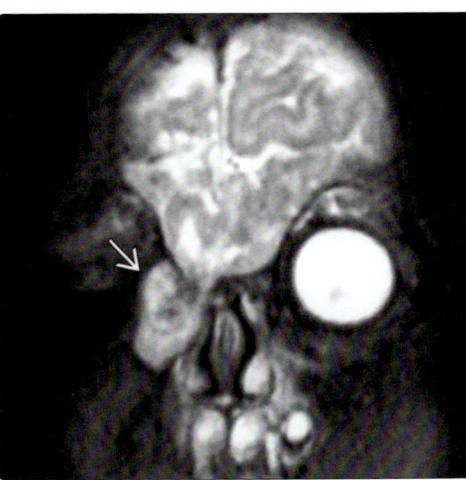

(Left) *Coronal bone CT reveals a bony defect in the anterior skull base ➡ and right nasal cavity soft tissue mass ➡ in this infant with a nasoethmoidal cephalocele.* (Right) *Coronal T2 MR shows the rarest type of frontoethmoidal cephalocele, the nasoorbital cephalocele ➡, herniating through a defect between the nasal and lacrimal bones.*

TERMINOLOGY

- Congenital nasal pyriform aperture stenosis (CNPAS): Congenital narrowing of anterior bony nasal passageway

IMAGING

- Best tool: Bone CT in axial & coronal planes
  - Medial deviation of anterior maxillae ± thickening of nasal processes
  - Abnormal maxillary dentition: **Solitary median maxillary central incisor (SMMCI)** (in up to 75%)
  - Triangle-shaped palate

TOP DIFFERENTIAL DIAGNOSES

- Nasolacrimal duct mucoceles
  - Intranasal component narrows anterior nasal cavity
- Nasal choanal stenosis/atresia
  - Narrow posterior nasal passage by membrane or bone

PATHOLOGY

- CNPAS without SMMCI is almost always isolated anomaly
- Solitary maxillary central incisor in 75% of cases
  - Associated with **holoprosencephaly**

CLINICAL ISSUES

- Respiratory distress in newborn/infant
  - Can mimic choanal atresia/stenosis
  - Breathing problems may be triggered by upper respiratory infection
  - Symptoms may be more pronounced with feeding
- Narrow nasal inlet on clinical exam
- CNPAS 1/5 to 1/3 as common as choanal atresia

DIAGNOSTIC CHECKLIST

- Bone CT recommended for diagnosis or bony narrowing & dental abnormalities
- Brain MR recommended in cases of SMMCI to exclude midline brain anomalies

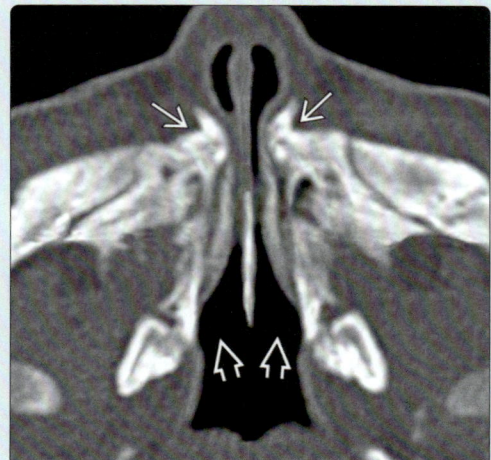
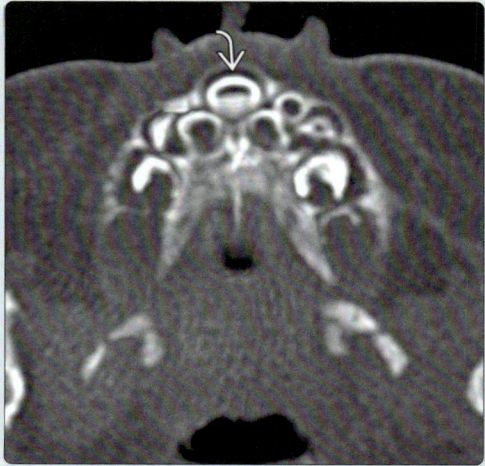

(Left) Axial bone CT in a newborn shows the typical features of congenital nasal pyriform aperture stenosis. There is overgrowth of the anterior maxillae ➡ with marked narrowing of the anterior nasal passages. There is no associated choanal atresia ➡. (Right) Axial bone CT at the level of the palate in the same patient shows a classic associated finding in patients with pyriform aperture stenosis: A solitary median maxillary central incisor, or megaincisor ➡.

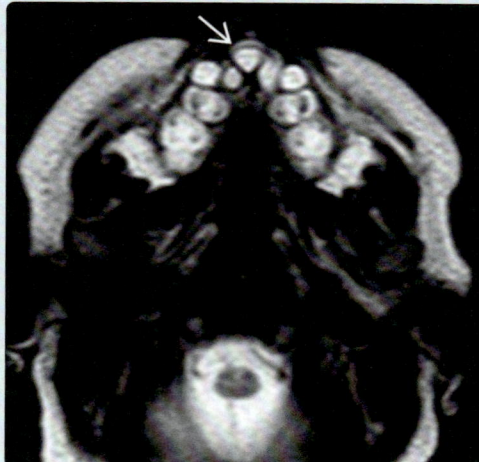
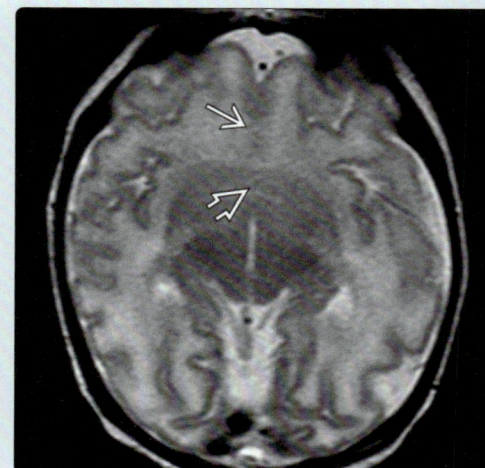

(Left) Axial T2 MR in a 3-day-old infant with congenital nasal pyriform aperture stenosis demonstrates associated solitary median maxillary central incisor ➡. (Right) Axial T2 MR in the same infant shows midline fusion of the inferior frontal lobes ➡, hypothalamus, and inferior basal ganglia ➡, consistent with semilobar holoprosencephaly.

TERMINOLOGY

Abbreviations

- Congenital nasal pyriform aperture stenosis (CNPAS)

Definitions

- Congenital narrowing of anterior bony nasal passageway/nasal aperture

IMAGING

General Features

- Best diagnostic clue
  - Medialization & thickening of anterior maxillae with narrowing of nasal airway
- Size
  - Pyriform aperture (PA) size in CNPAS
    - PA width < 11 mm in term infant is diagnostic (normal = 13.4-15.6 mm)

Imaging Recommendations

- Best imaging tool
  - Bone CT in axial & coronal planes

CT Findings

- Narrowed bony nasal inlet
  - Medial deviation of lateral wall of PA (anterior maxillae) ± thickening of nasal processes
- Triangle-shaped hard palate
  - Bony ridge along oral surface of hard palate on coronal images
- Abnormal maxillary dentition may occur
  - Fused or malaligned central & lateral incisors
  - Solitary median maxillary central incisor (SMMCI) syndrome (in up to 75%)
- Decreased width of nasal cavity, midface, & palate
- Thinning of anterior nasal septum
- Posterior choanae normal in caliber

DIFFERENTIAL DIAGNOSIS

Nasolacrimal Duct Mucocele

- Obstruction of distal nasolacrimal ducts → cysts at bilateral inferior meatus → narrow anterior nasal cavity
- Bony aperture is normal

Nasal Choanal Stenosis/Atresia

- Narrow or occluded posterior nasal passage: Membranous, osseous, or mixed
- Anterior nasal passage normal in caliber

PATHOLOGY

General Features

- Etiology
  - 3 theories of pathogenesis
    - Deficiency of primary palate derived from midline mesodermal tissue
      - Embryologically, medial maxillary swelling forms structures of primary palate, including 4 incisors
      - Mesoderm thought to have inductive effect on forebrain, hence association of SMMCI syndrome with holoprosencephaly
    - Overgrowth or dysplasia of nasal processes of maxilla
    - Premature ossification of midline palatal suture (recently proposed theory)
- Associated abnormalities
  - CNPAS without SMMCI is almost always isolated anomaly
  - Upper teeth anomalies
    - SMMCI syndrome (75% of CNPAS cases)
  - Semilobar or alobar holoprosencephaly
  - Endocrine dysfunction: Pituitary-adrenal axis

CLINICAL ISSUES

Presentation

- Most common signs/symptoms
  - Symptoms may be more pronounced with feeding
  - Respiratory distress, especially with feeding, as infants are obligate nasal breathers
    - Can mimic choanal atresia/stenosis
    - Breathing problems may be triggered by upper respiratory infection further compromising airway
  - Cyanosis
  - Nasogastric tube difficult to pass

Demographics

- Age
  - Newborns or infants in 1st few months of life
- Epidemiology
  - Congenital airway obstruction affects 1 in 5,000 infants
    - Majority are choanal atresia
    - CNPAS 1/5 to 1/3 as common as choanal atresia
      - 1 in 25,000 live births

Treatment

- Conservative with special feeding techniques
  - Nasal cavity eventually grows, & mild obstruction is relieved
- Surgical intervention in patients with persistent respiratory difficulty & poor weight gain
  - Resection of anteromedial maxilla ± anterior aspect inferior turbinates & reconstruction of anterior nasal orifice
  - PA width < 5.7 mm in neonate may correlate with need for surgical intervention
  - Recent literature suggests dilatation without bone removal successful in some patients

DIAGNOSTIC CHECKLIST

Image Interpretation Pearls

- Brain MR recommended in cases of solitary maxillary central incisor to exclude midline brain anomalies

SELECTED REFERENCES

1. Adil E et al: Congenital pyriform aperture stenosis: not all patients require open repair. Otolaryngol Head Neck Surg. 172(2):629-34, 2025
2. Rosi-Schumacher M et al: Comparison of surgical techniques for the treatment of congenital nasal pyriform aperture stenosis: a systematic review. Ann Otol Rhinol Laryngol. 133(7):639-46, 2024
3. Shivnani D et al: Neonatal nasal obstruction: a comprehensive analysis of our 20 years' experience. Indian J Otolaryngol Head Neck Surg. 76(3):2490-501, 2024
4. Wine TM et al: Congenital nasal pyriform aperture stenosis: evidence of premature fusion of the midline palatal suture. AJNR Am J Neuroradiol. 42(6):1163-6, 2021

Acute Rhinosinusitis

TERMINOLOGY

- Acute rhinosinusitis (ARS) = inflammatory sinonasal process lasting < 4 weeks in adults & < 12 weeks in children
- Acute bacterial rhinosinusitis (ABRS)
- Viral rhinosinusitis (VRS)

IMAGING

- **ARS is clinical diagnosis, & imaging is rarely necessary**
- Radiography: Inaccurate; **no** role in medical practice
- NECT: Can suggest ARS but lacks specificity & should not be performed routinely for diagnosis
  - May be considered to evaluate complications or if diagnosis remains uncertain on clinical grounds
  - Axial < 1-mm slice thickness with coronal & sagittal reconstructions
  - Best sign = air-fluid level (nonspecific) ± bubbly secretions with mucosal thickening
  - Most common in ethmoid & maxillary sinuses
  - Often asymmetric sinus involvement

- MR: Indicated for suspected complications

TOP DIFFERENTIAL DIAGNOSES

- Pseudo-fluid level from large maxillary polyp/cyst
- Posttraumatic blood level
- Postobstructive noninfected secretions

PATHOLOGY

- Most cases follow viral upper respiratory infection

CLINICAL ISSUES

- **Signs/symptoms of ARS**: < 4 weeks of **purulent** nasal drainage, nasal obstruction, & facial pain, pressure, fullness
- VRS usually self-limited
- ARS complications rare but critically important to identify
  - Orbital cellulitis, subperiosteal abscess, meningitis, subdural empyema, brain abscess, venous sinus thrombosis

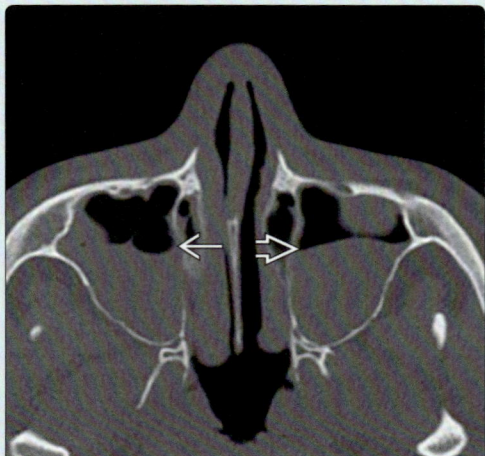
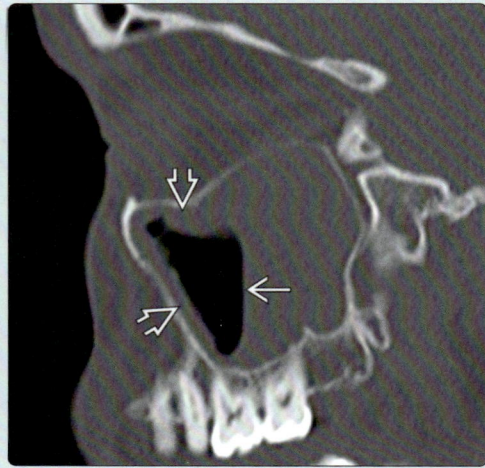

(Left) Axial NECT in a patient clinically diagnosed with acute rhinosinusitis (ARS) shows a bubbly air-fluid level ➡ in right maxillary sinus from layering secretions. In contrast, note rounded contour ⇨ & lack of true meniscus in partially opacified left maxillary sinus due to mucosal thickening & retention cyst. (Right) Sagittal NECT in a patient clinically diagnosed with ARS shows an air-fluid level ➡ in maxillary sinus & diffuse mucosal thickening ⇨. Layering fluid is nonspecific & can also be seen with recent sinus irrigation.

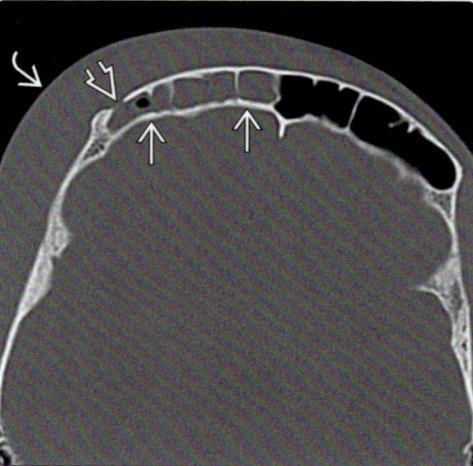
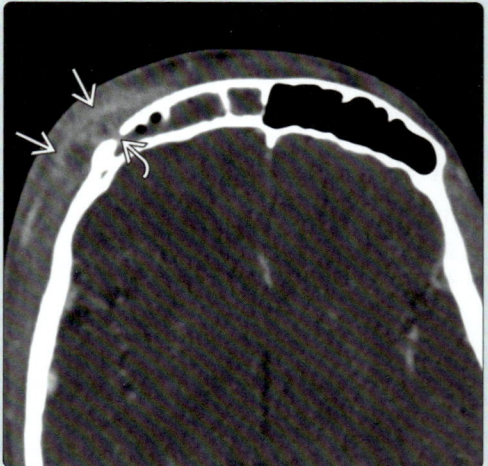

(Left) Axial NECT in a patient with complicated ARS shows a near-complete opacified right frontal sinus ➡ with focal bone dehiscence along the outer cortex ⇨. Note diffuse swelling of the right frontal scalp ➡, indicating underlying cellulitis & necessitating further imaging with CECT. (Right) Axial CECT in the same patient shows right frontal sinusitis complicated by cortical dehiscence ➡ & development of an overlying abscess ➡ along with cellulitis of the scalp.

Acute Rhinosinusitis

TERMINOLOGY

Abbreviations

- Acute rhinosinusitis (ARS)

Definitions

- Adult ARS: Sinonasal inflammation lasting < 4 weeks & demonstrating sudden onset of symptoms
  - Symptoms: **Both** nasal congestion/obstruction **or** nasal discharge & facial pain/pressure **or** reduced smell
- Pediatric ARS: Sinonasal inflammation lasting < 12 weeks & demonstrating sudden onset of symptoms
  - Symptoms: 2 or more of nasal congestion/obstruction, discolored nasal discharge, or cough
- ARS is **clinical** diagnosis, which does not require imaging or endoscopy to make initial diagnosis
  - Image to assess for complications, surgical planning, or unclear clinical diagnosis (uncommon)
- Classified into viral rhinosinusitis (VRS) vs. acute bacterial rhinosinusitis (ABRS) based on clinical presentation

IMAGING

General Features

- Best diagnostic clue
  - **Imaging findings are imperfect & lack specificity; needs appropriate clinical history!**
  - Air-fluid level (nonspecific) ± bubbly/frothy secretions within sinus with mucosal thickening
- Location
  - Ethmoid & maxillary most common, typically asymmetric

Radiographic Findings

- Radiography
  - **Inaccurate; no role in evaluation**

CT Findings

- NECT
  - **Air-fluid level**, bubbly or frothy-appearing secretions
    - Air-fluid level is nonspecific finding, which can be seen with recent sinus irrigation
    - Bubbly/frothy secretions also nonspecific, which may be due to nose blowing
  - Moderate mucosal thickening, generally > 1 cm in sinus cavity, ostium, or nasal cavity
  - May see polypoid inflammatory tissue obstructing drainage pathways
- CECT
  - Indicated when orbital or intracranial complications suspected clinically
  - Inflamed sinus mucosa enhances, but thin linear soft tissue deep to mucosa does not
  - Central secretions do not enhance
- Bone CT
  - Bone destruction not typical for acute infection
    - If present, suspect aggressive invasive sinus infection or neoplasm
  - Osteoneogenesis, sinus wall sclerosis & thickening, usually indicates chronic inflammation

MR Findings

- T1WI

- Mucosal thickening isointense to other soft tissue
  - Air-fluid level
  - Hyperintense secretions when chronic sinusitis present
- T2WI
  - Thickened edematous mucosa, especially in maxillary & ethmoids
  - Air-fluid level
  - Low signal intensity secretions if proteinaceous, chronic
- T1WI C+
  - Enhancing mucosa lining sinus cavity
  - Central secretions do not enhance

Imaging Recommendations

- Best imaging tool
  - **ARS is 100% clinical diagnosis**
  - Radiographs inaccurate; play no role in patient evaluation!
  - CT: Consider only if evaluating for complications, failed medical therapy, alternative diagnoses, or surgical candidate
    - NECT delineates anatomic variants prior to endoscopic sinus surgery
    - CECT indicated if concern for complications
  - MR superior for evaluating orbital or intracranial complications, invasive fungal disease, neoplasm
- Protocol advice
  - Bone CT
    - Axial ≤ 1-mm slice thickness with coronal, sagittal reconstructions to evaluate drainage pathways
  - MR
    - Multiplanar T1 & T2 sequences necessary
    - C+ T1 with fat suppression best for intracranial/orbital complications

DIFFERENTIAL DIAGNOSIS

Pseudofluid Level

- Mucus retention cyst mimics air-fluid level
- Rounded contour with incomplete fluid level

Posttraumatic Blood Level

- Clinical history of recent facial injury
- Increased attenuation of layering fluid (blood)
- Associated sinus wall fractures

Postobstructive Secretions

- Lesion obstructs sinus drainage pathway, resulting in noninfected trapped sinus cavity fluid
- MR differentiates tumor from obstructed secretions
  - Neoplasm generally lower T2 signal compared to hyperintense secretions; frequently hypoenhancing relative to sinonasal mucosa

PATHOLOGY

General Features

- Etiology
  - ABRS uncommonly follows VRS (0.5-2.0% of cases) in adults but more commonly follows upper respiratory infection (URI) in children (4-7%)
    - URI (typically viral) → mucosal swelling → sinus outflow obstruction → static secretions → bacterial infection

- Viral symptoms usually improve in 7-10 days
- Symptoms > 10 days or worsening after 5-7 days suggest bacterial superinfection
  □ Common organisms: *Streptococcus pneumonia*, *Haemophilus influenzae*, *Moraxella catarrhalis*
  ○ **Odontogenic rhinosinusitis**: Apical periodontitis with dehiscence or transosseous spread of infection into maxillary sinus
    - Likely underdiagnosed (reported prevalence 10-15%, but may be as high as 45%)
- Genetics
  ○ Cystic fibrosis (autosomal recessive disorder) predisposes to rhinosinusitis & polyps
- Associated abnormalities
  ○ Structural abnormalities may narrow drainage pathways
    - Anatomic variants of septum, uncinate process, middle turbinate, frontal recess, ethmoid sinuses
    - Polyps, either isolated or associated with allergic sinusitis with diffuse polyposis
    - Benign or malignant neoplasms
  ○ Predisposing systemic disorders: Allergies, immunoglobulin deficiency, immotile cilia syndrome, cystic fibrosis, vitamin D deficiency

Staging, Grading, & Classification

- Can be classified according to etiology: Viral, bacterial, vasomotor

Gross Pathologic & Surgical Features

- Edematous, erythematous mucosa with ostial obstruction, purulent secretions

Microscopic Features

- Tissue-invasive bacteria
- Luminal exudate of neutrophils, eosinophils

CLINICAL ISSUES

Presentation

- Most common signs/symptoms
  ○ **Cardinal signs/symptoms of ARS**: < 4 weeks of **purulent** nasal drainage & obstruction, facial pain, or pressure
    - VRS: Signs/symptoms last < 10 days, does not progress
    - ABRS: Signs/symptoms fail to improve within 10 days **or** worsen within 10 days after initial improvement
- Other signs/symptoms
  ○ Fever, cough, malaise, hyposmia, anosmia, dental pain, ear pressure/fullness
    - Facial/dental pain predicts ABRS, but location correlates poorly with site of involvement
- Clinical profile
  ○ Nasal discharge & obstruction following viral URI lasting < 4 weeks (adult) or < 12 weeks (child)
  ○ Laboratory results
    - Nasal/nasopharynx cultures poorly correlate with sinus cultures; do not differentiate ABRS from VRS
    - Endoscopic middle meatus aspiration more specific but generally not necessary in uncomplicated ARS

Demographics

- Age

○ Generally adult disease but can be seen in children
    - Typically follows viral URI in children
- Epidemiology
  ○ Sinonasal inflammatory disease is ubiquitous
  ○ Rhinosinusitis affects nearly 31 million patients in USA annually
    - 12% (1 in 8 adults) of USA population annually
    - > 1 billion physician visits & > $3 billion in ARS healthcare expenditures/year
  ○ VRS & ARS often follow/coexist with common cold

Natural History & Prognosis

- VRS usually self-limited
- ABRS may resolve without antibiotics
- ABRS course may be shortened by medical therapy, surgical drainage, & possibly saline irrigation
- If ABRS untreated, rarely **complications** may ensue
  ○ Orbital cellulitis, subperiosteal abscess, meningitis, subdural empyema, brain abscess, venous sinus thrombosis

Treatment

- Medical therapy
  ○ Antibiotics (in uncomplicated cases with worsening after 7 days, earlier if extenuating circumstances)
  ○ Intranasal corticosteroids
  ○ Topical saline irrigation (adjunct to antibiotics for ABRS)
- Surgical therapy
  ○ More often performed for chronic rhinosinusitis
  ○ Drainage procedures performed in acute disease (frontal & sphenoid) to prevent development of complications

DIAGNOSTIC CHECKLIST

Consider

- Bone CT if suspect alternative diagnoses, failed therapy, complications, or surgical candidate
  ○ Acquire ≤ 1-mm axial slices with coronal & sagittal reformations
- CT limitations
  ○ Cannot differentiate viral from bacterial disease
  ○ High incidence of sinus mucosal abnormalities in asymptomatic patients

Image Interpretation Pearls

- Air-fluid level is not always present; not highly specific indicator
- In correct clinical setting, even severe mucosal thickening can indicate ABRS
- Normal nasal mucosal cycle may be impossible to distinguish from ARS mucosal thickening
- Look for signs of invasive fungal sinusitis if immunocompromised patient

SELECTED REFERENCES

1. Butler FM et al: Acute rhinosinusitis: rapid evidence review. Am Fam Physician. 111(1):47-53, 2025
2. Hallak B et al: Management strategy of intracranial complications of sinusitis: our experience and review of the literature. Allergy Rhinol (Providence). 13:21526575221125031, 2022
3. Bleier BS et al: Acute and chronic sinusitis. Med Clin North Am. 105(5):859-70, 2021
4. McCann MR et al: Emergency radiologic approach to sinus disease. Emerg Radiol. 28(5):1003-10, 2021

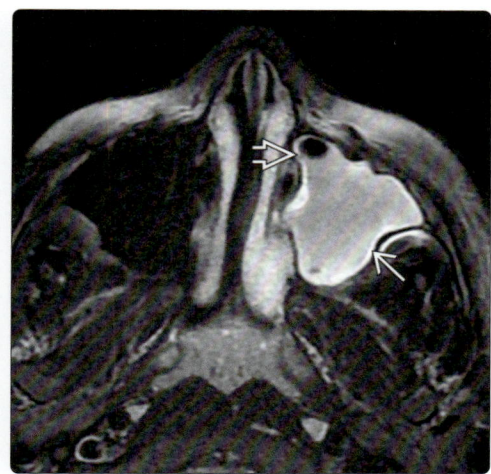

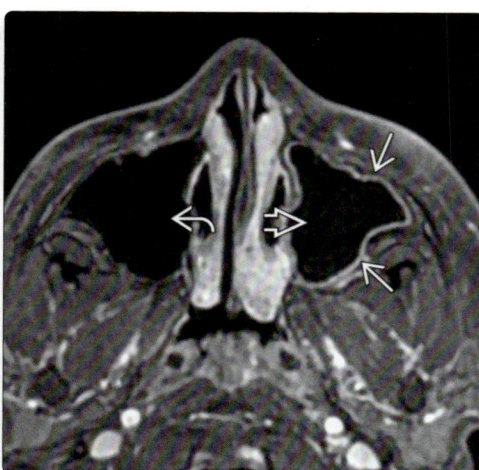

(Left) *Axial T2 FS MR in a patient with fever, facial pain, & nasal discharge shows a near-complete fluid opacified* ⮕ *left maxillary sinus with discrete air-fluid level* ⮕. (Right) *Axial T1 SPGR C+ MR in the same patient shows circumferential mucosal thickening* ⮕ *in the left maxillary sinus, which enhances avidly. Note the left maxillary sinus is subtly hyperintense* ⮕ *relative to the normally aerated right maxillary sinus* ⮕*, indicating fluid opacification.*

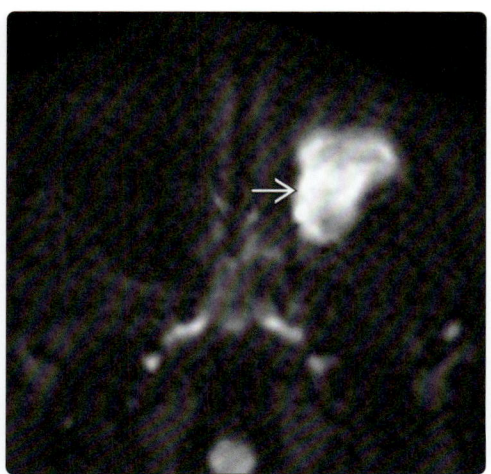

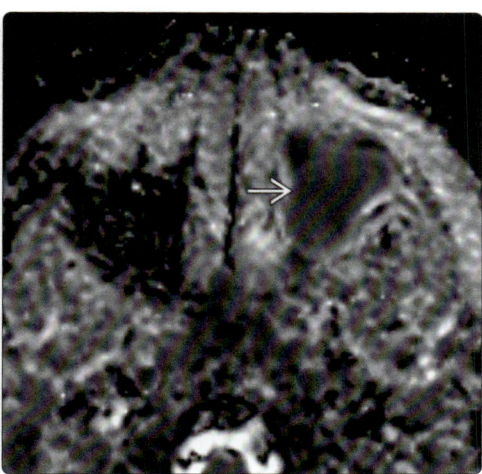

(Left) *Axial DWI trace in a patient with acute left maxillary sinusitis shows an almost completely opacified left maxillary sinus* ⮕*, which is markedly hyperintense on the DWI trace sequence.* (Right) *Axial ADC map in the same patient shows reduced diffusivity of the purulent fluid, manifesting as dark ADC signal intensity* ⮕*. The reduced diffusivity of water molecules is likely due to a combination of proteinaceous fluid & inflammatory cellular infiltrate.*

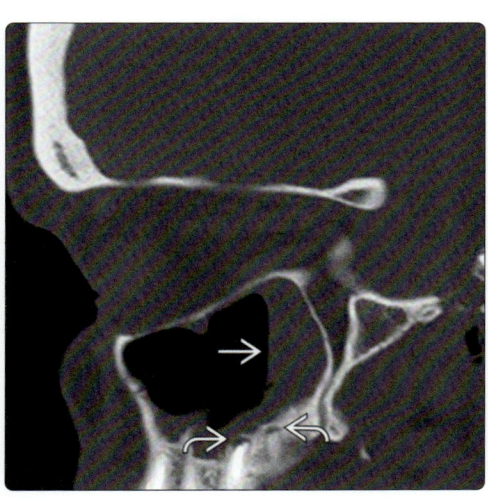

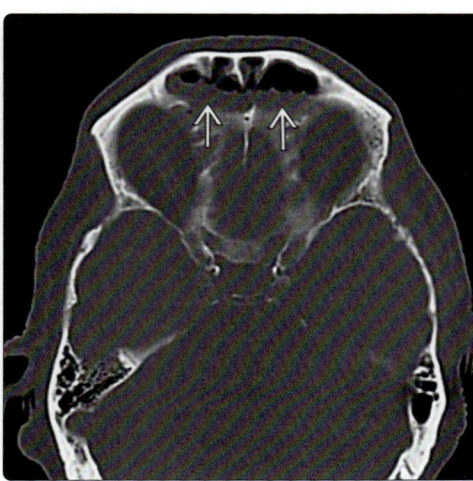

(Left) *Sagittal reconstruction NECT in a patient with clinical ARS shows corroborating air-fluid level* ⮕ *in the maxillary sinus. Careful inspection reveals periapical lucencies of the maxillary teeth* ⮕*, an easily overlooked finding that may contribute an odontogenic component to the maxillary sinusitis.* (Right) *Axial NECT performed for headache & fever reveals frothy air-fluid levels* ⮕ *in both frontal sinuses. Although ARS is a clinical diagnosis, imaging may be performed to rule out suspected complications.*

Chronic Rhinosinusitis

TERMINOLOGY

- Group of disorders characterized by inflammation of nose & sinuses ≥ 12 consecutive weeks
  - This broad definition is based on signs & symptoms & does not restrict to specific etiology
- CRS generally divided into 2 major clinical phenotypes: Chronic rhinosinusitis (CRS) with nasal polyps & CRS without nasal polyps

IMAGING

- Nonenhanced bone CT is gold standard for evaluation
  - Sinus mucosal thickening & opacification with thickening & sclerosis of bony walls
  - Involved sinus normal or decreased volume
  - Intrasinus hyperdensity or calcifications common
  - Mucus retention cysts & polyps are common
  - May show established pattern of obstructive sinus disease

TOP DIFFERENTIAL DIAGNOSES

- Granulomatosis with polyangiitis, allergic fungal sinusitis, sinonasal polyposis, fungal mycetoma, sarcoidosis

PATHOLOGY

- Causes of CRS are numerous, disparate, & frequently overlapping
- Many factors & processes play role in etiology of chronic rhinosinusitis

CLINICAL ISSUES

- Affects 12-14% of USA adult population
- Often associated conditions, such as allergy, underlying anatomic variations

DIAGNOSTIC CHECKLIST

- CT best for evaluating changes in bone & identifying anatomic variants that may predispose to recurrent disease
- There is lack of correlation between symptomatology & imaging findings

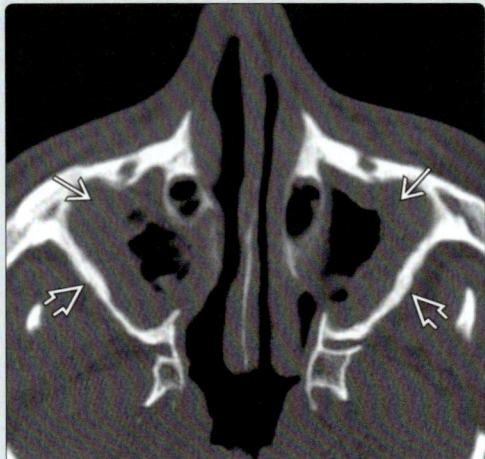
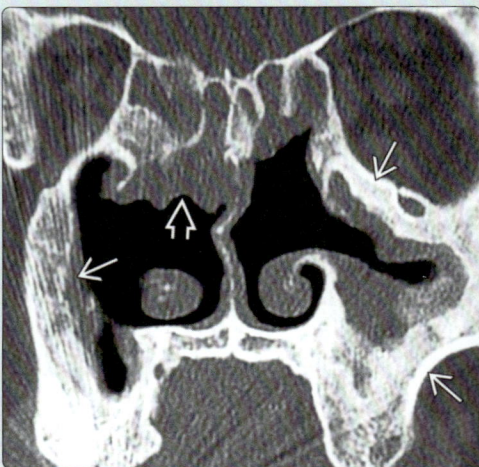

(Left) Axial bone CT in a cystic fibrosis patient shows bilateral maxillary sinus mucosal thickening ➡ and thickening of the bony sinus walls (osteitis) ➡, consistent with chronic inflammatory disease. (Right) Coronal bone CT shows marked diffuse chronic osteitis of the sinus walls ➡ in a patient with chronic rhinosinusitis (CRS) and sinonasal polyposis ➡. Extensive changes from prior endoscopic surgery are present.

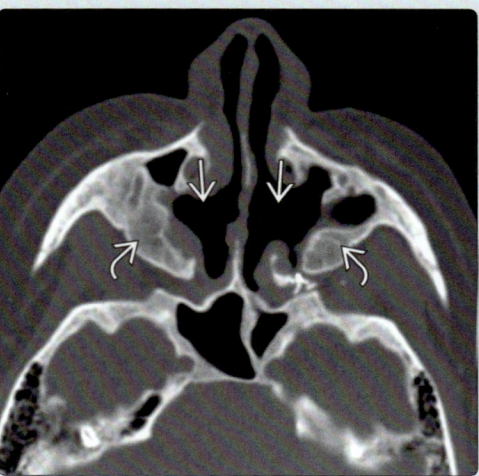
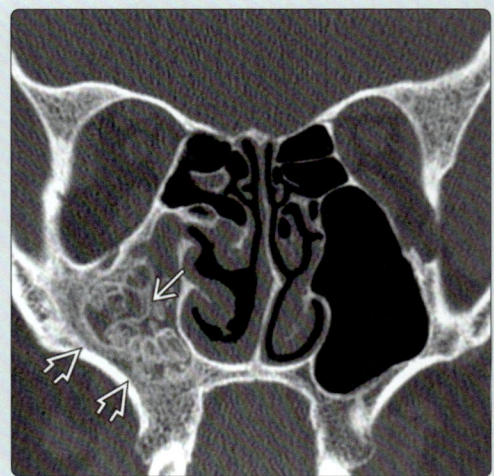

(Left) Axial bone CT shows marked chronic osteitis ➡ of the walls of both maxillary sinuses. The volume of the sinuses is diminished, and there is patchy mucosal thickening. Changes are noted from prior surgery with bilateral antrostomy defects ➡. (Right) Coronal bone CT in a patient with longstanding right maxillary inflammation shows prominent calcifications ➡ within the inspissated right maxillary sinus secretions. Osteitis of the walls of the sinus ➡ is also present.

TERMINOLOGY

Abbreviations
- Chronic rhinosinusitis (CRS)

Definitions
- Group of disorders characterized by inflammation of nose & sinuses **≥ 12 consecutive weeks** of duration
  - This broad definition is based on signs & symptoms & does not restrict to specific etiology

IMAGING

General Features
- Best diagnostic clue
  - Sinus cavity opacification or mucosal thickening with hyperostosis/sclerosis of bony walls
- Location
  - Maxillary & ethmoid sinuses > frontal & sphenoid sinuses
- Size
  - Involved sinus normal or decreased volume
    - No sinus expansion in uncomplicated cases
- Morphology
  - Disease can be localized or diffuse & may occur in particular pattern (i.e., ostiomeatal unit) in cases caused by obstruction

Radiographic Findings
- Radiography
  - Can demonstrate opacification, mucosal thickening, bony sclerosis, & air-fluid levels
  - Lower sensitivity & specificity than CT

CT Findings
- CECT
  - Enhancement of inflamed mucosa may be seen
  - Contrast **not** necessary in uncomplicated cases
- Bone CT
  - Mucosal thickening or opacification of sinus without expansion of sinus
  - Air fluid levels occur with superimposed acute sinusitis
  - Variable density of secretions
    - Isodense to hyperdense depending on protein, water, fungal content
    - Hyperdense secretions may be secondary to inspissated mucus or fungal sinusitis
  - Occasional calcification may be present
  - Bony walls of sinus thickened & sclerotic (osteitis)
  - Mucus retention cysts & polyps are common

MR Findings
- T1WI
  - Thickened mucosa isointense to other soft tissue
  - Variable signal of retained secretions depending on variable water & protein content
    - Higher protein content causes higher T1 signal
- T2WI
  - Mucosa typically hyperintense
  - Retained secretions range from hyperintense (↑ water content) to hypointense (↓ water, desiccated)
  - Thickened sinus walls evident on T2 MR
- T1WI C+
  - Mucosal enhancement typical
  - Contrast not necessary in uncomplicated cases

Imaging Recommendations
- Best imaging tool
  - Thin-section axial bone CT with coronal reformatted images
  - Mucosal thickening, opacification, & osseous changes are well depicted
- Protocol advice
  - 0.625- to 1.25-mm-thick axial CT in bone algorithm with coronal ± sagittal reformatted images

DIFFERENTIAL DIAGNOSIS

Fungal Sinusitis, Mycetoma
- Sinus opacified; hyperdensity/calcifications common
- Often seen in clinical setting of CRS
  - Bony changes may mimic CRS

Allergic Fungal Sinusitis
- Form of CRS in patients with asthma, allergy
- Involved sinuses opacified & expanded with central high-attenuation material

Sinonasal Polyposis
- Multiple, variable-density polypoid soft tissue masses in nasal cavity & sinuses
- Expansion, remodeling of bony walls may be present
- Generally occurs in setting of CRS with background of chronic mucosal thickening & opacification

Acute Rhinosinusitis
- Clinical course of shorter duration often following viral URI
- Air-fluid levels & bubbly secretions in addition to mucosal thickening
- No bone changes

Sinonasal Granulomatosis with Polyangiitis
- Nodular soft tissue thickening ± bone erosion
- Tends to affect nasal cavity > sinuses
  - Involves septum & turbinates

Sinonasal Sarcoidosis
- Nodular soft tissue thickening ± bone erosion
- Sinonasal involvement less common than granulomatosis with polyangiitis
- Predilection for nasal cavity with septal involvement

PATHOLOGY

General Features
- Etiology
  - Definition of CRS is symptom based & does not include specific etiology
  - Causes of CRS are numerous, disparate, & frequently overlapping
    - Inflammation plays greater role than infection
    - Biofilms (antibiotic-resistant bacterial colonies) decrease antibiotic efficacy & release inflammatory mediators
  - Many factors & processes play role in etiology of CRS

– Systemic host factors: Allergic, immunodeficiency, genetic/congenital, mucociliary dysfunction, endocrine, neuromechanism
– Local host factors: Anatomic variants, neoplastic, acquired mucociliary dysfunction
– Environmental: Microorganisms, noxious chemicals, medications, trauma, surgery
- Genetics
  o Sporadic disease in most cases
  o Genetics play role when underlying systemic disorder present
    – Cystic fibrosis, primary ciliary dysmotility, immunodeficiency
- Associated abnormalities
  o Asthma, allergy (> 50% of CRS patients)
  o Dental disease (maxillary)
  o Sinonasal polyposis

Staging, Grading, & Classification

- Rhinosinusitis: 5 clinical categories
  o Acute, subacute, chronic, recurrent acute, acute exacerbation of CRS
- CRS may be bacterial, allergic, or fungal in nature
  o **Bacterial CRS**
    – Bacteria may initiate CRS, cause disease persistence, or exacerbate noninfectious inflammation
    – Common organisms: *Staphylococcus aureus*, coagulase-negative *Staphylococcus*, anaerobic & gram-negative bacteria
  o **Allergic CRS**
    – Cytokines & allergic mediators → nasal allergic inflammation → mucosal swelling → obstruction of ostia
  o **Allergic fungal sinusitis**
    – Eosinophilic response to presence of noninvasive fungal elements

Gross Pathologic & Surgical Features

- Mucosal swelling, purulent discharge, polypoid changes, erythema

Microscopic Features

- Mixed inflammatory infiltrate of lymphocytes, plasma cells, eosinophils, interleukin-8, & interferon-γ
- Changes in adjacent bone similar to osteomyelitis

CLINICAL ISSUES

Presentation

- Most common signs/symptoms
  o Nasal obstruction, nasal discharge, hyposmia, anosmia
- Other signs/symptoms
  o Facial pain & pressure, headache
- CRS definition: Sinonasal infection/inflammation **> 12 weeks of duration**
- Nasal endoscopy & CT performed to quantify mucosal disease & target culturing

Demographics

- Age
  o All ages affected
- Epidemiology

o CRS results in 18-22 million office visits in USA annually
o Prevalence of CRS difficult to determine due to heterogeneity of disease & diagnostic imprecision

Natural History & Prognosis

- Persistent, recurrent sinusitis often refractory to medical therapy
- Often associated conditions, such as allergy, underlying anatomic variations
  o Patients with mucosal eosinophilia have poorer outcomes
- Nasal endoscopy best objective indicator of early recurrent disease

Treatment

- **Pharmacologic therapy**: Intranasal saline irrigation & intranasal steroids thought to be 1st line; may also require antibiotics, antifungals, decongestants, antihistamines
- Treatment of comorbid conditions (inhalant sensitivities, polyps, infections, immune deficiencies) critical for treatment success of CRS
- Surgery reserved for cases recalcitrant to medical therapy
  o **Functional endoscopic sinus surgery** current surgical treatment of choice

DIAGNOSTIC CHECKLIST

Consider

- CT study of choice in CRS
  o Evaluates changes in bone & identifies anatomic variants that may predispose to recurrent disease

Image Interpretation Pearls

- Mucosal thickening or opacification in nonexpanded sinus with associated bone thickening/sclerosis most consistent with CRS
- CT yields little information about etiology of mucosal changes
- There is lack of correlation between symptomatology & imaging findings

SELECTED REFERENCES

1. Keating MK et al: Chronic rhinosinusitis. Am Fam Physician. 108(4):370-7, 2023
2. Cho SH et al: Medical management strategies in acute and chronic rhinosinusitis. J Allergy Clin Immunol Pract. 8(5):1559-64, 2020
3. Fokkens WJ et al: European position paper on rhinosinusitis and nasal polyps 2020. Rhinology. 58(Suppl S29):1-464, 2020
4. Yip J et al: Endotypes of chronic rhinosinusitis. Curr Opin Otolaryngol Head Neck Surg. 27(1):14-9, 2019
5. Koskinen A et al: Diagnostic accuracy of symptoms, endoscopy, and imaging signs of chronic rhinosinusitis without nasal polyps compared to allergic rhinitis. Am J Rhinol Allergy. 32(3):121-31, 2018
6. Orlandi RR et al: International consensus statement on allergy and rhinology: Rhinosinusitis. Int Forum Allergy Rhinol. 6 Suppl 1:S22-209, 2016
7. Huang BY et al: Current trends in sinonasal imaging. Neuroimaging Clin N Am. 25(4):507-25, 2015
8. Joshi VM et al: Imaging in sinonasal inflammatory disease. Neuroimaging Clin N Am. 25(4):549-68, 2015
9. Hamilos DL: Chronic rhinosinusitis: epidemiology and medical management. J Allergy Clin Immunol. 128(4):693-707; quiz 708-9, 2011
10. Chan Y et al: An update on the classifications, diagnosis, and treatment of rhinosinusitis. Curr Opin Otolaryngol Head Neck Surg. 17(3):204-8, 2009
11. Nair S: Correlation between symptoms and radiological findings in patients of chronic rhinosinusitis: a modified radiological typing system. Rhinology. 47(2):181-6, 2009
12. Mafee MF et al: Imaging of rhinosinusitis and its complications: plain film, CT, and MRI. Clin Rev Allergy Immunol. 30(2):165-86, 2006

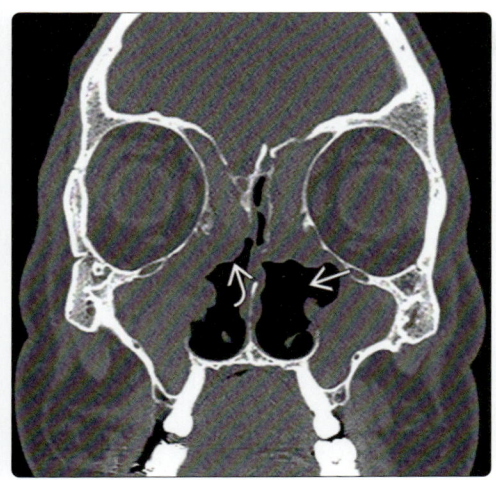
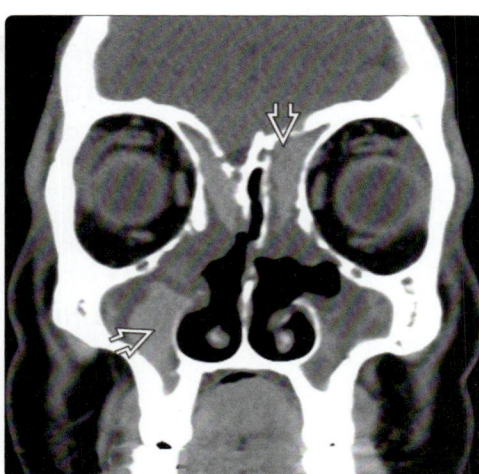

(Left) Coronal bone CT in a 34-year-old man with underlying cystic fibrosis and CRS shows postsurgical changes related to bilateral antrostomies ➡. There is extensive mucosal thickening of the paranasal sinuses. Some areas appear nodular or polypoid, suggesting underlying polyps ➡. (Right) Soft tissue windows in the same patient show multifocal areas of relative hyperdensity ➡. This appearance can be seen with inspissated secretions or fungal colonization.

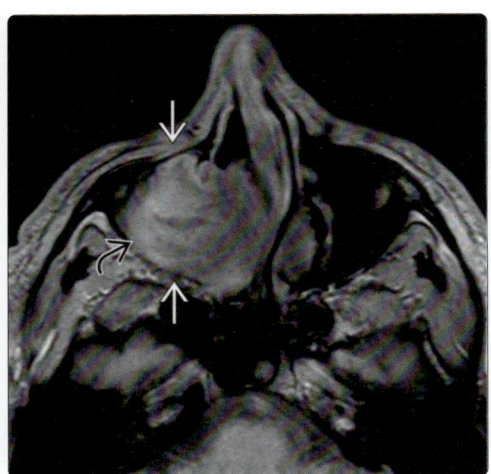
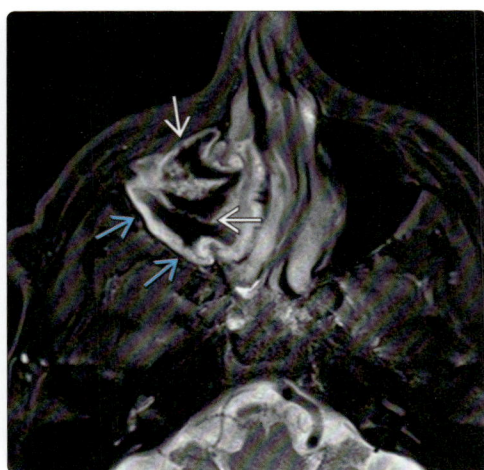

(Left) Axial T1 MR shows complete opacification of the right maxillary sinus with heterogeneous signal intensity ➡. Areas of higher signal ➡ correlate with more highly inspissated secretions. (Right) Axial T2 FS MR in the same patient again shows complete opacification of the right maxillary sinus with marked central dark signal correlating with highly inspissated secretions ➡. Note the normal hyperintense mucosa. ➡.

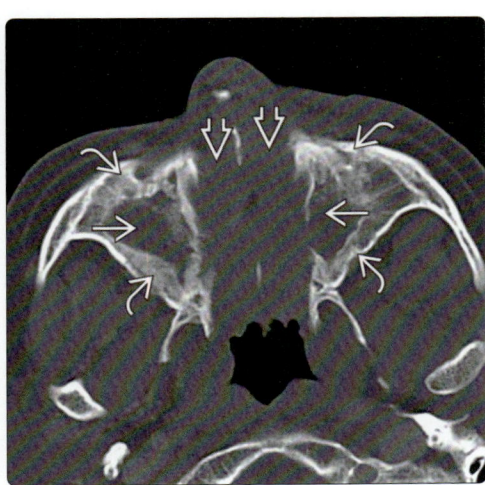
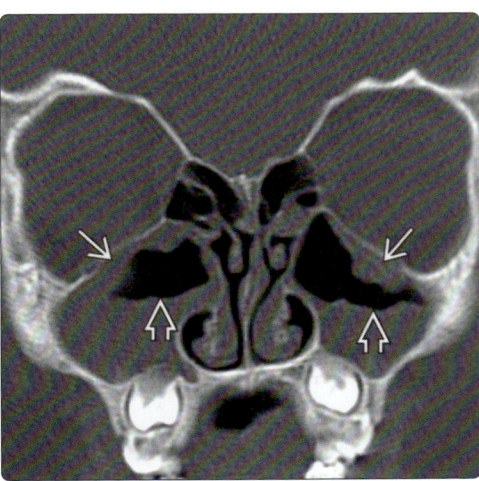

(Left) Axial bone CT in a granulomatosis with polyangiitis patient shows typical changes of CRS involving maxillary sinuses. Soft tissue opacifies the sinuses ➡ and nasal cavity ➡. There is prominent osteitis involving the sinus walls ➡. (Right) Coronal bone CT in a child with cystic fibrosis shows lobular mucosal thickening in both maxillary sinuses ➡. Fluid levels ➡ are present, suggesting acute infection superimposed on chronic inflammation. Osteitis has not yet developed in this young patient.

TERMINOLOGY

- Superficial complications: Osteomyelitis, subgaleal abscess (Pott puffy tumor), septic thrombophlebitis
- Orbital complications: Preseptal cellulitis/abscess, orbital (postseptal) cellulitis, subperiosteal postseptal abscess (SPA), orbital abscess, septic thrombophlebitis
- Intracranial complications: Meningitis, epidural abscess, subdural empyema (SDE), cerebritis, brain abscess, cavernous sinus thrombosis (CST)

IMAGING

- CECT for orbital complications
- Contrast-enhanced MR with diffusion imaging for intracranial & extracranial complications

TOP DIFFERENTIAL DIAGNOSES

- SPA: Orbital pseudotumor, extraconal neoplasm
- CST: Pseudotumor of cavernous sinus (Tolosa-Hunt), cavernous sinus neoplasm

- SDE: Subdural hygroma/hematoma
- Cerebritis or cerebral abscess: Tumefactive MS, glioblastoma, solitary metastasis, radiation necrosis

PATHOLOGY

- Orbital & intracranial complications more likely in acute rhinosinusitis
- Superficial complications more common in chronic rhinosinusitis
- Orbital complications most often from ethmoid sinusitis
- Intracranial complications most often from frontal sinusitis

CLINICAL ISSUES

- Orbital complications more common in children
- Intracranial complications more common from adolescence to 2nd & 3rd decades
- Intracranial complications more common in male patients
- Intracranial complications → 50-80% mortality if not diagnosed & treated early

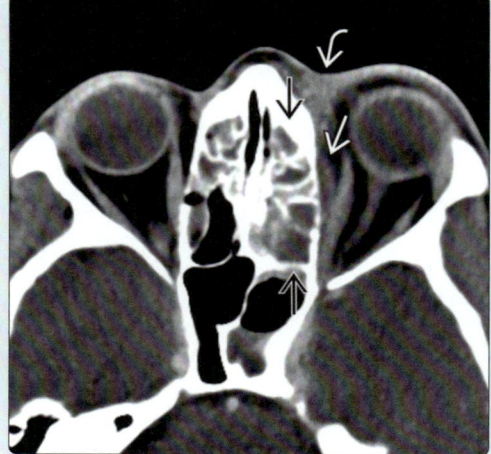
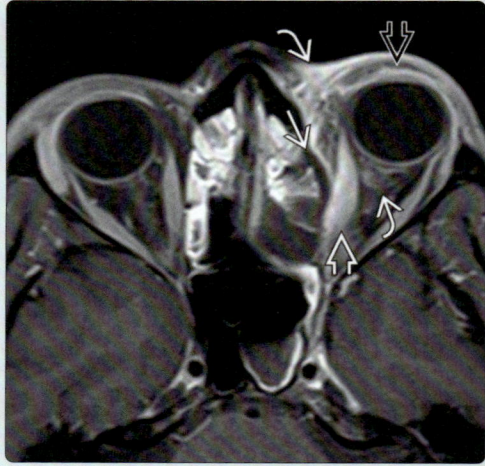

(Left) *Axial CECT demonstrates a thin crescentic collection ⟶ along the left medial extraconal space adjacent to opacified left ethmoid air cells ⟶, compatible with subperiosteal postseptal abscess (SPA). Note mild fat stranding in left preseptal soft tissues ⟶.*
(Right) *Axial T1 C+ FS MR in the same patient shows the thin medial SPA ⟶ with adjacent preseptal and postseptal fat stranding ⟶ ⟶ and medial rectus myositis ⟶. Even small SPA may result in proptosis ⟶, as seen in this case.*

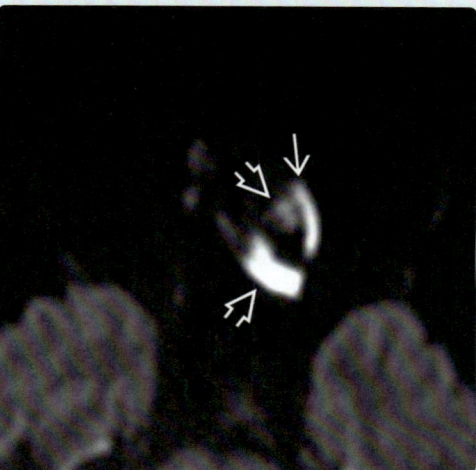
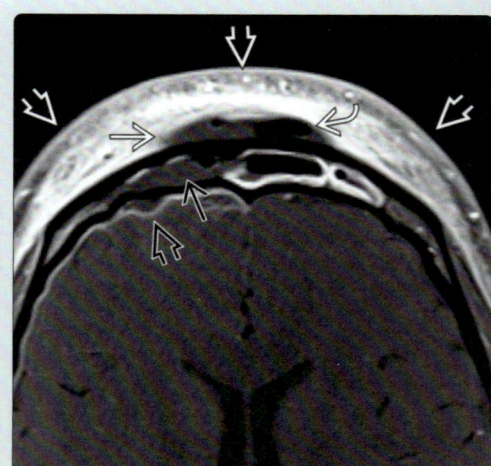

(Left) *Axial DWI MR in the same patient demonstrates reduced diffusivity within the SPA ⟶. Note reduced diffusivity in the adjacent ethmoid sinuses ⟶ corresponding with purulent material of acute sinusitis.*
(Right) *Axial T1 C+ FS MR shows a large, rim-enhancing collection ⟶ with internal gas ⟶ and extensive soft tissue inflammation ⟶, consistent with subgaleal abscess (Pott puffy tumor) complicating right frontal sinusitis ⟶. Note an additional small right frontal epidural abscess ⟶.*

Complications of Rhinosinusitis

TERMINOLOGY

Abbreviations
- Rhinosinusitis (RS)

Definitions
- Complications of acute rhinosinusitis (ARS) or chronic rhinosinusitis (CRS) may affect bone & overlying soft tissues, orbit, or intracranial cavity
  - **Superficial complications**: Osteomyelitis, subgaleal abscess (Pott puffy tumor), septic thrombophlebitis
  - **Orbital complications**: Preseptal cellulitis/abscess, orbital (postseptal) cellulitis, subperiosteal postseptal abscess (SPA), orbital abscess, septic thrombophlebitis
  - **Intracranial complications**: Meningitis, epidural abscess (EDA), subdural empyema (SDE), cerebritis, brain abscess, cavernous sinus thrombosis (CST)

IMAGING

General Features
- Best diagnostic clue
  - Orbital SPA: Rim-enhancing, central low-density mass in extraconal space; edema of adjacent fat
  - CST: Heterogeneous or ↓ enhancement in enlarged cavernous sinus; often enlarged or thrombosed superior ophthalmic vein (SOV)
  - EDA & SDE: Extraaxial fluid collection in epidural or subdural space, respectively, with reduced diffusivity & enhancing adjacent meninges
  - Cerebral abscess: Ring-enhancing mass in brain parenchyma with uniformly thick walls, central reduced diffusivity, & surrounding vasogenic edema
- Location
  - Orbital SPA: Superior (frontal sinusitis), medial (ethmoid sinusitis), or inferior (maxillary sinusitis) extraconal space near superior, medial, or inferior rectus muscles, respectively
  - EDA & SDE: Subfrontal (frontal or ethmoid sinusitis) or above planum sphenoidale (sphenoid sinusitis); often overlies bone dehiscence/erosion
  - Cerebral abscess: Most often in frontal lobes related to frontal sinusitis
  - Subgaleal abscess: Soft tissues anterior to frontal sinuses; often overlies bone dehiscence/erosion
- Morphology
  - SPA: Lentiform with base along orbital roof, lamina papyracea, or orbital floor
  - CST: Convex lateral margin of enlarged cavernous sinus
  - EDA: Lenticular pus collection adjacent to infected sinus
  - SDE: Crescentic pus collection conforming to shape of adjacent cerebrum
  - Cerebritis: Ill-defined edema within brain
  - Cerebral abscess: Round or ovoid parenchymal collection

CT Findings
- CECT
  - SPA
    - Peripherally enhancing, central low-attenuation collection in extraconal space; broadly abuts underlying bone
    - Edema of surrounding fat with swelling of affected extraocular muscle(s) ± dehiscence of sinus wall
  - CST
    - Heterogeneous or ↓ enhancement in sinus compared to contralateral side
    - Convex lateral margins (swollen) cavernous sinus
    - Enlargement ± thrombosis of SOV
  - SDE
    - Extraaxial subdural collection with low attenuation centrally & adjacent enhancing dura
  - Cerebral abscess
    - Ring-enhancing lesion with uniform wall & surrounding low-density vasogenic edema
  - Skull osteomyelitis/subgaleal abscess
    - Focal bone lysis, sequestrum formation, reactive bone sclerosis
      - May lead to giant frontal sinus appearance with lucent cavity exceeding prior sinus size & lacking normal thin sclerotic bone margin
    - Focal, rim-enhancing fluid collection with subgaleal abscess

MR Findings
- SPA
  - Peripherally enhancing extraconal collection with central reduced diffusivity, low to intermediate T1 signal, & ↑ T2 signal
- CST
  - Enlarged, heterogeneous enhancing cavernous sinus
  - Enlarged or thrombosed SOV (absence of flow void)
  - Extraocular muscles may be enlarged from venous engorgement
  - Cavernous carotid artery may be narrowed
- SDE
  - Crescentic, rim-enhancing extraaxial subdural collection with central reduced diffusivity, low T1 signal, & ↑ T2 signal
  - Adjacent enhancing dura
- EDA
  - Lenticular, rim-enhancing extraaxial epidural collection with central reduced diffusivity, low T1 signal, & ↑ T2 signal
  - Typically subjacent to affected sinus
- Cerebritis
  - Amorphous high-signal area of brain on T2 or FLAIR
  - No ring enhancement on T1 C+ sequences
- Cerebral abscess
  - Ring-enhancing lesion with uniform wall thickness
  - Central reduced diffusivity, ↓ T1, & ↑ T2 signal
  - Rim may be ↓ T2 signal surrounded by ↑ T2 signal vasogenic edema

Imaging Recommendations
- Best imaging tool
  - CECT for orbital complications; contrast-enhanced MR with diffusion-weighted imaging for intracranial complications
- Protocol advice
  - Orbital complications: Thin-section (1-mm) axial CT through sinuses/orbits post contrast with coronal reformats

- CST: Multiplanar gadolinium-enhanced MR; post contrast with fat suppression; thin-slice axial & coronal through cavernous sinuses/orbits; SPGR C+ to assess CST
- Intracranial complications: Multiplanar MR with gadolinium; diffusion-weighted imaging imperative

DIFFERENTIAL DIAGNOSIS

Subperiosteal Postseptal Abscess

- Idiopathic orbital inflammation (pseudotumor)
- Extraconal neoplasm
  - Orbital lymphoproliferative lesions
  - Rhabdomyosarcoma

Cavernous Sinus Thrombosis

- Idiopathic inflammatory pseudotumor, apical subtype (Tolosa-Hunt syndrome)
- Cavernous sinus neoplasm
  - Meningioma
  - Sinonasal non-Hodgkin lymphoma
  - Masticator space CNV3 perineural tumor

Subdural Empyema

- Subdural hygroma
- Chronic subdural hematoma

Cerebritis or Cerebral Abscess

- Cerebral contusion
- Multiple sclerosis
- Glioblastoma
- Radiation & chemotherapy effects on brain

PATHOLOGY

General Features

- Etiology
  - Intraorbital & intracranial complications more likely in ARS; osseous complications more common in CRS
    - Most complications result from bacterial infections; less likely fungal sources
    - Sinocutaneous fistulae reported with frontal CRS
  - SPA: Valveless ethmoidal veins allow access of ethmoid infection into orbit through thin lamina papyracea
    - Can result from extension from any sinus; most commonly due to ethmoid sinusitis
  - CST: Septic thrombophlebitis of ophthalmic veins
    - Can spread from maxillary sinus via inferior ophthalmic vein or sphenoid sinus via pterygoid plexus
  - Subgaleal abscess (Pott puffy tumor): Osteothrombophlebitis from frontal sinusitis
  - Intracranial complications: Most often from frontal sinusitis because of emissary vein network (Behçet plexus) connecting sinus mucosa with meninges
    - Frontal > > sphenoid > ethmoid > maxillary
- Associated abnormalities
  - Meningitis/meningoencephalitis, ± infarct

CLINICAL ISSUES

Presentation

- Most common signs/symptoms

- Orbital cellulitis/SPA/orbital abscess: Proptosis, chemosis, ↓ visual acuity, limited ocular motility
- Subgaleal abscess: Forehead swelling
- CST: Extremely ill patients with retroorbital pain, cranial nerve palsies, & signs of meningitis
- SDE/EDA: Headache, fever, signs of mass effect
- Cerebral abscess: Headache, seizure, focal deficits depending on location

Demographics

- Age
  - Orbital complications of RS more common in children
  - Intracranial complications more common from adolescence to 2nd & 3rd decades
- Sex
  - Intracranial complications more common in males
- Epidemiology
  - 3% of sinusitis patients experience preseptal or orbital inflammation
    - Permanent ocular sequelae in 4.5% of sinogenic orbital infections
    - 15-20% of optic neuritis due to posterior ethmoid & sphenoid sinusitis (rhinogenic optic neuritis)
  - 3% of headaches related to sinusitis
  - 3% of intracranial abscesses secondary to sinusitis

Natural History & Prognosis

- Potential progression of orbital & intracranial complications if untreated
  - Prognosis excellent with appropriate antibiotic therapy & surgical drainage
- Intracranial complications → 50-80% mortality if not diagnosed & treated early

Treatment

- Appropriate antibiotic therapy in all cases
- Surgical intervention for SPA (functional endoscopic sinus surgery), some SDE, & cerebral abscesses

DIAGNOSTIC CHECKLIST

Consider

- Imaging valuable in patients with uncertain diagnosis, deteriorating condition despite treatment
- Multiplanar contrast-enhanced MR with diffusion imaging advantageous for evaluating intracranial complications

Image Interpretation Pearls

- Diffusion imaging is helpful in differentiating SPA from phlegmon; improves sensitivity for detecting intracranial & extracranial complications of RS
- Compare size & shape of affected cavernous sinus to contralateral side to diagnose CST

SELECTED REFERENCES

1. Lohnherr V et al: Orbital complications of sinusitis in children - retrospective analysis of an 8.5 year experience. Int J Pediatr Otorhinolaryngol. 177:111865,, 2024
2. Yu AJ et al: Complicated odontogenic sinusitis: extrasinus infectious spread. Otolaryngol Clin North Am. 57(6):1019-30, 2024
3. Expert Panel on Neurological Imaging et al: ACR Appropriateness Criteria® Sinonasal Disease: 2021 update. J Am Coll Radiol. 19(5S):S175-93, 2022
4. Snidvongs K et al: Risk factors of orbital complications in outpatients presenting with severe rhinosinusitis: a case-control study. Clin Otolaryngol. 46(3):587-93, 2021

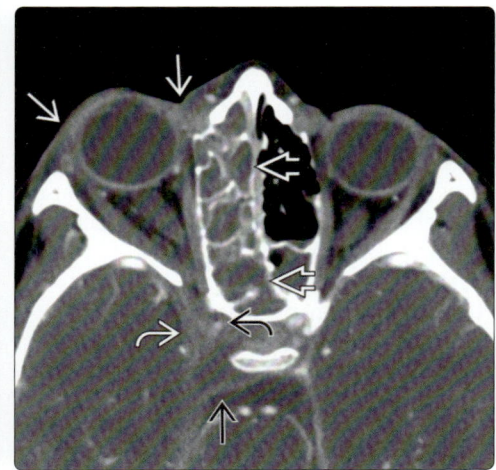

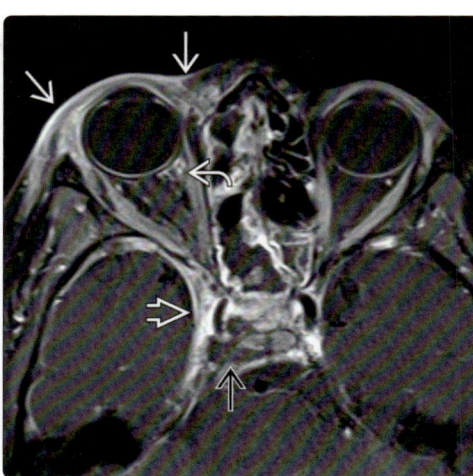

(Left) *Axial CECT of a child with complicated rhinosinusitis shows proptosis, diffuse opacification of the right ethmoid and sphenoid sinuses ➡, periorbital/preseptal edema ➡, and an enlarged right cavernous sinus ➡ from thrombus and retroclival abscess ➡. The right carotid artery is narrowed ➡ from vasospasm.* (Right) *Axial T1 C+ FS MR better delineates the preseptal ➡ and postseptal ➡ phlegmon, heterogeneously enhancing cavernous sinus thrombosis ➡ and retroclival abscess ➡.*

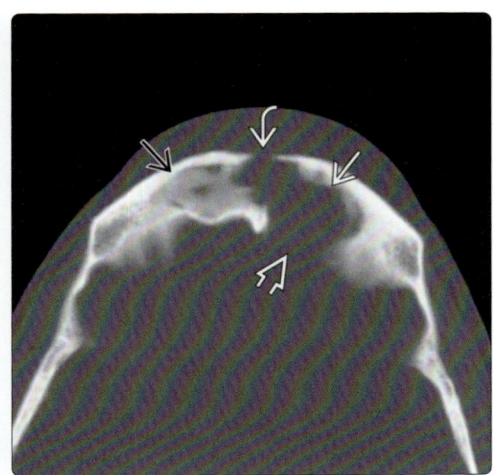

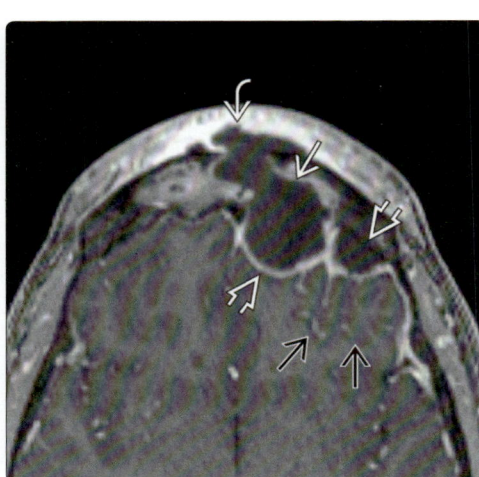

(Left) *Axial NECT in a patient with altered mental status and forehead swelling shows an opacified left frontal sinus ➡ with dehiscent outer ➡ and inner ➡ cortices. Mixed lucency and sclerosis of the right frontal bone ➡ indicate chronic osteomyelitis changes.* (Right) *Axial T1 SPGR C+ MR shows an opacified, expanded left frontal sinus ➡ with overlying subperiosteal abscess ➡ (Pott puffy tumor) and subjacent epidural abscesses ➡ with dural thickening. Note leptomeningeal enhancement ➡ from meningitis.*

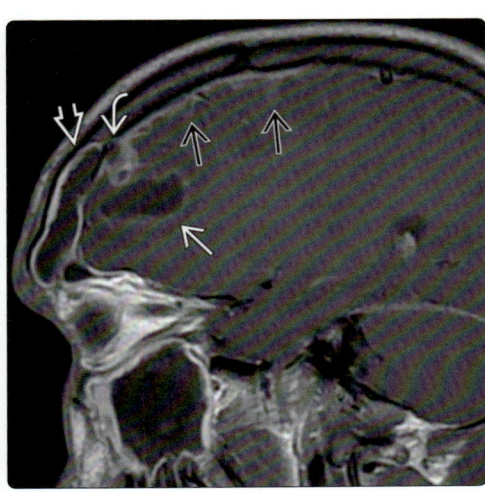

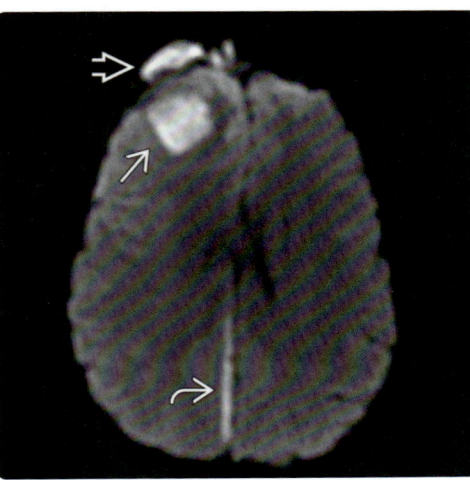

(Left) *Sagittal T1 C+ MR shows right frontal sinus disease ➡ with adjacent small epidural abscess ➡ and right frontal cerebral abscess ➡ Additional meningeal enhancement corresponds to meningitis ➡ in this patient with intracranial complications of acute sinusitis.* (Right) *Axial DWI MR in the same patient demonstrates reduced diffusivity within the right frontal cerebral abscess ➡ and adjacent infected right frontal sinus ➡. Note additional thin right posterior parafalcine subdural empyema ➡.*

KEY FACTS

TERMINOLOGY

- Fungus ball, aspergilloma
- Chronic, noninvasive form of fungal sinus infection
- Fungal colonization of material within sinus cavity

IMAGING

- Single paranasal sinus containing high-density material
  - Fine, round-to-linear matrix calcifications
- Maxillary > sphenoid > > frontal > ethmoid sinuses
  - Sinus often normal size & nonexpanded
  - May conform to sinus shape or be ball-shaped
- T1-hypointense signal in solid, mycetomatous mass
- T2-hypointense signal may be mistaken for air

TOP DIFFERENTIAL DIAGNOSES

- Chronic rhinosinusitis
- Allergic fungal sinusitis
- Sinonasal mucocele
- Invasive fungal sinusitis

PATHOLOGY

- Saprophytic fungal growth within paranasal sinus
  - Usually *Aspergillus fumigatus*
- No tissue invasion (mucosa, blood vessel, bone)
- Tightly packed fungal hyphae without allergic mucin

CLINICAL ISSUES

- Asymptomatic or mild pressure sensation overlying sinuses
- Immunocompetent, nonatopic, otherwise healthy patient
  - Most common in older female patients
  - Indolent course for up to years
- Surgical curettage is treatment of choice & is curative
- Antifungal therapy not effective

DIAGNOSTIC CHECKLIST

- Do not mistake low T2 signal for air
- Check for any signs of invasive disease
- May coexist with other forms of chronic rhinosinusitis

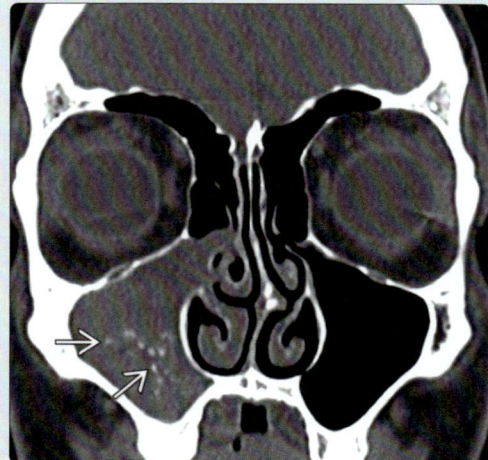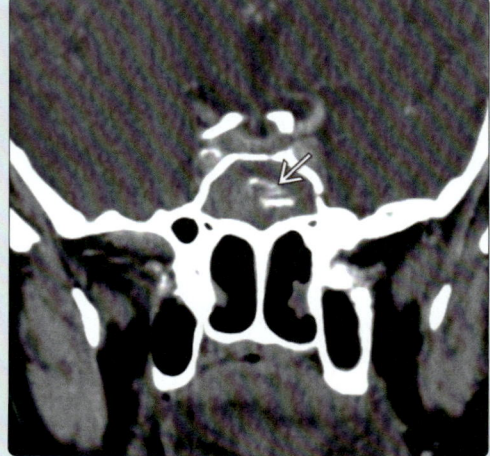

(Left) Coronal bone CT shows the classic features of a mycetoma within the right maxillary sinus. The sinus is opacified but not expanded. Mixed-density material consistent with fungal elements and calcium deposits ➡ are present in the sinus. (Right) Coronal CECT in a patient with a sphenoid sinus mycetoma demonstrates multiple foci of calcification ➡ within the fungus ball. The sinus is opacified, and there is mild periosteal thickening that does not show expansion.

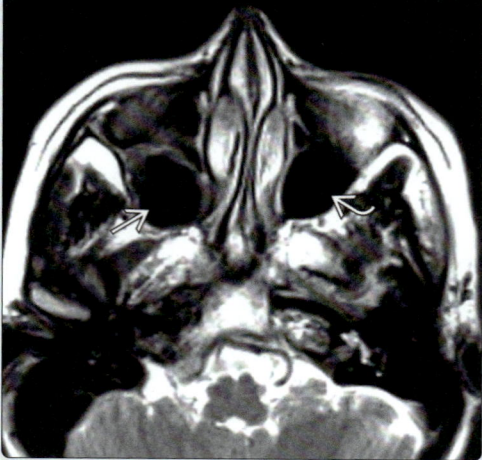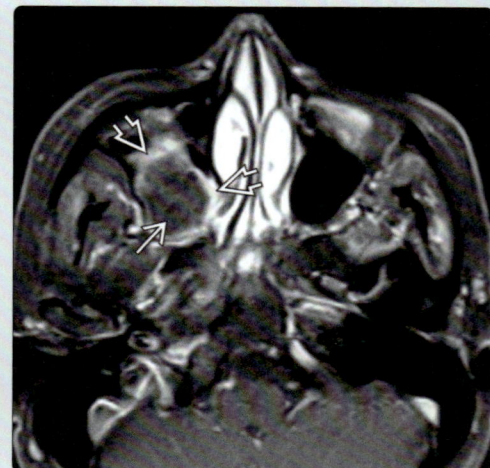

(Left) Axial T2 MR in a middle-aged woman with mild facial pressure sensation shows a normally aerated left maxillary sinus ➡ and opacification of the right maxillary sinus ➡ with material that is nearly as dark in signal as air. (Right) Axial T1 C+ FS MR shows intermediate signal within the right maxillary sinus ➡, confirming that the cavity is opacified and not air-filled. The material within the sinus is nonenhancing with rim enhancement evident in the surrounding mucosa ➡.

TERMINOLOGY

Synonyms

- Fungus ball, aspergilloma

Definitions

- Chronic, **noninvasive** form of fungal sinus infection
- Fungal **colonization** of material within sinus cavity

IMAGING

General Features

- Best diagnostic clue
  - Single paranasal sinus containing **high-density** opacification
    - Fine, round-to-linear intrinsic calcifications
- Location
  - Usually affects **single sinus**
  - **Maxillary** > sphenoid > > frontal > ethmoid sinuses
- Size
  - Sinus often normal size & **nonexpanded**
- Morphology
  - May conform to sinus shape; can be ovoid or rounded (so-called fungus ball) within sinus lumen

CT Findings

- CECT
  - Thickened mucosa at periphery of sinus may enhance
- Bone CT
  - Opacification or focal mass within sinus lumen
  - Central areas of **high density** ± calcification (70%)
  - Chronic mucoperiosteal change may be present

MR Findings

- T1WI
  - Variable signal material in affected sinus
  - **T1-hypointense signal** due to absence of free water in thick, solid, mycetomatous mass
- T2WI
  - **Hypointense** signal due to macromolecular protein binding may be mistaken for air
- T1WI C+
  - Inflamed peripheral mucosa may enhance

Imaging Recommendations

- Best imaging tool
  - NECT diagnostic typically; better for detecting calcification

DIFFERENTIAL DIAGNOSIS

Chronic Rhinosinusitis

- Less likely to appear mass-like
- Calcification less likely

Allergic Fungal Sinusitis

- Atopic patient with chronic polypoid rhinosinusitis
- Multiple sinus involvement with expansion & erosion
- High-density (CT) & low T1/T2 (MR) inspissated contents

Sinonasal Mucocele

- Sinus opacified & expanded
- Frontal & ethmoid > > maxillary & sphenoid

Invasive Fungal Sinusitis

- Immunocompromised patient
- Bone destruction & soft tissue invasion

Sinonasal Inverted Papilloma

- Mass in nasal cavity centered at middle meatus
- Convoluted, cerebriform architecture

PATHOLOGY

General Features

- Etiology
  - Saprophytic fungal growth within paranasal sinus
  - Usually *Aspergillus fumigatus*

Gross Pathologic & Surgical Features

- Thick, cheesy, gray-green, semisolid material

Microscopic Features

- Tightly packed fungal hyphae without allergic mucin
- No tissue invasion (mucosa, blood vessel, bone) compared to acute invasive fungal sinusitis

CLINICAL ISSUES

Presentation

- Most common signs/symptoms
  - Asymptomatic or mild pressure sensation over sinuses
- Clinical profile
  - Immunocompetent, nonatopic, otherwise healthy patient with no or minimal symptoms

Demographics

- Age
  - Most common in older patients but may occur in all ages
- Sex
  - Female predilection

Natural History & Prognosis

- Indolent course for up to years

Treatment

- Surgical curettage is treatment of choice & is curative
- Antifungal therapy rarely necessary

DIAGNOSTIC CHECKLIST

Consider

- Patient only mildly symptomatic & immunocompetent with single sinus involved
- May coexist with other forms of chronic rhinosinusitis

SELECTED REFERENCES

1. Dagher R et al: Imaging approach for fungal sinusitis. Curr Opin Otolaryngol Head Neck Surg. 33(1):56-63, 2025
2. Lee DH et al: Computed tomography-based differential diagnosis of fungus balls in the maxillary sinus. Oral Surg Oral Med Oral Pathol Oral Radiol. 129(3):277-81, 2020
3. Deutsch PG et al: Invasive and non-invasive fungal rhinosinusitis-a review and update of the evidence. Medicina (Kaunas). 55(7): 319, 2019
4. Chen JC et al: The significance of computed tomographic findings in the diagnosis of fungus ball in the paranasal sinuses. Am J Rhinol Allergy. 26(2):117-9, 2012
5. Robey AB et al: The changing face of paranasal sinus fungus balls. Ann Otol Rhinol Laryngol. 118(7):500-5, 2009
6. Palacios E et al: Sinonasal mycetoma. Ear Nose Throat J. 87(11):606-8, 2008

TERMINOLOGY

- Severe form of chronic rhinosinusitis (CRS) with polyposis
- Allergic response to fungi characterized by eosinophilic mucin with noninvasive fungal hyphae

IMAGING

- Imaging is part of diagnostic criteria: Look for hyperdense opacification & bony expansion of multiple sinuses
- Centrally hyperdense & peripherally hypodense on CT
- Expansion of sinus with bony remodeling & erosion
- Hypointense on T2WI MR; may mimic air

TOP DIFFERENTIAL DIAGNOSES

- Sinonasal polyposis
- Eosinophilic mucin rhinosinusitis
- Sinus fungal mycetoma
- Sinonasal solitary polyp
- Sinonasal mucocele
- Sinonasal non-Hodgkin lymphoma

PATHOLOGY

- **Type 1**, IgE-mediated hypersensitivity
- Immune response to fungal antigens
- Viscous, eosinophilic mucin with fungal hyphae
- **Absence** of tissue invasion

CLINICAL ISSUES

- Symptoms: Nasal obstruction, rhinorrhea
- Immunocompetent patient with longstanding CRS
- Serum eosinophilia, elevated IgE
- Cutaneous sensitivity to fungal antigens
- Topical steroids 1st-line medical therapy
- Surgical debridement + perioperative systemic steroids
- Topical & systemic antifungal agents & biologics

DIAGNOSTIC CHECKLIST

- Consider allergic fungal sinusitis in polyposis patient with increased density & expansion involving multiple sinuses

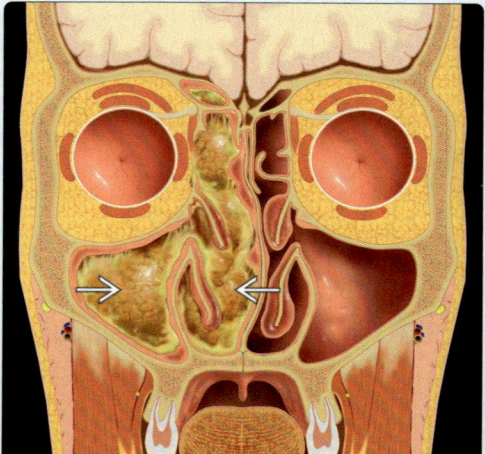
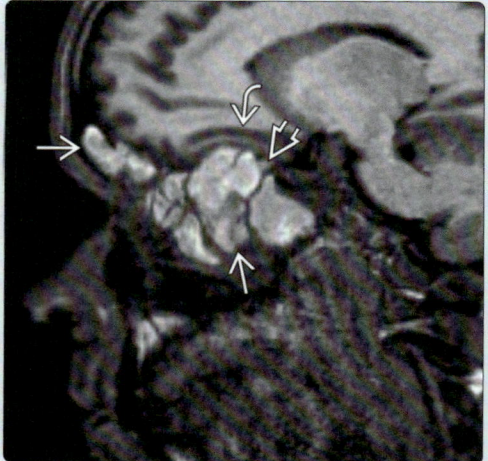

(Left) Coronal graphic shows classic features of allergic fungal sinusitis (AFS), including opacification and expansion of multiple paranasal sinuses and the nasal cavity. Centrally inspissated material ➡ is surrounded by peripheral edematous mucosa. (Right) Sagittal T1 MR shows expansile opacification of the paranasal sinuses with hyperintense secretions ➡. Mass effect on the optic nerve ➡ resulted in progressive left-sided vision loss. There is mild compression of the frontal lobe parenchyma ➡.

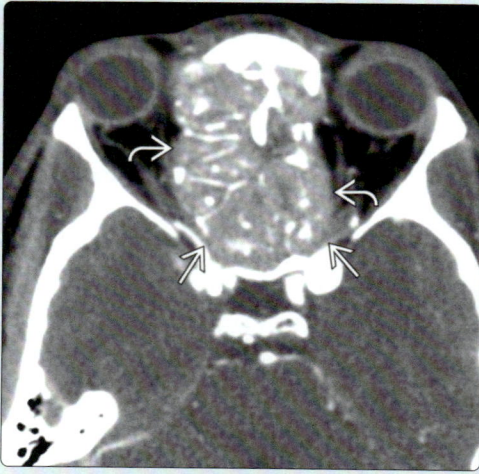
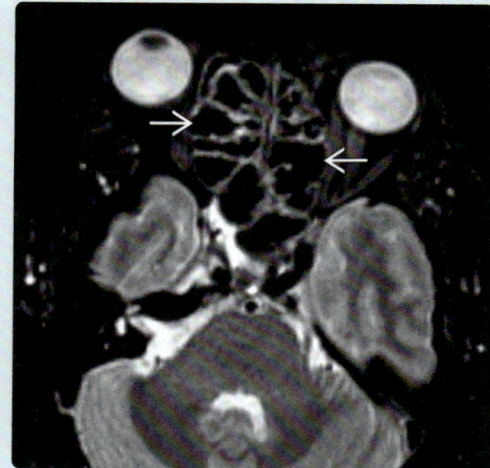

(Left) Axial CTA done for preoperative planning in the same patient shows hyperdense sinus secretions in multiple sinuses due to thick eosinophilic mucin that is typical of AFS. Bony expansion erodes into the left greater than right optic canals ➡ and both medial orbits ➡. Bone changes can be reversible after treatment. (Right) Axial T2 FS MR in the same patient shows hypointense secretions in the paranasal sinuses ➡ that mimic normal aeration.

TERMINOLOGY

Abbreviations

- Allergic fungal sinusitis (AFS)

Definitions

- Severe form of chronic rhinosinusitis (CRS) with polyposis
  - Allergic response to fungi in susceptible individuals
- Characterized by production of eosinophilic mucin-containing **noninvasive fungal hyphae**

IMAGING

General Features

- Best diagnostic clue
  - Imaging forms part of diagnostic criteria
  - **Opacification & expansion** of multiple sinuses
  - Centrally **hyperdense** & peripherally **hypodense** on CT
  - Hypointense on T2WI MR; may **mimic air**
- Location
  - Involves **multiple sinuses**
  - Often **unilateral** or bilateral (50/50); R > L

CT Findings

- NECT
  - Hyperdense material **centrally** within opacified sinuses
  - Hypodense **rim of mucosa**
  - **Expansion** of sinus with bony remodeling

MR Findings

- T1WI
  - Signal **variable** (water, protein, & fungal content)
- T2WI
  - **Hypointense** signal **centrally** due to dense fungal concretions & heavy metals; may mimic air
- T1WI C+
  - Peripheral inflamed mucosa enhances

DIFFERENTIAL DIAGNOSIS

Sinonasal Polyposis

- Common form of CRS with polyposis
- Absence of specific antigenic or atopic etiology

Eosinophilic Mucin Rhinosinusitis

- Similar to AFS but without identifiable hyphae; unclear if distinct entity or variant of AFS
- Resembles severe CRS with polyposis with more submucosal edema & less hyperdense mucin

Sinus Fungal Mycetoma

- Noninvasive fungal colonization without hyperimmunity
- Isolated, especially maxillary; hyperdense with Ca++

Sinonasal Solitary Polyp

- Low-density mass with rim enhancement
- Classic antrochoanal polyp (ACP)

Sinonasal Mucocele

- Isolated postobstructive lesion
- Chronic, expansile features with bony remodeling

Sinonasal Non-Hodgkin Lymphoma

- Sinonasal mass with bone destruction or remodeling

PATHOLOGY

General Features

- Etiology
  - **Type 2** immune response characterized by antifungal IgE-mediated hypersensitivity with eosinophil-rich mucin

Gross Pathologic & Surgical Features

- Viscous brown or greenish-black mucus with peanut butter/cottage cheese consistency

Microscopic Features

- Viscous, eosinophilic mucin with fungal hyphae
- Organisms: *Aspergillus &* dematiaceous species
- **Absence** of tissue invasion

CLINICAL ISSUES

Presentation

- Most common signs/symptoms
  - Nasal obstruction, rhinorrhea
- Clinical profile
  - **Immunocompetent** patient with longstanding CRS
  - Polyposis history
  - Serum eosinophilia, elevated IgE
  - Cutaneous sensitivity to fungal antigens

Demographics

- Age
  - Primarily young adults (mean: ~ 30 years)
- Sex
  - Male predominance
- Epidemiology
  - Asthma history in ~ 65%
  - Higher incidence in patients of African descent
  - Predilection for warm, humid climates

Natural History & Prognosis

- Slow, indolent course in face of CRS & allergy
- Rarely vision loss when sphenoid sinuses involved
- Uncommon progression to chronic invasive fungal sinusitis

Treatment

- Topical steroids 1st-line medical therapy
- Surgical debridement + perioperative systemic steroids
- Topical & systemic antifungal agents may be beneficial
- Increasing use of biologics (immunotherapies)

DIAGNOSTIC CHECKLIST

Consider

- AFS in polyposis patient with increased density & expansion involving multiple sinuses

Image Interpretation Pearls

- Hypointense on T2WI MR; may **mimic air**

SELECTED REFERENCES

1. Alsalem S et al: Value of MRI signal intensity in evaluation of allergic fungal rhinosinusitis compared with CT Hounsfield units: retrospective study. Medicine (Baltimore). 103(28):e38951, 2024
2. Xu T et al: Consideration of the clinical diagnosis of allergic fungal sinusitis: a single-center retrospective study. Ear Nose Throat J. 1455613231167247, 2023

KEY FACTS

TERMINOLOGY

- Acute invasive fungal rhinosinusitis (AIFRS): Rapidly progressive (hours to days) transmucosal fungal sinus infection with vascular, bone, soft tissue, orbit, & intracranial invasion → "dry gangrene"
  - Immunocompromised & diabetics most vulnerable

IMAGING

- AIFRS: Commonly starts at middle turbinate, then spreads to maxillary & ethmoid sinuses > sphenoid sinus
- Sinus opacification with focal bone erosion, adjacent soft tissue infiltration, & nonenhancing mucosa
  - CT: Sinus opacification with focal bone erosion & soft tissue infiltration: **Soft tissue where it should not be!**
  - MR: Superior for evaluating intraorbital & intracranial extension, **nonenhancing sinonasal mucosa**

TOP DIFFERENTIAL DIAGNOSES

- Acute rhinosinusitis with complication

- Sinonasal granulomatosis with polyangiitis
- Sinonasal squamous cell carcinoma
- Sinonasal non-Hodgkin lymphoma

PATHOLOGY

- 3 distinct clinical/pathologic subgroups of invasive fungal rhinosinusitis (IFRS)
  - **Acute (fulminant) invasive** FRS (AIFRS)
  - **Chronic** IFRS (CIFRS)
  - **Granulomatous** IFRS (GIFRS)

CLINICAL ISSUES

- AIFRS: Facial swelling, fever, nasal congestion, orbital symptoms, headache, &/or cranial nerve palsy
  - **Mortality 30-80%**
  - Treatment: Radical debridement ± immune stimulating therapy
- CIFRS: Sinus pain, nasal discharge, epistaxis, fever, polyposis
- GIFRS: Enlarging cheek, orbit, or sinonasal mass

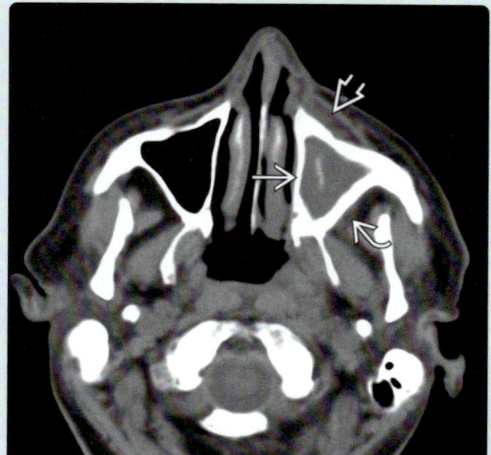
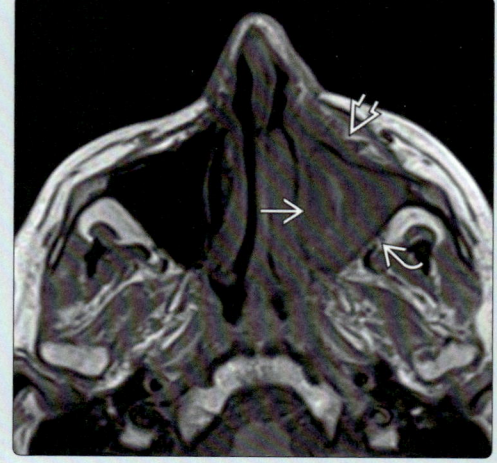

(Left) Axial NECT for a recalcitrant headache in a patient with B-cell lymphoma status post stem cell transplant shows opacification of the left maxillary sinus ➡ with mucoperiosteal reaction. Note subtle, but alarming, infiltration of the premaxillary ➡ & retroantral ➡ fat. (Right) Axial T1 MR in the same patient again shows heterogeneous opacification of the left maxillary sinus ➡ but better delineates the premaxillary ➡ & retromaxillary ➡ soft tissue infiltration, which in this case is due to Aspergillus AIFRS.

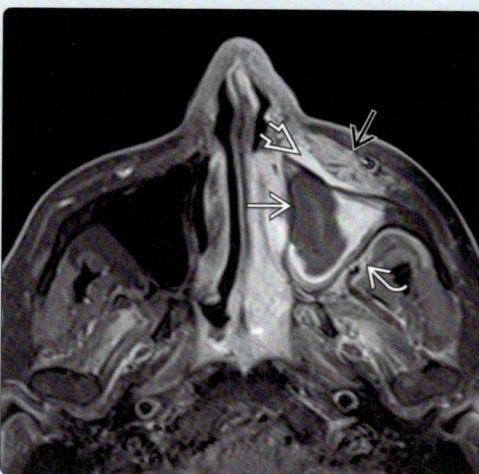
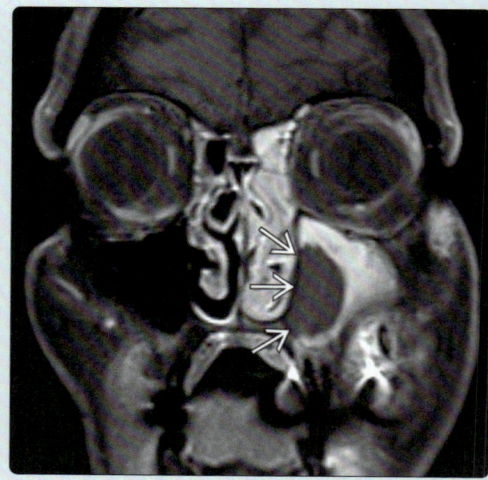

(Left) Axial T1 C+ FS MR of Aspergillus AIFRS shows loss of contrast enhancement (LOCE) involving the left maxillary mucosa ➡, signifying dry gangrene. Note infiltration of the pre- ➡ & retromaxillary fat ➡ with enhancing soft tissue as well as myositis of the superficial musculoaponeurotic system ➡. (Right) Coronal T1 C+ FS MR shows characteristic LOCE lesion ➡ of the maxillary sinus mucosa, corresponding to black eschar seen on endoscopy. Preoperative MR can help delineate gangrenous & viable mucosa.

TERMINOLOGY

Synonyms

- Acute invasive fungal rhinosinusitis (AIFRS): Acute necrotizing fungal rhinosinusitis (FRS)
- Granulomatous invasive FRS (GIFRS): Primary paranasal granuloma, indolent fungal sinusitis

Definitions

- AIFRS: Rapidly progressive (hours to days) transmucosal fungal sinus infection in immunocompromised patients (usually) with vascular, bone, soft tissue, orbit, & intracranial invasion, resulting in "dry gangrene"
- Chronic invasive FRS (CIFRS): Indolent (weeks to months) infection with dematiaceous > hyaline molds or mucormycoses; associated with less severe immunocompromise than AIFRS
- GIFRS: Indolent (weeks to months) infection with fungal invasion of orbit, nose, paranasal sinuses, or maxilla with characteristic noncaseating granulomas; often mass-like
  - Primarily in Sudan, India, Pakistan, & Saudi Arabia; occasionally patients without travel to endemic regions

IMAGING

General Features

- Best diagnostic clue
  - Sinus opacification with focal bone erosion, adjacent soft tissue infiltration, & nonenhancing mucosa
  - 7-variable CT model with ≥ 2 positive variables yielded 100% specificity & 100% positive predictive value
    - Periantral fat, orbit, pterygopalatine fossa, nasolacrimal duct, lacrimal sac invasion, nasal septal ulceration, bone dehiscence
- Location
  - AIFRS: Commonly starts at middle turbinate, then spreads to maxillary & ethmoid sinuses > sphenoid sinus
    - Spread from sinuses can extend in any direction & invade contiguous structures
  - CIFRS: Most common in ethmoid & sphenoid sinuses
- Morphology
  - Ill-defined or mass-like soft tissue lesion

CT Findings

- NECT
  - Earliest finding = unilateral nasal soft tissue thickening
  - Complete or partial soft tissue opacification of affected sinus; mucosal thickening
  - Focal areas of sinus wall erosion
    - **Subtle bone erosion** as fungi extend along vessels
  - Infiltration of adjacent fat & soft tissues
    - Maxillary sinus: **Perimaxillary fat infiltration** (anterior, premaxillary, or retroantral fat)
    - Can be present without bone destruction due to spread via perivascular channels
    - May be due to edema from vascular congestion, tissue infiltration by fungal elements
- CECT
  - Periantral soft tissues, adjacent musculature may enhance
- CTA

  - Arterial narrowing/occlusion; defines extent of territorial ischemia; identifies pseudoaneurysm
- CTV: Better for identifying cavernous sinus thrombosis

MR Findings

- T1WI
  - Variable signal of material within involved sinus
    - Depends on protein/water content, presence of fungal elements
  - ↓ signal (similar to soft tissue) within periantral or orbital fat
    - **Key sequence** for identifying infiltration of fat planes
- T2WI
  - Variable signal of sinus secretions
    - Fungal elements may cause hypointense T2 signal
  - High-signal edema with fat suppression
- T1WI C+
  - Loss of contrast-enhancing lesions
    - Nonenhancing, hypointense mucosa (black turbinate sign), corresponds with necrotic eschar
  - Enhancement of involved soft tissues
  - Leptomeningeal enhancement
- MRA
  - Vascular involvement (narrowing, dissection, thrombosis)

Angiographic Findings

- Narrowing, dissection, thrombosis, or pseudoaneurysm

Imaging Recommendations

- Best imaging tool
  - CECT with soft tissue & bone windows to evaluate soft tissue infiltration & bone erosion
  - MR superior for evaluating intraorbital & intracranial extension, defining extent of nonenhancing lesions

DIFFERENTIAL DIAGNOSIS

Complicated Rhinosinusitis

- Patient may not be immunocompromised
- Bone erosion less likely
- Air-fluid level, peripheral mucosal thickening in sinus
- Complications of subperiosteal postseptal abscess, cavernous sinus thrombosis, meningitis, & cerebral abscess may appear similar to AIFRS

Sinonasal Granulomatosis With Polyangiitis

- Usually involves nasal cavity (septum & turbinates)
- Less mass-like soft tissue, prominent bone erosion
- Orbit & skull base involvement possible

Sinonasal Squamous Cell Carcinoma

- Typically immunocompetent patient
- Maxillary antrum most common site
- Solid mass with bone destruction

Sinonasal Non-Hodgkin Lymphoma

- B-cell lymphoma: Solid, homogeneous mass in nasal cavity
  - ↓ T2 signal due to ↑ N:C ratio could mimic fungus
- NK-/T-cell lymphoma: May show loss of contrast enhancement & destruction

PATHOLOGY

General Features

- Etiology
  - Vascular & soft tissue invasion by fungi in high-risk patients with **neutropenia/dysfunctional neutrophils**
    - Poorly controlled diabetes mellitus (48%), 1/2 of patients present with diabetic ketoacidosis
    - Hematologic malignancy (39%)
    - Corticosteroid use (28%)
    - Renal or liver failure (7%); solid organ transplant (6%)
    - HIV/AIDS (2%); autoimmune disease (1%)
  - Rare in patients with normal immune function
  - Spread from sinuses via vascular invasion
  - **Conversion of allergic fungal sinusitis to invasive fungal sinus disease is extraordinarily rare**

Staging, Grading, & Classification

- 3 distinct clinical/pathologic subgroups of IFRS
  - **Acute (fulminant) invasive** FRS
  - **Chronic invasive** FRS
  - **Granulomatous invasive** FRS
- Diagnosis requires identification of invasive fungi from biopsy samples of mucosa, submucosa, bone

Gross Pathologic & Surgical Features

- AIFRS: Necrotic, discolored tissue due to fungus

Microscopic Features

- AIFRS
  - Hyphal invasion of mucosa, submucosa, & blood vessels
  - Prominent tissue infarction & neutrophilic infiltrates
- CIFRS
  - Dense accumulation of hyphae with occasional vascular invasion
  - Sparse inflammatory reaction; > 50% *Aspergillus fumigatus*
- GIFRS
  - Noncaseating granulomatous response with considerable fibrosis & scant hyphae
  - Vasculitis, vascular proliferation, perivascular fibrosis
  - *A. flavus* most common

CLINICAL ISSUES

Presentation

- Most common signs/symptoms
  - AIFRS: Facial swelling (65%), fever (63%), nasal congestion (52%), orbital symptoms (50%), headache (46%), cranial nerve palsy (42%)
  - CIFRS: Pain, nasal discharge, epistaxis, fever, polyposis
  - GIFRS: Enlarging cheek, orbit, or sinonasal mass: **May exactly mimic malignancy on imaging!**
- Clinical profile
  - AIFRS: Rapidly progressive (hours to days) invasive fungal infection in immunocompromised patient
  - CIFRS: Slowly destructive process (> 12 weeks) seen in patients with AIDS, diabetes mellitus, or those on corticosteroids
    - Can be seen in immunocompetent patient
    - May take months/years to develop, persist, recur

- GIFRS: Immunocompetent host with > 12-week course of enlarging cheek, orbit, or sinonasal mass

Demographics

- Age
  - Typically in adults, mean age = 42 years
- Epidemiology
  - **Diabetic** or **immunocompromised** patients with predisposing conditions
  - GIFRS: Geographic predilection, primarily in Sudan, India, Pakistan, & Saudi Arabia

Natural History & Prognosis

- AIFRS: Can be rapidly progressive & fatal in hours to days without appropriate surgical-medical therapy
  - **Mortality 30-80%**
  - Best prognosis: Limited to sinus & proximal tissues, diabetes (with higher hemoglobin A1c %, which may signify more reversible cause of immunosuppression), lack of extrasinonasal nonenhancing lesions, & surgical debridement
  - Poor prognosis: Orbital, skull base, & intracranial involvement; persistent, nonenhancing lesions after debridement; active hematologic disease; recent chemotherapy; recent bone marrow transplant; atypical fungi
  - AIFRS of sphenoid sinus can lead to cavernous sinus thrombosis, carotid occlusion, mycotic aneurysm formation, cranial nerve dysfunction, cerebral infarction

Treatment

- Radical debridement until histopathologically normal tissue reached
  - Use preoperative identification of nonenhancing lesions as general prediction of surgical margins
- Antifungal therapy with amphotericin B
  - *Mucor* species not sensitive to "azole" antifungal
- Treat underlying condition responsible for immunocompromised state

DIAGNOSTIC CHECKLIST

Consider

- AIFRS in diabetic/immunocompromised patient with maxillary sinus disease & "dirty" periantral fat, even if no bone erosion present

Image Interpretation Pearls

- Do not confuse normal variability in volume of periantral fat or normal musculature with fat infiltration
- Evaluate orbit, intracranial cavities for involvement
- Closely examine cavernous sinus & internal carotid & basilar arteries in sphenoid AIFRS
- Identify nonenhancing foci on pre- & postoperative scans
- **Do not confuse or conflate allergic fungal sinusitis with AIFRS: These are vastly different diseases with different morbidity & mortality!**

SELECTED REFERENCES

1. Baqays A et al: Systematic review of granulomatous invasive fungal sinusitis management. Laryngoscope Investig Otolaryngol. 10(1):e70086, 2025
2. Wu MJ et al: Paediatric acute invasive fungal sinusitis outcomes over a 13-year period. Clin Otolaryngol. 50(4):728-32, 2025

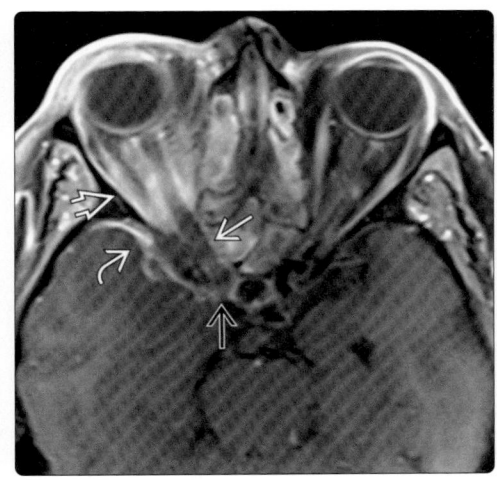

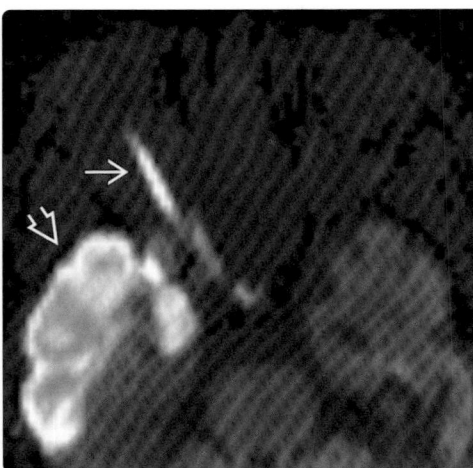

(Left) Axial T1 C+ FS MR in a case of AIFRS shows loss of enhancement in right orbital apex ⬦ with inflammatory enhancement ⮆ in remaining orbital soft tissues & adjacent dural thickening ⮥. Note ↑ signal in right internal carotid artery (ICA) corresponding to thrombosis ⮥. (Right) Axial DTI in the same patient shows diffusion restriction in right optic nerve ⮆ & temporal lobe ⮆ corresponding to posterior ischemic optic neuropathy & right middle cerebral artery territory infarct from angioinvasion & occlusion of right ICA.

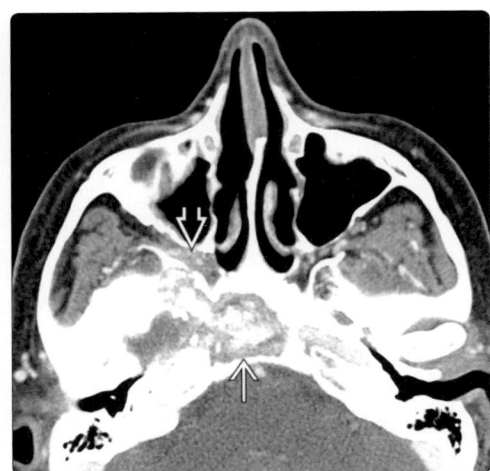

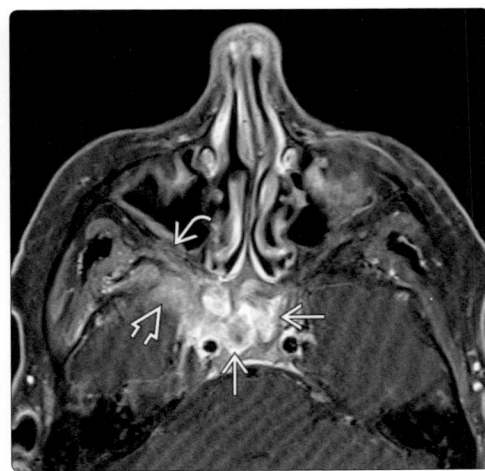

(Left) Axial CECT in a patient with 4 months of headache & congestion shows a lytic clival lesion ⮆ with soft tissue replacement of the pterygopalatine fossa (PPF) ⮆. Biopsy found chronic invasive fungal rhinosinusitis (CIFRS) of sphenoid sinus origin. (Right) Axial T1 C+ FS MR in the same patient shows opacified sphenoid sinuses ⮆, abnormal marrow enhancement involving the clivus & right greater wing of sphenoid ⮆, & infiltration of the PPF & retromaxillary fat ⮆ with enhancing soft tissue.

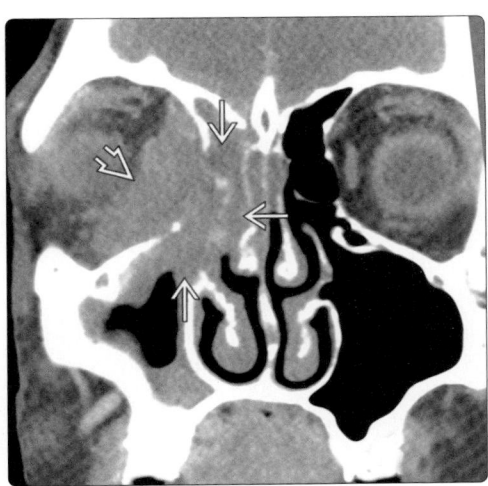

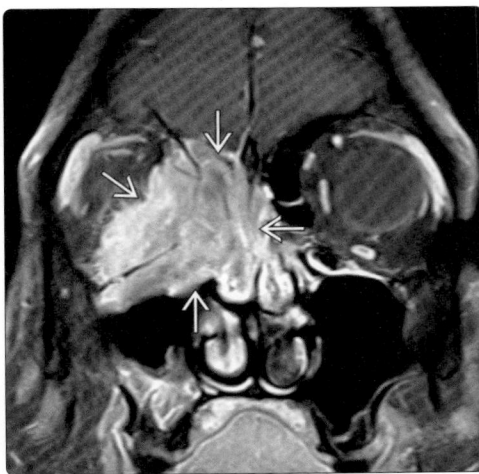

(Left) Coronal CECT of an otherwise healthy young adult with 4 months of progressive proptosis shows a large, infiltrating sinonasal mass ⮆ with orbital invasion ⮆. Biopsy demonstrated granulomatosis invasive fungal rhinosinusitis (GIFRS). (Right) Coronal T1 C+ FS MR in the same patient shows the "mass" ⮆ to enhance heterogeneously, but less avidly, than the normal sinonasal mucosa, mimicking malignancy on imaging. Note that the clinical presentation & imaging appearance are unlike that of typical AIFRS.

KEY FACTS

TERMINOLOGY

- Nonneoplastic, inflammatory swelling of sinonasal mucosa that buckles to form "polyps"

IMAGING

- Involves nasal cavity and paranasal sinuses (vs. retention cysts mainly within sinuses)
  - Predominantly along lateral nasal wall and nasal cavity roof
  - Commonly involves middle turbinate, sparing inferior turbinate
  - Anterior > posterior
  - Primarily mucoid or soft tissue density
  - Remodeling of sinonasal bones common in severe cases
- MR complementary to CT for assessing intraorbital and intracranial extension and for differentiation of sinonasal polyposis (SNP) from neoplasm

TOP DIFFERENTIAL DIAGNOSES

- Allergic fungal sinusitis
- Cystic fibrosis: mucous retention cyst
- Solitary polyp
- Granulomatosis with polyangiitis
- Respiratory epithelial adenomatoid hamartoma (REAH)

PATHOLOGY

- Formal pathogenesis of SNP has not been clarified
  - Chronic inflammation is major factor
  - Associated with allergy, asthma, primary ciliary dyskinesia, aspirin sensitivity, and cystic fibrosis

CLINICAL ISSUES

- Although not life threatening, chronic SNP unresponsive to therapy can be chronic, debilitating disease
- Medical therapy is treatment of choice
- Surgery reserved for symptomatic relief and correction of cosmetic deformities, orbital and intracranial involvement

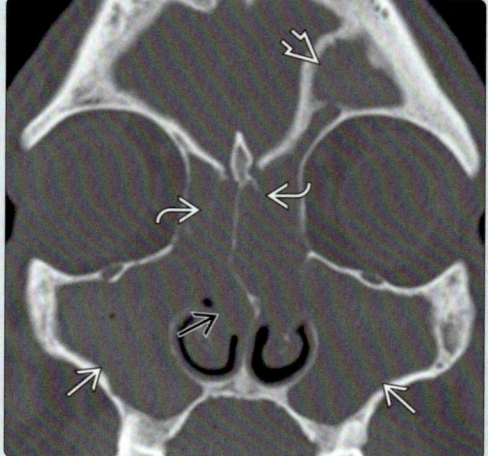
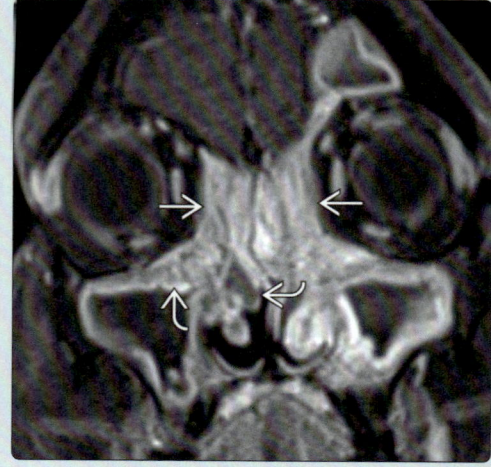

(Left) Coronal NECT in a patient with aspirin sensitivity and sinonasal polyposis shows a bilateral middle meatus pattern of obstruction with opacified maxillary sinuses ➡ bilaterally and opacified left frontal sinus ➡. Note rarefaction and truncation of the remnant ethmoid septa ➡ as well as lobular soft tissue along the nasal septum ➡. (Right) Coronal T1 C+ FS MR in the same patient shows diffuse lobular mucosal thickening ➡, including areas of submucosal nonenhancement ➡.

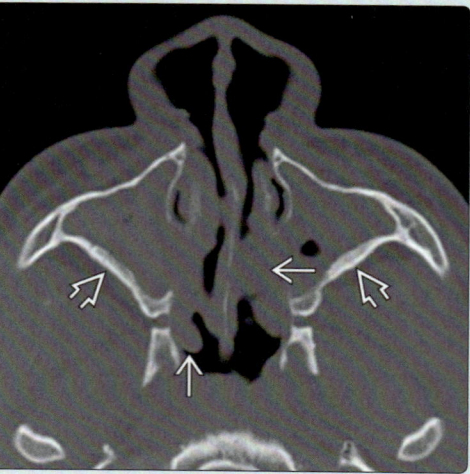
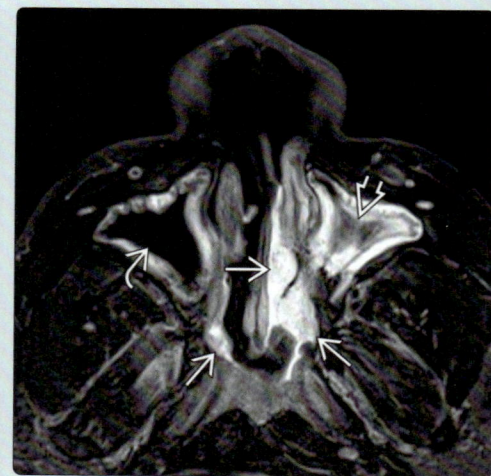

(Left) Axial NECT in the same patient shows lobular mucosal thickening ➡ along the nasal septum and inferior turbinates, corresponding with polyps. Note wall thickening ➡ of the opacified maxillary sinuses from chronic obstruction. (Right) Axial T2 FS MR in the same patient shows bright polyps ➡ along the nasal septum and inferior turbinates. Left maxillary sinus is opacified by heterogeneous signal intensity mucus ➡. Right maxillary sinus is not aerated; rather, it is filled with T2 dark inspissated mucus ➡, which mimics air.

Sinonasal Polyposis

TERMINOLOGY

Abbreviations

- Sinonasal polyposis (SNP)

Synonyms

- Chronic rhinosinusitis with polyposis (CRSwP)

Definitions

- Nonneoplastic, inflammatory swelling of sinonasal mucosa that buckles to form polyps
- SNP is general term for nonspecific majority of cases
- Specific minority forms of CRSwP are classified separately

IMAGING

General Features

- Best diagnostic clue
  - Polypoid masses involving nasal cavity and paranasal sinuses mixed with chronic inflammatory secretions
- Location
  - Predominantly along lateral nasal wall (near middle meatus), roof of nasal cavity, and ethmoids
  - Commonly involves middle turbinate, sparing inferior turbinate
    - May reflect differences in VCAM1 and CysLT1R protein receptor expression in turbinates
  - Anterior sinonasal cavities > posterior
  - Involves nasal cavity and paranasal sinuses (vs. retention cysts mainly within sinuses)
  - Usually **multiple and bilateral**; may be unilateral
- Size
  - Variable; up to several centimeters
- Morphology
  - Polypoid, lobular

CT Findings

- NECT
  - Primarily mucoid or soft tissue density
    - May be hyperdense with ↑ protein, ↓ water content, &/or colonization with fungal elements
- CECT
  - Mucosal enhancement at periphery of polyps
    - **No central enhancement** (as seen with neoplasms)
- Bone CT
  - Multiple, polypoid, soft tissue masses within nasal cavity and paranasal sinuses
  - **Remodeling** of sinonasal **bones** common in severe cases
    - May have areas of **bone erosion**
    - Often associated with rarefaction of adjacent bone
  - Other findings
    - Ethmoid sinus remodeling with trabecular loss and convex lateral walls bulging into orbits
    - **Air-fluid levels** nonspecific and may signal superinfection or trapped fluid
    - Truncation of bulbous, bony, inferior portion of middle turbinates

MR Findings

- T1WI
  - Fresh mucus (high water content) is hypointense
  - Bizarre mixture of layered signals seen in sinuses and nose
    - Results from polyps mixed with various ages of mucus
- T2WI
  - Fresh mucus is hyperintense
  - Chronic, inspissated mucus can appear **low signal** (mimics air)
- T1WI C+
  - Thin mucosal enhancement between polypoid soft tissue lesions without central enhancement

Imaging Recommendations

- Best imaging tool
  - NECT (bone) with multiplanar reconstructions
- Protocol advice
  - Consider frameless stereotaxy acquisition for routine sinus CT protocol in CRSwP patients, as many are surgical candidates
  - MR complementary to CT for assessing intraorbital and intracranial extension and for differentiating SNP from neoplasm

DIFFERENTIAL DIAGNOSIS

Allergic Fungal Sinusitis

- Severe chronic rhinosinusitis with allergic response to fungi
- Eosinophilic mucin containing noninvasive fungal hyphae
- Associated with sinonasal polyps; considered specific minority subtype of SNP
- Multiple unilateral or pansinus involvement
- CT shows high-density central material with low-density rim in expanded sinuses
- MR shows low signal, particularly on T2 (can mimic air)

Cystic Fibrosis

- Marked paranasal sinus hypoplasia with severe SNP
- Frontal sinus aplasia and sphenoid hypoplasia predictive

Sinonasal Retention Cyst

- Clinically asymptomatic or sinusitis history
- Lesions within sinuses with relative sparing of nasal cavity
- Difficult to distinguish from polyps based on density/signal intensity alone
  - Fluid density/signal on CT/MR; no central enhancement

Sinonasal Solitary Polyps

- Unilateral, solitary lesion
- Extends from antrum through widened infundibulum into nasal cavity

Granulomatosis With Polyangiitis

- Multisystem granulomatous disease involving lung and kidney
- Nodular soft tissue most often involving septum, inferior turbinates, and lateral nasal wall
- Bony destruction (septal perforation) rather than remodeling
- Orbital invasion relatively common

Sinonasal Sarcoidosis

- Multisystem granulomatous disease
- Nodular soft tissue most often involving septum and turbinates

Respiratory Epithelial Adenomatoid Hamartoma

- Benign sinonasal glandular inflammatory lesion that can mimic neoplasm or polyp on imaging
  - May occur in isolation or in setting of CRSwP
- CT shows opacification and smooth widening of olfactory recess, often bilateral
- MR shows bright T2 signal and uniform enhancement

PATHOLOGY

General Features

- Etiology
  - Inflammatory swelling of unstable respiratory mucosa
  - Formal pathogenesis of SNP has not been clarified; chronic persistent inflammation is major factor
    - Principal hypothesis: Allergy and inflammation cause unstable mucosa with epithelial cell proliferation and morphologic changes
    - Other factors implicated
      - Cytokines (*IL-5*, *IL-10*, HLA-G, granulocyte-macrophage colony-stimulating factor, tumor necrosis factor)
      - Mechanical forces in areas of contact between opposing mucosal membranes
      - Potential role of bacterial biofilms
- Associated abnormalities
  - Associated with chronic rhinosinusitis, allergy, asthma, primary ciliary dyskinesia, aspirin sensitivity, and cystic fibrosis
  - Polyposis and allergic fungal sinusitis (AFS) are **frequently** seen in association (~ 66% of cases)

Gross Pathologic & Surgical Features

- Pinkish, fleshy, pedunculated polypoid sinonasal masses with glistening mucoid surface

Microscopic Features

- Intact surface respiratory epithelium
- Underlying stroma is edematous with inflammatory cellular infiltrate and variable vascularity, glands, and goblet cells
- Eosinophil-dominated inflammation with component of neutrophils and mast cells
- May show squamous, cartilaginous, or osseous metaplasia ± surface ulceration and granuloma formation
  - Superinfecting bacteria include *Pseudomonas aeruginosa*, *Bacteroides fragilis*, *Staphylococcus aureus*

CLINICAL ISSUES

Presentation

- Most common signs/symptoms
  - Progressive nasal stuffiness and obstruction
  - Sensation of secretions that cannot be expelled
- Other signs/symptoms
  - Rhinorrhea, facial pain, headaches, anosmia, and nasal quality of voice
  - Cosmetic deformity, hypertelorism in cases of "polypoid mucocele"
- Clinical profile
  - Allergic patient with progressive nasal stuffiness
  - Polyps identified with nasal endoscopy

Demographics

- Age
  - Most common in adults > 20 years
  - Rare in children < 5 years
- Epidemiology
  - Frequency of polyps
    - 1-2% of normal population
    - 5% of extrinsic asthma patients
    - 13% of intrinsic bronchial asthma patients
    - 16% of "dental" sinusitis patients
    - 20% of cystic fibrosis patients
    - > 50% of aspirin-intolerant patients

Natural History & Prognosis

- Often waxing and waning; chronic, relentless disease
- Eosinophilic-type CRSwP more likely to have postoperative recurrence, shorter disease-free interval
- If left unattended, may become highly deforming in central facial region
- Although not life threatening, chronic SNP unresponsive to therapy can be chronic, debilitating disease with substantial decline in quality of life

Treatment

- Medical therapy is treatment of choice
- Topical and oral corticosteroids to reduce rhinitis symptoms, ↓ polyp size, and reduce recurrence
- Antibiotics when superinfected
- Surgery reserved for symptomatic relief and correction of cosmetic deformities, orbital and intracranial involvement
  - Endoscopic polypectomy, functional endoscopic sinus surgery, sphenoethmoidectomy, or balloon sinuplasty
  - Usually only temporary relief
- Increasing role of disease-modifying drugs, monoclonal antibodies, and biologics to treat predisposing diseases

DIAGNOSTIC CHECKLIST

Consider

- If density of expansile polyps is ↑ ± signal heterogeneous on MR, then AFS in setting of polyposis is likely

Image Interpretation Pearls

- Polyps occur in sinuses **and** nasal cavity
  - Mucous retention cysts typically located in sinuses only
- Individual polyps cannot be differentiated from mucous retention cysts based on density or signal characteristics alone
- Do not be alarmed if areas of **bone erosion** are present in addition to remodeling
  - If predominant pattern is aggressive-appearing bone destruction, must rule out malignancy or granulomatous disease
  - If disease burden is asymmetric, must exclude occult sinonasal malignancy

SELECTED REFERENCES

1. Kim DH et al: Comparative effectiveness of dupilumab versus sinus surgery for chronic rhinosinusitis with polyps: systematic review and a meta-analysis. Am J Rhinol Allergy. 38(6):428-36, 2024
2. Chen T et al: Association of sinonasal computed tomography scores to patient-reported outcome measures: a systematic review and meta-analysis. Otolaryngol Head Neck Surg. 168(4):628-34, 2023

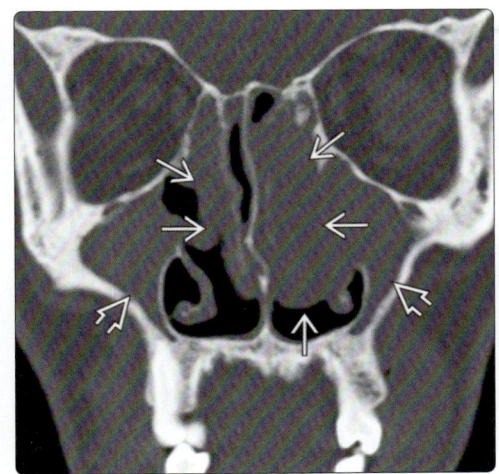

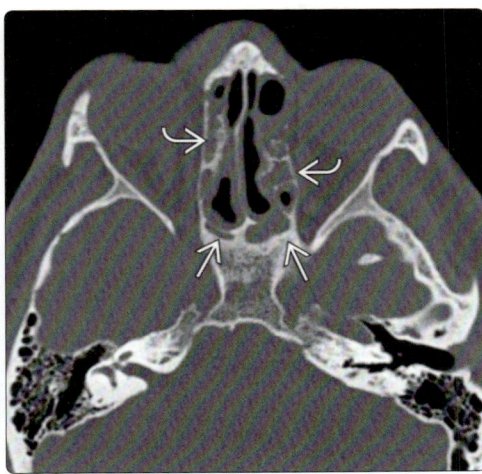

(Left) *Coronal CECT of a cystic fibrosis (CF) patient shows diffuse lobular mucosal thickening ➡ within the middle meatus and ethmoidectomy beds (left > right) corresponding to sinonasal polyposis. Note obstruction of the hypoplastic maxillary sinuses ➡. (Right) Axial NECT in the same patient shows a characteristic CF finding: Hypoplastic sphenoid sinuses ➡, which do not aerate dorsal to the anterior clinoid process. Note diffuse sinus mucosal thickening ➡. CF patients are prone to develop sinonasal polyposis.*

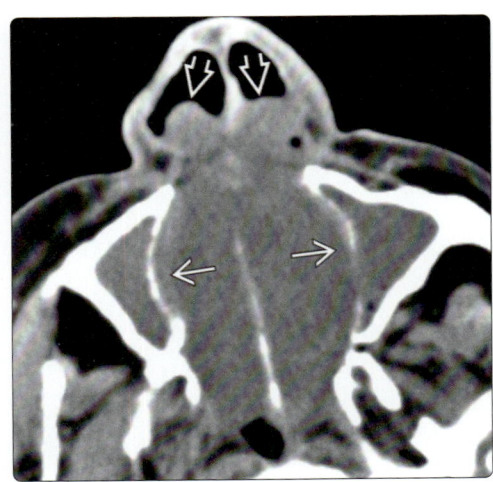

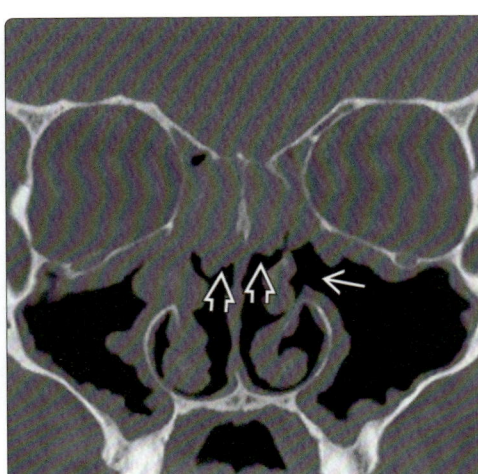

(Left) *Axial NECT shows opacification of the nasal cavities and maxillary sinuses. Nasal polyps extend into the bilateral nasal vestibules ➡. Note osseous remodeling and expansion of the nasal cavities ➡, a consequence of longstanding sinonasal polyposis. (Right) Coronal bone CT demonstrates sequela of prior endoscopic sinus surgery ➡ with extensive polypoid mucosal thickening throughout the sinnonasal cavity. Note nasal polyps in the olfactory recesses ➡ in this patient with anosmia from sinonasal polyposis.*

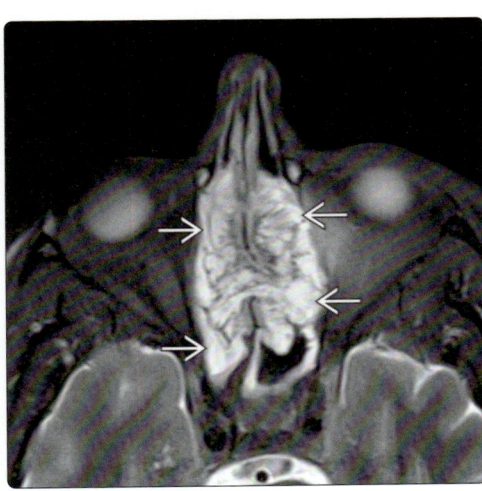

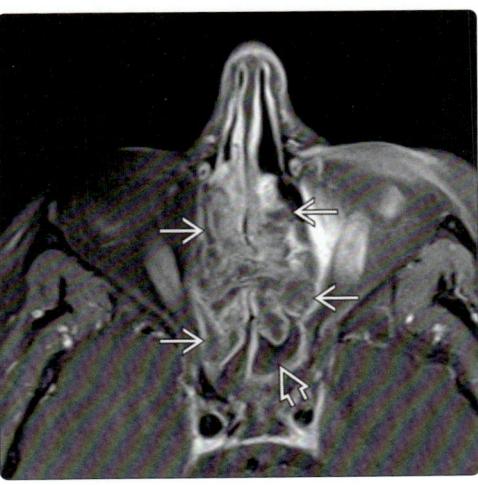

(Left) *Axial T2 FS MR in a patient with sinonasal polyposis shows extensive, lobular, T2 bright mucosal thickening ➡ throughout the ethmoid and sphenoid sinuses bilaterally. (Right) Axial T1 C+ FS MR in the same patient shows the characteristic postcontrast T1 appearance of sinonasal polyposis with lobular, superficially enhancing mucosal thickening but defined submucosal nonenhancement ➡. Left sphenoid sinus ➡ is hypointense but not as dark as air, indicating inspissated mucus rather that aeration.*

Solitary Sinonasal Polyp

IMAGING

- Most common type is **antrochoanal**
  - Polypoid mass extends from maxillary antrum → enlarged maxillary ostium or accessory ostium → nasal cavity
- Peripheral enhancement with **no** central enhancement
- Bone surrounding infundibulum/accessory ostium smoothly remodeled, not destroyed
- Large lesions extend into nasopharyngeal airway

TOP DIFFERENTIAL DIAGNOSES

- Nasal glioma (intranasal type)
- Nasoethmoidal cephalocele
- Juvenile angiofibroma
- Inverted papilloma
- Olfactory neuroblastoma
- Sinonasal mucocele

PATHOLOGY

- **Inflammatory polyp** resulting from edematous hypertrophy of respiratory epithelium
- Postobstructive inflammatory disease is often present
  - Greater when antrochoanal polyp exits antrum via natural ostium vs. accessory ostium

CLINICAL ISSUES

- 4-6% of all sinonasal polyps
- Most common in **teenagers** and young adults
- Typical symptoms: Unilateral nasal obstruction, worse on expiration
- Complete surgical removal of nasal and antral components is treatment of choice

DIAGNOSTIC CHECKLIST

- Begin imaging evaluation with coronal bone CT
- If bone CT or endoscopy appearance is atypical, then consider MR with contrast to rule out neoplasm

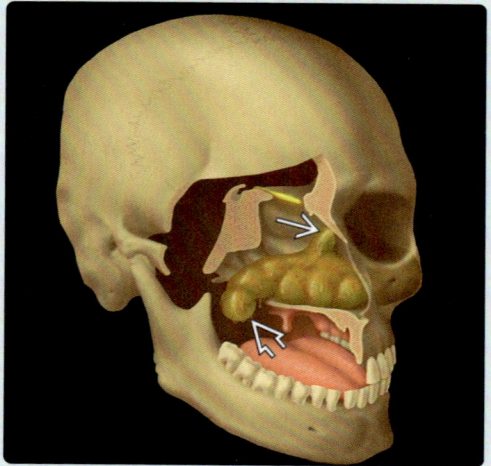
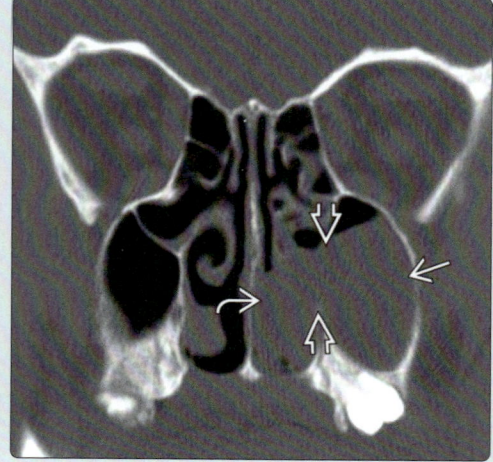

(Left) Longitudinal oblique graphic shows an antrochoanal polyp (ACP) extending from maxillary antrum through a posterior fontanelle ➡ into the nasal cavity. Note the posterior extension of the polyp into the nasopharynx ➡. (Right) Coronal bone CT shows a typical ACP extending from the left maxillary antrum ➡ into the nasal cavity ➡ via a secondary ostium ➡ located posterior to the ostiomeatal complex.

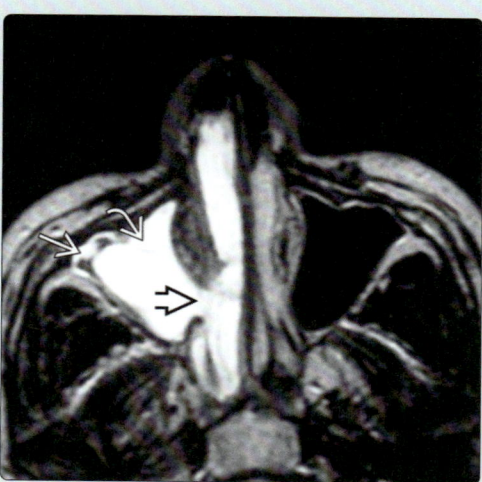
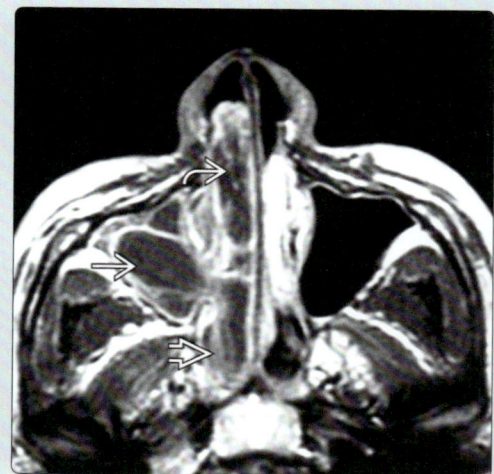

(Left) Axial T2 MR shows diffuse, homogeneous, hyperintense signal ➡ within an ACP. The polyp extends into the nasal cavity via a secondary ostium ➡. A small amount of trapped secretions ➡ is noted lateral to the lesion. (Right) Axial T1 C+ MR shows the antral ➡, nasal ➡, and nasopharyngeal ➡ components of this ACP. Note that there is thin, peripheral, but no central or nodular, enhancement of the lesion, which helps to distinguish it from a neoplasm.

Solitary Sinonasal Polyp

TERMINOLOGY

Abbreviations
- Antrochoanal polyp (ACP)

Synonyms
- Killian polyp

Definitions
- ACP: Inflammatory polyp arising from maxillary sinus antrum, herniating through major or accessory ostium into nasal cavity ± prolapsing into nasopharynx
  - Other solitary polyps named based on site of origin → site of termination

IMAGING

General Features
- Best diagnostic clue
  - **Dumbbell-shaped lesion** with maxillary antral origin connected by narrow stalk from maxillary infundibulum/accessory ostium → nasal cavity
- Location
  - Most common type: Antrochoanal polyp
    - Solitary polypoid mass fills maxillary antrum, then spills through enlarged maxillary ostium and infundibulum or accessory ostium into nasal cavity
      - □ Large lesions extend through choana into nasopharyngeal airway
  - Nasochoanal, sphenochoanal, frontochoanal, and ethmochoanal polyps are less common
- Size
  - Typically large
    - May reach > 5 cm in size
- Morphology
  - Dumbbell-shaped polypoid mass
  - Bulbous nasopharyngeal component in larger lesions

Radiographic Findings
- Lateral radiography: Polypoid soft tissue density resting on nasal surface of soft palate surrounded by air

CT Findings
- CECT
  - Peripheral enhancement of surrounding mucosa with **no central enhancement**
- Bone CT
  - Well-defined, dumbbell-shaped, low-mucoid-density mass
    - Arises from maxillary antrum, then extends through widened maxillary ostium or accessory ostium into ipsilateral nasal cavity
      - □ Bone surrounding infundibulum/accessory ostium smoothly remodeled, not destroyed
      - □ Stalk or midportion of dumbbell may be difficult to see on coronal sinus CT
    - Large lesions extend into nasopharyngeal airway
    - May have ↑ density centrally depending on chronicity ± fungal colonization
    - Metaplastic ossification rarely occurs with polyps

MR Findings
- T1WI

- Low signal most common due to ↑ water content
  - Variable signal intensity with chronicity
- T2WI
  - High-intensity polyp (near water signal intensity)
- T1WI C+
  - No enhancement of central portion of lesion
  - Thin, peripheral enhancement of mucosa

Imaging Recommendations
- Best imaging tool
  - If endoscopic examination clearly reveals ACP, then unenhanced coronal bone CT alone may be sufficient
- Protocol advice
  - Thin-slice axial bone CT with coronal and sagittal reformats
  - MR with contrast may be used in some cases to confirm polyp vs. neoplasm

DIFFERENTIAL DIAGNOSIS

Nasal Glioma
- Intranasal type: Soft tissue mass in nasal cavity
  - Maxillary antrum uninvolved except via secondary obstruction
- Tract through septum to skull base; rare in nasopharynx

Cephalocele, Frontoethmoidal
- Nasoethmoidal type: Polypoid mass in nose
- Intracranial origin with connection to brain parenchyma
- Defect in cribriform plate

Juvenile Angiofibroma
- Adolescent boys with **enhancing mass** centered in posterior nasal cavity near sphenopalatine foramen
- Often extends into pterygopalatine fossa
- May obstruct maxillary sinus but only extends into this sinus when very large

Sinonasal Inverted Papilloma
- Men with **enhancing mass** along lateral nasal wall near middle meatus
- Often herniates into maxillary sinus, causing ostiomeatal unit pattern of obstructive sinus opacification
- Convoluted, cerebriform architecture

Olfactory Neuroblastoma
- Diffusely **enhancing mass** in superior nasal cavity
- Aggressive, destructive lesion passes through cribriform plate into anterior cranial fossa
- Maxillary involvement unusual

Sinonasal Mucocele
- Expanded, opacified sinus with smooth osseous remodeling
- No central enhancement

PATHOLOGY

General Features
- Etiology
  - Inflammatory polyp (retention cyst) of maxillary sinus resulting from edematous hypertrophy of respiratory epithelium

– Fluid accumulates in lamina propria with polypoid distention, rather than glandular distention
– Allergy and repeated bouts of sinusitis thought to play role in etiology
– ↓ lipoxygenase pathway products might be involved in pathogenesis
– Urokinase-type plasminogen activator and plasminogen activator 1 may also have role
○ Passage of antral polyp into nose can occur via 2 different routes
– Through maxillary infundibulum
– Through **accessory ostium** of maxillary sinus
○ Sphenochoanal polyp route
– Sphenoid sinus → sphenoid ostium → sphenoethmoidal recess → choana → nasopharynx
• Associated abnormalities
○ Postobstructive inflammatory disease
– Greater when ACP exits antrum via natural ostium vs. accessory ostium

Gross Pathologic & Surgical Features

• Glistening, pale, mucosa-covered, grape-like mass
• Superficially looks like any other nasal polyp
○ Careful inspection reveals **stalk** leading laterally through maxillary sinus primary or accessory ostium

Microscopic Features

• Edematous hypertrophy of respiratory epithelium of maxillary antrum
○ No distention of mucous glands of sinus
• Loose mucoid stroma and mucous glands covered by respiratory epithelium
○ Reactive atypical stromal cells or cysts may be seen
• Few inflammatory cells with no eosinophils

CLINICAL ISSUES

Presentation

• Most common signs/symptoms
○ Unilateral nasal obstruction, worse on expiration
– When large, protrudes into nasopharyngeal airway
– May mimic nasopharyngeal tumor
• Other signs/symptoms
○ Nasal discharge
○ Mouth breathing, snoring with sleep apnea
○ Cheek pain, sore throat, headache
• Clinical profile
○ Teenager with unilateral nasal obstruction due to unilateral nasal polyp
○ Rhinoscopic examination: Polyp occludes nasal airway
– Obstruction of nasopharynx may be clinically confused with primary nasopharyngeal tumor

Demographics

• Age
○ Most common in teenagers and young adults
– **Mean: ~ 10 years**
– 2nd smaller group presents in 3rd-5th decades
• Sex
○ M > F
• Epidemiology
○ 4-6% of all sinonasal polyps

○ Antrochoanal > > sphenochoanal > ethmochoanal polyp
○ Much more prevalent in pediatric population
○ 40% of patients have allergies but no etiologic link to allergies

Natural History & Prognosis

• Herniation of ACP into nasal cavity may take years to occur
• Surgical removal of both components creates surgical cure
○ If surgical removal of nasal portion of ACP is completed without removal of antral base, then recurrence can be expected
– Mean time to recurrence: 45 months

Treatment

• Complete surgical removal of nasal and antral components is treatment of choice
○ Surgical procedures
– Intranasal avulsion, Caldwell-Luc antrostomy, and endoscopic removal through middle meatus
• Corticosteroids are ineffective

DIAGNOSTIC CHECKLIST

Consider

• Begin imaging evaluation with coronal bone CT
• If bone CT or endoscopy appearance is atypical, consider MR with contrast to rule out central enhancement (neoplasm)

Image Interpretation Pearls

• Mucoid density/signal antrochoanal mass with thin rim of peripheral enhancement **only** is highly characteristic of ACP
• Do not mistake nasopharyngeal component for nasopharyngeal neoplasm
○ Look for ipsilateral opacification of maxillary antrum even if stalk is difficult to see
• Differential diagnosis of ACP in atypical location on coronal sinus CT should include inverting papilloma

SELECTED REFERENCES

1. Perić A et al: Clinical and histological differences between choanal polyps in children and adults: a 15-year retrospective study. OTO Open. 8(4):e70004, 2024
2. Galluzzi F et al: Recurrences of surgery for antrochoanal polyps in children: a systematic review. Int J Pediatr Otorhinolaryngol. 106:26-30, 2018
3. Bakshi SS et al: Antrochoanal polyp. J Allergy Clin Immunol Pract. 5(3):806-7, 2017
4. Lee DH et al: Difference of antrochoanal polyp between children and adults. Int J Pediatr Otorhinolaryngol. 84:143-6, 2016
5. Thompson LD et al: Update on select benign mesenchymal and meningothelial sinonasal tract lesions. Head Neck Pathol. 10(1):95-108, 2016
6. Choudhury N et al: Endoscopic management of antrochoanal polyps: a single UK centre's experience. Eur Arch Otorhinolaryngol. 272(9):2305-11, 2015
7. Kizil Y et al: Analysis of choanal polyps. J Craniofac Surg. 25(3):1082-4, 2014
8. Yaman H et al: Evaluation and management of antrochoanal polyps. Clin Exp Otorhinolaryngol. 3(2):110-4, 2010
9. Frosini P et al: Antrochoanal polyp: analysis of 200 cases. Acta Otorhinolaryngol Ital. 29(1):21-6, 2009
10. Yuca K et al: Evaluation and treatment of antrochoanal polyps. J Otolaryngol. 35(6):420-3, 2006
11. Maldonado M et al: The antrochoanal polyp. Rhinology. 42(4):178-82, 2004
12. Chung SK et al: Surgical, radiologic, and histologic findings of the antrochoanal polyp. Am J Rhinol. 16(2):71-6, 2002
13. Pruna X et al: Antrochoanal polyps in children: CT findings and differential diagnosis. Eur Radiol. 10(5):849-51, 2000
14. Weissman JL et al: Sphenochoanal polyps: evaluation with CT and MR imaging. Radiology. 178(1):145-8, 1991

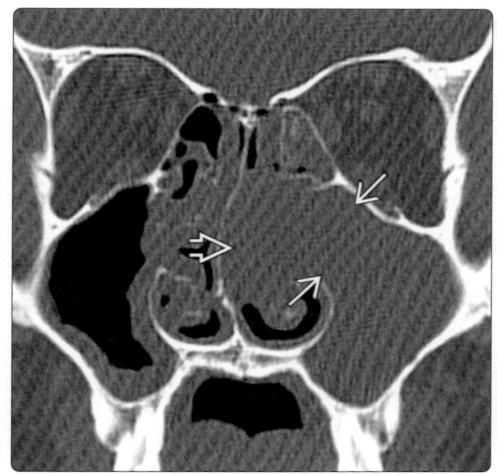

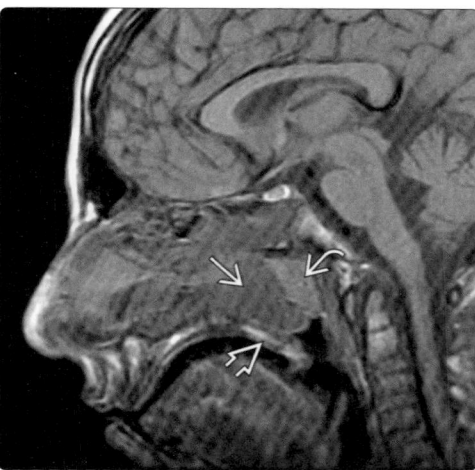

(Left) *Coronal bone CT shows an opacified left maxillary sinus. The maxillary ostium is widened ➡, and a large solitary polyp ➡ extends through the ostium into the nasal cavity. The polyp obstructs the middle meatus.* (Right) *Sagittal T1 MR shows a large, intermediate-signal polyp ➡ extending from the nasal cavity into the nasopharynx. Note normal high signal intensity in the palate ➡ below the polyp. The adenoidal tissue ➡ is slightly hyperintense compared to the polyp.*

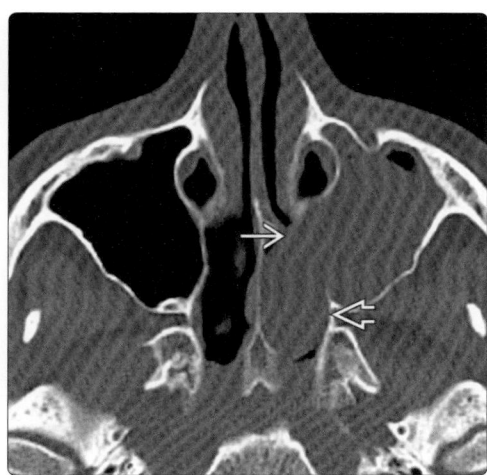

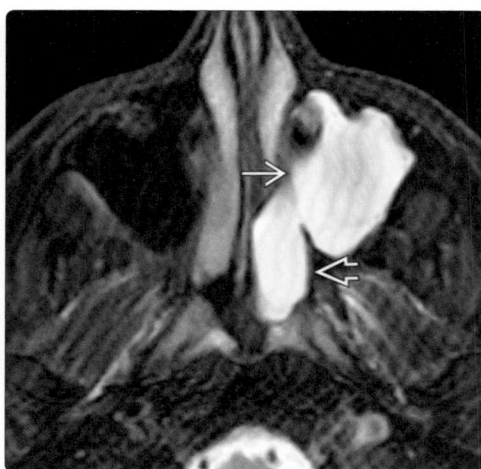

(Left) *Axial bone CT shows near-complete opacification of the left maxillary sinus with extension of polypoid tissue into the nasal cavity ➡ and posteriorly through the choana ➡. This is a typical appearance of an ACP.* (Right) *Axial T2 FS MR in the same patient shows a markedly T2-hyperintense ACP filling the left maxillary sinus and extending into the nasal cavity ➡ and into the nasopharynx via the choana ➡.*

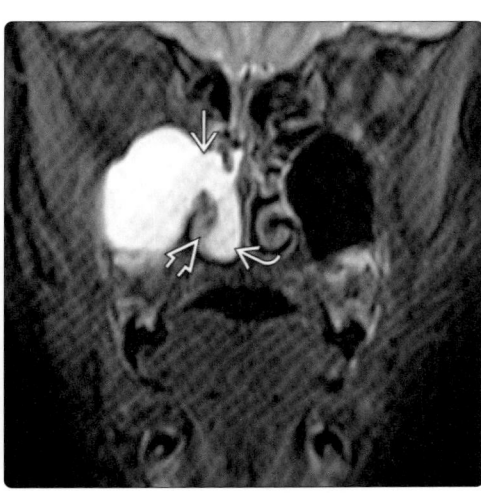

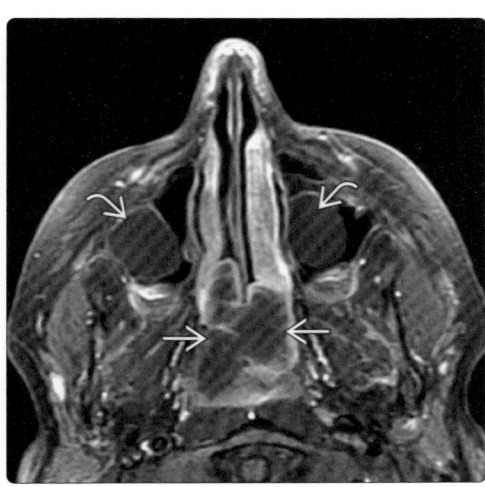

(Left) *Coronal STIR MR demonstrates a typical ACP extending through the ostium ➡ between the maxillary sinus into the nasal cavity. The intranasal component ➡ is seen medial to the lower signal intensity inferior turbinate ➡.* (Right) *Axial T1 C+ FS MR shows a dumbbell-shaped nasochoanal polyp ➡ occluding the choanal openings and filling the nasopharynx. Only peripheral enhancement is seen around the lesion. Note the retention cysts ➡ in the maxillary antra.*

KEY FACTS

IMAGING

- Opacified, **expanded** sinus with **smooth remodeling** of walls
  - May occur in septated sinuses & pneumatized anatomic variant air cells
  - **Frontal (60-65%)** > **ethmoid (25%)** > maxillary (5-10%) > sphenoid (2-5%)
- CT: Thin-section CT with coronal & sagittal reformat helpful for surgical planning & delineation of adjacent normal anatomy
  - Low-density or soft tissue density opacification of sinus with expansion
  - Bony sinus walls remodeled
  - No central enhancement; ± minimal peripheral enhancement
- MR: Enhanced MR recommended for detection of intracranial involvement & identifying potential obstructing neoplasm as underlying cause
  - High-water-content mucus typically shows ↓ T1 signal, ↑ T2 signal, but signal varies with protein content

TOP DIFFERENTIAL DIAGNOSES

- Allergic fungal sinusitis
- Sinonasal polyposis
- Solitary sinonasal polyp

PATHOLOGY

- Cause is obstructed drainage pathway of affected sinus or air cell

CLINICAL ISSUES

- Most common expansile lesion of paranasal sinuses
- Slowly progressive symptoms that vary depending on lesion location without signs of acute infection
  - > 90% have ophthalmic symptoms & signs
- Surgical cure is goal & expected result when mucocele is present

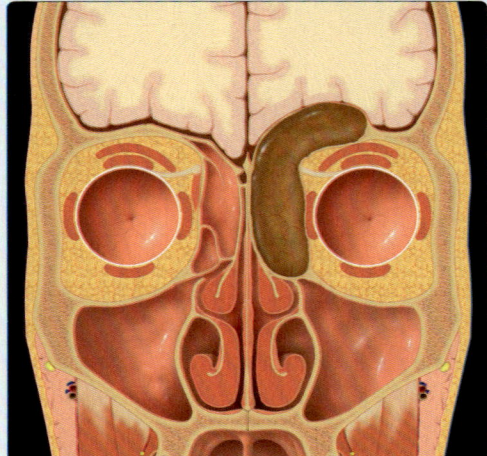
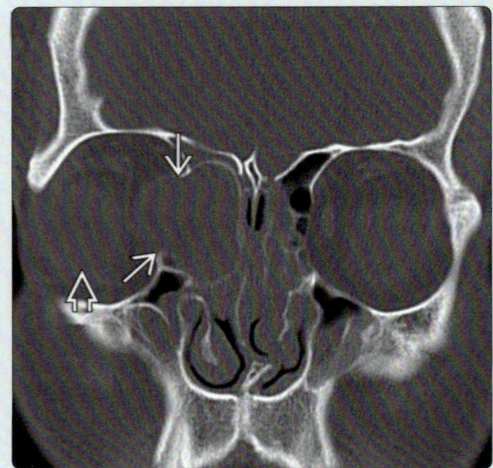

(Left) Coronal graphic shows a large left anterior ethmoid mucocele extending into the left frontal sinus. The affected sinuses are expanded without evidence of aggressive bone destruction. (Right) Coronal bone CT shows the typical features of a right ethmoid mucocele. The sinus is opacified, and there is remodeling of the surrounding bony walls with erosion of the lamina papyracea ➡. Note the mass effect on the orbit with lateralization of the globe ➡.

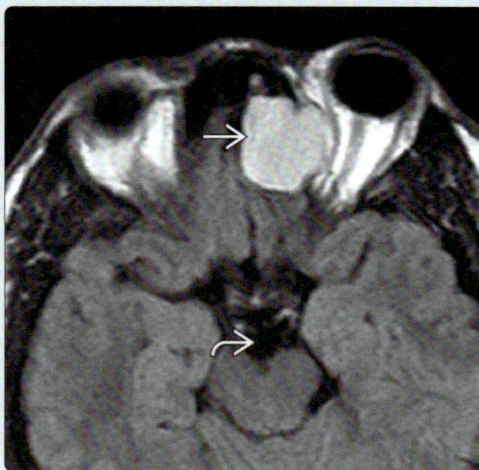
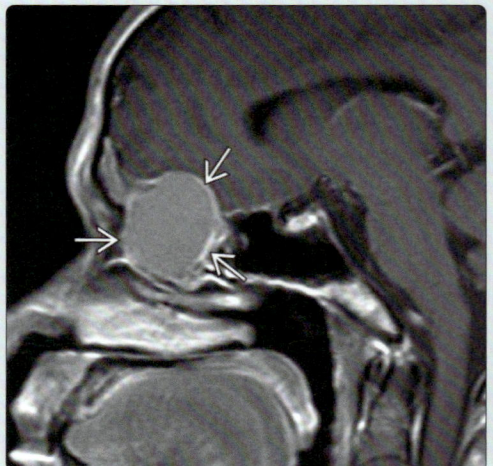

(Left) Axial FLAIR MR in a patient with proptosis and diplopia shows a homogeneous, expansile left ethmoid mucocele. Note that the material within the mucocele ➡ is hyperintense compared to CSF ➡. This likely reflects the high protein content within the mucocele. (Right) Sagittal T1 C+ MR demonstrates increased T1 signal in the mucocele, likely related to elevated protein content. There is no central enhancement within the mucocele with only minimal peripheral enhancement ➡.

TERMINOLOGY

Definitions

- Expanded, chronically obstructed sinus, lined by normal respiratory epithelium & completely filled with mucus

IMAGING

General Features

- Best diagnostic clue
  - **Opacified, expanded sinus** with smooth remodeling of walls
- Location
  - > 90% in frontal & ethmoid sinuses
    - **Frontal (60-65%)** > ethmoid (25%) > maxillary (5-10%) > sphenoid (2-5%)
  - May occur in septated sinuses & pneumatized anatomic variant air cells
  - Ethmoid mucoceles have greatest potential for intraorbital extension
  - Sphenoid mucoceles have greatest potential for intracranial extension
- Morphology
  - Frontal mucocele: Expands anteriorly into skin of forehead or posteriorly into anterior cranial fossa
    - May also expand orbital roof & contact superior rectus/levator complex
  - Ethmoid mucocele: Thins & remodels lamina papyracea (lateral ethmoid air cell wall), bowing it into orbit
  - Maxillary mucocele: Expands into ipsilateral nasal cavity, usually in area of secondary ostium of maxillary sinus or into premaxillary soft tissues
  - Sphenoid sinus mucocele: Expands anterolaterally into posterior ethmoids & orbital apex

Radiographic Findings

- Radiography
  - Frontal & maxillary sinus mucocele can be suggested from plain film findings
    - "Clouding" of expanded sinus with loss of normal mucoperiosteal line of sinus wall
  - Ethmoid & sphenoid mucocele may be missed

CT Findings

- CECT
  - No central enhancement; ± minimal peripheral enhancement
    - Thick peripheral enhancement raises suspicion of superinfection (mucopyocele)
- Bone CT
  - Low-density or soft tissue density opacification of sinus with **expansion**
    - High-density areas related to desiccation of secretions or fungal colonization
  - Bony sinus walls remodeled
    - May be thinned, focally absent, or normal thickness
    - Lacks aggressive osseous destruction

MR Findings

- T1WI
  - High water content of mucus interior yields ↓ T1 signal
    - When protein content high, ↑ T1 signal
- T2WI
  - High water content of mucus interior yields ↑ T2 signal
    - When areas of inspissated mucus exist, may be ↓ T2 signal
- DWI
  - Central diffusion restriction helpful in distinguishing mucopyocele from mucocele
    - ADC map < 0.78 ×10^{-3} mm²/s (100% sensitive for mucopyocele)
- T1WI C+
  - No central enhancement; ± minimal peripheral enhancement
    - Thickened peripheral mucosa suggests infected mucocele (mucopyocele)
    - Consider tumor obstruction of sinus with secondary mucocele if associated nodular enhancement

Imaging Recommendations

- Best imaging tool
  - Small mucocele may require only unenhanced bone CT
  - Larger mucocele with significant regional compression may benefit from enhanced MR & multiplanar bone CT
- Protocol advice
  - Thin-section CT with coronal & sagittal reformats aids surgical planning & delineation of adjacent normal anatomy
  - Enhanced MR recommended for detection of intracranial involvement & identifying obstructing neoplasm as cause of mucocele

DIFFERENTIAL DIAGNOSIS

Allergic Fungal Sinusitis

- Involves multiple sinuses (key distinguishing feature)
- Typically expansile, especially if seen with polyps
- High central density on CT; low central T2 MR signal

Sinonasal Polyposis

- Involves multiple sinuses **&** nasal cavity
- May have multiple small mucoceles associated

Solitary Sinonasal Polyp

- "Dumbbell" cystic mass fills maxillary antrum, herniates through sinus ostium into adjacent nasal cavity

Slow-Growing Benign or Malignant Tumor

- May mimic mucocele when seen on bone/unenhanced CT
- Central, nodular enhancement on CT/MR differentiates from mucocele

PATHOLOGY

General Features

- Etiology
  - Results from **obstruction of primary ostium** of affected sinus
    - Obstruction from inflammation, trauma, functional endoscopic sinus surgery, or any space-occupying, sinonasal mass
    - Secretion of mucus into obstructed sinus creates mucocele

— Sinus expansion from pressure necrosis with slow erosion of inner surface of bony sinus wall matched by new bone formation on outer periosteal surface

- Associated abnormalities
  o Obstructing mass at ostium may cause secondary mucocele

Gross Pathologic & Surgical Features

- Mucocele lumen filled with thick mucoid or gelatinous secretions

Microscopic Features

- Histologically indistinguishable from polyps & retention cysts
- Flattened, pseudostratified, ciliated columnar epithelium = mucus-secreting respiratory epithelium
  o Squamous metaplasia can be seen in longstanding cases
- Retained mucous secretions are sterile
  o Purulent exudate present in cases of mucopyocele
- Reactive bone formation or bony remodeling of adjacent sinus walls may be present

CLINICAL ISSUES

Presentation

- Most common signs/symptoms
  o > 90% have ophthalmic signs & symptoms
  o Principal presenting symptoms depend on site of involvement
    — Frontal mucocele: Forehead bossing, proptosis, diplopia, & mass in superomedial orbit
    — Ethmoid mucocele: Proptosis, blurred vision ± visual loss, periorbital swelling
    — Maxillary mucocele: Nasal obstruction from medial projection with cheek pressure, rhinorrhea
    — Sphenoid mucocele: Visual loss, oculomotor palsy, headache
- Other signs/symptoms
  o Epiphora, decreased color vision, hypoglobus (downward displaced eye)
  o If pain present, consider mucopyocele
- Clinical profile
  o Slowly progressive symptoms that vary depending on lesion location without signs of acute infection
  o Diagnosis requires correlation between clinical, radiographic, & pathologic findings, as diagnosis on histopathology alone can be difficult

Demographics

- Age
  o Most common in adults
    — Occurs in all age groups
  o In children, look for obstructing mass or underlying disorder (cystic fibrosis, immotile cilia syndrome)
- Epidemiology
  o Most common expansile lesion of paranasal sinuses
  o Although rare, sphenoid mucocele has highest complication rate due to proximity of vital structures

Natural History & Prognosis

- Gradual, clinically silent enlargement over months to years
- Cranial neuropathy (CNII-CNVI) may not recover following surgery if chronic at time of presentation

- Complications in untreated cases
  o Include superimposed infection (mucopyocele), meningitis ± brain abscess

Treatment

- Surgical cure is goal & expected result when mucocele is present
  o Endoscopic sinus surgery
    — Reserved for uncomplicated maxillary or ethmoid mucocele
  o Most frontal mucoceles treated with osteoplastic flap ± obliteration
  o Transfacial surgical approaches
    — Reserved for deeper posterior ethmoid or sphenoid mucocele
  o Transcranial surgical approach
    — Reserved for mucoceles with intracranial extension or causing compression of bone structures with optic pathway neurologic symptoms

DIAGNOSTIC CHECKLIST

Consider

- Extensive peripheral enhancement may suggest **mucopyocele**
- If central enhancement present, consider neoplasm

Image Interpretation Pearls

- Look for thin peripheral rim of expanded bone
- No central enhancement on postcontrast CT or MR

SELECTED REFERENCES

1. Adewole V et al: Diffusion-weighted MRI over standard MRI for differential diagnosis between mucopyocele and mucoceles. Laryngoscope. 135(3):1003-14, 2025
2. Magboul NA et al: Mucocele of the paranasal sinuses: retrospective analysis of a series of eight cases. Cureus. 15(7):e41986, 2023
3. Malik M et al: Ophthalmic presentation and outcome for sinonasal mucoceles. Ophthalmic Plast Reconstr Surg. 39(1):44-8, 2022
4. Plantier DB et al: Mucocele: clinical characteristics and outcomes in 46 operated patients. Int Arch Otorhinolaryngol. 23(1):88-91, 2019
5. Al-Qudah M: Image-guided sinus surgery in sinonasal pathologies with skull base/orbital erosion. J Craniofac Surg. 26(5):1606-8, 2015
6. Lee JT et al: Intracranial mucocele formation in the context of longstanding chronic rhinosinusitis: a clinicopathologic series and literature review. Allergy Rhinol (Providence). 4(3):e166-75, 2013
7. Scangas GA et al: The natural history and clinical characteristics of paranasal sinus mucoceles: a clinical review. Int Forum Allergy Rhinol. 3(9):712-7, 2013
8. Devars du Mayne M et al: Sinus mucocele: natural history and long-term recurrence rate. Eur Ann Otorhinolaryngol Head Neck Dis. 129(3):125-30, 2012
9. Soon SR et al: Sphenoid sinus mucocele: 10 cases and literature review. J Laryngol Otol. 124(1):44-7, 2010
10. Lee TJ et al: Extensive paranasal sinus mucoceles: a 15-year review of 82 cases. Am J Otolaryngol. 30(4):234-8, 2009
11. Sadiq SA et al: Ophthalmic manifestations of paranasal sinus mucocoeles. Int Ophthalmol. 29(2):75-9, 2009
12. Eggesbø HB: Radiological imaging of inflammatory lesions in the nasal cavity and paranasal sinuses. Eur Radiol. 16(4):872-88, 2006
13. Kosling S et al: Mucoceles of the sphenoid sinus. Eur J Radiol. 51(1):1-5, 2004
14. Landsberg R et al: Magnetic resonance imaging–aided navigation in endoscopic sinus surgery of a bone-destructive sphenoclinoid mucocele. Ann Otol Rhinol Laryngol. 112(8):740-4, 2003
15. Lloyd G et al: Optimum imaging for mucoceles. J Laryngol Otol. 114(3): 233-6, 2000
16. Rombaux P et al: Endoscopic endonasal surgery for paranasal sinus mucoceles. Acta Otorhinolaryngol Belg. 54(2): 115-22, 2000
17. Busaba NY et al: Maxillary sinus mucoceles: clinical presentation and long-term results of endoscopic surgical treatment. Laryngoscope. 109(9): 1446-9, 1999

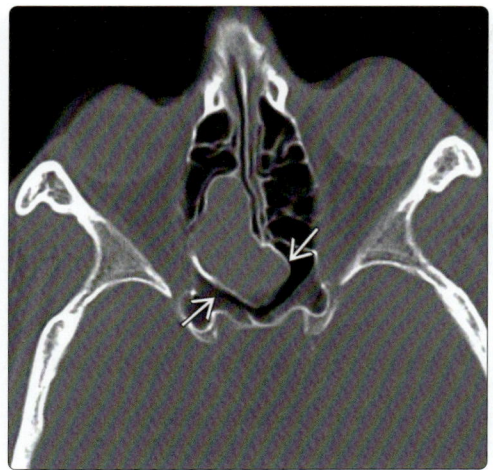
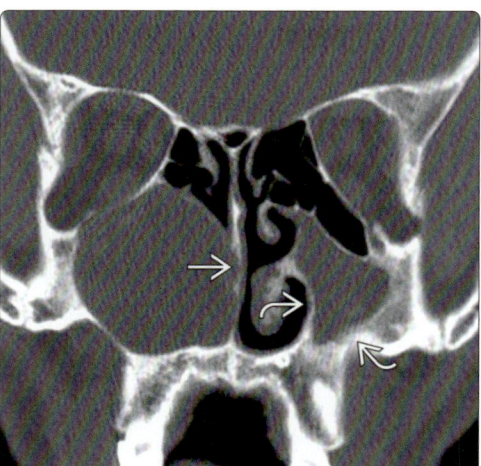

(Left) Axial bone CT demonstrates a posterior ethmoid mucocele that extends into the sphenoid sinuses ➡ rather than into the orbit. The bone surrounding the lesion is thinned and remodeled. (Right) Coronal bone CT shows a large mucocele arising within the right maxillary sinus, an unusual location for a mucocele. The lesion occludes the nasal airway ➡. Note the changes of chronic sinusitis of the left maxillary sinus with decreased volume and thickening of the walls ➡.

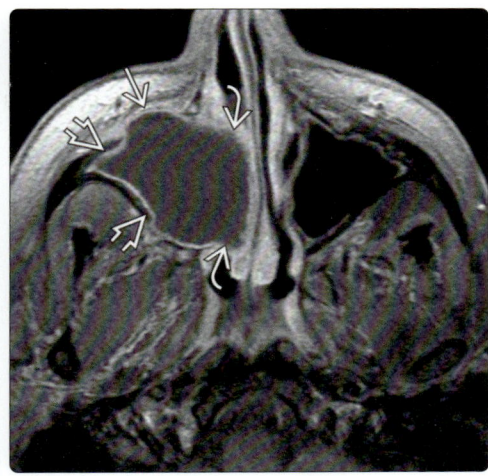
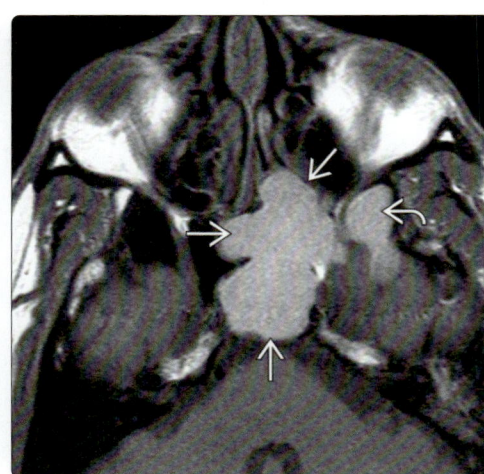

(Left) Axial T1 C+ FS MR shows a mucocele of the right maxillary sinus with erosion of the anterior wall ➡ and extension medially ➡ into the nasal cavity. There is peripheral mucosal enhancement ➡ but no central enhancement. This helps distinguish a mucocele from a neoplasm. (Right) Axial T1 MR demonstrates a large mucocele ➡ of the left sphenoid sinus. The lesion is homogeneously hyperintense, consistent with proteinaceous contents. Note the involvement of the lateral recess ➡.

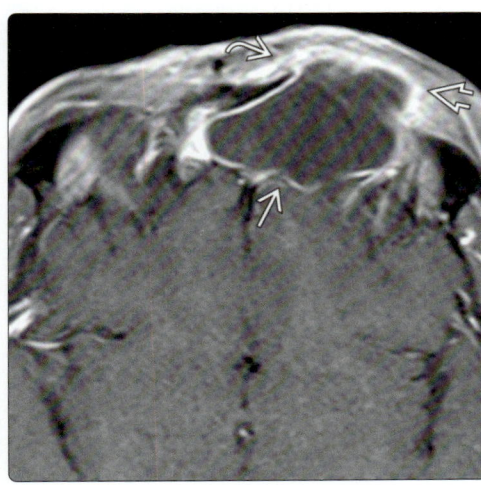
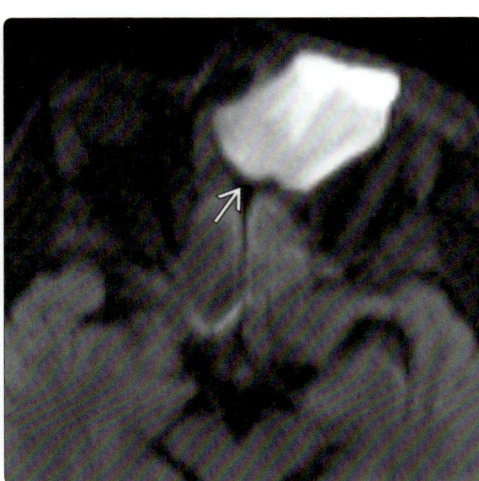

(Left) Axial T1 C+ FS MR shows expansion of the left frontal sinus with low central T1 signal and peripheral enhancement ➡. Note extension through the anterior table ➡ with inflammation in the frontal scalp soft tissues ➡, suggesting mucopyocele. (Right) Axial DWI MR in the same patient demonstrates high central diffusion signal ➡ in this case of left frontal sinus mucopyocele. Internal diffusion restriction (corresponding low ADC map value not shown) helps to differentiate mucopyocele from mucocele.

Sinonasal Organized Hematoma

TERMINOLOGY

- Sinonasal organized hematoma (SOH)
- **Rare**, nonneoplastic, expansile process from recurring hemorrhage within obstructed paranasal sinus; provokes proliferative fibrotic response with neovascularization
- Synonyms: Hematoma, hematocele, hemorrhagic pseudotumor, angiomatous polyp

IMAGING

- Maxillary sinus location accounts for majority of cases
  - Medial extension to nasal cavity and ethmoid sinus
- Bone CT
  - Expansile mass in unilateral maxillary sinus
  - Nasal cavity with smooth scalloping and erosion
- MR
  - Mixed T1 and T2 signal
  - Signal compatible with subacute and chronic hemorrhage

- Heterogeneous areas of irregular or nodular **enhancement** seen on both CT and MR can **mimic neoplasm**

TOP DIFFERENTIAL DIAGNOSES

- Solitary sinonasal polyp, mucocele
- Inverted papilloma, maxillary sinus carcinoma

CLINICAL ISSUES

- Middle-aged patient presents with epistaxis and nasal obstruction

DIAGNOSTIC CHECKLIST

- Subacute and chronic hemorrhage can result in mixed hyperdensity on CT and mixed signal on T2 MR
- Consider SOH when heterogeneous central enhancement occurs in what otherwise appears to represent benign mucocele or polyp
- Consider SOH as **rare** alternative to sinonasal neoplasm in radiologic differential

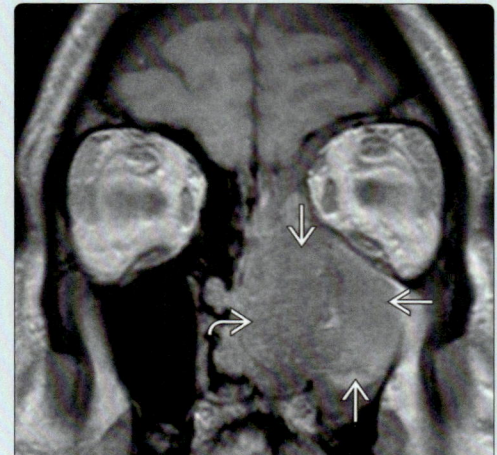
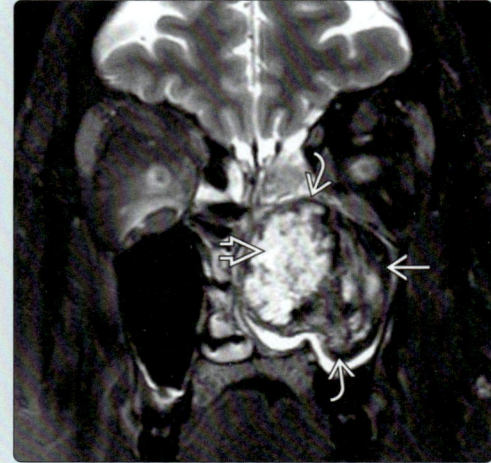

(Left) Coronal T1 MR in a patient presenting with recurrent epistaxis and nasal obstruction demonstrates mixed iso- to hyperintensity ➡ in the left maxillary sinus protruding into the left nasal cavity ➡. (Right) Coronal T2 FS MR in the same patient shows heterogeneous, expansile contents in the left maxillary sinus, predominantly low signal in its lateral aspect ➡ and high signal in its medial aspect ➡. Note a hypointense capsule around the mass ➡.

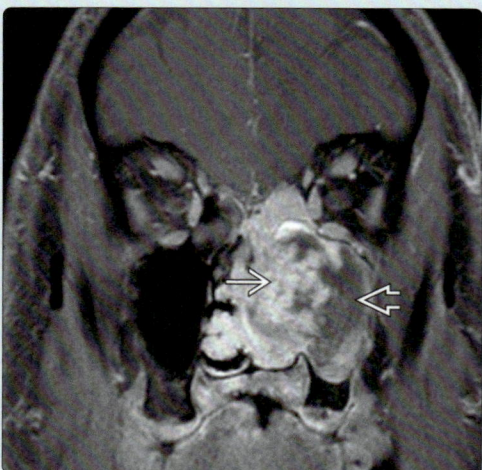
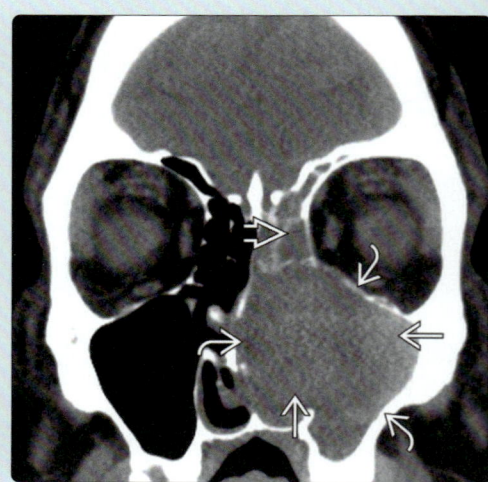

(Left) Coronal T1 C+ FS MR in the same patient show heterogeneous nodular enhancement medially ➡ and nonenhancing components laterally ➡. (Right) Coronal reformat of a preoperative NECT soft tissue window shows iso- to hyperdense soft tissue ➡ opacifying the left maxillary sinus with bony remodeling ➡. Note postobstructive opacification of left anterior ethmoid air cells ➡. Pathologic analysis revealed pockets of chronic hematoma with granulation tissue and fibrosis.

Sinonasal Organized Hematoma

TERMINOLOGY

Abbreviations
- Sinonasal organized hematoma (SOH)

Synonyms
- Hematoma, hematocele, hemorrhagic pseudotumor, angiomatous polyp

Definitions
- **Rare**, nonneoplastic, expansile process by which recurring hemorrhage within obstructed paranasal sinus provokes proliferative fibrotic response with neovascularization

IMAGING

General Features
- Best diagnostic clue
  o Solitary enhancing, expansile mass in maxillary sinus demonstrates smooth expansion and erosion of bony walls in patient with epistaxis and nasal obstruction
- Location
  o Maxillary sinus location accounts for nearly all cases, with medial extension to nasal cavity and ethmoid sinus
  o Isolated reports of nasal cavity, ethmoid, frontal, and sphenoid sinus origins
- Size
  o Usually large (4-5 cm)

CT Findings
- NECT
  o Isodense to hyperdense soft tissue opacification of maxillary sinus
  o Bony margins: Smooth scalloping and erosion indicative of underlying expansile process or mass
  o Bone erosion of medial wall of maxillary sinus and uncinate process common
- CECT
  o Heterogeneous areas of irregular and nodular enhancement

MR Findings
- T1WI
  o Soft tissue is predominantly isointense to normal mucosa with scattered areas of T1 hyperintensity
  o May be mostly **hyperintense** if recent hemorrhage
- T2WI
  o Heterogeneous signal, including areas of **marked hypointensity** and **hyperintensity**
  o T2-hypointense rim may be present
- T2* GRE
  o Areas of hemorrhage demonstrate hypointensity due to susceptibility artifact
- T1WI C+
  o Areas of moderate to marked irregular or nodular enhancement

Imaging Recommendations
- Best imaging tool
  o Unenhanced sinus CT in combination with focused enhanced MR of skull base and sinuses
    – CT best demonstrates bony changes related to underlying expanding mass
    – MR best differentiates enhancing portions of lesion and distinguishes SOH from adjacent obstructed secretions

DIFFERENTIAL DIAGNOSIS

Solitary Sinonasal Polyp
- Polypoid or dumbbell-shaped cystic mass extends from maxillary antrum to nasal cavity through enlarged ostium

Mucocele
- Opacified, expanded sinus with smooth remodeling of walls and no central enhancement

Inverted Papilloma
- Most commonly occurs along lateral nasal cavity wall, involves middle turbinate and maxillary ostium, and can extend to maxillary antrum with smooth bony remodeling

Maxillary Sinus Carcinoma
- Malignant epithelial tumor occurs most often in maxillary antrum with aggressive bone destruction

PATHOLOGY

General Features
- Lobulated mass with mixed areas of organized subacute and chronic hemorrhage, fibrin clots, fibrosis, inflammation, and neovascularization

CLINICAL ISSUES

Presentation
- Middle-aged patient presents with epistaxis and nasal obstruction

Demographics
- M > F (2:1)

Treatment
- Complete excision of lesion is curative

DIAGNOSTIC CHECKLIST

Consider
- Consider SOH when heterogeneous central enhancement occurs in what otherwise appears to represent benign mucocele or polyp
- Consider SOH as **rare** alternative to sinonasal neoplasm in radiologic differential

SELECTED REFERENCES

1. Jiao A et al: Sinonasal organized hematoma. Radiographics. 45(1):e240215, 2025
2. Park MJ et al: Sinonasal organizing hematoma: demographics, diagnosis, and treatment outcomes of 112 patients. Laryngoscope. 134(4):1581-90, 2024
3. Sharma R et al: Sinonasal organized hematoma: a preoperative & intraoperative diagnostic evaluation of two cases. Indian J Otolaryngol Head Neck Surg. 76(6):5972-7, 2024
4. Barros EF et al: A destructive sinonasal organizing hematoma mimicking malignancy. Oral Oncol. 147:106619, 2023
5. Goyal A et al: Sinonasal organized hematoma: case report and review of the literature. Radiol Case Rep. 18(12):4569-73, 2023
6. Min HJ et al: Sinonasal organized hematoma mimicking nasal polyposis. Ear Nose Throat J. 100(8):NP381-3, 2020

Silent Sinus Syndrome

TERMINOLOGY

- Acquired asymptomatic process by which walls of maxillary sinus retract, causing reduced volume of sinus, depression of ipsilateral orbital floor, enophthalmos, and hypoglobus

IMAGING

- Diminished volume of maxillary antrum with retraction (concavity) of all walls
- Increase in ipsilateral orbital volume with inferior position ("depression") of orbital floor
- Lateralized uncinate and expanded middle meatus
- Opacification of affected sinus

TOP DIFFERENTIAL DIAGNOSES

- Maxillary sinus hypoplasia
- Posttraumatic or postsurgical change

PATHOLOGY

- Occult chronic obstruction of maxillary ostium → negative pressure within sinus → stagnant mucus fills sinus → osteolysis thins/remodels bony walls → retraction of sinus walls, including orbital floor

CLINICAL ISSUES

- Process is typically painless, usually asymptomatic ("silent")
- Adult with **unilateral** enophthalmos or hypoglobus in absence of trauma
- Diplopia is most common visual symptom

DIAGNOSTIC CHECKLIST

- Evaluate extent of pneumatization into malar eminence and superior alveolus to differentiate silent sinus syndrome (SSS) from hypoplasia
  - SSS: Antrum fully pneumatized
  - Sinus hypoplasia: Not fully pneumatized

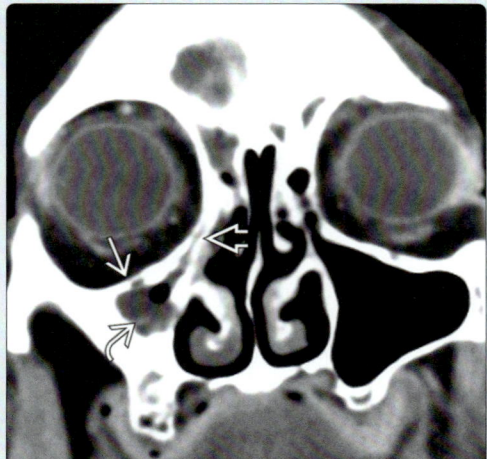
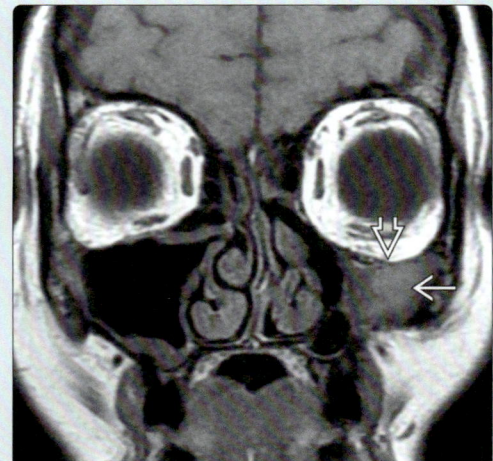

(Left) Coronal MPR of a maxillofacial CECT demonstrates atelectasis of the right maxillary sinus with mucosal thickening ⟍. Note a lateralized uncinate process obstructing the maxillary infundibulum ⟶ and downward bowing of the floor of the right orbit ⟶ with enophthalmos (not shown). (Right) Coronal noncontrast T1 MR of the paranasal sinus shows hypoplastic left maxillary sinus with internal hyperintense proteinaceous contents ⟶ and ↑ volume of the left orbit with downward bowing of the floor ⟹.

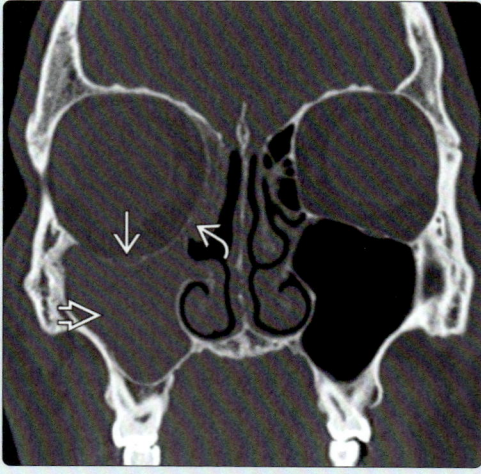
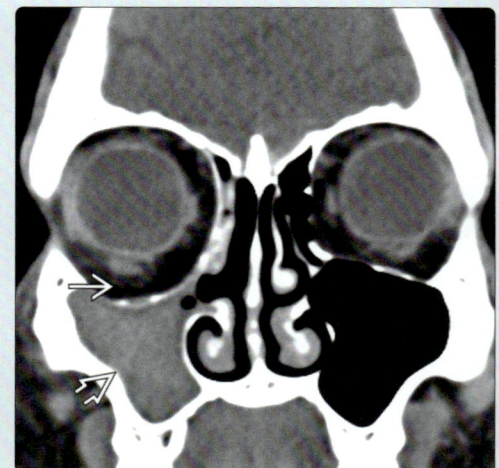

(Left) Coronal MPR of a preoperative high-resolution bone window NECT shows complete opacification of the right maxillary sinus ⟹ with bony remodeling and downward bowing of the right orbital floor ⟶, suggesting silent sinus syndrome. Note a lateralized uncinate process and obstruction of the infundibulum ⟹. (Right) Coronal MPR soft tissue window NECT in same patient shows ↓ maxillary volume ⟹ and ↑ orbital volume ⟹.

Silent Sinus Syndrome

TERMINOLOGY

Abbreviations

- Silent sinus syndrome (SSS)

Definitions

- Painless, asymptomatic retraction of maxillary sinus walls, causing ↓ volume of involved maxillary sinus, depression of ipsilateral orbital floor, ipsilateral enophthalmus, and hypoglobus

IMAGING

General Features

- Best diagnostic clue
  - Retraction of maxillary sinus walls with diminished sinus volume
- Location
  - Maxillary sinus, typically unilateral
- Size
  - Diminished volume of maxillary antrum
- Morphology
  - Inward bowing of all or most antral walls

CT Findings

- Bone CT
  - Diminished volume of maxillary antrum with retraction (concavity) of all walls
    - Compensatory increase in ipsilateral orbital volume with inferior position of orbital floor
  - Near to complete opacification of affected sinus
  - Lateralized uncinate and expanded middle meatus with variable retraction of middle turbinate and nasal septal deviation
  - Demineralization of sinus walls

MR Findings

- T1WI
  - Opacified sinus with mixed-signal contents and diminished volume
  - Prominence of inferior extraconal orbital fat
- T2WI
  - Mixed-signal central secretions with ↑ signal peripheral mucosa
  - Enophthalmos measured in axial plane typically measures 2-6 mm

Imaging Recommendations

- Best imaging tool
  - Axial bone CT with coronal reformats

DIFFERENTIAL DIAGNOSIS

Maxillary Sinus Hypoplasia

- Incomplete pneumatization into malar eminence and maxillary alveolar ridge
- Sinus may be aerated

Posttraumatic or Postsurgical Change

- Look for surgical changes or fractures
- Sinus may not have mucosal disease

PATHOLOGY

General Features

- Etiology
  - Occult chronic obstruction of maxillary ostium → negative pressure within sinus → stagnant mucus fills sinus → osteolysis thins and remodels bony walls → retraction of sinus walls, including orbital floor
- Associated abnormalities
  - Ipsilateral enophthalmos

Gross Pathologic & Surgical Features

- Thin or absent orbital floor bone, mucoid material in maxillary sinus, edematous sinus mucosa

Microscopic Features

- Similar to chronic sinusitis with inflammatory debris, but cultures typically negative

CLINICAL ISSUES

Presentation

- Most common signs/symptoms
  - Eye asymmetry or "sagging," diplopia, enophthalmos
  - Symptoms of chronic rhinosinusitis (CRS) typically absent (i.e., "silent")
- Other signs/symptoms
  - Hypoglobus, malar depression, upper lid retraction, vague dental or facial pain
  - Widened middle meatus with retracted uncinate process on nasal endoscopy
- Clinical profile
  - Adult with painless enophthalmos or facial asymmetry ± diplopia with no history of prior trauma

Demographics

- Age
  - Adults: 25-75 years

Treatment

- Functional endoscopic sinus surgery and transconjunctival reconstruction of orbital floor

DIAGNOSTIC CHECKLIST

Image Interpretation Pearls

- Evaluate extent of pneumatization into malar eminence and superior alveolus to differentiate SSS from hypoplasia
  - SSS: Antrum fully pneumatized
  - Sinus hypoplasia: Not fully pneumatized

SELECTED REFERENCES

1. Chernov ES et al: Pediatric silent sinus syndrome: a case report and literature review. Ann Otol Rhinol Laryngol. 134(4):284-90, 2025
2. Amin D et al: A novel staging system to consolidate silent sinus syndrome and chronic maxillary atelectasis: a systematic review and case series. Int Forum Allergy Rhinol. 14(8):1378-81, 2024
3. Khatoon M et al: Silent sinus syndrome of the frontal sinus: a case report. Cureus. 16(12):e75516, 2024
4. Tousidonis M et al: Contemporary treatment of silent sinus syndrome: a case report and literature review. Cureus. 16(4):e57577, 2024
5. Salari S et al: Silent sinus syndrome: a case report. Clin Case Rep. 11(11):e8095, 2023
6. Albadr FB: Silent sinus syndrome: interesting computed tomography and magnetic resonance imaging findings. J Clin Imaging Sci. 10:38, 2020

Granulomatosis With Polyangiitis (Wegener)

TERMINOLOGY

- Idiopathic, autoimmune **necrotizing granulomatous vasculitis** that preferentially involves upper and lower respiratory tracts, kidneys, skin, and joints

IMAGING

- Nodular soft tissue in nose with **septal and nonseptal cartilaginous and bone destruction**
  - **Orbital invasion** most common extrasinonasal H&N site
  - When severe, dura may be involved
- Multiplanar bone CT is best tool for initial evaluation
- Add enhanced MR; best if orbital or intracranial involvement suspected

TOP DIFFERENTIAL DIAGNOSES

- Sinonasal sarcoidosis
- Nasal cocaine necrosis
- Chronic rhinosinusitis
- Invasive fungal sinusitis

- Sinonasal non-Hodgkin lymphoma

CLINICAL ISSUES

- H&N involvement in 72-100% of granulomatosis with polyangiitis (GPA) patients
  - Rhinologic symptoms in > 80%
- Symptoms mimic chronic rhinosinusitis
  - Diagnosis often delayed because symptoms mistaken for chronic rhinosinusitis
- Typically 40-60 years
  - Males more commonly affected than females
- Generally indolent disease
  - May transition to fulminating disease

DIAGNOSTIC CHECKLIST

- Consult with clinician for history of other organ system involvement (GPA vs. sarcoidosis) or cocaine abuse
- Can be impossible to differentiate from sinonasal sarcoidosis or lymphoma on imaging

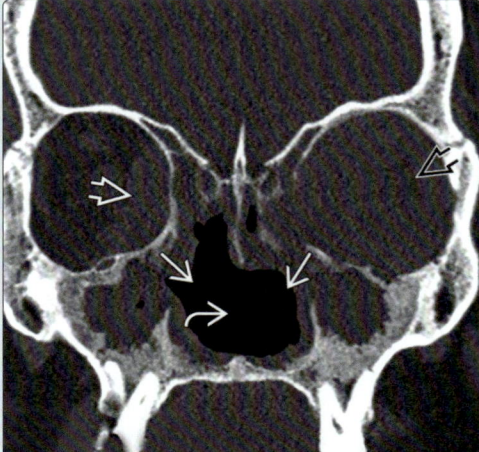
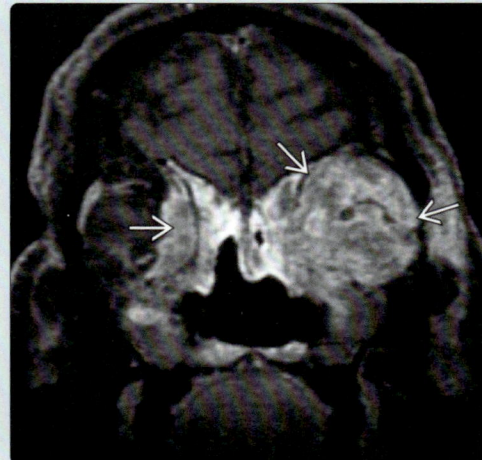

(Left) Coronal bone CT in severe granulomatosis with polyangiitis (GPA) shows extensive soft tissue thickening in the maxillary & ethmoid sinuses & nasal cavity. There is destruction of the nasal septum ➡ & bilateral inferior & middle turbinates ➡, diffuse soft tissue infiltration of left orbit ➡, & milder disease of the right orbit ➡. (Right) Coronal T1 C+ FS MR in the same patient shows marked enhancement of soft tissue in the orbits ➡, L > R, contiguous with mucosal thickening in the nasal cavity & paranasal sinuses.

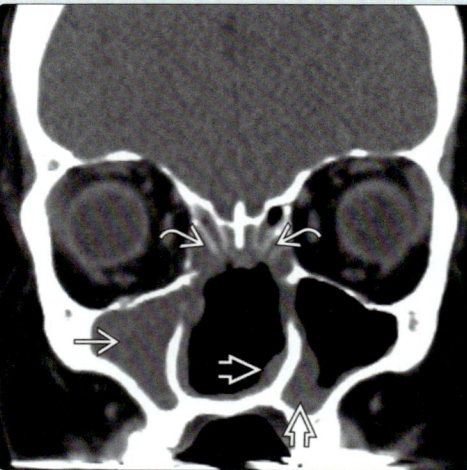
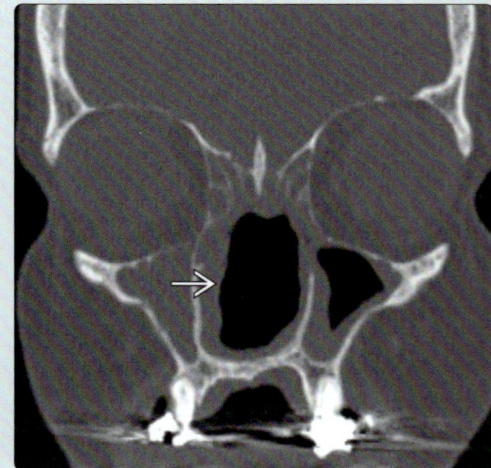

(Left) Coronal MPR of NECT soft tissue window image in the same patient shows opacification of right maxillary sinus ➡, bilateral ethmoids ➡, & mild soft tissue thickening in the left maxillary sinus & the nasal cavity ➡. (Right) Coronal MPR NECT bone window image in a patient with proteinase 3-anti-neutrophil cytoplasmic antibody (ANCA)-positive GPA shows complete destruction of nasal septum ➡ & bilateral middle & inferior turbinates. GPA typically presents between ages 40 & 60 with slight male predominance.

Granulomatosis With Polyangiitis (Wegener)

TERMINOLOGY

Abbreviations
- Anti-neutrophil cytoplasmic antibody (ANCA)
- ANCA-associated vasculitis (AAV)
- Granulomatosis with polyangiitis (GPA)

Synonyms
- Wegener granulomatosis

Definitions
- Idiopathic, autoimmune small vessel **necrotizing granulomatous vasculitis**
- Preferentially affects upper and lower respiratory tracts, kidneys, skin, and joints

IMAGING

General Features
- Best diagnostic clue
  - Severe chronic rhinosinusitis (mucosal thickening and hyperostosis) with additional features of soft tissue mass/nodularity and septal/nonseptal cartilaginous and osseous destruction
- Location
  - Nasal cavity (septum > turbinates) > sinuses (maxillary > ethmoid > frontal > sphenoid)
  - Other H&N sites
    - Orbital invasion most common extrasinonasal site
    - Nasopharynx, subglottic larynx, oral cavity, temporal bone, and salivary glands
    - Progressive bone erosion of anterior and central skull base can lead to intracranial extension and pachymeningitis
- Morphology
  - Ulcerative ± nodular disease

CT Findings
- NECT
  - Chronic rhinosinusitis with localized mucosal nodularity and masses centered in nasal cavity
  - Periantral soft tissue infiltration
  - Orbital extension often 1st extrasinonasal site of invasion
  - Less commonly involves skull base, pterygopalatine fossa, retromaxillary region, and nasopharynx
- CECT
  - Enhancing nodular and mass-like mucosal thickening
  - Enhancing soft tissue may extend into orbit
- Bone CT
  - Chronic obstruction and inflammation of adjacent sinuses may result in nonspecific hyperostosis of sinus walls
  - **Osseous/cartilaginous erosion** often affects nasal septum primarily, causing **perforation**
  - Destruction then involves turbinates and lateral nasal wall (uncinate process and medial wall maxillary sinus)
  - May affect hard palate, leading to sinonasal-oral fistula

MR Findings
- T1WI
  - Low- to intermediate-signal nodular masses
- T2WI
  - ↓ signal nodular masses (compared to inflamed mucosa with ↑ T2 signal)
  - ↑ signal edema of soft tissues during acute exacerbations with extension into adjacent soft tissues
- T1WI C+
  - Nodular and mass-like enhancing tissue along mucosa
  - **Orbital involvement** presents with enhancing infiltrating mass within orbit, often with contiguous sinonasal disease
  - **Meningeal thickening** with enhancement < 5% (late finding in those with skull base invasion)
    - Pachymeningitis typically seen in anterior or central skull base as part of contiguous sinonasal extension, but can be seen independently

Imaging Recommendations
- Best imaging tool
  - Bone-only coronal sinus CT is best tool for initial evaluation
    - Axial MDCT with reformats also very helpful for identifying bone erosion
- Protocol advice
  - If orbital, deep facial, skull base, or meningeal involvement suspected from CT or clinical symptoms, then use enhanced, fat-saturated MR

DIFFERENTIAL DIAGNOSIS

Sinonasal Sarcoidosis
- Systemic granulomatous disease
  - Sinonasal involvement less common than GPA
- May be indistinguishable from GPA on imaging

Nasal Cocaine Necrosis
- Septal perforation with nasal inflammatory changes
- May be less nodular than GPA

Chronic Rhinosinusitis
- Symptoms of GPA mimic chronic sinusitis
- Bone thickening and sclerosis, **not** destruction
- No systemic disease

Invasive Fungal Sinusitis
- Rapidly progressive sinonasal destructive process in immunocompromised patient
- Sinus > nasal cavity is site of origin; destroys any adjacent bone

Sinonasal Non-Hodgkin Lymphoma
- Midline soft tissue mass with septal and nonseptal bone destruction or remodeling
  - NK/T-cell type lymphoma (a.k.a. lethal midline granuloma)
- May exactly mimic GPA on imaging

PATHOLOGY

General Features
- Etiology
  - AAV is necrotizing vasculitis affecting small vessels and is associated with either myeloperoxidase-ANCA or proteinase 3-ANCA

– 3 types of AAV: GPA, eosinophilic GPA, and microscopic polyangiitis
- Associated abnormalities
  - Secondary sinus bacterial infections common (e.g., *Staphylococcus aureus*)
  - Other organ system involvement
    – **Lungs (95%), kidneys (85%)**, joints (65%)
    – Intracranial abnormalities include **pachymeningitis** and brain infarcts

Gross Pathologic & Surgical Features

- Initial appearance: Diffuse mucosal ulcerations with crusting
- Advanced disease: Cartilaginous and osseous septal destruction leads eventually to saddle nose deformity

Microscopic Features

- Noncaseating, necrotizing, multinucleated, and giant cell granulomas
- Acute ± chronic inflammatory cell infiltrate
- Fibrinoid necrosis of small- to medium-sized vessels

CLINICAL ISSUES

Presentation

- Most common signs/symptoms
  - Nasal obstruction and epistaxis
- Other signs/symptoms
  - Pain, anosmia, purulent rhinorrhea
  - Septal ulcerations and perforation can lead to saddle nose deformity
  - Hoarseness (larynx), stridor (trachea), hearing loss, and ear pain (temporal bone)
  - Constitutional symptoms: Fatigue, night sweats, weight loss
- Clinical profile
  - Classic clinical triad
    – Necrotizing granulomas of upper and lower respiratory tracts
    – Necrotizing vasculitis of both arteries and veins
    – Glomerulonephritis
  - Diagnosis made by biopsy of affected area (nose, sinus, lung, kidney)
    – Multiple biopsies may be inconclusive
      □ Nasal biopsies positive in ~ 40%
  - Laboratory findings
    – ↑ **c-ANCA** (85-98% specificity for GPA)
      □ c-ANCA titers followed for disease response to therapy
    – ↑ ESR
    – ↑ serum creatinine signals presence of renal GPA

Demographics

- Age
  - Typically 40-60 years
- Sex
  - M > F [except laryngeal form (M < F)]
    – May be slightly more prevalent in women when presenting at younger age
- Epidemiology
  - Rare disease
  - H&N involvement in 72-100%

○ Rhinologic symptoms in > 80%

Natural History & Prognosis

- 3-year lag in diagnosis common because initially mistaken for chronic sinusitis
  - Better prognosis if diagnosed at younger age
- Generally indolent disease
  - "Limited disease," localized to nose or orbit
    – Treated appropriately, associated with good to excellent prognosis
  - May transition to fulminating fatal disease
    – Fulminant sinonasal disease may result in complete nasal destruction (autorhinectomy)
    – Untreated, aggressive disease can be fatal secondary to renal failure or sepsis (major cause of morbidity and mortality)
- Long-term remissions have been achieved
  - Length of remission difficult to predict
  - Spontaneous remissions have been reported

Treatment

- Medical treatments include immunosuppressive agents, cyclophosphamide, and other cytotoxic drugs
  - Fulminant disease treated with high-dose prednisone followed by cyclophosphamide
- Surgery reserved for selected H&N manifestations, such as saddle nose deformity and subglottic stenosis
  - Surgical manipulation may exacerbate neoosteogenesis in sinonasal cavities

DIAGNOSTIC CHECKLIST

Consider

- GPA should be considered when **destructive process** centered **in nasal cavity**, particularly when septal perforation is present
- Consult with clinician for history of other organ system involvement (GPA vs. sarcoidosis) or cocaine abuse

Image Interpretation Pearls

- Can be impossible to differentiate from nongranulomatous rhinosinusitis, sinonasal malignancy, or sarcoid

SELECTED REFERENCES

1. Ryoo I et al: Comparison of imaging findings between granulomatosis with polyangiitis and eosinophilic granulomatosis with polyangiitis on sinus CT: importance of high-density opacification of the paranasal sinuses. AJNR Am J Neuroradiol. 46(2):355-61, 2025
2. Falde SD et al: Proteinase 3-specific antineutrophil cytoplasmic antibody-associated vasculitis. Lancet Rheumatol. 6(5):e314-27, 2024
3. Holle JU et al: [Update on treatment of ANCA-associated vasculitis.] Z Rheumatol. 83(10):787-99, 2024
4. Sharma P et al: ANCA-associated vasculitis. Adv Kidney Dis Health. 31(3):194-205, 2024
5. Tateyama K et al: Sinonasal manifestations of granulomatosis with polyangiitis: a retrospective analysis. Auris Nasus Larynx. 51(4):625-30, 2024
6. Zhu Y et al: Granulomatosis with polyangiitis. IDCases. 36:e01970, 2024
7. Junek ML et al: Ocular manifestations of ANCA-associated vasculitis. Rheumatology (Oxford). 62(7):2517-24, 2023
8. Garlapati P et al: Granulomatosis with polyangiitis. StatPearls, 2022
9. Coates ML et al: Updates in antineutrophil cytoplasmic antibody (ANCA) associated vasculitis for the ENT surgeon. Clin Otolaryngol. 45(3):316-26, 2020
10. Puéchal X: Granulomatosis with polyangiitis (Wegener's). Joint Bone Spine. 87(6):572-8, 2020

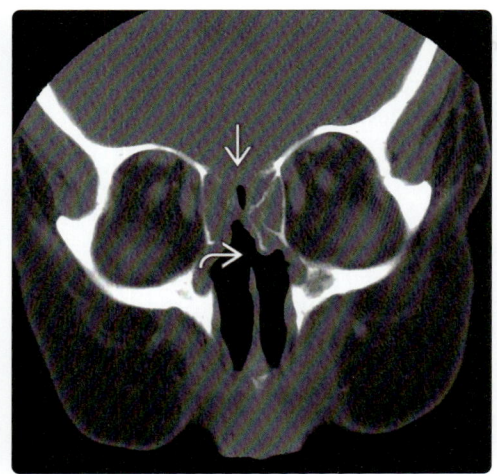

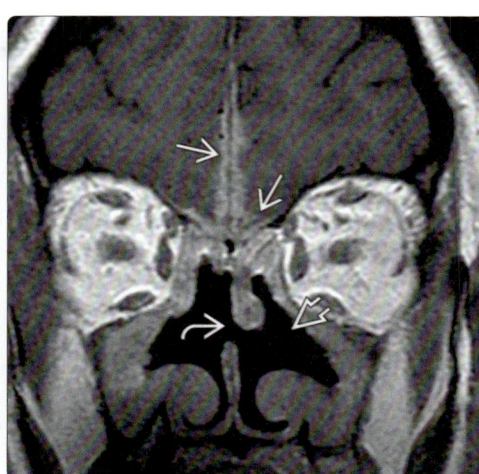

(Left) Coronal MPR NECT bone window image in a GPA patient with chronic rhinosinusitis shows perforation of the septum ➜. Note confluent opacification of the ethmoid sinuses bilaterally, associated with destruction of the cribriform plate ➜. (Right) Coronal MR in the same patient shows diffuse mucosal thickening in maxillary & ethmoid sinuses, perforation of the septum ➜, & bilateral destruction of the turbinates & lateral nasal cavity walls ➜. Note the contiguous pachymeningitis in the anterior cranial fossa ➜.

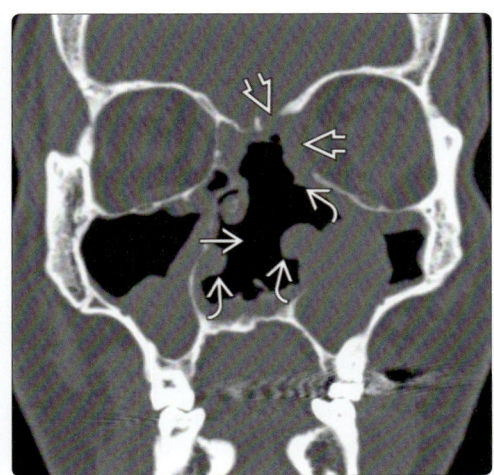

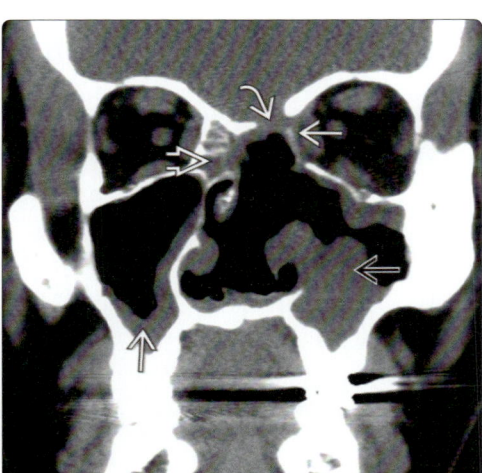

(Left) Coronal MPR of NECT bone window image in a patient with GPA with headache shows destruction of nasal septum ➜ & left middle & bilateral inferior turbinates ➜. Note erosions along the cribriform plate & lamina papyracea on left side ➜. (Right) Coronal MPR NECT soft tissue window image in the same patient shows soft tissue in the bilateral maxillary sinuses (L > R) ➜, right ethmoid ➜, & at the roof of left ethmoid ➜. Note thin sleeve of soft tissue thickening along the medial extraconal compartment of left orbit ➜.

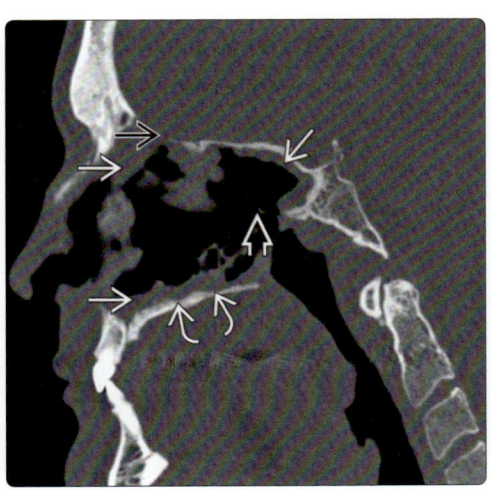

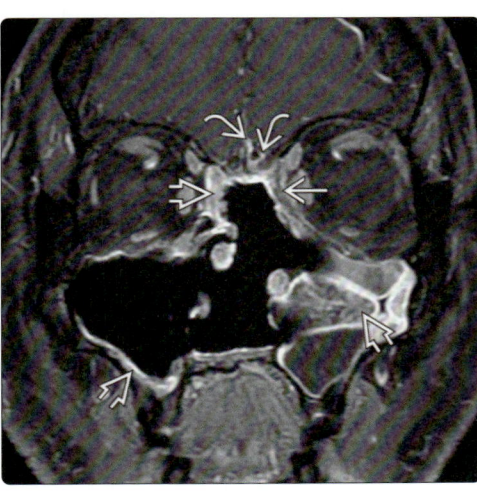

(Left) Sagittal MPR of high-resolution NECT bone window image shows erosive changes along the cribriform plate ➜, hard palate ➜, & bony destruction along the floor of sphenoid sinus ➜. Note associated soft tissue thickening in sinonasal region ➜. (Right) Coronal T1 C+ FS MR in the same patient shows heterogeneously enhancing soft tissue in maxillary (L > R) & ethmoid region ➜. Note dural thickening & enhancement ➜ as well as minimal soft tissue in the medial left orbit ➜.

Nasal Cocaine Necrosis

TERMINOLOGY

- Destruction of osteocartilaginous structures of nose, sinuses, and palate induced by chronic inhalation of cocaine

IMAGING

- Perforation of osteocartilaginous nasal septum ± turbinates/palate **without** soft tissue mass
  - 75% occur in quadrangular cartilage; 25% involve vomer-perpendicular ethmoidal lamina
- Thin-section CT with multiplanar reformat recommended to fully delineate extent of bone destruction

TOP DIFFERENTIAL DIAGNOSES

- Traumatic nasal septal perforation
- Granulomatosis with polyangiitis
- Sinonasal sarcoidosis
- Sinonasal non-Hodgkin lymphoma
- Other drug-related septal perforation

PATHOLOGY

- Nasal septal destruction results from combined effects of chemical irritation, ischemic necrosis from vasoconstriction, and direct trauma from autoinstrumentation
- Chemical agents (i.e., levamisole) added to cocaine to enhance its appearance, add weight, and produce additional psychoactive effects may contribute to necrosis

CLINICAL ISSUES

- Nasal obstruction and discharge are most common symptoms of acquired septal lesions
- ~ 1.75 million Americans ≥ 12 years old are regular (at least once per month) cocaine users
- Antineutrophilic cytoplasmic antibodies directed against human neutrophil elastase may discriminate cocaine-related necrosis from granulomatosis with polyangiitis

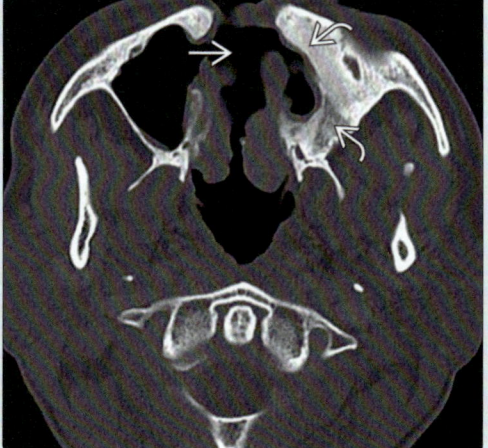
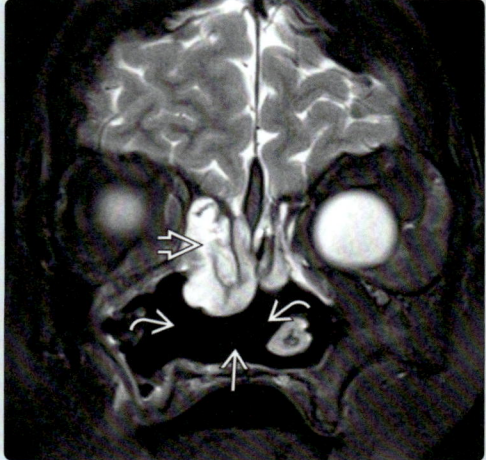

(Left) Axial NECT, high-resolution bone window image, in a 35-year-old man with history of longstanding nasal cocaine abuse shows complete destruction of the nasal septum ➡ with saddle nose deformity (not shown). Note reactive chronic osteitis changes in the left maxilla ➡. (Right) Coronal T2 MR shows osteocartilaginous nasal septal destruction ➡ along with destruction of middle and inferior turbinates and lateral nasal walls ➡. Polypoidal mucosal thickening in the right nasoethmoidal region ➡ is shown.

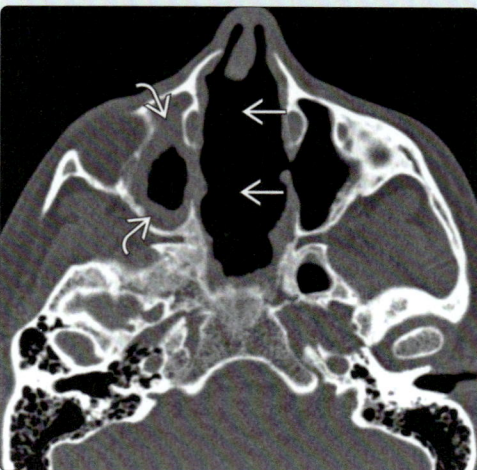
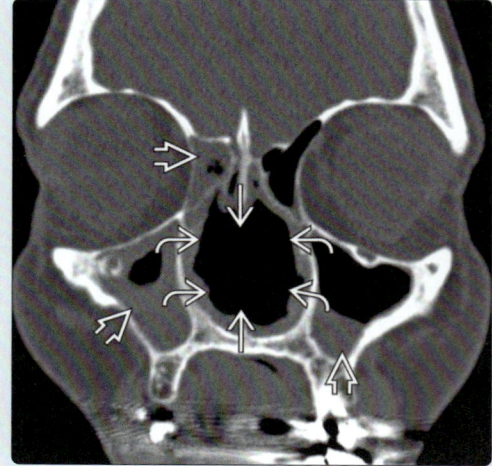

(Left) Axial NECT, high-resolution bone window image, reveals near-total nasal septal destruction ➡. Mild mucosal thickening in right maxillary sinus ➡ is shown. (Right) Coronal MPR NECT, high-resolution bone window image, reveals destruction of nasal septum ➡, middle and inferior turbinates ➡, and paranasal sinus mucosal thickening ➡. Levamisole added to cocaine to enhance its appearance, add weight, and produce additional psychoactive effects also contributes to nasal necrosis.

TERMINOLOGY

Abbreviations

- Nasal cocaine necrosis (NCN)

Synonyms

- Cocaine-induced midline destructive lesions

Definitions

- Destruction of osteocartilaginous structures of nose, sinuses, and palate induced by chronic inhalation of cocaine

IMAGING

General Features

- Best diagnostic clue
  - Perforation of osteocartilaginous nasal septum ± turbinates/palate **without** soft tissue mass
- Location
  - Nasal septal mucosa and cartilage

Imaging Recommendations

- Best imaging tool
  - Bone CT optimal for evaluating extent of bone destruction

CT Findings

- Bone CT
  - **Nasal septum erosion**
  - Erosion of portions of 1 or both inferior turbinates in > 50%
  - Bone destruction may extend to lateral nasal wall, palate, or orbit

DIFFERENTIAL DIAGNOSIS

Traumatic Nasal Septal Perforation

- Septal necrosis secondary to hematoma in cartilaginous septum leading to ischemia
- Rhinotillexomania (chronic nose picking) causes septal injury due to repetitive trauma/inflammation
  - Imaging findings include septal perforation, absence of anterior/inferior septum

Granulomatosis With Polyangiitis, Sinonasal

- Necrotizing granulomatous vasculitis
- Nodular soft tissue lesions
- Predilection for nasal septum and turbinates

Sarcoidosis, Sinonasal

- Systemic granulomatous disease [less frequent sinonasal involvement than granulomatosis with polyangiitis (GPA)]
- Predilection for nasal septal and inferior turbinate involvement

Non-Hodgkin Lymphoma, Sinonasal

- Predilection for nasal cavity site of origin with frequent destruction of septum
- Large soft tissue mass in nasal cavity

Fungal Sinusitis, Invasive

- Occurs in immunocompromised population
- Maxillary and sphenoid sinuses more common location of origin than nasal cavity

Other Drug-Related Septal Perforation

- Intranasal opioid/acetaminophen or corticosteroids, bevacizumab

PATHOLOGY

General Features

- Etiology
  - Nasal septal destruction results from combined effects of chemical irritation, ischemic necrosis from vasoconstriction, and direct trauma from autoinstrumentation
  - Perforation results with chronic (> 3 months) intranasal use

Staging, Grading, & Classification

- Diagnosis can be made by identifying cocaine metabolites in urine

Gross Pathologic & Surgical Features

- Atrophic, irritated mucosa with necrosis

Microscopic Features

- Ranges from fibrosis with mild inflammation and necrosis to dense inflammatory infiltrate with extensive necrosis

CLINICAL ISSUES

Presentation

- Most common signs/symptoms
  - Nasal obstruction and discharge are most common symptoms of acquired septal lesions

Demographics

- Age
  - Adolescent to adult age groups
- Sex
  - M > F
- Epidemiology
  - ~ 1.75 million Americans ≥ 12 years old are regular (at least once per month) cocaine users
  - Prevalence of cocaine-induced sinonasal complications ~ 5%

Natural History & Prognosis

- Continued intranasal cocaine use may result in disintegration of nasal cartilage and loss of structural integrity

DIAGNOSTIC CHECKLIST

Consider

- Clinical history of cocaine use is key to diagnosis

SELECTED REFERENCES

1. Iorio L et al: Cocaine- and levamisole-induced vasculitis: defining the spectrum of autoimmune manifestations. J Clin Med. 13(17):5116, 2024
2. Hansen FV et al: Damage to the nose and midface from cocaine abuse. Ugeskr Laeger. 185(40):V07230473, 2023
3. Ruffer N et al: [Cocaine-induced vasculitis and mimics of vasculitis.] Z Rheumatol. 82(7):606-14, 2023
4. Nitro L et al: Distribution of cocaine-induced midline destructive lesions: systematic review and classification. Eur Arch Otorhinolaryngol. 279(7):3257-67, 2022

TERMINOLOGY

- Fibroosseous lesion in which normal medullary bone is replaced by weak osseous & fibrous tissue

IMAGING

- Classic appearance: **Ground-glass** density on NECT
  - Density varies with amount of fibrous tissue
  - Variable enhancement of fibrous component
  - Variable presence of lucent/lytic foci
- MR signal & enhancement are highly variable
  - **Expansion of medullary space** is key feature of fibrous dysplasia (FD)
  - **Low T2 signal** characteristic but often not present
  - When T2 hyperintense & enhancing: Neoplasm mimic
- Best imaging tool: Thin-section **bone-algorithm NECT**

TOP DIFFERENTIAL DIAGNOSES

- Ossifying fibroma; osteoma; neoosteogenesis

PATHOLOGY

- Etiology: Defective gene in bone-forming cells in early fetal life: ↑ osteogenesis in bone marrow
- Can obstruct sinus → recurrent infection, mucocele formation
- 3 forms of FD: Monostotic, polyostotic, & McCune-Albright syndrome

CLINICAL ISSUES

- Headache, pain, sinonasal obstruction, & recurrent sinusitis
- Monostotic form most common, 25% in H&N
- Highest incidence: 3-15 years
  - Disease quiescent after cessation of skeletal growth

DIAGNOSTIC CHECKLIST

- MR appearance can be somewhat confusing: Fibrous component **enhances intensely**
  - **Mimics aggressive neoplasm** without comparison CT
  - **NECT critical** to establish correct diagnosis

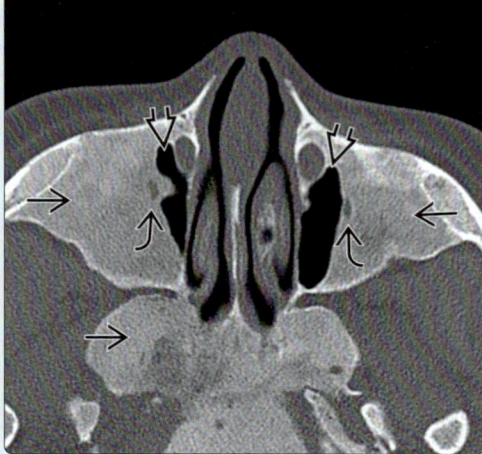
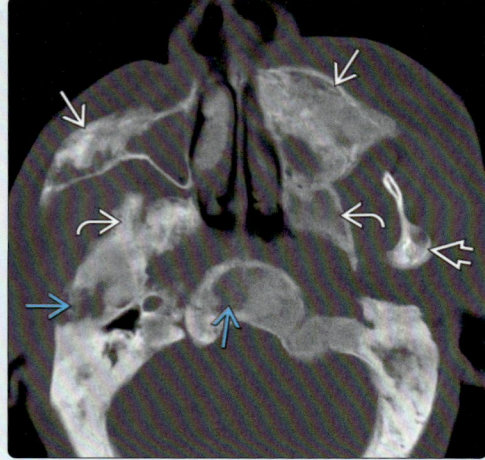

(Left) *Axial bone CT shows ground-glass expansion of the maxilla and skull base, consistent with polyostotic fibrous dysplasia ➡ in this case of McCune-Albright syndrome. Note decreased volume of the maxillary sinuses ➡ and medial displacement of the infraorbital canals ➡. (Right) Axial bone CT shows extensive polyostotic fibrous dysplasia of the maxilla ➡, sphenoid ➡, and left mandibular condyle ➡. Lytic changes ➡ may represent predominantly fibrous elements or cystic degeneration.*

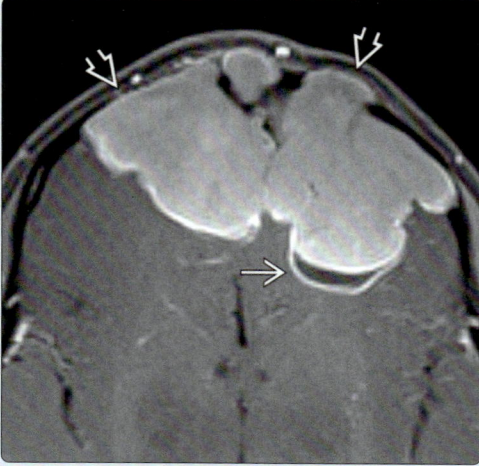
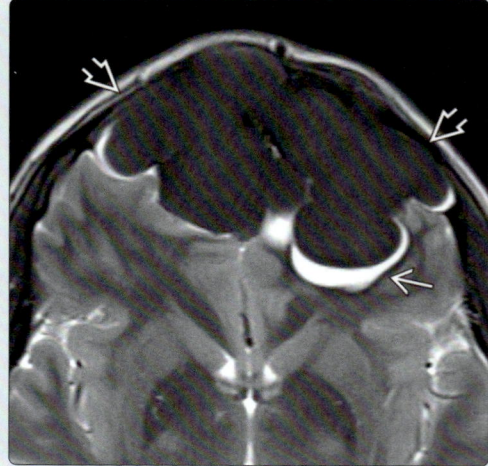

(Left) *Axial T1 C+ FS MR demonstrates an expansile, enhancing mass ➡ projecting from the frontal sinuses into the anterior cranial fossa, which can be mistaken for an aggressive neoplasm. The posterior rim-enhancing hypointensity ➡ corresponds to trapped secretions from the frontal sinuses. (Right) Axial T2 MR in the same patient shows diffuse low signal ➡, characteristic of fibrous dysplasia. Peripheral T2 hyperintensity corresponds to trapped secretions ➡ from the expanded frontal sinuses.*

TERMINOLOGY

Abbreviations
- Fibrous dysplasia (FD)

Synonyms
- Jaffe-Lichtenstein syndrome: FD with café-au-lait spots
- Cherubism: Hereditary form, polyostotic, bilateral
- Leontiasis ossea: Lion-like facial appearance

Definitions
- Normal medullary bone replaced by fibroosseous tissue with varying degree of osseous metaplasia

IMAGING

General Features
- Best diagnostic clue
  - Ill-defined, expansile, ground-glass diploic space
- Location
  - Maxilla > mandible > frontal > ethmoid & sphenoid
- Morphology
  - Generally ill defined, **expansile**, unilateral or asymmetric

CT Findings
- CECT
  - Variable enhancement of fibrous component
- Bone CT
  - **Ground-glass**, expansile lesion with rim of intact cortex
    - Density varies with amount of fibrous tissue

MR Findings
- T1WI
  - **Expanded medullary space with** intermediate to ↓ signal
  - Hypointense peripheral cortical bone
- T2WI
  - Variable: Hyperintense, intermediate, or hypointense
- T1WI C+
  - Homogeneous or heterogeneous
  - Fibrous component **may enhance intensely**
    - **Mimics aggressive neoplasm** without comparison CT

Nuclear Medicine Findings
- PET
  - Can be variably **hot** on FDG PET

Imaging Recommendations
- Best imaging tool
  - Thin-section bone-algorithm NECT

DIFFERENTIAL DIAGNOSIS

Sinonasal Ossifying Fibroma
- Solitary, well defined, expansile
- Mixed bone & soft tissue density

Sinonasal Osteoma
- Solitary, well defined; projects into sinus lumen
- Densely ossified

Neoosteogenesis
- Slightly thickened, sclerotic sinus walls

- Near site of surgery or chronic inflammation

Meningioma, Skull Base
- Hyperostosis may mimic FD, but enhancing intracranial dural tail distinguishes from FD

PATHOLOGY

General Features
- Genetics
  - Cherubism: Autosomal dominant, *SH3BP2* mutation > 80%
- Associated abnormalities
  - Can cause sinus obstruction → recurrent infection, mucocele formation, nasal airway obstruction

Microscopic Features
- Immature (woven), poorly organized osseous component arises metaplastically from fibrous stroma

CLINICAL ISSUES

Presentation
- Most common signs/symptoms
  - Painless facial deformity, nasal obstruction

Demographics
- Age
  - 75% < 30 years
- Sex
  - M < F in polyostotic form (1:3)
- Epidemiology
  - Monostotic (70-80%): H&N involved in 25%
  - Polyostotic (20-30%): Bones of H&N involved in ≥ 50%
  - McCune-Albright syndrome (3-10% of FD) with endocrine anomalies

Natural History & Prognosis
- Becomes quiescent with cessation of skeletal growth
- Progression after age 16 years is uncommon & minimal
- Malignant transformation (< 1%), often osteosarcoma
  - More common if patient is polyostotic or has McCune-Albright syndrome

Treatment
- Clinical & imaging follow-up if minimally symptomatic
- Surgical excision if functional compromise

DIAGNOSTIC CHECKLIST

Consider
- Consider FD if **expansile, enhancing intraosseous lesion on MR**, particularly if **T2 hypointense**, & perform NECT

Image Interpretation Pearls
- MR appearance (signal & enhancement pattern) highly variable & can mimic aggressive neoplasm
  - NECT critical to problem solve

SELECTED REFERENCES

1. Liu L et al: Malignant transformation of craniofacial fibrous dysplasia: a clinicopathological, immunohistochemical and molecular analysis of 15 cases in one single institution. J Stomatol Oral Maxillofac Surg. 126(3):102098, 2024

TERMINOLOGY

- Benign, well-defined, slow-growing, bone-forming tumor

IMAGING

- Well-marginated bone density lesion that arises from wall of paranasal sinus & protrudes into sinus lumen
- Location: Frontal & ethmoid > > > maxillary & sphenoid
- Larger osteomas may be associated with following findings
  - Sinus opacification or mucocele formation from ostial obstruction
  - Orbital mass effect from extraconal extension
  - Pneumocephalus or intraparenchymal tension pneumatocele
  - Brain abscess ± subdural empyema
- CT density depends on "ivory" vs. "mature" components

TOP DIFFERENTIAL DIAGNOSES

- Sinonasal fibrous dysplasia
- Sinonasal ossifying fibroma

- Sinonasal osteosarcoma

PATHOLOGY

- If multiple osteomas are discovered, consider Gardner syndrome
- Etiology not well established; theories include developmental, traumatic, & infectious causes
- Microscopic classifications in literature tend to distinguish between ivory, mature, & mixed types

CLINICAL ISSUES

- Most common benign tumor of paranasal sinuses
- Usually asymptomatic, incidental finding
  - Found in 1% of patients on radiographs & 3% on CT done for sinonasal symptoms
  - < 5% of all osteomas are symptomatic
- M:F ~ 1.5-2.6:1.0
- Symptomatic lesions typically treated surgically

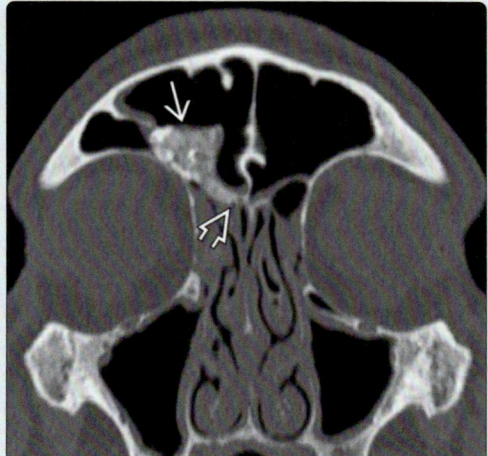
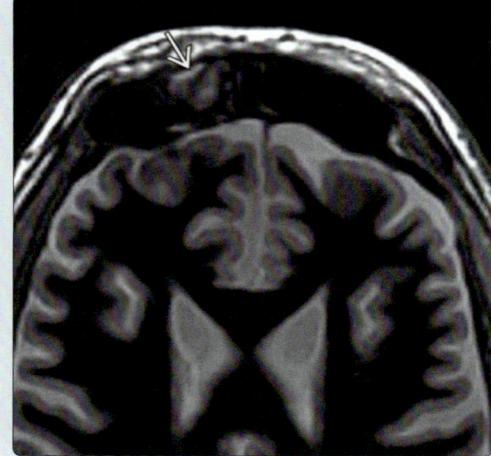

(Left) Oblique coronal CT in a 63-year-old man with essential tremor undergoing imaging for preoperative planning to place deep electrodes is shown. There is an incidental ossified frontal sinus mass ➡. This osteoma is pedunculated from its attachment site at the lateral aspect of the right cribriform plate ⬅. (Right) Axial T2 MR in the same patient shows heterogeneous areas of increased signal ➡ within the frontal osteoma. The hyperintense areas may represent fibrous stroma.

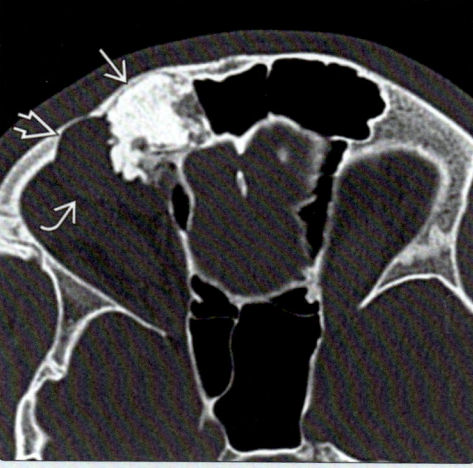
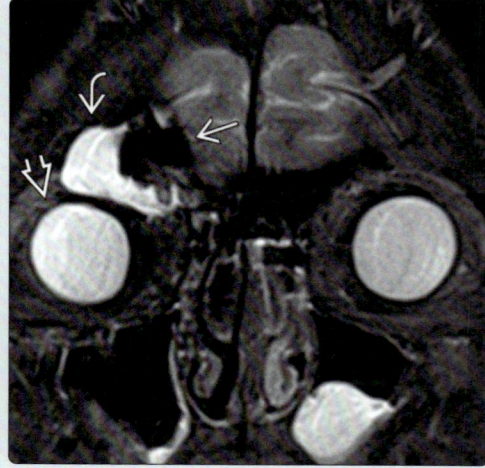

(Left) Axial bone CT demonstrates a dense osseous lesion ➡ occupying the right frontal sinus, compatible with osteoma. There is obstruction of the right frontal sinus with associated mucocele ➡ projecting into the right orbit and scalloping the right frontal bone ➡. (Right) Coronal STIR MR in the same patient shows the hypointense right frontal sinus osteoma ➡ with hyperintense mucocele ➡, resulting in mass effect upon the right globe ➡.

TERMINOLOGY

Synonyms
- Hamartoma of bone

Definitions
- Benign, well-defined, slow-growing, bone-forming tumor

IMAGING

General Features
- Best diagnostic clue
  - Well-marginated bone density lesion that arises from wall of paranasal sinus & protrudes into sinus lumen
- Location
  - Almost exclusively in craniofacial skeleton; paranasal sinuses most common
    - Frontal & ethmoid > > > maxillary & sphenoid
    - Extensive 2009 study concluded: 55.0% ethmoid, 37.5% frontal, 6.0% maxillary, 1.5% sphenoid
  - Traditionally named for sinus lumen invaded by osteoma, not bone of origin (unlike cranial osteomas)
  - May extend intracranially or into orbit
  - Other areas of reported involvement
    - Skull, maxilla, mandible, & temporal bone (especially bony external auditory canal)
- Size
  - Range from few millimeters to several centimeters (typically 1.5-40.0 mm)
    - Majority < 10 mm
    - > 30 mm = "giant" osteoma
- Morphology
  - Sessile or pedunculated, projecting off wall of sinus

Radiographic Findings
- Radiography
  - Well-defined bone density lesion within sinus lumen ± associated inflammatory mucosal disease

CT Findings
- CECT
  - No appreciable enhancement due to high density of lesion
- Bone CT
  - Ivory type has homogeneous, well-defined, **bone-based, high-density mass**
  - Non-ivory-type osteomas may contain areas of soft tissue density
  - Larger osteoma may be associated with
    - Sinus opacification or mucocele formation from ostial obstruction
    - Orbital mass effect from extraconal extension
    - **Pneumocephalus** or intraparenchymal tension pneumatocele
    - Brain abscess ± subdural empyema

MR Findings
- T1WI
  - Low signal on all sequences; often not seen
  - Can be confused with air
  - Yellow marrow areas may be high signal
- T2WI
  - Hypointense or follows marrow signal
  - May have hypointense cortical rim
  - Fibrous portions have ↑ signal
- T1WI C+
  - No appreciable enhancement (except in fibrous areas)
  - Intracranial complications (e.g., mucocele, abscess) better evaluated with contrast

Imaging Recommendations
- Best imaging tool
  - Thin-slice bone CT without contrast
- Protocol advice
  - When larger osteoma involves dural surface, MR may be warranted before surgery
    - Enhanced MR best for assessing adjacent orbital & intracranial structures

DIFFERENTIAL DIAGNOSIS

Sinonasal Fibrous Dysplasia
- Expansile lesion of bone typically with ground-glass matrix
- Small foci may mimic osteoma

Sinonasal Ossifying Fibroma
- Thick, mature bony wall transitioning to immature woven bone centrally
- Most of center of lesion is low density on CT (fibroosseous)

Sinonasal Osteosarcoma
- Bone-forming, invasive, malignant tumor of bone
- Periosteal elevation, permeative margins present
- Soft tissue component often present

Osteoblastoma
- Uncommon in craniofacial skeleton
- Benign, but can have more aggressive imaging features (surrounding bone edema & periosteal reaction)

PATHOLOGY

General Features
- Etiology
  - Remains controversial
    - Linked to trauma, infection, or abnormal embryologic development
      - Occurs often at embryologic junction of cartilaginous ethmoid & membranous frontal bones, supporting developmental source
    - Some experts believe osteoma is actually end-stage of fibroosseous lesion, not true benign neoplasm
- Genetics
  - Usually sporadic, solitary lesions
  - If multiple osteomas are discovered, consider **Gardner syndrome** (GS): Rare autosomal dominant disorder
    - Multiple craniofacial osteomas
    - Intestinal colorectal polyposis progresses to adenocarcinoma
    - Lesions of soft tissues: Fibromatosis, cutaneous epidermoid cysts, lipomas, desmoid tumors, & leiomyomas
    - Clinically evident osteomas develop ~ 17 years before GS diagnosis
- Associated abnormalities

- ~ 37% accompanied by pathologic sinonasal findings
  - Focal obstruction & inflammation, generalized inflammation, polyposis

Staging, Grading, & Classification

- Osteomas composed of dense, mature bone without fibrous stroma
  - Ivory
  - Compact
  - Eburnated osteomas
- Osteomas composed of trabeculae of mature bone separated by fibrous stroma
  - Mature
  - Cancellous
  - Spongy
  - Spongious
- Mixed

Gross Pathologic & Surgical Features

- Hard, pale, ossified mass within sinus lumen
- Rock hard, lobulated mass with ivory-like appearance protruding into sinus lumen

Microscopic Features

- Ivory osteomas composed of dense, mature lamellar bone, & little fibrous stroma
- Mature osteomas composed of large trabeculae of mature lamellar bone & more abundant fibrous stroma
  - ± osteoblastic rimming
- Those with osteoblastoma-like features more aggressive

CLINICAL ISSUES

Presentation

- Most common signs/symptoms
  - Usually asymptomatic, incidental finding
    - Found incidentally in 1% of patients on radiographs & 3% on CT performed for sinonasal symptoms
    - < 5% of all osteomas are symptomatic
- Other signs/symptoms
  - Sinusitis related to obstruction of sinus ostium
  - Headache, facial pain, swelling, or asymmetry
  - Proptosis & diplopia from intraorbital extension
  - Loss of visual acuity from sphenoethmoidal lesions compressing optic nerve
  - Rarely, dizziness, meningitis, or seizure from pneumocephalus, intracranial mucocele, or abscess
- Clinical profile
  - Asymptomatic adult with incidental finding of osteoma on CT performed for other sinonasal complaints

Demographics

- Age
  - Reported in all ages > 20 years
    - > 50% between 50-70 years; rare under age 10
- Sex
  - M:F ~ 1.5-2.6:1.0
- Epidemiology
  - Very common lesion in general population (3% prevalence)
  - Most common primary craniofacial bone tumor
    - Almost all osteomas occur in craniofacial skeleton

- Most common benign tumor of paranasal sinuses

Natural History & Prognosis

- Benign tumor, slowly ↑ in size by continuous bone formation (0.4-6.0 mm/year)
  - Growth rate greatest at puberty
- Becomes symptomatic when large, obstructs sinus drainage, or extends intracranially or into orbit
- Degeneration into osteosarcoma has not been reported
- Prognosis is excellent
  - Cure with complete resection, if necessary

Treatment

- If asymptomatic, can treat with watchful waiting
- Complete surgical removal for following indications
  - Unrelenting symptoms
  - Located near frontal sinus ostium
  - > 50% of volume of frontal sinus filled by osteoma
  - Extends intraorbitally or intracranially
  - CT evidence of significant enlargement
- Traditionally removed with open surgical procedures
- Endonasal endoscopic resection possible
  - Small size
  - Frontoethmoidal or orbitoethmoidal in location

DIAGNOSTIC CHECKLIST

Consider

- Other fibroosseous lesions if soft tissue density is major component of lesion
- Be sure to evaluate for affect of osteoma on adjacent structures
  - Patency of sinus drainage pathways; mass effect on orbit, meninges, & brain

Image Interpretation Pearls

- Dense, ossified sinus mass should be considered osteoma until proven otherwise
- If multiple craniofacial osteomas, consider possibility of GS

SELECTED REFERENCES

1. Dewantoro D et al: Endoscopically managed giant frontoethmoidal osteoma with orbital extension. BMJ Case Rep. 17(6):e259236, 2024
2. Movio G et al: Paranasal osteoma: the importance of surveillance. Cureus. 15(9):e44696, 2023
3. Değer HM et al: Clinical experience and treatment approaches in sinonasal osteomas from a tertiary care hospital in Turkey. Auris Nasus Larynx. 49(1):84-91, 2022
4. Giotakis E et al: Gigantic paranasal sinuses osteomas: clinical features, management considerations, and long-term outcomes. Eur Arch Otorhinolaryngol. 278(5):1429-41, 2021
5. Bedard T et al: Atypical enostoses-series of ten cases and literature review. Medicina (Kaunas). 56(10):534, 2020
6. Watley DC et al: Surgical approach to frontal sinus osteoma: a systematic review. Am J Rhinol Allergy. 33(5):462-9, 2019
7. Yu D et al: Bone and dental abnormalities as first signs of familial Gardner's syndrome in a Chinese family: a literature review and a case report. Med Sci (Paris). 34 Focus issue F1:20-5, 2018
8. Erdogan N et al: A prospective study of paranasal sinus osteomas in 1,889 cases: changing patterns of localization. Laryngoscope. 119(12):2355-9, 2009
9. McHugh JB et al: Sino-orbital osteoma: a clinicopathologic study of 45 surgically treated cases with emphasis on tumors with osteoblastoma-like features. Arch Pathol Lab Med. 133(10):1587-93, 2009
10. Alexander AA et al: Paranasal sinus osteomas and Gardner's syndrome. Ann Otol Rhinol Laryngol. 116(9):658-62, 2007
11. de Chalain T et al: Ivory osteoma of the craniofacial skeleton. J Craniofac Surg. 14(5): 729-35, 2003

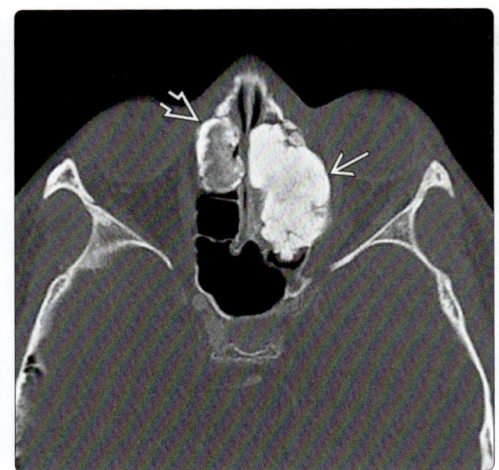

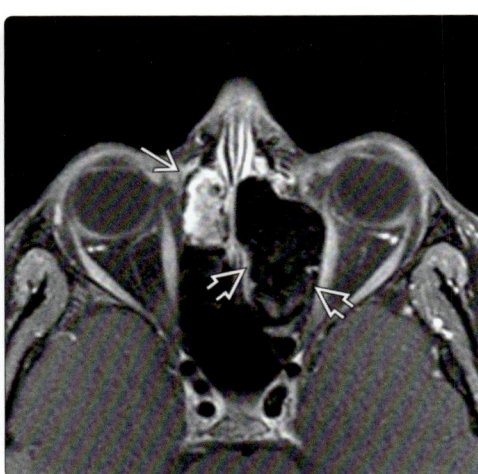

(Left) Axial bone window CECT in a 15-year-old boy who underwent contrast CT for a desmoid tumor in the left neck shows bilateral L > R ethmoid osteomas, which are a manifestation of Gardner syndrome in this patient. The left-sided lesion ➡ is much denser than the right ➡. (Right) Axial T1 C+ FS MR in the same patient demonstrates mild, heterogeneous enhancement in the right osteoma ➡, consistent with fibrous content. The larger, more sclerotic/ossified left-sided lesion ➡ does not enhance.

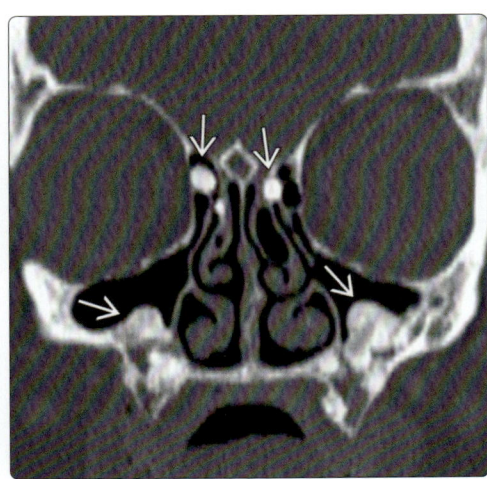

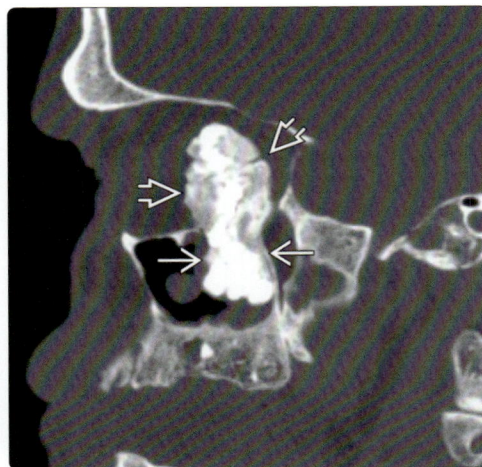

(Left) Coronal bone CT shows multifocal osteomas involving the sinonasal cavity ➡ in this patient with Gardner syndrome. (Right) Sagittal CT reformation in a different patient shows a large, lobulated ivory osteoma involving the right maxillary sinus ➡. The mass extends into the posterior aspect of the orbit ➡ and caused proptosis in this patient.

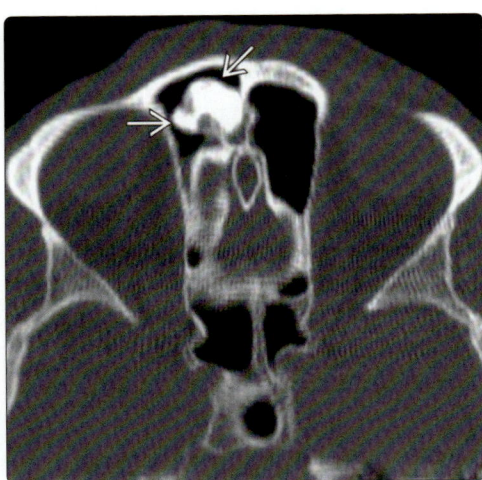

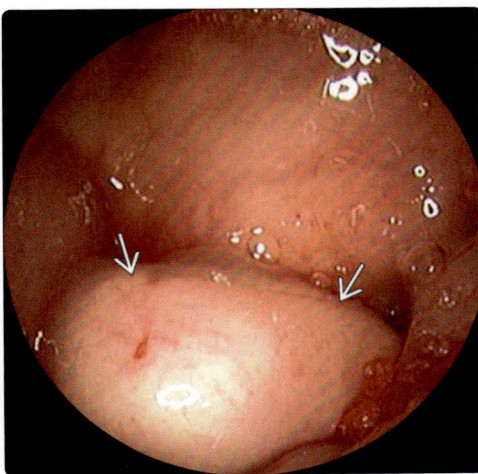

(Left) Axial CT reconstruction shows the classic appearance of an ivory compact osteoma ➡ arising within the right frontal sinus. This mass did not occlude the frontal recess, and there is no associated mucosal disease or mucocele formation. (Right) Intraoperative photograph of the frontal sinus shows a smooth, mucosa-covered pale osteoma ➡ along the floor of the sinus. The osteoma was encroaching upon the frontal sinus ostium.

Sinonasal Ossifying Fibroma

TERMINOLOGY

- Benign fibroosseous lesion composed of fibrous tissue & mature bone

IMAGING

- Imaging appearance varies (↑ ossification with age)
  - Classic appearance: Thick, bony peripheral rim surrounding fibrous center
- CT
  - **Expansile mass** with **soft tissue density** (fibrous) **central** area surrounded by **ossified rim**
  - May be indistinguishable from fibrous dysplasia & osteoma
- MR
  - T1: Intermediate to low signal throughout tumor
  - T2: Mixed low- & high-signal areas
  - Inhomogeneous enhancement of fibrous components
- MR appearance variable & may appear aggressive
- Important to correlate with CT appearance

TOP DIFFERENTIAL DIAGNOSES

- Sinonasal fibrous dysplasia
- Sinonasal osteoma
- Sinonasal osteosarcoma

PATHOLOGY

- Likely origin is mesenchyme of periodontal ligament

CLINICAL ISSUES

- Generally asymptomatic & found incidentally
- Age: 20-40 years most common
- Sex: M:F = 1:5
- Benign but locally aggressive
  - May obstruct sinus drainage, cause cosmetic deformity & ocular dysfunction
- Complete surgical excision is treatment of choice
- Lesions with benign behavior that do not produce deformity may be treated with curettage & ostectomy
  - High rate of recurrence with incomplete resection

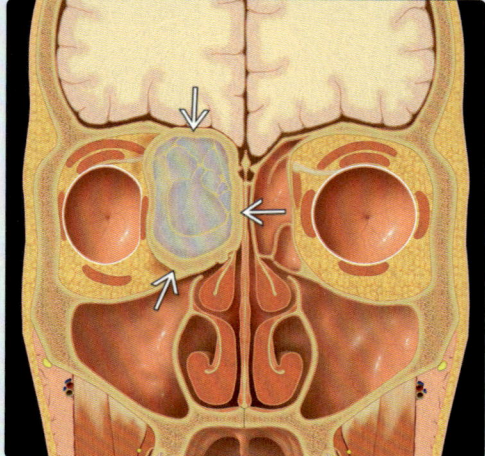
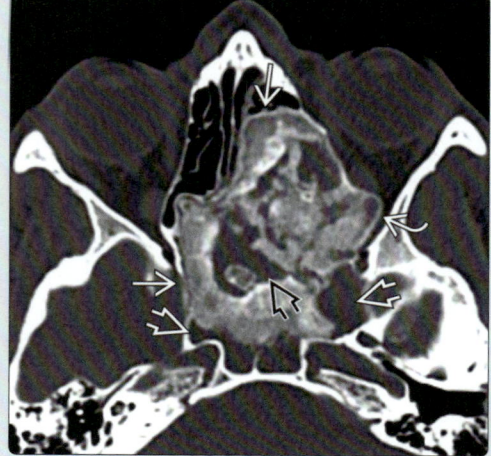

(Left) Coronal graphic shows an ossifying fibroma (OsFib) of the ethmoid region with dense osseous material peripherally ➡ and a fibrous center. The margins are well defined. There is mass effect on the orbital contents. (Right) Axial bone CT shows an expansile lesion centered in the posterior sinonasal cavity extending into the left orbit ➡. This lesion demonstrates predominant peripheral ossification ➡ with a central fibrotic core ➡, typical for OsFib. Note obstructed secretion in the sphenoid sinuses ➡.

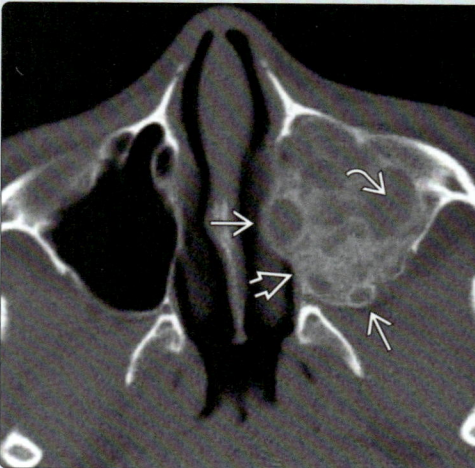
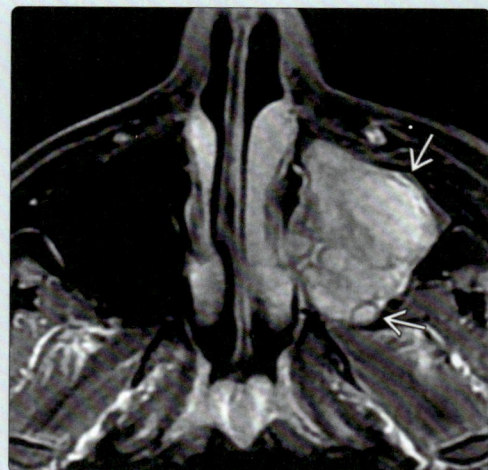

(Left) Axial bone CT demonstrates a circumscribed mass within the left maxillary sinus with expansile margins ➡ containing both ossified ➡ and soft tissue components ➡ in this case of trabecular juvenile OsFib. (Right) Axial T1 C+ FS MR in the same patient demonstrates heterogeneous enhancement of the left maxillary sinus mass. Note that enhancement is more pronounced in fibrous components ➡, which showed soft tissue attenuation on comparison CT.

TERMINOLOGY

Abbreviations
- Ossifying fibroma (OsFib)

Synonyms
- Cemento-OsFib, psammomatoid juvenile OsFib, trabecular juvenile OsFib

Definitions
- Benign fibroosseous lesion composed of encapsulated mixture of fibrous tissue & mature bone

IMAGING

General Features
- Best diagnostic clue
  - Well-demarcated, expansile mass with soft tissue density (fibrous) central area surrounded by ossified rim
- Location
  - 10-20% of craniofacial OsFib arise from maxilla
    - Most common craniofacial site is mandible (75%)
  - Characteristically **monostotic**
- Size
  - 0.5-10 cm
- Morphology
  - Well circumscribed, expansile

CT Findings
- NECT
  - Well-circumscribed, expansile mass with mixed soft tissue & bone density
  - Most often unilobular
- CECT
  - Fibrous areas may show subtle to more avid enhancement
- Bone CT
  - Imaging appearance depends on age of OsFib (↑ ossified portions with age)
  - Classic appearance
    - **Thick, bony peripheral rim** surrounding **low-attenuation fibrous center**
  - Other appearance
    - Scattered foci of soft tissue among ossified areas
    - Thin, eggshell appearance of peripheral bone
  - CT appearance may be indistinguishable from fibrous dysplasia & osteoma
  - May absorb maxillary tooth roots

MR Findings
- T1WI
  - Intermediate to low signal throughout tumor
    - Fibrous areas intermediate signal (classically central)
    - Ossified areas hypointense (classically peripheral)
- T2WI
  - Mixed low- & high-signal areas
    - Fibrous areas hyperintense (usually lesion center)
    - Ossified areas hypointense (usually lesion periphery)
  - Obstructed secretions behind lesion & associated mucocele are hyperintense
  - Fluid-fluid levels in portions of tumors may be seen
- T1WI C+
  - Inhomogeneous enhancement of fibrous portions of tumor matrix
  - Enhancement of outer shell & septa may be seen

Imaging Recommendations
- Best imaging tool
  - Fibroosseous lesions of craniofacial area best studied with bone algorithm CT
- Protocol advice
  - Thin-slice bone CT in axial plane with coronal ± sagittal reformatted images
  - Enhanced T1 fat-saturated MR provides complete presurgical roadmap of surrounding soft tissues at risk

DIFFERENTIAL DIAGNOSIS

Sinonasal Fibrous Dysplasia
- Poorly defined expansion of maxillofacial bones
- Classic ground-glass appearance
- Mixed pattern of less active ground-glass & more active fibrous areas
- May be monostotic (70%) or polyostotic (30%)
- Encompasses rather than absorbs healthy tooth roots

Sinonasal Osteoma
- Mass composed of mostly solid lamellar bone
- Frontal sinus common location

Sinonasal Osteosarcoma
- Destructive, aggressive lesion of craniofacial bones
- Tumor "new bone" in mass matrix
- Sunburst periosteal reaction
- Most common in adolescent boys or as long-term complication of XRT

Cementoblastoma
- Benign tumor of cementum in young males
- Dense mass associated with tooth root
- Not located in frontal, ethmoid, or sphenoid sinuses

PATHOLOGY

General Features
- Etiology
  - Thought to arise from **mesenchyme of periodontal ligament** (related to cemento-OsFib), but not all tooth related
    - Presumed to originate from mesenchymal blast cells
    - Closely related to fibrous dysplasia & ameloblastoma
  - Densely cellular, well-defined, fibrous tumor with ossification progressing from periphery toward center
    - Early stage: Primarily fibrous
    - Late stage: Fills in with mature bone
- Associated abnormalities
  - Large lesions may result in cosmetic deformity, ocular dysfunction
  - May obstruct sinus drainage pathways & lead to mucocele formation
  - Intracranial extension complicated by tension pneumocephalus has been reported

Staging, Grading, & Classification
- Subtypes described

- ○ Cemento-OsFib
- ○ Juvenile OsFib
  - – Psammomatoid
  - – Trabecular

Gross Pathologic & Surgical Features

- Gritty, gray to white, hard lesion

Microscopic Features

- Islands of osteoid rimmed by osteoblast-forming lamellar bone
- Central OsFib contains immature (woven) bone, whereas periphery has more mature (lamellar) bone
- Fibrous stroma shows parallel & whorl arrangement of collagen & fibroblasts
  - ○ May be densely cellular with hemorrhage, inflammation, & giant cells
- OsFib may be histologically indistinguishable from active form of fibrous dysplasia

CLINICAL ISSUES

Presentation

- Most common signs/symptoms
  - ○ Generally **asymptomatic** & found incidentally
- Other signs/symptoms
  - ○ Chronic sinusitis symptoms: Rhinorrhea, pain, cheek swelling, nasal obstruction
  - ○ Displaced teeth
  - ○ Exophthalmos, diplopia, visual acuity loss due to orbital mass effect
- Clinical profile
  - ○ **20- to 40-year-old woman** with mixed soft tissue-ossified sinus lesion incidentally detected on CT performed for other reasons
  - ○ Appearance mimics other fibroosseous lesions, & diagnosis not made on basis of imaging alone
    - – Based on combination of clinical, radiologic, & pathologic criteria
  - ○ Hyperparathyroidism-jaw tumor syndrome rare association
    - – Autosomal dominant disease with parathyroid adenoma or carcinoma & OsFib of jaws
    - – Occasionally renal & uterine tumors

Demographics

- Age
  - ○ 1st appears in young adult
    - – 20-40 years most common
  - ○ Wide range reported
- Sex
  - ○ M:F = 1:5
- Epidemiology
  - ○ 10-20% of craniofacial OsFib arise in maxilla
  - ○ < 0.5% risk of malignant degeneration

Natural History & Prognosis

- Slow growing but may be locally aggressive
  - ○ OsFib of paranasal sinuses are more aggressive than OsFib of mandible
  - ○ Juvenile subtypes of OsFib may have aggressive, locally destructive behavior

- Prognosis excellent after complete resection
- High rate of recurrence if incompletely resected

Treatment

- Complete surgical excision is treatment of choice as permitted by OsFib location
- Lesions with benign behavior that do not produce deformity may be treated with curettage & ostectomy
  - ○ Recurrence rates higher with this approach

DIAGNOSTIC CHECKLIST

Consider

- May not have classic bony rim with fibrous center
  - ○ Densities may be patchy & randomly distributed

Image Interpretation Pearls

- MR appearance of OsFib highly variable, & lesion may appear more aggressive
  - ○ Careful correlation with CT important
- May be **indistinguishable from fibrous dysplasia**
  - ○ Refer to more generically as "fibroosseous lesion"
  - ○ If polyostotic process, fibrous dysplasia more likely

Reporting Tips

- Describe position in relation to sinus drainage pathways
- Be sure to describe mass effect on adjacent structures, such as orbit, neural foramina, & intracranial cavity

SELECTED REFERENCES

1. Lo Casto A et al: Uncommon nasal mass presentation: a radiological case series. J Pers Med. 14(12):1145, 2024
2. Ma J et al: Prognostic factors in transnasal endoscopic surgery for paediatric patients with ossifying fibroma of the paranasal sinuses and skull base. J Otolaryngol Head Neck Surg. 52(1):48, 2023
3. Cortes-Santiago N et al: Review of pediatric head and neck neoplasms that raise the possibility of a cancer predisposition syndrome. Head Neck Pathol. 15(1):16-24, 2021
4. Dong D et al: Fibro-osseous lesions of paranasal sinus and craniofacial region: a retrospective study of 282 cases. Laryngoscope. 131(1):E1-7, 2020
5. Ibrahem HMt Ossifying fibroma of the jaw bones in hyperparathyroidism-jaw tumor syndrome: analysis of 24 cases retrieved from literatures. J Dent Sci. 15(4):426-32, 2020
6. Liu JJ et al: Ossifying fibroma of the maxilla and sinonasal tract: case series. Allergy Rhinol (Providence). 8(1):32-6, 2017
7. Ciniglio Appiani M et al: Ossifying fibromas of the paranasal sinuses: diagnosis and management. Acta Otorhinolaryngol Ital. 35(5):355-61, 2015
8. MacDonald DS: Maxillofacial fibro-osseous lesions. Clin Radiol. 70(1):25-36, 2015
9. McCarthy EF: Fibro-osseous lesions of the maxillofacial bones. Head Neck Pathol. 7(1) 5-10, 2013
10. MacDonald-Jankowski DS: Ossifying fibroma: a systematic review. Dentomaxillofac Radiol. 38(8):495-513, 2009
11. Boudewyns AN et al: Sinonasal fibro-osseous hamartoma: case presentation and differential diagnosis with other fibro-osseous lesions involving the paranasal sinuses. Eur Arch Otorhinolaryngol. 263(3):276-81, 2006
12. Eller R et al: Common fibro-osseous lesions of the paranasal sinuses. Otolaryngol Clin North Am. 39(3):585-600, x, 2006
13. Mehta D et al: Paediatric fibro-osseous lesions of the nose and paranasal sinuses. Int J Pediatr Otorhinolaryngol. 70(2):193-9, 2006
14. Kendi AT et al: Sinonasal ossifying fibroma with fluid-fluid levels on MR images. AJNR Am J Neuroradiol. 24(8):1639-41, 2003
15. Alawi F: Benign fibro-osseous diseases of the maxillofacial bones. A review and differential diagnosis. Am J Clin Pathol. 118 Suppl:S50-70, 2002
16. Khoury NJ et al: Juvenile ossifying fibroma: CT and MR findings. Eur Radiol. 12 Suppl 3:S109-13, 2002
17. Engelbrecht V et al: CT and MRI of congenital sinonasal ossifying fibroma. Neuroradiology. 41(7):526-9, 1999
18. Thompson J et al: Nasopharyngeal nonossifying variant of ossifying fibromyxoid tumor: CT and MR findings. AJNR Am J Neuroradiol. 16(5):1132-4, 1995

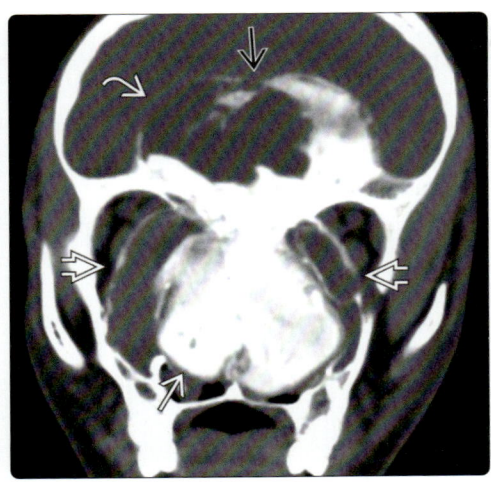

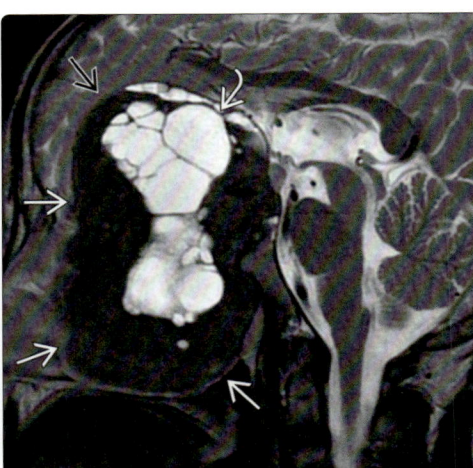

(Left) Coronal bone CT shows an expansile mass in the sinonasal cavity, which shows regions of dense ossification ➡ and hypodense ➡ components. There is expansion into anterior cranial fossa ➡ and bilateral orbits ➡. (Right) Sagittal T2 MR in the same patient shows peripheral T2-hypointense signal ➡ corresponding to ossification on CT and central multiloculated cystic component ➡. Intracranial extension causes mass effect in the anterior cranial fossa ➡ in this patient with juvenile OsFib.

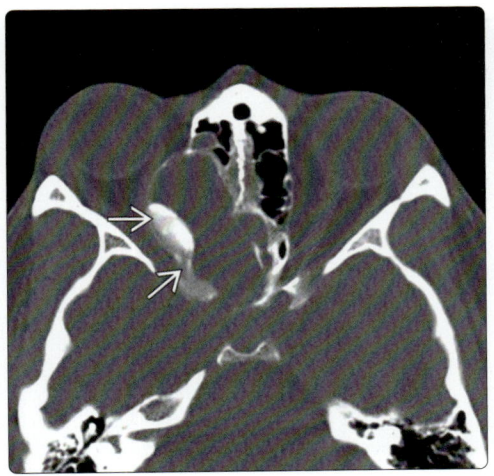

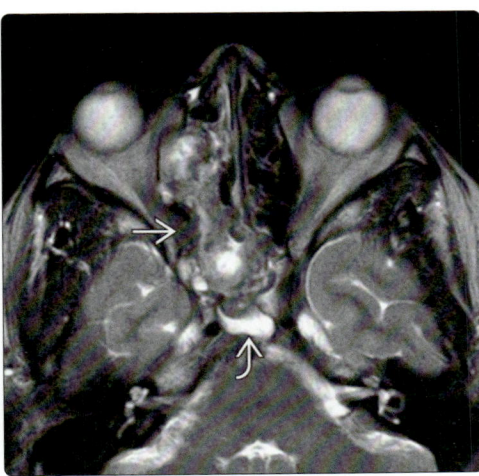

(Left) Axial bone CT demonstrates an expansile, predominantly soft tissue density mass within the posterior ethmoid region. A focus of peripheral ossification ➡ along the lateral margin suggests that this is a fibroosseous lesion, in this case, an OsFib. (Right) Axial T2 MR in the same patient shows hypointense signal in the ossified portion ➡ of the lesion. Note the hyperintense obstructed secretions ➡ in the sphenoid sinus posterior to the lesion.

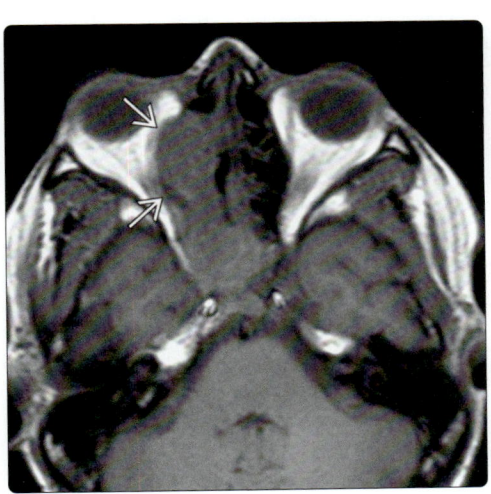

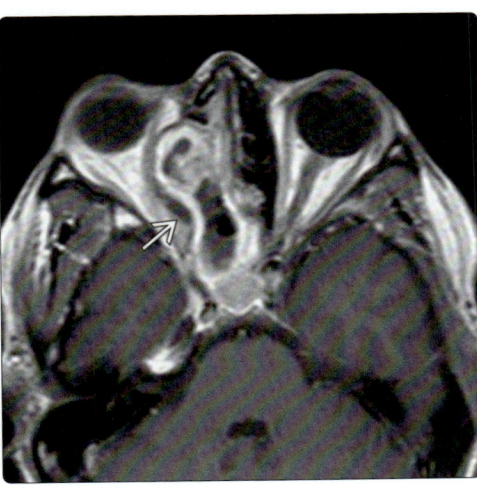

(Left) Axial T1 MR in the same patient shows signal intensity similar to that of muscle within the majority of the OsFib. The margins are well defined. Note the mass effect on the right orbital contents ➡, causing diplopia in this patient. (Right) Axial T1 C+ MR in the same patient reveals heterogeneous enhancement throughout the lesion. The fibrous portions of OsFib typically enhance, and there is little or no enhancement in the ossified ➡ portions.

TERMINOLOGY

- Benign, vascular, nonencapsulated, locally invasive mass originating in nasal cavity

IMAGING

- Centered in posterior nasal cavity arising at sphenopalatine foramen; extends into nasopharynx, sphenoid sinus, pterygopalatine fossa, masticator space, orbit, skull base
- CT findings
  - Heterogeneous vs. diffuse, avid enhancement
  - Bone remodeling and destruction
    - Posterior wall of maxillary sinus bowed anteriorly
    - ± skull base invasion, intracranial extension
- MR findings
  - Tubular signal voids on spin-echo-based sequences due to fast flow in enlarged vessels
  - Intense enhancement, diffuse or heterogeneous
- Angiography typically performed at time of preoperative embolization; shows tumor blush

- Most common feeding artery: Internal maxillary branch of external carotid artery

TOP DIFFERENTIAL DIAGNOSES

- Rhabdomyosarcoma
- Childhood nasopharyngeal carcinoma
- Antrochoana. polyp
- Olfactory neuroblastoma

CLINICAL ISSUES

- Unilateral nasal obstruction (90%), epistaxis (60%)
  - Occurs almost exclusively in adolescent males
- Preferred treatment: Complete surgical resection using preoperative embolization to ↓ blood loss
  - ± adjuvant radiation therapy after surgery or as primary treatment in some cases

DIAGNOSTIC CHECKLIST

- Look for extension into surrounding structures
- Consider other diagnoses (or genetic testing) in females

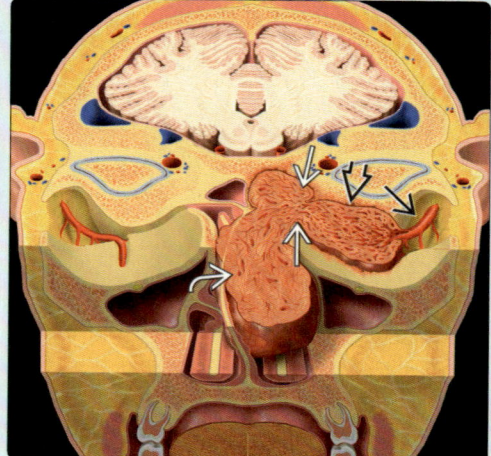
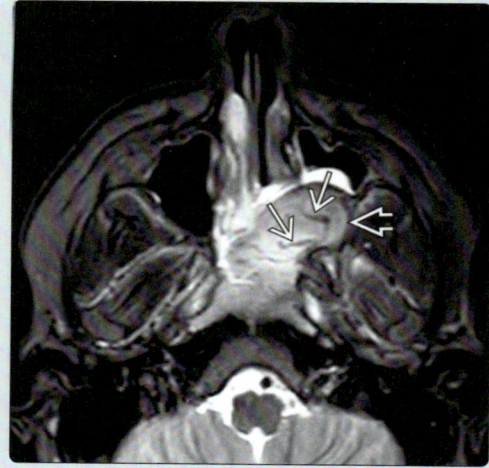

(Left) Graphic shows the classic features and location of juvenile angiofibroma (JAF). The site of origin is the sphenopalatine foramen (SPF) ➡ with tumoral extension into the pterygopalatine fossa (PPF) ➡ and nasal cavity ➡. The internal maxillary artery ➡ is the dominant feeding vessel. (Right) Axial STIR MR in a teenage patient shows a well-defined mass with intralesional flow voids ➡ widening the left PPF, deviating the posterior wall of the maxillary sinus forward and extending into the left infratemporal fossa ➡.

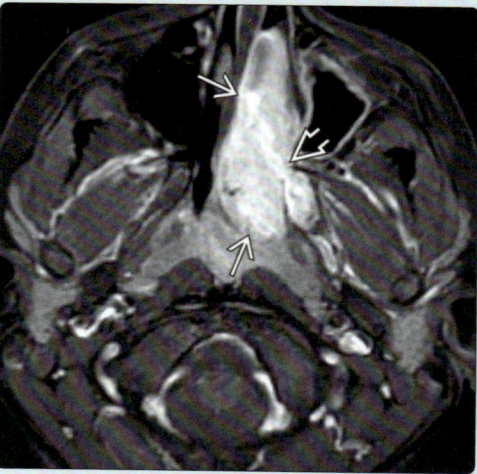
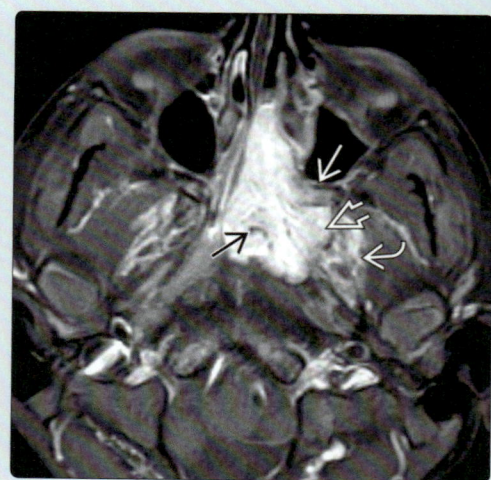

(Left) Axial T1 C+ FS MR in a 15-year-old patient with nasal obstruction shows an enhancing JAF ➡ filling the left nasal cavity and extending into the nasopharynx. The presumed site of origin is the SPF ➡. (Right) Axial T1 C+ FS MR in the same patient shows a few intralesional high-flow vessels ➡ with extension of the JAF into the widened PPF ➡. There is destruction of the left pterygoid ➡ with extension of the mass into the masticator space ➡.

Juvenile Angiofibroma

TERMINOLOGY

Abbreviations
- Juvenile angiofibroma (JAF)

Synonyms
- Juvenile nasopharyngeal angiofibroma (JNA); fibromatous or angiofibromatous hamartoma
  - JAF of nasal cavity more correct terminology
  - JNA commonly used term, but tumor begins in nasal cavity, not in nasopharynx

Definitions
- Benign, vascular, nonencapsulated, locally invasive nasal cavity mass

IMAGING

General Features
- Best diagnostic clue
  - Intensely enhancing soft tissue mass originating at sphenopalatine foramen (SPF) in adolescent male
- Location
  - Centered in posterior wall of nasal cavity off-midline, at margin of SPF
    - SPF is medial opening of pterygopalatine fossa (PPF) into superior meatus of nose
    - Extends anteriorly into nasal cavity, posteriorly into nasopharynx, and laterally into PPF
      □ Penetrates PPF early (90%) with involvement of upper medial pterygoid lamina
    - Sphenoid sinus extension (60%)
    - May extend into maxillary (43%) and ethmoid sinuses (35%), masticator space, and inferior orbital fissure
    - 5-20% extend into middle cranial fossa via vidian canal or foramen rotundum
  - Extranasopharyngeal angiofibroma, entity showing pathologic findings of JAF but with other differences
    - Located at nasal septum, turbinate, etc.
    - M:F = 2.1:1; mean age: 28.7 years
    - Mainly nasal obstruction; epistaxis only 25%
    - Female sex or normal vascularity does not exclude
- Size
  - Usually 2-6 cm but may become massive
- Morphology
  - Lobular, usually well-circumscribed mass
    - Large lesions have infiltrating margins

Radiographic Findings
- Lateral skull radiograph shows anterior displacement of posterior wall of maxillary antrum
  - Called antral sign, bow sign, or Holman-Miller sign
  - Nonspecific sign, denotes any slow-growing mass
- Associated with nasal cavity opacification
- ± nasal cavity/nasopharyngeal soft tissue mass

CT Findings
- CECT
  - Heterogeneous vs. diffuse, avid enhancement of soft tissue mass in nasal cavity originating near SPF
  - Frequent extension into adjacent nasopharynx and PPF
  - ± opacified sphenoid sinus (obstructed nonenhancing secretions vs. enhancing tumor infiltration)
  - ± intracranial or orbital extension
- Bone CT
  - Bone remodeling ± destruction
    - Antral sign; nonspecific
    - Ipsilateral nasal cavity and PPF enlarged
    - ± skull base invasion; pterygoid lamina erosion specific
- CTA
  - Enlarged ipsilateral external carotid artery (ECA) and internal maxillary (IMAX) artery

MR Findings
- T1WI: Heterogeneous, intermediate signal
  - Signal voids represent flow in enlarged vessels
- T2WI: Heterogeneous, intermediate to high signal
  - Punctate and serpentine flow voids within tumor
- T1WI C+ FS: Intense enhancement ± flow voids
  - Coronal plane shows cavernous sinus, sphenoid sinus, or skull base extension
- MRA: Enlarged ipsilateral ECA and IMAX artery
  - Lesional vessels may be too small to evaluate with MRA

Angiographic Findings
- Conventional angiography typically performed at time of preoperative embolization
- Intense capillary tumor blush is fed by enlarged feeding vessels from ECA
  - Most common feeding vessels: IMAX and ascending pharyngeal arteries from ECA
  - If skull base or cavernous sinus extension, then internal carotid artery (ICA) supply common
  - ± supply from contralateral ECA branches

Imaging Recommendations
- Best imaging tool
  - Maxillofacial bone-only NECT in axial and coronal planes for evaluating bone remodeling vs. destruction
  - Postcontrast MR optimal for mapping lesion extent and determining vascularity
  - Catheter angiography of both ECA and ICA
    - Often in conjunction with embolization therapy
    - Helps plan surgery and ↓ intraoperative blood loss
- Protocol advice
  - Maxillofacial MR with T1 C+ FS in axial and coronal planes
    - Multiplanar imaging for evaluating extension into sphenoid sinus, orbit, skull base
  - Precontrast non-fat-suppressed T1 vital in evaluating infiltration of normal fat in PPF and adjacent bone
  - CECT may be helpful for evaluating residual disease in postoperative period

DIFFERENTIAL DIAGNOSIS

Rhabdomyosarcoma
- Intermediate- to mildly high-signal mass with variable enhancement (often mild to moderate) ± bone destruction
- Can arise in many locations (not necessarily nasal cavity)
- Rarely penetrates SPF into PPF

Childhood Nasopharyngeal Carcinoma
- Mostly EBV-related, undifferentiated carcinoma

- Invasive mass of lateral nasopharynx
- Mild to moderate enhancement
- 90% + nodal metastases, diagnosed at advanced stage

Antrochoanal Polyp

- Maxillary antrum opacified
- Homogeneous mass herniates into anterior nasal cavity, then nasopharynx; PPF not involved
- Peripheral enhancement only

Encephalocele

- Nasoethmoidal type presents as intranasal mass
- Connection to intracranial cavity seen on imaging
- No enhancement
- Usually more anterior in position

Olfactory Neuroblastoma

- 1st incidence peaks in 2nd decade; F > M
- Presenting symptoms same as JAF
- Nasal cavity mass near cribriform plate
- Cystic intracranial components characteristic

PATHOLOGY

General Features

- Etiology
  - Unknown: Recent consideration as vasoproliferative tumor, positive staining for markers that may promote angiogenesis and proliferation

Staging, Grading, & Classification

- Staging systems based on tumor size (< or > 6 cm), invasion to PPF anterior &/or posterior to pterygoid plates, and skull base/intracranial invasion

Microscopic Features

- Unencapsulated, highly vascular polypoid mass of angiomatous tissue in fibrous stroma
- Myofibroblast thought to be cell of origin
- ± estrogen, testosterone, or progesterone receptors

CLINICAL ISSUES

Presentation

- Most common signs/symptoms
  - Unilateral nasal obstruction (90%), epistaxis (60%)
- Other signs/symptoms
  - Nasal voice, nasal discharge, anosmia, pain or swelling in cheek, proptosis, serous otitis media
- Clinical profile
  - Adolescent male with nasal obstruction and epistaxis
  - Nasal endoscopy: Vascular-appearing nasal cavity mass
    - Biopsy in outpatient setting should be avoided due to risk of hemorrhage

Demographics

- Age
  - 10-25 years; average age at onset: 15 years
- Sex
  - Almost exclusively occurs in male patients
    - If found in female, may have genetic mosaicism
- Epidemiology
  - 0.5% of all H&N neoplasms

Natural History & Prognosis

- May rarely spontaneously regress
- Local recurrence rate with surgery: 6-24%
  - Local recurrence more common with large lesions (> 6 cm), intracranial spread, previous treatment

Treatment

- Preferred: Complete surgical resection using preoperative embolization to ↓ blood loss
  - Transarterial embolization most often, direct puncture embolization in some centers
- Multiple surgical approaches
  - Open resection (midface degloving) vs. endoscopic or endoscopic-assisted removal ± laser assistance
  - Endoscopic resection associated with ↓ bleeding and shorter hospital stay
- Radiation therapy (RT)
  - Adjuvant to surgery for unresectable intracranial disease and cavernous sinus involvement
    - 78% control rates reported
  - Used with caution in young patients due to potential to induce malignancies
- Hormonal therapy (estrogen) controversial
  - Not routine; complete tumor regression not achieved
  - Feminization side effects undesirable in adolescent male
- Recent reports of some success with sirolimus

DIAGNOSTIC CHECKLIST

Consider

- JAF in adolescent male patient with epistaxis and enhancing posterior nasal cavity mass
- Consider other diagnoses (or genetic testing) in female patients

Image Interpretation Pearls

- Evaluate JAF extension into surrounding structures
  - Orbit, infratemporal fossa, sphenoid sinus, and skull base
  - Failure to identify subtle deep growth will result in incomplete surgical resection

SELECTED REFERENCES

1. Kasai S et al: Dose-dependent tumor regression during sirolimus therapy in an advanced juvenile nasopharyngeal angiofibroma case. Pediatr Int. 66(1):e15807, 2024
2. Baba A et al: MRI features of sinonasal tract angiofibroma/juvenile nasopharyngeal angiofibroma: case series and systematic review. J Neuroimaging. 33(5):675-87, 2023
3. Diaz A et al: Embolization in juvenile nasopharyngeal angiofibroma surgery: a systematic review and meta-analysis. Laryngoscope. 133(7):1529-39, 2023
4. Jurlina M et al: Endoscopic, endoscopic-assisted and open approaches in the treatment of juvenile angiofibroma: what has been new in the past decade (and 1586 cases)? Eur Arch Otorhinolaryngol. 280(5):2081-9, 2023
5. Kothari DS et al: Preoperative embolization techniques in the treatment of juvenile nasopharyngeal angiofibroma: a systematic review. Otolaryngol Head Neck Surg. 169(3):454-66, 2023
6. Mamlouk MD: Solid and vascular neck masses in children. Neuroimaging Clin N Am. 33(4):607-21, 2023
7. Scholfield DW et al: Midfacial degloving for juvenile angiofibroma: a case-series of 21 adult males: an alternative to the endoscopic approach and when it should be considered. Clin Otolaryngol. 46(3):659-64, 2021
8. Fernández KS et al: Sirolimus for the treatment of juvenile nasopharyngeal angiofibroma. Pediatr Blood Cancer. 67(4):e28162, 2020
9. Bertazzon G et al: Contemporary management of juvenile angiofibroma. Curr Opin Otolaryngol Head Neck Surg. 27(1):47-53, 2019
10. Rodriguez DP et al: Masses of the nose, nasal cavity, and nasopharynx in children. Radiographics. 37(6):1704-30, 2017

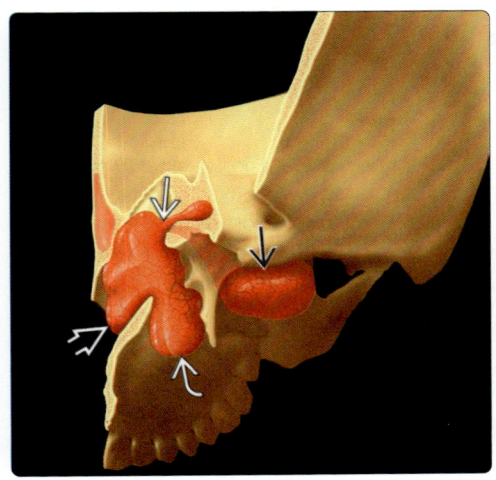

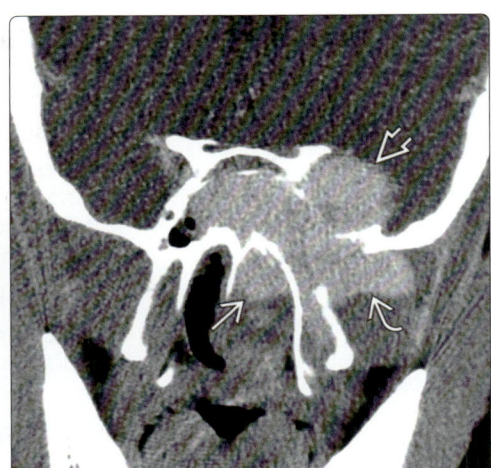

(Left) Posterior oblique sagittal graphic shows the spread patterns of JAF. The lesion originates at the SPF ➡ and extends into the nasal cavity ➡, nasopharynx/oropharynx ➡, and infratemporal fossa ➡. (Right) Coronal CECT shows a large JAF extending into the nasopharynx ➡, infratemporal fossa ➡, and middle cranial fossa ➡. The sphenoid sinus is replaced by the tumor. As seen in this case, JAF classically shows avid enhancement.

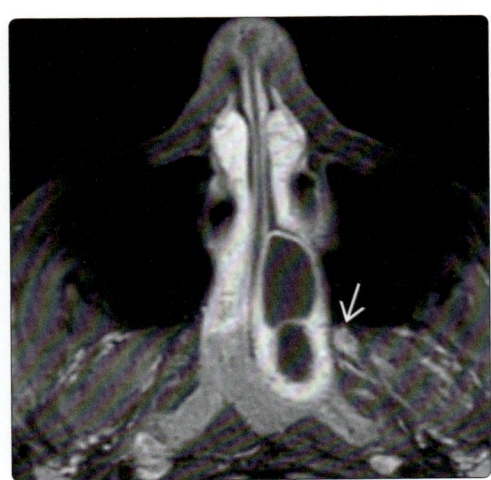

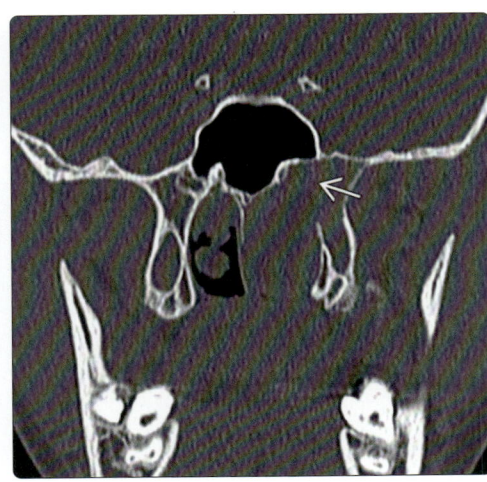

(Left) Axial T1 C+ FS MR in a 13-year-old boy with epistaxis shows an enhancing mass obstructing the left nasal cavity, extending into the left nasopharynx, compressing the adenoids, with minimal enhancement in the left pterygoid ➡. Cystic areas are uncommon in JAF, but the location is typical. (Right) Coronal bone CT in the same patient shows an intact but thin floor of the left sphenoid sinus and floor of the middle cranial fossa, but destruction and infiltration of the left pterygoid plate ➡, typical of JAF.

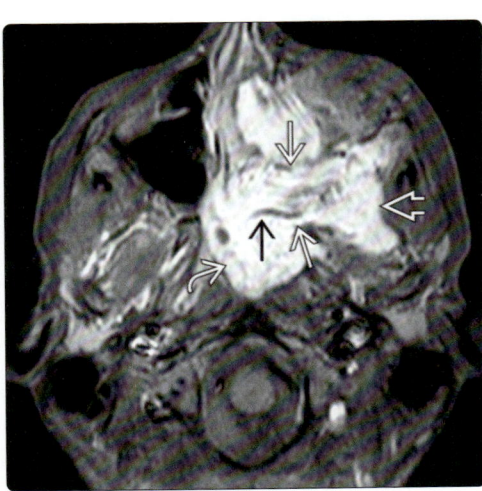

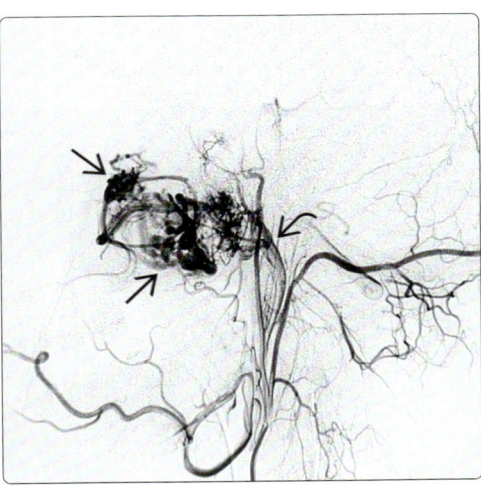

(Left) Axial T1 C+ FS MR shows avid enhancement throughout JAF. The mass enlarges the PPF ➡ and extends laterally into the masticator space ➡ and medially into the nasopharynx ➡. Several serpiginous flow voids ➡ are noted, consistent with enlarged feeding vessels. (Right) Lateral DSA from an external carotid artery injection shows areas of dense tumor blush ➡ within JAF prior to embolization. As is typical, the main arterial feeding vessel for this JAF is the internal maxillary artery ➡.

KEY FACTS

IMAGING

- Typical location: Along lateral nasal wall **centered at middle meatus** ± extension into antrum
- CT findings
  - Focal bony hyperostosis suggests point of tumor origin
  - Osseous destruction suggests squamous cell carcinoma-inverted papilloma (SCCa-IPap)
- MR findings
  - T2: Predominantly hyperintense to skeletal muscle
  - T2 & T1 C+ FS: Curvilinear striations or convoluted, cerebriform pattern are characteristic
  - T2 FS differentiates tumor from obstructed secretions
- PET cannot reliably distinguish benign IPap & SCCa
- Best imaging tool: Multiplanar MR best maps tumor & differentiates tumor from obstructed secretions
- T2 FS & T1 C+ FS MR best show internal architecture
- Loss of convoluted, cerebriform pattern ± extrasinus invasion ↑ concern for SCCa-IPap

TOP DIFFERENTIAL DIAGNOSES

- Solitary sinonasal (antrochoanal) polyp
- Sinonasal SCCa
- Sinonasal polyposis

PATHOLOGY

- Hyperplastic squamous epithelium replaces seromucinous ducts & glands in stroma with endophytic growth pattern
- **10%** either degenerate into or **coexist with SCCa**
  - SCCa may be synchronous (7%) or metachronous (4%)

CLINICAL ISSUES

- Typically 40-70 years
- M > F (3.4:1)
- High rate of local recurrence if incompletely resected

DIAGNOSTIC CHECKLIST

- Deeply invasive disease may alter surgical approach
- Look for additional masses: 4% are multifocal

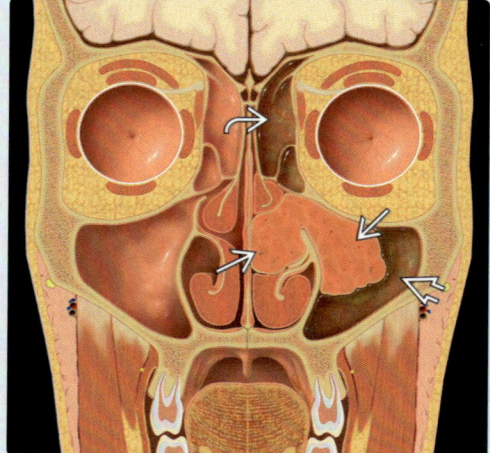
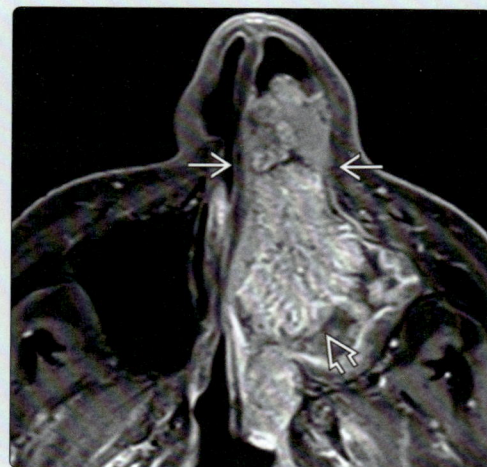

(Left) Coronal graphic shows an inverted papilloma (IPap) ➡ originating near the middle meatus and extending into the maxillary sinus. Blocked secretions are noted in the ethmoid ➡ and maxillary ➡ sinuses. (Right) Axial T1 C+ FS MR shows a left nasal cavity and maxillary sinus polypoid mass with convoluted, cerebriform enhancement pattern ➡ characteristic of IPap. This mass expands the left nasal cavity ➡ without osseous destruction.

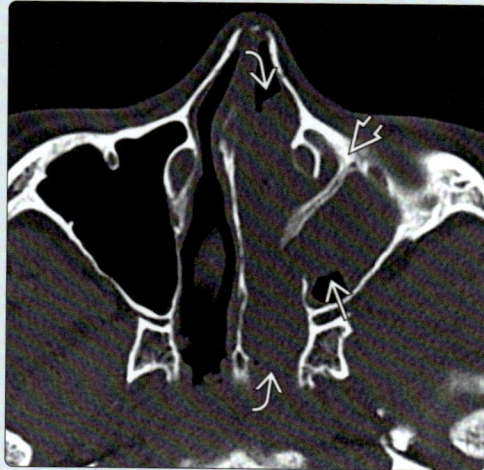
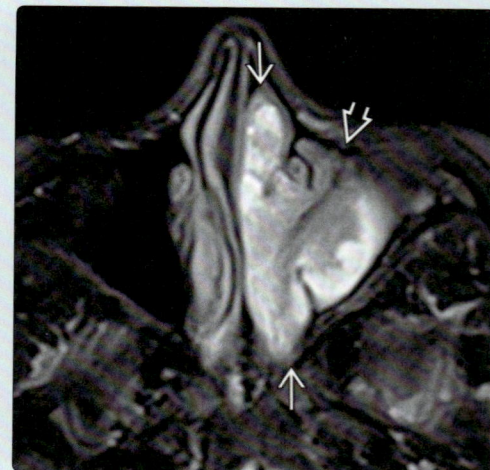

(Left) Axial bone CT demonstrates a polypoid mass within the left maxillary sinus ➡ and left nasal cavity ➡. A large osseous stalk ➡ projects from the left anterior maxillary sinus wall, the attachment site of this IPap. (Right) Axial T2 FS MR in the same patient shows the convoluted, cerebriform pattern ➡ of signal emanating from the hypointense osseous stalk ➡ attached to the left anterior maxillary sinus wall in this case of IPap.

Sinonasal Inverted Papilloma

TERMINOLOGY

Abbreviations
- Inverted papilloma (IPap)

Synonyms
- Sinonasal papilloma, schneiderian papilloma, squamous cell papilloma, endophytic papilloma

Definitions
- Benign epithelial tumor of nasal mucosa with histology showing epithelium proliferating into underlying stroma

IMAGING

General Features
- Best diagnostic clue
  - Mass along lateral nasal wall **centered at middle meatus** ± extension into antrum with local bone remodeling & obstructive sinus disease
- Location
  - Most commonly originates along lateral nasal wall near middle meatus
  - Spreads into adjacent sinuses
    - Maxillary (69%), ethmoid (50-90%), sphenoid (10-20%), frontal (10-15%), orbit & CNS (~ 30%)
  - Uncommonly originates in maxillary antrum, sphenoid, frontal, or ethmoid sinuses
- Size
  - Small IPap: < 3-cm mass centered in middle meatal region of lateral wall of nose
  - Large IPap: > 3-cm mass that remodels nasal cavity, invades or obstructs ipsilateral sinuses

CT Findings
- NECT
  - Soft tissue mass along lateral nasal wall at middle meatus ± extension into maxillary sinus
    - 40% show entrapped bone
    - 10% show tumoral calcification
    - Focal hyperostosis of adjacent bone (plaque- or cone-shaped) may indicate point of tumor origin
  - Unilateral obstruction yields ostiomeatal unit (OMU) pattern of inflammatory sinus disease
  - Small IPap may show no bone changes, making identification of tumor difficult
  - Larger IPap shows bone remodeling & mass effect in middle meatal region
- CECT
  - IPap enhances, whereas obstructed sinus secretions do not
    - Variable enhancement pattern from diffuse to heterogeneous
    - **Convoluted, cerebriform appearance** is classic
    - Consider synchronous squamous cell carcinoma (SCCa) if bony destruction ± focal loss of cerebriform morphology

MR Findings
- T1WI
  - Isointense to slightly hyperintense to soft tissue & muscle
- T2WI
  - Heterogeneous, predominantly hyperintense to skeletal muscle
    - Curvilinear striations or convoluted, cerebriform pattern are classic
  - Loss of convoluted, cerebriform pattern raises concern for SCCa-IPap
- DWI
  - ADC values lower in SCCa-IPap than IPap
- T1WI C+
  - Enhancement may have convoluted, cerebriform appearance
  - If portion of tumor appears invasive or necrosis present, then consider synchronous SCCa

Imaging Recommendations
- Best imaging tool
  - Tumor usually 1st detected on sinus CT performed for evaluation of "sinusitis" symptoms
  - When mass is found on CT, MR completed for preoperative tumor mapping
- Protocol advice
  - Multiplanar MR optimal for tumor mapping & differentiating tumor from obstructed secretions
  - T2 FS & T1 C+ FS sequences best show internal architecture

Nuclear Medicine Findings
- PET/CT
  - High FDG uptake typical in IPap with higher standardized uptake value in associated SCCa
    - PET cannot reliably distinguished benign IPap & SCCa

DIFFERENTIAL DIAGNOSIS

Sinonasal Solitary Polyps
- Antrochoanal polyp: Dumbbell-shaped lesion involving maxillary antrum & ipsilateral nasal cavity
- Peripheral, **not central**, enhancing lesion with mucus or fluid density (CT) or intensity (MR) contents

Sinonasal Polyposis
- Polypoid lesions in nasal cavity & paranasal sinuses
- Bone remodeling & sinus expansion

Sinonasal Squamous Cell Carcinoma
- Destroys, rather than remodels, bones in most cases
- Typically originates within maxillary antrum > nasal cavity

Juvenile Angiofibroma
- Adolescent boys with nosebleeds
- Mass centered at margin of sphenopalatine foramen in posterior nasal cavity
- Intense enhancement of this highly vascular mass is typical

Olfactory Neuroblastoma
- Typically centered in superior nasal cavity near cribriform plate
- Intense enhancement; more likely to invade orbit/anterior skull base

PATHOLOGY

General Features
- Etiology

- Originates in lateral nasal wall or medial maxillary wall from schneiderian sinonasal epithelium
- Neither etiology nor factors responsible for malignant transformation are fully elucidated
  - Viral origin has been postulated (e.g., HPV > > EBV)
- Associated abnormalities
  - **10%** either degenerate into or **coexist with SCCa**
    - SCCa may be either synchronous (7%) or metachronous (4%)

Staging, Grading, & Classification

- 3 sinonasal (schneiderian) papilloma types arise from nasal mucosa
  - IPap (~ 50-80%)
  - Exophytic papilloma (~ 20-50%): Occurs on nasal septum in young males; rarely imaged prior to surgical treatment
  - Oncocytic papilloma (~ 3-5%)
- No widely accepted, clinically relevant staging system

Gross Pathologic & Surgical Features

- Endoscopic or surgical observations
  - Bulky, opaque, polypoid mucosal mass with red-gray color characteristic of lobulated tumor surface

Microscopic Features

- Hyperplastic squamous epithelium replacing seromucinous ducts & glands in underlying stroma
  - Mucosal infoldings into stroma without interrupting basement membrane
- Surrounding nasal mucosa often shows squamous metaplasia

CLINICAL ISSUES

Presentation

- Most common signs/symptoms
  - Similar to recurrent sinusitis with nasal obstruction & discharge
- Other signs/symptoms
  - Epistaxis, anosmia, headache, pain
- Clinical profile
  - Adult **male** patient with symptoms similar to chronic rhinosinusitis

Demographics

- Age
  - Typically 40-70 years
- Sex
  - M > F (3.4:1)
- Epidemiology
  - 0.5-7% of all tumors of nasal cavity
  - Involves at least 1 paranasal sinus 82% of time
  - Typically unifocal; causes unilateral "sinusitis"
    - Multifocal in 4% of cases
  - Bilateral in up to 13% due to transseptal extension

Natural History & Prognosis

- Benign but locally aggressive tumor
  - Strong potential for local recurrence if incompletely resected
  - When SCCa is associated, prognosis changes to survival rates associated with nasal SCCa

Treatment

- Type of surgery depends on location & size of lesion as well as involvement of critical structures
  - Surgical resection using variety of methods
    - Endoscopic resection is effective for most smaller tumors
    - Midfacial degloving & sublabial approaches for larger lesions
    - Medial maxillectomy through lateral rhinotomy + wide en bloc excision in more extensive IPap
  - Electrocautery &/or high-speed drilling of bone at attachment site

DIAGNOSTIC CHECKLIST

Consider

- T1 C+ FS MR used to search for convoluted, cerebriform appearance
- MR used to evaluate for extension beyond sinonasal cavities & differentiate tumor from secretions

Image Interpretation Pearls

- Identify invasion of deeper areas (ethmoid sinuses, pterygopalatine fossa, orbit) at imaging, as this may alter surgical approach
- Areas of necrosis or frank bony destruction should raise suspicion for coexistent SCCa
- Look for additional masses, as 4% are multifocal

SELECTED REFERENCES

1. Sun K et al: Development of a clinical prediction model to predict malignant transformation of sinonasal inverted papilloma based on hematological indices and clinical features. Laryngoscope Investig Otolaryngol. 10(1):e70075, 2025
2. Cho SW et al: Treatment outcome and prognostic factors of inverted papilloma involving the frontal sinus. Laryngoscope Investig Otolaryngol. 9(1):e1206, 2024
3. Talati V et al: Computed tomography imaging patterns of sinonasal inverted papillomas: comparison of primary and recurrent disease. Laryngoscope. 134(4):1591-6, 2024
4. Paehler Vor der Holte A et al: Impact of human papillomaviruses (HPV) on recurrence rate and malignant progression of sinonasal papillomas. Cancer Med. 10(2):634-41, 2021
5. Yan CH et al: Imaging predictors for malignant transformation of inverted papilloma. Laryngoscope. 129(4):777-82, 2019
6. Vorasubin N et al: Schneiderian papillomas: comparative review of exophytic, oncocytic, and inverted types. Am J Rhinol Allergy. 27(4):287-92, 2013
7. Jeon TY et al: 18F-FDG PET/CT findings of sinonasal inverted papilloma with or without coexistent malignancy: comparison with MR imaging findings in eight patients. Neuroradiology. 51(4):265-71, 2009
8. Karkos PD et al: Computed tomography and/or magnetic resonance imaging for pre-operative planning for inverted nasal papilloma: review of evidence. J Laryngol Otol. 123(7):705-9, 2009
9. Jeon TY et al: Sinonasal inverted papilloma: value of convoluted cerebriform pattern on MR imaging. AJNR Am J Neuroradiol. 29(8):1556-60, 2008
10. Lee DK et al: Focal hyperostosis on CT of sinonasal inverted papilloma as a predictor of tumor origin. AJNR Am J Neuroradiol. 28(4):618-21, 2007
11. Shojaku H et al: Positron emission tomography for predicting malignancy of sinonasal inverted papilloma. Clin Nucl Med. 32(4):275-8, 2007
12. Yousuf K et al: Site of attachment of inverted papilloma predicted by CT findings of osteitis. Am J Rhinol. 21(1):32-6, 2007
13. Phillips PP et al: The clinical behavior of inverting papilloma of the nose and paranasal sinuses: report of 112 cases and review of the literature. Laryngoscope. 100(5):463-9, 1990

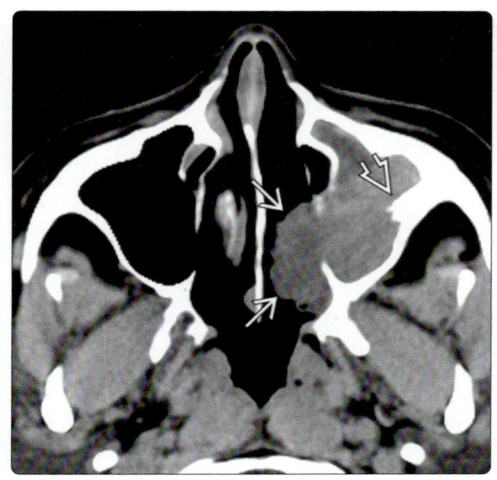
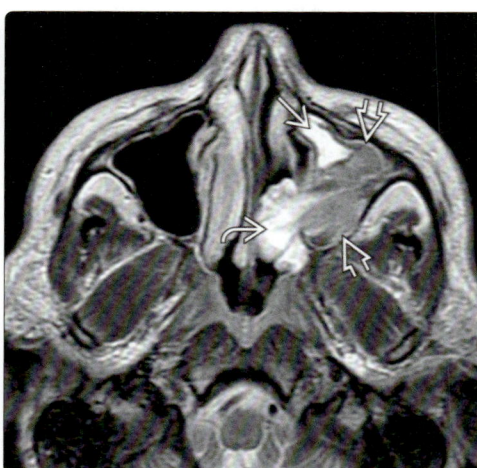

(Left) *Axial NECT shows a slightly lobular soft tissue mass within the left nasal cavity ➡ with extension into the left maxillary sinus with osseous thickening at the site of attachment ➡. It is difficult to differentiate the mass from obstructed secretions on the CT.* (Right) *Axial T2 MR shows a heterogeneous IPap ➡ that occupies most of the maxillary antrum. The mass is hypointense compared to secretions ➡ trapped anteromedially. The nasal component of this papilloma ➡ is hyperintense.*

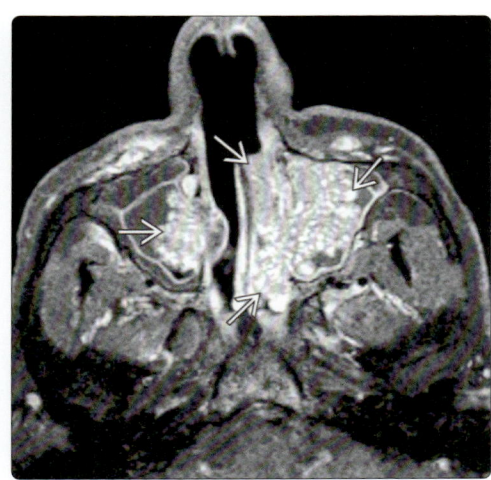
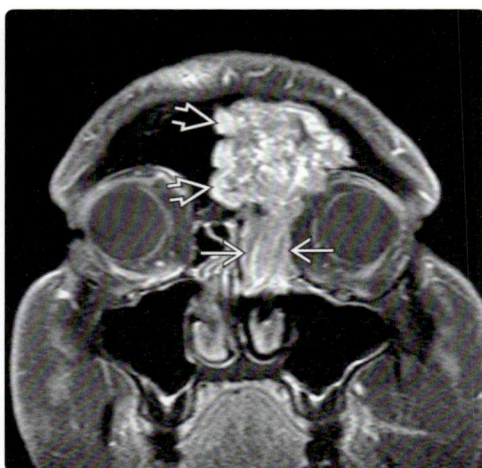

(Left) *Axial T1 C+ MR shows an unusual case of bilateral IPap ➡ due to transseptal extension involving the maxillary sinuses. The larger lesion on the left nearly fills the nasal cavity. Both lesions demonstrate the typical convoluted morphology.* (Right) *Coronal T1 C+ FS MR shows IPap involving the ethmoid sinuses ➡ in addition to the frontal sinus. Trapped secretions ➡ along the margin of the frontal tumor component are proteinaceous with intrinsic T1 shortening.*

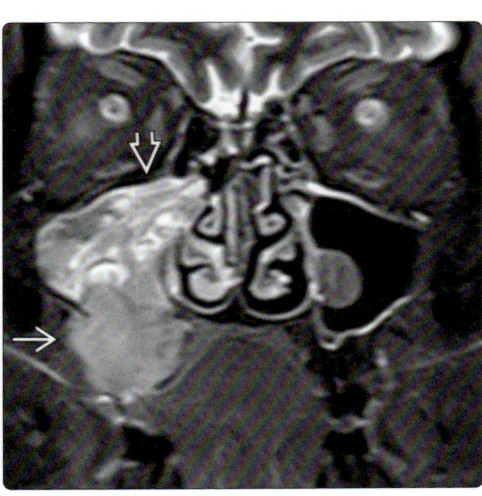
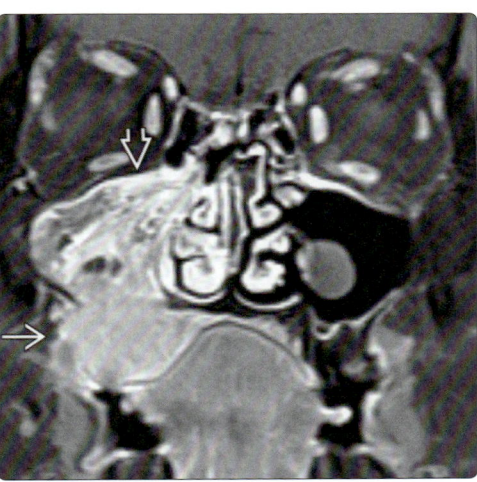

(Left) *Coronal STIR MR shows a mass filling the right maxillary sinus with predominant convoluted, cerebriform pattern ➡. However, an inferior portion with homogeneous intermediate signal intensity ➡ destroys the maxillary sinus floor, consistent with squamous cell carcinoma (SCCa) arising from IPap.* (Right) *Coronal T1 C+ FS MR in the same patient shows convoluted, cerebriform enhancement pattern ➡ of the IPap with loss of this pattern ➡ in the destructive SCCa portion of the mass.*

Sinonasal Hemangioma

TERMINOLOGY

- Lobular capillary hemangioma (LCH): Benign capillary proliferation with distinct lobular architecture

IMAGING

- Location: LCH: Nasal septum (50%) & inferior turbinate (30%)
- Typically ≤ 2 cm
- CT
  - Central areas of lobular enhancement surrounded by iso- to hypodense "cap" of variable thickness
  - May cause bone remodeling
- MR
  - Usually **T2 hyperintense**
  - Homogeneous, **avid enhancement ± flow voids**
- Lobular areas of capillary blush on angiography
  - Preoperative embolization ↓ intraoperative bleeding

TOP DIFFERENTIAL DIAGNOSES

- Venous malformation (old term: Cavernous hemangioma)
  - No central avid enhancement or flow voids
  - Centripetal pattern of enhancement with delayed filling
  - Variable T2 signal
- Juvenile angiofibroma
- Sinonasal melanoma
- Sinonasal pleomorphic adenoma
- Angiomatous polyp

PATHOLOGY

- Predisposing factors include trauma & hormonal influences

CLINICAL ISSUES

- Symptoms: Epistaxis & nasal obstruction
- Peak incidence in 5th decade with slight F > M

DIAGNOSTIC CHECKLIST

- Multiplanar MR if lesion near skull base

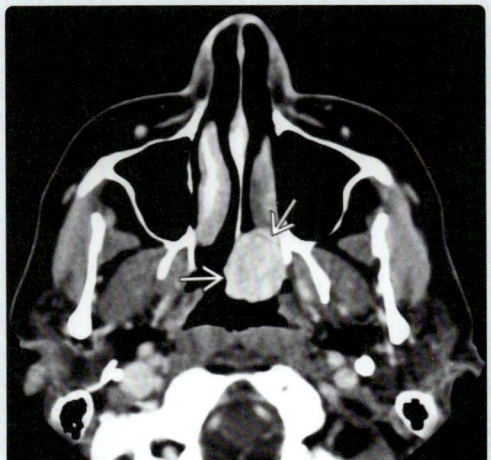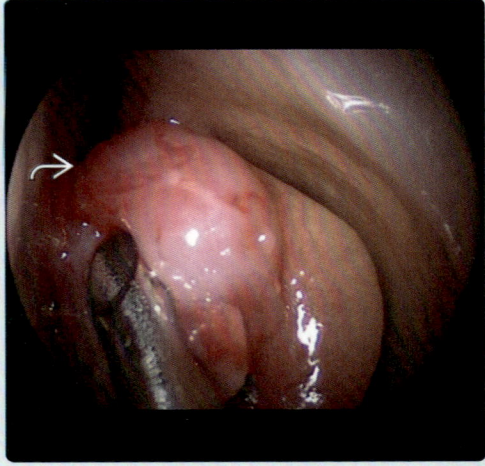

(Left) Axial CECT demonstrates an avidly enhancing, well-circumscribed soft tissue mass ➡ in the posterior nasal cavity and protruding into the nasopharynx. No bony destructive changes were seen. This lobular hemangioma arose from the inferior turbinate; the patient presented with nasal bleeding. (Right) Endoscopic view of a lobular capillary hemangioma shows a lobulated, epithelial-lined, red, hypervascular mass ➡.

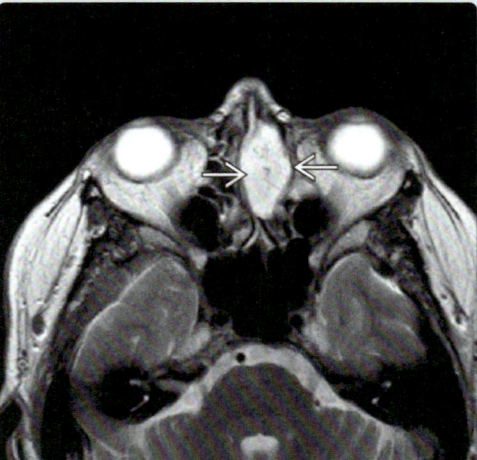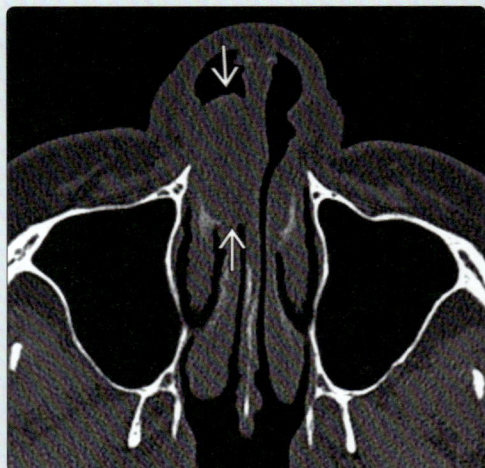

(Left) Axial T2 MR demonstrates a well-defined, ovoid soft tissue mass ➡ in the superior aspect of the left nasal cavity in an adult patient with intermittent epistaxis. The lesion is homogeneously hyperintense on this sequence, typical of hemangioma. No orbital invasion is appreciated. (Right) Axial bone CT in a patient presenting with right nasal obstruction and epistaxis shows a circumscribed mass ➡ in the right anterior nasal cavity without osseous destruction in this case of sinonasal hemangioma.

TERMINOLOGY

Abbreviations
- Lobular capillary hemangioma (LCH)

Synonyms
- Pyogenic granuloma is old term; no evidence for infectious origin & no granulation tissue

Definitions
- Benign capillary proliferation with microscopically distinct lobular architecture affecting lip, nose, oral mucosa, & tongue

IMAGING

General Features
- Best diagnostic clue
  - Well-defined, enhancing nasal cavity mass arising from **anterior septum or turbinates**
- Location
  - LCH: Nasal septum most common (50%), followed by inferior turbinate (30%)
- Size
  - Typically ≤ 2 cm (capillary hemangioma is generally larger than LCH)
- Morphology
  - Well defined, lobulated

CT Findings
- NECT
  - Isodense to slightly hypodense, lobular or polypoid soft tissue mass
- CECT
  - **Avid enhancement**
  - Central areas of lobular enhancement surrounded by iso- to hypodense "cap" of variable thickness
- Bone CT
  - Bones may be normal or show benign remodeling

MR Findings
- T1WI
  - Low- to intermediate-signal mass (compared to muscle)
- T2WI
  - Most often **hyperintense**
  - Larger lesions may show signal voids (**flow voids**)
- T1WI C+
  - Intense homogeneous enhancement > nasal turbinate

Imaging Recommendations
- Best imaging tool
  - Multiplanar enhanced MR
  - If large, bone CT for bone changes

DIFFERENTIAL DIAGNOSIS

Venous Malformation
- Old term is cavernous hemangioma; historical misnomer applies to nonneoplastic **venous malformation**
- May mimic LCH clinically (& even pathologically), but imaging differs
- Lateral nasal wall typical location

- Centripetal-lobular & mild contrast enhancement or multifocal nodular
  - Fills in centrally on delayed imaging
- Heterogeneous & variable T2 signal: Mixed hypo- & hyperintensity
- May cause bone erosion changes

Juvenile Angiofibroma
- Occurs exclusively in males, usually adolescents
- Posteriorly, nasal cavity near sphenopalatine foramen

Sinonasal Melanoma
- Clinical: Middle-aged patient
- ↑ precontrast T1 signal, ↓ T2 signal

Sinonasal Pleomorphic Adenoma
- Circumscribed, enhancing mass arising from minor salivary gland rests
- Typically arises from nasal septum

PATHOLOGY

General Features
- Etiology
  - Predisposing factors include **trauma** (nose picking, nasal packing) & **hormonal factors** (pregnancy, oral contraceptives)

Gross Pathologic & Surgical Features
- Solitary, red to purple, hypervascularized nasal mass ± superficial ulceration
- Pedunculated with stalk or sessile with broad base

Microscopic Features
- Lobular growth pattern of capillary proliferation

CLINICAL ISSUES

Presentation
- Most common signs/symptoms
  - **Epistaxis** & nasal obstruction

Demographics
- Age
  - Peak incidence in 5th decade
- Sex: Slight female predominance

Natural History & Prognosis
- "Pregnancy tumor" may regress after parturition

Treatment
- Local surgical excision

DIAGNOSTIC CHECKLIST

Consider
- Multiplanar MR for tumor mapping if lesion extends superiorly toward skull base

SELECTED REFERENCES

1. Lozano-Burga Y et al: Nasal lobular capillary hemangioma during pregnancy: a systematic review. Ear Nose Throat J. ePub, 2024
2. Valencia-Sanchez BA et al: Pediatric intranasal lobular capillary hemangioma: a scoping review and multimedia case presentation. Ann Plast Surg. 93(5):637-42, 2024

Sinonasal Nerve Sheath Tumor

TERMINOLOGY

- Slow-growing, benign tumors arising from nerve sheath (schwannoma) or peripheral nerve tissue (neurofibroma)
- Peripheral nerve sheath tumor (PNST)

IMAGING

- Well-defined, **expansile** soft tissue mass arising in nasoethmoid region with adjacent bone remodeling
- MR shows extent & differentiates obstructed secretions
  - Hypo- to hyperintense ± **intramural cysts**
  - Schwannoma: **Whorled** pattern of enhancement
- NECT best shows **benign osseous remodeling**

TOP DIFFERENTIAL DIAGNOSES

- Inverted papilloma
- Sinonasal pleomorphic adenoma
- Sinonasal mucocele
- Sinonasal solitary polyp
- Sinonasal hemangioma

PATHOLOGY

- Several PNST types: Schwannoma, neurofibroma, perineurioma (rare in sinonasal region), & malignant PNST
- ↑ incidence of sinonasal neurofibromas in *NF1*
- ↑ incidence of sinonasal schwannomas in *NF2*
- FNA may confuse schwannoma with spindle cell sarcoma

CLINICAL ISSUES

- Rare sinonasal benign tumor
- Nonspecific symptoms may mimic inflammatory disease
  - Nasal obstruction, epistaxis, anosmia
- < 4% of H&N schwannomas arise in sinonasal cavities
- Treatment: Surgical excision is curative

DIAGNOSTIC CHECKLIST

- Imaging role: Direct biopsy, accurately map extent of lesion, & look for orbital/intracranial extension
- Imaging features usually not specific enough to make histologic diagnosis

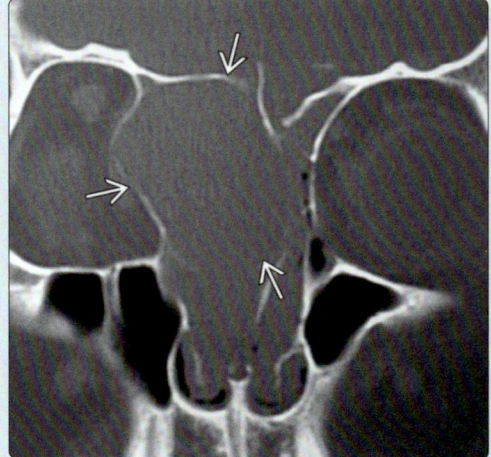
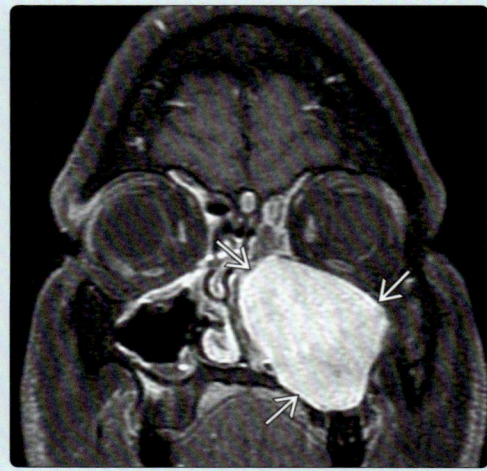

(Left) Coronal bone CT demonstrates an expansile mass involving the right nasal cavity and ethmoid region ➡. Note the smooth remodeling of the bone surrounding the lesion, suggestive of a benign mass. This schwannoma could be confused with a mucocele on CT alone. (Right) Coronal T1 C+ FS MR shows diffuse enhancement throughout a neurofibroma ➡, easily distinguishing this solid enhancing tumor from mucocele, a more common expansile paranasal sinus lesion.

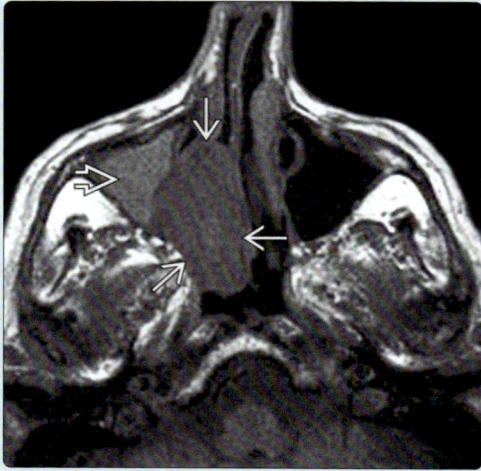
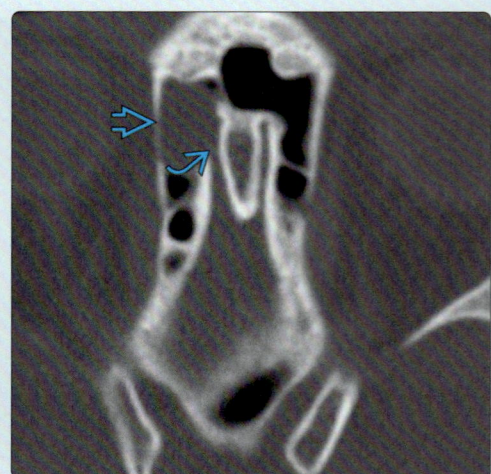

(Left) Axial T1 MR shows a schwannoma in the right nasal cavity ➡ deviating the septum to the left. Trapped secretions with high T1 signal are noted lateral to the mass in the maxillary sinus ➡. (Right) Axial CT shows a small, well-defined mass ➡ in the nasofrontal recess underneath the ethmoid roof, associated with erosion of the lateral wall of the lateral lamella ➡.

Sinonasal Nerve Sheath Tumor

TERMINOLOGY

Synonyms
- Peripheral nerve sheath tumor (PNST)
  - Schwannoma = neurilemoma

Definitions
- Slow-growing, benign tumors of nerve sheath (schwannoma) or peripheral nerve tissue (neurofibroma)

IMAGING

General Features
- Best diagnostic clue
  - Well-defined, expansile soft tissue mass arising in nasoethmoid region with adjacent bone remodeling
- Location
  - Schwannomas most common in nasal cavity & ethmoids
  - Rare cases extend into orbit or intracranially
- Size
  - Can reach large size
- Morphology
  - Usually ovoid-round, smooth margin

Imaging Recommendations
- Best imaging tool
  - MR for extent & differentiate from obstructed secretions
  - Bone CT best shows benign pattern of bone remodeling
- Protocol advice
  - Multiplanar MR with T1, STIR/T2 FS, & T1 C+ FS

CT Findings
- NECT
  - Schwannoma: Isodense to other soft tissue
  - Neurofibroma: May show homogeneous ↓ attenuation
- CECT
  - Variable enhancement but usually mild
- Bone CT
  - **Expansile** mass with **bone remodeling**, not destruction

MR Findings
- T1WI
  - Intermediate signal typical
- T2WI
  - Hypo- to hyperintense ± **intramural cysts**
- T1WI C+ FS
  - Schwannoma: **Whorled** pattern of enhancement

DIFFERENTIAL DIAGNOSIS

Sinonasal Inverted Papilloma
- Convoluted or cerebriform architecture

Sinonasal Pleomorphic Adenoma
- Imaging looks benign but is nonspecific

Sinonasal Mucocele
- Peripheral **(no central) enhancement** with contrast

Solitary Sinonasal Polyps
- Homogeneous ↓ T1 & ↑ T2 MR signal
- Peripheral **(no central) enhancement**

Sinonasal Hemangioma
- Benign enhancing lesion along anterior nasal septum
- Increased incidence during pregnancy

Juvenile Angiofibroma
- Adolescent boys with nasal obstruction & epistaxis
- Highly vascular with avid enhancement & flow voids on MR

Sinonasal Non-Hodgkin Lymphoma
- Malignant lymphoid neoplasm with nasal cavity predilection

Sinonasal Melanoma
- Malignancy typically arising in septum/turbinates
- ↑ T1 & ↓ T2 MR signal typical of highly melanotic lesions

PATHOLOGY

General Features
- Etiology
  - Schwannomas arise from Schwann cells of CNV1 & V2 & autonomic nerves to septal vessels & mucosa
    - Olfactory nerve lacks Schwann cells
- Genetics
  - ↑ incidence of sinonasal neurofibromas in *NF1*
  - ↑ incidence of sinonasal schwannomas in *NF2*

Microscopic Features
- Schwannoma: Compact spindle cell proliferations of hypercellular (Antoni A) & myxoid (Antoni B) areas

CLINICAL ISSUES

Presentation
- Most common signs/symptoms
  - Symptoms often nonspecific; mimics inflammation
  - Nasal obstruction, epistaxis, anosmia

Demographics
- Age
  - Children to older adults
  - Most schwannomas present in 4th-6th decades
- Epidemiology
  - 45% of PNSTs arise in H&N
  - < 4% of H&N schwannomas are sinonasal

Natural History & Prognosis
- Prognosis excellent for benign nerve sheath tumors
- Malignant transformation: Neurofibroma > schwannoma

Treatment
- Surgical excision is curative
- Adjuvant radiotherapy reserved for malignant lesions

DIAGNOSTIC CHECKLIST

Image Interpretation Pearls
- Role of imaging is to direct biopsy, accurately map extent of lesion, and evaluate for orbital/intracranial extension

SELECTED REFERENCES

1. Liao JY et al: Nasal cavity schwannoma-a case report and review of the literature. Ear Nose Throat J. 103(1):19-24, 2024

Sinonasal Pleomorphic Adenoma

TERMINOLOGY

- Pleomorphic adenoma (PA)
- Benign, histologically heterogeneous tumor with epithelial, myoepithelial, & stromal components

IMAGING

- Originates in nasal cavity (septum > lateral nasal) > paranasal sinuses
- CT findings
  - Well-demarcated soft tissue mass in anterior nasal cavity often arising from septum
  - Bone remodeled rather than destroyed
- MR findings
  - Typically **very high T2 signal** and low T1 signal
  - Variable enhancement; heterogeneous in larger lesions

TOP DIFFERENTIAL DIAGNOSES

- Sinonasal solitary polyp
- Sinonasal hemangioma
- Sinonasal inverted papilloma
- Juvenile angiofibroma
- Sinonasal nerve sheath tumor

PATHOLOGY

- Thought to arise from minor salivary rests
  - Nasal septal PA tends to be highly cellular with little stromal component (compared to salivary gland tumors)

CLINICAL ISSUES

- Presentation
  - Nasal obstruction ± epistaxis
  - Most present at 30-60 years
  - More common in women
- Slow growing with excellent prognosis
- Treatment is local surgical excision
- Consider PA in adult patient with benign-appearing anterior nasal mass

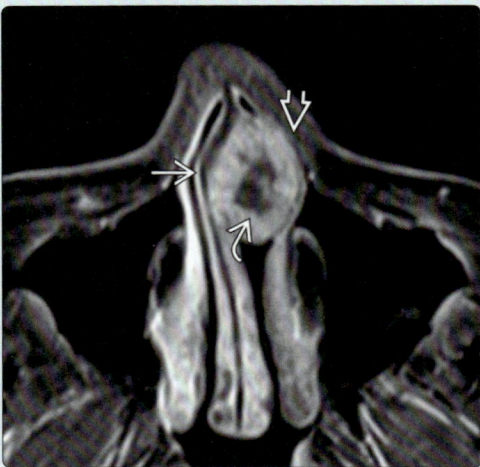
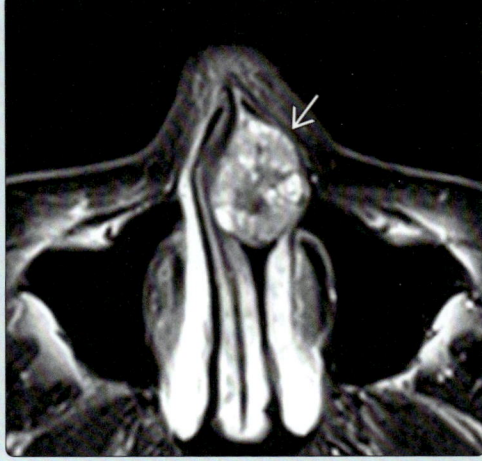

(Left) *Axial T1 C+ FS MR shows a circumscribed, enhancing mass arising from the left anterior nasal septum* ➡ *with smooth osseous remodeling* ➡ *in this case of sinonasal pleomorphic adenoma (PA). Larger lesions may demonstrate heterogeneous internal enhancement* ➡. (Right) *Axial T2 FS MR in the same patient demonstrates heterogeneous, predominantly hyperintense T2 signal intensity* ➡ *within the sinonasal PA.*

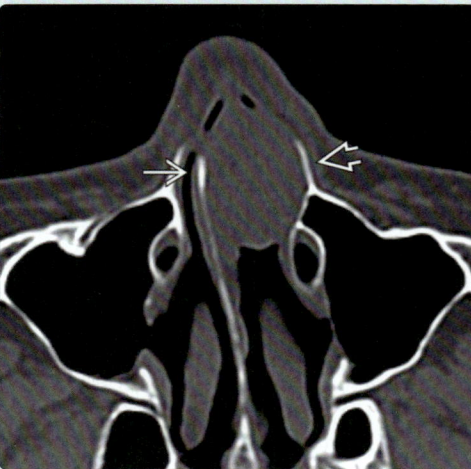
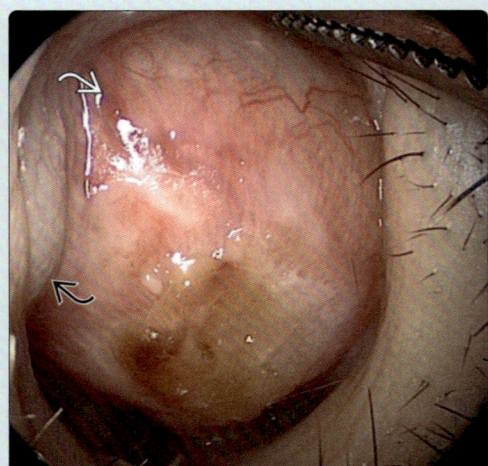

(Left) *Axial bone CT in the same patient demonstrates the circumscribed PA in the left nasal cavity adjacent to the nasal septum with osseous remodeling, but not destruction, of the nasal septum* ➡ *and lateral nasal wall* ➡, *which is typical of a benign lesion.* (Right) *Nasal endoscopic view demonstrates a well-circumscribed, round PA* ➡ *in the anterior nasal cavity originating from the anterior nasal septum* ➡.

TERMINOLOGY

Abbreviations

- Pleomorphic adenoma (PA)

Synonyms

- Benign mixed tumor

Definitions

- Benign, histologically heterogeneous tumor with epithelial, myoepithelial, & stromal components

IMAGING

General Features

- Best diagnostic clue
  - Sharply marginated, round-ovoid soft tissue mass ± adjacent bone remodeling
- Location
  - Nasal cavity (septum > lateral nasal) > paranasal sinuses
    - Maxillary sinus & nasopharynx less common
- Size
  - Most < 2 cm
- Morphology
  - Round or ovoid with well-defined margins
  - Larger lesions may have lobular margins

Imaging Recommendations

- Best imaging tool
  - CECT vs. multiplanar enhanced MR
- Protocol advice
  - Bone window images helpful for evaluating bone remodeling

CT Findings

- NECT
  - Well-demarcated soft tissue mass in anterior nasal cavity often arising from septum
- CECT
  - Variable enhancement; heterogeneous in larger lesions
- Bone CT
  - Bone **remodeling** rather than destruction

MR Findings

- T1WI
  - Well-circumscribed, low-signal mass
- T2WI
  - Typically **very high T2** signal
    - Heterogeneous signal in larger lesions
- DWI
  - No diffusion restriction: High ADC value
- T1WI C+ FS
  - Small lesions enhance homogeneously
  - Heterogeneous enhancement in larger PA

DIFFERENTIAL DIAGNOSIS

Sinonasal Solitary Polyp

- Low attenuation with peripheral enhancement only
- Usually arises in maxillary antrum & extends into nasal cavity

Sinonasal Hemangioma

- Circumscribed, enhancing mass presenting with epistaxis

- Typically arises from nasal septum

Sinonasal Inverted Papilloma

- Arises along lateral nasal wall near middle meatus
- Convoluted, cerebriform architecture ± calcification

Juvenile Angiofibroma

- Adolescent male patient with nasal obstruction & epistaxis
- Arises in posterior nasal cavity near sphenopalatine foramen
- Vascular lesion with avid enhancement & flow voids

Sinonasal Nerve Sheath Tumor

- Rare, benign mass
- Usually arises in superior nasal cavity

PATHOLOGY

General Features

- Etiology
  - Thought to arise from **minor salivary rests**

Microscopic Features

- Lobular architecture of loose chondromyxoid stroma & cellular component of rounded epithelial & spindle-shaped myoepithelial cells

CLINICAL ISSUES

Presentation

- Most common signs/symptoms
  - Nasal obstruction or intermittent epistaxis
- Other signs/symptoms
  - Swelling or mass of nose

Demographics

- Age
  - Most present at 30-60 years but can occur at any age
- Sex
  - F > M
- Epidemiology
  - 8% of PAs arise from minor salivary rests in aerodigestive tract

Natural History & Prognosis

- Slow growing with excellent prognosis
- Tendency to recur if incompletely resected
- ~ 6% risk of malignant transformation (carcinoma ex pleomorphic adenoma)

Treatment

- Local surgical excision with clear margins generally curative

DIAGNOSTIC CHECKLIST

Consider

- Benign-appearing anterior nasal cavity mass

SELECTED REFERENCES

1. Konsulov S et al: Diagnostic challenges of sinonasal pleomorphic adenoma. Cureus. 16(2):e54010, 2024
2. Karligkiotis A et al: Endoscopic endonasal resection of sinonasal and nasopharyngeal pleomorphic adenomas: a case series. Turk Arch Otorhinolaryngol. 58(3):186-92, 2020

Sinonasal Hamartomas

TERMINOLOGY

- REAH: Most common; overgrowth of surface epithelium-derived, medium-sized, ciliated glands surrounded by thickened basement membrane
- SMH: Benign proliferation of small eosinophilic glands arising in sinonasal tract
- CMH: Benign mesenchymal sinonasal tract tumor composed of cysts lined by respiratory epithelium associated with cartilaginous nodules and variably myxoid spindle cell stroma

IMAGING

- Nonaggressive sinonasal mass with little to no enhancement
- Expanded olfactory cleft without bony erosion
- 3 variants may appear similar on imaging
  - REAH: Nasal cavity, especially posterior septum & olfactory cleft, ± ethmoids
    - Commonly bilateral
  - SMH: Typically posterior nasal septum & nasopharynx
  - CMH: Often bilateral, sinonasal ± skull base extension

TOP DIFFERENTIAL DIAGNOSES

- Sinonasal inflammatory polyp
- Inverted papilloma
- Olfactory neuroblastoma

PATHOLOGY

- CMH is associated with *DICER1* pathogenic variants

CLINICAL ISSUES

- Clinical presentation: Nasal obstruction, anosmia, headache, epistaxis, often with chronic rhinosinusitis
- Male predominance, median age 6th decade (11-86 years)
- Treatment: Complete resection

DIAGNOSTIC CHECKLIST

- Discoid or polypoid shape on sagittal MPR
- Isolated olfactory cleft opacification, uni- or bilateral

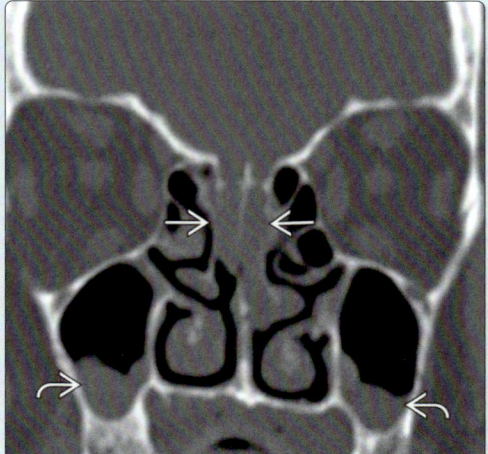
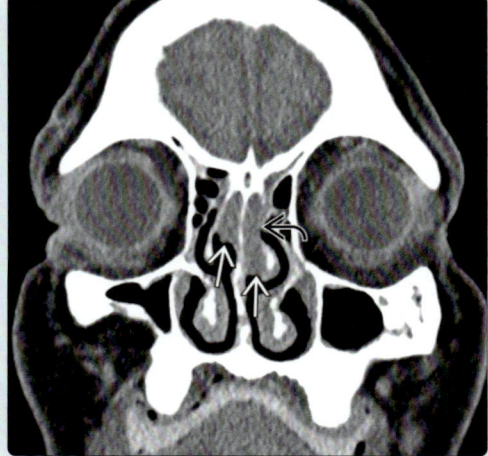

(Left) Coronal bone CT shows typical findings in REAH with opacification of both olfactory clefts ➡. There appears to be mild bone expansion, and the bony septum appears thinned without overt bone destruction. Additional areas of mucosal thickening ➡ are noted. (Right) Coronal CT in a patient with allergies and rhinosinusitis presenting with intermittent epistaxis shows bilateral olfactory cleft hypodense soft tissue opacification due to REAH ➡. Mild osseous erosive changes ➡ are noted. Bilateral involvement is typical.

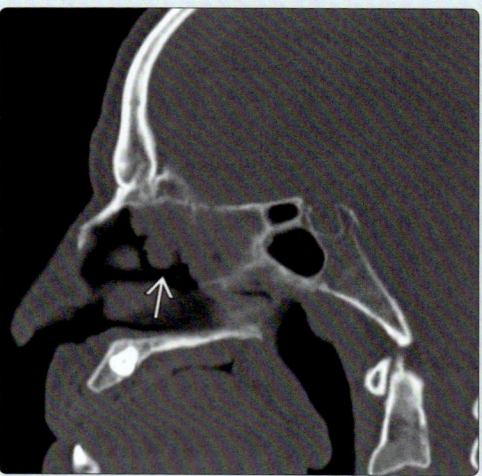
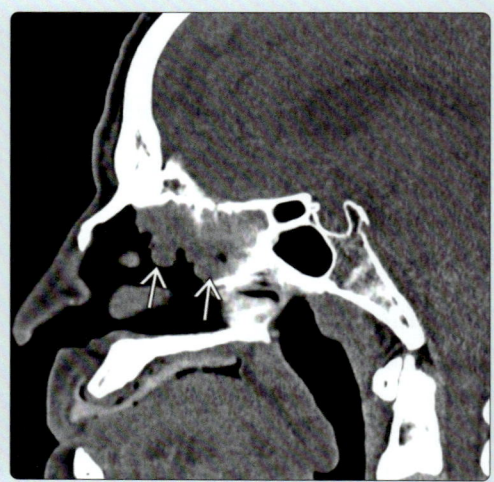

(Left) Sagittal bone CT shows polypoid soft tissue opacification below the planum sphenoidale ➡ due to REAH. No osseous destructive changes are present. This appearance is similar to sinonasal polyposis and requires direct visualization and biopsy to confirm. (Right) Sagittal CT in the same patient shows low-density, lobulated polypoid soft tissue opacification ➡ abutting the anterior skull base in the olfactory cleft due to REAH.

TERMINOLOGY

Definitions

- **3 subtypes**
  - Respiratory epithelial adenomatous hamartoma (REAH): Most common; overgrowth of surface epithelium-derived ciliated glands
  - Seromucinous hamartoma (SMH): Benign proliferation of sinonasal tract eosinophilic glands
  - Chondromesenchymal hamartoma (CMH): Benign sinonasal tract tumor composed of respiratory epithelial-lined cysts associated with cartilaginous nodules in myxoid stroma

IMAGING

General Features

- Best diagnostic clue
  - Nonaggressive soft tissue mass of nasal cavity or paranasal sinuses with little to no enhancement
  - 3 variants may appear similar on imaging
- Location
  - REAH: Nasal cavity, especially posterior septum & olfactory cleft, ± ethmoids
    - Commonly bilateral
  - SMH: Nasal cavity and paranasal sinuses, typically posterior nasal septum & nasopharynx
  - CMH: Frequently bilateral (~ 25%), tumors involve paranasal sinuses (mostly ethmoid) & nasal cavity, sometimes with skull base extension
- Morphology
  - Expansion of olfactory cleft without bony erosion

CT Findings

- REAH: Lobulated soft tissue expanding olfactory cleft(s)
  - May have bone expansion/remodeling
- SMH: Well circumscribed & homogeneous
- CMH: Complex, solid & cystic, heterogeneous soft tissue mass, frequent calcification, & bone erosion

MR Findings

- REAH: Little to no enhancement
- SMH: Well circumscribed & homogeneous

Imaging Recommendations

- Best imaging tool
  - CT

DIFFERENTIAL DIAGNOSIS

Sinonasal Inflammatory Polyp

- No bone expansion, erosion, or solid enhancement

Inverted Papilloma

- Solid-appearing, enhancing sinonasal mass

Olfactory Neuroblastoma

- Erosion of cribriform plate, intracranial extension

PATHOLOGY

General Features

- CMH is associated with *DICER1* pathogenic variants

Gross Pathologic & Surgical Features

- REAH: Polypoid or exophytic with rubbery consistency, tan-white to reddish brown, up to 60 mm
- SMH: Polypoid mass, ranging 4-60 mm
- CMH: Polypoid, fleshy soft tissue masses

Microscopic Features

- REAH: Polypoid glandular proliferation expanding from surface epithelium into stroma
- SMH: Polypoid lesion lined by respiratory ciliated epithelium with eosinophilic stromal glands
- CMH: Cysts lined by respiratory epithelium with cartilaginous nodules in bland spindled cell stroma

CLINICAL ISSUES

Presentation

- Most common signs/symptoms
  - REAH: Nasal obstruction, anosmia, headache, epistaxis, often with chronic rhinosinusitis
    - Male predominance, median age 6th decade
  - SMH: Nasal obstruction, purulent rhinorrhea, epistaxis
    - Wide age range (11-86 years)
  - CMH
    - Part of *DICER1*
    - < 1% of pleuropulmonary blastoma patients have CMH
- Other signs/symptoms
  - REAH may be incidental isolated finding or in association with polyps, inverted papilloma, or adenocarcinomas

Demographics

- Associated with allergy & sinonasal inflammatory disorders

Natural History & Prognosis

- Good prognosis, considered benign
- REAH & SMH: Rare recurrence after resection
- CMH: ~ 25% recur locally if incompletely resected

Treatment

- Complete resection

DIAGNOSTIC CHECKLIST

Consider

- Isolated olfactory cleft opacification, uni- or bilateral

Image Interpretation Pearls

- Discoid or polypoid shape on sagittal MPR

SELECTED REFERENCES

1. Schemel AF et al: Respiratory epithelial adenomatoid hamartoma. Head Neck Pathol. 17(2):498-501, 2023
2. WHO Classification of Tumours Online: Head and neck tumours. 9th version. Published 2023. Accessed March 31, 2025. https://tumourclassification.iarc.who.int/chapters/52
3. Hawley KA et al: CT findings of sinonasal respiratory epithelial adenomatoid hamartoma: a closer look at the olfactory clefts. AJNR Am J Neuroradiol. 34(5):1086-90 2013

Sinonasal Glomangiopericytoma

TERMINOLOGY

- Rare benign sinonasal vascular neoplasm of pericytes
- Older term hemangiopericytoma not preferred

IMAGING

- Markedly enhancing nasal cavity mass
- Mean size: 3 cm
- Morphology: Usually unilateral, round or lobulated
- CT: Soft tissue density mass ± calcification
- MR: T1 iso- to hypointense, T2 iso- to hyperintense
- C+ MR: Intense enhancement
- DCE show rapid wash-in & wash-out of contrast

TOP DIFFERENTIAL DIAGNOSES

- Sinonasal melanoma
- Solitary fibrous tumor
- Sinonasal tract angiofibroma
- Lobular capillary hemangioma

PATHOLOGY

- Gross: Polypoid mass, red to pink with hemorrhage
- Microscopic: Ovoid to spindled syncytium of myoid-type cells within richly vascularized stroma
  - Intact surface epithelium
- Immunohistochemistry: Positive for α-smooth muscle actin
- Molecular genetics: *CTNNB1* mutations

CLINICAL ISSUES

- Peak incidence: 6th-7th decades
- Symptoms: Nasal obstruction, epistaxis, facial pain
- Treatment: Surgical resection
- Good prognosis, rare nodal or distant metastases

DIAGNOSTIC CHECKLIST

- Consider if nasal cavity mass in older patient with epistaxis having benign bone changes & avid enhancement
- Consider preoperative embolization to ↓ bleeding

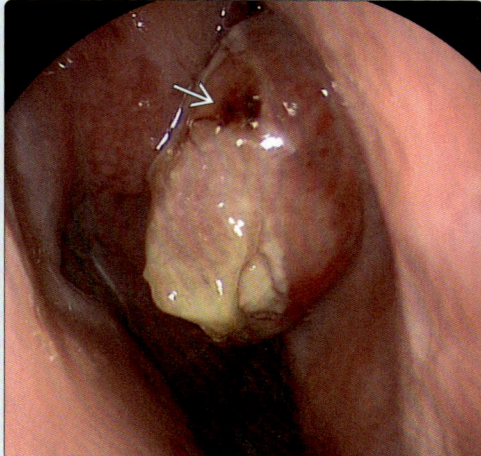
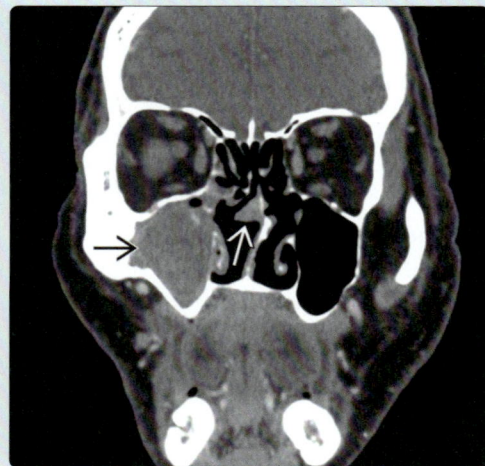

(Left) *Nasal endoscopy in a patient with epistaxis and a history of oral anticoagulation shows a vascular nasal cavity mass with focal bleeding ➡.* (Right) *Coronal CECT in the same patient shows a small, irregular, triangular-shaped, enhancing mass arising along the nasal septum ➡. Enhancement/density and shape are clues to the diagnosis of a neoplasm because a benign polyp would be rounded and have water density. There are unrelated obstructed secretions in the right maxillary sinus ➡.*

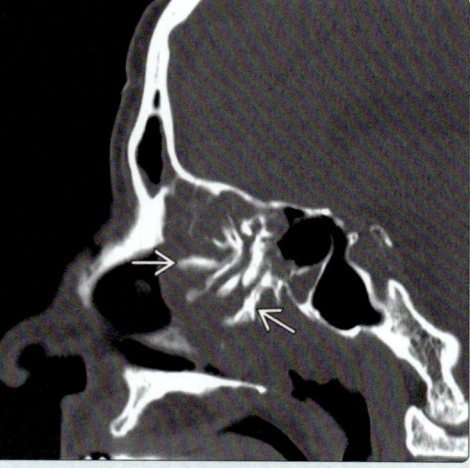
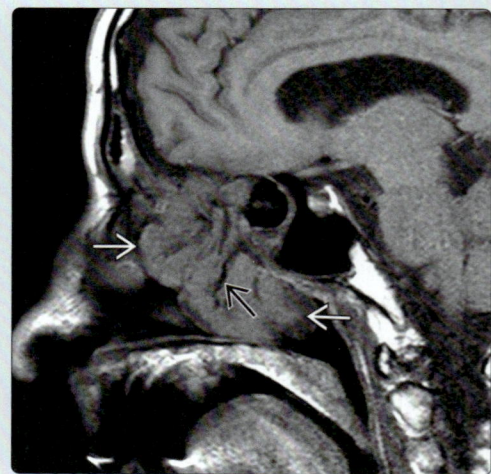

(Left) *Sagittal bone CT in a patient with symptoms of unilateral nasal obstruction and clinical signs of sinusitis shows dense foci of calcification within a nasal cavity mass ➡. Fragments of mature bone were present in the pathology specimen.* (Right) *Sagittal T1 MR in the same patient shows a soft tissue mass iso- to hypointense relative to gray matter in the posterior nasal cavity and ethmoids ➡ with linear foci of intratumoral hypointensity ➡ correlating to calcifications on CT.*

TERMINOLOGY

Abbreviations
- Glomangiopericytoma (GPC)

Synonyms
- Sinonasal-type hemangiopericytoma & myopericytoma are older terms, not preferred

Definitions
- Rare benign vascular neoplasm of pericytes

IMAGING

General Features
- Best diagnostic clue
  - Markedly enhancing nasal cavity mass
- Location
  - Nasal cavity ± sinuses (ethmoid, maxillary, sphenoid)
- Size
  - Variable, 1-5 cm (mean 3 cm)
- Morphology
  - Unilateral (< 5% bilateral), round or lobulated

CT Findings
- Soft tissue density mass ± Ca^{++} or bone formation

MR Findings
- T1 iso- to hypointense ± calcifications
- T2 iso- to hyperintense, heterogeneous
- T1 C+ shows intense enhancement
- DCE show rapid wash-in & wash-out of contrast
- Flow voids uncommon but possible
- High mean ADC value

Imaging Recommendations
- Best imaging tool
  - CT & MR complementary
- Consider preoperative embolization, may ↓ bleeding at surgery

DIFFERENTIAL DIAGNOSIS

Sinonasal Melanoma
- Intrinsic T1 hyperintensity may be clue, if present

Solitary Fibrous Tumor
- Imaging mimic; immunohistochemical panels (&/or molecular genetics) differentiate solitary fibrous tumor (SFT) from GPC

Sinonasal Tract Angiofibroma
- Centered at sphenopalatine foramen, flow voids typical
- Younger demographic: Teen males with epistaxis

Lobular Capillary Hemangioma
- Imaging appearance is similar, flow voids

PATHOLOGY

General Features
- 1% of all sinonasal tract neoplasms
- Borderline benign to low-grade malignant tumor

Staging, Grading, & Classification
- Follows 8th edition AJCC sinonasal tumor staging

Gross Pathologic & Surgical Features
- Polypoid mass, beefy red to grayish pink with hemorrhage
- Endoscopically mass appears submucosal on exam

Microscopic Features
- Intact overlying respiratory epithelium
- Ovoid to spindled syncytium of myoid-type cells within richly vascularized stroma

Immunohistochemistry
- Positive for α-smooth muscle actin
- Typically CD34 (-) differentiates from SFT, which is CD34 (+)
- Nuclear signal transducer & activator of transcription (STAT) 6 (-) differentiates from SFT, which is STAT (+)

Molecular Genetics
- *CTNNB1* mutations

CLINICAL ISSUES

Presentation
- Most common signs/symptoms
  - Nasal obstruction, epistaxis, facial pain
- Other signs/symptoms
  - Headaches, anosmia or hyposmia, proptosis
  - Rare osteomalacia: ↓ serum phosphate & ↑ alkaline phosphatase
- < 0.5% incidence of all sinonasal tract neoplasms

Demographics
- Peak incidence: 6th-7th decades
- Slight female predominance

Natural History & Prognosis
- Good prognosis, rare nodal or distant metastases
- 5-year survival rate: 88%

Treatment
- Surgical resection, often done endoscopically

DIAGNOSTIC CHECKLIST

Consider
- Slow-growing, intensely enhancing nasal cavity mass

Image Interpretation Pearls
- Unilateral nasal mass with nonaggressive bone changes

Reporting Tips
- Consider preoperative embolization

SELECTED REFERENCES

1. Lo Casto A et al: Uncommon nasal mass presentation: a radiological case series. J Pers Med. 14(12):1145, 2024
2. WHO Classification of Tumours Editorial Board: WHO Classification of Tumours: Head and Neck Tumours, 5th ed. IARC, 2024
3. Agarwal A et al: Update from the 5th Edition of the WHO Classification of Nasal, Paranasal, and Skull Base Tumors: imaging overview with histopathologic and genetic correlation. AJNR Am J Neuroradiol. 44(10):1116-25, 2023
4. Suh CH et al: CT and MRI findings of glomangiopericytoma in the head and neck: case series study and systematic review. AJNR Am J Neuroradiol. 41(1):155-9, 2020

TERMINOLOGY

- Malignant epithelial tumor with squamous cell or epidermoid differentiation

IMAGING

- Location: Maxillary antrum involved in > 80%
- CT findings
  - Soft tissue density mass with irregular margins
  - Aggressive **bone destruction**
- MR findings
  - ↓ T2 signal due to ↑ nuclear:cytoplasmic ratio
  - Enhances to lesser degree than other sinonasal malignancies
- Multiplanar enhanced MR optimal for tumor mapping, detection of perineural tumor spread & nodes

TOP DIFFERENTIAL DIAGNOSES

- Sinonasal adenocarcinoma
- Sinonasal undifferentiated carcinoma
- Invasive fungal sinusitis
- Sinonasal non-Hodgkin lymphoma
- Granulomatosis with polyangiitis (Wegener)
- Adenoid cystic carcinoma

PATHOLOGY

- Risk factors: Inhaled wood dust, metallic particles (nickel & chromium), chemicals, HPV, inverted papilloma
  - Formaldehyde, arsenic, & asbestos exposure may ↑ risk
  - HPV, pre- or coexisting inverted papilloma ↑ risk

CLINICAL ISSUES

- Symptoms mimic chronic sinusitis & delay diagnosis
- Age at presentation: 50-70 years old
- Most common malignancy of sinonasal area
- 15% of maxillary sinus squamous cell carcinomas have malignant adenopathy
- Overall **5-year survival: 60%**
- Combined surgery & XRT most common treatment

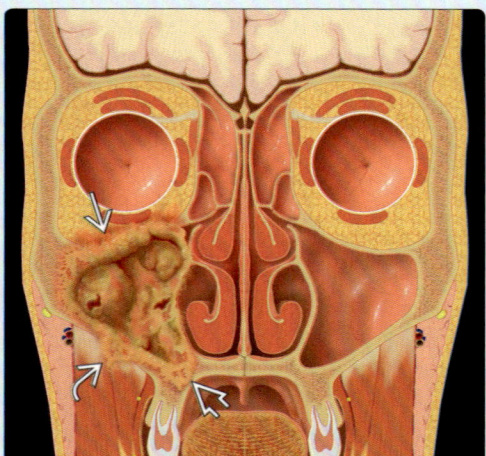
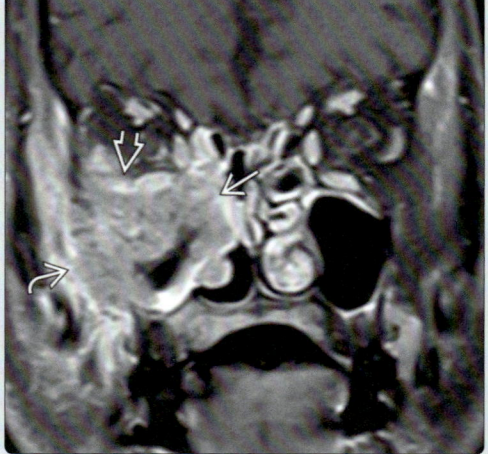

(Left) Coronal graphic shows the typical features of an aggressive right maxillary squamous cell carcinoma (SCCa) with destruction of the maxillary sinus walls. Extension into the orbit ➡, maxillary alveolus ➡, and buccal space ➡ is noted. (Right) Coronal T1 C+ FS MR shows an enhancing mass in the right maxillary sinus ➡ extending into the adjacent orbit ➡ and masticator spaces ➡ in this case of sinonasal SCCa.

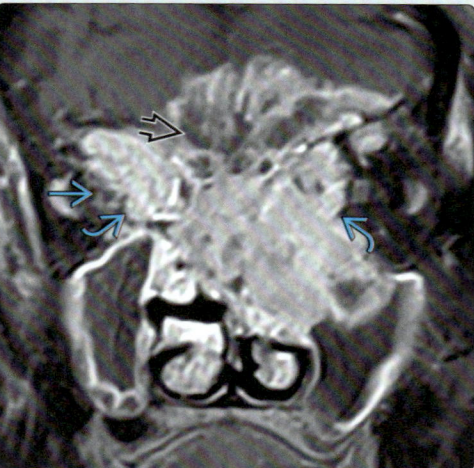
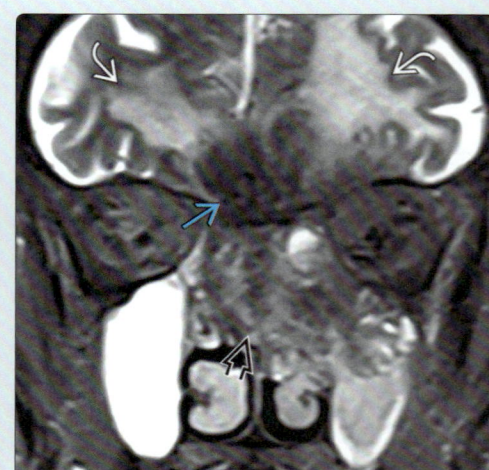

(Left) Coronal T1 C+ FS MR shows a large sinonasal mass with gross intracranial ➡ and bilateral orbital extension ➡. Notice that the right optic nerve/sheath complex is involved ➡. (Right) Coronal T2 FS MR shows a large, infiltrative sinonasal mass ➡ with intracranial extension. Extensive vasogenic edema ➡ is noted in the bilateral frontal lobe. Marked hypointensity in the intracranial component likely reflects a hypercellular nature ➡.

Sinonasal Squamous Cell Carcinoma

TERMINOLOGY

Abbreviations
- Squamous cell carcinoma (SCCa)

Synonyms
- Epidermoid carcinoma, transitional carcinoma, nonkeratinizing carcinoma, respiratory mucosal carcinoma

Definitions
- Malignant epithelial tumor growing from sinus surface epithelium into sinus lumen with squamous cell or epidermoid differentiation

IMAGING

General Features
- Best diagnostic clue
  - Aggressive antral soft tissue mass with invasion & destruction of sinus walls
- Location
  - 75% arise in sinuses; 25% arise primarily in nasal cavity
    - **Maxillary antrum (85%)**, ethmoid (10%), frontal/sphenoid (< 5%)
  - Radiologist creates presurgical tumor map of spread
    - Medial: Nasal cavity → ethmoid sinuses
    - Anterior: Premaxillary soft tissues of cheek → V2 nerve involvement at infraorbital foramen
    - Posterior: Retroantral fat pad, pterygopalatine fossa (PPF), & masticator space
    - Lateral: Malar eminence & subcutaneous tissues
    - Superior: Through orbital floor into orbit proper or via PPF → inferior orbital fissure → orbit
    - Inferior: Maxillary alveolar ridge, buccal space, & hard palate
    - Perineural tumor spread (PNTS): Infraorbital nerve or PPF → V2 (foramen rotundum) → cavernous sinus
- Size
  - Usually fills maxillary antrum
- Morphology
  - Often irregular & **spiculated margins**

CT Findings
- CECT
  - Solid, moderately enhancing mass with aggressive bone destruction
  - Enhancement tends to be heterogeneous
  - Nonenhancing areas may represent necrosis
- Bone CT
  - **Bone destruction** is characteristic
  - Soft tissue density mass with irregular margins

MR Findings
- T1WI
  - Intermediate-signal mass, similar to muscle signal: Look for displacement of adjacent fat
  - Areas of intratumoral hemorrhage may show ↑ T1 signal
- T2WI
  - Intermediate to high signal compared to musculature but lower than other sinonasal malignancies
    - **↓ T2 signal** due to ↑ cellularity

  - T2 differentiates high-signal obstructed sinus secretions from tumor
- DWI
  - Mildly ↓ ADC due to ↑ N:C ratio
- T1WI C+
  - Enhancement typically mild to moderate; diffuse but heterogeneous
    - **Enhances to lesser degree** than adenocarcinoma, olfactory neuroblastoma, melanoma
  - Areas of necrosis do not enhance
  - T1 C+ FS images optimal for detecting PNTS

Nuclear Medicine Findings
- PET
  - Avid uptake of F-18 FDG due to hypermetabolism
    - Useful in staging to identify metastatic disease
    - High sensitivity for detection of recurrent disease
  - If SCCa arose in inverted papilloma, both may show FDG-avid uptake

Imaging Recommendations
- Best imaging tool
  - Most are initially diagnosed on routine NECT for evaluation of "sinusitis" symptoms
  - Multiplanar enhanced MR optimal for tumor mapping, detection of PNTS, & retropharyngeal nodes
- Protocol advice
  - Precontrast T1 & postcontrast T1 MR with fat suppression from sellar floor to hyoid bone

DIFFERENTIAL DIAGNOSIS

Sinonasal Adenocarcinoma
- Imaging features can be similar to SCCa
- Predilection for ethmoid sinus
- Tends to enhance more than SCCa

Sinonasal Undifferentiated Carcinoma
- Can be impossible to distinguish from SCCa
- Rapidly growing

Invasive Fungal Sinusitis
- Immunocompromised patient
- Rapidly progressive destructive lesion
- Internal carotid artery (ICA) invasion and thrombosis may be associated

Sinonasal Non-Hodgkin Lymphoma
- Bulky, homogeneous sinonasal mass (B-cell type)
- Tendency to cause nasal septum destruction (NKTL type)
- May exactly mimic Wegener granulomatosis

Granulomatosis With Polyangiitis (Wegener Granulomatosis)
- Septal & nonseptal bone destruction in nose
- Chronic sinusitis associated
- Sinonasal disease associated with tracheobronchial & renal disease

PATHOLOGY

General Features
- Etiology

o Risk factors: Inhaled wood dust, metallic particles (nickel, chromium), & chemicals used in leather & textile industries; Thorotrast exposure
  – Formaldehyde & asbestos exposure may ↑ risk
  – HPV, pre- or coexisting inverted papilloma ↑ risk
  – No direct link to alcohol or tobacco use

Staging, Grading, & Classification

- Staging taken from American Joint Committee on Cancer (AJCC) staging tables (8th edition)
- **Maxillary sinus** primary tumor (T) staging criteria
  o **T1**: Maxillary antrum only; **no bone destruction**
  o **T2**: Bone invasion (hard palate, nasal wall); **not** involving posterior wall maxillary sinus or pterygoid plates
  o **T3**: Invades bone of posterior wall ± subcutaneous tissues ± floor of medial orbital wall ± pterygoid fossa ± ethmoid sinuses
  o **T4a** (resectable): Invades anterior orbit, skin, infratemporal fossa, pterygoid plates, cribriform plate, frontal or sphenoid sinuses
  o **T4b** (unresectable): Involves orbital apex, dura, brain, middle fossa, clivus, nasopharynx, non-V2 cranial nerves

Gross Pathologic & Surgical Features

- Friable, polypoid, papillary, or fungating soft tissue mass
- Aggressive spread into adjacent structures

Microscopic Features

- 2 main subtypes: Keratinizing (80%) & nonkeratinizing (20%)
  o Keratinizing: Papillary or inverted architectural patterns; dyskeratosis, poorly to well differentiated
  o Nonkeratinizing: Exophytic pattern; interconnecting ribbon-like growth, hypercellular, pleomorphism; used to be called transitional cell carcinoma
- Papillary variant of SCCa uncommon

CLINICAL ISSUES

Presentation

- Most common signs/symptoms
  o **Symptoms mimic chronic sinusitis** & delay diagnosis
  o Nasal cavity primaries present earlier with nasal obstruction, bleeding
- Other signs/symptoms
  o Larger maxillary tumors: Unilateral nasal obstruction, epistaxis, & cheek numbness
  o Tooth pain or loosening, proptosis & diplopia, trismus, facial asymmetry
- Clinical profile
  o Older male patient presenting with unilateral sinusitis refractory to medical therapy

Demographics

- Age
  o 50-70 years old
- Epidemiology
  o 3% of H&N neoplasms
  o **Most common malignancy** of sinonasal area
    – SCCa accounts for 80% of malignant tumors of sinonasal area
  o 15% of maxillary sinus SCCa have malignant adenopathy

  – Retropharyngeal or level I & II nodes
  – Parotid nodes when primary tumor involves facial skin
o ↑ incidence if history of radiation therapy
o 20-25% sinonasal SCCa are HPV(+); more common in nasal cavity & ethmoid → younger patients & better prognosis than HPV(-) SCCa

Natural History & Prognosis

- Overall **5-year survival: 60%**
- Survival statistics heavily influenced by tumor stage
  o T1 SCCa treated aggressively have 100% survival (rarely diagnosed at T1 primary stage)
  o 5-year survival rates for T4a primary SCCa drop to 34%
- Better prognosis: Nasal cavity SCCa, low tumor stage, HPV(+) tumor, & history of inverted papilloma
- Worse prognosis: Extension beyond sinus walls, regional nodal disease, PNTS, large primary tumor size
- Recurrence rate: 10-30%
- Relapse occurs at primary site > regional lymph nodes
  o If tumor recurs, 90% < 1-year survival

Treatment

- Combined treatment with surgery & XRT
  o En bloc resection vs. endoscopic resection depending on tumor size & structures involved
  o XRT may be conventional, 3D conformal, or IMRT
- Chemotherapy gaining popularity as genetics of SCCa are better understood
  o Induction chemotherapy prior to definitive surgery improves survival of locoregionally advanced primary disease
  o Immune checkpoint inhibitors in combination with chemotherapy improve survival for recurrent/metastatic SCCa

DIAGNOSTIC CHECKLIST

Consider

- SCCa primary diagnosis in adult male with aggressive soft tissue mass in maxillary antrum

Image Interpretation Pearls

- ↓ T2 signal & tendency to enhance less than other sinonasal malignancies

Reporting Tips

- Evaluate for extension into orbit, masticator space, palate
  o Check PPF & foramen rotundum for V2 PNTS
  o Check for retropharyngeal & level I & II lymph nodes

SELECTED REFERENCES

1. Patel SD et al: Comparison of surveillance modalities in the surveillance of sinonasal squamous cell carcinoma recurrence: a multi-institutional study. Int Forum Allergy Rhinol. 15(4):384-94, 2025
2. Qian Y et al: Pembrolizumab with chemotherapy for patients with recurrent or metastatic nasal cavity and paranasal sinus squamous cell carcinoma: a prospective phase II study. Clin Cancer Res. 31(9):1636-43, 2025
3. Abiri A et al: Induction chemotherapy for locoregionally advanced sinonasal squamous cell carcinoma. J Neurol Surg B Skull Base. 85(Suppl 2):e153-60, 2024
4. Wang L et al: Patterns of lymph node metastasis in 441 patients with sinonasal squamous cell carcinoma. Ther Adv Med Oncol. 16:17588359241299331, 2024
5. Ramkumar SP et al: High-risk human papillomavirus 16/18 associated with improved survival in sinonasal squamous cell carcinoma. Cancer. 129(9):1372-83, 2023

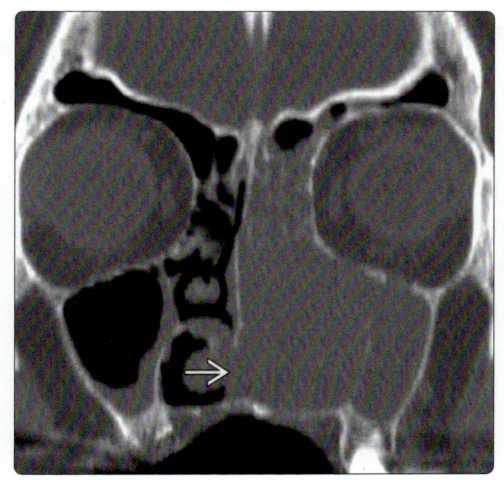

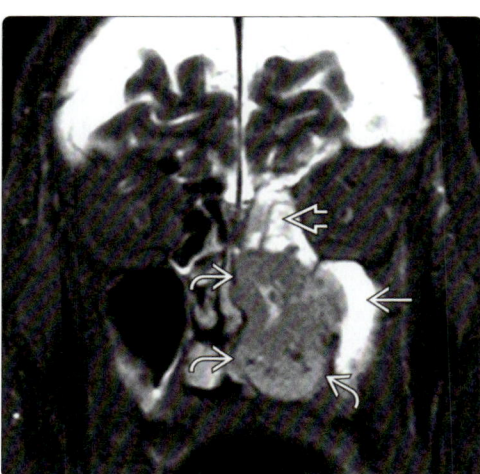

(Left) Coronal CT reconstruction shows a large mass filling the left nasal cavity with erosion of ipsilateral turbinates. This SCCa eroded the inferior nasal septum ➡. The margins of the mass are difficult to delineate here. (Right) Coronal STIR MR defines hypointense signal intensity tumor margins ➡. Obstructed secretions within the maxillary ➡ and ethmoid sinuses ➡ are hyperintense compared to the tumor. The low T2 tumor signal may be related to its high N:C ratio.

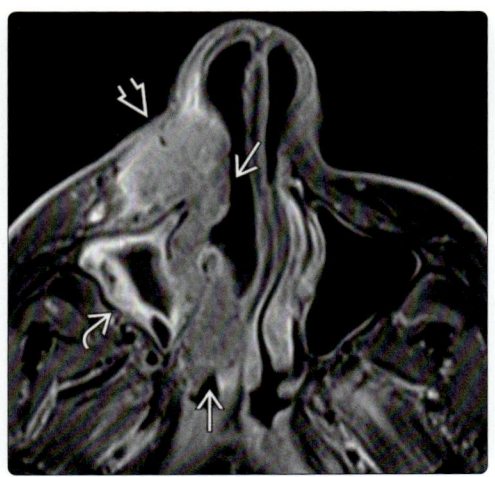

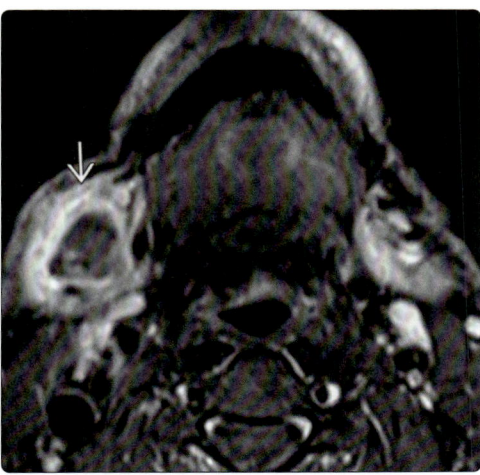

(Left) Axial T1 C+ FS MR demonstrates a right nasal cavity mass ➡ extending into the premaxillary soft tissues ➡, which enhances less than the normal sinus mucosa ➡ in this case of sinonasal SCCa. (Right) Axial T1 C+ FS MR in the same patient shows a centrally necrotic metastatic lymph node in the right cervical level IB ➡. Metastatic lymphadenopathy from sinonasal SCCa typically involves the retropharyngeal space or cervical levels I or II and is a poor prognostic factor.

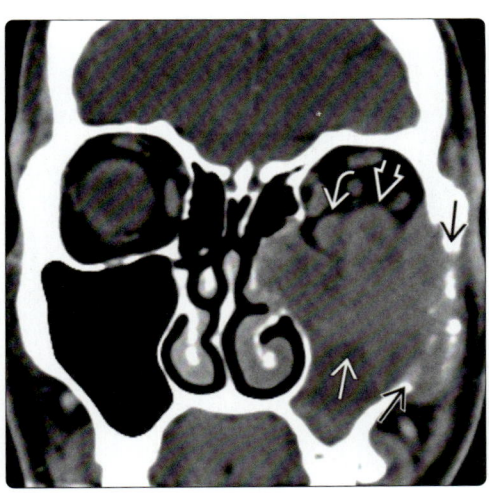

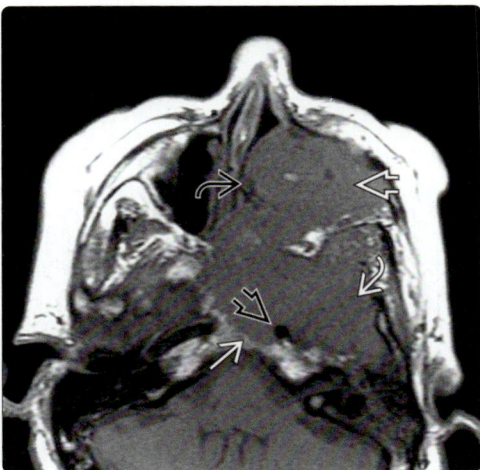

(Left) Coronal CECT shows an enhancing lesion filling the left maxillary sinus ➡ invading the orbit ➡ with mass effect upon the inferior rectus ➡. Note multifocal osseous destruction of the lateral maxillary sinus wall and zygoma ➡. The maxillary sinus is the most common site of origin of sinonasal SCCa. (Right) Axial T1 MR shows a very large antral SCCa ➡ with extension into the nasal cavity ➡, infratemporal fossa ➡, and clivus ➡. The mass encases the left internal carotid artery ➡, but the flow void is preserved.

KEY FACTS

TERMINOLOGY

- Malignant neuroectodermal tumor arising from **olfactory neuroepithelium** in superior nasal cavity

IMAGING

- Enhanced MR and bone CT best delineate ONB for en bloc craniofacial surgery
- **Dumbbell-shaped** mass with "waist" at cribriform plate
- Bone CT: Bone remodeling mixed with bone destruction, especially of cribriform plate
- CECT/T1 C+ MR: Homogeneously enhancing mass
  - **Peritumoral cysts** at intracranial tumor-brain margin
- T2 MR sequences best differentiate tumor from sinus secretions

TOP DIFFERENTIAL DIAGNOSES

- Sinonasal adenocarcinoma
- Anterior skull base meningioma
- Sinonasal squamous cell carcinoma

- Sinonasal non-Hodgkin lymphoma
- Sinonasal melanoma
- Sinonasal undifferentiated carcinoma

PATHOLOGY

- No etiologic, genetic, or risk factors elucidated
- Staging: **Kadish classification**; good predictor of outcome
- Histologic grading: Hyams system

CLINICAL ISSUES

- **Middle-aged** patient with unilateral nasal obstruction and mild epistaxis
  - Slight male predilection
- Combined surgical resection and radiotherapy is treatment of choice
- Excellent prognosis vs. other sinonasal malignancies
  - 5-year survival rates: 75-77% overall
  - Recurrence in ~ 30%
  - Metastases in 10-30% of patients

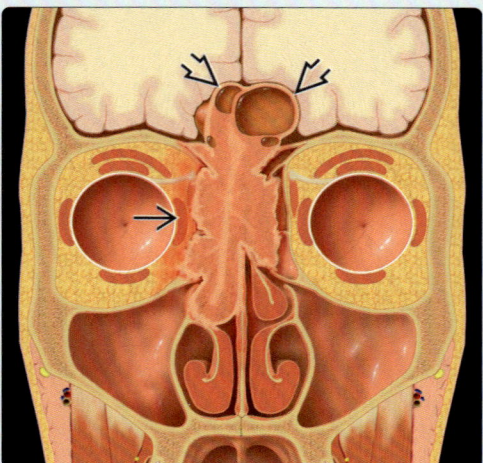
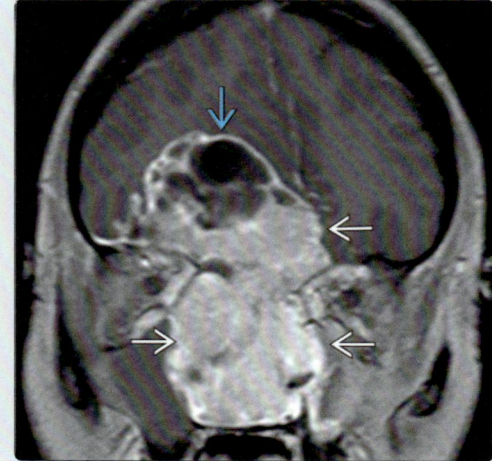

(Left) Coronal graphic shows the classic features of olfactory neuroblastoma (ONB) centered below the cribriform plate and extending into the anterior cranial fossa and right orbit ➡. Cyst formation ➥ is noted at the tumor-brain interface. *(Right)* Coronal T1 C+ MR shows a large sinonasal mass eroding through the anterior skull base intracranially to the anterior cranial fossa with pronounced mass effect on the brain parenchyma ➡. Note the characteristic peritumoral cysts at the brain-tumor interface ➡.

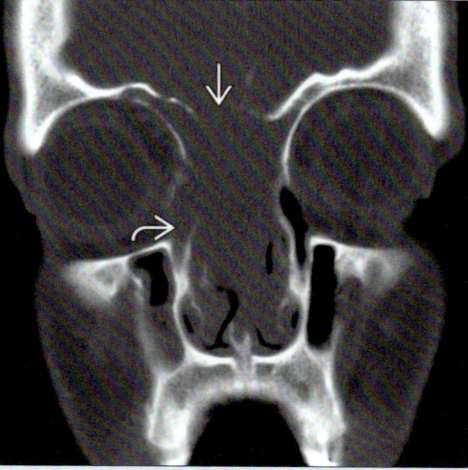
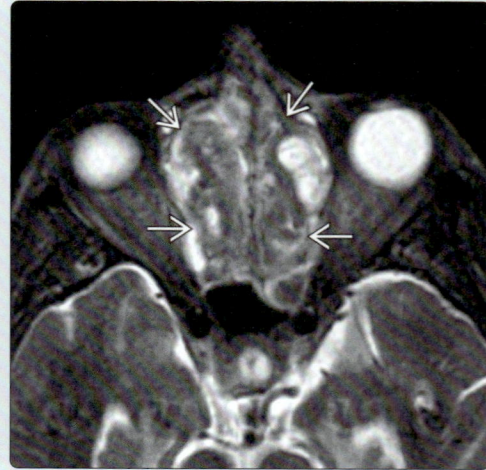

(Left) Coronal bone CT shows an ONB filling the upper nasal cavity and ethmoid sinuses. The lesion extends through the anterior skull base ➡. The lamina papyracea on the right is thinned and laterally displaced ➡. *(Right)* Axial STIR MR demonstrates a large, heterogeneous ONB ➡ centered in the midline below the skull base and occupying the nasal cavity and ethmoid sinuses. The mass is predominantly hypointense in this case and causes hypertelorism.

Olfactory Neuroblastoma

TERMINOLOGY

Abbreviations

- Olfactory neuroblastoma (ONB)

Synonyms

- Esthesioneuroblastoma, pleomorphic olfactory neuroblastoma

Definitions

- Rare, malignant, neuroectodermal sinonasal (SN) tumor

IMAGING

General Features

- Best diagnostic clue
  - Dumbbell-shaped mass with upper portion in anterior cranial fossa, lower portion in upper nasal cavity, and "waist" at level of cribriform plate
  - **Peripheral tumor cysts** at intracranial tumor-brain margin are highly suggestive of diagnosis of ONB
- Location
  - Superior nasal cavity **at olfactory recess with erosion of cribriform plate**
    - Intranasal ONB: Unilateral nasal expansile mass centered at olfactory recess; local spread in nose and sinuses
    - Extranasal ONB: Tumor in anterior cranial fossa with parenchymal and dural infiltration, extension into orbits
- Size
  - Range from < 1-cm nodule to mass filling entire nasal cavity and lower anterior cranial fossa
- Morphology
  - Polypoid mass when small; dumbbell-shaped when large

CT Findings

- NECT
  - Bone CT
    - Bone remodeling causing enlargement of olfactory recess with bone erosion at cribriform plate
    - Speckled pattern of calcification within tumor matrix unusual
- CECT
  - Homogeneously enhancing mass
  - When large, may see nonenhancing areas of necrosis with intracranial peritumoral cyst

MR Findings

- T1WI
  - Hypointense to intermediate signal intensity mass compared to brain
  - Areas of hemorrhage can be hyperintense
- T2WI
  - Tumor is intermediate to hyperintense to brain with areas of cystic degeneration
    - Obstructed secretions in adjacent sinuses often hyperintense (provide inherent contrast to tumor)
  - Hemorrhagic foci are hypo- to hyperintense depending on age of blood
  - Intracranial cysts at tumor-brain interface are hyperintense
- DWI
  - Average mean ADC ~ 1.2×10^{-3} mm²/s
  - ONB considered small round blue cell tumor (SRBCT); however, mean ADC map value typically higher than other sinonasal malignancies
- T1WI C+
  - **Avid homogeneous tumor enhancement**
  - Enhancement heterogeneous in areas of necrosis

Nuclear Medicine Findings

- FDG PET positive, higher sensitivity of detecting nodal and distant metastases
- Somatostatin-receptor PET imaging (i.e., DOTATATE) may also be helpful in detecting metastatic disease

Imaging Recommendations

- Best imaging tool
  - Enhanced MR with bone CT best delineates ONB for en bloc craniofacial surgery
- Protocol advice
  - Bone CT shows precise extent of bone destruction and may alter extent of craniofacial resection
  - T2 MR best differentiates tumor from sinus secretions
  - Multiplanar T1 C+ FS MR for evaluating tumor extension beyond SN cavities

DIFFERENTIAL DIAGNOSIS

Sinonasal Adenocarcinoma

- **Wood dust and occupational exposures** are risk factors
- Predilection for ethmoid origin with nasal cavity involvement
- Enhances less avidly and more heterogeneously than ONB

Anterior Skull Base Meningioma

- May cause hyperostosis in adjacent skull base
- Not often associated with cyst formation at tumor-brain interface

Sinonasal Squamous Cell Carcinoma

- More common in **maxillary antrum** than nasal cavity
- Does not enhance to same degree as ONB

Non-Hodgkin Lymphoma

- Dense on NECT, low ADC map value
- Does not enhance to same degree as ONB
- Rarely breaches skull base

Sinonasal Melanoma

- Favors **lower nasal cavity** as site of origin (septum and turbinates)
- Increased T1 & decreased T2 signal in melanotic type

Sinonasal Undifferentiated Carcinoma

- Difficult to distinguish from ONB on imaging
- Not typically confined to cribriform plate/superior nasal cavity

PATHOLOGY

General Features

- Etiology
  - No etiologic basis or risk factors elucidated

- Tumor of neural crest origin and **begins in olfactory neuroepithelium** in superior nasal cavity at cribriform plate
- Associated abnormalities
  - ONB patients occasionally present with paraneoplastic symptoms
    - Adrenocorticotropic hormone → Cushing syndrome
    - Syndrome of inappropriate antidiuretic hormone secretion → antidiuretic hormone secretion → hyponatremia

Staging, Grading, & Classification

- Staging criteria: Modified **Kadish classification**; good predictor of outcome; stage C is most common
  - Stage A: Localized to nasal cavity
  - Stage B: Localized to nasal cavity and sinuses
  - Stage C: Orbital and intracranial extension
  - Stage D: Cervical and distant metastases
- Histologic grading: Hyams system; stronger prediction of prognosis
  - Grades 1-4 based on architectural pleomorphism, neurofibrillary matrix, rosette formation, mitoses, necrosis, presence of gland formation, and calcifications

Gross Pathologic & Surgical Features

- Clinically appears as firm, nonpulsatile mass covered by intact respiratory mucosa
  - Tumor may bleed profusely on biopsy
- Broad-based, pedunculated, lobulated, mucosal-covered mass at cribriform plate; soft, glistening
  - May show engorged, red appearance due to rich, vascular stroma

Microscopic Features

- Submucosal lesion with prominent nested appearance
  - Neurofibrillary intercellular matrix and rosette formations
  - Mild nuclear pleomorphism with low mitotic activity most common
- Frequently contains areas of necrosis and calcification
- Electron microscopy
  - Shows neurosecretory granules
  - May help make correct diagnosis when light microscopy is inconclusive
- ONB is type of SRBCT; may be difficult to differentiate from other SRBCTs
  - Lymphoma, Ewing sarcoma, melanoma, rhabdomyosarcoma, Merkel cell carcinoma

CLINICAL ISSUES

Presentation

- Most common signs/symptoms
  - Nasal obstruction and **epistaxis**
    - Symptoms usually predate diagnosis by 6-12 months
- Other signs/symptoms
  - Anosmia, rhinorrhea
  - Hypertelorism, proptosis, diplopia, and epiphora
  - Headache
  - Cranial neuropathies suggest skull base/cavernous sinus involvement
- Clinical profile

- **Middle-aged patient** with unilateral nasal obstruction and mild epistaxis

Demographics

- Age
  - Recent evidence suggests **unimodal distribution** with peak in 4th-6th decades
    - Previously thought **bimodal distribution** with peaks in 2nd and 6th decades
- Sex
  - Slight male predominance
- Epidemiology
  - 2-3% of all intranasal neoplasms

Natural History & Prognosis

- **5-year survival rates: 75-77% overall**
  - Staging and tumor grade are significant prognostic indicators
    - 5-year disease-free survival
      - Kadish stage A: > 90%; stage B: 70-90%; stage C: 35-70%; stage D: < 35%
- Negative prognostic indicators
  - Female sex, age < 20 or > 50 years at presentation
  - Higher tumor histology grade, higher staging (Kadish C and D)
- Recurrence in ~ 30% up to 15 years after primary diagnosis
- Metastases in 10-30% of patients
  - Nodal &/or distant metastases to lung, bone, liver

Treatment

- Combined therapy using craniofacial resection and radiotherapy is treatment of choice
  - Radiotherapy offers better local control because negative resection margins often difficult to achieve
  - Low-stage resectable tumors may be approached endoscopically in selected patients
- Chemotherapy reserved for larger, high-grade ONB and disseminated disease

DIAGNOSTIC CHECKLIST

Consider

- Using both preoperative CT and MR
  - CT for detection of extent of bone destruction
  - MR for precise mapping of tumor soft tissue extent

Image Interpretation Pearls

- Dumbbell-shaped mass with "waist" at cribriform plate + intracranial marginal cysts are characteristic of ONB

SELECTED REFERENCES

1. Yamauchi H et al: Assessing the histological malignancy grade of olfactory neuroblastoma using the apparent diffusion coefficient histogram analysis. Cureus. 16(8):e66718, 2024
2. Agarwal A et al: Update from the 5th Edition of the WHO Classification of nasal, paranasal, and skull base tumors: imaging overview with histopathologic and genetic correlation. AJNR Am J Neuroradiol. 44(10):1116-25, 2023
3. Berger MH et al: Characteristics and overall survival in pediatric versus adult esthesioneuroblastoma: a population-based study. Int J Pediatr Otorhinolaryngol. 144:110696, 2021
4. Zlochower AB et al: Doing great with DOTATATE: update on GA-68 DOTATATE positron emission tomography/computed tomography and magnetic resonance imaging for evaluation of sinonasal tumors. Top Magn Reson Imaging. 30(3):151-8, 2021

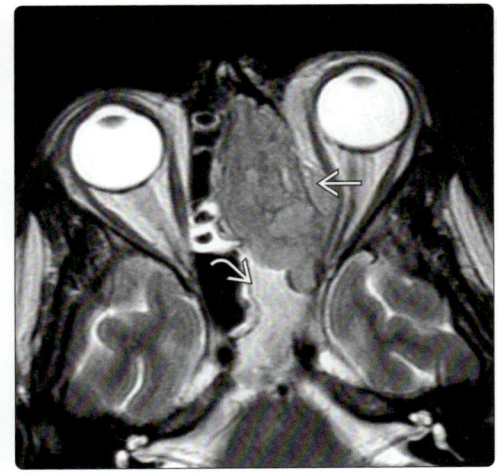

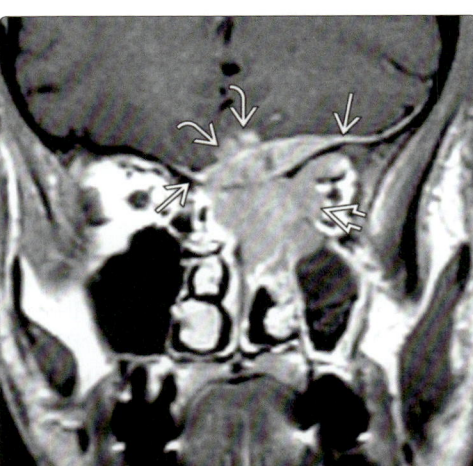

(Left) Axial T2 FS MR shows diffuse intermediate to low signal within an ONB centered in the left nasal cavity. Extension into the left orbit ⮕ is seen. Trapped secretions ⮕ are noted in the left sphenoid sinus. (Right) Coronal T1 C+ MR shows intracranial extension of a left nasal cavity ONB. The tumor avidly enhances and invades dura, causing a dural tail ⮕. Invasion into the left frontal lobe ⮕ and left orbit ⮕ is also present.

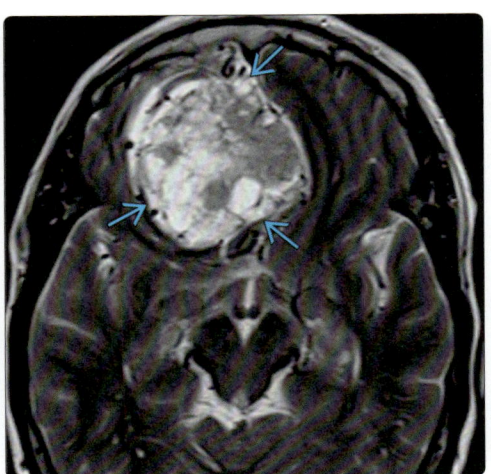

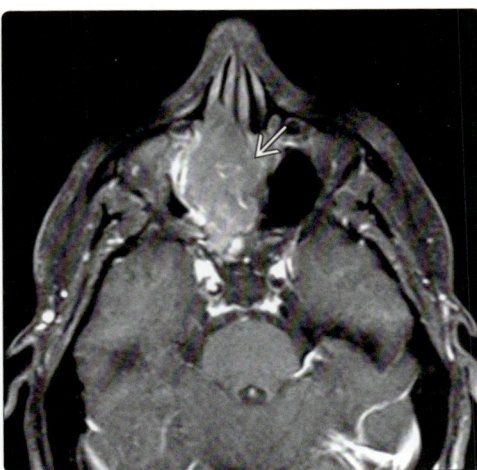

(Left) Axial T2 MR shows the large intracranial portion of an ONB exerting pronounced mass effect upon the brain parenchyma. Note the classic peritumoral cysts ⮕. (Right) Axial T1 C+ MR shows mild, diffuse, homogeneous enhancement throughout an ONB centered in the right nasal cavity. This ONB crossed the midline ⮕ through the nasal septum.

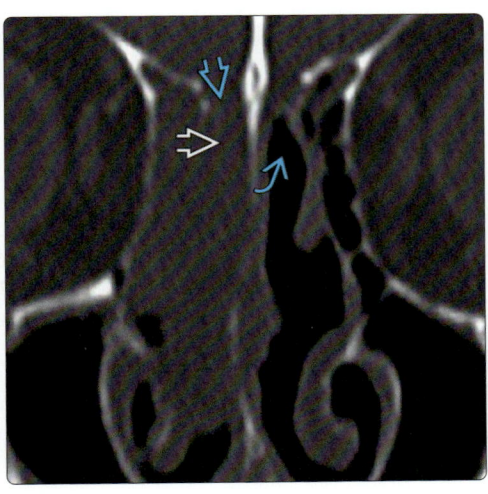

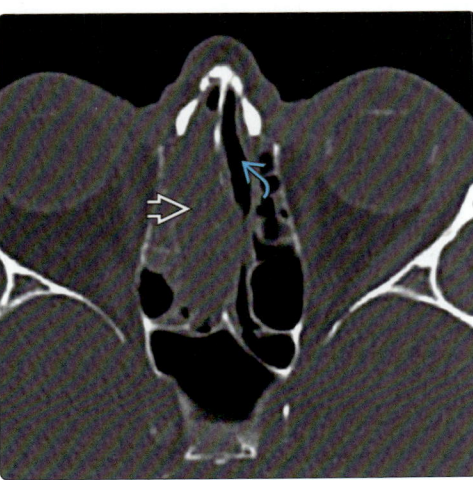

(Left) Coronal bone CT shows a unilateral expansile mass in the right nasal cavity with expansion of the olfactory recess ⮕ and erosion at the cribriform plate ⮕. No intracranial extension is noted. The left nasal cavity olfactory recess is normal ⮕. This was proven to be an intranasal ONB. (Right) Axial bone CT shows an expansile mass centered in the olfactory recess ⮕. Notice the contralateral normal olfactory recess ⮕.

TERMINOLOGY

- Arises from melanocytes migrated from **neural crest origin** to sinonasal epithelium

IMAGING

- Soft tissue mass in nasal cavity > paranasal sinuses with bone destruction ± remodeling
  - Predilection for nasal septum, lateral nasal wall, and inferior turbinate
- MR (melanotic melanoma)
  - **↑ T1 and ↓ T2 signal** results from melanin, free radicals, metal ions, and hemorrhage
  - T2* GRE may show **blooming** when hemorrhage present in sinonasal melanoma (SNM)
  - Avidly enhances due to vascularity; enhancement may not be visible due to intrinsic high T1 signal

TOP DIFFERENTIAL DIAGNOSES

- Squamous cell carcinoma
- Sinonasal adenocarcinoma
- Non-Hodgkin lymphoma

CLINICAL ISSUES

- Adult with nasal stuffiness, epistaxis, and pigmented mass identified at nasal endoscopy
  - 5th-8th decades most common
  - > 85% occurs in White patients, M = F
- Poor prognosis with 20-40% chance of 5-year survival
  - Mean survival: ~ 24 months
  - Systemic metastatic disease typically precedes death
- SNM < 2% of melanomas and 4-12% of sinonasal malignancies

DIAGNOSTIC CHECKLIST

- Look for hemorrhagic mass arising in lower nasal cavity with ↑ T1 and ↓ T2 signal
- Consider SNM for pigmented appearance on nasal endoscopy

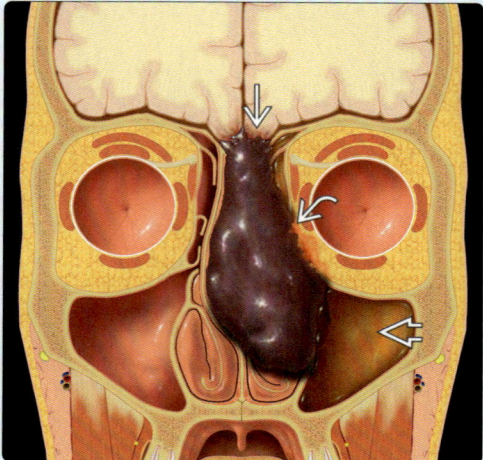

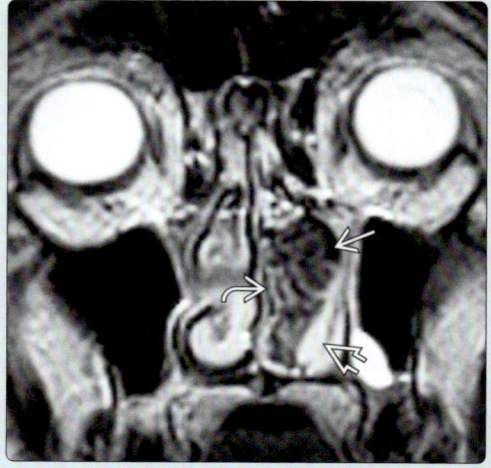

(Left) Coronal graphic shows a darkly pigmented (highly melanotic) mass centered in the nasal cavity. Invasion of the skull base ➡, orbit ➡, and lateral nasal wall is seen, but the septum is deviated rather than invaded. Trapped secretions ➡ are noted in the left maxillary sinus. (Right) Coronal T2 MR shows hypointense signal in the left nasal melanoma ➡ compared to the adjacent hyperintense turbinate ➡. The mass does not invade the nasal septum ➡.

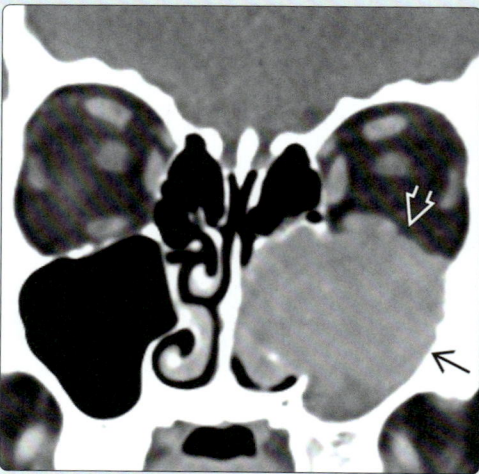

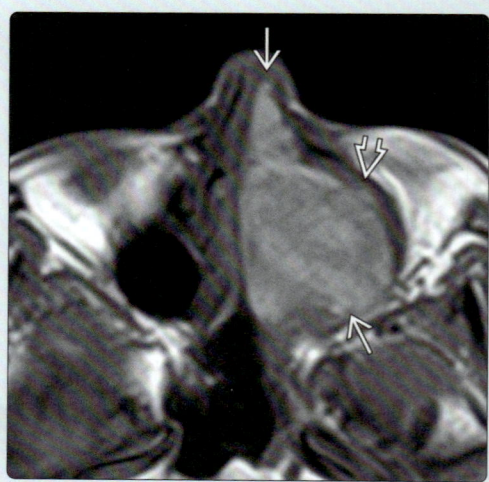

(Left) Coronal CECT shows an enhancing, aggressive mass centered in the left maxillary sinus ➡ with left orbital invasion ➡. The imaging appearance of this sinonasal melanoma is indistinguishable from other aggressive sinonasal malignancies, such as squamous cell carcinoma. (Right) Axial T1 MR demonstrates a left nasal cavity mass extending into the left orbit ➡. Diffuse intrinsic T1 hyperintensity ➡ comes from melanin within this sinonasal melanoma.

Sinonasal Melanoma

TERMINOLOGY

Abbreviations

- Sinonasal melanoma (SNM)

Definitions

- Malignant transformation of melanocytes migrating from neural crest in sinonasal cavity

IMAGING

General Features

- Best diagnostic clue
  - ↑ T1 MR signal mass in nasal cavity
- Location
  - **Nasal cavity** > sinuses
    - Nasal septum, lateral wall, and inferior turbinate
- Size
  - Large polypoid sinonasal mass

CT Findings

- Bone CT
  - Lobular soft tissue mass in nasal cavity
  - Bone destruction ± remodeling

MR Findings

- T1WI
  - **Melanotic** melanoma: ↑ **signal** due to melanin, free radicals, metal ions, hemorrhage
  - **Amelanotic** melanoma: Intermediate signal (20-25%)
- T2WI
  - **Melanotic** melanoma: ↓ **signal**
  - Amelanotic melanoma: Variable signal
- T2* GRE
  - Areas of hemorrhage may show blooming
- T1WI C+
  - Avid enhancement

Imaging Recommendations

- Best imaging tool
  - Multiplanar MR with contrast

DIFFERENTIAL DIAGNOSIS

Sinonasal Squamous Cell Carcinoma

- Arises in maxillary antrum > nasal cavity
- Aggressive bone destruction; heterogeneous with variable enhancement

Sinonasal Adenocarcinoma

- Arises in nasal cavity and ethmoid sinuses
- Intestinal-type associated with occupational wood dust exposure

Sinonasal Non-Hodgkin Lymphoma

- Sinonasal mass with bone destruction ± remodeling
- Homogeneous; ↓ T2 signal; ↓ ADC

Olfactory Neuroblastoma

- Mass near cribriform plate with bone destruction

Sinonasal Undifferentiated Carcinoma

- Rare aggressive sinonasal mass

- Most commonly in superior nasal cavity and ethmoid sinuses

PATHOLOGY

General Features

- Etiology
  - Neuroectodermal tumor arising from melanocytes in nasal cavity and sinuses

Gross Pathologic & Surgical Features

- Pink to dark colored, soft vascular nasal mass arising from septum and lateral nasal wall

Microscopic Features

- Epithelioid, spindle, and mixed cell types
- Melanin heavily deposited, limited, or absent

CLINICAL ISSUES

Presentation

- Most common signs/symptoms
  - Nasal obstruction, epistaxis, pain, hyposmia
- Physical exam
  - Bulky, brownish black, friable vascular nasal mass

Demographics

- Age
  - 5th-8th decades most common (range: 30-85 years)
- Epidemiology
  - SNM < 2% of melanomas and 4-7% of sinonasal malignancies
  - 85% occur in White patients
- Sex: M = F

Natural History & Prognosis

- Poor prognosis with 20-40% chance of 5-year survival
- Metastasis to lungs, lymph nodes, and brain typically precedes death

Treatment

- Radical surgery with adjuvant radiotherapy

DIAGNOSTIC CHECKLIST

Consider

- May appear similar to polyp if low melanin content
- Consider SNM for pigmented appearance on nasal endoscopy

Image Interpretation Pearls

- Look for mass arising in lower nasal cavity with ↑ T1 and ↓ T2 signal

SELECTED REFERENCES

1. Kshirsagar RS et al: Outcomes of immunotherapy treatment in sinonasal mucosal melanoma. Am J Rhinol Allergy. 39(2):102-8, 2025
2. Foreman RK et al: Sinonasal mucosal melanoma: a contemporary review. Surg Pathol Clin. 17(4):667-82, 2024
3. Rojas-Lechuga MJ et al: Survival outcomes in sinonasal mucosal melanoma: systematic review and meta-analysis. J Pers Med. 14(12):1120, 2024
4. Ding W et al: Pattern and prognostic value of lymph node metastasis in sinonasal mucosal melanoma. Ear Nose Throat J. 104(5):NP278-86, 2022

TERMINOLOGY

- Malignant neoplasm with glandular differentiation arising from surface respiratory epithelium or seromucinous glands

IMAGING

- Predilection for nasal cavity & ethmoid sinuses
- May reach large size due to delay in diagnosis
  - 75% with involvement of > 1 sinonasal (SN) region at diagnosis
- CT
  - Well- to poorly defined mass with bone destruction or remodeling ± calcifications
- MR
  - Typically intermediate to hyperintense T2 signal
  - Diffuse, heterogeneous enhancement
- Goals of imaging: Determine malignant characteristics & orbital or intracranial extension

TOP DIFFERENTIAL DIAGNOSES

- Sinonasal squamous cell carcinoma
- Olfactory neuroblastoma
- Sinonasal undifferentiated carcinoma
- Sinonasal non-Hodgkin lymphoma

PATHOLOGY

- 2 major subtypes
  - Intestinal (related to wood dust exposure): Most frequent form colonic > solid > papillary > mucinous & mixed type
  - Nonintestinal: Unrelated to wood dust exposure
- Accounts for 15% of all SN cancers

CLINICAL ISSUES

- 6th decade most common; M > F (~ 3:1)
- Poor prognosis with higher grades, incomplete resection, & intracranial involvement; 5-year survival rates ~ 50%
- Complete surgical excision for cure

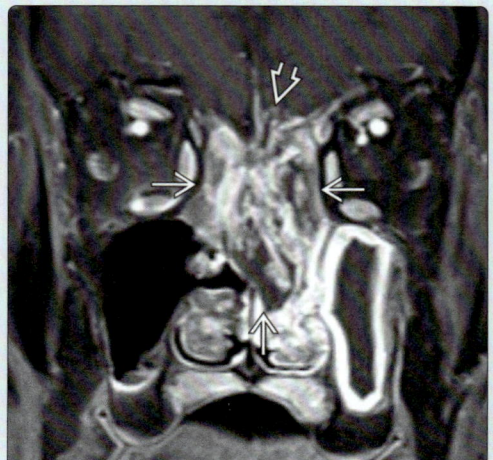
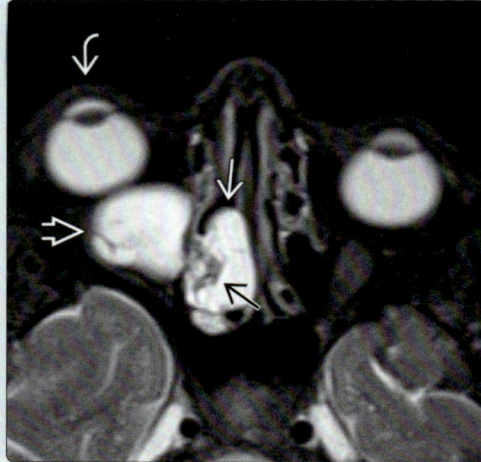

(Left) Coronal T1 C+ FS MR shows a heterogeneously enhancing mass ➡ in the superior nasal cavity and ethmoid sinuses with subtle extension through the anterior skull base ➡ in sinonasal adenocarcinoma (SN AdenoCa). (Right) Axial T2 FS MR shows T2-hyperintense mass ➡ in right posterior ethmoid sinuses invading right orbit ➡ with exophthalmos ➡ in low-grade nonintestinal-type SN AdenoCA. Regions of internal hypointense signal ➡ corresponded with calcifications on CT (not shown).

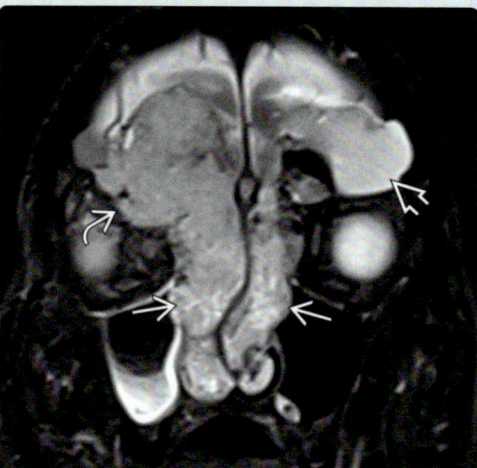
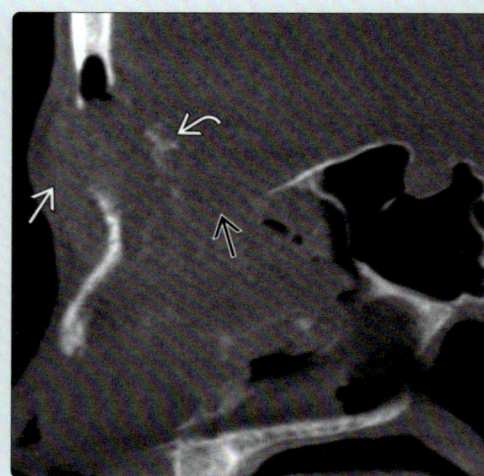

(Left) Coronal T2 FS MR shows an intermediate signal intensity mass involving the nasal cavity bilaterally ➡ and invading the right orbit ➡. Postobstructive frontal sinus secretions are noted ➡. This was nonintestinal-type AdenoCa. (Right) Midline sagittal bone CT in the same patient shows the soft tissue mass invading through the anterior frontal sinus into the scalp soft tissues ➡. There is destruction of the anterior skull base ➡ with calcified tumor extending intracranially ➡.

Sinonasal Adenocarcinoma

TERMINOLOGY

Abbreviations

- Sinonasal adenocarcinoma (SN AdenoCa)

Definitions

- Malignant neoplasm with glandular differentiation arising from surface respiratory epithelium or seromucinous glands

IMAGING

General Features

- Best diagnostic clue
  - Poorly defined, enhancing SN mass with ethmoid sinus, nasal cavity, & skull base involvement
- Location
  - Predilection for **nasal cavity & ethmoid sinuses**
- Size
  - May reach large size due to **delay in diagnosis**

CT Findings

- CECT
  - Diffuse, often heterogeneous enhancement
  - May be invasive; look for dural or orbit invasion
- Bone CT
  - Bone destruction > remodeling

MR Findings

- T1WI
  - Intermediate signal; ↑ signal in foci of hemorrhage
- T2WI
  - Variable; typically intermediate to hyperintense
- T1WI C+
  - Diffuse, heterogeneous enhancement

Imaging Recommendations

- Best imaging tool
  - Multiplanar enhanced MR
- Protocol advice
  - C+ FS MR to map tumor extension & detect perineural spread

DIFFERENTIAL DIAGNOSIS

Sinonasal Squamous Cell Carcinoma

- Usually in maxillary antrum; more ill defined

Olfactory Neuroblastoma

- Adolescent or middle-aged
- Near cribriform plate; intense enhancement

Sinonasal Undifferentiated Carcinoma

- Can look very similar to SN AdenoCa
- Aggressive with rapid growth

Sinonasal Non-Hodgkin Lymphoma

- Homogeneous, ↓ T2 signal & ADC map value
- NK/T-cell lymphoma has predilection for nasal cavity

Sinonasal SWI/SNF Complex-Deficient Carcinoma

- Rare, highly aggressive sinonasal malignancy
- Glandular subtype may mimic nonintestinal-type SN AdenoCa on histopathology

PATHOLOGY

General Features

- Etiology
  - **Wood dust exposure** has strong link to intestinal-type AdenoCa
    - Other exposure: Inhaled metal dust, cork, & leather & textile industry chemicals

Staging, Grading, & Classification

- American Joint Committee on Cancer (AJCC) TNM staging system most frequently used for lesions originating in nasal cavity & ethmoids
- Subtypes include
  - Intestinal: Most frequent form is colonic (40%) followed by solid (20%), papillary (18%), & mucinous & mixed type (together 22%)
  - Nonintestinal: Unrelated to wood dust exposure

Gross Pathologic & Surgical Features

- Tan-white-pink; flat, exophytic, or papillary; friable to firm

Microscopic Features

- Well differentiated
  - Unencapsulated tumor, uniform glands with cystic spaces, no stroma
- Poorly differentiated
  - Invasive, solid growth pattern, pleomorphism, ↑ mitoses

CLINICAL ISSUES

Presentation

- Most common signs/symptoms
  - Nasal stuffiness & obstruction
  - Epistaxis

Demographics

- Age
  - **6th decade most common** (mean: 64 years)
- Sex
  - **M > F** (~ 3:1)
- Epidemiology
  - 15% of all SN cancers

Natural History & Prognosis

- Prognosis excellent for low grade, poor for high grade
- 5-year survival: ~ 50%

Treatment

- Complete surgical excision for cure
- Radiation therapy & chemotherapy used alone or in conjunction with surgery

DIAGNOSTIC CHECKLIST

Consider

- SN AdenoCa if history of occupational exposure & involvement of nasal cavity & ethmoid sinuses

SELECTED REFERENCES

1. Arcovito G et al: Sinonasal adenocarcinomas: an update. Surg Pathol Clin. 17(4):653-66, 2024
2. Baptista Freitas M et al: Sinonasal adenocarcinoma: clinicopathological characterization and prognostic factors. Cureus. 16(3):e56067, 2024

Sinonasal Non-Hodgkin Lymphoma

TERMINOLOGY

- Sinonasal non-Hodgkin lymphoma: Extranodal lymphoproliferative malignancy

IMAGING

- Appearance can mimic variety of neoplasms & aggressive inflammatory disorders
- CT: Homogeneous mass ± bone remodeling or destruction
  - May be hyperdense due to high N:C ratio
- Imaging modality of choice: Multiplanar MR with T1 C+ FS
- MR: ↓ T2 signal & ↓ ADC map value
- PET for initial staging & treatment response

TOP DIFFERENTIAL DIAGNOSES

- Sinonasal squamous cell carcinoma
- Sinonasal granulomatosis with polyangiitis (Wegener granulomatosis)
- Olfactory neuroblastoma
- Sinonasal adenocarcinoma

PATHOLOGY

- 2 pathologic subgroups
  - B-cell (Western) phenotype
  - T-cell (Asian) phenotype
    - Natural killer/T-cell lymphoma (Asian): Subtype of T cell

CLINICAL ISSUES

- Male patient in 6th decade with nonspecific symptoms of nasal obstruction & discharge
- Local radiotherapy (XRT) is primary treatment ± combination chemotherapy

DIAGNOSTIC CHECKLIST

- NHL could be included in DDx for almost any aggressive adult nasal soft tissue mass
- Imaging clue to diagnosis: Presence of enlarged cervical nodes & Waldeyer ring lymphatic mass

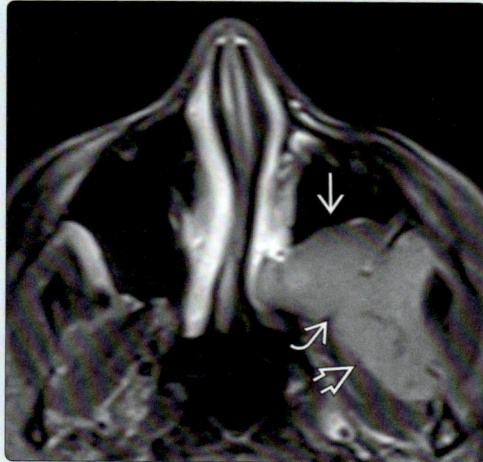
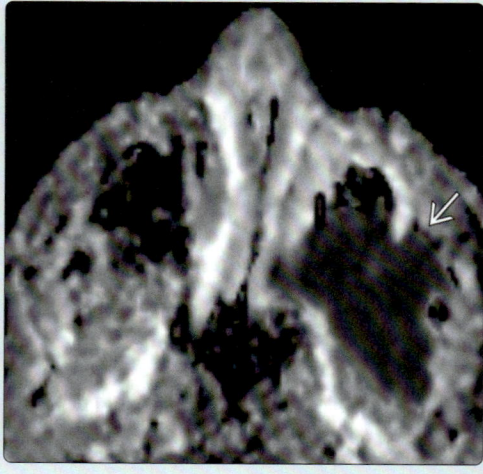

(Left) Axial T2 FS MR shows a left maxillary sinus mass ➡ with homogeneous intermediate T2 signal intensity breaking through the left posterior maxillary sinus wall ➡ and extending into the left masticator space ➡ in this case of diffuse large B-cell lymphoma (DLBCL). (Right) Axial ADC map in the same patient demonstrates diffuse low ADC map value ➡ of the tumor, a characteristic imaging feature of lymphoma given high cellularity and high N:C ratio.

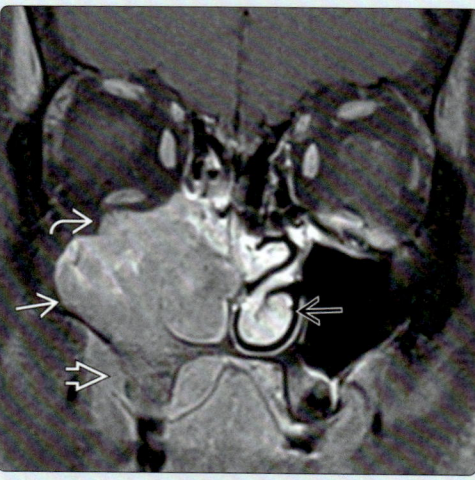
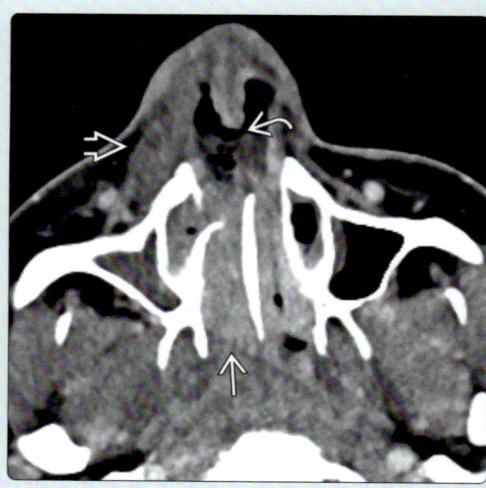

(Left) Coronal T1 C+ FS MR shows enhancing mass ➡ in right maxillary sinus extending to right infraorbital canal ➡ and maxillary alveolus ➡. Note mass enhancement is less than normal sinonasal mucosa ➡, typical for NHL-SN. (Right) Axial CECT shows ill-defined, enhancing nasal cavity mass ➡ extending into right nasal soft tissues ➡ and associated anterior septal destruction ➡ in natural killer/T-cell lymphoma (NKTL). These imaging features mimic inflammatory conditions like granulomatosis with polyangiitis.

Sinonasal Non-Hodgkin Lymphoma

TERMINOLOGY

Abbreviations

- Sinonasal non-Hodgkin lymphoma (NHL-SN)

Definitions

- NHL-SN: Extranodal lymphoproliferative malignancy
  - Diffuse large B-cell lymphoma (DLBCL): Most common B-cell subtype of NHL-SN
  - Natural killer/T-cell lymphoma (NKTL): Most common T-cell subtype of NHL-SN
    - Previously called lethal midline granuloma, polymorphic reticulosis, angiocentric T-cell lymphoma

IMAGING

General Features

- Best diagnostic clue
  - **Homogeneous soft tissue mass** with predilection for nasal cavity ± bone destruction
  - Very nonspecific imaging features
    - NHL-SN **can mimic** variety of neoplasms & aggressive inflammatory disorders
- Location
  - **DLBCL**: **Maxillary** > nasal cavity > ethmoid > sphenoid > frontal sinuses
  - **NKTL**: **Nasal cavity** > > maxillary > ethmoid sinuses
    - NKTL may have simultaneous involvement of nasopharynx & oropharynx in addition to sinonasal cavities
- Morphology
  - Variable: Diffusely infiltrative & ill-defined, nodular, or bulky mass

CT Findings

- NECT
  - Bulky, lobular, soft tissue mass in nasal cavity ± sinuses
  - May be **hyperdense** compared to soft tissue due to high N:C ratio
  - NKTL: Infiltrative > polypoid soft tissue mass in nasal cavity ± ulceration/necrosis/bone destruction
    - Used to be called midline lethal granuloma
- CECT
  - Moderate **homogeneous enhancement**
- Bone CT
  - Tends to remodel &/or erode bone
  - B-cell (Western) type: Soft tissue & osseous destruction
    - More likely to invade orbit
  - T-cell (Asian) type: Nasal septal destruction & perforation

MR Findings

- T1WI
  - Intermediate, homogeneous signal similar to or slightly higher than muscle
- T2WI
  - **Low to intermediate** homogeneous signal
    - Due to highly cellular nature & ↑ N:C ratio
- DWI
  - Restricted diffusion, significantly lower ADC values compared with squamous cell carcinomas
- T1WI C+
  - Variable but diffuse & homogeneous enhancement
    - Typically > muscle but < mucosa
  - Nonenhancing areas of necrosis more common in NKTL than in other NHL-SN
    - May mimic mucosal nonenhancement of invasive fungal sinusitis

Nuclear Medicine Findings

- PET
  - May show avid uptake
  - Valuable for initial staging & treatment response evaluation

Imaging Recommendations

- Best imaging tool
  - Multiplanar MR with T1 C+ FS
    - MR better delineates tumor margins & differentiates tumor from mucosal thickening & secretions
- Protocol advice
  - Begin with thin-section axial & coronal T1 & T2 sequences without FS
  - Follow with T1 C+ FS MR in same planes through sinonasal area

DIFFERENTIAL DIAGNOSIS

Sinonasal Squamous Cell Carcinoma

- Most common in maxillary sinus
- More heterogeneous with frank bone destruction

Granulomatosis With Polyangiitis (Wegener Granulomatosis)

- **Can be indistinguishable** from NHL-SN on imaging
- Favors nasal cavity (septum & turbinates)
- Cytoplasmic antineutrophil cytoplasmic antibody, c-ANCA(+)

Olfactory Neuroblastoma

- Adolescent or middle-aged adult
- Superior nasal cavity near cribriform plate
- Typically higher T2 signal, more prominent enhancement

Sinonasal Adenocarcinoma

- More likely to originate in sinuses, particularly ethmoids
- May be related to occupational exposure (wood dust)

Invasive Fungal Sinusitis

- Transmucosal fungal sinus infection in immunocompromised patient
- Loss of mucosal enhancement (black turbinate sign)
- May mimic NKTL

PATHOLOGY

General Features

- Etiology
  - Malignant lymphoproliferative disorder arising from variety of immune cell types
  - 2 subgroups
    - **B-cell (Western) phenotype**: Most frequent type in paranasal sinuses; less aggressive
      - ☐ DLBCL most common
    - **T-cell (Asian) phenotype**: More common in nasal cavity; more aggressive

□ NKTL most common
□ EBV likely has role in pathogenesis of NKTL
- Associated abnormalities
  ○ Lymph nodes **infrequently** involved
  ○ Distant metastases seen in stage IV: Liver, spleen, brain, & bone marrow

Staging, Grading, & Classification

- Multiple staging systems: Lugano classification, Ann Arbor staging system, Murphy staging system
  ○ Lugano classification is modified update of Ann Arbor staging system, most commonly used
- Histologic classification: WHO system for lymphoid neoplasms (1999)
  ○ Multiple additional classification systems: Rappaport, Luke-Collins, Revised European American Lymphoma (REAL)
- Large tumors & those with extranasal extension represent higher tumor stage

Gross Pathologic & Surgical Features

- Polypoid, soft to rubbery mass with homogeneous pink-tan or bluish color
- Locally destructive & ulcerative

Microscopic Features

- Monomorphous malignant cellular infiltrate of various types
- Various types are characterized immunophenotypically
- NKTL: Polymorphous cellular infiltrate of mononuclear cells growing in angiocentric, angiodestructive growth pattern
  ○ Mucosal ulceration, pseudoepitheliomatous hyperplasia, & inflammatory infiltrate may be seen
  ○ EBV(+) in nearly all cases

CLINICAL ISSUES

Presentation

- Most common signs/symptoms
  ○ Nasal obstruction & discharge
    – **Symptoms mimic sinusitis**, which leads to delay in diagnosis
  ○ Bleeding more common in NKTL due to ulceration & necrosis
- Other signs/symptoms
  ○ Unilateral facial swelling, otitis media, cervical adenopathy, headache
  ○ NKTL: Septal cartilage destruction leads to saddle nose deformity
- Clinical profile
  ○ Male patient in 6th decade with nonspecific symptoms of nasal obstruction & discharge

Demographics

- Age
  ○ DLBCL: 6th-8th decades
  ○ NKTL: 5th-6th decades
- Sex
  ○ DLBCL: M:F = 1.2:1
  ○ NKTL: M:F = 2:1
- Ethnicity
  ○ B-cell type more common in USA & Europe

– Accounts for 55-85% of SN lymphomas in Western populations
  ○ T-cell type more common in **East Asia & Latin America**
- Epidemiology
  ○ < 1% of all H&N malignancies
    – 0.2-2% of all lymphomas arise in SN cavities
    – Malignant lymphoma is **most common nonepithelial SN malignancy**
  ○ < 50% of NHL occurs in H&N
    – 60% of H&N NHL is extranodal (sinonasal, oral cavity, laryngopharynx, salivary glands)
    – **44%** of H&N extranodal lymphomas occur **in sinonasal cavities**

Natural History & Prognosis

- B-cell type can have slow, indolent course if left untreated
  ○ Prognosis of DLBCL generally good with 50-75% 5-year survival
- NKTL has worse prognosis; can be rapidly fatal
  ○ Worse prognosis than DLBCL even though usually manifests as local disease in nasal cavity
  ○ 30-50% 5-year survival

Treatment

- Primary treatment: Local radiotherapy (XRT)
- Intermediate or more aggressive NHL-SN usually treated with combination chemotherapy or combination of radiation & chemotherapy
- NKTL: XRT for local disease; XRT & chemotherapy for multifocal or disseminated disease

DIAGNOSTIC CHECKLIST

Consider

- NHL-SN can be **difficult to distinguish** from other neoplasms, chronic sinusitis, & granulomatous disorders
  ○ NHL could be included in DDx for almost any aggressive adult nasal soft tissue mass
- Differentiation from granulomatous disease requires biopsy & laboratory studies

Image Interpretation Pearls

- Presence of enlarged homogeneous cervical nodes may be clue to diagnosis
- Simultaneous involvement of nasopharynx & oropharynx in addition to SN cavities is suggestive of NKTL, particularly in Asian patients
- Be sure to evaluate for extension beyond sinonasal cavities

SELECTED REFERENCES

1. Agarwal A et al: Extranodal natural killer/T-cell lymphoma, nasal type, misdiagnosed as fungal sinusitis. Radiol Imaging Cancer. 5(4):e230054, 2023
2. Bitner BF et al: Sinonasal lymphoma: a primer for otolaryngologists. Laryngoscope Investig Otolaryngol. 7(6):1712-24, 2022
3. Lehrich BM et al: Treatment modalities and survival outcomes for sinonasal diffuse large B-cell lymphoma. Laryngoscope. 131(11):E2727-35, 2021
4. Chen Y et al: Differential diagnosis of sinonasal extranodal NK/T cell lymphoma and diffuse large B cell lymphoma on MRI. Neuroradiology. 62(9):1149-55, 2020
5. He M et al: Differentiation between sinonasal natural killer/T-cell lymphomas and diffuse large B-cell lymphomas by RESOLVE DWI combined with conventional MRI. Magn Reson Imaging. 62:10-17, 2019
6. Harnsberger HR et al: Non-Hodgkin's lymphoma of the head and neck: CT evaluation of nodal and extranodal sites. AJR Am J Roentgenol. 149(4):785-91, 1987

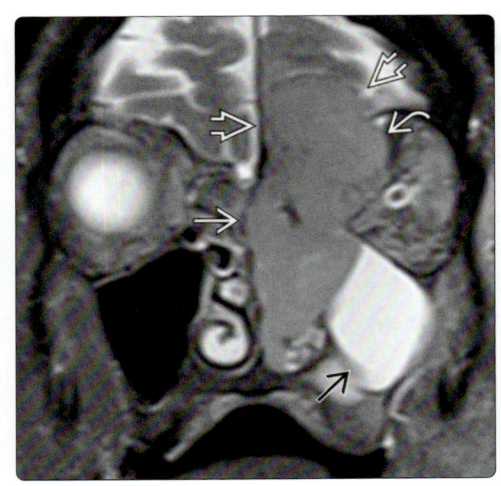

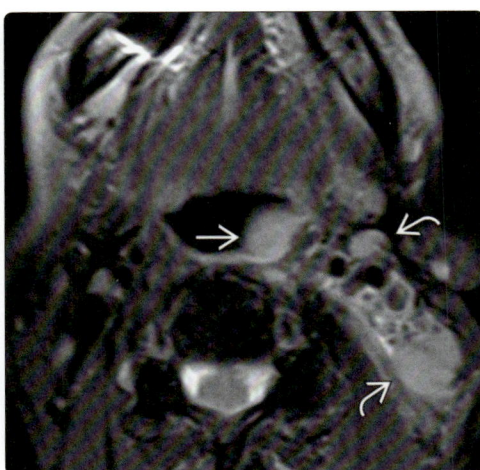

(Left) *Coronal STIR MR demonstrates a left sinonasal mass* ➡️ *with homogeneous low STIR signal intensity in this case of DLBCL. This mass invades the left anterior cranial fossa* ➡️ *and left orbit* ➡️. *Note left maxillary sinus hyperintense trapped secretions* ➡️. (Right) *Axial T2 FS MR in the same patient shows additional involvement of the left palatine tonsil* ➡️ *and multiple left cervical lymph nodes* ➡️, *suggesting the imaging diagnosis of NHL-SN.*

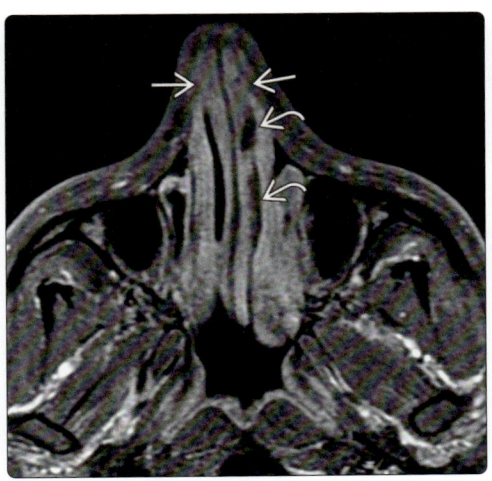

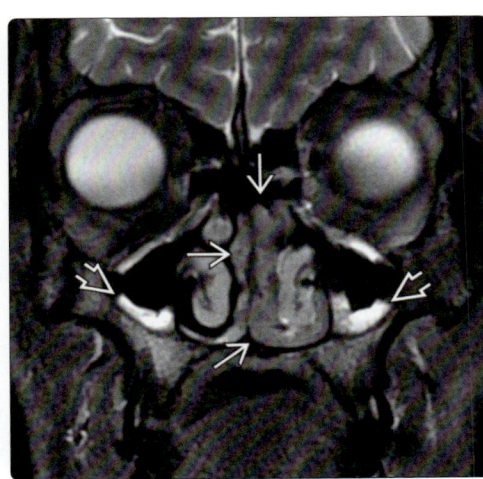

(Left) *Axial T2 FS MR demonstrates thickening of the nasal septum* ➡️ *with regions of nonenhancing necrosis* ➡️ *in this case of NKTL. The mucosal nonenhancement may mimic the imaging appearance of invasive fungal sinusitis.* (Right) *Coronal T2 FS MR in the same patient shows hypointense soft tissue thickening* ➡️ *of the nasal septum and left nasal cavity walls at the sites of involvement of NKTL. Note the more hyperintense normal sinus mucosa* ➡️.

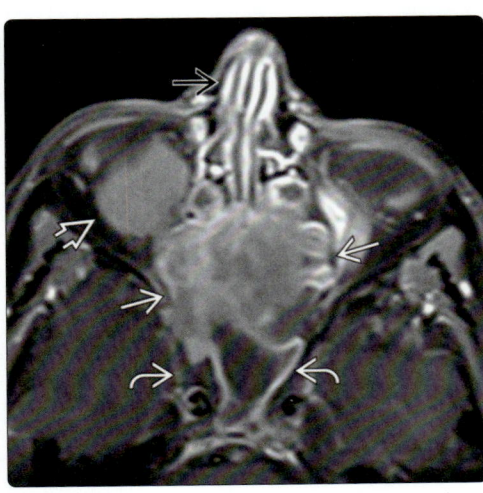

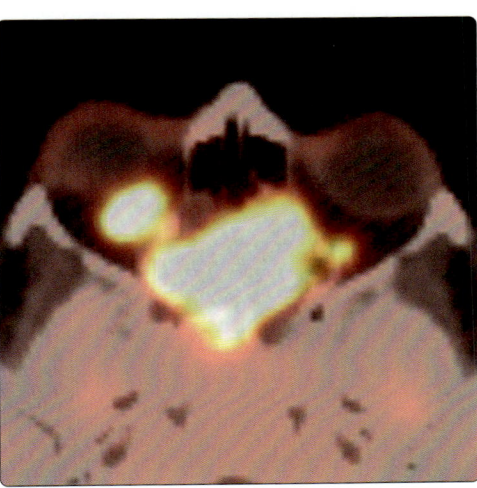

(Left) *Axial T1 C+ FS MR shows an enhancing mass in the posterior sinonasal cavity* ➡️ *with extension into the right orbit* ➡️ *in this case of DLBCL. The mass enhances less than the normal sinonasal mucosa* ➡️. *Note trapped secretions in the sphenoid sinuses* ➡️. (Right) *Axial FDG PET/CT in the same patient demonstrates diffuse FDG avidity within the lesion. FDG PET is useful in initial staging and monitoring treatment response of NHL-SN.*

Sinonasal Neuroendocrine Carcinoma

TERMINOLOGY

- Rare malignancy of epithelial origin expressing neuroendocrine markers
- Pathologically distinguishable from other sinonasal neuroectodermal tumors: Olfactory neuroblastoma (ONB), sinonasal undifferentiated carcinoma (SNUC), small cell neuroendocrine carcinoma (SCNEC)

IMAGING

- Sinonasal neuroectodermal tumors **cannot** reliably be distinguished with radiologic criteria
- Predilection for superior **nasal cavity** & **ethmoid sinuses**
- Variably enhancing, ill-defined mass; bone destruction & invasion of adjacent compartments

TOP DIFFERENTIAL DIAGNOSES

- Olfactory neuroblastoma
- Sinonasal undifferentiated carcinoma
- Sinonasal squamous cell carcinoma

- Sinonasal adenocarcinoma

PATHOLOGY

- Sinonasal neuroendocrine neoplasms range from more differentiated (ONB) to less differentiated (SNEC) to poorly differentiated (SCNEC)
- 2/3 (+) for epithelial markers (low molecular weight cytokeratins & epithelial membrane antigen)
- Immunoreactive for neuroendocrine markers (chromogranin, synaptophysin, S100, CD57)

CLINICAL ISSUES

- Wide age range; average: ~ 50 years
- Usually present with locally advanced disease
  - **60%** present as **stage IV disease**
- Management of these rare neoplasms often based on analogous treatment principles for neuroendocrine carcinoma of other anatomic sites (lung & larynx) & treatment of SNUC
- Overall 5-year survival: ~ 70%

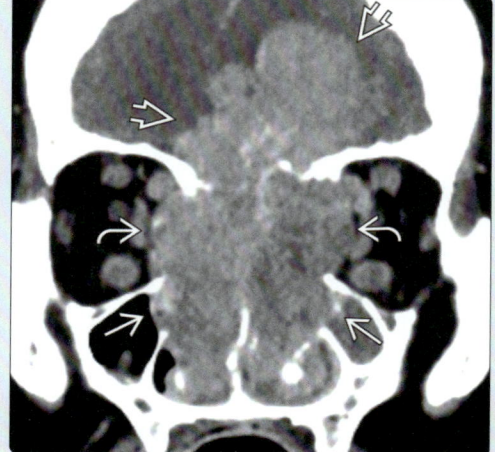
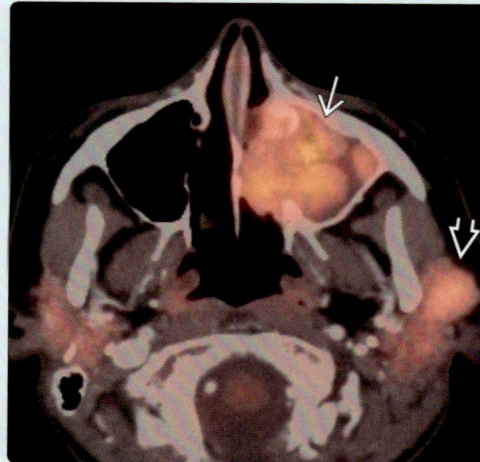

(Left) Coronal CECT shows a large, enhancing, destructive sinonasal mass ➡ with intracranial ⇗ and bilateral orbital ➚ extension in this case of pathologically proven SNEC. The nonspecific imaging appearance overlaps with most aggressive sinonasal malignancies. (Right) Axial FDG PET/CT shows an enhancing and FDG-avid mass ➡ centered in the left maxillary sinus in this patient with SNEC. Note metastatic lymphadenopathy in the left parotid gland ⇨. Both FDG and DOTATATE PET can be useful in staging SNEC.

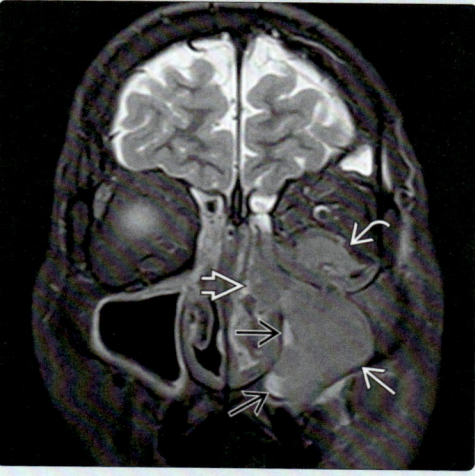
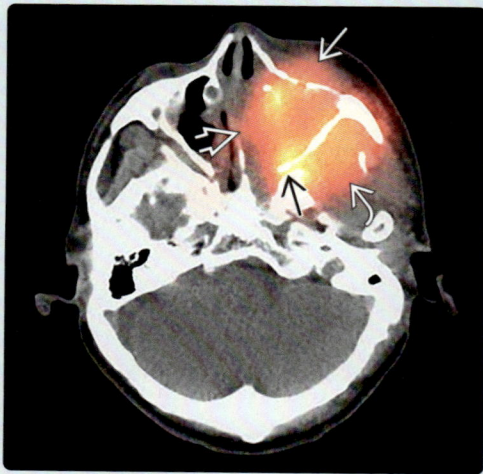

(Left) Coronal T2 FS MR demonstrates a hypointense soft tissue mass filling the left maxillary sinus ➡ with extension into the left nasal cavity ➡ and orbit ➚. Note hyperintense trapped secretion in the medial left maxillary sinus ➡. (Right) Axial In-111 pentetreotide-fused SPECT/CT in the same patient shows increased radiotracer uptake of the left maxillary sinus SNEC. There is extension into the left premaxillary soft tissues ➡, nasal cavity ➡, retromaxillary fat ➚, and pterygopalatine fossa ➡.

TERMINOLOGY

Abbreviations

- Sinonasal neuroendocrine carcinoma (SNEC)

Definitions

- Rare malignancy of epithelial origin expressing neuroendocrine markers
  - Pathologically distinguishable from other sinonasal neuroectodermal tumors: Olfactory neuroblastoma (ONB), sinonasal undifferentiated carcinoma (SNUC), small cell neuroendocrine carcinoma (SCNEC)

IMAGING

General Features

- Best diagnostic clue
  - Sinonasal neuroectodermal tumors cannot generally be distinguished by clinical or radiologic criteria
- Location
  - Predilection for superior **nasal cavity** & **ethmoid sinuses**
  - In H&N, more common in larynx

CT Findings

- CECT
  - Variably enhancing soft tissue mass with ill-defined borders & invasion of adjacent compartments
- Bone CT
  - Aggressive bone destruction

MR Findings

- T1WI
  - Ill-defined soft tissue mass; isointense to musculature
- STIR
  - Heterogeneous, low to intermediate long TR signal
- T1WI C+ FS
  - Variable, typically diffuse enhancement

Nuclear Medicine Findings

- In-111 pentetreotide scintigraphy
  - ↑ uptake in well- & moderately differentiated SNEC
- Ga-68 DOTATATE PET/CT
  - ↑ uptake, binds to somatostatin receptors with greater affinity than In-111 pentetreotide

Imaging Recommendations

- Best imaging tool
  - Multiplanar gadolinium-enhanced MR with fat suppression best delineates tumor extent

DIFFERENTIAL DIAGNOSIS

Olfactory Neuroblastoma

- Arises near cribriform plate; highly vascular with avid enhancement ± flow voids

Sinonasal Undifferentiated Carcinoma

- Aggressive, ill-defined mass; often with necrosis
- Least differentiated of neuroectodermal tumors with tenuous neuroendocrine differentiation

Sinonasal Adenocarcinoma

- Nonspecific imaging features; ethmoid predilection; rare < 40-50 years of age

Sinonasal Squamous Cell Carcinoma

- Most common sinonasal malignancy; commonly arises in maxillary antrum (~ 70%)

Small Cell Neuroendocrine Carcinoma

- Rare; nonspecific features; cannot distinguish from SNEC or SNUC on imaging
- Poorly differentiated, small cell variant of neuroendocrine carcinoma

PATHOLOGY

General Features

- Etiology
  - Cell of origin not clearly known
    - Derived from endocrine cells of dispersed neuroendocrine system vs. basal progenitor cells in olfactory mucosa

Staging, Grading, & Classification

- SNEC is **part of spectrum of neuroendocrine tumors**
  - ONB (most differentiated) → SNEC → SCNEC → SNUC
- SNEC is morphologically distinct from SCNEC & immunohistochemically distinct from SNUC

Microscopic Features

- 2/3 (+) for epithelial markers (low-molecular-weight cytokeratins & epithelial membrane antigen)
- Neurosecretory granules
  - Immunoreactive for neuroendocrine markers (chromogranin, synaptophysin, S100, CD57)

CLINICAL ISSUES

Presentation

- Most common signs/symptoms
  - Nasal obstruction, discharge, & epistaxis

Demographics

- Age
  - Wide range (20-70 years); average: ~ 50 years

Natural History & Prognosis

- Usually present with locally advanced disease
  - **60%** present as **stage IV disease**

Treatment

- Management of these rare neoplasms often based on analogous treatment principles for neuroendocrine carcinoma of other anatomic sites (lung & larynx) & treatment of SNUC
  - Multimodality approach utilized at most institutions (surgery + chemotherapy & XRT)
  - Lu-177 DOTATATE & Y-90 DOTATATE can provide targeted XRT in tumors avid on Ga-68 DOTATATE PET/CT

SELECTED REFERENCES

1. Keilin CA et al: Sinonasal neuroendocrine carcinoma: 15 years of experience at a single institution. J Neurol Surg B Skull Base. 84(1):51-9, 2023
2. Issa K et al: Survival outcomes in sinonasal carcinoma with neuroendocrine differentiation: a NCDB analysis. Am J Otolaryngol. 42(2):102851, 2021
3. Lin N et al: Small cell neuroendocrine carcinoma of paranasal sinuses: radiologic features in 14 cases. J Comput Assist Tomogr. 45(1):135-41, 2021

Sinonasal Undifferentiated Carcinoma

TERMINOLOGY

- Sinonasal undifferentiated carcinoma (**SNUC**)
- Rare, aggressive sinonasal nonsquamous cell epithelial or nonepithelial malignant neoplasm of varying histogenesis

IMAGING

- Aggressive sinonasal mass with bone destruction & rapid growth
- Large, typically > 4 cm at presentation
- Origin most common in nasal cavity & extending into paranasal sinuses; ethmoid sinus origin more common than maxillary sinus
- Bone CT: Poorly defined soft tissue sinonasal mass with aggressive bone destruction
- MR: Isointense to muscle on T1
  - Low to intermediate T2 signal
  - Heterogeneous enhancement with necrosis
- PET: ↑ avidity
  - Helpful in detection of metastatic disease

TOP DIFFERENTIAL DIAGNOSES

- Sinonasal squamous cell carcinoma
- Olfactory neuroblastoma
- Sinonasal adenocarcinoma
- Sinonasal non-Hodgkin lymphoma

CLINICAL ISSUES

- Distant metastases to bone, brain & dura, liver, & cervical nodes more common than other sinonasal malignancies
- Aggressive multimodality therapy treatment, including craniofacial resection & adjuvant chemotherapy ± XRT
- Poor prognosis despite aggressive treatment

DIAGNOSTIC CHECKLIST

- Imaging features are nonspecific
- Tumor growth rate & presence of nodes/distant metastases helpful for suggesting SNUC
- Consider extending coverage to evaluate for intracranial (particularly dural) & cervical nodal disease

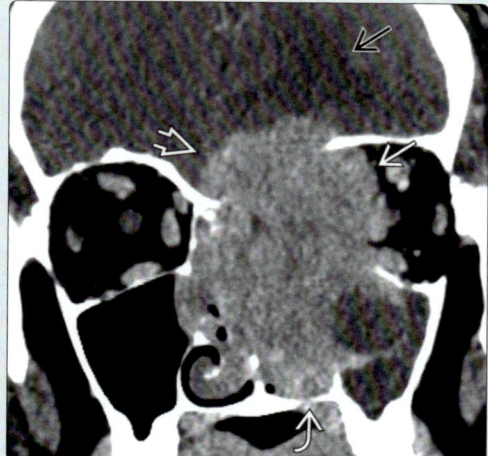
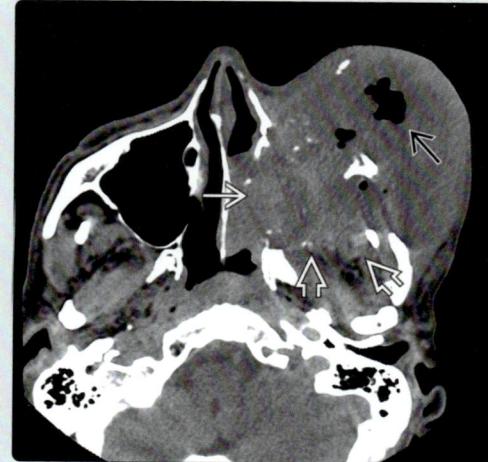

(Left) Coronal CECT shows a destructive, enhancing mass in the sinonasal cavity with left orbital ➡ & intracranial ➡ invasion resulting in left frontal lobe vasogenic edema ➡ in this case of SNUC. Additional subtle destruction affects the left nasal cavity floor ➡. (Right) Axial NECT demonstrates a large mass in the left maxillary antrum with marked bone destruction & extension into the nasal cavity ➡, masticator space ➡, & soft tissues of the cheek. Foci of air ➡ are seen within the necrotic portion of this rapidly growing lesion.

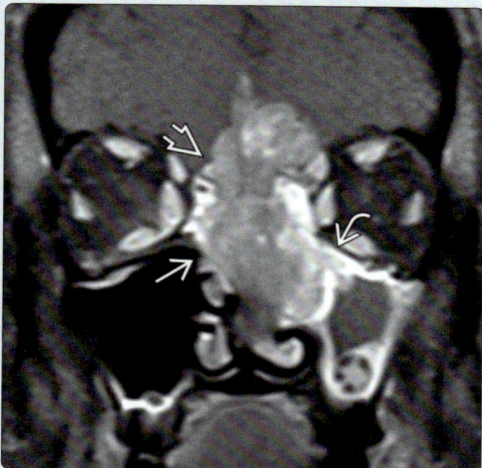
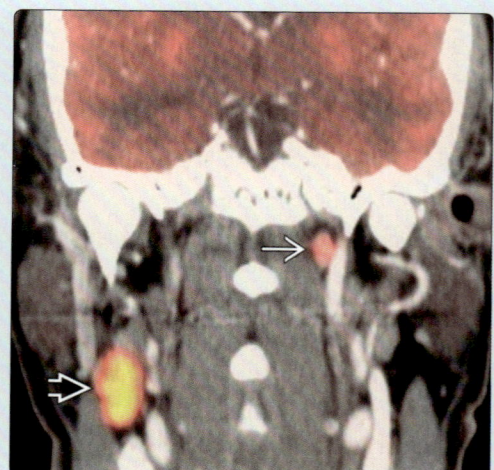

(Left) Coronal T1 C+ FS MR shows an aggressive mass centered in the nasal cavity & ethmoid sinuses ➡, extending intracranially through the anterior skull base ➡ in this patient with SNUC. Tumor is also noted extending into the left extraconal orbit ➡. (Right) Coronal PET/CT in the same patient demonstrates FDG avidity in the left retropharyngeal ➡ & right cervical ➡ lymph nodes, compatible with metastatic lymphadenopathy.

Sinonasal Adenoid Cystic Carcinoma

KEY FACTS

TERMINOLOGY

- Malignant neoplasm arising from minor salivary gland tissue

IMAGING

- Location: **Maxillary** > nasal cavity
- Low grade: Solidly enhancing, well-defined soft tissue mass
- High grade: Poorly defined, heterogeneous + bone destruction ± perineural tumor spread (PNTS)
- Bone CT variable: Smooth remodeling in low-grade tumors to aggressive destruction for high-grade tumors
- Multiplanar, **gadolinium-enhanced MR with fat suppression** recommended
  - Improves detection of PNTS

TOP DIFFERENTIAL DIAGNOSES

- Sinonasal squamous cell carcinoma
- Sinonasal adenocarcinoma (intestinal type)
- Olfactory neuroblastoma
- Sinonasal undifferentiated carcinoma

PATHOLOGY

- Not associated with inhalation exposures
- 3 histologic types
  - Cribriform (52%)
  - Tubular (20%)
  - Solid (29%); worst outcome; higher tendency for PNTS
- Most patients present with **T4 disease (65%)**

CLINICAL ISSUES

- Sinonasal adenoid cystic carcinoma (ACCa) accounts for 10-25% of H&N ACCa
  - Most common sinonasal salivary tumor
- Symptoms mimic sinusitis
  - **Facial pain ± numbness** (CNV2) → PNTS
- More common in White patients
- Overall 5-year survival rate: 50-86%
  - Late recurrences are not uncommon even > 15 years after initial therapy
- Treatment: Resection and postop radiation

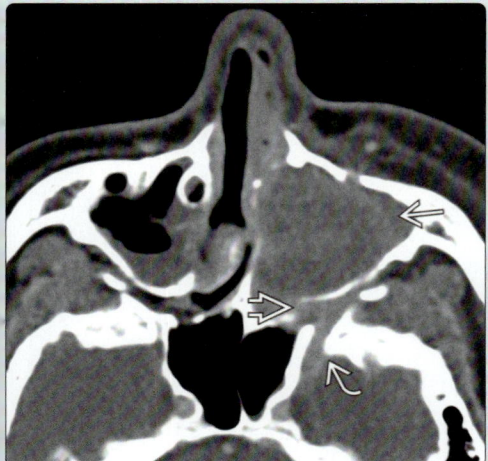
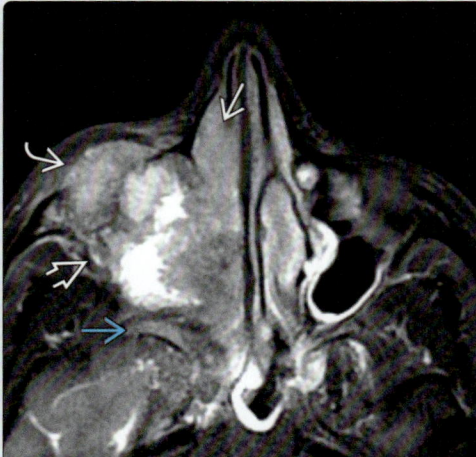

(Left) Axial CECT shows a mass filling the left maxillary sinus ➡. Note enhancing soft tissue expanding the left pterygopalatine fossa ➡ and foramen rotundum ➡, compatible with perineural tumor spread from the left maxillary sinus adenoid cystic carcinoma (ACCa). (Right) Axial T2 FS MR shows an intermediate T2 signal intensity mass in the right nasal cavity ➡ and maxillary sinus ➡ with premaxillary soft tissue extension ➡ in this case of ACCa. Note perineural tumor spread within the right pterygopalatine fossa ➡.

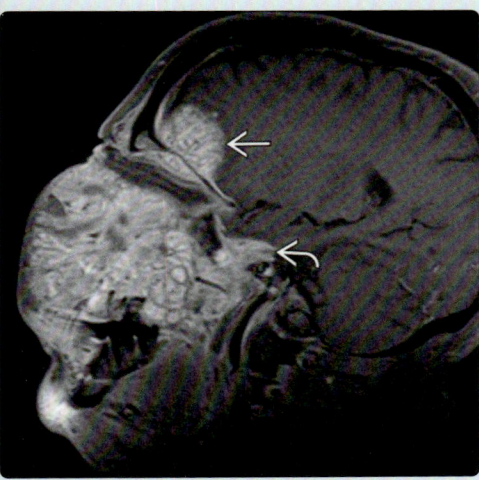
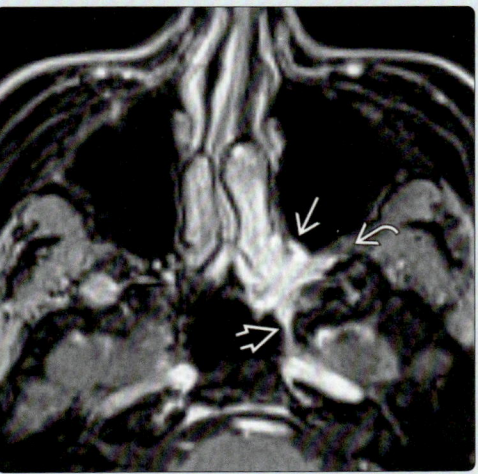

(Left) Sagittal T1 C+ FS MR shows a heterogeneous enhancing ACCa involving the paranasal sinuses and orbit with intradural extension through the orbital roof ➡. Note gross perineural tumor spread into the cavernous sinus ➡. (Right) Axial T1WI C+ FS MR shows an enhancing mass centered in the left sphenopalatine foramen ➡, compatible with ACCa. There is enhancement extending into the left pterygopalatine fossa ➡ and vidian canal ➡, consistent with perineural tumor spread.

IMAGING

- Arises from maxilla, nasal septum, and skull base
  - Nasal septum location: Posterosuperior vomer
- Bone CT: **Chondroid matrix calcification** and narrow bony transition zone
  - 50% with chondroid matrix
- MR: ↑ T2 signal, ↓ T1
- ↑ ADC value (≈ 2,000 x 10^{-6} mm²/s)
- Heterogeneous variegated enhancement
- CT best tool for identifying characteristic matrix calcifications and bone destruction

TOP DIFFERENTIAL DIAGNOSES

- Sinonasal osteosarcoma
- Skull base meningioma
- Sinonasal ossifying fibroma
- Sinonasal fibrous dysplasia
- Olfactory neuroblastoma

PATHOLOGY

- Malignant neoplasm arising from chondrocytes, embryonal rests, or mesenchymal cells
- May complicate Ollier and Maffucci syndromes

CLINICAL ISSUES

- Presents in 5th-7th decades
  - Onset of symptoms to diagnosis: 3 months to 1 year
- Accounts for only 0.1% of H&N cancers
- Surgical resection is primary treatment modality
  - Difficult to achieve oncologic resection due to proximity of vital structures
  - Late recurrences after long disease-free periods are reported; long-term follow-up advised
- Overall 5-year survival: 54-81%

DIAGNOSTIC CHECKLIST

- Sinonasal mass with **arc** or **ring-like calcified matrix** on CT and ↑ T2/↑ ADC value on MR suggests chondrosarcoma

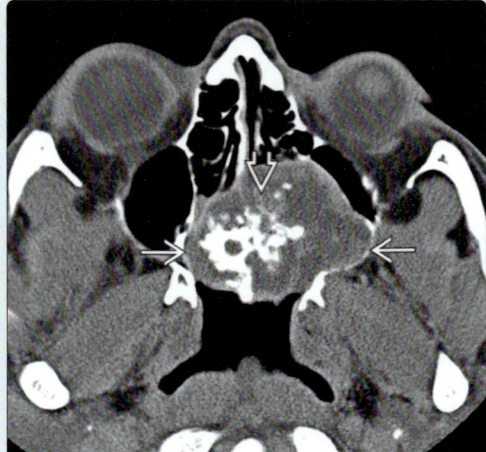
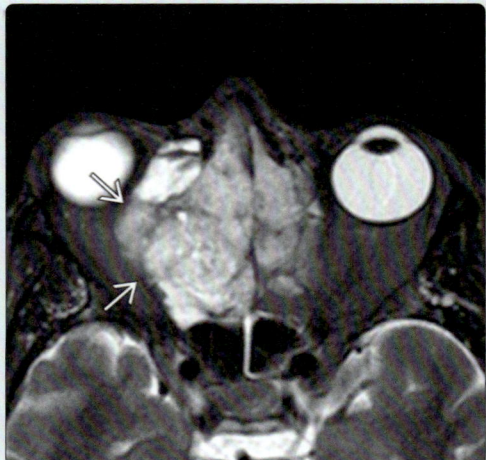

(Left) *Axial NECT in a young adult with 3-4 years of difficulty breathing through her nose shows a mass ➡ arising from posterior nasal septum, causing remodeling of the sinus walls. Note the characteristic ring and arc appearance of chondroid matrix ➡. (Right) Axial STIR MR demonstrates a large chondrosarcoma involving the ethmoid sinuses bilaterally. There is extension into the right orbit ➡. High signal on T2-weighted images is a common feature of this histology.*

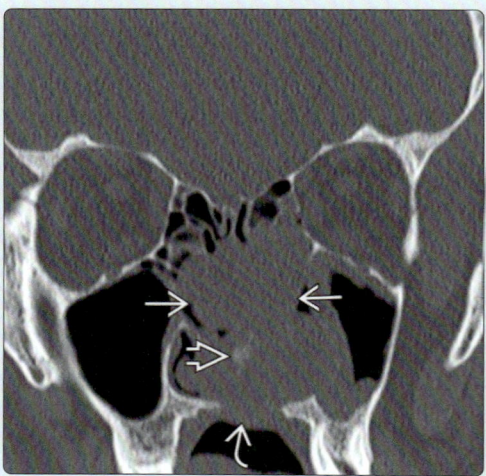
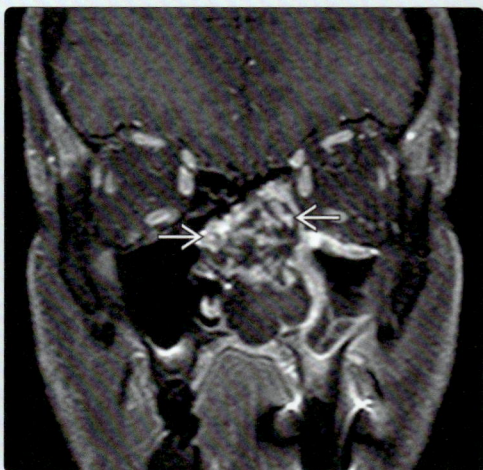

(Left) *Coronal bone CT shows a mass destroying the nasal septum with tumor filling the L > R nasal cavity ➡. A small focus of chondroid matrix ➡ is noted. Tumor erodes through the floor of the nasal cavity, creating a small submucosal bulge beneath the hard palate ➡. (Right) Coronal T1 C+ FS MR in the same patient shows a tumor with generally low signal intensity with a typical variegated enhancement pattern ➡ within this nasal septum chondrosarcoma.*

Sinonasal Osteosarcoma

KEY FACTS

TERMINOLOGY

- Rare, malignant bone tumor arising from **primitive bone-forming mesenchyma**

IMAGING

- > 50% of craniofacial osteosarcoma (OSa) arise in jaw
  - Mandible > maxilla
  - < 50% involve extragnathic bones
- CT best for osteoid matrix & cortical involvement
  - **Hyperdense mass** with osteoid matrix & **sunburst** periosteal reaction
- MR best evaluates extent in marrow & adjacent structures

TOP DIFFERENTIAL DIAGNOSES

- Chondrosarcoma
- Ossifying fibroma
- Osteoma
- Fibrous dysplasia
- Metastasis

PATHOLOGY

- Up to 25% are 2nd malignancy in **prior radiation field**
- Higher incidence in hereditary retinoblastoma & Li Fraumeni syndrome
- May arise in bone affected by Paget disease, fibrous dysplasia, multiple exostoses, enchondromatosis

CLINICAL ISSUES

- Common symptoms
  - Painful facial swelling
  - Nasal obstruction & epistaxis
  - Change in maxillary tooth position ± tooth loosening
- Most present in 3rd-4th decades
  - Older than classical OSa of long bones
- No strong sex predilection
- Craniofacial OSa accounts for 6-13% of all OSa
- Complete surgical resection is mainstay of treatment
- Worse prognosis in radiation-induced OSa & extragnathic locations

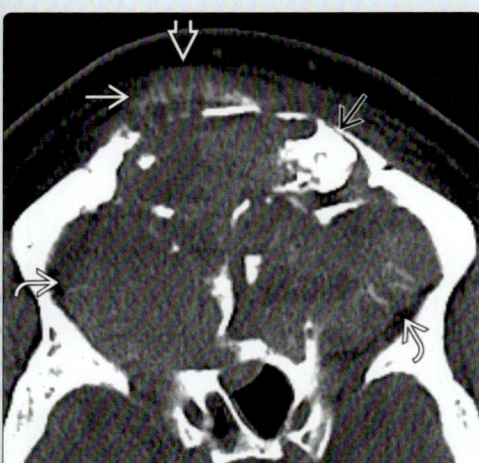

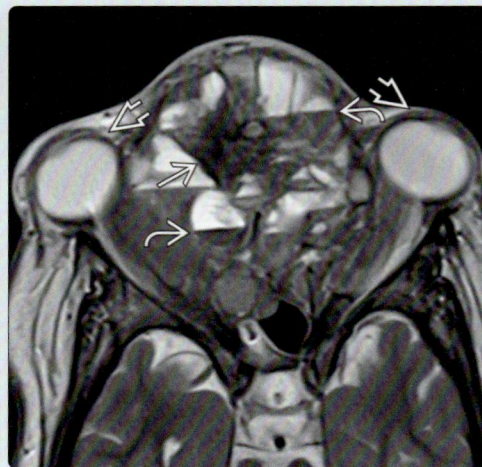

(Left) Axial bone CT shows an expansile, destructive sinonasal mass extending into the orbits ⊅ and prefrontal soft tissues ⊅. Note linear "sunburst" periosteal reaction ⊅ and dense calcification ⊅ in this pathology-proven case of osteoblastic osteosarcoma. (Right) Axial T2 MR in the same patient shows regions of low T2 signal ⊅ corresponding with enhancing soft tissue (not shown). Multilocular cysts with fluid-fluid levels ⊅ correspond with an associated aneurysmal bone cyst. There is resultant severe telecanthus ⊅.

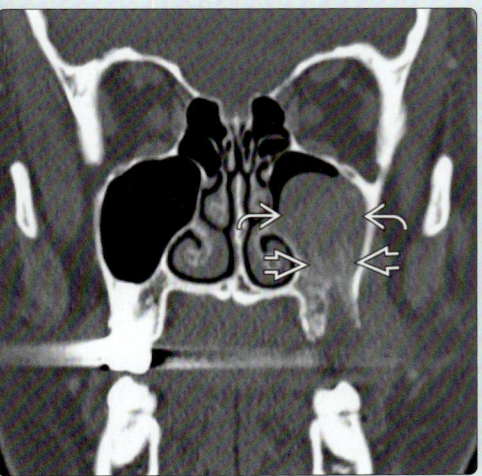

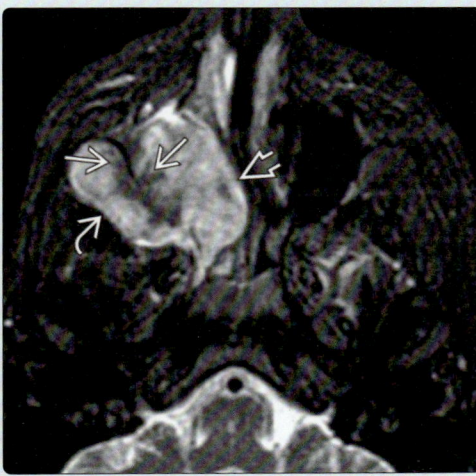

(Left) Coronal bone CT shows a soft tissue mass in the left maxillary sinus ⊅. Spicules of bone indicating periosteal reaction radiate from the tumor origin in the maxillary alveolus ⊅. (Right) Axial T2WI FS MR demonstrates a large osteosarcoma centered near the lateral wall of the right maxillary sinus. There is medial extension into the nasal cavity ⊅ and lateral extension into the masticator space ⊅. Linear, hypointense radiating periosteal reaction ⊅ is noted along the bone of origin.

Sinonasal SWI/SNF Complex-Deficient Carcinoma

KEY FACTS

TERMINOLOGY

- SWItch/sucrose nonfermentable (SWI/SNF)-related matrix-associated actin-dependent regulator of chromatin subfamily B member 1
- *SMARCB1*: Loss of *SMARCB1*::*INI1* protein expression on immunohistochemistry
- *SMARCA4*: BRG1 stain negative on immunohistochemistry

IMAGING

- Destructive sinonasal mass
- *SMARCB1* involves sinuses (especially ethmoids)
- *SMARCA4* typically nasal origin
- May invade skull base & orbits
- CT may show calcified matrix (50%) ± "hair-on-end" periosteal reaction
- MR shows variable T2 hyperintensity, intense enhancement, & low ADC
- FDG PET usually highly avid
- Staging follows 8th edition AJCC sinonasal tumors

- Recommended imaging tools: Sinus NECT for bones, calcified tumor matrix, periosteal reaction
- Enhanced MR for local invasion & perineural spread
- FDG PET for distant metastases

TOP DIFFERENTIAL DIAGNOSES

- Sinonasal undifferentiated carcinoma
- Neuroendocrine tumor
- Olfactory neuroblastoma
- HPV-associated multiphenotypic sinonasal carcinoma

PATHOLOGY

- Undifferentiated carcinoma with *SMARCB1* (INI1) or *SMARCA4* (BRG1) loss on immunohistochemistry

CLINICAL ISSUES

- *SMARCB1* has aggressive clinical course with 56% of patients deceased at median of 16 months
- *SMARCA4* also highly aggressive clinically; 2/3 of patients deceased within 1 year

(Left) *Axial bone CT in a patient with SMARCB1-deficient sinonasal tumor shows a maxillary sinus mass with aggressive bone destruction of the posterior wall ➡ with tumor extending into the masticator space. Note faintly mineralized, calcified tumor matrix along the peripheral tumor borders ➡.* (Right) *Axial T2 MR in the same patient shows heterogeneous tumor in the maxillary sinus invading the nasal cavity ➡ and masticator space ➡. Imaging cannot differentiate this from other aggressive malignancies.*

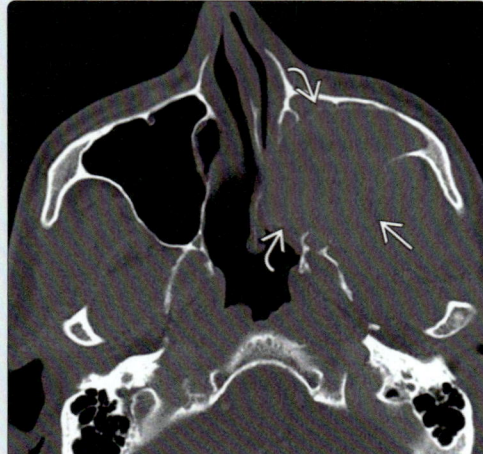
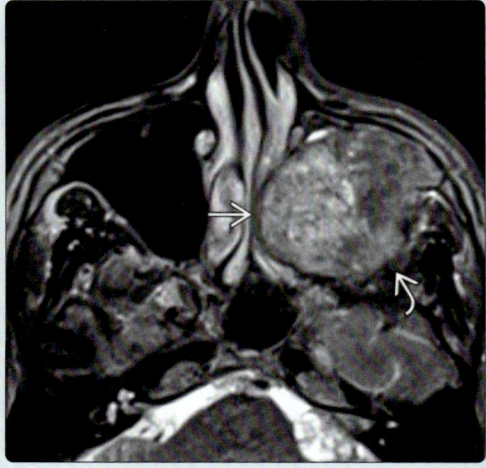

(Left) *Coronal T1 C+ FS MR shows heterogeneous solid enhancement of this SMARCB1-deficient carcinoma involving the nasal cavity ➡, maxillary sinus, maxillary alveolus ➡, and inferior extraconal orbit ➡.* (Right) *Sagittal bone CT shows an aggressive pattern of osseous destruction with tumor invading through the outer table of the frontal sinus into the scalp subcutaneous tissues ➡ and intracranial compartment ➡. Tumor matrix calcifications ➡ are noted.*

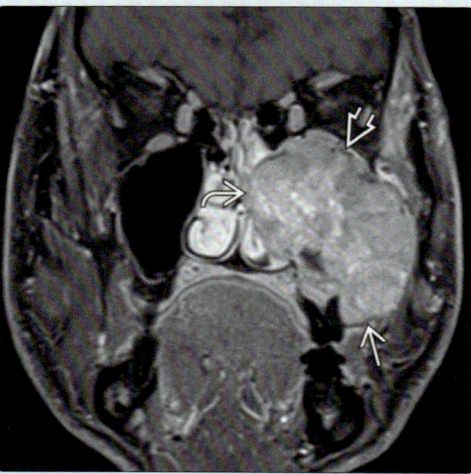
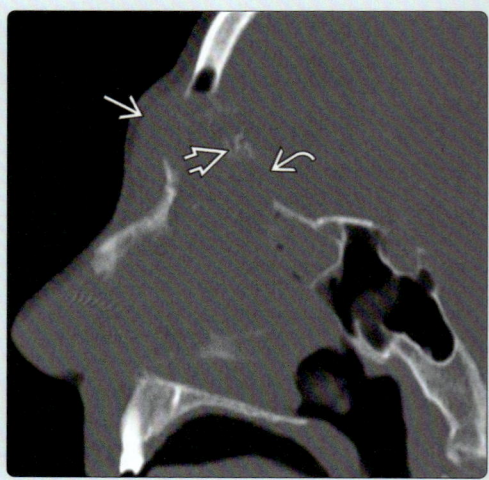

TERMINOLOGY

Abbreviations

- SWItch/sucrose nonfermentable (SWI/SNF)

Definitions

- SWI/SNF-related matrix-associated actin-dependent regulator of chromatin subfamily B member 1
- SWI/SNF subtypes distinguished immunohistochemically
  - *SMARCB1*: Loss of *SMARCB1::INI1* protein expression
  - *SMARCA4*: BRG1 stain negative

IMAGING

General Features

- Best diagnostic clue
  - Destructive nasal or ethmoid sinus mass
- Location
  - *SMARCB1* involves sinuses (especially ethmoids)
  - *SMARCA4* typically nasal
- Size
  - Usually large with extensive local tissue invasion

CT Findings

- Destructive; often invades skull base & orbits
- Calcified matrix (50%)
- ± "hair-on-end" periosteal reaction

MR Findings

- Variable T2 hyperintensity
- Intense enhancement
- Low ADC

Nuclear Medicine Findings

- High FDG uptake typical

Imaging Recommendations

- Best imaging tool
  - Sinus CT for bony margins, matrix, periosteal reaction
  - Enhanced MR for local invasion & perineural spread
  - FDG PET for distant metastases
- Protocol advice
  - NECT & enhanced MR ± PET for distant metastasis

DIFFERENTIAL DIAGNOSIS

Sinonasal Undifferentiated Carcinoma

- Diagnosis of exclusion; imaging is similar
- Heterogeneous, aggressive, & destructive

Sinonasal Neuroendocrine Tumor

- Imaging is similar
- Origin in ethmoids & superior nasal cavity
- Ill-defined margins, aggressive bone destruction

Olfactory Neuroblastoma

- Erosion lamina papyracea & anterior skull base
- Peritumoral cysts at brain interface

HPV-Associated Multiphenotypic Sinonasal Carcinoma

- Imaging is similar; high-risk HPV on molecular pathology
- Nasal cavity origin (89% arise in turbinate)

PATHOLOGY

General Features

- SWI/SNF complex-deficient carcinomas constitute 1-3% of sinonasal carcinomas & 3-20% of tumors previously diagnosed as sinonasal undifferentiated carcinoma

Staging, Grading, & Classification

- Follows 8th edition AJCC sinonasal tumor staging

Gross Pathologic & Surgical Features

- *SMARCB1* lacks gland formation, often nondescript basaloid > eosinophilic/oncocytoid morphology
- *SMARCB4* lacks glandular or squamous immunophenotypes

Immunohistochemistry

- *SMARCB1*
  - Defined by *SMARCB1* loss
- *SMARCB4*
  - Undifferentiated with loss of *SMARCB4*

CLINICAL ISSUES

Presentation

- Most common signs/symptoms
  - Nonspecific symptoms of nasal obstruction, sinusitis, epistaxis, & headache due to obstruction
  - Typically presents at high T stage (T4)
- Other signs/symptoms
  - Orbital complications (e.g., proptosis or diplopia)

Demographics

- Male predominance
- *SMARCB1* peaks 6th decade (11-89 years)
- *SMARCA4* lower median age: 44 years

Natural History & Prognosis

- *SMARCB1*-deficient sinonasal carcinoma has aggressive clinical course with 56% of patients deceased at median of 16 months
- *SMARCA4* also highly aggressive
  - 2/3 of patients deceased within 1 year

Treatment

- Complete surgical ± radiation ± chemotherapy

DIAGNOSTIC CHECKLIST

Image Interpretation Pearls

- Highly aggressive & invasive-appearing tumor

SELECTED REFERENCES

1. Xu X et al: Outcomes of SWI/SNF complex-deficient sinonasal carcinomas in a Southeast Asian cohort. Head Neck. 47(1):14-22, 2025
2. WHO Classification of Tumours Editorial Board: WHO Classification of Head and Neck Tumours. Vol 9. 5th ed. IARC, 2024
3. Agaimy A: SWI/SNF-deficient sinonasal carcinomas. Adv Anat Pathol. 30(2):95-103, 2023
4. Agarwal A et al: Update from the 5th Edition of the WHO Classification of nasal, paranasal, and skull base tumors: imaging overview with histopathologic and genetic correlation. AJNR Am J Neuroradiol. 44(10):1116-25, 2023

Sinonasal Biphenotypic Sarcoma

TERMINOLOGY

- Bland spindle cell malignancy showing neural & myogenic differentiation, exclusively affects sinonasal tract

IMAGING

- Location: Superior nasal cavity ± sinus invasion
  - Extension outside sinonasal tract in 27%, often orbit
- CT
  - Mixed lytic & sclerotic changes
  - Hyperostotic bone formation is common (80%)
  - Frequent erosion of nasal septum, lamina papyracea, &/or cribriform plate
- MR
  - T1: Isointense (relative to gray matter)
  - T2: Iso- to hyperintense (relative to gray matter)
  - T1 C+ MR: Homogeneous to heterogeneous enhancement
  - May have intratumoral cystic change or necrosis
- Best imaging tool: Enhanced MR for full disease extent

TOP DIFFERENTIAL DIAGNOSES

- Sinonasal squamous cell carcinoma
- Sinonasal adenocarcinoma
- Sinonasal melanoma
- Sinonasal non-Hodgkin lymphoma
- Olfactory neuroblastoma

PATHOLOGY

- Dual neural & myogenic features
- Rearrangements of *PAX3* gene hallmark

CLINICAL ISSUES

- Presents with nasal obstruction, congestion, epistaxis
- Mean age at presentation: 53 years (range: 24-87 years)
- F:M = 3:1
- **Slow-growing** mass; no reports of metastases
- Treatment: Surgical excision ± adjuvant radiochemotherapy
- Locally aggressive with recurrence in ~ 1/3 to 1/2

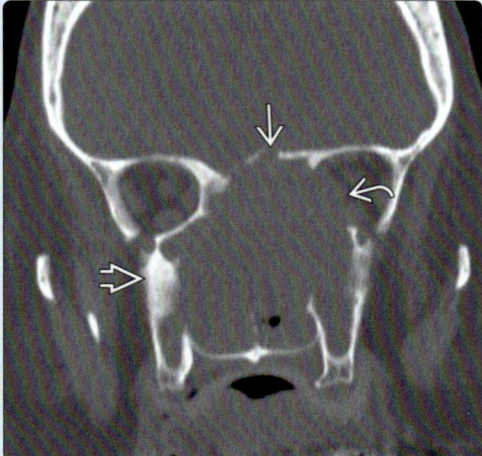
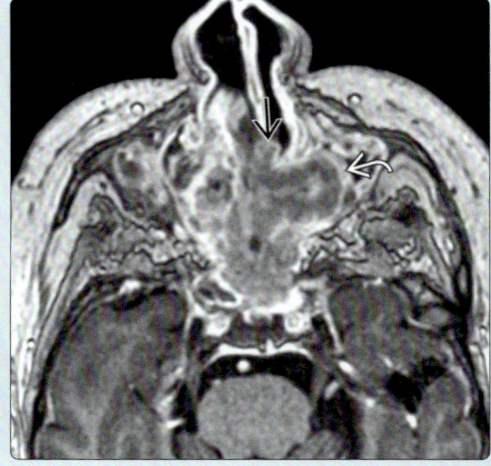

(Left) Coronal bone CT shows a soft tissue mass arising in the nasal cavity with bone erosion and invasion of the intracranial compartment ➡, orbit ➡, and diffuse erosion of the nasal septum and ethmoid septations. Bony hyperostosis ➡ is noted, which is frequently observed with biphenotypic sarcoma. (Right) Axial T1 C+ MR in the same patient shows a heterogeneously enhancing sinus mass destroying the nasal septum ➡ and involving the left maxillary sinus ➡ and orbit (not shown).

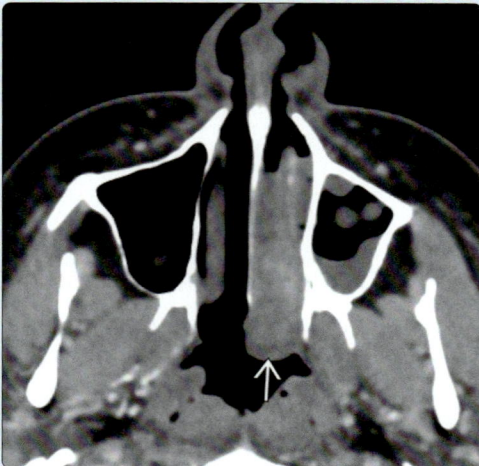
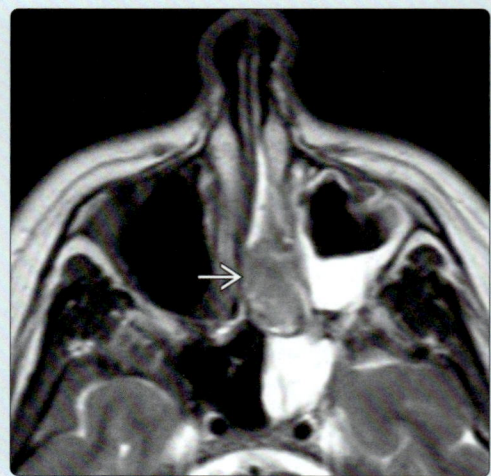

(Left) Axial CECT shows a heterogeneously enhancing mass mildly expanding left nasal cavity ➡ without bony destruction. CT features are nonspecific in this case. (Right) Axial T2 MR in the same patient shows a small, iso- to hypointense, obstructing left nasal cavity soft tissue mass ➡. Note trapped secretions in left maxillary and sphenoid sinuses. Imaging appearance is not specific in this small biphenotypic sinonasal sarcoma and could be seen with other neoplasms, such as squamous cell carcinoma, melanoma, or lymphoma.

TERMINOLOGY

Abbreviations

- Biphenotypic sinonasal sarcoma (BSNS)

Synonyms

- Low-grade sarcoma with neural & myogenic elements

Definitions

- Bland spindle cell malignancy showing neural & myogenic differentiation, exclusively affects sinonasal tract

IMAGING

General Features

- Best diagnostic clue
  - Superior nasal mass
  - Slow growth pattern but locally aggressive
  - **Bone erosion** present in 20-27%
    - Often nasal septum, lamina papyracea, &/or cribriform plate
- Location
  - Typically upper nasal cavity mass often invading ethmoids > ethmoid sinus > sphenoid sinuses, though can arise anywhere in sinonasal tract
  - Extension outside sinonasal tract in 27%, often orbital
- Size
  - Median tumor: 4 cm
- Morphology
  - Most unilateral, but can be bilateral

CT Findings

- Mixed lytic & sclerotic changes
- **Hyperostotic bone** formation is common (~ 80%)

MR Findings

- T1 shows isointense signal to (relative to gray matter)
- T2: Iso- to hyperintense signal (relative to gray matter)
- T1 C+ MR: Homogeneous to heterogeneous enhancement
- May have intratumoral cystic change or necrosis

Imaging Recommendations

- Best imaging tool
  - Enhanced MR to evaluate full disease extent
- Protocol advice
  - CT sinus & sinus MR ± contrast complimentary

DIFFERENTIAL DIAGNOSIS

Sinonasal Squamous Cell Carcinoma

- Arises in maxillary sinus more commonly

Sinonasal Adenocarcinoma

- May appear similar; often heterogeneous with hemorrhage

Sinonasal Melanoma

- Intrinsic T1 hyperintensity may be clue if present

Sinonasal Non-Hodgkin Lymphoma

- Homogeneous, diffusion-restricting

Olfactory Neuroblastoma

- May have cysts at brain-tumor interface

PATHOLOGY

General Features

- Dual neural & myogenic features

Staging, Grading, & Classification

- Staging AJCC 8th edition for nasal/ethmoid neoplasms
- Usually low grade with low mitotic rate

Gross Pathologic & Surgical Features

- Nonspecific tan-white or pink, firm mass; may be polypoid
- Tumors often large; median size 40 mm

Microscopic Features

- Spindle morphology with neural & myogenic differentiation, infiltrative, herringbone appearance

Immunohistochemistry

- Focal or patchy S100(+) (100%), focal or patchy SMA(+) (92%) may be β-catenin (+) (54%)
- Most stain positive for PAX3

Molecular Genetics

- Rearrangements of *PAX3* gene hallmark
- *PAX3::MAML3* most common gene fusion variant

CLINICAL ISSUES

Presentation

- Most common signs/symptoms
  - Mimics sinusitis: Congestion & mucopurulent drainage
  - Nasal obstruction, epistaxis, mucocele
- Other signs/symptoms
  - ± facial swelling, pain, & pressure

Demographics

- Mean age at presentation: 53 years (range: 24-87 years)
- F:M = 3:1

Natural History & Prognosis

- Local recurrence in ~ 1/3 to 1/2
  - May occur years after initial diagnosis
  - Median time to recurrence 11 months
- **Slow-growing** mass; no reports of metastases

Treatment

- Surgical excision ± adjuvant radiotherapy ± chemotherapy

DIAGNOSTIC CHECKLIST

Consider

- CT and enhanced MR are complementary

Image Interpretation Pearls

- Bony hyperostosis is common feature

SELECTED REFERENCES

1. WHO Classification of Tumours Online: Head and neck tumours. 9th version. Published 2023. Accessed February 27, 2025. https://tumourclassification.iarc.who.int/chapters/52
2. Dean KE et al: Imaging review of new and emerging sinonasal tumors and tumor-like entities from the fourth edition of the World Health Organization Classification of Head and Neck Tumors. AJNR Am J Neuroradiol. 40(4):584-90, 2019

TERMINOLOGY

- Epithelial sinonasal tract neoplasm with surface & minor salivary gland elements having transcriptionally active HPV

IMAGING

- CT: Enhancing soft tissue mass involving turbinate/nasal cavity ± bone destruction
  - Well-circumscribed mass ± regional bone invasion
  - Variable tumoral calcifications
- MR: Heterogeneous T1 &/or T2 hyperintensities
  - Heterogeneous enhancement
  - May have orbital &/or intracranial extension
- Suggests more aggressive tumor if seen
- Circumscribed margins ± regional bone invasion

TOP DIFFERENTIAL DIAGNOSES

- Sinonasal squamous cell carcinoma
- Sinonasal adenocarcinoma
- Sinonasal minor salivary gland malignancy
- Sinonasal undifferentiated carcinoma
- Olfactory neuroblastoma

PATHOLOGY

- Features of squamous cell dysplasia & salivary gland carcinoma; can mimic adenoid cystic carcinoma
- High-grade cellularity, high mitotic index, tumor necrosis, bone invasion are frequent
- **High-risk HPV** (**80% type 33**) by in situ hybridization or PCR

CLINICAL ISSUES

- Sinonasal obstructive symptoms &/or epistaxis
- Mean age: 54 (range 28-90) years
- Slight female predominance
- Indolent behavior despite high-grade histology
- Treatment: Surgical resection ± adjuvant radiation
- **Better prognosis** than non-HPV-associated carcinomas, similar to oropharyngeal squamous cell carcinomas
- Regional spread, metastases, death due to tumor are rare

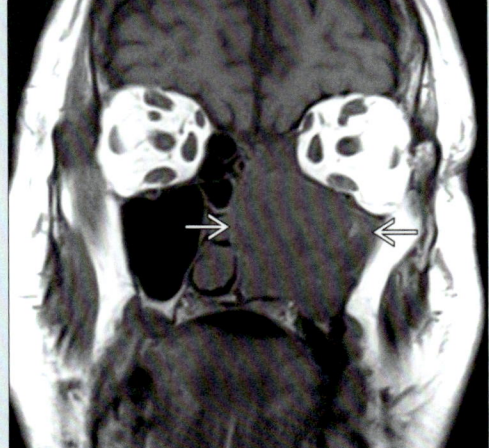
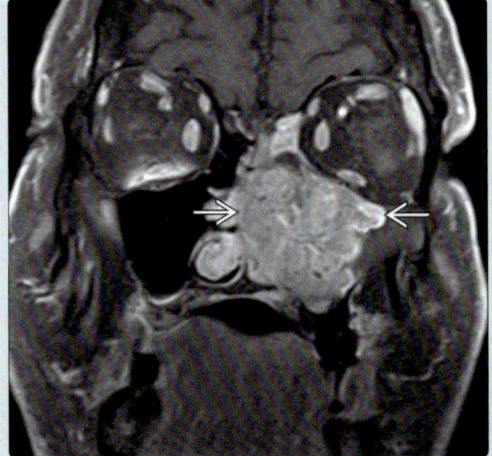

(Left) Coronal T1 MR in a patient with nasal congestion, epiphora, and blood-tinged mucus shows a heterogeneously enhancing mass involving the left nasal cavity and maxillary sinus ➡ with smooth borders. The mass appears to have pushing borders without orbital or intracranial invasion. (Right) Coronal T1 C+ FS MR shows a heterogeneously enhancing mass ➡ in the same patient. Tumor is inseparable from the middle turbinate and has sharply defined tumor borders without intracranial or orbital extension.

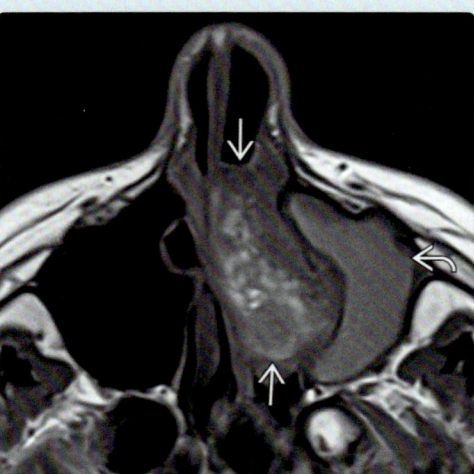
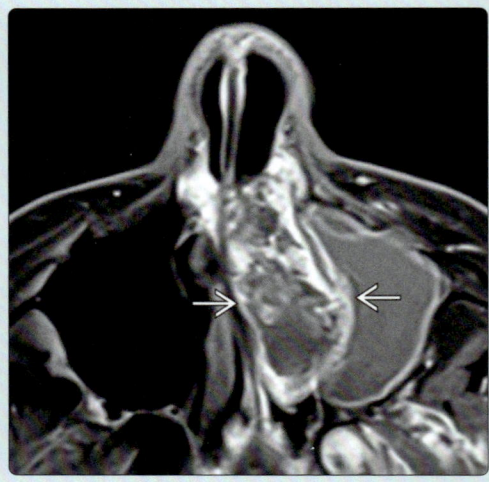

(Left) Axial T1 MR shows a typical heterogeneous HPV-MC expanding the left nasal cavity, inseparable from the turbinate ➡. Intrinsic hyperintensities may reflect hemorrhage; patients often present with epistaxis. Trapped secretions are noted in the left maxillary sinus ➡. (Right) Axial T1 C+ FS MR in the same patient shows patchy enhancement within the mass ➡. Tumor cannot be differentiated from other sinonasal malignancies, including SNUC or melanoma, among others.

TERMINOLOGY

Abbreviations

- HPV-associated multiphenotypic carcinoma (HPV-MC)

Definitions

- Epithelial sinonasal tract neoplasm with surface & minor salivary gland elements having transcriptionally active HPV

IMAGING

General Features

- Best diagnostic clue
  - Well-marginated, heterogeneous nasal cavity mass
- Location
  - Most arise in **nasal cavity** (~ 90%), especially from **turbinate**
  - ± paranasal sinus involvement (maxillary > ethmoid > frontal)
  - Rare cases affect paranasal sinuses alone
- Size
  - Mean long tumor diameter = 4.6 cm
- Morphology
  - Circumscribed margins ± regional bone invasion

CT Findings

- Enhancing soft tissue mass involving turbinate/nasal cavity ± bone destruction
- May have adjacent paranasal sinus invasion
- Mass effect on surrounding structures often seen
- May have orbital &/or intracranial extension
- Variable tumoral calcifications

MR Findings

- Well-defined mass with smooth tumor margins
- Heterogeneous T1 &/or T2 hyperintensities
- Heterogeneous enhancing soft tissue mass
- Perineural tumor spread uncommon
  - Suggests more aggressive tumor if seen

Imaging Recommendations

- Best imaging tool
  - Noncontrast sinus CT for screening
  - Enhanced sinus MR for staging

DIFFERENTIAL DIAGNOSIS

Sinonasal Squamous Cell Carcinoma

- Majority arise in maxillary sinus
- Typically lower T2 signal & aggressive bone destruction

Sinonasal Adenocarcinoma

- May appear very similar

Sinonasal Minor Salivary Gland Malignancy

- May appear similar; however, perineural spread often seen

Sinonasal Undifferentiated Carcinoma

- May appear very similar, however, typically more aggressive

Olfactory Neuroblastoma

- Centered at cribriform plate

PATHOLOGY

General Features

- Tumors have high-risk HPV, most commonly type 33 (~ 80%)

Staging, Grading, & Classification

- Staged according to AJCC TNM 8th edition for sinonasal tract tumors

Gross Pathologic & Surgical Features

- Tan-white, often polypoid, mass

Microscopic Features

- Features of both squamous cell dysplasia & salivary gland carcinoma; can mimic adenoid cystic carcinoma
- Tumors grow as solid sheets, lobules, & cribriform nests with basaloid cells
- High-grade cellularity, high mitotic index, tumor necrosis, bone invasion are frequent

Molecular Genetics

- **High-risk HPV (80% type 33)** by in situ hybridization or PCR

CLINICAL ISSUES

Presentation

- Most common signs/symptoms
  - Sinonasal obstructive symptoms &/or epistaxis

Demographics

- Mean age: 54 (range 28-90) years
- Slight female predominance

Natural History & Prognosis

- Indolent behavior despite high-grade histology
- **Better prognosis** than non-HPV-associated carcinomas, similar to oropharyngeal squamous cell carcinomas
- Local recurrences are common (~ 1/3 of cases), including some late recurrences
- Distant metastases are rare (5%)
- Regional spread & death due to tumor are rare

Treatment

- Complete surgical resection ± adjuvant radiation

DIAGNOSTIC CHECKLIST

Image Interpretation Pearls

- Consider HPV-MC in patients with well-circumscribed and heterogeneously enhancing nasal cavity mass

SELECTED REFERENCES

1. Fernandez-Pose M et al: Surgical treatment for uncommon malignancies of the paranasal sinuses and anterior cranial fossa: report of two cases and literature review. Int J Oral Maxillofac Surg. 54(5):404-10, 2025
2. Abi-Saab T et al: Morphologic spectrum of HPV-associated sinonasal carcinomas. Head Neck Pathol. 18(1):67, 2024
3. Beaumont C et al: HPV-related multiphenotypic sinonasal carcinoma: a clinicoradiological series of 3 cases with full endoscopic surgical outcome. Ear Nose Throat J. ePub, 2024
4. WHO Classification of Tumours Editorial Board: WHO Classification of Head and Neck Tumours. 5th ed. IARC, 2024
5. Baba A et al: Radiological features of human papillomavirus-related multiphenotypic sinonasal carcinoma: systematic review and case series. Neuroradiology. 64(10):2049-58, 2022

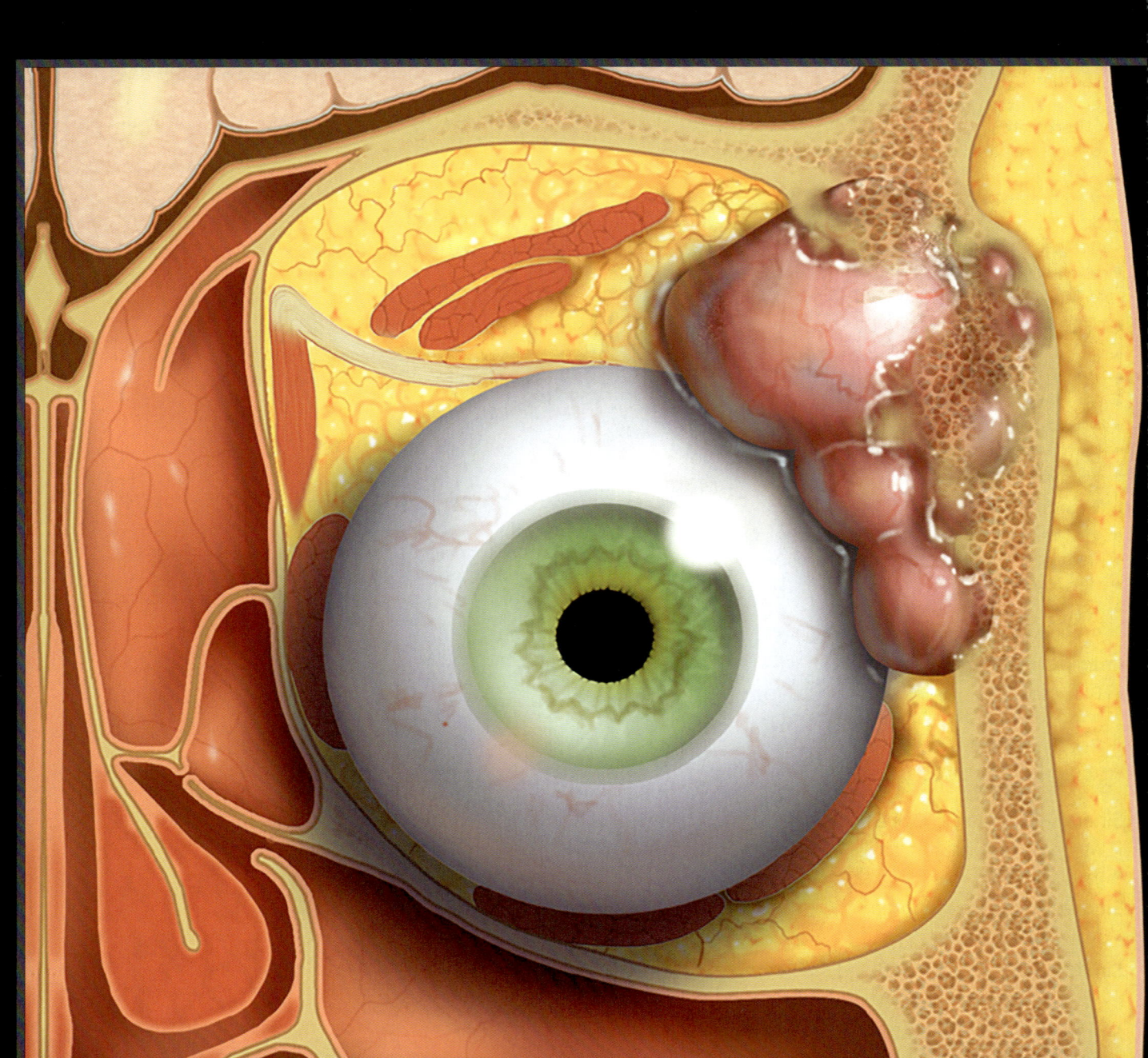

SECTION 22
Orbit

Imaging Approach and Indications

General Approach

Evaluation of the orbit involves evaluation of the eye (or globe) and the bony orbit, soft tissues, and periorbita.

- The term orbital refers to bony structures and soft tissues extrinsic to the globe, whereas the term ocular refers to the globe itself.

Imaging of the orbit and globe is complementary to the physical and ophthalmoscopic examination.

Ultrasound

Ultrasound of the eye is a readily available complement to funduscopic examination and is traditionally performed in the ophthalmology clinic. Transocular ultrasound provides a limited, high-resolution assessment of the globe and other intraorbital soft tissues.

CT

Because of its superior bony characterization, CT has advantages over MR for orbital lesions that arise from or directly affect the bones, such as epithelial inclusions, osteocartilaginous tumors with matrix, osteodystrophic processes, benign masses that cause bony scalloping, and aggressive malignancies that cause bony destruction.

The presence of calcification is a specific differentiating feature in some lesions, and CT can provide essential diagnostic information, even after an MR has been obtained. For example, an indeterminate diagnosis of perioptic nerve meningioma on MR might be confirmed with identification of calcification on CT.

In some instances, CT can provide enough information to allow for a definitive diagnosis and guide therapy without the need for MR. Examples include thyroid ophthalmopathy, clinically benign lacrimal mass, orbital cavernous malformation, and orbital disease that is secondary to a sinonasal process.

MR

For complex orbital disease, MR is the preferred modality. Superior soft tissue differentiation and enhancement make MR ideal for characterizing the extent of lesions, including extraocular tumors, vascular malformations, and complex infectious or inflammatory processes.

In particular, MR is the optimal modality for delineating the extent of malignant orbital disease. Important features visible on MR include optic nerve invasion, perineural extension of tumor to the orbit, intracranial extension of disease, and hematogenous or CSF disseminated metastases.

Although ultrasound is usually the 1st line for imaging the globe, MR can provide a more accurate visualization of retrobulbar extension of intraocular malignancy, including retinoblastoma, ocular melanoma, and ocular metastases.

Additionally, MR provides exquisite characterization of the globe itself, which is particularly useful in circumstances wherein funduscopic evaluation is obscured, such as swollen or injured eye, retinal detachment, large intraocular mass, vitreal hemorrhage, or opaque media from any cause.

Microscopy coil MR imaging has been shown to achieve a higher spatial resolution beyond conventional imaging.

Imaging Anatomy

Bony Orbit

Major components of the bony orbital walls are the frontal bone superiorly, zygomatic bone laterally and inferiorly, maxillary bone inferiorly and medially, and ethmoid bone medially. Smaller contributions medially include the lacrimal bone, nasal bone, and a tiny portion of the palatine bone. The sphenoid bone makes up a large portion of the orbit posteriorly and laterally, forming the complex foramina at the orbital apex.

Globe

The aqueous-filled anterior segment includes anterior and posterior chambers, both anterior to the lens. The vitreous-filled posterior segment occupies the bulk of the globe posteriorly. The layers, or tunica, of the eye include the inner retina, vascular choroid, and outer structural sclera. The anterior refractive constructs include the iris and ciliary body, which are specialized portions of the uvea, as well as the lens.

Orbital Septum

The orbital septum is composed of fascia arising from the orbital periosteum that inserts onto the aponeurosis of the lids' tarsal plates, providing a barrier between the anterior periorbita and intraorbital contents. Although the septum itself is often not discernible as a discrete structure on routine imaging, its presence is evident when a pathology, such as preseptal infection, is contained on 1 side of the barrier.

Lacrimal Apparatus

The lacrimal gland lies in a bony fossa at the anterior aspect of the superolateral orbit. Lacrimal drainage is via canaliculi and sac at the inferomedial orbit, and, from there, it passes through the nasolacrimal duct, which drains via the inferior meatus.

Extraocular Muscles

The 4 rectus muscles originate from the annulus of Zinn at the apex and insert on the corneoscleral surface. The superior oblique has similar origin and insertion but courses through the trochlea ("pulley") at the superomedial orbital rim (trochlea is made of hyaline cartilage, and its calcification is common). The inferior oblique has a short, more direct course originating from the anteroinferior orbital rim. The levator palpebrae superioris originates at the annulus, coursing just above the superior rectus, forming the superior muscle complex, and inserts at the upper eyelid.

- The muscles normally taper anteriorly at their tendinous insertions (which can be lost in some pathologies, such as pseudotumor, while preserved in others, such as thyroid ophthalmopathy).
- The 4 rectus muscles with their intervening septa form the cone, creating extraconal and intraconal compartments with certain lesions having predilection for 1 compartment.

Optic Nerve-Sheath Complex

The optic nerve (CNII) is actually a central nervous tract that traverses the optic canal and orbit to insert at the optic nerve head. The surrounding dural sheath is contiguous with the intracranial dura posteriorly and with the sclera anteriorly. A thin rim of CSF surrounding the nerve is typically visible on MR and is contiguous with CSF in the intracranial cisterns.

Peripheral Cranial Nerves

CNIII, CNIV, and CNVI supply motor innervation to the extraocular muscles (EOMs) and parasympathetics to the iris via CNIII. The individual branches of these nerves are not reliably distinguished within the orbit. However, knowledge of

Differential Diagnosis: Orbit

Congenital lesions (globe)	Infectious lesions (globe)	Benign tumors
Coloboma	Ocular toxocariasis	Lacrimal pleomorphic adenoma
Persistent hyperplastic primary vitreous	Acute endophthalmitis	Optic pathway glioma
Coats disease		Optic nerve sheath meningioma
Congenital lesions (orbit)	**Infectious lesions (orbit)**	**Malignant tumors (globe)**
Orbital dermoid and epidermoid	Orbital subperiosteal abscess	Retinoblastoma
Orbital neurofibromatosis, type 1	Orbital cellulitis	Uveal melanoma
Vascular malformations	**Inflammatory lesions**	**Malignant tumors (orbit)**
Orbital lymphatic malformation	Orbital idiopathic pseudotumor	Lacrimal epithelial carcinoma
Orbital varix	Orbital sarcoidosis	Lymphoproliferative lesions
Orbital cavernous malformation	Thyroid ophthalmopathy	Orbital Langerhans histiocytosis
Vascular neoplasms	Optic neuritis	Metastases
Orbital infantile hemangioma	IgG4-related disease	

their course through the cavernous sinus and superior orbital fissure (SOF) allows localization of pathology that involves these nerves.

Two CNV branches course through the orbit. V1 passes with other nerves through the SOF and exits the orbit through the supraorbital foramen. V2 passes through foramen rotundum and inferior orbital fissure and exits the orbit through the infraorbital foramen.

Vascular Structures

The ophthalmic artery enters the orbit alongside the optic nerve within the optic canal; it is frequently visible, as it diverges from the nerve near the apex. High-resolution angiography, CT, and MR show the artery originating as the 1st intradural branch of the internal carotid artery. The superior ophthalmic vein is variable but typically found coursing between the superior rectus muscle and the optic nerve.
- Medial orbital wall has canals for the anterior and posterior ethmoidal vessels (and nerves).

Orbital Fat

In addition to acting as a volume "filler" for the orbital cavity, orbital fat provides intrinsic imaging contrast, making other structures and disease processes more conspicuous.

Anatomy-based Imaging Issues

In approaching orbital lesions, it is useful to localize the process to a subregion of the orbit.
- **Globe**: Is the lesion entirely intraocular, or is there transscleral extension, particularly with regard to the optic nerve head?
- **Optic nerve**: Does the lesion arise within the nerve proper or involve primarily the dural sheath?
- **EOM**: Is the lesion intraconal or extraconal, or does it arise from the muscles themselves? Is muscle involvement symmetric or otherwise characteristic?
- **Lacrimal gland**: Is the lesion unilateral or bilateral, indicating a systemic process?
- **Bone**: Does the lesion arise from the bone itself? If the lesion is adjacent to bone, does the bone show benign scalloped remodeling or aggressive destruction?
- **Focality**: Is the lesion isolated or multiple, focal or diffuse? Does the lesion extend beyond the orbit?

Imaging Protocols

CT

Routine imaging of the orbit with CT does not require special discussion, except for 1 clinical circumstance: Intermittent proptosis due to orbital varix. This dynamic lesion enlarges with increases in venous pressures and is best demonstrated with provocation. A scan repeated with the breath held in Valsalva maneuver increases venous pressures and dynamically enlarges the varix.

MR

Routine orbit MR protocol includes 3 sequence types (coronal and axial) at 3-mm slice thickness and 18-cm FOV. Whole-brain imaging is added when indicated.
- Precontrast T1WI (without fat suppression)
- T2WI with fat suppression (alternatively STIR)
- Postcontrast T1WI (with fat suppression)

Pathologic Issues: Vascular Malformations

Vascular malformations: Congenital, nonneoplastic lesions with classification that reflects their histologic and hemodynamic features.

Orbital cavernous malformation: This common mass is unique to the orbit. It is encapsulated with low-flow venous channels. The term "hemangioma" is commonly used to refer to this lesion but is actually a misnomer.

Venolymphatic malformation: Lesions may have no flow (type 1), venous flow (type 2), or may be mixed. There may be a distensible component, resulting in varix. Outdated terminology to be avoided includes "lymphangioma" and "cystic hygroma."

Arteriovenous malformations (AVMs): True orbital AVMs are rare lesions with high-flow arterial (type 3) hemodynamics.

Selected References

1. Gotti Naves G et al: Practical approach to orbital lesions by anatomic compartments. Radiographics. 44(10):e240026, 2024
2. Dobbs NW et al: MR-eye: high-resolution microscopy coil MRI for the assessment of the orbit and periorbital structures, part 1: technique and anatomy. AJNR Am J Neuroradiol. 41(6):947-50, 2020
3. Yanoff M et al: Ophthalmology. 4th ed. Saunders, 2013
4. Rootman J: Diseases of the Orbit: A Multidisciplinary Approach. Lippincott, 2003

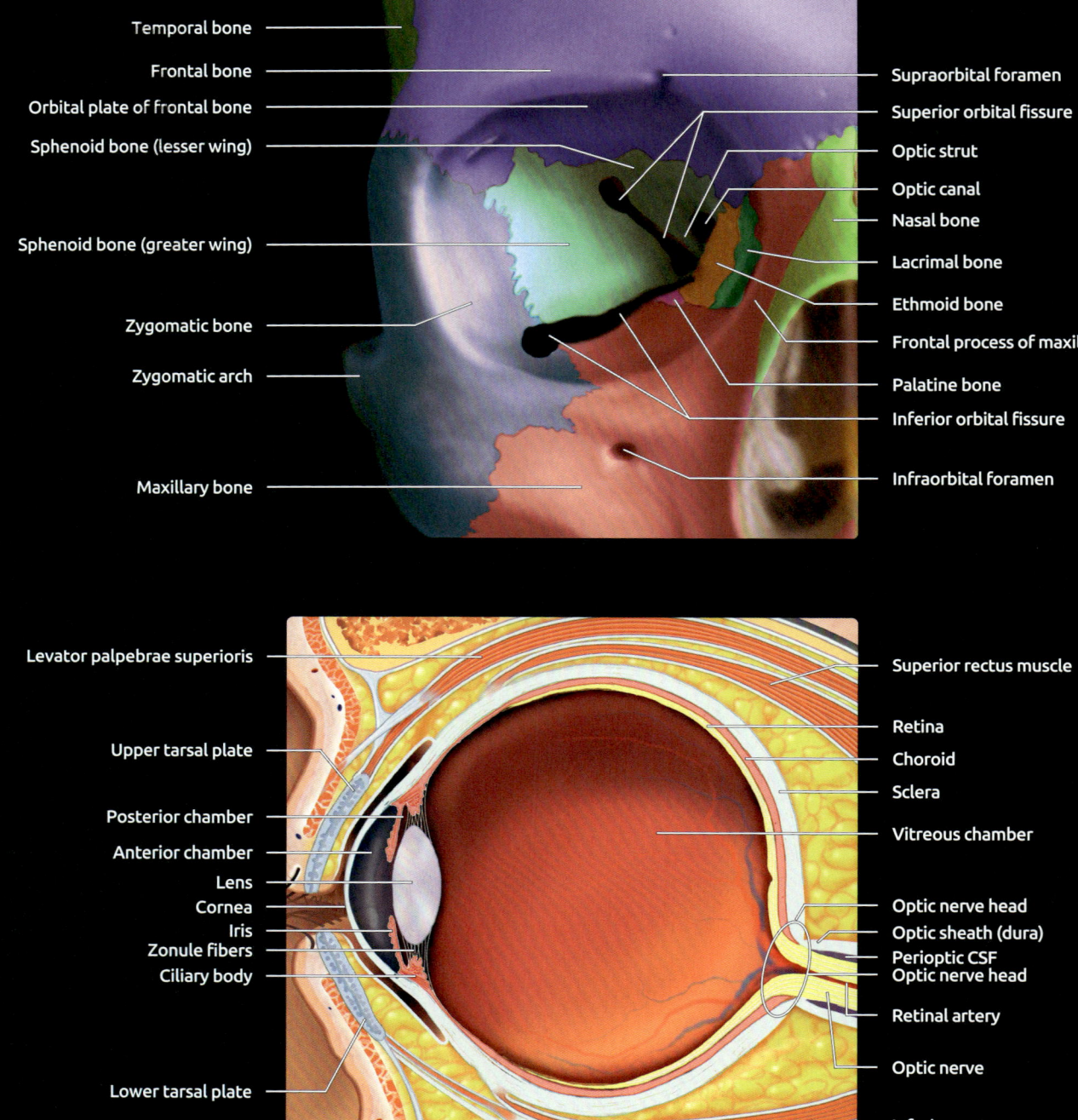

Top labels (left):
- Temporal bone
- Frontal bone
- Orbital plate of frontal bone
- Sphenoid bone (lesser wing)
- Sphenoid bone (greater wing)
- Zygomatic bone
- Zygomatic arch
- Maxillary bone

Top labels (right):
- Supraorbital foramen
- Superior orbital fissure
- Optic strut
- Optic canal
- Nasal bone
- Lacrimal bone
- Ethmoid bone
- Frontal process of maxilla
- Palatine bone
- Inferior orbital fissure
- Infraorbital foramen

Bottom labels (left):
- Levator palpebrae superioris
- Upper tarsal plate
- Posterior chamber
- Anterior chamber
- Lens
- Cornea
- Iris
- Zonule fibers
- Ciliary body
- Lower tarsal plate
- Inferior oblique

Bottom labels (right):
- Superior rectus muscle
- Retina
- Choroid
- Sclera
- Vitreous chamber
- Optic nerve head
- Optic sheath (dura)
- Perioptic CSF
- Optic nerve head
- Retinal artery
- Optic nerve
- Inferior rectus

(**Top**) *Frontal graphic demonstrates the complex anatomy of the bony orbit. The walls of the orbital cavity receive contributions from 7 different bones of the skull. The complex foramina and fissures at the apex are located primarily within the greater and lesser wings of the sphenoid bone and its junctions with adjacent bones. Superior orbital fissure (SOF) transmits the CNIII, CNIV, and CNVI, branches of V1 (lacrimal, frontal, nasociliary nerves) and ophthalmic veins. Inferior orbital fissure primarily transmits the infraorbital nerve and zygomatic nerve (V2) and infraorbital vessels. Optic canal contains optic nerve, ophthalmic artery, and sympathetic nerves. Optic strut separates the SOF and optic canal. (**Bottom**) Sagittal graphic demonstrates the anterior and posterior segments of the globe. The aqueous anterior segment is composed of the anterior chamber and very small posterior chamber. The much larger posterior segment is filled by the vitreous chamber. The layered tunicae of the retina, choroid, and sclera are demonstrated as well as the components of the optic nerve at its insertion. Some of the extraocular muscles and eyelid structures are also demonstrated.*

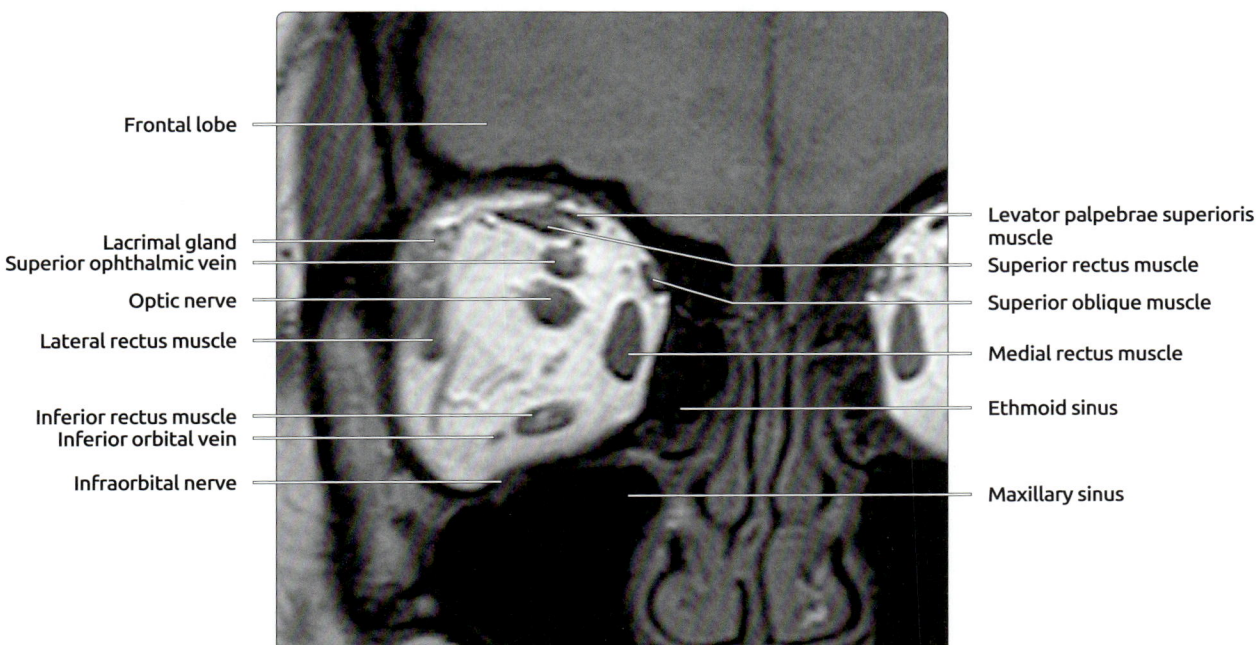

Frontal lobe

Lacrimal gland
Superior ophthalmic vein

Optic nerve

Lateral rectus muscle

Inferior rectus muscle
Inferior orbital vein

Infraorbital nerve

Levator palpebrae superioris muscle
Superior rectus muscle
Superior oblique muscle

Medial rectus muscle

Ethmoid sinus

Maxillary sinus

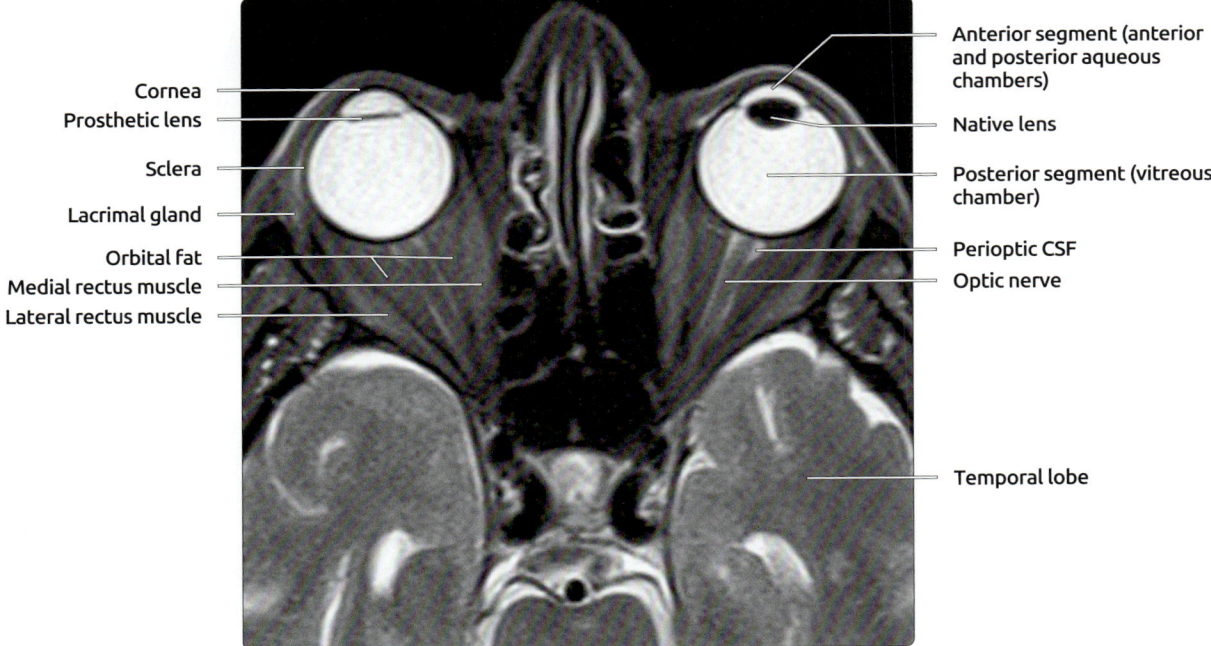

Cornea
Prosthetic lens

Sclera

Lacrimal gland

Orbital fat
Medial rectus muscle
Lateral rectus muscle

Anterior segment (anterior and posterior aqueous chambers)

Native lens

Posterior segment (vitreous chamber)

Perioptic CSF
Optic nerve

Temporal lobe

(Top) *Coronal T1WI MR demonstrates the "cone" of extraocular muscles, the optic nerve, and few vascular structures of the orbit. The hyperintense T1 fat signal provides excellent contrast for visualizing the infraorbital anatomy.* **(Bottom)** *Axial T2WI MR with fat suppression nearly eliminates signal from orbital fat, allowing for conspicuity of fluid signal structures. A small amount of CSF surrounding the optic nerve is usually visible on T2WI. The normal extraocular muscles show intermediate to low signal. A small portion of the lacrimal gland is seen, but the majority of the gland is located further superiorly. The anterior segment of the eye shows water signal, primarily representing the anterior chamber; the posterior chamber is not separately discernible on routine MR. The posterior segment also shows water signal composed of the vitreous chamber. Note that this patient has a prosthetic lens on the right.*

Coloboma

TERMINOLOGY

- Coloboma: Gap or defect of ocular tissue
- May involve any or all structures of embryonic cleft
- Types of posterior coloboma
  - Optic disc coloboma
  - Choroidoretinal coloboma
- Related but distinctly different anomalies
  - Morning glory disc anomaly
  - Peripapillary staphyloma

IMAGING

- Focal defect at posterior pole of globe
- Outpouching contiguous with vitreous
- Oriented posteriorly with long axis of globe
- Microphthalmos and retrobulbar cysts often present
- Isodense to vitreous on CT
- Isointense to vitreous on MR
- Bulging of posterior globe on prenatal MR

TOP DIFFERENTIAL DIAGNOSES

- Congenital microphthalmos
- Congenital glaucoma
- Neurofibromatosis type 1
- Degenerative staphyloma
- Axial myopia

PATHOLOGY

- Failure of embryonic fissure fusion
- Isolated, sporadic, and syndromic genetic etiologies
- Bilateral when syndromic

CLINICAL ISSUES

- ↓ visual acuity; leukocoria
- Treatment to address refractive errors, strabismus, amblyopia, retinal detachment

DIAGNOSTIC CHECKLIST

- Look for syndromic and systemic associations

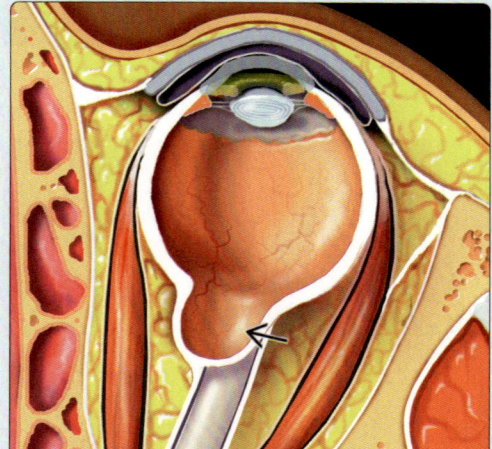
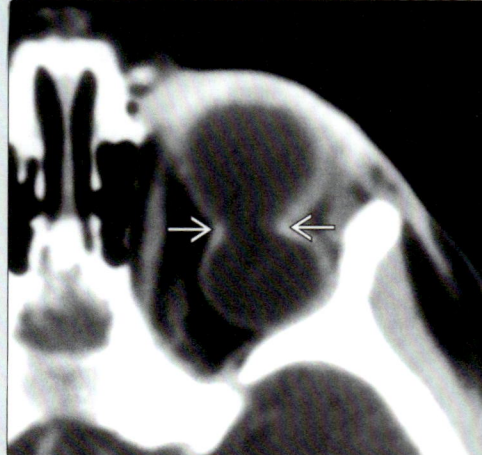

(Left) *Axial graphic of classic optic disc coloboma shows a focal defect in the posterior globe at the site of the optic nerve head insertion ➡.* (Right) *Axial CECT demonstrates a broad colobomatous defect ➡ centered on the upper margin of the optic disc. Note the vitreous appears contiguous with retrobulbar outpouching. Apart from the retrobulbar outpouching, the globe is small.*

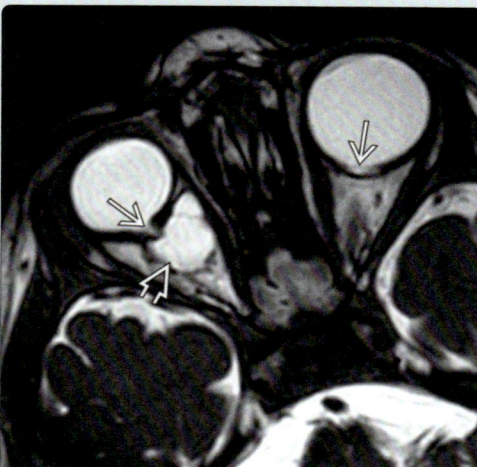
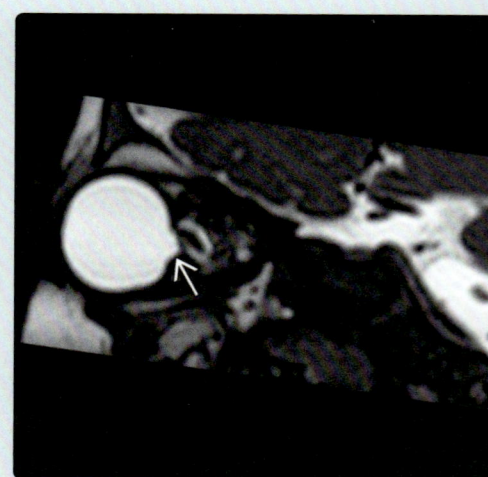

(Left) *Axial CISS MR in a 9-month-old baby with multiple congenital anomalies shows bilateral posterior globe defects ➡. The choroidoretinal coloboma on the right is associated with microphthalmia and retrobulbar cyst ➡ and optic nerve hypoplasia (not shown).* (Right) *Sagittal reformatted 3D T2 CISS MR in a 6-month-old with bilateral colobomas on clinical exam shows right optic disc coloboma ➡. Notice that fluid in the posterior outpouching is isointense and contiguous with the vitreous fluid.*

TERMINOLOGY

Abbreviations

- Optic disc coloboma (ODC)
- Choroidoretinal coloboma (CRC)

Definitions

- Coloboma: **Gap** or defect of ocular tissue
- Types of **posterior** coloboma
  - **ODC**: Excavation confined to **optic disc**
  - **CRC**: Defect separate from or extends **beyond disc**
- **Related but distinctly different anomalies**
  - Morning glory disc anomaly (**MGDA**): Defect with glial tissue and pigmented rim
  - Peripapillary staphyloma (**PPS**): Congenital scleral excavation at optic nerve head
- Other colobomatous lesions
  - May involve any or all structures of **embryonic cleft**
    - Iris, ciliary body, lens, or eyelid (in up to 50% of patients with Goldenhar syndrome)
  - Fuchs coloboma
    - Inferiorly tilted disc with crescent-shaped defect along inferonasal margin

IMAGING

General Features

- Best diagnostic clue
  - Focal defect with outpouching at posterior pole of globe; vitreous contiguous with defect
  - **Microphthalmos** and retrobulbar **cysts** often present
- Location
  - Posterior globe (usually inferomedial) at optic **nerve head** insertion
- Morphology
  - **Crater-shaped** excavation, contiguous with vitreous
  - Oriented posteriorly with **long axis** of globe
  - MGDA defect funnel-shaped with central glial tissue
  - PPS excavation encircles optic disc
- Laterality
  - Unilateral when sporadic, bilateral when syndromic
  - MGDA almost always unilateral, R > L
  - PPS usually unilateral

CT Findings

- NECT
  - Fluid in defect ± retrobulbar cyst **isodense to vitreous**
  - Subretinal hyperdensity if hemorrhage
- Bone CT
  - Ca++ may develop at margins of chronic defects

MR Findings

- T1WI and T2WI
  - **Isointense to vitreous**
  - Complex signal if retinal detachment, including hemorrhagic or proteinaceous fluid (T1 hyperintense)
  - MGDA: Funnel-shaped optic disc + adjacent ↑ T1/↓ T2 retinal surface elevation ± fat signal within adjacent distal optic nerve sheath ± optic nerve enlargement
- Enhancement
  - Sclera enhances; glial tuft in MGDA may enhance

- Otherwise no abnormal enhancement within defect
- Prenatal MR
  - Bulging of posterior globe profile

Ultrasonographic Findings

- Outpouching of posterior globe at optic nerve head
- Hypoechoic retrobulbar mass if cyst present

Imaging Recommendations

- Best imaging tool
  - MR or CT shows globe and extraocular features, especially if defects prevent direct visualization
  - CT provides reasonable depiction without sedation
  - MR of brain helpful if **syndromic** to evaluate for associated **intracranial abnormalities**

DIFFERENTIAL DIAGNOSIS

Congenital Microphthalmos

- Congenital severe ocular derangement
- Deformed, small globe with adjacent cyst

Congenital Glaucoma

- Present at birth, usually bilateral
- Enlarged globe

Neurofibromatosis Type 1

- Globe enlargement = buphthalmos
- May have associated optic glioma, sphenoid wing dysplasia, plexiform neurofibroma

Degenerative Staphyloma

- Degenerative ectasia of globe
- Thinning of posterior sclera-uveal rim
- Enlarged globe, associated with myopia
- Usually off center, temporal to disc (coloboma usually nasal to disc)

Axial Myopia

- Elongated anteroposterior dimension

Orbital Trauma

- Traumatic globe rupture results in globe deformity

PATHOLOGY

General Features

- Etiology
  - Embryologic considerations
    - Embryonic fissure extends along **inferonasal** aspect of optic cup and stalk
    - Fissure fusion (**5th-7th week**) required for normal globe and nerve formation
  - Coloboma (ODC/CRC)
    - Failure of embryonic fissure fusion superiorly
  - MGDA
    - Faulty scleral closure (4th week)
    - Mesoectodermal dysgenesis of optic nerve head
  - PPS
    - Incomplete differentiation of sclera
    - Diminished peripapillary structural support
- Genetics
  - **Sporadic** coloboma

– Noninherited
– Unilateral; especially isolated ODC
– Possible maternal environmental factors
□ Vitamin A deficiency, drug use, alcohol abuse
○ **Nonsyndromic** coloboma
– Typically **autosomal dominant**
– Identified with many specific mutations
□ *PAX2, PAX6, SHH, VSX2* (CHX10), *MAF*, SOX2, others
○ **Syndromic** coloboma
– Usually **autosomal recessive**
– Typically bilateral, especially CRC
– Associated with trisomies
– Dozens of syndromes (CHARGE, Aicardi, papillorenal, COACH, Meckel, Warburg, Lenz)
○ **MGDA**
– Typically sporadic; rare familial cases
– Unilateral, except when familial
○ **PPS**
– Typically sporadic
– Unilateral, usually isolated anomaly
• Associated abnormalities
○ Triad of major congenital globe anomalies
– Microphthalmos, anophthalmos, and coloboma (**MAC**)
○ Orbital
– Microphthalmia; optic tract and chiasm atrophy
– Retrobulbar colobomatous cyst
□ Frequently present, may be multiple
□ Typically retrobulbar but may project anteriorly
□ May be separate or communicate with globe
– Retinal detachment (25-40%) (ODC, MGDA)
– Congenital optic pit (ODC, MGDA)
– Cataract; hyaloid artery (ODC, MGDA)
– Iris coloboma (ODC)
– Persistent hyperplastic primary vitreous, aniridia (MGDA)
○ Systemic
– Renal, CNS, and many other systemic associations, particularly when bilateral
– MGDA: Basal cephaloceles, moyamoya, callosal agenesis, persistent craniopharyngeal canal, hypopituitarism, variable deformity of pituitary gland and infundibulum, ipsilateral optic nerve thickening, and tubular or nodular nasopharyngeal lesions
– PPS: Usually isolated; rare associated facial lesions, frontonasal dysplasia, facial capillary hemangioma

Staging, Grading, & Classification
• Simple coloboma (normal globe and cornea): ~ 15%
○ Best prognosis for vision
• Coloboma with microcornea (< 30 mm): ~ 40%
○ Better prognosis
• Coloboma with microcornea and microphthalmos: ~ 40%
○ Worse prognosis
• Coloboma with microphthalmos and cyst: ~ 5%
○ Worst prognosis for vision

CLINICAL ISSUES
Presentation
• Most common signs/symptoms
○ ↓ **visual acuity** (VA)

• Other signs/symptoms
○ **Leukocoria**
○ Iris involvement causes typical keyhole defect
○ Microphthalmia or anophthalmia in severe cases
○ Associated **syndromic** features
• Clinical profile
○ Vision depends on extent of optic disc involvement and retinal detachment
– Strabismus and nystagmus secondary to poor VA
– Reduced visual evoked potentials
• Funduscopic examination
○ ODC: Enlarged disc with excavation
– May resemble glaucomatous cupping
○ CRC: White with pigmented margins
– Extends inferiorly from or inferior to disc
○ MGDA: Enlarged, excavated disc; central core of tissue
– Central tuft of tissue with surrounding ring of pigment; resembles morning glory blossom
○ PPS: Central crater with recessed optic nerve
– Optic disc sunken, otherwise normal; atrophy of surrounding pigment epithelium

Demographics
• Sex
○ No predilection, except MGDA: M < F = 1:2
• Epidemiology
○ Coloboma (nonsyndromic): 1:12,000
– Accounts for up to 10% of childhood blindness
○ MGDA and PPS: Rare

Natural History & Prognosis
• Visual acuity correlates with retinal status
○ Detachment leads to precipitous vision loss
○ Nerve atrophy and cataracts may lead to more insidious vision loss

Treatment
• Address refractive errors, strabismus, amblyopia
• Retinal detachment management

DIAGNOSTIC CHECKLIST
Consider
• Coloboma is ophthalmoscopic diagnosis
• Imaging confirms ocular features, identifies retrobulbar findings, such as cyst, and evaluates coexistent anomalies

Image Interpretation Pearls
• Look for **syndromic** and systemic associations

SELECTED REFERENCES

1. Fang F et al: Ocular manifestations and pathological features in goldenhar syndrome a 10-year retrospective study. Ophthalmol Ther. 14(4):643-57, 2025
2. Firouzabadi FD et al: Morning glory disc anomaly: expanding the MR phenotype. AJNR Am J Neuroradiol. 45(8):1070-5, 2024
3. Gotti Naves G et al: Practical approach to orbital lesions by anatomic compartments. Radiographics. 44(10):e240026, 2024
4. Nguyen DT et al: Optic nerve abnormalities in morning glory disc anomaly: an MRI study. J Neuroophthalmol. 42(2):199-202, 2022
5. Lingam G et al: Ocular coloboma-a comprehensive review for the clinician. Eye (Lond). 35(8):2086-109, 2021

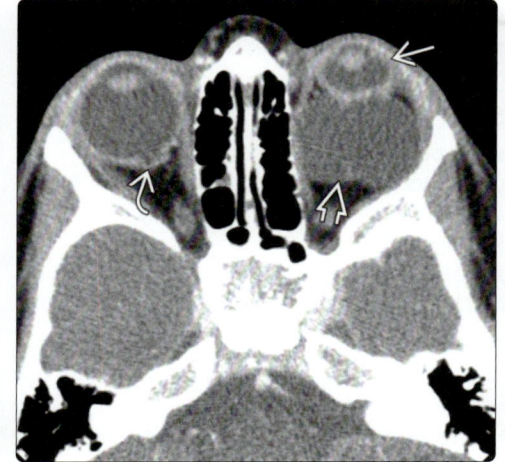
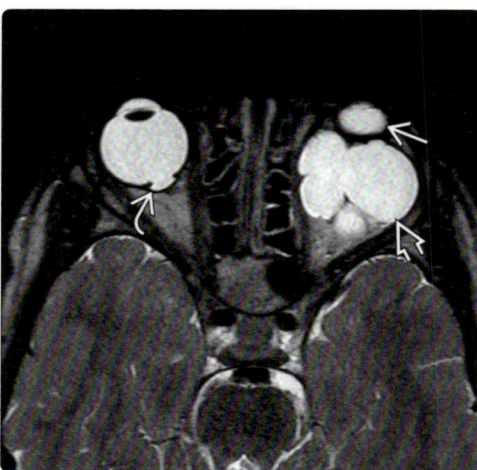

(Left) Axial CECT in a 4-year-old boy with bilateral colobomas demonstrates microphthalmia ➡ with a large, lobulated retrobulbar cyst ⊃ on the left, and optic disc coloboma ⊅ on the right. (Right) Axial T2 MR in the same patient shows to better advantage the microphthalmic left globe ➡, the large multiloculated left retrobulbar cyst ⊃, and the right optic disc coloboma ⊅. Bilateral colobomas are most common in patients with syndromic conditions.

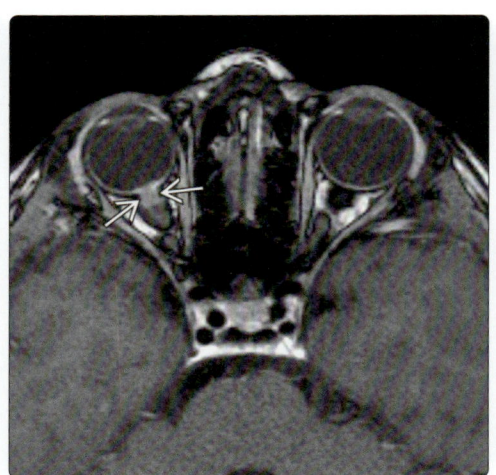
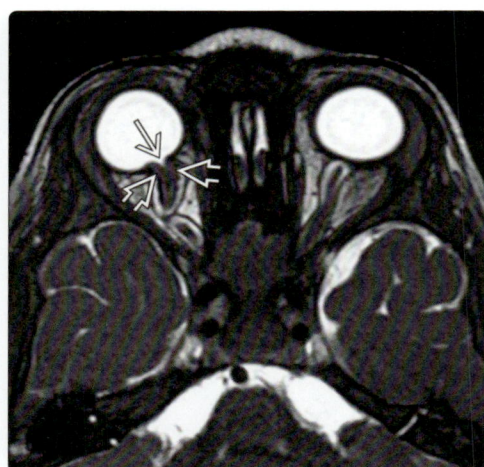

(Left) Axial T1 C+ FS MR in a 4-year-old child with morning glory anomaly, which is a distinctly different anomaly than coloboma but in a similar location, demonstrates microphthalmia and an enhancing glial tuft ➡ at the site of the dorsal globe defect. (Right) Axial CISS MR in an 18-month-old boy shows the typical funnel-shaped defect ➡ and surrounding hypointense glial tuft ⊃ that is typical of morning glory disc anomaly.

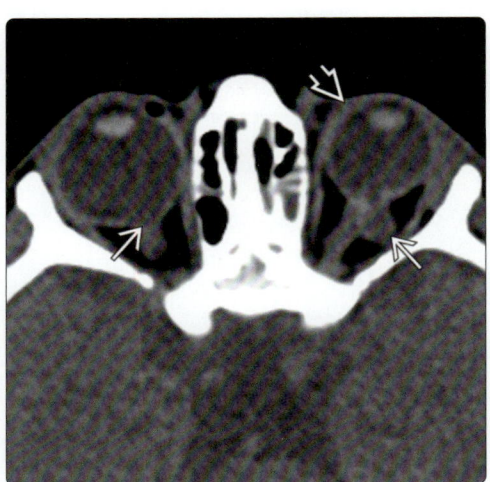
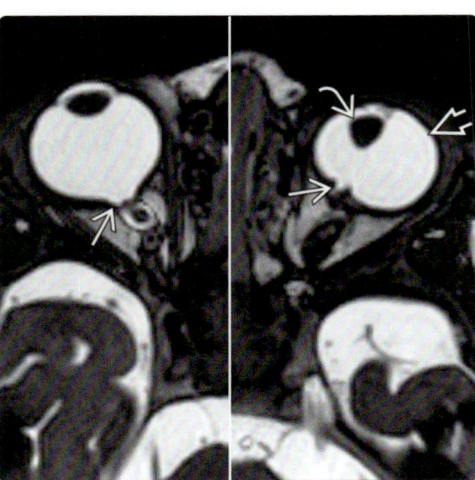

(Left) Axial NECT of the internal auditory canal in a patient with CHARGE syndrome shows bilateral colobomas ➡ and left microphthalmia ⊃. (Right) Axial CISS MR merged images of right and left globes in a 6-month-old with bilateral chorioretinal colobomas on clinical exam demonstrates bilateral dorsal globe colobomas ➡, left microphthalmia ⊃ and subluxed/malrotated left ocular lens ⊅. Bilateral colobomas should raise the question of an associated syndromic condition.

Persistent Hyperplastic Primary Vitreous

TERMINOLOGY

- Persistent fetal vasculature = preferred term
- Congenital lesion incomplete regression of embryonic primary vitreous & hyaloid fetal vasculature

IMAGING

- **Martini glass shape** of enhancing soft tissue
  ○ Triangular retrolental vascular tuft of tissue
  ○ Central tissue stalk of hyaloid remnant
- Retinal detachment common
- Small globe, hyperdense vitreous
- Calcification rare
- Hyperintense blood with layering debris

TOP DIFFERENTIAL DIAGNOSES

- Retinoblastoma
- Congenital cataract
- Coats disease
- Retinopathy of prematurity

PATHOLOGY

- Normal fetal primary vitreous involutes by birth
- **Failure of hyaloid regression** causes remnant to persist in Cloquet canal

CLINICAL ISSUES

- **Leukocoria** with poor vision and small eye
- Anterior type has better prognosis for vision
- Surgical options include lensectomy, vitrectomy
- Long-term management
  ○ Amblyopia therapy and refractive correction
  ○ Management of glaucoma and detachments

DIAGNOSTIC CHECKLIST

- Primary vitreous may be incompletely regressed and normally visible in premature infant
- Persistent hyperplastic primary vitreous is most common intraocular abnormality to be confused with retinoblastoma

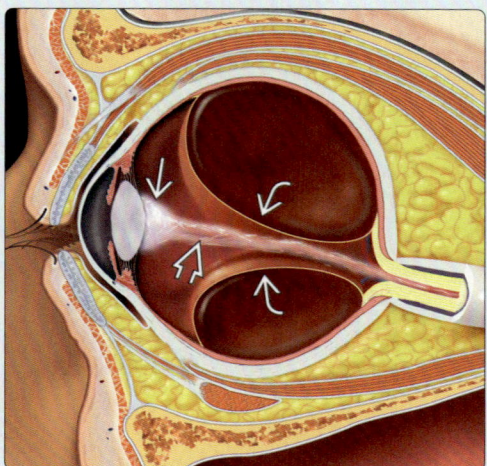
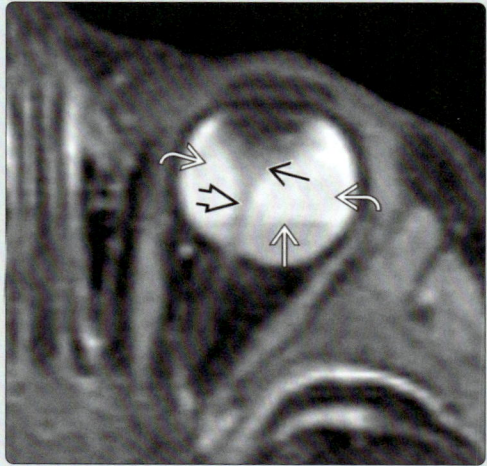

(Left) Sagittal graphic depicts persistent hyperplastic primary vitreous ➡. A triangular retrolental soft tissue mass is present with a stalk-like hyaloid remnant ➡. Note the large, V-shaped retinal detachment ➡. (Right) Axial T1WI C+ FS MR shows the martini glass appearance of a retrolental tuft of tissue ➡ with a stalk ➡ extending to the optic nerve head. A large, hyperintense detachment is present ➡ with associated hemorrhage and fluid level ➡.

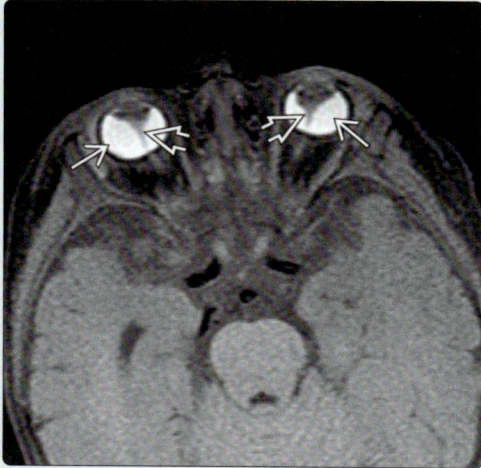
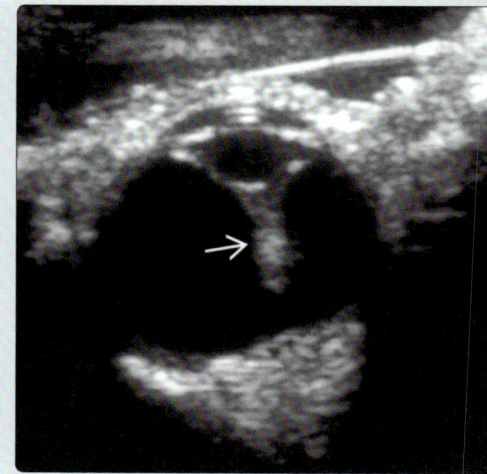

(Left) Axial T1WI FS MR shows bilateral microphthalmia and abnormal hyperintense, hemorrhagic retinal detachments within the bilateral posterior globes ➡. The hypointense signal intensity extending from the lens to the optic disc represents the hyaloid remnant ➡. (Right) Transverse ultrasound in an infant with Walker-Warburg syndrome shows a linear echogenicity ➡ extending posteriorly from the lens to the optic nerve, representing the fibrovascular remnant containing the hyaloid artery.

TERMINOLOGY

Abbreviations

- Persistent hyperplastic primary vitreous (**PHPV**)

Definitions

- **Persistent fetal vasculature** = preferred term
- Congenital: **Incomplete regression of embryonic primary vitreous and hyaloid fetal vasculature of globe**

IMAGING

General Features

- Best diagnostic clue
  - **Retrolental soft tissue** and **stalk**
  - **Hyperdense or hyperintense small globe**
- Location
  - Isolated posterior form (15-25%)
  - Isolated anterior form (5-25%)
  - Mixed anterior and posterior (50-80%)
  - **Unilateral >> bilateral**
    - Bilateral in systemic or syndromic conditions: Norrie disease, Walker-Warburg syndrome, trisomy 13
- Morphology
  - **Martini glass shape** of enhancing soft tissue
    - Triangular retrolental vascular tuft of tissue
    - Central tissue stalk of hyaloid remnant
  - **Retinal detachment** common
- Enhancement
  - Retrolental tissue enhances, as does vitreous depending on degree of persistent vascularity

CT Findings

- Small globe, linear retrolental density &/or vitreous hemorrhage, retinal detachment
- Calcification rare

MR Findings

- Retrolental martini glass-shaped enhancing soft tissue
- Small globe, vitreous abnormally hyperintense on both T1WI and T2WI
- Hemorrhage and layering debris in vitreous &/or retinal detachment common: Signal varies with age of blood

Ultrasonographic Findings

- Lens displacement, hyperechoic retrolental stalk
- Internal vascularity on color Doppler = persistent hyaloid artery
- ± retinal detachment

Imaging Recommendations

- Best imaging tool
  - **MR superior for differentiating noncalcified retinoblastoma from other causes of leukocoria**
- Protocol advice
  - Contrast enhancement is essential

DIFFERENTIAL DIAGNOSIS

Retinoblastoma

- Calcification differentiates from PHPV

Congenital Cataract

- Malformed lens due to prenatal insult

Coats Disease

- Exudative retinopathy with detachments

Retinopathy of Prematurity

- Retrolental fibroplasia; small, dense globe

PATHOLOGY

General Features

- Etiology
  - Primary vitreous = embryonic hyaloid vasculature of developing globe
  - Normal fetal primary vitreous involutes by 8th month of gestation
  - Failure of hyaloid regression causes remnant to persist in Cloquet canal

Microscopic Features

- Fibrovascular loose connective tissue
- Hyaloid artery remnant

CLINICAL ISSUES

Presentation

- Most common signs/symptoms
  - Leukocoria with poor vision and small globe
- Other signs/symptoms
  - Cataract, strabismus, nystagmus, uveitis

Natural History & Prognosis

- Anterior: Best prognosis for vision
- Posterior: May have light/motion perception only
- Risk of secondary glaucoma

Treatment

- Goals: Salvage vision, avoid glaucoma, pupil cosmesis
- Surgical options
  - Anterior: Lensectomy, intraocular prosthetic lens
  - Posterior: Vitrectomy, removal of hyaloid stalk
- Long-term management
  - Amblyopia therapy and refractive correction
  - Management of glaucoma and detachments

DIAGNOSTIC CHECKLIST

Consider

- Primary vitreous may be incompletely regressed and normally visible in premature infant, or on fetal MR before 25-weeks gestation

Image Interpretation Pearls

- PHPV is most common intraocular abnormality to be confused with retinoblastoma

SELECTED REFERENCES

1. Gerrie SK et al: Pediatric orbital lesions: ocular pathologies. Pediatr Radiol. 54(6):876-96, 2024
2. Rumboldt Z et al: Retinoblastoma and beyond: pediatric orbital mass lesions. Neuroradiology. 67(2):469-92, 2024
3. Prakhunhungsit S et al: Diagnostic and management strategies in patients with persistent fetal vasculature: current insights. Clin Ophthalmol. 14:4325-35, 2020

Coats Disease

TERMINOLOGY

- Retinal telangiectasias, exudative retinopathy
- Abnormal retinal capillary development, leading to subretinal accumulation of exudate

IMAGING

- Subretinal exudate with retinal detachment
- Unilateral in 90%; bilateral when syndromic
- Affected eye normal or slightly smaller than normal eye
- Typical V-shaped contour of retinal detachment
- CT: Hyperdense exudate, calcification very uncommon
- MR: Hyperintense proteinaceous, hemorrhagic exudate
  - Retinal detachment ± small size of globe
  - Subfoveal enhancing nodules
  - Intraretinal macrocysts
  - Nerve enhancement in advanced disease
- Ultrasound
  - Linear detached retina & tiny cholesterol crystals

TOP DIFFERENTIAL DIAGNOSES

- Retinoblastoma
- Persistent hyperplastic primary vitreous
- Retinopathy of prematurity
- Ocular toxocariasis

CLINICAL ISSUES

- Presents with leukocoria, vision loss
- Tortuous & dilated capillaries with tiny aneurysms
- Male predominance; usually onset within 1st decade
- Treatment
  - Laser photocoagulation & cryotherapy
  - Intravitreal antivascular endothelial growth factor (VEGF) therapy as adjunct treatment to inhibit angiogenesis
- Vitrectomy & retinal reattachment when advanced

DIAGNOSTIC CHECKLIST

- Retinoblastoma is most important differential consideration

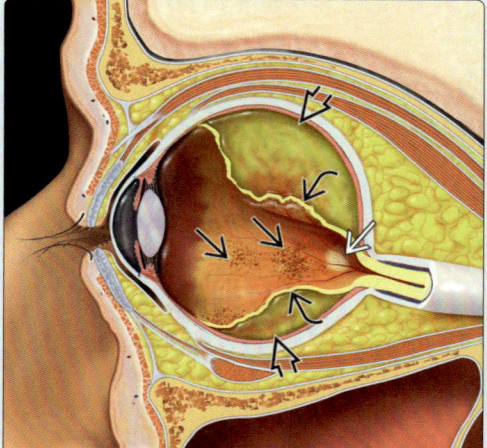
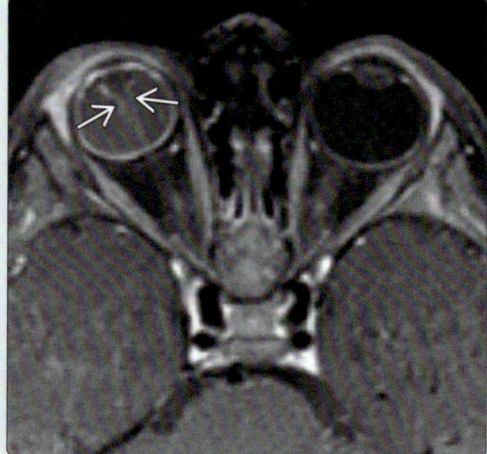

(Left) Sagittal graphic depicts both dilatation & tiny aneurysms of retinal capillaries ➡ with associated large subretinal exudates ➡ & retinal detachments ➡. A subfoveal nodule ➡ is also demonstrated. (Right) Axial T1 C+ FS MR in a 10-month-old boy with leukocoria shows a small right globe with near-complete Y-shaped retinal detachment ➡ without an intraocular mass. The mildly hyperintense subretinal fluid is consistent with subretinal exudates. Unilateral involvement is almost universal in Coats disease.

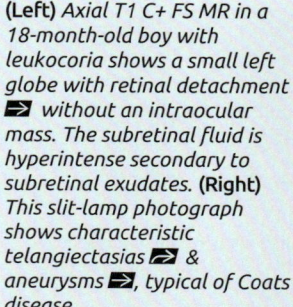
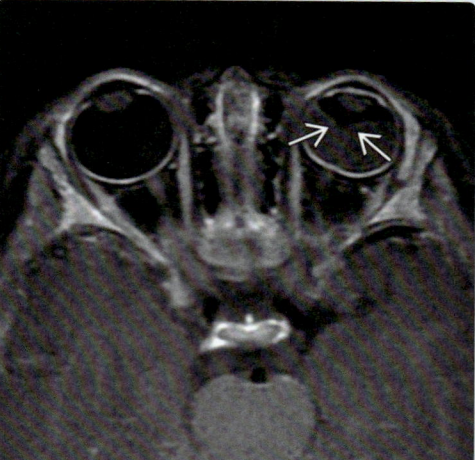
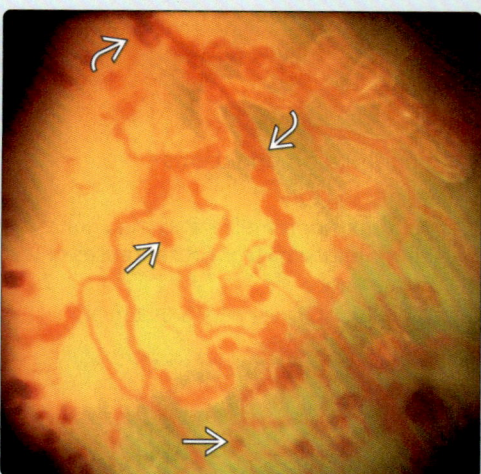

(Left) Axial T1 C+ FS MR in a 18-month-old boy with leukocoria shows a small left globe with retinal detachment ➡ without an intraocular mass. The subretinal fluid is hyperintense secondary to subretinal exudates. (Right) This slit-lamp photograph shows characteristic telangiectasias ➡ & aneurysms ➡, typical of Coats disease.

Coats Disease

TERMINOLOGY

Synonyms
- **Retinal telangiectasias**
- Exudative retinitis, **exudative retinopathy**

Definitions
- Abnormal retinal capillary development, leading to subretinal accumulation of exudate

IMAGING

General Features
- Best diagnostic clue: **Subretinal exudate**, typical **V-shape** of **retinal detachment**
- Location: **Unilateral** in 90%; bilateral when syndromic
- Size: Affected eye **slightly smaller** than normal eye, or normal-sized globe

Imaging Recommendations
- Protocol advice
  - Check CT &/or susceptibility-weighted images for calcification (almost always absent in Coats disease, present in most retinoblastomas)
  - Always include contrast enhancement

CT Findings
- Hyperdense exudate, calcification very **uncommon**

MR Findings
- T1WI & T2WI: Hyperintense proteinaceous, hemorrhagic exudate
  - Retinal detachment ± small size of globe
- T1WI C+ FS: Subfoveal enhancing nodules
  - Intraretinal macrocysts

Ultrasonographic Findings
- Grayscale ultrasound
  - Linear detached retina & tiny cholesterol crystals

DIFFERENTIAL DIAGNOSIS

Retinoblastoma
- Most common ocular tumor in children
- **Calcification** present in vast majority

Persistent Hyperplastic Primary Vitreous
- Normal fetal hyaloid vasculature fails to regress
- **Retrolental tissue** & stalk in small eye

Retinopathy of Prematurity
- Fibrovascular proliferation of immature retina, related to hyperoxia of extrauterine NICU environment
- Retinal detachment common
- **Small globe**, hyperdense, bilateral
- Calcification rare except in advanced stages (phthisis bulbi)

Ocular Toxocariasis
- Parasitic infection, typically *Toxocara canis*
  - Larval death → immunoallergic reaction to antigens → sclerosing endophthalmitis
- Intravitreal membranes, uveoscleral thickening/nodularity & retinal detachments
- Enhancing retinal nodule

PATHOLOGY

General Features
- Etiology
  - Breakdown of blood-retinal endothelial barrier
  - Leakage of exudate into subretinal space
- Associated abnormalities
  - Usually isolated but some syndromic associations
  - Norrie disease
    - X-linked recessive, mutation of *NDP* gene
    - Bilateral, infantile onset, more severe
  - Coats plus syndrome: Skeletal defects, growth failure, movement disorder, seizures

CLINICAL ISSUES

Presentation
- Most common signs/symptoms
  - **Leukocoria**, vision loss, strabismus
- Other signs/symptoms
  - Tortuous & dilated capillaries with tiny aneurysms on funduscopy

Demographics
- Age: Onset within 1st decade most common
  - Uncommon variation presents in adults
- Sex: Male predominance

Natural History & Prognosis
- Vision spared in early stages
- Increasing exudate leads to retinal detachment
- Secondary glaucoma & blindness in late stages
- Adult variation shows limited involvement, slower progression, & tendency to hemorrhage

Treatment
- Laser photocoagulation & cryotherapy
- Intravitreal antivascular endothelial growth factor (VEGF) therapy as adjunct to ablation treatment to inhibit angiogenesis
- Vitrectomy & retinal reattachment when advanced

DIAGNOSTIC CHECKLIST

Consider
- Retinoblastoma is most important differential consideration

Image Interpretation Pearls
- Lack of calcification & enhancement distinguish Coats disease from retinoblastoma
- Smaller size of affected globe may help distinguish Coats disease from noncalcifying retinoblastoma

SELECTED REFERENCES

1. Gerrie SK et al: Pediatric orbital lesions: ocular pathologies. Pediatr Radiol. 54(6):876-96, 2024
2. Hansraj S et al: Clinical presentation and treatment outcomes of adult-onset Coats disease. J Vitreoretin Dis. ePub, 2024
3. Rumboldt Z et al: Retinoblastoma and beyond: pediatric orbital mass lesions. Neuroradiology. 67(2):469-92, 2024
4. Tsai ASH et al: Clinical characteristics and treatment outcomes in unilateral Coats disease - a global collaborative study. Ophthalmol Retina. 9(6):570-9, 2024

Orbital Dermoid and Epidermoid

TERMINOLOGY

- Congenital orbital ectodermal inclusion lesion resulting in choristomatous cyst
- Dermoid: Includes dermal appendages
- Epidermoid: Dermal adnexal structures absent

IMAGING

- Cystic, well-demarcated, extraconal mass with lipid, fluid, or mixed contents
- Adjacent to orbital periosteum, near suture lines
- Superolateral at frontozygomatic suture most common
- May contain debris or fluid levels
- Osseous remodeling in majority of lesions with smooth, scalloped margins and thinning or dehiscence
- Distinguishing features
  - Dermoid: Typically but not exclusively contains fat; more heterogeneous, complex signal on MR, DWI variable
  - Epidermoid: Density and intensity similar to fluid; more homogeneous; diffusion restriction on MR

TOP DIFFERENTIAL DIAGNOSES

- Dermolipoma
- Frontal or ethmoid sinus mucocele
- Lacrimal gland cyst

PATHOLOGY

- Congenital inclusion of trapped ectoderm at suture site
- Fibrous capsule lined by squamous epithelium

CLINICAL ISSUES

- Firm, nontender mass; fixed to underlying bone
- Slowly progressive; may rupture with acute inflammation
- Presentation typically in childhood; deeper lesions in adults
- Surgical resection curative

DIAGNOSTIC CHECKLIST

- Features distinctive, but deep or inflamed lesions may present diagnostic challenge
- Fat presence essentially pathognomonic for dermoid cyst

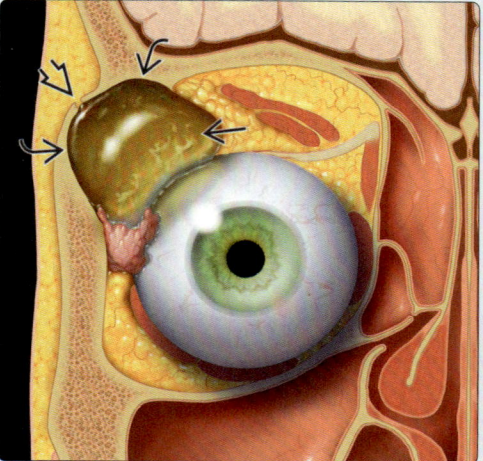
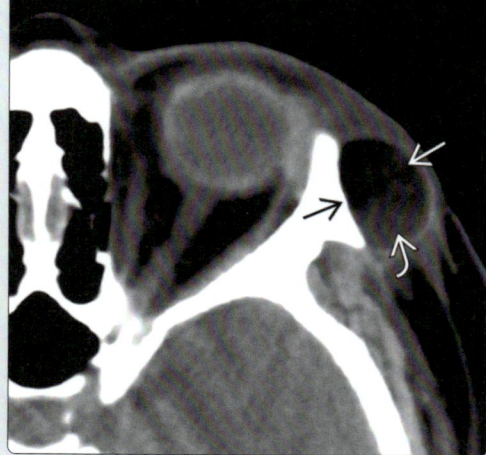

(Left) Coronal graphic depicts a superotemporal dermoid cyst ➡ located adjacent to the frontozygomatic suture of the right orbit ➡. There is resultant mass effect on the globe with remodeling of the bony orbit ➡. (Right) Axial NECT shows an ovoid mass in the temporal fossa adjacent to the lateral orbit near the "frontozygomatic" suture ➡. This dermoid cyst shows fat density with slightly more dense debris layering dependently ➡. Note the broad, scalloped remodeling of the adjacent bone ➡.

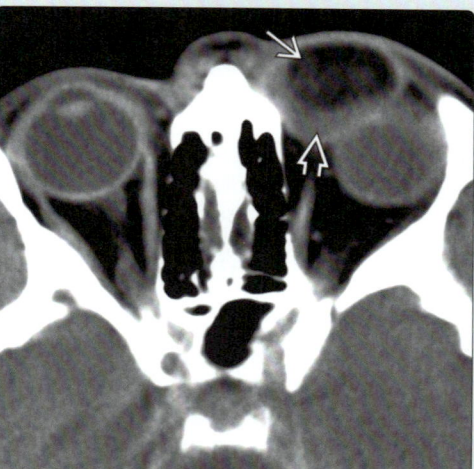
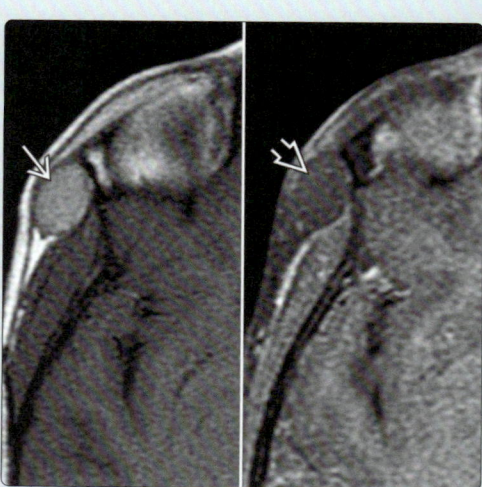

(Left) Axial NECT shows a dermoid cyst ➡ located medially in the orbit, near the location of the "frontolacrimal" suture. The cyst has fat-density contents as well as dependent soft tissue density debris ➡. (Right) Axial MR shows a right "pterional" dermoid cyst lateral to the orbit in the temporal fossa on T1 noncontrast ➡ and T1 fat-saturated postcontrast ➡ MR. Signal suppression with fat saturation indicates lipid content.

Orbital Dermoid and Epidermoid

TERMINOLOGY

Synonyms
- Congenital orbital **ectodermal inclusion cyst**

Definitions
- Cystic, **choristomatous** mass lesion of orbit resulting from congenital epithelial **inclusion**
- Dermoid lesions
  - Epithelial elements + dermal substructure, including **dermal appendages**
- Epidermoid lesions
  - Epithelial elements **without adnexal structures**

IMAGING

General Features
- Best diagnostic clue
  - Cystic, well-demarcated, anterosuperior extraconal mass with **lipid, fluid,** or **mixed contents**
- Location
  - Adjacent to orbital periosteum, near **suture lines**
  - Majority extraconal in **superolateral** aspect of anterior orbit, at **frontozygomatic** suture (65-75%)
  - Remainder mostly in **superonasal** aspect, at frontolacrimal suture, but can occur anywhere
- Size
  - Typically < 1-2 cm in superficial lesions
  - Larger in deep, complicated lesions
- Morphology
  - Ovoid, **well-demarcated** cystic mass
  - Most show thin, definable wall (75%)
  - No nodular soft tissue outside cyst (80%)
- Subtypes
  - **Superficial** (simple, exophytic)
    - Typically smaller, discrete, rounded
    - Present in early childhood
  - **Deep** (complicated, endophytic)
    - More insidious, extensive bony changes
    - Rarely intradiploic
- Contents
  - Lipid components evident in 40-50% of lesions
  - May contain mixed **fluid** or **debris**
  - **Fluid-fluid levels** in 5-10% of lesions
- Distinguishing features
  - Dermoid: Typically but not exclusively contains **fat**; more heterogeneous
  - Epidermoid: Density and intensity similar to **fluid**; more homogeneous

Radiographic Findings
- Radiography
  - Scalloped bony lucency with sclerotic margins

CT Findings
- NECT
  - **Hypodense fat** in ~ 1/2
    - Density -30 to -80 HU
  - **Calcification** in 15%
    - Fine or punctate, in cyst wall
- CECT

- Mild, thin rim enhancement
  - Irregular margins and enhancement indicate rupture with inflammatory reaction
- Bone CT
  - **Osseous remodeling** in majority of lesions (85%)
    - Pressure excavation; smooth, **scalloped** margins
    - **Thinning** of bone, may cause focal dehiscence
    - Bony tunnel, cleft, or pit in up to 1/3, leading to dumbbell appearance

MR Findings
- T1WI
  - Strongly **hyperintense** if **fatty** contents
  - Isointense or slightly hyperintense otherwise
- T2WI
  - Isointense or mildly hypointense
  - Heterogeneous **debris**
  - May show fluid-fluid levels
- DWI
  - Epidermoid shows diffusion restriction
    - Spatial restriction of diffusion of water molecules between keratin layers within cyst
  - Dermoid cysts DWI variable depending upon contents; may or may not restrict diffusion
    - Ectodermal components, such as fat and hair, may cause decreased water diffusion within cyst
- T1WI C+
  - Thin **rim enhancement**
  - More extensive **inflammation if ruptured**
- Fat-saturation techniques
  - Dermoid shows **suppression** of lipid signal

Ultrasonographic Findings
- Grayscale ultrasound
  - Adequate for evaluation of simple superficial lesions without posterior extension
  - High internal **reflectivity**, variable attenuation
  - Debris may impair determination of cystic nature

Imaging Recommendations
- Best imaging tool
  - CT without contrast often adequate for diagnosis
- Protocol advice
  - Pursue MR with contrast if features not characteristic, particularly with lesion growth

DIFFERENTIAL DIAGNOSIS

Orbital Dermolipoma
- Clinical: Soft, solid, lateral canthus mass
- Imaging: Homogeneous episcleral fat

Frontal or Ethmoid Sinus Mucocele
- Clinical: Chronic obstructive sinusitis
- Imaging: Expansile, obstructed sinus space

Lacrimal Gland Cyst
- Clinical: Lacrimal swelling and inflammation
- Imaging: Fluid density and intensity within gland

Orbital Cellulitis
- Clinical: May mimic ruptured dermoid

- Imaging: Preseptal or intraorbital infiltration

Orbital Rhabdomyosarcoma

- Clinical: Enlarging orbital mass in child
- Imaging: Variably enhancing, aggressive orbital mass

Lacrimal Gland Neoplasm

- Clinical: Minor salivary tumors
  - Pleomorphic adenoma; adenoid cystic carcinoma
- Imaging: Benign or invasive lacrimal mass with **enhancing solid components**

PATHOLOGY

General Features

- Etiology
  - **Congenital inclusion** of dermal elements
  - Sequestration of trapped surface **ectoderm**
  - Typically at site of embryonic **suture** closure
  - Acquired epidermoid may occur after remote surgery or trauma (**implantation** cyst)

Gross Pathologic & Surgical Features

- Tethered to orbital **periosteum** by fibrovascular tissue
- Oily or cheesy tan, yellow, or white material

Microscopic Features

- Dermoid
  - **Sebaceous** glands and hair **follicles**, blood vessels, **fat**, and collagen; sweat glands in minority (20%)
  - Contains keratin, sebaceous secretions, lipid metabolites, and hair
- Epidermoid
  - **No adnexal** structures
  - Filled with **keratinaceous** debris and cholesterol

CLINICAL ISSUES

Presentation

- Most common signs/symptoms
  - Firm, rounded mass at **lateral eyebrow**
  - **Nontender**, slowly progressive
- Other signs/symptoms
  - Painless in 90% but **inflamed if ruptured**
    - May rarely present as orbital cellulitis
  - Relatively **fixed** to underlying bone
- Clinical profile
  - Childhood presentation
    - More common than adult
    - **Subcutaneous** nodule near orbital rim
    - Smaller, little globe displacement
  - May present with **rupture** (10-15%)
    - Secondary to **trauma** or **spontaneous**
    - Acute inflammation **mimics cellulitis** or inflammatory tumor
    - Can result in entrapment, neuropathy
  - Mass effect if very large
    - Diplopia due to restricted movement
    - Compromise of globe or optic nerve

Demographics

- Age

  - Usually presents in **childhood** and teenage years
  - Simple, superficial lesions often present in infancy
  - May present or **grow at any age**
  - Occasionally will appear in adult and grow significantly over several months
- Sex
  - Equal or slight male predominance
- Epidemiology
  - Most common noninflammatory, nonneoplastic, space-occupying lesion of orbit
    - 1/2 of childhood orbital lesions
    - 90% of cystic orbital lesions
  - 10% of head and neck dermoid and epidermoid cysts periorbital in location

Natural History & Prognosis

- Benign lesion, usually cosmetic considerations
- Very **slow growth**, usually dormant for years
  - Present during childhood but small and dormant
  - May become symptomatic during **rapid growth** phase in **young adult**
- Sudden growth or change following **rupture**
  - Significant **inflammation** and increased size
- Dermoid cysts along scalp midline have higher potential of intracranial extension
- Dermoid cysts in more lateral areas of skull/scalp rarely associated with intracranial extension
  - But temporal dermoid cysts have higher rate of intracranial extension

Treatment

- **Surgical resection** curative
  - Entire cyst must be removed to prevent recurrence
    - Including growth center at periosteal interface
  - **Brow** or **eyelid crease** incision most common
    - Approach depends on location in orbit
  - Lesions evident in early childhood should be removed to avoid traumatic rupture
- Steroids or nonsteroidal drugs to calm inflammation in ruptured lesions
- Asymptomatic small lesions may be observed expectantly
  - Particularly small epidermoid with less inflammatory response in event of rupture

DIAGNOSTIC CHECKLIST

Consider

- Features of typical lesions distinctive, but deep or inflamed lesions may present diagnostic challenge
- Dermoid cyst distinct from dermolipoma

Image Interpretation Pearls

- Presence of fat essentially **pathognomonic**
- Posterior extent of **complex lesions** may not be clinically apparent; therefore, imaging is warranted

SELECTED REFERENCES

1. Ng JJ et al: Surgical management of 2350 pediatric dermoid cysts. Plast Reconstr Surg. 156(1):120-9, 2025
2. Menousek JP et al: A unique case of frontotemporal dermoid cyst presenting as orbital cellulitis. Cureus. 15(4):e37050, 2023
3. Oh HJ et al: Craniofacial epidermoid and dermoid cysts. J Craniofac Surg. 34(8):2405-9, 2023

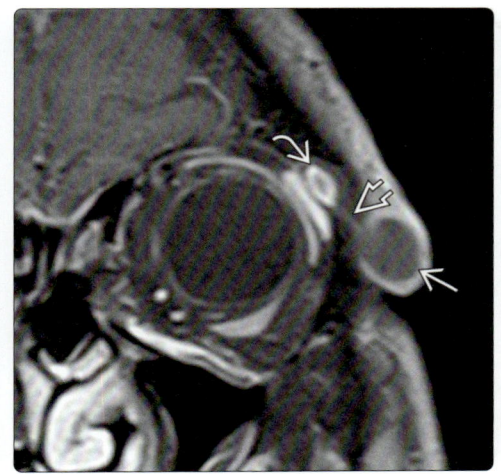

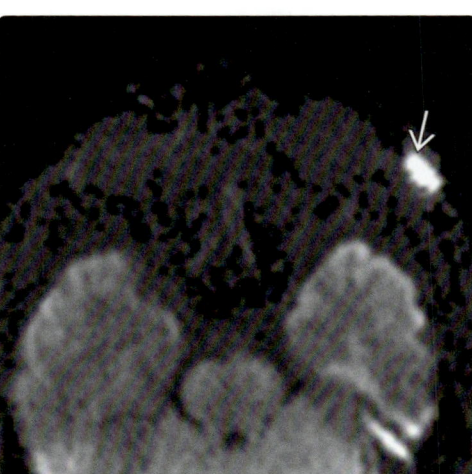

(Left) *Coronal T1 postcontrast MR shows an epidermoid cyst with thin marginal enhancement* ⇨ *lateral to the left orbital rim. A smaller intraorbital component is seen along the inner margin of the orbital wall* ⇨ *with scalloping of the bone at the lacrimal fossa. A small connecting stalk is visible near the frontozygomatic suture* ⇨. *(Right) Axial DWI MR shows diffusion restriction in the same lesion at the left lateral orbital rim* ⇨, *suggesting an epidermoid cyst. Note that dermoid cysts may sometimes restrict diffusion.*

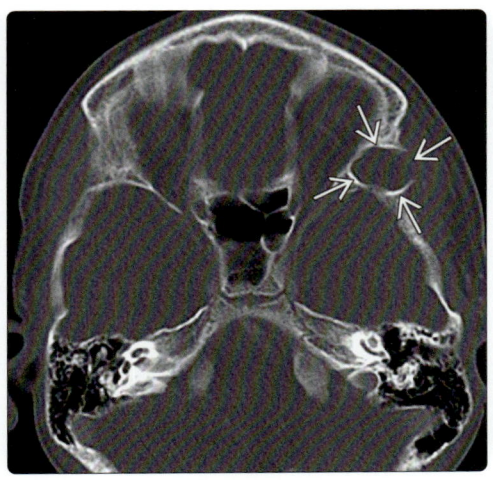

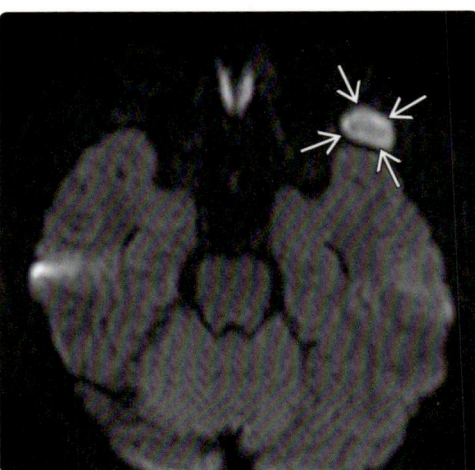

(Left) *Axial NECT bone window shows a left pterional expansile intradiploic dermoid cyst* ⇨ *lateral to the orbit, projecting toward the temporal fossa. No definite fatty contents are detected on imaging. (Right) Axial DWI MR in the same patient shows diffusion restriction* ⇨ *of the cyst contents. Even though the presence of diffusion restriction and the absence of fatty contents should favor epidermoid, this lesion was proven to be a dermoid cyst. Remember, dermoid cysts may also restrict diffusion.*

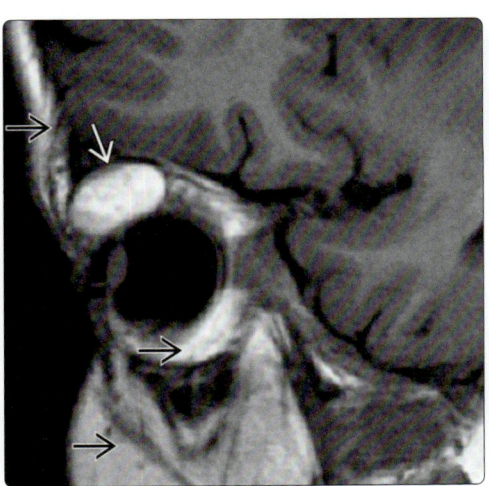

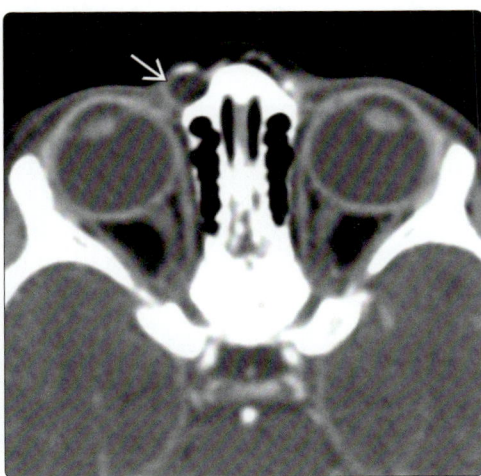

(Left) *Sagittal oblique unenhanced T1 MR without fat suppression shows a hyperintense superior orbital dermoid cyst* ⇨ *due to fatty contents. Note similar signal intensity of normal fat in the scalp, orbit, and face* ⇨. *If T1 hyperintensity is due to proteinaceous or hemorrhagic contents, it will not suppress in fat-saturated sequences. (Right) Axial CECT in a child with a right medial periorbital dermoid cyst shows a well-defined, nonenhancing cyst* ⇨ *deep to right angular artery, causing mild scalloping of the underlying bone.*

TERMINOLOGY

- Neurofibromatosis type 1 (NF1): Neurocutaneous disorder (inherited tumor syndrome) with distinct orbitocranial manifestations

IMAGING

- Constellation of features pathognomonic of NF1
  - Plexiform neurofibroma (PNF)
  - Optic pathway glioma (OPG)
  - Sphenoid dysplasia (SD)
  - Buphthalmos (ox eye)
  - Optic nerve sheath ectasia
- Orbitofacial NF1 typically unilateral
- OPG in NF1 shows variable enhancement
  - OPG without NF1 often shows more enhancement

TOP DIFFERENTIAL DIAGNOSES

- **PNF**: Rhabdomyosarcoma, infantile hemangioma, Langerhans cell histiocytosis, venolymphatic malformation

- **OPG with NF1**: OPG without NF1, optic neuritis, optic nerve sheath meningioma
- **SD**: Congenital cephalocele, traumatic cephalocele
- **Buphthalmos**: Congenital glaucoma, coloboma
- **Optic nerve sheath ectasia**: Normal variant, intracranial hypertension

PATHOLOGY

- Autosomal dominant, 50% new mutations

CLINICAL ISSUES

- Presentation: Periorbital masses, proptosis, and ptosis
- Natural history: Progressive orbitofacial deformity and progressive visual and ophthalmologic dysfunction

DIAGNOSTIC CHECKLIST

- Although NF1 is inherited disorder, orbital manifestations are progressive and develop over time
- Rapid change in PNF concerning for malignant sarcomatous degeneration

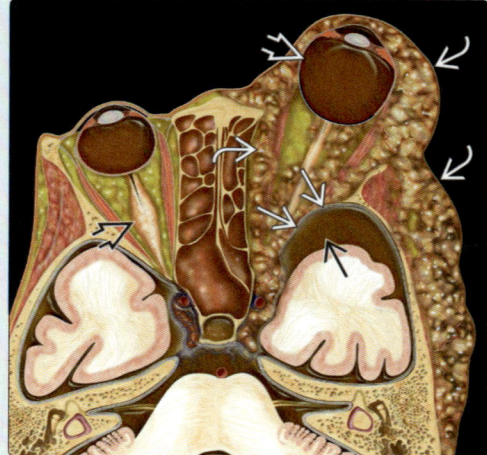
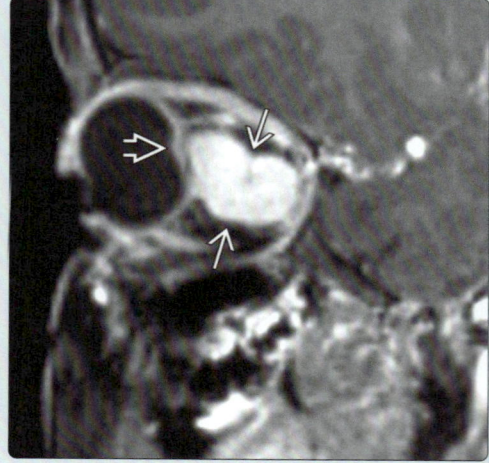

(Left) Axial graphic shows orbital neurofibromatosis type 1 (NF1), including sphenoid wing dysplasia ➡ with enlarged CSF space protruding through the bony defect ➡. Note plexiform neurofibromas ➡ & buphthalmos ➡. An optic nerve glioma is also evident ➡. (Right) Sagittal T1 C+ FS MR shows an enhancing intraorbital optic nerve glioma ➡. Note a tiny focus of enhancement at the elevated optic papilla due to papilledema ➡ (not tumor), which disappeared after chemotherapy when the glioma shrunk (not shown).

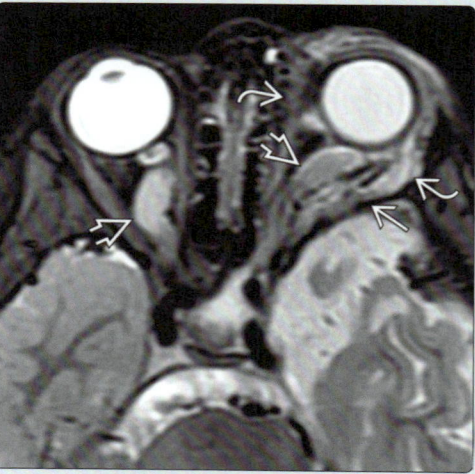
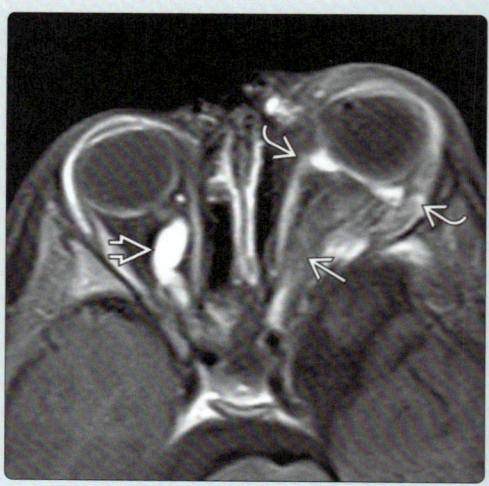

(Left) Axial T2 FS MR shows typical features of NF1 with bilateral optic nerve gliomas ➡, an infiltrative, T2-hyperintense mass in the left orbit ➡, consistent with plexiform neurofibroma and left sphenoid dysplasia ➡. (Right) Corresponding axial T1 C+ FS MR shows that the right optic nerve glioma ➡ and left plexiform neurofibroma ➡ enhance, while the left optic nerve glioma does not ➡. Optic nerve gliomas in NF1 show variable enhancement. Optic nerve glioma in patients without NF1 often show more enhancement.

TERMINOLOGY

Abbreviations
- Neurofibromatosis type 1 (NF1), optic nerve (ON)

Synonyms
- von Recklinghausen disease

Definitions
- **Neurocutaneous disorder** (inherited tumor syndrome) with distinct orbitofacial and cranial manifestations

IMAGING

General Features
- Best diagnostic clue
  - Constellation of orbital, skull base, and intracranial features **pathognomonic** of NF1
- Location
  - Orbitofacial NF1 typically **unilateral**
- Morphology
  - **Plexiform neurofibroma** (PNF)
    - Serpentine, unencapsulated, infiltrative masses
    - May involve intraorbital branches of cranial nerves (III, IV, V1, VI) and sclera
    - Associated enlargement of skull base foramina
    - Frequently transspatial with contiguous tumors in preseptal orbit, temporal fossa, and skull base
  - **Optic pathway glioma** (OPG)
    - Tubular or lobular enlargement of ON
    - May involve any segment of ON, chiasm, tracts &/or radiations
  - **Sphenoid dysplasia** (SD)
    - Bony defects, decalcification, or remodeling of greater wing and lateral orbital wall
    - Enlargement of middle fossa with herniation of intracranial contents into orbit
    - Associated enlargement of CSF space anterior middle fossa common
    - Almost always associated with orbital PNF
  - **Buphthalmos (ox eye)**
    - Increased axial AP globe diameter
    - Remodeling and enlargement of anterior orbital rim
    - Thickening of uveal/scleral layer
    - May be associated with anterior orbit PNF
  - **ON sheath ectasia**
    - Nontumorous enlargement of dural sheath allowing increased CSF signal around ON

Radiographic Findings
- Radiography
  - **Bare orbit** sign: Absence of innominate line (superior border of greater wing of sphenoid in frontal view)
  - Enlarged, **egg-shaped** anterior orbital rim
  - **Harlequin eye** appearance: Innominate line appears as elevated dense ridge; rarely in NF1 SD
    - Classically, sign of coronal craniostenosis
  - Optic canal &/or superior/inferior orbital fissure enlargement when filled with PNF

CT Findings
- **PNF**: Hypodense, **infiltrative** soft tissue masses with variable enhancement
  - Increased overall orbital fat density due to small PNF of cranial nerve branches
- **OPG** or **dural ectasia**: Enlarged nerve/sheath contour
- **SD**: Bony **defect** with **herniation** of middle fossa into orbit; proptosis may be marked

MR Findings
- T1WI
  - **PNF**: Hypointense, **ill-defined** soft tissue masses
  - **OPG**: Isointense ON mass ± **cystic** hypointensity
- T2WI
  - **PNF**: Hyperintense nodular masses with central low-signal **target sign**
  - **OPG**: Hyperintense **fusiform** ON mass
    - **Perineural arachnoid gliomatosis (PAG)**: Hyperintense astrocytic proliferation in subarachnoid space
  - **Buphthalmos**: Enlarged globe, thickened sclera
  - **Nerve sheath ectasia**: Increased **perioptic fluid**
- T1WI C+
  - **PNF**: Irregular infiltrative **serpentine** masses; variable enhancement, may be intense
  - **OPG**: Variably enhancing ON mass, PAG show moderate enhancement
    - Isolated tumors without NF1 often show more enhancement
    - Papilledema may produce tiny focus of enhancement at elevated optic papilla without OPG tumor infiltration into eye globe
      - May disappear after chemotherapy when OPG shrinks

Ultrasonographic Findings
- **PNF**: Irregular, compressible, **highly** reflective
- **OPG**: Smooth nerve enlargement, **minimally** reflective
- **SD**: Defect of posterior bony orbital wall
- **Buphthalmos**: Increased eye diameter

Imaging Recommendations
- Best imaging tool
  - MR ideal for assessment of orbital, extracranial, and intracranial lesions
  - CT to assess skull base defects and surgical planning

DIFFERENTIAL DIAGNOSIS

Plexiform Neurofibroma
- Rhabdomyosarcoma
- Infantile hemangioma
- Langerhans cell histiocytosis
- Leukemia
- Venolymphatic malformation

Optic Pathway Glioma
- OPG without NF1
- Optic neuritis
- ON sheath meningioma

Sphenoid Dysplasia

- Congenital or posttraumatic sphenorbital cephalocele

Buphthalmos

- Congenital glaucoma
- Coloboma

Optic Nerve Sheath Ectasia

- Normal variant
- Idiopathic intracranial hypertension
- ON sheath meningioma

PATHOLOGY

General Features

- Etiology
  - Disorder of histogenesis, classified as neurocutaneous inherited tumor syndrome
  - Orbital features of NF1 have interrelated underlying pathology
    - In particular, SD and PNF intimately associated
- Genetics
  - **Autosomal dominant**; variable expression
  - 50% **new mutations**; gene locus = 17q11.2
  - Loss of NF1 **tumor suppressor** gene function
  - Loss of NF1 gene activates 3 distinct Ras effector pathways (PI3K/AKT/mTOR, MEK/ERK, and cAMP pathways) that mediate OPG tumorigenesis
    - Nonneoplastic cells from tumor microenvironment like microglia, T cells, and neurons also contribute via various soluble factors
- Associated abnormalities
  - **CNS tumors** on brain imaging
  - Nonneoplastic foci of abnormal signal intensity **(FASI)**
  - Diffuse soft tissue neurofibromas; skeletal deformities

Staging, Grading, & Classification

- Diagnostic criteria for NF1 established by NIH consensus statement on NF

Gross Pathologic & Surgical Features

- **PNF**: Worm-like, infiltrating, tortuous masses
  - May involve eyelid, anterior periorbita, scalp, orbit, temporal fossa, and skull base
- **OPG**: Diffuse nerve enlargement; tan-white tumor
  - Cystic component with mucinous changes
  - 2 growth patterns: Intraneural and perineural forms; rarely both coexist
  - **Intraneural form** shows fusiform enlargement of nerve
  - **PAG** shows astrocytic proliferation in subarachnoid space surrounding relatively preserved ON
- **SD**: Bony defect of posterior lateral orbit
  - Middle cranial fossa expansion with enlarged CSF space
- **Buphthalmos**: Associated with PNF in anterior orbit

Microscopic Features

- **PNF**: Myxoid endoneural accumulation early
  - Schwann cell proliferation, collagen accumulation
- **OPG**: Spindle-shaped astrocytes with hyperplasia of fibroblasts and meningothelial cells
- **SD**: Bone decalcification; premature suture closure
- **Buphthalmos**: Periscleral infiltration by plexiform tumors

CLINICAL ISSUES

Presentation

- Most common signs/symptoms
  - PNF
    - Bulky soft tissue masses; **bag-of-worms** texture
    - PNF anywhere indicative of NF1
  - OPG
    - Visual deficit, often relatively **mild**
    - Proptosis associated with poor vision
  - SD
    - **Pulsatile exophthalmos** due to orbital encroachment by middle fossa contents
  - Buphthalmos
    - Enlarged eye; impaired vision, glaucoma

Demographics

- Age
  - Findings may not be evident at birth
  - Cutaneous signs present at birth or 1st year
  - Tumors begin to appear in childhood
- Epidemiology
  - NF1 **most common** inherited tumor syndrome
  - Orbital involvement in up to 1/3 of NF1

Natural History & Prognosis

- PNF may undergo **sarcomatous degeneration** to malignant peripheral nerve sheath tumor (2-16%)
- Decreased life expectancy
  - Malignancy most common cause of death

Treatment

- PNF
  - Generally not surgically curable due to infiltrative nature
  - Debulking may be required for vision or cosmesis
  - Radiation therapy not effective
- OPG
  - Observation unless vision threatened
  - Chemotherapy when progression occurs
  - Surgery challenging; done when no useful vision or to treat corneal exposure or proptosis
  - Radiation not recommended in children
    - Risk of secondary tumors, moyamoya syndrome, and neurocognitive sequelae
- SD
  - Transcranial reconstruction with bone grafts
- Buphthalmos
  - Medical ± surgical therapy for glaucoma

DIAGNOSTIC CHECKLIST

Consider

- Although NF1 is inherited disorder, orbital manifestations are progressive and develop over time

Image Interpretation Pearls

- Rapid change in PNF; consider sarcomatous degeneration

SELECTED REFERENCES

1. Chen Y et al: An overview of optic pathway glioma with neurofibromatosis type 1: pathogenesis, risk factors, and therapeutic strategies. Invest Ophthalmol Vis Sci. 65(6):8, 2024

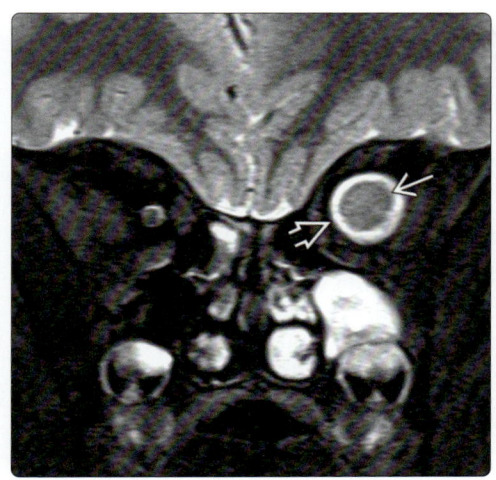

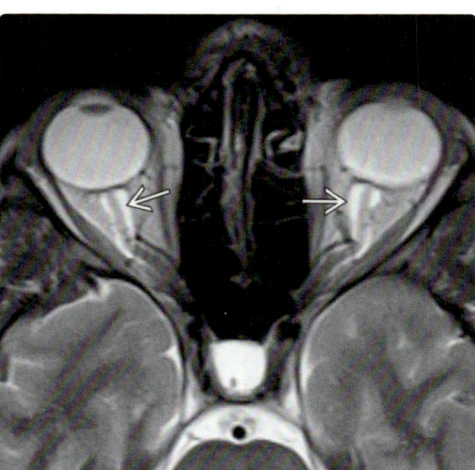

(Left) *Coronal T2 FS MR in a patient with NF1 shows a fusiform left optic nerve glioma* ➡️ *involving the intraorbital segment. Ectasia of the optic nerve sheath allows for increased CSF signal intensity around the nerve* ➡️.
(Right) *Axial T2 FS MR in a patient with NF1, but no orbital masses, shows ectasia of the optic dural sheaths, which manifests as increased CSF signal surrounding the intraorbital segments of the optic nerves bilaterally* ➡️, *and mild tortuosity of the optic nerves without enlargement.*

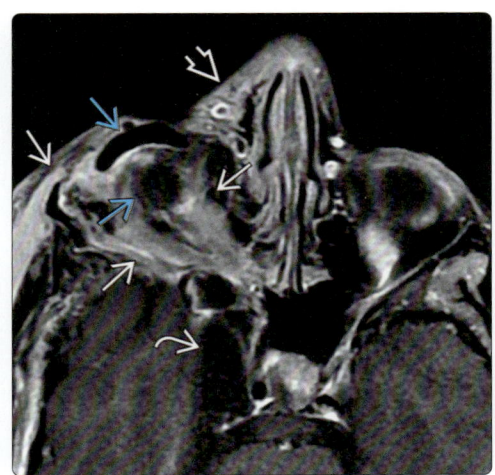

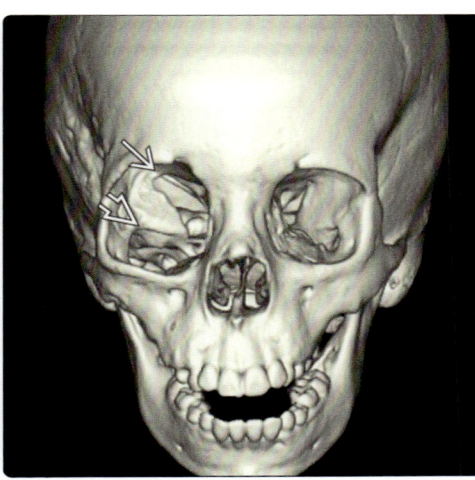

(Left) *Axial T1 C+ FS MR shows a transspatial orbitotemporal plexiform neurofibroma* ➡️ *involving the nasal soft tissues* ➡️. *There is ipsilateral dilatation of the Meckel cave* ➡️. *The patient also has a 2-piece globe prosthesis* ➡️, *placed after enucleation.*
(Right) *Anterior 3D surface rendering cone CT in a child with NF1 shows diffuse enlargement of the right orbit. There is associated enlargement of the superior* ➡️ *and inferior* ➡️ *orbital fissures in this child with extensive associated plexiform neurofibroma.*

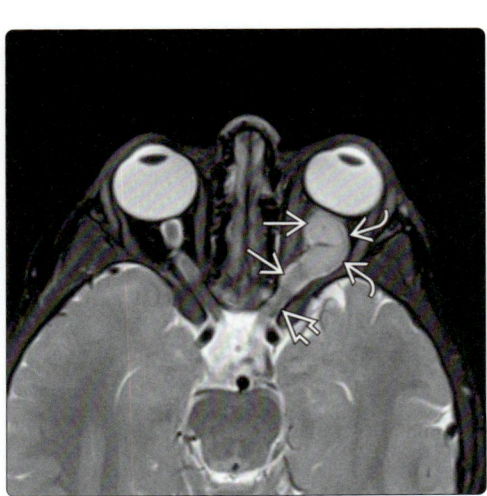

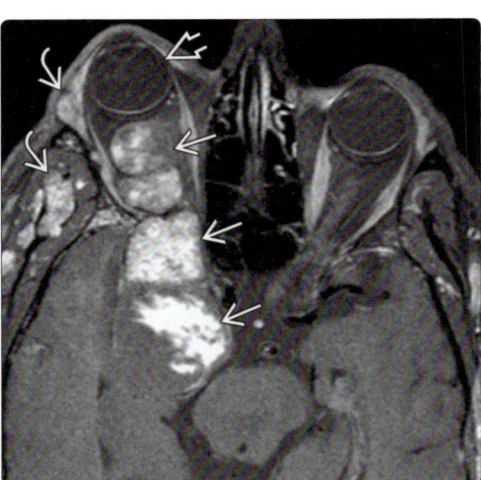

(Left) *Axial T2 FS MR shows a tortuous fusiform left optic nerve glioma involving the intraorbital* ➡️ *and canalicular* ➡️ *segments. Notice a thin layer of slightly T2-hyperintense perineural arachnoid gliomatosis (PAG)* ➡️. (Right) *Axial T1 C+ FS MR shows patchy enhancement of lobulated, massively enlarged right optic nerve, involving the intraorbital, intracanalicular, and prechiasmatic portions* ➡️. *The right globe is severely proptotic* ➡️. *Extracranial plexiform tumors in the orbitotemporal regions are also evident* ➡️.

Orbital Lymphatic Malformation

TERMINOLOGY

- Congenital vascular malformation with isolated lymphatic (lymphatic malformation) or mixed venous and lymphatic (venolymphatic malformation) elements

IMAGING

- Lobulated, transspatial mass
- Multiloculated cystic features with fluid-fluid levels, blood products, and minimal enhancement
- Variants: Superficial vs. deep, macrocystic vs. microcystic
- CT: Irregular, cystic hypodense mass with mixed hyperdense blood products
- MR: Variable signal resulting from mixed-age hemorrhagic, lymphatic, or proteinaceous fluid
- May show minimal enhancement, typically at margins, more pronounced if prominent venous components
- US: Hypoechoic with heterogeneous internal echoes
- Best imaging tool
  - Dedicated orbital MR to include fluid-sensitive (T2 FS or STIR) and T1 C+ FS series

TOP DIFFERENTIAL DIAGNOSES

- Orbital varix; orbital cavernous venous malformation; infantile hemangioma; plexiform neurofibroma

PATHOLOGY

- Congenital, nonneoplastic vascular malformation
- Dilated dysplastic lymphatic ± venous channels

CLINICAL ISSUES

- Mass effect with proptosis in pediatric patient
- May rapidly ↑ in size due to acute hemorrhage
- Conservative therapy preferred due to surgical risk
- Percutaneous sclerotherapy for suitable lesions
- Surgical resection difficult; recurrence common

DIAGNOSTIC CHECKLIST

- Blood products and fluid-fluid levels highly suggestive

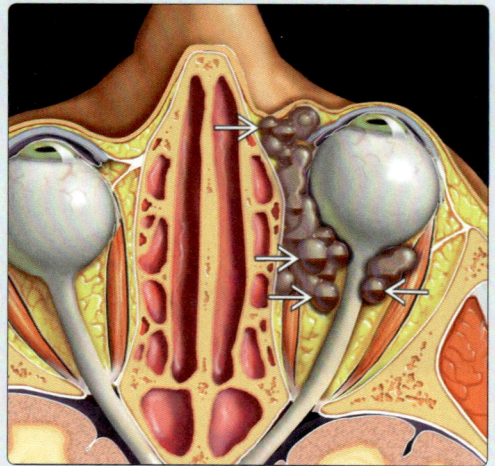 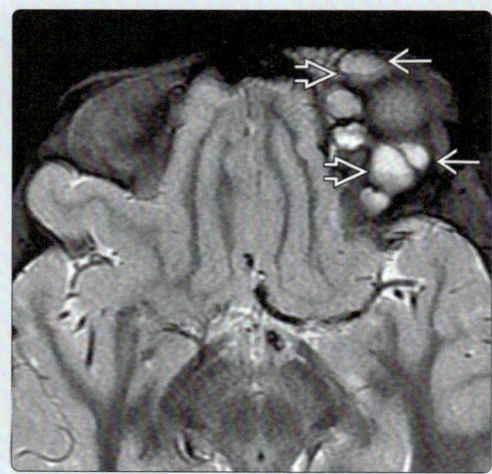

(Left) Axial graphic depicts typical features of orbital lymphatic malformation (LM), including transspatial extension and characteristic fluid-fluid levels within loculations ➡. (Right) Axial T2 FS MR shows a multilocular transspatial lesion ➡ involving the preseptal and postseptal orbit with fluid levels ➡, consistent with LM. Distinct and well-defined segments of the lesion are characteristic.

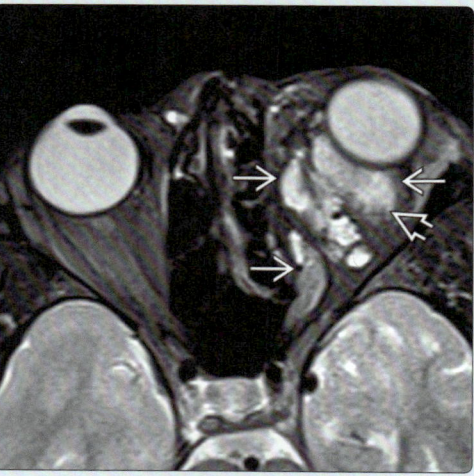 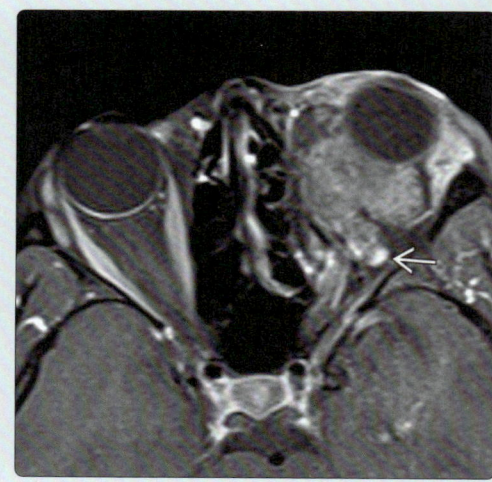

(Left) Axial T2 FS MR in a patient presenting with painless proptosis demonstrates a multilocular, macrocystic postseptal mass ➡ with heterogeneous proteinaceous or hemorrhagic contents. There is a fluid level consistent with intralesional hemorrhage ➡. (Right) Axial T1 C+ FS MR in the same patient demonstrates only trace foci of enhancement ➡ at the posterior periphery of the lesion. The lesion is large but results in only mild proptosis.

TERMINOLOGY

Abbreviations

- Orbital lymphatic malformation (LM or OLM)
- Orbital venolymphatic malformation (VLM or OVLM)

Synonyms

- Avoid incorrect terms: Cystic hygroma and lymphangioma
- Vascular malformation, lymphatic type; lymphatic anomaly

Definitions

- Congenital vascular malformation with variable **lymphatic** ± venous vascular elements
- LM: Subtype of slow-/low-flow congenital vascular malformation of embryonic lymphatic sacs; not neoplastic
  - No communication with normal lymphatics
  - Composed of macrocysts > 1 cm &/or microcysts < 1 cm
- VLM: Combined elements of venous malformation (VM) and LM

IMAGING

General Features

- Best diagnostic clue
  - Lobulated, multiloculated **transspatial** mass; insinuates between vessels and other normal structures
  - Macrocystic LM: Multiloculated cystic neck mass with imperceptible wall, thin septations, and fluid-fluid levels
  - Microcystic LM: Ill-defined, infiltrative, &/or solid-appearing
- Location
  - **Superficial**: Often confined to conjunctiva
  - **Deep**: Extending into orbit
    - Extraconal > intraconal but often transspatial
- Morphology
  - **Irregular** margins, **multilocular cysts** with fluid levels
  - Macrocystic (> 1 cm), microcystic (< 1 cm), or mixed
  - Posterior venous lesions with more well-defined margins may mimic orbital cavernous venous malformation

CT Findings

- NECT
  - Irregular, multicystic, **hypodense** mass ± fluid-fluid levels
  - Hemorrhage with mixed hyperdense **blood products**
  - ± phleboliths in VM components of VLM
- CECT
  - Cystic structures with minimal **rim &/or septal enhancement** ± fluid-fluid levels
  - More diffuse, patchy, and gradual enhancement suggests **venous components** in mixed VLM ± phleboliths in VM components of VLM

MR Findings

- T1WI
  - **Lobulated**, hypointense unless prior hemorrhage
  - **Fluid-fluid levels** with variable signal due to mixed-age hemorrhagic, lymphatic, or proteinaceous fluid in multilocular cystic spaces
  - Different ages of **blood products**; subacute blood characteristically **hyperintense**
- T2WI FS
  - Lobulated, **very hyperintense** fluid signal
  - **Fluid-fluid levels** show signal corresponding to age of blood products
  - No vascular flow voids (unlike infantile hemangioma)
  - Transspatial lesions often poorly marginated
- T1WI C+ FS
  - No significant enhancement, ± minimal rim enhancement at margins of cysts
  - Patchy enhancement suggests VLM or microcystic LM
  - Nonenhancing **thrombus** may be visible with acute exacerbation

Ultrasonographic Findings

- Grayscale ultrasound
  - Unilocular vs. septated and multilocular transspatial mass
  - **Hypoechoic**/anechoic blood and lymph-filled cystic spaces
  - **Heterogeneous** internal echoes ± swirling debris &/or layering fluid-debris levels
  - No true vascular flow in cysts by Doppler
  - ± flow (from encased normal vessels) in septations

Imaging Recommendations

- Best imaging tool
  - Dedicated orbital MR to include fluid-sensitive (T2 FS or STIR) and T1 C+ FS series
- Protocol advice
  - Include brain imaging for intracranial abnormalities

DIFFERENTIAL DIAGNOSIS

Orbital Varix

- Clinical: **Intermittent** pain and **proptosis**
- Imaging: Similar to LM or VLM, but **dynamic expansion** demonstrated with **Valsalva**
- Pathology: Often considered part of **VLM spectrum** but with **distensible** venous component

Orbital Cavernous Venous Malformation

- Clinical: Slowly growing, **painless** mass, most **common** benign orbital mass in **adults**
- Imaging: Circumscribed, ovoid, **intraconal** solid mass with **dynamic** fill-in enhancement
- Pathology: **Pseudoencapsulated** venous malformation, unique to orbit

Infantile Hemangioma

- Clinical: Highly vascular tumor of **infancy**; typically increases in size, and then **regresses** spontaneously
- Imaging: Well-defined, intensely enhancing orbitofacial mass with **flow voids**
- Pathology: Vascular **neoplasm**, **not** vascular malformation

Plexiform Neurofibroma

- Clinical: Associated with **neurofibromatosis** type 1
- Imaging: Infiltrative, transspatial masses, associated with **sphenoid dysplasia**, orbitofacial deformity, proptosis, and buphthalmos
- Pathology: Nerve sheath tumor of neurocutaneous syndrome

PATHOLOGY

General Features

- Etiology
  - Congenital, **nonneoplastic, low-flow vascular malformation**
  - Arise from pluripotent venous anlage
  - Lymphatic tissue not normally found in orbit
- Associated abnormalities
  - Malformations in other regions of head and neck
  - Generalized lymphatic anomaly (lymphangiomatosis)
  - Noncontiguous **intracranial** vascular malformations
    - 70% of patients with periorbital VLM have intracranial vascular and parenchymal anomalies
      - Developmental venous anomaly, cerebral cavernous malformation, dural arteriovenous malformation (AVM), pial AVM, sinus pericranii

Staging, Grading, & Classification

- General classification of orbital vascular malformations
  - **Type 1**: No flow (LM)
  - **Type 2**: Venous flow (VLM or venous malformation)
    - Nondistensible vs. distensible (associated with varix)
  - **Type 3**: Arterial flow (high flow, AVM)
- General classification of LM: Microcystic or macrocystic

Microscopic Features

- **Unencapsulated** mass of irregularly shaped sinuses; infiltrates into adjacent stroma
- Dilated **dysplastic** venous ± lymphatic channels lined with flattened endothelial cells
- **Cystic** spaces + lymphatic fluid or chronic blood products
- **Lymphoid follicles** and lymphocyte infiltration
- Positive **lymphatic** IHC **markers** confirms lymphatic origin
  - PROX1 and VEGFR3 most sensitive, specific
- Recent recommendation: Use IHC panel of PROX1, D2-40, VEGFR3, CD31, and CD34 antibodies to differentiate LM from other vascular malformations

CLINICAL ISSUES

Presentation

- Most common signs/symptoms
  - Progressive **proptosis** with **sudden episodic worsening**
- Other signs/symptoms
  - Mass effect; compressive optic neuropathy
  - Diplopia, restricted extraocular muscles, ptosis
  - Periorbital ecchymosis associated with hemorrhage
- Clinical profile
  - Lesions may **rapidly ↑** in size due to **acute intralesional hemorrhage**
    - Recurrent hemorrhages in 50%
    - Associated with lesion **recurrence** after surgery
    - **Thrombosis** may precipitate hemorrhage; related to stasis, congestion, and inflammation
  - Lesions may intermittently ↑ and ↓ in size in conjunction with upper respiratory infection
    - Related to presence of **lymphatic tissue**

Demographics

- Age: **Infants to young adults**
  - 40% present by age 6; 60% present by age 16

Natural History & Prognosis

- **Progressive slow growth** during childhood, through puberty and into early adulthood, with **episodic acute enlargement** due to **hemorrhage**
- Infiltrating nature results in frequent **recurrence**
- Refractory visual problems and disfigurement common
- Poor visual acuity with multiple surgical resections
- Optic nerve compromise with recurrent large lesions

Treatment

- Options, risks, complications
  - Conservative therapy
    - **Observation** preferred if vision is not threatened due to hazards of surgery
    - Systemic **steroids** may ↓ pain, swelling, and proptosis, especially in younger patients
    - 45% of smaller lesions show **regression**
    - Sirolimus recently reported as effective treatment of orbital LM and VLMs, especially microcystic LMs
  - Image-guided sclerotherapy
    - Percutaneous **intralesional** injection of sclerosing agent, particularly for macrocystic lesions
  - Surgery
    - Difficult resection due to complex **insinuation** with normal orbital structures
    - **Recurrence** after surgery common (~ 50%)
    - Acute mass effect due to hemorrhage may require emergent **decompression**
    - Indications include optic nerve dysfunction, corneal compromise, and intractable amblyopia

DIAGNOSTIC CHECKLIST

Consider

- Deep circumscribed lesions in adults may mimic orbital cavernous venous malformation
- VLM and orbital varix are related lesions
  - VLM is hemodynamically isolated
  - Varix has systemic drainage, which accounts for pressure-dependent distensibility

Image Interpretation Pearls

- Presence of blood products with **fluid-fluid levels** is highly suggestive of LM or VLM

SELECTED REFERENCES

1. Azizinik F et al: Vascular lesions of head and neck region: a pictorial review. Eur J Radiol. 189:112190, 2025
2. Gerrie SK et al: Pediatric orbital lesions: non-neoplastic extraocular soft-tissue lesions. Pediatr Radiol. 54(6):910-21, 2024
3. International Society for the Study of Vascular Anomalies: ISSVA Classification for Vascular Anomalies. Reviewed 2024. Accessed May 28, 2025. https://www.issva.org/classification
4. Booth TN: Congenital cystic neck masses. Neuroimaging Clin N Am. 33(4):591-605, 2023
5. Mamlouk MD: Solid and vascular neck masses in children. Neuroimaging Clin N Am. 33(4):607-21, 2023
6. Wiegand S et al: Efficacy of sirolimus in children with lymphatic malformations of the head and neck. Eur Arch Otorhinolaryngol. 279(8):3801-10, 2022
7. Shoji MK et al: The use of sirolimus for treatment of orbital lymphatic malformations: a systematic review. Ophthalmic Plast Reconstr Surg. 36(3):215-21, 2020
8. Merrow AC et al: 2014 revised classification of vascular lesions from the International Society for the Study of Vascular Anomalies: radiologic-pathologic update. Radiographics. 36(5):1494-516, 2016

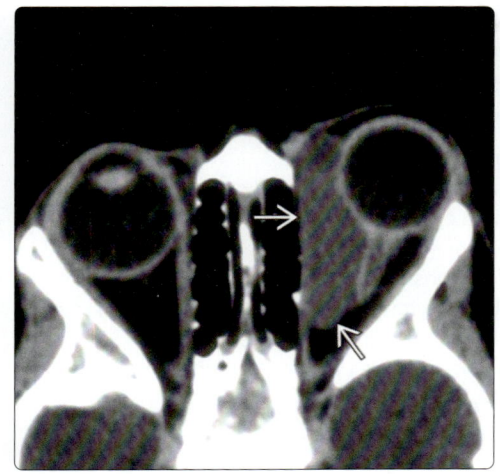
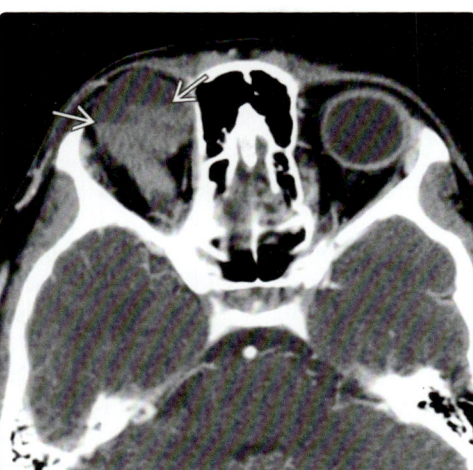

(Left) Axial CECT shows a cystic, well-defined, nonenhancing mass with an imperceptible wall in the medial left orbit ➡. The mass has a simple, unilocular appearance but is transspatial with intraconal, extraconal, and preseptal components. Soft mass conforms to and does not distort globe. (Right) Axial CECT shows multiple loculations within the mass and demonstrates fluids of varying density with discrete fluid-fluid levels ➡. The more dense chronic hemorrhagic products are seen layering dependently.

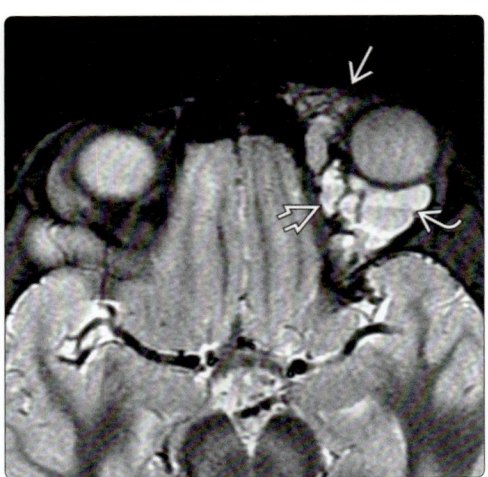
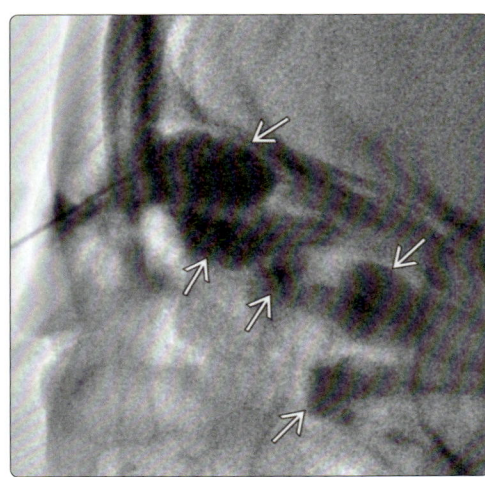

(Left) Axial STIR MR shows a preseptal ➡ and postseptal ➡ cystic mass of the right orbit causing proptosis and containing internal fluid-fluid levels ➡, consistent with OLM. Note the soft appearance without deformation of globe. (Right) The patient underwent sclerosis of the LM with doxycycline. Sagittal fluoroscopic image during the procedure shows filling of each of the macrocysts ➡ of the LM with contrast.

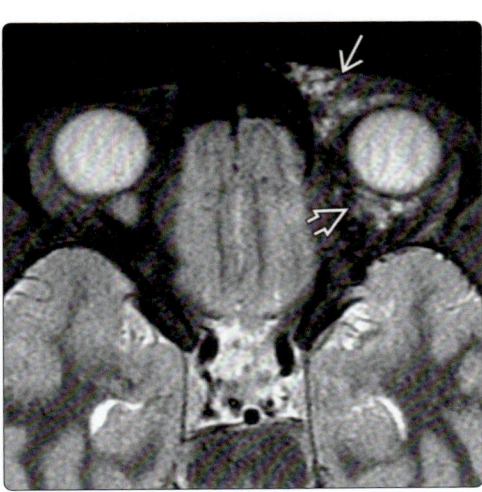
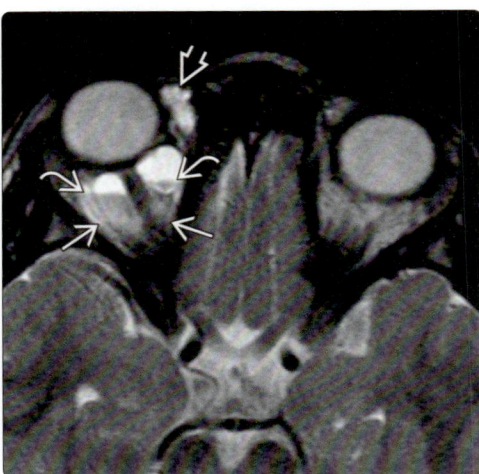

(Left) Axial STIR MR follow-up after sclerosis shows significant decrease in the size of preseptal ➡ and postseptal ➡ components of LM. Proptosis has also resolved. (Right) Axial T2 MR in a 5-year-old child with painful proptosis shows a multiloculated LM in the retrobulbar intraconal ➡ and anteromedial extraconal ➡ spaces, causing moderate right proptosis. Combination of macrocystic and microcystic components, associated with fluid-fluid levels ➡, is essentially diagnostic of LM.

Orbital Venous Varix

TERMINOLOGY

- Low-flow venous malformation with systemic venous connection & dynamically distensible varix

IMAGING

- Intensely enhancing orbital mass that distends with ↑ venous pressure
- Nonenhancing foci of flow, hemorrhage, thrombosis, or cystic lymphatic spaces
- Best imaging tool: Dynamic CT ± provocation maneuver

TOP DIFFERENTIAL DIAGNOSES

- Orbital lymphatic malformation
  - Multiloculated with fluid levels; no systemic venous connection
- Orbital cavernous venous malformation
  - Common adult orbital mass, "cavernous hemangioma"
- Orbital infantile hemangioma
  - Benign neoplasm of infancy that typically regresses

PATHOLOGY

- Congenital venous malformation with slow flow, distensible component, & systemic venous connection
- Dilated venous channels with fibrotic walls ± phleboliths

CLINICAL ISSUES

- Intermittent, reversible proptosis
- Proptosis elicited by change in head position or Valsalva
- Variable pain & ophthalmoplegia
- Sudden worsening due to thrombosis or hemorrhage
- **Treatment options**
  - Observation if symptoms mild & stable (majority)
  - Transcatheter embolization or sclerosis
  - Surgery for intractable pain or threatened vision

DIAGNOSTIC CHECKLIST

- Routine imaging may be negative unless provocative test performed (e.g., Valsalva)

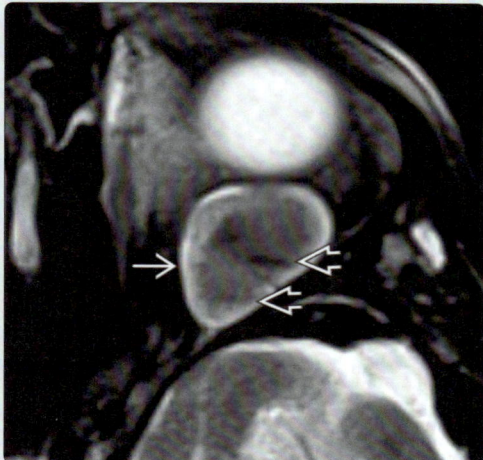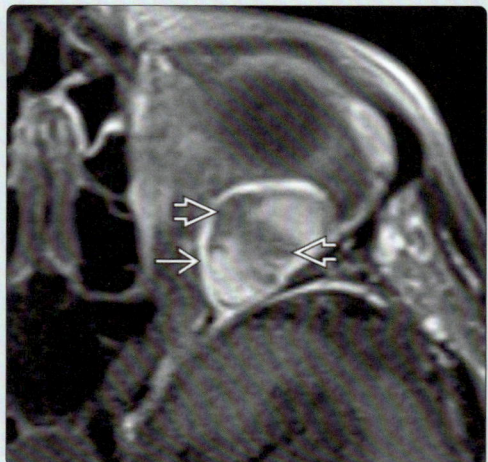

(Left) *Axial T2 FS MR in a patient with intermittent left proptosis shows a heterogeneously T2-hypointense mass ⇒ with multiple internal fluid levels ⇒.* (Right) *Axial T1 C+ FS MR in the same patient shows intense, heterogeneous enhancement of the retrobulbar mass ⇒. Nonenhancing regions ⇒ may reflect cystic or lymphatic spaces or thrombus. Intermittent proptosis is key history and typical of orbital venous varix.*

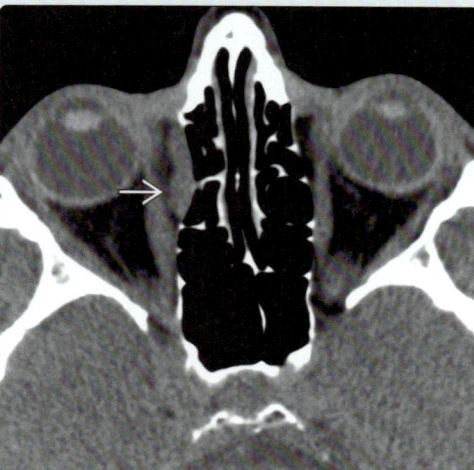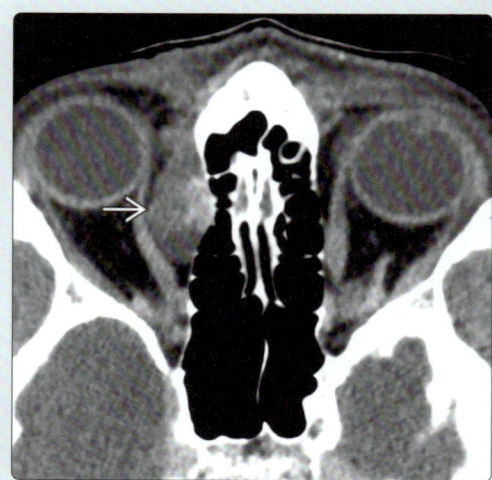

(Left) *Axial NECT acquired during quiet respiration shows a low-density extraconal mass in the medial right orbit ⇒.* (Right) *Axial CECT performed after Valsalva maneuver shows increase in the size of the mass ⇒ with partial enhancement, indicating varix with systemic venous communication. Imaging during provocative maneuver (Valsalva or prone positioning) is frequently required to demonstrate orbital venous varices.*

TERMINOLOGY

Synonyms

- **Distensible** orbital venous malformation

Definitions

- **Low-flow** venous malformation with **systemic venous connection** & dynamically **distensible** varix

IMAGING

General Features

- Best diagnostic clue
  - Intensely enhancing orbital mass that **distends** with ↑ **venous pressure**
- Location
  - May occur anywhere in orbit; usually retrobulbar & extraconal, often superolateral
- Size
  - Changes **dynamically** with venous pressure
    - ↑ in size with prone position or Valsalva maneuver, leading to "stress proptosis"
  - May be undetectable unless elicited
- Morphology
  - Well-defined margins but may have irregular or lobulated contours; often **tubular** or **tortuous**

CT Findings

- NECT: Well-defined, tubular or tortuous soft tissue density lesion in retrobulbar space; may contain **phleboliths**
- CECT: Intense enhancement; ↑ **in size on Valsalva**

MR Findings

- T1WI & T2WI: Complex signal, blood products, fluid levels
- T1WI C+: **Intense enhancement**
  - Variable areas of nonenhancement
    - Heterogeneous fast or turbulent **flow void**
    - Areas of **thrombosis** or acute **hemorrhage**
    - Cystic or lymphatic spaces

Ultrasonographic Findings

- **Hypoechoic**; slow flow on Doppler; dynamically ↑ with Valsalva; circumscribed & mass-like when thrombosed

Imaging Recommendations

- Best imaging tool
  - **Dynamic** CECT or MR with **provocation** maneuver
  - MR indicated if thrombosis or hemorrhage suspected
- Protocol advice
  - CECT ± provocation maneuver (dynamic MR also useful)
    - Valsalva for 10-15 seconds
    - Varix will distend when venous pressure raised
  - US useful for bedside provocative challenge

DIFFERENTIAL DIAGNOSIS

Orbital Lymphatic Malformation

- May also present with acute proptosis due to hemorrhage
- Multiloculated spaces, fluid levels, no enhancement unless associated with component of venous malformation

Orbital Cavernous Venous Malformation

- Most common isolated orbital mass in adults

- Well-defined, intense dynamic "fill-in" enhancement

Orbital Infantile Hemangioma

- Infant lesion; frequently regresses spontaneously
- Intense enhancement & flow voids

PATHOLOGY

General Features

- Etiology
  - Primary: **Congenital** vascular malformation with slow flow, distensible component, & **systemic** venous connection
  - Secondary: In association with dural arteriovenous (AV) fistula, cavernous carotid (CC) fistula or intracranial AV malformation (AVM)
- Associated abnormalities
  - May **coexist** with **lymphatic malformation**
  - Varicosities due to AV fistulae are not considered primary malformations
  - Associated with blue rubber bleb nevus syndrome

Gross Pathologic & Surgical Features

- Single or multiple dilated valveless, thin-walled vessels
- Acute hemorrhage or thrombosis may be present

Microscopic Features

- Dilated venous channels with fibrotic walls ± **phleboliths**

CLINICAL ISSUES

Presentation

- Most common signs/symptoms
  - Intermittent **reversible proptosis**
- Other signs/symptoms
  - Variable pain & ophthalmoplegia

Natural History & Prognosis

- **Congenital** nonprogressive lesion
- Sudden worsening due to **thrombosis** or **hemorrhage** often prompts attention or intervention

Treatment

- Observation if symptoms mild & stable (majority of cases)
- Transcatheter **embolization** or **sclerosis rarely needed**
- Surgery for intractable pain or threatened vision
  - Jugular vein compression during surgery may be helpful to distend lesion during excision

DIAGNOSTIC CHECKLIST

Image Interpretation Pearls

- Routine imaging may be negative unless provocative test performed (e.g., Valsalva, or image in prone position)
- Exclude secondary varix (AVM, dural AV fistula, CC fistula)

SELECTED REFERENCES

1. Liu J et al: A jugular venous compression adjunct for surgical excision of distensible orbital venous malformations. Orbit. 44(1):39-48, 2025
2. Kaneko N et al: Intermittent orbital pain due to hemodynamic collapse of an orbital varix: a case report. Case Rep Ophthalmol. 14(1):353-7, 2023
3. Pichayawat C et al: Acute unilateral orbital varix thrombosis in preexisting bilateral orbital varices: illustrative case. J Neurosurg Case Lessons. 5(25), 2023

Orbital Cavernous Venous Malformation (Hemangioma)

TERMINOLOGY

- Venous vascular malformation of orbit characterized by endothelial-lined cavernous spaces
- Pseudoencapsulated morphology distinguishes orbital cavernous venous malformation from venous malformations elsewhere in head and neck
- Synonymous with cavernous "hemangioma" (misnomer)

IMAGING

- Solid, enhancing intraorbital mass
  - Most intraconal, usually lateral
  - Ovoid or round, sharply marginated
  - Pseudocapsule of compressed surrounding tissue
- CT
  - Benign remodeling of bone in larger lesions
- MR
  - T2 hyperintense; internal septations may be visible
  - Characteristic dynamic enhancement
    - Heterogeneous, early, patchy central enhancement
    - Fills in homogeneously on delayed images

PATHOLOGY

- Slowly growing vascular malformation
- ISSVA classification as slow-flow venous lesion
- Dilated vascular channels of thin-walled sinusoidal spaces, flattened endothelial cells, scant fibrous connective stroma
- Pseudocapsule with surrounding compressed tissue
- No evidence of cellular proliferation

CLINICAL ISSUES

- Slowly progressive, painless proptosis
- Most common isolated orbital mass in adults
- Female predominance; faster growth during pregnancy
- Excellent prognosis; rare recurrence after surgery

DIAGNOSTIC CHECKLIST

- Often discovered incidentally during brain MR
- "Hemangioma" is common term but misnomer
- Patchy, dynamic enhancement is characteristic

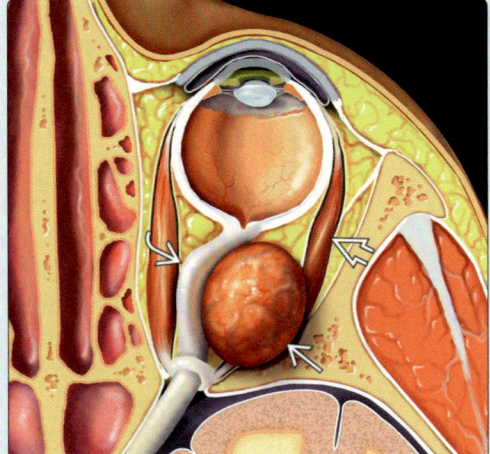 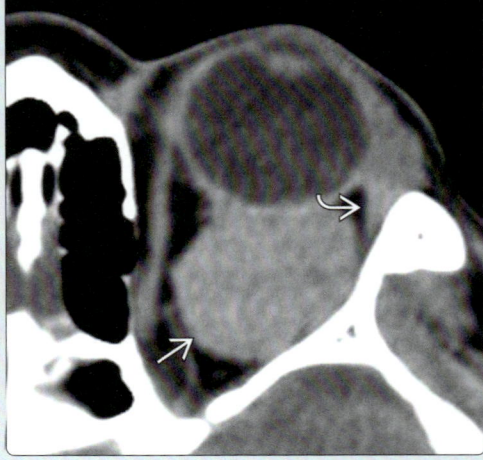

(Left) Axial graphic through the orbit shows an ovoid, well-demarcated intraconal mass ➡ that displaces the optic nerve ➡ and adjacent lateral rectus muscle ➡. Note the lack of adjacent structure invasion. (Right) Axial NECT shows a well-demarcated, ovoid, slightly hyperdense mass centered in the lateral aspect of the left orbit ➡. The lateral rectus muscle is seen draping around the lateral margin of this intraconal mass ➡.

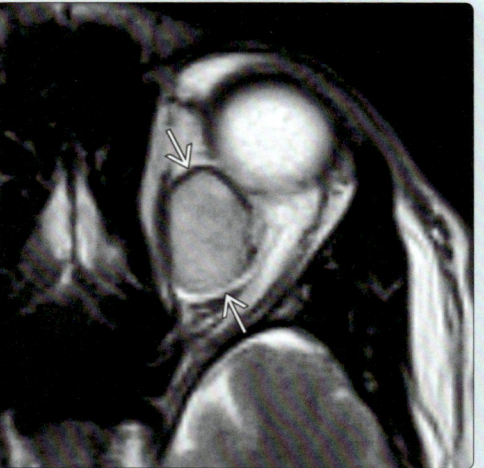 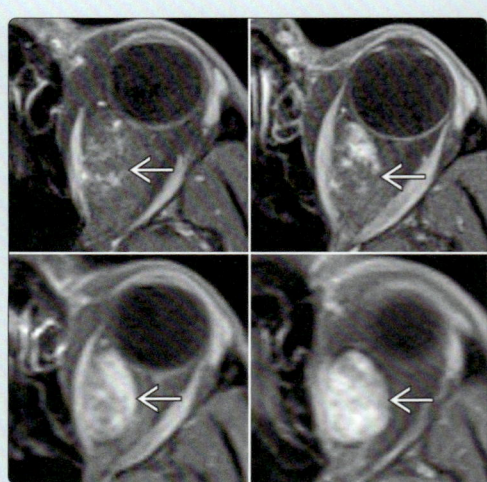

(Left) Axial T2 MR reveals a sharply marginated, ovoid, hyperintense intraconal mass. A thin rim of variable signal ➡ represents the pseudocapsule, accentuated by a chemical shift artifact. (Right) Axial T1 C+ FS MR images demonstrate progressive enhancement of a vascular mass in the medial left orbit ➡. Serial scans were obtained over the course of several minutes, from earliest (top left) to latest (bottom right), following contrast injection.

Orbital Cavernous Venous Malformation (Hemangioma)

TERMINOLOGY

Abbreviations
- Orbital cavernous venous malformation (**OCVM**)

Synonyms
- Cavernous hemangioma (misnomer)
- **Encapsulated** cavernous lesion of orbit

Definitions
- Venous vascular **malformation** of orbit characterized by endothelial-lined **cavernous** spaces

IMAGING

General Features
- Best diagnostic clue
  - Well-demarcated, ovoid, enhancing **intraconal** mass
  - Avid **dynamic** enhancement
    - Initially patchy, homogeneous on delayed images
- Location
  - Most (> 75%) **intraconal**, usually lateral
  - Involves orbital fissures or optic canal in 10-20%
  - Intramuscular or exclusively extraconal lesions also occur
- Size
  - Ranging from few millimeters (incidental) to very large (with mass effect)
- Morphology
  - **Ovoid** or round, sharply **marginated**
  - **Pseudocapsule** of compressed surrounding tissue
  - Indents rather than conforms to globe
  - Does not expand with Valsalva

CT Findings
- NECT
  - Homogeneously isodense
  - Benign remodeling of bone in large lesions
- CECT
  - Avid enhancement

MR Findings
- T1WI
  - Homogeneous and isointense to hypointense
  - Pseudocapsule may be visible as hypointense rim
- T2WI
  - Hyperintense; internal septations may be visible, particularly in larger lesions
  - Chemical shift artifact visible in frequency-encoded direction
- DWI
  - Bright on DWI with mean ADC values ranging from 1.23-1.39 x 10^{-3} mm²/s
    - Schwannomas shown to have statistically higher mean ADC of 1.92 x 10^{-3} mm²/s
    - Lymphoma typically shows lower ADC < 0.6 × 10^{-3} mm²/s
- T1WI C+
  - Characteristic fill-in pattern on dynamic enhancement
    - Heterogeneous, early, patchy central enhancement
    - Diffuse enhancement in venous phase
    - Homogeneous on delayed postcontrast images
- MRA
  - Does not show high-flow characteristics
  - Not visible on routine MRA

Ultrasonographic Findings
- Grayscale ultrasound
  - Well-demarcated, hyperechoic retrobulbar mass
  - Highly reflective borders representing pseudocapsule

Angiographic Findings
- Contrast puddles extending into late venous phase
- No distinct tumor blush

Nuclear Medicine Findings
- SPECT shows delayed focal uptake on Tc-99m RBC scintigraphy

Imaging Recommendations
- Best imaging tool
  - Enhanced thin-section dedicated orbital MR
    - Specific MR features include patchy dynamic enhancement, septations, and pseudocapsule
- Protocol advice
  - CT usually diagnostic in appropriate clinical setting
  - MR appearance is characteristic
    - Use fat-suppressed FSE or STIR for T2WI
    - Use fat-suppressed T1WI post contrast
    - Include dynamic enhanced scan to show characteristic enhancement pattern
      - FSE T1 or spoiled gradient pulse sequence
      - Serial images every 30 s for 2 min
      - Delayed scans to 10 min for large lesions

DIFFERENTIAL DIAGNOSIS

Lymphoproliferative Lesion
- Spectrum from polyclonal reactive to lymphoma (MALT)
- Infiltrative or "plastic" homogeneously enhancing mass
  - Can involve any area of orbit

Orbital Metastasis
- Muscles and globe more common
- May involve any area of orbit or extend from bone

Optic Nerve Sheath Meningioma
- Fusiform, enhancing mass surrounding optic nerve
- Tram-track calcification and enhancement

Optic Nerve Glioma
- Minor association with neurofibromatosis type 1 (NF1)
- Tubular mass indistinguishable from optic nerve

Orbital Varix
- Uniformly enhancing vascular mass
- Distensible, enlarges with Valsalva maneuver

Orbital Lymphatic Malformation
- Prone to hemorrhage with sudden proptosis
- Multilocular mass, transspatial, fluid levels

Solitary Fibrous Tumor
- Uncommon; may mimic OCVM
- Intense enhancement; margins less well defined

Schwannoma

- Uncommon in orbit
- Ovoid to fusiform, homogeneously or peripherally enhancing mass

Neurofibroma

- Diagnostic feature of NF1
- Irregular, lobulated, or serpentine masses

PATHOLOGY

General Features

- Etiology
  - Slowly growing vascular malformation
  - Slow-flow venous lesion with dilated vascular spaces
  - Nonneoplastic; not true hemangioma
- Associated abnormalities
  - Multiple lesions associated with systemic disorders
    - e.g., blue rubber bleb nevus syndrome

Staging, Grading, & Classification

- International Society for the Study of Vascular Anomalies (ISSVA) classification of vascular malformations
  - OCVM classified as slow-flow venous lesion
  - Some arterial imaging features have been observed; however, no arterial elements present histologically, and OCVM is considered essentially venous lesion

Gross Pathologic & Surgical Features

- Round, well-defined, reddish mass; vascular channels
- Fibrous pseudocapsule, distinct from surrounding compressed tissue
- Apical vascular tag frequently present

Microscopic Features

- Network of dilated vascular channels, larger than capillaries, filled with red blood cells
- Thin-walled sinusoidal spaces lined with mature, flattened endothelial cells, surrounded by few layers of smooth muscle, separated by scant fibrous connective stroma
- No evidence of cellular proliferation
  - Lack of GLUT1, desmin, and Ki-67 immunohistochemical markers supports malformative over neoplastic pathophysiology

CLINICAL ISSUES

Presentation

- Most common signs/symptoms
  - Slowly progressive, painless proptosis
- Other signs/symptoms
  - Headache or retrobulbar pain
  - Vision loss due to compressive optic neuropathy
- Clinical profile
  - Diplopia, visual impairment, increased intraocular pressure with large lesions
- Funduscopic examination
  - Choroidal striae, optic nerve elevation, and posterior indentation with large lesions

Demographics

- Age
  - Range: 10-60 years; mean: 40 years

- Sex
  - Female predominance, ~ 2:1
- Ethnicity
  - No known predilection
- Epidemiology: Most common isolated orbital mass in adults (5% of orbital masses)

Natural History & Prognosis

- Slow, progressive enlargement over years
  - On average, 10-15% volume growth per year
- Faster growth during pregnancy
- Eventually compress and displace orbital structures
- Excellent prognosis; very low recurrence rate

Treatment

- Surgical resection indicated for visual disturbance, cosmesis, or other significant mass effect
  - Lateral orbitotomy is conventional surgical approach
  - Transconjunctival techniques may be option
  - More extensive surgery for apex lesions
    - Higher complication rate
- Pseudocapsule promotes easy extraction
- Observation alone for stable lesions, lesions without significant symptoms, or poor surgical candidates
- Endovascular sclerotherapy may be useful
- Intralesional laser, cryosurgical, and radiosurgical techniques are alternatives

DIAGNOSTIC CHECKLIST

Consider

- Most common adult orbital mass lesion
  - Often discovered incidentally during brain MR
- Hemangioma is common term but misnomer
  - OCVM is malformation, not neoplasm
- Solitary fibrous tumor is rare but has similar imaging appearance
- Distinct lesion from infantile ("capillary") hemangioma, neoplastic tumor of infancy

Image Interpretation Pearls

- Patchy, dynamic enhancement is characteristic feature reminiscent of cavernous malformations seen elsewhere
- Macroscopic calcifications or phleboliths are not typical, unlike venous malformations elsewhere
- MR appearance showing septations on T2WI is more specific than CT in distinguishing from other orbital masses

Reporting Tips

- Radiologist should be confident diagnosing this common benign adult lesion with characteristic appearance

SELECTED REFERENCES

1. ISSVA Classification of Vascular Anomalies 2025. International Society for the Study of Vascular Anomalies. Published 2018. Updated 2025. Accessed April 2, 2025. http://issva.org/classification
2. Roelofs KA et al: Radiologic features of well-circumscribed orbital tumors with histopathologic correlation: a multi-center study. Ophthalmic Plast Reconstr Surg. 40(4):380-7, 2024
3. Bonavolontà P et al: Epidemiological analysis of venous malformation of the orbit. J Craniofac Surg. 31(3):759-61, 2020
4. Rootman DB et al: Cavernous venous malformations of the orbit (so-called cavernous haemangioma): a comprehensive evaluation of their clinical, imaging and histologic nature. Br J Ophthalmol. 98(7):880-8, 2014

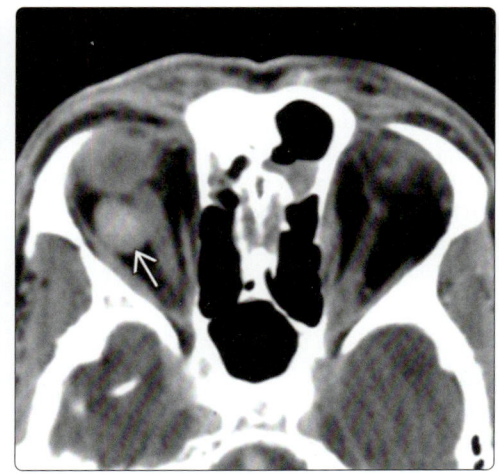

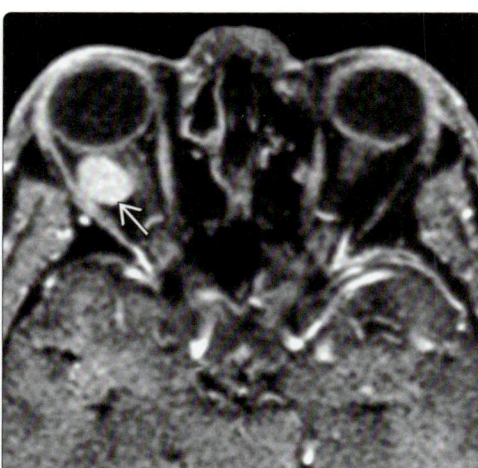

(Left) *Axial CECT shows an ovoid, well-circumscribed, enhancing mass ➡ within the intraconal fat of the right orbit, abutting the optic nerve and lateral rectus muscle.* (Right) *Axial T1 C+ FS MR demonstrates avid enhancement of an intraconal mass ➡. The mass is relatively small with little mass effect and no aggressive features. Such lesions are frequently asymptomatic or have gradual changes that may go unnoticed by the patient.*

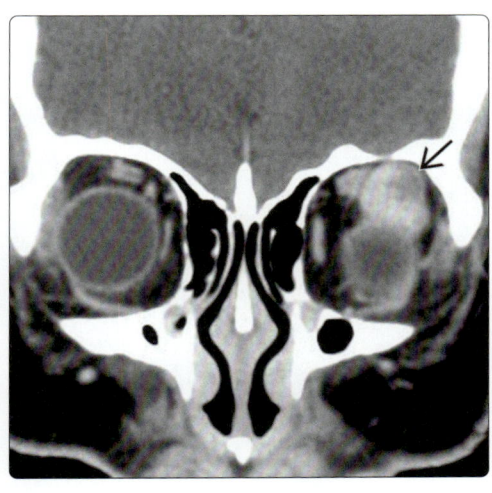

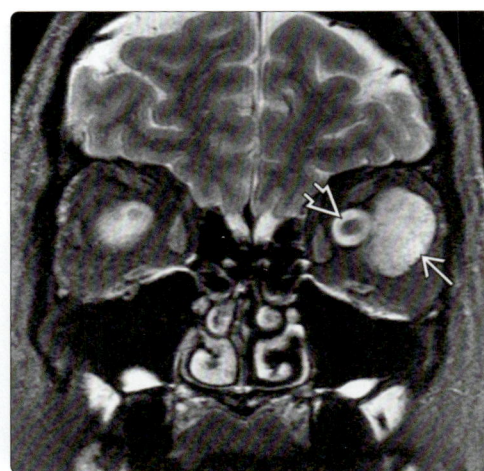

(Left) *Coronal CECT shows an intraconal mass ➡ with a patchy, early enhancement pattern, highly suggestive of orbital cavernous malformation. Although the lesion extends to the periphery of the orbit, its center is intraconal.* (Right) *Coronal STIR MR shows a large intraconal cavernous malformation ➡. The mass shows high signal similar to the CSF that surrounds the displaced optic nerve ➡.*

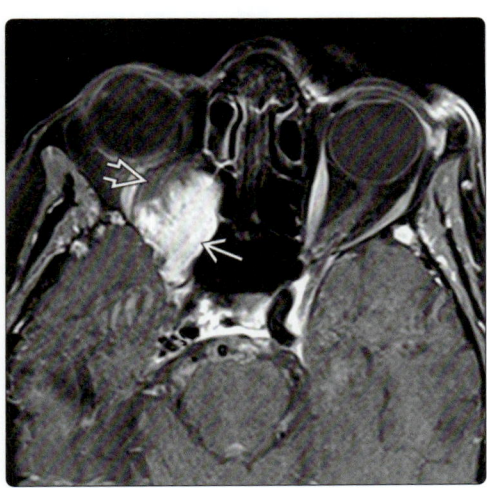

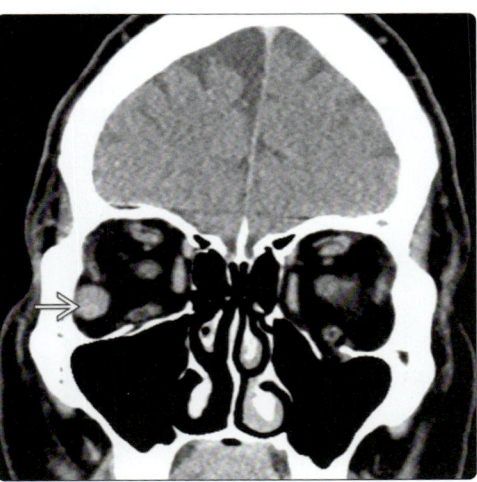

(Left) *Axial T1 FS MR shows incomplete but intense enhancement of the large orbital cavernous malformation that involves the apex ➡. The nonenhancing portions ➡ would be expected to fill in on delayed images.* (Right) *Coronal CECT of the head demonstrates an enhancing lesion, a cavernous venous malformation in the right orbit in a less common extraconal location ➡. The most common location for orbital cavernous venous malformation is intraconal.*

TERMINOLOGY

- Ocular larva migrans (OLM)
- Sclerosing endophthalmitis
- Granulomatous retinal nematode infection

IMAGING

- Enhancing granulomatous nodule posteriorly in eye with inflammatory features
- Posterior pole of eye; almost always unilateral
- CT: Nodular mass without calcification
  o Vitreal hyperdensity due to retinal detachment
- MR: Intravitreal membranes, retinal detachments
  o Enhancing retinal nodule
- US: Echogenic nodular granuloma
  o Vitreous membranes and retinal folds

TOP DIFFERENTIAL DIAGNOSES

- Retinoblastoma
- Coats disease
- Persistent hyperplastic primary vitreous
- Retinopathy of prematurity
- Acute endophthalmitis

PATHOLOGY

- *Toxocara* species of roundworm parasites
- Humans are paratenic (accidental) hosts
- Larvae migrate from intestine to eye
- Disease due to **immunoallergic** reaction to antigens following larval death → sclerosing endophthalmitis with small eosinophilic abscess

CLINICAL ISSUES

- Progressive forms of disease
  o Chronic endophthalmitis
  o Posterior granuloma
  o Peripheral granuloma

DIAGNOSTIC CHECKLIST

- May closely mimic retinoblastoma

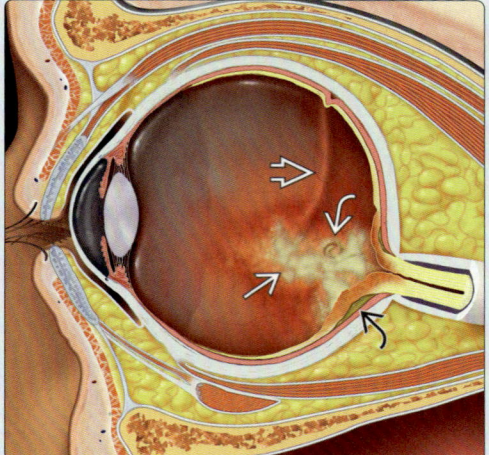
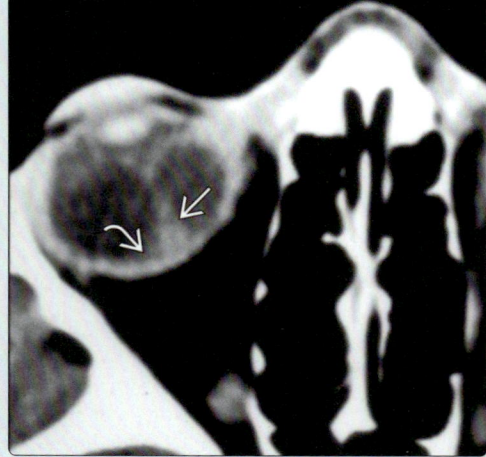

(Left) Sagittal graphic demonstrates a granulomatous reaction ⇒ secondary to a dead Toxocara larva ⇒. A retinal fold ⇒ is present due to postinflammatory changes and traction as well as a small subretinal fluid collection ⇒. (Right) Axial CECT shows a mildly enhancing nodule posteriorly in the right eye ⇒. Adjacent chorioretinal thickening ⇒ represents inflammatory changes, postinflammatory membranes, retinal folds, &/or subretinal fluid collection.

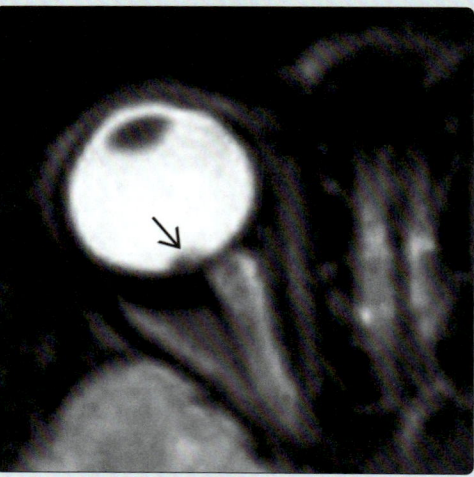
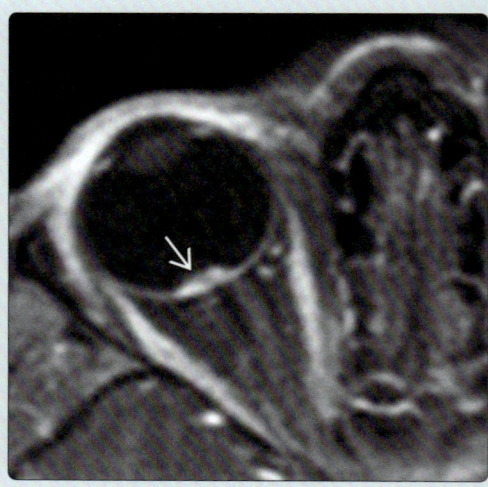

(Left) Axial T2 FS MR shows a small, retinal-based mass at the posterior pole of the globe ⇒, representing granulomatous reaction at the site of the expired nematode larva. There was no calcification on CT. No other retinal complications are evident. (Right) Axial T1 C+ FS MR shows moderate enhancement of a retinal-based nodule at the posterior pole of the right globe ⇒, representing granulomatous reaction at the site of the expired nematode larva.

Ocular Toxocariasis

TERMINOLOGY

Synonyms
- Ocular larva migrans (OLM)
- Sclerosing **endophthalmitis**

Definitions
- Granulomatous retinal nematode infection

IMAGING

General Features
- Best diagnostic clue
  - Enhancing granulomatous **nodule** posteriorly in eye with **inflammatory** and postinflammatory features
- Location
  - **Posterior pole** of eye; almost always **unilateral**
- Morphology
  - Retinal-based **nodular mass**

Imaging Recommendations
- Best imaging tool
  - CT and MR adjuncts to ultrasound and funduscopy

CT Findings
- Moderately enhancing retinal posterior nodular mass **without calcification**
- Vitreal hyperdensity due to **retinal detachment**

MR Findings
- T2WI: Isointense or hypointense to vitreous
  - Higher T2 signal than retinoblastoma
  - Intravitreal **membranes** and retinal **detachments**
  - Variable signal subretinal fluid
- T1WI C+: **Enhancing retinal nodule**

Ultrasonographic Findings
- Grayscale ultrasound: Echogenic **nodular** granuloma
  - Vitreous membranes and **retinal folds**, extend out from granulomatous nodule

Optical Coherence Tomography
- Retinal mass above pigmented layer

DIFFERENTIAL DIAGNOSIS

Retinoblastoma
- Most **common** ocular tumor in children
- **Calcification** present in vast majority

Coats Disease
- Retinal telangiectasias with **exudative retinopathy**
- Retinal **detachments** with large complex exudates

Persistent Hyperplastic Primary Vitreous
- Normal fetal hyaloid **fails to regress**
- **Retrolental tissue** and stalk in small eye

Retinopathy of Prematurity
- **Retrolental fibroplasia** related to excess **oxygen**
- Small globe, hyperdense, **bilateral**

Acute Endophthalmitis
- **Bacterial** or **fungal** infection of eye

- **Uveoscleral** enhancement

PATHOLOGY

General Features
- Etiology
  - Ingestion of **contaminated** food or geophagia
  - Disease due to **immunoallergic** reaction to antigens following larval death → sclerosing endophthalmitis with small eosinophilic abscess

Parasitology
- *Toxocara* species of **roundworm parasites**
  - *Toxocara canis* (dog host) and *Toxocara cati* (cat host)
- Humans are paratenic (accidental) hosts
  - Ingestion of eggs from ova-laden **pet feces**
  - Larvae migrate from intestine to eye

Laboratory Tests
- Serum ELISA for anti-*Toxocara* antibodies
  - **Low titers** in ocular compared to visceral disease

CLINICAL ISSUES

Presentation
- Most common signs/symptoms
  - Loss of visual acuity, **leukocoria**
- Other signs/symptoms
  - Squinting, perceived light flashes
  - Chorioretinitis, optic papillitis, endophthalmitis

Demographics
- Epidemiology
  - Ocular infection rare in developed world
  - Majority of **pets** are infested (33-100%)
- Age: Mean: 8 years (may occur in young adults)
- Sex: 60% male, 40% female

Natural History & Prognosis
- Ocular disease **months to years** after initial infection
- Chronic endophthalmitis
- Posterior granuloma
- Peripheral granuloma

Treatment
- Pharmaceutical
  - Antihelmintic (mebendazole, albendazole)
  - Corticosteroids
- Surgical
  - Vitrectomy and subretinal surgery
  - Photocoagulation

DIAGNOSTIC CHECKLIST

Image Interpretation Pearls
- May closely mimic retinoblastoma
- Lack of calcification on CT helps differentiate

SELECTED REFERENCES

1. Gerrie SK et al: Pediatric orbital lesions: ocular pathologies. Pediatr Radiol. 54(6):876-96, 2024
2. Curi ALL et al: Pediatric posterior infectious uveitis. Ocul Immunol Inflamm. 31(10):1944-54, 2023

Orbital Cellulitis

TERMINOLOGY

- Preseptal cellulitis
  - Infection limited to superficial periorbita
- Orbital (postseptal) cellulitis
  - Infection posterior to orbital septum
- Orbital septum
  - Connective tissue plane that acts as diaphragm

IMAGING

- Superficial periorbital or deep intraorbital soft tissue infiltration with mass effect & enhancement
- Enhanced CT adequate for uncomplicated cases
- MR shows diffusion restriction if abscess is present

TOP DIFFERENTIAL DIAGNOSES

- Orbital subperiosteal abscess
- Invasive fungal infection
- Idiopathic orbital inflammatory disease
- Orbital sarcoidosis

PATHOLOGY

- Etiology
  - Preseptal cellulitis: Trauma, insect bites common
  - Intraorbital cellulitis: Sinusitis most common
- Microbiology
  - Related to traumatic & sinogenic etiologies
  - Adults more likely polymicrobial & less responsive

CLINICAL ISSUES

- Presentation
  - Preseptal cellulitis
    - Periorbital edema & erythema
  - Intraorbital cellulitis
    - Axial (forward) displacement of globe
- Treatment
  - Targeted antimicrobials with cultures
  - Concomitant corticosteroids to reduce inflammation
  - Surgical drainage may be required if abscess develops

(Left) Axial T1 C+ FS MR shows abnormal enhancement within the orbit ➡ adjacent to ethmoid sinusitis. Note perineural extension of infection along the 2nd division trigeminal nerve in the foramen rotundum ➤. (Right) Coronal T1 C+ FS MR shows bilateral orbital cellulitis with extensive, enhancing, ill-defined orbital enhancement ➡. Filling defects with both superior ophthalmic veins indicate thrombosis ➡. Cavernous sinus thrombosis was also present (not shown). Both optic nerves ➔ are displaced inferiorly.

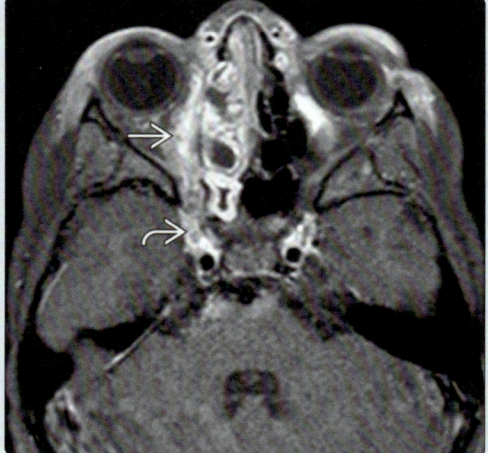
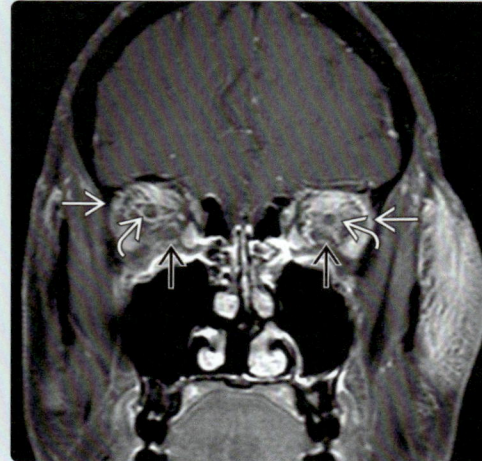

(Left) Axial CECT shows pre- ➔ and postseptal ➡ cellulitis in a patient without sinusitis. A clue to its origin is suggested with asymmetric nasolacrimal duct soft tissue ➡. This patient had clinical dacryocystitis requiring antibiotics and endoscopic dacryocystorhinostomy. (Right) Coronal CECT shows findings of sinusitis and ill-defined soft tissue in the medial orbit, consistent with orbital cellulitis ➡. A nasal septal abscess ➡ is partly imaged along with intracranial spread noted with epidural abscess ➡.

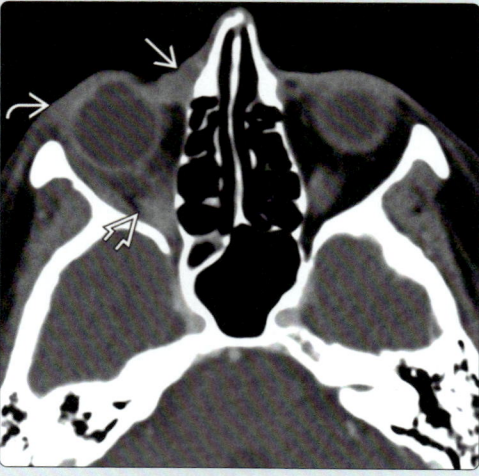
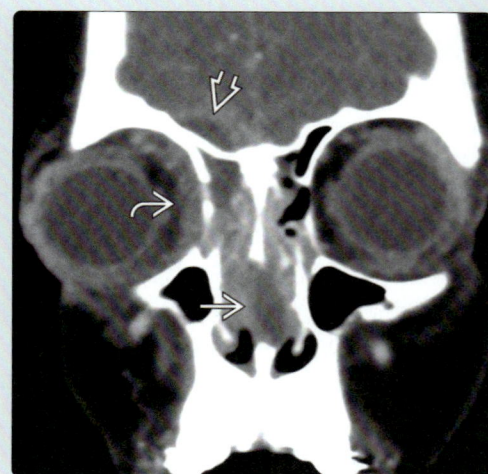

Orbital Cellulitis

TERMINOLOGY

Synonyms
- **Preseptal cellulitis**
  - Infection limited to superficial periorbita
- **Orbital (postseptal) cellulitis**
  - Infection posterior to orbital septum
  - Extraconal &/or intraconal

Definitions
- **Orbital septum**
  - Connective tissue plane that acts as **diaphragm** at anterior boundary of orbit
- **Phlegmon**
  - Infectious infiltrate **without** discrete **abscess**
- **Subperiosteal abscess**
  - Complication of cellulitis

IMAGING

General Features
- Best diagnostic clue
  - Superficial or deep orbital **soft tissue infiltration & inflammation** with **mass effect & enhancement**
- Location
  - **Preseptal**: Anterior periorbital soft tissues
  - **Orbital**: Extraconal &/or intraconal
- Morphology
  - **Infiltrative** & ill defined with **mass effect**

Imaging Recommendations
- Best imaging tool
  - CECT adequate for uncomplicated cases
    - Note: MR is more sensitive than CT
  - MR with contrast for difficult or aggressive cases
- Protocol advice
  - Serial CECT useful if treatment response indeterminate

CT Findings
- CECT
  - **Infiltration** of periorbital &/or intraorbital fat
  - Diffuse, heterogeneous **enhancement**

MR Findings
- T1WI
  - Hypointense infiltration of normal fat
- T2WI FS
  - Heterogeneous hyperintensity
- DWI
  - Restriction demonstrated if abscess is present
- T1WI C+ FS
  - Diffuse, heterogeneous enhancement

DIFFERENTIAL DIAGNOSIS

Orbital Subperiosteal Abscess
- Progressive complication of sinogenic orbital cellulitis

Invasive Fungal Infection
- Opportunistic sinus infection with orbital extension

Idiopathic Orbital Inflammatory Pseudotumor
- Mass-like features, multifocal involvement

Orbital Sarcoidosis
- Multifocal, mass-like involvement, especially lacrimal

PATHOLOGY

General Features
- Etiology
  - **Preseptal** cellulitis
    - Trauma #1 cause; insect bites also common
    - Less often dental infection & dacryocystitis
  - **Orbital** cellulitis
    - Sinusitis most common cause
    - May be secondary to foreign bodies
- Associated abnormalities
  - Underlying **sinus disease**
    - Sinonasal polyposis or obstructive lesion

Microbiology
- Bacterial
  - **Preseptal**: *Staphylococcus*, *Streptococcus*, & *H. influenzae*
  - **Intraorbital**: Polymicrobial, including anaerobes

CLINICAL ISSUES

Presentation
- Most common signs/symptoms
  - **Preseptal** cellulitis
    - Periorbital edema & erythema
  - **Orbital** cellulitis
    - Axial (forward) displacement of globe
- Other signs/symptoms
  - **Fever**, pain, chemosis, malaise
  - **Loss of vision** & movement are ominous signs

Natural History & Prognosis
- **Preseptal** cellulitis
  - Responds well to antibiotics
  - Postseptal extension uncommon
- **Orbital** cellulitis
  - Potential complications: Orbital/periorbital abscess, optic neuritis/perineuritis, intracranial spread, dacryoadenitis, & cavernous sinus thrombophlebitis or thrombosis

Treatment
- Targeted **antimicrobials** with cultures
  - IV therapy when fulminant or aggressive
- Concomitant **corticosteroids** to reduce inflammation
- Surgical drainage may be required if abscess develops
  - Younger children usually respond without surgery

DIAGNOSTIC CHECKLIST

Image Interpretation Pearls
- Serial imaging to assess treatment response
- Check for venous & intracranial complications

SELECTED REFERENCES

1. Tajima S et al: A case of bisphosphonate-related osteonecrosis of the maxilla with orbital cellulitis. Ear Nose Throat J. 104(1):22-4, 2025
2. Ang T et al: Radiological differentiation between bacterial orbital cellulitis and invasive fungal sino-orbital infections. Int Ophthalmol. 44(1):319, 2024
3. Winegar BA: Imaging of painful ophthalmologic disorders. Neurol Clin. 40(3):641-60, 2022

Orbital Subperiosteal Abscess

TERMINOLOGY

- **Purulent** accumulation between bony **orbital wall** and orbital **periosteum**

IMAGING

- Lentiform, rim-enhancing collection along orbital wall
  - Loculated fluid density/signal on CT/MR
  - Adjacent sinusitis
- Demineralization &/or dehiscence of orbital wall
- Diffusion restriction within abscess on MR
- **Imaging recommendations**
  - CT with contrast for diagnosis and monitoring
  - MR with contrast for complications or to avoid radiation

TOP DIFFERENTIAL DIAGNOSES

- Orbital cellulitis
- Idiopathic orbital inflammation
- Sinonasal mucocele
- Nasolacrimal duct mucocele

PATHOLOGY

- Due to sinusitis > trauma, foreign body, odontogenic
- Upper respiratory microbes: Simple and aerobic in children; polymicrobial and anaerobic in adults

CLINICAL ISSUES

- Presentation and natural history
  - Eye swelling, erythema, gaze restriction
  - Rapidly progressive, potentially blinding disease
  - Venous thrombosis, intracranial extension complications
- Treatment
  - Targeted IV antibiotics
  - Surgical drainage for larger abscesses and older patients
  - Factors that may indicate surgical drainage
    - \> 10 years, mass effect, or visual compromise
    - Large volume abscess or frontal sinus origin

DIAGNOSTIC CHECKLIST

- Risk of blindness, which requires immediate attention

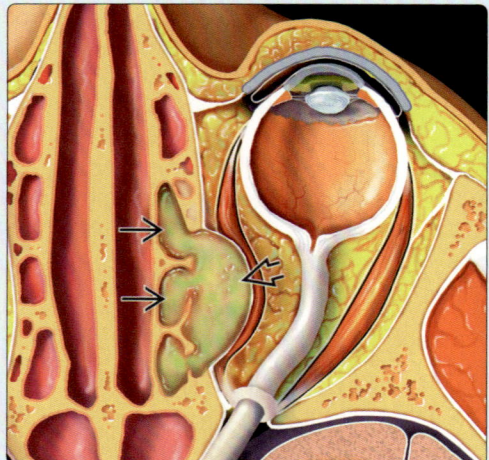 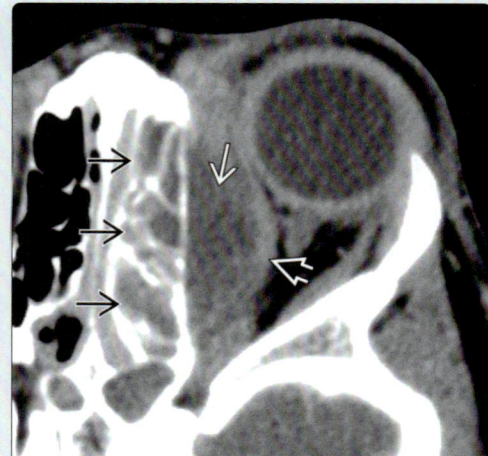

(Left) Axial graphic depicts spread of infection from the left ethmoid sinuses ➡ through the lamina papyracea into the medial orbit. Resultant subperiosteal abscess ➡ causes mass effect, displacing the adjacent muscle cone and putting the optic nerve at risk. (Right) Axial CECT shows asymmetric opacification of the left ethmoid sinuses ➡ with a large subperiosteal abscess extending into the medial extraconal orbit ➡. Displacement of the medial rectus ➡ is a typical finding.

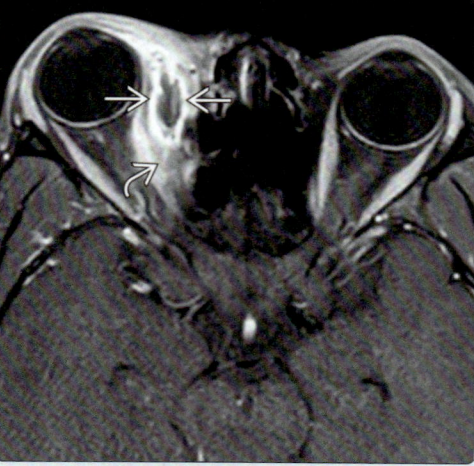 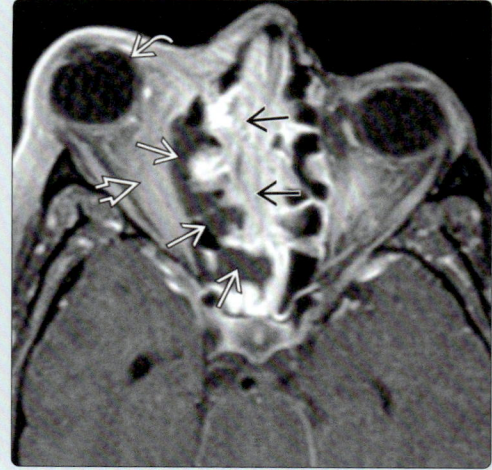

(Left) Axial T1 C+ FS MR shows an irregularly shaped, rim-enhancing abscess ➡ in the medial orbit with adjacent soft tissue enhancement related to cellulitis ➡. This abscess resulted from a retained wooden foreign body. (Right) Axial T1 C+ FS MR shows a large subperiosteal abscess ➡ extending through the lamina papyracea with findings of acute sinusitis ➡ and extensive right orbital cellulitis ➡. Marked proptosis ➡ is evident. Posterior extension of the abscess implies a higher risk of vision loss.

TERMINOLOGY

Abbreviations
- Orbital subperiosteal abscess (SPA)

Definitions
- Purulent accumulation between bony orbital wall and orbital periosteum

IMAGING

General Features
- Best diagnostic clue
  - **Lentiform**, **rim-enhancing**, low-density fluid collection along orbital wall
    - Adjacent **sinusitis**, particularly ethmoid
- Location
  - **Medial extraconal** orbit, along lamina papyracea
    - More common; associated ethmoid/maxillary sinusitis
  - **Superior, lateral, inferior** locations less common
    - Superior may be associated with frontal sinusitis
    - Tendency toward more advanced disease than medial SPA, more likely to require surgery
    - Inferior or lateral collections are less common and may suggest odontogenic origin, which requires treating offending dental source
- Size
  - Surgery indicated for larger volume SPA
  - SPA may appear small relative to degree of orbital **edema** and **proptosis**
- Morphology
  - Flat or **lenticular** collection bowing into extraconal space
  - **Displacement** of adjacent **rectus** muscle

CT Findings
- NECT
  - Hypodense orbital fluid collection, medial most common
  - Opacified ethmoid, maxillary, &/or frontal sinuses
  - Inflammatory stranding of orbital fat (**"dirty" fat**)
- CECT
  - **Rim-enhancing**, hypodense **fluid** collection
  - Prominently enhancing paranasal sinus mucosa
  - Displaced, enlarged, irregular rectus muscle
- Bone CT
  - **Demineralization** &/or **dehiscence** of orbital wall, particularly lamina papyracea

MR Findings
- T1WI
  - Hypointense **fluid** signal within abscess
  - Infiltrative inflammatory hypointensity in orbital fat
- T2WI FS
  - Hyperintense **fluid** signal within abscess
  - Infiltrative inflammatory hyperintensity in orbital fat
  - Opacified ethmoid, maxillary, &/or frontal sinuses
- DWI
  - Diffusion **restriction** within abscess, due to viscosity and dense cellular material within pus
- T1WI C+
  - **Rim-enhancing**, orbital fluid collection, especially medial
  - Prominently enhancing paranasal sinus mucosa
  - Irregular infiltrative enhancement of orbital fat

Ultrasonographic Findings
- Grayscale ultrasound
  - Fusiform fluid collection between bone and highly reflective **periosteum**, adjacent to muscle

Imaging Recommendations
- Best imaging tool
  - CT with contrast for diagnosis and monitoring
    - Abscess volume measurements aid surgical decision
- Protocol advice
  - Serial CTs helpful for monitoring response
  - MR with contrast for problem solving
    - Evaluate for potential intracranial complications
    - More sensitive than CT and should be pursued when strong clinical suspicion
  - Low-dose CT technique or consider MR in children

DIFFERENTIAL DIAGNOSIS

Orbital Cellulitis
- Infiltration and enhancement without discrete collection
- Trauma or sinusitis; may be preseptal or intraorbital

Idiopathic Orbital Inflammation
- Inflammatory pseudotumor, without fever/leukocytosis

Sinonasal Mucocele
- Chronic paranasal sinus obstruction with expansion and osseous remodeling and hyperdense contents

Nasolacrimal Duct Mucocele
- Cystic mass in enlarged lacrimal sac with enlarged and opacified nasolacrimal duct

Subperiosteal Hematoma
- Extraconal collection, hyperdense on NECT if acute

Dermoid/Epidermoid
- Developmental epithelial inclusion
- May show localized inflammation if ruptured

PATHOLOGY

General Features
- Etiology
  - Secondary to adjacent **sinusitis** most often
    - Hematogenous transmission of bacteria through valveless **orbital veins**
    - Direct extension through congenital or acquired **dehiscence**, particularly in lamina papyracea
    - Orbital **cellulitis** precedes SPA
  - Microbiology
    - **Upper respiratory** flora, varies by age group
      - Children: Commonly single **aerobes**
      - Adolescents: Mixed, mostly aerobes
      - Adults: **Mixed aerobes** and **anaerobes**
    - Emergence of more aggressive aerobes, including methicillin-resistant *Staphylococcus aureus* (**MRSA**), over recent decades
  - Abscess formation
    - Sinusitis leads to orbital **periostitis**

- – Relatively **avascular** subperiosteal space promotes accumulation of pus
- Associated abnormalities
  - Underlying sinus disease
    - – Polyposis, mechanical sinonasal obstruction
    - – Cystic fibrosis, ciliary dyskinesia
  - Uncommonly etiology is odontogenic
    - – Especially inferior orbital abscesses
    - – Look for dental source

Staging, Grading, & Classification

- Chandler grouping of sinus-related orbital disease (does not necessarily imply order of disease progression)
  - **I**: Preseptal cellulitis
  - **II**: Orbital (postseptal) cellulitis
  - **III**: Subperiosteal abscess
  - **IV**: Large intraorbital abscess
  - **V**: Extraorbital complications
    - – Cavernous sinus thrombosis, intracranial extension

Gross Pathologic & Surgical Features

- Pocket of yellow-green fluid in expanded space between bone and periosteum

Microscopic Features

- Necrotic debris with inflammatory cell and microorganisms

CLINICAL ISSUES

Presentation

- Most common signs/symptoms
  - Orbital **edema** and painful **proptosis** with **fever**
  - Proptosis &/or limitation of extraocular movements are high risk for orbital SPA; should undergo imaging
- Other signs/symptoms
  - Eye swelling, erythema, gaze restriction
  - Visual disturbance in 15-30%
    - – Optic neuritis due to intraconal extension
    - – Retinal ischemia from central artery occlusion
- Clinical profile
  - Associated with acute or chronic sinusitis
  - Preceded by upper respiratory infection in children

Demographics

- Age
  - Most common in children
  - More severe in adults
- Sex
  - Male patients more likely to require surgical drainage

Natural History & Prognosis

- Rapidly progressive, **potentially blinding** disease
- IV antibiotics with surgical drainage when indicated results in **excellent prognosis** in most cases
- Progression of SPA leads to frank intraorbital abscess
  - Increased proptosis, increased pressure
  - Worsening vision, ophthalmoplegia
- Other complications
  - **Superior ophthalmic vein** thrombosis
  - **Cavernous sinus thrombosis**, rare but devastating
  - **Intracranial** extension
    - – Meningitis, empyema, cerebritis, brain abscess

Treatment

- Medical therapy (IV antibiotics)
  - Manageable with antibiotics alone in 25-50%
    - – Children under 10 years of age
      - □ Majority of small SPA manageable without surgery
      - □ Simple aerobic microbes responsive to antibiotics
    - – Absence of visual signs or surgical indications
    - – Phlegmon with small or no abscess
  - Antibiotic regimen
    - – Broad polymicrobial coverage, targeted with cultures
    - – Add anaerobe coverage when indicated
- Surgical indications
  - **Emergent** (immediate drainage)
    - – Optic nerve or retinal compromise
    - – Intracranial involvement
  - **Urgent** (antibiotics alone inadequate)
    - – Age 10 years or older or immunocompromised
    - – Visual compromise or disproportionate pain
    - – Proptosis, muscle restriction, elevated pressure
    - – Frontal sinus origin
    - – Superior or inferior extension of abscess
    - – Larger volume (> 3.8 mL or > 1.25 mL if superior)
    - – Gas in collection (suggests anaerobic infection)
    - – Bone destruction
  - **Expectant** (after failed medical therapy)
    - – Visual changes at any time
    - – Persistent fever after 36 hours
    - – Clinical deterioration after 24-48 hours
    - – No improvement after 72 hours
- Surgical options
  - Endoscopic drainage
    - – Generally preferred for small SPA
  - External drainage
    - – Larger abscesses, abscesses extending along roof or floor of orbit or originating from frontal sinus

DIAGNOSTIC CHECKLIST

Consider

- Orbital disease may be **1st sign** of sinusitis

Image Interpretation Pearls

- Superior location and larger abscess volume increase likelihood of surgical drainage
- Presence of diffusion restriction on MR increases diagnostic confidence when contrast cannot be administered

Reporting Tips

- Requires immediate attention (may cause blindness)

SELECTED REFERENCES

1. Alsughayer L et al: Subperiosteal abscess volume; an objective indication for surgical management in pediatrics. Eur Arch Otorhinolaryngol. 281(12):€405-13, 2024
2. Yu AJ et al: Complicated odontogenic sinusitis: extrasinus infectious spread. Otolaryngol Clin North Am. 57(6):1019-30, 2024
3. Guerin JB et al: Infectious and inflammatory processes of the orbits in children. Neuroimaging Clin N Am. 33(4):685-97, 2023
4. Houle AN et al: Odontogenic subperiosteal abscess of the lateral orbit: timely recognition and management. Eur J Dent. 15(4):802-5, 2021
5. Abtahi SMB et al: Non-medial infectious orbital cellulitis: etiology, causative organisms, radiologic findings, management and complications. J Ophthalmic Inflamm Infect. 10(1):22, 2020

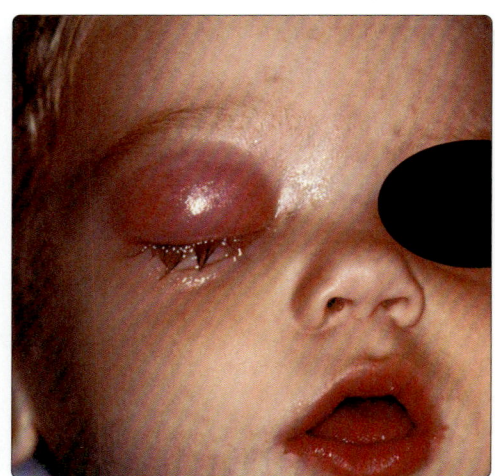
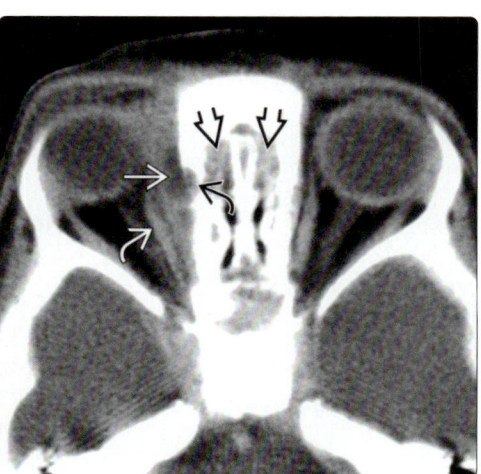

(Left) *Clinical photograph of a young child with sinusitis and cystic fibrosis shows a swollen eyelid but relatively minor periorbital edema, indicating postseptal disease.* (Right) *Axial CECT in the same child shows opacification of the ethmoid sinuses ⊳ with dehiscence of the right lamina papyracea ⊿. A small subperiosteal abscess ⇒ is present with displacement of the adjacent medial rectus ⇗. The patient responded well to IV antibiotics without surgery.*

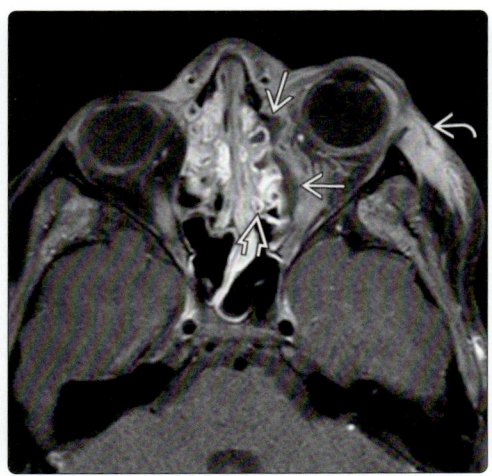
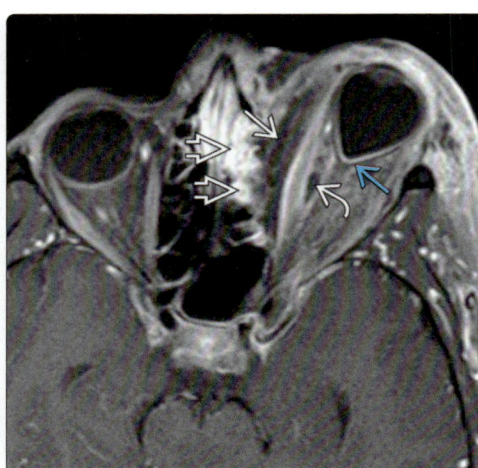

(Left) *Axial T1 C+ FS MR shows a subperiosteal abscess ⇒ immediately adjacent to ethmoid sinusitis ⊳. Note associated proptosis and extraorbital soft tissue enhancement ⊿.* (Right) *Axial T1 C+ FS MR demonstrates a low-intensity extraconal ⇒ and intraconal ⇗ abscess with rim enhancement. Ethmoid sinusitis ⊳ with mucosal enhancement is evident. Tenting of the posterior globe (guitar pick sign) ⇨ is noted from orbital compartment syndrome, and this patient suffered total vision loss in the left eye.*

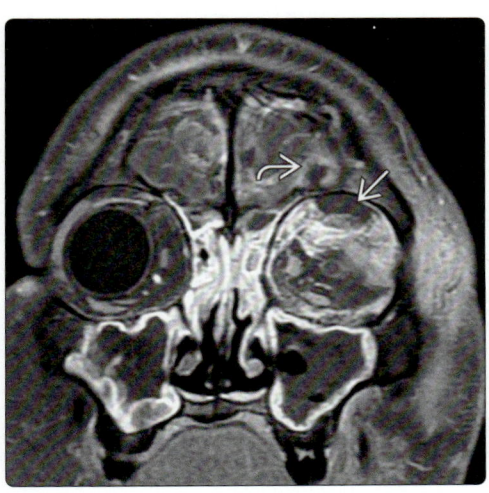
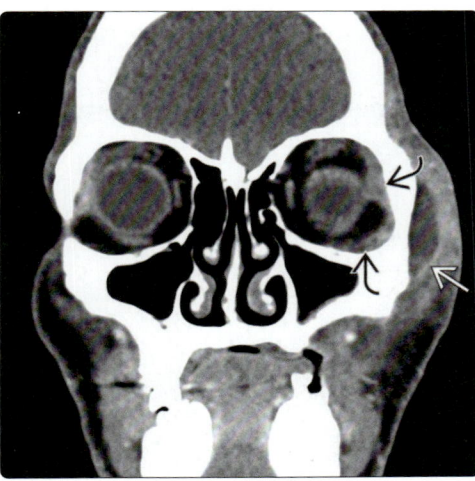

(Left) *Coronal T1 C+ FS MR shows subperiosteal abscess in the superior orbit ⇒ extending from frontal sinusitis. Note associated intracranial spread of infection ⊿.* (Right) *Coronal CECT shows abscess lateral to the orbit ⇒ extending superiorly from maxillary dental decay. Subperiosteal abscess in the inferolateral orbit ⊿ is an unusual location and suggests a source outside the sinuses. Odontogenic etiologies are a less common source of orbital infection, but are important to recognize to allow appropriate treatment.*

Idiopathic Orbital Inflammation (Pseudotumor)

TERMINOLOGY

- Nonspecific orbital inflammation, not due to any known etiology or systemic illness

IMAGING

- Poorly marginated, mass-like, or infiltrative, enhancing inflammatory tissue involving any area of orbit
  - **Lacrimal** (lacrimal gland)
  - **Myositic** (extraocular muscles)
  - **Anterior** (globe, retrobulbar orbit)
  - **Diffuse** (multifocal intraconal ± extraconal)
  - **Apical** (orbital apex, intracranial extension)
- Moderate to marked diffuse irregularity, enlargement, and enhancement of involved structures
- Best imaging tool: Enhanced MR with fat suppression
- Disease variants
  - Tolosa-Hunt syndrome: Orbital apex into cavernous sinus
  - Sclerosing: More often bilateral, may extend into sinuses

TOP DIFFERENTIAL DIAGNOSES

- Lymphoproliferative lesions, especially lymphoma
- Thyroid ophthalmopathy
- Sarcoidosis
- Granulomatosis with polyangiitis (Wegener)
- Orbital cellulitis
- IgG4-related disease

PATHOLOGY

- Polymorphous chronic inflammation and fibrosis

CLINICAL ISSUES

- Acute to subacute orbital pain, swelling, restricted motion, diplopia, proptosis, and impaired vision
- Steroid treatment effective in most patients
- Most common painful orbital mass in adults

DIAGNOSTIC CHECKLIST

- Diagnosis of exclusion

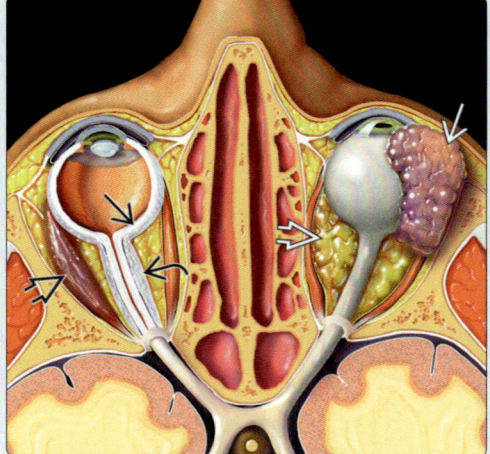

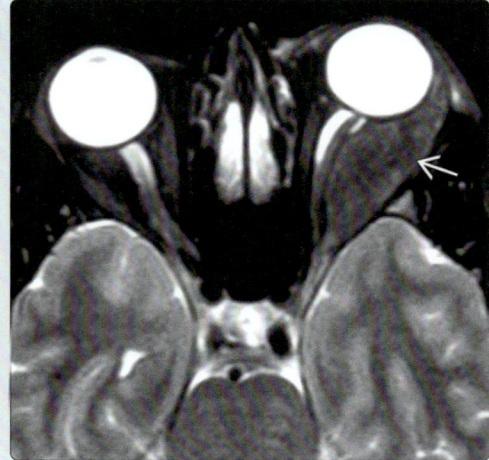

(Left) Axial graphic depicts the numerous, varied potential patterns of idiopathic orbital inflammation involvement, including extraocular muscle enlargement ➡, orbital fat infiltration ➡, lacrimal gland ➡, sclera ➡, and optic sheath ➡ involvement. (Right) Axial STIR MR shows tumefactive enlargement of the left lateral rectus muscle ➡, resulting in proptosis. The relatively low signal of the mass may reflect cellularity &/or fibrosis. Isolated lateral rectus muscle enlargement is a characteristic appearance for idiopathic orbital inflammation.

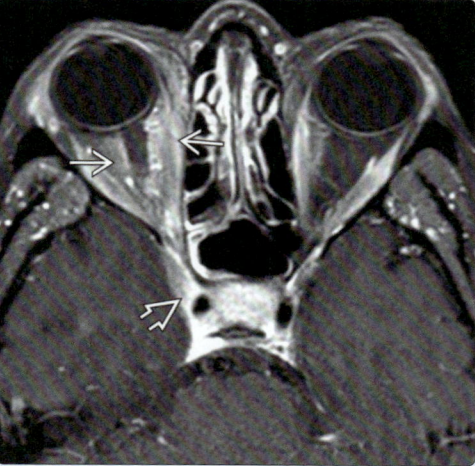

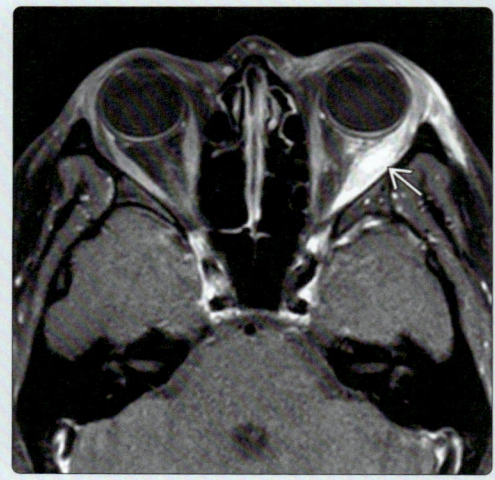

(Left) Axial T1 C+ FS MR shows ill-defined orbital enhancement ➡ in a patient with painful right ophthalmoplegia and vision loss. Enhancement extends through the orbital apex into the cavernous sinus ➡, typical of Tolosa-Hunt syndrome. (Right) Axial T1 C+ FS MR in a patient with 5 days of left eye swelling, erythema and pain on eye movement shows enlargement of the left lateral rectus muscle involving the tendinous insertion with intense enhancement ➡. Symptoms resolved after steroids.

Idiopathic Orbital Inflammation (Pseudotumor)

TERMINOLOGY

Abbreviations
- Idiopathic orbital inflammation (IOI)

Synonyms
- Orbital pseudotumor (or simply "**pseudotumor**")

Definitions
- **Tolosa-Hunt syndrome**
  - Variant **apical** form extending into cavernous sinus
- **Sclerosing** orbital inflammatory pseudotumor
  - Variant form with chronic progressive **fibrosis**

IMAGING

General Features
- Best diagnostic clue
  - Poorly marginated, mass-like, **enhancing inflammatory** soft tissue involving any area of orbit
- Location
  - Typically unilateral, bilateral in 10-25% of cases
  - Categorized by area(s) of involvement
    - **Lacrimal** (lacrimal gland) dacryoadenitis
      - Most common pattern (~ 20% overall)
      - Diffuse enlargement of 1 or both (~ 20%) glands
      - Cannot differentiate from lymphoproliferative lesions or sarcoidosis by imaging alone
    - **Myositic** [extraocular muscles (EOMs)]
      - 2nd most common pattern
      - Any muscle affected; lateral rectus and superior complex most frequent
      - Involves tendinous insertions (unlike thyroid disease), tubular configuration, shaggy margins
    - **Anterior** (globe, retrobulbar orbit)
      - 3rd most common pattern
      - Uveal-scleral (episcleritis or sclerotenonitis): Thickened sclera with shaggy enhancement
      - Variable retrobulbar fat, optic nerve and sheath involvement
    - **Diffuse** (multifocal intraconal ± extraconal)
      - Overlaps with other patterns
      - Often mass-like; tends not to distort globe or erode bone
    - **Apical** (orbital apex, intracranial extension)
      - Less common; involves orbital apex with posterior extension through fissures
  - Disease variants
    - **Tolosa-Hunt syndrome**: Apical disease that extends through orbital fissures into cavernous sinus
    - **Sclerosing**: More often bilateral, may involve sinuses
- Morphology
  - May be focally mass-like or diffuse
  - Irregular margins, **infiltrative** features

CT Findings
- NECT
  - Lacrimal, EOM, or other orbital mass
  - **Multifocal** or **infiltrative** soft tissue
- CECT
  - Moderate diffuse irregularity and enhancement of involved structures
- Bone CT
  - May rarely remodel or erode bone

MR Findings
- T1WI
  - Hypointense, particularly sclerosing disease
- T2WI FS
  - Varies: Isointense or slightly hyperintense to muscle
  - **Hypointense** compared to many orbital lesions due to **cellular infiltrate** and **fibrosis**
    - Particularly in chronic or sclerosing disease
    - Portends worse treatment response
- DWI
  - Higher ADC favors IOI, while lower ADC suggests lymphoproliferative disorder, but overlap exists
- T1WI C+
  - Moderate to marked diffuse irregularity, enlargement, and enhancement of involved structures
  - Tolosa-Hunt syndrome: Enhancement and fullness of anterior cavernous sinus and orbital fissures

Imaging Recommendations
- Best imaging tool
  - Contrast-enhanced thin-section MR with fat suppression

DIFFERENTIAL DIAGNOSIS

Lymphoproliferative Lesions
- Non-Hodgkin lymphoma, usually mucosa-associated lymphoid tissue (MALT)
  - Lower ADC than IOI
- Pliable mass, involving lacrimal gland, multifocal or diffusely in orbit; often bilateral

Thyroid Ophthalmopathy
- Thyroid dysfunction clinically; less often painful
- Bilateral, characteristic pattern of EOM involvement; affects muscle bellies, spares tendons

Sarcoidosis
- Orbit involved in 20% of patients with systemic sarcoidosis
- Granulomatous enhancement of multiple orbital structures, particularly lacrimal gland

Granulomatosis With Polyangiitis (Wegener)
- Necrotizing vasculitis of multiple organs
- Paranasal sinus and orbital involvement with bone destruction; commonly bilateral

Orbital Cellulitis
- Secondary to adjacent sinusitis (ethmoid) or trauma
- Phlegmonous periorbital and intraconal infiltration; may be accompanied by subperiosteal abscess

Carotid-Cavernous Fistula
- Presents with pulsatile exophthalmos, chemosis
- Enlarged arterialized venous structures (signal voids) without discrete orbital mass

IgG4-Related Disease
- Considered systemic disease with multiorgan involvement

- Any part of orbit may be involved with predilection for lacrimal gland and trigeminal nerve
- Increased serum IgG4(+) in 60-70% of patients
- Steroid responsive

PATHOLOGY

General Features

- Etiology
  - Pathogenesis unknown; probably related to underlying **immune-mediated** processes
  - Not due to infection, granulomatous disease, thyroid orbitopathy, lymphoproliferative disease, or other specific systemic illness
- Associated abnormalities
  - Secondary angle-closure glaucoma
  - **Autoimmune** disorders

Gross Pathologic & Surgical Features

- Typically soft, compressible mass
- Occasionally hard, fibrotic; particularly chronic

Microscopic Features

- Polymorphous infiltration of **chronic inflammatory** cells with variable fibrosis
- Proliferating fibroblastic **connective tissue**
- Capillary proliferation with perivasculitis
- Histologic variations
  - **Sclerosing**: Disproportionate connective tissue and early fibrosis with sclerosis
  - **Granulomatous**: Histiocytes, multinucleated giant cells, and granuloma formation
  - **Vasculitic**: Small vessel inflammatory infiltrate
  - **Eosinophilic**: Infiltration of eosinophilia without vasculitis; more common in children

CLINICAL ISSUES

Presentation

- Most common signs/symptoms
  - Acute-onset orbital **pain, inflammation,** and **edema**
  - Restricted eye motion, **diplopia,** and **proptosis**
- Other signs/symptoms
  - Impaired vision (perineuritis)
- Clinical profile
  - **Lacrimal**
    - Enlarged, tender gland
    - Proptosis and globe displacement
    - More likely to have systemic disorder
  - **Myositic**
    - Diplopia; painful limitation of ocular movement
    - Conjunctival injection at muscle insertions
  - **Anterior**
    - Proptosis, ptosis, lid swelling, injection
    - Uveitis, sclerotenonitis, retinal detachments
    - Decreased vision and limited movement
  - **Apical**
    - Milder signs of inflammation
    - Decreased vision; optic neuropathy
  - **Tolosa-Hunt**
    - Painful ophthalmoplegia (CNIII, IV, V, VI)

- Diagnosis
  - Biopsy for confirmation indicated in patients unresponsive to or relapse after 1st-line therapy
  - Serologic studies indicated for IgG and subtypes, including IgG4

Demographics

- Age
  - Any may be affected; Mean onset 52 years
- Sex
  - Overall: F = M; myositic form: F > M (2:1)
- Epidemiology
  - Most common painful orbital mass in adults
    - 10% of all orbital masses
  - 3rd most common orbital disorder
    - After thyroid and lymphoproliferative lesions

Natural History & Prognosis

- 5-10% **resolve spontaneously**
- Pattern of involvement affects prognosis
  - Recurrence more likely with multifocal disease
  - Poorer visual outcome in apical and diffuse disease
- Intermittent disease more likely in younger patients
- Chronic sclerosing disease not as responsive, but therapy may slow progression
- Rarely, severe cases progress to fixed, painless, sightless eye requiring exenteration
- **Risk factors** include low socioeconomic status, elevated BMI, and bisphosphonate therapy

Treatment

- **Systemic steroids** are 1st-line therapy
  - **80-85%** of patients respond
  - Dramatic and rapid improvement typical
  - Recurrence after initial response in **25-40%**
- 2nd-line therapies for nonresponsive or refractory cases or when steroids contraindicated
  - Low-dose radiotherapy
  - Cytotoxic chemotherapy
  - Other immunosuppressive agents

DIAGNOSTIC CHECKLIST

Consider

- **Diagnosis of exclusion**
- Atypical onset, poor response, or recurrence should prompt biopsy to confirm and exclude lymphoma
- Consider other **systemic causes** with bilateral, multifocal, lacrimal, or apical involvement
- Consider cellulitis and cavernous-carotid fistula if acute

Image Interpretation Pearls

- Isolated **lateral rectus** enlargement most likely IOI

SELECTED REFERENCES

1. Ang T et al: Differentiation of bacterial orbital cellulitis and diffuse non-specific orbital inflammation on magnetic resonance imaging. Eur J Ophthalmol. 35(2):727-33, 2025
2. Ang T et al: Magnetic resonance imaging of idiopathic orbital myositis. Ophthalmic Plast Reconstr Surg. 40(5):544-51, 2024
3. Gupta L et al: Diffusion-weighted imaging of the orbit: a case series and systematic review. Ophthalmic Plast Reconstr Surg. 39(5):407-18, 2023
4. Ferreira TA et al: CT and MR imaging of orbital inflammation. Neuroradiology. 60(12):1253-66, 2018

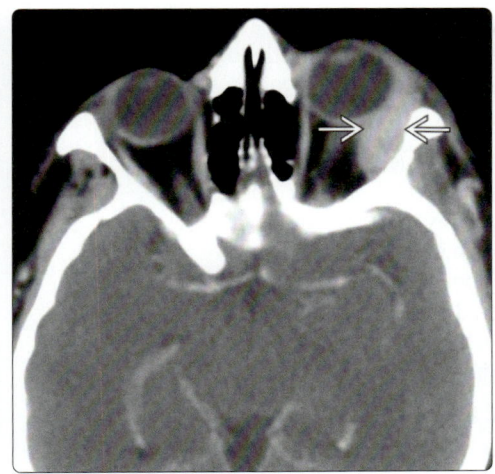

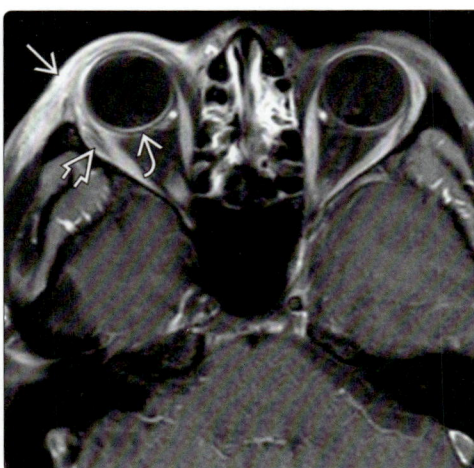

(Left) Axial CECT shows unilateral lacrimal gland enlargement and enhancement ➡ that was due to idiopathic orbital inflammation. Although neoplasm cannot be excluded, note the globe is displaced without deformation. Adjacent bones appear normal. (Right) Axial T1 C+ FS MR in a patient with right eyelid swelling and pain shows preseptal soft tissue ➡ and extraconal ➡ enhancement in this patient with recurring orbital inflammation. Thin, asymmetric uveoscleral enhancement ➡ is noted.

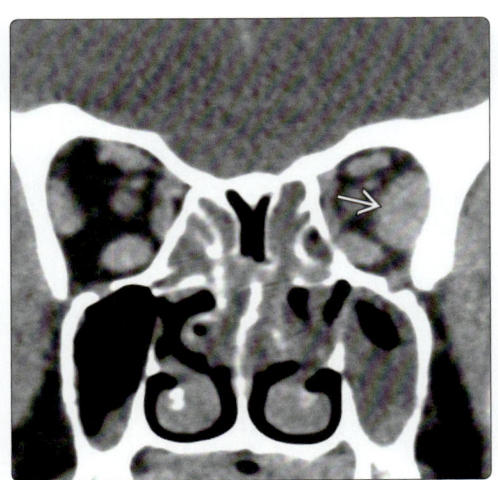

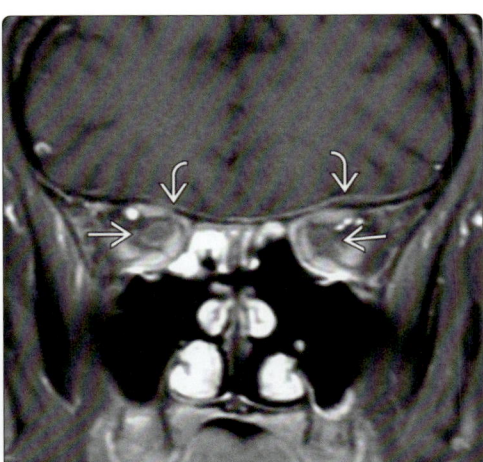

(Left) Coronal CECT shows enlargement and enhancement of the left lateral rectus muscle in idiopathic orbital inflammation ➡. An isolated lateral rectus muscle is typical of idiopathic orbital inflammation and not characteristic of thyroid associated orbitopathy. (Right) Coronal T1 C+ FS MR shows hazy, ill-defined enhancement in the posterior orbits ➡ and thin pachymeningeal thickening ➡ and enhancement in this patient with idiopathic orbital inflammation.

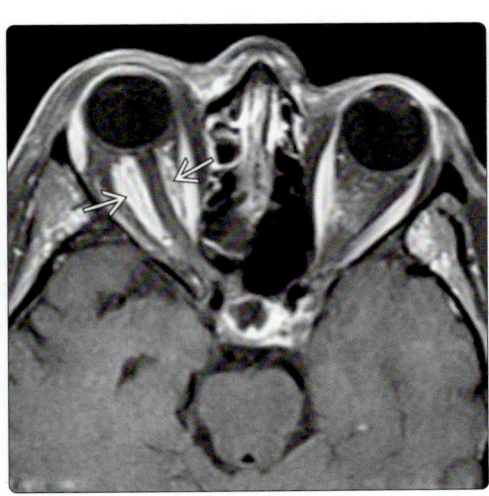

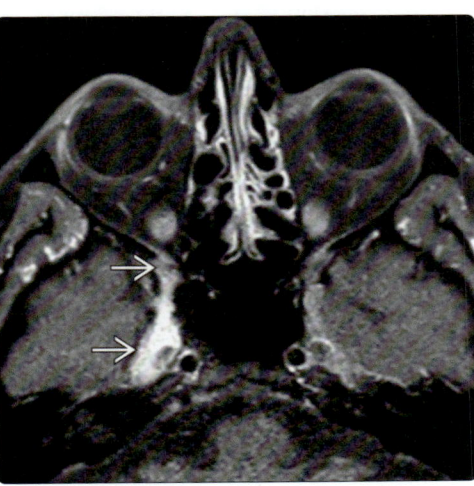

(Left) Axial T1 C+ FS MR in an older woman with optic neuropathy shows an intraconal mass encasing the optic nerve sheath ➡. A presumptive diagnosis of meningioma was made based on the initial clinical presentation. (Right) Axial T1 C+ FS MR shows asymmetric enhancement of the right cavernous sinus extending to the orbital apex ➡ in this patient with Tolosa-Hunt syndrome who presented with right trigeminal distribution numbness and abducens nerve palsy, which improved with steroids.

Orbital Sarcoidosis

TERMINOLOGY

- Noncaseating granulomatous inflammation of orbit

IMAGING

- Multiple sites of orbital involvement
  - Diffuse lacrimal gland infiltration
  - Optic nerve sheath thickening, enhancement
  - Asymmetric extraocular muscle infiltration
  - Intraorbital enhancing soft tissue masses
  - Eyelid and periorbital preseptal infiltration
  - Uveitis, especially anterior, but also posterior
- Best imaging tool: T1 and T1 C+ MR
- Ga-67 scintigraphy supportive but nonspecific

TOP DIFFERENTIAL DIAGNOSES

- Idiopathic orbital inflammatory disease
- Lymphoproliferative lesions
- Granulomatosis with polyangiitis
- Thyroid ophthalmopathy

PATHOLOGY

- Unknown etiology
- Noncaseating granulomas are pathologic hallmark
- Elevated ACE levels support diagnosis

CLINICAL ISSUES

- Most common signs/symptoms
  - Uveitis, lacrimal mass, and dacryoadenitis
  - Swelling, ptosis, and globe displacement
- Other signs/symptoms
  - Eye pain, conjunctivitis, vitreous and retinal changes
  - Vision loss, diplopia, perineuritis, papillitis
- Associated with systemic sarcoidosis
- Female predilection

DIAGNOSTIC CHECKLIST

- Imaging appearance similar to that of idiopathic inflammation and lymphoproliferative lesions

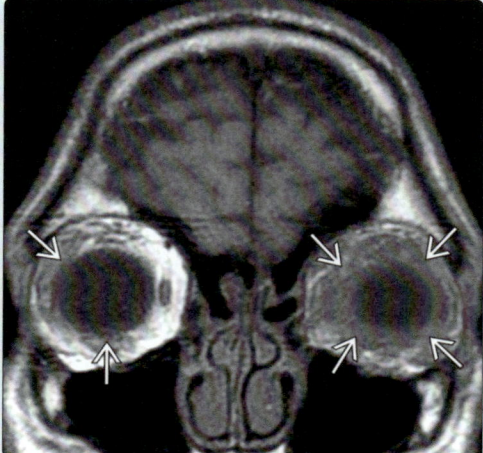
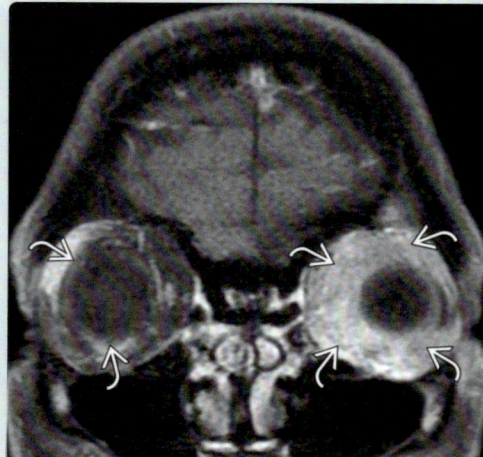

(Left) Coronal T1 MR in a 52-year-old woman with history of systemic sarcoidosis who presented with left globe proptosis and pain shows diffuse infiltration of soft tissue ➡ in bilateral orbits (left >> right) involving extra- & intraconal compartments, extraocular muscles, and surrounding the globs. (Right) Coronal T1 C+ FS MR in the same patient shows diffuse avid enhancement of the infiltrating soft tissue in both orbits (left >> right) ➡. Complete resolution was noted after a course of steroids (not shown).

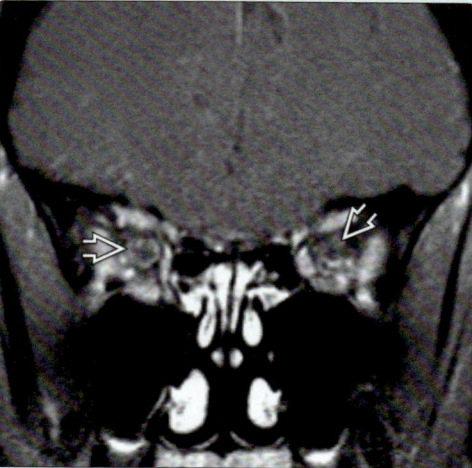
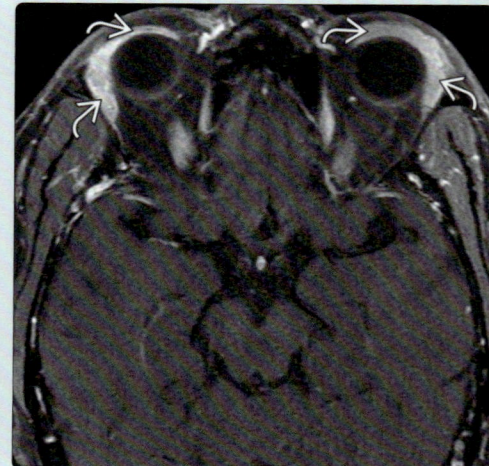

(Left) Coronal T1 C+ FS MR in a patient with known history of sarcoidosis who presented with bilateral retrobulbar pain shows mild thickening and circumferential enhancement of bilateral optic nerve sheaths ➡. (Right) Axial T1 C+ FS MR shows diffuse enlargement and enhancement of bilateral lacrymal glands (left > right) ➡. CT chest showed bilateral hilar lymph nodes (not shown). Nodal biopsy revealed noncaseating granulomas, consistent with sarcoidosis.

TERMINOLOGY

Definitions

- **Noncaseating, granulomatous** inflammation of orbit

IMAGING

General Features

- Best diagnostic clue
  - Infiltrative, nodular or mass-like, enhancing soft tissue that affects extraocular structures of orbit
- Location
  - Diffuse **lacrimal gland** infiltration
    - Most common extraocular site of involvement (~ 60%)
  - Optic **nerve sheath** thickening, enhancement
  - Asymmetric **extraocular muscle** (EOM) infiltration
  - Intraorbital enhancing **soft tissue masses**
  - Eyelid and **periorbital preseptal** infiltration

CT Findings

- CECT
  - Abnormal soft tissue typically enhances

MR Findings

- T1WI
  - **Hypointensity** of involved orbital structures or masses
- T2WI
  - Variable **hyperintensity** of involved orbital structures or masses
- T1WI C+
  - Diffuse **enlargement** and homogeneous **enhancement** of involved structures
    - Lacrimal gland, muscles, optic nerve ± sheath
  - Enhancing intraorbital soft tissue **masses**

Nuclear Medicine Findings

- Ga-67 scintigraphy
  - Increased uptake; supportive but nonspecific

Imaging Recommendations

- Best imaging tool
  - High-resolution T1 and T1 C+ FS MR in axial and coronal planes

DIFFERENTIAL DIAGNOSIS

Idiopathic Orbital Inflammatory Disease

- Nonspecific inflammation, protean manifestations

Lymphoproliferative Lesions

- Soft, homogeneous orbital masses

Thyroid Ophthalmopathy

- Predictable medial/inferior EOM enlargement pattern

Granulomatosis With Polyangiitis (Wegener)

- Necrotizing vasculitis, sinonasal and orbital disease

PATHOLOGY

General Features

- Etiology
  - Unknown
- Laboratory

- Elevated CSF and serum **ACE levels** support diagnosis
- Serum **lysozyme** is more sensitive but less specific

Microscopic Features

- **Noncaseating** granulomas are pathologic hallmark

CLINICAL ISSUES

Presentation

- Most common signs/symptoms
  - Uveitis, lacrimal mass, and dacryoadenitis
  - Swelling, ptosis, and globe displacement
- Clinical profile
  - Associated with **systemic** sarcoidosis
    - Orbital disease common **initial presentation**
    - 30-60% of patients with sarcoidosis have ophthalmic disease
      - Most often in form of bilateral, granulomatous, intraocular inflammation
  - Can be associated with neurosarcoidosis
    - Leptomeningeal, dural, and parenchymal brain and spinal lesions

Demographics

- Age
  - 20-40 years most common
- Sex
  - **Female** predominance (2:1)
- Ethnicity
  - Highest in African & Northern European descent
- Epidemiology
  - Prevalence: 2-60 per 100,000

Treatment

- Observation for mild disease, although orbital involvement typically warrants treatment
- Oral **corticosteroids** are treatment of choice
- Other immunosuppressants for recalcitrant disease

DIAGNOSTIC CHECKLIST

Image Interpretation Pearls

- Imaging appearance similar to that of **idiopathic inflammation** and **lymphoproliferative** lesions
- Follow-up studies generally demonstrate improvement with steroid treatment
- Correlative imaging, including chest x-ray (CXR) or chest CT, may demonstrate bilateral hilar lymphadenopathy (BHL)
  - From studies of uveitis patients with proven sarcoidosis, 63-83% showed BHL on CXR and 86-100% showed BHL on CT chest

SELECTED REFERENCES

1. Salim S et al: Orbital and adnexal sarcoidosis: clinical presentations and management outcomes. Indian J Ophthalmol. 73(2):214-20, 2025
2. Simakurthy S et al: Ocular sarcoidosis. StatPearls, 2025
3. Rosenbaum JT et al: Ocular sarcoidosis. Clin Chest Med. 45(1):59-70, 2024
4. Barbera SC et al: Orbital sarcoidosis with invasion of the lacrimal gland. Ear Nose Throat J. ePub, 2023
5. Stevens SM et al: Orbital sarcoidosis masquerading as late postoperative blepharoplasty complication: a case report. Ophthalmic Plast Reconstr Surg. 38(4):e113-6, 2022
6. Babu K et al: Orbital sarcoidosis in a high TB endemic country - a case series from south India. Ocul Immunol Inflamm. 29(5):957-62, 2021

Thyroid-Associated Orbitopathy

TERMINOLOGY

- Graves ophthalmopathy, thyroid eye disease
- Autoimmune orbital inflammation associated with autoimmune thyroid dysfunction
- Typical patient is middle-aged woman with lid retraction, periorbital edema, proptosis, and restricted gaze

IMAGING

- Bilateral extraocular muscle (EOM) enlargement
  - Nonuniform, symmetric involvement
  - I'M SLO mnemonic for sites of predilection
  - Enlargement of muscle bellies; typically spares tendons
- Heterogeneous areas of internal lower density
- Exophthalmos and increased orbital fat
- T2/STIR signal correlates with disease activity
  - High signal acutely due to edema and inflammation
  - Low-signal chronic disease due to fibrosis
- Decreased EOM enhancement compared to normal

TOP DIFFERENTIAL DIAGNOSES

- Idiopathic orbital inflammation
- Orbital sarcoidosis
- Orbital cellulitis
- Lymphoproliferative disease
- IgG4-related disease

PATHOLOGY

- Autoimmune inflammation due to thyrotropin receptor autoantigens present in both thyroid gland and orbit
- Orbital fibroblasts and adipocytes involved in T-cell lymphocyte cytokine-mediated inflammation
- Associated with other autoimmune diseases

CLINICAL ISSUES

- Orbital disease may not be concordant with thyroid disease
- Corticosteroids 1st line of therapy in acute disease
- Surgery for decompression in severe cases

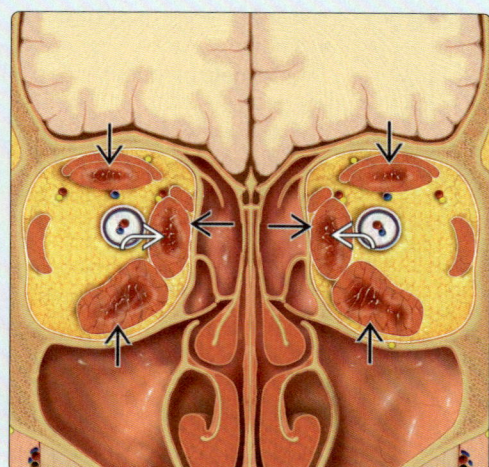
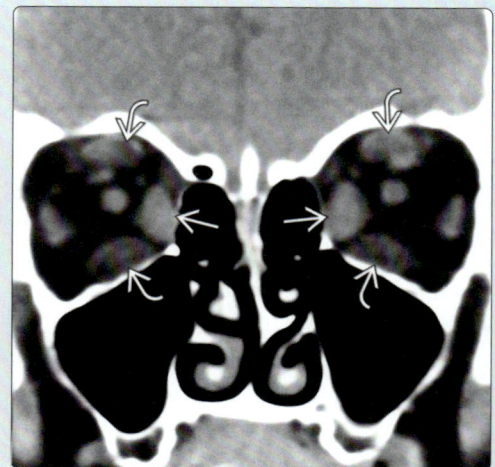

(Left) Coronal graphic shows bilateral symmetric enlargement of extraocular muscles (EOMs) ➡. Heterogeneity within the muscles ➡ represents accumulation of lymphocytes and mucopolysaccharide deposition. (Right) Coronal NECT demonstrates symmetric bilateral EOM enlargement, particularly in the medial rectus muscles ➡. The inferior and superior rectus muscles appear symmetrically enlarged and demonstrate typical foci of patchy low fat attenuation ➡.

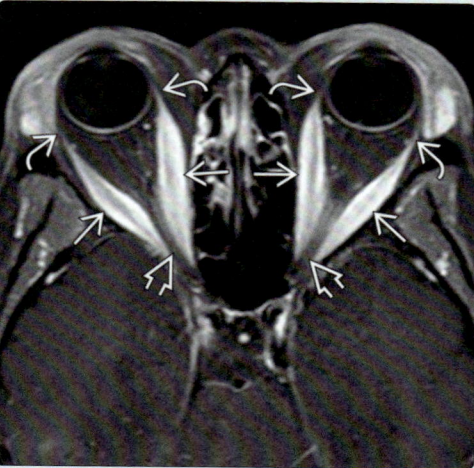
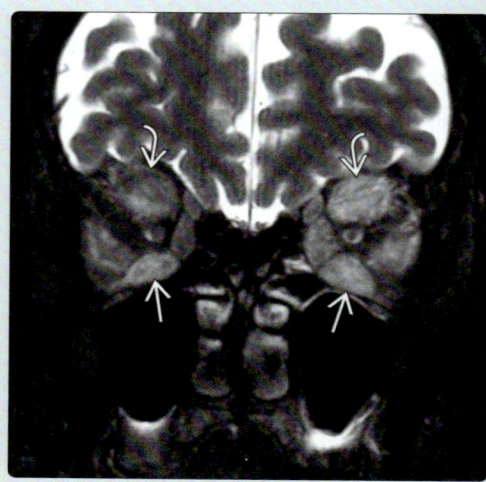

(Left) Axial T1 C+ FS MR demonstrates characteristic symmetric findings of thyroid-associated orbitopathy (TAO) with bilateral rectus muscle belly enlargement ➡. Note the slender appearance of tendinous insertions, which are spared ➡. Muscles impinge on both optic nerves at the orbital apex ➡. (Right) STIR MR shows marked asymmetrical enlargement of bilateral rectus muscles ➡, L > R. The superior rectus-levator muscle complex is disproportionately involved ➡, and muscle hyperintensity supports active inflammation.

Thyroid-Associated Orbitopathy

TERMINOLOGY

Synonyms

- **Graves** ophthalmopathy, thyroid eye disease

Definitions

- **Autoimmune** orbital inflammatory condition associated with autoimmune thyroid dysfunction

IMAGING

General Features

- Best diagnostic clue
  - Bilateral **extraocular muscle** (EOM) enlargement
- Location
  - Nonuniform, symmetric EOM involvement
    - Bilateral in 90%; symmetrical in 70%
    - **I'M SLO** mnemonic for sites of predilection
    - Inferior ≥ medial ≥ superior > lateral ≥ oblique
    - Isolated muscle involvement in 5%
    - Superior ophthalmic vein (SOV) periphlebitis in ~ 5%
      - □ SOV enlargement ≥ 2x diameter of uninvolved side
      - □ Perivenular inflammation and wall thickening
      - □ May signal more active disease
- Size
  - EOM enlargement varies with disease severity
  - Thickness > 5 mm considered abnormal
    - Midbelly thickness correlates with muscle volume
  - Normative EOM thickness (mm) at midbelly (CT data)
    - Inferior: 4.8; medial: 4.2; superior: 4.6; lateral: 3.3
- Morphology
  - Enlargement of **muscle bellies**; typically **spares tendons** but may be involved in acute phase
  - Increased **orbital fat**, especially in patients < 40 years

CT Findings

- NECT
  - Enlargement of EOM bellies
  - Heterogeneous areas of internal lower density
    - Due to glycosaminoglycan deposition
  - Exophthalmos
    - Line drawn between lateral orbital rims demonstrates degree of exophthalmos
  - Other features
    - Straightened ("stretched") optic nerve
    - Lacrimal glands enlarged in ~ 30% (10% asymmetric)

MR Findings

- T1WI
  - Isointense enlargement of EOM bellies
  - ± fat signal in EOMs centrally
- T2WI FS
  - Increased EOM signal in acute disease
    - Increased water due to edema and inflammation
  - Decreased EOM signal in chronic disease
    - Involutional changes with fibrosis
  - Decreased optic nerve diameter posteriorly
- STIR
  - Signal intensity ratio correlates with clinical activity
    - Correlates with increased muscle volume
- T1WI C+

  - Decreased EOM enhancement compared to normal
    - Impaired microcirculation, decreased perfusion
    - Secondary to intraorbital mass effect
  - Superior ophthalmic vein periphlebitis

Ultrasonographic Findings

- Grayscale ultrasound
  - Enlarged EOM bellies, spares tendons
  - Internal reflectivity lower in acute disease
    - Edema and inflammation
  - Internal reflectivity higher in chronic disease
    - End-stage changes and fibrosis

Imaging Recommendations

- Best imaging tool
  - CT for uncomplicated disease and surgical planning
  - MR to assess disease activity in deciding therapy, assessing optic nerve compromise, and atypical thyroid-associated orbitopathy (TAO) to exclude other pathology
- Protocol advice
  - Imaging not routinely necessary in patients with mild disease if diagnosis is established clinically
  - Volumetric analysis (EOM)
    - Can be used to monitor treatment response
    - Transverse diameter correlates with volume

DIFFERENTIAL DIAGNOSIS

Idiopathic Orbital Inflammation

- Inflammatory changes with proptosis and ophthalmoplegia, **pain** common feature
- Unilateral > bilateral, often involves **lateral rectus**; may involve other orbital structures (especially lacrimal gland)

Sarcoidosis

- Orbital disease in 20% of patients with systemic sarcoid
- Granulomatous multifocal orbital enhancement

Orbital Cellulitis

- Proptosis, fever, associated sinus infection (ethmoid)
- Fat infiltration, subperiosteal abscess, myositis

Lymphoproliferative Lesions

- Non-Hodgkin lymphoma, primary to orbit or with systemic disease; MALT variety typical
- Pliable, homogeneously enhancing mass may originate from or infiltrate EOM

Metastasis

- History of known primary
- Isolated or multiple masses in soft tissues or bone

IgG4-Related Disease

- EOM enlargement with sinus mucosal thickening
- **Trigeminal nerve** enlargement and enhancement

PATHOLOGY

General Features

- Etiology
  - Autoimmune inflammation of orbital structures
  - Thyrotropin receptor-like autoantigens present in both thyroid gland and orbital fibroblasts

- Orbital fibroblasts react to lymphocyte (T-cell) infiltration and cytokine-mediated inflammation
  - Glycosaminoglycan (Hyaluron) deposition
  - Fibroblast proliferation, differentiation into adipocytes, and adipogenesis
- Associated abnormalities
  - May be seen with autoimmune (Hashimoto) thyroiditis
  - Increased incidence of myasthenia gravis
    - Potential confounding cause of EOM dysfunction
  - Associated with other autoimmune diseases
  - Marine-Lenhart syndrome = TAO + functional thyroid nodules
    - Occurs ~ 0.8-2.7% of TAO

Staging, Grading, & Classification

- Functional classification (clinical severity and risk)
  - Mild: Eyelid lag and retraction with proptosis in setting of active hyperthyroidism
  - Moderate: Soft tissue inflammation, intermittent myopathy, stabilizes without major sequelae
  - Severe: Rapid and fulminant, greater mass effect, severe sequelae, including optic nerve compromise
- VISA scheme
  - **Vision**: Specifically, optic neuropathy
  - **Inflammation**: Indicated by pain and swelling
  - **Strabismus**: Limitations in motility
  - **Appearance**: Proptosis, lid function, and exposure

Gross Pathologic & Surgical Features

- Gross enlargement of EOM, increased orbital fat

Microscopic Features

- Mixed cellular infiltration with lymphocytes, plasma cells, macrophages, and eosinophils
- Glycosaminoglycan (Hyaluron) deposition
- Enlargement of fibroblasts, increased collagen
- Fibrosis and muscle degeneration in chronic phase

CLINICAL ISSUES

Presentation

- Most common signs/symptoms
  - Eyelid retraction, periorbital edema, proptosis, pain, restricted gaze
- Other signs/symptoms
  - Eyelid lag on downgaze, incomplete closure
  - Dry eyes, chemosis, and corneal ulceration
  - Diplopia, restricted EOM movement, strabismus
  - Dysthyroid optic neuropathy in severe cases
    - Vision loss due to optic nerve compression at apex
- Clinical profile
  - Orbitopathy common in systemic Graves disease
    - 30-50% have clinically evident orbital symptoms
    - 70-90% have orbital disease, including subclinical
    - 5% have severe orbital disease
  - Associated with systemic thyroid disease
    - 80-90% hyperthyroid
    - 10-20% hypothyroid or euthyroid
    - Orbit symptoms precede systemic disease in 20%; coincident in 40%; afterwards in 40%

Demographics

- Age
  - Young and middle-aged adults (30-50 years)
  - Orbitopathy more severe in older patients
  - Graves disease uncommon in children
- Sex
  - F > > M (3-6x more common)
  - More severe and later onset in males
- Ethnicity
  - ↑ frequency and severity in patients of European ancestry
- Epidemiology
  - Incidence: 1:2,000 to 1:5,000
  - Most common cause of exophthalmos in adults
  - 25-50% of Graves patients develop TAO

Natural History & Prognosis

- Orbitopathy often self-limited, favorable outcome
- Significant chronic disease in 10-15%; severe in 5%
- Treatment of systemic thyroid disease may worsen orbitopathy, particularly radioiodine treatment
- Smoking exacerbates orbital disease

Treatment

- Supportive therapy for early and mild cases
  - Corneal care; observation for vision impairment
- More aggressive therapy for patients with severe inflammation or optic nerve compromise
- Medical therapy
  - Corticosteroids 1st-line therapy in acute disease
    - 85% stabilization and 40% reduction of disease
- Radiation therapy
  - Rapid palliation with 60-70% response
- Surgical therapy
  - Decompression for uncontrolled mass effect
    - Chronic disease, failed medical therapy
    - Resection of lateral orbital walls/orbital floors
    - Muscle volumes may increase following decompression, unrelated to disease reactivation
  - Restoration of eyelid position and function
  - Correction of strabismus

DIAGNOSTIC CHECKLIST

Consider

- Most common cause of exophthalmos in adult
- Typical patient is middle-aged woman

Image Interpretation Pearls

- Fluid-sensitive MR sequence can help differentiate acute edema from late-change fibrosis
- MR shows optic nerve compression better than CT

Reporting Tips

- Consider other diagnoses if isolated to lateral rectus

SELECTED REFERENCES

1. Hu Z et al: Evaluation of inflammatory activity of extraocular muscles in thyroid associated orbitopathy by [(68)Ga]DOTATATE PET/CT. Mol Imaging Biol. 27(1):120-30, 2025
2. Goodyear K et al: Prevalence, clinical and imaging characteristics of superior ophthalmic vein periphlebitis in thyroid eye disease. Ophthalmic Plast Reconstr Surg. 40(4):399-402, 2024

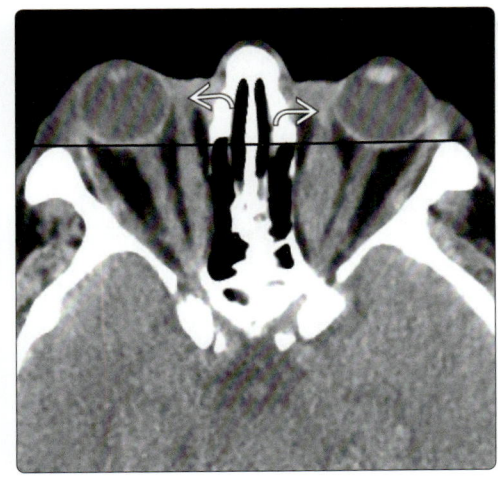
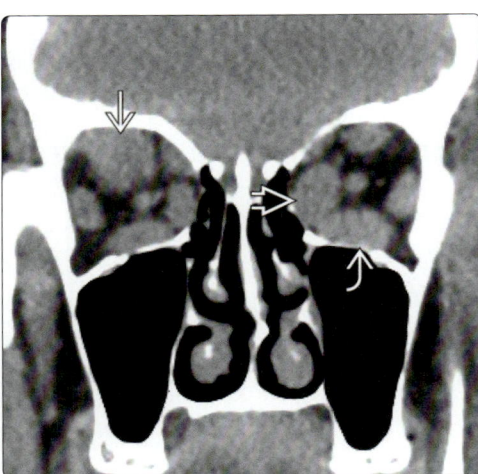

(Left) *Axial NECT demonstrates bilateral proptosis, which can be estimated by the degree of anterior displacement relative to the black horizontal line. There is asymmetrical involvement by TAO with bilateral medial rectus enlargement sparing the tendinous insertions* ➡. **(Right)** *Coronal NECT in the same patient demonstrates asymmetrical findings of TAO: The right superior rectus-levator complex* ➡ *and left medial* ➡ *and inferior* ➡ *rectus muscles are disproportionately involved.*

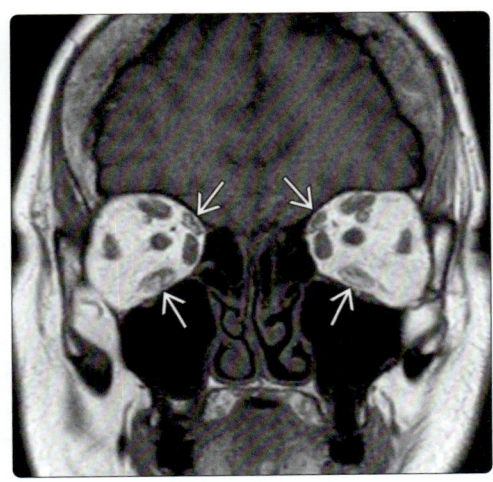
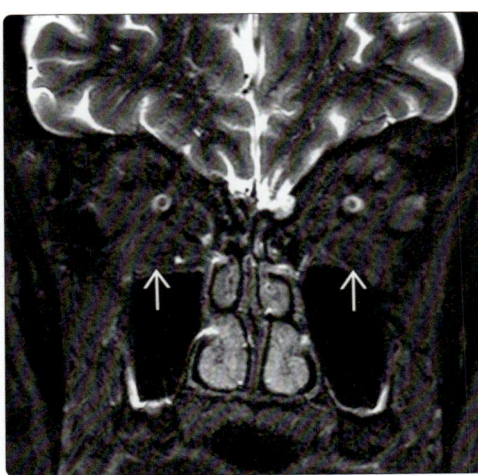

(Left) *Coronal T1 MR shows diffuse and relatively symmetric bilateral EOM enlargement in chronic TAO with associated fatty infiltration, particularly involving the inferior rectus and superior oblique muscles* ➡. **(Right)** *Coronal STIR MR in the same patient shows the hypointense appearance of the EOMs, likely due to a combination of chronic fibrosis and technical signal suppression of intrinsically hyperintense fat with inactive disease* ➡. *Consequently, the muscles are difficult to identify on this STIR image.*

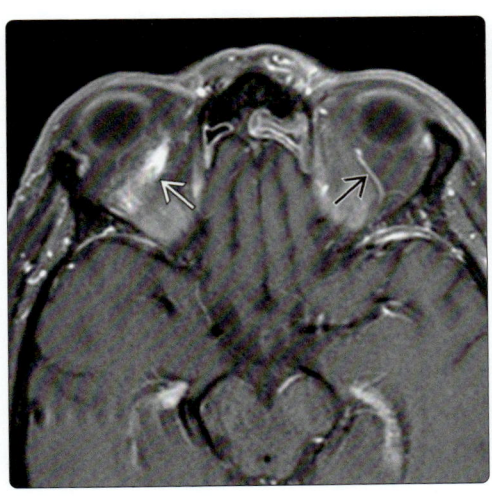
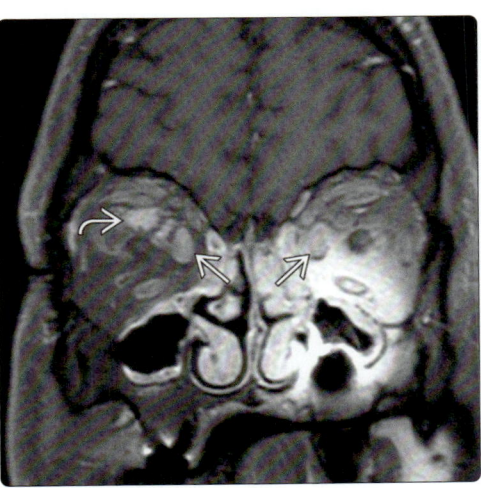

(Left) *Axial T1 C+ FS MR in a patient with TAO demonstrates enlargement and poor border delineation of the right superior ophthalmic vein due to periphlebitis* ➡, *an uncommonly recognized complication. Note the normal-appearing contralateral superior ophthalmic vein* ➡ *for comparison.* **(Right)** *Coronal T1 C+ FS MR in the same patient shows superior ophthalmic vein periphlebitis* ➡ *along with right greater than left medial rectus enlargement* ➡ *in active TAO.*

KEY FACTS

IMAGING

- Focal or segmental T2 hyperintensity of optic nerve
- Central or diffuse optic nerve enhancement
- Optic nerve diffuse & mild enlargement
- Variant peripheral sheath enhancement pattern
  - Less likely to be associated with multiple sclerosis (MS)
- Image brain & spinal cord

TOP DIFFERENTIAL DIAGNOSES

- Ischemic optic neuropathy
- Infectious optic neuritis
- Idiopathic perineuritis (pseudotumor)
- Granulomatous optic neuropathy (sarcoid)
- Optic nerve sheath meningioma
- Optic nerve glioma

PATHOLOGY

- Autoimmune demyelination in susceptible patients
- Triggered by infection, systemic disease, other stressor

CLINICAL ISSUES

- Symptoms
  - Acute loss of visual acuity & color vision, eye pain
- Distinct clinical profiles & different treatment implications
  - MS
  - Acute demyelinating encephalomyelitis (ADEM)
  - Neuromyelitis optica spectrum disorder (NMOSD)
  - Antimyelin oligodendrocyte glycoprotein (MOGAD)
  - GFAP-associated meningoencephalomyelitis (GFAP)
  - CRMP5-IgG-associated optic neuritis (CRMP5)
  - Chronic relapsing inflammatory optic neuritis (CRION)

DIAGNOSTIC CHECKLIST

- Critical role to identify CNS demyelinating lesions
  - High incidence of MS, brain findings predict MS
  - NMOSD or MOGAD if longitudinally extensive myelitis
  - GFAP & CRMP5 optic neuritis unlikely to enhance
  - GFAP: Perivascular radial white matter enhancement

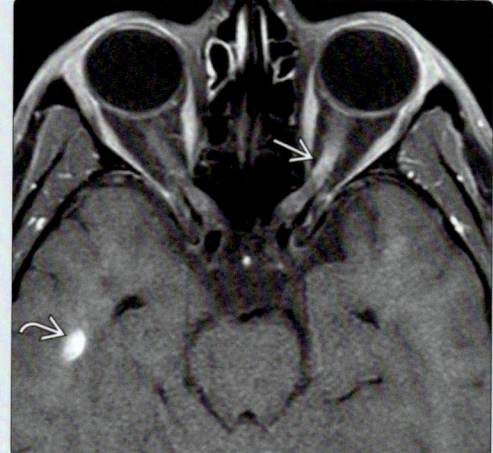
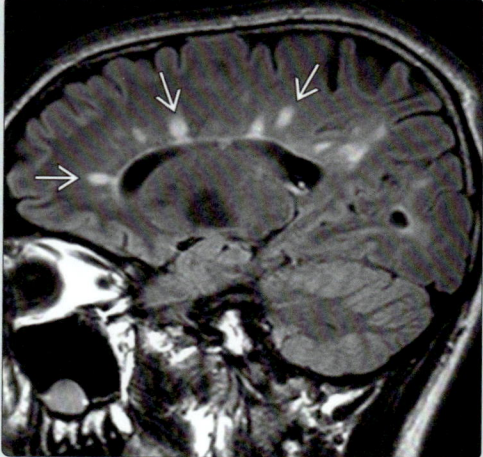

(Left) Axial T1 C+ FS MR shows typical short-segment enhancement of the intraorbital optic nerve ➡ in optic neuritis. It is important to identify additional lesions in the brain &/or spinal cord, as these help to characterize a systemic disorder, such as multiple sclerosis (MS). The enhancing temporal lobe plaque ➡ indicates active disease in this patient with MS. (Right) Parasagittal FLAIR MR in the same patient shows multiple ovoid hyperintensities ➡ in a classic pericallosal orientation and distribution for MS.

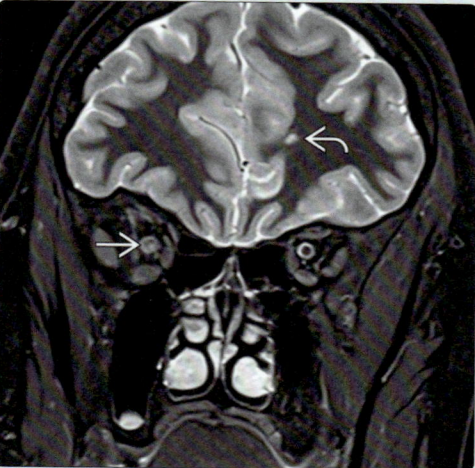
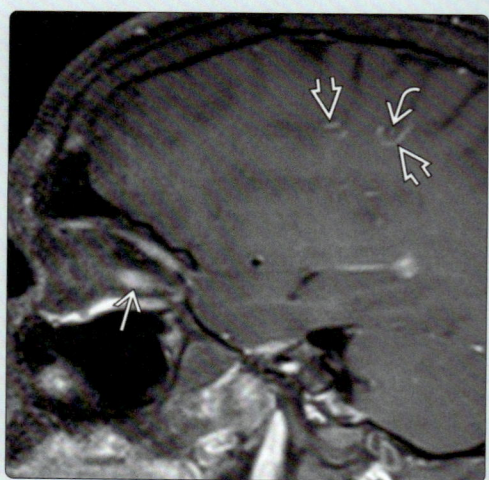

(Left) Coronal STIR MR in a patient with right optic neuritis shows abnormal hyperintensity ➡. Note the presence of a juxtacortical white matter hyperintensity ➡, raising concern for MS, subsequently confirmed clinically. (Right) Sagittal T1 C+ FS MR in the same patient demonstrates enhancement along the right optic nerve ➡ along with multiple enhancing intracranial lesions. Several juxtacortical plaques showed a classic incomplete enhancing ring ➡ &/or presence of a central vein sign ➡, classic findings in MS.

TERMINOLOGY

Abbreviations
- Optic neuritis (ON)

IMAGING

General Features
- Best diagnostic clue
  - **Enhancement** & mild **enlargement** of optic nerve
  - Enhancement uncommon in glial fibrillary acidic protein astrocytopathy (GFAP), collapsin-response mediator protein antibody (CRMP5)
- Location
  - **Unilateral** in 70%
    - More commonly bilateral in children
  - Segment(s) of nerve involvement
    - Anterior intraorbital: 45%
    - Midintraorbital: 60%
    - Intracanalicular: 35%
    - Prechiasmatic & chiasm: 10%
- Size
  - Optic nerve diffusely, mildly **enlarged**

CT Findings
- CECT
  - Normal ± enlarged, enhancing optic nerve

MR Findings
- T1WI
  - Optic nerve diffuse mild **enlargement**
- T2WI
  - Focal or segmental **hyperintensity** of optic nerve
    - Typical: Focal, short segment, favors multiple sclerosis (MS)
    - Atypical: Long segment, favors neuromyelitis optica spectrum disorder (NMOSD) or myelin oligodendrocyte glycoprotein antibody disorder (MOGAD)
    - Atypical: Posterior or chiasm location favors NMOSD
  - ± coexistent brain & spinal cord lesions
- STIR
  - Hyperintensity of optic nerves similar to T2WI
- FLAIR
  - ± coexistent **white matter** lesions in brain
    - Presence is **predictor** for **MS**
    - Especially if increased on early follow-up brain scan
- T1WI C+
  - **Nerve enhancement** centrally or diffusely > 90%
    - Consistent with active demyelination
  - Variant peripheral sheath enhancement pattern
    - Atypical pattern more common in MOGAD
    - Less likely to be associated with MS
    - May mimic nerve sheath meningioma

Imaging Recommendations
- Best imaging tool
  - Enhanced MR is imaging tool of choice
- Protocol advice
  - Image entire neuraxis (brain & cord)
  - **Whole-brain** thin sagittal FLAIR
  - **Orbits**: T2 FSE or STIR & T1 C+ FS

DIFFERENTIAL DIAGNOSIS

Ischemic Optic Neuropathy
- Restricted diffusion at nerve head, otherwise often normal
- More likely in **male**, advanced age
- Visual acuity does **not** improve, unlike acute ON

Infectious Optic Neuritis
- Nerve enlargement more pronounced
- May be indistinguishable from typical ON on imaging

Idiopathic Perineuritis (Pseudotumor)
- Enlarged, enhancing optic nerve sheath complex
- Inflammation may involve any orbital structure
- **Painful proptosis**; mobility restriction & diplopia

Granulomatous Optic Neuropathy (Sarcoid)
- Enlarged, enhancing optic nerve similar to ON
- Extraocular muscle & lacrimal gland involvement
- **Intracranial disease** with leptomeningeal enhancement

Optic Nerve Sheath Meningioma
- Thickened, enhancing optic nerve sheath
- Tram-track **calcifications** are diagnostic
- Progressive vision loss, **lack of pain**

Optic Nerve Glioma
- **Tubular enlarged, variably enhancing** optic nerve
- Neurofibromatosis type 1 often present
- Rare malignant optic glioma in adults

Radiation-Induced Optic Neuropathy
- Bilateral optic nerve enhancement
- 1-3 years following radiation
- Pituitary, parasellar, & skull base tumors

Toxic Optic Neuropathy
- Methanol, carbon monoxide, many pharmaceuticals

Other Systemic or Inflammatory Conditions
- Systemic lupus erythematosus, Sjögren syndrome, rheumatoid arthritis, antiphospholipid antibody, paraneoplastic syndrome

PATHOLOGY

General Features
- Etiology
  - **Autoimmune** process
- Genetics
  - HLA alleles associated with risk of developing ON & MS

Staging, Grading, & Classification
- Subtypes of ON
  - Neuroretinitis
  - Papillitis
  - Retrobulbar neuritis
  - Perineuritis
- McDonald criteria based on clinical, imaging, & CSF

Microscopic Features
- Acute: Macrophages, lymphocytes, & plasma cells

- Myelin loss, axonal damage, cholesterol droplets
- Chronic: Atrophy, gliosis, astrocytic scar
  - Axonal loss, little remyelination, may cavitate

CLINICAL ISSUES

Presentation

- Most common signs/symptoms
  - Acute loss of visual acuity & eye pain
- Other signs/symptoms
  - Dyschromatopsia (impaired color vision)
  - Vision worse in bright light
  - Phosgenes (light flashes)
  - Eye tenderness or pain with movement
  - Uhthoff symptom: Exertion-induced vision loss
  - Relative afferent pupillary defect
  - Swollen optic disc (papillitis) in 33%
  - Delayed visual evoked potential (VEP) latency
- Clinical profile
  - Typical acute ON
    - May present as clinically isolated syndrome (CIS)
    - High risk of developing clinically definite MS
    - May be infectious or parainfectious
  - NMOSD
    - Acute ON, typically bilateral, with myelitis
    - ON more likely to relapse, worse outcome
    - Seropositive autoantibody to aquaporin-4
  - MOGAD
    - ~ 20-50% of ON in children, 5% in adults
    - No ethnicity or sex predilection
    - Seropositive autoantibody marker, antibodies to MOG
    - Better vision prognosis
    - ON often bilateral
    - Nerve sheath enhancement more typical
  - Chronic relapsing inflammatory ON (CRION)
    - Recurrent, steroid-responsive/-dependent ON
    - Any age, sex, & ethnicity, but most often young to middle-aged women
    - Rare idiopathic ON; diagnosis of exclusion
  - Acute demyelinating encephalomyelitis (ADEM)
    - **Monophasic** demyelinating disorder
    - May involve optic nerves primarily or exclusively
  - GFAP astrocytopathy
    - Paraneoplastic in 20-34%
    - Perivascular radial white matter enhancement
  - CRMP5-IgG-associated autoimmunity
    - Paraneoplastic syndromes
    - 20% have ON, enhancement uncommon
    - 70% have underlying cancer (#1 is small-cell lung)
  - Pediatric ON
    - Rare, ≤ 5% of cases
    - More frequently bilateral (40-60%)
    - Less likely to develop MS (15-35%)
    - May follow viral illness or vaccination
    - More frequently attributable to ADEM
  - Isolated ON
    - May be solitary, recurrent, or chronic relapsing

Demographics

- Age

- MS presentation: 15-50 years; mean: early 30s
- Sex
  - M:F = 1:2
- Ethnicity
  - Highest prevalence among Northern European ancestry
  - Moderately high with Mediterranean ancestry
  - Low with African or Asian ancestry
- Epidemiology
  - Incidence MS: 4-6 per 100,000 in USA & Europe
  - 40-60% of ON patients ultimately develop MS
    - Up to 75% of women, 35% of men
  - MR findings highly correlated with subsequent MS
    - Up to 75% of patients with brain lesions
    - 25% of patients with normal brain MR
  - 70-90% of MS patients develop ON at some point

Natural History & Prognosis

- Acute symptom onset over hours to days
- Spontaneous **recovery of vision** characteristic of MS
  - Begins in 2 weeks, continues for months to years
  - Acuity: 70% ≥ 20/25; 80% ≥ 20/30; 90% ≥ 20/40
- ON frequently **initial demyelinating event** in MS
- Recurrent ON is common
  - Overall 35%, seen in MS, NMOSD, MOGAD
  - Recurs in same eye in 20-30%

Treatment

- Dependent on etiology; MS by far most common
- Corticosteroid treatment (IV with PO taper) for MS
  - Accelerates short-term recovery
  - Does not alter long-term vision outcome
- Immunomodulatory therapy for steroid failures
  - Differentiate MS from other etiologies
  - Immunomodulation may worsen NMOSD & MOGAD

DIAGNOSTIC CHECKLIST

Consider

- Spontaneous **recovery** of vision is typical if MS
  - Consider other etiologies if vision remains poor
  - Ischemic neuropathy more likely in older patients

Image Interpretation Pearls

- Identifying CNS demyelinating lesions in CNS is critical neuroimaging task in setting of ON
  - High incidence of MS in patients with ON
  - Concurrent MR brain findings strongly predict MS
  - NMOSD or MOGAD with longitudinally extensive myelitis
  - GFAP if perivascular radial white matter enhancement

SELECTED REFERENCES

1. Guier CP et al: Optic neuritis. StatPearls, 2025
2. Shetty D et al: Glial fibrillary acidic protein astrocytopathy: review of pathogenesis, imaging features, and radiographic mimics. AJNR Am J Neuroradiol. 45(10):1394-402, 2024
3. Bennett JL et al: Optic neuritis and autoimmune optic neuropathies: advances in diagnosis and treatment. Lancet Neurol. 22(1):89-100, 2023

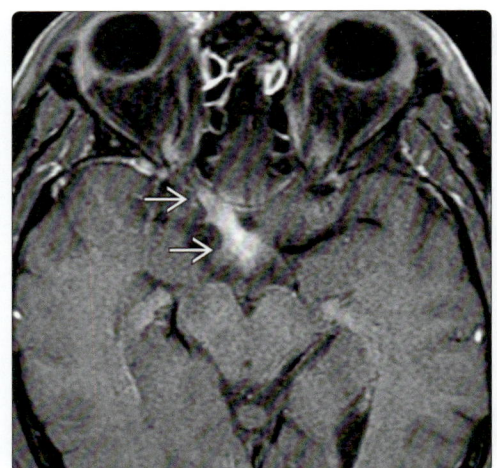

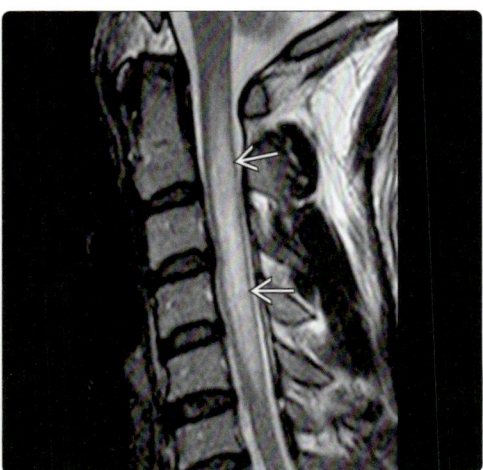

(Left) Axial T1 C+ FS MR in a patient with severe acute vision loss shows marked enhancement of the right optic nerve, involving the cisternal segment and extending from the optic canal to the chiasm ➡. (Right) Sagittal T2 MR in the same patient also with acute myelopathy shows a long segment of cervical cord enlargement with T2 hyperintensity ➡. MR of the brain was normal, and CSF did not show oligoclonal bands. Serum antibody testing confirmed neuromyelitis optica.

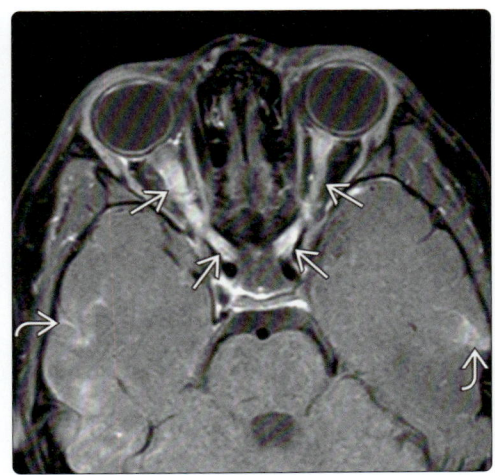

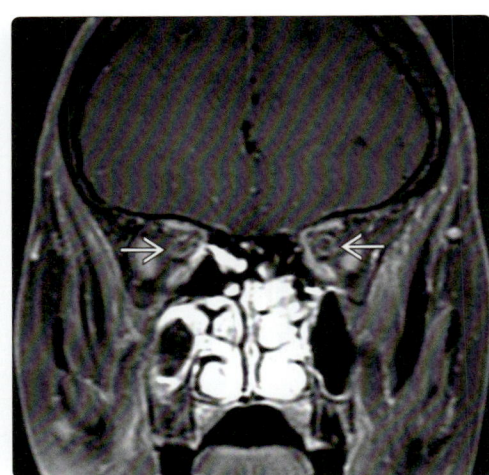

(Left) Axial T1 C+ FS MR shows typical long-segment bilateral optic neuritis MOGAD ➡. The longitudinally extensive nature and bilateral occurrence favors MOGAD over MS. Areas of abnormal parenchymal enhancement ➡ were also present. (Right) Coronal T1 C+ FS MR shows bilateral optic nerve sheath enhancement ➡ due to optic perineuritis in NMOSD. This atypical pattern of optic neuritis is more often seen with NMOSD and MOGAD and may mimic other inflammatory disorders &/or meningioma.

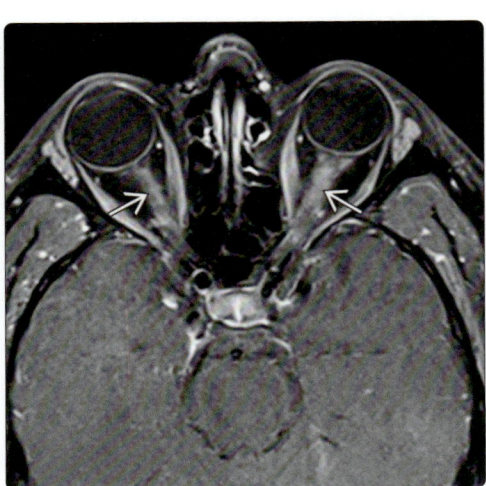

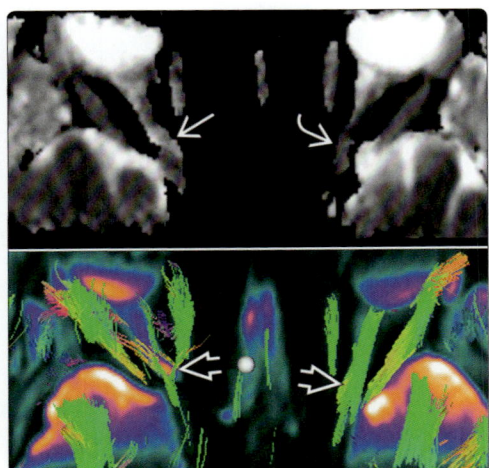

(Left) Axial T1 C+ FS MR in a young male patient with blurry vision and eye pain shows patchy enhancement and mild enlargement of the optic nerves ➡, worse on the left. CSF and clinical course were consistent with ADEM. (Right) Axial diffusivity image (top) in a patient with optic neuritis shows increased mean diffusivity in the right optic nerve ➡ compared to the left ➡. Tractography (bottom) shows corresponding loss of fiber bundle distinction of the right compared to left optic nerves ➡.

Orbital Langerhans Cell Histiocytosis

TERMINOLOGY

- Langerhans cell histiocytosis (LCH): Spectrum of disease caused by neoplastic clonal proliferations of CD1a, CD207, & S100 protein (+) dendritic cells
- Single system (SS) (unifocal or multifocal) vs. multisystem (MS) disease
  - Most frequently involved: Bone (80-90%) & skin (40-50%)
  - Risk organ (RO) involvement: Liver, spleen, marrow; confers worse prognosis (high risk)
  - Others: Lymph nodes, lung, pituitary, thymus, GI tract
- Historic categorization
  - Eosinophilic granuloma: Unifocal, SS; isolated bone or lung involvement
  - Hand-Schüller-Christian: Chronic disseminated form
  - Letterer-Siwe: Acute disseminated form

IMAGING

- Orbital disease typically unifocal SS but may occur in conjunction with multifocal SS or MS disease

- Anterior or lateral orbitofrontal skull most common; greater sphenoid wing common in multifocal disease
- Punched-out or geographic lytic bone lesion
- Associated soft tissue mass with heterogeneous enhancement
- MR to assess orbital extension & intracranial involvement
- PET/CT vs. whole-body STIR or whole-body DWI MR for multifocal or MS disease

TOP DIFFERENTIAL DIAGNOSES

- Rhabdomyosarcoma
- Metastasis
- Leukemia

CLINICAL ISSUES

- Periorbital pain & swelling, proptosis
- Local curettage & intralesional corticosteroid injection
  - Excellent prognosis for localized lesions
- Systemic chemotherapy for extensive disease

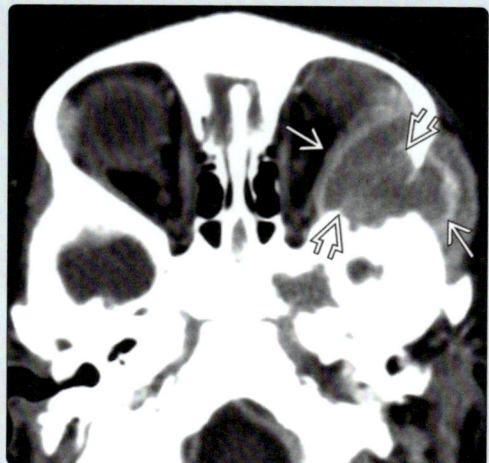
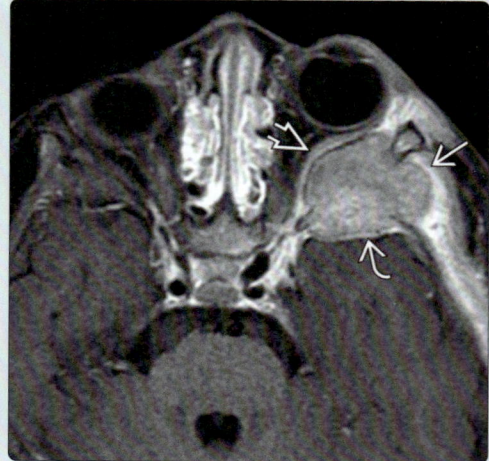

(Left) Axial CECT in a child with proptosis shows a large, heterogeneously enhancing mass ➡ associated with a large lytic lesion involving the lateral orbital wall and greater wing of the left sphenoid ⮕ without aggressive periosteal reaction. (Right) Axial T1 C+ MR in the same patient shows moderate contrast enhancement of the soft tissue mass ➡ medially deviating the left lateral rectus muscle ⮕ and resulting in proptosis. Note extension also into the left middle cranial fossa with dural thickening/enhancement ➡.

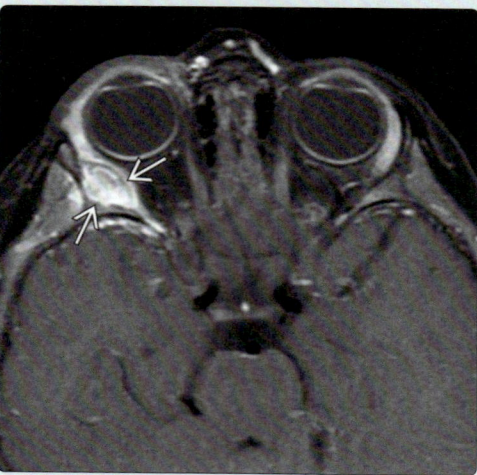
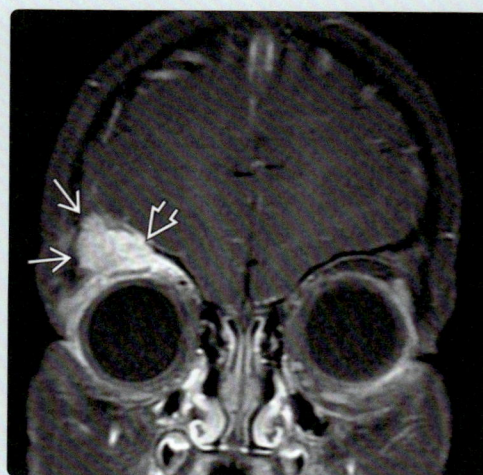

(Left) Axial T1 C+ FS MR in a 2-year-old girl shows a well-defined, homogeneously enhancing mass ➡ in the greater wing of the right sphenoid without aggressive periosteal reaction. There is mild extraconal intraorbital extension without proptosis. (Right) Coronal T1 C+ FS MR in the same child shows a well-defined, homogeneously enhancing mass ➡ with sharply outlined osseous destruction of the superolateral orbital wall ⮕. There is mild extraconal extension into the orbit.

TERMINOLOGY

Definitions

- Neoplastic clonal proliferation of CD1a, CD207, & S100 protein (+) dendritic cells
- Single system (SS) (unifocal or multifocal) vs. multisystem (MS) disease
  - Bone (80-90%) & skin (40-50%) are most frequent
  - Risk organ (RO) involvement: Liver, spleen, marrow; confers worse prognosis (high risk)
  - Other organs: Lymph nodes, pituitary, thymus, GI tract
  - CNS-risk lesion: Skull base & many facial lesions
    - Diabetes insipidus (25% overall, 50% with MS disease), growth hormone deficiency (10%), parenchymal mass lesions (1%), & delayed neurodegenerative changes

IMAGING

General Features

- Best diagnostic clue
  - Geographic, **lytic** lesion of skull/orbit with associated enhancing **soft tissue mass**
- Location
  - Orbital disease typically **unifocal** but may occur in conjunction with multifocal or MS disease
  - **Anterior** or **lateral** orbitofrontal skull most common
  - Lateral orbital wall & greater sphenoid wing also common, particularly multifocal disease

CT Findings

- CT: Well-defined, lytic orbital wall &/or greater wing sphenoid lesion + enhancing soft tissue mass
  - Calvarial lesions classically described as beveled edge due to greater inner than outer table involvement
  - No matrix, calcification, or periosteal new bone

MR Findings

- T1WI: Isointense to hypointense soft tissue mass
  - May have signal ↑ due to lipid-laden histiocytes
- T2WI: Isointense to hyperintense soft tissue mass
- STIR: Whole-body STIR to assess for multifocal disease
- DWI: Whole-body DWI (recent literature reports similar accuracy to FDG PET for staging & treatment)
- T1WIC+ FS: **Diffusely enhancing** soft tissue mass
  - Frequently mildly heterogeneous
  - ± intracranial extension with dural involvement

Nuclear Medicine Findings

- FDG PET/CT: Highly sensitive for active LCH

Imaging Recommendations

- Best imaging tool
  - MR to assess orbital ± intracranial involvement

DIFFERENTIAL DIAGNOSIS

Rhabdomyosarcoma

- Soft tissue mass, frequently without aggressive bone destruction when occurs in orbit

Metastasis

- Particularly neuroblastoma in young children, usually with aggressive periosteal reaction

Leukemia

- Acute myeloid leukemia, chronic lymphotic leukemia, or granulocytic sarcoma
- Enhancing soft tissue orbital masses ± bone destruction

PATHOLOGY

General Features

- Etiology
  - Reactive vs. neoplastic (neoplastic currently favored)
  - Unknown cause: Infectious agents (especially viruses), immune system dysfunction, neoplastic mechanisms, genetic factors, cellular adhesion molecules proposed

Staging, Grading, & Classification

- **Unifocal, SS**
  - Bony lesions; older patient population; best prognosis
- **Multifocal, SS**
  - Bone, skin, viscera; younger patient population
- **Multifocal, MS involvement**
  - Disseminated, fulminant; infants; worst prognosis

CLINICAL ISSUES

Presentation

- Most common signs/symptoms
  - Periorbital pain & swelling, proptosis
- Other signs/symptoms
  - Diplopia or nerve palsies due to mass effect
  - Effects on visual acuity may → amblyopia in younger patients

Demographics

- Sex: M:F 1.2-3:1
- Age: 90% of cases are < 15 years at presentation
  - Median 3 years of age at diagnosis

Natural History & Prognosis

- Excellent prognosis for localized lesions
- High mortality with disseminated disease

Treatment

- SS disease
  - Unifocal bone disease: Observation vs. curettage & local steroid injection
  - Multifocal bone disease or CNS-risk lesion: Chemotherapy & steroids x 6-12 months
- MS disease (± RO): Multiagent chemotherapy x 12 months
- Recent success with MAPK pathway inhibitors: BRAF inhibitors & MEK inhibitors

DIAGNOSTIC CHECKLIST

Reporting Tips

- Skeletal imaging to exclude multifocal disease

SELECTED REFERENCES

1. Degar BA et al: Clinical characteristics and treatment of histiocytic disorders in children. Hematol Oncol Clin North Am. 39(3):513-29, 2025
2. Malakooti Shijani SM et al: Orbital and ocular adnexal histiocytic tumors; a multidisciplinary literature review. Orbit. 1-13, 2025
3. Baratto L et al: Comparison of whole-body DW-MRI with 2-[(18)F]FDG PET for staging and treatment monitoring of children with Langerhans cell histiocytosis. Eur J Nucl Med Mol Imaging. 50(6):1689-98, 2023

Orbital Infantile Hemangioma

TERMINOLOGY

- Widespread misuse of term hemangioma in literature
- Definition: **Benign vascular tumor** of infancy

IMAGING

- Location: Preseptal &/or postseptal orbit
- CT findings
  - Lobular, slightly hyperdense, homogeneous
  - Intense enhancement, decreases with involution
- MR findings
  - T1 intermediate; prominent internal **flow voids**
  - Moderate **T2 hyperintensity** (high cellularity)
- US: High vessel density, absent arteriovenous shunting, high peak arterial Doppler shift

TOP DIFFERENTIAL DIAGNOSES

- Rhabdomyosarcoma
- Metastatic neuroblastoma
- Orbital cellulitis
- Orbital Langerhans cell histiocytosis
- Orbital venolymphatic malformation
- Plexiform neurofibroma
- Orbital non-Hodgkin lymphoma

PATHOLOGY

- **Proliferation** of vascular endothelium; cellular hyperplasia

CLINICAL ISSUES

- **Distinguish** from **vascular malformations**
  - Present at birth; grow in monophasic fashion
- 3 distinct phases
  - **Proliferative phase**: Appears few weeks after birth & grows rapidly for year 1 or 2
  - **Involuting phase**: Regression over 3-5 years
  - **Involuted phase**: Complete regression by late childhood

DIAGNOSTIC CHECKLIST

- T2-hyperintense enhancing mass with flow voids in infant

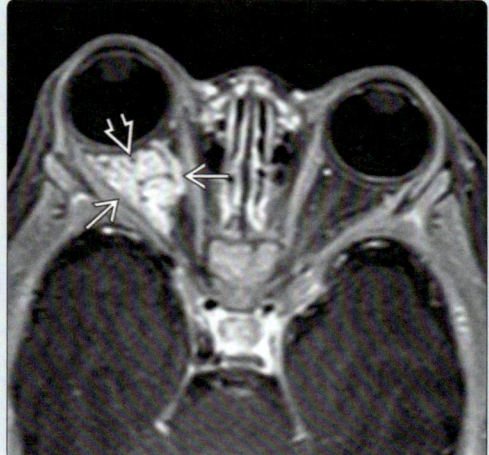
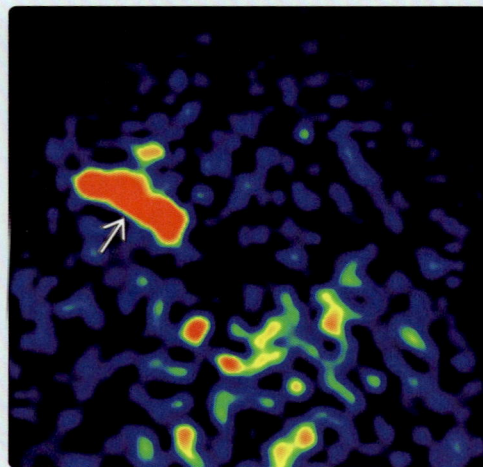

(Left) Axial T1 C+ FS MR in a 3-month-old with proptosis demonstrates an intensely enhancing intraconal mass in the right orbit ⮥ with multiple intralesional flow voids ⮕, resulting in moderate proptosis. The degree of enhancement and intralesional flow voids in a child of this age is typical of infantile hemangioma (IH). (Right) Axial arterial spin label MR in the same patient shows increased signal ⮕ corresponding to the enhancing orbital mass, typical of IHs.

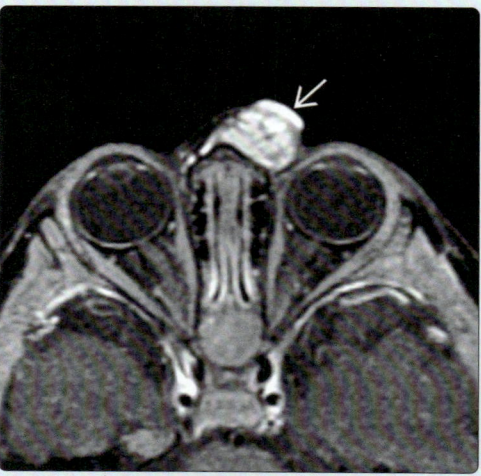
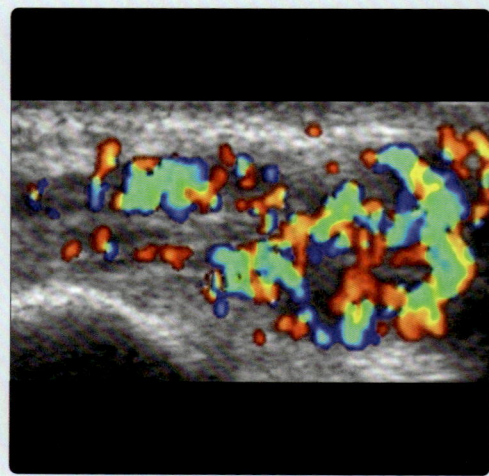

(Left) Axial T1 C+ FS MR depicts a well-delineated, intensely enhancing IH ⮕ with internal septations &/or flow voids in a typical preseptal, periorbital location, without adjacent bone destruction. Once again, postseptal extension is absent. (Right) Color Doppler US in the same patient shows high vessel density, consistent with the proliferating phase of an IH. However, remember that, if imaging appearance, timeline, or physical exam findings are atypical for IH, biopsy is indicated.

TERMINOLOGY

Synonyms
- Capillary hemangioma

Definitions
- **Benign vascular tumor** of infancy
- **Not** vascular malformation (congenital errors of vessel development)
- Widespread misuse of term hemangioma in literature
- 2025 revised classification by International Society for Study of Vascular Anomalies (ISSVA) retains 2 main categories
  - Vascular tumors: True neoplasms with cellular proliferation; grow out of proportion to patient
  - Vascular malformation: Congenital errors of vessel development; grow commensurate with patient

IMAGING

General Features
- Best diagnostic clue
  - Lobular, well-defined, **hypervascular, intensely enhancing** mass in infant
- Location
  - May involve multiple contiguous areas
  - Predilection for eyelids, supranasal periorbita
  - Sites of orbital involvement
    - Most commonly superficial, superomedial, extraconal
    - May extend postseptal into superior orbital fissure or intraconal space
    - Exclusively retrobulbar in 10%
- Size
  - Variable; small, superficial lesions rarely imaged
- Morphology
  - Ranges from lobular to infiltrative
    - Infiltrative pattern typical in postseptal component

CT Findings
- Well-circumscribed, lobulated mass with diffuse, intense contrast enhancement in proliferative phase (PP)
  - Prominent vessels in/adjacent to mass
  - No internal calcification or surrounding edema
  - Decreases with involution
- Progressive fatty infiltration of mass + decreased size in involuting phase (IP)

MR Findings
- T1: Iso- to slightly hyperintense to muscle in PP, hyperintense from fatty replacement during IP
  - Internal flow voids
- T2: Moderate signal intensity reflects high cellularity
  - **Flow voids** frequently visible
- T1 C+ FS: Diffuse, **intense enhancement in PP**
  - Enhancement may appear heterogeneous, particularly in involuting phase
- MRA: Generally not necessary for diagnosis but helpful in assessing associated arterial abnormalities in **PHACE** syndrome: **P**osterior fossa anomalies, **h**emangioma, **a**rterial, **c**ardiac, **e**ye
  - Stenosis, occlusion, agenesis, aneurysm of craniocervical vessels
- MPGR: Intralesional high-flow vessels

- DWI: ADC values are higher in infantile hemangiomas (IHs) vs. pediatric soft tissue malignancies
  - IH: $1.3\text{-}1.5 \times 10^{-3}$ mm²/sec
  - Sarcomas: $0.67\text{-}0.78 \times 10^{-3}$ mm²/sec

Ultrasonographic Findings
- Lobular soft tissue mass with high vessel density on color Doppler (> 5 vessels/cm²)
- High systolic Doppler shift (> 2 kHz): Many arterial tracings with low resistive index but no arterialized veins

Imaging Recommendations
- Best imaging tool
  - When small & superficial, US may be sufficient to confirm clinical diagnosis
  - MR best to map larger, deeper, more complex lesions
- Protocol advice
  - Enhanced MR in multiple planes with fat suppression best for tumor mapping

DIFFERENTIAL DIAGNOSIS

Rhabdomyosarcoma
- Rapidly progressive invasive orbital mass
- Bone destruction present when large
- Mean ADC value of rhabdomyosarcomas significantly lower compared with infantile hemangiomas

Metastatic Neuroblastoma
- Rapidly progressive osseous metastatic mass
  - Spiculated/sunburst periosteal reaction
- Predilection for greater sphenoid wing

Orbital Cellulitis
- Inflammatory changes ± abscess formation

Orbital Langerhans Cell Histiocytosis
- Well-defined, lytic bone lesion with enhancing soft tissue mass in children

Orbital Venolymphatic Malformation
- Fluid signal intensity mass with delayed/gradual patchy enhancement of venous component
- ± phleboliths in venous component
- Nonenhancing lymphatic components
- ± fluid-fluid levels

Plexiform Neurofibroma
- Infiltrative, contrast-enhancing mass + sphenoid dysplasia
- Plus other stigmata of neurofibromatosis type 1

Orbital Non-Hodgkin Lymphoma
- Multicompartmental, infiltrating mass

Orbital Leukemia
- Homogeneous masses that mold to orbital walls ± periosteal reaction, usually without frank bone destruction

PATHOLOGY

General Features
- Etiology
  - **Proliferation** of vascular endothelium

– Proposed theory: Clonal expansion of angioblasts with high expression of basic fibroblast growth factors & other angiogenesis markers
- ○ **Distinguish from vascular malformation**: Localized defect of vascular morphogenesis
  - – With quiescent endothelium
- Genetics
  - ○ Most cases sporadic
  - ○ Some associated with pleiotropic genetic syndromes
  - ○ Small percent autosomal dominant
- Associated abnormalities
  - ○ Large lesions may involve ectodermal structures of face, neck, & airway
    - – Parotid involvement common
  - ○ **PHACE** syndrome

Staging, Grading, & Classification

- Classification by location
  - ○ Deep: Within deep tissues of lid & anterior orbit, or entirely retrobulbar
  - ○ Superficial: Confined to dermis
  - ○ Combined: Both dermal & deep components
- Proliferating, involuting & involuted phases

Microscopic Features

- Prominent endothelial cells forming small vascular channels (PP), flat endothelial cells + fibrofatty replacement

Immunohistochemical Features

- GLUT-1 positive during all phases of proliferation & regression

CLINICAL ISSUES

Presentation

- Most common signs/symptoms
  - ○ Unilateral eyelid, brow, or nasal growing superficial soft tissue mass in young infant (PP)
  - ○ Ophthalmologic symptoms common: Amblyopia, astigmatism, proptosis, & decreased visual acuity
    - – Risk of amblyopia highest when diffuse, > 1 cm in size, & associated with PHACE syndrome
- Clinical profile
  - ○ Rubbery, soft mass
  - ○ **Reddish or strawberry-like discoloration of skin**
    - – **Blanche with pressure** (unlike port-wine stain)
    - – Occasionally deeper lesions show bluish skin
  - ○ Enlarge with Valsalva or crying in 50%
  - ○ Occasional periorbital fat excess following involution

Demographics

- Age
  - ○ Typically inapparent at birth; most appear within 1st few weeks; majority by 1-3 months
  - ○ Up to 1/3 nascent at birth (i.e., pale or erythematous macule, telangiectasia, pseudoecchymotic patch or red spot)
- Sex
  - ○ M:F = 1:2-3
  - ○ Even higher female predominance in genetic syndromes
- Epidemiology

- ○ Infantile hemangiomas all sites: Affects ~ 5% of neonates, up to 10% of premature infants

Natural History & Prognosis

- 3 distinct phases
  - ○ **PF**: Appears few weeks after birth & grows rapidly for year 1 or 2
  - ○ **Involuting phase**: Regression over several years
  - ○ **Involuted phase**: Usually complete regression by late childhood, 90% resolve by 9 years of age
- Distinguish from vascular malformations: Present at birth & grow in monophasic fashion with age
- Distinguish from noninvoluting congenital hemangioma (**NICH**) & rapidly involuting congenital hemangioma (**RICH**)
  - ○ Present at or before birth, GLUT1 negative

Treatment

- Expectant observation unless complications
- Indications for treatment
  - ○ Ophthalmologic: Visual disturbance, nerve compromise, proptosis
  - ○ Dermatologic: Ulceration, infection, cosmesis
- Propranolol (β-blocker) has replaced oral steroids as 1° therapy
- Corticosteroids: Intralesional, systemic, or topical

DIAGNOSTIC CHECKLIST

Consider

- Remember, differential diagnosis for rapidly growing mass in infant includes malignancy
  - ○ If imaging appearance, timeline, or physical exam findings are atypical for infantile hemangioma, exclude other lesions by biopsy

Image Interpretation Pearls

- US can provide easy bedside evaluation
- In appropriate age group, T2-hyperintense cellular, enhancing mass with prominent flow voids nearly diagnostic

Reporting Tips

- Map lesion with particular reference to critical structures in orbit & intracranial compartment

SELECTED REFERENCES

1. International Society for the Study of Vascular Anomalies: 2025 ISSVA Classification for Vascular Anomalies. Published 2018. Updated 2025. Accessed October 5, 2024. https://www.issva.org/classification
2. Soliman SE et al: Ophthalmic involvement in PHACES syndrome: prevalence, spectrum of anomalies, and outcomes. J AAPOS. 26(3):129.e1-7, 2022
3. Proisy M et al: PHACES syndrome and associated anomalies: risk associated with small and large facial hemangiomas. AJR Am J Roentgenol. 217(2):507-14, 2021
4. Mamlouk MD et al: Arterial spin-labeling perfusion for PHACE syndrome. AJNR Am J Neuroradiol. 42(1):173-7, 2020
5. Kralik SF et al: Orbital infantile hemangioma and rhabdomyosarcoma in children: differentiation using diffusion-weighted magnetic resonance imaging. J AAPOS. 22(1):27-31, 2018
6. Merrow AC et al: 2014 revised classification of vascular lesions from the International Society for the Study of Vascular Anomalies: radiologic-pathologic update. Radiographics. 36(5):1494-516, 2016
7. Meltzer DE et al: Enlargement of the internal auditory canal and associated posterior fossa anomalies in PHACES association. AJNR Am J Neuroradiol. 36(11):2159-62, 2015
8. Judd CD et al: Intracranial infantile hemangiomas associated with PHACE syndrome. AJNR Am J Neuroradiol. 28(1):25-9, 2007

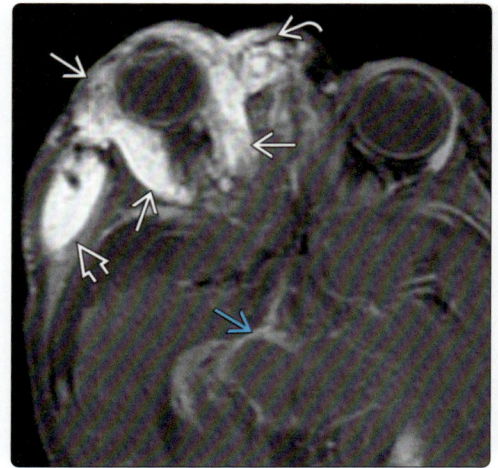

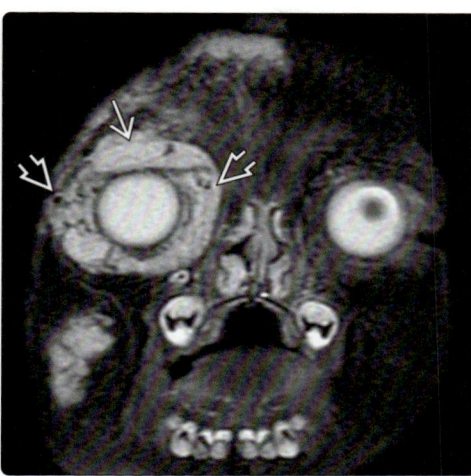

(Left) *Axial T1 C+ FS MR in a 3-month-old girl with PHACE syndrome shows an enhancing mass involving the preseptal and postseptal right orbit* ➡️. *There is involvement of the suprazygomatic masticator space* ➡️ *and the medial canthus* ➡️. *Abnormal enhancement at the surface of the midbrain may represent venous engorgement or an additional hemangioma* ➡️. (Right) *Coronal T2 FS MR in the same patient shows intermediate signal of the orbital hemangioma* ➡️. *There are flow voids* ➡️ *within the mass.*

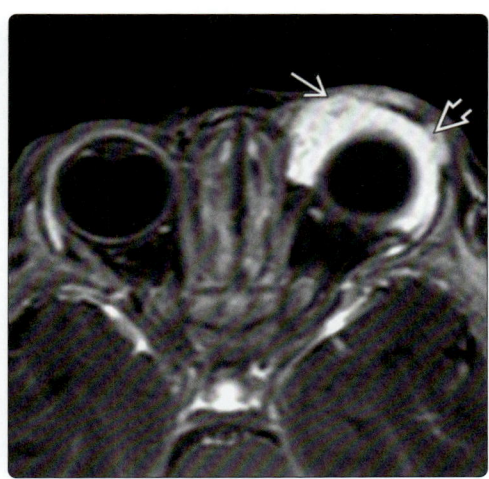

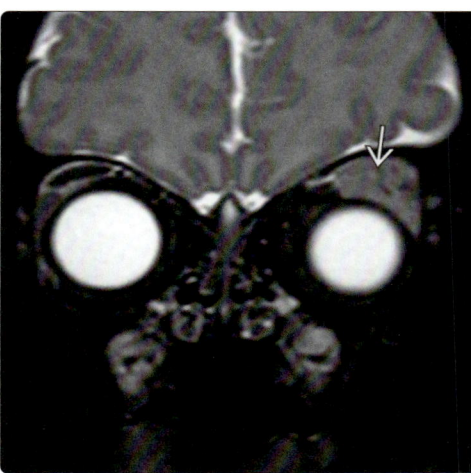

(Left) *Axial T1 C+ FS MR in a 1-month-old girl shows an intensely enhancing mass occupying the medial* ➡️ *and lateral* ➡️ *aspects of the left periorbital soft tissues. While the mass has postseptal extension, it remains extraconal. The globe is mildly displaced posteriorly.* (Right) *Coronal T2 FS MR in the same patient shows intermediate signal intensity of the orbital mass with abnormal flow voids* ➡️, *consistent with an orbital IH. There is downward displacement of the globe.*

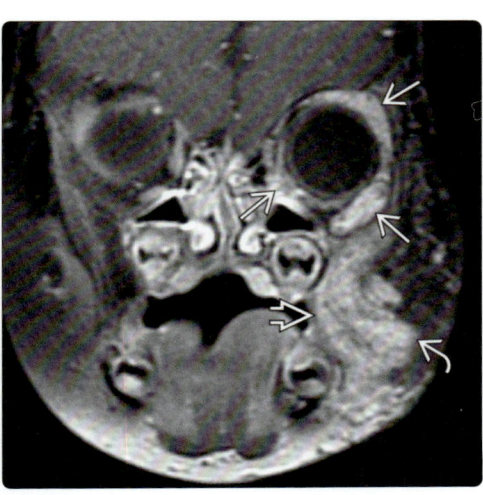

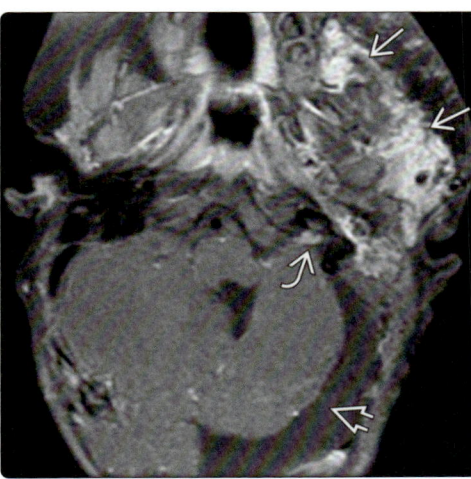

(Left) *Coronal T1 C+ FS MR in a 9-month-old girl with PHACE shows an enhancing mass circumferentially involving the left orbit* ➡️. *There are additional components of hemangioma in the left deep face involving the gingivobuccal* ➡️ *and parotid* ➡️ *spaces.* (Right) *Axial T1 C+ FS MR in the same patient shows the inferior extent of the tumor in the parotid and masticator spaces* ➡️. *There is ipsilateral cerebellar hypoplasia* ➡️ *and abnormal enhancement in the internal auditory canal* ➡️.

KEY FACTS

TERMINOLOGY

- Optic pathway glioma (OPG)
- Primary neuroglial tumor of optic pathway
- 3 broad subtypes
  - Childhood syndromic [neurofibromatosis type 1 (NF1)], childhood sporadic, adult

IMAGING

- Fusiform optic nerve (ON) mass with variable posterior pathway involvement
  - Sporadic lesions tend to be larger and cause more distortion of normal morphology than syndromic lesions
- MR is preferred imaging modality
  - Isointense to mildly hypointense on T1WI
  - Variably hyperintense on T2WI
  - Enhancement varies from minimal to intense
- Associated neuroimaging findings in NF1
  - Increased T2 foci in brain, other CNS tumors, sphenoid dysplasia, buphthalmos

TOP DIFFERENTIAL DIAGNOSES

- Optic neuritis
- ON sheath meningioma
- Idiopathic orbital inflammatory pseudotumor
- Sarcoidosis

PATHOLOGY

- Childhood OPG: Low-grade glioma
- Adult OPG: Anaplastic astrocytoma or glioblastoma multiforme

CLINICAL ISSUES

- Decreased vision, proptosis; often asymptomatic
- Childhood OPG: Onset 0.5-15.0 years
- 30-40% of patients with OPG have NF1
- 11-30% of patients with NF1 have OPG
- Natural history highly variable, but generally indolent in childhood OPG

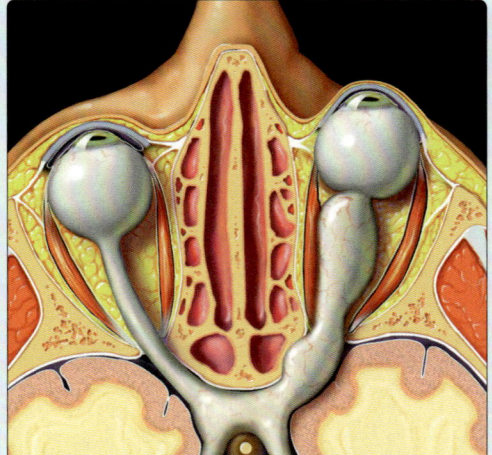
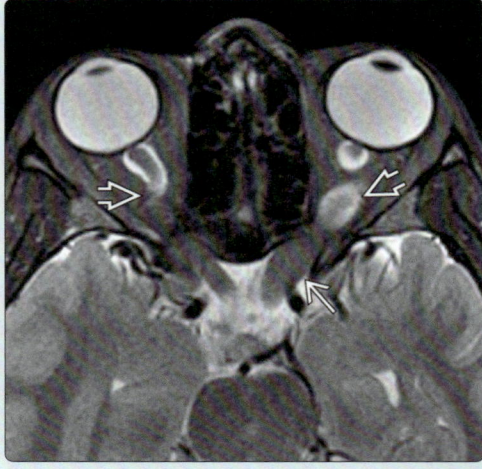

(Left) Axial graphic depicts a left optic pathway glioma (OPG) extending along the length of the intraorbital nerve, through the enlarged optic canal, and into the prechiasmatic segment. The fusiform pattern of enlargement is typical. (Right) Axial T2 MR in a 9-year-old girl with neurofibromatosis type 1 (NF1) and mild left proptosis shows abnormal thickening of the intracranial left optic nerve (ON) ➡, consistent with an ON glioma. There is bilateral tortuosity of the ON sheaths ➡; however, no right ON mass was visible.

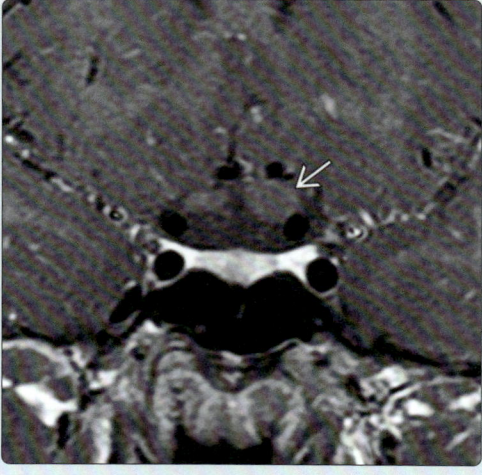
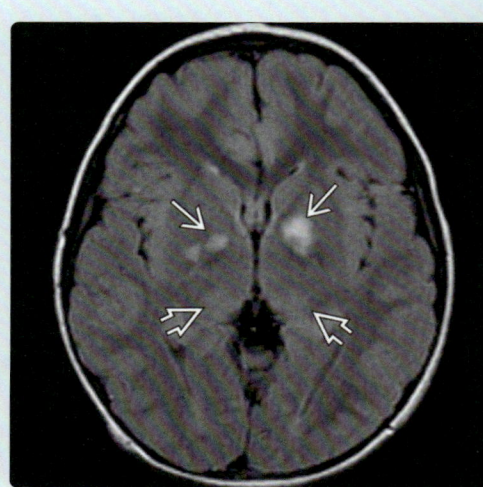

(Left) Coronal T1 C+ FS MR in the same patient shows abnormal thickening of the prechiasmatic portion of the left ON ➡. There is no abnormal enhancement of the affected segment of the left ON. (Right) Axial FLAIR MR in a 7-year-old child with NF1 shows typical hyperintense foci in the bilateral globus pallidus ➡ and thalamus ➡. When present in a patient with OPG, this supports the diagnosis of NF1. Lesions are also common in cerebellar white matter and the brainstem.

TERMINOLOGY

Abbreviations
- Optic pathway glioma (OPG)

Synonyms
- Optic nerve (ON) glioma; anterior visual pathway glioma

Definitions
- Primary neuroglial tumor of optic pathway
- 3 broad subtypes
  - Childhood benign tumors: **With** neurofibromatosis type 1 (**NF1**), syndromic 30-40%
  - Childhood benign tumors: **Without** NF1 (sporadic)
  - Adult tumors: Typically malignant

IMAGING

General Features
- Best diagnostic clue
  - Fusiform ON mass with variable posterior pathway involvement
- Location
  - **Childhood lesions with NF1 (syndromic)**
    - Anterior pathways, unilateral or bilateral
    - Bilateral highly associated with NF1
    - 50% extend to chiasm, hypothalamus, and retrochiasmal optic pathways
    - Optic radiation involvement is rare
  - **Childhood lesions without NF1 (sporadic)**
    - Chiasm and retrochiasmal segment > intraorbital ON
  - **Adult lesions**
    - Unilateral ON with posterior extension
- Morphology
  - General
    - Diffuse, **sausage-shaped or fusiform** enlargement of nerve and chiasm
    - Characteristic kinking or buckling of nerve
  - Syndromic: Smooth, tubular, tortuous ON enlargement
  - Sporadic: Smooth, nodular with cystic components
  - Adult: Diffuse ON enlargement, invasive features
- Associated neuroimaging findings if NF1 present: Increased T2 foci in brain, other CNS tumors, sphenoid dysplasia, buphthalmos, plexiform neurofibromas

CT Findings
- NECT
  - Isodense fusiform nerve enlargement; focal hypodensity if cystic spaces
- Bone CT
  - Calcification rare (unlike ON sheath meningioma)
  - Enlargement of bony optic canal if intracranial extension

MR Findings
- T1WI
  - Enlargement of portion, or all of ON, chiasm, &/or tract
  - Isointense to mildly hypointense compared to brain
  - Focal hypointensity if cystic spaces present
- T2WI
  - Signal is variable but moderate hyperintensity typical
  - Peripheral hyperintensity surrounding ON
    - Some authors believe this is perineural arachnoid gliomatosis (PAG), usually in NF1
  - Focally hyperintense cystic spaces of mucinous degeneration in sporadic cases
- DWI
  - Elevated mean ADC values have been demonstrated
- T1WI C+
  - Enhancement varies from minimal to intense
    - Syndromic: Often little enhancement
    - Sporadic: Often moderate to intense enhancement
    - Adult: Usually moderate heterogeneous enhancement
  - DCE MR: Increased mean permeability values demonstrated in clinically aggressive tumors

Imaging Recommendations
- Best imaging tool
  - MR is preferred imaging modality
    - Defines involvement of proximal optic pathways
    - Allows assessment of related intracranial findings in patients with NF1

DIFFERENTIAL DIAGNOSIS

Optic Neuritis
- Acute-onset pain and vision loss
- Enhancing ON with minimal nerve enlargement

Optic Nerve Sheath Meningioma
- Slow-onset proptosis and decreased vision in adult
- Perineural mass, may be calcified

Idiopathic Orbital Inflammatory Pseudotumor
- Painful proptosis, mass-like inflammation
- Can involve any structure in orbit
- Variable imaging appearance, including perineural enhancement

Sarcoidosis
- Systemic illness, orbital inflammation
- Predilection for lacrimal gland
- ON, orbital, and intracranial enhancement

PATHOLOGY

General Features
- Genetics
  - NF1 (if present): Autosomal dominant with variable penetrance and variable clinical expressivity
  - *BRAF* duplication and MAPK pathway activation common
- Associated abnormalities
  - Focal brain T2/FLAIR hyperintensities in NF1 patients
    - Seen in 80-90% of NF1 patients who have OPG
    - Seen in 50-70% of all NF1 patients
  - Other CNS tumors in NF1 patients (most commonly low-grade astrocytoma)
  - Recent advanced MR techniques are exploring abnormal subventricular zone of 3rd ventricle as origin of OPG

Staging, Grading, & Classification
- Low-grade gliomas
  - Vast majority of childhood lesions
  - 60% WHO grade 1 pilocytic astrocytoma

- 40% WHO grade 2 fibrillary astrocytoma
- High-grade gliomas
  - Most adult lesions, occasionally childhood lesions
  - Anaplastic astrocytoma, glioblastoma multiforme
- Dodge classification defines locoregional extent of tumor
  - Stage A: Limited to 1 ON
  - Stage B: Involves chiasm ± ON
  - Stage C: Extends toward hypothalamus or posterior visual pathways

Gross Pathologic & Surgical Features

- Diffuse ON enlargement; tan-white tumor
- Cystic component: Mucinous degeneration or infarction

Microscopic Features

- Circumferential perineural infiltration with arachnoid gliomatosis, usually with NF1
  - Central nerve sparing (relatively preserved vision)
- Sporadic: Expansile intraneural infiltration

CLINICAL ISSUES

Presentation

- Most common signs/symptoms
  - Decreased vision
- Other signs/symptoms
  - Proptosis, optic atrophy
  - Nystagmus
  - Intracranial mass effect
- Clinical profile
  - Childhood OPG
    - Syndromic: Frequently asymptomatic; lesions detected on routine imaging
    - Sporadic: Larger, more aggressive
  - Adult OPG
    - Aggressive course with rapid deterioration of vision

Demographics

- Age
  - Childhood: Onset 0.5-15.0 years (mean: 5 years)
  - Adult: Onset 20-80 years (mean: 50 years)
- Sex
  - Slight female predominance in childhood OPG
- Epidemiology
  - Childhood benign lesions
    - 3% of orbital tumors; 5% of intracranial tumors
    - 30-40% of patients with OPG have NF1
    - 11-30% of patients with NF1 have OPG
  - Adult malignant lesions: Very rare

Natural History & Prognosis

- Natural history highly variable
  - Ranges from spontaneous regression to progressive visual and neurologic impairment, culminating in death
- Syndromic: Generally indolent course, progression typically stops by age 6, though can continue to age 12
  - Progression most frequent first 2 years following diagnosis
  - Spontaneous regression can occur
- Sporadic: Less indolent, more intervention required
  - Shorter time to relapse
- Adult: Poor prognosis, rapidly fatal

- Specific location impacts prognosis
  - Rate of complications and death
    - Optic chiasm/retrochiasmal gliomas > ON gliomas

Treatment

- Childhood lesions with NF1
  - Biopsy generally not required; **presumptive diagnosis**
  - Observation unless vision threatened
  - Chemotherapy is 1st line for tumor progression
  - Radiation therapy (XRT) and surgery reserved for patients with bulky tumor or older children with progressive disease
    - XRT complications: Secondary tumors, radiation necrosis, moyamoya disease, impaired growth, cognitive deficits
- Childhood lesions without NF1
  - Biopsy typically indicated
  - Surgical debulking for large tumors when there is severe visual loss and proptosis
  - Adjunctive XRT, including proton therapy ± chemotherapy
- Adult OPG
  - Multimodality therapy

DIAGNOSTIC CHECKLIST

Consider

- Clinical and imaging features vary with specific subtype: Syndromic, sporadic, adult
- Bilateral intraorbital lesions indicate syndrome (NF1)

SELECTED REFERENCES

1. Chen Y et al: An overview of optic pathway glioma with neurofibromatosis type 1: pathogenesis, risk factors, and therapeutic strategies. Invest Ophthalmol Vis Sci. 65(6):8, 2024
2. Packer RJ: Optic pathway gliomas: long-term outcomes and challenges. Neuro Oncol. 26(7):1325-6, 2024
3. Boonzaier NR et al: Quantitative MRI demonstrates abnormalities of the third ventricle subventricular zone in neurofibromatosis type-1 and sporadic paediatric optic pathway glioma. Neuroimage Clin. 28:102447, 2020
4. Pisapia JM et al: Predicting pediatric optic pathway glioma progression using advanced magnetic resonance image analysis and machine learning. Neurooncol Adv. 2(1):vdaa090, 2020
5. de Blank PMK et al: Optic pathway gliomas in neurofibromatosis type 1: an update: surveillance, treatment indications, and biomarkers of vision. J Neuroophthalmol. 37 Suppl 1:S23-32, 2017
6. Friedrich RE et al: Optic pathway glioma and cerebral focal abnormal signal intensity in patients with neurofibromatosis type 1: characteristics, treatment choices and follow-up in 134 affected individuals and a brief review of the literature. Anticancer Res. 36(8):4095-121, 2016
7. Aquilina K et al: Optic pathway glioma in children: does visual deficit correlate with radiology in focal exophytic lesions? Childs Nerv Syst. 31(11):2041-9, 2015
8. Shofty B et al: The effect of chemotherapy on optic pathway gliomas and their sub-components: a volumetric MR analysis study. Pediatr Blood Cancer. 62(8):1353-9, 2015
9. Rodriguez FJ et al: BRAF duplications and MAPK pathway activation are frequent in gliomas of the optic nerve proper. J Neuropathol Exp Neurol. 71(9):789-94, 2012
10. Nicolin G et al: Natural history and outcome of optic pathway gliomas in children. Pediatr Blood Cancer. 53(7):1231-7, 2009
11. Jost SC et al: Diffusion-weighted and dynamic contrast-enhanced imaging as markers of clinical behavior in children with optic pathway glioma. Pediatr Radiol. 38(12):1293-9, 2008
12. Pereira LS et al: Perineural arachnoidal gliomatosis: case report. Arq Bras Oftalmol. 71(4):595-8, 2008
13. Zeid JL et al: Orbital optic nerve gliomas in children with neurofibromatosis type 1. J AAPOS. 10(6):534-9, 2006

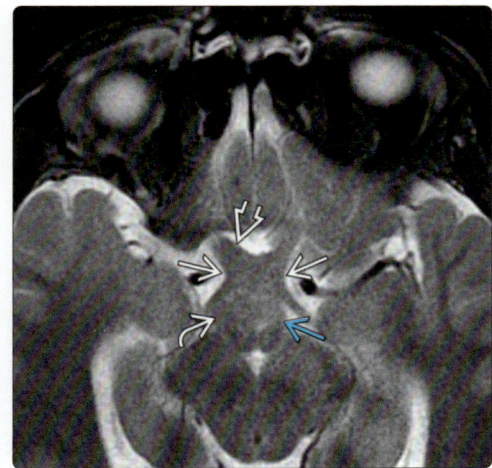

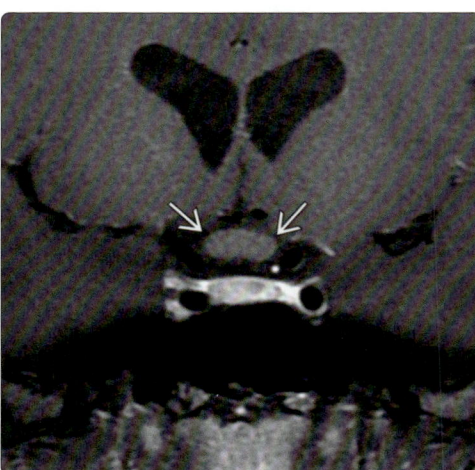

(Left) Axial T2 FS MR in an 12-year-old girl with NF1 shows diffuse, bilateral enlargement of the optic chiasm ➡ and the right prechiasmatic ON ➡. The angle of this image allows visualization of tumor involving the right hypothalamus in the area of the tuber cinereum ➡. Note the contralateral normal tuber cinereum ➡. (Right) Coronal T1 C+ FS MR in the same patient shows diffuse, nonenhancing expansion of the optic chiasm ➡.

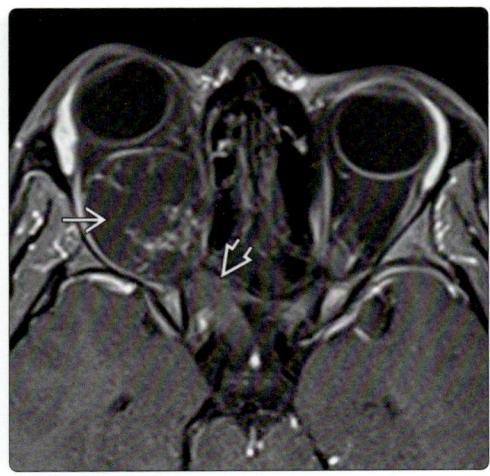

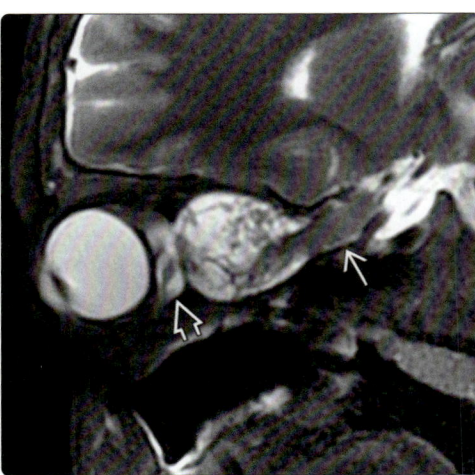

(Left) Axial T1 C+ FS MR in a 17-year-old boy with NF1 demonstrates a heterogeneously enhancing mass in the intraorbital portion of the right ON ➡. There is a relatively nonenhancing component extending through the optic canal ➡. (Right) Oblique sagittal T2 FS MR in the same patient shows the mass to be heterogeneously hyperintense with relatively hypointense signal intensity where it passes through the optic canal ➡. There is ectasia of the ON sheath more anteriorly ➡.

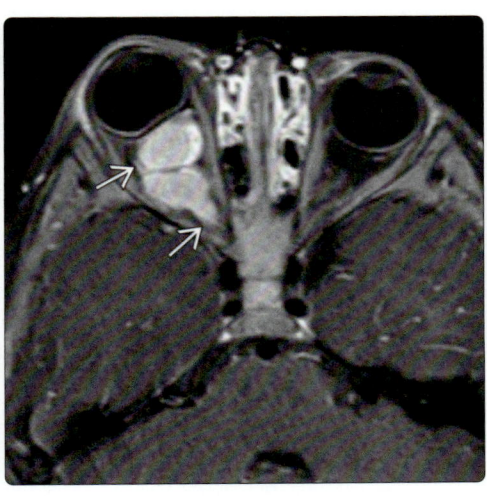

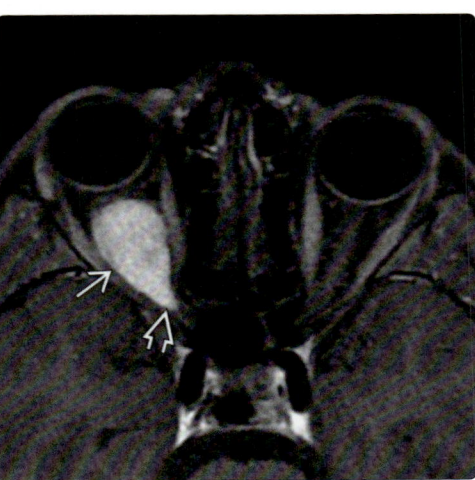

(Left) Axial T1 C+ FS MR in a 2-year-old with NF1 shows diffuse enlargement, tortuosity, and contrast enhancement involving the entire intraorbital right ON ➡, resulting in flattening of the posterior aspect of the globe and proptosis. (Right) Axial T1 C+ FS MR in a 10-year-old boy without NF1 but who has proptosis and decreased vision in the right eye shows diffuse enlargement and enhancement of the intraorbital ➡ and intracanalicular ➡ segments of the right ON.

Optic Nerve Sheath Meningioma

TERMINOLOGY

- Optic nerve sheath meningioma
  - a.k.a. perioptic meningioma
- Benign, slow-growing tumor of optic nerve sheath
- Distinct entity from intracranial (sphenoorbital) meningioma that extends through orbital apex

IMAGING

- Uniformly enhancing mass surrounding intraorbital optic nerve with calcification in 1/3 to 1/2 of cases
- Tram-track pattern of enhancement or calcification around optic nerve
- Variably hyperintense to hypointense on T2WI

TOP DIFFERENTIAL DIAGNOSES

- Optic nerve glioma
- Orbital pseudotumor
- Orbital sarcoidosis
- Metastasis
- Orbit lymphoproliferative lesions

PATHOLOGY

- Benign tumor arising from arachnoid "cap" cells within optic nerve sheath
- Histologic subtypes and degree of calcification affect signal intensity on T2WI MR

CLINICAL ISSUES

- Classic triad: Visual loss, optic atrophy, optociliary venous shunting
- Fractionated radiotherapy currently 1st-line therapy; radiosurgery also being explored

DIAGNOSTIC CHECKLIST

- MR is preferred imaging modality, but look for calcification on CT when diagnosis in doubt
- Look for other findings of neurofibromatosis type 2, especially in pediatric patients

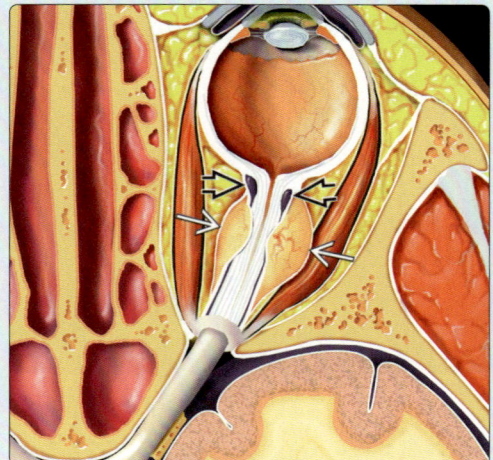
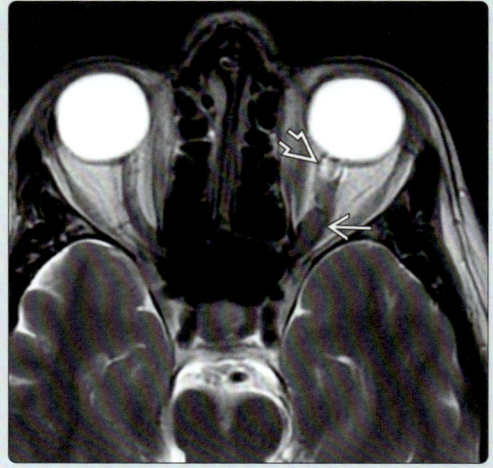

(Left) Axial graphic depicts a fusiform meningioma ➡ arising from the optic nerve (ON) sheath. A characteristic perioptic cyst ➡ behind the globe represents trapped CSF within the nerve sheath. (Right) Axial T2 MR in a 50-year-old woman with progressive, painless vision loss shows a fusiform mass extending along the ON sheath ➡. There is relative sparing of the anterior segment of the optic nerve sheath complex, posterior to the globe, with small areas of trapped CSF ➡.

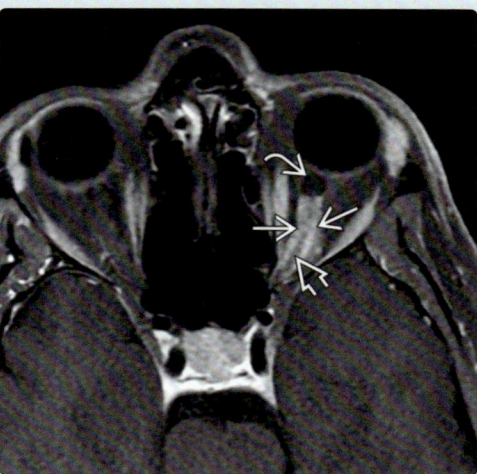
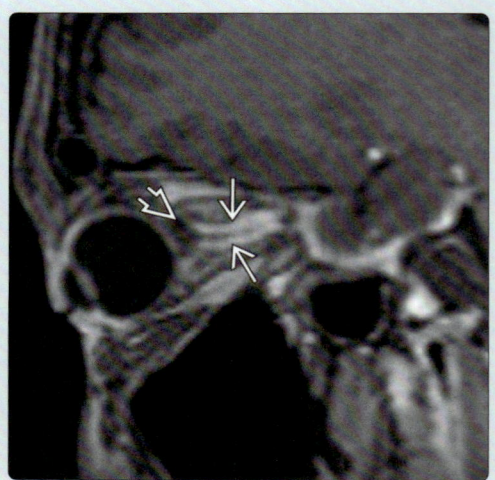

(Left) Axial T1+ FS MR in the same patient shows enhancement of the thickened sheath ➡, sparing the nerve ➡. Again seen are small areas of trapped CSF posterior to the globe ➡. (Right) Reformatted oblique sagittal T1+ FS MR in the same patient shows curvilinear enhancement along the ON sheath ➡. There is relative sparing of the anterior segment of the optic nerve sheath complex, posterior to the globe, with adjacent trapped CSF ➡.

TERMINOLOGY

Abbreviations
- Optic nerve sheath meningioma (ONSM)

Synonyms
- Perioptic meningioma

Definitions
- Benign, slow-growing neoplasm of optic nerve (ON) dural sheath
- Distinct entity from intracranial (sphenoorbital) meningioma that extends through orbital apex
  - 90% of meningiomas that involve orbit are secondary lesions rather than primary ONSM

IMAGING

General Features
- Best diagnostic clue
  - Enhancing mass surrounding intraorbital ON with calcification
- Location
  - Intraconal or orbital apex mass that arises from ON sheath complex
- Size
  - Intraorbital ONSM relatively small at presentation because of early symptoms
  - Sphenoorbital tumors typically have larger intracranial component
- Morphology
  - Solid, well-defined enlargement of ON sheath
  - Encases ON in circumferential pattern but may be eccentric or pedunculated
  - Tubular shape (65%) > pedunculated (25%) > fusiform (10%)
    - Diffuse thickening more common than segmental
    - En plaque variants may occur

CT Findings
- NECT
  - Linear or punctate calcification seen in 1/3-1/2 cases
    - Typically spares distal ON at nerve head insertion
  - If no calcification, tumor is isodense to other soft tissue
- CECT
  - Uniform, moderately intense enhancement
  - **Tram-track** appearance: Tumor enhancement or calcification around ON
    - Although relatively specific, tram-track enhancement **not** pathognomonic
      - □ Pseudotumor, lymphoma, and sarcoid may have peripheral perioptic enhancement

MR Findings
- T1WI
  - Isointense to other soft tissue
- T2WI
  - Variably hyperintense to hypointense depending on degree of calcification and histologic subtype
  - **Perioptic cysts** are specific feature
    - Defined as increased CSF within nerve sheath surrounding distal ON between tumor and globe

- STIR
  - Similar to T2 but lesions more conspicuous because of suppression of orbital fat signal
- T1WI C+
  - Uniform moderate to marked enhancement of tumor with central nonenhancing ON
  - Tumor best demonstrated with fat suppression

Imaging Recommendations
- Best imaging tool
  - Contrast-enhanced MR with fat suppression
    - MR better than CT for characterizing tumor relative to adjacent orbital structures
    - MR best shows extent of disease involving orbital apex, optic canal, ON chiasm, and intracranial structures
  - CT better demonstrates calcification in indeterminate cases
  - 68Ga-DOTATATE-PET may be useful to confirm diagnosis
- Protocol advice
  - Postcontrast, fat-suppressed T1WI delineates tumor margins best
  - Perioptic cysts best demonstrated on T2WI with fat saturation

DIFFERENTIAL DIAGNOSIS

Optic Pathway Glioma
- Fusiform enlargement of ON
  - Variable contrast enhancement
- No tram-track enhancement, calcification, or perioptic cysts
- Typically low-grade pediatric tumor (ONSM usually adult tumor)
- May be associated with neurofibromatosis type 1 (NF1); ONSM associated with NF2

Optic Neuritis
- T2-hyperintense, enhancing ON with minimal nerve enlargement or patchy sheath enhancement
- Often associated with inflammatory and demyelinating processes, such as multiple sclerosis

Orbital Idiopathic Inflammatory Pseudotumor
- Ill defined and usually not isolated to ON sheath
  - May involve many of intraorbital structures: Extraocular muscles, ON sheath, lacrimal glands, globe, &/or orbital apex
- Presents with painful exophthalmos

Orbital Sarcoidosis
- When no systemic disease, can be indistinguishable from ONSM on enhanced CT and MR
- Predilection for lacrimal glands

Metastasis
- Breast and lung most common primaries
- Often involve choroid and extraocular muscles

Orbit Lymphoproliferative Lesions
- Usually not isolated to ON sheath
- Typically well-defined, pliable mass
- Decreased T2 signal due to high cellularity

PATHOLOGY

General Features

- Etiology
  - Benign tumor arising from **arachnoid "cap" cells** within ON sheath
- Genetics
  - **NF2** present in 4-12% of patients
    - 28% of juveniles diagnosed with ONSM are concomitantly diagnosed with NF2
- Associated abnormalities
  - Patients with NF2 show other characteristic findings, such as bilateral vestibular schwannoma
    - Multiple inherited schwannomas, meningiomas, and ependymomas

Staging, Grading, & Classification

- Same WHO classification as for intracranial meningiomas
  - Majority WHO grade 1 but varies depending on meningioma subtype

Gross Pathologic & Surgical Features

- Sharply circumscribed, unencapsulated
- Circumferential to ON
- Tightly adherent to perineural pial microvascular structures
  - Rarely invades ON

Microscopic Features

- Histologic features similar to intracranial meningiomas
  - Multiple meningioma subtypes
  - WHO grades 1-3, majority WHO grade 1
- Meningothelial subtype most common in orbit
- Transitional (54%) and meningotheliomatous (38%) subtypes most common in children
- Positive for progesterone receptors in 40-80%
  - More common in women
- Fibroblastic and transitional subtypes tend to be hypointense to cerebral cortex on T2WI MR

CLINICAL ISSUES

Presentation

- Most common signs/symptoms
  - Slow, usually painless progressive unilateral vision loss and proptosis
  - Central vision preserved until late in disease
- Other signs/symptoms
  - Diplopia, transient visual obscuration, headache
  - Funduscopic examination
    - Optic disc pallor and swelling typical
    - Optociliary venous shunting in association with optic disc changes very suggestive of ONSM
- Clinical profile
  - Classic triad
    - Visual loss, optic atrophy, optocilliary venous shunting

Demographics

- Age
  - Broad age range, typically 4th and 5th decades
  - ONSM in juvenile patients has distinct natural history
    - Average age at presentation: 10 years
    - More likely associated with NF2

- Sex
  - F:M ~ 2:1 to 4:1
    - In children, slightly more common in boys
- Epidemiology
  - ~ 5% of primary orbital tumors
  - Only 2% of meningiomas are ONSM
  - Radiation exposure, hereditary predisposition, and hormonal influence are cited risk factors

Natural History & Prognosis

- Progressive but slow vision loss expected in most untreated patients
- More aggressive behavior in juvenile patients
  - Relative increased size, growth, recurrence rates, and incidence of malignant degeneration
- Postoperative visual impairment inevitable as tumor tightly adherent to pia and shares blood supply

Treatment

- **Fractionated stereotactic radiotherapy** (and more recently radiosurgery) used when vision still present but visual loss progressive
- Observation with regular visual testing and MR surveillance recommended if vision normal and stable
- Surgical excision indicated if intracranial extension or if vision preservation impossible
  - Generally poor results with optic canal or ON sheath decompression

DIAGNOSTIC CHECKLIST

Consider

- ON glioma is major differential consideration in young patients
- When imaging appearance characteristic, radiation therapy without biopsy may provide best chance of vision preservation

Image Interpretation Pearls

- MR is preferred imaging modality for tumor assessment
  - CT shows calcification when diagnosis in doubt

SELECTED REFERENCES

1. Tang T et al: The treatment efficacy of radiotherapy for optic nerve sheath meningioma. Eye (Lond). 38(1):89-94, 2024
2. Vosoughi AR et al: Presumed optic nerve sheath meningioma presenting with relapsing-remitting course and periorbital pain. J Neuroophthalmol. 44(1):e103-4, 2024
3. Horowitz T et al: Optic nerve sheath meningiomas: solving diagnostic challenges with (68)Ga-DOTATOC PET/CT. Diagnostics (Basel). 13(13):2307, 2023
4. Zohdy YM et al: A compartmentalized classification for sphenoorbital meningiomas. World Neurosurg. 182:217-8, 2023
5. Arnold AC et al: Dilation of the perioptic subarachnoid space anterior to optic nerve sheath meningioma. J Neuroophthalmol. 41(1):e100-2, 2020
6. Interlandi E et al: Optical coherence tomography angiography findings in optic nerve sheath meningioma. Case Rep Ophthalmol. 11(2):364-9, 2020
7. Vanikieti K et al: Pediatric primary optic nerve sheath meningioma. Int Med Case Rep J. 8:159-63, 2015
8. Shapey J et al: Diagnosis and management of optic nerve sheath meningiomas. J Clin Neurosci. 20(8):1045-56, 2013
9. Milker-Zabel S et al: Fractionated stereotactic radiation therapy in the management of primary optic nerve sheath meningiomas. J Neurooncol. 94(3):419-24, 2009
10. Jackson A et al: Intracanalicular optic nerve meningioma: a serious diagnostic pitfall. AJNR Am J Neuroradiol. 24(6):1167-70, 2003

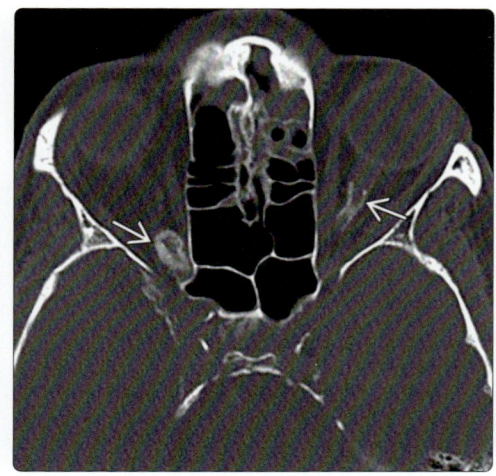

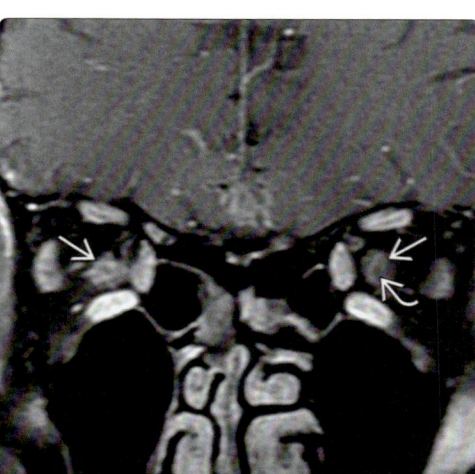

(Left) *Axial bone CT in a 70-year-old man with visual deficits and suspected stroke demonstrates tram-track calcifications along the bilateral intraorbital ON sheaths ➡. (Right) Coronal T1 C+ FS MR in the same patient shows concentric enhancement of the ON sheaths ➡, corresponding to the CT calcifications, consistent with bilateral ON sheath meningioma. There is no significant enhancement of the ONs, located centrally ➡ within the thickened, enhancing sheaths.*

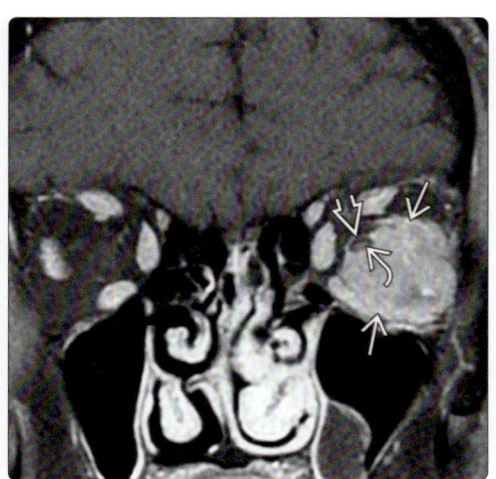

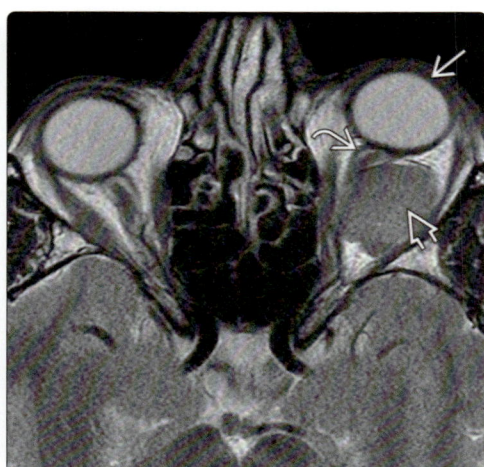

(Left) *Coronal T1 C+ FS MR in a 40-year-old man with progressive left proptosis and blurry vision shows an enhancing mass ➡ arising from the ON sheath. Note the spared CSF ➡ and ON ➡. (Right) Axial T2 MR in the same patient shows proptosis ➡ due to the eccentric ON sheath mass ➡. There is sparing of the anterior segment of the nerve and sheath ➡. This ON sheath meningioma (ONSM) has intermediate T2 signal intensity, similar to gray matter.*

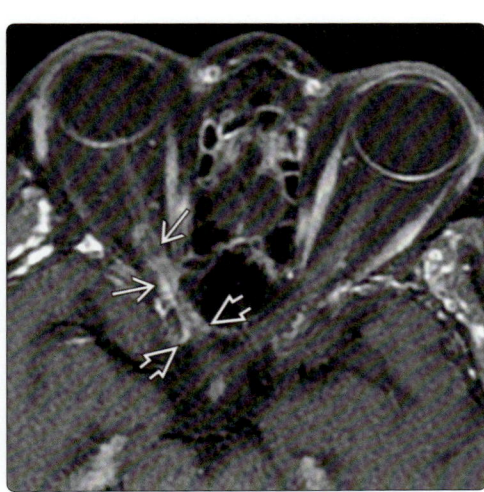

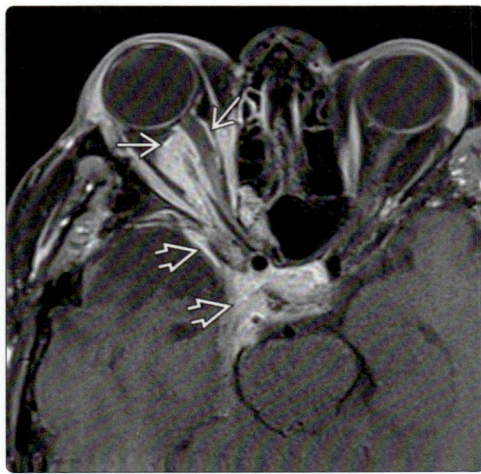

(Left) *Axial T1 C+ FS MR in a 65-year-old woman with progressive right vision loss shows thin linear enhancement of the ON sheath ➡ extending through the optic canal to involve the prechiasmatic ON ➡. (Right) T1C+ FS MR in a 56-year-old woman shows intraorbital tumor involving the ON sheath ➡. There is an intracranial component in the cavernous sinus area ➡. It is difficult to say if this is an ONSM that extended intracranially or a sphenoorbital meningioma involving the orbit.*

Lacrimal Gland Pleomorphic Adenoma

TERMINOLOGY

- Pleomorphic adenoma (PA) of lacrimal gland
  - a.k.a. benign mixed tumor
- Benign epithelial neoplasm of lacrimal gland

IMAGING

- Unilateral circumscribed lacrimal fossa mass with **scalloped bony remodeling**
- Anterior superotemporal extraconal orbit
  - Majority originate in orbital lobe of lacrimal gland
- CT: Mild heterogeneity; occasional punctate calcifications
- MR: Iso- to hyperintense T2 MR signal; ↑ ADC map value
- Moderate to marked enhancement on CECT and T1 MR

TOP DIFFERENTIAL DIAGNOSES

- Lacrimal gland lymphoproliferative lesion
- Lacrimal gland carcinoma
- Orbital dermoid/epidermoid
- Orbital idiopathic inflammatory pseudotumor

- Dacryoadenitis
- Lacrimal cyst

CLINICAL ISSUES

- Most common lacrimal gland tumor
  - Up to 90% of benign tumors of lacrimal gland
  - Up to 50% of primary epithelial tumors of lacrimal gland
- Cumulative low risk of malignant transformation
  - 5% at 10 years; 10% at 20 years; 20% at 30 years
  - Carcinoma ex PA accounts for ~ 10% of lacrimal gland carcinoma
- Occurs in 2nd to 5th decades
- Presents with slowly progressive, painless proptosis
- Complete surgical excision is curative
  - If capsular disruption, need long-term follow-up

DIAGNOSTIC CHECKLIST

- Scalloped bony remodeling on CT is characteristic
- Small cystic elements may be seen on CT or MR

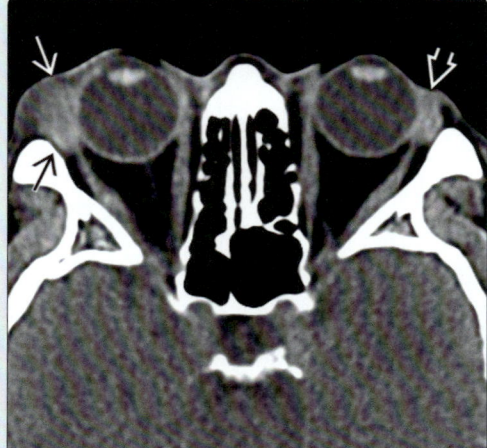
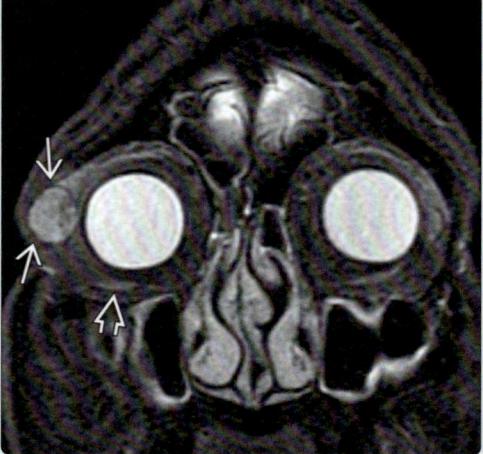

(Left) Axial NECT in a 40-year-old man with prior trauma and a suspected hematic cyst of the right orbit shows the right lacrimal gland is enlarged ➡ and relatively hypodense to the normal left lacrimal gland ➡. There is subtle scalloping of the lateral orbital wall ➡. Pathology showed a pleomorphic adenoma (PA). (Right) Coronal T2 FS MR in the same patient shows a well-circumscribed mass in the palpebral portion of the lacrimal gland ➡. Mass has a mildly "bosselated" shape, reminiscent of parotid PA, and is isointense to muscle ➡.

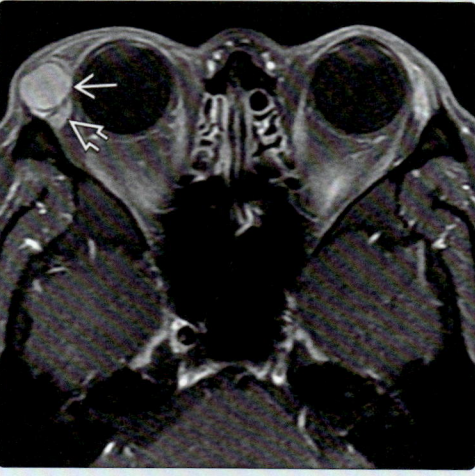
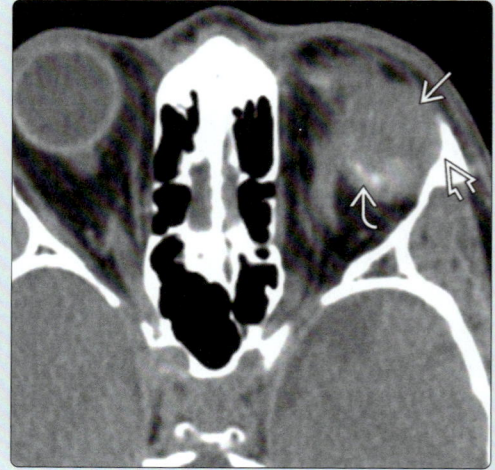

(Left) Axial T1 C+ FS MR in the same patient shows brisk enhancement of the well-circumscribed and mildly bosselated lacrimal gland mass ➡. The enhancement is similar to the adjacent lacrimal gland tissue ➡. (Right) Axial NECT shows a well-defined, lobular mass of the left lacrimal gland ➡ with internal calcifications ➡ and slight osseous scalloping of the lateral orbital wall ➡ in this case of a PA. Note that internal calcifications are not pathognomonic for a PA.

Lacrimal Gland Pleomorphic Adenoma

TERMINOLOGY

Abbreviations
- Pleomorphic adenoma (PA) of lacrimal gland

Synonyms
- Benign mixed tumor of lacrimal gland

Definitions
- Benign epithelial neoplasm of lacrimal gland

IMAGING

General Features
- Best diagnostic clue
  - Unilateral lacrimal mass with scalloped bony remodeling
- Location
  - Anterior **superotemporal extraconal** orbit
    - Majority originate in orbital lobe of gland
- Morphology
  - Solid, round or oval, circumscribed

CT Findings
- CECT
  - Moderate to marked enhancement
  - Small cystic elements common
- Bone CT
  - Soft tissue mass, **remodeling** of **lacrimal fossa**
  - Occasional punctate calcification (33%)

MR Findings
- T1WI
  - Hypointense to isointense compared to muscle; mild heterogeneity
- T2WI
  - Isointense to hyperintense compared to muscle
  - ↑ conspicuity of cystic elements
- DWI
  - Higher ADC value favors PA over malignancy
- T1WI C+
  - Moderate to marked enhancement

Imaging Recommendations
- Best imaging tool
  - Enhanced MR to confirm circumscribed nature
  - Coronal bone CT to assess bony remodeling

DIFFERENTIAL DIAGNOSIS

Orbital Lymphoproliferative Lesions
- Homogeneous enlargement of gland; molds around globe
- ↑ density on NECT; ↓ T2 MR signal; ↓ ADC map value; homogeneous enhancement

Lacrimal Gland Carcinoma
- Ill-defined margins, invasion of adjacent bone/soft tissue
- Imaging features can be nonspecific

Orbital Dermoid and Epidermoid
- Well-circumscribed, extraconal, at frontozygomatic suture
- DWI high signal if epidermoid; presence of fat = dermoid; scalloping of adjacent bone

Orbital Idiopathic Inflammatory Pseudotumor
- Palpably enlarged, tender gland
- Diffuse anterior-posterior enlargement of gland with stranding of fat at margins

Dacryoadenitis
- Tender, enlarged gland often with overlying cellulitis
- Infiltration and stranding in surrounding fat

Lacrimal Cyst
- Well-defined, fluid density/signal within parenchyma

PATHOLOGY

Staging, Grading, & Classification
- Follows WHO classification for salivary neoplasms

Microscopic Features
- "Pleomorphic": Diverse epithelial and myoepithelial components

CLINICAL ISSUES

Presentation
- Most common signs/symptoms
  - Slowly progressive painless proptosis
  - Inferomedial globe displacement

Demographics
- Age
  - 2nd to 5th decades
    - Generally younger age than malignant neoplasms
- Epidemiology
  - **~ 1-2%** of orbital tumors; most common epithelial neoplasm of lacrimal gland

Natural History & Prognosis
- Cumulative low risk of malignant transformation
  - 5% at 10 years; 10% at 20 years; 20% at 30 years
  - Carcinoma ex pleomorphic adenoma may be any type, but adenocarcinoma, not otherwise specified and mucoepidermoid most common

Treatment
- Complete surgical excision is curative
  - Lateral orbitotomy for wide exposure
  - Intact removal without rupture or incision
    - Capsular disruption requires long-term follow-up for possible seeding, which may lead to recurrence with risk of malignancy

DIAGNOSTIC CHECKLIST

Image Interpretation Pearls
- Scalloped bony remodeling is characteristic but not pathognomonic

SELECTED REFERENCES

1. Aryasit O et al: Clinical characteristics, radiologic features, and histopathology of biopsied lacrimal gland tumors. Sci Rep. 13(1):16615, 2023
2. Fakhril-Din Z et al: Adenocarcinoma in situ (ductal type) ex pleomorphic adenoma of the lacrimal gland. Am J Ophthalmol Case Rep. 31:101855, 2023

TERMINOLOGY

- Retinoblastoma (RB)
- Malignant primary retinal neoplasm
- Trilateral/quadrilateral RB: Bilateral ocular RB plus pineal ± suprasellar tumors

IMAGING

- Unilateral in 60%, bilateral in 40%
- Trilateral or quadrilateral disease rare
- **Extraocular extension** in **< 10%**
  - Indicates poor prognosis
- CT: **Calcification** in **> 90%**
- MR: Assess extent of intraocular tumor and presence of optic nerve, orbital, or intracranial involvement
  - T1: Mild hyperintensity
  - T2: Moderate to marked hypointensity
  - Moderate to marked heterogeneous enhancement

TOP DIFFERENTIAL DIAGNOSES

- Persistent hyperplastic primary vitreous
- Coats disease
- Retinopathy of prematurity
- Orbital toxocariasis

PATHOLOGY

- **Primitive neuroectodermal tumor**
- Inherited (germline): Multilateral > unilateral

CLINICAL ISSUES

- Most common intraocular tumor of childhood
- **Leukocoria** in 50-60%
- 90-95% diagnosed by age 5 years

DIAGNOSTIC CHECKLIST

- Calcified intraocular mass in child is RB until proven otherwise

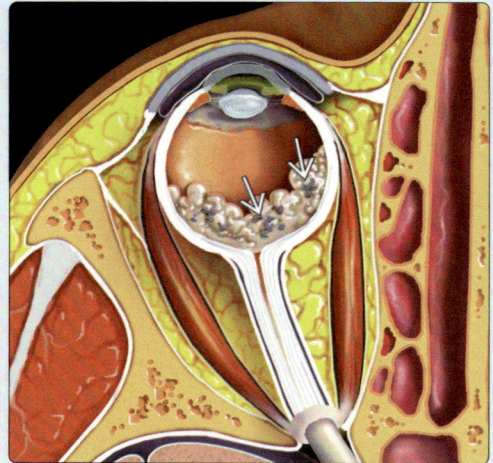
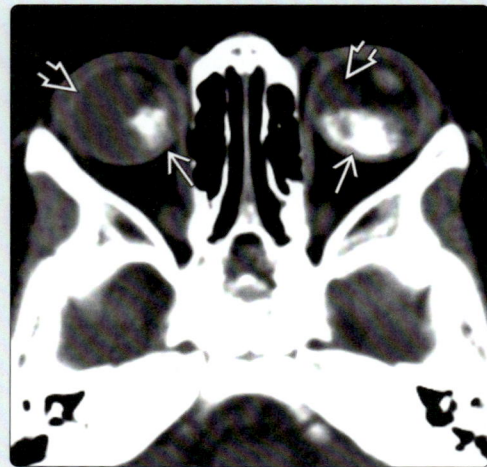

(Left) *Axial graphic depicts retinoblastoma (RB) with lobulated tumor extending through the limiting membrane into the vitreous. Punctate Ca++ ➡ are characteristic.* (Right) *Axial NECT in a 14-month-old with decreased vision and falling while ambulating shows bilateral, intraocular, partially calcified masses ➡, consistent with RB. Intraocular areas of intermediate attenuation ⇨ may represent noncalcified portions of the mass or mildly hyperdense subretinal or vitreous fluid.*

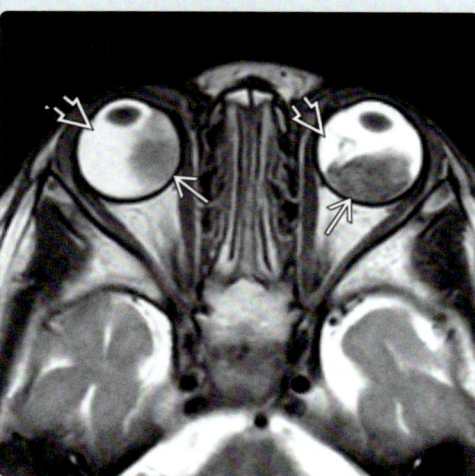
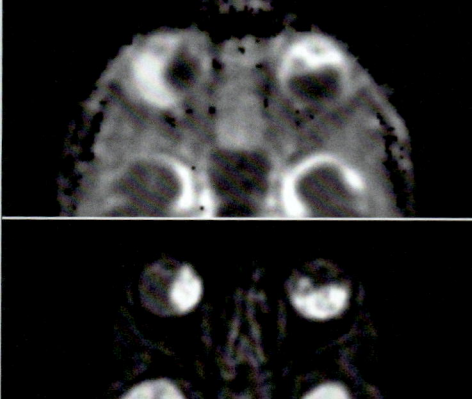

(Left) *Axial T2 MR in the same patient demonstrates hypointense T2 signal within the known calcified intraocular masses ➡ and mild associated bilateral subretinal fluid ⇨. Retinal detachment is a common finding in patients with RB.* (Right) *Axial ADC (top) and DWI (bottom) images in the same patient show the expected restricted diffusion in the bilateral RB.*

TERMINOLOGY

Abbreviations
- Retinoblastoma (RB)

Definitions
- Malignant primary retinal neoplasm
- **Trilateral** RB: Bilateral ocular tumors plus midline intracranial neuroblastic tumor, typically pineal
- **Quadrilateral** (tetralateral) RB: Bilateral disease plus pineal and suprasellar tumors

IMAGING

General Features
- Best diagnostic clue
  - Intraocular **calcified** mass in child
- Location
  - Diagnosis typically with ophthalmoscopy and ultrasound
    - MR for tumor mapping and prognostication
  - Unilateral in 60%, **bilateral in 40%**
  - Trilateral or quadrilateral disease rare
    - 5-15% of familial lesions
  - Extraocular extension in < 10%
    - Spreads along scleral vessels into orbit and along optic nerve to subarachnoid space
  - Predictors for metastatic disease: Involvement of optic nerve, choroid, anterior chamber or orbit
    - Anterior chamber enhancement reflects neoangiogenesis and is associated with more aggressive tumor behavior
  - Role of MR: Exclude pseudoneoplastic lesions
    - Intraocular (choroid, sclera, prelaminar optic nerve), extraocular (postlaminar optic nerve, orbital), intracranial (pineal, parasellar, metastatic) involvement
- Growth patterns
  - **Endophytic** form (45%)
    - Inward protrusion into vitreous
    - Associated with vitreous seeding
  - **Exophytic** form (45%)
    - Outward growth into subretinal space, typically with hemispherical configuration
    - Associated retinal detachment and subretinal exudate
  - **Mixed** endophytic and exophytic (10%)
  - **Diffuse infiltrating** form (rare, older children)
    - Plaque-like growth along retina; often no Ca^{++}
    - Simulates inflammatory or other conditions

CT Findings
- Punctate or finely speckled **Ca^{++}** (> 90-95%)
- Moderate to marked heterogeneous enhancement

MR Findings
- T1WI: Variable, mildly hyperintense (vs. vitreous)
- T2WI: Moderate to markedly hypointense (vs. vitreous)
  - Helps distinguish from other hyperintense lesions (persistent hyperplastic primary vitreous, Coats)
  - Best sequence for subretinal fluid ± vitreous hemorrhage
  - Best to assess extent of intraocular disease and presence of optic nerve or extraocular invasion

- Choroidal invasion: Localized thickening and heterogeneous contrast enhancement near tumor
  - **Scleral invasion**: Interruption in thin, hypointense zone surrounding enhancing choroid
  - **Optic nerve invasion**: Thickening of optic disc (prelaminar), enhancement of nerve (postlaminar)
    - MR shown to have low sensitivity and specificity in assessing optic nerve invasion
- T1WI C+: Moderate to marked heterogeneous enhancement
- Imaging of orbital prosthesis
  - Fibrovascularization (indicated by heterogeneous enhancement) secures prosthesis and provides surface for muscular attachment
- DWI: Diffusion restriction with ADC $(0.619 \pm 0.22) \times 10^{-3}$ mm2/s

Ultrasonographic Findings
- A scan: Highly reflective spikes at Ca^{++}
- B scan: Echodense, irregular mass with focal shadows

Imaging Recommendations
- Best imaging tool
  - Enhanced MR with fat-saturated T1- and T2-weighted imaging best for tumor mapping
  - Ca^{++} on CT relatively specific
- Protocol advice
  - Include whole brain to assess for trilateral disease

DIFFERENTIAL DIAGNOSIS

Persistent Hyperplastic Primary Vitreous
- Small globe, hyperdense; no Ca^{++}
- Hyperintense on T2WI; retrolental tissue stalk

Coats Disease
- Normal-sized globe, hyperdense; no Ca^{++}
- Hyperintense on T1WI and T2WI

Retinopathy of Prematurity
- Retrolental fibroplasia; associated with excess oxygen and premature retinal vessels
- Small globe, hyperdense, bilateral; Ca^{++} if advanced

Retinal Astrocytoma
- Rare lesion, associated with tuberous sclerosis; ± Ca^{++}

Toxocariasis, Orbit
- Uveoscleral enhancement; no Ca^{++} acutely
- Moderately enhancing retinal nodule
- Intravitreal membranes & retinal detachment

Other Causes of Leukocoria
- Retinal detachment
  - Subretinal hemorrhage, retinal folds
- Choroidal osteoma
- Choroidal hemangioma (hamartoma)
- Retinal dysplasia

PATHOLOGY

General Features
- Etiology
  - Primitive neuroectodermal tumor

- o **Sporadic** (nongermline): **60%** of RB
  - – Majority (85%) of unilateral disease
- o **Inherited** (germline): **40%** of RB
  - – Essentially all bilateral and multilateral disease
    - □ Minority (15%) of unilateral disease
  - – Autosomal dominant with 90% penetrance
  - – Positive family history in 5-10%
  - – New germline mutations in 30-35%
- • Genetics
  - o *RB1* gene: Chromosome 13, q14 band
  - o Somatic mosaicism in 10-20% of RB patients
- • Associated abnormalities
  - o Risk of 2nd malignancy ↑ in germline disease
    - – Sarcoma, melanoma, CNS tumors, epithelial tumors (lung, bladder, breast)
    - – 20-30% in nonirradiated patients
    - – 50-60% in irradiated patients
    - – Occur within 30 years, average 10-13 years
  - o 13q deletion syndrome: RB, multiple organ anomalies

Staging, Grading, & Classification

- • Reese-Ellsworth classification
  - o Groups 1-5
  - o Based on size, location, and multifocality
  - o More useful in radiation therapy management
- • International (Murphree) classification of RB (ICRB); newer
  - o Groups A through E
  - o Based on size, retinal location, subretinal or vitreous seeding, and several specific prognostic features
  - o More useful in chemotherapy management

Microscopic Features

- • Small round cells, scant cytoplasm, and large nuclei
- • Flexner-Wintersteiner rosettes and fleurettes

CLINICAL ISSUES

Presentation

- • Most common signs/symptoms
  - o **Leukocoria** (50-60%)
- • Other signs/symptoms
  - o Severe vision loss
  - o Strabismus if macular involvement or retinal detachment
  - o Proptosis if significant orbital disease
  - o Rubeosis iridis (redness of iris secondary to neovascularization) correlates with anterior chamber enhancement on MR
  - o Inflammatory signs in 10%
  - o Less common: Anisocoria, heterochromia, glaucoma, cataract, nystagmus

Demographics

- • Age
  - o RB is congenital but usually not apparent at birth
  - o Average age at diagnosis: 18 months
    - – Unilateral: 24 months, bilateral: 13 months
    - – Earlier with family history and routine screening
  - o 90-95% diagnosed by age 5 years
- • Epidemiology
  - o Most common intraocular tumor of childhood
  - o Incidence 1:17,000 live births, ↑ in past 60 years

- o 3% of cancers in children < 15
- o 1% of cancer deaths; 5% of childhood blindness

Natural History & Prognosis

- • Degree of nerve involvement correlates with survival
  - o Superficial or no invasion: 90%
  - o Invasion to lamina cribrosa (prelaminar): 70%
  - o Invasion beyond lamina cribrosa (postlaminar): 60%
  - o Involvement at surgical margin: 20%
- • Poor prognosis for extraocular disease: < 10% 5-year disease-free survival
- • Poor prognosis for trilateral disease or CSF spread
  - o < 24-month survival

Treatment

- • > 95% children with RB in United States cured with modern techniques; challenge is maintaining eye and vision
- • Based on tumor volume and localization, intraocular tumor extension, and extraocular stage of disease
- • Enucleation: Advanced disease, no chance to preserve useful vision
- • External beam radiation therapy: Bulky tumors with seeding
  - o Unfavorable complications (arrested bone growth and radiation-induced tumors)
- • Chemotherapy (chemoreduction): Currently favored 1st-line therapy for lower-grade intraocular tumors
  - o Limits need for external radiation and enucleation
  - o Combine with other local modalities to achieve cure
  - o Intraarterial chemotherapy
- • Plaque radiotherapy: Locally directed, I-125 or other isotope for selected solitary or small tumors
- • Cryotherapy: Primary local treatment of small anterior tumors
- • Photocoagulation: Primary local treatment of small posterior tumors

DIAGNOSTIC CHECKLIST

Consider

- • Assess for intraocular and extraocular spread, including optic nerve
  - o Check for intracranial trilateral or quadrilateral disease in pineal and suprasellar regions

Image Interpretation Pearls

- • Calcified intraocular mass in child is RB until proven otherwise

SELECTED REFERENCES

1. Jansen RW et al: Correlation of gene expression with magnetic resonance imaging features of retinoblastoma: a multi-center radiogenomics validation study. Eur Radiol. 34(2):863-72, 2024
2. Onishi T et al: Outcomes of five cases of retinoblastoma with optic nerve invasion on imaging. Jpn J Ophthalmol. 68(6):741-50, 2024
3. Pai V et al: Diagnostic imaging for retinoblastoma cancer staging: guide for providing essential insights for ophthalmologists and oncologists. Radiographics. 44(4):e230125, 2024
4. Rumboldt Z et al: Retinoblastoma and beyond: pediatric orbital mass lesions. Neuroradiology. 67(2):469-92, 2024
5. Zhao J et al: Multimodal imaging for the differential diagnosis and efficacy evaluation of intraocular retinoblastoma in children with selective ophthalmic artery infusion. Transl Pediatr. 13(7):1022-32, 2024
6. Gui T et al: Clinical and magnetic resonance imaging features of 14 patients with trilateral retinoblastoma. Quant Imaging Med Surg. 11(4):1458-69, 2021

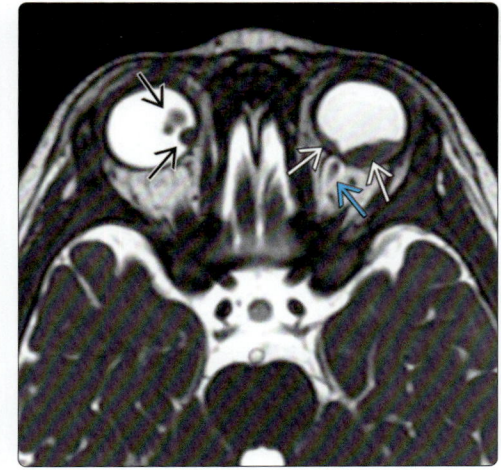

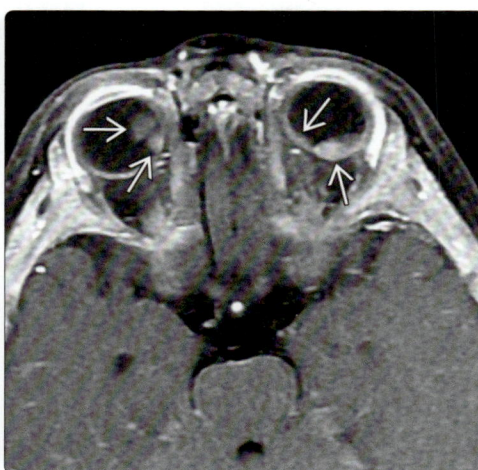

(Left) Axial T2WI MR in a 7-month-old with RB shows bilateral irregular masses in the right ➡ and left ➡ ocular globes. The tumor has T2 signal that is markedly hypointense compared to vitreous. Although the left-sided tumor is along the posterior globe, the visualized optic nerve sheath complex ➡ appears normal. (Right) Axial T1 C+ FS MR in the same patient shows moderate heterogeneous enhancement ➡ of the masses in the bilateral ocular globes.

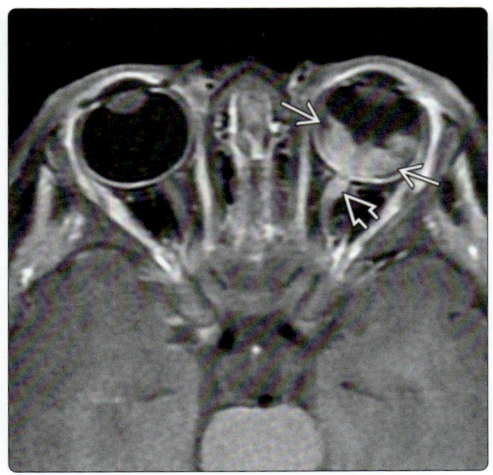

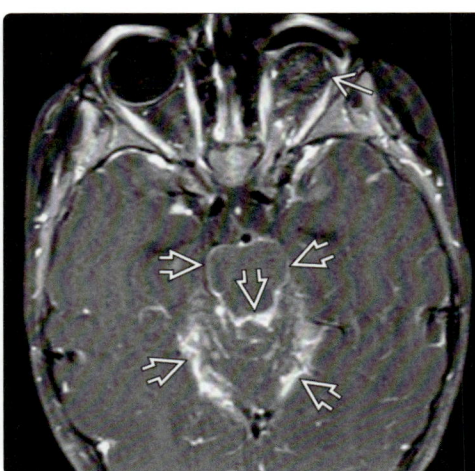

(Left) Axial T1 C+ FS MR in a 17-month-old with RB shows a moderately enhancing mass in the left posterior ocular globe ➡ with apparent extension into the optic nerve ➡. Pathology proved RB invasion of the optic nerve. (Right) Axial T1 C+ FS MR in the same patient acquired 7 months later shows interval left ocular enucleation and prosthesis placement ➡. There is now extensive abnormal leptomeningeal enhancement ➡, consistent with CNS metastatic disease.

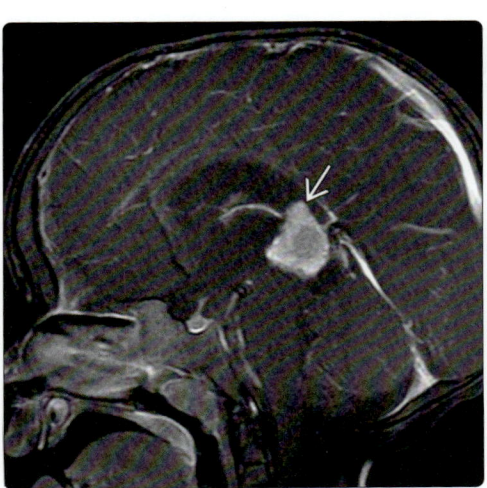

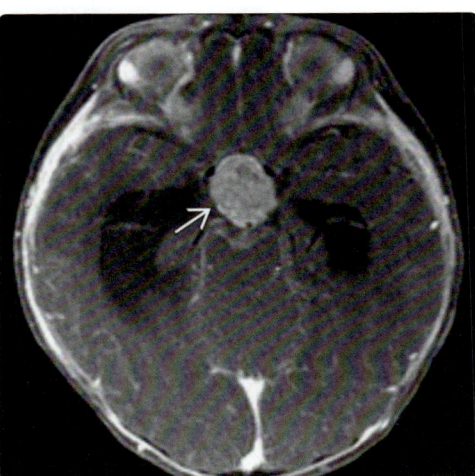

(Left) Sagittal T1 C+ FS MR in a 3-year-old with bilateral RB (not shown) demonstrates a lobulated enhancing mass ➡ in the region of the pineal gland, in the typical location of trilateral RB. (Right) Axial T1 C+ FS MR in a 3-month-old with vomiting found to have bilateral retinoblastoma (not shown) and hydrocephalus secondary to an enhancing suprasellar mass ➡ that proved to be a rare location of trilateral RB.

TERMINOLOGY

- Synonyms: Uveal melanoma, choroidal melanoma, ciliary body melanoma, iris melanoma
- Malignancy arising from melanocytes
  - Most often in choroid

IMAGING

- Choroid > ciliary > iris
- Dome- or mushroom-shaped with broad choroidal base
- Often with associated retinal detachment
- **Ultrasound** is primary imaging modality for evaluation of intraocular disease
- **Enhanced MR** with fat suppression to assess extraocular disease
  - Mildly to strongly T1 hyperintense to vitreous
  - T2 hypointense
  - Moderate, diffuse tumor enhancement
- Ocular coherence tomography emerging as valuable modality for ophthalmologists

TOP DIFFERENTIAL DIAGNOSES

- Choroidal metastasis
- Choroidal hemangioma
- Retinal detachment
- Choroidal osteoma

PATHOLOGY

- Sun exposure, light-colored irides ↑ risk

CLINICAL ISSUES

- **Painless vision disturbance**
- Blurred vision, scotoma, field loss, floaters
- Most common primary intraocular tumor in adults
- Globe-sparing treatment options for small/medium tumors
- Prognosis worsens with extraocular invasion, extension through Bruch membrane, and ↑ in size
- Death from systemic metastases; liver most common

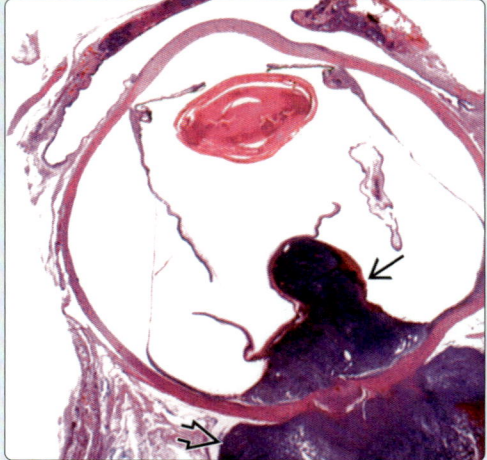
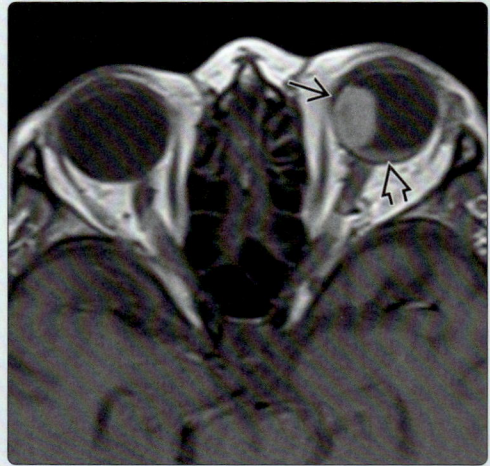

(Left) Micropathology at low power shows a mushroom-shaped ocular melanoma ➡ penetrating through the Bruch membrane. Bulky extraocular tumor is seen extending posteriorly through the optic nerve head ➡. (Right) Axial T1 MR shows an intrinsically T1-hyperintense mass ➡ along the left posteromedial ocular wall, consistent with choroidal melanoma. Hyperintense T1 signal is a consequence of high melanin content. An associated retinal detachment ➡ is also present.

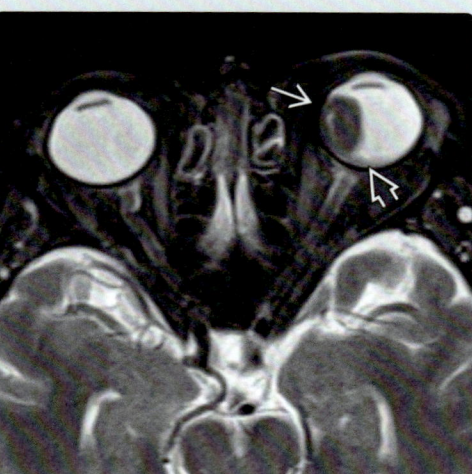
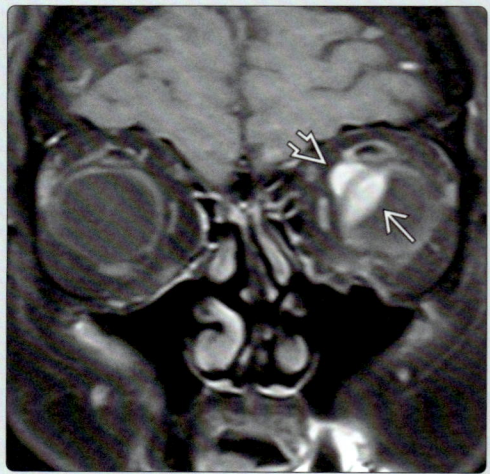

(Left) Axial T2 FS MR in the same patient shows hypointense T2 signal ➡ of the mass relative to vitreous, which is typical of ocular melanoma. There is an adjacent retinal detachment ➡, often associated with ocular melanoma. (Right) Coronal T1 C+ FS MR in the same patient demonstrates avid enhancement of the mass along the posteromedial left ocular wall ➡. Extraocular extension ➡ of > 5 mm places this mass in the highest T stage (T4e) for choroidal melanoma according to the AJCC TNM staging system.

Ocular Melanoma

TERMINOLOGY

Synonyms
- **Uveal melanoma**, choroidal melanoma, ciliary body melanoma, iris melanoma

Definitions
- Primary malignancy of uveal tract (iris, ciliary body, choroid)

IMAGING

General Features
- Best diagnostic clue
  - Enhancing intraocular mass in adult, ↑ **T1WI MR signal**
- Location
  - Temporal hemisphere posterior to equator most common site of origin
  - Posterior uvea
    - **Choroidal lesions (85%)**
      - ▫ Posterior segment peripheral mass
      - ▫ Transscleral/optic nerve extension when advanced
  - Anterior uvea
    - Ciliary body (10%)
    - Iris lesions (5%)
- Size
  - Criteria for therapeutic decisions
    - Small: 5- to 16-mm diameter, < 3-mm depth
    - Medium: 5- to 16-mm diameter, 3- to 10-mm depth
    - Large: > 16-mm diameter, > 10-mm depth
- Morphology
  - Dome- or mound-shaped, broad choroidal base
  - **Mushroom shape** implies penetration through Bruch membrane (separates choroid from retina)
  - Diffuse, laterally spreading form in 5%
  - Typically solid; cavitary variant appears cystic

CT Findings
- NECT
  - Solid soft tissue density mass
  - Ca++ rare; may occur after therapy
- CECT
  - Diffuse moderate enhancement

MR Findings
- T1WI
  - Mildly to strongly **hyperintense** compared with vitreous
    - Signal ↑ with ↑ melanotic pigmentation
  - **Retinal detachments** with subretinal fluid: Variably hyperintense due to blood products or protein
- T2WI
  - Strongly **hypointense** compared with vitreous
  - Subretinal fluid: Signal varies with content
- T1WI C+
  - Moderate, diffuse tumor enhancement
  - No enhancement of retinal detachment/subretinal fluid

Ultrasonographic Findings
- A scan
  - Low to medium internal reflectivity
  - Spike at tumor surface; vascular oscillations
- B scan
  - Domed, lobulated, or mushroom-shaped mass
  - Choroidal excavation/scleral bowing indicate invasion

Nuclear Medicine Findings
- PET/CT
  - Limited utility at primary site, sensitive for metastases
  - Higher tumor SUV correlated with chromosome 3 loss and larger tumor size (poor prognostic signs)
- I-123 IMP SPECT
  - May help diagnose atypical or indeterminate lesions

Other Modality Findings
- Ocular coherence CT (OCT) and OCT angiography (OCTA) becoming important in recent years
  - OCT shows promise in assessing changes in ocular nevi that could signal malignancy
  - OCTA helps assess retinal vascular abnormalities caused by choroidal melanoma

Imaging Recommendations
- Best imaging tool
  - Ultrasound for intraocular tumor evaluation
  - Enhanced MR of orbits with fat suppression to assess extraocular disease

DIFFERENTIAL DIAGNOSIS

Choroidal Metastasis
- Breast and lung primaries most common
  - Located on temporal side of macula

Choroidal Hemangioma (Hamartoma)
- Benign vascular lesion
- Circumscribed form in adults ± retinal detachment
- Diffuse form in infants associated with Sturge-Weber
- > T2 signal and enhancement than melanoma

Retinal Detachment
- Serous, exudative, or hemorrhagic
- Myriad etiologies, including trauma, inflammation, underlying tumor, or systemic disease
- Does not enhance but may obscure underlying mass

Choroidal Osteoma
- Tendency to occur in young women
- Often asymptomatic, found incidentally
- Curvilinear, plaque-like calcified lesion along posterior globe

Conjunctival Melanoma
- Melanoma arising from bulbar conjunctiva
- ~ 5% of ocular melanomas
- Similar to skin melanoma; most commonly regional lymph node metastasis

Idiopathic Orbital Inflammation
- May affect any orbital structure
  - Globe/scleral involvement → endophthalmitis
- Painful, inflammatory presentation

Retinoblastoma
- Most common intraocular tumor in children
- Rarely occurs in adults, Ca++ in 95%

PATHOLOGY

General Features

- Etiology
  - Primary malignancy arising from choroidal melanocytes
- Genetics
  - Several mutations/familial melanoma syndromes known
- Associated abnormalities
  - Ocular melanocytosis, dysplastic nevus syndrome, xeroderma pigmentosum
- Risk factors
  - Genetic factors have greatest influence on risk
  - Sun exposure, light-colored irides ↑ risk

Staging, Grading, & Classification

- Modified Callender classification
  - Spindle cell nevus: Premalignant
  - Spindle cell melanoma: A and B cell types
  - Fascicular: Palisaded B cells (spindle subtype)
  - Necrotic: Significant necrosis prior to treatment
  - Mixed: Spindle and epithelioid cells
  - Epithelioid: Predominantly epithelioid cells

Gross Pathologic & Surgical Features

- Range from heavily pigmented to amelanotic
- Discoloration and atrophy of overlying retina

Microscopic Features

- 3 cell types used for classification
  - Spindle A: Elongated nuclei, few mitoses
  - Spindle B: Plump nuclei, more prominent nucleoli
  - Epithelioid: Ovoid nuclei, anaplastic, poor prognosis

CLINICAL ISSUES

Presentation

- Most common signs/symptoms
  - **Painless vision disturbance**
  - Frequent coexisting retinal detachment
- Other signs/symptoms
  - Blurred vision, scotoma, field loss, floaters
  - Pain rare (due to ciliary nerve involvement)
- Clinical profile
  - **Frequently asymptomatic**
    - Often discovered on routine eye exam
    - Presentation more advanced when located farther from fovea and nerve head
- Ophthalmoscopy
  - Dome-shaped mass of variable pigmentation
  - Orange discoloration of overlying retina; exudative detachment may obscure mass

Demographics

- Age
  - Peak incidence: **6th decade**
    - Iris melanoma presents slightly younger
- Ethnicity
  - **Northern European descent highest risk**
  - Latino, Asian uncommon; African descent rare
- Epidemiology
  - **Most common primary intraocular tumor in adults**

- Incidence 6-8 per 1 million, 5% of all melanomas

Natural History & Prognosis

- Appears to be systemic disease at presentation with treatment of primary disease curative in some patients
- Death from systemic metastases (liver most common)
  - 5-year cumulative metastasis rate: 25%
  - 10-year cumulative metastasis rate: 34%
  - No effective treatment for metastatic disease
- Worse prognosis if any of following
  - Large size, anterior location, extension through Bruch membrane, transscleral/nerve invasion
  - Amelanotic, epithelioid pattern, highly mitotic

Treatment

- Protocols largely driven by results of Collaborative Ocular Melanoma Study (COMS) Group
  - Multicenter NIH/National Eye Institute trial
- Observation
  - Suitable for indeterminate stable small nevi
  - Sequential ultrasound to document stability
- Transpupillary thermotherapy
  - Option for small tumors; preserves vision
  - Tumor heating by infrared radiation
- Surgical block excision (sclerouvectomy)
  - Option for small tumors < 1/3 of globe circumference
  - Preserves some vision
- Plaque brachytherapy
  - Common option for medium-sized tumors
  - Isotope plaque (I-125) sutured over tumor site
- External beam irradiation
  - Alternative for medium-sized tumors
  - Charged particles (protons, helium ions)
  - Gamma knife radiosurgery
- Surgical enucleation
  - Standard for large tumors, treatment failures
  - Radical exenteration for widespread tumor

DIAGNOSTIC CHECKLIST

Consider

- Most common ocular tumor in adults
- Ultrasonography remains most frequently utilized diagnostic modality for intraocular disease
- MR more accurate than ultrasound for extraocular spread

Image Interpretation Pearls

- Enhancement reliably distinguishes tumor from associated retinal detachment on MR

SELECTED REFERENCES

1. Kulbay M et al: Uveal melanoma: comprehensive review of its pathophysiology, diagnosis, treatment, and future perspectives. Biomedicines. 12(8):1758, 2024
2. Mirshahvalad SA et al: A systematic review and meta-analysis on the diagnostic and prognostic values of (18)F-FDG PET in uveal melanoma and its hepatic metastasis. Cancers (Basel). 16(9):1712, 2024
3. Jaarsma-Coes MG et al: Magnetic resonance imaging in the clinical care for uveal melanoma patients-a systematic review from an ophthalmic perspective. Cancers (Basel). 15(11):2995, 2023
4. Foti PV et al: Diagnostic methods and therapeutic options of uveal melanoma with emphasis on MR imaging-part I: MR imaging with pathologic correlation and technical considerations. Insights Imaging. 12(1):66, 2021

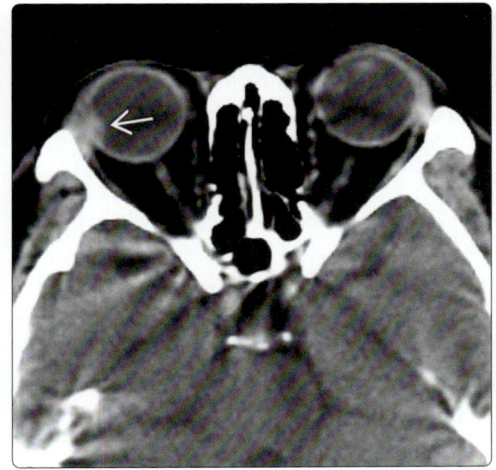
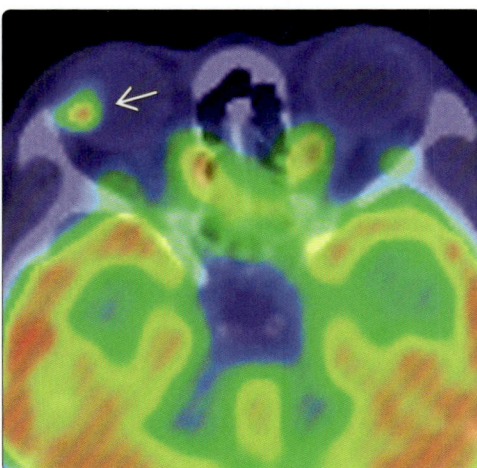

(Left) Axial CT from a PET/CT study done for staging in a 57-year-old woman with right ocular melanoma shows intermediate density of the dome-shaped mass along the right lateral aspect of the uveal tract ➡️. (Right) Axial FDG PET/CT in the same patient shows increased uptake of FDG in the ocular melanoma ➡️. The mass had a maximum SUV of 7.4. FDG PET has low sensitivity but high specificity for the intraocular primary. Larger lesions tend to have higher FDG uptake.

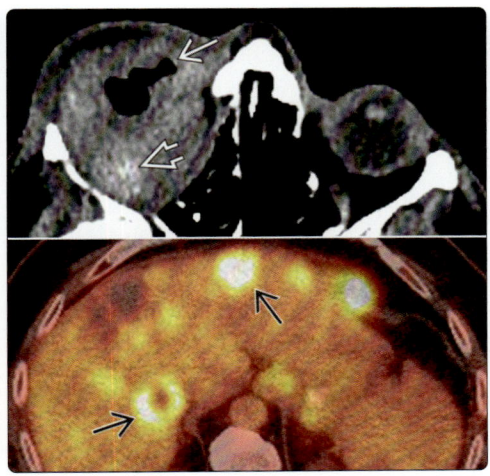
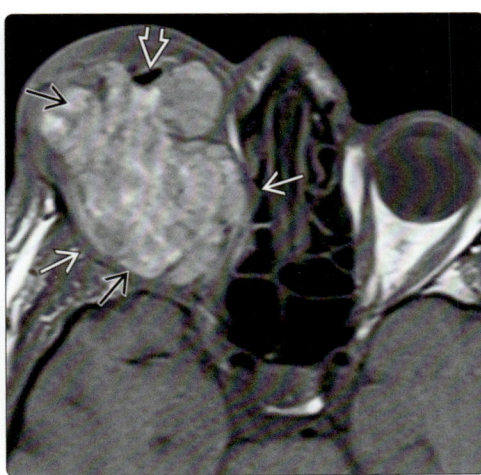

(Left) Axial CT (top) shows a large, heterogeneously hyperdense ➡️ right orbital mass with an ill-defined globe. Intralesional gas ➡️ is from recent biopsy proving uveal melanoma. The axial PET/CT (bottom) shows multifocal liver metastases ➡️. (Right) Axial T1 MR in the same patient shows heterogeneous, predominantly hyperintense T1 signal ➡️, compatible with high melanin content. Again noted is expansion of the orbit ➡️ and a small volume of residual postprocedural gas ➡️.

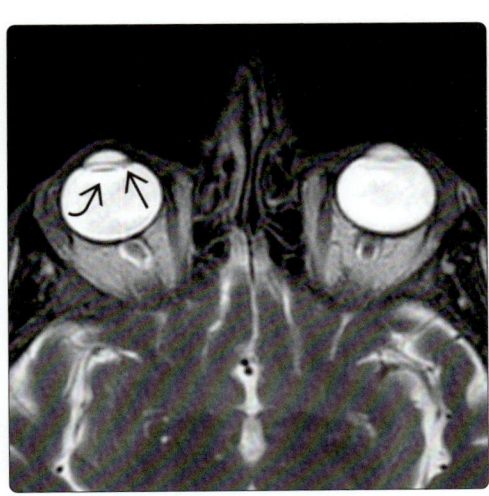
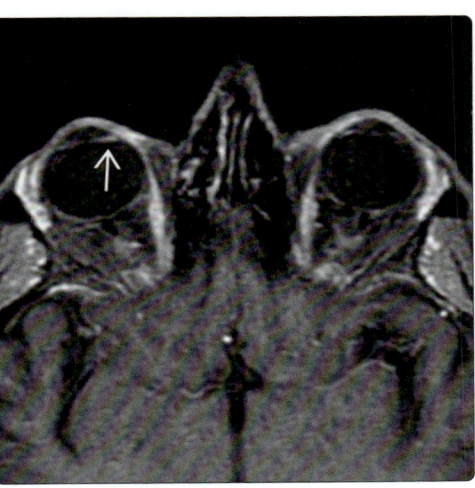

(Left) Axial T2 MR in a case of iris melanoma demonstrates subtle thickening of the medial right iris ➡️ with posterolateral displacement of the artificial intraocular lens ➡️. Although more easily diagnosed on ophthalmologic exam, MR is helpful in determining extent of disease. (Right) Axial T1 C+ FS MR demonstrates slight thickening of enhancement along the medial right iris ➡️ in keeping with known iris melanoma. AJCC 8th edition T staging differs for iris origin of uveal melanoma.

Orbital Lymphoproliferative Lesions

TERMINOLOGY

- Spectrum of lesions ranging from benign lymphoid hyperplasia to malignant lymphoma

IMAGING

- Solid, pliable, homogeneously enhancing tumor
  - Can involve any part of orbit; lacrimal predilection
- Mass with lobulated margins
  - Molds to adjacent structures in "plastic" fashion
- Mildly T2 hyperintense to muscle (high cellularity)
- Decrease ADC, particularly in true lymphoma
- Moderate to marked, homogeneous enhancement

TOP DIFFERENTIAL DIAGNOSES

- IgG4-related disease
- Idiopathic orbital inflammation
- Orbital sarcoidosis
- Orbital Sjögren syndrome
- Lacrimal gland epithelial tumor

PATHOLOGY

- Spectrum of lymphocytic proliferation
  - Benign **lymphoid hyperplasia**
    - Reactive, polyclonal; indeterminate when atypical
  - Non-Hodgkin **lymphoma**
    - Low-grade MALT/ENMZL most common

CLINICAL ISSUES

- Presentation: Insidious anterior orbital/eyelid swelling
- Long-term risk of developing systemic lymphoma
- Lymphoid hyperplasia responsive to steroids
- Lymphoma responsive to radiation therapy

DIAGNOSTIC CHECKLIST

- Benign hyperplasia vs. malignant lymphoma
  - **Hyperplasia**: Well defined, bilateral, flow void sign, higher enhancement ratio, sinusitis, less older patients
  - **Lymphoma**: Irregular, unilateral, diffusion restriction, lower enhancement ratio, more older patients

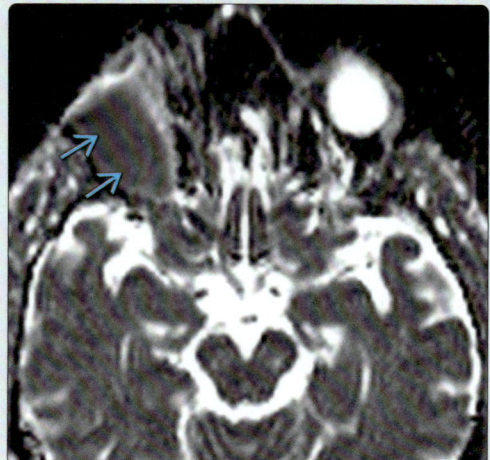
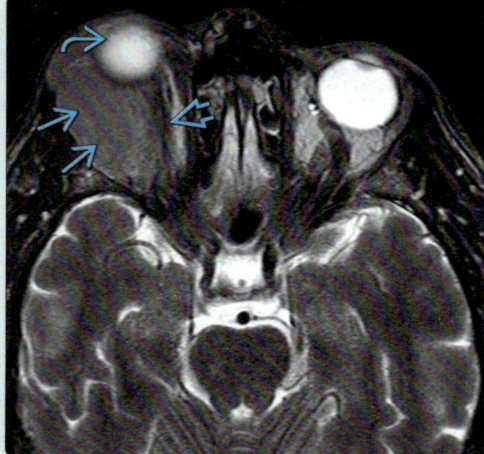

(Left) Axial ADC map in a 65-year-old man with restricted right globe movements shows a solid intraorbital mass with a low ADC value ➡, indicating high cellularity due to extranodal marginal zone lymphoma. (Right) Axial T2 FS MR in the same patient shows a well-circumscribed solid right orbital mass, which is slightly hyperintense ➡ compared to extraocular muscle. Note mild right globe proptosis ➡. Note medial displacement of the right optic nerve intraorbital segment ➡.

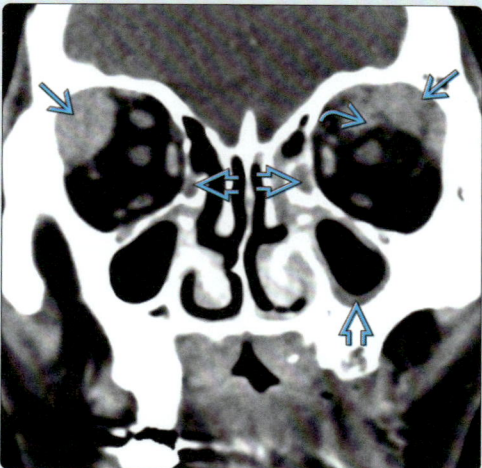
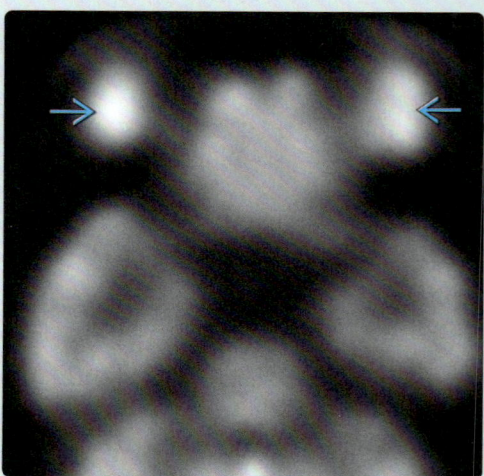

(Left) Coronal MPR orbit CECT in a patient with bilateral eyelid swelling shows near symmetric enlargement of bilateral lacrimal glands ➡. The fat planes between adjacent extraocular muscles and left orbital mass is effaced ➡. Note mild sinus mucosal disease in bilateral ethmoids and left maxillary sinuses ➡. (Right) Axial FDG PET in the same patient shows mild increased FDG activity in bilateral lacrimal gland masses ➡. Biopsy revealed lymphoid hyperplasia. It showed complete resolution on a course of steroids.

Orbital Lymphoproliferative Lesions

TERMINOLOGY

Abbreviations
- Orbital lymphoproliferative lesions (OLPL)

Synonyms
- Mucosa-associated lymphoid tissue (MALT) lymphoma = extranodal marginal zone lymphoma (ENMZL)

Definitions
- OLPL represents **spectrum** of lesions ranging from benign lymphoid hyperplasia (LH) to malignant non-Hodgkin lymphoma (NHL)

IMAGING

General Features
- Best diagnostic clue
  - **Solid**, **pliable**, **homogeneously enhancing** tumor that molds to and encases orbital structures
- Location
  - Can involve **any part of orbit**
    - Predilection for **lacrimal gland**, which may be only site of involvement
    - Anterior extraconal orbit, often centered in **superotemporal** quadrant
    - **Conjunctival** disease frequent; isolated in 20%
    - May present with primary **extraocular** muscle involvement, simulating thyroid orbitopathy
    - **Diffuse infiltrative** form may occur with intraconal, muscular, or perineural involvement
  - **Unilateral** in most cases of 1° **lymphoma** (60-75%)
  - **Bilateral** in most cases of **benign** OLPL (50-80%)
- Morphology
  - Mass with **lobulated** margins
    - Margins more **well-defined** in **benign** OLPL
    - Margins more **irregular** in true **lymphoma**
  - Often molds to adjacent structures in "**plastic**" fashion
  - May have infiltrative or inflammatory appearance
- Associated findings
  - Concomitant **sinusitis** associated with **benign** OLPL

CT Findings
- NECT
  - Isodense to slightly **hyperdense** due to highly **cellular** nature and nuclear:cytoplasmic ratio
- CECT
  - Moderate, diffuse, **homogeneous** enhancement
  - Dynamic enhancement pattern helps distinguish from inflammatory disease
- Bone CT
  - Bone destruction indicates aggressive histology
    - Molding associated with more indolent disease

MR Findings
- T1WI
  - Mildly hyperintense to muscle; homogeneous
- T2WI
  - Only **mildly hyperintense** to muscle (high **cellularity**)
  - Adjacent vessel flow void associated with benign OLPL
- DWI
  - **Decrease ADC**, particularly in true **lymphoma**
- T1WI C+
  - Moderate to marked, **homogeneous enhancement**
  - Enhancement ratio (to muscle) higher with benign OLPL

Nuclear Medicine Findings
- PET/CT
  - Limited value in assessing orbital disease due to high activity in extraocular muscles and typical small volume of disease
  - Useful in screening for systemic lymphoma

Imaging Recommendations
- Best imaging tool
  - MR modality of choice for evaluating location and extent of disease
- Protocol advice
  - Axial and coronal MR: T1, T2, diffusion, and C+ FS

DIFFERENTIAL DIAGNOSIS

IgG4-Related Disease
- Infiltrative masses with subacute presentation
- Accounts for significant number of previously diagnosed LH
- Characteristic T2 hypointensity
- Predilection for lacrimal and perineural involvement

Idiopathic Orbital Inflammation (Pseudotumor)
- Presentation typically more acute and painful
- Similar wide range of imaging appearances

Orbital Sarcoidosis
- Painless masses anywhere in orbit
- Predilection for lacrimal glands; may be bilateral

Orbital Sjögren Syndrome
- Lacrimal involvement with keratoconjunctivitis sicca
- Look for bilateral parotid enlargement, cysts, Ca^{++}

Thyroid Eye Disease
- Painless, often bilateral symmetric proptosis
- Characteristic pattern of extraocular muscle enlargement

Orbital Cellulitis
- Pain, erythema, fever; associated with sinusitis
- Discrete orbital masses are less common

Lacrimal Gland Epithelial Tumor
- Unilateral lacrimal mass, painless when benign
- T2 MR signal more hyperintense

Orbital Metastasis
- Can occur anywhere in orbit
- Breast and lung carcinoma are common primaries

PATHOLOGY

General Features
- Etiology
  - **Reactive** or **malignant** lymphocytic proliferation
- Genetics
  - Hyperplasia = **polyclonal**
  - Lymphoma = **monoclonal**
  - ENMZL markers often indeterminate
- Associated abnormalities

- Systemic conditions: Collagen vascular disease, Sjögren disease, hematologic malignancy
- Immunocompromised status: AIDS, transplant patients

Staging, Grading, & Classification

- Classification of OLPL spectrum
  - **Benign LH**: 10-40%
    - Reactive hyperplasia, polyclonal
    - Atypical hyperplasia; indeterminate
  - **NHL**: 60-90%
    - Low-grade MALT/ENMZL most common
    - Other: Follicular, diffuse large B-cell, mantle cell, NK/T cell, Burkitt, and other lymphomas
- Staging of orbital lymphomas
  - Ann Arbor system: Stages I-IV; (E) if extranodal disease
    - Subclassification: (A) without, or (B) with systemic symptoms (weight loss, fever, night sweats)
  - Most MALT/ENMZL stage IE-A or IIE-A at presentation

Microscopic Features

- Common feature of all OLPL subtypes: Cellular lymphocytic infiltration
- Hyperplasia: Polymorphous infiltrate of lymphocytes, follicle formation, endothelial proliferation
- Small B-cell lymphoma: Small, round lymphocytes; vaguely nodular plasma cells
  - Characteristic **marginal zone** cells in ENMZL

CLINICAL ISSUES

Presentation

- Most common signs/symptoms
  - **Insidious** anterior orbital/eyelid swelling
    - Fleshy mass visible if conjunctiva involved
  - Intraorbital **mass** effect with **proptosis, diplopia**
    - Globe **displacement** (nonaxial, inferior) in 50%
- Other signs/symptoms
  - Fever, night sweats, weight loss
- Clinical profile
  - 4 basic clinical syndromes
    - Indolent painless orbital mass (most common)
    - Fulminant orbital mass (immunocompromised)
    - Regional bony mass (secondary orbit extension)
    - Neuroophthalmic (CNS disease)

Demographics

- Age
  - Older patients (5th-8th decades)
    - **Benign** OLPL in **younger** patients
    - **Lymphoma** in **older** patients
- Epidemiology
  - 5-10% of orbital masses; most common adult neoplasm
  - Constitutes 1-2% of NHL, 8% of extranodal lymphoma
  - Orbit involvement develops in 5% of systemic NHL
  - Systemic lymphoma in up to 50% at presentation

Natural History & Prognosis

- **Indolent** course for primary low-grade and low-stage (IE-A) tumors
- Major long-term **risk** of developing **systemic lymphoma**
  - Systemic relapse in 25-75%
  - Typically abdominal, pelvic, or neck lymph nodes

- Histology affects risk of systemic disease
  - Small B cell (atypical hyperplasia, MALT, etc.): 25-50%
  - All others (large B cell, mantle cell, T cell, etc.): 50-75%
- Orbital site affects risk of systemic disease
  - Eyelid: 67%; orbit: 35%; conjunctiva: 20%
  - Increased risk of systemic disease if bilateral
- **Excellent prognosis** for **MALT/ENMZL** with radiotherapy
  - Survival: 5 years = 90-100%, 10 years = 70-90%
  - Local control approaches 100%
  - Indolent course even after relapse
- Good local control for other types of lymphoma but poorer long-term survival with systemic disease

Treatment

- LH
  - Responsive to **steroids**, given systemically or injected locally
- Low-grade small B-cell lymphoma (MALT/ENMZL)
  - Excellent response to **radiation** therapy alone
- High-grade diffuse B-cell lymphoma
  - Systemic chemotherapy or immunotherapy
  - Local radiation treatment may be beneficial in selected areas

DIAGNOSTIC CHECKLIST

Consider

- Whole-body **staging** and **surveillance** indicated due to risk of development of systemic lymphoma
- Tumor location has significant impact on eventual risk of systemic lymphoma

Image Interpretation Pearls

- **Broad range** of imaging manifestations
  - Carefully examine anterior compartment structures, including orbital septum, conjunctiva, and lids
  - May involve any portion of orbit
- Consider OLPL in differential for any orbital mass
- Features that help distinguish benign hyperplasia from true lymphoma
  - **Benign**: Well defined, bilateral, flow void sign, higher enhancement ratio, and sinusitis; less older patients
  - **Lymphoma**: Irregular, unilateral, diffusion restriction, and lower enhancement ratio; more older patients

SELECTED REFERENCES

1. Yazici G et al: The role of radiotherapy in indolent ocular adnexal and orbital lymphomas. Head Neck. 47(3):891-8, 2025
2. Ang T et al: Evaluation of orbital lesions with DCE-MRI: a literature review. Orbit. 43(3):408-16, 2024
3. Boltezar L et al: Ocular adnexal lymphoma - a retrospective study and review of the literature. Radiol Oncol. 58(3):416-24, 2024
4. Ishak F et al: Orbital lymphoma presenting as recurrent orbital cellulitis: a diagnostic challenge. Cureus. 16(10):e70759, 2024
5. Urrutia YA et al: Case series of orbital lymphoma: cardinal presentations. Plast Reconstr Surg Glob Open. 12(6):e5913, 2024
6. Bennassi A et al: Orbital follicular lymphoma with large cell component treated with low-dose radiotherapy: a case report and review of literature. Cancer Radiother. 27(4):337-40, 2023
7. Keren S et al: Paediatric orbital lymphoma; a case series and review of the literature. Eye (Lond). 37(5):1002-8, 2023
8. Singh S et al: Lymphoproliferative tumors involving the lacrimal drainage system: a major review. Orbit. 39(4):276-84, 2020
9. Olsen TG et al: Orbital lymphoma. Surv Ophthalmol. 64(1):45-66, 2019

Orbital Lymphoproliferative Lesions

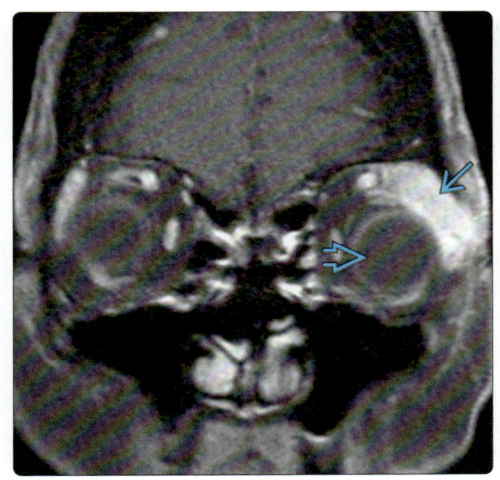

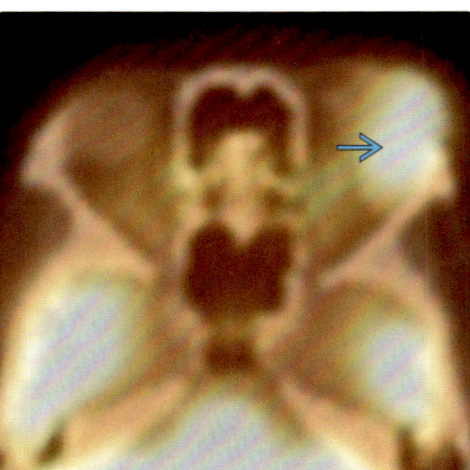

(Left) Coronal T1 C+ FS MR in a 70-year-old man with diplopia and left globe proptosis shows an avid, homogeneously enhancing mass in the left lacrimal gland ➡. Note inferior and medial displacement of the left globe due to mass effect ➡. (Right) Axial FDG PET/CT in the same patient shows significant FDG avidity ➡ in the left lacrimal gland, suggesting high-grade lymphoma. FDG PET has limited value in assessing orbital disease due to very high activity in extraocular muscles, and typically small volume disease.

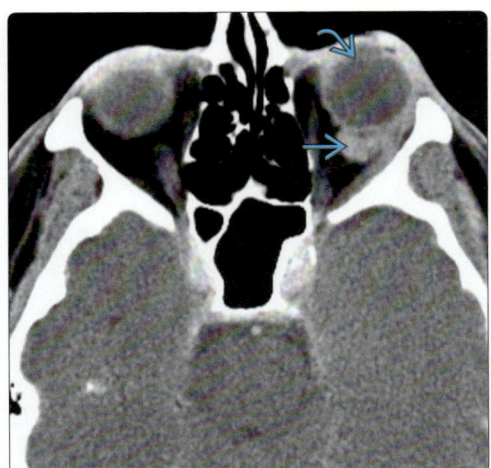

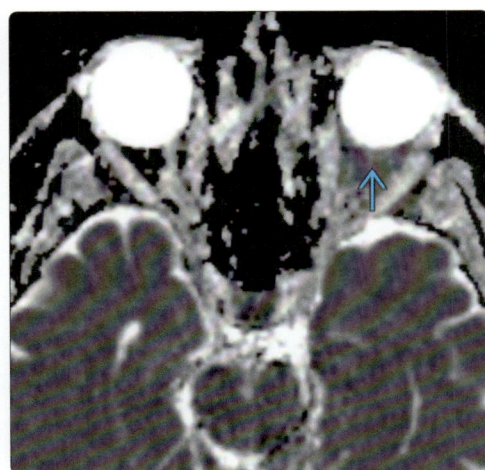

(Left) Axial orbit CECT in a patient with left globe swelling shows a small amount of homogeneously enhancing, well-circumscribed mass ➡ conforming to the posterior surface of the left globe in the intraconal compartment. Note mild left globe proptosis ➡. (Right) Axial ADC map in the same patient shows low ADC values in this left retrobulbar mass ➡. Biopsy was consistent with mucosa-associated lymphoid tissue (MALT) lymphoma, and the patient was treated with radiation therapy.

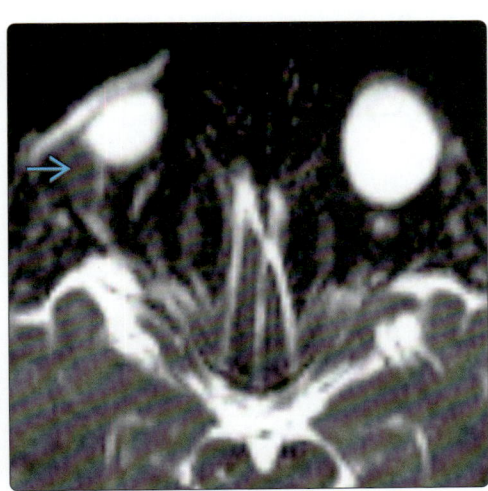

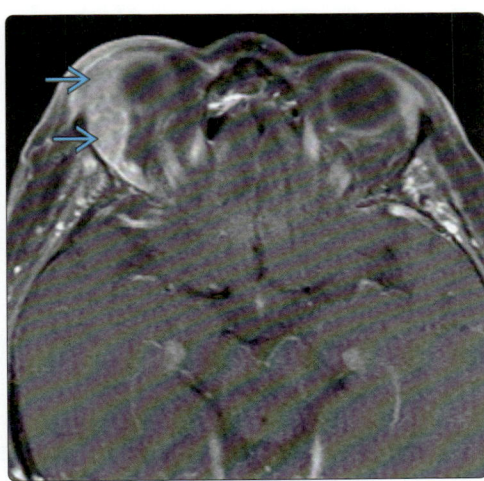

(Left) Axial ADC map in a 53-year-old woman with biopsy-proven extranodal marginal zone lymphoma of the right lacrimal gland shows a mass with a low ADC value ➡, suggesting high cellularity. (Right) Axial T1 C+ MR in the same patient shows a homogeneously enhancing solid mass involving both deep and palpebral segments of the right lacrimal gland ➡. Low-grade lymphomas are highly radiosensitive, whereas high-grade tumors benefit from systemic chemotherapy or immunotherapy.

Lacrimal Gland Carcinoma

TERMINOLOGY

- Malignant epithelial neoplasm of lacrimal gland
  - Subtypes include adenoid cystic carcinoma (ACCa), carcinoma ex pleomorphic adenoma, adenocarcinoma, mucoepidermoid carcinoma, and squamous cell carcinoma

IMAGING

- Irregular or lobular lacrimal gland mass
  - Bone destruction seen in 70%; best imaging indicator of malignancy
- CT: Isodense with moderate enhancement
  - Bone algorithm CT to delineate bone erosion
- MR: Isointense to hyperintense T2 signal and enhancement
  - T1 C+ FS images best for tumor mapping and perineural spread
- PET/CT: FDG uptake variable

TOP DIFFERENTIAL DIAGNOSES

- Orbital lymphoproliferative lesion
- Lacrimal pleomorphic adenoma
- Idiopathic orbital inflammation
- Dacryoadenitis
- Orbital sarcoidosis
- Orbital Sjögren syndrome

PATHOLOGY

- Parallels that of salivary gland neoplasms
- Divided into low and high grade based on WHO classification of salivary tumors

CLINICAL ISSUES

- ~ 1-2% of orbital neoplasms
- ACCa most common malignant lacrimal tumor
  - Must assess for perineural spread
  - Pain → bone/perineural involvement

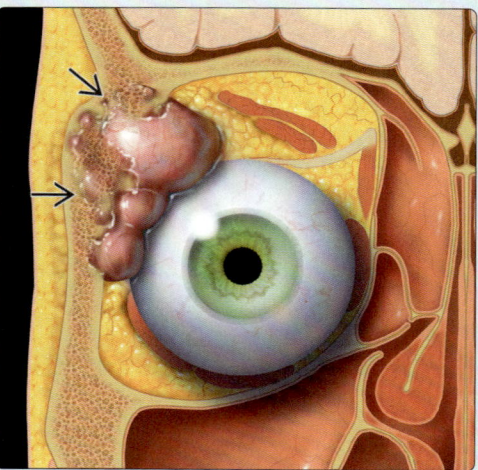
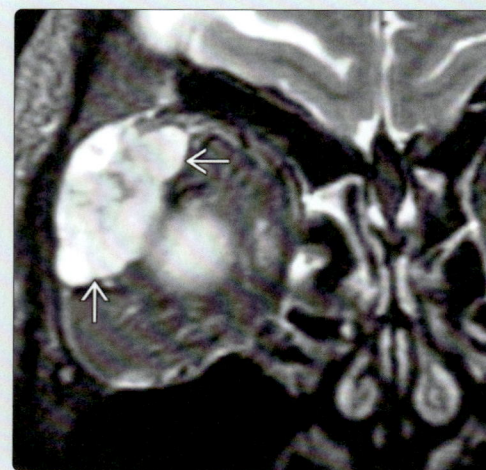

(Left) Coronal graphic depicts an infiltrating mass of the right lacrimal gland. The superolateral bony orbit is invaded ➡ by this lacrimal gland carcinoma, and the globe is displaced inferomedially. (Right) Coronal T2 FS MR shows a markedly hyperintense, somewhat heterogeneous mass ➡ with lobulated, circumscribed borders centered in the right lacrimal fossa. In the absence of bone destruction, this adenoid cystic carcinoma cannot be distinguished from a benign lacrimal tumor.

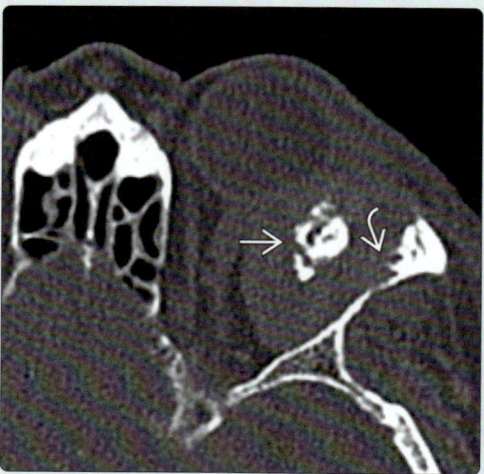
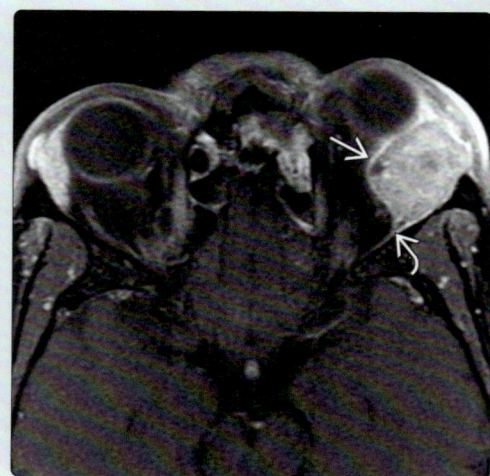

(Left) Axial bone CT shows a large left lacrimal gland mass with internal dystrophic calcification ➡ and osseous erosion ➡. Along with osseous erosion, this longstanding mass exhibited interval growth and pain consistent with carcinoma ex pleomorphic adenoma. (Right) Axial T1 C+ FS MR shows an enhancing left lacrimal mass ➡, pathology-proven mucoepidermoid carcinoma, in this patient presenting with 2 weeks of left-sided headache and proptosis. A posterior tail or wedge sign ➡ suggests a malignant lesion.

Lacrimal Gland Carcinoma

TERMINOLOGY

Synonyms

- Subtypes include adenoid cystic carcinoma (ACCa), carcinoma ex pleomorphic adenoma, adenocarcinoma, mucoepidermoid carcinoma, and squamous cell carcinoma

Definitions

- Malignant epithelial neoplasm of lacrimal gland

IMAGING

General Features

- Best diagnostic clue
  - Irregular lacrimal fossa mass **with bone erosion**
- Location
  - Superior temporal quadrant of orbit
  - Contiguous or perineural spread to surrounding structures and skull base
- Morphology
  - Lobular and marginated to irregular and infiltrative
  - Wedge or tail sign: Tumor confined by septa between superior and lateral recti, takes on triangular shape with posterior extension

CT Findings

- NECT
  - Lobular or infiltrative, isodense mass
- CECT
  - Moderate to marked enhancement
- Bone CT
  - Bone destruction in 70%; **best indicator of malignant nature**

MR Findings

- T1WI
  - Isointense to mildly hypointense to muscle
- T2WI
  - Isointense to hyperintense to muscle
- DWI
  - Low ADC map value (compared to pleomorphic adenoma)
- T1WI C+
  - Moderate to marked enhancement

Imaging Recommendations

- Best imaging tool
  - T1 C+ FS MR best for mapping tumor extent and perineural spread
- Protocol advice
  - Bone algorithm CT to identify osseous erosion

DIFFERENTIAL DIAGNOSIS

Orbital Lymphoproliferative Lesion

- Typically shows **lower T2 signal** intensity and **ADC map value**

Lacrimal Pleomorphic Adenoma

- Slow-growing mass; scalloped, bone remodeling

Idiopathic Orbital Inflammation

- Steroid-responsive, noninfectious inflammation
- Painful and may be bilateral

Dacryoadenitis

- Acute to subacute onset of painful swelling

Orbital Sarcoidosis

- Granulomatous process ± concurrent sinusitis

Orbital Sjögren Syndrome

- Autoimmune sialadenitis

PATHOLOGY

Staging, Grading, & Classification

- American Joint Committee on Cancer (AJCC) 8th edition staging based primarily on size of lesion, periosteal involvement, and osseous invasion
- Histology based on WHO classification
  - Multiple histologic categories divided into 2 broad categories: Low-grade and high-grade tumors

CLINICAL ISSUES

Presentation

- Most common signs/symptoms
  - Inferomedial globe displacement (75%)
- Other signs/symptoms
  - Diplopia
  - **Pain → bone/perineural involvement**
  - Sensory loss in distribution of lacrimal nerve

Demographics

- Epidemiology
  - Rare: ~ 1-2% of orbital neoplasms
  - ACCa most common malignant epithelial lacrimal neoplasm (~ 60%)

Natural History & Prognosis

- Low grade: Good prognosis following local resection
- High grade: Local/distant recurrence common, especially ACCa
  - Disease-free survival rate: 50% at 10 years for ACCa
  - Incidence of distant failure independent of degree of local control
  - Lung and bone most common metastatic sites

Treatment

- Primarily surgical, ranging from local resection to exenteration ± bone removal
- Adjuvant radiation therapy for high-grade lesions

DIAGNOSTIC CHECKLIST

Consider

- Malignant if unilateral lacrimal mass + bone destruction

Image Interpretation Pearls

- Perineural spread is important feature of ACCa, most common lacrimal gland carcinoma

SELECTED REFERENCES

1. Goldberg H et al: Lacrimal gland adenocarcinoma clinicopathologic features and outcomes compared with those of lacrimal gland adenoid cystic carcinoma. Ophthalmic Plast Reconstr Surg. 40(4):419-25, 2024

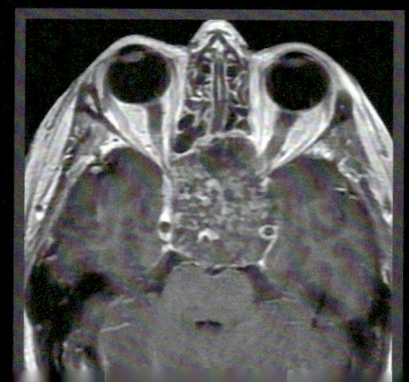
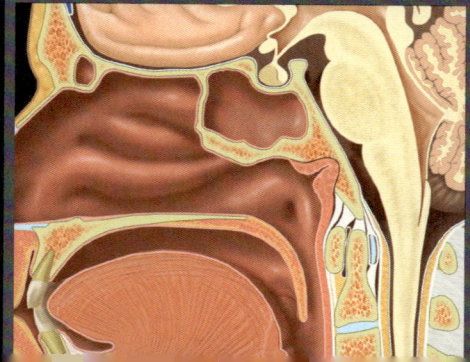
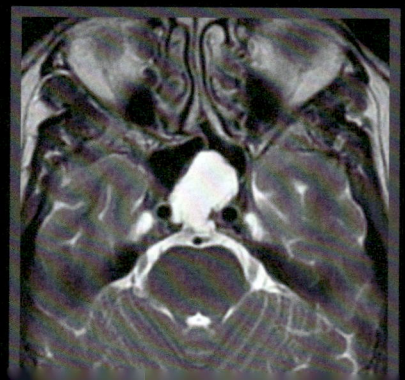

Diffuse or Multifocal Skull Base Disease

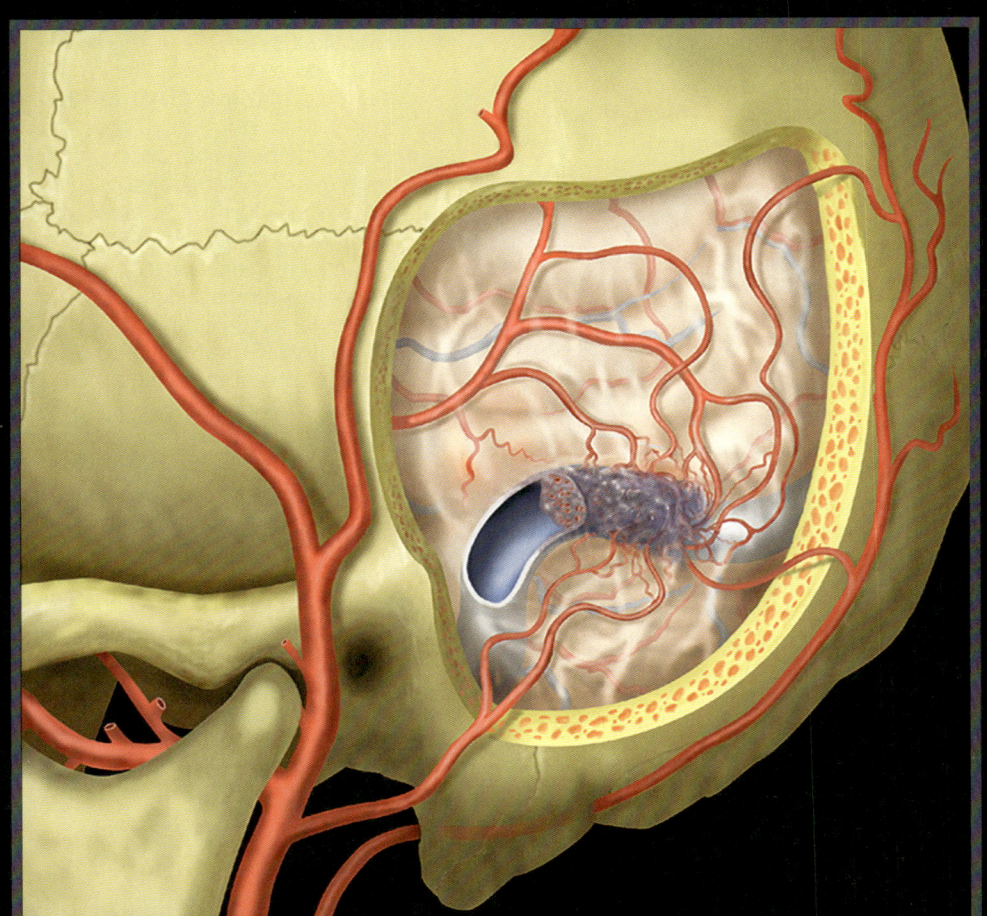

Imaging Approaches and Indications

CT is the primary imaging tool for evaluating the bony details of the skull base (SB). Multislice CT scanners allow thin slices (≤ 1 mm) and provide excellent multiplanar reformatted images. These function as the mainstay for evaluating bony changes associated with SB diseases as well as providing evidence for calcific or bony matrices of these lesions. CTA is optimum for suspected arterial abnormality or to determine arterial relationships to soft tissue lesions.

MR is an essential partner to bone CT in evaluating SB lesions, as it provides the best understanding of lesion soft tissue extent. T1 precontrast images show lesion margins against the contrast of SB marrow fat. T1 also reveals high-signal subacute blood and intralesion high-velocity flow voids to best advantage. Enhanced, fat-saturated T1 sequences define enhancement characteristics of the lesion in question. GRE may show blooming if hemorrhage or venous sinus thrombosis is present. DWI hyperintensity in a focal SB lesion suggests the diagnosis of epidermoid. MRA and MRV are important sequences to acquire if internal carotid (ICA) and vertebral artery or venous sinus involvement is suspected.

Imaging Anatomy

The SB is made up of 5 bones: The paired frontal and temporal bones (T-bones) and the unpaired ethmoid, sphenoid, and occipital bones. Two major surfaces of the SB can be described: The **endocranial surface**, which faces the brain, cisterns, cranial nerves (CNs) and intracranial vessels, and the **exocranial surface**, which faces the extracranial head and neck. The exocranial surface has numerous interfaces with the sinus, nose, orbits, masticator (MS), parotid (PS), parapharyngeal (PPS), pharyngeal mucosal (PMS), carotid (CS), retropharyngeal (RPS), and perivertebral spaces (PVS).

The **endocranial surface** can be further divided into 3 regions: The anterior (ASB), central (CSB), and posterior SB (PSB).

- **ASB**: Floor of anterior cranial fossa, comprised of orbital plate of frontal bone, ethmoid bone cribriform plate and ethmoid sinus roof, and planum sphenoidale and lesser wing of sphenoid bone (LWS); important ASB foramina include **foramen cecum (FC)** and **cribriform plate foramina**
- **CSB**: Floor of middle cranial fossa, made up of **basisphenoid**, **greater wing** of sphenoid bone (GWS), and **T-bone** anterior to petrous ridge; bony landmarks of CSB include sella turcica, tuberculum sellae, and posterior clinoid process; important CSB foramina and fissures are optic canal, superior orbital fissure (SOF), inferior orbital fissure (IOF), foramen rotundum, foramen ovale, foramen spinosum, vidian canal, carotid canal, and foramen lacerum
- **PSB**: Bony bowl that makes up floor of posterior cranial fossa, made up of **posterior wall** of **T-bone** and **occipital bone**; occipital bone has 3 parts: Basilar part (lower clivus/basiocciput), condylar part lateral to foramen magnum, including occipital condyles, and squamous part (large bony plate posterosuperior to foramen magnum); important PSB foramina and fissures include internal auditory canal (IAC), jugular foramen (JF), hypoglossal canal, stylomastoid foramen, and foramen magnum

Skull Base Foramina/Fissures and Contents

Anterior Skull Base
- **Foramen cecum**: Midline, anterior to crista galli; embryologic remnant of anterior neuropore, which normally involutes in early childhood
- **Cribriform plate foramina**: Roof of nasal cavity; transmits afferent fibers from nasal mucosa to olfactory bulbs of **CNI**

Central Skull Base
- **Optic canal**: Medial LWS; transmits **CNII** to **globe**, dura, arachnoid and pia, CSF, ophthalmic artery
- **SOF**: Between LWS and GWS; transmits **CNIII**, **CNIV**, **CNVI**, **CNV1**, and superior ophthalmic vein
- **IOF**: Cleft between maxilla body and GWS; transmits inferior orbital artery, vein, and nerve
- **Foramen rotundum**: Conduit to pterygopalatine fossa (PPF) within sphenoid bone superolateral to vidian canal; transmits **CNV2** to **PPF**, artery of foramen rotundum, emissary veins from cavernous sinus to pterygoid plexus
- **Foramen ovale**: Within GWS; transmits **CNV3** into **MS**, lesser petrosal nerve, and accessory meningeal branch of internal maxillary artery
- **Foramen spinosum**: Within GWS posterolateral to foramen ovale; transmits middle meningeal artery and vein and recurrent branch of CNV3
- **Vidian canal**: Inferolateral to foramen rotundum within GWS; connects foramen lacerum to PPF; transmits vidian nerve and artery
- **Carotid canal**: In T-bone and GWS; transmits petrous (C2) and lacerum (C3) segments of ICA and **sympathetic plexus**
- **Foramen lacerum**: Gap in bone filled by cartilaginous plate

Posterior Skull Base
- **IAC**: In posterior wall of T-bone; medial opening = porus acusticus; transmits **CNVII**, **CNVIII**, and labyrinthine artery
- **JF**: Cleft between temporal and occipital bones with 2 parts (pars nervosa and vascularis); pars nervosa transmits **CNXI** into **CS**, Jacobson nerve, inferior petrosal vein; pars vascularis transmits **CNX**, **CNXI**, Arnold nerve, posterior meningeal artery, jugular bulb
- **Hypoglossal canal**: Found with condylar occipital bone inferomedial to JF; transmits **CNXII** into **CS**
- **Stylomastoid foramen**: Exocranial surface of T-bone between medial mastoid tip and styloid process; transmits **CNVII** into **PS**
- **Foramen magnum**: Occipital bone inferior ring; transmits medulla oblongata, vertebral arteries, and **CNXI** (ascending spinal component)

Embryology

ASB embryology is key to understanding disease in this area (anterior neuropore anomaly, cephalocele, nasal glioma). The **prenasal space** is a transient prenatal region separating nasal bones and the cartilaginous nasal capsule. The anterior neuropore extends from intracranial space to prenasal space and briefly contacts skin at the bridge of the nose but involutes prior to birth. The prenasal space reduces to a small canal anterior to the crista galli called the **foramen cecum**. The newborn FC diameter is ~ 4 mm. The FC should be completely ossified by 2 years of age.

Skull Base DDx: Tumors & Tumor-Like Lesions by Site

Skull base, anterior, central, or posterior	Melanoma, N
Meningioma	Lacrimal gland carcinoma, O
Giant cell tumor	**Central skull base**
Solitary fibrous tumor	Sella: Pituitary macroadenoma
Metastases	Clivus: Chordoma, benign notochordal cell tumor
Multiple myeloma	Petrooccipital fissure: Chondrosarcoma
Plasmacytoma	Meckel cave: Trigeminal schwannoma
Osteosarcoma	Temporal bone: Tumor
Rhabdomyosarcoma, parameningeal	Endolymphatic sac tumor
Langerhans cell histiocytosis	Temporal bone: Tumor-like lesions
Tumor-like lesions	Acquired cholesteatoma
Fibrous dysplasia	Congenital cholesteatoma
Paget disease	Cholesterol granuloma
Idiopathic extraorbital inflammation (pseudotumor)	**Posterior skull base**
Anterior skull base	Clivus (occipital bone): Chordoma
Mucocele, SN	Jugular foramen
Osteoma, SN	Jugular paraganglioma
Olfactory neuroblastoma, N	Jugular foramen schwannoma
Squamous cell carcinoma, SN	Jugular foramen meningioma
Non-Hodgkin lymphoma, SN or O	Hypoglossal canal: Hypoglossal schwannoma
SN = sinonasal; N = nasal; O = orbit.	

As the ASB originates largely from cartilaginous precursors, the process of ossification can be confusing on imaging. The ASB ossifies from posterior to anterior and lateral to medial. At birth, ASB is composed of cartilage, which progressively ossifies. Ossification of the crista galli and cribriform plate begins at 2 months and is complete by 24 months. The crista galli contains fat at 12 months (**do not** call it a dermoid). The area of the FC ossifies last, reaching its adult configuration by 2 years (**do not** overcall an anterior neuropore anomaly).

The CSB forms from ~ 24 ossification centers. Major centers include the presphenoid (planum sphenoidale), postsphenoid (basisphenoid containing sella, dorsum, sphenoid sinus), alisphenoid (GWS), and orbitosphenoid (LWS). The **sphenooccipital synchondrosis** lies between the basisphenoid and basiocciput. It is the site of most postnatal SB growth and one of the last sutures to fuse (completed by 20 years of age). Persistence of the **craniopharyngeal canal** (remnant of Rathke pouch) may occur between the presphenoid and basisphenoid. Persistence of the **median basal canal** may be seen between the basioccipital ossification centers.

Approaches to Skull Base Imaging Issues

Creating SB lesion DDx can be difficult because some lesions can occur anywhere along the SB. Understanding the DDx list of the lesions that can occur anywhere in the SB is essential. Adding this group to a site-specific DDx can yield a near-complete set of possible lesions to be considered. ASB, CSB, and PSB DDx lists can be constructed. The CSB can be further refined into shorter site-specific DDx lists for the sella, clivus, petrooccipital fissure, and Meckel cave. The PSB has 1 important site-specific DDx for the JF.

Knowledgeable reports about SB lesions require the radiologist to understand the interface relationships between the SB and the extracranial head and neck. The ASB sits atop the frontal and ethmoid sinuses, orbit, and nose. Many of the ASB lesions originate in these structures. The CSB resides superior to the MS, PS, and PMSs. Nasopharyngeal carcinoma directly accesses the intracranial compartment via the foramen lacerum (perivascular spread). MS and PS malignancies may reach the intracranial compartment via perineural spread along CNV3 and CNVII, respectively. The PSB directly interacts with the CS, RPS, and PVSs. When JF lesions exit the SB inferiorly, they plunge directly into the nasopharyngeal CS.

Without a clear understanding of perineural tumor (PNT) SB spread, the radiologist may not identify this key imaging finding. PNT from PS malignancy enters the stylomastoid foramen and climbs the CNVII mastoid segment. MS malignancy at CNV3 PNT traverses foramen ovale on its way to Meckel cave. Cheek skin, palate, sinus, or orbit carcinoma can access CNV2 via the infraorbital nerve or PPF, following CNV2 through the foramen rotundum into the middle cranial fossa. PPF malignancy may also show PNT spread via the vidian nerve to the foramen lacerum. PNT also connects between CNV and CNVII along the greater superficial petrosal nerve on the superior ridge of the petrous T-bone.

Selected References

1. Wang W et al: Imaging of congenital anomalies and defects of the skull base and calvarium. Br J Radiol. 97(1157):902-12, 2024
2. Yamano A et al: Preoperative vascular and cranial nerve imaging in skull base tumors. Cancers (Basel). 17(1):62, 2024
3. Battal B et al: Imaging of skull base tumors. Tomography. 9(4):1196-235, 2023

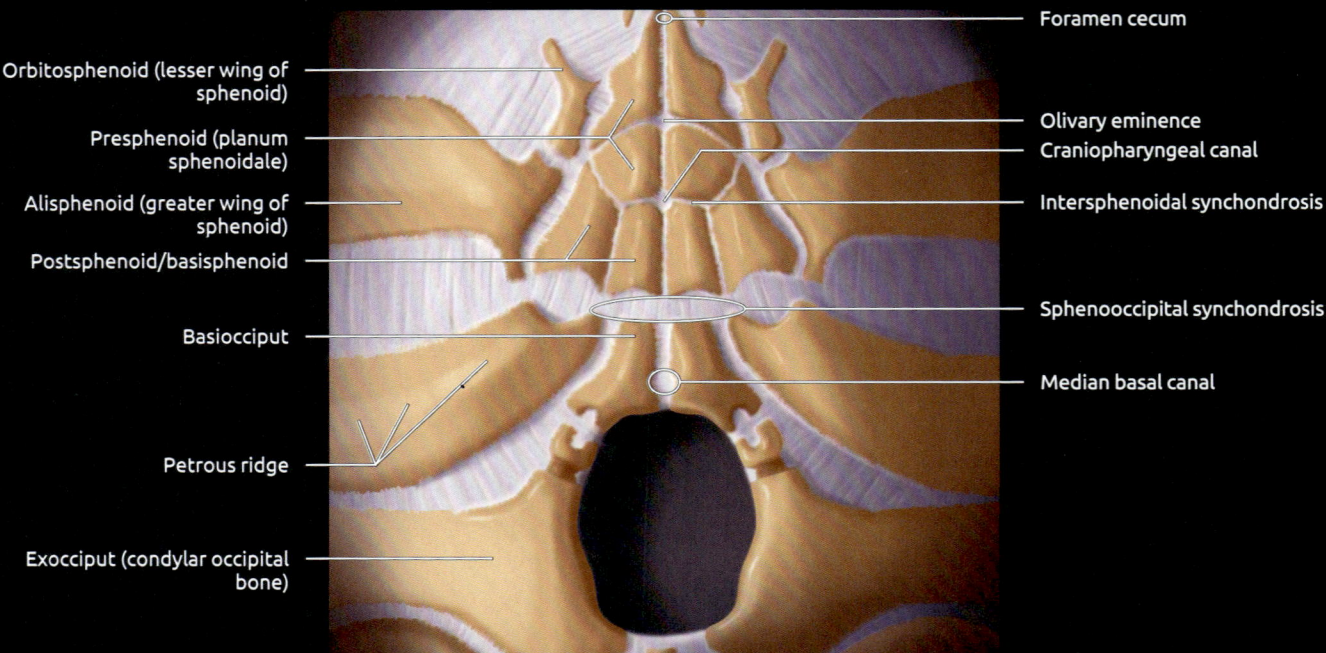

Foramen cecum

Orbitosphenoid (lesser wing of sphenoid)

Presphenoid (planum sphenoidale)

Olivary eminence

Craniopharyngeal canal

Alisphenoid (greater wing of sphenoid)

Intersphenoidal synchondrosis

Postsphenoid/basisphenoid

Basiocciput

Sphenooccipital synchondrosis

Median basal canal

Petrous ridge

Exocciput (condylar occipital bone)

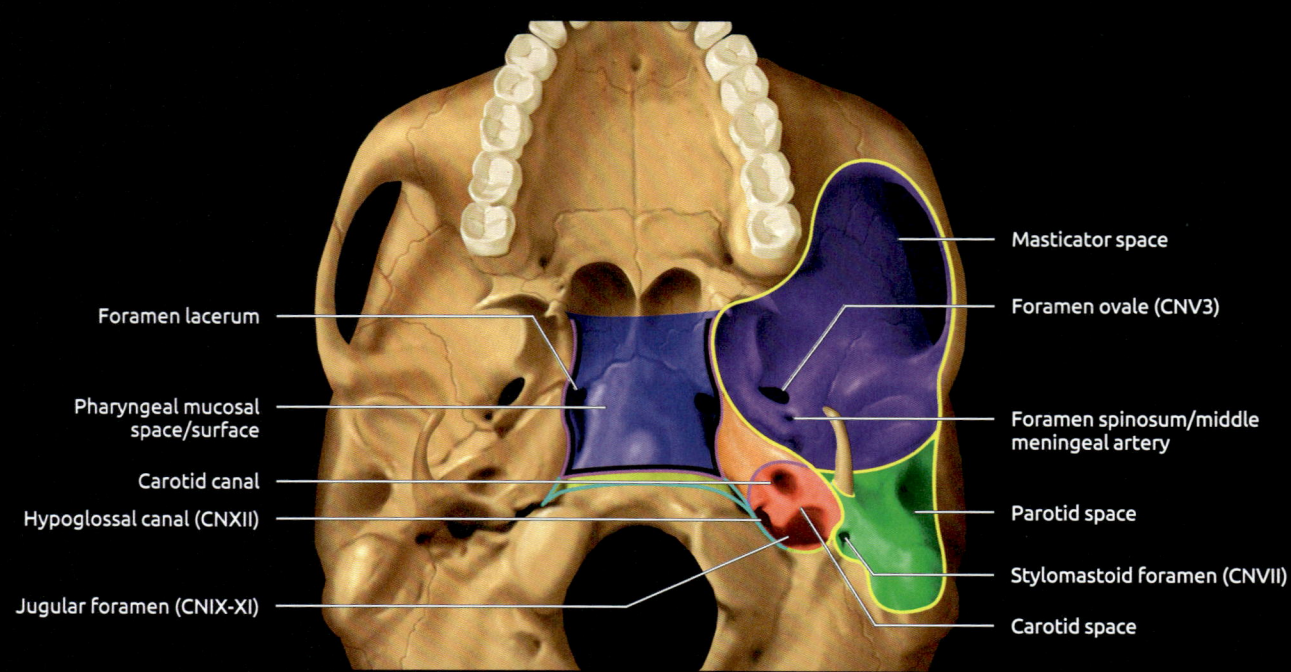

Masticator space

Foramen lacerum

Foramen ovale (CNV3)

Pharyngeal mucosal space/surface

Carotid canal

Foramen spinosum/middle meningeal artery

Hypoglossal canal (CNXII)

Parotid space

Jugular foramen (CNIX-XI)

Stylomastoid foramen (CNVII)

Carotid space

(Top) *Graphic of the skull base shows many ossification centers. Between the ossification centers of presphenoid is a cartilaginous gap called the olivary eminence, which is obliterated shortly after birth. In the midline, note the craniopharyngeal canal, sphenooccipital synchondrosis, and median basal canal. The sphenooccipital synchondrosis fuses over the first 20 years of life, while the craniopharyngeal and median basal canals are rarely persistent into childhood. When persistent, these 2 canals can rarely be the source of meningitis.* **(Bottom)** *Graphic of the skull base viewed from below shows the relationship of spaces of the suprahyoid neck to the skull base. Four spaces have key interactions with the skull base: Masticator, parotid, carotid, and pharyngeal mucosal spaces. Parotid space (green) malignancy can follow CNVII into the stylomastoid foramen. Masticator space (purple) receives CNV3, while CNIX-XII enter the carotid space (red). The pharyngeal mucosal space abuts the foramen lacerum, which is covered by fibrocartilage in life.*

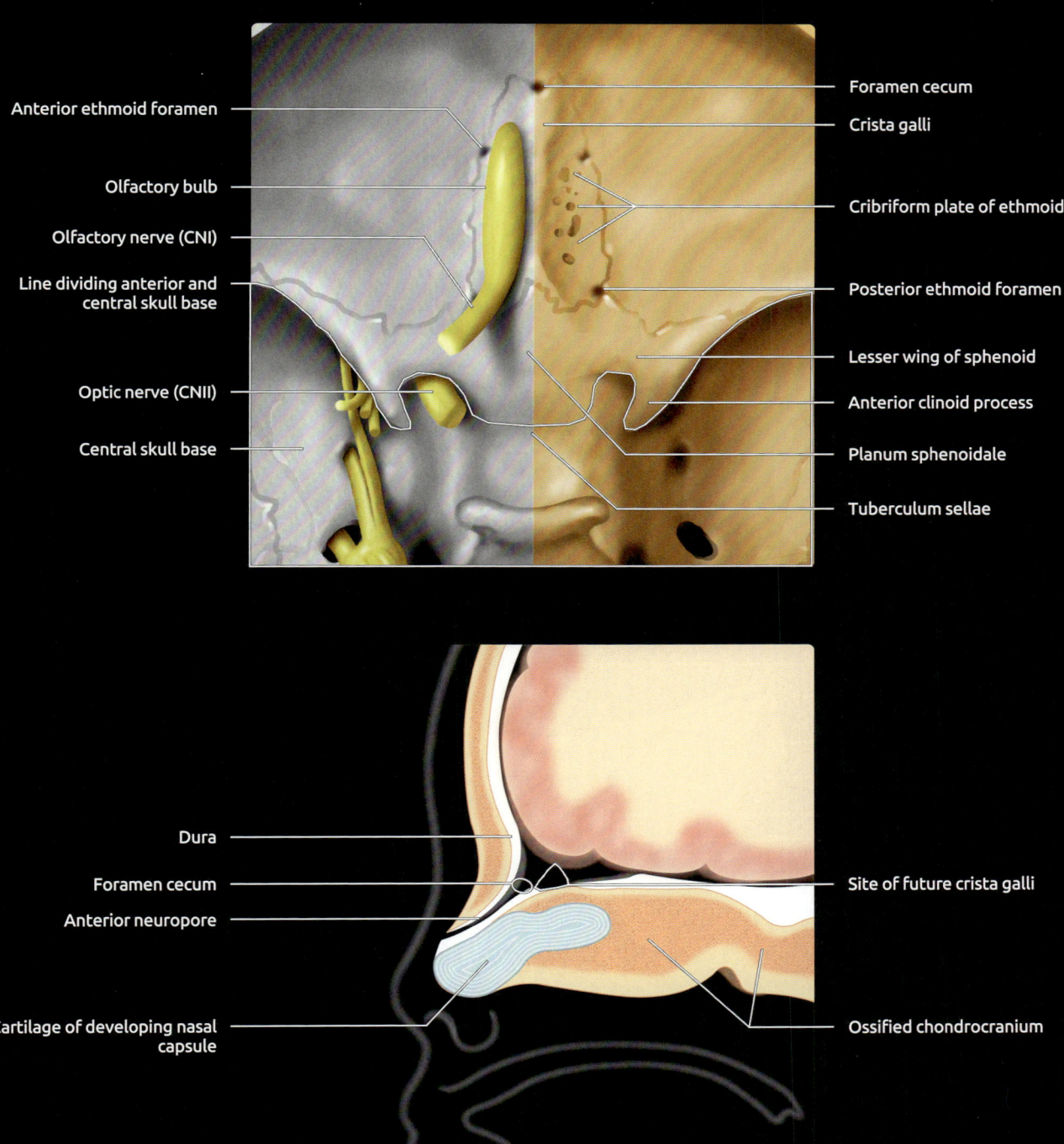

Anterior ethmoid foramen

Olfactory bulb

Olfactory nerve (CNI)

Line dividing anterior and central skull base

Optic nerve (CNII)

Central skull base

Foramen cecum

Crista galli

Cribriform plate of ethmoid

Posterior ethmoid foramen

Lesser wing of sphenoid

Anterior clinoid process

Planum sphenoidale

Tuberculum sellae

Dura

Foramen cecum

Anterior neuropore

Cartilage of developing nasal capsule

Site of future crista galli

Ossified chondrocranium

(Top) *Graphic of the anterior skull base seen from above shows the olfactory bulb of CNI lying on the cribriform plate. Neural structures have been removed on the right, allowing visualization of numerous perforations in the cribriform plate, through which afferent fibers from olfactory mucosa pass to form the olfactory bulb. The posterior margin of the anterior skull base is formed by the lesser wing of sphenoid and planum sphenoidale. Note the foramen cecum, a small pit anterior to the crista galli, bounded anteriorly by frontal bone and posteriorly by ethmoid bone. If the anterior neuropore persists, an enlarged foramen cecum, bifid crista galli, and epidermoid along the neuropore tract are possible. **(Bottom)** Sagittal graphic of the anterior skull base during development shows ossification of the chondrocranium proceeding from posterior to anterior. The prenasal space is now encased in bone and has become the foramen cecum. A normal stalk of dura extends through the foramen cecum to skin (anterior neuropore).*

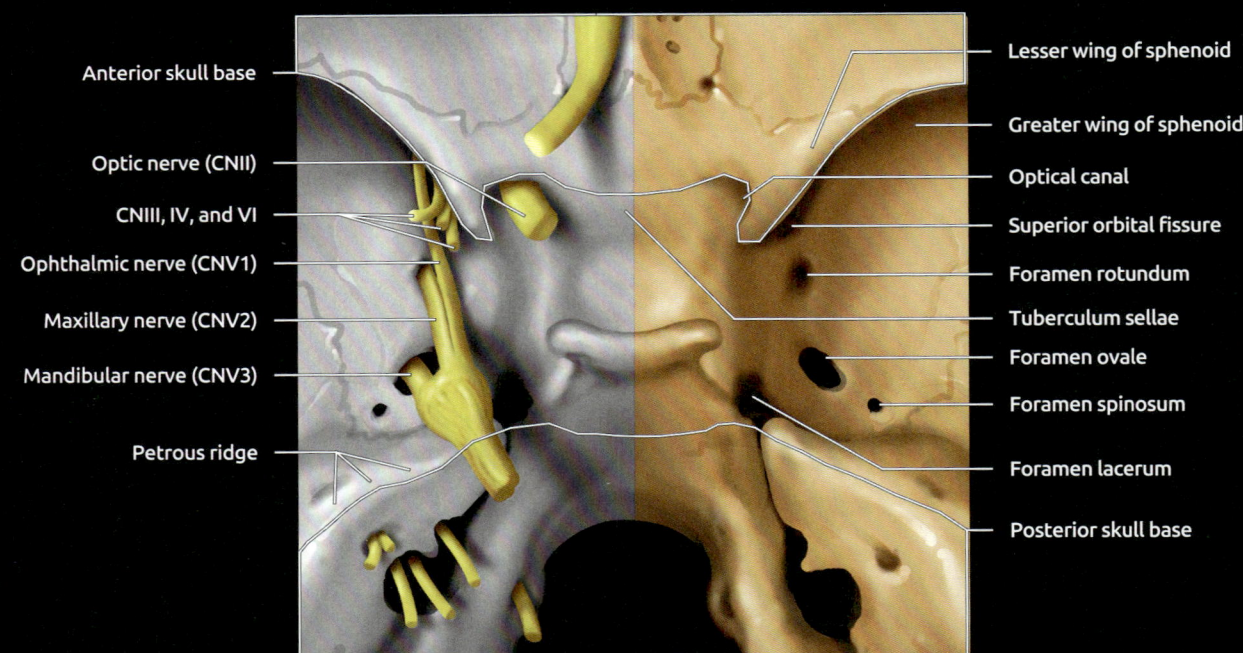

Anterior skull base

Optic nerve (CNII)

CNIII, IV, and VI

Ophthalmic nerve (CNV1)

Maxillary nerve (CNV2)

Mandibular nerve (CNV3)

Petrous ridge

Lesser wing of sphenoid

Greater wing of sphenoid

Optical canal

Superior orbital fissure

Foramen rotundum

Tuberculum sellae

Foramen ovale

Foramen spinosum

Foramen lacerum

Posterior skull base

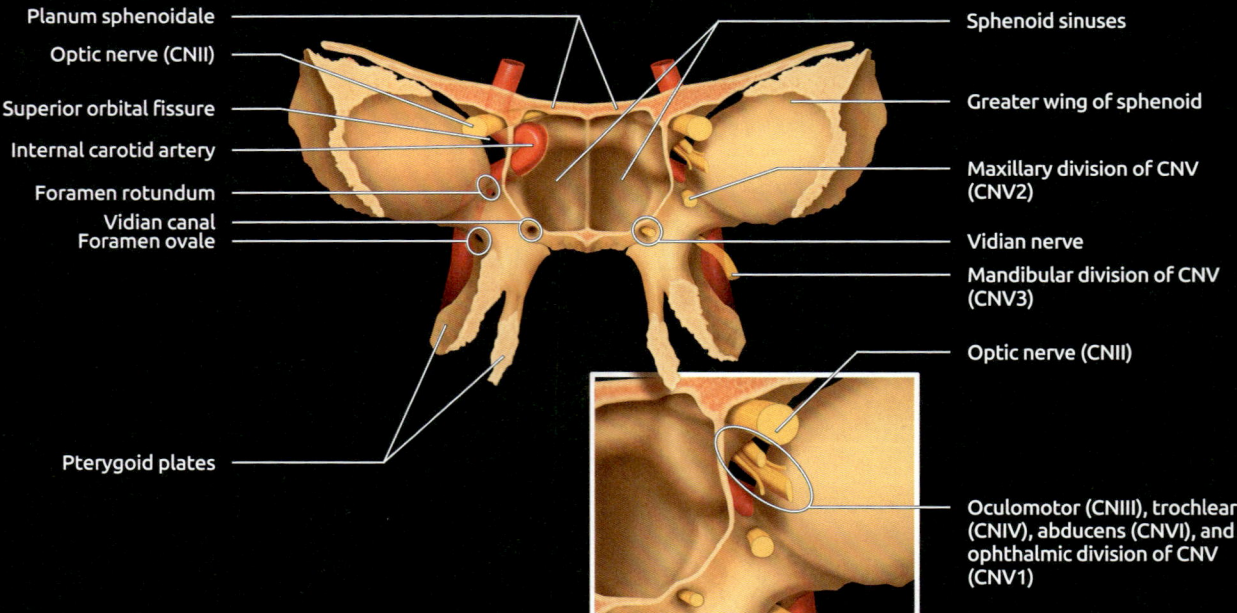

Planum sphenoidale

Optic nerve (CNII)

Superior orbital fissure

Internal carotid artery

Foramen rotundum

Vidian canal
Foramen ovale

Pterygoid plates

Sphenoid sinuses

Greater wing of sphenoid

Maxillary division of CNV (CNV2)

Vidian nerve

Mandibular division of CNV (CNV3)

Optic nerve (CNII)

Oculomotor (CNIII), trochlear (CNIV), abducens (CNVI), and ophthalmic division of CNV (CNV1)

(Top) *Graphic of the central skull base seen from above shows the important nerves on the left and the numerous fissures and foramina on the right. The greater wing of the sphenoid forms the anterior wall of the middle cranial fossa. The posterior limit of the central skull base is the dorsum sella medially and the petrous ridge laterally.* **(Bottom)** *Coronal graphic shows the important anatomy of the central skull base/sphenoid bone. The cavernous portions of the internal carotid arteries lie lateral and posterior to the sinuses. At the orbital apex, the optic nerve can be seen traversing the optic canal. Multiple cranial nerves pass through the superior orbital fissure into the orbit, including CNIII, IV, and VI, as well as the ophthalmic division on CNV. The maxillary division of CNV in foramen rotundum and the vidian nerve are positioned lateral and inferior to the sinus, respectively.*

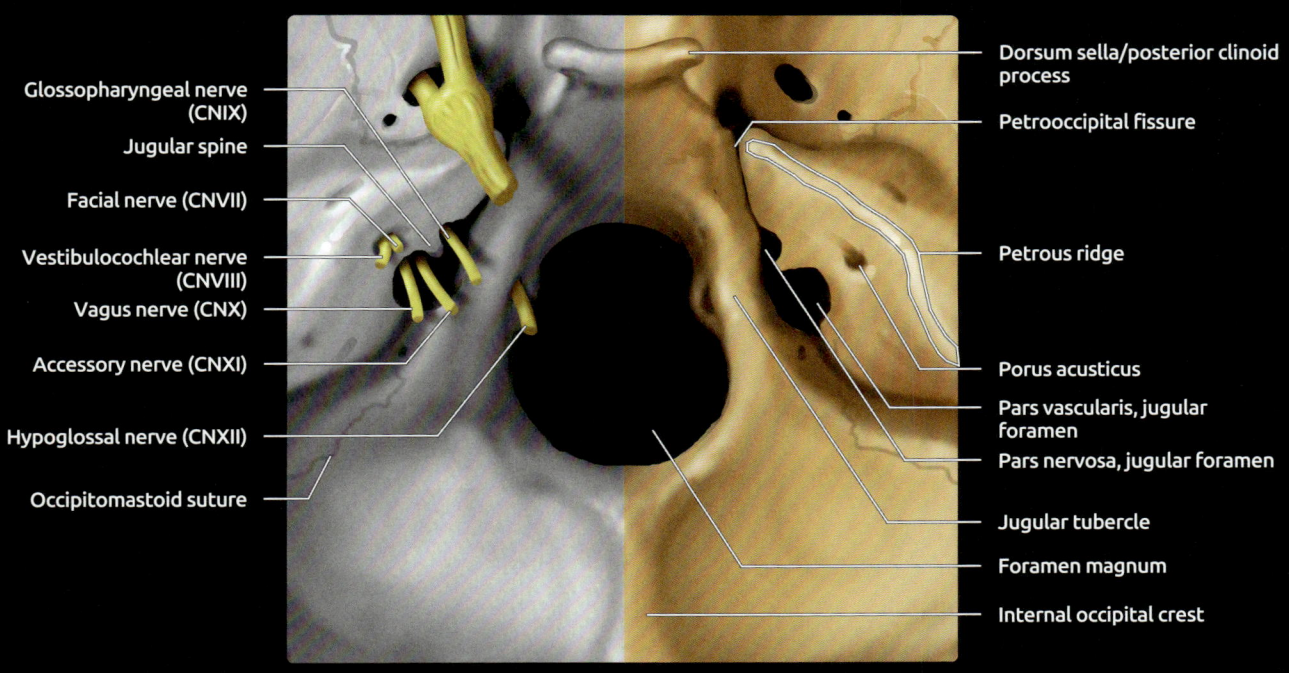

Glossopharyngeal nerve (CNIX)

Jugular spine

Facial nerve (CNVII)

Vestibulocochlear nerve (CNVIII)

Vagus nerve (CNX)

Accessory nerve (CNXI)

Hypoglossal nerve (CNXII)

Occipitomastoid suture

Dorsum sella/posterior clinoid process

Petrooccipital fissure

Petrous ridge

Porus acusticus

Pars vascularis, jugular foramen

Pars nervosa, jugular foramen

Jugular tubercle

Foramen magnum

Internal occipital crest

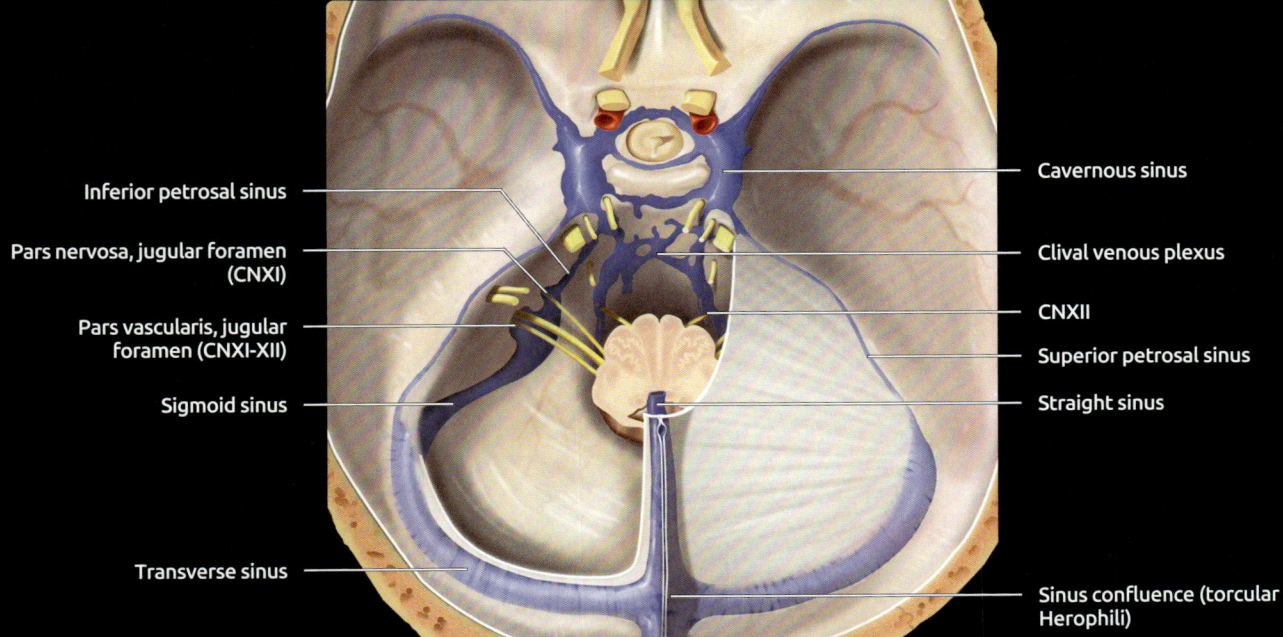

Inferior petrosal sinus

Pars nervosa, jugular foramen (CNXI)

Pars vascularis, jugular foramen (CNXI-XII)

Sigmoid sinus

Transverse sinus

Cavernous sinus

Clival venous plexus

CNXII

Superior petrosal sinus

Straight sinus

Sinus confluence (torcular Herophili)

(Top) *Graphic shows the posterior skull base as seen from above. The neural structures are shown on the left, while the bony landmarks are seen on the right. The anterior boundary of posterior skull base is the clivus medially and petrous ridge laterally. The major foramina are the foramen magnum, porus acusticus, jugular foramen, and hypoglossal canal. Notice that the jugular foramen connects anteriorly with the petrooccipital fissure.* **(Bottom)** *Graphic of the posterior skull base shows the major dural venous sinuses and jugular foramen from above. The midbrain and pons, as well as the left 1/2 of the tentorium cerebelli, have been removed. Notice the transverse sinus is in the wall of the occipital bone, while the sigmoid sinus is in the medial wall of the temporal bone. The 2 portions of the jugular foramen are also visible. The anterior pars nervosa receives the glossopharyngeal nerve (CNIX), while the pars vascularis has the vagus (CNX) and accessory (CNXI) nerves passing through it.*

TERMINOLOGY

- Benign, **cystic mass arising dorsal to clivus with intradural component in prepontine cistern**
  - Considered to be benign or low-grade tumor

IMAGING

- CT: Prepontine intradural mass connected by osseous stalk or pedicle to clivus
  - Most will appear as well-marginated, scalloped lesion of clivus with sclerotic margins
- MR: Provides best depiction of lesion, stalk, and intradural component
  - Uniformly T2 hyperintense
  - Clival component hypointense compared to normal marrow
  - Restricted diffusion may be noted
  - **Lack of enhancement** helps to favor benign tumor (previously ecchordosis physalifora); now considered on continuum with chordoma histologically

- Beware of enhancement on postcontrast delayed FLAIR imaging

TOP DIFFERENTIAL DIAGNOSES

- Chordoma
- Skull base metastasis
- Dermoid or epidermoid
- Arachnoid cyst

PATHOLOGY

- Few clear cells (**physaliphorous cells**) surrounded by chondromyxoid stroma

CLINICAL ISSUES

- Asymptomatic, and usually found incidentally on head MR
  - Found in 2% of autopsies and 1.6% of MR studies
- Indolent lesion, which does not appear to grow
- Typically not managed surgically unless significant brainstem compression or symptoms are present

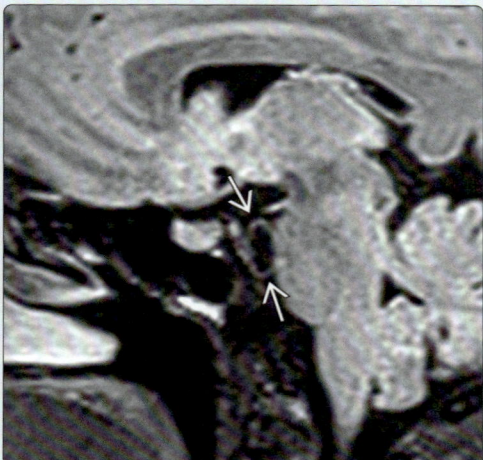
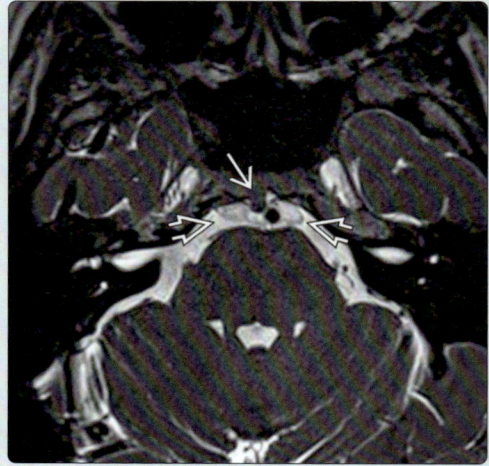

(Left) Sagittal T2 FLAIR MR demonstrates the intradural component of a classic benign notochordal cell tumor (BNCT) with a notable thin-walled ➡ cyst, which is otherwise isointense with CSF. The clival portion of the lesion is not well seen. (Right) Axial 3D T2 MR SSFSE demonstrates a small bony strut ➡ of classic BNCT and the intradural cystic component of the lesion ➡, which is surrounding the basilar artery. The cystic lesion within the clivus is not apparent on this section.

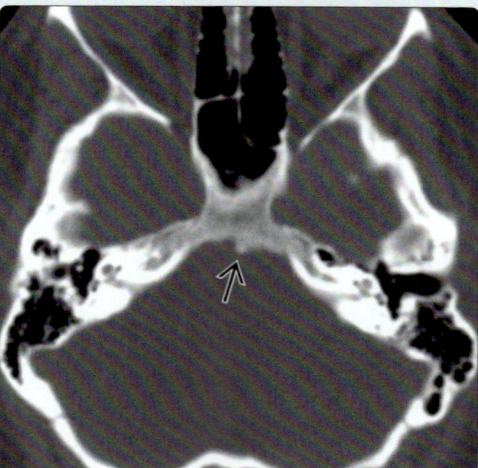
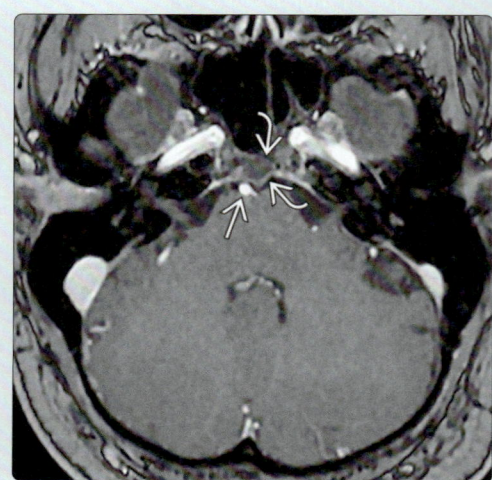

(Left) Axial bone CT from an asymptomatic patient with incidental BNCT shows a bony spicule ➡, which often accompanies the sclerotic margins of these lesions on CT. The intradural component may not be appreciated on CT. (Right) Axial T1 MR after contrast administration in a different patient demonstrates the intradural component of the ecchordosis as a near CSF signal intensity lobular lesion ➡ in the prepontine cistern adjacent to the basilar artery ➡, Lack of enhancement helps differentiate from chordoma.

TERMINOLOGY

Abbreviations
- Benign notochordal cell tumor (BNCT)

Definitions
- Benign, cystic mass arising from dorsal clivus, considered to be **benign notochordal tumor**

IMAGING

General Features
- Best diagnostic clue
  - Well-defined lesion of clivus with prepontine intradural cystic mass connected by stalk or pedicle to clival lesion
- Location
  - **Prepontine cistern** along dorsal midline clivus most common; occasionally paramedian
  - Recently proposed classification system depends on BNCT appearance; clivus alone or clivus and intradural component
- Morphology
  - Well defined, lobular ± bony stalk

Imaging Recommendations
- Best imaging tool
  - MR provides best depiction of lesion, stalk, and intradural component
- Protocol advice
  - Sagittal images and 3D T2 best for identifying osseous stalk attaching lesion to clivus and cyst

CT Findings
- NECT
  - CT may not identify intradural component (similar density to CSF)
- Bone CT
  - Variable osseous stalk or pedicle connecting basisphenoid portion of clivus to intradural component
  - Well-marginated, scalloped clival component with sclerotic margins

MR Findings
- T1WI
  - Intradural component may be nearly isointense to CSF
  - Intraclival component (if present) hypointense compared to normal clivus marrow
- T2WI
  - Uniformly hyperintense in most cases
- DWI
  - **Restricted diffusion** often noted
- T1WI C+
  - No enhancement noted (differentiates from chordoma)

DIFFERENTIAL DIAGNOSIS

Clivus Chordoma
- Malignant clival mass that typically remains extradural
- Variable enhancement; destroys bone
- Aggressive and symptomatic

Skull Base Metastasis
- Multiple lesions, enhancement is common

Dermoid and Epidermoid
- Rarely located in clivus but may closely resemble imaging characteristics

Arachnoid Cyst
- Follows CSF density/signal intensity exactly

PATHOLOGY

General Features
- Etiology
  - Benign, congenital malformation arising from ectopic notochordal tissue

Gross Pathologic & Surgical Features
- Small cystic or gelatinous mass, which has intradural component and is attached to clivus by stalk

Microscopic Features
- Few clear cells (physaliphorous cells) surrounded by chondromyxoid stroma

CLINICAL ISSUES

Presentation
- Most common signs/symptoms
  - Asymptomatic lesion may be found incidentally on head MR or CT
- Other signs/symptoms
  - Rare brainstem compressive symptoms, pontine hemorrhage, CSF fistulae with rhinorrhea

Demographics
- Epidemiology
  - Found in 2% of autopsies and 1.6% of MR studies

Natural History & Prognosis
- Indolent lesion, which **does not** appear to **grow**

Treatment
- Typically not managed surgically unless significant brainstem compression or symptoms are present

DIAGNOSTIC CHECKLIST

Image Interpretation Pearls
- Identification of stalk arising from clivus with intradural extension of lesion into prepontine cistern is characteristic

SELECTED REFERENCES

1. Peels J et al: Delayed FLAIR-enhancement of benign notochordal remnant (ecchordosis physaliphora). Neuroradiol J. 38(2):220-3, 2024
2. Stevens AR et al: Ecchordosis physaliphora: does it even exist? AJNR Am J Neuroradiol. 44(8):889-93, 2023
3. Kogue R et al: Evaluation of intradural ecchordosis physaliphora with three-dimensional fluid-attenuated inversion recovery. J Comput Assist Tomogr. 44(5):699-703, 2020
4. Lin E et al: Prognostic implications of gadolinium enhancement of skull base chordomas. AJNR Am J Neuroradiol. 39(8):1509-14, 2018
5. Golden LD et al: Benign notochordal lesions of the posterior clivus: retrospective review of prevalence and imaging characteristics. J Neuroimaging. 24(3):245-9, 2014
6. Chihara C et al: Ecchordosis physaliphora and its variants: proposed new classification based on high-resolution fast MR imaging employing steady-state acquisition. Eur Radiol. 23(10):2854-60, 2013
7. Alkan O et al: A case of ecchordosis physaliphora presenting with an intratumoral hemorrhage. Turk Neurosurg. 19(3):293-6, 2009

TERMINOLOGY

- Fossa navicularis magna (FNM)
  - Congenital defect resulting from minor pharyngeal formation miscue, creating ventral cortical concavity of clivus defect in ventral surface of midclivus

IMAGING

- Sagittal bone CT
  - FNM appears as **ventral cortical concavity of clivus, corticated divot** of **midline, ventral, and midclivus**
- Sagittal MR
  - Nasopharyngeal **adenoids/mucosa** project into FNM lumen

TOP DIFFERENTIAL DIAGNOSES

- Persistent craniopharyngeal canal (P-CPC)
- Median basal canal (MBC)
- Extraosseous chordoma
- Benign notochordal cell tumor

PATHOLOGY

- Best etiology hypothesis
  - During notochord ascent, focal adhesions form between notochord and foregut endoderm
  - Pharyngeal mucosa is then carried along with notochord toward developing skull base
  - Final result is midline divot (FNM) in ventral midclivus lined with pharyngeal mucosa/adenoidal tissue

CLINICAL ISSUES

- **Asymptomatic, incidental finding, rarely infected**

DIAGNOSTIC CHECKLIST

- **Location comparison** of congenital lesions in area
  - P-CPC anterior to sphenoccipital synchondrosis
  - FNM and MBC posterior to sphenoccipital synchondrosis
  - FNM affects ventral cortex of midclivus
  - MBC is most commonly transclival in lower clivus

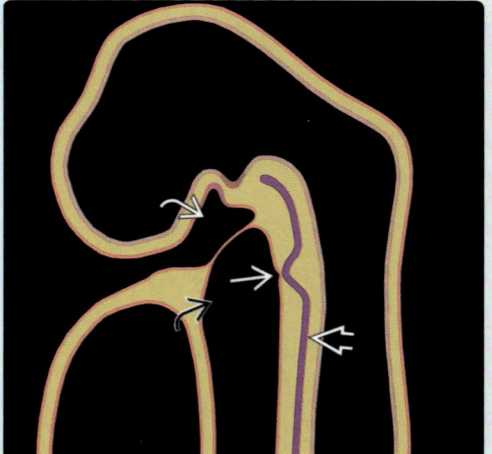
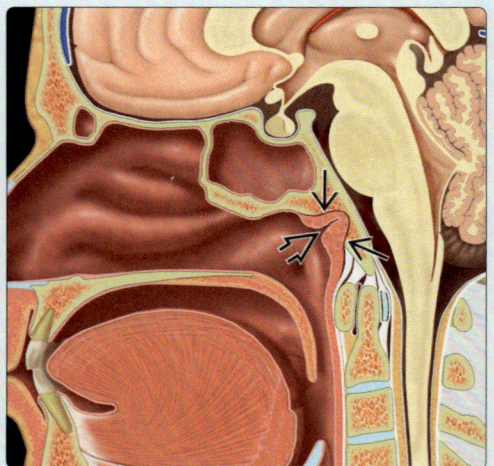

(Left) Sagittal graphic of a 4- to 5-week-old fetus shows that, as the notochord ➡ ascends, it forms focal adhesions with the foregut endoderm ➡, and a portion of pharyngeal mucosa is carried along with notochord to the developing skull base. A diverticulum (FNM) lined with pharyngeal mucosa/adenoids will appear in the midline; see stomodeum ➡ and foregut ⬈. (Right) Sagittal graphic of an adult FNM shows the lesion ➡ is boat-shaped, midline, in the ventral midclivus, and filled with mucosa and adenoidal tissue ⬈.

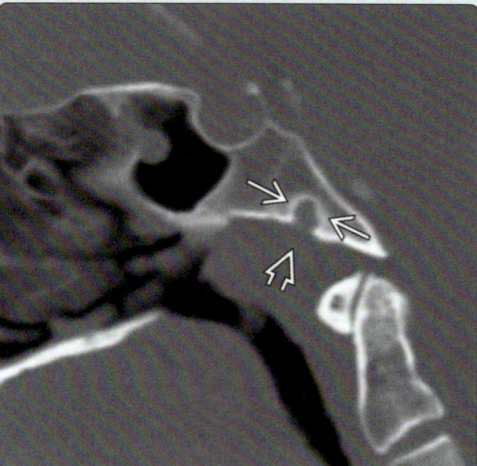
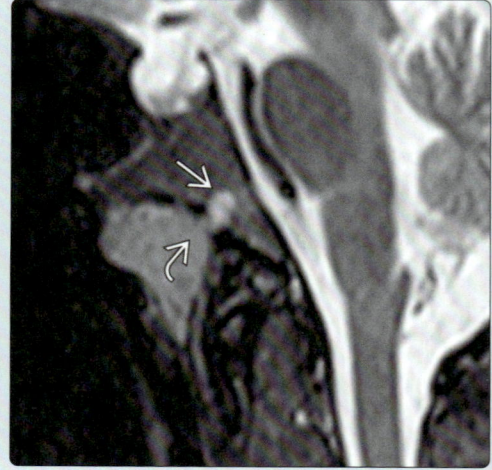

(Left) Sagittal bone CT reformation in a patient scanned for neck pain reveals an incidental, boat-shaped FNM ➡ with nasopharyngeal adenoids/mucosa projecting into its lumen ➡. (Right) Sagittal T2 MR in the same patient demonstrates a defect in the ventral clivus ➡ with contiguous nasopharyngeal mucosa/adenoidal tissue ➡.

Fossa Navicularis Magna

TERMINOLOGY

Abbreviations

- Fossa navicularis magna (FNM)

Synonyms

- Pharyngeal bursa or pharyngeal fossa

Definitions

- Congenital, ventral cortical concavity of clivus defect in ventral surface of midclivus

IMAGING

General Features

- Best diagnostic clue
  - Sagittal bone CT: **Ventral cortical concavity of clivus, corticated divot of midline, ventral, and midclivus**
  - Sagittal MR: **Nasopharyngeal adenoids/mucosa project into FNM lumen**
- Location
  - Defect found in ventral midline surface of clivus
  - Posterior to sphenoccipital synchondrosis
- Size
  - Variable: Barely visible to 15 mm
- Morphology
  - Ovoid on axial view; ventral cortical concavity of clivus on sagittal view

CT Findings

- Bone CT
  - Axial: Ovoid, corticated lesion of midclivus
  - Sagittal: Ventral cortical concavity of clivus lesion; ventral clival surface
  - Air may be trapped in adenoidal tissue within FNM
  - Distance between deepest point of FNM and intracranial contents helps assessing risk of infection

MR Findings

- T1WI FS
  - Mucosa/adenoidal tissue project into FNM
- T1WI C+ FS
  - Mild enhancement of adenoidal tissue in FNM
  - If significant enhancement ± adjacent skull base bone abnormalities, consider infection
    - Infected FNM is extremely rare

DIFFERENTIAL DIAGNOSIS

Persistent Craniopharyngeal Canal

- Persistent bony canal between anterior floor of sella and nasopharyngeal roof
- Results from developmental nonobliteration of adenohypophyseal stalk
- May be intermediate in size and contain ectopic pituitary
- May be large and contain cephalocele, tumors, or both

Median Basal Canal

- Persistent bony canal spanning lower clivus inner cortex to posterior nasopharynx
- Notochordal track remnant
- Very rare lesion

Extraosseous Chordoma

- Midline nasopharyngeal chordoma with soft tissue and bony components
- May have median basal canal (MBC) component

Benign Notochordal Cell Tumor

- Superior dorsal clival cortex scalloping lesion
- Benign congenital malformation arising from ectopic notochordal tissue

PATHOLOGY

General Features

- Most common hypothesis regarding development of this anatomic variant
  - During notochord ascent, **focal adhesions** form **between notochord and foregut endoderm**
  - Pharyngeal mucosa will be carried along with notochord toward developing skull base
  - Midline divot in ventral midclivus lined with pharyngeal mucosa/lymphoid tissue results (FNM)

CLINICAL ISSUES

Presentation

- Most common signs/symptoms
  - **Asymptomatic; incidental finding**
  - Rarely infected ± meningitis

Demographics

- Age
  - Present at birth; age of discovery based on incidental lesion discovery while imaging for another reason
- Epidemiology
  - ~ 5% if count smaller fossa navicularis and FNM

Natural History & Prognosis

- Incidental finding; very rarely may cause skull base osteomyelitis ± meningitis

Treatment

- No treatment required unless infected

DIAGNOSTIC CHECKLIST

Consider

- FNM is **not** associated with Tornwaldt cyst
- **Differentiate between other congenital lesions in this area based on location**
  - Persistent craniopharyngeal canal anterior to sphenoccipital synchondrosis (SOS)
  - FNM and MBC posterior to SOS
  - FNM affects ventral cortex of midclivus
  - MBC is most commonly transclival in lower clivus

SELECTED REFERENCES

1. Deopujari CE Et al: Endonasal Endoscopic Skull Base Surgery in Children: Anatomical and Technical Considerations. In Kanaan IN et al: Neuroanatomy Guidance to Successful Neurosurgical Interventions. Springer, 2024
2. Adanir SS et al: Radiologic evaluation of the fossa navicularis on dry skull: a comparative CBCT study. J Craniofac Surg. 34(3):1085-8, 2023

Invasive Pituitary Macroadenoma (Pituitary Neuroendocrine Tumor)

TERMINOLOGY

- Invasive, benign pituitary adenoma with inferior extension into skull base
- Redefined as pituitary neuroendocrine tumor (PitNET)

IMAGING

- Multiplanar gadolinium-enhanced MR is imaging modality of choice
- Mass invading central skull base **contiguous with and inseparable from soft tissue mass in sella**
- Ill-defined soft tissue mass centered in sella with invasion of surrounding bone and soft tissue
- Intense enhancement may be heterogeneous as tumor enlarges
- May **extend into cavernous sinus**
- DWI can help predict biological aggressive lesions

TOP DIFFERENTIAL DIAGNOSES

- Clival chordoma

- Skull base meningioma
- Skull base metastasis
- Petrooccipital chondrosarcoma
- Skull base plasmacytoma

CLINICAL ISSUES

- Mean age at presentation: ~ 40 years
- 25% visual field defect or other cranial nerve palsy
- Treatment: Multimodality therapy required for best outcome
  - Surgery often indicated for decompression of optic apparatus
  - Resection often incomplete and leads to recurrences
  - ↑ morbidity due to proximity to vital structures

DIAGNOSTIC CHECKLIST

- Look at sagittal images for normal pituitary gland, and, if absent, invasive adenoma should be at top of DDx

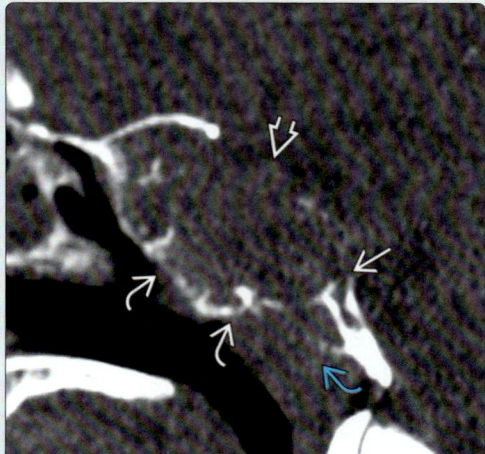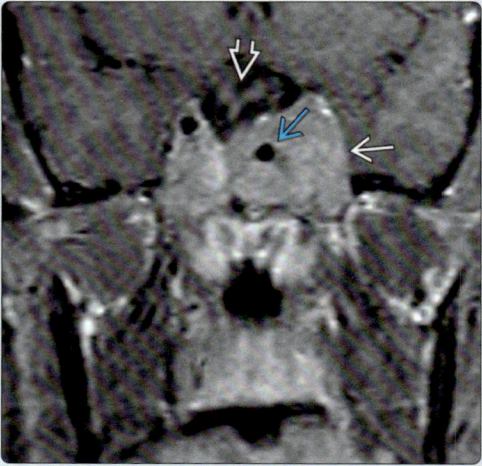

(Left) *Sagittal CT in a 50-year-old man with headaches demonstrates a large macroadenoma with predominantly downward growth. There is destruction of the sellar floor and extension into the sphenoid sinus ⊇ and clivus ⊇. Note irregularity of the sphenoid floor ⊅ and involvement of nasopharynx ⊇.* (Right) *Coronal T1 FS C+ MR in the same patient shows a solidly enhancing macroadenoma ⊇ merging with the pituitary gland. The left ICA is encased by the mass ⊇. Note deformed optic chiasm and pituitary stalk ⊇.*

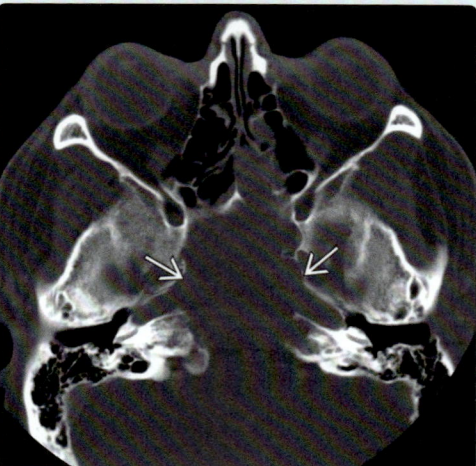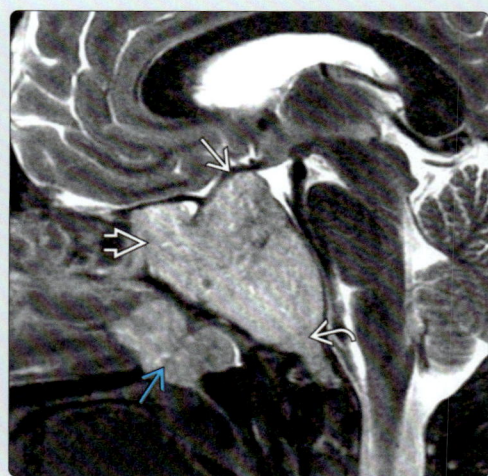

(Left) *Axial bone CT of invasive pituitary macroadenoma shows extensive bone erosion of the central skull base and dorsal clivus. The sella and basisphenoid are largely destroyed. Tumor extends to the medial aspects of the petrous internal carotid artery canals ⊇.* (Right) *Sagittal T2WI MR in the same patient shows suprasellar extension ⊇ and invasion anteriorly into the basisphenoid ⊇ and inferiorly into the clivus ⊇. Tumor also extends anteroinferiorly into the nasopharynx and posterior nasal cavity ⊇.*

Invasive Pituitary Macroadenoma (Pituitary Neuroendocrine Tumor)

TERMINOLOGY

Definitions

- Invasive benign pituitary macroadenoma with inferior extension into skull base

IMAGING

General Features

- Best diagnostic clue
  - Mass invading central skull base **contiguous with and inseparable from soft tissue mass in sella**
- Size
  - Generally > 5 cm, although small tumors can be invasive

CT Findings

- NECT
  - Mass centered in sella with invasion of surrounding bone and soft tissue
  - Hemorrhage in 10%; Ca^{++} in 2%

MR Findings

- T1WI
  - Mass typically isointense to gray matter, although heterogeneity is common
- T2WI
  - Variable signal on long TR images; may be heterogeneous
- T1WI C+
  - Intense heterogeneous enhancement
    - Dural tail may be seen and mimic meningioma
    - May **extend into cavernous sinus**

Imaging Recommendations

- Best imaging tool
  - Multiplanar gadolinium-enhanced MR

DIFFERENTIAL DIAGNOSIS

Clival Chordoma

- Midline clival mass
- ↑ **T2 signal** characteristic

Skull Base Meningioma

- Centered along lateral margin of cavernous sinus or tentorium
- Avidly enhancing ± dural tail, tumoral Ca^{++}

Skull Base Metastasis

- Destructive mass that can be anywhere in skull base

Chondrosarcoma (Petrooccipital Fissure)

- Centered along lateral margin of clivus in petrooccipital fissure
- **Chondroid Ca**$^{++}$ (50%)

Skull Base Plasmacytoma

- T2 signal is low to intermediate
- > 50% have concurrent multiple myeloma

PATHOLOGY

General Features

- Etiology

- Hypothesis for pituitary tumor formation
  - Hypophysiotrophic hormone excess, suppressive hormone insufficiency, or growth factor excess → hyperplasia
  - Hyperplasia predisposes to genetic instability → cell transformation → adenoma formation

Staging, Grading, & Classification

- Radioanatomic classification of adenomas
  - Stage I: Microadenoma < 1 cm without sellar expansion
  - Stage II: Macroadenoma ≥ 1 cm and may be suprasellar
  - Stage III: Macroadenoma with enlargement and invasion of floor or suprasellar extension
  - Stage IV: Destruction of sella

Microscopic Features

- Monotonous sheets of uniform cells

CLINICAL ISSUES

Presentation

- Most common signs/symptoms
  - **Pituitary hormonal abnormality** (symptoms depend on which hormone secreted)
- Other signs/symptoms
  - 25% visual field defect or other cranial nerve palsy

Demographics

- Age
  - Mean age at presentation: ~ 40 years
- Epidemiology
  - Pituitary adenoma: 15% of intracranial tumors
  - Invasive adenomas account for 35% of all pituitary neoplasms

Natural History & Prognosis

- Adenomas typically slow growing
- > 1/3 behave in more aggressive manner with high recurrence rate
- Tumor markers like Ki-67 can potentially predict unfavorable treatment outcomes

Treatment

- Multimodality therapy and long-term follow-up required for best outcome
- Surgical resection is treatment of choice, if possible
  - Surgery often followed by radiation ± chemotherapy

DIAGNOSTIC CHECKLIST

Image Interpretation Pearls

- **Look at sagittal images for normal pituitary gland**; if absent, invasive adenoma should be at top of DDx

SELECTED REFERENCES

1. Xu D et al: Advancements in molecular diagnosis and pharmacotherapeutic strategies for invasive pituitary adenomas. Immun Inflamm Dis. 12(12):e70098, 2024
2. Ho KKY et al: Pituitary adenoma or neuroendocrine tumour: the need for an integrated prognostic classification. Nat Rev Endocrinol. 19(11):671-8, 2023
3. Shih RY et al: Primary tumors of the pituitary gland: radiologic-pathologic correlation. Radiographics. 41(7):2029-46, 2021
4. Chapman PR et al: Neuroimaging of the pituitary gland: practical anatomy and pathology. Radiol Clin North Am. 58(6):1115-33, 2020

Chordoma

TERMINOLOGY

- Rare, locally aggressive tumor of clivus arising from cranial end of primitive notochord remnant

IMAGING

- Location: **Clivus**; sphenooccipital synchondrosis
  - Can occur anywhere along primitive notochord
- CT findings
  - **Midline**, expansile, multilobulated, well-circumscribed mass narrowing prepontine cistern
  - Lytic bone destruction with intratumoral Ca^{++}
  - Variable enhancement
- MR findings
  - T1: Intermediate to low signal compared to brain
  - T2: Classically ↑ ↑ signal
  - T1WI C+: Moderate to marked enhancement
  - DWI: Mean ADC value $1474 \pm 117 \times 10^{-6}$ mm²/s, generally less than chondrosarcoma

- FDG PET for metastases & to monitor post radiation response

TOP DIFFERENTIAL DIAGNOSES

- Invasive pituitary macroadenoma (pituitary neuroendocrine tumor)
- Benign notochordal cell tumor (ecchordosis physaliphora)
- Skull base chondrosarcoma, skull base plasmacytoma
- Skull base metastasis, skull base meningioma

CLINICAL ISSUES

- **35%** of all chordomas arise in **skull base**
- Common symptoms: Headache & diplopia (CNVI)
- Most common age: 30-50 years; M:F = 1:1
- Treatment: Should be managed by multidisciplinary skull base team; surgical resection (conventional vs. endonasal endoscopic)
  - Proton beam RT: Postop & unresectable tumors
- Brachyury: Molecular marker distinctive for chordoma

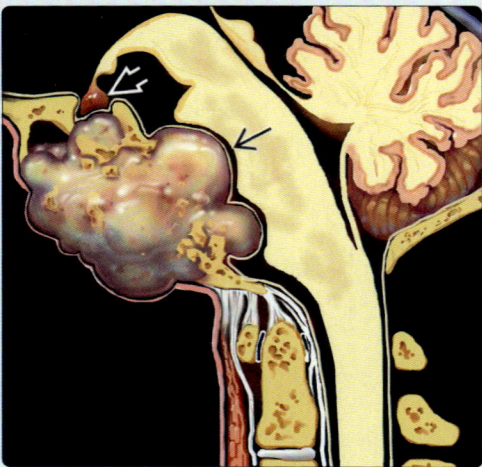
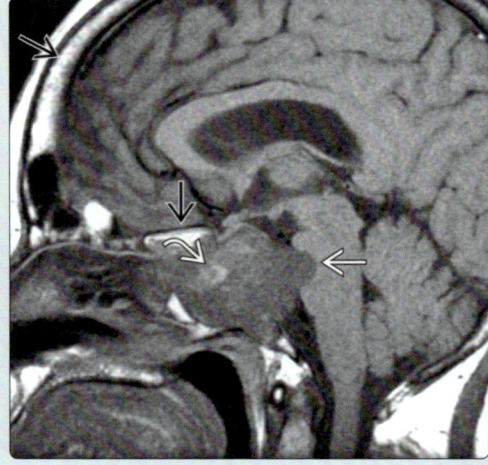

(Left) Sagittal graphic shows an expansile, destructive mass originating from the clivus, "thumbing" pons ⇨ & elevating the pituitary gland ⇨. Note bone fragments floating in chordoma. (Right) Sagittal T1 MR shows near-complete involvement of the clivus with expansile low-signal tumor compared to hyperintense normal marrow ⇨. Note the classic "thumb" ⇨ of tumor compressing the pons and small foci of high signal ⇨ from intratumoral hemorrhage, Ca^{++}, or mucin.

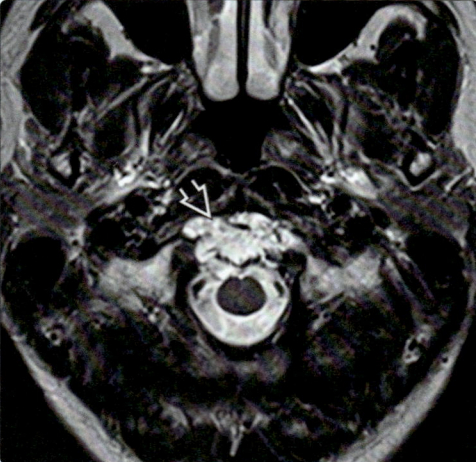
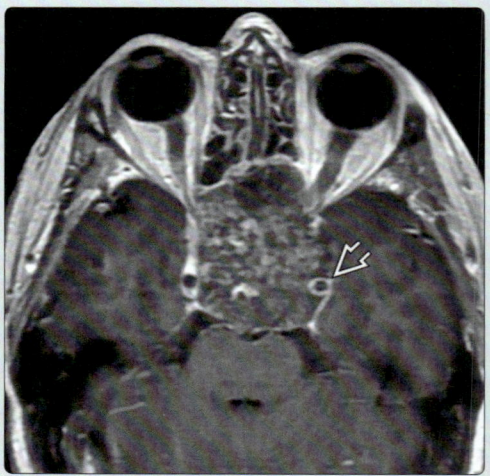

(Left) Axial T2 MR shows characteristic marked, diffuse hyperintensity of this mildly expansile clival chordoma with signal intensity close to CSF and with an internal matrix ⇨. (Right) Axial T1 C+ MR shows minimal heterogeneous intratumoral enhancement. There is tumor extension into the left cavernous sinus with encasement of the internal carotid artery (ICA) ⇨. Angiographic balloon occlusion testing of the left ICA may be warranted should surgery be considered in this patient.

Chordoma

TERMINOLOGY

Abbreviations
- Clival chordoma (CCh)

Synonyms
- Basicranial chordoma

Definitions
- Rare, locally aggressive tumor of clivus arising from cranial end of primitive notochord remnant

IMAGING

General Features
- Best diagnostic clue
  - **Destructive, expansile, midline clival mass** with ↑ T2 signal
- Location
  - Can occur anywhere along primitive notochord
    - Clivus near sphenooccipital synchondrosis
    - Commonly found in midline from sella to coccyx
  - Other rare locations in head & neck
    - Sella, paranasal sinuses, nasopharynx, maxilla
- Size
  - Usually 2-5 cm at presentation
- Morphology
  - Expansile, multilobulated, well-circumscribed mass
  - Expanding tumor **invades or displaces** local structures

CT Findings
- NECT
  - Midline, well-circumscribed, expansile soft tissue mass
  - Hyperdense relative to adjacent neural axis
- CECT
  - Variable enhancement
  - Low density foci represent myxoid/gelatinous material
- Bone CT
  - Mass causes lytic bone destruction
  - **Intratumoral Ca^{++}** = sequestra from destroyed bone > dystrophic Ca^{++}

MR Findings
- T1WI
  - Intermediate to low signal compared to brain
    - Low signal distinguishes from adjacent fatty marrow
  - Small foci high signal: Hemorrhage or mucoid material
  - Tumor "thumb" **indents anterior pons** on sagittal images
- T2WI
  - Classically high **T2 signal**
    - Secondary to high fluid content
  - Foci of low signal from Ca^{++}, hemorrhage, & mucoid
  - Low signal septations separate high signal lobules
- T2* GRE
  - Foci of hemorrhage or Ca^{++} have hypointense signal
- DWI
  - Mean ADC value $1474 \pm 117 \times 10^{-6}$ mm²/s
  - Generally lower than chondrosarcoma
- T1WI C+
  - Moderate to marked enhancement

- Marked enhancement is risk factor for tumor progression/recurrence post resection
  - **Honeycomb enhancement pattern** secondary to intratumoral areas of low signal intensity
  - Subtle or no enhancement reflects necrosis ± ↑ volume mucinous material
- MRA
  - Vessel encasement/displacement frequent
    - Arterial narrowing rare; MRA less useful than MR

Angiographic Findings
- Avascular mass
- Propensity to displace & encase internal carotid arteries & vertebrobasilar system
- Balloon test occlusion evaluates risk of neurologic impairment with vessel sacrifice

Nuclear Medicine Findings
- 18F-FDG PET for metastases & to monitor treatment response after radiation

Imaging Recommendations
- Best imaging tool
  - Both CT & MR usually needed for treatment planning
  - MR ± contrast best confirms diagnosis & extent of tumor
- Protocol advice
  - Focused-enhanced MR of skull base
  - Thin-section axial skull base CT with coronal ± sagittal MPR

DIFFERENTIAL DIAGNOSIS

Invasive Pituitary Macroadenoma (Pituitary Neuroendocrine Tumor)
- Originates in sella & involves pituitary gland
- Extends into sphenoid sinus, not prepontine cistern

Benign Notochordal Cell Tumor (Ecchordosis Physaliphora)
- Now considered on continuum with chordoma
- Histologically benign notochord remnant lesion
- Nonenhancing, T2-hyperintense clival or retroclival mass
- Includes both extraosseous & intraosseous lesions

Skull Base Chondrosarcoma
- Arises off midline at petrooccipital fissure
- Similar T1 & T2 characteristics to CCh
- Chondroid Ca^{++} more common
- ADC values $2051 \pm 261 \times 10^{-6}$ mm²/s
  - Higher than in chordoma
- *IDH1* mutations common but not seen in chordoma

Skull Base Plasmacytoma
- Can be midline destructive mass of clivus
- T2 signal usually intermediate to low, low ADC

Skull Base Metastasis
- Destructive lesion; smaller extraosseous component
- Known primary neoplasm
- T2 signal usually intermediate to low, low ADC

Skull Base Meningioma
- Sclerosis/hyperostosis of adjacent bone

- Homogeneous enhancement with dural tails
- Commonly causes narrowing of encased vessels
- T2 signal usually intermediate (close to brain)

PATHOLOGY

General Features
- Etiology
  - Arises from remnants of primitive notochord
- Genetics
  - Familial chordoma rarely reported
  - Brachyury gene: Molecular marker distinctive for chordoma
    - Represents transcription factor in notochord development
    - Potential use for target in chordoma therapy

Staging, Grading, & Classification
- Low to intermediate malignancy, slow growing but locally aggressive
- 2 histopathologic subtypes
  - Typical (classic) chordoma & chondroid chordoma

Gross Pathologic & Surgical Features
- Gross appearance: Multilobulated, gelatinous, gray mass

Microscopic Features
- Classic chordoma: Cords of physaliphorous cells with areas of necrosis, hemorrhage, & entrapped bone
  - **Physaliphorous cells** have bubbly appearance & confirm diagnosis
    - Large cell containing mucin & glycogen vacuoles
- Chondroid chordoma: Stroma resembles hyaline cartilage with neoplastic cells in lacunae
  - Term "chondroid" in chondroid chordoma is misnomer; refers to histologic mimic
  - Lesion does not contain cartilage or cartilage origin cells
- Classic & chondroid chordomas immunopositive for epithelial markers cytokeratin & EMA
  - Chondrosarcoma is negative for these markers
- Transcription factor **brachyury**: Recently described as specific for chordoma

CLINICAL ISSUES

Presentation
- Most common signs/symptoms
  - Headaches & diplopia from CNVI involvement
- Other signs/symptoms
  - Ophthalmoplegia results from tumor proximity to cranial nerves
    - CNIII, IV, & VI in cavernous sinus
    - CNVI in Dorello canal
  - Visual loss (optic nerve, chiasm, optic tracts involved)
  - Facial pain (CNV2)
  - Lateral growth can injure CNVII or VIII in cerebellopontine angle-internal auditory canal
  - Large chordoma may reach jugular foramen, inferolaterally affecting CNIX-XII
  - Headache likely related to stretching of dura
- Clinical profile
  - Slow onset of ophthalmoplegia & headache in adult

Demographics
- Age
  - 30-50 years, but can occur at any age
- Sex
  - M:F = 1:1
- Ethnicity
  - White > Black patients
- Epidemiology
  - **35%** of all chordomas arise in **skull base**
  - 50% are sacrococcygeal
  - 15% arise from vertebral body

Natural History & Prognosis
- Begins as expansile destructive bone lesion
  - Infiltrates/transgresses dura, encases cranial nerves & vessels, & compresses brain/brainstem
  - Rarely begins as intradural/intracranial
- Better prognosis if young age at presentation
- Chondroid chordoma has better prognosis than classic
- Poorer 5-year survival than chondrosarcoma
- Local recurrence is common despite combined therapy
  - Rarely tumor recurrence along surgical tract
- Distant metastasis rare: Lymph nodes, bone, lung, liver
  - Distant metastases more common in recurrent CCh
- "Drop" metastasis with subarachnoid seeding rare

Treatment
- Should be managed by multidisciplinary skull base team
- Surgical resection (conventional vs. endonasal endoscopic)
  - Complete excision difficult due to proximity of adjacent critical structures
- Proton beam RT: Postop & unresectable tumors

DIAGNOSTIC CHECKLIST

Consider
- Destructive midline mass originating from clivus; **hyperintense on T2** is most common presentation

Image Interpretation Pearls
- T1WI C+ MR best for tumor characteristics & extent
- Bone CT can better characterize bony destruction
- Look for encasement of internal carotid artery & vertebrobasilar system

Reporting Tips
- Comment on involvement of adjacent vital structures
- ADC values $1474 \pm 117 \times 10^{-6}$ mm²/s differentiates from higher ADC values of chondrosarcoma
  - Must exclude hemorrhage/Ca^{++}, cystic areas/necrosis from region of interest when measuring ADC

SELECTED REFERENCES

1. Alshammari D et al: Image guided endonasal endoscopic approach to different clivus pathologies. Int J Surg Case Rep. 127:110806, 2025
2. Hong S et al: Predicting the need for occipitocervical fusion for patients with lower clival chordoma: a single-center retrospective study. World Neurosurg. 187:e321-30, 2024
3. Stevens AR et al: Ecchordosis physaliphora: does it even exist? AJNR Am J Neuroradiol. 44(8):889-93, 2023
4. Mark IT et al: MRI enhancement patterns in 28 cases of clival chordomas. J Clin Neurosci. 99:117-22, 2022
5. Olson JT et al: Chordoma: 18F-FDG PET/CT and MRI imaging features. Skeletal Radiol. 50(8):1657-66, 2021

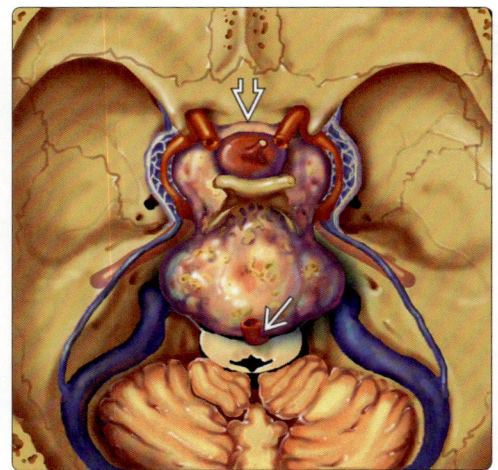

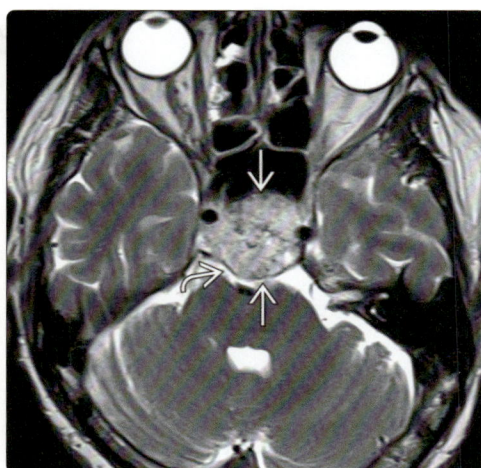

(Left) *Axial graphic illustrates a large clival chordoma pushing posteriorly to indent the low pons and basilar artery ➡. Basisphenoid invasion ⇶ is also seen lifting the pituitary gland in the sella.* **(Right)** *Axial T2 MR shows a heterogeneous mixed signal intensity clival chordoma ➡. Although not as hyperintense as many chordomas, it is relatively bright compared to brain. There is typical expansion of the clivus with tumor borders extending into the prepontine cistern ➡ and partly effacing the CSF.*

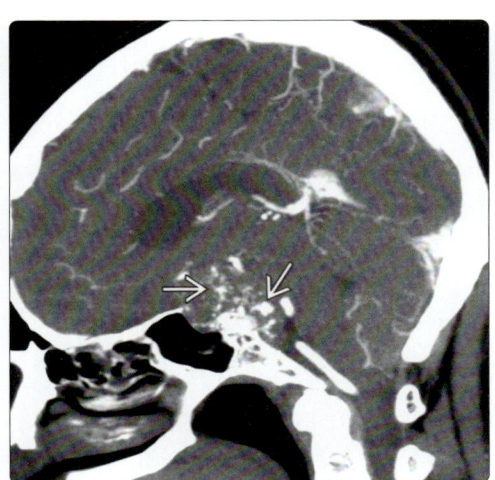

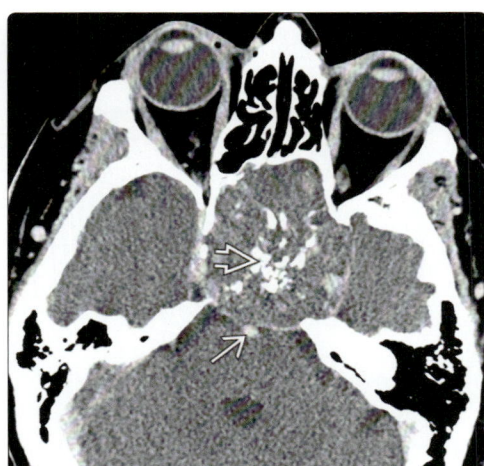

(Left) *Sagittal CTA performed for preoperative planning shows extensive intratumoral matrix Ca++ ➡ in this clival chordoma. Calcified matrix is seen in ~ 50% of chordomas.* **(Right)** *Axial CECT in a different patient demonstrates a typical midline clival chordoma with irregular intratumoral calcifications ⇶, representing associated calcified matrix &/or bone fragments. This tumor compresses the pons and basilar artery ➡ posteriorly.*

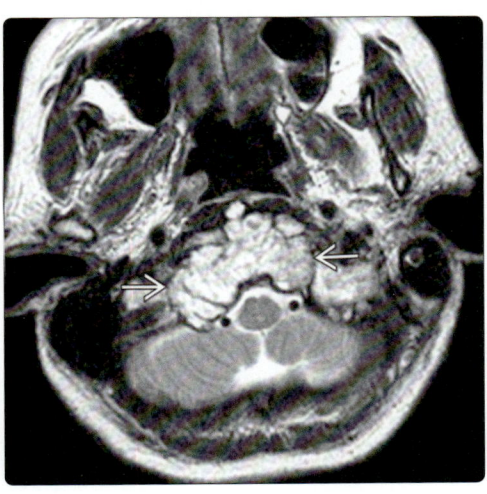

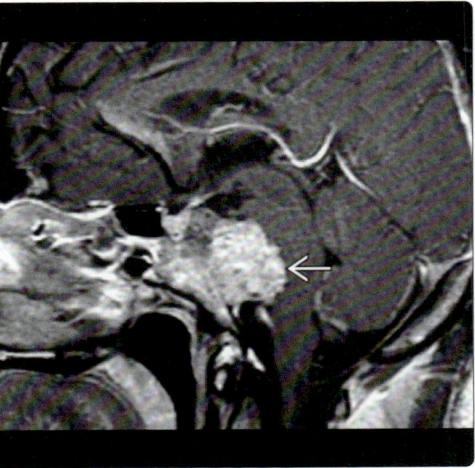

(Left) *Axial T2 MR shows a large, hyperintense clival chordoma involving the occipital condyles ➡. Marked hyperintense T2 signal is a classic feature of chordoma. Surgical excision would also require stabilization of craniocervical junction given the extent of occipital condylar involvement.* **(Right)** *Sagittal T1 C+ MR shows heterogeneous enhancement of chordoma. Note posterior extension with "thumbing" of pons ➡. Increased enhancement is a risk factor for progression/recurrence post resection.*

Persistent Craniopharyngeal Canal

TERMINOLOGY

- Persistent craniopharyngeal canal (PCPC)
- Synonyms: Transsphenoidal canal, craniopharyngeal duct, hypophyseal canal, basipharyngeal canal, persistent hypophyseal canal
- Developmental anomaly with persistent tract from nasopharynx to pituitary fossa
- Believed by many to be persistent Rathke duct

IMAGING

- Skull base bone CT
  - Midline, well-marginated tract from sella to roof of nasopharynx
  - Anterior to sphenooccipital synchondrosis
  - Typically < 1.5 mm in diameter
- Multiplanar MR
  - Smoothly marginated cylindrical "canal" extending from sella to nasopharynx
  - Variable signal intensity in canal itself

- MR best to evaluate pituitary & suprasellar structures for associated abnormality
- Coronal sections reveal adenohypophysis perched on craniopharyngeal canal like **ball on tee**

TOP DIFFERENTIAL DIAGNOSES

- Skull base cephalocele
- Sphenobasilar synchondrosis
- Persistent medial basal canal

PATHOLOGY

- Associations with pituitary abnormalities, cephaloceles, midline craniofacial anomalies

CLINICAL ISSUES

- Typically incidental finding
- Seen in 0.42% of population
- Usually obliterated by 12th week of gestation
- **"Leave alone" lesion** when isolated finding
- Rare cause for recurrent meningitis in children

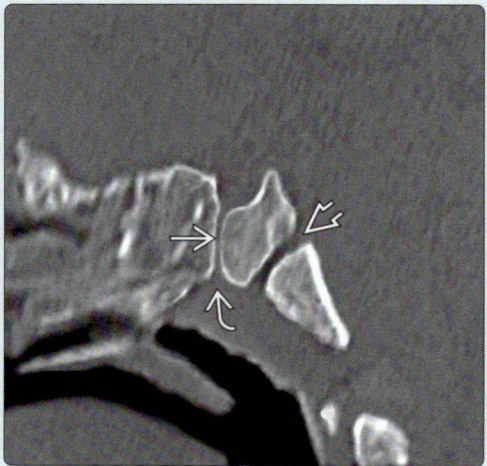
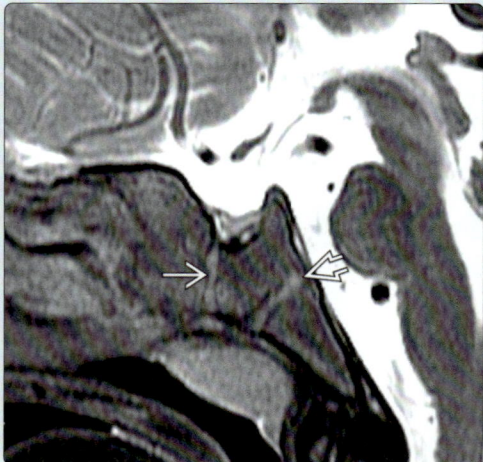

(Left) *Sagittal reformatted CT shows a bony tract originating in the floor of the sella turcica ➡, extending to the roof of the nasopharynx ➡. Note unfused sphenooccipital synchondrosis ➡ posteriorly in this child.* (Right) *Sagittal T2 MR in the same patient shows a persistent craniopharyngeal canal ➡ evident as a small tract with central intermediate signal and hypointense margins extending from the pituitary fossa to the nasopharynx. Normal sphenooccipital synchondrosis ➡ is posterior to the craniopharyngeal canal.*

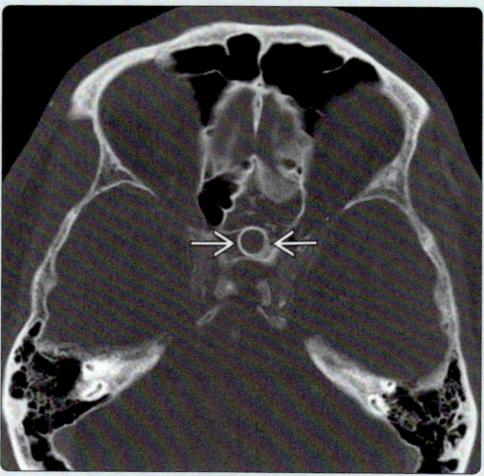
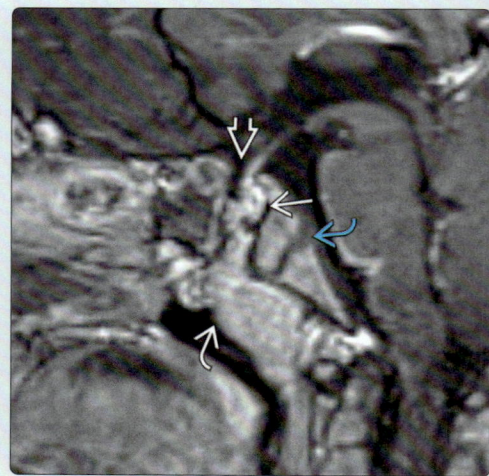

(Left) *Axial bone CT shows an incidental well-defined, sclerotic, ovoid "lesion" in the sphenoid bone ➡, consistent with the midsegment of a persistent craniopharyngeal canal. This smooth canal should be demonstrated in contiguity with the sella and nasopharynx.* (Right) *Sagittal T1 C+ MR in a patient with a persistent craniopharyngeal canal ➡ demonstrates pituitary and glioneuronal heterotopic tissue ➡ herniation into the nasopharynx ➡. Note sphenooccipital synchondrosis ➡.*

Persistent Craniopharyngeal Canal

TERMINOLOGY

Abbreviations
- Persistent craniopharyngeal canal (PCPC)

Synonyms
- Transsphenoidal canal, craniopharyngeal duct, hypophyseal canal, basipharyngeal canal, persistent hypophyseal canal

Definitions
- Developmental anomaly with **persistent tract from nasopharyngeal roof to pituitary fossa**
  - May represent persistent Rathke duct
    - Alternative hypothesis: Persistent vascular channel unrelated to Rathke duct

IMAGING

General Features
- Best diagnostic clue
  - Midline, well-marginated, cylindrical to ovoid tract from sella to nasopharyngeal roof
- Location
  - Extends between superior surface of nasopharynx to sella turcica floor in oblique fashion
    - Terminates in nasopharynx near junction of vomer & sphenoid rostrum
  - Lies anatomically between presphenoid & basisphenoid
    - **Anterior to sphenooccipital synchondrosis**
- Size
  - Typically < 1.5 mm in diameter
    - When larger, evaluate carefully for **associated pituitary abnormality**
- Morphology
  - Tubular canal
    - Occasionally ends blindly without communication with sella

Imaging Recommendations
- Best imaging tool
  - High-resolution skull base CT
  - Multiplanar MR to exclude pituitary abnormality or cephalocele
- Protocol advice
  - Sagittal & coronal CT reconstructions

CT Findings
- Bone CT
  - Smoothly marginated cylindrical-to-ovoid **midline bony "canal"** extending from sella to nasopharynx
  - **Oblique orientation** to nasopharynx
  - May rarely contain air if communication with pharyngeal lumen exists

MR Findings
- Smoothly marginated tubular canal in sphenoid
- Variable signal intensity in canal
- May demonstrate central enhancement on postcontrast T1W images
- Coronal sections reveal adenohypophysis perched on craniopharyngeal canal like **ball on tee**
- Evaluate pituitary & suprasellar structures for potential associated abnormality

DIFFERENTIAL DIAGNOSIS

Skull Base Cephalocele
- Nasopharyngeal or basioccipital nasopharyngeal cephalocele types in similar location
- Contain variable meningeal-lined CSF/brain parenchyma

Sphenooccipital Synchondrosis
- Linear cleft between basisphenoid & basiocciput
- Conspicuity decreases from childhood to adulthood

Persistent Medial Basal Canal (Basilaris Medianus)
- Developmental variant of lower midline clivus
- Posteroinferior to sphenooccipital synchondrosis

PATHOLOGY

General Features
- Etiology
  - Developmental anomaly with persistent tract from nasopharynx to pituitary fossa
    - Most believe it to be persistence of Rathke duct
- Associated abnormalities
  - Pituitary abnormalities, cephaloceles, midline craniofacial anomalies
  - Association of other abnormalities may lead to increased size of craniopharyngeal canal
  - Cysts within PCPC

CLINICAL ISSUES

Presentation
- Most common signs/symptoms
  - Typically **incidental finding**
- Other signs/symptoms
  - Pituitary dysfunction or uncommon/rare meningitis
  - Rare CSF leak via PCPC
  - Rarely, pituitary tissue may present as nasopharyngeal mass with PCPC

Demographics
- Epidemiology: Seen in 0.42% of population

Natural History & Prognosis
- Usually obliterated by 12th week of gestation
- Rarely reported to cause upper airway obstruction (during infancy), CSF leak, meningitis, sinusitis, hydrocephalus

Treatment
- **"Leave alone" lesion** when isolated finding

DIAGNOSTIC CHECKLIST

Image Interpretation Pearls
- Evaluate hypothalamic-pituitary axis for associated abnormality
- Infant or young child with midline nasopharyngeal polyp, particularly if associated with hypertelorism, should have skull base imaging

SELECTED REFERENCES

1. Wang W et al: Imaging of congenital anomalies and defects of the skull base and calvarium. Br J Radiol. 97(1157):902-12, 2024

Sphenoid Benign Fatty Lesion

TERMINOLOGY

- Synonym: Arrested pneumatization of sphenoid
- Definition: Well-corticated, fat-containing lesion of sphenoid bone
  - Occurs in regions where primary or accessory pneumatization known to occur
  - Usually adjacent to posterior sinus wall

IMAGING

- Bone CT findings
  - Thin-section axial images best for depicting uniform cortical bone rim
  - Well-defined, **low-attenuation** (fat density), nonexpansile lesion with **sclerotic rim**
  - May have occasional curvilinear calcification or soft tissue density
- MR
  - Can help delineate smaller lesions

- **Central ↑ T1**, variable T2, and ↓ T1 signal post fat suppression
  - Hypointense rim
  - Minimal, if any, enhancement (normal marrow)

TOP DIFFERENTIAL DIAGNOSES

- Fibrous dysplasia
- Venous malformation
- Chordoma
- Ossifying fibroma

CLINICAL ISSUES

- Common incidental "leave alone" lesions on CT or MR depicting skull base

DIAGNOSTIC CHECKLIST

- Identification of internal fat and sclerotic margin is essentially pathognomonic
- Nonexpansile on CT and no uptake on FDG-PET

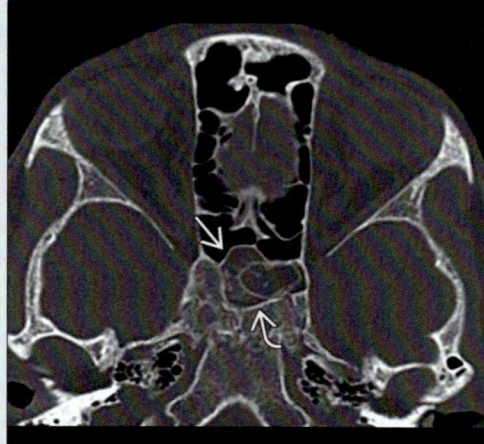
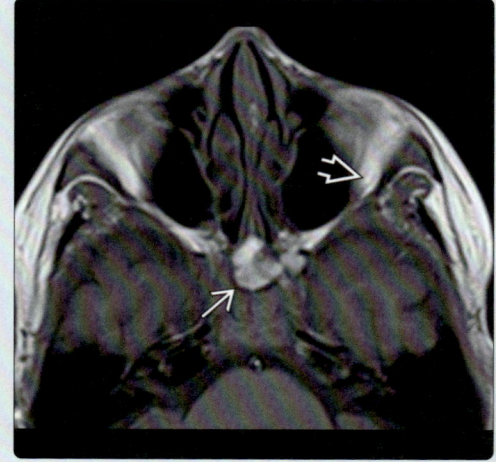

(Left) Axial bone CT shows characteristic features of an incidentally discovered fatty lesion of the sphenoid. The lesion ➡ bulges into the left sphenoid sinus ➡ and has well-defined sclerotic margins and predominantly low-density (fat) centrally. (Right) Axial T1WI MR in the same patient demonstrates a homogeneously hyperintense, nonexpansile lesion ➡ in the left aspect of the basisphenoid similar in signal to subcutaneous or orbital fat ➡. MR may be useful to confirm internal fatty contents.

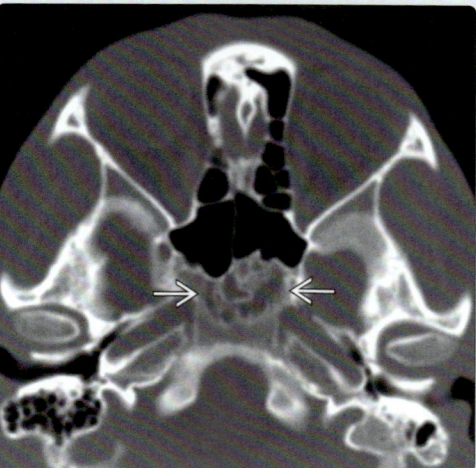
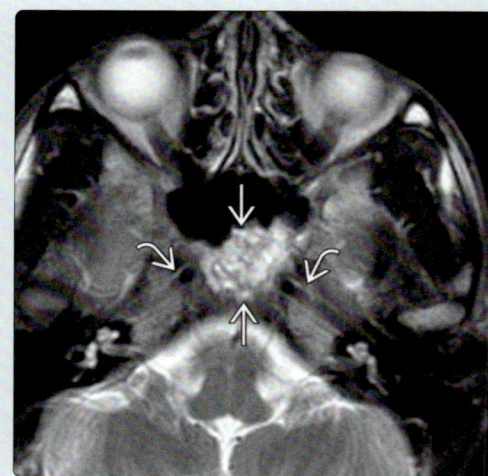

(Left) Axial bone CT demonstrates a typical benign, fatty lesion of the sphenoid ➡ with well-defined margins and a low-density central component, confirmed on MR to represent fat. (Right) Axial T2WI MR in the same patient confirms predominantly hyperintense (paralleling fat) signal with a lobulated contour to the lesion ➡. There is no significant distortion of skull base foramina or normal structures, such as petrous segments of internal carotid arteries ➡.

Central Skull Base Trigeminal Schwannoma

TERMINOLOGY

- Synonyms: Giant trigeminal schwannoma (TS), "dumbbell" TS

IMAGING

- Tubular mass along course of trigeminal nerve
  - Can involve preganglionic (cisternal) segment, Meckel cave, CNV1 (superior orbital fissure), CNV2 (foramen rotundum), CNV3 (foramen ovale)
  - May extend extracranially via CNV exit foramina
- Size: Small to giant
- Morphology: Dumbbell shape secondary to constriction at porus trigeminus or skull base foramen
- CT: Soft tissue mass with smooth, bony erosion of central skull base, ± foraminal widening
- MR: T1 iso- to hypointense, T2 hyperintense, variable enhancement
  - Cystic change is common

TOP DIFFERENTIAL DIAGNOSES

- Meningioma
- CNV3 perineural tumor
- CNV2 perineural tumor
- Non-Hodgkin lymphoma

PATHOLOGY

- Benign nerve sheath tumor
  - 2nd most common intracranial schwannoma next to vestibular schwannoma
- May occur in setting of neurofibromatosis type 2

DIAGNOSTIC CHECKLIST

- Dumbbell-shaped or tubular mass along course of trigeminal nerve is characteristic
- Enhanced MR best to identify intracranial and extracranial extent of lesion
- Search for additional intracranial schwannomas, which may indicate neurofibromatosis type 2

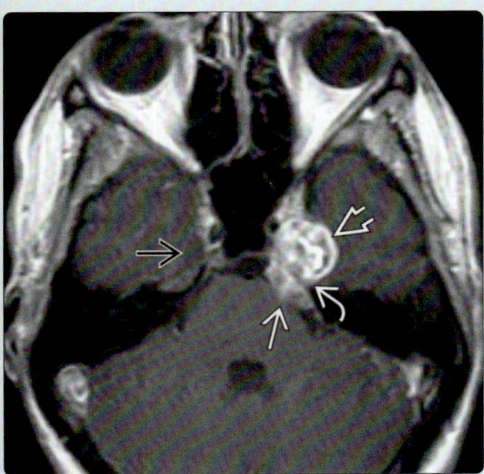
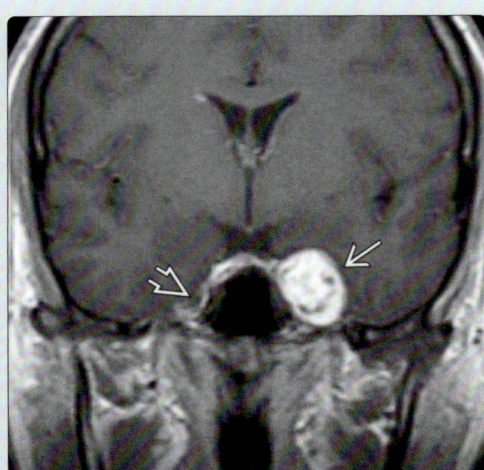

(Left) Axial T1 C+ MR of a 29-year-old woman with headaches shows an extraaxial enhancing mass extending from the left trigeminal root entry zone ➡ to the Meckel cave ➡. There is narrowing of the mass as it traverses the porus trigeminus ➡. Notice the normal contralateral Meckel cave ➡. (Right) Coronal T1 C+ MR of same 29-year-old woman shows the Meckel cave component of the tumor ➡. Notice the normal contralateral Meckel cave ➡.

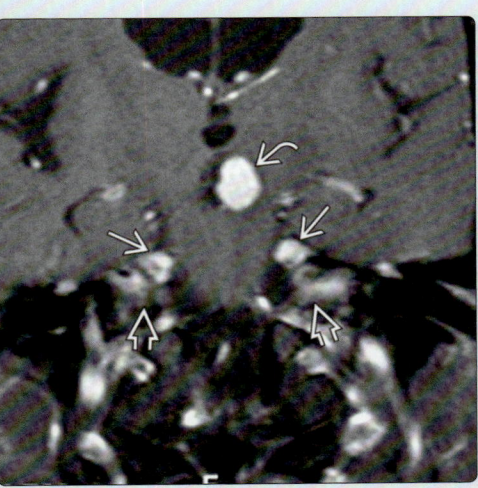
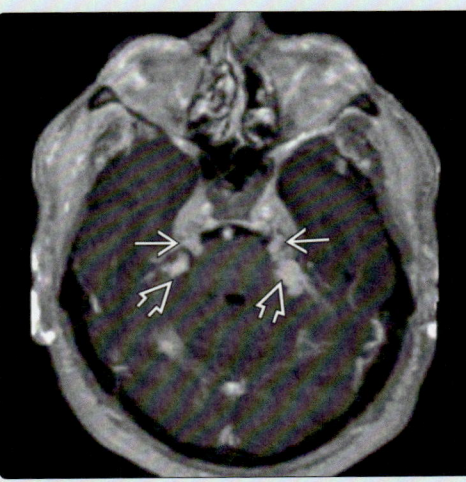

(Left) T1 C+ MR of a 47-year-old man with a history of NF2. There are bilateral extraaxial masses at the root entry zones of the trigeminal nerves ➡. There are similar findings in the bilateral IACs ➡ (vestibular schwannomas), and there is a mass in the interpeduncular cistern ➡, consistent with a schwannoma of CNIII. (Right) Axial T1 C+ MR of same 47-year-old NF2 patient. There are bilateral extraaxial masses extending from the trigeminal root entry zones to the Meckel caves ➡. Bilateral vestibular schwannomas are visible ➡.

Hypoglossal Nerve Schwannoma

TERMINOLOGY

- Benign tumor of differentiated Schwann cells surrounding CNXII

IMAGING

- Multiplanar contrast-enhanced MR with bone CT for delineation of bone margins
- CT findings
  - Sharply marginated fusiform mass with enlarged hypoglossal canal (HC)
  - Coronal plane: Remodeling of undersurface of jugular tubercle
  - Tongue muscle atrophy with fatty replacement
- MR: Homogeneous, enhancing mass following course of CNXII
  - Cephalad growth toward preolivary sulcus
  - Caudal growth into nasopharyngeal carotid space
- Distal lesions may present in carotid space, submandibular space, or in tongue

TOP DIFFERENTIAL DIAGNOSES

- Asymmetric HC venous drainage
- Skull base metastasis
- Persistent hypoglossal artery
- Jugular foramen meningioma
- Jugular paraganglioma

PATHOLOGY

- Smooth, encapsulated mass arising eccentrically from CNXII
- Multiple schwannomas are associated with neurofibromatosis type 2 (NF2)

CLINICAL ISSUES

- Hypoglossal neuropathy results in unilateral tongue denervation
- Larger lesions may produce multiple lower cranial neuropathies
- Surgical removal in single operation is curative
- Gamma Knife radiosurgery is alternative treatment option

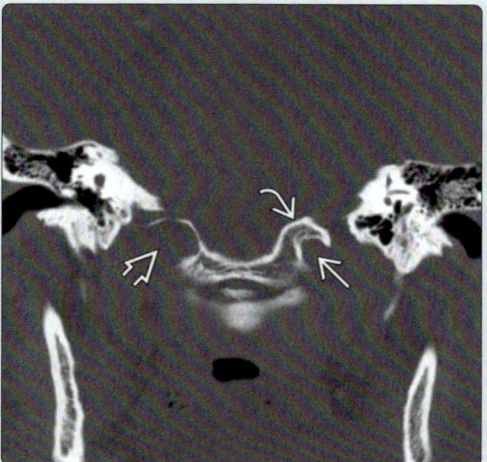
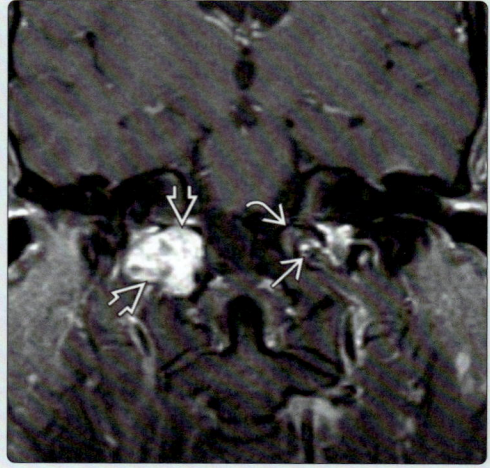

(Left) Coronal bone CT shows a markedly expanded hypoglossal canal (HC) on the right ➡, eroding the undersurface of the "eagle's beak." Contrast this with the normal left HC ➡ and jugular tubercle ➡. (Right) Coronal T1 C+ FS MR in the same patient reveals heterogeneous enhancement of the schwannoma ➡ with marked scalloping of the adjacent occipital bone and obliteration of the normal "eagle's beak," as seen on CT. The normal HC ➡ and jugular tubercle ➡ are identified on the left.

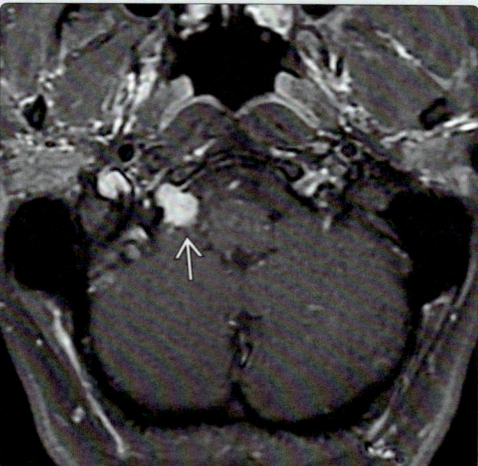
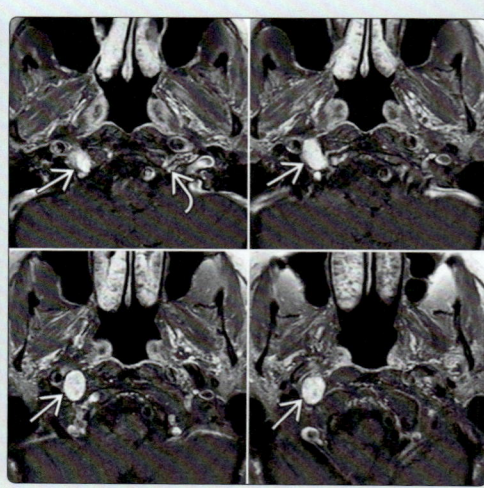

(Left) Axial T1 C+ FS MR shows a well-defined, uniformly enhancing, dumbbell-shaped lesion arising from the right HC with an intracranial component ➡, consistent with a schwannoma. There is no mass effect on brain parenchyma. (Right) Contiguous axial T1 C+ FS MR slices (superior to inferior) through the HC show a lobular enhancing schwannoma ➡ extending from the HC into the upper carotid space on the right. Note the normal left HC ➡. In this case, there was no significant intracranial component.

Hypoglossal Nerve Schwannoma

TERMINOLOGY

Abbreviations
- Hypoglossal nerve schwannoma (HNS)

Definitions
- Extremely rare, benign tumor of differentiated Schwann cells surrounding CNXII

IMAGING

General Features
- Best diagnostic clue
  - Fusiform, well-defined soft tissue mass along expected course of CNXII
- Location
  - May occur anywhere along course of CNXII
    - Distal lesions may present in carotid space, submandibular space, or in tongue
- Size
  - Usually large at presentation
- Morphology
  - Fusiform lesions that may attain **dumbbell shape**

CT Findings
- NECT
  - Sharply marginated soft tissue density mass along course of CNXII
  - Fatty attenuation in ipsilateral hemitongue secondary to chronic denervation atrophy
- CECT
  - Uniformly enhancing ± intramural cysts
- Bone CT
  - Smooth, sharply marginated & enlarged hypoglossal canal (HC)
  - Coronal plane: Enlargement, remodeling of undersurface of jugular tubercle (below "eagle's beak")

MR Findings
- T1WI
  - Typically isointense to gray matter
  - Associated denervation may cause ipsilateral tongue muscle atrophy & fatty replacement with ↑ signal
- T2WI
  - Typically ↑ signal
  - Large HNS may have ↑ T2 signal **intramural cysts**
- T1WI C+
  - Uniform enhancement when small

Imaging Recommendations
- Best imaging tool
  - Enhanced multiplanar MR with bone CT providing detail on bony remodeling of HC

DIFFERENTIAL DIAGNOSIS

Asymmetric Hypoglossal Canal Venous Drainage (Pseudolesion)
- Nonenlarged HC with normal cortical margins
- Linear transcanalicular venous enhancement surrounding normal nerve

Skull Base Metastasis
- Bony margins of HC are lytic or permeative
- Enhancing, invasive mass

Persistent Hypoglossal Artery
- MR + MRA: Flow void passes through enlarged HC to basilar artery

Jugular Foramen Meningioma
- Dural-based mass with enhancing dural tail; secondarily involves HC
- Permeative-sclerotic bony changes or hyperostosis

Jugular Paraganglioma
- Permeative-destructive bone margins of jugular foramen
- Multiple flow voids are characteristic on MR

PATHOLOGY

Gross Pathologic & Surgical Features
- Smooth, tan, ovoid, encapsulated, & lobulated mass
- Arises eccentrically from CNXII nerve sheath

CLINICAL ISSUES

Presentation
- Most common signs/symptoms
  - Hypoglossal neuropathy results in **unilateral tongue denervation**
    - Tongue deviates toward side of lesion on protrusion

Demographics
- Epidemiology
  - Extremely rare schwannoma (much less common than CNV, VII, IX or X)

Natural History & Prognosis
- Slowly growing, benign tumor

Treatment
- Surgical removal of tumor in single operation is optimal
  - Proposed tumor grading system for operative care
    - Type A, intradural; type B, dumbbell; type C, extracranial; type D, peripheral

DIAGNOSTIC CHECKLIST

Consider
- HNS if well-defined fusiform mass identified along expected course of CNXII

Reporting Tips
- Be sure to follow entire craniocaudal extent of lesion

SELECTED REFERENCES

1. Byeon Y et al: Radiographic and neurological outcomes of Gamma Knife radiosurgery for lower cranial nerve schwannomas: a single-institution experience. J Neurosurg. 142(2):488-97, 2025
2. Gennaro P et al: Hypoglossal nerve palsy misdiagnosed as tongue tumor: a rare case of calcified hypoglossal schwannoma. Indian J Otolaryngol Head Neck Surg. 76(1):1240-3, 2024
3. de Sousa Costa R et al: The hypoglossal nerve. Semin Ultrasound CT MR. 44(2):104-14, 2023
4. Di Pascuale I et al: Hypoglossal nerve schwannoma: case report and literature review. World Neurosurg. 135:205-8, 2020

Skull Base Lesions

TERMINOLOGY

- 2- to 6-mm soft tissue nodule posterior/posterolateral to vertebral artery (VA), attached to spinal accessory nerve (SAN) at foramen magnum (FM) level

IMAGING

- CT
  - Enhancing nodule on CECT
  - Filling defect on CT myelogram
- MR
  - FLAIR hyperintense (higher signal than brainstem & cerebellum); enhancing on postcontrast T1WI
  - Occult on routine T2WI (indistinct from adjacent CSF), but hypointense to CSF on 3D heavily T2WI
  - Also occult on precontrast T1WI, DWI, SWI/GRE
  - May see faint linear enhancement extending cranial or caudal from benign enhancing FM lesion

TOP DIFFERENTIAL DIAGNOSES

- Meningioma & dural-based inflammatory/metastatic lesion
- Schwannoma (SAN or C1 nerve root)
- VA aneurysm
- Cystic lesions, such as arachnoid, neurenteric, & synovial cysts

PATHOLOGY

- Solid cystic lesion with deeper solid component adherent to SAN, covered by yellow membrane
- Benign fibrotic arachnoid nodule attached to SAN

CLINICAL ISSUES

- Incidental benign "do not touch" lesion

DIAGNOSTIC CHECKLIST

- Best imaging tool: 3D FLAIR, thin-section 3D postcontrast (MPRAGE, FSPGR, TFE etc.), & 3D heavily T2WI MR (FIESTA, CISS, bFFE, etc.)

(Left) Axial FLAIR MR in a patient with headaches shows an incidental hyperintense lesion ⮕ posterior & lateral to the right vertebral artery (VA) ⮕ at the level of the foramen magnum (FM), suggesting a benign enhancing FM lesion (BEFML). (Right) Axial T1WI C+ MR in the same patient shows that the enhancing lesion ⮕ is distinct from the VA ⮕. BEFMLs are incidental benign "do not touch" lesions seen in 3.4% of brain MRs, stable in 90%, & best detected on 3D FLAIR, thin-section 3D postcontrast, & 3D heavily T2WI MR.

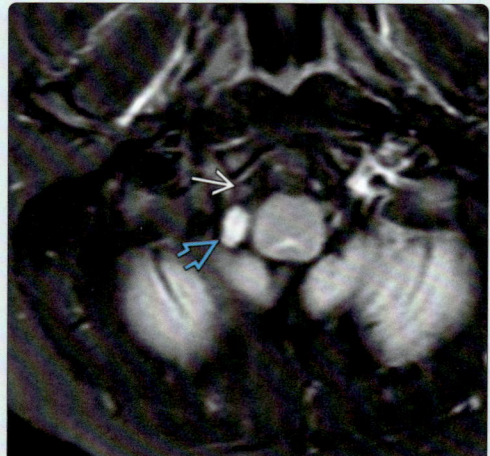
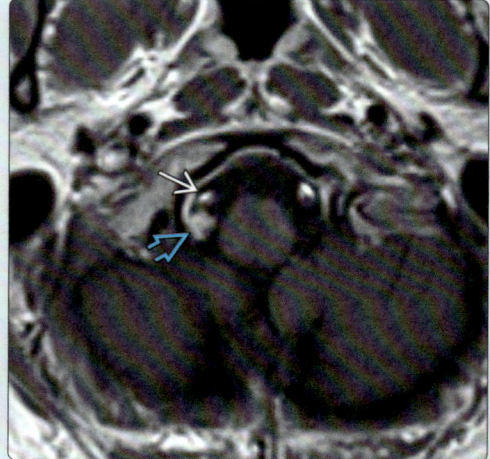

(Left) Axial CT myelogram in the same patient shows a filling defect ⮕ in the contrast-filled CSF posterolateral to right VA ⮕, corresponding to the BEFML. (Right) Axial 3D heavily T2WI CISS MR in a patient with left facial numbness shows an incidental nodule ⮕ abutting the left spinal accessory nerve (SAN) ⮕ at the FM level, distinct from the left VA ⮕. Compare the right SAN ⮕. Note that the BEFML can be occult on routine T2WI, somewhat indistinguishable from the adjacent CSF.

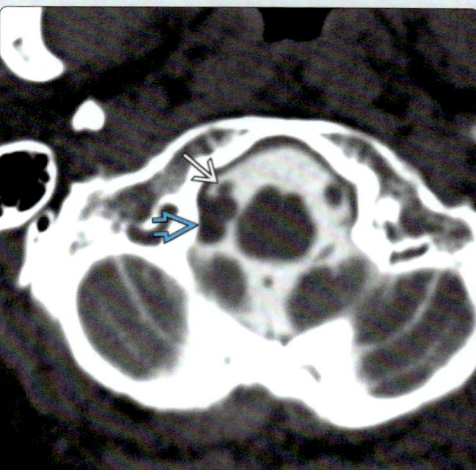
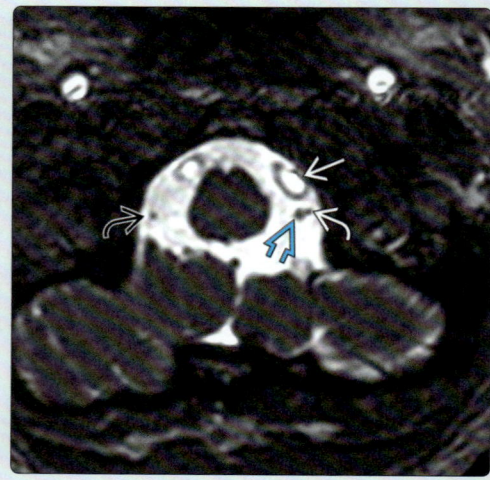

Benign Enhancing Foramen Magnum Lesion

TERMINOLOGY

Abbreviations
- Benign enhancing foramen magnum lesion (BEFML)

Definitions
- Intradural extramedullary enhancing foramen magnum (FM) lesion posterior or posterolateral to vertebral artery (VA) just distal to its dural penetration

IMAGING

General Features
- Best diagnostic clue
  - Small FLAIR hyperintense lesion adjacent to VA just after dural penetration by artery, stable on follow-up
- Location
  - Posterior/posterolateral to VA, connected to spinal accessory nerve (SAN), at level of FM & below jugular foramen
- Size
  - Average: 3.8 mm (usual range: 2-6 mm)
- Morphology
  - Round or ovoid soft tissue nodule

CT Findings
- NECT
  - Isodense to white matter (25 HU), barely perceptible
- CECT
  - Small enhancing nodule, similar in attenuation to upper cervical epidural venous plexus (85-90 HU)
- CT myelogram: Filling defect posterior/posterolateral to VA

MR Findings
- FLAIR
  - 3D FLAIR preferred over 2D FLAIR due to thinner sections & better CSF suppression
    - Hyperintense ↑↑ signal than brainstem & cerebellum
  - 35% BEFML abuts ipsilateral VA, while 100% connected with SAN
- T1WI C+
  - 92% BEFML enhance
  - Linear faintly enhancing structure seen up to BEFML in 1/3, extending cranially or rostrally
    - Corresponds to SAN (leptomeninges containing small vessels connecting to SAN in cadaveric studies)
- Other sequences
  - Isointense & not distinctly seen on T2WI, precontrast T1WI, or DWI
  - Hypointense to CSF & hyperintense to SAN on 3D heavily T2WI (FIESTA, CISS, bFFE, etc.)
  - No susceptibility on SWI/GRE & occult on time-of-flight MRA

Angiographic Findings
- No arterial or venous structure to explain BEFML

DIFFERENTIAL DIAGNOSIS

Meningioma & Dural-Based Inflammatory or Metastatic Lesion
- Peripherally located at FM with broad dural base (BEFML does not abut dura)

- Distinctly seen on T2WI

Schwannoma
- Can arise from SAN or C1 nerve root
- T2 hyperintense, slow progressive growth

Aneurysm
- Arises from VA or posterior inferior cerebellar artery
- Patent aneurysm: Follows artery signal on all sequences
- Thrombosed aneurysm: ↑ on T1WI, blooming ↓ on SWI

Arachnoid, Neuroenteric, & Synovial Cysts
- Nonenhancing, T2 hyperintense; suppresses on FLAIR
- Neurenteric cyst can be T1 hyperintense

PATHOLOGY

Gross Pathologic & Surgical Features
- Surgical features: Solid cystic lesion with deeper solid component adherent to SAN, covered by yellow membrane
- Histopathology: Similar to arachnoid tissue composed of hypocellular dense fibrotic nodules, arachnoid cells, focal nests of meningothelial cap cells & psammoma bodies

Older theories
- Vascular: Varix of bridging vein coursing along SAN
- Neural: Focal bulge from ectopic glial rests or heterotopias within the leptomeninges around SAN

CLINICAL ISSUES

Presentation
- Most common signs/symptoms
  - Asymptomatic incidental finding

Demographics
- No age or sex predilection
- Mean lesion size does not vary among different ages

Natural History & Prognosis
- Seen in 3.4% of brain MR images; 91% of BEFMLs stable at 3 years
- Usually solitary (90%), multiple (2-3) BEFMLs seen in 10% of cases

Treatment
- "Do not touch" lesion

DIAGNOSTIC CHECKLIST

Consider
- 2- to 6-mm benign-looking FLAIR hyperintense lesions posterior/posterolateral to VA at FM

Image Interpretation Pearls
- Occult on T2WI, precontrast T1WI, DWI & SWI/GRE
- Best sequences: 3D FLAIR, 3D T1 C+, & 3D heavily T2WI MR
- 3D FLAIR superior in detecting relations with SAN

SELECTED REFERENCES

1. Mark IT et al: Benign enhancing foramen magnum lesions. AJNR Am J Neuroradiol. 44(9):999-1001, 2023
2. Kogue R et al: Small high-signal lesions posterior to the intracranial vertebral artery incidentally identified by 3D FLAIR: retrospective study of 127 patients. Neuroradiology. 60(6):591-7, 2018

Jugular Bulb Pseudolesion

TERMINOLOGY

- Asymmetric, large jugular bulb (JB) flow phenomenon simulates neoplasm or thrombosis on MR sequences

IMAGING

- Best diagnostic clue: Complex MR signal in JB with normal jugular foramen (JF) cortex & jugular spine
  - Complex MR signal does not persist on all MR sequences
  - Normal bony margins of JB on temporal bone CT

TOP DIFFERENTIAL DIAGNOSES

- High JB
- JB diverticulum
- Dehiscent JB
- Sigmoid sinus-JB thrombosis
- Jugular paraganglioma
- JF schwannoma
- JF meningioma

CLINICAL ISSUES

- Found incidentally on brain MR during work-up for unrelated symptoms
- Surgical exploration must be avoided by radiologist making correct diagnosis
- No treatment or follow-up required

DIAGNOSTIC CHECKLIST

- JB pseudolesion is most common JB "lesion"
- Once abnormality is seen in JF on MR, first question to ask is, "Am I looking at JB pseudolesion?"
  - Do not mistake JB pseudolesion for schwannoma or venous sinus thrombosis
- If JB pseudolesion is observed while patient is in imaging center, add MRV to protocol to clarify
- Use bone CT or CTA/CTV to evaluate bony margins of JF if MR diagnosis uncertain

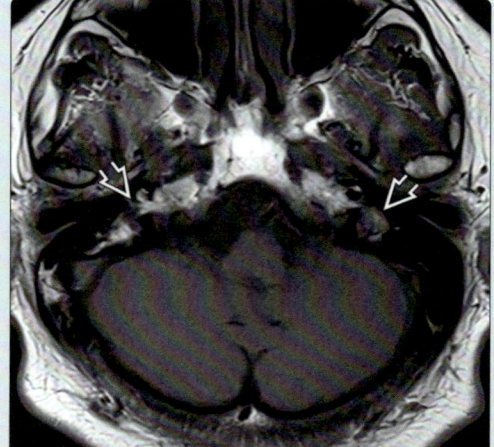
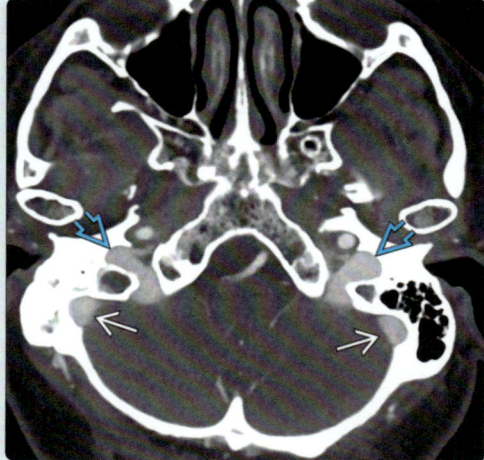

(Left) *Axial T1WI MR shows heterogeneous signal in the jugular foramen (JF) ➡, concerning for pathology in a patient with vertigo. Pseudolesions of the JF are common, often related to an asymmetric, large jugular bulb and turbulent flow or a high-riding jugular bulb.* (Right) *Axial CTA in the same patient shows normal enhancement of the jugular bulbs ➡. The enhancement is similar to the enhancement of the normal sigmoid sinuses ➡. Other sequences, such as MRA/MRV, can confirm this as a jugular bulb pseudolesion.*

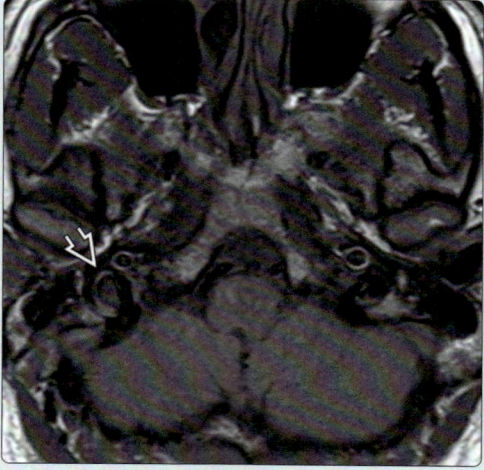
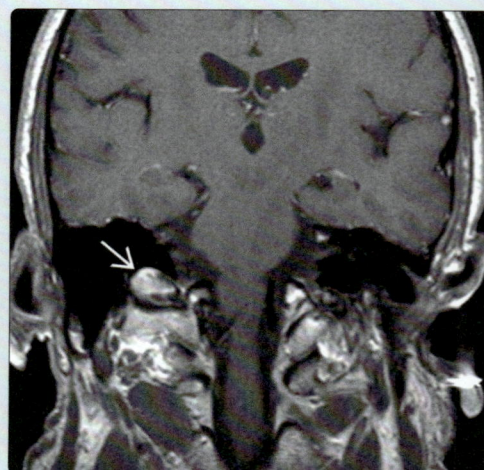

(Left) *Axial T1WI MR shows heterogeneous signal intensity within the right JF ➡, concerning for pathology. Other MR sequences proved this to be a jugular bulb pseudolesion, related to an asymmetric, large jugular bulb and turbulent flow.* (Right) *Coronal T1WI C+ MR shows a jugular bulb pseudolesion ➡ related to turbulent flow in a mildly asymmetric right jugular bulb. This pseudolesion may be mistaken for a schwannoma or venous thrombosis. Other MR sequences confirmed this pseudolesion.*

Jugular Bulb Pseudolesion

TERMINOLOGY

Synonyms
- Jugular bulb (JB) pseudomass; "leave alone" lesion of jugular foramen (JF)

Definitions
- Asymmetric, large JB flow phenomenon simulates neoplasm or thrombosis on MR sequences

IMAGING

General Features
- Best diagnostic clue
  - **Complex MR signal** intensity in **JB** with normal JF cortex & jugular spine
- Location
  - JF bulb
    - Prominent JB more commonly **right-sided**
- Size
  - Typical JB measures 1.0-1.5 cm
- Morphology
  - Rounded area of heterogeneous signal intensity centered on JF

CT Findings
- CECT
  - Normal enhancing sigmoid sinus (SS) & JB
    - No filling defect to suggest thrombosis
- Bone CT
  - Asymmetric JB with **intact cortical margins** & jugular spine
- CTV: Asymmetric JB shows same enhancement as internal jugular vein (IJV) & SS

MR Findings
- T1WI
  - Variable signal; may have soft tissue intensity or heterogeneous signal
- T2WI
  - Heterogeneous signal intensity
    - Usually conspicuous when iso- to hyperintense
- FLAIR
  - Heterogeneous signal intensity, often hyperintense
- T2* GRE
  - No significant blooming or susceptibility artifact
- T1WI C+
  - Avid enhancement of JB
    - Identical enhancement to adjacent IJV & SS
- MRV
  - JB shows asymmetric enlargement without evidence of thrombosis
    - Phase-contrast MRV: Shows normal flow in JB & SS
- SWI
  - No significant hypointense signal

Angiographic Findings
- Catheter venography: Normal, asymmetrically large SS & JB fill with contrast
  - JB often "high-riding"

DIFFERENTIAL DIAGNOSIS

High Jugular Bulb
- Most cephalad portion of JB extends superior to floor of internal auditory canal ± basal turn of cochlea
- Bone CT: JB cortical margins intact; no middle ear extension

Jugular Bulb Diverticulum
- Focal polypoid mass extending from cephalad JB into middle ear
- Smooth bone margins, intact sigmoid plate

Dehiscent Jugular Bulb
- Usually present with vascular "mass" behind intact tympanic membrane
- Sigmoid plate dehiscence on CT

Sigmoid Sinus-Jugular Bulb Thrombosis
- NECT: Hyperdense SS/JB, normal bony margins
- CECT/CTA/CTV: Look for intraluminal thrombus
  - Vasa vasorum of vein wall may enhance as thin white rim (empty delta sign)
- MRV: Filling defect or lack of flow

Jugular Paraganglioma
- Permeative bony changes along JF
- T1 MR: JF mass with high-velocity flow voids
- Vector of spread: Superolateral from JB to middle ear

Jugular Foramen Schwannoma
- Smoothly scalloped, enlarged JF
- T1 C+ MR: Dumbbell-shaped, enhancing mass in JF
- Vector of spread: Superomedial along CNIX-XI

Jugular Foramen Meningioma
- Permeative-sclerotic or hyperostotic bony change around JF
- T1 C+ MR: Enhancing dural tails along margins
- Vector of spread: Centrifugal along dural surfaces

PATHOLOGY

General Features
- Etiology
  - Normal developmental variant

CLINICAL ISSUES

Presentation
- Most common signs/symptoms
  - **Asymptomatic**
    - Found incidentally on brain MR during work-up for unrelated symptoms

Demographics
- Epidemiology
  - Most common "lesion" of JF found on MR imaging

SELECTED REFERENCES

1. Alves IS et al: Imaging of vertigo and dizziness: a site-based approach, part 1 (middle ear, bony labyrinth, and temporomandibular joint). Semin Ultrasound CT MR. 45(5):360-71, 2024
2. Expert Panel on Neurological Imaging et al: ACR Appropriateness Criteria® tinnitus: 2023 update. J Am Coll Radiol. 20(11S):S574-91, 2023

Skull Base Lesions

TERMINOLOGY

- High jugular bulb (JB): Superior aspect of JB extends above floor of internal auditory canal (IAC) with **no** middle ear connection
  - If dehiscence into middle ear present, use "dehiscent JB" not "high JB" to describe

IMAGING

- Most cephalad portion of JB extends superior to **floor of IAC** ± at level of basal turn of cochlea
  - Jugular foramen cortical margins intact
- Axial: JB at level of IAC or cochlea
- Coronal: JB medial ± inferior to semicircular canals
- T1 C+: High JB enhances same as jugular vein
- MRV: Same signal as surrounding venous structures
- High JB occurs most commonly on **right**
- Best imaging tool: Temporal bone CT

TOP DIFFERENTIAL DIAGNOSES

- JB pseudolesion; JB diverticulum; dehiscent JB
- Jugular paraganglioma
- Jugular foramen schwannoma
- Jugular foramen meningioma

PATHOLOGY

- High JB is more commonly seen with poorly aerated mastoid air cells
- JB diverticulum present in 35% of cases with high JB

CLINICAL ISSUES

- High JB is typically **incidental**
  - May increase risk of inadvertently entering JB during mastoidectomy, so include in report!
- Otoscopic exam: Normal
- Conservative management most common treatment
- Reported to be associated with pulsatile tinnitus or Ménière disease; causality uncertain

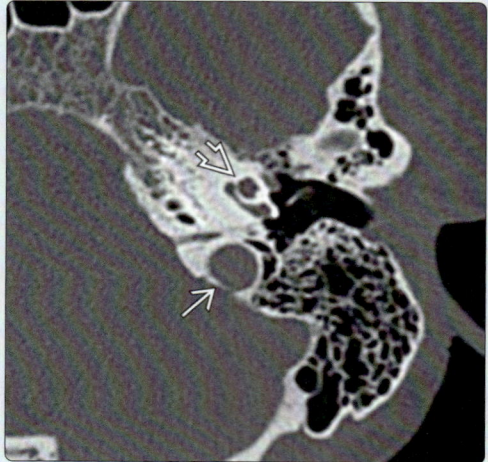
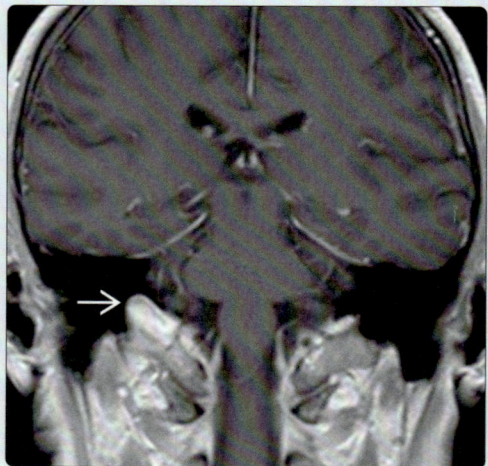

(Left) Axial T-bone CT of the left ear shows a high jugular bulb (JB) ➡ at level of the cochlea ➡ with intact cortical margins. These congenital lesions are typically incidental but may be associated with pulsatile tinnitus or other symptoms. (Right) Coronal T1 C+ MR shows a high JB ➡ that was connected inferiorly to a large internal jugular vein. The top of the high JB reaches the level of the floor of the internal auditory canal. On axial images, this may mimic an inner ear lesion if the connection to the jugular vein is not seen.

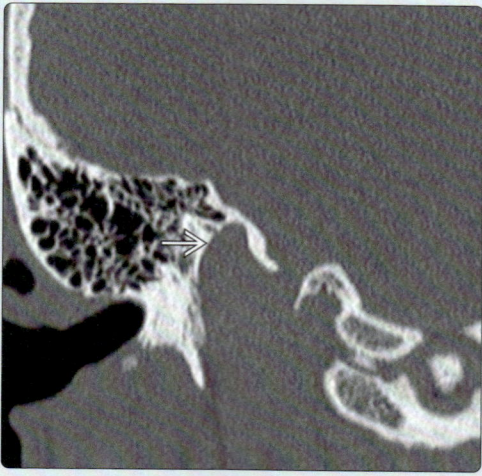
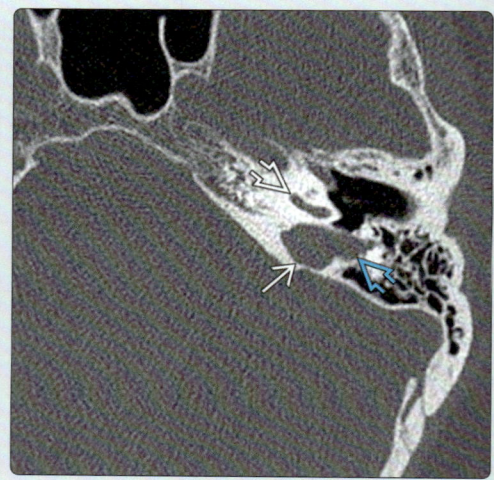

(Left) Coronal T-bone CT shows a high JB ➡ as a cephalad extension of the jugular foramen. A high JB occurs most commonly on the right side. This congenital lesion can be associated with JB dehiscence or a JB diverticulum. (Right) Axial T-bone CT of the left ear shows a high JB ➡ present at the level of the basal turn of the cochlea ➡. There is a lateral diverticulum ➡ associated with this high JB. A JB diverticulum is present in 35% of cases with a high-riding JB.

TERMINOLOGY

Abbreviations
- High jugular bulb (JB)

Synonyms
- High-riding JB

Definitions
- Superior aspect of JB extends above floor of internal auditory canal (IAC) with **no** connection to middle ear
  - If dehiscent JB into middle ear, use "dehiscent JB" not "high JB" to describe
  - May be associated with JB diverticulum

IMAGING

General Features
- Best diagnostic clue
  - Bone CT: Most cephalad portion of JB extends superior to floor of IAC ± at level of basal turn of cochlea
- Location
  - When JB reaches or exceeds floor of IAC
  - Occurs most commonly on right
- Size
  - Variable; JB typically 1.0-1.5 cm
- Morphology
  - Superior extension of JB with smooth bony margins

Imaging Recommendations
- Best imaging tool: Temporal bone CT

CT Findings
- NECT
  - Axial: JB at level of IAC, often at cochlea basal turn
  - Coronal: JB medial ± inferior to semicircular canals
- Bone CT: Jugular foramen (JF) cortical margins intact, including sigmoid plate

MR Findings
- T1: May be heterogeneous
- T2: Most commonly hypointense (invisible), may be heterogeneous
- T1 C+: High JB enhances same as internal jugular vein (IJV)
  - Coronal: Extends to level of IAC
- MRV: Same signal as surrounding venous structures

DIFFERENTIAL DIAGNOSIS

Jugular Bulb Pseudolesion
- MR shows asymmetric large JB with mass-like signal
- Usually found incidentally in skull base work-up
- Bone CT: Intact jugular spine & JB cortical margins

Jugular Bulb Diverticulum
- Bone CT: Focal projection extending off JB margin superiorly into deep temporal bone just behind IAC
- T1 C+ MR: Enhancing middle ear mass connects to enhancing JB

Dehiscent Jugular Bulb
- Vascular retrotympanic mass
- Protruding mass extends into posteroinferior middle ear cavity
- Bone CT: Sigmoid plate shows focal dehiscence
- T1 C+ MR: Enhancing mass connects to enhancing JB

Jugular Paraganglioma
- Enhancing mass in JF
- Bone CT: Permeative destructive JF bony changes
- T1 MR: High-velocity flow voids ("pepper")

Jugular Foramen Schwannoma
- Dumbbell-shaped mass along CNIX-XI
- Bone CT: Smoothly scalloped, enlarged JF
- T1 C+ MR: Fusiform, enhancing JF mass

Jugular Foramen Meningioma
- Mass in JF spreading centrifugally along dural planes
- Bone CT: Permeative-sclerotic or hyperostotic margins
- T1 C+ MR: Avidly enhancing mass with dural tails

PATHOLOGY

General Features
- Etiology
  - Congenital abnormality, benign vascular variant
  - High JB is more commonly seen with poorly aerated mastoid & perilymphatic structures

CLINICAL ISSUES

Presentation
- Most common signs/symptoms
  - Most commonly **incidental** finding
  - Reported to be associated with pulsatile tinnitus or Ménière disease; causality uncertain

Demographics
- Age: May be discovered at any age
- Sex: Slight female predominance
- Epidemiology: **5%** of temporal bone specimens
  - JB diverticulum present in 35% of cases with high JB

Treatment
- Conservative management

DIAGNOSTIC CHECKLIST

Consider
- High JB is typically incidental
- Increased risk of entering JB during mastoidectomy, so include in report!

Image Interpretation Pearls
- MR: Complex or increased signal of high JB does not persist on all MR sequences

SELECTED REFERENCES

1. D'Souza WP et al: Characterization of jugular bulb position on computed tomography (CT) with implications for excision of vestibular schwannomas. Neurosurg Rev. 48(1):54, 2025
2. Alves IS et al: Imaging of vertigo and dizziness: a site-based approach, part 1 (middle ear, bony labyrinth, and temporomandibular joint). Semin Ultrasound CT MR. 45(5):360-71, 2024
3. Page JC et al: Lateral temporal bone resection with a high-riding jugular bulb. Otol Neurotol. 45(8):e617, 2024

Dehiscent Jugular Bulb

TERMINOLOGY

- Normal venous variant with superior & lateral extension of jugular bulb (JB) into middle ear (ME) cavity through dehiscent sigmoid plate

IMAGING

- Soft tissue mass in ME contiguous with JB through **dehiscent sigmoid plate**
  - **Lateral outpouching** from JB best seen on coronal CT
  - Enhances to same degree as adjacent venous structures on C+ CT & MR
  - CTV or MRV may be performed in equivocal cases

TOP DIFFERENTIAL DIAGNOSES

- Asymmetrically large JB
- High-riding JB
- Aberrant internal carotid artery
- Jugular paraganglioma
- Jugular foramen schwannoma

- Jugular foramen meningioma

CLINICAL ISSUES

- Dehiscent JB (DJB) has been reported as linked to pulsatile tinnitus, hearing loss, Ménière disease
- Otoscopy: **Vascular blue "mass"** behind intact tympanic membrane may prompt imaging
- Otoscopic + bone CT findings make correct diagnosis
  - Correct DJB diagnosis provides warning to surgeons when surgery contemplated for other indications

DIAGNOSTIC CHECKLIST

- DJB in differential diagnosis list of any vascular retrotympanic mass
- Coronal temporal bone CT will show direct continuity of ME mass with JB
- Important to exclude communication of any vascular lesion with adjacent petrous carotid canal, which would indicate aberrant or lateralized internal carotid artery

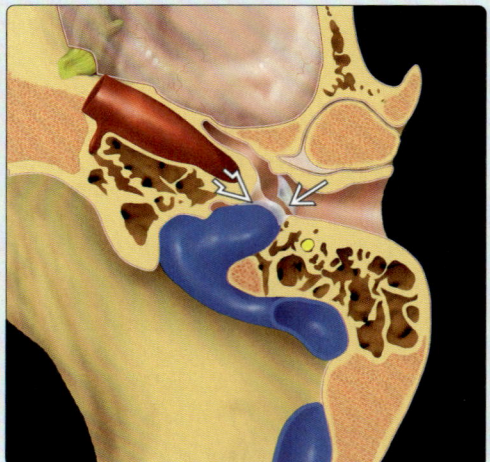
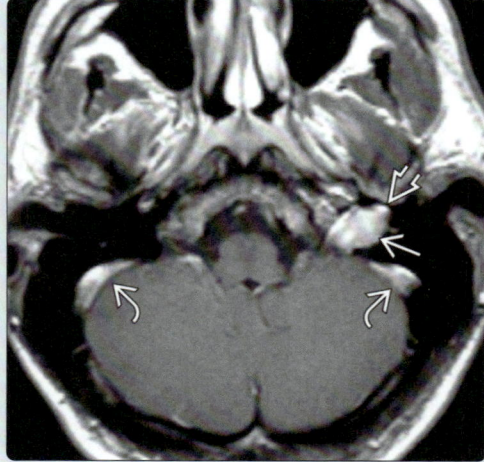

(Left) Axial graphic depicts a dehiscent jugular bulb projecting superolaterally into the middle ear through the dehiscent sigmoid plate ➡. Typically, a blue-colored vascular "mass" is identified behind the posteroinferior quadrant of the intact tympanic membrane ➡. (Right) Axial T1WI C+ MR shows enhancement of the prominent jugular bulb ➡ contiguous with the dehiscent component in the middle ear ➡. Enhancement is identical to the sigmoid sinuses ➡.

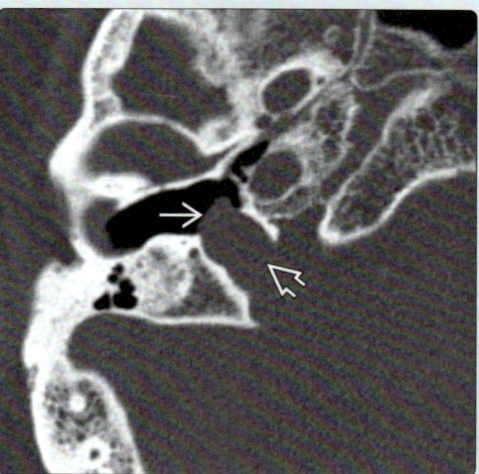
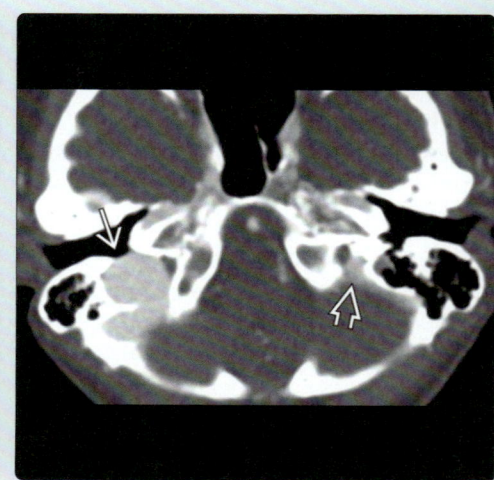

(Left) Axial bone CT demonstrates the jugular bulb ➡ and a soft tissue density mass ➡ within the inferior right middle ear cavity contiguous through the widely dehiscent jugular plate. The bone changes are smooth with no aggressive features. (Right) Axial CECT shows a prominent right jugular bulb ➡ with dehiscence of the sigmoid plate. Compare this with the left jugular bulb ➡ and intact sigmoid plate. Jugular bulb dehiscence is more common on the right.

TERMINOLOGY

Abbreviations

- Dehiscent jugular bulb (DJB)

Definitions

- Normal venous variant with superior & lateral extension of JB into middle ear (ME) through dehiscent sigmoid plate

IMAGING

CT Findings

- CECT
  - Protruding mass enhances to same degree as JB
- Bone CT
  - Soft tissue mass in posteroinferior ME
    - Sigmoid plate dehiscent
- CTV
  - Enhancement pattern mirrors sigmoid sinus & internal jugular (IJ) vein

MR Findings

- T1WI
  - May have heterogeneous intensity or flow void
- T2WI
  - May have heterogeneous intensity or flow void
- T1WI C+
  - ME "mass" may show enhancement or flow characteristics similar to adjacent JB
- MRV
  - Coronal images show **lateral lobulation** best

Imaging Recommendations

- Best imaging tool
  - High-resolution CT of temporal bone is complementary to MR in evaluating possible vascular lesion of jugular foramen or ME

DIFFERENTIAL DIAGNOSIS

High Jugular Bulb

- Defined by superior portion extending to floor of IAC
- Bone CT: JB cortical margins intact, including sigmoid plate

Jugular Bulb Diverticulum

- Bone CT: Focal polypoid mass extending from superior JB
- Sigmoid plate is intact

Aberrant Internal Carotid Artery

- Vascular lesion in ME is contiguous with petrous internal carotid artery

Jugular Paraganglioma

- Bone CT: Permeative-destructive bony changes along JB superolateral margins
- Unenhanced T1 MR: Jugular foramen mass with high-velocity flow voids ("pepper")
- Vector of spread: Superolateral from JB through ME floor into hypotympanum

PATHOLOGY

General Features

- Etiology

- Congenital lesion
- May be more common in underpneumatized temporal bone
- Associated abnormalities
  - Most often associated with high-riding JB

CLINICAL ISSUES

Presentation

- Most common signs/symptoms
  - **Asymptomatic** incidental finding
- Other signs/symptoms
  - DJB has been reported as linked to many symptoms, though causality disputed
    - Hearing loss, Ménière disease
    - Rhythmic pulsatile tinnitus that changes with exercise or IJ compression
- **Otoscopy**: Blue-colored vascular mass behind intact TM, prompting imaging
  - Seen in **posteroinferior TM quadrant**

Demographics

- Age
  - Discovered on otoscopic or radiologic exam at any age
- Epidemiology
  - Most common vascular variant of petrous bone
  - More common on right side
    - Dural venous sinuses & jugular vein are larger on right in 75% of population

Natural History & Prognosis

- Renders JB vulnerable to trauma
  - Important to warn surgeons of presence of DJB when surgery is contemplated for other indications

DIAGNOSTIC CHECKLIST

Consider

- DJB in differential diagnosis list of any vascular retrotympanic mass

Image Interpretation Pearls

- Coronal TB CT will show direct continuity of ME mass with JB
- Smooth bony margins exclude more aggressive processes, such as tumor or infection

SELECTED REFERENCES

1. Tudose RC et al: Anatomical variations of the jugular bulb: a critical and comprehensive review. Medicina (Kaunas). 60(9):1408, 2024
2. Dai C et al: CT evaluation of unilateral pulsatile tinnitus with jugular bulb wall dehiscence. Eur Radiol. 33(6):4464-71, 2023
3. Hu J et al: Value of CT and three-dimensional reconstruction revealing specific radiological signs for screening causative high jugular bulb in patients with Meniere's disease. BMC Med Imaging. 20(1):103, 2020
4. Lee SY et al: Jugular bulb resurfacing with bone cement for patients with high dehiscent jugular bulb and ipsilateral pulsatile tinnitus. Otol Neurotol. 40(2):192-9, 2019
5. Atmaca S et al: High and dehiscent jugular bulb: clear and present danger during middle ear surgery. Surg Radiol Anat. 36(4):369-74, 2014
6. Ball M et al: Beware the silent presentation of a high and dehiscent jugular bulb in the external ear canal. J Laryngol Otol. 124(7):790-2, 2010
7. El-Begermy MA et al: A novel surgical technique for management of tinnitus due to high dehiscent jugular bulb. Otolaryngol Head Neck Surg. 142(4):576-81, 2010

TERMINOLOGY

- Jugular bulb diverticulum (JBD): Congenital vascular anomaly of jugular bulb (JB) with **focal, finger-like projection extending from JB** into surrounding skull base

IMAGING

- T-bone CT: Focal projection extending off JB margin **superiorly** into deep T-bone just behind IAC
- Other directions of extension: **Lateral, medial, anterior, or posterior**
- Imaging protocol: Start with thin-section T-bone CT
  - If concern lingers, MR with contrast & MRV

TOP DIFFERENTIAL DIAGNOSES

- JB pseudolesion
- High JB
- Dehiscent JB
- Jugular paraganglioma
- Jugular foramen schwannoma or meningioma

PATHOLOGY

- JBD thought to represent expansion of high JB into surrounding bone but hindered by dense otic capsule

CLINICAL ISSUES

- **Asymptomatic**, incidental finding commonly
- Many symptoms have been linked to JBD
- JBD present in 35% of cases with high-riding JB

DIAGNOSTIC CHECKLIST

- JBD in differential of medial T-bone mass with smooth margins on CT
- Turbulent flow makes JB & JBD difficult to evaluate by MR
- Look for smooth, bony remodeling on bone CT & continuity with JB
- On axial T1 C+ MR, enhancing foci behind IAC may be mistaken for schwannoma
- Include in radiology report to warn surgeon if ear surgery planned!

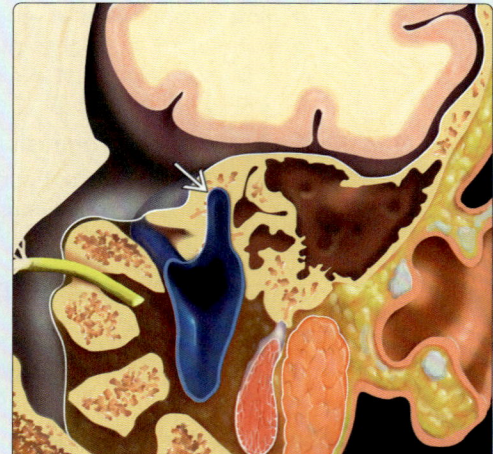
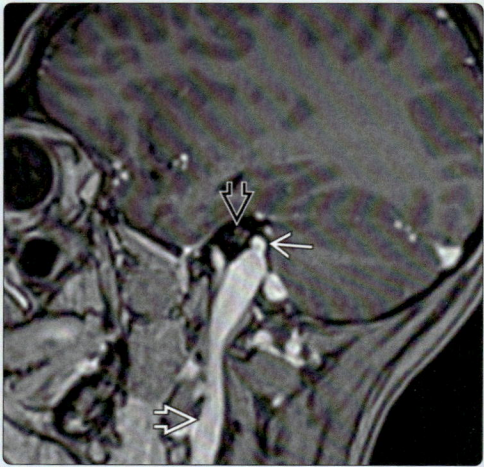

(Left) Coronal graphic depicts a jugular bulb diverticulum (JBD) as a finger-like, superior projection off the jugular bulb (JB) into the petrous T-bone ➡ without extension into the middle ear. (Right) Sagittal T1 C+ SPGR MR shows a superior projecting enhancing JBD ➡. This polypoid extension from the JB has similar enhancement characteristics as the JB & jugular vein ➡. Note the internal auditory canal ➡ anterior to the JBD. This JB lesion is more common on the left side. JBDs are present in 35% of cases with a high-riding JB.

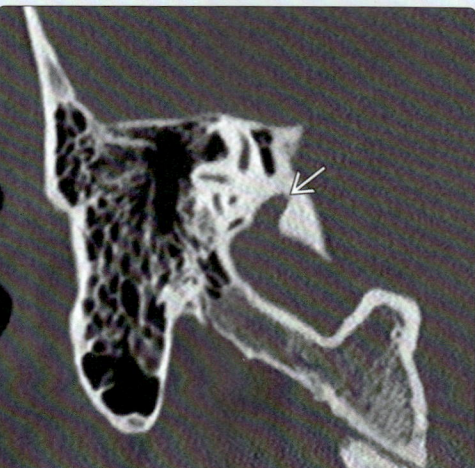
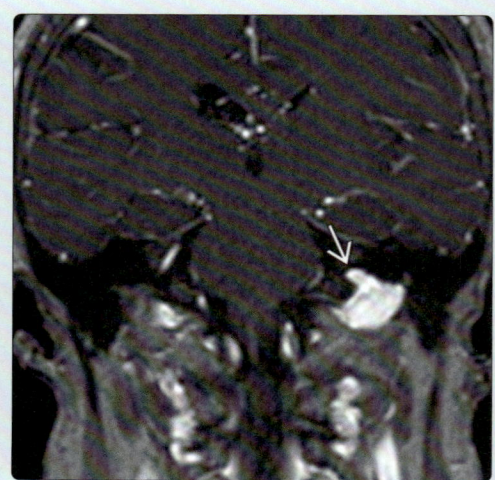

(Left) Coronal right ear CT shows a JBD ➡ as a thumb-like projection arising from the superior JB margin. Continuity with the normal JB & smooth bony margins helps confirm the diagnosis. Patients are asymptomatic as a rule, though many symptoms have been associated with a JBD. Include in radiology report to warn surgeon if ear surgery is planned! (Right) Coronal T1 C+ SPGR MR shows a superior & medially projecting enhancing JBD ➡. This polypoid extension from the JB has similar enhancement as the JB & jugular vein.

Jugular Bulb Diverticulum

TERMINOLOGY

Abbreviations
- Jugular bulb diverticulum (JBD)

Synonyms
- Jugular diverticulum, petrous jugular malposition

Definitions
- **Congenital vascular anomaly** of jugular bulb (JB) with focal, **finger-like projection** extending from JB into surrounding skull base

IMAGING

General Features
- Best diagnostic clue
  - T-bone CT: **Focal polypoid projection** extending off JB margin superiorly into deep T-bone just behind internal auditory canal (IAC)
- Location
  - JBD most commonly extends superiorly
  - Other directions of extension
    - Lateral, medial, anterior, or posterior
    - Lateral extension is often through dehiscent sigmoid plate = dehiscent JB
  - JB itself may be **high** or, less commonly, in normal position
- Size
  - Typical JB measures 1.0-1.5 cm
  - Diverticulum smaller than JB, typically < 1 cm in diameter & length
- Morphology
  - Lobulated outpouching arising from JB
  - May be finger-like or broad based

CT Findings
- Bone CT: JBD is **well-corticated, smooth polypoid extension** off JB margin
  - Axial: Most commonly seen behind IAC
  - Coronal: Finger-like projection off top of JB
- CECT: Uniform enhancement of JB & JBD
- CTA: Contiguous with JB, similar enhancement

MR Findings
- T1WI: Heterogeneous signal intensity
- T2WI: Low signal from high-velocity flow (invisible)
  - Turbulent flow, heterogeneous high intensity (uncommon)
- T1WI C+: Avid enhancement, similar to JB & internal jugular vein (IJV)
  - May mimic schwannoma, meningioma, or paraganglioma
- MRV: Finger-like projection off JB

Imaging Recommendations
- Protocol advice: Start with thin-section T-bone CT
  - If concern lingers, MR with contrast & MRV

DIFFERENTIAL DIAGNOSIS

Jugular Bulb Pseudolesion
- MR shows asymmetric large JB with mass-like signal
- Usually found incidentally in skull base work-up

- Bone CT: Intact jugular spine & JB cortical margins

High Jugular Bulb
- Defined by most as cephalad portion of JB extending superior to floor of IAC ± at level of basal turn of cochlea
- CT: Jugular foramen (JF) cortical margins intact, including sigmoid plate
- MR: Complex or increased signal does not persist on all MR sequences

Dehiscent Jugular Bulb
- Vascular retrotympanic mass
- Protruding mass extends into posteroinferior middle ear cavity
- CT: Sigmoid plate shows focal dehiscence
- T1 C+ MR: Avidly enhancing middle ear mass connects to avidly enhancing JB

Jugular Paraganglioma
- Enhancing mass in JF
- CT: Permeative destructive JF margin bony changes
- T1 MR: High-velocity flow voids ("pepper")

Jugular Foramen Schwannoma
- Dumbbell-shaped mass along CNIX-XI
- CT: Smoothly scalloped bony margins of enlarged JF
- T1 C+ MR: Fusiform, enhancing mass in JF

Jugular Foramen Meningioma
- CT: Permeative-sclerotic or hyperostotic JF margins
- T1 C+ MR: Avidly enhancing mass with dural tails

PATHOLOGY

General Features
- Etiology
  - May be secondary to hemodynamic factors
  - More commonly seen with high-riding JB
  - Thought to represent expansion of high JB into surrounding bone, hindered by dense otic capsule

CLINICAL ISSUES

Presentation
- Most common signs/symptoms
  - **Asymptomatic**, incidental finding
- Many symptoms have been linked to JBD, based on direction of diverticulum extension: Sensorineural hearing loss, tinnitus, vertigo
- Symptoms reported have tenuous link to JBD

Demographics
- Epidemiology
  - Present in 8% of T-bone specimen studies
  - More common on left side

Treatment
- Conservative management of symptoms
- **Caveat**: Include in radiology report to warn surgeon if ear surgery planned!

SELECTED REFERENCES

1. Daou BJ et al: Causes of pulsatile tinnitus and treatment options. Neurosurg Clin N Am. 35(3):293-303, 2024

TERMINOLOGY

- Benign tumor arising from paraganglia located in & around jugular foramen (JF)

IMAGING

- Bone CT: **Permeative-destructive** bone changes along JF margins
  - Jugular spine erosion is common
  - Floor of middle ear cavity dehisced
- MR: Lesions > 2 cm demonstrate characteristic **salt & pepper** appearance
- CTA/angiography: Main arterial supply is from **ascending pharyngeal artery**
- **Paraganglia rests** occur in 3 distinct bodies around JF: Jugular bulb (JB), tympanic branch of CNIX (Jacobson nerve), & auricular branch of CNX (Arnold nerve)
- Vector of spread: **Superolateral** through floor of middle ear is typical

TOP DIFFERENTIAL DIAGNOSES

- Tympanic paraganglioma
- JF schwannoma
- JF meningioma
- JF metastasis
- Dehiscent JB

CLINICAL ISSUES

- Presentation: Objective pulsatile tinnitus most common
  - Other symptoms: CNIX-XI ± CNXII cranial neuropathy
  - CNVII or CNVIII neuropathy less often
- Otoscopic exam: **Red, pulsatile** retrotympanic mass
- M:F = 1:4
- Jugular paraganglioma (JP) is most common JF tumor
- JP & carotid body paraganglioma account for 80% of H&N paragangliomas
- Treatment: Surgical resection ± radiation
  - Radiosurgery may be used as primary therapy

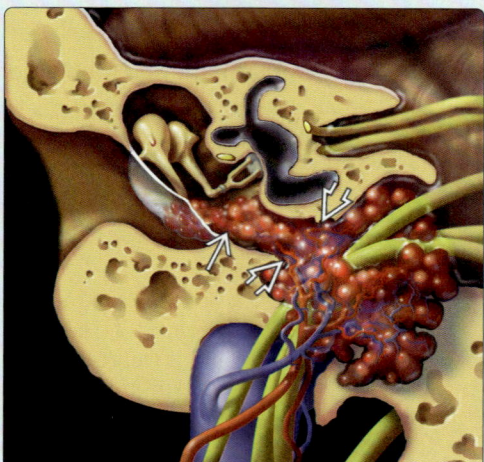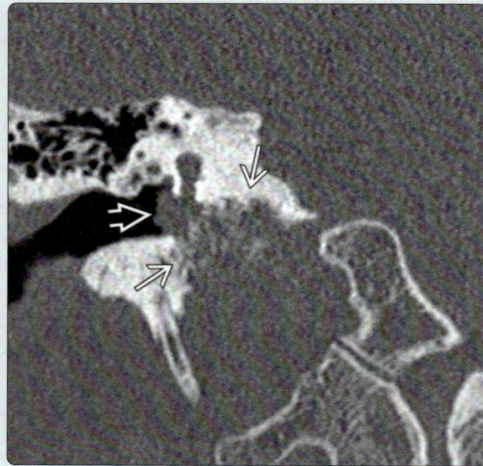

(Left) Coronal graphic shows a jugular paraganglioma (JP) centered in the jugular foramen (JF) dehiscing the middle ear floor ➡ to reach the middle ear cavity ➡. The main arterial supply for this vascular tumor is the ascending pharyngeal artery. (Right) Coronal temporal bone CT of the right ear shows the classic permeative-destructive margins ➡ of a JP. Note the typical vector of spread superolateral from the JF to the middle ear ➡, seen as a vascular retrotympanic mass at otoscopy.

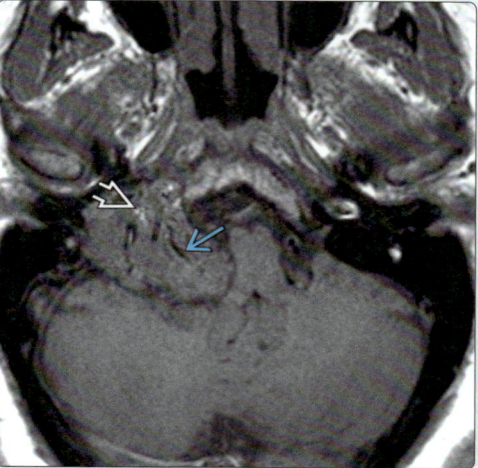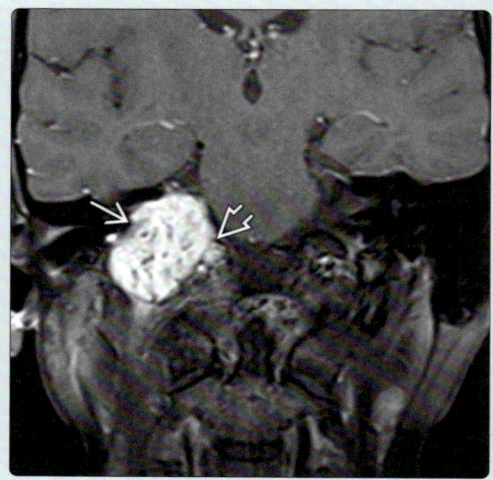

(Left) Axial T1WI MR shows a large mass arising from the JF with multiple areas of salt & pepper. The "salt" ➡ represents blood products or slow flow, while the "pepper" ➡ represents high-velocity arterial branch flow voids that help differentiate this tumor from other lesions in this location. (Right) Coronal T1 C+ MR shows a large enhancing mass in the JF ➡ with destruction & enhancement of the jugular tubercle ➡. A JP is the most common tumor of the JF.

Jugular Paraganglioma

TERMINOLOGY

Abbreviations
- Jugular paraganglioma (JP) [new WHO terminology (2022)]

Synonyms
- Former terminology: Glomus jugulare paraganglioma (GJP), glomus jugulotympanicum paraganglioma, chemodectoma

Definitions
- Benign tumor arising from paraganglia located in & around jugular foramen (JF)

IMAGING

General Features
- Best diagnostic clue
  - Mass in JF with **permeative-destructive** change of adjacent bone on CT
  - Multiple black dots (**"pepper"**) in tumor indicate high-velocity flow voids from feeding arterial branches on MR
- Location
  - Paraganglia rests occur in 3 distinct bodies around JF
    - Jugular bulb (JB), tympanic branch of CNIX (Jacobson nerve), & auricular branch of CNX (Arnold nerve)
  - Vector of spread: **Superolateral** through floor of middle ear (most common)
- Size
  - Large at presentation: 2-6 cm most common
- Morphology
  - Poorly marginated JF tumor with adjacent bone invasion

CT Findings
- NECT
  - Poorly defined soft tissue mass centered over JF
- CECT
  - Diffuse, intense enhancement
- Bone CT
  - **Permeative-destructive** bone changes along superolateral margin of JF mark extent of tumor
    - Jugular spine erosion is common
    - Vertical segment of petrous internal carotid artery (ICA) posterior wall often dehiscent
    - Mastoid segment of facial nerve may be engulfed
  - Mimics malignancy

MR Findings
- T1WI
  - Lesions > 2 cm show characteristic **salt & pepper appearance**
    - "Salt" refers to hyperintense foci within tumor related to hemorrhage or slow flow
      - Hyperintense foci relatively rare MR finding
    - "Pepper" refers to numerous hypointense foci within tumor, representing high-velocity arterial flow voids
      - Hypointense foci common MR finding
- T2WI
  - Mixed hyperintense mass with hypointense foci ("pepper")
- T1WI C+
  - Intense enhancement is characteristic
  - Delineates tumor extent in skull base & middle ear
  - Tumor may extend intraluminal within internal jugular vein or sigmoid sinus
  - Coronal: May show tongue of tumor curving up from JF, through middle ear floor, terminating on cochlear promontory
- MRV: Delineates sigmoid sinus & jugular vein status
- DCE MRP: Elevated Vp may be present

Angiographic Findings
- **Hypervascular** mass with enlarged feeding arteries, rapid, intense tumor blush, & early draining veins
  - Main arterial supply is from **ascending pharyngeal artery** that supplies inferomedial territory
  - Caroticotympanic branches of ICA & meningeal branches of vertebral artery may contribute
  - Anterior tympanic artery from external carotid artery (ECA) supplies anterior compartment
  - Stylomastoid artery from ECA supplies posterolateral compartment

Nuclear Medicine Findings
- PET
  - Paragangliomas show **avid** F-18 FDG uptake & Ga-68 DOTATATE uptake
    - Ga-68 DOTATATE: Somatostatin analog radiotracer: Images neuroendocrine tumors
  - Useful in staging, detecting metastasis, or monitoring response to therapy

Imaging Recommendations
- Best imaging tool
  - Combination of bone CT & enhanced MR
- Bone CT, MR, & angiography all done before surgery
- Bone CT delineates areas of bone destruction
  - Shows bony landmarks less well seen on MR
- MR reveals exact soft tissue extent of tumor
- Angiography provides vascular roadmap for surgeon
  - Embolization used for preoperative hemostasis

DIFFERENTIAL DIAGNOSIS

Tympanic Paraganglioma
- Bone CT: Globoid mass on cochlear promontory
  - Middle ear floor intact
- T1 C+ MR: Mass enhances
  - May differentiate location of tympanic paraganglioma (TP) from obstructed secretions
- Otoscopy: Larger TP may mimic JP, vascular retrotympanic mass

Jugular Foramen Schwannoma
- Bone CT: Smooth remodeling, enlargement of JF
- T1 C+ MR: Fusiform, enhancing mass ± cysts
- Angiography: Absence of tumor blush or enlarged feeding arteries; "puddling" on venous phase
- Vector of spread: Superomedial along CNIX-XI course

Jugular Foramen Meningioma
- Bone CT: Permeative-sclerotic bony JF margins
- T1 C+ MR: Enhancing mass with dural tails
- Angiography: Prolonged but mild tumor blush
- Vector of spread: Centrifugal spread along dural surfaces

Jugular Foramen Metastasis

- Bone CT: Destructive bone changes on JF margins
- T1 C+ MR: Heterogeneously enhancing, invasive mass
- Vector of spread: Irregular, centrifugal spread pattern

Dehiscent Jugular Bulb

- Bone CT: Sigmoid plate is focally dehiscent
- Coronal CT or MR: Superolateral extension of JB into middle ear
- Otoscopy: Blue-black posteroinferior quadrant retrotympanic mass

PATHOLOGY

General Features

- Etiology
  - Benign tumor arising from JF **paraganglia**
  - Paraganglia: Chemoreceptors that respond to changes in blood oxygen, carbon dioxide
- Genetics
  - Familial prevalence ~ 40% for all paragangliomas
  - Germline *SDHB* & *SDHD* mutations
    - Higher risk of malignant paraganglioma
    - Multiple lesions common
- Associated abnormalities
  - Increased risk of thyroid malignancy
  - Increased risk of paragangliomas in multiple endocrine neoplasia type 2, neurofibromatosis type 1, multiple mucocutaneous neuromas

Staging, Grading, & Classification

- **Glasscock-Jackson classification** of JP: Correlates tumor extent with surgical approach
  - I: Small tumor involving JB, middle ear, mastoid
  - II: Tumor extends under internal auditory canal (IAC); may have intracranial extension
  - III: Extends into petrous apex (PA); may have intracranial extension
  - IV: Extends beyond PA, into clivus or infratemporal fossa; ± intracranial extension
- **Fisch classification**: Anatomic classification
  - A: Tumor limited to middle ear
  - B: Limited to tympanomastoid area, no infralabyrinthine involvement
  - C: Invades infralabyrinthine compartment & PA
    - C1: Limited involvement of vertical carotid canal
    - C2: Invades vertical carotid canal
    - C3: Invades horizontal carotid canal
  - D1: Intracranial extension < 2 cm
  - D2: Intracranial extension > 2 cm
- **Modified Fisch classification**: Added V to indicate vertebral artery involvement

Gross Pathologic & Surgical Features

- Lobulated solid mass with fibrous pseudocapsule
- Cut surface shows multiple enlarged feeding arteries

Microscopic Features

- Biphasic cell pattern composed of chief cells & sustentacular cells surrounded by fibromuscular stroma
  - Chief cells arranged in characteristic compact cell nests or balls of cells (zellballen)

- Electromicroscopy: Shows neurosecretory granules

CLINICAL ISSUES

Presentation

- Most common signs/symptoms
  - Objective **pulsatile tinnitus**
  - Otoscopic exam: **Red, pulsatile** retrotympanic mass
  - Other symptoms: CNIX-XI ± CNXII cranial neuropathy; CNVII or CNVIII cranial neuropathy less often
  - Otologic symptoms predominate initially with cranial nerve palsies occurring late
- Clinical profile
  - 50-year-old woman with progressive pulsatile tinnitus & red, pulsatile retrotympanic mass

Demographics

- Age
  - 40-60 years
- Sex
  - M:F = 1:4
- Epidemiology
  - JP & carotid body paraganglioma account for 80% of H&N paragangliomas
  - JP is most common JF tumor
  - Multifocal 5-10% in sporadic JPs
  - Multifocal 25-50% in familial JPs

Natural History & Prognosis

- Slow-growing tumor can be watched in older patients
- 60% have postoperative cranial neuropathy
- Aggressive behavior is seen in 2-13% of cases
  - Increased in patients with familial tumor syndromes
- Mortality rates are estimated at 15%

Treatment

- Surgery: Infratemporal fossa approach
- Larger lesions may require surgery & radiation
- XRT/radiosurgery may be used as primary therapy

DIAGNOSTIC CHECKLIST

Consider

- Look for multifocal lesions when evaluating JP
- JP & JF metastases: Permeative bone destruction
- Vascular schwannoma may mimic JP on CT/MR

Image Interpretation Pearls

- JP diagnosed when mass shows
  - Bone CT: Permeative-destructive bone invasion
  - MR: JF mass with prominent flow voids ("pepper")
  - Vector of spread: Superolateral → JF into middle ear

SELECTED REFERENCES

1. Lamas C et al: Current management of head and neck paragangliomas: a multicenter series with long-term follow-up. Otolaryngol Head Neck Surg. 172(1):176-83, 2025
2. Hartmann K et al: 68 Ga-DOTATATE PET to characterize lesions in the neuroaxis. Clin Nucl Med. 49(1):9-15, 2024
3. Ota Y et al: Precise differentiation between jugular foramen paragangliomas and metastases: utility of diffusion-weighted and dynamic contrast-enhanced magnetic resonance imaging. Neuroradiology. 65(4):805-13, 2023

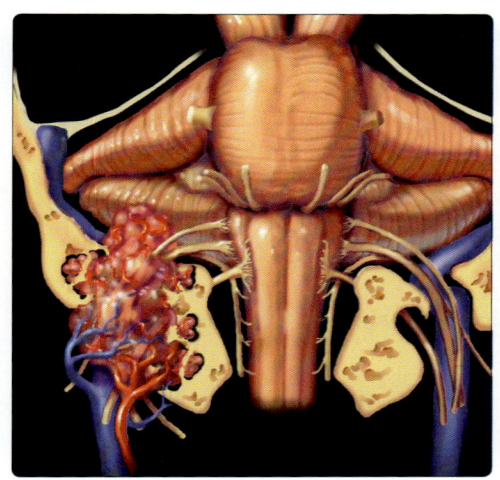

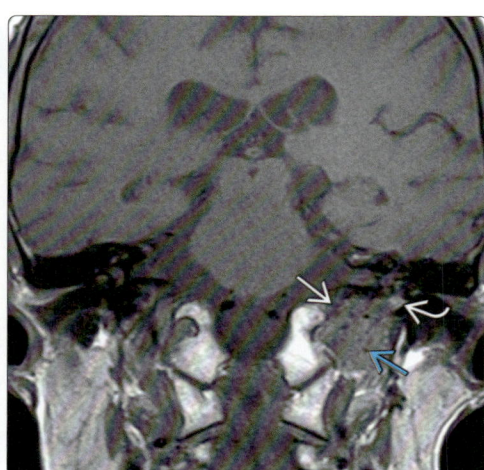

(Left) Coronal graphic shows a large JP arising from the JF, engulfing the jugular vein and CNIX-XII, & infiltrating the adjacent skull base. (Right) Coronal T1 MR shows a large skull base mass ➡ centered in the JF. Note the multiple high-velocity flow voids ("pepper") ➡, characteristic of a paraganglioma. A JP is the most common JF tumor and 2nd most common tumor of the temporal bone. Pulsatile tinnitus is the most common presenting symptom. Extension ➡ to the middle ear is common in large lesions.

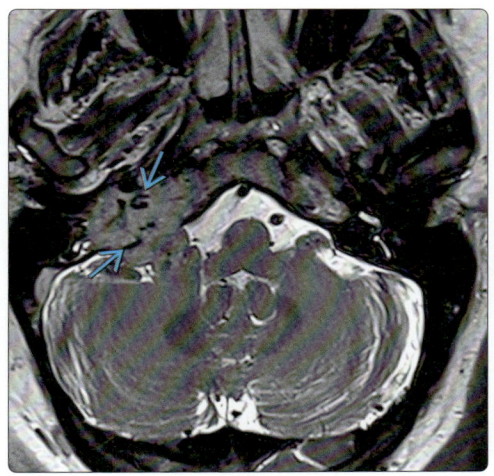

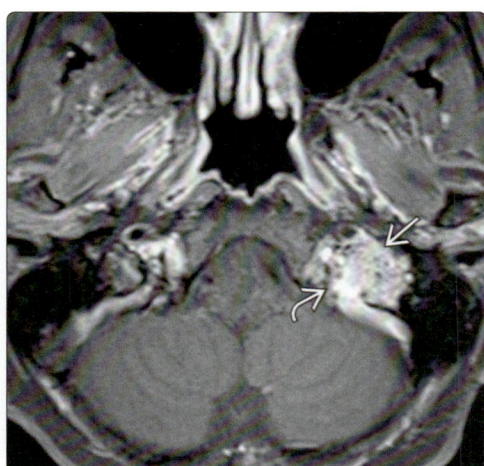

(Left) Axial T2 SPACE MR in a 47-year-old woman shows a large mass arising from the JF with multiple high-velocity flow voids ➡ that help differentiate this tumor from other lesions in this location, such as schwannoma and meningioma. (Right) Axial T1WI C+ FS MR shows an enhancing JP ➡ involving the JF, engulfing the jugular bulb (JB) ➡ in a patient with an SDHB mutation. These patients are at risk for a more aggressive paraganglioma and metastatic disease. A Ga-68 DOTATATE scan is often helpful.

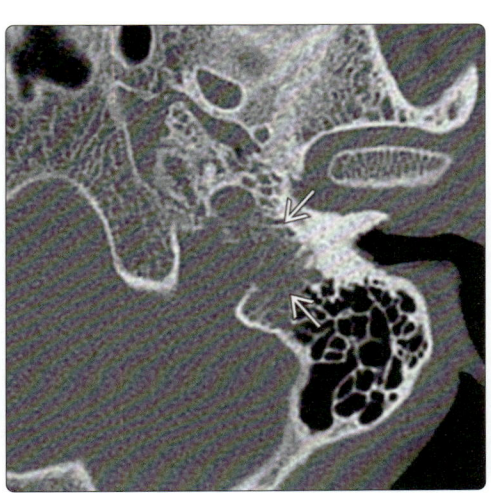

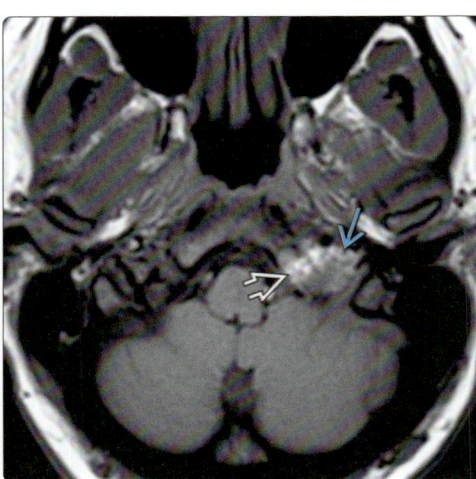

(Left) Axial temporal bone CT of the left ear shows a JP with typical bony permeative-destructive margins ➡. These tumors may present in a patient with pulsatile tinnitus. (Right) Axial T1 MR in a patient with hearing loss & tinnitus shows a heterogeneous JF mass with a salt & pepper appearance with hyperintense foci ➡ & vascular flow voids ➡. Larger tumors may show both. Paraganglia rests occur in 3 locations around JF: JB, tympanic branch of CNIX (Jacobson nerve), & auricular branch of CNX (Arnold nerve).

Skull Base Lesions

TERMINOLOGY

- Benign tumor of differentiated Schwann cells wrapping around CNIX, X, or XI within jugular foramen (JF)

IMAGING

- Bone CT: Sharply marginated, enlarged JF
- T1WI C+ MR
  - Tubular or dumbbell-shaped, uniformly enhancing
  - No flow voids ("pepper") (vs. paraganglioma)
  - Nonenhancing cystic areas in large lesions
- T2WI hyperintense
- Superomedial vector of tumor growth
  - Follows craniocaudal course of CNIX-XI
  - Grows cephalad from JF through basal cistern toward retroolivary sulcus of lateral medulla
  - Grows inferiorly from JF into nasopharyngeal carotid space
- MRV: Dural sinus compressed, not occluded

TOP DIFFERENTIAL DIAGNOSES

- JF pseudolesion
- Jugular paraganglioma
- JF meningioma
- Skull base metastasis

CLINICAL ISSUES

- Mean age: 45 years old
- **Sensorineural hearing loss** in 90% at presentation
  - May present clinically like vestibular schwannoma
- 2nd most common JF tumor
  - **Glossopharyngeal nerve** (CNIX) most common nerve of origin
- Complete surgical removal of tumor in single procedure is goal
  - May be complicated by lower cranial neuropathy
- Radiosurgery as primary or adjuvant therapy

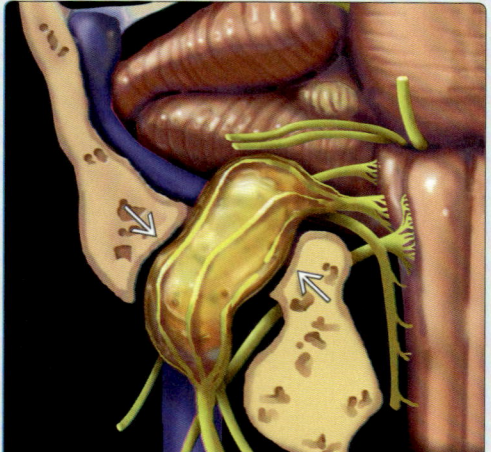
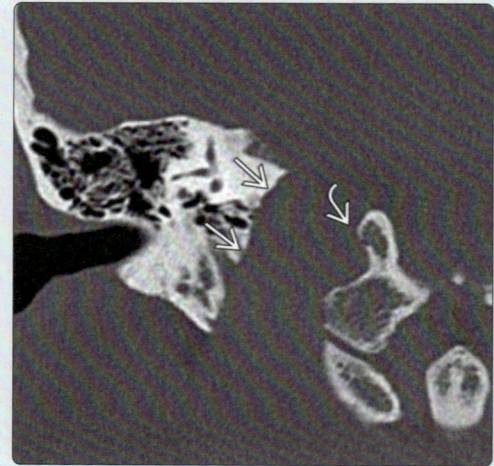

(Left) Coronal graphic depicts a classic jugular foramen (JF) schwannoma as a fusiform mass arising on one of the cranial nerves (IX-XI) within the JF. Note the vector of spread is superomedial. The JF ➡ is smoothly enlarged with an intact cortex. (Right) Coronal bone CT shows a sharply marginated, enlarged JF with amputation of the lateral jugular tubercle "bird's beak" ➡. The smooth enlargement ➡ with sclerotic margins is characteristic of JF schwannoma and can help differentiate a schwannoma from a paraganglioma.

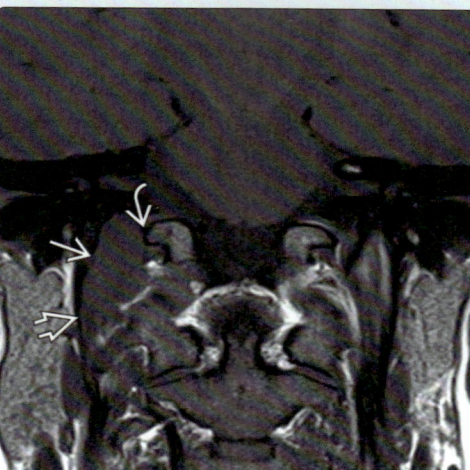
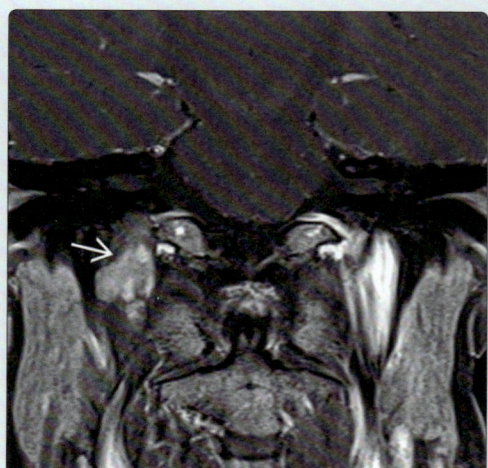

(Left) Coronal T1 MR shows a JF schwannoma ➡ projecting superomedially from the JF toward the brainstem. Inferiorly, the schwannoma extends into the nasopharyngeal carotid space ➡. There is amputation of the lateral aspect of the jugular tubercle ➡. Lack of flow voids helps differentiate this schwannoma from the more common jugular paraganglioma. (Right) Coronal T1 C+ MR in the same patient shows avid enhancement of the JF schwannoma ➡.

Jugular Foramen Schwannoma

TERMINOLOGY

Abbreviations
- Jugular foramen schwannoma (JFS)

Synonyms
- Neuroma, neurilemoma, neurinoma

Definitions
- Benign tumor of differentiated Schwann cells wrapping around CNIX, X, or XI within jugular foramen (JF)
  - Glossopharyngeal nerve (CNIX) most common nerve of origin in JF

IMAGING

General Features
- Best diagnostic clue
  - Sharply marginated, enlarged JF on bone CT
  - Fusiform, enhancing mass enlarging JF on T1WI C+ MR
- Location
  - JF
    - Vector of tumor growth
      □ Follows general craniocaudal course of CNIX-XI
      □ Grows cephalad from JF through basal cistern toward retroolivary sulcus of lateral medulla
      □ Grows inferiorly from JF into nasopharyngeal carotid space
- Size
  - Often large at presentation (> 3 cm)
- Morphology
  - Fusiform or "dumbbell" mass
    - Waist is within JF

CT Findings
- NECT
  - Well-defined soft tissue mass isodense to brain, occasionally hypodense
- CECT
  - Dense contrast enhancement is typical
  - Larger JFS often show nonenhancing intramural cysts
- Bone CT
  - **Smooth JF enlargement** with thin, sclerotic margins
  - Coronal plane may show amputation of lateral jugular tubercle ("bird's beak")
  - Multilobular intraosseous extension into adjacent skull base may be marked

MR Findings
- T1WI
  - Tubular or dumbbell-shaped JF mass
  - Typically isointense to brain
  - Internal carotid artery characteristically displaced over anteromedial margin of JFS in nasopharyngeal carotid space
  - **No flow voids** ("pepper") or hyperintensity related to blood products ("salt") even when large
- T2WI
  - High signal relative to white matter
  - ↑ signal **cystic areas** can be seen in large JFS
    - 25% of JFS show intramural cysts
  - Hypointense blood products extremely rare

- DWI
  - No diffusion restriction
  - May be mildly hyperintense related to T2 shine-through
- T1WI C+
  - Uniformly enhancing JF mass
  - Nonenhancing intramural cystic components in larger tumors may be seen
  - When small, may be difficult to differentiate enhancing normal jugular bulb (JB) from small JFS
    - Tissue-intensity mass seen better on unenhanced T1 and T2WI
- MRV
  - Dural sinuses usually compressed, not occluded
    - Occlusion can be evaluated with phase-contrast MRV employing low-velocity encoding setting

Angiographic Findings
- Tumor is moderately vascular
- Feeding vessels are tortuous but not enlarged
- Scattered contrast "puddles" are characteristic in venous phase
- No arteriovenous shunting or vascular encasement

Imaging Recommendations
- Best imaging tool
  - Enhanced brain/skull base MR best delineates internal architecture and soft tissue extent of JFS
  - Bone CT is best for assessing JF cortex for typical **smooth, sclerotic** margins

DIFFERENTIAL DIAGNOSIS

Jugular Foramen Pseudolesion
- Venous flow phenomenon mimics schwannoma or other lesion
- Asymmetric large JB with complex MR signal
- Asymmetric large JF with normal margins on CT
- T1 C+ MR: Slow flow in JF enhances
- MRV: Normal dural sinuses and jugular bulb

Jugular Paraganglioma
- Permeative-destructive JF bone margins on bone CT
- High-velocity flow voids ("pepper") on unenhanced MR sequences
- Rapid tumor blush with early draining veins on angiography
- Growth vector: Superolateral from JF into middle ear

Jugular Foramen Meningioma
- Permeative-sclerotic bone margins of JF on CT
- Intermediate to low signal on T2WI
- Dural-based mass with enhancing dural tails
- Prolonged blush into capillary phase on angiography
- Growth vector: Centrifugally along dural surfaces

Skull Base Metastasis
- Bony margins of JF are destructive on CT
- Heterogeneously enhancing, invasive JF mass
- Growth vector: All directions from JF
- Multiple lesions commonly seen

PATHOLOGY

General Features

- Etiology
  - Arises from differentiated neoplastic Schwann cells wrapping around CNIX, X, or XI
- Genetics
  - **90%** are solitary and sporadic
  - 4% arise in setting of neurofibromatosis type 2 (NF2)
  - < 5% associated with schwannomatosis
- Associated abnormalities
  - Multiple schwannomas are associated with NF2 or schwannomatosis
  - Increased incidence with prior irradiation

Staging, Grading, & Classification

- WHO grade 1
- Kaye and Pellet surgical classification (used by some surgeons)
  - Type A: Extends to cerebellopontine angle (CPA)
  - Type B: Within JF
  - Type C: Nasopharyngeal carotid space &/or JF
  - Type D: Intracranial and extracranial (cisternal and carotid space)

Gross Pathologic & Surgical Features

- Smooth, lobulated mass arising from nerve sheath
  - Arises eccentrically from nerve sheath
- Tan, round/ovoid, encapsulated mass

Microscopic Features

- Differentiated neoplastic Schwann cells
- Spindle cells with elongated nuclei
  - Antoni A: Areas of compact, elongated cells
  - Antoni B: Areas of less cellular, loosely arranged tumor, ± clusters of lipid-laden cells
- Immunochemistry: Strong, diffuse immunostaining for S100 protein = neural crest marker antigen present in supporting cells of nervous system and SOX10
- No necrosis but may have intratumoral cysts ± hemorrhage

CLINICAL ISSUES

Presentation

- Most common signs/symptoms
  - **Sensorineural hearing loss** (SNHL) in 90% at presentation
    - May present clinically like vestibular schwannoma
- Other signs/symptoms
  - CNIX-XI neuropathy occurs late in disease progression
  - Hoarseness, aspiration (recurrent laryngeal nerve, branch of CNX)
  - Dizziness may be related to cerebellar compression
  - Pulsatile tinnitus may be related to dural sinus thrombosis and dural arteriovenous fistula
  - Hemifacial spasm (mass effect on CNVII in CPA)
- Clinical profile
  - Middle-aged (~ 45 years old) individual with unilateral SNHL

Demographics

- Age

- Mean: 45 years; typically 4th-6th decades
- Sex
  - No predilection
- Epidemiology
  - Schwannomas represent 8% of intracranial tumors
    - 85-90% of CPA tumors are schwannoma
  - 2nd most common JF tumor
    - Jugular paraganglioma > > schwannoma > meningioma
    - Nonvestibular schwannoma incidence: CNV > > CNIX > CNX > CNVII > CNXI > CNXII > CNIII > CNIV > CNVI
  - **Glossopharyngeal nerve** (CNIX) most common nerve of origin of JFS

Natural History & Prognosis

- Benign, slow-growing tumor
- Advanced disease or treatment may result in late CNVII-XII neuropathy

Treatment

- Complete surgical removal of tumor in single procedure is goal
- Surgical approach dictated by presence or absence of cisternal or nasopharyngeal carotid space extension
  - Surgical cure may be complicated by lower cranial neuropathy, often CNIX and CNX
- Stereotactic radiosurgery is used more frequently as primary or adjuvant therapy

DIAGNOSTIC CHECKLIST

Consider

- JFS most likely when smooth, scalloped margins seen around JF soft tissue mass on CT

Image Interpretation Pearls

- Lack of flow voids help differentiate JF schwannoma from more common jugular paraganglioma

Reporting Tips

- Be sure to describe extension below skull base into carotid space and other soft tissues of the neck

SELECTED REFERENCES

1. Siempis T et al: Gamma-Knife radiosurgery for jugular foramen schwannomas. A systematic review and meta-analysis. World Neurosurg X. 25:100411, 2025
2. Vasireddi AK et al: The "outline sign": thin hyperenhancing perimeter as an MR imaging feature of meningioma. a useful tool in the temporal bone region for differentiating meningiomas from schwannomas and paragangliomas. AJNR Am J Neuroradiol. 46(2):349-54, 2025
3. Carlstrom LP et al: Lower cranial nerve schwannomas: cohort study and systematic review. Neurosurgery. 94(4):745-55, 2024
4. Bal J et al: Management of non-vestibular schwannomas in adult patients: a systematic review and consensus statement on behalf of the EANS skull base section part III: lower cranial nerve schwannomas, jugular foramen (CN IX, X, XI) and hypoglossal schwannoma (XII). Acta Neurochir (Wien). 164(2):321-9, 2022
5. Ota Y et al: MR diffusion and dynamic-contrast enhanced imaging to distinguish meningioma, paraganglioma, and schwannoma in the cerebellopontine angle and jugular foramen. J Neuroimaging. 32(3):502-10, 2022
6. Pires A et al: Differentiation of jugular foramen paragangliomas versus schwannomas using golden-angle radial sparse parallel dynamic contrast-enhanced MRI. AJNR Am J Neuroradiol. 42(10):1847-52, 2021
7. Eldevik OP et al: Imaging findings in schwannomas of the jugular foramen. AJNR Am J Neuroradiol. 21(6):1139-44, 2000

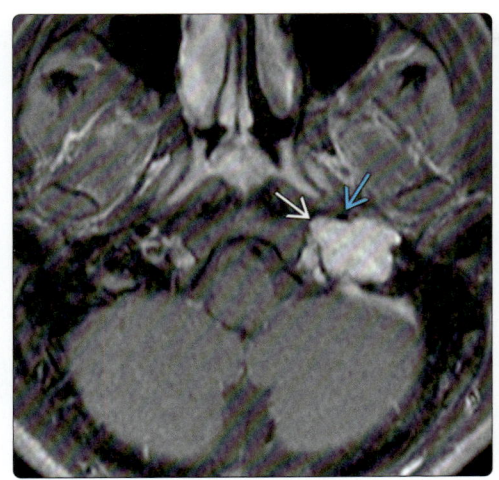

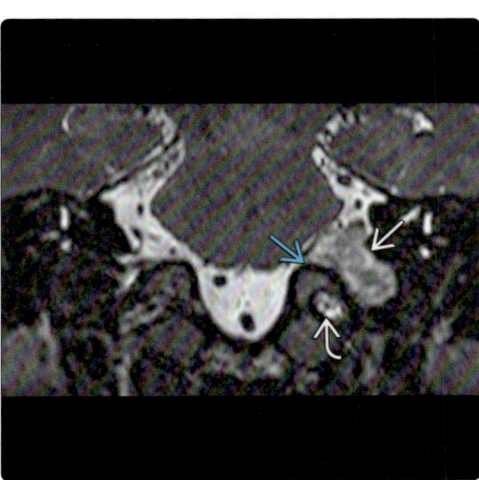

(Left) Axial T1 C+ MR shows typical avid homogeneous enhancement of the JF schwannoma ➡️. Note the anterior location of the IAC ➡️. The adjacent venous structures are compressed, but patent. Occlusion is rarely present. (Right) Coronal SPACE MR shows a heterogeneous, lobulated mass arising from the JF ➡️. Note the typical superomedial vector of spread toward the brainstem. The jugular tubercle appears intact ➡️. The normal hypoglossal canal ➡️ is present beneath the jugular tubercle, "bird's beak."

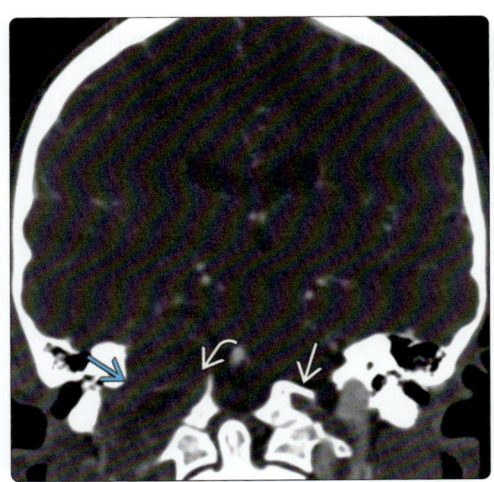

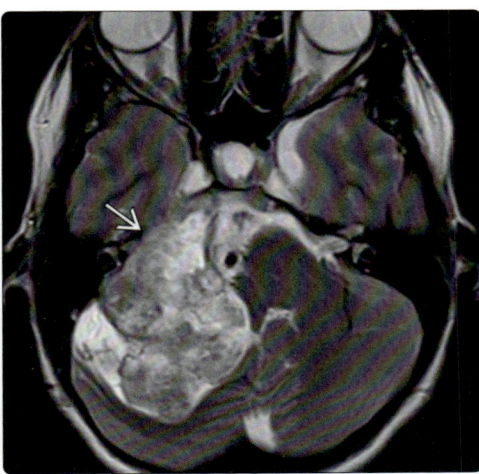

(Left) Coronal CTA in a 20-year-old patient with headaches shows a large right JF mass ➡️ with smooth erosion of the JF bony margins. Note the right lateral jugular tubercle is completely eroded ➡️. A normal left jugular tubercle ➡️ is present. (Right) Axial T2 MR in the same patient shows a large, heterogeneous, hyperintense mass ➡️ with a typical lack of high-velocity flow voids, which helps differentiate this complex schwannoma from the more common jugular paraganglioma.

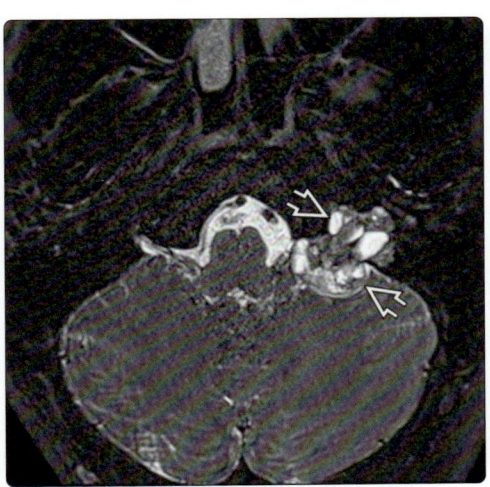

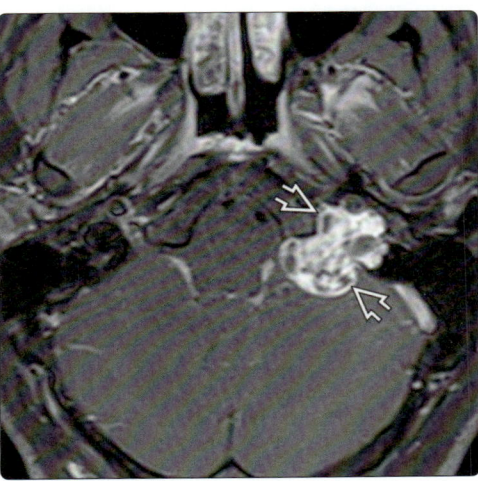

(Left) Axial T2 SPACE MR in a 40-year-old patient with sensorineural hearing loss shows a left JF schwannoma ➡️ with heterogeneous signal related to blood products and cystic changes. Hemorrhage within schwannomas is rare. The glossopharyngeal nerve (CNIX) is the most common nerve of origin in JF schwannomas. (Right) Axial T1 C+ MR in the same patient shows heterogeneous enhancement ➡️ related to intramural cysts and blood products. Schwannomas are typically T2 hyperintense and enhance homogeneously.

KEY FACTS

TERMINOLOGY

- Benign neoplasm arising from arachnoid cap cells found along cranial nerves (CNs) within jugular foramen (JF)

IMAGING

- Bone CT: **Permeative-sclerotic** JF margins
- T1WI C+ MR: Enhancing JF mass spreading along dural surfaces
  - Enhancing **dural tails** may be seen
  - No high-velocity flow voids
- **Centrifugal** vector of spread: Extends in all directions from JF along dural surfaces and through surrounding bones
  - May protrude into basal cisterns or nasopharyngeal carotid space

TOP DIFFERENTIAL DIAGNOSES

- Jugular paraganglioma
- JF schwannoma
- JF metastasis

- JF pseudolesion
- Dehiscent jugular bulb

PATHOLOGY

- Proliferation of arachnoid meningothelial cap cells along CNIX-XI in JF

CLINICAL ISSUES

- CNIX-XI neuropathy most common presentation
- Risk factors
  - Prior nasopharynx, skull base, or brain radiation; neurofibromatosis type 2; female sex hormones
- Meningioma is 3rd most common JF mass
  - Paraganglioma > > schwannoma > meningioma
- Treatment: Complete surgical removal is goal
  - Surgical cure often results in multiple lower cranial neuropathies
  - Radiotherapy for older adult patients, poor surgical risk or subtotal resection

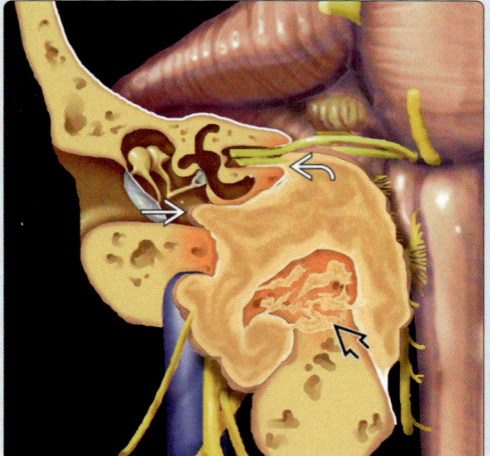
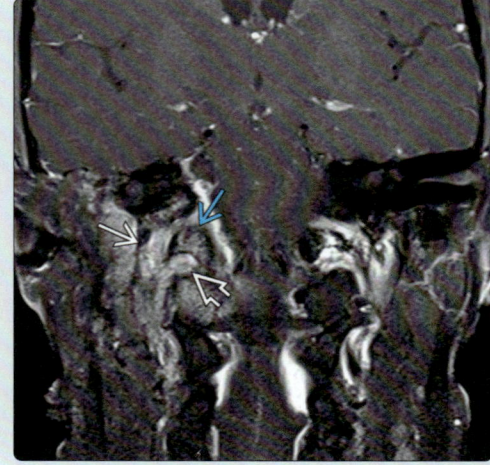

(Left) *Coronal graphic shows a large jugular foramen (JF) meningioma invading the middle ear ➡, skull base marrow ⮕ of the jugular tubercle, and internal auditory canal ➡. Note the cranial nerves (CNs) of the JF (CNIX-XI) are engulfed.* (Right) *Coronal T1WI C+ FS MR shows a large JF meningioma ➡ with extension to the hypoglossal canal ⮕ with bony involvement of the jugular tubercle ➡. JF meningiomas often extend along dural surfaces and through the surrounding bones.*

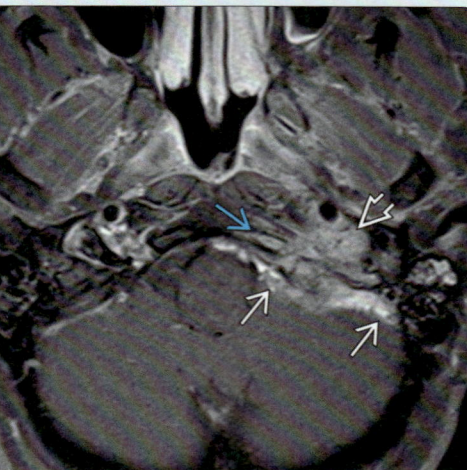
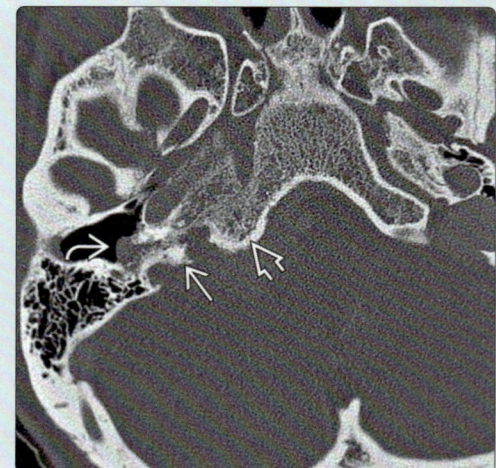

(Left) *Axial T1WI C+ FS MR shows a JF meningioma ⮕ as an enhancing mass with dural tails ➡ and skull base infiltration ➡. The lack of flow voids and dural tails helps differentiate this from the more common jugular paraganglioma.* (Right) *Axial bone CT shows the characteristic permeative sclerotic changes along the JF ➡ and lateral clivus ⮕ of this JF meningioma. The meningioma extends into the middle ear ⮕ and may present clinically as a vascular or white retrotympanic mass on otoscopy.*

Jugular Foramen Meningioma

TERMINOLOGY

Definitions

- Benign neoplasm arising from arachnoid cap cells found along cranial nerves (CNs) within jugular foramen (JF)

IMAGING

General Features

- Best diagnostic clue
  - **Permeative-sclerotic** involvement of bone around JF on CT
  - Enhancing JF mass spreading **centrifugally** along dural surfaces on enhanced MR
- Location
  - Centered within JF
  - Vector of spread: Centrifugal pattern (away from center)
    - Extends in all directions from JF along dural surfaces and through surrounding bones
      - □ Dural-based spread into basal cisterns most common
    - May extend into nasopharyngeal carotid space below
- Morphology
  - Poorly circumscribed mass

CT Findings

- NECT
  - Hyperdense JF mass
- Bone CT
  - **Permeative-sclerotic** JF margins
  - ± hyperostosis of adjacent cortex

MR Findings

- T1WI
  - Hypo- to isointense JF mass compared to brain parenchyma
  - **No** high-velocity flow voids
- T2WI
  - Relative T2 hypointensity suggests dense histology
- T1WI C+
  - Dense, uniform contrast enhancement
  - Enhancing **dural tails** may be visible along adjacent dural surfaces of basal cisterns
- MRV
  - May occlude dural sinuses and jugular bulb
    - Patency of adjacent dural sinuses should be documented prior to surgery

Angiographic Findings

- Supply primarily from dural branches of external carotid artery and vertebral artery
- Angiography provides vascular roadmap for surgeon
  - Evaluates collateral arterial and venous circulation
  - Embolization used for preoperative hemostasis

DIFFERENTIAL DIAGNOSIS

Jugular Paraganglioma

- **Permeative-destructive** JF bony margins on CT
- High-velocity flow voids ("pepper") characteristic on MR
- Vector of spread: Superolateral into middle ear

Jugular Foramen Schwannoma

- **Smooth** enlargement of JF on CT
- Tubular JF mass on MR ± intramural cysts when large
- Vector of spread: Superomedial along CNIX-XI

Jugular Foramen Metastasis

- **Destructive** bone margins of JF on CT
- Heterogeneously enhancing invasive JF mass on MR

Jugular Foramen Pseudolesion

- Asymmetric JF MR signal suggests lesion
- JF bony margins intact on CT
- Complex JF signal does not persist on all MR sequences

Dehiscent Jugular Bulb

- Superolateral extension of jugular bulb into middle ear
- Sigmoid plate focally dehiscent on CT

PATHOLOGY

General Features

- Etiology
  - Meningioma arises from proliferation of arachnoidal cap cells of meninges
- Genetics
  - Sporadic: Isolated defect on chromosome 22
  - Inherited: Associated with neurofibromatosis type 2 (NF2) and systemic chromosome 22 abnormality
  - Non-NF2 mutations: *TRAF7, SMO, AKT1, PIK3CA, KLF4*

Staging, Grading, & Classification

- Typical meningioma (90%): WHO grade 1
- Atypical meningioma (7%): WHO grade 2
- Anaplastic (malignant) meningioma (3%): WHO grade 3

CLINICAL ISSUES

Presentation

- Most common signs/symptoms
  - CNIX-XI neuropathy

Demographics

- Age
  - Typically 40-60 years
- Sex
  - F > M = 2:1

DIAGNOSTIC CHECKLIST

Image Interpretation Pearls

- Large JF meningioma may mimic jugular paraganglioma

SELECTED REFERENCES

1. Vasireddi AK et al: The "outline sign": thin hyperenhancing perimeter as an MR imaging feature of meningioma. A useful tool in the temporal bone region for differentiating meningiomas from schwannomas and paragangliomas. AJNR Am J Neuroradiol. 46(2):349-54, 2025
2. Ota Y et al: Utility of dynamic susceptibility contrast MRI for differentiation between paragangliomas and meningiomas in the cerebellopontine angle and jugular foramen region. Clin Imaging. 96:49-55, 2023
3. Han JJ et al: Clinicoradiologic characteristics of temporal bone meningioma: multicenter retrospective analysis. Laryngoscope. 131(1):173-8, 2021
4. Hamilton BE et al: Imaging and clinical characteristics of temporal bone meningioma. AJNR Am J Neuroradiol. 27(10):2204-9, 2006

Skull Base Lesions

TERMINOLOGY

- Arachnoid granulation (AG): Defined as enlarged arachnoid villi projecting into major dural venous sinus (DVS) lumen
- When large (1-1.5 cm in diameter) or occupy significant portion of dural sinus lumen → giant AG
- Vermiform giant AG: Giant AG with worm-like appearance
- Aberrant AG (AbAG): Arachnoid pit
  - Defined as AG that penetrates dura but fails to reach DVS, typically in sphenoid or temporal bone

IMAGING

- Intrasinus AG: Well-circumscribed, discrete filling defect in venous sinus ± inner calvarial table erosion
  - CECT: Nonenhancing; CSF density
  - MR: T2 like CSF, often ↑ FLAIR, SWI isointense to brain
- AbAG: Multiple focal outpouchings in inner table
  - Sphenoid bone location: Greater wing
  - Temporal bone location: Posterior wall or tegmen

TOP DIFFERENTIAL DIAGNOSES

- Brain herniations into DVS or calvarium
- DVS thrombosis, dural arteriovenous fistula

PATHOLOGY

- Normal variant enlarged arachnoid villi
- Brain tissue may herniate into DVS; usually in giant AG

CLINICAL ISSUES

- AG: Asymptomatic; rarely cause or consequence of BIH
- AbAG: Mostly asymptomatic; may be seen in BIH
  - If large with rupture, **CSF leak** ± meningitis possible
  - Large AG may have associated **cephalocele** (± seizure)
  - **Meningitis** may complicate CSF leak

DIAGNOSTIC CHECKLIST

- Sphenoid bone: CSF leak into sphenoid sinus → rhinorrhea
- Temporal bone: CSF leak into middle ear-mastoid → otorrhea

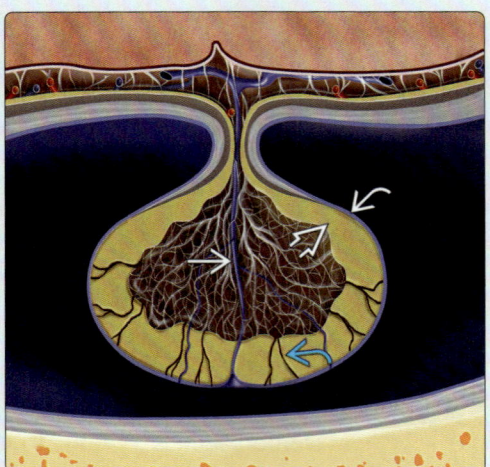
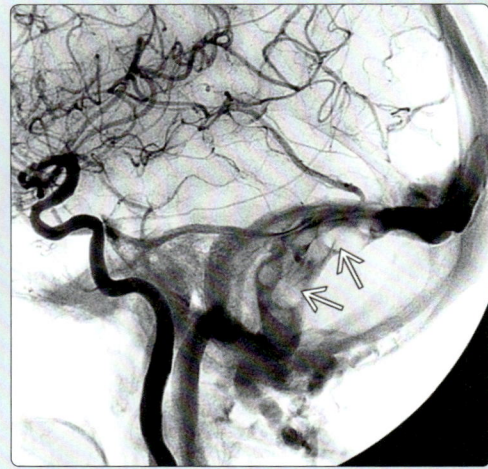

(Left) Graphic shows a large arachnoid granulation (AG) projecting into dural venous sinus (DVS). CSF core extends into the AG & is separated by arachnoid cap cells ⇒ from the venous sinus endothelium ⇒. Large AGs often contain prominent venous channels ⇒ & septations. Channels ⇒ in the arachnoid cap drain CSF into the DVS. (Right) Lateral internal carotid angiogram shows an incidental giant multilobulated AG ⇒ in the right sigmoid sinus. No intrasinus pressure gradient was present across the lesion.

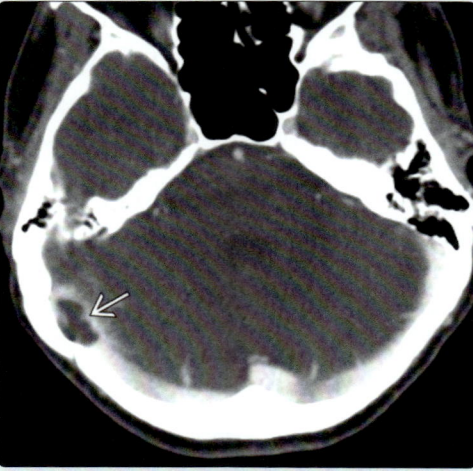
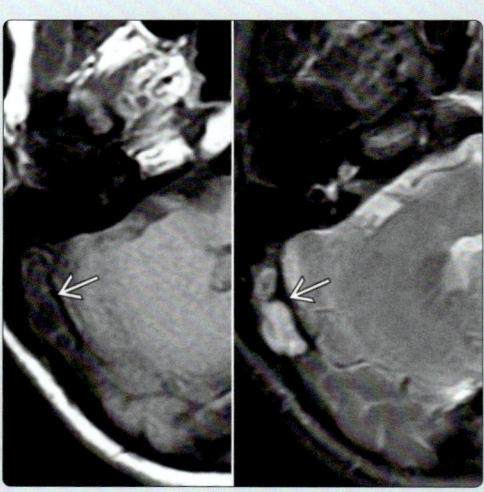

(Left) Axial CECT through the posterior fossa in the same patient shows a lobulated filling defect ⇒ at the junction of transverse & sigmoid sinus. The central low density of this AG is caused by the core of CSF. (Right) Axial T1 C+ & T2 FS MR images through the posterior fossa in the same patient show the vermiform giant AG ⇒ to have some internal septations, no significant enhancement, & central hyperintensity similar to CSF. Despite the conspicuous imaging appearance, this was deemed an incidental finding.

Dural Sinus and Aberrant Arachnoid Granulations

TERMINOLOGY

Abbreviations
- Arachnoid granulation (AG)
- Aberrant AG (AbAG)

Synonyms
- Pacchionian depressions, granulations, or bodies
- When large (1-1.5 cm in diameter) or occupy a significant portion of the dural sinus lumen → giant AG
- When in sphenoid bone and temporal bone → AbAG (arachnoid pit)

Definitions
- Arachnoid villi: Term used to describe smaller AG
- **AG**: Enlarged arachnoid villi projecting from subarachnoid space (SAS) into major dural venous sinus (DVS) lumen
- **AbAG**: AG that penetrates dura but fails to reach DVS, typically in sphenoid or temporal bone
  - Rarely other bones, such as parietal, occipital bone
  - a.k.a. **arachnoid pits** or osteodural defects
- **Vermiform giant AG**: Giant AG with worm-like appearance
  - Can mimic other pathology like DVS thrombosis, DVS cavernomas or brain tumors

IMAGING

General Features
- Best diagnostic clue
  - Intrasinus AG: Discrete filling defect in DVS ± inner calvarial table erosion
    - CECT: Nonenhancing; similar density to CSF
    - MR: T1/T2 intensity like CSF; often ↑ FLAIR
      - Signal intensity not following CSF on at least 1 sequence in 80%, usually FLAIR
    - Brain tissue may herniate into DVS, usually as part of giant AG
  - AbAG: Multiple focal outpouches in inner table of bone
    - Bone CT: Multiple smooth arachnoid pits in bone
    - MR: T1 and T2 intensity follows CSF
- Location
  - Most common location: Transverse sinus
  - Other locations: Sigmoid, sagittal, or straight sinus
  - AbAG most common location
    - Sphenoid bone, often greater wing, or lateral sphenoid sinus wall
    - Temporal bone: Posterior wall or tegmen tympani
- Size
  - 5-15 mm
  - If > 10-15 mm, called giant AG
- Morphology
  - AG project from SAS into major DVS lumen
  - CSF core from SAS extends into AG and is separated from DVS endothelium by arachnoid cap cells
  - Giant AGs often contain prominent venous channels and septations in CSF core
  - Channels in arachnoid cap **drain CSF** into DVS

CT Findings
- NECT
  - Intrasinus AG isodense with CSF
  - CSF pulsations may result in erosion or scalloping of inner table
  - AbAG: Focal osseous erosions in sphenoid bone
    - If large, may be multilocular; mimic cystic bone lesion
- CECT
  - Nonenhancing, ovoid focal filling defect within DVS
- CT venogram
  - Focal filling defect within DVS

MR Findings
- T1WI
  - AG iso- to slightly more intense than CSF
- T2WI
  - Hyperintense (like CSF)
  - Surrounded by normal flow void of major DVS
  - AbAG: High-signal outpouching into skull bone inner table
    - If large, may see arachnoid pouch bulging into sphenoid sinus lumen
      - Arachnoid strands: Low-signal lines within pouch
    - Larger lesions may have **CSF leak** into sphenoid sinus
      - Fluid levels seen in sphenoid sinus if leak present
    - Larger lesions may have associated **cephalocele**
- DWI
  - Facilitated diffusion: DWI hypointense and ADC bright similar to CSF
- T1WI C+
  - Intrasinus AG: Ovoid without enhancement surrounded by enhancing blood in dural sinus
    - Veins, septa may enhance
  - AbAG: Nonenhancing foci in sphenoid bone
- MRV
  - Intrasinus AG
    - Source images show focal signal loss in location of AG
    - MRV reformation shows focal defect in affected sinus
- SWI
  - Isointense to brain with internal venous flow voids

Imaging Recommendations
- Best imaging tool
  - Intrasinus AG: Enhanced MR with 3D T1 MR sequences like MPRAGE, and MRV
  - AbAG: Bone CT of skull base
    - Enhanced MR and high-resolution 3D T2 MR sequences like CISS/SPACE/FIESTA focused to sphenoid bone area

DIFFERENTIAL DIAGNOSIS

Brain Herniations With Surrounding CSF Into Dural Venous Sinus or Calvarium
- Filling defects in DVS mimicking AG
- Asymptomatic with normal signal intensity of brain and CSF
- Temporal lobe → transverse sinus; cerebellum → skull; cerebellum → sigmoid sinus

Sternberg (Lateral Craniopharyngeal) Canal
- Membranous space in lateral sphenoid sinus wall
- Controversial, extremely rare cause of lateral sphenoid sinus spontaneous CSF leak/cephalocele
- Should be medial to foramen rotundum (CNV2) in sphenoid sinus wall

- Arachnoid pits usually lateral to foramen rotundum, much more common with CSF leak/cephalocele

Transverse-Sigmoid Sinus Pseudolesion

- Asymmetric complex flow phenomenon in DVS

Dural Sinus Thrombosis

- NECT: Hyperdense if acute, later iso- to hypodense when subacute to chronic
- CECT: Nonenhancing clot in venous sinus lumen
- MR: Iso- to hyperintense on T1, or lack of flow void on T2
  - SWI: Dark clot (vs. isointense to brain AG)
  - T1 C+: Nonenhancing clot in venous sinus lumen
  - Postcontrast MRV best to show nonenhancing clot as filling defect
  - Phase contrast MRV (without gadolinium) also shows clot as filling defect
  - Time-of-flight MRV may miss clot if it is hyperintense, mimicking normal flow signal

Dural Arteriovenous Fistula

- MR: Recanalized, irregular transverse-sigmoid sinuses
  - MRA: Enlarged, feeding external carotid artery branches; early venous drainage

PATHOLOGY

General Features

- Etiology
  - Intrasinus AG: Normal variant enlarged arachnoid villi
    - Penetrates dura overlying venous sinus
    - Arachnoid cap cells in margin of AG responsible for CSF resorption
    - Giant AGs can regress after therapeutic CSF removal in **benign intracranial hypertension (BIH)**
      - □ Giant AG could be **consequence** of intracranial hypertension, buffering CSF compartment
  - AbAG: AG that penetrates dura but fails to reach venous sinus in sphenoid or temporal bone
    - CSF pulsations enlarge AbAG → arachnoid pouch bulging
    - Bulging arachnoid pouch penetrates subjacent structures (dura, then underlying bone)
    - If pouch stretches and ruptures, CSF enters air cells
      - □ Sphenoid bone-sphenoid sinus: CSF leak → sphenoid sinus fluid → rhinorrhea
      - □ Temporal bone-air cells: CSF leak → middle ear-mastoid fluid → otorrhea
      - □ Cephalocele possible in larger AbAG

Microscopic Features

- Enlarged arachnoid villi
- Central core of loose connective tissue with CSF
- Peripheral zone of dense connective tissue
- Projects through dura of venous sinus wall

CLINICAL ISSUES

Presentation

- Most common signs/symptoms
  - Intrasinus AG: Asymptomatic with rare exception

- If suspect giant AG in venous sinus **causing BIH** (venous hypertension) with headache, conventional angiography with pressure measurements needed
- In most cases, no pressure gradient across giant AG in DVS found
  - AbAG: Mostly asymptomatic
    - If CSF pulsations enlarge AbAG in sphenoid sinus or temporal bone wall, CSF leak ± meningitis possible
      - □ Sphenoid sinus wall rupture: Rhinorrhea
      - □ Temporal bone-air cell rupture: Otorrhea
    - If significant cephalocele occurs, seizure possible
- Other signs/symptoms
  - **BIH** in obese, middle-aged women with rhinorrhea
    - Look for AbAG (arachnoid pits) in sphenoid bone adjacent to sphenoid sinus

Demographics

- Age
  - ↑ in frequency with ↑ age; ≥ 40 years
- Epidemiology
  - Intrasinus AG: 25% CECT or T2 MR
  - AbAG: Sphenoid bone: < 2%; temporal bone: < 1%

Natural History & Prognosis

- Intrasinus AG: Remains asymptomatic
- AbAG: May remain small
  - If enlarge in response to CSF pulsations, may penetrate dura, bone, and air cells
    - CSF leak, cephalocele, or meningitis may result

Treatment

- Intrasinus AG: No treatment required
- AbAG: No treatment needed unless enlarged with resulting CSF leak
  - If CSF leak present into sphenoid sinus or temporal bone, surgical dural repair necessary
    - Surgical repair prevents meningitis possibility

DIAGNOSTIC CHECKLIST

Consider

- If **intrasinus giant AG** with history of headache, consider angiogram to look for intrasinus pressure gradient
- If **AbAG** presents in lateral wall **sphenoid bone**, look for fluid in sphenoid sinus as evidence for CSF leak
  - MR to evaluate for possible associated cephalocele
- If **AbAG** found in posterior wall of **temporal bone**, look for fluid in mastoid air cells as evidence for CSF leak

Image Interpretation Pearls

- Intrasinus AG
  - Confirm AG remains CSF density (on CECT or CT angiogram) and intensity (on T1 and T2 MR)
  - Make sure proximal venous sinus and DVS are normal from imaging perspective
- AbAG in lateral sphenoid sinus wall or posterior wall temporal bone
  - If large or multiple, look for evidence of CSF leak

SELECTED REFERENCES

1. Guevara Tirado OA et al: Neuroimaging of vermiform giant arachnoid granulations in children. Children (Basel). 11(7):763, 2024

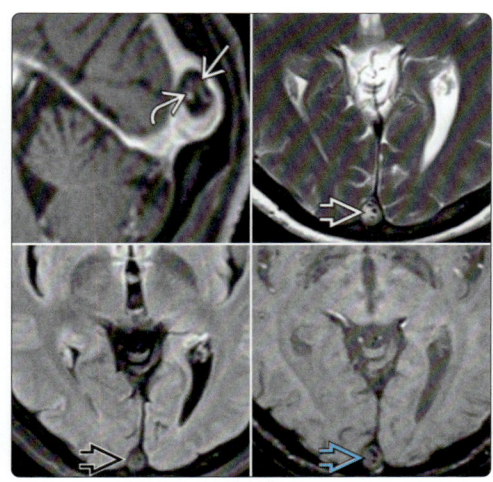

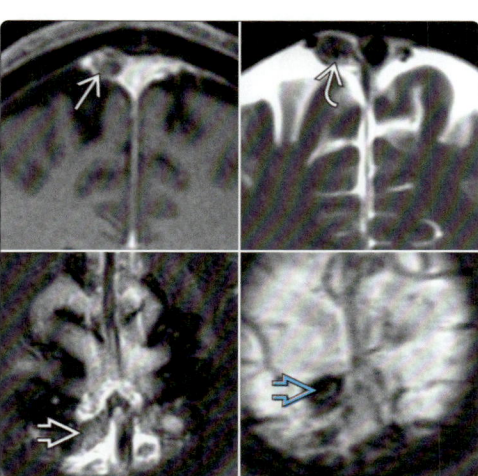

(Left) *Sagittal T1 C+ MPRAGE MR (top left) shows a nonenhancing giant AG* ➡ *in enhancing torcula. Note the enhancing internal veins* ➡ *in AG. Note bright CSF-like T2 (top right)* ➡*, iso- to bright FLAIR* ➡ *(bottom left), & isointense SWI* ➡ *(bottom right) signals with internal venous flow voids.* (Right) *Clot mimicking AG is shown. Coronal T1 C+ MPRAGE MR (top left) shows nonenhancing clot* ➡ *in superior sagittal sinus. Clot has dark T2* ➡ *(top right), mixed bright FLAIR* ➡ *(bottom left), & dark SWI (bottom right) signals* ➡*.*

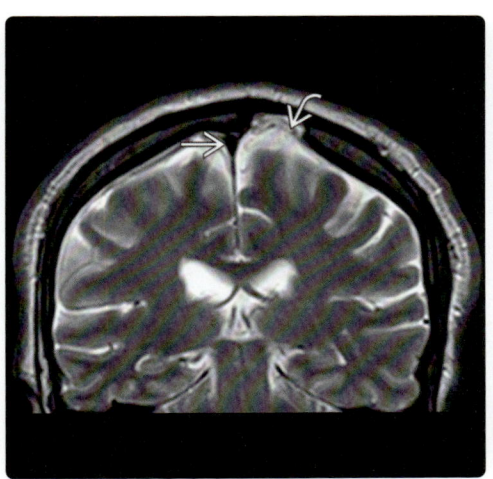

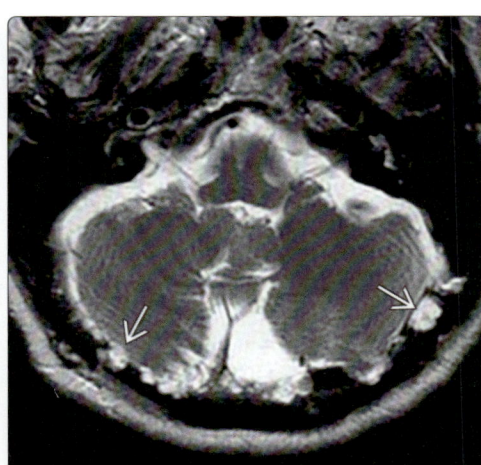

(Left) *Coronal T2 MR shows an aberrant AG (AbAG) seen as a high-signal outpouching smoothly scalloping the inner table of the left parietal calvarium* ➡*. The AbAG has penetrated the dura but failed to reach the adjacent superior sagittal sinus DVS* ➡*. Note the low-signal strands within the AbAG due to veins & septations.* (Right) *Axial T2 MR in another patient shows focal defects of posterior fossa occipital calvarial inner table showing predominantly CSF signal, typical of multiple AGs* ➡*, an incidental finding in this patient.*

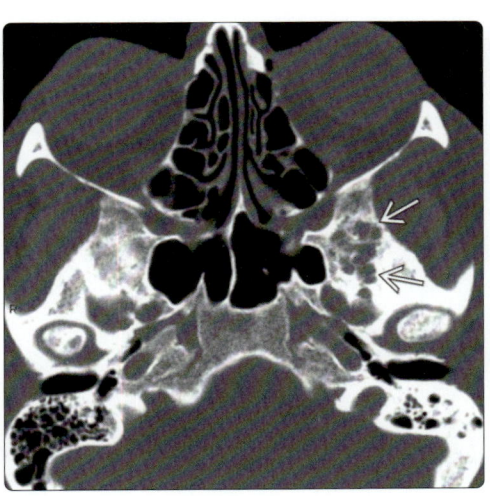

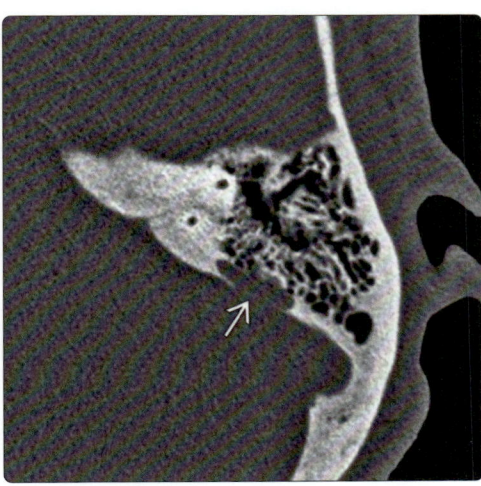

(Left) *Axial bone CT through the midsphenoid sinus shows multiple ovoid bony defects in the greater wing of sphenoid bone* ➡ *representing AbAGs (arachnoid pits). These AGs may enlarge from CSF pulsations.* (Right) *Axial left ear temporal bone CT reveals an example of an incidental AbAG* ➡ *in the posteromedial tegmen mastoideum. No CSF in the mastoid is present.*

TERMINOLOGY

- Dural sinus thrombosis (DST)

IMAGING

- MR with MRV is best single imaging exam for DST & parenchymal complications
- CT findings, acute
  - ↑ **density** thrombus in affected dural sinus on NECT
  - Conforms to shape of sinus; fusiform enlargement
  - CECT → enhancing dura surrounding less dense thrombus
- MR findings
  - ↓ **signal** (blooming) on **T2*** sequences in thrombus
  - Acute thrombus isointense on T1WI and hypointense on T2WI can mimic normal flow void
  - Parenchymal hemorrhage more common than arterial infarct
  - MRV shows lack of flow-related enhancement

TOP DIFFERENTIAL DIAGNOSES

- Arachnoid granulation
- Physiologic sinus flow asymmetry
- Dural sinus hypoplasia-aplasia
- Subdural hematoma

PATHOLOGY

- Wide variety of causes (> 100 identified)
  - Otomastoiditis most common
  - Pregnancy & oral contraceptives
  - Trauma (temporal bone fracture)
  - Metabolic (dehydration, thyrotoxicosis, cirrhosis)

CLINICAL ISSUES

- Headache most common symptom (70-90%)
- Young female patients most common (autoimmune, oral contraceptives)
- ≤ **50%** of DSTs progress to venous **infarction**

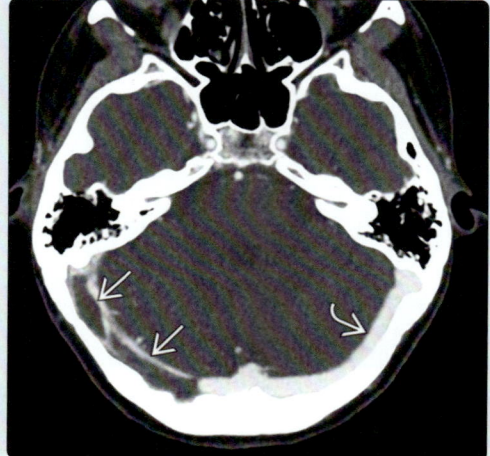
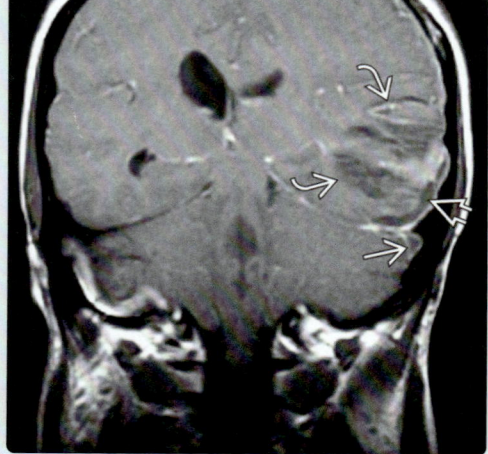

(Left) Axial venous-phase CT in a 21-year-old woman with coagulopathy shows a near-occlusive hypodense clot in the right transverse sinus (TS) ➡. The linear marginal enhancement represents a combination of dural enhancement and residual peripheral flow. Note the normal left TS ➡. (Right) Coronal T1 C+ MR demonstrates a clot as a hypointense filling defect in the TS ➡. Enlarged, clot-filled vein of Labbé can be seen tracking cephalad ➡ toward the patient's temporal lobe infarction ➡.

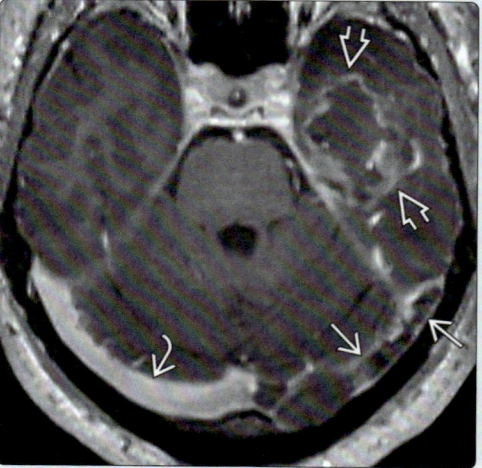
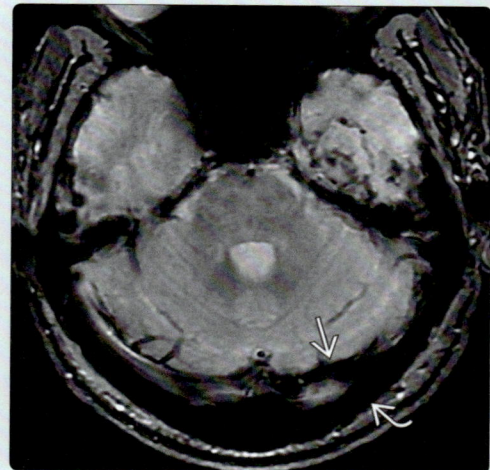

(Left) Axial T1 C+ MR in a 64-year-old man with headaches and confusion shows filling defect in the left TS ➡, consistent with thrombosis. Note the left temporal intraaxial mass ➡ and normal right TS ➡. Left temporal mass later confirmed glioma. (Right) Axial T2* GRE in the same patient shows increased hypointensity or "blooming" in the left TS ➡. This finding usually seen in acute/subacute thrombus can be difficult to separate from the hypointensity of the normal adjacent bone ➡.

TERMINOLOGY

Abbreviations

- Dural sinus thrombosis (DST)

Synonyms

- Cerebral venous sinus thrombosis, sinovenous thrombosis

Definitions

- In situ thrombosis of posterior fossa dural venous sinus due to variety of causes

IMAGING

General Features

- Best diagnostic clue
  - ↑ density (CT) or abnormal signal intensity (MR) in affected dural sinus of posterior fossa
- Location
  - Thrombophlebitis most commonly starts at transverse-sigmoid confluence
  - DST may involve ≥ 1 of following posterior fossa sinuses: Torcular Herophili, transverse sinus (TS) ± vein of Labbé, sigmoid sinus (SS), jugular bulb
- Size
  - In acute thrombosis, affected sinus may be enlarged
    - **Caveat**: TS size typically asymmetric from side to side in individual
- Morphology
  - Conforms to shape of dural sinus affected
    - Fusiform enlargement of venous structure acutely
    - Important for distinguishing DST from arachnoid granulation (focal filling defect)

CT Findings

- NECT
  - ↑ **density** thrombus in affected dural sinus
  - Dense triangle of thrombus, **δ** sign, when sinus seen in cross section
    - Phrase typically used to describe sagittal sinus thrombosis
    - Sagittal CT reconstruction of TS or coronal reconstruction of SS could show **δ** sign
  - Parenchymal venous infarction may be associated (~ 1/3 of cases)
    - Parenchymal hypodensity (edema ± infarction)
      - Temporal or occipital lobe location with TS thrombosis
      - Cerebellar hemisphere location with distal TS & SS thrombosis
      - Cortical/subcortical hemorrhages (may be petechial or parenchymal)
- CECT
  - Reverse or empty delta sign, enhancing dural leaves surrounding less dense thrombus (25% of cases)
  - **Filling defect** in TS ± SS; may extend into jugular bulb or vein
  - Shaggy, dilated, irregular cortical veins (collateral channels)
  - CECT alone unreliable for diagnosis of DST extent (high-density clot may appear like patent enhancing sinus)
- CTA

  - When performed per arterial protocol, enhancement phase too early to evaluate venous sinuses
  - Hyperdense sinus could potentially be confused with venous contrast
- CTV
  - 10- to 15-second delay beyond CTA image acquisition allowing venous timing for CT venogram
  - Filling defect in dural venous sinus with surrounding accentuated dural enhancement

MR Findings

- T1WI
  - Acute DST: Absent flow void with isointense clot (similar to gray matter)
  - **Subacute DST: Hyperintense clot** (methemoglobin)
  - Chronic DST: Isointense clot
- T2WI
  - Acute DST: Hypointense clot (deoxyhemoglobin)
  - **Subacute DST: Hyperintense clot**
  - Chronic DST: Hyperintense clot
  - Additional findings if parenchymal infarction present
    - Gyral swelling, sulcal effacement in temporal lobe
- T2* GRE
  - Profound hypointense signal or **blooming** on T2* sequences with acute or subacute thrombosis
    - May be difficult to discern against bone, air (in adjacent temporal bone)
  - Parenchymal hemorrhage in venous infarct ↓ signal in acute stage
- DWI
  - Acute & subacute clot may demonstrate restricted diffusion
  - Acute parenchymal venous infarct shows restricted diffusion
    - Parenchymal DWI abnormalities are more likely reversible compared to arterial ischemic insults
- T1WI C+
  - Filling defect may nearly completely fill dural sinuses
  - **Peripheral enhancement** may be reactive dura or residual flow around clot
  - Chronic DST may enhance intensely & should be correlated with MRV findings
    - Irregular, enhancing venous channels may be seen with incomplete recanalization; enhancement within recanalized clot may mimic normal sinus enhancement
  - Associated parenchymal venous infarction may show patchy enhancement
- MRV
  - Lack of flow-related signal in TS-SS, ± jugular bulb

Angiographic Findings

- Late venous-phase images critical
  - Complete lack of flow in affected dural sinuses
  - Central filling defect with surrounding contrast

Imaging Recommendations

- Best imaging tool
  - MR with MRV is best single imaging exam for DST
    - Almost all MR sequences show signal abnormality in dural sinuses

- – Complications (venous infarct, hemorrhage) easily identified
- – Susceptibility weighted imaging (SWI) may prove to be useful technique
  - ○ CT/CTV diagnoses DST but less sensitive for complications
- Protocol advice
  - ○ Coronal & sagittal CTV reconstructions ± MRV sequences very helpful for TS & SS thrombosis evaluation
  - ○ Contrast-enhanced MRV ↓ false-positive DST in small but patent dural sinus
  - ○ Use MRV with multiple encoding gradients to distinguish physiologic flow asymmetry from thrombus

DIFFERENTIAL DIAGNOSIS

Arachnoid Granulation

- Focal ovoid filling defect extending into TS-SS
- CSF density (CT) & intensity (MR)

Physiologic Sinus Flow Asymmetry

- Slow or asymmetric flow creates MR variable signal

Normal Dural Sinus

- Flowing blood in normal, asymmetric dural sinus
- Slightly more dense than brain on NECT (hematocrit dependent)

Dural Sinus Hypoplasia-Aplasia

- 33% of normal individuals have unilateral hypoplastic TS
- Congenitally small TS may show no flow or enhancement on MRV
- Sagittal T1 shows no TS structure along posterior tentorium

Subdural Hematoma

- Subdural blood adjacent to TS-SS mimics clot within dural sinus; false reverse (empty) delta sign

PATHOLOGY

General Features

- Etiology
  - ○ Most common cause: **Otomastoiditis ± subdural empyema → dural sinus thrombophlebitis**
    - – Wide variety of causes (> 100 identified)
      - □ Pregnancy, oral contraceptives
      - □ Trauma (temporal, occipital bone fracture adjacent to sinus); variable rate of DST depending on sinus involved
      - □ Metabolic (dehydration, thyrotoxicosis, cirrhosis)
      - □ Hematologic (coagulopathy)
- Associated abnormalities
  - ○ DST with arterial infarctions in patients with Behçet disease

CLINICAL ISSUES

Presentation

- Most common signs/symptoms
  - ○ Headache (70-90%)
  - ○ May be confused clinically with idiopathic intracranial hypertension (pseudotumor cerebri)

- – No diagnosis of **pseudotumor cerebri** should be made without venous evaluation
- Other signs/symptoms
  - ○ Nausea, vomiting, & papilledema
  - ○ Neurologic deficits & seizures
- Clinical profile
  - ○ Young woman with sudden-onset unrelenting headache &/or ear infection ± oral contraceptive use

Demographics

- Age
  - ○ May be seen at any age
  - ○ Young female most common (autoimmune, oral contraceptives)
- Sex
  - ○ F > M
- Epidemiology
  - ○ **1% of acute stokes** arise from **DST**

Natural History & Prognosis

- **≤ 50% of DSTs** progress to venous **infarction**
  - ○ Extension to straight sinus or vein of Labbé dramatically ↑ complication risk
    - – Temporal lobe infarction ± parenchymal hemorrhage

Treatment

- Anticoagulation (heparin) is mainstay of therapy
- Endovascular thrombolysis may be utilized for subacute or chronic thrombosis or if lack of improvement with anticoagulation
- Treat inciting cause of thrombosis

DIAGNOSTIC CHECKLIST

Image Interpretation Pearls

- Use contralateral cortical veins, dural sinuses, or arterial structures for density comparison on NECT
- CECT may be misleading, may mask clot

Reporting Tips

- Identify cause of DST if possible
- Identify which veins are secondarily involved
- Identify complications

SELECTED REFERENCES

1. Nguyen VN et al: Cerebral venous sinus thrombosis. Neurosurg Clin N Am. 35(3):343-53, 2024
2. Saposnik G et al: Diagnosis and management of cerebral venous thrombosis: a scientific statement from the American Heart Association. Stroke. 55(3):e77-90, 2024
3. Ghoneim A et al: Imaging of cerebral venous thrombosis. Clin Radiol. 75(4):254-64, 2020
4. Pai V et al: Pearls and pitfalls in the magnetic resonance diagnosis of dural sinus thrombosis: a comprehensive guide for the trainee radiologist. J Clin Imaging Sci. 10:77, 2020
5. van Dam LF et al: Current imaging modalities for diagnosing cerebral vein thrombosis - a critical review. Thromb Res. 189:132-9, 2020
6. Yeo LL et al: Deep cerebral venous thrombosis treatment : endovascular case using aspiration and review of the various treatment modalities. Clin Neuroradiol. 30(4):661-70, 2020
7. Leach JL et al: Partially recanalized chronic dural sinus thrombosis: findings on MR imaging, time-of-flight MR venography, and contrast-enhanced MR venography. AJNR Am J Neuroradiol. 28(4):782-9, 2007
8. Leach JL et al: Imaging of cerebral venous thrombosis: current techniques, spectrum of findings, and diagnostic pitfalls. Radiographics. 26 Suppl 1:S19-41; discussion S42-3, 2006

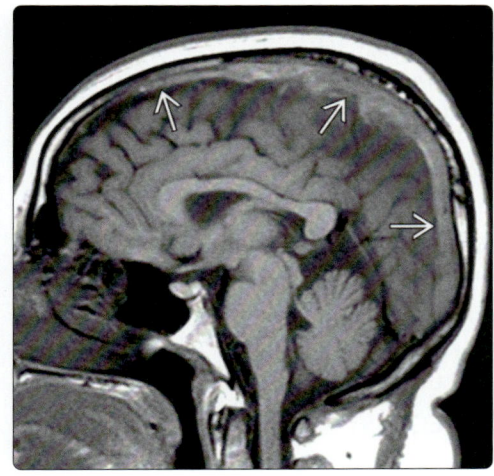

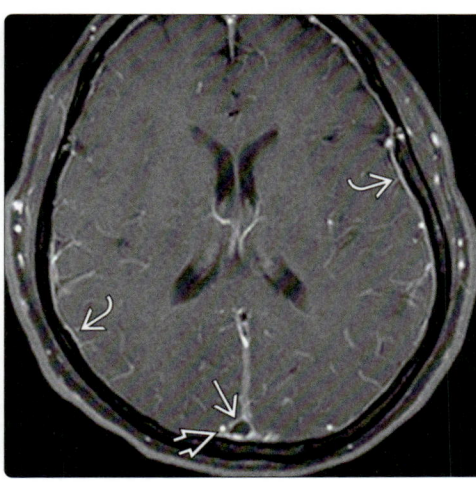

(Left) *Sagittal T1 MR demonstrates subacute clot as heterogeneous increased T1 signal in entirety of thrombosed superior sagittal sinus (SSS) ➡. Another MR clue may be loss of normal-phase artifact on the sagittal midline image.* (Right) *Postgadolinium T1 FS MR is notable for accentuated diffuse meningeal thickening & enhancement ➡, the empty delta sign of the thrombosed SSS ➡, & a prominent collateral vein ➡ adjacent to the SSS.*

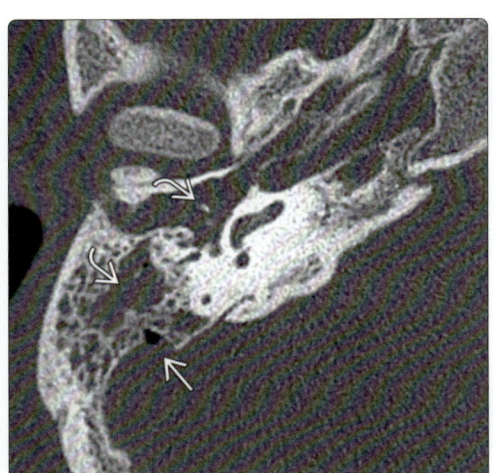

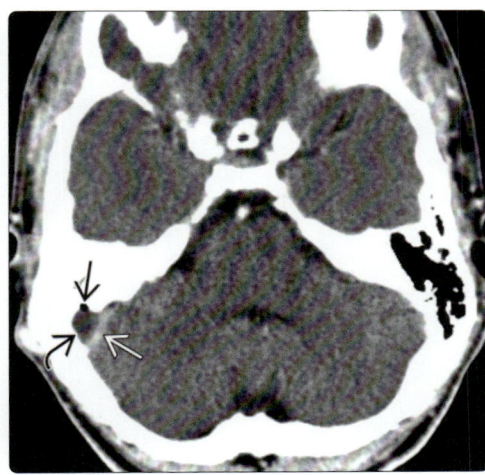

(Left) *Axial bone CT in a patient with acute coalescent otomastoiditis ➡ with opacification of the middle ear & mastoids shows thinning of the sigmoid plate & a small focus of air in the expected location of the sigmoid sinus ➡.* (Right) *Axial CECT in the same patient depicts only compressed & displaced sigmoid sinus ➡. Intracranial air ➡ is again noted adjacent to a hypodense epidural abscess ➡ lateral to the compressed sigmoid sinus.*

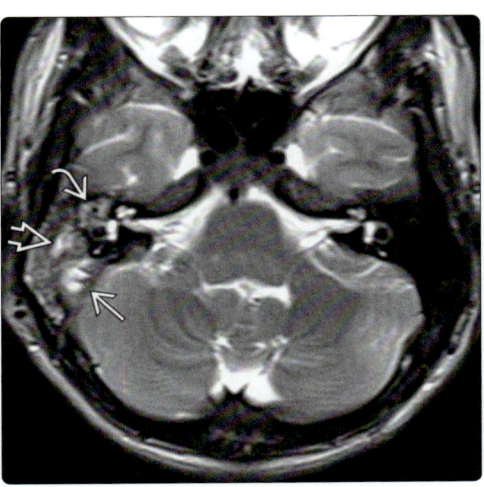

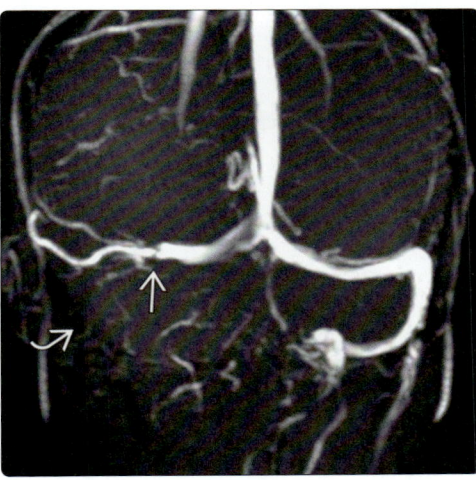

(Left) *Axial T2 MR in the same patient shows inflammatory material in the right mastoid ➡ & middle ear ➡ as well as a high-signal epidural abscess & compressed &/or thrombosed sigmoid sinus ➡. Note the normal appearance of the right temporal lobe & cerebellum.* (Right) *Anteroposterior MIP of phase-contrast MRV in the same patient demonstrates abrupt occlusion ➡ of the right TS and lack of flow-related signal in the right sigmoid sinus ➡ & jugular bulb/vein.*

Cavernous Sinus Thrombosis

TERMINOLOGY

- Cavernous sinus thrombosis/thrombophlebitis (CST)
- CST: Blood clot in cavernous sinus (CS) ± infection/thrombophlebitis

IMAGING

- Relevant anatomy
  - CS = trabeculated venous cavities
  - Receive blood from multiple valveless veins
  - Blood flows in any direction (depending on pressure gradient)
- CECT or MR
  - CT findings often subtle or negative in CST
  - Enlarged CS with convex margins
  - Filling defects in cavernous sinus
  - Enlarged superior ophthalmic vein ± clot, proptosis
  - Enlarged extraocular muscles
  - Intracavernous carotid artery: Rarely stenosis, thrombosis, or pseudoaneurysm formation

TOP DIFFERENTIAL DIAGNOSES

- Cavernous sinus neoplasm
  - Meningioma, lymphoma, metastasis
- Cavernous carotid aneurysm, fistula
- Infection/inflammation
  - Idiopathic inflammatory orbital pseudotumor, sarcoidosis, granulomatosis with polyangiitis (Wegener)

PATHOLOGY

- Often complication of sinusitis/midface infection
  - *Staphylococcus aureus* most common pathogen

CLINICAL ISSUES

- Headache most common early symptom
- Orbital pain, ophthalmoplegia, visual loss

DIAGNOSTIC CHECKLIST

- Clinical setting + high index of suspicion
- Negative CT → MR/MRV or CTA

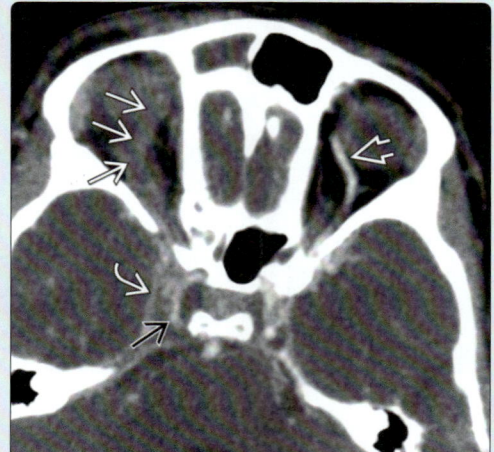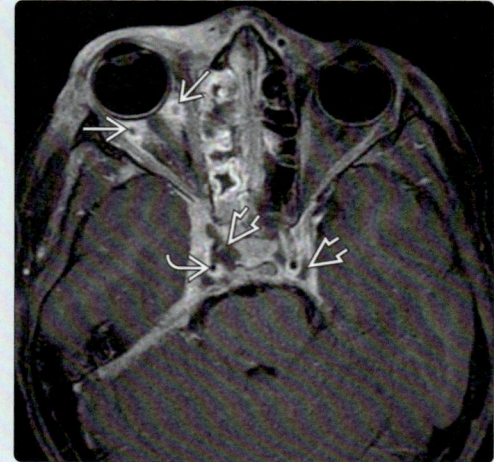

(Left) Axial CECT in a 10-year-old with right periorbital cellulitis and sinusitis shows nonenhancement of the enlarged, thrombosed right SOV ➡, normal enhancement of left SOV ➡, and enlargement/decreased enhancement in the right cavernous sinus ➡. Notice also narrowing/spasm of the right cavernous ICA ➡. (Right) Axial T1 C+ FS MR in the same patient shows nonenhancing thrombus in the orbital veins ➡, right greater than the left cavernous sinuses ➡, and asymmetric narrowing of the right ICA ➡.

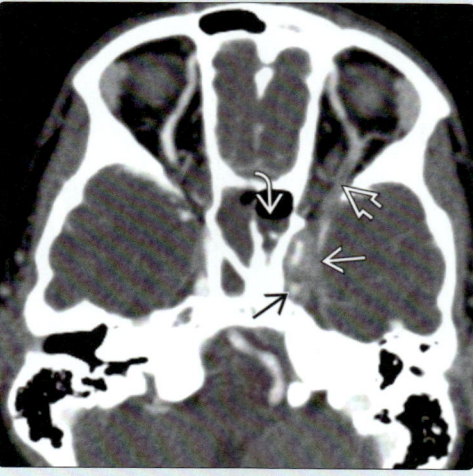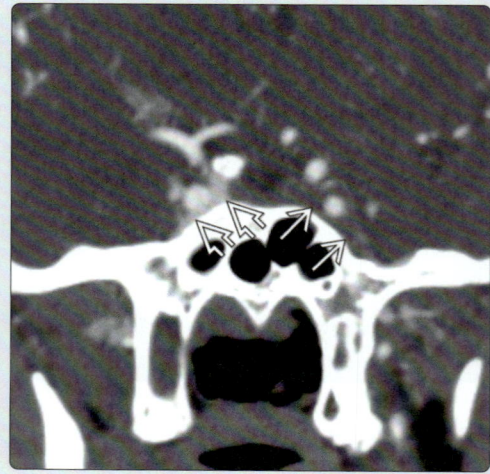

(Left) Axial CECT in a teenager with headache and fever shows enlargement and hypoenhancement of the left cavernous sinus ➡, an intraluminal filling defect in the posterior aspect of the left SOV ➡, and bilateral sphenoid sinus disease with an air-fluid level on the left ➡. Notice also narrowing of the cavernous segment of the left ICA ➡. (Right) Coronal CECT in a patient with periorbital swelling & ophthalmoplegia shows absent enhancement in the left cavernous sinus ➡ and normal enhancement in the right ➡.

TERMINOLOGY

Abbreviations
- Cavernous sinus thrombosis/thrombophlebitis (CST)

Definitions
- CST: Blood clot in cavernous sinus (CS)
  - ± infection/thrombophlebitis

IMAGING

General Features
- Best diagnostic clue
  - Appropriate clinical setting + high index of suspicion
- Location
  - Relevant anatomy
    - CS = trabeculated venous cavities, not single pool of blood, with multiple venous interconnections
    - Receive blood from multiple valveless veins
      □ Facial veins via superior ophthalmic vein (SOV) and inferior ophthalmic vein (IOV)
      □ Sphenoid, deep middle cerebral veins
    - CSs drain into
      □ Inferior petrosal sinuses → internal jugular veins (IJVs)
      □ Superior petrosal sinuses → sigmoid sinuses
    - Blood flow is in variable direction, depending on pressure gradient

Imaging Recommendations
- Best imaging tool
  - CTA: 1- to 3-mm sections through orbits and CSs
  - MR + contrast, MRA/MRV

CT Findings
- NECT: Findings often subtle or negative
- CECT: Nonenhancing filling defects in involved CS
  - CS margins convex laterally, not flat/concave
  - Orbits: SOVs ↑ ± clot
    - Proptosis, enlarged extraocular muscles
    - Diffuse orbital edema
  - Intracavernous carotid artery: ± narrowing; rarely stenosis, thrombosis, or pseudoaneurysm formation
- CTA/CTV: Filling defects in 1 or both CSs
  - ± narrowing; rarely stenosis, thrombosis, or pseudoaneurysm formation

MR Findings
- Enlarged CS with convex lateral margins
- Isointense to gray matter on T1WI, heterogeneous high signal intensity on T2WI
- Variable contrast enhancement, filling defects in CS
- May see hyperintense clot in CS or SOV on DWI

DIFFERENTIAL DIAGNOSIS

Cavernous Sinus Neoplasm
- Meningioma, schwannoma
- Metastasis, lymphoma, invasive carcinomas

Cavernous Carotid Aneurysm, Fistula
- Dilates SOV & CS, ↑ enhancement of extraocular muscles, patchy enhancement of intraorbital fat, flow voids

Infection/Inflammation
- Idiopathic inflammatory orbital pseudotumor, sarcoidosis, granulomatosis with polyangiitis (Wegener)

PATHOLOGY

General Features
- Etiology
  - Complication of sinusitis or other infection
    - Skin infection, orbital complication of sinusitis, odontogenic disease, or otomastoiditis
  - Other causes
    - Trauma; underlying malignancy
  - Most common infectious agents
    - *Staphylococcus aureus* ~ 70% of infections
    - *Streptococcus pneumoniae*, gram rods, anaerobes
    - Fungi (*Aspergillus*, *Rhizopus*) rare

CLINICAL ISSUES

Presentation
- Most common signs/symptoms
  - Headache and fever most common early symptoms
    - Often localized to regions innervated by V1 and V2
  - Orbital pain, facial and periorbital edema, chemosis
  - Proptosis, ophthalmoplegia (involvement of CNIII, IV, and VI), visual loss
- Other signs/symptoms
  - Hypoesthesia or hyperesthesia in V1 and V2 dermatomes
  - ↓ pupillary responses
  - Signs/symptoms in contralateral eye diagnostic of CST
  - Meningeal signs
  - Systemic signs indicative of sepsis are late findings

Natural History & Prognosis
- Without therapy → signs in contralateral eye in 24-48 hours
  - Spread via communicating veins to contralateral CS
- Can be fatal (death from sepsis or CNS involvement)
- Incidence/fatality significantly ↓ with early antibiotics
  - Even with antibiotics, mortality rate can be as high as 30%
- Complete recovery infrequent
  - Permanent visual impairment (15%)
  - Cranial nerve deficits (50%)

Treatment
- IV antibiotics
- Supportive care, hydration, steroids ± anticoagulation

DIAGNOSTIC CHECKLIST

Image Interpretation Pearls
- Maintain high clinical suspicion
- Negative CT → MR/MRV or CTA

SELECTED REFERENCES

1. Singh S et al: Pediatric head and neck emergencies. Neuroradiology. 66(11):2053-70, 2024
2. Winegar BA: Imaging of painful ophthalmologic disorders. Neurol Clin. 40(3):641-60, 2022
3. Nagaraj UD et al: Imaging of orbital infectious and inflammatory disease in children. Pediatr Radiol. 51(7):1149-61, 2021

Dural Arteriovenous Fistula

TERMINOLOGY

- Dural arteriovenous fistula (DAVF)
- Acquired direct shunt between dural artery and dural venous sinus or cortical vein

IMAGING

- Best imaging modality: DSA
- Most common site: Transverse sinus (TS)
- CECT findings in DAVF
  - Tortuous enhancing dural feeders with enlarged dural sinus
  - Enlarged cortical draining veins → aggressive DAVF
  - ± flow-related aneurysms
- MR findings in DAVF
  - Localized or generalized venous dilatation
  - Focal T2 hyperintensity in adjacent white matter (venous congestion)
- Dynamic contrast-enhanced MRA and arterial spin-labeling sequences improves detection of intracranial DAVF

TOP DIFFERENTIAL DIAGNOSES

- Hypoplastic TS-sigmoid sinus (TS-SS)
- Jugular bulb pseudolesion
- Dural sinus thrombosis
- Pial arteriovenous malformation

CLINICAL ISSUES

- Accounts for 35% of infratentorial vascular malformations
- TS-SS DAVF presents with pulsatile tinnitus
- Usually present in middle-aged, older adult patients
- Prognosis depends on location, venous drainage pattern

DIAGNOSTIC CHECKLIST

- If patient has objective pulsatile tinnitus and no other vascular lesion on cross-sectional imaging, angiography necessary to completely exclude DAVF
- Single pedicle or small DAVF may not be seen on MR or MRA
- Newer MRA sequences can help select patients for DSA

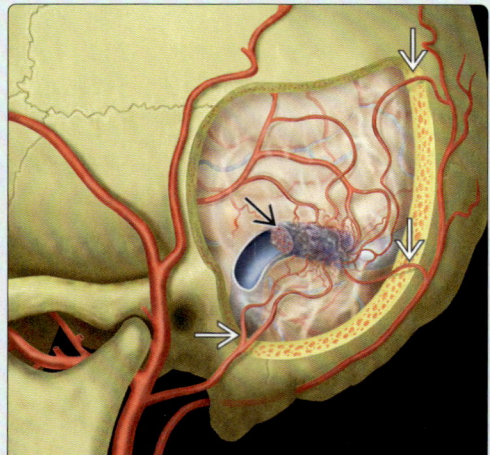 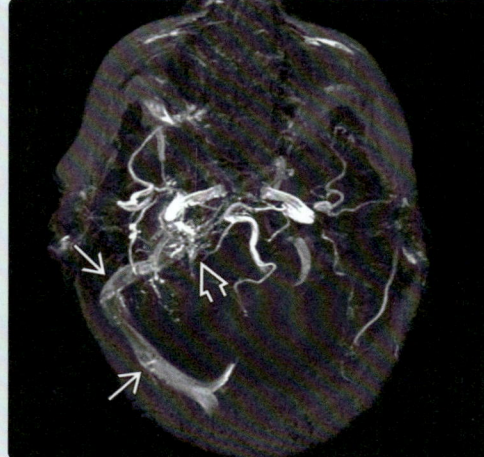

(Left) Graphic of typical dural arteriovenous fistula (DAVF) with a short segment of a thrombosed transverse sinus (TS) ➡ shows DAVF consisting of multiple dural vessels in the wall of thrombosed segment. Multiple dural & transosseous feeders arise from external ➡ (ECA) & internal carotid arteries (ICA). *(Right)* MRA shows extensive, prominent vascularity in the right skull base ➡ from a DAVF. Source images from MRA should be reviewed for correlation with MIP images. Dural sinuses ➡ remain patent in this case. Thrombosis is often seen.

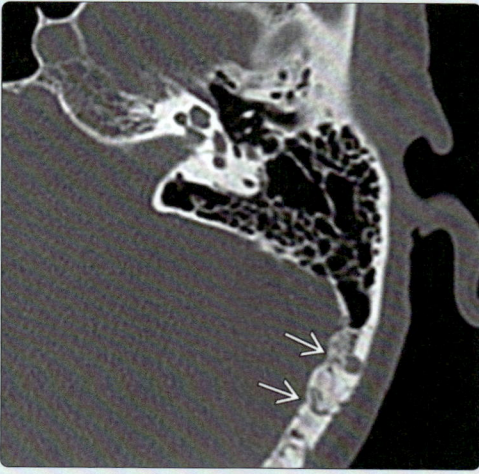 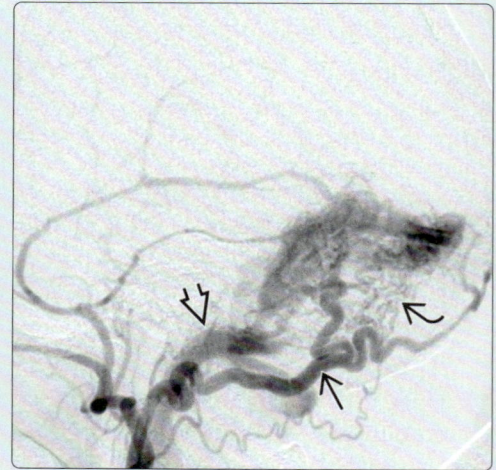

(Left) Axial bone CT of the left temporal bone demonstrates the left posterior squamous temporal bone is permeated with multiple prominent serpiginous canals ➡ secondary to DAVF transosseous collaterals. *(Right)* Midarterial lateral image from a left ECA DSA reveals an enlarged occipital artery ➡ terminating in a network of transosseous collaterals ➡ & shunting into the sigmoid sinus. Notice the sigmoid sinus ➡ is partially & irregularly recanalized post thrombosis.

Dural Arteriovenous Fistula

TERMINOLOGY

Abbreviations
- Dural arteriovenous fistula (DAVF)

Synonyms
- Dural arteriovenous (AV) shunt, dural fistula

Definitions
- Abnormal acquired direct shunt between dural artery and dural venous sinus or cortical vein
  - Heterogeneous group of lesions with common angioarchitecture (AV shunts within dura)
  - Distinct from true AV malformation because most DAVFs are acquired
    - Exception is vein of Galen malformation

IMAGING

General Features
- Best diagnostic clue
  - Network of tiny vessels in wall of thrombosed dural venous sinus
- Location
  - Skull base dural venous sinuses
    - Most common site → transverse sinus (TS)
    - 2nd most common site → cavernous sinus (CS)
- Size
  - Variable size, but actual shunt nidus is usually < 2 cm
- Morphology
  - Innumerable, serpiginous AV shunts in wall of dural sinus

CT Findings
- NECT
  - Usually normal in cases presenting without hemorrhage
  - Subarachnoid, subdural, or parenchymal hemorrhage may be seen in cases presenting acutely with hemorrhage
    - Parenchymal hemorrhage not in typical location for hypertensive bleed
- CECT
  - If small, CECT may be normal
  - Larger DAVFs show tortuous dural feeders with enlarged dural sinus ± flow-related aneurysms
  - Dilated vessels in proximity to parenchymal hemorrhage (if present); enlarged, tortuous cortical draining veins
- Bone CT
  - Transosseous collateral channels may be seen in skull base, squamous temporal bone

MR Findings
- T1WI
  - May be normal
  - Isointense thrombosed dural sinus ± flow voids
- T2WI
  - Isointense thrombosed sinus ± flow voids
  - Localized or generalized venous dilatation
  - Focal T2 hyperintensity in adjacent white matter (venous congestion)
- T2* GRE
  - Usually normal in uncomplicated DAVF
  - May show parenchymal hemorrhage in DAVF with cortical venous drainage
  - Thrombosed dural sinus will bloom
- DWI
  - Normal unless venous infarct or ischemia present
- T1WI C+
  - Chronically thrombosed sinus enhances intensely
  - Rare: Diffuse dural enhancement, parenchymal enhancement
- MRA
  - Time-resolved contrast-enhanced MRA useful for depiction of angioarchitecture and dynamics
  - TOF MRA positive in larger DAVF
  - Arterial spin-labeled imaging may be sensitive examination
- MRV
  - Occluded involved sinus, collateral flow
  - 3D phase-contrast MRA with low-velocity encoding can identify fistula, feeding arteries, flow reversal in draining veins

Angiographic Findings
- Conventional
  - Most common site = wall of TS or sigmoid sinus (SS) (35-40%)
    - Multiple arterial feeders are typical with dural/transosseous branches from external carotid artery (ECA), most commonly followed by internal carotid artery (ICA) and vertebral artery tentorial/dural branches
    - Arterial inflow into parallel venous channel common
    - Involved dural sinus often thrombosed
    - Flow reversal in dural sinus/cortical veins correlates with ↑ symptoms, hemorrhage risk
    - Tortuous engorged pial veins with venous congestion/hypertension (clinically aggressive)
    - High flow may result in high-flow vasculopathy with progressive stenoses, outlet occlusion, bizarre vascular appearance

Imaging Recommendations
- Best imaging tool
  - DSA with superselective catheterization of involved dural supply

DIFFERENTIAL DIAGNOSIS

Dural Sinus Hypoplasia-Aplasia
- Congenitally small TS-SS may have low flow on MRV, no enhancement on T1 C+ MR
- Sagittal T1WI shows no or very small sinus in normal anatomic location
- No signal abnormalities on T2, FLAIR, or GRE

Sigmoid Sinus-Jugular Bulb Pseudolesion
- Slow or asymmetric flow creates variable signal on MR sequences; use MRV to clarify

Thrombosed Dural Sinus
- Collateral/congested venous drainage can mimic DAVF

Pial Arteriovenous Malformation
- Congenital lesion with intraaxial nidus

PATHOLOGY

General Features

- Etiology
  - Adult DAVFs are usually **acquired**, not congenital
    - May be idiopathic
    - Can occur in response to **trauma**, **craniotomy**, **venous occlusion**, or **venous hypertension**
- Associated abnormalities
  - Cortical drainage may lead to edema, encephalopathy, hemorrhage

Staging, Grading, & Classification

- **Cognard classification** of intracranial DAVFs correlates venous drainage pattern with clinical course
  - Type I: Located in sinus wall; normal antegrade venous drainage; benign clinical course
  - Type IIA: Located in main dural sinus; reflux into sinus but not cortical veins
  - Type IIB: Reflux (retrograde drainage) into cortical veins; 10-20% hemorrhage
  - Type III: Direct cortical drainage; no venous ectasia; 40% hemorrhage
  - Type IV: Direct cortical drainage; venous ectasia; 65% hemorrhage
  - Type V: Spinal perimedullary venous drainage; progressive myelopathy

CLINICAL ISSUES

Presentation

- Most common signs/symptoms
  - 2 major modes of presentation
    - Hemorrhage (parenchymal, multicompartmental)
    - Venous hypertension/congestion (pulsatile tinnitus, dementia, seizures, encephalopathy)
  - Symptoms vary with site, type of shunt
    - TS-SS → pulsatile tinnitus
    - CS → pulsatile exophthalmos, chemosis, retroorbital pain
    - Brainstem DAVF → quadriparesis, lower cranial nerve palsies
- Clinical profile
  - Middle-aged patient with pulse-synchronous tinnitus

Demographics

- Age
  - DAVFs usually present in middle-aged or older adult patients
- Epidemiology
  - Rare, acquired lesions
  - Account for 6% of supratentorial and 35% of infratentorial vascular malformations
  - Account for 10-15% of all cerebrovascular malformations with AV shunting

Natural History & Prognosis

- Prognosis, clinical course depends on location, venous drainage pattern
  - 98% of DAVFs without retrograde venous drainage have benign course

- DAVFs draining into major dural sinus usually follow benign clinical course
  - DAVFs with retrograde cortical venous drainage have aggressive clinical course
- Overall risk of hemorrhage from DAVF = 2% per year (depends on location and hemodynamics)
- Spontaneous closure rare
- Acute deterioration has been reported after lumbar puncture

Treatment

- Observation in selected cases
- Treatment options if hemorrhage risk exists
  - Endovascular → embolization
  - Surgical resection → skeletonization of involved sinus
  - Stereotactic radiosurgery
- Recurrences common

DIAGNOSTIC CHECKLIST

Consider

- DAVFs are rare but treatable, so consider in patient with hemorrhage in atypical location for hypertensive bleed and no other cause
- If patient has objective pulsatile tinnitus and no other vascular lesion on cross-sectional imaging, DSA necessary to completely exclude DAVF

Image Interpretation Pearls

- Single pedicle or small DAVF may not be seen on MR or MRA
- Venous collateral flow in dural sinus thrombosis can become very prominent and mimic DAVF

Reporting Tips

- Evaluate both ICA/ECA and vertebral arteries when performing angiography in patient with spontaneous intracranial hemorrhage
- Identification of associated venous varix is important, as this finding signals ↑ risk of hemorrhage

SELECTED REFERENCES

1. Qedair J et al: Dural arteriovenous fistulas at the craniocervical junction: a systematic review and meta-analysis. Neurosurg Rev. 47(1):812, 2024
2. Alkhaibary A et al: Intracranial dural arteriovenous fistula: a comprehensive review of the history, management, and future prospective. Acta Neurol Belg. 123(2):359-66, 2023
3. Chen X et al: Overview of multimodal MRI of intracranial dural arteriovenous fistulas. J Interv Med. 5(4):173-9, 2022
4. Dissaux B et al: Assessment of 4D MR angiography at 3T compared with DSA for the follow-up of embolized brain dural arteriovenous fistula: a dual-center study. AJNR Am J Neuroradiol. 42(2):340-6, 2020
5. Grossberg JA et al: The use of contrast-enhanced, time-resolved magnetic resonance angiography in cerebrovascular pathology. Neurosurg Focus. 47(6):E3, 2019
6. Haller S et al: Arterial spin labeling perfusion of the brain: emerging clinical applications. Radiology. 281(2):337-56, 2016
7. Josephson CB et al: Computed tomography angiography or magnetic resonance angiography for detection of intracranial vascular malformations in patients with intracerebral haemorrhage. Cochrane Database Syst Rev. 9:CD009372, 2014
8. Kobayashi A et al: Prognosis and treatment of intracranial dural arteriovenous fistulae: a systematic review and meta-analysis. Int J Stroke. 9(6):670-7, 2014
9. Lin N et al: Non-galenic arteriovenous fistulas in adults: transarterial embolization and literature review. J Neurointerv Surg. 7(11):835-40, 2014

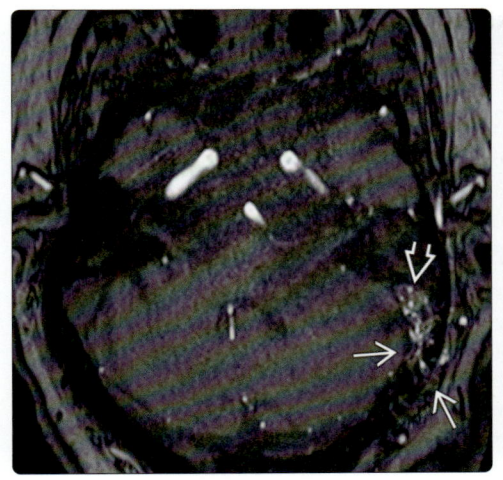

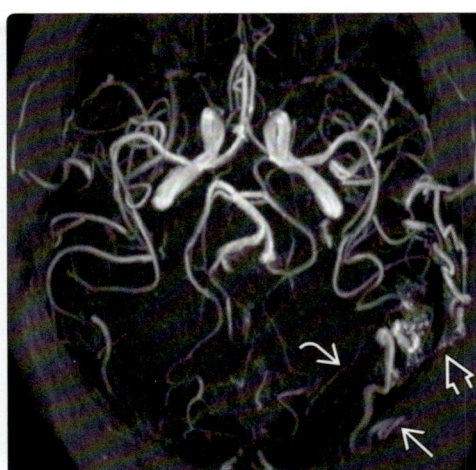

(Left) Axial MRA source image in a patient with left pulsatile tinnitus demonstrates linear & punctate areas of flow-related signal in the left occipital bone ➡ extending into a thrombosed left sigmoid sinus ➡. (Right) Axial MRA MIP in the same patient shows a prominent distal occipital artery ➡. Note the feeder from the superficial temporal artery ➡. The transverse sinus ➡ is not recanalized. Flow-related MRA artifacts can mimic partial flow/recanalization.

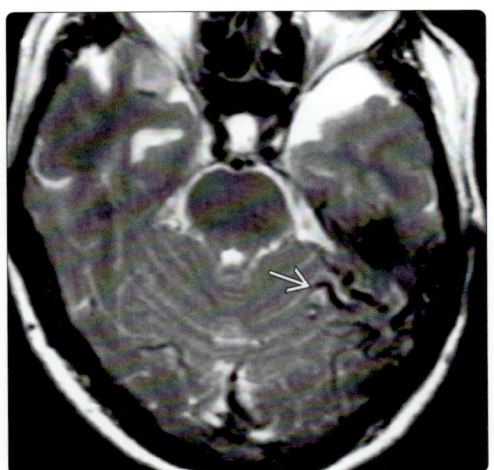

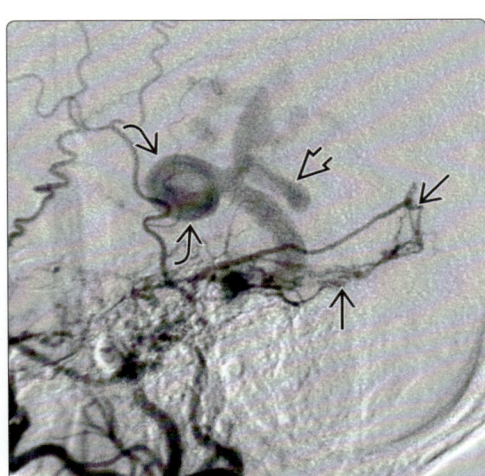

(Left) Axial T2WI MR in patient with DAVF shows enlargement of multiple prominent cerebellar veins ➡. Lesions with enlarged cortical veins have an increased incidence of intracranial hemorrhage. White matter edema from venous congestion may also be evident. (Right) Lateral ECA angiography in the same patient shows enlarged dural feeders ➡ to DAVF. Deep cortical venous drainage ➡ is well seen, & venous varix ➡ is displayed. Tentorial DAVFs may have particularly complex anatomy.

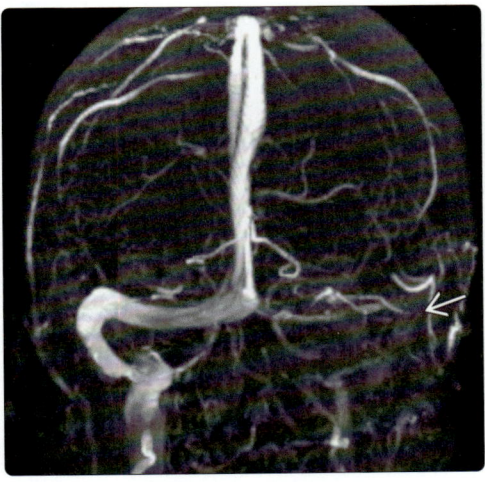

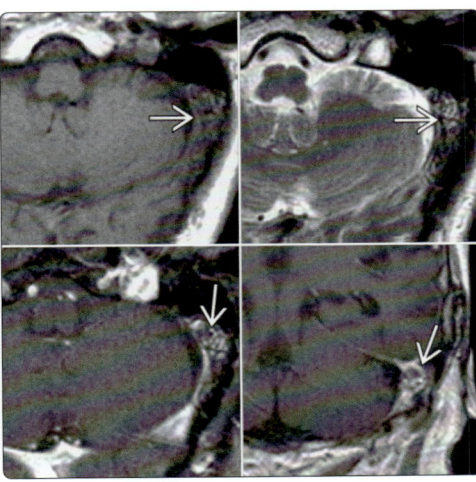

(Left) AP MRV reveals that the left TS and sigmoid sinus are smaller than the right with distal TS occlusion ➡. The distal TS-proximal sigmoid sinus confluence is the most common site for DAVFs of the posterior skull base. (Right) Composite MR shows an atypical DAVF with innumerable small flow voids ➡ in the thrombosed segment of TS-sigmoid sinus junction. MRA may show flow-related enhancement of vessels, but angiography is often necessary to confirm.

Skull Base Cephalocele

TERMINOLOGY

- Basal cephalocele = congenital extracranial herniation of meninges, CSF, ± brain tissue through mesodermal defect in sphenoid, ethmoid, or basiocciput

IMAGING

- Nasopharyngeal
  - Transethmoid: Defect in cribriform plate
  - Sphenoethmoid: Bony defect junction of cribriform plate and planum sphenoidale
  - Sphenonasopharyngeal = transsphenoid: Defect in body of sphenoid bone
    - Most common
  - Basioccipital-nasopharyngeal (transbasioccipital): Bony defect parallel & inferior to sphenooccipital synchondrosis
    - Area of median basal canal
- Sphenoorbital
- Sphenomaxillary

- Best imaging tool
  - MR best identifies meninges, CSF, brain, pituitary, & optic nerves/chiasm position
  - Bone CT defines osseous defects prior to surgery

TOP DIFFERENTIAL DIAGNOSES

- Nasal glioma
- Nasal dermal sinus
- Teratoma

CLINICAL ISSUES

- Most common signs/symptoms
  - May be clinically occult
  - Hypertelorism, nasal mass, nasal stuffiness, endocrine dysfunction
  - Recurrent meningitis
- Combined surgical procedure may involve neurosurgery, otolaryngology, &/or plastic surgery

(Left) *Sagittal T1 MR in a child with transphenoid cephalocele shows a large CSF-filled sac extending through the floor of the sella/midline sphenoid bone ➡. No identifiable pituitary tissue was present.* (Right) *Axial T1 MR in the same patient shows typical appearance of morning glory disc anomaly as hyperintense T1 fat within the distal optic nerve sheath ➡. This patient did not have associated moyamoya vasculopathy, as can sometimes be seen.*

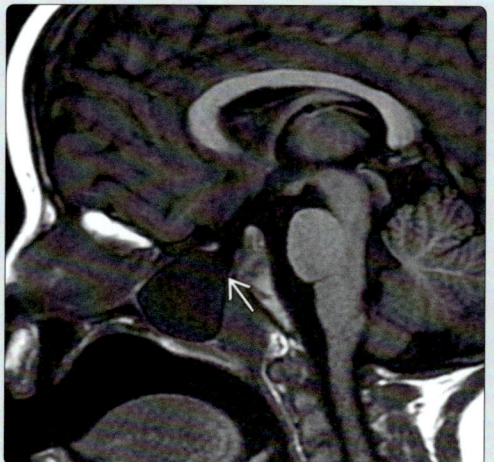
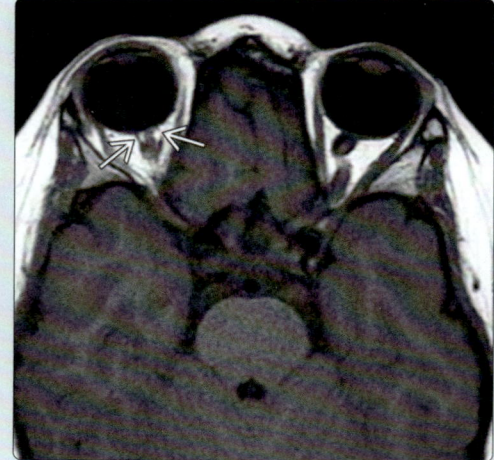

(Left) *Sagittal T1 MR in a 9-month-old demonstrates a large CSF-filled cephalocele ➡, extending via a defect in the midline sphenoid, anterior to the sphenooccipital synchondrosis ➡, and associated callosal agenesis ➡.* (Right) *Sagittal T1 MR in a child with nasal mass shows a transethmoid cephalocele ➡ containing a portion of the inferior left frontal lobe ➡.*

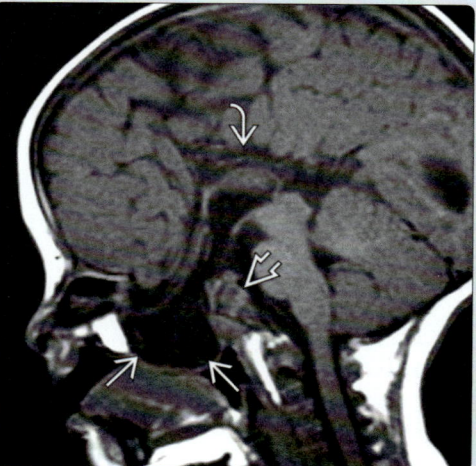
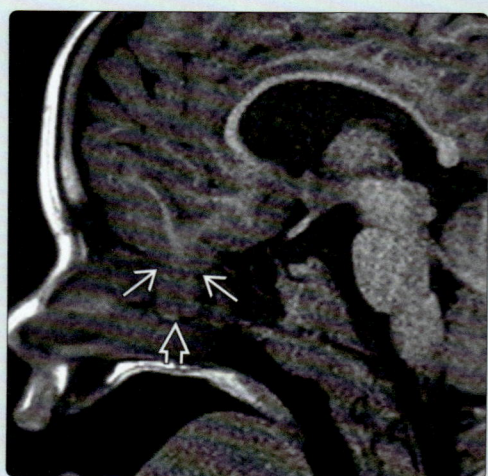

TERMINOLOGY

Synonyms

- Basal cephaloceles
- "Occult" cephaloceles

Definitions

- Basal cephalocele = congenital extracranial herniation of **meninges, CSF ± brain tissue** through mesodermal defect in **sphenoid, ethmoid,** or **basiocciput**
  - Nasopharyngeal
    - Transethmoid
    - Sphenoethmoid
    - Sphenonasopharyngeal = transsphenoid (large craniopharyngeal canal)
    - Basioccipital-nasopharyngeal (transbasioccipital)
  - Sphenoorbital
  - Sphenomaxillary

IMAGING

General Features

- Best diagnostic clue
  - Midline inferior herniation of CSF ± brain or pituitary gland into nasopharynx through defect in skull base
- Location
  - **Nasopharyngeal**
    - Transethmoid: Bone defect in cribriform plate
    - Sphenoethmoid: Bony defect at junction of cribriform plate & planum sphenoidale
    - Sphenonasopharyngeal = transsphenoid = **craniopharyngeal canal**
      □ Bony defect in midline body of sphenoid bone
    - Basioccipital-nasopharyngeal (transbasioccipital)
      □ Bony defect parallel & 1.0-1.5 cm inferior to sphenooccipital synchondrosis
      □ In area of persistent **median basal canal**
      □ May simulate patent sphenooccipital synchondrosis
      □ Communicates with prepontine cistern
  - **Sphenoorbital**
    - Posterior orbital cephaloceles communicate with **middle cranial fossa** through optic foramen, superior orbital fissure, or orbital wall defect
  - **Sphenomaxillary**
    - Extend through **superior orbital fissure** into posterior orbit ± extension through inferior orbital fissure & pterygopalatine fossa
- Size
  - Variable
- Morphology
  - Well circumscribed, round or ovoid

Imaging Recommendations

- Best imaging tool
  - MR best identifies meninges, CSF, brain, pituitary, & optic nerves/chiasm position
  - Bone CT complimentary to define osseous defects prior to surgery
- Protocol advice
  - Thin (3-mm) multiplanar T1 & T2 MR
  - CT with multiplanar reformations for surgical planning

CT Findings

- NECT
  - Variable attenuation mass protruding into nasopharynx (or orbit)
    - Most commonly CSF attenuation
- Bone CT
  - Depicts osseous defect in skull base

MR Findings

- Mass with variable signal intensity protruding into nasopharynx, oropharynx, or orbit
  - Depends on content of cephalocele: CSF, meninges, brain
  - Pituitary gland variable location within cephalocele
    - Frequently lines posterior wall of cephalocele
- No abnormal enhancement
  - Presence of enhancement may suggest infection/inflammation

DIFFERENTIAL DIAGNOSIS

Nasal Glioma

- Well-defined soft tissue mass
- No intracranial extension

Nasal Dermal Sinus

- Nasal dorsum skin pit ± cyst tip of nose to foramen cecum
- ± bifid crista galli

Teratoma

- Oropharyngeal location
- Mixed cystic/solid mass with soft tissue, fat, & calcium

PATHOLOGY

General Features

- Etiology
  - **Majority congenital**; rarely after trauma or surgery
    - Osseous defect secondary to faulty separation of neurectoderm from surface ectoderm during neural tube formation
      □ Prevents mesodermal tissue, which should form bone, from interposing between 2 germ layers
- Genetics
  - Sporadic
  - No well-defined genetic link
- Associated abnormalities
  - Callosal dysgenesis
  - Eye abnormalities: Optic pits or posterior coloboma
  - Midline facial clefts: Lip, nose, palate
  - Rare triad: Morning glory disc anomaly, moyamoya vasculopathy, & transsphenoidal cephalocele
  - Rare reports
    - Internal carotid artery (ICA) dysgenesis
    - Epignathus teratoma
    - Hypothalamic hamartoma
    - Tornwaldt cyst & enterogenous cyst reported with median canalis basilaris

Staging, Grading, & Classification

- Cephaloceles classified **by contents** of sac
  - Meningocele: Leptomeninges & CSF

- Meningoencephalocele (encephalocele): Leptomeninges, CSF, & brain
- Atretic cephalocele is forme fruste of cephaloceles, i.e., small, noncystic, flat nodules in scalp
  - Parietal are near vertex, occipital are cephalic to external occipital protuberance
- Cephaloceles classified **by site** of osseous defect
  - Calvarium
    - Occipitocervical, occipital, parietal, lateral, interfrontal, temporal
  - Skull base
    - Frontoethmoidal = sincipital
      □ Nasofrontal, nasoethmoidal, & nasoorbital
    - Basal cephaloceles
      □ Nasopharyngeal: Transethmoid, sphenoethmoid, sphenonasopharyngeal (transsphenoid or craniopharyngeal canal), basioccipital-nasopharyngeal (transbasioccipital)
      □ Sphenoorbital
      □ Sphenomaxillary
- Craniopharyngeal canal classification
  - Type 1: Small, incidental canal
  - Type 2: Medium-sized canals + ectopic pituitary tissue
  - Type 3: Large canals containing cephaloceles &/or tumors
    - 3A: Contain cephaloceles
    - 3B: Contain tumors
    - 3C: Contain cephaloceles & tumors

Gross Pathologic & Surgical Features

- Well-defined, meningeal-lined mass containing CSF ± brain tissue

Microscopic Features

- Meningoceles: Leptomeninges & CSF
- Meningoencephaloceles: Leptomeninges, CSF, & brain
- Atretic cephaloceles: Dura, fibrous tissue, & degenerated brain tissue

CLINICAL ISSUES

Presentation

- Most common signs/symptoms
  - May be clinically **occult**
  - Hypertelorism
  - Nasal mass & nasal stuffiness
  - Endocrine dysfunction
- Other signs/symptoms
  - **Recurrent meningitis**
    - Highest incidence in patients with basioccipital-nasopharyngeal cephalocele
  - Developmental delay primarily related to associated malformations

Demographics

- Age
  - Congenital lesion
    - May be recognized on prenatal US/MR or present after birth

Natural History & Prognosis

- Present at birth

- May not be diagnosed at birth due to occult location
- May increase in size rapidly if CSF-filled
- Prognosis depends in part on associated abnormalities

Treatment

- Combined surgical procedure may involve neurosurgery, otolaryngology, &/or plastic surgery
- Continued increase in success with endoscopic repair

DIAGNOSTIC CHECKLIST

Consider

- Look for cephalocele in patients with recurrent meningitis history
- High-resolution sagittal & coronal T1 & T2 images
  - Optimal evaluation of contents of mass and contiguity with intracranial space
- Bone CT with multiplanar reformations defines osseous defect prior to surgical repair

Reporting Tips

- Identify lesion contents and osseous defect prior to surgical repair
- Recognize associated intracranial and craniofacial abnormalities

SELECTED REFERENCES

1. Kameda-Smith MM et al: Pediatric congenital anterior skull base encephaloceles and surgical management: a comparative review of 22 patients treated with transnasally, transcranially, or combined approach with a review of the literature. Neurosurgery. 95(4):859-76, 2024
2. Wang W et al: Imaging of congenital anomalies and defects of the skull base and calvarium. Br J Radiol. 97(1157):902-12, 2024
3. Pavanello M et al: A rare triad of morning glory disc anomaly, moyamoya vasculopathy, and transsphenoidal cephalocele: pathophysiological considerations and surgical management. Neurol Sci. 42(12):5433-9, 2021
4. Thompson HM et al: Current management of congenital anterior cranial base encephaloceles. Int J Pediatr Otorhinolaryngol. 131:109868, 2020
5. Keshri AK et al: Transnasal endoscopic repair of pediatric meningoencephalocele. J Pediatr Neurosci. 11(1):42-5, 2016
6. Abele TA et al: Craniopharyngeal canal and its spectrum of pathology. AJNR Am J Neuroradiol. 35(4):772-7, 2014
7. Morabito R et al: Pharyngeal enterogenous cyst associated with canalis basilaris medianus in a newborn. Pediatr Radiol. 43(4):512-5, 2013
8. Lohman BD et al: Not the typical Tornwaldt's cyst this time? A nasopharyngeal cyst associated with canalis basilaris medianus. Br J Radiol. 84(1005):e169-71, 2011
9. Borges A: Imaging of the central skull base. Neuroimaging Clin N Am. 19(4):669-96, 2009
10. Castelnuovo P et al: Endoscopic endonasal management of encephaloceles in children: an eight-year experience. Int J Pediatr Otorhinolaryngol. 73(8):1132-6, 2009
11. Lesavoy MA et al: Nasopharyngeal encephalocele: report of transcranial and transpalatal repair with a 25-year follow-up. J Craniofac Surg. 20(6):2251-6, 2009
12. Schuknecht B et al: Nontraumatic skull base defects with spontaneous CSF rhinorrhea and arachnoid herniation: imaging findings and correlation with endoscopic sinus surgery in 27 patients. AJNR Am J Neuroradiol. 29(3):542-9, 2008
13. Ekinci G et al: Transsphenoidal (large craniopharyngeal) canal associated with a normally functioning pituitary gland and nasopharyngeal extension, hyperprolactinemia, and hypothalamic hamartoma. AJR Am J Roentgenol. 180(1):76-7, 2003
14. Koch BL et al: Congenital malformations causing skull base changes. Neuroimaging Clin N Am. 4(3):479-98, 1994
15. Naidich TP et al: Cephaloceles and related malformations. AJNR Am J Neuroradiol. 13(2):655-90, 1992
16. Currarino G: Canalis basilaris medianus and related defects of the basiocciput. AJNR Am J Neuroradiol. 9(1):208-11, 1988
17. Nager GT: Cephaloceles. Laryngoscope. 97(1):77-84, 1987
18. Currarino G et al: Transsphenoidal canal (large craniopharyngeal canal) and its pathologic implications. AJNR Am J Neuroradiol. 6(1):39-43, 1985

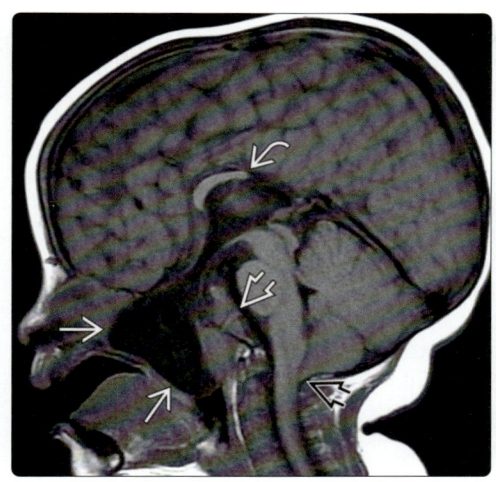

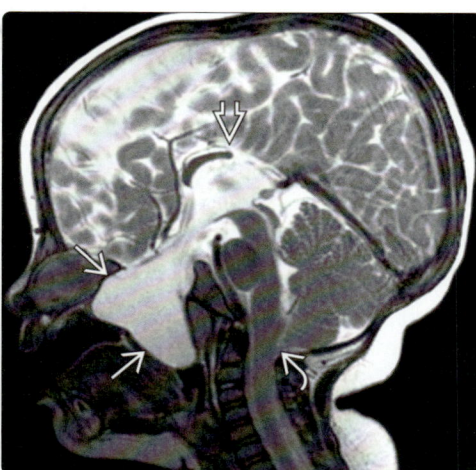

(Left) Sagittal T1 MR in an 18-month-old boy shows a large transsphenoidal cephalocele ➡ occluding the nasopharynx anterior to the sphenooccipital synchondrosis ➡. The pituitary gland is not identifiable; the corpus callosum is dysplastic ➡. There is associated Chiari 1 configuration of the cerebellar tonsil ➡. (Right) Sagittal T2 MR in the same patient shows similar findings of skull base cephalocele ➡, corpus callosum dysgenesis ➡, and low-lying cerebellar tonsil ➡.

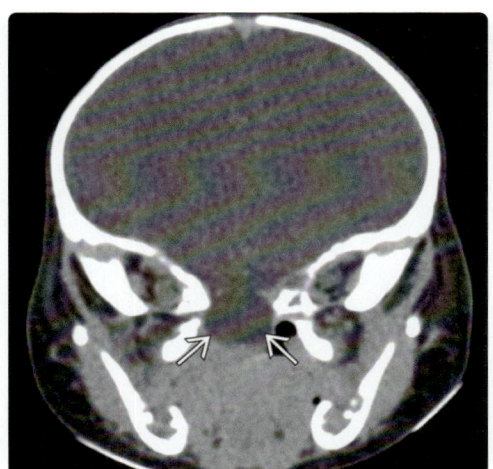

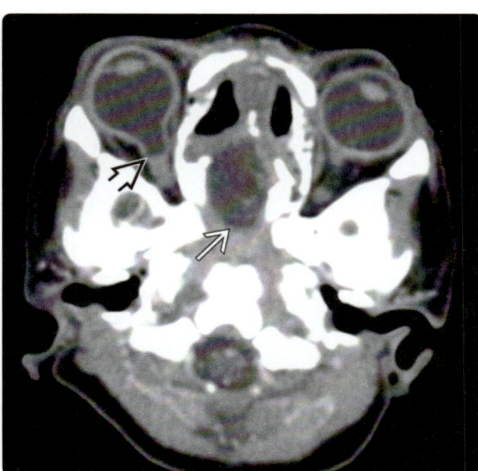

(Left) Coronal CECT in a 5-day-old infant with a nasal mass shows a transsphenoidal cephalocele ➡ extending into the nasopharynx via a large skull base defect. On this image, the contents of the cephalocele appear to be predominantly CSF. MR is better for determining the nature of the contents. (Right) Axial CECT in the same child shows hypertelorism secondary to the cephalocele extending through the skull base defect ➡ and a well-defined optic nerve coloboma ➡.

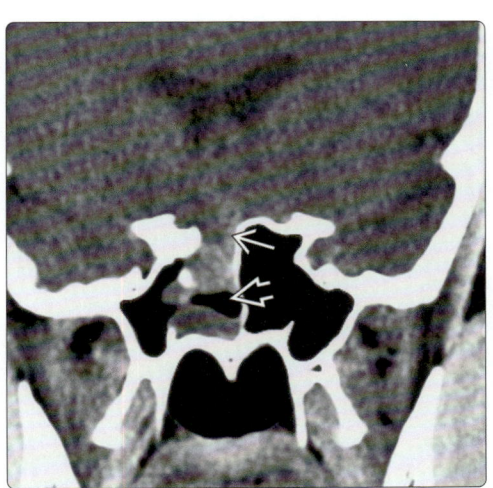

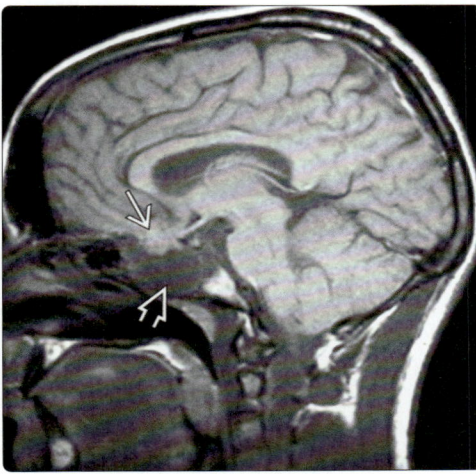

(Left) Coronal NECT defines a defect ➡ in the roof of the partially opacified right sphenoid sinus ➡ in a teenager. In this case, the skull defect was related to previous head trauma, and the patient had a posttraumatic CSF leak. (Right) Sagittal T1 MR in the same patient better defines the nature of the cephalocele herniating through a skull base defect into the sphenoid sinus. It contains posterior inferior frontal lobe tissue ➡ and a large amount of CSF ➡.

IMAGING

- Best clue: Anterior or central **skull base (SB) defect** on bone CT with **positive β2-transferrin** test on nasal secretions
- Anterior SB bone CT findings
  - Bone defect in horizontal **cribriform plate** & vertical **lateral lamella** of cribriform plate at ethmoid roof
  - Other evidence for fracture, endoscopic sinus surgery, congenital cephalocele
- Central SB bone CT findings
  - Bone defect in sellar floor (transnasal pituitary surgery), lateral wall sphenoid (osseous dural defect)
- Multiple defects often present in obese patient with **idiopathic intracranial hypertension**
- MR used if cephalocele suspected

TOP DIFFERENTIAL DIAGNOSES

- Vasomotor rhinitis
- SB defect without CSF leak

PATHOLOGY

- Congenital CSF leak
  - Cribriform defect ± congenital cephalocele, persistent craniopharyngeal canal
- Acquired leak: Spontaneous leak from osseous dural defect
  - Lateral roof of sphenoid sinus
- Posttraumatic leak: Can occur with any facial or SB fracture or even closed head injury
  - Roof or lateral wall of sphenoid sinus, or cribriform plate/ethmoid roof
- Postoperative defect: After functional endoscopic sinus surgery (FESS) or transnasal SB surgery
  - **Middle turbinate-cribriform plate** attachment, deep **olfactory fossa**, & anteroposterior **SB slope** important

CLINICAL ISSUES

- Rhinorrhea with Valsalva or head down maneuvers
- **β2-transferrin** best test to confirm fluid from nose as CSF
- Persistent CSF leaks endoscopically repaired

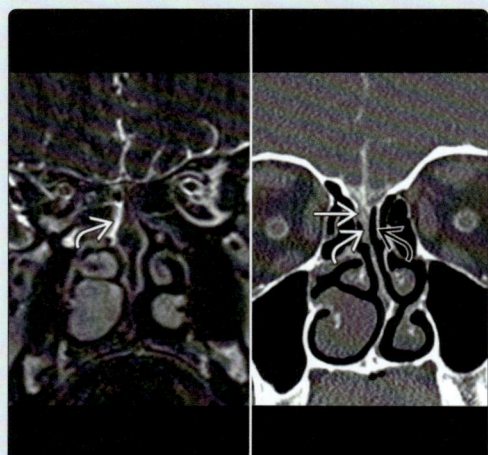
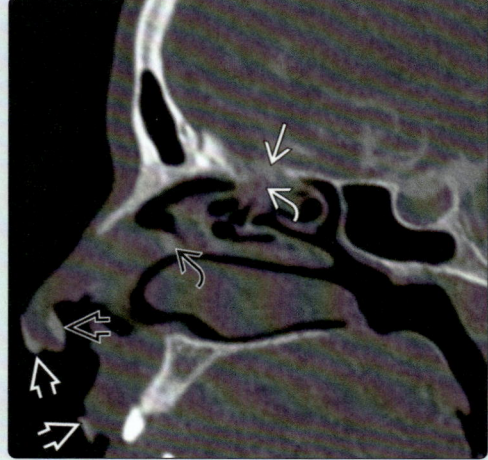

(Left) Coronal heavily T2WI SPACE MR (left) in right-sided CSF rhinorrhea shows bright signal suggesting CSF leak into right superior meatus ⤵. Coronal CT cisternogram (right) shows contrast-filled, bright CSF extending into right superior meatus through a cribriform plate defect ➡. Note air in normal left superior meatus ⤴. (Right) Sagittal reformat of CT cisternogram in prone position shows cribriform plate defect ➡ with bright CSF in superior meatus ⤵, nasal cavity ⤵, anterior nares ⤵, and on external nose and lip ⤵.

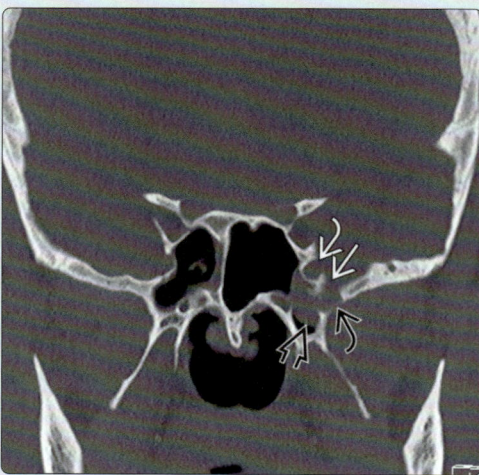
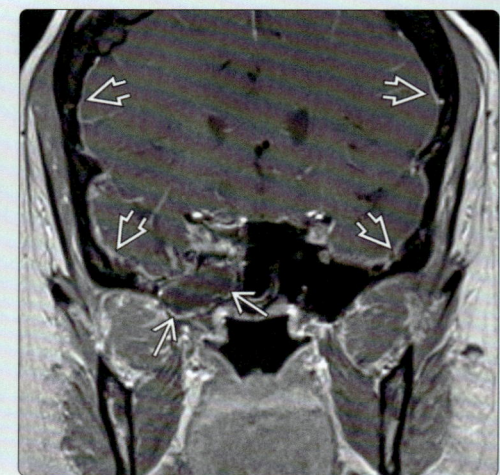

(Left) Coronal bone CT shows left sphenoid sinus lateral wall defect ➡ lateral to foramen rotundum (FR) ⤵ with cephalocele ⤵. Note another arachnoid pit scalloping left greater sphenoid wing inferolaterally ⤵. Sternberg canal is controversial (should be medial to FR to comply with Sternberg's original description). (Right) Coronal T1 C+ MR shows peripheral enhancement ➡ of right lateral sphenoid cephalocele. Note bilateral, diffuse dural enhancement ⤵, including at defect, even without infection.

TERMINOLOGY

Definitions

- Osseous dural defect or osteodural defect (ODD): Focal gap though dura & underlying skull base (SB) bone
  - Acquired; seen commonly with intracranial hypertension
  - May result from underlying congenital fissures, bone thinning, or **arachnoid pits** due to aberrant arachnoid granulations (AbAG)
- AbAG: Arachnoid granulations that penetrate dura but fail to reach dural venous sinus
  - Typically at lateral edges of cribriform plate or in floor of middle cranial fossa involving sphenoid or temporal bone from lateral wall of sella to tegmen tympani
  - Rarely between transverse sinus & bony labyrinth or jugular foramen region

IMAGING

Imaging Recommendations

- Best imaging tool
  - Bone CT with multiplanar reformations
    - Large defects easily visualized on multiplanar CT, obviating need for CT cisternography
  - MR used if cephalocele suspected
  - **CT/MR cisternogram**: Small defects > 1 potential leak
    - Positive study much more likely if active leak
    - Be sure to scan SB prior to intrathecal contrast, as osteoneogenesis can mimic contrast in sinus cavity
    - After lumbar puncture (LP) & intrathecal contrast placed, do maneuvers that increase rhinorrhea
    - CT cisternogram far more commonly used; MR cisternogram may be more accurate

CT Findings

- Bone CT
  - Anterior SB
    - Bone defect in horizontal **cribriform plate** & vertical **lateral lamella** of cribriform plate at ethmoid roof
  - Central SB
    - Bone defect in sellar floor (transnasal pituitary surgery), lateral wall sphenoid near (usually lateral to) foramen rotundum (FR), especially in obese patient
    - Persistent Sternberg canal as etiology of lateral sphenoid cephalocele controversial
      - □ As per original description, should be medial to FR & vidian canal, entering nasopharynx

MR Findings

- T2WI
  - Osseous defect, fluid in sinus cavity
  - Traction encephalomalacia at leak site, especially if cephalocele present
- T1WI C+
  - Defect dural enhancement common, even if no infection
  - **Bilateral diffuse dural enhancement** may be seen with **CSF** leak/**hypotension**

DIFFERENTIAL DIAGNOSIS

Vasomotor Rhinitis

- Rhinorrhea from sinuses with negative β2-transferrin

Skull Base Defect Without CSF Leak

- Not all bony defects leak CSF

PATHOLOGY

General Features

- Etiology
  - **Congenital** CSF leak: **Cribriform** plate defect, congenital cephalocele, persistent **craniopharyngeal canal**
  - **Acquired** leak: Spontaneous leak from **ODD**
    - Most common at lateral roof of sphenoid sinus near FR in obese patient
    - Usually secondary to **idiopathic intracranial hypertension (IIH)** → gradual SB thinning → SB defect
  - **Posttraumatic** leak: Can occur after facial or SB fracture or closed head injury
    - Most commonly seen at roof or lateral wall of sphenoid sinus or cribriform plate/ethmoid roof
  - **Postoperative** defect: After functional endoscopic sinus surgery (FESS) or transnasal SB surgery
  - Important to take special care at FESS not to detach vertical portion of basal lamella of **middle turbinate** delicate attachment to **cribriform plate** of ethmoid
  - **Keros classification** of ethmoid roof/olfactory fossa into 3 types according to increasing vertical height of lateral lamella & resultant depth of olfactory fossa
    - 1-3 mm in Keros type I, 4-7 mm in type II, & 8-16 mm in type III
    - Deepest Keros type III has maximum risk for iatrogenic injury to lateral lamella & CSF leak during FESS
  - Following transnasal transsphenoidal hypophysectomy
    - **SB slopes** downward variably in anterior to posterior direction in sagittal plane, from frontal recess to planum sphenoidale along ethmoid roof
    - Back-to-front technique during transnasal SB surgery helps reduce CSF leak
    - Lower-lying posterior SB level located first after identifying superior meatus & sphenoid sinus ostium

CLINICAL ISSUES

Presentation

- Most common signs/symptoms
  - Rhinorrhea ipsilateral to SB defect usually
  - Rare paradoxical CSF rhinorrhea in nose not connected directly to CSF: From eustachian tube or contralateral SB
  - **β2-transferrin** best 1st test to confirm nasal fluid as CSF

Natural History & Prognosis

- Posttraumatic CSF leaks: Usually resolve spontaneously due to scarring at SB defect
- Spontaneous CSF leak: Usually secondary to IIH, gradual SB thinning → frank defect

Treatment

- Persistent CSF leaks endoscopically repaired
- Treated spontaneous leaks from IIH may recur unless bariatric surgery or medical therapy

SELECTED REFERENCES

1. Scoffings DJ et al: Intrathecal contrast-enhanced computed tomography and MR cisternography for skull base cerebrospinal fluid leaks and other intracranial applications. Neuroimaging Clin N Am. 35(1):105-21, 2025

Skull Base Fibrous Dysplasia

TERMINOLOGY

- Fibrous dysplasia (FD)
- Congenital disorder with defect in osteoblastic differentiation and maturation, resulting in progressive replacement of normal cancellous bone by mixture of fibrous tissue and immature woven bone

IMAGING

- May affect calvarium, skull base, and facial bones
- Density (CT) and signal (MR) appearance highly variable
- CT findings
  - Expansile lesion centered in medullary space with variable attenuation
  - Sclerotic FD: Ground-glass density
  - Pagetoid FD: Mixed lucent and sclerotic areas
  - Cystic FD: Centrally lucent with thin sclerotic borders
- MR findings
  - Low signal in ossified ± fibrous portions of lesion
  - Variable enhancement depending on lesion pattern
- PET findings
  - Can be variably hypermetabolic on FDG PET

TOP DIFFERENTIAL DIAGNOSES

- Paget disease
- Ossifying fibroma
- Meningioma
- Skull base metastasis

PATHOLOGY

- Contains fibrous tissue with interspersed trabeculae of immature woven bone that resemble Chinese characters
- Sporadic mutation of *GNAS* gene; is not inherited
- Associated abnormalities include aneurysmal bone cyst, multiple endocrine disorders in McCune-Albright syndrome

CLINICAL ISSUES

- Indications for surgical intervention include diplopia, proptosis, compression of optic nerve, and cranial nerve palsies

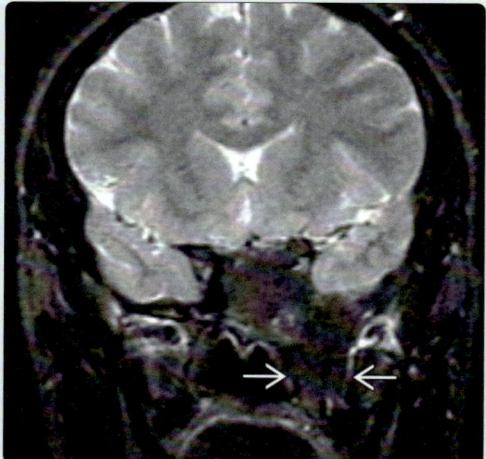
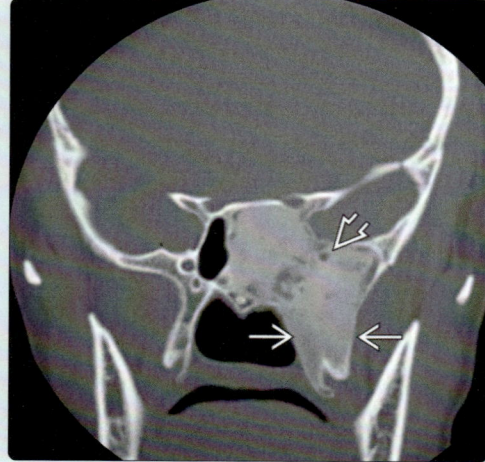

(Left) Coronal T2WI MR in a patient with fibrous dysplasia (FD) of the skull base shows expanded bone and marked hypointensity on T2 images extending into pterygoid processes ➡. Heterogeneity may suggest malignancy in some cases. (Right) Coronal CT in the same patient shows expansion of body and greater wing of the sphenoid with obliteration of left sphenoid sinus. Left foramen rotundum ➡ is narrowed and laterally displaced. Note the marked expansion of left pterygoid process and medial and lateral pterygoid plates ➡.

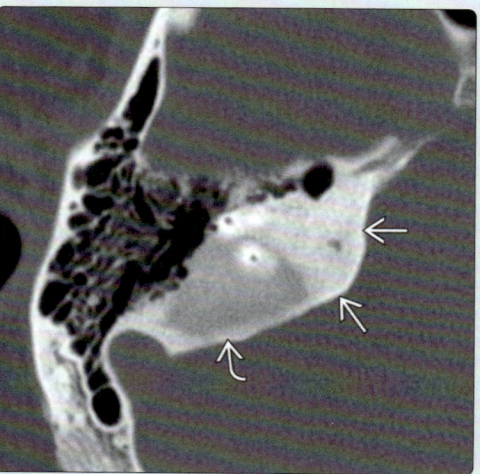
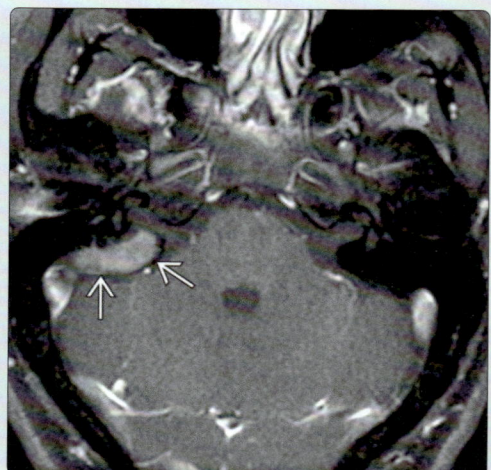

(Left) Axial bone CT shows FD involving the temporal bone with smooth, expanded appearance of the bone ➡. Petrous temporal bone is extensively involved with sparing of the inner ear structures. More posterior-lateral component ➡ shows the classic ground-glass density. (Right) Axial T1WI C+ FS MR in the same patient demonstrates enhancement of the entire extent of the involved petrous bone ➡. In this case, enhancement is diffuse and homogeneous.

Skull Base Fibrous Dysplasia

TERMINOLOGY

Abbreviations
- Fibrous dysplasia (FD)

Synonyms
- Craniofacial FD (CFD), osteitis fibrosa, osteodystrophy fibrosa, McCune-Albright syndrome

Definitions
- Congenital disorder with **defect in osteoblastic differentiation and maturation**, resulting in progressive replacement of normal cancellous bone by mixture of fibrous tissue and immature woven bone

IMAGING

General Features
- Best diagnostic clue
  - **Ground-glass matrix** in **expansile bone** lesion on bone CT
- Location
  - May affect any bone, including skull, skull base, and facial bones
  - Often > 1 bone involved (polyostotic)
- Size
  - Polyostotic lesions can be massive
- Morphology
  - Expanded bone

Radiographic Findings
- Radiography
  - Expanded, thickened bone with ground-glass density
  - May be accompanied by areas of sclerosis or lucency

CT Findings
- NECT
  - Appearance varies with relative content of fibrous vs. osseous tissue
  - Expansile lesion with abrupt transition zone between lesion and normal bone typical
- CECT
  - Enhancement often difficult to appreciate except in areas of lucent bone
- Bone CT
  - **Expansile** lesion centered in **medullary space** with variable attenuation
    - **Pagetoid (mixed) pattern** (50%): Mixed radiopacity and radiolucency
    - **Sclerotic FD** (25%): Ground-glass density
    - **Cystic FD** (25%): Centrally lucent lesions with thinned but sclerotic borders

MR Findings
- T1WI
  - Expansile mass with ↓ signal in ossified ± fibrous portions of lesion
- T2WI
  - **Low signal** in ossified ± fibrous portions of lesion
  - In active phase, heterogeneous signal pattern often present
- T1WI C+
  - Variable enhancement depending on lesion pattern
    - None, rim, or diffuse
  - Impressive enhancement may also be seen in fibrous areas
- MRA
  - Vascular narrowing or displacement where affected bone encroaches on arterial vascular canals/foramina
- MRV
  - Vascular narrowing or displacement where affected bone encroaches on venous vascular canals/foramina

Nuclear Medicine Findings
- Bone scan
  - Nonspecific; sensitive to extent of skeletal lesions in polyostotic FD
  - ↑ radionuclide accumulation, perfusion, and delayed bone phase
- PET
  - Hypermetabolic on FDG PET; accumulation of C-11 methyl-L-methionine on PET

Imaging Recommendations
- Best imaging tool
  - Bone CT best for most cases
- Protocol advice
  - T1 C+ FS MR in complicated cases (cranial neuropathy, suspected malignant transformation)

DIFFERENTIAL DIAGNOSIS

Paget Disease
- Typically presents in older adults
- Involves temporal bone and calvarium more frequently than craniofacial area
- Cotton wool CT appearance

Ossifying Fibroma
- May mimic cystic form of FD
- Thick, bony rim and lower density center
- Tends to appear more mass-like and localized than FD

Meningioma
- Intraosseous meningioma may mimic FD
- En plaque soft tissue mass may be evident on enhanced MR

Skull Base Metastasis
- Mixed sclerotic-destructive may mimic FD
- Prostate and breast carcinoma most common primary tumors to metastasize to skull base

Chondrosarcoma
- Centered on petrooccipital fissure
- Arc or ring-like matrix calcifications on bone CT
- Hyperintense on T2WI MR

Giant Cell Tumor
- May mimic sclerotic FD
- Hypointense on T2 MR due to hemosiderin deposition
- More intense enhancement on MR than FD

PATHOLOGY

General Features
- Etiology

- o **Benign, tumor-like lesion** of bone with local arrest of normal structural/architectural development
- Genetics
  - o Sporadic mutation of *GNAS* gene; is not inherited
  - o All cells descended from mutated cell line can manifest features of monostotic or polyostotic FD
- Associated abnormalities
  - o Aneurysmal bone cysts
  - o Multiple endocrine disorders may be seen in McCune-Albright syndrome

Staging, Grading, & Classification

- **Monostotic vs. polyostotic**
- Specific lesion type relates to disease activity
  - o Pagetoid
  - o Sclerotic
  - o Cystic

Gross Pathologic & Surgical Features

- Tan-yellow to white mass
- Rubbery to gritty consistency depending on fibrous vs. osseous content

Microscopic Features

- Fibrous tissue with interspersed trabeculae of immature woven bone that resemble Chinese characters

CLINICAL ISSUES

Presentation

- Most common signs/symptoms
  - o Symptoms depend on lesion location
    - Temporal bone: Congenital hearing loss (CHL), external auditory canal (EAC) stenosis, CNVII weakness
    - Orbital: Proptosis, optic neuropathy
    - Sinonasal: Ostial obstruction → mucocele formation
- Other signs/symptoms
  - o Pain, focal swelling, tenderness
  - o Leontiasis ossea (lion facies) with extensive facial bone involvement
    - Alters facial and calvarial contours
    - Obstructs sinuses
    - Complex cranial neuropathy possible from foraminal encroachment
- Clinical profile
  - o 3 presentations: Monostotic, polyostotic, and McCune-Albright syndrome
  - o **Monostotic FD (70%)**
    - Single osseous site affected
    - Older children and young adults (75% present before age 30)
    - Skull base and face involved in 25%; maxilla (especially zygomatic process) and mandible (molar area) > > frontal bone > ethmoid and sphenoid bones > temporal bone
    - May be asymptomatic, incidental finding
  - o Polyostotic FD (25%)
    - Involves ≥ 2 separate osseous sites
    - Skull base and face involved in 50%
    - Younger patients (mean age at diagnosis 8 years)
      - □ 2/3 have symptoms, including craniofacial asymmetry, by age 10

- o McCune-Albright syndrome (3-5%)
  - Polyostotic FD (usually unilateral)
  - Associated with endocrine dysfunction (precocious puberty) and cutaneous hyperpigmentation (café au lait spots)
  - Appears earlier and affects more bones more severely

Demographics

- Age
  - o **Most < 30 years**
- Sex
  - o M:F = 1:2
  - o McCune-Albright syndrome: Female predominance
- Epidemiology
  - o One of most common fibroosseous lesions
  - o Monostotic FD 6x more common than polyostotic FD
  - o Polyostotic form more likely to have calvarial involvement

Natural History & Prognosis

- Monostotic CFD has excellent prognosis
  - o Often ceases to progress after puberty
- Polyostotic FD rarely life threatening but has poor prognosis
  - o May progress beyond 3rd decade
- Malignant (sarcomatous) transformation of FD is rare (< 0.5% of cases)
  - o Osteosarcoma most common

Treatment

- Aggressive surgical management typically not recommended
- Radiation therapy generally avoided (may cause malignant transformation)
- Bisphosphonate therapy may ameliorate course (↓ pain and fractures)

DIAGNOSTIC CHECKLIST

Image Interpretation Pearls

- Classic appearance → **ground-glass on bone CT**; ↓ signal on T2WI MR

SELECTED REFERENCES

1. Papargyriou GE et al: Benign bony lesions of paranasal sinuses and skull base: from osteoma to fibrous dysplasia. Curr Opin Otolaryngol Head Neck Surg. 32(2):81-8, 2024
2. Szymczuk V et al: Craniofacial fibrous dysplasia: clinical and therapeutic implications. Curr Osteoporos Rep. 21(2):147-53, 2023
3. Chapurlat R et al: Bisphosphonates for the treatment of fibrous dysplasia of bone. 143:115784, 2021
4. Chattopadhyay A et al: Craniofacial fibrous dysplasia. J Clin Rheumatol. 26(7):e214, 2020
5. Davidova LA et al: An analysis of clinical and histopathologic features of fibrous dysplasia of the jaws: a series of 40 cases and review of literature. Head Neck Pathol. 14(2):353-61, 2020
6. Hwang D et al: Radiographic follow-up of fibrous dysplasia in 138 patients. AJR Am J Roentgenol. 215(6):1430-5, 2020
7. Lee SE et al: The diagnostic utility of the GNAS mutation in patients with fibrous dysplasia: meta-analysis of 168 sporadic cases. Hum Pathol. 43(8):1234-42, 2012
8. Wei YT et al: Fibrous dysplasia of skull. J Craniofac Surg. 21(2):538-42, 2010
9. Hullar TE et al: Paget's disease and fibrous dysplasia. Otolaryngol Clin North Am. 36(4):707-32, 2003
10. Chong VF et al: Fibrous dysplasia involving the base of the skull. AJR Am J Roentgenol. 178(3):717-20, 2002

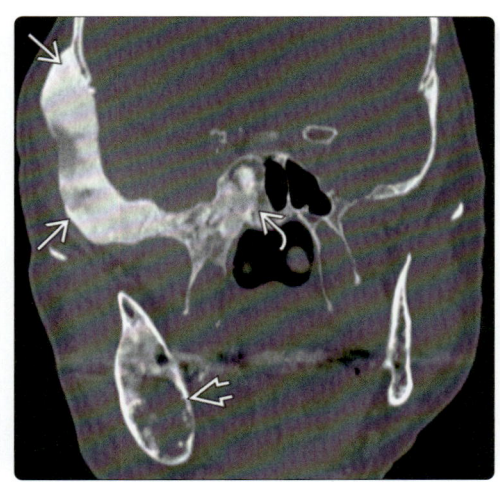

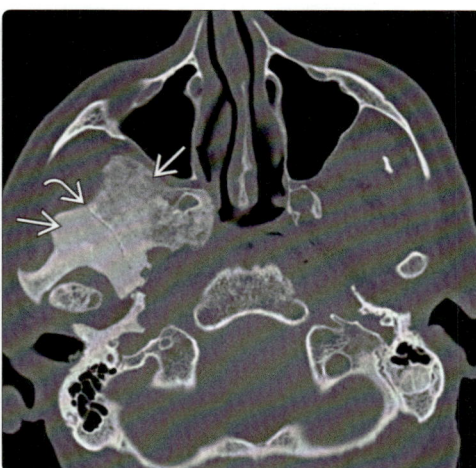

(Left) Coronal bone CT shows expanded mixed density within a squamous temporal bone ➡. Mixed density involvement of the sphenoid bone is also noted with expansion ➡. A predominantly cystic low-density focus of FD involvement is seen in the mandibular body ➡ near the ramus. (Right) Axial bone CT in the same patient with polyostotic FD shows mixed lucent and sclerotic pattern of bone involvement ➡. Note abrupt transition of the imaging appearance at a suture ➡, a characteristic of FD.

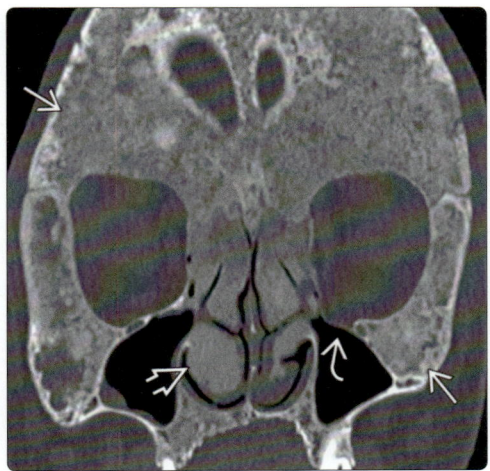

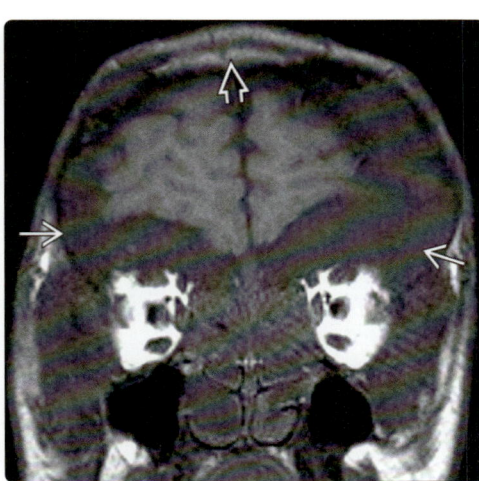

(Left) Coronal bone CT in a 27-year-old man shows an extensive pagetoid type of FD ➡ involving the craniofacial region. Note sclerotic changes ➡ in the nasal turbinates. Defect in the floor of the left orbit ➡ is secondary to previous orbital decompression. (Right) Coronal T1WI MR in the same patient shows expansion of bone and marked diffuse hypointensity ➡ replacing the normal marrow signal. Compare this with the normal marrow signal ➡ in the vertex.

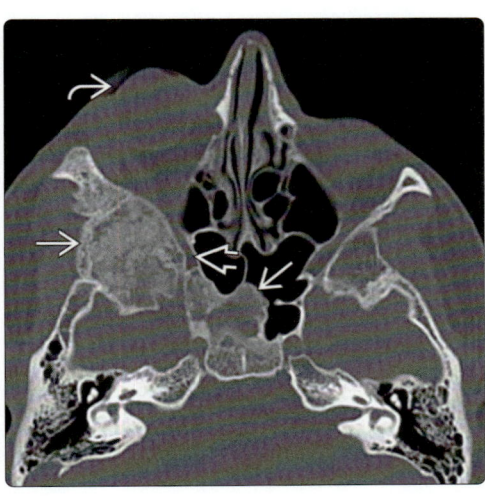

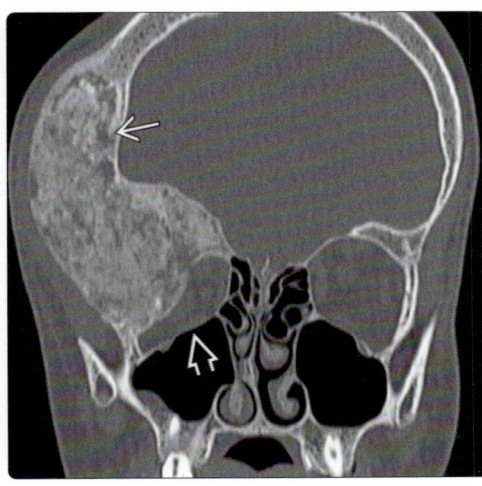

(Left) Axial bone window NECT shows a mixed sclerotic and lucent bone FD ➡ affecting the right sphenoid bone. Note narrowing of the right inferior orbital fissure ➡ and right proptosis ➡. (Right) Coronal CT in the same patient shows the degree of bone expansion and the mixed sclerotic and lucent pattern of bone changes ➡. The right orbital structures ➡ are compressed. This patient underwent surgery to reduce the orbital compression and preserve vision.

Skull Base Paget Disease

TERMINOLOGY

- Primary metabolic bony disease of unknown etiology

IMAGING

- CT findings
  - Bone CT most demonstrative of mixed sclerosis and lysis
  - Well-defined, lytic regions with expansion of bone in early-phase disease
  - Cotton wool appearance in later lytic-sclerotic phase
- MR findings
  - T1WI: Hypointense signal due to fibrovascular replacement of marrow space
  - Heterogeneous enhancement due to hypervascular nature of new bone
  - Basilar invagination from bone softening and expansion
- FDG PET/CT: ↑ FDG uptake in active phase

TOP DIFFERENTIAL DIAGNOSES

- Fibrous dysplasia; skull base metastasis

- Osteopetrosis
- Osteogenesis imperfecta

PATHOLOGY

- Cases may have autosomal dominant transmission
  - Some consistent mutations identified in familial cases and some sporadic cases
- Both environmental and genetic causes likely
- Histologic mosaic bone pattern in final stage of disease

CLINICAL ISSUES

- Common presentation: Expansile, lytic, and sclerotic bony disease of axial skeleton and skull in older adult male patient
  - Hearing loss if temporal bone involvement
  - May be incidental finding
- Malignant transformation in < 1% of cases
- Treatment: Lasting response to bisphosphonate agents

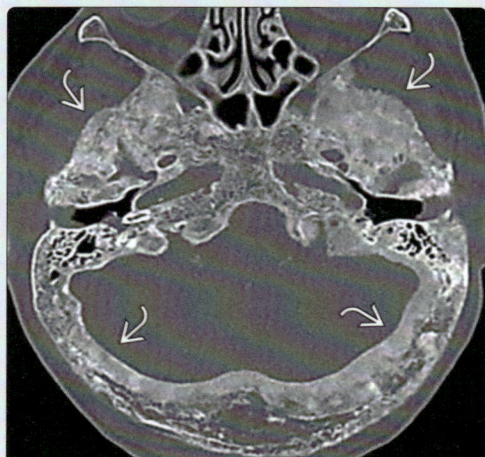
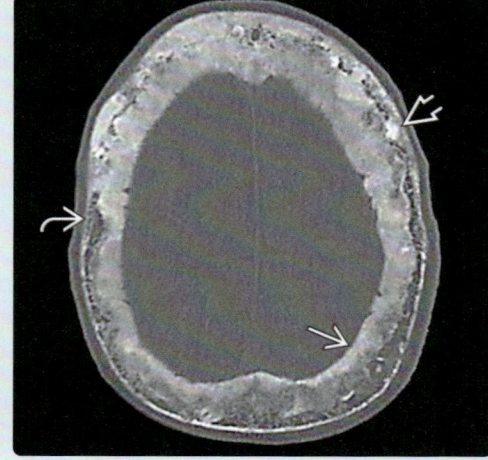

(Left) *Axial bone CT in an older adult performed for collapse and no significant past history shows diffuse skull base and temporal bone Paget disease with irregular demineralization and expansion of the bone* ➡. (Right) *Axial bone CT through the vertex in the same patient demonstrates the extensive nature of calvarial disease with diffuse, irregular calvarial cortical thickening* ➡, *patchy foci of osteolysis* ➡, *and islands of sclerotic bone* ➡, *representing so-called cotton wool lesions.*

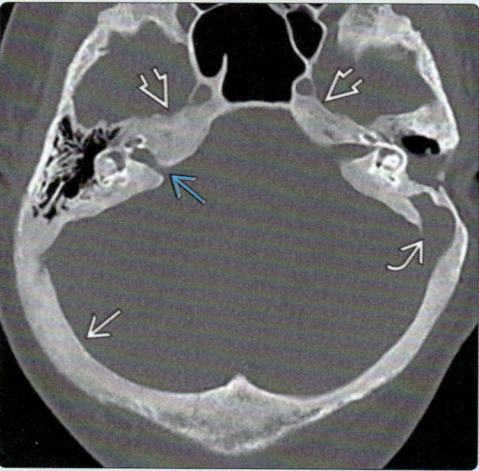
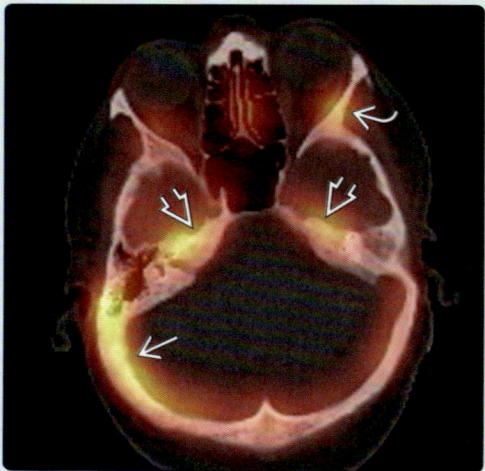

(Left) *Axial NECT in a patient with bilateral hearing loss shows focal involvement of right occipital bone* ➡. *There is also involvement of petrous apex* ➡ *with narrowing of the right internal auditory canal and otic capsule* ➡. *Note evidence of previous surgery for left cholesteatoma* ➡. (Right) *Axial Tc-99m SPECT CT in the same patient to assess the extent of bone changes shows increased tracer uptake in the right occipital bone* ➡ *petrous apex* ➡ *as well as the lateral wall of left orbit* ➡. *There was no further skeletal involvement.*

Skull Base Paget Disease

TERMINOLOGY

Abbreviations

- Paget disease (PD)

Synonyms

- Osteitis deformans

Definitions

- Primary metabolic bony disease of unknown etiology caused by waves of osteoclastic and osteoblastic activity

IMAGING

General Features

- Best diagnostic clue
  - Mixed **expansile, lytic, and sclerotic** bony disease of axial skeleton and skull in older adult male patient

Imaging Recommendations

- Best imaging tool
  - Bone CT most demonstrative of mixed sclerosis and lysis

CT Findings

- Bone CT
  - Characteristic stages of bone remodeling with progression from bony lysis to sclerosis
    - Well-defined lytic regions with expansion of bone in early phase of disease
    - **Cotton wool** appearance in later mixed lytic-sclerotic phase
  - Basilar invagination from bone softening and expansion

MR Findings

- T1WI
  - **Hypointense signal** due to fibrovascular replacement of fat in marrow space
  - Patchy ↑ signal possible with hemorrhage, slow flow in vascular channels
- T2WI
  - Heterogeneous, occasional hyperintense signal
- T1WI C+
  - Heterogeneous enhancement due to vascular channels in involved bone

DIFFERENTIAL DIAGNOSIS

Fibrous Dysplasia

- Classic ground-glass appearance and expansion in segments of diseased bone
- Can have more focal areas of soft tissue and sclerosis → mimics PD

Skull Base Metastasis

- Investigate for history of known malignancy
- Associated soft tissue mass more common

Osteopetrosis

- Presents in childhood
- Uniform bony sclerosis, diffuse involvement

Osteogenesis Imperfecta

- Age of onset usually much younger

PATHOLOGY

General Features

- Etiology
  - Admixture of environmental and genetic factors seem responsible for PD
- Genetics
  - Some cases have clear autosomal dominant transmission
  - Mutations in *SQSTM1* and *OPTN* locus of chromosome 10p13 have been discovered

Staging, Grading, & Classification

- 1st stage of disease is lysis
- Progresses to mixed lytic and sclerotic disease
- Final stage of disease is dense sclerosis

Microscopic Features

- Histologic mosaic bone pattern in final stage of disease

CLINICAL ISSUES

Presentation

- Most common signs/symptoms
  - Occasional incidental finding
  - Pagetic bone pain is uncommon
    - Constant, boring character
  - Hearing loss with temporal bone involvement
    - **Conductive hearing loss** may result from involvement of ossicles
    - **Sensorineural hearing loss** may result from bony compression of CNVIII or cochlear involvement
- Other signs/symptoms
  - Wide range of other presentations, including
    - Skull deformity and fractures
    - Cranial neuropathies
    - Brainstem and cerebellar dysfunction
    - ↑ alkaline phosphatase levels

Demographics

- Age
  - Typically disease of older adults (uncommon < age 55)
- Sex
  - M:F = 3:2

Natural History & Prognosis

- Generally benign course
- Malignant transformation to osteosarcoma in < 1% of cases

Treatment

- Newly described treatments with bisphosphonates result in sustained remission in most patients

SELECTED REFERENCES

1. Oflas M et al: Paget's disease mimicking prostate cancer metastasis with (68)Ga-PSMA PET/CT. Mol Imaging Radionucl Ther. 33(3):199-202, 2024
2. Üstün F et al: Paget's disease of the bone found incidentally on F-18 FDG PET/CT: clinical significance and differential diagnostic criteria. Acta Endocrinol (Buchar). 19(3):292-300, 2023
3. Tilden W et al: An update on imaging of Paget's sarcoma. Skeletal Radiol. 50(7):1275-90, 2021
4. Reid IR: Management of Paget's disease of bone. Osteoporos Int. 31(5):827-37, 2020
5. Gruener G et al: Paget's disease of bone. Handb Clin Neurol. 119:529-40, 2014

TERMINOLOGY

- Langerhans cell histiocytosis (LCH): Spectrum of disorders caused by neoplastic clonal proliferations of CD1a, CD207, S100 (+) dendritic cells
  - Single system (SS) (unifocal or multifocal) vs. multisystem (MS) disease
  - Bone & skin most frequently involved
  - High-risk organ involvement: Liver, spleen, marrow = worse prognosis
  - Other organs: Lymph nodes, pituitary, thymus, gastrointestinal tract, CNS
  - 70% have involvement of H&N: Skull base, temporal bone, craniofacial

IMAGING

- CT findings
  - Geographic, lytic lesion of skull base/temporal bone
  - Associated with enhancing soft tissue mass
- MR findings
  - Heterogeneous, strongly enhancing soft tissue mass ± intracranial/dural extension
- PET/CT: FDG avid useful for multisystem involvement

TOP DIFFERENTIAL DIAGNOSES

- Acute coalescent otomastoiditis
- Rhabdomyosarcoma, acquired cholesteatoma

CLINICAL ISSUES

- Typical presentation: Young male patient with otalgia, otorrhea, & postauricular mass
  - Usually presents in 1st decade
  - M:F = 1.2-3:1
  - Otologic symptoms may be only initial sign of disease
  - More common among White patients
- 90% cure rate for unifocal disease of temporal bone
- Usually responds well to medical management
- Curettage or mastoidectomy for localized temporal bone disease

(Left) Axial CECT in Langerhans cell histiocytosis (LCH) demonstrates involvement of the ossicles, otic capsule, and mastoid bilaterally with well-defined destruction ➮. Note involvement of the right occipital bone ➮. Normal bone margins are beveled and clearly defined. (Right) Axial T1 C+ FS MR in the same patient demonstrates intense enhancement of LCH in both the middle ears and mastoid ➮. There is involvement of the soft tissue over the right occipital region ➮ as well as the left sigmoid sinus ➮.

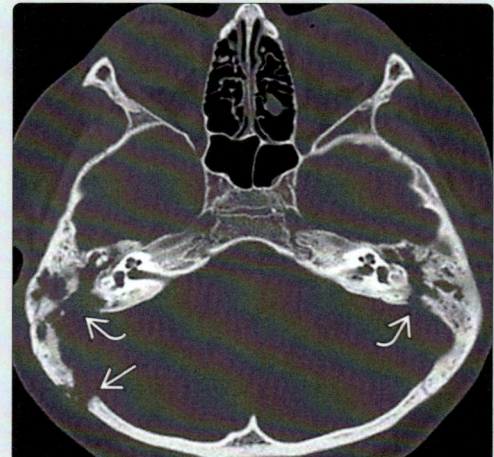
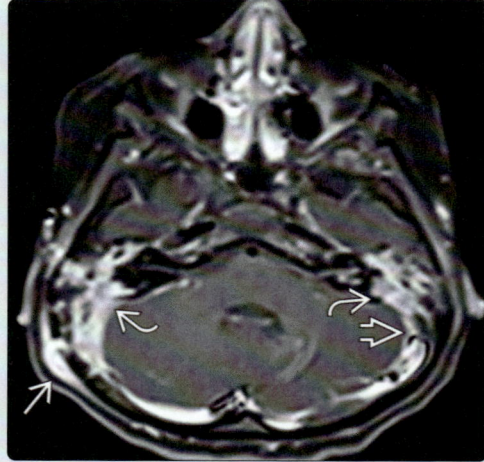

(Left) Axial bone CT shows multiple foci of lytic osseous destruction associated with soft tissue masses involving the central skull base ➮, occipital bone ➮, and right squamous temporal bone ➮. Note the characteristic beveled edge with differential involvement of the outer and inner tables ➮. (Right) Midline sagittal T1 C+ MR in the same patient shows heterogeneously enhancing masses arising within the clivus and sphenoid ➮ and occipital bones ➮ in this patient with multifocal LCH.

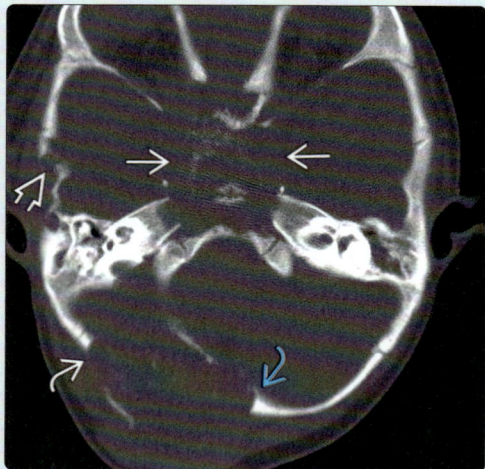
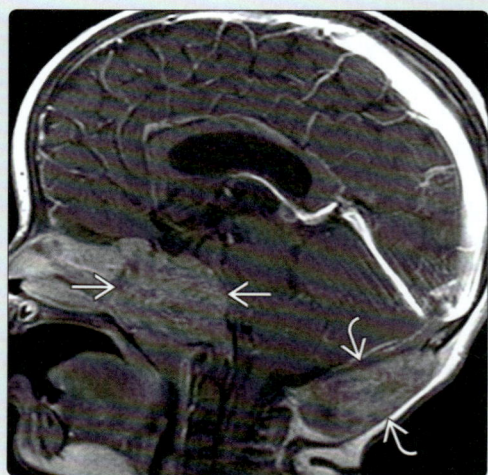

Skull Base Langerhans Cell Histiocytosis

TERMINOLOGY

Abbreviations
- Langerhans cell histiocytosis (LCH)

Synonyms
- Eosinophilic granuloma, histiocytosis X, Hand-Schüller-Christian disease, Letterer-Siwe disease

Definitions
- LCH: Spectrum of disorders caused by neoplastic clonal proliferations of CD1a, CD207, S100 (+) dendritic cells
- Single system (SS) (unifocal or multifocal) vs. multisystem (MS) disease
  - Bone & skin most frequently involved
  - Worse prognosis: Organs at high risk are liver, spleen, marrow
  - Other organs: Lymph nodes, pituitary, thymus, gastrointestinal tract, CNS
  - H&N: Skull base, temporal bone, craniofacial

IMAGING

General Features
- Best diagnostic clue
  - Well-marginated, **geographic, lytic lesion** of skull base/temporal bone + enhancing soft tissue mass
- Location
  - **Mastoid portion** of temporal bone common site for H&N disease
    - Petrous apex less common
  - Skull lesions (frontal & parietal bones) more common than skull base
  - Mandible, maxilla, & vertebral body lesions also may occur
  - Unifocal 50-75%; multifocal SS 10-20%; all others multifocal/MS disease
- Size
  - Varies from small, punched-out lesion to total diffuse bony involvement
- Morphology
  - Destructive, marginated lesion most often

Radiographic Findings
- Radiography
  - Lytic bone lesion with punched-out borders
  - "Button sequestrum" occasionally noted in skull lesions

CT Findings
- CECT
  - Variably enhancing soft tissue mass with mastoid destruction
  - May involve contiguous dura
- Bone CT
  - Bony lesions of variable appearance, typically lytic
    - Most have sharply defined, punched-out appearance
    - Geographic bone destruction in mastoid temporal bone
      - □ Ossicular & otic capsule destruction
    - Lytic lesions with beveled margins, ± sclerosis (common appearance in skull)
    - May have more diffuse bone destructive change

MR Findings
- T1WI
  - Iso- to hypointense bone lesion ± soft tissue mass
  - ↑ signal in proliferative LCH lesions due to lipid-laden macrophages
- T2WI
  - Hyper- to isointense mass
  - Rarely blood products in soft tissue mass
- STIR
  - Similar findings to T2WI
  - Whole-body STIR to assess for multifocal disease
    - More sensitive for skeletal & extraskeletal LCH than radiographs or bone scan
    - Limited ability to distinguish active vs. residual disease
- T1WI C+
  - Heterogeneous, strongly enhancing soft tissue mass
  - May show defined or infiltrative borders
  - ± intracranial extension/dural enhancement

Nuclear Medicine Findings
- Bone scan: Most lesions ↑ radiotracer uptake, few ↓ or absent radiotracer uptake
- PET/CT: FDG highly sensitive for active LCH (↑ radiotracer uptake)

Imaging Recommendations
- Best imaging tool
  - Bone CT delineates geographic pattern of temporal bone/skull base involvement
  - Gadolinium-enhanced MR best for depicting soft tissue extent & intracranial involvement
  - CECT or MR help differentiate inflammatory mastoid lesions from LCH
  - Whole-body DWI MR and PET/CT for staging
- Protocol advice
  - C+ FS MR

DIFFERENTIAL DIAGNOSIS

Acute Coalescent Otomastoiditis
- Acutely ill patient; responsive to antibiotics
- Trabecular loss, cortical dehiscence usually less extensive than in LCH
- No soft tissue component unless abscess present

Rhabdomyosarcoma
- Aggressive unilateral soft tissue mass with bone destruction
- More common in petrous apex & middle ear than mastoid
- Biopsy may be required to differentiate from LCH

Acquired Cholesteatoma
- Tympanic membrane perforation with white mass on otoscopy
- Bone destruction involves scutum & ossicles; usually less extensive than LCH
- Does not enhance; + diffusion restriction

Congenital Cholesteatoma
- White, retrotympanic mass on otoscopy
- Does not enhance; + diffusion restriction

Cholesterol Granuloma

- Preceded by history of chronic ear infections
- More common in petrous apex & middle ear than mastoid
- Hyperintense on T1 MR

Fibrous Dysplasia

- Lytic phase lesions may mimic LCH
- Typically causes bone expansion & areas of ground-glass attenuation

PATHOLOGY

General Features

- Genetics
  - Monoclonality of pathologic Langerhans cell
  - > 50% carry mutations in *BRAF*

Staging, Grading, & Classification

- Location of LCH lesion & SS vs. MS involvement → treatment decisions & prognosis
  - Young age, multifocal involvement, multiorgan dysfunction, relapse
  - Low-risk organs: Skin, bone, lungs, lymph nodes, gastrointestinal tract, pituitary gland, & CNS
  - High-risk organs: Liver, spleen, & bone marrow
- Formerly classified into 1 of 3 overlapping forms
  - Unifocal LCH (eosinophilic granuloma)
  - Hand-Schüller-Christian disease
    - Multifocal bone, skin, viscera, & brain involvement
  - Letterer-Siwe disease
    - Acute, fulminant, disseminated multiorgan disease, including liver, spleen, lymphatic, lung, & bone

Microscopic Features

- Active lesion: Granuloma of dendritic Langerhans cells > inflammatory cells
- Later stages: Macrophages > Langerhans cells + fibrotic & xanthomatous changes
- Birbeck granule: Classic "tennis racquet" organelle found by electron microscopy in up to 40% of Langerhans cells
  - Diagnostic importance diminished due to immunostaining of specific markers now available (CD1a, CD207, S100 protein)

CLINICAL ISSUES

Presentation

- Most common signs/symptoms
  - **Otologic symptoms** may be only initial sign of disease
    - Initial presentation with otologic symptoms in 25%
    - Conductive hearing loss & otorrhea
      - □ Otorrhea from secondary infection with granulation tissue formation
- Other signs/symptoms
  - Otalgia, vertigo
  - Otitis externa/media
  - Postauricular swelling
  - Facial nerve palsy, sensorineural hearing loss
  - Aural polyp from erosion of external auditory canal wall by lesion
  - Proptosis, ptosis with orbital involvement
- Clinical profile
  - Male child or adolescent with otalgia, otorrhea, & postauricular mass

Demographics

- Age
  - 90% of cases < 15 years at presentation
  - SS, unifocal (70% of cases); peak age: 5-15 years
  - SS, multifocal (20% of cases); peak age: 1-5 years
  - MS high-risk organ-positive (10% of cases); peak age: 0-2 years
- Sex
  - **M:F = 2:1**
- Epidemiology
  - Rare (0.2-2.0 cases per 100,00 children)
  - **70% have involvement of H&N**
    - Bilateral disease in up to 45% of cases
  - Bone lesions most common manifestation of disease (80-95% of children with LCH)

Natural History & Prognosis

- 90% cure rate for unifocal disease of temporal bone
- Soft tissue component resolves initially, then reossification of lytic bone lesion
- Local recurrence may occur

Treatment

- SS disease
  - Unifocal bone disease: Watchful waiting vs. curettage & local steroid injection
  - Multifocal bone disease or CNS-risk lesion: Chemotherapy & steroids x 6-12 months
- MS disease (± high-risk organ): Multiagent chemotherapy x 12 months

DIAGNOSTIC CHECKLIST

Consider

- Consider LCH when destructive temporal bone lesion does not respond to antibiotics & tympanostomy tubes

Reporting Tips

- Differentiation of LCH lesion from rhabdomyosarcoma essential

SELECTED REFERENCES

1. An R et al: The value of 18F-FDG PET/CT in Langerhans cell histiocytosis. Ann Nucl Med. 38(3):238-45, 2024
2. Baratto L et al: Comparison of whole-body DW-MRI with 2-[(18)F]FDG PET for staging and treatment monitoring of children with Langerhans cell histiocytosis. Eur J Nucl Med Mol Imaging. 50(6):1689-98, 2023
3. Chugh A et al: Unisystem Langerhans cell histiocytosis in maxillofacial region in pediatrics: comprehensive and systematic review. Oral Maxillofac Surg. 25(4):429-44, 2021
4. Gargan ML et al: Langerhans cell histiocytosis in children under 12 months of age: the spectrum of imaging and clinical findings: experience in an Irish tertiary referral centre. Eur J Radiol. 134:109375, 2021
5. Iaremenko O et al: Clinical presentation, imaging and response to interferon-alpha therapy in Erdheim-Chester disease: case-based review. Rheumatol Int. 40(9):1529-36, 2020
6. Rajakulasingam R et al: Skeletal staging in Langerhans cell histiocytosis: a multimodality imaging review. Skeletal Radiol. 50(6):1081-93, 2020
7. Chevallier KM et al: Differentiating pediatric rhabdomyosarcoma and Langerhans cell histiocytosis of the temporal bone by imaging appearance. AJNR Am J Neuroradiol. 37(6):1185-9, 2016
8. Egeler RM et al: Langerhans cell histiocytosis is a neoplasm and consequently its recurrence is a relapse: In memory of Bob Arceci. Pediatr Blood Cancer. 63(10):1704-12, 2016

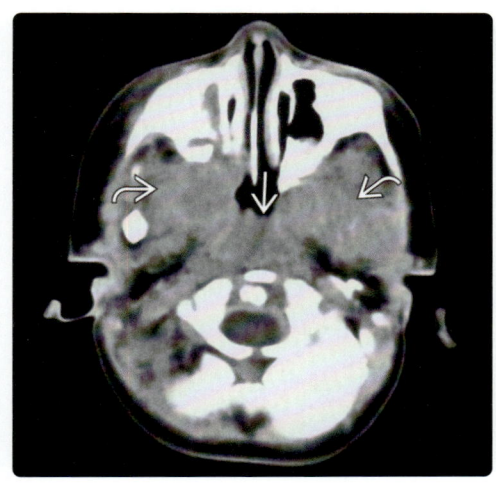

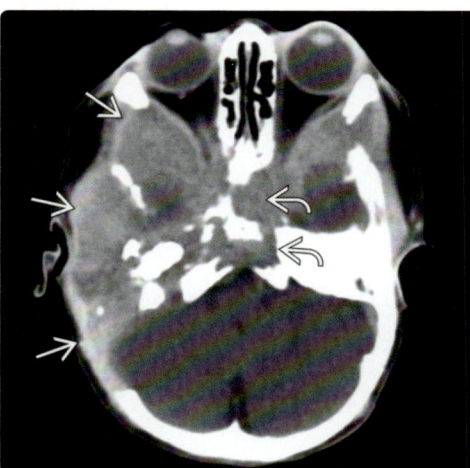

(Left) Axial CECT demonstrates an extensive LCH lesion with considerable soft tissue involvement. LCH extends into the nasopharynx ➡ and bilateral nasopharyngeal masticator space ➡. (Right) Higher section axial CECT demonstrates a large LCH lesion of the central skull base ➡ and temporal bone ➡ with relatively homogeneous enhancement. The mass results in extensive destruction of the right temporal bone, sphenoid wings, and clivus.

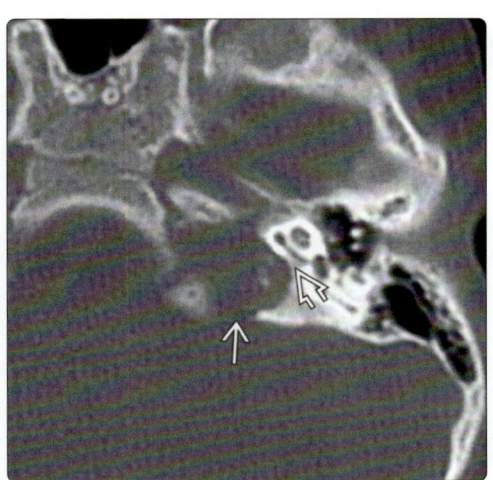

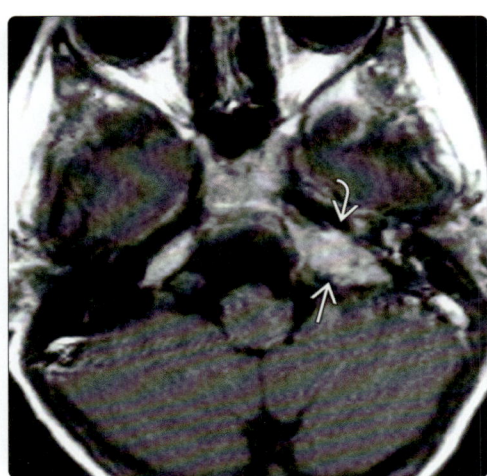

(Left) Axial bone CT demonstrates an LCH lesion in the left petrous apex ➡ with scalloping of the otic capsule ➡. The lesion is also contiguous with the petrous segment of the internal carotid artery (ICA) along the anterior margin. (Right) Axial T1 C+ MR in the same patient demonstrates uniform enhancement of the LCH lesion in the petrous apex ➡. Contiguity with the petrous ICA ➡ is evident.

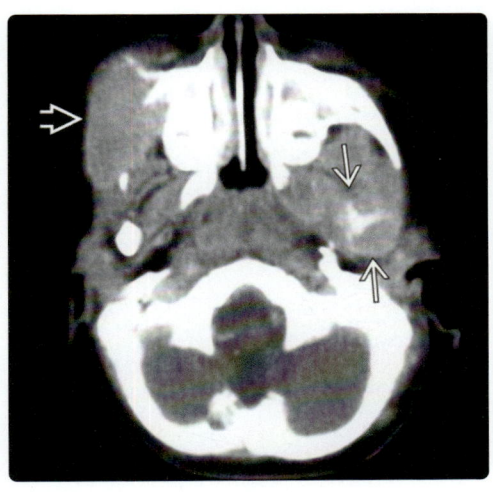

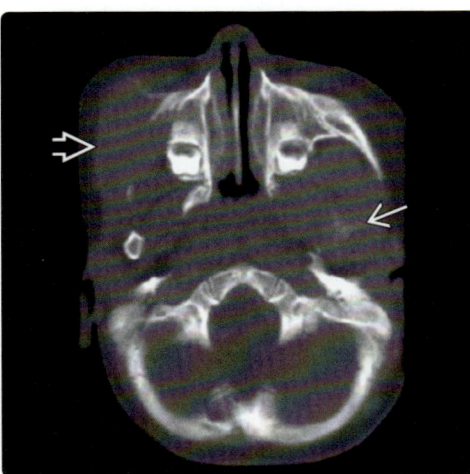

(Left) Axial CECT shows expansile, uniformly enhancing soft tissue lesions presenting as a cheek mass that results in bony destruction of the right zygoma ➡ and a 2nd mass in the left masticator space destroying the subcondylar mandible ➡. (Right) Axial bone window CT in the same patient demonstrates midface bone destruction involving the right zygoma ➡ and marked demineralization and destruction of the subcondylar mandible on the left ➡. Other midfacial and skull lesions were present but not depicted.

TERMINOLOGY

- Rare, heritable metabolic bone disease with defective bone remodeling, resulting in overproduction of immature bone
- **Autosomal recessive osteopetrosis** (AROP): Childhood severe form
- **Autosomal dominant osteopetrosis** (ADOP): Adult benign, less severe form

IMAGING

- **AROP**: CT findings seen in **infancy**
  - Diffuse ↑ in overall bone density
  - Temporal bone: Internal auditory canal (IAC) & internal carotid artery canal stenoses, middle ear encroachment
  - Skull base: Foraminal & dural sinus stenoses
- **ADOP type 1**: Adult CT findings
  - Universal otosclerosis
    - Spares spine
  - **Dense sclerosis of calvarium**
- **ADOP type 2**: Adult CT findings

- Dense sclerosis of skull base, spine, pelvis
  - **Spares calvarium**
- Generalized ↑ density of entire skull base
- Endobones (unresorbed primary ossification centers) = bone within bone appearance
- Sclerotic otic capsule beyond normal bony labyrinth margins
- IAC short & trumpet-shaped

TOP DIFFERENTIAL DIAGNOSES

- Skull base Paget disease
- Skull base fibrous dysplasia

PATHOLOGY

- Hereditary disorder: *CLCN7* gene mutation

CLINICAL ISSUES

- **AROP** apparent in infancy; **ADOP** manifests later in life
- Radiographic skeletal survey is recommended when osteopetrosis is suspected clinically

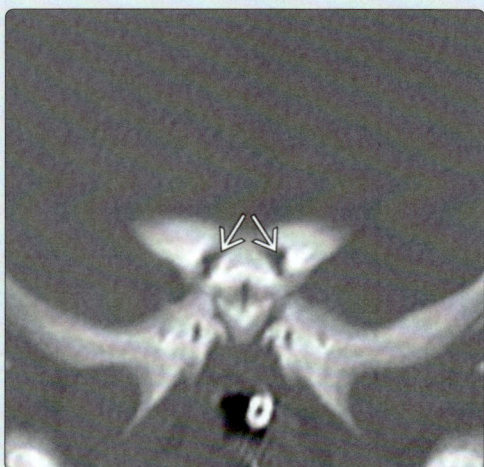
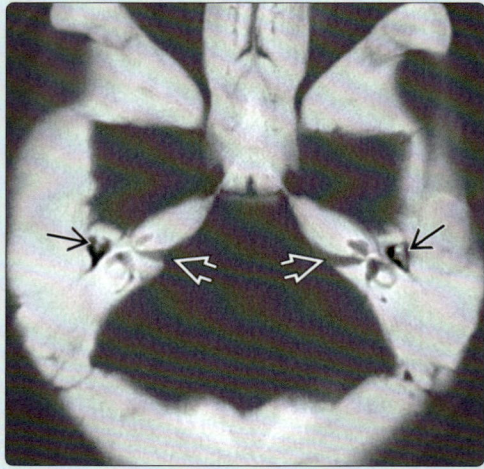

(Left) Coronal bone CT in a 6-month-old boy with autosomal recessive osteopetrosis (AROP) shows diffuse sclerosis involving all visualized osseous structures of the face and skull base. Thickening and sclerosis result in significant bilateral optic canal stenosis ➡ and subsequent optic atrophy. (Right) Axial skull base bone CT shows diffuse sclerosis of entire cranial base. There is narrowing of both middle ear cavities ➡. Note also compromise of each internal auditory canal (IAC) ➡. This child has AROP.

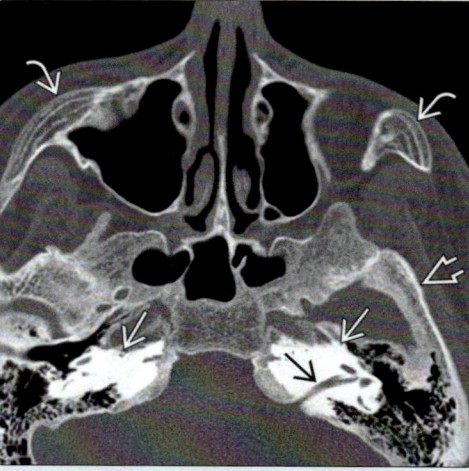
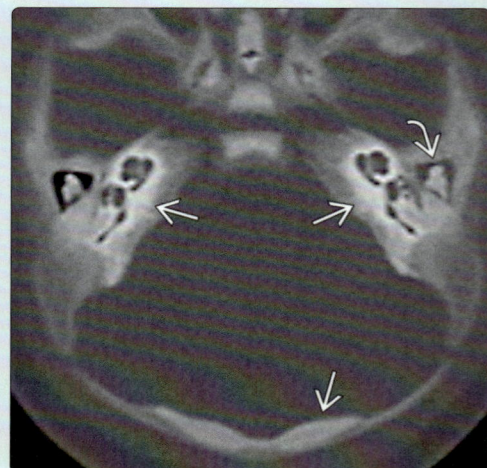

(Left) Axial bone CT in a young adult with autosomal dominant osteopetrosis (ADOP) shows bilateral dense sclerosis of temporal bones ➡, narrow left IAC ➡, & thickening of calvarium ➡ without increased density. Notice endobone appearance of both malar eminences ➡ from unresorbed primary ossification centers. (Right) Axial bone CT in a patient with AROP shows dense sclerosis of the cranial base and temporal bones ➡ with compromised middle ear cavity and encroachment on the left ossicular mass ➡.

Skull Base Osteopetrosis

TERMINOLOGY

Synonyms
- Marble bone disease

Definitions
- Rare, heritable metabolic bone disease with defective bone remodeling, resulting in overproduction of immature bone
- **Autosomal recessive osteopetrosis** (AROP)
  - Childhood severe form; malignant infantile osteoporosis
- **Autosomal dominant osteopetrosis** (ADOP), type 2
  - Adult less severe form; Albers-Schönberg disease

IMAGING

General Features
- Best diagnostic clue
  - Dense, sclerotic bones (chalk bones)
- Location
  - Temporal bone, calvarium, & skull base

Radiographic Findings
- Radiography
  - Dense bone is easily appreciated in AROP

CT Findings
- NECT
  - **AROP**: Ca^{++} within basal ganglia, thalami, dentate nuclei, & white matter
    - From renal tubular acidosis secondary to associated carbonic anhydrase II deficiency
- Bone CT
  - **AROP**: CT findings seen in **infancy**
    - Diffuse ↑ in overall bone density
    - Temporal bone: Internal auditory canal (IAC) & internal carotid artery (ICA) canal stenoses, middle ear encroachment
    - Skull base: Foraminal & dural sinus stenoses
  - **ADOP**: Adult CT findings
    - **Type 1**: Dense sclerosis of calvarium
      - Universal otosclerosis; spares spine
    - **Type 2**: Dense sclerosis of skull base, spine, pelvis; spares calvarium
      - Generalized ↑ density of entire skull base
      - Endobones (unresorbed primary ossification centers)= bone within bone appearance
      - Sclerotic otic capsule beyond normal bony labyrinth margins; IAC short & trumpet-shaped
      - Enlarged subarcuate fossa possible

MR Findings
- T1WI
  - AROP: Thickening of calvarium, skull base, & temporal bone
- T2* GRE
  - ADOP type 2: Blooming of Ca^{++} in basal ganglia, thalami, dentate nuclei, & white matter
- T1WI C+
  - AROP: C+ in suprahyoid neck = extramedullary hematopoiesis
- MRA: Petrous ICA stenosis (AROP)
- MRV: Dural venous sinus stenosis (AROP)

DIFFERENTIAL DIAGNOSIS

Skull Base Paget Disease
- Clinical: Older adult patients
- Usually seen as diffuse, cotton wool appearance
- Demineralized otic capsule correlates with sensorineural hearing loss (SNHL)

Skull Base Fibrous Dysplasia
- Clinical: < 30 years old
- Relative sparing of otic capsule
- Lytic, sclerotic, or mixed with characteristic ↑ bone volume

Renal Osteodystrophy
- Osteomalacia & secondary hyperparathyroidism related to chronic kidney disease
- Salt & pepper skull or diffuse calvarial sclerosis

PATHOLOGY

General Features
- Etiology
  - Hereditary disorder: *CLCN7* gene mutation
- Genetics
  - Autosomal recessive or dominant
- Overproduction of immature bone
  - Osteoclast function is defective

Microscopic Features
- Persistent primary bony spongiosa

CLINICAL ISSUES

Presentation
- Most common signs/symptoms
  - AROP
    - Cranial neuropathies, poor bone growth, petrous ICA, & dural venous sinus stenoses
    - Marrow replaced: Anemia & neutropenia
      - Extramedullary hematopoiesis possible
    - Fragile bones: **Fractures** with minor trauma
  - ADOP
    - Asymptomatic to progressive symptoms
    - Eustachian tube obstruction with otitis media
    - Facial nerve, other cranial nerve deficits
    - External auditory canal stenosis

Demographics
- Age
  - **AROP** apparent in infancy; **ADOP** manifests later in life

Natural History & Prognosis
- Children with AROP rarely survive childhood
- Progressive bilateral hearing loss in ADOP type 2

SELECTED REFERENCES

1. McLuckey MN et al: Osteopetrosis in the pediatric patient: what the radiologist needs to know. Pediatr Radiol. 54(7):1105-15, 2024
2. Polgreen LE et al: Autosomal dominant osteopetrosis. Bone. 170:116723, 2023
3. Calder AD et al: Imaging in osteopetrosis. Bone. 165:116560, 2022
4. Spinnato P et al: Spectrum of skeletal imaging features in osteopetrosis: inheritance pattern and radiological associations. Genes (Basel). 13(11):1965, 2022

Skull Base Giant Cell Tumor

TERMINOLOGY

- Giant cell tumor (GCT)
- Benign intraosseous neoplasm arising from **multinucleated giant cells**

IMAGING

- CT: **Expansile**, intraosseous soft tissue mass with thinned surrounding **cortical shell**
  - Overlying cortical shell may be focally dehiscent
- MR: T1/T2 **hypointense rim** and prominent internal enhancement
- Sphenoid bone > temporal bone > > frontal bone

TOP DIFFERENTIAL DIAGNOSES

- Aneurysmal bone cyst
- Chordoma
- Chondrosarcoma
- Fibrous dysplasia
- Plasmacytoma

PATHOLOGY

- Hemorrhage/hemosiderin deposition common
- Overlap with other giant cell-containing tumors: Giant cell lesion, aneurysmal bone cyst, brown tumor, diffuse-type tenosynovial GCT
- Major neoplastic component of GCT comprised by stromal cells, not multinucleated giant cells
- 96% of GCTs have mutations in the histone *H3-3A* gene

CLINICAL ISSUES

- Rare lesion: 2% of all GCTs arise in skull base
- Peak incidence: 3rd-4th decades
- Metastases in 2% of cases
- Recurrence rate 40-60% after resection

DIAGNOSTIC CHECKLIST

- Make sure lesion arises in sphenoid bone vs. sphenoid sinus
- Is lesion margin expansile (GCT) or purely lytic (malignancy)?
- Consider fibrous dysplasia if lytic with ground-glass foci

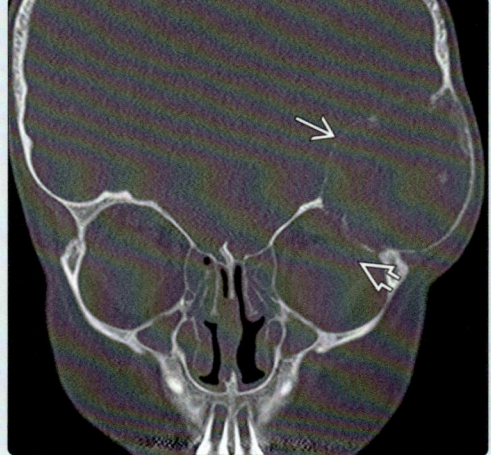
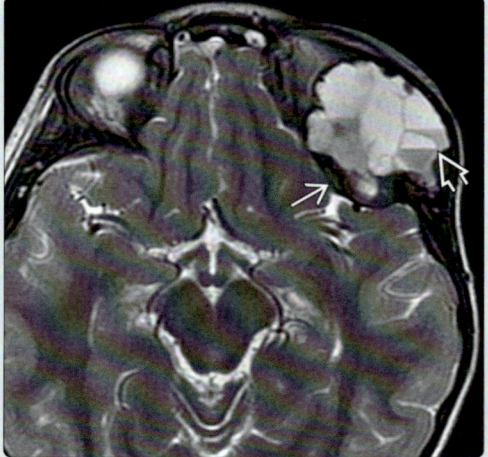

(Left) Coronal NECT in a 3-year-old boy with left ocular ptosis and supraorbital mass shows a thin, peripheral, calcified border of the supraorbital mass ➡. There is inferior displacement of the ocular globe ➡. (Right) Axial T2 MR in the same patient shows peripheral low signal of the mass ➡, which may represent hemosiderin combined with the calcified shell. Pathology proved giant cell tumor (GCT). There are prominent internal fluid/debris levels ➡, consistent with a component of aneurysmal bone cyst.

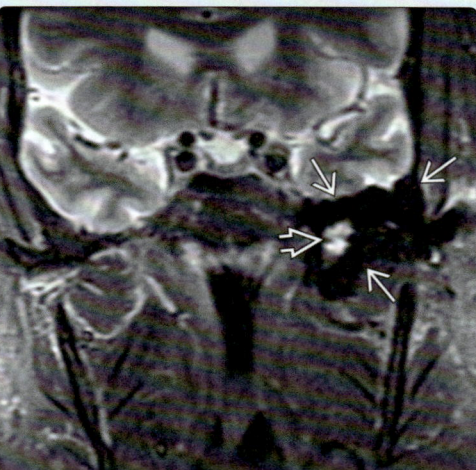
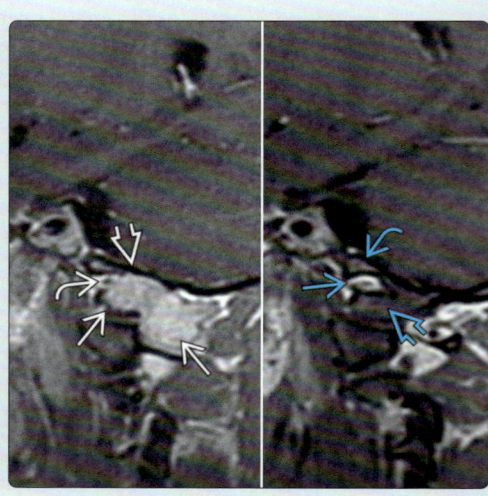

(Left) Coronal T2 FS MR of a 69-year-old man with pain in the left TMJ area shows a peripherally hypointense mass in the left temporal bone ➡. There is an area with intense high signal ➡ within this GCT. (Right) Composite sagittal T1 C+ MR of an 18-year-old man shows an expansile enhancing GCT of the occipital condyle ➡ and the posterior part of the jugular tubercle ➡, also in the hypoglossal canal, next to the hypoglossal nerve ➡. Right panel shows the contralateral hypoglossal canal ➡, occipital condyle ➡, and jugular tubercle ➡.

TERMINOLOGY

Abbreviations
- Giant cell tumor (GCT)

Synonyms
- Osteoclastoma

Definitions
- Benign intraosseous neoplasm featuring **multinucleated giant cells**

IMAGING

General Features
- Best diagnostic clue
  - CT: **Expansile**, intraosseous soft tissue mass with thin surrounding cortical shell
  - MR: **Hypointense rim**, robust internal enhancement
- Location
  - Sphenoid bone > temporal bone > > frontal bone
- Size
  - Variable, usually > 3 cm

CT Findings
- NECT
  - Mildly hyperdense soft tissue mass
- CECT
  - Marked enhancement
- Bone CT
  - Overlying **cortical shell** may be focally dehiscent
  - Occasional scant matrix calcification

MR Findings
- T1WI
  - Mixed iso- to hyperintense to gray matter
  - **Hypointense rim** common
- T2WI
  - Mixed iso- to hyperintense to gray matter
    - Occasionally diffusely hypointense (due to hemosiderin, calcification)
  - Markedly hypointense rim
  - Fluid levels with aneurysmal bone cyst component
- T1WI C+
  - Marked enhancement

DIFFERENTIAL DIAGNOSIS

Aneurysmal Bone Cyst
- Soap bubble appearance with blood-fluid levels
- May arise secondarily from GCT

Chordoma
- Destructive midline clival mass with bone fragments

Chondrosarcoma
- Eccentric erosive mass, chondroid calcifications

Fibrous Dysplasia
- Diffuse ground-glass density, hypointense on T2WI
- < 30 years old, rarely progressive

Plasmacytoma
- Homogeneous soft tissue mass
- Solitary or seen in association with multiple myeloma

PATHOLOGY

General Features
- Etiology
  - Unknown
  - Can arise secondarily in pagetoid bone

Microscopic Features
- Multinucleated osteoclastic giant cells, often with hemorrhage/hemosiderin
- Light microscopy resembles other lesions with giant cells
  - Patient demographics, lesion location, and radiographic features often necessary to arrive at specific diagnosis
    - Giant cell lesion (formerly known as giant cell reparative granuloma)
    - Brown tumor
    - Aneurysmal bone cyst
    - Diffuse-type tenosynovial GCT (formerly called pigmented villonodular synovitis)

Molecular Genetics
- 96% of GCTs have mutations in histone *H3-3A* gene

CLINICAL ISSUES

Presentation
- Most common signs/symptoms
  - Headache and local pain, cranial nerve palsies
- Other signs/symptoms
  - Sphenoid GCT: Diplopia, ophthalmoplegia
  - Temporal bone GCT: Otalgia, hearing loss, facial palsy, TMJ dysfunction

Demographics
- Age
  - Peak incidence: 3rd-4th decades
- Sex
  - Female predominance
- Epidemiology
  - Only 2% of all GCTs in skull base

Natural History & Prognosis
- Rare sarcomatous transformation, usually post RT
- Metastases in 2% of cases

Treatment
- Preoperative embolization, surgical resection/curettage
- Radiation therapy for inoperable lesions

SELECTED REFERENCES

1. Amoodi H et al: Giant cell tumor of the temporal bone and skull base. J Craniofac Surg. 34(7):e628-30, 2023
2. Rekhi B et al: Giant cell tumor of bone: an update, including spectrum of pathological features, pathogenesis, molecular profile and the differential diagnoses. Histol Histopathol. 38(2):139-53, 2023
3. Zhao SS et al: Image findings of tendon sheaths affected by diffuse tenosynovial giant cell tumors of the skull base. Eur Rev Med Pharmacol Sci. 27(6):2571-9, 2023
4. Huang Q et al: Diffuse-type tenosynovial giant cell tumor invading the temporal bone: three cases. Ear Nose Throat J. 104(7):NP450-5, 2022
5. Li X et al: Imaging features, staging system, and surgical management of giant cell lesions of the temporal bone. Acta Otolaryngol. 142(7-8):553-61, 2022

Skull Base Meningioma

TERMINOLOGY

- Benign extraaxial neoplasm arising from arachnoid cap cells

IMAGING

- Anterior skull base: Olfactory groove, planum sphenoidale, tuberculum sella, and sphenoid wing
- Central skull base: Petroclival and pericavernous
- Posterior skull base: Lower clival and foramen magnum
- Morphology: Sessile (en plaque)/lentiform > globose/spherical
- CT findings
  o Hyperdense, homogeneously enhancing mass
  o 25% intramural calcification
  o Hyperostosis > permeative sclerotic
- MR findings
  o Isointense to gray matter with prominent enhancement
  o Enhancing reactive dural tail in 60%
  o CSF-vascular cleft between tumor and parenchyma

TOP DIFFERENTIAL DIAGNOSES

- Skull base metastasis
- Giant pituitary macroadenoma (pituitary neuroendocrine tumor)
- Trigeminal schwannoma
- Clival chordoma, chondrosarcoma, plasmacytoma

CLINICAL ISSUES

- Most common primary intracranial tumor
- Middle-aged to older adult patients
- M:F = 1:3
- Proximity to neurovascular structures makes treatment challenging

DIAGNOSTIC CHECKLIST

- Assess involvement of critical skull base structures: Optic canal, vessels, cavernous sinus, Meckel cave, internal auditory canal, foramen magnum

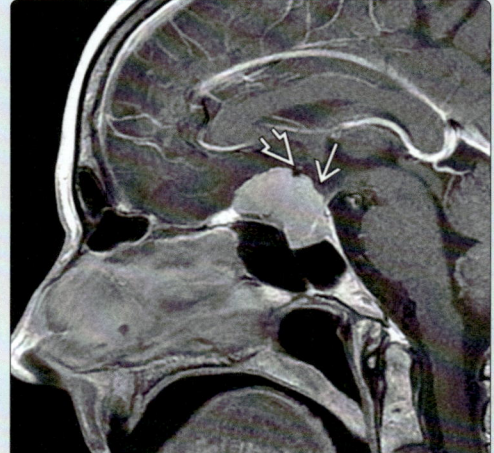
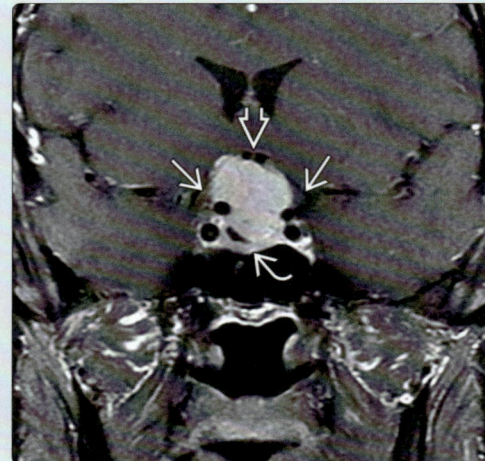

(Left) Sagittal T1 C+ MR of a 63-year-old woman with a visual deficit shows an enhancing mass extending from the planum sphenoidale, across the tuberculum sella, into the sella. The chiasm is displaced posteriorly ➡. The anterior cerebral arteries (ACAs) are displaced superiorly ➡. (Right) Coronal T1 C+ MR of same 63-year-old woman shows the sellar component of the mass splaying the optic nerves ➡. The ACAs are displaced superiorly ➡. The mass is separate from the pituitary in this coronal image ➡.

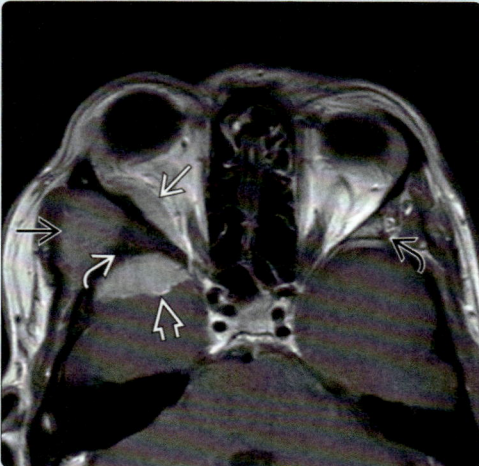
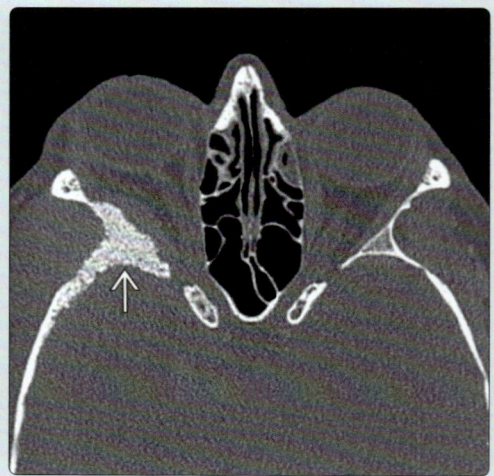

(Left) Axial T1 C+ MR shows meningioma resulting in hyperostosis of the greater sphenoid wing ➡. Intense enhancement is noted in the intracranial dural component ➡. Soft tissue component is noted in the temporal fossa ➡. Orbital tumor extension ➡ results in proptosis. Note normal size and fatty marrow signal ➡ of the normal left greater sphenoid wing for comparison. (Right) Axial bone CT shows enlargement and increased density of the greater sphenoid wing from hyperostosis ➡ due to meningioma infiltration.

TERMINOLOGY

Definitions

- Benign extraaxial neoplasm arising from arachnoid cap cells

IMAGING

General Features

- Best diagnostic clue
  - Avidly enhancing, extraaxial **dural-based mass with enhancing tails**
- Location
  - **Anterior skull base** (40% of intracranial meningiomas)
    - 50% in olfactory groove and tuberculum sella
      - □ Olfactory groove involves sinonasal cavity in 15%
      - □ Tuberculum sella may involve optic canals
    - 50% in sphenoid wing
      - □ Clinoidal (medial sphenoid wing)
      - □ Sphenoorbital (lateral sphenoid wing); most frequently symptomatic
  - **Central skull base**
    - Petroclival: Arise from upper 2/3 of clivus, ~ 2% posterior fossa meningiomas
      - □ Extension to posterior fossa, posterior cavernous sinus and Meckel cave, and middle cranial fossa
    - Cavernous sinus meningioma can involve neurovascular foramina, orbital apex
  - **Posterior skull base**
    - Lower clival, foramen magnum
      - □ Foramen magnum lesions may be posterior, anterior, or lateral
  - Additional skull base locations: Cerebellopontine angle/internal auditory canal (IAC), temporal bone, jugular foramen
- Morphology
  - Sessile/lentiform > globose/spherical
  - Occasional en plaque configuration
    - Carpet-like tumor overlying hyperostotic bone
    - Common in sphenotemporal buttress lesions

CT Findings

- NECT
  - **75% hyperdense** compared with brain parenchyma
  - **25%** intramural **calcification**
    - May occasionally be entirely calcified
- CECT
  - 90% show strong, uniform enhancement
- Bone CT
  - Hyperostotic > permeative, sclerotic adjacent bone
    - **Hyperostotic bone** may or may not be invaded
    - Upward "blistering" at sphenoid/ethmoid roof
      - □ **Pneumosinus dilatans** of adjacent sinus

MR Findings

- T1WI
  - Hypo- to isointense to gray matter
    - May be low or absent signal in heavily calcified areas
  - Rare increased signal in foci of hemorrhage
- T2WI
  - Hypo- to isointense to gray matter
  - 25% atypical: Necrosis, cysts

- **CSF-vascular cleft** at periphery of large lesions
  - Thin space between tumor and brain containing CSF and vessels
- Peritumoral edema correlates with pial blood supply
  - Increased surgical morbidity and early recurrence
- Narrowing of internal carotid artery (ICA) in cavernous sinus more likely than with pituitary mass
- May have spoke-wheel or sunburst linear hypointensities due to arterial feeders near point of dural attachment
- T2* GRE
  - If significantly calcified, may bloom
- PWI
  - Elevated rCBV typical
- T1WI C+
  - **Prominent enhancement in 95%**
    - Enhancing dural tail in 60%
  - Meningioma within cavernous sinus typically enhances to lesser degree than uninvolved sinus
  - Enhancing vessels in CSF-vascular cleft may be visible

Angiographic Findings

- Dural vessels supply center, pial vessels supply periphery
- Sunburst or spoke-wheel pattern of enlarged dural feeders
- Prolonged vascular "stain" into venous phase

Nuclear Medicine Findings

- DOTATATE PET shows uptake in meningioma
  - Can be used for imaging surveillance after treatment
- 177Lu-DOTATATE in clinical trials as treatment alternative for patients failing surgical &/or radiotherapeutic options

Imaging Recommendations

- Best imaging tool
  - Enhanced T1 FS MR generally best for tumor mapping

DIFFERENTIAL DIAGNOSIS

Skull Base Metastasis

- Variable appearance depending on histology of primary and whether metastases are to skull base marrow or dura
  - Multiple dural-based, enhancing masses

Giant Pituitary Macroadenoma (Pituitary Neuroendocrine Tumor)

- Large, invasive mass with skull base invasion
- No identifiable normal pituitary tissue

Trigeminal Schwannoma

- Parasellar mass, often with cystic components
- May extend into exiting foramina, prepontine cistern

Clival Chordoma

- Midline destructive mass
- High T2 signal; heterogeneous enhancement

Chondrosarcoma

- Eccentric mass with chondroid matrix
- Increased T2 signal with bone destruction
- Location typically at petroclival junction

Plasmacytoma

- Lytic destructive mass of clivus
- Iso- to hypointense T2 signal

- May be solitary or multiple in setting of multiple myeloma

Neurosarcoid
- Multifocal, dural-based, enhancing foci
- Look for infundibular stalk enhancement and enlargement

Solitary Fibrous Tumor
- Heterogeneous with flow voids
- May have ring-like peripheral high signal on DWI

Rosai-Dorfman Disease
- a.k.a. sinus histiocytosis with massive lymphadenopathy
- Rare histiocytic proliferative disease
- May have multiple dural-based, T2-hypointense masses

PATHOLOGY

General Features
- Etiology
  - Most are sporadic
  - Multiple inherited schwannomas, meningiomas, and ependymomas in neurofibromatosis type 2 (NF2)
  - Increased incidence following radiotherapy
    - More commonly over convexities than skull base
    - Develop 20-35 years following radiation
- Genetics
  - Most common mutation is functional loss of NF2 gene on chromosome 22 (~ 60% of sporadic meningiomas)

Staging, Grading, & Classification
- WHO classification (2016)
  - Grade 1: Benign (90%), e.g., meningothelial
  - Grade 2: Atypical (7%), e.g., clear cell
  - Grade 3: Anaplastic/malignant (2%), e.g., rhabdoid
- Grade 2 and 3 meningiomas are less common at skull base than along convexities
- Poor correlation of histologic grade to imaging features

Gross Pathologic & Surgical Features
- Semilunar or en plaque > round or globose
- Sharply circumscribed
- Adjacent dural thickening (tail)
  - **Not specific for meningioma**; may accompany any dural-based process
  - Usually reactive, not neoplastic

Microscopic Features
- Arise from meningothelial (arachnoid cap) cells
  - Relatively uniform cells with tendency to form whorls
  - Fibrous content correlates with T2 signal hypointensity
  - Attached to dura
- Psammoma bodies (laminated calcific concretions)
- Highly vascularized

CLINICAL ISSUES

Presentation
- Most common signs/symptoms
  - May be incidental finding
    - 33% of incidental intracranial neoplasms
  - Symptoms often nonspecific
    - Headache
    - Dizziness

    - Syncope
- Other signs/symptoms
  - Anterior skull base: Anosmia, visual loss, proptosis
  - Central skull base: Ophthalmoplegia
  - Posterior skull base: Myelopathy, lower cranial neuropathy

Demographics
- Age
  - Middle-aged to older adult patients
    - Peak age: 60 years
- Sex
  - M:F = 1:3
- Epidemiology
  - Most common primary intracranial tumor
  - Most common extraaxial tumor
  - 15-25% of primary intracranial tumors
  - 10% multiple (NF2; multiple meningiomatosis)

Natural History & Prognosis
- Indolent course is typical
- More aggressive course in WHO grade 2/3 lesions
- Those with peritumoral brain edema have **higher surgical complication and recurrence rates**

Treatment
- Surgery most likely to achieve cure but often requires complex combined approach with significant morbidity risk
  - Preoperative angiography/embolization may be employed to reduce intraoperative blood loss
  - Simpson grading system used to estimate completeness of resection
    - Grade I (complete removal, including dura and underlying bone) → grade IV (subtotal resection)
  - Prognosis for cure depends on location more than grade
- Radiotherapy/radiosurgery may be used primarily or adjunctive when resection is incomplete

DIAGNOSTIC CHECKLIST

Consider
- Solitary, enhancing, dural-based extraaxial mass is usually meningioma in adults without known malignancy

Reporting Tips
- Assess caliber of ICA, basilar, or vertebral arteries if surrounded by tumor
  - Meningioma often narrows ICA
    - Other parasellar lesions, such as schwannoma, macroadenoma, and lymphoma, typically will not
- Assess for Meckel cave or optic canal involvement
- Always **search for 2nd meningioma**
  - Multiple meningiomas in 10% of sporadic cases
- Report brain edema: Correlates with surgical morbidity & recurrence

SELECTED REFERENCES

1. Kurz SC et al: Evaluation of the SSTR2-targeted radiopharmaceutical 177Lu-DOTATATE and SSTR2-specific 68Ga-DOTATATE PET as imaging biomarker in patients with intracranial meningioma. Clin Cancer Res. 30(4):680-6, 2024
2. Nadeem A et al: Intracranial intricacies: comprehensive analysis of rare skull base meningiomas-a single-center case series. Clin Case Rep. 12(1):e8376, 2024

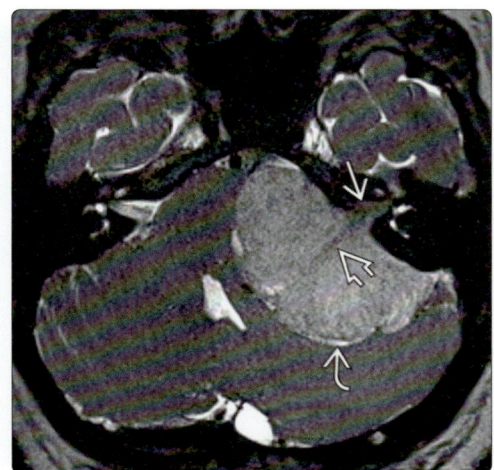

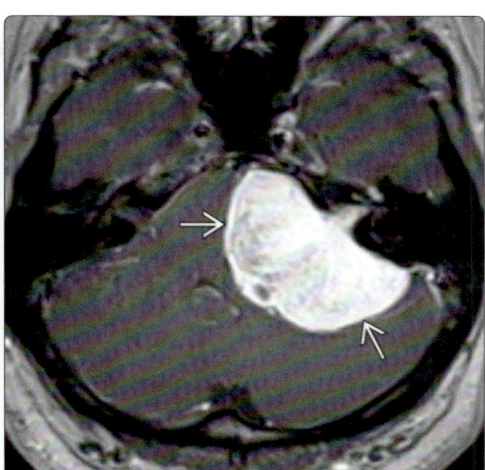

(Left) Axial T2 SSFP MR shows mildly hyperintense meningioma of the cerebellopontine angle (CPA) with mild expansion of internal auditory canal (IAC) by tumor ➡. Thin CSF cleft is noted ➡, and linear radiating hypointense bands are related to spoke-wheel appearance of tiny arterial feeders that can be seen (usually best seen at angiography) with meningioma ➡. (Right) Axial T1 C+ FS MR in the same patient shows relatively intense and mildly heterogeneous enhancement of this meningioma ➡.

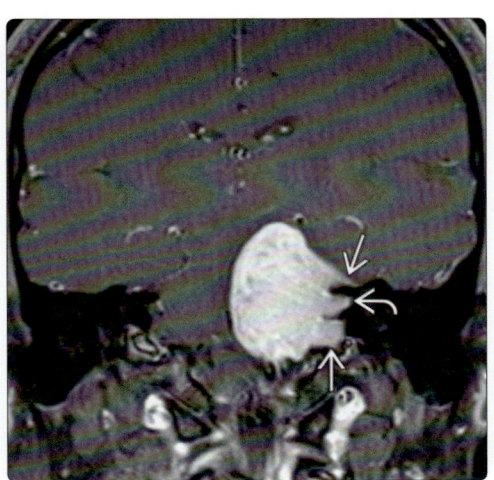

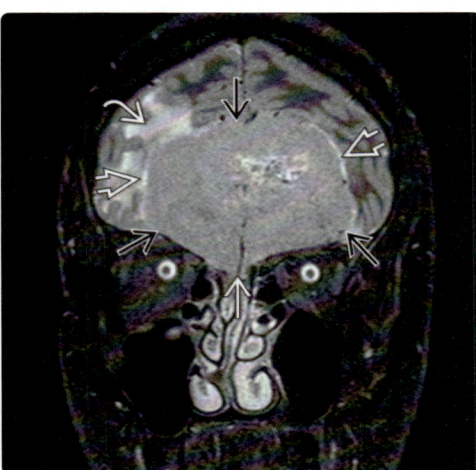

(Left) Coronal T1 C+ FS MR shows the dural-based attachments ➡ of this tumor, along with extension into the IAC ➡. The spoke-wheel appearance of fine linear vasculature is noted. (Right) Coronal STIR MR in a patient imaged for papilledema shows a large mildly heterogeneous isointense mass ➡ arising in the olfactory fossa ➡ bilaterally, displacing both frontal lobes. A thin CSF cleft ➡ indicates the extraaxial nature of this tumor. Associated brain edema ➡ predicts higher surgical morbidity.

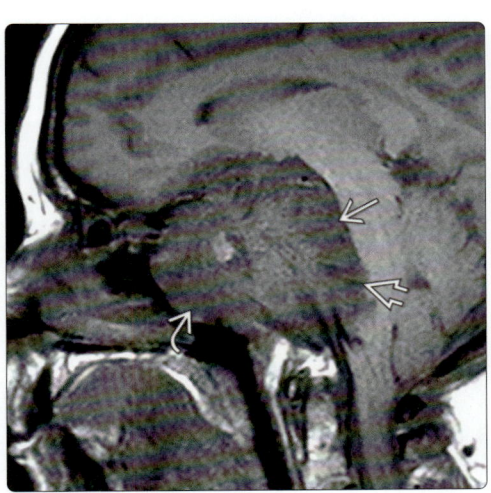

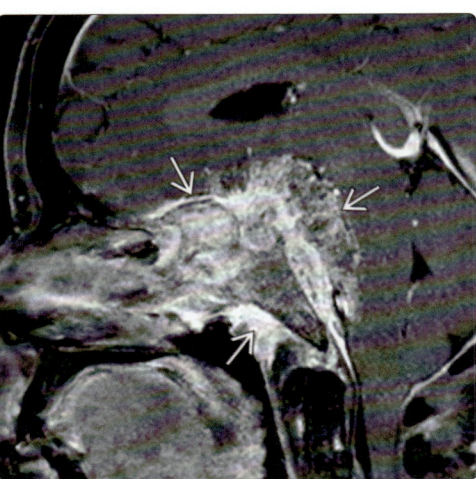

(Left) Sagittal T1 MR shows an unusually aggressive-appearing giant central skull base meningioma ➡, completely invading the clivus and extending into the sphenoid sinus and nasopharynx ➡. A sunburst pattern of vascularity ➡ is noted within the tumor. (Right) Sagittal T1 C+ FS MR in the same patient shows heterogeneous enhancement of the giant central skull base meningioma ➡. Tumor obliterates normal marrow and invades the sella, nasopharynx, and posterior fossa.

TERMINOLOGY

- Abbreviations: Solitary bone plasmacytoma (SBP), extramedullary plasmacytoma (EMP), multiple myeloma (MM)
- Definition: Isolated intramedullary or extramedullary neoplasm of plasma cells in absence of clinical or radiographic findings of MM

IMAGING

- CT findings
  - SBP: Solitary intraosseous, **lytic mass with nonsclerotic margins**
  - EMP: Sinonasal mass with secondary osseous invasion of skull base
- MR findings
  - Homogeneously enhancing intraosseous/extraosseous skull base mass
  - More sensitive for marrow space involvement and excluding additional small/early lesions

- Bone CT best defines trabecular and cortical destruction
- MR best defines marrow extent and extraosseous soft tissue tumor

TOP DIFFERENTIAL DIAGNOSES

- MM
- Skull base metastasis
- Non-Hodgkin lymphoma
- Invasive pituitary macroadenoma (pituitary neuroendocrine tumor)
- Chordoma, skull base meningioma

PATHOLOGY

- Monoclonal proliferation of immunoglobulin-secreting plasma cells

CLINICAL ISSUES

- Symptoms: Local pain, headache, cranial nerve deficits
- If skull base plasmacytoma diagnosed, complete clinical and radiologic work-up for MM required

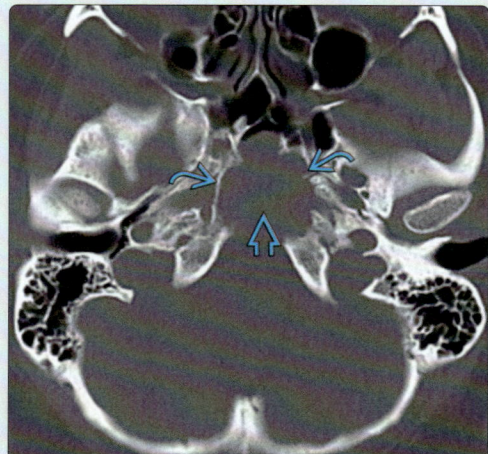
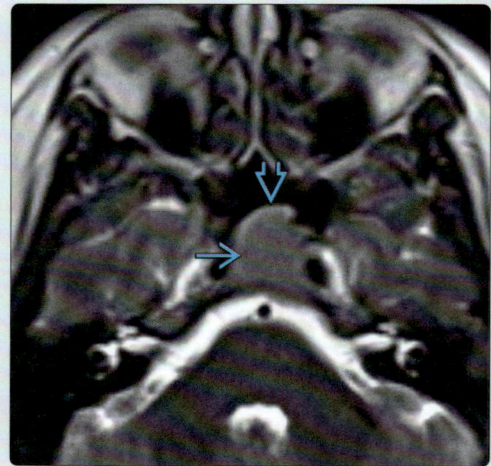

(Left) Axial NECT bone window in a 52-year-old man shows a well-circumscribed lytic central skull base lesion ➡ with nonsclerotic margins ➡. (Right) Axial T2 MR in the same patient shows central skull base mass with signal intensity isointense to gray matter ➡. Mild protrusion into the sphenoid sinus anteriorly ➡ is noted. Top differential diagnoses include plasmacytoma, multiple myeloma, metastasis, and invasive pituitary macroadenoma (pituitary neuroendocrine tumor).

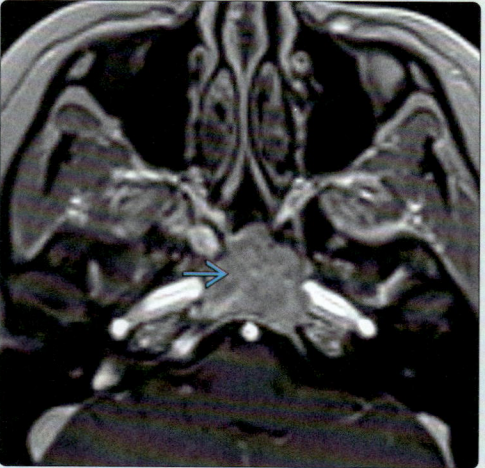
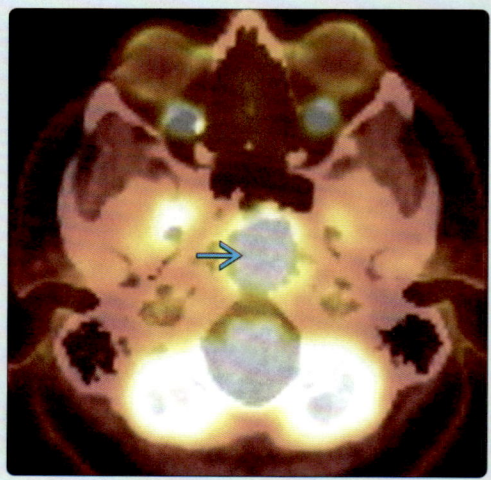

(Left) Axial 3D T1 C+ SPGR MR in the same patient shows homogeneous moderate enhancement ➡. (Right) Axial FDG PET/CT in the same patient shows avid FDG activity within the central skull base mass ➡. No other lesion was identified elsewhere in the body. Biopsy was consistent with plasmacytoma. Solitary bone plasmacytoma (SBP) accounts for 5% of plasmacytomas. SBP is defined by a single lytic lesion of bone due to monoclonal plasma cell neoplasm.

TERMINOLOGY

Abbreviations
- Solitary bone plasmacytoma (SBP), extramedullar plasmacytoma (EMP)

Synonyms
- Solitary plasmacytoma, skull base plasmacytoma

Definitions
- Plasmacytoma in broad sense consists of localized or focal soft tissue infiltrate or mass that consists of neoplastic monoclonal plasma cells
- Plasma cell neoplasms present in several pathologic and clinical forms and include multiple lesion variants and solitary lesion variants
- Malignant plasmacytoma in context of **multiple myeloma (MM)**
  - Focal intramedullary or extramedullary tumor in context of criteria that establish diagnosis of MM
  - This is most common form of monoclonal plasma cell infiltrate or mass
  - > 90% of patients with plasma cell tumor will meet criteria for MM, and most will have multiple lesions
  - Majority of plasma cell lesions of skull base are seen in context of multiple additional bony lesions and fulfill established criteria for MM
- **Solitary plasmacytoma** is rare and exists in 2 basic forms: Solitary bone plasmacytoma (SBP) and extramedullary plasmacytoma (EMP)
  - SBP
    - Defined by presence of **single lytic lesion of bone** due to monoclonal plasma cell neoplasm, ± soft tissue extension
    - Seen in absence of systemic disease, end organ damage, or other criteria to fulfill diagnosis of MM
    - In skull base, predilection for sphenoid bone and petrous apex
    - Accounts for 5% of plasmacytomas
  - EMP
    - Solitary extraosseous or soft tissue plasma cell proliferation in absence of other criteria to fulfill diagnosis of MM
    - Though closely related to SBP and MM, appears to be distinct entity
    - Soft tissue mass often associated with mucosal surface of sinonasal cavity or nasopharynx with secondary skull base erosion
    - Rarely arises as primary dural-based lesion
    - Accounts for ~ 2% of plasmacytomas
- Solitary plasmacytomas can be further classified based on histologic evaluation of bone marrow aspirate remote from lesion
  - Solitary plasmacytoma without bone marrow plasmacytosis (normal bone marrow distant from lesion)
    - Progression of solitary plasmacytomas to MM in 10% of cases
  - Solitary plasmacytoma with minimal bone marrow plasmacytosis (monoclonal infiltration < 10%)
    - 60% of SBPs will develop into MM
    - 20% of EMPs will transform into MM

IMAGING

General Features
- Best diagnostic clue
  - CT shows solitary intraosseous mass causing **lytic destruction** of skull base
  - MR demonstrates expansile, homogeneously enhancing mass of skull base
  - Imaging features of solitary plasmacytoma is identical to that of individual lesions in MM
- Location
  - SBP: Epicenter is marrow space of sphenoid, temporal (petrous), or occipital bones
    - Soft tissue mass may be isolated to bone
    - Can have significant extraosseous soft tissue component
  - EMP: Involves skull base secondarily when lesion originates in sinonasal cavities, orbit, or nasopharynx
    - Sinonasal region is most common site of origin
    - Predominantly extraosseous with secondary skull base erosion or scalloping
      □ Some authors require absence of bone involvement to classify as EMP
    - EMPs that occur in nasopharynx or sphenoid sinus can invade clivus and be indistinguishable from SBPs
    - Rarely affects dura or leptomeninges primarily
- Size
  - Variable, often large at presentation
- Morphology
  - SBP: Intraosseous mass with biconvex expansion of involved bone, ± extraosseous mass
  - EMP: Infiltrative soft tissue mass adjacent to skull base with secondary osseous erosion

Radiographic Findings
- Radiography
  - SBP: Lucent osseous lesion with nonsclerotic margins
  - EMP: Nonspecific sinus opacification with expansion, bony erosion

CT Findings
- NECT
  - Hyperdense (relative to muscle or brain) soft tissue attenuation
- CECT
  - Mild to moderate, homogeneous enhancement
- Bone CT
  - SBP: Lytic lesion with **scalloped, nonsclerotic margins**
    - No tumoral calcification, but peripherally displaced osseous fragments may be seen

MR Findings
- T1WI
  - Homogeneous, iso- to hypointense to gray matter (GM)
- T2WI
  - Homogeneous, isointense to GM most often
- STIR
  - Homogeneous, iso- or hyperintense to GM
- FLAIR
  - Homogeneous, iso- or hyperintense to GM
- T1WI C+

- Moderate, homogeneous enhancement

Nuclear Medicine Findings
- Bone scan
  - No Tc-99m pertechnetate uptake (cold lesion)
- PET/CT
  - Moderate to marked FDG uptake

Imaging Recommendations
- Best imaging tool
  - Bone CT best defines trabecular and cortical destruction
  - MR best defines marrow extent and extraosseous soft tissue tumor
- Protocol advice
  - MR of skull base to include **multiplanar T1, followed by T1 C+ FS** in same planes for direct comparison
  - Follow with bone CT without contrast to assess bony margins and extent of bone destruction
  - **Whole-body work-up** necessary to confirm isolated nature of solitary plasmacytoma and exclude MM

DIFFERENTIAL DIAGNOSIS

Multiple Myeloma
- Key is identifying additional lesions
- Multiple radiolucent lesions on radiographs and CT
- MR shows additional focal bone marrow lesions or diffuse marrow replacement

Skull Base Metastasis
- Known primary tumor
- Multiple lesions common

Invasive Pituitary Macroadenoma (Pituitary Neuroendocrine Tumor)
- Expansile mass of clivus indistinguishable from pituitary gland
- Predominant growth vector of macroadenoma is inferior into clivus and sphenoid sinus

Chordoma
- Solitary midline clivus lesion
- May contain calcifications or ossific fragments on CT
- Typically very hyperintense on T2 MR

Non-Hodgkin Lymphoma
- Soft tissue mass with bony destruction of skull base
- Secondary invasion of skull base from nasal cavity site of origin

Skull Base Meningioma
- Dural meningioma can invade bony skull base secondarily
- Rarely meningioma originates from intraosseous location
- Permeative, sclerotic expansile, intraosseous mass on CT
- Avid enhancement on CT and MR

Nasopharyngeal Carcinoma
- Mass originates in nasopharyngeal mucosal space
- Destructive upward invasion of basisphenoid and basiocciput

Giant Cell Tumor
- Expansile, intraosseous clival neoplasm arising from multinucleated giant cells

CLINICAL ISSUES

Presentation
- Most common signs/symptoms
  - Highly dependent on lesion location
  - Local pain and headache
  - Various cranial neuropathies

Demographics
- Age
  - Most present in 5th-9th decades
- Sex
  - M > F
  - EMP: Occurs predominately in male patients
- Ethnicity
  - More common in Black patients
- Epidemiology
  - SBP: From all locations, represent only 3-5% of plasma cell neoplasms
  - EMP: **80%** of primary EMPs occur in head & neck

Treatment
- Radiation therapy is mainstay of treatment for solitary lesions
- Follow-up critical to monitor for evolution of MM

DIAGNOSTIC CHECKLIST

Consider
- When plasmacytoma diagnosed, patient needs complete work-up for MM
- **If no MM is present**, then lesion considered **solitary plasmacytoma**
  - Routine follow-up is then employed to watch for possible emergence of MM

Image Interpretation Pearls
- SBP: CT shows solitary intraosseous, osteolytic soft tissue mass with nonsclerotic margins
- Use enhanced MR with fat suppression to exclude additional lesions in commonly overlooked regions
  - Mandibular condyle, greater wing of sphenoid, occipital condyle, calvarium, upper cervical spine

Reporting Tips
- Include broad differential for solitary, expansile clival lesion
- Recommend whole-body work-up, including skeletal survey, MR, or PET/CT to exclude additional lesions

SELECTED REFERENCES

1. Welsh CT et al: Cytology to more clearly distinguish solitary plasmacytoma at the skull base. Diagn Cytopathol. 53(5):E75-9, 2025
2. Elsabah H et al: Skull base plasmacytoma in young patients aged below 40 years: radiological perspectives and clinical outcomes. Cancer Rep (Hoboken). 7(7):e2106, 2024
3. Huang TR et al: Solitary bone plasmacytoma of the skull base with an unusual presentation. Ear Nose Throat J. ePub, 2024
4. Mansouri H et al: Solitary plasmacytoma of the skull base: a case report and literature review. Radiol Case Rep. 18(11):3894-8, 2023
5. Wang J et al: A solitary skull base plasmacytoma mimicking paraganglioma on 68Ga-DOTATATE PET/CT. Clin Nucl Med. 46(1):e18-20, 2021
6. Hillengass J et al: International myeloma working group consensus recommendations on imaging in monoclonal plasma cell disorders. Lancet Oncol. 20(6):e302-12, 2019

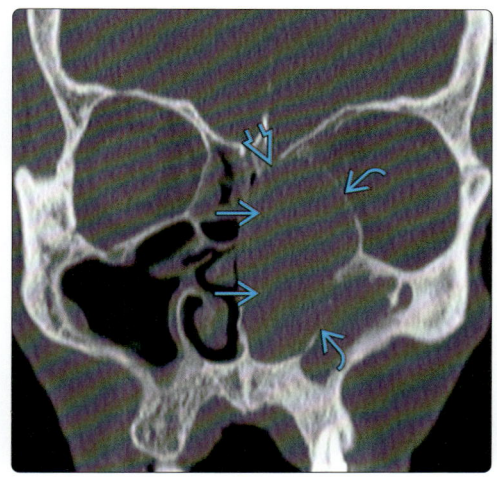

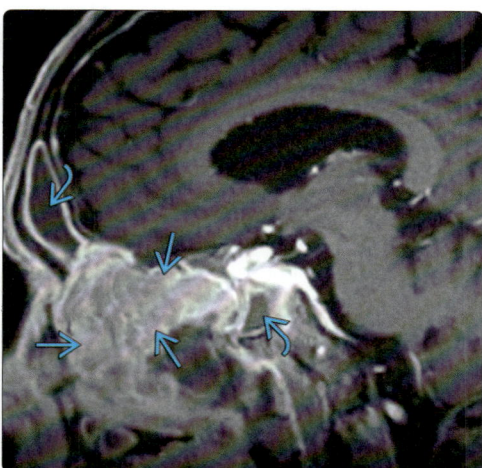

(Left) Coronal MPR NECT bone window shows a large, expansile soft tissue mass centered in the left nasal cavity ➡ with extension to the left ethmoid sinus. Note surrounding bone expansion and remodeling ➡ and erosion of anterior skull base ➡. (Right) Sagittal 3D T1 C+ SPGR MR in the same patient shows moderately enhancing mass at the anterior skull base in the sinonasal region ➡. Note postobstructive secretions in frontal and sphenoid sinus ➡. Biopsy confirmed extramedullary plasmacytoma (EMP).

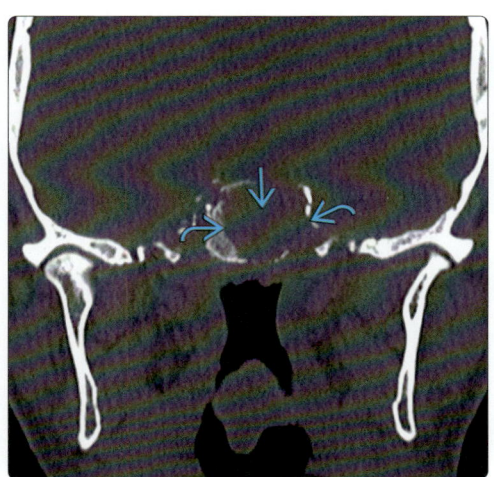

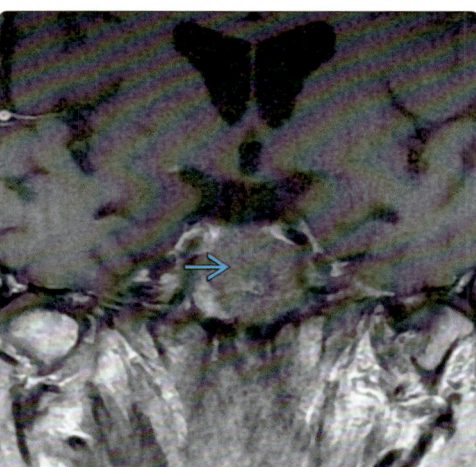

(Left) Coronal MPR NECT bone window in a 65-year-old woman shows a well-delineated lytic lesion ➡ with nonsclerotic margins ➡ involving basisphenoid. (Right) Coronal T1 C+ MR in the same patient shows a moderately enhancing mass ➡ in the central skull base corresponding to lytic lesion seen on CT. Biopsy was consistent with plasmacytoma. SBPs are seen in the absence of systemic disease, end-organ damage, or other criteria to fulfill the diagnosis of multiple myeloma.

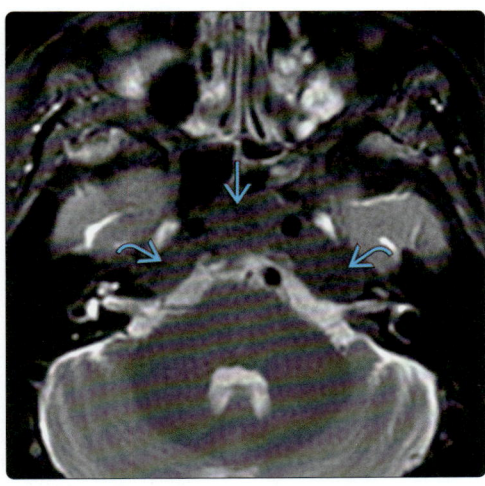

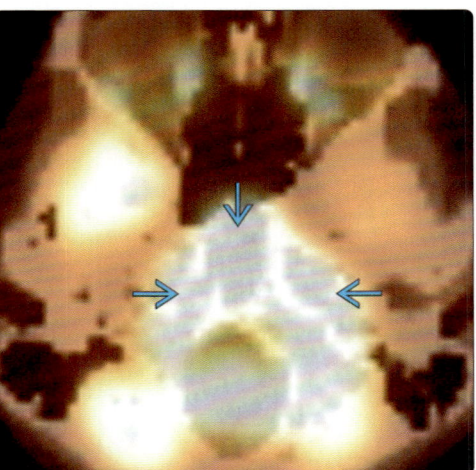

(Left) Axial T2 FS MR in a 68-year-old man shows an iso- to hypointense mass centered in the central skull base along the clivus ➡ extending to adjacent petrous apices bilaterally ➡. (Right) Axial FDG PET/CT in the same patient shows avid FDG uptake in this mass ➡. No other lesion was identified elsewhere in the body. Histopathology revealed plasmacytoma. SBP has a predilection to sphenoid bone and petrous apex.

Skull Base Multiple Myeloma

TERMINOLOGY

- Malignant monoclonal plasma cell proliferation

IMAGING

- CT shows osteolytic lesion(s) of skull base with additional skeletal lesions of calvarium, facial bones, cervical spine, etc.
- MR is most sensitive for evaluation of marrow involvement and assessing soft tissue characteristics
  - Homogeneous, isointense to gray matter on T1 and T2 MR with moderate, diffuse enhancement

TOP DIFFERENTIAL DIAGNOSES

- Skull base metastases
- Non-Hodgkin lymphoma
- Chordoma
- Chondrosarcoma
- Invasive pituitary macroadenoma (pituitary neuroendocrine tumor)

CLINICAL ISSUES

- Most patients > 40 years of age (average: 62)
- M > F (70% vs. 30%)
- Patients have localized pain and cranial neuropathy depending on lesion location
- Systemic symptoms related to anemia, renal failure, hypercalcemia

DIAGNOSTIC CHECKLIST

- Key to imaging diagnosis: Demonstrating multiple marrow-replacing, **osteolytic lesions** on CT or plain films
- **T1 C+ FS MR** to evaluate commonly overlooked regions of skull base and face
  - Clivus, petrous apex, occipital condyle, greater wing of sphenoid, mandibular condyle
- Whole-body imaging is recommended to evaluate for extracranial disease

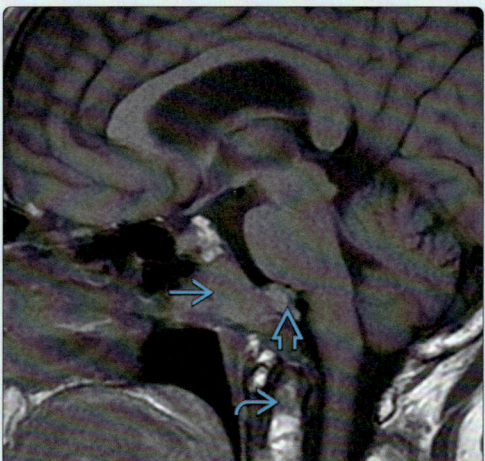
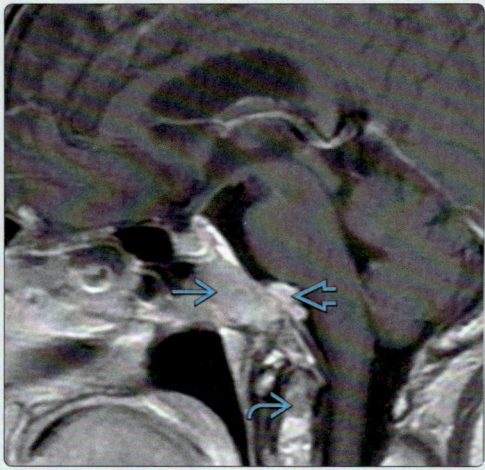

(Left) Sagittal T1 MR in a patient with recurrent multiple myeloma who presented with diplopia shows an infiltrating mass in the clivus ➡ with a small soft tissue bulging into the prepontine/medullary cistern ➡. Note an additional T1-hypointense lesion ➡ in the odontoid process. (Right) Sagittal T1 C+ MR in the same patient shows moderate homogeneous enhancement of the clival mass ➡ extending posteriorly in the prepontine/medullary cistern ➡ and odontoid lesion ➡.

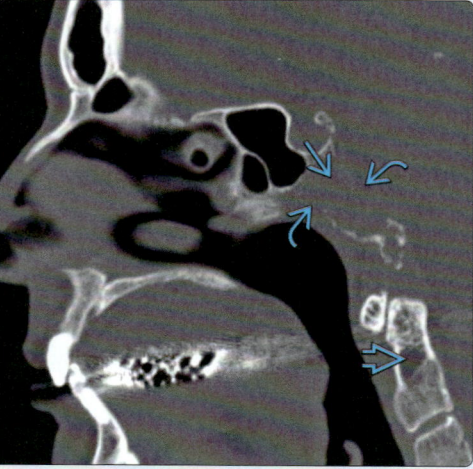
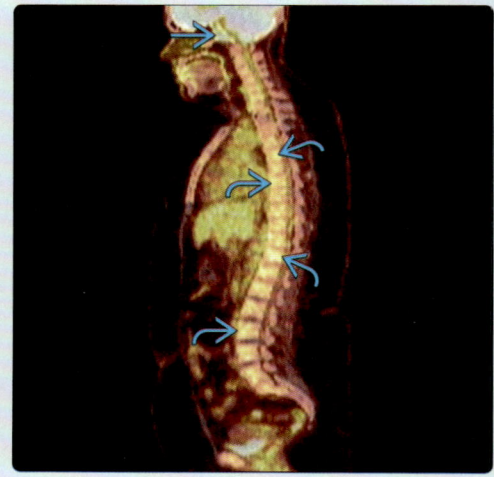

(Left) Sagittal MPR NECT bone window shows a lytic lesion involving the clivus ➡ with cortical bone destruction ➡. Also note an additional lytic lesion in the odontoid process ➡. (Right) Sagittal MPR FDG PET/CT in the same patient shows marked FDG avidity in the skull base mass ➡. Also note numerous foci of FDG uptake through out the spine ➡. These findings are consistent with skull base involvement in a patient with known multiple myeloma.

Skull Base Multiple Myeloma

TERMINOLOGY

Abbreviations
- Multiple myeloma (MM)

Definitions
- Malignant monoclonal plasma cell neoplasm of bone marrow

IMAGING

Imaging Recommendations
- Best imaging tool
  - CT optimally shows **lytic lesions** in osseous skull base and calvarium
  - MR best for detection of marrow-replacing lesions and to evaluate extraosseous soft tissue
- Protocol advice
  - MR of skull base to include multiplanar **T1WI, followed by T1WI C+ FS** in same planes for direct comparison

Radiographic Findings
- Limited value in evaluating skull base
- Classic punched-out lytic lesions of calvaria

CT Findings
- Bone CT
  - Multiple **intraosseous lytic lesions** with nonsclerotic margins

MR Findings
- T1WI
  - Homogeneous, isointense to gray matter (GM)
- T2WI
  - Homogeneous, typically isointense to GM
- DWI
  - Sensitive to marrow malignancy (low ADC)
- T1WI C+ FS
  - Moderate, homogeneous enhancement ± soft tissue extension

Nuclear Medicine Findings
- Bone scan
  - Often little or no uptake of Tc-99m pertechnetate (cold lesion)
- PET
  - Can detect bone marrow lesions and extramedullary lesions with high sensitivity and specificity
  - FDG avidity indicates active disease and can be used to assess treatment response
- PET/CT
  - 90% sensitive and specific for focal MM
- Tc-99m MIBI
  - Radiotracer accumulates inside plasma cells infiltrating bone marrow
  - > 90% sensitivity and specificity for marrow and extramedullary lesions

DIFFERENTIAL DIAGNOSIS

Skull Base Metastases
- Often late stage with known primary extracranial neoplasm

Non-Hodgkin Lymphoma
- Lymphoproliferative neoplasm with focal or multifocal, osseous &/or extraosseous involvement of skull base

Chordoma
- Solitary, expansile clival mass with marked T2 hyperintensity

Chondrosarcoma
- Solitary, expansile, destructive paramidline or midline skull base mass, typically with significant T2 hyperintensity

Invasive Pituitary Macroadenoma (Pituitary Neuroendocrine Tumor)
- Benign lesion with invasion inferiorly into clivus

CLINICAL ISSUES

Presentation
- Most common signs/symptoms
  - Pain at site of lesion
  - Site-dependent cranial neuropathy
  - Diplopia, compressive optic neuropathy

Demographics
- Age
  - Majority > 40 years (average: 62)
- Sex
  - M > F (70% vs. 30%)
- Epidemiology
  - Associated with exposure to radiation and agricultural agents (pesticides)

Treatment
- Oral regimen of melphalan and prednisone has been mainstay of therapy
  - Newer treatments include thalidomide, bortezomib, lenalidomide
- Autologous stem cell transplantation prolongs survival

DIAGNOSTIC CHECKLIST

Image Interpretation Pearls
- T1 C+ FS MR to evaluate commonly overlooked regions of skull base and face
  - Petrous apex, mandibular condyle, occipital condyle, greater wing of sphenoid

Reporting Tips
- Can be difficult to differentiate MM from metastatic disease
- If skull base and calvarial lesions identified, whole-body imaging recommended to evaluate for additional lesions

SELECTED REFERENCES

1. Chen Y et al: Immunoglobulin D-lambda multiple myeloma initially presenting in the sphenoid sinus, orbital apex, and skull base: a systematic review with a case report. J Neurol Surg Rep. 85(3):e144-55, 2024
2. Lesar U et al: Multiple myeloma in a young female presenting as an aggressive skull-base tumour. SA J Radiol. 28(1):2883, 2024
3. Lin CH et al: Current novel targeted therapeutic strategies in multiple myeloma. Int J Mol Sci. 25(11), 2024
4. Virk J et al: Imaging in multiple myeloma. Presse Med. 54(1):104263, 2024

TERMINOLOGY

- Metastatic disease affecting osseous skull base &/or adjacent dura

IMAGING

- Enhancing, destructive mass of osseous skull base in patient with **known extracranial primary malignancy**
- Often dominant lesion seen in context of multiple additional skeletal lesions affecting skull base, calvarium, spine, etc.
- MR most sensitive modality
  - **Osseous metastasis**: Enhancing marrow space mass ± extraosseous extension
  - **Dural metastasis**: Enhancing, infiltrating, dural-based lesion
- Noncontrast T1 & T1 C+ FS MR best sequences
- CT shows variable pattern of cortical and trabecular bone involvement: Lytic, permeative, sclerotic

TOP DIFFERENTIAL DIAGNOSES

- Multiple myeloma
- Non-Hodgkin lymphoma
- Skull base meningioma
- Solitary central skull base mass
  - Invasive pituitary adenoma, chordoma, chondrosarcoma

PATHOLOGY

- Cancer sources: Breast (40%) > lung (14%) > prostate (12%)

CLINICAL ISSUES

- Skull base metastases from extracranial primaries occur in 4% of cancer patients

DIAGNOSTIC CHECKLIST

- Consider metastatic disease if skull base lesion seen in patient with known malignancy who develops craniofacial pain or cranial neuropathy
- Look for additional skeletal/osseous lesions of cervical spine, skull base, calvarium

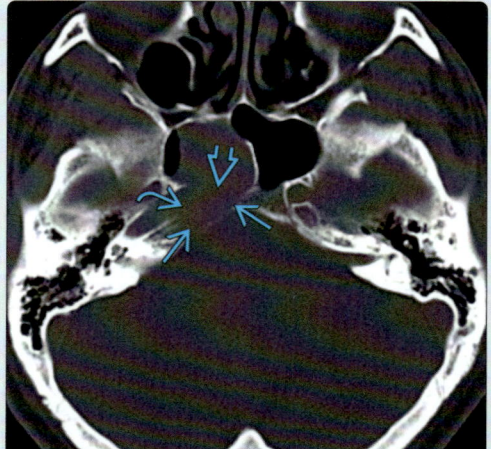
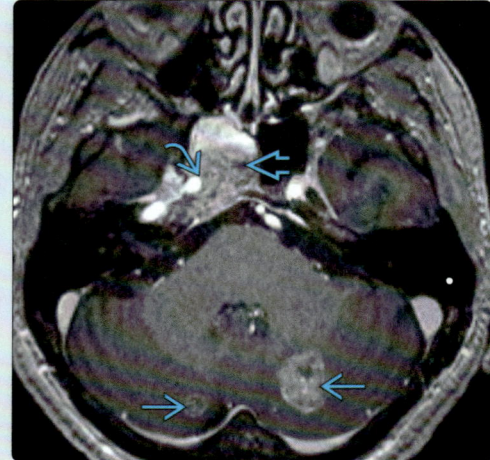

(Left) Axial NECT bone window in a patient with renal cell carcinoma shows a lytic lesion ⇨ involving the right petrous apex and adjacent clivus ⇨. There is erosion of the carotid canal and posterior wall of sphenoid sinus ⇨. (Right) Axial 3D T1 C+ SPGR MR in the same patient shows enhancing mass in the skull base with soft tissue protruding into sphenoid sinus ⇨ and partially encasing right petrous internal carotid artery (ICA) ⇨. Additional enhancing lesions in both cerebellar hemispheres ⇨ are consistent with metastasis.

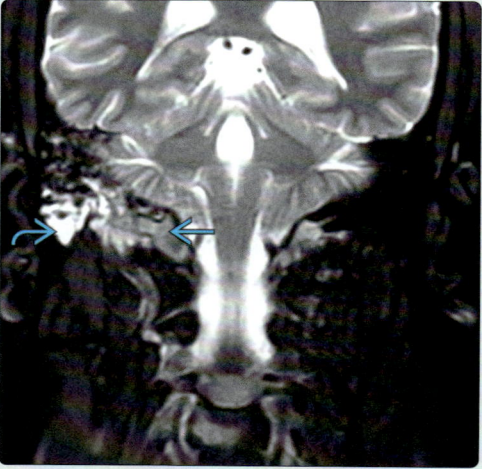
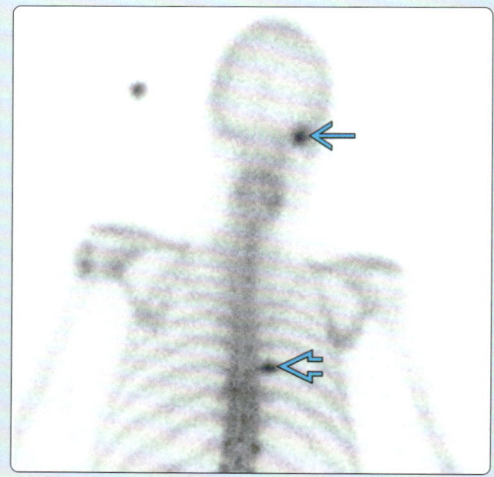

(Left) Coronal T2 FS MR in a 52-year-old woman with a history of breast cancer shows hyperintense focal marrow signal in the right occipital condyle ⇨ and adjacent petrous temporal bone. Also note right mastoid effusion ⇨. (Right) Posterior whole-body planar Tc-99m bone scan in the same patient shows focal radiotracer uptake at the right skull base corresponding to a lesion seen on MR ⇨. Additional focal tracer activity in the right posterior 7th rib ⇨ is consistent with metastasis.

Skull Base Metastasis

TERMINOLOGY

Definitions

- Metastatic disease affecting osseous skull base &/or adjacent soft tissue structures, including dura

IMAGING

General Features

- Best diagnostic clue
  - Enhancing, destructive mass of osseous skull base in patient with **known extracranial primary malignancy**
  - Often dominant lesion seen in context of multiple osseous lesions affecting skull base, calvarium, spine, etc.
- Location
  - Osseous
    - Occurs where bone marrow is most abundant: Clivus, nonpneumatized petrous apex, and greater wing of sphenoid
  - Dural
    - Occurs anywhere along dura of anterior, central, or posterior skull base
- Size
  - Often large, dominant, symptomatic lesion with subsequent detection of **additional lesions**
  - Small, "strategically located" lesions can affect cranial nerves and produce neurologic deficit

Imaging Recommendations

- Best imaging tool
  - CT and MR are complimentary
    - Enhanced MR best evaluates marrow signal abnormality and enhancement and soft tissue involvement
    - Bone CT is variable, ranging from destructive, lytic lesions to sclerotic lesions
- Protocol advice
  - Axial and coronal **precontrast T1 MR without FS** identifies low-signal marrow lesions
  - **T1 C+ FS MR** in identical planes to demonstrate osseous and extraosseous tumor

CT Findings

- Bone CT
  - Variable pattern of cortical and trabecular bone involvement: Lytic, permeative, sclerotic, mixed patterns

MR Findings

- T1WI
  - Hypointense marrow lesion **replaces high-signal fat**
- T2WI
  - Variable marrow signal depending on cellularity &/or sclerosis
- T1WI C+ FS
  - Enhancing marrow space mass ± extraosseous extension
  - Pearl: Without FS, ↑ signal of enhancing tumor may be inconspicuous against background of ↑ signal from normal fat

Nuclear Medicine Findings

- PET/CT
  - Combination of lytic-destructive lesions on CT with moderate to marked FDG uptake

DIFFERENTIAL DIAGNOSIS

Multiple Myeloma

- Plasma cell neoplasm
- Multiple enhancing lytic lesions of skull base & calvarium

Non-Hodgkin Lymphoma

- Lymphoproliferative neoplasm
- Can have multifocal extranodal & extralymphatic lesions of skull base and dura

Skull Base Meningioma

- Primary dural-based, enhancing neoplasm(s) with secondary sclerosis or invasion of skull base
- May be multiple & mimic metastatic disease

Solitary Central Skull Base Mass

- Invasive pituitary macroadenoma
- Chordoma
- Chondrosarcoma

Idiopathic Inflammatory Pseudotumor

- Enhancing, nonneoplastic fibroinflammatory process of orbital apex, cavernous sinus, or skull base

PATHOLOGY

General Features

- Etiology
  - Source of metastases: Breast cancer (40%) > lung cancer (14%) > prostate cancer (12%)

CLINICAL ISSUES

Presentation

- Most common signs/symptoms
  - Headache, craniofacial pain, & progressive unilateral cranial neuropathy

Demographics

- Epidemiology
  - Skull base metastasis from extracranial primaries occurs in 4% of cancer patients

Treatment

- Radiation therapy is mainstay of treatment for focal/isolated disease

DIAGNOSTIC CHECKLIST

Image Interpretation Pearls

- In metastatic evaluation of brain, remember to include osseous skull base and adjacent dura in search pattern

SELECTED REFERENCES

1. Wang Y et al: Skull base metastasis of uterine carcinosarcoma mimicking primary carcinoma of the middle ear. Clin Nucl Med. 50(5):419-20, 2025
2. Cheung IHW et al: Case report of large solitary skull base metastasis from renal cell carcinoma as initial clinical presentation: radiological findings and differentials. Radiol Case Rep. 19(11):5376-9, 2024
3. Dutta S et al: Metastasis to the skull base involving the sphenoid and cavernous sinus in hepatocellular carcinoma. J R Coll Physicians Edinb. 54(3):221-4, 2024

Skull Base Chondrosarcoma

TERMINOLOGY

- Skull base chondrosarcoma (CSa-SB): Chondroid malignancy of skull base

IMAGING

- Typical location **off-midline**, centered on **petrooccipital fissure**
- CT
  - Characteristic **chondroid tumor matrix calcification in 50%**
  - Arc or ring-like calcifications
  - Sharp, narrow, nonsclerotic transition zone to adjacent normal bone
- MR
  - High T2 signal with scattered hypointense foci (calcifications)
  - Heterogeneously enhancing
  - Whorls of enhancing lines within tumor matrix often seen

TOP DIFFERENTIAL DIAGNOSES

- Chordoma
- Skull base metastasis
- Plasmacytoma
- Nasopharyngeal carcinoma (invasive)
- Meningioma
- Benign petrous apex lesions

CLINICAL ISSUES

- Typically, middle-aged patient with insidious onset of headache and cranial nerve palsies (especially CNVI)

DIAGNOSTIC CHECKLIST

- Is lesion **off-midline** (CSa) or in midline (chordoma)?
- Do calcifications represent **arc-whorl intralesional calcifications** (CSa) or fragmented destroyed bone (chordoma)?
- Consider MR angiography or CTA for preoperative characterization of vessel involvement

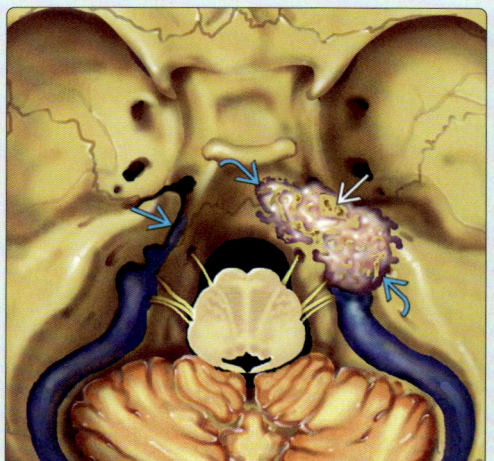
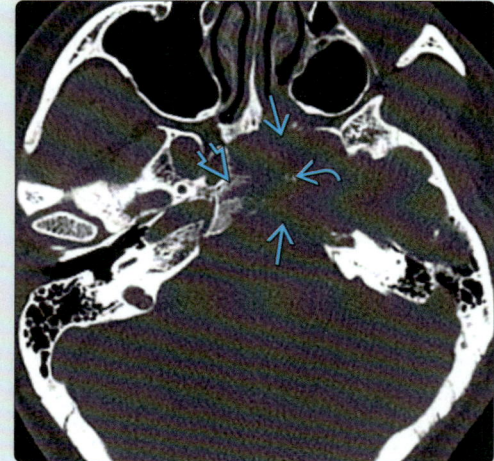

(Left) Axial graphic depicts the classic location of a chondrosarcoma of the skull base centered in the left petrooccipital fissure ➡. Note the normal right petrooccipital fissure ➡. Chondroid calcifications, depicted in yellow, are present within the lesion ➡. (Right) Axial bone window NECT in a 58-year-old man with diplopia shows a large soft tissue mass centered left of the midline in the region of petroclival fissure ➡. Note subtle internal calcifications ➡ and a normal right petroclival fissure ➡.

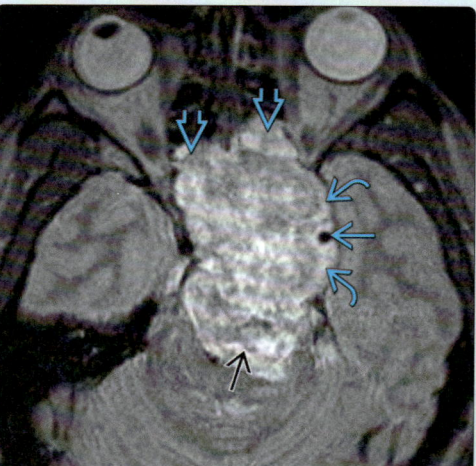
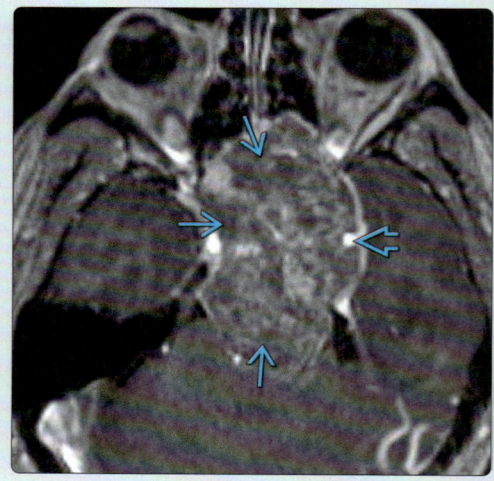

(Left) Axial 3D T2 SPACE MR in the same patient shows a large, well-circumscribed, heterogeneous hyperintense mass with extension to the left cavernous sinus ➡ encasing the interior auditory canal (IAC) ➡ anteriorly into the ethmoids ➡ and posteriorly to the prepontine cistern ➡ with mass effect on the pons. (Right) Axial 3D T1 C+ SPGR MR in the same patient shows heterogeneous, mild enhancement of the mass ➡ with normal enhancement of left ICA ➡.

TERMINOLOGY

Abbreviations
- Skull base chondrosarcoma (CSa-SB)

Definitions
- CSa-SB: Rare, slow-growing but locally aggressive chondroid tumors of skull base

IMAGING

General Features
- Best diagnostic clue
  - Solitary enhancing osteolytic soft tissue mass, centered at petrooccipital fissure (POF) ± chondroid matrix
- Location
  - Off-midline at **POF** (2/3)
  - Anterior basisphenoid (1/3)
- Size
  - Variable, usually > 3 cm at time of diagnosis
- Morphology
  - Well-circumscribed, lobulated margins

CT Findings
- NECT
  - Soft tissue component is relatively dense
- CECT
  - Variable, heterogeneous enhancement
- Bone CT
  - Expansile mass at POF producing erosive or destructive bone changes in clivus and petrous apex
  - ~ 50% will have radiographically classic chondroid matrix with **"rings and arcs" calcification**
  - Sharp, narrow, nonsclerotic transition zone to adjacent normal bone

MR Findings
- T1WI
  - Low to intermediate signal intensity relative to gray matter
    - ↓ signal foci within tumor may suggest underlying coarse matrix mineralization or fibrocartilaginous elements
- T2WI
  - Variable, usually **high signal**
  - Hypointense foci (calcifications) less conspicuous than on CT
- T1WI C+
  - Heterogeneous enhancement

Angiographic Findings
- Avascular or hypovascular mass
- Internal carotid artery displacement ± encasement

Imaging Recommendations
- Best imaging tool
  - Combination of multiplanar, gadolinium-enhanced MR and high-resolution bone CT
- Protocol advice
  - High-resolution axial bone CT for evaluation of chondroid matrix and pattern of bone destruction
  - MR of skull base to include T2WI and multiplanar T1WI, followed by T1WI C+ FS in same planes for direct comparison
  - MRA and MRV, or CTA helpful to assess vascular involvement preoperatively
    - Carotid injury risk higher for endoscopic resection of CSa-SB

DIFFERENTIAL DIAGNOSIS

Chordoma
- Destructive clival lesion; bone fragments within matrix
- Midline > lateral location
- Low T1 and markedly high T2 MR signal; enhancing mass
- Chondroid chordomas more aggressive and worse prognosis
- May be impossible to distinguish chordoma from chondrosarcoma on routine imaging

Skull Base Metastasis
- Bone CT: Destructive mass that can be anywhere in skull base
- MR: Often multiple enhancing, invasive lesions
- Typically low to intermediate T2 signal
- Known primary tumor

Plasmacytoma & Multiple Myeloma
- Usually more midline, within clivus
- **T2 signal is low** to intermediate
- > 50% have concurrent multiple myeloma
  - Multiple lesions of skull base or calvarium generally exclude CSa-SB

Nasopharyngeal Carcinoma
- Primary mass in nasopharyngeal mucosal space
- Tumor invades superiorly to clivus, foramen lacerum, and POF

Meningioma
- Calcification in meningioma can mimic chondroid matrix
- Hyperostosis possible; not typically destructive in absence of invasion
- Low to intermediate T2 MR signal; enhancing with dural tails

Non-Hodgkin Lymphoma
- Lymphoproliferative neoplasm with focal or multifocal, osseous &/or extraosseous involvement of skull base
- Low to intermediate T2 MR signal, may restrict on DWI

Chondromyxoid Fibroma
- Rare, expansile, noninfiltrating skull base mass
- Areas of ground-glass density may be seen

PATHOLOGY

General Features
- Etiology
  - Arises from remnants of embryonal cartilage, endochondral bone, or from primitive mesenchymal cells in meninges
    - May arise from metaplasia of meningeal fibroblasts
- Genetics
  - May complicate Ollier disease and Maffucci syndrome

o *IDH1* and *IDH2* gene mutations seen in 50% of cases
o *TP53* mutations common

Staging, Grading, & Classification

- Classification
  o Conventional CSa: Hyaline (7%), myxoid (30%), or mixed (63%)
  o Clear cell
  o Mesenchymal
  o Dedifferentiated
- WHO grading from 1 to 3
  o Based on degree of cellularity, pleomorphism, mitoses, and multinucleated cells

Microscopic Features

- Hypercellular tumor composed of chondrocytes with hyperchromatic, pleomorphic nuclei and prominent nucleoli
  o Binucleate or multinucleate cells are rule
- Hyaline matrix may calcify in "ringlets"
  o Intercellular matrix is solid in hyaline type compared to mucinous/gelatinous matrix in myxoid or mixed types
- Histology may overlap with or be confused with that of chordoma
  o Histology particularly confusing in chondroid chordoma, myxoid CSa
  o Differentiation facilitated by immunohistochemical staining

CLINICAL ISSUES

Presentation

- Most common signs/symptoms
  o **Abducens (CNVI) palsy** due to proximity of Dorello canal
  o **Headache**
  o Mean duration of symptoms at diagnosis = 27 months
- Other signs/symptoms
  o Other cranial nerve palsies (CNIII, V, VII, VIII)
- Clinical profile
  o Middle-aged patient with insidious onset of headaches and cranial nerve palsies

Demographics

- Age
  o Range: 10-80 years
  o Mean: 40 years
- Epidemiology
  o 6% of all skull base tumors
  o 75% of all cranial CSa occur in skull base

Natural History & Prognosis

- Prognosis depends on extent at diagnosis, histologic grade, and completeness of surgical resection
  o Disease-specific 10-year survival rates of 99% recently reported
  o Most central CSa-SBs are well to moderately differentiated
  o High-grade CSa metastasizes to bones and lung more frequently
- Conventional CSa: Indolent growth pattern
  o Most are slow growing, locally invasive, but rarely metastasize

- Mesenchymal and dedifferentiated forms: Aggressive behavior; poor prognosis

Treatment

- Maximal safe surgical resection treatment of choice
  o Often via expanded endoscopic endonasal approach ± multilayer skull base repair
  o Basal subfrontal approach used for tumor that invades clivus and extends anteriorly into sphenoid and ethmoid sinuses
  o Subtemporal and preauricular infratemporal approach used when CSa extends laterally beyond petrous internal carotid artery
- Combined radical resection and postoperative, high-dose, fractionated precision conformal radiation therapy most often utilized
  o Postoperative adjuvant radiation therapy frequently administered, usually with particle therapy, such as proton beam therapy (PBT)
  o Compared with photon therapy, PBT enables dose escalation while limiting damage to dose-limiting neurologic structures, particularly brainstem and optic apparatus
    – Due to energy deposition being delivered at high maximum with rapid decrease at end of penetration range (Bragg peak phenomenon)
  o Essential requirements for PBT following gross total or maximal safe resection
    – Tissue diagnosis, minimal residual tumor after resection, and adequate clearance from PBT dose-limiting structures (≥ 3 mm from brainstem and ≥ 5 mm from optic apparatus)

DIAGNOSTIC CHECKLIST

Consider

- Is lesion in off-midline (CSa) vs. midline (chordoma)?
- Do calcifications represent arc-whorl intralesional calcifications (CSa) or fragmented destroyed bone (chordoma)?
- Does patient have known primary neoplasm (metastasis), myeloma (plasmacytoma), or nasopharyngeal mass (nasopharyngeal carcinoma)?

Image Interpretation Pearls

- Classic appearance: Heterogeneously enhancing tumor located at **POF** with hyperintense signal on T2 MR
  o CT shows chondroid mineralization and bone destruction
- When no tumor matrix found, difficult to tell from CSa plasmacytoma, focal metastasis, or chondromyxoid fibroma

SELECTED REFERENCES

1. Yu J et al: Asymptomatic chondrosarcoma of the skull base: a case report. Ear Nose Throat J. 104(1):NP29-33, 2025
2. Miladinovic V et al: Robust IMPT and follow-up toxicity in skull base chordoma and chondrosarcoma-a single-institution clinical experience. Strahlenther Onkol. 200(12):1066-73, 2024
3. Nakamura M et al: A systematic review and meta-analysis of radiotherapy and particle beam therapy for skull base chondrosarcoma: TRP-chondrosarcoma 2024. Front Oncol. 14:1380716, 2024
4. Potter GM et al: Skull base chordoma and chondrosarcoma: neuroradiologist's guide to diagnosis, surgical management, and proton beam therapy. Radiographics. 44(10):e240036, 2024

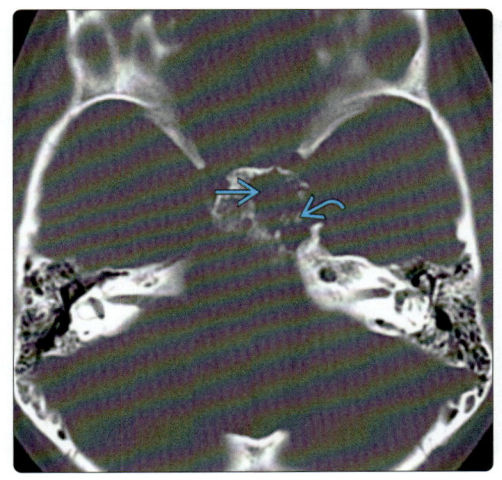

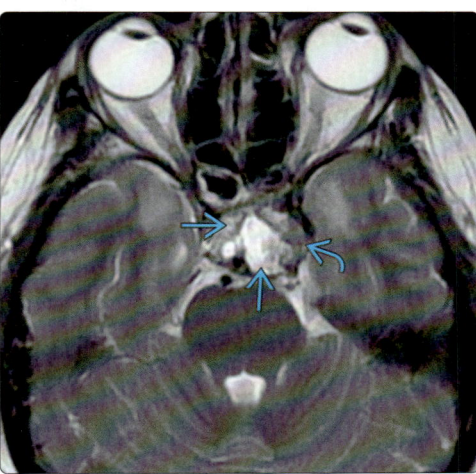

(Left) Axial bone window NECT shows a lytic lesion ➡ with internal calcific densities ➡ centered left of the midline in the petroclival fissure region. Approximately 50% of these tumors show chondroid matrix calcifications, typically described as the rings and arc type of calcifications. (Right) Axial T2 MR in the same patient shows an expansile, heterogeneous, hyperintense mass ➡ corresponding to a lytic lesion on CT. Note mild extension to the left cavernous sinus ➡.

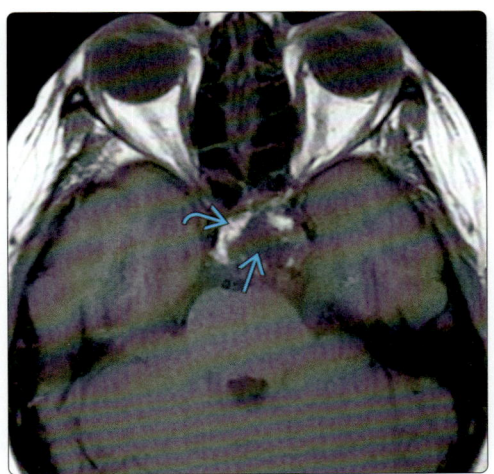

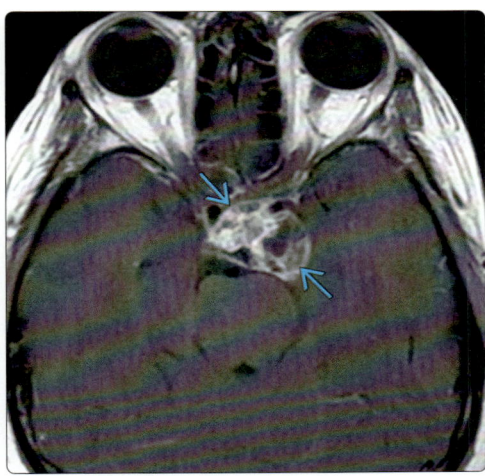

(Left) Axial T1 MR in the same patient shows the mass is predominantly hypointense ➡ and shows patchy areas of internal hyperintensities ➡. Common clinical presentations include CNVI palsy and headache. (Right) Axial T1 C+ MR in the same patient shows heterogeneous enhancement of the mass ➡. Biopsy revealed low-grade chondrosarcoma. This patient underwent maximal safe resection followed by proton beam radiation.

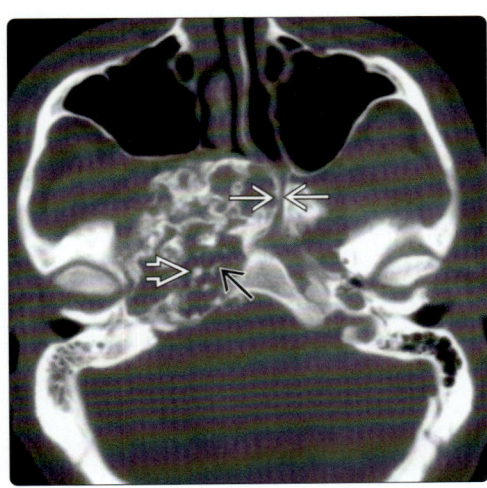

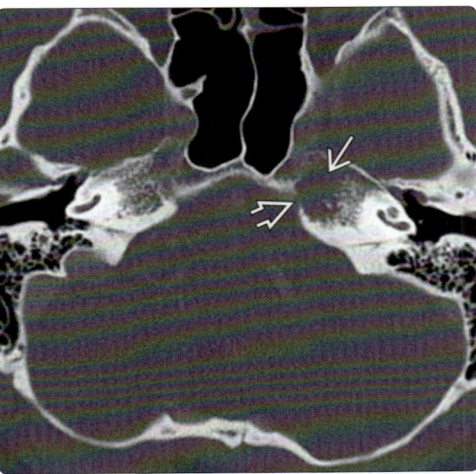

(Left) Axial bone CT shows rounded ➡ and arc-like ➡ calcified foci in this large chondrosarcoma centered at the petrooccipital fissure. Up to 50% of chondrosarcomas demonstrate matrix calcification. Note slight narrowing of the left vidian canal ➡. (Right) Axial bone window CT shows subtle bone destruction ➡ with cortical erosion ➡ in this small left petrous apex chondrosarcoma. No calcified matrix is seen. MR showed a corresponding T2-hyperintense and enhancing mass in this location.

Skull Base Osteosarcoma

TERMINOLOGY

- Neoplasm composed of malignant cells producing osteoid matrix or immature bone

IMAGING

- Very rare in skull base → clivus, parasellar, sphenoid wing, and anterior skull base
- CT findings
  - Often destructive and expansile
  - May be **lytic** or **blastic**
  - May show **tumor bone formation** and periosteal reaction
- MR findings
  - Heterogeneous low to intermediate T1 signal
  - Intermediate to high T2 signal; bone components ↓ T2 signal
  - Marrow/soft tissue enhancement

TOP DIFFERENTIAL DIAGNOSES

- Chordoma
- Chondrosarcoma
- Metastatic disease
- Plasmacytoma
- Non-Hodgkin lymphoma
- Invasive macroadenoma

PATHOLOGY

- May occur as late effect of previous irradiation
- Associated with Paget disease, fibrous dysplasia, giant cell tumor, Ollier disease, chronic osteomyelitis

CLINICAL ISSUES

- Nonspecific symptoms: Swelling, pain
- Present in 3rd-4th decades; M = F
- Difficult to completely resect due to proximity to critical structures within skull base
- Relatively resistant to XRT

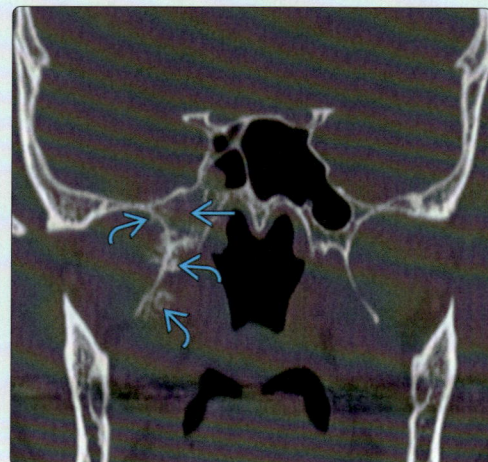
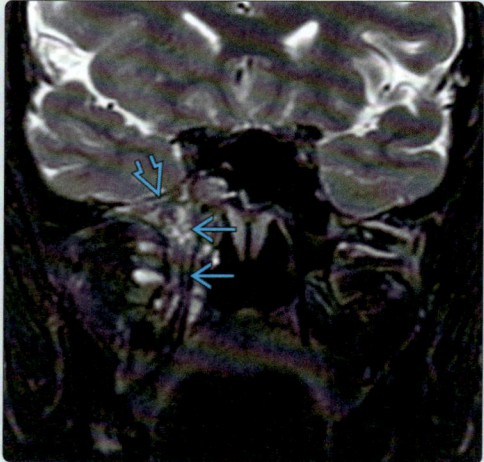

(Left) Coronal NECT MPR bone window in a patient with a remote history of nasopharyngeal cancer treated with radiation therapy and now presenting with biopsy-proven radiation-induced osteogenic sarcoma shows permeative changes in the root of the right pterygoid ➡ and hairy periosteal reaction ➡ extending to the lateral pterygoid plate. (Right) Coronal T2 FS MR in the same patient shows altered marrow signal in the right pterygoid ➡ and greater wing of sphenoid ➡.

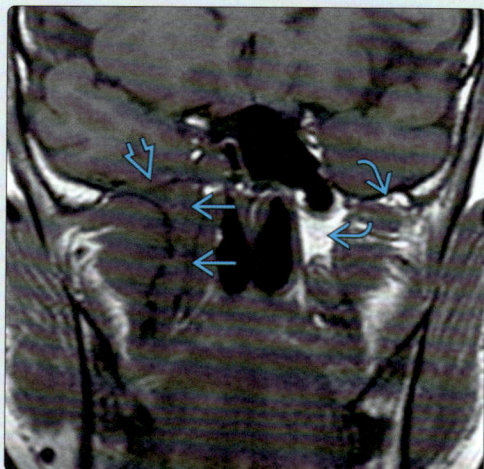
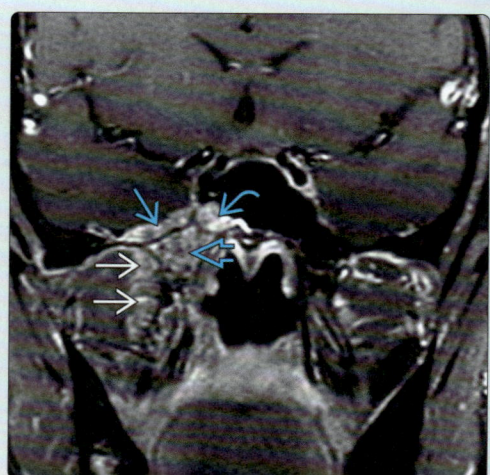

(Left) Coronal T1 MR in the same patient shows marrow replacement process in the right pterygoid ➡ and adjacent greater wing of sphenoid ➡. Note normal fatty marrow in the left pterygoid and greater wing of sphenoid ➡. (Right) Coronal T1 C+ MR in the same patient shows heterogeneous marrow enhancement in the right pterygoid and greater wing of sphenoid ➡. Note enhancing soft tissue along the dura ➡, sphenoid sinus ➡ and skull base soft tissues ➡.

TERMINOLOGY

Abbreviations

- Osteosarcoma of skull base (OSa-SB)

Definitions

- Neoplasm composed of malignant spindle cells producing osteoid matrix or immature bone

IMAGING

General Features

- Best diagnostic clue
  - Aggressive, ill-defined mass arising from bone with soft tissue and **osteoid matrix**
- Location
  - Occurs rarely in skull base: Clivus, sphenoid-sella, greater sphenoid wing, anterior skull base

Imaging Recommendations

- Best imaging tool
  - Multiplanar contrast-enhanced MR best for evaluating marrow space and soft tissue involvement
  - Bone CT shows internal osteoid matrix and periosteal reaction to better advantage

CT Findings

- Bone CT
  - Expansile mass may be **lytic** or **blastic**
  - May show **tumor bone formation** or malignant periosteal reaction (sun burst/hairy pattern)

MR Findings

- T1WI
  - Heterogeneous, low to intermediate signal
- T2WI
  - Heterogeneous, intermediate to high T2 signal with densely ossified components showing ↓ signal
- T1WI C+ FS
  - Marrow/soft tissue components show enhancement

DIFFERENTIAL DIAGNOSIS

Chordoma

- Midline clival mass; hyperintense on T2WI MR

Chondrosarcoma

- Expansile mass at petrooccipital fissure (POF) producing erosive or destructive bone changes in clivus and petrous apex
- 50% will have radiographically classic chondroid matrix with **rings and arcs** of calcification

Skull Base Metastasis

- Patient has known primary neoplasm; lesions often multiple

Plasmacytoma

- Solitary or multiple if in setting of multiple myeloma
- Homogeneous, lytic, and well defined

Invasive Macroadenoma

- Can be significantly or predominantly invasive to clivus
- Cannot distinguish pituitary gland from mass

PATHOLOGY

General Features

- Etiology
  - Primary etiology unknown
  - May occur secondary to **prior irradiation**
- Associated abnormalities
  - May be associated with Paget disease, fibrous dysplasia, giant cell tumor, solitary or multiple osteochondroma, enchondroma, Ollier disease

Staging, Grading, & Classification

- Classification based upon histology: Osteoblastic, chondroblastic, fibroblastic, telangiectatic, and juxtacortical types
- Grading (low, intermediate, high) based on degree of cellular atypia and recognizable histologic architecture

Microscopic Features

- Osteoid production by atypical neoplastic osteoblasts

CLINICAL ISSUES

Presentation

- Most common signs/symptoms
  - Swelling, mass, and pain
- Other signs/symptoms
  - Cranial nerve deficits

Demographics

- Age
  - 3rd-4th decades
- Sex
  - M = F
- Epidemiology
  - Most common primary bone malignancy overall but only 6-10% in head & neck

Natural History & Prognosis

- Poor overall survival

Treatment

- Maximal safe surgical resection with adjuvant radiation

SELECTED REFERENCES

1. Khalil Y et al: A rare case of osteoblastic osteosarcoma of the temporal bone and comprehensive review of the literature. Otol Neurotol. 46(5):e198-201, 2025
2. Matsuda Y et al: A case of radiation-induced osteosarcoma with RB1 gene alteration treated by skull base surgery and craniofacial reconstruction. Acta Med Okayama. 77(1):85-90, 2023
3. Sharin F et al: Management of osteosarcoma of the head and neck. Curr Opin Otolaryngol Head Neck Surg. 31(4):269-75, 2023
4. Machoň V et al: Reconstruction of temporomandibular joint and skull base defect following osteosarcoma resection. J Craniofac Surg. 33(7):e667-9, 2022
5. Bin Alamer O et al: Primary and radiation induced skull base osteosarcoma: a systematic review of clinical features and treatment outcomes. J Neurooncol. 153(2):183-202, 2021
6. Kappel AD et al: Radiation-induced intracranial osteosarcoma of the anterior skull base after treatment of esthesioneuroblastoma. BMJ Case Rep. 14(1), 2021
7. Merna C et al: Determinants of survival in skull base osteosarcoma: a national cancer database study. World Neurosurg. 151:e828-38, 2021
8. Washington NR et al: Osteosarcoma of the skull base presenting as a petrocavernous pseudoaneurysm and masquerading as an intracranial abscess: illustrative case. J Neurosurg Case Lessons. 2(1):CASE20148, 2021

Skull Base Osteomyelitis

TERMINOLOGY

- Skull base osteomyelitis (SBO)
- Severe infection of temporal, sphenoid, ± occipital bone causing bone destruction
- Typical SBO: Temporal bone involved initially, most often from necrotizing external otitis (NEO)
- Atypical SBO: Usually secondary to invasive sinusitis or deep face infection; can be idiopathic

IMAGING

- Ill-defined, infiltrative process involving temporal bone &/or central skull base
  - CT demonstrates cortical erosion and destruction
  - MR shows abnormal marrow signal and enhancement
  - Extraosseous inflammation mimics neoplasm

TOP DIFFERENTIAL DIAGNOSES

- Metastatic disease of skull base
- Nasopharyngeal carcinoma
- Non-Hodgkin lymphoma of skull base

PATHOLOGY

- **Pseudomonas** #1 pathogen (in typical SBO/NEO)
- **Bacterial or fungal** (*Mucor* and *Aspergillus*) in atypical SBO

CLINICAL ISSUES

- Most often seen in **immunocompromised** patients, especially **older adult diabetic patients**
- Elevated erythrocyte sedimentation rate (ESR)
- Indolent course and nonspecific symptoms, difficult to diagnose clinically
- High morbidity and mortality despite intensive antibiotic therapy

DIAGNOSTIC CHECKLIST

- **Bone CT and enhanced MR** best evaluate osseous destruction and marrow involvement
- Consider SBO for any infiltrative skull base process if **biopsies negative for malignancy**

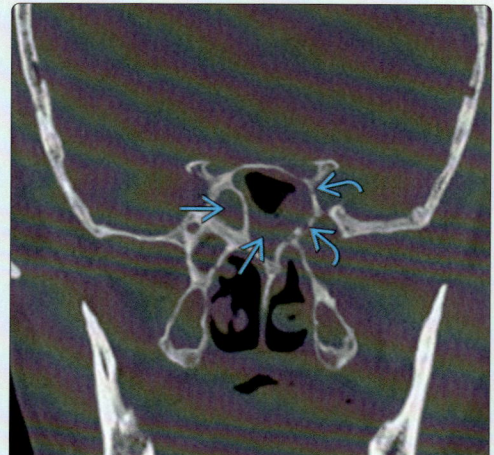
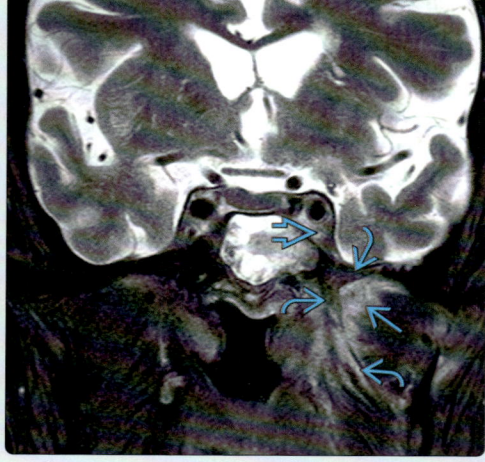

(Left) Coronal MPR NECT bone window in a patient with a history of uncontrolled diabetes with worsening headaches and new-onset diplopia shows mucosal thickening in the sphenoid sinus ➡ with subtle cortical erosive changes in the left lateral and inferolateral walls ⮕. (Right) Coronal T2 FS MR in the same patient shows marrow edema along the left pterygoid and adjacent greater wing of the sphenoid ⮕. Note soft tissue edema at the skull base ➡ and fullness of the left cavernous sinus ➡.

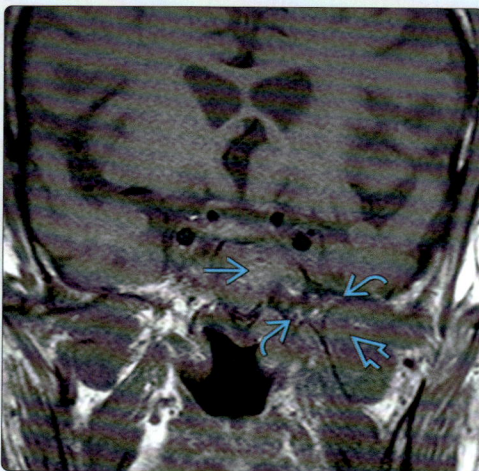
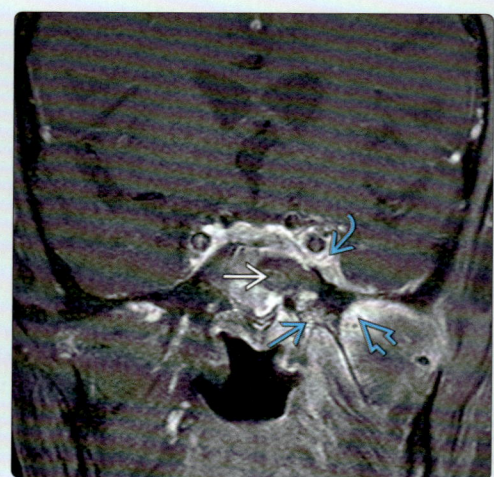

(Left) Coronal T1 MR in the same patient shows low signal in the left pterygoid and greater wing of sphenoid ⮕. Note subtle hyperintensity in the sphenoid sinus ➡ with loss of fat plane at skull base soft tissues ⮕. (Right) Coronal T1 C+ FS MR shows heterogeneous marrow enhancement ⮕ and skull base soft tissues ⮕. Note phlegmonus changes in left cavernous sinus ➡ and a nonenhancing area in sphenoid sinus ➡ due to fungal elements. Biopsy = skull base osteomyelitis (SBO) due to invasive aspergillosis.

TERMINOLOGY

Abbreviations

- Skull base osteomyelitis (SBO)

Definitions

- SBO: Severe infection of temporal, sphenoid, &/or occipital bone that results in osseous destruction &/or marrow space involvement
- **Typical SBO**: Infection involves temporal bone initially, occurs most often as result of **necrotizing external otitis** (NEO)
  - Many authors consider part of spectrum of NEO
  - SBO can occur secondary to other infections related to temporal bone, including otomastoiditis or petrous apicitis
  - Can occur secondary to trauma or surgery of temporal bone
  - *Pseudomonas aeruginosa* is most common pathogen
- **Atypical SBO**: Occurs secondary to **invasive sinusitis** or deep face infections, not temporal bone
  - No recent history of NEO or otomastoiditis
  - a.k.a. central skull base osteomyelitis
  - Less common than typical SBO
  - Can be idiopathic, without specific localized head & neck infection

IMAGING

General Features

- Best diagnostic clue
  - Ill-defined, infiltrative process of skull base with osseous erosion and destruction on CT, abnormal marrow signal and enhancement on MR, usually with extraosseous inflammation of intracranial &/or extracranial soft tissues
- Location
  - Temporal bone and central skull base
- Morphology
  - Ill defined and infiltrative with osseous and extraosseous abnormalities

Radiographic Findings

- Opacified mastoid air cells, external auditory canal (EAC) soft tissue fullness, or sphenoid sinus opacification with cortical erosions of skull base

CT Findings

- Typical SBO
  - Early: Swollen EAC soft tissues with localized bone erosion and adjacent cellulitis or abscess
  - Destruction of petrous apex and central skull base occurs with advanced or inadequately treated disease
- Atypical SBO
  - Early: Sphenoid sinus opacification
  - Late: Cortical erosion, trabecular demineralization, and late osteolysis of central skull base

MR Findings

- T1WI
  - Soft tissue opacification, thickened EAC, temporal bone, or sphenoid sinus
  - Low signal replaces normal T1-hyperintense marrow fat
- STIR
  - High signal within inflamed EAC, auricle, adjacent soft tissues, and infected marrow
- DWI
  - ADC values tend to be higher with SBO than malignancy
- T1WI C+ FS
  - Abnormal marrow enhancement and infiltrative extraosseous enhancing soft tissue
  - Soft tissue infiltration in nasopharyngeal soft tissues may mimic neoplasm, such as nasopharyngeal carcinoma
  - MR may show combination of enhancing soft tissue and nonenhancing areas of devitalized tissue in *Mucor*

Nuclear Medicine Findings

- 3-phase Tc-99m methylene diphosphonate (MDP) bone scan
  - Highly sensitive study for early detection of SBO with sensitivity approaching 100%
- Ga-67 scan
  - Higher specificity compared to MDP 3-phase bone scan
- FDG PET
  - Can be used as complementary study to determine extent of infection

Imaging Recommendations

- Best imaging tool
  - Combined bone CT and enhanced MR best evaluate cortical and trabecular integrity, marrow space and soft tissue cellulitis, phlegmon, or abscess
- Protocol advice
  - CT performed using high-resolution thin-slice technique with bone algorithm
  - MR performed using **multiplanar precontrast T1 (without FS)** and **corresponding T1 C+ FS**, and STIR
    - MR more sensitive than CT for early marrow involvement in nonpneumatized petrous apex, basisphenoid, and basiocciput

DIFFERENTIAL DIAGNOSIS

Metastatic Disease of Skull Base

- Usually known primary tumor
- Multiple lesions common
- SBO may be mistaken for metastatic disease in neutropenic cancer patients

Nasopharyngeal Carcinoma

- Mass originates in nasopharyngeal mucosal space
  - Usually mucosal primary is visible clinically
- Destructive upward invasion of basisphenoid and basiocciput
- May mimic SBO when advanced skull base invasion is present

Non-Hodgkin Lymphoma of Skull Base

- Soft tissue mass with bony destruction of skull base
- Secondary invasion of skull base from nasal cavity site of origin
- Other hematologic malignancies (e.g., leukemia) can appear similar

Granulomatosis With Polyangiitis

- Rare mimic of SBO due to destructive changes

- Other granulomatous diseases (e.g., TB, sarcoid) also rarely can mimic SBO

Idiopathic Skull Base Inflammation (Inflammatory Pseudotumor)

- Noninfectious source of inflammation may appear identical
- May primarily involve skull base or extend secondarily from idiopathic orbital inflammation
- Diagnosis of exclusion

Bone Dysplasias

- Fibrous dysplasia, skull base
  - MR mimic of SBO; CT shows ground-glass opacification and bone expansion with variable lytic foci
- Paget disease, skull base
  - MR mimic of SBO; CT shows osseous expansion with lytic lesion (osteoporosis circumscripta) or mixed lytic-sclerotic foci having cotton wool appearance

PATHOLOGY

General Features

- **Necrotizing otitis externa = typical SBO**
  - Infection starts in external ear and surrounding soft tissues, spreads lateral to medial in temporal bone
  - Occurs most often in **diabetic patients**
  - Partially treated NOE may create confusing clinical and imaging picture of relatively normal EAC but persistent SBO (may spread to central skull base)
  - *Pseudomonas aeruginosa* identified in 98% of cases
- **Atypical SBO** usually due to invasive sinusitis, which spreads to central skull base
  - Also occurs most often in **immunocompromised** (diabetes, HIV, chronic steroid use)
  - Typical pathogens: Gram-positive bacteria; fungal: **Zygomycetes** (*Mucor* in ketoacidosis) and *Aspergillus* (neutropenia)
  - **Angioinvasion** is common in invasive fungal disease, often affecting cavernous sinuses &/or intracranial vessels
    - May result in intracranial infarcts

Gross Pathologic & Surgical Features

- Specimens contain variable inflammatory changes ranging from edema to frank purulence
- Tissue demonstrates variable necrosis, particularly with fungal etiology
- Specimens may not demonstrate microorganisms at histology
- Cultures important for definitive treatment

CLINICAL ISSUES

Presentation

- Most common signs/symptoms
  - Typical SBO: Otalgia, otorrhea, and hearing loss in diabetic patient
  - Atypical SBO: Sinusitis, headache, fever, malaise, cranial neuropathies in immunocompromised patient
- Other signs/symptoms
  - **Elevated sedimentation rate**
    - Helps distinguish infection from malignancy
  - Elevated WBC

- Fever and generalized signs of infection
- Purulent sinusitis or otorrhea
- Cranial nerve deficits

Demographics

- Most commonly seen in older adult patients with diabetes
- Seen in other immunosuppressed patients all ages

Natural History & Prognosis

- Associated with high morbidity and mortality despite intensive antibiotic therapy

Treatment

- Intensive pathogen-specific antibiotic therapy, including IV antibiotics
- Surgical approaches
  - Biopsy and culture for definitive diagnosis and organism identification
  - Surgical debridement of necrotic bone and soft tissue, especially for fungal disease
  - Drainage of pneumatized spaces
  - Drainage of abscesses

DIAGNOSTIC CHECKLIST

Consider

- Radiologic and clinical diagnosis of SBO requires high index of suspicion
  - SBO is more common than reported
  - Delay in diagnosis is common
- Consider SBO for any infiltrative skull base process if **biopsies are negative for malignancy**

Image Interpretation Pearls

- High-resolution bone CT of skull base necessary to identify **early cortical erosion**
- Multiplanar MR, including **precontrast T1 without FS** and **T1 C+ FS** images, required to identify marrow space involvement
  - High-yield target areas: Nonpneumatized petrous apex, basisphenoid, and basiocciput

Reporting Tips

- Improvement in soft tissue abnormalities best indicator of early radiologic improvement
- Abnormalities of bone and bone marrow may persist for weeks to months despite response to treatment

SELECTED REFERENCES

1. Eustace MB et al: Central skull base osteomyelitis in Queensland, Australia, 2010-2020. Open Forum Infect Dis. 11(10):ofae614, 2024
2. Khanum I et al: Skull base osteomyelitis (SBO): a dreaded clinical entity. J Pak Med Assoc. 74(10):1767-72, 2024
3. Krishnakumar L et al: Skull base osteomyelitis- marauders of the skull. Indian J Otolaryngol Head Neck Surg. 76(2):1770-4, 2024
4. Simon M et al: Skull base osteomyelitis: HBO as a therapeutic concept effects on clinical and radiological results. Eur Arch Otorhinolaryngol. 282(4):1835-42, 2024
5. bYew Toong L et al: Skull base osteomyelitis: a 5-year review and prognostic outcome in a single tertiary institution. OTO Open. 8(3):e70001, 2024
6. Chapman PR et al: Skull base osteomyelitis: a comprehensive imaging review. AJNR Am J Neuroradiol. 42(3):404-13, 2021
7. Clark MP et al: Central or atypical skull base osteomyelitis: diagnosis and treatment. Skull Base. 19(4):247-54, 2009
8. Carfrae MJ et al: Malignant otitis externa. Otolaryngol Clin North Am. 41(3):537-49, viii-ix, 2008

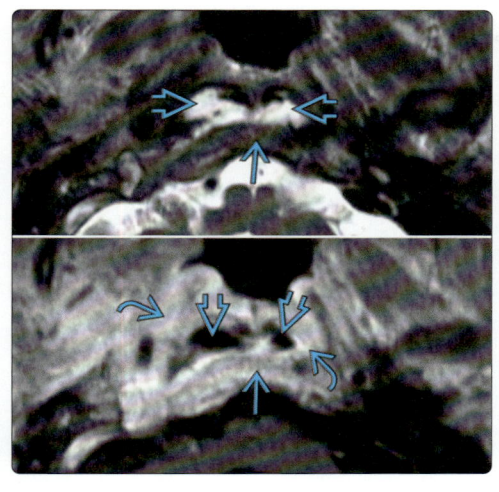
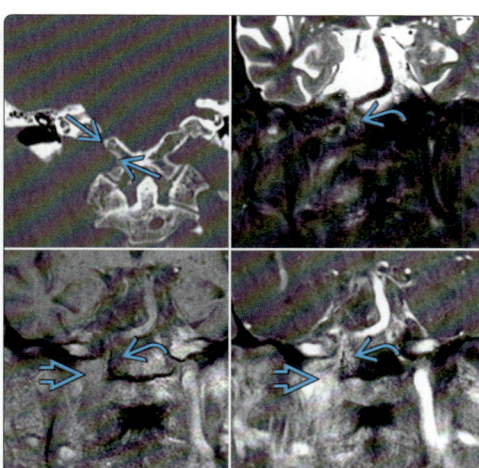

(Left) Axial T2 FS (top) and T1 C+ (bottom) MR images show marrow edema and enhancement in clivus ➡, soft tissue inflammation extending to the nasopharynx ➡, and abscess in longus colli muscles ➡. Findings are consistent with SBO. (Right) Coronal NECT (top left) shows cortical erosions in the right occipital condyle ➡. Coronal T2 (top right), T1 (bottom left), and T1 C+ (bottom right) MR images show marrow edema and enhancement in the right occipital condyle and adjacent clivus ➡ with soft tissue phlegmon ➡, suggesting SBO.

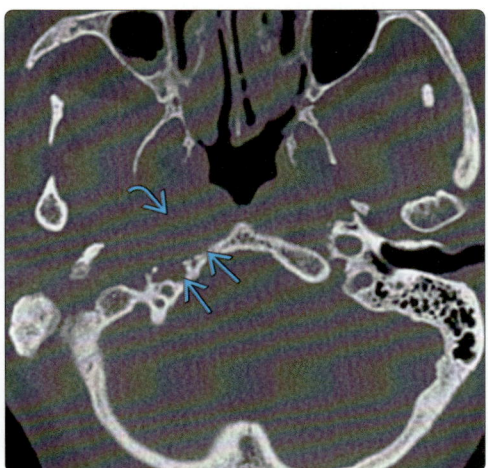
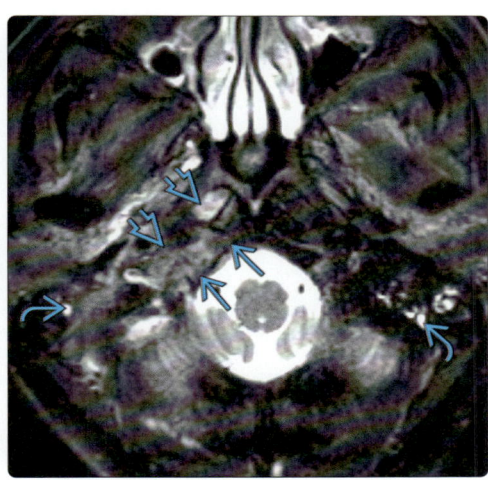

(Left) Axial bone window NECT in a 70-year-man with longstanding diabetes and recent-onset right ear pain and discharge shows cortical erosive changes in the right occipital condyle ➡ and adjacent soft tissue fullness ➡. (Right) Axial T2 FS MR in the same patient shows marrow edema in the right occipital condyle ➡ and adjacent soft tissue edema ➡. Small bilateral mastoid effusions ➡ can be noted.

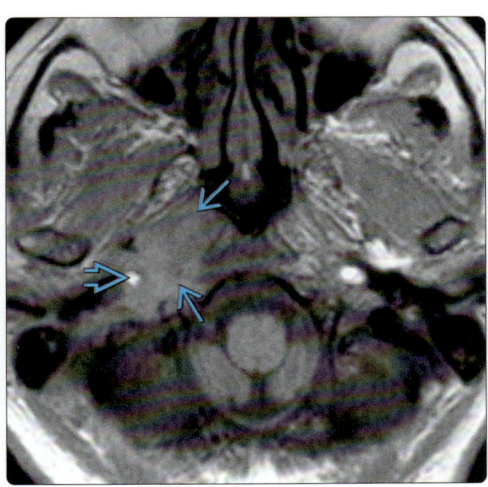
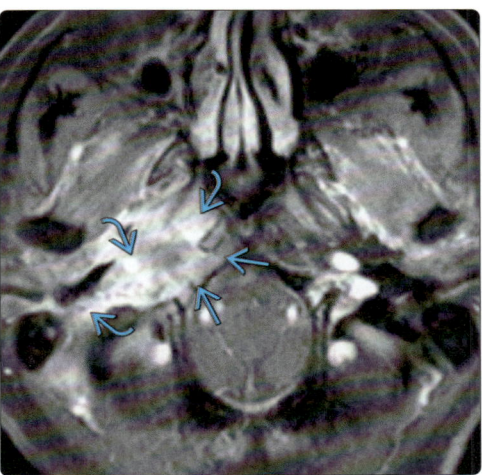

(Left) Axial T1 MR in the same patient shows soft tissue signal intensity with loss of fat plane in the right skull base region extending to the right carotid space ➡. Mild narrowing of right carotid ➡ also can be noted. (Right) Axial T1 C+ MR in the same patient shows marrow enhancement involving the right occipital condyle ➡ with adjacent phlegmon in the soft tissue extending to the nasopharynx, carotid space, and stylomastoid foramen ➡. Findings are consistent with SBO and culture was positive for Pseudomonas.

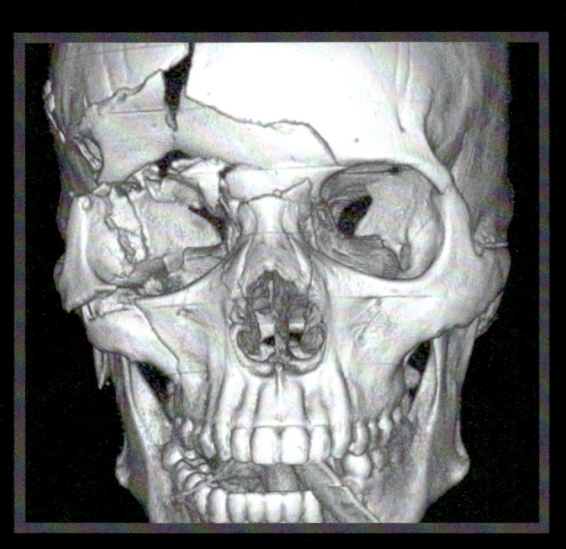

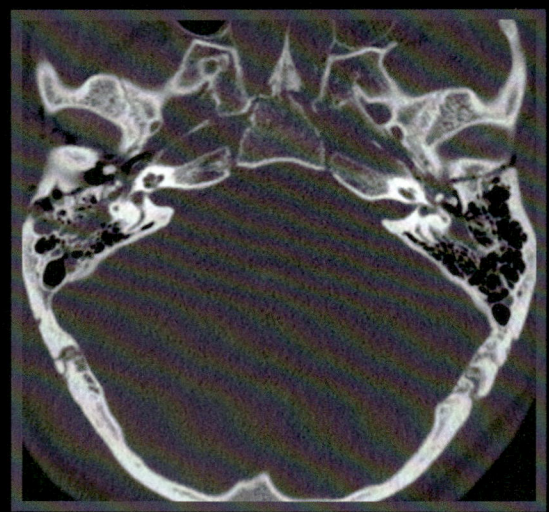

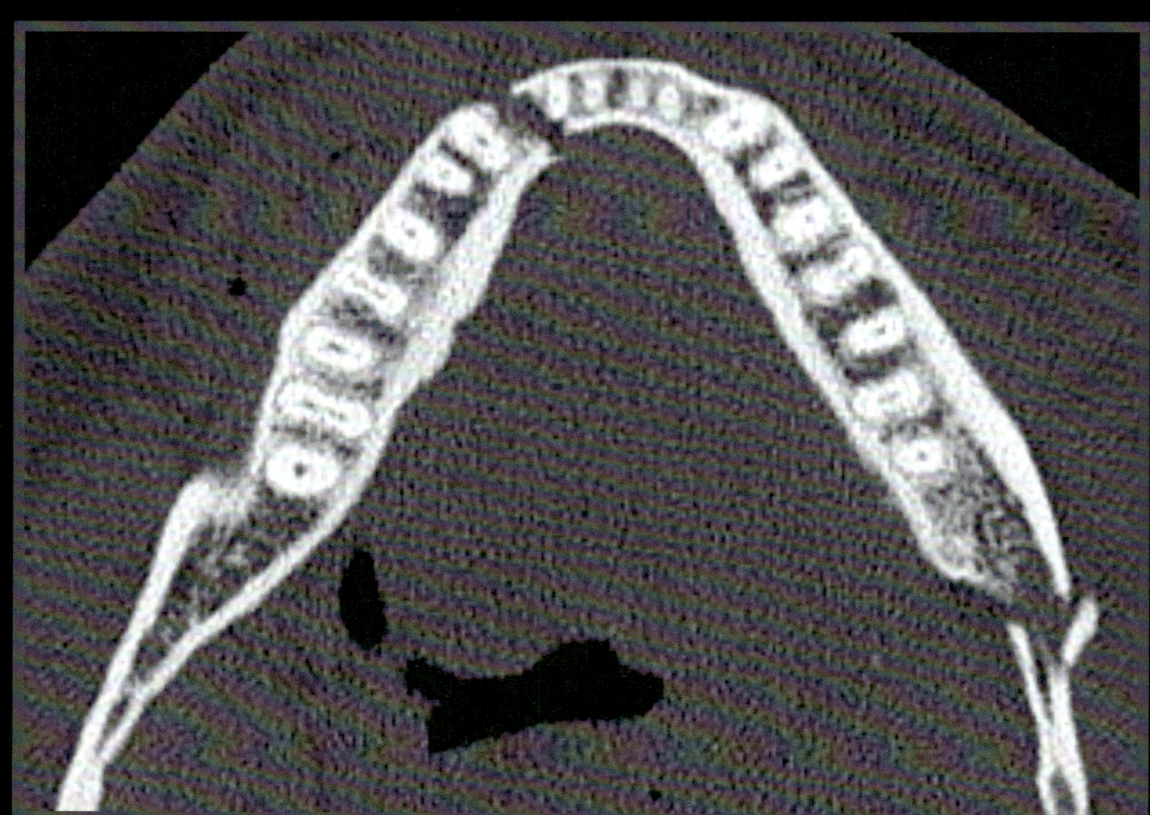

SECTION 24
Skull Base, Facial, and Temporal Bone Trauma

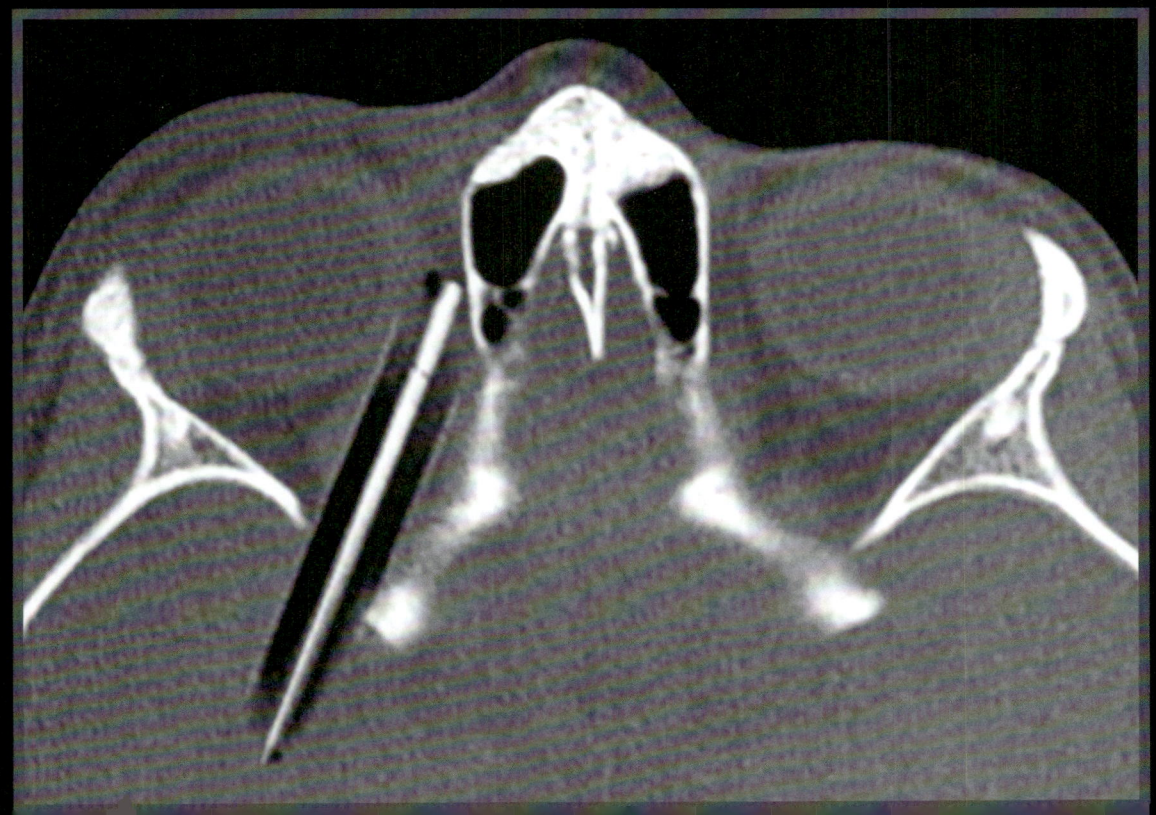

Summary Thoughts: Skull Base & Facial Trauma

Skull base fractures (fxs) require considerable force & are often associated with other craniofacial injuries. Blunt trauma is responsible for > 90% of skull base & facial fxs & is frequently related to vehicular accidents. Injuries may range from a solitary linear fx to complex injuries involving the craniofacial skeleton. Associated intracranial injuries, such as cerebral contusion, intra-/extraaxial hemorrhage, dural tears, & vascular injuries, are common in these cases. The objective of imaging in these trauma patients is to depict the location & extent of fxs & to recognize associated injuries to vital structures. Accurate imaging interpretation also aids in surgical planning & in preventing complications.

Imaging Approaches & Indications

High-resolution bone algorithm CT is the modality of choice for imaging skull base & facial trauma. Thin-slice (0.6- to 1.0-mm) axial images extend from the skull vertex through the facial bones with coronal & sagittal reformatted images generated from the axial dataset. Sagittal reformatted images are helpful for assessing injuries to the anterior & central skull base (ASB & CSB), particularly in patients with CSF leak. **3D reformatted** images of facial fxs are beneficial for surgical planning as they provide a more anatomic representation of fx malalignment prior to reconstruction.

Patients with **CSF leak** or **recurrent meningitis** usually have visible defects in the ASB & CSB that are demonstrated with high-resolution bone CT. If a defect is not identified on bone CT or there are multiple fxs & it is unclear which is the source of the leak, CT cisternography may better delineate the leak site.

Arterial vascular injuries may be seen with CSB fxs that traverse the carotid canals. CTA can be performed in these patients to assess for **dissection**, traumatic **pseudoaneurysm**, or presence of **carotid-cavernous fistula**. Fxs of the petrous temporal bones & posterior fossa may extend into the major venous sinuses, resulting in posterior fossa epidural hematoma or posttraumatic venous thrombosis. CTV or MRV may be obtained in such cases. Conventional angiography is typically not necessary but used for treating vascular complications.

Cerebral injuries are often seen in high-impact trauma. Although MR is not performed initially, it is more sensitive for assessing the degree of parenchymal injury.

Approaches to Imaging Issues in Skull Base & Facial Trauma

Anterior Skull Base

ASB, or frontobasal, trauma is frequently associated with injury to the sinonasal cavities & orbits. The majority of these patients have facial injuries, including fxs of the frontal bone, orbital roofs, & cribriform plates (CP). Imaging analysis should address the following questions.
- Do fx lines involve CP or traverse anterior or posterior walls of frontal sinuses?
- Do fxs involve orbital apex or optic canals?

Central Skull Base

CSB, or lateral basal, trauma may involve the sphenoid sinus walls, cavernous sinuses, & clivus & may present with carotid vascular injury or cranial nerves (CNs) III, IV, VI, or CNVI-III

deficits. Imaging analysis should address the following questions.
- Are walls of sphenoid sinuses, carotid canals, & clivus intact?
- Do cavernous sinuses appear symmetric?

Temporal Bone

Petrous temporal fxs typically have a longitudinal or transverse trajectory. The longitudinal type more often spares the otic capsule traversing the mastoid & middle ear cavities & squamous portion, & may result in ossicular chain disruption. Transverse fxs more often involve the otic capsule extending into the occipital bone after traversing the inner ear. Imaging analysis should address the following questions.
- Does main fx line involve or spare otic capsule?
- Is ossicular chain intact?
- Does fx traverse inner ear or CNVII canal?
- Does fx traverse tegmen?

Posterior Skull Base

Fxs of the occipital bones may be isolated or associated with transverse petrous ridge fxs. The fx may extend into a dural venous sinus, jugular foramen (CNIX-XI), or CNXII canal. Craniocervical junction injuries should also be suspected in these patients. Imaging analysis should address the following questions.
- Does fx extend into transverse sinus, sigmoid sinus, or jugular foramen?
- Does fx involve internal auditory canal or hypoglossal canal?

Orbital Trauma

Orbital fxs are classified as: (1) Those involving the orbital walls, frequently the inferior orbital rim, & (2) the orbital "blowout" fx. Blowout fxs may involve the orbital floor or medial orbital wall, but the inferior orbital rim remains intact. Imaging analysis should address the following questions.
- Is there **entrapment** of inferior ± medial rectus muscles & fat; how large & displaced are fx fragments?
- Is fx isolated or are other orbital or facial fxs present [zygomaticomaxillary complex (ZMC) fx, nasoorbitalethmoid (NOE) fx, Le Fort]?

Transfacial Fracture (Le Fort)

There are 3 types of Le Fort fxs, & a consistent feature of all 3 types is the presence of bilateral pterygoid plate fxs. Le Fort I is a horizontal fx through the maxilla involving the piriform aperture. Le Fort II is a pyramidal fx involving the nasofrontal junction, infraorbital rims, medial orbital walls & orbital floors, & zygomaticomaxillary suture lines. Le Fort III (craniofacial separation) consists of fxs at the nasofrontal junction extending laterally through the lateral orbital walls & zygomatic arches. Le Fort fxs are rarely pure & are often seen in combination with other fxs. Imaging analysis should address the following questions.
- Which Le Fort types are involved; are fxs same on each side of face?
- Are other facial fx patterns present (ZMC, NOE)?

Zygomaticomaxillary Complex Fracture

The prominent position of the zygomatic arch makes it susceptible to trauma. This fx type was formerly referred to as the tripod fx; however, that is a misnomer as the zygoma has 4 involved articulations, & 5 distinct fxs are evident. Imaging analysis should address the following questions.
- How displaced & comminuted is ZMC fx?

Temporal Bone, Skull Base, & Facial Trauma Complications

Fracture Locations/Type	Potential Complications
Skull Base Trauma	
Anterior skull base	Posterior wall frontal sinus contaminated fx; cribriform plate fx: CSF leak/cephalocele/meningitis, CNI injury; orbital apex or optic canal fx: CNII injury
Central skull base	Internal carotid artery injury: Thrombosis, dissection, pseudoaneurysm, carotid-cavernous fistula; sphenoid sinus superior wall fx: CSF leak/cephalocele if dural tear; CNs at risk: CNIII, IV, VI, CNVI-III
Posterior skull base	Transvenous sinus fx: Venous sinus thrombosis, epidural hematoma; CNs at risk: CNVII-VIII (internal auditory canal); CNIX-XI (jugular foramen); CNXII (hypoglossal canal)
Temporal bone	Tegmen mastoideum/tympani fx: CSF leak/cephalocele if dural tear; CNs at risk: CNVII (facial nerve canal fx), CNVIII (transcochlear fx)
Orbital Trauma	
Medial blowout	Medial rectus entrapment; diplopia, enophthalmos
Inferior blowout	Inferior rectus entrapment; infraorbital nerve injury, diplopia, enophthalmos
Foreign body	Globe rupture; CNII laceration/transection; infection
Facial Trauma	
Transfacial (Le Fort I-III), zygomaticomaxillary complex fx, complex midfacial, nasoorbitalethmoid fxs	Traumatic telecanthus, nasolacrimal apparatus injury, epiphora, inferior orbital nerve injury (CNV2), malocclusion, mucocele
Mandibular fx	Trismus, inferior alveolar nerve injury, infection, loss of teeth

- What is extent of involvement of orbital floor, orbital apex, & lamina papyracea?
- How is lateral orbital wall displaced & is pterygoid plate fractured?

Complex Midfacial Fracture

The complex midfacial fx or "facial smash injury" consists of multiple facial fxs that cannot be classified as one of the named patterns (Le Fort, ZMC, NOE). Imaging analysis should address where the fxs are concentrated & the presence of associated orbital or skull base injuries.

Nasoorbitalethmoid Fracture

High-force trauma to the nasal bones is transmitted to the ethmoid sinuses & orbits in NOE fxs. The **medial canthal tendon** (MCT) may be disrupted in these cases & fxs may extend into the lacrimal apparatus. Imaging analysis should address the following questions.
- Is bone fragment to which MCT attaches displaced or comminuted?
- Is nasal bridge displaced posteriorly into ethmoids or superiorly into anterior fossa?
- Are there injuries to CP, frontal recess, or globes?

Mandible Fracture

Mandible fxs may occur within the alveolus (parasymphysis, body, or angle) or posterior to the teeth (ascending ramus, subcondylar region, condyle, or coronoid process). The mandible is essentially a ring of bone & multiple fxs are common, often bilaterally. Fx fragment displacement is affected by muscular attachments to the bone. Imaging analysis should address the following questions.
- Where are fxs located & what is degree & direction of displacement?
- Is inferior alveolar foramen or canal involved?
- Are condyles subluxed or dislocated?
- Do fxs involve periodontal ligament space (tooth socket)?

Clinical Implications

Understanding the mechanisms & complications of injury is essential for managing skull base trauma. The objective of treatment in patients with facial trauma is to stabilize & restore facial anatomy & to provide skeletal support for the function of mastication. Treatment is also directed toward relief of early & prevention of late complications.

Clinical signs of ASB injury include epistaxis, proptosis, chemosis, rhinorrhea, anosmia, & visual deficits. In addition to CSF leak, patients with fxs of the posterior frontal sinus wall or CP are at risk for subsequent meningitis. Fxs at the orbital apex & optic canal may cause visual deficits. Signs of temporal bone trauma may include postauricular hematoma (Battle sign), hemotympanum, otorrhea, conductive or sensorineural hearing loss, vertigo, or facial weakness. Clinical signs of posterior skull base trauma include symptoms of mass effect from epidural hematoma related to dural sinus trauma or lower CN deficits.

In patients with midfacial trauma, injuries to the palate, maxilla, & mandible should be assessed at imaging, as lack of appropriate repair can result in malocclusion. Depending on the degree, orbital floor involvement in patients with a ZMC fx will likely require surgical reduction. Orbital wall fxs will be treated if there is entrapment of the extraocular muscles, impingement upon the orbital apex or middle cranial fossa, or to prevent globe malposition that is resulting in diplopia or enophthalmos. Traumatic telecanthus & damage to the lacrimal drainage pathway are complications of NOE fxs that require surgical intervention.

Selected References

1. Bai J et al: Imaging of cerebrovascular complications from blunt skull base trauma. Emerg Radiol. 31(4):529-42, 2024
2. Omami G et al: Imaging of maxillofacial injuries. Dent Clin North Am. 68(2):393-407, 2024
3. Adams A: Imaging of skull base trauma: fracture patterns and soft tissue injuries. Neuroimaging Clin N Am. 31(4):599-620, 2021

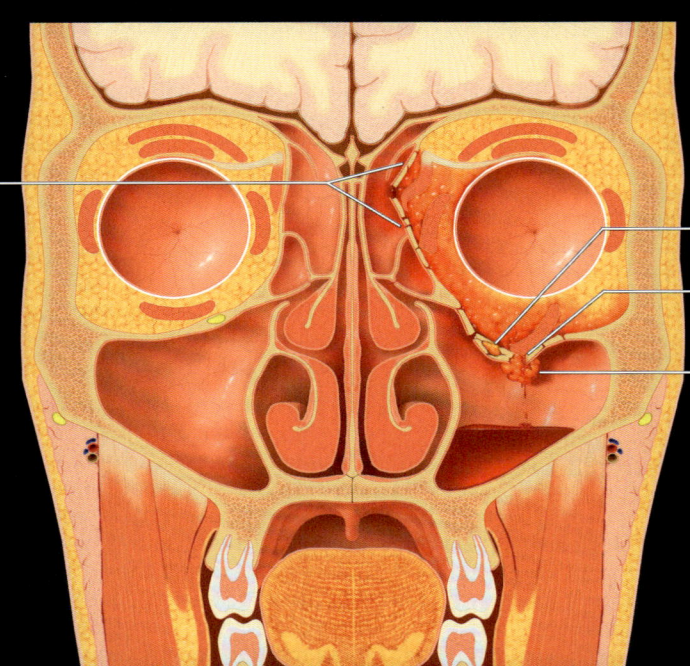

Frontal bone fracture with extension across cribriform plate

Temporal bone fracture of squamous portion & petrous ridge traversing petrous carotid canal

Occipital bone fracture extending into transverse sinus & jugular foramen

Posterior fossa (venous) epidural hematoma

Fracture extends through lesser sphenoid wing involving optic canal with optic nerve injury

Linear fracture through clivus with posterior extension into hypoglossal canal (CNXII)

Medial blowout fracture (lamina papyracea)

Injured infraorbital nerve (CNV2)

Entrapped inferior rectus muscle

Orbital fat herniating into maxillary sinus

(Top) *Graphic of endocranial view of the skull base shows multiple fractures with expected complications. An anterior skull base fracture crosses the cribriform plate & extends into the optic canal. A fracture through the right middle fossa extends through the petrous apex involving the petrous carotid canal. An oblique clival fracture extends into the hypoglossal canal. A posterior fossa occipital fracture damages the transverse sinus & causes an extraaxial hemorrhage.* **(Bottom)** *Coronal graphic illustrates a medial & an inferior blowout fracture on the left. The medial blowout fracture displaces the lamina papyracea medially into the ethmoid sinus. An inferior blowout fracture of the floor of the orbit (maxillary sinus roof) with infraorbital nerve injury is depicted. Herniation of the inferior rectus muscle & orbital fat into the maxillary sinus may occur with variably sized floor fractures. A blow to the anterior orbit/globe, such as from a baseball, may cause either one or both of these fractures.*

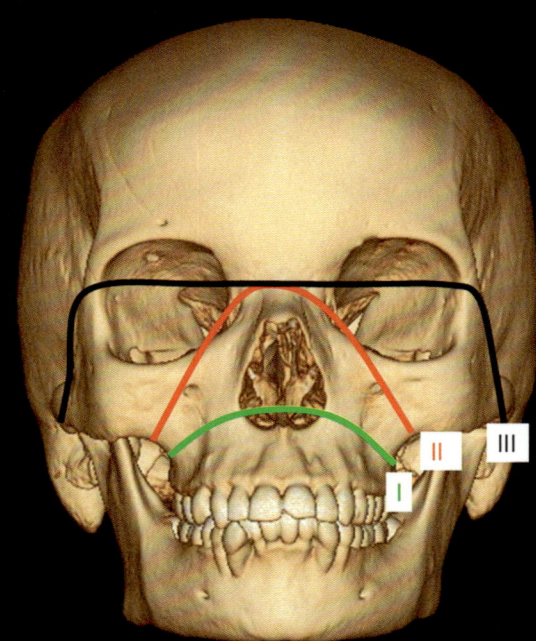

Nasoorbitalethmoid fracture

Zygomaticomaxillary complex fracture shows fracture lines through lateral orbital wall, zygomatic arch, & anterior maxillary wall with orbital floor involvement

Nasoorbitalethmoid fracture with dominant fracture fragment attached to medial canthal tendon

Mandibular body fracture crosses inferior alveolar canal

Inferior alveolar nerve injury from transmandibular fracture

II

III

I

(Top) *Frontal graphic demonstrates fractures of the midface.* **(Bottom)** *Coronal graphic shows lines defining the 3 types of Le Fort fractures. Le Fort I (green) involves the nasal aperture & essentially separates the maxilla & palate from the remaining midface. Le Fort II (red) traverses the inferior orbital rim & is also known as the pyramidal fracture due to its configuration. Le Fort III (black), or craniofacial separation, extends through the zygomatic arches. A common feature of all 3 Le Fort fracture types is involvement of the pterygoid plates (not shown).*

KEY FACTS

IMAGING

- Bone algorithm MDCT with coronal reconstructions, CTA/MRA for suspected vascular injury
  - Dedicated brain imaging critical to evaluate for intracranial injuries (present in up to 90%)
- **Longitudinal fractures**: Vertical plane parallels long axis of petrous ridge (PR)
  - External auditory canal (EAC), middle ear (ME)/ossicular involvement common; otic capsule (OC) involvement rare
- **Transverse fractures**: Perpendicular to PR long axis
  - OC involvement, facial nerve (CNVII) injury very common; EAC/ME involvement rare
- **Oblique fractures**: Mixed features, typically horizontal and parallel to PR long axis
- OC-violating vs. OC-sparing classification better predicts complications, such as sensorineural hearing loss, CNVII injury, and CSF leak

- **Ossicular injuries**: **Dislocations** > > fractures, incus most commonly involved
- **CNVII injuries**: Most commonly at **geniculate ganglion**; symptoms often resolve spontaneously
- All varieties: Assess for tegmen fracture (CSF leak), carotid canal injury, extension to central skull base, intracranial, and cervical spine injury

TOP DIFFERENTIAL DIAGNOSES

- Pseudofractures: Sutures, fissures, canaliculi, aqueducts
- Incus interposition procedure

DIAGNOSTIC CHECKLIST

- Always assess most clinically relevant structures: CNVII canal, otic capsule, tegmen, carotid canal, ossicles
- Do not misdiagnose pseudofracture
- Consider CTA/MRA if carotid canal fracture and CTV/MRV if dural sinus/jugular foramen region fracture

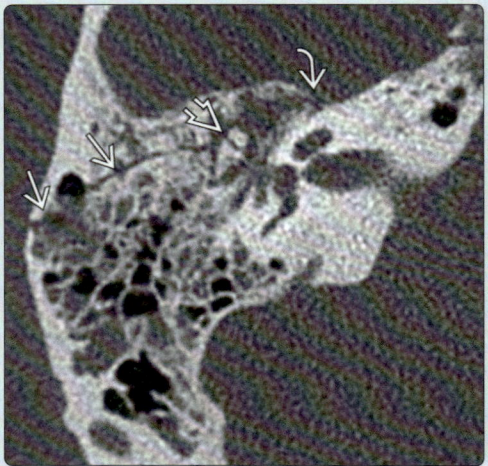
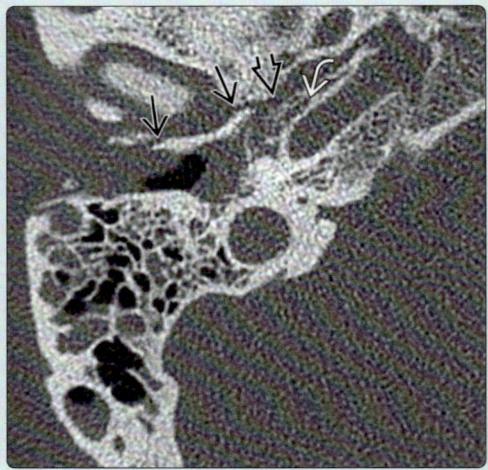

(Left) Axial NECT of the right temporal bone in a 37-year-old man who was assaulted shows a longitudinal fracture plane ➡ causing subtle widening of the incudostapedial joint ➡ and propagating through the anterior wall of the epitympanum ➡. (Right) Axial NECT in the same patient shows an inferior continuation of the longitudinal fracture through the posterior wall of the TMJ fossa ➡ and eustachian tube ➡, and questionably into the carotid canal ➡. A follow-up CTA was negative for carotid injury.

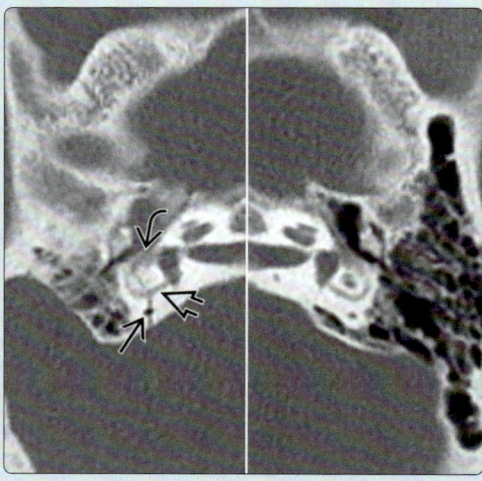
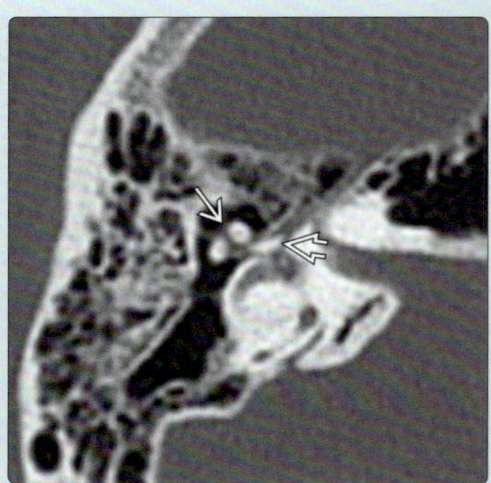

(Left) Composite mirrored axial NECTs in a 34-year-old man show an otic capsule violating (OCV) fracture that traverses the posterior semicircular canal (SCC) ➡ as well as the anterior ➡ and posterior ➡ limbs of lateral SCC. Normal anatomy is visible in the right-hand panel. (Right) Axial NECT in a 57-year-old man who inserted a cotton swab through the tympanic membrane shows disruption of the incudostapedial joint ➡. There is also a fragment of the otic capsule displaced medially into the tympanic facial nerve canal ➡.

TERMINOLOGY

Definitions

- Traumatic injury of temporal bone ± ossicle injury

IMAGING

General Features

- Best diagnostic clue
  - Bone CT shows fracture line
  - Secondary signs include **hemotympanum**, **pneumolabyrinth**, intracranial (IC) or extracranial air/hemorrhage near mastoid
    - Unexplained **parapharyngeal space air** should prompt search for **mastoid fracture**
- Morphology
  - **Classification best correlating with outcome: Otic capsule violating (OCV)** vs. **OC sparing (OCS)**
    - **OCS fractures**: Majority of fractures; commonly extend to middle ear and cause conductive hearing loss (CHL) or mixed
    - **OCV fractures**: Minority (5-20%) have increased incidence of **sensorineural hearing loss** (SNHL), **CNVII injury**, and **CSF leak**
  - Older classification is longitudinal vs. transverse (relative to long axis of petrous ridge)
    - Roughly corresponds to OCS vs. OCV
    - Many fractures actually oblique or mixed

CT Findings

- Bone CT
  - **OCS fractures**
    - Often involve temporal squamosa, external auditory canal (EAC), tympanic membrane (TM), and middle ear (ME); usually spare otic capsule
      - Hemotympanum and ossicular disruption common
    - CNVII canal involvement most often occurs at geniculate or tympanic segments
      - CNVII injury less common than with OCV fractures
  - **OCV fractures**
    - Often extend from occipital area (foramen magnum) through petrous pyramid and otic capsule
      - May involve jugular foramen, foramen lacerum, internal auditory canal (IAC)
    - Frequent CNVII injury, often at geniculate or IAC
    - Labyrinthine structures (cochlea, vestibule, semicircular canals) more often affected than in OCS fracture; CSF leak, SNHL, IC complications common
    - EAC, TM, and ME involved less commonly than in longitudinal fractures
  - **Ossicular injuries**
    - **Dislocations** > > fractures
      - Incus most commonly fractured ossicle
    - Incudostapedial > incudomalleolar > complete incus dislocation
      - Penetrating injury may also affect ossicular chain
    - Stapediovestibular disruption: Increasingly diagnosed with high-resolution MDCT
    - Malleus dislocation rare (supported by malleal ligaments, TM attachments)

- **Perilymph fistula (PLF)**: Oval or round window rupture, communication between ME and membranous labyrinth
  - Subtle findings include pneumolabyrinth and fluid at oval/round windows
- All fracture types: Assess for tegmen fractures, carotid canal injuries, propagation to central skull base, and IC and cervical spine injuries
  - Up to 90% of patients with temporal bone fractures have concomitant IC injury and up to 9% have cervical spine injury
- CTA
  - Consider CTA if fracture extends to carotid canal
    - Carotid canal fracture only moderately associated with internal carotid artery (ICA) injury
      - Risk similar to other findings not typically associated with ICA injury (e.g., subdural hematoma)
- CTV
  - Consider CTV if fracture extends to dural venous sinus or jugular bulb
  - Both carotid and dural venous sinus injuries are rare

MR Findings

- T1WI
  - Hemotympanum, hemolabyrinth (low signal acutely, high signal subacutely)
  - ICA injury: Dissection (fried-egg sign) or occlusion (loss of ICA flow void)
- T2WI
  - ME and mastoid debris appears hyperintense
  - Look for hypointense line of intact dura over tegmen on coronal images if CSF leak suspected
  - Loss of expected high signal in labyrinth may indicate hemolabyrinth, pneumolabyrinth, or posttraumatic labyrinthitis ossificans if subacute imaging
- T1WI C+
  - Most valuable for suspected subacute IC complications (meningitis, abscess)
  - CNVII, membranous labyrinth may enhance when involved by fracture
- MRA
  - ICA occlusion or dissection, carotid cavernous fistula
- MRV
  - Sigmoid sinus or jugular vein thrombosis

Imaging Recommendations

- Best imaging tool
  - Temporal bone CT
- Protocol advice
  - Bone algorithm MDCT with reconstructed coronal images
    - 3D CT reconstructions helpful for clarifying fracture orientation, ossicular alignment
  - Routine brain CT or MR for IC complications
  - Consider CTA/MRA if involves carotid canal, CTV/MRV if involves dural sinus or jugular foramen

DIFFERENTIAL DIAGNOSIS

Pseudofractures

- Sclerotic, well-corticated margins, typically bilateral and symmetric

- Sutures/fissures
  - External: Temporoparietal, petrooccipital, sphenopetrosal (angular), occipitomastoid
  - Internal: Petrotympanic, petrosquamosal, tympanosquamous, tympanomastoid
- Canaliculi
  - Mastoid, inferior tympanic, subarcuate (petromastoid canal), singular canaliculi
- Aqueducts
  - Cochlear, vestibular aqueducts

Incus Interposition Procedure

- Surgical remodeling/realignment of incus to bridge deficient ossicular chain and correct CHL
- Mimics chronic incus dislocation

Mastoiditis/Mastoid Effusion

- Preexisting mastoid or ME opacification may not reflect hemotympanum or CSF leak

PATHOLOGY

General Features

- Etiology
  - Temporal bone fracture requires application of great force, typically high-velocity impact
    - Motor vehicle accident (MVA) most common etiology
  - Longitudinal fractures due to lateral impact
  - Transverse fracture due to occipital or frontal impact
  - Tympanic plate fracture due to blow on chin

CLINICAL ISSUES

Presentation

- Most common signs/symptoms
  - Physical findings: Periauricular swelling and ecchymosis (Battle sign), EAC hemorrhage, hemotympanum
  - **CHL**: Initially may reflect hemotympanum ± TM injury
    - If persistent, must evaluate for ossicular injury
  - **SNHL**: Injury to OC, IAC, brainstem, or PLF
    - If fracture absent, may reflect labyrinthine concussion
    - Intralabyrinthine hemorrhage may ultimately lead to labyrinthitis ossificans
  - **Facial nerve dysfunction**: CNVII injuries represent spectrum from stretching/crushing/compression to complete transection
    - Delayed paresis often reflects reversible injury; typically managed conservatively
    - Immediate, complete paralysis: Poor prognosis for recovery; may be managed surgically
  - **CSF leak**: Most resolve spontaneously within 7 days
    - Surgery for persistent leak
    - ≤ 10% develop meningitis
  - **Vertigo**: Common after even minor head trauma
    - When severe/persistent, may reflect brainstem injury, labyrinthine concussion, benign paroxysmal positional vertigo, Ménière syndrome (endolymphatic hydrops), PLF
  - **Perilymphatic fistula**: Symptoms often vague; dizziness, vertigo, imbalance, fluctuating SNHL
    - Early detection facilitates surgical repair, hearing preservation

- Chronic presentations
  - Acquired cephalocele
  - Acquired cholesteatoma
    - Squamous invasion of fracture site
  - EAC stenosis
- Other signs/symptoms
  - IC pathology on CT in up to 90%
    - Extracerebral (epidural, subdural, subarachnoid) or intracerebral (contusion, diffuse axonal injury)
  - CNVI injury
  - Trismus if glenoid fossa is involved

Demographics

- Age
  - All ages; CNVII paralysis less common in pediatric temporal bone fractures
- Sex
  - M > F
- Epidemiology
  - Most common fractures of skull base
  - Incidence is increasing, likely reflecting increasing traffic and population

Natural History & Prognosis

- Related to presence or absence of facial nerve injury, ossicular injury, PLF, IC complications

Treatment

- Management of severe head injury is priority
- Anticoagulation ± endovascular therapy for carotid injury
- Antibiotics if CSF leak is present
- Management of CNVII injuries remains controversial; most advocate observation ± steroids for paresis
  - Surgical decompression or CNVII repair may be performed in patients with immediate paralysis

DIAGNOSTIC CHECKLIST

Consider

- Systematically assess most clinically relevant structures: CNVII canal, otic capsule, tegmen, carotid canal, ossicles
- Do not forget to evaluate IC contents

Image Interpretation Pearls

- Check contralateral side to exclude pseudofracture

Reporting Tips

- Classify fractures with regard to both anatomic (longitudinal/transverse/oblique) and OCV/sparing criteria

SELECTED REFERENCES

1. Steele JL et al: Long-term outcomes of adult temporal bone fractures with hearing loss: results of a multinational database analysis. Laryngoscope. ePub, 2025
2. Kohler R et al: Temporal bone fractures and related complications in pediatric and adult cranio-facial trauma: a comparison of MDCT findings in the acute emergency setting. Tomography. 10(5):727-37, 2024
3. Han S et al: Two cases of multiple ossicular chain disruption after penetrating injury and tympanic membrane healing. J Audiol Otol. 27(4):246-50, 2023
4. Yimam EW et al: Imaging patterns of temporal bone fracture among patients with head injury at Tikur Anbessa Specialized Hospital, Ethiopia. Ethiop J Health Sci. 33(6):979-86, 2023
5. Kurihara YY et al: Temporal bone trauma: typical CT and MRI appearances and important points for evaluation. Radiographics. 40(4):1148-62, 2020

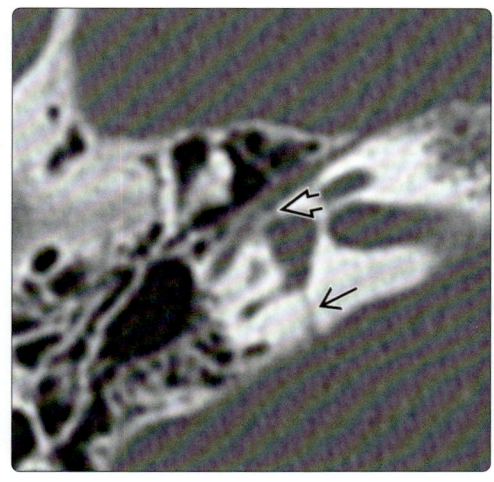
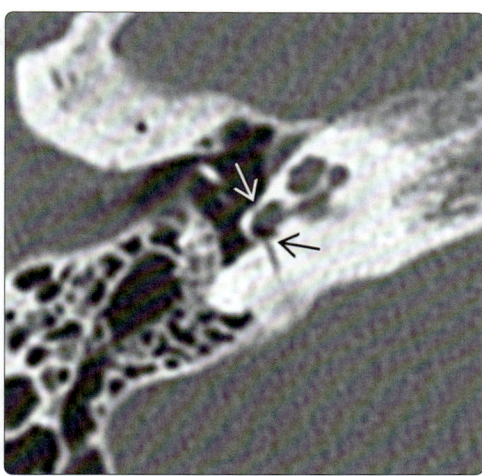

(Left) Axial NECT in a 73-year-old man with trauma shows a transverse OCV fracture plane ⇨ extending through the vestibule. The fracture reaches the tympanic segment of the facial nerve ⇨ more anteriorly. (Right) Axial NECT in the same patient shows the fracture plane reaching the round window niche ⇨. More anteriorly, the fracture is extending through the lateral aspect of the basal turn of the cochlea ⇨ to the anterior aspect of the otic capsule.

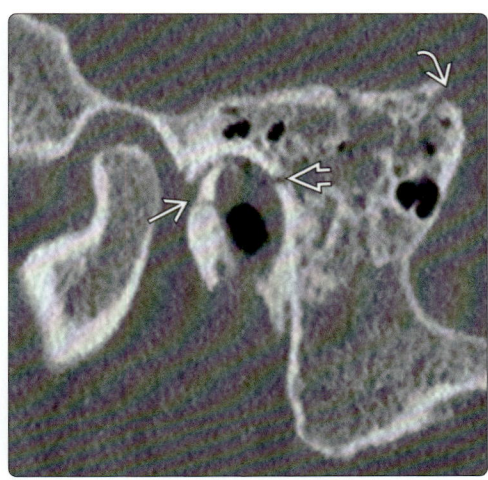
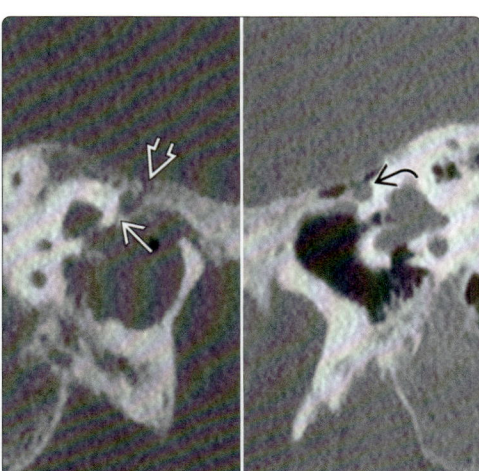

(Left) Sagittal CT in a 47-year-old man with trauma shows a fracture involving anterior ⇨ and posterior ⇨ walls of the external auditory canal. There is a more posterior component of the fracture breaching the tegmen mastoideum ⇨. (Right) Composite mirrored sagittal images of the right and left temporal bones in the same patient show extension of a fracture plane through the right facial nerve genu ⇨ and tegmen tympani ⇨ in the left-hand panel. The normal left facial nerve genu ⇨ is visible for comparison in the right-hand panel.

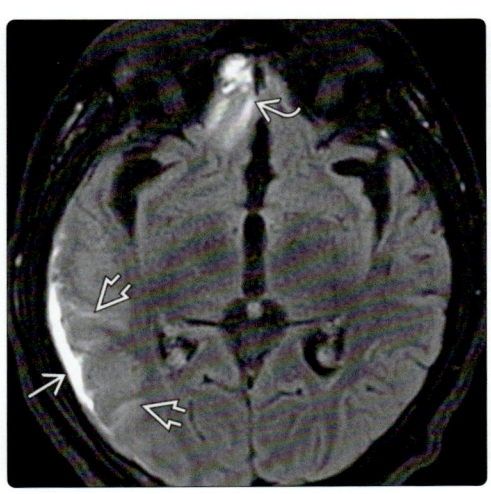
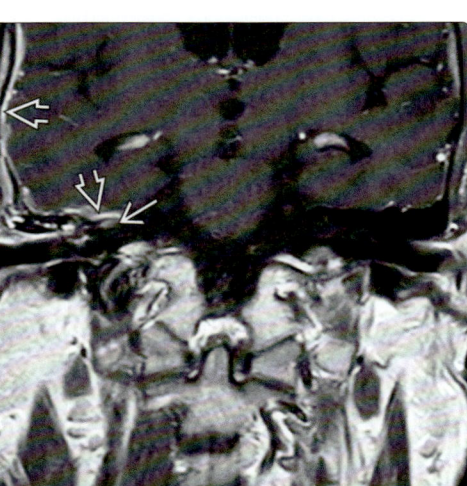

(Left) Axial FLAIR MR in the same patient shows an acute subdural hematoma ⇨, subarachnoid hemorrhage ⇨, and a hemorrhagic contusion ⇨ of the inferomedial frontal lobe. (Right) Coronal T1 C+ FS MR in the same patient shows abnormal signal in the superior internal auditory canal ⇨. Considering the fracture through the genu seen on CT, this signal may represent T1-intense blood products, reactive enhancement, or both. There is reactive dural enhancement along the periphery of the right temporal lobe ⇨.

KEY FACTS

TERMINOLOGY

- Injury to middle ear ossicles; dislocation or subluxation > > fracture

IMAGING

- **Malalignment or dislocation** of ossicle articulations
- **Incudostapedial** > incudomalleolar > complete incus dislocation > stapediovestibular disruption > malleus dislocation
- **Incudostapedial dislocation**
  - Incus lenticular process anterior or posterior to stapes head
- **Incudomalleolar dislocation/disruption**
  - Axial CT: Ice cream falling off of cone appearance
  - Sagittal CT: Disruption of "molar tooth"
- **Incus dislocation**
  - Disrupted incudomalleolar and incudostapedial joints → incus dissociating from malleus and stapes
- **Stapes dislocation/stapediovestibular disruption**

- Suspect if transverse fracture through oval window
- Actual disruption difficult to see; < 1-mm images may identify stapes fragments or footplate malalignment
- **Malleus dislocation**
  - Rare traumatic ossicle injury

TOP DIFFERENTIAL DIAGNOSES

- **Congenital ossicular anomalies and fixation**
  - Abnormal shape, size, or orientation; fixation of ossicles to wall of middle ear cavity
- **Ossicular prosthesis**
  - Stapes prosthesis: Missing all or part of stapes superstructure
  - Incus interposition graft: Mimics chronic incus dislocation
- **Chronic otomastoiditis with ossicular erosions**
  - Erosive ossicular changes in absence of cholesteatoma in patient with history of chronic otitis media
- **Congenital cholesteatoma with ossicular erosions**
- **Acquired cholesteatoma with ossicular erosions**

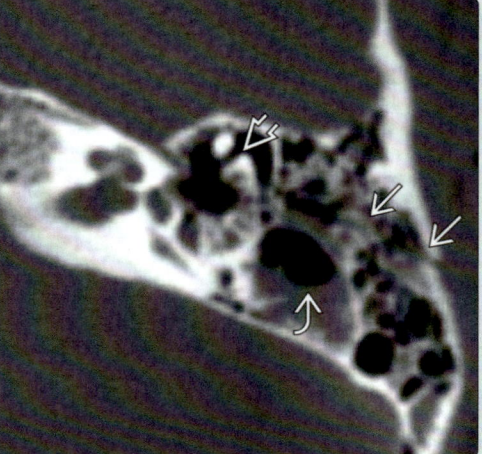
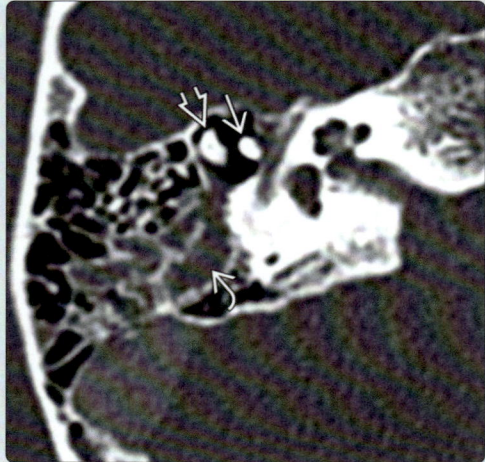

(Left) Axial bone CT in a 7-year-old child who fell 8 feet shows a longitudinal, otic capsule-sparing temporal bone fracture ➡, mild widening of the incudomalleolar joint ➡, and blood in the antrum ➡. (Right) Axial bone CT in a 14-year-old girl status post all-terrain vehicle accident shows findings of incus dislocation with increased distance between a medially dislocated malleus head ➡ and a laterally positioned/rotated incus ➡. The incudostapedial joint was also disrupted (not shown). Note mastoid hemorrhage ➡.

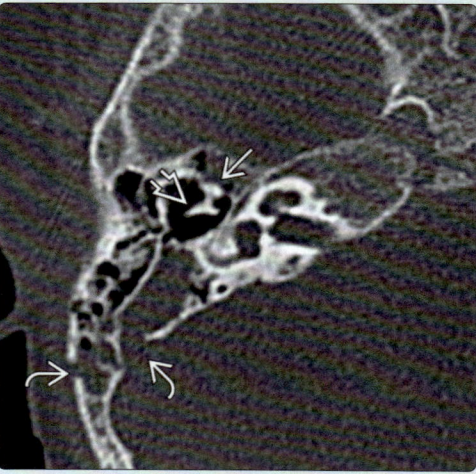
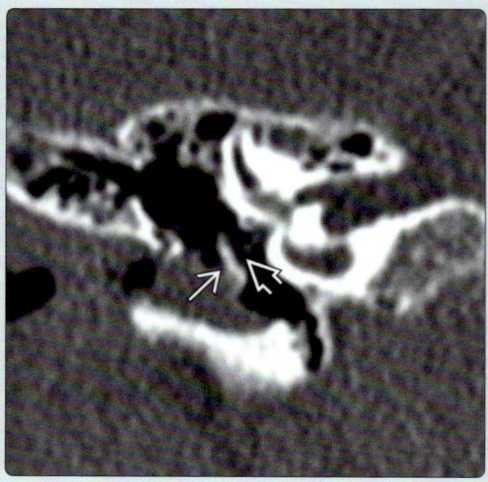

(Left) Axial bone CT in an 18-month-old child after a TV fell on his head shows malposition and malrotation of the malleus head ➡ and the incus body ➡ as well as a diastatic otic capsule-sparing mastoid fracture ➡. (Right) Coronal reformat bone CT in the same child also shows the inferior position of the incus long process ➡ relative to the stapes head ➡, consistent with incus dislocation secondary to incudomalleolar and incudostapedial joint disruption.

Ossicular Dislocations and Disruptions

TERMINOLOGY

Definitions

- Injury to middle ear ossicles
  - Dislocation or subluxation > > fracture

IMAGING

General Features

- Best diagnostic clue
  - **Malalignment or dislocation** of ossicle articulations
- Location
  - **Incudostapedial** > incudomalleolar > complete incus dislocation > stapediovestibular disruption > malleus dislocation
- Morphology
  - **Incudostapedial** dislocation difficult to diagnose on CT, oblique reconstructions helpful
    - **Incus lenticular process anterior or posterior to stapes head**
  - **Incudomalleolar** dislocation/disruption
    - Axial CT: **Malleus head offset** from incus short process looks like **ice cream falling off of cone**
    - Sagittal CT: **Disruption of molar tooth**
  - **Incus** dislocation
    - **Incudomalleolar and incudostapedial joints disrupted** → incus dissociates from malleus and stapes
  - **Stapes** dislocation/stapediovestibular disruption rare
    - Suspect if **transverse fracture line passing through oval window**
    - Actual disruption difficult to see; < 1-mm images may identify stapes fragments or footplate malalignment
  - **Malleus** dislocation **rare**

Imaging Recommendations

- Best imaging tool
  - High-resolution temporal bone CT
    - 0.50- to 0.75-mm slice thickness
- Protocol advice
  - Bone algorithm MDCT with reconstructed coronal ± oblique &/or sagittal images
    - 3D CT reconstructions helpful for clarifying ossicular alignment

DIFFERENTIAL DIAGNOSIS

Congenital Ossicular Anomalies and Fixation

- Ossicular fixation: **Rigid bar or fibrous band** connects ossicle to wall of middle ear cavity
- Ossicular malformation: Abnormal **shape, size, or orientation**

Ossicular Prosthesis

- Surgical reconstruction of malfunctioned portions of ossicular chain to improve hearing
  - Stapes prosthesis
    - **Missing all or part of stapes superstructure**
  - Incus interposition graft
    - **Mimics chronic incus dislocation**
  - Partial ossicular replacement prosthesis (PORP)
  - Total ossicular replacement prosthesis (TORP)

Chronic Otomastoiditis With Ossicular Erosions

- Erosive ossicular changes in absence of cholesteatoma in patient with history of chronic otitis media

Congenital Cholesteatoma With Ossicular Erosions

- Smooth, well-circumscribed middle ear mass ± ossicular erosions

Acquired Cholesteatoma With Ossicular Erosions

- Soft tissue mass in Prussak space with scutum, ossicle, &/or lateral epitympanum wall erosion

PATHOLOGY

General Features

- Etiology
  - Disruption of ossicle support: Ligaments and tendons; tetanic contraction of stapedius and tensor tympani muscles contribute to many injuries
    - Head trauma > > blast injury; rarely secondary to foreign body insertion or lightning strike
    - Incus involved in most posttraumatic ossicular disruptions; weaker ligamentous support compared to malleus and stapes
    - Malleus support: Anterior, lateral, & superior malleolar ligaments; tensor tympani tendon; embedded in tympanic membrane
    - Stapes support: Stapedius tendon (stapes hub); stapediovestibular articulation (stapes footplate and annular ligament)
- Associated abnormalities
  - Temporal bone fractures
    - **Otic capsule violating or otic capsule sparing** (preferred classification)
    - **Longitudinal, transverse, or mixed**
  - **Pneumolabyrinth** secondary to posttraumatic perilymph fistula
  - Middle ear/mastoid opacification/**hemotympanum**
  - **Intracranial injury**: Extraaxial hematoma, parenchymal contusion, pneumocephalus, cerebral edema, diffuse axonal injury
  - **Facial nerve canal fracture** with facial nerve injury
  - **CSF leak**
  - **Carotid artery canal &/or jugular foramen fracture**

CLINICAL ISSUES

Presentation

- Most common signs/symptoms
  - Posttraumatic **conductive hearing loss**
    - Secondary to hemotympanum &/or injury to tympanic membrane, tympanic ring, or ossicles
    - Suspect ossicular injury if persistent hearing loss ≥ 30 decibels lasting **≥ 2 months following trauma**

Treatment

- Ossicular reconstruction with repositioning or interpositioning of various materials: Ossicles, cortical bone grafts, bone cement, PORP, or TORP

SELECTED REFERENCES

1. Johns JD et al: Temporal bone trauma. Otolaryngol Clin North Am. 56(6):1055-67, 2023

Skull Base Trauma

TERMINOLOGY

- Traumatic injury of bony anterior, middle, or posterior cranial fossa

IMAGING

- Noncorticated, noninterdigitating lucency and pneumocephalus or intraorbital emphysema
- Location
  - Anterior fossa: Frontal bone-sinus, cribriform plate
  - Middle fossa: Greater sphenoid wing, sphenoid sinus, clivus
  - Posterior fossa: Petrous temporal bone, occiput
- Protocol advice
  - Bone CT: Skull, facial bones, and cervical spine
  - NECT: Brain and neck soft tissues
  - CTA or MRA: Suspected neurovascular injury
  - MR brain: Suspected cerebral injury
  - DSA following CTA or MRA for vascular injuries

TOP DIFFERENTIAL DIAGNOSES

- Pseudofractures
  - Sutures, fissures, canals, and foramina
  - Emissary veins and venous sinuses

PATHOLOGY

- Associated abnormalities
  - Intracranial contusion, hematoma, pneumocephalus
  - Neurovascular injury
  - CSF fistula/leak
  - Cranial nerve deficits

CLINICAL ISSUES

- Results from high-velocity impact: Motor vehicle accident, gunshot/missile
- Management triaged according to degree/severity of intracranial injury
- Blunt and penetrating vascular injuries of skull base can be life-threatening emergencies

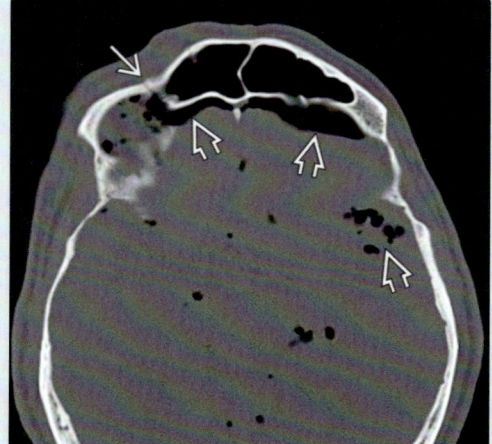
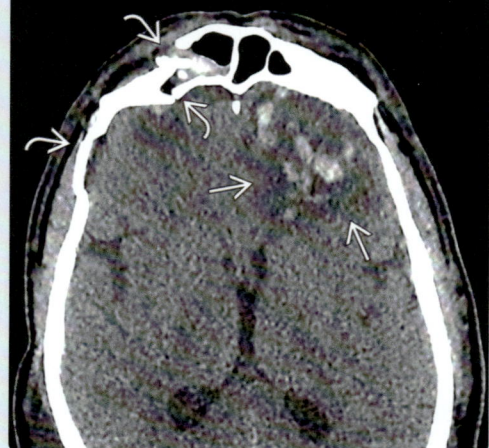

(Left) Axial bone CT shows an anterior skull base or type I/II frontobasal fracture with a fracture line extending through the superomedial orbit ⇨ just lateral to the frontal sinus. There is significant associated pneumocephalus ⇨. (Right) Axial CT shows multiple fractures through the anterior and posterior walls of the right frontal sinus and right frontal bone ⇨. Note the hemorrhagic contusion in the frontal lobe of the brain with surrounding edema ⇨. Review of brain parenchyma is critical in skull base trauma.

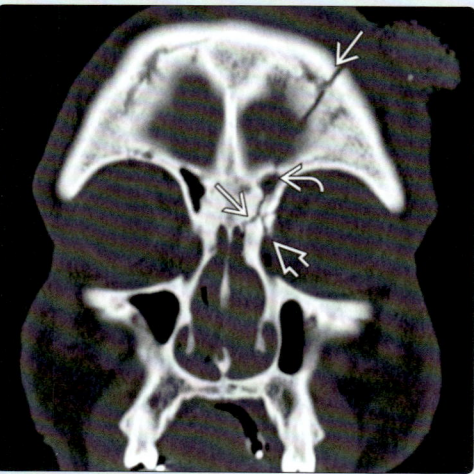
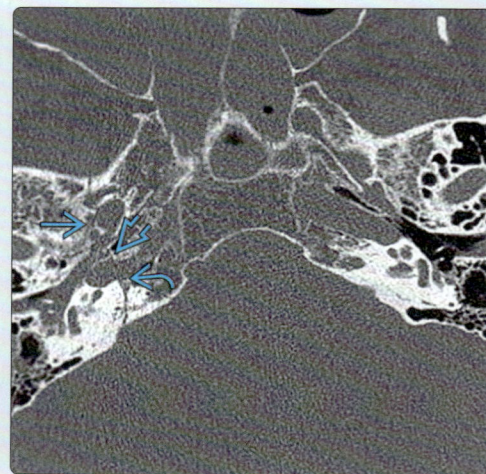

(Left) Coronal bone CT shows an anterior skull base/type III frontobasal fracture with a large fracture ⇨ extending through the left frontal bone to the nasoorbitoethmoid complex. The fracture traverses the left frontal sinus ⇨ terminating in the region of the left lacrimal sac ⇨. (Right) Axial bone CT shows a middle cranial fossa fracture extending through the greater wing of the sphenoid, traversing the foramen ovale, foramen spinosum ⇨, and carotid canal ⇨. Notice the step-off in the carotid canal ⇨, necessitating CTA.

TERMINOLOGY

Definitions

- Traumatic injury of anterior, middle, or posterior skull base

IMAGING

General Features

- Best diagnostic clue
  - Noncorticated, noninterdigitating lucency in skull base bone ± pneumocephalus or intraorbital emphysema
- Location
  - Anterior cranial fossa (ACF)
    - Frontal bone, ethmoid bone, and anterior sphenoid bone
    - Includes frontal sinus, medial 1/3 superior orbital rim, nasoethmoid, cribriform plate, and planum sphenoidale
  - Middle cranial fossa (MCF): Greater wing of sphenoid (GWS) bone, sphenoid sinus, clivus
    - Includes cavernous sinus, horizontal and vertical petrous carotid canals
  - Posterior cranial fossa (PCF): Petrous temporal bone and occiput
- Size
  - Fractures involving cribriform plate, fovea ethmoidalis, carotid canal **may be subtle**
- Morphology
  - Linear
    - Longitudinal, transverse, or oblique
      - May be vertical or horizontal
      - ACF longitudinal fractures run **parallel to cribriform plate**
      - ACF transverse or oblique fractures usually extend to involve orbit and sphenoid
      - MCF fractures typically **transverse or oblique**
  - Comminuted
    - Often associated skull or midface fractures

Imaging Recommendations

- Best imaging tool
  - Thin-slice axial bone CT with multiplanar reconstruction
- Protocol advice
  - Bone CT: Head and facial bones
    - Multidetector CT (MDCT) higher accuracy for detection of fracture
    - Thin-section axial acquisition with 1-mm coronal and sagittal reformats
    - 3D volumetric reconstruction for assessment of deformity, fracture orientation, and reconstruction planning
  - NECT: Head and facial bones
    - Assess **associated intracranial injury**
    - Assess soft tissue injury of orbit, face, upper neck
  - CTA or MRA: **Suspected carotid/vertebral dissection, thromboembolism, carotid-cavernous fistula (CCF)**
    - Fracture involves carotid canal or extends through clivus
    - Enlarged superior ophthalmic vein, significant air in cavernous sinus
  - Brain MR: Suspected **cerebral parenchymal injury**

CT Findings

- NECT
  - Associated intracranial injury
    - Epidural, subdural hematoma, parenchymal contusion, subarachnoid blood, infarct
  - Associated intraorbital soft tissue injury
    - Globe rupture or tenting; intraocular hemorrhage
    - Lens dislocation
    - Retrobulbar or subperiosteal hematoma
  - Paranasal sinus hemorrhage or hematoma
- Bone CT
  - Noncorticated, noninterdigitating lucency
    - May have associated diastasis of sutures
  - Comminution of bone typically mild to moderate
    - Displacement of bone fragments
    - Highly comminuted cribriform or ethmoid fractures usually associated with complex facial fractures
  - Associated pneumocephalus, intraorbital emphysema
  - Air-fluid levels in frontal, ethmoid, sphenoid sinuses
- CTA
  - Arterial occlusion/**dissection**
    - Vessel wall irregularity, luminal narrowing, pseudoaneurysm
    - Lack of contrast opacification
      - Segmental, high-grade, flame-shaped or tapered narrowing/string sign → dissection
    - 16-slice or greater MDCT: **92% negative predictive value** for carotid/vertebral occlusion, dissection
  - CCF
    - Focal bulging, asymmetric distention of involved cavernous sinus
    - Enlargement of ipsilateral superior ophthalmic vein
    - Fistula tract between cavernous carotid and cavernous sinus

MR Findings

- T1WI FS
  - Consider without contrast for cervical dissection
- T1WI/T2WI/FLAIR/DWI: Hemorrhage, infarction, shear injury
  - Loss of flow void in internal carotid artery (ICA)/vertebral or fried egg/crescent sign → occlusion or dissection
- MRA: Carotid/vertebral occlusion or dissection, CCF

DIFFERENTIAL DIAGNOSIS

Pseudofractures of Skull Base

- Sutures and fissures
  - Sphenofrontal suture and metopic suture
  - Sphenooccipital synchondroses
  - Petrooccipital fissure
  - Sphenopetrosal synchondrosis and sphenosquamosal suture
  - Tympanosquamous suture and petrotympanic fissure
  - Occipitomastoid suture
- Canals and foramina
  - Anterior, posterior ethmoidal artery canal
  - Supraorbital artery foramen; vidian canal
  - Neurovascular channels from foramen rotundum and ovale

– Inferior and lateral rotundal canals
– Accessory meningeal artery canal and foramen of Vesalius
- Emissary veins and venous sinuses
  o Mastoid, occipital, petrosquamosal, posterior condylar
  o Superior petrosal sinus

PATHOLOGY

General Features

- Etiology
  o ACF: Results from frontal bone impact
    – **Predominately** secondary to **motor vehicle accident** (MVA)
    – Low-velocity frontal bone injuries → linear fractures of anterior ± central skull base
    – High-velocity lateral or inferior frontal bone/glabella, supraorbital region and zygoma → anterior and central skull base involvement
  o MCF: High-velocity impact to lateral frontal bone, zygoma, temporal or parietal bone
- Associated abnormalities
  o Intracranial contusion, hematoma
  o Pneumocephalus
  o CSF fistula/leak
    – ↑ probability with linear or comminuted fractures involving ACF, central anterior skull base
  o Carotid or vertebrobasilar dissection, thromboembolism
    – Fracture involving sphenoid sinus or carotid canal → ↑ probability of neurovascular injury
  o Dural AV fistula
    – CCF: ↑ **incidence of CCF with sphenoid, carotid canal fracture**
  o Cranial nerve deficits
    – Frontobasal: CNI, less commonly CNIII, IV, VI
    – MCF: CNIII-VI
  o Horner syndrome

Staging, Grading, & Classification

- AOCMF classification divides skull base into 9 regions: Left and right frontal, central, middle, and PCF
  o Anterior skull base: Frontal bone and LWS
  o Central skull base
    – Central anterior: Cribriform plate and planum sphenoidale
    – Central middle: Sella and parasellar compartments
    – Central posterior: Clivus
  o Middle: Sphenoid, GWS, and temporal bone
  o Posterior: Parietal and occipital bone
- Other classifications
  o Frontobasal: Type I-III
    – Types I and II are linear fractures involving frontal bone, nasoorbitoethmoid, cribriform plate or planum sphenoidale (type I) or extend through orbit and squamous temporal bone (type II)
    – Type III: Combined comminuted type I and type II fractures

CLINICAL ISSUES

Presentation

- Most common signs/symptoms

  o Frontal or temporal scalp laceration, hematoma
    – Periorbital hematoma ("raccoon eyes")
  o Proptosis, other orbital injuries
  o Altered mental status, loss of consciousness, and neurological deficit
- Other signs/symptoms
  o Nausea, vomiting, seizure, drowsiness

Demographics

- Age
  o All ages; less common in pediatric populations
- Sex
  o M > F
- Epidemiology
  o High-velocity impact predominately MVA, gunshot/missile
  o Lower velocity blunt trauma more often following falls, assault/nonaccidental trauma

Natural History & Prognosis

- ACF/type II and III frontobasal
  o Higher risk for intracranial injuries
  o Higher risk for CSF leak
- MCF fractures
  o Higher risk for intracranial injuries
  o Higher risk for neurovascular injuries
  o Higher risk for cranial nerve deficits

Treatment

- Management triaged according to degree/severity of intracranial injury
- Endovascular treatment for neurovascular injury
- Antibiotic coverage for meningitis/CSF leak
- Management of orbital injuries
- CSF leak repair

SELECTED REFERENCES

1. Jung G et al: Clinical features and management of skull base fractures in the pediatric population: a systematic review. Children (Basel). 11(5):564 2024
2. Bischof GN et al: Brain trauma imaging. J Nucl Med. 64(1):20-9, 2023
3. Rodriguez A et al: Vascular injuries in head and neck trauma. Radiol Clin North Am. 61(3):467-77, 2023
4. Schulze M et al: Flat panel CT versus multidetector CT in skull base imaging: are there differences in image quality? Head Face Med. 19(1):50, 2023
5. Dreizin D et al: CT of skull base fractures: classification systems, complications, and management. Radiographics. 41(3):762-82 2021
6. Quirk B et al: Skull base imaging, anatomy, pathology and protocols. Pract Neurol. 20(1):39-49, 2020
7. Varshneya K et al: Risks, costs, and outcomes of cerebrospinal fluid leaks after pediatric skull fractures: a MarketScan analysis between 2007 and 2015. Neurosurg Focus. 47(5):E10, 2019
8. Bobinski M et al: Basic imaging of skull base trauma. J Neurol Surg B Skull Base. 77(5):381-7, 2016
9. Baugnon KL et al: Skull base fractures and their complications. Neuroimaging Clin N Am. 24(3):439-65, vii-viii, 2014
10. Di Ieva A et al: The comprehensive AOCMF classification: skull base and cranial vault fractures - level 2 and 3 tutorial. Craniomaxillofac Trauma Reconstr. 7(Suppl 1):S103-13, 2014
11. Lin DT et al: Surgical treatment of traumatic injuries of the cranial base. Otolaryngol Clin North Am. 46(5):749-57, 2013
12. Mithani SK et al: Predictable patterns of intracranial and cervical spine injury in craniomaxillofacial trauma: analysis of 4786 patients. Plast Reconstr Surg. 123(4):1293-301, 2009
13. Atabaki SM et al: A clinical decision rule for cranial computed tomography in minor pediatric head trauma. Arch Pediatr Adolesc Med. 162(5):439-45, 2008
14. Feiz-Erfan I et al: Incidence and pattern of direct blunt neurovascular injury associated with trauma to the skull base. J Neurosurg. 107(2):364-9, 2007

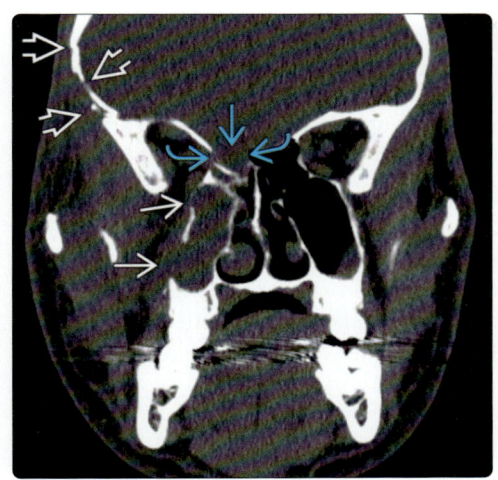

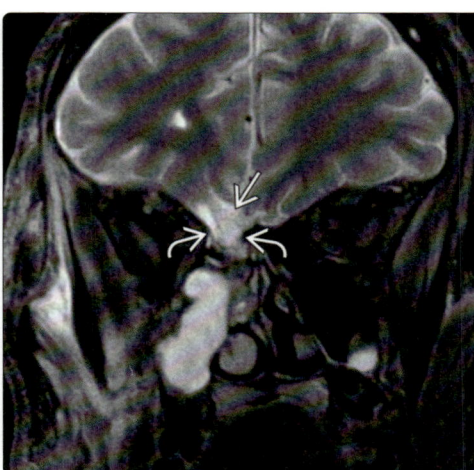

(Left) Coronal NECT demonstrates numerous subacute to chronic facial ⇨ and skull fractures ⇨ in a patient presenting with rhinorrhea. A dehiscent depressed fracture of the right planum sphenoidale ⇨ with fluid opacification of the right ethmoid air cells ⇨ is seen. (Right) Coronal T2 FS MR in the same patient shows gliotic right frontal parenchyma and CSF (meningoencephalocele ⇨) herniated into the depressed right planum sphenoidale fracture ⇨, the source of the CSF rhinorrhea.

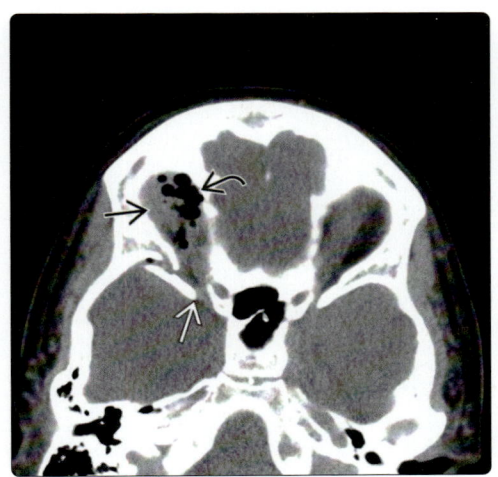

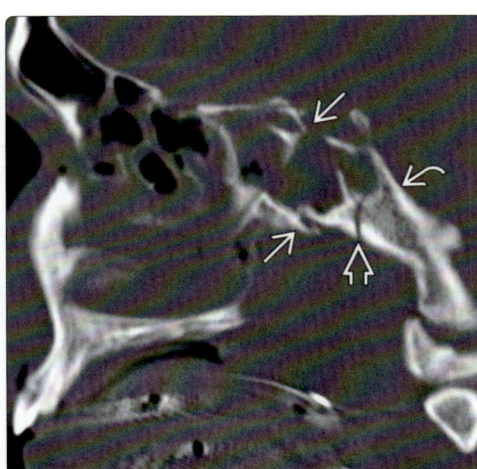

(Left) Axial NECT shows a displaced fracture through the posterior rim of the right lesser wing of the sphenoid bone with orbital emphysema ⇨ and a subperiosteal hematoma ⇨. Note that slight rotation of the sphenoid wing fracture fragment impinges on the superior orbital fissure ⇨. (Right) Sagittal bone CT in a patient following a motor vehicle accident (MVA) shows multiple comminuted sphenoid ⇨ and clival ⇨ fractures. The posterior clivus is intact ⇨, reducing the probability of vertebral artery injury.

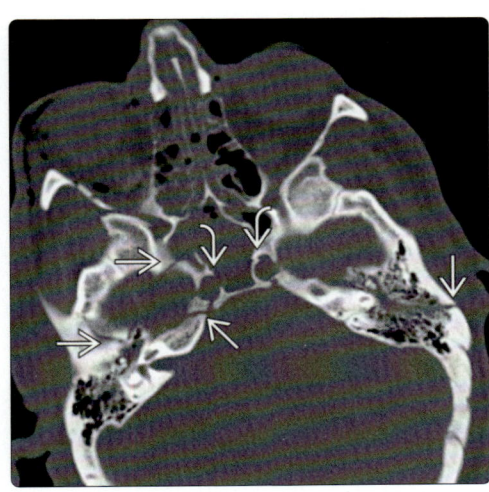

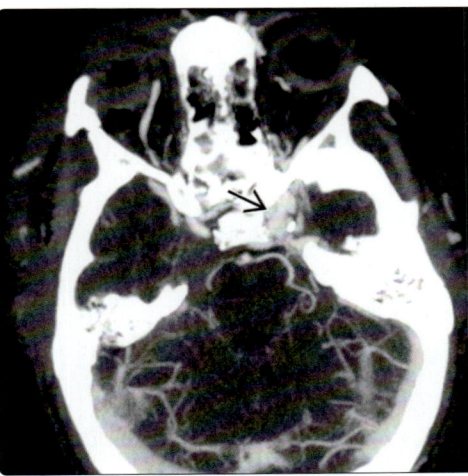

(Left) Axial bone CT in a patient following a high-speed MVA shows multiple temporal, petrous temporal bone and sphenoid fractures ⇨. Both carotid canals are fractured ⇨, increasing the probability of carotid injury. (Right) Axial CTA shows asymmetric abnormal venous enhancement in conjunction with arterial enhancement in this traumatic carotid-cavernous fistula (CCF) ⇨ in the left cavernous carotid. The superior ophthalmic vein was also enlarged (not shown). The CCF was confirmed on digital subtraction angiography.

KEY FACTS

TERMINOLOGY

- Definition: Fracture complex with fracture lines involving zygomatic arch, lateral orbital wall & rim, anterior & lateral walls of maxillary sinus, & orbital floor & inferior orbital rim
  - Previous called **trimalar** or **tripod** fracture, ZMC fracture terminology most accurate as fracture involves lateral orbital wall along zygomaticosphenoid suture

IMAGING

- Fracture lines through or near sutures of zygoma
- Modality of choice: Thin-slice axial bone algorithm CT
  - Can be reformatted in coronal plane
  - 3D reformatted images very helpful for demonstrating degree of fracture displacement & angulation for surgical planning

TOP DIFFERENTIAL DIAGNOSES

- Complex midfacial fracture
- Transfacial (Le Fort) fractures

- Zygomatic arch fracture

PATHOLOGY

- Most common mechanism of injury: Direct blow to cheek (malar eminence)
- Classification systems not often used to plan treatment since advent of miniplates & microplates

CLINICAL ISSUES

- Teenage to young adult males most commonly affected
- Signs & symptoms
  - Loss of cheek projection with ↑ facial width
  - Impaired sensation or anesthesia of cheek/upper lip
    - Infraorbital nerve injury
  - Enophthalmos
    - Displaced or angulated fracture may ↑ orbital volume
  - Trismus
- Excellent prognosis for restored cosmesis after surgical fixation

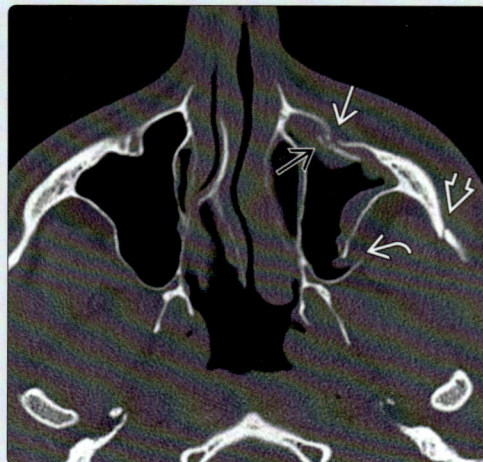
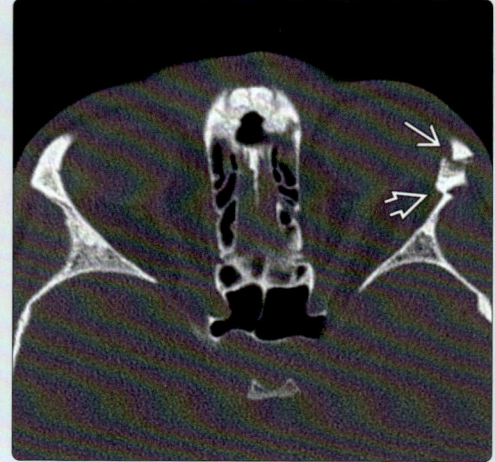

(Left) Axial bone CT shows the typical fracture patterns of a zygomaticomaxillary complex (ZMC) fracture. Fracture extends through the zygomatic arch ➡ with additional comminuted fractures involving the left anterior ➡ and lateral ➡ maxillary sinus walls. Note fracture also involves the infraorbital canal ➡. (Right) Axial bone CT through the orbits in the same patient shows additional typical ZMC fracture components through the lateral orbital rim ➡ and wall ➡.

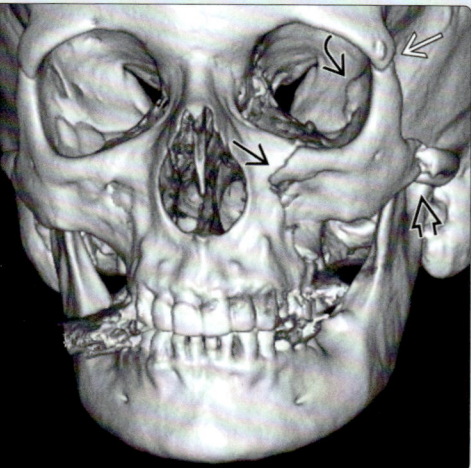
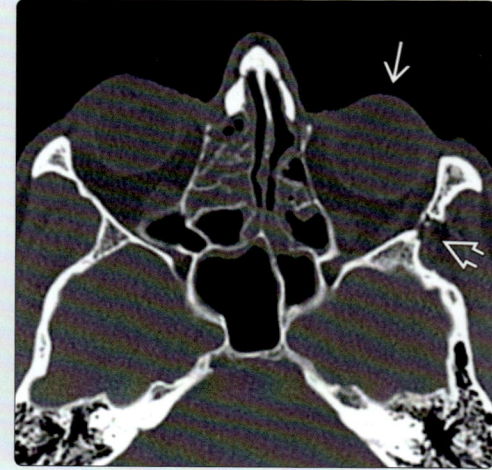

(Left) 3D reconstruction shows the classic features of a ZMC fracture. Fractures involve the walls of the left maxillary sinus ➡, the left zygomatic arch ➡, lateral orbital wall ➡, and lateral orbital rim ➡. (Right) Axial bone CT shows left enophthalmos ➡ from increased orbital volume, resulting from a prior left ZMC fracture, with remote fracture of the left lateral orbital wall at the zygomaticosphenoid suture ➡. Remaining ZMC fracture components are not shown.

Zygomaticomaxillary Complex Fracture

TERMINOLOGY

Abbreviations

- Zygomaticomaxillary complex (ZMC) fracture

Synonyms

- Trimalar fracture; tripod fracture; displaced ZMC fracture = quadripod or quadramalar fracture
- **ZMC fracture terminology most universally accepted**

Definitions

- Fracture complex with fracture lines involving zygomatic arch, lateral orbital wall & rim, anterior & lateral walls of maxillary sinus, & orbital floor & inferior orbital rim

IMAGING

General Features

- Best diagnostic clue
  - Fracture complex with fracture lines involving zygomatic arch, lateral orbital wall & rim, anterior & lateral walls of maxillary sinus, & orbital floor & inferior orbital rim
- Location
  - **Fracture lines through or near sutures of zygoma**

CT Findings

- Bone CT
  - Lucent fracture line locations
    - Along lateral orbital wall & rim (**frontozygomatic & zygomaticosphenoid sutures**)
    - From inferior orbital fissure to orbital floor (**near infraorbital canal**)
    - Down anterior maxilla (**near zygomaticomaxillary suture**)
    - Up posterior maxillary wall to inferior orbital fissure
    - Also fracture through **zygomatic arch** (**near zygomaticotemporal suture**)

Imaging Recommendations

- Best imaging tool
  - Thin-slice (0.6-1.0 mm) axial bone algorithm CT

DIFFERENTIAL DIAGNOSIS

Complex Midfacial Fracture

- Multiple markedly comminuted fractures not fitting into classification
- Bilateral

Transfacial (Le Fort) Fractures

- All 3 Le Fort types involve pterygoid processes
- Le Fort II is only type involving inferior orbital rim
- Le Fort III is only type involving zygomatic arch

Zygomatic Arch Fracture

- Isolated zygomatic arch fracture(s) without maxillary wall or orbital wall involvement

Inferior Orbital (Blowout) Fracture

- Pure inferior orbital blowout fractures involve orbital floor sparing orbital rim
- Sparing of zygomatic arch, lateral orbital wall & rim, maxillary sinus walls

PATHOLOGY

General Features

- Etiology
  - Most commonly occurs after **direct blow to cheek** (malar eminence) during assault
  - Zygomas have 2 attachments to cranium & 2 to midface, creating portions of inferior & lateral orbital walls
    - **ZMC fracture + ipsilateral nasoorbitoethmoidal fracture**, higher incidence of postop complications/deformities

Staging, Grading, & Classification

- Classification systems not often used to plan treatment with use of miniplates & microplates
- 1 of more complete classification systems based upon type, frequency, & postreduction stability of malar fractures

CLINICAL ISSUES

Presentation

- Most common signs/symptoms
  - Loss of cheek projection with ↑ facial width
  - **Impaired sensation** or anesthesia of cheek/upper lip
    - Infraorbital nerve injury (**> 90% of cases**)
  - Trismus
    - Impingement of **temporalis muscle** or **coronoid process** of mandible by depressed zygomatic arch
  - Enophthalmos
    - Displaced or angulated fracture may ↑ orbital volume

Demographics

- Age
  - Teenage to young adults most common
- Sex
  - More common in males
- Epidemiology
  - Zygomatic fractures are common, accounting for 17% of facial fractures

Natural History & Prognosis

- Excellent prognosis for restored cosmesis after surgical fixation
- Surgical results depend somewhat upon degree of comminution, fracture displacement, & angulation

Treatment

- Surgical exposure indicated if angulated or severely comminuted
- Surgery goals
  - Correct 3D position of malar prominence
  - Restore orbital volume by correcting alignment of zygoma & sphenoid
- Intraoperative CT &/or augmented reality helpful in fixation of displaced/angulated ZMC fracture or with displaced orbital floor

SELECTED REFERENCES

1. Kim TH et al: Enhancing surgical approach: breakthrough markerless surface registration with augmented reality for zygomatic complex fracture surgeries. Ann Plast Surg. 93(1):70-3, 2024
2. Winegar BA et al: Spectrum of critical imaging findings in complex facial skeletal trauma. Radiographics. 33(1):3-19, 2013

TERMINOLOGY

- **Central upper midface fracture** complex involving confluence of medial and upper maxillary buttresses and their posterior extensions
  - Disruption of medial canthal regions, ethmoids, and medial orbital walls

IMAGING

- Bone CT: Nasal bone fracture in combination with fractures of medial orbital wall and frontal process of maxilla

TOP DIFFERENTIAL DIAGNOSES

- Complex midfacial fracture
- Nasal bone fracture
- Medial orbital blowout fracture

PATHOLOGY

- Force transmitted through nasal bones and involves ethmoid sinuses and medial orbits

- May involve frontal recess resulting in impaired frontal sinus drainage
- May involve cribriform plate → CSF leak, meningoencephalocele, intracranial infection
- Manson classification
  - Type I: Medial canthal insertion on large fracture fragment
  - Type II: Canthal tendon attached to small bone fragment
  - Type III: Complete avulsion of medial canthal tendon

CLINICAL ISSUES

- Symptoms and signs
  - Loss of nasal projection in profile
  - Increased distance between inner corners of eyes (telecanthus)
- Nasoorbitalethmoidal fractures can be among most difficult facial fracture patterns to accurately repair
- Treatment goals: Restore intercanthal distance, collapsed nasal projection, and orbital volumes

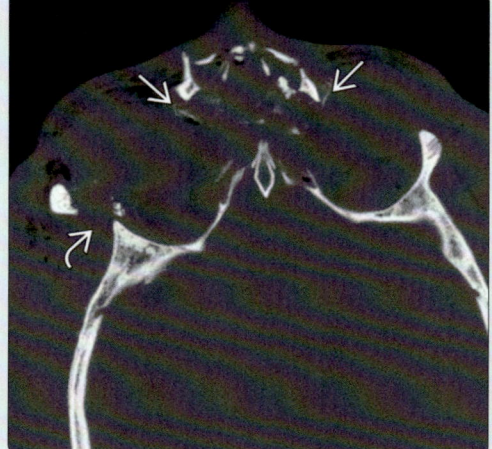
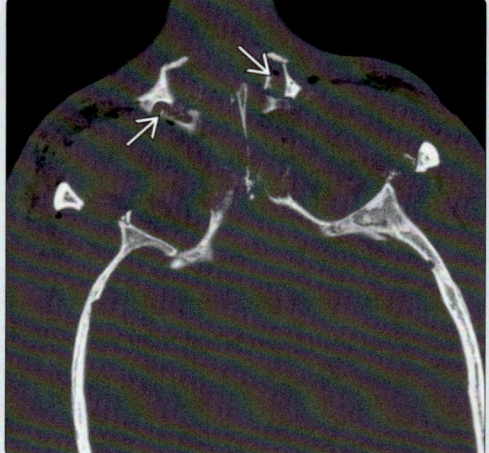

(Left) Axial bone CT shows markedly comminuted fractures involving the nasoorbitalethmoidal (NOE) complex. Multiple small fracture fragments are noted in the medial canthal regions ➡, and there is a degree of telecanthus. Soft tissue swelling, emphysema, and a lateral orbital fracture ➡ are noted. (Right) Axial bone CT viewed inferiorly in the same patient shows that the fractures involve both nasolacrimal ducts ➡. In such a patient, epiphora would be an expected complication of the injury.

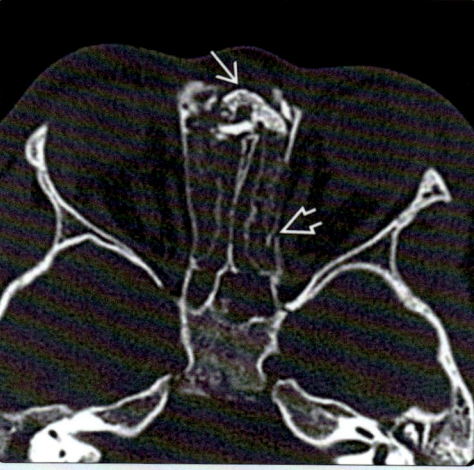
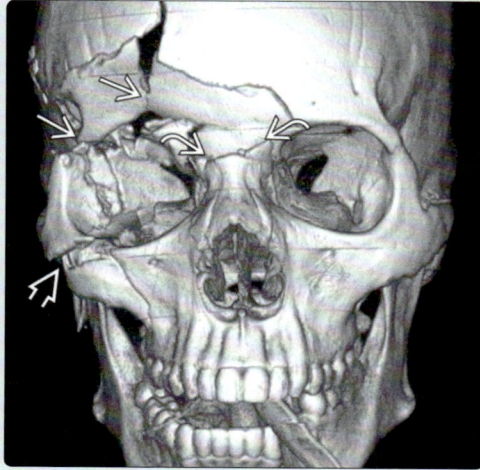

(Left) Axial bone CT demonstrates comminuted fractures involving the NOE complex with retropulsion of the nasal bridge ➡ and fracture of the left lamina papyracea ➡. Patient will require surgery to restore collapsed nasal projection. (Right) Anterior 3D reconstructed bone CT in a 20-year-old patient demonstrates highly comminuted fractures involving the NOE ➡, orbit ➡, and maxilla ➡. Patient will require surgery to repair the comminuted fractures and restore right orbital volume.

Nasoorbitoethmoid (NOE) Fracture

TERMINOLOGY

Abbreviations
- Nasoorbitalethmoidal (NOE) fracture

Definitions
- **Central upper midface fracture** complex
  - Involving confluence of medial and upper maxillary buttresses and their posterior extensions along medial orbital wall and floor
  - Distinguished from simple nasal fractures by posterior disruption of medial canthal regions, ethmoids, and medial orbital walls

IMAGING

General Features
- Best diagnostic clue
  - Nasal bone fracture in combination with fractures of medial orbital wall and frontal process of maxilla
- Location
  - Central upper midface; nasal dorsum and medial orbits
  - Includes damage to ethmoid sinus and walls

Imaging Recommendations
- Best imaging tool
  - Thin-section bone algorithm CT + multiplanar reformats

CT Findings
- Bone CT
  - Nasal bone fractures in combination with fractures of medial orbital wall and frontal process of maxilla
  - Frontal recess involvement likely if there is displaced anterior table fracture medial to supraorbital notch involving frontal sinus floor

DIFFERENTIAL DIAGNOSIS

Complex Midfacial Fracture
- Severe injury with fracture pattern not falling into other classifications

Nasal Bone Fracture
- Intact medial orbital walls and frontal process of maxilla

Medial Orbital Blowout Fracture
- Orbital rims spared

PATHOLOGY

General Features
- Etiology
  - NOE = facial unit composed of nasal bones, medial orbital walls, and frontal process of maxillary bones
  - **High-force trauma**
    - Thin nasal bones, ethmoid sinus walls, & medial orbits act as "crumple zone," allow force to be dissipated
    - Critical structures (brain and optic nerve) lie in stronger bone posteriorly and are relatively protected
- Associated abnormalities
  - Fractures through **frontal recess** with disruption of frontal sinus drainage
  - Associated fractures of **cribriform plate**
  - Severe **ocular injuries**
  - Orbital hematoma
  - Contiguous skull fractures
  - Cervical spine injuries
  - Intracranial injuries

Staging, Grading, & Classification
- Manson classification system (3 major subsets based on degree of injury to medial canthal attachment)
  - Type I: Fractured piece is large, and medial canthal insertion on it is intact
  - Type II: Comminution of bony buttress and canthus is attached to small bone fragment
  - Type III: Avulsion of medial canthal tendon from its osseous insertion (clinical diagnosis, not with imaging)

CLINICAL ISSUES

Presentation
- Most common signs/symptoms
  - Loss of nasal projection in profile
  - ↑ distance between inner corners of eyes (telecanthus)
- Other signs/symptoms
  - Epiphora (5-31% of NOE fracture patients)
  - Globe malposition; vision loss

Natural History & Prognosis
- Significant cosmetic and functional deficits may arise from high-force NOE injury
  - Midface retrusion and nasal shortening
    - From telescoping of nasal bones
  - Telecanthus from disruption of medial canthal tendons
    - From bony insertion or displacement of medial canthal tendon fragment
  - Epiphora from injury to lacrimal puncta, canaliculi, sac, or nasolacrimal duct

Treatment
- Goals: Restore intercanthal distance, collapsed nasal projection, & orbital volumes
- Recent advances in minimally invasive surgical techniques and multidisciplinary approach may improve outcomes

DIAGNOSTIC CHECKLIST

Reporting Tips
- Imaging description should include
  - **Degree of comminution** of medial vertical maxillary buttress in region of medial canthal tendon attachment
  - Distance between 2 lacrimal fossae in coronal plane
  - Involvement of frontal sinus drainage pathway and orbit
- Also report degree of comminution of surrounding nasal, maxillary, and orbital walls for surgical planning purposes

SELECTED REFERENCES

1. Butchy MV et al: The clinical value of computed tomography of facial bone injuries in pediatric trauma patients. Am Surg. 91(2):253-8, 2025
2. Kochkine S et al: Facial fractures: the "bottom-up" approach. Clin Imaging. 101:167-79, 2023
3. Zhang Y et al: Introduction of digital-assisted multidisciplinary treatment in the functional and morphological reconstruction of naso-orbital-ethmoid fractures. J Craniofac Surg. 33(7):1991-5, 2022
4. Yesantharao PS et al: The association of zygomaticomaxillary complex fractures with naso-orbitoethmoid fractures in pediatric populations. Plast Reconstr Surg. 147(5):777e-86e, 2021

TERMINOLOGY

- Fractures disrupting **pterygomaxillary junction**, disjoining portions of face (maxilla) from skull

IMAGING

- Best diagnostic clue: Pterygoid process & pterygoid plate fractures in patients with clinically mobile facial skeleton
- **Le Fort I**: Pyriform rim + medial & lateral walls of maxillary sinus or alveolus + nasal septum
- **Le Fort II**: Medial orbital wall, including frontomaxillary suture + nasofrontal junction; inferior orbital wall, including zygomaticomaxillary suture + inferior rim
- **Le Fort III**: Medial orbital wall, including frontomaxillary suture + nasofrontal junction; lateral orbital wall, including zygomaticofrontal suture + zygomaticosphenoid suture + zygomatic arch
- Facial skeleton divided into 4 subunits (more practical classification of injuries): Frontal, upper midface, lower midface, & mandible

TOP DIFFERENTIAL DIAGNOSES

- Zygomaticomaxillary complex fracture
- Nasoorbitalethmoidal fracture
- Pterygoid plate avulsion

PATHOLOGY

- **Type I**: Floating palate
  - Inferior portions of medial & lateral maxillary buttresses
- **Type II**: Pyramidal fracture
  - Superior portion of medial maxillary buttress + inferior portion of lateral maxillary buttress
- **Type III**: Craniofacial dissociation
  - Superior portions of lateral & medial maxillary buttresses + upper transverse maxillary buttress

DIAGNOSTIC CHECKLIST

- Pterygoid process frature key feature of Le Fort fractures
- Patterns of fracture can be unilateral, bilateral, or combination

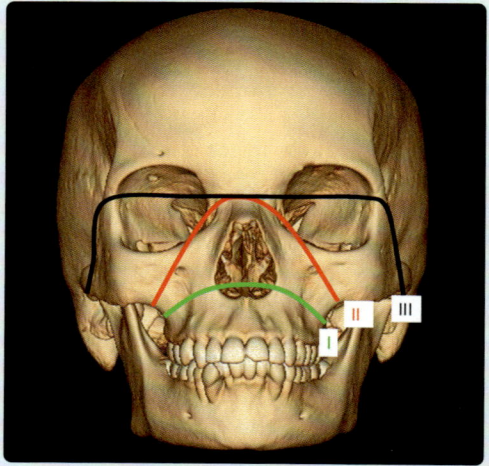
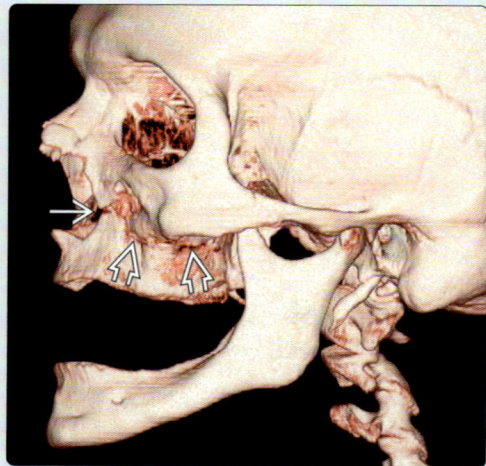

(Left) Frontal graphic demonstrates the 3 types of Le Fort fractures. Le Fort I (green) involves the nasal aperture & piriform rim; Le Fort II (red) traverses the inferior & medial orbital walls; & Le Fort III (black) extends through the zygomatic arches & lateral & medial orbital walls. (Right) Lateral bone CT 3D reformation shows a horizontal Le Fort I fracture ⇗ separating the maxillary alveolus from the midface. Note the involvement of the nasal aperture ⇗. The inferior orbital rim & zygomatic arch are intact.

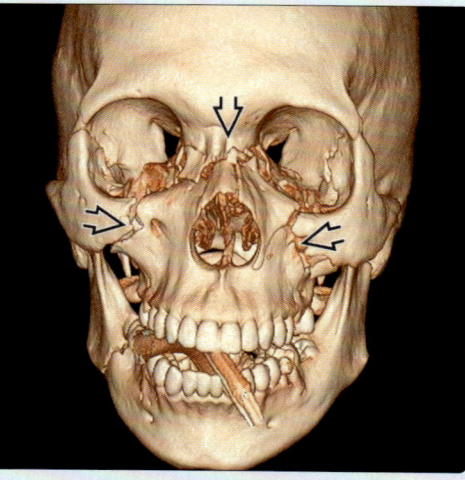
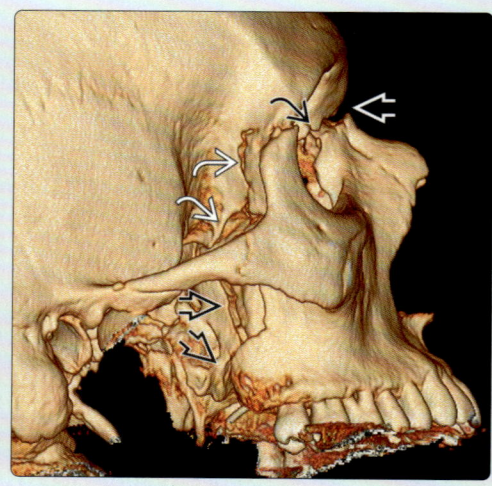

(Left) AP CT 3D reformation shows a Le Fort II fracture ⇗ with subtle clockwise rotation of the midface & an asymmetric bite. Note the bilateral inferior orbital rim involvement with sparing of the nasal aperture. (Right) Lateral bone CT 3D reformation shows a right Le Fort III fracture with nasofrontal diastasis ⇗, medial ⇗ & lateral ⇗ orbital wall fractures, & pterygoid plate fractures ⇗. The inferior orbital rim is spared.

Transfacial Fractures (Le Fort)

TERMINOLOGY

Synonyms

- Le Fort fracture

Definitions

- Fractures disrupting **pterygomaxillary junction (posterior vertical maxillary buttress)**, disjoining portions of face (maxilla) from skull

IMAGING

General Features

- Best diagnostic clue
  - **Pterygoid process & pterygoid plate fractures** in patients with clinically mobile facial skeleton

Imaging Recommendations

- Best imaging tool
  - Thin-section bone CT
- Protocol advice
  - Noncontrast helical CT (slice thickness ≤ 1 mm) in bone algorithm with multiplanar & 3D reformations
  - Shaded surface 3D renderings facilitate Le Fort fracture analysis & assist in surgical planning

CT Findings

- Le Fort I
  - Fracture involving **pyriform rim** + **medial & lateral walls of maxillary sinus** or alveolus + nasal septum
- Le Fort II
  - Fracture involving **medial orbital wall**, including **frontomaxillary suture** + **nasofrontal junction**
  - Fracture involving involving **inferior orbital wall**, including **zygomaticomaxillary suture** + **inferior rim**
- Le Fort III
  - Fracture involving **medial orbital wall**, including **frontomaxillary suture** + **nasofrontal junction**
  - Fracture involving **lateral orbital wall**, including **zygomaticofrontal suture** + **zygomaticosphenoid suture** + **zygomatic arch**

DIFFERENTIAL DIAGNOSIS

Zygomaticomaxillary Complex Fracture

- Spares pterygoid process/plates
- Involves zygomaticofrontal, zygomaticomaxillary, zygomaticosphenoid, & zygomaticotemporal sutures

Nasoorbitalethmoidal Fracture

- Spares pterygoid processes/plates
- Depression of nasal pyramid ± telecanthus due to displacement of medial canthal ligament

Complex Facial Fracture

- Highly comminuted midface fracture
- In pure form, spares pterygoid processes/plates but frequently coexists with Le Fort patterns

Pterygoid Plate Avulsion

- Associated with violent trauma to mandible
- Lateral pterygoid plate typically involved, pterygoid process proper usually spared

PATHOLOGY

Staging, Grading, & Classification

- **Type I: Floating palate**
  - Pterygomaxillary disjunction + fractures of inferior portions of medial & lateral maxillary buttresses
- **Type II: Pyramidal fracture**
  - Pterygomaxillary disjunction + fractures of superior portion of medial maxillary buttress + inferior portion of lateral maxillary buttress
- **Type III: Craniofacial dissociation**
  - Pterygomaxillary disjunction + fractures of superior portions of lateral & medial maxillary buttresses + upper transverse maxillary buttress
- **Combinations of Le Fort types**
  - Unilateral/asymmetric Le Fort fracture & combinations of Le Fort fracture with other facial fracture types (zygomaticomaxillary complex, nasoorbitoethmoid) are common

CLINICAL ISSUES

Presentation

- Most common signs/symptoms
  - "Mobile face"
    - Maxillary alveolus/hard palate, midface, or entire face
- Other signs/symptoms
  - Enophthalmos, diplopia (Le Fort II)
  - Infraorbital nerve injury with facial sensory loss (Le Fort II)
  - Periorbital ecchymosis (Le Fort II & III)
  - Lacrimal apparatus injury with epiphora (Le Fort II & III)
  - Dental malocclusion

Natural History & Prognosis

- Long-term complications may include
  - Facial deformity, breathing difficulty, & masticatory problems/malocclusion
  - Telecanthus, visual loss, diplopia, & epiphora
  - Anosmia, facial numbness, & headaches

Treatment

- Surgical reduction & fixation of facial fractures
  - Starts with frontal bone "bar"
  - Other facial bones "suspended" from frontal bar
  - Zygomaticofrontal injuries repaired 1st, palatoalveolar complex last
  - Orbital fractures repaired after horizontal & vertical buttresses surgically reconstituted

DIAGNOSTIC CHECKLIST

Image Interpretation Pearls

- Involvement of **pterygoid processes/plates** is key feature of Le Fort fractures

SELECTED REFERENCES

1. Omami G et al: Imaging of maxillofacial injuries. Dent Clin North Am. 68(2):393-407, 2024
2. Lin C et al: Classifying and standardizing panfacial trauma according to anatomic categories and facial injury severity scale: a 10-year retrospective study. BMC Oral Health. 21(1):557, 2021
3. Gómez Roselló E et al: Facial fractures: classification and highlights for a useful report. Insights Imaging. 11(1):49, 2020

(Left) Oblique bone CT 3D reformation shows a right Le Fort I fracture ➡ mobilizing the right hemimaxilla, which is rotated inferiorly ➯. In addition, there are multiple nasal bone fractures ➡ & comminuted left maxillary fractures ➡. (Right) Sagittal bone CT reformation shows the utility of sagittal reformats for demonstrating the maxillary disjunction of a Le Fort I with fracture extending from the lateral aspect of the nasal aperture ➡ through the pterygoid process ➡.

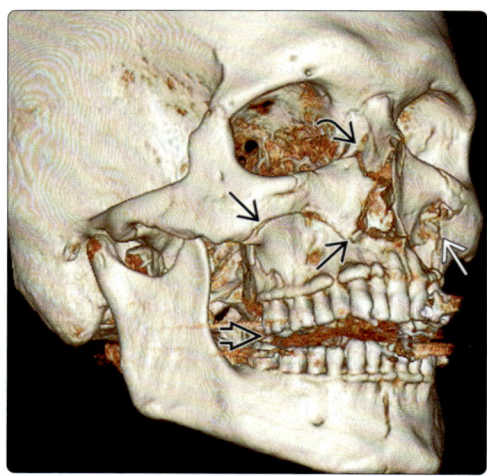
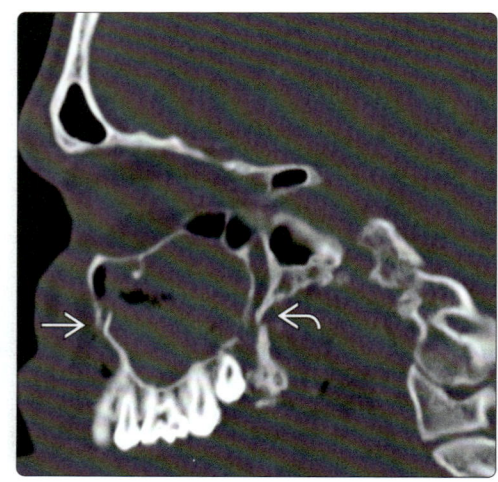

(Left) Frontal bone CT 3D reformation shows a left Le Fort II fracture extending from the nasal bones ➡ through the ethmoid complex & anteroinferiorly to the inferior orbital rim ➯. Note the associated bilateral Le Fort I fractures ➯. Microplate fixation is evident from an old zygomaticomaxillary repair ➡. (Right) Lateral bone CT 3D reformation shows a Le Fort II fracture involving the nasal bones ➡ & inferior orbital rim ➯. There is an associated Le Fort I fracture ➯. The fractured pterygoid plate is obscured by the mandible.

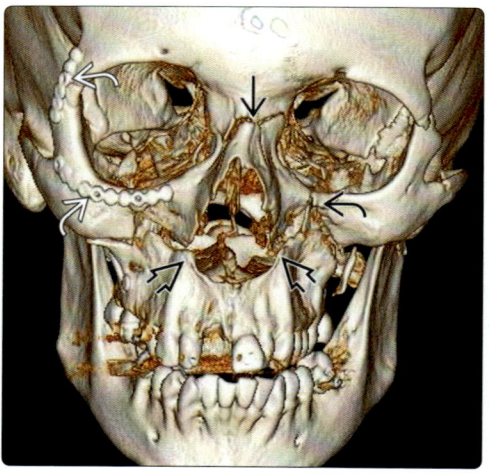
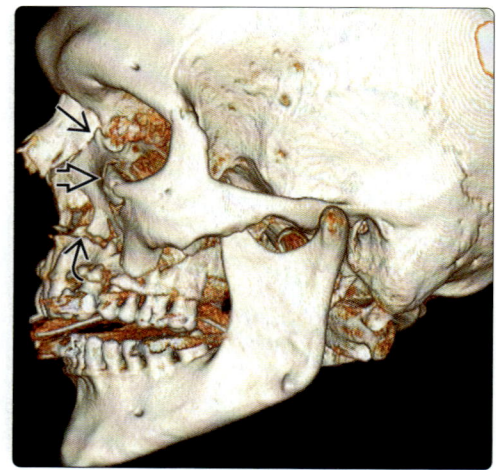

(Left) Oblique bone CT 3D reformation displays features of a right Le Fort III fracture with craniofacial disjunction, including depressed nasal fracture ➯, zygoma fractures ➡, & a depressed zygomatic arch fracture ➯. Note accompanying comminuted orbital & maxillary smash fractures ➯. (Right) Axial bone CT of a Le Fort I & II fracture shows bilateral nasal bone ➡, anterior & posterolateral maxillary walls ➡, & pterygoid plates fractures ➡. Note fracture of the right mandibular condyle ➯ & air in the soft tissues ➯.

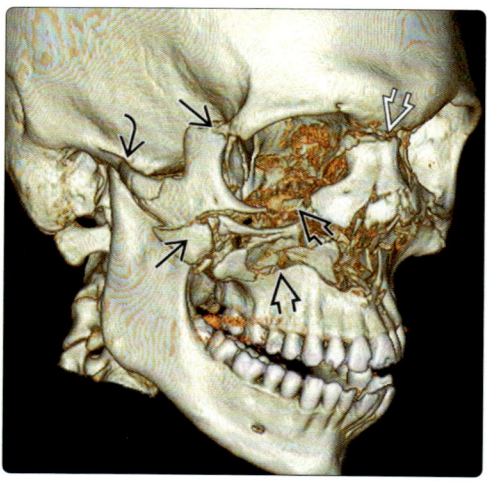
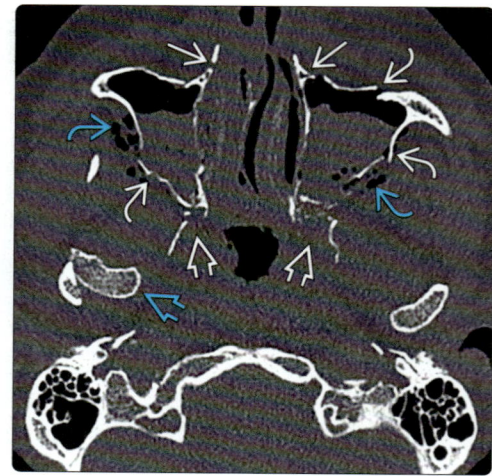

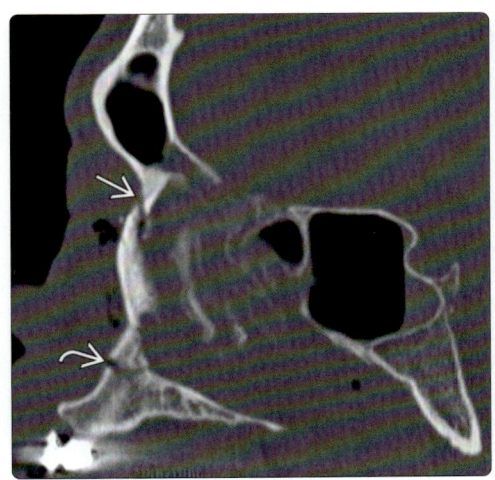

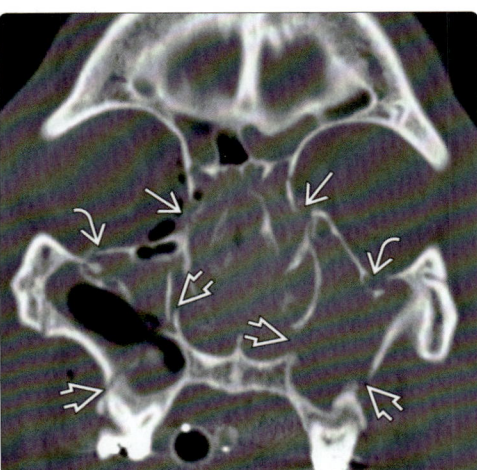

(Left) Bone CT reformation shows combined Le Fort I & II features with a nasofrontal junction fracture ➡, representing Le Fort II pattern, & a medial maxillary buttress fracture ➡, representing Le Fort I pattern. (Right) Coronal bone CT reformation shows fractures involving inferomedial orbital walls ➡ extending from nasofrontal junction. Fractures go through the upper transverse maxillary buttresses (orbital rim & floors) ➡ as well as inferior medial & lateral maxillary buttresses ➡. This constitutes Le Fort I & II patterns.

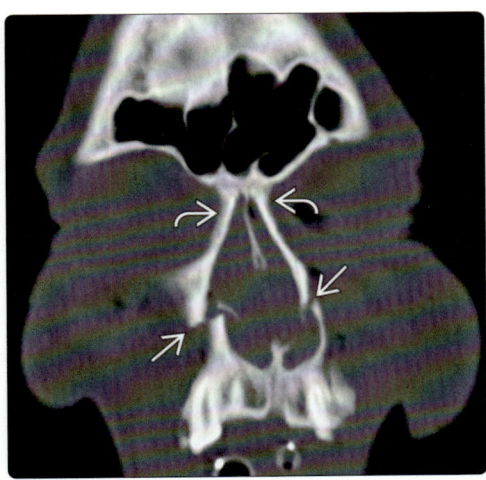

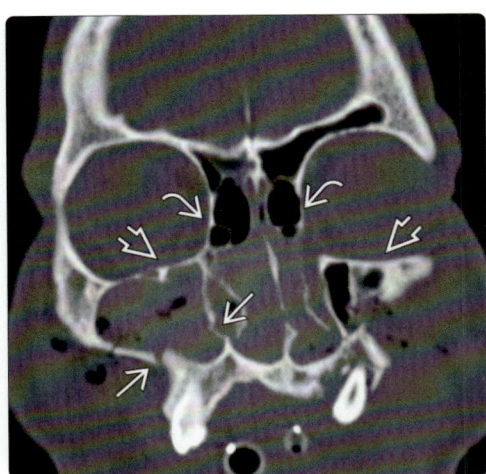

(Left) Coronal bone CT reformation illustrates the transverse & vertical buttresses. There are fractures through the inferior medial (lower transverse) maxillary buttress ➡, representing a component of the Le Fort I pattern. Note that the vertical medial maxillary buttress ➡ is preserved. (Right) Coronal bone CT reformation shows fractures through the right lower transverse medial & lateral maxillary buttresses ➡ in a Le Fort I pattern. The upper transverse ➡ & vertical ➡ buttresses are intact.

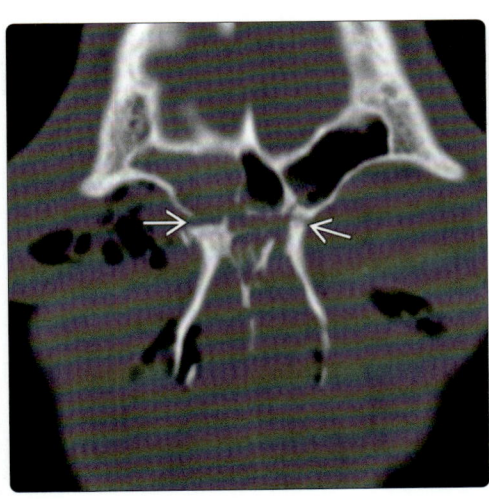

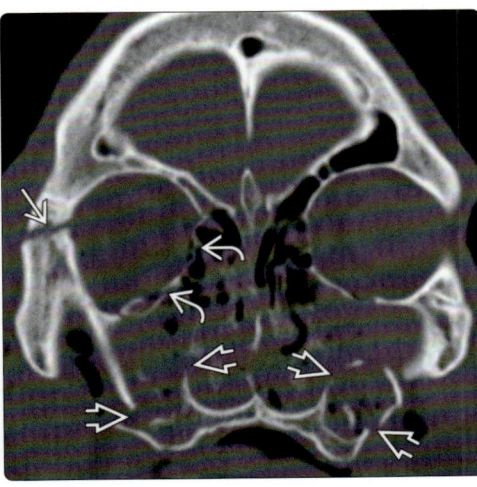

(Left) Coronal bone CT reformation shows fractures through nasofrontal junction ➡ common to Le Fort II & III patterns. This fracture site is at the confluence of the vertical (medial maxillary) & transverse (upper maxillary) buttresses, forming the anterior point of midfacial (craniofacial) disjunction. (Right) Coronal bone CT reformation shows a fracture of the right upper transverse buttresses ➡ & zygomaticofrontal suture ➡, representing Le Fort II & III patterns. Also present is a complete Le Fort I fracture ➡.

Complex Facial Fracture

TERMINOLOGY

- Synonyms: Facial smash injury, panfacial fracture
- No widely accepted definition
  - Severely comminuted fractures of multiple facial bones
  - Does not follow pattern described for traditional transfacial (Le Fort) fracture

IMAGING

- Thin-section axial bone CT with multiplanar & 3D reconstructions is modality of choice
  - 3D CT reformatted images improve appreciation of disrupted facial architecture for surgical planning
- Fractures may involve frontal, nasoethmoid, midfacial, or craniofacial regions
  - May also involve mandible
- CTA may be necessary to exclude carotid artery injury
- MR helps assess associated intracranial & orbital injuries

TOP DIFFERENTIAL DIAGNOSES

- Transfacial (Le Fort) fracture
- Zygomaticomaxillary complex fracture
- Nasoorbitalethmoidal fracture

PATHOLOGY

- High association with intracranial injuries

CLINICAL ISSUES

- Signs/symptoms include gross facial deformity, telecanthus, cerebrospinal fluid leak, visual loss
- Soft tissue injuries & loss of bone structure may lead to malocclusion, "dish" face deformity, & enophthalmos
- Treatment often delayed for other life-threatening injuries
- Reconstruction often performed in multiple stages
- Preoperative CT, virtual surgical planning, intraoperative navigation, & 3D reconstructions aid in planning & execution of complex craniofacial fracture reconstruction
- Intraoperative CT reduces risk of revision surgery

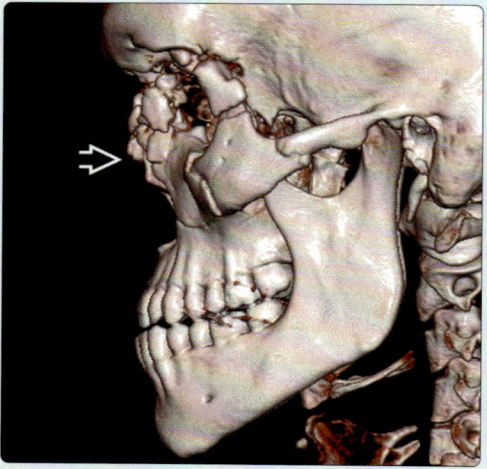
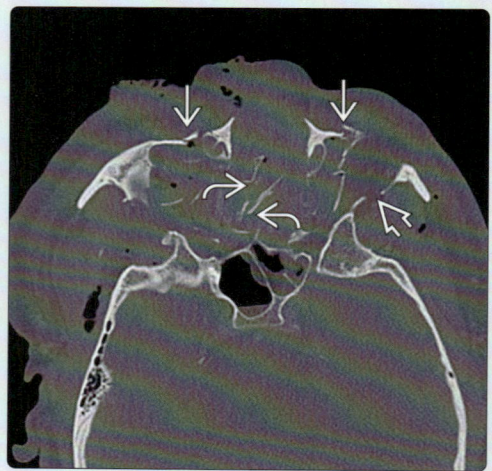

(Left) Lateral 3D reformation of facial CT demonstrates extensive comminuted midface fractures with concave anteroposterior facial dimension ("dish" face deformity) ➡. (Right) Axial bone CT in the same patient demonstrates extensive injuries to the facial soft tissues & underlying facial skeleton. Lacerations with soft tissue emphysema are noted. Severely comminuted fractures involve the maxillae ➡, orbital walls ➡, & nasal septum ➡. The entire face is depressed.

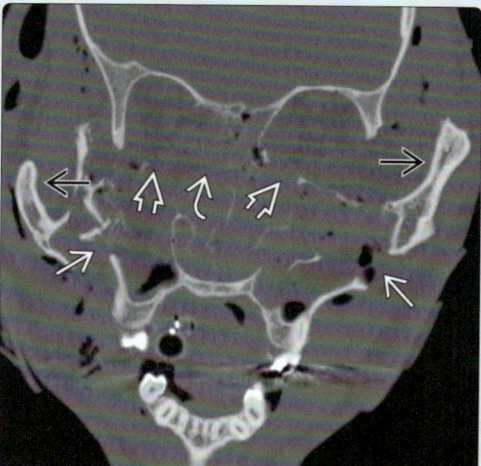
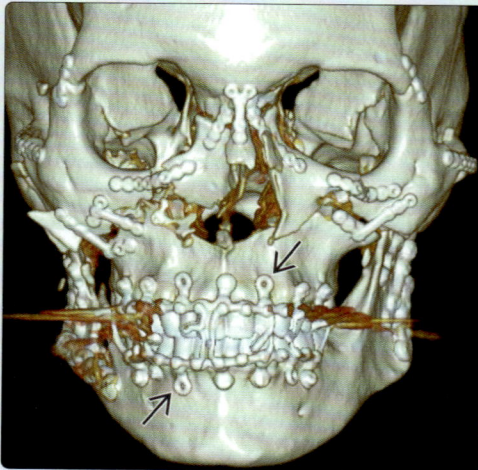

(Left) Coronal bone CT demonstrates extensive displaced fractures of the midface, including maxillary sinus walls ➡, orbits ➡, and ethmoid sinuses ➡. Lateral displacement of the zygomas results in increased facial width ➡. The fractures do not conform to a classic Le Fort fracture pattern. (Right) Anteroposterior bone CT 3D surface rendering in the same patient shows improved alignment of panfacial fractures with multifocal malleable plate and screw fixation & maxillomandibular fixation hardware ➡.

Complex Facial Fracture

TERMINOLOGY

Abbreviations
- Complex facial fracture (CFFx)

Synonyms
- Facial smash injury, panfacial fracture

Definitions
- No widely accepted definition of CFFx or panfacial fracture
- Definitions include
  - Severely comminuted fractures involving multiple facial bones that do not follow pattern described for traditional transfacial (Le Fort) fracture
  - Fractures involving upper, middle, & lower face (nasoorbitalethmoidal, zygomaticomaxillary complex, central midface, & mandible)
  - Fracture patterns involving both midface & mandible

IMAGING

General Features
- Best diagnostic clue
  - Numerous markedly comminuted fractures from high-energy impact that cannot be classified as traditional transfacial types
- Location
  - May involve frontal, nasoethmoid, midfacial, or craniofacial regions; may also involve mandible

Imaging Recommendations
- Best imaging tool
  - Thin-section axial bone CT with multiplanar & 3D reconstruction
- Protocol advice
  - 3D CT reformatted images improve appreciation of disrupted facial architecture for surgical planning
  - CTA may be necessary to exclude carotid artery injury
  - MR helps assess associated intracranial & orbital injuries

CT Findings
- Bone CT
  - Multiple severely comminuted fractures
  - Fractures do not follow classic facial trauma patterns

DIFFERENTIAL DIAGNOSIS

Transfacial (Le Fort) Fractures
- Fractures occur along 3 lines of weakness in facial skeleton
- Bilateral pterygoid plate fractures required

Zygomaticomaxillary Complex Fracture
- Lateral midface fracture complex from blunt trauma to malar eminence
- Fractures involve zygomatic arch, lateral orbital wall & rim, anterior & lateral walls of maxillary sinus, & orbital floor

Nasoorbitalethmoidal Fracture
- Comminuted fractures from high-impact force to nasal bridge
- Frequently involve frontal recess, cribriform plate, nasolacrimal duct, & medial canthal tendon

PATHOLOGY

General Features
- Etiology
  - High-energy impact to face causes highly comminuted fractures
- Associated abnormalities
  - High association with intracranial injuries
  - CFFx involving frontal & nasoethmoid regions have ↑ incidence of dural tears
  - CFFx of nasoethmoid region may have associated injuries to lacrimal apparatus, medial canthal tendon, frontal recess, & cribriform plate

Staging, Grading, & Classification
- No widely accepted definition or classification of CFFx
  - Some describe as involving both midface & mandible
  - Others describe them as involving upper, middle, & lower face (nasoorbitalethmoidal, zygomaticomaxillary complex, central midface, & mandible)
  - Some authors divide panfacial (smash) fractures into 4 types: Frontal smash, nasoethmoid smash, central midface smash, craniofacial smash

CLINICAL ISSUES

Presentation
- Most common signs/symptoms
  - Gross facial deformity
- Other signs/symptoms
  - Telecanthus, cerebrospinal fluid leak, visual loss

Demographics
- Age
  - Most common in adolescents & young adults
- Sex
  - Predominantly male patients

Natural History & Prognosis
- Soft tissue injuries & loss of bone structure may lead to malocclusion, "dish" face deformity, & enophthalmos
- Difficult to completely repair, & patients often left with cosmetic deformity & functional deficits

Treatment
- Goal of treatment → restore function & facial contour
  - Multispecialty surgical team often required for best intracranial & extracranial outcome
- Advantages of early treatment include reduced risk of postop infection & maintained soft tissue expansion
- Intraoperative CT reduces risk of revision surgery

SELECTED REFERENCES

1. Pham TD et al: A review on artificial intelligence for the diagnosis of fractures in facial trauma imaging. Front Artif Intell. 6:1278529, 2023
2. Alasraj A et al: Does intraoperative computed tomography scanning in maxillofacial trauma surgery affect the revision rate? J Oral Maxillofac Surg. 79(2):412-9, 2021
3. Cuddy K et al: Management of zygomaticomaxillary complex fractures utilizing intraoperative 3-dimensional imaging: the ZYGOMAS protocol. J Oral Maxillofac Surg. 79(1):177-82, 2021
4. Massenburg BB et al: Management of panfacial trauma: sequencing and pitfalls. Semin Plast Surg. 35(4):292-8, 2021

Orbital Foreign Body

TERMINOLOGY

- Foreign material introduced into orbit via trauma

IMAGING

- CT sensitive & safe modality for detecting foreign body (FB)
  - Density and shape indicate nature of object
  - **Metal** density > 1,000-2,000 HU attenuation artifact
    - Firearms, workplace materials
    - Button battery → caustic injury
  - **Glass** denser than bone; wide variation
    - Pane shards or safety glass fragments
  - **Wood** typically low density, similar to air when dry
    - Pencils with dense stylus core, tree branches
  - **Miscellaneous** objects of any origin
    - Plastic or sponge very low density, similar to air
    - Sand or gravel: Dense, granular material
- Consider MR for possible FB if CT negative
  - Contraindicated if unknown ferromagneticity
  - Inflammation or granulation suggest organic material

TOP DIFFERENTIAL DIAGNOSES

- Ophthalmic surgical device; phthisis bulbi
- Dystrophic calcification

PATHOLOGY

- Most FB occur with high-velocity or projectile injury
  - Hammering, occupational, assault, MVA
  - May occur after apparently trivial trauma

CLINICAL ISSUES

- Organic FB more likely to incite cellulitis and abscess
- All puncture wounds require exploration
- Surgical decision depends on type and location of FB

DIAGNOSTIC CHECKLIST

- CT is study of choice and should be performed 1st
- Occult FB discoveries are surprisingly common
- Assess for globe rupture and optic nerve injury

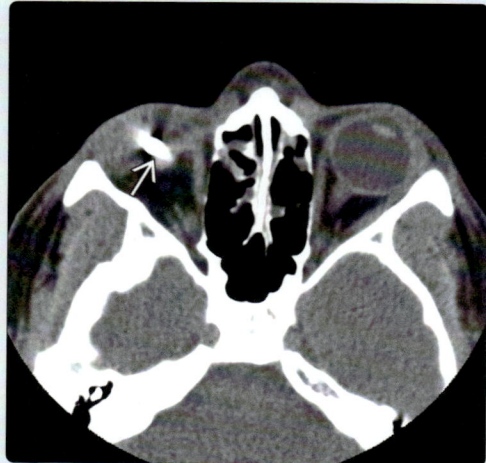
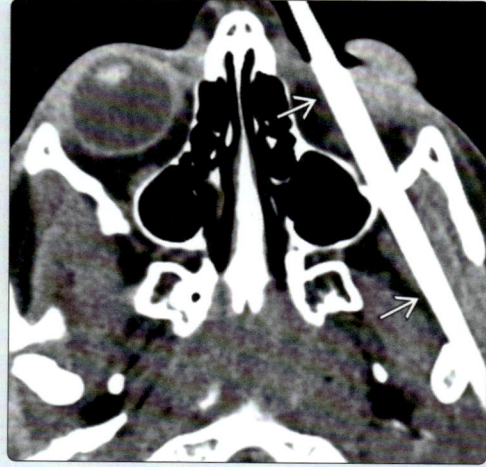

(Left) Axial NECT in a child who was accidentally shot with a BB gun demonstrates streak artifact from the metallic BB within the ruptured right globe ➡ with moderate adjacent soft swelling. (Right) Axial NECT in a child shows an orbital impalement injury by a fishing rod, which is similar to bone attenuation ➡, traversing the left inferolateral extraocular orbit and masticator space.

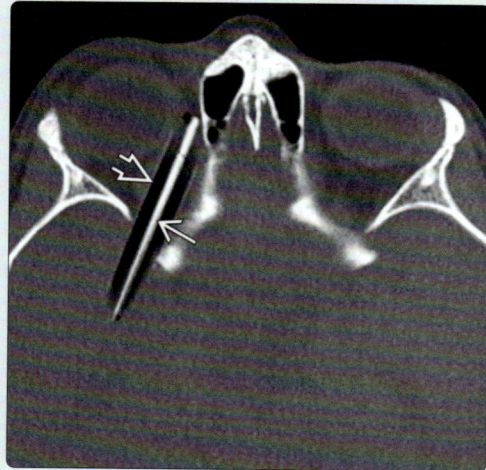
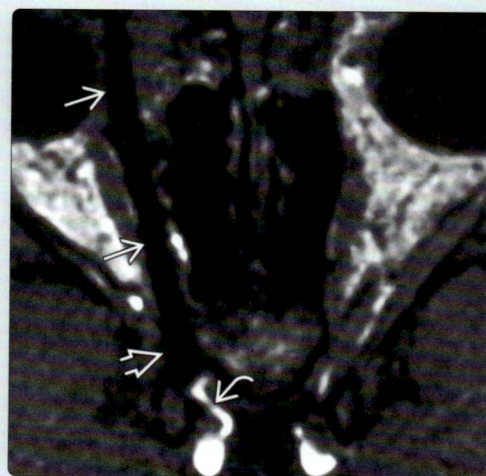

(Left) Axial bone CT shows a piece of a broken pencil within the right orbit. The center dense core represents the pencil stylus ("lead") ➡. The outer casing of wood is low density ➡. (Right) Axial source image from 3D time of flight MRA shows a long, hypointense, intraorbital foreign body, known to represent a twig ➡, paralleling the right medial orbital wall and impaling the optic nerve within the optic canal ➡ just proximal to the ophthalmic artery ➡. The twig was similar to air in attenuation on CT.

Orbital Foreign Body

TERMINOLOGY

Abbreviations
- Foreign body (FB)

Definitions
- Foreign material introduced into orbit via trauma

IMAGING

General Features
- Size: Larger FB easier to detect
  - Glass: > 90% if ≥ 1.5 mm; < 50% if ≤ 0.5 mm

Imaging Recommendations
- Best imaging tool
  - **CT** most sensitive modality for detecting FB
    - Safe in presence of metallic object
  - Consider **MR** to assess for possibility of plastic, wooden, or other organic FB if CT negative
    - Contraindicated if unknown ferromagneticity

CT Findings
- NECT
  - **Metal** FB very high density (> 1,000-2,000 HU)
    - Streak artifact due to **beam-hardening** effect
    - Firearm projectiles, workplace materials
    - **Button battery**: Caustic injury due to hydroxide radical production in tissues adjacent to negative pole
  - **Glass** FB denser than bone, varies with type
    - High-density glass (e.g., crystal) easiest to detect
  - **Wood** FB varies with water content and type of wood
    - Range from -550 HU to +289 HU
    - Pencils (with dense stylus core) and tree branches similar to air attenuation
    - With time, absorption of fluid → loss of air attenuation
  - **Miscellaneous** FB range from ordinary to bizarre
    - **Plastic** or **sponge** very low density, similar to air
    - **Sand** or **gravel** appear as dense, granular material

MR Findings
- Wood may be similar to air on all sequences
- STIR: Hyperintense inflammatory response surrounding FB, particularly organic material
- T1WI C+ FS: Enhancement of inflammatory or granulation tissue suggests organic origin

DIFFERENTIAL DIAGNOSIS

Ophthalmic Surgical Device
- Intraocular lens (refractive correction)
- Scleral band (sponge, rubber, or plastic)
- Intraocular retinopexy tamponade (oil or gas)
- Ocular prosthesis (following enucleation)
- Glaucoma drainage valve

Phthisis Bulbi
- Shrunken, disfigured, calcified globe
- Chronic end-stage due to severe eye injury

Dystrophic Calcification
- Drusen (punctate calcification at optic disc)
- Rectus muscle insertion, trochlear sling

- Nonspecific senile scleral calcification

PATHOLOGY

General Features
- Etiology
  - Most FB occur with **high-velocity** or **projectile** injury
    - Hammering is common mechanism (metal on metal)
    - Occupational hazard (nail gun, glass workers)
    - Assault (knives, gunshot, BB pellets)
    - Motor vehicle collision (glass, metallic fragments)
  - May occur after apparently trivial trauma
- Associated abnormalities
  - **Fractures** and **globe injury** in path of introduced object
  - More complications with heavier and posterior FB

CLINICAL ISSUES

Presentation
- Most common signs/symptoms
  - Sharp, stabbing pain at time of injury
  - Pain on eye movement, ↓ visual acuity
  - Hyphema, vitreal hemorrhage
- Other signs/symptoms
  - Orbital mass, cellulitis, or abscess
  - Optic neuropathy
  - Orbital wall fracture

Demographics
- Epidemiology
  - Penetrating injury is component of 50% of trauma to eye
  - Intraocular FB present in 20-40% of open globe injuries

Natural History & Prognosis
- **Organic** FB more likely to incite **cellulitis and abscess** compared with metallic FB

Treatment
- All puncture wounds require surgical exploration
- Inorganic FB may be treated conservatively
- Surgical removal depends on **type and location** of FB
  - Anterior metallic FB may be removed to prevent infection, motility impairment, ptosis, or fistula formation
  - FB at orbital apex adjacent to optic nerve may require optic canal decompression

DIAGNOSTIC CHECKLIST

Image Interpretation Pearls
- CT is **study of choice** and should be performed 1st
- **Occult** FB discoveries are surprisingly common

Reporting Tips
- Assess for **globe rupture** and **optic nerve** injury

SELECTED REFERENCES

1. Chen L et al: Prolonged button battery exposure leading to severe ocular injury without heavy metal poisoning. Case Rep Ophthalmol. 15(1):170-5, 2024
2. Farahvash A et al: A computed tomography scan near miss of an intraorbital wooden foreign body. Plast Surg (Oakv). 32(1):158-61, 2024
3. Hötte GJ et al: Ocular injury and emergencies around the globe. Atlas Oral Maxillofac Surg Clin North Am. 29(1):19-28, 2021

TERMINOLOGY

- Traumatic deformity of orbital floor or medial wall resulting from impact of blunt object larger than orbital aperture

IMAGING

- High-resolution axial bone CT with coronal & sagittal reconstructions is modality of choice
- 2 broad categories of blowout fractures
  - Open door: Large, displaced, frequently comminuted
  - Trapdoor: Linear, hinged, minimally displaced
- Associated findings
  - Herniation of orbital contents through bony defect
  - Involvement of infraorbital canal
  - Orbital soft tissue injury
  - May occur in combination with other facial fractures
    - Nasal, transfacial, zygomaticomaxillary complex
- Orbital emphysema may have mass effect
  - Compression/stretch of optic nerve insertion ("tenting" of globe)

TOP DIFFERENTIAL DIAGNOSES

- Dehiscent lamina papyracea
- Orbital decompression surgery
- Nasoorbitalethmoidal fracture

CLINICAL ISSUES

- Most common symptoms
  - Diplopia: Typically related to entrapment
  - Enophthalmos: Due to prolapse of orbital contents into sinuses
  - Hypesthesia of cheek & upper gum: Due to infraorbital nerve injury

DIAGNOSTIC CHECKLIST

- Entrapment is clinical, not radiographic diagnosis
  - Note abnormal position & morphology of extraocular muscles
- In children, minimally displaced but highly symptomatic trapdoor fractures are common

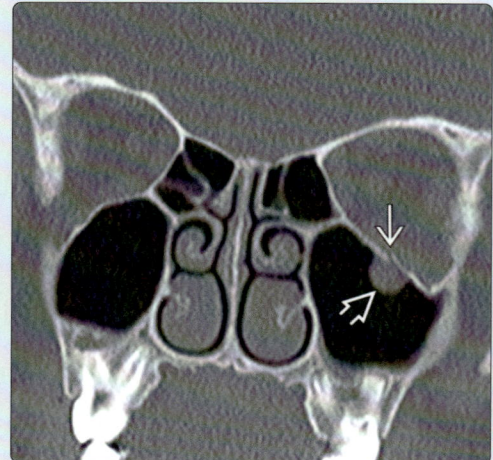
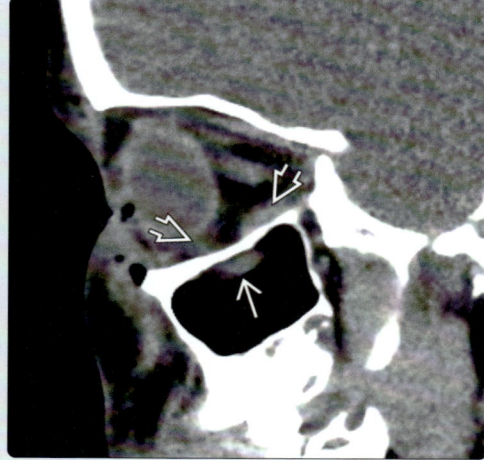

(Left) Coronal bone window NECT in an 8-year-old boy shows a minimally displaced fracture of the left orbital floor ➡. There is subjacent abnormal soft tissue suspicious for herniated fat &/or inferior rectus muscle ➡. (Right) Sagittal soft tissue NECT in the same patient shows the inferior rectus muscle herniating through the orbital floor defect ➡. The portions of the muscle on either side of the herniation ➡ are visible on this image.

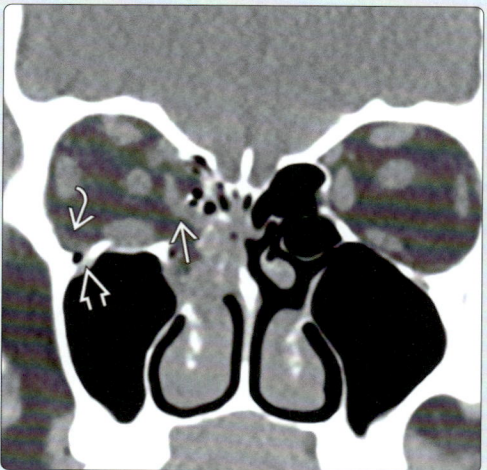
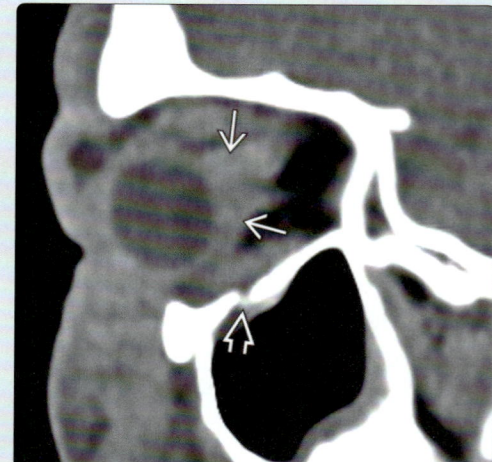

(Left) Coronal NECT in a 32-year-old man shows herniation of the abnormally shaped right medial rectus muscle into a comminuted acute fracture of the lamina papyracea ➡. Notice also an associated fracture of the orbital floor ➡ and minimal adjacent extraconal soft tissue edema/hemorrhage ➡. (Right) Sagittal NECT in a 32-year-old man shows a retrobulbar hematoma ➡ in association with an acute fracture of the orbital floor ➡.

Orbital Blowout Fracture

TERMINOLOGY

Abbreviations

- Orbital blowout fracture (OBF)

Definitions

- Orbital floor or medial wall fracture resulting from impact of blunt object of diameter greater than orbital aperture
  - Pure: Without orbital rim fracture
  - Impure: With orbital rim fracture

IMAGING

General Features

- Best diagnostic clue
  - Deformity of orbital floor/medial wall ± herniation of orbital contents through bony defect
- Location
  - Floor fractures: Middle 1/3, near infraorbital canal
  - In younger patients (< 50 years), mostly assault, so left side more common
- Morphology
  - Open door: Large, displaced, frequently comminuted
  - Trapdoor: Linear, hinged, minimally displaced
    - High frequency of extraocular muscle (EOM) entrapment despite scant external signs of trauma
      - Term "white-eyed OBF" coined because of minimal orbital swelling/ecchymoses
    - May be difficult to diagnose radiographically because of minimal displacement
    - Many pediatric blowout fractures are trapdoor type
      - Fracture fragments recoil back to original position, may entrap extraconal fat, muscle &/or fascia

CT Findings

- Fracture of orbital floor/medial wall
  - ± herniation of orbital contents (fat, EOMs)
  - ± fracture through infraorbital &/or nasolacrimal canal
  - ± injury to orbital soft tissues (globe rupture, retrobulbar hematoma)
- Orbital emphysema may have mass effect
  - Stretch of optic nerve insertion ("tenting" of globe)
- May occur in combination with other facial fractures: Nasal, Le Fort types, zygomaticomaxillary complex (ZMC)
- Soft tissue algorithm also important for evaluation of orbital contents; complementary to bone windows for evaluation of orbital contents

Imaging Recommendations

- Best imaging tool
  - Thin-slice bone algorithm MDCT in axial plane with coronal, sagittal reconstructions
    - Involvement of infraorbital canal best in coronal plane
    - Involvement of orbital rim best in sagittal plane
- Protocol advice
  - Include soft tissue images for orbital contents

DIFFERENTIAL DIAGNOSIS

Dehiscent Lamina Papyracea

- Medial wall deformity may reflect congenital dehiscence &/or is associated with ethmoid hypoplasia

Orbital Decompression Surgery

- Resection of medial orbital wall, for thyroid orbitopathy

Nasoorbitalethmoidal Fracture

- Fractures also involve nasal bridge with nasal depression & traumatic telecanthus

Zygomaticomaxillary Complex Fracture

- Fractures also seen in zygomatic arch, lateral orbital wall, maxillary sinus walls

CLINICAL ISSUES

Presentation

- Most common signs/symptoms
  - Diplopia
    - Typically secondary to EOM ± fat entrapment
    - May be due to edema/hemorrhage ± entrapment
  - Enophthalmos
    - Secondary to prolapse of orbital contents into maxillary (or ethmoid) sinus
  - Hypesthesia of cheek & upper gum
    - Secondary to fracture through infraorbital canal
- Other signs/symptoms
  - Visual loss
    - Secondary to globe/optic nerve injury
  - Oculocardiac reflex

Natural History & Prognosis

- Small, uncomplicated fractures: No treatment
- Urgent surgery recommended for nonresolving oculocardiac reflex, white-eyed OBF with severe gaze restriction, early enophthalmos
- Timing otherwise controversial
  - Most advocate surgery within 2 weeks for diplopia, herniation of orbital contents, large floor defect (> 50% floor area) that may cause delayed enophthalmos

Treatment

- Orbital floor reconstruction typically performed with alloplast (titanium mesh, porous polyethylene)

DIAGNOSTIC CHECKLIST

Consider

- In children, minimally displaced but highly symptomatic trapdoor fractures are common

Image Interpretation Pearls

- Entrapment is clinical, not radiographic, diagnosis

Reporting Tips

- Check position, orientation, configuration of EOMs; entrapment can occur without significant displacement
- Check for mass effect on optic nerve insertion from retrobulbar hematoma or emphysema

SELECTED REFERENCES

1. Nikunen M et al: Orbital blowout fractures: manifestations and missed diagnoses in 207 surgically treated patients. Med Oral Patol Oral Cir Bucal. 29(5):e598-605, 2024
2. Voss JO et al: Diagnostic pitfalls in pediatric orbital entrapment fractures. J Craniomaxillofac Surg. 52(2):228-33, 2024
3. Hassan B et al: Pediatric orbital fractures. Oral Maxillofac Surg Clin North Am. 35(4):585-96, 2023

KEY FACTS

IMAGING

- Mandible simulates bony ring: **2 breaks** common (50%)
  - Parasymphyseal fracture often associated with contralateral angle/body or subcondylar fracture
  - Bilateral condylar process fractures after direct impact to symphysis
- CT has largely replaced plain film evaluation of facial trauma
  - Thin-slice axial bone algorithm CT with coronal & 3D reformat
- Bone CT appearance
  - Lucent, noncorticated lines with variable diastasis, angulation, & comminution
  - Fracture tends to follow long axis of teeth
  - In condylar neck fracture, condylar head pulled anteromedially by lateral pterygoid muscle
  - Empty TMJ sign when TMJ dislocated

TOP DIFFERENTIAL DIAGNOSES

- Pseudofractures: Nutrient canal, inferior alveolar nerve canal, mandibular lingula, mental foramen

PATHOLOGY

- Causes of mandibular fracture
  - Motor vehicle accidents: 40%
  - Assault: 40%
  - Fall: 10%
  - Sports-related injury: 5%
- 15% have ≥ 1 other facial bone fracture

CLINICAL ISSUES

- 2nd most commonly fractured facial bone
- Goals of treatment are restoration of normal occlusion & complete bony union
- Wound infection is potential complication of fracture to tooth-bearing portion of mandible

(Left) Axial bone CT shows right parasymphyseal ➡ and left mandibular angle ⇨ fractures involving the left inferior alveolar canal ➡. A fracture through the teeth is considered open, requiring antibiotics. Two fractures are often present, as the mandible is essentially a fixed ring of bone. (Right) Coronal bone CT demonstrates bilateral angulated mandibular condylar neck fractures ➡. No TMJ dislocation is present ➡. A concurrent parasymphyseal mandibular fracture is not shown.

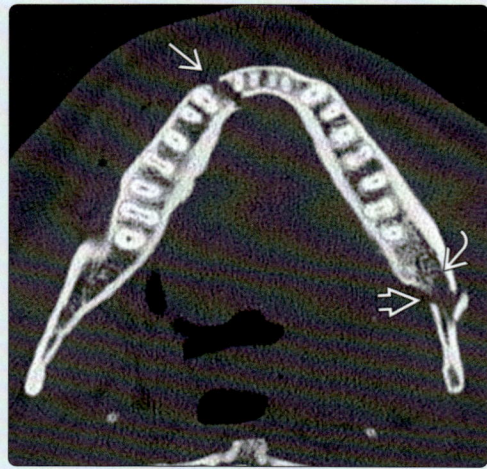
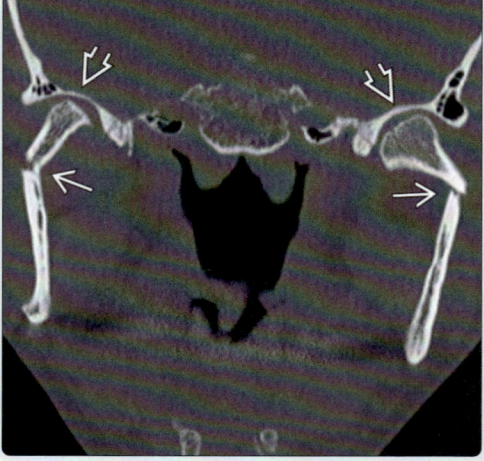

(Left) Axial bone CT demonstrates a left empty TMJ sign ➡ due to an inferiorly displaced left mandibular condyle. The right mandibular condyle ➡ is normally positioned. (Right) Axial bone CT in the same patient shows a displaced fracture of the left mandibular condylar neck ➡. The left condylar head fragment ➡ is anteromedially displaced due to forces from the lateral pterygoid muscle, resulting in TMJ dislocation.

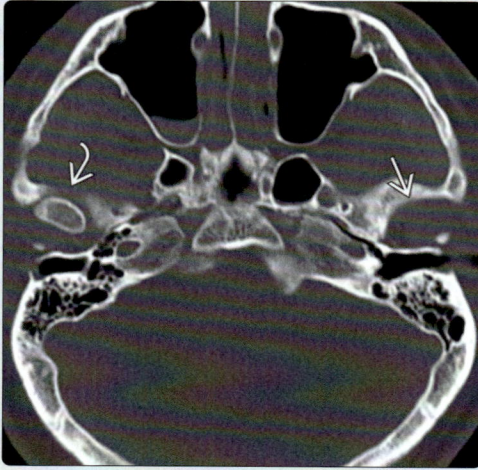
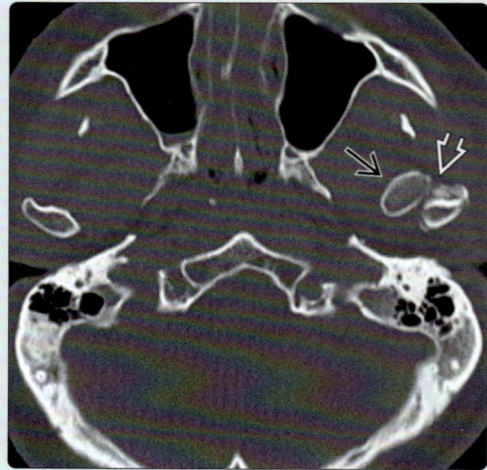

TERMINOLOGY

Abbreviations

- Fracture of mandible

Definitions

- Traumatic break in mandibular cortex

IMAGING

General Features

- Best diagnostic clue
  - Focal, noncorticated lucency in mandibular cortex
- Location
  - Mandible simulates bony ring
    - **2 breaks in ring common** (50%) & bilateral fracture result
      - Parasymphyseal fracture on one side often associated with contralateral angle/body or condyle/subcondylar fracture
      - Bilateral condylar process fractures after direct impact to symphysis
    - Alternatively, unilateral mandibular fracture may occur with **contralateral TMJ dislocation**

CT Findings

- Bone CT
  - Lucent, noncorticated fracture lines with variable diastasis, angulation, & comminution
  - Fracture lines tend to follow long axis of teeth
  - In condylar neck fracture, **condylar head pulled anteromedially** by lateral pterygoid muscle
  - **Empty TMJ sign** may be seen on axial CT images when TMJ dislocated

MR Findings

- T1WI
  - ↓ marrow signal intensity from edema
  - May see discrete, well-defined, hypointense fracture line
  - Hypointense joint effusion if TMJ affected
- T2WI
  - ↑ marrow signal due to edema
    - Surrounding edema on MR may be more extensive than fracture length
  - Hypointense fracture line
  - Surrounding ↑ signal soft tissue edema

Imaging Recommendations

- Best imaging tool
  - Thin-slice axial bone CT through mandible & TMJs

DIFFERENTIAL DIAGNOSIS

Nutrient Canal

- Pseudofracture caused by radiolucent channels extending through osseous structures
- Commonly mistaken for fracture lines

Inferior Alveolar Nerve Canal (V3)

- Normally located inferior & medial within mandibular body running parallel to body
- Corticated, begins at mandibular foramen & ends at mental foramen

Mandibular Lingula

- Small bony projection extending from medial mandible at mandibular foramen for inferior alveolar nerve
- Usually symmetric and triangular in shape

PATHOLOGY

General Features

- Etiology
  - Fracture causes
    - Motor vehicle accidents: 40%
    - Assault: 40%
    - Fall: 10%
    - Sports-related injury: 5%
- Associated abnormalities
  - 15% of cases with mandibular fracture have ≥ 1 other facial bone fracture

CLINICAL ISSUES

Presentation

- Most common signs/symptoms
  - Jaw pain or trismus (normal opening > 40 mm)
  - Abnormal mobility on palpation & mouth opening
- **Flail mandible**
  - Bilateral parasymphyseal or body fractures with posterior displacement of central fragment & tongue → **airway compromise**

Demographics

- Epidemiology
  - Mandible is **2nd most commonly fractured facial bone**
    - Account for ~ 25% of facial fractures
  - Mandibular fracture frequencies
    - Angle: 25%
    - Body: 25%
    - Condylar process: 20%
    - Symphyseal/parasymphyseal: 20%
    - Ramus: 5%
    - Alveolar border: 3%
    - Coronoid process: 2%

Treatment

- Goals are restoring normal occlusion & complete bony union

DIAGNOSTIC CHECKLIST

Consider

- Mandible is considered ring of bone → look for 2nd fracture, TMJ dislocation (empty TMJ sign), malocclusion, or additional facial fracture
- **Flail mandible** → emergency, which may compromise airway

SELECTED REFERENCES

1. van Nistelrooij N et al: Detecting mandible fractures in CBCT scans using a 3-stage neural network. J Dent Res. 103(13):1384-91, 2024
2. Mittermiller PA et al: The comprehensive AO CMF classification system for mandibular fractures: a multicenter validation study. Craniomaxillofac Trauma Reconstr. 12(4):254-65, 2019
3. Dreizin D et al: Multidetector CT of mandibular fractures, reductions, and complications: a clinically relevant primer for the radiologist. Radiographics. 36(5):1539-64, 2016

KEY FACTS

TERMINOLOGY

- Internal derangement (ID) of TMJ
- Abnormal positional and functional relationship between articular disc and articulating surfaces

IMAGING

- Best imaging tool: Oblique corrected sagittal PD or T1 and T2 MR
- Articular disc most commonly positioned **anterior** to mandibular condyle
- Normal or dysmorphic disc morphology

TOP DIFFERENTIAL DIAGNOSES

- Rheumatoid arthritis
- Synovial chondromatosis
- Calcium pyrophosphate deposition disease
- Tenosynovial giant cell tumor

CLINICAL ISSUES

- Very prevalent: 20-30% of population
  - Majority asymptomatic
  - **ID** seen in **> 80% of symptomatic TMJ patients**
  - Symptoms: Trismus, preauricular pain, limited range of motion
- Most prevalent from 20-40 years
- Symptomatic joints: F:M = 4:1
  - More common in males if 2° to trauma
- Treatment
  - Conservative: Bite splint
  - Surgical: Arthrocentesis and discectomy

DIAGNOSTIC CHECKLIST

- Report anterior disc displacement ± reduction
- Report associated effusion or synovitis

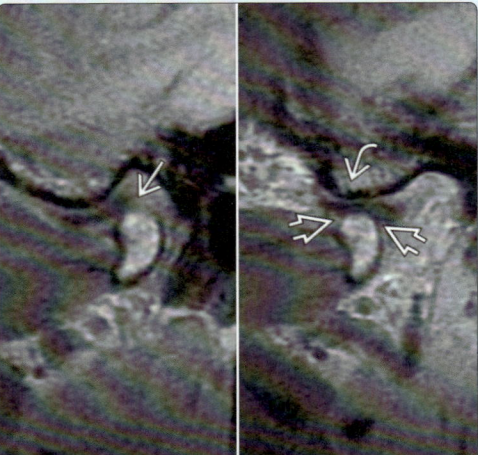
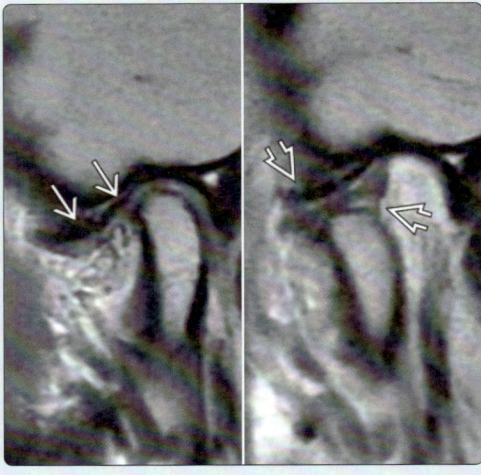

(Left) Sagittal oblique PD MR images in a 72-year-old man show normal alignment of the condyle and disc ➡ in the closed-mouth position. There is normal condyle movement and normal alignment of condyle and disc ➡ at the articular eminence ➡ (open mouth). (Right) Sagittal oblique PD MR in a 30-year-old woman with TMJ painful clicking shows anterior dislocation of the disc ➡. In the open-mouth position, the disc is positioned normally between condyle and articular eminence ➡ (anterior displacement with reduction).

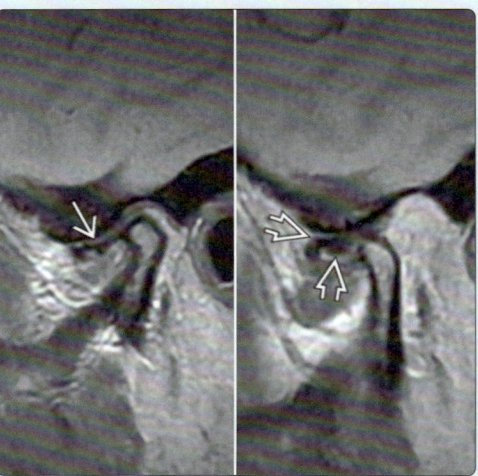
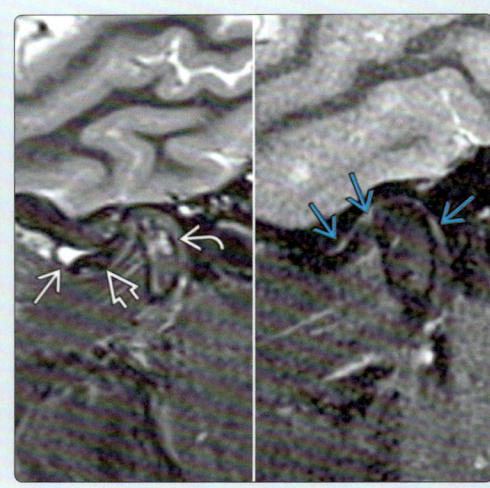

(Left) Oblique sagittal PD MR in a 46-year-old woman shows anterior dislocation of the irregular disc in the closed-mouth position ➡. In the open-mouth position, the articular disc stays anterior to the condyle ➡ (anterior displacement without reduction). (Right) Oblique sagittal STIR MR images in 2 different patients show TMJ effusions. In the left panel, there is an effusion ➡ along the displaced disc ➡. There is condylar flattening with subchondral edema ➡. On the right, the other effusion ➡ is more subtle.

TMJ Disc Displacement

TERMINOLOGY

Synonyms

- Internal derangement (ID) of TMJ

Definitions

- Abnormal positional and functional relationship between articular disc and articulating surfaces

IMAGING

General Features

- Best diagnostic clue
  - Articular disc positioned anterior to mandibular condyle
- Location
  - Usually intracapsular
  - Unilateral or bilateral
- Morphology
  - Normal disc shape or dysmorphic

Imaging Recommendations

- Best imaging tool
  - Thin-section oblique corrected sagittal and coronal MR in **closed** and **open-mouth positions**
- Protocol advice
  - MR sequences should include sagittal PD or T1 and T2
  - Cine images provide more functional information

MR Findings

- T1WI
  - Displacement: Anterior, medial, lateral, combination
    - Posterior band of articular disc **anterior to 11-12 o'clock position** relative to mandibular condyle
    - Anterior displacement = angle > 10° between posterior band and vertical orientation of condyle
    - Posterior disc displacement is rare
    - Lateral displacement seen on coronal images
    - Open-mouth images assess reduction of displacement
  - Displaced disc may be perforated, fibrotic, or have dysmorphic contours or adhesions
- T2WI
  - Superior or inferior joint space **effusion** with ↑ **signal**
  - ↑ signal in condyle if associated marrow edema
- T1WI C+
  - Disc nonenhancing
  - Associated acute synovitis will enhance

DIFFERENTIAL DIAGNOSIS

Rheumatoid Arthritis

- Proliferating, inflamed synovial tissue ("pannus")
- Enhancing, enlarged synovium
- Moderate to significant osteoarthritis often present as well

Synovial Chondromatosis

- Chondrometaplasia of synovial membrane
- Cartilaginous nodules detach from synovium and calcify

Calcium Pyrophosphate Dihydrate Deposition Disease

- Metabolic disease associated with chondrocalcinosis
- Uncommon in TMJ

- Calcified, enhancing intracapsular mass

Tenosynovial Giant Cell Tumor

- Rare in TMJ, locally aggressive
- Tumefactive proliferation of synovium

Synovial Cyst

- Rare in TMJ, arises from synovium

PATHOLOGY

General Features

- Etiology
  - Multifactorial; dysfunctional remodeling
    - ↓ adaptivity of articular surface ± overloading
    - Ligamentous laxity
    - Inflammatory changes are secondary
  - May occur secondary to trauma (condylar fracture/dislocation)

Gross Pathologic & Surgical Features

- Hyperemic, deformed articular disc

Microscopic Features

- Connective tissue hyalinization, hyperplasia, ↑ vascularity

CLINICAL ISSUES

Presentation

- Most common signs/symptoms
  - **Majority asymptomatic**
  - Trismus
  - Preauricular pain
- Other signs/symptoms
  - Limited range of motion on opening
  - "Clicking" or locking

Demographics

- Age
  - Adults: Most prevalent from 20-40 years
- Sex
  - Symptomatic: **F:M = 4:1**
- Epidemiology
  - 20-30% of population
  - ID seen in > 80% of symptomatic TMJ patients

Treatment

- Conservative treatment with bite splint
- Surgical options: Arthrocentesis, arthroscopy
  - End-stage TMJ disease may be treated with joint replacement, polymer or alloy

SELECTED REFERENCES

1. Larheim TA et al: Temporomandibular joint pathologies: pictorial review. Br J Radiol. 97(1153):53-67, 2024
2. Millón Cruz A et al: Reliability of magnetic resonance for temporomandibular joint disc perforation: a 12 years retrospective study. J Craniomaxillofac Surg. 52(5):548-57, 2024
3. Pollard R: [Imaging in temporomandibular joint disorders.] Ned Tijdschr Tandheelkd. 131(5):217-21, 2024
4. Minervini G et al: Temporomandibular joint disk displacement: etiology, diagnosis, imaging, and therapeutic approaches. J Craniofac Surg. 34(3):1115-21, 2023
5. Luo D et al: A magnetic resonance imaging study on the temporomandibular joint disc-condyle relationship in young asymptomatic adults. Int J Oral Maxillofac Surg. 51(2):226-33, 2021

Petrous Apex

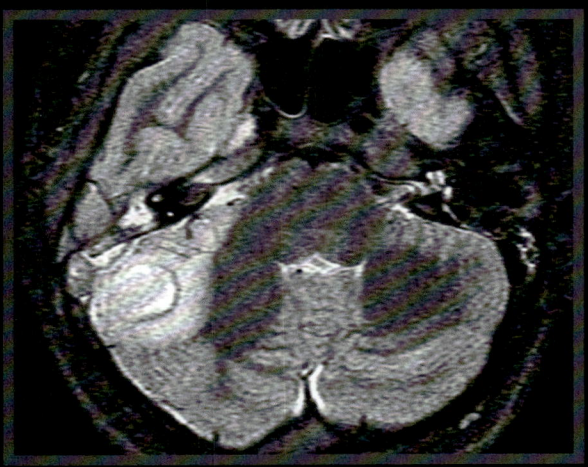

Intratemporal Facial Nerve

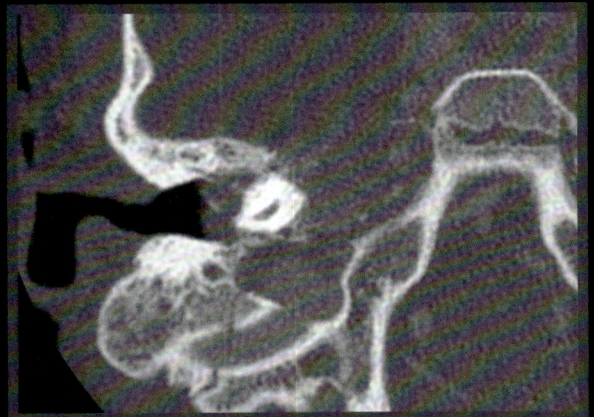

Temporal Bone, No Specific Anatomic Location

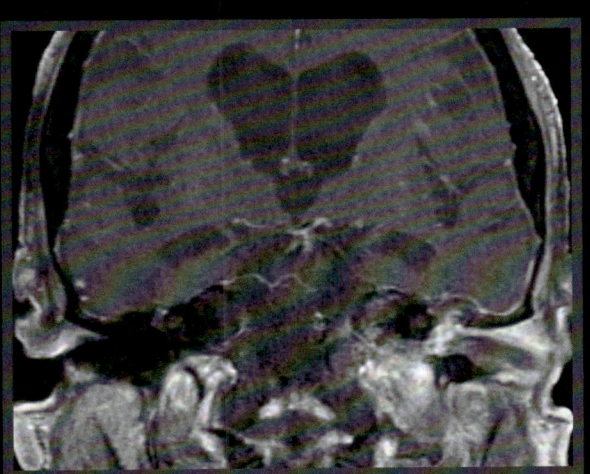

Summary Thoughts: Temporal Bone

The temporal bone is one of the most complex and intriguing areas of the head and neck. Understanding normal anatomy is key to accurate temporal bone image interpretation. Incorporating the otologic findings of a middle ear mass also helps the radiologist to arrive at a correct preoperative diagnosis. If the clinical question is conductive hearing loss (CHL), an abnormality on CT is almost always present and should be extensively searched for, especially in children.

Cholesteatoma is a very common clinical concern in most ear, nose, throat (ENT) practices. The following questions should be addressed in a patient with a cholesteatoma: (1) Is the tegmen tympani intact? (2) Is there potential for a fistula into the membranous labyrinth? (3) Is the facial nerve canal adjacent to or eroded by the cholesteatoma? (4) Is there tissue in the sinus tympani? (5) What is the relationship of the mass to the ossicles?

Imaging Techniques & Indications

CT is the primary imaging tool for evaluating the fine bony detail of the temporal bone. Current multislice CT scanners allow thin slices (≤ 1 mm) and provide excellent multiplanar reformatted images, which have become the mainstay for diagnosis of temporal bone disease. Current protocols include direct axial and reformatted coronal views, vestibular oblique or short-axis views (Pöschl plane), and cochlear oblique or long-axis views (Stenver plane). A window width of 4,000 HU is ideal.

CT is the imaging study of choice when the clinical question is CHL, external auditory canal (EAC) atresia/stenosis, or possible cholesteatoma.

MR is best for evaluation of inner ear pathology, particularly sensorineural hearing loss (SNHL). High-resolution 3D MR cisternographic sequences provide an excellent screening examination for patients with SNHL. These thin-section (≤ 1-mm) T2-weighted MR sequences (SPACE, FIESTA, etc.) in the axial and coronal planes can help identify mass lesions of the internal auditory canal (IAC), particularly a vestibular schwannoma. Sagittal oblique planes are excellent for evaluation of a child with SNHL to easily identify the 4 nerves within the IAC.

The gold standard for imaging patients with acquired SNHL is enhanced thin-section (≤ 3-mm) axial and coronal images through the temporal bone with fat-saturated, postcontrast images. Precontrast T1-weighted images are helpful to evaluate for T1-hyperintense lesions, such as hemorrhage or lipoma.

When the clinical question is SNHL, a petrous apex lesion, or possible IAC or cerebellopontine angle (CPA) lesion, MR is the imaging study of choice.

Embryology

The otocyst buds from the neuroectoderm migrate to the location of the inner ear and become the membranous labyrinth. The EAC forms from the 1st branchial groove or cleft. The middle ear (tympanic) cavity forms from the 1st branchial (pharyngeal) pouch. The tympanic membrane (TM) forms where the EAC (1st branchial cleft) and middle ear (1st branchial pouch) meet. The middle ear cavity and the eustachian tube form from the same 1st branchial pouch. The middle ear cavity envelops the ossicles.

The **ossicles** form primarily from the 1st and 2nd branchial arches, separately from the inner ear. The endolymphatic system forms from the otocyst. The perilymphatic space and otic capsule form from surrounding mesenchyme.

In nonsyndromic EAC atresia, the inner ear is spared, as it forms from migration of the otocyst, which is independent from the 1st and 2nd branchial groove-pouch-arch interaction. Therefore, inner ear anomalies in most cases form without EAC or middle ear anomalies. A combination of external, middle, and inner ear anomalies suggests a syndromic etiology or teratogenic insult.

Consider the following questions when evaluating a patient with **EAC atresia**: (1) Is the EAC atresia plate thick, thin, or part membranous in nature? (2) How small is the middle ear cavity? (3) What is the status of the ossicles? (4) Is the facial nerve canal anomalous in its course or dehiscent? (5) What is the status of the oval and round windows? (6) Is there a congenital cholesteatoma? (7) Are the inner ear structures normal?

Imaging Anatomy

The temporal bone is located in the middle cranial fossa posterolateral floor. Its boundaries include the sphenoid bone anteriorly, occipital bone posteriorly and medially, and parietal bone superiorly and laterally.

There are **5 bony parts** of the adult temporal bone: Squamous, mastoid, petrous, tympanic, and styloid portions. The squamous portion forms the lateral wall of the middle cranial fossa. The mastoid process represents the postnatal development of the posteroinferior mastoid. The petrous portion of the temporal bone contains the middle and inner ear, IAC, and petrous apex. The tympanic segment is a U-shaped bone that forms most of the bony external ear. The styloid portion forms the styloid process after birth.

The **petrous portion** of the temporal bone includes 2 important structures anteriorly. The tegmen tympani (Latin for "roof of the cavity") serves as the roof of the tympanic cavity. The arcuate eminence is the bony prominence over the superior semicircular canal (SCC) and serves as an important surgical landmark along the middle cranial fossa floor.

There are **5 major anatomic** components of the temporal bone: EAC, middle ear-mastoid (ME-M), inner ear, petrous apex, and facial nerve. These anatomic components help define the various differential diagnosis lists of the temporal bone.

The **EAC** is made up of the tympanic bone medially and fibrocartilage laterally. The medial border of the EAC is formed by the TM, which attaches to the scutum superiorly and the tympanic anulus inferiorly. The nodal drainage of the EAC and the adjacent scalp is to the parotid lymph nodes.

The **middle ear** includes the epitympanum, mesotympanum, and hypotympanum. The **epitympanum** (attic) is defined superiorly by the tegmen tympani, which forms the roof. The inferior margin is defined by a line between the scutum and the tympanic segment of the facial nerve. The tegmen tympani is the thin, bony roof between the epitympanum and the middle cranial fossa dura. **Prussak space** represents the lateral epitympanic recess and is a classic location for acquired (pars flaccida) **cholesteatoma**. The malleus head and body and the short process of the incus are present within the epitympanum.

The **mesotympanum** is the middle ear area between the epitympanum above and the hypotympanum below. It is defined superiorly by a line between the scutum and tympanic segment of the facial nerve and inferiorly by a line between the tympanic anulus and the base of the cochlear promontory. The remainder of the ossicles (manubrium of the malleus, long and lenticular process of the incus, and stapes) are located in the mesotympanum. The 2 muscles of the middle ear, the **tensor tympani** and **stapedius** muscles, are also in the mesotympanum and function to dampen sound. The posterior wall of the mesotympanum has 3 important structures: Facial nerve recess, pyramidal eminence, and sinus tympani. The **facial nerve recess** contains the mastoid facial nerve and may be dehiscent or have a bony covering. The **pyramidal eminence** contains the belly and tendon of the stapedius muscle. The **sinus tympani** is a clinical blind spot during a standard mastoid surgical approach to the temporal bone, where cholesteatomas may hide. The medial wall contains the lateral SCC, the tympanic segment of the facial nerve, and the oval and round windows. The **hypotympanum** is a shallow trough on the floor of the middle ear cavity.

The **mastoid** sinus contains 3 important anatomic structures. The **mastoid antrum** (Latin for "cave") is the large, central mastoid air cell. The **aditus ad antrum** (Latin for "entrance to the cave") connects the epitympanum of the middle ear to the mastoid antrum. **Körner septum** is part of the petrosquamosal suture running posterolaterally through the mastoid air cells. This septum functions as an important surgical landmark within the mastoid air cells and also serves as a barrier to the extension of infection from the lateral mastoid air cells to the medial mastoid air cells. The mastoid temporal bone continues to develop after birth. As the mastoid eminence protects the facial nerve, this nerve is relatively unprotected until the eminence is formed. This is why the facial nerve is vulnerable to birth trauma.

The **inner ear** contains the **membranous labyrinth**, which is housed within the bony labyrinth (otic capsule). The membranous labyrinth consists of the fluid spaces within the bony labyrinth, including the fluid and soft tissues within the vestibule, SCCs and cochlea, the endolymphatic duct and sac, and cochlear duct. The vestibule houses the largest part of the membranous labyrinth, consisting of the utricle and saccule. The utricle is the more cephalad portion, and the saccule is the more caudal portion of the vestibule. The vestibule is separated laterally from the middle ear by the oval window niche. The SCCs project off the superior, posterior, and lateral aspects of the vestibule. The lateral (or horizontal) SCC is at risk for fistula formation from an epitympanic cholesteatoma, as it projects into the epitympanum. The endolymphatic duct and sac contain endolymph, whereas the cochlear duct contains perilymph.

The **bony labyrinth** (otic capsule) forms the cochlea, vestibule, SCCs, and vestibular and cochlear aqueducts. The **cochlea** has ~ 2.5 turns. The entire cochlea encircles a central bony axis, the **modiolus**. The modiolus houses the spiral ganglion, cell bodies of the cochlear nerve. The 3 spiral chambers of the cochlea are the scala tympani (posterior chamber), scala vestibuli (anterior chamber), and scala media (contains organ of Corti = hearing apparatus).

The **SCCs** project off the superior, lateral, and posterior aspects of the vestibule. The superior SCC projects cephalad. The bony ridge over the superior SCC in the roof of the petrous pyramid is the arcuate eminence, an important surgical landmark. The lateral (or horizontal) SCC projects into the middle ear. The tympanic segment of the facial nerve is on the undersurface of the lateral SCC. The posterior SCC projects posteriorly along the petrous ridge. The crus communis is the common origin of the superior and posterior SCCs.

The **petrous apex** is anteromedial to the inner ear and lateral to the petrooccipital fissure. It is pneumatized in ~ 33% of people. The abducens nerve (CNVI) passes along the medial surface of the petrous apex and through the Dorello canal. The trigeminal nerve (CNV) passes through the porus trigeminus into Meckel cave on the cephalad-medial surface of the petrous apex. In petrous apicitis, CNV and CNVI are commonly affected.

The petrous **internal carotid artery** (ICA) includes the vertical and horizontal segments within the petrous temporal bone. The vertical segment rises to the genu beneath the cochlea. The horizontal segment projects anteromedially to turn cephalad as the cavernous segment.

The **intratemporal facial nerve (CNVII)** is composed of the IAC and labyrinthine, tympanic, and mastoid segments. The IAC segment is located anterosuperiorly within the IAC. The labyrinthine segment extends from the IAC fundus to the geniculate ganglion. The geniculate ganglion is also known as the anterior genu, and the greater superficial petrosal nerve originates here. The tympanic segment leaves the geniculate ganglion and passes under the lateral SCC. The posterior genu is the portion where the tympanic segment bends inferiorly to become the mastoid segment. The mastoid segment leaves the posterior genu to pass inferiorly to the stylomastoid foramen. It first gives off the motor nerve to the stapedius muscle, then the chorda tympani nerve. The facial nerve then exits the skull base through the stylomastoid foramen.

The **motor root of CNVII** innervates the muscles of facial expression, stapedius, platysma, and the posterior belly of the digastric muscles. The sensory-parasympathetic root (nervus intermedius) contains special sensory visceral afferent fibers that convey taste to the anterior 2/3 of the tongue; the parasympathetic portion provides general visceral efferent secretomotor fibers to lacrimal, submandibular, and sublingual glands.

CNVII has **4 major functions** that help localize a lesion along its course. Lacrimation is via the greater superficial petrosal nerve. The stapedius nerve provides the stapedius reflex, which creates sound dampening. Taste to the anterior 2/3 of the tongue is via the chorda tympani nerve to the lingual nerve to the oral tongue. Motor branches supply muscles of facial expression.

The 2 muscles of the temporal bone, the **tensor tympani** and **stapedius** muscles, function to dampen sound. When dysfunctional, the patient presents with hyperacusis. The tensor tympani is innervated by a trigeminal nerve (CNV3) branch. It is located in the anteromedial wall of the mesotympanum. The tensor tympani muscle tendon goes through the cochleariform process and turns laterally to attach to the manubrium of the malleus. The stapedius muscle is innervated by CNVII. The stapedius muscle belly is located in the pyramidal eminence. The stapedius tendon attaches to the head of the stapes.

There are 3 ossicles of the middle ear: **Malleus**, **incus**, and **stapes**. The malleus is the most anterior ossicle and is

Differential Diagnosis: Location

External auditory canal	Inner ear
External auditory canal atresia/stenosis	Superior semicircular canal dehiscence
Cholesteatoma	Labyrinthitis and labyrinthine ossificans
Squamous cell carcinoma	Large endolymphatic sac anomaly
Exostoses (surfer's ear)	Fenestral and cochlear otosclerosis
Osteoma	Intralabyrinthine schwannoma
Medial canal fibrosis	Endolymphatic sac tumor
Keratosis obturans	Intralabyrinthine hemorrhage
Necrotizing otitis externa	Labyrinthine malformations
Middle ear-mastoid	**Petrous apex**
Acquired cholesteatoma	Trapped fluid
Congenital cholesteatoma	Cholesterol granuloma
Cholesterol granuloma	Congenital cholesteatoma
Acute coalescent mastoiditis	Cephalocele
Chronic otitis media ± tympanosclerosis	Apical petrositis
Dehiscent jugular bulb	Mucocele
Aberrant internal carotid artery	**Intratemporal facial nerve**
Tympanic paraganglioma	Herpetic facial neuritis (Bell palsy)
Jugular paraganglioma	Facial nerve venous malformation (hemangioma)
Meningioma	Facial nerve schwannoma
Rhabdomyosarcoma	Perineural parotid malignancy

composed of the umbo, manubrium, and head. The incus is located posteriorly and consists of the short process, body, long process, and lenticular process. The stapes is located medially and consists of the head, crura, and footplate.

Imaging Issues of the Temporal Bone

When faced with a temporal bone study, use a systematic approach through the 5 major functional components (EAC, ME-M, inner ear, petrous apex, and facial nerve). Evaluate and report on the location of the ICA, status of the ossicles, location of CNVII, integrity of the facial nerve canal, presence of the oval window, and integrity of the fissula ante fenestram (anterior margin of the oval window). If a lesion of the temporal bone is found, its location and clinical findings help refine the differential diagnosis list.

CHL is caused by a disruption of the conductive chain, which may be due to diseases of the EAC, TM, ossicles, or oval window. Typical lesions to consider in a patient with CHL include acquired cholesteatoma, chronic otitis media, EAC atresia/stenosis, fenestral otosclerosis, and cholesterol granuloma. Less common etiologies include oval window atresia, congenital cholesteatoma, ossicular fixation, and medial canal fibrosis.

SNHL involves lesions of the cochlea, modiolus, or cochlear nerve. These lesions may occur in the temporal bone, IAC, CPA, or brainstem. Inner ear abnormalities in congenital SNHL may provide clues to a specific syndromic etiology. Positive findings help direct genetic testing and affect patient management. The most common lesion to present with acquired unilateral SNHL is vestibular schwannoma (~ 90% of lesions). Other much less common etiologies include meningioma, otosclerosis, facial nerve schwannoma, metastases, and labyrinthitis.

Whenever the temporal bone is imaged, the entire facial nerve canal should be visualized and inspected. If a lesion of CNVII is found, it should be precisely localized to 1 of the CNVII segments: Cisternal segment (brainstem to porus acousticus), IAC (canalicular) segment, labyrinthine segment, tympanic segment, mastoid segment, or parotid segment.

Some lesions of the temporal bone may result in **facial nerve paralysis**, including Bell palsy, temporal bone fractures, cholesteatoma, schwannoma, venous malformation, jugular paraganglioma, meningioma, metastases, middle ear rhabdomyosarcoma, and Langerhans cell histiocytosis.

Clinical Implications

When a middle ear lesion is present, correlation with **otoscopic findings** provides critical clues to precise preoperative diagnosis. If a ruptured TM is present, a cholesteatoma may be seen through the defect. Most retrotympanic lesions have a distinctive hue and location. When the ENT surgeon sees a **white** middle ear lesion behind an intact TM, diagnoses to consider include a congenital cholesteatoma or schwannoma. If there is a **red** hue, the list includes a paraganglioma or aberrant ICA. If there is **blue**, cholesterol granuloma, chronic otitis media with hemorrhage, or a dehiscent jugular bulb should be considered.

Peripheral facial nerve paralysis is defined as unilateral facial nerve injury with involvement of the entire face, including the forehead. This type of CNVII injury includes loss of the 4 facial nerve functions: Lacrimation (parasympathetic), stapedius reflex (sound dampening), taste to the anterior 2/3 of the tongue, and facial expression. Injury to CNVII at any point as it winds through the temporal bone results in peripheral facial nerve paralysis.

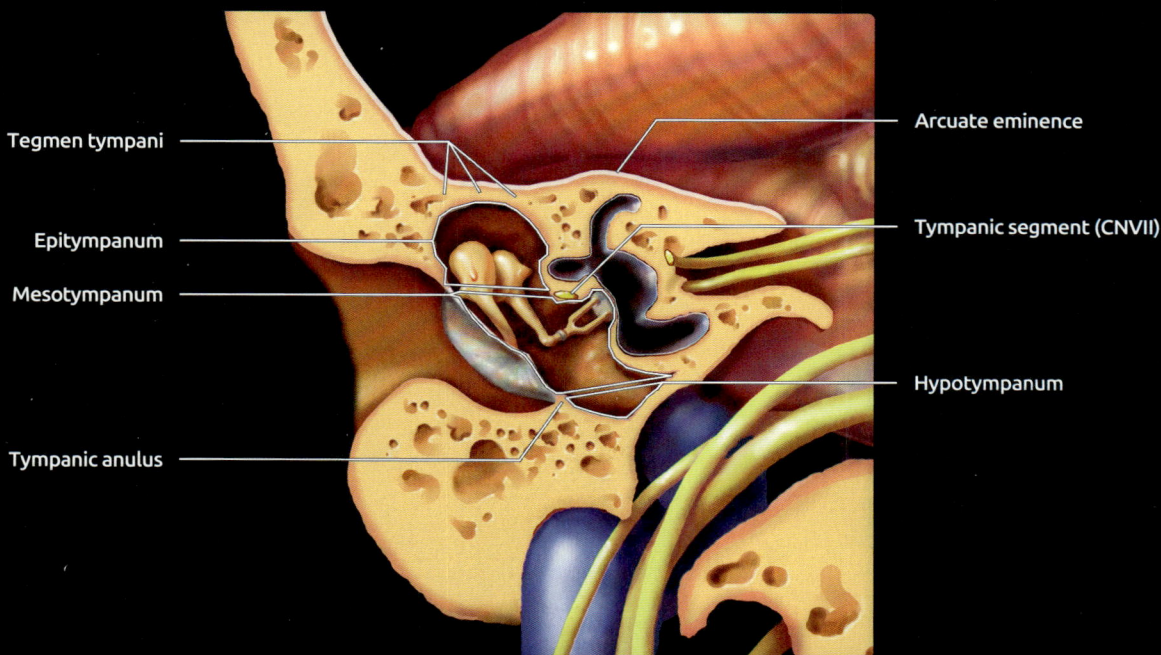

Tegmen tympani

Epitympanum

Mesotympanum

Tympanic anulus

Arcuate eminence

Tympanic segment (CNVII)

Hypotympanum

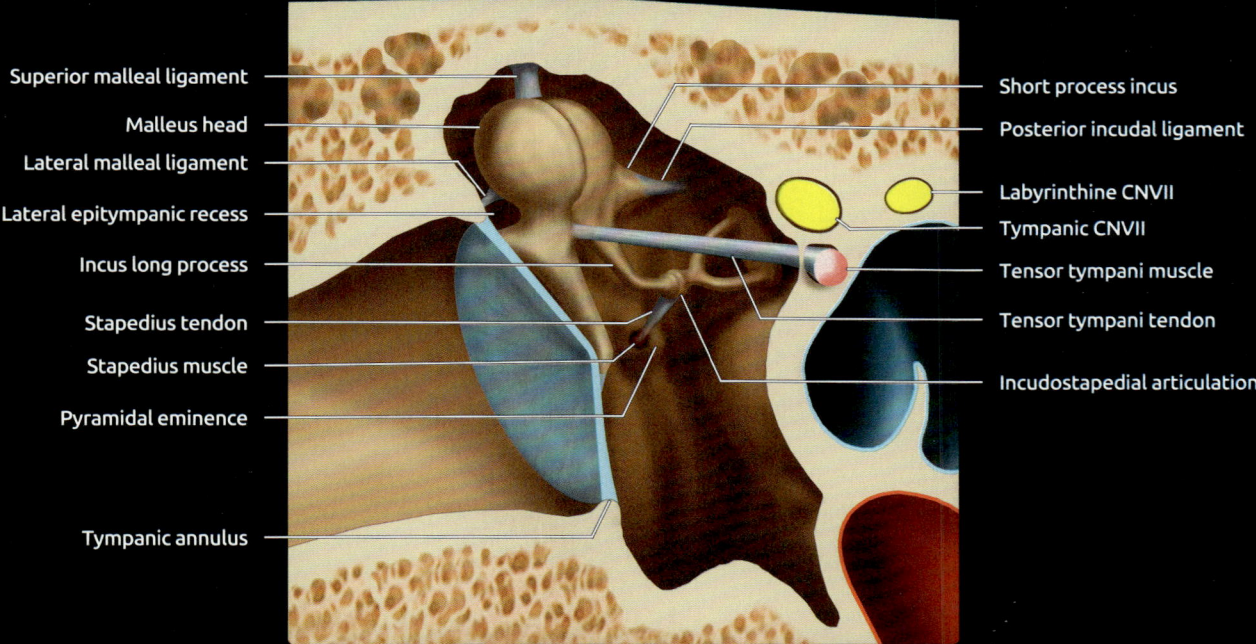

Superior malleal ligament

Malleus head

Lateral malleal ligament

Lateral epitympanic recess

Incus long process

Stapedius tendon

Stapedius muscle

Pyramidal eminence

Tympanic annulus

Short process incus

Posterior incudal ligament

Labyrinthine CNVII

Tympanic CNVII

Tensor tympani muscle

Tensor tympani tendon

Incudostapedial articulation

(Top) *Coronal magnified graphic shows the middle ear. The middle ear is divided into 3 portions: Epitympanum, mesotympanum, and hypotympanum. The epitympanum is defined as the middle ear cavity above a line drawn from the tip of the scutum to the tympanic segment of CNVII. The epitympanic roof is called the tegmen tympani. The mesotympanum extends from this line inferiorly to a line connecting the tympanic anulus to the base of the cochlear promontory. **(Bottom)** Coronal graphic highlights the middle ear ossicles, ligaments, and tendons. The malleus is the most lateral ossicle. The Prussak space is the lateral tympanic recess, where acquired (pars flaccida) cholesteatomas arise. The tensor tympani tendon crosses the medial middle ear and attaches to the malleus body. The stapedius tendon emerges from the pyramidal eminence to attach to the stapes hub region. The tympanic membrane attaches to the scutum superiorly and the tympanic annulus inferiorly.*

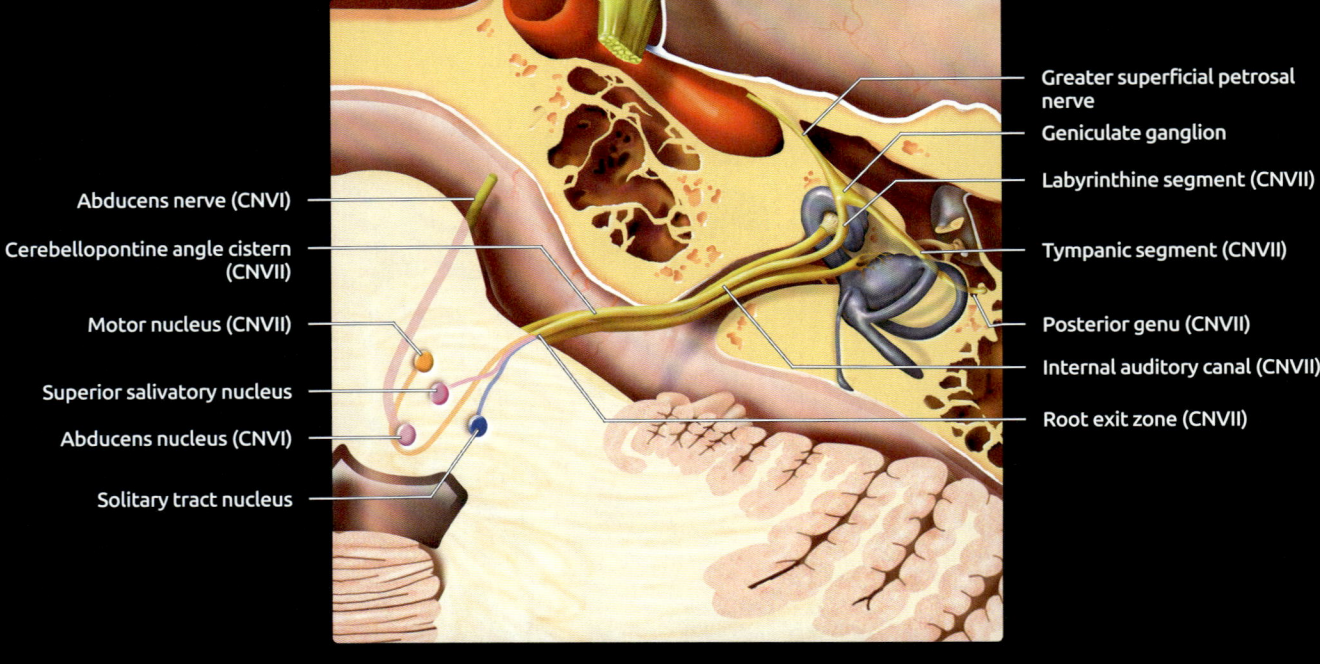

Greater superficial petrosal nerve

Geniculate ganglion

Labyrinthine segment (CNVII)

Tympanic segment (CNVII)

Posterior genu (CNVII)

Internal auditory canal (CNVII)

Root exit zone (CNVII)

Abducens nerve (CNVI)

Cerebellopontine angle cistern (CNVII)

Motor nucleus (CNVII)

Superior salivatory nucleus

Abducens nucleus (CNVI)

Solitary tract nucleus

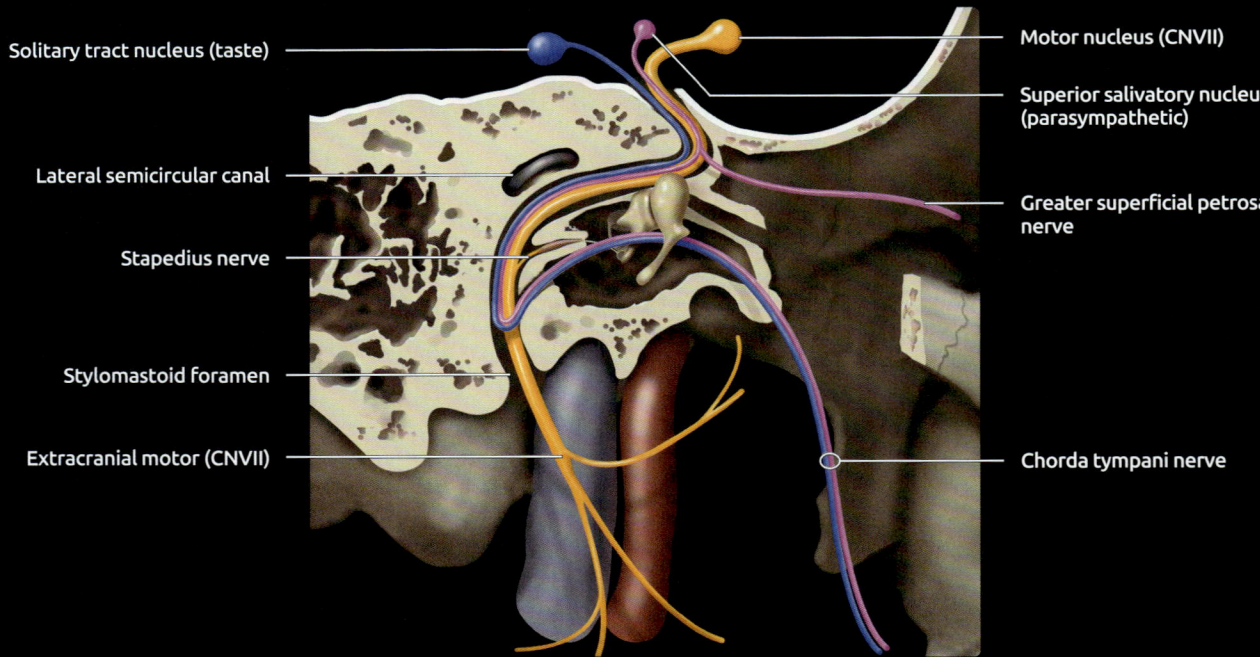

Solitary tract nucleus (taste)

Lateral semicircular canal

Stapedius nerve

Stylomastoid foramen

Extracranial motor (CNVII)

Motor nucleus (CNVII)

Superior salivatory nucleus (parasympathetic)

Greater superficial petrosal nerve

Chorda tympani nerve

(Top) *Axial graphic shows the facial nerve from the brainstem nuclei to the posterior genu in the temporal bone. The motor nucleus sends out fibers, which encircle the CNVI nucleus before reaching the root exit zone at the pontomedullary junction. Superior salivatory nucleus sends parasympathetic secretomotor fibers to the lacrimal, submandibular, and sublingual glands. The solitary tract nucleus receives the anterior 2/3 of tongue taste information, via the chorda tympani nerve, to the lingual nerve, to the oral tongue.* (Bottom) *Sagittal graphic depicting CNVII within the temporal bone [temporal motor fibers pass through the temporal bone, giving off the stapedius nerve to the stapedius muscle, then exit via the stylomastoid foramen to the extracranial CNVII (entirely motor)]. Parasympathetic fibers from the superior salivatory nucleus reach the lacrimal gland via the greater superficial petrosal nerve and the submandibular-sublingual glands via the chorda tympanic nerve. The anterior 2/3 of tongue taste fibers come via the chorda tympani nerve.*

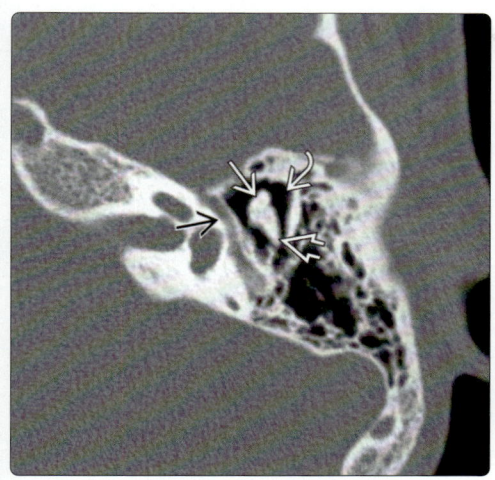

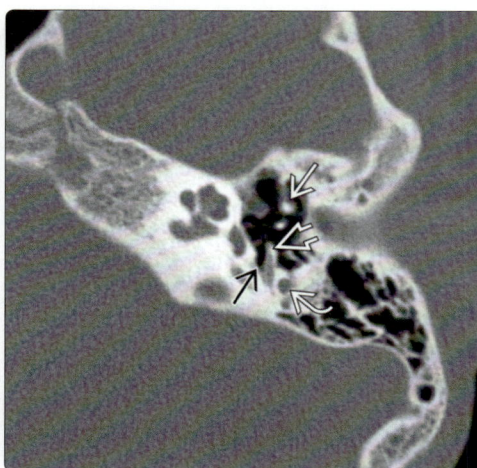

(Left) *Axial temporal bone CT through the epitympanum shows the malleus head ➡ anterior to the incus short process ➡. Prussak space is the lateral epitympanic recess ➡ and is a typical location for acquired cholesteatoma. Tympanic segment CNVII is well seen ➡.* (Right) *Axial temporal bone CT through the mesotympanum shows the posterior wall sinus tympani ➡ and pyramidal eminence ➡, which contain the stapedius muscle and mastoid CNVII ➡. The most anterior ossicle is the malleus ➡. The posterior ossicle is the incus.*

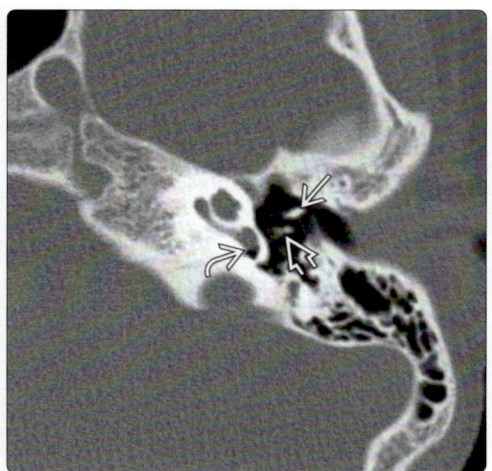

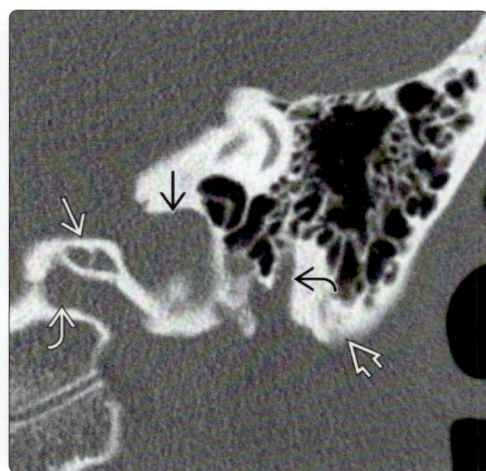

(Left) *Axial temporal bone CT through the low mesotympanum shows the normal manubrium of malleus ➡ and the incudostapedial articulation ➡. Basal turn of the cochlea ends at the round window ➡.* (Right) *Coronal temporal bone CT through the posterior mastoid region shows the mastoid segment of CNVII ➡, which then exits at the stylomastoid foramen. The mastoid tip ➡ helps protect this portion of CNVII. The jugular foramen ➡ and the hypoglossal canal ➡ are separated by the jugular tubercle ➡.*

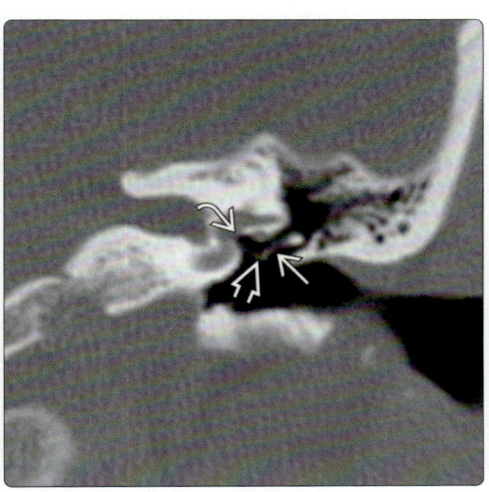

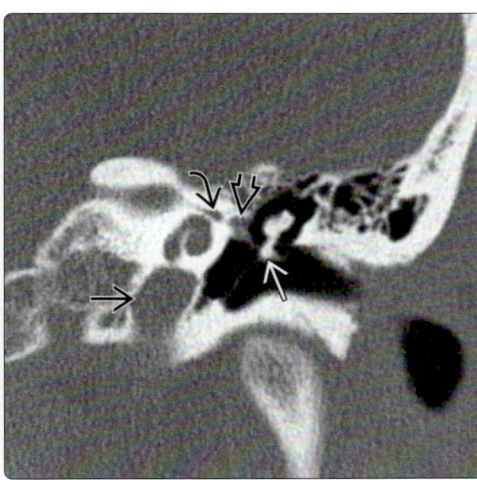

(Left) *Coronal temporal bone CT through the oval window shows the long process of the incus ➡ and lenticular process ➡. Notice the absence of bone evident in the normal oval window niche ➡. The oval window is best visualized in the coronal plane.* (Right) *Coronal temporal bone CT through the anterior middle ear shows the malleus ➡, labyrinthine ➡, and tympanic ➡ facial nerve segments. Notice the horizontal petrous internal carotid artery (ICA) ➡ below the cochlea.*

Temporal Bone Overview

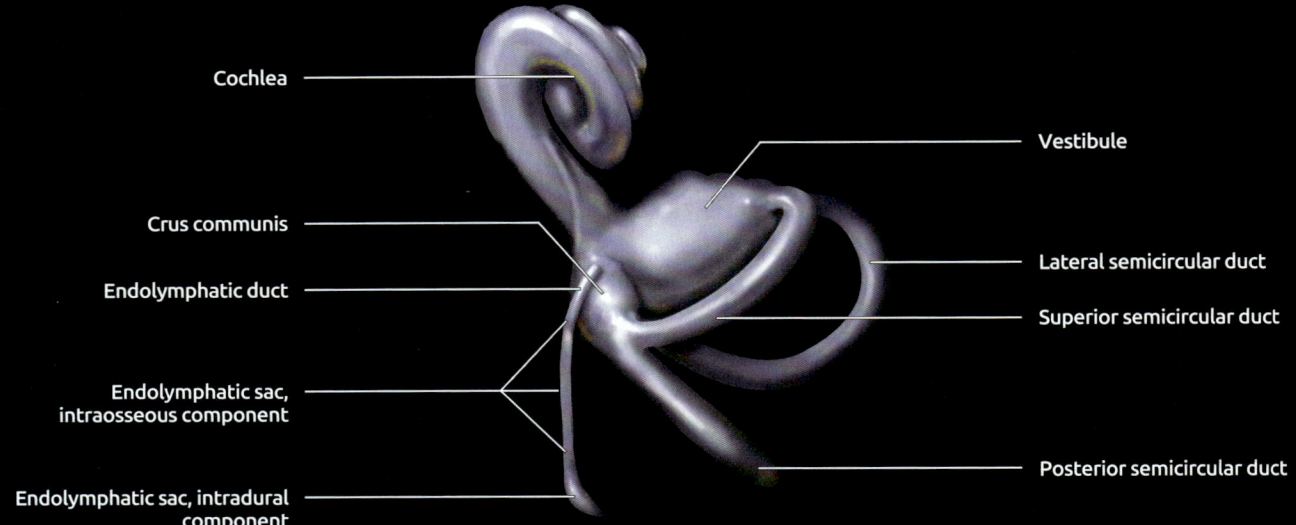

Cochlea

Vestibule

Crus communis

Endolymphatic duct

Lateral semicircular duct

Superior semicircular duct

Endolymphatic sac, intraosseous component

Endolymphatic sac, intradural component

Posterior semicircular duct

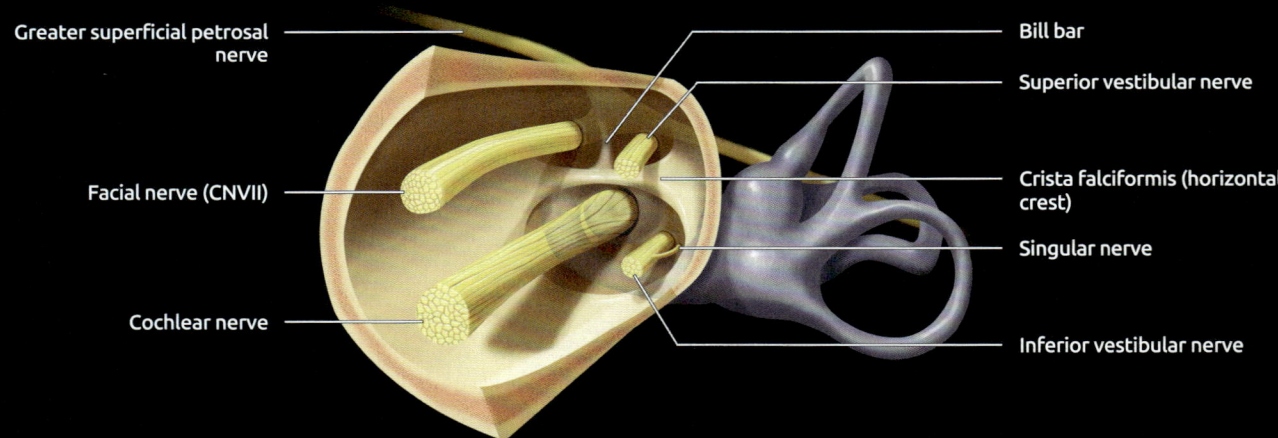

Greater superficial petrosal nerve

Bill bar

Superior vestibular nerve

Facial nerve (CNVII)

Crista falciformis (horizontal crest)

Singular nerve

Cochlear nerve

Inferior vestibular nerve

(Top) *Graphic shows membranous labyrinth seen from above. Key elements of the membranous labyrinth to consider include ~ 2.5 turns of the cochlea, the meeting point of the superior and posterior semicircular ducts (crus communis), and endolymphatic duct and sac. Note that the endolymphatic duct has intraosseous and intradural components.* (Bottom) *Graphic depicts cranial nerve relationships in the fundus of the internal auditory canal (IAC). Notice that the horizontal crista falciformis separates the cochlear nerve and inferior vestibular nerve below from CNVII and superior vestibular nerve above. Also note the vertical Bill bar separating CNVII from the superior vestibular nerve. Bill bar is not visible on CT or MR.*

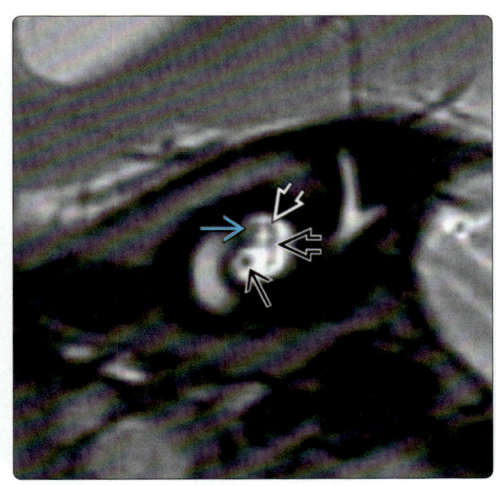

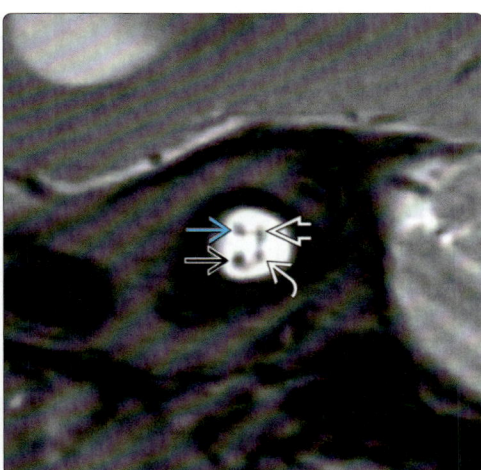

(Left) Sagittal oblique T2 MR of the lateral IAC shows the anterosuperior facial nerve ➡ and the anteroinferior cochlear nerve ➡. The crista falciformis ➡ is seen as a low-signal line dividing facial and superior vestibular ➡ nerves from the cochlear and inferior vestibular nerves. (Right) In the mid-IAC, 4 discrete nerves are visible. The anterosuperior facial nerve ➡ is normally slightly smaller than the anteroinferior cochlear nerve ➡. The superior ➡ and inferior ➡ vestibular nerves are often joined by connecting fibers.

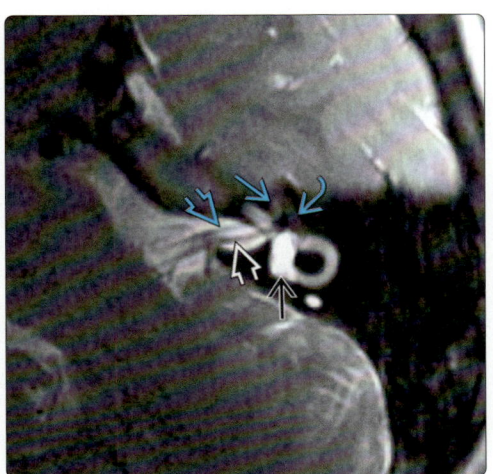

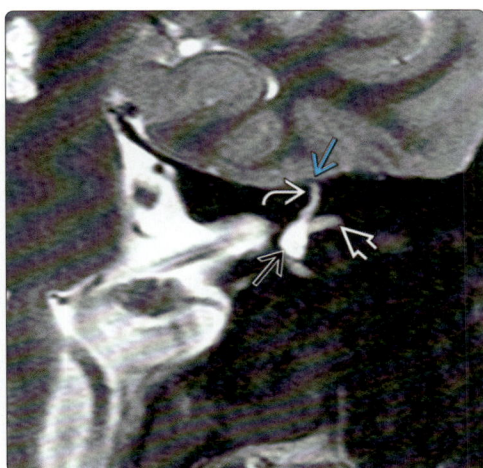

(Left) Axial T2 MR shows the labyrinthine ➡ and anterior tympanic ➡ segments of the facial nerve. As they are not surrounded by CSF, as is CNVII in the IAC ➡, they are more difficult to see. Note the superior vestibular nerve ➡ and vestibule ➡. (Right) Coronal T2 MR shows the inner ear membranous labyrinth as high-signal fluid. Note the superior ➡ and lateral ➡ semicircular canals (SCCs) and the vestibule ➡. The bony ridge over the superior SCC is the arcuate eminence ➡, an important surgical landmark.

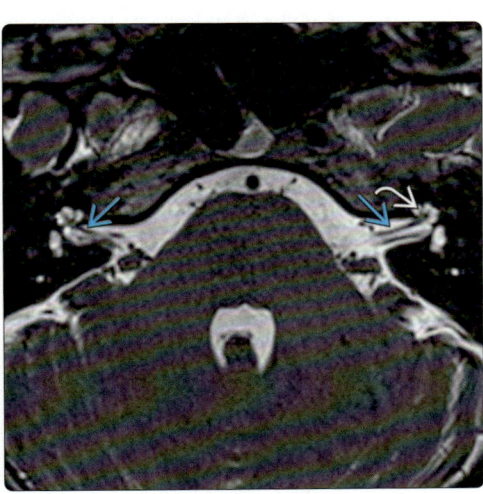

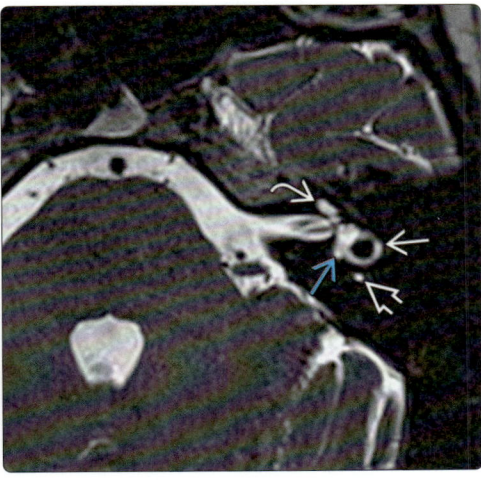

(Left) Axial T2 SPACE MR at the level of the cochlear nerve canal shows the cochlear nerve ➡ anteriorly in the inferior IAC. The bony modiolus ➡ of the cochlea is seen as a low-signal structure at the hub of the cochlea. The modiolus houses the spiral ganglion and cell bodies of the cochlear nerve. (Right) Axial T2 SPACE MR at the level of the vestibule ➡ shows the lateral ➡ and posterior ➡ semicircular canals. The basal (1st) turn of the cochlea ➡ is also well seen. The cochlea has ~ 2.5 turns.

Foramen Tympanicum

TERMINOLOGY

- Synonyms: Foramen of Huschke; tympanic bone dehiscence
- Definition: Developmental ossification defect in anteroinferior aspect of bony external auditory canal (EAC)
  - Should be considered normal EAC variant

IMAGING

- Axial T-bone CT: ~ 4- to 6-mm bony dehiscence in medial, anteroinferior aspect of bony EAC
- Axial diameter: Variable; 2-8 mm (mean: ~ 4 mm)

TOP DIFFERENTIAL DIAGNOSES

- 1st branchial cleft cyst
- EAC cholesteatoma
- EAC squamous cell carcinoma

PATHOLOGY

- Foramen tympanicum is formed in tympanic plate of T-bone before 1 year of age

- Usually closes before 5 years of age
- Persistence seen on bone CT after 5 years of age in ~ 7 % of patients
- Pathology associated with foramen tympanicum
  - **Spontaneous herniation of TMJ soft tissues** into EAC
  - Parotid gland and synovial TMJ fistulas into EAC
  - Foramen tympanicum may facilitate ear injury during TMJ arthroscopy

CLINICAL ISSUES

- **Asymptomatic** normal variant found incidentally during T-bone CT
- Otorrhea with otalgia possible if dehiscence is large
  - Physical examination reveals polypoid lesion in anteroinferior bony EAC
  - If patient opens mouth, polypoid lesion disappears
- Gustatory otorrhea (occurs with eating)
  - Sialo-aural fistula from parotid gland through foramen tympanicum to EAC

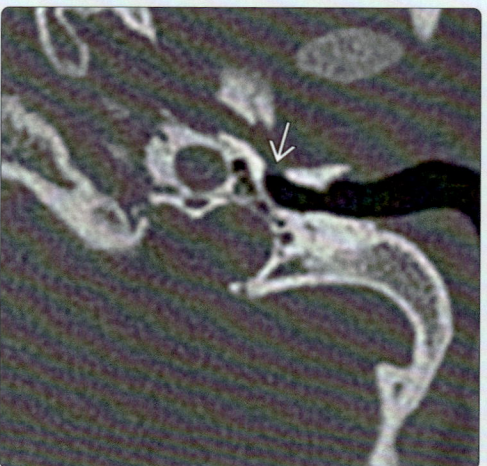
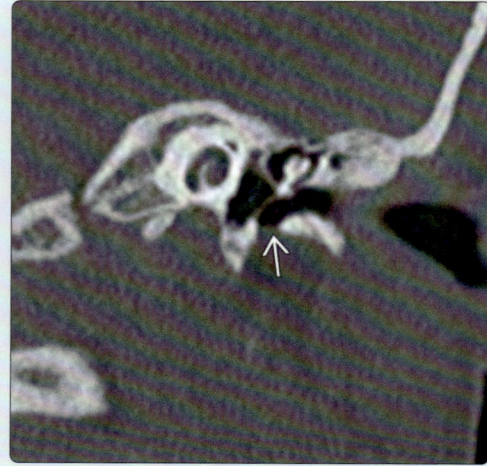

(Left) Axial T-bone CT of the left ear shows the appearance of an incidental foramen tympanicum ➡ in a 7-year-old child. Notice the tympanic bone dehiscence at the anteroinferior osseous external auditory canal (EAC) that normally closes by 5 years of age, but is present after 5 years of age in 7% of patients. (Right) Coronal T-bone CT in the same patient demonstrates the well-defined area of incomplete ossification in the anterior medial aspect of the osseous EAC ➡.

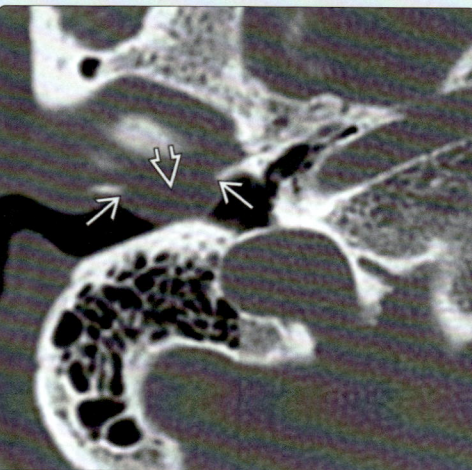
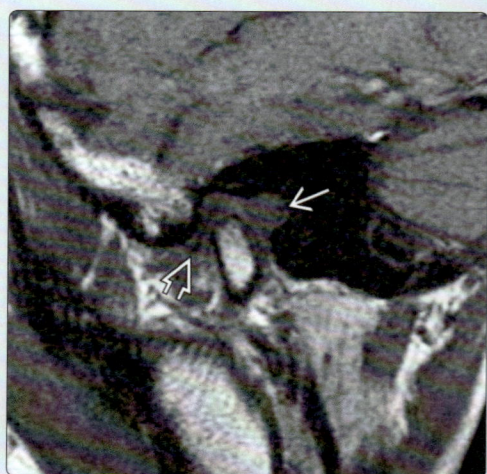

(Left) Axial bone CT through the EAC reveals a large (14-mm) foramen tympanicum in the anteroinferior bony EAC ➡. The posterior TMJ soft tissues have prolapsed through a dehiscence ➡ into the EAC lumen. (Right) Sagittal T1 MR in the closed-mouth position shows posterior TMJ soft tissues filling the lumen of the EAC ➡. Meniscus ➡ is in normal position. With the mouth open (not shown), the soft tissue in the EAC diminishes considerably, suggesting it is the joint capsule that has prolapsed into the EAC.

TERMINOLOGY

Synonyms
- Foramen of Huschke
- Tympanic bone dehiscence

Definitions
- Foramen tympanicum
  - Developmental ossification defect in anteroinferior aspect of bony external auditory canal (EAC)

IMAGING

General Features
- Best diagnostic clue
  - Axial T-bone CT: ~ 4- to 6-mm bony dehiscence in medial, anteroinferior aspect of bony EAC
- Location
  - Located at anteroinferior aspect of EAC, posteromedial to TMJ
- Size
  - Axial diameter: Variable; 2-8 mm (mean: ~ 4 mm)
  - Mean sagittal diameter: 3.5 mm

CT Findings
- Bone CT
  - Focal dehiscence visible on axial bone CT in medial, anteroinferior aspect of bony EAC
    - In bony wall, shared in common with TMJ
  - **Dehiscence** found in **~ 7%** of normal T-bones
    - **Focal thinning** of bone in this location: **35%**
  - Bilateral > unilateral
  - Larger lesions have additional findings
    - Polypoid mass in anteroinferior EAC
      - □ From **prolapse of TMJ retrodiscal soft tissues**
      - □ Rarely results from **parotid prolapse**

MR Findings
- Only positive in case of larger dehiscence when TMJ soft tissues or parotid prolapse is present

Imaging Recommendations
- Best imaging tool
  - T-bone CT defines extent of foramen tympanicum
  - When large with prolapsing tissue, TMJ MR is used to define tissue type

DIFFERENTIAL DIAGNOSIS

1st Branchial Cleft Cyst
- Cyst intraparotid or periauricular

External Auditory Canal Cholesteatoma
- Bony EAC destruction with bone fragments

External Auditory Canal Squamous Cell Carcinoma
- Begins as obvious auricular squamous cell carcinoma
- After multiple treatments, invades EAC ± focal bony wall destruction

PATHOLOGY

General Features
- Etiology

- Foramen tympanicum is formed in tympanic plate of T-bone at ~ 1 year of age
  - Usually closes before 5 years of age
  - Persistence after 5 years of age seen on bone CT in ~ 7% of patients
- Foramen is defined by traversing structure
  - Foramen tympanicum is **not** true foramen
  - More appropriate term than foramen tympanicum is **tympanic bone dehiscence**
  - Considered **normal variant**
- Pathology associated with foramen tympanicum
  - Spontaneous herniation of TMJ soft tissues into EAC
  - Foramen tympanicum may facilitate ear injury during TMJ arthroscopy
  - Parotid gland and synovial TMJ fistulas into EAC
  - Infection spread through foramen tympanicum from EAC outward or from TMJ inward

CLINICAL ISSUES

Presentation
- Most common signs/symptoms
  - **Asymptomatic** bony defect found incidentally during T-bone CT
- Other signs/symptoms
  - Otorrhea with otalgia possible if dehiscence is large
    - Physical examination reveals polypoid lesion in anteroinferior bony EAC
    - If patient opens mouth, polypoid lesion disappears
  - Salivary fistula formation with **gustatory otorrhea** and otalgia
    - Extremely rare lesion
    - Sialo-aural fistula from parotid gland through foramen tympanicum to EAC
    - Otorrhea fluid tests positive for amylase
    - Gustatory otorrhea occurs when eating
  - Complication during TMJ arthroscopy
    - Inadvertent passage of arthroscope into EAC or middle ear
    - Resultant otologic complications possible
  - TMJ/masticator space infection or EAC infection may spread in either direction

Demographics
- Sex
  - Persistence seen in F > M

Natural History & Prognosis
- Persistent foramen tympanicum at 5 years of age
  - May continue to close with increasing age in some patients
  - Newer literature suggests ↑ in age-related thinning may lead to ↑ in prevalence with older age

SELECTED REFERENCES

1. Pazardzhikliev D et al: Foramen tympanicum (foramen of Huschke) as a cause of unexplained spontaneous otorrhea: a case report. Cureus. 16(8):e66658, 2024
2. Rabuel V et al: Foramen tympanicum: tomographic study of a large cohort of Europeans. Surg Radiol Anat. 47(1):38, 2024
3. Lacout A et al: Foramen tympanicum, or foramen of Huschke: pathologic cases and anatomic CT study. AJNR Am J Neuroradiol. 26(6):1317-23, 2005

Congenital External and Middle Ear Malformation

KEY FACTS

TERMINOLOGY

- Congenital external & middle ear malformation (CEMEM)

IMAGING

- Auricle: Anotia or microtia
- External auditory canal (EAC) stenosis: Narrow EAC, tympanic plate (TP) hypoplasia
  - Normal or thickened tympanic membrane (TM)
  - Small middle ear cavity (MEC)
  - Subtle ossicular anomaly
- EAC atresia: Absent EAC, TP, & TM; moderate or severe CEMEM + middle ear findings
- Moderate CEMEM middle ear findings
  - Small MEC ± low tegmen tympani
  - Fusion, malformation, & rotation of malleus & incus
  - Oval window atresia (35%) ± aberrant CNVII tympanic segment
  - Mastoid CNVII more anterolateral than normal
- Severe CEMEM middle ear findings
  - Tiny or absent MEC, low tegmen tympani
  - Ossicles absent or rudimentary
  - Oval window atresia (35%) ± aberrant CNVII tympanic segment
  - Aberrant facial nerve canal course
- Erosive opacity in stenotic EAC or MEC suggests congenital cholesteatoma

TOP DIFFERENTIAL DIAGNOSES

- Acquired EAC stenosis (surfer's ear)
- EAC osteoma
- Tympanosclerosis

CLINICAL ISSUES

- Conductive hearing loss = most common symptom
- Severity of microtia approximates severity of CEMEM

DIAGNOSTIC CHECKLIST

- EAC atresia = clinical diagnosis
- CT provides preoperative roadmap

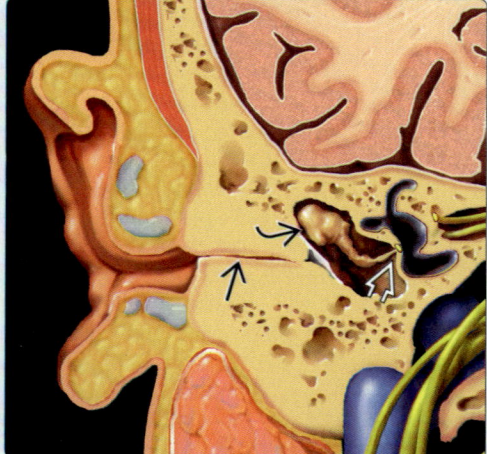
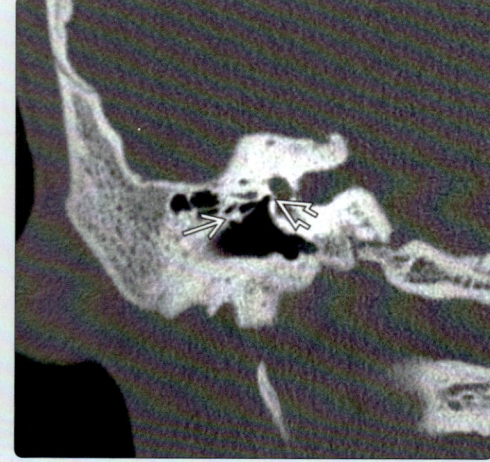

(Left) Coronal graphic of the right ear shows a deformed auricle with an absent external auditory canal (EAC) ➡. Ossicular fusion mass ➡ and rotation with oval window atresia ➡ are also present. (Right) Coronal bone CT in this patient with congenital external ear malformation shows an absent EAC and a thick atretic plate with the ossicular fusion mass ➡ ankylosed to the lateral wall of the middle ear cavity. Oval window atresia is present. Note narrowed oval window niche and thin bone covering the oval window ➡ itself.

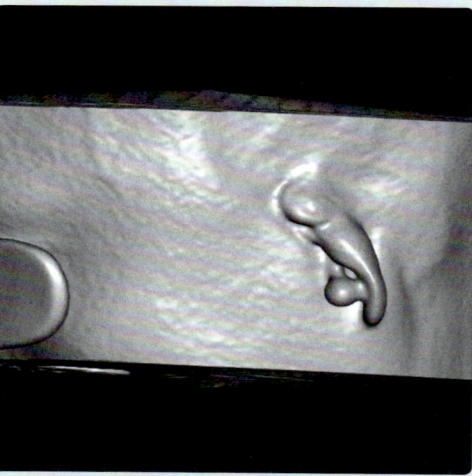
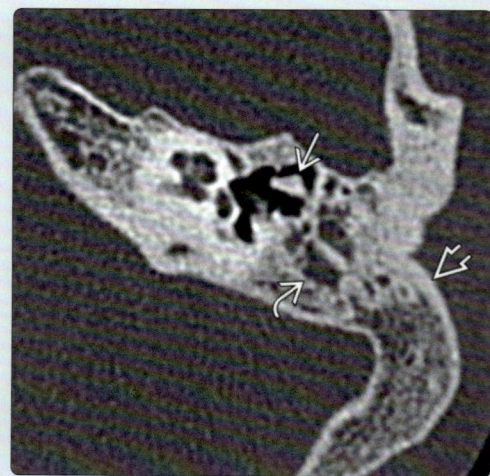

(Left) Lateral 3D soft tissue surface-rendered NECT reformation shows a dysplastic auricle in a teenager with nonsyndromic unilateral microtia and EAC atresia. (Right) Axial bone CT in the same patient shows a boomerang appearance of the malformed, fused malleus and incus ➡. Note also a small middle ear cavity and underdeveloped ➡, opacified mastoid air cells ➡. A low-lying tympanic segment and anteriorly positioned mastoid segment facial nerve canal were also noted (not shown).

Congenital External and Middle Ear Malformation

TERMINOLOGY

Abbreviations
- Congenital external & middle ear malformation (CEMEM)

Synonyms
- Congenital aural atresia or dysplasia

Definitions
- Anotia: Absent auricle
- Microtia: Small, malformed auricle
- External ear malformation [auricle & external auditory canal (EAC)]
  - EAC atresia: Absent EAC, tympanic plate (TP), & tympanic membrane (TM)
  - EAC stenosis: Narrow EAC, TP hypoplasia, TM present
  - EAC duplication: Duplication of part or all of EAC
- Middle ear cavity (MEC) malformation: Aplasia or hypoplasia MEC + ossicular anomaly

IMAGING

General Features
- Best diagnostic clue
  - Microtia or anotia + absent EAC
  - Microtia or normal pinna + narrow EAC
- Location
  - EAC & MEC; unilateral or bilateral
- Morphology
  - Small, malformed auricle (microtia) or anotia
  - Mildest CEMEM has narrowed EAC
  - More severe CEMEM has no identifiable EAC or TP
  - Hypoplastic MEC
  - Dysmorphic ossicles, especially malleus & incus

CT Findings
- Bone CT
  - Auricle & EAC in CEMEM
    - Dysmorphic auricle: Anotia or microtia
    - EAC stenosis
      - □ Narrow or blind-ending EAC
      - □ TP present but small; TM thickened ± Ca^{++}
      - □ Erosive opacity suggests keratosis obturans or EAC cholesteatoma
    - EAC atresia
      - □ Absent EAC
      - □ Absent TP & TM
      - □ Membranous ± (thick or thin) bony atresia plate
    - Duplicated EAC
      - □ Duplication of membranous or entire EAC
  - Middle ear malformation
    - Mild CEMEM: EAC stenosis
      - □ MEC: Mild hypoplasia, shallow facial recess
      - □ Oval window: Normal or stenotic ± anomalous course of tympanic segment CNVII
      - □ Ossicles: Variable malformation, rotation, fusion to lateral MEC, fusion of malleolar-incudal articulation
      - □ Mastoid segment CNVII: Near normal in location
    - Moderate CEMEM: EAC stenosis or atresia
      - □ MEC: Moderate hypoplasia ± low tegmen tympani
      - □ Oval window: Atresia (35%) ± anomalous course ± dehiscent tympanic segment CNVII
      - □ Round window: Atresia (5%)
      - □ Ossicles: Malformed, rotated, fused (malleus & incus > stapes); malleus-incus fusion may have boomerang appearance on axial images
      - □ Mastoid CNVII: More anterolateral than normal
      - □ Rounded or erosive opacity = associated congenital cholesteatoma (2%)
    - Severe CEMEM: EAC atresia
      - □ MEC: Tiny or absent, low tegmen tympani
      - □ Oval & round windows: Atresia
      - □ Ossicles: Absent or rudimentary
      - □ CNVII: ± hypoplasia; anomalous/bizarre course
  - Facial nerve canal findings
    - Aberrant tympanic & mastoid segments common
    - Tympanic segment may be dehiscent, overlying oval or round windows
    - Mastoid segment usually anterolaterally displaced
    - May exit skull base into glenoid fossa or lateral to styloid process
  - Mastoid pneumatization: Normal to absent
  - Inner ear & IAC: < 30% anomaly = syndromic
  - Mandible: Micrognathia + low-set pinna = syndromic

MR Findings
- Limited utility, e.g., large congenital cholesteatoma

Imaging Recommendations
- Best imaging tool
  - High-resolution CT
- Protocol advice
  - 0.6-mm axial CT with coronal & oblique reformats

DIFFERENTIAL DIAGNOSIS

Acquired External Auditory Canal Stenosis (Surfer's Ear)
- Bilateral acquired lesions + normal auricle
- Exostosis of EAC, often presenting with history of cold water swimming or other local EAC trauma

External Auditory Canal Osteoma
- Unilateral, acquired, benign bony growth obliterates EAC

External Auditory Canal Cholesteatoma
- Erosive opacity in normal or stenotic EAC
- May have bone fragments in soft tissue mass

Tympanosclerosis
- EAC normal in size
- Inflammatory calcifications of TM, ossicles, MEC

Keratosis Obturans, External Auditory Canal
- Keratin debris opacifies & erodes stenotic EAC

PATHOLOGY

General Features
- Etiology
  - Variety of causes of CEMEM, often unknown
  - Known syndromic/genetic causes

○ Epithelial cells of 1st branchial groove fail to split & canalize, resulting in CEMEM
- Genetics
  ○ 14% have positive prior family history
  ○ Infrequently linked to chromosome 18 mutations
  ○ May be associated with various syndromes
    – Hemifacial microsomia spectrum
    – Branchiootorenal syndrome
    – Treacher Collins syndrome
- Associated abnormalities
  ○ Isolated or part of craniofacial syndrome
    – Suggested by micrognathia + low-set pinna
    – Branchial cleft anomalies
  ○ Inner ear anomalies uncommon unless syndromic
    – Inner ear forms earlier from otocyst
- Embryology-anatomy in CEMEM
  ○ 1st & 2nd branchial arches & 1st pharyngeal pouch develop at same time during embryogenesis
  ○ Branchial groove & 1st pharyngeal pouch give rise to EAC
    – Initially, solid core of epithelial cells
    – In 3rd trimester, cell core canalizes into EAC
    – Failure of canalization leads to CEMEM
  ○ 1st branchial arch forms malleus head, incus body & short process, & tensor tympani tendon
  ○ 2nd branchial arch forms manubrium of malleus, long process of incus, stapes (except footplate), & stapedial muscle & tendon
    – Ossicular fusion mass very common in CEMEM
    – Oval window atresia may be associated with CEMEM
  ○ Inner ear forms earlier than EAC; anomalies unusual in CEMEM unless syndromic

Staging, Grading, & Classification

- Jahrsdoerfer scale & surgical outcomes
  ○ Score of ≥ 7 points → predicts better surgical outcome
  ○ Ideally, cochlear function should be present & inner ear structures normal on imaging
- Scoring system; best possible score = 10 points
  ○ Stapes present: 2
  ○ Oval window open: 1
  ○ Middle ear space present: 1
  ○ Facial nerve course identified: 1
  ○ Malleus-incus complex present: 1
  ○ Incus-stapes connection present: 1
  ○ Mastoid pneumatization present: 1
  ○ Round window present: 1
  ○ External ear present: 1
- Recommendations
  ○ Operate on unilateral CEMEM score ≥ 7
  ○ Operate on bilateral CEMEM score ≥ 5-6

CLINICAL ISSUES

Presentation

- Most common signs/symptoms
  ○ Conductive hearing loss = most common symptom
  ○ Physical exam
    – Absent, small ± low-set auricle
      □ Severity of microtia approximates severity of CEMEM & MEC malformation
    – EAC is stenotic or absent

Demographics

- Age
  ○ Present at birth
- Epidemiology
  ○ 1 in 10,000-20,000 live births
  ○ Unilateral:bilateral cases = 4:1
    – Nonsyndromic CEMEM usually unilateral
    – Bilateral CEMEM common when syndromic
- Sex: Occurs more commonly in males

Natural History & Prognosis

- Static clinical course, unless associated MEC cholesteatoma or syndromic
- In unilateral atresia, other ear typically has normal hearing
- Bilateral atresia: Bilateral conductive hearing loss
  ○ After surgery, hearing is adequate but not normal
- Auricle reconstruction may require 4-5 staged surgeries

Treatment

- Cosmetic reconstruction of auricle usually in adolescence
- CT to assess course of CNVII & oval window & inner ear status prior to surgery
- Bilateral atresia is treated at 5-6 years of age, when head has reached 90% of adult size
  ○ Auricle reconstruction precedes surgical treatment of MEC & ossicles
  ○ Surgical reconstruction of ear with mildest EAC atresia
  ○ Both auricles are repaired for cosmetic reasons
- Normal morphology & location of stapes important for surgical reconstruction & ossicular function

DIAGNOSTIC CHECKLIST

Consider

- EAC atresia = clinical diagnosis
  ○ CT provides preoperative roadmap
  ○ CT scoring systems suggest when to operate

Reporting Tips

- Preoperative CT checklist used for surgical planning
  ○ Atresia plate: Bony vs. membranous; note thickness
  ○ Report size of MEC as normal or small
  ○ Status of ossicles: Presence, morphology, & ankylosis
  ○ Oval window present? Stapes?
    – If no stapes, ossicular reconstruction is difficult
  ○ Trace course of CNVII; aberrant CNVII = risk at surgery
  ○ Survey for erosive opacity suggesting cholesteatoma

SELECTED REFERENCES

1. Vangrinsven G et al: Beyond the otoscope: an imaging review of congenital cholesteatoma. Insights Imaging. 15(1):194, 2024
2. Robson CD: Conductive hearing loss in children. Neuroimaging Clin N Am. 33(4):543-62, 2023
3. Gautam R et al: Congenital aural atresia: what the radiologist needs to know? Curr Probl Diagn Radiol. 51(4):599-616, 2022
4. Gautam R et al: High-resolution computed tomography evaluation of congenital aural atresia - how useful is this? J Laryngol Otol. 134(7):610-22, 2020
5. Metwally MI et al: Ear malformations: what do radiologists need to know? Clin Imaging. 66:42-53, 2020
6. Mukherjee S et al: The "boomerang" malleus-incus complex in congenital aural atresia. AJNR Am J Neuroradiol. 35(11):2181-5, 2014
7. Shonka DC Jr et al: The Jahrsdoerfer grading scale in surgery to repair congenital aural atresia. Arch Otolaryngol Head Neck Surg. 134(8):873-7, 2008

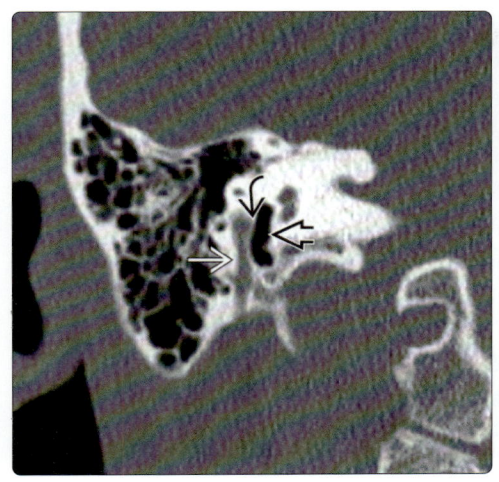

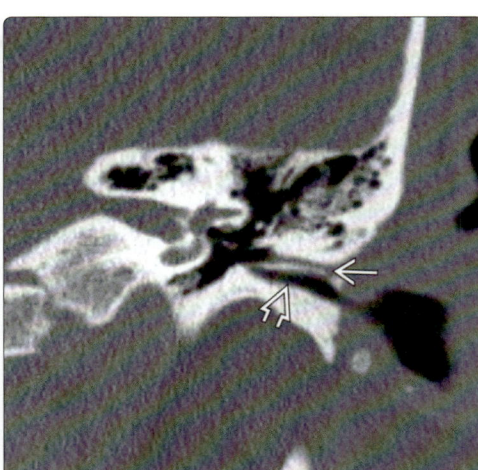

(Left) Coronal bone CT in a patient with congenital external ear malformation through the pyramidal eminence ⮕ demonstrates the mastoid segment of the facial nerve canal ⮕ at the same level as the sinus tympani ⮕. This is anterior to its normal location. (Right) Coronal bone CT in a patient with bilateral EAC malformation shows that the left narrowed EAC canal has 2 channels: 1 aerated ⮕ and 1 with a membranous plug ⮕. Such a duplicated EAC is a rare variant seen in EAC atresia.

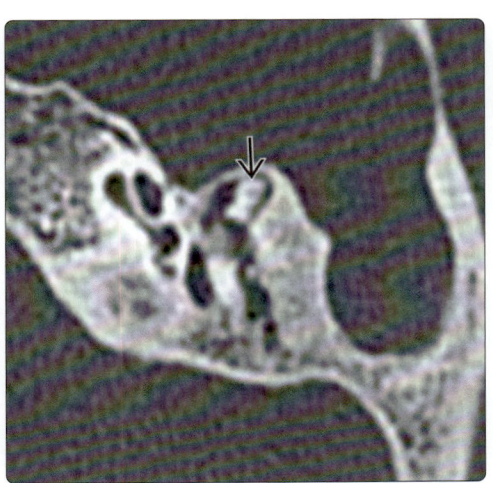

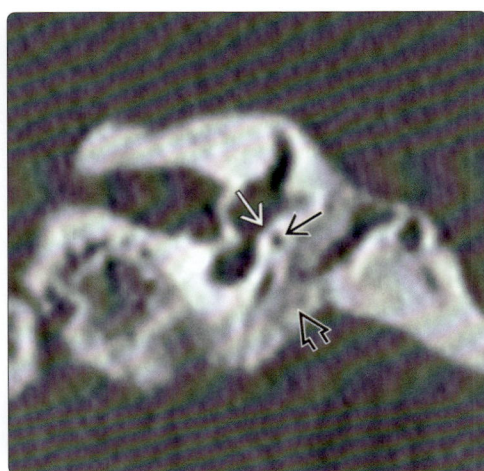

(Left) Axial bone CT in a patient with severe microtia and congenital external ear malformation shows a very small, opacified middle ear cavity with an ossicular fusion mass located laterally in the epitympanum ⮕. (Right) Coronal bone CT in the same patient shows the diminutive middle ear cavity and a thick, bony atretic plate ⮕. In addition, there is an aberrant course of the tympanic segment of CNVII ⮕, which courses over an atretic oval window ⮕.

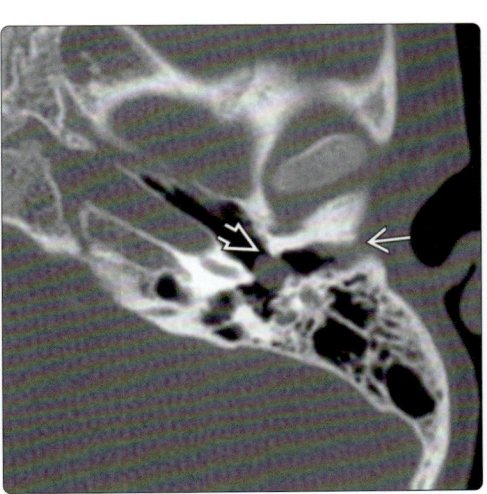

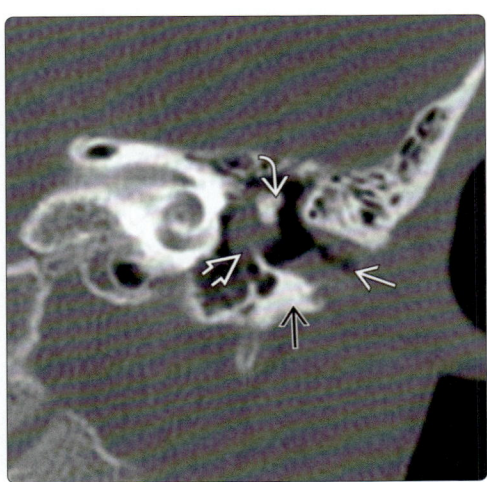

(Left) Axial bone CT in a 9-year-old boy with left conductive hearing loss reveals EAC stenosis ⮕ with partial EAC opacification. There is a rounded opacity ⮕ within the mildly hypoplastic middle ear cavity, consistent with a congenital cholesteatoma. (Right) Coronal bone CT in a 9-year-old boy with EAC stenosis ⮕ is shown. The congenital cholesteatoma ⮕ surrounds and erodes the malleus ⮕, which also has an abnormal orientation. Note the small tympanic plate ⮕.

Necrotizing External Otitis

TERMINOLOGY

- Necrotizing external otitis (NEO): Severe **invasive infection** of external auditory canal (EAC), adjacent soft tissues, and skull base
- a.k.a. malignant otitis externa; often used synonymously with skull base osteomyelitis

IMAGING

- Bone CT/ CECT
  - High-resolution bone CT best demonstrates bone erosion and demineralization
  - CECT: Soft tissue thickening of EAC with abnormal enhancement, infiltration of fat planes beyond EAC, including phlegmon and abscess
- MR
  - Study of choice for determining soft tissue extent, marrow involvement, and intracranial complications
- Nuclear medicine
  - Bone and gallium scans often done together
    - If both positive, with gallium scan showing larger activity area, high correlation with NEO

TOP DIFFERENTIAL DIAGNOSES

- EAC squamous cell carcinoma
- EAC cholesteatoma
- Postinflammatory medial canal fibrosis
- EAC keratosis obturans

PATHOLOGY

- **Pseudomonas aeruginosa**: 95% of NEO infections
- Other pathogens include *Staphylococcus* and fungal infections, such as *Aspergillus*

CLINICAL ISSUES

- Classic: Older adult diabetic patient presents with severe otalgia and otorrhea
- Can present in other immunocompromised patients, including HIV, chemotherapy, transplant immunosuppression

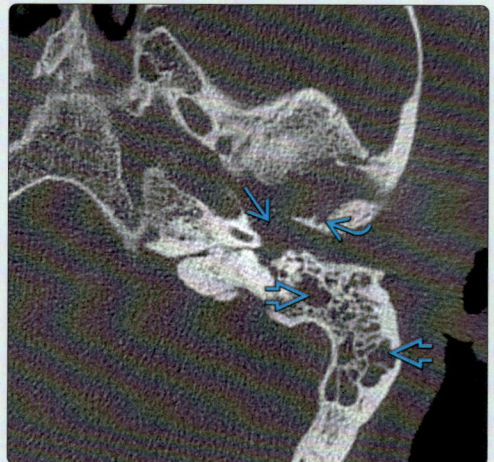
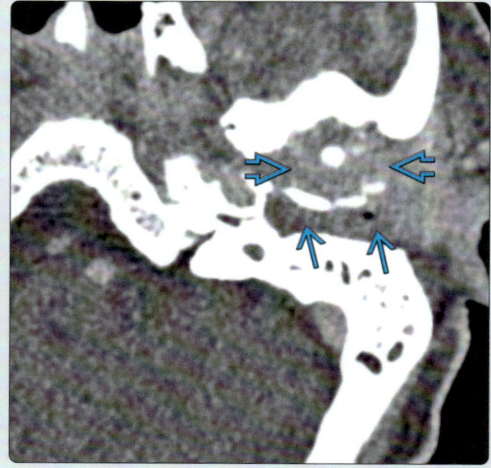

(Left) Axial high-resolution bone window CECT shows erosive changes along the anterior wall of the left external auditory canal (EAC) ➡ and left TMJ ➡. Note opacification of mastoid air cells ➡. (Right) Axial soft tissue window MPR CECT shows opacification of the EAC ➡ extending to the left TMJ ➡. These findings are consistent with necrotizing external otitis (NEO). Culture was positive for pseudomonas aeruginosa. Patient was treated with aggressive debridement and systemic antibiotic therapy.

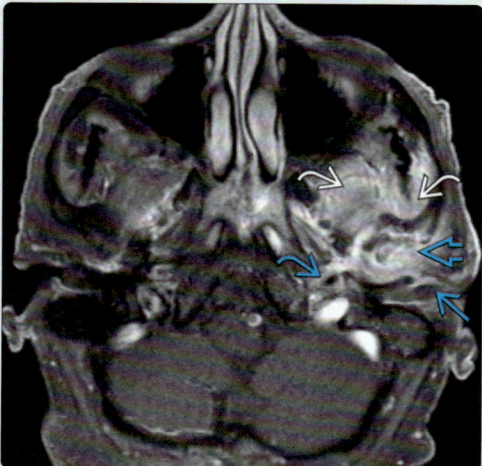
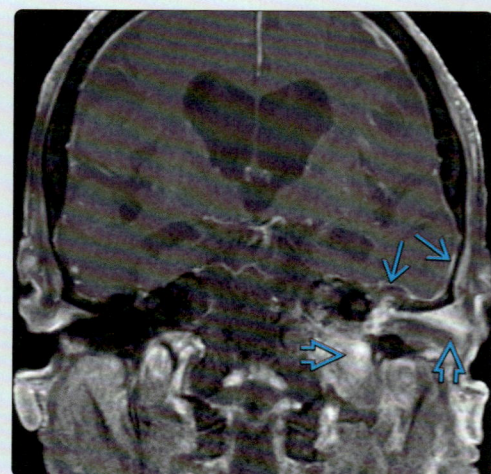

(Left) Axial T1 C+ FS MR in the same patient shows fluid signal with rim enhancement in the left EAC ➡. There are extensive phlegmonous changes in the left TMJ ➡ extending to the masticator space ➡ and jugular foramen ➡. (Right) Coronal T1 C+ FS MR in the same patient shows local pachymeningeal enhancement in the left temporal region ➡, suggesting intracranial extension of infection. Phlegmonous changes in the EAC and adjacent skull base soft tissues ➡ are noted.

TERMINOLOGY

Abbreviations
- Necrotizing external otitis (NEO)

Synonyms
- Malignant external otitis, malignant otitis externa

Definitions
- NEO: Severe **invasive infection** of external auditory canal (EAC), adjacent soft tissues, and skull base

IMAGING

General Features
- Best diagnostic clue
  - Abnormal soft tissue thickening, enhancement, opacification, and cortical erosion of EAC

CT Findings
- **High-resolution bone CT:** Best demonstrates cortical bone erosion and trabecular demineralization of EAC, adjacent temporal bone, TMJ, or clivus
- **CECT:** Can readily demonstrate soft tissue thickening and opacification of EAC with abnormal enhancement, infiltration of fat planes beyond EAC, and phlegmon or abscess

MR Findings
- Study of choice for determining soft tissue extent, marrow involvement, and intracranial complications
- T1WI best demonstrates fat signal within tissue planes, local fat pads, and marrow signal of bones; infection causes loss of signal in these regions
- STIR demonstrates increased signal in areas of cellulitis, osteomyelitis, and abscess formation
- T1WI C+ FS best shows enhancement of affected soft tissue and marrow involvement; ring enhancement of abscess
- DWI can show diffusion restriction of abscess in soft tissues

Nuclear Medicine Findings
- Bone scan (Tc-99m MDP) is highly sensitive for bone involvement but not specific
- Gallium scan (Ga-67) more specific for osteomyelitis and useful for following therapeutic response

Imaging Recommendations
- Best imaging tool
  - Best diagnostic tool is combination of high-resolution bone CT and MR performed ± gadolinium contrast
  - Given high specificity, gallium scan correlates well with treatment response
  - SUVmax on 18 F FDG PET is preferred parameter for treatment response evaluation of NEO at end-of-treatment scan

DIFFERENTIAL DIAGNOSIS

External Auditory Canal Squamous Cell Carcinoma
- Known, often treated auricle squamous cell carcinoma
- CT-MR: Imaging mimics NEO

External Auditory Canal Cholesteatoma
- Submucosal EAC mass
- CT: Unilateral EAC mass with bony erosion (intramural bony "flakes" in 50%)

Postinflammatory Medial Canal Fibrosis
- CT: Fibrous crescent in medial EAC
  - No underlying bony erosion

PATHOLOGY

General Features
- Etiology
  - *Pseudomonas aeruginosa*: 95% of NEO infections
  - *Aspergillus fumigatus*, in immunosuppressed/AIDS patients

CLINICAL ISSUES

Presentation
- Most common signs/symptoms
  - Severe otalgia and otorrhea
- Other signs/symptoms
  - Cranial nerve palsies herald skull base osteomyelitis
  - WBC normal or mildly increased, ESR invariably increased

Demographics
- Age
  - Diabetic patients older (> 60 years)
  - Nondiabetic, immunocompromised patients younger
- Epidemiology
  - **95%** of adults with NEO have **diabetes**

Natural History & Prognosis
- Begins as soft tissue EAC infection
  - Spreads into adjacent osseous and soft tissue structures
  - May progress to skull base osteomyelitis
  - May progress to deep spatial abscess
- 20% recurrence rate

Treatment
- Glucose control, aggressive granulation debridement
- Systemic (ciprofloxacin) and topical antibiotic therapy or systemic antifungals
- Surgical drainage if deep facial abscess

DIAGNOSTIC CHECKLIST

Consider
- EAC squamous cell carcinoma can mimic NEO on imaging
  - Auricle squamous cell carcinoma clinically obvious
- Extension to nasopharyngeal soft tissues can mimic nasopharyngeal carcinoma radiographically

SELECTED REFERENCES

1. Al Aaraj MS et al: Necrotizing (malignant) otitis externa. StatPearls, 2025
2. Jansen RW et al: Treatment response evaluation in necrotizing otitis externa using 18 F-FDG-PET imaging. Otol Neurotol. 46(3):295-302, 2025
3. Thabet W et al: Fungal necrotizing otitis externa: clinical and therapeutic features. Ear Nose Throat J. ePub, 2025
4. Sideris G et al: Fungal malignant otitis externa: a systematic review. Cureus. 16(10):e71345, 2024

Keratosis Obturans

TERMINOLOGY

- Keratosis obturans (KO): Mass-like soft tissue density and obstruction of bony external auditory canal (EAC) resulting from accumulation of desquamated keratin; can cause generalized internal auditory canal (IAC) enlargement, but focal bony erosion and periostitis are unusual

IMAGING

- Temporal bone CT findings
  - Benign-appearing soft tissue lesion partially or completely filling EAC
  - May diffusely enlarge EAC
  - **No** bony erosive change (unlike EAC cholesteatoma)
  - Bilateral (50%)
  - Middle ear spared unless KO neglected

TOP DIFFERENTIAL DIAGNOSES

- Benign EAC debris
- EAC cholesteatoma
- Medial canal fibrosis
- Necrotizing external otitis
- EAC squamous cell carcinoma

CLINICAL ISSUES

- Clinical presentation
  - Acute **severe otalgia**; conductive hearing loss
- KO treatment
  - Excision of keratin "plug"
  - Removal of reaccumulated debris often required

DIAGNOSTIC CHECKLIST

- "KO" and "EAC cholesteatoma" terms often confused
  - KO: EAC luminal lesion **without** bony erosions
    - If large, may involve middle ear through damaged tympanic membrane
  - EAC cholesteatoma: Submucosal lesion with EAC erosions ± bony flecks (50%)
    - If large, may involve mastoid air cells

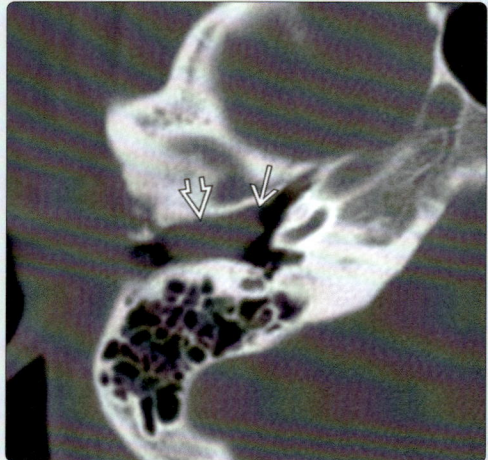
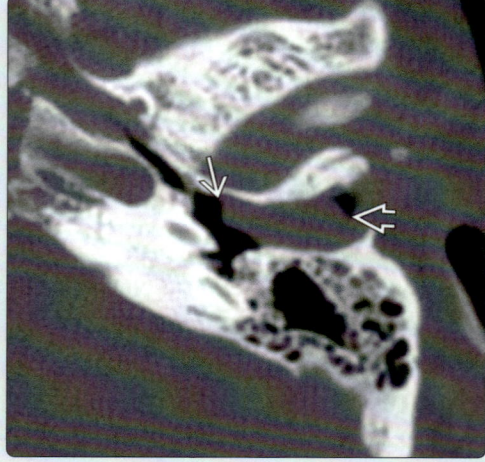

(Left) Axial bone CT in a patient with otoscopic evidence of an external auditory canal (EAC) obstruction shows a soft tissue "plug" ⇨ in the EAC extending laterally from the tympanic membrane ➡. Note absence of underlying bony changes. (Right) Axial bone CT in a patient with conductive hearing loss demonstrates a benign-appearing soft tissue lesion in the left EAC extending from the tympanic membrane ➡ to the lateral bony EAC margin ➡. The middle ear and underlying EAC bone are not involved.

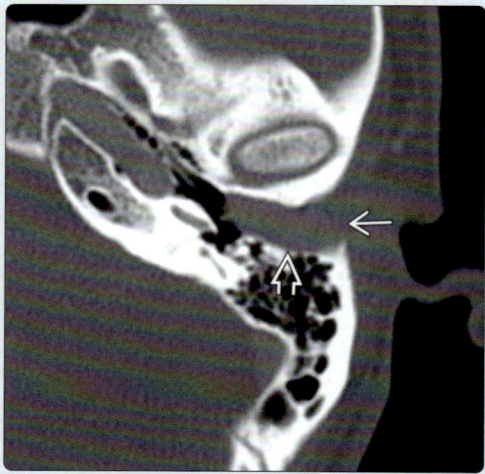
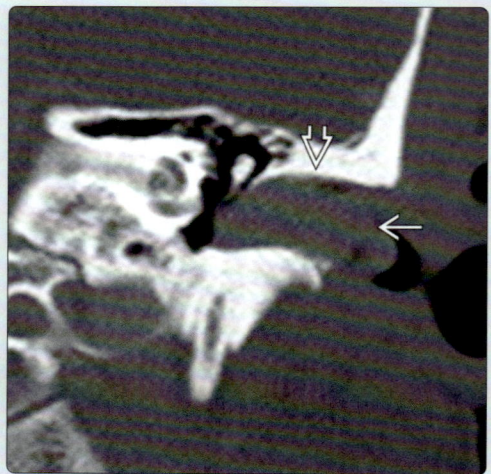

(Left) Axial bone CT shows soft tissue completely filling the left EAC ➡ from the tympanic membrane into both the bony and cartilaginous portions of the EAC. There is associated smooth bony remodeling ➡. (Right) Coronal bone CT in the same patient again shows soft tissue completely filling the left EAC ➡ with associated smooth bony remodeling ➡, consistent with keratosis obturans. No bony erosions are present, which would be expected with EAC cholesteatoma.

TERMINOLOGY

Abbreviations
- Keratosis obturans (KO)

Synonyms
- Laminated epithelial "plug;" keratin "plug"

Definitions
- KO: Abnormal accumulation and obstruction of bony external auditory canal (EAC) from desquamated keratin without erosive bony changes

IMAGING

General Features
- Best diagnostic clue
  - KO appears as homogeneous soft tissue filling EAC
    - Mild EAC enlargement common
    - Focal bony erosion **not** present
- Morphology
  - Soft tissue conforms to EAC

CT Findings
- Bone CT
  - Benign-appearing soft tissue filling EAC
    - May diffusely enlarge EAC
    - **No** bony erosive change (cf. EAC cholesteatoma)
  - Bilateral (50%)
  - Middle ear spared unless KO neglected

MR Findings
- T1WI
  - Homogeneous, low to intermediate signal soft tissue filling EAC
- T2WI
  - Isointense or low signal intensity
- T1WI C+
  - May rim enhance

Imaging Recommendations
- Best imaging tool
  - Temporal bone CT

DIFFERENTIAL DIAGNOSIS

Benign External Auditory Canal Debris
- CT: Partially filled EAC; no bony erosion
- Clinical: Waxy debris visible

External Auditory Canal Cholesteatoma
- CT: Unilateral EAC soft tissue with bony erosion
  - Bony intramural flakes (50%)
- Clinical: Mucosal irregularity; submucosal mass

Medial Canal Fibrosis
- CT: Soft tissue filling medial EAC with lateral concave margin; no bony erosion
- Clinical: Prior inflammation, surgery, or trauma

Necrotizing External Otitis
- CT: EAC swelling ± bone erosion ± abscess
- Clinical: Diabetic patient; otorrhea

External Auditory Canal Squamous Cell Carcinoma
- CT: Irregular mass ± bony erosion
  - Extends from external ear to involve EAC
- Clinical: Known squamous cell carcinoma on auricle

PATHOLOGY

General Features
- Etiology
  - 2 common theories
    - Abnormal epithelial migration with keratinaceous debris build-up
    - Sympathetic reflex stimulation of ceruminous glands in EAC causes hyperemia and epidermal plugging
  - Radiation dermatitis can also produce radiation KO
- Associated abnormalities
  - Chronic sinusitis and bronchiectasis

Gross Pathologic & Surgical Features
- Marked inflammation in subepithelial tissue
- Benign keratin "plug" fills EAC without focal bony erosion

Microscopic Features
- Desquamated keratin tissue
- Keratin tightly organized in lamellar pattern in KO
  - EAC cholesteatoma organized in random keratin pattern

CLINICAL ISSUES

Presentation
- Most common signs/symptoms
  - Acute **severe otalgia**
  - Conductive hearing loss

Demographics
- Age
  - Younger patients (< 40 years old)
- Epidemiology
  - Rare EAC lesion

Treatment
- Excision of keratin "plug" is mainstay of treatment
  - Some studies have shown promise with topical treatments
- Direct treatment of granulations when present
  - Excision, cauterization, topical steroids
- Removal of reaccumulated debris often required

DIAGNOSTIC CHECKLIST

Image Interpretation Pearls
- "KO" and "EAC cholesteatoma" terms often confused
  - KO: EAC luminal lesion **without** bony erosions
  - EAC cholesteatoma: Submucosal lesion with EAC erosions ± bony flecks (50%)
  - Both lesions consist of exfoliated keratin

SELECTED REFERENCES

1. Harounian JA et al: Contemporary management of keratosis obturans: a systematic review. J Laryngol Otol. 135(9):759-64, 2021
2. Zwemstra M et al: A novel topical treatment for keratosis obturans. Otol Neurotol. 42(10):e1503-6, 2021

Medial Canal Fibrosis

TERMINOLOGY

- Medial canal fibrosis (MCF)
  - Discrete clinicopathologic disease characterized by formation of fibrous tissue in medial aspect of bony external auditory canal (EAC)

IMAGING

- **Early-stage MCF**
  - Thickened tympanic membrane (TM) with mildly edematous medial EAC walls
- **Late-stage MCF**
  - Thick tissue "crescent" overlying lateral TM surface
  - TM **cannot** be resolved as separate from MCF fibrous mass
  - No underlying bony changes present

TOP DIFFERENTIAL DIAGNOSES

- Benign EAC debris
- Keratosis obturans

- EAC cholesteatoma, EAC exostoses (surfer's ear)
- EAC squamous cell carcinoma
- Necrotizing external otitis

PATHOLOGY

- MCF is final common pathophysiologic pathway for multiple mechanisms of injury to EAC
  - Chronic otitis externa: Most common etiology
  - Secondary to surgical procedure or trauma
  - Suppurative otitis media
  - Radiotherapy to EAC

CLINICAL ISSUES

- Common presentation
  - 50-year-old woman with bilateral otorrhea, conductive hearing loss (CHL), history of chronic otitis
- Treatment options
  - Early phase: Topical steroids
  - Late phase: Surgery corrects CHL; recurrence frequent

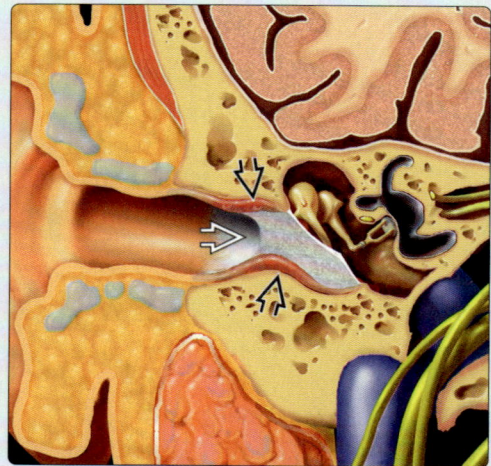
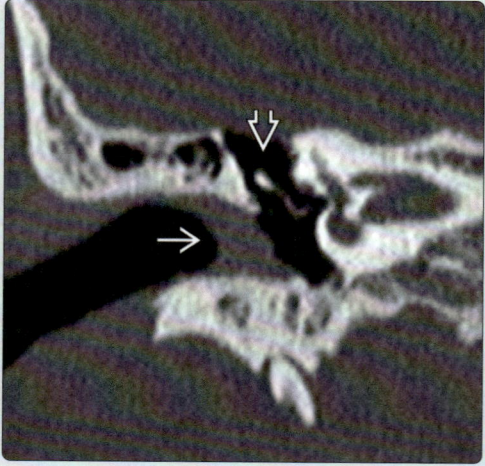

(Left) Coronal graphic of the right ear shows medial canal fibrosis (MCF) as a thick, fibrous crescent ⮞ overlying the tympanic membrane (TM) and filling the medial external auditory canal (EAC). Inflammatory changes ⮞ of medial EAC walls are also depicted. (Right) Coronal bone CT shows a crescentic soft tissue plug ⮞ in the right bony EAC indistinguishable from the TM, compatible with MCF. Note the lack of middle ear or mastoid disease extension ⮞.

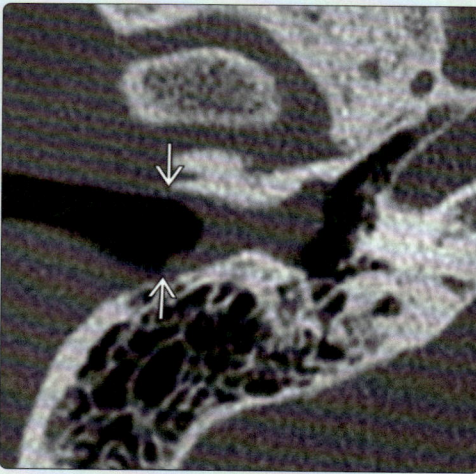
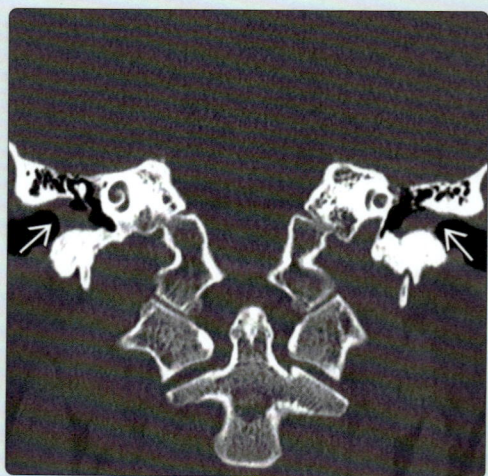

(Left) Axial bone CT in a patient with right conductive hearing loss shows MCF. Note that the lateral margin does not extend beyond the bony-cartilaginous junction of the EAC ⮞. (Right) Coronal bone CT shows soft tissue filling the medial EACs, the lateral crescent shape ⮞, indistinguishable from the TMs, and without osseous erosion or expansion. Bilateral involvement occurs in ~ 50% of MCF cases.

TERMINOLOGY

Abbreviations

- Medial canal fibrosis (MCF)

Synonyms

- Idiopathic inflammatory medial meatal fibrotizing otitis (IMFO)
- Postinflammatory MCF, acquired MCF, acquired atresia, chronic stenosing external otitis

Definitions

- Discrete clinicopathologic disease characterized by formation of fibrous tissue in medial aspect of bony external auditory canal (EAC)

IMAGING

General Features

- Best diagnostic clue
  - Crescent-shaped, fibrous tissue overlying lateral surface of tympanic membrane (TM)
- Location
  - Medial EAC, adjacent to TM
  - ~ 50% bilateral
- Size
  - Variable
    - May have mild thickening of TM with edematous EAC walls early
    - More advanced cases show near-complete opacification of EAC
- Morphology
  - Homogeneous soft tissue conforming to medial EAC

CT Findings

- CECT
  - May see slight enhancement of edematous EAC thickened walls
- Bone CT
  - Unilateral or bilateral medial EAC fibrous plug
  - **Early-stage MCF**
    - Thickened TM with mildly edematous soft tissue thickening of medial EAC walls
  - **Late-stage MCF**
    - Thick crescent of tissue filling EAC and overlying lateral surface of TM
    - Typically does not extend lateral to bony-cartilaginous junction of EAC
    - TM cannot be resolved as separate from MCF fibrous mass
    - No underlying bony changes present
    - Middle-ear mastoid uninvolved

MR Findings

- T1WI
  - Homogeneous, low-signal soft tissue in medial EAC
- T2WI
  - Intermediate- to low-signal soft tissue in medial EAC
  - More fibrous tissue present = lower signal
- T1WI C+
  - Enhancement of thickened, inflamed/edematous EAC walls and TM common

Imaging Recommendations

- Best imaging tool
  - Temporal bone CT
- Protocol advice
  - Temporal bone thin-section (≤ 1-mm), nonenhanced, bone algorithm CT
    - Acquire in axial plane; reconstruct coronal plane
    - Be sure to include entire EAC in magnified images

DIFFERENTIAL DIAGNOSIS

Benign External Auditory Canal Debris

- Clinical: Usually obvious on otoscopic exam
- Temporal bone CT: Luminal soft tissue in EAC without osseous erosion
  - Air often present in clefts and interstices of EAC debris

Keratosis Obturans

- Clinical: Younger patients with sinusitis and bronchiectasis
- Temporal bone CT: Bilateral keratin plugs filling EAC
  - Mild, diffuse EAC enlargement seen without focal bony erosions
  - Spares middle ear cavity

External Auditory Canal Cholesteatoma

- Clinical: Otorrhea and EAC mass in older patient population
- Temporal bone CT: Unilateral EAC soft tissue with underlying bony destruction
  - Bony "flakes" seen within mass in 50% of cases

External Auditory Canal Exostoses

- Clinical: Younger patients with repetitive exposure to cold water (surfer's ear)
- Temporal bone CT: Bilateral osseous encroachment of EAC canal
  - Diffuse, broad-based overgrowth of osseous EAC with normal skin surfaces
  - Usually begins at medial osseous EAC

External Auditory Canal Squamous Cell Carcinoma

- Clinical: Ulcerating lesion affects external ear
  - Spreads to involve EAC surfaces
- CT: Irregular, ill-defined mass with underlying aggressive bony erosion
  - Can mimic EAC cholesteatoma

Necrotizing External Otitis

- Clinical: Older adult diabetics with *Pseudomonas aeruginosa* EAC infection
- Temporal bone CT: EAC skin thickening ± underlying bone erosion ± deep space abscess (extension of disease inferiorly)
  - Diagnosis confirmed with biopsy and culture

PATHOLOGY

General Features

- Etiology
  - Chronic inflammation of medial EAC heals via granulation tissue formation
    - Granulation tissue slowly matures into mature fibrous plug

- MCF is final common pathophysiologic pathway for multiple mechanisms of injury to EAC
  - Chronic otitis externa
    - □ Most common underlying etiology
  - Secondary to surgical procedure or trauma
  - Suppurative otitis media
  - Radiotherapy to EAC
  - Ectopic apocrine glands in medial canal
- Autoimmune mechanism suspected

Staging, Grading, & Classification

- Early (wet) stage
  - Chronic otitis (externa or media with TM perforation) with otorrhea and conductive hearing loss (CHL)
- Late (dry) stage (mature MCF)
  - Medial EAC fibrous plug with CHL

Gross Pathologic & Surgical Features

- Inflamed, edematous margins to fibrous plug covering TM

Microscopic Features

- Early stage
  - Granulation tissue
  - May demonstrate lymphocyte infiltration
- Late stage
  - Layered fibrous connective tissue
  - May demonstrate focal areas of calcification

CLINICAL ISSUES

Presentation

- Most common signs/symptoms
  - CHL
    - Typically 20-40 decibels
  - Other signs/symptoms
    - Chronic otitis externa
    - Chronic dermatitis (eczema or psoriasis)
    - Tinnitus
    - Otorrhea
  - Early stage
    - Chronic otitis with otorrhea and CHL (wet)
  - Late stage
    - Mature fibrous plug present with CHL (dry)
- Clinical profile
  - 50-year-old woman with bilateral otorrhea, CHL, and history of chronic otitis

Demographics

- Age
  - Mean: 50 years old
  - Range: 5-80 years old
    - Usually rare in pediatric population
- Sex
  - M:F = 1:2
- Epidemiology
  - Rare lesion

Natural History & Prognosis

- Surgical complication
  - Clinically relevant recurrence following surgery (~ 7-40%)
  - Restenosis may occur years after treatment

Treatment

- Surgical intervention alone corrects CHL
- Early phase
  - Topical steroids
- Late phase
  - Surgical intervention required to correct CHL
  - Excision of all fibrous tissue and involved skin
    - Wide canaloplasty
    - Meatoplasty followed by reconstruction by split skin graft
- Squamous epithelium may be needed to repopulate EAC and lateral TM
  - Skin grafts may be needed from posterior pinna

DIAGNOSTIC CHECKLIST

Consider

- Differentiate MCF from keratosis obturans and EAC cholesteatoma
  - MCF: Look for medial EAC tissue plug with no EAC bone changes
  - Keratosis obturans: Look for complete opacification and subtle EAC bony widening
  - EAC cholesteatoma: Look for focal EAC soft tissue mass with underlying bony erosion ± intramural bone flecks

Image Interpretation Pearls

- Crescentic soft tissue plug against TM highly suggestive of MCF
- No role for MR imaging in MCF diagnosis or imaging evaluation
- Long-term follow-up is recommended to evaluate risk of recurrence

SELECTED REFERENCES

1. Kamaruzaman F et al: A rare case of idiopathic bilateral medial canal fibrosis. Cureus. 15(7):e41830, 2023
2. Mantsopoulos K et al: Postinflammatory medial meatal fibrosis: histopathologic features and outcomes of surgical management. Ear Nose Throat J. 102(6):391-6, 2023
3. Karkas A et al: Acquired medial external auditory canal stenosis, anterior tympanomeatal angle blunting, and lateralized tympanic membrane: nosology, diagnosis, and treatment. Eur Ann Otorhinolaryngol Head Neck Dis. 136(2):93-7, 2019
4. Keller RG et al: Postinflammatory medial canal fibrosis: an institutional review and meta-analysis of short- and long-term outcomes. Laryngoscope. 127(2):488-95, 2017
5. Moser G et al: Ectopic apocrine glands as a predisposing factor for postinflammatory medial meatal fibrosis: a clinicopathologic study. Otol Neurotol. 36(1):191-7, 2015
6. Ghani A et al: Postinflammatory medial meatal fibrosis: early and late surgical outcomes. J Laryngol Otol. 127(12):1160-8, 2013
7. Ursick JA et al: Medial canal fibrosis. Ear Nose Throat J. 92(9):414, 2013
8. Hopsu E et al: Idiopathic inflammatory medial meatal fibrotizing otitis presenting in children. Otol Neurotol. 29(3):350-2, 2008
9. Lin VY et al: Medial canal fibrosis: surgical technique, results, and a proposed grading system. Otol Neurotol. 26(5):825-9, 2005
10. Luong A et al: Acquired external auditory canal stenosis: assessment and management. Curr Opin Otolaryngol Head Neck Surg. 13(5):273-6, 2005
11. Hopsu E et al: Idiopathic inflammatory medial meatal fibrotizing otitis. Arch Otolaryngol Head Neck Surg. 128(11):1313-6, 2002
12. Lavy J et al: Chronic stenosing external otitis/postinflammatory acquired atresia: a review. Clin Otolaryngol. 25(6):435-9, 2000
13. el-Sayed Y: Acquired medial canal fibrosis. J Laryngol Otol. 112(2):145-9, 1998
14. Slattery WH 3rd et al: Postinflammatory medial canal fibrosis. Am J Otol. 18(3):294-7, 1997

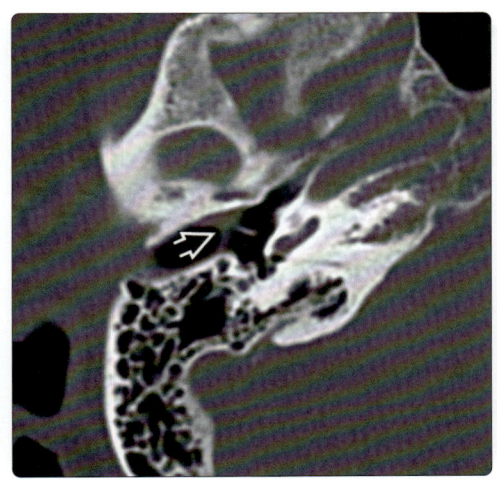

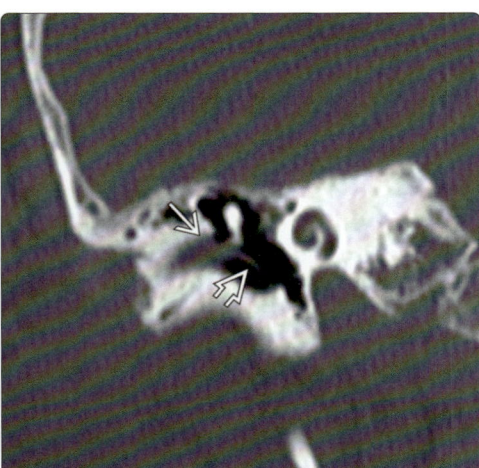

(Left) Axial bone CT of the right ear shows the early findings of MCF as thin, crescentic TM thickening ⮕. Clinical diagnosis at this stage is necessary as CT will not differentiate this appearance from other causes of TM thickening. (Right) Coronal bone CT in the same patient reveals that the upper TM ⮕ is thicker than the lower portion ⮕. As the lesion progresses, the fibrous crescent will affect the whole lateral TM surface.

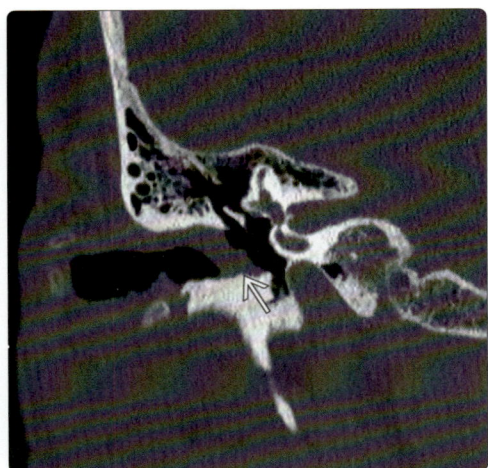

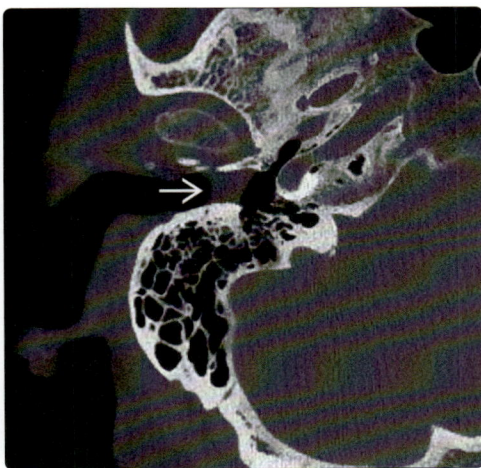

(Left) Coronal bone CT in a 76-year-old with conductive hearing loss on the right and findings of MCF shows typical soft tissue density of the medial canal in MCF ⮕. The middle ear cavity is spared. (Right) Axial bone CT in the same patient again shows the fibrotic plug ⮕ in the medial canal against the TM. No bony changes are present.

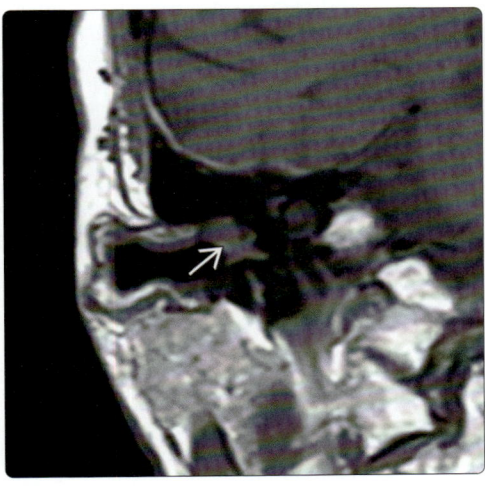

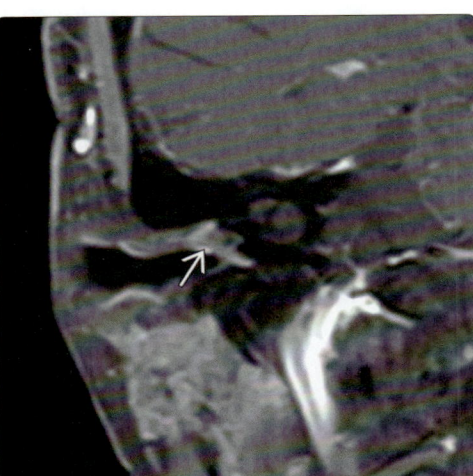

(Left) Coronal T1 MR in same patient shows T1 soft tissue signal lesion in the medial canal ⮕. No definite abnormality within the middle ear is identified. (Right) Coronal T1 C+ FS MR depicts enhancing fibrotic tissue in the medial canal abutting the TM ⮕, consistent with MCF.

EAC-Acquired Cholesteatoma

TERMINOLOGY

- External auditory canal cholesteatoma (EACC)
- EACC: EAC erosive lesion composed of exfoliated keratin within stratified squamous epithelium

IMAGING

- **Unilateral** (usually) scalloping soft tissue bony EAC mass
- **Bone fragments** within soft tissue mass (50%)
- May extend locally into subjacent bony structures
- Tympanic membrane intact; middle ear spared

TOP DIFFERENTIAL DIAGNOSES

- Medial canal fibrosis
- Necrotizing external otitis
- Squamous cell carcinoma of EAC
- Keratosis obturans

PATHOLOGY

- Spontaneous: Abnormal migration of EAC ectoderm

- Secondary: Postoperative or posttraumatic
- Congenital: Ectodermal rest within EAC wall (rare)
  - May also be associated with congenital EAC stenosis

CLINICAL ISSUES

- Presentation
  - Primary symptoms: Otorrhea & otalgia
- Demographics
  - Older population: 40-75 years old
- Natural history: Relentless increase in size & erosion of EAC bony wall
  - May show less aggressive behavior in pediatric patients
- Treatment options
  - Surgical excision for larger lesions with bony invasion

DIAGNOSTIC CHECKLIST

- Focal, unilateral (usually) EAC mass + EAC bony scalloping ± bony flecks = EACC

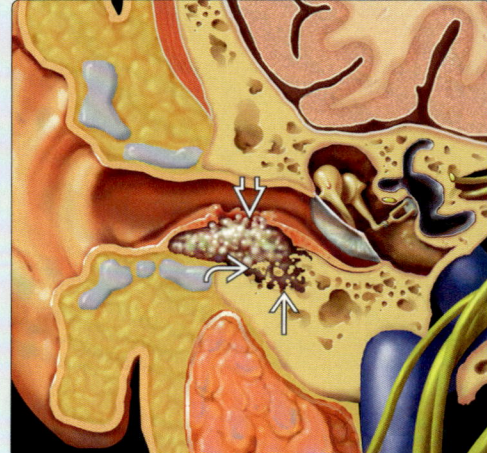
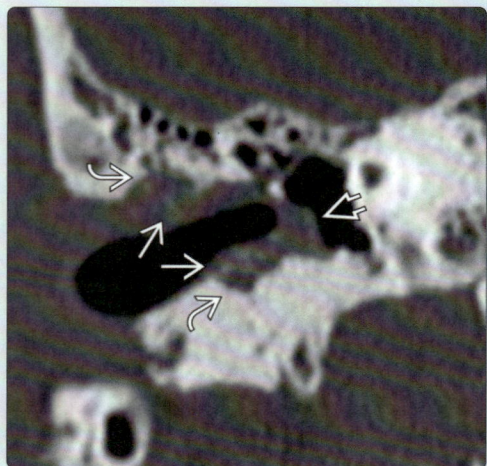

(Left) Coronal graphic shows an external auditory canal cholesteatoma (EACC) as an erosive, scalloping subepithelial mass ⇨ in the inferior bony EAC. Note bone erosion ➡ with bony flecks ⇗ within the cholesteatoma matrix. (Right) Coronal bone CT shows soft tissue thickening of the medial EAC walls extending to the tympanic membrane ➡ with multifocal regions of osseous erosions ⬈ and internal bony flecks ➡ compatible with EAC cholesteatoma.

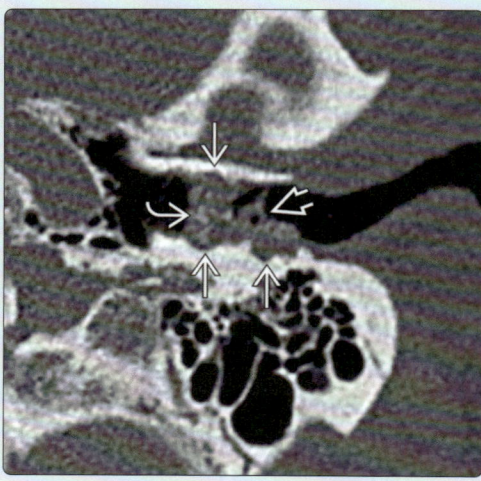
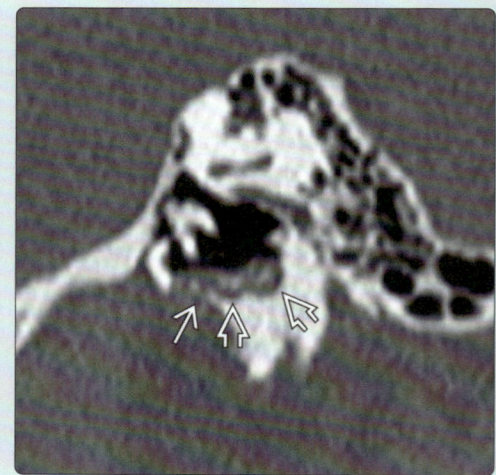

(Left) Axial NECT through the level of the floor of the EAC shows a lobular soft tissue mass ➡ with subtle scalloping of the bony EAC margins ➡. Note the speckled density of the mass with prominent bone flecks ➚ within the EACC. (Right) Sagittal NECT in the same patient highlights the importance of multiplanar reformats in EACC imaging. Note complete erosion through the anterior floor of EAC ➡ as well as additional areas of scalloping ➡. Bone flecks are evident in the cholesteatoma.

TERMINOLOGY

Abbreviations

- External auditory canal cholesteatoma (EACC)

Definitions

- EAC erosive lesion composed of exfoliated keratin within stratified squamous epithelium

IMAGING

General Features

- Best diagnostic clue
  - Erosive EAC soft tissue mass ± internal bony flecks
    - Typically **unilateral**; bilateral disease is rare

CT Findings

- Bone CT
  - **Unilateral** (usually) scalloping soft tissue bony EAC mass
  - **Bone fragments** within soft tissue mass (50%)
  - May extend locally into subjacent bony structures
  - Tympanic membrane intact; middle ear spared

MR Findings

- T1WI
  - Soft tissue intensity mass in EAC
- T2WI
  - Intermediate signal intensity
- DWI
  - Reduced diffusivity
- T1WI C+
  - Cholesteatoma itself is nonenhancing
  - ± thin, enhancing rim of granulation tissue/inflammation

Imaging Recommendations

- Best imaging tool
  - Temporal bone CT with multiplanar reformats
  - Consider MR with non-EPI DWI if CT equivocal

DIFFERENTIAL DIAGNOSIS

Medial Canal Fibrosis

- CT: Obstructive fibrous tissue within medial EAC
  - ~ 50% **bilateral**; lateral convex margin; no bony erosion

Necrotizing External Otitis

- Diabetic patients with *Pseudomonas* infection
- **CT**: **Unilateral** inflammatory soft tissue changes
  - Bony osteomyelitis changes

Squamous Cell Carcinoma of External Auditory Canal

- Older patients with enhancing EAC mass
- **CT**: **Unilateral** invasive soft tissue mass

Keratosis Obturans

- Younger patients with sinusitis & bronchiectasis
- **CT**: Keratin plug filling EAC
  - ~ 50% **bilateral**; can diffusely enlarge EAC without erosion

PATHOLOGY

General Features

- Etiology

- Spontaneous: Abnormal migration of EAC ectoderm
- Secondary: Postoperative or posttraumatic
- Congenital: Ectodermal rest within EAC wall (rare)
  - ± congenital external ear malformation

Staging, Grading, & Classification

- Staging criteria (histopathology + clinical stage)
  - Stage I: Superficial; hyperplasia of canal epithelium
  - Stage II: Periosteitis; localized to ear pocket
  - Stage III: Extension into bony canal
  - Stage IV: Extension into adjacent bony structures

Gross Pathologic & Surgical Features

- Different type of cholesteatoma; not pearly white
- Waxy material discolored by inflammatory change
- Intramural bony fragments possible

Microscopic Features

- Similar to epidermoid inclusion cyst
- Stratified squamous epithelium with progressive exfoliation of keratinous material

CLINICAL ISSUES

Presentation

- Most common signs/symptoms
  - Otorrhea & otalgia
- Other signs/symptoms
  - Conductive hearing loss

Demographics

- Age
  - Older population: 40-75 years
- Epidemiology
  - 0.1% incidence in new ENT patients

Natural History & Prognosis

- Relentless increase in size & erosion of EAC bony wall
  - May show less aggressive behavior in pediatric patients
- Typical vector of spread = EAC bony wall into mastoid cavity
- Recurrences more common with increasing lesion size & invasion of surrounding osseous structures

Treatment

- Most controlled with periodic office debridement
- Surgical excision for larger lesions with bony invasion

DIAGNOSTIC CHECKLIST

Consider

- EAC cholesteatoma is usually **unilateral** lesion
  - Medial canal fibrosis & keratosis obturans often bilateral

Image Interpretation Pearls

- Focal, unilateral (usually) EAC mass + EAC bony scalloping ± bony flecks = EACC

SELECTED REFERENCES

1. Chan CY et al: Cholesteatoma in congenital aural atresia and external auditory canal stenosis: a systematic review. Otolaryngol Head Neck Surg. 169(3):449-53, 2023
2. He G et al: Primary external auditory canal cholesteatoma of 301 ears: a single-center study. Eur Arch Otorhinolaryngol. 279(4):1787-94, 2021

EAC Osteoma

TERMINOLOGY

- Osteoma: Rare, benign, focal, pedunculated, bony overgrowth of osseous external auditory canal (EAC) with normal overlying mucosa

IMAGING

- Most common site: Bony-cartilaginous EAC junction
- Bone CT: Benign-appearing, focal, **pedunculated**, bony overgrowth of osseous EAC
  - Wax, squamous debris, or **secondary cholesteatoma** possible with large, lateral lesions

TOP DIFFERENTIAL DIAGNOSES

- EAC exostoses (surfer's ear)
- EAC cholesteatoma
- Medial canal fibrosis
- Benign EAC debris
- Hyperdense foreign body

PATHOLOGY

- Irregularly oriented, **lamellated bone** with surrounding discrete, fibrovascular channels
- Osteoma found in other temporal bone sites
  - Ossicles, mastoid, internal auditory canal

CLINICAL ISSUES

- Asymptomatic, usually incidental finding
- Larger lesions may be associated with conductive hearing loss &/or cholesteatoma
- Treatment
  - Permanent cure with adequate surgical excision

DIAGNOSTIC CHECKLIST

- Differentiate from EAC exostoses
  - EAC osteoma: Narrow-based, single lesion, lateral EAC; **unilateral**
  - EAC exostosis: Broad-based, circumferential, multilobular, medial EAC; **bilateral**

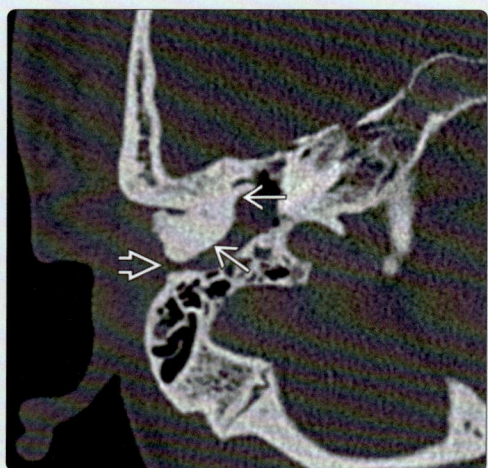
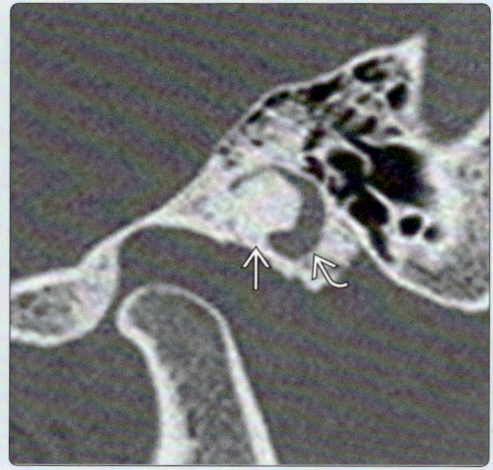

(Left) Axial bone CT shows a pedunculated osseous mass arising from the anterior wall of the right external auditory canal (EAC) ➡ with resultant severe narrowing and cerumen/debris filling the medial EAC ➡. (Right) Sagittal bone CT in the same patient shows the same bony mass arising from a relatively narrow stalk ➡. The severely narrowed EAC is filled with cerumen/debris ➡. This EAC osteoma was unilateral in this patient with a completely normal left EAC (not shown).

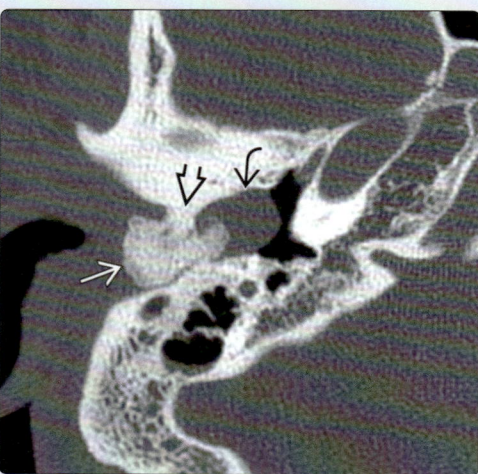
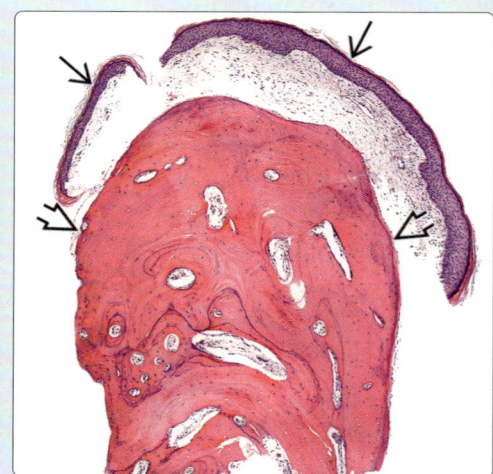

(Left) Axial bone CT in a patient whose clinical exam showed occlusion of the EAC reveals a pedunculated osteoma ➡ arising from the anterior EAC bony wall ➡. Note the secondary cholesteatoma ➡ within the medial EAC. (Right) H&E micrograph reveals surface squamous epithelium ➡ is uninvolved by the osteoma ➡. There is well-formed, mature compact bone within the osteoma. This osteoma expanded from the adjacent bony EAC cortex, creating an obstructing submucosal mass. (From DP: H&N.)

TERMINOLOGY

Abbreviations

- External auditory canal (EAC) osteoma

Definitions

- Rare, benign, focal, pedunculated, bony overgrowth of osseous EAC with normal overlying soft tissues

IMAGING

General Features

- Best diagnostic clue
  - Unilateral, solitary, **pedunculated**, bony overgrowth of EAC without aggressive features
- Location
  - Unilateral EAC, single lesion typical
  - Most common site: Bony cartilaginous junction EAC
- Size
  - Variable, usually small (< 1 cm)
- Morphology
  - Variable, usually oval

CT Findings

- Bone CT
  - Benign-appearing, focal, **pedunculated**, bony overgrowth of osseous EAC
  - Wax, squamous debris, or secondary cholesteatoma possible with large, lateral lesions

Imaging Recommendations

- Best imaging tool
  - Multiplanar temporal bone CT
  - MR not useful in this setting, unless there are complications related to obstruction, including cholesteatoma

DIFFERENTIAL DIAGNOSIS

External Auditory Canal Exostoses (Surfer's Ear)

- Broad-based, **bilateral** bony EAC overgrowths
- Circumferential, multilobular
- Associated with chronic cold water exposure

External Auditory Canal Cholesteatoma

- Unilateral EAC destructive mass
- Intramural bony flakes (50%)

Medial Canal Fibrosis

- Fibrous mass in medial EAC without bony erosion
- Follows otitis externa or surgical procedure

Benign External Auditory Canal Debris

- Soft tissue density in EAC without bony changes

Foreign Body

- May be hyperdense on CT; no direct attachment to bony wall of EAC

PATHOLOGY

General Features

- Etiology
  - Likely spontaneous bony growth
  - Reaction to repeated external insult
- Embryology/anatomy
  - May be attached to tympanosquamous or tympanomastoid suture line

Gross Pathologic & Surgical Features

- Osteoma connected to underlying EAC bone

Microscopic Features

- Pathologically similar to exostoses
- Irregularly oriented, **lamellated bone** with surrounding discrete, fibrovascular channels

CLINICAL ISSUES

Presentation

- Most common signs/symptoms
  - Asymptomatic, usually incidental finding
  - Other signs/symptoms
    - If large, conductive hearing loss or cholesteatoma
    - If associated with cholesteatoma, serous otitis media

Demographics

- Age
  - Broad range
- Epidemiology
  - Unilateral and solitary
  - EAC osteoma is less common than exostoses
  - 20% prevalence in surfers (possible early exostoses)

Natural History & Prognosis

- Permanent cure with adequate surgical excision
- Possible surgical complications
  - EAC stenosis
  - TMJ prolapse

Treatment

- Medical therapy is adequate without surgical excision for symptomatic lesions
- Surgical removal may be performed through EAC under local anesthesia

DIAGNOSTIC CHECKLIST

Image Interpretation Pearls

- Differentiate from EAC exostoses
  - EAC osteoma: Narrow-based, single lesion, lateral EAC; **unilateral**
  - EAC exostosis: Broad-based, circumferential, multilobular, medial EAC; **bilateral**

SELECTED REFERENCES

1. Hu CY et al: Factors related to cholesteatoma formation in external auditory canal osteomas and treatment algorithm. Ear Nose Throat J. ePub, 2024
2. Chen CK et al: Endoscopic transcanal removal of external auditory canal osteomas. Biomed J. 44(4):489-94, 2020
3. Iaccarino I et al: A case of external auditory canal osteoma complicated with cholesteatoma, mastoiditis, labyrinthitis and internal auditory canal pachymeningitis. Acta Otorhinolaryngol Ital. 39(5):358-62, 2019
4. Ata N et al: External auditory canal osteoma with cholesteatoma and sinus thrombosis. J Craniofac Surg. 26(7):2234-5, 2015
5. Spielmann PM et al: Surgical management of external auditory canal lesions. J Laryngol Otol. 127(3):246-51, 2013
6. Carbone PN et al: External auditory osteoma. Head Neck Pathol. 6(2):244-6, 2012

EAC Exostoses

TERMINOLOGY

- Definition: Benign overgrowth of bony external auditory canal (EAC) in response to chronic cold water exposure

IMAGING

- Temporal bone CT
  - **Bilateral** lesions in all cases
  - Broad-based or more focal circumferential bony overgrowth of osseous EAC
  - Variable EAC stenosis results

TOP DIFFERENTIAL DIAGNOSES

- EAC osteoma
- EAC cholesteatoma
- Medial canal fibrosis

CLINICAL ISSUES

- Most common symptom
  - Conductive hearing loss

- Other signs/symptoms
  - Otitis externa, tinnitus, otalgia
- Patient profile
  - 20-50 years old
  - Male predominance
  - 70% prevalence in surfers
    - Increased incidence with increased time of exposure
- Treatment options
  - Often require no treatment
  - May require surgical excision

DIAGNOSTIC CHECKLIST

- Image interpretation pearls
  - Most common differential diagnosis: EAC osteoma
  - EAC osteoma: Unilateral, lateral bony EAC focal osseous protuberance
  - EAC exostoses: Bilateral midbony EAC circumferential, multilobular narrowing

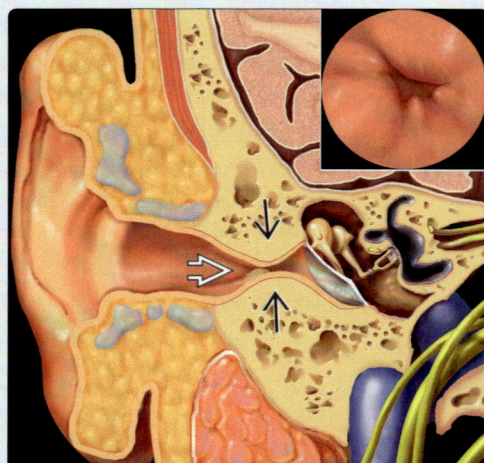
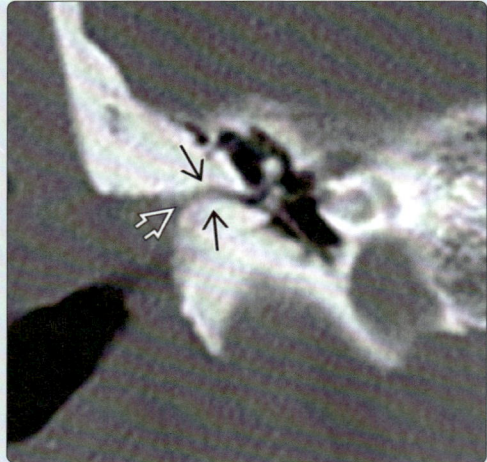

(Left) Coronal graphic shows benign-appearing bony overgrowth of the right external auditory canal (EAC) ➡ in a case of EAC exostoses. Insert shows an otoscopic view of circumferential submucosal EAC narrowing ⇨. (Right) Coronal bone CT of the right temporal bone shows severe EAC stenosis ⇨ secondary to circumferential exostoses ➡ that developed bilaterally as a result of chronic cold water exposure from surfing.

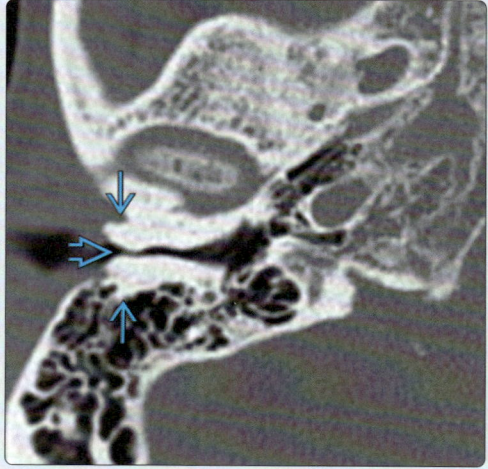
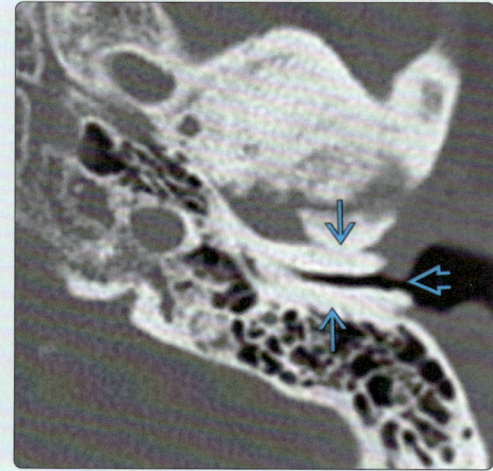

(Left) Magnified axial CT shows broad-based osseous overgrowth ➡ of the right EAC in a patient with conductive hearing loss. There is severe narrowing ⇨ of the lumen of the EAC. (Right) Magnified axial CT of the left external auditory canal in the same patient shows similar findings of broad-based osseous overgrowth ➡ with narrowing of the EAC ➡.

TERMINOLOGY

Synonyms

- Surfer's ear; cold water ear

Definitions

- Benign overgrowth of bony external auditory canal (EAC) in response to chronic cold water exposure

IMAGING

General Features

- Best diagnostic clue
  - Benign overgrowth of osseous EAC with normal overlying soft tissues
- Location
  - Bony EAC; **bilateral**
  - Usually located medial to EAC isthmus
    - EAC osteoma usually located lateral to isthmus
- Size
  - Variable; narrowing of EAC
- Morphology
  - Broad-based or focal; circumferential

CT Findings

- CECT
  - Normal soft tissues overlying stenotic EAC
- Bone CT
  - Broad-based or more focal circumferential bony overgrowth of osseous EAC
  - Bilateral; variable EAC stenosis results

Imaging Recommendations

- Best imaging tool
  - Temporal bone CT
  - MR of no help with this diagnosis

DIFFERENTIAL DIAGNOSIS

External Auditory Canal Osteoma

- Unilateral focal, pedunculated, bony overgrowth

External Auditory Canal Cholesteatoma

- Unilateral, bone flakes (50%)
- Underlying bony scalloping

Medial Canal Fibrosis

- Soft tissue filling medial EAC with lateral concave margin
- No bony expansion or overgrowth

PATHOLOGY

General Features

- Etiology
  - Bony EAC reaction to cold water exposure
  - Theory: Irritation of EAC results in increased vascular flow
  - Occurs exclusively in humans

Gross Pathologic & Surgical Features

- Benign, bony overgrowth of osseous EAC

Microscopic Features

- Pathologically similar to osteoma
- Parallel, concentric layers of subperiosteal bone
  - Broad-based lamellar bone

CLINICAL ISSUES

Presentation

- Most common signs/symptoms
  - Conductive hearing loss (CHL)
  - Other signs/symptoms
    - Otitis externa, tinnitus, otalgia
  - Although bilateral, 80% present with unilateral symptoms
- Clinical profile
  - CHL in adult male with history of prolonged cold water exposure (swimmers, surfers, divers)

Demographics

- Age
  - 20-50 years
- Sex
  - Male predominance
- Ethnicity
  - Lesion not usually found in Black patients
- Epidemiology
  - 70% prevalence in surfers
  - Increasing incidence with increasing time of exposure

Natural History & Prognosis

- Complete occlusion of EAC is rare
- Normal hearing and normal epithelial migration patterns seen postoperatively
- 5% surgical complication rate
  - Canal stenosis, TMJ prolapse, sensorineural hearing loss, and persistent tympanic membrane (TM) perforation

Treatment

- Often requires no treatment
- May require surgical excision
  - Complications of superior EAC drilling
    - TM perforation
    - TMJ dehiscence
  - Drilling excision along posterior, inferior, and anterior walls performed with less risk of complications
    - Allows preservation of canal skin, leading to permanent cure

DIAGNOSTIC CHECKLIST

Image Interpretation Pearls

- Most common differential diagnosis: EAC osteoma
  - Osteoma: Unilateral, focal osseous protuberance
  - Exostoses: Bilateral circumferential, multilobular bony EAC narrowing

SELECTED REFERENCES

1. Swisher AR et al: Complication rates in osteotome and drill techniques in external auditory canal exostoses: a systematic review and meta-analysis. Ann Otol Rhinol Laryngol. 132(10):1249-60, 2023
2. Landefeld K et al: Surfer's ear. StatPearls, 2020
3. Simas V et al: Australian surfers' awareness of 'surfer's ear'. BMJ Open Sport Exerc Med. 6(1):e000641, 2020
4. Simas V et al: Lifetime prevalence of exostoses in New Zealand surfers. J Prim Health Care. 11(1):47-53, 2019

EAC Skin Squamous Cell Carcinoma

TERMINOLOGY

- Squamous cell carcinoma (SCCa) most common malignancy of external auditory canal (EAC)

IMAGING

- Bone destruction or soft tissue invasion indicates aggressive malignancy
- Temporal bone CT best predicts osseous invasion
- Enhanced MR superior for intracranial, parotid, and perineural spread
- Either CECT or enhanced MR of neck for adenopathy

TOP DIFFERENTIAL DIAGNOSES

- Benign EAC debris, EAC cholesteatoma
- Necrotizing external otitis
- Osteoradionecrosis

PATHOLOGY

- Disease of older adults (median age: 65 years)

- ↑ incidence in patients with otologic diseases

CLINICAL ISSUES

- Biopsy critical as early SCCa appears identical to other Dx on imaging
- Secondary EAC involvement from regional primary skin SCCa more common than primary EAC SCCa
- EAC SCCa 1st destroys bony canal, then invades surrounding anatomic structures
- **5-year survival** for early stage (T1/T2) = 70%; advanced stage (T3) = 41%
- With small tumors, en bloc resection often curative

DIAGNOSTIC CHECKLIST

- Soft tissue extent, bone or parotid invasion, intracranial extension, CNVII perineural spread
- CT/MR should include parotid for 1st-order nodes
- Look for intraparotid nodes, pre- and postauricular nodes, then levels II and VA

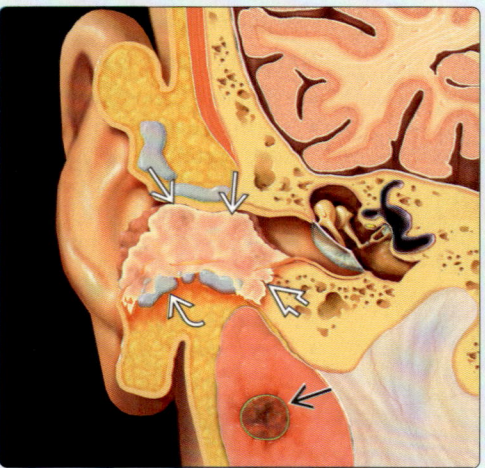
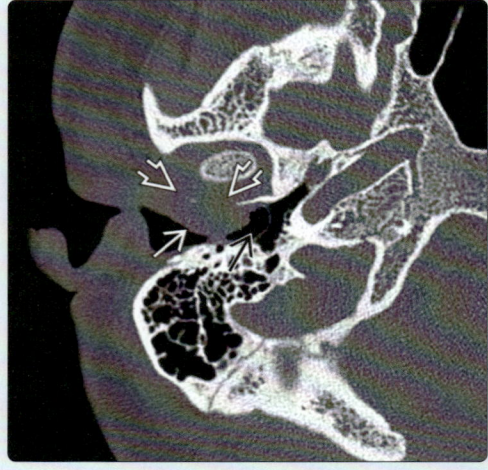

(Left) Graphic illustrates large external auditory canal (EAC) squamous cell carcinoma (SCCa) presenting as a mass ⇨ filling the canal. Note aggressive features with infiltration of auricle and its cartilages ⇨, invasion of temporal bone ⇨, and metastatic intraparotid node ⇨. (Right) Axial CT of the temporal bone reveals SCCa of right EAC with a prominent soft tissue mass ⇨ filling EAC. Osseous invasion through the posterior wall of TMJ condylar fossa ⇨ is present. Distal EAC at the tympanic membrane ⇨ is clear of tumor.

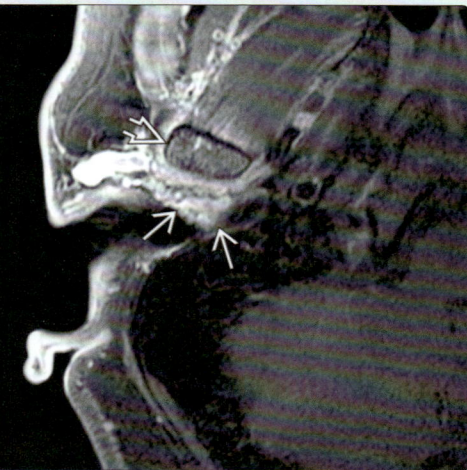
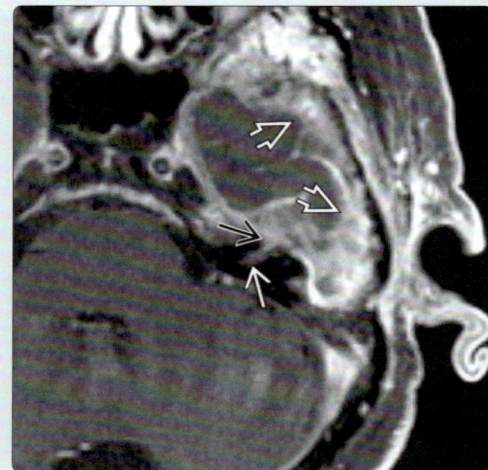

(Left) Axial T1WI C+ FS MR shows a solidly enhancing EAC SCCa ⇨ filling the canal and invading anteriorly into the TMJ. Note the soft tissue tumor ⇨ around the right condylar head. (Right) Axial T1WI C+ FS MR shows more advanced EAC SCCa with gross transdural ⇨ extension into the left middle cranial fossa. There is marked thickening and enhancement along CNVII of the geniculate ganglion ⇨ and in the internal auditory canal ⇨, representing perineural tumor spread.

EAC Skin Squamous Cell Carcinoma

TERMINOLOGY

Definitions

- Squamous cell carcinoma (SCCa) involving external auditory canal (EAC)

IMAGING

General Features

- Best diagnostic clue
  - EAC mass ± aggressive, underlying bony changes
- Relevant anatomy
  - EAC, auricle, and adjacent scalp
  - Nodal drainage to parotid, pre- and postauricular nodes

CT Findings

- CECT
  - Heterogeneously enhancing EAC lesion
  - Intraparotid and periauricular nodes at risk
- Bone CT
  - Early: EAC soft tissue mass without bony destruction
  - EAC nonossified cartilage invasion difficult to diagnose
  - EAC bone destruction early sign of progressing disease

MR Findings

- T2WI
  - Heterogeneous high signal
- T1WI C+
  - Homogeneous or heterogeneous enhancement
  - Rarely, advanced disease spreads to middle ear, CNVII, or intracranial
    - Posterior cranial fossa invasion can involve sigmoid sinus

Nuclear Medicine Findings

- PET
  - Useful for detecting residual/recurrent disease post treatment

DIFFERENTIAL DIAGNOSIS

Benign External Auditory Canal Debris

- CT: Soft tissue debris in EAC without bony erosion

External Auditory Canal Cholesteatoma

- Unilateral EAC mass ± bony "flakes" with underlying bony destruction

Necrotizing External Otitis

- Older **diabetic** patients with *Pseudomonas* infection
- CT: Granulation tissue with possible bony erosion at inferior bony-cartilaginous junction

Osteoradionecrosis

- Disruption of mastoid air cells septa superimposed on radiation-induced otomastoiditis

PATHOLOGY

General Features

- Etiology
  - Auricle skin SCCa spreads into EAC > > 1° EAC carcinoma

Staging, Grading, & Classification

- T1: Tumor limited to EAC without bony erosion or soft tissue invasion
- T2: Tumor with limited EAC bone or soft tissue involvement
- T3: Tumor with osseous EAC erosion and limited soft tissue/middle ear/mastoid involvement
- T4: Tumor erodes inner ear structures/TMJ/extensive soft tissue, or CNVII paresis

CLINICAL ISSUES

Presentation

- Most common signs/symptoms
  - Early, small lesions mimic benign processes both clinically and imaging
  - Ulcerating auricle: EAC skin lesion
    - Presentation may **mimic otitis externa** or **EAC cholesteatoma**
  - Otorrhea, otalgia, and conductive hearing loss

Demographics

- Age
  - Disease of older adults (median: 65 years)
- Epidemiology
  - Malignant tumors of EAC are very rare
    - 85% of all malignant tumors of EAC are SCCa

Natural History & Prognosis

- EAC SCCa destroys osseous EAC, then invades surrounding anatomic structures
  - Posterior extension into mastoid bone
  - Anterior extension into TMJ
- Lymph node metastases rare, poor prognostic indicator

Treatment

- En bloc resection nearly always performed
- T1-T2 tumors: Surgery or radiation therapy (RT)
- T3-T4 tumors: Surgery & RT ± chemo-/immunotherapy

DIAGNOSTIC CHECKLIST

Consider

- Secondary EAC involvement from adjacent skin SCCa much more common than 1° EAC SCCa
- Evaluate surrounding structures for disease spread
  - Parotid gland (direct invasion or nodes)
  - TMJ
  - Mastoid temporal bone

Image Interpretation Pearls

- Look for osseous destructive changes
- CT/MR should include parotid for 1st-order nodes

Reporting Tips

- Soft tissue extent, bone or parotid invasion, regional nodal disease, intracranial extension, CNVII perineural spread

SELECTED REFERENCES

1. Gone J et al: Squamous cell carcinoma of the external auditory canal presenting as a persistent ear infection: a case report and imaging features. Cureus. 16(8):e66188, 2024
2. Cazzador D et al: Survival outcomes in squamous cell carcinoma of the external auditory canal: a systematic review and meta-analysis. J Clin Med. 12(7):2490, 2023

KEY FACTS

TERMINOLOGY

- Congenital middle ear cholesteatoma (CMEC)
  - Cholesteatoma in ME behind intact TM in patient with no history of surgery, recurrent otitis media, or otorrhea

IMAGING

- Temporal bone CT findings
  - Small: Well-circumscribed soft tissue ME mass medial to ossicles
  - Large: Erodes ossicles, ME wall, lateral semicircular canal, or tegmen tympani
  - Long process of incus and stapes superstructure most commonly eroded ossicles
  - If aditus ad antrum occluded, mastoid air cells opacify with retained secretions
- MR findings
  - T1WI C+: Rim-enhancing ME mass
  - Non-echo-planar DWI sequences recommended
    - Minimize susceptibility artifacts

- ↑ sensitivity for detection of smaller lesions (2 mm)
- High signal on DWI + corresponding low signal on ADC
  - Highly specific due to high keratin content

TOP DIFFERENTIAL DIAGNOSES

- Pars flaccida-acquired cholesteatoma
- Pars tensa-acquired cholesteatoma
- Tympanic paraganglioma
- Facial nerve schwannoma of tympanic segment
- ME cholesterol granuloma

CLINICAL ISSUES

- Younger patient (< 20 years old)
- **Often incidental** avascular ME mass behind **intact TM**
- Unilateral conductive hearing loss (30%)
- Complete surgical excision = treatment of choice

DIAGNOSTIC CHECKLIST

- Consider CMEC when avascular mass seen behind intact TM in younger patient (< 20 years old)

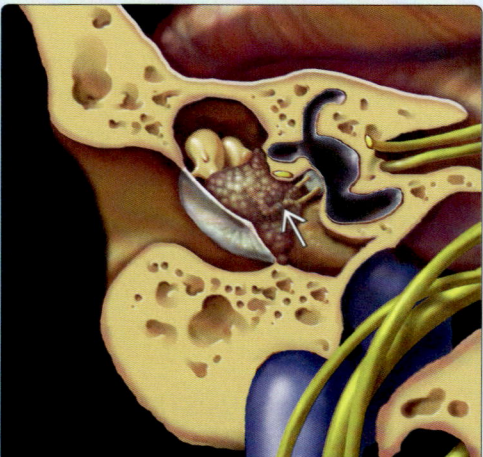
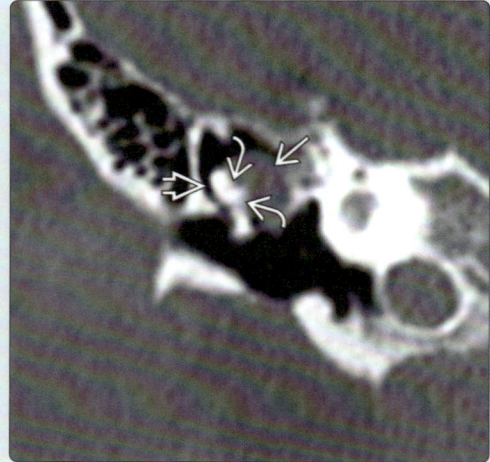

(Left) Coronal graphic shows congenital middle ear cholesteatoma (CMEC). Notice that the lesion surrounds and is medial to the ossicles ➡. The tympanic membrane is intact. (Right) Coronal temporal bone CT of the right ear in a child without a history of ear infections or tympanic membrane perforation shows a lobulated mass in the medial epitympanic cavity that proved to be a congenital cholesteatoma ➡. There are mild erosions along the medial aspect of the malleus and incus ➡. Notice that the lateral attic is clear ➡.

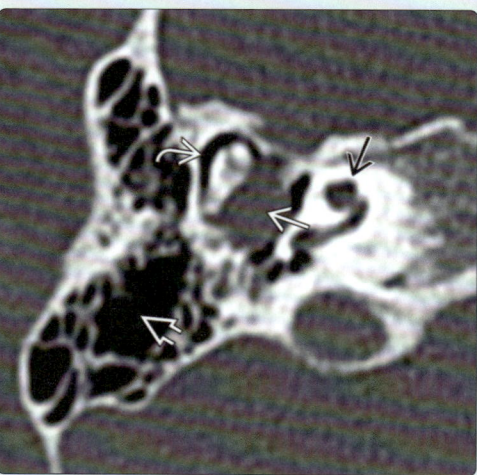
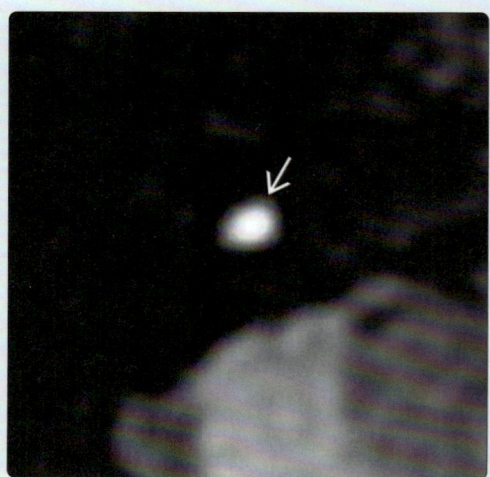

(Left) Axial bone CT of the right ear in the same patient reveals the well-circumscribed medial epitympanic congenital cholesteatoma ➡. The lateral attic ➡ and mastoid air cells ➡ are clear. Notice also the unwound appearance of the cochlea ➡, with the middle and apical turns offset, in this patient with branchiootorenal syndrome. (Right) Axial DWI MR in the same patient demonstrates characteristic hyperintense signal, consistent with reduced diffusivity within the medial epitympanic congenital cholesteatoma ➡.

Congenital Middle Ear Cholesteatoma

TERMINOLOGY

Abbreviations
- Congenital middle ear cholesteatoma (CMEC)

Synonyms
- Primary cholesteatoma, epidermoid

Definitions
- Cholesteatoma in middle ear (ME) behind intact tympanic membrane (TM) with no history of surgery, recurrent otitis media, or otorrhea

IMAGING

General Features
- Best diagnostic clue
  - Temporal bone CT shows smooth, well-circumscribed ME mass ± ossicular erosions
- Location
  - Multiple ME locations
    - Anterosuperior quadrant of tympanic cavity near eustachian tube
    - Posterior epitympanum at tympanic isthmi (area between ME cavity and attic)
    - Epitympanum medial to ossicles
- Size
  - Usually small because identified on otoscopic exam
  - Entire ME cavity not involved if small at presentation
- Morphology
  - Lobular, discrete ME mass

CT Findings
- Bone CT
  - Temporal bone CT appearance depends on size of lesion
  - Small: Detected early, appears as well-circumscribed soft tissue ME mass
  - Large: Larger CMEC may erode ossicles, ME wall, lateral semicircular canal, or tegmen tympani
    - Long process of incus and stapes superstructure most commonly eroded ossicles
    - Bone erosion less common than in acquired cholesteatoma
    - Labyrinthine extension may occur but late in disease process
    - Associated inflammatory changes infrequent
      - Mastoid pneumatization often normal
      - If aditus ad antrum occluded, mastoid air cells may opacify with retained secretions
  - Common ME locations
    - **Anterosuperior quadrant** of ME, adjacent to eustachian tube and anterior tympanic ring
      - Inferior but adjacent to tensor tympani muscle
    - Posterior epitympanum at tympanic isthmi (area between ME cavity and attic)
    - Epitympanum medial to ossicles

MR Findings
- T1WI
  - Iso- to hypointense ME mass
- T2WI
  - Intermediate-intensity ME mass
  - With larger lesions, aditus ad antrum obstruction seen as high-signal-retained secretions in mastoid
- DWI
  - Non-echo-planar DWI sequences recommended
    - Minimize susceptibility artifacts
    - ↑ sensitivity for detection of smaller lesions (2 mm)
    - High signal on DWI + corresponding low signal on ADC
      - Highly specific due to high keratin content
- T1WI C+
  - Peripherally enhancing ME mass
    - CMEC is nonenhancing material with subtle rim enhancement
  - If lesion is longstanding, associated scar may be seen as thickened area of enhancement adjacent to CMEC

Imaging Recommendations
- Best imaging tool
  - Temporal bone CT = exam of choice
  - T1WI C+ MR is complementary exam in certain circumstances
    - Recommended if recurrent or large CMEC
    - Recommended if diagnosis uncertain with tympanic paraganglioma or facial nerve schwannoma possible considerations
      - Glomus tumor and CNVII schwannoma enhance
- Protocol advice
  - If large CMEC, DWI sequence diagnostic

DIFFERENTIAL DIAGNOSIS

Pars Flaccida-Acquired Cholesteatoma
- Otoscopy shows **pars flaccida TM perforation**
  - Upper 1/3 of TM
- CT findings
  - Scutum erosion with lesion in lateral epitympanum
  - Ossicular chain and lateral semicircular canal erosion
  - Chronic inflammatory changes present
    - Mastoid underpneumatized

Pars Tensa-Acquired Cholesteatoma
- Otoscopy shows **pars tensa TM perforation**
  - Lower 2/3 of TM
- CT findings
  - Lesion enlarges medial to ossicles
  - Ossicular erosion common

Tympanic Paraganglioma
- Otoscopy shows pulsatile, vascular mass behind TM
  - Unusual in pediatric or adolescent patient
- CT findings
  - Sessile mass on cochlear promontory
  - No bony erosion
- MR findings
  - Focal enhancing mass on T1WI C+ MR

Facial Nerve Schwannoma of Tympanic Segment
- Otoscopy shows avascular mass behind intact TM
  - Appearance can closely mimic CMEC
- CT findings
  - Tubular mass emanating from tympanic CNVII canal
  - Enlarged bony facial nerve canal
  - Enlarged geniculate fossa

- MR findings
  - Tubular enhancing mass on T1WI C+ MR
  - Extends from geniculate ganglion along tympanic segment of facial nerve

Middle Ear Cholesterol Granuloma

- Otoscopy reveals blue TM
  - History of prior surgery or recurrent ME infection
- CT findings
  - ME mass with ossicular erosions common
- MR findings
  - T1 unenhanced MR shows high signal in ME mass

PATHOLOGY

General Features

- Etiology
  - 2 principal theories
    - Congenital **ectodermal rest** in ME cavity left behind with closure of neural tube (3rd-5th weeks of fetal life)
    - Lack of regression of epidermoid formation
      - Epidermoid formation: Point of epithelial transformation between tympanic cavity and eustachian tube
      - If it does not regress, becomes mass-like ME accumulation of stratified epithelial squamous cells
      - **Anterosuperior** CMEC results
  - Neither theory is unifying
- Associated abnormalities
  - External auditory canal (EAC) atresia can present with associated congenital cholesteatoma: In EAC or ME
  - Rarely associated with 1st branchial cleft remnant
- Other locations of congenital cholesteatoma in temporal bone: Petrous apex, mastoids, EAC, facial nerve canal

Staging, Grading, & Classification

- CMEC staging system
  - Stage 1: Single quadrant; no ossicular involvement or mastoid extension
  - Stage 2: Multiple quadrants; no ossicular involvement or mastoid extension
  - Stage 3: Ossicular involvement; no mastoid extension
  - Stage 4: Mastoid extension

Gross Pathologic & Surgical Features

- Circumscribed, pearly white mass with capsular sheen

Microscopic Features

- Identical to epidermoid inclusion cyst
- Stratified squamous epithelium with progressive exfoliation of keratinous material
- Contents rich in cholesterol crystals

CLINICAL ISSUES

Presentation

- Most common signs/symptoms
  - **Often incidental** avascular ME mass behind **intact TM**
- Other signs/symptoms
  - Unilateral conductive hearing loss (30%)
  - Large CMEC can obstruct eustachian tube with resultant ME-mastoid effusion and infection

Demographics

- Age
  - Average age of presentation or detection
    - Anterior or anterosuperior: 4 years
    - Posterosuperior and mesotympanum: 12 years
    - Attic and mastoid antrum involvement: 20 years
- Sex
  - M:F = 3:1
- Epidemiology
  - Accounts for 5% of all temporal bone cholesteatomas

Natural History & Prognosis

- Smaller, anterior lesions have better outcome with complete surgical resection
  - Smaller lesions may be encapsulated and easily removed
- If untreated, keratin debris accumulates over time with resultant larger lesion
  - Enlarging, cyst-like lesion may rupture, extending throughout ME
  - If eustachian tube obstructed, otomastoid opacification may occur
  - Larger lesions with infection may be difficult to differentiate from acquired cholesteatoma
- Large lesions or posterior epitympanic cholesteatoma have recurrence rates as high as 20%

Treatment

- Complete surgical excision = treatment of choice
  - Tympanoplasty for small, well-encapsulated CMEC
  - Tympanoplasty with canal wall up mastoidectomy for large CMEC
  - Tympanoplasty with canal wall down mastoidectomy for very large CMEC
- Ossicle chain reconstruction often necessary

DIAGNOSTIC CHECKLIST

Consider

- CMEC when avascular mass seen behind **intact TM**
- CMEC when no history of repeated ME infections
- CMEC when ME is opacified with wall erosion in congenital EAC atresia

Image Interpretation Pearls

- Younger patient + CT lesion medial to ossicles + normal mastoid pneumatization = CMEC

SELECTED REFERENCES

1. Vangrinsven G et al: Beyond the otoscope: an imaging review of congenital cholesteatoma. Insights Imaging. 15(1):194, 2024
2. Wei B et al: Congenital cholesteatoma clinical and surgical management. Int J Pediatr Otorhinolaryngol. 164:111401, 2023
3. Kennedy KL et al: Middle ear cholesteatoma. StatPearls. 2021
4. Shekdar KV et al: Imaging of pediatric hearing loss. Neuroimaging Clin N Am. 29(1):103-15, 2019
5. Juliano AF et al: Imaging review of the temporal bone: part II. Traumatic, postoperative, and noninflammatory nonneoplastic conditions. Radiology. 276(3):655-72, 2015
6. Bacciu A et al: Open vs closed type congenital cholesteatoma of the middle ear: two distinct entities or two aspects of the same phenomenon? Int J Pediatr Otorhinolaryngol. 78(12):2205-9, 2014
7. Más-Estellés F et al: Contemporary non-echo-planar diffusion-weighted imaging of middle ear cholesteatomas. Radiographics. 32(4):1197-213, 2012
8. Kutz JW Jr et al: Congenital middle ear cholesteatoma. Ear Nose Throat J. 86(11):654, 2007

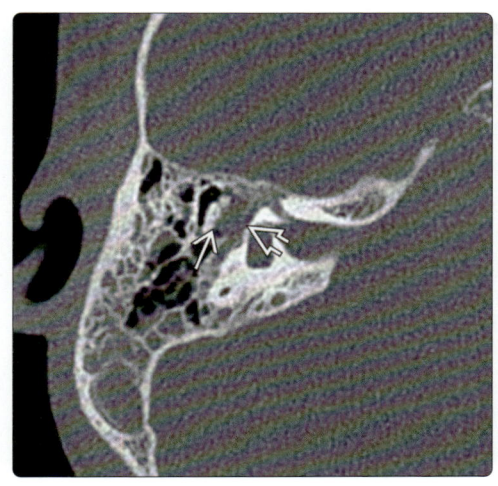

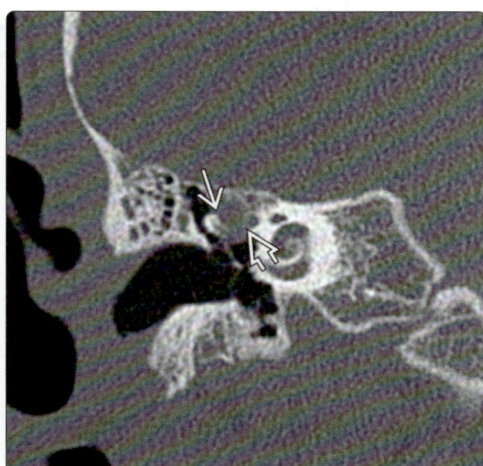

(Left) Axial bone CT of the right ear in a patient presenting clinically with recurrent otomastoiditis and conductive hearing loss reveals a soft tissue mass in the medial epitympanum eroding the medial surface of the head of the malleus and short process of the incus ➡. The anterior tympanic CNVII canal is also dehiscent ➡. (Right) Coronal bone CT in the same patient shows erosion of medial malleus head ➡ and lateral margin of anterior tympanic segment of CNVII canal ➡ by this medial epitympanic CMEC.

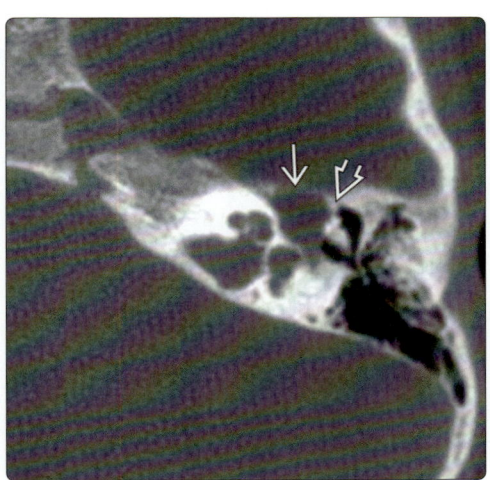

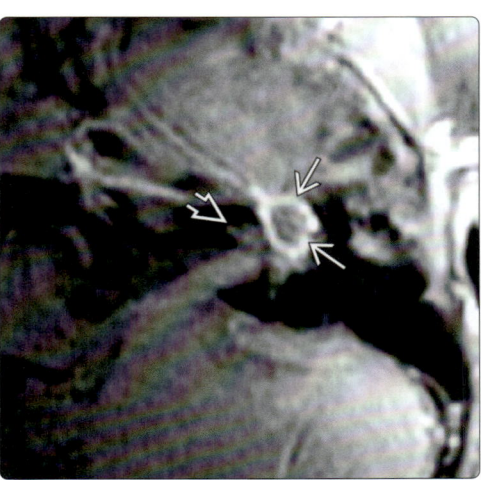

(Left) Axial bone CT of the left ear reveals a CMEC in the anterior epitympanic recess scalloping the middle ear wall ➡ and bowing the epitympanic cog posteriorly ➡. The malleus head abuts the posterior margin of the CMEC. (Right) Axial T1WI C+ MR in the same patient reveals typical rim enhancement ➡ along the peripheral margins of this anterior epitympanic CMEC. Notice the normal signal within the more medial cochlea ➡. If available, DWI would demonstrate reduced diffusivity.

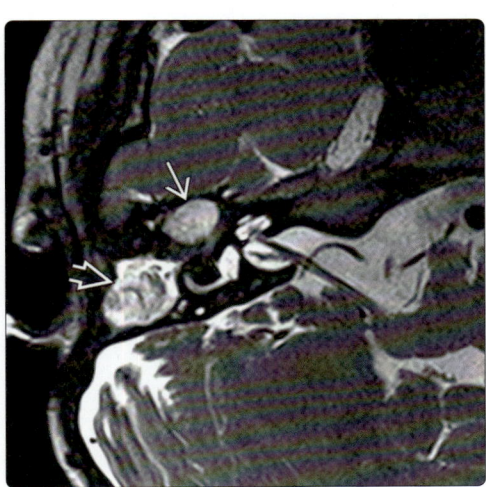

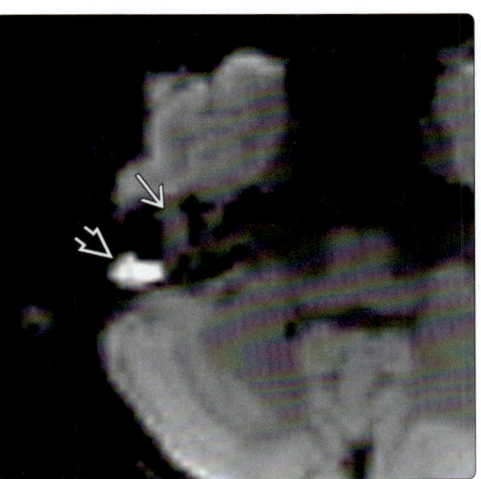

(Left) Axial T2WI MR in a 5-year-old boy previously operated on for CMEC reveals material in middle ear cavity ➡ and mastoid antrum ➡. Differentiating postoperative changes from recurrent cholesteatoma is not possible on this image. (Right) Axial DWI MR in the same patient shows the mastoid collection with reduced diffusivity ➡, indicating recurrent congenital cholesteatoma. However, the middle ear collection does not demonstrate diffusion restriction ➡ and is not a recurrent cholesteatoma.

Congenital Mastoid Cholesteatoma

TERMINOLOGY

- Definition: Cholesteatoma in mastoid secondary to epithelial rest

IMAGING

- Bone CT findings
  - Expansile soft tissue mass
  - Smooth erosion of mastoid bone
- MR findings
  - T1 low, T2 high
  - T1WI C+ nonenhancing; bows sigmoid sinus
  - **Reduced diffusion** (high DWI, low ADC)
- Mastoid locations
  - Anywhere in mastoid area
  - Medial mastoid ± internal auditory canal ± petrous apex

TOP DIFFERENTIAL DIAGNOSES

- Large pars flaccida-acquired cholesteatoma
- Mastoid cholesterol granuloma
- Temporal bone fibrous dysplasia
- Temporal bone Langerhans cell histiocytosis

PATHOLOGY

- Microscopic: Stratified squamous epithelium with progressive exfoliation of keratinous material

CLINICAL ISSUES

- Presentations
  - Older patient group (20-40 years)
    - Compared to middle ear cholesteatoma
  - Retroauricular swelling & pain; ± headache
  - May be **incidentally found** on imaging
- Treatment
  - Surgical resection is treatment of choice
  - Sigmoid sinus preservation important

DIAGNOSTIC CHECKLIST

- DWI **reduced diffusion** confirms congenital mastoid cholesteatoma diagnosis

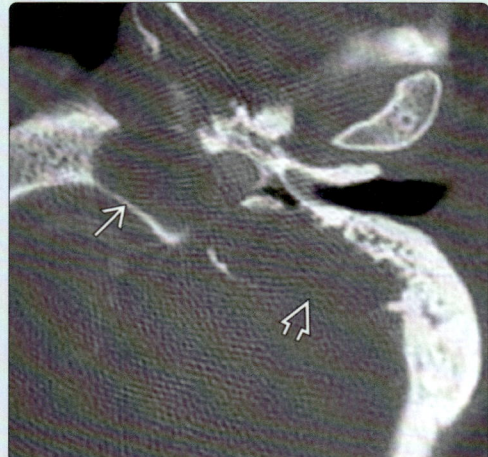
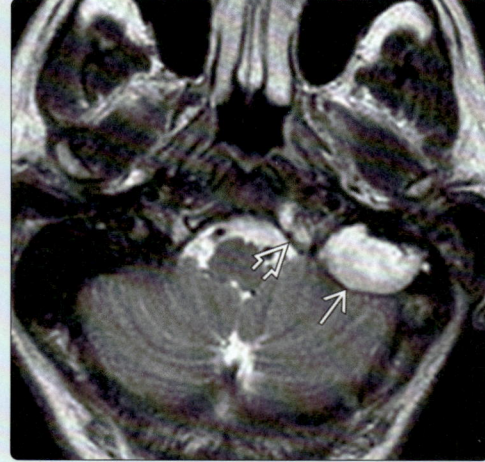

(Left) Axial bone CT shows a multilobular congenital cholesteatoma involving the lateral clivus ➡ & the medial mastoid ➡. The expansile bony margins are suggestive of this diagnosis. (Right) Axial T2WI MR in the same patient reveals a giant temporal bone congenital mastoid cholesteatoma as a high-signal, sharply marginated mass ➡ with involvement of the lateral clivus ➡, corresponding to the osseous destruction on CT.

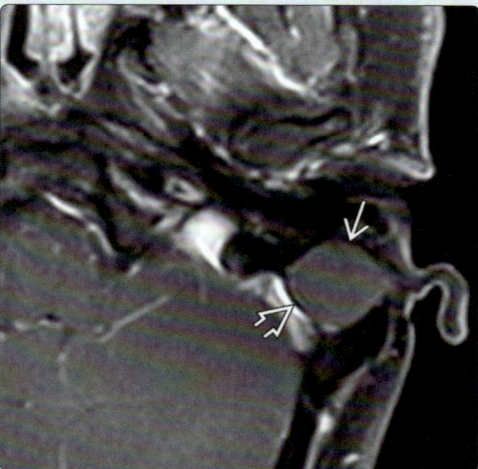
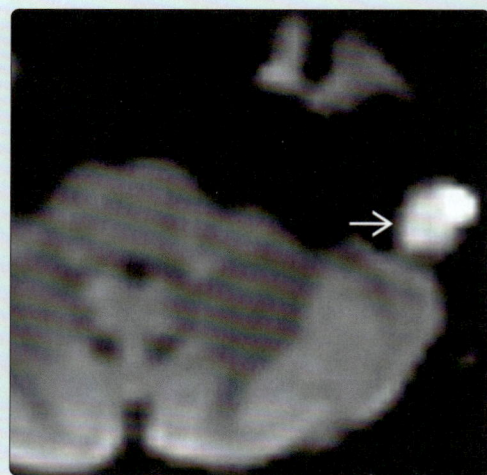

(Left) Axial T1WI C+ FS MR of the left ear reveals a nonenhancing, intermediate signal intensity soft tissue mass ➡ (congenital mastoid cholesteatoma) centered in the lateral mastoid air cells. Note the enhancing sigmoid sinus lateral margin is bowed inward by the the cholesteatoma ➡. (Right) Axial DWI MR in the same patient shows high signal ➡ in the location of the congenital mastoid cholesteatoma. Restricted diffusion within the lesion is highly suggestive of the diagnosis of cholesteatoma.

Congenital Mastoid Cholesteatoma

TERMINOLOGY

Abbreviations
- Congenital mastoid cholesteatoma (CMC)

Synonyms
- Primary mastoid cholesteatoma or epidermoid

Definitions
- Congenital cholesteatoma in mastoid secondary to epithelial rest

IMAGING

General Features
- Best diagnostic clue
  - Bone CT: Smooth erosion of mastoid bone
  - MR: T1 low, T2 high, nonenhancing, DWI high signal
- Location
  - Anywhere in mastoid area
    - Medial mastoid ± internal auditory canal (IAC) ± petrous apex
    - Occipitomastoid suture
- Size
  - Usually large (> 3 cm) as clinically silent
- Morphology
  - Lobular, ovoid

CT Findings
- Bone CT
  - Lobular soft tissue mastoid mass erodes trabeculae, thin or dehiscent cortex
    - May exit mastoid → external auditory canal (EAC), parotid space, carotid space

MR Findings
- T1WI
  - Iso- to hyperintense mastoid area mass
- T2WI
  - Intermediate to high intensity
- DWI
  - High signal (reduced diffusion)
- T1WI C+ FS
  - Subtle rim enhancement; CMC itself is nonenhancing

Imaging Recommendations
- Best imaging tool
  - Temporal bone CT = initial exam of choice
  - MR helpful in diagnosis & assessing extramastoid spread
    - Transverse-sigmoid sinus status
    - Extracranial spread

DIFFERENTIAL DIAGNOSIS

Large Pars Flaccida-Acquired Cholesteatoma
- Middle ear & mastoid affected; erosive
- MR: T1 low, T2 & DWI high signal

Mastoid Cholesterol Granuloma
- Middle ear & mastoid affected; erosive
- MR: T1 high, T2 high signal

Temporal Bone Fibrous Dysplasia
- Expansile bony process
- MR: Variable; usually T1 low, T2 low

Temporal Bone Langerhans Histiocytosis
- Destructive + soft tissue mass: mastoid > petrous apex & middle ear cavity
- MR: T1 low, T2 high signal; enhancing

Temporal Bone Rhabdomyosarcoma
- Soft tissue mass with bone destruction: Petrous apex & middle ear cavity > mastoid

PATHOLOGY

General Features
- Etiology
  - Congenital ectodermal rest in mastoid or occipitomastoid suture

Microscopic Features
- Same as epidermoid inclusion cyst
- Stratified squamous epithelium with progressive exfoliation of keratinous material

CLINICAL ISSUES

Presentation
- Most common signs/symptoms
  - Retroauricular swelling & pain ± headache
  - May be found incidentally on imaging
- Other signs/symptoms
  - When large, involving medial mastoid/IAC, may present with meningitis; retroauricular abscess

Demographics
- Age
  - Older patient group compared to middle ear congenital cholesteatoma; presents in 20-40 year olds

Natural History & Prognosis
- If untreated, keratin debris accumulates → increase size

Treatment
- Surgical resection treatment of choice; mastoidectomy

DIAGNOSTIC CHECKLIST

Consider
- Suspect CMC if globular nonenhancing mastoid area mass
  - DWI reduced diffusion confirms diagnosis

Reporting Tips
- In all lesions of mastoid area, comment on status of transverse-sigmoid sinus

SELECTED REFERENCES

1. Vangrinsven G et al: Beyond the otoscope: an imaging review of congenital cholesteatoma. Insights Imaging. 15(1):194, 2024
2. Wei B et al: Congenital cholesteatoma clinical and surgical management. Int J Pediatr Otorhinolaryngol. 164:111401, 2023
3. Chevallier KM et al: Differentiating pediatric rhabdomyosarcoma and Langerhans cell histiocytosis of the temporal bone by imaging appearance. AJNR Am J Neuroradiol. Jun;37(6):1185-9, 2016

Oval Window Atresia

TERMINOLOGY

- Oval window atresia (OWA): Absent space between lateral semicircular canal above & cochlear promontory below
- Majority also have anomalous stapes & malpositioned CNVII

IMAGING

- Temporal bone CT findings
  - Normal OW replaced by ossific "web" or plate
  - **Inferomedially positioned** tympanic segment **CNVII**
    - May completely overlie OW
    - May reside on superior or inferior OW margin
- Key surgical finding on CT = facial nerve location impacts safe surgical correction
- Best imaging tool: Multiplanar temporal bone CT
  - OW niche best seen in coronal & Pöschl planes
  - CNVII relative to OW best seen in coronal plane
  - Stapes crura best seen in axial plane
- Bony plate over OW + inferomedial tympanic CNVII = OWA
  - If both findings present, no differential diagnosis present

TOP DIFFERENTIAL DIAGNOSES

- Tympanosclerosis
- Fenestral otosclerosis
- Congenital external ear malformation

PATHOLOGY

- Best hypothesis for OWA etiology
  - Primitive stapes fails to fuse with primitive vestibule during 7th week of gestation

CLINICAL ISSUES

- Clinical presentation
  - Nonprogressive conductive hearing deficit from birth
  - Lack of history of otomastoiditis; normal external auditory canal

DIAGNOSTIC CHECKLIST

- Thickened bone over OW + inferomedially displaced tympanic CNVII = OWA

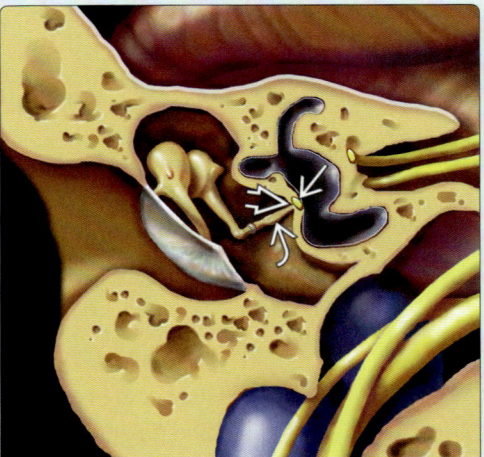
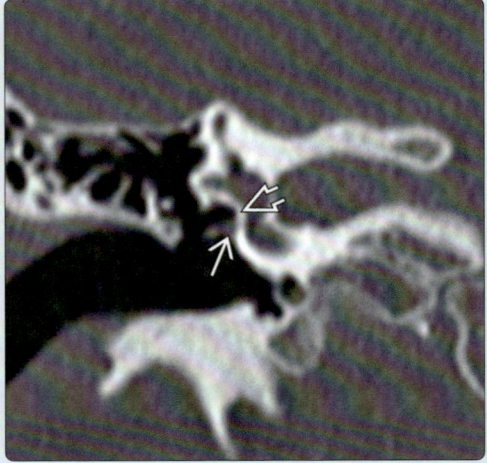

(Left) Coronal graphic illustrates features of oval window atresia ➡, including malformation of the stapes crura and footplate ➡, and the tympanic segment of the facial nerve in an abnormal location ➡. (Right) Coronal bone CT in an adolescent with conductive hearing loss reveals a bony plate along the atretic oval window ➡. Notice that the tympanic segment of CNVII is present along the inferior margin of the oval window niche ➡.

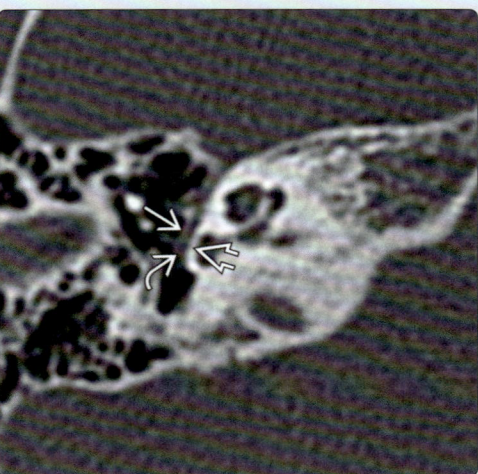
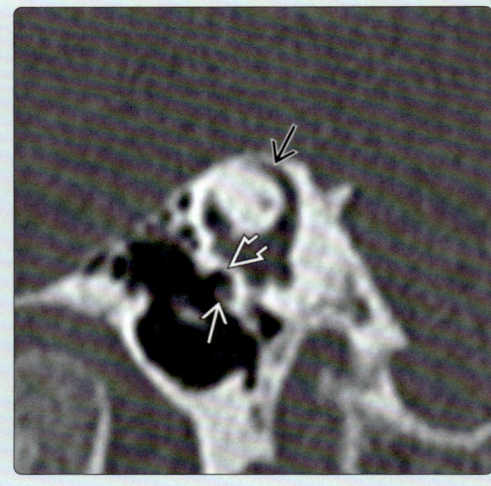

(Left) Axial bone CT in the same patient shows bony oval window atresia ➡. The tympanic segment of CNVII ➡ courses along the inferior margin of the atretic oval window, adjacent to an otherwise normal-appearing stapes ➡. (Right) Coronal oblique bone CT (Pöschl view) in plane with the superior semicircular canal ➡ in the same patient reveals the bony plate along the atretic oval window ➡. The tympanic segment of CNVII ➡ is visible inferior to the atretic oval window.

TERMINOLOGY

Abbreviations
- Oval window atresia (OWA)

Synonyms
- Congenital absence of oval window (OW)

Definitions
- Absent space between lateral semicircular canal above & cochlear promontory below
- Majority also have anomalous stapes & malpositioned CNVII

IMAGING

General Features
- Best diagnostic clue
  - Absence of OW lucency with bony plate at its location between vestibule & middle ear (ME)

CT Findings
- Bone CT
  - Normal OW replaced by ossific web
  - Malformed stapes superstructure (absence of normal paired crura) & distal incus
    - Soft tissue connecting shortened long process to stapes head may be inapparent on CT
  - **Inferomedially positioned** tympanic segment **CNVII**
    - May reside on superior or inferior margin of OW
    - May completely overlie expected location of OW
      - □ **Critical surgical importance** (associated in > 60%)
      - □ OW drill-out may be contraindicated if present
  - External auditory canal (EAC) usually normal

Imaging Recommendations
- Best imaging tool
  - Multiplanar high-resolution temporal bone CT
    - OW niche best seen in coronal & Pöschl planes
    - CNVII relative to OW best seen in coronal plane
    - Stapes crura best seen in axial plane

DIFFERENTIAL DIAGNOSIS

Tympanosclerosis
- Clinical: Chronic otomastoiditis
- Imaging: Stapes may be thickened, including footplate
  - Ossific deposits on ossicle surface may be seen
  - ME debris/sclerotic mastoid = chronic otomastoiditis
  - Facial nerve normal

Fenestral Otosclerosis
- Clinical: Rare in childhood
- Imaging: Lucent lesions anterior to OW
  - Obliterative variety (< 10%) results in similar appearance to OWA but stapes and facial nerve normal

Congenital External Ear Malformation
- Clinical: Microtia, EAC malformation
- Imaging: Variable EAC narrowing or absence
  - Ossicle fusion, rotation; CNVII anomalous course
  - OWA may be associated

PATHOLOGY

General Features
- Etiology
  - Best hypothesis: Primitive stapes fails to fuse with primitive vestibule during 7th week of gestation
  - Alternate hypothesis: Developing facial nerve displaced & interposed between primitive stapes & otic capsule
  - If stapes forms but annular ligament does not, stapes footplate is ankylosed (**congenital stapes fixation**)
    - Caution: May result in congenital conductive hearing loss in absence of imaging findings

Gross Pathologic & Surgical Features
- Tympanic segment of CNVII abnormal in many cases
  - Inferomedially positioned
- Abnormal incus lenticular process associated
  - Expected since distal incus & stapes superstructure are both formed from 2nd branchial arch

CLINICAL ISSUES

Presentation
- Most common signs/symptoms
  - Profound conductive hearing deficit in child
    - Nonprogressive; air-bone gap > 40 dB

Demographics
- Epidemiology
  - OWA **bilateral** in ~ **40%**
  - May be associated with EAC atresia/stenosis
  - May be seen in various syndromes, **CHARGE** syndrome most common
- Age: Usually discovered in children
- Sex: M > F

Natural History & Prognosis
- Surgical correction results are modest over long term

Treatment
- Vestibulotomy with ossiculoplasty
  - Stapes or total ossicular replacement prosthesis
  - Difficult as landmarks for vestibule are few; risk of ectopic facial nerve injury
- Fenestration above OWA & piston prosthesis placement
- Alternative treatment (**round** window vibroplasty)
  - Version of active ME implants (vibrant sound bridge)

DIAGNOSTIC CHECKLIST

Image Interpretation Pearls
- Thickened bone over OW + inferomedially displaced tympanic CNVII = OWA

SELECTED REFERENCES

1. Chen X et al: Imaging findings of isolated congenital middle ear malformation on high-resolution computed tomography. Neuroradiology. 66(11):2043-52, 2024
2. Robson CD: Conductive hearing loss in children. Neuroimaging Clin N Am. 33(4):543-62, 2023
3. D'Arco F et al: Temporal bone and intracranial abnormalities in syndromic causes of hearing loss: an updated guide. Eur J Radiol. 123:108803, 2020
4. Zeifer B et al: Congenital absence of the oval window: radiologic diagnosis and associated anomalies. AJNR Am J Neuroradiol. 21(2):322-7, 2000

KEY FACTS

TERMINOLOGY

- Lateralized internal carotid artery (Lat-ICA)
- Rare temporal bone vascular variant

IMAGING

- CTA best shows ICA entering anterior middle ear cavity lateral to normal position
- Petrous ICA genu lateral to line drawn perpendicular to midpoint cochlea basal turn on axial images
- Dehiscent lateral ICA often associated
- Coronal bone CT: Tympanic canaliculus not enlarged
- On maximal intensity projection, CTA/MRA vessel contour mimics aberrant ICA
- Source images best for clarifying exact anomalous course of ICA through temporal bone

TOP DIFFERENTIAL DIAGNOSES

- Aberrant ICA
- Tympanic paraganglioma
- Jugular paraganglioma
- ICA aneurysm at petrous apex

PATHOLOGY

- Developmental anomaly
- Not associated with persistent stapedial artery

CLINICAL ISSUES

- Often asymptomatic; incidental on CT or otoscopy
- Patient may present with pulsatile tinnitus
- Important finding to avoid inadvertent surgical injury

DIAGNOSTIC CHECKLIST

- Differentiate from aberrant ICA
  - Aberrant ICA: Inferior tympanic canaliculus enlarged, vertical carotid canal hypoplastic or absent, courses across cochlear promontory
  - Lat-ICA: Inferior tympanic canaliculus and vertical carotid canal normal, courses in anterior middle ear cavity at level of cochlear basal turn

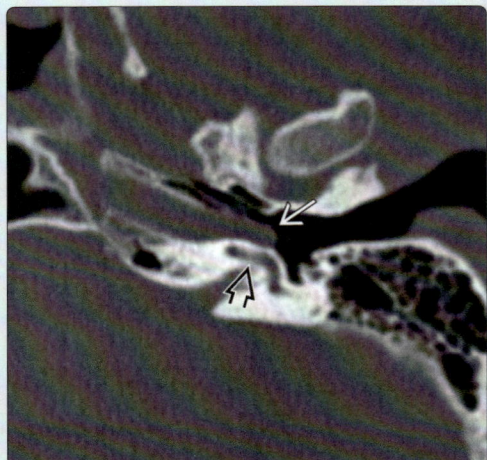
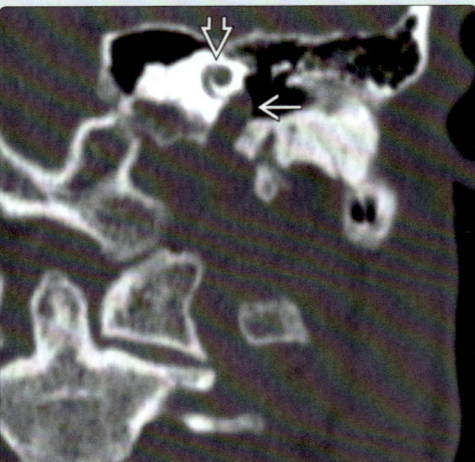

(Left) Axial left ear temporal bone CT shows a lateralized petrous internal carotid artery (ICA) with its genu ➡ located lateral to a line drawn perpendicular to the midportion of the cochlear basal turn ➡. The position in the anterior middle ear is typical. Inferior tympanic canaliculus was normal (not shown), helping to differentiate from an aberrant ICA. (Right) Coronal bone CT shows a left ICA ➡ extending more lateral to the cochlea ➡ than expected within the anterior hypo- and mesotympanum.

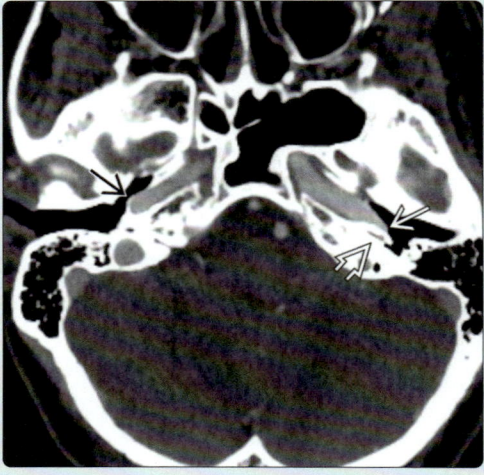
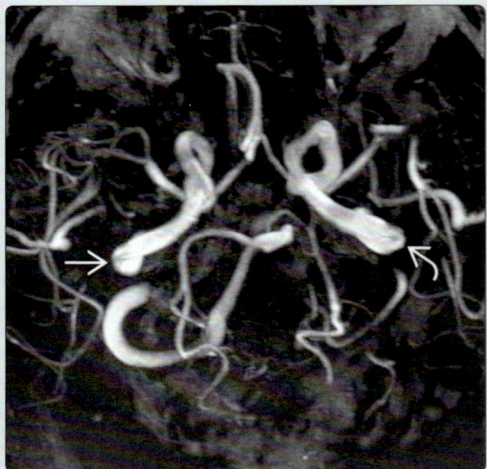

(Left) Axial CTA depicts the left petrous ICA genus projecting laterally into the anterior middle ear cavity, beyond the midpoint of the basal turn of the cochlea ➡. Compare to the normal right side ➡. There is associated lateral wall dehiscence ➡, a common finding in a lateralized ICA. (Right) MRA MIP shows asymmetry of the ICAs with the posterior genu (where ascending carotid becomes petrous portion) appearing more posterior on the right ➡ and slightly more lateral than on left ➡, which is a lateralized ICA.

TERMINOLOGY

Abbreviations
- Lateralized internal carotid artery (Lat-ICA)

Definitions
- Anomalous intratemporal course of ICA
  - Enters anterior mesotympanum
  - Often has dehiscent lateral ICA bony wall

IMAGING

General Features
- Best diagnostic clue
  - Lateral course of ICA in mesotympanum
- Location
  - ICA lies in anteromedial aspect of middle ear cavity as it turns medially to petrous segment

CT Findings
- Bone CT
  - Protrusion of ICA into anterior aspect of middle ear
    - Dehiscence usually near basal turn of cochlea
  - Coronal temporal bone CT shows laterally displaced ICA at level of cochlear promontory
- CTA
  - Intermediate window/level setting shows course and contour of Lat-ICA projecting into middle ear
  - Bone window shows lateral wall dehiscence

MR Findings
- MRA
  - On MIP, mimics aberrant ICA
  - Source images show lateral position of genu of vertical and horizontal portions of petrous ICA
  - Basilar projection reveals bulbous, posterolaterally placed petrous ICA
- Routine MR sequences
  - ± "invisible" Lat-ICA due to low-signal mastoid air/bone

Imaging Recommendations
- Best imaging tool
  - Temporal bone CT/CTA best show course and distinguish from aberrant ICA
  - MRA source images key to clarify anomalous course
- Protocol advice
  - CTA most readily confirms diagnosis
  - Carefully evaluate coronal and axial planes

DIFFERENTIAL DIAGNOSIS

Aberrant Internal Carotid Artery
- Aberrant ICA enters hypotympanum through enlarged inferior tympanic canaliculus, courses through middle ear across cochlear promontory

Tympanic Paraganglioma
- Focal mass on cochlear promontory
- No tubular shape; normal ICA on MRA/CTA

Jugular Paraganglioma
- Mass arising in jugular foramen and projecting superolaterally into middle ear

- Permeative-destructive bony changes on CT

Internal Carotid Artery Aneurysm at Petrous Apex
- Focal or fusiform expansion of petrous ICA canal
- MRA and CTA show focal vascular mass

PATHOLOGY

General Features
- Etiology
  - Developmental variation
    - No etiology known
- Associated abnormalities
  - Lat-ICA appears to be isolated finding
  - Not associated with persistent stapedial artery

CLINICAL ISSUES

Presentation
- Most common signs/symptoms
  - Often asymptomatic; incidental finding on CT or otoscopy
  - Patient may present for imaging with objective or subjective pulsatile tinnitus or with retrotympanic mass

Demographics
- Sex
  - No sex predilection known
- Epidemiology
  - Rare temporal bone vascular lesion

Natural History & Prognosis
- Developmental anomaly
- No long-term sequelae reported

Treatment
- None; probably incidental developmental anomaly
- Important radiologic observation
- **Inadvertent surgical vascular injury can result in significant neurologic deficits**

DIAGNOSTIC CHECKLIST

Consider
- Must differentiate from aberrant ICA
  - Lat-ICA does not enter middle ear through enlarged inferior tympanic canaliculus
  - ICA does not course across cochlear promontory
- Important normal vascular variant to recognize and report to avoid surgical injury to ICA

Image Interpretation Pearls
- Always check course of ICA on temporal bone CT or CTA
- Always check integrity of lateral wall of temporal ICA

SELECTED REFERENCES

1. Tames HLVC et al: Postoperative imaging of the temporal bone. Radiographics. 41(3):858-75, 2021
2. Glastonbury CM et al: Lateralized petrous internal carotid artery: imaging features and distinction from the aberrant internal carotid artery. Neuroradiology. 54(9):1007-13, 2012
3. Vattoth S et al: A compartment-based approach for the imaging evaluation of tinnitus. AJNR Am J Neuroradiol. 31(2):211-8, 2010

Aberrant Internal Carotid Artery

TERMINOLOGY

- Aberrant internal carotid artery (AbICA): Congenital vascular anomaly resulting from failure of formation of extracranial ICA with arterial collateral pathway

IMAGING

- Appearance of AbICA on thin-section (< 1-mm) temporal bone CT is diagnostic
- AbICA appears as **tubular** lesion crossing middle ear from posterior to anterior
- Enlarged inferior tympanic canaliculus important observation
- Caution: Do not mistake AbICA for tympanicum paraganglioma

TOP DIFFERENTIAL DIAGNOSES

- Vascular middle ear lesion
  - Tympanic paraganglioma
  - Dehiscent jugular bulb
  - Lateralized ICA

PATHOLOGY

- Best explanation: "Alternative blood flow" theory
  - Persistence of pharyngeal artery system means C1 portion of ICA is absent
  - Mature arterial collateral system compensates for absent C1 and vertical petrous ICA segments
  - Ascending pharyngeal artery → inferior tympanic artery → caroticotympanic artery → posterolateral aspect of horizontal petrous ICA
- 30% of AbICAs have persistent stapedial artery

CLINICAL ISSUES

- Typically asymptomatic and discovered at time of routine physical exam, during middle ear surgery, or as incidental imaging finding
- Associated symptoms: Pulsatile tinnitus and conductive hearing loss
- No treatment is best treatment

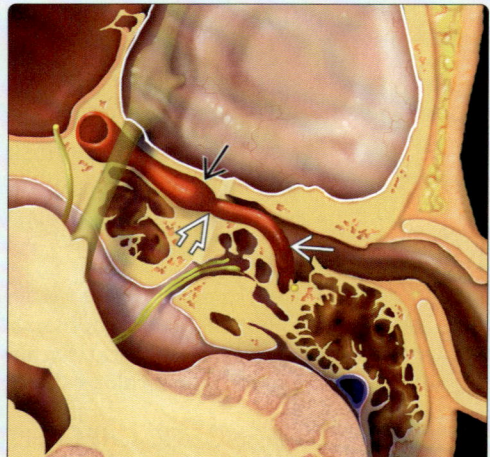
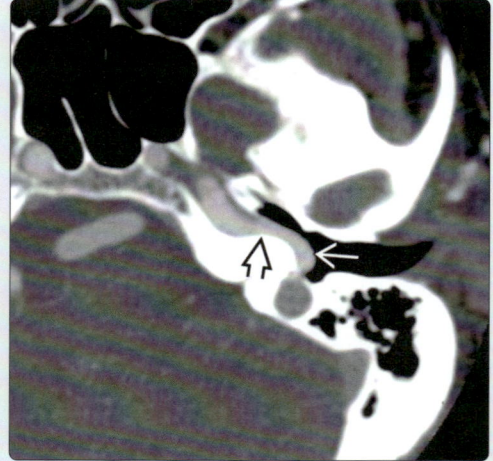

(Left) Axial graphic of the left temporal bone illustrates a classic aberrant internal carotid artery (AbICA) ➡ rising along the posterior cochlear promontory and crossing along the medial middle ear wall to rejoin the horizontal petrous ICA ➡. At the point of reconnection to the horizontal petrous ICA, stenosis ➡ is often present. (Right) Axial CTA through the middle ear shows the looping AbICA ➡ on the low cochlear promontory. Note the caliber change ➡ as the AbICA rejoins the normal horizontal segment of the ICA.

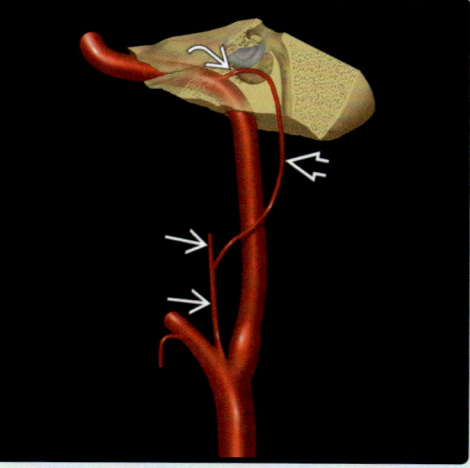
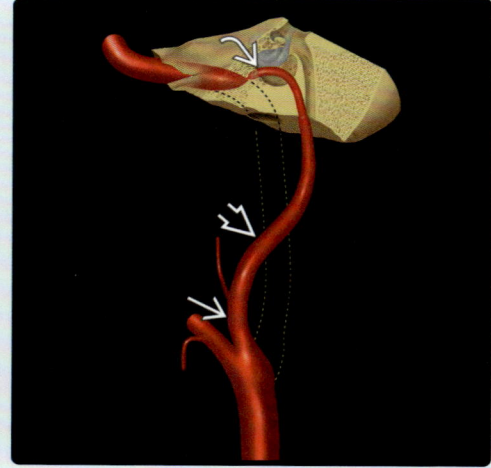

(Left) Lateral graphic of normal adult cervical and petrous ICA shows the inferior tympanic artery ➡ branching off the ascending pharyngeal artery ➡, passing into the temporal bone to anastomose with the very small caroticotympanic artery ➡ on the cochlear promontory. (Right) Lateral graphic shows failure of the cervical ICA to develop (dotted lines) with the ascending pharyngeal ➡, inferior tympanic ➡, and caroticotympanic ➡ arteries providing an alternative collateral arterial channel, resulting in an AbICA.

Aberrant Internal Carotid Artery

TERMINOLOGY

Abbreviations

- Aberrant internal carotid artery (AbICA)

Synonyms

- Aberrant carotid artery

Definitions

- Congenital vascular anomaly resulting from failure of formation of extracranial ICA with arterial collateral pathway

IMAGING

General Features

- Best diagnostic clue
  - Tubular structure running horizontally through middle ear cavity from posterior to anterior
- Location
  - Enters posterior middle ear through enlarged inferior tympanic canaliculus
    - Posterior and lateral to expected site of petrous carotid canal
  - Courses anteriorly across cochlear promontory to join horizontal petrous ICA through dehiscent carotid plate
  - Most commonly unilateral
- Size
  - Smaller than horizontal petrous ICA
- Morphology
  - Tubular morphology is key observation

CT Findings

- CECT
  - Enhancement equivalent to other arteries
    - **Caution**: Tympanic paraganglioma also enhances: Use morphology to differentiate tubular AbICA from ovoid paraganglioma
- Bone CT
  - Appearance of AbICA on thin-section (< 1 mm) temporal bone CT is diagnostic
  - Axial bone CT
    - AbICA appears as tubular lesion crossing middle ear from posterior to anterior
    - **Enlarged inferior tympanic canaliculus** is important observation
      - □ Anteromedial to stylomastoid foramen and mastoid segment of facial nerve
    - Smaller AbICA often stenotic at point of reconnection with horizontal petrous ICA
    - Carotid foramen and vertical segment of petrous ICA are absent
  - Coronal bone CT
    - AbICA appears as round soft tissue lesion on cochlear promontory
      - □ Single slice looks disturbingly like tympanic paraganglioma
      - □ **Caution**: Do not mistake AbICA for tympanic paraganglioma
      - □ Tubular nature of AbICA is key observation

- Inferior tympanic canaliculus is vertical tube posterolateral to normal location of vertical segment of petrous ICA
  - □ Rises at coronal level of round window niche
  - If **persistent stapedial artery** associated
    - Absent foramen spinosum
    - Enlarged anterior tympanic segment of CNVII canal
- CTA
  - Diagnostic for AbICA
  - Usually not necessary, as temporal bone CT alone is diagnostic

MR Findings

- Conventional MR does not reliably identify AbICA
- MRA source images and reformatted images show aberrant nature of vessel
  - AbICA enters skull base posterior and lateral compared to normal contralateral side
  - Frontal reformat: Petrous segment of ICA extends laterally instead of medially
    - In left ear, AbICA looks like 7
    - In right ear, AbICA looks like reverse 7

Angiographic Findings

- Frontal view: Petrous segment of ICA extends laterally instead of medially
- Lateral view: Absent extracranial course of suprabifurcation ICA (C1 segment)
  - Smaller caliber vessels arise from bifurcation posteriorly, looping back to horizontal segment of petrous ICA
    - Stenosis may be present at site of reconnection between AbICA and horizontal petrous ICA
- Conventional angiography no longer necessary to confirm imaging diagnosis
  - CTA or MRA sufficient if uncertainty arises from bone CT

Imaging Recommendations

- Best imaging tool
  - Temporal bone CT: Tubular morphology and posterolateral position diagnostic
    - Contrast CT or CTA not necessary
- Protocol advice
  - Bone CT: < 1-mm axial and coronal images
  - If MR is used, MRA is critical component

DIFFERENTIAL DIAGNOSIS

Tympanic Paraganglioma

- Otoscopy: Pink/red, pulsatile, retrotympanic mass
- Bone CT: Focal ovoid mass on cochlear promontory
- MR: T1WI C+ enhancing mass

Lateralized Internal Carotid Artery

- Otoscopy: Vague, vascular hue deep behind tympanic membrane
- Bone CT: Dehiscent lateral wall of petrous ICA genu

Petrous Internal Carotid Artery Aneurysm

- Otoscopy: Negative unless large
- Bone CT: Focal, smooth, petrous ICA canal expansion
  - ICA has normal course but focal ovoid, expansile portion
- CTA or MRA is diagnostic of nonthrombosed aneurysm

Dehiscent Jugular Bulb

- Otoscopy: Gray-blue retrotympanic mass in posteroinferior quadrant
- Bone CT: Focal absence of sigmoid plate
  - "Bud" from superolateral jugular bulb enters middle ear as "mass"

Cholesterol Granuloma in Middle Ear

- Otoscopy: Blue-black retrotympanic mass
- Bone CT: Appears identical to acquired cholesteatoma
- MR: High signal on T1 and T2 without contrast suggests diagnosis

Congenital Cholesteatoma in Middle Ear

- Otoscopy: White-tan retrotympanic mass
- Bone CT: Multilobular soft tissue middle ear mass medial to ossicles
- MR: Low T1, high T2 signal mass; DWI restricted diffusion

PATHOLOGY

General Features

- Etiology
  - Etiology of AbICA is controversial
  - Best explanation: "Alternative blood flow" theory
    - Persistence of pharyngeal artery system means C1 portion of ICA is absent
    - Mature arterial collateral system compensates for absent C1 and vertical petrous ICA segments
      - Ascending pharyngeal artery → inferior tympanic artery → caroticotympanic artery → posterolateral aspect of horizontal petrous ICA
  - Results of absent extracranial ICA C1 segment
    - Ascending pharyngeal, inferior tympanic, and caroticotympanic arteries enlarge
    - Inferior tympanic canaliculus enlarges to accommodate enlarged inferior tympanic artery
    - Bony margin of posterolateral horizontal petrous ICA canal is penetrated at site of caroticotympanic artery origin
- Associated abnormalities
  - 30% of AbICAs have **persistent stapedial artery**
    - Enlarged anterior tympanic segment of CNV2 canal
    - Absent ipsilateral foramen spinosum

Gross Pathologic & Surgical Features

- Pulsatile aberrant artery is found in middle ear cavity

Microscopic Features

- Histologically normal artery

CLINICAL ISSUES

Presentation

- Most common signs/symptoms
  - Most commonly **asymptomatic**
    - Discovered at time of routine physical exam, during middle ear surgery, or as incidental imaging finding
  - Associated symptoms
    - Pulsatile tinnitus (PT) (pulse-synchronous sound)
      - May be subjective (only patient hears) or objective (patient and clinician hear)

□ Subjective PT: Pulsatile sound may transmit directly through cochlear promontory to basal turn of cochlea
□ Objective PT: When stenosis present at junction of AbICA and normal horizontal petrous ICA
    - Conductive hearing loss
    - Vertigo, otalgia rare
  - Otoscopy: Retrotympanic pink-red mass
    - Inferior aspect of tympanic membrane
    - May mimic paraganglioma

Demographics

- Age
  - Average at presentation: 38 years
- Sex
  - M < F in single study (N = 16)
- Epidemiology
  - Very rare disorder

Natural History & Prognosis

- No long-term sequelae reported with AbICA
- Poor prognosis results only if misdiagnosis → biopsy
  - Pseudoaneurysm may require endovascular repair
- If tinnitus is loud, AbICA can be debilitating

Treatment

- **No treatment** is best treatment
- Greatest risk is misdiagnosis leading to biopsy
- Most patients have minor symptoms that do not require treatment
- Persistent stapedial artery does not require treatment

DIAGNOSTIC CHECKLIST

Image Interpretation Pearls

- Radiologist must remain firm on imaging diagnosis despite clinical impression of paraganglioma
  - Biopsy or attempted resection of misdiagnosed AbICA can be disastrous
    - Hemorrhage, stroke, or death may result from vessel injury
- Retropharyngeal cervical ICA is sometimes referred to as AbICA in literature

Reporting Tips

- Report diagnosis; offer no differential diagnosis
- Equivocal report, such as "cannot exclude paraganglioma," may lead to surgical intervention

SELECTED REFERENCES

1. Verbist B et al: ESR essentials: diagnostic strategies in tinnitus-practice recommendations by the European Society of Head and Neck Radiology. Eur Radiol. 35(3):1303-12, 2025
2. Lv S et al: Analysis of etiology, diagnosis, and treatment strategy and efficacy of pulsatile tinnitus caused by abnormal vascular anatomy. Curr Med Sci. 43(1):173-83, 2023
3. Benson JC et al: Temporal bone anatomy. Neuroimaging Clin N Am. 32(4):763-75, 2022
4. Wadhavkar N et al: Laceration of aberrant internal carotid artery following myringotomy: a case report and review of literature. Ann Otol Rhinol Laryngol. 131(5):555-61, 2022
5. Kumar R et al: Detecting causes of pulsatile tinnitus on CT arteriography-venography: a pictorial review. Eur J Radiol. 139:109722, 2021
6. Sullivan AM et al: Arterial anomalies of the middle ear: a pictorial review with clinical-embryologic and imaging correlation. Neuroimaging Clin N Am. 29(1):93-102, 2019

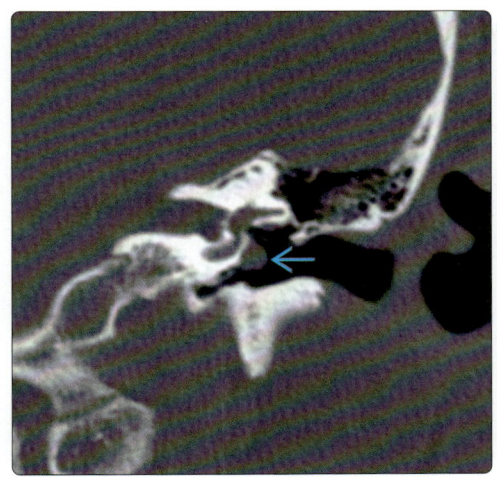

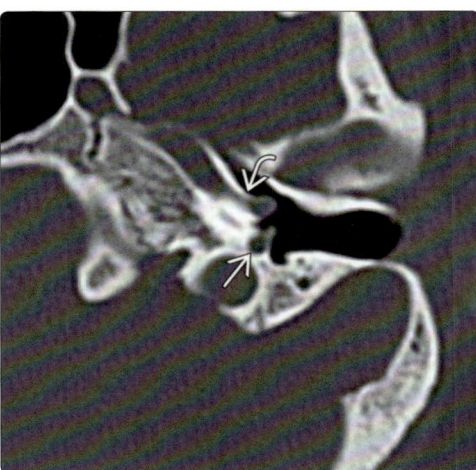

(Left) Coronal left temporal bone CT at the level of the oval window shows the AbICA ➡ as a "mass" located on the cochlear promontory, resembling a tympanic paraganglioma. Accidental biopsy of AbICA may have devastating consequences. (Right) Axial bone CT reveals a smaller caliber AbICA entering the middle ear cavity through an enlarged inferior tympanic canaliculus ➡, coursing across the middle ear on the cochlear promontory, and reentering the horizontal petrous ICA ➡.

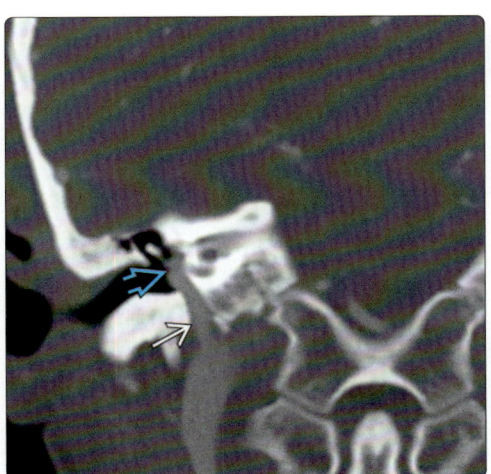

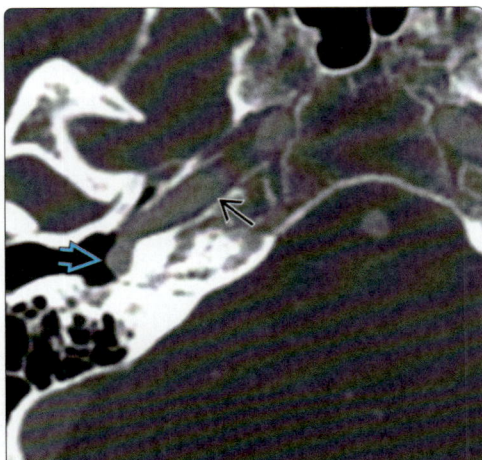

(Left) Coronal CTA of the right ear shows the posterior aspect of an AbICA with its enlarged inferior tympanic canaliculus ➡ and extension to the cochlear promontory ➡. On otoscopy, this appears as a vascular retrotympanic mass that mimics a paraganglioma. (Right) Axial CTA shows a right AbICA ➡ coursing across the middle ear cavity on the low cochlear promontory in the typical location for a tympanic paraganglioma. Its tubular shape can help prevent a misdiagnosis. Note the normal horizontal petrous segment ICA ➡.

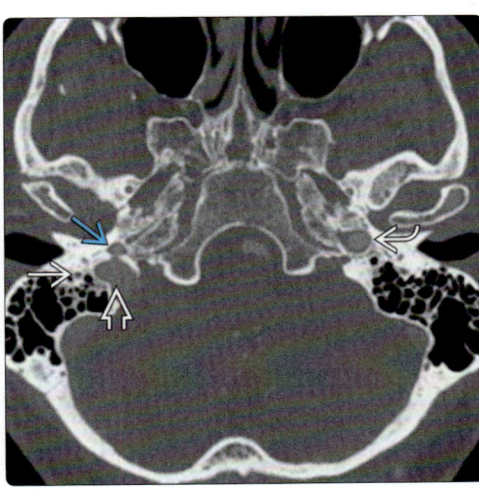

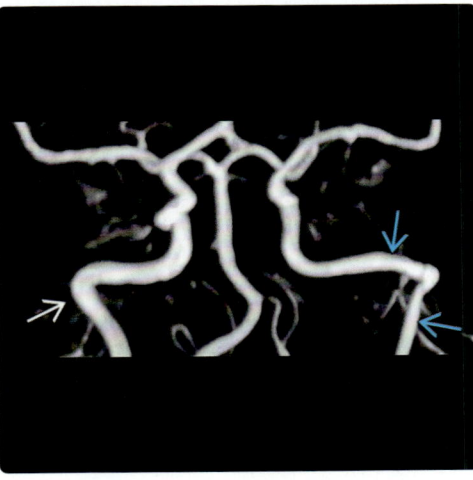

(Left) Axial CTA at the skull base shows an enlarged inferior tympanic canaliculus ➡ containing an AbICA located anterior and medial to the stylomastoid foramen and the mastoid segment of the facial nerve ➡. The caliber of an AbICA is smaller than a normal ICA ➡. Note the normal jugular bulb ➡. (Right) Anteroposterior reformat of a time-of-flight MRA shows the characteristic 7 sign ➡ as the left AbICA extends laterally into the middle ear. Compare this with the contralateral normal ICA ➡.

KEY FACTS

TERMINOLOGY

- Persistent stapedial artery (PSA): Rare congenital vascular anomaly in which embryologic stapedial artery persists

IMAGING

- **Temporal bone CT or CTA**
  - High-resolution imaging may allow identification of tiny linear vessel in medial aspect of middle ear
  - Absent foramen spinosum
  - Enlargement of anterior tympanic segment of facial nerve canal
  - Frequently bilateral
- **MRA**
  - Flow-related signal in PSA of middle ear and aberrant middle meningeal artery (MMA) origin

TOP DIFFERENTIAL DIAGNOSES

- Aberrant internal carotid artery
- Facial nerve schwannoma

- Facial nerve venous malformation ("hemangioma")
- Perineural parotid malignancy in CNVII canal

PATHOLOGY

- PSA results in **aberrant vessel** in middle ear cavity
- PSA runs over promontory, courses through obturator foramen of stapes, enters tympanic CNVII canal through gap in its wall posterior to cochleariform process, and exits anteriorly to give rise to MMA

CLINICAL ISSUES

- Most cases are asymptomatic; no treatment required
- Can be associated with pulsatile tinnitus and conductive hearing loss
- If encountered surgically, may limit exposure of stapes, and can lead to intraoperative hemorrhage
- Can be associated with aberrant ICA

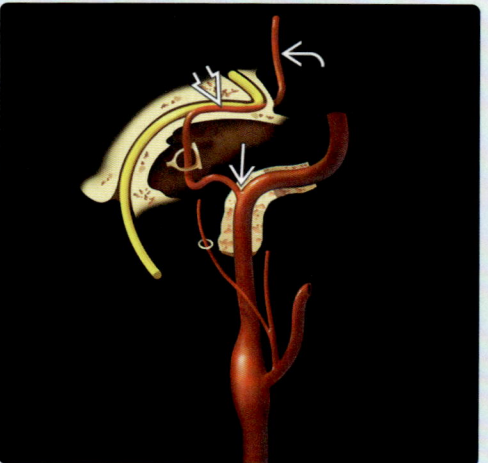
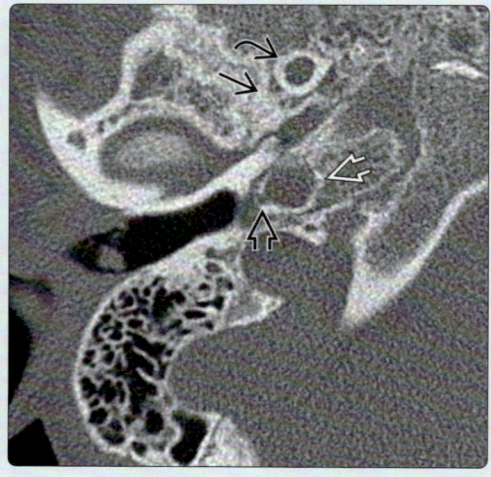

(Left) *Lateral graphic shows the persistent stapedial artery (PSA) arising from the vertical segment of the petrous internal carotid artery ➡, passing through the stapes, and traveling along the tympanic segment of the facial nerve ➡ to become the middle meningeal artery ➡.* (Right) *Axial bone CT shows absence of the right foramen spinosum ➡ posterolateral to the normal foramen ovale ➡. PSA ➡ is seen arising from the petrous carotid canal ➡, termed the hyoido-stapedial artery.*

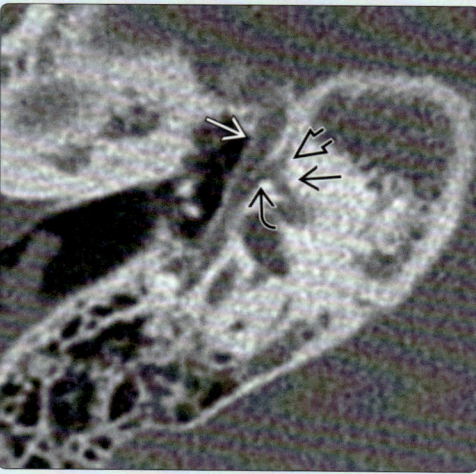
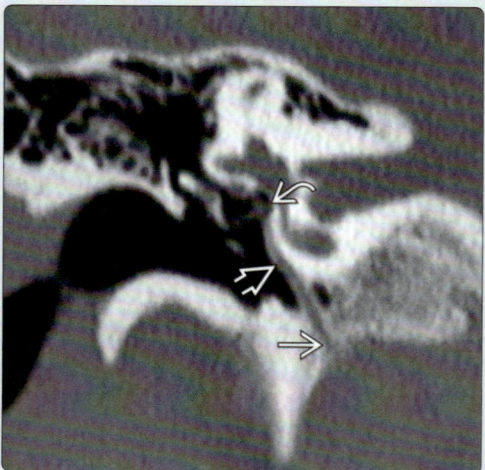

(Left) *Axial oblique bone CT shows the distal PSA ➡ extending from the anterior tympanic CNVII canal. The N sign is created by the PSA and inverse V of the labyrinthine ➡, geniculate ➡, and proximal tympanic ➡ CNVII canal.* (Right) *Coronal bone CT demonstrates the PSA arising from the genu of the petrous internal carotid artery ➡, ascending on the cochlear promontory ➡, and passing through the crura of the stapes ➡ on its way to join the tympanic segment of the facial nerve canal. (Courtesy K. Funk, MD.)*

TERMINOLOGY

Abbreviations

- Persistent stapedial artery (PSA)

Definitions

- Rare congenital vascular anomaly in which embryologic stapedial artery persists

IMAGING

General Features

- Best diagnostic clue
  - Absent foramen spinosum of skull base and enlargement of anterior tympanic segment facial nerve (CNVII) canal
- Location
  - PSA runs over promontory, courses through obturator foramen of stapes, enters tympanic CNVII canal through gap in its wall just posterior to cochleariform process, and exits middle ear to give rise to middle meningeal artery (MMA)
  - Frequently bilateral
- Size
  - PSA is typically ≤ 1 mm; requires high-resolution imaging and attention to detail

CT Findings

- Bone CT
  - **Absent** ipsilateral **foramen spinosum**
  - PSA leaves carotid through small canaliculus from posterior bony carotid canal (hyoido-stapedial artery)
  - PSA arises from inferior tympanic artery through inferior tympanic canaliculus (pharyngo-stapedial artery)
  - Curvilinear structure crosses over cochlear promontory
  - **Anterior tympanic segment** of CNVII canal enlarged; enlargement can be subtle
    - Separate parallel canal possible
    - N sign: On axial anterior tympanic canal of PSA combined with inverse V shape of CNVII canal near geniculate ganglion
    - 3-eyed snail sign: On coronal anterior tympanic canal of PSA lateral to tympanic and labyrinthine CNVII canal segments above cochlea
  - PSA seen in isolation or in conjunction with **aberrant internal carotid artery** (AbICA)

Angiographic Findings

- External carotid artery (ECA) arteriogram
  - Shows absence of normal proximal MMA
  - PSA may arise from inferior tympanic artery
- Internal carotid artery (ICA) arteriogram: PSA arising from infracochlear petrous ICA or from AbICA

Imaging Recommendations

- Best imaging tool
  - Axial and coronal temporal bone CT

DIFFERENTIAL DIAGNOSIS

Aberrant Internal Carotid Artery

- Absent carotid plate and vascular retrotympanic structure contiguous with ICA

Facial Nerve Venous Malformation ("Hemangioma")

- Bone CT: Intralesional ossification (50%)
- T1 C+ MR: Enhancing mass in geniculate fossa

Facial Nerve Schwannoma

- Bone CT: Tubular or focal enlargement of CNVII canal
- T1 C+ MR: Mass enhancing in CNVII canal

Perineural Parotid Malignancy, Mastoid CNVII

- Bone CT: Enlarged mastoid segment of CNVII canal
- T1 C+ MR: Enhancing tumor coming up from parotid

PATHOLOGY

General Features

- Etiology
  - Embryonic stapedial artery resides in middle ear cavity and forms communication between ICA and ECA branches
  - Stapedial artery **typically involutes** in 10th week of gestation
  - Failure to involute leads to persistent aberrant vessel in middle ear and represents abnormal arterial communication between ICA and MMA
- Associated abnormalities
  - **AbICA**

CLINICAL ISSUES

Presentation

- Most common signs/symptoms
  - Most cases are asymptomatic and discovered incidentally on imaging or at surgery
  - Can be associated with pulsatile tinnitus and conductive hearing loss
  - Can be associated with AbICA
  - If encountered surgically, may limit exposure of the stapes; can lead to intraoperative hemorrhage

Demographics

- Age
  - Congenital; may be discovered at any age
- Epidemiology
  - Very rare lesion: 0.02-0.48% of population

Treatment

- **No treatment** is best treatment
- Surgical ligation, coagulation, laser ablation may be considered

DIAGNOSTIC CHECKLIST

Consider

- If **AbICA** discovered, look for associated **PSA**
- Check for absence of foramen spinosum and subtle enlargement of tympanic CNVII canal
- High-resolution imaging and attention to detail required

SELECTED REFERENCES

1. Kumar R et al: Detecting causes of pulsatile tinnitus on CT arteriography-venography: a pictorial review. Eur J Radiol. 139:109722, 2021
2. LoVerde ZJ et al: The many faces of persistent stapedial artery: CT findings and embryologic explanations. AJNR Am J Neuroradiol. 42(1):160-6, 2021

TERMINOLOGY

- Acute coalescent otomastoiditis (ACOM): Acute middle ear-mastoid infection with progressive bony resorption and demineralization due to intramastoid empyema ± osteomyelitis

IMAGING

- Bone CT findings: Mastoid cortex ± trabecula erosions (coalescent otomastoiditis)
- CECT or enhanced MR findings of **ACOM complications**
  - **Subperiosteal abscess**: Periauricular fluid collection
  - **Bezold abscess**: Walled-off pus in and around sternocleidomastoid muscle
  - **Middle cranial fossa abscess** (epidural or temporal lobe abscess)
  - **Posterior fossa abscess** (epidural or cerebellar abscess)
  - **Thrombosed sigmoid sinus ± internal jugular vein**

TOP DIFFERENTIAL DIAGNOSES

- Acquired cholesteatoma
- Apical petrositis
- Temporal bone Langerhans histiocytosis
- Temporal bone rhabdomyosarcoma/metastasis

PATHOLOGY

- Common pathophysiology
  - Granulation tissue or cholesteatoma blocks aditus ad antrum and prevents mastoid air cell drainage
- Less common pathophysiology
  - Mastoid cortex remains intact with septic thrombophlebitis of **emissary veins** seeding periosteum

CLINICAL ISSUES

- Young child with days to weeks history of otalgia, postauricular swelling, fever, and otorrhea

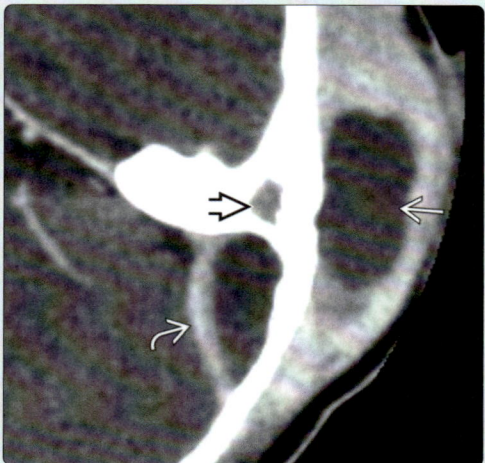
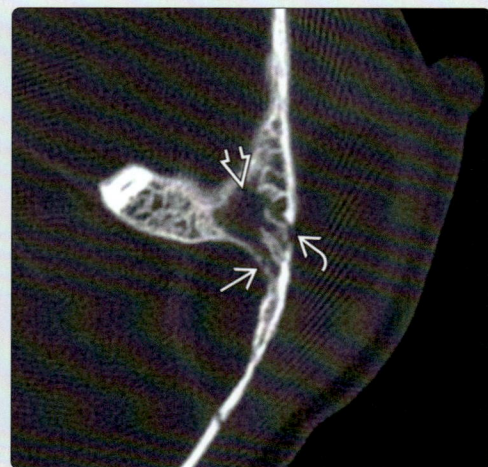

(Left) Axial CECT in a patient with a postauricular tender mass, headache, and fever reveals postauricular abscess ➡ and coalescent otomastoiditis ➡, resulting in epidural extension of infection with nonthrombosed sigmoid sinus ➡. (Right) Axial bone CT of the same patient shows loss of mastoid trabecula ➡ and demineralized sigmoid plate ➡, diagnostic of coalescent otomastoiditis. Subtle erosion of the lateral mastoid cortex ➡ indicates continuity of mastoid infection with the postauricular abscess.

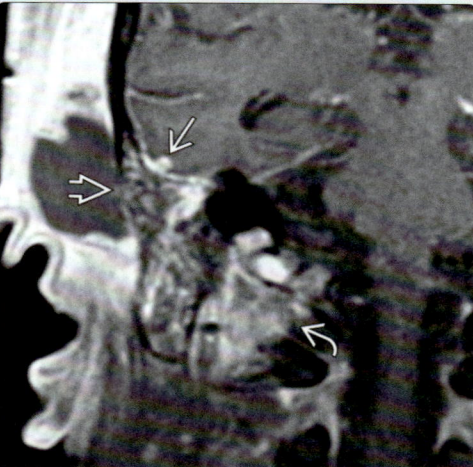
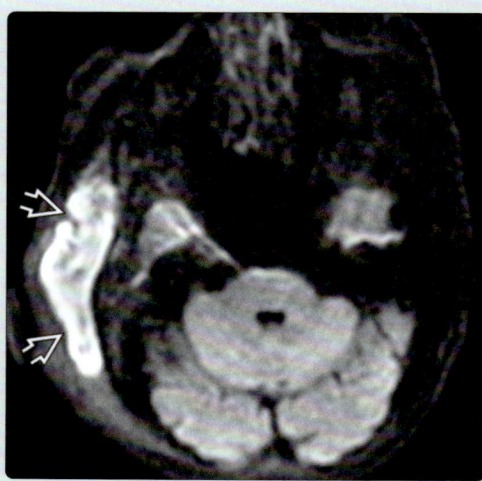

(Left) Coronal T1WI C+ FS MR reveals mastoid enhancement with a large periauricular abscess. Lateral mastoid is focally dehiscent ➡ with thick and enhancing proximal meninges ➡. Subjacent skull base demonstrates abnormal enhancement ➡, indicating extensive associated skull base osteomyelitis. (Right) Axial DWI MR of the same patient reveals restricted diffusion within the extensive periauricular abscess ➡. (Courtesy N. Fischbein, MD.)

Coalescent Otomastoiditis With Complications

TERMINOLOGY

Abbreviations
- Acute coalescent otomastoiditis (ACOM)
- Acute otomastoiditis (AOM)

Synonyms
- Coalescent otomastoiditis with abscess

Definitions
- ACOM: Acute middle ear-mastoid (ME-M) infection with progressive bony resorption and demineralization due to intramastoid empyema ± osteomyelitis
- ACOM + abscess: Coalescent otomastoiditis with resultant **intracranial** or **extracranial** abscess
- AOM: Acute infection in ME-M without destruction of mastoid septations or cortex

IMAGING

General Features
- Best diagnostic clue
  - Rim-enhancing fluid collection adjacent to eroded mastoid cortex + mastoid air cell opacification ± internal gas/air
- Location
  - Abscess adjacent to mastoid cortical dehiscence
    - **Lateral mastoid wall**
      - Postauricular (thin cortical bone) abscess
      - Pre- or periauricular abscess
    - **Inferior mastoid wall**
      - Mastoid tip → Bezold abscess
      - Other remaining inferior mastoid cortical dehiscence → transspatial abscess
    - **Tegmen mastoideum** → temporal lobe abscess
    - **Medial mastoid wall** → posterior fossa epidural abscess, cerebellar abscess
- Size
  - Variable; usually presents with > 1-cm fluid pocket
- Morphology
  - Crescentic, lentiform, or spherical

CT Findings
- CECT
  - **Subperiosteal abscess**: Periauricular fluid collection
    - Thick, enhancing lateral wall represents inflamed periosteum
  - **Bezold abscess**: Walled-off pus in and around sternocleidomastoid muscle
  - **Middle cranial fossa abscess**
    - Epidural or temporal lobe rim-enhancing fluid
  - **Posterior fossa abscess**
    - Epidural or cerebellar, rim-enhancing fluid
- Bone CT
  - ME-M opacification
  - Variable trabecular and cortical erosions (CT sign of coalescent otomastoiditis)
  - Subtle to grossly **dehiscent cortex** just deep to abscess
    - Lateral mastoid cortex → subperiosteal abscess
    - Mastoid tip cortex → Bezold abscess
    - Tegmen mastoideum cortex → epidural or temporal lobe abscess

- Medial mastoid cortex → epidural or cerebellar abscess
- CTV
  - May show thrombosed sigmoid sinus &/or internal jugular vein (IJV)

MR Findings
- T2WI FS
  - High signal fills ME-M, may be hypointense to CSF
  - High-signal fluid in epidural or parenchymal abscess
  - Low signal intensity in sigmoid sinus or IJV if thrombus present
- DWI
  - Decreased diffusion in abscess
- T1WI C+ FS
  - Variable enhancement of ME-M
  - Rim-enhancing pus in extracranial subperiosteal, intracranial epidural, or parenchymal abscess
  - Filling defect(s) in sigmoid sinus &/or IJV if thrombus present
- MRV
  - May show dural sinus/venous thrombosis (DST/DVT)

Imaging Recommendations
- Best imaging tool
  - Temporal bone CT defines bony changes (coalescence, cortical dehiscence)
    - CECT will define most infectious complications
  - Enhanced temporal bone MR more sensitive for intracranial complications (DST, meningitis, subdural empyema, parenchymal abscess)
- Protocol advice
  - Section thickness small (≤ 3 mm) for enhanced MR

DIFFERENTIAL DIAGNOSIS

Acquired Cholesteatoma
- Clinical: Retraction or rupture of tympanic membrane; may be superinfected
- Imaging: CT shows erosive mass; MR shows nonenhancing mass with decreased diffusion
- When associated with ACOM, may also cause extracranial or intracranial abscess

Apical Petrositis
- Clinical: CNVI palsy, retroauricular pain, AOM
- Imaging: CT shows coalescent changes in pneumatized petrous apex
  - T1WI C+ MR shows enhancing meninges and focal, walled-off fluid in petrous apex
- In young patients, may rarely see osteomyelitis in nonpneumatized petrous apex → marrow enhancement + narrowed, petrous internal carotid artery

Temporal Bone Langerhans Histiocytosis
- Clinical: Child with otorrhea and periauricular mass
- Imaging: Extensive, sometimes bilateral mastoid destruction with enhancing mass
  - Petrous apex &/or middle ear < mastoid

Temporal Bone Rhabdomyosarcoma
- Clinical: Neurologic deficits common, including CNVII palsy

- Imaging: CT shows lytic bone destruction ± intracranial extension
  - T1WI C+ MR shows enhancing soft tissue mass
  - Petrous apex & middle ear cavity > mastoid

Metastasis, Temporal Bone
- Clinical: Otorrhea, otalgia, and periauricular mass
- Imaging: Lytic bone destruction ± mass

PATHOLOGY

General Features
- Etiology
  - Inflammation, granulation tissue, or cholesteatoma blocks aditus ad antrum and prevents mastoid air cell drainage
  - Local hyperemia-acidosis creates enzymatic resorption of trabeculae (coalescent otomastoiditis)
  - Subtle or gross cortical dehiscence conveys infection into adjacent tissues
  - Less common pathophysiology: Mastoid cortex remains intact with septic thrombophlebitis of **emissary veins** seeding periosteum
- MacEwen triangle
  - Surgical access point to mastoid antrum at posterosuperior external auditory canal
  - Weakest bone, loose periosteum facilitates breakout of infection in postauricular location

Gross Pathologic & Surgical Features
- Pus in mastoid, mastoid osteomyelitis, adjacent abscess
- Granulation tissue or **cholesteatoma** occasionally identified in ME-M
  - More common in subacute-chronic disease; requires more extensive surgery

Microscopic Features
- Polymicrobial aerobes and anaerobes
- *Streptococcus* species common

CLINICAL ISSUES

Presentation
- Most common signs/symptoms
  - Otalgia (ear pain) ± otorrhea (ear drainage)
  - Postauricular pain ± swelling
  - Fever
  - Other temporal bone signs/symptoms
    - Lateralized auricle (ear pushed outward by abscess)
    - Hearing loss: Conductive > > sensorineural
  - Intracranial complications
    - Headache, mental status changes, nausea, vomiting, and seizures
    - Nuchal rigidity and photophobia
    - Papilledema
    - CNVI palsy
- Clinical profile
  - Child with days to weeks history of otalgia, postauricular swelling, fever, and otorrhea
  - 35-70% of patients already received antibiotics for AOM
  - Postauricular edema (Griesinger sign) common in uncomplicated AOM (85%)

- Rim-enhancing fluid collection = subperiosteal abscess

Demographics
- Age
  - Infants and young children
  - If complication of acquired cholesteatoma, often older age group affected
- Epidemiology
  - 0.24% of patients with AOM develop ACOM

Natural History & Prognosis
- Isolated extracranial subperiosteal abscess
  - Excellent prognosis with prompt therapy
  - Worse if prior incomplete antibiotic therapy, virulent organism, or immunocompromised host
- Intracranial abscess
  - Epidural abscess most common
  - If concomitant complications, worse prognosis
    - Venous sinus thrombosis
    - Subdural empyema or parenchymal abscess (temporal lobe most common)

Treatment
- IV antibiotics ± tympanocentesis with myringotomy tube placement
- Surgical treatment
  - Incision and drainage of extracranial subperiosteal abscess ± mastoidectomy
- Surgical therapy must be performed with hearing preservation in mind
  - Mastoidectomy for cholesteatoma

DIAGNOSTIC CHECKLIST

Consider
- Seek other complications of ACOM
  - Temporal bone findings (T1WI C+ MR)
    - Facial nerve paralysis shows as enhancing CNVII
    - Labyrinthitis shows as enhancement within membranous labyrinth
    - Apical petrositis (enhancing apical air cells on MR)
  - Intracranial findings (T1WI C+ MR)
    - Subdural empyema, meningitis, brain abscess ± dural sinus, or IJV thrombosis

Image Interpretation Pearls
- MR used to distinguish between hyperintense perisinus epidural abscess and hypointense DST
- Epidural abscess is elliptical; DST is rounded/triangular

SELECTED REFERENCES

1. Singh S et al: Pediatric head and neck emergencies. Neuroradiology. 66(11):2053-70, 2024
2. O'Brien WT Sr: Common neck and otomastoid infections in children. Neuroimaging Clin N Am. 33(4):661-71, 2023
3. Stein JM et al: Imaging of head and neck infections. Neuroimaging Clin N Am. 33(1):185-206, 2023
4. Saat R et al: Detection of coalescent acute mastoiditis on MRI in comparison with CT. Clin Neuroradiol. 31(3):589-97, 2020
5. Saat R et al: Comparison of MR imaging findings in paediatric and adult patients with acute mastoiditis and incidental intramastoid bright signal on T2-weighted images. Eur Radiol. 26(8):2632-9, 2016
6. Saat R et al: MR imaging features of acute mastoiditis and their clinical relevance. AJNR Am J Neuroradiol. 36(2):361-7, 2015

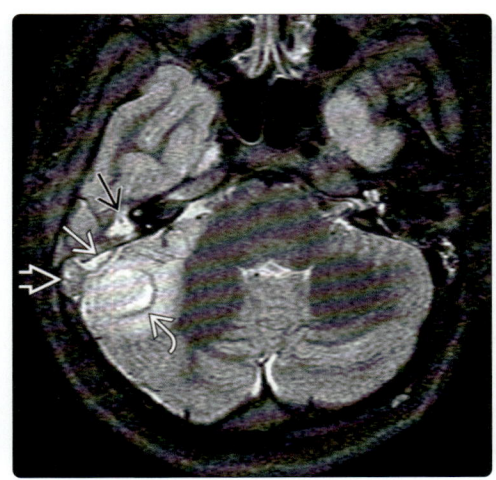
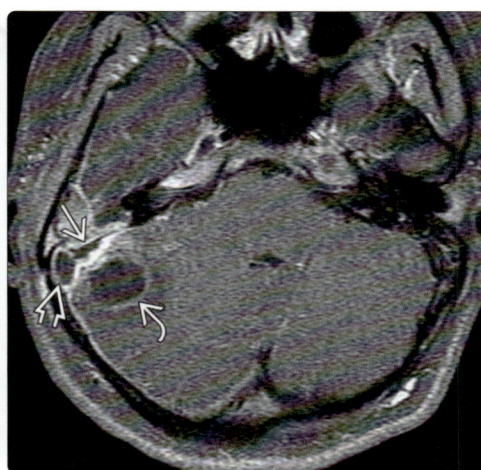

(Left) *Axial T2WI FS MR in a 15-year-old girl with mastoid tenderness and headache reveals a hyperintense epidural abscess ➡ adjacent to the mastoid cortex, hypointense sigmoid sinus thrombus ⇒, and cerebellar abscess ➡ with a hypointense rim and surrounding edema. There is fluid within adjacent mastoid air cells ⇨. **(Right)** Axial T1WI C+ MR in the same patient shows the epidural abscess ➡, sigmoid sinus thrombus ⇒, and cerebellar abscess ➡, all as hypointense with peripheral enhancement.*

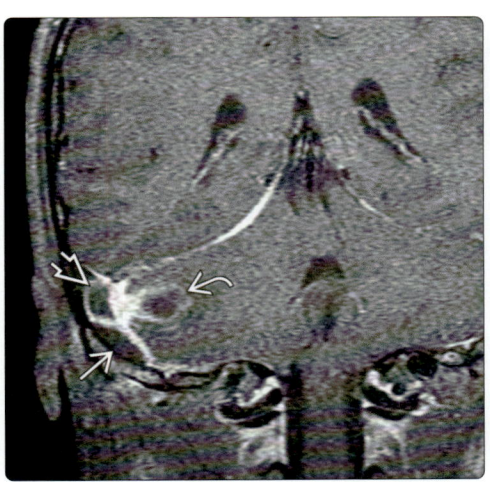
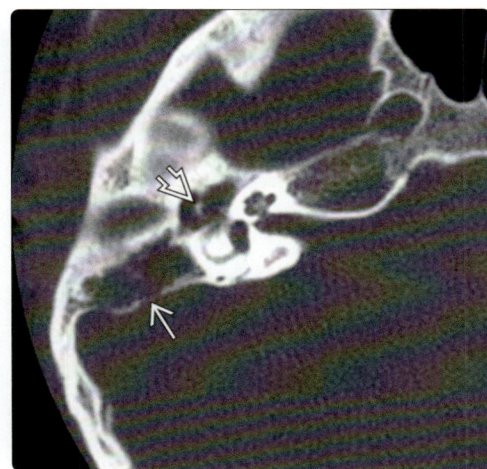

(Left) *Coronal T1WI C+ FS MR in the same patient shows the elliptical epidural abscess ➡ sitting beneath the oval thrombosed sigmoid sinus ⇒. The cerebellar abscess ➡ is again seen, as well as dural and tentorial enhancement. **(Right)** Axial temporal bone CT shows opacification of the middle ear space and mastoid air cells with erosion of the posterior mastoid cortex ➡ and ossicles ⇒, consistent with coalescent otomastoiditis and cholesteatoma, both confirmed at surgery.*

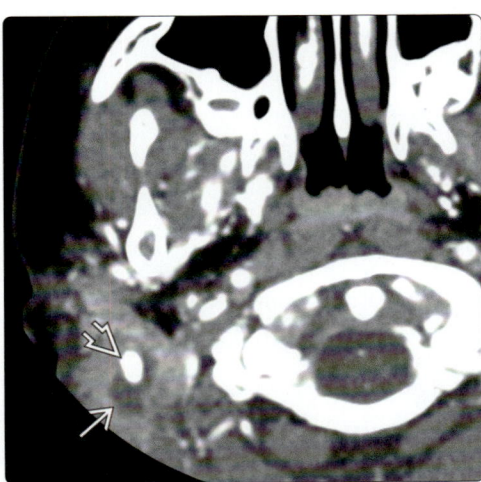
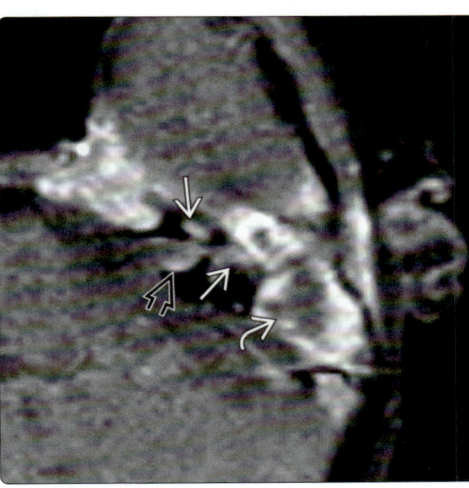

(Left) *Axial CECT in an 11-year-old girl with coalescent otomastoiditis shows low attenuation ➡ surrounding the mastoid process ⇒ and extending along the sternocleidomastoid muscle, which is consistent with a Bezold abscess. **(Right)** Axial T1WI C+ MR in a different patient reveals acute otomastoiditis with a coalescent area of mastoid suppuration ➡. There are areas of abnormal extracranial and intracranial enhancement to include within the IAC ⇨ and labyrinthine structures ➡.*

Chronic Otomastoiditis With Ossicular Erosions

TERMINOLOGY

- Synonyms: Noncholesteatomatous ossicular erosion; postinflammatory ossicular erosion
- Definition: Erosive changes involving ossicles in absence of cholesteatoma in patient with history of chronic otomastoiditis (COM)

IMAGING

- Axial bone CT
  - **Posterior line of "2 parallel lines" of ossicular chain is absent (subtotal or total)**
  - ± fibrous tissue replacement of incudostapedial joint
  - Incudostapedial joint appears widened on axial CT
  - Erosion of "cone" (incus body/short process) may occur
  - Associated findings of chronic otitis media
    - Underpneumatization of mastoid air cells
    - Inflammatory debris in middle ear and mastoid
- Coronal bone CT
  - **Vertical segment of "right angle" missing**

- – Long process of incus most commonly absent/eroded
  - Tympanic membrane retraction often present
- Limited role of MR in diagnosis/evaluation
  - Acute or complicated COM
  - Differentiation of cholesteatoma from inflammatory debris using non-EPI DWI if CT is equivocal

TOP DIFFERENTIAL DIAGNOSES

- Mild congenital external ear malformation, acquired cholesteatoma + ossicular erosion, congenital middle ear cholesteatoma + ossicular erosion, postoperative ossicular loss, posttraumatic ossicular dislocation

PATHOLOGY

- COM initially causes periostitis and osteitis
- Subsequent osteoclasia and decalcification → bone loss

CLINICAL ISSUES

- Clinical presentation: Chronic otitis media history
  - Postinflammatory conductive hearing loss

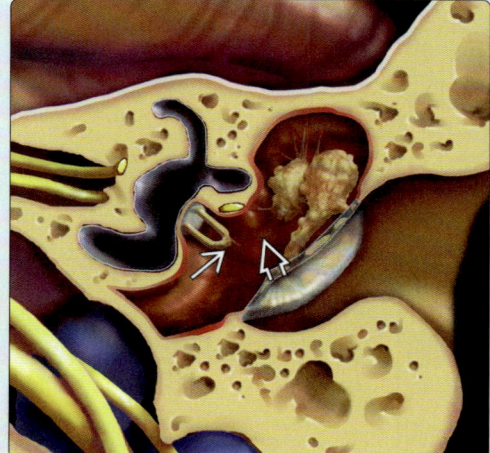
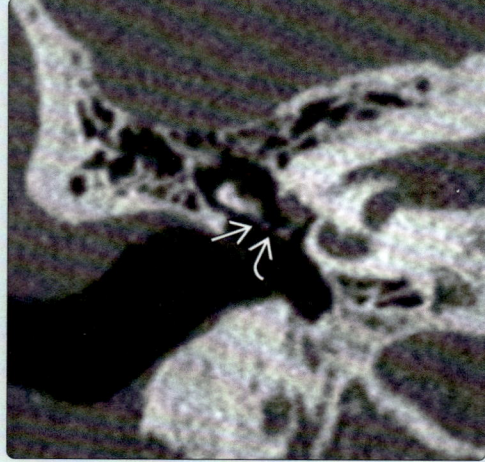

(Left) Coronal graphic of the left ear shows postinflammatory ossicular erosion of the incus long process ➡ and stapes hub ➡. Note tympanosclerosis changes of the tympanic membrane and remaining ossicles. (Right) Coronal bone CT shows thinning of the incus long process with distal resorption ➡, resulting in a missing vertical segment of the "right angle" ➡ between the incus and stapes. Ossicular chain discontinuity results in conductive hearing loss in this case of chronic otomastoiditis (COM) with ossicular erosion.

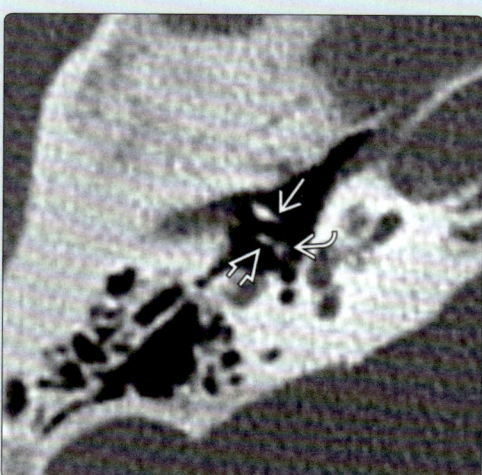
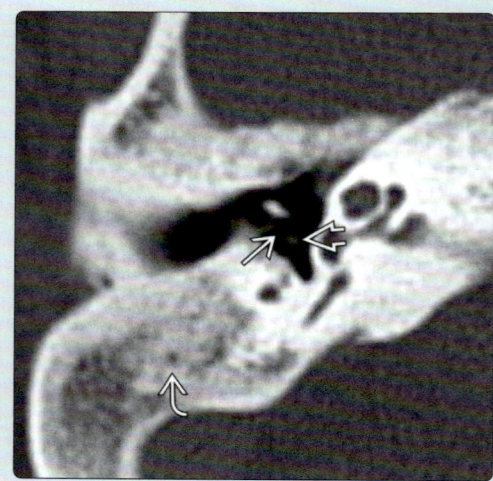

(Left) Axial bone CT through the mesotympanum shows a normal configuration of an ossicular chain with "2 parallel lines," representing a tensor tympani tendon attachment site at the malleus neck ➡ anteriorly and incus lenticular process ➡, incudostapedial joint, and head of stapes ➡ posteriorly. (Right) Axial bone CT in COM shows absent "parallel lines" with eroded long process of incus ➡ and thickened head of stapes ➡. Note a sclerotic, underpneumatized mastoid ➡, a secondary finding that can be seen with COM.

TERMINOLOGY

Abbreviations
- Chronic otomastoiditis (COM)

Synonyms
- Noncholesteatomatous ossicular erosion; postinflammatory ossicular erosion

Definitions
- Erosive changes involving ossicles in absence of cholesteatoma in patient with history of COM

IMAGING

CT Findings
- Bone CT
  - Understanding ossicular chain normal anatomy is critical for making this imaging diagnosis
    - Axial CT (epitympanum): **"Ice cream cone"**
      - Anterior "ice cream" = malleus head
      - Posterior "cone" = incus body/short process
    - Axial CT (mesotympanum): **"2 parallel lines"**
      - Anterior line = tensor tympani tendon leading to malleus neck
      - Posterior line = incus lenticular process, incudostapedial joint (ISJ), and stapes head
    - Coronal CT through long process incus: Ossicular **"right angle"**
      - Vertically oriented incus long process
      - Horizontally oriented incus lenticular process
  - Axial bone CT images
    - Absence of part of posterior line of "2 parallel lines"
      - ISJ may be replaced by fibrous tissue
      - ISJ appears widened on axial CT
    - Erosion of "cone" (incus body/short process)
  - Coronal bone CT images
    - Long process of incus most commonly absent
      - **Vertical segment of "right angle" missing**
    - Tympanic membrane retraction often present
    - ± tympanic segment facial nerve canal dehiscence
  - Mastoid underpneumatization common

Imaging Recommendations
- Best imaging tool
  - Axial and coronal temporal bone CT
  - MR imaging has niche roles in this setting
    - Complicated COM or acute otitis media is present
    - Differentiation of cholesteatoma from inflammatory debris using non-EPI DWI if CT is equivocal

DIFFERENTIAL DIAGNOSIS

Mild Congenital External Ear Malformation
- Congenital hearing loss; microtia
- CT: Rotation ± fusion of ossicles

Acquired Cholesteatoma + Ossicular Erosion
- CT: Nondependent soft tissue mass associated with bone erosion
  - Perforated or retracted tympanic membrane

Congenital Middle Ear Cholesteatoma + Ossicular Erosion
- CT: Soft tissue usually medial to ossicles
- Focal ossicular erosion associated

Postoperative Ossicular Loss
- Evidence for mastoidectomy/atticotomy
- CT: Stapedectomy for otosclerosis most commonly

Posttraumatic Ossicular Dislocation
- Fractured, dislocated ossicle may appear absent

PATHOLOGY

General Features
- Etiology
  - COM initiates ossicular loss; initial phase: Periostitis and osteitis
  - Subsequent **osteoclasia and decalcification → bone loss**
  - Incus is most vulnerable portion of ossicular chain due to anatomic position and tenuous blood supply

CLINICAL ISSUES

Presentation
- Most common signs/symptoms
  - Postinflammatory **conductive hearing loss**
    - Usually long history of chronic otitis media

Demographics
- Epidemiology: Very common clinical and CT entity

Natural History & Prognosis
- Surgical repair results variable
- Relates to severity of ossicular loss and associated tympanic membrane status
  - Involved malleus = predictor of postoperative hearing outcome, independent of stapes damage

Treatment
- Exploratory tympanotomy with ossicular reconstruction

DIAGNOSTIC CHECKLIST

Consider
- In patients with conductive hearing loss
  - Look for ossicular loss with COM
  - Then consider other diagnoses
    - **Cholesteatoma if nonenhancing soft tissue "mass" associated with ossicular erosion**
    - Ossicular malformation in **mild external auditory canal (EAC) malformation**

Image Interpretation Pearls
- Absence of segment of ossicular chain
  - Common CT finding; easily overlooked

SELECTED REFERENCES

1. Fadda G et al: Factors influencing audiologic outcomes in ossiculoplasty for chronic otitis media: a prospective multicentre study. Acta Otorhinolaryngol Ital. 44(6):400-11, 2024
2. Kuru A et al: Bone mineral density of the incus body and long process in patients with chronic otitis media and its relationship with functional outcome in type II tympanoplasty. Acta Otolaryngol. 144(3):233-6, 2024

Chronic Otomastoiditis With Tympanosclerosis

TERMINOLOGY

- Definition: Calcific, bony, or fibrous middle ear foci usually due to suppurative chronic otomastoiditis (COM)

IMAGING

- Bone CT: Common locations of tympanosclerotic **calcification**
  - Tympanic membrane
  - Ossicle surface
  - Stapes footplate
  - Muscle tendons
  - Ossicle ligaments
- Focal tympanosclerotic **ossifications**
  - May be seen anywhere in middle-ear mastoid
- COM findings associated

TOP DIFFERENTIAL DIAGNOSES

- Chronic otitis media
- COM with ossicular erosions
- COM with ossicular fixation
- Fenestral otosclerosis
- Ossicular prosthesis

PATHOLOGY

- Etiology: Healing response to repeated inflammatory events in middle-ear mastoid
- True tympanosclerosis: Diffuse hyalinization & deposition of calcium & phosphate crystals
- New bone formation (osteoneogenesis)

CLINICAL ISSUES

- Clinical presentation
  - Severe conductive hearing loss + history of COM
  - Conductive hearing loss out of proportion to inflammatory debris
- Treatment options
  - Atticotomy with mobilization of ossicles
  - Insertion of prosthesis or homograft device

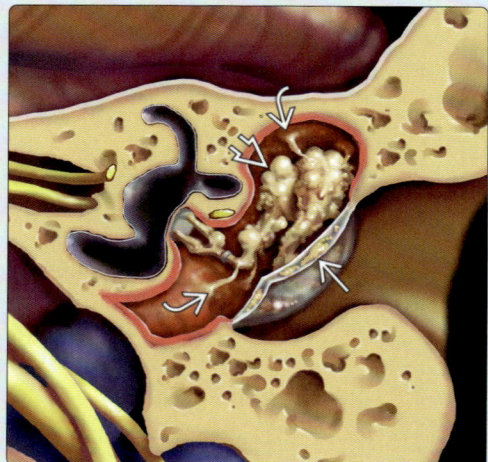
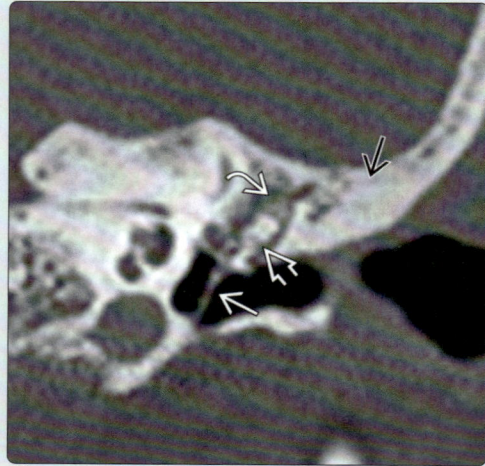

(Left) Coronal graphic shows severe tympanosclerosis in the setting of chronic otomastoiditis. Postinflammatory calcification can be seen in the tympanic membrane ➡, ossicles ➡, and ossicle suspensory ligaments ➡. (Right) Coronal bone CT shows amorphous calcific debris within the middle ear cavity ➡, irregular ossicular surfaces ➡, and partially calcified tympanic membrane ➡, consistent with tympanosclerosis. Note an underpneumatized mastoid ➡ in this patient with chronic otomastoiditis.

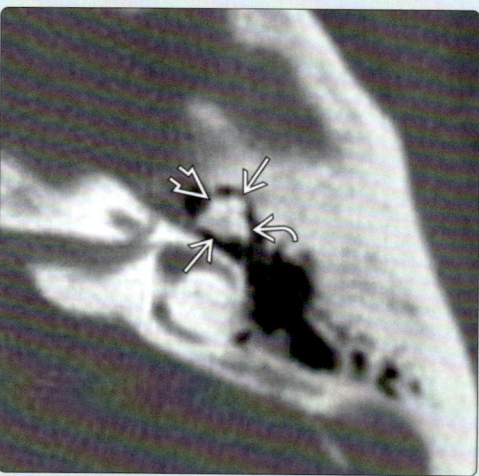
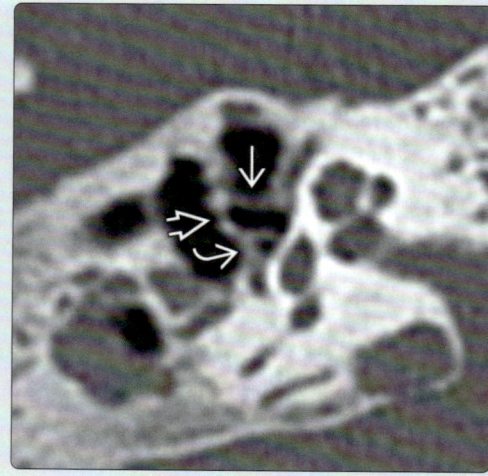

(Left) Axial bone CT in a patient with profound conductive hearing loss due to tympanosclerosis shows exuberant calcification ➡ along the malleus head ➡ and incus body/short process ➡, encasing the incudomallear joint. (Right) Axial bone CT demonstrates more subtle findings of tympanosclerosis, including increased density and thickening of the tensor tympani tendon ➡ and stapes crura ➡. There is an additional possible region of ankylosis ➡ between the malleus and incus.

Chronic Otomastoiditis With Tympanosclerosis

TERMINOLOGY

Abbreviations
- Chronic otomastoiditis (COM) with tympanosclerosis

Synonyms
- COM with focal calcification or ossification
- Postinflammatory ossicular fixation

Definitions
- Calcific, bony, or fibrous middle ear foci typically due to suppurative COM, much less commonly trauma

IMAGING

General Features
- Best diagnostic clue
  - Bone CT shows high-density foci in middle-ear mastoid (ME-M) associated with sporadic inflammatory debris
  - Calcific "**sprinkles**" on "**ice cream**" (malleus head) & "**cone**" (incus body/short process)

CT Findings
- Bone CT
  - Common locations of tympanosclerotic calcification
    - **Tympanic membrane**
    - **Ossicle surface**
    - **Stapes footplate**
      - □ Crura & footplate thickened
    - **Muscle tendons**
      - □ Stapedius & tensor tympani muscles
    - **Ossicle ligaments**
    - Mastoid air cells
  - Focal tympanosclerotic **ossifications**
    - Heaped-up new bone (osteoneogenesis)
    - May occur anywhere in ME-M
  - COM findings
    - Heterogeneous soft tissue (inflammatory) ME-M
    - Underpneumatized mastoid

DIFFERENTIAL DIAGNOSIS

Chronic Otitis Media
- Clinical: Conductive hearing loss (CHL) variable
  - COM history
- CT: Patchy, nondestructive middle ear debris
  - Debris not calcific or ossific

Chronic Otomastoiditis With Ossicular Erosions
- Clinical: COM + CHL
- CT: Ossicle loss ± inflammatory debris

Chronic Otomastoiditis With Ossicular Fixation
- Clinical: COM + CHL
- CT: Focal ossicle ankylosis
  - May have component of tympanosclerosis

Fenestral Otosclerosis
- Clinical: No history of COM (well-pneumatized mastoid)
- CT: Lucency at fissula ante fenestram
  - Thickened otic capsule anterior to oval window

PATHOLOGY

General Features
- Etiology
  - Healing response to repeated inflammatory events
    - Chronic inflammation → hypoxic ME-M environment → free radicals → local tissue injury → hyaline degeneration & calcification → tissue sclerosis
  - True calcific tympanosclerosis
    - Diffuse hyalinization & deposition of calcium & phosphate crystals
  - Ossific tympanosclerosis
    - New bone formation (osteoneogenesis)
- Associated abnormalities
  - Formed by fused collagenous fibers
    - Calcium & phosphate crystal deposits harden fibers

Staging, Grading, & Classification
- 3 types of **postinflammatory ossicular fixation**
  - **Fibrous tissue fixation**
    - No calcification
  - **True calcific tympanosclerosis**
    - Multiple small calcifications
  - **Ossific tympanosclerosis**
    - New bone formation (osteoneogenesis)

Microscopic Features
- Calcification of previously hyalinized mucoperiosteum
- Onion skin-like lamellar arrangement

CLINICAL ISSUES

Presentation
- Most common signs/symptoms
  - Severe CHL + COM history
- Other signs/symptoms
  - Otoscopy: Thick, opaque tympanic membrane

Demographics
- Age
  - Average age at diagnosis = 35 years
- Epidemiology
  - 10% of patients with **suppurative** COM develop tympanosclerosis

Treatment
- Atticotomy with mobilization of ossicles
  - Patients with less ossicular disease have better postsurgical hearing outcome
- Insertion of prosthesis or homograft device

DIAGNOSTIC CHECKLIST

Image Interpretation Pearls
- Look for calcific "**sprinkles**" on "**ice cream**" (malleus head) & "**cone**" (incus body/short process) in CHL patient

SELECTED REFERENCES

1. Larem A et al: Reliability of high-resolution CT scan in diagnosis of ossicular tympanosclerosis. Laryngoscope Investig Otolaryngol. 6(3):540-8, 2021
2. Yildiz S et al: Is ossicular chain fixation predictable for tympanosclerosis on preoperative temporal bone computed tomography? Eur Arch Otorhinolaryngol. 278(8):2789-94, 2021

Pars Flaccida Cholesteatoma

TERMINOLOGY

- Pars flaccida cholesteatoma (PFC)
- Attic or Prussak space cholesteatoma

IMAGING

- T-bone CT: Smaller PFC
  - Opacified Prussak space + scutum and ossicle erosions
- T-bone CT: Larger PFC
  - Look for lateral semicircular canal, facial nerve canal, and tegmen tympani ± mastoideum dehiscence
  - Exclude sinus tympani extension (associated with high postoperative recurrence rate)
- MR with non-echo-planar DWI most sensitive tool; troubleshoots issues raised by bone CT
  - Cholesteatoma is **light bulb bright** on DWI
  - Non-echo-planar DWI far superior to conventional echo-planar DWI
  - May obviate need for exploratory surgery in high-risk retraction pockets or 2nd-look revision surgery

TOP DIFFERENTIAL DIAGNOSES

- Acquired pars tensa cholesteatoma
- Congenital middle ear cholesteatoma
- Middle ear cholesterol granuloma
- Tympanic paraganglioma

PATHOLOGY

- Starts at pars flaccida of tympanic membrane (TM)
- Microscopically consists of exfoliated keratin within stratified squamous epithelium

CLINICAL ISSUES

- Most common type of cholesteatoma (**80%** of all acquired cholesteatomas)
- Patient with chronic middle ear inflammatory disease, conductive hearing loss, and TM abnormality
  - TM retraction: PFC **not** visible; CT makes diagnosis if ossicle or bone loss, light bulb bright on DWI MR
  - TM perforation: PFC visible; diagnosis known

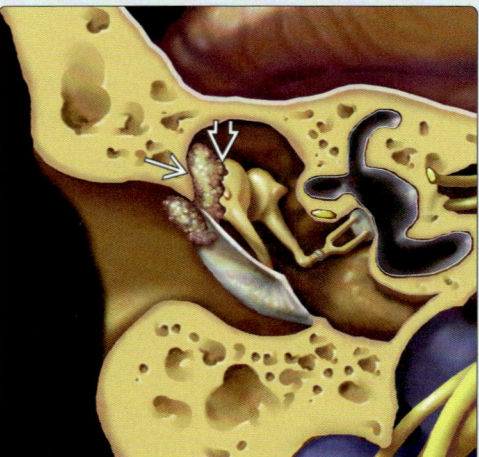
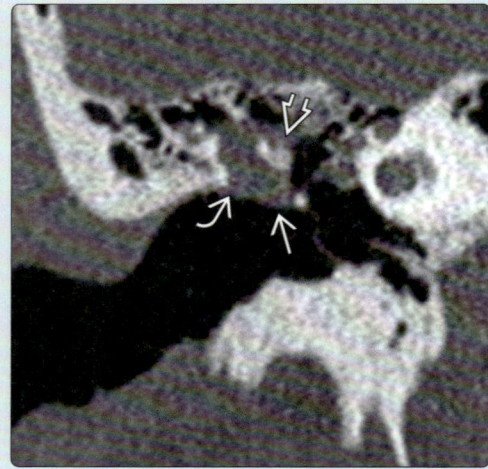

(Left) Coronal graphic shows small cholesteatoma originating at the pars flaccida portion of the tympanic membrane with filling of the Prussak space ➡. Slight erosion ➡ with medial displacement of the head of malleus is present. (Right) Coronal bone CT shows soft tissue within the Prussak space ➡ extending lateral to the ossicles. Note erosions of the scutum ➡ and ossicles ➡, the classic appearance of acquired pars flaccida cholesteatoma (PFC).

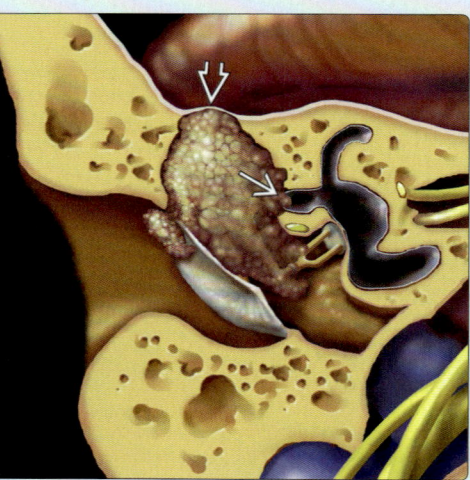
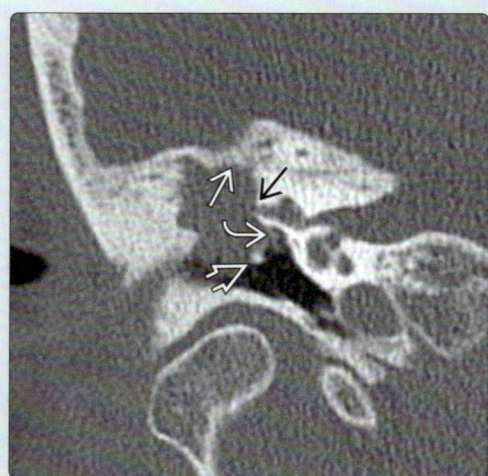

(Left) Coronal graphic shows a large PFC. Complications include erosion of ossicles, dehiscence of the lateral semicircular canal ➡, and scalloping of the tegmen tympani ➡. (Right) Coronal NECT shows a large PFC that fills the middle ear. There is irregular demineralization of the tegmen tympani ➡ as well as marked erosion and medialization of the remnant ossicles ➡. There is demineralization of the tympanic segment facial nerve canal ➡ and dehiscence of the lateral semicircular canal ➡.

Pars Flaccida Cholesteatoma

TERMINOLOGY

Abbreviations
- Pars flaccida cholesteatoma (PFC)

Synonyms
- Attic or Prussak space cholesteatoma
- Primary acquired cholesteatoma

Definitions
- Nonneoplastic mass-like accumulation of exfoliated keratin within stratified squamous epithelium, Prussak space origin

IMAGING

General Features
- Best diagnostic clue
  - Soft tissue mass starts in Prussak space with scutum, ossicle, or lateral epitympanum wall erosion
- Location
  - From Prussak space, spreads to posterior epitympanum, posterior mesotympanum and, less commonly, anterior epitympanum
- Size
  - From millimeters (early) to centimeters (late)
  - If neglected, may fill middle ear (ME) cavity and beyond
- Morphology
  - Lobular, well-circumscribed ME mass
  - Soft tissue density, nonenhancing
  - Large lesions often associated with scar and effusion; may be less well defined

CT Findings
- CECT
  - **No enhancement of cholesteatoma**
    - Surrounding granulation tissue may enhance
- Bone CT
  - **Small PFC**
    - Soft tissue mass starts in **Prussak space**
    - Ossicular chain erosion in 70%
      - Long process of incus erosion more common than incus body and malleus head erosion
    - Ossicles **medially** displaced
    - Scutum **erosion** common
    - Caveat: Small cholesteatoma without bone erosion can be nonspecific on bone CT
  - **Large PFC**
    - Local extension
      - Superior extension into Prussak space and remaining epitympanum
      - Posterolateral through aditus ad antrum into mastoid antrum
      - Expansion and scalloping of ME and mastoid cavity
    - Important potential bone erosions/complications
      - Lateral semicircular canal/labyrinthine fistula
      - Tegmentum tympani and mastoideum/intracranial extension ± infection
      - CNVII canal, tympanic segment CNVII injury
      - Focal erosions around oval or round window

MR Findings
- T1WI
  - Hypointense ME mass
- T2WI
  - Homogeneously hyperintense ME mass
    - Trapped mastoid secretions often brighter than PFC
- DWI
  - Characteristically **light bulb bright**: Hyperintense at high B values, may show true **reduced diffusivity**, as in other types of cholesteatoma or epidermoid
  - Non-echo-planar (e.g., HASTE) DWI and small FOV DWI preparations (e.g., ZOOMit or FOCUS) are superior to conventional echo-planar (EPI) DWI
    - May obviate need for exploratory surgery in high-risk retraction pockets or 2nd-look revision surgery
    - Traditional EPI DWI limited in T-bone by susceptibility, motion, and ghosting artifacts
    - Newer EPI DWI with segmented or multishot EPI prep (e.g., RESOLVE) superior to conventional EPI DWI
- T1WI C+
  - **PFC itself does not enhance** but commonly shows enhancing peripheral rind of granulation tissue/scar
  - If tegmen erosion present, dural thickening and enhancement overlies bony defect
  - Shows intracranial complications, such as meningitis

Imaging Recommendations
- Best imaging tool
  - T-bone CT with multiplanar reconstruction is 1st-line study; coronal best shows Prussak space, attic, scutum
  - T-bone MR with non-EPI DWI most sensitive and specific tool; complementary to CT
    - Confirm or exclude cholesteatoma with non-EPI DWI if CT is equivocal
    - T1 C+ MR to answer specific issues raised by bone CT
      - Enhancement of labyrinth suggests labyrinthitis
      - Temporal lobe extension, intracranial abscess, meningitis, dural sinus thrombosis
- Protocol advice
  - **Non-EPI DWI more sensitive than EPI DWI prep**
    - Reportedly detects lesion as small as 2 mm

DIFFERENTIAL DIAGNOSIS

Acquired Pars Tensa Cholesteatoma
- Otoscopy: Tympanic membrane (TM) rupture or retraction in posterosuperior pars tensa area
- Less common than pars flaccida (PF) type
- Bone CT: Sinus tympani and facial recess involvement = classic; ossicles pushed laterally

Middle Ear Congenital Cholesteatoma
- Otoscopy: Tan-white mass behind **intact** TM
- Bone CT: Nondependent ME mass
  - Medial to ossicles ± ossicle erosions

Middle Ear Cholesterol Granuloma
- Otoscopy: Retrotympanic "blue" mass
- Bone CT: Ossicular and bony erosions may be similar to cholesteatoma
- MR: **Hyperintense** on T1; no reduced diffusivity

Tympanic Paraganglioma
- Otoscopy: Retrotympanic red, pulsatile mass

- Bone CT: Mass on cochlear promontory; ME floor intact
- MR: T1 C+ shows avidly enhancing tumor

PATHOLOGY

General Features

- Etiology
  - Originates at PF portion of TM
    - PF = small posterosuperior portion of TM
  - Various theories on pathogenesis
    - Squamous metaplasia theory: ME inflammation transforms mucosa
    - Squamous immigration/invasion theory: Lateral TM squamous epithelium migrates to ME via TM perforation
    - Squamous basal hyperplasia/papillary ingrowth theory: Proliferating basal keratinocytes penetrate basement membrane with subepithelial spread
    - Squamous obstruction/vacuum retraction pocket theory: Eustachian tube dysfunction causes ME vacuum effect → retraction pocket and keratin accumulation
    - Mucosal traction theory (**new theory**): Apposition of medial TM surface and mucosa of lateral ossicles → coupling/adhesion, which retracts TM via ME mucociliary clearance yielding keratin accumulation
  - Squamous epithelium + keratin accumulation form cholesteatoma
  - Precursor retraction pocket not required for PF cholesteatoma formation, although commonly seen

Gross Pathologic & Surgical Features

- Pearly tumor composed of soft, waxy, white-gray or pale yellow material
- Chronic inflammatory change always present
- Erosion of ossicles, scutum, and upper part of bony tympanic annulus visible in most cases

Microscopic Features

- Stratified squamous epithelium with anucleated (dead) keratin squames
- Layer of granulation tissue always present when in contact with bone; seems to be cause of bone erosion

CLINICAL ISSUES

Presentation

- Most common signs/symptoms
  - Foul-smelling aural discharge
  - Conductive hearing loss (CHL)
  - Chronic ME inflammatory disease and TM retraction or perforation
- Other signs/symptoms
  - Noise- or pressure-induced vertigo (**Tullio phenomenon**) if lateral semicircular canal dehisced
- Otologic examination
  - TM retraction pocket or perforation at PF
    - If TM perforation: PFC visible by otoscopy
    - If TM retracted: PFC often not visible by otoscopy → imaging diagnosis

Demographics

- Age

  - May occur in children or adults
  - Unusual in children < 4 years
  - Cholesteatoma in children more aggressive
    - Extensive disease and recurrence common
- Epidemiology
  - Most common type of cholesteatoma (**80%** of all **acquired cholesteatomas**)

Natural History & Prognosis

- Progressive ↑ in size of cholesteatoma
  - Increasing destruction of surrounding structures, including ossicular chain, lateral semicircular canal, tegmen tympani
- CNVII involvement, venous sinus thrombosis, and intracranial extension are late complications
- Small cholesteatoma: Excellent for total eradication with normal long-term hearing
- Large cholesteatoma: Residual CHL is possible
- Recurrence rate: 5-10%

Treatment

- Early treatment of retraction pocket with tympanostomy tube may prevent cholesteatoma formation
- Surgeries include transcanal endoscopic ear surgery (TEES), canal-wall up mastoidectomy, & canal-wall down mastoidectomy
  - TM and ossicular reconstruction may be necessary
  - Treatment aimed at clearing cholesteatoma and infection to prevent further damage
  - Hearing improvement is secondary goal

DIAGNOSTIC CHECKLIST

Consider

- 2 clinical presentations for imaging possible cholesteatoma
  - Patient has **visible cholesteatoma**
    - Referrer wants to know extent/complications
  - Patient has **visible TM retraction pocket** + **CHL**
    - Referrer wants to know if cholesteatoma is present **and**, if so, extent of cholesteatoma
    - Caution: If ME soft tissue seen without bone or ossicle erosion, do not suggest cholesteatoma

Image Interpretation Pearls

- When ME and mastoid completely opacified with no ossicular erosion, most likely ME effusion, not cholesteatoma

Reporting Tips

- Sinus tympani extension associated with high postoperative recurrence rate
- Lateral semicircular canal fistula and CNVII canal dehiscence warrant cautious operation

SELECTED REFERENCES

1. Wojciechowski T et al: Radiologic evaluation and clinical assessment of facial sinus in adults and children - computed tomography study. Auris Nasus Larynx. 51(1):189-97, 2024
2. Noschang Lopes da Silva M et al: Residual cholesteatoma after endoscopic-assisted canal wall-up tympanomastoidectomy: a randomized controlled trial. Otol Neurotol. 43(7):803-7, 2022
3. Baba A et al: Preoperative predictive criteria for mastoid extension in pars flaccida cholesteatoma in assessments using temporal bone high-resolution computed tomography. Auris Nasus Larynx. 48(4):609-14, 2021

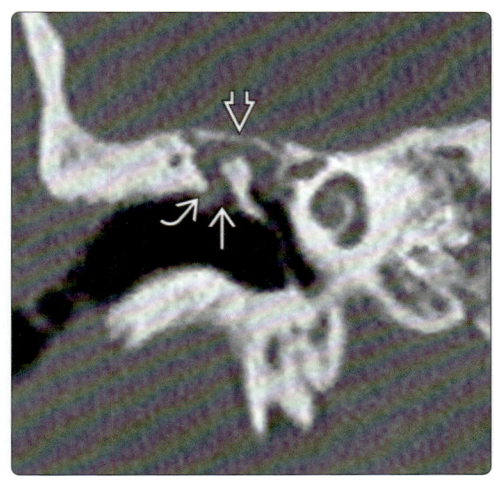

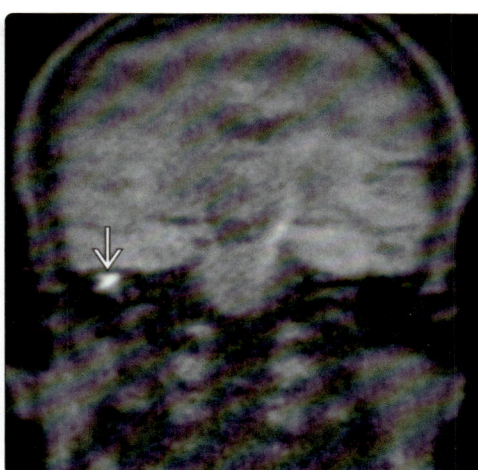

(Left) Coronal NECT in a patient with a retraction pocket on otoscopy shows opacification of the lateral epitympanic recess, Prussak space ➡, and attic. Note subtle blunting of the scutum ➡ and scalloping of tegmen tympani ➡, suspicious for PFC. (Right) Coronal non-echo-planar (EPI) DWI MR in the same patient removes any doubt: This patient has a PFC, which is light bulb bright ➡. Non-EPI DWI is superior to conventional EPI DWI preparations, which are subject to susceptibility, motion, and ghosting artifacts.

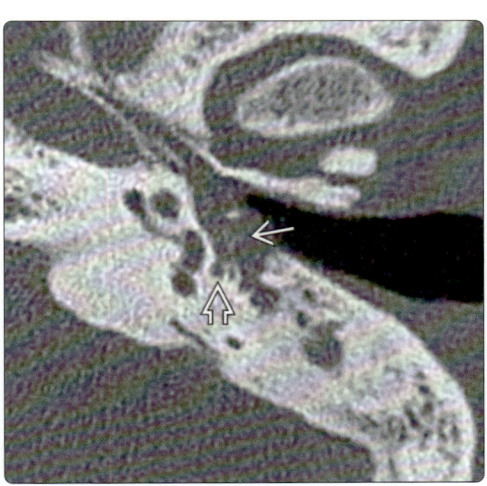

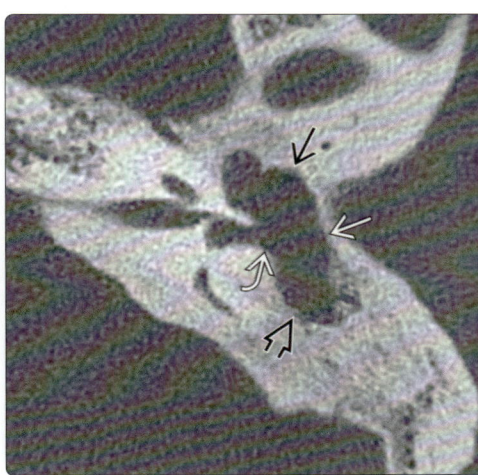

(Left) Axial bone CT demonstrates large PFC filling the mesotympanum with erosion of the incus long process ➡. Note extension into the sinus tympani ➡, which is associated with high postoperative recurrence rate. (Right) Axial bone CT in the same patient shows PFC filling the epitympanum ➡ and mastoid antrum ➡ with expansion of the aditus ad antrum ➡. Note lateral semicircular canal dehiscence ➡, which may lead to labyrinthine fistula.

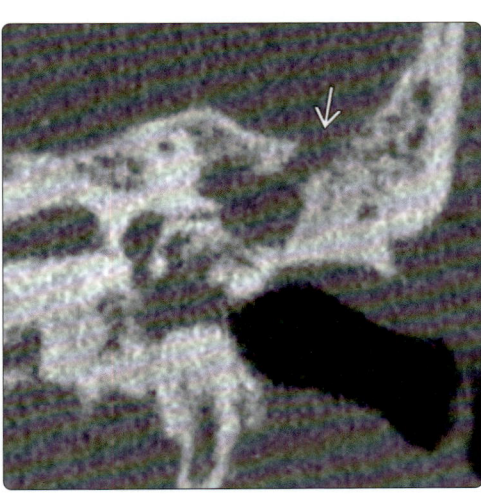

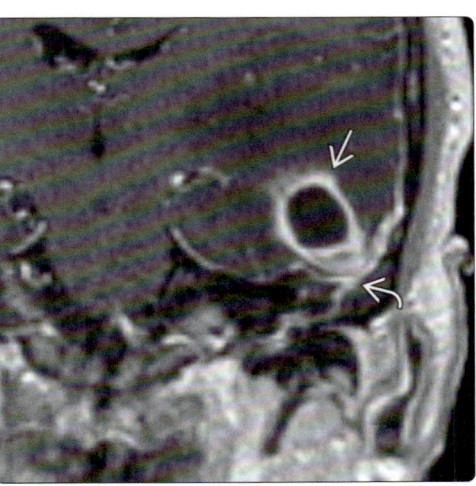

(Left) Coronal bone CT in a 55-year-old with chronic ear infections and new dysarthria shows soft tissue filling the tympanic cavity with dehiscence of the tegmen ➡. (Right) Coronal T1 C+ MR in the same patient shows a rim-enhancing collection ➡ with surrounding edema in the left temporal lobe adjacent to the tegmen dehiscence ➡. Pathology demonstrated infected cholesteatoma with associated cerebral abscess.

Pars Tensa Cholesteatoma

TERMINOLOGY

- Pars tensa cholesteatoma (PTC)
- Synonym: Secondary acquired cholesteatoma
- Definition
  - Nonneoplastic, mass-like accumulation of exfoliated keratin within stratified squamous epithelium at pars tensa tympanic membrane (TM), often at retraction pocket or site of prior perforation

IMAGING

- Temporal bone CT with multiplanar recons = 1st-line study
  - **Erosive** mass in **posterior mesotympanum**
  - Usually found **medial** to ossicles
  - May involve sinus tympani, facial recess, and aditus ad antrum ± mastoid
  - Ossicular **erosion** is common along medial incus long process, stapes superstructure, and malleus manubrium
- MR with **non-echo-planar DWI** most sensitive tool; troubleshoots issues raised by bone CT

- Cholesteatoma is **light bulb bright** on DWI
- Non-echo-planar DWI far superior to conventional echo-planar DWI
  - May obviate need for 2nd-look surgery

TOP DIFFERENTIAL DIAGNOSES

- Middle ear congenital cholesteatoma
- Pars flaccida cholesteatoma
- Middle ear cholesterol granuloma
- Tympanic paraganglioma

PATHOLOGY

- Mucosal traction theory (**new theory**): Apposition of medial TM surface and mucosa of lateral ossicles → coupling/adhesion, which retracts TM via middle ear mucociliary clearance, yielding keratin accumulation

CLINICAL ISSUES

- **10-20%** of all middle ear cholesteatomas
- Significantly less common than pars flaccida cholesteatoma

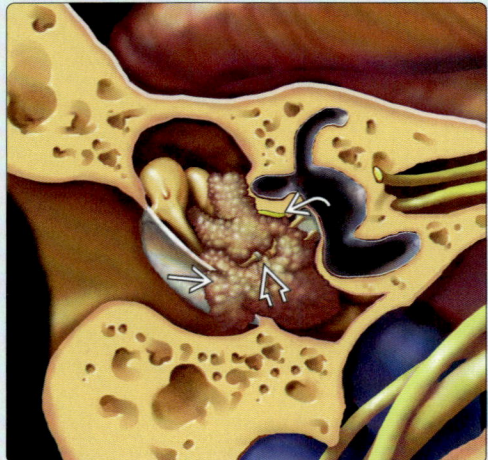
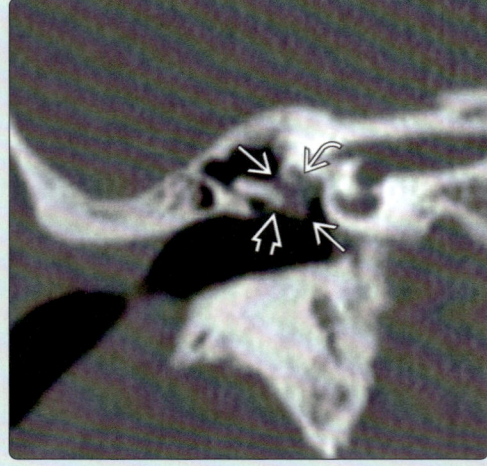

(Left) Coronal graphic of pars tensa cholesteatoma (PTC) shows cholesteatoma extending laterally through an inferior tympanic membrane (TM) rupture ➡. The middle ear PTC erodes ossicles ➡, invades and flattens the tympanic CNVII canal ➡, and is primarily medial to the ossicles. (Right) Coronal NECT shows PTC ➡ with TM perforation. Note soft tissue medial to the truncated ossicular chain ➡ and erosion of the tympanic facial nerve canal ➡. Bone erosion is a hallmark imaging finding of cholesteatoma on CT.

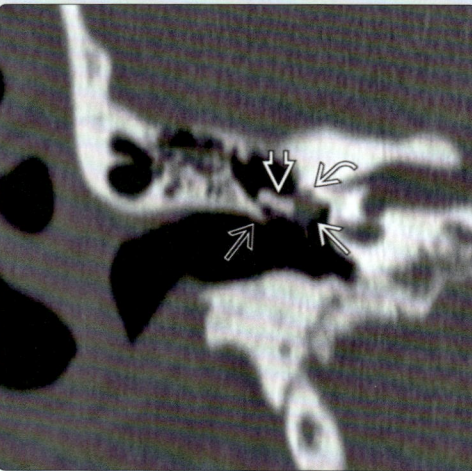
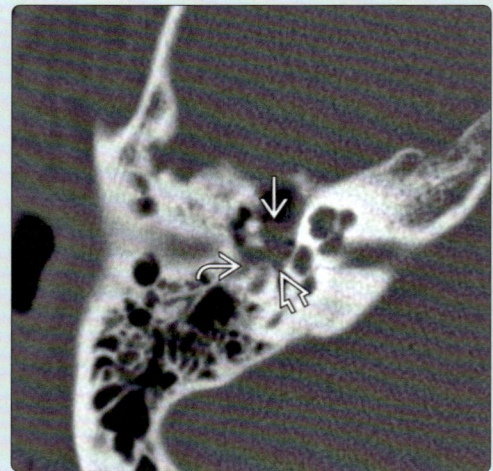

(Left) Coronal NECT in a patient with PTC shows mass-like middle ear soft tissue ➡ primarily located medial to the eroded ossicular chain ➡. Note associated erosion of the tympanic facial nerve canal ➡. A sharp scutum ➡ and clear lateral epitympanic recess differentiate PTC from pars flaccida cholesteatoma. (Right) Axial NECT in the same patient shows PTC ➡ medial to ossicles, involving the sinus tympani ➡ and facial recess ➡, potential surgical "blind spots" that must be scrutinized on imaging.

Pars Tensa Cholesteatoma

TERMINOLOGY

Abbreviations
- Pars tensa cholesteatoma (PTC)

Synonyms
- Sinus cholesteatoma due to involvement of sinus tympani
- Secondary acquired cholesteatoma

Definitions
- Nonneoplastic, mass-like accumulation of exfoliated keratin within stratified squamous epithelium at pars tensa tympanic membrane (TM), often at retraction pocket or site of prior perforation
  - "Tense" lower 3/4 of TM

IMAGING

General Features
- Best diagnostic clue
  - Erosive mass in posterior mesotympanum involving sinus tympani, facial nerve recess, and aditus ad antrum ± mastoid
- Location
  - Posterior mesotympanum
    - Spreads posteromedially
    - In part, **medial to ossicles**
- Size
  - Several millimeters to 2-3 cm [fills middle ear (ME) cavity]
- Morphology
  - Lobular, well-circumscribed, nonenhancing soft tissue density mass
  - Ossicular or bone erosion
    - Bone erosion has multiple causes
      □ Inflammatory enzymatic dissolution of bone
      □ Pressure-induced bone &/or ossicular resorption from enlarging PTC

CT Findings
- CECT
  - Nonenhancing soft tissue mass
- Bone CT
  - **Small PTC**
    - Soft tissue mass begins at **posterior mesotympanum**
    - Most commonly begins at or involves sinus tympani and facial nerve recess
    - Mass projects **medial** to ossicular chain
    - Subtle lateral displacement of ossicles
    - Early ossicular **erosion** from medial aspect
  - **Large PTC**
    - Fills ME cavity
    - Invades mastoid through widened aditus ad antrum
    - Ossicular **erosion** common
      □ Along medial incus long process, stapes superstructure, and manubrium of malleus
    - Posterior tegmen tympani and anterior tegmen mastoideum dehiscence may occur
    - May erode facial nerve canal

MR Findings
- T1WI
  - Hypointense ME mass
- T2WI
  - PTC usually high signal
    - Trapped secretions of mastoid higher signal than PTC
- DWI
  - Characteristically **light bulb bright**
    - Hyperintense at high B values; may show true **reduced diffusivity**, as in other types of cholesteatoma or epidermoid
  - Non-echo-planar (e.g., HASTE) DWI and small FOV DWI preparations (e.g., ZOOMit or FOCUS) are superior to conventional echo-planar (EPI) DWI; may obviate need for 2nd-look surgery
    - Traditional EPI DWI limited in temporal bone by susceptibility, motion, and ghosting artifacts
    - Newer EPI DWI with segmented or multishot EPI prep (e.g., RESOLVE) superior to conventional EPI DWI
- T1WI C+
  - **PTC itself does not enhance** but commonly shows enhancing peripheral rind of granulation tissue/scar
    - Delayed (45-60 minutes) imaging may help discriminate nonenhancing PTC from surrounding inflammation, granulation, or scar
  - If tegmen erosion present, dural thickening and enhancement overlies bony defect
  - Shows intracranial complications, such as meningitis

Imaging Recommendations
- Best imaging tool
  - Temporal bone bone CT with multiplanar recons = 1st-line study
  - Temporal bone MR with non-EPI DWI most sensitive and specific tool; complementary to CT
    - T1 C+ MR to answer specific issues raised by bone CT
      □ Confirm or exclude cholesteatoma if CT is equivocal
      □ Enhancement of labyrinth suggests labyrinthitis
      □ Temporal lobe extension, subperiosteal or intracranial abscess, meningitis, labyrinthitis, transverse sinus thrombosis

DIFFERENTIAL DIAGNOSIS

Middle Ear Congenital Cholesteatoma
- Otoscopy: White mass behind intact TM in children
- Bone CT: Often located posteriorly (like PTC)

Pars Flaccida Cholesteatoma
- Otoscopy: Pars flaccida perforation or retraction pocket
- Bone CT: Prussak space mass with eroded scutum, lateral body of incus and head of malleus; medialized ossicles

Middle Ear Cholesterol Granuloma
- Otoscopy: Blue mass behind intact TM
- Bone CT: Ossicular and bony erosions may mimic cholesteatoma
- T1 MR: Hyperintense mass

Tympanic Paraganglioma
- Otoscopy: Cherry red pulsatile mass behind intact TM
- Bone CT: Mass on cochlear promontory, no ossicular erosion
- T1 C+ MR: Intense enhancement of mass

PATHOLOGY

General Features

- Etiology
  - Squamous metaplasia theory: ME inflammation transforms mucosa
  - Squamous immigration/invasion theory: Lateral TM squamous epithelium migrates to ME via TM perforation
  - Squamous basal hyperplasia/papillary ingrowth theory: Proliferating basal keratinocytes penetrate basement membrane with subepithelial spread
  - Squamous obstruction/vacuum retraction pocket theory: Eustachian tube dysfunction causes ME vacuum effect → retraction pocket and keratin accumulation
  - Mucosal traction theory (**new theory**): Apposition of medial TM surface and mucosa of lateral ossicles → coupling/adhesion, which retracts TM via ME mucociliary clearance, yielding keratin accumulation

Gross Pathologic & Surgical Features

- Pearly tumor seen at surgery
- Well-circumscribed, soft, waxy, white material

Microscopic Features

- Stratified squamous epithelium with anucleated (dead) keratin squames
- Same histology as epidermoid and any cholesteatoma elsewhere in body

CLINICAL ISSUES

Presentation

- Most common signs/symptoms
  - Can be asymptomatic
  - History of chronic otitis media ± TM perforation
  - Progressive unilateral conductive hearing loss
  - Foul-smelling otorrhea due to infection
- Other signs/symptoms
  - Noise- or pressure-induced vertigo if labyrinthine fistula
    - Most common at basal turn of cochlea
  - Facial nerve paresis or palsy
    - Due to pressure effect (slow onset), infection (acute onset), CNVII canal erosion
      - CNVII canal erosion more common in PTC than pars flaccida cholesteatoma
  - Otalgia, headache
    - If infected ± intracranial complication
- Otologic examination
  - Retraction pocket, perforation, or visible cholesteatoma at pars tensa
  - Edema, granulation tissue, aural polyp representing chronic inflammation
  - Sensorineural hearing loss suspicious for complication with labyrinthine fistula

Demographics

- Age
  - Occurs in children and adults
- Sex
  - M = F
- Epidemiology
  - **10-20%** of all ME cholesteatomas

- Significantly less common than pars flaccida cholesteatoma

Natural History & Prognosis

- Progressive enlargement with growing symptom complex due to local extension
- Small lesion
  - Excellent for total eradication and normal hearing
- Large lesion
  - Residual conductive hearing loss common
- Postoperative recurrence rate ~ 10%

Treatment

- Potential surgical approaches for PTC removal
  - Transcanal endoscopic ear surgery (TEES): Assess middle ear through external auditory canal (EAC)
  - Canal-wall up mastoidectomy: Posterior wall EAC not removed
  - Canal-wall down mastoidectomy: Posterior wall EAC removed
- TM and ossicular reconstruction required for hearing restoration if ossicular chain involved

DIAGNOSTIC CHECKLIST

Consider

- PTC if CT shows that ME mass is **centered posteriorly**, extends **medial to ossicles**, and displaces ossicles laterally
- Consider PTC if bone CT shows medial ossicle **erosion**

Image Interpretation Pearls

- Axial and coronal CT show location, local extension, and telltale **erosions** best
  - Caution calling cholesteatoma on CT if no ossicular or bone erosions
    - Absent erosions, may be impossible to differentiate from ME fluid or noncholesteatoma debris
- **MR with non-EPI DWI is most sensitive and specific imaging tool for cholesteatoma**
  - MR differentiates PTC from effusion, granulation, cholesterol granuloma, and tympanic paraganglioma
    - T1 C+ MR shows intracranial complication or labyrinthitis, if suspected

Reporting Tips

- Sinus tympani involvement is often site of recurrence
- Presence of labyrinthine fistula, degree of posterior canal wall erosion and mastoid aeration/sclerosis affects choice of operation
- Facial nerve canal erosion and tegmen dehiscence important for preoperative planning
- Intracranial complication requires urgent attention

SELECTED REFERENCES

1. Marchioni D et al: Endoscopic transcanal surgery of pars tensa cholesteatoma: preliminary results. Acta Otorrinolaringol Esp (Engl Ed). 74(2):101-7, 2023
2. Stefanescu EH et al: High-resolution computed tomography in middle ear cholesteatoma: how much do we need it? Medicina (Kaunas). 59(10):1712, 2023
3. Baba A et al: Non-echoplanar diffusion weighed imaging and T1-weighted imaging for cholesteatoma mastoid extension. Auris Nasus Larynx. 48(5):846-51, 2021
4. Gulotta G et al: Facial nerve dehiscence and cholesteatoma: a comparison between decades. J Int Adv Otol. 16(3):367-72, 2020

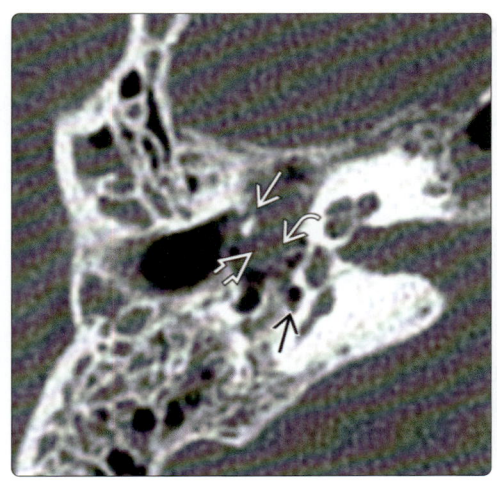
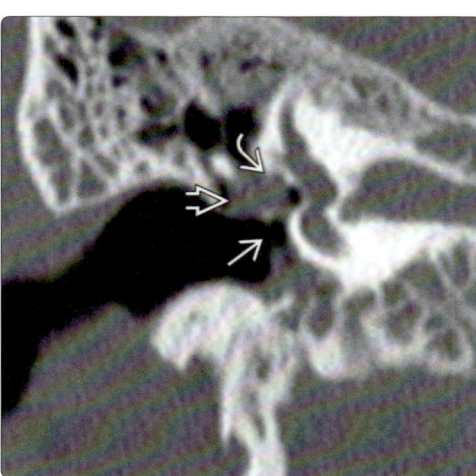

(Left) Axial bone CT shows a mesotympanic mass medial to the malleus ➡ and destroying the long process of the incus ⮕ and stapes superstructure ➡, compatible with PTC. This lesion does not extend into the sinus tympani ➡. (Right) Coronal bone CT demonstrates perforation of the inferior pars tensa ➡. Associated PTC ➡ is seen medial to the ossicles and destroying the incus and stapes. Also note osseous dehiscence of the tympanic facial nerve canal ➡.

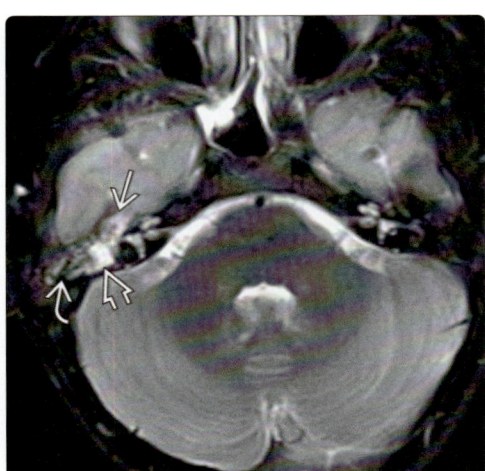
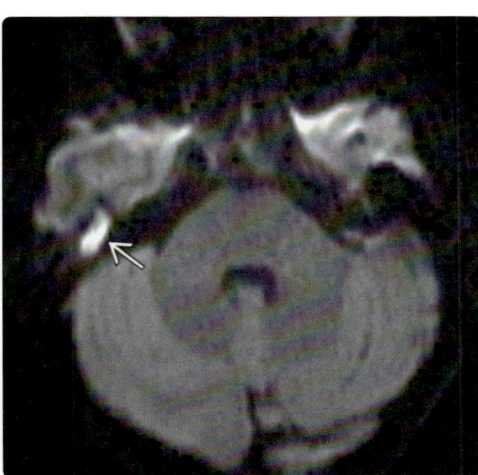

(Left) Axial T2 FS MR in a patient with chronic otitis media and PTC on otoscopy shows filling of the middle ear ➡ and mastoid antrum ➡ with T2 hyperintensity as well as high signal in the mastoid air cells ➡. T2 alone cannot differentiate ear effusion from cholesteatoma. (Right) Axial DTI trace MR in the same patient shows reduced diffusivity as marked bright signal within the middle ear and mastoid antrum ➡, differentiating cholesteatoma from mastoid effusion. DWI is an indispensable MR sequence for cholesteatoma imaging.

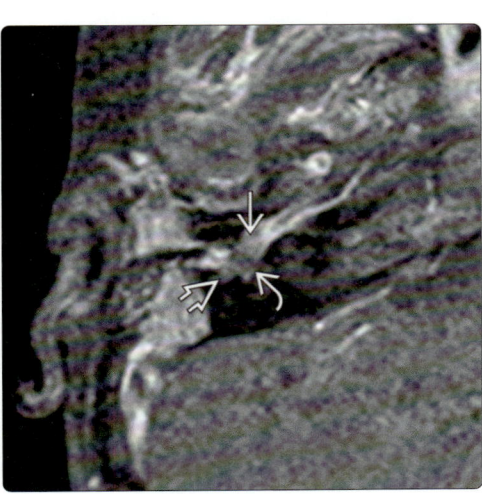
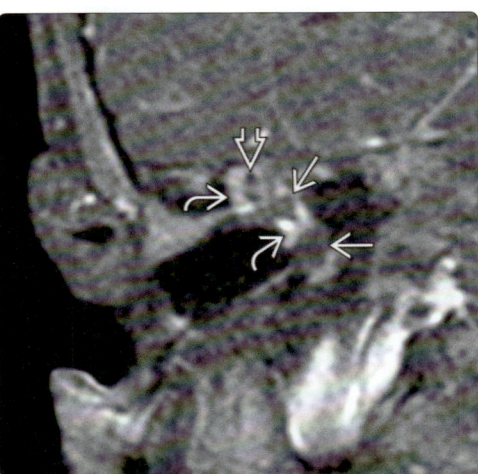

(Left) Axial T1 C+ FS MR in the same patient shows the characteristically nonenhancing PTC ➡, which involves the sinus tympani ➡ and facial recess ➡. Administration of IV contrast is helpful in cholesteatoma imaging, as it is reliably nonenhancing on MR. (Right) Coronal T1 C+ FS MR shows PTC in the middle ear to be characteristically nonenhancing ➡ and located predominantly medial to the hypointense ossicles ➡. Adjacent enhancing soft tissue ➡ represents granulation tissue and inflammation.

TERMINOLOGY

- Synonyms: Automastoidectomy; "shell" or "rind" cholesteatoma
- Rare variant of acquired cholesteatoma
- Definition: Residual cholesteatoma "rind" left behind after acquired middle ear-mastoid cholesteatoma extrudes central matrix through dehiscent **external auditory canal (EAC) bony wall**

IMAGING

- Temporal bone CT findings
  - Mastoidectomy cavity with residual soft tissue "rind" along cavity wall **without** history of mastoidectomy
  - Large lesion can fistulize any area of inner ear
  - Focal dehiscence of posterior or superior EAC wall
- Temporal bone MR findings
  - Residual rind of cholesteatoma shows reduced diffusivity
  - Enhancing soft tissue = granulation tissue

TOP DIFFERENTIAL DIAGNOSES

- Coalescent mastoiditis
- Mastoidectomy
- Keratosis obturans with automastoidectomy

PATHOLOGY

- "Rind" of tissue found along wall of cavity
- Only "lining" of cholesteatoma seen by pathologist

CLINICAL ISSUES

- Long history of chronic otitis media, ear drainage **without** mastoidectomy
- May report material "falling out of ear"

DIAGNOSTIC CHECKLIST

- CT suggests mastoidectomy but no prior surgery: Automastoidectomy
- Check for ossicle destruction, inner ear or CNVII canal dehiscence, EAC wall erosion

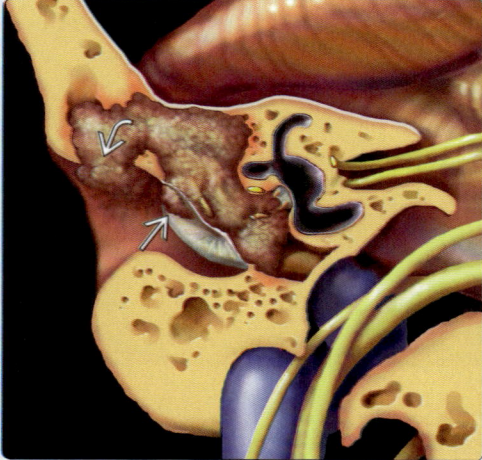
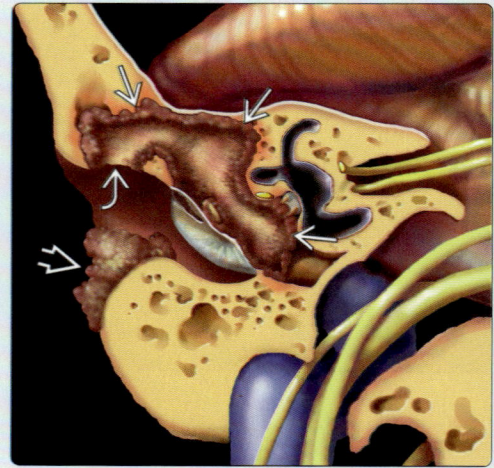

(Left) Coronal graphic shows a large cholesteatoma beginning at a pars flaccida perforation ➡. The lesion has eroded the middle ear walls, ossicles, mastoid cavity, and external auditory canal (EAC) bony walls ➡. (Right) Coronal graphic reveals that the large cholesteatoma has evacuated its central material through the EAC dehiscence ➡ and fallen into the external ear canal ➡. A mural cholesteatoma is left behind as a cholesteatoma "rind" along the walls of the middle ear and mastoid ➡.

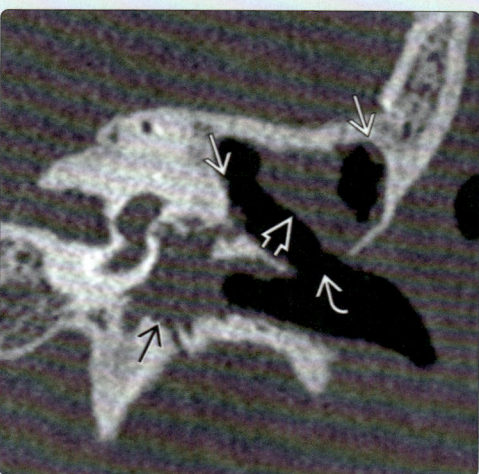
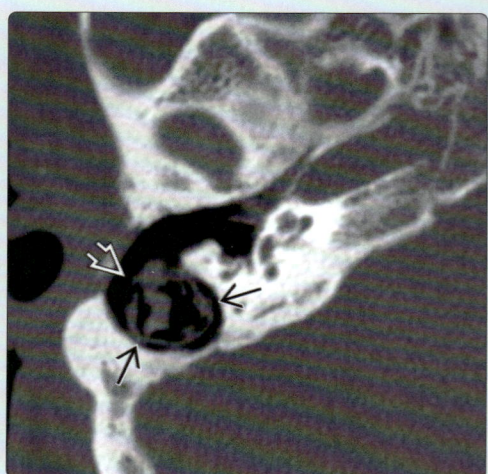

(Left) Coronal bone CT shows an automastoidectomy communicating with the bony EAC ➡ with persistent internal debris ➡. A thin rind of mural cholesteatoma ➡ lines the automastoidectomy bowl. In addition, persistent cholesteatoma fills the tympanic cavity ➡. (Right) Axial temporal bone CT reveals mural cholesteatoma as residual rind of tissue in a "hollowed out" mastoid bowl ➡. The lesion has eroded into the posterior bony EAC ➡.

Mural Cholesteatoma

TERMINOLOGY

Synonyms
- Automastoidectomy; "shell" or "rind" cholesteatoma

Definitions
- Residual cholesteatoma "rind" left behind after acquired middle ear-mastoid cholesteatoma extrudes central matrix through dehiscent **external auditory canal (EAC) bony wall**

IMAGING

General Features
- Best diagnostic clue
  - Mastoidectomy cavity with residual soft tissue along cavity wall **without** history of mastoidectomy
- Location
  - Middle ear & mastoid
- Size
  - Cholesteatoma "**rind**" of variable thickness

CT Findings
- Bone CT
  - "Hollowed out" middle ear-mastoid with residual **cholesteatoma "rind"** seen along walls of cavity
  - Common cavity connects middle ear & antrum
  - Ossicles destroyed; scutum truncated
  - Labyrinthine fistula may be present

MR Findings
- T1WI
  - Mastoid cavity appears similar to surgical defect
- DWI
  - Residual cholesteatoma markedly hyperintense
  - Non-echo-planar (EPI) DWI is more sensitive than traditional EPI diffusion for detecting residual cholesteatoma component
- T1WI C+
  - Peripheral enhancement along margin of cavity = granulation tissue **not** cholesteatoma

Imaging Recommendations
- Best imaging tool
  - Temporal bone CT is 1st-line modality
  - MR with non-EPI DWI is most sensitive for detecting residual cholesteatoma component
- Protocol advice
  - Temporal bone CT in axial & coronal planes
  - Temporal bone MR with T1 C+ & non-EPI DWI

DIFFERENTIAL DIAGNOSIS

Coalescent Mastoiditis
- Middle ear cavity not enlarged
- Mastoid air cells confluent with acute otitis media
- Middle ear & mastoid completely opacified

Mastoidectomy
- Canal wall down mastoidectomy: Posterior bony EAC wall resected; mastoidectomy bowl communicates with EAC
- Posterolateral wall of mastoid absent
- Surgical history is known

Keratosis Obturans With Automastoidectomy
- Soft tissue filling EAC ± osseous expansion
- Rare reported cases of dehiscence & automastoidectomy

PATHOLOGY

General Features
- Etiology
  - Acquired cholesteatoma begins in middle ear
  - Enlargement of cholesteatoma fills entire middle ear cavity ± mastoid antrum
  - Pressure built up with further cholesteatoma growth relieved by expulsion of content through EAC dehiscence or tympanic membrane (TM) perforation
  - Cholesteatoma matrix extrudes through perforated TM or directly into EAC
  - Outer shell/erosive membrane persists after drainage
  - Continued cavity growth from enzymatic activity

Gross Pathologic & Surgical Features
- Cholesteatoma "rind" found along wall of cavity

Microscopic Features
- Only "lining" of cholesteatoma viewable
- Aggressive keratinizing stratified squamous epithelium

CLINICAL ISSUES

Presentation
- Most common signs/symptoms
  - Long history of chronic otitis media
    - No history of mastoidectomy
    - May report material "falling out of ear"
  - Otologic exam: TM perforation or draining sinus through EAC wall

Demographics
- Age: Usually in older patient
- Epidemiology: Rare variant form of acquired cholesteatoma

Natural History & Prognosis
- Restoration of hearing difficult because of complete ossicle destruction & bone erosion

Treatment
- Surgery depends on lesion size & extent
  - Excision of tissue lining cavity is imperative

DIAGNOSTIC CHECKLIST

Consider
- Imaging findings suggest mastoidectomy has occurred
  - **No** history of mastoidectomy; hence term **automastoidectomy**

Image Interpretation Pearls
- EAC dehiscence along with "hollowed out" mastoid + mastoid "rind" = mural cholesteatoma

SELECTED REFERENCES

1. Çelebi İ et al: Multidetector computed tomography findings of auto-evacuated secondary acquired cholesteatoma: a morphologic and quantitative analysis. J Int Adv Otol. 14(3):464-71, 2018

KEY FACTS

TERMINOLOGY

- Cholesterol granuloma (CG): Recurrent hemorrhage into middle ear (ME) cavity causes inflammatory mass of granulation tissue

IMAGING

- Bone CT: Smoothly **expansile mass** of ME ± mastoid air cells
- MR: **High T1** and T2 signal in ME

TOP DIFFERENTIAL DIAGNOSES

- Dehiscent jugular bulb
- Aberrant internal carotid artery
- Chronic otitis media + hemorrhage
- Pars flaccida-acquired cholesteatoma
- Paraganglioma
  - Tympanic paraganglioma
  - Jugular paraganglioma
- Encephalocele of ME
- Traumatic hemotympanum

CLINICAL ISSUES

- Clinical presentation
  - Symptoms: Conductive hearing loss
  - Otoscopy: Nonpulsating bluish discoloration of tympanic membrane = "blue" eardrum
  - Symptoms arise years after initial otitis media
- Treatment options
  - Initial surgery: Resection of wall and contents
  - Intractable disease: Mastoidectomy + ventilation tube
- Natural history
  - Most ME CGs grow over decades
- Recurrence rates for ME CG are much lower than for petrous apex CG

DIAGNOSTIC CHECKLIST

- "Blue" tympanic membrane + **expansile** bone changes (on bone CT) + **high T1** (on MR) = CG of ME

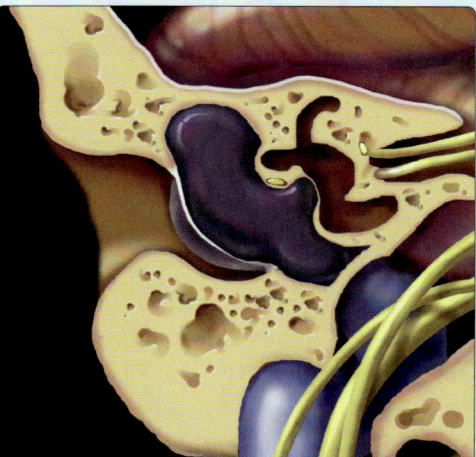
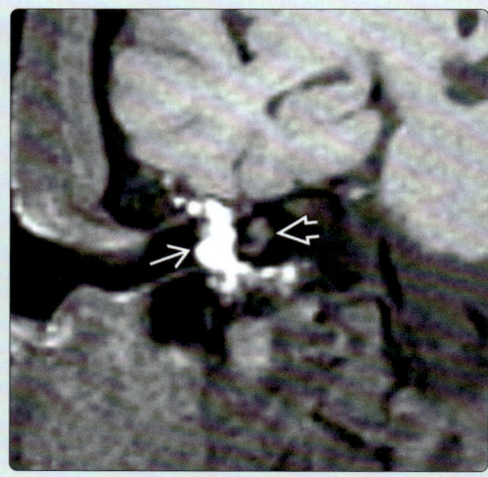

(Left) Coronal graphic depicts a large middle ear cholesterol granuloma. The entire middle ear is filled with dark brown ("chocolate") fluid with the ossicles no longer present. Otoscopy reveals a blue-black eardrum. (Right) Coronal T1WI MR demonstrates a retrotympanic high-signal cholesterol granuloma ➡ that causes the tympanic membrane to bulge into the external auditory canal. Notice the signal of the cochlea medially ➨. The cholesterol granuloma fills the entire middle ear cavity.

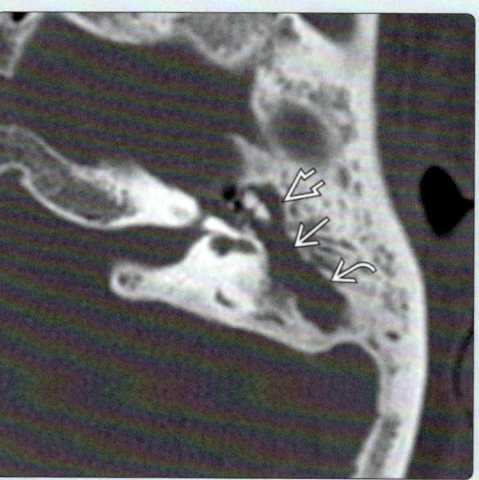
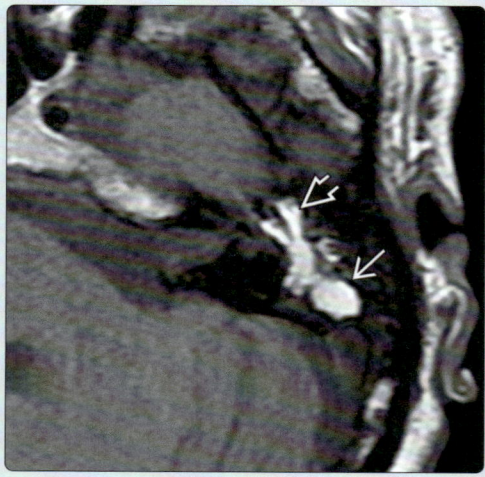

(Left) Axial bone CT shows a soft tissue mass in the epitympanum ➨, widened aditus ad antrum ➡, and mastoid antrum ➚. There is no way to tell that this is a cholesterol granuloma on CT. (Right) Axial T1WI MR in the same patient reveals the high-signal cholesterol granuloma in the middle ear ➨ and mastoid antrum ➨. The high signal of this lesion along with the enlarged aditus ad antrum on CT is highly suggestive of the diagnosis of cholesterol granuloma.

Middle Ear Cholesterol Granuloma

TERMINOLOGY

Abbreviations
- Cholesterol granuloma (CG)

Synonyms
- Cholesterol cyst, chocolate cyst, blue-dome cyst

Definitions
- Recurrent hemorrhage into middle ear (ME) cavity causes inflammatory mass of granulation tissue

IMAGING

General Features
- Best diagnostic clue
  - Bone CT: Smoothly **expansile mass** of ME ± mastoid cells
  - MR: **High T1** and T2 signal in ME
- Location
  - CG most commonly arises in ME
    - Also occurs in petrous apex (PA) and orbit
- Size
  - Depends on chronicity; millimeters to centimeters
- Morphology
  - Expansile nature critical to diagnosis

CT Findings
- CECT
  - May be useful to distinguish small CG from tympanic paraganglioma, which enhances briskly
- Bone CT
  - Early CG-ME bone CT findings
    - Small ME mass
    - No ossicular loss or bone remodeling
    - Difficult to make specific diagnosis
  - Late CG-ME bone CT findings
    - Opacified ME and mastoid
    - **Expansile bony changes** with scalloping
    - Ossicular displacement ± destruction

MR Findings
- T1WI
  - ↑ **signal** from paramagnetic effect of **methemoglobin**
- T2WI
  - Central ↑ signal from granulation tissue
  - Peripheral ↓ signal from hemosiderin deposition
- STIR
  - Follows T2 signal
- T1WI C+ FS
  - Inherent high T1 signal confused with enhancement
    - Compare to unenhanced T1WI
- MRA
  - May be useful to distinguish CG from vascular anomalies [e.g., aberrant internal carotid artery (ICA)]
    - CT preferred to eliminate vascular lesions

Imaging Recommendations
- Best imaging tool
  - Temporal bone CT initially
    - MR used in larger lesions
- Protocol advice
  - Remember to use axial and coronal T1 MR prior to contrast when CG-ME suspected

DIFFERENTIAL DIAGNOSIS

Dehiscent Jugular Bulb
- Otoscopy: Blue-black mass in ME
- Bone CT: Absence of thin bone between jugular bulb and hypotympanum
  - Diverticulum of jugular vein extends into ME
- Thin-section CT needed for diagnosis
  - Both axial and reconstructed coronal planes useful

Aberrant Internal Carotid Artery
- Otoscopy: Pink, pulsatile mass in ME
- Bone CT: Tubular mass crosses ME cavity to rejoin horizontal petrous ICA
  - Large inferior tympanic canaliculus
- Enlarged collateral vessel traverses ME when ICA fails to develop

Chronic Otitis Media + Hemorrhage
- Otoscopy: Inflammatory tissue and blood in ME ± ruptured tympanic membrane (TM)
- Bone CT: Inflammatory tissue and blood fill ME **without** expansile bony changes
- MR: Variable T1 and T2 signal

Pars Flaccida-Acquired Cholesteatoma
- Otoscopy: TM retraction-rupture ± visible cholesteatoma
- Bone CT: Erosive ME-mastoid mass with ossicle loss
- MR: Usually low T1 and high T2
  - Rim enhances on T1 C+
  - DWI restriction
- Associated with recurrent prior infections ± effusions, similar to CG-ME
- Microscopic: Cholesteatoma lined by squamous epithelium
  - CG-ME lined with fibrous connective tissue

Paraganglioma
- Otoscopy: Red mass in ME
- Bone CT
  - Tympanic paraganglioma
    - On cochlear promontory
  - Jugular paraganglioma
    - Permeative bone changes, jugular foramen to ME

Encephalocele of Middle Ear
- Surgical view: Can mimic CG-ME strongly
- Bone CT: Dehiscent tegmen tympani with brain herniation into ME or mastoid cavity
- MR: Coronal T2 may define contents
- Usually posttraumatic or postsurgical

Traumatic Hemotympanum
- Otoscopy: Blood in ME from recent trauma
- Bone CT: Associated temporal bone fractures
- MR: High T1 methemoglobin does not expand ME
  - No obstruction as with CG-ME

PATHOLOGY

General Features

- Etiology
  - Still not definite
  - Obstruction-vacuum hypothesis
    - Chronic otitis media, cholesteatoma, or previous surgery obstructs air cells of ME ± mastoid air cells
    - Resorption of gas in obstructed air cells creates relative vacuum
    - ↓ in pressure → mucosal engorgement → blood vessel rupture
    - Anaerobic RBC degradation to cholesterol crystals incites multinucleated foreign giant cell response → inflammation with small vessel proliferation → vessel rupture
    - Granulation tissue forms from repeated hemorrhage, expanding ME ± mastoid
  - Exposed marrow hypothesis
    - In young adulthood, enlarging mucosa creates bony defects into hematopoietic marrow of temporal bone
    - Recurrent microhemorrhage → accumulation of RBC degradation products
    - Anaerobic RBC degradation to cholesterol crystals incites multinucleated foreign giant cell response
    - Obstruction secondary to inflammation, rather than obstruction as primary cause
- Associated abnormalities
  - Recurrent otitis media or effusion
  - Cholesteatoma
  - Benign granulation tissue
- Differences between CG-ME and CG-PA
  - CG-ME presents with conductive hearing loss
  - CG-PA presents with facial pain, headache
  - CG-ME not associated with history of cranial neuropathies
  - CG-PA associated with neuropathies of CNV-VII
  - CG-ME has history of recurrent infections
  - CG-PA has no history of infection
  - CG-ME has bone erosion late
  - CG-PA may have extensive bone erosion
  - CG-ME occurs in poorly pneumatized temporal bone (result of prior infections)
  - CG-PA occurs in highly pneumatized temporal bone

Gross Pathologic & Surgical Features

- Cystic mass with fibrous capsule, filled with brownish liquid containing old blood and cholesterol crystals
- Fluid described as "crankcase oil" or chocolate cyst

Microscopic Features

- Lined by fibrous connective tissue
- RBCs
- Multinucleated giant cells surrounding cholesterol crystals embedded in connective tissue
- Hemosiderin-laden macrophages, chronic inflammatory cells, and blood vessels

CLINICAL ISSUES

Presentation

- Most common signs/symptoms
  - Slowly progressive conductive hearing loss
  - Other signs/symptoms
    - Pulsatile tinnitus
    - "Pressure on ear"
    - Otoscopy: Nonpulsating bluish discoloration of TM = "blue" eardrum
- Clinical profile
  - Younger to middle-aged patient with "blue" eardrum and conductive hearing loss
  - Easily confused clinically with vascular malformation or vascular tumor
  - History of recurrent ME infection helpful for diagnosis

Demographics

- Age
  - Broad age range, beginning in 2nd decade
- Epidemiology
  - CG-ME much more common than CG-PA

Natural History & Prognosis

- Great variability in growth rate of CG-ME
  - Depends on frequency and severity of microhemorrhages within lesion
- Most CG-ME grow over decades
  - Symptoms arise years after initial otitis media
- Recurrence rates for CG-ME much lower than for CG-PA
  - Easier surgical exposure
- Clinical prognostic indicator
  - Protruding TM: Poorer treatment outcome
  - Retracted TM: Better treatment outcome

Treatment

- Initial surgery: Resection of wall and contents
- Intractable disease: Mastoidectomy + ventilation tube

DIAGNOSTIC CHECKLIST

Consider

- "Blue" TM + expansile changes (CT) + high T1 (MR) = CG-ME

Image Interpretation Pearls

- Do not mistake high T1 signal for enhancement
  - Compare with unenhanced T1

Reporting Tips

- Note if extension into eustachian tube or mastoid
- Comment on ossicle status

SELECTED REFERENCES

1. Lin LJ et al: Ossicular reconstruction with various degrees of malleus preservation in patients with chronic otitis media. Ear Nose Throat J. ePub, 2024
2. Robson CD: Conductive hearing loss in children. Neuroimaging Clin N Am. 33(4):543-62, 2023
3. Angeletti D et al: Tympanic cholesterol granuloma and exclusive endoscopic approach. Am J Case Rep. 21:e925369, 2020

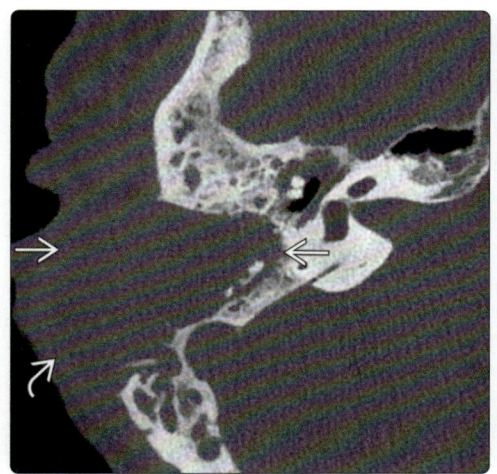

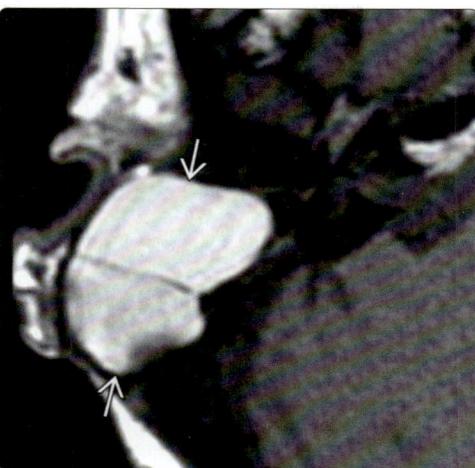

(Left) Axial bone CT shows wide expansion of the mastoid and middle ear due to a large cholesterol granuloma ➡. CT features are not specific, however. The osseous lateral wall is markedly thinned, making it appear dehiscent ➡. (Right) Axial T1 MR in the same patient shows a large, expansile, hyperintense cholesterol granuloma involving the middle ear and mastoids ➡. There was no signal suppression on fat-saturated T1 MR (not shown).

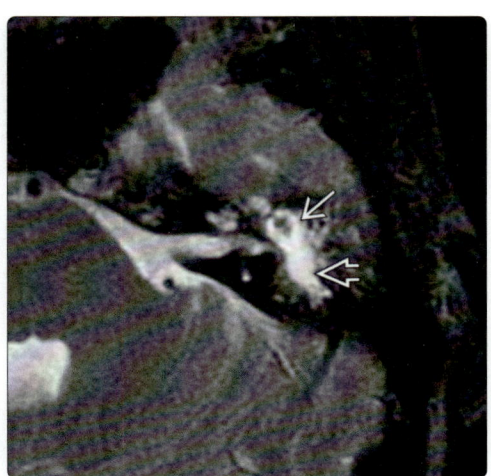

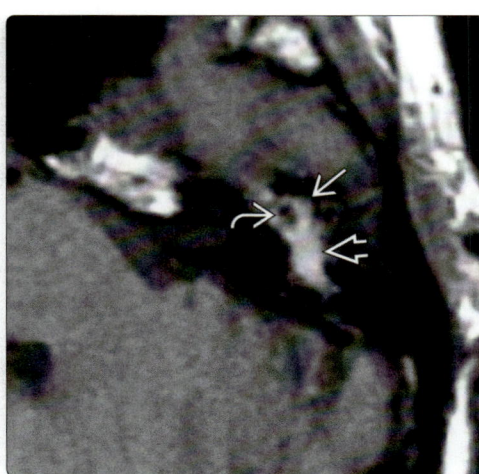

(Left) Axial T2WI fat-saturated MR in the same patient reveals hyperintense cholesterol granuloma in the epitympanum ➡ and mastoid antrum ➡. Early-phase disease preserves the ossicles and shows no evidence of bony scalloping. (Right) Axial T1WI MR in a patient with a blue-black retrotympanic lesion shows a high-signal cholesterol granuloma filling the middle ear ➡ and mastoid antrum ➡. Note the low-signal head of the malleus and short process of incus ➡ visible within the lesion.

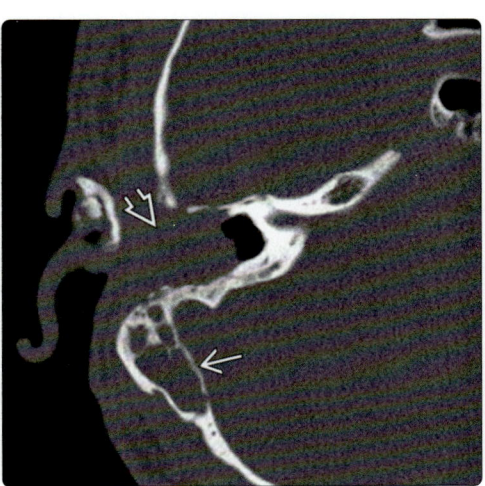

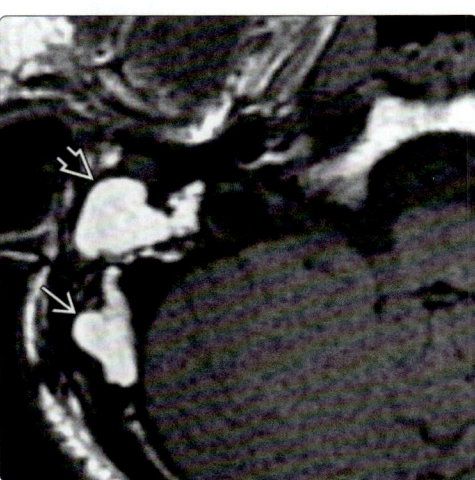

(Left) Axial bone CT reveals a postoperative temporal bone with soft tissue in the mastoid bowl and middle ear ➡ as well as in the posterior mastoid air cells ➡. The nature of the soft tissue cannot be determined on CT images. (Right) Axial T1 nonenhanced MR in the same patient shows a bilobed high-signal cholesterol granuloma filling the mastoid bowl ➡ and the posterior mastoid air cells ➡.

Tympanic Paraganglioma

TERMINOLOGY

- Tympanic paraganglioma (TPG)
- Benign tumor arising from paraganglia situated on **cochlear promontory**

IMAGING

- Best imaging study: Bone CT without contrast
- CT: Mass with flat base on cochlear promontory
- MR: Enhancing mass with flat base on cochlear promontory
- Floor of middle ear cavity is **intact** (if dehiscent, consider jugular paraganglioma)

TOP DIFFERENTIAL DIAGNOSES

- Jugular paraganglioma
- Aberrant internal carotid artery (AbICA)
- Dehiscent jugular bulb
- Congenital cholesteatoma, middle ear
- Facial nerve schwannoma, tympanic segment

PATHOLOGY

- Arise from paraganglia found along tympanic nerve (Jacobson nerve) on cochlear promontory
- TPG is most common tumor of middle ear

CLINICAL ISSUES

- Clinical presentation
  - 40- to 60-year-old woman
  - Vascular retrotympanic mass & pulsatile tinnitus
- Screening
  - Genetic and biochemical testing is recommended for every patient with head and neck paraganglioma
- Treatment options
  - Surgical resection
  - Approach depends on extent of TPG
- TPG may be clinically indistinguishable from jugular paraganglioma or AbICA

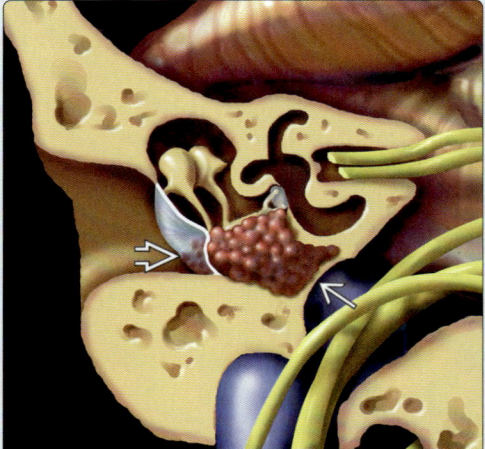
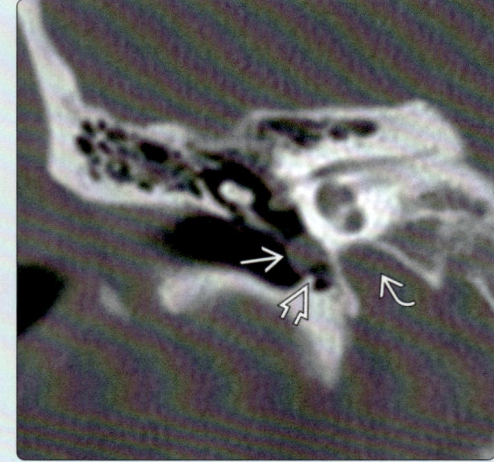

(Left) Coronal graphic shows a vascular tympanic paraganglioma (TPG) over cochlear promontory & filling inferior middle ear cavity. The bony floor of the middle ear cavity is intact ➡. Otoscopy reveals this tumor as a reddish, pulsatile mass behind lower tympanic membrane ➡. (Right) Coronal bone CT shows a classic small TPG ➡ located on the cochlear promontory just cephalad to the tympanic annulus ➡. On a single coronal image, the TPG looks remarkably like an aberrant ICA, but this case shows a normal ICA ➡.

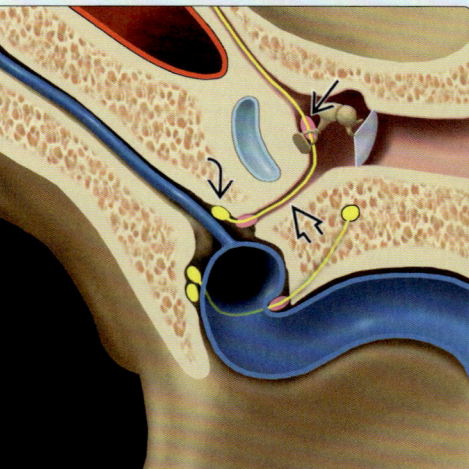
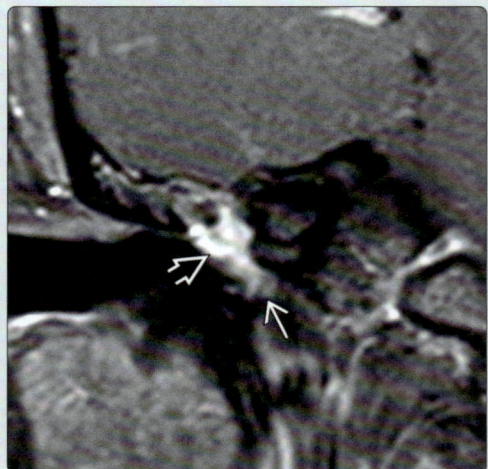

(Left) Axial graphic shows paraganglia ➡ along the course of the tympanic nerve ➡ (branch of glossopharyngeal nerve ➡) on the cochlear promontory. TPGs arise from this normal cellular collection. (Right) Coronal T1 C+ FS MR demonstrates a large, solidly enhancing TPG filling the middle ear cavity ➡. The floor is intact ➡, separating the tumor from the jugular bulb below.

Tympanic Paraganglioma

TERMINOLOGY

Abbreviations
- Tympanic paraganglioma (TPG)

Synonyms
- Middle ear paraganglioma
- Former terminology: Glomus tympanicum, chemodectoma, nonchromaffin paraganglioma

Definitions
- Benign tumor arising from paraganglia situated on cochlear promontory

IMAGING

General Features
- Best diagnostic clue
  - CT: Mass with flat base on cochlear promontory without significant osseous destruction
  - MR: Enhancing mass on cochlear promontory
- Location
  - Primary location: **Cochlear promontory**
  - Variant locations
    - Anteriorly beneath cochleariform process
    - Inferiorly in recess beneath cochlea basal turn
- Size
  - Millimeters to ~ 2 cm, usually found < 1 cm in size when clinically present with pulsatile tinnitus (PT)
  - May be so small that nonfocused imaging, or lack of clinical information with history of PT, causes radiologist to miss lesion altogether
- Morphology
  - Round mass with flat base most common
  - Larger lesions may fill middle ear cavity

CT Findings
- CECT
  - Difficult to identify enhancing middle ear mass
- Bone CT
  - Focal mass with flat base on cochlear promontory is characteristic
  - Small TPG
    - Subtle soft tissue bump may be present on cochlear promontory
    - Extends from cochlear promontory into lower mesotympanum &/or hypotympanum
    - May reach as far lateral as lower tympanic membrane (TM)
  - Large TPG
    - Fills middle ear cavity, creating attic block, resulting in fluid collection in mastoid
    - Tumor margins may not be discernible on CT
    - Jugular plate is **intact** (if dehiscent or permeative, diagnosis may be jugular paraganglioma with lesion centered in jugular foramen with superolateral extension into middle ear cavity)
    - Larger lesions may show permeative bone changes with destruction of medial wall of middle ear cavity ± ossicles
    - Rare involvement of air cells along inferior cochlear promontory may be mistaken for invasion

MR Findings
- T1WI
  - Soft tissue intensity mass on cochlear promontory
  - Small TPG will not have high-velocity flow voids in mass
    - These lesions often present clinically with PT when small; therefore, it is rare to see flow voids within TPG
- T2WI
  - TPG has lower signal intensity compared to bright obstructed fluid
- T1WI C+
  - Focal, enhancing mass on cochlear promontory
  - With larger obstructing TPG, contrast helps differentiate tumor from obstructed secretions
  - Utilized to determine tumor of hypotympanum
- MRA
  - Does not show enlarged vessels

Angiographic Findings
- TPG arterial supply
  - **Ascending pharyngeal artery** & its inferior tympanic branch, via inferior tympanic canaliculus

Imaging Recommendations
- Best imaging tool
  - Bone CT: Dedicated temporal bone CT with thin sections without contrast best if TPG suspected clinically
  - MR: Used if TPG suspected from CT findings
    - Small TPG may be missed if slice thickness > 3 mm
    - May be used to confirm hypotympanic TPG
  - Angiography: Unnecessary if TPG CT diagnosis
- Protocol advice
  - Keep enhanced MR slice thickness ≤ 3 mm

DIFFERENTIAL DIAGNOSIS

Jugular Paraganglioma
- Imaging: CT shows permeative change in bony floor of middle ear, mass centered in jugular foramen with superolateral extension into hypotympanum
- Clinical: Red-pink mass behind TM ± PT
  - Otoscopic exam identical to TPG

Aberrant Internal Carotid Artery
- Imaging: Tubular mass crosses middle ear cavity, connecting to horizontal internal carotid artery (ICA)
  - Large inferior tympanic canaliculus
- Clinical: Red-pink mass behind TM ± PT

Dehiscent Jugular Bulb
- Imaging: CT shows dehiscent jugular or sigmoid plate
  - Venous protrusion into middle ear cavity from superolateral jugular bulb
- Clinical: May be asymptomatic; purple/blue mass behind posteroinferior intact TM

Middle Ear Congenital Cholesteatoma
- Imaging: T1 C+ MR shows no enhancement of lesion, may have peripheral enhancement, bright signal on diffusion, & dark signal on ADC
- Clinical: White mass behind intact TM

Facial Nerve Schwannoma, Tympanic Segment
- Imaging: Pedunculated tympanic segment mass

- Clinical: Tan-white mass behind superior intact TM

PATHOLOGY

General Features

- Etiology
  - Arises from paraganglia found along tympanic nerve (Jacobson nerve) on cochlear promontory
    - Primitive neural crest-derived chemoreceptor cells
  - Nonchromaffin (nonsecretory) in this location
- Genetics
  - Hereditary predisposition in ~ 40%, most commonly associated with succinate dehydrogenase (SDH) gene mutations
    - *SDHD* is most common mutation for head & neck paragangliomas (~ 47% of hereditary cases)
    - *SDHB* mutation most commonly associated with metastatic disease
    - Rare association with mutations of *VHL*, *RET*, and *NF1*

Staging, Grading, & Classification

- Glasscock-Jackson classification of TPG
  - Type I: Small mass limited to cochlear promontory
  - Type II: Tumor completely filling middle ear cavity
  - Type III: Tumor filling middle ear & extending into mastoid air cells
  - Type IV: Tumor filling middle ear & extending into mastoid ± through TM to fill external auditory canal (EAC) ± extension anterior to ICA

Gross Pathologic & Surgical Features

- Glistening, red, polypoid mass on cochlear promontory
- Fibrous pseudocapsule

Microscopic Features

- All paragangliomas have same histopathology
- Biphasic cell pattern composed of chief cells & sustentacular cells surrounded by fibromuscular stroma
- Chief cells arranged in characteristic compact cell nests or "balls" of cells, referred to as **zellballen**
- Immunohistochemistry: Diffuse chromogranin reaction in chief cells
- Electron microscopy: Shows neurosecretory granules

CLINICAL ISSUES

Presentation

- Most common signs/symptoms
  - Vascular, pulsatile retrotympanic mass
    - If small: Anteroinferior quadrant of TM
    - Pneumatic otoscopy will cause blanching of mass known as Brown sign
  - Other signs/symptoms
    - PT (90%), conductive hearing loss (CHL) (50%), facial nerve (FN) paralysis (5%)
- Clinical profile
  - 50-year-old woman, PT, vascular retrotympanic mass

Demographics

- Age
  - 66% between 40-60 years of age at diagnosis
- Sex
  - M:F = 1:3

- Epidemiology
  - TPG is most common tumor of middle ear
  - TPG may be associated with hereditary paraganglioma-pheochromocytoma syndromes

Natural History & Prognosis

- Slow-growing, noninvasive tumor
- Average time from onset of symptoms to surgical treatment is 3 years
- Complete resection with goal of hearing and facial function preservation yields permanent surgical cure
- Recommended that all head and neck paraganglioma patients undergo screening for SDH gene mutations
  - 40% of head and neck paraganglioma patients have germline mutation
    - Most commonly *SDHD* mutation
  - 25% of patients with *SDHB* pathogenic variants have metastatic lesions

Treatment

- Smaller TPG lesions
  - Removed via tympanostomy through EAC
- Larger TPG lesions
  - Often require mastoidectomy
- Both endoscopic middle ear surgery (EMES) and microscopic middle ear surgery (MMES) demonstrate favorable surgical outcomes with low complication rates
- Preoperative selective embolization not necessary
- Stereotactic radiosurgery used when conventional surgical resection is contraindicated or incomplete

DIAGNOSTIC CHECKLIST

Consider

- Be careful with initial diagnosis
  - TPG may be clinically indistinguishable from jugular paraganglioma or aberrant ICA
  - If TPG is diagnosed when jugular paraganglioma is present, incomplete surgery will result
  - If TPG is diagnosed when aberrant ICA is present, biopsy could be fatal
- Preoperative imaging must differentiate these diagnoses

Image Interpretation Pearls

- Ask clinician color & location of retrotympanic mass
  - Red anteroinferior mass: TPG
  - Blue posteroinferior mass: Dehiscent jugular bulb
  - Red mass crossing behind inferior TM: Aberrant ICA
  - White mass: Congenital cholesteatoma (inferior) or facial nerve schwannoma (superior)

Reporting Tips

- Report if tumor in mesotympanum only vs. hypotympanum or epitympanum
  - Difference between tympanostomy or mastoidectomy

SELECTED REFERENCES

1. Chaushu H et al: Success and safety of endoscopic versus microscopic resection of temporal bone paraganglioma: a meta-analysis. Eur Arch Otorhinolaryngol. 281(10):5119-27, 2024
2. Yilala MH et al: Long-term surgical outcome of class A and B tympanomastoid paragangliomas. Cancers (Basel). 16(8):1466, 2024
3. Lee SJ et al: Treatment outcomes of patients with glomus tympanicum tumors presenting with pulsatile tinnitus. J Clin Med. 10(11):2348, 2021

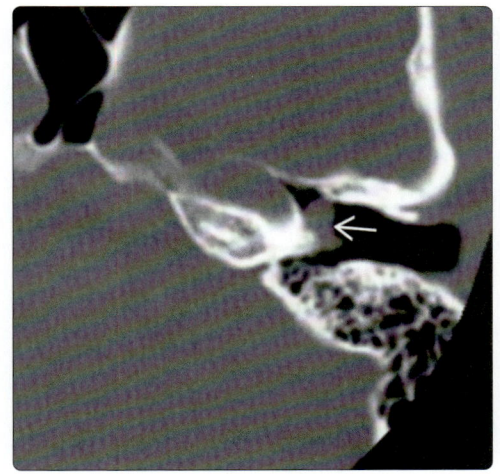

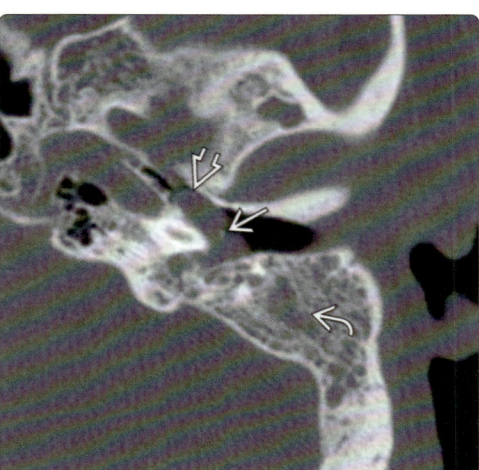

(Left) Axial left temporal bone CT shows a multilobular soft tissue mass on the low cochlear promontory ➡, consistent with a diagnosis of TPG. (Right) Axial bone CT shows a large TPG in the middle ear cavity. The lesion bulges the tympanic membrane laterally around the umbo of the manubrium ➡. Note extension into the proximal bony eustachian tube ➡ & opacification of mastoid air cells ➡ secondary to aditus ad antrum obstruction.

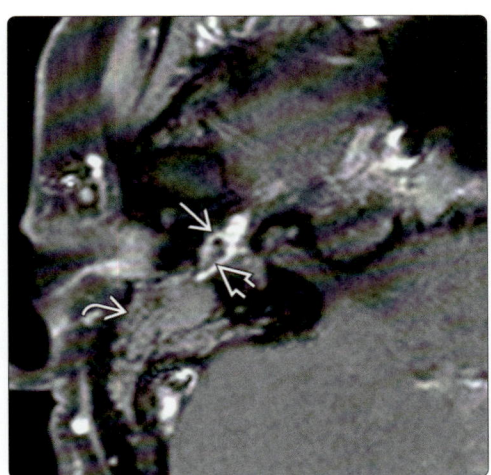

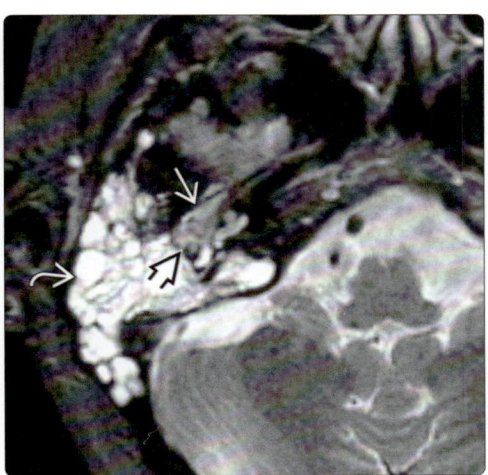

(Left) Axial T1 C+ FS MR of the right temporal bone shows an enhancing TPG ➡ filling the middle ear. Note the dark ossicles embedded within the tumor ➡. The aditus ad antrum is obstructed, causing nonenhancing fluid ➡ to back up within the mastoid air cells. (Right) Axial T2 FS MR reveals the TPG to be an intermediate signal intensity lesion in the middle ear ➡ compared to the very high signal obstructed mastoid secretions ➡. Note that the posterior margin of the mass obstructs the aditus ad antrum ➡.

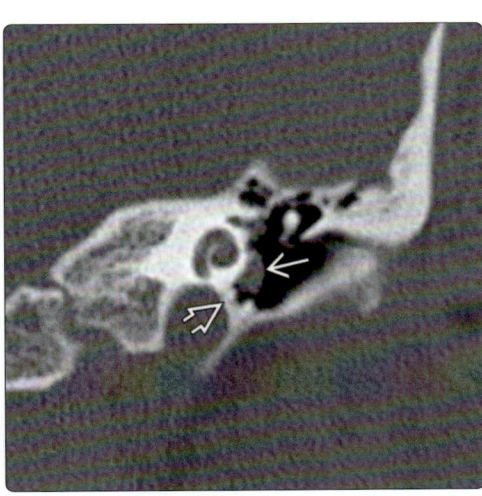

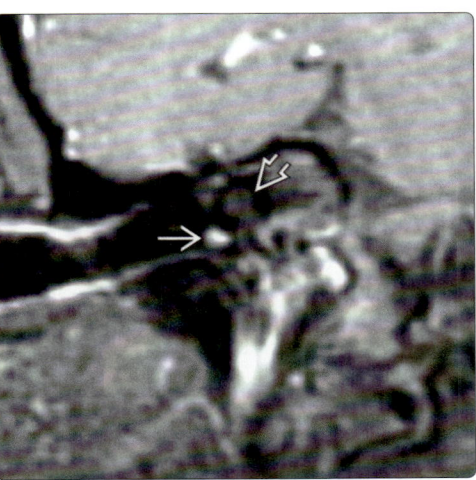

(Left) Coronal bone CT shows a sessile soft tissue lesion on the cochlear promontory ➡. This, in combination with the otoscopic report of a red, pulsatile, retrotympanic mass, is highly suggestive of TPG. Note the floor of the middle ear cavity is intact ➡, excluding the diagnosis of an aberrant ICA. (Right) Coronal T1 C+ FS MR reveals a TPG ➡ focus of enhancement inferolateral to the cochlea ➡. It would be easy to overlook such a small TPG without direction from the clinical history.

TERMINOLOGY

- Synonym: Intratympanic meningioma
- Definition: Meningioma involving middle ear (ME) or inner ear of temporal bone

IMAGING

- Morphology: Dural-based globular or en plaque mass
  - Extends into temporal bone via tegmen, internal carotid artery, or jugular foramen
- Bone CT findings
  - Permeative-sclerotic or **hyperostotic** changes
  - May underestimate extent of tumor
  - Intratumoral **calcification** common
  - **Ossicles intact** without destruction typically
- MR findings
  - Avidly enhancing mass involving temporal bone
  - If dural **tail** present, helps make diagnosis
  - Outline hyperenhancing rim sign favors meningioma
- 3 principal sites of origin + specific vector of spread

- Tegmen tympani tumor grows inferiorly into ME
  - Jugular foramen tumor grows centrifugally into ME if superolateral spread present
  - Internal auditory canal (IAC) tumor grows into inner ear
- Imaging protocol suggestion
  - Thin T1 C+ FS IAC MR best shows tumor extent
  - Especially with extensive intraosseous component

CLINICAL ISSUES

- Hearing loss patterns
  - Conductive: Tegmen tympani meningioma
  - Sensorineural: IAC meningioma
  - Mixed: Jugular foramen meningioma
- Otoscopy: Vascular retrotympanic mass if extends to ME
- Treatment: Surgical removal

DIAGNOSTIC CHECKLIST

- Identify site of origin, vector of spread, & extent
- Dural tails (MR) ± permeative sclerotic bone changes (CT)

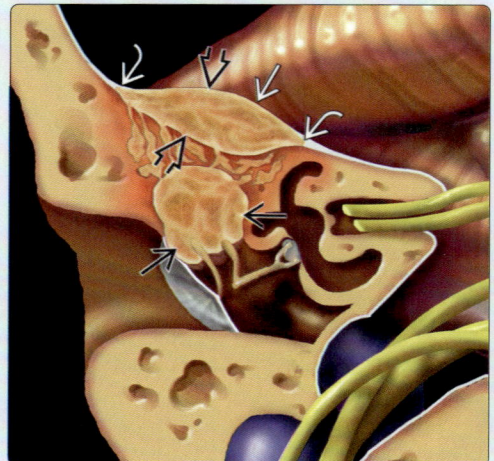
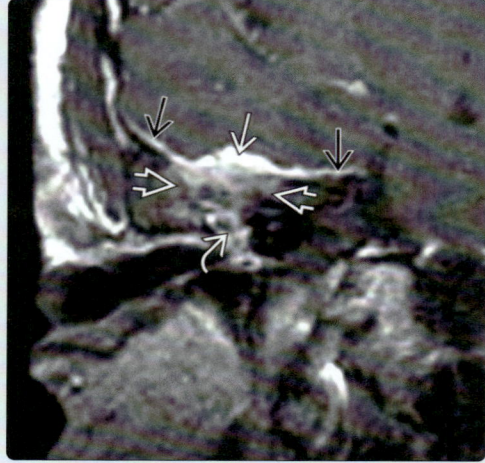

(Left) Coronal graphic of a tegmen tympani meningioma reveals en plaque dural origin of the tumor ➡ with spread through the tegmen ⊟ thickened by hyperostosis into the superior middle ear cavity. The ossicles have been engulfed by the tumor ➡. Dural tails are visible along the tumor margins ➡. (Right) Coronal T1 C+ FS MR shows an en plaque meningioma arising along the middle cranial fossa floor ➡. Note the enhancing dural tails ➡. Transosseous tegmen tumor ➡ spreads into the middle ear cavity & engulfs the ossicles ➡.

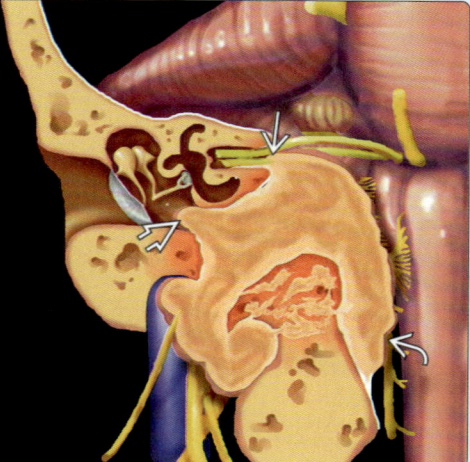
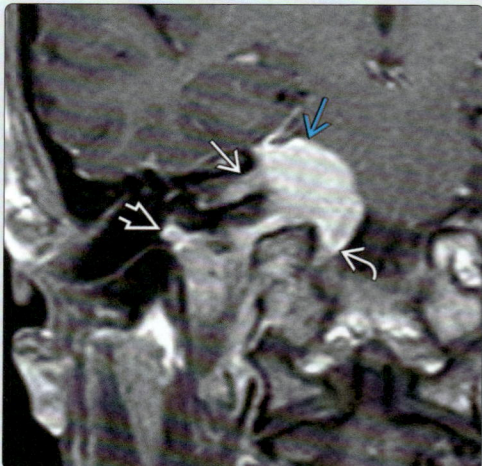

(Left) Coronal graphic of a jugular foramen (JF) meningioma depicts centrifugal spread pattern reaching the internal auditory canal (IAC) ➡, middle ear ⊟, & basal cistern ➡. When a JF meningioma reaches middle ear, it can mimic glomus jugulare paraganglioma. (Right) Coronal T1 C+ FS MR shows an extensive JF meningioma that spreads to IAC ➡, middle ear ⊟, & basal cistern ➡. Centrifugal spread pattern, dural-based morphology, & absence of flow voids with the outline sign ⊟ suggest meningioma.

TERMINOLOGY

Synonyms

- Temporal bone meningioma, intratympanic meningioma, middle ear (ME) meningioma

Definitions

- Meningioma involving temporal bone
  - May extend to ME, inner ear (IE), mastoid air cells, petrous apex air cells, internal auditory canal (IAC) &/or external auditory canal (EAC)

IMAGING

General Features

- Best diagnostic clue
  - Well-defined, **avidly enhancing** temporal bone mass
    - Best seen on T1 C+ FS MR
    - **Dural tails** highly suggestive of diagnosis
  - Bone CT shows **permeative-sclerotic** bone change
    - **Hyperostosis** is characteristic, if present
  - **Outline sign**: When seen, increases diagnostic confidence for meningioma
    - Thin, curvilinear, hyperenhancing line that may be seen along margin of meningioma on spin-echo postcontrast T1-weighted image
    - Can be complete enhancing line all around mass or incomplete & seen along parts of mass
    - Thought to reflect enhancement of hypervascular meningioma tumor capsule
- Location
  - From 3 principal sites of origin
    - Tegmen tympani
    - Jugular foramen
    - Cerebellopontine angle (CPA)/IAC
- Size
  - ME & IE component small (< 15 mm)
    - Involvement of temporal bone & beyond can be large
- Morphology
  - Dural component appears **globular** or **en plaque**
  - ME-mastoid components usually small, lobular, soft tissue masses
  - Transosseous/intraosseous component can be lobular or irregular with osseous enlargement
- **Vector of spread** characteristics from each site
  - **Tegmen tympani meningioma** spreads **inferiorly** to ME
  - **Jugular foramen meningioma** spreads **centrifugally** along dural surfaces in all directions
    - Enters ME via **superolateral** route
    - Mimics jugular paraganglioma when ME involvement occurs
  - **IAC meningioma** spreads from **CPA → IAC → intralabyrinthine structures** laterally

CT Findings

- CECT
  - 90% show strong, uniform enhancement
- Bone CT
  - General bone change findings
    - When transosseous: **Permeative-sclerotic** appearance, variable mild expansile changes

- When adjacent to bone: Sclerotic or **hyperostotic**
  - Intratumoral **calcification** common

MR Findings

- T1WI
  - Isointense to brain gray matter
- T2WI
  - Isointense or slightly higher signal than gray matter
  - If calcifications present, scattered low-intensity foci
- DWI
  - Characteristic low ADC signal intensity
- T1WI C+
  - 90% of temporal bone meningiomas strongly enhance
  - Dural component & ME/IE component enhance more strongly than intra-/transosseous components
  - If dural tail is present, may allow precise diagnosis
  - Outline sign
    - Thin, curvilinear, hyperenhancing line that may be seen along margin of meningioma

Angiographic Findings

- Vascular tumor with immediate tumor "blush"
- **Prolonged** vascular "stain" into venous phase
- Sunburst pattern of enlarged dural feeders may occur with large tumors
- ME component may be obscured by subtraction artifact

Imaging Recommendations

- Best imaging tool
  - Combined focused imaging of temporal bone with bone algorithm CT & thin-section T1 C+ FS MR
    - Temporal bone CT
      - Gives precise information about ossicles, CNVII
      - In larger lesions, pattern of bone change distinguishes meningioma from other pathologies
      - CT may underestimate tumor extent
    - Thin-section focused MR with T1 C+ fat saturated
      - Best to show tumor within bone, dura, & ME-IE
- Protocol advice
  - Bone CT: < 1-mm axial unenhanced sections with multiplanar reformations
  - MR: ≤ 3-mm T1 FS C+ axial & coronal sequences
  - Do not ignore precontrast T1 sequences for replacement of normal fat of temporal bone
    - Do **not** use fat saturation on precontrast T1 series

DIFFERENTIAL DIAGNOSIS

Jugular Paraganglioma

- Clinical: Red-vascular retrotympanic mass
- Temporal bone CT: Permeative-destructive bone erosion along superolateral margin of jugular bulb
- T1 MR: Jugular foramen mass with flow voids ("pepper") ± hyperintense foci ("salt") ± ME extension

Tympanic Paraganglioma

- Clinical: Red-vascular retrotympanic mass
- Temporal bone CT: Globular mass on cochlear promontory
  - Bony floor of ME cavity intact
- T1 C+ MR: Enhancing mass on cochlear promontory

Dehiscent Jugular Bulb

- Clinical: Blue-vascular posteroinferior retrotympanic mass
- Temporal bone CT: Dehisced bony plate between jugular bulb & ME

Aberrant Internal Carotid Artery

- Clinical: Red-vascular retrotympanic mass crosses cochlear promontory
- Temporal bone CT: Tubular mass crosses ME cavity to join horizontal petrous internal carotid artery (ICA)
  - Enlarged inferior tympanic canaliculus
- MRA: Asymmetric aberrant vessel

Middle Ear Cholesterol Granuloma

- Clinical: Blue-black retrotympanic mass
- Temporal bone CT: ME opacified ± ossicle destruction
- T1 MR: High signal from methemoglobin

PATHOLOGY

General Features

- Etiology
  - Arise from **arachnoid "cap" cells**
    - Embryonic migration anomaly
- Genetics
  - Long-arm deletions of chromosome 22 common if associated with multiply inherited schwannomas, meningiomas, & ependymomas (MISME) (neurofibromatosis type 2)
    - *NF2* gene inactivated in 60% of sporadic cases

Gross Pathologic & Surgical Features

- Sharply circumscribed, **unencapsulated**
- Adjacent dural thickening (collar or **tail**) is usually **reactive**, not neoplastic
- Globular (most common) or en plaque types

Microscopic Features

- Wide range of histology with little bearing on outcome
  - Meningothelial, fibrous, transitional, psammomatous, angiomatous, miscellaneous other (microcystic, chordoid, clear cell, secretory)
- Nests & whorls of meningiomatous cells
- Psammoma bodies: Calcifications

CLINICAL ISSUES

Presentation

- Most common signs/symptoms
  - Hearing loss
    - Conductive: Tegmen tympani meningioma
    - Sensorineural: IAC meningioma
    - Mixed: Jugular foramen meningioma
  - Facial neuropathy rare
  - Otoscopic examination: Vascular retrotympanic mass
    - ME component may represent "tip of iceberg" for larger intracranial component
- Other signs/symptoms
  - Symptoms from larger intracranial component
    - Skull base/CPA/IAC: Complex cranial neuropathy may involve V, VII, & VIII
    - Jugular foramen: IX-XII cranial neuropathy possible

- Clinical profile
  - Middle-aged woman with conductive hearing loss

Demographics

- Age
  - Average age at presentation = 45 years
- Sex
  - M:F = 1:3
- Epidemiology
  - 7% of intracranial meningiomas originate from anterior or posterior surface of petrous bone

Natural History & Prognosis

- Slow-growing benign tumor
- Relatively high recurrence rate due to difficulty of complete excision
- Prognosis relates to surgical outcome & complications
  - Hearing usually preserved at preoperative level
  - Facial nerve function good to acceptable
  - Chance of cranial nerve function restoration is low
  - Risk of new lower cranial nerve injury

Treatment

- Complete surgical excision
- Aggressive surgery advocated because bone invasion hard to see at surgery
- Endoscopic techniques are increasingly integrated with microsurgery
  - Endoscopy provides access to hard-to-reach areas within temporal bone
  - Offers clearer view of tumor & surrounding anatomy
- Radiotherapy can be considered if critical structures, such as cavernous sinus, ICA, or important cranial nerves, are involved

DIAGNOSTIC CHECKLIST

Image Interpretation Pearls

- Identify site of origin (tegmen, jugular foramen, or IAC)
- Use imaging findings to make meningioma diagnosis
  - Morphology: Dural-based globular or en plaque mass
  - Bone CT: Permeative-sclerotic, sclerotic, or hyperostotic
  - MR: Enhancing tumor with dural tail
- Use combination of CT & MR findings to define full tumor extent

SELECTED REFERENCES

1. Vasireddi AK et al: The "outline sign": thin hyperenhancing perimeter as an MR imaging feature of meningioma. A useful tool in the temporal bone region for differentiating meningiomas from schwannomas and paragangliomas. AJNR Am J Neuroradiol. 46(2):349-54, 2025
2. Burato A et al: En plaque meningioma of the temporal bone: a systematic review on the imaging and management of a rare tumor. Cancer Treat Res Commun. ePub, 2024
3. Han JJ et al: Clinicoradiologic characteristics of temporal bone meningioma: multicenter retrospective analysis. Laryngoscope. 131(1):173-8, 2021
4. Zeleník K et al: Temporal bone meningiomas: emphasizing radiologic signs to improve preoperative diagnosis. Eur Arch Otorhinolaryngol. 278(1):271-3, 2021
5. Stevens KL et al: Middle ear meningiomas: a case series reviewing the clinical presentation, radiologic features, and contemporary management of a rare temporal bone pathology. Am J Otolaryngol. 35(3):384-9, 2014
6. Hamilton BE et al: Imaging and clinical characteristics of temporal bone meningioma. AJNR Am J Neuroradiol. 27(10):2204-9, 2006

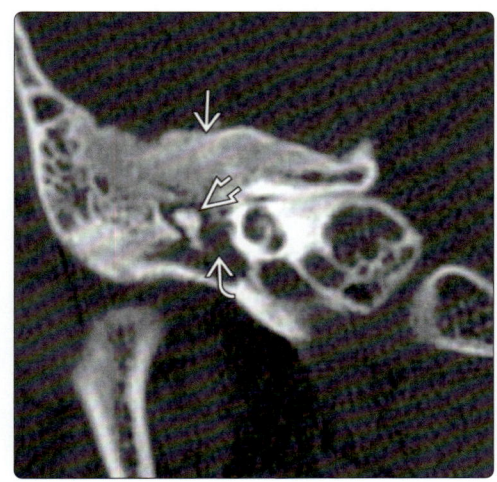

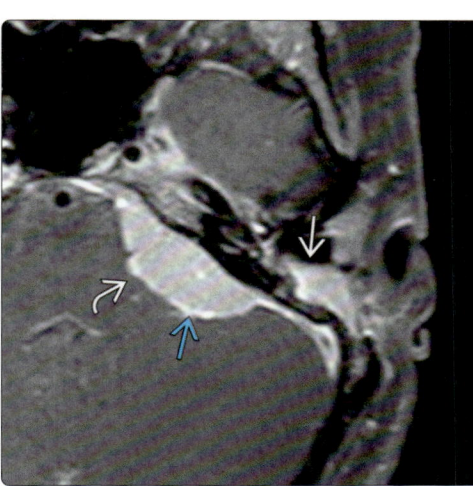

(Left) Coronal bone CT shows a thickened, sclerotic tegmen tympani ➡. Soft tissue density fills the middle ear ➡. The ossicles ➡ are encased but not eroded by this meningioma involving the middle ear. (Right) Axial T1 C+ FS MR shows an enhancing, dural-based meningioma in the cerebellopontine angle (CPA) cistern ➡ & tympanic cavity ➡. Note the presence of an outline sign ➡ (a thin, hyperenhancing tumor rim), which improves diagnostic confidence for a meningioma.

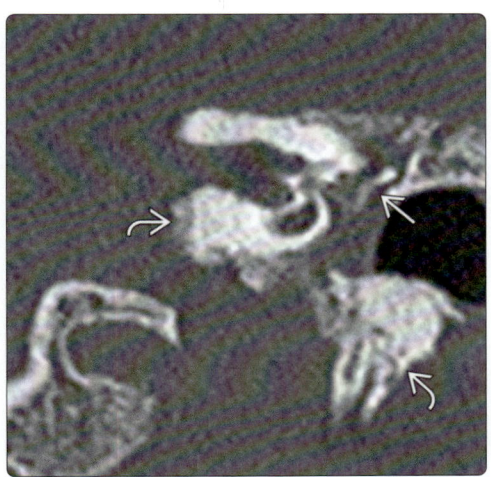

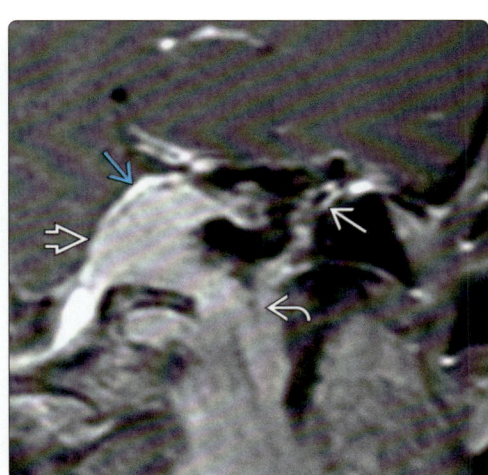

(Left) Coronal bone CT shows opacification of the middle ear by meningioma involvement without ossicular erosion ➡. Permeative-sclerotic changes are noted involving the temporal bone ➡. (Right) Coronal T1 C+ FS MR in the same patient shows the dural-based enhancing mass ➡ in the CPA-IAC extending through the jugular foramen ➡ into the upper neck. The ossicles are surrounded by enhancing middle ear meningioma ➡. An outline sign ➡ (hyperenhancing tumor rim) is present, characteristic of meningioma.

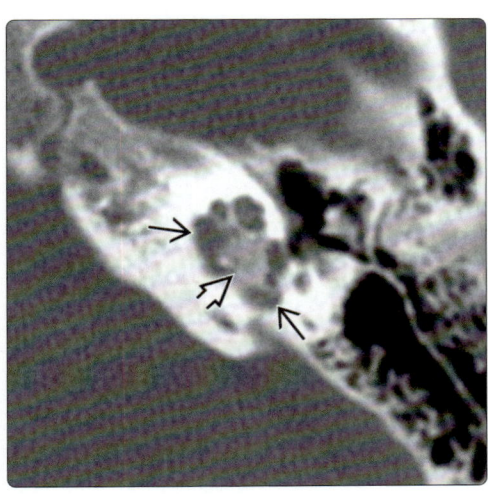

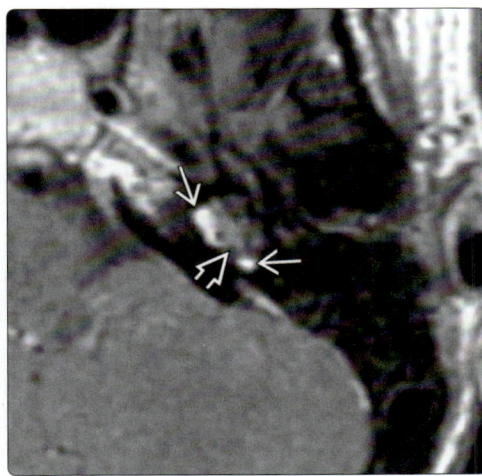

(Left) Axial bone CT shows a rare inner ear meningioma with both lucent ➡ & sclerotic ➡ components. The lesion involves the area of the vestibule & basal turn of the cochlea. (Courtesy R. Wallace, MD.) (Right) Axial T1 C+ MR demonstrates a rare inner ear meningioma with enhancement ➡ of corresponding radiolucent areas on CT & relative lack of enhancement in the corresponding CT radiodense areas ➡.

Middle Ear Schwannoma

TERMINOLOGY

- **Primary schwannoma**: Primary to middle ear (ME) cavity
  - Tympanic segment CNVII > > tympanic nerve (CNIX branch), chorda tympani nerve (CNVII branch)
- **Secondary schwannoma**: Arises outside ME
  - Jugular foramen schwannoma involves ME
  - Translabyrinthine CNVIII schwannoma
  - Primary inner ear schwannoma → ME

IMAGING

- Bone CT findings
  - **CNVII schwannoma**: Well-marginated mass emanating from CNVII canal
  - **Transotic intralabyrinthine schwannoma** (spread from inner ear with ME protrusion): Labyrinth erosions with mass protruding into ME via round or oval window

- **ME schwannoma** (from chorda tympani or tympanic nerve): Focal mass filling ME without involving CNVII canal; inferior tympanic canaliculus expanded in tympanic nerve schwannoma
- T1 C+ MR findings
  - CNVII schwannoma: Enhancing mass contiguous with tympanic or mastoid CNVII
  - Transotic intralabyrinthine schwannoma: Enhancing mass contiguous with IAC & inner ear spaces

TOP DIFFERENTIAL DIAGNOSES

- Congenital ME cholesteatoma
- Tympanic paraganglioma
- Pars flaccida-acquired cholesteatoma
- ME neuroendocrine tumor

CLINICAL ISSUES

- Presentation: Conductive hearing loss
- Otoscopy: Fleshy-white mass behind intact tympanic membrane

(Left) Axial bone CT in a patient presenting with left facial weakness shows a soft tissue mass in the epitympanum displacing ossicles laterally ➡. The patient also had conductive hearing loss due to mass effect on the ossicular chain. Note the dehiscence along the lateral aspect of the tympanic segment of facial nerve canal ➡, suggesting the tumor origin. (Right) Axial T1 C+ FS MR in the same patient shows corresponding enhancement in this facial schwannoma ➡.

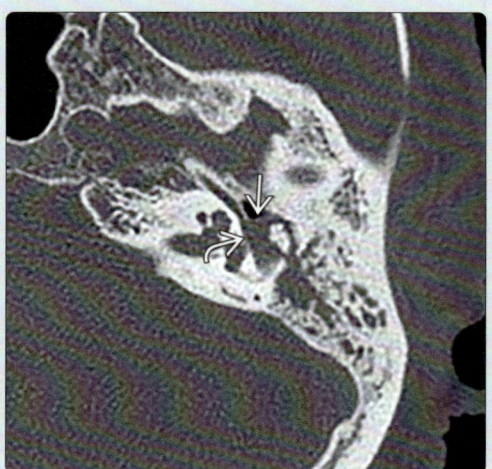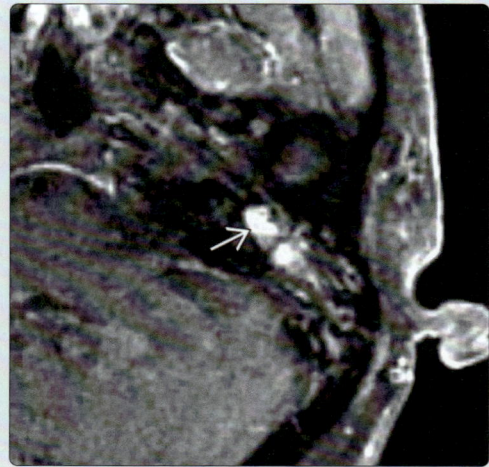

(Left) Axial bone CT shows facial nerve schwannoma protruding from the posterior genu into the posterior mesotympanum ➡. Note that the tumor abuts the short process of incus ➡, causing subtle erosion in this area. (Right) Axial T1 C+ MR reveals homogeneous enhancement of facial nerve schwannoma ➡ protruding from the posterior genu into the posterior mesotympanum. The patient presented with conductive hearing loss and a tan-white mass behind an intact tympanic membrane.

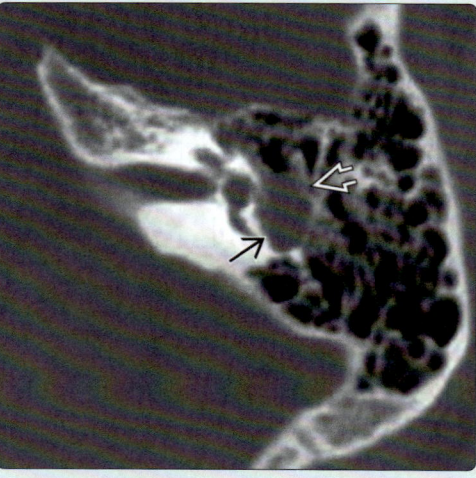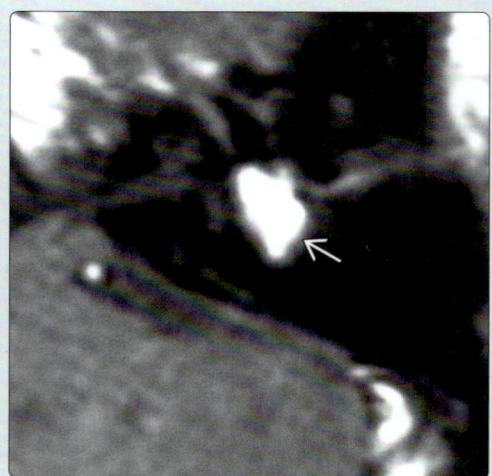

TERMINOLOGY

Synonyms

- Facial nerve schwannoma, tympanic nerve schwannoma, chorda tympani schwannoma

Definitions

- **Primary schwannoma**: Tumor primary to middle ear (ME)
  - Tympanic segment CNVII > > tympanic nerve (tympanic branch of CNIX or Jacobson nerve), chorda tympani nerve
- **Secondary schwannoma**: Arises outside ME
  - Large CNIX-XI jugular foramen schwannoma eroding into ME
  - Translabyrinthine CNVIII schwannoma
    - Cerebellopontine angle-internal auditory canal (CPA-IAC) → inner ear → ME
  - Primary inner ear schwannoma → ME

IMAGING

General Features

- Best diagnostic clue
  - T1 C+ MR shows enhancing mass in ME
- Size
  - Variable, usually < 15 mm
- Morphology
  - Well-marginated, lobular mass

CT Findings

- CECT
  - Lesion enhances with contrast
- Bone CT
  - **Facial nerve schwannoma**
    - Well-marginated mass emanating from CNVII canal
      - □ Tympanic or mastoid segments
  - **Transotic intralabyrinthine schwannoma** (spread from inner ear with ME protrusion)
    - Labyrinth erosions with mass protruding into ME via round or oval window
  - **ME schwannoma** (chorda tympani or tympanic nerve)
    - Well-marginated ME mass sparing CNVII canal
    - Bony expansion when large

MR Findings

- T1WI C+
  - Lobulated, enhancing mass (differentiates from cholesteatoma)
    - Facial nerve schwannoma: Contiguous with tympanic or mastoid CNVII
    - Transotic intralabyrinthine schwannoma: Enhancing mass contiguous with IAC & inner ear
    - ME schwannoma: Mass primary to ME cavity
  - **Intramural cysts** may be visible when large

Imaging Recommendations

- Best imaging tool
  - T1 C+ MR thin sections through temporal bone
- Protocol advice
  - Thin-section T1 C+ MR with diffusion differentiates schwannoma from cholesteatoma
  - Thin-section bone CT in axial & coronal planes

DIFFERENTIAL DIAGNOSIS

Congenital Middle Ear Cholesteatoma

- Child or young adult with conductive hearing loss
- Otoscopy: Tan-white mass behind **intact tympanic membrane (TM)**
- Bone CT: Lobulated mass, medial to ossicles
- MR: Nonenhancing ME mass
  - DWI: High signal from restricted diffusion

Tympanic Paraganglioma

- Adult patient population
- Otoscopy: Pink-red, pulsatile mass behind intact TM
- Bone CT: Cochlear promontory mass; ME floor intact
- MR: Enhancing mass

Middle Ear Neuroendocrine Tumor

- Rare ME tumor (formerly termed ME adenoma)
- Otoscopy: Tan mass behind intact TM
- Bone CT: Remodeling or invasive-appearing ME mass
- MR: Enhancing ME mass

PATHOLOGY

General Features

- Etiology
  - Neuroectodermal origin
  - Slow-growing, encapsulated, benign lesion

Gross Pathologic & Surgical Features

- Encapsulated tan or gray neoplasm

CLINICAL ISSUES

Presentation

- Most common signs/symptoms
  - Conductive hearing loss (especially tympanic)
  - Facial nerve weak (↑ in women, labyrinthine/tympanic)
  - Otoscopy: Fleshy-white mass behind intact TM

Treatment

- Surgical removal, radiation, or imaging surveillance

DIAGNOSTIC CHECKLIST

Consider

- If ME schwannoma diagnosis is considered
  - Is tumor from facial nerve canal?
    - Pedunculated facial nerve schwannoma
  - Is tumor primary to ME cavity?
    - ME schwannoma
    - Tympanic paraganglioma
    - ME congenital cholesteatoma
    - ME neuroendocrine tumor

SELECTED REFERENCES

1. Rehal O et al: Chorda tympani schwannoma: a rare nerve sheath tumor of the middle ear cleft. Otol Neurotol. 45(4):e359-61, 2024
2. Maccarrone F et al: Features and management of a schwannoma of the chorda tympani and review of the literature. Neuroradiol J. 36(4):486-90, 2023
3. Wiggins RH 3rd et al: The many faces of facial nerve schwannoma. AJNR Am J Neuroradiol. 27(3):694-9, 2006

Middle Ear Neuroendocrine Tumor

TERMINOLOGY

- Middle ear (ME) neuroendocrine tumor (MeNET)
  - Very rare, benign tumor of mixed exocrine and neuroendocrine origin
  - Formerly termed middle ear adenoma

IMAGING

- Soft tissue mass in ME
- Temporal bone CT findings
  - ME mass behind intact tympanic membrane (TM)
  - Indistinguishable on bone CT from tympanic paraganglioma and pedunculated ME schwannoma
  - Well-pneumatized mastoid (no history of chronic otitis media)
  - May show areas of local bone invasion
  - May show new bone formation in tympanic cavity or around eustachian tube opening
- MR findings
  - If large adenoma present, T1WI C+ MR may be helpful in defining lesion extent
  - MeNET enhances like tympanic paraganglioma and pedunculated CNVII schwannoma

TOP DIFFERENTIAL DIAGNOSES

- Tympanic paraganglioma
- Pedunculated facial nerve schwannoma
- ME congenital cholesteatoma

CLINICAL ISSUES

- Otoscopy appearance
  - Tan-pink soft tissue mass behind intact TM
- Principal symptoms
  - Tinnitus and conductive hearing loss
  - "Ear fullness"
- Mean age at presentation: 45 years
- Natural history of tumor
  - If aggressive type, facial nerve injury possible

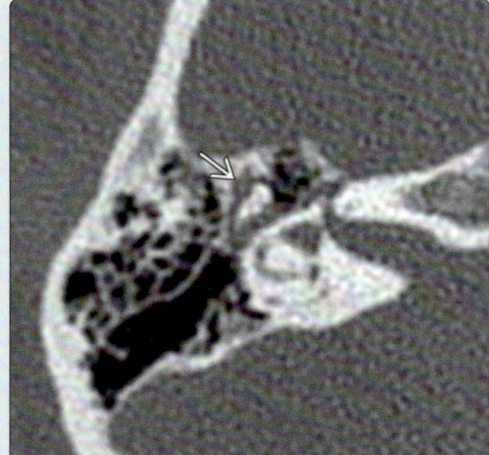
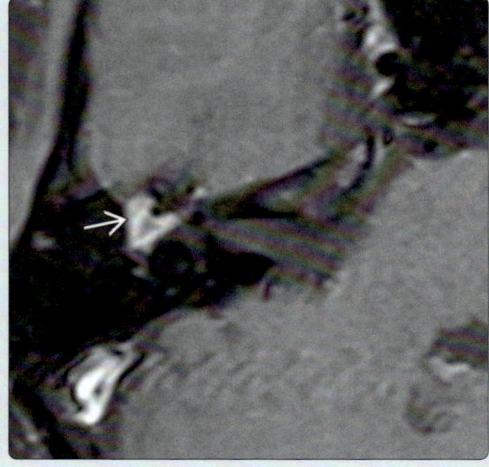

(Left) Axial bone algorithm CT of the right middle ear in a patient who presented with conductive hearing loss and a white mass behind an intact tympanic membrane (TM) shows abnormal soft tissue density ➡ surrounding ossicles without osseous destruction. (Right) Axial T1 FS MR in the same patient shows abnormal enhancing soft tissue ➡ surrounding the right ossicles at the level of the epitympanum, found to be a middle ear neuroendocrine tumor. No restricted diffusion was seen to suggest a cholesteatoma.

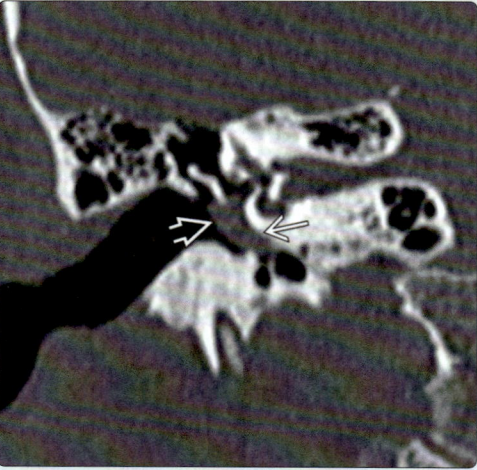
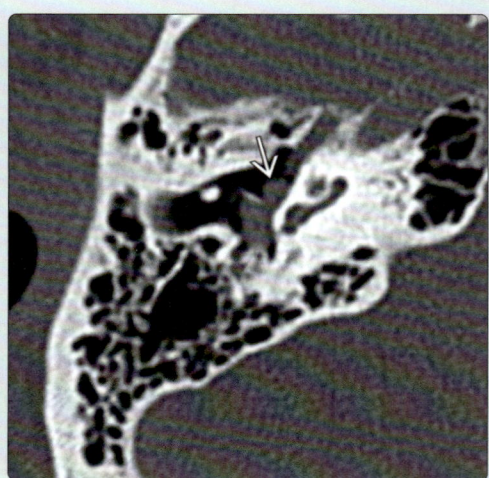

(Left) Coronal bone CT through the middle ear cavity shows a soft tissue mass on the cochlear promontory ➡ within the hypotympanum and mesotympanum and posterior to the TM ➡, found to be a noninvasive middle ear neuroendocrine tumor. (Right) Axial bone CT through the low mesotympanum shows a noninvasive middle ear neuroendocrine tumor ➡ over the cochlear promontory without osseous destruction and behind an intact TM.

TERMINOLOGY

Abbreviations

- Middle ear (ME) neuroendocrine tumor (MeNET)

Synonyms

- Formerly ME adenoma (MEA); terminology changed to MeNET in WHO Classification of Head and Neck Tumors, 5th edition (2022)
- Numerous acronyms: Mixed epithelial and neuroendocrine tumor (MENET), neuroendocrine adenoma of ME (NAME), ME adenoma with neuroendocrine differentiation (MEA-ND), ME adenomatous tumors (MEAT), ME adenomatous neuroendocrine tumors (MEANTs)

Definitions

- Very rare, benign tumor arising from mucosal cells of ME having variable mixed epithelial and neuroendocrine differentiation

IMAGING

General Features

- Best diagnostic clue
  - Soft tissue mass + well-pneumatized mastoid (no chronic otitis media findings)
- Location
  - ME cavity proper (mesotympanum); can be found around eustachian tube opening
- Size
  - Early symptoms: Small (< 10 mm) at diagnosis
- Morphology
  - Often irregularly marginated

CT Findings

- CECT
  - Enhances but difficult to see
- Bone CT
  - Mass within ME behind intact tympanic membrane (TM)
    - Indistinguishable on bone CT from tympanic paraganglioma and pedunculated ME schwannoma
    - May rarely show areas of local bone invasion

MR Findings

- DWI
  - Typically do not have restricted diffusion
- T1WI C+
  - Enhancing soft tissue mass in ME

Imaging Recommendations

- Best imaging tool
  - Temporal bone CT
- Protocol advice
  - Axial and coronal bone CT without contrast
    - If large adenoma present, T1WI C+ MR may be helpful in defining lesion extent

DIFFERENTIAL DIAGNOSIS

Tympanic Paraganglioma

- Otoscopy: Pulsatile, red, retrotympanic mass
- CT: Noninvasive cochlear promontory mass
- T1WI C+ MR: Enhancing mass

Pedunculated Facial Nerve Schwannoma

- Otoscopy: Avascular mass mimics congenital cholesteatoma
- T1WI C+ MR: Enhancing mass connected to CNVII

Middle Ear Congenital Cholesteatoma

- Clinical: Child; no history of chronic otitis media
- CT: When large, typically erosive
- T1WI C+ MR: No enhancement

PATHOLOGY

General Features

- Etiology
  - Benign, indolent epithelial tumors of ME that rarely invade bone
    - **Mixed exocrine and neuroendocrine** differentiation
  - MeNET arises from modified respiratory mucosa

Gross Pathologic & Surgical Features

- Pink, yellow, gray, or reddish-brown, firm tissue mass

CLINICAL ISSUES

Presentation

- Most common signs/symptoms
  - Otoscopy: Tan-pink soft tissue mass behind intact TM
  - Conductive hearing loss

Demographics

- Age
  - Mean at presentation: 45 years
- Sex
  - M = F
- Epidemiology
  - Very rare ME tumor

Natural History & Prognosis

- Slow-growing, benign tumor
- If aggressive type, facial nerve injury possible
- Recurrence of tumor common problem
- May progress to become malignant adenocarcinoma

Treatment

- Complete surgical excision is treatment of choice

DIAGNOSTIC CHECKLIST

Image Interpretation Pearls

- Otoscopic examination and imaging findings both nonspecific

Reporting Tips

- Describe extension outside of ME
  - Follow-up required: 20% recurrence rate

SELECTED REFERENCES

1. You D et al: Clinical predilection features of middle ear adenomatous neuroendocrine tumors: a review of 10 patients and a special case is attached. Ear Nose Throat J. ePub, 2024
2. Mete O et al: Update from the 5th edition of the World Health Organization Classification of Head and Neck Tumors: overview of the 2022 WHO classification of head and neck neuroendocrine neoplasms. Head Neck Pathol. 16(1):123-42, 2022

Temporal Bone Rhabdomyosarcoma

TERMINOLOGY

- **Rhabdomyosarcoma (RMS): Rare, destructive, pediatric T-bone lesion**
  - Arises from embryonic skeletal muscle precursor cells or pluripotential mesenchymal cells

IMAGING

- Middle ear-mastoid or petrous apex destructive mass with variable contrast enhancement
  - Middle ear RMS often with associated external auditory canal extension (aural polyp)
  - Petrous apex RMS may be primary or spread from parameningeal RMS
  - Skull base and cranial nerve involvement common
- Both CT and MR recommended to stage skull base destruction and middle ear and intracranial extension
- T1 C+ FS MR best to detect intracranial extension via tegmen, mastoid roof, ± skull base foramina
- T2 MR helpful to differentiate obstructed mastoid secretions (more hyperintense than RMS)

TOP DIFFERENTIAL DIAGNOSES

- Acquired cholesteatoma
- Langerhans cell histiocytosis of T-bone
- Acute otomastoiditis with coalescence
- Metastatic neuroblastoma
- Cholesterol granuloma of middle ear

CLINICAL ISSUES

- Clinical presentation
  - Child (< 6 years old) with chronic otitis media
  - Other symptoms: Otorrhea, ear pain, external auditory canal polyp
- Most common soft tissue sarcoma in children
- Up to 40% of RMSs in children occur in H&N
  - 7% of H&N RMSs occur in T-bone

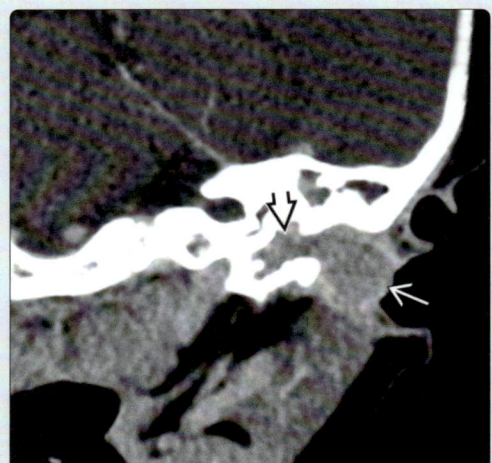
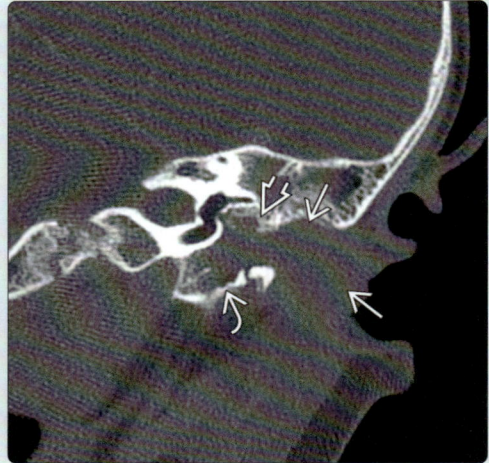

(Left) Coronal CECT in a 2-year-old child with an external auditory canal (EAC) polyp and bleeding shows a lobulated mass filling and protruding from the left EAC ➡. There is also involvement of middle ear cavity ⊡. This was a rapidly growing rhabdomyosarcoma (RMS), as the clinician reported visualization of tympanic membrane 3 weeks prior. (Right) Coronal bone CT in the same patient shows rapidly growing RMS of the left EAC ➡, middle ear cavity ⊡, and mastoid air cells. This tumor causes osseous erosion of floor of hypotympanum ⊡.

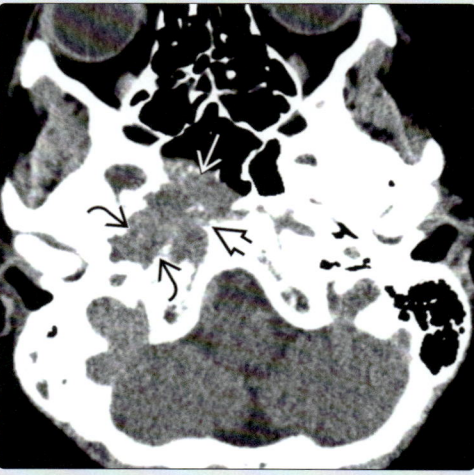
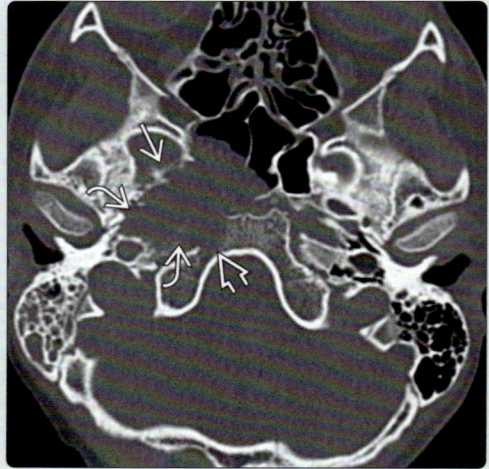

(Left) Axial NECT of the skull base in an 11-year-old boy with nasopharyngeal RMS shows superior extension of the mass into the sphenoid sinus ➡, adjacent skull base/clivus ⊡, and inferior aspect of the petrous apex ⊡. (Right) Axial bone CT in the same patient clearly defines erosion of the petrous apex ➡, clivus ⊡, and middle cranial fossa floor ➡ in a patient with RMS of the nasopharynx. This is a characteristic pattern of spread in parameningeal RMS.

TERMINOLOGY

Abbreviations

- Rhabdomyosarcoma (RMS)

Definitions

- Rare, **destructive**, **pediatric T-bone lesion**
  - Arises from embryonic skeletal muscle precursor cells or pluripotential mesenchymal cells

IMAGING

General Features

- Best diagnostic clue
  - T-bone CT: Destructive middle ear-mastoid or petrous apex (PA) mass + variable contrast enhancement
  - T1 FS C+ MR: Irregular, invasive, enhancing middle ear-mastoid or PA mass in child
- Location
  - Middle ear ± mastoid or PA
    - Or direct extension from other parameningeal sites: Nasopharynx, masticator space, pterygopalatine fossa, or parapharyngeal space
  - Possible areas of extension with T-bone involvement
    - Lateral into external auditory canal (EAC)
    - Medial into internal auditory canal (IAC) via CNVII canal
    - Cephalad into middle cranial fossa via mastoid or tympanic tegmen
    - Posterior into posterior cranial fossa: Direct extension or perineural spread (CNVII canal → IAC → posterior fossa)
    - Inferior into carotid space via carotid canal or jugular foramen
    - Anteroinferior into TMJ, masticator, or parotid spaces
- Size
  - Depends on tumor location; most > 3 cm
  - Fills middle ear-mastoid complex with intracranial extension
- Morphology
  - Poorly defined, locally destructive mass

CT Findings

- Middle ear-mastoid or PA destructive mass
  - Lytic, destructive bone and ossicle changes
  - Soft tissue mass with variable contrast enhancement
    - Mass may be hemorrhagic and necrotic
  - Often with associated EAC extension
  - Skull base and cranial nerve foraminal involvement common
- Nodal metastases rare at presentation unless intracranial or extracranial extension present

MR Findings

- **Iso**- to hypointense **T1**; **hyper**- to isointense **T2** mass
- Variable contrast enhancement
  - Coronal images best to detect intracranial extension via tegmen, mastoid roof ± skull base foramina
- Intracranial extension in parameningeal RMS → meningeal thickening and enhancement
  - ± enhancing intracranial mass
- T2 helpful to differentiate obstructed mastoid secretions (more hyperintense than RMS)

Nuclear Medicine Findings

- PET
  - Intense FDG uptake by soft tissue tumor
  - Helpful for staging and posttreatment surveillance
    - Nodal staging
    - Distant metastases staging

Imaging Recommendations

- Best imaging tool
  - Both CT and MR recommended to stage primary mass, skull base destruction, and intracranial extension
  - Coronal T1 C+ FS MR best to identify intracranial and extracranial extension
- Protocol advice
  - Complex skull base mass with potential for intracranial extension, distant metastases, and cervical adenopathy requires careful multimodality work-up
    - Thin-section T-bone CT in axial plane with coronal and sagittal reformations
    - Multiplanar MR pre- and post contrast
    - Cervical adenopathy can be staged with either CECT, MR, or **PET/CT**

DIFFERENTIAL DIAGNOSIS

Pars Flaccida-Acquired Cholesteatoma

- Clinical: Pars flaccida tympanic membrane (TM) perforation or retraction ± visible cholesteatoma
- Bone CT: Scutum and ossicle erosion; soft tissue in Prussak space
  - Unless large, less extensive bone changes than RMS

Pars Tensa-Acquired Cholesteatoma

- Clinical: Pars tensa TM perforation with visible cholesteatoma
- Bone CT: Soft tissue medial to ossicles with erosions

T-Bone Langerhans Cell Histiocytosis

- Clinical: Pediatric patient with middle ear mass
  - Usually no cranial nerve palsy
- Bone CT: Destructive, enhancing T-bone mass
  - Often bilateral or with other osseous lesions

Acute Otomastoiditis With Coalescence

- Clinical: Fever, mastoid tenderness in child
- Bone CT: Opacified middle ear-mastoid
  - Mastoid trabecular breakdown mimics tumor

Metastatic Neuroblastoma

- Metastatic disease to skull base frequently bilateral with enhancing masses, aggressive osseous erosion, and spiculated periosteal reaction

Middle Ear Cholesterol Granuloma

- Clinical: Retrotympanic "vascular" blue hue
  - Past history of multiple prior ear infections
- Imaging: MR shows **high-T1-** and high-T2-signal mass in middle ear ± mastoid

PATHOLOGY

General Features

- Etiology

- Malignant tumor of **embryologic skeletal muscle cells** or **pluripotential mesenchymal cells**
- Rarely radiation-induced 2nd primary neoplasm
- Genetics
  - Most cases are sporadic
  - Increased incidence in children with *Tp53* tumor suppressor gene mutation, Noonan syndrome, Beckwith-Wiedemann syndrome, hereditary retinoblastoma

Staging, Grading, & Classification

- **T-bone RMS** considered **parameningeal**
- Clinical group system (International Rhabdomyosarcoma Study Group) based on surgical resection prior to chemo/RT
  - Group I: Completely resected localized disease, no regional nodes
  - Group II: Total gross resection + completely resected regional disease or microscopic residual disease
  - Group III: Gross residual disease
  - Group IV: Distant metastases; worst prognosis
- TNM staging based on clinical and radiologic findings prior to any treatment

Gross Pathologic & Surgical Features

- Variable: Smooth, lobulated necrotic or hemorrhagic **or** infiltrative mass with poorly defined margins

Microscopic Features

- **Rhabdomyoblasts** in varying stages of differentiation
- Immunohistochemistry positive for desmin, vimentin, MSA, antimyogenin, and MYOD1
- 3 subtypes: Embryonal, alveolar, and pleomorphic
  - **Embryonal** (**ERMS**): Most common (55%)
    - Occurs in younger children
    - Accounts for > 50% of all RMSs; 70-90% occur in H&N or genitourinary tract
  - **Alveolar** (**ARMS**): 2nd most common (20%)
    - Usually occurs in older patients (15-25 years of age)
    - Most common in extremities and trunk
  - **Pleomorphic** (**anaplastic**): Least common (20%)
    - Very rare; generally adults 40-60 years of age
    - Most common in extremities, rare in H&N

CLINICAL ISSUES

Presentation

- Most common signs/symptoms
  - Mimics chronic otitis media with chronic otorrhea (sometimes bloody) and ear pain
  - Other signs/symptoms
    - Aural (EAC) polyp
    - Facial nerve palsy
    - Postauricular mass
- Other signs/symptoms
  - Hearing loss, headache, cervical lymph nodes
- Clinical profile
  - **Child < 6 years of age** with chronic otitis media, otorrhea, and ear pain with EAC polyp unresponsive to medical management

Demographics

- Age
  - **Bimodal**; children (2-5 years) and late teens (15-19 years)

- Rarely occurs in adults
- Epidemiology
  - RMS is most common soft tissue sarcoma in children
    - Most common pediatric T-bone malignancy
  - Up to **40% of RMSs occur in H&N**
    - **Orbit**: Most common H&N site
    - **Parameningeal sites**: Middle ear, paranasal sinus, nasopharynx, masticator space, pterygopalatine fossa, parapharyngeal space
      - □ Intracranial extension in up to 55%
  - 7% of H&N RMSs occur in T-bone

Natural History & Prognosis

- Delay to diagnosis common
  - Child initially treated for acute or chronic otitis media
- T-bone RMS has **high probability of meningeal extension** at time of diagnosis
  - Extremely poor prognosis if intracranial spread and distant metastases present
- Embryonal type better prognosis than ARMS
- Distant metastases: Lungs > > bone, liver, brain

Treatment

- T-bone RMSs are rarely resectable
  - Surgery: Biopsy or debulking
  - Multidrug chemotherapy + adjuvant radiation

DIAGNOSTIC CHECKLIST

Consider

- Clinical: Consider T-bone RMS if aural polyp or CNVII palsy found in child with chronic otitis media
- Imaging: Consider T-bone RMS if unilateral destructive T-bone mass in child
  - **Caveat**: Langerhans cell histiocytosis of T-bone can exactly mimic T-bone RMS

Image Interpretation Pearls

- Both CT and MR important for staging primary site, local disease, and nodal metastases
- Coronal plane needed to assess integrity of skull base and detect intracranial extension
  - MR is preferred modality
- PET/CT: Nodal, distant metastases and surveillance
  - Replacing bone scan in RMS work-up

Reporting Tips

- Describe location and extent of osseous destruction
  - Note intra- and extracranial extension
  - Note perivascular and perineural spread

SELECTED REFERENCES

1. Li Y et al: Rhabdomyosarcoma of the middle ear and mastoid in children: experience of the Beijing Children's Hospital-BCH. Otol Neurotol. 46(3):314-320, 2025
2. Markov SS et al: Rhabdomyosarcoma of the middle ear case report. Children (Basel). 11(12):1496, 2024
3. Crane JN et al: Clinical group and modified TNM stage for rhabdomyosarcoma: a review from the Children's Oncology Group. Pediatr Blood Cancer. 69(6):e29644, 2022
4. Robson CD: Imaging of head and neck neoplasms in children. Pediatr Radiol. 40(4):499-509, 2010

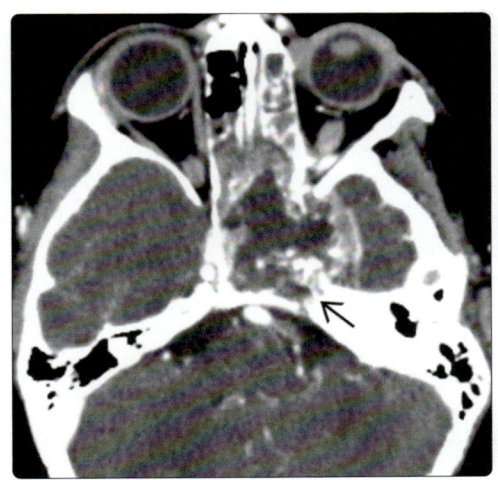

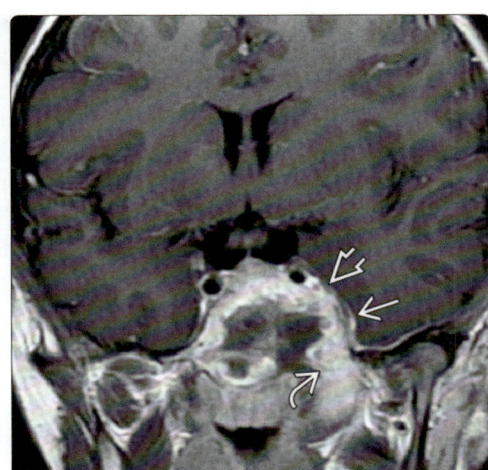

(Left) Axial CECT in a 6-year-old boy with left facial nerve palsy shows superior extension of a large, necrotic left parapharyngeal RMS invading the sphenoid sinus, cavernous sinus, and middle cranial fossa with erosion of the left petrous apex ➡. (Right) Coronal T1WI C+ MR in a patient with parapharyngeal RMS shows extension of the mass into the middle cranial fossa ➡ by direct skull base destruction ➡ as well as involvement of the left cavernous sinus ➡. Smooth interface with brain suggests no intradural extension.

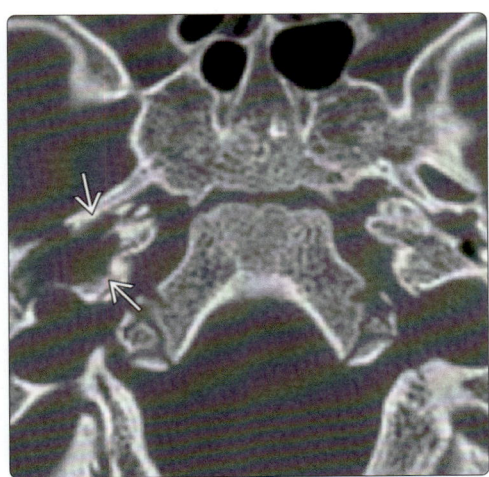

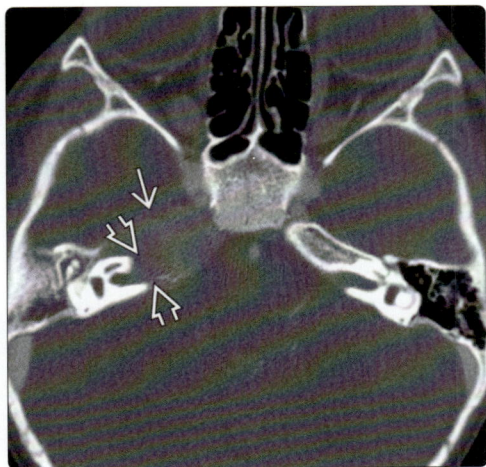

(Left) Axial bone CT in a 2-year-old child with chronic otitis media shows a lytic lesion in the right petrous apex ➡. Initial biopsy showed no evidence of malignancy or Langerhans cell histiocytosis. T-bone RMS remained stable for 8 months. (Right) Axial bone CT in the same patient (with prior biopsy negative), presenting now with growing right petrous apex lesion and right facial nerve palsy, shows marked destruction of the right petrous apex ➡ with complete erosion of the walls of the right internal auditory canal ➡.

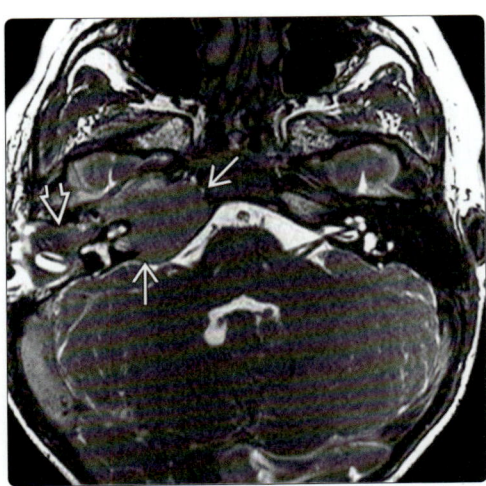

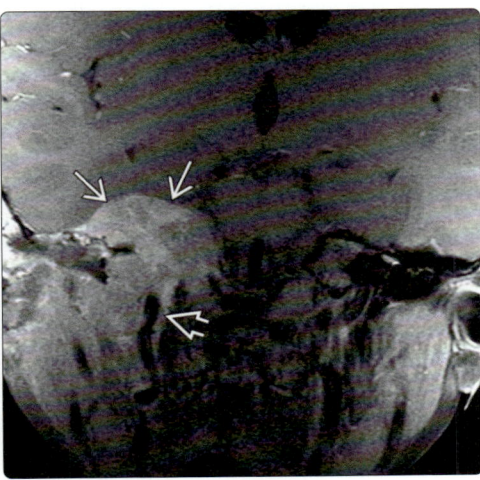

(Left) Axial T2 FSE MR shows an expansile, hypointense mass, typical of a very cellular lesion. The lesion involves the middle ear cavity ➡ and petrous apex ➡. RMS was confirmed at repeat biopsy in this 3-year-old child. (Right) Coronal T1WI C+ FS MR defines the intracranial extension ➡, which is common in patients with parameningeal RMS. Note also extension along the vertical segment of the petrous internal carotid artery ➡.

TERMINOLOGY

- Cephalocele is broad term that includes meningocele, encephalocele, or meningoencephalocele
- Temporal bone cephalocele: Protrusion of cranial contents into middle ear (ME) or mastoid through dehiscence of tegmen

IMAGING

- CT: Dehiscence of **tegmen tympani** &/or **tegmen mastoideum** with associated soft tissue opacification of epitympanum that is inseparable form intracranial soft tissue density
- MR: Downward protrusion of meninges &/or temporal lobe brain tissue through tegmen

TOP DIFFERENTIAL DIAGNOSES

- Large cholesteatoma with tegmen dehiscence
- ME cholesterol granuloma
- Temporal bone arachnoid granulation

PATHOLOGY

- Temporal bone cephalocele has multiple etiologies
  - Congenital
  - Acquired
    - Postsurgical or posttraumatic
    - ME disease ± cholesteatoma
    - Chronic **idiopathic intracranial hypertension**
    - Spontaneous
      - Anatomic predisposition: Thin tegmen

CLINICAL ISSUES

- Clinical presentation
  - 85% conductive or mixed hearing loss
  - Broad range of symptomatology depends on size of defect, contents, chronicity, & presence of CSF leak
- Treatment options
  - Surgical repair of tegmen generally advised to clear ME & minimize risk of meningitis
  - Treat idiopathic intracranial hypertension if present

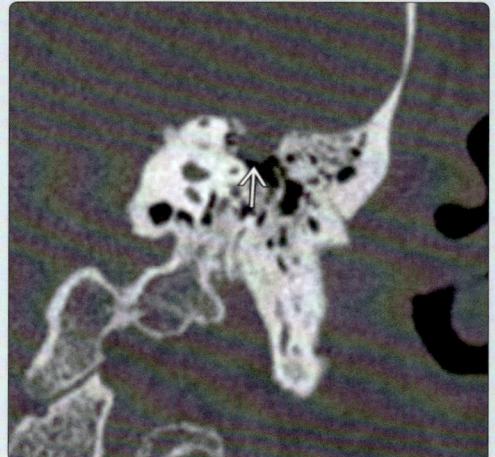
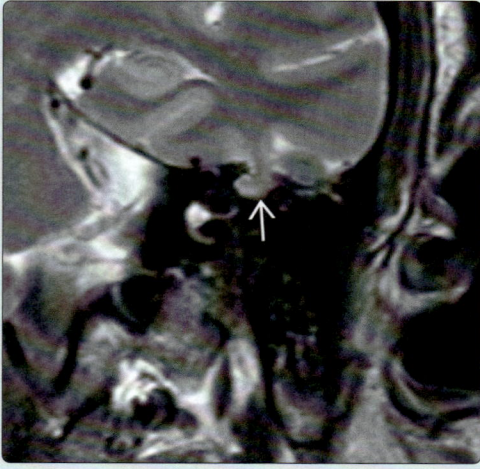

(Left) Coronal bone CT in a 69-year-old man who presented with bilateral conductive hearing loss through the left temporal bone shows polypoid soft tissue density ➡ protruding through a large defect in the posterior tegmen tympani. The soft tissue density is contiguous with intracranial tissues. (Right) Coronal T2 MR in the same patient demonstrates focal temporal bone encephalocele ➡ with a small volume of temporal lobe cortex extending through the defect of the posterior tegmen tympani.

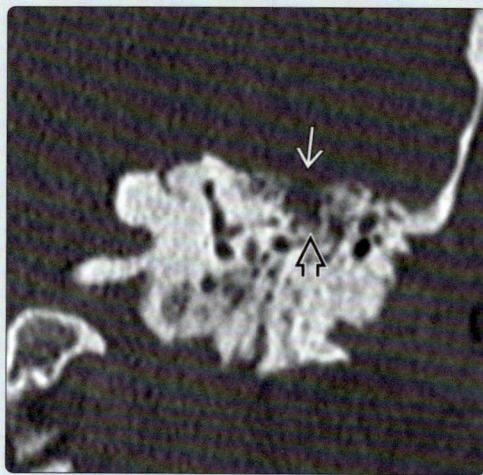
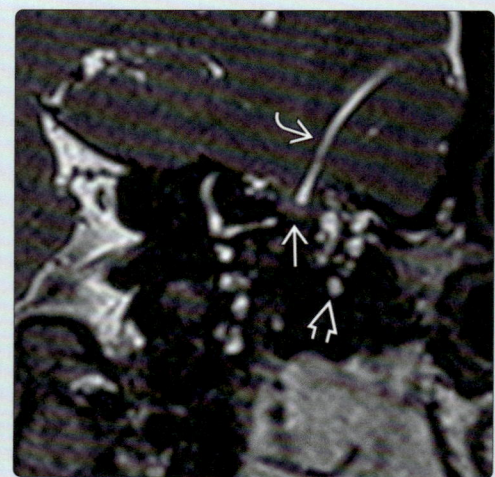

(Left) Coronal bone CT in a 52-year-old woman presenting with left conductive hearing loss shows a defect in the tegmen ➡ with underlying soft tissue ⬈ suspicious for a cephalocele. (Right) Coronal 3D T2 TSE in the same patient shows the temporal bone cephalocele ➡ herniating through the tegmen defect. Note the extension of a left temporal sulcus ➡ into the defect with the cephalocele. Fluid in the mastoid air cells ➡ correlated with a CSF leak in this patient.

TERMINOLOGY

Synonyms

- Temporal lobe meningocele, encephalocele, or meningoencephalocele; defined by content

Definitions

- Protrusion of cranial contents into middle ear (ME) or mastoid through dehiscence of tegmen ± CSF leak

IMAGING

General Features

- Best diagnostic clue
  - CT: **Tegmen tympani** (ME roof) or **mastoideum** (mastoid roof) dehiscence
  - MR: Downward protrusion of meninges &/or temporal lobe brain tissue through tegmen
- Location
  - Tegmen tympani, tegmen mastoideum, or both
  - Lesions may be unilateral or bilateral
- Size
  - Gap of few millimeters to centimeter or more
- Morphology
  - Hourglass or hammock shapes possible

Imaging Recommendations

- Best imaging tool
  - Temporal bone CT used initially to define bony dehiscence
  - Focused coronal T2 MR best for cephalocele contents
    - T1 C+ MR shows intracranial complication
  - Both CT & MR **coronal** views are key

CT Findings

- Bone CT
  - **Focal bone defect** in tegmen tympani or mastoideum
  - Other associated findings possible
    - ME-mastoid soft tissue underlying osseous defect
    - Mastoidectomy or other surgical findings
    - Acute or chronic complex fractures
    - If sporadic, superior semicircular canal dehiscence may also be present
  - Opacified ME-mastoid air cells if **CSF leak**
    - CT cisternography: May be useful in localizing CSF leak

MR Findings

- T2WI
  - Small defects have dural defect → meningocele
  - Large defects may contain meningoencephalocele
    - Brain parenchyma, sulcus, CSF cleft, ± temporal horn extending into ME/mastoid
    - Dura may be thin, or dural rent may be present
  - If associated dural leakage, high-signal CSF in ME-mastoid
- T1WI C+
  - Possible rim enhancement
    - Occasionally, there is enhancement in ME in setting of chronic ME disease

DIFFERENTIAL DIAGNOSIS

Large Cholesteatoma With Tegmen Dehiscence

- Imaging: Nondependent soft tissue mass with ossicular erosion (on CT)
  - Restricted diffusion on DWI if large on MR

Middle Ear Cholesterol Granuloma

- Imaging: High T1 & T2 MR signal characteristic

Temporal Bone Arachnoid Granulation

- If large, may create cephalocele ± CSF leak
- Imaging: Focal cortical defect on CT
  - Enhances on T1 C+ MR

PATHOLOGY

General Features

- Etiology
  - Congenital
  - Acquired
    - Traumatic
      - □ Surgically induced: Post mastoidectomy
      - □ Posttraumatic
    - Nontraumatic
      - □ Chronic ME disease ± cholesteatoma
    - Related to idiopathic intracranial hypertension (IIH)
    - Spontaneous
      - □ Anatomic predisposition: Thin tegmen

CLINICAL ISSUES

Presentation

- Most common signs/symptoms
  - 85% conductive or mixed hearing loss
  - Broad range of symptomatology depends on size of defect, contents, chronicity, & presence of CSF leak

Demographics

- Age
  - Usually presents > 50 years
  - Cholesteatoma & IIH groups may present earlier

Natural History & Prognosis

- Tegmen defect does not always result in cephalocele
- Delayed presentation of cephalocele develops over time with CSF pulsation, increased intracranial pressure, & low-grade inflammation

Treatment

- Surgical osteodural repair of tegmen generally recommended due to risk of **meningitis**
- Treat IIH if present

SELECTED REFERENCES

1. Spinos D et al: The association between obesity and spontaneous temporal bone CSF leak outcomes: a systematic review and meta-analysis. Laryngoscope. 134(5):2012-8, 2024
2. Srinivasan R et al: MRI features to aid the identification of lateral temporal bone cephaloceles. Br J Radiol. 96(1150):20230014, 2023
3. Hernandez-Montero E et al: Surgical management of middle cranial fossa bone defects: meningoencephalic herniation and cerebrospinal fluid leaks. Am J Otolaryngol. 41(4):102560, 2020
4. Worrall DM et al: Temporal bone encephaloceles: utility of preoperative imaging. Otolaryngol Head Neck Surg. 163(3):577-81, 2020

TERMINOLOGY

- Ossicular replacement prosthesis (ORP)
- **Ossiculoplasty**: Surgical reconstruction of malfunctioned ossicular chain to improve or to maintain residual conductive hearing function
- Common ORP types
  - Stapes prosthesis
  - Incus interposition graft or strut
  - Partial ORP (PORP)
  - Total ORP (TORP)

IMAGING

- Temporal bone CT = best imaging tool
  - All or part of ossicular chain, replaced by tissue graft (autograft, homograft, autolograft) or allograft
  - CT may over- or underestimate (< 1 mm) size of metallic ORP due to metal artifacts
    - Ultrahigh-resolution CT promising, more accurate assessment of metallic prosthesis size

- CT may underestimate fluoroplastic portion of ORP if surrounded by soft tissue
- Allow leeway for mediolateral ORP position
- **Prosthesis malfunction** findings on CT
  - Displacement, dislocation, protrusion, extrusion
  - Native residual ossicular erosion or necrosis
  - Abnormal soft tissue-embedded ORP
  - Recurrent/progressive primary disease
    - Cholesteatoma, otosclerosis, tympanosclerosis
- Prosthetic MR safety
  - Most modern ossicular replacement prostheses are tested safe or conditional at 1.5T or 3T
  - Check specific device against known MR safety record

TOP DIFFERENTIAL DIAGNOSES

- Chronic otitis media with tympanosclerosis
- Posttraumatic incus dislocation
- Foreign body in middle ear
- Semiimplantable direct drive hearing device

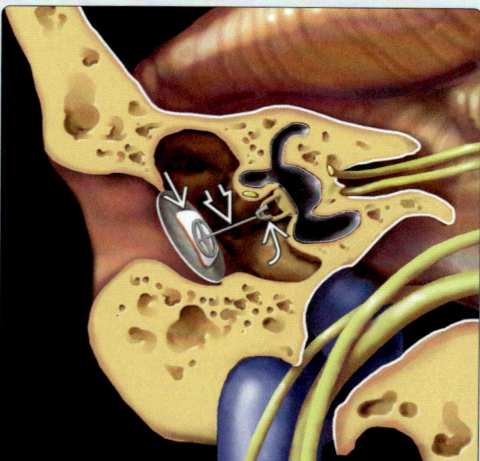
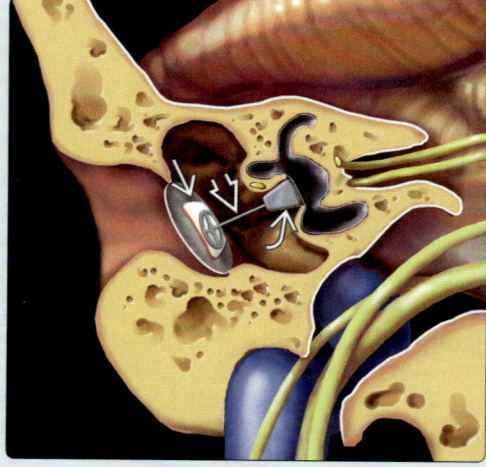

(Left) Coronal graphic shows a titanium partial ORP (PORP) ➡ connecting the tympanic membrane (TM) to capitulum of stapes ➡. A cartilage graft ➡ is often placed between the TM and head of prosthesis to reduce incidence of implant extrusion. Prostheses connecting any part of ossicular chain to capitulum are called PORP. *(Right)* Coronal graphic shows a total ORP (TORP) ➡ connecting TM to the oval window. A piston-based TORP ➡ is used with stapedectomy. Intervening cartilage cap ➡ is between TM and prosthesis head.

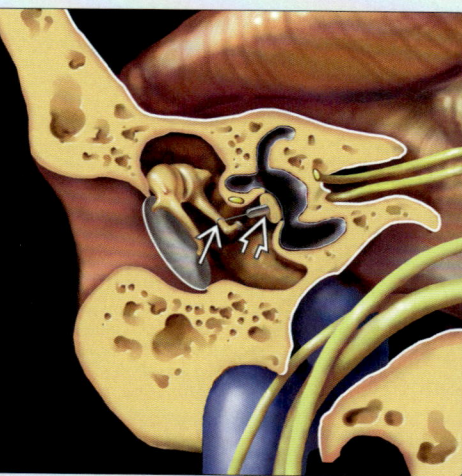
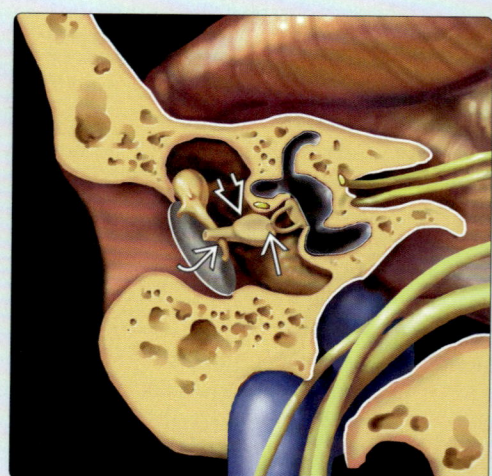

(Left) Coronal graphic shows a type of stapes piston prosthesis. The incus end ➡ hooks to the incus long process. The piston base ➡ connects to the oval window via stapedotomy. *(Right)* Coronal graphic shows an incus interposition graft where the incus ➡ is sculpted and rotated to connect the handle of the malleus to capitulum of the stapes. A groove ➡ is created in the remaining long process of incus to anchor it to the manubrium. A hole ➡ is drilled in the incus body to accommodate the stapes capitulum.

Ossicular Prosthesis

TERMINOLOGY

Synonyms
- Ossicular replacement prosthesis (ORP)

Definitions
- Ossiculoplasty: Surgical reconstruction of malfunctioned part of ossicular chain (OC) to improve or maintain conductive hearing function
- Materials: Allograft > autograft > > homograft
  - **Allograft**: Synthetic ossicular replacements (titanium)
  - **Autograft**: Patient's own ossicle used
  - **Homograft**: Radiated, frozen human ossicles
    - Homograft use ↓ ↓ in 1990s over concern of risk for disease transmission (e.g., AIDS)
  - **Autologous**: Patient's own pinna cortical bone and cartilage

4 Common Ossicular Replacement Prosthesis Types
- Stapes prosthesis
- Incus interposition graft
- Partial ORP (PORP)
- Total ORP (TORP)

IMAGING

General Features
- Best diagnostic clue
  - All or part of OC replaced by tissue graft (autograft, homograft, autolograft) or allograft
    - Auto-, homo-, autolograft: Ossicular bone density
    - Allograft: Metallic, soft tissue density, or combination
  - Prosthetic malfunction suggested by displacement, presence of abnormal soft tissue ± recurrence of conductive hearing loss (CHL)
  - Findings of underlying disease (e.g., otosclerosis), its complications [e.g., middle ear (ME) erosion in cholesteatoma], or related surgery (mastoidectomy) may be seen
- Location
  - Mesotympanum (ME cavity proper)

CT Findings
- Bone CT
  - **Stapes prosthesis**
    - Most commonly seen in otosclerosis setting
    - Stapes allograft connects long process of incus to stapes footplate of oval window (OW)
      - "Missing" all or part of stapes superstructure
      - OW interaction usually through hole in stapes footplate (stapedotomy)
      - OW insertion need not be central to function normally
    - Allograft materials variably visible
      - **Metallic** (titanium, stainless steel, platinum), soft tissue density (fluoroplastic), or combination
      - 5 main types: Wire loop, stapes piston > > bucket handle, ball socket, or homemade
      - Anatomic parts are designated as incus end (hook/clip/bucket handle) and shaft/base (wire loop/piston)

- Ultrahigh-resolution CT (0.25-mm slice thickness) more accurately depicts prosthesis length
  - Incus interposition graft or strut
    - Most commonly seen in chronic otitis media (COM)
    - Incus **rotated and resculpted** to connect malleus with stapes capitulum
      - Normal incus is "missing"
      - Typically patient's own incus body (autograft)
      - Malleus head, cortical bone, or cartilage graft may be used if incus not available
      - Looks like dislocated incus if history of surgery is not known
    - Interposition hydroxylapatite strut alternative that can be positioned between malleus handle and stapes
  - TORP or PORP
    - More commonly seen in advanced COM or cholesteatoma
    - TORP: Replace entire OC, connect **tympanic membrane (TM) to OW**
      - Anatomically, TORP head on TM, shaft and base on OW
      - Shaft is straight from TM to OW
    - PORP: Replace **part of OC** to **articulate with stapes superstructure**
      - Straight if connects TM to capitulum
      - Short and angled if only incudostapedial joint replaced
    - Materials: Metallic (titanium), bone density (ceramic), plastic, or combination
    - Wide variety of designs available
      - Specific name depends on manufacturer
    - TM looks thickened due to use of cartilage cap
- Prosthetic malfunction on bone CT
  - General CT findings
    - Dislocation/subluxation: Most commonly occurs in early postoperative period (< 6 weeks)
      - Before fibrosis secures ORP
    - Lateralization: Prosthesis drifts away, widened gap with OW
    - Protrusion: Prosthesis protrudes into vestibule (vertigo)
      - Length of prosthesis can be inaccurate to estimate on conventional MDCT at 0.5- to 0.6-mm slice thickness
      - Ultrahigh-resolution CT (0.25-mm slice thickness, matrix 1024 x 1024) has good accuracy but is not widely available
    - Abnormal soft tissue visible on scan
      - Embedded ORP: Represents granulation, fibrosis, or recurrent cholesteatoma
      - At OW: Granulation-fibrosis; soft tissue develops 4-6 weeks after surgery (excessive stapedectomy)
    - Ankylosis with ME wall
      - Higher risk if ossicle touches ME wall and with Gelfoam (used with TORP)
    - Recurrent/progressive COM, cholesteatoma, otosclerosis
    - Surgical complications: Rare, occur early
      - Pneumolabyrinth or unexplained fluid in ME may suggest perilymph fistula

□ ME wall thickening and soft tissue may suggest postoperative otitis media
- Specific stapes prosthesis malfunction findings
  – Necrosis of long process of incus: Related to manipulation and crimping
  – Malleoincudal joint subluxation: Abnormal torque from too long/malpositioned prosthesis
  – Medialization with vestibular penetration
- Specific incus interposition malfunction findings
  – Incus necrosis or recurrent cholesteatoma
- Specific TORP/PORP malfunction findings
  – Extrusion of prosthesis through TM
    □ Incidence reduced with interposing cartilage cap between TM and ORP head
  – Rare medialization with vestibular penetration

Imaging Recommendations

- Best imaging tool
  - Temporal bone CT axial and coronal ~ 0.6-mm slices best for evaluating ossicle status and prosthesis complications
    – Ossicle relationships best seen on coronal CT
- TORP and PORP **MR safety**
  - Many modern prostheses are tested safe or conditional at 1.5T or 3T
  - Modern (post 1987) stapes prostheses do not pose risk in vivo when exposed to MR magnetic fields
  - Check specific product against known MR safety

DIFFERENTIAL DIAGNOSIS

Chronic Otitis Media With Tympanosclerosis

- If history of ossicular surgery unknown, misdiagnosis possible
- Must know normal prosthesis appearances

Posttraumatic Incus Dislocation

- Temporal bone trauma history is key
- May appear identical to incus interposition graft
- Incus may be found anywhere in ME or external auditory canal

Middle Ear Foreign Body

- Clinical history is crucial

Semiimplantable Direct Drive Hearing Device

- Synonym: Active ME implantation devices
- Designed for moderate to severe sensorineural hearing loss with **intact ME ossicles**
  - May soon be used for CHL
- Implantable components consist of floating mass transducer **anchored to incus**
- Receiver in retroauricular subcutaneous layer [called vibrating ORP (VORP)]
  - Connecting wire visible

PATHOLOGY

General Features

- Etiology
  - Need for OC surgery driven by multiple clinical scenarios
    – COM and cholesteatoma account for **80%** of ossicular injuries
    – Fenestral otosclerosis

– COM with tympanosclerosis
– Trauma
– Congenital or idiopathic ossicle fusion

Gross Pathologic & Surgical Features

- Incus erosion = most commonly encountered defect
  - Incudostapedial joint erosion > absent incus > absent incus and stapes superstructure
- Stapes foot plate fixation due to otosclerosis, tympanosclerosis, or congenital stapes fixation
- Malleoincudal fixation may be congenital or due to tympanosclerosis

CLINICAL ISSUES

Presentation

- Most common signs/symptoms
  - CHL
- Other signs/symptoms
  - Postoperative symptoms suggesting **prosthesis malfunction**
    – Recurrent CHL, new sensorineural hearing loss, dizziness, &/or vertigo weeks to months after surgery

Demographics

- Age: All

Natural History & Prognosis

- Early postoperative malfunction relates to surgical error or graft subluxation/dislocation
- Delayed prosthetic malfunction from mechanical failure, scarring, or recurrent/progressive disease

Treatment

- Treat recurrent otitis media ± cholesteatoma first
- Prosthesis malfunction requires replacement

DIAGNOSTIC CHECKLIST

Consider

- Consider prosthesis subluxation if recurrent CHL or vertigo

Image Interpretation Pearls

- Must have clinical and surgical history (including type of prosthesis used)
- Must have knowledge of the following prior to evaluation
  - Normal ossicular anatomy
  - Normal prosthesis appearance
  - Detailed surgical history

SELECTED REFERENCES

1. Gluth MB et al: A multi-center study of ossiculoplasty hearing outcomes and a grading scale of ear environment risk. Laryngoscope. 135 Suppl 2(Suppl 2):S1-11, 2025
2. Boukhzer S et al: Ultra-high-resolution CT of the temporal bone: the end of stapes prosthesis dimensional error and correlation with patient symptoms. Eur J Radiol. 175:111467, 2024
3. Daher GS et al: MRI safety of stapes prostheses: a systematic review. Otol Neurotol. 45(5):469-74, 2024
4. Bhatt PR et al: Imaging of the postoperative temporal bone. Neuroimaging Clin N Am. 32(1):175-92, 2022
5. Panda A et al: Beyond tympanomastoidectomy: a review of less common postoperative temporal bone CT findings. AJNR Am J Neuroradiol. 42(1):12-21, 2021
6. Tames HLVC et al: Postoperative imaging of the temporal bone. Radiographics. 41(3):858-75, 2021

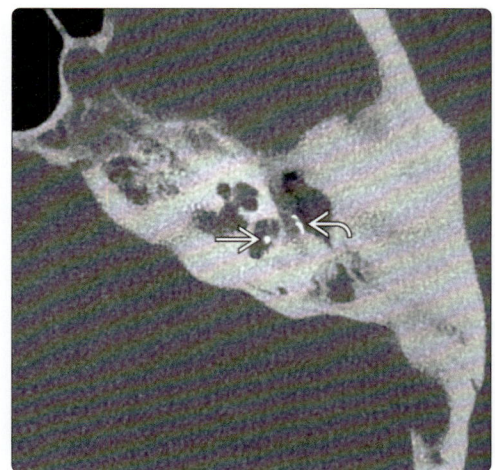

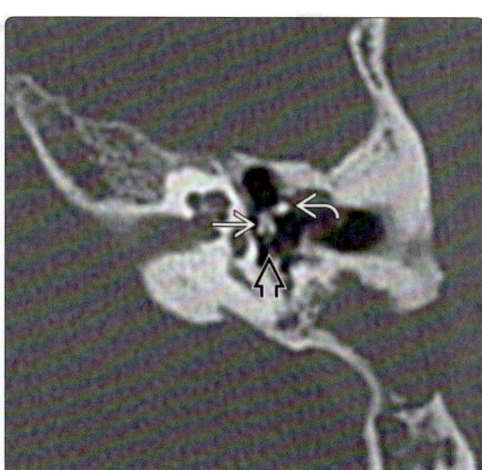

(Left) Axial bone CT shows a rare complication of TORP placement with medial migration of the distal prosthesis into the vestibule ➡, resulting in postoperative severe vertigo and dizziness. The head of the prosthesis ➡ is partly embedded in middle ear soft tissue. (Right) Axial bone CT shows a Kartush hydroxylapatite interposition strut ➡ placed between the malleus handle ➡ and partly visualized stapes ➡. Reviewing the medical record and confirming prosthesis type aids in interpretation of the postoperative CT.

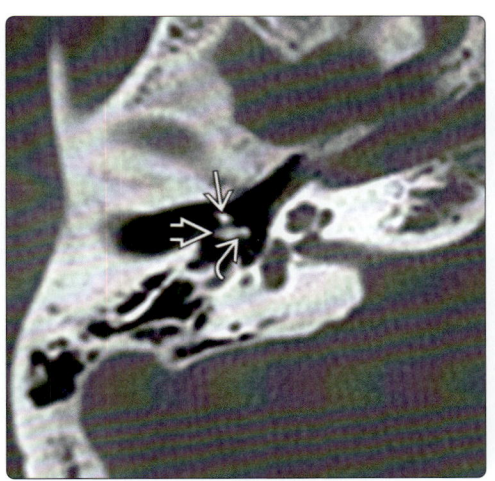

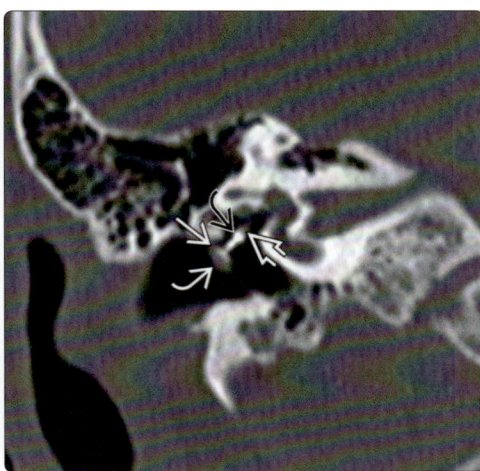

(Left) Axial bone CT demonstrates an incus interposition graft ➡. The incus is rotated to connect the manubrium of the malleus ➡ with the capitulum of the stapes. A hole ➡ has been drilled in the incus body to receive the capitulum. (Right) Coronal bone CT shows a metallic PORP. The head ➡, shaft, and base ➡ project straight across to the stapes capitulum ➡. Focal soft tissue thickening at the TM represents the cartilage cap ➡ commonly used with PORP and TORP to reduce the risk of extrusion.

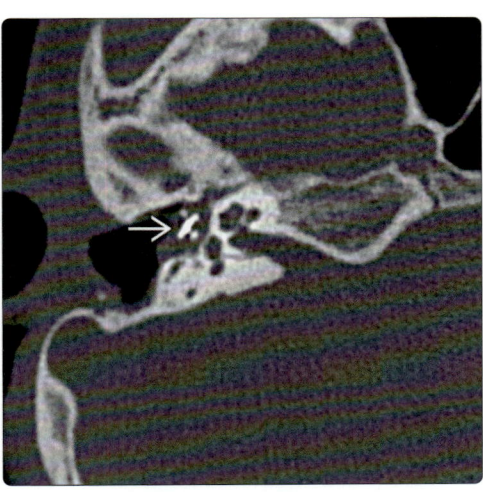

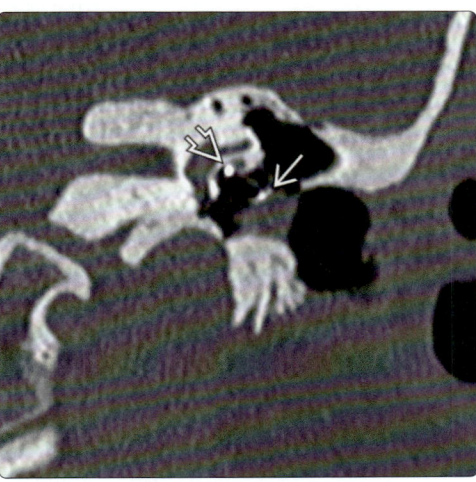

(Left) Axial bone CT in a patient with conductive hearing loss shows a PORP encased in recurrent cholesteatoma ➡ and displaced posteriorly, migrated out of the oval window. (Right) Coronal bone CT in a patient with recurrent left conductive hearing loss shows a malpositioned TORP, angulated due to soft tissue thickening along the TM ➡. The distal prosthesis is dislocated from the oval window niche and abuts the medial aspect of the tympanic segment of the facial nerve ➡.

TERMINOLOGY

- Petromastoid canal (PMC) definition: Normal temporal bone osseous canal that passes through arch of superior semicircular canal conveying subarcuate artery to otic capsule
- Synonyms: Subarcuate canal or canaliculus

IMAGING

- Osseous canal passing beneath superior semicircular canal
  - Infant: Globoid to tubular + CSF in subarachnoid space
    - Best seen on axial high-resolution T2 MR
  - Adult: Linear with sclerotic margins on CT; usually not seen on MR

TOP DIFFERENTIAL DIAGNOSES

- Large vestibular aqueduct (incomplete partition type II)
- Prominent cochlear aqueduct
- Temporal bone fracture, otic capsule-involving

PATHOLOGY

- Maximum size of PMC occurs at week 21 of embryonic development
  - Then ↓ in size to form subarcuate fossa & PMC
- Contains subarcuate artery & vein
- PMC in child < 2 years of age
  - **Dural-lined subarachnoid space** connected to cerebellopontine angle cistern
- PMC in child > 2 years of age
  - Involutes with disappearance of dura, subarachnoid space, and CSF

DIAGNOSTIC CHECKLIST

- PMC may be mistaken for pathology
  - In infant: Inner ear or petrous apex lesion
  - In adult: Temporal bone fracture
- PMC is potential route of spread of infection

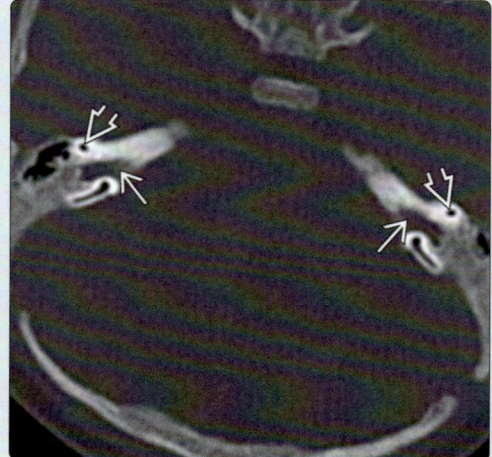 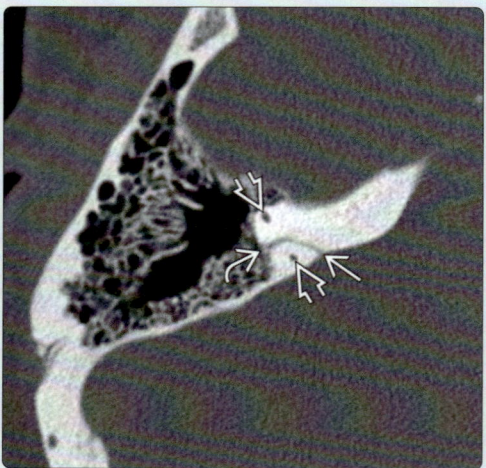

(Left) Axial bone CT in a 7-week-old infant shows normal prominence of the bilateral petromastoid canals ➡ extending inferior to the arch of the superior semicircular canals ➡. (Right) Axial temporal bone CT of an adult right ear shows a normal, linear, arching petromastoid canal passing from the medial petrous ridge ➡ under the superior semicircular canal ➡ to the lateral wall of the mastoid antrum ➡. Occasionally, this will be straighter in configuration and simulate a fracture.

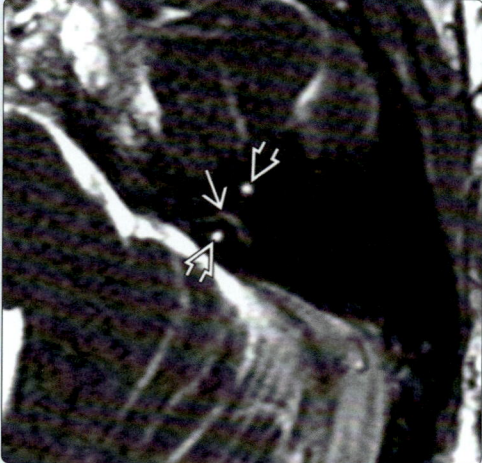 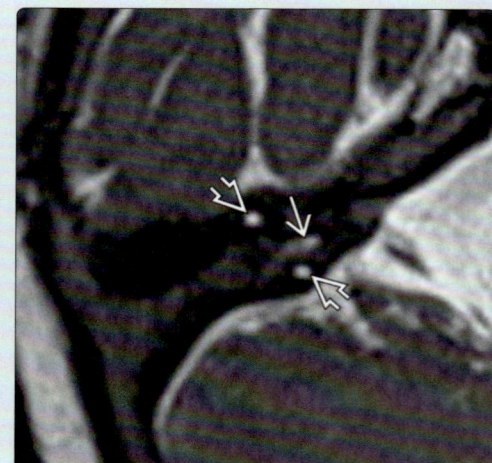

(Left) Axial 3D FIESTA MR shows a fluid-filled petromastoid canal ➡ passing beneath the superior semicircular canal ➡. This is a common incidental finding on MR as well as CT. (Right) Axial 3D T2 CUBE MR in a 4-month-old shows a more tubular appearance of the petromastoid canal ➡ just before it passes under the superior semicircular canal ➡. Tubular appearance of the petromastoid canal is more typical in infancy.

TERMINOLOGY

Abbreviations

- Petromastoid canal (PMC)

Synonyms

- Subarcuate canal or canaliculus, subarcuate channel or tract, subarcuate artery canal

Definitions

- PMC: Normal temporal bone osseous canal that passes through arch of superior semicircular canal (SSC) conveying subarcuate artery to otic capsule

IMAGING

General Features

- Best diagnostic clue
  - Osseous canal passing through superior SSC
  - < 2 years of age: Globoid to tubular + CSF in subarachnoid space
  - Adult: Linear (< 1 mm wide) + sclerotic margins on CT

CT Findings

- Bone CT
  - Infant under 2 years of age
    - PMC passes under SSC
    - Measures 2-3x cross-sectional SSC dimension
  - Child > 2 years of age
    - Adult: PMC seen as dark line passing under SSC
    - Measures ≤ cross-sectional SSC dimension

MR Findings

- T2WI
  - Infant < 2 years of age
    - CSF intensity passage from subarcuate fossa medially to lateral wall of mastoid antrum
    - Passes under SCC
  - Child > 2 years of age
    - PMC sometimes faintly visible in adult

Imaging Recommendations

- Best imaging tool
  - Noncontrast temporal bone CT best shows PMC

DIFFERENTIAL DIAGNOSIS

Large Vestibular Aqueduct (Incomplete Partition Type II)

- CT: Large bony vestibular aqueduct posterior to internal auditory canal (IAC)
  - Connects to crus communis; orthogonal to PMC course
- MR: Large endolymphatic sac & duct

Prominent Cochlear Aqueduct

- May be mistaken for fracture or PMC
- CT: Parallel & inferior to IAC

Temporal Bone Fracture

- Clinical history of significant head trauma
- CT: Lacks sclerotic margins of subarcuate canaliculus
  - Air-fluid levels in middle ear cavity ± mastoid air cells
  - Pneumolabyrinth possible

PATHOLOGY

General Features

- Embryology/anatomy
  - Maximum size of subarcuate sinus occurs at week 21 of embryonic development
  - Then ↓ in size to form subarcuate fossa & PMC
    - Contains subarcuate artery & vein
    - PMC in child < 2 years of age is **dural-lined subarachnoid space** connected to cerebellopontine angle (CPA) cistern
    - After 2 years of age, PMC involutes with disappearance of dura, subarachnoid space, and CSF
  - Adult PMC
    - Mean length: 10.5 mm
    - ~ 50% of canals 0.5-1.0 mm wide
    - Other 50% > 1-2 mm
  - **Subarcuate artery**
    - Subarcuate artery arises from labyrinthine artery medial to IAC
    - Labyrinthine artery arises from basilar artery or anterior inferior cerebellar artery (AICA)
    - Subarcuate artery may arise directly from AICA
    - Enters subarcuate fossa to travel in PMC
    - Supplies otic capsule, SCCs, & posterior wall vestibule
    - Distal branches anastomose with branches from superficial petrosal, stylomastoid, posterior meningeal, & occipital arteries

CLINICAL ISSUES

Presentation

- Most common signs/symptoms
  - Asymptomatic normal variant
- Clinical profile
  - Conspicuous structure in infants
  - May be incorrectly identified as **petrous apex or inner ear lesion**

Natural History & Prognosis

- Normal anatomic variant
- No treatment required

DIAGNOSTIC CHECKLIST

Consider

- PMC may be mistaken for pathology
  - In infant: Petrous apex or inner ear anomaly
  - In adult: Temporal bone fracture
- PMC is potential route of spread of infection

SELECTED REFERENCES

1. Benson JC et al: Temporal bone anatomy. Neuroimaging Clin N Am. 32(4):763-75, 2022
2. Mena-Domínguez EA et al: Petromastoid canal. Acta Otorrinolaringol Esp. 66(3):180, 2015
3. Koral K et al: MRI of the petromastoid canal in children. J Magn Reson Imaging. 39(4):966-71, 2014
4. Migirov L et al: Radiology of the petromastoid canal. Otol Neurotol. 27(3):410-3, 2006
5. Krombach GA et al: The petromastoid canal on computed tomography. Eur Radiol. 12(11):2770-5, 2002

KEY FACTS

TERMINOLOGY

- Synonyms for cochlear cleft
  - Localized pericochlear hypoattenuating foci
  - Cochlear capsule space
- Cochlear cleft definition
  - Developmental lucency attributed to nonosseous otic capsule space adjacent to cochlea in children

IMAGING

- Bone CT (< 1-mm thick images)
  - Bilateral > unilateral
  - C-shaped, thin, sharply defined lucency in otic capsule
  - Adjacent to middle & apical portions of cochlear turns
    - Lateral > medial aspect of cochlea
  - May extend to apical turn on axial images
  - Anterior to oval window, does not extend to oval window
- Parallel to cochlea on coronal images
  - Lucency curved, in shape of cochlear promontory

TOP DIFFERENTIAL DIAGNOSES

- Fenestral otosclerosis
- Cochlear otosclerosis
- Temporal bone Paget disease
- Temporal bone fibrous dysplasia
- Temporal bone osteoradionecrosis
- Temporal bone osteogenesis imperfecta

CLINICAL ISSUES

- Clinical presentation
  - Incidental finding in child
- Becomes less conspicuous & disappears with age
  - Medial lucency disappears first
- Age vs. incidence of cochlear cleft
  - **< 4 years**: Present in **~ 60%**
  - 4-7 years: Present in ~ 45%
  - 7-10 years: Present in ~ 25%
  - 10-19 years: Present in ~ 20%

(Left) Normal temporal bone CT in a 2-month-old girl with sensorineural hearing loss demonstrates well-defined curvilinear lucency ➡ within the otic capsule bone parallel to the cochlear turns. The lucency is more pronounced laterally than medially. These findings are characteristic of developmental cochlear cleft. (Right) Right ear coronal reformatted bone CT reveals the curvilinear lucency ➡ within the otic capsule bone parallel to the cochlea, just deep to the surface of the cochlear promontory.

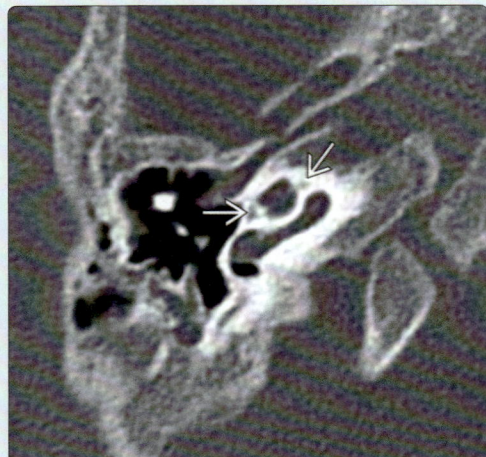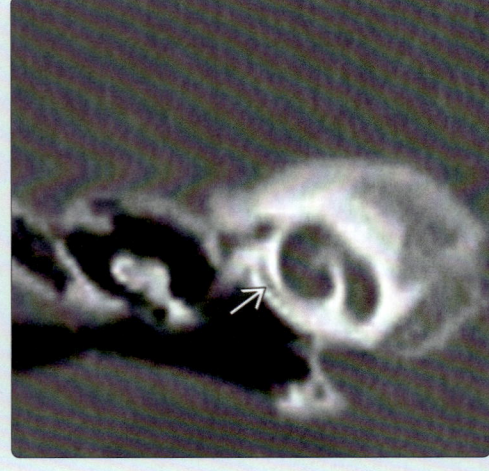

(Left) Axial bone CT in a 7-year-old girl shows a linear lucency ➡ medial & lateral to the apical portions of the cochlea, most prominent laterally. (Right) Coronal bone CT reformation in the same patient shows a faint cochlear cleft ➡ lateral to the cochlea. There is now histologic proof in the literature that this represents fatty marrow, not yet ossified. Cochlear cleft is most common in infants & young children but may persist into adulthood & should not be mistaken for temporal bone pathology.

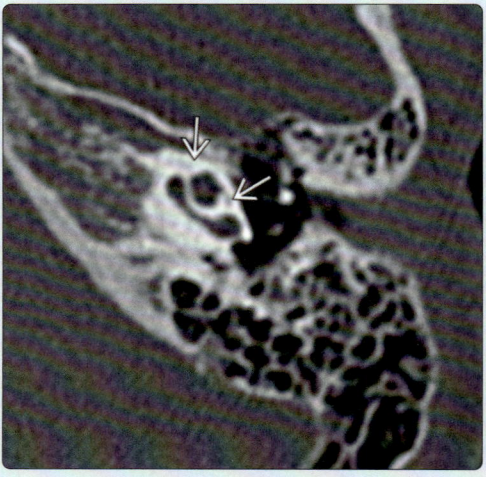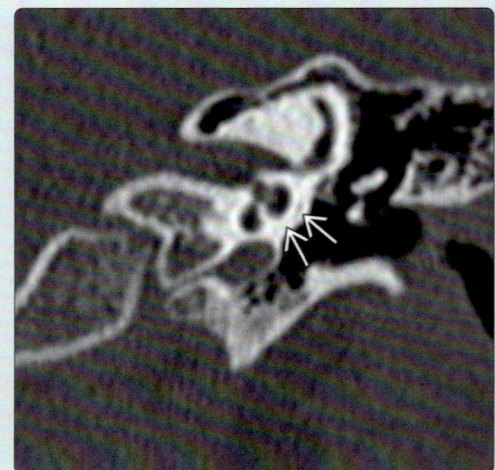

TERMINOLOGY

Abbreviations

- Cochlear cleft (CC)

Synonyms

- Localized pericochlear hypoattenuating foci
- Cochlear capsule space

Definitions

- Developmental **lucency** = not yet ossified residual fatty marrow, in otic capsule space adjacent to cochlea in children

IMAGING

General Features

- Best diagnostic clue
  - Sharply defined, thin, curvilinear lucency on bone CT
- Location
  - Adjacent to apical portion 1st cochlear turn

CT Findings

- Bone CT: Bilateral > unilateral
  - C-shaped, thin, sharply defined lucency in otic capsule
    - Adjacent to middle & apical portions of first 2 cochlear turns; rarely adjacent to basal portion of 1st turn
    - Adjacent lateral > medial aspect of cochlea
    - May extend to apical turn on axial images
    - Anterior to oval window, does not extend to oval window
  - Parallel to cochlea on coronal images
    - Follows shape of cochlear promontory

MR Findings

- High-resolution T2 MR may be normal
  - Faint intermediate T1, large plaques ↑ T2 signal, enhancing on T1WI C+ in active phase

Imaging Recommendations

- Best imaging tool: Bone CT
- Protocol advice: < 1-mm images

DIFFERENTIAL DIAGNOSIS

Fenestral Otosclerosis

- Rare in children
- Conductive hearing loss
- CT: Focal smudgy hypodensity begins at fissula ante fenestram
  - Expands otic capsule anterior to the oval window
  - May spread to involve round window margin, cochlear otic capsule

Cochlear Otosclerosis

- Rare in children
- Mixed hearing loss
- CT: Lucency in pericochlear bony labyrinth

Temporal Bone Paget Disease

- Most patients > 50 years
- Diffuse involvement of bony labyrinth, not confined to lateral wall → diffuse cotton wool appearance

Temporal Bone Fibrous Dysplasia

- Most patients < 30 years
- Involves all parts of temporal bone, usually spares inner ear, sclerotic/ground-glass appearance most common

Temporal Bone Osteoradionecrosis

- Radiation history; uncommon complication
- CT: Heterogeneous, permeative lucency otic capsule bone

Temporal Bone Osteogenesis Imperfecta

- Generalized hypodensity, multiple skeletal fractures
- CT: Lucency of otic capsule bone, looks like severe cochlear otosclerosis

PATHOLOGY

Staging, Grading, & Classification

- CC scoring
  - 0: Cleft not present
  - 1: No definite cleft
  - 2: Small cleft
  - 3: Moderate cleft
  - 4: Large cleft

Microscopic Features

- Histopathologic proof that this = areas of residual fatty marrow, related to incomplete marrow ossification

CLINICAL ISSUES

Presentation

- Usually incidental finding

Demographics

- Age
  - **< 4 years**: Present in **~ 60%**
  - 4-7 years: Present in ~ 45%
  - 7-10 years: Present in ~ 25%
  - 10-19 years: Present in ~ 20%
  - May persist well into adult life

Natural History & Prognosis

- Becomes less conspicuous with age
- Medial lucency disappears first

DIAGNOSTIC CHECKLIST

Image Interpretation Pearls

- Sharply defined, thin, linear lucency around cochlea, typically in infant/young child
  - May persist into adulthood
- Often bilateral

Reporting Tips

- Do not mistake for otosclerosis
  - Fenestral otosclerosis tends to expand otic capsule anterior to oval window

SELECTED REFERENCES

1. Pucetaite M et al: The cochlear cleft: CT correlation with histopathology. Otol Neurotol. 41(6):745-9, 2020
2. Chadwell JB et al: The cochlear cleft. AJNR Am J Neuroradiol. 25(1):21-4, 2004

Labyrinthine Aplasia

TERMINOLOGY

- Synonyms: Complete labyrinthine aplasia (CLA); Michel anomaly (old synonym)

IMAGING

- Bilateral or unilateral anomaly
- Temporal bone CT findings
  - Otic capsule bone: Aplasia/hypoplasia
  - Absent cochlea, vestibule, semicircular canals, and vestibular aqueduct
  - Cochlear promontory: Absent/flattened
  - Ossicles: Normal or malformed stapes
  - Tegmen tympani: Normal, low, or defective
  - Facial nerve canal: Aberrant course
  - Petrous apex: Hypoplasia
  - Internal auditory canal: Aplasia/hypoplasia
  - Carotid canal: Normal or absent
- MR: Absent vestibular and cochlear nerves

TOP DIFFERENTIAL DIAGNOSES

- Cochlear aplasia
- Common cavity
- Labyrinthine ossification, obliterative type

PATHOLOGY

- Genetic mutation: *FGF3* mutations [LAMM (CLA, microtia, microdontia) syndrome], *HOXA1* mutations, thalidomide exposure, or unknown etiology
- **Otic placode** development arrest **before 3rd week**

CLINICAL ISSUES

- Extremely rare anomaly
- Congenital sensorineural hearing loss
- Horizontal gaze palsy (*HOXA1*) or abnormal teeth (LAMM) suggest underlying syndrome

DIAGNOSTIC CHECKLIST

- Often asymmetric: Contralateral common cavity, inner ear hypoplasia, or cochlear incomplete partition type I anomaly

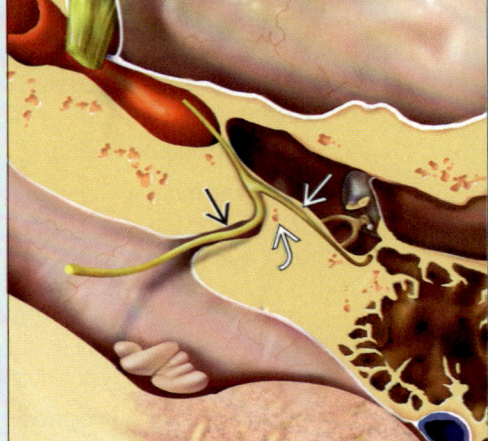
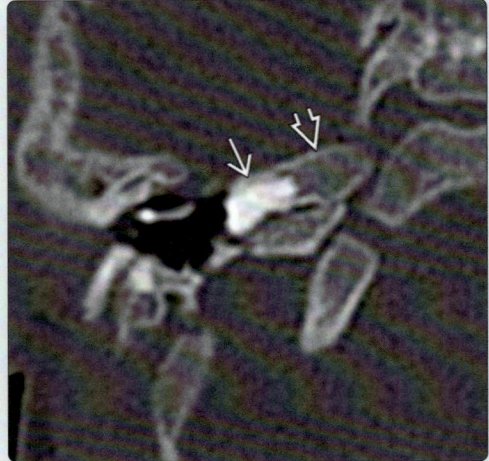

(Left) *Axial graphic depicts labyrinthine aplasia. Note complete absence of all inner ear structures* ⇨ *with the exception of a small IAC with only CNVII* ⇨*. The lateral wall of the inner ear (promontory) is flattened* ⇨*.* (Right) *Axial bone CT in a 2-month-old girl with profound bilateral sensorineural hearing loss (SNHL) shows complete absence of labyrinthine structures in a hypoplastic otic capsule* ⇨ *and mildly small petrous apex* ⇨*. Patients with labyrinthine aplasia may have a small or normal-sized otic capsule and petrous bone.*

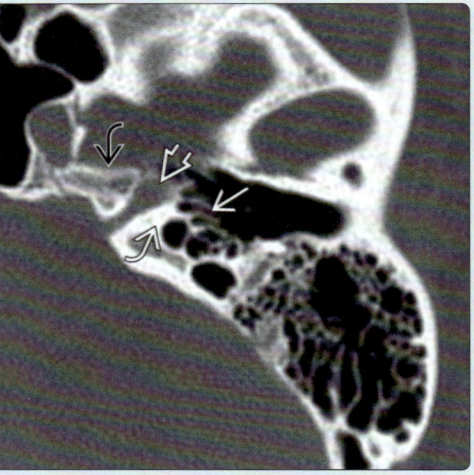
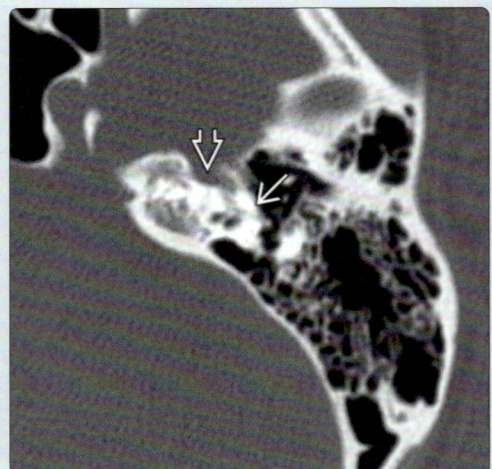

(Left) *Axial bone CT in 21-year-old woman with SNHL shows severe hypoplasia of the otic capsule bone with air cells in the expected location of the promontory* ⇨*. The inner ear structures are absent* ⇨*. CNVII canal is present with a broadened anterior genu* ⇨*. Note the petrous apex is hypoplastic* ⇨*, narrow in width.* (Right) *Axial bone CT in the same patient at a more cephalad level shows hypoplastic otic capsule bone* ⇨*. The anterior genu and proximal tympanic segment of the anomalous CNVII canal* ⇨ *are visible.*

TERMINOLOGY

Synonyms

- **Complete labyrinthine aplasia** (CLA)
- Old synonym: Michel anomaly

Definitions

- **Absent cochlea, vestibule, and semicircular canals** (SCCs)

IMAGING

General Features

- Best diagnostic clue
  - Complete absence of inner ear structures
- Morphology
  - **3 subgroups** based on radiologic findings
  - **CLA with hypoplastic or aplastic petrous bone**
    - Middle ear could be adjacent to posterior fossa
  - **CLA without otic capsule**
    - Hypo-/aplastic otic capsule but normal petrous bone
  - **CLA with otic capsule**
    - Normal otic capsule and petrous bone
    - Labyrinthine segment of facial canal in normal location only in this subgroup
    - Otic capsule essential for normal facial canal location

CT Findings

- Bone CT
  - Otic capsule bone: Aplasia/hypoplasia
  - Absent cochlea, vestibule, SCC, vestibular aqueduct
  - Cochlear promontory: Absent/flattened
  - Ossicles: Normal usually or malformed stapes
  - Tegmen tympani: Normal, low, or defective (suggesting encephalocele)
  - Middle ear and mastoid: Normal or hypoplastic
  - Facial nerve canal: Aberrant course
  - Petrous apex: Normal or hypoplasia
  - Internal auditory canal (IAC): Aplasia/hypoplasia
  - Jugular bulb/vein: Normal, dehiscent or stenotic + large emissary veins
  - Carotid canal: Normal or absent
  - Clivus: Normal or narrowed
  - Cervical spine: Normal or ± anomalies

MR Findings

- T2WI
  - Absent membranous labyrinth
  - Absent vestibular and cochlear nerves
    - IAC contain only facial nerve
  - Large cerebellopontine angle cistern/arachnoid cyst
  - ± pontine anomaly

Imaging Recommendations

- Best imaging tool
  - High-resolution temporal bone CT
  - Heavily T2WI 3D (CISS, FIESTA) MR IAC/temporal bones

DIFFERENTIAL DIAGNOSIS

Cochlear Aplasia

- Absent cochlea, dysmorphic vestibule, and SCC

Common Cavity

- Ovoid globular sac of cochlea + vestibule

Labyrinthine Ossificans

- Postmeningitic ossification, promontory well formed

PATHOLOGY

General Features

- Etiology
  - Genetic mutation, thalidomide exposure, or unknown
- Genetics
  - *FGF3* mutations: LAMM (CLA, microtia, microdontia)
  - *HOXA1* mutations: Bosley-Salih-Alorainy syndrome (BSAS) and Athabaskan brainstem dysgenesis (ABDS)
- Associated abnormalities
  - BSAS and ABDS: Congenital heart disease, horizontal gaze palsy, absent internal carotid arteries

Gross Pathologic & Surgical Features

- Failure of bony and membranous labyrinth formation

CLINICAL ISSUES

Presentation

- Most common signs/symptoms
  - Congenital sensorineural hearing loss (SNHL)
- **Audiologic evaluation findings**
  - No response
  - May show findings of profound SNHL on low frequencies

Demographics

- Epidemiology
  - Extremely rare, < 1% of inner ear malformations

Treatment

- Unilateral CLA: Assess contralateral side for cochlear implantation if bilateral SNHL
- Bilateral CLA: Auditory brainstem implantation (ABI)

DIAGNOSTIC CHECKLIST

Consider

- CLA if cochlea, vestibule, & SCC are absent

Image Interpretation Pearls

- Often asymmetric: Contralateral common cavity, inner ear hypoplasia, or cochlear incomplete partition type I anomaly

Reporting Tips

- Variable pathognomonic flattening of cochlear promontory: Subtle to marked
- Evaluate tegmen tympani integrity on coronal reformats

SELECTED REFERENCES

1. Lewis M et al: Syndromic hearing loss in children. Neuroimaging Clin N Am. 33(4):563-80, 2023
2. O'Brien WT et al: Nonsyndromic congenital causes of sensorineural hearing loss in children: an illustrative review. AJR Am J Roentgenol. 216(4):1048-55, 2021
3. D'Arco F et al: The link between inner ear malformations and the rest of the body: what we know so far about genetic, imaging and histology. Neuroradiology. 62(5):539-44, 2020
4. Sennaroğlu L et al: Classification and current management of inner ear malformations. Balkan Med J. 34(5):397-411, 2017

TERMINOLOGY

- Absent cochlea, but vestibule, semicircular canals (SCC), & internal auditory canal (IAC) are present in some form

IMAGING

- Cochlea: **Absent** bilaterally or unilaterally
- Cochlear nerve canal & cochlear nerve: **Absent**
- Cochlear promontory: Hypoplastic, **flattened**
- Vestibule & SCC: Dilated **[cochlear aplasia with dilated vestibule (CADV)]** or hypoplastic or normal
- Vestibular aqueduct: **Normal**
- Facial nerve canal: **Anomalous**, obtuse angle anterior genu
- IAC: **Hypoplastic**
- Middle ear: Normal size
- Ossicles: Normal or malformed stapes
- Oval window: Normal or stenotic/atretic

TOP DIFFERENTIAL DIAGNOSES

- Labyrinthine aplasia
  - Cochlea, vestibule, & SCC absent
- Common cavity deformity
  - Dilated cochlea & vestibule form common cavity
- Cochlear hypoplasia: 4 types
- Cystic cochleovestibular anomaly
  - Cochlea & vestibule are cystic with no internal architecture
- Labyrinthine ossificans
  - Acquired sensorineural hearing loss (SNHL), postmeningitic, normal promontory

CLINICAL ISSUES

- Extremely rare, congenital SNHL, usually bilateral

DIAGNOSTIC CHECKLIST

- Cochlear aplasia if no cochlea is seen on CT or T2 MR but rest of membranous labyrinth is present
- Distinguish CADV (Tx auditory brainstem implantation) from common cavity (Tx cochlear implant)

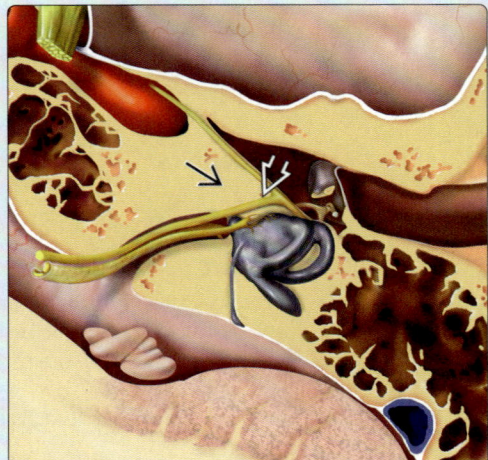
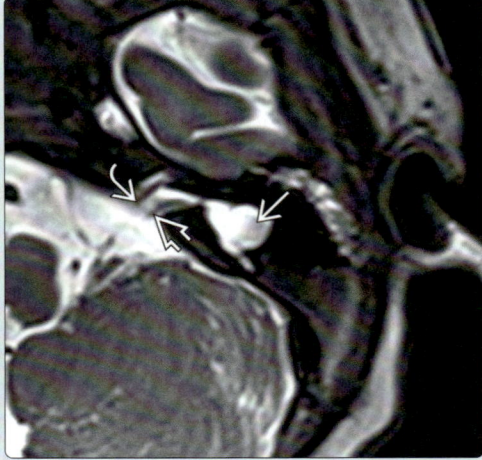

(Left) Axial graphic shows cochlear aplasia, including a small IAC with absence of the cochlear nerve, an absent cochlea ⇨, vestibular & semicircular canal (SCC) malformation, & flattening of CNVII anterior genu ⇨. The facial nerve canal occupies the normal cochlear location. (Right) Axial T2 SPACE MR in a 4-month-old girl with congenital SNHL reveals cochlear absence. There is a globular vestibule-horizontal SCC anomaly ⇨. A short, narrow IAC contains vestibular ⇨ & facial ⇨ nerves. No cochlear nerve was seen.

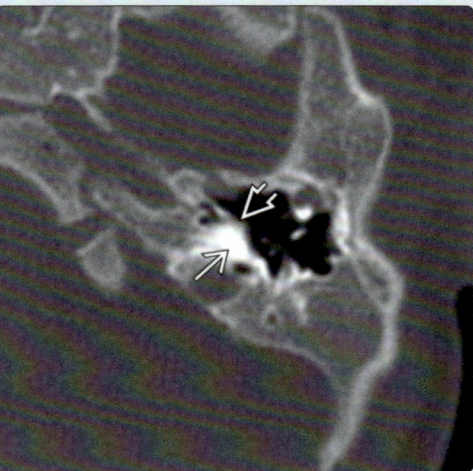
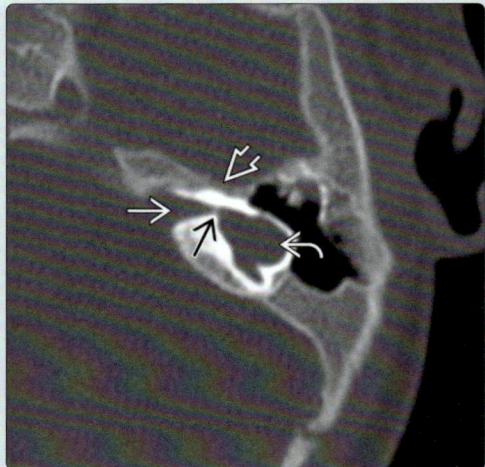

(Left) Axial bone CT in the same patient demonstrates absence of the cochlea ⇨ and mild flattening of the cochlear promontory ⇨. (Right) Axial bone CT in the same patient shows the cochlear aplasia with a dilated vestibule. The dilated vestibule ⇨ is at the posterolateral aspect of the IAC fundus ⇨ (a differentiating feature from common cavity malformation where the IAC fundus opens at middle of the cavity medially). A shortened, narrowed IAC is seen ⇨. An obtuse anterior genu of the facial nerve canal is partially visualized ⇨.

TERMINOLOGY

Definitions

- Absent cochlea, but vestibule, semicircular canals (SCCs), & internal auditory canal (IAC) are present in some form

IMAGING

General Features

- Best diagnostic clue
  - Absent cochlea, usually dysmorphic vestibule & SCC
- Morphology
  - 2 subgroups according to vestibular system
  - **Cochlear aplasia with normal labyrinth**
    - Normally developed vestibule and SCCs
  - **Cochlear aplasia with dilated vestibule (CADV)**
    - Dilated vestibule and normal or dilated SCCs
  - Extremely important to **distinguish CADV from common cavity (CC)** malformation
    - Cochlear implant (CI) contraindicated in cochlear aplasia
    - CI can be done in CC if cochleovestibular nerve present
    - In CADV, **IAC fundus** opens into anteromedial aspect of dilated vestibule
    - In CC, IAC fundus opens into center of CC medially

CT Findings

- Bone CT
  - Cochlea: Absent, bilaterally or unilaterally
  - Cochlear nerve canal: Absent
  - Cochlear promontory: Hypoplastic, flattened
  - Vestibule & SCC: Often malformed, globular, & dilated, or hypoplastic or normal
  - Vestibular aqueduct: Usually normal
  - Facial nerve canal: Anteriorly displaced occupying normal location of cochlea; obtuse angle anterior genu
  - IAC: Usually hypoplastic
  - Middle ear: Normal size
  - Ossicles: Normal or malformed stapes
  - Oval window: Normal or stenotic/atretic
  - Round window: Atretic

MR Findings

- T2WI
  - Cochlea & cochlear nerve: Absent
  - Vestibule & SCC: Variable abnormality

Imaging Recommendations

- Best imaging tool
  - Temporal bone CT or heavily T2W 3D (CISS, FIESTA) MR

DIFFERENTIAL DIAGNOSIS

Labyrinthine Aplasia

- Cochlea, vestibule, & SCC absent

Common Cavity Malformation

- Dilated cochlea & vestibule form CC
- IAC fundus opens at center of CC medially

Cochlear Hypoplasia: 4 Types

- Cochlear hypoplasia (CH)-I (bud-like cochlea)

- CH-II (cystic hypoplastic cochlea): Recurrent meningitis due to defective stapes footplate
- CH-III (cochlea with < 2 turns)
- CH-IV (cochlea with hypoplastic middle and apical turns)

Cystic Cochleovestibular Anomaly

- Cochlea & vestibule are cystic with no internal architecture; figure 8 or snowman appearance

Labyrinthine Ossificans

- Acquired sensorineural hearing loss (SNHL), usually following meningitis
- Ossified membranous labyrinth, **normal promontory**

PATHOLOGY

General Features

- Associated abnormalities
  - Vestibule & SCC may be normal or dilated

Gross Pathologic & Surgical Features

- Absent cochlea, remaining inner ear present but abnormal

CLINICAL ISSUES

Presentation

- Most common signs/symptoms
  - Congenital SNHL, usually bilateral
- Audiologic evaluation findings
  - No hearing level; only stimulation is vibrotactile

Demographics

- Epidemiology
  - < 1% of all inner ear congenital lesions

Treatment

- Auditory brainstem implantation (ABI)

DIAGNOSTIC CHECKLIST

Consider

- Cochlear aplasia diagnosed if **no** cochlea is seen on CT or T2 MR but rest of membranous labyrinth is present
  - Distinguish **cochlear aplasia (flat promontory)** from **labyrinthine ossificans (normal promontory)**
- If differentiation of **CADV (ABI)** from **CC (CI)** difficult at imaging, audiology should be analyzed critically
  - Audiologically no hearing in CADV; profound hearing loss in CC malformation

SELECTED REFERENCES

1. Lewis M et al: Syndromic hearing loss in children. Neuroimaging Clin N Am. 33(4):563-80, 2023
2. Robson CD et al: Non-syndromic sensorineural hearing loss in children. Neuroimaging Clin N Am. 33(4):531-42, 2023
3. Kim BJ et al: Long-term audiologic outcomes and potential outcome predictors of cochlear implantation in cochlear aplasia with dilated vestibule: a case series. Clin Otolaryngol. 47(5):599-605, 2022
4. O'Brien WT et al: Nonsyndromic congenital causes of sensorineural hearing loss in children: an illustrative review. AJR Am J Roentgenol. 216(4):1048-55, 2021
5. D'Arco F et al: The link between inner ear malformations and the rest of the body: what we know so far about genetic, imaging and histology. Neuroradiology. 62(5):539-44, 2020
6. Sennaroğlu L et al: Classification and current management of inner ear malformations. Balkan Med J. 34(5):397-411, 2017

Cochlear Hypoplasia

TERMINOLOGY

- Small, underdeveloped cochlea; 4 types

IMAGING

- Cochlear hypoplasia (CH) of variable severity
  - **CH-I** (bud-like cochlea)
  - **CH-II** (cystic hypoplastic cochlea)
  - **CH-III** (cochlea with < 2 turns)
  - **CH-IV** (cochlea with hypoplastic middle & apical turns)
- Cochlear nerve canal: Absent, narrow, normal, wide
- Cochlear nerve: Often absent or hypoplastic
- Facial nerve canal: Aberrant course ± dehiscence
- Internal auditory canal: Normal or narrow/anomalous
- Vestibule: Normal, dilated, or hypoplastic
- Semicircular canals: Normal, dilated, hypoplastic, or absent
- Vestibular aqueduct: Normal or large

TOP DIFFERENTIAL DIAGNOSES

- **CHARGE syndrome**
  - Small/absent semicircular canal, variable CH, ± funnel-shaped, large vestibular aqueduct
- **Cochlear incomplete partition type II (IP-II)**
  - Deficient modiolus, absent interscalar septum between plump apical & middle turns, usually with large vestibular aqueduct
- **Branchiootorenal syndrome**
  - Hypoplastic offset middle & apical turns, ± funnel-shaped, large vestibular aqueduct
- **Dwarf cochlea (miniature cochlea)**
  - Normal number but smaller diameter of turns
- **Cochlear incomplete partition type III (IP-III)**
  - Cochlea size is normal to large; interscalar septum present but absent modiolus

DIAGNOSTIC CHECKLIST

- Consider CHARGE & branchiootorenal syndromes if distinctive associated findings are present

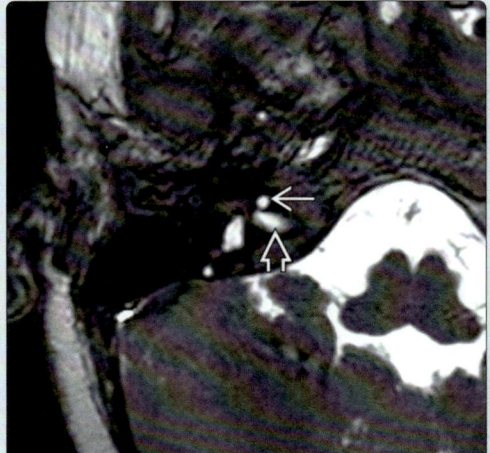
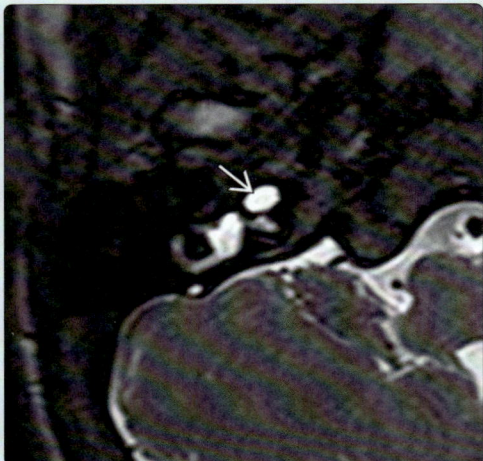

(Left) Axial T2 MR shows a small, bud-like structure consistent with cochlear hypoplasia type I (CH-I; bud-like cochlea) ➡ arising from the internal auditory canal ⊒. (Right) 3D T2 SPACE MR in an infant boy with bilateral profound sensorineural hearing loss (SNHL) shows CH-II (cystic hypoplastic cochlea) with a single, rounded cochlear turn ➡ without modiolus and interscalar septa. Note that the cochlea has smaller dimensions but with normal external outline. CSF gusher and recurrent meningitis may occur in CH-II.

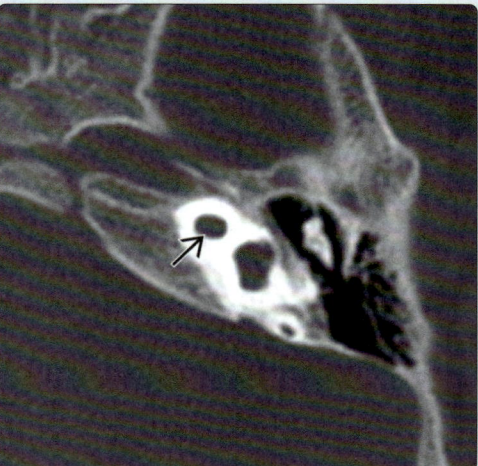
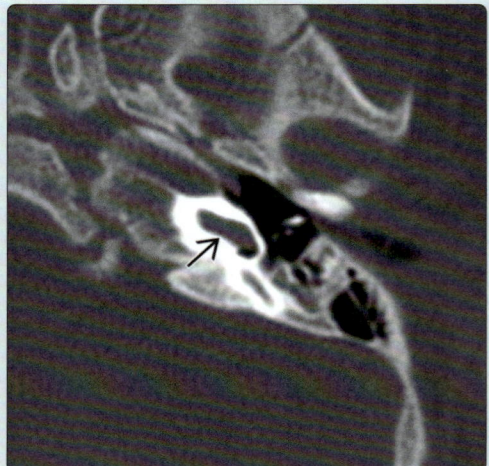

(Left) Axial bone CT in a 10-month-old girl with profound SNHL shows CH-IV (cochlea with hypoplastic middle and apical turns). The middle and apical turns ➡ are severely hypoplastic and located anteromedially (instead of their normal central position). (Right) Axial bone CT in the same patient shows a relatively normal-appearing basal turn of the left cochlea ➡.

TERMINOLOGY

Abbreviations

- Cochlear hypoplasia (CH)

Definitions

- Cochlear underdevelopment: External dimensions < normal cochlea with internal architecture deformities
- Term "cochlea with 1.5 turns" used to define CH (especially CH type III; cochlea with < 2 turns)
  - Avoid this term for cochlear incomplete partition type II

IMAGING

General Features

- Best diagnostic clue
  - Small cochlea; CH classified into 4 types

CT Findings

- Bone CT
  - **CH-I (bud-like cochlea)**: Small, ovoid/round, bud-shaped cochlea arising from internal auditory canal (IAC)
    - Severely deformed internal architecture with no modiolus & interscalar septa (ISS)
  - **CH-II (cystic hypoplastic cochlea)**: Small cochlea with defective modiolus & ISS but normal external outline
    - Modiolus may be totally absent with large communication with IAC → **CSF gusher** at surgery
    - Cochlear implant **electrode misplacement** into IAC
    - Vestibular aqueduct may enlarge & vestibule dilate
    - **Stapes footplate** may be defective → **recurrent meningitis**
  - **CH-III (cochlea with < 2 turns)**: Small cochlea, short modiolus, & reduced overall length of ISS
    - Vestibule & semicircular canals (SCCs) usually hypoplastic
    - Cochlear aperture (CA) may be hypoplastic or aplastic
  - **CH-IV (cochlea with hypoplastic middle & apical turns)**: Small cochlear middle & apical turns
    - Located **anteromedially** (instead of normal central position) over **normal basal turn**
    - Facial nerve labyrinthine segment usually located anterior to cochlea
  - Round window: Absent or present
  - Cochlear nerve canal (CNC): Absent, narrow, or wide
  - IAC: Normal or narrow/anomalous
  - Vestibule: Normal, dilated, or hypoplastic
  - SCCs: Normal, dilated, hypoplastic, or absent
  - Vestibular aqueduct: Normal or large
  - **Facial nerve canal**: **Aberrant course** due to associated SCC (especially lateral SCC) abnormalities ± dehiscence
  - Middle ear space & contents: Usually normal but **stapedial fixation** may occur, especially in CH-III & CH-IV
  - **Cochlear promontory may lack normal protuberance**
    - Difficult to identify promontory & round window through facial recess during cochlear implantation (CI)
    - Additional transcanal approach may be required to expose hypoplastic cochlea

MR Findings

- Cochlea: Small, internal structure present or absent

- **Cochlear nerve (CN)**: Often absent or hypoplastic, especially when CA hypoplasia/aplasia

DIFFERENTIAL DIAGNOSIS

CHARGE Syndrome

- CH, flattened apical turn or normal; stenotic CNC

Cochlear Incomplete Partition Type II (IP-II)

- Cochlear modiolus deficient ± plump apical & middle turns
- Deficient septation between apical & middle turns

Branchiootorenal Syndrome

- Tapered cochlear basal turn
- Hypoplastic, offset middle & apical cochlear turns

Dwarf Cochlea (Miniature Cochlea)

- Normal-appearing cochlea with normal number of turns but with reduced diameter of turns

Cochlear Incomplete Partition Type III (IP-III)

- Cochlea normal to large in size

CLINICAL ISSUES

Presentation

- Most common signs/symptoms
  - Congenital sensorineural hearing loss (SNHL)
  - Stapedial fixation may produce conductive hearing loss (CHL), especially in CH-III & CH-IV

Treatment

- Hearing aids only: Mild or moderate SNHL; stapes surgery: Pure CHL; both: Mixed hearing loss
- CI: Profound SNHL if CN present
- Auditory brainstem implantation (ABI): Profound SNHL if CN deficient (frequent)
- CI on side with better developed CN/better audiologic findings
- Contralateral ABI if limited language development with CI
- Simultaneous CI & ABI if 2-3 years of age & barely visible CN
  - To avoid losing valuable time for language development

DIAGNOSTIC CHECKLIST

Consider

- CH if small cochlea with < 2 turns

SELECTED REFERENCES

1. D'Arco F et al: Subtle malformation of the cochlear apex and genetic abnormalities: beyond the "thorny" cochlea. AJNR Am J Neuroradiol. 44(1):79-81, 2023
2. Lewis MA et al: The spectrum of cochlear malformations in CHARGE syndrome and insights into the role of the CHD7 gene during embryogenesis of the inner ear. Neuroradiology. 65(4):819-34, 2023
3. Lewis M et al: Syndromic hearing loss in children. Neuroimaging Clin N Am. 33(4):563-80, 2023
4. Robson CD et al: Non-syndromic sensorineural hearing loss in children. Neuroimaging Clin N Am. 33(4):531-42, 2023
5. Pao J et al: Re-examining the cochlea in branchio-oto-renal syndrome: genotype-phenotype correlation. AJNR Am J Neuroradiol. 43(2):309-14, 2022
6. O'Brien WT et al: Nonsyndromic congenital causes of sensorineura hearing loss in children: an illustrative review. AJR Am J Roentgenol. 216(4):1048-55, 2021
7. Robson CD: Conductive hearing loss in children. Neuroimaging Clin N Am. 33(4):543-62, 2023

Common Cavity Malformation

TERMINOLOGY

- Common cavity (CC) is cystic space representing undifferentiated cochlea & vestibule

IMAGING

- **Cochlea, vestibule, & horizontal semicircular canal (SCC)**: CC, variable size
- Posterior & superior SCC: Usually absent or malformed
- IAC: Variable size, anomalous course, deficient fundus
  - Small CC: Stenotic IAC; large CC: Widened IAC
- CNVIII: Small or absent components
- Facial nerve canal: Anomalous course
- Vestibular aqueduct: Not dilated, may be absent; ossicles: Normal or anomalous stapes & stenotic oval window

TOP DIFFERENTIAL DIAGNOSES

- Cystic cochleovestibular anomaly: **Figure 8 or snowman**
- Cochlear aplasia with dilated vestibule: **IAC fundus opens into anteromedial aspect of vestibule**

PATHOLOGY

- Arrested **otocyst** development at **4th** gestational **week**
- *HOXA1* mutations: Bosley-Salih-Alorainy syndrome

CLINICAL ISSUES

- Congenital sensorineural hearing loss
- Cochlear implantation if cochleovestibular nerve (CVN) with enough cochlear nerve fibers (size/hearing aid trial)
- Auditory brainstem implantation if cochlear fibers questionable, as in nondemonstrated or small CVN in MR
- Potential risk of recurrent meningitis for large CC & large IAC with associated perilymph fistula

DIAGNOSTIC CHECKLIST

- CC if cochlea, vestibule, & horizontal SCC form single cavity without differentiation
  - In CC, **IAC fundus usually opens into center of cavity**
- Consider cystic cochleovestibular anomaly if differentiated into separate but featureless cochlea & vestibule

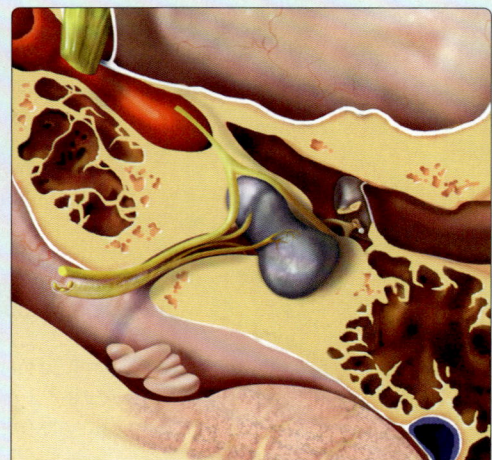
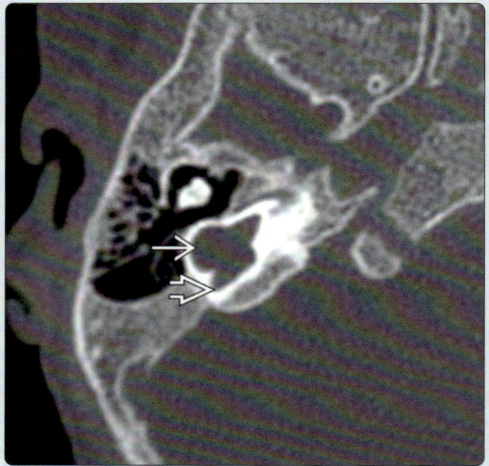

(Left) *Axial graphic shows features of a common cavity (CC) malformation. Note that the cochlea & vestibule are merged into a common cyst. Semicircular canals are not distinct from cystic vestibular component.* (Right) *Axial bone CT in a 6-month-old boy with unilateral sensorineural hearing loss reveals a CC anomaly of the inner ear with a cystic structure, representing the rudimentary cochlea bud, vestibule, & horizontal semicircular canal ➡. A dilated posterior semicircular canal ⇨ is seen.*

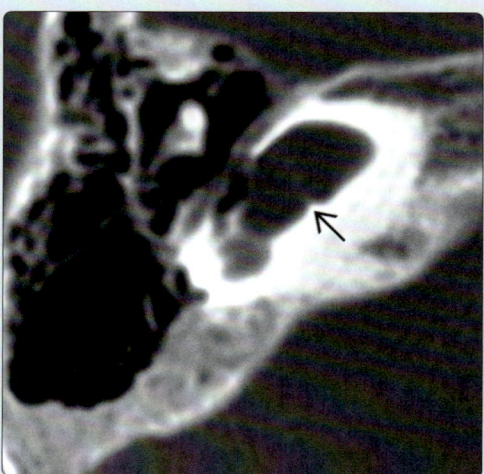
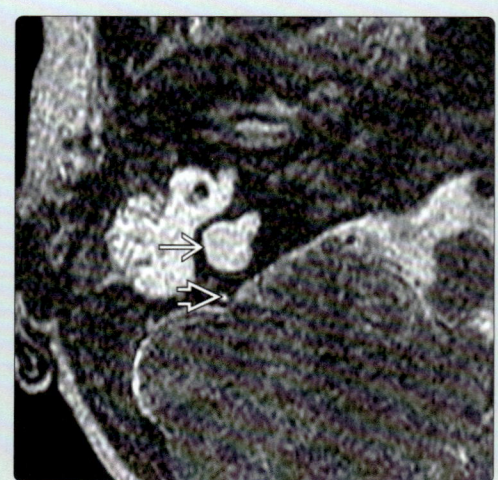

(Left) *Axial bone CT shows a featureless cochlea, vestibule, & semicircular canals as a single cystic structure ➡. The ossicular chain, middle ear, & mastoid air cells are normal.* (Right) *Axial 3D FIESTA MR in an 18-month-old child with bilateral congenital sensorineural hearing loss demonstrates a CC anomaly with a cystic structure, representing the vestibule, rudimentary cochlear bud, & horizontal semicircular canal ➡. There is a small posterior semicircular canal ⇨.*

TERMINOLOGY

Definitions

- Common cavity (CC) is cystic space representing **undifferentiated cochlea & vestibule**

IMAGING

General Features

- Best diagnostic clue
  - Featureless CC represents rudimentary cochlea, vestibule, & semicircular canals (SCCs)

CT Findings

- Bone CT
  - Unilateral or bilateral & often asymmetric
  - **Cochlea, vestibule, & horizontal SCC**: CC, variable size
  - Posterior & superior SCC: Usually absent or malformed
  - Internal auditory canal (IAC)
    - Small CC: Stenotic IAC; large CC: Widened IAC
    - Defective fundus
    - Course may be anomalous
    - **IAC fundus** may **enter center of CC medially**
    - If open at anterior aspect of CC, difficult to discriminate cochlear aplasia with dilated vestibule (CADV)
  - Facial nerve canal: Anomalous labyrinthine segment & anterior genu
  - Middle ear space & ossicles: Normal or anomalous stapes & stenotic oval window
  - Vestibular aqueduct: Not dilated, may be absent

MR Findings

- T2WI
  - High signal intensity fluid within CC
  - Posterior & superior SCC: Usually absent or malformed
  - IAC: Single common **cochleovestibular nerve (CVN)** ± anomalous course of CNVII
  - Normally, cochlear & vestibular nerves originate from brainstem as CVN & separate in IAC
    - Into cochlear, superior, & inferior vestibular nerves
    - In **CC, unbranched CVN** enters CC
  - **Cochlear nerve fiber content in CVN** impossible to assess with current imaging; considered normal if
    - Size similar to contralateral normal CVN, or 1.5-2.0x that of ipsilateral facial nerve

Imaging Recommendations

- Best imaging tool
  - Temporal bone CT or MR
- Protocol advice
  - Heavily T2W 3D (CISS, FIESTA) oblique sagittal MR through IAC used to assess presence & size of CVN

DIFFERENTIAL DIAGNOSIS

Cystic Cochleovestibular Malformation

- Imaging: Cochlea & vestibule are usually enlarged & cystic without internal architecture; figure 8 or snowman

Cochlear Aplasia

- Imaging: Absent cochlea, normal or dilated vestibule

- Cochlear aplasia with dilated vestibule has IAC fundus opening at its anteromedial aspect

Rudimentary Otocyst

- **No IAC** connection (unlike CC)

Incomplete Partition Type III (IP-III)

- Modiolus absent but interscalar septa present, giving corkscrew appearance of cochlea
- Contiguous with bulbous IAC

PATHOLOGY

General Features

- Etiology
  - Unknown or genetic mutation
  - *HOXA1* mutations: Bosley-Salih-Alorainy syndrome

CLINICAL ISSUES

Presentation

- Most common signs/symptoms
  - Congenital sensorineural hearing loss (SNHL)
  - Potential risk of recurrent meningitis for large CC & large IAC with associated perilymph fistula
- **Audiologic evaluation findings**
  - Profound hearing loss

Treatment

- **Cochlear implantation (CI)** if **CVN with enough cochlear nerve fibers**
- **Hearing aid trial**: If behavioral audiometric response or language development occurs with hearing aid use
  - Enough cochlear fibers possibly exist in CVN
- **Auditory brainstem implantation (ABI)** if cochlear fibers questionable, as in nondemonstrated or small CVN in MR
- Contralateral ABI if limited language development with CI

DIAGNOSTIC CHECKLIST

Consider

- CC if cochlea & vestibule form single cavity without differentiation

Image Interpretation Pearls

- Oblique sagittal IAC 3D T2 MR to determine presence & size (cochlear fiber content) of CVN

Reporting Tips

- Can be difficult to distinguish CC from CADV, audiology helps differentiate
  - Profound hearing loss in CC; no hearing in CADV
- Consider cystic cochleovestibular anomaly if differentiated into separate but featureless cochlea & vestibule

SELECTED REFERENCES

1. Lewis M et al: Syndromic hearing loss in children. Neuroimaging Clin N Am. 33(4):563-80, 2023
2. Robson CD et al: Non-syndromic sensorineural hearing loss in children. Neuroimaging Clin N Am. 33(4):531-42, 2023
3. Al-Mahboob A et al: Cochlear implantation in common cavity deformity: a systematic review. Eur Arch Otorhinolaryngol. 279(1):37-48, 2022
4. O'Brien WT et al: Nonsyndromic congenital causes of sensorineura hearing loss in children: an illustrative review. AJR Am J Roentgenol. 216(4):1048-55, 2021

Cystic Cochleovestibular Malformation

TERMINOLOGY

- Cochlear **incomplete partition type I (IP-I)** + dilated vestibule & horizontal semicircular canal (SCC)

IMAGING

- Cochlea: Absent internal septation & modiolus (IP-I)
- Vestibule & SCC: Dilated vestibule & lateral (horizontal) SCC form single cavity, wide communication with cochlea
- CNVII canal: Normal or mildly obtuse anterior genu angle; normal or dehiscent tympanic segment
- Internal auditory canal: Small or dilated, defective fundus
- CNVIII: Nerves hypoplastic or absent
- Vestibular aqueduct: Usually normal
- Oval window: Normal or stenotic + stapedial anomaly

TOP DIFFERENTIAL DIAGNOSES

- Cochlear aplasia
- Common cavity
- Cochlear hypoplasia type II (cystic hypoplastic cochlea)

- Incomplete partition type III (IP-III)

CLINICAL ISSUES

- Congenital sensorineural hearing loss
  - Severe to profound in majority of patients
- CSF leak & meningitis from translabyrinthine fistula
  - Middle ear exploration to excise & repair stapes footplate/oval window cyst & defect
- Cochlear implant (CI) or auditory brainstem implant (ABI) (if deficient cochlear nerve)
- Contralateral ABI if limited language development with CI

DIAGNOSTIC CHECKLIST

- **Cystic cochleovestibular malformation (IP-I)**
  - Figure 8 cochlea & vestibule lacking internal architecture
  - Defective IAC fundus: Risk of CSF gusher at surgery
  - Stapes footplate defect: Spontaneous CSF fistula & recurrent meningitis
- MR to detect hypoplasia/aplasia of CNVIII components

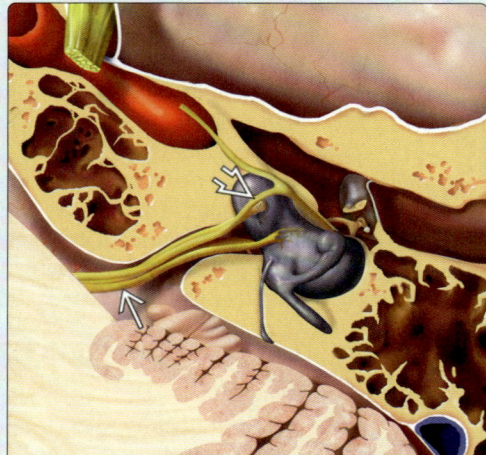
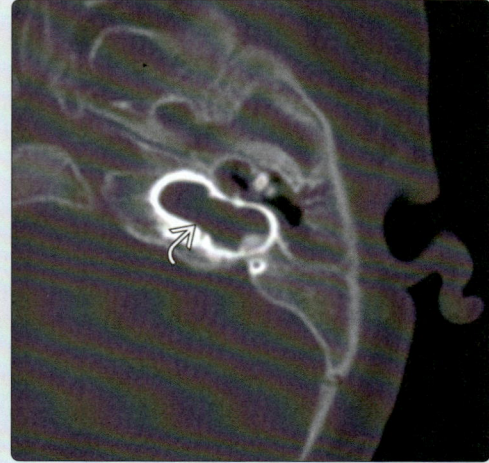

(Left) Figure 8 morphology of a featureless cochlea & vestibule is shown. The cochlear interscalar septum & modiolus are absent. CNVIII components are hypoplastic ➡. IAC is narrow & shortened. CNVII labyrinthine segment has lost its anteriorly curving shape & appears straightened ➡ as it ends at the geniculate ganglion. (Right) Axial bone CT in a 6-month-old girl with unilateral sensorineural hearing loss (SNHL) & multiple congenital anomalies shows typical figure 8 morphology of cystic cochleovestibular malformation (CCVM) ➡.

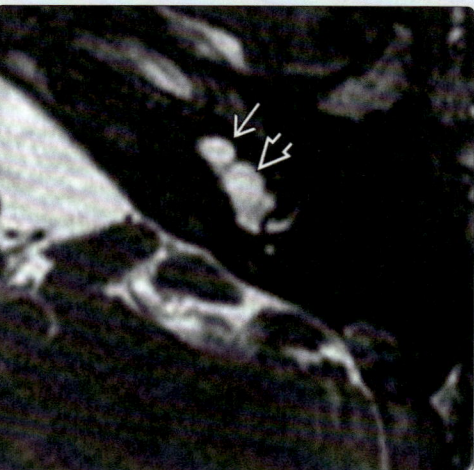
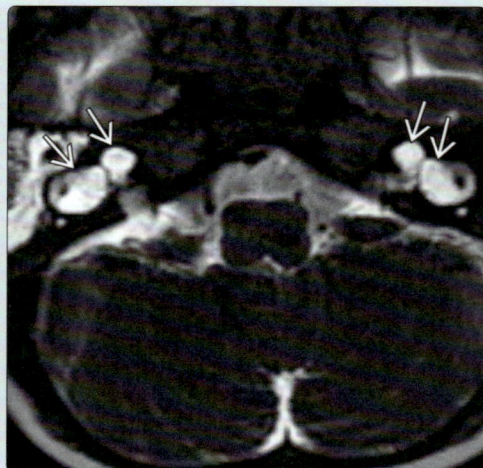

(Left) Axial FIESTA MR in a child with left SNHL shows a cochlea that lacks internal architecture ➡ (IP-I) and an enlarged vestibule ➡, forming nearly a figure 8 or snowman configuration. (Right) Axial T2 FIESTA MR in a 1-year-old child with 2 episodes of meningitis & otorrhea shows bilateral CCVM ➡ & right middle ear hyperintensity that may represent serous fluid or CSF, as these patients are at increased risk of CSF leak.

Cystic Cochleovestibular Malformation

TERMINOLOGY

Abbreviations
- Cystic cochleovestibular malformation (CCVM)

Synonyms
- Cystic cochleovestibular anomaly
- Cochlear **incomplete partition type I (IP-I)**

Definitions
- Cochlea lacks interscalar septum & modiolus (IP-I) + dilated vestibule & lateral (horizontal) semicircular canal (SCC)

IMAGING

General Features
- Best diagnostic clue
  - Cystic, featureless cochlea + dilated vestibule/lateral SCC
- Morphology
  - Cochlea & vestibule: **Figure 8** or **sloping snowman**

CT Findings
- Bone CT
  - Cochlea: **Absent internal septation & modiolus (IP-I)**, variable size
  - Vestibule: **Dilated, large cochlear communication**
  - SCC: **Dilated, lateral SCC** forms common cavity with vestibule, anterior limb superior SCC ± dilated
  - Internal auditory canal (IAC): Small or dilated
    - **Defect between IAC fundus** & cochlea due to cochlear aperture defect & absent modiolus
      - □ CSF may completely fill cochlea
  - CNVII canal: Normal or mildly obtuse anterior genu angle; normal or dehiscent tympanic segment
  - Vestibular aqueduct: Usually normal
  - Oval window: Normal or stenotic + stapedial anomaly
  - **Stapes footplate defect** & CSF filling cochlea with **cystic structure** in stapes footplate
    - **Endosteal** developmental anomaly
    - Easily infected during otitis media attack
    - **Spontaneous CSF fistula & recurrent meningitis**

MR Findings
- T2WI
  - Cochlea + vestibule: Figure 8 contour
  - Cochlea: Lacks internal septation & modiolus
  - Vestibule & horizontal SCC: Dilated
  - CNVIII: Nerves hypoplastic or absent

Imaging Recommendations
- Best imaging tool
  - MR for CNVIII components, mainly cochlear nerve (**CN**)
- Protocol advice
  - 3D T2 (CISS, FIESTA): Axial & oblique sagittal

DIFFERENTIAL DIAGNOSIS

Cochlear Aplasia
- **Absent cochlea**; vestibule & SCC variable

Common Cavity
- **Cystic cochlea & vestibule** form undifferentiated or minimally differentiated common cavity

Cochlear Hypoplasia Type II (Cystic Hypoplastic Cochlea)
- Defective cochlear modiolus & interscalar septa
- **Endosteal** developmental anomaly with **defective stapes footplate** development (like IP-I)
- Recurrent meningitis more common than IP-I (CCVM)

Incomplete Partition Type III (IP-III)
- Modiolus absent but interscalar septa present, giving corkscrew appearance of cochlea
- Contiguous with bulbous IAC; predisposes to high-volume CSF **gusher** during cochlear implant (CI) surgery
- **Outer** periosteal & enchondral **layers defective** but with thick endosteal layer & **normal stapes footplate**
  - Meningitis rare (unlike IP-I & cochlear hypoplasia type II)

PATHOLOGY

Gross Pathologic & Surgical Features
- Cochlea & vestibule lack internal architecture

CLINICAL ISSUES

Presentation
- Most common signs/symptoms
  - Congenital sensorineural hearing loss (SNHL)
  - CSF leak & meningitis from translabyrinthine fistula
  - Risk of labyrinthine ossification from meningitis
- **Audiologic evaluation findings**
  - Severe to profound SNHL in majority

Treatment
- CI: Risks in CCVM: CSF gusher (deficient IAC fundus), facial nerve damage (dehiscent)
  - CSF leakage from cochleostomy should be sealed; then only subtotal petrosectomy to seal middle ear from nose
- Auditory brainstem implantation (ABI) if aplastic CN
- Contralateral ABI if limited language development with CI
- IP-I with recurrent meningitis & normal tympanic membranes, & fluid filling middle ear & mastoid
  - Middle ear exploration to excise & repair stapes footplate/oval window cyst & defect

DIAGNOSTIC CHECKLIST

Consider
- CCVM: **Figure 8** or **sloping snowman** cochlea & vestibule

Image Interpretation Pearls
- MR to detect hypoplasia/aplasia of CNVIII components

SELECTED REFERENCES

1. Lewis M et al: Syndromic hearing loss in children. Neuroimaging Clin N Am. 33(4):563-80, 2023
2. Robson CD et al: Non-syndromic sensorineural hearing loss in children. Neuroimaging Clin N Am. 33(4):531-42, 2023
3. O'Brien WT et al: Nonsyndromic congenital causes of sensorineura hearing loss in children: an illustrative review. AJR Am J Roentgenol. 216(4):1048-55, 2021
4. D'Arco F et al: The link between inner ear malformations and the rest of the body: what we know so far about genetic, imaging and histology. Neuroradiology. 62(5):539-44, 2020
5. Sennaroğlu L et al: Classification and current management of inner ear malformations. Balkan Med J. 34(5):397-411, 2017

TERMINOLOGY

- Incomplete partition type I (IP-I) spectrum of anomalies: Mild (cochlea lacks modiolus and interscalar septum) to severe [cystic cochleovestibular malformation (CCVM)]
- Cochlear IP-I: Milder form of IP-I; cochlea has some external structure, variable anomaly vestibule, & semicircular canal (SCC)
- CCVM: Least differentiated manifestation of IP-I involving cochlea, vestibule, & SCC

IMAGING

- IP-I has absent interscalar septum & modiolus
- Spectrum of IP-I severity
  - Amorphous sac, wide communication between cochlea & vestibule; figure 8 morphology (CCVM)
  - Some external structure, dilated vestibule, & horizontal SCC (most common)
  - External indentations suggesting cochlear turns, ± normal vestibule (rare)

- Cochlear nerve canal & internal auditory canal: Normal, wide (most common), or narrow; absent macula cribrosa
- Cochlear nerve: Usually hypoplastic or absent
- Vestibule & horizontal SCC: Usually dilated
- Vestibular aqueduct: Usually normal

TOP DIFFERENTIAL DIAGNOSES

- **Cochlear hypoplasia**: Small cochlea, 4 subtypes
- **Cochlear incomplete partition type II (IP-II)**
  - Defective septation between middle & apical cochlear turns, normal basal turn
  - ± large vestibular aqueduct/endolymphatic sac
- **Common cavity malformation**
  - Single cystic structure = cochlea + vestibule

CLINICAL ISSUES

- When profound bilateral sensorineural hearing loss: Cochlear implantation variably successful
  - Risk of CSF gusher

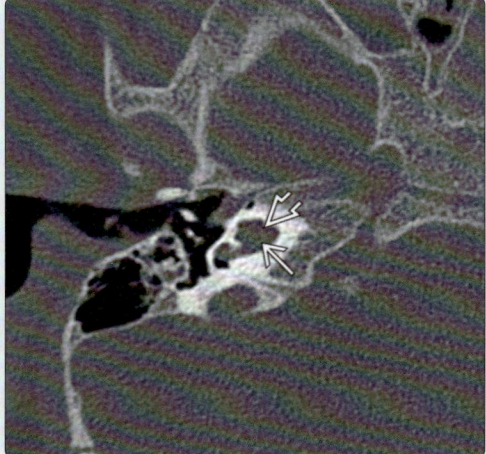
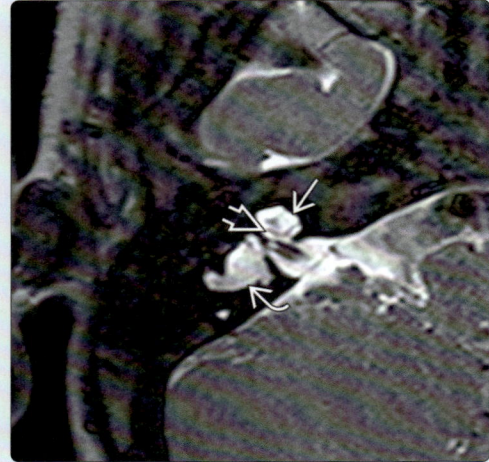

(Left) Axial bone CT in a 9-month-old girl with right SNHL shows complete absence of the cochlear modiolus ➡ & interscalar septum ➡. The anomaly affects entire cochlea. In this relatively mild & uncommon manifestation of IP-I, there is some external "shape" to the cochlea. (Right) Axial T2 MR in a 1-year-old boy with SNHL shows a large, amorphous cochlea ➡. The modiolus & osseous interscalar septum are absent. Curvilinear internal hypointensity presumably represents the spiral lamina ➡. The vestibule ➡ & lateral SCCs are dilated.

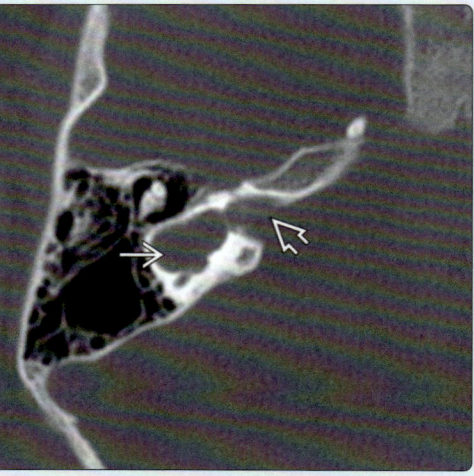
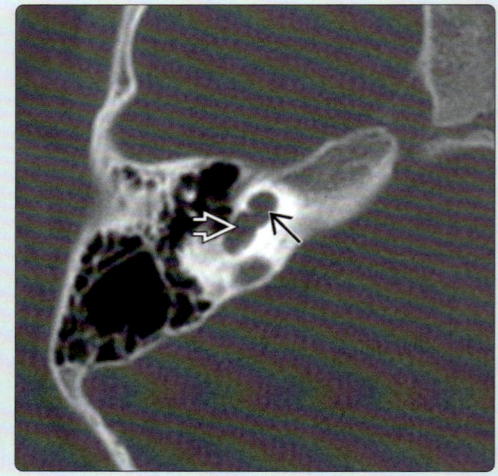

(Left) Axial bone CT in a 4-year-old boy with right SNHL shows dilatation of the vestibule & horizontal SCC ➡. The vestibular aqueduct is not enlarged. The internal auditory meatus is widened ➡. (Right) Axial bone CT in the same patient shows cystic cochlea that lacks internal structure ➡. Note wide communication between the cochlea & vestibule ➡. This is the more common form of IP-I, with a cystic cochlea & dilatation of the vestibule & horizontal SCC, also referred to as cystic cochleovestibular malformation.

TERMINOLOGY

Abbreviations
- Cochlear incomplete partition type I (IP-I)

Definitions
- Cochlear IP-I: Absent internal structure of entire cochlea
  - Cochlear IP-I
    - Milder form of IP-I confined to cochlea without internal structure, normal to large in size
  - Cystic cochleovestibular malformation (CCVM)
    - Least differentiated manifestation of IP-I involving cochlea without internal structure, malformed vestibule, & semicircular canals (SCCs)

IMAGING

General Features
- Best diagnostic clue
  - Cochlea lacks **interscalar septum** between basal, middle, & apical turns
    - Absent modiolus
- Size
  - Normal-sized or large cochlea
- Morphology
  - Variable morphology, unilateral or bilateral
  - Most differentiated IP-I
    - Visible external cochlear turns lacking internal interscalar septum & modiolus
    - **Normal** vestibule & SCCs
  - Least differentiated IP-I
    - Cystic featureless cochlea with cystic vestibular malformation
    - Figure 8 morphology

CT Findings
- Bone CT
  - Cochlea
    - **Malformation affects entire cochlea**
    - **Absent interscalar septum**
    - **Absent modiolus**
    - Variable external contour
      - Amorphous sac or external indentations suggesting cochlear turns
  - Cochlear nerve canal and internal auditory canal
    - Normal, wide, or narrow; absent macula cribrosa
  - Vestibule & horizontal SCC
    - Grossly dilated or normal
  - Vestibular aqueduct (VA)
    - Rarely enlarged
  - Middle ear & ossicles
    - Normal or oval window stenosis/atresia + abnormal stapes

MR Findings
- 3D T2 SPACE, FIESTA, or equivalent
  - Cochlea: Lacks modiolus & interscalar septum; internal curvilinear hypointensity may represent spiral lamina in mildest IP-I
  - Vestibule & horizontal SCC: Usually dilated
  - Cochlear nerve: Usually hypoplastic or aplastic

Imaging Recommendations
- Best imaging tool
  - MR: To evaluate presence & size of cochlear nerve

DIFFERENTIAL DIAGNOSIS

Cochlear Incomplete Partition Type II (IP-II)
- Normal basal turn, deficient interscalar septum between cochlear middle & apical turns
- Modiolus deficient or absent
- ± large VA, large endolymphatic sac

Cochlear Hypoplasia
- Small cochlea, 4 subtypes

CHARGE Syndrome
- Stenotic/atretic cochlear nerve canal
- Variable cochlear anomaly
- Small vestibule & small/absent SCCs
- Funnel-shaped VA

Common Cavity Malformation
- Single cystic structure represents undifferentiated cochlea + vestibule

CLINICAL ISSUES

Presentation
- Most common signs/symptoms
  - Sensorineural hearing loss (SNHL)

Natural History & Prognosis
- Congenital SNHL
- Absent macula cribrosa & modiolus
  - Risk of CSF gusher at cochleostomy or stapedectomy
  - Risk of meningitis & postmeningitic labyrinthitis ossificans

Treatment
- Profound bilateral SNHL: Cochlear implantation with variable success
  - CSF gusher is most common surgical complication
  - Cochlear implantation more successful in IP-II group compared to IP-I group

SELECTED REFERENCES

1. D'Arco F et al: Incomplete partition type II in its various manifestations: isolated, in association with EVA, syndromic, and beyond; a multicentre international study. Neuroradiology. 66(8):1397-403, 2024
2. Lewis M et al: Syndromic hearing loss in children. Neuroimaging Clin N Am. 33(4):563-80, 2023
3. Robson CD et al: Non-syndromic sensorineural hearing loss in children. Neuroimaging Clin N Am. 33(4):531-42, 2023
4. O'Brien WT et al: Nonsyndromic congenital causes of sensorineura hearing loss in children: an illustrative review. AJR Am J Roentgenol. 216(4):1048-55, 2021
5. Sennaroğlu L: Radiological features and pathognomonic sign of stapes footplate fistula in inner ear malformations. Turk Arch Otorhinolaryngol. 59(2):95-102, 2021
6. D'Arco F et al: The link between inner ear malformations and the rest of the body: what we know so far about genetic, imaging and histology. Neuroradiology. 62(5):539-44, 2020
7. Sennaroğlu L et al: Classification and current management of inner ear malformations. Balkan Med J. 34(5):397-11, 2017
8. Suk Y et al: Surgical outcomes after cochlear implantation in children with incomplete partition type I: comparison with deaf children with a normal inner ear structure. Otol Neurotol. 36(1):e11-7, 2015

Cochlear Incomplete Partition Type II (IP-II)

TERMINOLOGY

- Incomplete partition type II (IP-II): Incomplete partition due to deficient interscalar septum (ISS) between middle & apical cochlear turns
- Mondini anomaly (historic terminology): IP-II + large vestibular aqueduct (LVA)

IMAGING

- Cochlea: Absent ISS between plump middle & apical turns
  - Do not mistake osseous spiral lamina for ISS on MR
  - Smooth external contour between middle & apical turns posterolaterally ("baseball cap" cochlea)
  - Asymmetric scalar chambers, deficient or absent modiolus
- Vestibular aqueduct/endolymphatic sac
  - Typically large > borderline large & flared; rarely normal
- Vestibule: Normal or large
- Semicircular canal (SCC): Normal or mildly plump anterior limb lateral SCC

TOP DIFFERENTIAL DIAGNOSES

- Cochlear IP-I, cochlear hypoplasia
- CHARGE syndrome
- X-linked stapes gusher (DFNX2)

PATHOLOGY

- *SLC26A4* mutation most common
- Syndromic deafness: Pendred syndrome
- Nonsyndromic deafness: DFNB4
- ~ 20% of temporal bones with LVA have IP-II anomaly

CLINICAL ISSUES

- Bilateral or unilateral, severe or profound sensorineural hearing loss (SNHL)
- SNHL precipitated by minor trauma
- Fluctuating, progressive SNHL (or mixed hearing loss)
- LVA: Avoid concussive-prone contact sports (controversial)
- Profound bilateral SNHL: Treatment is cochlear implantation

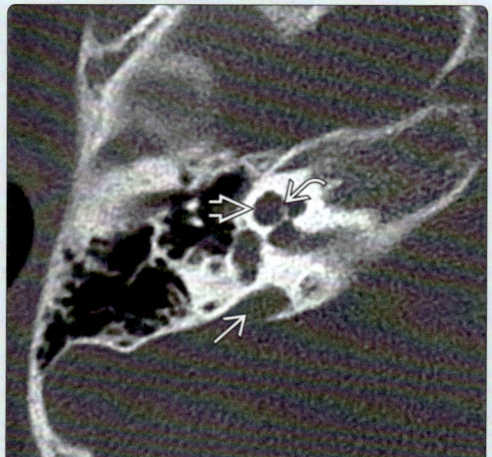
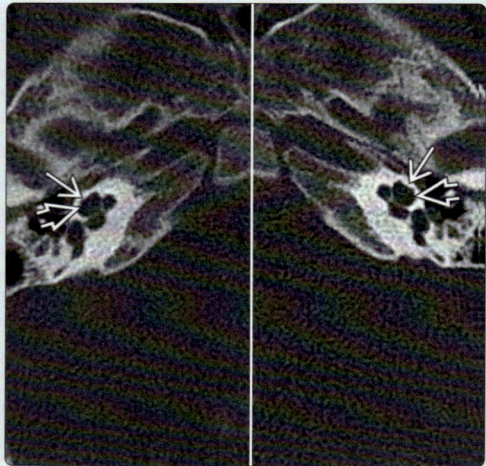

(Left) Axial bone CT in 4-year-old girl with mixed hearing loss shows a large vestibular aqueduct (VA) ➡ & incomplete partition type II (IP-II) cochlear anomaly with smooth contour laterally & deficiency of the interscalar septum (ISS) between apical & middle turns ➡. The modiolus ➡ is malformed. (Right) Axial bone CT in a 4-year-old boy with severe bilateral sensorineural hearing loss shows bilateral IP-II cochlear anomaly with "baseball cap" configuration of the middle/apical turns ➡ & deficient ISS ➡.

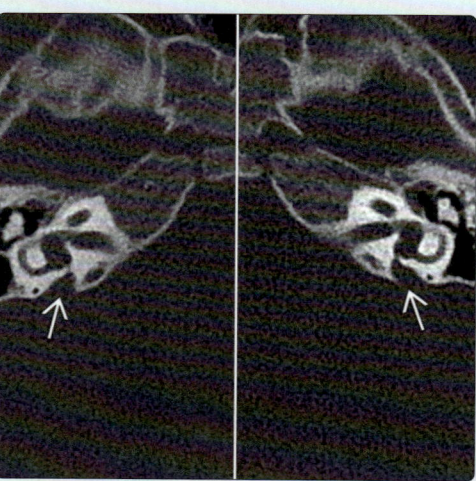
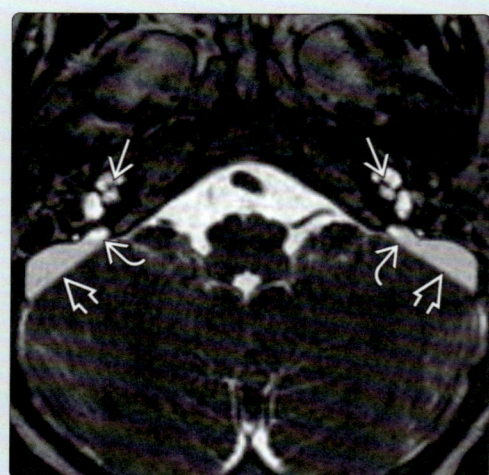

(Left) Axial bone CT in the same patient shows enlargement of the bilateral vestibular aqueducts, each of which measured 2.5 mm at the operculum ➡. (Right) Axial T2 FIESTA MR in the same patient shows bilateral modiolar deficiency ➡ & bilateral enlargement of the extraosseous ➡ & intraosseous ➡ portions of the endolymphatic sacs. The patient was subsequently tested for Pendred syndrome, with SLC26A4 variant documented; therefore, thyroid function tests will also be followed closely.

Cochlear Incomplete Partition Type II (IP-II)

TERMINOLOGY

Abbreviations

- Cochlear incomplete partition type II (IP-II)

Synonyms

- Mondini anomaly (historic terminology): IP-II + large vestibular aqueduct (LVA)

Definitions

- IP-II: Incomplete partition due to deficient interscalar septum (ISS) between middle & apical cochlear turns

IMAGING

General Features

- Best diagnostic clue
  - Temporal bone CT & T2 MR: Absent ISS between plump middle & apical cochlear turns
  - ± associated LVA/large endolymphatic sac (ES)

CT Findings

- Bone CT
  - Cochlea: Normal basal turn, **deficient ISS** between **plump middle** & **apical turns**, asymmetric scalar chambers
    - Smooth external contour between middle & apical turns posterolaterally ("baseball cap" cochlea)
    - Deficient or absent modiolus
  - Cochlear nerve canal: Normal (most) or mild stenosis
  - Vestibular aqueduct: Typically large (most) or borderline large & flared; rarely normal
  - Vestibule: Normal or large
  - Semicircular canals (SCCs): Normal or plump anterior limb lateral SCCs

MR Findings

- 3D FIESTA, T2 SPACE, FIESTA, CISS or equivalent
  - Cochlea: Normal basal turn, deficient ISS between plump middle & apical turns, asymmetric scalar chambers
    - Deficient or absent modiolus
  - Cochlear nerve: Usually normal
  - ES & duct: Typically large, triangular morphology
  - Vestibule & SCC: Normal or mildly enlarged vestibule; normal or plump lateral SCC

DIFFERENTIAL DIAGNOSIS

Cochlear Incomplete Partition Type I (IP-I)

- Entire cochlea lacks internal structure

Cochlear Hypoplasia

- Small cochlea, 4 types

CHARGE Syndrome

- ± deficient cochlear septation; flattened/absent apical turn, cochlear nerve canal stenosis/atresia
- Funnel-shaped LVA, large ES, small vestibule, & hypoplastic/absent SCC

X-Linked Stapes Gusher (DFNX2)

- Deficient cochlear internal septation; corkscrew cochlear morphology; absent modiolus

- Widened internal auditory canal fundus & cochlear nerve canal

PATHOLOGY

General Features

- Etiology
  - Genetic ± environmental factors produce hearing loss
  - Cochlea has microscopic infrastructural deficiencies
  - Enlarged scala media & hair cell damage
  - Susceptible to injury from mild trauma
- Genetics
  - *SLC26A4* mutation (PDS gene, chromosome 7q22.3)
    - Autosomal recessive; encodes pendrin protein (anion exchanger)
    - Syndromic deafness: Pendred syndrome (bilateral LVA + thyroid organification defect ± goiter); homozygous or compound heterozygous mutations
    - Nonsyndromic deafness: DFNB4 (enlarged vestibular aqueduct syndrome) heterozygous mutations, autosomal recessive
      - □ 2nd most common cause of nonsyndromic deafness after *GJB2* mutation
  - Targeted gene panel tests for multiple genes, rather than single gene testing for most common (*GJB2*, *SLC26A4*, & *CDH23*)

CLINICAL ISSUES

Presentation

- Most common signs/symptoms
  - Bilateral or unilateral, severe or profound sensorineural hearing loss (SNHL) precipitated by minor trauma
- Other signs/symptoms
  - Vestibular symptoms
  - Pendred syndrome: Hypothyroidism ± goiter

Natural History & Prognosis

- Fluctuating, progressive SNHL (or mixed hearing loss)

Treatment

- LVA: Avoid concussive-prone contact sports & try to prevent head trauma (controversial)
- Profound bilateral SNHL: **Cochlear implantation**

DIAGNOSTIC CHECKLIST

Image Interpretation Pearls

- Plump apical & middle cochlear turns form single chamber; deficient or absent modiolus
- **Do not mistake osseous spiral lamina for ISS on MR**

SELECTED REFERENCES

1. D'Arco F et al: Incomplete partition type II in its various manifestations: isolated, in association with EVA, syndromic, and beyond; a multicentre international study. Neuroradiology. 66(8):1397-403, 2024
2. Rajput K et al: Etiology of childhood profound sensorineural hearing loss: the role of hearing loss gene panel testing. Otolaryngol Head Neck Surg. 171(5):1518-25, 2024
3. Lewis MA et al: The spectrum of cochlear malformations in CHARGE syndrome and insights into the role of the CHD7 gene during embryogenesis of the inner ear. Neuroradiology. 65(4):819-34, 2023
4. Lewis M et al: Syndromic hearing loss in children. Neuroimaging Clin N Am. 33(4):563-80, 2023

Large Vestibular Aqueduct

TERMINOLOGY

- Large vestibular aqueduct (LVA)
- **Incomplete partition type II (IP-II)** between middle & apical cochlear turns; **often seen with LVA**
- IP-II + LVA + minimally dilated vestibule: **Mondini** deformity

IMAGING

- Axial CT: **Midpoint of vestibular aqueduct** between posterior labyrinth & operculum **> 1.5 mm**
- MR: Enlarged endolymphatic sac & duct
- Cochlea: Abnormal in ~ 75% of LVA cases
  - Absent septation & modiolus between middle & apical turns (**IP-II**); enlarged **scala vestibuli > 1.2 mm**
- 2nd interscalar ridge notch **angle > 114°, depth ≤ 0.31 mm**
- Vestibule & semicircular canal: Normal or mildly enlarged

TOP DIFFERENTIAL DIAGNOSES

- Cystic cochleovestibular malformation (IP-I)
- Cochlear hypoplasia

- CHARGE syndrome (funnel-shaped LVA)
- Branchiootorenal syndrome (funnel-shaped LVA)

PATHOLOGY

- *SLC26A4* mutations in ~ 50% of LVA patients
- **IP-II**: Arrested development at **7th** gestational **week**
- Modiolar defects in IP-II may be from **transmission of high CSF pressure** into inner ear **due to LVA**

CLINICAL ISSUES

- Most common imaging abnormality in pediatric SNHL
- Bilateral anomaly (most); **initially normal hearing**
- **Progressive/fluctuating SNHL** due to high pulsating CSF pressure or head trauma
- Avoid contact sports & try to prevent head trauma
- **Hearing aid first, cochlear implantation** later
- All IP-II have cochlear nerve, ABI not indicated

DIAGNOSTIC CHECKLIST

- LVA diagnosis: Look for associated cochlear IP-II anomaly

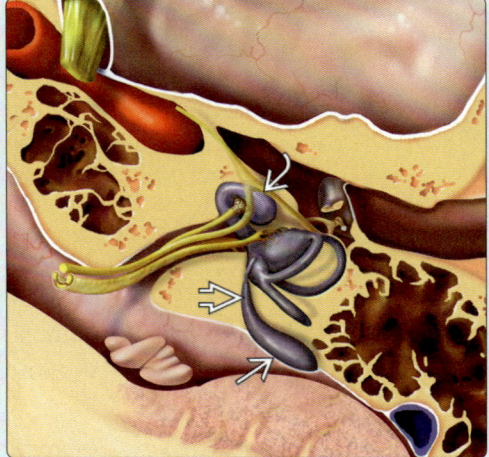
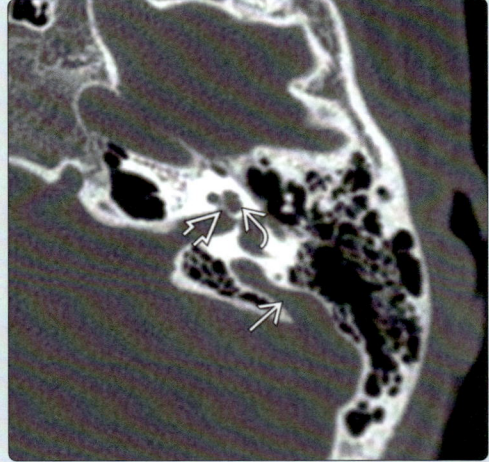

(Left) *In the left inner ear, large endolymphatic sac (ES) epidural ⇨ & intraosseous ⇨ components are shown. Cochlea is malformed with absent septation between middle & apical turns, which appear bulbous ⇨. (Right) Axial temporal bone CT in a 15-year-old boy with sensorineural hearing loss (SNHL) shows a large vestibular aqueduct (LVA) ⇨. The modiolus is defective toward apex & present at base ⇨. Note that the scalar chambers are asymmetric (anterior scala vestibuli > posterior scala tympani) ⇨.*

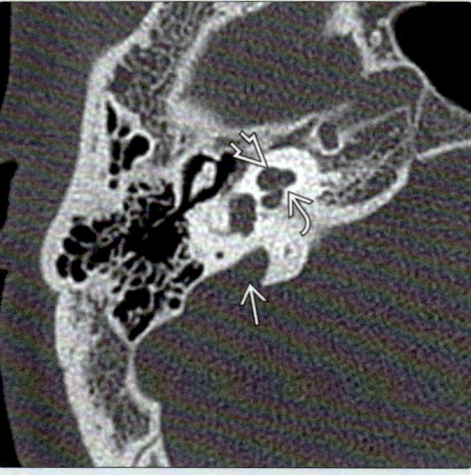
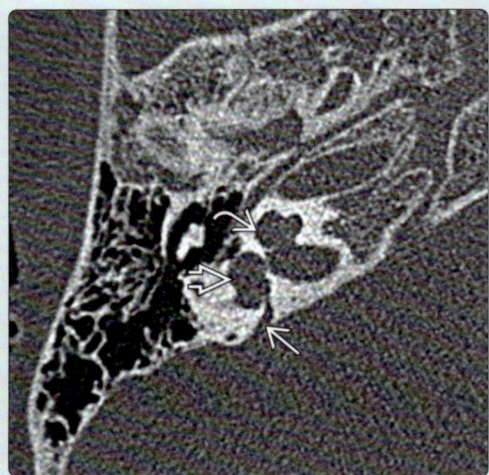

(Left) *Axial temporal bone CT in a 17-year-old girl with Pendred syndrome shows an LVA ⇨ & absent septation between the middle & apical cochlear turns ⇨ with a deficient modiolus ⇨. This is typical of incomplete partition type II (IP-II), which results in a baseball cap-shaped cochlea. (Right) Axial bone CT in a 3-year-old boy with SNHL shows Mondini deformity with LVA ⇨, typical IP-II cochlear anomaly ⇨ with plump cochlear middle & apical turns, absent modiolus, & no apical septation, and the vestibule is mildly enlarged ⇨.*

TERMINOLOGY

Abbreviations

- Large vestibular aqueduct (LVA)

Synonyms

- Large endolymphatic sac anomaly (**LESA**): T2 MR term
- Enlarged vestibular aqueduct (**EVA**): CT term
- **Mondini** deformity (historic terminology): LVA + minimally dilated vestibule + incomplete partition type II (IP-II)

Definitions

- LVA: Enlarged bony vestibular aqueduct (VA) houses large endolymphatic sac (ES) & duct
  - Associated with variable cochlear malformation
- **IP-II**: Deficient modiolus & interscalar septum (ISS) between **middle & apical** cochlear turns; often seen with LVA
- IP-II: Normal cochlear external dimensions
  - Not correct to classify IP-II as cochlea with 1.5 turns
  - Term cochlea with 1.5 turns should be used only for cochlear hypoplasia (CH) (especially CH-III)

IMAGING

General Features

- Best diagnostic clue
  - CT: EVA ± IP-II; 3D T2 MR: LESA ± IP-II
- Location
  - **Endolymphatic duct (ELD) & sac (ELS)** located within bony **VA**
  - Connects crus communis [meeting point of posterior & superior semicircular canals (SCCs)] to fovea
    - **Fovea**: Cup-shaped area at posterior temporal bone margin; **operculum**: Opening of VA into fovea
  - ELD: Short, proximal part connected to crus communis
  - ELS: Longer, distal part with both intraosseous & intradural (fovea area) components
  - ELD transition to ELS defined by change in wall cell architecture (not seen at imaging)
  - Normal ELS & ELD barely visible on heavily T2WI 3D MR
- Size
  - **Cincinnati** criteria: Axial temporal bone CT: **LVA ≥ 1 mm at midpoint**, ± ≥ 2 mm at opercular margin perpendicular to long axis of VA
  - Literature variable for LVA; vertical & axial VA width **> 1.5 mm at midpoint** of labyrinth & operculum (classic **Valvassori** criteria)
  - Transverse oblique reformat (**Pöschl view**) parallel to plane of superior SCC: LVA **≥ 0.8-0.9 mm at midpoint**
- Morphology
  - Axial bone CT: V-shaped, enlarged bony VA
  - Axial T2 MR: Large ELS along posterior wall of petrous bone, lateral to dural reflection

CT Findings

- Bone CT
  - LVA: May scallop posterior margin of petrous bone
  - Cochlea: Abnormal on CT in ~ 75% of LVA cases
    - Normal or **deficient septation** between **plump apical & middle turns** (IP-II); normal basal turn
    - **Asymmetric scalar chambers**: Anterior > posterior

- **Deficient** (typical), absent, or normal **modiolus**
  - Vestibule: Normal or mildly enlarged
  - SCC: Normal or mildly dilated
    - Reduced size of lateral SCC bone island with enlargement of lateral SCC may be seen in IP-II
  - Middle ear space & ossicles: Normal

MR Findings

- 3D T2 SPACE, FIESTA, CISS or equivalent
  - ELS & ELD: Enlarged, variable hyperintense signal
  - Cochlea: **Deficient septation** between **plump apical & middle turns (IP-II)** or normal in LVA only
  - **Asymmetric perilymphatic scalar chambers**: Anterior **scala vestibuli larger** than posterior scala tympani
    - Intervening scala media (endolymph) not seen on MR
    - Scala media has anterior vestibular (Reissner) & posterior basilar membranes with organ of Corti
    - **Spiral lamina**: Thin, bony plate tapers laterally connecting to medial aspect of basilar membrane
      □ Separates scala media from posterior scala tympani (osseous spiral lamina-basilar membrane complex)
    - Cochlear nerve fibers traverse modiolus, branching onto spiral lamina-basal membrane & organ of Corti
    - In 3D T2 MR, **spiral lamina-basilar membrane complex** seen as **thin, hypointense**, transverse **line**
      □ **Between scala vestibuli** anteriorly & **scala tympani** posteriorly in each cochlear turn
  - **ISS**: Membranous bony struts extending toward modiolus: **Thin, hypointense lines** in MR; **separates** basal, middle, & apical **turns of cochlea**
  - ISS continuous, has 3 parts, & forms 3 interscalar ridges or notches (R1, R2, R3) along outer margin of cochlea
  - 1st part (enchondral ossification) divides lower basal turn & lower middle turn (posterior medial)
  - 2nd/3rd parts (membranous ossification) faulty in IP-II
  - 2nd divides upper basal & upper middle turns (lateral)
  - 3rd part divides lower middle & apical turns (medial)
  - **R2 notch** formed by 2nd part located along **lateral margin of cochlea**; best seen on 3D T2 **MR**
  - R2 notch **angle > 114°** & **depth ≤ 0.31 mm** suggest **IP-II & scala communis**
  - **Scala communis**: Due to defect of osseous ISS, which separates cochlear turns
  - In IP-II, 2nd part of **ISS bulges anteriorly** due to **enlarged scala vestibuli** in 3D T2 MR
    - **> 1.2 mm** between **spiral lamina-basilar membrane complex** of upper basal turn & 2nd part of **ISS**
    - **Spiral lamina-basilar membrane thin line** denotes apparent posterior margin of its scala vestibuli
    - 1st signal void anteriorly represents 2nd part of **ISS**; denotes anterior margin of scala vestibuli
  - **Deficient**/absent (IP-II), or normal **modiolus**

Imaging Recommendations

- Protocol advice
  - Temporal bone CT or heavily T2WI 3D (CISS, FIESTA) MR

DIFFERENTIAL DIAGNOSIS

Cystic Cochleovestibular Malformation (IP-I)

- Cystic cochlea & vestibule without internal structure

Cochlear Hypoplasia

- Small cochlea; usually < 2 turns

CHARGE Syndrome

- Funnel-shaped LVA, small vestibule, & small/absent SCC
- Cochlear nerve canal stenosis/atresia & thickened modiolus; occasional cochlear hypoplasia

Branchiootorenal Syndrome

- Funnel-shaped LVA, tapered basal turn, & small, offset middle & apical turns

High-Riding Jugular Bulb

- Communicates with jugular foramen, not vestibule

PATHOLOGY

General Features

- Etiology
  - LVA + large ELS/ELD occur during embryogenesis
  - IP-II may be from **transmission of high CSF pressure** into inner ear **due to LVA**
  - Mild: May be EVA only, or EVA & mild vestibule dilation
  - Transmission of CSF pressure into cochlea → spectrum of anomalies: Dilated scala vestibuli, scala communis, &
    - **Modiolar defects**: Superior (cystic apex), partial, subtotal, or rarely complete
  - **ISS bulging** upward due to high **pressure in scala vestibuli** constant finding in IP-II
  - **Cochlea "fragile"** & susceptible to injury from mild trauma due to microscopic infrastructure deficiencies
  - **Conductive** component of mixed hearing loss (MHL) due to **"3rd window" effect of EVA** on sound transmission
- Genetics
  - *SLC26A4* mutations (chromosome 7)
    - ~ **50%** of **LVA** patients have *SLC26A4* mutations
    - Autosomal recessive inheritance
  - *SLC26A4* gene encodes **pendrin protein** (chloride/bicarbonate anion exchanger)
    - ↑ endolymphatic pH by bicarbonate secretion
  - ↓ or **absent pendrin** expression → **acidification** & **abnormal expansion** of developing inner ear
  - Acidification → ↓ **endolymphatic potassium** concentration with loss of endocochlear potential
  - Acidification → ↑ **endolymphatic calcium** concentration, which is toxic to stria vascularis & organ of Corti; *FOXI1* mutations (less common): *SLC26A4* transcriptional **activator gene**
  - **Syndromic deafness: Pendred syndrome**
    - Sensorineural hearing loss (**SNHL**) + thyroid organification defect ± **goiter**
    - Autosomal recessive; biallelic *SLC26A4* mutation; ~ 10% of hereditary deafness
  - **Nonsyndromic deafness (Nsd)**: Deafness autosomal recessive 4 (**DFNB4**)
    - Isolated familial SNHL; ~ 4% of Nsd; 2nd most common cause of Nsd after *GJB2* mutation
- Associated abnormalities
  - **Pendred syndrome**: Goiter (2nd decade)
  - Distal renal tubular acidosis (rare)
- Embryology: **IP-II**: Arrested development at **7th** gestational **week**

- Mondini deformity described in association with thalidomide, rubella, Pendred syndrome, CHARGE syndrome, Klippel-Feil syndrome, DiGeorge syndrome, & Wildervanck syndrome (cervico-ocular-acoustic dysplasia)

Gross Pathologic & Surgical Features

- Enlarged VA houses large ES found in dural sleeve in fovea in posterior wall of temporal bone

CLINICAL ISSUES

Presentation

- Most common signs/symptoms
  - SNHL (or MHL due to "3rd window" effect)
    - Fluctuating or **progressive course** ± linear relationship between VA width & progressive SNHL; SNHL precipitated by minor head trauma
- Other signs/symptoms
  - Tinnitus, vertigo, dizziness
  - Pendred syndrome: Hypothyroidism in ~ 50%, ± goiter in adolescence
- **Audiologic evaluation findings**
  - Varies from normal to profound hearing loss
  - Air bone gap due to "3rd window" effect from EVA; may resemble superior SCC dehiscence syndrome

Demographics

- Epidemiology
  - LVA: Most common CT/MR abnormality in pediatric SNHL; bilateral (most) or unilateral anomaly

Treatment

- Avoid contact sports & try to prevent head trauma
- **Hearing aid** first, **cochlear implantation** later
- All IP-II have cochlear nerve, auditory brainstem implant (ABI) not indicated
- **CSF oozing/gusher** occasionally at cochlear implant (CI) surgery in IP-II: Due to modiolar defects from high CSF pressure transmission
- **Pulsating round window** at CI surgery in IP-II: "3rd window" effect of EVA transmitting CSF pressure into cochlea

DIAGNOSTIC CHECKLIST

Consider

- Known *SLC26A4* mutation/Pendred syndrome: Look for EVA/LESA
- EVA/LESA: Recommend *SLC26A4* testing, US thyroid, thyroid function tests, ± perchlorate discharge test
- Obtain MR if borderline VA measurements on CT

Image Interpretation Pearls

- LVA diagnosis: Look for associated cochlear anomaly

Reporting Tips

- Reformatted coronal CT or transverse oblique view differentiates LVA from high-riding jugular bulb

SELECTED REFERENCES

1. Yu K et al: The correlation between deafness progression and SLC26A4 mutations in enlarged vestibular aqueduct patients. Eur Arch Otorhinolaryngol. 281(2): 649-54, 2024
2. Connor SEJ et al: Is CT or MRI the optimal imaging investigation for the diagnosis of large vestibular aqueduct syndrome and large endolymphatic sac anomaly? Eur Arch Otorhinolaryngol. 276(3):693-702, 2019

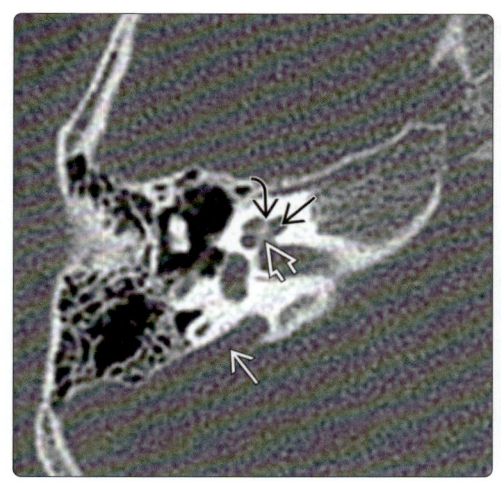
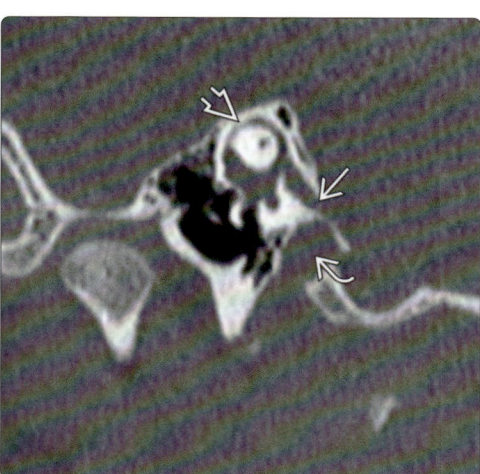

(Left) Axial temporal bone CT in a 3-year-old girl with SNHL shows LVA ➡. Cochlea is normal with interscalar septum (R2) ➡ separating the cochlear turns, spiral lamina ➡ separating scala vestibuli from scala tympani inside a turn, & normal modiolus ➡. (Right) Reformatted short-axis oblique (Pöschl view) temporal bone CT in a 3-year-old girl with SNHL demonstrates the right LVA ➡ in its entirety. The reconstructed image is parallel to the plane of the superior semicircular canal ➡. The jugular bulb ➡ lies inferior to the LVA.

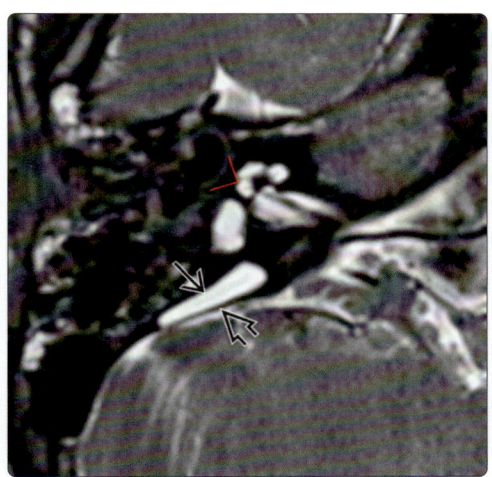
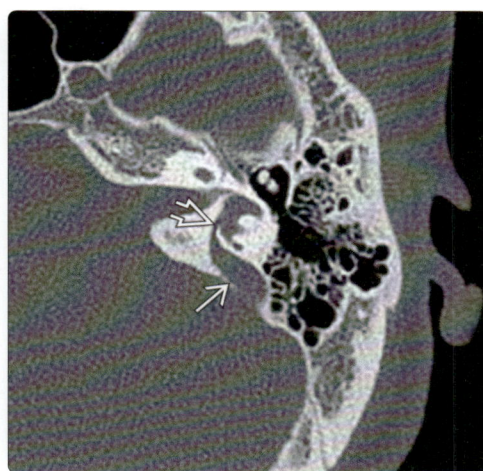

(Left) Axial T2 MR shows hyperintense LESA ➡ lying anterolateral to hypointense dura ➡. Note normal lateral R2 notch angle (red) & depth (from lateral tangential line along cochlear turns to angle vertex) associated with the 2nd part of interscalar septum (ISS) between upper basal & upper middle cochlear turns. (Right) Axial temporal bone CT in 17-year-old girl with Pendred syndrome reveals the entirety of the left LVA ➡ extending from the crus communis ➡ of the vestibule to the operculum at posterior aspect of the petrous bone.

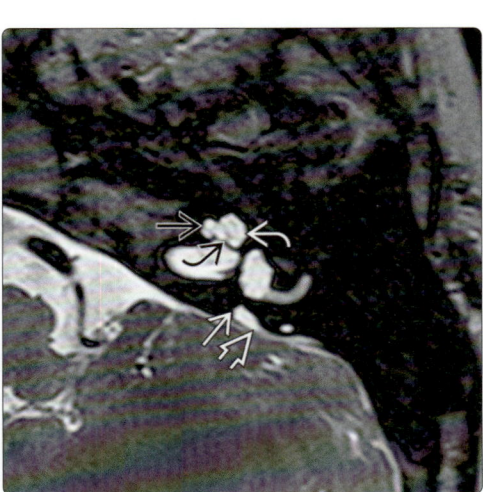
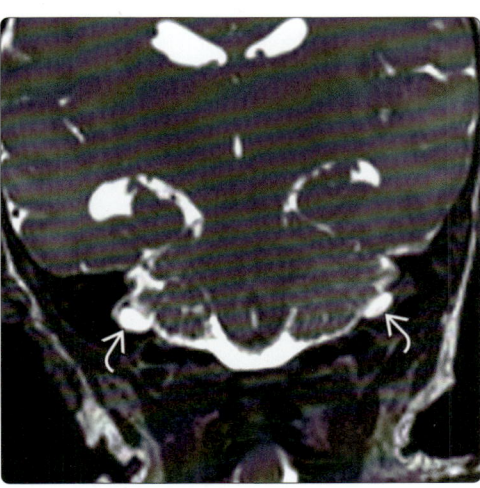

(Left) Axial 3D FIESTA MR in a 3-year-old boy with SNHL shows a large ES ➡ lateral to hypointense dura ➡. There is a deficient 2nd part of ISS, & the lateral R2 notch angle between the distal cochlear turns is abnormally wide with narrowed depth ➡. Note the modiolar deficiency ➡. The hypointense line in the center of each cochlear turn is the normal osseous spiral lamina-basilar membrane complex ➡. (Right) Coronal 3D T2 MR through posterior petrous bone margins in another child shows bilateral large ESs ➡.

KEY FACTS

TERMINOLOGY

- Stenosis or atresia of cochlear nerve canal (CNC)
- Cochlear nerve deficiency (CND): Cochlear nerve (CN) hypoplasia/aplasia

IMAGING

- CNC or cochlear aperture (CA) extends from internal auditory canal (IAC) fundus to modiolus
  - Diameter measured at narrowest point
  - **CNC (CA) stenosis: < 1.4 mm**
- Cochlea (spectrum of findings)
  - Normal
  - Normal modiolus + mildly stenotic CNC
  - Thickened modiolus + stenotic/atretic CNC
  - Cochlear anomaly + stenotic/atretic CNC
- IAC: Normal, small, absent or "duplicated" (separate CNVII canal)
- CND: CN smaller than normal ipsilateral facial nerve (hypoplasia) or absent (aplasia)

- Normal CN almost similar size of facial nerve or slightly larger, & larger than vestibular nerves

TOP DIFFERENTIAL DIAGNOSES

- CHARGE syndrome
- Cochlear aplasia or hypoplasia

PATHOLOGY

- CN size correlates with spiral ganglion cell population, but thin CN may still transmit impulses for hearing

CLINICAL ISSUES

- Presents with congenital sensorineural hearing loss (SNHL)
- 2% of congenital profound deafness due to CND
- Treat with cochlear implantation (CI), ABI if CI fails

DIAGNOSTIC CHECKLIST

- Most cases of CND have normal cochlea ± modiolar thickening ± CNC stenosis or atresia
- Assess CNs on axial & **oblique sagittal** heavily T2W 3D MR

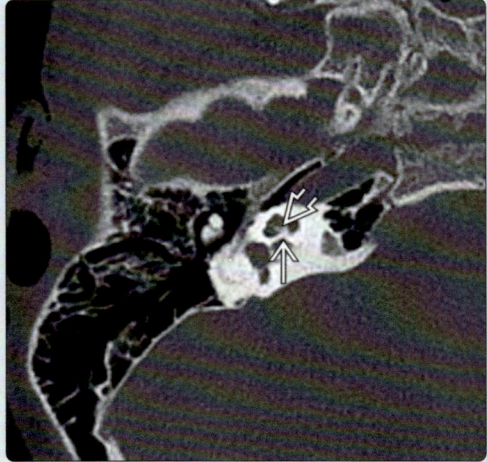
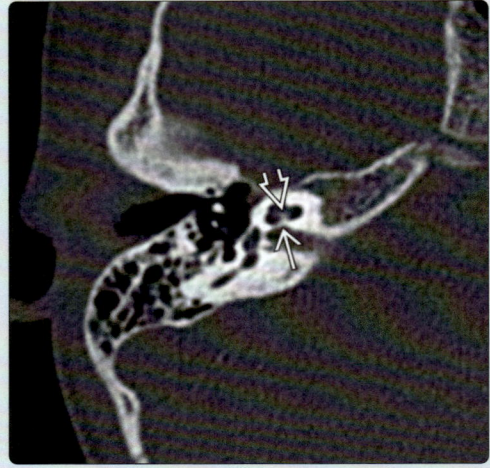

(Left) Axial bone CT in a 4-year-old girl with profound right sensorineural hearing loss (SNHL) is shown. There is absence of the cochlear nerve canal (CNC) ➡ and marked thickening of the modiolus ➡. (Right) Axial bone CT in a 7-year-old girl with profound right SNHL demonstrates absence of the CNC ➡ and thickening of the modiolus ➡. The vestibule, vestibular aqueduct, and semicircular canals were otherwise normal (not shown).

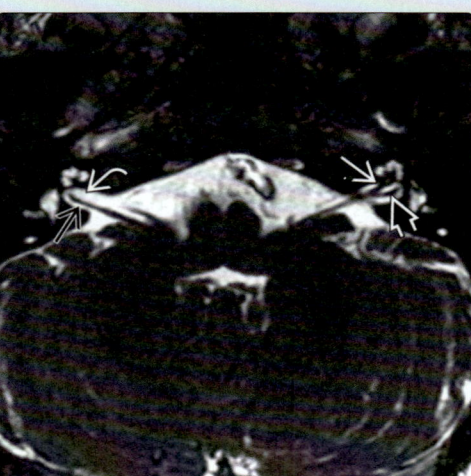
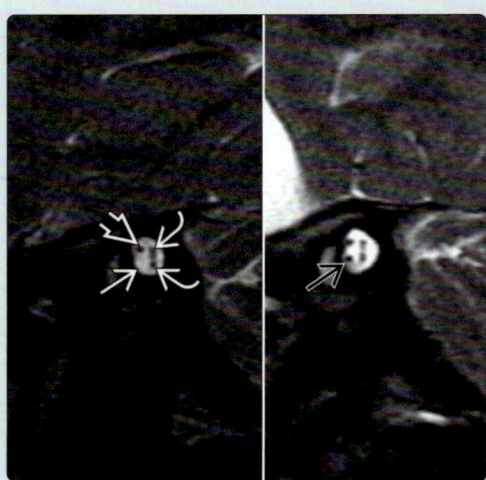

(Left) Axial T2 FIESTA MR in a 7-year-old boy with profound right SNHL shows a normal left cochlear nerve (CN) ➡ and normal left inferior vestibular nerve ➡. The right CN ➡ is absent, and the right inferior vestibular ➡ is normal. (Right) Sagittal oblique high-resolution T2 FSE MR in the same patient shows right CN aplasia ➡, a normal facial nerve ➡, normal vestibular nerves ➡ compared to the normal left CN ➡, and intact facial and superior/inferior vestibular nerves.

TERMINOLOGY

Abbreviations

- **Cochlear nerve canal (CNC)**

Synonyms

- **Cochlear aperture (CA)** (a.k.a. cochlear fossette or bony CNC) stenosis or atresia
- **Isolated cochlea**: CNC (CA) absent & filled with bone

Definitions

- CNC hypoplasia-aplasia: Narrowing or absence of CNC
- Cochlear nerve (CN) deficiency (CND): Hypoplasia or aplasia

IMAGING

General Features

- Best diagnostic clue
  - Normal CN is larger than either superior vestibular nerves (SVNs) or inferior vestibular nerves (IVNs) in 90%
  - Normal CN similar or larger than CNVII in 64%
  - CND: CN smaller than normal CNVII (hypoplasia) or absent (aplasia) on MR
  - CNC (CA) width: Narrowest diameter between internal auditory canal (IAC) fundus & modiolus on axial images
  - CNC (CA) hypoplasia: CNC width < 1.4 mm
- Location
  - CNC extends from IAC fundus to modiolus
  - CNVII anterosuperior; **CN anteroinferior** ("7-up, Coke down"); SVN posterosuperior; IVN posteroinferior **in IAC**

Imaging Recommendations

- Protocol advice
  - Sagittal oblique 3D T2 MR perpendicular to plane of CN

CT Findings

- Bone CT
  - CNC (CA): Seen on axial midmodiolar section
    - Normal: In some cases of CND on MR
    - Stenosis: Severity varies
    - Atresia: Complete absence of CNC
  - Cochlea variable appearance
    - Normal turns & modiolus with normal or mildly stenotic CNC
    - Normal turns & **thickened modiolus** with moderate to severe stenosis of CNC
    - Abnormal cochlea with stenotic/atretic CNC (less common) (e.g., cochlear hypoplasia)
  - Vestibule & semicircular canal (SCC): Normal (most); less commonly abnormal (e.g., syndromic etiology)
  - IAC: Normal or small, rarely separate CNVII canal ("duplicated IAC")
    - **Narrow IAC**: **< 2.5 mm** at midpoint of IAC
  - CNVII canal: Normal (most) or anomalous (rare)

MR Findings

- CN: Hypoplasia or aplasia
  - CNC (CA) normal: Occasional CND
  - CNC (CA) mildly stenotic: CN normal or CND
  - CNC (CA) stenotic < 1.4 mm ± thickened modiolus: CND
  - CNC (CA) stenosis + IAC narrowing: CND difficult to see on MR because of ↓ CSF around CNVIII & CNVII
  - CNC (CA) aplasia: CN absent (nonvisualization may be severe hypoplasia or true aplasia)
- Vestibular nerves (VNs)
  - Normal IAC: VN usually normal
  - Narrow IAC: VN normal or deficient

DIFFERENTIAL DIAGNOSIS

CHARGE Syndrome

- CNC stenosis/atresia, CNVIII deficiency, hypoplastic vestibule, absent/hypoplastic SCC

Cochlear Aplasia

- Cochlea absent

Cochlear Hypoplasia

- Small cochlea, 4 subtypes

CLINICAL ISSUES

Presentation

- Most common signs/symptoms
  - Congenital sensorineural hearing loss (SNHL)
- Audiologic evaluation findings: Neural-type SNHL typical of isolated CND
  - Otoacoustic emissions or cochlear microphonics present (intact cochlea with outer hair cell function)
    - May pass newborn hearing screening if automated auditory brainstem response (ABR) not obtained
  - Absent ABR

Treatment

- Hearing aids do not provide enough amplification in CNC (CA) hypoplasia/aplasia
- Bilateral hypoplastic CNC (CA) with hypoplastic CN, hearing aid trial necessary
  - If no functional hearing after trial, do cochlear implantation (CI)
- MR differentiation of CN hypoplasia from aplasia difficult, especially if IAC narrow
  - Absence of identifiable nerve on MR, does not equal complete absence, may be some fibers still present
- Do full audiometric test battery even if MR appears to be CN aplasia
  - Evidence of hearing sometimes detected, then CI
- Auditory brainstem implantation (ABI) when CI contraindicated or fails
- ABI 1st-line therapy for CNC (CA) aplasia
- Simultaneous CI & ABI if barely visible CN in children between 2-3 years age: To avoid losing valuable time for language development

SELECTED REFERENCES

1. Lewis M et al: Syndromic hearing loss in children. Neuroimaging Clin N Am. 33(4):563-80, 2023
2. Robson CD et al: Non-syndromic sensorineural hearing loss in children. Neuroimaging Clin N Am. 33(4):531-42, 2023
3. Dewyer NA et al: Pediatric single-sided deafness: a review of prevalence, radiologic findings, and cochlear implant candidacy. Ann Otol Rhinol Laryngol. 131(3):233-8, 2021
4. O'Brien WT et al: Nonsyndromic congenital causes of sensorineura hearing loss in children: an illustrative review. AJR Am J Roentgenol. 216(4):1048-55, 2021

KEY FACTS

TERMINOLOGY

- Definition: Hypoplasia/aplasia of 1 or multiple semicircular canals (SCCs) ± hypoplastic vestibule

IMAGING

- Hypoplastic vestibule + hypoplasia/aplasia of all SCCs in CHARGE syndrome
  - Oval window stenosis/atresia and anomalous CNVII
  - Cochlea: Variable malformation; thickened modiolus, flattened apical ± middle turns or single turn/hypoplasia
  - Cochlear nerve canal (CNC): Stenosis/atresia
  - Vestibular aqueduct: Dilated, funnel-shaped
- Hypoplasia of single SCC + normal (or large) vestibule
  - Posterior SCC (PSCC) + normal or flattened cochlear apical turn: Waardenburg and Alagille syndromes
  - PSCC + hypoplastic unwound or "thorny" cochlea: Branchiootorenal (BOR) syndrome
  - Lateral SCC (LSCC) + dense stapes superstructure, incomplete partition type II: 22q11.2 deletion (DiGeorge)

- LSCC: Oval window stenosis/atresia and anomalous ± dehiscent tympanic segment CNVII

TOP DIFFERENTIAL DIAGNOSES

- **Down syndrome**
  - Small or absent LSCC bone island; globular SCC-vestibule (anlage) anomaly
  - CNC stenosis, IAC stenosis, LVA variable
- **Labyrinthine ossificans**: Prior meningitis or surgery

DIAGNOSTIC CHECKLIST

- **CHARGE** if hypoplasia vestibule + SCC
- Consider **BOR** for hypoplastic unwound or "thorny" cochlea; look for PSCC anomaly
- Consider Waardenburg syndrome for PSCC anomaly and Hirschsprung disease
- Consider Alagille syndrome for PSCC anomaly, peripheral pulmonary artery stenosis, and cholestatic liver disease
- Consider sporadic, 22q11.2 deletion or Down syndrome for LSCC anomalies

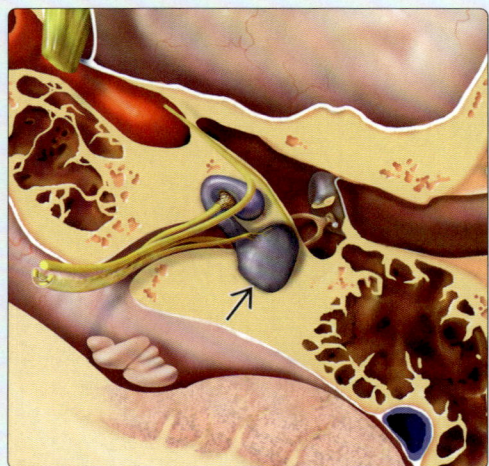
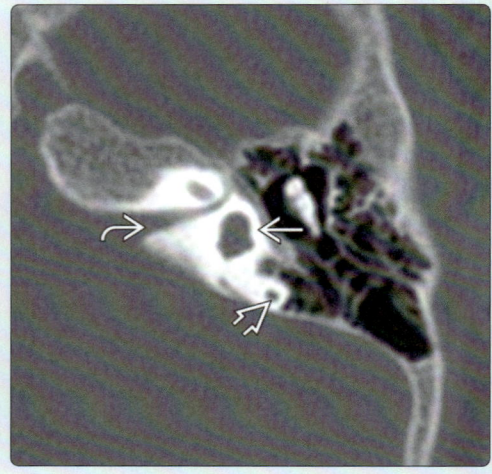

(Left) Axial graphic depicts a severe syndromic type of semicircular canal (SCC) anomaly with complete absence of all SCCs, cochlear malformation, and a dysmorphic small vestibule ➡. (Right) Axial bone CT in a 12-month-old boy with profound sensorineural hearing loss (SNHL) shows complete absence of the horizontal (lateral) SCC ➡ at the level of the vestibule. A normal posterior SCC ➡ is seen. The internal auditory canal (IAC) ➡ is narrow.

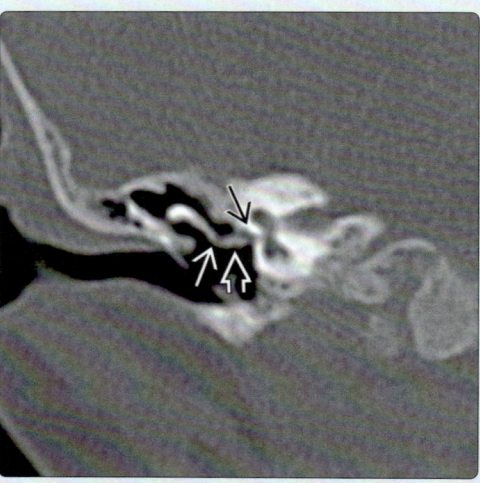
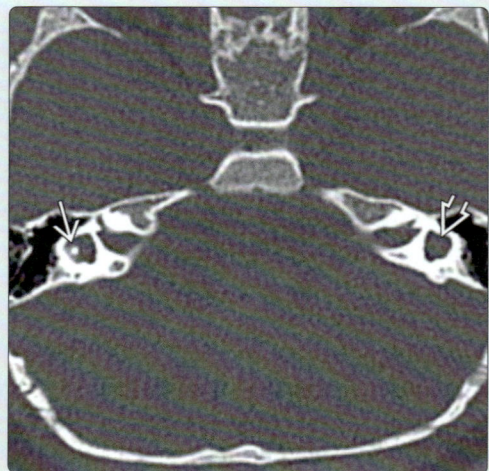

(Left) Coronal bone CT in a patient with CHARGE syndrome shows absence of SCCs and bone covering the oval window ➡. Note characteristic lack of lenticular process of incus ➡ and thick stapes ➡. (Right) Axial bone CT in a 6-year-old girl with Waardenburg syndrome shows small bone island for right lateral SCC ➡ and a globular SCC-vestibule anomaly with absence of the bone island between the lateral SCC and vestibule ➡. Bilateral posterior SCCs are absent, and the superior SSCs are mildly dilated (not shown).

TERMINOLOGY

Synonyms

- Semicircular canal (SCC)-vestibule malformation

IMAGING

General Features

- Best diagnostic clue
  - Hypoplasia/aplasia of 1 or multiple SCCs ± hypoplastic vestibule
- Location
  - Posterior membranous labyrinth
- Size
  - Varies from aplasia of all SCCs + hypoplastic vestibule to hypoplasia of 1 SCC and normal vestibule
- Morphology
  - SCCs are short or aplastic; small bone island
  - Vestibule normal or small

CT Findings

- Bone CT
  - Hypoplastic vestibule + hypoplasia/aplasia of **all SCCs**
    - Oval window stenosis/atresia
    - Anomalous ± dehiscent tympanic segment CNVII
    - Cochlea: Thickened modiolus, flattened apical ± middle turns, deficient cochlear septation [incomplete partition type I (IP-I)], cochlear hypoplasia
    - Cochlear nerve canal (CNC): Stenosis or atresia
    - Vestibular aqueduct: Dilated, funnel-shaped
    - Associated findings of **CHARGE syndrome** (**c**oloboma, **h**eart disease, **a**tresia choanae, growth and developmental **r**estriction, **g**enital hypoplasia, **e**ar anomalies)
  - Hypoplasia **single SCC** + normal or large vestibule
    - Posterior SCC (PSCC) hypoplasia (uncommon)
      □ Small bone island with small, globular or rudimentary/absent PSCC
      □ Anomalous origin PSCC from horizontal SCC (HSCC) and superior SCC (SSCC)
      □ Syndromic etiology: Waardenburg (WS), Alagille, and **branchiootorenal (BOR) syndromes**
      □ Anomaly often overlooked on CT
      □ Cochlea: Flattened apical turn (WS); hypoplastic unwound or "thorny" cochlea (BOR)
    - HSCC or lateral SCC (LSCC) hypoplasia/aplasia
      □ Hypoplasia: Small bone island with small or globular LSCC: **Trisomy 21, 22q11.2 deletion (DiGeorge)**
      □ Aplasia: Absent part/all LSCC (rare) + oval window stenosis/atresia
      □ Anomalous ± dehiscent tympanic segment CNVII
      □ Cochlea: Typically normal depending on syndromic etiology

MR Findings

- T2WI
  - Hypoplastic or absent SCC fluid signal
  - Normal or small vestibule
  - Cochlea: Normal or abnormal (e.g., CHARGE, BOR)

Imaging Recommendations

- Best imaging tool
  - Temporal bone CT or MR
- Protocol advice
  - Axial and reconstructed coronal images

DIFFERENTIAL DIAGNOSIS

Sporadic Semicircular Canal Dysplasia

- Dilated vestibule and dysmorphic LSCC forming confluent common sac
- Normal or mildly dysplastic PSCC and SSCC

CHARGE Syndrome

- Small vestibule + hypoplasia/aplasia of all SCCs
- Variable cochlear anomaly
  - Flattened apical turn; normal middle and basal turns
  - Flattened middle and apical turns
  - Single globular cochlear turn, absent internal structure
  - Cochlear hypoplasia: Range from normal → hypoplastic upper cochlea → dysmorphic second 1/2 of basal turn + hypoplastic upper cochlear → abnormal first 1/2 of basal turn + severely hypoplastic second 1/2 of basal turn & remainder of cochlea
- Funnel-shaped large vestibular aqueduct (LVA)
- Ossicular malformation

Branchiootorenal Syndrome

- Hypoplasia/absence of PSCC, normal vestibule
- Characteristic cochlear anomalies: Hypoplastic unwound or "thorny" cochlea
- Funnel-shaped LVA
- Ossicular malformation

Down Syndrome

- Small LSCC bone island, small or globular LSCC, CNC ± internal auditory canal (IAC) stenosis, ± LVA

Labyrinthine Ossificans

- Fibrosis and ossification of membranous labyrinth
- When affects SCCs, may mimic hypoplasia

Waardenburg Syndrome

- Characterized by deafness and pigmentation abnormalities
- 4 distinct subtypes involving several genes
- All showing deafness and pigmentary disturbance
- Sensorineural hearing loss (SNHL) due to absent melanocyte-derived intermediate cells of stria vascularis
  - Endolymphatic collapse and secondary agenesis of organ of Corti (cochleosaccular degeneration)
- PSCC agenesis most frequent, followed by SSCC and LSCC anomalies
- Normal or large vestibule
- Normal or flattened cochlear apical turn
- Normal, hypoplastic or absent cochlea nerve
- Normal VA or LVA

Alagille Syndrome (Arteriohepatic Dysplasia)

- PSCC anomaly/hypoplasia
- Peripheral pulmonary artery stenosis
- Paucity or stenosis of intrahepatic bile ducts → cholestatic liver disease, cirrhosis, hepatic failure

22q11.2 Deletion Syndrome (DiGeorge/Velocardiofacial Syndrome)

- Malformed LSCC with small bony island (33%)
- LSCC and vestibule fused to be single cavity (29%)
- Dense stapes superstructure (36%); IP-II (23%)

Goldenhar Syndrome (Oculoauriculovertebral Dysplasia)

- Rare, unilateral aplasia of all SCCs reported

PATHOLOGY

General Features

- Etiology
  - SCC begins to develop from utricle segment of otocyst at 6-8 gestational weeks
  - Development completed between 19th and 22nd weeks
  - Otic vesicle ventral pars inferior develops into vestibular sacculus and cochlear canal; fully formed by week 9
  - Otic vesicle dorsal pars superior develops into utricle and then SCC by week 8
  - SSCC forms 1st, followed by PSCC, and then LSCC
    - Isolated LSCC anomalies are therefore most common
  - Cochlear and vestibular development may be dependent or independent mechanisms
- Genetics
  - SCC aplasia or hypoplasia usually **syndromic**, rarely isolated
    - **CHARGE syndrome**: *CHD7* mutation
    - **BOR syndrome** (ear malformations, branchial and renal anomalies): *EYA1* or *SIX1* mutations
    - **WS**: Several genes *PAX3, MITF, EDN3, EDNRB, SOX10*
      - □ *SOX10* mutations cause 15% of type 2 WS and 50% of type 4 WS (type 2 WS + Hirschsprung disease)
      - □ *SOX10* mutation patients may also show impaired myelination of CNS and PNS
      - □ **P**eripheral/**c**entral dysmyelinating leukodystrophy, **W**S, **H**irschsprung disease (PCWH)
    - **Alagille syndrome** (arteriohepatic dysplasia): *JAG1* (90%) or *NOTCH2* (1-2%) mutations
    - 22q11.2 deletion syndrome (DiGeorge/velocardiofacial syndrome): Most common chromosomal microdeletion disorder
      - □ De novo nonhomologous meiotic recombination events
- Associated abnormalities
  - Common and varies with syndromic etiology

Gross Pathologic & Surgical Features

- SCC atresia, hypoplasia ± anomalous origin
- HSCC hypoplasia/atresia: Oval window hypoplasia/atresia common
- Tympanic segment CNVII anomalous course ± dehiscent
- Cochlea, endolymphatic duct and sac anomaly varies with syndrome

CLINICAL ISSUES

Presentation

- Most common signs/symptoms
  - SNHL
    - Common even when cochlea appears normal on imaging
  - Conductive hearing loss from oval window atresia and ossicular anomalies
  - Vestibular symptoms
    - Vestibular function variable, even with SCC aplasia
    - Caloric responses may be absent
    - Positional vertigo
  - Facial nerve weakness/palsy

Demographics

- Age
  - Congenital
- Epidemiology
  - Uncommon inner ear anomaly
  - Typically syndromic etiology: CHARGE and BOR most common syndromes

DIAGNOSTIC CHECKLIST

Consider

- CHARGE syndrome: Hypoplastic vestibule and SCC
- BOR: Hypoplastic unwound or "thorny" cochlea; look for PSCC anomaly
- WS type IV (rare): Constipation and SNHL; look for PSCC anomaly
- Alagille syndromes (rare): Liver disease and pulmonary stenosis; look for PSCC anomaly

Image Interpretation Pearls

- Axial and coronal temporal bone to assess oval window and CNVII tympanic segment

SELECTED REFERENCES

1. Lewis MA et al: The spectrum of cochlear malformations in CHARGE syndrome and insights into the role of the CHD7 gene during embryogenesis of the inner ear. Neuroradiology. 65(4):819-34, 2023
2. Lewis M et al: Syndromic hearing loss in children. Neuroimaging Clin N Am. 33(4):563-80, 2023
3. Robson CD: Conductive hearing loss in children. Neuroimaging Clin N Am. 33(4):543-62, 2023
4. Feraco P et al: Imaging of inner ear malformations: a primer for radiologists. Radiol Med. 126(10):1282-95, 2021
5. O'Brien WT et al: Nonsyndromic congenital causes of sensorineura hearing loss in children: an illustrative review. AJR Am J Roentgenol. 216(4):1048-55, 2021
6. D'Arco F et al: Temporal bone and intracranial abnormalities in syndromic causes of hearing loss: an updated guide. Eur J Radiol. 123:108803, 2020
7. Verheij E et al: Anatomic malformations of the middle and inner ear in 22q11.2 deletion syndrome: case series and literature review. AJNR Am J Neuroradiol. 39(5):928-34, 2018
8. Green GE et al: CHD7 mutations and CHARGE syndrome in semicircular canal dysplasia. Otol Neurotol. 35(8):1466-70, 2014
9. Elmaleh-Bergès M et al: Spectrum of temporal bone abnormalities in patients with Waardenburg syndrome and SOX10 mutations. AJNR Am J Neuroradiol. 34(6):1257-63, 2013
10. Intrapiromkul J et al: Inner ear anomalies seen on CT images in people with Down syndrome. Pediatr Radiol. 42(12):1449-55, 2012
11. Joshi VM et al: CT and MR imaging of the inner ear and brain in children with congenital sensorineural hearing loss. Radiographics. 32(3):683-98, 2012
12. Blaser S et al: Inner ear dysplasia is common in children with Down syndrome (trisomy 21). Laryngoscope. 116(12):2113-9, 2006
13. Koch B et al: Partial absence of the posterior semicircular canal in Alagille syndrome: CT findings. Pediatr Radiol. 36(9):977-9, 2006
14. Morimoto AK et al: Absent semicircular canals in CHARGE syndrome: radiologic spectrum of findings. AJNR Am J Neuroradiol. 27(8):1663-71, 2006
15. Lemmerling MM et al: Unilateral semicircular canal aplasia in Goldenhar's syndrome. AJNR Am J Neuroradiol. 21(7):1334-6, 2000

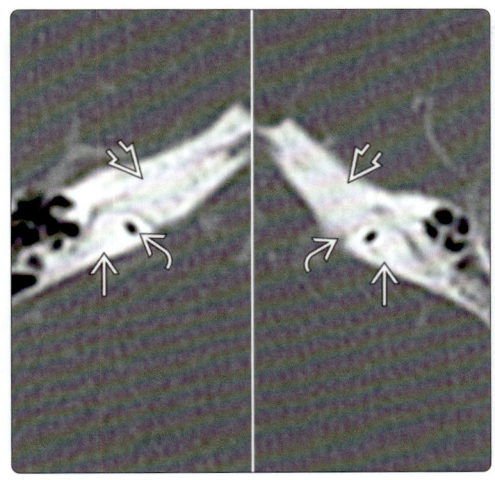

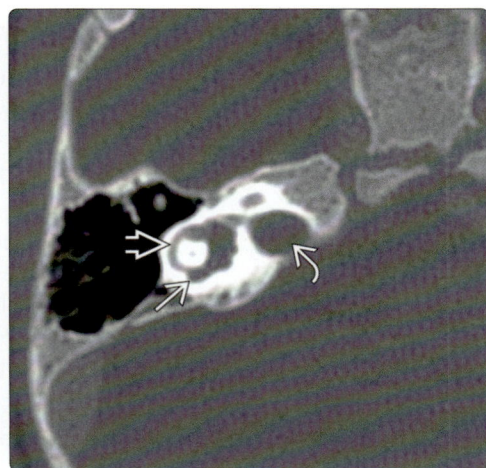

(Left) Axial CT angiogram with bone algorithm in a child with Alagille syndrome demonstrates bilateral absence of the posterior SCCs ➡ and absence of the anterior limb of the superior SCCs ➡. Notice the normal posterior limb of the superior SCCs ➡. (Right) Axial bone CT in a 19-month-old boy with branchiootorenal syndrome (BOR) shows an underdeveloped and anomalous posterior SCC ➡ alongside a normal horizontal SCC ➡. Note the bulbous IAC ➡.

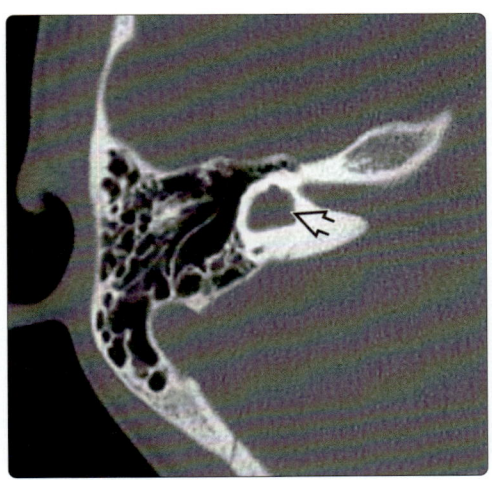

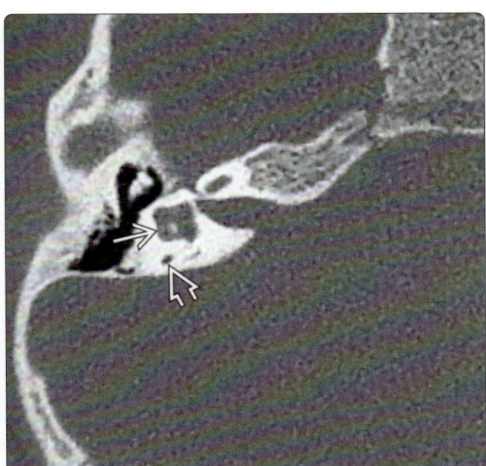

(Left) Axial bone CT in a child with Down syndrome (trisomy 21) shows a globular SCC-vestibule anomaly with absence of the bone island between the lateral SCC and vestibule ➡. This anomaly may be subtle and overlooked when the bone island is present but small. (Right) Axial bone HRCT of temporal bones shows nonsyndromic right lateral SCC hypoplasia with a shorter radius of its semicircle ➡ and an underdeveloped tiny bone island between it and the vestibule. The right posterior SCC ➡ is normal. The left SCCs are normal.

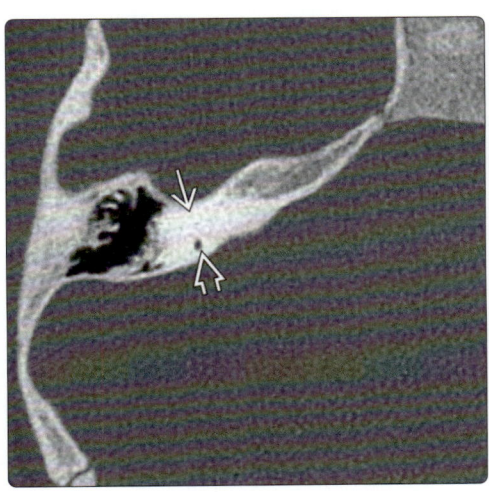

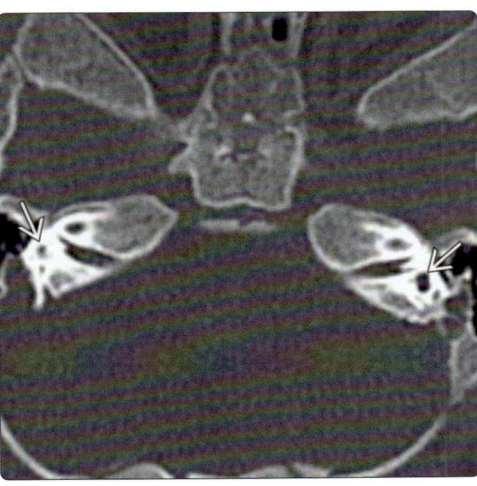

(Left) Axial bone HRCT at a higher level in the same nonsyndromic patient shows absence of the anterior limb/apex ➡ of the right superior SCC, but its posterior limb ➡ is intact. (Right) Axial bone CT in an 18-month-old child with CHARGE syndrome shows typical findings of severe hypoplasia of the bilateral vestibules ➡ (right smaller than left), absence of the bilateral SCCs, and bilateral narrowing of the IACs.

Semicircular Canal-Vestibule Globular Anomaly

TERMINOLOGY

- Dilatation of semicircular canal (SCC) and globular vestibule
- Bone island between vestibule and affected SCC is small or absent (persistent SCC anlage anomaly)

IMAGING

- Most frequently seen SCC and vestibular anomaly
- Usually affects lateral SCC (LSCC): Last to develop
- Isolated finding or with other temporal bone anomalies
- SCC: Widened lumen of 1 limb or entire SCC; small or absent bone island
- Vestibule: Normal or large, less commonly small
- Cochlea: Normal or malformed

TOP DIFFERENTIAL DIAGNOSES

- **Large vestibular aqueduct (LVA)**
  - LVA, ± IP-II anomaly, ± globular vestibule/LSCC
- **Apert syndrome**
  - Craniosynostosis, polysyndactyly, LSCC anlage anomaly

- **Trisomy 21**
  - Vestibule normal or small; small LSCC bone island or persistent SCC anlage anomaly
- **22q11.2 deletion syndrome**
  - Vestibule normal, large or small; small LSCC bone island or persistent SCC anlage anomaly

CLINICAL ISSUES

- Mild form may be asymptomatic
- Vestibular symptoms: Normal or imbalance, vertigo
- Caloric testing: Absent or decreased caloric responses
- Hearing: Normal, sensorineural, mixed, or conductive hearing loss (ossicular or inner ear origin)

DIAGNOSTIC CHECKLIST

- LSCC + external and middle ear malformation
  - Syndromic or chromosomal/genetic anomaly
  - Craniofacial anomaly (most)
  - Toxic exposure

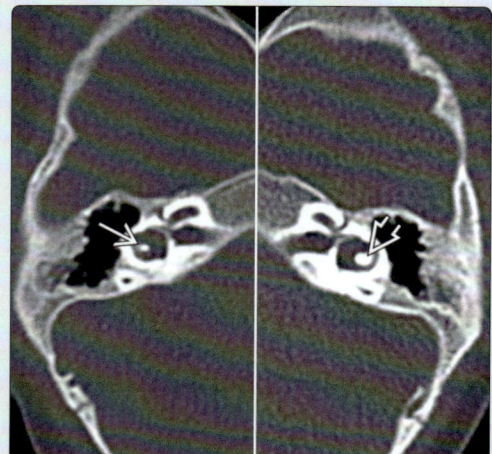
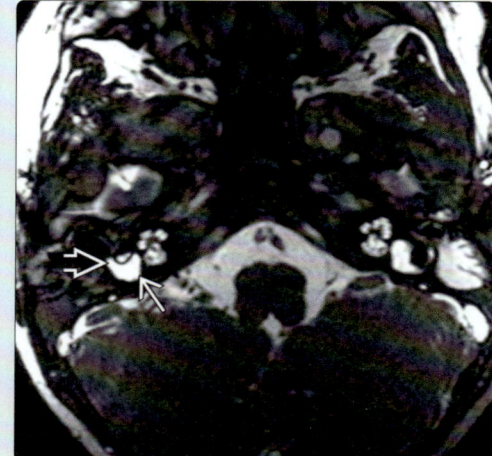

(Left) Axial temporal bone CT in a 20-month-old child with bilateral conductive hearing loss showed bilateral fusion of the malleus head to the attic wall (not shown) & a small bone island ➡ between the right lateral semicircular canal (SCC) & the vestibule. Compare to normal left bone island ➡. (Right) Axial FIESTA MR in a 7-month-old infant demonstrates a dilated right vestibule ➡ forming a globular anomaly with the lateral SCC ➡ and absence of the normal lateral SCC bone island. Compare to normal left-sided structures.

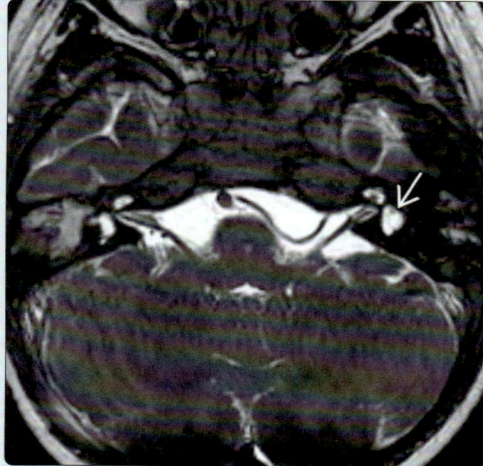
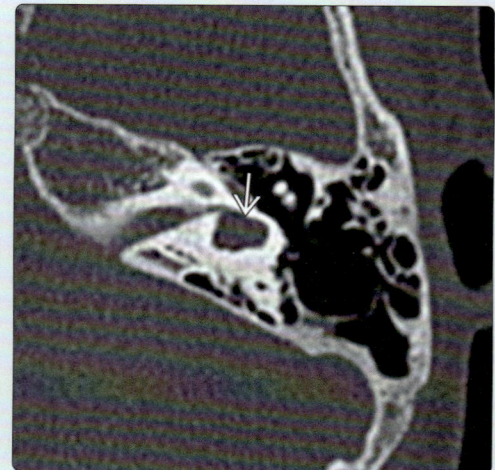

(Left) Axial FIESTA MR through the temporal bones in a 4-year-old child shows absence of the bone island between the left lateral SCC and the vestibule, resulting in a globular anomaly ➡. All other inner ear structures were normal. (Right) Axial bone CT in a 10-year-old boy with right-sided external auditory canal atresia (not shown) and left-sided absence of the bone island between the lateral SCC and the vestibule shows the resulting globular anomaly ➡.

TERMINOLOGY

Synonyms

- Persistent semicircular canal (SCC) anlage anomaly

Definitions

- Dilatation of SCC and globular vestibule
- Small or absent bone island between vestibule and affected SCC

IMAGING

General Features

- Best diagnostic clue
  - Most frequently encountered anomaly of SCC and vestibule
  - Globular appearance of SCC ± globular vestibule
  - **Lateral SCC** (LSCC) **most frequently affected** (embryologically last to develop)
  - Isolated anomaly or associated with other inner/middle/external ear anomalies
- Location
  - Posterior membranous labyrinth
- Morphology
  - **Superior** SCC (SSCC) and **posterior** SCC (PSCC) develop from 1 pouch of utricle by **19-weeks** gestation
  - **LSCC** develops from separate pouch of utricle by **22-weeks** gestation
  - Developing pouches flatten and central portions fuse, leaving SCC
  - Failure of central absorption leads to globular anomaly

CT Findings

- Bone CT
  - SCC
    - Widened SCC lumen: May affect only 1 limb of SCC or entire SCC
    - Small or absent bone island
  - Vestibule: Normal or large, less commonly small
  - Cochlea: Normal or malformed
  - Vestibular aqueduct: Normal or large
  - Oval window: Stenosis or atresia if LSCC involved
  - Middle ear space and ossicles: Normal (most) or malformed
  - External ear: Normal (most) or stenotic/atretic

Imaging Recommendations

- Best imaging tool
  - High-resolution temporal bone CT or MR

DIFFERENTIAL DIAGNOSIS

Large Vestibular Aqueduct

- Large vestibular aqueduct, cochlear modiolar deficiency ± incomplete partition type II anomaly

Apert Syndrome

- Syndromic craniosynostosis + widened sagittal suture, polysyndactyly, globular vestibule/LSCC

Trisomy 21

- Vestibule normal to small; small LSCC bone island or anlage anomaly

22q11.2 Deletion Syndrome (Velocardiofacial Syndrome)

- Vestibule normal, large or small; small LSCC bone island or anlage anomaly

PATHOLOGY

General Features

- Genetics
  - Candidate genes with SCC anomalies in mice: *Otx1*, *Prx1*, *Prx2*, and *Hmx3*

CLINICAL ISSUES

Presentation

- Most common signs/symptoms
  - Mild form may be asymptomatic
  - Vestibular symptoms: Normal or imbalance, tinnitus, vertigo
  - Caloric testing: Absent or decreased caloric responses
  - Hearing: Normal, sensorineural, mixed, or conductive hearing loss (ossicular or inner ear origin)

DIAGNOSTIC CHECKLIST

Consider

- LSCC anomaly + external and middle ear malformation
  - Craniofacial anomaly (most) (e.g., hemifacial microsomia, Treacher Collins syndrome)
  - Syndromic or chromosomal/genetic anomaly
  - Toxic exposure

SELECTED REFERENCES

1. Lewis M et al: Syndromic hearing loss in children. Neuroimaging Clin N Am. 33(4):563-80, 2023
2. Robson CD et al: Non-syndromic sensorineural hearing loss in children. Neuroimaging Clin N Am. 33(4):531-42, 2023
3. O'Brien WT et al: Nonsyndromic congenital causes of sensorineura hearing loss in children: an illustrative review. AJR Am J Roentgenol. 216(4):1048-55, 2021
4. D'Arco F et al: Temporal bone and intracranial abnormalities in syndromic causes of hearing loss: an updated guide. Eur J Radiol. 123:108803, 2020
5. Tahir E et al: Inner-ear malformations as a cause of single-sided deafness. J Laryngol Otol. 134(6):509-18, 2020
6. Intrapiromkul J et al: Inner ear anomalies seen on CT images in people with Down syndrome. Pediatr Radiol. 42(12):1449-55, 2012
7. Lan MY et al: Measurements of normal inner ear on computed tomography in children with congenital sensorineural hearing loss. Eur Arch Otorhinolaryngol. 266(9):1361-4, 2009
8. Zhou G et al: Inner ear anomalies and conductive hearing loss in children with Apert syndrome: an overlooked otologic aspect. Otol Neurotol. 30(2):184-9, 2009
9. Dallan I et al: Bilateral, isolated, lateral semicircular canal malformation without hearing loss. J Laryngol Otol. 122(8):858-60, 2008
10. Blaser S et al: Inner ear dysplasia is common in children with Down syndrome (trisomy 21). Laryngoscope. 116(12):2113-9, 2006
11. Quintero-Rivera F et al: Intracranial anomalies detected by imaging studies in 30 patients with Apert syndrome. Am J Med Genet A. 140(12):1337-8, 2006
12. Matsunaga T et al: Familial lateral semicircular canal malformation with external and middle ear abnormalities. Am J Med Genet A. 116A(4):360-7, 2003
13. Purcell D et al: Establishment of normative cochlear and vestibular measurements to aid in the diagnosis of inner ear malformations. Otolaryngol Head Neck Surg. 128(1):78-87, 2003
14. Johnson J et al: Sensorineural and conductive hearing loss associated with lateral semicircular canal malformation. Laryngoscope. 110(10 Pt 1):1673-9, 2000

TERMINOLOGY

- Labyrinthitis: Subacute inflammatory or infectious disease of fluid-filled spaces of inner ear

IMAGING

- **No imaging** necessary if classic presentation [unilateral sudden-onset sensorineural hearing loss (SNHL)]
- MR findings
  - T1 C+ FS: Normal to moderately enhanced inner ear
  - T2: Normal high fluid signal preserved in acute/subacute
    - Lose fluid signal in chronic disease 2° to fibrous/osseous replacement
  - T1: Normal to mild ↑ signal; if hemorrhage, ↑ signal
- Temporal bone CT findings
  - Normal in acute/subacute labyrinthitis; labyrinthine ossificans possible if prior suppurative labyrinthitis

TOP DIFFERENTIAL DIAGNOSES

- Labyrinthine ossificans

- Intralabyrinthine schwannoma
- Intralabyrinthine hemorrhage
- Cochlear otosclerosis

PATHOLOGY

- Labyrinthitis classification
  - Viral labyrinthitis: Unilateral
  - Bacterial labyrinthitis: Meningogenic (bilateral) > > tympanogenic (unilateral)
  - Posttraumatic/postsurgical: Unilateral
  - Autoimmune: Related to systemic disease (bilateral)

CLINICAL ISSUES

- Viral: Sudden-onset unilateral SNHL ± vertigo & tinnitus
- Bacterial: Labyrinthitis ossificans possible
  - Meningogenic: Child with bacterial meningitis → bilateral, progressive SNHL
  - Tympanogenic: Acute bacterial otomastoiditis → direct spread through round or oval window

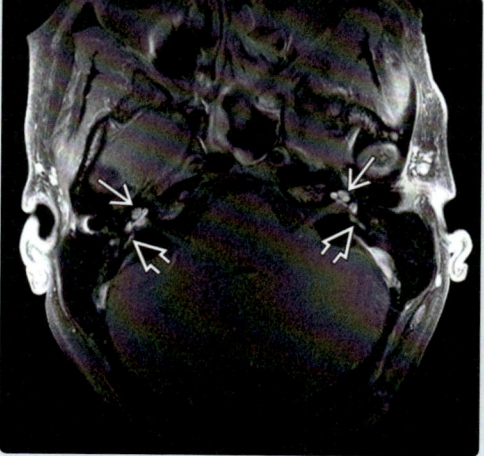
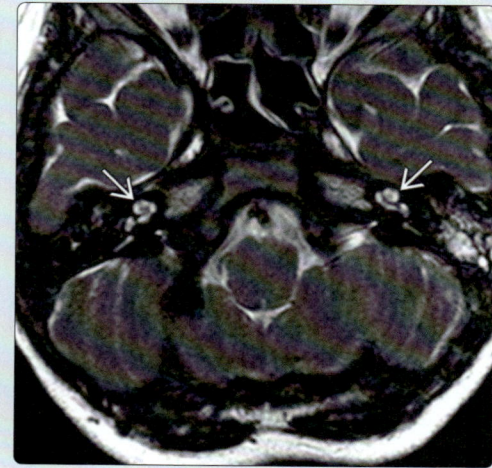

(Left) *Axial T1 C+ FS MR in an 8-year-old child with meningogenic labyrinthitis shows intense bilateral enhancement of the cochlea ➡ & posterior semicircular canals ➡. Additional images (not shown) also demonstrated bilateral enhancement of the vestibules & all semicircular canals.* (Right) *Axial T2 FSE MR in a patient with bilateral labyrinthitis shows normal hyperintense fluid within the cochlea bilaterally ➡. Normal to slightly decreased fluid signal is typical of acute/subacute labyrinthitis.*

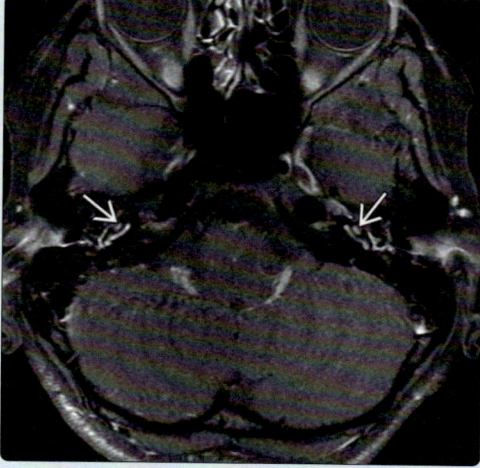
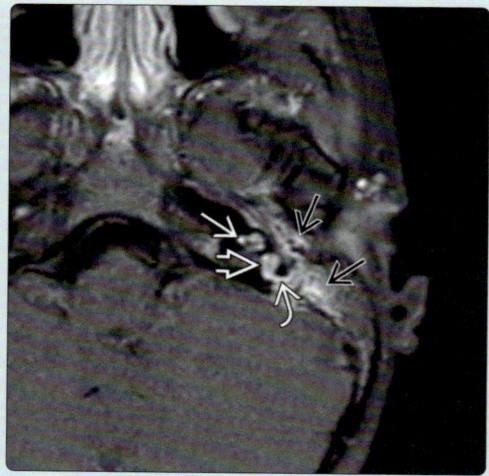

(Left) *Axial T1 C+ FS MR in a patient with sudden-onset bilateral sensorineural hearing loss shows enhancement in the bilateral cochlea ➡. Axial FIESTA MR images (not shown) revealed ↓ fluid signal, consistent with the chronic stage of labyrinthitis.* (Right) *Axial T1 C+ FS MR in a child with meningogenic labyrinthitis shows abnormal enhancement involving the left cochlea ➡, vestibule ➡, & lateral semicircular canal ➡. Note also extensive abnormal enhancement in the left middle ear cavity & mastoid air cells ➡.*

TERMINOLOGY

Synonyms

- Subacute labyrinthitis

Definitions

- Subacute inflammatory or infectious disease of fluid-filled spaces of inner ear (IE)
  - Labyrinthitis causes secondary changes within membranous labyrinth of IE

IMAGING

General Features

- Best diagnostic clue
  - T1 C+ MR shows **faint to moderate enhancement** within normally fluid-filled spaces of **IE**

CT Findings

- Bone CT: Normal in acute & subacute phases
  - If suppurative labyrinthitis (bacterial, pus producing) → **labyrinthine ossificans** (LO)
    - Initially fibrous, then ossific over weeks or years

MR Findings

- T1WI: Signal often normal
  - In severe, diffuse membranous labyrinthitis, may show subtle ↑ in signal
  - If intralabyrinthine hemorrhage present, ↑ in IE signal
- T2WI: Normal high-signal IE fluid in acute/subacute phases
  - T2 may differentiate acute/subacute labyrinthitis from intralabyrinthine schwannoma (hypointense IE fluid)
  - Chronic disease → LO → replacement of hyperintense T2 signal with hypointense signal
  - Focal/diffuse, faint to moderate enhancement within normally fluid-filled spaces of cochlea, vestibule, & semicircular canals
- T1WI C+: Acute/subacute phases may be normal
  - Enhancement may persist after symptoms resolve

Imaging Recommendations

- Best imaging tool
  - If classic clinical presentation, no imaging necessary
  - Atypical presentation: Thin-section T1 C-, T1 C+, & T2 MR are key sequences

DIFFERENTIAL DIAGNOSIS

Labyrinthine Ossificans

- Bone CT: Ossification of membranous labyrinth
- T1 C+ MR: Early phase, IE enhancement
- T2 MR: Hypointensity replaces normal hyperintense IE fluid

Intralabyrinthine Schwannoma

- T1 C+ MR: Enhancement more intense & localized than labyrinthitis
- T2 MR: Focal ↓ signal = area of enhancement

Intralabyrinthine Hemorrhage

- Underlying coagulopathy or trauma history
- T1 MR: Hyperintense precontrast T1 signal

Cochlear Otosclerosis

- Temporal bone CT: Characteristic areas of focal demineralization in otic capsule
- T1 C+ MR: When enhancement present, involves bony labyrinth (not membranous labyrinth)

CLINICAL ISSUES

Presentation

- Most common signs/symptoms
  - Sudden onset of sensorineural hearing loss (SNHL), vertigo, & tinnitus
- Labyrinthitis classification
  - **Viral labyrinthitis**
    - Sudden unilateral SNHL ± upper respiratory illness
    - Not imaged if classic presentation
    - Probably hematogenous spread
  - **Bacterial labyrinthitis**
    - Often progresses to permanent SNHL
    - **Meningogenic**: Bilateral; secondary to meningitis
      - □ Primary cause of acquired childhood deafness
      - □ Spreads from fundus of internal auditory canal (IAC) through lamina cribrosa → vestibule **or** cochlear nerve canal → cochlea **or** cochlear aqueduct → cochlear basal turn
    - **Tympanogenic**: Unilateral; 2° to bacterial otomastoiditis
      - □ Acute bacterial otomastoiditis → direct spread through round or oval window
  - **Posttraumatic/postsurgical**: Unilateral
    - Hemorrhage likely incites enhancement
    - Healing → granulation tissue ± LO
  - **Autoimmune**: Very rare, related to systemic disease
    - Granulomatosis with polyangiitis (Wegener), Cogan, polyarteritis nodosa, relapsing polychondritis, systemic lupus erythematosus, rheumatoid arthritis

Demographics

- Any age may be affected
  - Meningogenic labyrinthitis is disease of childhood
- Epidemiology: Viral > > bacterial labyrinthitis

Natural History & Prognosis

- Hearing loss recovery common in viral labyrinthitis
  - May be recurrent & debilitating
- Persistent SNHL common in bacterial labyrinthitis
- Labyrinthine ossification more frequent with meningogenic labyrinthitis and *Streptococcus pneumoniae* infection

Treatment

- Viral etiology: Steroids, vestibular suppressants, & vestibular exercises
- Bacterial: Topical & IV antibiotics
  - Surgical intervention when severe

SELECTED REFERENCES

1. Baba A et al: Advanced imaging of head and neck infections. J Neuroimaging. 33(4):477-92, 2023
2. Robson CD et al: Non-syndromic sensorineural hearing loss in children. Neuroimaging Clin N Am. 33(4):531-42, 2023
3. Benson JC et al: MRI of the internal auditory canal, labyrinth, and middle ear: how we do it. Radiology. 297(2):252-65, 2020

Otosyphilis

TERMINOLOGY

- Sexually transmitted inner ear disease caused by bacterium spirochete *Treponema pallidum*

IMAGING

- Bone CT: **Moth-eaten permeative demineralization** of temporal bone (syphilitic osteitis)
  - Inner ear, middle ear-mastoid, ossicles
- T1 C+ MR: Enhancement of CNVII & CNVIII in internal auditory canal ± fluid-filled labyrinth (syphilitic labyrinthitis-meningitis)

TOP DIFFERENTIAL DIAGNOSES

- Cochlear otosclerosis
  - Patchy radiolucent foci throughout otic capsule
- Temporal bone osteogenesis imperfecta
  - Cochlear otosclerosis mimic but more severe
- Temporal bone Paget disease
  - Diffuse otic capsule & skull base demineralization

- Temporal bone fibrous dysplasia
  - Ground-glass expansile bone
- Postirradiated temporal bone
  - Moth-eaten otic capsule ± skull base & EAC involvement

PATHOLOGY

- Sexually transmitted spirochete *T. pallidum*
- **Osteitis**: Inflammatory resorptive osteitis
- **Labyrinthitis**: Obliterative endarteritis

CLINICAL ISSUES

- Diagnosis made when otologic symptoms are present with positive serology
- Hearing loss (90%), tinnitus (73%), & vertigo (53%)
- Clinical mimic: Ménière disease

DIAGNOSTIC CHECKLIST

- Consider: If HIV patient with hearing loss & permeative inner ear demineralization, test for positive syphilis serology before diagnosing otosyphilis

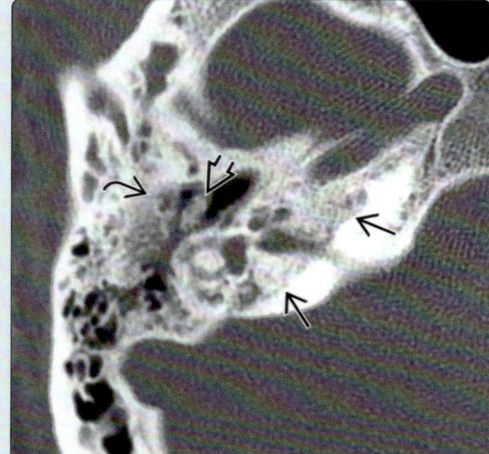
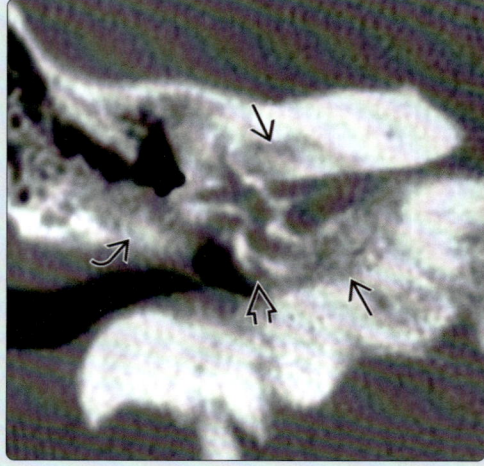

(Left) Axial temporal bone CT shows typical findings of advanced middle and inner ear otosyphilis. There are extensive moth-eaten permeative bony changes of the inner ear ➡, middle ear-mastoid ➡, and ossicles ➡ that are individually well marginated. (Courtesy M. Sandlin, MD.) (Right) Coronal temporal bone CT of right ear shows severe otosyphilis as permeative demineralization of otic capsule ➡, cochlear promontory ➡, and bones of the middle ear wall ➡.

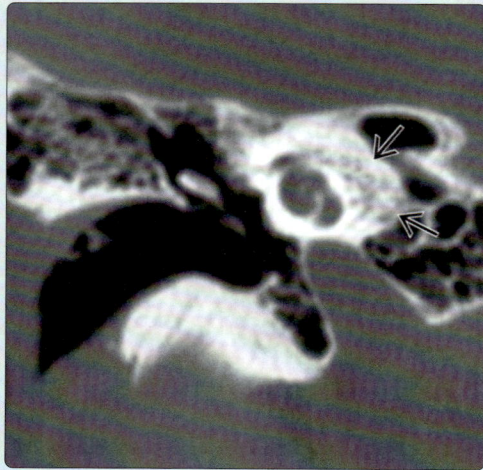
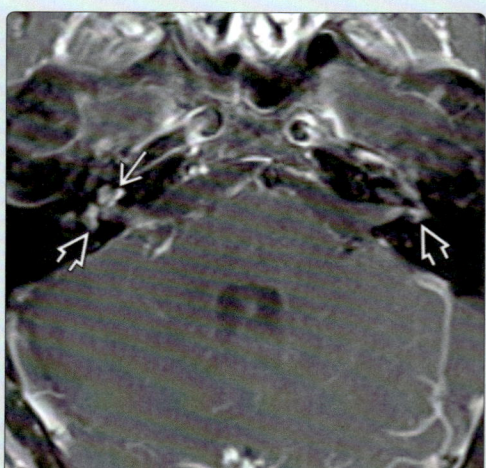

(Left) Coronal temporal bone CT shows subtle permeative demineralization of otic capsule ➡ from otosyphilis. Small foci are different from larger cochlear otosclerosis plaque-like demineralization. (Right) Axial T1 C+ FS MR through the posterior fossa in an HIV(+) patient with hearing loss and vertigo shows typical findings of the labyrinthitis form of otosyphilis. There is striking abnormal enhancement in the right cochlea ➡ and bilateral vestibules ➡, representing infectious/inflammatory disease.

TERMINOLOGY

Synonyms

- Luetic labyrinthitis, osteitis, & meningitis

Definitions

- Sexually transmitted inner ear disease caused by bacterium spirochete *Treponema pallidum*

IMAGING

General Features

- Best diagnostic clue
  - Moth-eaten permeative demineralization of temporal bone
- Location
  - Otic capsule, internal auditory canal (IAC), & cerebellopontine angle meninges

CT Findings

- **Osteitis**: Moth-eaten permeative bone change
  - Inner ear, middle ear-mastoid, ossicles
- **Labyrinthitis**: Not seen on temporal bone CT
- If contrast contemplated, do MR with contrast instead

MR Findings

- T1WI
  - Osteitis: Patchy areas of intermediate signal
- T2WI
  - Osteitis: If severe, patchy high signal in otic capsule
  - IAC meningeal infection: Thickened CNVII-VIII
- T1WI C+
  - Osteitis: **Patchy, enhancing foci** in otic capsule
  - Labyrinthitis: Enhancing fluid-filled spaces of inner ear
  - IAC meningitis: Enhancement of leptomeninges within IAC, including CNVII & CNVIII

Imaging Recommendations

- Best imaging tool
  - Osteitis: Temporal bone CT
  - Labyrinthitis & IAC meningitis: T1 C+ MR

DIFFERENTIAL DIAGNOSIS

Cochlear Otosclerosis

- Clinical: Mixed hearing loss
- Imaging: Patchy radiolucent foci throughout otic capsule
  - Ossicles not involved

Temporal Bone Osteogenesis Imperfecta

- Clinical: Children with brittle bones & blue sclera
- Imaging: Cochlear otosclerosis mimic but more severe

Temporal Bone Paget Disease

- Clinical: Affects older adults
- Imaging: Otic capsule demineralization is diffuse, involves entire skull base

Temporal Bone Fibrous Dysplasia

- Clinical: < 30-year-old patient group
- Imaging: Ground-glass expansile bone

Postirradiated Temporal Bone

- Clinical: Post temporal bone irradiation

- Imaging: Also moth-eaten otic capsule

PATHOLOGY

General Features

- Etiology
  - Sexually transmitted spirochete *T. pallidum*

Gross Pathologic & Surgical Features

- Endolymphatic duct rarely obstructed by gumma

Microscopic Features

- Osteitis: Inflammatory resorptive osteitis
- Labyrinthitis: Obliterative endarteritis

CLINICAL ISSUES

Presentation

- Most common signs/symptoms
  - **Hearing loss** (90%), tinnitus (73%), & vertigo (53%)
  - Facial palsy; meningeal signs
- Clinical profile
  - Diagnosis made when otologic symptoms are present with positive serology
  - Otosyphilis is late manifestation

Demographics

- Epidemiology
  - Incidence began to ↑ in 1980s due to AIDS
  - Early disease incidence ↑ 71% from 2014 to 2018 in USA
- Age: Older patients
- Sex: M > F
- Ethnicity: Black > White patients

Natural History & Prognosis

- After therapy, hearing loss improves in 25% of patients
- After therapy, tinnitus & vertigo improve in 75% of patients
- Best response when symptoms are fluctuating, hearing loss is < 5-year duration, & patient is < 60 years old

Treatment

- Antibiotics & corticosteroids

DIAGNOSTIC CHECKLIST

Consider

- If HIV patient with permeative inner ear demineralization, test for syphilis serology

Image Interpretation Pearls

- Permeative demineralization of otic capsule = **syphilitic osteitis**
- T1 C+ MR enhancement of CNVII & CNVIII in IAC ± fluid-filled labyrinth = **syphilitic labyrinthitis-meningitis**

SELECTED REFERENCES

1. Chandrasekharan R et al: Magnetic resonance imaging in otosyphilis: a rare manifestation of neurosyphilis. Indian J Radiol Imaging. 32(2):278-84, 2022
2. Ramchandani MS et al: Otosyphilis: a review of the literature. Sex Transm Dis. 47(5):296-300, 2020
3. Kivekäs I et al: Bilateral temporal bone otosyphilis. Otol Neurotol. 35(2):e90-1, 2014
4. Ogungbemi A et al: Computed tomography features of luetic osteitis (otosyphilis) of the temporal bone. J Laryngol Otol. 128(2):185-8, 2014
5. Swartz JD: The otodystrophies: diagnosis and differential diagnosis. Semin Ultrasound CT MR. 25(4):305-18, 2004

Labyrinthine Ossificans

TERMINOLOGY

- **Membranous labyrinth ossification**: Healing response to inner ear infection, inflammation, trauma, or surgery

IMAGING

- Varies with severity
  - Mild: "Enlarged" modiolus; subtle inner ear new bone
  - Severe: All inner ear fluid replaced by bone
- Temporal bone CT: **High-density** bone deposition within membranous labyrinth
- T2 MR: **Low-intensity** foci within high-signal fluid of membranous labyrinth

TOP DIFFERENTIAL DIAGNOSES

- Labyrinthine aplasia
- Cochlear aplasia
- Intravestibular lipoma
- Cochlear otosclerosis
- Labyrinthine schwannoma

PATHOLOGY

- **Fibrous stage**: Fibroblast proliferation
- **Ossific stage**: Osteoblasts forming abnormal bony trabeculae within membranous labyrinthine spaces

CLINICAL ISSUES

- Most common: Bilateral sensorineural hearing loss (SNHL) in child weeks to months after acute meningitis episode
- Less common: Unilateral SNHL with prior history of surgery, trauma, middle ear-mastoid infection
- Cochlear implantation used for SNHL correction if cochlear nerve is still present
- Bilateral cochlear labyrinthine ossificans (LO) is serious detriment to cochlear implantation

DIAGNOSTIC CHECKLIST

- Precochlear implant evaluation of temporal bone in children: Look for LO & inner ear congenital anomalies
- Describe LO as **cochlear** or **noncochlear**

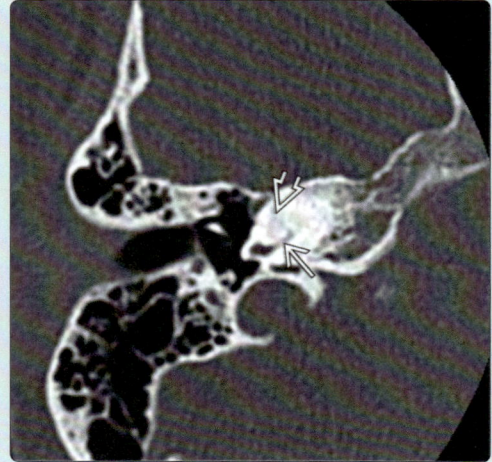
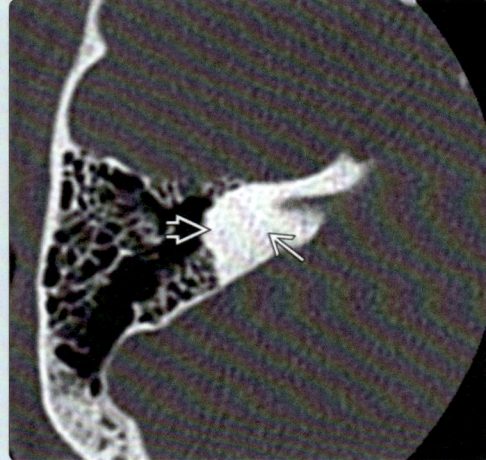

(Left) Axial bone CT in a 13-year-old girl with prior history of meningitis shows subtotal ossification of the basal turn of the cochlea ➡ and complete ossification of the middle and apical turns ➡. (Right) Axial bone CT in the same patient shows complete ossification of the otic capsule without identifiable labyrinthine structures at the expected site of vestibule ➡ or lateral semicircular canal ➡. Study obtained at the time of meningitis 8 years prior demonstrated normal inner ear structures (not shown).

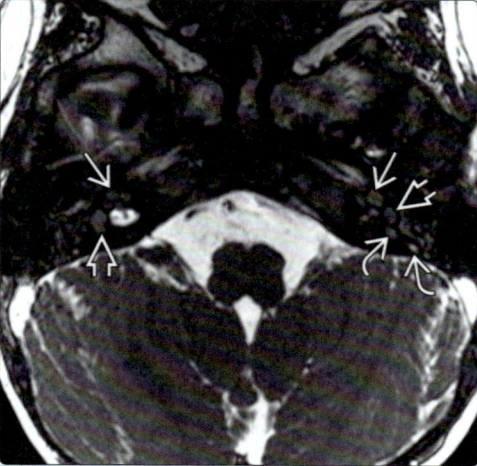
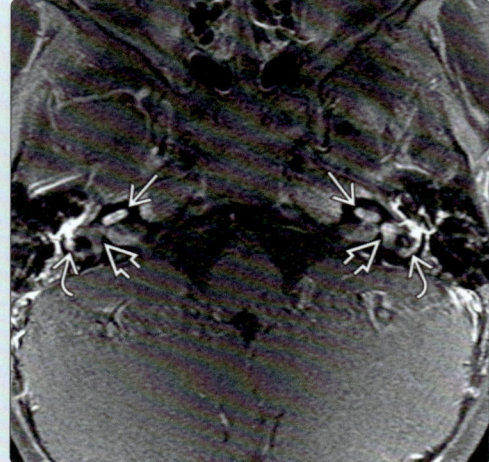

(Left) Axial thin-section T2WI MR in a 2-year-old child with bacterial meningitis 3 weeks prior shows diffuse, bilateral decrease in normal hyperintense inner ear fluid involving the cochlea ➡, vestibule ➡, and visualized portions of semicircular canals ➡. These findings are consistent with early fibroosseous replacement of normal inner ear fluid. (Right) Axial T1WI C+ FS MR in the same patient shows bilateral abnormal inner ear enhancement in the cochlea ➡, vestibule ➡, and lateral semicircular canal ➡.

Labyrinthine Ossificans

TERMINOLOGY

Abbreviations

- Labyrinthine ossificans (LO)

Synonyms

- Labyrinthine ossification, ossifying labyrinthitis, labyrinthitis ossificans, chronic labyrinthitis

Definitions

- Membranous labyrinth ossification as healing response to **infectious, inflammatory, traumatic, or surgical** insult to inner ear

IMAGING

General Features

- Best diagnostic clue
  - Temporal bone CT: High-density bone deposition within membranous labyrinth
  - T2 MR: Low-intensity foci within high-signal fluid of membranous labyrinth
- Location
  - **Membranous labyrinth** fluid spaces
  - **Cochlear LO**: Fluid spaces of cochlea affected
  - **Noncochlear LO**: Fluid spaces of semicircular canals (SCCs) or vestibule affected
- Morphology
  - Focal ossific plaques or diffuse ossification of membranous labyrinth

CT Findings

- CECT
  - No role in making LO diagnosis
- Bone CT
  - **Mild LO**: Fibroosseous changes result in hazy increased density within fluid spaces of membranous labyrinth & prominent-appearing modiolus
  - **Moderate LO**: Focal areas of bony encroachment on fluid spaces of membranous labyrinth
    - May be **cochlear**, **noncochlear**, or both
  - **Severe LO**: Membranous labyrinth completely obliterated by bone, replacing fluid spaces

MR Findings

- T2WI
  - **Mild LO**: Intermediate- & low-signal fibroosseous material partially replaces high-signal fluid spaces of membranous labyrinth
    - Associated with apparent "enlargement" of modiolus
  - **Moderate LO**: Focal areas of low-signal bone encroaching on high-signal fluid spaces of membranous labyrinth
    - May be cochlear, noncochlear, or both
  - **Severe LO**: High-signal membranous labyrinth absent, completely replaced by low-signal bone
    - Cochlear nerve often severely atrophied
- T1WI C+
  - **Membranous labyrinthitis** secondary to **infection** is usual precursor to LO
    - In this pre-LO phase, membranous labyrinth enhances, signifying active labyrinthitis

- Enhancement may be hololabyrinthine or segmental
- Enhancement may persist in ossifying stage of LO

Imaging Recommendations

- Best imaging tool
  - ≤ 1-mm thick axial & reformatted coronal temporal bone CTs are easiest imaging tools to diagnose LO
- High-resolution T2 MR makes diagnosis
  - Careful inspection for absent inner ear fluid spaces
  - T2 MR can show fibrous obliteration of membranous labyrinth, whereas CT cannot
  - T1 C+ MR very useful in showing enhancing inner ear in pre-LO phase with labyrinthitis

DIFFERENTIAL DIAGNOSIS

Labyrinthine Aplasia

- Clinical: Congenital sensorineural hearing loss (SNHL)
- Bone CT: **Flattening of cochlear promontory**
  - Labyrinthine aplasia: Absent cochlea, vestibule, SCCs

Cochlear Aplasia

- Clinical: SNHL present from birth
- Bone CT: Absent cochlea; flattening of cochlear promontory

Intravestibular Lipoma

- Clinical: Mild, high frequency SNHL often present
- MR: **T1 high-signal** foci in vestibule
  - Cerebellopontine angle/internal auditory canal lipoma may be associated

Cochlear Otosclerosis

- Clinical: Disease of young adults
- Bone CT: Radiolucent foci in **bony labyrinth**
  - Does not encroach on membranous labyrinth, even in healing phase

Labyrinthine Schwannoma

- Clinical: Protracted history of slowly progressive unilateral SNHL
- MR: T1 C+ focal intralabyrinthine enhancement
  - T2 MR shows hypointense material within enhancing portion of membranous labyrinth

PATHOLOGY

General Features

- Etiology
  - Suppurative membranous labyrinthitis → cascading inflammatory response in membranous labyrinth
    - Begins with fibrosis, progresses to ossification (as early as 4 weeks)
  - LO caused by suppurative labyrinthitis from multiple sources
    - **Meningogenic** LO: From meningitis; bilateral
    - **Tympanogenic** LO: From middle ear infection; unilateral
    - **Hematogenic** LO: From blood-borne infection, such as measles or mumps (rare); bilateral
  - LO may also arise after severe trauma or temporal bone surgery

- LO also identified as cause of SNHL in children with sickle cell anemia
  - Hypothesis: Sequelae of arterial vasoocclusive ischemia &/or venous obstruction to inner ear
- Labyrinthitis progresses to LO when suppurative
- LO seen on temporal bone CT as early as 4 weeks after episode of meningitis

Gross Pathologic & Surgical Features

- Gross pathology of inner ear with LO shows new bone formation in membranous labyrinth
- At surgery for cochlear implantation, bony obstruction to implant entry through round window niche is observed

Microscopic Features

- **Fibrous stage**: Fibroblast proliferation
- **Ossific stage**: Osteoblasts form abnormal bony trabeculae within membranous labyrinthine spaces
  - Scala tympani in basal turn is most frequent area of ossification in all causes of LO
  - Meningitis → suppurative labyrinthitis associated with greatest amount of ossification

CLINICAL ISSUES

Presentation

- Most common signs/symptoms
  - Unilateral or bilateral SNHL
  - Other signs/symptoms
    - Severe vertigo is infrequent but devastating
    - Vertigo may be serious enough to require labyrinthectomy
- Clinical profile
  - Bilateral SNHL in child weeks to months after acute meningitis episode
- Other possible patient histories
  - Suppurative middle ear infection (tympanogenic LO)
  - Severe bout of mumps, measles, or other viral illness (hematogenic LO)
  - Profound head & skull base trauma (posttraumatic LO)
  - Previous temporal bone surgery (postsurgical LO)

Demographics

- Age
  - Pediatric malady
- Epidemiology
  - Meningogenic labyrinthitis is most common cause of acquired childhood deafness
    - Most commonly from *Streptococcus pneumoniae* or *Haemophilus influenzae*
  - 6-30% have some degree of hearing loss following meningitis

Natural History & Prognosis

- Gradual deterioration of hearing following ear infection (unilateral) or meningitis, blood-borne infection, head trauma, or temporal bone surgery (bilateral)
- Prognosis for SNHL is defined by response to cochlear implantation
- High-resolution axial T2WI MR shows high negative predictive value in predicting intraoperative cochlear obstruction

Treatment

- **Cochlear implantation** used for SNHL correction if cochlear nerve is still present
  - Bilateral cochlear LO is serious detriment to cochlear implantation
    - **Presurgical** identification of cochlear LO is key
    - Allows planning for "drill-out" of obstructed cochlea & modifications of implant device
- "Drill-out," newer cochlear implant devices available for obstructed cochlea
  - Scala vestibuli insertion is 1 alternative
- Labyrinthectomy used in cases of intractable vertigo

DIAGNOSTIC CHECKLIST

Consider

- In precochlear implant evaluation of temporal bone in children, look for LO & inner ear congenital anomalies
  - Both of these diagnoses will often force surgical plan to be individualized
- LO may be contraindication to cochlear implantation or complicate surgery

Image Interpretation Pearls

- Radiologist should describe LO as **cochlear** or **noncochlear**
  - Only describing LO of inner ear does not help cochlear implant surgeon decide what can be done
    - Cochlear LO makes implant problematic
  - Be specific about which noncochlear portions of membranous labyrinth are involved

SELECTED REFERENCES

1. Baba A et al: Advanced imaging of head and neck infections. J Neuroimaging. 33(4):477-92, 2023
2. Robson CD et al: Non-syndromic sensorineural hearing loss in children. Neuroimaging Clin N Am. 33(4):531-42, 2023
3. Orman G et al: Accuracy of MR imaging for detection of sensorineural hearing loss in infants with bacterial meningitis. AJNR Am J Neuroradiol. 41(6):1081-6, 2020
4. Chandrasekhar SS et al: Clinical practice guideline: sudden hearing loss (update) executive summary. Otolaryngol Head Neck Surg. 161(2):195-210, 2019
5. Bloch SL et al: Labyrinthitis ossificans: on the mechanism of perilabyrinthine bone remodeling. Ann Otol Rhinol Laryngol. 124(8):649-54, 2015
6. Jiang ZY et al: Utility of MRIs in adult cochlear implant evaluations. Otol Neurotol. 35(9):1533-5, 2014
7. Lin HY et al: The incidence of tympanogenic labyrinthitis ossificans. J Laryngol Otol. 128(7):618-20, 2014
8. Young JY et al: Preoperative imaging of sensorineural hearing loss in pediatric candidates for cochlear implantation. Radiographics. 34(5):E133-49, 2014
9. Kopelovich JC et al: Early prediction of postmeningitic hearing loss in children using magnetic resonance imaging. Arch Otolaryngol Head Neck Surg. 137(5):441-7, 2011
10. Durisin M et al: Cochlear osteoneogenesis after meningitis in cochlear implant patients: a retrospective analysis. Otol Neurotol. 31(7):1072-8, 2010
11. Saito N et al: Clinical and radiologic manifestations of sickle cell disease in the head and neck. Radiographics. 30(4):1021-34, 2010
12. Isaacson B et al: Labyrinthitis ossificans: how accurate is MRI in predicting cochlear obstruction? Otolaryngol Head Neck Surg. 140(5):692-6, 2009
13. Ozgen B et al: Complete labyrinthine aplasia: clinical and radiologic findings with review of the literature. AJNR Am J Neuroradiol. 30(4):774-80, 2009
14. Berrettini S et al: Scala vestibuli cochlear implantation in patients with partially ossified cochleas. J Laryngol Otol. 116(11):946-50, 2002
15. Glastonbury CM et al: Imaging findings of cochlear nerve deficiency. AJNR Am J Neuroradiol. 23(4):635-43, 2002
16. Swartz JD et al: Labyrinthine ossification: etiologies and CT findings. Radiology. 157(2):395-8, 1985

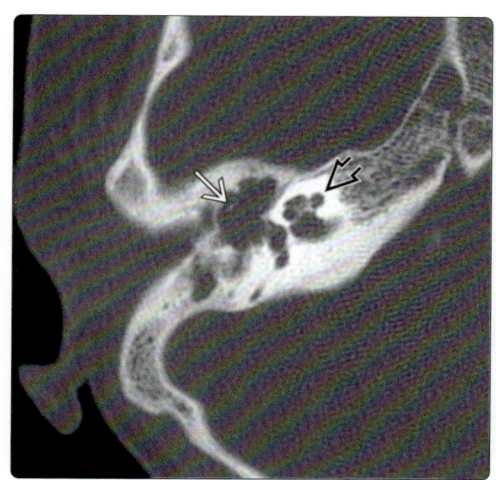
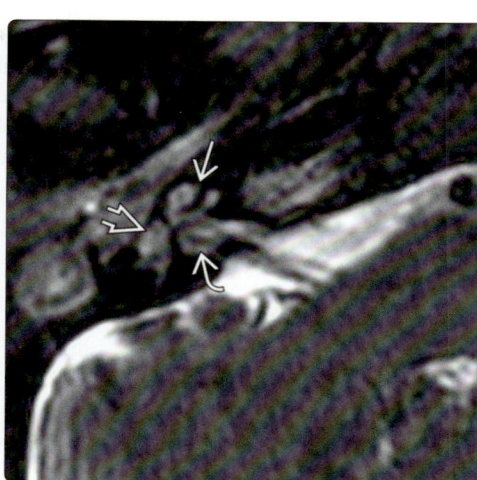

(Left) Axial bone CT in a 10-year-old boy with otomastoiditis with ossicular destruction ➡ shows a normal appearance of the cochlea ➡. (Right) Axial T2WI FS MR in the same patient 5 days later demonstrates abnormal hypointense signal within the cochlea ➡, vestibule ➡, and internal auditory canal ➡, consistent with early fibroosseous replacement of normal inner ear fluid.

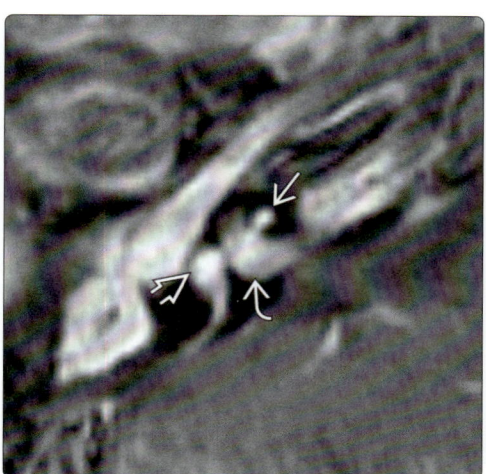
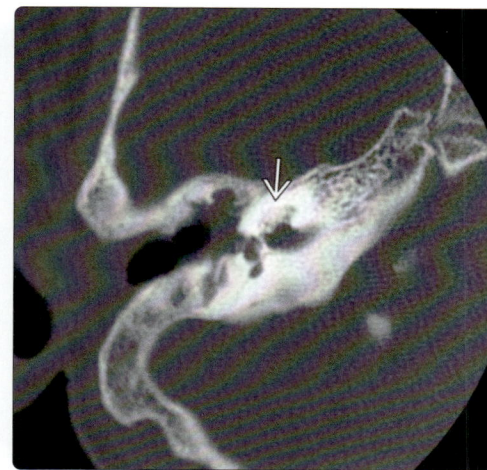

(Left) Axial T1WI C+ FS MR in the same patient shows corresponding abnormal enhancement in the middle ear and mastoid as well as in the cochlea ➡, vestibule ➡, and internal auditory canal (IAC) ➡. (Right) Axial bone CT in the same patient 1 year after the infection shows interval near-complete cochlear ossification ➡, consistent with labyrinthine ossificans (LO).

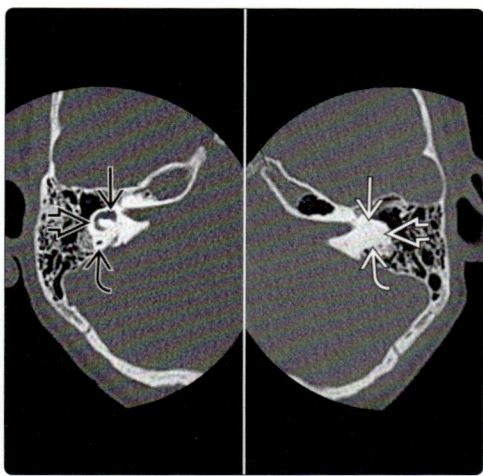
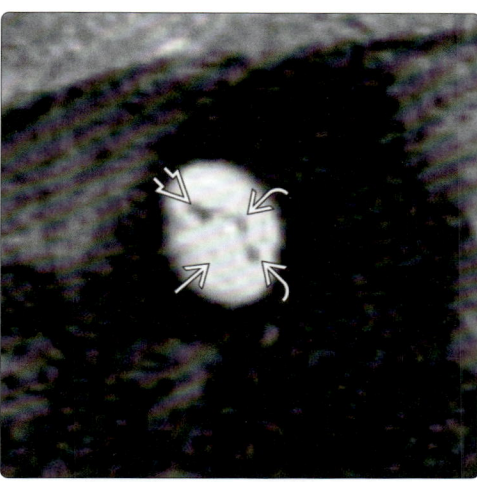

(Left) Axial bone CT in an 8-year-old child with left sensorineural hearing loss shows complete ossification of the left vestibule ➡, lateral semicircular canal ➡, and posterior limb of the posterior semicircular canal ➡. Compare to the normal right side ➡, ➡, ➡, respectively. (Right) Sagittal T2WI MR through the IAC in a patient with ipsilateral severe cochlear LO shows severe atrophy of cochlear nerve ➡ compared with normal facial nerve ➡ and vestibular nerves ➡, a common associated finding in severe LO.

TERMINOLOGY

- Synonym: **Otospongiosis**
- Types: Fenestral (FOto) or cochlear otosclerosis (COto)
  - COto also called retrofenestral otosclerosis
- Pathologic appearance of lytic, spongy bone foci in bony labyrinth of unknown cause
  - Starts perifenestral (FOto), progresses to surround cochlea (FOto + COto)
- **Fissula ante fenestram**: Cleft of fibrocartilaginous tissue between inner & middle ears just anterior to oval window

IMAGING

- Best diagnostic clue: Temporal bone CT shows **lytic (otospongiotic) foci** involving bony labyrinth
- FOto: Lucency limited to anterior margin of oval window (fissula ante fenestram)
  - "Heaped up" new bone may narrow, or later, occlude oval & round windows (obliterative otosclerosis)
- COto: Lucency affects pericochlear bony labyrinth

TOP DIFFERENTIAL DIAGNOSES

- Chronic otitis media with tympanosclerosis
- Temporal bone Paget disease
- Temporal bone fibrous dysplasia
- Temporal bone osteoradionecrosis
- Temporal bone osteogenesis imperfecta

PATHOLOGY

- Enchondral layer of bony labyrinth displays spongy, vascular, decalcified, irregular bone formation

CLINICAL ISSUES

- Young adult with conductive or mixed hearing loss

DIAGNOSTIC CHECKLIST

- Typical otosclerosis is **lytic** & affects **bony** labyrinth
- Report obliterative otosclerosis & anatomic findings impacting surgery: Facial nerve prolapse, semicircular canal dehiscence, vascular anomalies, findings predisposing to gusher

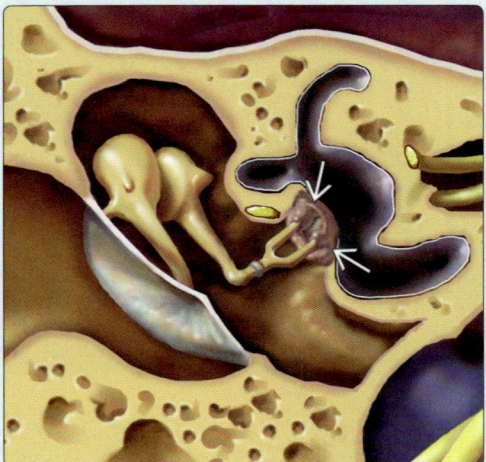
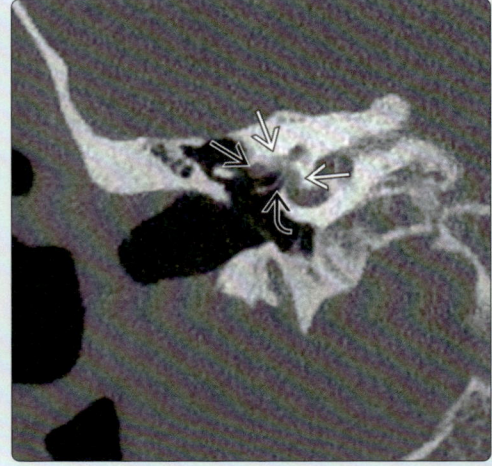

(Left) Coronal graphic illustrates findings of fenestral otosclerosis with a "donut" otospongiotic plaque ➡ surrounding the stapes footplate in the oval window. The crisp margins of the oval window are obscured by plaque. (Right) Coronal bone CT shows a large lucent plaque of fenestral otosclerosis encroaching on the anterior margin of the oval window niche ➡. Stapes is evident ➡ in the oval window. The facial nerve tympanic segment ➡ is normally positioned.

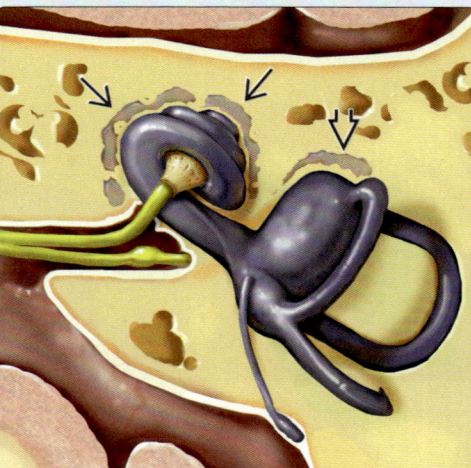
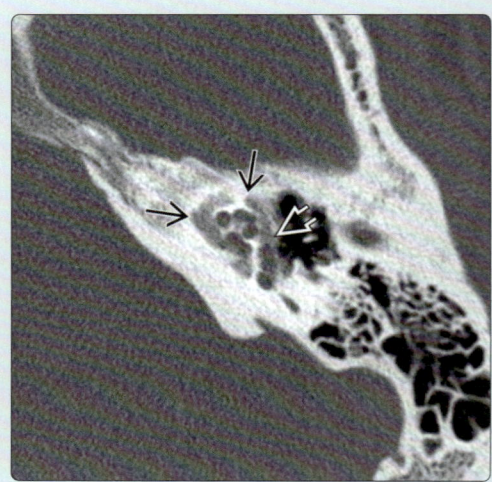

(Left) Axial graphic demonstrates a classic example of cochlear otosclerosis. Note otospongiotic plaques in a halo configuration around the cochlea ➡ with concurrent fenestral otosclerosis ➡. (Right) Axial left temporal bone CT shows cochlear otosclerosis as diffuse osteolytic foci surrounding the cochlea ➡. Concurrent fenestral otosclerosis is noted as bony lucency along cochlear promontory extending from the fissula ante fenestram ➡.

Otosclerosis

TERMINOLOGY

Abbreviations

- Fenestral otosclerosis (FOto), cochlear otosclerosis (COto)

Synonyms

- Otospongiosis; COto also called retrofenestral otosclerosis

Definitions

- Pathologic appearance of **lytic, spongy bone foci** in bony labyrinth of unknown cause
  - Starts perifenestral (FOto), progresses to surround cochlea (FOto + COto)
- **Fissula ante fenestram**: Cleft of fibrocartilaginous tissue between inner & middle ears just anterior to oval window
- Cochlear cleft is fatty marrow due to incomplete ossification that parallels cochlea rather than localizing to fissula antefenestram
  - May normally be present in children & adults, should be differentiated from otosclerosis

IMAGING

General Features

- Best diagnostic clue
  - Temporal bone CT: Lucent (otospongiotic) foci involving bony labyrinth
  - Usually in context of normally aerated middle ear
- Location
  - FOto: Starts at anterior margin of oval window (fissula ante fenestram)
    - Involves any bony area along medial wall middle ear
  - COto: Affects pericochlear bony labyrinth
    - May involve any portion of bony labyrinth
- Size
  - Millimeter punctate or linear foci; may become confluent
- Morphology
  - FOto: Ovoid plaques most common
  - COto: Ovoid to linear (confluent foci)

CT Findings

- CECT
  - No role for CECT in diagnosis of otosclerosis
- Bone CT
  - **Early** temporal bone CT findings
    - Begins as radiolucency at oval window anterior margin (FOto)
    - Spreads to involve all margins of oval & round windows
    - Abnormal thickening of otic capsule bone near oval window (> 2.3 mm) with bulging contour
    - Progressive disease involving any part of bony labyrinth, including internal auditory canal (IAC) lateral walls
    - May spread to inner ear otic capsule (COto)
  - **Late**, chronic (healing phase) temporal bone CT findings
    - FOto: "Heaped up" new bone may narrow or occlude oval & round windows (obliterative otosclerosis)
      - Increases surgical risk & requires drilling to place prosthesis
    - COto: Mixed radiolucent-radiodense foci present in bony labyrinth
      - Double ring sign or "halo" of radiolucency surrounds cochlea in severe COto
  - Associated findings in otosclerosis
    - Facial nerve prolapse (2.7-29.5%) predicts higher surgical complexity
    - IAC diverticulae more common in otosclerosis

MR Findings

- T1WI
  - Faint intermediate T1 signal of plaques
- T2WI
  - Thin-section, high-resolution T2 may not visualize otosclerosis, even when extensive
  - Large plaques can show increased signal
- T1WI C+
  - Enhancing punctate foci in medial wall of middle ear (FOto) ± pericochlear bony labyrinth (COto)
    - Most obvious when FOto & COto combined
  - Enhancing lesions may be seen anywhere in bony labyrinth in severe cases

Imaging Recommendations

- Best imaging tool
  - Temporal bone CT
- Protocol advice
  - T1 C+ MR shows enhancing foci in active phase
  - High-resolution T2 MR may miss otosclerosis

DIFFERENTIAL DIAGNOSIS

Chronic Otitis Media With Tympanosclerosis

- Clinical: Obvious chronic middle ear-mastoid inflammatory disease
- Imaging: Postinflammatory new bone deposition is not limited to oval & round windows as with most FOto
  - Seen in tympanic membrane, middle ear, ossicles, & mastoids
  - New bone deposition is irregular, not smooth, in oval window area

Temporal Bone Paget Disease

- Clinical: Bone disease of old age (> 50 years)
- Imaging: Diffuse skull base involvement is rule
  - Diffuse involvement of bony labyrinth, not only lateral wall
  - Usually diffuse temporal bone cotton wool appearance

Temporal Bone Fibrous Dysplasia

- Clinical: Bone disease of young (age < 30 years)
- Imaging: Involves all parts of temporal bone
  - Relative sparing of inner ear is rule
  - Usually sclerotic, ground-glass appearance

Temporal Bone Osteoradionecrosis

- Clinical: Prior skull base or nasopharynx radiation therapy
- CT: Diffuse, permeative otic capsule lucencies

Temporal Bone Osteogenesis Imperfecta

- Clinical: Blue sclera
- Imaging: Looks like severe COto with more generalized demineralization of bony labyrinth

PATHOLOGY

General Features

- Genetics
  - Sporadic or autosomal dominant gene transmission
- Bony otic capsule development: 3 layers
  - Thin inner endosteal layer
  - **Middle layer** of combined endochondral & intrachondral bone (**otosclerosis occurs here**)
  - Outer periosteal layer
- Normal otosclerosis progression
  - Begins at fissula ante fenestram (FOto)
  - Disease spreads from fissula ante fenestram posteriorly along oval window margins to round window
  - Continued active disease spreads to otic capsule (both FOto & COto present)
- Active **FOto fixes stapes footplate** in oval window niche
  - This "donut" FOto ankyloses stapes footplate
  - Pathophysiology of **conductive hearing loss**
- COto leads to sensorineural hearing loss
  - Best hypothesis: Spiral ligament becomes compromised
  - Secondary hypothesis: Toxic proteases affect cochlear nerve cells
- Etiology: Unknown

Staging, Grading, & Classification

- Symons/Fanning CT grading system of otosclerosis (2005) has high intra- & interobserver agreement
  - Grade 1: Solely fenestral
  - Grade 2: Patchy localized cochlear disease (± FOto)
    - To basal cochlear turn (grade 2A)
    - To middle/apical turns (grade 2B)
  - Grade 3: Diffuse confluent cochlear involvement (± FOto)

Gross Pathologic & Surgical Features

- Otoscopic vascular hue behind tympanic membrane (TM) = **Schwartze sign**
  - Active otosclerotic areas along margins of oval & round windows or beneath cochlear promontory
- Bony ankylosis of stapes footplate is reflected as stapes immobilization when pulled on by surgeon

Microscopic Features

- Enchondral layer of bony labyrinth displays spongy, vascular, decalcified, irregular bone formation
- 3 pathologic phases of otosclerosis
  - Acute phase: Deposition of islets of osteoid tissue
  - Subacute phase: Spongiotic remodeling with osteoclasts causing focal bone resorption
  - Chronic-sclerotic phase: Osteoblasts create new bone with irregular features resembling mosaic
- **Otospongiosis** better describes active disease process
- Chronic, healing phase appears truly **sclerotic**
- May be histologically indistinguishable from Paget disease

CLINICAL ISSUES

Presentation

- Most common signs/symptoms
  - Bilateral progressive conductive (FOto) or mixed (FOto + COto) hearing loss

- Other signs/symptoms
  - Tinnitus (ringing in ears)
  - Otoscopy: Vascular hue behind TM = Schwartze sign
- Clinical profile
  - Young adult presenting with unexplained **bilateral progressive** conductive or **mixed hearing loss**

Demographics

- Epidemiology
  - Occurs in 1% of population
  - Most common type is **FOto alone (85%)**; COto in 15%
  - **FOto** causes ~ **90% conductive hearing loss in adults**
- Sex: M:F = 1:2
- Age: Appears in 2nd to 3rd decades of life

Natural History & Prognosis

- FOto: Conductive hearing loss is progressive
- COto: Untreated, will evolve to profound hearing loss

Treatment

- FOto: **Stapedectomy** with stapes prosthesis
  - Results negatively impacted by concurrent COto
  - If round window is obliterated, stapes prosthesis will fail
  - If narrow oval window niche height (< 1.4 mm on coronal CT reformat), stapes surgery more challenging
- Cochlear implantation
  - Used when severe FOto & COto present bilaterally, resulting in profound mixed hearing loss
  - If round window obliteration present bilaterally, cochlear implantation may be more challenging
- **Fluoride** treatment if COto present
  - Early treatment can arrest progression

DIAGNOSTIC CHECKLIST

Consider

- Always check oval window anterior margin for FOto in CT evaluation of conductive hearing loss
  - Common blind spot; CT findings can be subtle
- If COto present, FOto also is present, so look for it
- MDCT sometimes shows normal fissula ante fenestram on pediatric temporal bone exams as focal radiolucency

Image Interpretation Pearls

- Lucencies within bony labyrinth is typical of otosclerosis
- Bone in membranous labyrinth is **labyrinthine ossificans**

Reporting Tips

- Report findings predicting poor surgical outcome: Obliterative otosclerosis, facial nerve prolapse, semicircular canal dehiscence, aberrant internal carotid artery or persistent stapedial artery, & findings predisposing to stapes gusher

SELECTED REFERENCES

1. Bouatay R et al: Interest of computer tomography in the study of prognostic factors of otosclerosis. Eur Arch Otorhinolaryngol. 281(8):4113-9, 2024
2. Bassiouni M et al: Missed radiological diagnosis of otosclerosis in high-resolution computed tomography of the temporal bone-retrospective analysis of imaging, radiological reports, and request forms. J Clin Med. 12(2):630, 2023
3. Mangia LRL et al: Imaging studies in otosclerosis: an up-to-date comprehensive review. Int Arch Otorhinolaryngol. 25(2):e318-27, 2021

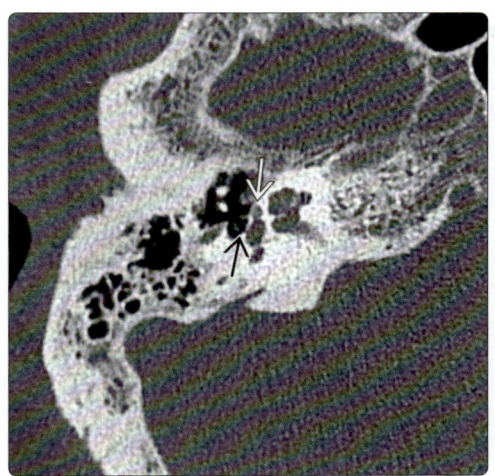
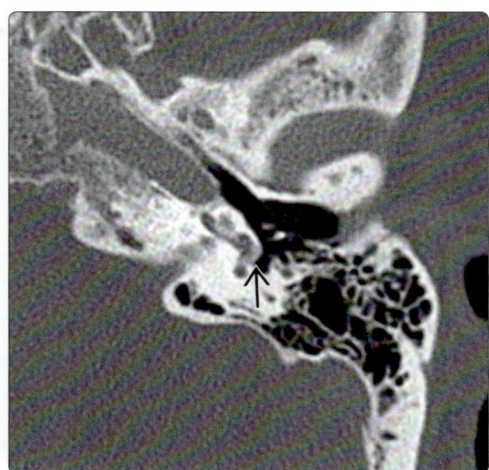

(Left) Axial bone CT shows a well-defined focal lucent plaque isolated to the fissula ante fenestrum typical of fenestral otosclerosis ➡. Stapes crura are visible in the oval window niche ➡. (Right) Axial left temporal bone CT demonstrates mixed lucent and sclerotic otospongiotic plaque overgrowing the round window ("obliterative" otosclerosis) ➡. This makes surgery more challenging, predisposing to stapes prosthesis failure and making cochlear implantation more challenging.

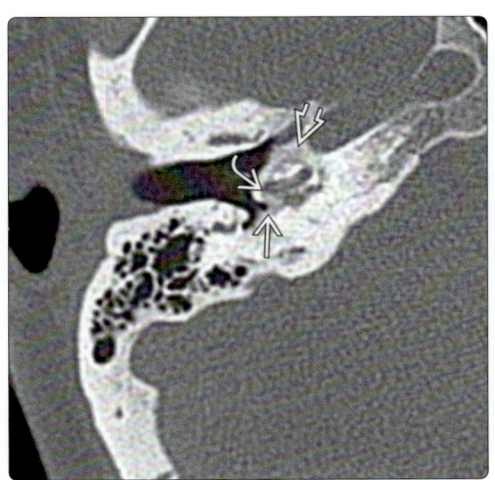
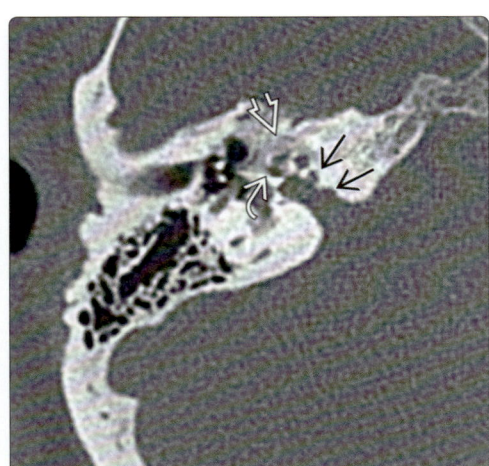

(Left) Axial bone CT shows diffuse pericochlear halo of cochlear otosclerosis ➡ with narrowing of round window due to thickened plaque ➡. Endosteal involvement is indicated by lucency extending membranous cochlea margin ➡. (Right) Axial bone CT shows diffuse pericochlear halo of cochlear otosclerosis ➡. Small internal auditory canal diverticulae ➡ are noted, seen with greater frequency in otosclerosis, and endosteal involvement is seen with lucency extending to the outer margin of the membranous labyrinth ➡.

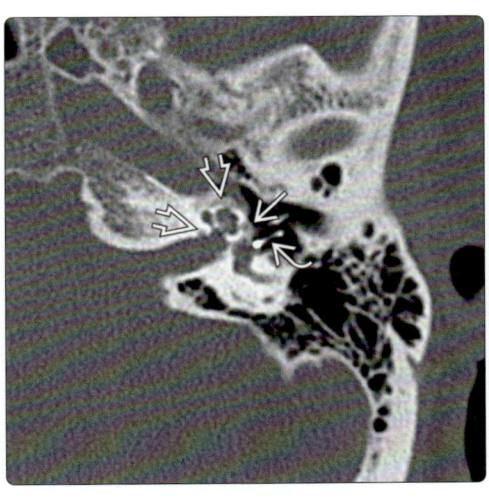
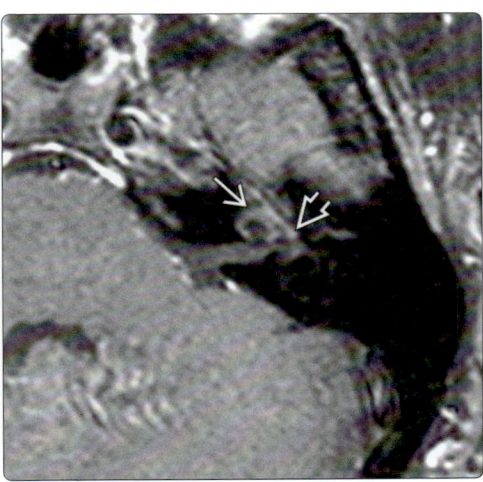

(Left) Axial left temporal bone CT shows typical lytic plaques of combined fenestral ➡ and cochlear otosclerosis ➡. The patient has undergone stapedectomy with insertion of a stapes prosthesis. Note the metallic density stapes prosthesis ➡ at the oval window. (Right) Axial T1WI C+ FS MR in the same patient reveals enhancement anterior to the oval window (fissula ante fenestram) ➡ and surrounding the cochlea ➡, representing active fenestral and cochlear otosclerosis, respectively.

TERMINOLOGY

- Osteogenesis imperfecta (OI): Genetic disorder of collagen & bone that can affect temporal bone & inner ear

IMAGING

- Inner ear: Normal or **progressive otic capsule demineralization** (OI type I)
  - Early: Band-like pericochlear lucency (CT)
  - Late: Lucent otic capsule bone (CT), enhances on MR
- Mastoid & ossicles: Tendency to fracture, deformity
- Skull base & cranium: Diffuse demineralization, **wormian bones**, fractures
- ± jugular vein stenosis & large mastoid emissary veins

TOP DIFFERENTIAL DIAGNOSES

- **Otosclerosis**: Demineralized otic capsule bone, may be indistinguishable from OI
- **Cochlear cleft**: Incidental pericochlear lucency in child

PATHOLOGY

- Most OI is **autosomal dominant** (AD); *COL1A1* or *COL1A2* mutations (95%) → **defective collagen**
- OI type I (AD): **Mild ± later onset; fractures**, ± minimal deformity, **blue sclerae, hearing loss**
- OI type II [AD, autosomal recessive (AR)]: **Perinatal lethality**; osteopenia, severe deformity, multiple fractures
- OI type III (AD, AR): Progressive deformity, short stature, dentinogenesis imperfecta, ± blue sclerae
- OI type IV (AD): Mild/moderate deformity & fracture, mild blue sclerae, dentinogenesis imperfecta, hearing loss

CLINICAL ISSUES

- OI represents heterogeneous group of diseases characterized by bone fragility, fractures, & deformity
- Other manifestations of OI include short stature, blue sclerae, dentinogenesis imperfecta, & **hearing loss (HL)**
- HL in ~ 60%: Conductive, sensorineural HL, or mixed ± vertigo

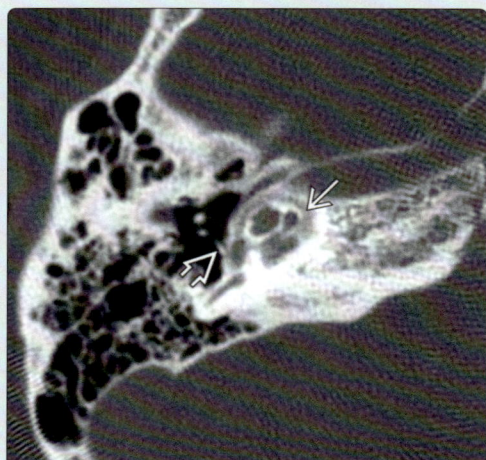
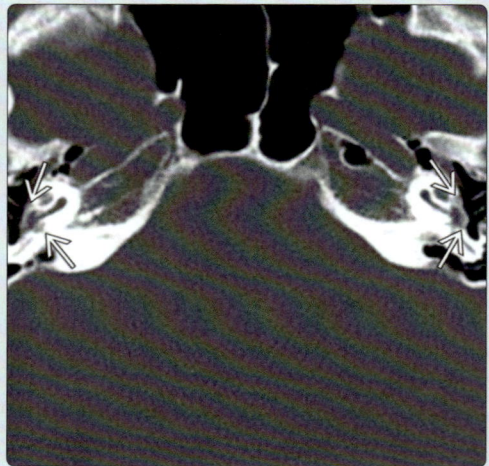

(Left) *Axial right temporal bone CT shows extensive pericochlear otic capsule bony demineralization* ➡ *of the inner ear in a patient with osteogenesis imperfecta (OI). The posterior crus of the stapes is also thickened* ➡. (Right) *Axial bone CT in an adult with known OI shows bilateral, symmetric pericochlear otic capsule demineralization* ➡, *typical of OI, but indistinguishable from otosclerosis by imaging alone.*

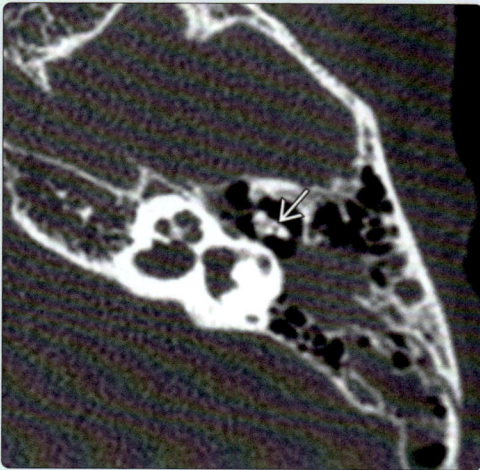
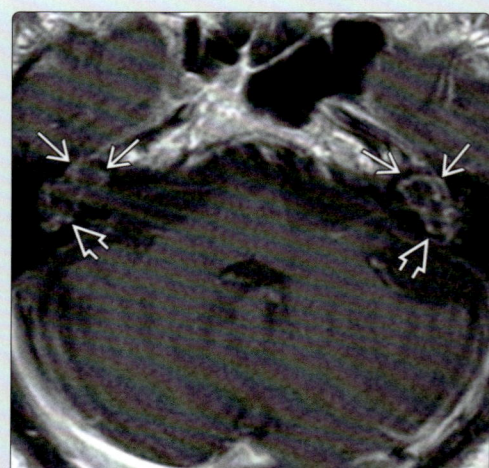

(Left) *Axial bone CT in a 13-year-old boy with OI who fell and hit his head on the ground shows a fracture of the short process of the incus* ➡. *In addition, there were tympanic plate and mastoid fractures.* (Right) *Axial T1 C+ MR in an adult with OI demonstrates left greater than right pericochlear* ➡ *and perivestibular* ➡ *contrast enhancement. There was also corresponding hyperintense signal on T2-weighted images (not shown).*

TERMINOLOGY

Abbreviations
- Osteogenesis imperfecta (OI)

Definitions
- Inherited connective tissue disorder that affects collagen type I biosynthesis
- Heterogeneous group of diseases → by bone fragility, fractures, & deformity
- Other manifestations of OI include blue sclerae, dentinogenesis imperfecta, & hearing loss

IMAGING

General Features
- Best diagnostic clue: Multiple fractures in patient with blue sclerae
  - Demineralization of otic capsule bone indistinguishable from retrofenestral otosclerosis

Imaging Recommendations
- Best imaging tool
  - Temporal bone CT for OI with hearing loss

CT Findings
- Bone CT
  - Skull: Normal or undermineralized ± deformity/fractures, wormian bones, basilar impression
  - External auditory canal (EAC): Normal or mildly stenotic
  - Ossicles: Tendency to fracture
    - Normal or demineralized/deformed stapedial crura
    - Normal or thinning of distal incus long process
  - Inner ear: Normal or progressive otic capsule demineralization (OI type I)
    - Early: Band-like pericochlear lucency
    - Late: Lucent otic capsule bone around cochlea, facial nerve canal, vestibule, & semicircular canal (SCC)
  - ± large mastoid emissary foramina

MR Findings
- Normal or enhancement of abnormal otic capsule bone
- ± hydrocephalus, craniocervical junction (CCJ) stenosis, basilar impression, &/or large emissary veins

DIFFERENTIAL DIAGNOSIS

Nonaccidental Injury
- Unexplained fractures, ± skeletal osteopenia due to nutritional deprivation

Cochlear Otosclerosis
- Demineralization of otic capsule bone, localized without systemic bony involvement

Cochlear Cleft
- Faintly lucent ring around cochlea in patients < 3 years of age; gradually disappears

Paget Disease, Temporal Bone
- ± asymmetric petrous bone demineralization in association with other skull & skeletal findings

Otosyphilis
- Moth-eaten permeative inflammatory resorptive osteitis, labyrinthitis, internal auditory canal (IAC) gummatous lesion, demineralized ossicles

PATHOLOGY

General Features
- Etiology
  - Genetic mutation → ↓ amount of structurally normal collagen ± ↑ in structurally abnormal collagen
  - Mutations involve genes responsible for synthesis or intracellular processing of collagen
- Genetics
  - Autosomal dominant (AD), de novo genetic mutation, or autosomal recessive (AR)
  - *COL1A1* (chromosome 17) or *COL1A2* (chromosome 7) mutations (95%)
    - Encodes type I collagen: Most abundant protein in body, major bone protein; OI types I-IV (AD ± AR)
  - Mutations in encoding genes (e.g., *CRTAP*) that modify intracellular processing of collagen: AR, severe or lethal
    - OI types VII & VIII

Staging, Grading, & Classification
- **OI type I** (AD): **Fractures**, minimal to no deformity, **blue sclerae** ± normal stature, **hearing loss**
  - **Mild phenotype**: Fractures peak in **childhood**, post menopausal (women), & 6th decade (men)
- **OI type II** (AD, AR): Osteopenia, severe deformity, multiple fractures, platyspondyly, beaded ribs, hearing loss
  - **Severe lethal** perinatal **form**
- **OI type III** (AD, AR): Progressive deformity, very short stature, dentinogenesis imperfecta, variable scleral hue
  - **Evident at birth**
- **OI type IV** (AD): Mild/moderate deformity & fracture, variable short stature, mild blue sclerae, dentinogenesis imperfecta, hearing loss
  - **Milder phenotype**
- **OI type V** (AD): Like type IV, Ca^{++} forearm interosseous membrane, dislocated radial head, hyperplastic callus

Microscopic Features
- Deficient & abnormal ossification: Otic capsule, middle ear walls, mastoid septa & ossicles

CLINICAL ISSUES

Presentation
- Most common signs/symptoms
  - **Multiple fractures from minimal trauma**
  - Osteopenia & deformity; short stature, joint laxity
  - Blue sclerae
  - Hearing loss in 2/3 patients; multifactorial
    - Imaging abnormalities have poor correlation with presence or absence of hearing loss

SELECTED REFERENCES

1. Cannalire G et al: Osteoporosis and bone fragility in children: diagnostic and treatment strategies. J Clin Med. 13(16):4951, 2024
2. Gazzotti S et al: Imaging in osteogenesis imperfecta: where we are and where we are going. Eur J Med Genet. 68:104926, 2024

KEY FACTS

TERMINOLOGY

- Intralabyrinthine schwannoma (ILS): Benign tumor arising from Schwann cells within structures of membranous labyrinth

IMAGING

- T1 C+ MR: Focal enhancing mass in membranous labyrinth
- High-resolution T2 MR: Filling defect within hyperintense perilymph
- Focal intralabyrinthine mass named by location
  - **Intracochlear**: Schwannoma within cochlea
  - **Intravestibular**: Within vestibule of inner ear
  - **Vestibulocochlear**: Involves both vestibule & cochlea
  - **Transmodiolar**: Crosses modiolus from cochlea to fundus of internal auditory canal (IAC)
  - **Transmacular**: Crosses from vestibule into fundus of IAC
  - **Transotic**: Involves inner ear, fundus of IAC to middle ear
- Use focused T1 C+ or high-resolution T2 imaging (SPACE, CISS, FIESTA, 3D-TSE) of CPA-IAC to make diagnosis of ILS

TOP DIFFERENTIAL DIAGNOSES

- Labyrinthitis, labyrinthine ossificans
- Intralabyrinthine hemorrhage
- Facial nerve schwannoma with inner ear dehiscence
- Intralabyrinthine lipoma

CLINICAL ISSUES

- Tumor location-specific symptoms
  - When in vestibule: Tinnitus, episodic vertigo with nausea & vomiting, mixed hearing loss
  - When in cochlea: Slowly progressive sensorineural hearing loss
- Conservative management vs. surgical resection
  - Removal if disabling symptoms (intractable vertigo)

DIAGNOSTIC CHECKLIST

- When visually interrogating MRs to "rule out acoustic schwannoma," remember to carefully evaluate inner ear fluid spaces for ILS

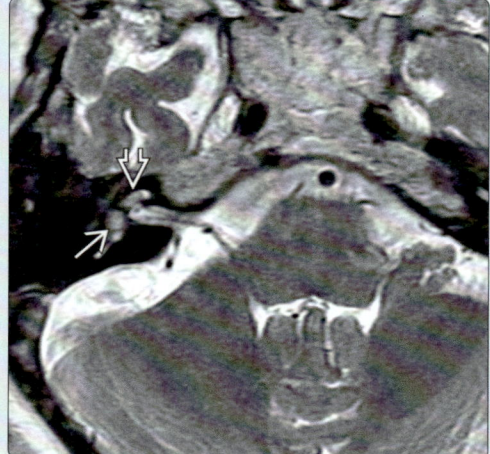
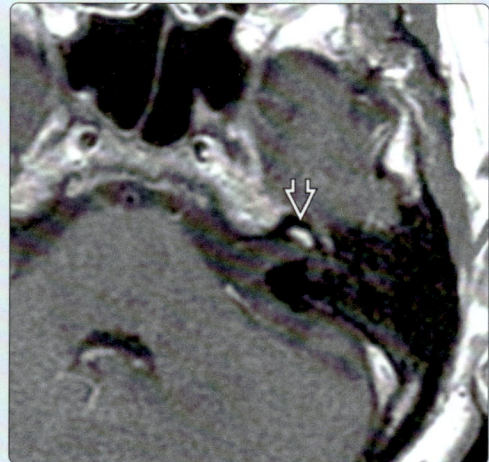

(Left) Axial T2WI MR shows a classic example of an intralabyrinthine schwannoma (ILS). This is a vestibulocochlear type, as it involves both the vestibule ➡ and cochlea ⮕. Note soft tissue intensity replacing the normal fluid signal of the membranous labyrinth. (Right) Axial T1WI C+ MR shows an intracochlear schwannoma as focal enhancement of the cochlea ⮕. It is important to review precontrast T1 & T2 images to exclude intralabyrinthine hemorrhage, lipoma, & labyrinthitis, which may mimic this tumor.

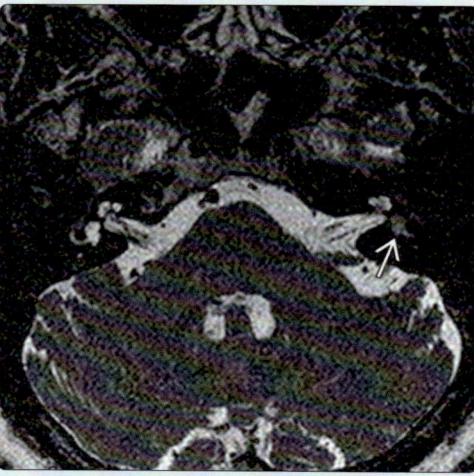
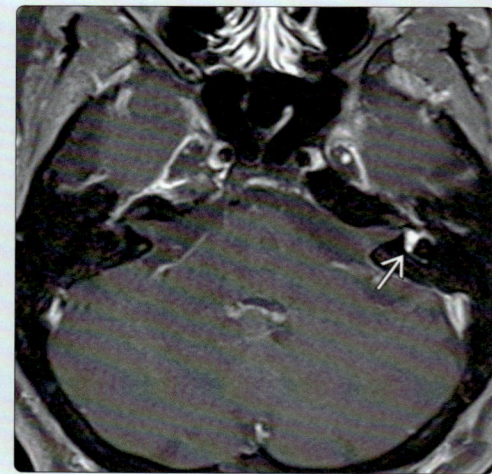

(Left) Axial T2 SPACE MR shows a soft tissue filling defect ➡ in the left vestibule replacing the normal high-intensity perilymphatic fluid. This intravestibular type of ILS often presents with vertigo or tinnitus. (Right) Axial T1WI C+ MR in the same patient shows intense enhancement of this intravestibular schwannoma ➡. When these tumors are small, they may be treated conservatively unless the patient has intractable vertigo or the tumor shows signs of interval growth.

Intralabyrinthine Schwannoma

TERMINOLOGY

Abbreviations
- Intralabyrinthine schwannoma (ILS)

Synonyms
- Inner ear schwannoma

Definitions
- ILS: Benign tumor arising from Schwann cells within structures of membranous labyrinth
  - Includes schwannomas of cochlea, vestibule, or both as well as tumors of inner ear extending to internal auditory canal (IAC) or middle ear

IMAGING

General Features
- Best diagnostic clue
  - T1 C+ MR: Focal enhancing mass in membranous labyrinth
  - High-resolution T2 MR: Filling defect within hyperintense perilymph
- Location
  - Focal intralabyrinthine mass named by location
    - **Intracochlear**: Schwannoma within cochlea
    - **Intravestibular**: Schwannoma within vestibule of inner ear
    - **Vestibulocochlear**: Schwannoma involves both vestibule & cochlea
    - **Transmodiolar**: Schwannoma crosses modiolus from cochlea to fundus of IAC
    - **Transmacular**: Schwannoma crosses from vestibule into fundus of IAC
    - **Transotic**: Schwannoma crosses entire inner ear from fundus of IAC to middle ear
- Size
  - Usually remains in millimeter range within membranous labyrinth
  - Larger lesions extend extralabyrinthine
- Morphology
  - Early, small lesions are ovoid to round
  - Older, larger lesions take on shape of portion of membranous labyrinth affected

CT Findings
- NECT
  - Typically normal, ILS not seen
- CECT
  - ILS not visible on CECT even if thin sections obtained
- Bone CT
  - Normal, unless mass projects into middle ear through round window niche
  - In very large lesions (transmodiolar, transmacular, transotic), bone erosion may be visible
  - Bone CT usually not helpful in making this diagnosis

MR Findings
- T1WI
  - Soft tissue intensity material in inner ear
  - May be mildly hyperintense to fluid of labyrinth
  - Not seen unless larger lesion is present & thinner sections are obtained
- T2WI
  - Focal low-signal mass within high-signal fluid of membranous labyrinth
- FLAIR
  - Hyperintense signal on delayed 3D-FLAIR
- T1WI C+
  - Homogeneous enhancement of ILS
  - ILS may project multiple directions from inner ear
    - Through round window into middle ear
    - Along vestibular nerve branches into fundus of IAC = transmacular ILS
    - Through modiolus & cochlear nerve canal into IAC = transmodiolar ILS

Imaging Recommendations
- Use focused T1 C+ or high-resolution T2 imaging (i.e., SPACE, CISS, FIESTA, 3D-TSE) of cerebellopontine angle (CPA)-IAC to make diagnosis of ILS
- Careful examination of all "rule out acoustic schwannoma" MR scans for presence of intralabyrinthine mass is critical
- Observe precise location of tumor
  - Consider if it involves vestibule, cochlea, or both
  - Consider if it projects into middle ear or IAC fundus
- All patients undergoing surgery for Ménière disease should undergo preoperative focused MR to exclude ILS

DIFFERENTIAL DIAGNOSIS

Labyrinthitis
- Clinical: Acute onset of sensorineural hearing loss (SNHL) ± vertigo & facial neuropathy
- High-resolution T2 MR: No soft tissue intensity mass seen within high-signal inner ear fluid
- T1 C+ MR: Enhancement of most or all of membranous labyrinth

Labyrinthine Ossificans
- Clinical: History of previous meningitis or suppurative middle ear-mastoiditis
- High-resolution T2 MR: Focal low-signal areas within high-signal inner ear fluid; when fibroosseous, may mimic ILS
- T1 C+ MR: Minimal or no inner ear enhancement
- Bone CT: Encroachment on fluid of membranous labyrinth by bone

Intralabyrinthine Hemorrhage
- Clinical: Unilateral sudden onset of SNHL
- T1 MR: High-signal fluid within membranous labyrinth

Facial Nerve Schwannoma With Dehiscence Into Inner Ear
- Clinical: SNHL with associated facial neuropathy
- T1 C+ MR: Enhancing tubular mass follows course of intratemporal facial nerve canal
  - Involvement of inner ear is secondary finding
- Bone CT: Smooth enlargement of intratemporal facial nerve canal

Intralabyrinthine Lipoma
- Clinical: Hearing loss or asymptomatic
- T1 MR: High-signal fat in vestibule or cochlea

PATHOLOGY

General Features

- Etiology
  - Tumor arises from Schwann cells wrapping distal vestibular or cochlear nerve axons within membranous labyrinth
  - Secondary endolymphatic hydrops explains Ménière symptoms
- Same pathology as other schwannomas in human body
- Intracochlear is most common type of ILS

Gross Pathologic & Surgical Features

- Tan-gray, encapsulated mass found within labyrinth

Microscopic Features

- Differentiated neoplastic Schwann cells
- Antoni A: Areas of compact, elongated cells
- Antoni B: Less densely cellular areas with tumor loosely arranged, ± clusters of lipid-laden cells
- Strong, diffuse expression of S100 protein

CLINICAL ISSUES

Presentation

- Most common signs/symptoms
  - Unilateral SNHL
    - Sudden onset of SNHL is extremely rare
  - Tumor location-specific symptoms
    - When in vestibule: Tinnitus, episodic vertigo with nausea & vomiting, mixed hearing loss (tumor impedes stapes footplate, creating element of conductive hearing loss)
    - When in cochlea: Slowly progressive SNHL
- Clinical profile
  - Unilateral SNHL that develops over decades

Demographics

- Age
  - Adults > 40
- Sex
  - No sex predilection
- Epidemiology
  - Rare lesion
  - Perhaps 100x less common than CPA-IAC vestibular schwannoma

Natural History & Prognosis

- Very slow-growing, benign tumor of membranous labyrinth
- History of progressive hearing loss may date back 20 years
- Often grows to fill inner ear, then stops growing
- Total deafness in ear will result eventually if untreated
- Deafness certain if tumor removed

Treatment

- Conservative management
  - Watchful waiting
  - Applied when symptoms are minor (serviceable hearing maintained) & tumor is confined to inner ear
- Surgical removal
  - Translabyrinthine surgery removes tumor in vestibule
- Transotic surgery completed for tumors involving cochlea or middle ear
- Completed if symptoms are disabling
  - Usually when there is intractable vertigo
- If transmodiolar or transmacular extension is significant, middle cranial fossa approach may be used
- Cochlear implantation in patients with severe hearing loss
- Placement of cochlear implant
  - May be done ± tumor removal with positive results

DIAGNOSTIC CHECKLIST

Consider

- ILS may be missed by excellent radiologists because they are not aware of its existence
- ILS now being diagnosed more often with high-resolution T2 imaging (CISS, FIESTA, 3D-TSE)
  - Increased diagnosis in part secondary to increased awareness of this lesion
  - Some ILS do not enhance robustly but can be seen on high-resolution T2 MR

Image Interpretation Pearls

- When visually interrogating MRs to "rule out acoustic schwannoma," remember to carefully evaluate inner ear fluid spaces for ILS
  - Unless radiologists specifically look at inner ear for focal lesions, ILS will be missed
- Once ILS is suspected, use high-resolution T2 MR to differentiate ILS from labyrinthitis
  - ILS will appear as soft tissue intensity lesion within high-signal inner ear fluid
  - Labyrinthitis will show no focal mass within high-signal inner ear fluid

SELECTED REFERENCES

1. Plontke SK et al: Revised classification of inner ear schwannomas. Otol Neurotol. 46(1):3-9, 2025
2. Hershey E et al: Changing management of intravestibular schwannomas in the era of cochlear implantation for single-sided deafness. Otol Neurotol. 45(4):e337-41, 2024
3. Liaci E et al: Pediatric intracochlear schwannoma: case series and review of the literature. J Int Adv Otol. 20(6):484-8, 2024
4. Wang K et al: Cochlear implant outcomes in patients with intralabyrinthine schwannoma: a scoping review. Laryngoscope. 134(9):3910-20, 2024
5. Kurata N et al: Advanced magnetic resonance imaging sheds light on the distinct pathophysiology of various types of acute sensorineural hearing loss. Otol Neurotol. 44(7):656-63, 2023
6. Bagattini M et al: Histopathologic evaluation of intralabyrinthine schwannoma. Audiol Neurootol. 26(4):265-72, 2021
7. Totten DJ et al: Management of vestibular dysfunction and hearing loss in intralabyrinthine schwannomas. Am J Otolaryngol. 42(4):102984, 2021
8. Cho SJ et al: Diagnostic assessment of magnetic resonance imaging for patients with intralabyrinthine schwannoma: a systematic review. J Neuroradiol. 49(1):41-6, 2020
9. Choudhury B et al: Intralabyrinthine schwannomas: disease presentation, tumor management, and hearing rehabilitation. J Neurol Surg B Skull Base. 80(2):196-202, 2019
10. Bae YJ et al: Differentiation between intralabyrinthine schwannoma and contrast-enhancing labyrinthitis on MRI: quantitative analysis of signal intensity Characteristics. Otol Neurotol. 39(8):1045-52, 2018
11. Gosselin É et al: Meta-analysis on the clinical outcomes in patients with intralabyrinthine schwannomas: conservative management vs. microsurgery. Eur Arch Otorhinolaryngol. 273(6):1357-67, 2015
12. Salzman KL et al: Intralabyrinthine schwannomas: imaging diagnosis and classification. AJNR Am J Neuroradiol. 33(1):104-9, 2012

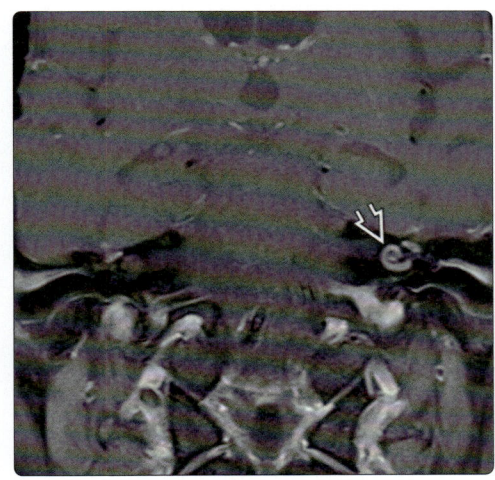
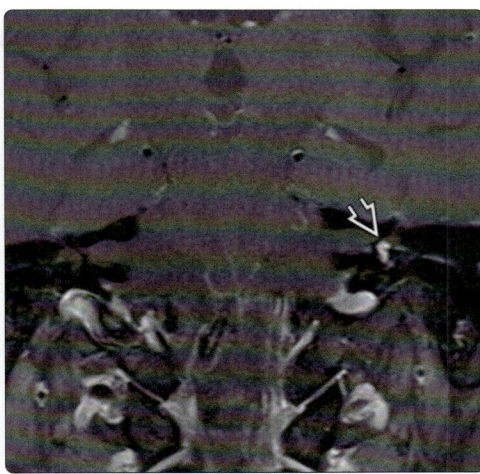

(Left) *Coronal T1WI C+ FS MR shows enhancement of the cochlea ➥, suggesting an intracochlear schwannoma, the most common type of ILS. It is important to review precontrast T1 images to exclude intralabyrinthine hemorrhage or lipoma.* **(Right)** *Coronal T1WI C+ FS MR in the same patient shows enhancement of the vestibule ➥, revealing this to be a vestibulocochlear schwannoma. These rare tumors may result in hearing loss &/or vestibular symptoms.*

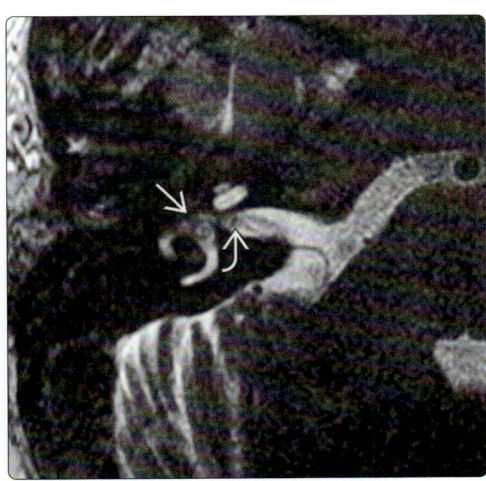
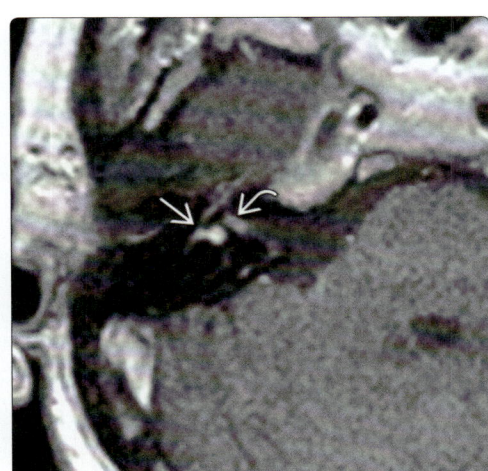

(Left) *Axial T2WI MR shows a transmacular type of ILS as soft tissue intensity material filling the vestibule ➥ & coursing along the vestibular nerve branches into the distal fundus ➥ of the internal auditory canal (IAC).* **(Right)** *Axial T1WI C+ MR in the same patient shows enhancement of both the intravestibular ➥ & distal intracanalicular portion ➥ of this transmacular schwannoma. The slight difference in enhancement characteristics is related to volume averaging.*

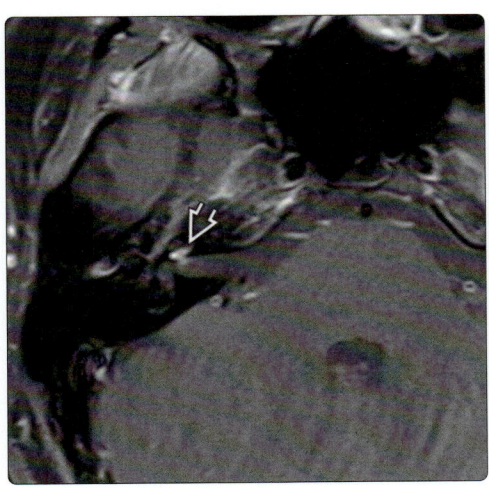
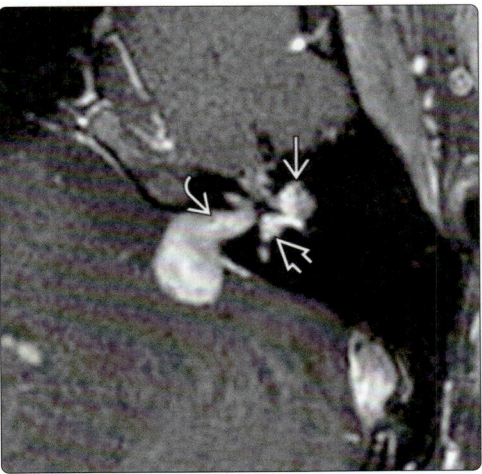

(Left) *Axial T1WI C+ MR shows enhancement of the cochlea ➥ & distal IAC fundus in this transmodiolar type of ILS. This tumor grew from the cochlea through the modiolus & cochlear nerve canal to reach the IAC fundus. These tumors are being recognized more frequently with the use of high-resolution T2 MR & increased awareness of the lesion.* **(Right)** *Axial T1WI C+ FS MR shows the very rare transotic type of ILS. Note the enhancing tumor extends from the cerebellopontine angle through the IAC ➥, involving inner ear ➥ & middle ear ➥.*

Endolymphatic Sac Tumor

TERMINOLOGY

- Endolymphatic sac tumor (ELST)
- Papillary cystadenomatous tumor of ELS
  - Originates from epithelium of endolymphatic sac

IMAGING

- Location: Centered in **fovea of ELS** in presigmoid, posterior surface petrous T-bone
- CT findings
  - **Permeative-destructive** retrolabyrinthine mass
  - Central, spiculated tumor **Ca^{++}** (100%)
  - Thin, **calcified rim** at posterior tumor margin
- MR findings
  - T1-hyperintense foci in 80%
  - Inhomogeneous T2 signal
  - Heterogeneous enhancement
- Angiographic findings
  - Tumors < 3 cm supplied by ECA branches
  - Tumors > 3 cm also recruit ICA branches

TOP DIFFERENTIAL DIAGNOSES

- Petrous apex cholesterol granuloma
- Jugular paraganglioma
- Petrous apex meningioma
- T-bone metastasis

PATHOLOGY

- Sporadic occurrence more common than von Hippel-Lindau disease (VHL)-associated ELST
  - **15% of VHL patients** develop **ELST**, 30% bilateral
- VHL
  - Cerebellar & spinal cord hemangioblastoma, renal cell carcinoma, pheochromocytoma
  - Kidney & pancreas cysts

CLINICAL ISSUES

- Sensorineural hearing loss most common symptom
- Treatment: Complete surgical resection
- If sporadic ELST, check patient & family for VHL

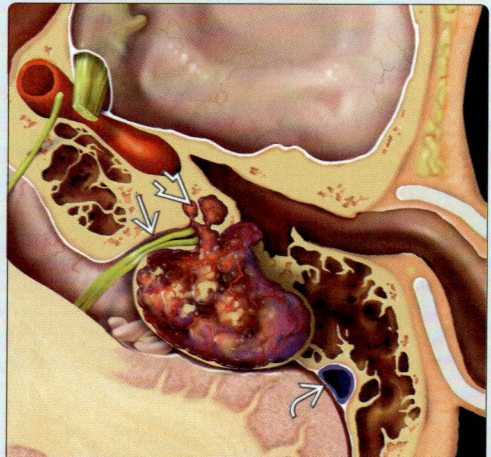
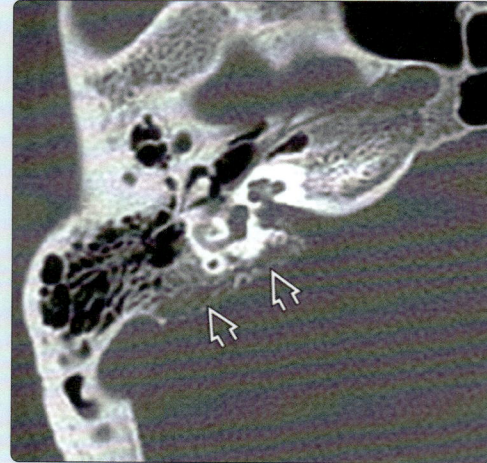

(Left) Axial graphic of T-bone illustrates typical appearance of endolymphatic sac tumor (ELST). Important features include its vascular nature, tendency to fistulize in inner ear ➡, & bone fragments within tumor matrix. Note the classic retrolabyrinthine location between the internal auditory canal (IAC) ➡ and sigmoid sinus ➡. (Right) Axial bone CT shows imaging features of ELST, including tumor centered in posterior T-bone in area of fovea of the endolymphatic sac, spiculated tumor matrix Ca^{++} ➡, and permeative bone changes.

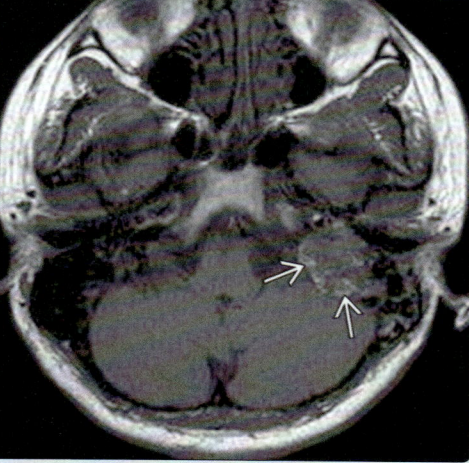
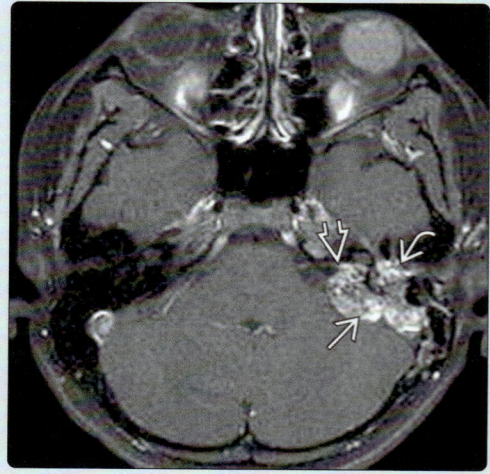

(Left) Axial T1WI MR shows an expansile, lobular mass centered in the left T-bone with areas of ↑ T1 signal, which are common in ELST and are typically peripheral in location ➡. (Right) Axial T1WI C+ FS MR in the same patient reveals the typical intense, heterogeneous contrast enhancement ➡ expected in ELST. This tumor has also grown into the left IAC ➡, middle ear ➡, & mastoid. Note diffuse abnormal signal in the left globe, indicating retinal angioma with detachment seen in von Hippel-Lindau disease.

Endolymphatic Sac Tumor

TERMINOLOGY

Abbreviations

- Endolymphatic sac tumor (ELST)

Synonyms

- Adenomatous tumor of ELS, Heffner tumor

Definitions

- Papillary cystadenomatous tumor of ELS
  - Originates from epithelium of ELS & duct

IMAGING

General Features

- Best diagnostic clue
  - Bone CT: Central intratumoral **bone spicules** & **posterior rim Ca++**
  - MR: **High-signal** foci on **unenhanced T1**
- Location
  - **Retrolabyrinthine**: Posteromedial T-bone
  - Centered in **fovea of ELS** in presigmoid, posterior surface petrous T-bone
- Size
  - Variable but often small & detected earlier with von Hippel-Lindau disease (VHL) screening
- Morphology
  - Infiltrative, poorly circumscribed lesion

CT Findings

- Bone CT
  - **Permeative-destructive** retrolabyrinthine mass
    - Central, spiculated tumor **Ca++ (100%)**
    - Thin, **calcified rim**, posterior margin tumor

MR Findings

- T1WI
  - **Hyperintense foci** in **80%**
    - Hemorrhage, cholesterol cleft
  - Tumors > 2 cm may have **flow voids**
- T2WI
  - Inhomogeneous signal from bone fragments & cysts
- T1WI C+
  - Heterogeneous enhancement

Angiographic Findings

- Tumors < 3 cm supplied by external carotid artery branches
- Tumors > 3 cm also recruit internal carotid artery (ICA) branches

Nuclear Medicine Findings

- Ga-68 DOTATATE PET/CT: Tumor may show ↑ uptake secondary to somatostatin receptors

Imaging Recommendations

- Best imaging tool
  - Bone CT & T1 C+ MR (both necessary)

DIFFERENTIAL DIAGNOSIS

Petrous Apex Cholesterol Granuloma

- Bone CT: Smooth, expansile margins
- MR: Entire lesion has ↑ signal on T1 & T2

Petrous Apex Meningioma

- Bone CT: Scalloped margins ± hyperostosis ± permeative sclerotic bones
- MR: T1 C+ homogeneous enhancement; dural tail; ↓ T2 signal intensity

Jugular Paraganglioma

- Bone CT: Permeative-destructive bone invasion without spicules
- MR: ↑ T1 foci rare; T2 flow voids very common

T-Bone Metastasis

- History of primary tumor

PATHOLOGY

General Features

- Genetics
  - Sporadic > VHL ELST
  - *VHL* tumor suppressor gene mutated in both
- Associated abnormalities
  - VHL disease
  - 15% of VHL patients develop ELST, 30% bilateral

Gross Pathologic & Surgical Features

- Heaped up tumor on posterior wall of T-bone

CLINICAL ISSUES

Presentation

- Most common signs/symptoms
  - Sensorineural hearing loss > tinnitus
- Other signs/symptoms
  - Vertigo (mimics Ménière disease), ataxia
  - Facial nerve palsy

Demographics

- Age
  - Sporadic: 40-50 years; VHL: 30 years

Natural History & Prognosis

- Prognosis excellent with complete surgical resection
  - VHL ELST found earlier (annual MR screening)
- Late recurrence possible so follow-up imaging recommended

Treatment

- Complete surgical resection
  - Preoperative embolization for larger lesions
- Radiation therapy if unresectable or nonsurgical candidate

DIAGNOSTIC CHECKLIST

Consider

- Bilateral ELST = VHL diagnosis
- If sporadic ELST, check patient & family for VHL

Image Interpretation Pearls

- Posterior wall T-bone **tumor with ↑ T1 foci = ELST**

SELECTED REFERENCES

1. Blandino A et al: Endolymphatic sac tumor. Post-radiosurgery evaluation using time-resolved imaging of contrast kinetics MR angiography. Ear Nose Throat J. ePub, 2025

Intralabyrinthine Hemorrhage

TERMINOLOGY

- Blood within normally fluid-filled spaces of labyrinth

IMAGING

- T1 MR: **High signal** within normally fluid-filled space of labyrinth
  - Shortened T1 relaxation time caused by intra-/extracellular methemoglobin
- FLAIR: Abnormal ↑ signal in labyrinth
- T2 MR: Variable depending on age of hemorrhage
- T1 C+: High signal, not to be confused with enhancement
- T1 FS: High inner ear signal remains on fat-saturated images, excludes rare intralabyrinthine lipoma

TOP DIFFERENTIAL DIAGNOSES

- Labyrinthitis
- Vestibular schwannoma
- Intralabyrinthine schwannoma
- Congenital intralabyrinthine lipoma

CLINICAL ISSUES

- Presentation: Acute onset of unilateral sensorineural hearing loss
  - May be accompanied by vertigo
- History: Anticoagulant therapy, sickle cell disease, hematologic disorder or trauma
- Prognosis: Recovery of hearing is generally poor
- Treatment: IV or intratympanic steroids may be of benefit

DIAGNOSTIC CHECKLIST

- Always perform unenhanced T1 MR and evaluate for evidence of intralabyrinthine hyperintensity
- Differentiate from intralabyrinthine lipoma with fat-saturated images
- For patients with sudden sensorineural hearing loss, MR findings, including intralabyrinthine hemorrhage, are rare

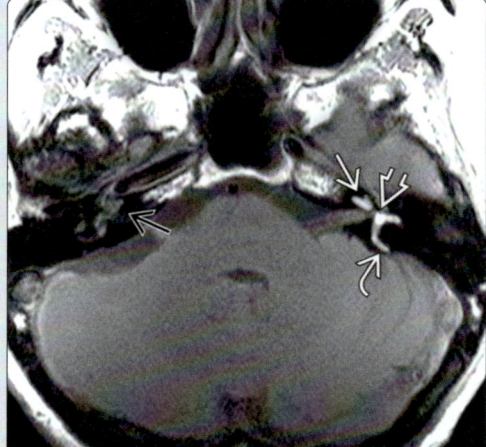
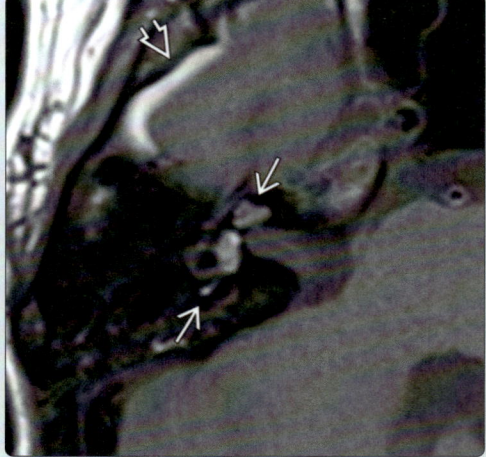

(Left) Axial T1 MR at the level of the internal auditory canals shows hyperintense signal in the left cochlea ➡, vestibule ➡, and semicircular canals ➡, representing intralabyrinthine hemorrhage (ILH). Compare to normal T1-hypointense fluid signal in the right labyrinth ➡. (Right) Axial T1 MR shows increased T1 hyperintensity within the right labyrinthine ➡, consistent with ILH. Note additional T1-hyperintense subdural hematoma ➡ in this patient with traumatic ILH.

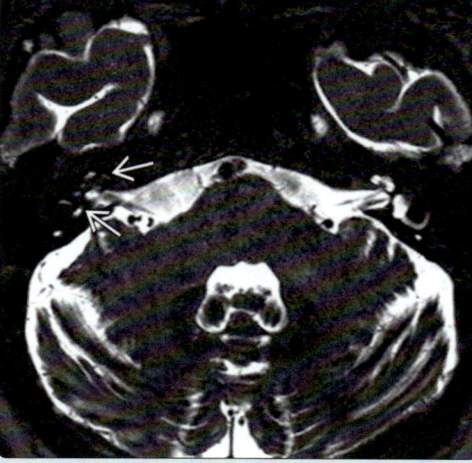
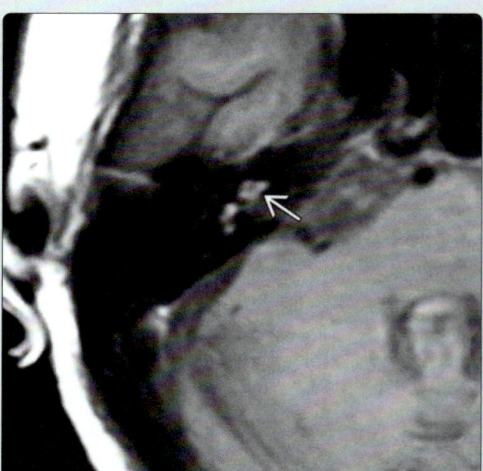

(Left) Axial T2 MR in a 76-year-old with multiple myeloma and sudden right sensorineural hearing loss and vertigo shows patchy loss of signal ➡ in the right cochlea, vestibule, and semicircular canals. (Right) Axial T1 MR in the same patient shows diffuse hyperintensity ➡ of the cochlea and vestibule, compatible with ILH. FLAIR images (not shown) also demonstrated patchy, abnormal, hyperintense signal of the right inner ear.

TERMINOLOGY

Abbreviations

- Intralabyrinthine hemorrhage (ILH)

Synonyms

- Inner ear (IE) hemorrhage, labyrinthine hemorrhage

Definitions

- Blood within normally fluid-filled spaces of labyrinth

IMAGING

General Features

- Best diagnostic clue
  - **Hyperintense signal** on T1 unenhanced MR of IE
    - IE fluid normally isointense with CSF
    - Highly proteinaceous IE contents may have identical appearance

MR Findings

- T1WI
  - High signal within normally fluid-filled space of labyrinth on unenhanced T1
    - IE normally low signal (fluid intensity)
  - T1 hyperintensity generally resolves by 3-4 months
- T2WI
  - Variable: May be high or low depending on hemorrhage age
- FLAIR
  - Hyperintense signal within labyrinth is identified
- T1WI C+
  - Hyperintense signal in IE is generally unchanged compared to unenhanced T1

Imaging Recommendations

- Protocol advice
  - If abnormal hyperintensity in IE is encountered on postcontrast imaging, correlation with unenhanced T1 images recommended to evaluate for intrinsic T1 hyperintense lesion, such as subacute hemorrhage, proteinaceous fluid related to labyrinthitis, or rare intralabyrinthine lipoma

DIFFERENTIAL DIAGNOSIS

Labyrinthitis

- T1 C+ MR high signal (enhancement)
  - Focal or diffuse, usually faint
- Unenhanced T1 usually normal
- Some infectious or inflammatory processes in IE might actually cause hemorrhage

Vestibular Schwannoma

- Intralabyrinthine ↑ signal on unenhanced T1 MR from high protein content
  - Postoperative cochlear FLAIR hyperintensity correlates with worse hearing outcomes

Intralabyrinthine Schwannoma

- T1 C+ MR ↑ signal (focal intense enhancement)

Congenital Intralabyrinthine Lipoma

- Unenhanced T1 ↑ signal may appear identical

- T1 fat saturated: Lesion no longer seen (saturates)

PATHOLOGY

General Features

- Etiology
  - Trauma or surgery
  - Anticoagulant therapy
  - Hematologic conditions: Leukemia, sickle cell anemia, other hyperviscosity syndromes
  - Neoplasm: Endolymphatic sac tumors, sporadic or von Hippel-Lindau related

CLINICAL ISSUES

Presentation

- Symptoms: **Acute-onset unilateral sensorineural hearing loss (SNHL)**
  - Sudden hearing loss: Hearing loss that has evolved over hours to days
  - At least 30-decibel ↓ in threshold in 3 contiguous test frequencies over 24- to 72-hour period
- Other signs/symptoms: Vertigo, tinnitus

Demographics

- Age
  - Possible at any age
- Ethnicity
  - Spontaneous ILH more common in Black patients due to ↑ incidence in sickle cell disease

Natural History & Prognosis

- ILH is generally associated with profound SNHL with unsatisfactory recovery

Treatment

- Early treatment with IV corticosteroid may have some benefit
- Intratympanic corticosteroids advocated by some as potential salvage therapy

DIAGNOSTIC CHECKLIST

Consider

- **Intravestibular lipoma** also has ↑ unenhanced T1 signal
  - Will lose its signal (saturate) on fat-saturated images

Image Interpretation Pearls

- Always perform unenhanced T1 and evaluate for evidence of intralabyrinthine high signal

SELECTED REFERENCES

1. Laredo J et al: Vestibular dysfunction in patients with sickle cell disease: a systematic review. Otol Neurotol. 45(10):1098-107, 2024
2. Kim MB et al: Anatomical and pathological findings of magnetic resonance imaging in idiopathic sudden sensorineural hearing loss. J Audiol Otol. 24(4):198-203, 2020
3. Young YH: Contemporary review of the causes and differential diagnosis of sudden sensorineural hearing loss. Int J Audiol. 59(4):243-53, 2020
4. Chen K et al: Audiological outcomes in sudden sensorineural hearing loss with presumed inner ear hemorrhage. Am J Otolaryngol. 40(2):274-8, 2019
5. Chen XH et al: The natural history of labyrinthine hemorrhage in patients with sudden sensorineural hearing loss. Ear Nose Throat J. 98(5):E13-20, 2019
6. Vivas EX et al: Spontaneous labyrinthine hemorrhage: a case series. Otolaryngol Head Neck Surg. 159(5):908-13, 2018

Semicircular Canal Dehiscence

TERMINOLOGY

- Semicircular canal dehiscence (SCCD): Defined as extreme thinning or absence of bony roof over superior SCC
- Posterior SCC (PSCC) may also be dehiscent

IMAGING

- Coronal T-bone CT: ≥ 2-mm dehiscence of roof of SSCC
  - Thinning of **tegmen tympani** may be associated
- Transverse oblique (Pöschl) T-bone CT reformats
  - Optimal view of SSCC dehiscent roof
- Axial T-bone CT
  - In-plane view of dehiscent PSCC

PATHOLOGY

- Unknown; developmentally thinned ± acquired component
- Results in "unphysiologic motion" of endolymph
- Best hypothesis for clinical findings
  - Dehiscence creates **3rd mobile window** into inner ear

- 3rd window allows canal to respond to sound & pressure changes in membranous labyrinth

CLINICAL ISSUES

- Presenting signs & symptoms
  - Sound ± pressure-induced vestibular symptoms ± eye movements
  - Conductive hearing loss
  - Chronic disequilibrium may be debilitating
  - Oscillopsia (oscillating vision)
- **Tullio phenomenon**
  - Vertigo ± nystagmus related to sound
- Treatable form of vestibular disturbance

DIAGNOSTIC CHECKLIST

- Vestibular symptoms + positive bone CT = SCCD syndrome
- Use opposite SCC to compare with suspicious side; however, dehiscences can be bilateral

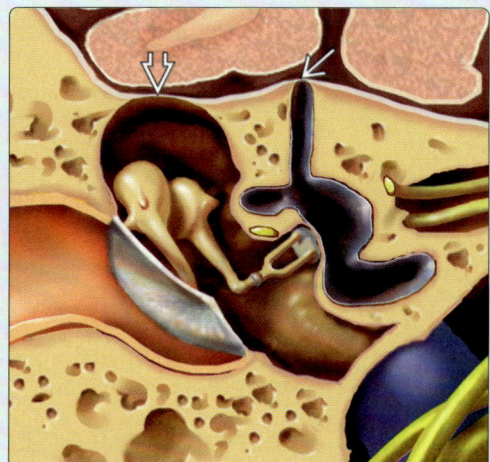
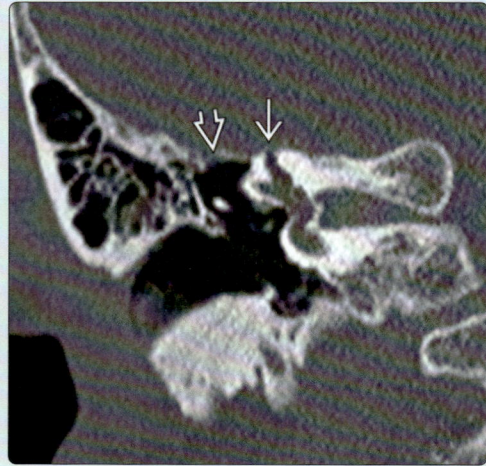

(Left) Coronal graphic illustrates the principal findings of superior semicircular canal dehiscence (SCCD): Absence of bone overlying the superior semicircular canal ➡ and associated thinning of tegmen tympani ➡. (Right) Coronal bone CT shows dehiscence of the right superior semicircular canal ➡ in a patient presenting with classical symptoms of sound-induced dizziness (Tullio phenomenon). The tegmen ➡ is thinned but appears intact.

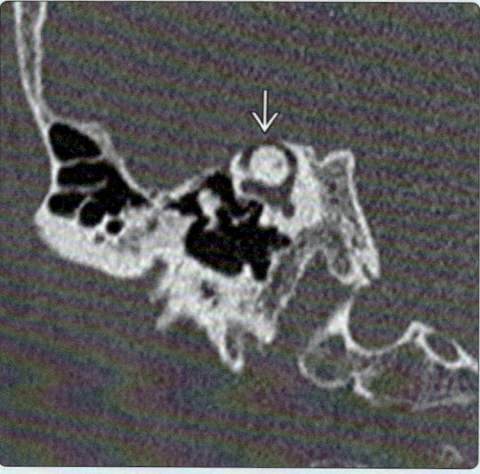
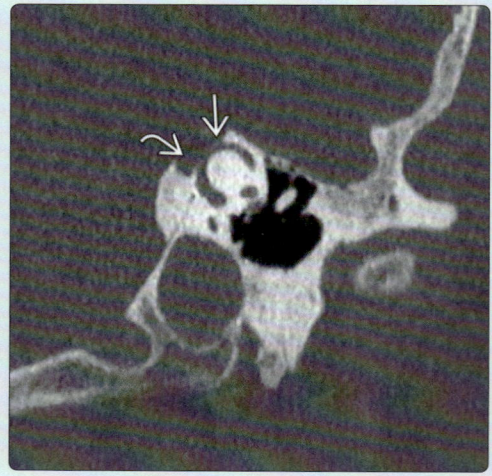

(Left) Oblique Pöschl bone CT shows broad SCCD ➡ in this patient presenting with debilitating dizziness due to loud noises who experienced dizziness with pneumatic otoscopy and pressure on the ipsilateral side of the head. Contralateral SCCD was also noted. (Right) Oblique Pöschl bone CT shows a broad dehiscence of the superior semicircular canal ➡ with associated erosion into the superior petrosal sinus ➡. This is a less common variant of SCCD that may also present with pulsatile tinnitus.

Semicircular Canal Dehiscence

TERMINOLOGY

Abbreviations
- Semicircular canal dehiscence (SCCD)

Definitions
- Extreme thinning or absence of bone roof over superior or posterior SCC

IMAGING

General Features
- Best diagnostic clue
  - T-bone CT shows dehiscence of bone covering superior (SSCC) or posterior (PSCC) SCC
- Location
  - May be bilateral
- Size
  - 2- to 4-mm dehiscent segment

CT Findings
- Bone CT
  - Coronal T-bone CT
    - ≥ 2-mm dehiscence of roof of SSCC
    - Thinned **tegmen tympani** may be associated
  - Transverse oblique (Pöschl) T-bone CT reformats
    - Ideal view of SSCC dehiscent roof
  - Axial T-bone CT
    - ≥ 2-mm dehiscence of superficial bony wall of PSCC

MR Findings
- T2WI
  - Thin-section high-resolution T2 MR
    - Coronal: Absent arcuate eminence bone over SSCC
    - Axial: Best shows segmental absence of PSCC
  - Can overestimate SCCD; T-bone CT to confirm
- T1WI C+
  - Look for acoustic schwannoma as alternative explanation for vertigo

Imaging Recommendations
- High-resolution T-bone CT best test
  - Transverse oblique (Pöschl) MPR best shows SCCD
  - Unenhanced high-resolution (< 1-mm) T-bone CT
- High-resolution ≤ 0.6-mm T2 SSFP MR effective to rule out SCCD, but positive cases need high-resolution CT to confirm

DIFFERENTIAL DIAGNOSIS

Normal Thinning of Superior Semicircular Canal or Posterior Semicircular Canal Wall
- Asymptomatic thinning of bony over SSCC or PSCC
- Usually seen on only 1 coronal or axial CT

PATHOLOGY

General Features
- Etiology
  - Unknown; developmental ± acquired component
    - Head injury or change in intracranial pressure (ICP) (barotrauma) may fracture thin bone or destabilize dura over preexistent dehiscence
    - De novo SSCD development by CT is reported
- Best hypothesis for clinical findings
  - Bony opening overlying SCC creates **3rd mobile window** into inner ear, allowing canal to respond to sound & pressure changes in membranous labyrinth
  - Motion at oval window (from loud noises) or ↑ ICP may bow thin cover over SSCC or PSCC
  - "**Unphysiologic motion**" of endolymph in SCC
  - Similar clinical findings described with cholesteatomas eroding horizontal SCC

Gross Pathologic & Surgical Features
- Surgical view shows absent bony cover over SSCC or PSCC

CLINICAL ISSUES

Presentation
- Most common signs/symptoms
  - Sound ± pressure-induced vestibular symptoms ± eye movements
  - Conductive hearing loss
    - Low-frequency air-bone gap at audiometry
  - Other symptoms & signs
    - **Tullio sign**: Vertigo ± nystagmus related to sound
    - Chronic disequilibrium may be debilitating
    - Oscillopsia (oscillating vision)

Demographics
- Age
  - Mean: 50 years; range: 20-70 years
- Epidemiology
  - ~ 2% of population have thinning or dehiscence of bone over SSCC on autopsy; 50% bilateral
  - Prevalence of incidental SCCD on (64-slice) MDCT = 2%
  - Frequently associated with tegmen underdevelopment
  - SSCC dehiscence > > PSCC dehiscence

Natural History & Prognosis
- Slowly progressive symptoms

Treatment
- Treatable form of vestibular disturbance
- Earplugs & avoidance of provoking stimuli
- Surgical resurfacing of affected SCC beneficial

DIAGNOSTIC CHECKLIST

Consider
- Vestibular symptoms + positive CT = **SCCD syndrome**

Image Interpretation Pearls
- Use opposite SCC to compare, but may be bilateral

SELECTED REFERENCES

1. Matari NH et al: Pöschl Reformations created from high-resolution noncontrast enhanced CT head exams can be used to detect and classify superior semicircular canal abnormalities. Otol Neurotol. 46(2):176-82, 2025
2. Khandalavala KR et al: Third window lesions of the inner ear: a pictorial review. Am J Otolaryngol. 45(2):104192, 2024
3. Shankar A et al: Superior canal dehiscence and the risk of additional dehiscences: a retrospective CT cohort study. Otol Neurotol. 45(7):e525-31, 2024
4. Motasaddi Zarandy M et al: Prevalence of otic capsule dehiscence in temporal bone computed tomography scan. Eur Arch Otorhinolaryngol. 280(1):125-30, 2023

Cochlear Implant

TERMINOLOGY

- Cochlear implant (CI)
  - Multicomponent electronic device that provides auditory information by directly stimulating cochlear nerve

IMAGING

- Postoperative CI evaluation: Temporal bone CT
- Stimulation wire tip typically in basal & 2nd cochlear turns
  - Variants include split electrode & apical turn insertion
- Complications: Extracochlear migration, basal/tip fold over, under-/overinsertion, pinching, scalar translocation
  - No wire in cochlea ("empty cochlea") is malpositioned
  - Wire fracture or kinking may cause malfunction
- Modified Stenver view to best show CI position

CLINICAL ISSUES

- Torque in 1.5T MR is sufficient to cause implant movement
  - Most CI patients should **not** undergo MR
  - Some may have MR with special precautions

DIAGNOSTIC CHECKLIST

- **Contraindications** to CI placement
  - Cochlear or labyrinthine aplasia
  - Absent cochlear nerve (no longer absolute contraindication)
- Key **relative contraindications** to CI placement
  - Labyrinthine ossificans
  - Malformed cochlea (common cavity, cystic cochleovestibular anomaly)
- Key findings that may complicate surgery
  - Hypoplastic mastoid process
  - Aberrant facial nerve
  - Otosclerosis
  - Otomastoiditis
  - Dehiscent jugular bulb
  - Aberrant internal carotid artery
  - Persistent stapedial artery
  - Enlarged endolymphatic sac anomaly

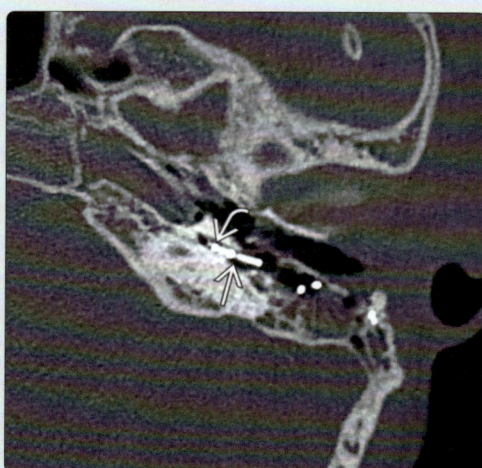
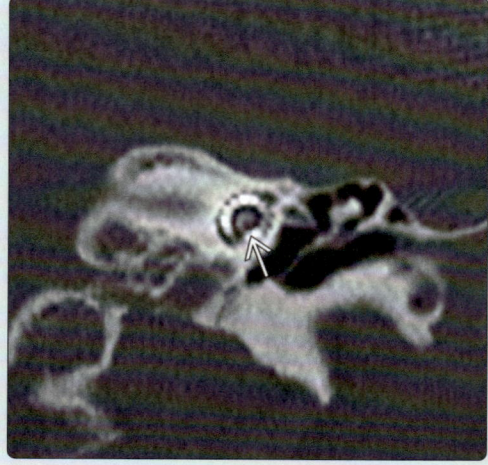

(Left) Axial bone CT demonstrates the normal position of a multichannel cochlear implant insertion site through the oval window ➡. Individual electrodes are seen as individual buttons with a beaded appearance in the basal turn of the cochlea ➡. (Right) Coronal bone CT MPR in the same patient shows the multichannel electrode array positioned in the distal middle turn of cochlea ➡, close to the cochlear apex. Individual electrodes are better seen by their beaded appearance on this MPR.

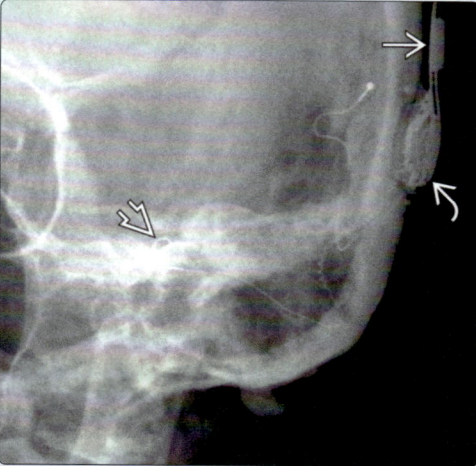
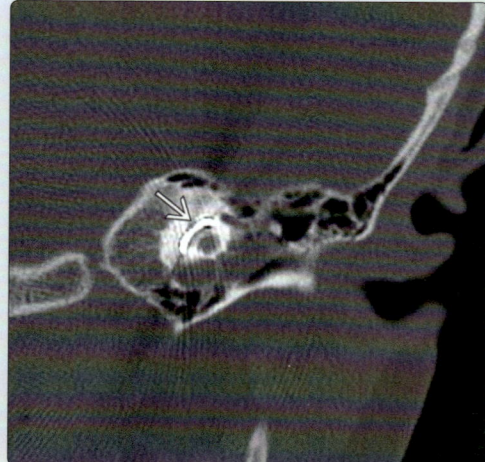

(Left) Modified Stenvers view of the left temporal bone shows the normal configuration of the distal cochlear implant wire spiraling within the cochlea ➡. The receiver ➡ and magnet ➡ are seen in profile in the subcutaneous tissues. (Right) Coronal left temporal bone CT shows a normally positioned cochlear implant wire ➡ in the basal turn of the cochlea.

Cochlear Implant

TERMINOLOGY

Abbreviations
- Cochlear implant (CI)

Synonyms
- Cochlear electrode

Definitions
- CI: Multicomponent electronic device that provides auditory information by directly stimulating auditory fibers in cochlea
  - **Microphone**
    - External component that resides behind ear
    - Receives sound from environment
    - Transforms sound to electrical impulse
    - Transmits impulse to speech processor
  - **Speech processor**
    - External component that may be attached to microphone or worn separately in clothing
    - Custom programmed computer that emphasizes speech over other sounds
    - Digitally encodes sounds from human speech frequencies
    - Encoding strategy depends on manufacturer
  - **Transmitter**
    - External component that resides behind ear, atop subcutaneous receiver
    - Transcutaneously sends magnetic impulses from speech processor to receiver
    - Held in place by magnet in subcutaneous receiver
  - **Receiver**
    - Thin, subcutaneous component behind external ear
    - Surgically implanted
    - Converts magnetic impulses from transmitter to electrical signal for stimulator wire
  - **Stimulator**
    - Wire placed inside cochlea directly stimulates spiral ganglion cells & cochlear axons
    - Stimulator wire enters cochlea via round window
    - Electrode wire array looks like tiny buttons on CT

IMAGING

General Features
- Best diagnostic clue
  - Thin, metallic wire (stimulator) with tiny beads (electrodes) extending into cochlea
  - Stimulator wire is connected to subcutaneous receiver behind ear
- Location
  - Stimulator wire usually enters basal turn of cochlea, typically extending into 2nd, & sometimes, apical turn
  - Enters cochlea via round window in most (preferred)
  - Split electrodes (may be used in otosclerosis) can have separate electrodes entering at round window & middle turn of cochlea via cochleostomy
  - Some patients undergo retrograde approach via cochleostomy at apical turn (e.g., due to round window atresia)
- Size
  - Submillimeter thickness
- Morphology
  - Curvilinear with small beads on intracochlear simulator

Radiographic Findings
- Modified Stenver view of temporal bone shows CI best
  - Head rotated 45° from direct AP, away from implanted ear; slight head flexion

CT Findings
- Bone CT
  - Identify preoperative contraindications to implantation &/or postoperative complications
    - Key preoperative absolute contraindication: Cochlear aplasia alone or in labyrinthine aplasia
    - Key preoperative relative contraindications: Labyrinthitis ossificans, other inner ear dysplasias
  - Preimplant CT: Findings that may complicate surgery
    - Hypoplastic mastoid process
    - Aberrant facial nerve course, otomastoiditis
    - Fenestral ± cochlear otosclerosis
    - Persistent stapedial artery
    - Dehiscent jugular bulb
    - Aberrant internal carotid artery
    - Enlarged endolymphatic sac & duct
  - Postoperative search for complications
    - Key postoperative complication: **Misplaced wire** (not in cochlea)
    - Wire penetrates only partway into cochlea
    - **Broken wire**
    - Wire penetration out of inner ear
  - Nonoptimal postsurgical findings
    - Basal or tip fold over (electrode folds over on itself)
    - Underinsertion (electrode buttons outside of cochlea)
    - Overinsertion (electrode buttons > 3-4 mm beyond round window)
    - Kinking or pinching
  - Modified Stenver MPR to show CI position
  - Cone beam CT &/or ultrahigh-resolution CT best

MR Findings
- T2WI
  - Must include high-resolution fluid sequence
  - Preoperative setting: Look for absolute & relative contraindications
    - Key preoperative (now considered relative) contraindication: **Absence of cochlear nerve**
    - Absent fluid signal in cochlea (e.g., labyrinthitis ossificans): Confirm osseous nature with CT
    - Relative contraindications
      - Ipsilateral brainstem infarct, superficial siderosis
  - Postoperatively, traditional CI **not** routinely **safe** for MR
    - CT, not MR, to evaluate postoperative complications
    - Magnetic torque may dislodge CI
    - Embedded magnet causes marked field distortion
    - Some success with careful precautions & bandaging magnet allows MR, but complications still occur

Imaging Recommendations
- Preoperative high-resolution temporal bone CT & high-resolution T2 MR are complimentary

- Preoperative evaluation
  - Temporal bone CT
    - Adequately evaluates round window patency
    - Identifies bony labyrinthitis ossificans in cochlea
    - Shows inner anomalies & anatomic variants
  - Temporal bone MR
    - Identifies fibrous & ossific cochlear obstruction
    - Can see absent or hypoplastic cochlear nerve
- Postoperative evaluation
  - Modified CT Stenvers view shows CI misplacement
  - High-resolution or cone beam CT now superior tool

DIFFERENTIAL DIAGNOSIS

Major Lesions to Identify in Preoperative Cochlear Implant Candidate

- Contraindication diagnoses
  - Cochlear nerve & cochlear nerve canal aplasia
  - Atretic cochlea
    - Labyrinthine aplasia, cochlear aplasia
    -
- Relative contraindication diagnoses
  - Cochlear nerve hypoplasia/deficiency
  - Malformed cochlea
    - Common cavity malformation
    - Cystic cochleovestibular malformation (incomplete partition type I)
  - Severe labyrinthine ossificans (can undergo drill-out/cochleostomy)

Cochlear Nerve & Cochlear Nerve Canal Aplasia-Hypoplasia

- Imaging: Absent cochlear nerve with small internal auditory canal (congenital type)
- Embryogenesis: Cochlear nerve fails to form

Labyrinthine Aplasia

- Imaging: No cochlea or vestibule present
- Embryogenesis: Developmental arrest, 3rd gestational week (GW)

Cochlear Aplasia

- Imaging: No cochlea present
- Embryogenesis: Developmental arrest, late 3rd GW

Common Cavity Malformation

- Imaging: Coalesced cystic cochlea & vestibule form common cavity
- Embryogenesis: Developmental arrest, 4th GW

Cystic Cochleovestibular Malformation (IP-I)

- Imaging: Cochlea & vestibule cystic with no internal architecture
- Embryogenesis: Developmental arrest, 5th GW

PATHOLOGY

General Features

- Etiology
  - Primary causes of hearing loss = congenital, infection

Gross Pathologic & Surgical Features

- Placement of CI requires partial mastoidectomy

CLINICAL ISSUES

Presentation

- Most common signs/symptoms
  - Severe bilateral sensorineural hearing loss (SNHL)
- Clinical profile
  - Candidates usually **> 2 years old** with severe SNHL
  - No benefit from conventional hearing aids

Demographics

- Epidemiology
  - National Health Interview Survey found 21.0% of American adults had hearing loss in 2014

Natural History & Prognosis

- Postlingually deafened patients (those who have already learned to speak, usually > 5 years old) have best outcome
- Postoperative complications (5%)
  - Transient CNVII paresis, imbalance, perilymph fistula, hardware failure, & skin flap problems
- 90% of CI patients report understanding basic sentences after 6 months
- Torque experienced by CI in 1.5T MR is sufficient to cause implant movement; traditional CI patients should not undergo 1.5T MR
  - MR-compatible CI is now available
  - External components should be removed

Treatment

- CI is effective rehabilitation method for profoundly hearing-impaired patients who do not benefit from hearing aids
- CI users should return to clinic at least 1x per year for speech processor adjustments
- Postoperative results depend on number of intracochlear electrodes
- Alternative hearing augmentation options
  - Hearing aid
  - Ossicular prosthesis
  - Auditory brainstem implant

DIAGNOSTIC CHECKLIST

Consider

- Are there any contraindications to CI placement?
- Are there any findings that might complicate surgery?
- Which side would be easier for surgeon?
- Postoperative patients: Is CI in appropriate location (within cochlea)?

SELECTED REFERENCES

1. Malhotra V et al: Morphometric analysis of temporal bone radiology for cochlear implant candidacy. Indian J Otolaryngol Head Neck Surg. 76(1):702-11, 2024
2. Shakhtour LB et al: Evaluation of cochlear implantation in children with cochlear nerve absence or deficiency. Otolaryngol Head Neck Surg. 171(4):1197-204, 2024
3. Cheung LL et al: Misplaced cochlear implant electrodes outside the cochlea: a literature review and presentation of radiological and electrophysiological findings. Otol Neurotol. 43(5):567-79, 2022
4. Dewyer NA et al: Pediatric single-sided deafness: a review of prevalence, radiologic findings, and cochlear implant candidacy. Ann Otol Rhinol Laryngol. 31(3):233-8, 2021

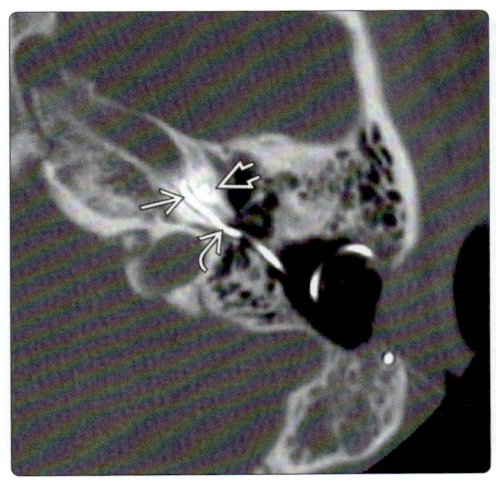

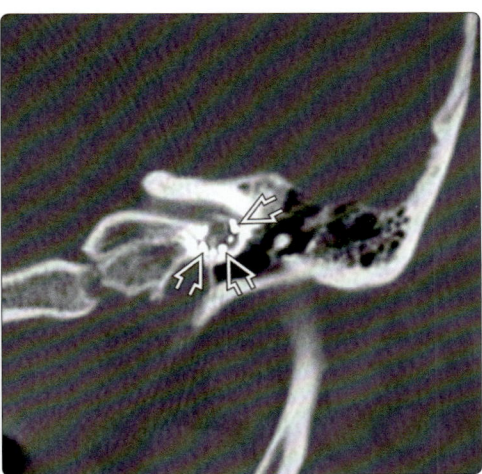

(Left) *Axial left temporal bone CT demonstrates a normal cochlear implant. The wire enters the round window ⇨ on its way to the basal turn of the cochlea ⇨, extending well into the cochlear 2nd turn ⇨. There is no evidence of wire kinking or breaking.* (Right) *Coronal temporal bone CT in the same patient reveals the cochlear implant wire appropriately positioned within the cochlea. The normal beaded appearance from electrodes on the distal cochlear implant wire ⇨ is well appreciated on this image.*

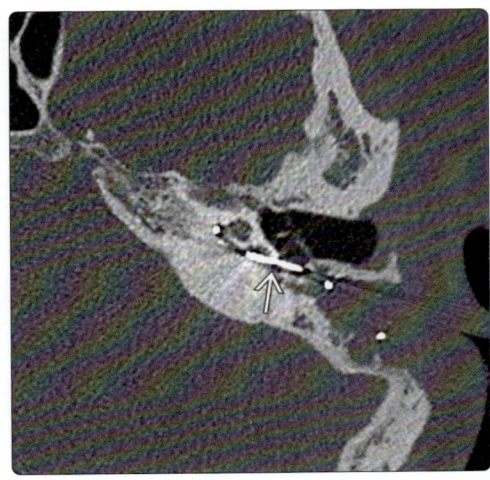

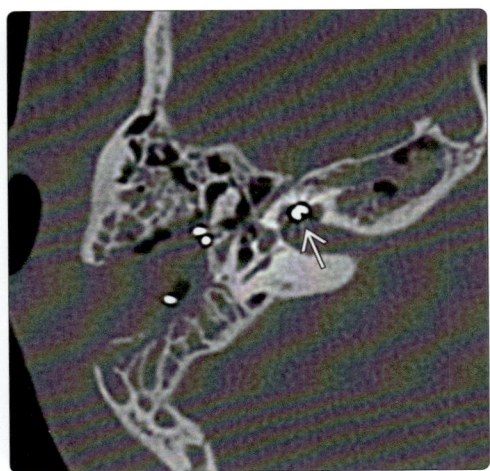

(Left) *Axial temporal bone CT shows several of the button electrodes ⇨ of a multichannel implant proximal to the basal turn of the cochlea (underinsertion).* (Right) *Axial bone CT shows fold over of the distal cochlear electrode tip within a cystic-appearing cochlea ⇨. Tip fold over is not usually identifiable with electrophysiologic monitoring and requires imaging confirmation. Deactivating involved electrodes can be helpful; however, some cases require revision surgery.*

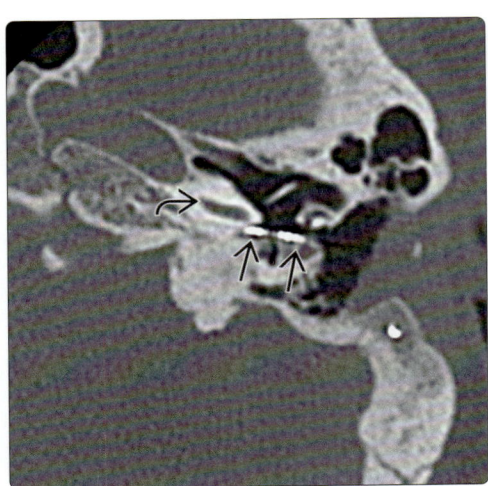

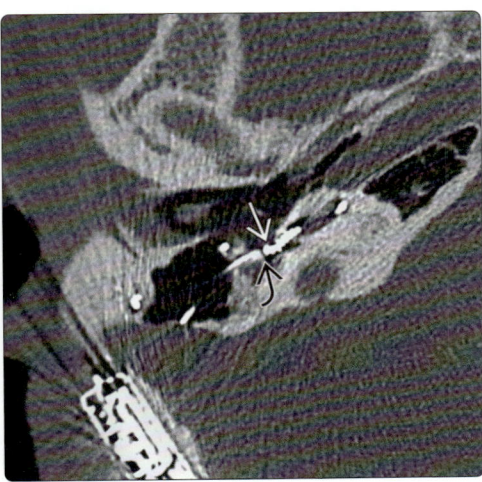

(Left) *Axial bone CT shows abnormal dislocation of this patients' cochlear implant. The electrodes leads ⇨ are displaced into the tympanic cavity. Note the basal turn of cochlea ⇨ is empty.* (Right) *Axial bone CT shows slight pinching of the electrode array proximal to the round window. Several electrode buttons extend outside the basal turn of cochlea ⇨, lateral to the round window (underinsertion). The radiolucent gap ⇨ at the wire-electrode junction should not be mistaken for lead fracture on MDCT.*

Petrous Apex Asymmetric Marrow

TERMINOLOGY

- Petrous apex (PA) asymmetric marrow: Asymmetric pneumatization of PA with nonpneumatized marrow space in opposite PA simulating mass lesion
- Synonym: PA pseudolesion

IMAGING

- Temporal bone CT findings
  - Normal PA marrow space
  - Normal air cells visible in contralateral PA
  - **No expansile changes** present
- MR findings
  - Nonpneumatized PA contains normal fatty marrow, hyperintense on T1WI
  - Mimics cholesterol granuloma
  - Fat-saturated sequences confirm fatty nature of lesion

TOP DIFFERENTIAL DIAGNOSES

- PA trapped fluid

- PA cholesterol granuloma
- PA congenital cholesteatoma
- Apical petrositis

PATHOLOGY

- Congenital normal variant in PA pneumatization-marrow space spectrum
- Embryology-anatomy
  - **33%** have pneumatized petrous apices
  - 5% are asymmetrically pneumatized

CLINICAL ISSUES

- Clinical presentation
  - **Asymptomatic** by definition
- Patient undergoing brain MR for unrelated symptoms
  - Incidental MR finding
- Requires no treatment or follow-up
- If mentioned in radiology report, be certain to convey incidental nature

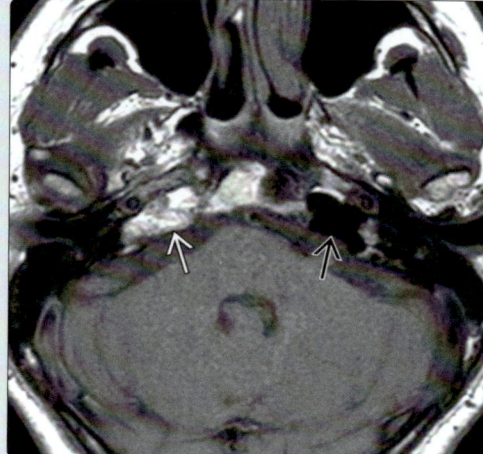
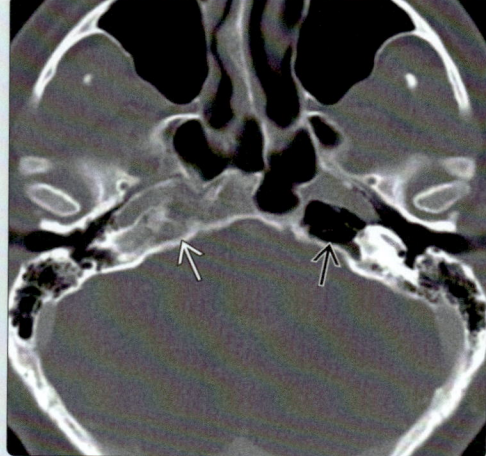

(Left) Axial T1 MR in a patient imaged for tinnitus shows asymmetric, hyperintense marrow in the right petrous apex ➡. Note the heterogeneous signal appearance of normal marrow (similar to marrow elsewhere). Lack of signal in the left petrous apex is due to developmental pneumatization ➡. (Right) Axial bone CT in the same patient confirms normal fatty marrow in the right petrous apex ➡ and developmentally pneumatized air cells on the left ➡.

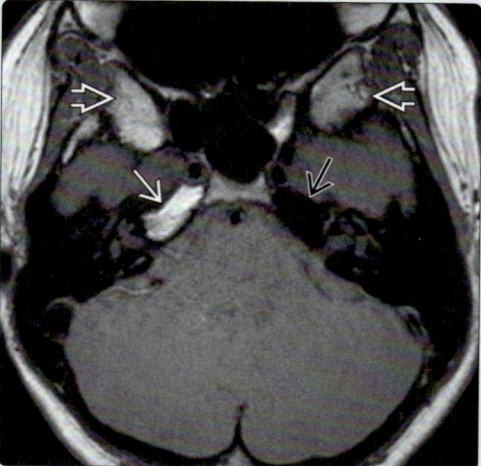
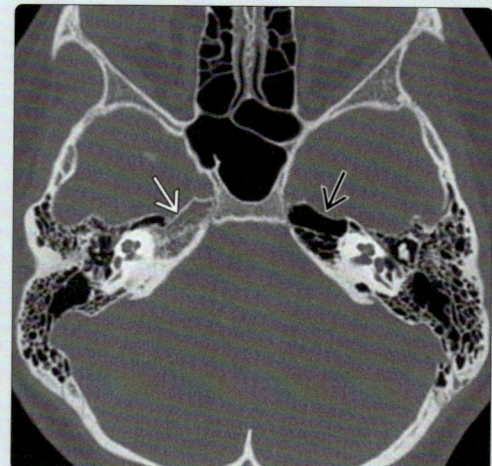

(Left) Axial T1 MR in a patient referred for evaluation of suspected cholesterol granuloma shows asymmetric, hyperintense signal in the right petrous apex ➡ due to fatty marrow. The left petrous apex is pneumatized ➡. Note how signal is similar to the greater sphenoid wing marrow ➡. (Right) Axial bone CT in the same patient confirms normal asymmetric marrow in the right petrous apex ➡. The left petrous apex shows normal development pneumatization ➡.

TERMINOLOGY

Abbreviations
- Petrous apex (PA)

Synonyms
- PA pseudolesion

Definitions
- PA asymmetric marrow: Asymmetric pneumatization of PA with nonpneumatized marrow space in opposite PA simulating mass lesion

IMAGING

General Features
- Best diagnostic clue
  - Asymmetric, pneumatized PA across from opposite normal PA bone marrow in absence of expansile changes

CT Findings
- CECT
  - No abnormal enhancement present
- Bone CT
  - Normal PA marrow space juxtaposed with contralateral normal PA air cells
  - **No expansile changes** present

MR Findings
- T1WI
  - Nonpneumatized PA contains normal fatty marrow, hyperintense on T1WI in adults
- T2WI
  - When fatty, PA marrow will be hyperintense, similar to subcutaneous fat
  - Look for signal paralleling marrow elsewhere
- T1WI C+
  - Fat-saturated sequences remove fatty marrow high signal, confirming diagnosis of normal PA

Imaging Recommendations
- Best imaging tool
  - Most commonly **incidental finding** on brain MR
    - Fat saturation confirms benign fat (due to marrow); cholesterol granuloma will not suppress
  - Temporal bone CT used to confirm marrow in PA
    - Ensures no worrisome changes to trabeculae, lack of expansile or erosive bone changes
- Protocol advice
  - Lesion is 1st suspected on MR without fat saturation
  - Use fat-saturated sequences to confirm fatty nature

DIFFERENTIAL DIAGNOSIS

Petrous Apex Trapped Fluid
- Bone CT: Nonexpansile, opacified PA air cells
  - Preserved septations, simple effusion
- MR: Low or intermediate T1, high T2 signal in most cases

Petrous Apex Cholesterol Granuloma
- Bone CT: Smooth, expansile PA mass
  - Loss of normal internal septations
- MR: High signal on T1 and T2

Petrous Apex Congenital Cholesteatoma
- Bone CT: Smooth, expansile PA lesion
- MR: Low T1, high T2 signal; nonenhancing
  - DWI high signal

Apical Petrositis
- Bone CT: Destruction of PA trabecula and cortex
- MR: Thick, enhancing walls with focal fluid ± dural enhancement

Petrous Apex Mucocele
- Bone CT: Smooth, expansile PA lesion
- MR: Low T1, high T2 signal; DWI low signal

PATHOLOGY

General Features
- Etiology
  - Congenital normal variant in PA pneumatization-marrow space spectrum
- Embryology-anatomy
  - **33%** have pneumatized PAs
  - 5% are asymmetrically pneumatized
  - PA pneumatization amount correlates with amount of mastoid aeration

CLINICAL ISSUES

Presentation
- Most common signs/symptoms
  - **Asymptomatic** by definition
- Clinical profile
  - Patient undergoing brain MR for unrelated symptoms
  - Incidental MR finding
    - PA marrow may be described as suspicious for cholesterol granuloma in radiology report
    - Patient may be referred for surgical assessment

Natural History & Prognosis
- PA marrow remains unchanged over time
- Multiple possible morbidities from treatment of this "leave alone" lesion of PA

Treatment
- Requires no treatment or follow-up

DIAGNOSTIC CHECKLIST

Consider
- PA asymmetric marrow is **common incidental finding** on brain MR
- May be misdiagnosed as PA cholesterol granuloma or high T1 signal trapped PA fluid
- One of **"leave alone"** lesions of PA
  - Trapped PA fluid is also "leave alone" lesion
- Misdiagnosis creates clinical confusion and potential for unnecessary treatment

SELECTED REFERENCES

1. Gupta N et al: Pediatric petrous apex lesions: a radiological classification and diagnostic algorithm. Can Assoc Radiol J. 73(4):655-71, 2022
2. Huang JH et al: Skull base tumor mimics. Neuroimaging Clin N Am. 32(2):327-44, 2022

Petrous Apex Cephalocele

TERMINOLOGY

- Definition: Cystic- or lytic-appearing lesion of petrous apex (PA) caused by dehiscence of PA roof & localized inferior herniation of floor of Meckel cave (MC)

IMAGING

- Bone CT findings
  - Unilateral or bilateral expansile PA lesions
  - Enlarges porus trigeminus PA notch
- MR findings
  - CSF-intensity, ovoid PA lesion on all sequences
  - Directly communicates with MC
  - Appears to "spill out" of patulous MC

TOP DIFFERENTIAL DIAGNOSES

- PA cholesterol granuloma
- PA congenital cholesteatoma
- PA mucocele
- PA effusion

- Skull base chondrosarcoma

CLINICAL ISSUES

- Most commonly **incidental, asymptomatic** MR finding
- Rare clinical presentation
  - Symptomatic (CSF otorrhea, trigeminal neuralgia, meningitis); lesion breaks into temporal bone air cells
  - Headache from idiopathic intracranial hypertension
    - Consider if empty sella, enlarged optic nerve CSF spaces with PA cephalocele (PAC)
- **No treatment** in most cases
- Surgical treatment
  - If lesion communicates with PA air cells

DIAGNOSTIC CHECKLIST

- PAC = "leave alone" lesion of PA; convey incidental nature in radiologic report
- PAC requires **no further work-up** or surgical intervention in most cases

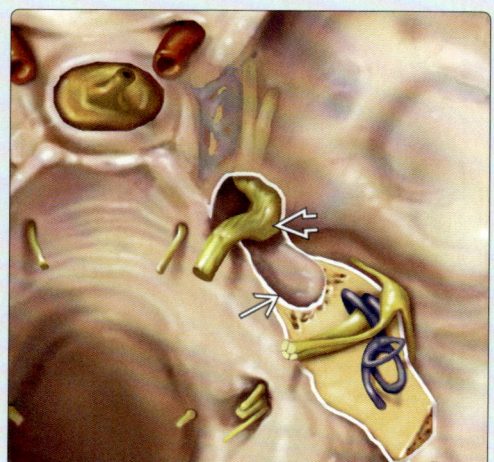
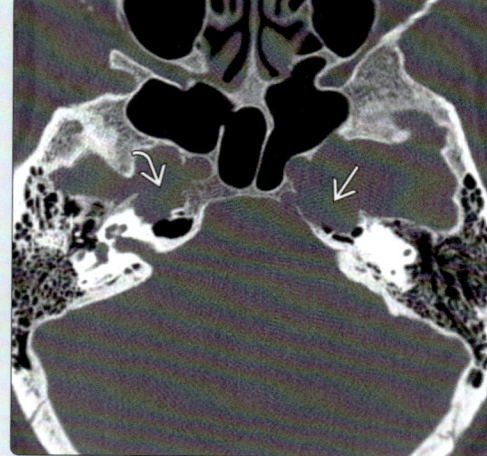

(Left) Axial graphic illustrates herniation of a cephalocele from the Meckel cave into the petrous apex (PA) ➡. A portion of the trigeminal ganglion is depicted protruding into the cephalocele ➡. (Right) Axial bone CT demonstrates large left ➡ and smaller right ➡ PA cephaloceles. The lesions project into the PAs from posteromedial Meckel caves and produce a scalloped, lytic appearance in the bone.

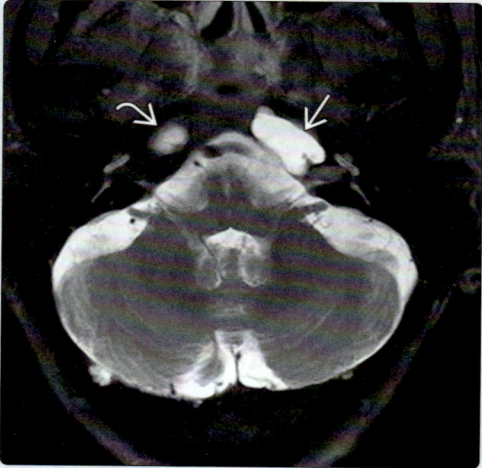
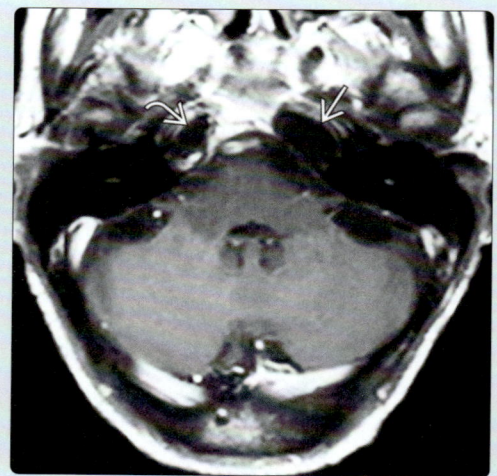

(Left) Axial T2 MR shows a fluid-filled structure ➡ in the left PA. A smaller cystic structure is identified on the right ➡. These lesions were shown on other slices to communicate with Meckel caves bilaterally, consistent with PA cephalocele. (Right) Axial T1 C+ MR in the same patient shows no enhancement in the left ➡ or right ➡ PA cephaloceles that consist of CSF signal. Occasionally, nerve rootlets can be found in the cephalocele. Otherwise, there is no solid tissue present within the cephalocele.

Petrous Apex Cephalocele

TERMINOLOGY

Abbreviations
- Petrous apex (PA) cephalocele (PAC)

Synonyms
- PA arachnoid cyst, cavum trigeminale cephalocele

Definitions
- Congenital or acquired dehiscence of PA roof & localized herniation of floor of Meckel cave (MC)

IMAGING

General Features
- Best diagnostic clue
  - CSF density/intensity lesion of PA that directly communicates with MC
  - Appears to "spill out" of patulous MC
- Location
  - Anteromedial PA directly adjacent to MC

CT Findings
- Bone CT
  - Unilateral (more common) or bilateral **smooth, expansile** PA lesion(s)
  - **Enlarged** PA **porus trigeminus notch**
- CT cisternography
  - Contrast fills MC & PAC
  - When CSF otorrhea present, may define PAC connection to temporal bone air cells

MR Findings
- T1WI
  - Low signal, isointense to CSF
- T2WI
  - High signal, isointense to CSF
  - Coronal best shows connection to MC
- FLAIR
  - Fluid in PAC attenuates with CSF
- T1WI C+
  - No enhancement vs. mild rim enhancement
  - If gasserian ganglion within cephalocele, will appear as enhancing component within ovoid, nonenhancing lesion
    - Periganglionic venous plexus also enhances

Imaging Recommendations
- Best imaging tool
  - Focused multiplanar T2 MR makes diagnosis
  - Temporal bone CT confirms impression
  - CT cisternography if CSF otorrhea present

DIFFERENTIAL DIAGNOSIS

Petrous Apex Cholesterol Granuloma
- CT: Expansile PA lesion
- MR: T1 & T2 high signal, no FLAIR suppression

Petrous Apex Congenital Cholesteatoma
- CT: Smooth, expansile PA mass
- MR: T1 low, T2 high signal, high FLAIR; DWI restricts

Petrous Apex Mucocele
- CT: Smooth, expansile PA lesion
- MR: T1 low, T2 high signal; DWI negative

Petrous Apex Effusion
- CT: Nonexpansile, aerated PA cell opacification
- MR: T1 low, T2 high signal; DWI negative

Skull base chondrosarcoma
- CT: Expansile mass, erosive/destructive changes in PA/clivus, 50% chondroid matrix calcifications
- MR: High T2 with scattered low T2 (calcifications), heterogenous enhancement

PATHOLOGY

General Features
- Etiology
  - Congenital hypothesis
    - Developmental anomaly results in deficient dural & osseous covering of PA
    - Defect allows MC herniation into PA
  - Acquired hypothesis
    - Chronic CSF pulsations against thin anterior wall of pneumatized PA results in dehiscence
    - Eventual prolapse of meninges into PA defect
    - Idiopathic intracranial hypertension (IIH) may accelerate dehiscence
- Associated abnormalities
  - Consider IIH if empty sella (~ 54% of PAC cases), enlarged optic nerve CSF spaces

Microscopic Features
- 1 or all 3 meningeal layers may be present

CLINICAL ISSUES

Presentation
- Most common signs/symptoms
  - **Incidental asymptomatic** MR brain finding
  - More commonly reported in female patients
  - May be complicated by CSF otorrhea, trigeminal neuralgia, or meningitis if cephalocele erodes into temporal bone air cells

Treatment
- **No treatment** in most cases
- Surgical treatment if air cell communication exists
  - Recurrent meningitis & CSF leak require surgery
  - Middle cranial fossa extradural approach
    - Repair dural defect; obliterate PA defect

SELECTED REFERENCES

1. Reecher HM et al: Resolution of refractory trigeminal neuralgia after endoscopic decompression of the foramina rotundum and ovale in a patient with bilateral petrous apex cephaloceles: illustrative case. J Neurosurg Case Lessons. 9(8):CASE24283, 2025
2. Brotis A et al: Incidental petrous apex cephalocele presenting with transient global amnesia: a case report and rapid literature review. Cureus. 16(1):e51778, 2024
3. Martínez JL et al: Trigeminal neuralgia secondary to Meckel's cave meningoencephaloceles: a systematic review and illustrative case. Neurol India. 70(3):857-63, 2022
4. Alkhaibary A et al: Bilateral petrous apex cephaloceles: is surgical intervention indicated? Int J Surg Case Rep. 72:373-6, 2020

Congenital Petrous Apex Cholesteatoma

TERMINOLOGY

- Petrous apex (PA) cholesteatoma (epidermoid): Ectopic ectodermal tissue in petrous bone ultimately gives rise to expansile, cystic mass lined by stratified squamous epithelium and filled with keratinous debris

IMAGING

- Bone CT: **Expansile** mass with smooth, lobular bone remodeling and lytic change
  - Shows smooth, expansile, lobulated lesion of PA
- MR: Expansile PA lesion with low T1, high T2 signal but **without** enhancement
  - **Restricted diffusion** (high signal on DWI) is **characteristic**
- May simultaneously involve adjacent areas
  - Horizontal petrous internal carotid artery (ICA) canal
  - Inner ear structures (otic capsule)
  - Internal auditory canal
  - Meckel cave
  - Medial mastoid air cells
  - Facial nerve canal (labyrinthine and anterior tympanic segments)

TOP DIFFERENTIAL DIAGNOSES

- PA cholesterol granuloma
- Petrooccipital fissure chondrosarcoma
- PA cephalocele
- PA effusion
- Apical petrositis
- PA mucocele

PATHOLOGY

- Growth occurs from progressive internal desquamation of epithelium combined with surrounding bone demineralization

CLINICAL ISSUES

- Clinical profile: 40-year-old adult with unilateral sensorineural hearing loss

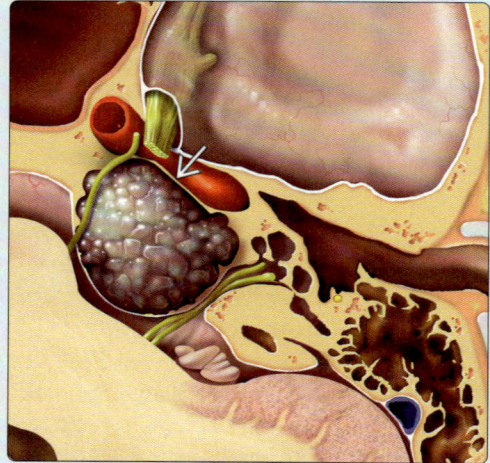
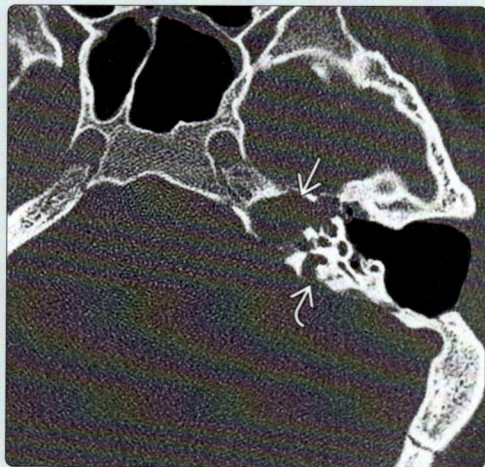

(Left) *Axial graphic depicts typical petrous apex (PA) congenital cholesteatoma. Notice the benign expansile nature of the PA bone as it responds to the growing cholesteatoma. The horizontal petrous internal carotid artery (ICA) posterior wall is thinned ➡ by cholesteatoma growth.* (Right) *Axial CT through temporal bone shows a well-circumscribed, lytic lesion in the left PA, pathologically confirmed to represent cholesteatoma ➡. Bony erosion extends also along the posterior wall of the petrous ridge ➡ as well.*

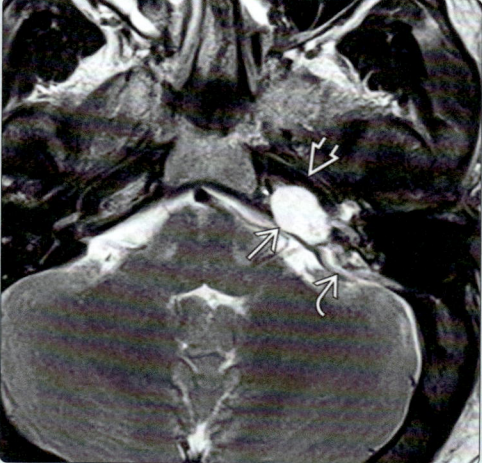
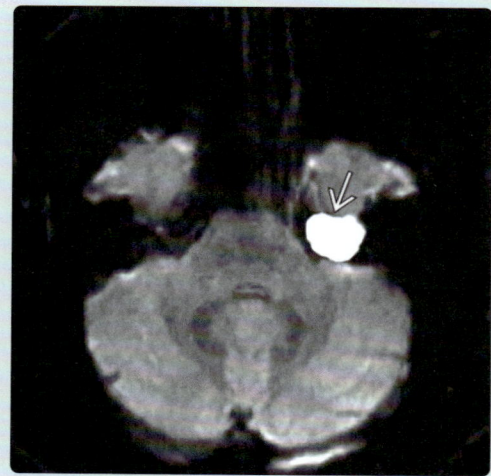

(Left) *Axial T2 MR in the same patient shows a hyperintense lesion in the left PA ➡ with posterolateral extension along the posterior wall of the petrous ridge ➡. The lesion displaces the petrous carotid slightly anteriorly ➡.* (Right) *Axial DWI MR in the same patient shows diffusion restriction throughout the lesion ➡. The lesion was also shown to be nonenhancing on other sequences. The combination of CT and MR findings with diffusion restriction is characteristic of PA cholesteatoma.*

Congenital Petrous Apex Cholesteatoma

TERMINOLOGY

Abbreviations

- Petrous apex (PA) cholesteatoma (PA-Chol)

Synonyms

- Congenital cholesteatoma, epidermoid or epidermoid cyst

Definitions

- PA-Chol (epidermoid): Ectopic ectodermal tissue in petrous bone ultimately gives rise to expansile, cystic mass lined by stratified squamous epithelium and filled with keratinous debris

IMAGING

General Features

- Best diagnostic clue
  - Bone CT: **Expansile** mass with **smooth**, **lobular bone remodeling**
  - MR: Expansile PA lesion with low T1, high T2 signal but without central parenchymal enhancement
    - DWI MR sequence shows cholesteatoma as predominantly hyperintense
- Location
  - PA (may involve more than PA)
    - Medial inner ear and internal auditory canal (IAC)
    - Medial mastoid
  - May simultaneously involve adjacent areas
    - Horizontal petrous internal carotid artery (ICA) canal
    - Inner ear structures (otic capsule); sensorineural hearing loss (SNHL)
    - IAC (vertigo, SNHL)
    - Meckel cave
    - Medial mastoid air cells
    - Facial nerve canal (labyrinthine and anterior tympanic segments); produce facial nerve paralysis
- Size
  - May become very large before discovered
  - 2-10 cm in maximum diameter
- Morphology
  - Ovoid to round, lobulated
  - When involves medial inner ear and mastoid with PA, may have "**dumbbell**" morphology

CT Findings

- CECT: PA-Chol will **not** enhance
- Bone CT: Shows smooth, expansile, lobulated lesion of PA
  - Margins are sharply demarcated
  - No intrinsic calcification, bone matrix, or hyperostosis

MR Findings

- T1WI: **Low** signal
  - May be homogeneous or heterogeneous
- T2WI: **High** signal predominantly, can be heterogeneous
- FLAIR: Does not attenuate on FLAIR
  - Partial attenuation (mixed intermediate to low signal) may be seen
- DWI: **Restricted diffusion** is **characteristic**
- T1WI C+: **No** intrinsic enhancement; peripheral linear enhancement

Imaging Recommendations

- Best imaging tool
  - As with most skull base lesions, CT and C+ MR are complementary and both are recommended for complete evaluation
  - Temporal bone CT is best initial exam
    - No contrast necessary
    - Best assessment of bony involvement
  - MR in axial and coronal planes used to confirm diagnosis and obtain soft tissue roadmap for surgery
    - Especially useful in large lesions
    - T1 C+ MR confirms lack of enhancement
    - Use **DWI sequence** to confirm diagnosis

DIFFERENTIAL DIAGNOSIS

Petrous Apex Cholesterol Granuloma

- Clinical: Previous history of chronic otomastoiditis common
- Bone CT: Smooth, lobular, expansile mass
- MR: High signal on T1 and T2
  - DWI shows no restricted diffusion

Petrooccipital Fissure Chondrosarcoma

- Can produce lytic mass in PA on CT
- T2 hyperintensity could be mistaken for cystic change
- Typically enhances

Petrous Apex Cephalocele

- Can have smooth, lytic appearance on CT
- MR: Nonenhancing and T2 hyperintensity may suggest cystic lesion
- Clue to diagnosis is identifying communication with CSF

Petrous Apex Trapped Fluid

- Clinical: Asymptomatic incidental finding on T2 MR
- Bone CT: Nonexpansile, opacified PA air cells
- MR: Low or intermediate T1 + high T2 signal in most cases
  - Can be high signal on T1

Apical Petrositis

- Clinical: Septic patient unless already partially treated with antibiotics
- Bone CT: Destructive PA lesion with trabecular and cortical loss
- MR: Thick, enhancing walls with focal fluid
  - Dural thickening and enhancement

Petrous Apex Mucocele

- Bone CT: Smooth, expansile lesion
- MR: Low T1, high T2 signal
- May exactly mimic cholesteatoma of PA
  - Except **no** diffusion restriction seen on DWI MR sequence

PATHOLOGY

General Features

- Etiology
  - **Aberrant PA epithelial rest** of **exfoliated keratin** within stratified squamous epithelium
    - Growth from **progressive desquamation of epithelium**

- – PA-Chol congenital, primary to PA or along labyrinthine segment of CNVII
- – PA-Chol may be part of large, multilobular lesion involving inner ear, IAC, medial mastoid
- Embryology-anatomy
  - Rests of epithelial tissue can occur in multiple locations in and around temporal bone
    - – Middle ear > cerebellopontine angle (CPA) > mastoid > PA > facial nerve canal

Gross Pathologic & Surgical Features

- Pearly white tissue within "eggshell" bone

Microscopic Features

- Sheets of stratified, keratinizing, squamous epithelium
  - No evidence of abnormal mitosis present
  - Granulation tissue and fibrosis often surround them
- Rich in cholesterol crystals
- Identical to epidermoid cyst

CLINICAL ISSUES

Presentation

- Most common signs/symptoms
  - SNHL when large
- Other signs/symptoms
  - Peripheral facial nerve paralysis
  - Abducens nerve paralysis
  - Headache
- Clinical profile
  - 40-year-old patient with unilateral SNHL

Demographics

- Age
  - 20-50 years
- Epidemiology
  - Very rare (< 1% of PA lesions)
    - – Trapped fluid > > apical petrositis, cholesterol granuloma, metastases > PA congenital cholesteatoma

Natural History & Prognosis

- Very slow-growing lesion
- Complete surgical removal arrests symptom progression

Treatment

- Surgical approaches
  - Removal via transpetrous approach
  - Middle fossa approach also used

DIAGNOSTIC CHECKLIST

Consider

- Once discovery of PA **expansile lesion** occurs, sort into benign expansile and invasive expansile groups
  - Invasive group includes chondrosarcoma, apical petrositis, metastases, plasmacytoma, and Langerhans cell histiocytosis
  - Benign group includes cholesteatoma, cholesterol granuloma, mucocele, petrous ICA aneurysm, and PA cephalocele

Image Interpretation Pearls

- MR helpful in differentiating benign-appearing expansile PA lesions on CT
  - Congenital cholesteatoma of PA
    - – T1 low, T2 high signal
    - – T1 C+ shows no enhancement
    - – FLAIR shows partial or absent attenuation
    - – DWI shows **restricted diffusion**
  - Cholesterol granuloma of PA
    - – T1 high, T2 high signal
  - Chondrosarcoma
    - – May show fairly well-circumscribed, expansile, lytic lesion of PA, usually in contact with petrooccipital fissure (POF)
    - – Can show intrinsic "arcs and whorls," but often no intrinsic matrix
    - – T2 hyperintensity can be variable; can be striking and appear cystic
    - – Central parenchymal enhancement of chondrosarcoma is differentiating feature
  - PA cephalocele
    - – Look for connection to patulous Meckel cave

Reporting Tips

- Be precise about which surrounding structure are involved by PA-chol
  - Is horizontal petrous or cavernous ICA involved?
  - Are CPA-IAC facial or vestibulocochlear nerves compressed?
  - Is inner ear eroded?
  - Is either jugular foramen or sigmoid sinus involved?
  - Examine bony facial nerve canal throughout its course for erosion

SELECTED REFERENCES

1. Vangrinsven G et al: Beyond the otoscope: an imaging review of congenital cholesteatoma. Insights Imaging. 15(1):194, 2024
2. Shimanuki MN et al: Imaging of temporal bone mass lesions: a pictorial review. Diagnostics (Basel). 13(16), 2023
3. Gupta N et al: Pediatric petrous apex lesions: a radiological classification and diagnostic algorithm. Can Assoc Radiol J. 73(4):655-71, 2022
4. Potter GM et al: Imaging of petrous apex lesions. Neuroimaging Clin N Am. 31(4):523-40, 2021
5. Maxwell AK et al: Congenital cholesteatoma of the sphenoid, occipital, and temporal bones: 54-year follow up. Otol Neurotol. 41(5):e593-6, 2020
6. Casazza GC et al: Primary petrous apex epidermoids with skull base erosion. Otol Neurotol. 40(5):e556-61, 2019
7. Orhan KS et al: Endoscope-assisted surgery for petrous bone cholesteatoma with hearing preservation. J Int Adv Otol. 15(3):391-5, 2019
8. Iannella G et al: Giant petrous bone cholesteatoma: combined microscopic surgery and an adjuvant endoscopic approach. J Neurol Surg Rep. 77(1):e46-9, 2016
9. MacKeith SA et al: Recurrent aseptic meningitis as a rare but important presentation of congenital petrous apex cholesteatoma: the value of appropriate imaging. BMJ Case Rep. 2014
10. Radhakrishnan R et al: Petrous apex lesions in the pediatric population. Pediatr Radiol. 44(3):325-39; quiz 323-4, 2014
11. Chapman PR et al: Petrous apex lesions: pictorial review. AJR Am J Roentgenol. 196(3 Suppl):WS26-37 Quiz S40-3, 2011
12. De Foer B et al: Diffusion-weighted magnetic resonance imaging of the temporal bone. Neuroradiology. 52(9):785-807, 2010
13. Moffat D et al: Petrous temporal bone cholesteatoma: a new classification and long-term surgical outcomes. Skull Base. 18(2):107-15, 2008
14. Kojima H et al: Congenital cholesteatoma clinical features and surgical results. Am J Otolaryngol. 27(5):299-305, 2006
15. Profant M et al: Petrous apex cholesteatoma. Acta Otolaryngol. 120(2):164-7, 2000

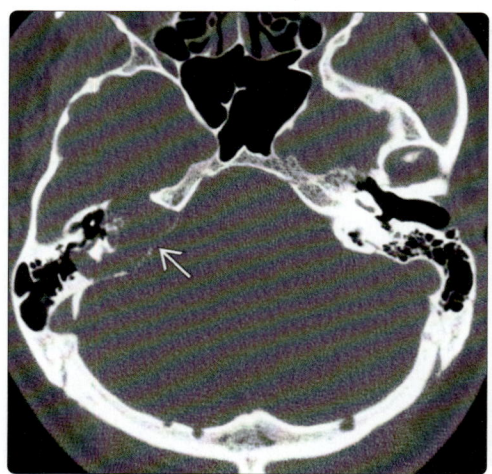
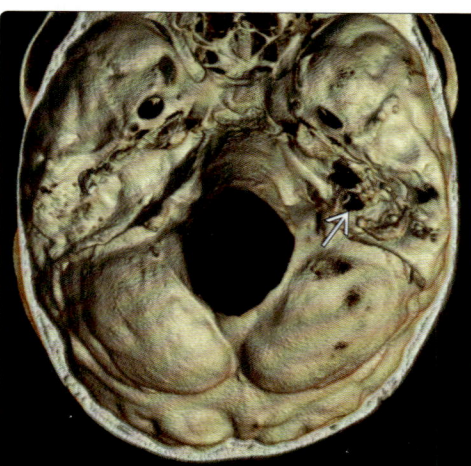

(Left) Axial CT in a 32-year-old with chronic right hearing loss and facial nerve palsy demonstrates a large, lytic, and expansile cholesteatoma ➡ in the right petrous bone affecting the apex and the middle ear. The lesion has destroyed much of the otic capsule and bony facial nerve canal. (Right) 3D CT of skull base in the same patient shows the extensive destruction of the right petrous bone ➡ with excavation of the roof.

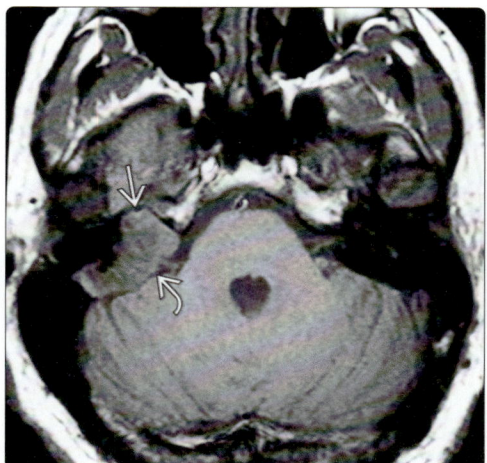
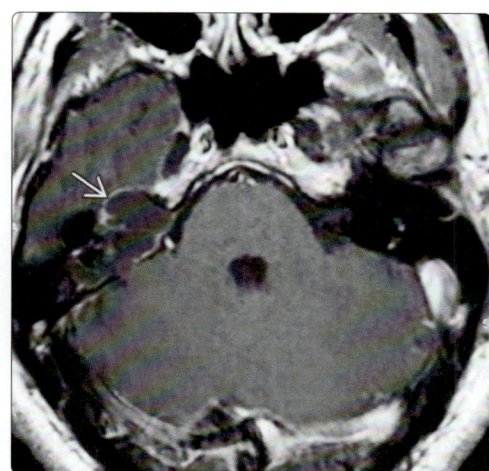

(Left) Axial T1 MR in the same patient shows low to intermediate signal in the expansile mass ➡ of the right PA. The cholesteatoma is encroaching upon the right cerebellopontine angle ➡, and the IAC is completely obscured. (Right) Axial T1 C+ MR shows some peripheral linear enhancement ➡ but no central enhancement of this congenital cholesteatoma of the right petrous bone.

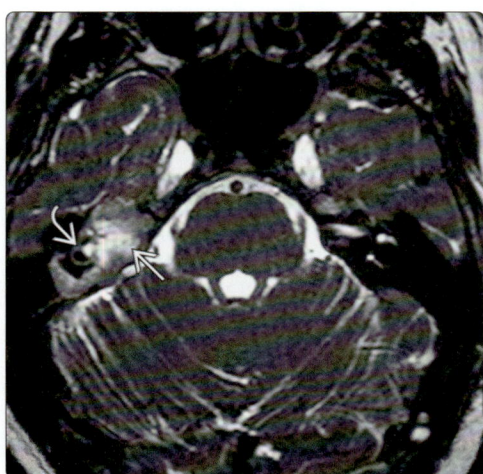
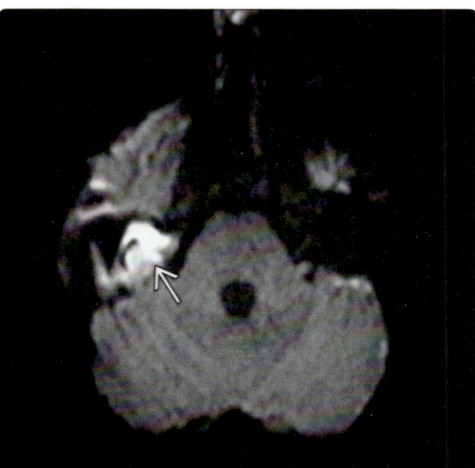

(Left) High-resolution 3D T2 MR shows mixed signal in the expansile mass of the right petrous bone ➡. Some fluid-filled remnants of the labyrinth ➡ can be seen laterally. (Right) Axial DWI MR shows characteristic high signal compatible with diffusion restriction ➡, a typical feature of cholesteatomas or epidermoids.

TERMINOLOGY

- Definition: Sterile fluid in petrous apex (PA) air cells
- a.k.a. PA effusion

IMAGING

- Bone CT findings
  - Opacified PA air cells
  - **No** PA expansion
  - **No** trabecular loss or cortical erosion
- MR findings
  - T1 intermediate to high signal in PA most common
  - High T2 signal in PA
  - No enhancement (sterile fluid)
- Middle ear & mastoid air cells usually clear

TOP DIFFERENTIAL DIAGNOSES

- PA cholesterol granuloma
- PA congenital cholesteatoma
- Apical petrositis

PATHOLOGY

- Sterile fluid in PA air cell
- Pathophysiology
  - May occur as normal developmental variant within pneumatized PA
  - May also follow remote otomastoiditis

CLINICAL ISSUES

- Principal presenting symptom: **None**
- Nonexpansile & nondestructive fluid in unilateral PA requires no further work-up
- Incidental finding on brain MR or CT for unrelated symptoms
  - Most common lesion found in PA
  - Residual fluid in PA air cells present in 1% of all head MR images
  - Seen in > 10% of ICU patients
- Do thin temporal bone CT if atypical on MR
- Treatment: **None**

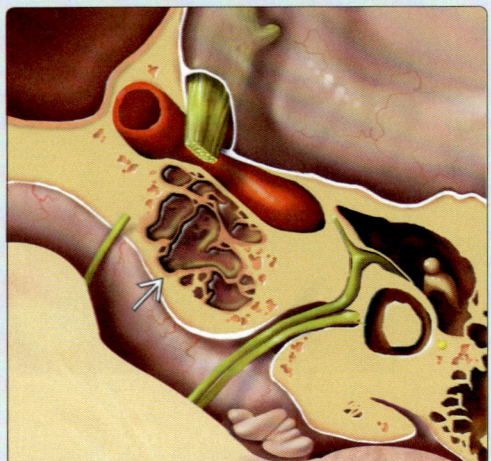
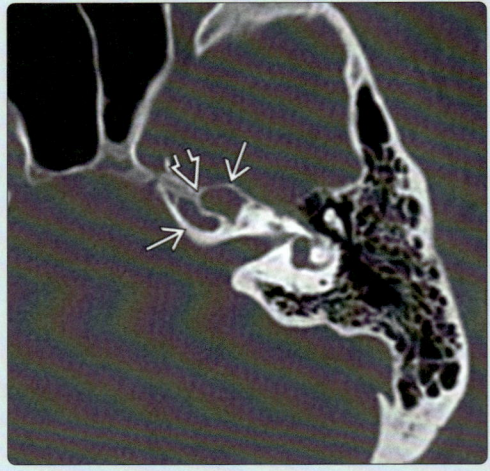

(Left) Axial graphic of the left temporal bone demonstrates fluid-filled petrous apex air cells ➡. Notice that trapped fluid in the petrous apex has no associated expansion or trabecular breakdown. (Right) Axial bone CT demonstrates a typical example of petrous apex trapped fluid as a group of nonexpansile, opacified petrous apex air cells ➡ with preservation of the trabecula ⇒ and cortical margins. Also notice the absence of fluid opacification of the middle ear and mastoid air cells.

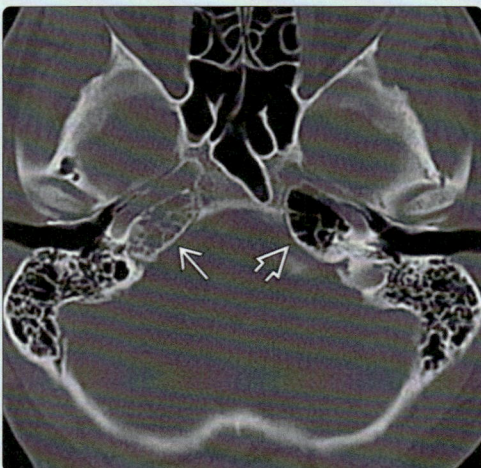
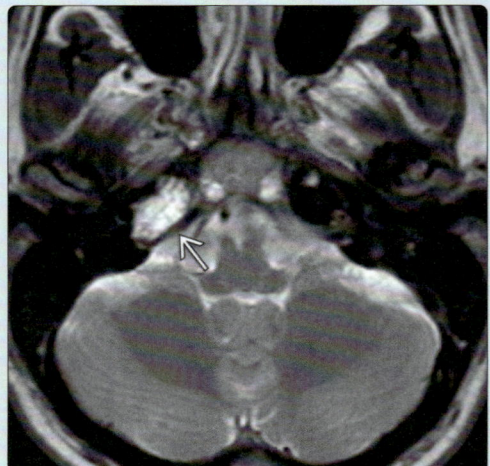

(Left) Axial bone CT shows opacified right petrous apex air cells ➡ with intact trabeculae and cortex, similar in appearance to multiple prior exams, and consistent with trapped fluid in the petrous apex. Note the normal aerated left petrous apex ⇒ for comparison. (Right) Axial T2 MR in the same patient demonstrates hyperintense fluid within the right petrous apex ➡ with intact trabeculae and cortex.

TERMINOLOGY

Abbreviations

- Trapped fluid within petrous apex (TF-PA)

Synonyms

- PA effusion

IMAGING

General Features

- Best diagnostic clue
  - Bone CT showing opacified PA air cells **without** trabecular loss or expansion
  - High T2 signal fluid in PA on MR without expansion

CT Findings

- CECT
  - No enhancement of PA or adjacent meninges
  - Absence of middle ear or mastoid inflammation
- Bone CT
  - Unilateral opacification of PA air cells
  - **No cortical or trabecular erosions** of PA
  - **Not expansile** lesion
  - Sclerotic air cell margins from presumed remote inflammation (~ 50%) or developmental variant

MR Findings

- T1WI
  - Variable; intermediate to high signal in PA most common (proteinaceous fluid)
    - Heterogeneous T1 signal possible
- T2WI
  - **High T2 signal** fluid
  - Intact PA trabeculae (linear hypointensity)
- DWI
  - No diffusion restriction
- T1WI C+
  - No enhancement of PA or adjacent meninges

Imaging Recommendations

- Best imaging tool
  - Bone CT after TF-PA is discovered on brain MR

DIFFERENTIAL DIAGNOSIS

Petrous Apex Cholesterol Granuloma

- Bone CT: Expansile lesion of PA air cells
  - Loss of PA bony trabeculae
- MR: High T1, high T2 signal

Petrous Apex Congenital Cholesteatoma

- Bone CT: Expansile lesion of PA air cells
  - Loss of PA bony trabeculae
- MR: Low T1, high T2 signal
  - Diffusion restriction

Apical Petrositis

- Bone CT: Trabecular & cortical erosion
- MR: Low T1 signal, high T2 signal
  - T1 C+ shows thickened, enhancing meninges with spread to adjacent structures
- Clinical setting of otomastoiditis or post mastoidectomy

PATHOLOGY

General Features

- Etiology
  - May occur as normal developmental variant
  - May also follow remote otomastoiditis
  - Sterile PA air cell fluid
- Embryology-anatomy
  - PA pneumatization required for TF-PA to occur

Microscopic Features

- Clear to xanthochromic fluid discovered at surgery
- No microorganisms or tumor cells present

CLINICAL ISSUES

Presentation

- Most common signs/symptoms
  - **Asymptomatic** (usually incidental finding on brain MR for unrelated symptoms)

Demographics

- Epidemiology
  - Residual fluid in PA air cells present in 1% of all head MR images
  - Seen in > 10% of ICU patients
  - TF-PA is most common lesion found in PA

Natural History & Prognosis

- TF-PA remains unchanged throughout patient's life
- Rarely, fluid becomes superinfected with TF-PA, transforming into apical petrositis

Treatment

- No therapy is warranted for classic TF-PA
  - No follow-up needed

DIAGNOSTIC CHECKLIST

Image Interpretation Pearls

- Nonexpansile & nondestructive benign fluid in unilateral PA requires **no** further work-up
- Consider thin-slice temporal bone CT to evaluate for intact trabeculae & cortex if atypical findings on MR
- Imaging findings suspicious for other PA etiology: PA expansion, cortical irregularity, or adjacent meningeal enhancement/thickening
  - Contrast enhancement & fat saturation on MR may also be helpful in differentiating TF-PA from other PA lesions

SELECTED REFERENCES

1. Eugine R et al: Patterns of pneumatization of parts of temporal bone in high-resolution computed tomography and its implications. Otol Neurotol. 46(4):405-12, 2025
2. Huang JH et al: Skull base tumor mimics. Neuroimaging Clin N Am. 32(2):327-44, 2022
3. Huyett P et al: Radiographic mastoid and middle ear effusions in intensive care unit subjects. Respir Care. 62(3):350-6, 2017
4. Razek AA et al: Lesions of the petrous apex: classification and findings at CT and MR imaging. Radiographics. 32(1):151-73, 2012
5. Chapman PR et al: Petrous apex lesions: pictorial review. AJR Am J Roentgenol. 196(3 Suppl):WS26-37 Quiz S40-3, 2011
6. Leonetti JP et al: Incidental petrous apex findings on magnetic resonance imaging. Ear Nose Throat J. 80(4):200-2, 205-6, 2001
7. Moore KR et al: 'Leave me alone' lesions of the petrous apex. AJNR Am J Neuroradiol. 19(4):733-8, 1998

TERMINOLOGY

- Mucus-containing, expanded petrous apex (PA) air cell(s) lined by secretory epithelium, resulting from chronic ostial obstruction

IMAGING

- Fluid-filled, **expanded** PA air cell(s)
- CT: Smooth, expansile PA, intact cortex
- MR: T1 low, T2 high-signal fluid usually
  - Nonenhancing, no diffusion restriction

TOP DIFFERENTIAL DIAGNOSES

- PA cholesterol granuloma
- PA trapped fluid
- PA congenital cholesteatoma
- PA cephalocele
- Temporal bone internal carotid artery aneurysm

PATHOLOGY

- Results from **obstruction to PA air cell drainage**
- Secretion of mucus into obstructed air cells from previous middle ear-mastoid infection, trauma, surgery
- Air cell expansion from pressure remodeling of wall

CLINICAL ISSUES

- Often incidental and asymptomatic
- Rare lesion
- Headache or rare cranial neuropathy from compression
- Treatment issues: Controversial if patient asymptomatic
  - Consider follow-up CT to see if mucocele increases in size
  - Surgical obliteration if enlarges and symptomatic

DIAGNOSTIC CHECKLIST

- When bone CT shows fluid-filled expansile PA lesion with intact cortex, MR can further characterize lesion
  - PA mucocele can look similar to PA cholesterol granuloma but has more consistently low T1

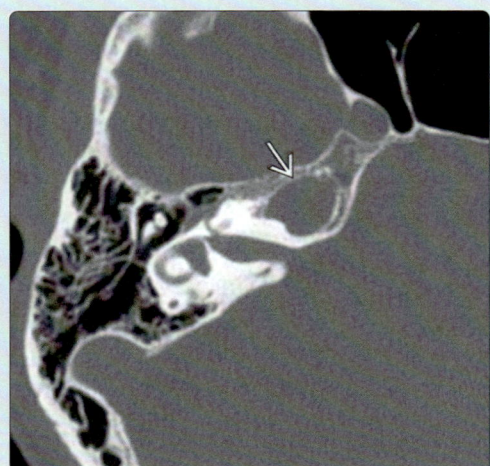
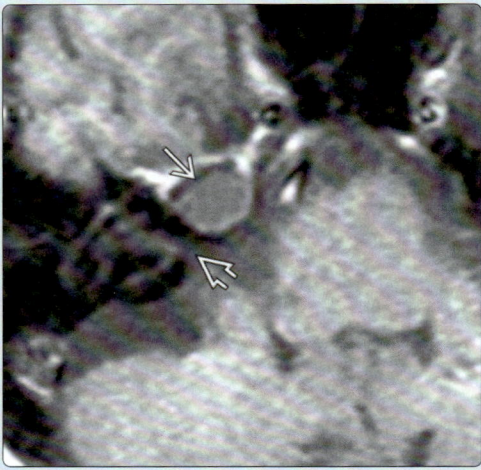

(Left) Axial bone CT shows an expansile right petrous apex (PA) lesion ➡ with loss of the normal air cell trabeculations. The differential diagnosis is congenital cholesteatoma, cholesterol granuloma, and mucocele. (Right) Axial T1WI MR in the same patient demonstrates an expansile PA mucocele ➡ with minimally higher signal than CSF. Note low-signal CSF of the internal auditory canal ➡ just posterolateral to the lesion. Low signal on T1WI excludes a cholesterol granuloma.

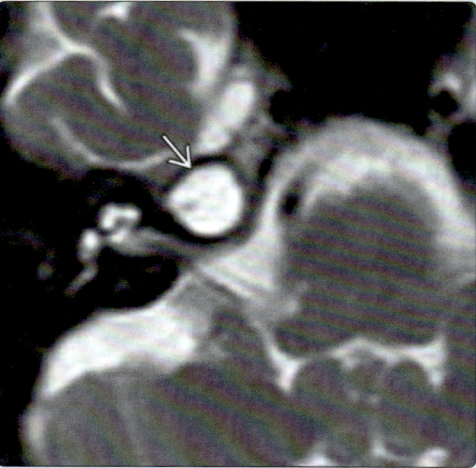
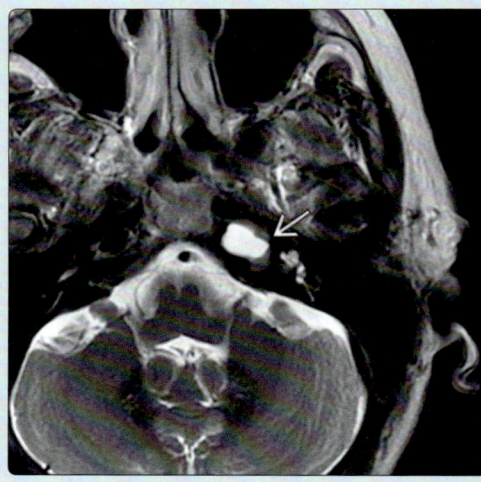

(Left) Axial T2WI MR in the same patient demonstrates the PA mucocele is uniformly hyperintense ➡. DWI (not shown) had no restricted diffusion. An expansile PA lesion with low T1, high T2, and no restricted diffusion is highly suggestive of mucocele. (Right) Axial T2WI MR demonstrates bright T2 signal in an expanded PA mucocele ➡. T1 signal was low (not a cholesterol granuloma) and there was no restricted diffusion (not a congenital cholesteatoma).

Petrous Apex Mucocele

TERMINOLOGY

Definitions

- Mucus-containing, expanded petrous apex (PA) air cell(s) lined by secretory epithelium resulting from chronic ostial obstruction

IMAGING

General Features

- Best diagnostic clue
  - CT: Fluid-filled, **expanded** PA air cell(s)
  - MR: T1 low, T2 high signal, DWI without restricted diffusion, nonenhancing

Imaging Recommendations

- Best imaging tool
  - Temporal bone or skull base CT: Fluid-filled, expanded PA
  - Enhanced MR if atypical CT features
    - MR will differentiate PA mucocele from congenital cholesteatoma

CT Findings

- Bone CT
  - **Expanded**, opacified PA air cell(s)
  - PA walls **remodeled** ± thinned or focally absent

MR Findings

- T1WI
  - **Usually low signal**; increased signal if proteinaceous
- T2WI
  - Usually high signal
    - If inspissated mucus exists, decreased signal
- DWI
  - No restricted diffusion
- T1WI C+ FS
  - May have minimal peripheral rim enhancement

DIFFERENTIAL DIAGNOSIS

Petrous Apex Cholesterol Granuloma

- Bone CT: Expansile PA air cells
- MR: High T1, high T2 signal with low rim

Petrous Apex Trapped Fluid

- Bone CT: Nonexpansile air cells
- MR: T1 variable but usually increased signal, high T2

Petrous Apex Congenital Cholesteatoma

- Bone CT: Expansile PA air cells
- MR: T1 low, T2 high, **diffusion restriction**

Petrous Apex Cephalocele

- Bone CT: Communicates with intracranial subarachnoid space or Meckel cave
  - PA wall interrupted, often superiorly or posteriorly
- MR: Follows CSF on all sequences

Temporal Bone Internal Carotid Artery Aneurysm

- CT: Expansile bony petrous internal carotid artery canal
- MR: Complex signal

PATHOLOGY

General Features

- Etiology
  - Results from **obstruction of PA air cell drainage**
    - Obstruction from middle ear-mastoid infection, trauma, previous surgery
    - Secretion of mucus into obstructed air cells
    - PA air cell expansion from pressure remodeling of wall

Microscopic Features

- Flattened, pseudostratified, ciliated columnar epithelium = mucus-secreting respiratory epithelium
- Reactive bone formation or bone remodeling of air cell wall may be present

CLINICAL ISSUES

Presentation

- Most common signs/symptoms
  - Often incidental finding on CT or MR in asymptomatic patient
  - May have headache
  - Rare cranial neuropathy from compression

Demographics

- Age
  - Most common in adults, rare in pediatrics
- Epidemiology
  - Extremely **rare** lesion

Natural History & Prognosis

- Requires pneumatized PA
- Gradual enlargement over time

Treatment

- Controversial, especially in asymptomatic patient
- Consider follow-up CT to see if mucocele increases in size
- Surgical obliteration if enlarges and symptomatic

DIAGNOSTIC CHECKLIST

Consider

- When bone CT shows opacified, expansile PA lesion
  - Consider **mucocele** if **T1 is low**, T2 is high, no restricted diffusion
  - Consider **cholesterol granuloma** if **T1 is high**
  - Consider **congenital cholesteatoma** if **restricted diffusion**

SELECTED REFERENCES

1. Verma RR et al: Endoscopic transsphenoidal drainage of petrous apex mucocele. Ear Nose Throat J. 102(1):13-14, 2020
2. Campion T et al: Imaging of temporal bone inflammations in children: a pictorial review. Neuroradiology. 61(9):959-70, 2019
3. Razek AA et al: Lesions of the petrous apex: classification and findings at CT and MR imaging. Radiographics. 32(1):151-73, 2012
4. Chapman PR et al: Petrous apex lesions: pictorial review. AJR Am J Roentgenol. 196(3 Suppl):WS26-37 Quiz S40-3, 2011
5. Le BT et al: Petrous apex mucocele. Otol Neurotol. 29(1):102-3, 2008
6. Isaacson B et al: Lesions of the petrous apex: diagnosis and management. Otolaryngol Clin North Am. 40(3):479-519, viii, 2007
7. Muckle RP et al: Petrous apex lesions. Am J Otol. 19(2):219-25, 1998

TERMINOLOGY

- Petrous apex (PA) cholesterol granuloma (CG): **Expansile** PA lesion resulting from foreign body giant cell reaction to deposition of cholesterol crystals in apical air cells with fibrosis and vascular proliferation
- a.k.a. cholesterol cyst, "chocolate" cyst

IMAGING

- Temporal bone CT findings
  - **Sharply marginated**, **expansile** PA lesion
  - Trabecular breakdown of PA
  - Cortical thinning of PA ± focal bony wall dehiscence when large
- Temporal bone MR findings
  - **High T1 internal signal**
  - High T2 internal signal
  - Peripheral low T2 signal hemosiderin ring
  - No internal enhancement

TOP DIFFERENTIAL DIAGNOSES

- PA asymmetric marrow
- PA trapped fluid
- PA congenital cholesteatoma
- PA internal carotid artery aneurysm
- PA mucocele
- Apical petrositis

PATHOLOGY

- Pneumatized PA air cells required
- Obstruction-vacuum pathogenesis (classic hypothesis)
- Exposed bone marrow pathogenesis (recent alternative hypothesis)

CLINICAL ISSUES

- May be incidental asymptomatic lesion
- Most common symptoms: Headache, dizziness
- If CNV-VIII affected, facial pain/weakness, diplopia, or hearing loss, then surgical drainage

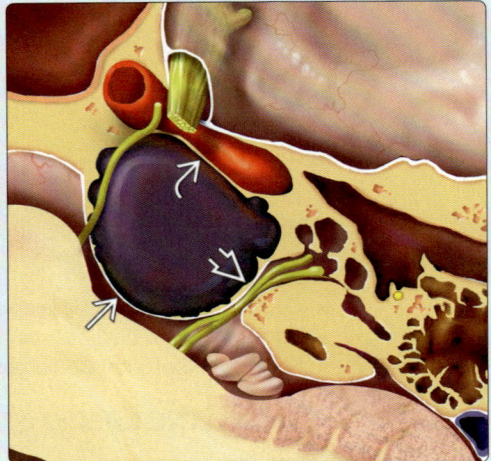
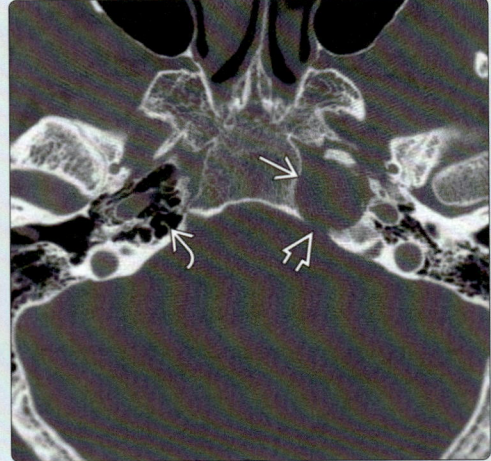

(Left) *Axial graphic shows a cholesterol granuloma (CG) of the petrous apex (PA) (PA-CG). The lesion is expansile with air cell trabecular loss and "eggshell" medial cortex ➡. The lesion compresses the internal auditory canal (IAC) ➡ and thins the posterior wall of the horizontal petrous internal carotid artery (ICA) canal ➡. (Right) Axial bone CT reveals an expansile CG in the left PA ➡ with marginal bone dehiscence ➡ present. The right PA is well pneumatized ➡. PA-CG most frequently occurs in pneumatized PA.*

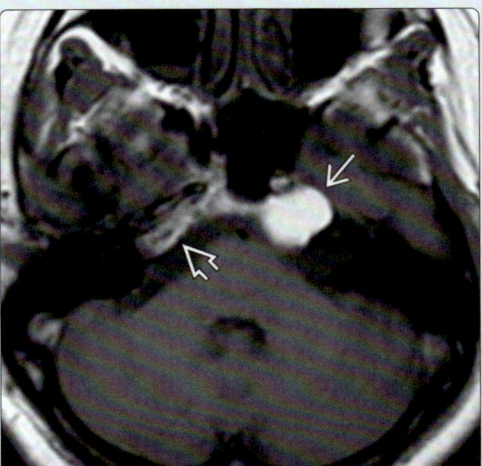
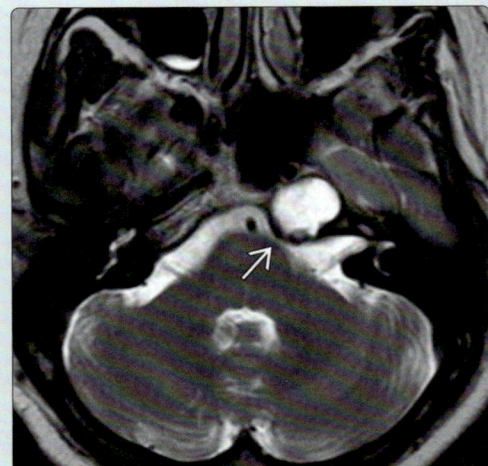

(Left) *Axial T1WI nonenhanced MR demonstrates a hyperintense, smoothly expansile lesion ➡ involving the left PA. Note the heterogeneous appearance of normal fatty marrow in the right PA ➡ for comparison. (Right) Axial T2WI MR in the same patient shows a smoothly expansile, hyperintense lesion with peripheral hypointense rim ➡ (due to internal methemoglobin and peripheral hemosiderin from prior chronic bleeding).*

TERMINOLOGY

Abbreviations

- Petrous apex (PA) cholesterol granuloma (CG) (PA-CG)

Synonyms

- Cholesterol cyst, "chocolate" cyst

Definitions

- **PA-CG:** **Expansile** PA lesion resulting from foreign body giant cell reaction to deposition of cholesterol crystals in apical air cells with fibrosis and vascular proliferation

IMAGING

General Features

- Best diagnostic clue
  - **High T1** and high T2 signal in expansile PA mass
- Location
  - PA air cells
  - When large, expands into adjacent structures
- Size
  - Ranges from small lesions confined to PA to large, lobulated masses
- Morphology
  - Smooth, sharply marginated; lobulated when large

CT Findings

- Bone CT
  - **Sharply marginated**, **expansile** PA lesion
  - **Trabecular breakdown** of PA
  - **Cortical thinning** of PA ± focal bony wall dehiscence when large
  - When large, expands regionally
    - Anteriorly to involve horizontal petrous internal carotid artery (ICA) canal
    - Medially into clivus, sphenoid sinus
    - Lateral to inner and middle ear, facial nerve canal
    - Posterior to internal auditory canal and cerebellopontine angle

MR Findings

- T1WI
  - **High internal signal**
    - Secondary to presence of hemorrhage, blood breakdown products, and cholesterol crystals
    - Most likely due to presence of paramagnetic intracellular methemoglobin
- T2WI
  - High internal signal
  - **Peripheral low-signal hemosiderin ring**
- FLAIR
  - High signal does not attenuate (remains high)
- T1WI C+
  - **No** internal enhancement
  - If no T1 precontrast imaging, may be mistaken for enhancing lesion
- MRA
  - Useful in surgical planning; assess for involvement of petrous ICA
  - Beware: Lesions with high T1 signal will appear bright on time-of-flight MRA; mimics aneurysm

Imaging Recommendations

- Best imaging tool
  - Combination bone CT and MR
    - Temporal bone CT evaluates trabecular destruction and expansion into adjacent structures
    - MR characteristic high T1 signal confirms diagnosis
- Protocol advice
  - Remember: Include **precontrast T1** sequence on MR
    - Contrast is not as helpful in delineating diagnosis of PA-CG from other PA lesions
  - MRA can evaluate possible involvement of petrous ICA in large lesions
  - Postoperative MR is more sensitive than CT for evaluation of recurrence
    - ↑ T1 signal in postoperative PA = recurrence
      - ☐ Beware of surgical fat packing (use fat saturation)

DIFFERENTIAL DIAGNOSIS

Petrous Apex Asymmetric Marrow

- CT: Nonexpansile, fat-density marrow
- MR: T1 high signal, T2 intermediate to high signal
  - Suppresses on fat-saturated MR

Petrous Apex Trapped Fluid

- CT: Nonexpansile; opacified air cells with intact cortex and trabeculae
- MR: Variable T1 signal, T2 high signal
  - No contrast enhancement of lesion or meninges

Petrous Apex Congenital Cholesteatoma

- CT: Expansile, smooth margins
- MR: T1 low signal, T2 intermediate to high signal
  - DWI: Restricted diffusion (high signal)

Petrous Apex Internal Carotid Artery Aneurysm

- CT: Smooth expansion of petrous ICA canal
- MR: Heterogeneous signal with internal flow void
  - T1 C+ MR: Heterogeneous internal enhancement

Petrous Apex Mucocele

- CT: Single expansile air cell area in PA
- MR: Low T1, high T2, facilitated diffusion

Apical Petrositis

- CT: Permeative destructive changes of cortex and trabeculae
- MR: T1 low signal, T2 high signal
  - Enhancing rim and meninges

PATHOLOGY

General Features

- Etiology
  - Obstruction-vacuum pathogenesis (classic hypothesis)
    - Otitis media creates mucosal obstruction of PA air cells, causing development of vacuum
    - Vacuum phenomena leads to rupture of blood vessels and hemorrhage in PA air cells
    - Anaerobic degradation of RBCs forms **cholesterol crystals**, which **incite foreign body giant cell infiltration**

- Granulation tissue forms secondary to repeated hemorrhage, leading to expansile PA lesion
  - Exposed bone marrow pathogenesis (recent alternative hypothesis)
    - Begins with mucosal penetration into PA in young adulthood
    - Marrow exposed, which leads to sustained/repeated microhemorrhage
    - Marrow provides lipids broken down into cholesterol crystals
- Embryology anatomy
  - Pneumatized PA air cells required
  - PA pneumatization occurs normally in 33% of people

Gross Pathologic & Surgical Features

- Cystic mass **without** epithelial lining
- Fibrous capsule filled with blue-brown liquid containing old blood and cholesterol crystals = "chocolate" cyst
- Fluid described as crankcase oil

Microscopic Features

- RBCs in various stages of degradation
- Multinucleated giant cells surrounding cholesterol crystals embedded in fibrous connective tissue
- Hemosiderin-laden macrophages
- Chronic inflammatory cells and blood vessels

CLINICAL ISSUES

Presentation

- Most common signs/symptoms
  - May be incidental asymptomatic lesion
  - Headache and dizziness most common presenting symptoms
- Other signs/symptoms
  - Facial pain, hearing loss, or diplopia if CNV-VIII involved
- Clinical profile
  - Otoscopy normal unless middle ear involved
    - Blue-black retrotympanic mass
  - Audiometric exam: Sensorineural hearing loss or mixed pattern
  - Typically unilateral lesion, but bilateral PA-CG reported in context of familial hypercholesterolemia

Demographics

- Age
  - Young to middle-aged adults
- Epidemiology
  - Most common surgical lesion in PA
  - Middle ear-CG more common than PA-CG

Natural History & Prognosis

- Growth rate highly variable
  - Most stable, or slow growing over decades
  - Rapid growth or sudden onset of new symptoms rare
  - Depends on frequency and severity of microhemorrhages
- Can be asymptomatic; if symptomatic, then surgery
  - Symptoms can show up years after initial bout of chronic otitis media
- Excellent prognosis if adequately drained surgically

Treatment

- Asymptomatic patients can be safely followed with imaging
- Surgical treatment tailored for each patient based on extent of lesion, etc.
  - Traditional surgery: Drainage and stent placement to reestablish PA aeration via transtemporal approach
    - Reported recurrence rate as high as 60%
  - Anterior endonasal approaches (e.g., selective transsphenoidal endoscopic drainage)
  - Extended middle cranial fossa approach with extradural removal of PA-CG and obliteration of its cavity
    - Significant ↓ in recurrence rates

DIAGNOSTIC CHECKLIST

Consider

- Consider PA-CG in any **expansile PA** lesion with **high T1** and T2 signal
- CT, MR, and MRA in preoperative planning, particularly in large lesions
- MR best for evaluating postoperative recurrence

Image Interpretation Pearls

- Characteristic appearance of **expansile, high T1** and T2 lesion differentiates from other PA lesions
- CT most useful to evaluate bony destruction and involvement of adjacent otic capsule and carotid canal
- Make sure to evaluate for internal flow &/or pulsation artifact to avoid misdiagnosing petrous ICA aneurysm

Reporting Tips

- Specifically comment on integrity of adjacent critical structures for presurgical planning
  - Facial nerve canal
  - Petrous ICA canal
  - Internal auditory canal
  - Inner ear otic capsule

SELECTED REFERENCES

1. Noy R et al: Surgical approaches to petrous apex cholesterol granulomas: a systematic review and network meta-analysis. Laryngoscope. 134(4):1540-50, 2024
2. Fieux M et al: Petrous apex cholesterol granuloma revealed by facial palsy. Ann Neurol. 89(2):414-15, 2021
3. Albakheet N et al: Familial hypercholesterolemia with bilateral cholesterol granuloma: a case series. Int J Surg Case Rep. 62:135-9, 2019
4. Campion T et al: Imaging of temporal bone inflammations in children: a pictorial review. Neuroradiology. 61(9):959-70, 2019
5. Stevens SM et al: Long-term symptom-specific outcomes for patients with petrous apex cholesterol granulomas: surgery versus observation. Otol Neurotol. 38(2):253-9, 2017
6. Sweeney AD et al: The natural history and management of petrous apex cholesterol granulomas. Otol Neurotol. 36(10):1714-9, 2015
7. Juliano AF et al: Imaging review of the temporal bone: part I. Anatomy and inflammatory and neoplastic processes. Radiology. 269(1):17-33, 2013
8. Hoa M et al: Petrous apex cholesterol granuloma: maintenance of drainage pathway, the histopathology of surgical management and histopathologic evidence for the exposed marrow theory. Otol Neurotol. 33(6):1059-65, 2012
9. Sanna M et al: Otoneurological management of petrous apex cholesterol granuloma. Am J Otolaryngol. 30(6):407-14, 2009
10. Castillo MP et al: Petrous apex cholesterol granuloma aeration: does it matter? Otolaryngol Head Neck Surg. 138(4):518-22, 2008
11. Oyama K et al: Petrous apex cholesterol granuloma treated via the endoscopic transsphenoidal approach. Acta Neurochir (Wien). 149(3):299-302; discussion 302, 2007
12. Jackler RK et al: A new theory to explain the genesis of petrous apex cholesterol granuloma. Otol Neurotol. 24(1): 96-106; discussion 106, 2003

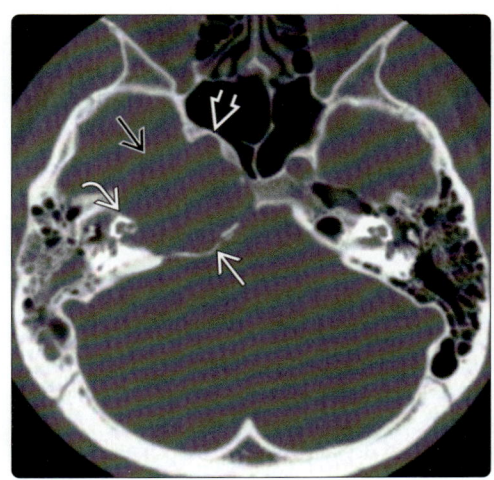

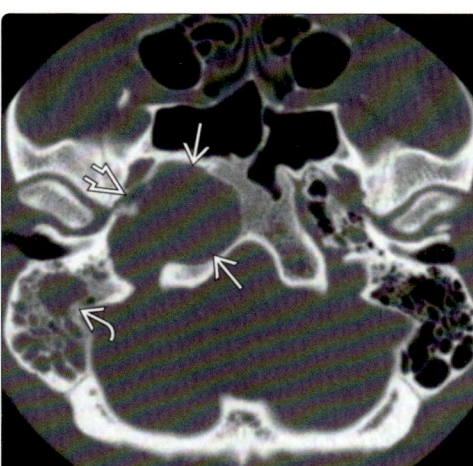

(Left) *A large PA-CG is seen on bone CT as an expansile mass ➡ with a fully dehiscent anterolateral margin ➡. The lesion extends into the IAC and is eroding the otic capsule ➡. The cavernous ICA ➡ is displaced anteriorly.* (Right) *A more inferior axial bone CT in the same patient again shows the PA-CG ➡ compressing the bony eustachian tube ➡. Fluid in the mastoid ➡ is secondary to eustachian tube obstruction.*

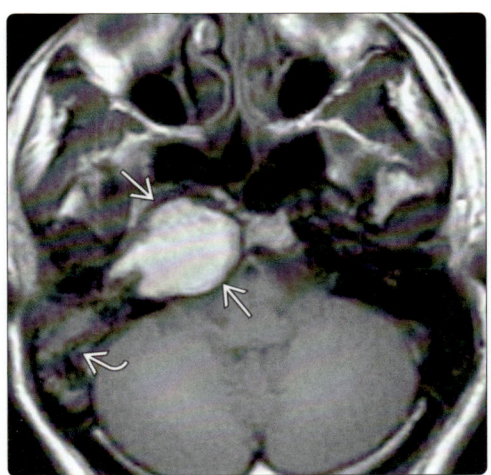

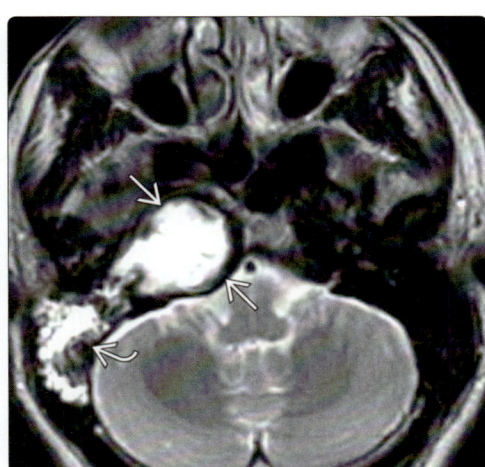

(Left) *Axial T1WI MR in the same patient reveals the expansile, high-signal PA-CG ➡. The mastoid fluid ➡ is of intermediate signal, most likely due to protein in the fluid.* (Right) *Axial T2WI MR in the same patient shows a high-signal, expansile PA mass ➡. A few low-signal foci are seen within the mass, secondary to hemosiderin deposits. In classic CG, there is high signal on both T1 and T2. Obstructed fluid in the mastoid ➡ is also high signal.*

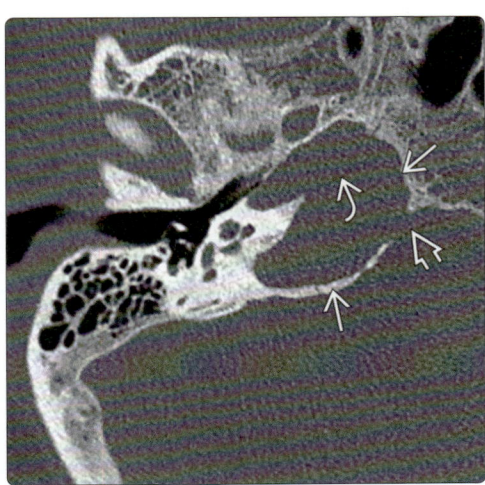

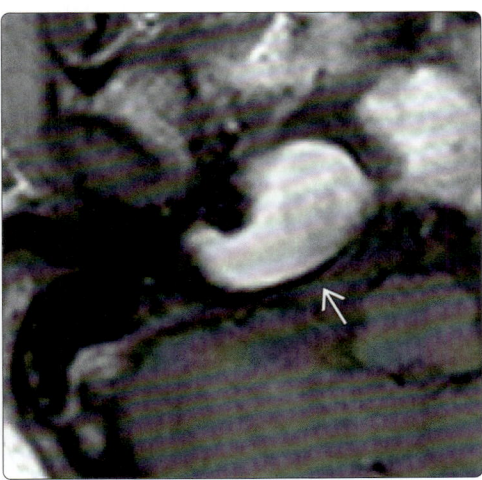

(Left) *Axial temporal bone CT shows an expansile mass of the PA ➡. There is focal bony thinning or dehiscence ➡. Erosion into the foramen lacerum ➡ is important to report so the surgeon is aware of the mass relationship with the ICA.* (Right) *Axial T1WI MR in the same patient shows a hyperintense mass expanding the PA ➡. This PA-CG was discovered incidentally when the patient was imaged for a possible stroke.*

TERMINOLOGY

- Definition: Extension of otomastoiditis (OM) infection into pneumatized petrous apex (PA) with resulting suppurative apical petrositis (or petrous apicitis)

IMAGING

- Bone CT: **Trabecular breakdown ± cortical erosions** in opacified PA air cells
- Early disease
  - **Rim-enhancing, fluid-filled PA**
  - Adjacent **meningeal thickening/enhancement**
- Advanced disease
  - Thickened, enhancing Meckel cave & cavernous sinus
  - Enhancing cranial nerves, especially CNV & CNVI
  - Skull base osteomyelitis (enhancing clival marrow)
  - Pachymeningitis with epidural or brain abscess
  - Petrous ± cavernous internal carotid artery spasm
  - Cavernous or sigmoid thrombosis possible

TOP DIFFERENTIAL DIAGNOSES

- PA trapped fluid
- PA congenital cholesteatoma
- PA metastasis
- PA cholesterol granuloma
- Petrooccipital fissure chondrosarcoma

PATHOLOGY

- Pathophysiology: Suppurative OM infection spreads via air cells or venous channels to PA

CLINICAL ISSUES

- **Gradenigo syndrome**
  - Classic triad of symptoms: Acute OM, deep facial pain (CNV), & lateral rectus palsy (CNVI)
  - Rare clinical presentation
- Treatment: Antibiotics alone are usually sufficient
  - If severe symptoms at presentation, surgical intervention with mastoidectomy

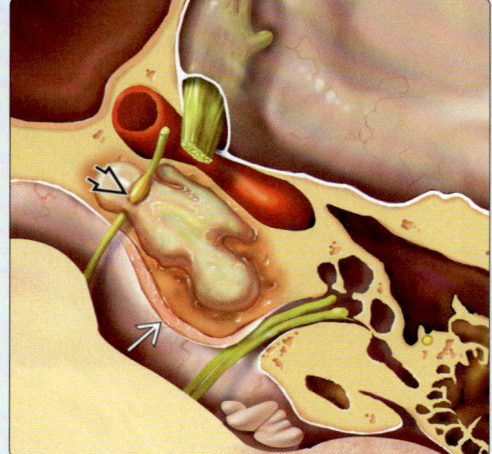
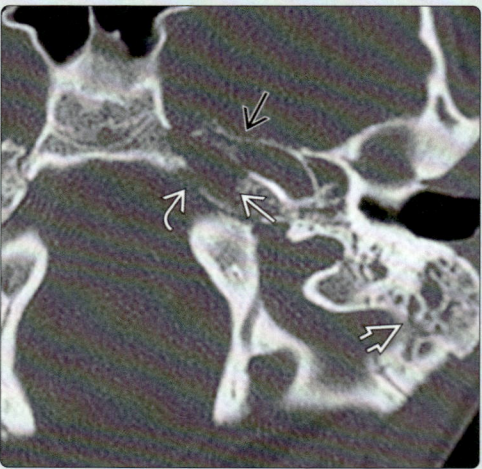

(Left) *Axial graphic of the left petrous apex (PA) shows confluent apical petrositis with PA abscess formation. Pus surrounds CNVI ➡, & associated inflammation thickens adjacent meninges ➡. (Right) Axial temporal bone CT in a young patient with petrous apicitis demonstrates left PA opacification & trabecular destruction ➡ as well as cortical disruption ➡. Note accompanying mastoid opacification ➡. Cortical irregularity of the petrous carotid canal raises suspicion of spread into the canal ➡.*

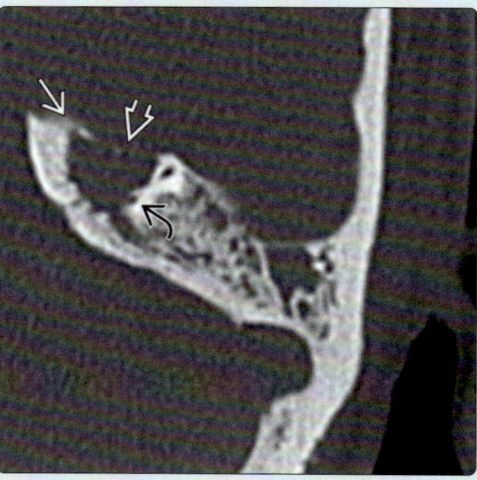
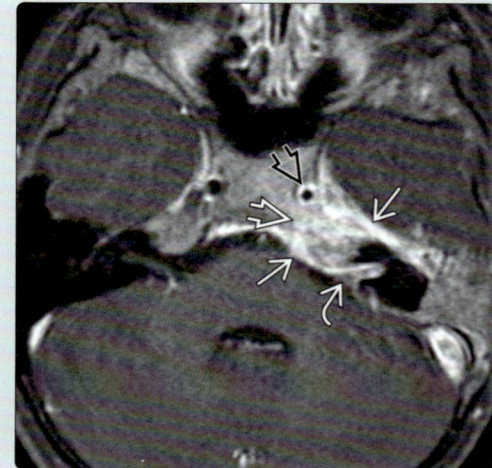

(Left) *Axial temporal bone CT shows an opacified PA ➡ and associated trabecular & anterior cortical erosion ➡, consistent with petrous apicitis; complicated by fistula with the medial aspect of the superior semicircular canal ➡. (Right) Axial T1WI C+ FS MR in the same patient shows infection of the PA with adjacent involvement of the clivus ➡, dura ➡, & internal auditory canal (IAC) ➡. Note the narrowing of the ICA ➡ secondary to associated infectious arteritis &/or spasm.*

Apical Petrositis

TERMINOLOGY

Synonyms
- Petrous apicitis, confluent apical petrositis

Definitions
- Extension of otomastoiditis (OM) into pneumatized petrous apex (PA), resulting in suppurative apical petrositis

IMAGING

General Features
- Best diagnostic clue
  - Bone CT: **Trabecular breakdown ± cortical erosions** in opacified PA air cells
- Location
  - Early disease: Infection within PA of temporal bone
    - Mastoid air cells can be simultaneously involved
  - Advanced disease: Spreads to adjacent meninges, skull base, Meckel cave, & cavernous sinus
    - Result in meningitis, epidural or brain abscess, skull base osteomyelitis, or cavernous sinus thrombosis
- Morphology
  - Irregular phlegmon confined to PA with cortical breakthrough & meningeal involvement

CT Findings
- CECT
  - Peripherally enhancing fluid (pus) in PA
  - Thickened & enhancing meninges
  - Advanced disease
    - Epidural or subdural abscess
    - Cavernous sinus phlegmon ± thrombosis
- Bone CT
  - Opacification of PA air cells
    - Mastoid air cell opacification usually associated
  - Destructive changes of PA = **coalescent apical petrositis**
    - PA **trabeculae lysis** & focal **cortical destruction**
  - Advanced disease
    - Fistulization to bony labyrinth

MR Findings
- T1WI
  - Asymmetric low to intermediate signal in PA
- T2WI
  - **High-signal** fluid in PA (± mastoid air cells)
- DWI
  - **Diffusion restriction** centrally in PA (pus)
- T1WI C+
  - **Rim-enhancing fluid** in PA
  - Adjacent avidly **enhancing meningeal thickening**
  - Advanced disease
    - Epidural, subdural, or brain rim-enhancing abscess
    - Perineural enhancement (especially CNV, CNVI)
    - Skull base osteomyelitis: Enhancing marrow in clivus
    - Nonenhancing cavernous sinus thrombosis
- MRA
  - Advanced disease may involve adjacent internal carotid artery (ICA)
    - Petrous ± cavernous ICA arteritis/spasm
    - Petrous carotid pseudoaneurysm is rare

- MRV
  - Advanced disease may involve adjacent veins
    - Cavernous-petrosal thrombosis
    - Sigmoid sinus-jugular bulb thrombosis possible

Nuclear Medicine Findings
- Bone scan
  - Asymmetric uptake in PA on Tc-99m bone scan or gallium scan
- PET/CT
  - Avid uptake possible; do not mistake for tumor

Imaging Recommendations
- Best imaging tool
  - Initial diagnosis with thin-section **temporal bone CT**
  - Axial & coronal skull base T1 C+ MR with fat saturation important in evaluating intracranial complications in advanced disease

DIFFERENTIAL DIAGNOSIS

Petrous Apex Trapped Fluid
- Clinical: Usually asymptomatic incidental finding
- CT: PA trabeculae & cortex maintained; nonexpansile
- MR: High T2 signal; no rim or meningeal enhancement

Petrous Apex Congenital Cholesteatoma
- Clinical: No acute infectious symptoms
- CT: Smooth cortical expansion; PA trabecular breakdown
- MR: Low T1 MR signal; restricted diffusion
  - No meningeal enhancement

Petrous Apex Metastasis
- Clinical: Systemic malignancy known, no acute infection
- CT: Permeative destructive mass of PA
- MR: Infiltrative, heterogeneously enhancing PA mass

Petrous Apex Cholesterol Granuloma
- CT: PA trabecular breakdown & cortical expansion
- MR: High T1 signal, no meningeal enhancement

Petrooccipital Fissure Chondrosarcoma
- Clinical: No acute infectious symptoms
- CT: Destructive mass of petrooccipital fissure, often Ca++
- MR: Infiltrative, heterogeneously enhancing mass

PATHOLOGY

General Features
- Etiology
  - Acute or chronic suppurative OM infection spreads via mastoid air cells or venous channels to PA
  - Infection of PA air cells causes coalescence with breakdown of trabeculae ± cortical loss
  - Direct extension of infection to adjacent structures (meninges, Meckel cave, & cavernous sinus)
- Embryology-anatomy
  - Pneumatized PA present in ~ 33% of patients
    - PA pneumatization required for apical petrositis to occur in most cases
  - In rare nonpneumatized PA, spread via fascial planes, vascular channels, or directly through osteomyelitic bone

Gross Pathologic & Surgical Features

- Soft osteomyelitic bone with pockets of purulent material within confluent PA air cells
- Air cell tracks from mastoid to PA filled with pus & granulation tissue
- Phlegmon thickens & inflames adjacent meninges

Microscopic Features

- Offending organism often not cultured secondary to preoperative broad-spectrum antibiotics
  - Flora of acute infection similar to OM
    - Acute pathogens: *Haemophilus influenzae*
  - Chronic apical petrositis associated with chronic suppurative OM
    - Chronic pathogens: *Pseudomonas aeruginosa, Proteus* spp.

CLINICAL ISSUES

Presentation

- Most common signs/symptoms
  - Otorrhea with deep facial, ear, or retroorbital pain
- Other signs/symptoms
  - Symptoms variable; may be subtle or prominent, appearing acutely or gradually
    - Acute onset of deep facial pain & otorrhea following acute OM
    - Insidious onset of cranial neuropathy (especially CNV) & otorrhea with chronic suppurative ear
    - Other cranial neuropathies (CNVI, VII, & VIII)
    - Fever, hearing loss, & diplopia
- Clinical profile
  - **Gradenigo syndrome**
    - Classic clinical triad: Acute OM, deep facial pain (CNV), & lateral rectus palsy (CNVI)
      - □ Via direct extension of infection involving Meckel cave (CNV) & Dorello canal (CNVI)
    - Characteristic but rare presentation

Demographics

- Age
  - Child or adolescent with acute OM
  - Adult with chronic suppurative ear or complication following mastoidectomy
- Epidemiology
  - Rare in postantibiotic era

Natural History & Prognosis

- Prognosis excellent if diagnosed early & given adequate surgical drainage & aggressive antibiotics
  - OM symptoms with new cranial nerve deficits suggestive
  - Delayed diagnosis/treatment increases morbidity due to infectious complications (e.g. meningitis, abscess, etc.)
- If untreated, progresses to obtundation & death (common in preantibiotic era)
- Rare presentation of Lemierre syndrome can occur as complication of apical petrositis
  - Fusobacterium necrophorum otic infection with associated thrombosis of cavernous &/or sigmoid sinus

Treatment

- Antibiotics alone usually sufficient

- When severe symptoms not yet present
- Addition of tympanostomy tube may improve symptoms
- If severe symptoms at presentation, surgical intervention with mastoidectomy
  - Surgery follows air cell tracks to PA
- Multiple surgical options have been described
  - Simple vs. radical mastoidectomy & middle cranial fossa approach

DIAGNOSTIC CHECKLIST

Consider

- Initial imaging with thin-section nonenhanced temporal bone CT
- MR with multiplanar fat-saturated enhanced images are most effective way to evaluate for intracranial complications

Image Interpretation Pearls

- Temporal bone CT can evaluate for trabecular ± cortical erosion, & involvement of middle & inner ear
- Contrast-enhanced MR with fat saturation can evaluate for adjacent intracranial & skull base infection
  - Describe extent & location(s) of involvement for presurgical planning
- Differentiate from other PA lesions
  - Rim-enhancing, diffusion restricting fluid in PA
  - Adjacent meningeal enhancement
  - Correlate findings with clinical history
- Evaluate vascular structures adjacent to PA for involvement &/or potential complications: ICA, dural venous sinuses, cavernous sinus

SELECTED REFERENCES

1. Horache K et al: Insights into Gradenigo syndrome: case presentation and review. Radiol Case Rep. 19(11):5442-6, 2024
2. Shareef M et al: Critical infections in the head and neck: a pictorial review of acute presentations and complications. Neuroradiol J. 37(4):402-17, 2024
3. Chengazi HV et al: Emergency radiologic approach to mastoid air cell fluid. Emerg Radiol. 28(3):633-40, 2021
4. McLaren J et al: How well do we know Gradenigo? A comprehensive literature review and proposal for novel diagnostic categories of Gradenigo's syndrome. Int J Pediatr Otorhinolaryngol. 132:109942, 2020
5. Campion T et al: Imaging of temporal bone inflammations in children: a pictorial review. Neuroradiology. 61(9):959-70, 2019
6. Gadre AK et al: The changing face of petrous apicitis-a 40-year experience. Laryngoscope. 128(1):195-201, 2018
7. Choi KY et al: Petrositis with bilateral abducens nerve palsies complicated by acute otitis media. Clin Exp Otorhinolaryngol. 7(1):59-62, 2014
8. Kong SK et al: Acute otitis media-induced petrous apicitis presenting as the Gradenigo syndrome: successfully treated by ventilation tube insertion. Am J Otolaryngol. 32(5):445-7, 2011
9. Ibrahim M et al: Diffusion-weighted MRI identifies petrous apex abscess in Gradenigo syndrome. J Neuroophthalmol. 30(1):34-6, 2010
10. Fournier HD et al: Surgical anatomy of the petrous apex and petroclival region. Adv Tech Stand Neurosurg. 32:91-146, 2007
11. Lee YH et al: CT, MRI and gallium SPECT in the diagnosis and treatment of petrous apicitis presenting as multiple cranial neuropathies. Br J Radiol. 78(934):948-51, 2005
12. Park SN et al: Cavernous sinus thrombophlebitis secondary to petrous apicitis: a case report. Otolaryngol Head Neck Surg. 128(2):284-6, 2003
13. Price T et al: Abducens nerve palsy as the sole presenting symptom of petrous apicitis. J Laryngol Otol. 116(9):726-9, 2002

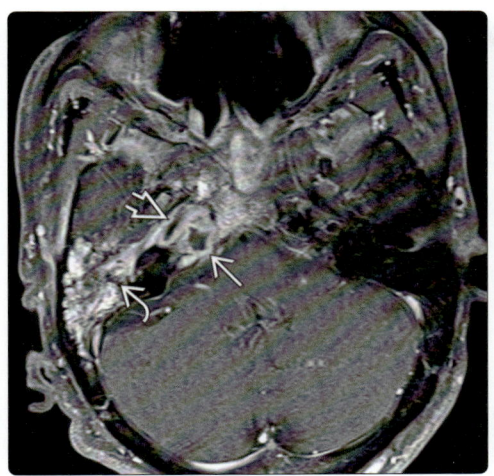
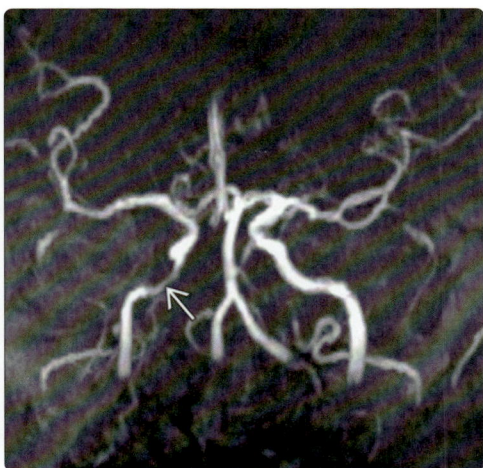

(Left) Axial T1WI C+ FS MR in a patient with severe headache associated with suppurative otomastoiditis ⇒ shows rim-enhancing pus in confluent PA air cells ⇒. The horizontal petrous ICA has thick, enhancing phlegmon along its margins ⇒. (Right) Coronal MRA in the same patient reveals a long segment of horizontal-cavernous ICA narrowing ⇒ secondary to carotid canal phlegmon associated with the confluent apical petrositis & suppurative otomastoiditis.

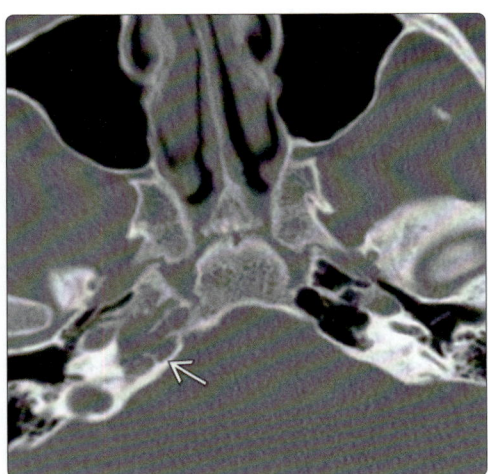
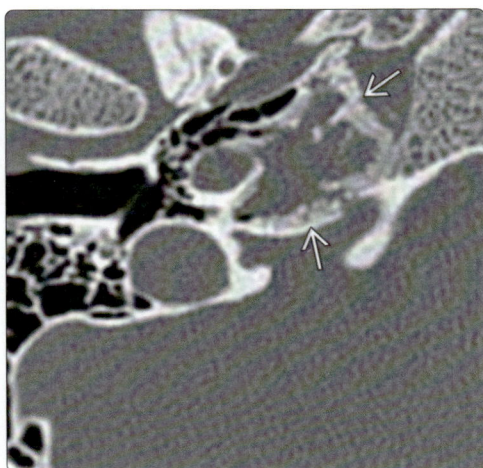

(Left) Axial bone CT in a patient with suspected trapped fluid in the PA on head MR shows opacification of PA air cells ⇒ without overt trabecular loss. The imaging diagnosis was uncomplicated trapped fluid. (Right) Axial bone CT in the same patient, now with new severe headache 2 years after initial diagnosis of trapped fluid, shows loss of PA trabeculae & cortical thickening ⇒. The presumptive imaging diagnosis of superinfection of trapped fluid was made, & symptoms responded to antibiotics.

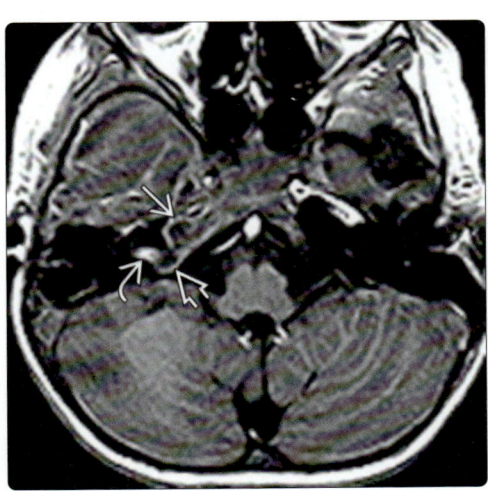
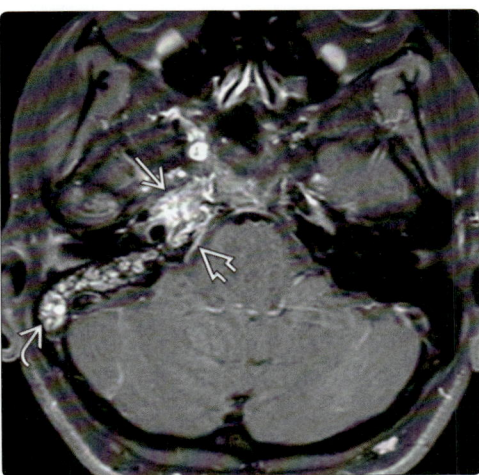

(Left) Axial T1WI C+ MR in a child presenting with headache & fever demonstrates rim-enhancing pus ⇒ in the right PA & area of the porus acusticus ⇒. Focal enhancement in the right IAC ⇒ indicates that the infection has caused focal meningitis. (Right) Axial T1 C+ FS MR shows abnormal enhancement in the right mastoids ⇒ & right PA due to petrous apicitis ⇒. There is localized early spread of infection to the adjacent intracranial dura ⇒.

TERMINOLOGY

- Rare congenital or acquired aneurysm of petrous internal carotid artery (ICA)

IMAGING

- Rarity and variable appearance make errors in initial imaging diagnosis relatively common
- Complex, expansile mass of petrous ICA canal with internal enhancement or flow on CTA, MRA, or angiogram
  - Variable size: 1-5 cm
  - Shape: Focal ovoid, fusiform, or cauliflower-like
- Bone CT findings
  - **Ovoid** or **fusiform** enlargement of petrous ICA canal
  - **Curvilinear calcifications** in aneurysm wall
  - Lesion can erode adjacent bone and appear to be invasive mass
  - Combination of peripheral calcification in wall and marginal bone erosion and fragmentation might suggest primary skull base lesion, such as chondrosarcoma

- CTA: **Patent fusiform or saccular aneurysm** of petrous ICA is **diagnostic**
- MR findings
  - Signal and enhancement complex and highly variable dependent on size, morphology, calcification, degree of thrombosis, and vascular flow pattern
  - Pulsation "ghosting" in phase-encoding direction

TOP DIFFERENTIAL DIAGNOSES

- Petrous apex cholesterol granuloma
- Petrooccipital fissure chondrosarcoma
- Skull base chordoma
- Skull base metastasis

CLINICAL ISSUES

- Sensorineural hearing loss, Horner syndrome, pulsatile tinnitus, stroke
- Gradual enlargement; progressive risk of rupture
- **Endovascular therapy**: Obliteration or stent placement

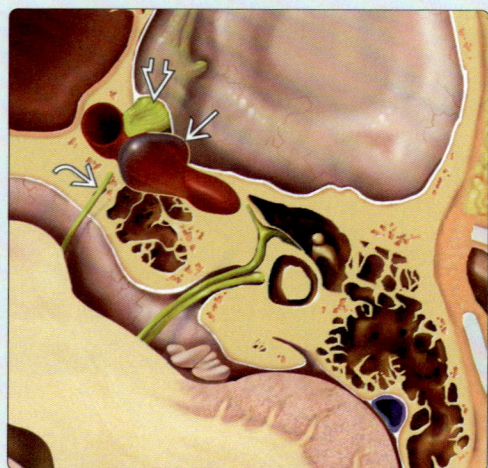
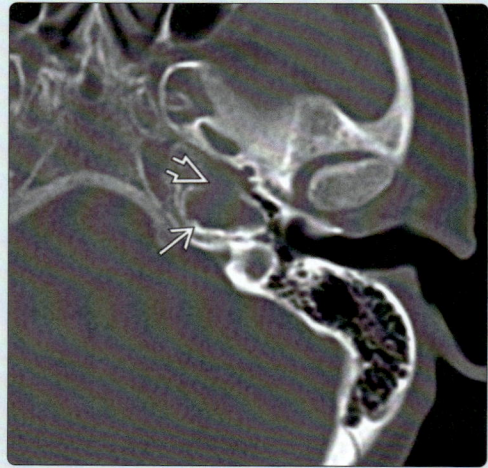

(Left) Axial graphic through the left temporal bone shows focal aneurysmal dilation ⇨ of the horizontal petrous internal carotid artery (ICA). Note the proximity to the trigeminal nerve ⇨ and the abducens nerve ⇨ to the petrous ICA aneurysm. (Right) Axial bone CT in a patient presenting with recurrent transient ischemic attacks shows an expansile ovoid lesion ⇨ in the left petrous apex (PA). Note the anterior wall dehiscence ⇨ where the aneurysm connects to the horizontal petrous ICA.

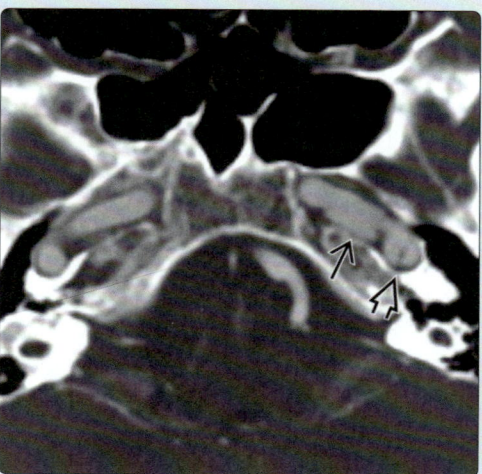
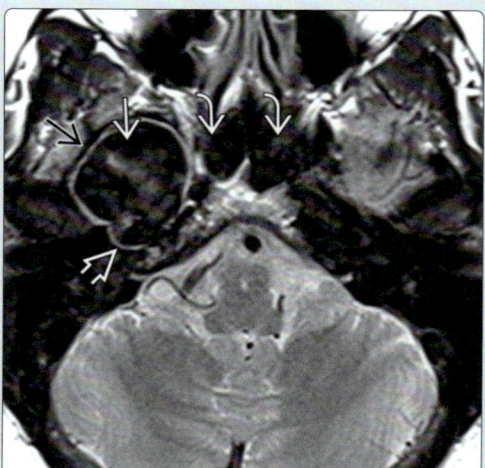

(Left) Axial CT angiogram in a patient with pulsatile tinnitus demonstrates broad-based outpouching from the left petrous ICA ⇨ with an associated dissection flap ⇨, compatible with a dissecting pseudoaneurysm. (Right) Axial T2 MR shows a predominantly hypointense mass ⇨ projecting from the PA, which communicates with the petrous ICA ⇨. Flow within this giant petrous ICA aneurysm results in complex internal signal ⇨ and pulsation artifact ⇨.

TERMINOLOGY

Definitions

- Rare congenital or acquired aneurysm of petrous internal carotid artery (ICA)

IMAGING

General Features

- Best diagnostic clue
  - Complex, expansile mass of petrous ICA canal with internal arterial flow on CTA, MRA, or angiogram
- Location
  - **Horizontal petrous ICA** most common location
- Size
  - Variable: 1-5 cm

CT Findings

- Bone CT
  - **Ovoid** or **fusiform** enlargement of petrous ICA canal
  - May appear **destructive**
    - Bone erosion and remodeling of petrous bone
  - **Curvilinear calcifications** in aneurysm wall
  - Combination of expansile mass showing areas of bone erosion/lysis and variable calcification can create appearance suggestive of chordoma or chondrosarcoma
- CTA
  - **Aneurysmal dilation** of petrous ICA is **diagnostic**
  - CTA can demonstrate relationship of aneurysm to parent petrous ICA vessel
  - Degree of lumen enhancement is determined by presence of aneurysm clot
  - Dissection flap → dissecting pseudoaneurysm

MR Findings

- T1WI
  - **Complex and variable signal mass**
    - High signal: Intraluminal clot, slow flow
    - Low signal: Wall calcification, high flow
  - Pulsation artifact with "ghosting" in phase-encoded direction
- T2WI
  - Complex signal mass with peripheral hemosiderin
  - Internal flow voids produce vascular swirl pattern
  - Pulsation artifact with "ghosting" in phase-encoded direction
- T1WI C+
  - Enhancement is highly variable dependent on size, clot, and flow pattern
- MRA
  - Enlarged, irregular, fusiform or saccular outpouching of ICA

Angiographic Findings

- DSA allows for identification of flow pattern, morphology of aneurysm, and point of origin of aneurysm from petrous ICA

Imaging Recommendations

- Best imaging tool
  - CTA is best exam
    - Diagnostic of aneurysm with precise localization along petrous ICA
    - Bone CT from CTA shows skull base anatomy

DIFFERENTIAL DIAGNOSIS

Petrous Apex Cholesterol Granuloma

- Bone CT: Expansile petrous apex (PA) mass
- MR: Hyperintense T1 and T2 signal in PA

Chondrosarcoma

- Classically appears as expansile mass of petrooccipital fissure but can be eccentric
- Invariably encroaches upon petrous ICA
- Bone CT: Expansile petrooccipital fissure mass

Chordoma

- Classically expansile, enhancing midline clivus mass
- But can be eccentric, involving PA and parasellar regions

CLINICAL ISSUES

Presentation

- Most common signs/symptoms
  - Often asymptomatic incidental finding
- Other signs/symptoms
  - Headache
  - Horner syndrome
  - Pulsatile tinnitus
  - Cranial neuropathies (CNV-CNXI)

Demographics

- Age
  - Congenital aneurysm: Childhood or adolescence
  - Acquired pseudoaneurysm: Any age
- Epidemiology
  - Relatively rare lesion: **Errors in diagnosis common**

Natural History & Prognosis

- Gradual enlargement; progressive risk of rupture
- Spontaneous thrombosis can occur in some

Treatment

- **Endovascular therapy**
  - Allows for pretreatment ICA occlusion trial
  - Balloon trapping or aneurysmal obliteration with ICA preservation
  - **Endovascular stent, including flow diverter stent** placement across aneurysm is viable option
- Surgical therapy no longer preferred 1st approach
  - When necessary, includes ICA sacrifice ± external carotid artery-ICA bypass

SELECTED REFERENCES

1. Charan BD et al: Reconstructive endovascular treatment of petrous ICA pseudoaneurysm in skull base osteomyelitis: a hidden catastrophe. BMJ Case Rep. 17(2), 2024
2. Murai Y et al: Petrous internal carotid artery aneurysms: a systematic review. J Nippon Med Sch. 87(4):172-83, 2020
3. Ghali MGZ et al: Flow diversion for the treatment of petrous internal carotid artery aneurysms. Asian J Neurosurg. 14(4):1058-62, 2019
4. Shapiro M et al: Toward an endovascular internal carotid artery classification system. AJNR Am J Neuroradiol. 35(2):230-6, 2014

TERMINOLOGY

- **Normal** contrast enhancement (CE) along course of intratemporal facial nerve (CNVII); typically subtle, symmetric with contralateral facial nerve and without bone changes or facial nerve symptoms
- Prominent perineural arteriovenous plexus responsible for normal enhancement

IMAGING

- T1 C+ MR enhancement along CNVII
  - Mastoid, tympanic, and geniculate ganglion segments generally show CE
  - CE variable, dependent on technique and field strength but normally symmetric bilaterally
  - Facial nerve within internal auditory canal should not enhance normally

TOP DIFFERENTIAL DIAGNOSES

- Bell palsy

- Ramsay Hunt syndrome
- Perineural parotid tumor of intratemporal CNVII
- Facial nerve schwannoma within temporal bone
- Facial nerve venous malformation

CLINICAL ISSUES

- Normal nerve enhancement **asymptomatic** by definition

DIAGNOSTIC CHECKLIST

- **Asymmetric** intratemporal facial nerve CE should be viewed with suspicion
  - Correlation with facial nerve paralysis or hemifacial spasm important if abnormal CE suspected
  - Any previous history of H&N cancer should alert to possibility of perineural tumor spread
- High-resolution T1 C+ FS MR through temporal bone should cover from brainstem through parotid glands to evaluate for facial nerve pathology
- Bone CT complementary in evaluation to exclude underlying bony changes

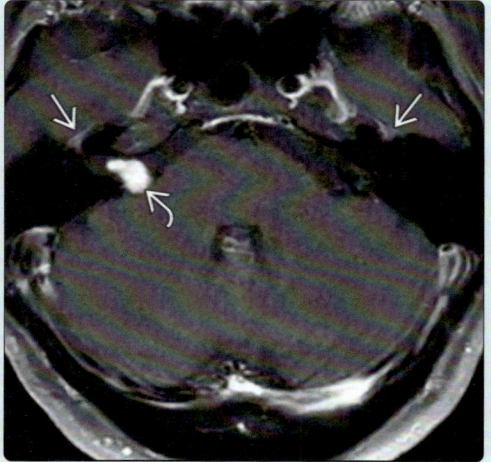
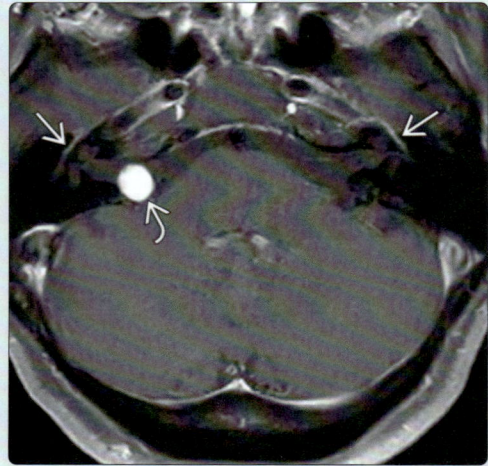

(Left) *Typical normal enhancement pattern of facial intratemporal facial nerves in a patient with vestibular schwannoma is shown. On this axial MR, the geniculate ganglia (triangular structures superolateral to the IAC) ➡️ demonstrate moderate symmetric enhancement. Right vestibular schwannoma ➡️ is noted.* (Right) *Axial MR slightly lower shows mild to moderate symmetric enhancement of the tympanic portions of the facial nerves ➡️. Aside from the vestibular schwannoma ➡️, no IAC enhancement is identified.*

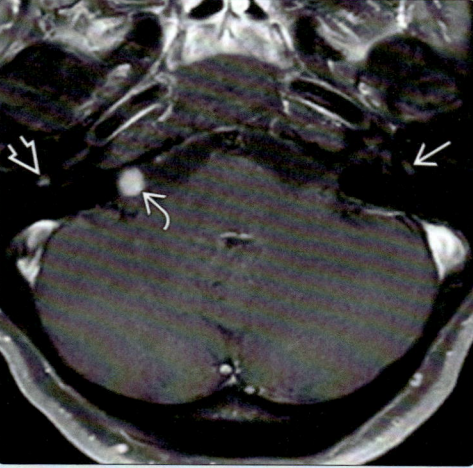
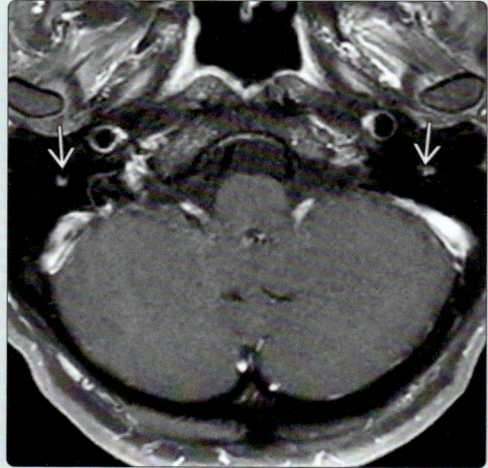

(Left) *Axial (slightly oblique) MR in the same patient demonstrates little or no enhancement of the posterior genu ➡️ of the left facial nerve and subtle normal enhancement of the proximal mastoid segment ➡️ of the right facial nerve. The lower vestibular schwannoma ➡️ is noted.* (Right) *Axial MR in the same patient shows moderate, normal linear enhancement of the lower mastoid segments ➡️ of the facial nerves. Contrast enhancement of mastoid segment CNVII is usually more robust distally.*

TERMINOLOGY

Definitions

- **Normal** contrast enhancement (CE) along course of intratemporal facial nerve (CNVII); typically mild to moderate, **symmetric** with contralateral facial nerve and without bone changes or facial nerve symptoms
- Prominent perineural arteriovenous plexus responsible for normal enhancement

IMAGING

General Features

- Best diagnostic clue
  - T1 C+ MR CE along CNVII geniculate ganglion, tympanic and mastoid segments without bony CNVII canal changes
  - CE variable, dependent on technique and field strength but **normally symmetric** bilaterally
  - Facial nerve within internal auditory canal (IAC) least likely to enhance normally

CT Findings

- Bone CT
  - Normal bony intratemporal CNVII canal

MR Findings

- T1WI
  - Normal CNVII can be seen as isointense signal that can appear prominent compared with surrounding low signal of adjacent osseous or pneumatized structures
- T1WI C+
  - Normal CE along portions of CNVII (1.5T spin-echo CE T1)
    - Mastoid > geniculate ganglion > tympanic segments
    - Usually symmetric side to side
- MR field strength and sequence summary
  - 1.5T MR: CE of CNVII canalicular and labyrinthine segments not seen
  - 3T MR: CE of CNVII
    - Mastoid (100%), geniculate (75%), tympanic (40%)
    - Subtle enhancement can even be seen in canalicular (15%) and labyrinthine (5%) segments
  - Comparing CE spin-echo to CE inversion recovery-prepared fast spoiled gradient-echo (IR-FSPGR)
    - IR-FSPGR: Greater CNVII signal intensity in all segments
  - CE 3D T1W FSE (CUBE and SPACE)
    - Geniculate (98%), tympanic (45%), mastoid (38%), fundal canalicular (16%)
  - CE T1 VIBE FS
    - CNVII enhancement in all segments on both 1.5T and 3T
    - Mastoid (100%), tympanic (99%), labyrinthine (88%), intraparotid (87%), canalicular (70%)

DIFFERENTIAL DIAGNOSIS

Bell Palsy

- Clinical: Acute onset of unilateral peripheral CNVII paralysis
- T1 C+ MR: Intense enhancement of intratemporal CNVII
  - "Tuft" of IAC fundal enhancement highly suggestive

Ramsay Hunt Syndrome

- Reactivation of herpes zoster from geniculate ganglion
- Typically robust enhancement of intratemporal facial nerve with typical vesicular rash of ear or soft palate

Perineural Parotid Tumor of Intratemporal CNVII

- T1 C+ MR: Nodular, asymmetric enhancement of facial nerve usually extending from intraparotid segment into mastoid segment and beyond
- May occur from primary parotid neoplasm or local spread of cutaneous malignancy

Facial Nerve Schwannoma of Intratemporal CNVII

- Most frequently found in geniculate fossa
- T1 C+ MR: Focal, enhancing mass along CNVII course
- Bone CT: Enlargement of intratemporal CNVII canal

Facial Nerve Venous Malformation (Hemangioma) Within Temporal Bone

- Most frequent location = geniculate fossa
- T1 C+ MR: Enhancing mass enlarges geniculate fossa
- Bone CT: Honeycomb bony changes ~ 50%

CLINICAL ISSUES

Presentation

- Most common signs/symptoms
  - **Asymptomatic** by definition
  - CNVII normal enhancement seen incidentally during T1 C+ MR work-up for unrelated clinical findings

DIAGNOSTIC CHECKLIST

Consider

- If facial nerve is normal in size, and enhancement is symmetric to corresponding contralateral facial nerve segment, probably normal
- **Asymmetric** intratemporal facial nerve CE should be viewed with suspicion
  - Correlation with facial nerve paralysis or hemifacial spasm important if abnormal CE suspected
  - Any previous history of H&N cancer should alert to possibility of perineural tumor spread
- **Normal** CNVII CE variable and dependent on field strength and MR sequence
- If fundal vestibular schwannoma present, labyrinthine segment of CNVII may enhance normally
  - Arteriovenous plexus congestion is likely cause
- Evaluation of tympanic or mastoid segments difficult if opacification, inflammation, or infection of middle ear and mastoid air cells
- Significant CE along cisternal, labyrinthine segment or extracranial mastoid CNVII segments **not** normal

SELECTED REFERENCES

1. Nawaz N et al: Normal facial nerve enhancement on volumetric interpolated breath-hold examination MRI sequence. AJNR Am J Neuroradiol. 46(6):1268-71, 2025
2. Warne R et al: Enhancement patterns of the normal facial nerve on three-dimensional T1W fast spin echo MRI. Br J Radiol. 94(1122):20201025, 2021
3. Radhakrishnan R et al: Comparison of normal facial nerve enhancement at 3T MRI using gadobutrol and gadopentetate dimeglumine. Neuroradiol J. 30(6):554-60, 2017

Middle Ear Prolapsing Facial Nerve

TERMINOLOGY

- Definition: Midtympanic facial nerve (CNVII) segment protrudes through bony dehiscence
  - **CNVII dehiscence** refers only to segmental absence of bony covering of CNVII
  - **Prolapsing CNVII**: CNVII protrudes through dehiscence in tympanic CNVII canal

IMAGING

- **Incidental finding** on temporal bone CT
  - Tubular soft tissue extends from midtympanic CNVII into oval window niche
- Coronal bone CT
  - Soft tissue mass in oval widow niche
  - Along undersurface of lateral semicircular canal
  - Contiguous with midtympanic segment of CNVII
- Axial bone CT
  - Hammock-like CNVII spanning middle ear cavity under lateral semicircular canal

TOP DIFFERENTIAL DIAGNOSES

- Intratemporal facial nerve schwannoma
- Oval window atresia
- Persistent stapedial artery
- Congenital cholesteatoma in facial nerve canal

CLINICAL ISSUES

- Clinical presentation
  - Most commonly **asymptomatic**
  - Rarely, conductive hearing loss present from impingement on stapes
  - Prolapsed facial nerve can be injured during surgical exposure of stapes or oval window

DIAGNOSTIC CHECKLIST

- Warning to radiologist
  - Prolapsed CNVII in peril during stapedectomy
    - Report & call this finding to ear surgeon

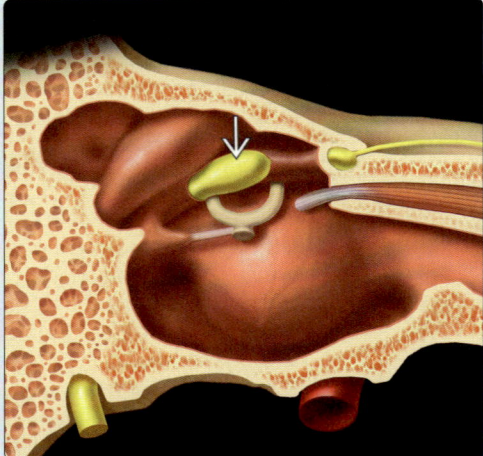
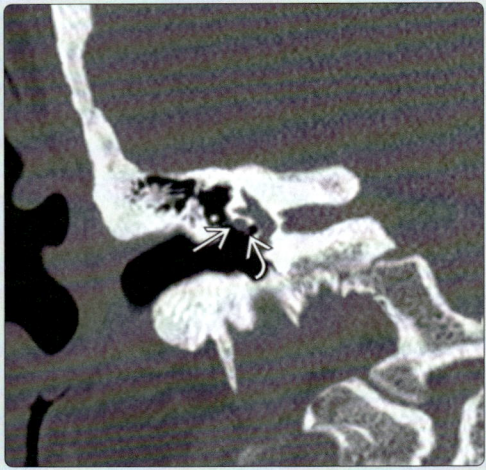

(Left) Graphic of medial wall of the right ear (anterior to the right) shows loss of bone covering the midtympanic segment of the facial nerve canal ➡ with associated mild enlargement and prolapse of tympanic facial nerve into oval window niche. (Right) Coronal bone CT of the right ear in a patient with sensorineural hearing loss (SNHL) shows incidental prolapse of the tympanic portion of the facial nerve ➡. The nerve is slightly larger than normal and devoid of a bony canal. A tiny density just below the facial nerve is a portion of the stapes crus ➡.

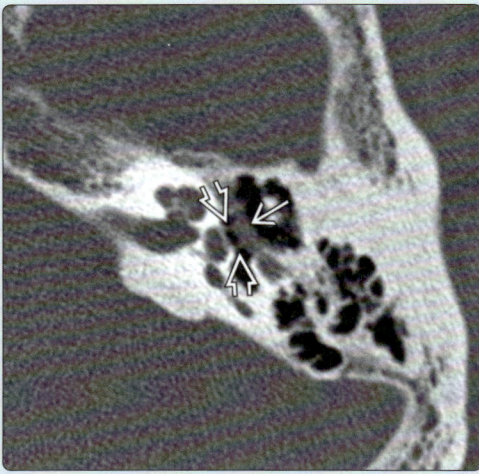
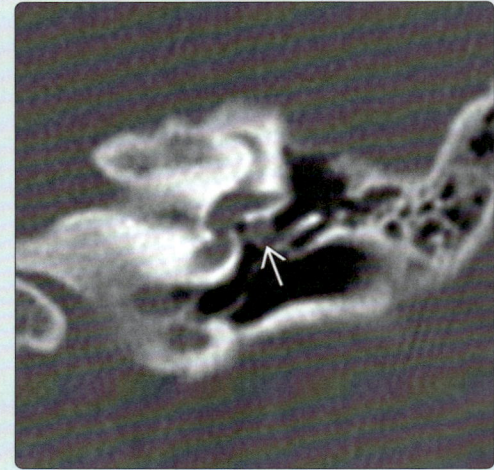

(Left) Axial CT in a patient with conductive hearing loss shows the protruding tympanic segment of CNVII ➡ is strung across the middle ear cavity. Notice that CNVII is prominent in size and touches the crura ➡ of the stapes, explaining conductive hearing loss presentation. (Right) Coronal left ear temporal bone CT shows the enlarged, prolapsed tympanic segment of CNVII in cross section ➡. Enhanced MR can differentiate protrusion of CNVII (no enhancement) vs. facial nerve schwannoma (enhancement).

TERMINOLOGY

Definitions

- Midtympanic facial nerve (CNVII) segment protrudes through bony dehiscence
- **CNVII dehiscence** refers only to segmental absence of bony covering of CNVII
- **Prolapsing CNVII**: CNVII protrudes through dehiscence

IMAGING

General Features

- Best diagnostic clue
  - Tubular soft tissue extends from midtympanic CNVII into oval window niche (CT)
- Location
  - Undersurface of lateral semicircular canal (LSCC) → oval window niche
- Size
  - Variable; may be subtle or appear mass-like (2-3 mm) within oval window niche
- Morphology
  - Smooth, tubular appearance

CT Findings

- Bone CT
  - Coronal: Soft tissue mass in oval widow niche
    - Along undersurface of LSCC
    - Contiguous with midtympanic segment of CNVII
  - Axial: Hammock-like CNVII spanning middle ear cavity under LSCC
  - Simple dehiscence (uncovered CNVII) poorly seen unless CNVII prolapsed through dehiscence

MR Findings

- No abnormality identified
- T1 C+ is normal, excluding facial nerve schwannoma

Imaging Recommendations

- Best imaging tool
  - Axial & coronal thin-section temporal bone CT
    - Best seen on **coronal** at level of oval window
- Protocol advice
  - When protruding CNVII is mass-like, use contrast-enhanced MR to exclude CNVII schwannoma
    - Facial nerve schwannoma enhances

DIFFERENTIAL DIAGNOSIS

Intratemporal Facial Nerve Schwannoma

- Clinical: Hearing loss > > facial nerve palsy
- CT: Tubular enlargement of CNVII canal
  - Geniculate fossa > tympanic > mastoid segments
- MR: Enhancing tubular mass enlarges CNVII canal

Oval Window Atresia

- Clinical: Conductive hearing loss
- ± external auditory canal (EAC) atresia
- CT: Facial nerve tympanic segment ectopic
  - Tympanic CNVII in oval window niche

Persistent Stapedial Artery

- Asymptomatic vascular variant
- CT: Absent foramen spinosum
  - Tubular lesion on cochlear promontory
  - Large anterior tympanic segment CNVII

Congenital Cholesteatoma in Facial Nerve Canal

- Rare congenital cholesteatoma type
- CT: Enlargement of CNVII bony canal
  - Most commonly geniculate ganglion area

PATHOLOGY

General Features

- Etiology
  - Congenital/developmental; can be acquired from cholesteatoma

CLINICAL ISSUES

Presentation

- Most common signs/symptoms
  - **Asymptomatic** most commonly
  - Rarely, conductive hearing loss from impingement on stapes
- Clinical profile
  - **Incidental finding** on temporal bone CT
    - Critical to communicate its presence to surgeon prior to middle ear exploration
    - Easy to injure facial nerve during stapedectomy if CNVII prolapse is present

Demographics

- Epidemiology
  - Simple dehiscence without protrusion ~ 50% of cases
  - Prolapsing facial nerve is rare (~ 1% of cases)
- Age: All

Natural History & Prognosis

- Excellent if left alone

Treatment

- Careful avoidance at time of middle ear surgery

DIAGNOSTIC CHECKLIST

Image Interpretation Pearls

- Prolapse often associated with absence of notch defect along undersurface of LSCC
- If notch is seen, consider alternative explanation

Reporting Tips

- Caveat: Prolapsed CNVII in peril during stapedectomy
  - Report & call this finding to ear surgeon

SELECTED REFERENCES

1. Cleland JB et al: Unusual case of multi-etiology conductive hearing loss from cephalocele and prolapsed facial nerve. Laryngoscope. 135(7):2492-6, 2025
2. Soloperto D et al: Endoscopic findings on facial nerve anatomy during exclusive endoscopic stapedotomy: clinical considerations and impact on surgical results. J Int Adv Otol. 19(6):503-10, 2023
3. Hernandez-Trejo AF et al: Prevalence of facial canal dehiscence and other bone defects by computed tomography. Eur Arch Otorhinolaryngol. 277(10):2681-6, 2020
4. Amadei EM et al: Revision stapes surgery after stapedotomy: a retrospective evaluation of 75 cases. Ear Nose Throat J. 97(6):E1-4, 2018
5. Swartz JD: The facial nerve canal: CT analysis of the protruding tympanic segment. Radiology. 153(2):443-7, 1984

Bell Palsy

TERMINOLOGY

- Bell palsy (BP): Herpetic peripheral facial nerve paralysis secondary to herpes simplex virus

IMAGING

- T1WI C+ FS MR: Fundal tuft and labyrinthine segment CNVII show intense asymmetric enhancement
  - Entire intratemporal CNVII may enhance
- Thin T2 MR: Smooth CNVII thickening is common but lacks focal nodularity
- Imaging usually not required in classic rapid-onset BP
  - Routine MR identifies nonidiopathic cause in 6.7%
- If **atypical BP**, search with imaging for underlying lesion

TOP DIFFERENTIAL DIAGNOSES

- Normal enhancement of intratemporal CNVII
- Ramsay Hunt syndrome
- Facial nerve schwannoma
- Facial nerve venous malformation (hemangioma)

- Perineural tumor from parotid

PATHOLOGY

- Etiology-pathogenesis (current hypothesis)
  - Latent **herpes simplex** infection of geniculate ganglion with reactivation and spread of inflammation along proximal and distal intratemporal facial nerve fibers

CLINICAL ISSUES

- Classic clinical presentation
  - Acute-onset peripheral CNVII paralysis (36-hour onset)
- Medical therapy for BP
  - Tapering course of prednisone; begin within 3 days of symptoms for best result
  - Antiviral agents no longer used
- Surgical therapy for BP is controversial
  - Profound denervation (> 95%) treated with facial nerve decompression from internal auditory canal fundus to stylomastoid foramen

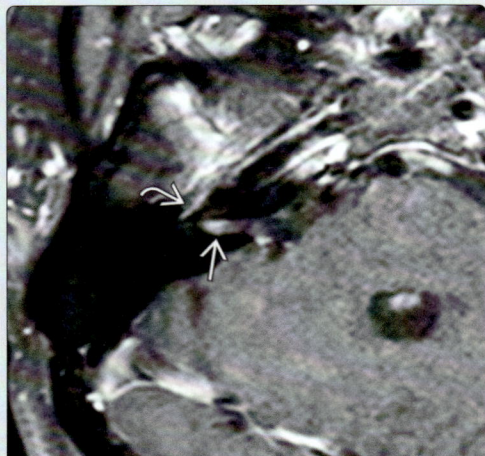
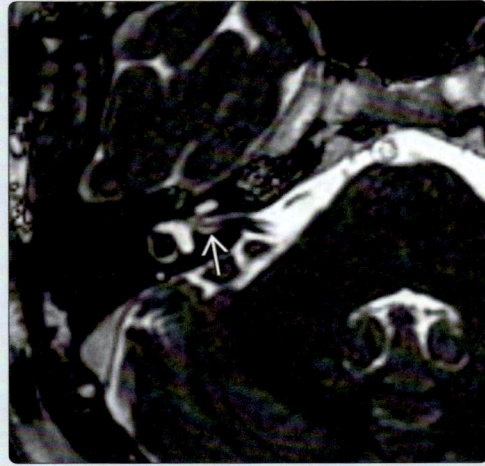

(Left) Axial T1 C+ FS MR in this 43-year-old man with right Bell palsy shows enhancement in the internal auditory canal (IAC) fundus ➡. The tympanic segment ➡ also shows mildly prominent enhancement. (Right) Axial enhanced thin T2 MR in the same patient shows mild thickening of the distal intracanalicular facial nerve ➡ without nodular expansion in the area of previously seen enhancement. Nerve edema and thickening are often seen with Bell palsy, but the nerve would not typically show corresponding nodularity as with schwannoma.

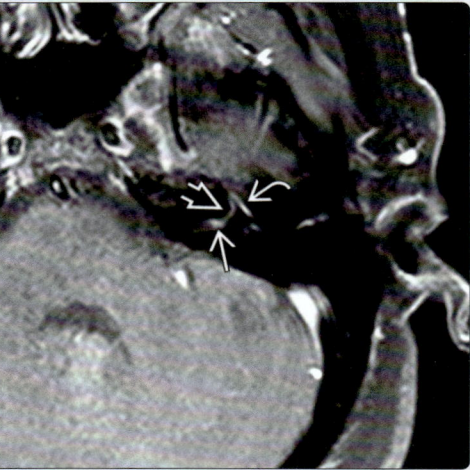
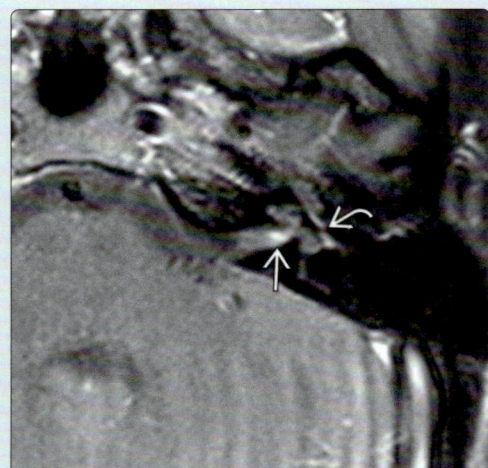

(Left) Axial T1 C+ FS MR shows classic findings of Bell palsy with the IAC fundal tuft sign ➡, labyrinthine ➡, and tympanic ➡ facial nerve segment enhancement. (Right) Axial T1 C+ FS MR in the same patient again shows the IAC fundal tuft sign ➡ and tympanic segment of the facial nerve enhancement ➡. Remember that the geniculate ganglion and posterior genu/upper mastoid segment of the facial nerve may normally enhance.

TERMINOLOGY

Abbreviations
- Bell palsy (BP)

Synonyms
- Herpetic facial paralysis

Definitions
- BP (original definition): Idiopathic acute onset of lower motor neuron facial paralysis
- BP (modern definition): Herpetic facial paralysis secondary to herpes simplex virus

Other Facts
- Named after Sir Charles Bell (1774-1842), who first described BP syndrome

IMAGING

General Features
- Best diagnostic clue
  - Fundal **tuft** and labyrinthine segment CNVII intense asymmetric enhancement on T1WI C+ MR
- Location
  - Fundal and labyrinthine segment CNVII most affected
  - Often involves entire intratemporal CNVII
    - Intraparotid segment less commonly affected
- Size
  - CNVII swells within facial nerve canal

CT Findings
- Bone CT
  - Normal facial nerve canal (if expansion present, **not** BP)

MR Findings
- T2WI
  - Brain normal; no high-signal lesions
  - High-resolution T2 C+ SSFP shows entire nerve enhances
    - Smooth, linear thickening along internal auditory canal (IAC) CNVII segment common without focal nodularity
- T1WI C+
  - Uniform, contiguous CNVII enhancement
    - CNVII: Normal in size within bony canal
    - CNVII: Conspicuous high signal appears slightly enlarged
    - Enhancement pattern is linear, not nodular
  - Enhancement usually present from distal IAC through labyrinthine segment, geniculate ganglion, and anterior tympanic segment
    - **Tuft** of enhancement in IAC fundus (premeatal segment) along with C+ of labyrinthine segment of CNVII are distinctive MR findings
    - Mastoid CNVII enhances less frequently
    - Enhancement of intraparotid CNVII infrequent

Imaging Recommendations
- Best imaging tool
  - Thin-section fat-saturated T1WI C+ MR focused to IAC and temporal bone
  - Temporal bone CT: Only used if MR creates suspicion of enlarged CNVII canal or focal lesion

- Classic rapid-onset BP requires **no imaging** in initial stages
  - 90% of BP patients recover spontaneously in < 2 months
  - If decompressive surgery is anticipated, MR imaging is warranted to ensure that no other lesion is causing CNVII paralysis
- If **atypical BP**, search for underlying lesion
  - Atypical BP
    - Slowly progressive CNVII palsy
    - Facial hyperfunction (spasm) preceding BP
    - Recurrent CNVII palsies
    - BP with any other associated cranial neuropathies
    - CNVII paralysis persisting or deepening > 2 months
    - History of skin cancer = higher risk of occult tumors

DIFFERENTIAL DIAGNOSIS

Normal Enhancement of Intratemporal CNVII
- Clinical: No facial nerve symptoms
- T1WI C+ MR: Mild, linear, discontinuous enhancement of anterior and posterior genus of intratemporal CNVII
  - IAC and labyrinthine CNVII segments normal

Ramsay Hunt Syndrome
- Clinical: Peripheral CNVII paralysis with CNVIII associated symptoms
  - External auditory canal (EAC) hemorrhagic vesicular rash
  - Varicella-zoster virus infection = cause
- T1WI C+ MR: Linear, continuous enhancement of fundal IAC and intratemporal CNVII
  - Enhancement of inner ear structures, vestibulocochlear nerve (CNVIII), IAC wall variable

Facial Nerve Schwannoma
- Clinical: Hearing loss more common than CNVII palsy
- T1WI C+ MR: Well-circumscribed, tubular, C+ mass within enlarged CNVII canal most commonly centered on geniculate ganglion

Facial Nerve Venous Malformation ("Hemangioma")
- Clinical: CNVII paralysis occurs when lesion is small
- Bone CT: May show intratumoral bone spicules
- T1WI C+ MR: Poorly circumscribed, enhancing mass commonly found in geniculate fossa

Perineural Tumor From Parotid
- Clinical: Parotid malignancy usually palpable
- Imaging: Invasive parotid mass is present
  - Tissue-filled stylomastoid foramen
  - CNVII is enlarged from distal to proximal with associated mastoid air cell invasion

PATHOLOGY

General Features
- Etiology
  - Etiology-pathogenesis (current hypothesis)
    - Latent herpes simplex infection of geniculate ganglion with reactivation and spread of inflammatory process along proximal and distal CNVII fibers
    - Pathophysiology: Formation of intraneural edema in neuronal sheaths caused by breakdown of blood-nerve barrier and venous congestion in epineural and perineural venous plexus

Brackman Facial Nerve Grading System

Grade	Description of Facial Paralysis	Measurement**	Function %	Estimated Function %
I	Normal	8/8	100	100
II	Slight	7/8	76-99	80
III	Moderate	5/8-6/8	51-75	60
IV	Moderately severe	3/8-4/8	26-50	40
V	Severe	1/8-2/8	1-25	20
VI	Total	0/8	0	0

* Facial nerve injury is measured by the superior movement of the midportion of the upper eyebrow and the lateral movement of the oral commissure. For each 0.25 cm of upward motion for both eyebrow and oral commissure, a scale of 1 is assigned up to 1 cm. The points are then added together. A total of 8 points can be obtained if both the eyebrow and the oral commissure both move 1 cm. Adapted from House JW et al: Facial nerve grading system.

House JW et al: Otolaryngol Head Neck Surg. 93(2):146-7, 1985.

- Intratemporal CNVII normal anatomy
  - CNVII normal C+ at its anterior and posterior genus
  - C+ from robust circumneural arteriovenous plexus
  - Familiarity with normal patterns of intratemporal CNVII enhancement allows radiologist to identify abnormal enhancement seen with BP

Gross Pathologic & Surgical Features

- CNVII edema peaks at 3 weeks after symptom onset

Microscopic Features

- Herpes simplex DNA recovered from CNVII

CLINICAL ISSUES

Presentation

- Most common signs/symptoms
  - Acute-onset peripheral CNVII paralysis (36-hour onset)
- Clinical profile
  - Healthy adult with acute unilateral CNVII paralysis
- Other signs/symptoms
  - Viral prodrome often reported before BP onset
  - 70%: Taste alterations days before CNVII paralysis
  - 50%: Pain around ipsilateral ear (not severe)

Demographics

- Age
  - All ages affected; incidence peaks in 5th decade
- Epidemiology
  - Herpetic facial paralysis thought to be responsible for ~ 75% of peripheral CNVII paralysis cases
  - Annual BP incidence: 10-50/100,000 persons

Natural History & Prognosis

- 80% of BP patients spontaneously recover all of CNVII function without therapy in first 2 months
  - 15% partially recover; 5% show no recovery
  - Recovery of function less likely with ↑ BMI
- Lower volume labyrinthine segment meatal foramen on CT predicts poor functional recovery

Treatment

- Test for diabetes and Lyme disease
- Medical therapy for BP

- Tapering course of prednisone; begin within 3 days of symptoms for best result
  - Acyclovir or valacyclovir (antivirals) no longer used
- Surgical therapy for BP is controversial
  - Profound denervation (> 95%) treated with CNVII decompression, fundus to stylomastoid foramen
  - Decompression performed within 2 weeks of onset of total paralysis for maximal effect
- Intensity, pattern ± location of enhancement on T1WI C+ MR **not** helpful in predicting individual patient outcome
- Older patients: Lower rate of complete CNVII recovery

DIAGNOSTIC CHECKLIST

Consider

- MR not necessary for typical BP, but routine MR has shown added value (controversial)
  - Confirms diagnosis in 93.3%
  - Shows cause of nonidiopathic facial paralysis in 6.7%
    - Some are potentially life-threatening and change management
- MR imaging important for **atypical** BP
- Abnormal CNVII C+ on MR may persist well beyond clinical improvement or full recovery
- Not all intratemporal facial nerves enhance in BP
  - < 10 days following onset of BP, CNVII often normal

Image Interpretation Pearls

- Tuft of IAC fundal + labyrinthine segment CNVII enhancement without associated focal lesion is highly suggestive of BP
- High-resolution T2 SSFP often shows CNVII thickening and edema but without focal nodularity

Reporting Tips

- Remember to comment on parotid as normal
- Note absence of focal CNVII lesions

SELECTED REFERENCES

1. Ross BC et al: Beyond the AJR: routine MRI may provide utility in identifying secondary causes in adult patients with suspected Bell palsy at initial presentation. AJR Am J Roentgenol. 222(2):e2329811, 2024
2. Savary T et al: Incidence of underlying abnormal findings on routine magnetic resonance imaging for Bell palsy. JAMA Netw Open. 6(4):e239158, 2023

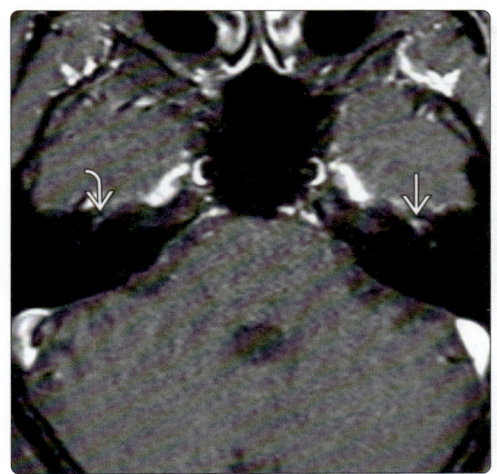

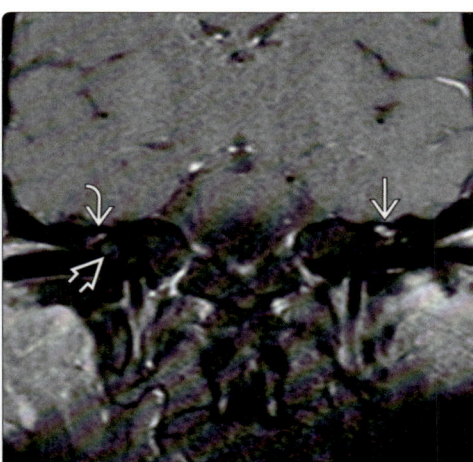

(Left) Axial T1 C+ FS MR shows asymmetrical enhancement involving the anterior genu of facial nerve on the left ➡ compared to normal enhancement on the right ➡. The entire left intratemporal CNVII enhanced. (Right) Coronal T1 C+ FS MR in the same patient shows intense left-sided enhancement of the 2 adjacent dots ➡ ("snake eyes," representing the CNVII anterior labyrinthine and tympanic segments). Normal faint enhancing "snake eyes" are seen on the right ➡ just above the shadow of the cochlea ("snail") ➡.

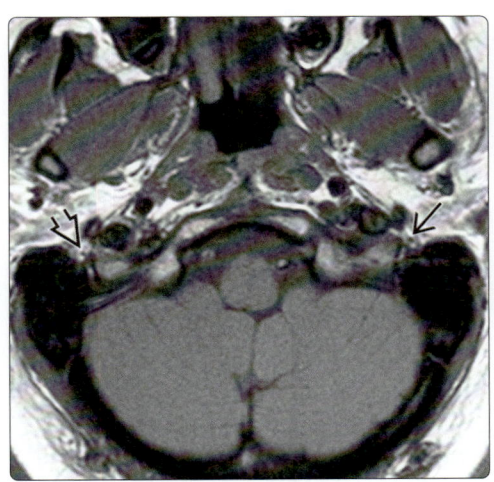

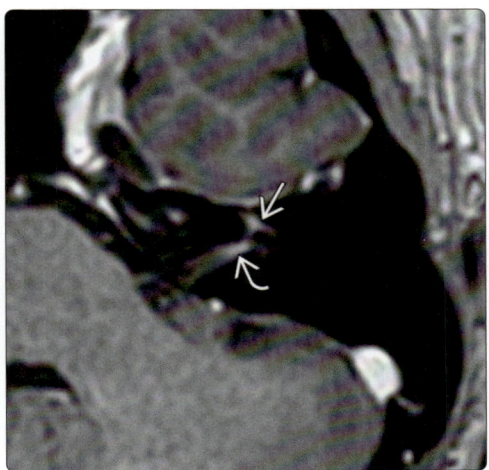

(Left) Axial T1 MR in a patient with left Bell palsy reveals that the left facial nerve in the stylomastoid foramen ➡ is larger than the right ➡. The injured left facial nerve swells when it is not confined by the intratemporal bony facial nerve canal. (Right) Axial T1 C+ MR shows enhancement of the left geniculate fossa and anterior tympanic segment of the facial nerve ➡ along with a tuft of enhancement in the distal IAC ➡, consistent with Bell palsy. The patient's facial nerve paralysis resolved on follow-up.

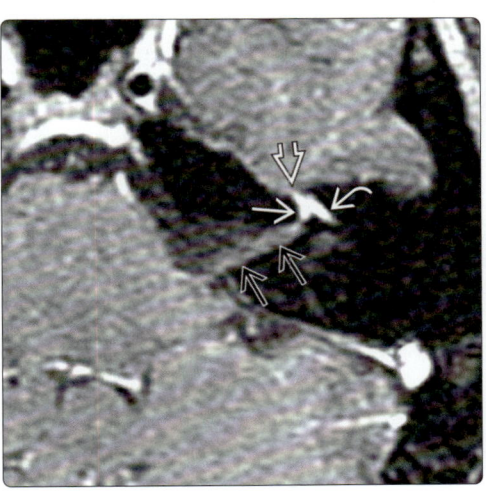

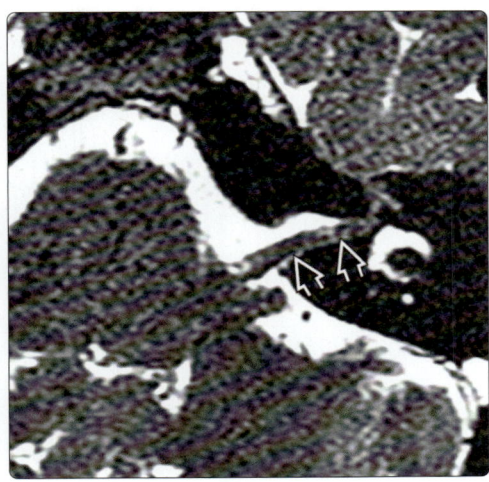

(Left) Axial T1 C+ FS MR in a patient with profound, unremitting Bell palsy shows intense enhancement of the labyrinthine ➡, geniculate ganglion ➡, and anterior tympanic portions ➡ of the facial nerve. The IAC tuft spreads along the IAC facial nerve as more subtle enhancement ➡, reaching the porus acusticus. (Right) Axial thin-section (1-mm) T2 FS MR in the same patient reveals a swollen intracanalicular facial nerve ➡ through the IAC.

Temporal Bone Facial Nerve Venous Malformation (Hemangioma)

KEY FACTS

TERMINOLOGY

- Facial nerve venous malformation (FNVM)
- Older terms: Facial nerve hemangioma/ossifying hemangioma
- Definition: Benign developmental lesion near intratemporal CNVII in geniculate fossa area

IMAGING

- Bone CT
  - **Honeycomb high-density matrix** lesion (50%)
  - Most commonly located in geniculate fossa
- T1 C+ FS MR
  - Enhancing geniculate ganglion area lesion
  - Usually with irregular margins

TOP DIFFERENTIAL DIAGNOSES

- Normal intratemporal facial nerve enhancement
- Intratemporal facial nerve schwannoma
- Bell palsy

- Perineural parotid malignancy on intratemporal CNVII
- Congenital cholesteatoma within intratemporal CNVII canal

PATHOLOGY

- **Immunohistochemical markers** critical to correct venous malformation (hemangioma) diagnosis
  - Endothelial lining of vascular channels stain negatively for hemangioma-associated markers (**GLUT1 & LeY**)
  - **Podoplanin** staining utilizing D2-40 antibody **negativity** excludes lymphatic malformation

CLINICAL ISSUES

- Intratemporal FNVM produces **peripheral CNVII paralysis** early in its natural history
  - Caveat: May be described as "**atypical Bell palsy**"
- Treatment: Perform surgery as soon as possible
  - Final CNVII function depends on duration of preoperative CNVII deficit
  - Smaller lesion are extraneural, larger lesion invade CNVII

(Left) Axial graphic illustrates a classic example of a medium-sized facial nerve venous malformation (FNVM) centered in the geniculate fossa ➡ of the temporal bone. Notice the honeycomb bone within the lesion matrix. (Right) Axial T1 C+ MR with fat saturation in a patient with left atypical Bell palsy reveals a classic left geniculate fossa enhancing FNVM ➡. Punctate areas of high density on bone CT (not shown) confirmed this imaging impression.

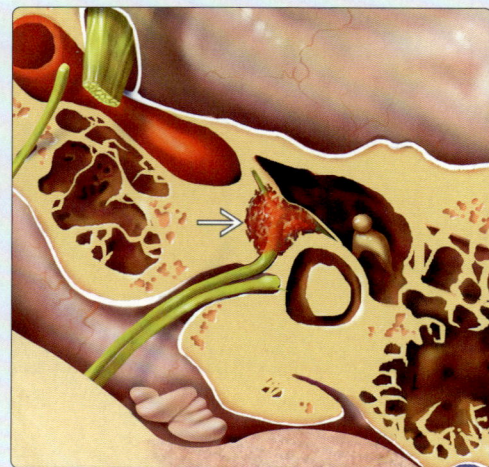
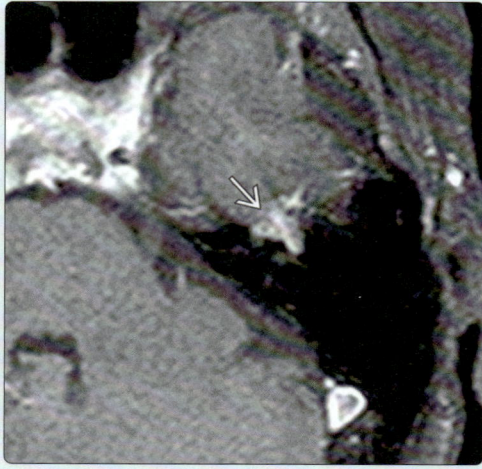

(Left) Axial bone CT demonstrates the honeycombing appearance of FNVM centered in the geniculate fossa ➡. Note extension of the lesion along the proximal tympanic CNVII segment ➡. (Right) Axial T1 C+ MR in the same patient shows a poorly marginated, avidly enhancing lesion in the geniculate fossa ➡. Note extension along the tympanic segment of CNVII ➡ and into the fundus of the internal auditory canal (IAC) ➡. IAC extension occurred via the labyrinthine segment of CNVII (not shown).

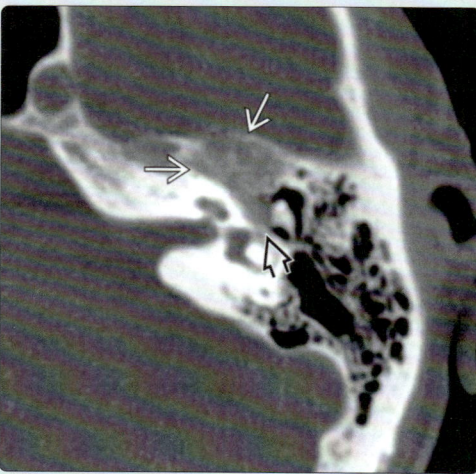
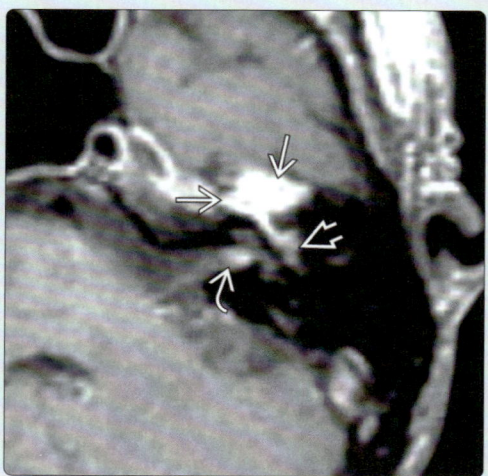

TERMINOLOGY

Abbreviations

- Facial nerve venous malformation (FNVM)

Synonyms

- Facial nerve hemangioma/ossifying hemangioma
  - Historic terms for FNVM

Definitions

- FNVM: Benign developmental lesion near intratemporal facial nerve in geniculate fossa area

IMAGING

General Features

- Best diagnostic clue
  - **Honeycomb high-density matrix** lesion in geniculate fossa area (bone CT)
  - Enhancing geniculate ganglion area lesion with irregular margins on T1 C+ MR
- Location
  - **Geniculate fossa** > > internal auditory canal (IAC), tympanic, labyrinthine & mastoid segments
- Size
  - Range: 2 mm to 2 cm
  - Small at presentation, **often < 1 cm**
- Morphology
  - Irregular, invasive-appearing margins typical

CT Findings

- Bone CT
  - Poorly marginated lesion of geniculate fossa
  - Expansile lucent lesion with intact bony cortex
  - Larger lesions affect adjacent temporal bone
    - Anteromedial to geniculate fossa
    - Labyrinthine segment CNVII → IAC
      - □ Dumbbell lesion appearance
  - Amorphous **honeycomb (or soap bubble) bone changes** are distinctive
    - Present in 50% of all lesions
    - Seen in 100% of larger lesions
  - Punctate high-density foci possible due to bony trabeculations or phleboliths; phleboliths less often seen with intraosseous VM compared to soft tissue VM

MR Findings

- T1WI
  - Mixed signal lesion with foci of low signal within lesion matrix (ossific matrix)
  - High signal foci may be present with hemorrhage &/or in situ thrombosis
- T2WI
  - Heterogeneous high-signal lesion with foci of low signal (bony trabeculae) within lesion matrix
- FLAIR
  - Mixed intermediate- & high-signal lesion
- T1WI C+
  - **Avid progressive lesion enhancement** is rule
    - Delayed-enhanced T1 MR typically shows more enhancement

- Dynamic T1-enhanced imaging shows progressive filling of lesion
  - Perineural spread from geniculate ganglion
    - Posterolateral along tympanic segment CNVII
    - Posteromedial along labyrinthine segment CNVII → IAC
      - □ **Dumbbell** appearance possible
  - Fundal IAC FNVM, exactly mimics vestibular schwannoma
    - Ovoid, well-demarcated, enhancing IAC mass
    - Low-signal foci may distinguish FNVM from vestibular schwannoma

Imaging Recommendations

- Best imaging tool
  - Imaging indicates CNVII (**facial nerve paresis**) or CNVIII (hearing loss) dysfunction
  - 1st exam: Thin-section **T1 C+ MR** focused to cerebellopontine angle (CPA)-IAC-inner ear
  - If MR negative or shows equivocal small area of enhancement along intratemporal CNVII, recommend **temporal bone CT**
    - Bone CT may show small FNVM in geniculate fossa
    - Inspect intratemporal CNVII canal carefully for 1- to 2-mm FNVM

DIFFERENTIAL DIAGNOSIS

Normal Intratemporal Facial Nerve Enhancement

- Clinical: Asymptomatic
- Imaging: T1 C+ MR shows normal enhancement of geniculate ganglion, anterior tympanic CNVII, &/or mastoid segment CNVII
- Sometimes mistaken for facial nerve pathology

Intratemporal Facial Nerve Schwannoma

- Clinical: Hearing loss ± gradual onset of CNVII paralysis
- Imaging: T1 C+ MR reveals tubular enhancing mass, smoothly enlarging CNVII canal (bone CT)
- Most commonly centered in geniculate ganglion similar to FNVM

Bell Palsy

- Clinical: Acute onset of peripheral CNVII paralysis
- Imaging: T1 C+ MR shows prominent enhancement of all or most of intratemporal CNVII
  - IAC enhancing tuft often present
- No focal mass; bone CT normal

Perineural Parotid Malignancy on Intratemporal CNVII

- Clinical: Parotid malignancy in history, palpable or subclinical
- Imaging: T1 C+ MR shows invasive parotid mass
  - Stylomastoid foramen is tissue-filled
  - CNVII enlarged & enhancing from distal to proximal
  - CNVII may be involved to CPA-IAC
  - Mastoid air cell invasion also possible
- Continuous linear nature different from focal FNVM

Congenital Cholesteatoma Within Intratemporal CNVII Canal

- Clinical: Avascular mass behind intact tympanic membrane

- Imaging: T1 C+ MR shows nonenhancing middle ear mass tracking along CNVII canal
- Involvement of facial nerve canal rare with this lesion

PATHOLOGY

General Features

- Etiology
  - Benign congenital VM arising from anastomotic sites between feeding arteries in temporal bone

Staging, Grading, & Classification

- Classification for vascular lesions based on clinical, histopathologic, & cytologic features introduced by Mulliken & Glowacki in 1982
  - **Malformation** term used for errors of vascular morphogenesis that develop in utero & persist postnatally
  - **Hemangioma** term reserved for benign vascular tumors that arise by cellular hyperplasia

Gross Pathologic & Surgical Features

- Richly vascular lesion without large feeding vessels

Microscopic Features

- H&E: Nonencapsulated venous malformation composed of dilated vascular channels of varying sizes
  - Widely ectatic vascular channels rimmed by thin, smooth muscle coats without evident elastic laminae
  - Flattened & mitotically quiescent endothelial cells
- Venous malformations = low-flow lesions
- Ossifying type: Lesion has spicules of lamellar bone
  - When seen, called **ossifying venous malformation**
- **Immunohistochemical markers** critical to make correct venous malformation diagnosis
  - Endothelial lining of vascular channels stain negatively for hemangioma markers (**GLUT1 & LeY antigen**)
  - CD31 (+) endothelial lining & smooth muscle component, consistent with venous malformation
  - Venous vs. lymphatic malformation endothelial differentiation
    - **Podoplanin** staining utilizing D2-40 antibody **negative** for endothelial cells confirms lack of lymphatic differentiation

CLINICAL ISSUES

Presentation

- Most common signs/symptoms
  - Intratemporal FNVM produces **peripheral CNVII paralysis** early in its natural history
    - Occurs early because of intimate relationship between CNVII & FNVM
    - Onset of CNVII paralysis usually acute: May be slowly progressive or intermittent
    - Caveat: May be described as "**atypical Bell palsy**"
  - IAC FNVM
    - Sensorineural hearing loss may be more prominent
    - IAC lesion with CNVII symptoms, consider FNVM
- Other signs/symptoms
  - Hemifacial spasm may progress to CNVII paralysis

Demographics

- Age
  - Wide range but usually adults
- Epidemiology
  - Rare lesion
    - 0.7% of all temporal bone lesions
  - Slightly less common than CNVII schwannoma

Natural History & Prognosis

- FNVM = slowly growing lesion
  - Proportional growth is norm
  - Disproportionate growth can occur secondary to infection, trauma, hormonal influences, or progressive hemodynamic forces
- Prognosis related to size at diagnosis, severity, & duration of preoperative CNVII paralysis
- After surgery, full CNVII function rarely regained

Treatment

- Surgery done as soon as possible
  - Final facial nerve function depends on duration of preoperative CNVII deficit
- Small FNVMs are extraneural
  - Resection with preservation of CNVII function = goal
    - Even with small lesions, rarely achieved
- Larger FNVM invades facial nerve
  - Segmental facial nerve resection completed
  - Followed by primary or cable graft repair of CNVII
  - When necessary, yields poorer outcome
- Surgical alternatives
  - Middle cranial fossa (MCF) approach if only geniculate
  - MCF-transmastoid approach for lesion of geniculate fossa & tympanic segment CNVII
  - Stereotactic radiosurgery
  - Cable graft or facial nerve reanimation
  - Observation may be considered if asymptomatic

DIAGNOSTIC CHECKLIST

Consider

- FNVM presents with CNVII dysfunction when small
  - Since early removal is best chance at CNVII preservation, radiologist must make diagnosis of subtle lesions
  - Caveat: **Small FNVM** may be **subtle** on T1 C+ **MR**
    - Use CT liberally in negative or equivocal MR

Image Interpretation Pearls

- Poorly circumscribed, enhancing lesion in geniculate fossa in setting of CNVII paralysis is most likely FNVM

SELECTED REFERENCES

1. Dandinarasaiah M et al: Characteristics and management of facial nerve schwannomas and hemangiomas. Otol Neurotol. 45(1):83-91, 2024
2. Jiang M et al: Differentiation of geniculate ganglion venous malformation from schwannoma: dynamic T1-weighted imaging provides unique diagnostic value. Eur Radiol. 33(11):7934-41, 2023
3. Strauss SB et al: Intraosseous venous malformations of the head and neck. AJNR Am J Neuroradiol. 43(8):1090-8, 2022

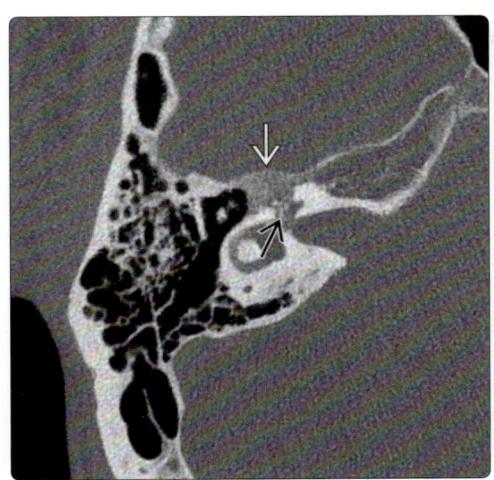

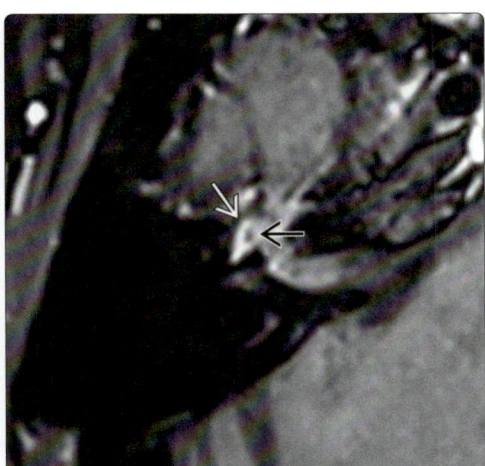

(Left) Axial bone CT in a patient with right facial nerve paralysis shows a mildly expansile lucency with a fine honeycomb appearance and intact overlying cortex in the geniculate fossa region ➡ and punctate calcifications ➡, typical of a VM. (Right) Axial T1 C+ FS MR in the same patient shows heterogeneous enhancement with a punctate hypointensity ➡ in the geniculate ganglion region ➡. This patient with longstanding facial paralysis was treated with facial nerve reanimation surgery.

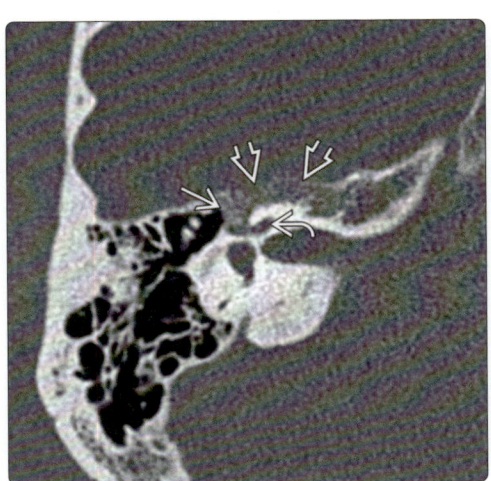

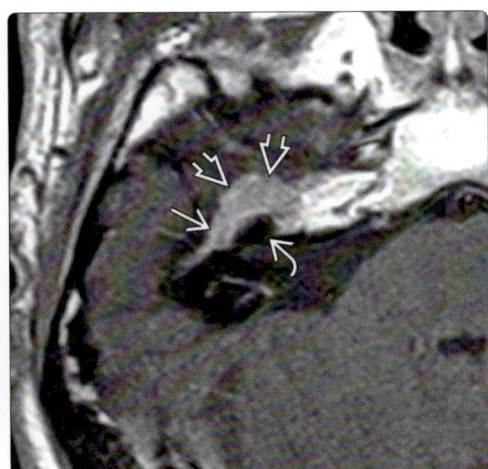

(Left) Axial bone CT through the right temporal bone demonstrates a medium-sized FNVM in the geniculate fossa ➡ with extension along the anteromedial surface of the temporal bone ➡. The crescentic shape of this lesion arching around the cochlea ➡ medially on the anterior temporal bone surface is typical of FNVM. (Right) Axial T1 C+ MR in the same patient shows diffuse FNVM enhancement in the geniculate fossa ➡, arching around the cochlea ➡ along the anteromedial temporal bone surface ➡.

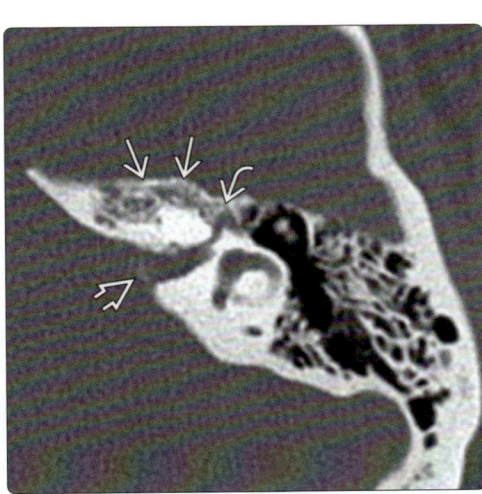

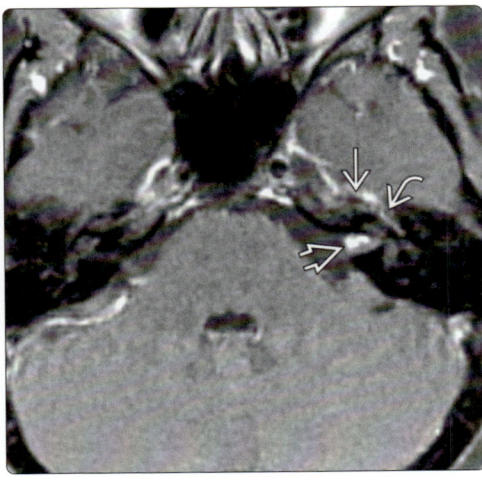

(Left) Axial bone CT shows an FNVM within the anteromedial temporal bone ➡ and in the bone surrounding the geniculate fossa ➡. Subtle foci of increased density ➡ are also seen in the IAC. (Right) Axial T1 C+ FS MR in the same patient shows the VM enhancing in the anteromedial temporal bone ➡, around the geniculate ganglion ➡, and in the IAC ➡. The IAC lobe of FNVM occurs due to extension along the labyrinthine segment of CNVII (not shown).

Temporal Bone Facial Nerve Schwannoma

TERMINOLOGY

- Facial nerve schwannoma (FNS): Rare benign tumor of Schwann cells that invests intratemporal facial nerve (CNVII)

IMAGING

- Temporal bone CT: Tubular mass spanning multiple intratemporal CNVII segments with smooth enlargement of bony CNVII canal
  - **> 90%** of FNS span ≥ 3 intratemporal CNVII segments
  - Most common location: Geniculate ganglion
- Temporal bone CT appearance dictated by specific location
  - **Geniculate fossa FNS**: Ovoid, smooth enlargement of geniculate fossa with projections into labyrinthine ± anterior tympanic segments of CNVII
  - **Tympanic segment FNS**: Pedunculated FNS emanates from tympanic CNVII into middle ear
  - **Mastoid segment FNS**: Tubular with sharp margins or globular with irregular margins into mastoids; look for intraparotid extension

- ○ **Greater superficial petrosal nerve (GSPN) schwannoma**: Enlargement of GSPN canal; middle cranial fossa mass
- T1 C+ MR: Homogeneously enhancing tubular mass ± intramural cysts

TOP DIFFERENTIAL DIAGNOSES

- Normal intratemporal facial nerve enhancement
- Bell palsy (herpetic facial paralysis)
- Intratemporal facial nerve venous malformation
- Intratemporal CNVII perineural malignancy

CLINICAL ISSUES

- Symptoms: Hearing loss (70%), CNVII paresis (50%)
  - Sensorineural (IAC); conductive loss if tympanic
- Treatment options
  - Conservative: Observation
  - Surgical treatment: Complete removal is goal
  - Radiotherapy: Nerve edema and hearing loss limit utility

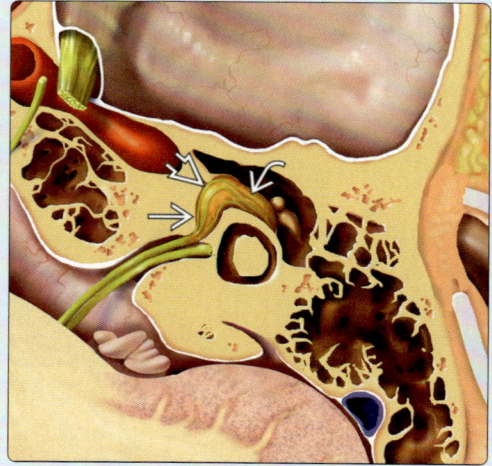
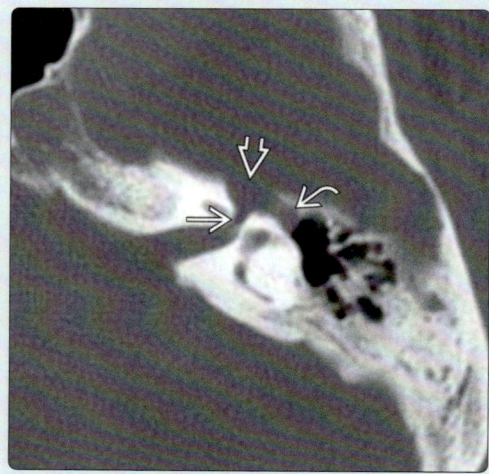

(Left) *Axial graphic shows a tubular facial nerve schwannoma (FNS) involving the labyrinthine ➡ segment, geniculate ganglion ➡, and anterior tympanic segment ➡ of the intratemporal facial nerve.* (Right) *Axial bone CT in a patient with CNVII paresis shows tubular enlargement of the distal labyrinthine segment ➡, geniculate fossa ➡, and anterior tympanic segment ➡ of the CNVII canal. Involvement of multiple segments of the facial nerve, as in this case, is highly suggestive of FNS.*

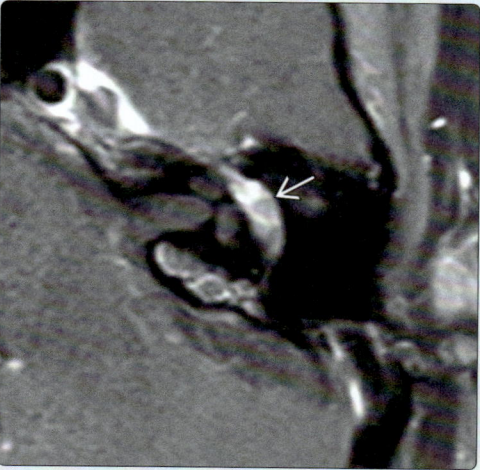
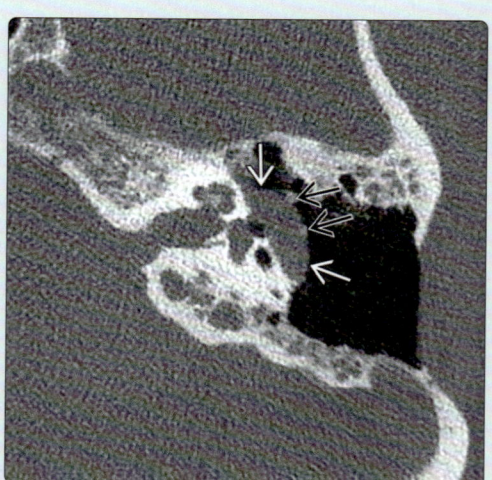

(Left) *Axial T1 C+ FS MR in a patient with left mixed conductive and sensorineural hearing loss and intermittent episodes of facial weakness shows expansion and enhancement of the tympanic segment of the facial nerve due to schwannoma ➡. (Right) Axial bone CT in the same patient shows marked expansion of the tympanic segment of facial nerve bony canal ➡. Patient underwent prior mastoidectomy and middle ear exploration for decompression of this facial schwannoma. Remnants of the ossicular chain ➡ are noted.*

Temporal Bone Facial Nerve Schwannoma

TERMINOLOGY

Abbreviations
- Facial nerve schwannoma (FNS)

Synonyms
- Facial neuroma, facial neurilemmoma

Definitions
- Rare benign tumor of Schwann cells that invests intratemporal facial nerve (CNVII)

IMAGING

General Features
- Best diagnostic clue
  - Temporal bone CT: Tubular mass spanning multiple intratemporal CNVII segments with smooth enlargement of bony CNVII canal
  - T1 C+ MR: Homogeneously enhancing tubular mass ± intramural cysts
- Location
  - Most common location: Geniculate ganglion
  - **> 90%** of FNS span **≥ 3 intratemporal CNVII segments**
- Size
  - Often long (multiple centimeters)
  - Cross-sectional measurement usually < 1 cm
- Morphology
  - Location dependent
    - Geniculate fossa: Ovoid or triangular
    - Greater superficial petrosal nerve (GSPN): Ovoid, projects into middle cranial fossa
    - Tympanic CNVII: Lobulates into middle ear
    - Mastoid CNVII: Irregular margin if breaks into surrounding air cells
    - Parotid CNVII: Tubular or ovoid mass along CNVII intraparotid course
  - **Tubular shape** along multiple CNVII segments

CT Findings
- CECT
  - No role for CECT in this diagnosis
  - Use enhanced MR instead
- Bone CT
  - General temporal bone CT appearances
    - Tubular enlargement of CNVII canal
    - Bony margins are smooth, benign-appearing
  - Temporal bone CT appearance is dictated by specific location of FNS along CNVII
    - **Geniculate fossa FNS**: Ovoid, smooth enlargement of geniculate fossa
      - □ Tumor projects into labyrinthine ± anterior tympanic segments of CNVII
    - **Tympanic segment FNS**: Pedunculated FNS emanates from tympanic segment of CNVII into middle ear cavity
    - **Mastoid segment FNS**: Either tubular with sharp margins or globular with irregular margins
      - □ Shape depends on whether FNS breaks into surrounding mastoid air cells
    - **GSPN schwannoma**: Ovoid enlargement of GSPN canal anteromedial to geniculate fossa

MR Findings
- T1WI
  - Intermediate- to low-signal lesion
- T2WI
  - High-signal lesion
- T1WI C+
  - **Geniculate ganglion FNS**: Ovoid, enhancing mass in enlarged geniculate fossa
    - Tumor tails project into labyrinthine ± anterior tympanic segments of CNVII
  - **Tympanic segment FNS**: Pedunculates into middle ear cavity
  - **Mastoid segment FNS**
    - Either tubular with sharp margins or globular with irregular margins
    - Depends on whether it breaks into surrounding mastoid air cells
  - **GSPN schwannoma**
    - Diagnosed when enhancing mass is seen in location of GSPN
    - Just anteromedial to geniculate fossa
    - Middle cranial fossa enhancing mass with connection to geniculate fossa
    - May be difficult to establish extraaxial nature of this schwannoma

Imaging Recommendations
- Best imaging tool
  - Patient presents with hearing loss ± CNVII paresis
    - Start with thin-section T1 C+ fat-saturated MR in axial and coronal plane through internal auditory canal (IAC) and temporal bone
    - If intratemporal, tubular enhancing mass is diagnosed on MR, then temporal bone CT helps delineate nature of lesion based on bone changes

DIFFERENTIAL DIAGNOSIS

Normal Intratemporal Facial Nerve Enhancement
- Clinical: Asymptomatic
- Temporal bone CT: Intratemporal CNVII canal is normal
- T1 C+ MR: Geniculate ganglion, anterior tympanic ± mastoid segments enhance normally
  - Labyrinthine CNVII does not enhance normally

Bell Palsy (Herpetic Facial Paralysis)
- Clinical: Sudden onset of peripheral CNVII paralysis
- Temporal bone CT: Normal intratemporal CNVII canal
- T1 C+ MR: Intratemporal + IAC fundal CNVII enhancement

Intratemporal Facial Nerve Venous Malformation
- Clinical: Sudden unilateral peripheral CNVII paralysis
- Temporal bone CT: Intratumoral honeycomb or bone spicules
- T1 C+ MR: Poorly circumscribed, geniculate fossa enhancing mass

Intratemporal CNVII Perineural Malignancy
- Clinical: Known or recurrent parotid malignancy
- Temporal bone CT: Mastoid CNVII canal is enlarged but less than in FNS
- T1 C+ MR: Infiltrating parotid mass is present

PATHOLOGY

General Features

- Etiology
  - Slow-growing benign tumor from Schwann cells investing intratemporal CNVII
- Genetics
  - If multiple schwannomas ± meningiomas, think neurofibromatosis type 2 (NF2)
- Associated abnormalities
  - NF2: Bilateral vestibular schwannomas; other schwannoma and meningioma possible

Gross Pathologic & Surgical Features

- Tan, ovoid-tubular, encapsulated mass
- Arises from outer nerve sheath layer of CNVII, expanding eccentrically away from nerve

Microscopic Features

- Benign, encapsulated tumor made up of bundles of spindle-shaped Schwann cells forming whorled pattern
- Cellular architecture consists of densely cellular (Antoni A) areas ± loose, myxomatous (Antoni B) areas
- S100 protein stain: Strongly and diffusely positive in both nucleus and cytoplasm
- May display **intramural cystic changes**

CLINICAL ISSUES

Presentation

- Most common signs/symptoms
  - Hearing loss present in ~ 70%
    - Preoperative functional testing may be helpful for IAC schwannomas medial to labyrinthine segment
    - Sensorineural hearing better in facial compared to vestibular schwannomas, particularly low frequencies
  - Facial nerve symptoms present in ~ 50%
    - CNVII weakness or paralysis > involuntary facial movements
    - Bell palsy-like CNVII paralysis is rare
  - Ear ± facial pain
- Other signs/symptoms
  - Cerebellopontine angle (CPA)-IAC FNS: Sensorineural hearing loss, vertigo, and tinnitus
  - Larger tympanic and mastoid segments FNS
    - Avascular retrotympanic mass
    - Conductive hearing loss

Demographics

- Age
  - Mean age at presentation: 50 years
- Epidemiology
  - FNS is rare tumor (< 1% of intrapetrous tumors)
    - Within temporal bone > > intraparotid > CPA-IAC

Natural History & Prognosis

- Slow-growing benign tumor
- Eventually enlarges sufficiently to cause hearing loss and other cranial neuropathy
- Some tumors (< 10%) do not grow or become symptomatic
- Risk of facial weakness ↑ with intratemporal involvement

- Risk for facial weakness and hearing loss ↑ with more segments involved
- Risk for hearing loss ↑ with more proximal tumor

Treatment

- **Conservative management**
  - If CNVII paralysis is absent or mild when diagnosed, surgical cure can be worse than disease
    - Incomplete recovery of full CNVII function may occur despite surgical restoration of CNVII continuity
  - Follow until CNVII symptoms begin to develop
  - Treatment used in older adult patients
- **Surgical treatment**
  - Goal = complete FNS removal with preservation of hearing and CNVII function restoration
    - Surgical decompression option to relieve pressure
  - Size-specific surgical techniques
    - Large FNS: Remove tumor + CNVII cable graft
    - Small FNS (< 1 cm): CNVII transposition with primary anastomosis
  - Location-specific surgery
    - Labyrinthine or geniculate FNS: Middle cranial fossa and transmastoid approaches combined
    - Tympanic-mastoid FNS: Transmastoid alone
- **Radiotherapy**
  - Stereotactic radiotherapy is possible but generally contraindicated for temporal bone location due to
    - Postradiation edema and nerve swelling
    - Risk of hearing loss

DIAGNOSTIC CHECKLIST

Consider

- Older patients with FNS often followed, not operated
- Younger patients without CNVII paresis often followed

Image Interpretation Pearls

- Intratemporal FNS: Segmental, tubular enlargement of CNVII canal
  - Distinctive imaging findings depending on segment of CNVII involved
- CPA-IAC FNS: Exactly mimics vestibular schwannoma if no extension into labyrinthine segment CNVII occurs
  - If present, labyrinthine segment tail makes imaging diagnosis
- Intraparotid FNS: Tubular mass in parotid coursing lateral to retromandibular vein
  - Enlarged mastoid segment is suggestive if present
  - Differentiate from perineural parotid malignancy

SELECTED REFERENCES

1. Cho YS et al: Long-term follow-up results of facial nerve schwannoma with good facial nerve function: a multicenter study. Eur Arch Otorhinolaryngol. 281(9):4719-25, 2024
2. Jiang M et al: Differentiation of geniculate ganglion venous malformation from schwannoma: dynamic T1-weighted imaging provides unique diagnostic value. Eur Radiol. 33(11):7934-41, 2023
3. Lewis D et al: Intraoperative diagnosis of facial schwannomas: a multicenter summation of clinical experience, preoperative avoidance, and intraoperative management protocol. J Neurosurg. 139(4):972-83, 2023
4. Libell JL et al: Facial nerve schwannoma: case report and brief review of the literature. Radiol Case Rep. 18(10):3442-7, 2023
5. Shapey J et al: Diffusion MRI of the facial-vestibulocochlear nerve complex: a prospective clinical validation study. Eur Radiol. 33(11):8067-76, 2023

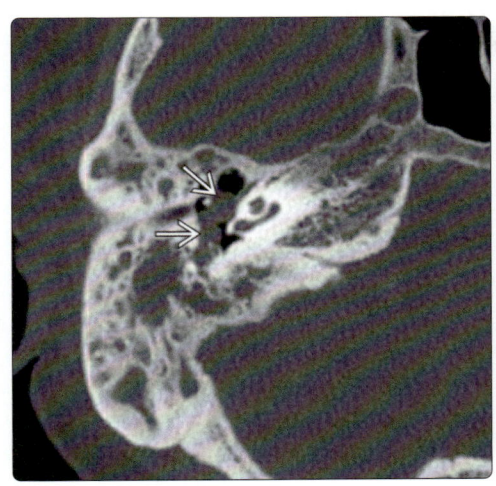

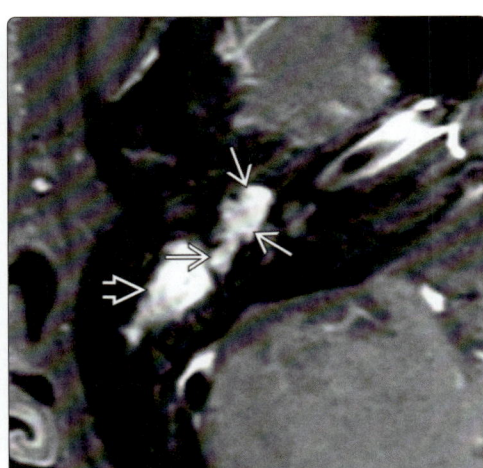

(Left) *Axial temporal bone CT in a patient with a history of hearing loss and tinnitus shows a lobulated FNS extending along the course of the tympanic segment of CNVII* ➡️. *The patient developed subjective right facial weakness not reproducible on clinical exam.* (Right) *Axial T1 C+ FS MR in the same patient shows corresponding soft tissue enhancement* ➡️ *along the tympanic segment of CNVII. Adjacent intrinsic mastoid hyperintensity* ⇨ *was due to T1-hyperintense secretions, not enhancing tumor.*

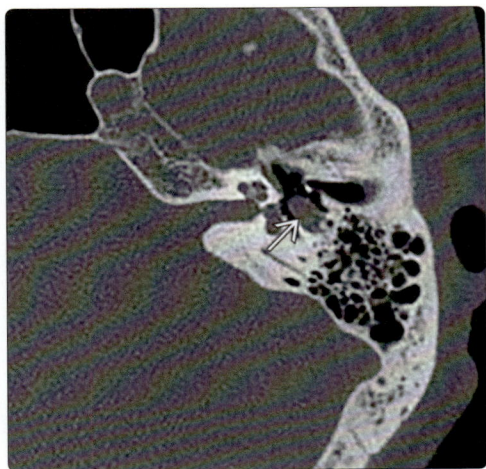

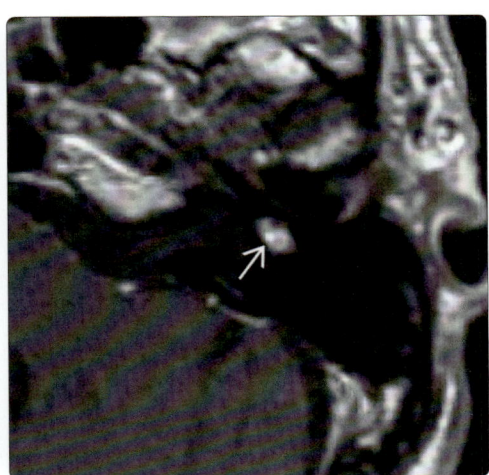

(Left) *Axial temporal bone CT in a patient with progressive partial left facial nerve paralysis associated with episodes of ipsilateral otalgia shows localized expansile enlargement of the tympanic segment of the facial nerve* ➡️. *The patient was initially treated with steroids for presumed Bell palsy, but subsequently underwent imaging when he did not respond.* (Right) *Axial T1 C+ MR in the same patient shows enhancing schwannoma* ➡️ *corresponding to the area of smooth osseous expansion on CT.*

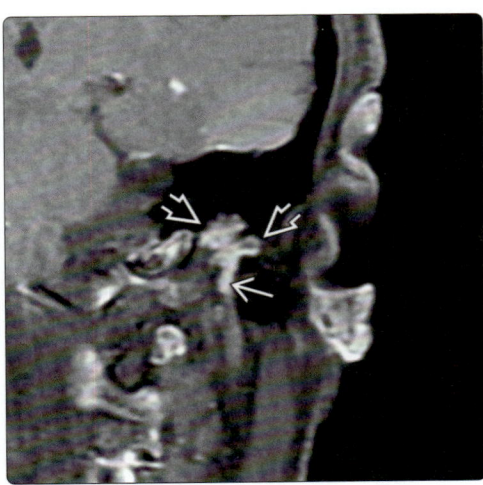

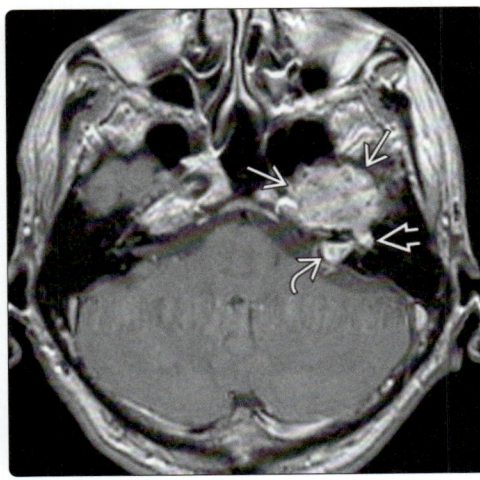

(Left) *Coronal T1 C+ FS MR in a patient with conductive hearing loss and facial twitching shows a multilobular, enhancing FNS* ⇨ *that has broken into mastoid air cells and projects inferiorly along the mastoid CN segment* ➡️. (Right) *Axial T1 C+ MR shows an enhancing mass* ➡️ *projecting into the medial middle cranial fossa from the greater superficial petrosal nerve. FNS diagnosis is suggested if the projections along the tympanic CNVII* ➡️ *and along the labyrinthine CNVII into the internal auditory canal* ➡️ *are seen.*

Temporal Bone Perineural Parotid Malignancy

TERMINOLOGY

- Perineural tumor (PNT) on CNVII in temporal bone: Local extension of malignant tumor along intratemporal CNVII

IMAGING

- Best clue: Poorly circumscribed, enhancing, tubular lesion extending from intraparotid tumor through stylomastoid foramen (SMF) to involve at least mastoid CNVII segment
  - **Contiguous spread** or **skip lesions** along CNVII
  - Image entire CNVII from end organ to brainstem
- Temporal bone CT findings
  - Intratemporal CNVII PNT may be difficult to detect
  - Mastoid CNVII canal may be slightly enlarged
  - Adjacent air cell opacification
- MR findings
  - Loss of SMF fat best seen on axial T1 MR
  - Axial images best delineate tympanic, geniculate ganglion, & labyrinthine CNVII PNT

- Coronal & sagittal images through temporal bone best show PNT extending through SMF into mastoid CNVII segment

TOP DIFFERENTIAL DIAGNOSES

- Bell palsy; temporal bone CNVII venous malformation ("hemangioma")
- Temporal bone CNVII schwannoma
- Transmodiolar cochlear nerve schwannoma
- Ramsay Hunt syndrome

CLINICAL ISSUES

- Clinical presentation
  - Asymptomatic (60%) but with imaging findings
  - Progressive peripheral CNVII paresis or paralysis in adult
- Treatment options
  - Surgery combined with postoperative radiation therapy
  - Primary radiation therapy with proton beam may be indicated for surgically unresectable tumors

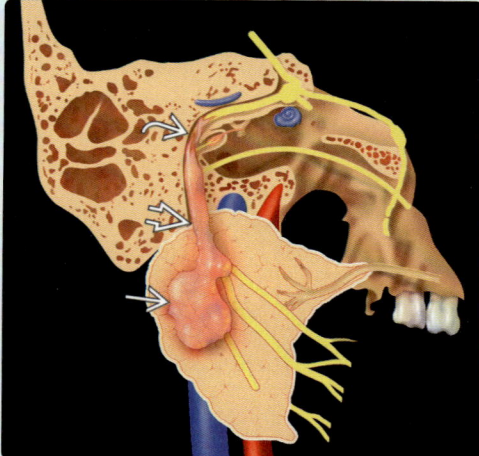
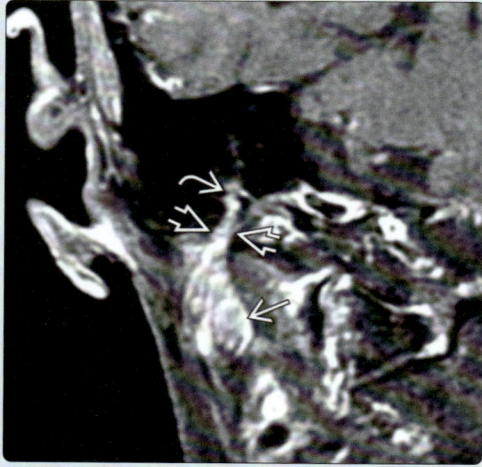

(Left) Sagittal graphic depicts an intraparotid neoplasm ➡ spreading along CNVII through the stylomastoid foramen ➡. Note that it travels superiorly along the mastoid segment of CNVII to the posterior genu ➡. (Right) Coronal T1WI C+ MR shows parotid adenoid cystic carcinoma ➡ spreading along proximal extracranial CNVII through the stylomastoid foramen ➡ then up the mastoid segment of CNVII ➡.

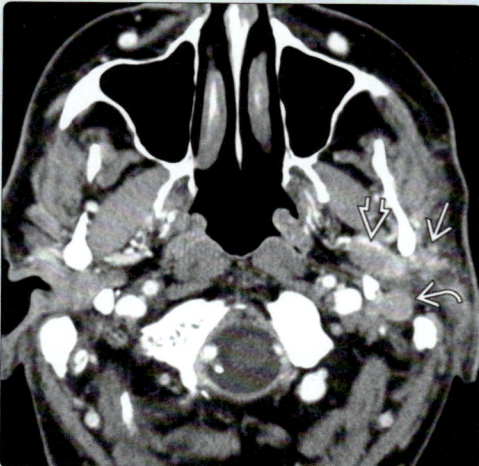
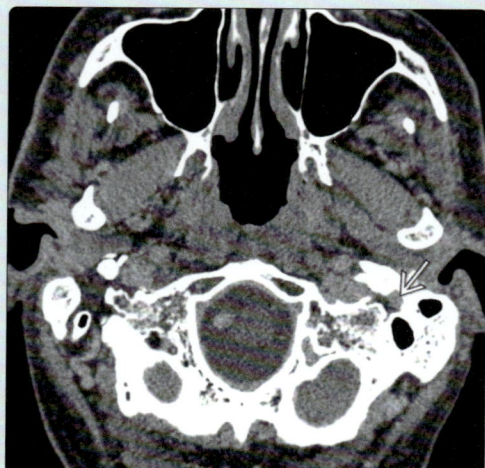

(Left) Axial CECT shows infiltrating parotid adenoid cystic carcinoma ➡ with perineural spread along the auriculotemporal nerve (branch of V3) ➡. Perineural spread along intraparotid CNVII is seen as a round lesion ➡ in the fat just below the stylomastoid foramen. (Right) Axial CECT demonstrates an enlarged facial nerve from a perineural tumor ➡ in the left stylomastoid foramen in this patient with primary parotid adenoid cystic carcinoma.

Temporal Bone Perineural Parotid Malignancy

TERMINOLOGY

Synonyms
- Neurotropic spread on intratemporal facial nerve (CNVII)

Definitions
- Local tumor extension along intratemporal CNVII

IMAGING

General Features
- Best diagnostic clue
  - Poorly circumscribed, enhancing, invasive mass arising within parotid gland extending through stylomastoid foramen (SMF) to involve mastoid CNVII segment
- Location
  - Extracranial & intracranial
  - Malignant primary parotid tumor or parotid metastasis can cause CNVII perineural tumor (PNT)
  - PNT can extend along entire course CNVII from end organ to nucleus in brainstem
- Size
  - Cross section size: Variable but larger than normal nerve
  - Length: May be many centimeters in length
- Morphology
  - Tubular enlargement of intratemporal CNVII
    - Contiguous spread along CNVII on histology but may appear as radiographic **skip lesions**

CT Findings
- CECT
  - Delineates intraparotid malignancy
  - Tumor replacing SMF fat pad
  - Intratemporal CNVII PNT may be difficult to detect
  - Chronic denervation atrophy of muscles of facial expression
    - Early & subacute denervation not seen on CT
- Bone CT
  - Asymmetric widening of SMF & mastoid CNVII canal
  - Adjacent mastoid air cells may show tumor invasion

MR Findings
- T1WI
  - Infiltrating parotid malignancy
  - Loss of fat in "bell" of SMF
    - Best seen on axial T1 MR images
  - ↑ signal in chronic denervated muscles of facial expression
- T2WI
  - High-resolution (≤ 3-mm slice thickness) T2 defines internal auditory canal (IAC) PNT if present
    - Fundal CNVII appears thickened
      - May connect to enlarged labyrinthine segment CNVII
    - ↑ T2 signal in intratemporal segment
- T2WI FS
  - ↑ T2 signal in subacute muscle denervation
    - Acute denervation not recognized because muscles too small
- T1WI C+
  - **Abnormally enlarged & enhancing intratemporal CNVII**
  - PNT may involve mastoid & tympanic segments of CNVII, geniculate ganglion, & labyrinthine segment CNVII
  - PNT may extend into IAC fundus as enhancing nodule
  - PNT can travel along CNVII → CNVIII via **auriculotemporal nerve**
- MR tractography
  - Emerging technique in evaluating PNT along CNVII

Nuclear Medicine Findings
- PET/CT rarely detects PNT
  - Because small volume of tumor along nerve or tumor itself is not classically FDG avid [e.g., adenoid cystic carcinoma (ACCa)]

Imaging Recommendations
- Best imaging tool
  - Enhanced multiplanar MR ± fat saturation
    - Defines scope of intraparotid malignancy
    - Best depicts intratemporal CNVII PNT
    - Shows denervation atrophy in muscles of facial expression
  - Temporal bone CT is best to evaluate osseous SMF & intratemporal CNVII canal
    - Also helpful in evaluating subtle involvement of adjacent structures
      - Adjacent middle ear & mastoid air cells
      - Medial external auditory canal
- Protocol advice
  - Beware that some 3T sequences exaggerate artifact with fat-saturation images & may render images of intratemporal CNVII uninterpretable
  - Scan must include entire course CNVII from nucleus → end organ

DIFFERENTIAL DIAGNOSIS

Bell Palsy
- Abrupt onset of peripheral CNVII paralysis
  - Self-limiting process: Generally resolves in 6 weeks
- Imaging: Intratemporal facial nerve asymmetric enhancement ± IAC fundal tuft on T1 C+ MR

Temporal Bone CNVII Venous Malformation ("Hemangioma")
- CNVII paralysis early in disease process
- Imaging: Infiltrating, focal, enhancing CNVII lesion in geniculate fossa on T1 C+ MR
  - Temporal bone CT: 50% with honeycomb bone pattern

Temporal Bone CNVII Schwannoma
- Hearing loss > > CNVII paralysis
- Imaging: Tubular, enhancing mass along course of intratemporal CNVII on T1 C+ MR
  - Temporal bone CT: Fusiform enlargement of intratemporal CNVII canal; most commonly at geniculate ganglion

Transmodiolar Cochlear Nerve Schwannoma
- Slowly progressive sensorineural hearing loss; no CNVII paralysis
- Imaging: Dumbbell-shaped, enhancing mass extending from cochlea through cochlear aperture into IAC fundus on T1 C+ MR

Ramsay Hunt Syndrome

- CNVII palsy + painful vesicles about ear
- Imaging: Enhancement of intratemporal CNVII

PATHOLOGY

General Features

- Etiology
  - Any parotid malignancy → PNT via direct invasion CNVII
  - Skin cancer [squamous cell carcinoma (SCCa), melanoma] → PNT
    - Direct extension along CNVII
    - More commonly CNV → CNVII via **auriculotemporal nerve**
  - Neurotropic tumors
    - ACCa: Salivary
    - SCCa: Skin
      - □ Less neurotropic but most common H&N cancer
    - Desmoplastic melanoma: Skin
    - Lymphoma
- Associated abnormalities
  - PNT is generally **retrograde** (toward CNS) **> antegrade** (away from CNS)
  - PNT CNVII: **Contiguous** or radiographic **skip areas**

Staging, Grading, & Classification

- Staging criteria: Salivary gland tumor with PNT on facial nerve
  - **T4**: Tumor **invades CNVII**
  - Stage IV: T4, any nodes, any metastases

Gross Pathologic & Surgical Features

- PNT can occur early in H&N cancers
- PNT can be extensive without local invasion of adjacent structures or significant lymphadenopathy

Microscopic Features

- Tumor first grows along CNVII sheath; eventually invades nerve

CLINICAL ISSUES

Presentation

- Most common signs/symptoms
  - Asymptomatic (60%) but with imaging findings
  - **Progressive peripheral CNVII paresis or paralysis**
    - Often preceded by facial twitching
  - Palpable parotid mass (not always)
- Other signs/symptoms
  - Burning or stinging facial or ear pain
  - Formication (sensation of ants crawling)
- Clinical profile
  - Adult + parotid mass + ipsilateral CNVII paralysis
  - May confuse with Bell palsy
    - High index of suspicion if parotid or skin cancer history

Demographics

- Age
  - 40-60 years old
- Epidemiology
  - ACCa is most common parotid malignancy to show PNT along CNVII

- Other malignancies with CNVII PNT
  - SCCa or melanoma directly from skin primary or nodal metastases
  - Non-Hodgkin lymphoma
  - Mucoepidermoid carcinoma

Natural History & Prognosis

- PNT presence = ↑ risk local recurrence of primary tumor
- Carcinomas with PNT usually have relentless progression
- CNVII PNT can lead to serious physical deformity
- H&N neoplasms can exist within nerves for years without symptoms
  - Especially true in low-grade ACCa
- Diagnosis is frequently delayed, & outcome is poor once clinical manifestations arise
- 5-year overall survival: Poor
- Parotid ACCa has distinct clinical behavior
  - Overall 10-year survival rate: 65%
  - Recurrence depends on stage > histologic grade
  - Often indolent & slow growing
  - Long-term (> 10-year) imaging follow-up is recommended given tendency of ACCa to recur late

Treatment

- Treatment & prognosis altered by PNT
- Surgery combined with postoperative radiation therapy
- Primary radiation therapy with proton beam may be indicated for surgically unresectable tumors

DIAGNOSTIC CHECKLIST

Consider

- Imaging findings of PNT may be subtle
  - **Caveat**: If radiologist does not think to search for PNT when suspected parotid malignancy is seen, diagnosis of PNT is usually missed
    - Identification of PNT & its extent on imaging is critical to patient's chances of cure
  - Beware Bell palsy diagnosis

Image Interpretation Pearls

- If invasive parotid space lesion seen on imaging, radiologist must search for intratemporal PNT on CNVII
- MR more sensitive than CECT in detecting PNT along intratemporal CNVII
- If SMF fat is invaded, dedicated temporal bone CT & enhanced MR to assess extent of CNVII PNT is recommended
- There may be radiologic **skip areas** along CNVII
  - Visually interrogate entire course of CNVII from nucleus/brainstem → end organ

SELECTED REFERENCES

1. Daloiso A et al: Temporal-parotid resection for malignant parotid tumors: a systematic review. Laryngoscope. ePub, 2025
2. Abdullaeva U et al: Diagnostic accuracy of MRI in detecting the perineural spread of head and neck tumors: a systematic review and meta-analysis. Diagnostics (Basel). 14(1):113, 2024
3. Hsieh KJ et al: Perineural spread of tumor in the skull base and head and neck. Oral Maxillofac Surg Clin North Am. 35(3):399-412, 2023
4. Van der Cruyssen F et al: Magnetic resonance neurography of the head and neck: state of the art, anatomy, pathology and future perspectives. Br J Radiol. 94(1119):20200798, 2021

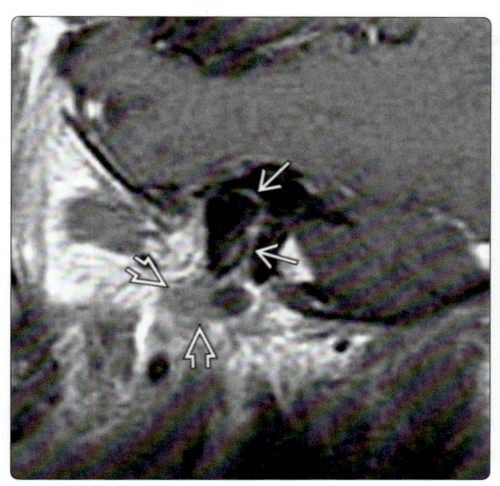

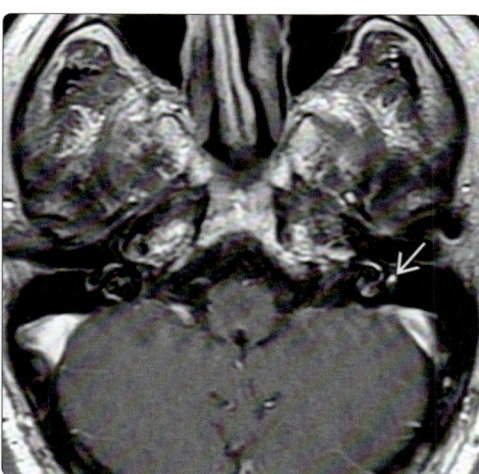

(Left) *Sagittal T1WI MR shows subtle, diffuse enlargement and enhancement of the left intratemporal facial nerve* ➡ *from primary parotid acinic cell carcinoma* ➡ *noted adjacent to the stylomastoid foramen.* (Right) *Axial T1WI C+ MR shows subtle, asymmetric enlargement and enhancement of the mastoid segment of CNVII* ➡ *from left parotid acinic cell carcinoma.*

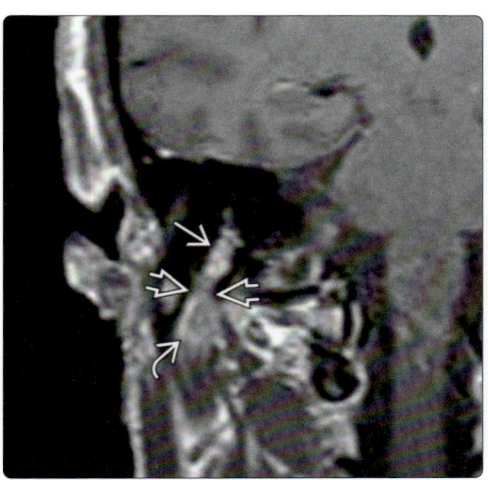

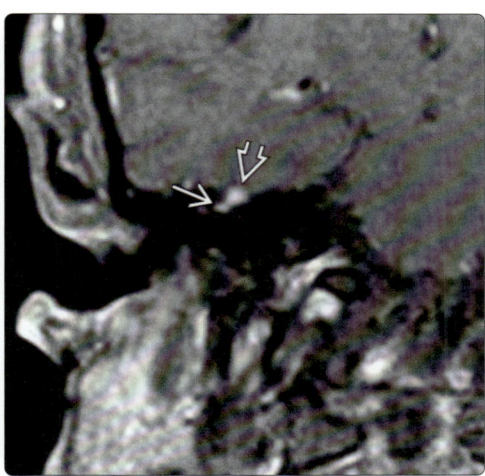

(Left) *Coronal T1WI C+ MR demonstrates primary parotid malignancy* ➡ *entering the right stylomastoid foramen* ➡ *and extending along the mastoid segment of CNVII* ➡. (Right) *Coronal T1WI C+ MR reveals a skip lesion of perineural tumor involving the right anterior tympanic* ➡ *and labyrinthine* ➡ *segments of CNVII in a patient with primary parotid malignancy. The intervening tympanic segment (not shown) appeared normal, hence the term skip lesion.*

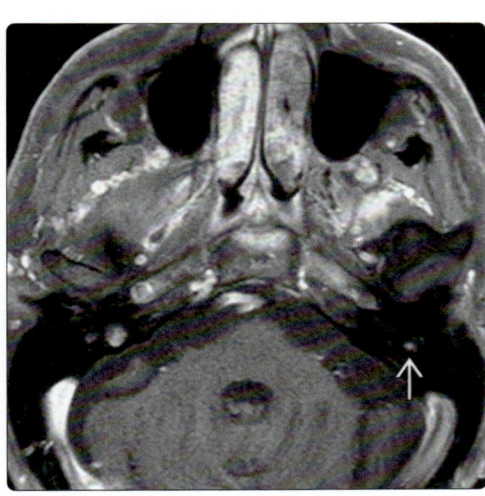

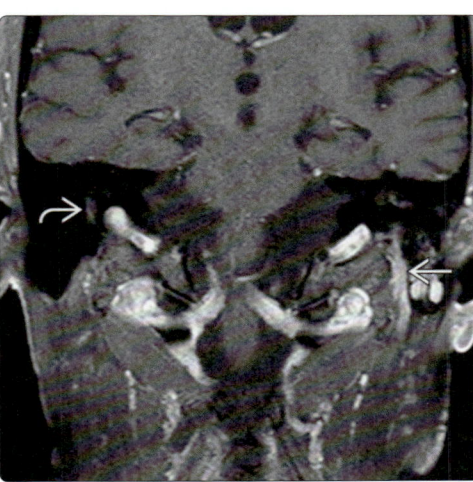

(Left) *Axial T1 C+ FS MR in a patient post resection for parotid adenoid cystic carcinoma shows abnormal asymmetric enhancement of the left mastoid segment of facial nerve* ➡ *due to perineural tumor spread.* (Right) *Coronal T1 C+ FS MR in the same patient shows a thickened, enhancing left descending/mastoid segment of the facial nerve as it exits the stylomastoid foramen* ➡. *In comparison, the normal mastoid segment right facial nerve* ➡ *is nonenhancing.*

TERMINOLOGY

- CSF leak into middle ear (ME) cavity
- Leak of CSF either from acquired tegmen, postsurgical T-bone, or congenital inner ear (IE) defect

IMAGING

- Axial bone CT (≤ 1 mm) + coronal reformats
  - Coronal best shows tegmen defect
- Bone CT findings
  - Opacified ME-mastoid air cells
  - Tegmen defect: Isolated or with cephalocele
  - Possible associated findings: Fracture, arachnoid granulation or osseous dural defect, postsurgical findings, IE malformation (IEM)
  - **Congenital IEM**: Most commonly, fistula around oval window, including stapes footplate & annular ligament
  - Cochlear aplasia with dilated vestibule, incomplete partition types I & II, IAC defects, modiolar defects
- MR findings if cephalocele suspected

- T2 coronal: Meningocele (fluid-filled sac) or encephalocele (brain)
  - Extends through tegmen defect into ME
- Imaging recommendations
  - CT: Include all paranasal sinuses & both T-bones

TOP DIFFERENTIAL DIAGNOSES

- Rhinorrhea without CSF leak
- Otorrhea without CSF leak

CLINICAL ISSUES

- Watery fluid leaking from nose (**paradoxic CSF rhinorrhea**) or external auditory canal
- Fluid positive for CSF **β2-transferrin** or β trace protein
- Obesity with ↑ intracranial hypertension (IIH) ↑ in frequency

DIAGNOSTIC CHECKLIST

- Multiple & bilateral defects common in posttraumatic or IIH patients

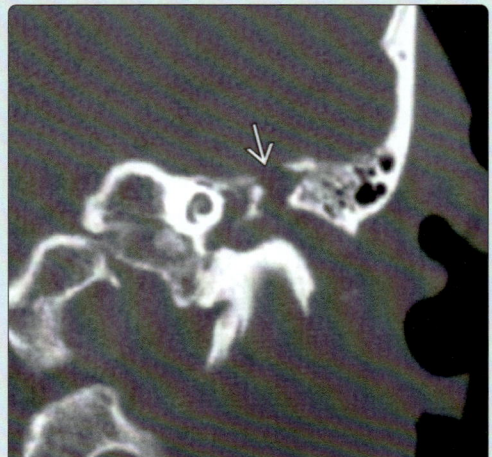
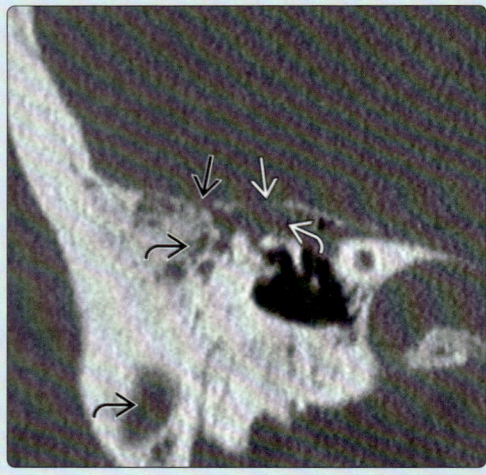

(Left) Coronal bone CT reveals a left temporal bone fracture with a large tegmen tympani defect ➡. The patient had left-sided CSF otorrhea after a motor vehicle accident. (Right) Longitudinal oblique (Stenver view) reconstruction of right temporal bone HRCT in another patient with CSF leak shows bony defects in tegmen tympani ➡ & tegmen mastoideum ➡, with opacification of epitympanum ➡ & mastoid air cells ➡. Epitympanum had a small cephalocele along with CSF on MR (not shown), & mastoid air cells showed only CSF.

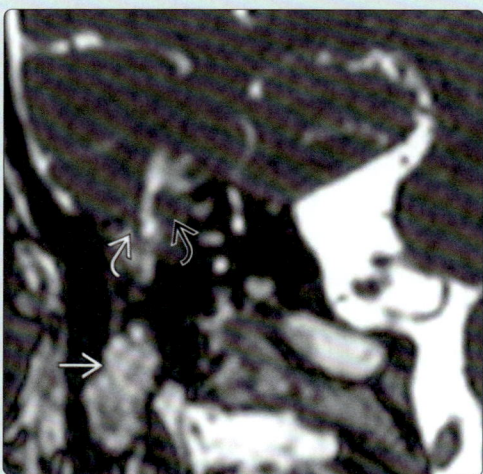
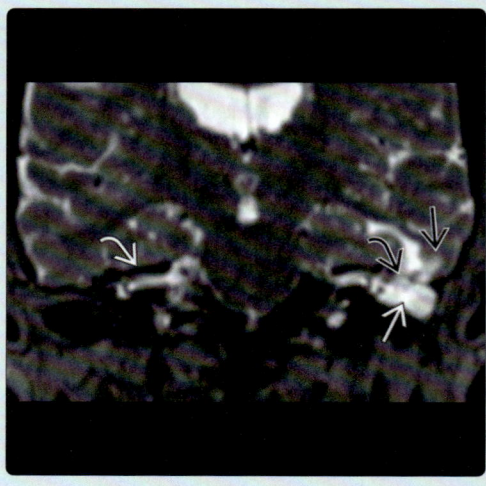

(Left) Coronal heavily T2WI CISS MR shows spontaneous right middle ear meningoencephalocele with part of inferior temporal gyrus ➡ and fusiform gyrus ➡ with intervening sulcus herniating into the middle ear cavity. Note bright CSF in mastoid air cells ➡. (Right) Coronal heavily T2WI SPACE MR shows a large left tegmen tympani osteodural defect ➡ with CSF leak into left middle ear cavity ➡. There is encephalomalacia in adjacent left temporal lobe ➡. Note normal hypointense osseous dural lining along the right tegmen tympani ➡.

TERMINOLOGY

Definitions

- CSF leak: Congenital or acquired
- Acquired **tegmen tympani** or **mastoideum** defect, resulting in leak of CSF into middle ear (ME) cavity
  - Traumatic or idiopathic intracranial hypertension (IIH)
- Acquired postsurgical T-bone defects
- Congenital inner ear malformation (IEM) with **perilymph fistula & CSF leak** into ME

IMAGING

General Features

- Location
  - Tegmen tympani or mastoideum
  - Congenital IEM: Most commonly fistula around oval window, including stapes footplate & annular ligament
    - Other sites: Tympanic opening of eustachian tube, or ventral defect in internal auditory canal (IAC), or enlarged vestibular aqueduct

CT Findings

- Bone CT
  - Opacified ME-mastoid from CSF
  - Possible causal findings: Previous T-bone surgery or fracture; osseous dural defect (pit, arachnoid granulation) of tegmen or posterior wall common in IIH
    - Congenital IEM: Cochlear aplasia with dilated vestibule, incomplete partition types I & II
      - Absent modiolus, semicircular canal anomalies, IAC enlargement or defects, including at lamina cribrosa

MR Findings

- T2WI
  - Fluid-filled ME-mastoid complex with dehiscent tegmen ± **cephalocele**; meningocele (CSF) or encephalocele (brain); traction encephalomalacia of adjacent brain from sag into bone defect common secondary finding
- T1WI C+
  - Thin dural enhancement at site of bone defect common even without infection/meningitis

Imaging Recommendations

- Protocol advice
  - Axial MDCT (≤ 1 mm); reformat coronals
  - Include all paranasal sinuses & both T-bones as multiple defects (common post trauma & in IIH) can occur
  - Heavily T2-weighted multiplanar, especially coronal, sequences best show associated cephalocele
  - Rarely, CT/MR cisternography if CT normal or multiple bone defects could be source of leak

DIFFERENTIAL DIAGNOSIS

Rhinorrhea Without CSF Leak

- Vasomotor rhinitis, posttraumatic autonomic dysfunction

Otorrhea Without CSF Leak

- Otitis media with tympanic membrane perforation, otitis externa, or external auditory canal (EAC) foreign body may all mimic CSF leak

PATHOLOGY

General Features

- Etiology
  - **Traumatic**: Most T-bone CSF leaks are traumatic (motor vehicle accident, gunshot wound)
  - **Spontaneous**: Tegmen defects ↑ due to ↑ obesity & IIH, rarely posterior T-bone posterior fossa defects
  - **Postsurgical**: Usually cholesteatoma resection with tegmen leak developing after surgery; stapes surgery: Perilymph gusher from oval window
  - **Congenital**: IEM + perilymph fistula
  - Inner ear dysplasia with abnormal otic capsule → weak stapes footplate or annular ligament with fistula
  - CSF pressure fluctuations → stapes footplate thinning or cracks in annular ligament
    - Inner ear dysplasia subjects more susceptible to CSF rhinorrhea post trauma/barotrauma
  - Narrow cochlear conduit in normal population prevent CSF from entering perilymphatic space during CSF pressure fluctuation

CLINICAL ISSUES

Presentation

- Most common signs/symptoms
  - Watery fluid leaking from nose or EAC
- Other signs/symptoms
  - Temporal lobe cephalocele may present with epilepsy
  - CSF lab tests: **β2-transferrin** (immunofixation or immunoblotting), & newer, faster, & cheaper **β trace protein** (immunoelectrophoresis or laser-nephelometry)
  - Ascending meningitis less common now due to early recognition & imaging after trauma
  - Posttraumatic: CNVII, CNVIII injuries

Demographics

- Epidemiology: 2-9% of patients with head injury have CSF leak; obese, middle-aged women with IIH

Natural History & Prognosis

- Posttraumatic: Up to 85% resolve spontaneously within 7 days; most within 6 months
- IIH: May require skull base repair, followed by treatment for ↑ intracranial pressure & weight reduction

Treatment

- Posttraumatic: Bed rest, lumbar drain
- IIH: Middle fossa or mastoid approach for T-bone

DIAGNOSTIC CHECKLIST

Consider

- **Paradoxic CSF rhinorrhea**: ME CSF → eustachian tube → nasopharynx → posterior choana → nasal cavity

SELECTED REFERENCES

1. Zhou DJ et al: Clinical characteristics and surgical outcomes of epilepsy associated with temporal encephalocele: a systematic review. Epilepsy Behav. 158:109928, 2024
2. Cooper T et al: Comparison of spontaneous temporal bone cerebrospinal fluid leaks from the middle and posterior fossa. Otol Neurotol. 41(2):e232-7, 2020

TERMINOLOGY

- Temporal bone arachnoid granulation (AG): **Nonvenous sinus-related** (aberrant) pseudopodial **pia-arachnoid projection** into tegmen tympani or posterior wall of temporal bone

IMAGING

- Bone CT findings
  - Ovoid/tubular scalloping erosion in temporal bone wall
- MR findings
  - Nonenhancing low signal (T1 C+)
  - High T2 signal lesion
- Locations
  - Lateral 1/3 of posterior temporal bone wall
    - Between posterior semicircular canal & anterior margin of sigmoid sinus
  - Tegmen tympani & mastoideum: Hard to see on CT/MR
- Size variation of posterior wall AG
  - Few millimeters to 2-3 centimeters (**giant AG**)

TOP DIFFERENTIAL DIAGNOSES

- Endolymphatic sac tumor
- Large vestibular aqueduct (incomplete partition type II)
- Temporal bone cephalocele
- Skull base dural arteriovenous fistula

PATHOLOGY

- CSF pulsations cause enlargement of aberrant AG that does not communicate directly with venous sinus

CLINICAL ISSUES

- **Incidental asymptomatic** finding
  - Rarely, CSF leak associated ± meningitis
- Posterior wall AG **prevalence ↑ with age**
- May be associated with obesity & idiopathic intracranial hypertension
- On bone CT, posterior wall AG seen in **2.5%** of patients
- Treatment: None unless CSF leak associated

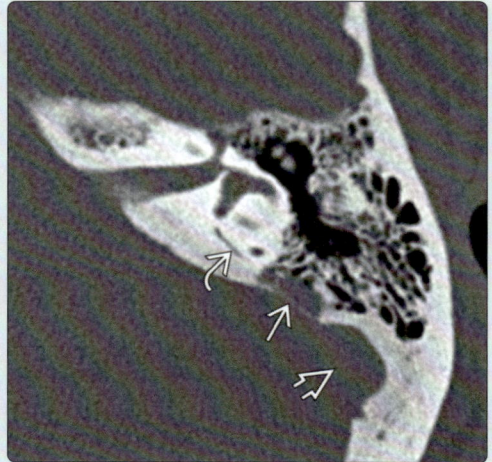
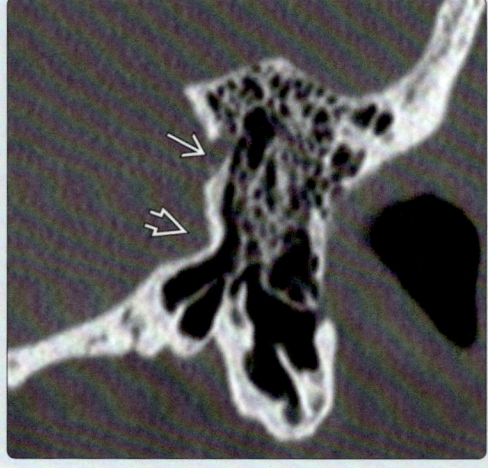

(Left) Axial bone CT of the left ear in a patient with right ear symptoms shows a medium-sized incidental arachnoid granulation (AG) in the medial mastoid wall ➡ projecting into the mastoid air cells. Note the proximity of the sigmoid sinus ➡ and bony vestibular aqueduct ➡. (Right) Short-axis oblique bone CT of the left temporal bone reveals a small AG ➡ in the medial mastoid wall. Note that the lesion is on the superior margin of the sigmoid sinus ➡.

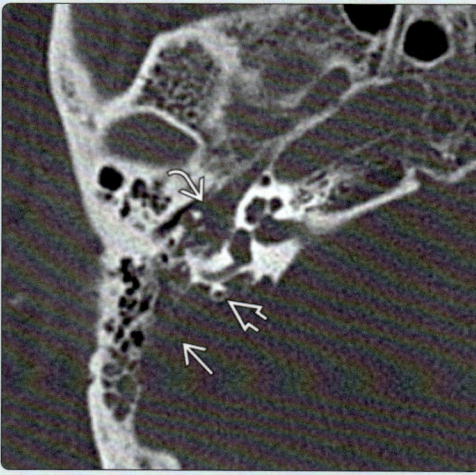
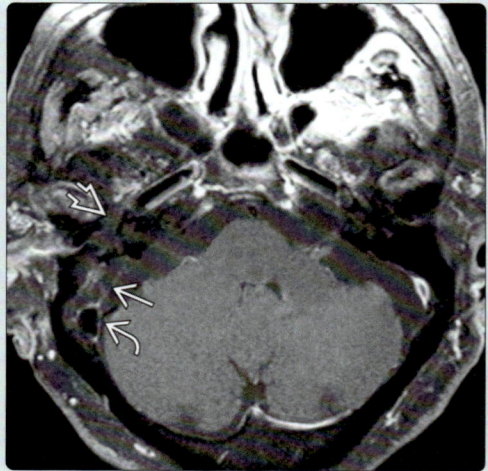

(Left) Axial bone CT of the right temporal bone in a patient with a clinically obvious CSF leak demonstrates a giant AG eroding the medial mastoid wall ➡. The posterior semicircular ➡ canal appears to float in the AG. The middle ear is full of fluid (CSF) ➡. (Right) Axial T1 C+ FS MR in the same patient reveals the giant AG ➡ as a lobular fluid signal structure with subtle rim enhancement. The middle ear fluid is low signal ➡. Note the proximity of the sigmoid sinus ➡ to the giant AG.

TERMINOLOGY

Abbreviations

- Arachnoid granulation (AG)

Synonyms

- Aberrant AG, osteodural defects
- When > 1 cm → giant AG

Definitions

- Temporal bone AG: **Nonvenous sinus-related** (aberrant) pseudopodial **pia-arachnoid projection** into tegmen tympani or posterior wall of temporal bone

IMAGING

General Features

- Best diagnostic clue
  - Bone CT: Scalloped lucency in temporal bone wall; ovoid or tubular; multilobular when large
  - MR: Nonenhancing low signal (T1 C+), high T2 signal lesion
- Location
  - Tegmen tympani
  - Lateral 1/3 of posterior temporal bone wall
    - Between posterior semicircular canal & anterior margin of sigmoid sinus
    - At axial level of crus communis
- Size
  - Tegmen tympani AG: Millimeters
  - Posterior wall AG: Few millimeters to 2-3 centimeters (**giant AG**)

CT Findings

- Bone CT
  - Tegmen tympani AG
    - Small size & variable ossification of normal tegmen makes it **difficult to see** with CT
  - Posterior wall AG
    - Ovoid or tubular lucency in medial mastoid wall
      - Multilobular when large
    - Mastoid cortex with focal erosion
    - AG may project into medial mastoid air cells

MR Findings

- T2WI
  - High signal similar to CSF
    - Possible thin internal septations
- T1WI C+ FS
  - Ovoid or tubular fluid signal lesion
  - No or subtle rim enhancement
    - No nodular enhancement

Imaging Recommendations

- Best imaging tool
  - High-resolution bone CT in combination with enhanced MR

DIFFERENTIAL DIAGNOSIS

Endolymphatic Sac Tumor

- Centered in fovea of endolymphatic sac, posterior wall
- CT: Spiculated or coarse calcifications within tumor matrix
  - Thin calcification along posterior margin
- MR: T1 high-signal foci from trapped blood products

Large Vestibular Aqueduct (Incomplete Partition Type II)

- CT: Enlarged bony vestibular aqueduct
- MR: Enlarged endolymphatic sac

Dural Arteriovenous Fistula, Skull Base

- CT: Transosseous collaterals traverse posterior mastoid
- MR: Recanalized, irregular transverse-sigmoid sinus

Temporal Bone Cephalocele

- Most often affects tegmen
- May contain meninges with CSF &/or brain

PATHOLOGY

General Features

- Etiology
  - **Temporal bone AG** = form of **aberrant AG**
    - Defined as AG that penetrates dura but **fails to reach venous sinus**
    - CSF pulsations suspected to enlarge AG, causing arachnoid pouch to bulge into temporal bone
      - Idiopathic intracranial hypertension (IIH) may facilitate AG growth
    - Rarely with arachnoid pouch enlargement, rupture results in CSF leak into mastoid temporal bone

Gross Pathologic & Surgical Features

- **Osteodural defect** with arachnoid pouch

CLINICAL ISSUES

Presentation

- Most common signs/symptoms
  - **Incidental asymptomatic** finding
- Other signs/symptoms
  - Rarely, CSF leak associated ± meningitis
  - May be associated with IIH

Demographics

- Epidemiology
  - Tegmen tympani AG > > posterior wall AG
  - Posterior wall AG **prevalence ↑ with age**
  - Can see posterior wall AG on CT in **~ 2.5%** of patients
  - May be associated with obesity & IIH

Treatment

- None unless CSF leak associated
- CSF leak treatment
  - Canal wall up mastoidectomy with repair of dural defect with tissue graft

SELECTED REFERENCES

1. Yancey KL et al: Impact of obesity and obstructive sleep apnea in lateral skull base cerebrospinal fluid leak repair. Laryngoscope. 130(9):2234-40, 2020
2. Deep NL et al: Giant posterior temporal bone arachnoid granulations: CT and MRI findings. Otol Neurotol. 37(7):963-6, 2016

Temporal Bone Fibrous Dysplasia

TERMINOLOGY

- Fibrous dysplasia (FD): Congenital disorder with **defect in osteoblastic differentiation & maturation**, resulting in progressive replacement of normal cancellous bone by mixture of **fibrous tissue & immature woven bone**

IMAGING

- Bone CT shows **expansile, ground-glass** bony matrix
  - Expansile lesion centered in medullary space with variable attenuation
  - **Pagetoid (mixed) pattern (50%)**: Mixed radiopacity & radiolucency
  - **Sclerotic FD (25%)**: Ground-glass density
  - **Cystic FD (25%)**: Centrally lucent lesions with thinned but sclerotic borders
- T1 MR: Expansile lesion with decreased signal
- T2 MR: Decreased signal in ossified ± fibrous areas
- T1 C+ FS MR: Diffuse, rim, or no enhancement possible

TOP DIFFERENTIAL DIAGNOSES

- Temporal bone Paget disease
- Temporal bone meningioma
- Temporal bone metastasis

PATHOLOGY

- Benign **tumor-like lesion** of bone with local arrest of normal structural/architectural development
  - Contains fibrous tissue (spindle cell stroma) with intramural woven bone trabeculae

CLINICAL ISSUES

- Clinical setting
  - Young patients affected (< 30 years)
  - Often asymptomatic lesion when small
  - Hearing loss in temporal bone FD is common; typically conductive & mild
- Natural history
  - Most spontaneously cease to grow by age 25-30 yr old

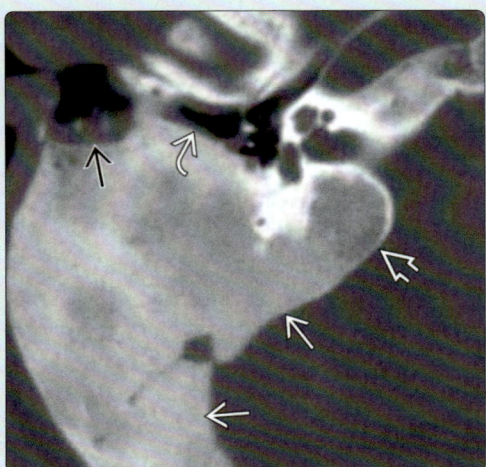
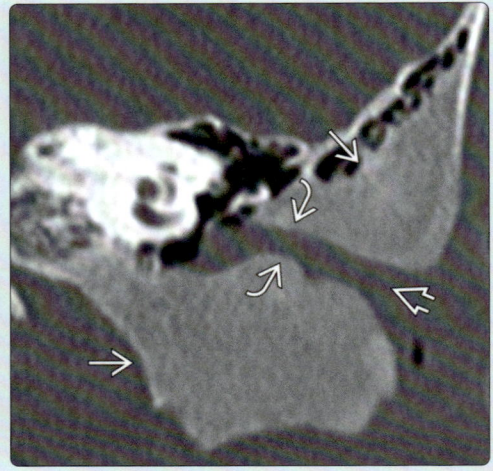

(Left) Axial bone CT reveals the common sclerotic variety of fibrous dysplasia (FD) involving the mastoid ⮕ and inner ear ⮕ and encroaching on the posterior middle ear. FD expansion causes external auditory canal (EAC) stenosis ⮕. Anterolaterally, note the previous biopsy site ⮕. (Right) Coronal bone CT shows left temporal bone expansion and a ground-glass appearance ⮕, consistent with FD, resulting in narrowing of the EAC ⮕ with cerumen impaction ⮕ leading to conductive hearing loss.

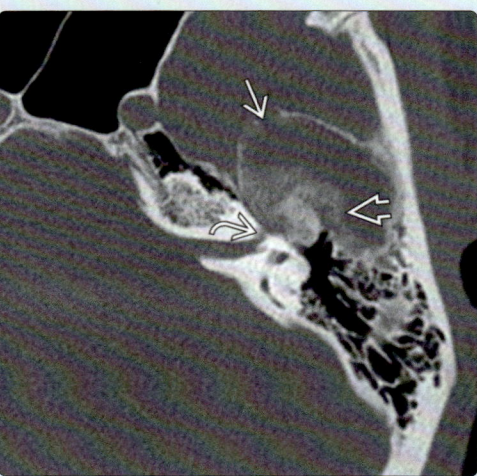
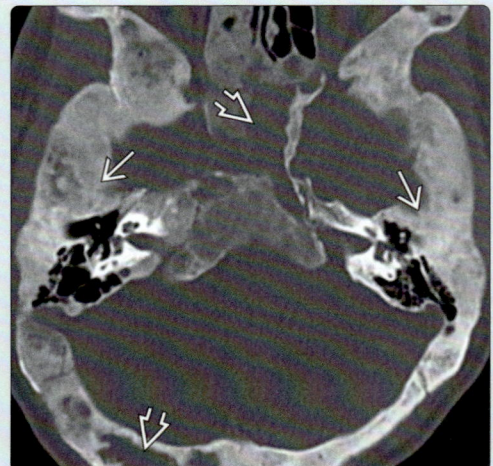

(Left) Axial left temporal bone CT reveals an aggressive-appearing anterior left temporal bone foci of cystic FD ⮕. A subtle ground-glass component ⮕ is visible within the lesion. Note that the labyrinthine segment ⮕ of the facial nerve canal is visible, but the lesion involves the geniculate fossa. (Right) Axial bone CT shows extensive osseous expansion of the temporal bones, skull base, and calvarium with a combination of ground-glass attenuation ⮕ and cystic changes ⮕, compatible with polyostotic FD.

TERMINOLOGY

Abbreviations

- Fibrous dysplasia (FD)

Definitions

- Congenital disorder with **defect in osteoblastic differentiation & maturation**, resulting in progressive replacement of normal cancellous bone by mixture of **fibrous tissue & immature woven bone**

IMAGING

General Features

- Best diagnostic clue
  - Bone CT shows **expansile, ground-glass** bony matrix
- Morphology
  - FD conforms to general shape of affected bone

CT Findings

- Bone CT
  - **Expansile lesion** centered in medullary space with variable attenuation
    - **Pagetoid (mixed) pattern (50%)**: Mixed radiopacity & radiolucency
    - **Sclerotic FD (25%)**: Ground-glass density
    - **Cystic FD (25%)**: Centrally lucent lesions with thinned but sclerotic borders

MR Findings

- T1WI
  - Expansile lesion with decreased signal
- T2WI
  - Decreased signal in ossified ± fibrous areas
- T1WI C+
  - Diffuse, rim, or limited enhancement possible
  - Active phase: Heterogeneous enhancement typical
    - May appear aggressive when present

Nuclear Medicine Findings

- Bone scan
  - Increased radionuclide accumulation, perfusion, & delayed phase
  - Nonspecific; sensitive to locations in polyostotic FD
- PET
  - Can be variably hypermetabolic on FDG PET

Imaging Recommendations

- Best imaging tool
  - Bone CT is key to making correct diagnosis

DIFFERENTIAL DIAGNOSIS

Temporal Bone Paget Disease

- Presents in older adult patients
- Cotton wool CT appearance
- Pagetoid ground-glass FD mimics Paget disease
- Involves temporal bone & calvarium, not craniofacial area

Temporal Bone Meningioma

- Intraosseous meningioma mimics FD on bone CT
- En plaque soft tissue mass seen on MR

Temporal Bone Metastasis

- Mixed sclerotic-destructive metastasis mimics FD
- Prostate & breast carcinoma most common

PATHOLOGY

General Features

- Etiology
  - Benign **tumor-like lesion** of bone with local arrest of normal structural & architectural development
- Genetics
  - Sporadic gene mutation of *GNAS* (GNAS1) gene
- Associated abnormalities
  - McCune-Albright syndrome = FD with café au lait spots, endocrine dysfunction with precocious puberty
  - Mazabraud syndrome = FD & intramuscular myxomas

Staging, Grading, & Classification

- Monostotic vs. polyostotic
- Specific lesion type relates to disease activity
  - Pagetoid (50%): Mixed sclerotic & fibrous
  - Sclerotic (25%): Predominantly sclerotic
  - Cystic (25%): Predominantly fibrous

Microscopic Features

- FD lesion contains fibrous tissue (spindle cell stroma) with intramural woven bone trabeculae

CLINICAL ISSUES

Presentation

- Most common signs/symptoms
  - Bulging of temporal area
  - Stenosis of external auditory canal with recurrent otitis
  - Hearing loss: Conductive, sensorineural, or mixed
    - Hearing loss in temporal bone FD is common; typically mild & nonprogressive

Demographics

- Age
  - Active in young patients (< 30 years); typically quiescent after puberty
- Sex
  - M:F = 1:3
- Epidemiology
  - Monostotic FD is 6x more common than polyostotic

DIAGNOSTIC CHECKLIST

Image Interpretation Pearls

- CT: Ground-glass appearance of lesion is classic, but cystic or lucent areas can occur & make diagnosis more challenging

SELECTED REFERENCES

1. Tuompo S et al: Craniofacial fibrous dysplasia: a review of current literature. Bone. ePub, 2024
2. Lianou AD et al: Fibrous dysplasia of the temporal bone: a demanding entity for radiologists and ENT surgeons. Maedica (Bucur). 17(2):524-7, 2022
3. Mohammed S et al: Fibrous dysplasia of temporal bone. Indian J Otolaryngol Head Neck Surg. 74(Suppl 3):4350-5, 2022
4. Sbai AA et al: Otalgia revealing McCune-Albright syndrome: a case report. Ann Med Surg (Lond). 82:104706, 2022

Temporal Bone Paget Disease

TERMINOLOGY

- **Paget disease (PD)**: Bone dysplasia of unknown etiology caused by alternating waves of unbalanced osteoclastic and osteoblastic activity; leads to abnormal bone remodeling, bone expansion, loss of structural integrity, and abnormal mineralization of affected bone

IMAGING

- **Temporal bone CT**
  - Temporal bone usually involved as part of diffuse/polyostotic involvement of calvarium and skull base
  - Demineralization, expansion, and disorganized trabecular bone is most common finding
  - Mixed lytic-sclerotic change occurs as disease progresses
  - Petrous apex (PA) most commonly involved region of temporal bone; disease begins in PA and proceeds posterolateral
  - Otic capsule demineralization and thinning occurs late and proceeds from peripheral (periosteal) layer to inner (endochondral) layer
  - Ossicles and ossicular ligaments occasionally demonstrate thickening and sclerosis
  - Bone expansion may reduce volume of middle ear (ossicular crowding) as well as narrowing of internal auditory canal
- **MR:** Bone often expanded with heterogeneous marrow signal and avid enhancement

TOP DIFFERENTIAL DIAGNOSES

- Temporal bone fibrous dysplasia
- Temporal bone osteoradionecrosis
- Otosclerosis
- Temporal bone meningioma

CLINICAL ISSUES

- Progressive **bilateral sensorineural hearing loss (SNHL) or mixed hearing loss** in older adult patient

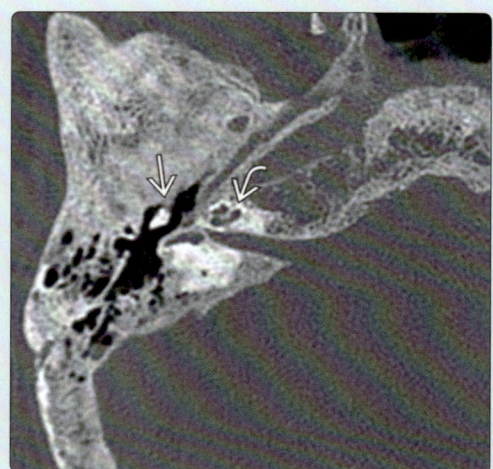
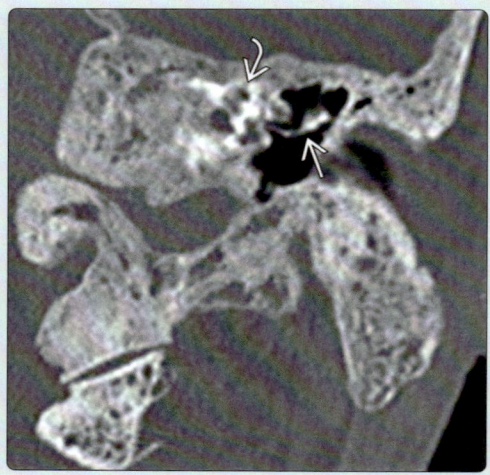

(Left) Axial CT shows Paget disease of the right temporal bone causing diffusely thickened bones of the clivus and petrous bone. Notice the thickened ligament ➡ connected to the malleus and the marked thinning and demineralization of the otic capsule ➡. (Right) Coronal bone CT in the opposite ear in the same patient reveals diffuse bony enlargement of all bones of the skull base and temporal bone. Marked demineralization of the otic capsule ➡ and thickening of the ossicles ➡ are evident.

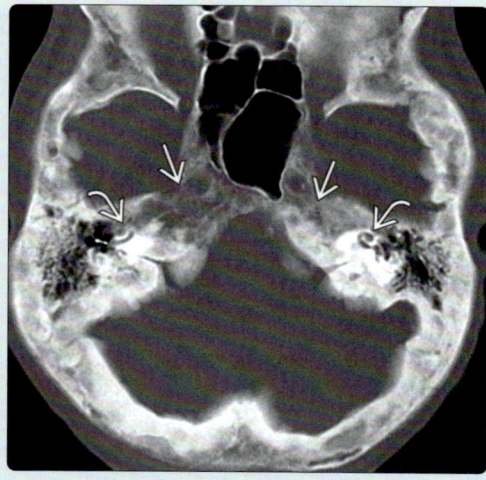
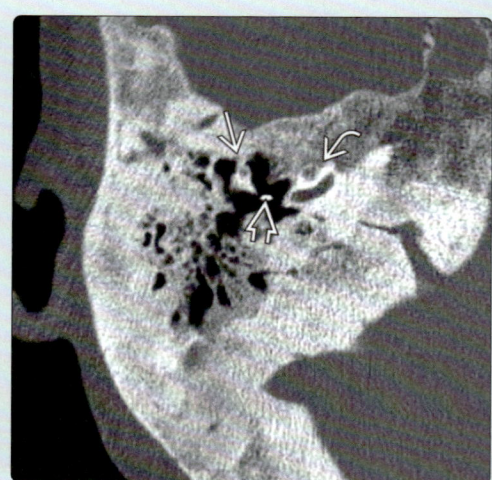

(Left) Axial bone CT shows diffuse, enlarged bones of the skull base with a cotton wool appearance. The petrous apices ➡ are enlarged but demineralized, which indicates that earlier, more active disease is present. The anteromedial otic capsules are eroded ➡. (Right) Axial bone CT in a patient with hearing loss shows malleal ligament ossification ➡ as well as the subacute erosive phase of Paget disease affecting the otic capsule ➡. Stapes prosthesis ➡ is noted.

TERMINOLOGY

Abbreviations
- Paget disease (PD)

Synonyms
- Osteitis deformans

Definitions
- Bone dysplasia characterized by abnormal bone remodeling, resulting from alternating waves of unbalanced osteoclastic and osteoblastic hyperactivity

IMAGING

General Features
- Best diagnostic clue
  - Temporal bone CT: Demineralization, bone expansion, and mixed lytic-sclerotic regions

CT Findings
- **Temporal bone CT**
  - Findings of bone depend on phase of disease
    - Early phase: Demineralization (osteolysis)
    - Intermediate phase: Mixed lytic-sclerotic changes with potential ground-glass appearance
    - Late phase: Extreme bone thickening with diploic heterogeneity
  - Temporal bone usually involved as part of polyostotic involvement of calvarium and skull base; rarely in isolation
  - Demineralization, expansion, and disorganized trabecular bone is most common finding
  - Petrous apex (PA) most commonly involved region of temporal bone; disease begins in PA and proceeds posterolateral
  - **Inner ear/otic capsule**
    - Otic capsule demineralization (peripheral to central) **involves all 3 layers**
      - □ Periosteum → endochondral → endosteum
  - **Internal auditory canal** (IAC)
    - Enlarging bone narrows IAC
    - Cochlear nerve canal and macula cribrosa of vestibule affected
  - **External auditory canal** (EAC) and **middle ear**
    - EAC tortuosity and stenosis
    - Middle ear cavity narrowing
    - Ossicles and ligaments with pagetoid changes

MR Findings
- T1WI
  - Diminished T1 signal
    - Marrow replacement by fibrous tissue
  - Heterogeneous, patchy, T1-hyperintense signal
- T1WI C+
  - Heterogeneous enhancement within thickened calvarium, skull base ± temporal bone possible
    - Secondary to hypervascular nature

Imaging Recommendations
- Best imaging tool
  - Temporal bone CT with characteristic changes in older adult patient

DIFFERENTIAL DIAGNOSIS

Temporal Bone Fibrous Dysplasia
- Clinical: Younger patient
- CT: ↑ bone volume
  - Commonly involves facial bones

Temporal Bone Osteoradionecrosis
- CT: Unilateral demineralization similar to acute PD
  - Not thickened or diffuse like in PD

Otosclerosis
- Clinical: Much younger patient compared with PD
- CT: Multifocal otic capsule demineralization
  - Usually bilateral, symmetric
  - Adjacent skull base and calvarium normal

Temporal Bone Meningioma
- Clinical: Middle-aged woman
- CT: Permeative-sclerotic and hyperostotic
  - Soft tissue in middle ear when transosseous

PATHOLOGY

General Features
- Etiology
  - Unknown; nuclear viral inclusions suggest possible viral etiology
  - Progressive osteodystrophy with **monostotic** and **polyostotic** varieties
- Associated abnormalities
  - Characteristic involvement of calvarium, skull base, vertebrae, pelvis, and long bones

CLINICAL ISSUES

Presentation
- Most common signs/symptoms
  - Bilateral progressive sensorineural hearing loss (SNHL) or mixed hearing loss in older adult patient
- Other signs/symptoms
  - Vertigo, tinnitus
- Laboratory abnormalities
  - ↑ serum alkaline phosphatase
  - ↑ urinary hydroxyproline

Demographics
- Age
  - > 40 years of age
- Sex
  - M:F = 4:1

Natural History & Prognosis
- Disorder usually progressive despite therapy
- Progressive bilateral mixed hearing loss → deafness

Treatment
- Bisphosphonates are among 1st-line medications
  - Acts by reducing bone resorption and turnover

SELECTED REFERENCES
1. Andreu-Arasa VC et al: Otosclerosis and dysplasias of the temporal bone. Neuroimaging Clin N Am. 29(1):29-47, 2019

Temporal Bone Langerhans Cell Histiocytosis

TERMINOLOGY

- Neoplastic clonal proliferation of CD1a, CD207, & S100 protein (+) dendritic cells
- Single system (SS) (unifocal or multifocal) vs. multisystem (MS) disease
  - Most frequently involved: Bone (80-90%) & skin (40-50%)
  - Risk organ (RO) involvement: Liver, spleen, marrow; confers worse prognosis (high risk)
  - Others: Lymph nodes, lung, pituitary, thymus, GI tract
- Historic categorization
  - Eosinophilic granuloma: Unifocal, SS; isolated bone or lung involvement
  - Hand-Schüller-Christian: Chronic disseminated form
  - Letterer-Siwe: Acute disseminated form

IMAGING

- Well-defined lytic lesions of T-bone with associated enhancing soft tissue masses
  - **Squamous & mastoid bones** > petrous apex

- Both enhanced CT & MR often performed in complex cases
  - Bone CT best for evaluating osseous structures
  - MR best for soft tissue evaluation

TOP DIFFERENTIAL DIAGNOSES

- Coalescent otomastoiditis
  - Resorption mastoid osseous septa
- T-bone rhabdomyosarcoma
  - Heterogeneous soft tissue mass with bone destruction
- T-bone metastasis
  - Destructive bone lesion (e.g., neuroblastoma)

CLINICAL ISSUES

- Otologic symptoms in **25%** of T-bone cases
  - **Conductive hearing loss ± otorrhea**
- T-bone presents in **1st decade** of life
- Other symptoms: Otalgia, vertigo, otitis media ± externa, periauricular soft tissue swelling, CNVII palsy, sensorineural hearing loss, aural polyp

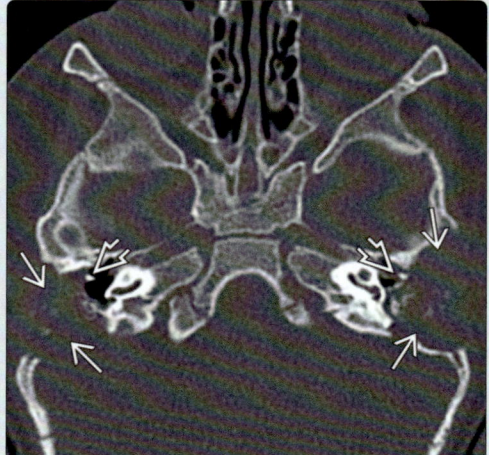 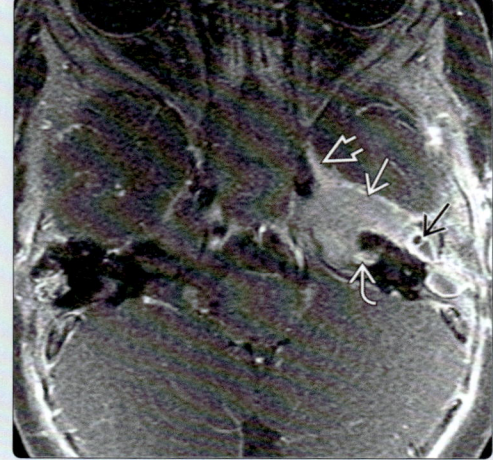

(Left) CT in a 2-year-old girl with bilateral otorrhea shows well-defined, destructive lesions of Langerhans cell histiocytosis (LCH) involving bilateral mastoid & left squamous temporal bones ➡, opacified middle ear cavities, & near-complete ossicular destruction ➡. Lesions lack typical aggressive periosteal reaction of metastatic neuroblastoma. (Right) Axial T1 C+ FS MR shows enhancing LCH extending into the left middle cranial fossa ➡, cavernous sinus ➡, & internal auditory canal ➡. Ossicles ➡ are encased by tumor.

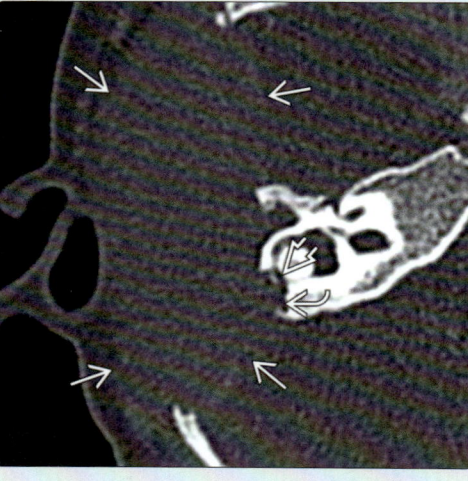 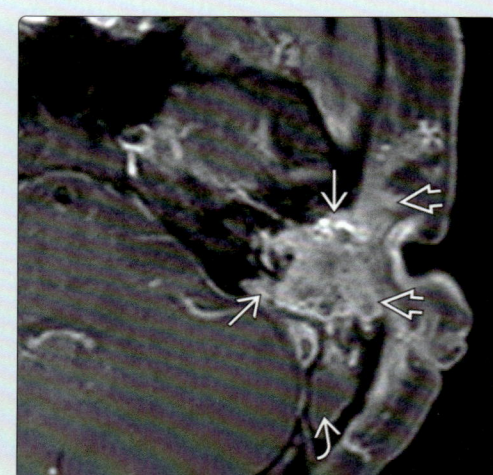

(Left) Axial bone CT in a child shows a large soft tissue mass ➡, smooth bone destruction of the right mastoid & squamosal T-bone, and extension into the right lateral ➡ & posterior ➡ semicircular canals. Otic capsule involvement reossified within 3 months following treatment for LCH (not shown). (Right) Axial T1 C+ FS MR shows extensive enhancement within the left T-bone ➡ due to involvement by LCH with extension into the adjacent extracranial soft tissues ➡. Trapped mastoid fluid ➡ is noted posteriorly.

TERMINOLOGY

Abbreviations

- Langerhans cell histiocytosis (LCH)

Synonyms

- Histiocytosis X, eosinophilic granuloma (EG), Hand-Schüller-Christian disease (HSCD), Letterer-Siwe disease, Abt-Letterer-Siwe disease (ALSD), Hashimoto-Pritzker

Definitions

- Neoplastic clonal proliferation of CD1a, CD207, & S100 protein (+) dendritic cells
- Single system (SS) (unifocal or multifocal) vs. multisystem (MS) disease
  - Bone (80-90%) & skin (40-50%) are most frequent
  - Risk organ (RO) involvement: Liver, spleen, marrow; confers worse prognosis (high risk)
  - Other organs: Lymph nodes, pituitary, thymus, GI tract
  - CNS-risk lesion: Skull base & many facial lesions
    - Diabetes insipidus (25% overall, 50% with MS disease), growth hormone deficiency (10%), parenchymal mass lesions (1%), & delayed neurodegenerative changes

IMAGING

General Features

- Best diagnostic clue
  - Well-defined **lytic bone** lesion, usually with **enhancing soft tissue** mass
- Location
  - Squamous & mastoid T-bone > petrous apex

CT Findings

- CECT: Variable lytic, punched-out lesions + enhancing soft tissue mass ± intracranial spread with dural enhancement
  - ± fluid-fluid levels
  - May involve ossicles, labyrinthine structures; may be bilateral
  - Beveled margins more common in calvarium LCH, sclerosis more common in skull base lesions
  - Posttreatment reossification of bony structures possible, including boundaries of bony labyrinth, petrous T-bone, skull, or orbits

MR Findings

- T1WI: Hypointense or isointense to muscle T-bone lesion ± soft tissue component
  - ± ↑ **T1** signal (lipid-laden macrophages)
  - ± **blood products** within soft tissue mass
- T2WI: Iso- to hyperintense soft tissue mass
  - **Fluid-fluid levels** may be present
- STIR: Iso- to hyperintense soft tissue mass
- T1WI C+ FS: Avid heterogeneous soft tissue enhancement
  - Well-defined or poorly defined margins
  - ± intracranial spread with dural enhancement

Nuclear Medicine Findings

- FDG PET/CT: Highly sensitive for active LCH

Imaging Recommendations

- Best imaging tool
  - Bone CT ± enhanced MR

DIFFERENTIAL DIAGNOSIS

Coalescent Otomastoiditis

- Acute infection of middle ear & mastoid air cells
- Progressive resorption of mastoid osseous septa

T-Bone Rhabdomyosarcoma

- Invasive heterogeneous soft tissue mass in child, usually with osseous destruction
- Lesions in anterior portion of temporal bone, including petrous apex & middle ear, more likely to be rhabdomyosarcoma

T-Bone Metastasis

- Destructive T-bone lesion (e.g., neuroblastoma)

PATHOLOGY

General Features

- Etiology
  - Reactive vs. neoplastic: Neoplastic currently favored
  - Unknown cause; infectious agents (especially viruses), immune system dysfunction, neoplastic mechanisms, genetic factors, & cellular adhesion molecules proposed
- Associated abnormalities
  - Hypothalamic-pituitary disease
    - Presents with symptoms of **diabetes insipidus**
      - Absent posterior pituitary hyperintensity on T1 MR
      - Thick, enhancing infundibulum

Staging, Grading, & Classification

- Unifocal, SS
  - Bony lesions; older patient population; best prognosis
- Multifocal, SS
  - Bone, skin, viscera; younger patient population
- Multifocal, MS
  - Disseminated, fulminant; infants; worst prognosis

CLINICAL ISSUES

Presentation

- Most common signs/symptoms: **Conductive hearing loss ± otorrhea**

Demographics

- Age: T-bone LCH typically presents in 1st decade
  - LCH in general: 90% are < 15 years at presentation

Natural History & Prognosis

- **90% cure** rate for **unifocal** disease of T-bone
- High mortality with disseminated disease

Treatment

- Depending on symptoms, location, & extent of disease: Observation, curettage, chemotherapy, BRAF & MEK inhibitors

SELECTED REFERENCES

1. Degar BA et al: Clinical characteristics and treatment of histiocytic disorders in children. Hematol Oncol Clin North Am. 39(3):513-29, 2025
2. Mayer S et al: Langerhans cell histiocytosis of the temporal bone. Ochsner J. 20(3):315-8, 2020
3. Chevallier KM et al: Differentiating pediatric rhabdomyosarcoma and Langerhans cell histiocytosis of the temporal bone by imaging appearance. AJNR Am J Neuroradiol. 37(6):1185-9, 2016

KEY FACTS

TERMINOLOGY

- Hematogenous spread from distant primary neoplasm
- Bony metastatic disease to petrous apex (PA) or middle ear-mastoid

IMAGING

- PA most common site
- Bone CT
  - Focal **lytic** or **permeative**, rarely **blastic** lesion
  - Commonly other bone metastases
  - Subtle appearance in pneumatized portions of temporal bone
  - Enhances significantly in most cases
  - CT differentiates benign lesions (i.e., fibrous dysplasia, osteoma)
- MR
  - T1: Lesion hypointense to normal fatty marrow
  - T1 C+ FS: Delineates tumor vs. normal fatty marrow

TOP DIFFERENTIAL DIAGNOSES

- Apical petrositis
- Cholesterol granuloma of PA
- Langerhans cell histiocytosis of temporal bone
- Plasmacytoma of temporal bone

CLINICAL ISSUES

- Often asymptomatic
  - Hearing loss if any symptoms
  - Cranial nerve (CN) palsy (CNVIII > CNVII > CNV or CNVI)
- Breast > lung > renal > prostate cancer origin
- Neuroblastoma & leukemia most common in children

DIAGNOSTIC CHECKLIST

- Remember background PA marrow/pneumatization is commonly asymmetric
- Isolated temporal bone lesion is less likely to be metastasis
- Look for dura, dural venous sinus, & brain invasion

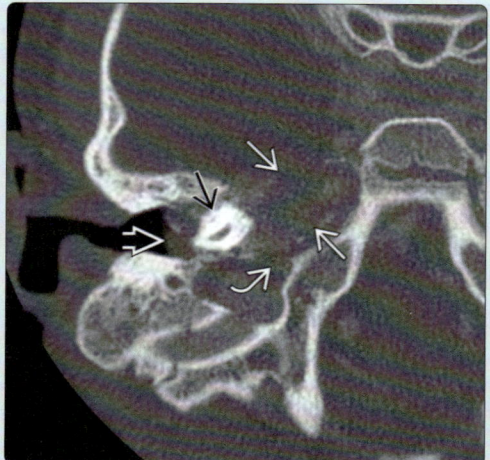
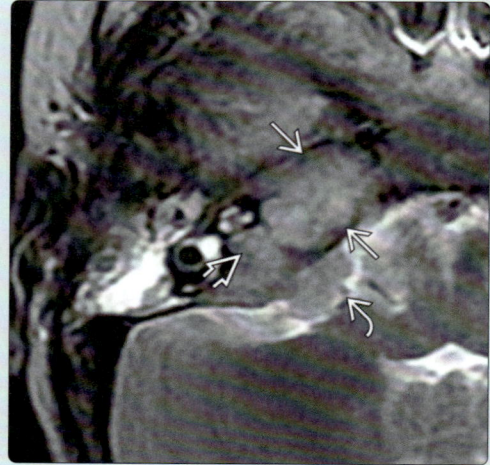

(Left) *Axial temporal bone CT in an infant with right CNVII palsy shows permeative, lytic petrous apex destruction ➡️ with sparing of dense otic capsule bone ➡️. Tumor extends into middle ear cavity ➡️ & erodes anterior wall of jugular foramen ➡️. (Right) Axial T2WI FS MR in the same patient shows a hypointense petrous apex mass ➡️, consistent with a cellular tumor. It extends into the right IAC ➡️ & cerebellopontine angle ➡️. Biopsy revealed neuroblastoma. Subsequent imaging revealed an adrenal primary.*

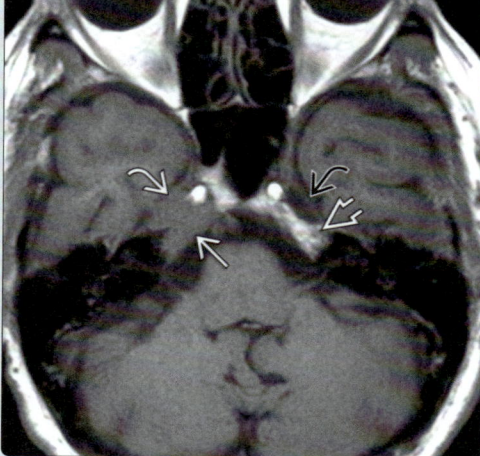
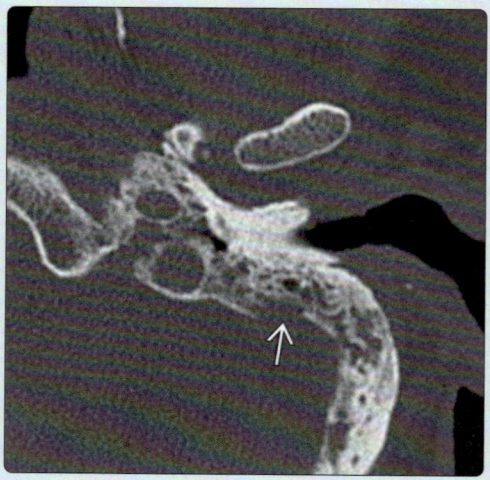

(Left) *Axial T1WI MR shows the typical appearance of right petrous apex metastasis replacing fatty marrow ➡️ with expansion into the right Meckel cave ➡️ in this patient with right facial numbness. On the left, note normal marrow signal in the petrous apex ➡️ & CSF in Meckel cave ➡️. (Right) Osseous mastoid bone metastasis with cortical destruction of the inner cortex/sigmoid plate ➡️ puts the sigmoid sinus at risk for invasion/thrombosis. Smaller metastases are easily missed, secondary to aerated/varied appearance of temporal bone.*

Temporal Bone Metastasis

TERMINOLOGY

Definitions

- Hematogenous spread to temporal bone from distant primary neoplasm
- Bony metastatic disease to petrous apex (PA) or middle ear-mastoid

IMAGING

General Features

- Best diagnostic clue
  - Bone CT shows focal destructive lesion of temporal bone
- Location
  - PA most common
- Size
  - Variable, 2-8 cm
- Morphology
  - Lytic, permeative destruction ± poorly defined margins

CT Findings

- CECT
  - Soft tissue component enhances significantly in most cases
- Bone CT
  - **Lytic or permeative**, rarely **blastic** lesion
    - Commonly has other bone metastases
  - Temporal bone cortex is destroyed
  - Subtle appearance in pneumatized portions of temporal bone

MR Findings

- T1WI
  - Nonspecific, low to intermediate signal
    - Lower signal metastasis easily distinguished from adjacent normal adult fatty marrow
- T2WI
  - Variable, may be hyper- or hypointense
    - Depends upon cellularity of primary lesion
- T1WI C+
  - Variable enhancement; may blend with normal fatty marrow
  - Fat saturation to exclude normal fatty marrow
  - Thin dural enhancement likely reactive
  - Thick, nodular or irregular dural enhancement is likely transdural tumor

Nuclear Medicine Findings

- Bone scan
  - Abnormal nonspecific ↑ radiotracer
- PET
  - Positive in temporal bone, other bones, & primary

Imaging Recommendations

- Best imaging tool
  - Both CT & MR necessary if surgical resection considered
- Protocol advice
  - T1 MR: Lesion hypointense to normal fatty marrow
  - T1 C+ FS MR: Differentiates tumor from normal fatty marrow & shows intracranial extension

DIFFERENTIAL DIAGNOSIS

Confluent Apical Petrositis

- Clinical: Infectious symptoms
- Imaging: Destructive lesion of PA + dural thickening

Petrous Apex Cholesterol Granuloma

- Clinical: History of chronic otitis media
- Imaging: Expansile PA lesion; high signal on T1

Temporal Bone Langerhans Cell Histiocytosis

- Clinical: Pediatric patient
- Imaging: Destructive middle ear-mastoid mass

Temporal Bone Plasmacytoma

- Clinical: Often with multiple myeloma
- Imaging: Destructive PA lesion

PATHOLOGY

General Features

- Etiology
  - Marrow-filled PA may predispose to metastases
- Must exclude direct extension from local primary (nasopharynx, parotid, maxillary sinus, external ear)

CLINICAL ISSUES

Presentation

- Most common signs/symptoms
  - Hearing loss most common symptom
  - Asymptomatic or skull base/ear pain
- Other signs/symptoms
  - Cranial nerve (CN) palsy (CNVIII > CNVII > CNV or CNVI)

Demographics

- Epidemiology
  - Breast > lung > renal > prostate cancer origin in adults
  - Neuroblastoma & leukemia most common in children

Natural History & Prognosis

- Poor, depends on primary tumor type

Treatment

- Surgery if tumor isolated to mastoid/middle ear
- Palliative depending on primary tumor type & other metastases

DIAGNOSTIC CHECKLIST

Image Interpretation Pearls

- Remember: PA marrow/pneumatization commonly asymmetric
- Isolated temporal bone lesion is less likely to be metastasis

Reporting Tips

- Look for dura, dural venous sinus, & brain invasion

SELECTED REFERENCES

1. Patil R et al: Facial nerve palsy from temporal bone metastasis in papillary carcinoma of thyroid: a case report. Radiol Case Rep. 20(6):2931-6, 2025
2. Epperson MV et al: Metastasis to the external auditory canal: a systematic review. Otol Neurotol. 45(8):e556-65, 2024
3. Jones AJ et al: Metastatic disease of the temporal bone: a contemporary review. Laryngoscope. 131(5):1101-9, 2021

TERMINOLOGY

- Radiation-induced injury to temporal bone

IMAGING

- Bone CT findings
  - **Moth-eaten destruction** of temporal bone and adjacent skull base ± **sequestrum**
- T2 MR findings
  - High-signal mucosal injury of external auditory canal (EAC), middle ear cavity, mastoid
  - High signal of adjacent brain → radiation necrosis
  - Meningitis, abscess, dural sinus thrombosis

TOP DIFFERENTIAL DIAGNOSES

- Malignant external otitis
- Coalescent mastoiditis
- Aggressive cholesteatoma
- EAC carcinoma
- Paget disease

PATHOLOGY

- **Avascular bone necrosis** from **obliterative endarteritis**
- Susceptible to infection, which accelerates ORN

CLINICAL ISSUES

- Presentation: Otalgia, otorrhea, hearing loss after regional radiation therapy (RT)
- Occurs few months to many years post RT (> 60 Gy)
  - Most common in setting of RT for parotid, EAC, or nasopharynx carcinoma
- Treatment options
  - Conservative management: 1st-line option
  - Surgical management and adjuvant therapy as indicated
  - Pentoxifylline, vitamin E, and clodronate (PENTOCLO) for prevention and treatment

DIAGNOSTIC CHECKLIST

- CT for bone changes, extent of involvement
- MR for complications

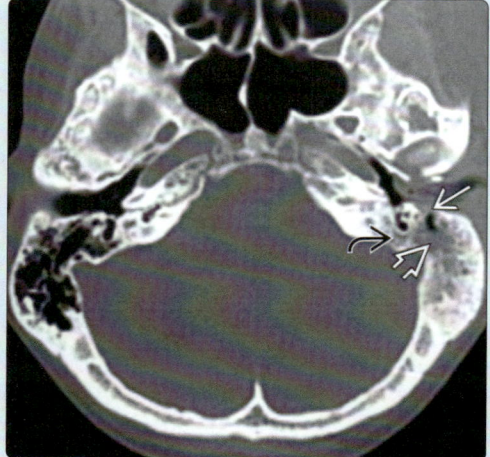
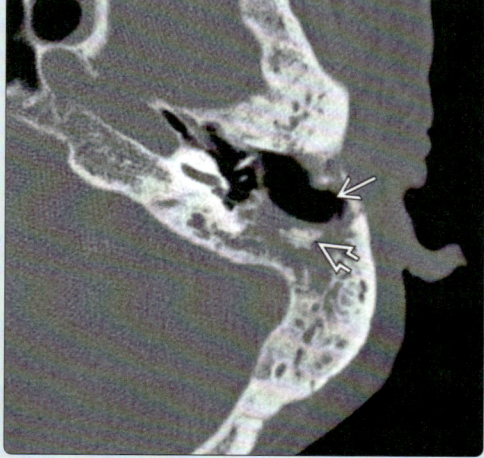

(Left) *Axial bone CT reveals abnormal soft tissue ⟶ filling the left external auditory canal (EAC) and mastoid air cells with obvious destruction of the posterior EAC wall and mastoid septations ⟶. Note mixed sclerotic and lytic ⟶ bone. Findings represent the classic appearance of temporal bone osteoradionecrosis (ORN).* (Right) *Axial bone CT shows radiation-induced necrosis of bony EAC ⟶ and confluent destruction of mastoid air cells. Note "floating" bony sequestrum ⟶, indicating severe ORN.*

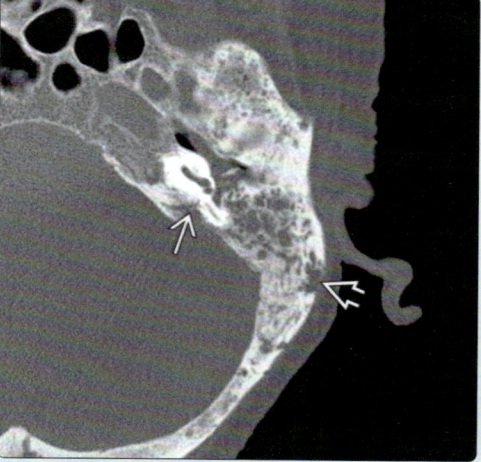
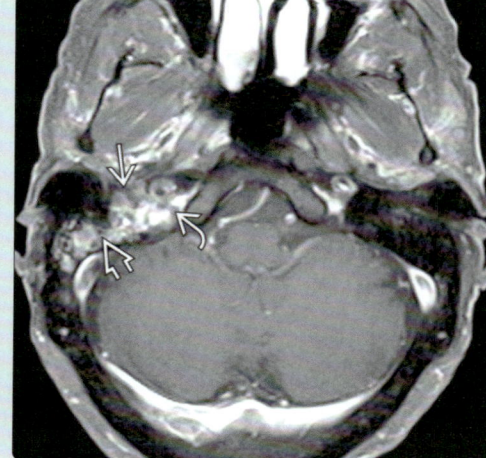

(Left) *Axial bone CT shows diffuse opacification of the middle ear and mastoid air cells in association with permeative-destructive bony changes in this previously radiated patient. Focal bone necrosis is seen in petrous bone ⟶ and lateral mastoid cortex ⟶.* (Right) *Axial T1 C+ FS MR in a previously radiated patient reveals nonspecific enhancing tissue in the middle ear ⟶, mastoid ⟶, and petrous apex ⟶. Although radiation changes can be suggested by MR, ORN of bone is a diagnosis best made by temporal bone CT.*

TERMINOLOGY

Abbreviations
- Osteoradionecrosis (ORN)

Synonyms
- Radiation osteitis, radiation necrosis, irradiation osteomyelitis, avascular bone necrosis

Definitions
- Radiation-induced injury to temporal bone
  - Localized (more common): Limited to external auditory canal (EAC)
  - Diffuse: Involves mastoid septations and middle ear cavity (MEC), possibly skull base

IMAGING

General Features
- Best diagnostic clue
  - Bone CT shows moth-eaten demineralization and destruction of temporal bone ± sequestrum

CT Findings
- CECT
  - Mucosal involvement may enhance
  - Contrast not needed to make diagnosis
- Bone CT
  - Diffuse mucosal thickening in EAC, MEC, and mastoid
  - **Permeative bone destruction** ± **sequestrum**

MR Findings
- T2WI
  - Nonspecific high signal in EAC, MEC, and mastoid
  - High-signal adjacent brain indicates **cerebral radiation necrosis**
- T1WI C+
  - Variable enhancement in osteitic bone
  - Mucosal injury will enhance

Imaging Recommendations
- Best imaging tool
  - Temporal bone CT
- Protocol advice
  - Thin-section axial and coronal bone CT
  - MR for complications
    - Cerebral radiation injury
    - Meningitis or abscess
    - Dural sinus thrombosis

DIFFERENTIAL DIAGNOSIS

Necrotizing External Otitis
- Immunocompromised, often diabetic patient; no radiation history
- EAC soft tissue and bone infection

Coalescent Mastoiditis
- Disruption of mastoid septa in acute/chronic otomastoiditis

Aggressive Cholesteatoma
- Cholesteatoma seen at otoscopy; no radiation history
- CT: Otic capsule invasion late finding

Paget Disease
- Bilateral sensorineural hearing loss
- Entire cranial base usually involved

External Auditory Canal Carcinoma
- Skin lesion of EAC
- No prior radiation therapy (RT)

PATHOLOGY

General Features
- Etiology
  - Radiation dose > 60 Gy
  - **Avascular bone necrosis** from obliterative endarteritis
  - Susceptible to infection, which accelerates ORN
- Temporal bone at higher risk for ORN
  - Poorly vascularized bone
  - Thin, protective overlying soft tissue
  - Exposure to respiratory pathogens via eustachian tube

Gross Pathologic & Surgical Features
- **Dead bone** and **soft tissue fibrosis**

CLINICAL ISSUES

Presentation
- Most common signs/symptoms
  - Purulent, foul-smelling otorrhea with spicules of exposed bone
  - Hearing loss
  - Otalgia
- Intracranial complications
  - Meningitis, abscess, sinus thrombosis, CSF leak

Natural History & Prognosis
- Occurs few months to many years post RT
  - More commonly in setting of parotid, EAC, or nasopharynx cancer
- Mastoid air cell destruction: Poor prognostic indicator

Treatment
- Conservative: Initial management for most patients
  - Local debridement of EAC
  - Antibiotics; otic prep (may need systemic treatment)
  - Pentoxifylline, vitamin E, and clodronate (PENTOCLO)
- Surgical: If conservative management fails
  - **Resect all necrotic tissue** ± repair with vascularized flap
  - Adjuvant PENTOCLO ± hyperbaric oxygen

DIAGNOSTIC CHECKLIST

Image Interpretation Pearls
- CT for bone changes; MR for soft tissue complications

SELECTED REFERENCES

1. Pathak S et al: What is the current management of osteoradionecrosis of the temporal bone following head and neck cancer radiotherapy? Laryngoscope. 135(8):2651-2, 2025
2. Herr MW et al: Radiation necrosis of the lateral skull base and temporal bone. Semin Plast Surg. 34(4):265-71, 2020
3. Yuhan BT et al: Osteoradionecrosis of the temporal bone: an evidence-based approach. Otol Neurotol. 39(9):1172-83, 2018
4. Ahmed S et al: CT findings in temporal bone osteoradionecrosis. J Comput Assist Tomogr. 38(5):662-6, 2014

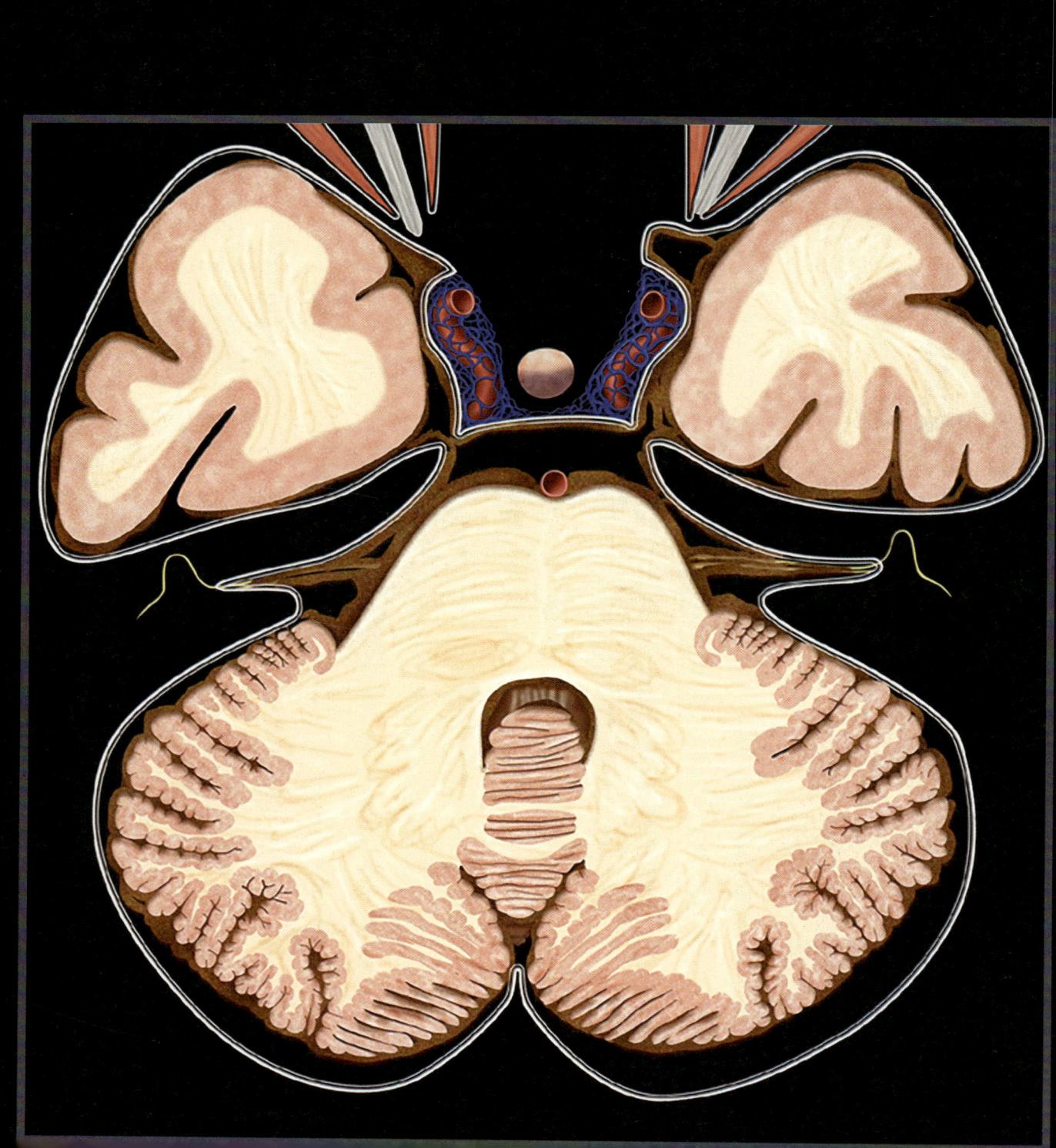

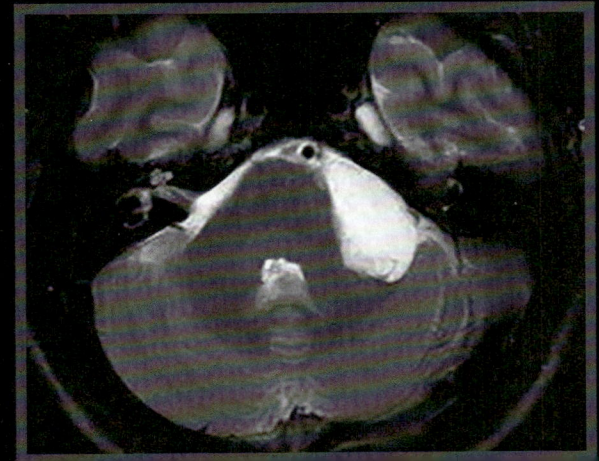

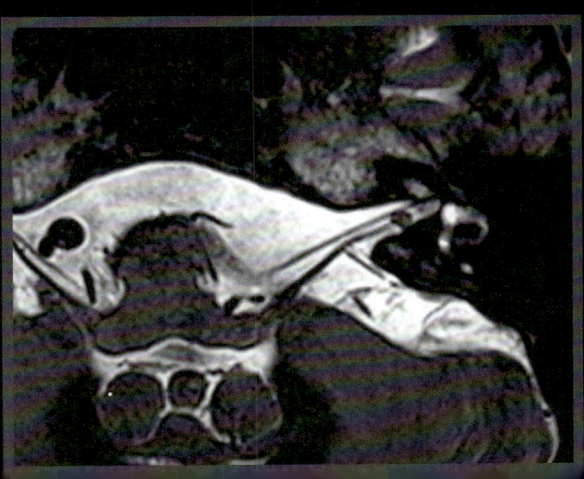

Terminology

The contents of the cerebellopontine angle (CPA) and internal auditory canal (IAC) cisterns include the facial nerve (CNVII), the vestibulocochlear nerve (CNVIII), and the anterior inferior cerebellar artery (AICA) loop. The bony IAC, its fundal crests (vertical and horizontal), and its opening in the porus acusticus are also included as part of this discussion.

Embryology

The temporal bone forms as 3 distinct embryologic events: (1) The external and middle ear, (2) the inner ear, and (3) the IAC. The practical implications of these 3 related but separate embryologic events are that the presence or absence of the IAC is independent of the development of the inner, middle, or external ear.

The IAC develops in response to formation and migration of the facial and vestibulocochlear nerves through this area. IAC size depends on the number of migrating nerve bundles. The fewer the nerve bundles, the smaller the IAC. If the IAC is very small and only 1 nerve is seen, it is usually the facial nerve.

Imaging Anatomy of Cochlea-IAC-CPA

The cochlear nerve portion of the vestibulocochlear nerve begins in the modiolus of the cochlea where the bipolar **spiral ganglia** are found. Distally projecting axons reach the organ of Corti within the scala media. Proximally projecting axons coalesce to form the cochlear nerve itself within the fundus of the IAC.

CNVIII in the IAC and CPA cisterns is made up of vestibular (balance) and cochlear (hearing) components. The cochlear nerve is located in the anteroinferior quadrant of the IAC. In the region of the porus acusticus, the cochlear nerve joins the superior and inferior vestibular nerve (SVN, IVN) bundles to become the vestibulocochlear nerve in the CPA cistern.

The vestibulocochlear nerve crosses the CPA cistern as the posterior nerve bundle (CNVII is the anterior nerve bundle) to enter the brainstem at the junction of the medulla and pons. The entering cochlear nerve fibers pierce the brainstem and bifurcate to form synapses with both the **dorsal** and the **ventral cochlear nuclei**. These 2 nuclei are found on the lateral surface of the inferior cerebellar peduncle. Their location can be accurately determined by looking at high-resolution T2 axial images and identifying the contour of the inferior cerebellar peduncle. The entering vestibular nerve fibers divide into 4 branches to form synapses with the superior, inferior, medial, and lateral nuclei. The vestibular nuclei are clustered in the inferior cerebellar peduncle just anteromedial to the cochlear nuclei.

Remembering the normal orientation of nerves within the IAC cistern is assisted by the mnemonic "7-Up, Coke down." CNVII is found in the anterosuperior quadrant, whereas the cochlear nerve is confined to the anteroinferior quadrant. Given this information, it is simple to remember that the SVN is posterosuperior, while the IVN is posteroinferior.

Other normal structures to be aware of in the IAC include the **horizontal crest** (crista falciformis) and the **vertical crest** ("Bill's bar"). The horizontal crest is a medially projecting horizontal bony shelf in the IAC fundus that separates the CNVII and SVN above from the cochlear nerve and IVN below. The vertical crest is found between CNVII and the SVN along the superior fundal bony wall. The horizontal crest is easily seen on both bone CT and high-resolution MR. The vertical crest is more readily seen on bone CT.

Openings from the IAC fundus into the inner ear are numerous. The largest is the anteroinferior **cochlear nerve canal**, which conveys the cochlear nerve from the modiolus to the IAC fundus. Anterosuperiorly, the **meatal foramen** opens into the labyrinthine segment of CNVII. The **macula cribrosa** is the multiply perforated bone that separates the vestibule of the inner ear from the IAC fundus.

Other nonneural normal anatomy of interest in the CPA cistern includes the AICA loop, flocculus, and choroid plexus. The **AICA** arises from the basilar artery, courses superolaterally into the CPA cistern, and then travels into the IAC cistern. Within the IAC, the AICA feeds the internal auditory artery of the cochlea. The AICA loop in the IAC or CPA cisterns may mimic a cranial nerve bundle on high-resolution T2WI MR. AICA vascular territory includes the cochlea, flocculus of the cerebellum, and anterolateral pons in the area of cranial nerve nuclei for CNV, CNVII, and CNVIII. The **flocculus** is a lobule of the cerebellum that projects into the posterolateral CPA cistern. The 4th ventricle **choroid plexus** typically passes through the foramen of Luschka in the CPA cistern.

Imaging Techniques & Indications

The principal clinical indication requiring radiologists to examine the CPA-IAC is **sensorineural hearing loss (SNHL)**. Three principal parameters must be satisfied when completing the MR study in SNHL: (1) Use contrast-enhanced T1 fat-saturated thin-section sequences through the CPA-IAC to identify enhancing lesions in this location, (2) utilize high-resolution T2-weighted sequences to answer presurgical questions when a mass lesion is found, and (3) screen the brain for intraaxial causes, such as multiple sclerosis.

The gold standard for imaging patients with acquired SNHL is enhanced thin-section (≤ 3-mm) axial and coronal fat-saturated MR through the CPA-IAC. With these enhanced sequences, it is highly unlikely that a lesion causing SNHL will be missed. Be sure to obtain an axial or coronal precontrast T1 sequence and use fat saturation when contrast is applied to avoid the rare but troublesome mistake of calling a CPA-IAC lipoma a vestibular schwannoma. In the absence of fat saturation, the inherent high signal of lipoma will appear to enhance, leading to the misdiagnosis of vestibular schwannoma.

High-resolution T2-weighted thin-section (≤ 1-mm) MR sequences (CISS, FIESTA, T2 space) in the axial and coronal planes without contrast can be used as a reasonable screening exam to identify patients with mass lesions in the CPA-IAC area. However, most radiologists, referring physicians, and patients prefer to have pre- and postcontrast images at the same session. High-resolution T2-weighted sequences are currently more commonly used as supplements when vestibular schwannoma is found on the enhanced T1 sequences to answer specific surgically relevant questions: What size is the fundal cap? What is the nerve of origin? Does the lesion enter the cochlear foramen?

Whenever MR is ordered for SNHL, remember to include whole-brain FLAIR, GRE, and DWI sequences. FLAIR will identify the rare multiple sclerosis patient presenting with SNHL as well as other intraaxial causes. GRE will demonstrate micro- or macrohemorrhage within a vestibular schwannoma

CPA Mass Differential Diagnosis

Pseudolesions	Vascular
Asymmetric cerebellar flocculus	Aneurysm (vertebrobasilar, posterior and anterior inferior cerebellar artery)
Asymmetric choroid plexus	Arteriovenous malformation
High jugular bulb	**Benign tumor**
Jugular bulb diverticulum	Choroid plexus papilloma
Marrow foci around internal auditory canal	Facial nerve schwannoma
Congenital	Hemangioblastoma, cerebellum
Arachnoid cyst	Internal auditory canal hemangioma (venous malformation)
Epidermoid cyst	Meningioma
Lipoma	Vestibular schwannoma
Neurofibromatosis type 2	**Malignant tumor**
Infectious	Brainstem glioma, pedunculated
Cysticercosis	Ependymoma, pedunculated
Meningitis	Melanotic schwannoma
Inflammatory	Metastases, systemic or subarachnoid spread ("drop")
Idiopathic intracranial pseudotumor	
Sarcoidosis	

and may help with aneurysm diagnosis when blooming of blood products or calcium in an aneurysm wall is seen. DWI helps evaluate for recent stroke and is useful for diagnosing epidermoid, a common CPA lesion that shows diffusion restriction.

Approaches to Imaging Issues of CPA-IAC

Approach to Sensorineural Hearing Loss in Adult

Unilateral SNHL in an otherwise healthy adult is evaluated with an enhanced thin-section fat-saturated T1WI MR of the CPA-IAC area with high-resolution T2WI sequences providing help in surgical planning if a lesion is identified. Despite audiometric and brainstem-evoked response testing in the otolaryngology clinic, positive MR studies for lesions causing the SNHL are infrequent (< 5% even in highly screened patient groups). **Vestibular schwannoma** is by far the most common cause of unilateral SNHL (~ 90% of lesions found with MR). It is important for the radiologist to become familiar with the wide range of appearances of vestibular schwannoma, including intramural cystic change, micro- and macroscopic hemorrhage, and associated arachnoid cyst.

Meningioma, epidermoid cyst, and CPA aneurysm are responsible for ~ 8% of lesions found in adult patients with SNHL. A long list of rare lesions, including otosclerosis, facial nerve, labyrinthine and jugular foramen schwannomas, IAC hemangioma, CPA metastases, labyrinthitis, sarcoidosis, lipoma, and superficial siderosis, make up < 2% of lesions causing unilateral SNHL in an adult that are found by MR.

Approach to Sensorineural Hearing Loss in Child

When a child presents with unilateral or bilateral SNHL, the emphasis in the imaging work-up veers away from the typical adult tumor causes. Instead, congenital inner ear or CPA-IAC lesions are sought as the cause of the hearing loss. Complications of suppurative labyrinthitis (labyrinthine ossificans) are also included in the differential diagnosis.

When the child's presentation is bilateral profound SNHL, imaging is usually obtained as part of the work-up for possible **cochlear implantation**. High-resolution T2 MR imaging is obtained in the axial and **oblique sagittal** planes to look for inner ear anomalies and labyrinthine ossificans as well as the presence or absence of a cochlear nerve in the IAC. If complex congenital inner ear disease is found, bone CT is often obtained to further define the inner ear fluid spaces and look for an absent cochlear nerve canal.

In reviewing the MR and CT in a child with SNHL, it is important to accurately describe any inner ear congenital anomaly, if present. If there is a history of meningitis, labyrinthine ossificans may be present. Look for bony encroachment on the fluid spaces of the inner ear. In particular, make sure the basal turn of the cochlea is open because occlusion by bony plaque may thwart successful cochlear implantation. Check the T2 oblique sagittal MR images for the presence of a normal cochlear nerve. If absent, cochlear implantation results may be negatively affected. Finally, look carefully at the IAC and CPA for signs of epidermoid cyst (restricted diffusion on DWI), lipoma (high signal on T1 precontrast sequences), and neurofibromatosis type 2 (bilateral CPA-IAC vestibular or facial schwannoma).

Selected References

1. Berry JM et al: A systematic review of cochlear implant-related magnetic resonance imaging artifact: implications for clinical imaging. Otol Neurotol. 45(3):204-14, 2024
2. Javed MA et al: CP angle medulloblastoma with supratentorial drop mets. J Ayub Med Coll Abbottabad. 36(2):443-6, 2024
3. Bächinger D et al: Internal auditory canal volume in normal and malformed inner ears. Eur Arch Otorhinolaryngol. 280(5):2149-54, 2023
4. Hyakusoku H et al: Pediatric internal auditory canal cavernous hemangioma with rapid progression of sensorineural hearing loss: illustrative case. J Neurosurg Case Lessons. 5(22):CASE23141, 2023
5. Palmisciano P et al: Transcanal transpromontorial approaches to the internal auditory canal: a systematic review. Laryngoscope. 133(11):2856-67, 2023
6. Totten DJ et al: Cerebellopontine angle and internal auditory canal lipomas: case series and systematic review. Laryngoscope. 131(9):2081-7, 2021

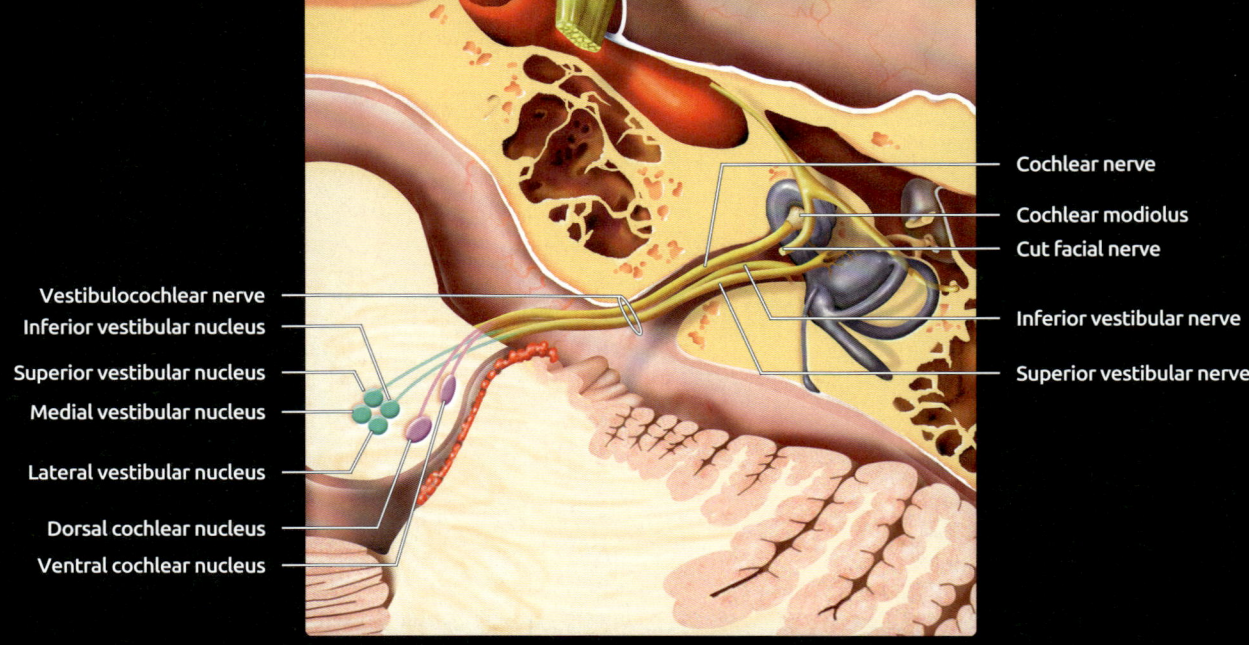

Vestibulocochlear nerve
Inferior vestibular nucleus
Superior vestibular nucleus
Medial vestibular nucleus
Lateral vestibular nucleus
Dorsal cochlear nucleus
Ventral cochlear nucleus

Cochlear nerve
Cochlear modiolus
Cut facial nerve
Inferior vestibular nerve
Superior vestibular nerve

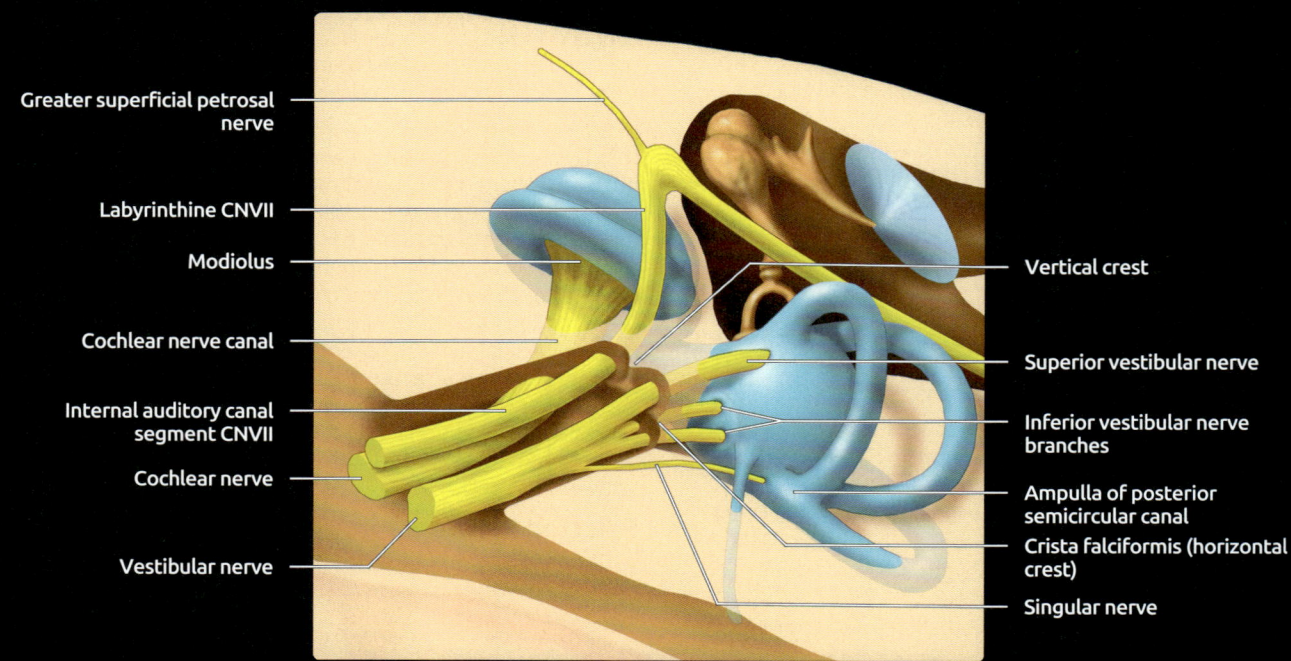

Greater superficial petrosal nerve
Labyrinthine CNVII
Modiolus
Cochlear nerve canal
Internal auditory canal segment CNVII
Cochlear nerve
Vestibular nerve

Vertical crest
Superior vestibular nerve
Inferior vestibular nerve branches
Ampulla of posterior semicircular canal
Crista falciformis (horizontal crest)
Singular nerve

(Top) *Axial graphic depicts the vestibulocochlear nerve (CNVIII). The cochlear component of CNVIII begins in bipolar cell bodies within the spiral ganglion in the modiolus. Central fibers run in the cochlear nerve to the dorsal and ventral cochlear nuclei on the lateral margin of the inferior cerebellar peduncle. Inferior and superior vestibular nerves begin in cell bodies in the vestibular ganglion; from there, they course centrally to 4 vestibular nuclei.* **(Bottom)** *Graphic shows the normal facial nerve and vestibulocochlear nerve in the internal auditory canal (IAC) and temporal bone. Notice that by the mid-IAC, there are 4 main nerves present, including the facial, cochlear, superior vestibular, and inferior vestibular nerves. The singular nerve branches off the inferior vestibular nerve midway through the IAC on its way to the ampulla of the posterior semicircular canal. Multiple inferior vestibular nerve branches pierce the macular cribrosa, as does the superior vestibular nerve, on their way to the vestibule.*

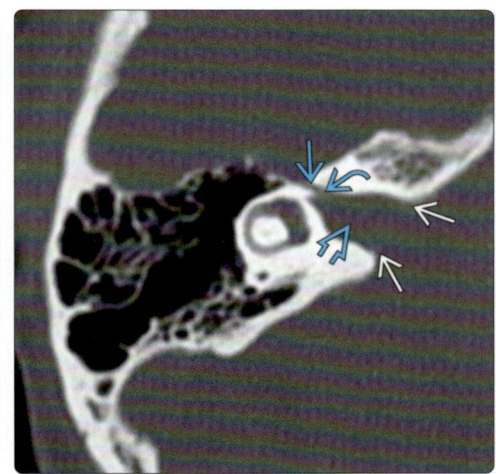

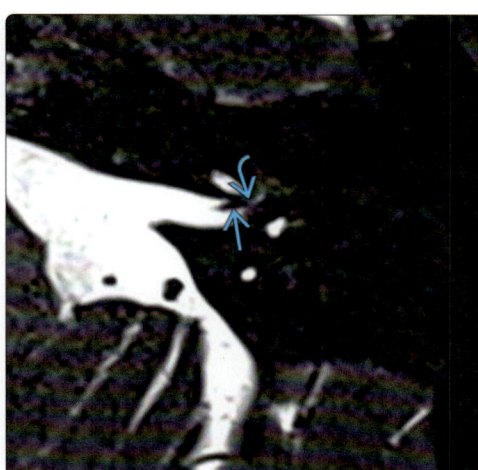

(Left) *Axial NECT MPR of the right temporal bone through the superior aspect of the IAC shows a labyrinthine segment of CNVII ⬅ communicating with the IAC ➡ through the meatal foramen ➡. The IAC communicates with the cerebellopontine angle through the porus acusticus ➡. (Right) Axial 3D T2 SPACE MR through the superior aspect of the left IAC shows CNVII ➡ at the fundus of the IAC entering the meatal foramen ➡. CVII runs the anterior and superior aspect of the IAC. The meatal foramen is better delineated on CT.*

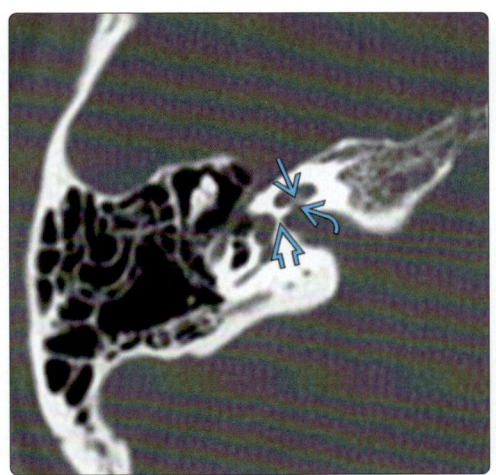

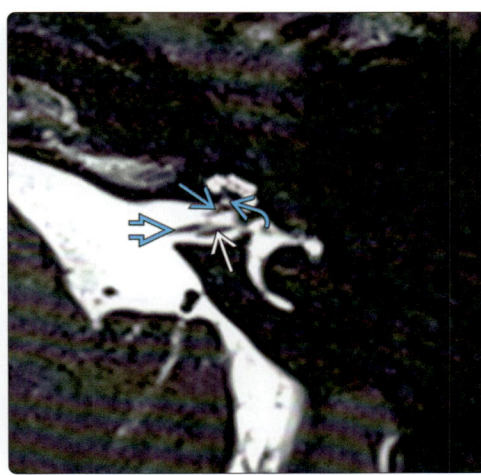

(Left) *Axial high-resolution NECT of the right temporal bone through the mid IAC shows the modiolus ➡, which houses the bipolar spiral ganglion in it. Proximal axons run through the cochlear canal ➡ to the cochlear nerve in the IAC fundus. The macula cribrosa transmits the vestibular nerve from the vestibule to the IAC ➡. (Right) Axial 3D T2 SPACE MR through mid left IAC shows the cochlear nerve ➡ entering the IAC through cochlear canal ➡. Note partially visualized CNVII ➡ and superior vestibular nerve ➡ in the IAC.*

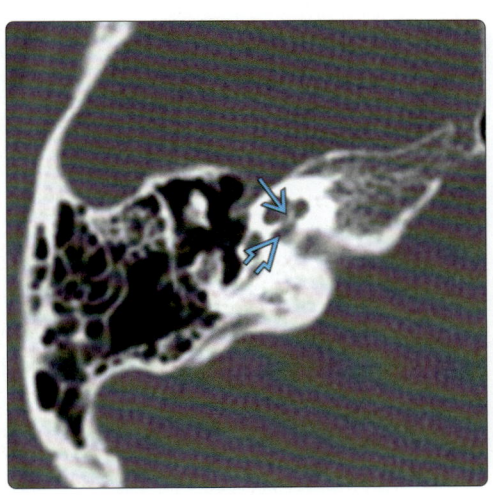

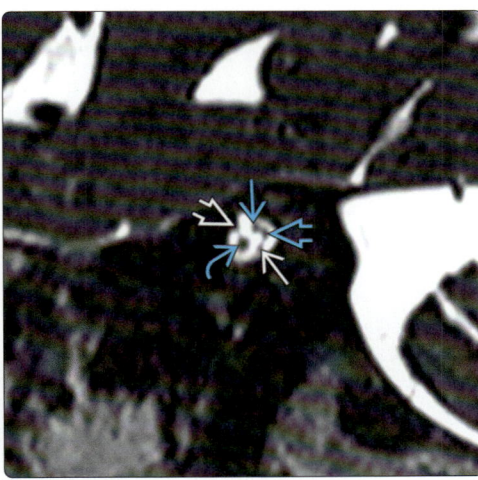

(Left) *Axial high-resolution NECT through the inferior aspect of the right IAC shows the modiolus ➡ in the cochlea, which communicates with the IAC ➡ through the cochlear canal. (Right) Sagittal oblique MPR of a 3D T2 SPACE MR of the left mid IAC shows CNII (anterior) ➡ and the superior vestibular nerve (posterior) ➡ in the upper 1/2 of the canal. In the inferior 1/2, the cochlear nerve (anterior) ➡ and inferior vestibular nerve (posterior) ➡ are seen. The upper and lower 1/2 of the canal is divided by the crista falciformis ➡.*

KEY FACTS

TERMINOLOGY

- Definition: Congenital inclusion of ectodermal epithelial elements during neural tube closure

IMAGING

- CPA cisternal **insinuating** mass with high signal on DWI MR
  - 90% intradural, 10% extradural
  - Margins usually scalloped or irregular
  - Cauliflower-like margins with "fronds" possible
- T1 and T2: Isointense or slightly hyperintense to CSF
- DWI: **Restricted diffusion** makes diagnosis

TOP DIFFERENTIAL DIAGNOSES

- Arachnoid cyst in CPA
- Cystic neoplasm in CPA
  - Cystic vestibular schwannoma
  - Cystic meningioma (uncommon)
  - Infratentorial ependymoma
  - Pilocytic astrocytoma
- Neurenteric cyst
- Neurocysticercosis in CPA

PATHOLOGY

- Surgical appearance: Pearly white CPA cistern mass
- Cyst wall: Internal layer of stratified squamous epithelium covered by fibrous capsule

CLINICAL ISSUES

- Clinical presentation
  - Principal presenting symptom: Dizziness and headache
    - Sensorineural hearing loss also common
  - If extends to lateral pons → trigeminal neuralgia
  - Rare symptoms: Facial palsy, seizure
- Treatment: Complete surgical removal is goal
  - If adherent to neural structures, complete removal may not be possible
  - If recurs, takes many years to grow
  - DWI MR key to diagnosing recurrence

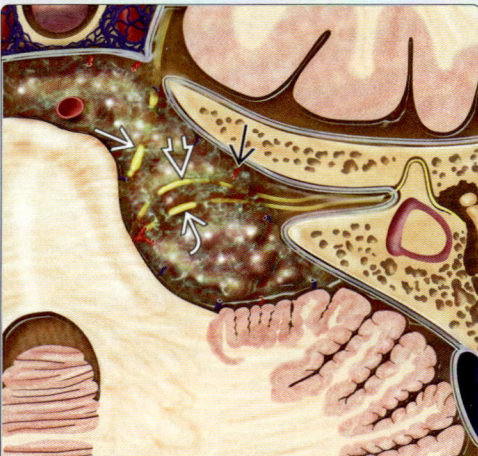
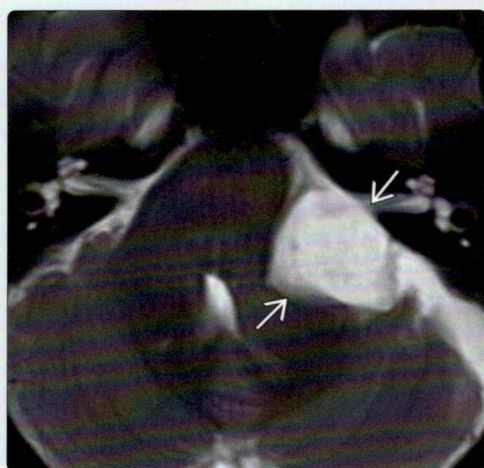

(Left) Graphic shows a large cerebellopontine angle (CPA) epidermoid cyst within a typical bed of pearls appearance. Note that CNV, ➡, CNVII ➡, and CNVIII ➡, along with the anterior inferior cerebellar artery loop ➡, are characteristically engulfed by this insinuating mass. (Right) Axial T2 FS shows a bright signal mass within the left CPA cistern ➡ with mass effect on the adjacent pons and middle cerebellar peduncle.

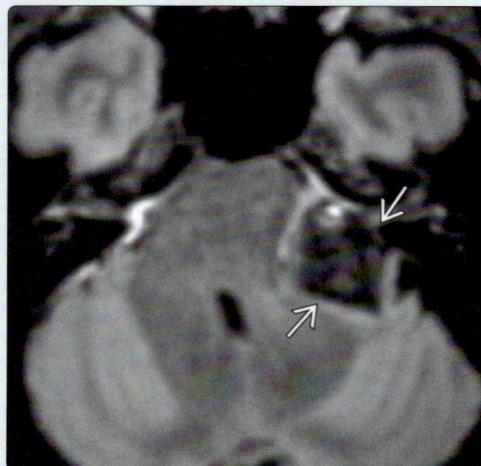
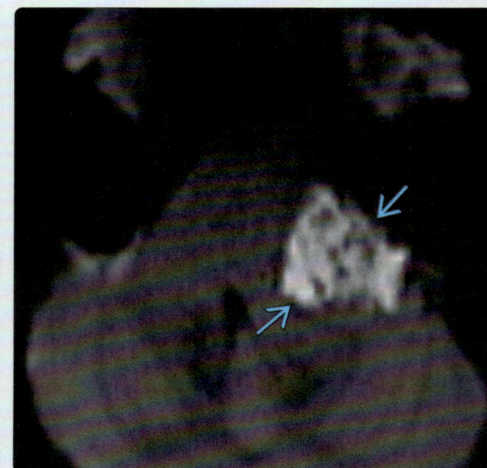

(Left) Axial FLAIR MR in the same patient shows incomplete signal suppression within the mass with heterogeneous, "dirty" signal ➡ within it. (Right) Axial DWI MR in the same patient shows striking hyperintense signal within the mass ➡, characteristic of an epidermoid cyst.

TERMINOLOGY

Synonyms

- Epidermoid tumor, primary cholesteatoma, or epithelial inclusion cyst

Definitions

- Congenital **inclusion** of ectodermal epithelial elements during neural tube closure

IMAGING

General Features

- Best diagnostic clue
  - Expansile, cystic-appearing, nonenhancing cerebellopontine angle (CPA) cistern mass with diffusion restriction on DWI MR
    - Engulfs CNVII, CNVIII, and anterior inferior cerebellar artery (AICA) loop
- Location
  - 50% of all intracranial epidermoids occur in CPA
- Size
  - Wide range: 1-8 cm or more in diameter
- Morphology
  - Insinuating mass in cisterns
  - Margins usually scalloped or irregular
    - Cauliflower-like margins with "fronds" possible
  - When large, compresses or invades brainstem ± cerebellum

CT Findings

- Similar density to CSF
- Calcification in 20%, usually margins
- Pressure erosion of temporal bone and skull base may occur
- No significant enhancement is rule
  - Occasional subtle linear enhancement along margin
- Rare variant: "Dense epidermoid"
  - 3% of intracranial epidermoids
  - Isodense or hyperdense to brain tissue
  - From protein, cyst debris saponification to calcium soaps or iron-containing pigment

MR Findings

- T1WI
  - Isointense or slightly hyperintense to CSF
  - If hyperintense, term "dirty" CSF has been applied
  - Rare variant: "White epidermoid" with high T1 compared to brain
    - Secondary to high triglycerides and unsaturated fatty acids
    - Caveat: If lesion in prepontine cistern, consider neuroepithelial cyst diagnosis
  - Epidermoid with hemorrhage
    - Mixed low- and high-signal areas
    - High signal secondary to methemoglobin
- T2WI
  - Isointense to hyperintense to CSF
  - "White epidermoid": Low T2 signal
- FLAIR
  - Does not null (attenuate) like CSF or arachnoid cyst
- DWI

- **Restricted diffusion** on DWI or DTI **makes diagnosis**
  - Secondary to high fractional anisotropy from diffusion along 2D geometric plane
    - Due to microstructure of parallel-layered keratin filaments and flakes
  - Apparent diffusion coefficient (ADC) = low signal
  - High-signal foci on DWI trace images in surgical bed indicates recurrence
- T1WI C+
  - No enhancement is rule
  - Subtle marginal enhancement may occur (25%)
- MRA
  - Vessels of CPA may be displaced or engulfed
  - Artery wall dimension not affected
- MRS
  - Resonances from lactate
  - No NAA, choline, or lipid

Imaging Recommendations

- Best imaging tool
  - Brain MR with FLAIR, DWI, and T1 C+ sequences
- Protocol advice
  - DWI sequence is most striking
  - If looking for recurrence, DWI (DTI) is best sequence

DIFFERENTIAL DIAGNOSIS

Arachnoid Cyst in CPA

- Displaces, does not engulf, adjacent structures
- Isointense to CSF on all standard MR sequences
  - T2 higher signal possible (if no CSF pulsations)
- Completely nulls on FLAIR (low signal)
- Hypointense (no restricted diffusion) on DWI trace MR
  - Contains highly mobile CSF
  - ADC = stationary water

Cystic Neoplasm in CPA

- Cystic vestibular schwannoma
- Cystic meningioma in CPA (uncommon)
- Infratentorial ependymoma
  - Pedunculates from 4th ventricle
- Pilocytic astrocytoma
  - Pedunculates from cerebellum
- All show some areas of enhancement on T1 C+ MR

Neurenteric Cyst

- Most common prepontine cistern in location
- T1 high signal (might mimic "white epidermoid")
- T2 signal often low

Neurocysticercosis in CPA

- Partially enhances
- Density/signal intensity does not precisely follow CSF
- Adjacent brain edema or gliosis common

PATHOLOGY

General Features

- Etiology
  - Congenital **inclusion of ectodermal elements** during neural tube closure
    - 3rd to 5th week of embryogenesis

○ CPA lesion derived from 1st branchial groove cells

Gross Pathologic & Surgical Features

- **Pearly white mass** in CPA
- Surgeons refer to it as "beautiful tumor"
- Lobulated, cauliflower-shaped surface features
- Insinuating growth pattern in cisterns
  ○ Engulfs cisternal vessels and nerves
    – May become adherent
- Lesion filled with soft, waxy, creamy, or flaky material

Microscopic Features

- Cyst wall: Internal layer of stratified squamous epithelium covered by fibrous capsule
- Cyst contents: Solid crystalline cholesterol, keratinaceous debris
  ○ **No** dermal appendages (hair follicles, sebaceous glands, or fat)
  ○ If any of these present, consider dermoid
- Grows in successive layers by desquamation of squamous epithelium from cyst wall
  ○ Conversion to keratin/cholesterol crystals forms concentric lamellae

CLINICAL ISSUES

Presentation

- Most common signs/symptoms
  ○ Principal presenting symptoms: Dizziness
  ○ Other symptoms depend on location, growth pattern
    – Sensorineural hearing loss: Common symptom
    – Trigeminal neuralgia (tic douloureux): If extends to lateral pontine CNV root entry zone
    – Seizures: If extends superiorly through incisura to temporomesial location
  ○ Symptoms usually present for > 4 years before diagnosis
- Clinical profile
  ○ 40-year-old patient with minor symptoms and large lesion discovered in CPA on MR
  ○ Asymptomatic patient shows incidental hyperintense lesion in CPA on DWI MR sequence

Demographics

- Age
  ○ Although congenital, presents in adult life
  ○ Broad presentation: 20-60 years
    – Peak age: 40 years
- Epidemiology
  ○ 3rd most common CPA mass
  ○ 1% of all intracranial tumors

Natural History & Prognosis

- Slow-growing congenital lesions that remain clinically silent for many years
- Smaller cisternal lesions are readily cured with surgery
- Larger lesions with upward supratentorial herniation are more difficult to completely remove
  ○ Larger lesions have more significant surgical complications
- Extremely rare malignant transformation to squamous cell carcinoma (SCCa)

○ Rapid clinical deterioration, failure to recover following surgery, or rapid lesion recurrence
○ Look for new tumor enhancement &/or leptomeningeal carcinomatosis

Treatment

- Complete surgical removal is goal
  ○ If large, near-total removal is prudent surgical choice
    – Aggressive total removal may cause significant cranial neuropathy
    – Used when capsule is adherent to brainstem and cranial nerves
- If recurs, takes many years to grow
  ○ DWI MR key to diagnosing recurrence

DIAGNOSTIC CHECKLIST

Consider

- MR diagnosis based on
  ○ Insinuating CPA lesion
  ○ Low signal on T1, high on T2 (similar but not identical to CSF)
  ○ No or partial nulling on FLAIR
  ○ Hyperintense on DWI trace images

Image Interpretation Pearls

- **Diffusion MR** imaging sequence is **key to correct diagnosis**

Reporting Tips

- Be sure to report prepontine or medial middle cranial fossa extension if present

SELECTED REFERENCES

1. Alsadi H et al: Intracranial epidermoid cyst with malignant degeneration and leptomeningeal carcinomatosis: illustrative case. J Neurosurg Case Lessons. 9(5):CASE24738, 2025
2. Kiss-Bodolay D et al: Intracranial epidermoid cyst: a volumetric study of a surgically challenging benign lesion. World Neurosurg. 185:e1129-35, 2024
3. Vernon V et al: Surgical management of cerebellopontine angle epidermoid cysts: an institutional experience of 10 years. Br J Neurosurg. 1-10, 2021
4. Shear BM et al: Extent of resection of epidermoid tumors and risk of recurrence: case report and meta-analysis. J Neurosurg. 1-11, 2019
5. Andica C et al: Spatial restriction within intracranial epidermoid cysts observed using short diffusion-time diffusion-weighted imaging. Magn Reson Med Sci. 17(3):269-72, 2018
6. Farhoud A et al: Surgical resection of cerebellopontine epidermoid cysts: limitations and outcome. J Neurol Surg B Skull Base. 79(2):167-72, 2018
7. Hasegawa M et al: Cerebellopontine angle epidermoid cysts: clinical presentations and surgical outcome. Neurosurg Rev. 39(2):259-66; discussion 266-7, 2016
8. Gopalakrishnan CV et al: Long term outcome in surgically treated posterior fossa epidermoids. Clin Neurol Neurosurg. 117:93-9, 2014
9. Schiefer TK et al: Epidermoids of the cerebellopontine angle: a 20-year experience. Surg Neurol. 70(6):584-90; discussion 590, 2008
10. Bonneville F et al: Imaging of cerebellopontine angle lesions: an update. Part 2: intra-axial lesions, skull base lesions that may invade the CPA region, and non-enhancing extra-axial lesions. Eur Radiol. 17(11):2908-20, 2007
11. Hamlat A et al: Malignant transformation of intra-cranial epithelial cysts: systematic article review. J Neurooncol. 74(2):187-94, 2005
12. Dutt SN et al: Radiologic differentiation of intracranial epidermoids from arachnoid cysts. Otol Neurotol. 23(1):84-92, 2002
13. Kobata H et al: Cerebellopontine angle epidermoids presenting with cranial nerve hyperactive dysfunction: pathogenesis and long-term surgical results in 30 patients. Neurosurgery. 50(2):276-85; discussion 285-6, 2002
14. Dechambre S et al: Diffusion-weighted MRI postoperative assessment of an epidermoid tumour in the cerebellopontine angle. Neuroradiology. 41(11):829-31, 1999

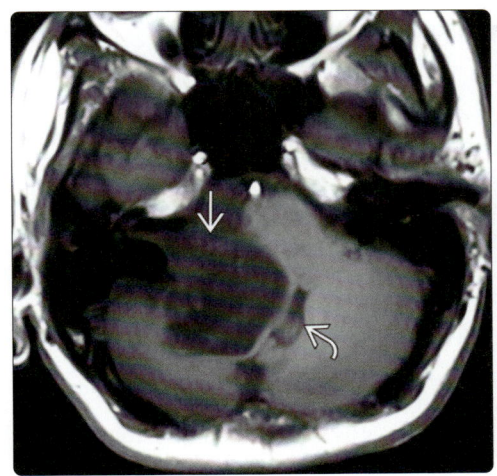
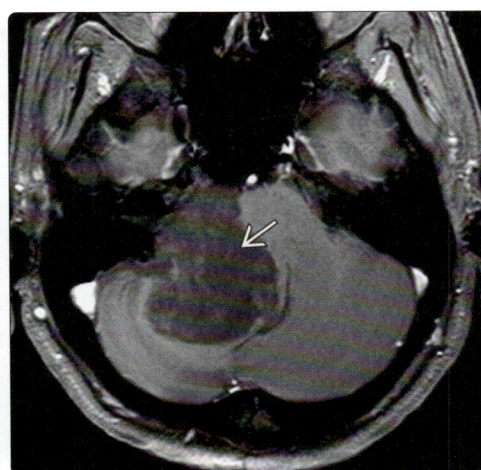

(Left) *Axial T1 MR in a 33-year-old woman with progressive dizziness and ataxia shows a large, lobulated epidermoid* ➡ *within the right CPA. There is expansion and encroachment into the right middle cerebellar peduncle and cerebellar hemisphere, deforming the 4th ventricle* ➡. *The lesion contains some areas of signal higher than CSF.* (Right) *Axial T1 C+ FS MR in the same patient demonstrates conspicuous lack of enhancement within the epidermoid* ➡.

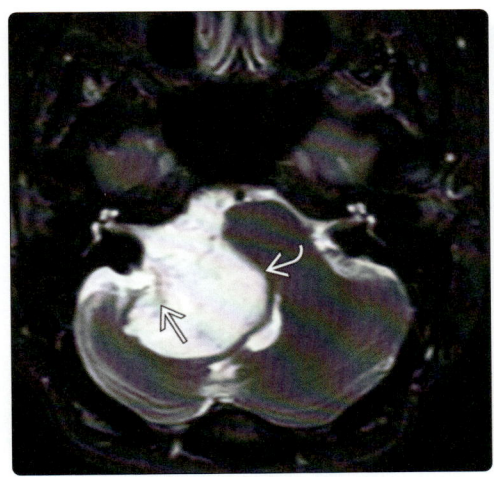
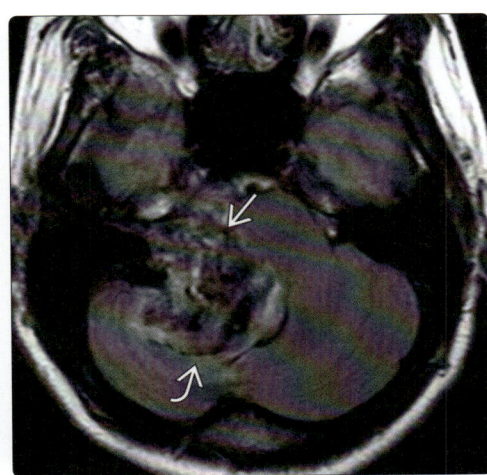

(Left) *Axial T2 FS MR in the same patient shows the epidermoid to have a predominantly cystic appearance with only scattered linear areas of lower signal* ➡. *The lesion "pushes" and displaces tissue of the cerebellar peduncle* ➡. (Right) *Axial FLAIR MR in the same patient shows the large right CPA epidermoid* ➡ *with complex signal that incompletely suppresses. This suggests intrinsic material not consistent with simple fluid or CSF. There is only subtle signal abnormality in cerebellum* ➡.

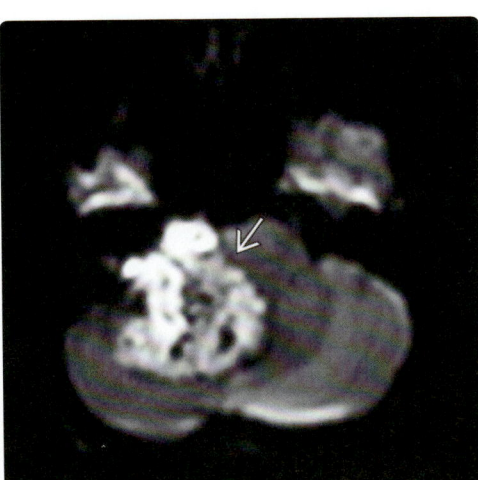
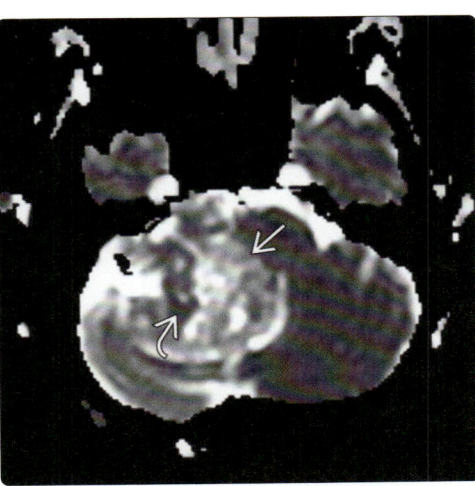

(Left) *Axial DWI MR through the large right CPA epidermoid* ➡ *in the same patient shows marked signal hyperintensity, helping differentiate this from arachnoid cyst.* (Right) *Corresponding axial ADC map shows heterogeneous signal with at least some areas of hypointensity* ➡, *suggesting diffusion restriction in this epidermoid* ➡.

CPA-IAC Arachnoid Cyst

TERMINOLOGY

- Arachnoid cyst (AC) definition: Developmental arachnoid duplication anomaly creating CSF-filled sac

IMAGING

- Sharply demarcated, ovoid, extraaxial cisternal cyst with imperceptible walls with CSF density (CT) or intensity (MR)
- AC signal parallels (isointense to) CSF on **all** MR sequences
- Complete fluid attenuation on FLAIR MR
- **No** diffusion restriction on DWI MR

TOP DIFFERENTIAL DIAGNOSES

- Epidermoid cyst in cerebellopontine angle (CPA)
- Cystic vestibular schwannoma
- Neurenteric cyst
- Cystic meningioma in CPA
- Cystic infratentorial ependymoma
- Cerebellar pilocytic astrocytoma

CLINICAL ISSUES

- Clinical presentation
  - Small AC: Asymptomatic incidental finding (MR)
  - Large AC: Mostly asymptomatic
    - Symptoms may arise from direct compression, hydrocephalus, ± ↑ intracranial pressure
- Natural history
  - Vast majority of ACs **do not** enlarge over time
- Treatment options
  - Most cases require **no** treatment
  - Treatment is highly selective process

DIAGNOSTIC CHECKLIST

- Differentiate AC from epidermoid cyst
- AC: No restriction on DWI = best clue
- Reporting tip: Since AC is usually not treated surgically, avoid offering any differential diagnosis when imaging findings diagnose AC

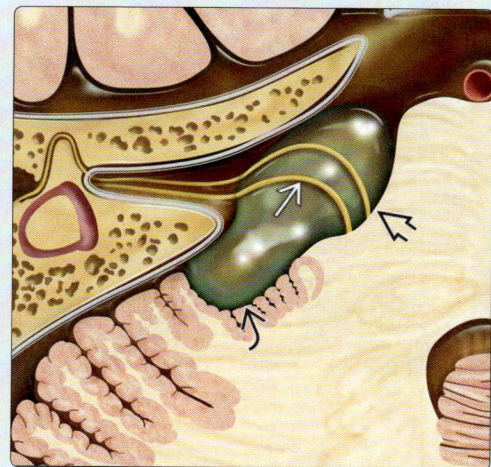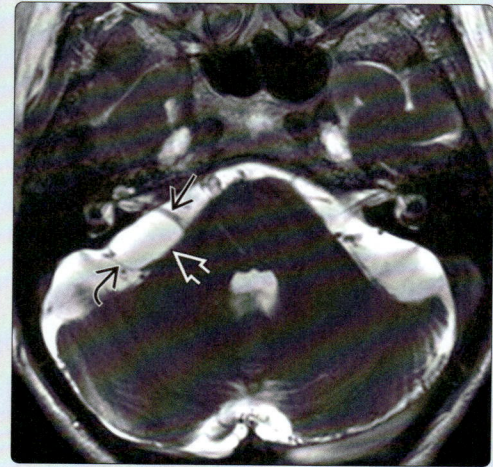

(Left) Axial graphic of an arachnoid cyst in the cerebellopontine angle (CPA) shows a thin, translucent wall. Notice the cyst bowing CNVII and CNVIII anteriorly ➡ and effacing of the brainstem ⇨ and cerebellum ⇨. (Right) Axial T2 MR reveals a right CPA arachnoid cyst causing bowing of the facial and vestibulocochlear nerves anteriorly ⇨, small bridging veins posteriorly ⇨, and flattening of the lateral margin of the brachium pontis ⇨.

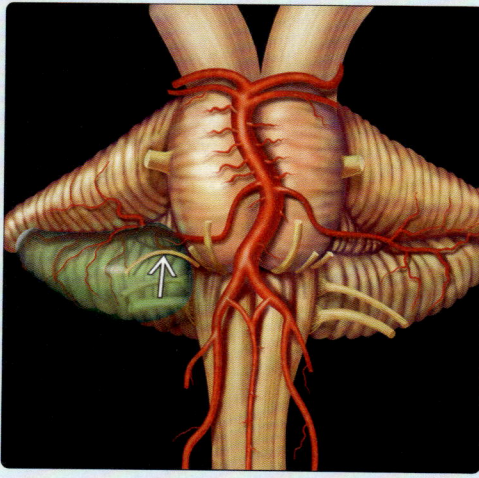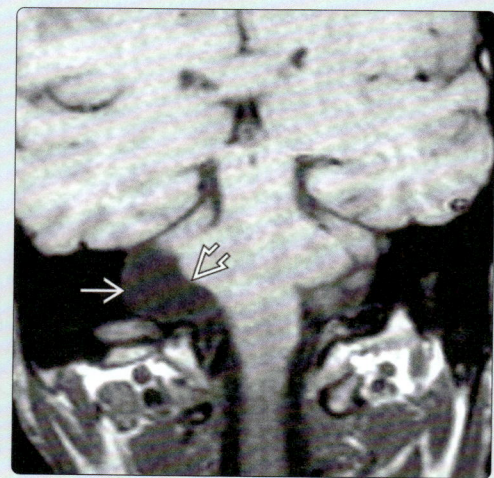

(Left) Coronal graphic of a CPA arachnoid cyst depicts a typical translucent cyst wall. CNVII and CNVIII are pushed by the cyst ➡ without being engulfed by it. In an epidermoid cyst, cranial nerves are usually engulfed. (Right) Coronal T1 MR demonstrates a small, CSF-intensity CPA arachnoid cyst ➡ with subtle mass effect on the adjacent brainstem ⇨. Complete fluid attenuation on FLAIR MR helps differentiate this lesion from an epidermoid cyst, which is the primary imaging differential diagnosis.

TERMINOLOGY

Abbreviations

- Arachnoid cyst (AC)

Synonyms

- Primary or congenital AC, subarachnoid cyst

Definitions

- Developmental arachnoid duplication anomaly creating **intraarachnoid** CSF-filled sac

IMAGING

General Features

- Best diagnostic clue
  - Sharply demarcated, ovoid or lentiform extraaxial cisternal cyst with imperceptible walls
  - CT: Lesion density = density of CSF
  - MR: Lesion signal = CSF signal on all sequences
    - **Complete fluid attenuation** on FLAIR
    - **No diffusion restriction** on DWI
- Location
  - 10-20% of all ACs occur in posterior fossa
    - Cerebellopontine angle (CPA) = most common infratentorial site
    - **10%** found in CPA
  - Spread patterns
    - Most remain confined to CPA (60%)
    - May spread dorsally along brainstem (25%)
    - Rarely spread into internal auditory canal (IAC)
- Size
  - Broad range: 1 cm to giant (> 8 cm)
  - When very large in posterior fossa, may be symptomatic
  - When large, will exert mass effect on vestibulocochlear and facial nerves, adjacent brainstem, and cerebellum
- Morphology
  - Sharply demarcated margins
  - Displaces, does not engulf, surrounding structures
  - Pushes cisternal structures but does not insinuate
    - Epidermoid cyst insinuates adjacent structures

CT Findings

- NECT
  - Density same as CSF
  - Rare high density from hemorrhage or proteinaceous fluid
- CECT
  - No enhancement of cavity or wall
- Bone CT
  - Rarely causes expansile remodeling of bone
    - Seen mostly in children
- CT cisternography
  - May show connection to subarachnoid space

MR Findings

- T1WI
  - Low-signal AC is isointense to CSF
- T2WI
  - High-signal lesion isointense to CSF
    - May have brighter signal than CSF
      - □ Cyst fluid generally lacks CSF pulsations
  - Well-circumscribed lesion
    - Compresses adjacent CNVII-VIII bundle, brainstem, and cerebellum when large
- FLAIR
  - Suppresses AC fluid completely
- DWI
  - No diffusion restriction
- T1WI C+
  - No enhancement seen
- High-resolution thin-section MR (CISS, FIESTA, T2 space)
  - Help define cyst wall, relationship to adjacent structures (CNVII, CNVIII, anterior inferior cerebellar artery, etc.)
- Phase-contrast cine MR
  - Flow quantification can sometimes distinguish AC from subarachnoid space
  - May rarely show connection between AC and cistern

Ultrasonographic Findings

- Grayscale ultrasound
  - Shows hypoechoic AC in infants < 1 year of age
  - Larger AC diagnosed in utero

Imaging Recommendations

- Best imaging tool
  - MR ± contrast
- Protocol advice
  - Add FLAIR (suppresses)
  - Add DWI (no restricted diffusion)

DIFFERENTIAL DIAGNOSIS

Epidermoid Cyst in CPA

- Major lesion of differential concern in setting of AC
- FLAIR: Incomplete fluid attenuation
- DWI: Restricted diffusion (high signal)
- Morphology: Insinuates into adjacent CSF spaces

Cystic Vestibular Schwannoma in CPA-IAC

- Intramural or marginal cysts seen in larger lesions
- Foci of enhancing tumor always present on T1WI C+ MR
- Rarely, larger lesions have associated AC

Cystic Meningioma in CPA-IAC

- Rare meningioma variant
- Dural tails, asymmetry to IAC still present with mixed enhancement on T1WI C+ MR

Neurenteric Cyst

- Rare prepontine cistern near midline
- Often contains proteinaceous fluid ($\uparrow$ on T1WI MR)

Cystic Infratentorial Ependymoma

- Ependymoma pedunculates from 4th ventricle via foramen of Luschka
- 50% calcified
- Cystic and solid enhancing components

Cerebellar Pilocytic Astrocytoma

- Cystic tumor in cerebellar hemisphere
- Enhancing mural nodule

PATHOLOGY

General Features

- Etiology
  - Embryonic meninges fail to merge
    - Remain separate as **duplicated** arachnoid
    - Split arachnoid contains CSF
  - 2 types
    - Noncommunicating; most common type
    - Communicating with subarachnoid space/cistern
- Genetics
  - Usually sporadic; rarely familial
  - Inherited disorders of metabolism
    - "Sticky" leptomeninges: Mucopolysaccharidoses
- Associated abnormalities
  - Vestibular schwannoma has AC associated in 0.5%

Gross Pathologic & Surgical Features

- Fluid-containing cyst with translucent membrane
- Displaces adjacent vessels or cranial nerves

Microscopic Features

- Thin wall of flattened but normal arachnoid cells

CLINICAL ISSUES

Presentation

- Most common signs/symptoms
  - Small AC: **Asymptomatic incidental** finding (MR)
  - Large AC: Symptoms from direct compression, hydrocephalus, ± ↑ intracranial pressure
  - Pediatric AC associated with higher symptom rate
- Other signs/symptoms
  - Defined by location and size
    - Headache
    - Dizziness, tinnitus ± sensorineural hearing loss
      □ Rarely facial nerve symptoms
    - Hemifacial spasm or trigeminal neuralgia
- Clinical profile
  - Adult undergoing brain MR for unrelated symptoms

Demographics

- Age
  - May be initially seen at any age
    - 75% of AC identified in childhood
- Sex
  - M:F = 3:1
- Epidemiology
  - Most common congenital intracranial cystic lesion
  - Accounts for 1% of intracranial masses

Natural History & Prognosis

- Most ACs **do not enlarge** over time
  - Infrequently enlarge via CSF pulsation through ball-valve opening into AC
  - Hemorrhage with subsequent ↓ in size reported
- If surgery is limited to AC where symptoms are clearly related, prognosis is excellent
- Radical cyst removal may result in cranial neuropathy ± vascular compromise

Treatment

- Most cases require **no treatment**
  - Pediatric AC more commonly treated than adult AC
- Surgical intervention is highly selective process
  - Reserved for cases where clear symptoms can be directly linked to AC anatomic location
  - Endoscopic cyst decompression via fenestration
    - Least invasive initial approach

DIAGNOSTIC CHECKLIST

Consider

- Differentiate AC from epidermoid cyst
  - AC: No restriction on DWI = best clue
- Determine if symptoms match location of AC before considering surgical treatment

Image Interpretation Pearls

- AC signal follows CSF on all MR sequences
  - Remember T2 signal may be higher than CSF from lack of CSF pulsation
- **DWI** sequence shows AC as **low signal**
- **FLAIR** sequence shows AC as **low signal**
- **No** enhancement of AC, including wall, is expected
  - Nodular enhancement suggests alternative diagnosis

Reporting Tips

- Since AC is usually not treated surgically, avoid offering any differential diagnosis when imaging findings diagnose AC

SELECTED REFERENCES

1. Lockard GM et al: Symptomatic and radiographic improvement following surgery for posterior fossa arachnoid cysts: meta-analysis and literature review. World Neurosurg. 192:e163-71, 2024
2. Quezada JJ et al: When is the radiology report of posterior fossa containing cyst/cystic-like CSF collection of clinical or surgical significance? J Neurosurg Pediatr. 1-6, 2024
3. Soleman J et al: Surgical treatment and outcome of posterior fossa arachnoid cysts in infants. J Neurosurg Pediatr. 28(5):544-52, 2021
4. Giordano M et al: Surgical management of cerebellopontine angle arachnoid cysts associated with hearing deficit in pediatric patients. J Neurosurg Pediatr. 21(2):119-23, 2018
5. Al-Holou WN et al: Prevalence and natural history of arachnoid cysts in adults. J Neurosurg. 118(2):222-31, 2013
6. Gangemi M et al: Endoscopy versus microsurgical cyst excision and shunting for treating intracranial arachnoid cysts. J Neurosurg Pediatr. 8(2):158-64, 2011
7. Olaya JE et al: Endoscopic fenestration of a cerebellopontine angle arachnoid cyst resulting in complete recovery from sensorineural hearing loss and facial nerve palsy. J Neurosurg Pediatr. 7(2):157-60, 2011
8. Boutarbouch M et al: Management of intracranial arachnoid cysts: institutional experience with initial 32 cases and review of the literature. Clin Neurol Neurosurg. 110(1):1-7, 2008
9. Helland CA et al: A population-based study of intracranial arachnoid cysts: clinical and neuroimaging outcomes following surgical cyst decompression in children. J Neurosurg. 105(5 Suppl):385-90, 2006
10. Osborn AG et al: Intracranial cysts: radiologic-pathologic correlation and imaging approach. Radiology. 239(3):650-64, 2006
11. Tang L et al: Diffusion-weighted imaging distinguishes recurrent epidermoid neoplasm from postoperative arachnoid cyst in the lumbosacral spine. J Comput Assist Tomogr. 30(3):507-9, 2006
12. Alaani A et al: Cerebellopontine angle arachnoid cysts in adult patients: what is the appropriate management? J Laryngol Otol. 119(5):337-41, 2005
13. Boltshauser E et al: Outcome in children with space-occupying posterior fossa arachnoid cysts. Neuropediatrics. 33(3):118-21, 2002
14. Dutt SN et al: Radiologic differentiation of intracranial epidermoids from arachnoid cysts. Otol Neurotol. 23(1):84-92, 2002
15. Gangemi M et al: Endoscopic surgery for large posterior fossa arachnoid cysts. Minim Invasive Neurosurg. 44(1):21-4, 2001

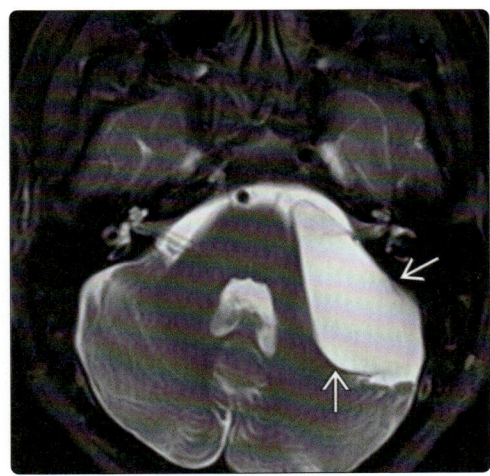

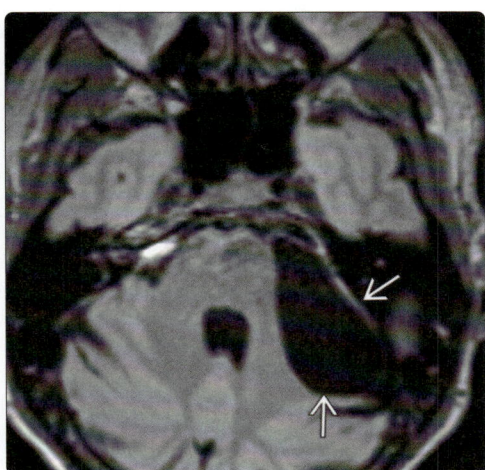

(Left) Axial T2 FS MR shows a large, circumscribed, hyperintense mass ➡ within the left CPA with local mass effect, consistent with an arachnoid cyst. (Right) Axial FLAIR in the same patient shows complete suppression of hyperintense signal within the mass ➡, consistent with CSF signal within an arachnoid cyst.

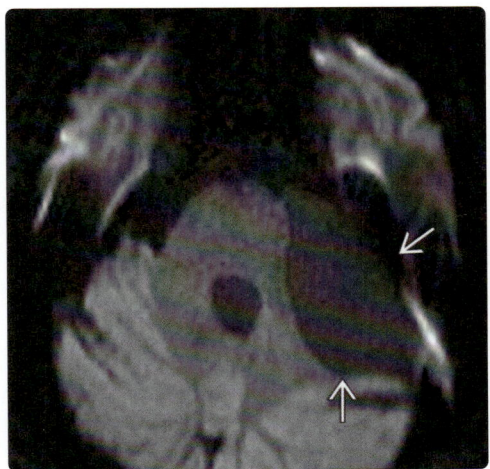

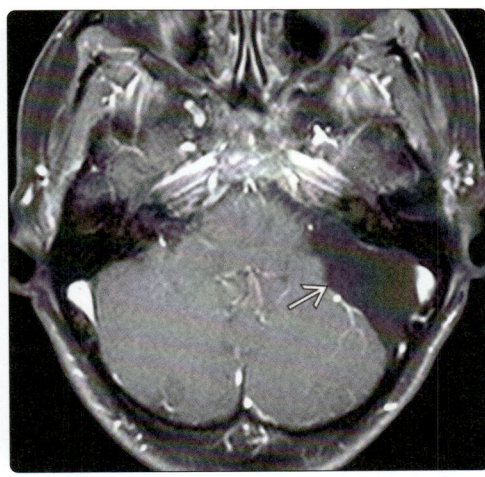

(Left) Axial DWI MR in the same patient shows no bright signal within the mass ➡, consistent with an arachnoid cyst, and helping to differentiate it from an epidermoid cyst, one of the main differential diagnosis considerations. (Right) Axial T1 C+ FS MR demonstrates a CPA arachnoid cyst ➡ that shows characteristic nonenhancement.

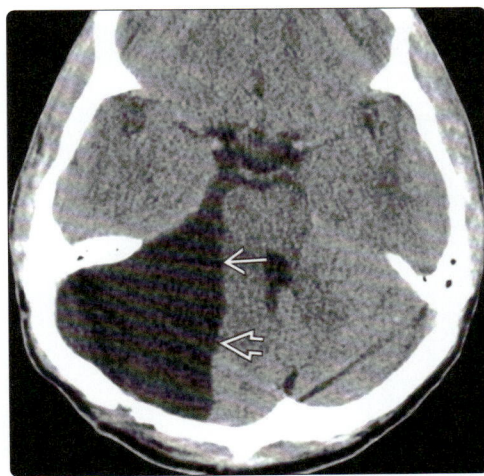

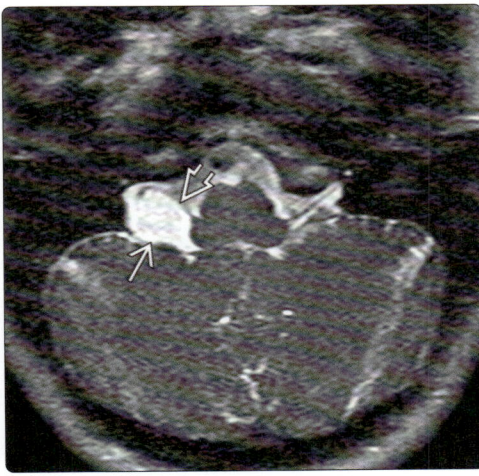

(Left) Axial NECT through the upper CPA cistern shows a large, low-density arachnoid cyst causing flattening of the lateral brachium pontis ➡ and cerebellar hemisphere ➡. (Right) Axial T2 FS MR demonstrates an incidental hyperintense CPA arachnoid cyst ➡ found at the time of imaging for headache. This lenticular-shaped lesion displaces the glossopharyngeal nerve (CNIX) anteriorly ➡. These small lesions require no additional imaging or treatment.

CPA-IAC Lipoma

TERMINOLOGY

- Lipoma in CPA-IAC: Nonneoplastic mass of adipose tissue in CPA-IAC area

IMAGING

- Focal, benign-appearing CPA-IAC mass, which follows fat density (CT) and intensity (MR)
- Concurrent intralabyrinthine deposit may be seen in association with CPA-IAC lipoma
- MR: Hyperintense CPA mass (parallels subcutaneous and marrow fat intensity)
  - Becomes **hypointense** with **fat saturation**
  - Caveat: Fat-saturated MR sequences avoid mistaking lipoma for "enhancing CPA mass"

TOP DIFFERENTIAL DIAGNOSES

- Hemorrhagic vestibular schwannoma
- Aneurysm in CPA-IAC
- Neurenteric cyst
- Ruptured dermoid cyst

PATHOLOGY

- Aberrant differentiation of embryonic meninx primitiva (meningeal precursor tissue)
- Lipoma composed of mature lipocytes (fat cells)

CLINICAL ISSUES

- Most common presentation: Adult presenting with unilateral sensorineural hearing loss
  - CNVIII compression: Tinnitus (40%), vertigo (45%)
  - Compression of CNV root entry zone: Trigeminal neuralgia (15%)
  - Compression of CNVII root exit zone: Hemifacial spasm, facial nerve weakness (10%)
  - Incidentally seen on brain CT or MR completed for unrelated reasons (33%)
- Treatment: **No treatment** is best treatment
  - If surgery required (cranial neuropathy), subtotal resection (debulking) only recommended

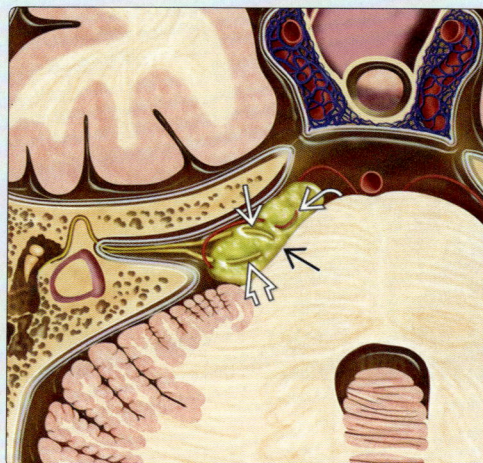
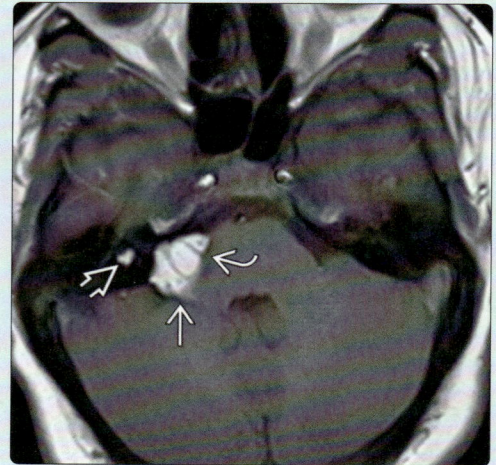

(Left) *Axial graphic shows a cerebellopontine angle (CPA) lipoma ⇨ abutting the lateral pons. Notice that the facial nerve ➡, vestibulocochlear nerve ⇛, and anterior inferior cerebellar artery (AICA) loop ⇗ all pass through the lipoma on their way to the internal auditory canal (IAC). (Right) Axial T1 MR shows an intrinsically hyperintense mass within the right CPA cistern ➡, which engulfs the AICA flow void ↗, consistent with a lipoma. Note the incidental 2nd lipoma within the vestibule ⇨.*

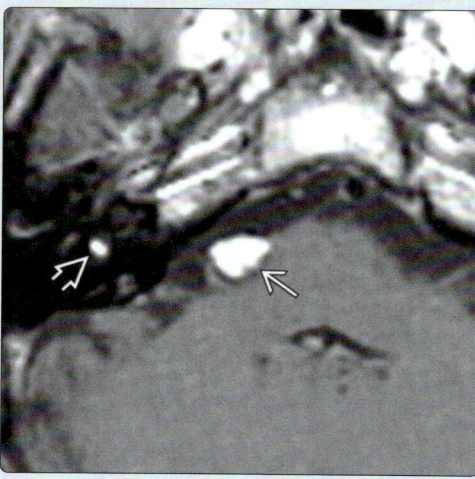
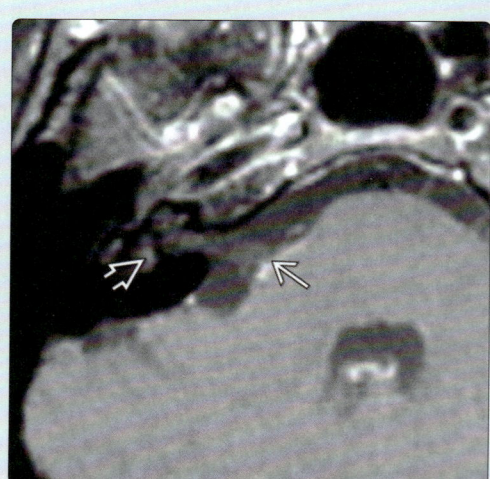

(Left) *Axial T1 MR reveals a hyperintense CPA lipoma ➡ abutting the lateral pons. Note the 2nd focus ⇨ of hyperintensity representing a small intravestibular lipoma. Such intralabyrinthine lipomas are very rare and may exist ± CPA lipoma. (Right) Axial T1 C+ FS MR in the same patient shows both lesions (vestibular ⇨ and CPA ➡) have lost signal. Fat-saturation MR sequences are key to confirming the diagnosis of lipoma and to avoid mistaking a lipoma for an enhancing CPA mass.*

TERMINOLOGY

Synonyms

- Lipochoristoma, lipomatous choristoma, congenital lipoma, lipomatous hamartoma

Definitions

- Lipoma in cerebellopontine angle (CPA)-internal auditory canal (IAC): **Nonneoplastic** mass of adipose tissue in CPA-IAC area
  - Congenital malformation; not true neoplasm

IMAGING

General Features

- Best diagnostic clue
  - Focal, benign-appearing CPA-IAC mass, which follows fat density (CT) and intensity (MR)
- Location
  - 20% of intracranial lipomas are infratentorial
  - Primary location = CPA cistern
    - May be in IAC only
    - Concurrent **intralabyrinthine lipoma** may be present
      □ Isolated intralabyrinthine lipoma also possible
- Size
  - Range: 0.5-5.0 cm in maximum diameter
    - May be as small as few millimeters
- Morphology
  - Lobulated, pial-based fatty mass
    - Characteristically encases facial nerve (CNVII), vestibulocochlear nerve (CNVIII), anterior inferior cerebellar artery (AICA) loop
  - Small lesions
    - Linear along course of CNVII and CNVIII in CPA
    - Ovoid within CPA cistern; tubular within IAC
  - Large lesions
    - Broad-based, hemispherical shape adherent to lateral pontine pial surface

CT Findings

- NECT
  - **Low-density** CPA-IAC mass
  - Measure mass using Hounsfield units (HU) if uncertain
    - Range: **-50 to -100 HU**
  - IAC lipoma may create bulbous bone CT appearance
- CECT
  - Lesion does **not** enhance

MR Findings

- T1WI
  - **Hyperintense** CPA-IAC mass (parallels subcutaneous and marrow fat intensity)
    - Noncontiguous 2nd fatty lesion in inner ear may be present
  - Becomes **hypointense** with fat-saturation MR sequences
- T2WI
  - Intermediate "fat-intensity" lesion
  - Conspicuous **chemical shift artifact** (frequency-encoding direction)
  - Signal parallels subcutaneous and marrow fat
- STIR
  - Hypointense due to STIR inherent fat suppression
  - STIR suppresses tissues with similar T1 relaxation times; may also suppress T1-hyperintense hemorrhage
- FLAIR
  - Hyperintense compared to cisternal CSF
  - Possible associated ipsilateral intralabyrinthine hyperintense signal
- T1WI C+
  - Lesion already hyperintense on precontrast images
  - Use **fat-saturated** T1WI C+ sequence
    - Lesion loses signal and **"disappears"** secondary to fat saturation
    - No enhancement in region of lesion is present

Imaging Recommendations

- Best imaging tool
  - **MR** is 1st study ordered when symptoms suggest possibility of CPA-IAC mass
  - CT can may be able to confirm diagnosis by measuring HU
- Protocol advice
  - When T1WI C+ MR focused to CPA area is anticipated, need at least 1 **precontrast T1 sequence**
    - Precontrast T1 sequence helps distinguish fatty and hemorrhagic lesions from enhancing lesions
    - Fatty lesions include lipoma and dermoid
    - Hemorrhagic lesions with methemoglobin high signal include aneurysm and venous varix
  - Once high signal is seen on precontrast T1 sequence, **fat-saturated sequences** distinguish fat from hemorrhage
    - **Caveat**: Fat saturation avoids mistaking lipoma for "enhancing CPA mass" (vestibular schwannoma)

DIFFERENTIAL DIAGNOSIS

Hemorrhagic Vestibular Schwannoma

- Rare manifestation of common lesion
- Patchy intraparenchymal hyperintensity on T1WI MR
- Hyperintensities persist with fat-saturated sequences
- T2* GRE shows blooming of intralesional hemorrhage

Aneurysm in CPA-IAC

- CPA aneurysm may have complex signal
  - Posterior inferior cerebellar artery aneurysm most common > vertebral artery > AICA
- Rarely enters IAC (AICA)
- Ovoid CPA mass with calcified rim (CT) and complex layered signal (MR)
- MR signal complex with high-signal areas from methemoglobin in aneurysm lumen or wall
  - Does not fat saturate

Neurenteric Cyst

- Most common in prepontine cistern
- Contains proteinaceous fluid (hyperintense on T1WI MR)
- Does not fat saturate

Ruptured Dermoid Cyst

- Ectodermal inclusion cyst
- Original location usually midline
- Rupture spreads fat droplets into subarachnoid space
- Rupture may lead to chemical meningitis

PATHOLOGY

General Features

- Etiology
  - Best hypotheses for congenital lipoma
    - Aberrant differentiation of meninx primitiva (neural crest derived mesenchymal anlage)
      □ Responsible for development of pia, arachnoid, dura, and subarachnoid cisterns
      □ Maldifferentiates into fat instead
    - Aberrant differentiation of mesenchyme associated with CNVIII
    - Hyperplasia of fat cells normally **within pia**
- Genetics
  - No known defects in sporadic CPA lipoma
  - Epidermal nevus syndrome has CPA lipomas as part of complex congenital anomalies
- Associated abnormalities
  - 2nd fatty lesion may occur in inner ear

Gross Pathologic & Surgical Features

- Soft, yellowish mass attached to leptomeninges
  - Sometimes adherent to lateral pontine pia
- May incorporate CNVII and CNVIII with dense adhesions
  - AICA loop may also be engulfed

Microscopic Features

- Histologically normal lipocytes in atypical location
- Highly vascularized adipose tissue
- Mature lipocytes; mitoses rare

CLINICAL ISSUES

Presentation

- Most common signs/symptoms
  - Unilateral sensorineural hearing loss (60%)
- Clinical profile
  - Adult presenting with slowly progressive unilateral sensorineural hearing loss
- Other signs/symptoms
  - Incidentally on brain CT or MR (33%)
  - CPA lipoma symptoms
    - CNVIII compression: Sensorineural hearing loss (60%), tinnitus (40%), vertigo (40%)
    - Compression of CNV root entry zone: **Trigeminal neuralgia** (15%)
    - Compression of CNVII root exit zone: **Hemifacial spasm**, facial nerve weakness (10%)
  - IAC lipoma symptoms
    - Sensorineural hearing loss, tinnitus, and vertigo only

Demographics

- Age
  - Range at presentation: 8-60 years
  - Mean at presentation: 45 years
- Epidemiology
  - Lipomas occur less frequently in CPA than epidermoid and arachnoid cysts
    - Epidermoid cyst > arachnoid cyst > > lipoma
  - CPA lipoma represents 10% of all intracranial lipomas

- Interhemispheric (45%), quadrigeminal/superior cerebellar (25%), suprasellar/interpeduncular (15%), sylvian cisterns (5%)

Natural History & Prognosis

- Usually does not grow over time
  - Lesion consists of mature lipocytes
  - Growth has been seen in pediatric lesions
  - Growth reported in obese or steroid-treated patients
- Stability confirmed with follow-up examinations

Treatment

- Primum non nocere ("first, do no harm") is guiding principle
  - **No treatment** is best treatment
- Conservative therapy recommendations
  - Medical therapy: Trigeminal neuralgia, hemifacial spasm
  - Discontinue steroid treatment if present; weight loss
- **Surgical removal is no longer recommended**
  - Injury to CNVII, CNVIII, or AICA common
  - Historically, 70% of postoperative patients had new postoperative deficits
- Surgical intervention if CNV or CNVII decompression needed
  - Subtotal removal (debulking) only recommended

DIAGNOSTIC CHECKLIST

Consider

- When high-signal lesion is seen in CPA-IAC on T1WI unenhanced MR, 3 explanations to consider
  - Fatty lesion
    - Lipoma most common (will fat saturate)
  - Hemorrhagic lesion
    - Aneurysm wall clot or clotted venous varix (dural arteriovenous fistula)
    - Rare hemorrhagic acoustic schwannoma
    - Hemorrhage will not fat saturate
  - Highly proteinaceous fluid
    - Neurenteric cyst (usually in prepontine cistern)
    - High protein hyperintensity will not fat saturate

Image Interpretation Pearls

- Once high-signal lesion is seen in CPA on precontrast T1WI MR, use **fat-saturation** sequences to confirm diagnosis

Reporting Tips

- Report size and extent of lipoma
  - Check inner ear for 2nd lesion
- Report CNVII, CNVIII, and AICA loop engulfed by lipoma

SELECTED REFERENCES

1. Benson JC et al: Inner ear signal abnormalities of adjacent intracranial lipochoristoma. AJNR Am J Neuroradiol. 46(5):1016-21, 2025
2. Totten DJ et al: Cerebellopontine angle and internal auditory canal lipomas: case series and systematic review. Laryngoscope. 131(9):2081-7, 2021
3. Uysal E et al: Internal auditory canal lipoma: an unusual intracranial lesion. World Neurosurg. 135:156-9, 2020
4. Bertot B et al: Diagnostic dilemma: cerebellopontine angle lipoma versus dermoid cyst. Cureus. 9(11):e1894, 2017
5. Scangas G et al: Lipochoristoma of the internal auditory canal. J Neurol Surg Rep. 76(1):e52-4, 2015
6. Bacciu A et al: Lipomas of the internal auditory canal and cerebellopontine angle. Ann Otol Rhinol Laryngol. 123(1):58-64, 2014
7. Filli L et al: Symptomatic lipoma of the internal auditory canal: CT and MRI findings. a case report. Neuroradiol J. 27(4):479-81, 2014

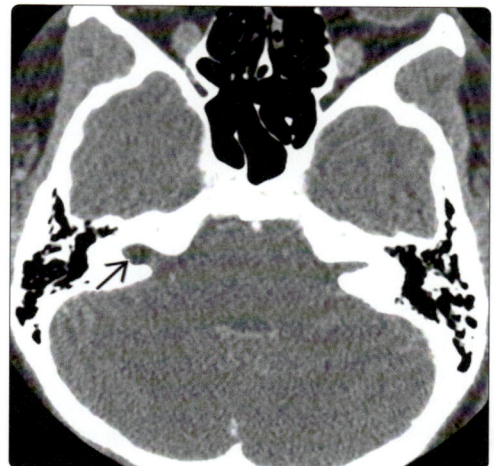

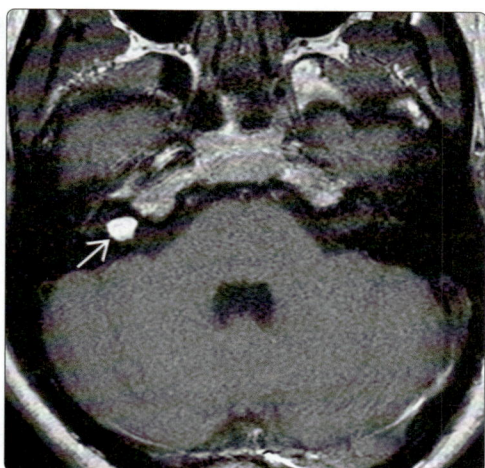

(Left) Axial CECT reveals a fat-density lesion ⊡ in the fundus of the right IAC. The bone shape in this area is bulbous in comparison to the opposite normal IAC, suggesting a congenital origin of the lesion. (Right) Axial T1 MR in the same patient shows the expected hyperintense fundal intracanalicular congenital lipoma ⊡. Lipoma of the CPA-IAC area may be found in the CPA, IAC, and, rarely, in the inner ear.

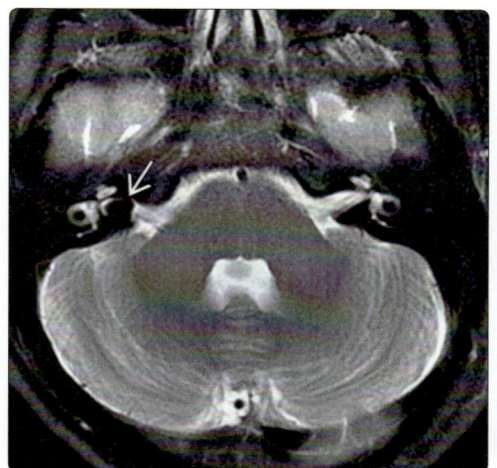

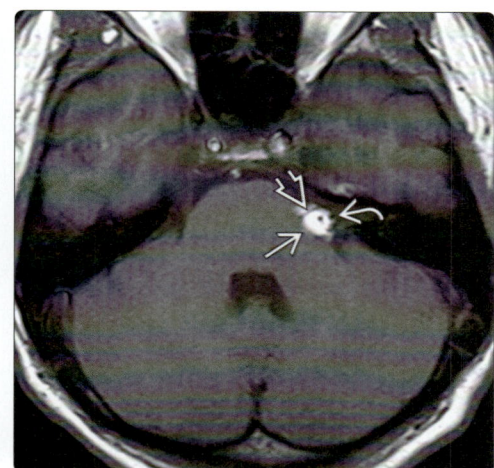

(Left) Axial T2 FS MR in the same patient shows the lipoma in the IAC fundus as a low-signal filling defect ⊡ in the high-signal surrounding CSF. (Right) Axial T1 MR in a 30-year-old patient with sensorineural hearing loss and trigeminal neuralgia shows a hyperintense CPA lipoma abutting the lateral pons ⊡. The linear hypointense line ⊡ is the proximal facial nerve (CNVII), while the hypointense dots within the lateral aspect of the lipoma ⊡ are AICA loops.

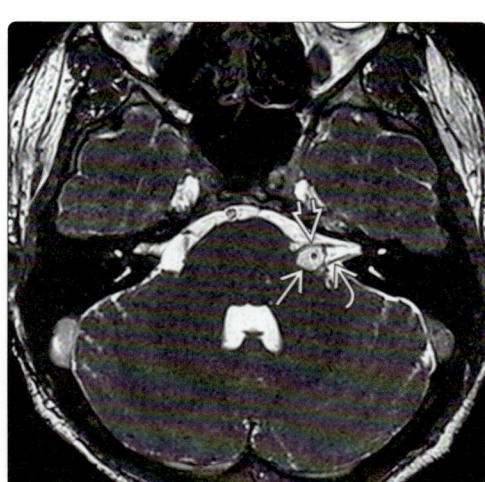

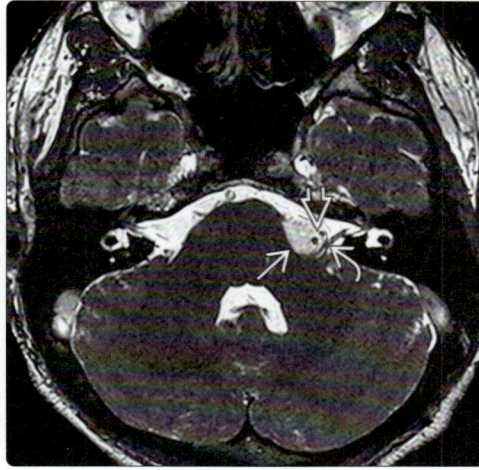

(Left) Axial CISS MR in the same patient better demonstrates the lipoma adherent to the lateral pons ⊡. Note the lesion engulfs the proximal CNVII ⊡ and superior vestibular CNVIII ⊡. The AICA loop is the hypointense dot in the center of the lipoma. (Right) Slightly inferior axial CISS MR in the same patient shows the lipoma ⊡ surrounding the AICA loops ⊡ and superior vestibular branch of the CNVIII ⊡. The possibility of CNVII and CNVIII injury and AICA stroke preclude surgery in this patient.

TERMINOLOGY

- Internal auditory canal venous malformation (IAC-VM): Rare, benign, developmental, nonneoplastic vascular lesion associated with perineural venous plexus of CNVII in IAC
- Historically and commonly referred to as "hemangioma" (misnomer)
  - **Venous malformation** (VM) preferred term

IMAGING

- Temporal bone CT findings
  - **Stippled/honeycomb ossification** in lesion matrix
- Enhanced T1 MR findings
  - Enhancing IAC mass (< 10 mm) in fundus
  - If extends along labyrinthine CNVII to geniculate ganglion, creates dumbbell appearance

TOP DIFFERENTIAL DIAGNOSES

- Cerebellopontine angle (CPA)-IAC meningioma
- Vestibular schwannoma
- CPA-IAC facial nerve schwannoma
- CPA-IAC metastases

PATHOLOGY

- Etiology
  - Benign, congenital, nonneoplastic VM involving perineural CNVII in IAC
- Microscopic features
  - Immunohistochemical markers critical to VM diagnosis
  - Endothelial lining of vascular channels **stains negatively** for hemangioma-associated markers (**GLUT1 and LeY** antigen)

DIAGNOSTIC CHECKLIST

- IAC enhancing mass + CNVII paralysis ± punctate ossifications = IAC-VM
- If infant or young child, consider infantile hemangioma, PHACE syndrome, and vascular anomaly syndromes

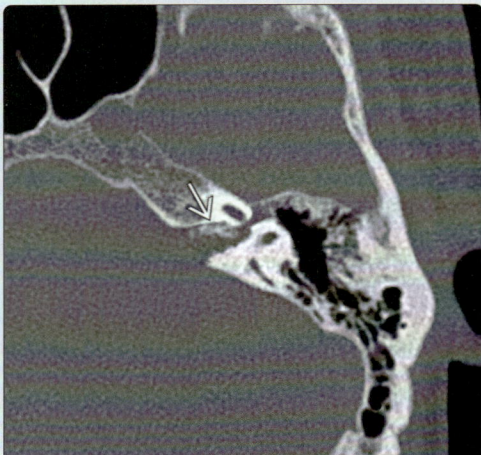
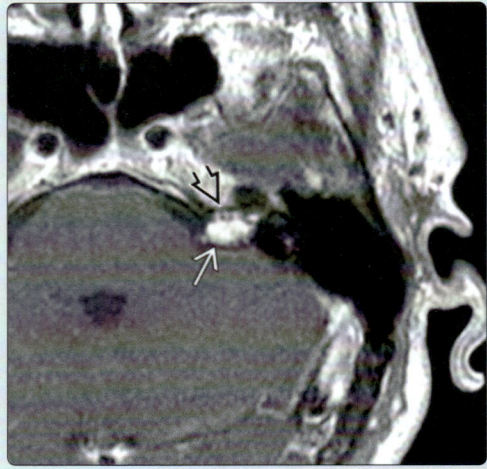

(Left) Axial bone CT shows typical CT stippled ossifications ➡ in the matrix of an internal auditory canal venous malformation (IAC-VM) ("hemangioma"). When found, ossifications help differentiate IAC-VM from IAC acoustic schwannoma. (Right) Axial T1 C+ MR in the same patient demonstrates an enhancing IAC-VM ➡. The low-signal foci ➡ along the anterior margin of the lesion are secondary to intratumoral ossifications.

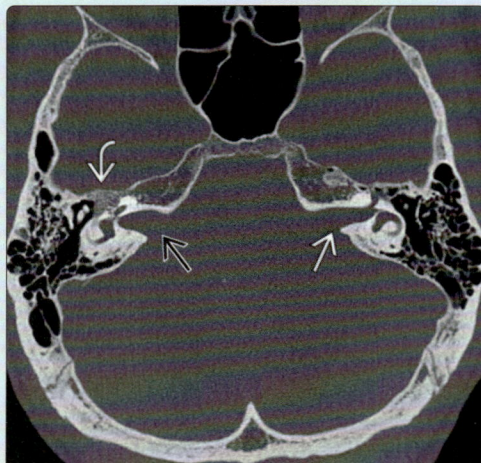
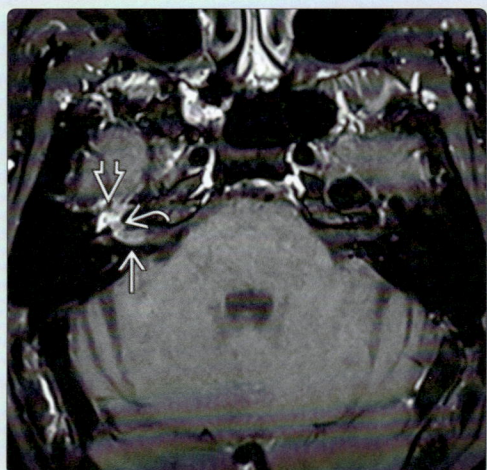

(Left) Axial bone CT shows asymmetrically smooth bony remodeling and widening of the right IAC ➡ compared to the left ➡. Classic matrix calcifications are not present in the IAC; however, the diagnosis is evident by classic lesion extension along the labyrinthine segment and geniculate fossa with expansile change and honeycomb matrix ➡. (Right) Axial T1 C+ FS MR in the same patient shows an enhancing VM in the IAC ➡, expanding the facial nerve labyrinthine segment ➡ and geniculate fossa ➡.

IAC Venous Malformation

TERMINOLOGY

Abbreviations

- Internal auditory canal venous malformation (IAC-VM)

Synonyms

- Hemangioma, cavernoma, cavernous hemangioma, cavernous malformation

Definitions

- IAC-VM: Rare, benign, developmental lesion associated with CNVII in IAC; may extend to geniculate ganglion

IMAGING

General Features

- Best diagnostic clue
  - **Stippled/honeycomb ossification** in lesion matrix
- Location
  - IAC ± labyrinthine CNVII ± geniculate ganglion
- Size
  - Small at presentation; **< 10 mm**
- Morphology
  - Ovoid to fusiform; may have irregular margins

CT Findings

- Bone CT
  - **Stippled calcification/ossification** often present
    - No hyperostosis of IAC bony walls
  - Rarely, IAC dilation from smooth osseous remodelling

MR Findings

- T1WI C+ FS
  - Enhancing IAC mass (< 10 mm) in fundus
  - Focal, intralesional, low-signal foci possible
  - If extends along labyrinthine CNVII to geniculate ganglion, creates **dumbbell** appearance

Imaging Recommendations

- Best imaging tool
  - High-resolution T2 bSSFP MR sequences (CISS, FIESTA)
  - Enhanced T1 FS MR; temporal bone CT to verify ossification

DIFFERENTIAL DIAGNOSIS

CPA-IAC Meningioma

- Most important lesion to differentiate from IAC-VM
- Enhancing IAC lesion ± **hyperostotic bony walls** ± calcification
- Dural-based enhancing mass (**dural tail**) with hyperperfusion

Vestibular Schwannoma

- Enhancing IAC lesion **without** ossification
- If larger, extends from porus acusticus to cerebellopontine angle (CPA) cistern

CPA-IAC Facial Nerve Schwannoma

- Enhancing CPA-IAC mass
- Facial nerve labyrinthine segment tail is key

CPA-IAC Metastases

- Pial type: Thickens CNVII and CNVII in IAC; enhances
- Dural type: Diffuse, smooth or nodular thickening of IAC-CPA dura; enhances

PATHOLOGY

General Features

- Etiology
  - Benign congenital VM arising in close approximation to IAC CNVII; "malformation" used for in utero **errors of vascular morphogenesis** that persist postnatally

Microscopic Features

- H&E: Nonencapsulated VM composed of dilated vascular channels of varying sizes
  - Widely ectatic vascular channels rimmed by smooth muscle coats without elastic laminae
  - Flattened and mitotically quiescent endothelial cells
  - Intralesional ossification often seen
- Immunohistochemical markers critical to VM diagnosis
  - Endothelial lining of vessels **stain negatively** for hemangioma-associated markers (**GLUT1 and LeY antigen**)
  - True IAC hemangiomas [GLUT1 (+)] also occur and are usually associated with PHACE syndrome; may be hard to distinguish from VM

CLINICAL ISSUES

Presentation

- Most common signs/symptoms
  - Hearing loss associated with **CNVII paralysis**
  - Hearing loss may come on rapidly

Demographics

- Epidemiology
  - **Rare** (< 1% of IAC masses)
  - 2nd most common site of VM along cranial nerves, after CN2

Natural History & Prognosis

- Adult-onset progressive hearing loss ± CNVII paralysis

Treatment

- Nerve-sparing surgical resection
- Rarely, CNVII graft necessary when CNVII invaded

DIAGNOSTIC CHECKLIST

Consider

- IAC enhancing mass + CNVII paralysis ± punctate ossifications = IAC-VM
- If infant or young child, consider infantile hemangioma, PHACE syndrome, and vascular anomaly syndromes

SELECTED REFERENCES

1. Putra J et al: Advances in vascular anomalies: refining classification in the molecular era. Histopathology. 86(7):1032-43, 2025
2. Li Z et al: Cavernous malformation from cranial nerves: a systematic review with a novel classification and patient-level analysis. Neurosurgery. 95(6):1274-84, 2024
3. Kunimoto K et al: ISSVA classification of vascular anomalies and molecular biology. Int J Mol Sci. 23(4):2358, 2022
4. Brinjikji W et al: Cervicofacial venous malformations are associated with intracranial developmental venous anomalies and dural venous sinus abnormalities. AJNR Am J Neuroradiol. 41(7):1209-14, 2020

CPA-IAC Meningitis

TERMINOLOGY

- Acute or chronic infectious infiltrate of pia, arachnoid, dura and CSF in vicinity of temporal bone, internal auditory canal (IAC), and cerebellopontine angle (CPA)

IMAGING

- CT may show underlying osteolytic defect and tympanomastoid effusion, suggesting subarachnoid space communication and possibly CSF leak
  - Acquired: **Bone erosion** (infection, cholesteatoma), **osseous tegmen defects** (fracture, surgery, intracranial hypertension), tegmen/posterior wall **ectopic arachnoid granulations**
  - Congenital: Inner ear lesions, cephalocele, patent petromastoid canal
- MR may show abnormal T2 FLAIR hyperintensity, enhancement, ± reduced diffusion in CPA, IAC, and adjacent cisterns
  - MR is specific but relatively insensitive

TOP DIFFERENTIAL DIAGNOSES

- Meningeal metastases
- Neurosarcoidosis, CPA-IAC
- ↑ FLAIR in CSF from subarachnoid bleed, artifact, ↑ O₂

PATHOLOGY

- Meningitis localized to temporal bone, CPA, or middle cranial fossa floor is secondary to temporal bone disease (otogenic) until proven otherwise
- Complications: Cerebritis, abscess, empyema, ventriculitis, otitic hydrocephalus, dural venous sinus thrombosis (DVST), arterial thrombosis

CLINICAL ISSUES

- Meningitis is clinical and laboratory (CSF sampling) diagnosis, **not** imaging diagnosis
- Imaging goal is to identify source and complications
- Treatment: IV antibiotics ± surgery

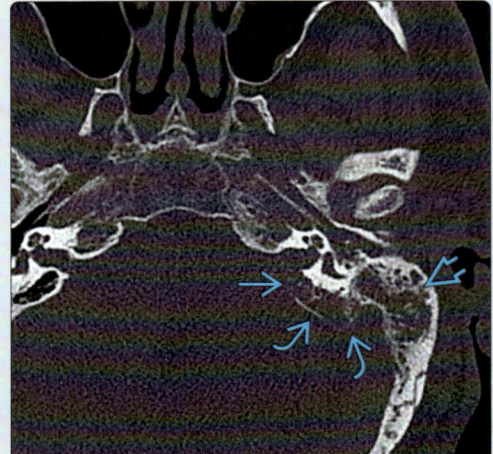 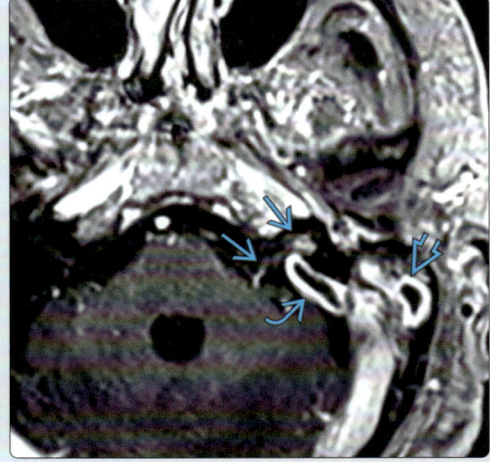

(Left) *Axial CT shows destructive osteolytic tympanomastoid opacification, cortical breakthrough, and septal erosions involving the internal auditory canal (IAC) and porus acusticus ⬌, retromeatal petrous face and sigmoid groove ⬌, and mastoid antrum ⬌.* (Right) *Axial 3D T1 C+ MR (same patient) shows enhancement within the left IAC fundus ⬌ and cranial nerves. Intraosseous rim-enhancing collections in the retromeatal Temporal bone ⬌ and mastoid ⬌ correspond to osteolysis on CT.*

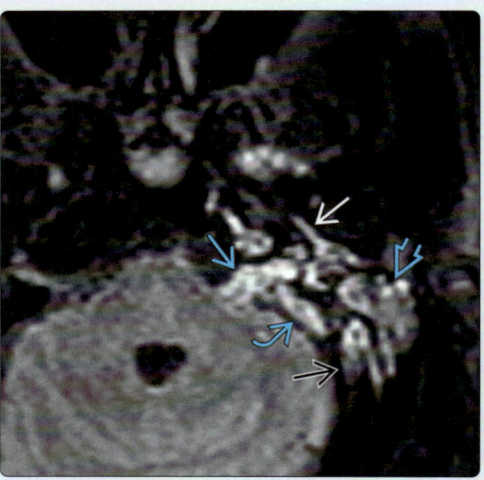 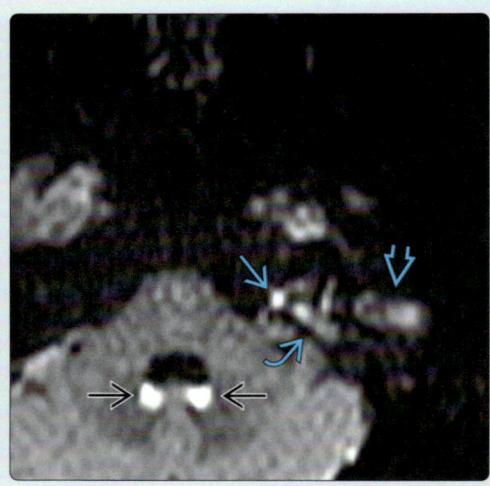

(Left) *Axial FLAIR C+ MR in the same patient shows abnormal hyperintensity in the IAC along CNVII/CNVIII ⬌, greater superficial petrosal nerve ➡, retromeatal T-bone ⬌, mastoid ⬌, and sigmoid dural venous sinus with preserved flow void ⬌.* (Right) *Axial non-EPI DWI in same patient shows reduced diffusion in IAC along CNVII/CNVIII ⬌, retromeatal T-bone ⬌, and mastoid ⬌. Retromeatal and mastoid collections are consistent with abscess. Dependent layering-reduced diffusion in 4th ventricle ⬌ reflects ventriculitis.*

TERMINOLOGY

Definitions

- Acute or chronic infectious infiltrate of pia, arachnoid, dura and CSF in vicinity of temporal bone, internal auditory canal (IAC), and cerebellopontine angle (CPA)
- Classified as acute pyogenic (bacterial), lymphocytic (viral), or chronic (tuberculous or granulomatous)

IMAGING

General Features

- Best diagnostic clue
  - Abnormal CSF by lumbar puncture combined with clinical findings of CNS infection is diagnostic standard
  - CT and MR are complementary in evaluation of possible meningitis related to temporal bone or CSF leak
    - High-resolution CT best shows osseous defects
    - MR best shows abnormal signal and enhancement in CPA and IAC

Imaging Recommendations

- Best imaging tool
  - MR has high specificity (strong positive predictive value) but only moderate sensitivity (limited negative predictive value) for meningitis
  - Lumbar puncture for CSF analysis usually indicated
- Protocol advice
  - High-resolution bone CT combined with whole-brain MR with FLAIR, DWI, and T1 C+

CT Findings

- Bone CT
  - Underlying osteolytic lesion causing abnormal tympanomastoid-subarachnoid space communication → meningitis ± CSF leak
  - Acquired predisposing lesions
    - Complicated or coalescent otomastoiditis, apical petrositis
    - Defects of tegmen tympani/mastoideum (fractures, surgery, idiopathic, intracranial hypertension, ectopic arachnoid granulations, CSF leak)
  - Congenital predisposing lesions
    - Congenital inner ear lesions, cephalocele, patent petromastoid canal

MR Findings

- T2WI
  - Meningitis: Hyperintense exudate lines CPA-IAC ± deep temporal bone meningeal surfaces
  - Temporal bone: High signal in middle ear if CSF leak
- FLAIR
  - Meningitis: **Hyperintense signal in sulci and cisterns** of posterior fossa and middle cranial fossa
  - Delayed C+ excellent for leptomeningeal infection
- DWI
  - **Detects complications**: Infarction, empyema, abscess
- T1WI C+
  - Meningitis: Meningeal exudate + brain surface
    - Thickened meninges: Local or diffuse
    - Dural thrombosis: Venous filling defect
  - Temporal bone: Focal meningeal thickening + enhancement within temporal bone may localize primary infection site
- CISS, FIESTA, or T2 space
  - Thin-section imaging may show predisposing arachnoid granulations, inner ear malformation, cephalocele

DIFFERENTIAL DIAGNOSIS

Meningeal Metastases

- Primary tumor usually known

Neurosarcoidosis

- Leptomeningeal nodular or lacy enhancement
- Temporal bone is uninvolved

Increased FLAIR Signal in CSF

- Nonspecific finding: Subarachnoid hemorrhage, artifact, acute stroke venous congestion, high inspired O_2

PATHOLOGY

General Features

- Etiology
  - Meningitis focused along deep surfaces of temporal bone or in floor of middle cranial fossa is secondary to temporal bone disease until proven otherwise

Gross Pathologic & Surgical Features

- Cisterns, sulci filled with cloudy CSF, then purulent exudate
- Pia-arachnoid thickened

CLINICAL ISSUES

Presentation

- Most common signs/symptoms
  - Meningitis is clinical and laboratory (CSF) diagnosis, **not** imaging diagnosis
  - Imaging goal is to identify source and complications
  - Signs and symptoms of complicated otomastoiditis: Fever, meningismus, cranial nerve deficits, labyrinthitis, otorrhea, CSF otorrhea, otitic hydrocephalus (rare)
- Clinical profile
  - CSF shows pleocytosis (↑ WBCs), ↑ CSF protein, ↓ glucose (infectious meningitis)

Natural History & Prognosis

- Effective antimicrobial agents have ↓ but not eliminated morbidity and mortality (~ 20%)

Treatment

- IV antibiotics
- Surgical treatment varies with cause and extent of complications

SELECTED REFERENCES

1. Sanjay P et al: Diagnostic performance of contrast-enhanced T2-FLAIR MRI in the detection of meningitis. SA J Radiol. 29(1):3018, 2025
2. Shabbir S et al: Positive predictive value of contrast-enhanced fluid-attenuated inversion recovery (FLAIR) magnetic resonance imaging in diagnosis of meningitis among pediatrics taking cerebrospinal fluid analysis as gold standard. Cureus. 16(11):e73356, 2024
3. Kralik SF et al: Diagnostic accuracy of MRI for detection of meningitis in infants. AJNR Am J Neuroradiol. 43(9):1350-5, 2022

Ramsay Hunt Syndrome

TERMINOLOGY

- Ramsay Hunt syndrome (RHS): Varicella-zoster virus infection involving sensory fibers of CNVII and CNVIII and portion of **external ear** supplied by auriculotemporal nerve

IMAGING

- Imaging diagnosis: Pathologic enhancement on T1 C+ MR of CNVII ± CNVIII in internal auditory canal (IAC) fundus along with all or part of membranous labyrinth
- Enhanced MR findings by location
  - IAC: Linear to nodular enhancement in IAC fundus
  - Intratemporal CNVII: Entire intratemporal CNVII enhancement typical
  - Membranous labyrinth: Fluid spaces of cochlea, vestibule, and semicircular canals may all be variably affected, particularly on delayed postcontrast FLAIR
  - External ear: Asymmetric cutaneous enhancement during active vesicular stage

TOP DIFFERENTIAL DIAGNOSES

- Bell palsy
- Vestibular schwannoma
- Meningitis
- Neurosarcoidosis in cerebellopontine angle-IAC

CLINICAL ISSUES

- Clinical presentation
  - CNVII palsy, vertigo, ear pain, and sensorineural hearing loss associated with external ear vesicular rash
  - RHS is 4th most common cause of facial nerve paralysis (2.4%), after Bell palsy (70%), stroke (18%), and head and neck cancer (2.6%)
  - Reserve MR for atypical clinical presentations
- Antiviral treatment and corticosteroids in combination generally recommended
  - Improves CNVII functional outcome
  - Improves symptoms and reduces duration of disease

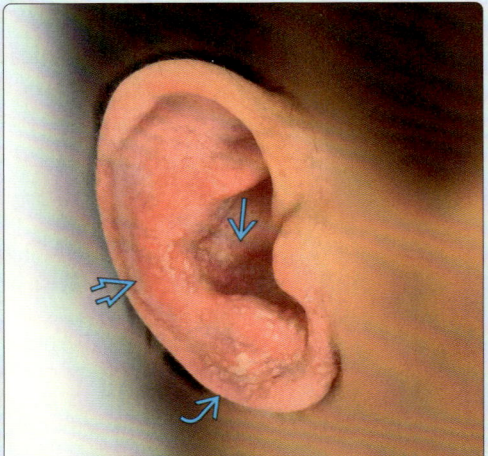
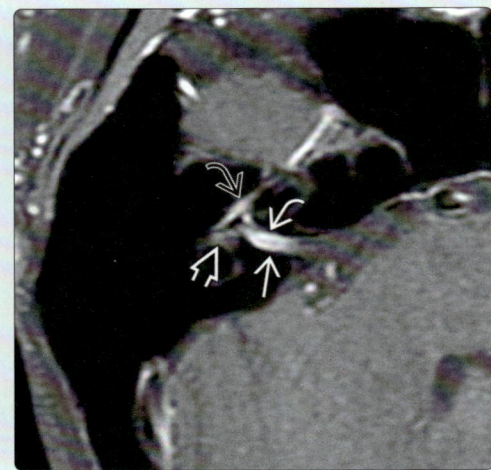

(Left) A herpetiform vesicular rash with surrounding erythema along the antihelix ⇨, concha →, and lobule ⇨ of the external ear is shown. In conjunction with ipsilateral peripheral facial nerve palsy in this immunocompromised patient, this is consistent with Ramsay Hunt syndrome (RHS). (Right) Axial T1 C+ FS MR in an RHS patient shows linear enhancement of CNVII in the IAC fundus ⇨ extending into the labyrinthine and tympanic segments ⇨. The superior vestibular nerve also enhances in the IAC fundus ⇨ and into the vestibule ⇨.

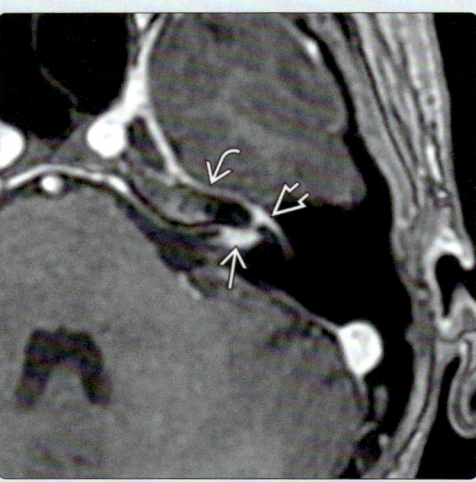
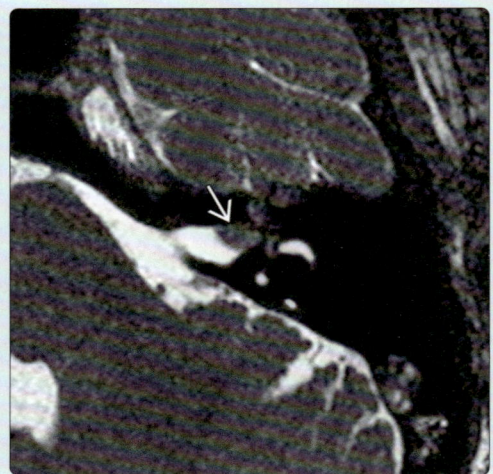

(Left) Axial C+ SPGR MR reveals enhancement of the left IAC fundus ⇨ as well as enhancement of the labyrinthine segment, geniculate ganglion, and anterior tympanic segment of CNVII ⇨. In addition, the greater superficial petrosal nerve branch of CNVII ⇨ enhances along the anterior margin of the petrous apex. (Right) Magnified axial T2 FS MR in the same patient shows nodular inflammatory tissue presenting as filling defect ⇨ in the fundus of the IAC.

TERMINOLOGY

Abbreviations

- Ramsay Hunt syndrome (RHS)

Definitions

- Syndrome of facial palsy, ear pain, vestibulocochlear symptoms, and rash of external ear produced by reactivation of varicella-zoster virus in geniculate ganglion of CNVII

IMAGING

General Features

- Best diagnostic clue
  - Pathologic linear or slightly nodular enhancement on T1 C+ MR of CNVII ± CNVII in internal auditory canal (IAC) fundus
  - Uncommonly, enhancement may include part or all of membranous labyrinth
  - 33-50% may have negative imaging studies

MR Findings

- T2WI
  - High-resolution (≤ 2-mm) T2
    - Fundal CNVII and CNVIII thickened
    - When severe, robust inflammation may produce ill-defined and nodular filling defect in IAC fundus and mimic vestibular schwannoma or other IAC mass
- FLAIR
  - Subtle abnormal signal in affected IAC &/or labyrinth
- T1WI C+
  - IAC
    - Linear to nodular enhancement in IAC fundus (CNVII and CNVIII)
    - IAC enhancement **not** always present (even with sensorineural hearing loss ± vertigo)
  - Intratemporal facial nerve
    - Entire intratemporal CNVII enhancement typical
      □ **Labyrinthine segment** CNVII and geniculate ganglion reliably enhance
  - Membranous labyrinth
    - Fluid spaces of cochlea, vestibule, and semicircular canals may all be variably affected, particularly on delayed postcontrast MR (especially FLAIR)
      □ Cochlear portion enhances most commonly
    - Membranous labyrinth enhancement may **not** be present (even when hearing loss and vertigo present)
  - External ear
    - Enhancing external ear vesicles and associated inflammation

Imaging Recommendations

- Best imaging tool
  - Whole-brain MR with enhanced sequences focused on cerebellopontine angle-IAC and temporal bone
  - Findings best seen on **fat-saturated** T1 C+ MR
- Protocol advice
  - If external ear vesicular rash is clinically apparent, **no imaging is necessary**

DIFFERENTIAL DIAGNOSIS

Bell Palsy

- Enhancement of CNVII; not membranous labyrinth or CNVIII
- Fundal CNVII enhancing "tuft"
- IAC enhancement usually less intense than in RHS

Meningitis

- Headache, stiff neck, fever
- Thickened, diffusely enhancing meninges
- CSF analysis may be revealing

PATHOLOGY

General Features

- Etiology
  - Classic hypothesis: Virus remains dormant within geniculate ganglion with periodic **reactivation**
    - Varicella-zoster virus can be cultured from vesicles or saliva

CLINICAL ISSUES

Presentation

- Most common signs/symptoms
  - Facial palsy, ear pain, vertigo, external ear vesicular rash
  - Hearing loss in patients with RHS as high as 85%, preferentially affecting high tones
- Other signs/symptoms
  - Fever, nausea, and vomiting

Natural History & Prognosis

- Ear pain followed in ~ 7 days by erythematous vesicular rash of external ear
- Cranial neuropathies appear after onset of ear pain
  - Appear before or after vesicular eruption
  - When before, imaging may be done to look for etiology of CNVII palsy

Treatment

- Pharmacologic treatment
  - Antiviral treatment with acyclovir and corticosteroids (↓ pain, improves CNVII function)

DIAGNOSTIC CHECKLIST

Consider

- Reserve MR for atypical clinical presentations

SELECTED REFERENCES

1. Hwang CJ et al: The epidemiology and treatment outcomes of facial nerve palsy using a population-based method. Ophthalmic Plast Reconstr Surg. ePub, 2025
2. Mandava S et al: A multi-institutional review of characteristics of idiopathic versus non-idiopathic facial paralysis. Laryngoscope. 135(8):2882-8, 2025
3. Han Y et al: Clinical analysis of 3D-fluid attenuated inversion recovery and T1 volume interpolated body examination sequences on delayed gadolinium-enhanced scanning in Ramsay Hunt syndrome. J Int Adv Otol. 19(5):407-13, 2023
4. Kim SH et al: Comparative prognosis in patients with Ramsay-Hunt syndrome and Bell's palsy. Eur Arch Otorhinolaryngol. 276(4):1011-6, 2019
5. Zimmermann J et al: Differential diagnosis of peripheral facial nerve palsy: a retrospective clinical, MRI and CSF-based study. J Neurol. 266(10):2488-94, 2019

TERMINOLOGY

- Neurosarcoidosis: Systemic disorder with **noncaseating epithelioid cell granulomas** of multiple organ systems

IMAGING

- MR findings
  - Multifocal enhancing meningeal masses
  - Other intracranial locations
    - Optic chiasm, hypothalamus, infundibulum
    - Cranial nerves (CNII > CNV > CNVII & CNVIII)
- **T2**: **Hypointense** or **hyperintense** meningeal foci
  - Hypointense: Fibrocollagenous tissue
  - Hyperintense: Inflammatory tissue
- T1 C+: Nodular or linear dural enhancing lesions

TOP DIFFERENTIAL DIAGNOSES

- Multiple meningiomas
- CPA-IAC metastases
- Meningitis

PATHOLOGY

- **Noncaseating granulomas** are characteristic
- Genetic polymorphisms of MHC have ↑ risk of disease

CLINICAL ISSUES

- Black patients affected more often than White patients
- Systemic sarcoidosis: Pulmonary symptoms
- CNS sarcoidosis symptoms
  - Visual loss & pituitary dysfunction
  - Cranial neuropathy: CNII > > CNV > **CNVII & VIII**
- Laboratory findings are confirmatory
  - Kveim-Siltzbach skin test positive in 85%
  - Serum ACE levels elevated in < 50%
  - Use modified Zajicek criteria for diagnosis
    - Divides into confirmed, probable, & possible
- Treatment options
  - Steroids ± immunomodulators
  - 50% of neurosarcoidosis progresses despite treatment

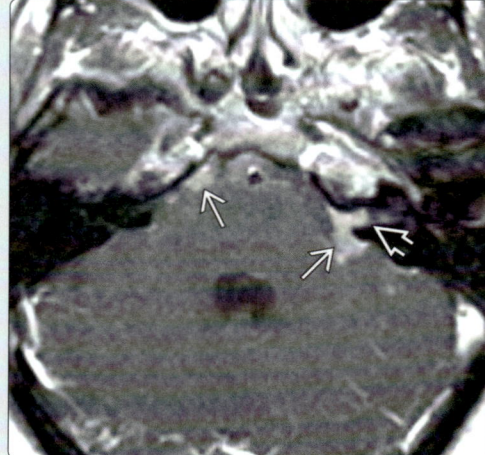
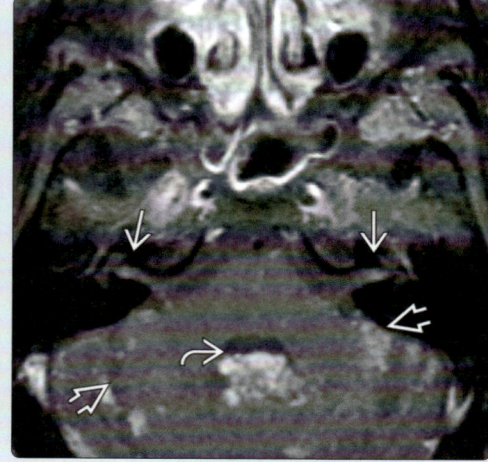

(Left) Axial T1 C+ MR shows multifocal enhancing meningeal nodules ⮥. The left CPA lesion enters the IAC ⮥. Inflammatory diseases (granulomatosis with polyangiitis, intracranial pseudotumor, granulomatous infection) & meningeal malignancies are part of the differential diagnosis. (Right) Axial T1 C+ FS MR shows enhancing foci in both IACs ➡ in this patient with sensorineural hearing loss due to sarcoidosis. The 4th ventricle ⮥ & cerebellar meninges ⮥ are also involved.

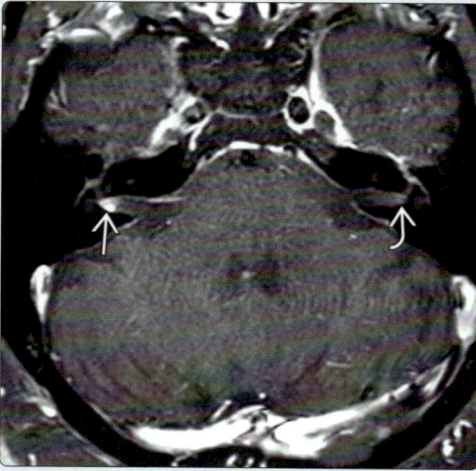
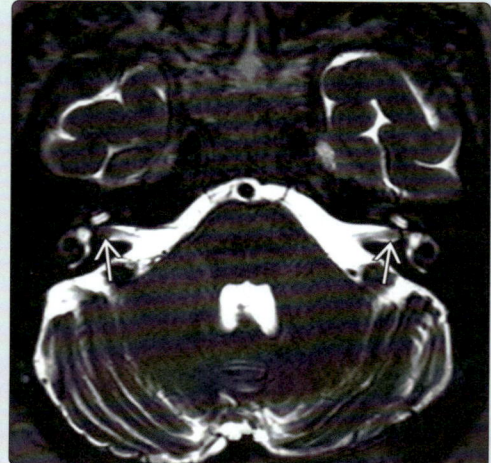

(Left) Axial T1 C+ FS MR shows nodular enhancement in the IAC ➡, mimicking a small schwannoma in this patient with uveitis & facial nerve palsy due to sarcoidosis. Faint contralateral IAC enhancement ⮥ was also noted, better imaged on a different slice (not shown). Characteristic bilateral hilar & right paratracheal adenopathy were noted on a chest CT (not shown). (Right) Axial thin SSFP T2 MR in the same patient shows nodular filling defects within the CSF of both IACs ➡, corresponding to enhancing nodules.

TERMINOLOGY

Definitions

- Systemic disorder with **noncaseating epithelioid cell granulomas** of multiple organ systems

IMAGING

General Features

- Best diagnostic clue
  - Solitary or multifocal enhancing meningeal mass(es) + abnormal CXR
- Location
  - **Dural** (~ 35%), **leptomeningeal** (~ 35%) > subarachnoid/perivascular spaces

MR Findings

- FLAIR
  - 50% have periventricular hyperintense lesions
    - Can infiltrate perivascular (Virchow-Robin) spaces
    - May cause vasculitis/angiitis of white matter
  - Hydrocephalus, lacunar infarcts
- T1WI C+
  - Nodular or linear dural enhancing lesions
  - Leptomeningeal disease spreads via perivascular spaces into brain
  - Cranial nerve (CN) enhancement

Imaging Recommendations

- Best imaging tool
  - MR with FLAIR & T1 C+ sequences
- Protocol advice
  - Include T1 C+ MR thin sections through cerebellopontine angle (CPA)

DIFFERENTIAL DIAGNOSIS

Multiple Meningiomas

- Clinical: Absent systemic manifestations of sarcoidosis
- Multifocal enhancing dural masses
- No parenchymal or subarachnoid space findings

CPA-IAC Metastases

- Clinical: Primary neoplasm usually known
- Nodular meningeal metastases < diffuse

Meningitis

- Clinical: Diagnosis based on CSF analysis

PATHOLOGY

General Features

- Etiology
  - Pathophysiology unknown
- Genetics
  - Sarcoidosis occurs in families
  - Genetic polymorphisms of MHC have ↑ risk of disease
- General pathology issues
  - Diagnosis often made after biopsy of skin lesions

Gross Pathologic & Surgical Features

- Granulomatous leptomeningitis (most common) or dural-based solitary mass (diffuse > nodular)

- May infiltrate along perivascular spaces

Microscopic Features

- **Noncaseating granulomas** are characteristic
  - Compact, radially arranged epithelioid cells

CLINICAL ISSUES

Presentation

- Most common signs/symptoms
  - CNS sarcoidosis
    - Visual loss
    - Pituitary/hypothalamic dysfunction
    - Cranial neuropathy: CNII > > CNV > CNVII & CNVIII
    - Headache, seizures, encephalopathy, dementia
    - Sensorineural hearing loss (SNHL) ± CNVII neuropathy
- Clinical profile
  - Adult with visual loss, central diabetes insipidus, & SNHL
- Laboratory findings are confirmatory
  - Kveim-Siltzbach skin test positive in 85%
  - Serum ACE levels elevated in < 50%
  - Use modified Zajicek criteria for diagnosis
    - Divides into confirmed, probable, & possible

Demographics

- Age
  - Bimodal: Initial peak 20-29 years; later peak > 50 years
- Ethnicity
  - USA: Risk in **Black patients** 3x that of White patients
- Epidemiology
  - CNS sarcoid: ~ **25%** of systemic sarcoidosis patients
  - One 1st-degree relative with sarcoid ↑ risk 3.7x

Natural History & Prognosis

- 2/3 have self-limited monophasic illness
  - Remainder have relapsing or chronic course
- > 50% recover without significant morbidity

Treatment

- No known cure; goal is alleviation of symptoms
- Prompt administration of steroids ± immunomodulators
  - Immunosuppressive therapy when disabling disease
- 50% of neurosarcoidosis progress despite therapy

DIAGNOSTIC CHECKLIST

Image Interpretation Pearls

- Consider sarcoid with multiple "meningiomas" in patient with systemic disease
- Consider sarcoid or metastases if bilateral IAC lesions in adult (not always neurofibromatosis type 2)

SELECTED REFERENCES

1. Cardoso O et al: Left-sided sensorineural hearing loss and facial weakness in a 35-year-old patient: a diagnostic challenge and case report. Cureus. 15(7):e41606, 2023
2. Cicilet S et al: Insights into neurosarcoidosis: an imaging perspective. Pol J Radiol. 88:e582-8, 2023
3. Kurokawa R et al: Dural and leptomeningeal diseases: anatomy, causes, and neuroimaging findings. Radiographics. 43(9):e230039, 2023
4. Nwebube CO et al: Facial nerve palsy in neurosarcoidosis: clinical course, neuroinflammatory accompaniments, ancillary investigations, and response to treatment. J Neurol. 269(10):5328-36, 2022
5. Pandey G et al: Primary presentation of sarcoidosis with profound bilateral sensorineural hearing loss. BMJ Case Rep. 14(8), 2021

TERMINOLOGY

- Vestibular schwannoma (VS): Benign tumor derived from Schwann cells of vestibular component of vestibulocochlear nerve (CNVIII) in cerebellopontine angle (CPA)-internal auditory canal (IAC) cistern

IMAGING

- VSs by far most common lesion found in CPA-IAC with imaging
- High-resolution T1WI fat-saturated enhanced MR represents gold standard for diagnosis
  - Focal, well-circumscribed, enhancing mass of CPA-IAC cistern
  - Small VS: Ovoid, enhancing intracanalicular mass
  - Large VS: Ice cream on cone shape in CPA and IAC
  - Most VSs are solid, but 15% have intramural cysts
- High-resolution T2 sequences: Tumor seen as "filling defect" (nodule or mass), isointense to brain, surrounded by hyperintense CSF signal

TOP DIFFERENTIAL DIAGNOSES

- Meningioma in CPA-IAC
- Facial nerve schwannoma in CPA-IAC
- Metastases in CPA-IAC
- Aneurysm in CPA
- Epidermoid cyst in CPA
- Arachnoid cyst in CPA

CLINICAL ISSUES

- Demographics and symptoms
  - Adults with unilateral sensorineural hearing loss
  - Other symptoms include unilateral tinnitus and vertigo
  - Larger tumors can cause brainstem compression and hydrocephalus
- Majority of tumors are unilateral & sporadic
- **Bilateral** VSs account for < 5% of cases; bilateral disease is hallmark of neurofibromatosis type 2 (NF2)

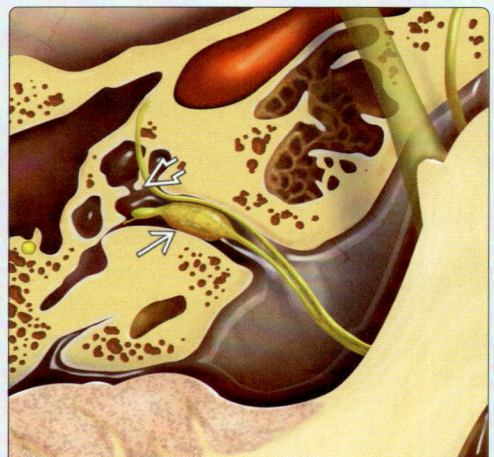
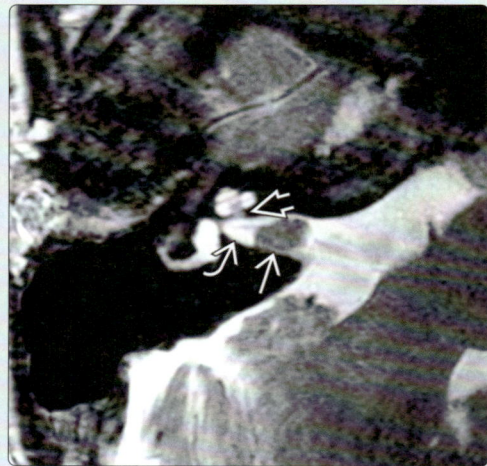

(Left) *Axial graphic shows a small intracanalicular vestibular schwannoma* ➡ *arising from the superior vestibular nerve. Notice that the cochlear nerve canal* ➡ *is uninvolved.* (Right) *Axial T2WI MR reveals a small intracanalicular vestibular schwannoma* ➡ *visualized as a soft tissue intensity mass surrounded by high-intensity CSF. The cochlear nerve canal* ➡ *is not involved, and an 8-mm fundal CSF cap* ➡ *is present.*

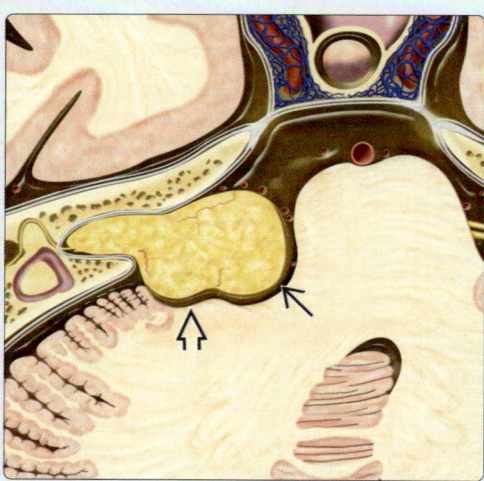
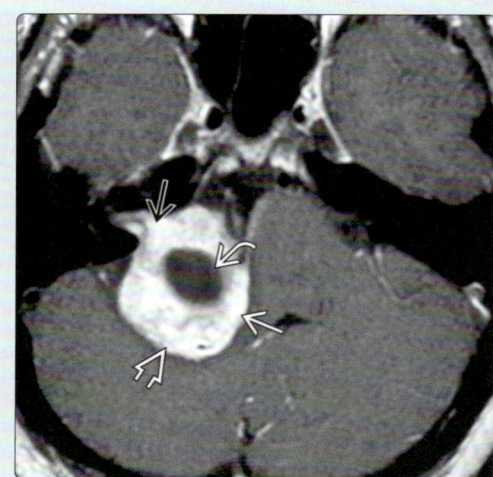

(Left) *Axial graphic of a large vestibular schwannoma reveals the typical ice cream on cone cerebellopontine angle (CPA)-internal auditory canal (IAC) morphology. Mass effect on the middle cerebellar peduncle* ➡ *and cerebellar hemisphere* ➡ *is evident.* (Right) *Axial T1WI C+ MR demonstrates a large CPA-IAC vestibular schwannoma compressing the middle cerebellar peduncle* ➡ *and cerebellar hemisphere* ➡. *Enhancement within the IAC* ➡ *and the large intramural cyst* ➡ *makes the imaging diagnosis certain.*

TERMINOLOGY

Abbreviations

- Vestibular schwannoma (VS)

Synonyms

- Acoustic schwannoma, acoustic neuroma, acoustic tumor
  - Uncommon names: Neurinoma, neurilemmoma

Definitions

- Benign tumor arising from Schwann cells of vestibular branches of CNVIII in cerebellopontine angle (CPA)-internal auditory canal (IAC)

IMAGING

General Features

- Best diagnostic clue
  - Avidly enhancing, well-circumscribed, ovoid or round nodule in IAC or CPA near porus acusticus; larger lesions often have classic **ice cream on cone** shape with CPA and IAC components
- Size
  - Small lesions: 2-10 mm
  - Larger lesions: Up to 5 cm in diameter
- Morphology
  - Small and intracanalicular VS: Round or ovoid mass
  - Large VS: "Ice cream" (CPA) on "cone" (IAC)

CT Findings

- CECT: Well-delineated, enhancing mass if large; sensitivity is dependent on technique, but smaller lesions (< 1 cm) can be missed by CECT
- Bone CT: IAC occasionally enlarged due to tumor; no intrinsic calcifications or hyperostosis, features that would suggest meningioma

MR Findings

- T1WI
  - Usually isointense with brain
  - ↑ intrinsic signal foci if rare macroscopic hemorrhage present
    - Microhemorrhages more common but not seen on T1
- T2WI FS
  - High-resolution, heavily T2-weighted through IAC (SPACE, DRIVE, CISS, FIESTA, etc.): Well-circumscribed nodule or mass, surrounded by hyperintense CSF signal of CPA-IAC cistern
- FLAIR
  - ↑ cochlear signal from ↑ perilymph protein
  - Large lesions can demonstrate edema or gliosis in adjacent brainstem or cerebellum
- T2* GRE
  - **Microhemorrhage** low-signal foci common on T2* GRE or SWI sequences; such microhemorrhage not generally seen in meningioma
- T1WI C+ FS
  - Focal, enhancing mass of CPA-IAC cistern centered on porus acusticus
  - 100% enhance strongly
  - **Most lesions are solid but 15%** have **intramural cysts** (low-signal foci)
  - Dural tails rare (compared to meningioma)
- Other MR findings
  - 0.5% with associated arachnoid cyst/trapped CSF

Imaging Recommendations

- Best imaging tool
  - Gold standard for evaluation of sensorineural hearing loss (SNHL) is whole-brain MR with dedicated high-resolution imaging through IACs, including axial and coronal thin-section T1WI C+ FS MR of CPA-IAC
- Protocol advice
  - Limited protocol with unenhanced sequences, including high-resolution T2 sequence (SPACE, CISS, or FIESTA) of CPA-IAC can be used as screening examination for VS
    - Used for uncomplicated unilateral SNHL in adult
    - Not useful for postoperative follow-up imaging

DIFFERENTIAL DIAGNOSIS

Meningioma in CPA-IAC

- Intracanalicular meningioma may mimic VS (rare)
- CECT: Dural-based mass eccentric to porus acusticus ± calcification
- T1WI C+ MR: Broad dural base with associated dural tails
- T2* GRE: Typically **no** microhemorrhages seen

Facial Nerve Schwannoma in CPA-IAC

- When confined to CPA-IAC, may exactly mimic VS
- Look for labyrinthine segment **tail** to differentiate

Metastases in CPA-IAC

- May have bilateral meningeal involvement
  - Beware of misdiagnosing as neurofibromatosis type 2 (NF2)

Aneurysm in CPA

- Ovoid to fusiform **complex signal** CPA mass

Epidermoid Cyst in CPA

- May mimic rare cystic VS
- Insinuating morphology
- T1WI C+ MR: Nonenhancing CPA mass
- DWI: **Diffusion restriction** characteristically present and generally diagnostic

Arachnoid Cyst in CPA

- Well-marginated CPA lesion: Does not enter IAC
- Follows CSF signal on all MR sequences
- DWI: No restricted diffusion

PATHOLOGY

General Features

- Genetics
  - Majority of VSs are unilateral and sporadic
  - Inactivating mutations of *NF2* tumor suppressor gene in majority of conventional VSs
  - Loss of chromosome 22q or *NF2* gene mutation seen in majority
  - NF2
    - Caused by pathogenic variants in *NF2* gene on chromosome 22q

- – Associated with multiple schwannomas, meningiomas, and ependymomas
- – 85% of NF2 cases demonstrate **bilateral** VSs
- Associated abnormalities
  - Arachnoid cyst (0.5%)
  - At surgery, may be arachnoid cyst or trapped CSF

Staging, Grading, & Classification

- WHO grade 1 lesion
- Koos grading scale: Defines tumor extension into CPA and brainstem compression
  - Grade I: Tumor confined to IAC
  - Grade II: Tumor extends to CPA without brainstem contact
  - Grade III: Tumor contacts brainstem without compression
  - Grade IV: Tumor compresses brainstem

Gross Pathologic & Surgical Features

- Tan, round-ovoid, encapsulated mass

Microscopic Features

- Differentiated Schwann cells in collagenous matrix
- Areas of compact, elongated cells = Antoni A
  - Most VSs composed mostly of Antoni A cells
- Areas less densely cellular with tumor loosely arranged ± clusters of lipid-laden cells = Antoni B
- Strong, diffuse expression of S100 protein
- No necrosis; instead intramural cysts
- < 1% hemorrhagic

CLINICAL ISSUES

Presentation

- Most common signs/symptoms
  - Adults with unilateral SNHL
- Clinical profile
  - Slowly progressive SNHL (90%)
  - Laboratory
    - – Brainstem electric response audiometry (BERA) most sensitive preimaging test for VS
    - – Screening MR could replace BERA
- Other symptoms
  - Small VS: Tinnitus (ringing in ear); disequilibrium
  - Large VS:
    - – Brainstem, cerebellar compression, hydrocephalus
    - – Trigeminal ± facial neuropathy possible

Demographics

- Age
  - Adults; VSs rare in children unless NF2
  - Peak = 40-60 years
  - Range = 30-70 years
- Epidemiology
  - Most common CPA-IAC mass (85-90%)
  - Most common lesion in unilateral SNHL **(> 90%)**
  - 3rd most common benign intracranial neoplasm following meningiomas and pituitary adenomas

Natural History & Prognosis

- No parameters reliably predict growth or growth rate in newly diagnosed VS

- Some tumors have higher growth rates (> 3-mm diameter/year) and more likely to proceed to significant hearing loss
- ~ 50% of tumors may be expected to grow over 5-year period

Treatment

- Observation appropriate in some cases of incidental or asymptomatic VS
  - 50% of patients will lose functional hearing at 3-4 years during observation
- **Surgical approach** depends on hearing status, size of VS, experience of surgeon, and patient factors
- **Retrosigmoid approach** when CPA or medial IAC component present
- **Translabyrinthine** resection if no hearing preservation possible
- **Middle cranial fossa** approach for intracanalicular VS
- Negative prognostic imaging findings for hearing preservation after surgery
  - Size > 2 cm
  - VS involves IAC fundus ± cochlear aperture
  - Persistent postoperative cochlear FLAIR hyperintensity
- **Stereotactic radiosurgery (SRS)**
  - Can be used primarily to treat small- to moderate-sized VSs without significant mass effect
  - Focused irradiation (12-14 Gy) with high conformity and precision in single fraction
  - 5-year control rates reported to range 90-99%
  - 5-year hearing preservation rates range 40-80%
  - Used when medical contraindications to surgery and residual postoperative VS
- For larger tumors, fractionated radiotherapy or hypofractionated stereotactic radiotherapy increasingly used

DIAGNOSTIC CHECKLIST

Image Interpretation Pearls

- Unilateral, well-circumscribed IAC or CPA-IAC mass should be considered VS until proven otherwise
- Always make sure there is no labyrinthine tail (tumor extending to geniculate ganglion) on all VSs to avoid misdiagnosing facial nerve schwannoma
- Bilateral VS pathognomonic of NF2

Reporting Tips

- Comment on tumor size ± CPA involvement
- Does VS involve cochlear nerve foramen or IAC fundus?
- How large in millimeters is fundal CSF cap?
- Is hemorrhage, intramural cyst, or arachnoid cyst/trapped CSF present within or associated with VS?
- When small, comment on nerve of origin if possible

SELECTED REFERENCES

1. Welby JP et al: Vestibular schwannoma-related increased labyrinthine postgadolinium 3D-FLAIR signal intensity and association with hearing impairment. AJNR Am J Neuroradiol. 46(3):567-71, 2025
2. Kujawa A et al: Automated Koos Classification of vestibular schwannoma. Front Radiol. 2:837191, 2022
3. Carlson ML et al: Vestibular schwannomas. N Engl J Med. 384(14):1335-48, 2021

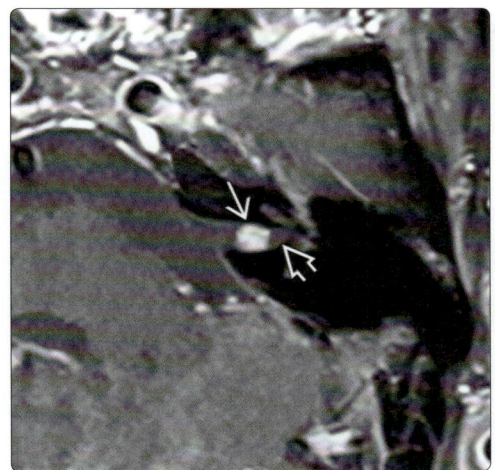
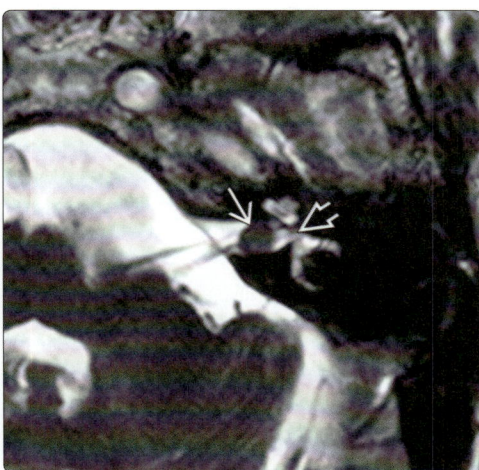

(Left) Axial T1WI C+ FS MR in a patient with left sensorineural hearing loss shows a small, enhancing vestibular schwannoma ➡ within the IAC with a 3-mm fundal CSF cap ➡ lateral to the tumor. (Right) Axial CISS MR in the same patient reveals a filling defect ➡ within the high-signal CSF in the IAC. The vestibular schwannoma is easily diagnosed with CISS imaging. The fundal CSF cap ➡ is more readily seen with T2 or CISS MR.

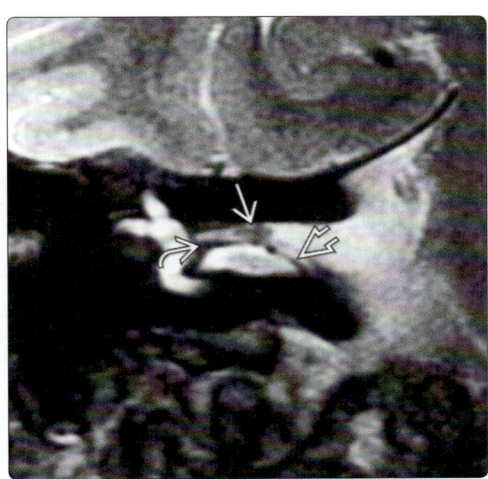
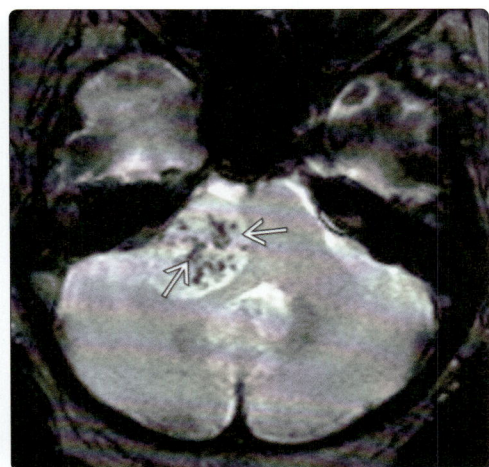

(Left) Coronal high-resolution thin-section T2WI MR demonstrates a 2-mm superior vestibular schwannoma ➡. The lesion is seen superior to the crista falciformis ➡ with the anterior inferior cerebellar artery loop ➡ visible in the lateral IAC. (Right) Axial T2* GRE MR reveals punctate microhemorrhages ➡ in the CPA component of a larger vestibular schwannoma. When present, this finding is highly suggestive of vestibular schwannoma.

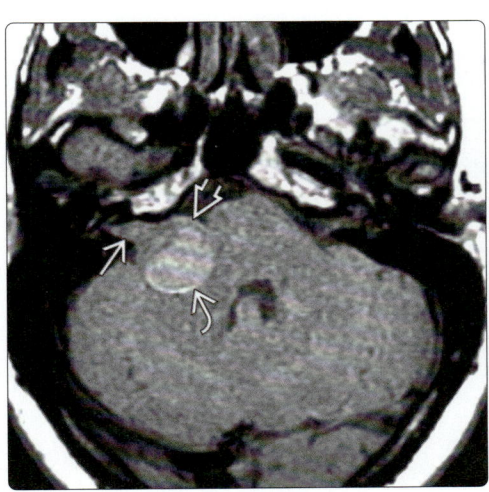
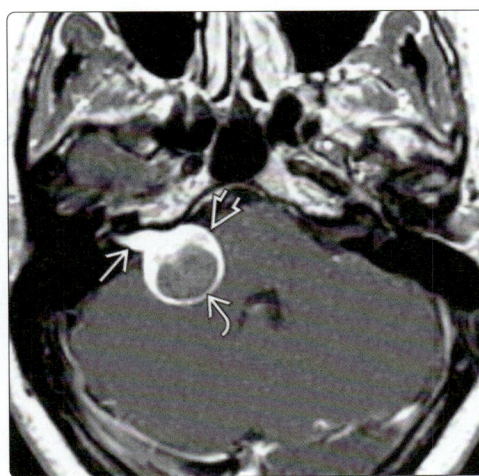

(Left) Axial T1WI MR reveals the IAC ➡ and CPA ➡ components of a larger vestibular schwannoma. Increased signal in the medial CPA portion of this tumor ➡ is due to methemoglobin from a subacute intratumoral hemorrhage. (Right) Axial T1WI C+ MR in the same patient shows an enhancing vestibular schwannoma with IAC ➡ and CPA ➡ components. The nonenhancing medial component ➡ is due to hemorrhage.

PHACE Syndrome

TERMINOLOGY

- **PHACE(S)**: Association of segmental craniofacial infantile hemangioma (IH) & 1 or more features listed in acronym
  - **P**osterior fossa malformations
  - **H**emangioma
  - **A**rterial lesions
  - **C**ardiac abnormalities/aortic coarctation
  - **E**ye abnormalities
  - **S**ternal defects or supraumbilical raphe
    - Deemphasized in recent literature

IMAGING

- Proliferating regional or midline cervicofacial IH: Lobulated or plaque-like, intense enhancement, prominent vascularity, increased perfusion on ASL
- Unilateral cerebellar hypoplasia & prominent retrocerebellar CSF space
- Widened internal auditory canal (IAC) ± IH ± persistent stapedial artery

- Hypoplasia, aplasia, aberrancy, ectasia, tortuosity, & stenoocclusive changes of major craniocervical arteries
- ± reduced perfusion (or infarction) in affected arterial territory

TOP DIFFERENTIAL DIAGNOSES

- Sturge-Weber syndrome
- Vestibular schwannoma
- Loeys-Dietz syndrome

CLINICAL ISSUES

- Cutaneous: Large regional or midline craniofacial IH (20% of these patients have PHACE)
  - IH appears at birth or in neonate
- Sex: 80-90% female incidence

DIAGNOSTIC CHECKLIST

- Look for ipsilateral cerebellar hemisphere anomaly of PHACE in patient clinically mistaken for Sturge-Weber syndrome with port-wine stain

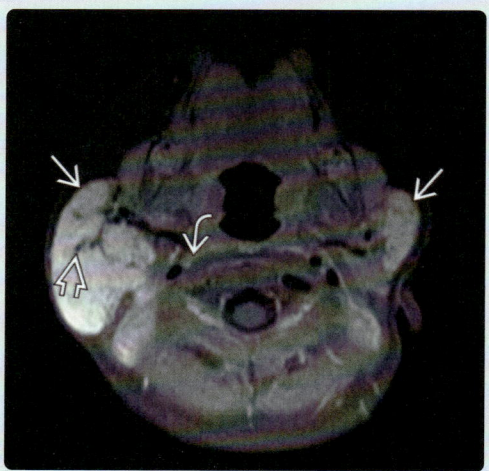
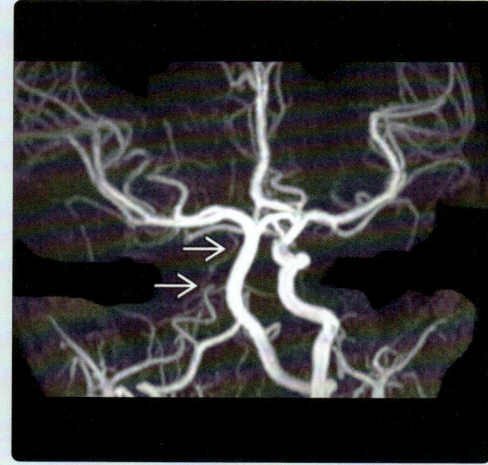

(Left) *Axial T1 C+ FS MR in an 8-month-old baby with PHACE syndrome shows right greater than left parotid/periparotid hemangiomas ➡ with typical intense enhancement, well-defined margins, & intralesional flow voids ➡. Note the absence of normal flow void in the expected location of the right internal carotid artery (ICA) ➡.* (Right) *Anterior 3D time-of-flight MRA in the same patient shows marked hypoplasia of the right ICA ➡. The patient also had hemangiomas in a bearded distribution as well as in the floor of mouth & airway.*

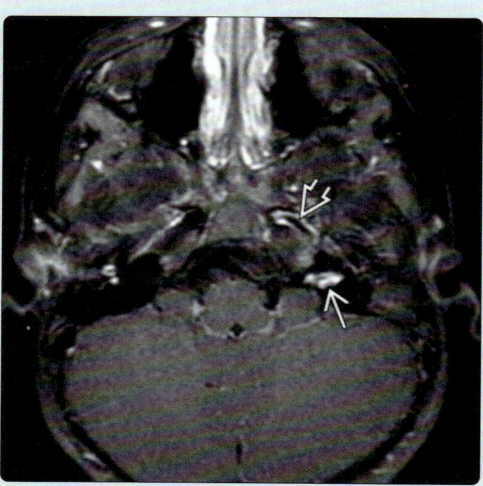
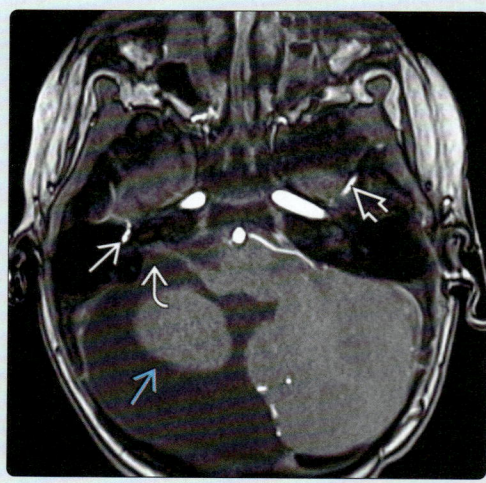

(Left) *Axial T1 C+ FS MR in a child with PHACE syndrome shows an enhancing left IAC lesion ➡, consistent with infantile hemangioma, which, along with extracranial hemangiomas, (not shown) involuted over time. A small left petrous ICA ➡ is also noted. MRA neck showed long-segment cervical ICA stenosis.* (Right) *Axial 3D time-of-flight MRA of an infant girl with PHACE & right cerebellar hypoplasia ➡ shows a right persistent stapedial artery ➡. Note the normal left middle meningeal artery ➡. The right IAC ➡ is widened.*

TERMINOLOGY

Synonyms

- PHACE association or syndrome, PHACES, PHACE(S)

Definitions

- Infantile hemangioma (IH): Most common benign vascular tumor of infancy; has predictable life cycle with proliferating & involuting phases
- **PHACE** acronym
  - **P**osterior fossa malformations
  - **H**emangioma (infantile)
  - **A**rterial lesions
  - **C**ardiac abnormalities/aortic coarctation
  - **E**ye abnormalities
- PHACE syndrome: Association of characteristic segmental or > 5-cm facial/scalp IHs + 1 major or 2 minor criteria
  - Major criteria are designated for brain, cerebrovascular, cardiovascular, ocular, & ventral/midline findings
- Possible PHACE: As above + 1 minor criterion or no IH + 2 major criteria

IMAGING

General Features

- Best diagnostic clue
  - Cervicofacial IH: Single or multiple; regional or midline
  - Posterior fossa anomaly: Unilateral (or bilateral) cerebellar hypoplasia ± malformation, prominent retrocerebellar CSF space
  - Cerebrovascular arterial abnormalities
  - Cardiovascular abnormalities
    - Aortic arch coarctation ± aneurysm, aberrant subclavian artery
  - Ocular anomalies

Imaging Recommendations

- Best imaging tool
  - MR/MRA for IH extent & CNS findings
- Protocol advice
  - Brain & orbits/face/neck MR/MRA; T1, T2 FS, ASL, T1 C+ FS MR; time-of-flight MRA

CT Findings

- IH: Enhances intensely; small, petrous internal carotid artery (ICA) canal; widened internal auditory canal (IAC) ipsilateral to cerebellar hypoplasia
- Persistent stapedial artery, absent foramen spinosum

MR Findings

- Proliferating IH: Lobulated, intermediate to high signal on T2 MR, prominent flow voids, intense uniform enhancement, increased perfusion on ASL
- Involuting IH: Smaller, less prominent flow voids, increased fibrofatty tissue, less enhancement
- Multiple IHs: Can involve CNS
  - Temporal bone locations: Pinna, external auditory canal, middle ear, & IAC (IAC IH simulates schwannoma)
  - Cavernous sinus IH
- Brain MR: Cerebellar hypoplasia ± malformation (unilateral > bilateral) & prominent retrocerebellar CSF space
  - True Dandy-Walker malformation is uncommon
  - Asymmetric Meckel cave enlargement
  - Agenesis/hypogenesis of corpus callosum ± lipoma
  - ± reduced perfusion (or infarction) in affected arterial territory
- MRA: Hypoplasia/aplasia, aberrant origin or course, kinking, tortuosity, loops, ectasia, or aneurysm of ICAs or vertebral arteries
  - Persistent fetal connections (e.g., persistent stapedial artery); stenoocclusive change with moyamoya-type collaterals; occasional intracranial arteriovenous fistula/arteriovenous malformation

DIFFERENTIAL DIAGNOSIS

Sturge-Weber Syndrome

- Facial capillary-venular port-wine stain

Vestibular Schwannoma

- Older child; enhancing tumor lacks marked vascularity

Loeys-Dietz Syndrome

- Tortuous ectatic craniocervical vessels & aortic root aneurysms

CLINICAL ISSUES

Presentation

- Most common signs/symptoms
  - Plaque-like cutaneous craniofacial IH: Typically supraorbital, malar, beard-like, or midline; L > R
- Other signs/symptoms
  - Neurologic: Developmental delay, seizures, headaches, stroke
  - Cardiac & aortic: Cardiac failure, cardiac tamponade

Demographics

- Precursor skin lesion is often present at birth with typical IH developing in neonatal period
  - Incidence ~ 5%; ~ 80-90% female incidence
  - PHACE syndrome is much less common

Natural History & Prognosis

- Variable prognosis, depends on type & severity of anomalies
- IH typically involutes by 5-7 years old
- Reports of progressive vascular phenomena leading to neurologic deficits from stroke
- Variable symptoms from cardiovascular manifestations

Treatment

- Propranolol: Accelerates involution
- Neurosurgical revascularization

SELECTED REFERENCES

1. ISSVA Classification of Vascular Anomalies: 2025 International Society for the Study of Vascular Anomalies. Published 2018. Updated 2025. Accessed May 2025. https://www.issva.org/classification
2. Keith L: PHACE syndrome: a review. Semin Pediatr Neurol. ePub, 2024
3. Proisy M et al: PHACES syndrome and associated anomalies: risk associated with small and large facial hemangiomas. AJR Am J Roentgenol. 1-8, 2021
4. Mamlouk MD et al: Arterial spin-labeling perfusion for PHACE syndrome. AJNR Am J Neuroradiol. 42(1):173-7, 2020
5. Wright JN et al: Asymmetric Meckel cave enlargement: a potential marker of PHACES syndrome. AJNR Am J Neuroradiol. 38(6):1223-7, 2017

CPA-IAC Meningioma

TERMINOLOGY

- Definition: Benign, unencapsulated neoplasm arising from meningothelial arachnoid cells of cerebellopontine angle (CPA)-internal auditory canal (IAC) dura

IMAGING

- 10% of meningiomas occur in posterior fossa
- When in CPA, asymmetric to IAC porus acusticus
- NECT: 25% calcified; 2 types seen
  - Homogeneous, sand-like (psammomatous)
  - Focal sunburst, globular, or rim pattern
- Bone CT: Hyperostotic or permeative sclerotic bone changes possible (en plaque type)
  - Bone CT indicated if bone invasion suspected on MR
- T2 MR: High-signal crescent from CSF ("CSF cleft")
  - Pial supply seen as flow voids between tumor & brain
- T1 C+ MR: Enhancing dural-based mass with dural tails centered along posterior petrous wall
  - IAC dural tail usually reactive, not tumor

TOP DIFFERENTIAL DIAGNOSES

- Vestibular schwannoma
- Dural metastases, CPA-IAC
- Epidermoid cyst, CPA-IAC
- Sarcoidosis, CPA-IAC

CLINICAL ISSUES

- Accounts for ~ 20% of primary intracranial tumors
  - Most common primary nonglial tumor
- 2nd most common CPA tumor
- Slow-growing tumor, displacing adjacent structures
- Often found as incidental brain MR finding
- < 10% symptomatic, usually no sensorineural hearing loss
- Treatment
  - Follow with imaging if smaller size and older patient
  - Preoperative embolization ↓ operative time & blood loss
  - Surgical removal if medically safe
  - Adjunctive radiation therapy with incomplete surgery

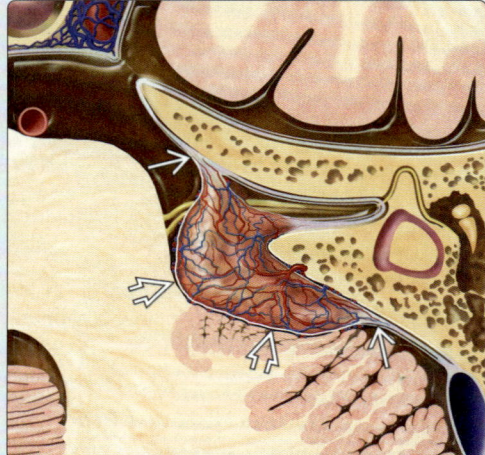
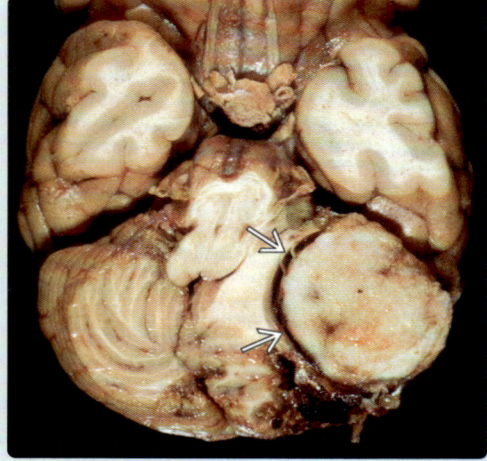

(Left) Axial graphic at the level of the IAC shows a large CPA meningioma causing mass effect on the brainstem and cerebellum. Notice the broad dural base creating the shape of a mushroom cap. Dural tails ➡ are present in ~ 60% of cases, typically representing reactive rather than neoplastic change. A CSF-vascular cleft ➡ is also visible. (Right) Gross pathologic section viewed from below shows a large CPA meningioma with a broad dural base compressing the cerebellum. The specimen demonstrates a CSF-vascular cleft ➡.

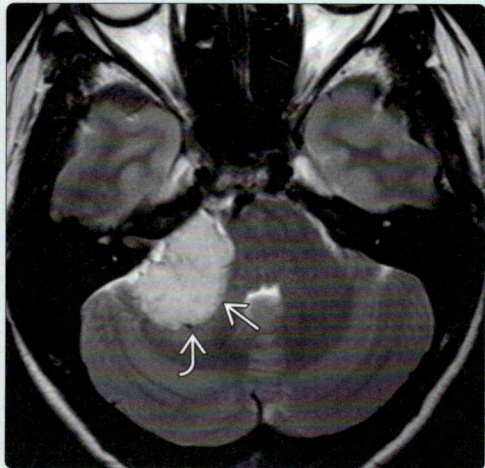
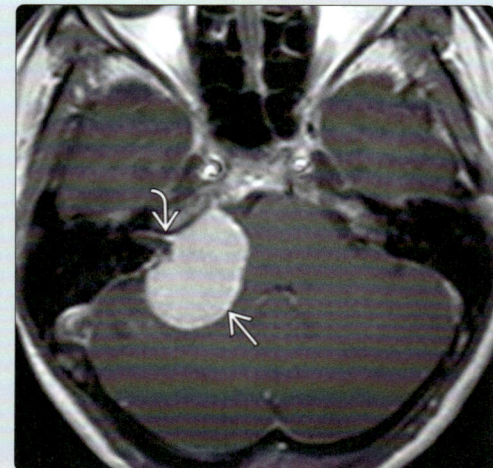

(Left) Axial T2 MR shows a mildly hyperintense meningioma in the right CPA ➡. Although centered over the IAC, there is no associated tumor involvement or flaring. Surface flow voids indicating pial supply are noted along the tumor-brain interface ➡. (Right) Axial T1 C+ MR shows homogeneous enhancement of this WHO grade I meningioma ➡ centered over the IAC. Note enhancement in the IAC is peripheral ➡, along the dura (dural tail), not along the expected course of the nerves, supporting the correct diagnosis of meningioma.

TERMINOLOGY

Definitions

- Benign, unencapsulated neoplasm arising from meningothelial arachnoid cells of cerebellopontine angle (CPA)-internal auditory canal (IAC) dura

IMAGING

General Features

- Best diagnostic clue
  - CPA dural-based enhancing mass with **dural tails**
- Location
  - 2–11% of meningiomas occur at CPA-IAC
  - When in CPA, **asymmetric** to IAC porus acusticus
- Size
  - Broad range; usually 1-8 cm but may be larger
  - Generally significantly larger than vestibular schwannoma at presentation
- Morphology
  - 3 distinct morphologies
    - Mushroom cap (hemispherical) with broad base towards posterior petrous wall (75%)
    - Plaque-like (en plaque) ± bone invasion with hyperostosis (20%)
    - Ovoid mass mimics vestibular schwannoma (5%)
  - Larger lesions often herniate superiorly through incisura into medial middle cranial fossa

CT Findings

- NECT
  - 25% isodense, 75% hyperdense
  - 25% calcified; 2 types seen
    - Homogeneous, sand-like (psammomatous)
    - Focal sunburst, globular, or rim pattern
- CECT
  - > 90% strong, uniform enhancement
- Bone CT
  - Hyperostotic or permeative sclerotic bone changes possible (en plaque type)
  - IAC flaring is rare (cf. vestibular schwannoma)

MR Findings

- T1WI
  - Isointense or minimally hyperintense to gray matter
  - When tumor has calcifications or is highly fibrous, hypointense areas are visible
- T2WI
  - Wide range of possible signals on T2 sequence
    - Isointense or hypointense CPA mass (compared to gray matter) is most likely meningioma
    - Focal or diffuse parenchymal low signal seen if calcified or highly fibrous
  - **CSF-vascular cleft**
    - Flow voids between tumor & brain indicate pial supply
    - High-signal crescent from CSF
  - Dural arterial feeders seen as arborizing flow voids
    - Spoke-wheel or sunburst pattern may be seen
  - High signal in adjacent brainstem or cerebellum
    - Represents peritumoral brain edema
    - Correlates with pial blood supply
    - Signals problems with safe removal
  - Thin hypointensity of tumor surface layer (peripheral rim) indicates low potential for tumor growth
- T2* GRE
  - Calcifications may bloom
- T1WI C+
  - Enhancing **dural-based mass** with **dural tails** centered along posterior petrous wall
    - > 95% enhance strongly
    - Heterogeneous enhancement when large
  - Dural tail in ~ 60%
    - More often **reactive** rather than neoplastic change
    - IAC component may mimic vestibular schwannoma
  - En plaque: Sessile, thickened, enhancing dura
- SWI
  - Foci of intratumoral blooming due to microhemorrhage
    - Typically present in schwannomas
    - Blooming in meningiomas rare, likely microcalcifications (phase images differentiate)

Angiographic Findings

- Digital subtraction angiography
  - Dural vessels supply tumor center
    - Dural feeders give sunburst or spoke-wheel appearance
  - **Pial vessels** supply **tumor rim**
  - Prolonged vascular "stain" into venous phase
- Interventional: Preoperative embolization
  - ↓ operative time and blood loss
  - Particulate agents favored (e.g., polyvinyl alcohol)
  - Optimal time between embolization & surgery: 7-9 days

Nuclear Medicine Findings

- DOTATATE PET
  - SSTR2 (somatostatin receptor 2) receptors present in nearly all meningiomas
  - Evolving role in posttreatment surveillance imaging

Imaging Recommendations

- Best imaging tool
  - Enhanced MR focused to posterior fossa
  - Bone CT if bone invasion suspected on MR
- Protocol advice
  - Whole-brain T2 ± FLAIR shows brain edema best

DIFFERENTIAL DIAGNOSIS

Vestibular Schwannoma

- Intracanalicular 1st, then CPA extension
- Intracanalicular meningioma may mimic

Dural Metastases, CPA-IAC

- May be bilateral in CPA area
- Multifocal meningeal involvement

Epidermoid Cyst, CPA-IAC

- Near CSF signal insinuating mass on MR
- DWI high signal is characteristic

Sarcoidosis, CPA-IAC

- Often multifocal, dural-based foci
- Look for infundibular stalk involvement

PATHOLOGY

General Features

- Etiology
  - Arises from arachnoid ("cap") meningothelial cells
  - Radiation therapy (XRT) predisposes
    - Most common radiation-induced tumor; latency 20-35 years
- Genetics
  - Long arm deletions of chromosome 22 are common
    - *NF2* gene inactivated in 60% of sporadic cases
  - May have progesterone, prolactin receptors; may express growth hormone
- Associated abnormalities
  - Neurofibromatosis type 2 (NF2)
    - 10% of multiple meningiomas have NF2
    - Meningioma + schwannoma = NF2
    - Multiple inherited schwannomas, meningiomas, and ependymomas (MISME)

Staging, Grading, & Classification

- WHO grading classification (grades 1-3)
  - Typical meningioma (grade 1, benign) = 90%
  - Atypical meningioma (grade 2) = 9%
  - Malignant (anaplastic) meningioma (grade 3) = 1%

Gross Pathologic & Surgical Features

- "Mushroom cap" (globose, hemispherical) morphology most common (75%)
- En plaque morphology (20%) also seen in CPA
- Sharply circumscribed, unencapsulated
- Adjacent dural tail is usually reactive, not neoplastic

Microscopic Features

- Subtypes (wide range of histology with little bearing on imaging appearance or clinical outcome)
  - Meningothelial (lobules of meningothelial cells)
  - Fibrous (parallel, interlacing fascicles of spindle-shaped cells)
  - Transitional (mixed; "onion bulb" whorls and lobules)
  - Angiomatous (↑ vascular channels), not equated with obsolete term angioblastic meningioma
  - Lipoblastic: Metaplasia into adipocytes; large triglyceride fat droplets
  - Miscellaneous forms (microcystic, chordoid, clear cell, secretory, lymphoplasmacyte rich, etc.)

CLINICAL ISSUES

Presentation

- Most common signs/symptoms
  - Incidental brain MR finding
  - < 10% symptomatic
  - Large tumors may present with hydrocephalus
- Clinical profile
  - Adult undergoing brain MR for unrelated indication

Demographics

- Age
  - Middle-aged, older adults; mean age 60 years
  - If found in children, consider possibility of NF2
- Sex
  - M:F = 1:1.5-3
- Ethnicity
  - More common in Black patients
- Epidemiology
  - Accounts for ~ 20% of primary intracranial tumors
    - Most common primary nonglial tumor
  - 1-1.5% prevalence at autopsy or imaging
  - 10% multiple (NF2; multiple meningiomatosis)
  - 2nd most common CPA-IAC mass
  - Risk factors: Ionizing radiation, 1st-degree family relative

Natural History & Prognosis

- Slow-growing tumor
- Compresses rather than invades structures
- Negative prognostic findings on MR
  - Peritumoral edema in adjacent brainstem
  - Significant subjacent bone invasion
- Positive prognostic finding on imaging
  - Thin, T2-hypointense tumor surface layer on MR
  - Heavily calcified tumor on CT suggests psammomatous (rare with low tendency towards growth or recurrence)
- Spontaneous meningioma regression may occur

Treatment

- Asymptomatic: Follow with serial imaging if smaller tumor or older patient
- Surgical removal if medically safe
  - Complete surgical removal possible in 95% when tumor does not invade skull base
- XRT
  - Adjunctive therapy with incomplete surgery
  - Primary therapy if extensive skull base invasion

DIAGNOSTIC CHECKLIST

Consider

- Meningioma when MR shows hemispherical, dural-based enhancing CPA mass with dural tails
- Meningioma when CPA mass is large but asymptomatic

Image Interpretation Pearls

- Dural tail in IAC suggests meningioma
- Focal or diffuse hypointensity on T2 in CPA mass typical
- T2-hypointense rim or calcified tumor have low growth rate
- Microbleeds on SWI favor schwannoma, not meningioma

Reporting Tips

- Report tumor extent, including intraosseous component
  - Mention cranial nerves in area of involvement
  - Note brain edema indicating pia-arachnoid involvement

SELECTED REFERENCES

1. Kurz SC et al: Evaluation of the SSTR2-targeted radiopharmaceutical 177Lu-DOTATATE and SSTR2-specific 68Ga-DOTATATE PET as imaging biomarker in patients with intracranial meningioma. Clin Cancer Res. 30(4):680-6, 2024
2. Mehta NH et al: Cerebellopontine angle meningiomas: a multi-institutional cohort study. Neurosurgery. 97(1):105-11, 2024
3. Shi Q et al: Imaging features of pediatric meningiomas: emphasis on unusual locations. Childs Nerv Syst. 40(12):3933-42, 2024
4. Smirniotopoulos JG et al: Differential diagnosis of intracranial masses. IDKD Springer Series, 2020

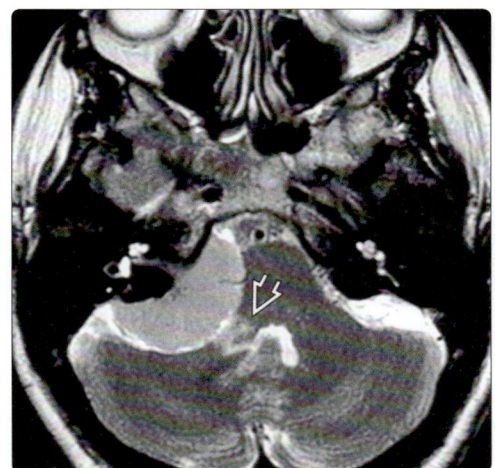
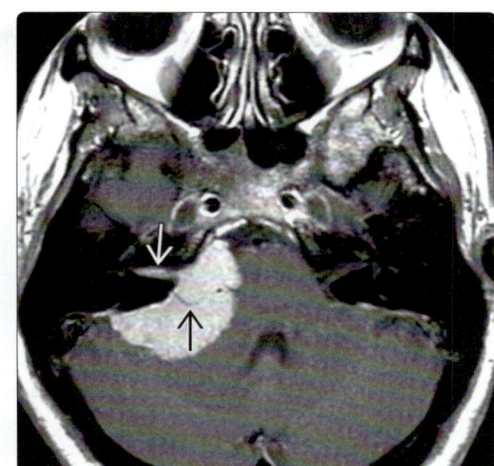

(Left) Axial T2 MR reveals high signal in the adjacent brachium pontis ➡. Pial invasion by the meningioma is likely. This MR finding is predictive of an increased risk of complications when surgical removal occurs. (Right) Axial T1 C+ MR in the same patient demonstrates the enhancing, large CPA meningioma with a small IAC component ➡. This degree and depth of IAC enhancement usually signifies a tumor rather than a dural reaction. Associated flow void is often seen with meningioma ➡.

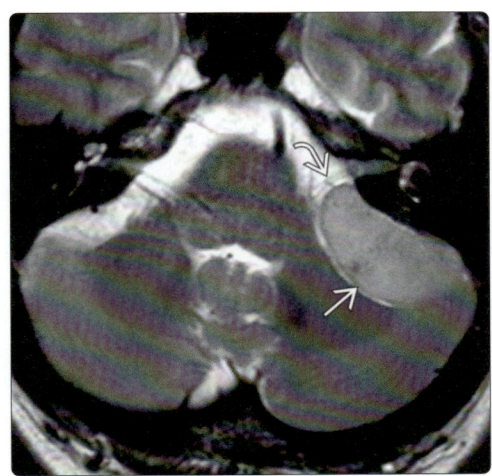
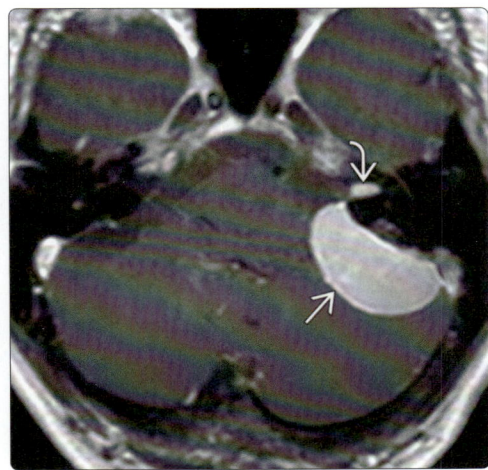

(Left) Axial T2 MR in a 60-year-old woman with left worse than right hearing loss shows an extraaxial mass nearly isointense to gray matter. A thin, peripheral, hypointense tumor margin ➡ predicts a low rate of future growth. The cisternal CNVII-VIII ➡ are displaced by the tumor. (Right) Axial T1 C+ FS MR in the same patient demonstrates the enhancing meningioma involving the left CPA ➡ with a broad dural base of attachment. The small, eccentric, intracanalicular component ➡ is better seen on enhanced MR.

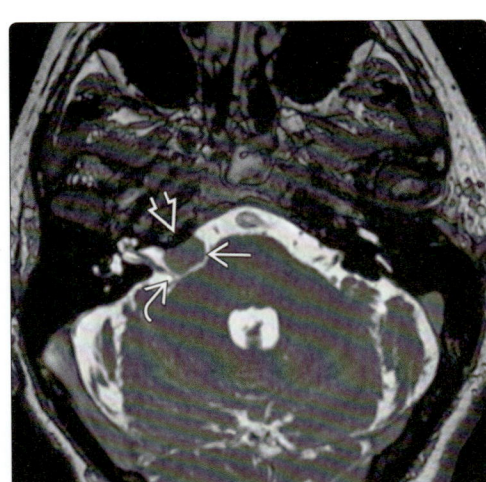
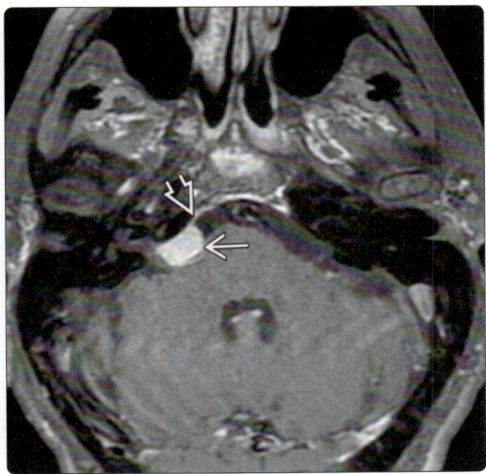

(Left) Axial SSFP MR shows a dural-based mass along the petrous ridge ➡. Note the hyperostosis evident by the outward displacement of the thickened petrous temporal bone ➡ adjacent to the site of dural attachment. The mass is eccentric to the IAC and displaces CNVII-VIII slightly posteriorly ➡. (Right) Axial T1 C+ FS MR shows homogeneous enhancement of this CPA meningioma ➡. A thin enhancing dural tail ➡ is evident.

CPA-IAC Facial Nerve Schwannoma

TERMINOLOGY

- Facial nerve schwannoma (FNS): Rare, benign tumor of Schwann cells that surround CNVII in CPA-IAC ± labyrinthine CNVII

IMAGING

- Temporal bone CT findings
  - Smoothly widened facial canal without destruction
- MR findings
  - T1 C+ MR: CPA-IAC-facial canal enhancing mass

TOP DIFFERENTIAL DIAGNOSES

- Bell palsy (herpetic facial paralysis)
- Vestibular schwannoma
- CPA-IAC meningioma

PATHOLOGY

- Tumor of Schwann cells lining CNVII, usually sporadic
- Neurofibromatosis type 2
  - Bilateral CPA-IAC schwannomas
  - May be of **vestibular** or **facial** nerve origin

CLINICAL ISSUES

- Clinical presentation
  - Sensorineural hearing loss (SNHL) if CPA-IAC
  - Facial nerve paralysis &/or conductive hearing loss if tympanic segment involved
  - SNHL & facial nerve paralysis similar in frequency
- Treatment options
  - Conservative management: Do nothing until CNVII paralysis present
  - Surgical management: Used when CNVII paralysis + other symptoms evolving
    - Debulking also effective
  - Stereotactic radiosurgery
    - Used for poor surgical candidates
    - Recent use in small- to medium-sized FNS with CNVII function & hearing relatively preserved

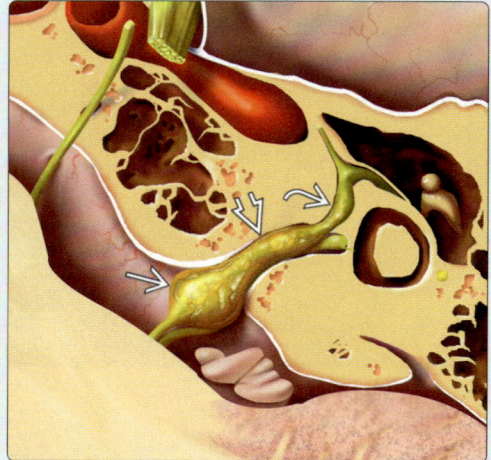

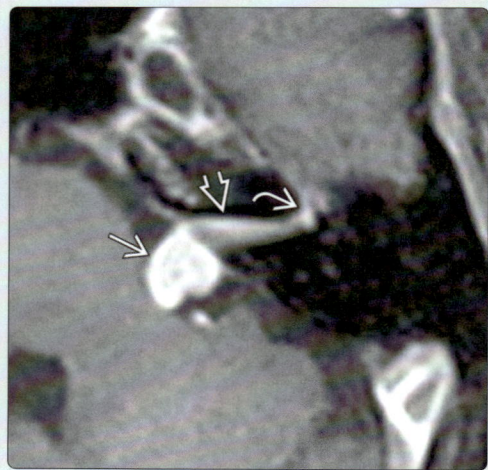

(Left) *Axial graphic of a larger facial nerve schwannoma (FNS) shows cerebellopontine angle (CPA) ("ice cream")* ➡️ *& internal auditory canal (IAC) ("cone")* ➡️ *components that mimic a vestibular schwannoma. The labyrinthine segment of facial nerve involvement* ➡️ *makes the diagnosis.* (Right) *Axial T1 C+ FS MR in a patient with unilateral sensorineural hearing loss shows FNS with CPA* ➡️ *& IAC* ➡️ *components. Note the labyrinthine segment facial nerve tail* ➡️*, which differentiates FNS from vestibular schwannoma.*

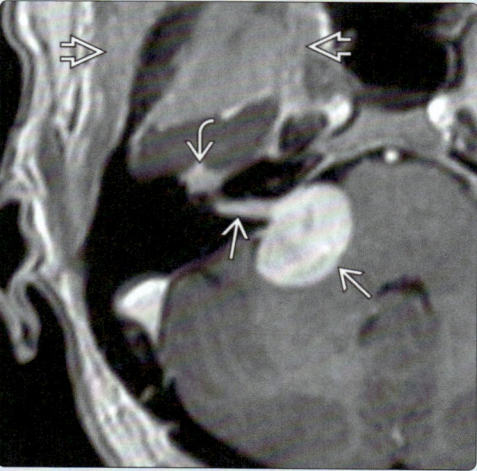

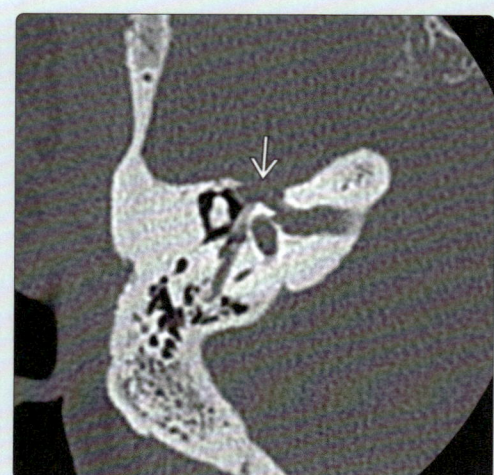

(Left) *Axial T1 C+ MR in a patient with NF2 shows a large, enhancing CPA-IAC mass* ➡️ *with extension to the geniculate fossa* ➡️*, compatible with facial schwannoma. Note large middle cranial fossa meningioma with transosseous extension also present* ➡️*.* (Right) *Axial bone CT in the same patient shows characteristic smooth, nondestructive osseous expansion of the anterior genu/geniculate fossa of facial nerve* ➡️ *due to schwannoma.*

TERMINOLOGY

Abbreviations

- Facial nerve schwannoma (FNS)

Synonyms

- Facial neuroma, facial neurilemmoma

Definitions

- Rare, benign tumor of Schwann cells that surround facial nerve in cerebellopontine angle (CPA)-internal auditory canal (IAC)

IMAGING

General Features

- Best diagnostic clue
  - CPA-IAC mass + **tail in labyrinthine CNVII canal**
- Location
  - CPA-IAC & labyrinthine segment of CNVII canal
  - Geniculate ganglion & tympanic segments most commonly involved in temporal bone
- Morphology
  - Large: CPA-IAC ice cream on cone shape with comma-shaped tail in labyrinthine segment CNVII
  - Small: IAC mass curves into labyrinthine tail (may be in IAC CNVII only mimicking vestibular schwannoma)

CT Findings

- Bone CT
  - ↑ size labyrinthine CNVII canal ± geniculate fossa

MR Findings

- PWI
  - Dynamic T1 C+ shows gradual, homogeneous enhancement of entire lesion
- T1WI C+
  - CPA-IAC-labyrinthine canal enhancing mass
    - ± **intramural cystic change**
- CISS, FIESTA, T2 SPACE
  - FNS CPA-IAC = low-signal mass displaces CSF signal
  - May identify nerve of origin for very tiny schwannomas

Imaging Recommendations

- Best imaging tool
  - CNVII or CNVIII symptoms: 1st study with T1 C+ FS MR
    - Axial ≤ 3-mm T1 C+ MR; axial & coronal of CPA-IAC
  - Bone CT: Smooth, scalloped widening of facial canal without destructive changes

DIFFERENTIAL DIAGNOSIS

Bell Palsy (Herpetic Facial Paralysis)

- T1 C+ MR: Prominent enhancement of intratemporal CNVII with IAC fundal tuft of enhancement

Vestibular Schwannoma

- T1 C+ MR: CPA-IAC enhancing mass without labyrinthine canal tail or other facial canal involvement

CPA-IAC Meningioma

- T1 C+ MR: Dural-based, eccentric CPA enhancing mass with dural tail projecting into IAC

PATHOLOGY

General Features

- Etiology
  - Tumor of Schwann cells investing CNVII
- Genetics
  - Multiple schwannomas = neurofibromatosis 2 (NF2)
- Associated abnormalities
  - **NF2**: Bilateral vestibular schwannoma; other cranial nerve schwannoma, meningiomas also seen

Gross Pathologic & Surgical Features

- Tumor arises from outer nerve sheath layer

Microscopic Features

- Encapsulated; bundles of spindle-shaped Schwann cells forming whorled pattern
- Cellular architecture: Densely cellular (**Antoni A**) areas ± loose, myxomatous (**Antoni B**) areas

CLINICAL ISSUES

Presentation

- Most common signs/symptoms
  - Transient or persistent facial palsy is most common symptom, followed by hearing loss
    - IAC or CPA FNS cause sensorineural hearing loss
    - Tympanic segment FNS tends to cause conductive hearing loss; more prone to develop facial palsy later
  - Other symptoms: Vertigo, hemifacial spasm

Demographics

- Age
  - Average age at presentation: ~ **50 years**
- Epidemiology
  - Rare tumor (CPA-IAC > temporal bone > parotid)

Natural History & Prognosis

- CNVII paralysis takes years to develop
- Surgical cure can be worse than disease

Treatment

- Conservative: Do nothing until CNVII paralysis present
  - Some do not grow; some never become symptomatic
- Surgery when CNVII paralysis + other symptoms evolving
  - Goal: Complete tumor removal + preservation of hearing & restoration of CNVII function
- Stereotactic radiosurgery
  - Primary treatment for small- to medium-sized FNS when CNVII function & hearing relatively preserved

DIAGNOSTIC CHECKLIST

Consider

- Thin-section imaging shows labyrinthine tail

Image Interpretation Pearls

- CPA-IAC FNS exactly mimics vestibular schwannoma if no labyrinthine tail or temporal bone component present

SELECTED REFERENCES

1. Rini JN et al: Somatostatin receptor-PET/CT/MRI of head and neck neuroendocrine tumors. AJNR Am J Neuroradiol. 44(8):959-66, 2023

TERMINOLOGY

- Definition: Systemic or CNS neoplasia involving CPA-IAC

IMAGING

- 4 major sites: Leptomeningeal (pia-arachnoid), dura, flocculus, and choroid plexus
- T1WI C+ MR most sensitive
  - **Leptomeningeal metastases**: Diffuse thickening and enhancement of cranial nerves in IAC
  - **Dural metastases**: Diffuse or focal, thick, enhancing dura
  - **Floccular metastases**: Enhancing floccular mass extending into CPA
  - **Choroid plexus metastases**: Enhancing choroid mass
  - Focal, enhancing brain metastases may be present
- FLAIR MR
  - Parenchymal brain metastases usually high signal

TOP DIFFERENTIAL DIAGNOSES

- Bilateral vestibular schwannoma (NF2)

- Sarcoidosis
- Meningitis
- Ramsay Hunt syndrome

PATHOLOGY

- Solid tumors, especially breast, lung, melanoma
- Lymphoproliferative malignancies (leukemia, lymphoma)
- CNS malignancies with CSF dissemination

CLINICAL ISSUES

- Rapidly progressive unilateral or bilateral facial nerve paralysis and sensorineural hearing loss
- Patient with past history of treated malignancy
- Usually found in late-stage malignancy
- CSF cytology gold standard but not mandatory

DIAGNOSTIC CHECKLIST

- Consider CPA metastasis > new adult NF2 diagnosis
- Rapid clinical progression + CPA mass suggests metastasis
  - Vestibular schwannoma rarely causes CNVII palsy

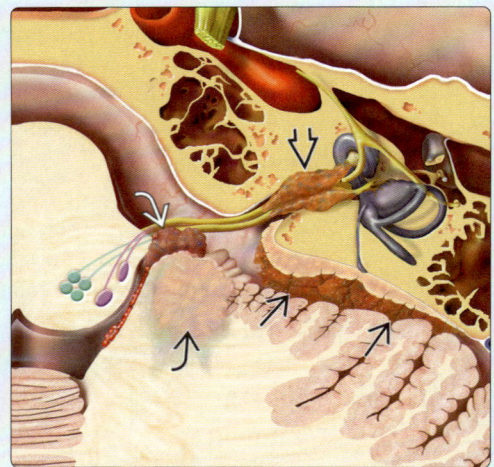
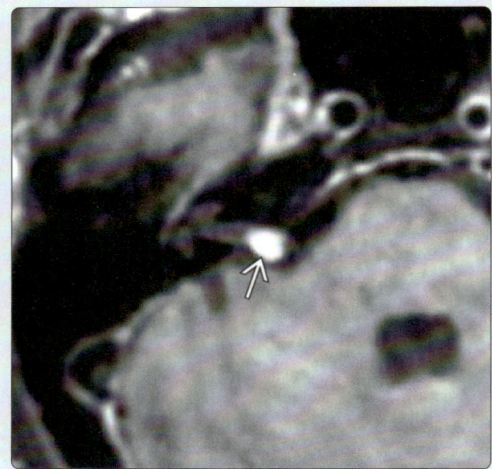

(Left) Axial graphic depicts the 4 major types of CPA-IAC area metastases. Along the posterolateral margin of the IAC, thickened dural metastases ⊟ are visible. Within the IAC, metastatic leptomeningeal (pia-arachnoid) ⊟ involvement is present. Choroid plexus ⊟ and floccular ⊟ metastases are also depicted. (Right) Axial T1 C+ FS MR shows an intensely enhancing CPA-IAC melanoma metastasis ⊟. The patient had widespread systemic & intracranial metastases.

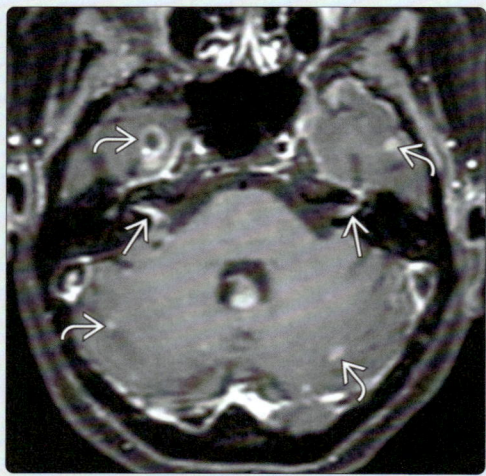
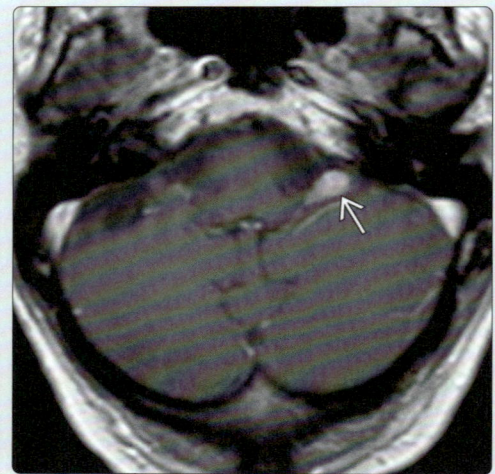

(Left) Axial T1 C+ FS MR shows bilateral IAC nodular enhancement ⊟ due to breast cancer leptomeningeal carcinomatosis. Numerous additional parenchymal brain metastases ⊟ are also noted. Most patients with IAC metastases have a known primary tumor. (Right) Axial T1 C+ FS MR shows an enhancing flocculus mass ⊟ due to CSF dissemination of glioblastoma. Spinal imaging and CSF sampling are indicated to evaluate for drop metastases.

TERMINOLOGY

Abbreviations

- Cerebellopontine angle (CPA)-internal auditory canal (IAC) metastases

Synonyms

- Leptomeningeal carcinomatosis, meningeal carcinomatosis, carcinomatous meningitis
  - All of above terms are misnomers for following reasons
    - Neoplasms are not always carcinomas
    - Pachymeninges (dura) and leptomeninges (pia + arachnoid) are often both involved
    - Usually does not contain inflammatory component
      □ "-itis" suffix makes no sense

Definitions

- CPA-IAC metastases: Systemic or CNS neoplasia affecting area of CPA-IAC

IMAGING

General Features

- Best diagnostic clue
  - Multiple enhancing masses on T1WI C+ MR
- Location
  - 4 major sites: **Leptomeningeal (pia-arachnoid), dura, flocculus, and choroid plexus**
  - Primary site locations
    - Primary malignancy: Breast, lung, and melanoma
      □ Found in 5-10% solid tumors
    - Meningeal lymphoproliferative malignancy
      □ Lymphoma and leukemia
    - Primary CNS malignancy seeds basal cisterns via CSF pathways: Drop metastases
  - CNVII and CNVIII are cranial nerves most often involved with leptomeningeal metastases
- Size
  - Often small (< 1 cm); metastases cause symptoms early
- Morphology
  - Leptomeningeal: Thickened CNVII and CNIII in IAC
  - Dura: Diffuse dural thickening (pachymeninges)
  - Flocculus: Enlarged flocculus with adjacent brain edema; mass extends into CPA cistern
  - Choroid plexus: Nodular thickening

CT Findings

- CECT
  - Unilateral or bilateral dural enhancement along CPA
  - CT shows metastases only when larger ± multiple

MR Findings

- T1WI
  - Focal dural thickening isointense to gray matter
  - Black-blood T1-enhanced technique ↑ sensitivity
- T2WI
  - High-resolution T2 MR
    - Leptomeningeal metastases: CNVII and CNVIII thickening
    - Floccular metastases: ↑ signal edema associated
- FLAIR

- Larger CPA-IAC metastases may cause ↑ signal in adjacent brainstem ± cerebellum
- Floccular metastases seen as ↑ signal
- Thin, linear, band-like surface enhancement may be seen along brainstem
  - Contrast-enhanced FLAIR improves visibility
  - Can be symmetric and diffuse
- DWI
  - May show diffusion restriction
- PWI
  - DCE-MR helps differentiate schwannomas vs. metastases
    - Higher plasma volume (Vp) most significant parameter
- T1WI C+
  - **Leptomeningeal metastases**: Diffuse thickening and enhancement of cranial nerves in IAC
    - Late finding shows plug of enhancing tissue in IAC
    - Unilateral or bilateral
  - **Dural metastases**: Thickened, enhancing dura
    - May be focal or diffuse
    - Associated with other dural or skull lesions
  - **Floccular metastases**: Enhancing floccular mass
  - **Choroid plexus metastases**: Enhancing nodular lesion along expected location of choroid plexus
    - Lateral recess 4th ventricle → foramen of Luschka → inferior CPA cistern
  - Focal, enhancing brain metastases may be present

Imaging Recommendations

- Best imaging tool
  - T1WI C+ MR posterior fossa best imaging tool and sequence
  - Whole-brain T1WI C+ for associated brain metastases
  - Enhanced FLAIR ↑ conspicuity of disease
- Protocol advice
  - Axial and coronal planes recommended

DIFFERENTIAL DIAGNOSIS

Bilateral Vestibular Schwannoma (Neurofibromatosis Type 2)

- Younger patients; no history of malignancy
- T1WI C+ MR shows bilateral CPA-IAC enhancing masses
  - Mimics bilateral leptomeningeal metastases
- Other cranial nerve schwannoma ± meningiomas possible

Sarcoidosis, CPA-IAC

- ↑ ESR and ACE
- T1WI C+ MR may be identical to metastases when multifocal meningeal type
  - May be bilateral CPA lesions mimicking neurofibromatosis 2 (NF2) or metastases
  - May be single, en plaque focus mimicking meningioma
- Look for infundibular stalk involvement

Meningitis, CPA-IAC

- Bacterial meningitis
- Fungal meningitis
- Tuberculous meningitis
- T1WI C+ MR may be identical to CPA-IAC metastases

- Clinical information and CSF evaluation are key

Ramsay Hunt Syndrome

- External ear vesicular rash
- T1WI C+ MR shows enhancement in IAC fundus and inner ear ± CNVII
  - Mimics unilateral leptomeningeal metastasis

PATHOLOGY

General Features

- Etiology
  - Metastatic tumor involves leptomeningeal or dural surfaces of CPA-IAC
    - Leptomeningeal metastases follow CNVII and CNVIII into IAC
  - Metastatic tumor deposits in flocculus or choroid plexus
  - Routes of spread
    - Extracranial neoplasm spreads hematogenously to meninges
    - CSF spread from intracranial or intraspinal neoplasm is less common
- Associated abnormalities
  - Multiple other pial or dural metastatic foci
  - Parenchymal brain metastases also possible
    - Pia + arachnoid = **leptomeninges**
- Key anatomy: Meninges has 3 discrete layers
  - **Dura** (pachymeninges): Dense connective tissue attached to calvarium
  - **Arachnoid**: Interposed between pia and dura
  - **Pia**: Clear membrane firmly attached to surface of brain; extends deeply into sulci

Gross Pathologic & Surgical Features

- Diffuse, nodular ± discrete

Microscopic Features

- Common tissue types found
  - Solid tumors = breast, lung, and melanoma
    - All involve both leptomeninges and pachymeninges
  - Lymphoproliferative malignancy = lymphoma and leukemia
    - Involve both leptomeninges and pachymeninges
  - Drop metastases from CNS malignancies
    - Medulloblastoma, ependymoma, glioblastoma
- CSF hematopathology gold standard but MR diagnosis with confirmatory clinical findings sufficient to establish diagnosis and initiate therapy
  - Excisional biopsy if diagnosis in question

CLINICAL ISSUES

Presentation

- Most common signs/symptoms
  - **Rapidly progressive** unilateral or bilateral facial nerve (CNVII) paralysis and sensorineural hearing loss (CNVIII)
- Other signs/symptoms
  - Vertigo and polycranial neuropathy
- Clinical profile
  - Patient with past history of treated malignancy

Demographics

- Age
  - Older adults
- Epidemiology
  - Increasingly seen complication of systemic cancer
    - Higher survival rate of cancer patients
    - Improved imaging techniques and ↑ surveillance

Natural History & Prognosis

- Meningeal metastases usually late-stage finding
- Poor prognosis as patients have advanced, incurable disease by definition

Treatment

- No curative treatments available
- Therapeutic goal is preserving neurologic function and improving quality of life
- Therapies are complex and individualized
- Primary tumor type + clinical, imaging, and cytologic findings guide treatment options
  - Radiotherapy ± systemic chemotherapy depending on tissue type; intrathecal chemotherapy
  - Multiple immunotherapies and targeted molecular therapies are under study; some have shown response &/or survival benefits
- Surgery will rarely play role at this stage
  - Solitary melanoma metastases may be exception

DIAGNOSTIC CHECKLIST

Consider

- Bilateral vestibular schwannoma in adult as NF2 may be more likely CPA metastases
  - Consider DCE PWI to better differentiate
- Rapid growth suggests metastasis
- CNVII palsy with CPA mass suggests metastasis
  - Vestibular schwannoma rarely causes CNVII palsy
- Absence of imaging findings indicating leptomeningeal metastasis does not rule it out

Image Interpretation Pearls

- If suspect CPA-IAC metastasis from T1WI C+ MR appearance or history of known malignancy, must review
  - Extracranial and calvarial structures for other lesions to confirm diagnosis
  - Look for involvement of other meningeal sites, such as parasellar, other basal meninges
  - Parenchymal brain for abnormal FLAIR high signal ± enhancing lesions on T1WI C+ sequences
- Include CPA-IAC in routine brain MR search pattern; recognized as site of perceptual skull base finding misses

SELECTED REFERENCES

1. Anamika A et al: Role of neuroradiological imaging in progressive sensorineural hearing loss: a retrospective study. Indian J Otolaryngol Head Neck Surg. 76(3):2474-9, 2024
2. Marzolino R et al: A case report of malignant cerebellopontine angle lesion highlighting the interdisciplinary diagnostic challenge in the case of unilateral progressive hearing loss. J Clin Med. 13(12):3483, 2024
3. Saeed L et al: A case of leptomeningeal carcinomatosis manifesting with vertigo in the setting of intracranial hypertension. Cureus. 15(10):e47431, 2023
4. Vaz MAS et al: Non-Hodgkin lymphoma mimicking vestibular schwannoma. Cureus. 15(12):e50965, 2023
5. Vong S et al: Analysis of perceptual errors in skull-base pathology. Neuroradiol J. 36(5):515-23, 2023

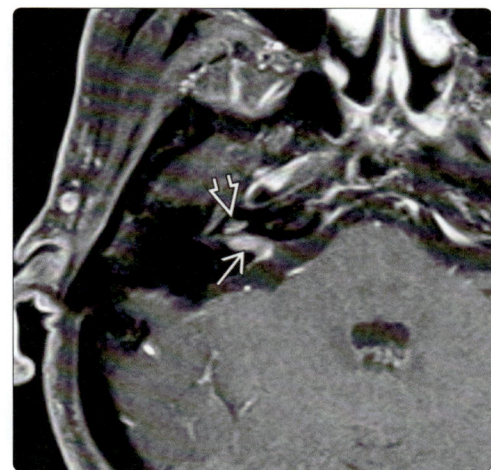

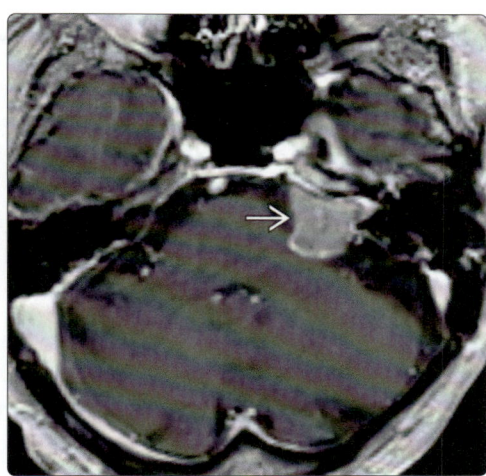

(Left) *Axial T1 C+ FS MR shows an enhancing metastasis in the right IAC ➡ with extension of enhancing tissue through the cochlear nerve canal, across the modiolus into the membranous labyrinth of the cochlea ➡. (Right) Axial T1 C+ MR shows a heterogeneous, enhancing mass in the CPA ➡ due to metastatic disease. While the appearance is similar to schwannoma, the patient had widespread systemic metastases, including multifocal intracranial disease due to non-small cell lung carcinoma metastases.*

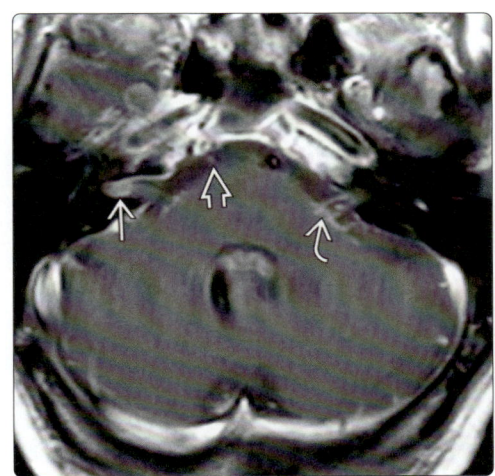

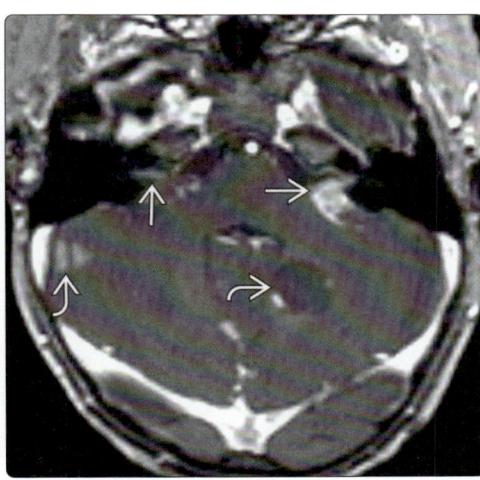

(Left) *Axial T1 C+ FS MR shows enhancing IAC nodules ➡ from lung adenocarcinoma metastasis in a patient with diplopia and hydrocephalus. Note subtle enhancing disease along the leptomeninges ➡ and right abducens nerve ➡. (Right) Axial T1 C+ MR shows nodular enhancement in the left > right CPA-IAC ➡ due to cerebrospinal dissemination of anaplastic pleomorphic xanthoastrocytoma. Multiple additional areas of spread ➡ are present. Spinal imaging is indicated to look for additional drop metastases.*

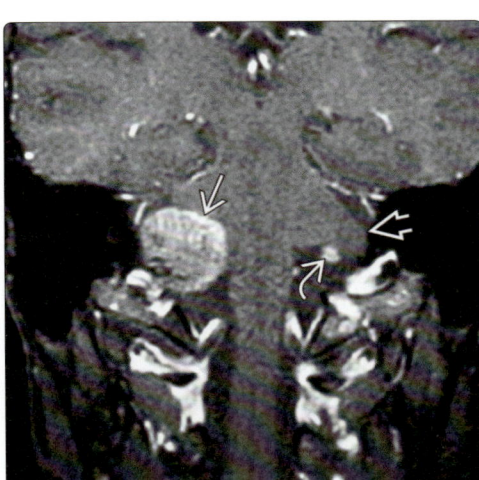

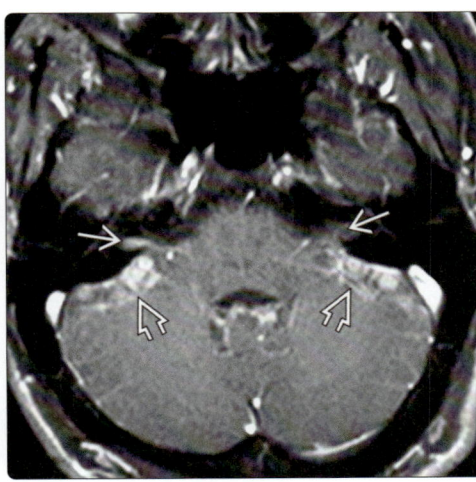

(Left) *Coronal T1 C+ MR depicts an enhancing breast carcinoma metastasis ➡ centered within the right flocculus. Note the normal flocculus ➡ and cisternal choroid plexus ➡. (Right) Axial T1 C+ FS MR reveals bilateral CPA-IAC drop metastases from a supratentorial glioblastoma. Bilateral IAC enhancing metastases ➡ are seen along with multiple leptomeningeal metastases on the cerebellar surface ➡.*

Trigeminal Neuralgia

TERMINOLOGY

- **Classic trigeminal neuralgia (TN)** causes recurrent, unilateral, electric shock-like pain ± facial spasms from vessel compressing ipsilateral CNV without other causes

IMAGING

- Artery (80-90%) or vein contacting cisternal CNV on high-resolution T2 MR
  - Arteries: **Superior cerebellar** (80-90%) most common > anterior inferior cerebellar > vertebral > basilar artery
- Location: Root entry zone (REZ) > trigeminal cave
- ↑ severity with CNV atrophy, displacement, deformity
- Rule out causes of secondary TN (mass, stroke, multiple sclerosis)
- Beware: Vascular contact alone can be normal variant

TOP DIFFERENTIAL DIAGNOSES

- CPA/IAC aneurysm, CPA-IAC arteriovenous malformation
- Posterior fossa developmental venous anomaly

PATHOLOGY

- Likely due to complex interplay of genetic susceptibility and environment with compression of CNV
- Compression → myelin loss → abnormal sensory impulses
- **Transition zone (TZ)** between central and peripheral myelin is vulnerable to demyelination
- REZ is proximal 6 mm of CNV from pons to TZ

CLINICAL ISSUES

- Primary TN can be classic (caused by vascular compression)
  - Vascular compression seen on imaging in 89%
- Secondary TN due to underlying lesion: CPA or skull base tumor, MS, perineural tumor spread
  - ↓ response to surgery if concurrent secondary cause

DIAGNOSTIC CHECKLIST

- Classic TN: High-resolution CSF bright sequences MR to identify compressing vessel and site
- ↑ severity predicts better surgical response

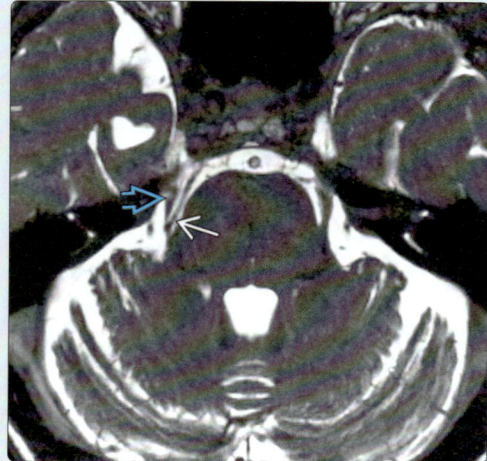
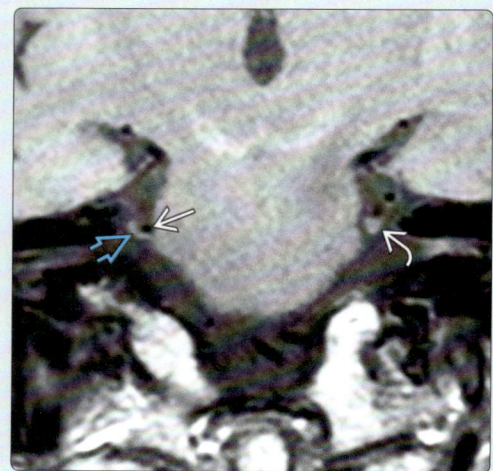

(Left) *Axial T2WI MR in this patient with right trigeminal neuralgia (TN) shows the low-signal superior cerebellar artery ➡ impinging on the root entry zone of the cisternal segment ➘ of the trigeminal nerve.* **(Right)** *Coronal T1WI MR in the same patient reveals the superior cerebellar artery ➡ compressing and deforming the cisternal right CNV at the root entry zone ➘. Notice the larger, normal left cisternal CNV ➚, indicating that atrophy is a feature of the affected right side.*

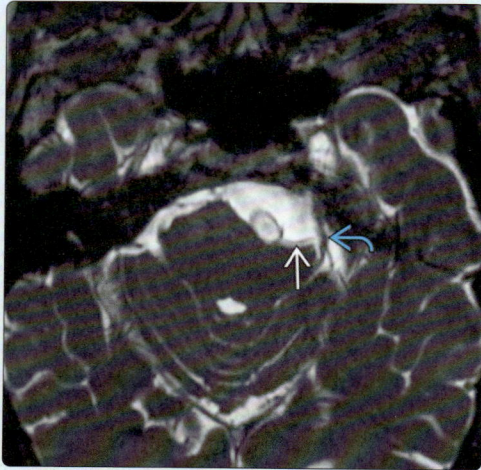
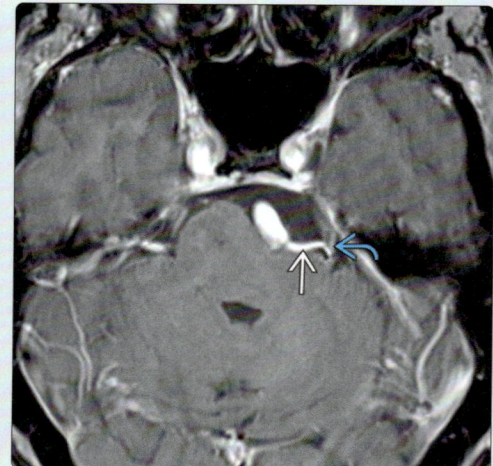

(Left) *Axial T2WI MR through the pons in an older patient with left classic TN shows a prominent anterior inferior cerebellar artery (AICA) ➡ on the left extending laterally to the root exit zone of the left CNV, compressing and deviating the proximal nerve ➘.* **(Right)** *Axial T1WI C+ FS MR in the same patient with classic TN shows a prominent AICA ➡ arising from a dolichoectatic basilar artery on the left extending to the root exit zone, compressing and deviating the proximal CNV ➘.*

TERMINOLOGY

Definitions

- **Classic trigeminal neuralgia (TN)**: Recurrent, unilateral, electric shock-like pain, ± facial spasms from vessel compressing CNV without other causes
- **Root entry zone (REZ)**: Proximal 6 mm of cisternal CNV from pons
  - Contains **transition zone (TZ)** between central and peripheral myelin, prone to demyelination

IMAGING

General Features

- Best diagnostic clue
  - Artery (80-90%) or vein contacting cisternal CNV on high-resolution T2 MR
    - **Superior cerebellar (SCA)** (80-90%) is most common > anterior inferior cerebellar (AICA) > vertebral > basilar artery
- Location
  - Cisternal portion of CNV
    - REZ most common affected location > trigeminal cave
- Morphology
  - ↑ severity with CNV nerve atrophy, deformity, and displacement
  - Vascular contact (lowest positive predictive value, worst response to surgery)
    - Can be normal variant, 67% asymptomatic

MR Findings

- **High-resolution 3D (SSFP) T2 MR**
  - Shows serpiginous low-signal (flow void) artery/vein contact
  - Atrophic, deformed, or displaced cisternal CNV
- MRA: Helps identify causative vessel
- Concurrent or secondary (nonvascular) causes of TN
  - FLAIR: Linear signal ↑ in pons from multiple sclerosis (MS)
    - MS plaque may precede symptoms by years
  - DWI: Brainstem infarct, cerebellopontine angle (CPA) epidermoid cyst
  - T1 FS C+: Enhancing mass or infiltrative process in CPA, skull base, leptomeninges, or cranial nerves
    - ± nerve enhancement after treatment, does not predict response

Imaging Recommendations

- Best imaging tool
  - High-resolution thin-section 3D T2 (SSFP) MR

DIFFERENTIAL DIAGNOSIS

Vertebrobasilar Dolichoectasia

- Common atherosclerotic finding in older adult patient
- Tortuous, dilated vertebrobasilar system
- Vertebral artery loop can unusually cause TN

CPA/IAC Aneurysm

- AICA or vertebral artery aneurysm
- Oval, complex signal mass
- Rarely causes TN

CPA/IAC Arteriovenous Malformation

- Much larger vessels (arteries and veins) with nidus
- Rare in posterior fossa

Posterior Fossa Developmental Venous Anomaly

- Larger vessels (veins)
- CPA rare as venous drainage route
- Rarely causes venous compression-induced TN

PATHOLOGY

General Features

- Etiology
  - ↑ evidence that TN is likely due to complex interplay of genetic susceptibility and environment
  - CNV compression causes loss of myelin of sensory fibers
  - Demyelination leads to abnormal sensory signals
  - TZ is prone to demyelination and vascular compression

CLINICAL ISSUES

Presentation

- Most common signs/symptoms
  - Recurrent, unilateral, electric shock-like pain most often affecting CNV2 ± CNV3 divisions

Demographics

- Age
  - 49-63 years old most common; M = F

Natural History & Prognosis

- 80% pain-free 5-10 years after surgery for severe neurovascular compression (NVC)
- 56% pain-free 5-10 years after surgery if mild NVC
- ↑ recurrence if concurrent MS, infarct
- Permanent surgical complications can include facial numbness (13%), deafness (5%)

Treatment

- Medical management is 1st-line therapy
- Microvascular decompression, nerve ablation if refractory

DIAGNOSTIC CHECKLIST

Image Interpretation Pearls

- Identify compressing vessel and site on high-resolution MR
- Describe severity, which predicts treatment response: Nerve atrophy > deformity > displacement > contact
- Identify concurrent or secondary (nonvascular) causes of TN, e.g., MS, CPA/IAC mass, perineural tumor spread (PNTS)
- If TN develops in patient with known history of head and neck cancer, be suspicious of PNTS
- Beware: Vascular contact alone can be normal variant

SELECTED REFERENCES

1. Kumar A et al: Radiological characteristics of the affected trigeminal nerve in cases of trigeminal neuralgia caused by pure venous conflict. World Neurosurg. 194:123500, 2025
2. Wamasing N et al: Magnetic resonance cisternography for trigeminal neuralgia: comparison between gradient-echo and spin-echo 3D sequences. Dentomaxillofac Radiol. 54(4):313-9, 2025
3. Bora N et al: A systematic review of the role of magnetic resonance imaging in the diagnosis and detection of neurovascular conflict in patients with trigeminal neuralgia. Cureus. 15(9):e44614, 2023

KEY FACTS

TERMINOLOGY

- Primary hemifacial spasm (HFS): **Neurovascular conflict** (NVC) of facial nerve at its **root exit zone** (REZ) within cerebellopontine angle (CPA) cistern causing ipsilateral HFS

IMAGING

- NVC: Tortuous or ectatic vessel impinging upon REZ
  - Thin-section high-resolution T2W bSSFP sequence (CISS, FIESTA) and coregistered MRA to best visualize
- Location: Anterior inferior cerebellar artery (AICA) (50%), posterior inferior cerebellar artery (PICA) (30%), vertebral artery (VA) (15%), vein (5%)

TOP DIFFERENTIAL DIAGNOSES

- Aneurysm, CPA-internal auditory canal
- Arteriovenous malformation, CPA
- Developmental venous anomaly, posterior fossa

PATHOLOGY

- Primary HFS: Vessel compression damages/irritates CNVII

- Secondary HFS: Nonvascular causes that may produce HFS syndrome

CLINICAL ISSUES

- Clinical presentation
  - Unilateral involuntary facial spasms; begins with orbicularis oculi spasms

DIAGNOSTIC CHECKLIST

- Determine if MRA source images or high-resolution T2 MR identify causal vessel
  - Positive MR findings present in ~ 50% HFS patients
  - Negative MR does not preclude surgical therapy
  - Preoperative high-resolution T2W bSSFP sequences (CISS, FIESTA) are associated with significantly higher surgical success rate
- First, look for cisternal mass lesions, multiple sclerosis, then follow CNVII distally into temporal bone and parotid
  - Exclude CNVII venous malformation, parotid malignancy

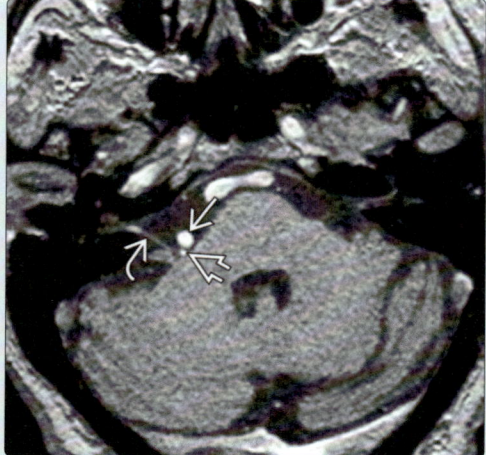
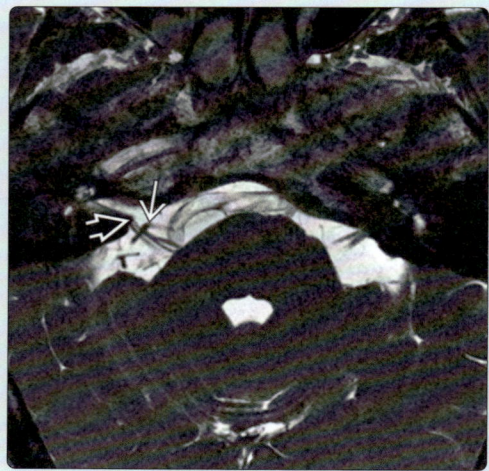

(Left) *Axial MRA in a patient with right hemifacial spasm (HFS) shows a tortuous right vertebral artery ➡ and associated posterior inferior cerebellar artery (PICA) ➡ pushing on the root exit zone (REZ) of the facial nerve. The facial nerve is visible in the cerebellopontine angle (CPA) cistern ➡.* (Right) *Axial CISS MR through the CPA cisterns in a patient with right HFS demonstrates a PICA loop ➡ pushing the cisternal CNVII and CNVII posteriorly, causing them to drape over the posterior margin of the porus acusticus ➡.*

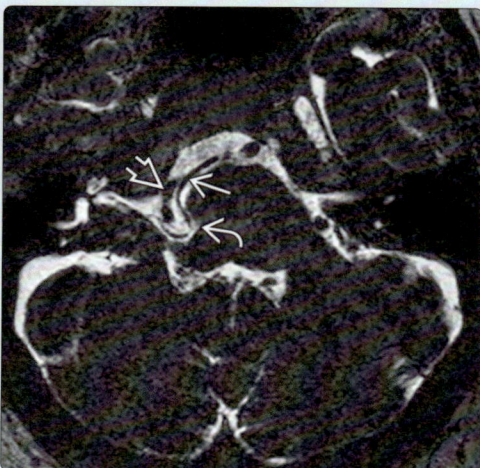
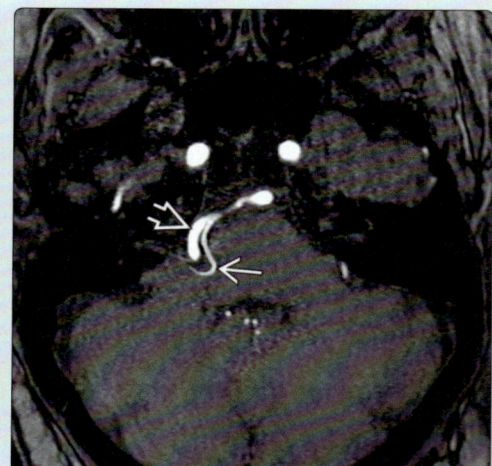

(Left) *Axial T2 MR in a 77-year-old woman with right HFS shows both a prominent ectatic right vertebral artery ➡ and tortuous right anterior inferior cerebellar artery (AICA) loop ➡ extending into the REZ of the right facial nerve. Note deformity of the lateral pontomedullary junction ➡.* (Right) *Axial 3D time-of-flight MR in the same patient shows an ectatic right vertebral artery ➡ as well as a tortuous AICA loop ➡ in the CPA cistern, effacing the REZ of a right facial nerve.*

TERMINOLOGY

Abbreviations
- Hemifacial spasm (HFS)

Synonyms
- Primary HFS, facial nerve vascular loop syndrome, facial nerve hyperactive dysfunction syndrome

Definitions
- Vascular compression of facial nerve at its root exit zone (REZ) within cerebellopontine angle (CPA) cistern causing ipsilateral hemifacial spasm

IMAGING

General Features
- Best diagnostic clue
  - High-resolution T2WI MR &/or MRA source images show asymmetric vessel (ectatic, tortuous, or lateralized) that impinges upon proximal facial nerve
- Location
  - Medial CPA cistern at CNVII root exit zone
- HFS-causative vessels: Anterior inferior cerebellar artery (AICA) (50%), posterior inferior cerebellar artery (PICA) (30%), vertebral artery (VA) (15%), vein (5%)

MR Findings
- T2WI
  - High-resolution T2 MR: Vessel best seen as tubular flow void coursing through high-signal CSF
  - MPR to demonstrate relationship of vessel to nerve
  - Can detect deformity of adjacent brainstem surface or deviation of proximal facial nerve
- MRA
  - Source images helpful in identifying arterial anatomy
- FLAIR
  - Adjacent brain most commonly normal
  - Multiple sclerosis (MS) may present with HFS

Imaging Recommendations
- Best imaging tool
  - Thin-section high-resolution T2-weighted bSSFP (CISS, FIESTA) best shows neurovascular conflict
  - Axial source images from time-of-flight imaging with coronal, sagittal, and 3D reformations provide excellent correlation and can help identify arterial anatomy
- Protocol advice
  - Whole-brain T2 or FLAIR MR to evaluate for MS
  - Include axial and coronal T1 C+ FS MR of brainstem and CPA cistern, including deep face
    - Look for asymmetric venous cause
    - Look for cisternal or perineural tumor, cranial neuritis

DIFFERENTIAL DIAGNOSIS

CPA-IAC Aneurysm
- PICA or VA aneurysm
- Oval complex signal mass

CPA Arteriovenous Malformation
- Larger vessels (arteries and veins) with nidus
- Rare in posterior fossa

Posterior Fossa Developmental Venous Anomaly
- Larger vessels (veins)
- CPA rare as venous drainage route or cause of HFS

PATHOLOGY

General Features
- Etiology
  - Neurovascular conflict (NVC) pathophysiology
    - Unclear, but most accepted hypothesis: Vascular compression in REZ → demyelination → nucleus hyperexcitability → CN symptoms
  - Primary HFS: CNVII bundle experiences "irritation" from vessel compression at REZ
  - Secondary HFS refers to nonvascular causes

CLINICAL ISSUES

Presentation
- Most common signs/symptoms
  - HFS: Unilateral, involuntary facial spasms

Demographics
- Age
  - Older patients (usually > 65 years)
- Epidemiology
  - < 1:100,000

Natural History & Prognosis
- 90% symptom-free ≥ 5 years after surgery

Treatment
- Local injections of botulinum toxin
  - 85% of patients get significant relief from local injections
  - Repeat treatment every 4 months
- **Microvascular decompression** as needed
  - Provides permanent relief in 90% of patients

DIAGNOSTIC CHECKLIST

Consider
- Positive MR findings present in ~ 50% of HFS patients

Image Interpretation Pearls
- Review MRA and high-resolution T2 MR for vessel that contacts, effaces, or displaces REZ of facial nerve
- After evaluating for vascular compression, exclude secondary causes of HFS

SELECTED REFERENCES

1. Ansari A et al: Fully endoscopic microvascular decompression for hemifacial spasm: a systematic review. Neurosurg Rev. 48(1):285, 2025
2. Kesumayadi I et al: Which surgical technique has a superior clinical outcome in microvascular decompression? A systematic review and meta-analysis study of transposition versus interposition for trigeminal neuralgia and hemifacial spasm. Neurosurg Rev. 48(1):408, 2025
3. Kaufmann AM: Hemifacial spasm: a neurosurgical perspective. J Neurosurg. 140(1):240-7, 2024
4. Busse S et al: Correlation of preoperative high-resolution neurovascular imaging and surgical success in neurovascular compression Syndromes. World Neurosurg. 172:e593-8, 2023
5. Haller S et al: Imaging of neurovascular compression syndromes: trigeminal neuralgia, hemifacial spasm, vestibular paroxysmia, and glossopharyngeal neuralgia. AJNR Am J Neuroradiol. 37(8):1384-92, 2016

TERMINOLOGY

- Aneurysm that arises from vertebrobasilar artery branches and may present radiologically as vascular or space-occupying lesion of CPA-IAC cistern

IMAGING

- CECT of partially thrombosed aneurysm
  - Complex mass with central or eccentric enhancing lumen, nonenhancing mural thrombus
  - Often has **calcified rim**
- CTA: Shows morphology of aneurysm lumen and relationship to parent vessel
- MR complex; possibly layered signal from Ca⁺⁺, clot, flow
  - T1: **Subacute luminal clot** is **hyperintense** secondary to **methemoglobin T1 shortening**
  - T2: Signal varies from hypointense flow void to **complex mixed signal** appearance
  - Vessel wall imaging: Vessel wall enhancement associated with increased risk of aneurysm rupture

- Angiogram: Visible lumen may be smaller than overall aneurysm if clot is present
  - May underestimate aneurysm size

TOP DIFFERENTIAL DIAGNOSES

- Vertebrobasilar dolichoectasia
- Dural arteriovenous fistula + venous varix
- Arteriovenous malformation

CLINICAL ISSUES

- Clinical presentation
  - Sensorineural hearing loss (70%)
  - Headache from subarachnoid hemorrhage (50%)
  - Hemifacial spasm or facial nerve palsy
- Larger, posterior circulation aneurysms rupture more often
- Treatment options
  - Surgical clipping
  - Endovascular coiling, stenting, or parent vessel occlusion depending on configuration

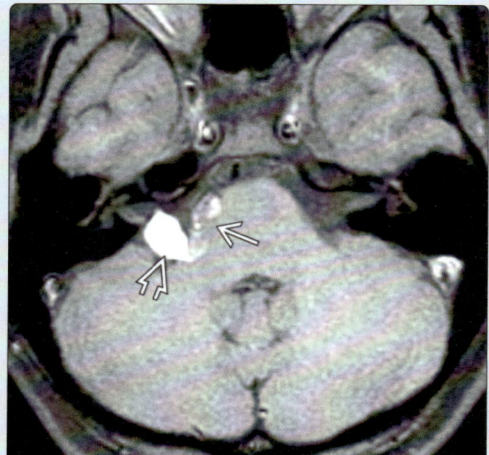
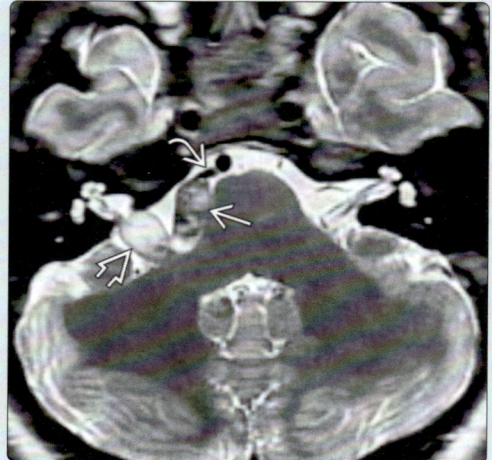

(Left) *Axial T1 MR shows a tubular, hyperintense mass extending laterally from the basilar artery into the CPA cistern. The more medial portion of the mass shows complex signal from flow and subacute clot ➡, while the more lateral component is completely thrombosed and filled with high-signal subacute clot ➡.* (Right) *Axial T2 MR in the same patient reveals the patent PICA-AICA complex takeoff from the basilar artery ➡ with an area of partial ➡ and complete thrombosis ➡ of the aneurysm.*

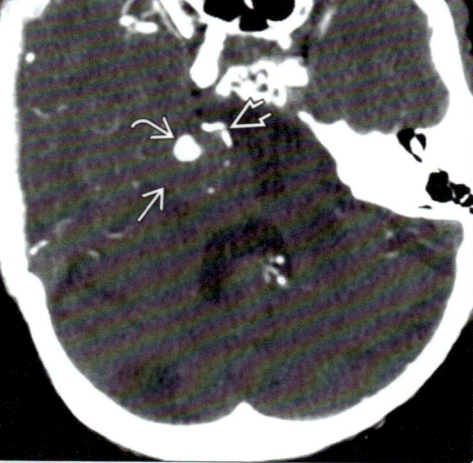
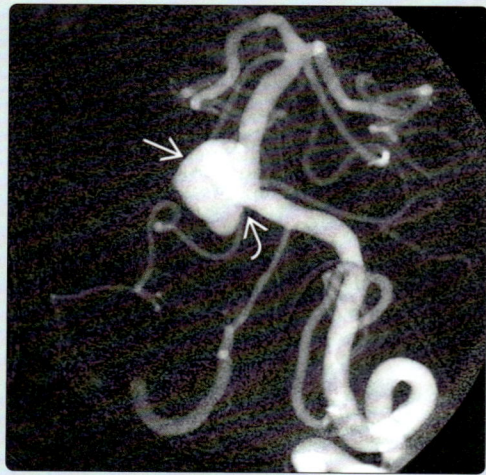

(Left) *Axial source image CTA in a 66-year-old woman presenting with stroke symptoms shows a large (2.5-cm), partially thrombosed aneurysm ➡ in the right CPA. The central lumen ➡ measures ~ 1 cm. Notice peripheral calcifications along the parent basilar artery ➡. Several chronic infarcts are noted.* (Right) *Anterior DSA in the same patient shows the saccular aneurysm ➡ arising near the origin of the right AICA ➡. Since thrombosed portions are not visualized, DSA can underestimate the total volume of lesion.*

TERMINOLOGY

Definitions

- Aneurysm that arises from vertebrobasilar artery branches and may present radiologically as space-occupying lesion of cerebellopontine angle (CPA)-internal auditory canal (IAC) cistern

IMAGING

General Features

- Best diagnostic clue
  - CPA mass with **calcified rim** (CT) or layered **complex signal** in wall (MR)
- Location
  - CPA aneurysms from posterior inferior cerebellar artery (PICA) > vertebral artery (VA) > anterior inferior cerebellar artery (AICA)
- Morphology: Round (saccular), ovoid, or fusiform-shaped

CT Findings

- CECT
  - Patent aneurysm: Well-delineated, iso- to hyperdense, extraaxial mass with strong, uniform enhancement
  - Thrombosis affects aneurysm appearance
    - Partial thrombosis: Complex mass with central or eccentric enhancing lumen, nonenhancing mural thrombus; often has **calcified rim**
    - Complete thrombosis: No enhancing lumen
- CTA
  - Aneurysm morphology and relationship to parent vessel

MR Findings

- T1WI
  - **Subacute luminal thrombus** is **T1 hyperintense** secondary to **methemoglobin** T1 shortening
- T2WI
  - Phase artifact from patent aneurysm common
  - Signal varies from hypointense **flow void** to **complex mixed signal** appearance
    - Varies with flow rate and age of luminal thrombus; complex signal from Ca^{++}, clot, flow
- T1WI C+
  - Aneurysm lumen enhances if slow flow present
- MRA
  - May delineate relationship with parent vessel
- Vessel wall imaging (VWI): Vessel wall enhancement associated with increased risk of aneurysm rupture

Angiographic Findings

- Visible lumen may be smaller than overall aneurysm if clot is present (angiogram may **underestimate** aneurysm size)
- Important for endovascular treatment planning
  - Angiography delineates precise vascular relationships

Imaging Recommendations

- Best imaging tool
  - If CT/MR suggests aneurysm, confirm with CTA or DSA

DIFFERENTIAL DIAGNOSIS

Vertebrobasilar Dolichoectasia

- MRA reprojections or source images show no aneurysm

Dural Atrioventricular Fistula + Venous Varix

- Angiogram delineates best
- MR venography may help delineate

Arteriovenous Malformation

- Large feeding arteries + nidus

PATHOLOGY

General Features

- Etiology
  - Inherited factors + hemodynamic-induced degenerative changes in vessel wall often combine to form aneurysm
- Genetics
  - Aneurysm propensity has hereditary driver

Gross Pathologic & Surgical Features

- Saccular: Berry-like outpouching of artery wall
- Fusiform: Enlarged, ectatic atherosclerotic artery

Microscopic Features

- Lacks internal elastic lamina and smooth muscle layers
- Degenerative changes in parent vessel common
- Thrombus, atherosclerosis are common

CLINICAL ISSUES

Presentation

- Most common signs/symptoms
  - Unilateral sensorineural hearing loss (SNHL) (70%)
- Other signs/symptoms
  - Headache from subarachnoid hemorrhage (50%), hemifacial spasm or facial nerve palsy, tinnitus, vertigo
- Clinical profile: Middle-aged patient, unilateral SNHL

Demographics

- Epidemiology
  - CPA aneurysms account for ≤ 1% of CPA masses
  - 10% of all intracranial aneurysms are vertebrobasilar
- Age: 40-60 years

Natural History & Prognosis

- Larger, posterior circulation aneurysms rupture more often
- Left unclipped, risk of aneurysm rupture increases

Treatment

- Endovascular coiling vs. surgical clipping

DIAGNOSTIC CHECKLIST

Image Interpretation Pearls

- CT: Rim Ca^{++} in CPA mass suggests aneurysm
- MR: Complex signal in CPA mass suggests aneurysm

SELECTED REFERENCES

1. Raz E et al: Neuroanatomy of the vertebrobasilar perforators: implications for aneurysm treatment. J Neurointerv Surg. jnis-2024-022144, 2024
2. Tjoumakaris SI et al: ARISE I consensus review on the management of intracranial aneurysms. Stroke. 55(5):1428-37, 2024
3. Tan S et al: Diagnostic performance of high-resolution vessel wall MR imaging combined with TOF-MRA in the follow-up of intracranial vertebrobasilar dissecting aneurysms after reconstructive endovascular treatment. AJNR Am J Neuroradiol. 44(4):453-9, 2023
4. Lakshmi M et al: Imaging of the cerebellopontine angle. Neuroimaging Clin N Am. 19(3):393-406, 2009

TERMINOLOGY

- Superficial siderosis (SS): Recurrent subarachnoid hemorrhage (SAH) causes hemosiderin deposits on surface of brain and cranial nerve leptomeninges

IMAGING

- NECT findings
  - Slightly hyperdense rim over brain surface
  - Brainstem high-density line most evident
  - **Caveat**: Do not mistake high-density rim on brain surfaces as SAH
- MR findings
  - Ventricle, brain, brainstem, cerebellum, and cervical spine surfaces may all have hypointense hemosiderin rim
  - Contours of brain and cranial nerves outlined by **hypointense rim** on T2, T2* GRE, or SWI MR
  - CNVIII appears darker and thicker than normal
  - GRE/SWI: Most sensitive to hemosiderin deposition on CNS surfaces (blooming dark signal)

- Once diagnosis of SS made, search for cause of recurrent SAH or spontaneous CSF leak is indicated
  - Whole-brain MR with contrast and MRA
  - Total-spine MR for dural defect
  - CT or MR myelography if CSF leak suspected

PATHOLOGY

- Hemosiderin deposits on infratentorial leptomeninges
- Affects brain, brainstem, cranial nerves, and spinal cord
- Causes bleeding from recurrent SAH or spinal CSF leak
  - **Spinal dural defect** with CSF leak #1 cause
  - Trauma: Nerve root avulsion, head injury, SDH
  - Bleeding neoplasm: Brain or spine
  - Arteriovenous or cavernous malformation
  - Aneurysm
  - Surgical sites (brain or spine)
  - Amyloid angiopathy
  - Vasculitis
  - Meningocele

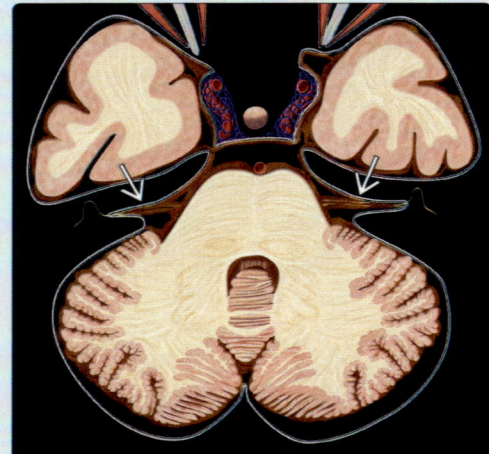
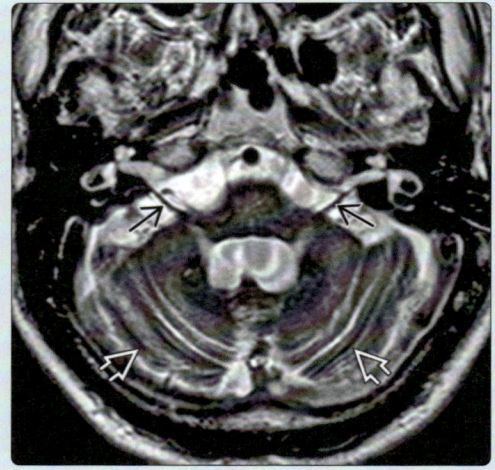

(Left) Axial graphic shows darker brown hemosiderin staining all surfaces of the brain, meninges, and cranial nerves (CNs). Notice that CNVII and CNVIII in the cerebellopontine angle (CPA)-internal auditory canal (IAC) ➡ are particularly affected. (Right) Axial T2 MR reveals superficial siderosis (SS) in the posterior fossa. Both vestibulocochlear nerves (CNVIII) are seen as very low-signal lines in the CPA cisterns ➡. Also observe the low signal along the surface of the cerebellar folia ➡.

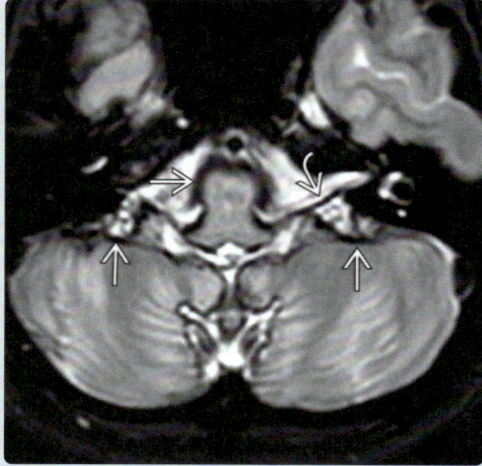
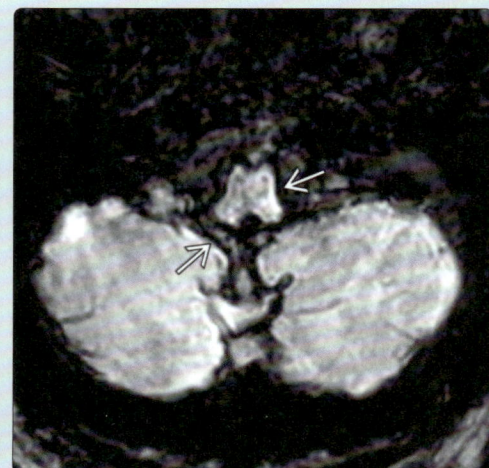

(Left) Axial T2 FS MR shows SS coating the posterior fossa leptomeninges ➡. Note SS along the left vestibulocochlear nerve ➡. SS can be seen on spin-echo sequences if extensive, but T2* GRE or SWI improves conspicuity. (Right) Axial T2* SWI MR shows diffuse SS involving the brainstem and cerebellum ➡. This patient had no intracranial source of hemorrhage identified. Spinal imaging showed a thoracic spine ventral dural defect (not shown), which was the likely source.

TERMINOLOGY

Abbreviations

- Cerebellopontine angle (CPA)
- Internadl auditory canal (IAC)
- Superficial siderosis (SS)

Synonyms

- Siderosis, CNS siderosis

Definitions

- Recurrent subarachnoid hemorrhage (SAH) causes **hemosiderin deposition** on surface of brain, **brainstem**, and **cranial nerve leptomeninges**
  - 1/3 of cases are idiopathic
- Primary (classic) SS: #1 cause is **spinal dural defects**
  - Dural tears: Most often ventral and typically due to osteophytes or calcified disc herniation
  - Dural ectasia (related to connective tissue disorder), traumatic nerve root avulsion, &/or postoperative pseudomeningocele leading to intracranial hypotension
    - Bleeding from fragile, leaky bridging veins with trabeculations around tears
- Secondary SS: Due to prior trauma, brain or spine surgery, tumors, &/or vascular lesions

IMAGING

General Features

- Best diagnostic clue
  - Contours of brain and cranial nerves outlined by thin, **hypointense rim** on T2, T2* GRE, or SWI MR
- Location
  - Cerebral hemispheres, cerebellum, brainstem, cranial nerves, and spinal cord may all be affected
- Size
  - Linear low signal along CNS surfaces varies in thickness but is usually ≤ 2 mm
- Morphology
  - Curvilinear dark lines on CNS surfaces

CT Findings

- NECT
  - Cerebral and **cerebellar atrophy**
    - Especially marked in posterior fossa
      - Cerebellar sulci often disproportionately large
  - **CNVIII** may be **hyperdense**
  - Slightly hyperdense rim over brain surface
    - Brainstem changes most evident
    - CT relatively insensitive to SS compared to MR
    - **Caveat**: High-density rim on brain surfaces may mimic SAH
- CECT
  - No enhancement typical

MR Findings

- T1WI
  - Hypointense signal may be seen on CNS surfaces
- T2WI
  - High-resolution thin-section T2 MR of CPA-IAC
    - **CNVIII** appears **hypointense**, thicker than normal
    - Adjacent cerebellar structures and brainstem show low-signal surfaces
    - Less easily seen than on T2* GRE images
  - Ventricle, brain, brainstem, cerebellum, and cervical spine surfaces all have hypointense hemosiderin rim
  - Vermian and cerebellar atrophy most prominent
- FLAIR
  - Thin, hypointense border on surfaces of brain, brainstem, cerebellum, and cranial nerves
- T2* GRE
  - More sensitive to hemosiderin deposition on CNS surfaces than T2 sequence
  - **Blooming** dark signal
    - Makes SS appear more conspicuous, thicker
- DWI
  - b0 can be used as "poor man's gradient-echo" sequence
  - Hypointensity may be seen in areas of SS
- T1WI C+
  - Surface of CNS does not enhance
- SWI
  - Highly sensitive to siderosis > T2* GRE
  - Blooming dark signal
    - Makes SS more conspicuous and larger
- MR findings do not correlate with severity of disease

Imaging Recommendations

- Best imaging tool
  - Brain MR with posterior fossa focus
    - Once diagnosis of SS is made, **search for cause** is indicated
    - Whole-brain MR with contrast and MRA
    - Total-spine MR &/or spinal CT myelography to evaluate for dural defect
- Protocol advice
  - Brain MR
    - Unenhanced MR with FLAIR initially
    - If suspect SS, add T2* GRE &/or SWI to confirm

DIFFERENTIAL DIAGNOSIS

Bounce Point Artifact

- Mismatch between repetition time and inversion time on inversion recovery T1 and FLAIR sequences
- Imaging clue: Not present on all sequences

Brain Surface Vessels

- Normal or abnormal surface veins
- Linear, focal area of low signal on brain surface

Neurocutaneous Melanosis

- Congenital syndrome
- Large or multiple congenital melanocytic nevi
- Benign or malignant pigment cell tumors of leptomeninges may be low signal on surface of brain
- T1 high signal diffusely in pia-arachnoid
- T2 low signal diffusely in pia-arachnoid

Meningioangiomatosis

- Hamartomatous proliferation of meningeal cells via intraparenchymal blood vessels into cerebral cortex
- Leptomeninges are thick and infiltrated with fibrous tissue
- May be calcified

PATHOLOGY

General Features

- Etiology
  - Repeated SAH deposits hemosiderin on CNS meninges
    - Brain, brainstem, cerebellum, cranial nerves, cord
  - Hemosiderin is cytotoxic to neurons
    - "Free" iron with excess production of hydroxyl radicals is best current hypothesis explaining cytotoxicity
  - CNVIII is extensively lined with CNS myelin, which is supported by hemosiderin-sensitive microglia
    - ↑ exposure in CPA cistern
  - SS and ependymal siderosis may occur in premature infants with germinal matrix bleeds
    - Related to germinal matrix bleed grade and intraventricular hematoma volume
- Associated abnormalities
  - Most due to **spinal dural defect**
    - Tear from disc herniation, trauma, or ectasia
    - 1/3 are idiopathic
  - **Causes of recurrent SAH**
    - Intradural surgical sites (brain or spine)
    - Traumatic
      - □ Cervical nerve root avulsion
      - □ Multiple episodes of head injury
      - □ Subdural hematoma (SDH)
    - Bleeding neoplasm (brain or spine)
    - Arteriovenous malformation (AVM)
    - Cavernous malformation
    - Aneurysm
    - Amyloid angiopathy
    - Vasculitis
    - Meningocele

Gross Pathologic & Surgical Features

- Dark brown discoloration of leptomeninges, ependyma, and subpial tissue
- Causes of recurrent SAH found in ~ 70%
  - Dural pathology (70%)
    - Traumatic cervical nerve root avulsion
    - Postsurgical due to "fragile" neovascularity
  - Bleeding neoplasms (15%)
    - Ependymoma, oligodendroglioma, astrocytoma, etc.
  - Vascular abnormalities (10%)
    - AVM or aneurysm
    - Multiple cavernous malformations near brain surface

Microscopic Features

- **Hemosiderin staining** of meninges and subpial tissues
- Thickened leptomeninges
- Cerebellar folia: Loss of Purkinje cells and Bergmann gliosis

CLINICAL ISSUES

Presentation

- Most common signs/symptoms
  - **Bilateral sensorineural hearing loss** (SNHL) in 95%
- Clinical profile
  - Past history of trauma or intradural surgery common
    - Past history of SAH rare

- Classic presentation is adult with bilateral SNHL and ataxia
  - Late complication of treated childhood cerebellar tumor
- Laboratory: CSF from lumbar puncture
  - High protein (100%), xanthochromic (75%)
- Other symptoms
  - **Ataxia** (88%)
  - **Myelopathy**
  - **Bilateral hemiparesis**
  - Anosmia: CNI very sensitive to hemosiderin deposition
  - Hyperreflexia, bladder disturbance, **dementia**, headache
  - Kinetic tremor, nystagmus &/or dysarthria
  - Presymptomatic phase averages 15 years

Demographics

- Age
  - Any but 4th-5th decades most common
- Epidemiology
  - Rare, chronic, progressive disorder
  - 0.15% of patients undergoing MR
- Sex: M:F = 3:1

Natural History & Prognosis

- Bilateral worsening SNHL and ataxia within 15 years
- Deafness almost certain if unrecognized
- 25% of patients bedridden within years after 1st symptom (adults) due to cerebellar ataxia, myelopathic syndrome, or both

Treatment

- Treat source of bleeding
  - Repair of spinal dural tears
    - Blood patch, sutures, muscle/fat grafts, or fibrin glue
  - Surgically remove source of bleeding
  - Endovascular therapy for AVM and aneurysm
- Cochlear implantation for SNHL

DIAGNOSTIC CHECKLIST

Consider

- Remember that SS is effect, not cause
- Spinal dural tear most common cause
- Look for source of recurrent SAH in spine or brain
- MR findings do not correlate with symptom severity
  - MR diagnosis may be made in absence of symptoms

Image Interpretation Pearls

- CNS surfaces and nerves look "outlined in black" on T2 MR
- SWI most sensitive sequence

Reporting Tips

- Describe individual findings of SS
- Describe any possible sites of chronic SAH
- Treatment may arrest progression of associated symptoms
- Image to identify dural defect if no intracranial source
  - Spine MR &/or CT myelography

SELECTED REFERENCES

1. Schievink WI: Superficial siderosis and the dura. Eur J Neurol. 31(3):e16182, 2024
2. Callen AL et al: Unusual neuroimaging findings in spontaneous intracranial hypotension. Neuroradiology. 65(5):875-82, 2023

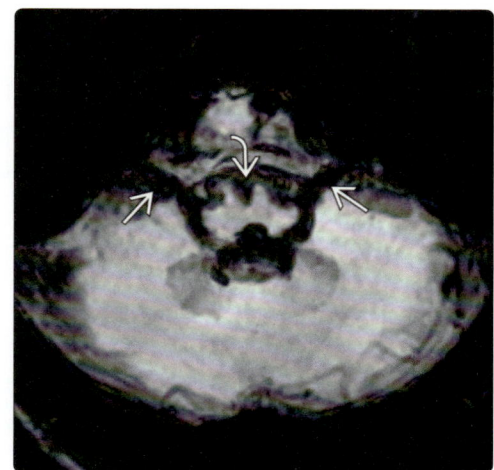

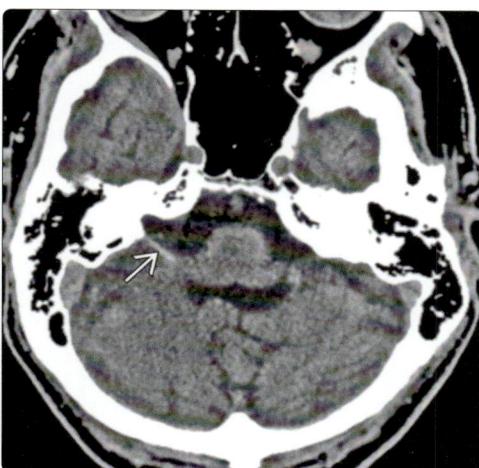

(Left) *Axial SWI MR shows thick hemosiderosis coating the medullary leptomeninges ➜ and bilateral 7th and 8th CNs ➜ in a patient with supratentorial neoplasm and a history of prior bleeding.* (Right) *Axial NECT demonstrates findings of SS as a high-density right vestibulocochlear nerve ➜. CT is often normal in patients with this disease, as the fine siderosis coating on the CNs, brain, and brainstem may not be dense enough to see.*

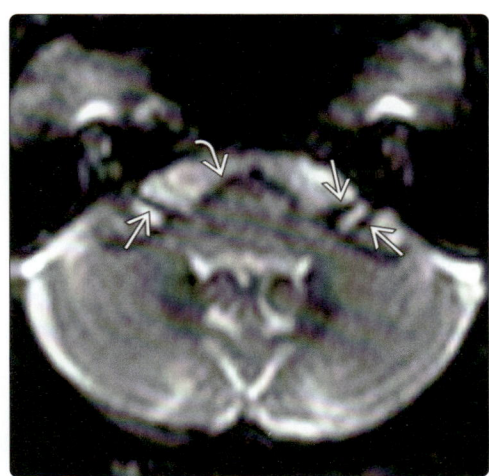

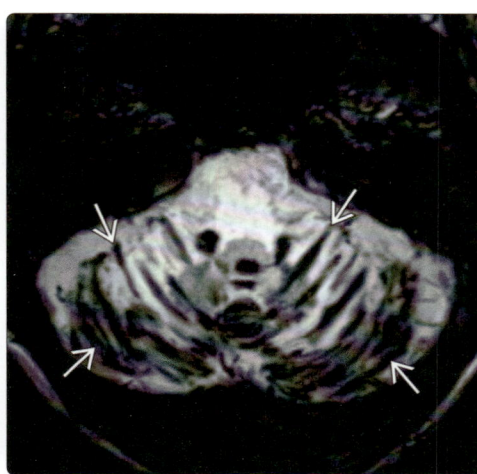

(Left) *Axial DWI-B0 image in a patient with vestibular dysfunction shows susceptibility along the vestibulocochlear and facial nerves traversing the CPA ➜. Siderosis is seen along the brainstem surfaces ➜. The B0 image is a useful "poor man's gradient-echo" if T2* or SWI sequences are not obtained.* (Right) *Axial SWI MR shows extensive thick, linear deposits of hemosiderin along cerebellar folia in the cerebellum ➜. SWI is the most sensitive sequence to detect siderosis.*

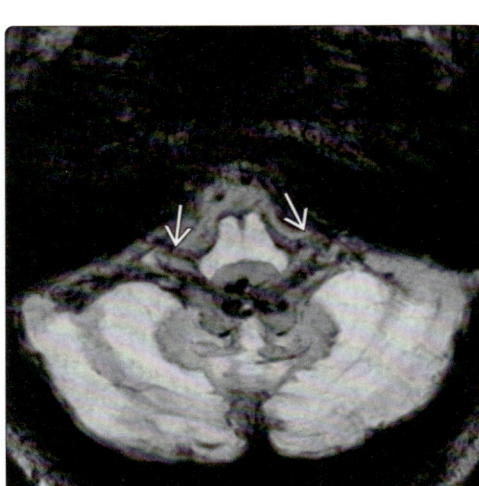

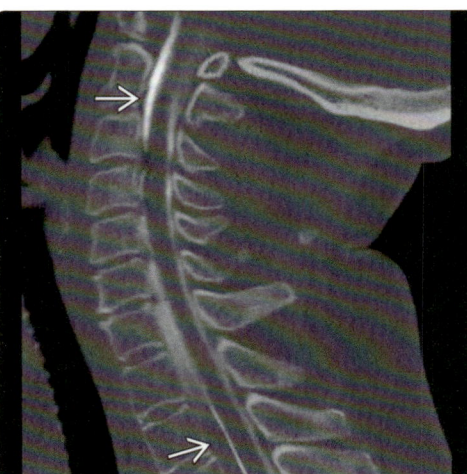

(Left) *Axial SWI MR shows SS involving the bilateral 7th and 8th CNs ➜.* (Right) *Sagittal dynamic CT myelogram in the same patient shows rapid filling of a ventral epidural collection ➜ due to suspected dural tear, which filled in on progressive imaging (not shown). Spinal dural defects are responsible for most cases of primary infratentorial SS and are usually ventral in location.*

INDEX

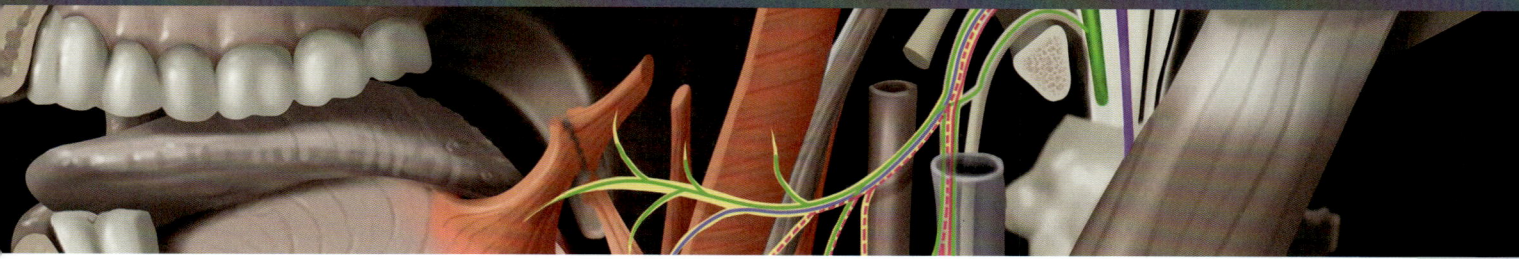

INDEX

INDEX

INDEX

INDEX

INDEX

INDEX

INDEX

INDEX

INDEX

INDEX

- periapical (radicular) cyst, **448–449**
  ameloblastoma vs., **473**
  dentigerous cyst vs., **451**
  diagnostic checklist, **449**
  differential diagnosis, **449**
  nasolabial cyst vs., **447**
  nasopalatine duct cyst vs., **459**
  odontogenic keratocyst vs., **453**
  prognosis, **449**
  simple bone cyst (traumatic) vs., **457**
- simple bone cyst (traumatic), **456–457**
  associated abnormalities, **457**
  diagnostic checklist, **456**
  differential diagnosis, **457**
  prognosis, **457**
- solitary median maxillary central incisor, **444–445**
  associated abnormalities, **445**
  diagnostic checklist, **445**
  differential diagnosis, **445**
  genetics, **445**
- TMJ tenosynovial giant cell tumor, **470–471**
  diagnostic checklist, **471**
  differential diagnosis, **471**
  genetics, **471**
  prognosis, **471**
Mandible metastasis, masticator space sarcoma vs., **65**
Mandibular alveolar ridge, **39, 394**
Mandibular division of CNV, **679**
Mandibular fibrous dysplasia, masticator space chondrosarcoma vs., **61**
Mandibular foramen, **38, 440**
Mandibular lingula, mandible fracture vs., **1015**
Mandibular main trunk, perineural tumor spread, **544**
Mandibular metastasis, masticator space chondrosarcoma vs., **61**
Mandibular nerve (CNV3), **20, 40, 441, 890**
Mandibular ossifying fibroma, masticator space chondrosarcoma vs., **61**
Mandibular osteomyelitis, **51**
- abscess, **419**
- masticator space sarcoma vs., **65**
Mandibular osteonecrosis, masticator space abscess vs., **51**
Mandibular osteosarcoma, masticator space chondrosarcoma vs., **61**
Mantle cell. *See* Non-Hodgkin lymphoma, pharyngeal mucosal space.
Mantle cell lymphoma, **366**
Manubrium, **222**
Marble bone disease. *See* Osteopetrosis, skull base.
Marfan syndrome, odontogenic keratocyst, **453**
Marginal zone lymphoma, **366**
MAS. *See* McCune-Albright syndrome.
Masseter muscle, **6, 38, 40, 72**
Mastication, muscle of, **38**
Masticator muscle hypertrophy
- benign, **44–45**
  CNV3 motor denervation vs., **47**
  diagnostic checklist, **45**
  differential diagnosis, **45**
  prognosis, **45**

- masticator space abscess vs., **52**
Masticator space, **6, 7, 13, 20, 47, 72, 395, 888**
- abscess, **50–53**
  benign masticator muscle hypertrophy vs., **45**
  CNV3 motor denervation vs., **47**
  diagnostic checklist, **52**
  differential diagnosis, **51–52**
  masticator space sarcoma vs., **65**
  prognosis, **52**
  retromolar trigone squamous cell carcinoma vs., **519**
- benign masticator muscle hypertrophy, **39, 44–45**
  CNV3 motor denervation vs., **47**
  diagnostic checklist, **45**
  differential diagnosis, **45**
  prognosis, **45**
- chondrosarcoma, **60–63, 64–67**
  diagnostic checklist, **62**
  differential diagnosis, **61**
  prognosis, **62**
  staging, grading, & classification, **62**
- CNV3 motor denervation, **46–49**
  associated abnormalities, **48**
  diagnostic checklist, **48**
  differential diagnosis, **47**
  prognosis, **48**
- CNV3 perineural tumor, **56–59**
  diagnostic checklist, **58**
  differential diagnosis, **57–58**
  prognosis, **58**
  rhinosinusitis complications vs., **712**
- CNV3 schwannoma, **54–55**
  CNV3 perineural tumor vs., **57**
  differential diagnosis, **55**
  prognosis, **55**
- common tumors, **5**
- denervation of muscles, **39**
- differential diagnosis, **39**
- infection, chondrosarcoma vs., **61**
- overview, **38–41**
- perineural tumor, CNV3 in masticator space, masticator space sarcoma vs., **65**
- progressive hemifacial atrophy syndrome, CNV3 motor denervation vs., **47**
- pseudolesion, benign masticator muscle hypertrophy vs., **45**
- pterygoid venous plexus asymmetry, **42–43**
  diagnostic checklist, **43**
  differential diagnosis, **43**
  masticator space CNV3 perineural tumor vs., **57**
  parapharyngeal space benign mixed tumor vs., **15**
  prognosis, **43**
- sarcoma, **64–67**
  benign masticator muscle hypertrophy vs., **45**
  CNV3 motor denervation vs., **47**
  diagnostic checklist, **66**
  differential diagnosis, **65**
  genetics, **66**
  masticator space abscess vs., **52**
  prognosis, **66**
  staging, grading, & classification, **66**

INDEX

INDEX

INDEX

INDEX

O

INDEX

INDEX

INDEX

INDEX

INDEX

INDEX

INDEX

INDEX

INDEX

INDEX

INDEX

INDEX

INDEX